MW00845700

SAVE UP TO 25%*

when you renew your coding essentials.

Buy 1–2 items, save 15%
Buy 3–5 items, save 20%
Buy 6+ items, save 25%

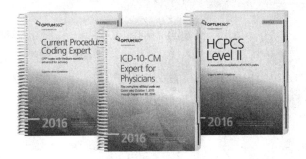

ITEM #	TITLE INDICATE THE ITEMS YOU WISH TO PURCHASE	QUANTITY	PRICE PER PRODUCT	TOTAL

	Subtotal	
(AK, DE, HI, MT, NH & OR are exempt)	Sales Tax	
1 item $10.95 • 2–4 items $12.95 • 5+ CALL	Shipping & Handling	
	TOTAL AMOUNT ENCLOSED	

Save up to 25% when you renew.

Visit **optumcoding.com** and enter the promo code below.

Call **1-800-464-3649, option 1,** and mention the promo code below.

Fax this order form with purchase order to **1-801-982-4033.** *Optum360 no longer accepts credit cards by fax.*

PROMO CODE
FOBA16WA

Mail this order form with payment and/or purchase order to:
Optum360, PO Box 88050, Chicago, IL 60680-9920.
Optum360 no longer accepts credit cards by mail.

Name _____

Address _____

_____

Customer Number _____   Contact Number _____

○ CHECK ENCLOSED (PAYABLE TO OPTUM360)

○ BILL ME ○ P.O.# _____

(_____) _____
Telephone
(_____) _____
Fax
_____@_____
E-mail

Optum360 respects your right to privacy. We will not sell or rent your email address or fax number to anyone outside Optum360 and its business partners. If you would like to remove your name from Optum360 promotions, please call 1-800-464-3649, option 1.

OPTUM360°™

PIONEER
THE NEW FRONTIER OF CODING
WITH A TRUSTED, INDUSTRY LEADER BY YOUR SIDE.

Navigate the changing landscape of coding and move forward with confidence.

With Optum360 tools and resources at your fingertips, you can open a world of opportunities and help build the foundation for greater efficiencies, financial gains, and competitive advantages. For over 30 years, our print resources have remained trusted tools for coding professionals, and our 2016 editions offer the same quality and reliability you have come to expect from us.

Eliminate roadblocks with web-based coding solutions. ICD-10 will have 668 percent more codes than ICD-9. Web-based coding solutions can help you experience a smooth, successful transition with fast access to ICD-10 codes, data and mapping tools, and can easily be used in conjunction with our ICD-10 books. Learn more about EncoderPro.com and RevenueCyclePro.com today by visiting **optumcoding.com/transitions**.

The new frontier of coding awaits.
Save up to 25% on the ICD-10, CPT®, and HCPCS coding resources you need.

 Visit OptumCoding.com and enter promo code **00000AD3** to save 25%

 Call 1.800.464.3649, option 1 and mention promo code **00000AD3** to save 20%

ICD-10-CM

Expert for Skilled Nursing Facilities, Inpatient Rehabilitation Services, and Inpatient Hospice

The Complete Official Code Set

2016

Publisher's Notice

ICD-10-CM Expert for Skilled Nursing Facilities, Inpatient Rehabilitation Services, and Inpatient Hospice: The Complete Official Code Set is designed to be an accurate and authoritative source regarding coding and every reasonable effort has been made to ensure accuracy and completeness of the content. However, Optum360 makes no guarantee, warranty, or representation that this publication is accurate, complete or without errors. It is understood that Optum360 is not rendering any legal or other professional services or advice in this publication and that Optum360 bears no liability for any results or consequences that may arise from the use of this book.

Our Commitment to Accuracy

Optum360 is committed to producing accurate and reliable materials.

To report corrections, please visit www.optumcoding.com/accuracy or email accuracy@optum.com. You can also reach customer service by calling 1.800.464.3649, option 1.

Acknowledgments

Lauri Gray, RHIT, CPC, AHIMA-Approved ICD-10-CM/PCS Trainer, *Product Manager*
Karen Schmidt, BSN, *Technical Director*
Anita Schmidt, BS, RHIT, AHIMA-Approved ICD-10-CM/PCS Trainer, *Clinical Technical Editor*
Peggy Willard, CCS, AHIMA-Approved ICD-10-CM/PCS Trainer, *Clinical Technical Editor*
Karen Krawzik, RHIT, CCS, AHIMA-Approved ICD-10-CM/PCS Trainer, *Clinical Technical Editor*
Stacy Perry, *Manager, Desktop Publishing*
Lisa Singley, *Project Manager*
Tracy Betzler, *Senior Desktop Publishing Specialist*
Hope M. Dunn, *Senior Desktop Publishing Specialist*
Katie Russell, *Desktop Publishing Specialist*
Kate Holden, *Editor*

Anita Schmidt, BS, RHIT, AHIMA-Approved ICD-10-CM/PCS Trainer

Ms. Schmidt has expertise in level I adult and pediatric trauma hospital coding, specializing in ICD-9-CM, DRG, and CPT coding. Her experience includes analysis of medical record documentation and assignment of ICD-9-CM codes and DRGs, and CPT code assignments for same-day surgery cases. She has conducted coding training and auditing, including DRG validation; conducted electronic health record training; and worked with clinical documentation specialists to identify documentation needs and potential areas for physician education. Ms. Schmidt is an active member of the American Health Information Management Association (AHIMA) and the Minnesota Health Information Management Association (MHIMA).

Peggy Willard, CCS, AHIMA-Approved ICD-10-CM/PCS Trainer

Ms. Willard has several years of experience in Level I Adult and Pediatric Trauma hospital coding, specializing in ICD-9-CM, DRG, and CPT coding. She has been extensively trained in ICD-10-CM and PCS. Her recent experience includes in-depth analysis of medical record documentation, ICD-10-CM code assignment, and DRG shifts based on ICD-10-CM code assignment. Ms. Willard's expertise includes conducting coding audits, conducting coding training for coding staff and clinical documentation specialists, and creating internal ICD-10-CM coding guidelines/tips. Ms. Willard is an active member of the American Health Information Management Association (AHIMA) and the Minnesota Health Information Management Association (MHIMA).

Karen Krawzik, RHIT, CCS, AHIMA-Approved ICD-10-CM/PCS Trainer

Ms. Krawzik has expertise in ICD-10-CM, ICD-9-CM, and CPT/HCPCS coding. Her coding experience includes inpatient, ambulatory surgery, and ancillary and emergency room records. She has served as a DRG analyst and auditor of commercial and government payer claims, and as a contract administrator. Most recently she was responsible for the conversion of the ICD-9-CM code set to ICD-10 and for analyzing audit results, identifying issues and trends, and developing remediation plans. Ms. Krawzik is credentialed by the American Health Information Management Association (AHIMA) as a Certified Coding Specialist (CCS) and is an AHIMA-approved ICD-10-CM/PCS trainer. She is an active member of AHIMA and the Missouri Health Information Management Association.

Contents

Contents

Preface

ICD-10-CM Official Preface

This 2016 update of the International Classification of Diseases, 10th revision, Clinical Modification (ICD-10-CM) is being published by the United States government in recognition of its responsibility to promulgate this classification throughout the United States for morbidity coding. The International Statistical Classification of Diseases and Related Health Problems, 10th Revision (ICD-10), published by the World Health Organization (WHO), is the foundation of ICD-10-CM. ICD-10 continues to be the classification used in cause-of-death coding in the United States. The ICD-10-CM is comparable with the ICD-10. The WHO Collaborating Center for the Family of International Classifications in North America, housed at the National Center for Health Statistics (NCHS), has responsibility for the implementation of ICD and other WHO-FIC classifications and serves as a liaison with the WHO, fulfilling international obligations for comparable classifications and the national health data needs of the United States. The historical background of ICD and ICD-10 can be found in the Introduction to the International Classification of Diseases and Related Health Problems (ICD-10), 2008, World Health Organization, Geneva, Switzerland.

ICD-10-CM is the United States' clinical modification of the World Health Organization's ICD-10. The term clinical is used to emphasize the modification's intent: to serve as a useful tool in the area of classification of morbidity data for indexing of medical records, medical care review, and ambulatory and other medical care programs, as well as for basic health statistics. To describe the clinical picture of the patient the codes must be more precise than those needed only for statistical groupings and trend analysis.

Characteristics of ICD-10-CM

ICD-10-CM far exceeds its predecessors in the number of concepts and codes provided. The disease classification has been expanded to include health-related conditions and to provide greater specificity at the sixth and seventh character level. The sixth and seventh characters are not optional and are intended for use in recording the information documented in the clinical record.

Introduction

History of ICD-10-CM

The ICD-10-CM classification system was developed by the National Center for Health Statistics (NCHS) as a clinical modification to the ICD-10 system developed by the World Health Organization (WHO), primarily as a unique system for use in the United States for morbidity and mortality reporting. Although ICD-10 replaced ICD-9 for use in coding and classifying mortality data from death certificates beginning January 1, 1999, ICD-10-CM implementation was postponed many years until legislation to replace ICD-9-CM, volumes 1 and 2, with ICD-10-CM was approved.

ICD-10 is the copyrighted product of the World Health Organization (WHO), which has authorized the development of a clinical modification (CM) of ICD-10 for use in the United States. However, all modifications to the ICD-10 must conform to WHO conventions for ICD. The development of ICD-10-CM included comprehensive evaluation by a Technical Advisory Panel and extensive consultation with physician groups, clinical coders, and other industry experts.

The ICD-10-CM draft and crosswalk between ICD-9-CM and ICD-10-CM were made available on the Centers for Medicare and Medicaid Services (CMS) website for public comment. The initial public comment period extended from December 1997 through February 1998. A field test for ICD-10-CM was conducted in the summer of 2003 jointly by The American Hospital Association (AHA) and the American Health Information Management Association (AHIMA). Public comments and suggestions were reviewed and additional modifications to ICD-10-CM were made. Revisions were made to ICD-10-CM based on the established update process for ICD-10-CM (the ICD-10-CM Coordination and Maintenance Committee) and the World Health Organization's ICD-10 (the Update and Revision Committee).

These revisions to ICD-10-CM have included:

- information relevant to ambulatory and managed care encounters
- expanded injury codes
- creation of combination diagnosis/symptom codes to reduce the number of codes needed to fully describe a condition
- the addition of 6th and 7th character classifications
- incorporation of common 4th and 5th character classifications
- classifications specific to laterality
- classification refinement for increased data granularity

This new structure allows for further expansion than was possible with the ICD-9-CM classification system.

The Department of Health and Human Services (HHS) published the final rule regarding the adoption of both ICD-10-CM and ICD-10-PCS in the January 16, 2009, Federal Register (45 CFR part 162 [CMS—0013—F]). The initial compliance date for implementation of ICD-10-CM and ICD-10-PCS as a replacement for ICD-9-CM was set at October 1, 2013. On April 17, 2012, the Department of Health and Human Services (HHS) released a notice to postpone the date by which certain health care entities have to comply with International Classification of Diseases, 10th Revision diagnosis and procedure codes (ICD-10). The compliance date for implementation of ICD-10-CM and ICD-10-PCS as a replacement for ICD-9-CM was changed to October 1, 2014. On April 1, 2014, Congress enacted the Protecting Access to Medicare Act of 2014, which contained a provision to delay the implementation of ICD-10-CM/PCS by at least one year, prohibiting the Department of Health and Human Services (HHS) from adopting the ICD-10-CM/PCS code sets as the mandatory standard until October 1, 2015.

ICD-10-CM: The Complete Official Code Set

ICD-10-CM: The Complete Official Code Set 2016 edition includes many of the enhancements described below in direct response to requests from our subscribers. Users will find many of the conventions, icons, color bars, and other enhancements familiar since many of these features are similar to the hallmark color coding and symbols of our ICD-9-CM code books.

As you review the content, you will find the following:

- Optum360 Exclusive feature — Check Placeholder Alert symbol, indicating the need for one or more "filler" x character assignments in the 5th and/or 6th character position, in order to appropriately assign a required character in the 7th character position
- Optum360 Exclusive feature — Key word differentiation by the use of a green font that highlights the differentiating terms in similar code descriptions in a given category
- Optum360 Exclusive color coding, symbols, and footnotes that alert coders to coding and reimbursement issues, including the majority of the Medicare code edits
- Optum360 Exclusive feature — Exclusive *following* references and Check Additional Character symbol in the indexes. The *following* references (designed and used exclusively by Optum360) help coders locate those alphanumeric codes that are out of sequence in the tabular section.
- Optum360 Exclusive feature — Exclusive shaded guides in the index help users easily follow the indent levels for the subterms under a main term.
- Illustrations at the back of the book feature anatomy and terminology included in the ICD-10-CM classification system
- Optum360 Exclusive feature — Detailed muscle/tendon tables that correspond to codes in chapters 13 and 19
- The complete ICD-10-CM official guidelines for coding and reporting, published by the U.S. Department of Health and Human Services and approved by the cooperating parties (American Health Information Management Association, National Center for Health Statistics, Centers for Medicare and Medicaid Services, American Hospital Association)
- Optum360 Exclusive feature —Official chapter-specific guidelines with coding examples at the beginning of each chapter
- All the official ICD-10-CM codes, indexes, notes, footnotes, and symbols
- Icons and definitions to differentiate between the two types of Excludes notes
- Check 4th, 5th, 6th, and 7th character symbols identify codes that require the addition of a 4th, 5th, 6th, or 7th character for code specificity and validity
- Color coding and symbol legend at the bottom of each page

Please review "How to Use *ICD-10-CM Expert for Skilled Nursing Facilities, Inpatient Rehabilitation Services, and Inpatient Hospice*" in this section to learn about the features that will help you assign and report correct codes, ensuring appropriate reimbursement.

How to Use ICD-10-CM Expert for Skilled Nursing Facilities, Inpatient Rehabilitation Services, and Inpatient Hospice 2016

This International Classification of Diseases, 10th Revision, Clinical Modification (ICD-10-CM) is being published by the United States Government in recognition of its responsibility to promulgate this classification throughout the United States for morbidity coding. This code book represents an adaptation of ICD-10 which was created specifically for use in the United States. Future revisions to ICD-10-CM will be made based on the established update process for ICD-10-CM (the ICD-10-CM Coordination and Maintenance Committee) and the World Health Organization's ICD-10 (the Update and Revision Committee). ICD-10-CM has been approved for implementation on October 1, 2015.

Steps to Correct Coding

1. Before beginning to use this code book, review section I.A., "Conventions for the ICD-10-CM" and section I.B., "General Coding Guidelines" of the ICD-10-CM Official Guidelines for Coding and Reporting 2016.

2. Look up the main term in the alphabetic index and scan the subterm entries as appropriate. Review continued lines and additional subterms that may appear in the next column or on the next page.

3. Note all parenthetical terms (nonessential modifiers) that help in code selection but do not affect code assignment. Shaded vertical guidelines in the Index are provided to help determine the indentation level for each subterm in relation to the main terms.

4. Pay close attention to the following instructions in the Index:

   - "see," "see also," and "see category" cross-references

   - "with"/"without" notes

   - "omit code" notes

   - "due to" subterms

   - other instructions found in note boxes, such as "code by site"

   - *Following* references and Check Additional Character symbol in the indexes. The *following* references (designed and used exclusively by Optum360) help coders locate those alphanumeric codes that are out of sequence in the tabular section.

5. Do not code from the alphabetic index without verifying the accuracy of the code in the tabular list. Locate the code in the alphanumerically arranged tabular list.

6. To determine the appropriateness of the code selection and proper coding, read all instructional material:

   - "includes" and both types of "excludes" notes

   - "use additional code" and "code first underlying disease" instructions

   - "code also"

   - 4th, 5th, and 6th character requirements and 7th character extension requirements

   - age and sex symbols

7. Consult the official ICD-10-CM guidelines, which govern the use of specific codes. These guidelines provide both general and chapter-specific coding guidance.

8. Confirm and assign the correct code.

Organization

This book is organized in the following manner:

Introduction

The introductory material in this book includes the ICD-10-CM Official Preface, the history of ICD-10-CM as well as an overview of the classification system.

Official ICD-10-CM Conventions and Guidelines

This section provides an explanation of the conventions and guidelines regulating the appropriate assignment and reporting of ICD-10-CM codes. This coding guidance is presented by the National Center for Health Statistics (NCHS), a governmental agency of the Centers for Disease Control and Prevention (CDC), within the United States Department of Health and Human Services (DHHS).

Alphabetic Index to Diseases

The alphabetic index to diseases is arranged in alphabetic order by disease — by specific illness, injury, eponym, abbreviation, or other descriptive diagnostic term. The Index also lists diagnostic terms for other reasons for encounters with health care professionals.

Neoplasm Table

The Neoplasm Table provides the proper code based upon histology of the neoplasm and site.

Table of Drugs and Chemicals

The Table of Drugs and Chemicals is also included within the alphabetic index.

The Table of Drugs and Chemicals lists the drug and the specific codes that identify the drug and the intent. No additional external cause of injury and poisoning code is assigned in ICD-10-CM.

Index to External Causes

The alphabetic index to external causes of injuries is arranged in alphabetic order by main term indicating the event.

Tabular List of Diseases

ICD-10-CM codes and descriptors are arranged numerically within the tabular list of diseases within 21 separate chapters according to body system or nature of injury and disease. Classifications which were previously considered supplemental to ICD-9-CM (e.g., V codes and E codes) are incorporated into the tabular listing of ICD-10-CM as individual chapters. Chapters 20 External Causes of Morbidity and 21 Factors Influencing Health Status and Contact with Health Services include chapter-specific guidelines.

Appendixes

The additional resources described below have been included as appendixes for the *ICD-10-CM Expert for Skilled Nursing Facilities, Inpatient Rehabilitation Services and Inpatient Hospice: The Complete Official Code Set.* These resources further instruct the professional coder on the appropriate application of the ICD-10-CM code set.

Appendix A: 10 Steps to Correct Coding

This step-by-step tutorial walks the coder through the process of locating the correct code in the Alphabetic Index and verifying it in the tabular section while following applicable conventions and guidelines. Detailed examples are provided and explained along with advice for proper sequencing.

Appendix B: Valid 3-character ICD-10-CM Codes
The user may consult this table to confirm that no further specificity, such as the use of 4th, 5th, 6th, or 7th characters or placeholders (x), is necessary. All ICD-10-CM codes that are valid at the three-character level are listed.

Appendix C: Pharmacology List 2016
This reference is provided to assist in accurate coding of drug classifications for adverse effects and poisonings, in addition to alerting the coder of potential chronic conditions in a patient record by identifying various medications used and their actions. This list is not all-inclusive but discusses many commonly used drugs.

Appendix D: Z Codes for Long-Term Drug Use with Associated Drugs
This resource correlates Z codes that are used to identify current long-term drug use with a list of drugs that are typically categorized to that class of drug.

Note: These tables are not all-inclusive but list some of the more commonly used drugs.

Appendix E: Z Code Only as Principal Diagnosis
Chapter 21, "Factors Influencing Health Status and Contact with Health Services," provides codes to deal with encounters for circumstances other than a disease or injury. Many of these codes may be reported *only* as the principal/first-listed diagnosis. This resource lists all of these codes in one table for quick and easy reference to ensure accurate reporting.

Appendix F: Hospice Criteria for Medicare Coverage on Noncancer Hospice Care
This resource provides the requirements that must be met for an individual to be recommended and covered for hospice care, in particular, when a patient does not have a cancer diagnosis.

Appendix G: Hospice Diagnosis and Quality Reporting Guidance
This resource provides an overview of the 2016 hospice proposed rule, including a summary of the major provisions regarding diagnosis reporting as well as quality measures and data submission requirements for the Hospice Quality Reporting Program.

Appendix H: Skilled Nursing Facility Resource Utilization Groups (RUG-IV) Classification System
Resource utilization (RUG-IV) groups are an element of Medicare's skilled nursing facility prospective payment system (SNF PPS). This resource describes the RUG-IV classification and its necessary elements as well as how this classification system is utilized within the SNF PPS.

Appendix I: Skilled Nursing Facility Active Diagnosis List
Although not all-inclusive this appendix provides a list of diseases and infections that should be reported on the MDS form, when present, as these active diagnoses can alter the plan of care for the resident.

Appendix J: Coding Issues for Long-Term Care (LTC)
This resource identifies coding and reporting issues that may be encountered in the long-term care setting. Specific case scenarios along with the applicable ICD-10-CM code(s) and rationale are provided.

Appendix K: Inpatient Rehabilitation Facility Prospective Payment System (PPS) Overview
The inpatient rehabilitation facility prospective payment system (IRF PPS) provides payment rates for rehabilitation facilities providing post-acute care for patients that require additional services to restore the patient's ability to live and work after a disabling injury or illness. This resource summarizes the revisions to the Quality Reporting Program, changes to the IRF-PAI instrument, the implementation of ICD-10-CM codes, and the proposed changes to the IRF PPS for FY 2016.

Appendix L: Rehabilitation Impairment Categories (RIC)
The intent of this resource was to provide a reference of all rehabilitation impairment categories (RIC) and the ICD-10-CM codes associated with each RIC. Although the specific RIC categories are listed, the ICD-10-CM code information was not available at the time of publication. Additional information on where to find future updates to this list is provided.

Appendix M: RIC Comorbid Conditions
Certain conditions when listed as a secondary diagnosis during a rehabilitation admission may qualify that stay for payment adjustment. All diagnoses that are considered comorbid conditions are identified in this resource in addition to any rehabilitation categories from which the comorbid condition would be exempt.

Illustrations
This section includes illustrations of normal anatomy with ICD-10-CM specific terminology.

Use of Official Sources
The *ICD-10-CM Expert for Skilled Nursing Facilities, Inpatient Rehabilitation Services, and Inpatient Hospice* contains the official U.S. Department of Health and Human Services, Tenth Revision, Clinical Modification, ICD-10-CM codes, effective for the current year.

The color-coding, footnotes and symbols, which identify coding and reimbursement issues, are derived from official federal government sources, including the Integrated Outpatient Code Edits (IOCE), version 16.2.

Overview of ICD-10-CM Official Conventions

This is an overview of the ICD-10-CM official conventions, which are general rules for the use of the classification system, independent of the guidelines. The official conventions and instructions of the classification, which take precedence over the guidelines, are incorporated within the Alphabetic Index and Tabular List as instructional notes and are applicable regardless of the health care setting. For the full version of the official conventions, see the ICD-10-CM Official Guidelines for Coding and Reporting 2016, section I.A., which is included in this book.

Format

ICD-10-CM is divided into two main parts: the Index, an alphabetical list of terms and their corresponding code, and the tabular list, a sequential, alphanumeric list of codes divided into chapters based on body system or condition. The Index contains the Index to Diseases and Injuries (main index) and the Index to External Causes of Injury. Also included in the main Index is the Neoplasm Table and a Table of Drugs and Chemicals.

The tabular list contains categories, subcategories, and valid codes. ICD-10-CM is an alphanumeric classification system. The 1st character of a three-character category is a letter. The 2nd and 3rd characters may be numbers or alpha characters. A three-character category without further subclassification is equivalent to a valid three-character code. Subcategories are either four or five characters. Subcategory characters include either letters or numbers. Codes may be three, four, five, six, or seven characters in length, in which each level of subdivision after a category is a subcategory. The final level of subdivision is a valid code. The final character in a code may be either a letter or a number.

The ICD-10-CM uses the letter "X" as a place-holder. A placeholder "X" is used as a 5th character place-holder at certain six-character codes to allow for future expansion, without disturbing the 6th character structure. For instance, an initial encounter for accidental poisoning by penicillin is coded to T36.0X1A. The "X" in the 5th character position is a place-holder, or filler character.

Similarly, certain categories have applicable 7th character extensions. In these cases, the 7th character extension is required for all codes within the category, or as otherwise instructed in the tabular list notations. 7th character extensions must always be the last character in the data field. If a code is not a full six characters in length, a dummy place-holder "X" must be used to fill in the empty characters when a 7th character extension is required.

Punctuation

[ ]   In the tabular list, brackets are used to enclose synonyms, alternative wording, or explanatory phrases. In the Index, brackets are used to identify manifestation codes.

( )   Parentheses are used in both the Index and tabular list to enclose nonessential modifiers; supplementary words that may be present or absent in the statement of a disease or procedure without affecting the code number to which it is assigned.

:   Colons are used in the tabular list after an incomplete term that needs one or more of the modifiers following the colon to make it assignable to a given category.

Abbreviations

NEC

The abbreviation NEC, "Not elsewhere classifiable" represents "other specified" in the ICD-10-CM. An index entry that states NEC directs the coder to an "other specified" code in the tabular list. Codes titled "Other" or "Other specified" in the tabular list (usually a code with a 4th or 6th character 8 and 5th character 9) are for use when the information in the medical record provides detail for which a specific code does not exist.

NOS

The abbreviation NOS, "Not otherwise specified," in the tabular list may be interpreted as "unspecified." Codes in the tabular list with "Unspecified" in the title (usually a code with a 4th or 6th character 9 and 5th character 0) are for use when the information in the medical record is insufficient to assign a more specific code.

Typeface

Boldface

Boldface type is used for main term entries in the alphabetic index, and all codes and descriptions in the tabular list.

General Notes

The following conventions and notes appear only in the tabular list of diseases:

Includes Notes

The word INCLUDES appears immediately under certain categories to further define, clarify, or give examples of the content of a code category.

Inclusion Terms

Lists of inclusion terms are included under certain codes. These terms indicate some of the conditions for which that code number may be used. Inclusion terms may be synonyms with the code title, or, in the case of "other specified" codes, the terms may also provide a list of various conditions included within a classification code. The inclusion terms are not exhaustive. The Index may provide additional terms that may also be assigned to a given code.

Excludes Notes

ICD-10-CM has two types of excludes notes. Each note has a different definition for use. However, they are similar in that they both indicate that codes excluded from each other are independent of each other.

Excludes 1

An EXCLUDES1 note is a "pure" excludes. It means "NOT CODED HERE!" An Excludes 1 note indicates mutually exclusive codes; two conditions that cannot be reported together. For example, a congenital form of a disease may not be reported with the acquired form of the same condition. The code excluded should never be reported with the applicable codes listed above the excludes notation.

Excludes 2

An EXCLUDES2 note means "NOT INCLUDED HERE." An Excludes 2 note indicates that although the excluded condition is not part of the condition it is excluded from, a patient may have both conditions at the same time. Therefore, when an Excludes 2 note appears under a code, it may be acceptable to use both the code and the excluded code together if supported by the medical documentation.

Default Codes

In the index, the default code is the code listed next to the main term. The default code represents the condition most commonly associated with the main term. This code may be assigned when documentation does not facilitate reporting a more specific code. Alternately, it may provide an unspecified code for the condition.

Syndromes

Follow the alphabetic index guidance when coding syndromes. In the absence of index guidance, assign codes for the documented manifestations of the syndrome.

And

When the term "and" is used in a narrative statement or code title it may be interpreted as "and/or."

With

The word "with" should be interpreted to mean "associated with" or "due to" when it appears in a code title, the Alphabetic Index, or an instructional note in the Tabular List.

Instructional Notes Used in the Tabular List

In the tabular section, the following instructional notes appear in red type for emphasis:

Code First/Use additional code:

These instructional notes provide sequencing instruction. They may appear independently of each other or to designate certain etiology/manifestation paired codes. These instructions signal the coder that an additional code should be reported to provide a more complete picture of that diagnosis.

In etiology/manifestation coding, ICD-10-CM requires the underlying condition to be sequenced first, followed by the manifestation. In these situations, codes with "In diseases classified elsewhere" in the code description are never permitted as a first-listed or principal diagnosis code and must be sequenced following the underlying condition code.

Code Also:

A code also note alerts the coder that more than one code may be required to fully describe the condition. Code sequencing is discretionary. Factors that may determine sequencing include severity and reason for the encounter.

Additional Conventions

Color-coding and symbols are included to alert the coder to important reimbursement issues affected by the diagnosis code assignment. Some codes may carry more than one color and/or symbol. For a quick reference to the color codes and their meanings, refer to the color/symbol legend located at the bottom of each page in the tabular listing.

Additional Characters Required

√4ᵗʰ This symbol indicates that the code requires a 4th character.

√5ᵗʰ This symbol indicates that the code requires a 5th character.

√6ᵗʰ This symbol indicates that the code requires a 6th character.

√7ᵗʰ This symbol indicates that the code requires a 7th character.

√x7ᵗʰ This symbol indicates that the code requires a 7th character following the placeholder "X". Codes with fewer than six characters that require a 7th character must contain placeholder "X" to fill in the empty character(s).

Italics

Italicized type is used for all exclusion notes and to identify manifestation codes, those codes that should note be reported as first-listed (principal) diagnoses.

Color Coding

Note

NOTE The term "Note" appears as an icon and precedes the instructional information. These notes function as an alert, to highlight coding instruction within the text.

Key Word

Green font is used throughout the Tabular List of Diseases to differentiate the key words that appear in similar code descriptions in a given category or subcategory.

For example, refer to the list of codes below from category C7A:

C7A.020   Malignant carcinoid tumor of the appendix

C7A.021   Malignant carcinoid tumor of the cecum

C7A.022   Malignant carcinoid tumor of the ascending colon

C7A.023   Malignant carcinoid tumor of the transverse colon

C7A.024   Malignant carcinoid tumor of the descending colon

C7A.025   Malignant carcinoid tumor of the sigmoid colon

C7A.029   Malignant carcinoid tumor of the large intestine, unspecified portion

The portion of the code description that appears in green font in the Tabular List, assists the coder in quickly identifying the key terms and in identifying the correct code. This convention is especially useful when the codes describe laterality, such as the following codes from category H40.22:

H40.221   Chronic angle-closure glaucoma, right eye

H40.222   Chronic angle-closure glaucoma, left eye

H40.223   Chronic angle-closure glaucoma, bilateral

H40.229   Chronic angle-closure glaucoma, unspecified eye

The key word convention is only used in those categories in which there are multiple codes with very similar descriptions with only a few words that differentiate them.

Medicare Code Edits

Medicare administrative contractors and many payers use Medicare code edits to check the coding accuracy on claims. The coding edit information in this manual, effective from October 1, 2015, to September 30, 2016, reflect those edits used for postacute care settings. This ICD-10 version of the Integrated Outpatient Code Editor (IOCE) is version 16.2.

Manifestation Code

These codes appear in italic type, with a **_blue color bar_** over the title. A manifestation code cannot be reported as a first-listed or principal diagnosis. By definition, a manifestation code represents a demonstration of some aspect of an underlying disease, which is separately classifiable. In the alphabetic index, these codes are listed as the secondary code in brackets. The underlying disease code is listed first.

Age and Sex Edit Symbols

The age and sex edits below are used to detect inconsistencies between the patient's age and/or sex and the patient's diagnosis. The following edit symbols appear in the Tabular List of diseases to the right of the code description.

Newborn Age: 0   N

> These diagnoses are intended for newborns and neonates and the patient's age must be 0 years.

Pediatric Age: 0-17   P

> These diagnoses are intended for children and the patient's age must between 0 and 17 years.

Maternity Age: 12-55   M

> These diagnoses are intended for childbearing patients between the age of 12 and 55 years.

Adult Age: 15-124   A

> These diagnoses are intended for the patients between the age of 15 and 124 years.

Male diagnosis only   ♂

Female diagnosis only   ♀

Other Notations in the Tabular

Rehabilitation Impairment Category   RIC

This symbol identifies a diagnosis that is recognized as a primary reason for inpatient rehabilitation grouping the case to a specific rehabilitation impairment category (RIC). Additional factors are involved in assigning a case to a specific case-mix group (CMG) within the RIC.

Alert: At the time of this publication CMS had not yet posted the list of ICD-10-CM codes that group to specific RIC. See appendix L, "Rehabilitation Impairment Categories (RIC)," for more information.

Comorbid Condition   CC

For some RIC certain comorbid conditions may qualify a case for payment adjustment when reported as a secondary diagnosis during admission. This symbol identifies those conditions recognized as having significant impact on the cost of furnishing inpatient rehabilitation services.

RIC Excl

Some CC conditions are excluded as qualifying secondary diagnoses for payment adjustment for specific RICs. If a CC condition is excluded from acting as a qualifying secondary condition the RIC exclusions are listed below the code. If no RIC exclusion is noted, then the condition may qualify regardless of the RIC assignment of the case.

Noncancer Diagnosis   `NC Dx`

This symbol indicates a noncancer diagnosis that may satisfy the medical necessity criteria for Medicare coverage of hospice care. The diagnosis alone does not support medical necessity but represents one of the many factors that establish medical necessity. For more detailed explanation of the noncancer diagnosis policies for hospice care please refer to appendix F, "Hospice Criteria for Medicare Coverage on Noncancer Hospice Care," located at the back of this book for further information.

RUG-IV Special Care High Diagnosis

A red color bar over the code description indicates a RUG-IV Special Care High Category diagnosis that may qualify a resident of a skilled nursing facility (SNF) for this clinical category. Before a resident is assigned to this category other qualifications must be met. Please refer to appendix H, "Skilled Nursing Facility Resource Utilization Groups (RUG-IV) Classification System," located at the back of this book for further information.

RUG-IV Special Care Low Diagnosis

A purple color bar over the code description indicates a RUG-IV Special Care Low Category diagnosis that may qualify a resident of a SNF for this clinical category. Before a resident is assigned to this category, other qualifications must be met. Please refer to appendix H, "Skilled Nursing Facility Resource Utilization Groups (RUG-IV) Classification System," located at the back of this book for further information.

RUG-IV Clinically Complex Diagnosis

A yellow color bar over the code description indicates a RUG-IV Clinically Complex Category diagnosis that may qualify a resident of a SN) for this clinical category. Before a resident is assigned to this category other qualifications must be met. Please refer to appendix H, "Skilled Nursing Facility Resource Utilization Groups (RUG-IV) Classification System," located at the back of this book for further information.

Other Specified Code

These codes will appear with a gray color bar over the code description. Use these codes when the documentation indicates a specified diagnosis, but the ICD-10-CM system does not have a specific code that describes the condition. These codes may be stated as "Other" or "Not elsewhere classified (NEC)."

Unspecified Code   ▽

These codes will have a blue icon in the shape of a yield sign at the right of the code description. Use these codes when neither the diagnostic statement nor the documentation provides enough information to assign a more specific diagnosis code. These codes may be stated as "Unspecified" or "Not otherwise specified (NOS)." Note: Do not assign these codes when a more specific diagnosis has been determined.

PDx Symbol   `PDx`

This symbol identifies a Z code that generally is for use as a first-listed (or primary) diagnosis only but may be used as an additional diagnosis if the patient has more than one encounter on the same day or there is more than one reason for the encounter.

The instructions for Z code use contained in the ICD-10-CM official coding guidelines identify those Z codes that can only be used as a PDx. All other Z codes may either be SDx or PDx, depending upon circumstances of the encounter, by meeting the definition of first-listed or principal diagnosis,

and by following any specific Z code guidelines in section I.C.21 a-c. The responsibility of those assigning the Z codes as PDx is to make sure the circumstances of the encounter meet the definition of first-listed or principal diagnosis, follow all coding instructions, and follow the Z code specific guidelines. Optum360 does not include any SDx edit since there is no official source for it and the Z code use is determined by circumstances of the encounter.

Note: Please note that the symbols indicating the Z code "principal or first-listed only" designation and the Z codes that may be principal or first-listed diagnoses included in the official coding guidelines [Section I.C.21.c.16] are consistent with reporting guidelines for health care encounters *excluding acute care inpatient admissions.* These Z code edits are often in conflict with the inpatient prospective payment system (IPPS) edits. For example, code Z34.90 Encounter for supervision of normal pregnancy, unspecified, unspecified trimester, may be an appropriate primary reason for an outpatient encounter. However, supervision for a normal pregnancy is not an acceptable principal diagnosis or reason for an inpatient admission and will have an unacceptable principal diagnosis edit under inpatient prospective payment system (IPPS).

Footnotes

All footnotes are identified by a numeric superscript that appears to the upper left of the code.

The following list identifies and explains the meaning of the numeric footnotes found in the tabular list:

1   Special Care High = With insulin injection and order changes

   This footnote indicates that this diagnosis code is a Special Care High category level diagnosis provided the resident is receiving insulin injection requiring physician order change on two or more days and provided other criteria are met.

2   Special Care High = With fever

   This footnote indicates that if this diagnosis code is assigned along with a diagnosis of fever, the case may qualify as a Special Care High category level, provided other criteria are met.

3   Special Care High = With pneumonia, weight loss, or vomiting

   This footnote indicates that if this diagnosis code is assigned along with a diagnosis of pneumonia, weight loss, or vomiting, the case may qualify as a Special Care High category level provided other criteria are met.

4   Special Care High = With 7th character indicating a subsequent encounter

   Only "subsequent" encounters are eligible for qualification into a Special Care High category level, provided other criteria are met.

5   Special Care Low = With oxygen therapy

   This footnote indicates that if this diagnosis code is assigned along with the resident's receiving oxygen therapy, the case may qualify as a Special Care Low category level, provided other criteria are met.

6   Special Care Low = Without insulin injection and order changes

   Insulin injection or physician order changes are not required for codes with this footnote to qualify as a Special Care Low category level; however, other criteria must also be met.

7   Clinically Complex = With 7th character indicating a subsequent encounter

   Only "subsequent" encounters are eligible for qualification into a Clinically Complex category level, provided other criteria are met.

8   Clinically Complex = Without fever

     A diagnosis of fever in addition to a code with this footnote is not
     necessary for a case to qualify as a Clinically Complex category level;
     however, other criteria must also be met.

9   Hospice Noncancer Diagnosis only when reported using an
     appropriate 7th character indicating a subsequent encounter or
     sequela.

     An appropriate 7th character may be **D** or **S**.

10   Hospice Questionable Admission Noncancer Diagnosis

     A code identified by this footnote, when used as the admitting
     diagnosis on a hospice encounter, may be viewed by Medicare as a
     questionable admission. The code may lack the specificity that
     would reasonably be contained in the medical record or the code
     conflicts with official coding guidelines and conventions. The
     patient's medical record and official coding guidelines should be
     reviewed carefully to ensure that a more appropriate diagnosis is not
     warranted.

11   This footnote identifies a code that, based on the Integrated
     Outpatient Code Editor, is considered a maternity diagnosis only
     when the code is reported using a 7th character A for an initial
     encounter.

Muscle and Tendon Table

ICD-10-CM categorizes certain muscles and tendons in the upper
and lower extremities by their action (e.g., extension or flexion) as
well as their anatomical location. The Muscle/Tendon Table is
provided at the beginning of chapter 13 and chapter 19 as a resource
to assist users when code selection is dependent depends on the
action of the muscle and/or tendon. The categories and/or
subcategories that relate to this table are identified by a purple
diamond icon ◆, which refers the user to a footnote at the bottom of
the page indicating the use of the table. Please note that this table is
not all-inclusive and proper code assignment should be based on
the provider's documentation.

Other Notations in the Alphabetic Indexes

▽   Subterms under main terms may continue to next column or page.
     This warning statement is a reminder to always check for additional
     subterms and information that may continue onto the next page or
     column before making a final selection.

Following References

The index includes *following* references to assist in locating
"out-of-sequence" codes in the tabular list. "Out-of-sequence" codes
contain an alphabetic character (letter) in the 3rd or 4th character
position. These codes are placed according to the classification rules —
the placement of the codes according to condition — not according to
alphabetic or numeric sequencing rules.

Example:

Carcinoma (malignant) (*see also,* Neoplasm, by site, malignant)
     neuroendocrine (*see also* Tumor, neuroendocrine)
          high grade, any site C7A.1 (*following* C75)
          poorly differentiated, any site C7A.1 (*following* C75)

In the tabular rubric, C7A is included after rubric C75 and before C76.

Gout, chronic (*see also* Gout, gouty) M1A.9
     drug-induced M1A.20 (*following* M08)
          ankle M1A.27-(*following* M08)
          elbow M1A.22-(*following* M08)

In the tabular rubric, M1A is included after rubric M08 and before M10.

ICD-10-CM Official Guidelines for Coding and Reporting 2016

Narrative changes appear in **bold** text.

Items <u>underlined</u> have been moved within the guidelines since the 2014 version.

Italics are used to indicate revisions to heading changes.

The Centers for Medicare and Medicaid Services (CMS) and the National Center for Health Statistics (NCHS), two departments within the U.S. Federal Government's Department of Health and Human Services (DHHS) provide the following guidelines for coding and reporting using the International Classification of Diseases, 10th Revision, Clinical Modification (ICD-10-CM). These guidelines should be used as a companion document to the official version of the ICD-10-CM as published on the NCHS website. The ICD-10-CM is a morbidity classification published by the United States for classifying diagnoses and reason for visits in all health care settings. The ICD-10-CM is based on the ICD-10, the statistical classification of disease published by the World Health Organization (WHO).

These guidelines have been approved by the four organizations that make up the Cooperating Parties for the ICD-10-CM: the American Hospital Association (AHA), the American Health Information Management Association (AHIMA), CMS, and NCHS.

These guidelines are a set of rules that have been developed to accompany and complement the official conventions and instructions provided within the ICD-10-CM itself. The instructions and conventions of the classification take precedence over guidelines. These guidelines are based on the coding and sequencing instructions in the Tabular List and Alphabetic Index of ICD-10-CM, but provide additional instruction. Adherence to these guidelines when assigning ICD-10-CM diagnosis codes is required under the Health Insurance Portability and Accountability Act (HIPAA). The diagnosis codes (Tabular List and Alphabetic Index) have been adopted under HIPAA for all healthcare settings. A joint effort between the healthcare provider and the coder is essential to achieve complete and accurate documentation, code assignment, and reporting of diagnoses and procedures. These guidelines have been developed to assist both the healthcare provider and the coder in identifying those diagnoses and procedures that are to be reported. The importance of consistent, complete documentation in the medical record cannot be overemphasized. Without such documentation accurate coding cannot be achieved. The entire record should be reviewed to determine the specific reason for the encounter and the conditions treated.

The term encounter is used for all settings, including hospital admissions. In the context of these guidelines, the term provider is used throughout the guidelines to mean physician or any qualified health care practitioner who is legally accountable for establishing the patient's diagnosis. Only this set of guidelines, approved by the Cooperating Parties, is official.

The guidelines are organized into sections. Section I includes the structure and conventions of the classification and general guidelines that apply to the entire classification, and chapter-specific guidelines that correspond to the chapters as they are arranged in the classification. Section II includes guidelines for selection of principal diagnosis for non-outpatient settings. Section III includes guidelines for reporting additional diagnoses in non-outpatient settings. Section IV is for outpatient coding and reporting. It is necessary to review all sections of the guidelines to fully understand all of the rules and instructions needed to code properly.

Section I. Conventions, general coding guidelines and chapter specific guidelines

The conventions, general guidelines and chapter-specific guidelines are applicable to all health care settings unless otherwise indicated. The conventions and instructions of the classification take precedence over guidelines.

A. Conventions for the ICD-10-CM

The conventions for the ICD-10-CM are the general rules for use of the classification independent of the guidelines. These conventions are incorporated within the Alphabetic Index and Tabular List of the ICD-10-CM as instructional notes.

1. **The Alphabetic Index and Tabular List**

   The ICD-10-CM is divided into the Alphabetic Index, an alphabetical list of terms and their corresponding code, and the Tabular List, a structured chronological list of codes divided into chapters based on body system or condition. The Alphabetic Index consists of the following parts: the Index of Diseases and Injury, the Index of External Causes of Injury, the Table of Neoplasms and the Table of Drugs and Chemicals.

   See Section I.C2. General guidelines

   See Section I.C.19. Adverse effects, poisoning, underdosing and toxic effects

2. **Format and Structure**

   The ICD-10-CM Tabular List contains categories, subcategories and codes. Characters for categories, subcategories and codes may be either a letter or a number. All categories are 3 characters. A three-character category that has no further subdivision is equivalent to a code. Subcategories are either 4 or 5 characters. Codes may be 3, 4, 5, 6 or 7 characters. That is, each level of subdivision after a category is a subcategory. The final level of subdivision is a code. Codes that have applicable 7th characters are still referred to as codes, not subcategories. A code that has an applicable 7th character is considered invalid without the 7th character.

   The ICD-10-CM uses an indented format for ease in reference.

3. **Use of codes for reporting purposes**

   For reporting purposes only codes are permissible, not categories or subcategories, and any applicable 7th character is required.

4. **Placeholder character**

   The ICD-10-CM utilizes a placeholder character "X". The "X" is used as a placeholder at certain codes to allow for future expansion. An example of this is at the poisoning, adverse effect and underdosing codes, categories T36-T50.

   Where a placeholder exists, the X must be used in order for the code to be considered a valid code.

5. **7th Characters**

   Certain ICD-10-CM categories have applicable 7th characters. The applicable 7th character is required for all codes within the category, or as the notes in the Tabular List instruct. The 7th character must always be the 7th character in the data field. If a code that requires a 7th character is not 6 characters, a placeholder X must be used to fill in the empty characters.

6. **Abbreviations**

   a. **Alphabetic Index abbreviations**
      NEC　　　"Not elsewhere classifiable"

This abbreviation in the Alphabetic Index represents "other specified". When a specific code is not available for a condition, the Alphabetic Index directs the coder to the "other specified" code in the Tabular List.

   NOS　　　"Not otherwise specified"

This abbreviation is the equivalent of unspecified.

   b. **Tabular List abbreviations**
      NEC　　　"Not elsewhere classifiable"

This abbreviation in the Tabular List represents "other specified". When a specific code is not available for a condition the Tabular List includes an NEC entry under a code to identify the code as the "other specified" code.

   NOS　　　"Not otherwise specified"

This abbreviation is the equivalent of unspecified.

7. **Punctuation**

   [ ]　Brackets are used in the Tabular List to enclose synonyms, alternative wording or explanatory phrases. Brackets are used in the Alphabetic Index to identify manifestation codes.

   ( )　Parentheses are used in both the Alphabetic Index and Tabular List to enclose supplementary words that may be present or absent in the statement of a disease or procedure without affecting the code number to which it is assigned. The terms within the parentheses are referred to as nonessential modifiers. The nonessential modifiers in the Alphabetic Index to Diseases apply to subterms following a main term except when a nonessential modifier and a subentry are mutually exclusive, the subentry takes precedence. For example, in the ICD-10-CM Alphabetic Index under the main term Enteritis, "acute" is a nonessential modifier and "chronic" is a subentry. In this case, the nonessential modifier "acute" does not apply to the subentry "chronic".

   :　Colons are used in the Tabular List after an incomplete term which needs one or more of the modifiers following the colon to make it assignable to a given category.

8. **Use of "and"**

   See Section I.A.14. Use of the term "And"

9. **Other and Unspecified codes**

   a. **"Other" codes**

      Codes titled "other" or "other specified" are for use when the information in the medical record provides detail for which a specific code does not exist. Alphabetic Index entries with NEC in the line designate "other" codes in the Tabular List. These Alphabetic Index entries represent specific disease entities for which no specific code exists so the term is included within an "other" code.

   b. **"Unspecified" codes**

      Codes titled "unspecified" are for use when the information in the medical record is insufficient to assign a more specific code. For those categories for which an unspecified code is not provided, the "other specified" code may represent both other and unspecified.

      See Section I.B.18 Use of Signs/Symptom/Unspecified Codes

10. **Includes Notes**

    This note appears immediately under a three character code title to further define, or give examples of, the content of the category.

11. **Inclusion Terms**

    List of terms is included under some codes. These terms are the conditions for which that code is to be used. The terms may be synonyms of the code title, or, in the case of "other specified" codes, the terms are a list of the various conditions assigned to that code. The inclusion terms are not necessarily exhaustive. Additional terms found only in the Alphabetic Index may also be assigned to a code.

12. **Excludes Notes**

    The ICD-10-CM has two types of excludes notes. Each type of note has a different definition for use but they are all similar in that they indicate that codes excluded from each other are independent of each other.

    a. **Excludes1**

       A type 1 Excludes note is a pure excludes note. It means "NOT CODED HERE!" An Excludes1 note indicates that the code excluded should never be used at the same time as the code above the Excludes1 note. An Excludes1 is used when two conditions cannot occur together, such as a congenital form versus an acquired form of the same condition.

b. **Excludes2**

A type 2 Excludes note represents "Not included here". An excludes2 note indicates that the condition excluded is not part of the condition represented by the code, but a patient may have both conditions at the same time. When an Excludes2 note appears under a code, it is acceptable to use both the code and the excluded code together, when appropriate.

13. **Etiology/manifestation convention ("code first", "use additional code" and "in diseases classified elsewhere" notes)**

Certain conditions have both an underlying etiology and multiple body system manifestations due to the underlying etiology. For such conditions, the ICD-10-CM has a coding convention that requires the underlying condition be sequenced first followed by the manifestation. Wherever such a combination exists, there is a "use additional code" note at the etiology code, and a "code first" note at the manifestation code. These instructional notes indicate the proper sequencing order of the codes, etiology followed by manifestation.

In most cases the manifestation codes will have in the code title, "in diseases classified elsewhere." Codes with this title are a component of the etiology/ manifestation convention. The code title indicates that it is a manifestation code. "In diseases classified elsewhere" codes are never permitted to be used as first-listed or principal diagnosis codes. They must be used in conjunction with an underlying condition code and they must be listed following the underlying condition. See category F02, Dementia in other diseases classified elsewhere, for an example of this convention.

There are manifestation codes that do not have "in diseases classified elsewhere" in the title. For such codes, there is a "use additional code" note at the etiology code and a "code first" note at the manifestation code and the rules for sequencing apply.

In addition to the notes in the Tabular List, these conditions also have a specific Alphabetic Index entry structure. In the Alphabetic Index both conditions are listed together with the etiology code first followed by the manifestation codes in brackets. The code in brackets is always to be sequenced second.

An example of the etiology/manifestation convention is dementia in Parkinson's disease. In the Alphabetic Index, code G20 is listed first, followed by code F02.80 or F02.81 in brackets. Code G20 represents the underlying etiology, Parkinson's disease, and must be sequenced first, whereas codes F02.80 and F02.81 represent the manifestation of dementia in diseases classified elsewhere, with or without behavioral disturbance.

"Code first" and "Use additional code" notes are also used as sequencing rules in the classification for certain codes that are not part of an etiology/ manifestation combination.

See Section I.B.7. Multiple coding for a single condition.

14. **"And"**

The word "and" should be interpreted to mean either "and" or "or" when it appears in a title.

For example, cases of "tuberculosis of bones", "tuberculosis of joints" and "tuberculosis of bones and joints" are classified to subcategory A18.0, Tuberculosis of bones and joints.

15. **"With"**

The word "with" should be interpreted to mean "associated with" or "due to" when it appears in a code title, the Alphabetic Index, or an instructional note in the Tabular List.

The word "with" in the Alphabetic Index is sequenced immediately following the main term, not in alphabetical order.

16. **"See" and "See Also"**

The "see" instruction following a main term in the Alphabetic Index indicates that another term should be referenced. It is necessary to go to the main term referenced with the "see" note to locate the correct code.

A "see also" instruction following a main term in the Alphabetic Index instructs that there is another main term that may also be referenced that may provide additional Alphabetic Index entries that may be useful. It is not necessary to follow the "see also" note when the original main term provides the necessary code.

17. **"Code also note"**

A "code also" note instructs that two codes may be required to fully describe a condition, but this note does not provide sequencing direction.

18. **Default codes**

A code listed next to a main term in the ICD-10-CM Alphabetic Index is referred to as a default code. The default code represents that condition that is most commonly associated with the main term, or is the unspecified code for the condition. If a condition is documented in a medical record (for example, appendicitis) without any additional information, such as acute or chronic, the default code should be assigned.

B. General Coding Guidelines

1. **Locating a code in the ICD-10-CM**

To select a code in the classification that corresponds to a diagnosis or reason for visit documented in a medical record, first locate the term in the Alphabetic Index, and then verify the code in the Tabular List. Read and be guided by instructional notations that appear in both the Alphabetic Index and the Tabular List.

It is essential to use both the Alphabetic Index and Tabular List when locating and assigning a code. The Alphabetic Index does not always provide the full code. Selection of the full code, including laterality and any applicable 7th character can only be done in the Tabular List. A dash (-) at the end of an Alphabetic Index entry indicates that additional characters are required. Even if a dash is not included at the Alphabetic Index entry, it is necessary to refer to the Tabular List to verify that no 7th character is required.

2. **Level of Detail in Coding**

Diagnosis codes are to be used and reported at their highest number of characters available.

ICD-10-CM diagnosis codes are composed of codes with 3, 4, 5, 6 or 7 characters. Codes with three characters are included in ICD-10-CM as the heading of a category of codes that may be further subdivided by the use of fourth and/or fifth characters and/or sixth characters, which provide greater detail.

A three-character code is to be used only if it is not further subdivided. A code is invalid if it has not been coded to the full number of characters required for that code, including the 7th character, if applicable.

3. **Code or codes from A00.0 through T88.9, Z00-Z99.8**

The appropriate code or codes from A00.0 through T88.9, Z00-Z99.8 must be used to identify diagnoses, symptoms, conditions, problems, complaints or other reason(s) for the encounter/visit.

4. **Signs and symptoms**

Codes that describe symptoms and signs, as opposed to diagnoses, are acceptable for reporting purposes when a related definitive diagnosis has not been established (confirmed) by the provider. Chapter 18 of ICD-10-CM, Symptoms, Signs, and Abnormal Clinical and Laboratory Findings, Not Elsewhere Classified (codes R00.0 - R99) contains many, but not all codes for symptoms.

See Section I.B.18 Use of Signs/Symptom/Unspecified Codes

5. **Conditions that are an integral part of a disease process**

Signs and symptoms that are associated routinely with a disease process should not be assigned as additional codes, unless otherwise instructed by the classification.

6. **Conditions that are not an integral part of a disease process**

Additional signs and symptoms that may not be associated routinely with a disease process should be coded when present.

7. **Multiple coding for a single condition**

In addition to the etiology/manifestation convention that requires two codes to fully describe a single condition that affects multiple body systems, there are other single conditions that also require more than one code. "Use additional code" notes are found in the Tabular List at codes that are not part of an etiology/manifestation pair where a secondary code is useful to fully describe a condition. The sequencing rule is the same as the etiology/manifestation pair, "use additional code" indicates that a secondary code should be added.

For example, for bacterial infections that are not included in chapter 1, a secondary code from category B95, Streptococcus, Staphylococcus, and Enterococcus, as the cause of diseases classified elsewhere, or B96, Other bacterial agents as the cause of diseases classified elsewhere, may be required to identify the bacterial organism causing the infection. A "use additional code" note will normally be found at the infectious disease code, indicating a need for the organism code to be added as a secondary code.

"Code first" notes are also under certain codes that are not specifically manifestation codes but may be due to an underlying cause. When there is a "code first" note and an underlying condition is present, the underlying condition should be sequenced first.

"Code, if applicable, any causal condition first", notes indicate that this code may be assigned as a principal diagnosis when the causal condition is unknown or not applicable. If a causal condition is known, then the code for that condition should be sequenced as the principal or first-listed diagnosis.

Multiple codes may be needed for sequela, complication codes and obstetric codes to more fully describe a condition. See the specific guidelines for these conditions for further instruction.

8. Acute and Chronic Conditions
If the same condition is described as both acute (subacute) and chronic, and separate subentries exist in the Alphabetic Index at the same indentation level, code both and sequence the acute (subacute) code first.

9. Combination Code
A combination code is a single code used to classify:

> Two diagnoses, or
>> A diagnosis with an associated secondary process (manifestation)
>> A diagnosis with an associated complication

Combination codes are identified by referring to subterm entries in the Alphabetic Index and by reading the inclusion and exclusion notes in the Tabular List.

Assign only the combination code when that code fully identifies the diagnostic conditions involved or when the Alphabetic Index so directs. Multiple coding should not be used when the classification provides a combination code that clearly identifies all of the elements documented in the diagnosis. When the combination code lacks necessary specificity in describing the manifestation or complication, an additional code should be used as a secondary code.

10. Sequela (Late Effects)
A sequela is the residual effect (condition produced) after the acute phase of an illness or injury has terminated. There is no time limit on when a sequela code can be used. The residual may be apparent early, such as in cerebral infarction, or it may occur months or years later, such as that due to a previous injury. Examples of sequela include: scar formation resulting from a burn, deviated septum due to a nasal fracture, and infertility due to tubal occlusion from old tuberculosis. Coding of sequela generally requires two codes sequenced in the following order: the condition or nature of the sequela is sequenced first. The sequela code is sequenced second.

An exception to the above guidelines are those instances where the code for the sequela is followed by a manifestation code identified in the Tabular List and title, or the sequela code has been expanded (at the fourth, fifth or sixth character levels) to include the manifestation(s). The code for the acute phase of an illness or injury that led to the sequela is never used with a code for the late effect.

See Section I.C.9. Sequelae of cerebrovascular disease

See Section I.C.15. Sequelae of complication of pregnancy, childbirth and the puerperium

See Section I.C.19. Application of 7th characters for Chapter 19

11. Impending or Threatened Condition
Code any condition described at the time of discharge as "impending" or "threatened" as follows:

> If it did occur, code as confirmed diagnosis.

> If it did not occur, reference the Alphabetic Index to determine if the condition has a subentry term for "impending" or "threatened" and also reference main term entries for "Impending" and for "Threatened."

> If the subterms are listed, assign the given code.

If the subterms are not listed, code the existing underlying condition(s) and not the condition described as impending or threatened.

12. Reporting Same Diagnosis Code More than Once
Each unique ICD-10-CM diagnosis code may be reported only once for an encounter. This applies to bilateral conditions when there are no distinct codes identifying laterality or two different conditions classified to the same ICD-10-CM diagnosis code.

13. Laterality
Some ICD-10-CM codes indicate laterality, specifying whether the condition occurs on the left, right or is bilateral. If no bilateral code is provided and the condition is bilateral, assign separate codes for both the left and right side. If the side is not identified in the medical record, assign the code for the unspecified side.

14. Documentation for BMI, Non-pressure ulcers, and Pressure Ulcer Stages
For the Body Mass Index (BMI), depth of non-pressure chronic ulcers and pressure ulcer stage codes, code assignment may be based on medical record documentation from clinicians who are not the patient's provider (i.e., physician or other qualified healthcare practitioner legally accountable for establishing the patient's diagnosis), since this information is typically documented by other clinicians involved in the care of the patient (e.g., a dietitian often documents the BMI and nurses often documents the pressure ulcer stages). However, the associated diagnosis (such as overweight, obesity, or pressure ulcer) must be documented by the patient's provider. If there is conflicting medical record documentation, either from the same clinician or different clinicians, the patient's attending provider should be queried for clarification.

The BMI codes should only be reported as secondary diagnoses. As with all other secondary diagnosis codes, the BMI codes should only be assigned when they meet the definition of a reportable additional diagnosis (see Section III, Reporting Additional Diagnoses).

15. Syndromes
Follow the Alphabetic Index guidance when coding syndromes. In the absence of Alphabetic Index guidance, assign codes for the documented manifestations of the syndrome.

Additional codes for manifestations that are not an integral part of the disease process may also be assigned when the condition does not have a unique code.

16. Documentation of Complications of Care
Code assignment is based on the provider's documentation of the relationship between the condition and the care or procedure. The guideline extends to any complications of care, regardless of the chapter the code is located in. It is important to note that not all conditions that occur during or following medical care or surgery are classified as complications. There must be a cause-and-effect relationship between the care provided and the condition, and an indication in the documentation that it is a complication. Query the provider for clarification, if the complication is not clearly documented.

17. Borderline Diagnosis
If the provider documents a "borderline" diagnosis at the time of discharge, the diagnosis is coded as confirmed, unless the classification provides a specific entry (e.g., borderline diabetes). If a borderline condition has a specific index entry in ICD-10-CM, it should be coded as such. Since borderline conditions are not uncertain diagnoses, no distinction is made between the care setting (inpatient versus outpatient). Whenever the documentation is unclear regarding a borderline condition, coders are encouraged to query for clarification.

18. Use of Sign/Symptom/Unspecified Codes
Sign/symptom and "unspecified" codes have acceptable, even necessary, uses. While specific diagnosis codes should be reported when they are supported by the available medical record documentation and clinical knowledge of the patient's health condition, there are instances when signs/symptoms or unspecified codes are the best choices for accurately reflecting the healthcare encounter. Each healthcare encounter should be coded to the level of certainty known for that encounter.

If a definitive diagnosis has not been established by the end of the encounter, it is appropriate to report codes for sign(s) and/or symptom(s) in lieu of a definitive diagnosis. When sufficient clinical information isn't known or available about a particular health condition to assign a more specific code, it is acceptable to report the appropriate "unspecified" code (e.g., a diagnosis of pneumonia has been determined, but not the specific type). Unspecified codes should be reported when they are the codes that most accurately reflects what is known about the patient's condition at the time of that particular encounter. It would be inappropriate to select a specific code that is not supported by the medical record documentation or conduct medically unnecessary diagnostic testing in order to determine a more specific code.

C. Chapter-Specific Coding Guidelines

In addition to general coding guidelines, there are guidelines for specific diagnoses and/or conditions in the classification. Unless otherwise indicated, these guidelines apply to all health care settings. Please refer to Section II for guidelines on the selection of principal diagnosis.

1. **Chapter 1: Certain Infectious and Parasitic Diseases (A00-B99)**
   a. **Human immunodeficiency virus (HIV) infections**
      1) **Code only confirmed cases**
         Code only confirmed cases of HIV infection/illness. This is an exception to the hospital inpatient guideline Section II, H.

         In this context, "confirmation" does not require documentation of positive serology or culture for HIV; the provider's diagnostic statement that the patient is HIV positive, or has an HIV-related illness is sufficient.

      2) **Selection and sequencing of HIV codes**
         (a) **Patient admitted for HIV-related condition**
            If a patient is admitted for an HIV-related condition, the principal diagnosis should be B20, Human immunodeficiency virus [HIV] disease followed by additional diagnosis codes for all reported HIV-related conditions.

         (b) **Patient with HIV disease admitted for unrelated condition**
            If a patient with HIV disease is admitted for an unrelated condition (such as a traumatic injury), the code for the unrelated condition (e.g., the nature of injury code) should be the principal diagnosis. Other diagnoses would be B20 followed by additional diagnosis codes for all reported HIV-related conditions.

         (c) **Whether the patient is newly diagnosed**
            Whether the patient is newly diagnosed or has had previous admissions/encounters for HIV conditions is irrelevant to the sequencing decision.

         (d) **Asymptomatic human immunodeficiency virus**
            Z21, Asymptomatic human immunodeficiency virus [HIV] infection status, is to be applied when the patient without any documentation of symptoms is listed as being "HIV positive," "known HIV," "HIV test positive," or similar terminology. Do not use this code if the term "AIDS" is used or if the patient is treated for any HIV-related illness or is described as having any condition(s) resulting from his/her HIV positive status; use B20 in these cases.

         (e) **Patients with inconclusive HIV serology**
            Patients with inconclusive HIV serology, but no definitive diagnosis or manifestations of the illness, may be assigned code R75, Inconclusive laboratory evidence of human immunodeficiency virus [HIV].

         (f) **Previously diagnosed HIV-related illness**
            Patients with any known prior diagnosis of an HIV-related illness should be coded to B20. Once a patient has developed an HIV-related illness, the patient should always be assigned code B20 on every subsequent admission/encounter. Patients previously diagnosed with any HIV illness (B20) should never be assigned to R75 or Z21, Asymptomatic human immunodeficiency virus [HIV] infection status.

         (g) **HIV infection in pregnancy, childbirth and the puerperium**
            During pregnancy, childbirth or the puerperium, a patient admitted (or presenting for a health care encounter) because of an HIV-related illness should receive a principal diagnosis code of O98.7-, Human immunodeficiency [HIV] disease complicating pregnancy, childbirth and the puerperium, followed by B20 and the code(s) for the HIV-related illness(es). Codes from Chapter 15 always take sequencing priority.

            Patients with asymptomatic HIV infection status admitted (or presenting for a health care encounter) during pregnancy, childbirth, or the puerperium should receive codes of O98.7- and Z21.

         (h) **Encounters for testing for HIV**
            If a patient is being seen to determine his/her HIV status, use code Z11.4, Encounter for screening for human immunodeficiency virus [HIV]. Use additional codes for any associated high risk behavior.

            If a patient with signs or symptoms is being seen for HIV testing, code the signs and symptoms. An additional counseling code Z71.7, Human immunodeficiency virus [HIV] counseling, may be used if counseling is provided during the encounter for the test.

            When a patient returns to be informed of his/her HIV test results and the test result is negative, use code Z71.7, Human immunodeficiency virus [HIV] counseling.

            If the results are positive, see previous guidelines and assign codes as appropriate.

   b. **Infectious agents as the cause of diseases classified to other chapters**
      Certain infections are classified in chapters other than Chapter 1 and no organism is identified as part of the infection code. In these instances, it is necessary to use an additional code from Chapter 1 to identify the organism. A code from category B95, Streptococcus, Staphylococcus, and Enterococcus as the cause of diseases classified to other chapters, B96, Other bacterial agents as the cause of diseases classified to other chapters, or B97, Viral agents as the cause of diseases classified to other chapters, is to be used as an additional code to identify the organism. An instructional note will be found at the infection code advising that an additional organism code is required.

   c. **Infections resistant to antibiotics**
      Many bacterial infections are resistant to current antibiotics. It is necessary to identify all infections documented as antibiotic resistant. Assign a code from category Z16, Resistance to antimicrobial drugs, following the infection code only if the infection code does not identify drug resistance.

   d. **Sepsis, severe sepsis, and septic shock**
      1) **Coding of sepsis and severe sepsis**
         (a) **Sepsis**
            For a diagnosis of sepsis, assign the appropriate code for the underlying systemic infection. If the type of infection or causal organism is not further specified, assign code A41.9, Sepsis, unspecified organism.

            A code from subcategory R65.2, Severe sepsis, should not be assigned unless severe sepsis or an associated acute organ dysfunction is documented.

            (i) Negative or inconclusive blood cultures and sepsis
               Negative or inconclusive blood cultures do not preclude a diagnosis of sepsis in patients with clinical evidence of the condition, however, the provider should be queried.

            (ii) Urosepsis
               The term urosepsis is a nonspecific term. It is not to be considered synonymous with sepsis. It has no default code in the Alphabetic Index. Should a provider use this term, he/she must be queried for clarification.

            (iii) Sepsis with organ dysfunction
               If a patient has sepsis and associated acute organ dysfunction or multiple organ dysfunction (MOD), follow the instructions for coding severe sepsis.

            (iv) Acute organ dysfunction that is not clearly associated with the sepsis
               If a patient has sepsis and an acute organ dysfunction, but the medical record documentation indicates that

the acute organ dysfunction is related to a medical condition other than the sepsis, do not assign a code from subcategory R65.2, Severe sepsis. An acute organ dysfunction must be associated with the sepsis in order to assign the severe sepsis code. If the documentation is not clear as to whether an acute organ dysfunction is related to the sepsis or another medical condition, query the provider.

(b) Severe sepsis

The coding of severe sepsis requires a minimum of 2 codes: first a code for the underlying systemic infection, followed by a code from subcategory R65.2, Severe sepsis. If the causal organism is not documented, assign code A41.9, Sepsis, unspecified organism, for the infection. Additional code(s) for the associated acute organ dysfunction are also required.

Due to the complex nature of severe sepsis, some cases may require querying the provider prior to assignment of the codes.

2) Septic shock

(a) Septic shock generally refers to circulatory failure associated with severe sepsis, and therefore, it represents a type of acute organ dysfunction.

For cases of septic shock, the code for the systemic infection should be sequenced first, followed by code R65.21, Severe sepsis with septic shock or code T81.12, Postprocedural septic shock. Any additional codes for the other acute organ dysfunctions should also be assigned. As noted in the sequencing instructions in the Tabular List, the code for septic shock cannot be assigned as a principal diagnosis.

3) Sequencing of severe sepsis

If severe sepsis is present on admission, and meets the definition of principal diagnosis, the underlying systemic infection should be assigned as principal diagnosis followed by the appropriate code from subcategory R65.2 as required by the sequencing rules in the Tabular List. A code from subcategory R65.2 can never be assigned as a principal diagnosis.

When severe sepsis develops during an encounter (it was not present on admission) the underlying systemic infection and the appropriate code from subcategory R65.2 should be assigned as secondary diagnoses.

Severe sepsis may be present on admission but the diagnosis may not be confirmed until sometime after admission. If the documentation is not clear whether severe sepsis was present on admission, the provider should be queried.

4) Sepsis and severe sepsis with a localized infection

If the reason for admission is both sepsis or severe sepsis and a localized infection, such as pneumonia or cellulitis, a code(s) for the underlying systemic infection should be assigned first and the code for the localized infection should be assigned as a secondary diagnosis. If the patient has severe sepsis, a code from subcategory R65.2 should also be assigned as a secondary diagnosis. If the patient is admitted with a localized infection, such as pneumonia, and sepsis/severe sepsis doesn't develop until after admission, the localized infection should be assigned first, followed by the appropriate sepsis/severe sepsis codes.

5) Sepsis due to a postprocedural infection

(a) Documentation of causal relationship

As with all postprocedural complications, code assignment is based on the provider's documentation of the relationship between the infection and the procedure.

(b) Sepsis due to a postprocedural infection

For such cases, the postprocedural infection code, such as T80.2, Infections following infusion, transfusion, and therapeutic injection, T81.4, Infection following a procedure, T88.0, Infection following immunization, or O86.0, Infection of obstetric surgical wound, should be coded first, followed by the code for the specific infection. If the patient has severe sepsis, the appropriate code from subcategory R65.2 should also be

assigned with the additional code(s) for any acute organ dysfunction.

(c) Postprocedural infection and postprocedural septic shock

In cases where a postprocedural infection has occurred and has resulted in severe sepsis the code for the precipitating complication such as code T81.4, Infection following a procedure, or O86.0, Infection of obstetrical surgical wound should be coded first followed by code R65.20, Severe sepsis without septic shock. A code for the systemic infection should also be assigned.

If a postprocedural infection has resulted in postprocedural septic shock, the code for the precipitating complication such as code T81.4, Infection following a procedure, or O86.0, Infection of obstetrical surgical wound should be coded first followed by code T81.12-, Postprocedural septic shock. A code for the systemic infection should also be assigned.

6) Sepsis and severe sepsis associated with a noninfectious process (condition)

In some cases a noninfectious process (condition), such as trauma, may lead to an infection which can result in sepsis or severe sepsis. If sepsis or severe sepsis is documented as associated with a noninfectious condition, such as a burn or serious injury, and this condition meets the definition for principal diagnosis, the code for the noninfectious condition should be sequenced first, followed by the code for the resulting infection. If severe sepsis is present, a code from subcategory R65.2 should also be assigned with any associated organ dysfunction(s) codes. It is not necessary to assign a code from subcategory R65.1, Systemic inflammatory response syndrome (SIRS) of non-infectious origin, for these cases.

If the infection meets the definition of principal diagnosis, it should be sequenced before the non-infectious condition. When both the associated non-infectious condition and the infection meet the definition of principal diagnosis, either may be assigned as principal diagnosis.

Only one code from category R65, Symptoms and signs specifically associated with systemic inflammation and infection, should be assigned. Therefore, when a non-infectious condition leads to an infection resulting in severe sepsis, assign the appropriate code from subcategory R65.2, Severe sepsis.

Do not additionally assign a code from subcategory R65.1, Systemic inflammatory response syndrome (SIRS) of non-infectious origin.

See Section I.C.18. SIRS due to non-infectious process

7) Sepsis and septic shock complicating abortion, pregnancy, childbirth, and the puerperium

See Section I.C.15. Sepsis and septic shock complicating abortion, pregnancy, childbirth and the puerperium

8) Newborn sepsis

See Section I.C.16. f. Bacterial sepsis of Newborn

e. Methicillin resistant *Staphylococcus aureus* (MRSA) conditions

1) Selection and sequencing of MRSA codes

(a) Combination codes for MRSA infection

When a patient is diagnosed with an infection that is due to methicillin resistant *Staphylococcus aureus* (MRSA), and that infection has a combination code that includes the causal organism (e.g., sepsis, pneumonia) assign the appropriate combination code for the condition (e.g., code A41.02, Sepsis due to Methicillin resistant *Staphylococcus aureus* or code J15.212, Pneumonia due to Methicillin resistant *Staphylococcus aureus*). Do not assign code B95.62, Methicillin resistant *Staphylococcus aureus* infection as the cause of diseases classified elsewhere, as an additional code because the combination code includes the type of infection and the MRSA organism. Do not assign a code from subcategory Z16.11, Resistance to penicillins, as an additional diagnosis.

See Section C.1. for instructions on coding and sequencing of sepsis and severe sepsis.

(b) **Other codes for MRSA infection**
When there is documentation of a current infection (e.g., wound infection, stitch abscess, urinary tract infection) due to MRSA, and that infection does not have a combination code that includes the causal organism, assign the appropriate code to identify the condition along with code B95.62, Methicillin resistant *Staphylococcus aureus* infection as the cause of diseases classified elsewhere for the MRSA infection. Do not assign a code from subcategory Z16.11, Resistance to penicillins.

(c) **Methicillin susceptible *Staphylococcus aureus* (MSSA) and MRSA colonization**
The condition or state of being colonized or carrying MSSA or MRSA is called colonization or carriage, while an individual person is described as being colonized or being a carrier. Colonization means that MSSA or MSRA is present on or in the body without necessarily causing illness. A positive MRSA colonization test might be documented by the provider as "MRSA screen positive" or "MRSA nasal swab positive".

Assign code Z22.322, Carrier or suspected carrier of Methicillin resistant *Staphylococcus aureus*, for patients documented as having MRSA colonization. Assign code Z22.321, Carrier or suspected carrier of Methicillin susceptible *Staphylococcus aureus*, for patient documented as having MSSA colonization. Colonization is not necessarily indicative of a disease process or as the cause of a specific condition the patient may have unless documented as such by the provider.

(d) **MRSA colonization and infection**
If a patient is documented as having both MRSA colonization and infection during a hospital admission, code Z22.322, Carrier or suspected carrier of Methicillin resistant *Staphylococcus aureus*, and a code for the MRSA infection may both be assigned.

2. **Chapter 2: Neoplasms (C00-D49)**

General guidelines

Chapter 2 of the ICD-10-CM contains the codes for most benign and all malignant neoplasms. Certain benign neoplasms, such as prostatic adenomas, may be found in the specific body system chapters. To properly code a neoplasm it is necessary to determine from the record if the neoplasm is benign, in-situ, malignant, or of uncertain histologic behavior. If malignant, any secondary (metastatic) sites should also be determined.

Primary malignant neoplasms overlapping site boundaries

A primary malignant neoplasm that overlaps two or more contiguous (next to each other) sites should be classified to the subcategory/code .8 ('overlapping lesion'), unless the combination is specifically indexed elsewhere. For multiple neoplasms of the same site that are not contiguous such as tumors in different quadrants of the same breast, codes for each site should be assigned.

Malignant neoplasm of ectopic tissue

Malignant neoplasms of ectopic tissue are to be coded to the site of origin mentioned, e.g., ectopic pancreatic malignant neoplasms involving the stomach are coded to pancreas, unspecified (C25.9).

The neoplasm table in the Alphabetic Index should be referenced first. However, if the histological term is documented, that term should be referenced first, rather than going immediately to the Neoplasm Table, in order to determine which column in the Neoplasm Table is appropriate. For example, if the documentation indicates "adenoma," refer to the term in the Alphabetic Index to review the entries under this term and the instructional note to "see also neoplasm, by site, benign." The table provides the proper code based on the type of neoplasm and the site. It is important to select the proper column in the table that corresponds to the type of neoplasm. The Tabular List should then be referenced to verify that the correct code has been selected from the table and that a more specific site code does not exist.

See Section I.C.21. Factors influencing health status and contact with health services, Status, for information regarding Z15.0, codes for genetic susceptibility to cancer.

a. **Treatment directed at the malignancy**
If the treatment is directed at the malignancy, designate the malignancy as the principal diagnosis.

The only exception to this guideline is if a patient admission/encounter is solely for the administration of chemotherapy, immunotherapy or radiation therapy, assign the appropriate Z51.- code as the first-listed or principal diagnosis, and the diagnosis or problem for which the service is being performed as a secondary diagnosis.

b. **Treatment of secondary site**
When a patient is admitted because of a primary neoplasm with metastasis and treatment is directed toward the secondary site only, the secondary neoplasm is designated as the principal diagnosis even though the primary malignancy is still present.

c. **Coding and sequencing of complications**
Coding and sequencing of complications associated with the malignancies or with the therapy thereof are subject to the following guidelines:

1) **Anemia associated with malignancy**
When admission/encounter is for management of an anemia associated with the malignancy, and the treatment is only for anemia, the appropriate code for the malignancy is sequenced as the principal or first-listed diagnosis followed by the appropriate code for the anemia (such as code D63.0, Anemia in neoplastic disease).

2) **Anemia associated with chemotherapy, immunotherapy and radiation therapy**
When the admission/encounter is for management of an anemia associated with an adverse effect of the administration of chemotherapy or immunotherapy and the only treatment is for the anemia, the anemia code is sequenced first followed by the appropriate codes for the neoplasm and the adverse effect (T45.1X5, Adverse effect of antineoplastic and immunosuppressive drugs).

When the admission/encounter is for management of an anemia associated with an adverse effect of radiotherapy, the anemia code should be sequenced first, followed by the appropriate neoplasm code and code Y84.2, Radiological procedure and radiotherapy as the cause of abnormal reaction of the patient, or of later complication, without mention of misadventure at the time of the procedure.

3) **Management of dehydration due to the malignancy**
When the admission/encounter is for management of dehydration due to the malignancy and only the dehydration is being treated (intravenous rehydration), the dehydration is sequenced first, followed by the code(s) for the malignancy.

4) **Treatment of a complication resulting from a surgical procedure**
When the admission/encounter is for treatment of a complication resulting from a surgical procedure, designate the complication as the principal or first-listed diagnosis if treatment is directed at resolving the complication.

d. **Primary malignancy previously excised**
When a primary malignancy has been previously excised or eradicated from its site and there is no further treatment directed to that site and there is no evidence of any existing primary malignancy, a code from category Z85, Personal history of malignant neoplasm, should be used to indicate the former site of the malignancy. Any mention of extension, invasion, or metastasis to another site is coded as a secondary malignant neoplasm to that site. The secondary site may be the principal or first-listed with the Z85 code used as a secondary code.

e. **Admissions/Encounters involving chemotherapy, immunotherapy and radiation therapy**

1) **Episode of care involves surgical removal of neoplasm**
When an episode of care involves the surgical removal of a neoplasm, primary or secondary site, followed by adjunct chemotherapy or radiation treatment during the same episode of care, the code for the neoplasm should be assigned as principal or first-listed diagnosis.

2) **Patient admission/encounter solely for administration of chemotherapy, immunotherapy and radiation therapy**
If a patient admission/encounter is solely for the administration of chemotherapy, immunotherapy or radiation therapy assign code Z51.0, Encounter for antineoplastic radiation therapy, or Z51.11, Encounter for antineoplastic chemotherapy, or Z51.12, Encounter for antineoplastic immunotherapy as the first-listed or principal diagnosis. If a patient receives more than one of these therapies during the same admission more than one of these codes may be assigned, in any sequence.

The malignancy for which the therapy is being administered should be assigned as a secondary diagnosis.

3) **Patient admitted for radiation therapy, chemotherapy or immunotherapy and develops complications**
When a patient is admitted for the purpose of radiotherapy, immunotherapy or chemotherapy and develops complications such as uncontrolled nausea and vomiting or dehydration, the principal or first-listed diagnosis is Z51.0, Encounter for antineoplastic radiation therapy, or Z51.11, Encounter for antineoplastic chemotherapy, or Z51.12, Encounter for antineoplastic immunotherapy followed by any codes for the complications.

f. **Admission/encounter to determine extent of malignancy**
When the reason for admission/encounter is to determine the extent of the malignancy, or for a procedure such as paracentesis or thoracentesis, the primary malignancy or appropriate metastatic site is designated as the principal or first-listed diagnosis, even though chemotherapy or radiotherapy is administered.

g. **Symptoms, signs, and abnormal findings listed in Chapter 18 associated with neoplasms**
Symptoms, signs, and ill-defined conditions listed in Chapter 18 characteristic of, or associated with, an existing primary or secondary site malignancy cannot be used to replace the malignancy as principal or first-listed diagnosis, regardless of the number of admissions or encounters for treatment and care of the neoplasm.
See section I.C.21. Factors influencing health status and contact with health services, Encounter for prophylactic organ removal.

h. **Admission/encounter for pain control/management**
See Section I.C.6. for information on coding admission/encounter for pain control/management.

i. **Malignancy in two or more noncontiguous sites**
A patient may have more than one malignant tumor in the same organ. These tumors may represent different primaries or metastatic disease, depending on the site. Should the documentation be unclear, the provider should be queried as to the status of each tumor so that the correct codes can be assigned.

j. **Disseminated malignant neoplasm, unspecified**
Code C80.0, Disseminated malignant neoplasm, unspecified, is for use only in those cases where the patient has advanced metastatic disease and no known primary or secondary sites are specified. It should not be used in place of assigning codes for the primary site and all known secondary sites.

k. **Malignant neoplasm without specification of site**
Code C80.1, Malignant (primary) neoplasm, unspecified, equates to Cancer, unspecified. This code should only be used when no determination can be made as to the primary site of a malignancy. This code should rarely be used in the inpatient setting.

l. **Sequencing of neoplasm codes**
1) **Encounter for treatment of primary malignancy**
If the reason for the encounter is for treatment of a primary malignancy, assign the malignancy as the principal/first-listed diagnosis. The primary site is to be sequenced first, followed by any metastatic sites.

2) **Encounter for treatment of secondary malignancy**
When an encounter is for a primary malignancy with metastasis and treatment is directed toward the metastatic (secondary) site(s) only, the metastatic site(s) is designated as the principal/first-listed diagnosis. The primary malignancy is coded as an additional code.

3) **Malignant neoplasm in a pregnant patient**
When a pregnant woman has a malignant neoplasm, a code from subcategory O9A.1-, Malignant neoplasm complicating pregnancy, childbirth, and the puerperium, should be sequenced first, followed by the appropriate code from Chapter 2 to indicate the type of neoplasm.

4) **Encounter for complication associated with a neoplasm**
When an encounter is for management of a complication associated with a neoplasm, such as dehydration, and the treatment is only for the complication, the complication is coded first, followed by the appropriate code(s) for the neoplasm.

The exception to this guideline is anemia. When the admission/encounter is for management of an anemia associated with the malignancy, and the treatment is only for anemia, the appropriate code for the malignancy is sequenced as the principal or first-listed diagnosis followed by code D63.0, Anemia in neoplastic disease.

5) **Complication from surgical procedure for treatment of a neoplasm**
When an encounter is for treatment of a complication resulting from a surgical procedure performed for the treatment of the neoplasm, designate the complication as the principal/first-listed diagnosis. See guideline regarding the coding of a current malignancy versus personal history to determine if the code for the neoplasm should also be assigned.

6) **Pathologic fracture due to a neoplasm**
When an encounter is for a pathological fracture due to a neoplasm, and the focus of treatment is the fracture, a code from subcategory M84.5, Pathological fracture in neoplastic disease, should be sequenced first, followed by the code for the neoplasm.

If the focus of treatment is the neoplasm with an associated pathological fracture, the neoplasm code should be sequenced first, followed by a code from M84.5 for the pathological fracture.

m. **Current malignancy versus personal history of malignancy**
When a primary malignancy has been excised but further treatment, such as an additional surgery for the malignancy, radiation therapy or chemotherapy is directed to that site, the primary malignancy code should be used until treatment is completed.

When a primary malignancy has been previously excised or eradicated from its site, there is no further treatment (of the malignancy) directed to that site, and there is no evidence of any existing primary malignancy, a code from category Z85, Personal history of malignant neoplasm, should be used to indicate the former site of the malignancy.
See Section I.C.21. Factors influencing health status and contact with health services, History (of)

n. **Leukemia, multiple myeloma, and malignant plasma cell neoplasms in remission versus personal history**
The categories for leukemia, and category C90, Multiple myeloma and malignant plasma cell neoplasms, have codes indicating whether or not the leukemia has achieved remission. There are also codes Z85.6, Personal history of leukemia, and Z85.79, Personal history of other malignant neoplasms of lymphoid, hematopoietic and related tissues. If the documentation is unclear, as to whether the leukemia has achieved remission, the provider should be queried.
See Section I.C.21. Factors influencing health status and contact with health services, History (of)

o. **Aftercare following surgery for neoplasm**
See Section I.C.21. Factors influencing health status and contact with health services, Aftercare

p. **Follow-up care for completed treatment of a malignancy**
See Section I.C.21. Factors influencing health status and contact with health services, Follow-up

q. **Prophylactic organ removal for prevention of malignancy**
See Section I.C. 21, Factors influencing health status and contact with health services, Prophylactic organ removal

r. **Malignant neoplasm associated with transplanted organ**
    A malignant neoplasm of a transplanted organ should be coded as a transplant complication. Assign first the appropriate code from category T86.-, Complications of transplanted organs and tissue, followed by code C80.2, Malignant neoplasm associated with transplanted organ. Use an additional code for the specific malignancy.

3. **Chapter 3: Disease of the blood and blood-forming organs and certain disorders involving the immune mechanism (D50-D89)**
    Reserved for future guideline expansion

4. **Chapter 4: Endocrine, Nutritional, and Metabolic Diseases (E00-E89)**
    a. Diabetes mellitus
    The diabetes mellitus codes are combination codes that include the type of diabetes mellitus, the body system affected, and the complications affecting that body system. As many codes within a particular category as are necessary to describe all of the complications of the disease may be used. They should be sequenced based on the reason for a particular encounter. Assign as many codes from categories E08 – E13 as needed to identify all of the associated conditions that the patient has.

    1) **Type of diabetes**
        The age of a patient is not the sole determining factor, though most type 1 diabetics develop the condition before reaching puberty. For this reason type 1 diabetes mellitus is also referred to as juvenile diabetes.

    2) **Type of diabetes mellitus not documented**
        If the type of diabetes mellitus is not documented in the medical record the default is E11.-, Type 2 diabetes mellitus.

    3) **Diabetes mellitus and the use of insulin**
        If the documentation in a medical record does not indicate the type of diabetes but does indicate that the patient uses insulin, code E11, Type 2 diabetes mellitus, should be assigned. Code Z79.4, Long-term (current) use of insulin, should also be assigned to indicate that the patient uses insulin. Code Z79.4 should not be assigned if insulin is given temporarily to bring a type 2 patient's blood sugar under control during an encounter.

    4) **Diabetes mellitus in pregnancy and gestational diabetes**
        See Section I.C.15. Diabetes mellitus in pregnancy.
        See Section I.C.15. Gestational (pregnancy induced) diabetes

    5) **Complications due to insulin pump malfunction**
        (a) **Underdose of insulin due to insulin pump failure**
            An underdose of insulin due to an insulin pump failure should be assigned to a code from subcategory T85.6, Mechanical complication of other specified internal and external prosthetic devices, implants and grafts, that specifies the type of pump malfunction, as the principal or first-listed code, followed by code T38.3x6-, Underdosing of insulin and oral hypoglycemic [antidiabetic] drugs. Additional codes for the type of diabetes mellitus and any associated complications due to the underdosing should also be assigned.

        (b) **Overdose of insulin due to insulin pump failure**
            The principal or first-listed code for an encounter due to an insulin pump malfunction resulting in an overdose of insulin, should also be T85.6-, Mechanical complication of other specified internal and external prosthetic devices, implants and grafts, followed by code T38.3X1-, Poisoning by insulin and oral hypoglycemic [antidiabetic] drugs, accidental (unintentional).

    6) **Secondary diabetes mellitus**
        Codes under categories E08, Diabetes mellitus due to underlying condition, E09, Drug or chemical induced diabetes mellitus, and E13, Other specified diabetes mellitus, identify complications/manifestations associated with secondary diabetes mellitus. Secondary diabetes is always caused by another condition or event (e.g., cystic fibrosis, malignant neoplasm of pancreas, pancreatectomy, adverse effect of drug, or poisoning).

        (a) **Secondary diabetes mellitus and the use of insulin**
            For patients who routinely use insulin, code Z79.4, Long-term (current) use of insulin, should also be assigned. Code Z79.4 should not be assigned if insulin is given temporarily to bring a patient's blood sugar under control during an encounter.

        (b) **Assigning and sequencing secondary diabetes codes and its causes**
            The sequencing of the secondary diabetes codes in relationship to codes for the cause of the diabetes is based on the Tabular List instructions for categories E08, E09 and E13.

            (i) **Secondary diabetes mellitus due to pancreatectomy**
                 For postpancreatectomy diabetes mellitus (lack of insulin due to the surgical removal of all or part of the pancreas), assign code E89.1, Postprocedural hypoinsulinemia. Assign a code from category E13 and a code from subcategory Z90.41-, Acquired absence of pancreas, as additional codes.

            (ii) **Secondary diabetes due to drugs**
                 Secondary diabetes may be caused by an adverse effect of correctly administered medications, poisoning or sequela of poisoning.
                 See section I.C.19.e for coding of adverse effects and poisoning, and section I.C.20 for external cause code reporting.

5. **Chapter 5: Mental, Behavioral and Neurodevelopmental disorders (F01 – F99)**
    a. Pain disorders related to psychological factors
    Assign code F45.41, for pain that is exclusively related to psychological disorders. As indicated by the Excludes 1 note under category G89, a code from category G89 should not be assigned with code F45.41.

    Code F45.42, Pain disorders with related psychological factors, should be used with a code from category G89, Pain, not elsewhere classified, if there is documentation of a psychological component for a patient with acute or chronic pain.
    See Section I.C.6. Pain

    b. Mental and behavioral disorders due to psychoactive substance use
    1) **In remission**
        Selection of codes for "in remission" for categories F10-F19, Mental and behavioral disorders due to psychoactive substance use (categories F10-F19 with -.21) requires the provider's clinical judgment. The appropriate codes for "in remission" are assigned only on the basis of provider documentation (as defined in the Official Guidelines for Coding and Reporting).

    2) **Psychoactive substance use, abuse and dependence**
        When the provider documentation refers to use, abuse and dependence of the same substance (e.g. alcohol, opioid, cannabis, etc.), only one code should be assigned to identify the pattern of use based on the following hierarchy:

        • If both use and abuse are documented, assign only the code for abuse
        • If both abuse and dependence are documented, assign only the code for dependence
        • If use, abuse and dependence are all documented, assign only the code for dependence
        • If both use and dependence are documented, assign only the code for dependence.

    3) **Psychoactive substance use**
        As with all other diagnoses, the codes for psychoactive substance use (F10.9-, F11.9-, F12.9-, F13.9-, F14.9-, F15.9-, F16.9-) should only be assigned based on provider documentation and when they meet the definition of a reportable diagnosis (see Section III, Reporting Additional Diagnoses). The codes are to be used only when the psychoactive substance use is associated with a mental or behavioral disorder, and such a relationship is documented by the provider.

6. **Chapter 6: Diseases of Nervous System (G00-G99)**

   a. **Dominant/nondominant side**

   Codes from category G81, Hemiplegia and hemiparesis, and subcategories, G83.1, Monoplegia of lower limb, G83.2, Monoplegia of upper limb, and G83.3, Monoplegia, unspecified, identify whether the dominant or nondominant side is affected. Should the affected side be documented, but not specified as dominant or nondominant, and the classification system does not indicate a default, code selection is as follows:

   - For ambidextrous patients, the default should be dominant.
   - If the left side is affected, the default is non-dominant.
   - If the right side is affected, the default is dominant.

   b. **Pain - Category G89**

   1) **General coding information**

   Codes in category G89, Pain, not elsewhere classified, may be used in conjunction with codes from other categories and chapters to provide more detail about acute or chronic pain and neoplasm-related pain, unless otherwise indicated below.

   If the pain is not specified as acute or chronic, post-thoracotomy, postprocedural, or neoplasm-related, do not assign codes from category G89.

   A code from category G89 should not be assigned if the underlying (definitive) diagnosis is known, unless the reason for the encounter is pain control/ management and not management of the underlying condition.

   When an admission or encounter is for a procedure aimed at treating the underlying condition (e.g., spinal fusion, kyphoplasty), a code for the underlying condition (e.g., vertebral fracture, spinal stenosis) should be assigned as the principal diagnosis. No code from category G89 should be assigned.

   (a) **Category G89 codes as principal or first-listed diagnosis**

   Category G89 codes are acceptable as principal diagnosis or the first-listed code:

   - When pain control or pain management is the reason for the admission/encounter (e.g., a patient with displaced intervertebral disc, nerve impingement and severe back pain presents for injection of steroid into the spinal canal). The underlying cause of the pain should be reported as an additional diagnosis, if known.

   - When a patient is admitted for the insertion of a neurostimulator for pain control, assign the appropriate pain code as the principal or first-listed diagnosis. When an admission or encounter is for a procedure aimed at treating the underlying condition and a neurostimulator is inserted for pain control during the same admission/encounter, a code for the underlying condition should be assigned as the principal diagnosis and the appropriate pain code should be assigned as a secondary diagnosis.

   (b) **Use of category G89 codes in conjunction with site specific pain codes**

   (i) **Assigning category G89 and site-specific pain codes**

   Codes from category G89 may be used in conjunction with codes that identify the site of pain (including codes from chapter 18) if the category G89 code provides additional information. For example, if the code describes the site of the pain, but does not fully describe whether the pain is acute or chronic, then both codes should be assigned.

   (ii) **Sequencing of category G89 codes with site-specific pain codes**

   The sequencing of category G89 codes with site-specific pain codes (including chapter 18 codes), is dependent on the circumstances of the encounter/admission as follows:

   - If the encounter is for pain control or pain management, assign the code from category G89 followed by the code identifying the specific site of pain (e.g., encounter for pain management for acute neck pain from trauma is assigned code G89.11, Acute pain due to trauma, followed by code M54.2, Cervicalgia, to identify the site of pain).

   - If the encounter is for any other reason except pain control or pain management, and a related definitive diagnosis has not been established (confirmed) by the provider, assign the code for the specific site of pain first, followed by the appropriate code from category G89.

   2) **Pain due to devices, implants and grafts**
   See Section I.C.19. Pain due to medical devices

   3) **Postoperative pain**

   The provider's documentation should be used to guide the coding of postoperative pain, as well as *Section III. Reporting Additional Diagnoses* and *Section IV. Diagnostic Coding and Reporting in the Outpatient Setting.*

   The default for post-thoracotomy and other postoperative pain not specified as acute or chronic is the code for the acute form.

   Routine or expected postoperative pain immediately after surgery should not be coded.

   (a) **Postoperative pain not associated with specific postoperative complication**

   Postoperative pain not associated with a specific postoperative complication is assigned to the appropriate postoperative pain code in category G89.

   (b) **Postoperative pain associated with specific postoperative complication**

   Postoperative pain associated with a specific postoperative complication (such as painful wire sutures) is assigned to the appropriate code(s) found in Chapter 19, Injury, poisoning, and certain other consequences of external causes. If appropriate, use additional code(s) from category G89 to identify acute or chronic pain (G89.18 or G89.28).

   4) **Chronic pain**

   Chronic pain is classified to subcategory G89.2. There is no time frame defining when pain becomes chronic pain. The provider's documentation should be used to guide use of these codes.

   5) **Neoplasm related pain**

   Code G89.3 is assigned to pain documented as being related, associated or due to cancer, primary or secondary malignancy, or tumor. This code is assigned regardless of whether the pain is acute or chronic.

   This code may be assigned as the principal or first-listed code when the stated reason for the admission/encounter is documented as pain control/pain management. The underlying neoplasm should be reported as an additional diagnosis.

   When the reason for the admission/encounter is management of the neoplasm and the pain associated with the neoplasm is also documented, code G89.3 may be assigned as an additional diagnosis. It is not necessary to assign an additional code for the site of the pain.

   See Section I.C.2 for instructions on the sequencing of neoplasms for all other stated reasons for the admission/encounter (except for pain control/pain management).

   6) **Chronic pain syndrome**

   Central pain syndrome (G89.0) and chronic pain syndrome (G89.4) are different than the term "chronic pain," and therefore codes should only be used when the provider has specifically documented this condition.

   See Section I.C.5. Pain disorders related to psychological factors

7. **Chapter 7: Diseases of Eye and Adnexa (H00-H59)**

   a. **Glaucoma**

   1) **Assigning glaucoma codes**

   Assign as many codes from category H40, Glaucoma, as needed to identify the type of glaucoma, the affected eye, and the glaucoma stage.

   2) **Bilateral glaucoma with same type and stage**

   When a patient has bilateral glaucoma and both eyes are documented as being the same type and stage, and there is a code for bilateral glaucoma, report only the code for the type of glaucoma, bilateral, with the seventh character for the stage.

When a patient has bilateral glaucoma and both eyes are documented as being the same type and stage, and the classification does not provide a code for bilateral glaucoma (i.e. subcategories H40.10, H40.11 and H40.20) report only one code for the type of glaucoma with the appropriate seventh character for the stage.

3) Bilateral glaucoma stage with different types or stages

When a patient has bilateral glaucoma and each eye is documented as having a different type or stage, and the classification distinguishes laterality, assign the appropriate code for each eye rather than the code for bilateral glaucoma.

When a patient has bilateral glaucoma and each eye is documented as having a different type, and the classification does not distinguish laterality (i.e. subcategories H40.10, H40.11 and H40.20), assign one code for each type of glaucoma with the appropriate seventh character for the stage.

When a patient has bilateral glaucoma and each eye is documented as having the same type, but different stage, and the classification does not distinguish laterality (i.e. subcategories H40.10, H40.11 and H40.20), assign a code for the type of glaucoma for each eye with the seventh character for the specific glaucoma stage documented for each eye.

4) Patient admitted with glaucoma and stage evolves during the admission

If a patient is admitted with glaucoma and the stage progresses during the admission, assign the code for highest stage documented.

5) Indeterminate stage glaucoma

Assignment of the seventh character "4" for "indeterminate stage" should be based on the clinical documentation. The seventh character "4" is used for glaucomas whose stage cannot be clinically determined. This seventh character should not be confused with the seventh character "0", unspecified, which should be assigned when there is no documentation regarding the stage of the glaucoma.

8. Chapter 8: Diseases of Ear and Mastoid Process (H60-H95)

Reserved for future guideline expansion

9. Chapter 9: Diseases of Circulatory System (I00-I99)

a. Hypertension

1) Hypertension with heart disease

Heart conditions classified to I50.- or I51.4-I51.9, are assigned to, a code from category I11, Hypertensive heart disease, when a causal relationship is stated (due to hypertension) or implied (hypertensive). Use an additional code from category I50, Heart failure, to identify the type of heart failure in those patients with heart failure.

The same heart conditions (I50.-, I51.4-I51.9) with hypertension, but without a stated causal relationship, are coded separately. Sequence according to the circumstances of the admission/encounter.

2) Hypertensive chronic kidney disease

Assign codes from category I12, Hypertensive chronic kidney disease, when both hypertension and a condition classifiable to category N18, Chronic kidney disease (CKD), are present. Unlike hypertension with heart disease, ICD-10-CM presumes a cause-and-effect relationship and classifies chronic kidney disease with hypertension as hypertensive chronic kidney disease.

The appropriate code from category N18 should be used as a secondary code with a code from category I12 to identify the stage of chronic kidney disease.

See Section I.C.14. Chronic kidney disease.

If a patient has hypertensive chronic kidney disease and acute renal failure, an additional code for the acute renal failure is required.

3) Hypertensive heart and chronic kidney disease

Assign codes from combination category I13, Hypertensive heart and chronic kidney disease, when both hypertensive

kidney disease and hypertensive heart disease are stated in the diagnosis. Assume a relationship between the hypertension and the chronic kidney disease, whether or not the condition is so designated. If heart failure is present, assign an additional code from category I50 to identify the type of heart failure.

The appropriate code from category N18, Chronic kidney disease, should be used as a secondary code with a code from category I13 to identify the stage of chronic kidney disease.

See Section I.C.14. Chronic kidney disease.

The codes in category I13, Hypertensive heart and chronic kidney disease, are combination codes that include hypertension, heart disease and chronic kidney disease. The Includes note at I13 specifies that the conditions included at I11 and I12 are included together in I13. If a patient has hypertension, heart disease and chronic kidney disease then a code from I13 should be used, not individual codes for hypertension, heart disease and chronic kidney disease, or codes from I11 or I12.

For patients with both acute renal failure and chronic kidney disease an additional code for acute renal failure is required.

4) Hypertensive cerebrovascular disease

For hypertensive cerebrovascular disease, first assign the appropriate code from categories I60-I69, followed by the appropriate hypertension code.

5) Hypertensive retinopathy

Subcategory H35.0, Background retinopathy and retinal vascular changes, should be used with a code from category I10 – I15, Hypertensive disease to include the systemic hypertension. The sequencing is based on the reason for the encounter.

6) Hypertension, secondary

Secondary hypertension is due to an underlying condition. Two codes are required: one to identify the underlying etiology and one from category I15 to identify the hypertension. Sequencing of codes is determined by the reason for admission/encounter.

7) Hypertension, transient

Assign code R03.0, Elevated blood pressure reading without diagnosis of hypertension, unless patient has an established diagnosis of hypertension. Assign code O13.-, Gestational [pregnancy-induced] hypertension without significant proteinuria, or O14.-, Pre-eclampsia, for transient hypertension of pregnancy.

8) Hypertension, controlled

This diagnostic statement usually refers to an existing state of hypertension under control by therapy. Assign the appropriate code from categories I10-I15, Hypertensive diseases.

9) Hypertension, uncontrolled

Uncontrolled hypertension may refer to untreated hypertension or hypertension not responding to current therapeutic regimen. In either case, assign the appropriate code from categories I10-I15, Hypertensive diseases.

b. Atherosclerotic coronary artery disease and angina

ICD-10-CM has combination codes for atherosclerotic heart disease with angina pectoris. The subcategories for these codes are I25.11, Atherosclerotic heart disease of native coronary artery with angina pectoris and I25.7, Atherosclerosis of coronary artery bypass graft(s) and coronary artery of transplanted heart with angina pectoris.

When using one of these combination codes it is not necessary to use an additional code for angina pectoris. A causal relationship can be assumed in a patient with both atherosclerosis and angina pectoris, unless the documentation indicates the angina is due to something other than the atherosclerosis.

If a patient with coronary artery disease is admitted due to an acute myocardial infarction (AMI), the AMI should be sequenced before the coronary artery disease.

See Section I.C.9. Acute myocardial infarction (AMI)

c. Intraoperative and postprocedural cerebrovascular accident

Medical record documentation should clearly specify the cause-and-effect relationship between the medical intervention and the cerebrovascular accident in order to assign a code for intraoperative or postprocedural cerebrovascular accident.

Proper code assignment depends on whether it was an infarction or hemorrhage and whether it occurred intraoperatively or postoperatively. If it was a cerebral hemorrhage, code assignment depends on the type of procedure performed.

d. Sequelae of cerebrovascular disease

1) Category I69, sequelae of cerebrovascular disease

Category I69 is used to indicate conditions classifiable to categories I60-I67 as the causes of sequela (neurologic deficits), themselves classified elsewhere. These "late effects" include neurologic deficits that persist after initial onset of conditions classifiable to categories I60-I67. The neurologic deficits caused by cerebrovascular disease may be present from the onset or may arise at any time after the onset of the condition classifiable to categories I60-I67.

Codes from category I69, Sequelae of cerebrovascular disease, that specify hemiplegia, hemiparesis and monoplegia identify whether the dominant or nondominant side is affected. Should the affected side be documented, but not specified as dominant or nondominant, and the classification system does not indicate a default, code selection is as follows:

- For ambidextrous patients, the default should be dominant.
- If the left side is affected, the default is non-dominant.
- If the right side is affected, the default is dominant.

2) Codes from category I69 with codes from I60-I67

Codes from category I69 may be assigned on a health care record with codes from I60-I67, if the patient has a current cerebrovascular disease and deficits from an old cerebrovascular disease.

3) Codes from category I69 and Personal history of transient ischemic attack (TIA) and cerebral infarction (Z86.73)

Codes from category I69 should not be assigned if the patient does not have neurologic deficits.

See Section I.C.21. 4. History (of) for use of personal history codes

e. Acute myocardial infarction (AMI)

1) ST elevation myocardial infarction (STEMI) and non ST elevation myocardial infarction (NSTEMI)

The ICD-10-CM codes for acute myocardial infarction (AMI) identify the site, such as anterolateral wall or true posterior wall. Subcategories I21.0-I21.2 and code I21.3 are used for ST elevation myocardial infarction (STEMI). Code I21.4, Non-ST elevation (NSTEMI) myocardial infarction, is used for non ST elevation myocardial infarction (NSTEMI) and nontransmural MIs.

If NSTEMI evolves to STEMI, assign the STEMI code. If STEMI converts to NSTEMI due to thrombolytic therapy, it is still coded as STEMI.

For encounters occurring while the myocardial infarction is equal to, or less than, four weeks old, including transfers to another acute setting or a postacute setting, and the patient requires continued care for the myocardial infarction, codes from category I21 may continue to be reported. For encounters after the 4 week time frame and the patient is still receiving care related to the myocardial infarction, the appropriate aftercare code should be assigned, rather than a code from category I21. For old or healed myocardial infarctions not requiring further care, code I25.2, Old myocardial infarction, may be assigned.

2) Acute myocardial infarction, unspecified

Code I21.3, ST elevation (STEMI) myocardial infarction of unspecified site, is the default for the unspecified term acute myocardial infarction. If only STEMI or transmural MI without the site is documented, query the provider as to the site, or assign code I21.3.

3) AMI documented as nontransmural or subendocardial but site provided

If an AMI is documented as nontransmural or subendocardial, but the site is provided, it is still coded as a subendocardial AMI.

See Section I.C.21.3 for information on coding status post administration of tPA in a different facility within the last 24 hrs.

4) Subsequent acute myocardial infarction

A code from category I22, Subsequent ST elevation (STEMI) and non ST elevation (NSTEMI) myocardial infarction, is to be used when a patient who has suffered an AMI has a new AMI within the 4 week time frame of the initial AMI. A code from category I22 must be used in conjunction with a code from category I21. The sequencing of the I22 and I21 codes depends on the circumstances of the encounter.

10. Chapter 10: Diseases of the Respiratory System (J00-J99)

a. Chronic Obstructive Pulmonary Disease [COPD] and Asthma

1) Acute exacerbation of chronic obstructive bronchitis and asthma

The codes in categories J44 and J45 distinguish between uncomplicated cases and those in acute exacerbation. An acute exacerbation is a worsening or a decompensation of a chronic condition. An acute exacerbation is not equivalent to an infection superimposed on a chronic condition, though an exacerbation may be triggered by an infection.

b. Acute Respiratory Failure

1) Acute respiratory failure as principal diagnosis

A code from subcategory J96.0, Acute respiratory failure, or subcategory J96.2, Acute and chronic respiratory failure, may be assigned as a principal diagnosis when it is the condition established after study to be chiefly responsible for occasioning the admission to the hospital, and the selection is supported by the Alphabetic Index and Tabular List. However, chapter-specific coding guidelines (such as obstetrics, poisoning, HIV, newborn) that provide sequencing direction take precedence.

2) Acute respiratory failure as secondary diagnosis

Respiratory failure may be listed as a secondary diagnosis if it occurs after admission, or if it is present on admission, but does not meet the definition of principal diagnosis.

3) Sequencing of acute respiratory failure and another acute condition

When a patient is admitted with respiratory failure and another acute condition, (e.g., myocardial infarction, cerebrovascular accident, aspiration pneumonia), the principal diagnosis will not be the same in every situation. This applies whether the other acute condition is a respiratory or nonrespiratory condition. Selection of the principal diagnosis will be dependent on the circumstances of admission. If both the respiratory failure and the other acute condition are equally responsible for occasioning the admission to the hospital, and there are no chapter-specific sequencing rules, the guideline regarding two or more diagnoses that equally meet the definition for principal diagnosis (Section II, C.) may be applied in these situations.

If the documentation is not clear as to whether acute respiratory failure and another condition are equally responsible for occasioning the admission, query the provider for clarification.

c. Influenza due to certain identified influenza viruses

Code only confirmed cases of influenza due to certain identified influenza viruses (category J09), and due to other identified influenza virus (category J10). This is an exception to the hospital inpatient guideline Section II, H. (Uncertain Diagnosis).

In this context, "confirmation" does not require documentation of positive laboratory testing specific for avian or other novel influenza A or other identified influenza virus. However, coding should be based on the provider's diagnostic statement that the patient has avian influenza, or other novel influenza A, for category J09, or has another particular identified strain of influenza, such as H1N1 or H3N2, but not identified as novel or variant, for category J10.

If the provider records "suspected" or "possible" or "probable" avian influenza, or novel influenza, or other identified influenza, then the appropriate influenza code from category J11, Influenza due to unidentified influenza virus, should be assigned. A code from category J09, Influenza due to certain identified influenza viruses, should not be assigned nor should a code from category J10, Influenza due to other identified influenza virus.

d. Ventilator associated pneumonia

1) Documentation of ventilator associated pneumonia

As with all procedural or postprocedural complications, code assignment is based on the provider's documentation of the relationship between the condition and the procedure.

Code J95.851, Ventilator associated pneumonia, should be assigned only when the provider has documented ventilator associated pneumonia (VAP). An additional code to identify the organism (e.g., Pseudomonas aeruginosa, code B96.5) should also be assigned. Do not assign an additional code from categories J12-J18 to identify the type of pneumonia.

Code J95.851 should not be assigned for cases where the patient has pneumonia and is on a mechanical ventilator and the provider has not specifically stated that the pneumonia is ventilator-associated pneumonia. If the documentation is unclear as to whether the patient has a pneumonia that is a complication attributable to the mechanical ventilator, query the provider.

2) Ventilator associated pneumonia develops after admission

A patient may be admitted with one type of pneumonia (e.g., code J13, Pneumonia due to Streptococcus pneu- monia) and subsequently develop VAP. In this instance, the principal diagnosis would be the appro- priate code from categories J12-J18 for the pneumonia diagnosed at the time of admission. Code J95.851, Ventilator assoc- iated pneumonia, would be assigned as an additional diagnosis when the provider has also documented the presence of ventilator associated pneumonia.

11. Chapter 11: Diseases of the Digestive System (K00-K95)

Reserved for future guideline expansion

12. Chapter 12: Diseases of the Skin and Subcutaneous Tissue (L00-L99)

a. Pressure ulcer stage codes

1) Pressure ulcer stages

Codes from category L89, Pressure ulcer, are combination codes that identify the site of the pressure ulcer as well as the stage of the ulcer.

The ICD-10-CM classifies pressure ulcer stages based on severity, which is designated by stages 1-4, unspecified stage and unstageable.

Assign as many codes from category L89 as needed to identify all the pressure ulcers the patient has, if applicable.

2) Unstageable pressure ulcers

Assignment of the code for unstageable pressure ulcer (L89.--0) should be based on the clinical documentation. These codes are used for pressure ulcers whose stage cannot be clinically determined (e.g., the ulcer is covered by eschar or has been treated with a skin or muscle graft) and pressure ulcers that are documented as deep tissue injury but not documented as due to trauma. This code should not be confused with the codes for unspecified stage (L89.--9). When there is no documentation regarding the stage of the pressure ulcer, assign the appropriate code for unspecified stage (L89.--9).

3) Documented pressure ulcer stage

Assignment of the pressure ulcer stage code should be guided by clinical documentation of the stage or documentation of the terms found in the Alphabetic Index. For clinical terms describing the stage that are not found in the Alphabetic Index, and there is no documentation of the stage, the provider should be queried.

4) Patients admitted with pressure ulcers documented as healed

No code is assigned if the documentation states that the pressure ulcer is completely healed.

5) Patients admitted with pressure ulcers documented as healing

Pressure ulcers described as healing should be assigned the appropriate pressure ulcer stage code based on the documentation in the medical record. If the documentation does not provide information about the stage of the healing pressure ulcer, assign the appropriate code for unspecified stage.

If the documentation is unclear as to whether the patient has a current (new) pressure ulcer or if the patient is being treated for a healing pressure ulcer, query the provider.

6) Patient admitted with pressure ulcer evolving into another stage during the admission

If a patient is admitted with a pressure ulcer at one stage and it progresses to a higher stage, assign the code for the highest stage reported for that site.

13. Chapter 13: Diseases of the Musculoskeletal System and Connective Tissue (M00-M99)

a. Site and laterality

Most of the codes within Chapter 13 have site and laterality designations. The site represents the bone, joint or the muscle involved. For some conditions where more than one bone, joint or muscle is usually involved, such as osteoarthritis, there is a "multiple sites" code available. For categories where no multiple site code is provided and more than one bone, joint or muscle is involved, multiple codes should be used to indicate the different sites involved.

1) Bone versus joint

For certain conditions, the bone may be affected at the upper or lower end, (e.g., avascular necrosis of bone, M87, Osteoporosis, M80, M81). Though the portion of the bone affected may be at the joint, the site designation will be the bone, not the joint.

b. Acute traumatic versus chronic or recurrent musculoskeletal conditions

Many musculoskeletal conditions are a result of previous injury or trauma to a site, or are recurrent conditions. Bone, joint or muscle conditions that are the result of a healed injury are usually found in chapter 13. Recurrent bone, joint or muscle conditions are also usually found in chapter 13. Any current, acute injury should be coded to the appropriate injury code from chapter 19. Chronic or recurrent conditions should generally be coded with a code from chapter 13. If it is difficult to determine from the documentation in the record which code is best to describe a condition, query the provider.

c. Coding of Pathologic Fractures

7th character A is for use as long as the patient is receiving active treatment for the fracture. Examples of active treatment are: surgical treatment, emergency department encounter, evaluation and continuing treatment by the same or a different physician. While the patient may be seen by a new or different provider over the course of treatment for a pathological fracture, assignment of the 7th character is based on whether the patient is undergoing active treatment and not whether the provider is seeing the patient for the first time.

7th character, D is to be used for encounters after the patient has completed active treatment. The other 7th characters, listed under each subcategory in the Tabular List, are to be used for subsequent encounters for treatment of problems associated with the healing, such as malunions, nonunions, and sequelae.

Care for complications of surgical treatment for fracture repairs during the healing or recovery phase should be coded with the appropriate complication codes.

See Section I.C.19. Coding of traumatic fractures.

d. Osteoporosis

Osteoporosis is a systemic condition, meaning that all bones of the musculoskeletal system are affected. Therefore, site is not a component of the codes under category M81, Osteoporosis without current pathological fracture. The site codes under category M80, Osteoporosis with current pathological fracture, identify the site of the fracture, not the osteoporosis.

1) Osteoporosis without pathological fracture

Category M81, Osteoporosis without current pathological fracture, is for use for patients with osteoporosis who do not currently have a pathologic fracture due to the osteoporosis, even if they have had a fracture in the past. For patients with a history of osteoporosis fractures, status code Z87.310, Personal history of (healed) osteoporosis fracture, should follow the code from M81.

2) Osteoporosis with current pathological fracture
Category M80, Osteoporosis with current pathological fracture, is for patients who have a current pathologic fracture at the time of an encounter. The codes under M80 identify the site of the fracture. A code from category M80, not a traumatic fracture code, should be used for any patient with known osteoporosis who suffers a fracture, even if the patient had a minor fall or trauma, if that fall or trauma would not usually break a normal, healthy bone.

14. Chapter 14: Diseases of Genitourinary System (N00-N99)
a. Chronic kidney disease
1) Stages of chronic kidney disease (CKD)
The ICD-10-CM classifies CKD based on severity. The severity of CKD is designated by stages 1-5. Stage 2, code N18.2, equates to mild CKD; stage 3, code N18.3, equates to moderate CKD; and stage 4, code N18.4, equates to severe CKD. Code N18.6, End stage renal disease (ESRD), is assigned when the provider has documented end-stage-renal disease (ESRD).

If both a stage of CKD and ESRD are documented, assign code N18.6 only.

2) Chronic kidney disease and kidney transplant status
Patients who have undergone kidney transplant may still have some form of chronic kidney disease (CKD) because the kidney transplant may not fully restore kidney function. Therefore, the presence of CKD alone does not constitute a transplant complication. Assign the appropriate N18 code for the patient's stage of CKD and code Z94.0, Kidney transplant status. If a transplant complication such as failure or rejection or other transplant complication is documented, see section I.C.19.g for information on coding complications of a kidney transplant. If the documentation is unclear as to whether the patient has a complication of the transplant, query the provider.

3) Chronic kidney disease with other conditions
Patients with CKD may also suffer from other serious conditions, most commonly diabetes mellitus and hypertension. The sequencing of the CKD code in relationship to codes for other contributing conditions is based on the conventions in the Tabular List.

See I.C.9. Hypertensive chronic kidney disease.

See I.C.19. Chronic kidney disease and kidney transplant complications.

15. Chapter 15: Pregnancy, Childbirth, and the Puerperium (O00-O9A)
a. General Rules for Obstetric Cases
1) Codes from chapter 15 and sequencing priority
Obstetric cases require codes from chapter 15, codes in the range O00-O9A, Pregnancy, Childbirth, and the Puerperium. Chapter 15 codes have sequencing priority over codes from other chapters. Additional codes from other chapters may be used in conjunction with chapter 15 codes to further specify conditions. Should the provider document that the pregnancy is incidental to the encounter, then code Z33.1, Pregnant state, incidental, should be used in place of any chapter 15 codes. It is the provider's responsibility to state that the condition being treated is not affecting the pregnancy.

2) Chapter 15 codes used only on the maternal record
Chapter 15 codes are to be used only on the maternal record, never on the record of the newborn.

3) Final character for trimester
The majority of codes in Chapter 15 have a final character indicating the trimester of pregnancy. The timeframes for the trimesters are indicated at the beginning of the chapter. If trimester is not a component of a code it is because the condition always occurs in a specific trimester, or the concept of trimester of pregnancy is not applicable. Certain codes have characters for only certain trimesters because the condition does not occur in all trimesters, but it may occur in more than just one.

Assignment of the final character for trimester should be based on the provider's documentation of the trimester (or number of weeks) for the current admission/encounter. This applies to the assignment of trimester for pre-existing conditions as well as

those that develop during or are due to the pregnancy. The provider's documentation of the number of weeks may be used to assign the appropriate code identifying the trimester.

Whenever delivery occurs during the current admission, and there is an "in childbirth" option for the obstetric complication being coded, the "in childbirth" code should be assigned.

4) Selection of trimester for inpatient admissions that encompass more than one trimesters
In instances when a patient is admitted to a hospital for complications of pregnancy during one trimester and remains in the hospital into a subsequent trimester, the trimester character for the antepartum complication code should be assigned on the basis of the trimester when the complication developed, not the trimester of the discharge. If the condition developed prior to the current admission/encounter or represents a pre-existing condition, the trimester character for the trimester at the time of the admission/encounter should be assigned.

5) Unspecified trimester
Each category that includes codes for trimester has a code for "unspecified trimester." The "unspecified trimester" code should rarely be used, such as when the documentation in the record is insufficient to determine the trimester and it is not possible to obtain clarification.

6) 7th character for fetus identification
Where applicable, a 7th character is to be assigned for certain categories (O31, O32, O33.3 - O33.6, O35, O36, O40, O41, O60.1, O60.2, O64, and O69) to identify the fetus for which the complication code applies.

Assign 7th character "0":

• For single gestations
• When the documentation in the record is insufficient to determine the fetus affected and it is not possible to obtain clarification.
• When it is not possible to clinically determine which fetus is affected.

b. Selection of OB principal or first-listed diagnosis
1) Routine outpatient prenatal visits
For routine outpatient prenatal visits when no complications are present, a code from category Z34, Encounter for supervision of normal pregnancy, should be used as the first-listed diagnosis. These codes should not be used in conjunction with chapter 15 codes.

2) Prenatal outpatient visits for high-risk patients
For routine prenatal outpatient visits for patients with high-risk pregnancies, a code from category O09, Supervision of high-risk pregnancy, should be used as the first-listed diagnosis. Secondary chapter 15 codes may be used in conjunction with these codes if appropriate.

3) Episodes when no delivery occurs
In episodes when no delivery occurs, the principal diagnosis should correspond to the principal complication of the pregnancy which necessitated the encounter. Should more than one complication exist, all of which are treated or monitored, any of the complications codes may be sequenced first.

4) When a delivery occurs
When a delivery occurs, the principal diagnosis should correspond to the main circumstances or complication of the delivery. In cases of cesarean delivery, the selection of the principal diagnosis should be the condition established after study that was responsible for the patient's admission. If the patient was admitted with a condition that resulted in the performance of a cesarean procedure, that condition should be selected as the principal diagnosis. If the reason for the admission/encounter was unrelated to the condition resulting in the cesarean delivery, the condition related to the reason for the admission/encounter should be selected as the principal diagnosis.

5) Outcome of delivery
A code from category Z37, Outcome of delivery, should be included on every maternal record when a delivery has occurred. These codes are not to be used on subsequent records or on the newborn record.

c. Pre-existing conditions versus conditions due to the pregnancy
Certain categories in Chapter 15 distinguish between conditions of the mother that existed prior to pregnancy (pre-existing) and those that are a direct result of pregnancy. When assigning codes from Chapter 15, it is important to assess if a condition was pre-existing prior to pregnancy or developed during or due to the pregnancy in order to assign the correct code.

Categories that do not distinguish between pre-existing and pregnancy-related conditions may be used for either. It is acceptable to use codes specifically for the puerperium with codes complicating pregnancy and childbirth if a condition arises postpartum during the delivery encounter.

d. Pre-existing hypertension in pregnancy
Category O10, Pre-existing hypertension complicating pregnancy, childbirth and the puerperium, includes codes for hypertensive heart and hypertensive chronic kidney disease. When assigning one of the O10 codes that includes hypertensive heart disease or hypertensive chronic kidney disease, it is necessary to add a secondary code from the appropriate hypertension category to specify the type of heart failure or chronic kidney disease.

See Section I.C.9. Hypertension.

e. Fetal conditions affecting the management of the mother

1) Codes from categories O35 and O36
Codes from categories O35, Maternal care for known or suspected fetal abnormality and damage, and O36, Maternal care for other fetal problems, are assigned only when the fetal condition is actually responsible for modifying the management of the mother, i.e., by requiring diagnostic studies, additional observation, special care, or termination of pregnancy. The fact that the fetal condition exists does not justify assigning a code from this series to the mother's record.

2) In utero surgery
In cases when surgery is performed on the fetus, a diagnosis code from category O35, Maternal care for known or suspected fetal abnormality and damage, should be assigned identifying the fetal condition. Assign the appropriate procedure code for the procedure performed.

No code from Chapter 16, the perinatal codes, should be used on the mother's record to identify fetal conditions. Surgery performed in utero on a fetus is still to be coded as an obstetric encounter.

f. HIV Infection in pregnancy, childbirth and the puerperium
During pregnancy, childbirth or the puerperium, a patient admitted because of an HIV-related illness should receive a principal diagnosis from subcategory O98.7-, Human immunodeficiency [HIV] disease complicating pregnancy, childbirth and the puerperium, followed by the code(s) for the HIV-related illness(es).

Patients with asymptomatic HIV infection status admitted during pregnancy, childbirth, or the puerperium should receive codes of O98.7- and Z21, Asymptomatic human immunodeficiency virus [HIV] infection status.

g. Diabetes mellitus in pregnancy
Diabetes mellitus is a significant complicating factor in pregnancy. Pregnant women who are diabetic should be assigned a code from category O24, Diabetes mellitus in pregnancy, childbirth, and the puerperium, first, followed by the appropriate diabetes code(s) (E08-E13) from Chapter 4.

h. Long term use of insulin
Code Z79.4, Long-term (current) use of insulin, should also be assigned if the diabetes mellitus is being treated with insulin.

i. Gestational (pregnancy induced) diabetes
Gestational (pregnancy induced) diabetes can occur during the second and third trimester of pregnancy in women who were not diabetic prior to pregnancy. Gestational diabetes can cause complications in the pregnancy similar to those of pre-existing

diabetes mellitus. It also puts the woman at greater risk of developing diabetes after the pregnancy. Codes for gestational diabetes are in subcategory O24.4, Gestational diabetes mellitus. No other code from category O24, Diabetes mellitus in pregnancy, childbirth, and the puerperium, should be used with a code from O24.4.

The codes under subcategory O24.4 include diet controlled and insulin controlled. If a patient with gestational diabetes is treated with both diet and insulin, only the code for insulin-controlled is required.

Code Z79.4, Long-term (current) use of insulin, should not be assigned with codes from subcategory O24.4.

An abnormal glucose tolerance in pregnancy is assigned a code from subcategory O99.81, Abnormal glucose complicating pregnancy, childbirth, and the puerperium.

j. Sepsis and septic shock complicating abortion, pregnancy, childbirth and the puerperium
When assigning a chapter 15 code for sepsis complicating abortion, pregnancy, childbirth, and the puerperium, a code for the specific type of infection should be assigned as an additional diagnosis. If severe sepsis is present, a code from subcategory R65.2, Severe sepsis, and code(s) for associated organ dysfunction(s) should also be assigned as additional diagnoses.

k. Puerperal sepsis
Code O85, Puerperal sepsis, should be assigned with a secondary code to identify the causal organism (e.g., for a bacterial infection, assign a code from category B95-B96, Bacterial infections in conditions classified elsewhere). A code from category A40, Streptococcal sepsis, or A41, Other sepsis, should not be used for puerperal sepsis. If applicable, use additional codes to identify severe sepsis (R65.2-) and any associated acute organ dysfunction.

l. Alcohol and tobacco use during pregnancy, childbirth and the puerperium

1) Alcohol use during pregnancy, childbirth and the puerperium
Codes under subcategory O99.31, Alcohol use complicating pregnancy, childbirth, and the puerperium, should be assigned for any pregnancy case when a mother uses alcohol during the pregnancy or postpartum. A secondary code from category F10, Alcohol related disorders, should also be assigned to identify manifestations of the alcohol use.

2) Tobacco use during pregnancy, childbirth and the puerperium
Codes under subcategory O99.33, Smoking (tobacco) complicating pregnancy, childbirth, and the puerperium, should be assigned for any pregnancy case when a mother uses any type of tobacco product during the pregnancy or postpartum. A secondary code from category F17, Nicotine dependence, or code Z72.0, Tobacco use, should also be assigned to identify the type of nicotine dependence.

m. Poisoning, toxic effects, adverse effects and underdosing in a pregnant patient
A code from subcategory O9A.2, Injury, poisoning and certain other consequences of external causes complicating pregnancy, childbirth, and the puerperium, should be sequenced first, followed by the appropriate injury, poisoning, toxic effect, adverse effect or underdosing code, and then the additional code(s) that specifies the condition caused by the poisoning, toxic effect, adverse effect or underdosing.

See Section I.C.19. Adverse effects, poisoning, underdosing and toxic effects.

n. Normal delivery, code O80

1) Encounter for full term uncomplicated delivery
Code O80 should be assigned when a woman is admitted for a full-term normal delivery and delivers a single, healthy infant without any complications antepartum, during the delivery, or postpartum during the delivery episode. Code O80 is always a principal diagnosis. It is not to be used if any other code from chapter 15 is needed to describe a current complication of the antenatal, delivery, or perinatal period. Additional codes from other chapters may be used with code O80 if they are not related to or are in any way complicating the pregnancy.

2) **Uncomplicated delivery with resolved antepartum complication**
Code O80 may be used if the patient had a complication at some point during the pregnancy, but the complication is not present at the time of the admission for delivery.

3) **Outcome of delivery for O80**
Z37.0, Single live birth, is the only outcome of delivery code appropriate for use with O80.

o. **The peripartum and postpartum periods**

1) **Peripartum and postpartum periods**
The postpartum period begins immediately after delivery and continues for six weeks following delivery. The peripartum period is defined as the last month of pregnancy to five months postpartum.

2) **Peripartum and postpartum complication**
A postpartum complication is any complication occurring within the six-week period.

3) **Pregnancy-related complications after 6 week period**
Chapter 15 codes may also be used to describe pregnancy-related complications after the peripartum or postpartum period if the provider documents that a condition is pregnancy related.

4) **Admission for routine postpartum care following delivery outside hospital**
When the mother delivers outside the hospital prior to admission and is admitted for routine postpartum care and no complications are noted, code Z39.0, Encounter for care and examination of mother immediately after delivery, should be assigned as the principal diagnosis.

5) **Pregnancy associated cardiomyopathy**
Pregnancy associated cardiomyopathy, code O90.3, is unique in that it may be diagnosed in the third trimester of pregnancy but may continue to progress months after delivery. For this reason, it is referred to as peripartum cardiomyopathy. Code O90.3 is only for use when the cardiomyopathy develops as a result of pregnancy in a woman who did not have pre-existing heart disease.

p. **Code O94, Sequelae of complication of pregnancy, childbirth, and the puerperium**

1) **Code O94**
Code O94, Sequelae of complication of pregnancy, childbirth, and the puerperium, is for use in those cases when an initial complication of a pregnancy develops a sequelae requiring care or treatment at a future date.

2) **After the initial postpartum period**
This code may be used at any time after the initial postpartum period.

3) **Sequencing of code O94**
This code, like all late effect codes, is to be sequenced following the code describing the sequelae of the complication.

q. *Termination of Pregnancy and Spontaneous abortions*

1) **Abortion with Liveborn Fetus**
When an attempted termination of pregnancy results in a liveborn fetus, assign code Z33.2, Encounter for elective termination of pregnancy and a code from category Z37, Outcome of Delivery.

2) **Retained Products of Conception following an abortion**
Subsequent encounters for retained products of conception following a spontaneous abortion or elective termination of pregnancy are assigned the appropriate code from category O03, Spontaneous abortion, or codes O07.4, Failed attempted termination of pregnancy without complication and Z33.2, Encounter for elective termination of pregnancy. This advice is appropriate even when the patient was discharged previously with a discharge diagnosis of complete abortion.

3) **Complications leading to abortion**
Codes from Chapter 15 may be used as additional codes to identify any documented complications of the pregnancy in conjunction with codes in categories in O07 and O08.

r. **Abuse in a pregnant patient**
For suspected or confirmed cases of abuse of a pregnant patient, a code(s) from subcategories O9A.3, Physical abuse complicating pregnancy, childbirth, and the puerperium, O9A.4, Sexual abuse complicating pregnancy, childbirth, and the puerperium, and O9A.5, Psychological abuse complicating pregnancy, childbirth, and the puerperium, should be sequenced first, followed by the appropriate codes (if applicable) to identify any associated current injury due to physical abuse, sexual abuse, and the perpetrator of abuse.
See Section I.C.19. Adult and child abuse, neglect and other maltreatment.

16. **Chapter 16: Certain Conditions Originating in the Perinatal Period (P00- P96)**
For coding and reporting purposes the perinatal period is defined as before birth through the 28th day following birth. The following guidelines are provided for reporting purposes

a. **General Perinatal Rules**

1) **Use of Chapter 16 codes**
Codes in this chapter are <u>never</u> for use on the maternal record. Codes from Chapter 15, the obstetric chapter, are never permitted on the newborn record. Chapter 16 codes may be used throughout the life of the patient if the condition is still present.

2) **Principal diagnosis for birth record**
When coding the birth episode in a newborn record, assign a code from category Z38, Liveborn infants according to place of birth and type of delivery, as the principal diagnosis. A code from category Z38 is assigned only once, to a newborn at the time of birth. If a newborn is transferred to another institution, a code from category Z38 should not be used at the receiving hospital.

A code from category Z38 is used only on the newborn record, not on the mother's record.

3) **Use of codes from other chapters with codes from Chapter 16**
Codes from other chapters may be used with codes from chapter 16 if the codes from the other chapters provide more specific detail. Codes for signs and symptoms may be assigned when a definitive diagnosis has not been established. If the reason for the encounter is a perinatal condition, the code from chapter 16 should be sequenced first.

4) **Use of Chapter 16 codes after the perinatal period**
Should a condition originate in the perinatal period, and continue throughout the life of the patient, the perinatal code should continue to be used regardless of the patient's age.

5) **Birth process or community acquired conditions**
If a newborn has a condition that may be either due to the birth process or community acquired and the documentation does not indicate which it is, the default is due to the birth process and the code from Chapter 16 should be used. If the condition is community-acquired, a code from Chapter 16 should not be assigned.

6) **Code all clinically significant conditions**
All clinically significant conditions noted on routine newborn examination should be coded. A condition is clinically significant if it requires:

- clinical evaluation; or
- therapeutic treatment; or
- diagnostic procedures; or
- extended length of hospital stay; or
- increased nursing care and/or monitoring; or
- has implications for future health care needs

Note: The perinatal guidelines listed above are the same as the general coding guidelines for "additional diagnoses", except for the final point regarding implications for future health care needs. Codes should be assigned for conditions that have been specified by the provider as having implications for future health care needs.

ICD-10-CM Official Guidelines for Coding and Reporting 2016

b. Observation and Evaluation of Newborns for Suspected Conditions not Found

Reserved for future expansion

c. Coding Additional Perinatal Diagnoses

1) Assigning codes for conditions that require treatment

Assign codes for conditions that require treatment or further investigation, prolong the length of stay, or require resource utilization.

2) Codes for conditions specified as having implications for future health care needs

Assign codes for conditions that have been specified by the provider as having implications for future health care needs.

Note: This guideline should not be used for adult patients.

d. Prematurity and Fetal Growth Retardation

Providers utilize different criteria in determining prematurity. A code for prematurity should not be assigned unless it is documented. Assignment of codes in categories P05, Disorders of newborn related to slow fetal growth and fetal malnutrition, and P07, Disorders of newborn related to short gestation and low birth weight, not elsewhere classified, should be based on the recorded birth weight and estimated gestational age. Codes from category P05 should not be assigned with codes from category P07.

When both birth weight and gestational age are available, two codes from category P07 should be assigned, with the code for birth weight sequenced before the code for gestational age.

e. Low birth weight and immaturity status

Codes from category P07, Disorders of newborn related to short gestation and low birth weight, not elsewhere classified, are for use for a child or adult who was premature or had a low birth weight as a newborn and this is affecting the patient's current health status.

See Section I.C.21. Factors influencing health status and contact with health services, Status.

f. Bacterial Sepsis of Newborn

Category P36, Bacterial sepsis of newborn, includes congenital sepsis. If a perinate is documented as having sepsis without documentation of congenital or community acquired, the default is congenital and a code from category P36 should be assigned. If the P36 code includes the causal organism, an additional code from category B95, Streptococcus, Staphylococcus, and Enterococcus as the cause of diseases classified elsewhere, or B96, Other bacterial agents as the cause of diseases classified elsewhere, should not be assigned. If the P36 code does not include the causal organism, assign an additional code from category B96. If applicable, use additional codes to identify severe sepsis (R65.2-) and any associated acute organ dysfunction.

g. Stillbirth

Code P95, Stillbirth, is only for use in institutions that maintain separate records for stillbirths. No other code should be used with P95. Code P95 should not be used on the mother's record.

17. Chapter 17: Congenital malformations, deformations, and chromosomal abnormalities (Q00-Q99)

Assign an appropriate code(s) from categories Q00-Q99, Congenital malformations, deformations, and chromosomal abnormalities when a malformation/deformation or chromosomal abnormality is documented. A malformation/deformation/or chromosomal abnormality may be the principal/first-listed diagnosis on a record or a secondary diagnosis.

When a malformation/deformation/or chromosomal abnormality does not have a unique code assignment, assign additional code(s) for any manifestations that may be present.

When the code assignment specifically identifies the malformation/deformation/or chromosomal abnormality, manifestations that are an inherent component of the anomaly should not be coded separately. Additional codes should be assigned for manifestations that are not an inherent component.

Codes from Chapter 17 may be used throughout the life of the patient. If a congenital malformation or deformity has been corrected, a personal history code should be used to identify the history of the malformation or deformity. Although present at birth, malformation/deformation/or chromosomal abnormality may not be identified until later in life. Whenever the condition is diagnosed by the physician, it is appropriate

to assign a code from codes Q00-Q99. For the birth admission, the appropriate code from category Z38, Liveborn infants, according to place of birth and type of delivery, should be sequenced as the principal diagnosis, followed by any congenital anomaly codes, Q00- Q99.

18. Chapter 18: Symptoms, signs, and abnormal clinical and laboratory findings, not elsewhere classified (R00-R99)

Chapter 18 includes symptoms, signs, abnormal results of clinical or other investigative procedures, and ill-defined conditions regarding which no diagnosis classifiable elsewhere is recorded. Signs and symptoms that point to a specific diagnosis have been assigned to a category in other chapters of the classification.

a. Use of symptom codes

Codes that describe symptoms and signs are acceptable for reporting purposes when a related definitive diagnosis has not been established (confirmed) by the provider.

b. Use of a symptom code with a definitive diagnosis code

Codes for signs and symptoms may be reported in addition to a related definitive diagnosis when the sign or symptom is not routinely associated with that diagnosis, such as the various signs and symptoms associated with complex syndromes. The definitive diagnosis code should be sequenced before the symptom code.

Signs or symptoms that are associated routinely with a disease process should not be assigned as additional codes, unless otherwise instructed by the classification.

c. Combination codes that include symptoms

ICD-10-CM contains a number of combination codes that identify both the definitive diagnosis and common symptoms of that diagnosis. When using one of these combination codes, an additional code should not be assigned for the symptom.

d. Repeated falls

Code R29.6, Repeated falls, is for use for encounters when a patient has recently fallen and the reason for the fall is being investigated.

Code Z91.81, History of falling, is for use when a patient has fallen in the past and is at risk for future falls. When appropriate, both codes R29.6 and Z91.81 may be assigned together.

e. Coma scale

The coma scale codes (R40.2-) can be used in conjunction with traumatic brain injury codes, acute cerebrovascular disease or sequelae of cerebrovascular disease codes. These codes are primarily for use by trauma registries, but they may be used in any setting where this information is collected. The coma scale codes should be sequenced after the diagnosis code(s).

These codes, one from each subcategory, are needed to complete the scale. The 7th character indicates when the scale was recorded. The 7th character should match for all three codes.

At a minimum, report the initial score documented on presentation at your facility. This may be a score from the emergency medicine technician (EMT) or in the emergency department. If desired, a facility may choose to capture multiple Glasgow coma scale scores.

Assign code R40.24, Glasgow coma scale, total score, when only the total score is documented in the medical record and not the individual score(s).

f. Functional quadriplegia

Functional quadriplegia (code R53.2) is the lack of ability to use one's limbs or to ambulate due to extreme debility. It is not associated with neurologic deficit or injury, and code R53.2 should not be used for cases of neurologic quadriplegia. It should only be assigned if functional quadriplegia is specifically documented in the medical record.

g. SIRS due to non-infectious process

The systemic inflammatory response syndrome (SIRS) can develop as a result of certain non-infectious disease processes, such as trauma, malignant neoplasm, or pancreatitis. When SIRS is documented with a noninfectious condition, and no subsequent infection is documented, the code for the underlying condition, such as an injury, should be assigned, followed by code R65.10, Systemic inflammatory response syndrome (SIRS) of non-infectious origin without acute organ dysfunction, or code R65.11, Systemic inflammatory response syndrome (SIRS) of non-infectious origin with acute organ dysfunction. If an associated acute organ dysfunction is documented, the appropriate code(s) for the specific type of organ dysfunction(s) should be assigned in addition to code R65.11. If acute organ dysfunction is documented, but it cannot be determined if the acute organ dysfunction is associated with SIRS or due to another condition (e.g., directly due to the trauma), the provider should be queried.

h. Death NOS

Code R99, Ill-defined and unknown cause of mortality, is only for use in the very limited circumstance when a patient who has already died is brought into an emergency department or other healthcare facility and is pronounced dead upon arrival. It does not represent the discharge disposition of death.

19. Chapter 19: Injury, poisoning, and certain other consequences of external causes (S00-T88)

a. Application of 7th Characters in Chapter 19

Most categories in chapter 19 have a 7th character requirement for each applicable code. Most categories in this chapter have three 7th character values (with the exception of fractures): A, initial encounter, D, subsequent encounter and S, sequela. Categories for traumatic fractures have additional 7th character values. While the patient may be seen by a new or different provider over the course of treatment for an injury, assignment of the 7th character is based on whether the patient is undergoing active treatment and not whether the provider is seeing the patient for the first time.

For complication codes, active treatment refers to treatment for the condition described by the code, even though it may be related to an earlier precipitating problem. For example, code T84.50XA, Infection and inflammatory reaction due to unspecified internal joint prosthesis, initial encounter, is used when active treatment is provided for the infection, even though the condition relates to the prosthetic device, implant or graft that was placed at a previous encounter.

7th character "A", initial encounter is used while the patient is receiving active treatment for the condition. Examples of active treatment are: surgical treatment, emergency department encounter, and evaluation and continuing treatment by the same or a different physician.

7th character "D" subsequent encounter is used for encounters after the patient has received active treatment of the condition and is receiving routine care for the condition during the healing or recovery phase. Examples of subsequent care are: cast change or removal, an x-ray to check healing status of fracture, removal of external or internal fixation device, medication adjustment, other aftercare and follow up visits following treatment of the injury or condition.

The aftercare Z codes should not be used for aftercare for conditions such as injuries or poisonings, where 7th characters are provided to identify subsequent care. For example, for aftercare of an injury, assign the acute injury code with the 7th character "D" (subsequent encounter).

7th character "S", sequela, is for use for complications or conditions that arise as a direct result of a condition, such as scar formation after a burn. The scars are sequelae of the burn. When using 7th character "S", it is necessary to use both the injury code that precipitated the sequela and the code for the sequela itself. The "S" is added only to the injury code, not the sequela code. The 7th character "S" identifies the injury responsible for the sequela. The specific type of sequela (e.g. scar) is sequenced first, followed by the injury code.

See Section I.B.10 Sequelae, (Late Effects)

b. Coding of injuries

When coding injuries, assign separate codes for each injury unless a combination code is provided, in which case the combination code is assigned. Code T07, Unspecified multiple injuries should not be assigned in the inpatient setting unless information for a more specific code is not available. Traumatic injury codes (S00-T14.9) are not to be used for normal, healing surgical wounds or to identify complications of surgical wounds.

The code for the most serious injury, as determined by the provider and the focus of treatment, is sequenced first.

1) Superficial injuries

Superficial injuries such as abrasions or contusions are not coded when associated with more severe injuries of the same site.

2) Primary injury with damage to nerves/blood vessels

When a primary injury results in minor damage to peripheral nerves or blood vessels, the primary injury is sequenced first with additional code(s) for injuries to nerves and spinal cord (such as category S04), and/or injury to blood vessels (such as category S15). When the primary injury is to the blood vessels or nerves, that injury should be sequenced first.

c. Coding of Traumatic Fractures

The principles of multiple coding of injuries should be followed in coding fractures. Fractures of specified sites are coded individually by site in accordance with both the provisions within categories S02, S12, S22, S32, S42, S49, S52, S59, S62, S72, S79, S82, S89, S92 and the level of detail furnished by medical record content.

A fracture not indicated as open or closed should be coded to closed. A fracture not indicated whether displaced or not displaced should be coded to displaced.

More specific guidelines are as follows:

1) Initial vs. Subsequent Encounter for Fractures

Traumatic fractures are coded using the appropriate 7th character for initial encounter (A, B, C) while the patient is receiving active treatment for the fracture. Examples of active treatment are: surgical treatment, emergency department encounter, and evaluation and continuing (ongoing) treatment by the same or different physician. The appropriate 7th character for initial encounter should also be assigned for a patient who delayed seeking treatment for the fracture or nonunion.

Fractures are coded using the appropriate 7th character for subsequent care for encounters after the patient has completed active treatment of the fracture and is receiving routine care for the fracture during the healing or recovery phase. Examples of fracture aftercare are: cast change or removal, an x-ray to check healing status of fracture, removal of external or internal fixation device, medication adjustment, and follow-up visits following fracture treatment.

Care for complications of surgical treatment for fracture repairs during the healing or recovery phase should be coded with the appropriate complication codes.

Care of complications of fractures, such as malunion and nonunion, should be reported with the appropriate 7th character for subsequent care with nonunion (K, M, N,) or subsequent care with malunion (P, Q, R).

Malunion/nonunion: The appropriate 7th character for initial encounter should also be assigned for a patient who delayed seeking treatment for the fracture or nonunion.

A code from category M80, not a traumatic fracture code, should be used for any patient with known osteoporosis who suffers a fracture, even if the patient had a minor fall or trauma, if that fall or trauma would not usually break a normal, healthy bone.

See Section I.C.13. Osteoporosis.

The aftercare Z codes should not be used for aftercare for traumatic fractures. For aftercare of a traumatic fracture, assign the acute fracture code with the appropriate 7th character.

2) Multiple fractures sequencing

Multiple fractures are sequenced in accordance with the severity of the fracture.

d. Coding of burns and corrosions

The ICD-10-CM makes a distinction between burns and corrosions. The burn codes are for thermal burns, except sunburns, that come from a heat source, such as a fire or hot appliance. The burn codes are also for burns resulting from electricity and radiation. Corrosions are burns due to chemicals. The guidelines are the same for burns and corrosions.

Current burns (T20-T25) are classified by depth, extent and by agent (X code). Burns are classified by depth as first degree (erythema),

ICD-10-CM Official Guidelines for Coding and Reporting 2016

second degree (blistering), and third degree (full-thickness involvement). Burns of the eye and internal organs (T26-T28) are classified by site, but not by degree.

1) Sequencing of burn and related condition codes
Sequence first the code that reflects the highest degree of burn when more than one burn is present.

    a.   When the reason for the admission or encounter is for treatment of external multiple burns, sequence first the code that reflects the burn of the highest degree.

    b.   When a patient has both internal and external burns, the circumstances of admission govern the selection of the principal diagnosis or first-listed diagnosis.

    c.   When a patient is admitted for burn injuries and other related conditions such as smoke inhalation and/or respiratory failure, the circumstances of admission govern the selection of the principal or first-listed diagnosis.

2) Burns of the same local site
Classify burns of the same local site (three-character category level, T20-T28) but of different degrees to the subcategory identifying the highest degree recorded in the diagnosis.

3) Non-healing burns
Non-healing burns are coded as acute burns.

Necrosis of burned skin should be coded as a non-healed burn.

4) Infected burn
For any documented infected burn site, use an additional code for the infection.

5) Assign separate codes for each burn site
When coding burns, assign separate codes for each burn site. Category T30, Burn and corrosion, body region unspecified is extremely vague and should rarely be used.

6) Burns and corrosions classified according to extent of body surface involved
Assign codes from category T31, Burns classified according to extent of body surface involved, or T32, Corrosions classified according to extent of body surface involved, when the site of the burn is not specified or when there is a need for additional data. It is advisable to use category T31 as additional coding when needed to provide data for evaluating burn mortality, such as that needed by burn units. It is also advisable to use category T31 as an additional code for reporting purposes when there is mention of a third-degree burn involving 20 percent or more of the body surface.

Categories T31 and T32 are based on the classic "rule of nines" in estimating body surface involved: head and neck are assigned nine percent, each arm nine percent, each leg 18 percent, the anterior trunk 18 percent, posterior trunk 18 percent, and genitalia one percent. Providers may change these percentage assignments where necessary to accommodate infants and children who have proportionately larger heads than adults, and patients who have large buttocks, thighs, or abdomen that involve burns.

7) Encounters for treatment of sequela of burns
Encounters for the treatment of the late effects of burns or corrosions (i.e., scars or joint contractures) should be coded with a burn or corrosion code with the 7th character "S" for sequela.

8) Sequelae with a late effect code and current burn
When appropriate, both a code for a current burn or corrosion with 7th character "A" or "D" and a burn or corrosion code with 7th character "S" may be assigned on the same record (when both a current burn and sequelae of an old burn exist). Burns and corrosions do not heal at the same rate and a current healing wound may still exist with sequela of a healed burn or corrosion.

See Section I.B.10 Sequela (Late Effects)

9) Use of an external cause code with burns and corrosions
An external cause code should be used with burns and corrosions to identify the source and intent of the burn, as well as the place where it occurred.

e. Adverse effects, poisoning, underdosing and toxic effects
Codes in categories T36-T65 are combination codes that include the substance that was taken as well as the intent. No additional external cause code is required for poisonings, toxic effects, adverse effects and underdosing codes.

1) Do not code directly from the Table of Drugs
Do not code directly from the Table of Drugs and Chemicals. Always refer back to the Tabular List.

2) Use as many codes as necessary to describe
Use as many codes as necessary to describe completely all drugs, medicinal or biological substances.

3) If the same code would describe the causative agent
If the same code would describe the causative agent for more than one adverse reaction, poisoning, toxic effect or underdosing, assign the code only once.

4) If two or more drugs, medicinal or biological substances
If two or more drugs, medicinal or biological substances are reported, code each individually unless a combination code is listed in the Table of Drugs and Chemicals.

5) The occurrence of drug toxicity is classified in ICD-10-CM as follows:

(a) Adverse effect
When coding an adverse effect of a drug that has been correctly prescribed and properly administered, assign the appropriate code for the nature of the adverse effect followed by the appropriate code for the adverse effect of the drug (T36-T50). The code for the drug should have a 5th or 6th character "5" (for example T36.0X5-) Examples of the nature of an adverse effect are tachycardia, delirium, gastrointestinal hemorrhaging, vomiting, hypokalemia, hepatitis, renal failure, or respiratory failure.

(b) Poisoning
When coding a poisoning or reaction to the improper use of a medication (e.g., overdose, wrong substance given or taken in error, wrong route of administration), first assign the appropriate code from categories T36-T50. The poisoning codes have an associated intent as their 5th or 6th character (accidental, intentional self-harm, assault and undetermined. Use additional code(s) for all manifestations of poisonings.

If there is also a diagnosis of abuse or dependence of the substance, the abuse or dependence is assigned as an additional code.

Examples of poisoning include:

    (i)   Error was made in drug prescription

        Errors made in drug prescription or in the administration of the drug by provider, nurse, patient, or other person.

    (ii) Overdose of a drug intentionally taken

        If an overdose of a drug was intentionally taken or administered and resulted in drug toxicity, it would be coded as a poisoning.

    (iii) Nonprescribed drug taken with correctly prescribed and properly administered drug

        If a nonprescribed drug or medicinal agent was taken in combination with a correctly prescribed and properly administered drug, any drug toxicity or other reaction resulting from the interaction of the two drugs would be classified as a poisoning.

    (iv) Interaction of drug(s) and alcohol

        When a reaction results from the interaction of a drug(s) and alcohol, this would be classified as poisoning.

        See Section I.C.4. if poisoning is the result of insulin pump malfunctions.

(c) Underdosing
Underdosing refers to taking less of a medication than is prescribed by a provider or a manufacturer's instruction. For underdosing, assign the code from categories T36-T50 (fifth or sixth character "6").

Codes for underdosing should never be assigned as principal or first-listed codes. If a patient has a relapse or exacerbation of the medical condition for which the drug is prescribed because of the reduction in dose, then the medical condition itself should be coded.

Noncompliance (Z91.12-, Z91.13-) or complication of care (Y63.61, Y63.8-Y63.9) codes are to be used with an underdosing code to indicate intent, if known.

(d) Toxic effects

When a harmful substance is ingested or comes in contact with a person, this is classified as a toxic effect. The toxic effect codes are in categories T51-T65.

Toxic effect codes have an associated intent: accidental, intentional self-harm, assault and undetermined.

f. Adult and child abuse, neglect and other maltreatment

Sequence first the appropriate code from categories T74.- (Adult and child abuse, neglect and other maltreatment, confirmed) or T76.- (Adult and child abuse, neglect and other maltreatment, suspected) for abuse, neglect and other maltreatment, followed by any accompanying mental health or injury code(s).

If the documentation in the medical record states abuse or neglect it is coded as confirmed (T74.-). It is coded as suspected if it is documented as suspected (T76.-).

For cases of confirmed abuse or neglect an external cause code from the assault section (X92-Y08) should be added to identify the cause of any physical injuries. A perpetrator code (Y07) should be added when the perpetrator of the abuse is known. For suspected cases of abuse or neglect, do not report external cause or perpetrator code.

If a suspected case of abuse, neglect or mistreatment is ruled out during an encounter code Z04.71, Encounter for examination and observation following alleged physical adult abuse, ruled out, or code Z04.72, Encounter for examination and observation following alleged child physical abuse, ruled out, should be used, not a code from T76.

If a suspected case of alleged rape or sexual abuse is ruled out during an encounter code Z04.41, Encounter for examination and observation following alleged physical adult abuse, ruled out, or code Z04.42, Encounter for examination and observation following alleged rape or sexual abuse, ruled out, should be used, not a code from T76.

See Section I.C.15. Abuse in a pregnant patient.

g. Complications of care

1) General guidelines for complications of care

(a) Documentation of complications of care

See Section I.B.16. for information on documentation of complications of care.

2) Pain due to medical devices

Pain associated with devices, implants or grafts left in a surgical site (for example painful hip prosthesis) is assigned to the appropriate code(s) found in Chapter 19, Injury, poisoning, and certain other consequences of external causes. Specific codes for pain due to medical devices are found in the T code section of the ICD-10-CM. Use additional code(s) from category G89 to identify acute or chronic pain due to presence of the device, implant or graft (G89.18 or G89.28).

3) Transplant complications

(a) Transplant complications other than kidney

Codes under category T86, Complications of transplanted organs and tissues, are for use for both complications and rejection of transplanted organs. A transplant complication code is only assigned if the complication affects the function of the transplanted organ. Two codes are required to fully describe a transplant complication: the appropriate code from category T86 and a secondary code that identifies the complication.

Pre-existing conditions or conditions that develop after the transplant are not coded as complications unless they affect the function of the transplanted organs.

See I.C.21. for transplant organ removal status

See I.C.2. for malignant neoplasm associated with transplanted organ.

(b) Kidney transplant complications

Patients who have undergone kidney transplant may still have some form of chronic kidney disease (CKD) because the kidney transplant may not fully restore kidney function. Code T86.1- should be assigned for documented complications of a kidney transplant, such as transplant failure or rejection or other transplant complication. Code T86.1- should not be assigned for post kidney transplant patients who have chronic kidney (CKD) unless a transplant complication such as transplant failure or rejection is documented. If the documentation is unclear as to whether the patient has a complication of the transplant, query the provider.

Conditions that affect the function of the transplanted kidney, other than CKD, should be assigned a code from subcategory T86.1, Complications of transplanted organ, Kidney, and a secondary code that identifies the complication.

For patients with CKD following a kidney transplant, but who do not have a complication such as failure or rejection, *see section I.C.14. Chronic kidney disease and kidney transplant status.*

4) Complication codes that include the external cause

As with certain other T codes, some of the complications of care codes have the external cause included in the code. The code includes the nature of the complication as well as the type of procedure that caused the complication. No external cause code indicating the type of procedure is necessary for these codes.

5) Complications of care codes within the body system chapters

Intraoperative and postprocedural complication codes are found within the body system chapters with codes specific to the organs and structures of that body system. These codes should be sequenced first, followed by a code(s) for the specific complication, if applicable.

20. Chapter 20: External Causes of Morbidity (V00-Y99)

The external causes of morbidity codes should never be sequenced as the first- listed or principal diagnosis.

External cause codes are intended to provide data for injury research and evaluation of injury prevention strategies. These codes capture how the injury or health condition happened (cause), the intent (unintentional or accidental; or intentional, such as suicide or assault), the place where the event occurred the activity of the patient at the time of the event, and the person's status (e.g., civilian, military).

There is no national requirement for mandatory ICD-10-CM external cause code reporting. Unless a provider is subject to a state-based external cause code reporting mandate or these codes are required by a particular payer, reporting of ICD-10-CM codes in Chapter 20, External Causes of Morbidity, is not required. In the absence of a mandatory reporting requirement, providers are encouraged to voluntarily report external cause codes, as they provide valuable data for injury research and evaluation of injury prevention strategies.

a. General External Cause Coding Guidelines

1) Used with any code in the range of A00.0-T88.9, Z00-Z99

An external cause code may be used with any code in the range of A00.0-T88.9, Z00-Z99, classification that is a health condition due to an external cause. Though they are most applicable to injuries, they are also valid for use with such things as infections or diseases due to an external source, and other health conditions, such as a heart attack that occurs during strenuous physical activity.

2) External cause code used for length of treatment

Assign the external cause code, with the appropriate 7th character (initial encounter, subsequent encounter or sequela) for each encounter for which the injury or condition is being treated.

Most categories in chapter 20 have a 7th character requirement for each applicable code. Most categories in this chapter have three 7th character values: A, initial encounter, D, subsequent encounter and S, sequela. While the patient may be seen by a new or different provider over the course of treatment for an injury or condition, assignment of the 7th character for external cause should match the 7th character of the code assigned for the associated injury or condition for the encounter.

3) **Use the full range of external cause codes**
Use the full range of external cause codes to completely describe the cause, the intent, the place of occurrence, and if applicable, the activity of the patient at the time of the event, and the patient's status, for all injuries, and other health conditions due to an external cause.

4) **Assign as many external cause codes as necessary**
Assign as many external cause codes as necessary to fully explain each cause. If only one external code can be recorded, assign the code most related to the principal diagnosis.

5) **The selection of the appropriate external cause code**
The selection of the appropriate external cause code is guided by the Alphabetic Index of External Causes and by Inclusion and Exclusion notes in the Tabular List.

6) **External cause code can never be a principal diagnosis**
An external cause code can never be a principal (first-listed) diagnosis.

7) **Combination external cause codes**
Certain of the external cause codes are combination codes that identify sequential events that result in an injury, such as a fall which results in striking against an object. The injury may be due to either event or both. The combination external cause code used should correspond to the sequence of events regardless of which caused the most serious injury.

8) **No external cause code needed in certain circumstances**
No external cause code from Chapter 20 is needed if the external cause and intent are included in a code from another chapter (e.g. T36.0X1- Poisoning by penicillins, accidental (unintentional)).

b. **Place of Occurrence Guideline**
Codes from category Y92, Place of occurrence of the external cause, are secondary codes for use after other external cause codes to identify the location of the patient at the time of injury or other condition.

Generally, a place of occurrence code is assigned only once, at the initial encounter for treatment. However, in the rare instance that a new injury occurs during hospitalization, an additional place of occurrence code may be assigned. No 7th characters are used for Y92.

Do not use place of occurrence code Y92.9 if the place is not stated or is not applicable.

c. **Activity code**
Assign a code from category Y93, Activity code, to describe the activity of the patient at the time the injury or other health condition occurred.

An activity code is used only once, at the initial encounter for treatment. Only one code from Y93 should be recorded on a medical record. An activity code should be used in conjunction with a place of occurrence code, Y92.

The activity codes are not applicable to poisonings, adverse effects, misadventures or sequela.

Do not assign Y93.9, Unspecified activity, if the activity is not stated.

A code from category Y93 is appropriate for use with external cause and intent codes if identifying the activity provides additional information about the event.

d. **Place of occurrence, activity, and status codes used with other external cause code**
When applicable, place of occurrence, activity, and external cause status codes are sequenced after the main external cause code(s). Regardless of the number of external cause codes assigned, there should be only one place of occurrence code, one activity code, and one external cause status code assigned to an encounter.

e. **If the reporting format limits the number of external cause codes**
If the reporting format limits the number of external cause codes that can be used in reporting clinical data, report the code for the

cause/intent most related to the principal diagnosis. If the format permits capture of additional external cause codes, the cause/intent, including medical misadventures, of the additional events should be reported rather than the codes for place, activity, or external status.

f. **Multiple external cause coding guidelines**
More than one external cause code is required to fully describe the external cause of an illness or injury. The assignment of external cause codes should be sequenced in the following priority:

If two or more events cause separate injuries, an external cause code should be assigned for each cause. The first-listed external cause code will be selected in the following order:

External codes for child and adult abuse take priority over all other external cause codes.

See Section I.C.19., Child and Adult abuse guidelines.

External cause codes for terrorism events take priority over all other external cause codes except child and adult abuse.

External cause codes for cataclysmic events take priority over all other external cause codes except child and adult abuse and terrorism.

External cause codes for transport accidents take priority over all other external cause codes except cataclysmic events, child and adult abuse and terrorism.

Activity and external cause status codes are assigned following all causal (intent) external cause codes.

The first-listed external cause code should correspond to the cause of the most serious diagnosis due to an assault, accident, or self-harm, following the order of hierarchy listed above.

g. **Child and adult abuse guideline**
Adult and child abuse, neglect and maltreatment are classified as assault. Any of the assault codes may be used to indicate the external cause of any injury resulting from the confirmed abuse.

For confirmed cases of abuse, neglect and maltreatment, when the perpetrator is known, a code from Y07, Perpetrator of maltreatment and neglect, should accompany any other assault codes.

See Section I.C.19. Adult and child abuse, neglect and other maltreatment

h. **Unknown or undetermined intent guideline**
If the intent (accident, self-harm, assault) of the cause of an injury or other condition is unknown or unspecified, code the intent as accidental intent. All transport accident categories assume accidental intent.

1) **Use of undetermined intent**
External cause codes for events of undetermined intent are only for use if the documentation in the record specifies that the intent cannot be determined.

i. **Sequelae (Late Effects) of External Cause Guidelines**
1) **Sequelae external cause codes**
Sequela are reported using the external cause code with the 7th character "S" for sequela. These codes should be used with any report of a late effect or sequela resulting from a previous injury.

See Section I.B.10 Sequela (Late Effects)

2) **Sequela external cause code with a related current injury**
A sequela external cause code should never be used with a related current nature of injury code.

3) **Use of sequela external cause codes for subsequent visits**
Use a late effect external cause code for subsequent visits when a late effect of the initial injury is being treated. Do not use a late effect external cause code for subsequent visits for follow-up care (e.g., to assess healing, to receive rehabilitative therapy) of the injury when no late effect of the injury has been documented.

j. **Terrorism guidelines**
1) **Cause of injury identified by the Federal Government (FBI) as terrorism**
When the cause of an injury is identified by the Federal Government (FBI) as terrorism, the first-listed external cause code should be a code from category Y38, Terrorism. The definition of terrorism employed by the FBI is found at the

inclusion note at the beginning of category Y38. Use additional code for place of occurrence (Y92.-). More than one Y38 code may be assigned if the injury is the result of more than one mechanism of terrorism.

2) **Cause of an injury is suspected to be the result of terrorism**
When the cause of an injury is suspected to be the result of terrorism a code from category Y38 should not be assigned. Suspected cases should be classified as assault.

3) **Code Y38.9, terrorism, secondary effects**
Assign code Y38.9, Terrorism, secondary effects, for conditions occurring subsequent to the terrorist event. This code should not be assigned for conditions that are due to the initial terrorist act.

It is acceptable to assign code Y38.9 with another code from Y38 if there is an injury due to the initial terrorist event and an injury that is a subsequent result of the terrorist event.

k. External cause status
A code from category Y99, External cause status, should be assigned whenever any other external cause code is assigned for an encounter, including an Activity code, except for the events noted below. Assign a code from category Y99, External cause status, to indicate the work status of the person at the time the event occurred. The status code indicates whether the event occurred during military activity, whether a non-military person was at work, whether an individual including a student or volunteer was involved in a non-work activity at the time of the causal event.

A code from Y99, External cause status, should be assigned, when applicable, with other external cause codes, such as transport accidents and falls. The external cause status codes are not applicable to poisonings, adverse effects, misadventures or late effects.

Do not assign a code from category Y99 if no other external cause codes (cause, activity) are applicable for the encounter.

An external cause status code is used only once, at the initial encounter for treatment. Only one code from Y99 should be recorded on a medical record.

Do not assign code Y99.9, Unspecified external cause status, if the status is not stated.

21. Chapter 21: Factors influencing health status and contact with health services (Z00-Z99)
Note: The chapter specific guidelines provide additional information about the use of Z codes for specified encounters.

a. Use of Z codes in any healthcare setting
Z codes are for use in any healthcare setting. Z codes may be used as either a first-listed (principal diagnosis code in the inpatient setting) or secondary code, depending on the circumstances of the encounter. Certain Z codes may only be used as first-listed or principal diagnosis.

b. Z Codes indicate a reason for an encounter
Z codes are not procedure codes. A corresponding procedure code must accompany a Z code to describe any procedure performed.

c. Categories of Z Codes

1) **Contact/Exposure**
Category Z20 indicates contact with, and suspected exposure to, communicable diseases. These codes are for patients who do not show any sign or symptom of a disease but are suspected to have been exposed to it by close personal contact with an infected individual or are in an area where a disease is epidemic.

Category Z77, Other contact with and (suspected) exposures hazardous to health, indicates contact with and suspected exposures hazardous to health.

Contact/exposure codes may be used as a first-listed code to explain an encounter for testing, or, more commonly, as a secondary code to identify a potential risk.

2) **Inoculations and vaccinations**
Code Z23 is for encounters for inoculations and vaccinations. It indicates that a patient is being seen to receive a prophylactic inoculation against a disease. Procedure codes are required to identify the actual administration of the injection and the type(s) of immunizations given. Code Z23 may be used as a

secondary code if the inoculation is given as a routine part of preventive health care, such as a well-baby visit.

3) **Status**
Status codes indicate that a patient is either a carrier of a disease or has the sequelae or residual of a past disease or condition. This includes such things as the presence of prosthetic or mechanical devices resulting from past treatment. A status code is informative, because the status may affect the course of treatment and its outcome. A status code is distinct from a history code. The history code indicates that the patient no longer has the condition.

A status code should not be used with a diagnosis code from one of the body system chapters, if the diagnosis code includes the information provided by the status code. For example, code Z94.1, Heart transplant status, should not be used with a code from subcategory T86.2, Complications of heart transplant. The status code does not provide additional information. The complication code indicates that the patient is a heart transplant patient.

For encounters for weaning from a mechanical ventilator, assign a code from subcategory J96.1, Chronic respiratory failure, followed by code Z99.11, Dependence on respirator [ventilator] status.

The status Z codes/categories are:

Z14　Genetic carrier

Genetic carrier status indicates that a person carries a gene, associated with a particular disease, which may be passed to offspring who may develop that disease. The person does not have the disease and is not at risk of developing the disease.

Z15　Genetic susceptibility to disease

Genetic susceptibility indicates that a person has a gene that increases the risk of that person developing the disease.

Codes from category Z15 should not be used as principal or first-listed codes. If the patient has the condition to which he/she is susceptible, and that condition is the reason for the encounter, the code for the current condition should be sequenced first. If the patient is being seen for follow-up after completed treatment for this condition, and the condition no longer exists, a follow-up code should be sequenced first, followed by the appropriate personal history and genetic susceptibility codes. If the purpose of the encounter is genetic counseling associated with procreative management, code Z31.5, Encounter for genetic counseling, should be assigned as the first-listed code, followed by a code from category Z15. Additional codes should be assigned for any applicable family or personal history.

Z16　Resistance to antimicrobial drugs

This code indicates that a patient has a condition that is resistant to antimicrobial drug treatment. Sequence the infection code first.

Z17　Estrogen receptor status

Z18　Retained foreign body fragments

Z21　Asymptomatic HIV infection status

This code indicates that a patient has tested positive for HIV but has manifested no signs or symptoms of the disease.

Z22　Carrier of infectious disease

Carrier status indicates that a person harbors the specific organisms of a disease without manifest symptoms and is capable of transmitting the infection.

Z28.3　Underimmunization status

Z33.1　Pregnant state, incidental

This code is a secondary code only for use when the pregnancy is in no way complicating the reason for visit. Otherwise, a code from the obstetric chapter is required.

ICD-10-CM Official Guidelines for Coding and Reporting 2016

Z66   Do not resuscitate

This code may be used when it is documented by the provider that a patient is on do not resuscitate status at any time during the stay.

Z67   Blood type

Z68   Body mass index (BMI)

Z74.Ø1   Bed confinement status

Z76.82   Awaiting organ transplant status

Z78   Other specified health status

Code Z78.1, Physical restraint status, may be used when it is documented by the provider that a patient has been put in restraints during the current encounter. Please note that this code should not be reported when it is documented by the provider that a patient is temporarily restrained during a procedure.

Z79   Long-term (current) drug therapy

Codes from this category indicate a patient's continuous use of a prescribed drug (including such things as aspirin therapy) for the long-term treatment of a condition or for prophylactic use. It is not for use for patients who have addictions to drugs. This subcategory is not for use of medications for detoxification or maintenance programs to prevent withdrawal symptoms in patients with drug dependence (e.g., methadone maintenance for opiate dependence). Assign the appropriate code for the drug dependence instead.

Assign a code from Z79 if the patient is receiving a medication for an extended period as a prophylactic measure (such as for the prevention of deep vein thrombosis) or as treatment of a chronic condition (such as arthritis) or a disease requiring a lengthy course of treatment (such as cancer). Do not assign a code from category Z79 for medication being administered for a brief period of time to treat an acute illness or injury (such as a course of antibiotics to treat acute bronchitis).

Z88   Allergy status to drugs, medicaments and biological substances

Except: Z88.9, Allergy status to unspecified drugs, medicaments and biological substances status

Z89   Acquired absence of limb

Z9Ø   Acquired absence of organs, not elsewhere classified

Z91.Ø-   Allergy status, other than to drugs and biological substances

Z92.82   Status post administration of tPA (rtPA) in a different facility within the last 24 hours prior to admission to a current facility

Assign code Z92.82, Status post administration of tPA (rtPA) in a different facility within the last 24 hours prior to admission to current facility, as a secondary diagnosis when a patient is received by transfer into a facility and documentation indicates they were administered tissue plasminogen activator (tPA) within the last 24 hours prior to admission to the current facility.

This guideline applies even if the patient is still receiving the tPA at the time they are received into the current facility.

The appropriate code for the condition for which the tPA was administered (such as cerebrovascular disease or myocardial infarction) should be assigned first.

Code Z92.82 is only applicable to the receiving facility record and not to the transferring facility record.

Z93   Artificial opening status

Z94   Transplanted organ and tissue status

Z95   Presence of cardiac and vascular implants and grafts

Z96   Presence of other functional implants

Z97   Presence of other devices

Z98   Other postprocedural states

Assign code Z98.85, Transplanted organ removal status, to indicate that a transplanted organ has been previously removed. This code should not be assigned for the encounter in which the transplanted organ is removed. The complication necessitating removal of the transplant organ should be assigned for that encounter.

See section I.C19. for information on the coding of organ transplant complications.

Z99   Dependence on enabling machines and devices, not elsewhere classified

Note: Categories Z89-Z9Ø and Z93-Z99 are for use only if there are no complications or malfunctions of the organ or tissue replaced, the amputation site or the equipment on which the patient is dependent.

4) **History (of)**

There are two types of history Z codes, personal and family. Personal history codes explain a patient's past medical condition that no longer exists and is not receiving any treatment, but that has the potential for recurrence, and therefore may require continued monitoring.

Family history codes are for use when a patient has a family member(s) who has had a particular disease that causes the patient to be at higher risk of also contracting the disease.

Personal history codes may be used in conjunction with follow-up codes and family history codes may be used in conjunction with screening codes to explain the need for a test or procedure. History codes are also acceptable on any medical record regardless of the reason for visit. A history of an illness, even if no longer present, is important information that may alter the type of treatment ordered.

The history Z code categories are:

Z8Ø   Family history of primary malignant neoplasm

Z81   Family history of mental and behavioral disorders

Z82   Family history of certain disabilities and chronic diseases (leading to disablement)

Z83   Family history of other specific disorders

Z84   Family history of other conditions

Z85   Personal history of malignant neoplasm

Z86   Personal history of certain other diseases

Z87   Personal history of other diseases and conditions

Z91.4-   Personal history of psychological trauma, not elsewhere classified

Z91.5   Personal history of self-harm

Z91.8-   Other specified personal risk factors, not elsewhere classified

Exception:

Z91.83, Wandering in diseases classified elsewhere

Z92   Personal history of medical treatment

Except: Z92.Ø, Personal history of contraception

Except: Z92.82, Status post administration of tPA (rtPA) in a different facility within the last 24 hours prior to admission to a current facility

5) **Screening**

Screening is the testing for disease or disease precursors in seemingly well individuals so that early detection and treatment can be provided for those who test positive for the disease (e.g., screening mammogram).

The testing of a person to rule out or confirm a suspected diagnosis because the patient has some sign or symptom is a diagnostic examination, not a screening. In these cases, the sign or symptom is used to explain the reason for the test.

A screening code may be a first-listed code if the reason for the visit is specifically the screening exam. It may also be used as an additional code if the screening is done during an office visit for other health problems. A screening code is not necessary if the screening is inherent to a routine examination, such as a pap smear done during a routine pelvic examination.

Should a condition be discovered during the screening then the code for the condition may be assigned as an additional diagnosis.

The Z code indicates that a screening exam is planned. A procedure code is required to confirm that the screening was performed.

The screening Z codes/categories:

Z11   Encounter for screening for infectious and parasitic diseases

Z12   Encounter for screening for malignant neoplasms

Z13   Encounter for screening for other diseases and disorders

       Except: Z13.9, Encounter for screening, unspecified

Z36   Encounter for antenatal screening for mother

6) **Observation**

There are two observation Z code categories. They are for use in very limited circumstances when a person is being observed for a suspected condition that is ruled out. The observation codes are not for use if an injury or illness or any signs or symptoms related to the suspected condition are present. In such cases the diagnosis/symptom code is used with the corresponding external cause code.

The observation codes are to be used as principal diagnosis only. Additional codes may be used in addition to the observation code but only if they are unrelated to the suspected condition being observed.

Codes from subcategory Z03.7, Encounter for suspected maternal and fetal conditions ruled out, may either be used as a first-listed or as an additional code assignment depending on the case. They are for use in very limited circumstances on a maternal record when an encounter is for a suspected maternal or fetal condition that is ruled out during that encounter (for example, a maternal or fetal condition may be suspected due to an abnormal test result). These codes should not be used when the condition is confirmed. In those cases, the confirmed condition should be coded. In addition, these codes are not for use if an illness or any signs or symptoms related to the suspected condition or problem are present. In such cases the diagnosis/symptom code is used.

Additional codes may be used in addition to the code from subcategory Z03.7, but only if they are unrelated to the suspected condition being evaluated.

Codes from subcategory Z03.7 may not be used for encounters for antenatal screening of mother. *See Section I.C.21.c.5, Screening.*

For encounters for suspected fetal condition that are inconclusive following testing and evaluation, assign the appropriate code from category O35, O36, O40 or O41.

The observation Z code categories:

Z03   Encounter for medical observation for suspected diseases and conditions ruled out

Z04   Encounter for examination and observation for other reasons

       Except: Z04.9, Encounter for examination and observation for unspecified reason

7) **Aftercare**

Aftercare visit codes cover situations when the initial treatment of a disease has been performed and the patient requires continued care during the healing or recovery phase, or for the long-term consequences of the disease. The aftercare Z code should not be used if treatment is directed at a current, acute disease. The diagnosis code is to be used in these cases. Exceptions to this rule are codes Z51.0, Encounter for antineoplastic radiation therapy, and codes from subcategory Z51.1, Encounter for antineoplastic chemotherapy and immunotherapy. These codes are to be first-listed, followed by the diagnosis code when a patient's encounter is solely to receive radiation therapy, chemotherapy, or immunotherapy for the treatment of a neoplasm. If the reason for the encounter is more than one type of antineoplastic therapy, code Z51.0 and a code from subcategory Z51.1 may be assigned together, in

which case one of these codes would be reported as a secondary diagnosis.

The aftercare Z codes should also not be used for aftercare for injuries. For aftercare of an injury, assign the acute injury code with the appropriate 7th character (for subsequent encounter).

The aftercare codes are generally first-listed to explain the specific reason for the encounter. An aftercare code may be used as an additional code when some type of aftercare is provided in addition to the reason for admission and no diagnosis code is applicable. An example of this would be the closure of a colostomy during an encounter for treatment of another condition.

Aftercare codes should be used in conjunction with other aftercare codes or diagnosis codes to provide better detail on the specifics of an aftercare encounter visit, unless otherwise directed by the classification. Should a patient receive multiple types of antineoplastic therapy during the same encounter, code Z51.0, Encounter for antineoplastic radiation therapy, and codes from subcategory Z51.1, Encounter for antineoplastic chemotherapy and immunotherapy, may be used together on a record. The sequencing of multiple aftercare codes depends on the circumstances of the encounter.

Certain aftercare Z code categories need a secondary diagnosis code to describe the resolving condition or sequelae. For others, the condition is included in the code title.

Additional Z code aftercare category terms include fitting and adjustment, and attention to artificial openings.

Status Z codes may be used with aftercare Z codes to indicate the nature of the aftercare. For example code Z95.1, Presence of aortocoronary bypass graft, may be used with code Z48.812, Encounter for surgical aftercare following surgery on the circulatory system, to indicate the surgery for which the aftercare is being performed. A status code should not be used when the aftercare code indicates the type of status, such as using Z43.0, Encounter for attention to tracheostomy, with Z93.0, Tracheostomy status.

The aftercare Z category/codes:

Z42   Encounter for plastic and reconstructive surgery following medical procedure or healed injury

Z43   Encounter for attention to artificial openings

Z44   Encounter for fitting and adjustment of external prosthetic device

Z45   Encounter for adjustment and management of implanted device

Z46   Encounter for fitting and adjustment of other devices

Z47   Orthopedic aftercare

Z48   Encounter for other postprocedural aftercare

Z49   Encounter for care involving renal dialysis

Z51   Encounter for other aftercare

8) **Follow-up**

The follow-up codes are used to explain continuing surveillance following completed treatment of a disease, condition, or injury. They imply that the condition has been fully treated and no longer exists. They should not be confused with aftercare codes, or injury codes with a 7th character for subsequent encounter, that explain ongoing care of a healing condition or its sequelae. Follow-up codes may be used in conjunction with history codes to provide the full picture of the healed condition and its treatment. The follow-up code is sequenced first, followed by the history code.

A follow-up code may be used to explain multiple visits. Should a condition be found to have recurred on the follow-up visit, then the diagnosis code for the condition should be assigned in place of the follow-up code.

The follow-up Z code categories:

Z08   Encounter for follow-up examination after completed treatment for malignant neoplasm

Z09   Encounter for follow-up examination after completed treatment for conditions other than malignant neoplasm

Z39   Encounter for maternal postpartum care and examination

9) Donor
Codes in category Z52, Donors of organs and tissues, are used for living individuals who are donating blood or other body tissue. These codes are only for individuals donating for others, not for self-donations. They are not used to identify cadaveric donations.

10) Counseling
Counseling Z codes are used when a patient or family member receives assistance in the aftermath of an illness or injury, or when support is required in coping with family or social problems. They are not used in conjunction with a diagnosis code when the counseling component of care is considered integral to standard treatment.

The counseling Z codes/categories:

Z30.0-   Encounter for general counseling and advice on contraception

Z31.5   Encounter for genetic counseling

Z31.6-   Encounter for general counseling and advice on procreation

Z32.2   Encounter for childbirth instruction

Z32.3   Encounter for childcare instruction

Z69   Encounter for mental health services for victim and perpetrator of abuse

Z70   Counseling related to sexual attitude, behavior and orientation

Z71   Persons encountering health services for other counseling and medical advice, not elsewhere classified

Z76.81   Expectant mother prebirth pediatrician visit

11) Encounters for obstetrical and reproductive services
See Section I.C.15. Pregnancy, Childbirth, and the Puerperium, for further instruction on the use of these codes.

Z codes for pregnancy are for use in those circumstances when none of the problems or complications included in the codes from the Obstetrics chapter exist (a routine prenatal visit or postpartum care). Codes in category Z34, Encounter for supervision of normal pregnancy, are always first-listed and are not to be used with any other code from the OB chapter.

Codes in category Z3A, Weeks of gestation, may be assigned to provide additional information about the pregnancy. The date of the admission should be used to determine weeks of gestation for inpatient admissions that encompass more than one gestational week.

The outcome of delivery, category Z37, should be included on all maternal delivery records. It is always a secondary code.

Z codes for family planning (contraceptive) or procreative management and counseling should be included on an obstetric record either during the pregnancy or the postpartum stage, if applicable.

Z codes/categories for obstetrical and reproductive services:

Z30   Encounter for contraceptive management

Z31   Encounter for procreative management

Z32.2   Encounter for childbirth instruction

Z32.3   Encounter for childcare instruction

Z33   Pregnant state

Z34   Encounter for supervision of normal pregnancy

Z36   Encounter for antenatal screening of mother

Z3A   Weeks of gestation

Z37   Outcome of delivery

Z39   Encounter for maternal postpartum care and examination

Z76.81   Expectant mother prebirth pediatrician visit

12) Newborns and Infants
See Section I.C.16. Newborn (Perinatal) Guidelines, for further instruction on the use of these codes.

Newborn Z codes/categories:

Z76.1   Encounter for health supervision and care of foundling

Z00.1-   Encounter for routine child health examination

Z38   Liveborn infants according to place of birth and type of delivery

13) Routine and administrative examinations
The Z codes allow for the description of encounters for routine examinations, such as, a general check-up, or, examinations for administrative purposes, such as, a pre-employment physical. The codes are not to be used if the examination is for diagnosis of a suspected condition or for treatment purposes. In such cases the diagnosis code is used. During a routine exam, should a diagnosis or condition be discovered, it should be coded as an additional code. Pre-existing and chronic conditions and history codes may also be included as additional codes as long as the examination is for administrative purposes and not focused on any particular condition.

Some of the codes for routine health examinations distinguish between "with" and "without" abnormal findings. Code assignment depends on the information that is known at the time the encounter is being coded. For example, if no abnormal findings were found during the examination, but the encounter is being coded before test results are back, it is acceptable to assign the code for "without abnormal findings." When assigning a code for "with abnormal findings," additional code(s) should be assigned to identify the specific abnormal finding(s).

Pre-operative examination and pre-procedural laboratory examination Z codes are for use only in those situations when a patient is being cleared for a procedure or surgery and no treatment is given.

The Z codes/categories for routine and administrative examinations:

Z00   Encounter for general examination without complaint, suspected or reported diagnosis

Z01   Encounter for other special examination without complaint, suspected or reported diagnosis

Z02   Encounter for administrative examination

Except: Z02.9, Encounter for administrative examinations, unspecified

Z32.0-   Encounter for pregnancy test

14) Miscellaneous Z codes
The miscellaneous Z codes capture a number of other health care encounters that do not fall into one of the other categories. Certain of these codes identify the reason for the encounter; others are for use as additional codes that provide useful information on circumstances that may affect a patient's care and treatment.

Prophylactic Organ Removal
For encounters specifically for prophylactic removal of an organ (such as prophylactic removal of breasts due to a genetic susceptibility to cancer or a family history of cancer), the principal or first-listed code should be a code from category Z40, Encounter for prophylactic surgery, followed by the appropriate codes to identify the associated risk factor (such as genetic susceptibility or family history).

If the patient has a malignancy of one site and is having prophylactic removal at another site to prevent either a new primary malignancy or metastatic disease, a code for the malignancy should also be assigned in addition to a code from subcategory Z40.0, Encounter for prophylactic surgery for risk factors related to malignant neoplasms. A Z40.0 code should not be assigned if the patient is having organ removal for treatment of a malignancy, such as the removal of the testes for the treatment of prostate cancer.

Miscellaneous Z codes/categories:

Z28   Immunization not carried out

Except: Z28.3, Underimmunization status

Z40   Encounter for prophylactic surgery

Z41   Encounter for procedures for purposes other than remedying health state

Except: Z41.9, Encounter for procedure for purposes other than remedying health state, unspecified

Z53   Persons encountering health services for specific procedures and treatment, not carried out

Z55   Problems related to education and literacy

Z56   Problems related to employment and unemployment

Z57   Occupational exposure to risk factors

Z58   Problems related to physical environment

Z59   Problems related to housing and economic circumstances

Z60   Problems related to social environment

Z62   Problems related to upbringing

Z63   Other problems related to primary support group, including family circumstances

Z64   Problems related to certain psychosocial circumstances

Z65   Problems related to other psychosocial circumstances

Z72   Problems related to lifestyle

Z73   Problems related to life management difficulty

Z74   Problems related to care provider dependency

Except: Z74.01, Bed confinement status

Z75   Problems related to medical facilities and other health care

Z76.0 Encounter for issue of repeat prescription

Z76.3 Healthy person accompanying sick person

Z76.4 Other boarder to healthcare facility

Z76.5 Malingerer [conscious simulation]

Z91.1- Patient's noncompliance with medical treatment and regimen

Z91.83 Wandering in diseases classified elsewhere

Z91.89 Other specified personal risk factors, not elsewhere classified

15) **Nonspecific Z codes**

Certain Z codes are so non-specific, or potentially redundant with other codes in the classification, that there can be little justification for their use in the inpatient setting. Their use in the outpatient setting should be limited to those instances when there is no further documentation to permit more precise coding. Otherwise, any sign or symptom or any other reason for visit that is captured in another code should be used.

Nonspecific Z codes/categories:

Z02.9 Encounter for administrative examinations, unspecified

Z04.9 Encounter for examination and observation for unspecified reason

Z13.9 Encounter for screening, unspecified

Z41.9 Encounter for procedure for purposes other than remedying health state, unspecified

Z52.9 Donor of unspecified organ or tissue

Z86.59 Personal history of other mental and behavioral disorders

Z88.9 Allergy status to unspecified drugs, medicaments and biological substances status

Z92.0 Personal history of contraception

16) **Z codes that may only be principal/first-listed diagnosis**

The following Z codes/categories may only be reported as the principal/first-listed diagnosis, except when there are multiple encounters on the same day and the medical records for the encounters are combined:

Z00   Encounter for general examination without complaint, suspected or reported diagnosis

Except: Z00.6

Z01   Encounter for other special examination without complaint, suspected or reported diagnosis

Z02   Encounter for administrative examination

Z03   Encounter for medical observation for suspected diseases and conditions ruled out

Z04   Encounter for examination and observation for other reasons

Z33.2 Encounter for elective termination of pregnancy

Z31.81 Encounter for male factor infertility in female patient

Z31.82 Encounter for Rh incompatibility status

Z31.83 Encounter for assisted reproductive fertility procedure cycle

Z31.84 Encounter for fertility preservation procedure

Z34   Encounter for supervision of normal pregnancy

Z39   Encounter for maternal postpartum care and examination

Z38   Liveborn infants according to place of birth and type of delivery

Z42   Encounter for plastic and reconstructive surgery following medical procedure or healed injury

Z51.0 Encounter for antineoplastic radiation therapy

Z51.1- Encounter for antineoplastic chemotherapy and immunotherapy

Z52   Donors of organs and tissues

Except: Z52.9, Donor of unspecified organ or tissue

Z76.1 Encounter for health supervision and care of foundling

Z76.2 Encounter for health supervision and care of other healthy infant and child

Z99.12 Encounter for respirator [ventilator] dependence during power failure

Section II. Selection of Principal Diagnosis

The circumstances of inpatient admission always govern the selection of principal diagnosis.

The principal diagnosis is defined in the Uniform Hospital Discharge Data Set (UHDDS) as "that condition established after study to be chiefly responsible for occasioning the admission of the patient to the hospital for care."

The UHDDS definitions are used by hospitals to report inpatient data elements in a standardized manner. These data elements and their definitions can be found in the July 31, 1985, Federal Register (Vol. 50, No, 147), pp. 31038-40.

Since that time the application of the UHDDS definitions has been expanded to include all non- outpatient settings (acute care, short term, long term care and psychiatric hospitals; home health agencies; rehab facilities; nursing homes, etc).

In determining principal diagnosis, coding conventions in the ICD-10-CM, the Tabular List and Alphabetic Index take precedence over these official coding guidelines.

(See Section I.A., Conventions for the ICD-10-CM)

The importance of consistent, complete documentation in the medical record cannot be overemphasized. Without such documentation the application of all coding guidelines is a difficult, if not impossible, task.

A. Codes for symptoms, signs, and ill-defined conditions

Codes for symptoms, signs, and ill-defined conditions from Chapter 18 are not to be used as principal diagnosis when a related definitive diagnosis has been established.

B. Two or more interrelated conditions, each potentially meeting the definition for principal diagnosis

When there are two or more interrelated conditions (such as diseases in the same ICD-10-CM chapter or manifestations characteristically associated with a certain disease) potentially meeting the definition of principal diagnosis, either condition may be sequenced first, unless the circumstances of the admission, the therapy provided, the Tabular List, or the Alphabetic Index indicate otherwise.

C. Two or more diagnoses that equally meet the definition for principal diagnosis

In the unusual instance when two or more diagnoses equally meet the criteria for principal diagnosis as determined by the circumstances of admission, diagnostic workup and/or therapy provided, and the Alphabetic Index, Tabular List, or another coding guidelines does not provide sequencing direction, any one of the diagnoses may be sequenced first.

D. Two or more comparative or contrasting conditions

In those rare instances when two or more contrasting or comparative diagnoses are documented as "either/or" (or similar terminology), they are coded as if the diagnoses were confirmed and the diagnoses are sequenced according to the circumstances of the admission. If no further determination can be made as to which diagnosis should be principal, either diagnosis may be sequenced first.

E. A symptom(s) followed by contrasting/ comparative diagnoses

GUIDELINE HAS BEEN DELETED EFFECTIVE OCTOBER 1, 2014

F. Original treatment plan not carried out

Sequence as the principal diagnosis the condition, which after study occasioned the admission to the hospital, even though treatment may not have been carried out due to unforeseen circumstances.

G. Complications of surgery and other medical care

When the admission is for treatment of a complication resulting from surgery or other medical care, the complication code is sequenced as the principal diagnosis. If the complication is classified to the T80-T88 series and the code lacks the necessary specificity in describing the complication, an additional code for the specific complication should be assigned.

H. Uncertain diagnosis

If the diagnosis documented at the time of discharge is qualified as "probable", "suspected", "likely", "questionable", "possible", or "still to be ruled out", or other similar terms indicating uncertainty, code the condition as if it existed or was established. The bases for these guidelines are the diagnostic workup, arrangements for further workup or observation, and initial therapeutic approach that correspond most closely with the established diagnosis.

Note: This guideline is applicable only to inpatient admissions to short-term, acute, long-term care and psychiatric hospitals.

I. Admission from observation unit

1. **Admission Following Medical Observation**

   When a patient is admitted to an observation unit for a medical condition, which either worsens or does not improve, and is subsequently admitted as an inpatient of the same hospital for this same medical condition, the principal diagnosis would be the medical condition which led to the hospital admission.

2. **Admission Following Post-Operative Observation**

   When a patient is admitted to an observation unit to monitor a condition (or complication) that develops following outpatient surgery, and then is subsequently admitted as an inpatient of the same hospital, hospitals should apply the Uniform Hospital Discharge Data Set (UHDDS) definition of principal diagnosis as "that condition established after study to be chiefly responsible for occasioning the admission of the patient to the hospital for care."

J. Admission from outpatient surgery

When a patient receives surgery in the hospital's outpatient surgery department and is subsequently admitted for continuing inpatient care at the same hospital, the following guidelines should be followed in selecting the principal diagnosis for the inpatient admission:

- If the reason for the inpatient admission is a complication, assign the complication as the principal diagnosis.

- If no complication, or other condition, is documented as the reason for the inpatient admission, assign the reason for the outpatient surgery as the principal diagnosis.

- If the reason for the inpatient admission is another condition unrelated to the surgery, assign the unrelated condition as the principal diagnosis.

K. Admissions/Encounters for Rehabilitation

When the purpose for the admission/encounter is rehabilitation, sequence first the code for the condition for which the service is being performed. For example, for an admission/encounter for rehabilitation for right-sided dominant hemiplegia following a cerebrovascular infarction, report code I69.351, Hemiplegia and hemiparesis following cerebral infarction affecting right dominant side, as the first-listed or principal diagnosis.

If the condition for which the rehabilitation service is no longer present, report the appropriate aftercare code as the first-listed or principal diagnosis. For example, if a patient with severe degenerative osteoarthritis of the hip, underwent hip replacement and the current encounter/admission is for rehabilitation, report code Z47.1, Aftercare following joint replacement surgery, as the first-listed or principal diagnosis.

See Section I.C.21.c.7, Factors influencing health states and contact with health services, Aftercare.

Section III. Reporting Additional Diagnoses

GENERAL RULES FOR OTHER (ADDITIONAL) DIAGNOSES

For reporting purposes the definition for "other diagnoses" is interpreted as additional conditions that affect patient care in terms of requiring:

> clinical evaluation; or
>
> therapeutic treatment; or
>
> diagnostic procedures; or
>
> extended length of hospital stay; or
>
> increased nursing care and/or monitoring.

The UHDDS item #11-b defines Other Diagnoses as "all conditions that coexist at the time of admission, that develop subsequently, or that affect the treatment received and/or the length of stay. Diagnoses that relate to an earlier episode which have no bearing on the current hospital stay are to be excluded." UHDDS definitions apply to inpatients in acute care, short-term, long term care and psychiatric hospital setting. The UHDDS definitions are used by acute care short-term hospitals to report inpatient data elements in a standardized manner. These data elements and their definitions can be found in the July 31, 1985, Federal Register (Vol. 50, No, 147), pp. 31038-40.

Since that time the application of the UHDDS definitions has been expanded to include all non-outpatient settings (acute care, short term, long term care and psychiatric hospitals; home health agencies; rehab facilities; nursing homes, etc).

The following guidelines are to be applied in designating "other diagnoses" when neither the Alphabetic Index nor the Tabular List in ICD-10-CM provide direction. The listing of the diagnoses in the patient record is the responsibility of the attending provider.

A. **Previous conditions**

   If the provider has included a diagnosis in the final diagnostic statement, such as the discharge summary or the face sheet, it should ordinarily be coded. Some providers include in the diagnostic statement resolved conditions or diagnoses and status-post procedures from previous admission that have no bearing on the current stay. Such conditions are not to be reported and are coded only if required by hospital policy.

   However, history codes (categories Z80-Z87) may be used as secondary codes if the historical condition or family history has an impact on current care or influences treatment.

B. **Abnormal findings**

   Abnormal findings (laboratory, x-ray, pathologic, and other diagnostic results) are not coded and reported unless the provider indicates their clinical significance. If the findings are outside the normal range and the attending provider has ordered other tests to evaluate the condition or prescribed treatment, it is appropriate to ask the provider whether the abnormal finding should be added.

   Please note: This differs from the coding practices in the outpatient setting for coding encounters for diagnostic tests that have been interpreted by a provider.

C. **Uncertain Diagnosis**

   If the diagnosis documented at the time of discharge is qualified as "probable", "suspected", "likely", "questionable", "possible", or "still to be ruled out" or other similar terms indicating uncertainty, code the condition as if it existed or was established. The bases for these guidelines are the diagnostic workup, arrangements for further workup or observation, and initial therapeutic approach that correspond most closely with the established diagnosis.

Note: This guideline is applicable only to inpatient admissions to short-term, acute, long-term care and psychiatric hospitals.

Section IV. Diagnostic Coding and Reporting Guidelines for Outpatient Services

These coding guidelines for outpatient diagnoses have been approved for use by hospitals/ providers in coding and reporting hospital-based outpatient services and provider-based office visits.

Information about the use of certain abbreviations, punctuation, symbols, and other conventions used in the ICD-10-CM Tabular List (code numbers and titles), can be found in Section IA of these guidelines, under "Conventions Used in the Tabular List." Section I.B. contains general guidelines that apply to the entire classification. Section I.C. contains chapter-specific guidelines that correspond to the chapters as they are arranged in the classification. Information about the correct sequence to use in finding a code is also described in Section I.

The terms encounter and visit are often used interchangeably in describing outpatient service contacts and, therefore, appear together in these guidelines without distinguishing one from the other.

Though the conventions and general guidelines apply to all settings, coding guidelines for outpatient and provider reporting of diagnoses will vary in a number of instances from those for inpatient diagnoses, recognizing that:

The Uniform Hospital Discharge Data Set (UHDDS) definition of principal diagnosis applies only to inpatients in acute, short-term, long-term care and psychiatric hospitals.

Coding guidelines for inconclusive diagnoses (probable, suspected, rule out, etc.) were developed for inpatient reporting and do not apply to outpatients.

A. Selection of first-listed condition

In the outpatient setting, the term first-listed diagnosis is used in lieu of principal diagnosis.

In determining the first-listed diagnosis the coding conventions of ICD-10-CM, as well as the general and disease specific guidelines take precedence over the outpatient guidelines.

Diagnoses often are not established at the time of the initial encounter/visit. It may take two or more visits before the diagnosis is confirmed.

The most critical rule involves beginning the search for the correct code assignment through the Alphabetic Index. Never begin searching initially in the Tabular List as this will lead to coding errors.

1. Outpatient surgery

When a patient presents for outpatient surgery (same day surgery), code the reason for the surgery as the first-listed diagnosis (reason for the encounter), even if the surgery is not performed due to a contraindication.

2. Observation stay

When a patient is admitted for observation for a medical condition, assign a code for the medical condition as the first-listed diagnosis.

When a patient presents for outpatient surgery and develops complications requiring admission to observation, code the reason for the surgery as the first reported diagnosis (reason for the encounter), followed by codes for the complications as secondary diagnoses.

B. Codes from A00.0 through T88.9, Z00-Z99

The appropriate code(s) from A00.0 through T88.9, Z00-Z99 must be used to identify diagnoses, symptoms, conditions, problems, complaints, or other reason(s) for the encounter/visit.

C. Accurate reporting of ICD-10-CM diagnosis codes

For accurate reporting of ICD-10-CM diagnosis codes, the documentation should describe the patient's condition, using terminology which includes specific diagnoses as well as symptoms, problems, or reasons for the encounter. There are ICD-10-CM codes to describe all of these.

D. Codes that describe symptoms and signs

Codes that describe symptoms and signs, as opposed to diagnoses, are acceptable for reporting purposes when a diagnosis has not been established (confirmed) by the provider. Chapter 18 of ICD-10-CM,

Symptoms, Signs, and Abnormal Clinical and Laboratory Findings Not Elsewhere Classified (codes R00-R99) contain many, but not all codes for symptoms.

E. Encounters for circumstances other than a disease or injury

ICD-10-CM provides codes to deal with encounters for circumstances other than a disease or injury. The Factors Influencing Health Status and Contact with Health Services codes (Z00-Z99) are provided to deal with occasions when circumstances other than a disease or injury are recorded as diagnosis or problems.

See Section I.C.21. Factors influencing health status and contact with health services.

F. Level of Detail in Coding

1. ICD-10-CM codes with 3, 4, 5, 6 or 7 characters

ICD-10-CM is composed of codes with 3, 4, 5, 6 or 7 characters. Codes with three characters are included in ICD-10-CM as the heading of a category of codes that may be further subdivided by the use of fourth, fifth, sixth or seventh characters to provide greater specificity.

2. Use of full number of *characters* required for a code

A three-character code is to be used only if it is not further subdivided. A code is invalid if it has not been coded to the full number of characters required for that code, including the 7th character extension, if applicable.

G. ICD-10-CM code for the diagnosis, condition, problem, or other reason for encounter/visit

List first the ICD-10-CM code for the diagnosis, condition, problem, or other reason for encounter/visit shown in the medical record to be chiefly responsible for the services provided. List additional codes that describe any coexisting conditions. In some cases the first-listed diagnosis may be a symptom when a diagnosis has not been established (confirmed) by the physician.

H. Uncertain diagnosis

Do not code diagnoses documented as "probable", "suspected," "questionable," "rule out," or "working diagnosis" or other similar terms indicating uncertainty. Rather, code the condition(s) to the highest degree of certainty for that encounter/visit, such as symptoms, signs, abnormal test results, or other reason for the visit.

Please note: This differs from the coding practices used by short-term, acute care, long-term care and psychiatric hospitals.

I. Chronic diseases

Chronic diseases treated on an ongoing basis may be coded and reported as many times as the patient receives treatment and care for the condition(s)

J. Code all documented conditions that coexist

Code all documented conditions that coexist at the time of the encounter/visit, and require or affect patient care treatment or management. Do not code conditions that were previously treated and no longer exist. However, history codes (categories Z80-Z87) may be used as secondary codes if the historical condition or family history has an impact on current care or influences treatment.

K. Patients receiving diagnostic services only

For patients receiving diagnostic services only during an encounter/visit, sequence first the diagnosis, condition, problem, or other reason for encounter/visit shown in the medical record to be chiefly responsible for the outpatient services provided during the encounter/visit. Codes for other diagnoses (e.g., chronic conditions) may be sequenced as additional diagnoses.

For encounters for routine laboratory/radiology testing in the absence of any signs, symptoms, or associated diagnosis, assign Z01.89, Encounter for other specified special examinations. If routine testing is performed during the same encounter as a test to evaluate a sign, symptom, or diagnosis, it is appropriate to assign both the Z code and the code describing the reason for the non-routine test.

For outpatient encounters for diagnostic tests that have been interpreted by a physician, and the final report is available at the time of coding, code any confirmed or definitive diagnosis(es) documented in the interpretation. Do not code related signs and symptoms as additional diagnoses.

Please note: This differs from the coding practice in the hospital inpatient setting regarding abnormal findings on test results.

L. Patients receiving therapeutic services only

For patients receiving therapeutic services only during an encounter/visit, sequence first the diagnosis, condition, problem, or other reason for encounter/visit shown in the medical record to be chiefly responsible for the outpatient services provided during the encounter/visit. Codes for other diagnoses (e.g., chronic conditions) may be sequenced as additional diagnoses.

The only exception to this rule is that when the primary reason for the admission/encounter is chemotherapy or radiation therapy, the appropriate Z code for the service is listed first, and the diagnosis or problem for which the service is being performed listed second.

M. Patients receiving preoperative evaluations only

For patients receiving preoperative evaluations only, sequence first a code from subcategory Z01.81, Encounter for pre-procedural examinations, to describe the pre-op consultations. Assign a code for the condition to describe the reason for the surgery as an additional diagnosis. Code also any findings related to the pre-op evaluation.

N. Ambulatory surgery

For ambulatory surgery, code the diagnosis for which the surgery was performed. If the postoperative diagnosis is known to be different from the preoperative diagnosis at the time the diagnosis is confirmed, select the postoperative diagnosis for coding, since it is the most definitive.

O. Routine outpatient prenatal visits

See Section I.C.15. Routine outpatient prenatal visits.

P. Encounters for general medical examinations with abnormal findings

The subcategories for encounters for general medical examinations, Z00.0-, provide codes for with and without abnormal findings. Should a general medical examination result in an abnormal finding, the code for general medical examination with abnormal finding should be assigned as the first-listed diagnosis. A secondary code for the abnormal finding should also be coded.

Q. Encounters for routine health screenings

See Section I.C.21. Factors influencing health status and contact with health services, Screening

Appendix I. Present on Admission Reporting Guidelines

Introduction

These guidelines are to be used as a supplement to the *ICD-10-CM Official Guidelines for Coding and Reporting* to facilitate the assignment of the Present on Admission (POA) indicator for each diagnosis and external cause of injury code reported on claim forms (UB-04 and 837 Institutional).

These guidelines are not intended to replace any guidelines in the main body of the *ICD-10-CM Official Guidelines for Coding and Reporting*. The POA guidelines are not intended to provide guidance on when a condition should be coded, but rather, how to apply the POA indicator to the final set of diagnosis codes that have been assigned in accordance with Sections I, II, and III of the official coding guidelines. Subsequent to the assignment of the ICD-10-CM codes, the POA indicator should then be assigned to those conditions that have been coded.

As stated in the Introduction to the *ICD-10-CM Official Guidelines for Coding and Reporting*, a joint effort between the healthcare provider and the coder is essential to achieve complete and accurate documentation, code assignment, and reporting of diagnoses and procedures. The importance of consistent, complete documentation in the medical record cannot be overemphasized. Medical record documentation from any provider involved in the care and treatment of the patient may be used to support the determination of whether a condition was present on admission or not. In the context of the official coding guidelines, the term "provider" means a physician or any qualified healthcare practitioner who is legally accountable for establishing the patient's diagnosis.

These guidelines are not a substitute for the provider's clinical judgment as to the determination of whether a condition was/was not present on admission. The provider should be queried regarding issues related to the linking of signs/symptoms, timing of test results, and the timing of findings.

General Reporting Requirements

All claims involving inpatient admissions to general acute care hospitals or other facilities that are subject to a law or regulation mandating collection of present on admission information.

Present on admission is defined as present at the time the order for inpatient admission occurs -- conditions that develop during an outpatient encounter, including emergency department, observation, or outpatient surgery, are considered as present on admission.

POA indicator is assigned to principal and secondary diagnoses (as defined in Section II of the Official Guidelines for Coding and Reporting) and the external cause of injury codes.

Issues related to inconsistent, missing, conflicting or unclear documentation must still be resolved by the provider.

If a condition would not be coded and reported based on UHDDS definitions and current official coding guidelines, then the POA indicator would not be reported.

Reporting Options

Y –	Yes
N –	No
U –	Unknown
W –	Clinically undetermined
	Unreported/Not used (or "1" for Medicare usage) – (Exempt from POA reporting)

Reporting Definitions

Y –	present at the time of inpatient admission
N –	not present at the time of inpatient admission
U –	documentation is insufficient to determine if condition is present on admission
W –	provider is unable to clinically determine whether condition was present on admission or not

Timeframe for POA Identification and Documentation

There is no required timeframe as to when a provider (per the definition of "provider" used in these guidelines) must identify or document a condition to be present on admission. In some clinical situations, it may not be possible for a provider to make a definitive diagnosis (or a condition may not be recognized or reported by the patient) for a period of time after admission. In some cases it may be several days before the provider arrives at a definitive diagnosis. This does not mean that the condition was not present on admission. Determination of whether the condition was present on admission or not will be based on the applicable POA guideline as identified in this document, or on the provider's best clinical judgment.

If at the time of code assignment the documentation is unclear as to whether a condition was present on admission or not, it is appropriate to query the provider for clarification.

Assigning the POA Indicator

Condition is on the "Exempt from Reporting" list

Leave the "present on admission" field blank if the condition is on the list of ICD-10-CM codes for which this field is not applicable. This is the only circumstance in which the field may be left blank.

POA Explicitly Documented

Assign "Y" for any condition the provider explicitly documents as being present on admission.

Assign "N" for any condition the provider explicitly documents as not present at the time of admission.

Conditions diagnosed prior to inpatient admission

Assign "Y" for conditions that were diagnosed prior to admission (example: hypertension, diabetes mellitus, asthma).

Conditions diagnosed during the admission but clearly present before admission

Assign "Y" for conditions diagnosed during the admission that were clearly present but not diagnosed until after admission occurred.

Diagnoses subsequently confirmed after admission are considered present on admission if at the time of admission they are documented as suspected, possible, rule out, differential diagnosis, or constitute an underlying cause of a symptom that is present at the time of admission.

Condition develops during outpatient encounter prior to inpatient admission

Assign "Y" for any condition that develops during an outpatient encounter prior to a written order for inpatient admission.

Documentation does not indicate whether condition was present on admission

Assign "U" when the medical record documentation is unclear as to whether the condition was present on admission. "U" should not be routinely assigned and used only in very limited circumstances. Coders are encouraged to query the providers when the documentation is unclear.

Documentation states that it cannot be determined whether the condition was or was not present on admission

Assign "W" when the medical record documentation indicates that it cannot be clinically determined whether or not the condition was present on admission.

Chronic condition with acute exacerbation during the admission

If a single code identifies both the chronic condition and the acute exacerbation, see POA guidelines pertaining to combination codes.

If a single code only identifies the chronic condition and not the acute exacerbation (e.g., acute exacerbation of chronic leukemia), assign "Y."

Conditions documented as possible, probable, suspected, or rule out at the time of discharge

If the final diagnosis contains a possible, probable, suspected, or rule out diagnosis, and this diagnosis was based on signs, symptoms or clinical findings suspected at the time of inpatient admission, assign "Y."

If the final diagnosis contains a possible, probable, suspected, or rule out diagnosis, and this diagnosis was based on signs, symptoms or clinical findings that were not present on admission, assign "N".

Conditions documented as impending or threatened at the time of discharge

If the final diagnosis contains an impending or threatened diagnosis, and this diagnosis is based on symptoms or clinical findings that were present on admission, assign "Y".

If the final diagnosis contains an impending or threatened diagnosis, and this diagnosis is based on symptoms or clinical findings that were not present on admission, assign "N".

Acute and Chronic Conditions

Assign "Y" for acute conditions that are present at time of admission and N for acute conditions that are not present at time of admission.

Assign "Y" for chronic conditions, even though the condition may not be diagnosed until after admission.

If a single code identifies both an acute and chronic condition, see the POA guidelines for combination codes.

Combination Codes

Assign "N" if any part of the combination code was not present on admission (e.g., COPD with acute exacerbation and the exacerbation was not present on admission; gastric ulcer that does not start bleeding until after admission; asthma patient develops status asthmaticus after admission).

Assign "Y" if all parts of the combination code were present on admission (e.g., patient with acute prostatitis admitted with hematuria).

If the final diagnosis includes comparative or contrasting diagnoses, and both were present, or suspected, at the time of admission, assign "Y".

For infection codes that include the causal organism, assign "Y" if the infection (or signs of the infection) was present on admission, even though the culture results may not be known until after admission (e.g., patient is admitted with pneumonia and the provider documents pseudomonas as the causal organism a few days later).

Same Diagnosis Code for Two or More Conditions

When the same ICD-10-CM diagnosis code applies to two or more conditions during the same encounter (e.g. two separate conditions classified to the same ICD-10-CM diagnosis code):

> Assign "Y" if all conditions represented by the single ICD-10-CM code were present on admission (e.g. bilateral unspecified age-related cataracts).

> Assign "N" if any of the conditions represented by the single ICD-10-CM code was not present on admission (e.g. traumatic secondary and recurrent hemorrhage and seroma is assigned to a single code T79.2, but only one of the conditions was present on admission).

Obstetrical conditions

Whether or not the patient delivers during the current hospitalization does not affect assignment of the POA indicator. The determining factor for POA assignment is whether the pregnancy complication or obstetrical condition described by the code was present at the time of admission or not.

If the pregnancy complication or obstetrical condition was present on admission (e.g., patient admitted in preterm labor), assign "Y".

If the pregnancy complication or obstetrical condition was not present on admission (e.g., 2nd degree laceration during delivery, postpartum hemorrhage that occurred during current hospitalization, fetal distress develops after admission), assign "N".

If the obstetrical code includes more than one diagnosis and any of the diagnoses identified by the code were not present on admission assign "N". (e.g., Category O11, Pre-existing hypertension with pre-eclampsia).

Perinatal conditions

Newborns are not considered to be admitted until after birth. Therefore, any condition present at birth or that developed in utero is considered present at admission and should be assigned "Y". This includes conditions that occur during delivery (e.g., injury during delivery, meconium aspiration, exposure to streptococcus B in the vaginal canal).

Congenital conditions and anomalies

Assign "Y" for congenital conditions and anomalies except for categories Q00-Q99, Congenital anomalies, which are on the exempt list. Congenital conditions are always considered present on admission.

External cause of injury codes

Assign "Y" for any external cause code representing an external cause of morbidity that occurred prior to inpatient admission (e.g., patient fell out of bed at home, patient fell out of bed in emergency room prior to admission).

Assign "N" for any external cause code representing an external cause of morbidity that occurred during inpatient hospitalization (e.g., patient fell out of hospital bed during hospital stay, patient experienced an adverse reaction to a medication administered after inpatient admission).

Categories and Codes Exempt from Diagnosis Present on Admission Requirement

Note: "Diagnosis present on admission" for these code categories are exempt because they represent circumstances regarding the healthcare encounter or factors influencing health status that do not represent a current disease or injury or are always present on admission.

B90–B94	Sequelae of infectious and parasitic diseases
E64	Sequelae of malnutrition and other nutritional deficiences
I25.2	Old myocardial infarction
I69	Sequelae of cerebrovascular disease
O09	Supervision of high risk pregnancy
O66.5	Attempted application of vacuum extractor and forceps
O80	Encounter for full-term uncomplicated delivery
O94	Sequelae of complication of pregnancy, childbirth, and the puerperium
P00	Newborn (suspected to be) affected by maternal conditions that may be unrelated to present pregnancy
Q00-Q99	Congenital malformations, deformations and chromosomal abnormalities

S00-T88.9	Injury, poisoning and certain other consequences of external causes with 7th character representing subsequent encounter or sequela
V00-V09	Pedestrian injured in transport accident
	Except:V00.81-, Accident with wheelchair (powered) V00.83-, Accident with motorized mobility scooter
V10-V19	Pedal cycle rider injured in transport accident
V20-V29	Motorcycle rider injured in transport accident
V30-V39	Occupant of three-wheeled motor vehicle injured in transport accident
V40-V49	Car occupant injured in transport accident
V50-V59	Occupant of pick-up truck or van injured in transport accident
V60-V69	Occupant of heavy transport vehicle injured in transport accident
V70-V79	Bus occupant injured in transport accident
V80-V89	Other land transport accidents
V90-V94	Water transport accidents
V95-V97	Air and space transport accidents
V98-V99	Other and unspecified transport accidents
W09	Fall on and from playground equipment
W14	Fall from tree
W15	Fall from cliff
W17.0	Fall into well
W17.1	Fall into storm drain or manhole
W18.01	Striking against sports equipment with subsequent fall
W21	Striking against or struck by sports equipment
W30	Contact with agricultural machinery
W31	Contact with other and unspecified machinery
W32-W34	Accidental handgun discharge and malfunction
W35-W40	Exposure to inanimate mechanical forces
W52	Crushed, pushed or stepped on by crowd or human stampede
W56	Contact with nonvenomous marine animal
W58	Contact with crocodile or alligator
W61	Contact with birds (domestic) (wild)
W62	Contact with nonvenomous amphibians
W89	Exposure to man-made visible and ultraviolet light
X02	Exposure to controlled fire in building or structure
X03	Exposure to controlled fire, not in building or structure
X04	Exposure to ignition of highly flammable material
X52	Prolonged stay in weightless environment
X71	Intentional self-harm by drowning and submersion
	Except: X71.0-, Intentional self-harm by drowning and submersion while in bath tub
X72	Intentional self-harm by handgun discharge
X73	Intentional self-harm by rifle, shotgun and larger firearm discharge
X74	Intentional self-harm by other and unspecified firearm and gun discharge
X75	Intentional self-harm by explosive material
X76	Intentional self-harm by smoke, fire and flames
X77	Intentional self-harm by steam, hot vapors and hot objects
X81	Intentional self-harm by jumping or lying in front of moving object
X82	Intentional self-harm by crashing of motor vehicle
X83	Intentional self-harm by other specified means
Y03	Assault by crashing of motor vehicle
Y07	Perpetrator of assault, maltreatment and neglect
Y08.8	Assault by strike by sports equipment
Y21	Drowning and submersion, undetermined intent
Y22	Handgun discharge, undetermined intent
Y23	Rifle, shotgun and larger firearm discharge, undetermined intent
Y24	Other and unspecified firearm discharge, undetermined intent
Y30	Falling, jumping or pushed from a high place, undetermined intent
Y32	Assault by crashing of motor vehicle, undetermined intent
Y36	Operations of war
Y37	Military operations
Y92	Place of occurrence of the external cause
Y93	Activity code
Y99	External cause status

Z00	Encounter for general examination without complaint, suspected or reported diagnosis
Z01	Encounter for other special examination without complaint, suspected or reported diagnosis
Z02	Encounter for administrative examination
Z03	Encounter for medical observation for suspected diseases and conditions ruled out
Z08	Encounter for follow-up examination following completed treatment for malignant neoplasm
Z09	Encounter for follow-up examination after completed treatment for conditions other than malignant neoplasm
Z11	Encounter for screening for infectious and parasitic diseases
Z11.8	Encounter for screening for other infectious and parasitic diseases
Z12	Encounter for screening for malignant neoplasms
Z13	Encounter for screening for other diseases and disorders
Z13.4	Encounter for screening for certain developmental disorders in childhood
Z13.5	Encounter for screening for eye and ear disorders
Z13.6	Encounter for screening for cardiovascular disorders
Z13.83	Encounter for screening for respiratory disorder NEC
Z13.89	Encounter for screening for other disorder
Z14	Genetic carrier
Z15	Genetic susceptibility to disease
Z17	Estrogen receptor status
Z18	Retained foreign body fragments
Z22	Carrier of infectious disease
Z23	Encounter for immunization
Z28	Immunization not carried out and underimmunization status
Z28.3	Underimmunization status
Z30	Encounter for contraceptive management
Z31	Encounter for procreative management
Z34	Encounter for supervision of normal pregnancy
Z36	Encounter for antenatal screening of mother
Z37	Outcome of delivery
Z38	Liveborn infants according to place of birth and type of delivery
Z39	Encounter for maternal postpartum care and examination
Z41	Encounter for procedures for purposes other than remedying health state
Z42	Encounter for plastic and reconstructive surgery following medical procedure or healed injury
Z43	Encounter for attention to artificial openings
Z44	Encounter for fitting and adjustment of external prosthetic device
Z45	Encounter for adjustment and management of implanted device
Z46	Encounter for fitting and adjustment of other devices
Z47.8	Encounter for other orthopedic aftercare
Z49	Encounter for care involving renal dialysis
Z51	Encounter for other aftercare
Z51.5	Encounter for palliative care
Z51.8	Encounter for other specified aftercare
Z52	Donors of organs and tissues
Z59	Problems related to housing and economic circumstances
Z63	Other problems related to primary support groupincluding family circumstances
Z65	Problems related to other psychosocial circumstances
Z65.8	Other specified problems related to psychosocial circumstances
Z67.1-Z67.9	Blood type
Z68	Body mass index (BMI)
Z72	Problems related to lifestyle
Z74.01	Bed confinement status
Z76	Persons encountering health services in other circumstances
Z77.110-Z77.128	Environmental pollution and hazards in the physical environment
Z78	Other specified health status
Z79	Long term (current) drug therapy
Z80	Family history of primary malignant neoplasm
Z81	Family history of mental and behavioral disorders
Z82	Family history of certain disabilities and chronic diseases (leading to disablement)
Z83	Family history of other specific disorders

Z84	Family history of other conditions		Z92	Personal history of medical treatment
Z85	Personal history of primary malignant neoplasm		Z93	Artificial opening status
Z86	Personal history of certain other diseases		Z94	Transplanted organ and tissue status
Z87	Personal history of other diseases and conditions		Z95	Presence of cardiac and vascular implants and grafts
Z87.828	Personal history of other (healed) physical injury and trauma		Z97	Presence of other devices
Z87.891	Personal history of nicotine dependence		Z98	Other postprocedural states
Z88	Allergy status to drugs, medicaments and biological substances		Z99	Dependence on enabling machines and devices, not elsewhere classified
Z89	Acquired absence of limb			
Z90.710	Acquired absence of both cervix and uterus			
Z91.0	Allergy status, other than to drugs and biological substances			
Z91.4	Personal history of psychological trauma, not elsewhere classified			
Z91.5	Personal history of self-harm			
Z91.8	Other specified risk factors, not elsewhere classified			

ICD-10-CM Index to Diseases and Injuries

A

Aarskog's syndrome Q87.1
Abandonment — *see* Maltreatment
Abasia (-astasia) (hysterical) F44.4
Abderhalden-Kaufmann-Lignac syndrome (cystinosis) E72.04
Abdomen, abdominal (*see also* condition)
  acute R10.0
  angina K55.1
  muscle deficiency syndrome Q79.4
Abdominalgia — *see* Pain, abdominal
Abduction contracture, hip or other joint — *see* Contraction, joint
Aberrant (congenital) (*see also* Malposition, congenital)
  adrenal gland Q89.1
  artery (peripheral) Q27.8
    basilar NEC Q28.1
    cerebral Q28.3
    coronary Q24.5
    digestive system Q27.8
    eye Q15.8
    lower limb Q27.8
    precerebral Q28.1
    pulmonary Q25.79
    renal Q27.2
    retina Q14.1
    specified site NEC Q27.8
    subclavian Q27.8
    upper limb Q27.8
    vertebral Q28.1
  breast Q83.8
  endocrine gland NEC Q89.2
  hepatic duct Q44.5
  pancreas Q45.3
  parathyroid gland Q89.2
  pituitary gland Q89.2
  sebaceous glands, mucous membrane, mouth, congenital Q38.6
  spleen Q89.09
  subclavian artery Q27.8
  thymus (gland) Q89.2
  thyroid gland Q89.2
  vein (peripheral) NEC Q27.8
    cerebral Q28.3
    digestive system Q27.8
    lower limb Q27.8
    precerebral Q28.1
    specified site NEC Q27.8
    upper limb Q27.8
Aberration
  distantal — *see* Disturbance, visual
  mental F99
Abetalipoproteinemia E78.6
Abiotrophy R68.89
Ablatio, ablation
  retinae — *see* Detachment, retina
Ablepharia, ablepharon Q10.3
Abnormal, abnormality, abnormalities (*see also* Anomaly)
  acid-base balance (mixed) E87.4
  albumin R77.0
  alphafetoprotein R77.2
  alveolar ridge K08.9
  anatomical relationship Q89.9
  apertures, congenital, diaphragm Q79.1
  auditory perception H93.29- ☑
    diplacusis — *see* Diplacusis
    hyperacusis — *see* Hyperacusis
    recruitment — *see* Recruitment, auditory
    threshold shift — *see* Shift, auditory threshold
  autosomes Q99.9
    fragile site Q95.5
  basal metabolic rate R94.8
  biosynthesis, testicular androgen E29.1
  bleeding time R79.1
  blood level (of)
    cobalt R79.0
    copper R79.0
    iron R79.0
    lithium R78.89

Abnormal, abnormality, abnormalities — *continued*
  blood level — *continued*
    magnesium R79.0
    mineral NEC R79.0
    zinc R79.0
  blood pressure
    elevated R03.0
    low reading (nonspecific) R03.1
  blood sugar R73.09
  blood-gas level R79.81
  bowel sounds R19.15
    absent R19.11
    hyperactive R19.12
  brain scan R94.02
  breathing R06.9
  caloric test R94.138
  cerebrospinal fluid R83.9
    cytology R83.6
    drug level R83.2
    enzyme level R83.0
    hormones R83.1
    immunology R83.4
    microbiology R83.5
    nonmedicinal level R83.3
    specified type NEC R83.8
  chemistry, blood R79.9
    C-reactive protein R79.82
    drugs — *see* Findings, abnormal, in blood
    gas level R79.81
    minerals R79.0
    pancytopenia D61.818
    PTT R79.1
    specified NEC R79.89
    toxins — *see* Findings, abnormal, in blood
  chest sounds (friction) (rales) R09.89
  chromosome, chromosomal Q99.9
    with more than three X chromosomes, female Q97.1
    analysis result R89.8
      bronchial washings R84.8
      cerebrospinal fluid R83.8
      cervix uteri NEC R87.89
      nasal secretions R84.8
      nipple discharge R89.8
      peritoneal fluid R85.89
      pleural fluid R84.8
      prostatic secretions R86.8
      saliva R85.89
      seminal fluid R86.8
      sputum R84.8
      synovial fluid R89.8
      throat scrapings R84.8
      vagina R87.89
      vulva R87.89
      wound secretions R89.8
    dicentric replacement Q93.2
    ring replacement Q93.2
    sex Q99.8
      female phenotype Q97.9
        specified NEC Q97.8
      male phenotype Q98.9
        specified NEC Q98.8
      structural male Q98.6
    specified NEC Q99.8
  clinical findings NEC R68.89
  coagulation D68.9
    newborn, transient P61.6
    profile R79.1
    time R79.1
  communication — *see* Fistula
  conjunctiva, vascular H11.41- ☑
  coronary artery Q24.5
  cortisol-binding globulin E27.8
  course, eustachian tube Q17.8
  creatinine clearance R94.4
  cytology
    anus R85.619
      atypical squamous cells cannot exclude high grade squamous intraepithelial lesion (ASC-H) R85.611
      atypical squamous cells of undetermined significance (ASC-US) R85.610

Abnormal, abnormality, abnormalities — *continued*
  cytology — *continued*
    anus — *continued*
      cytologic evidence of malignancy R85.614
      high grade squamous intraepithelial lesion (HGSIL) R85.613
      human papillomavirus (HPV) DNA test
        high risk positive R85.81
        low risk postive R85.82
      inadequate smear R85.615
      low grade squamous intraepithelial lesion (LGSIL) R85.612
      satisfactory anal smear but lacking transformation zone R85.616
      specified NEC R85.618
      unsatisfactory smear R85.615
    female genital organs — *see* Abnormal, Papanicolaou (smear)
  dark adaptation curve H53.61
  dentofacial NEC — *see* Anomaly, dentofacial
  development, developmental Q89.9
    central nervous system Q07.9
  diagnostic imaging
    abdomen, abdominal region NEC R93.5
    biliary tract R93.2
    breast R92.8
    central nervous system NEC R90.89
    cerebrovascular NEC R90.89
    coronary circulation R93.1
    digestive tract NEC R93.3
    gastrointestinal (tract) R93.3
    genitourinary organs R93.8
    head R93.0
    heart R93.1
    intrathoracic organ NEC R93.8
    limbs R93.6
    liver R93.2
    lung (field) R91.8
    musculoskeletal system NEC R93.7
    retroperitoneum R93.5
    site specified NEC R93.8
    skin and subcutaneous tissue R93.8
    skull R93.0
    urinary organs R93.4
  direction, teeth, fully erupted M26.30
  ear ossicles, acquired NEC H74.39- ☑
    ankylosis — *see* Ankylosis, ear ossicles
    discontinuity — *see* Discontinuity, ossicles, ear
    partial loss — *see* Loss, ossicles, ear (partial)
  Ebstein Q22.5
  echocardiogram R93.1
  echoencephalogram R90.81
  echogram — *see* Abnormal, diagnostic imaging
  electrocardiogram [ECG] [EKG] R94.31
  electroencephalogram [EEG] R94.01
  electrolyte — *see* Imbalance, electrolyte
  electromyogram [EMG] R94.131
  electro-oculogram [EOG] R94.110
  electrophysiological intracardiac studies R94.39
  electroretinogram [ERG] R94.111
  erythrocytes
    congenital, with perinatal jaundice D58.9
  feces (color) (contents) (mucus) R19.5
  finding — *see* Findings, abnormal, without diagnosis
  fluid
    amniotic — *see* Abnormal, specimen, specified
    cerebrospinal — *see* Abnormal, cerebrospinal fluid
    peritoneal — *see* Abnormal, specimen, digestive organs
    pleural — *see* Abnormal, specimen, respiratory organs
    synovial — *see* Abnormal, specimen, specified
    thorax (bronchial washings) (pleural fluid) — *see* Abnormal, specimen, respiratory organs
    vaginal — *see* Abnormal, specimen, female genital organs
  form
    teeth K00.2
    uterus — *see* Anomaly, uterus
  function studies
    auditory R94.120
    bladder R94.8

Abnormal, abnormality, abnormalities — *continued*
- function studies — *continued*
  - brain R94.09
  - cardiovascular R94.30
  - ear R94.128
  - endocrine NEC R94.7
  - eye NEC R94.118
  - kidney R94.4
  - liver R94.5
  - nervous system
    - central NEC R94.09
    - peripheral NEC R94.138
  - pancreas R94.8
  - placenta R94.8
  - pulmonary R94.2
  - special senses NEC R94.128
  - spleen R94.8
  - thyroid R94.6
  - vestibular R94.121
- gait — *see* Gait
  - hysterical F44.4
- gastrin secretion E16.4
- globulin R77.1
  - cortisol-binding E27.8
  - thyroid-binding E07.89
- glomerular, minor (*see also* N00-N07 with fourth character .0) N05.0
- glucagon secretion E16.3
- glucose tolerance (test) (non-fasting) R73.09
- gravitational (G) forces or states (effect of) T75.81 ☑
- hair (color) (shaft) L67.9
  - specified NEC L67.8
- hard tissue formation in pulp (dental) K04.3
- head movement R25.0
- heart
  - rate R00.9
    - specified NEC R00.8
  - shadow R93.1
  - sounds NEC R01.2
- hemoglobin (disease) (*see also* Disease, hemoglobin) D58.2
  - trait — *see* Trait, hemoglobin, abnormal
- histology NEC R89.7
- immunological findings R89.4
  - in serum R76.9
    - specified NEC R76.8
- increase in appetite R63.2
- involuntary movement — *see* Abnormal, movement, involuntary
- jaw closure M26.51
- karyotype R89.8
- kidney function test R94.4
- knee jerk R29.2
- leukocyte (cell) (differential) NEC D72.9
- liver
- loss of
  - height R29.890
  - weight R63.4
- mammogram NEC R92.8
  - calcification (calculus) R92.1
  - microcalcification R92.0
- Mantoux test R76.11
- movement (disorder) (*see also* Disorder, movement)
  - head R25.0
  - involuntary R25.9
    - fasciculation R25.3
    - of head R25.0
    - spasm R25.2
    - specified type NEC R25.8
    - tremor R25.1
- myoglobin (Aberdeen) (Annapolis) R89.7
- neonatal screening P09
- oculomotor study R94.113
- palmar creases Q82.8
- Papanicolaou (smear)
  - anus R85.619
    - atypical squamous cells cannot exclude high grade squamous intraepithelial lesion (ASC-H) R85.611
    - atypical squamous cells of undetermined significance (ASC-US) R85.610
    - cytologic evidence of malignancy R85.614
    - high grade squamous intraepithelial lesion (HGSIL) R85.613
    - human papillomavirus (HPV) DNA test
      - high risk positive R85.81
      - low risk positive R85.82

Abnormal, abnormality, abnormalities — *continued*
- Papanicolaou — *continued*
  - anus — *continued*
    - inadequate smear R85.615
    - low grade squamous intraepithelial lesion (LGSIL) R85.612
    - satisfactory anal smear but lacking transformation zone R85.616
    - specified NEC R85.618
    - unsatisfactory smear R85.615
  - bronchial washings R84.6
  - cerebrospinal fluid R83.6
  - cervix R87.619
    - atypical squamous cells cannot exclude high grade squamous intraepithelial lesion (ASC-H) R87.611
    - atypical squamous cells of undetermined significance (ASC-US) R87.610
    - cytologic evidence of malignancy R87.614
    - high grade squamous intraepithelial lesion (HGSIL) R87.613
    - inadequate smear R87.615
    - low grade squamous intraepithelial lesion (LGSIL) R87.612
    - non-atypical endometrial cells R87.618
    - satisfactory cervical smear but lacking transformation zone R87.616
    - specified NEC R87.618
    - thin preparaton R87.619
    - unsatisfactory smear R87.615
  - nasal secretions R84.6
  - nipple discharge R89.6
  - peritoneal fluid R85.69
  - pleural fluid R84.6
  - prostatic secretions R86.6
  - saliva R85.69
  - seminal fluid R86.6
  - sites NEC R89.6
  - sputum R84.6
  - synovial fluid R89.6
  - throat scrapings R84.6
  - vagina R87.629
    - atypical squamous cells cannot exclude high grade squamous intraepithelial lesion (ASC-H) R87.621
    - atypical squamous cells of undetermined significance (ASC-US) R87.620
    - cytologic evidence of malignancy R87.624
    - high grade squamous intraepithelial lesion (HGSIL) R87.623
    - inadequate smear R87.625
    - low grade squamous intraepithelial lesion (LGSIL) R87.622
    - specified NEC R87.628
    - thin preparation R87.629
    - unsatisfactory smear R87.625
  - vulva R87.69
  - wound secretions R89.6
- partial thromboplastin time (PTT) R79.1
- pelvis (bony) — *see* Deformity, pelvis
- percussion, chest (tympany) R09.89
- periods (grossly) — *see* Menstruation
- phonocardiogram R94.39
- plantar reflex R29.2
- plasma
  - protein R77.9
    - specified NEC R77.8
  - viscosity R70.1
- pleural (folds) Q34.0
- posture R29.3
- product of conception O02.9
  - specified type NEC O02.89
- prothrombin time (PT) R79.1
- pulmonary
  - artery, congenital Q25.79
  - function, newborn P28.89
  - test results R94.2
- pulsations in neck R00.2
- pupillary H21.56- ☑
  - function (reaction) (reflex) — *see* Anomaly, pupil, function
- radiological examination — *see* Abnormal, diagnostic imaging
- red blood cell(s) (morphology) (volume) R71.8
- reflex — *see* Reflex
- renal function test R94.4
- response to nerve stimulation R94.130

Abnormal, abnormality, abnormalities — *continued*
- retinal correspondence H53.31
- retinal function study R94.111
- rhythm, heart (*see also* Arrhythmia)
- saliva — *see* Abnormal, specimen, digestive organs
- scan
  - kidney R94.4
  - liver R93.2
  - thyroid R94.6
- secretion
  - gastrin E16.4
  - glucagon E16.3
- semen, seminal fluid — *see* Abnormal, specimen, male genital organs
- serum level (of)
  - acid phosphatase R74.8
  - alkaline phosphatase R74.8
  - amylase R74.8
  - enzymes R74.9
    - specified NEC R74.8
  - lipase R74.8
  - triacylglycerol lipase R74.8
- shape
  - gravid uterus — *see* Anomaly, uterus
- sinus venosus Q21.1
- size, tooth, teeth K00.2
- spacing, tooth, teeth, fully erupted M26.30
- specimen
  - digestive organs (peritoneal fluid) (saliva) R85.9
    - cytology R85.69
    - drug level R85.2
    - enzyme level R85.0
    - histology R85.7
    - hormones R85.1
    - immunology R85.4
    - microbiology R85.5
    - nonmedicinal level R85.3
    - specified type NEC R85.89
  - female genital organs (secretions) (smears) R87.9
    - cytology R87.69
      - cervix R87.619
        - human papillomavirus (HPV) DNA test
          - high risk positive R87.810
          - low risk positive R87.820
        - inadequate (unsatisfactory) smear R87.615
        - non-atypical endometrial cells R87.618
        - specified NEC R87.618
      - vagina R87.629
        - human papillomavirus (HPV) DNA test
          - high risk positive R87.811
          - low risk positive R87.821
        - inadequate (unsatisfactory) smear R87.625
      - vulva R87.69
    - drug level R87.2
    - enzyme level R87.0
    - histological R87.7
    - hormones R87.1
    - immunology R87.4
    - microbiology R87.5
    - nonmedicinal level R87.3
    - specified type NEC R87.89
  - male genital organs (prostatic secretions) (semen) R86.9
    - cytology R86.6
    - drug level R86.2
    - enzyme level R86.0
    - histological R86.7
    - hormones R86.1
    - immunology R86.4
    - microbiology R86.5
    - nonmedicinal level R86.3
    - specified type NEC R86.8
  - nipple discharge — *see* Abnormal, specimen, specified
  - respiratory organs (bronchial washings) (nasal secretions) (pleural fluid) (sputum) R84.9
    - cytology R84.6
    - drug level R84.2
    - enzyme level R84.0
    - histology R84.7
    - hormones R84.1
    - immunology R84.4
    - microbiology R84.5
    - nonmedicinal level R84.3
    - specified type NEC R84.8

Abnormal, abnormality, abnormalities — *continued*
  specimen — *continued*
    specified organ, system and tissue NOS R89.9
      cytology R89.6
      drug level R89.2
      enzyme level R89.0
      histology R89.7
      hormones R89.1
      immunology R89.4
      microbiology R89.5
      nonmedicinal level R89.3
      specified type NEC R89.8
    synovial fluid — *see* Abnormal, specimen, specified
    thorax (bronchial washings) (pleural fluids) — *see* Abnormal, specimen, respiratory organs
    vagina (secretion) (smear) R87.629
    vulva (secretion) (smear) R87.69
    wound secretion — *see* Abnormal, specimen, specified
  spermatozoa — *see* Abnormal, specimen, male genital organs
  sputum (amount) (color) (odor) R09.3
  stool (color) (contents) (mucus) R19.5
    bloody K92.1
    guaiac positive R19.5
  synchondrosis Q78.8
  thermography (*see also* Abnormal, diagnostic imaging) R93.8
  thyroid-binding globulin E07.89
  tooth, teeth (form) (size) K00.2
  toxicology (findings) R78.9
  transport protein E88.09
  tumor marker NEC R97.8
  ultrasound results — *see* Abnormal, diagnostic imaging
  umbilical cord complicating delivery O69.9 ☑
  urination NEC R39.19
  urine (constituents) R82.90
    bile R82.2
    cytological examination R82.8
    drugs R82.5
    fat R82.0
    glucose R81
    heavy metals R82.6
    hemoglobin R82.3
    histological examination R82.8
    ketones R82.4
    microbiological examination (culture) R82.7
    myoglobin R82.1
    positive culture R82.7
    protein — *see* Proteinuria
    specified substance NEC R82.99
      chromoabnormality NEC R82.91
    substances nonmedical R82.6
  uterine hemorrhage — *see* Hemorrhage, uterus
  vectorcardiogram R94.39
  visually evoked potential (VEP) R94.112
  white blood cells D72.9
    specified NEC D72.89
  X-ray examination — *see* Abnormal, diagnostic imaging
Abnormity (any organ or part) — *see* Anomaly
Abocclusion M26.29
  hemolytic disease (newborn) P55.1
  incompatibility reaction ABO — *see* Complication(s), transfusion, incompatibility reaction, ABO
Abolition, language R48.8
Aborter, habitual or recurrent — *see* Loss (of), pregnancy, recurrent
Abortion (complete) (spontaneous) O03.9
  with
    retained products of conception — *see* Abortion, incomplete
  attempted (elective) (failed) O07.4
    complicated by O07.30
      afibrinogenemia O07.1
      cardiac arrest O07.36
      chemical damage of pelvic organ(s) O07.34
      circulatory collapse O07.31
      cystitis O07.38
      defibrination syndrome O07.1
      electrolyte imbalance O07.33
      embolism (air) (amniotic fluid) (blood clot) (fat) (pulmonary) (septic) (soap) O07.2
      endometritis O07.0
      genital tract and pelvic infection O07.0
      hemolysis O07.1

Abortion — *continued*
  attempted — *continued*
    complicated by — *continued*
      hemorrhage (delayed) (excessive) O07.1
      infection
        genital tract or pelvic O07.0
        urinary tract tract O07.38
      intravascular coagulation O07.1
      laceration of pelvic organ(s) O07.34
      metabolic disorder O07.33
      oliguria O07.32
      oophoritis O07.0
      parametritis O07.0
      pelvic peritonitis O07.0
      perforation of pelvic organ(s) O07.34
      renal failure or shutdown O07.32
      salpingitis or salpingo-oophoritis O07.0
      sepsis O07.37
      shock O07.31
      specified condition NEC O07.39
      tubular necrosis (renal) O07.32
      uremia O07.32
      urinary tract infection O07.38
      venous complication NEC O07.35
        embolism (air) (amniotic fluid) (blood clot) (fat) (pulmonary) (septic) (soap) O07.2
  complicated (by) (following) O03.80
    afibrinogenemia O03.6
    cardiac arrest O03.86
    chemical damage of pelvic organ(s) O03.84
    circulatory collapse O03.81
    cystitis O03.88
    defibrination syndrome O03.6
    electrolyte imbalance O03.83
    embolism (air) (amniotic fluid) (blood clot) (fat) (pulmonary) (septic) (soap) O03.7
    endometritis O03.5
    genital tract and pelvic infection O03.5
    hemolysis O03.6
    hemorrhage (delayed) (excessive) O03.6
    infection
      genital tract or pelvic O03.5
      urinary tract O03.88
    intravascular coagulation O03.6
    laceration of pelvic organ(s) O03.84
    metabolic disorder O03.83
    oliguria O03.82
    oophoritis O03.5
    parametritis O03.5
    pelvic peritonitis O03.5
    perforation of pelvic organ(s) O03.84
    renal failure or shutdown O03.82
    salpingitis or salpingo-oophoritis O03.5
    sepsis O03.87
    shock O03.81
    specified condition NEC O03.89
    tubular necrosis (renal) O03.82
    uremia O03.82
    urinary tract infection O03.88
    venous complication NEC O03.85
      embolism (air) (amniotic fluid) (blood clot) (fat) (pulmonary) (septic) (soap) O03.7
  failed — *see* Abortion, attempted
  habitual or recurrent N96
    with current abortion — *see* categories O03-O06
    without current pregnancy N96
    care in current pregnancy O26.2- ☑
  incomplete (spontaneous) O03.4
    complicated (by) (following) O03.30
      afibrinogenemia O03.1
      cardiac arrest O03.36
      chemical damage of pelvic organ(s) O03.34
      circulatory collapse O03.31
      cystitis O03.38
      defibrination syndrome O03.1
      electrolyte imbalance O03.33
      embolism (air) (amniotic fluid) (blood clot) (fat) (pulmonary) (septic) (soap) O03.2
      endometritis O03.0
      genital tract and pelvic infection O03.0
      hemolysis O03.1
      hemorrhage (delayed) (excessive) O03.1
      infection
        genital tract or pelvic O03.0
        urinary tract O03.38
      intravascular coagulation O03.1
      laceration of pelvic organ(s) O03.34
      metabolic disorder O03.33

Abortion — *continued*
  incomplete — *continued*
    complicated — *continued*
      oliguria O03.32
      oophoritis O03.0
      parametritis O03.0
      pelvic peritonitis O03.0
      perforation of pelvic organ(s) O03.34
      renal failure or shutdown O03.32
      salpingitis or salpingo-oophoritis O03.0
      sepsis O03.37
      shock O03.31
      specified condition NEC O03.39
      tubular necrosis (renal) O03.32
      uremia O03.32
      urinary infection O03.38
      venous complication NEC O03.35
        embolism (air) (amniotic fluid) (blood clot) (fat) (pulmonary) (septic) (soap) O03.2
  induced (encounter for) Z33.2
    complicated by O04.80
      afibrinogenemia O04.6
      cardiac arrest O04.86
      chemical damage of pelvic organ(s) O04.84
      circulatory collapse O04.81
      cystitis O04.88
      defibrination syndrome O04.6
      electrolyte imbalance O04.83
      embolism (air) (amniotic fluid) (blood clot) (fat) (pulmonary) (septic) (soap) O04.7
      endometritis O04.5
      genital tract and pelvic infection O04.5
      hemolysis O04.6
      hemorrhage (delayed) (excessive) O04.6
      infection
        genital tract or pelvic O04.5
        urinary tract O04.88
      intravascular coagulation O04.6
      laceration of pelvic organ(s) O04.84
      metabolic disorder O04.83
      oliguria O04.82
      oophoritis O04.5
      parametritis O04.5
      pelvic peritonitis O04.5
      perforation of pelvic organ(s) O04.84
      renal failure or shutdown O04.82
      salpingitis or salpingo-oophoritis O04.5
      sepsis O04.87
      shock O04.81
      specified condition NEC O04.89
      tubular necrosis (renal) O04.82
      uremia O04.82
      urinary tract infection O04.88
      venous complication NEC O04.85
        embolism (air) (amniotic fluid) (blood clot) (fat) (pulmonary) (septic) (soap) O04.7
  missed O02.1
  spontaneous — *see* Abortion (complete) (spontaneous)
    threatened O20.0
  threatened (spontaneous) O20.0
  tubal O00.1
Abortus fever A23.1
Aboulomania F60.7
Abrami's disease D59.8
Abramov-Fiedler myocarditis (acute isolated myocarditis) I40.1
Abrasion T14.8
  abdomen, abdominal (wall) S30.811 ☑
  alveolar process S00.512 ☑
  ankle S90.51- ☑
  antecubital space — *see* Abrasion, elbow
  anus S30.817 ☑
  arm (upper) S40.81- ☑
  auditory canal — *see* Abrasion, ear
  auricle — *see* Abrasion, ear
  axilla — *see* Abrasion, arm
  back, lower S30.810 ☑
  breast S20.11- ☑
  brow S00.81 ☑
  buttock S30.810 ☑
  calf — *see* Abrasion, leg
  canthus — *see* Abrasion, eyelid
  cheek S00.81 ☑
    internal S00.512 ☑
  chest wall — *see* Abrasion, thorax
  chin S00.81 ☑
  clitoris S30.814 ☑

Abrasion — *continued*
- cornea S05.0- ☑
- costal region — *see* Abrasion, thorax
- dental K03.1
- digit(s)
  - foot — *see* Abrasion, toe
  - hand — *see* Abrasion, finger
- ear S00.41- ☑
- elbow S50.31- ☑
- epididymis S30.813 ☑
- epigastric region S30.811 ☑
- epiglottis S10.11 ☑
- esophagus (thoracic) S27.818 ☑
  - cervical S10.11 ☑
- eyebrow — *see* Abrasion, eyelid
- eyelid S00.21- ☑
- face S00.81 ☑
- finger(s) S60.41- ☑
  - index S60.41- ☑
  - little S60.41- ☑
  - middle S60.41- ☑
  - ring S60.41- ☑
- flank S30.811 ☑
- foot (except toe(s) alone) S90.81- ☑
  - toe — *see* Abrasion, toe
- forearm S50.81- ☑
  - elbow only — *see* Abrasion, elbow
- forehead S00.81 ☑
- genital organs, external
  - female S30.816 ☑
  - male S30.815 ☑
- groin S30.811 ☑
- gum S00.512 ☑
- hand S60.51- ☑
- head S00.91 ☑
  - ear — *see* Abrasion, ear
  - eyelid — *see* Abrasion, eyelid
  - lip S00.511 ☑
  - nose S00.31 ☑
  - oral cavity S00.512 ☑
  - scalp S00.01 ☑
  - specified site NEC S00.81 ☑
- heel — *see* Abrasion, foot
- hip S70.21- ☑
- inguinal region S30.811 ☑
- interscapular region S20.419 ☑
- jaw S00.81 ☑
- knee S80.21- ☑
- labium (majus) (minus) S30.814 ☑
- larynx S10.11 ☑
- leg (lower) S80.81- ☑
  - knee — *see* Abrasion, knee
  - upper — *see* Abrasion, thigh
- lip S00.511 ☑
- lower back S30.810 ☑
- lumbar region S30.810 ☑
- malar region S00.81 ☑
- mammary — *see* Abrasion, breast
- mastoid region S00.81 ☑
- mouth S00.512 ☑
- nail
  - finger — *see* Abrasion, finger
  - toe — *see* Abrasion, toe
- nape S10.81 ☑
- nasal S00.31 ☑
- neck S10.91 ☑
  - specified site NEC S10.81 ☑
  - throat S10.11 ☑
- nose S00.31 ☑
- occipital region S00.01 ☑
- oral cavity S00.512 ☑
- orbital region — *see* Abrasion, eyelid
- palate S00.512 ☑
- palm — *see* Abrasion, hand
- parietal region S00.01 ☑
- pelvis S30.810 ☑
- penis S30.812 ☑
- perineum
  - female S30.814 ☑
  - male S30.810 ☑
- periocular area — *see* Abrasion, eyelid
- phalanges
  - finger — *see* Abrasion, finger
  - toe — *see* Abrasion, toe
- pharynx S10.11 ☑
- pinna — *see* Abrasion, ear

Abrasion — *continued*
- popliteal space — *see* Abrasion, knee
- prepuce S30.812 ☑
- pubic region S30.810 ☑
- pudendum
  - female S30.816 ☑
  - male S30.815 ☑
- sacral region S30.810 ☑
- scalp S00.01 ☑
- scapular region — *see* Abrasion, shoulder
- scrotum S30.813 ☑
- shin — *see* Abrasion, leg
- shoulder S40.21- ☑
- skin NEC T14.8
- sternal region S20.319 ☑
- submaxillary region S00.81 ☑
- submental region S00.81 ☑
- subungual
  - finger(s) — *see* Abrasion, finger
  - toe(s) — *see* Abrasion, toe
- supraclavicular fossa S10.81 ☑
- supraorbital S00.81 ☑
- temple S00.81 ☑
- temporal region S00.81 ☑
- testis S30.813 ☑
- thigh S70.31- ☑
- thorax, thoracic (wall) S20.91 ☑
  - back S20.41- ☑
  - front S20.31- ☑
- throat S10.11 ☑
- thumb S60.31- ☑
- toe(s) (lesser) S90.416 ☑
  - great S90.41- ☑
- tongue S00.512 ☑
- tooth, teeth (dentifrice) (habitual) (hard tissues) (occupational) (ritual) (traditional) K03.1
- trachea S10.11 ☑
- tunica vaginalis S30.813 ☑
- tympanum, tympanic membrane — *see* Abrasion, ear
- uvula S00.512 ☑
- vagina S30.814 ☑
- vocal cords S10.11 ☑
- vulva S30.814 ☑
- wrist S60.81- ☑

Abrism — *see* Poisoning, food, noxious, plant

Abruptio placentae O45.9- ☑
- with
  - afibrinogenemia O45.01- ☑
  - coagulation defect O45.00- ☑
    - specified NEC O45.09- ☑
  - disseminated intravascular coagulation O45.02- ☑
  - hypofibrinogenemia O45.01- ☑
  - specified NEC O45.8- ☑

Abruption, placenta — *see* Abruptio placentae

Abscess (connective tissue) (embolic) (fistulous) (infective) (metastatic) (multiple) (pernicious) (pyogenic) (septic) L02.91
- with
  - diverticular disease (intestine) K57.80
    - with bleeding K57.81
    - large intestine K57.20
      - with
        - bleeding K57.21
        - small intestine K57.40
          - with bleeding K57.41
    - small intestine K57.00
      - with
        - bleeding K57.01
        - large intestine K57.40
          - with bleeding K57.41
  - lymphangitis — *code by* site under Abscess
- abdomen, abdominal
  - cavity K65.1
  - wall L02.211
- abdominopelvic K65.1
- accessory sinus — *see* Sinusitis
- adrenal (capsule) (gland) E27.8
- alveolar K04.7
  - with sinus K04.6
- amebic A06.4
  - brain (and liver or lung abscess) A06.6
  - genitourinary tract A06.82
  - liver (without mention of brain or lung abscess) A06.4
  - lung (and liver) (without mention of brain abscess) A06.5
  - specified site NEC A06.89

Abscess — *continued*
- amebic — *continued*
  - spleen A06.89
- anerobic A48.0
- ankle — *see* Abscess, lower limb
- anorectal K61.2
- antecubital space — *see* Abscess, upper limb
- antrum (chronic) (Highmore) — *see* Sinusitis, maxillary
- anus K61.0
- apical (tooth) K04.7
  - with sinus (alveolar) K04.6
- appendix K35.3
- areola (acute) (chronic) (nonpuerperal) N61
  - puerperal, postpartum or gestational — *see* Infection, nipple
- arm (any part) — *see* Abscess, upper limb
- artery (wall) I77.89
- atheromatous I77.2
- auricle, ear — *see* Abscess, ear, external
- axilla (region) L02.41- ☑
  - lymph gland or node L04.2
- back (any part, except buttock) L02.212
- Bartholin's gland N75.1
  - with
    - abortion — *see* Abortion, by type complicated by, sepsis
    - ectopic or molar pregnancy O08.0
  - following ectopic or molar pregnancy O08.0
- Bezold's — *see* Mastoiditis, acute
- bilharziasis B65.1
- bladder (wall) — *see* Cystitis, specified type NEC
- bone (subperiosteal) (*see also* Osteomyelitis, specified type NEC)
  - accessory sinus (chronic) — *see* Sinusitis
  - chronic or old — *see* Osteomyelitis, chronic
  - jaw (lower) (upper) M27.2
  - mastoid — *see* Mastoiditis, acute, subperiosteal
  - petrous — *see* Petrositis
  - spinal (tuberculous) A18.01
    - nontuberculous — *see* Osteomyelitis, vertebra
- bowel K63.0
- brain (any part) (cystic) (otogenic) G06.0
  - amebic (with abscess of any other site) A06.6
  - gonococcal A54.82
  - pheomycotic (chromomycotic) B43.1
  - tuberculous A17.81
- breast (acute) (chronic) (nonpuerperal) N61
  - newborn P39.0
  - puerperal, postpartum, gestational — *see* Mastitis, obstetric, purulent
- broad ligament N73.2
  - acute N73.0
  - chronic N73.1
- Brodie's (localized) (chronic) M86.8X- ☑
- bronchi J98.09
- buccal cavity K12.2
- bulbourethral gland N34.0
- bursa M71.00
  - ankle M71.07- ☑
  - elbow M71.02- ☑
  - foot M71.07- ☑
  - hand M71.04- ☑
  - hip M71.05- ☑
  - knee M71.06- ☑
  - multiple sites M71.09
  - pharyngeal J39.1
  - shoulder M71.01- ☑
  - specified site NEC M71.08
  - wrist M71.03- ☑
- buttock L02.31
- canthus — *see* Blepharoconjunctivitis
- cartilage — *see* Disorder, cartilage, specified type NEC
- cecum K35.3
- cerebellum, cerebellar G06.0
  - sequelae G09
- cerebral (embolic) G06.0
  - sequelae G09
- cervical (meaning neck) L02.11
  - lymph gland or node L04.0
- cervix (stump) (uteri) — *see* Cervicitis
- cheek (external) L02.01
  - inner K12.2
- chest J86.9
  - with fistula J86.0
  - wall L02.213
- chin L02.01
- choroid — *see* Inflammation, chorioretinal

Abscess — *continued*
circumtonsillar J36
cold (lung) (tuberculous) (*see also* Tuberculosis, abscess, lung)
  articular — *see* Tuberculosis, joint
colon (wall) K63.0
colostomy K94.02
conjunctiva — *see* Conjunctivitis, acute
cornea H16.31- ☑
corpus
  cavernosum N48.21
  luteum — *see* Oophoritis
Cowper's gland N34.0
cranium G06.0
cul-de-sac (Douglas') (posterior) — *see* Peritonitis, pelvic, female
cutaneous — *see* Abscess, by site
dental K04.7
  with sinus (alveolar) K04.6
dentoalveolar K04.7
  with sinus K04.6
diaphragm, diaphragmatic K65.1
Douglas' cul-de-sac or pouch — *see* Peritonitis, pelvic, female
Dubois A50.59
ear (middle) (*see also* Otitis, media, suppurative)
  acute — *see* Otitis, media, suppurative, acute
  external H60.0- ☑
entamebic — *see* Abscess, amebic
enterostomy K94.12
epididymis N45.4
epidural G06.2
  brain G06.0
  spinal cord G06.1
epiglottis J38.7
epiploon, epiploic K65.1
erysipelatous — *see* Erysipelas
esophagus K20.8
ethmoid (bone) (chronic) (sinus) J32.2
external auditory canal — *see* Abscess, ear, external
extradural G06.2
  brain G06.0
    sequelae G09
  spinal cord G06.1
extraperitoneal K68.19
eye — *see* Endophthalmitis, purulent
eyelid H00.03- ☑
face (any part, except ear, eye and nose) L02.01
fallopian tube — *see* Salpingitis
fascia M72.8
fauces J39.1
fecal K63.0
femoral (region) — *see* Abscess, lower limb
filaria, filarial — *see* Infestation, filarial
finger (any) (*see also* Abscess, hand)
  nail — *see* Cellulitis, finger
foot L02.61- ☑
forehead L02.01
frontal sinus (chronic) J32.1
gallbladder K81.0
genital organ or tract
  female (external) N76.4
  male N49.9
    multiple sites N49.8
    specified NEC N49.8
gestational mammary O91.11- ☑
gestational subareolar O91.11- ☑
gingival K05.21
gland, glandular (lymph) (acute) — *see* Lymphadenitis, acute
gluteal (region) L02.31
gonorrheal — *see* Gonococcus
groin L02.214
gum K05.21
hand L02.51- ☑
head NEC L02.811
  face (any part, except ear, eye and nose) L02.01
heart — *see* Carditis
heel — *see* Abscess, foot
helminthic — *see* Infestation, helminth
hepatic (cholangitic) (hematogenic) (lymphogenic) (pylephlebitic) K75.0
  amebic A06.4
hip (region) — *see* Abscess, lower limb
ileocecal K35.3
ileostomy (bud) K94.12

Abscess — *continued*
iliac (region) L02.214
  fossa K35.3
infraclavicular (fossa) — *see* Abscess, upper limb
inguinal (region) L02.214
  lymph gland or node L04.1
intestine, intestinal NEC K63.0
  rectal K61.1
intra-abdominal (*see also* Abscess, peritoneum) K65.1
  postoperative T81.4 ☑
    retroperitoneal K68.11
intracranial G06.0
intramammary — *see* Abscess, breast
intraorbital — *see* Abscess, orbit
intraperitoneal K65.1
intrasphincteric (anus) K61.4
intraspinal G06.1
intratonsillar J36
ischiorectal (fossa) K61.3
jaw (bone) (lower) (upper) M27.2
joint — *see* Arthritis, pyogenic or pyemic
  spine (tuberculous) A18.01
    nontuberculous — *see* Spondylopathy, infective
kidney N15.1
  with calculus N20.0
    with hydronephrosis N13.6
  puerperal (postpartum) O86.21
knee (*see also* Abscess, lower limb)
  joint M00.9
labium (majus) (minus) N76.4
lacrimal
  caruncle — *see* Inflammation, lacrimal, passages, acute
  gland — *see* Dacryoadenitis
  passages (duct) (sac) — *see* Inflammation, lacrimal, passages, acute
lacunar N34.0
larynx J38.7
lateral (alveolar) K04.7
  with sinus K04.6
leg (any part) — *see* Abscess, lower limb
lens H27.8
lingual K14.0
  tonsil J36
lip K13.0
Littre's gland N34.0
liver (cholangitic) (hematogenic) (lymphogenic) (pylephlebitic) (pyogenic) K75.0
  amebic (due to Entamoeba histolytica) (dysenteric) (tropical) A06.4
    with
      brain abscess (and liver or lung abscess) A06.6
      lung abscess A06.5
loin (region) L02.211
lower limb L02.41- ☑
lumbar (tuberculous) A18.01
  nontuberculous L02.212
lung (miliary) (putrid) J85.2
  with pneumonia J85.1
    due to specified organism (see Pneumonia, in (due to))
  amebic (with liver abscess) A06.5
    with
      brain abscess A06.6
      pneumonia A06.5
lymph, lymphatic, gland or node (acute) (*see also* Lymphadenitis, acute)
  mesentery I88.0
malar M27.2
mammary gland — *see* Abscess, breast
marginal, anus K61.0
mastoid — *see* Mastoiditis, acute
maxilla, maxillary M27.2
  molar (tooth) K04.7
    with sinus K04.6
  premolar K04.7
  sinus (chronic) J32.0
mediastinum J85.3
meibomian gland — *see* Hordeolum
meninges G06.2
mesentery, mesenteric K65.1
mesosalpinx — *see* Salpingitis
mons pubis L02.215
mouth (floor) K12.2
muscle — *see* Myositis, infective
myocardium I40.0

Abscess — *continued*
nabothian (follicle) — *see* Cervicitis
nasal J32.9
nasopharyngeal J39.1
navel L02.216
  newborn P38.9
    with mild hemorrhage P38.1
    without hemorrhage P38.9
neck (region) L02.11
  lymph gland or node L04.0
nephritic — *see* Abscess, kidney
nipple N61
  associated with
    lactation — *see* Pregnancy, complicated by, pregnancy — *see* Pregnancy, complicated by
nose (external) (fossa) (septum) J34.0
  sinus (chronic) — *see* Sinusitis
omentum K65.1
operative wound T81.4 ☑
orbit, orbital — *see* Cellulitis, orbit
otogenic G06.0
ovary, ovarian (corpus luteum) — *see* Oophoritis
oviduct — *see* Oophoritis
palate (soft) K12.2
  hard M27.2
palmar (space) — *see* Abscess, hand
pancreas (duct) — *see* Pancreatitis, acute
parafrenal N48.21
parametric, parametrium N73.2
  acute N73.0
  chronic N73.1
paranephric N15.1
parapancreatic — *see* Pancreatitis, acute
parapharyngeal J39.0
pararectal K61.1
parasinus — *see* Sinusitis
parauterine (*see also* Disease, pelvis, inflammatory) N73.2
paravaginal — *see* Vaginitis
parietal region (scalp) L02.811
parodontal K05.21
parotid (duct) (gland) K11.3
  region K12.2
pectoral (region) L02.213
pelvis, pelvic
  female — *see* Disease, pelvis, inflammatory
  male, peritoneal K65.1
penis N48.21
  gonococcal (accessory gland) (periurethral) A54.1
perianal K61.0
periapical K04.7
  with sinus (alveolar) K04.6
periappendicular K35.3
pericardial I30.1
pericecal K35.3
pericemental K05.21
pericholecystic — *see* Cholecystitis, acute
pericoronal K05.21
peridental K05.21
perimetric (*see also* Disease, pelvis, inflammatory) N73.2
perinephric, perinephritic — *see* Abscess, kidney
perineum, perineal (superficial) L02.215
  urethra N34.0
periodontal (parietal) K05.21
  apical K04.7
periosteum, periosteal (*see also* Osteomyelitis, specified type NEC)
  with osteomyelitis (*see also* Osteomyelitis, specified type NEC)
    acute — *see* Osteomyelitis, acute
    chronic — *see* Osteomyelitis, chronic
peripharyngeal J39.0
peripleuritic J86.9
  with fistula J86.0
periprostatic N41.2
perirectal K61.1
perirenal (tissue) — *see* Abscess, kidney
perisinuous (nose) — *see* Sinusitis
peritoneum, peritoneal (perforated) (ruptured) K65.1
  with appendicitis K35.3
  pelvic
    female — *see* Peritonitis, pelvic, female
    male K65.1
  postoperative T81.4 ☑
  puerperal, postpartum, childbirth O85
  tuberculous A18.31
peritonsillar J36

Abscess — *continued*
  perityphlic K35.3
  periureteral N28.89
  periurethral N34.0
    gonococcal (accessory gland) (periurethral) A54.1
  periuterine (*see also* Disease, pelvis, inflammatory) N73.2
  perivesical — *see* Cystitis, specified type NEC
  petrous bone — *see* Petrositis
  phagedenic NOS L02.91
    chancroid A57
  pharynx, pharyngeal (lateral) J39.1
  pilonidal L05.01
  pituitary (gland) E23.6
  pleura J86.9
    with fistula J86.0
  popliteal — *see* Abscess, lower limb
  postcecal K35.3
  postlaryngeal J38.7
  postnasal J34.0
  postoperative (any site) T81.4 ☑
    retroperitoneal K68.11
  postpharyngeal J39.0
  posttonsillar J36
  post-typhoid A01.09
  pouch of Douglas — *see* Peritonitis, pelvic, female
  premammary — *see* Abscess, breast
  prepatellar — *see* Abscess, lower limb
  prostate N41.2
    gonococcal (acute) (chronic) A54.22
  psoas muscle K68.12
  puerperal — *code by* site under Puerperal, abscess
  pulmonary — *see* Abscess, lung
  pulp, pulpal (dental) K04.0
  rectovaginal septum K63.0
  rectovesical — *see* Cystitis, specified type NEC
  rectum K61.1
  renal — *see* Abscess, kidney
  retina — *see* Inflammation, chorioretinal
  retrobulbar — *see* Abscess, orbit
  retrocecal K65.1
  retrolaryngeal J38.7
  retromammary — *see* Abscess, breast
  retroperitoneal NEC K68.19
    postprocedural K68.11
  retropharyngeal J39.0
  retrouterine — *see* Peritonitis, pelvic, female
  retrovesical — *see* Cystitis, specified type NEC
  root, tooth K04.7
    with sinus (alveolar) K04.6
  round ligament (*see also* Disease, pelvis, inflammatory) N73.2
  rupture (spontaneous) NOS L02.91
  sacrum (tuberculous) A18.01
    nontuberculous M46.28
  salivary (duct) (gland) K11.3
  scalp (any part) L02.811
  scapular — *see* Osteomyelitis, specified type NEC
  sclera — *see* Scleritis
  scrofulous (tuberculous) A18.2
  scrotum N49.2
  seminal vesicle N49.0
  septal, dental K04.7
    with sinus (alveolar) K04.6
  serous — *see* Periostitis
  shoulder (region) — *see* Abscess, upper limb
  sigmoid K63.0
  sinus (accessory) (chronic) (nasal) (*see also* Sinusitis)
    intracranial venous (any) G06.0
  Skene's duct or gland N34.0
  skin — *see* Abscess, by site
  specified site NEC L02.818
  spermatic cord N49.1
  sphenoidal (sinus) (chronic) J32.3
  spinal cord (any part) (staphylococcal) G06.1
    tuberculous A17.81
  spine (column) (tuberculous) A18.01
    epidural G06.1
    nontuberculous — *see* Osteomyelitis, vertebra
  spleen D73.3
    amebic A06.89
  stitch T81.4 ☑
  subarachnoid G06.2
    brain G06.0
    spinal cord G06.1
  subareolar — *see* Abscess, breast
  subcecal K35.3

Abscess — *continued*
  subcutaneous (*see also* Abscess, by site)
    pheomycotic (chromomycotic) B43.2
  subdiaphragmatic K65.1
  subdural G06.2
    brain G06.0
      sequelae G09
    spinal cord G06.1
  subgaleal L02.811
  subhepatic K65.1
  sublingual K12.2
    gland K11.3
  submammary — *see* Abscess, breast
  submandibular (region) (space) (triangle) K12.2
    gland K11.3
  submaxillary (region) L02.01
    gland K11.3
  submental L02.01
    gland K11.3
  subperiosteal — *see* Osteomyelitis, specified type NEC
  subphrenic K65.1
    postoperative T81.4 ☑
  suburethral N34.0
  sudoriparous L75.8
  supraclavicular (fossa) — *see* Abscess, upper limb
  suprapelvic, acute N73.0
  suprarenal (capsule) (gland) E27.8
  sweat gland L74.8
  tear duct — *see* Inflammation, lacrimal, passages, acute
  temple L02.01
  temporal region L02.01
  temporosphenoidal G06.0
  tendon (sheath) M65.00
    ankle M65.07- ☑
    foot M65.07- ☑
    forearm M65.03- ☑
    hand M65.04- ☑
    lower leg M65.06- ☑
    pelvic region M65.05- ☑
    shoulder region M65.01- ☑
    specified site NEC M65.08
    thigh M65.05- ☑
    upper arm M65.02- ☑
  testis N45.4
  thigh — *see* Abscess, lower limb
  thorax J86.9
    with fistula J86.0
  throat J39.1
  thumb (*see also* Abscess, hand)
    nail — *see* Cellulitis, finger
  thymus (gland) E32.1
  thyroid (gland) E06.0
  toe (any) (*see also* Abscess, foot)
    nail — *see* Cellulitis, toe
  tongue (staphylococcal) K14.0
  tonsil(s) (lingual) J36
  tonsillopharyngeal J36
  tooth, teeth (root) K04.7
    with sinus (alveolar) K04.6
    supporting structures NEC K05.21
  trachea J39.8
  trunk L02.219
    abdominal wall L02.211
    back L02.212
    chest wall L02.213
    groin L02.214
    perineum L02.215
    umbilicus L02.216
  tubal — *see* Salpingitis
  tuberculous — *see* Tuberculosis, abscess
  tubo-ovarian — *see* Salpingo-oophoritis
  tunica vaginalis N49.1
  umbilicus L02.216
  upper
    limb L02.41- ☑
    respiratory J39.8
  urethral (gland) N34.0
  urinary N34.0
  uterus, uterine (wall) (*see also* Endometritis)
    ligament (*see also* Disease, pelvis, inflammatory) N73.2
    neck — *see* Cervicitis
  uvula K12.2
  vagina (wall) — *see* Vaginitis
  vaginorectal — *see* Vaginitis

Abscess — *continued*
  vas deferens N49.1
  vermiform appendix K35.3
  vertebra (column) (tuberculous) A18.01
    nontuberculous — *see* Osteomyelitis, vertebra
  vesical — *see* Cystitis, specified type NEC
  vesico-uterine pouch — *see* Peritonitis, pelvic, female
  vitreous (humor) — *see* Endophthalmitis, purulent
  vocal cord J38.3
  von Bezold's — *see* Mastoiditis, acute
  vulva N76.4
  vulvovaginal gland N75.1
  web space — *see* Abscess, hand
  wound T81.4 ☑
  wrist — *see* Abscess, upper limb
Absence (of) (organ or part) (complete or partial)
  adrenal (gland) (congenital) Q89.1
    acquired E89.6
  albumin in blood E88.09
  alimentary tract (congenital) Q45.8
    upper Q40.8
  alveolar process (acquired) — *see* Anomaly, alveolar
  ankle (acquired) Z89.44- ☑
  anus (congenital) Q42.3
    with fistula Q42.2
  aorta (congenital) Q25.4
  appendix, congenital Q42.8
  arm (acquired) Z89.20- ☑
    above elbow Z89.22- ☑
      congenital (with hand present) — *see* Agenesis, arm, with hand present
        and hand — *see* Agenesis, forearm, and hand
    below elbow Z89.21- ☑
      congenital (with hand present) — *see* Agenesis, arm, with hand present
        and hand — *see* Agenesis, forearm, and hand
    congenital — *see* Defect, reduction, upper limb
    shoulder (following explantation of shoulder joint prosthesis) (joint) (with or without presence of antibiotic-impregnated cement spacer) Z89.23- ☑
      congenital (with hand present) — *see* Agenesis, arm, with hand present
  artery (congenital) (peripheral) Q27.8
    brain Q28.3
    coronary Q24.5
    pulmonary Q25.79
    specified NEC Q27.8
    umbilical Q27.0
  atrial septum (congenital) Q21.1
  auditory canal (congenital) (external) Q16.1
  auricle (ear), congenital Q16.0
  bile, biliary duct, congenital Q44.5
  bladder (acquired) Z90.6
    congenital Q64.5
  bowel sounds R19.11
  brain Q00.0
    part of Q04.3
  breast(s) (and nipple(s)) (acquired) Z90.1- ☑
    congenital Q83.8
  broad ligament Q50.6
  bronchus (congenital) Q32.4
  canaliculus lacrimalis, congenital Q10.4
  cerebellum (vermis) Q04.3
  cervix (acquired) (with uterus) Z90.710
    with remaining uterus Z90.712
    congenital Q51.5
  chin, congenital Q18.8
  cilia (congenital) Q10.3
    acquired — *see* Madarosis
  clitoris (congenital) Q52.6
  coccyx, congenital Q76.49
  cold sense R20.8
  congenital
    lumen — *see* Atresia
    organ or site NEC — *see* Agenesis
    septum — *see* Imperfect, closure
  corpus callosum Q04.0
  cricoid cartilage, congenital Q31.8
  diaphragm (with hernia), congenital Q79.1
  digestive organ(s) or tract, congenital Q45.8
    acquired NEC Z90.49
    upper Q40.8
  ductus arteriosus Q28.8
  duodenum (acquired) Z90.49
    congenital Q41.0

Absence — continued
  ear, congenital Q16.9
    acquired H93.8- ☑
    auricle Q16.0
    external Q16.0
    inner Q16.5
    lobe, lobule Q17.8
    middle, except ossicles Q16.4
      ossicles Q16.3
    ossicles Q16.3
  ejaculatory duct (congenital) Q55.4
  endocrine gland (congenital) NEC Q89.2
    acquired E89.89
  epididymis (congenital) Q55.4
    acquired Z90.79
  epiglottis, congenital Q31.8
  esophagus (congenital) Q39.8
    acquired (partial) Z90.49
  eustachian tube (congenital) Q16.2
  extremity (acquired) Z89.9
    congenital Q73.0
    knee (following explantation of knee joint prosthesis) (joint) (with or without presence of antibiotic-impregnated cement spacer) Z89.52- ☑
    lower (above knee) Z89.619
      below knee Z89.51- ☑
    upper — see Absence, arm
  eye (acquired) Z90.01
    congenital Q11.1
    muscle (congenital) Q10.3
  eyeball (acquired) Z90.01
  eyelid (fold) (congenital) Q10.3
    acquired Z90.01
  face, specified part NEC Q18.8
  fallopian tube(s) (acquired) Z90.79
    congenital Q50.6
  family member (causing problem in home) NEC (see also Disruption, family) Z63.32
  femur, congenital — see Defect, reduction, lower limb, longitudinal, femur
  fibrinogen (congenital) D68.2
    acquired D65
  finger(s) (acquired) Z89.02- ☑
    congenital — see Agenesis, hand
  foot (acquired) Z89.43- ☑
    congenital — see Agenesis, foot
  forearm (acquired) — see Absence, arm, below elbow
  gallbladder (acquired) Z90.49
    congenital Q44.0
  gamma globulin in blood D80.1
    hereditary D80.0
  genital organs
    acquired (female) (male) Z90.79
    female, congenital Q52.8
      external Q52.71
      internal NEC Q52.8
    male, congenital Q55.8
  genitourinary organs, congenital NEC
    female Q52.8
    male Q55.8
  globe (acquired) Z90.01
    congenital Q11.1
  glottis, congenital Q31.8
  hand and wrist (acquired) Z89.11- ☑
    congenital — see Agenesis, hand
  head, part (acquired) NEC Z90.09
  heat sense R20.8
  hip (following explantation of hip joint prosthesis) (joint) (with or without presence of antibiotic-impregnated cement spacer) Z89.62- ☑
  hymen (congenital) Q52.4
  ileum (acquired) Z90.49
    congenital Q41.2
  immunoglobulin, isolated NEC D80.3
    IgA D80.2
    IgG D80.3
    IgM D80.4
  incus (acquired) — see Loss, ossicles, ear
    congenital Q16.3
  inner ear, congenital Q16.5
  intestine (acquired) (small) Z90.49
    congenital Q41.9
      specified NEC Q41.8
    large Z90.49
      congenital Q42.9
        specified NEC Q42.8
  iris, congenital Q13.1

Absence — continued
  jejunum (acquired) Z90.49
    congenital Q41.1
  joint
    acquired
      hip (following explantation of hip joint prosthesis) (with or without presence of antibiotic-impregnated cement spacer) Z89.62- ☑
      knee (following explantation of knee joint prosthesis) (with or without presence of antibiotic-impregnated cement spacer) Z89.52- ☑
      shoulder (following explantation of shoulder joint prosthesis) (with or without presence of antibiotic-impregnated cement spacer) Z89.23- ☑
    congenital NEC Q74.8
  kidney(s) (acquired) Z90.5
    congenital Q60.2
      bilateral Q60.1
      unilateral Q60.0
  knee (following explantation of knee joint prosthesis) (joint) (with or without presence of antibiotic-impregnated cement spacer) Z89.52- ☑
  labyrinth, membranous Q16.5
  larynx (congenital) Q31.8
    acquired Z90.02
  leg (acquired) (above knee) Z89.61- ☑
    below knee (acquired) Z89.51- ☑
    congenital — see Defect, reduction, lower limb
  lens (acquired) (see also Aphakia)
    congenital Q12.3
    post cataract extraction Z98.4- ☑
  limb (acquired) — see Absence, extremity
  lip Q38.6
  liver (congenital) Q44.7
  lung (fissure) (lobe) (bilateral) (unilateral) (congenital) Q33.3
    acquired (any part) Z90.2
  menstruation — see Amenorrhea
  muscle (congenital) (pectoral) Q79.8
    ocular Q10.3
  neck, part Q18.8
  neutrophil — see Agranulocytosis
  nipple(s) (with breast(s)) (acquired) Z90.1- ☑
    congenital Q83.2
  nose (congenital) Q30.1
    acquired Z90.09
  organ
    of Corti, congenital Q16.5
    or site, congenital NEC Q89.8
      acquired NEC Z90.89
  osseous meatus (ear) Q16.4
  ovary (acquired)
    bilateral Z90.722
    congenital
      bilateral Q50.02
      unilateral Q50.01
    unilateral Z90.721
  oviduct (acquired)
    bilateral Z90.722
    congenital Q50.6
    unilateral Z90.721
  pancreas (congenital) Q45.0
    acquired Z90.410
      complete Z90.410
      partial Z90.411
      total Z90.410
  parathyroid gland (acquired) E89.2
    congenital Q89.2
  patella, congenital Q74.1
  penis (congenital) Q55.5
    acquired Z90.79
  pericardium (congenital) Q24.8
  pituitary gland (congenital) Q89.2
    acquired E89.3
  prostate (acquired) Z90.79
    congenital Q55.4
  pulmonary valve Q22.0
  punctum lacrimale (congenital) Q10.4
  radius, congenital — see Defect, reduction, upper limb, longitudinal, radius
  rectum (congenital) Q42.1
    with fistula Q42.0
    acquired Z90.49
  respiratory organ NOS Q34.9

Absence — continued
  rib (acquired) Z90.89
    congenital Q76.6
  sacrum, congenital Q76.49
  salivary gland(s), congenital Q38.4
  scrotum, congenital Q55.29
  seminal vesicles (congenital) Q55.4
    acquired Z90.79
  septum
    atrial (congenital) Q21.1
    between aorta and pulmonary artery Q21.4
    ventricular (congenital) Q20.4
  sex chromosome
    female phenotype Q97.8
    male phenotype Q98.8
  skull bone (congenital) Q75.8
    with
      anencephaly Q00.0
      encephalocele — see Encephalocele
      hydrocephalus Q03.9
        with spina bifida — see Spina bifida, by site, with hydrocephalus
      microcephaly Q02
  spermatic cord, congenital Q55.4
  spine, congenital Q76.49
  spleen (congenital) Q89.01
    acquired Z90.81
  sternum, congenital Q76.7
  stomach (acquired) (partial) Z90.3
    congenital Q40.2
  superior vena cava, congenital Q26.8
  teeth, tooth (congenital) K00.0
    acquired (complete) K08.109
      class I K08.101
      class II K08.102
      class III K08.103
      class IV K08.104
      due to
        caries K08.139
          class I K08.131
          class II K08.132
          class III K08.133
          class IV K08.134
        periodontal disease K08.129
          class I K08.121
          class II K08.122
          class III K08.123
          class IV K08.124
        specified NEC K08.199
          class I K08.191
          class II K08.192
          class III K08.193
          class IV K08.194
        trauma K08.119
          class I K08.111
          class II K08.112
          class III K08.113
          class IV K08.114
      partial K08.409
        class I K08.401
        class II K08.402
        class III K08.403
        class IV K08.404
        due to
          caries K08.439
            class I K08.431
            class II K08.432
            class III K08.433
            class IV K08.434
          periodontal disease K08.429
            class I K08.421
            class II K08.422
            class III K08.423
            class IV K08.424
          specified NEC K08.499
            class I K08.491
            class II K08.492
            class III K08.493
            class IV K08.494
          trauma K08.419
            class I K08.411
            class II K08.412
            class III K08.413
            class IV K08.414
  tendon (congenital) Q79.8
  testis (congenital) Q55.0
    acquired Z90.79

Absence — *continued*
   thumb (acquired) Z89.01- ☑
      congenital — *see* Agenesis, hand
   thymus gland Q89.2
   thyroid (gland) (acquired) E89.0
      cartilage, congenital Q31.8
      congenital E03.1
   toe(s) (acquired) Z89.42- ☑
      with foot — *see* Absence, foot and ankle
      congenital — *see* Agenesis, foot
      great Z89.41- ☑
   tongue, congenital Q38.3
   trachea (cartilage), congenital Q32.1
   transverse aortic arch, congenital Q25.4
   tricuspid valve Q22.4
   umbilical artery, congenital Q27.0
   upper arm and forearm with hand present, congenital
         — *see* Agenesis, arm, with hand present
   ureter (congenital) Q62.4
      acquired Z90.6
   urethra, congenital Q64.5
   uterus (acquired) Z90.710
      with cervix Z90.710
      with remaining cervical stump Z90.711
      congenital Q51.0
   uvula, congenital Q38.5
   vagina, congenital Q52.0
   vas deferens (congenital) Q55.4
      acquired Z90.79
   vein (peripheral) congenital NEC Q27.8
      cerebral Q28.3
      digestive system Q27.8
      great Q26.8
      lower limb Q27.8
      portal Q26.5
      precerebral Q28.1
      specified site NEC Q27.8
      upper limb Q27.8
   vena cava (inferior) (superior), congenital Q26.8
   ventricular septum Q20.4
   vertebra, congenital Q76.49
   vulva, congenital Q52.71
   wrist (acquired) Z89.12- ☑
Absorbent system disease I87.8
Absorption
   carbohydrate, disturbance K90.4
   chemical — *see* Table of Drugs and Chemicals
      through placenta (newborn) P04.9
         environmental substance P04.6
         nutritional substance P04.5
         obstetric anesthetic or analgesic drug P04.0
   drug NEC — *see* Table of Drugs and Chemicals
      addictive
         through placenta (newborn) P04.49
            cocaine P04.41
         medicinal
            through placenta (newborn) P04.1
      through placenta (newborn) P04.1
         obstetric anesthetic or analgesic drug P04.0
   fat, disturbance K90.4
      pancreatic K90.3
   noxious substance — *see* Table of Drugs and Chemicals
   protein, disturbance K90.4
   starch, disturbance K90.4
   toxic substance — *see* Table of Drugs and Chemicals
   uremic — *see* Uremia
Abstinence symptoms, syndrome
   alcohol F10.239
      with delirium F10.231
   cocaine F14.23
   neonatal P96.1
   nicotine — *see* Dependence, drug, nicotine, with,
         withdrawal
   opioid F11.93
      with dependence F11.23
   psychoactive NEC F19.939
      with
         delirium F19.931
         dependence F19.239
            with
               delirium F19.231
               perceptual disturbance F19.232
            uncomplicated F19.230
         perceptual disturbance F19.932
      uncomplicated F19.930

Abstinence symptoms, syndrome — *continued*
   sedative F13.939
      with
         delirium F13.931
         dependence F13.239
            with
               delirium F13.231
               perceptual disturbance F13.232
            uncomplicated F13.230
         perceptual disturbance F13.932
      uncomplicated F13.930
   stimulant NEC F15.93
      with dependence F15.23
Abulia R68.89
Abulomania F60.7
Abuse
   adult — *see* Maltreatment, adult
      as reason for
         couple seeking advice (including offender)
               Z63.0
   alcohol (non-dependent) F10.10
      with
         anxiety disorder F10.180
         intoxication F10.129
            with delirium F10.121
            uncomplicated F10.120
         mood disorder F10.14
         other specified disorder F10.188
         psychosis F10.159
            delusions F10.150
            hallucinations F10.151
         sexual dysfunction F10.181
         sleep disorder F10.182
         unspecified disorder F10.19
      counseling and surveillance Z71.41
   amphetamine (or related substance) — *see* Abuse,
         drug, stimulant NEC
   analgesics (non-prescribed) (over the counter) F55.8
   antacids F55.0
   antidepressants — *see* Abuse, drug, psychoactive NEC
   anxiolytic — *see* Abuse, drug, sedative
   barbiturates — *see* Abuse, drug, sedative
   caffeine — *see* Abuse, drug, stimulant NEC
   cannabis, cannabinoids — *see* Abuse, drug, cannabis
   child — *see* Maltreatment, child
   cocaine — *see* Abuse, drug, cocaine
   drug NEC (non-dependent) F19.10
      with sleep disorder F19.182
      amphetamine type — *see* Abuse, drug, stimulant
            NEC
      analgesics (non-prescribed) (over the counter)
            F55.8
      antacids F55.0
      antidepressants — *see* Abuse, drug, psychoactive
            NEC
      anxiolytics — *see* Abuse, drug, sedative
      barbiturates — *see* Abuse, drug, sedative
      caffeine — *see* Abuse, drug, stimulant NEC
      cannabis F12.10
         with
            anxiety disorder F12.180
            intoxication F12.129
               with
                  delirium F12.121
                  perceptual disturbance F12.122
               uncomplicated F12.120
            other specified disorder F12.188
            psychosis F12.159
               delusions F12.150
               hallucinations F12.151
            unspecified disorder F12.19
      cocaine F14.10
         with
            anxiety disorder F14.180
            intoxication F14.129
               with
                  delirium F14.121
                  perceptual disturbance F14.122
               uncomplicated F14.120
            mood disorder F14.14
            other specified disorder F14.188
            psychosis F14.159
               delusions F14.150
               hallucinations F14.151
            sexual dysfunction F14.181
            sleep disorder F14.182
            unspecified disorder F14.19
      counseling and surveillance Z71.51

Abuse — *continued*
   drug — *continued*
      hallucinogen F16.10
         with
            anxiety disorder F16.180
            flashbacks F16.183
            intoxication F16.129
               with
                  delirium F16.121
                  perceptual disturbance F16.122
               uncomplicated F16.120
            mood disorder F16.14
            other specified disorder F16.188
            perception disorder, persisting F16.183
            psychosis F16.159
               delusions F16.150
               hallucinations F16.151
            unspecified disorder F16.19
      hashish — *see* Abuse, drug, cannabis
      herbal or folk remedies F55.1
      hormones F55.3
      hypnotics — *see* Abuse, drug, sedative
      inhalant F18.10
         with
            anxiety disorder F18.180
            dementia, persisting F18.17
            intoxication F18.129
               with delirium F18.121
               uncomplicated F18.120
            mood disorder F18.14
            other specified disorder F18.188
            psychosis F18.159
               delusions F18.150
               hallucinations F18.151
            unspecified disorder F18.19
      laxatives F55.2
      LSD — *see* Abuse, drug, hallucinogen
      marihuana — *see* Abuse, drug, cannabis
      morphine type (opioids) — *see* Abuse, drug, opioid
      opioid F11.10
         with
            intoxication F11.129
               with
                  delirium F11.121
                  perceptual disturbance F11.122
               uncomplicated F11.120
            mood disorder F11.14
            other specified disorder F11.188
            psychosis F11.159
               delusions F11.150
               hallucinations F11.151
            sexual dysfunction F11.181
            sleep disorder F11.182
            unspecified disorder F11.19
      PCP (phencyclidine) (or related substance) — *see*
            Abuse, drug, hallucinogen
      psychoactive NEC F19.10
         with
            amnestic disorder F19.16
            anxiety disorder F19.180
            dementia F19.17
            intoxication F19.129
               with
                  delirium F19.121
                  perceptual disturbance F19.122
               uncomplicated F19.120
            mood disorder F19.14
            other specified disorder F19.188
            psychosis F19.159
               delusions F19.150
               hallucinations F19.151
            sexual dysfunction F19.181
            sleep disorder F19.182
            unspecified disorder F19.19
      sedative, hypnotic or anxiolytic F13.10
         with
            anxiety disorder F13.180
            intoxication F13.129
               with delirium F13.121
               uncomplicated F13.120
            mood disorder F13.14
            other specified disorder F13.188
            psychosis F13.159
               delusions F13.150
               hallucinations F13.151
            sexual dysfunction F13.181
            sleep disorder F13.182
            unspecified disorder F13.19

☑ **Additional Character Required** — **Refer to the Tabular List for Character Selection**   ▽ **Subterms under main terms may continue to next column or page**

Abuse — *continued*
  drug — *continued*
    solvent — *see* Abuse, drug, inhalant
    steroids F55.3
    stimulant NEC F15.10
      with
        anxiety disorder F15.180
        intoxication F15.129
          with
            delirium F15.121
            perceptual disturbance F15.122
          uncomplicated F15.120
        mood disorder F15.14
        other specified disorder F15.188
        psychosis F15.159
          delusions F15.150
          hallucinations F15.151
        sexual dysfunction F15.181
        sleep disorder F15.182
        unspecified disorder F15.19
    tranquilizers — *see* Abuse, drug, sedative
    vitamins F55.4
  hallucinogens — *see* Abuse, drug, hallucinogen
  hashish — *see* Abuse, drug, cannabis
  herbal or folk remedies F55.1
  hormones F55.3
  hypnotic — *see* Abuse, drug, sedative
  inhalant — *see* Abuse, drug, inhalant
  laxatives F55.2
  LSD — *see* Abuse, drug, hallucinogen
  marihuana — *see* Abuse, drug, cannabis
  morphine type (opioids) — *see* Abuse, drug, opioid
  non-psychoactive substance NEC F55.8
    antacids F55.0
    folk remedies F55.1
    herbal remedies F55.1
    hormones F55.3
    laxatives F55.2
    steroids F55.3
    vitamins F55.4
  opioids — *see* Abuse, drug, opioid
  PCP (phencyclidine) (or related substance) — *see* Abuse, drug, hallucinogen
  physical (adult) (child) — *see* Maltreatment
  psychoactive substance — *see* Abuse, drug, psychoactive NEC
  psychological (adult) (child) — *see* Maltreatment
  sedative — *see* Abuse, drug, sedative
  sexual — *see* Maltreatment
  solvent — *see* Abuse, drug, inhalant
  steroids F55.3
  vitamins F55.4
Acalculia R48.8
  developmental F81.2
Acanthamebiasis (with) B60.10
  conjunctiva B60.12
  keratoconjunctivitis B60.13
  meningoencephalitis B60.11
  other specified B60.19
Acanthocephaliasis B83.8
Acanthocheilonemiasis B74.4
Acanthocytosis E78.6
Acantholysis L11.9
Acanthosis (acquired) (nigricans) L83
  benign Q82.8
  congenital Q82.8
  seborrheic L82.1
    inflamed L82.0
  tongue K14.3
Acapnia E87.3
Acarbia E87.2
Acardia, acardius Q89.8
Acardiacus amorphus Q89.8
Acardiotrophia I51.4
Acariasis B88.0
  scabies B86
Acarodermatitis (urticarioides) B88.0
Acarophobia F40.218
Acatalasemia, acatalasia E80.3
Acathisia (drug induced) G25.71
Accelerated atrioventricular conduction I45.6
Accentuation of personality traits (type A) Z73.1
Accessory (congenital)
  adrenal gland Q89.1
  anus Q43.4
  appendix Q43.4
  atrioventricular conduction I45.6

Accessory — *continued*
  auditory ossicles Q16.3
  auricle (ear) Q17.0
  biliary duct or passage Q44.5
  bladder Q64.79
  blood vessels NEC Q27.9
    coronary Q24.5
  bone NEC Q79.8
  breast tissue, axilla Q83.1
  carpal bones Q74.0
  cecum Q43.4
  chromosome(s) NEC (nonsex) Q92.9
    with complex rearrangements NEC Q92.5
      seen only at prometaphase Q92.8
    13 — *see* Trisomy, 13
    18 — *see* Trisomy, 18
    21 — *see* Trisomy, 21
    partial Q92.9
    sex
      female phenotype Q97.8
  coronary artery Q24.5
  cusp(s), heart valve NEC Q24.8
    pulmonary Q22.3
  cystic duct Q44.5
  digit(s) Q69.9
  ear (auricle) (lobe) Q17.0
  endocrine gland NEC Q89.2
  eye muscle Q10.3
  eyelid Q10.3
  face bone(s) Q75.8
  fallopian tube (fimbria) (ostium) Q50.6
  finger(s) Q69.0
  foreskin N47.8
  frontonasal process Q75.8
  gallbladder Q44.1
  genital organ(s)
    female Q52.8
      external Q52.79
      internal NEC Q52.8
    male Q55.8
  genitourinary organs NEC Q89.8
    female Q52.8
    male Q55.8
  hallux Q69.2
  heart Q24.8
    valve NEC Q24.8
      pulmonary Q22.3
  hepatic ducts Q44.5
  hymen Q52.4
  intestine (large) (small) Q43.4
  kidney Q63.0
  lacrimal canal Q10.6
  leaflet, heart valve NEC Q24.8
  ligament, broad Q50.6
  liver Q44.7
    duct Q44.5
  lobule (ear) Q17.0
  lung (lobe) Q33.1
  muscle Q79.8
  navicular of carpus Q74.0
  nervous system, part NEC Q07.8
  nipple Q83.3
  nose Q30.8
  organ or site not listed — *see* Anomaly, by site
  ovary Q50.31
  oviduct Q50.6
  pancreas Q45.3
  parathyroid gland Q89.2
  parotid gland (and duct) Q38.4
  pituitary gland Q89.2
  preauricular appendage Q17.0
  prepuce N47.8
  renal arteries (multiple) Q27.2
  rib Q76.6
    cervical Q76.5
  roots (teeth) K00.2
  salivary gland Q38.4
  sesamoid bones Q74.8
    foot Q74.2
    hand Q74.0
  skin tags Q82.8
  spleen Q89.09
  sternum Q76.7
  submaxillary gland Q38.4
  tarsal bones Q74.2
  teeth, tooth K00.1
  tendon Q79.8
  thumb Q69.1

Accessory — *continued*
  thymus gland Q89.2
  thyroid gland Q89.2
  toes Q69.2
  tongue Q38.3
  tooth, teeth K00.1
  tragus Q17.0
  ureter Q62.5
  urethra Q64.79
  urinary organ or tract NEC Q64.8
  uterus Q51.2
  vagina Q52.10
  valve, heart NEC Q24.8
    pulmonary Q22.3
  vertebra Q76.49
  vocal cords Q31.8
  vulva Q52.79
Accident
  birth — *see* Birth, injury
  cardiac — *see* Infarct, myocardium
  cerebral I63.9
  cerebrovascular (embolic) (ischemic) (thrombotic) I63.9
    aborted I63.9
    hemorrhagic — *see* Hemorrhage, intracranial, intracerebral
    old (without sequelae) Z86.73
      with sequelae (of) — *see* Sequelae, infarction, cerebral
  coronary — *see* Infarct, myocardium
  craniovascular I63.9
  vascular, brain I63.9
Accidental — *see* condition
Accommodation (disorder) (*see also* condition)
  hysterical paralysis of F44.89
  insufficiency of H52.4
  paresis — *see* Paresis, of accommodation
  spasm — *see* Spasm, of accommodation
Accouchement — *see* Delivery
Accreta placenta O43.21- ☑
Accretio cordis (nonrheumatic) I31.0
Accretions, tooth, teeth K03.6
Acculturation difficulty Z60.3
Accumulation secretion, prostate N42.89
Acephalia, acephalism, acephalus, acephaly Q00.0
Acephalobrachia monster Q89.8
Acephalochirus monster Q89.8
Acephalogaster Q89.8
Acephalostomus monster Q89.8
Acephalothorax Q89.8
Acerophobia F40.298
Acetonemia R79.89
  in Type 1 diabetes E10.10
    with coma E10.11
Acetonuria R82.4
Achalasia (cardia) (esophagus) K22.0
  congenital Q39.5
  pylorus Q40.0
  sphincteral NEC K59.8
Ache(s) — *see* Pain
Acheilia Q38.6
Achilloburitis — *see* Tendinitis, Achilles
Achillodynia — *see* Tendinitis, Achilles
Achlorhydria, achlorhydric (neurogenic) K31.83
  anemia D50.8
  diarrhea K31.83
  psychogenic F45.8
  secondary to vagotomy K91.1
Achluophobia F40.228
Acholia K82.8
Acholuric jaundice (familial) (splenomegalic) (*see also* Spherocytosis)
  acquired D59.8
Achondrogenesis Q77.0
Achondroplasia (osteosclerosis congenita) Q77.4
Achroma, cutis L80
Achromat (ism), achromatopsia (acquired) (congenital) H53.51
Achromia, congenital — *see* Albinism
Achromia parasitica B36.0
Achylia gastrica K31.89
  psychogenic F45.8
Acid
  burn — *see* Corrosion
  deficiency
    amide nicotinic E52
    ascorbic E54
    folic E53.8

Acid — *continued*
  deficiency — *continued*
    nicotinic E52
    pantothenic E53.8
  intoxication E87.2
  peptic disease K30
  phosphatase deficiency E83.39
  stomach K30
    psychogenic F45.8
Acidemia E87.2
  argininosuccinic E72.22
  isovaleric E71.110
  metabolic (newborn) P19.9
    first noted before onset of labor P19.0
    first noted during labor P19.1
    noted at birth P19.2
  methylmalonic E71.120
  pipecolic E72.3
  propionic E71.121
Acidity, gastric (high) K30
  psychogenic F45.8
Acidocytopenia — *see* Agranulocytosis
Acidocytosis D72.1
Acidopenia — *see* Agranulocytosis
Acidosis (lactic) (respiratory) E87.2
  in Type 1 diabetes E10.10
    with coma E10.11
  kidney, tubular N25.89
  lactic E87.2
  metabolic NEC E87.2
    with respiratory acidosis E87.4
    late, of newborn P74.0
  mixed metabolic and respiratory, newborn P84
  newborn P84
  renal (hyperchloremic) (tubular) N25.89
  respiratory E87.2
    complicated by
      metabolic
        acidosis E87.4
        alkalosis E87.4
Aciduria
  argininosuccinic E72.22
  glutaric (type I) E72.3
    type II E71.313
    type III E71.5- ☑
  orotic (congenital) (hereditary) (pyrimidine deficiency)
    E79.8
    anemia D53.0
Acladiosis (skin) B36.0
Aclasis, diaphyseal Q78.6
Acleistocardia Q21.1
Aclusion — *see* Anomaly, dentofacial, malocclusion
Acne L70.9
  artificialis L70.8
  atrophica L70.2
  cachecticorum (Hebra) L70.8
  conglobata L70.1
  cystic L70.0
  decalvans L66.2
  excoriée des jeunes filles L70.5
  frontalis L70.2
  indurata L70.0
  infantile L70.4
  keloid L73.0
  lupoid L70.2
  necrotic, necrotica (miliaris) L70.2
  neonatal L70.4
  nodular L70.0
  occupational L70.8
  picker's L70.5
  pustular L70.0
  rodens L70.2
  rosacea L71.9
  specified NEC L70.8
  tropica L70.3
  varioliformis L70.2
  vulgaris L70.0
Acnitis (primary) A18.4
Acosta's disease T70.29 ☑
Acoustic — *see* condition
Acousticophobia F40.298
Acquired (*see also* condition)
  immunodeficiency syndrome (AIDS) B20
Acrania Q00.0
Acroangiodermatitis I78.9
Acroasphyxia, chronic I73.89
Acrobystitis N47.7
Acrocephalopolysyndactyly Q87.0

Acrocephalosyndactyly Q87.0
Acrocephaly Q75.0
Acrochondrohyperplasia — *see* Syndrome, Marfan's
Acrocyanosis I73.8 ☑
  newborn P28.2
    meaning transient blue hands and feet — *omit code*
Acrodermatitis L30.8
  atrophicans (chronica) L90.4
  continua (Hallopeau) L40.2
  enteropathica (hereditary) E83.2
  Hallopeau's L40.2
  infantile papular L44.4
  perstans L40.2
  pustulosa continua L40.2
  recalcitrant pustular L40.2
Acrodynia — *see* Poisoning, mercury
Acromegaly, acromegalia E22.0
Acromelalgia I73.81
Acromicria, acromikria Q79.8
Acronyx L60.0
Acropachy, thyroid — *see* Thyrotoxicosis
Acroparesthesia (simple) (vasomotor) I73.89
Acropathy, thyroid — *see* Thyrotoxicosis
Acrophobia F40.241
Acroposthitis N47.7
Acroscleriasis, acroscleroderma, acrosclerosis — *see* Sclerosis, systemic
Acrosphacelus I96
Acrospiroma, eccrine — *see* Neoplasm, skin, benign
Acrostealgia — *see* Osteochondropathy
Acrotrophodynia — *see* Immersion
ACTH ectopic syndrome E24.3
Actinic — *see* condition
Actinobacillosis, actinobacillus A28.8
  mallei A24.0
  muris A25.1
Actinomyces israelii (infection) — *see* Actinomycosis
Actinomycetoma (foot) B47.1
Actinomycosis, actinomycotic A42.9
  with pneumonia A42.0
  abdominal A42.1
  cervicofacial A42.2
  cutaneous A42.89
  gastrointestinal A42.1
  pulmonary A42.0
  sepsis A42.7
  specified site NEC A42.89
Actinoneuritis G62.82
Action, heart
  disorder I49.9
  irregular I49.9
    psychogenic F45.8
Activated protein C resistance D68.51
Active — *see* condition
Acute (*see also* condition)
  abdomen R10.0
  gallbladder — *see* Cholecystitis, acute
Acyanotic heart disease (congenital) Q24.9
Acystia Q64.5
Adair-Dighton syndrome (brittle bones and blue sclera, deafness) Q78.0
Adamantinoblastoma — *see* Ameloblastoma
Adamantinoma (*see also* Cyst, calcifying odontogenic)
  long bones C40.90
    lower limb C40.2- ☑
    upper limb C40.0- ☑
  malignant C41.1
    jaw (bone) (lower) C41.1
      upper C41.0
  tibial C40.2- ☑
Adamantoblastoma — *see* Ameloblastoma
Adams-Stokes (-Morgagni) disease or syndrome I45.9
Adaption reaction — *see* Disorder, adjustment
Addiction (*see also* Dependence) F19.20
  alcohol, alcoholic (ethyl) (methyl) (wood) (without remission) F10.20
    with remission F10.21
  drug — *see* Dependence, drug
  ethyl alcohol (without remission) F10.20
    with remission F10.21
  heroin — *see* Dependence, drug, opioid
  methyl alcohol (without remission) F10.20
    with remission F10.21
  methylated spirit (without remission) F10.20
    with remission F10.21

Addiction — *continued*
  morphine (-like substances) — *see* Dependence, drug, opioid
  nicotine — *see* Dependence, drug, nicotine
  opium and opioids — *see* Dependence, drug, opioid
  tobacco — *see* Dependence, drug, nicotine
Addison-Biermer anemia (pernicious) D51.0
Addisonian crisis E27.2
Addison's
  anemia (pernicious) D51.0
  disease (bronze) or syndrome E27.1
    tuberculous A18.7
  keloid L94.0
Addison-Schilder complex E71.528
Additional (*see also* Accessory)
  chromosome(s) Q99.8
    21 — *see* Trisomy, 21
  sex — *see* Abnormal, chromosome, sex
Adduction contracture, hip or other joint — *see* Contraction, joint
Adenitis (*see also* Lymphadenitis)
  acute, unspecified site L04.9
  axillary I88.9
    acute L04.2
    chronic or subacute I88.1
  Bartholin's gland N75.8
  bulbourethral gland — *see* Urethritis
  cervical I88.9
    acute L04.0
    chronic or subacute I88.1
  chancroid (Hemophilus ducreyi) A57
  chronic, unspecified site I88.1
  Cowper's gland — *see* Urethritis
  due to Pasteurella multocida (p. septica) A28.0
  epidemic, acute B27.09
  gangrenous L04.9
  gonorrheal NEC A54.89
  groin I88.9
    acute L04.1
    chronic or subacute I88.1
  infectious (acute) (epidemic) B27.09
  inguinal I88.9
    acute L04.1
    chronic or subacute I88.1
  lymph gland or node, except mesenteric I88.9
    acute — *see* Lymphadenitis, acute
    chronic or subacute I88.1
  mesenteric (acute) (chronic) (nonspecific) (subacute) I88.0
  parotid gland (suppurative) — *see* Sialoadenitis
  salivary gland (any) (suppurative) — *see* Sialoadenitis
  scrofulous (tuberculous) A18.2
  Skene's duct or gland — *see* Urethritis
  strumous, tuberculous A18.2
  subacute, unspecified site I88.1
  sublingual gland (suppurative) — *see* Sialoadenitis
  submandibular gland (suppurative) — *see* Sialoadenitis
  submaxillary gland (suppurative) — *see* Sialoadenitis
  tuberculous — *see* Tuberculosis, lymph gland
  urethral gland — *see* Urethritis
  Wharton's duct (suppurative) — *see* Sialoadenitis
Adenoacanthoma — *see* Neoplasm, malignant, by site
Adenoameloblastoma — *see* Cyst, calcifying odontogenic
Adenocarcinoid (tumor) — *see* Neoplasm, malignant, by site
Adenocarcinoma (*see also* Neoplasm, malignant, by site)
  acidophil
    specified site — *see* Neoplasm, malignant, by site
    unspecified site C75.1
  adrenal cortical C74.0- ☑
  alveolar — *see* Neoplasm, lung, malignant
  apocrine
    breast — *see* Neoplasm, breast, malignant
    in situ
      breast D05.8- ☑
      specified site NEC — *see* Neoplasm, skin, in situ
      unspecified site D04.9
    specified site NEC — *see* Neoplasm, skin, malignant
    unspecified site C44.99
  basal cell
    specified site — *see* Neoplasm, skin, malignant
    unspecified site C08.9
  basophil
    specified site — *see* Neoplasm, malignant, by site

Adenocarcinoma — *continued*
  basophil — *continued*
    unspecified site C75.1
  bile duct type C22.1
    liver C22.1
    specified site NEC — *see* Neoplasm, malignant, by
      site
    unspecified site C22.1
  bronchiolar — *see* Neoplasm, lung, malignant
  bronchioloalveolar — *see* Neoplasm, lung, malignant
  ceruminous C44.29- ☑
  cervix, in situ (*see also* Carcinoma, cervix uteri, in situ)
    D06.9
  chromophobe
    specified site — *see* Neoplasm, malignant, by site
    unspecified site C75.1
  diffuse type
    specified site — *see* Neoplasm, malignant, by site
    unspecified site C16.9
  duct
    infiltrating
      with Paget's disease — *see* Neoplasm, breast,
        malignant
      specified site — *see* Neoplasm, malignant, by
        site
      unspecified site (female) C50.91- ☑
        male C50.92- ☑
    specified site — *see* Neoplasm, malignant, by site
    unspecified site
      female C56.9
      male C61
  eosinophil
    specified site — *see* Neoplasm, malignant, by site
    unspecified site C75.1
  follicular
    with papillary C73
    moderately differentiated C73
    specified site — *see* Neoplasm, malignant, by site
    trabecular C73
    unspecified site C73
    well differentiated C73
  Hurthle cell C73
  in
    adenomatous
      polyposis coli C18.9
  infiltrating duct
    with Paget's disease — *see* Neoplasm, breast, ma-
      lignant
    specified site — *see* Neoplasm, by site, malignant
    unspecified site (female) C50.91- ☑
      male C50.92- ☑
  inflammatory
    specified site — *see* Neoplasm, by site, malignant
    unspecified site (female) C50.91- ☑
      male C50.92- ☑
  intestinal type
    specified site — *see* Neoplasm, by site, malignant
    unspecified site C16.9
  intracystic papillary
  intraductal
    breast D05.1- ☑
    noninfiltrating
      breast D05.1- ☑
      papillary
        with invasion
          specified site — *see* Neoplasm, by site,
            malignant
          unspecified site (female) C50.91- ☑
            male C50.92- ☑
        breast D05.1- ☑
        specified site NEC — *see* Neoplasm, in situ,
          by site
        unspecified site D05.1- ☑
      specified site NEC — *see* Neoplasm, in situ, by
        site
      unspecified site D05.1- ☑
    papillary
      with invasion
        specified site — *see* Neoplasm, malignant,
          by site
        unspecified site (female) C50.91- ☑
          male C50.92- ☑
      breast D05.1- ☑
      specified site — *see* Neoplasm, in situ, by site
      unspecified site D05.1- ☑
    specified site NEC — *see* Neoplasm, in situ, by site
    unspecified site D05.1- ☑

Adenocarcinoma — *continued*
  islet cell
    with exocrine, mixed
      specified site — *see* Neoplasm, malignant, by
        site
      unspecified site C25.9
    pancreas C25.4
    specified site NEC — *see* Neoplasm, malignant, by
      site
    unspecified site C25.4
  lobular
    in situ
      breast D05.0- ☑
      specified site NEC — *see* Neoplasm, in situ, by
        site
      unspecified site D05.0- ☑
    specified site — *see* Neoplasm, malignant, by site
    unspecified site (female) C50.91- ☑
      male C50.92- ☑
  mucoid (*see also* Neoplasm, malignant, by site)
    cell
      specified site — *see* Neoplasm, malignant, by
        site
      unspecified site C75.1
  nonencapsulated sclerosing C73
  papillary
    with follicular C73
    follicular variant C73
    intraductal (noninfiltrating)
      with invasion
        specified site — *see* Neoplasm, malignant,
          by site
        unspecified site (female) C50.91- ☑
          male C50.92- ☑
      breast D05.1- ☑
      specified site NEC — *see* Neoplasm, in situ, by
        site
      unspecified site D05.1- ☑
    serous
      specified site — *see* Neoplasm, malignant, by
        site
      unspecified site C56.9
  papillocystic
    specified site — *see* Neoplasm, malignant, by site
    unspecified site C56.9
  pseudomucinous
    specified site — *see* Neoplasm, malignant, by site
    unspecified site C56.9
  renal cell C64- ☑
  sebaceous — *see* Neoplasm, skin, malignant
  serous (*see also* Neoplasm, malignant, by site)
    papillary
      specified site — *see* Neoplasm, malignant, by
        site
      unspecified site C56.9
  sweat gland — *see* Neoplasm, skin, malignant
  water-clear cell C75.0
Adenocarcinoma-in-situ (*see also* Neoplasm, in situ, by
  site)
  breast D05.9- ☑
Adenofibroma
  clear cell — *see* Neoplasm, benign, by site
  endometrioid D27.9
    borderline malignancy D39.10
    malignant C56- ☑
  mucinous
    specified site — *see* Neoplasm, benign, by site
    unspecified site D27.9
  papillary
    specified site — *see* Neoplasm, benign, by site
    unspecified site D27.9
  prostate — *see* Enlargement, enlarged, prostate
  serous
    specified site — *see* Neoplasm, benign, by site
    unspecified site D27.9
  specified site — *see* Neoplasm, benign, by site
  unspecified site D27.9
Adenofibrosis
  breast — *see* Fibroadenosis, breast
  endometrioid N80.0
Adenoiditis (chronic) J35.02
  with tonsillitis J35.03
  acute J03.90
    recurrent J03.91
    specified organism NEC J03.80
      recurrent J03.81

Adenoiditis — *continued*
  acute — *continued*
    staphylococcal J03.80
      recurrent J03.81
    streptococcal J03.00
      recurrent J03.01
Adenoids — *see* condition
Adenolipoma — *see* Neoplasm, benign, by site
Adenolipomatosis, Launois-Bensaude E88.89
Adenolymphoma
  specified site — *see* Neoplasm, benign, by site
  unspecified site D11.9
Adenoma (*see also* Neoplasm, benign, by site)
  acidophil
    specified site — *see* Neoplasm, benign, by site
    unspecified site D35.2
  acidophil-basophil, mixed
    specified site — *see* Neoplasm, benign, by site
    unspecified site D35.2
  adrenal (cortical) D35.00
    clear cell D35.00
    compact cell D35.00
    glomerulosa cell D35.00
    heavily pigmented variant D35.00
    mixed cell D35.00
  alpha-cell
    pancreas D13.7
    specified site NEC — *see* Neoplasm, benign, by site
    unspecified site D13.7
  alveolar D14.30
  apocrine
    breast D24- ☑
    specified site NEC — *see* Neoplasm, skin, benign,
      by site
    unspecified site D23.9
  basal cell D11.9
  basophil
    specified site — *see* Neoplasm, benign, by site
    unspecified site D35.2
  basophil-acidophil, mixed
    specified site — *see* Neoplasm, benign, by site
    unspecified site D35.2
  beta-cell
    pancreas D13.7
    specified site NEC — *see* Neoplasm, benign, by site
    unspecified site D13.7
  bile duct D13.4
    common D13.5
    extrahepatic D13.5
    intrahepatic D13.4
    specified site NEC — *see* Neoplasm, benign, by site
    unspecified site D13.4
  black D35.00
  bronchial D38.1
    cylindroid type — *see* Neoplasm, lung, malignant
  ceruminous D23.2- ☑
  chief cell D35.1
  chromophobe
    specified site — *see* Neoplasm, benign, by site
    unspecified site D35.2
  colloid
    specified site — *see* Neoplasm, benign, by site
    unspecified site D34
  duct
  eccrine, papillary — *see* Neoplasm, skin, benign
  endocrine, multiple
    single specified site — *see* Neoplasm, uncertain
      behavior, by site
    two or more specified sites D44- ☑
    unspecified site D44.9
  endometrioid (*see also* Neoplasm, benign)
    borderline malignancy — *see* Neoplasm, uncertain
      behavior, by site
  eosinophil
    specified site — *see* Neoplasm, benign, by site
    unspecified site D35.2
  fetal
    specified site — *see* Neoplasm, benign, by site
    unspecified site D34
  follicular
    specified site — *see* Neoplasm, benign, by site
    unspecified site D34
  hepatocellular D13.4
  Hurthle cell D34
  islet cell
    pancreas D13.7
    specified site NEC — *see* Neoplasm, benign, by site
    unspecified site D13.7

▽ **Subterms under main terms may continue to next column or page**   ☑ **Additional Character Required — Refer to the Tabular List for Character Selection**   **11**

Adenocarcinoma — Adenoma

Adenoma — *continued*
  liver cell D13.4
  macrofollicular
    specified site — *see* Neoplasm, benign, by site
    unspecified site D34
  malignant, malignum — *see* Neoplasm, malignant,
    by site
  microcystic
    pancreas D13.7
    specified site NEC — *see* Neoplasm, benign, by site
    unspecified site D13.7
  microfollicular
    specified site — *see* Neoplasm, benign, by site
    unspecified site D34
  mucoid cell
    specified site — *see* Neoplasm, benign, by site
    unspecified site D35.2
  multiple endocrine
    single specified site — *see* Neoplasm, uncertain
      behavior, by site
    two or more specified sites D44- ☑
    unspecified site D44.9
  nipple D24- ☑
  papillary (*see also* Neoplasm, benign, by site)
    eccrine — *see* Neoplasm, skin, benign, by site
  Pick's tubular
    specified site — *see* Neoplasm, benign, by site
    unspecified site
      female D27.9
      male D29.20
  pleomorphic
    carcinoma in — *see* Neoplasm, salivary gland,
      malignant
    specified site — *see* Neoplasm, malignant, by
      site
    unspecified site C08.9
  polypoid (*see also* Neoplasm, benign)
    adenocarcinoma in — *see* Neoplasm, malignant,
      by site
    adenocarcinoma in situ — *see* Neoplasm, in situ,
      by site
  prostate — *see* Neoplasm, benign, prostate
  rete cell D29.20
  sebaceous — *see* Neoplasm, skin, benign
  Sertoli cell
    specified site — *see* Neoplasm, benign, by site
    unspecified site
      female D27.9
      male D29.20
  skin appendage — *see* Neoplasm, skin, benign
  sudoriferous gland — *see* Neoplasm, skin, benign
  sweat gland — *see* Neoplasm, skin, benign
  testicular
    specified site — *see* Neoplasm, benign, by site
    unspecified site
      female D27.9
      male D29.20
  tubular (*see also* Neoplasm, benign, by site)
    adenocarcinoma in — *see* Neoplasm, malignant,
      by site
    adenocarcinoma in situ — *see* Neoplasm, in situ,
      by site
    Pick's
      specified site — *see* Neoplasm, benign, by site
      unspecified site
        female D27.9
        male D29.20
  tubulovillous (*see also* Neoplasm, benign, by site)
    adenocarcinoma in — *see* Neoplasm, malignant,
      by site
    adenocarcinoma in situ — *see* Neoplasm, in situ,
      by site
  villous — *see* Neoplasm, uncertain behavior, by site
    adenocarcinoma in — *see* Neoplasm, malignant,
      by site
    adenocarcinoma in situ — *see* Neoplasm, in situ,
      by site
  water-clear cell D35.1
Adenomatosis
  endocrine (multiple) E31.20
    single specified site — *see* Neoplasm, uncertain
      behavior, by site
  erosive of nipple D24- ☑
  pluriendocrine — *see* Adenomatosis, endocrine
  pulmonary D38.1
    malignant — *see* Neoplasm, lung, malignant
  specified site — *see* Neoplasm, benign, by site

Adenomatosis — *continued*
  unspecified site D12.6
Adenomatous
  goiter (nontoxic) E04.9
    with hyperthyroidism — *see* Hyperthyroidism,
      with, goiter, nodular
    toxic — *see* Hyperthyroidism, with, goiter, nodular
Adenomyoma (*see also* Neoplasm, benign, by site)
  prostate — *see* Enlarged, prostate
Adenomyometritis N80.0
Adenomyosis N80.0
Adenopathy (lymph gland) R59.9
  generalized R59.1
  inguinal R59.0
  localized R59.0
  mediastinal R59.0
  mesentery R59.0
  syphilitic (secondary) A51.49
  tracheobronchial R59.0
    tuberculous A15.4
      primary (progressive) A15.7
  tuberculous (*see also* Tuberculosis, lymph gland)
    tracheobronchial A15.4
      primary (progressive) A15.7
Adenosalpingitis — *see* Salpingitis
Adenosarcoma — *see* Neoplasm, malignant, by site
Adenosclerosis I88.8
Adenosis (sclerosing) breast — *see* Fibroadenosis, breast
Adenovirus, as cause of disease classified elsewhere
  B97.0
Adentia (complete) (partial) — *see* Absence, teeth
Adherent (*see also* Adhesions)
  labia (minora) N90.89
  pericardium (nonrheumatic) I31.0
    rheumatic I09.2
  placenta (with hemorrhage) O72.0
    without hemorrhage O73.0
  prepuce, newborn N47.0
  scar (skin) L90.5
  tendon in scar L90.5
Adhesions, adhesive (postinfective) K66.0
  with intestinal obstruction K56.5
  abdominal (wall) — *see* Adhesions, peritoneum
  appendix K38.8
  bile duct (common) (hepatic) K83.8
  bladder (sphincter) N32.89
  bowel — *see* Adhesions, peritoneum
  cardiac I31.0
    rheumatic I09.2
  cecum — *see* Adhesions, peritoneum
  cervicovaginal N88.1
    congenital Q52.8
    postpartal O90.89
      old N88.1
  cervix N88.1
  ciliary body NEC — *see* Adhesions, iris
  clitoris N90.89
  colon — *see* Adhesions, peritoneum
  common duct K83.8
  congenital (*see also* Anomaly, by site)
    fingers — *see* Syndactylism, complex, fingers
    omental, anomalous Q43.3
    peritoneal Q43.3
    tongue (to gum or roof of mouth) Q38.3
  conjunctiva (acquired) H11.21- ☑
    congenital Q15.8
  cystic duct K82.8
  diaphragm — *see* Adhesions, peritoneum
  due to foreign body — *see* Foreign body
  duodenum — *see* Adhesions, peritoneum
  ear
    middle H74.1- ☑
  epididymis N50.8
  epidural — *see* Adhesions, meninges
  epiglottis J38.7
  eyelid H02.59
  female pelvis N73.6
  gallbladder K82.8
  globe H44.89
  heart I31.0
    rheumatic I09.2
  ileocecal (coil) — *see* Adhesions, peritoneum
  ileum — *see* Adhesions, peritoneum
  intestine (*see also* Adhesions, peritoneum)
    with obstruction K56.5
  intra-abdominal — *see* Adhesions, peritoneum

Adhesions, adhesive — *continued*
  iris H21.50- ☑
    anterior H21.51- ☑
    goniosynechiae H21.52- ☑
    posterior H21.54- ☑
    to corneal graft T85.89 ☑
  joint — *see* Ankylosis
    knee M23.8X ☑
    temporomandibular M26.61
  labium (majus) (minus), congenital Q52.5
  liver — *see* Adhesions, peritoneum
  lung J98.4
  mediastinum J98.5
  meninges (cerebral) (spinal) G96.12
    congenital Q07.8
    tuberculous (cerebral) (spinal) A17.0
  mesenteric — *see* Adhesions, peritoneum
  nasal (septum) (to turbinates) J34.89
  ocular muscle — *see* Strabismus, mechanical
  omentum — *see* Adhesions, peritoneum
  ovary N73.6
    congenital (to cecum, kidney or omentum) Q50.39
  paraovarian N73.6
  pelvic (peritoneal)
    female N73.6
      postprocedural N99.4
    male — *see* Adhesions, peritoneum
    postpartal (old) N73.6
    tuberculous A18.17
  penis to scrotum (congenital) Q55.8
  periappendiceal (*see also* Adhesions, peritoneum)
  pericardium (nonrheumatic) I31.0
    focal I31.8
    rheumatic I09.2
    tuberculous A18.84
  pericholecystic K82.8
  perigastric — *see* Adhesions, peritoneum
  periovarian N73.6
  periprostatic N42.89
  perirectal — *see* Adhesions, peritoneum
  perirenal N28.89
  peritoneum, peritoneal (postinfective) (postprocedu-
    ral) K66.0
    with obstruction (intestinal) K56.5
    congenital Q43.3
    pelvic, female N73.6
      postprocedural N99.4
    postpartal, pelvic N73.6
    to uterus N73.6
  peritubal N73.6
  periureteral N28.89
  periuterine N73.6
  perivesical N32.89
  perivesicular (seminal vesicle) N50.8
  pleura, pleuritic J94.8
    tuberculous NEC A15.6
  pleuropericardial J94.8
  postoperative (gastrointestinal tract) K66.0
    with obstruction K91.3
    due to foreign body accidentally left in wound —
      see Foreign body, accidentally left during a
      procedure
    pelvic peritoneal N99.4
    urethra — *see* Stricture, urethra, postprocedural
    vagina N99.2
  postpartal, old (vulva or perineum) N90.89
  preputial, prepuce N47.5
  pulmonary J98.4
  pylorus — *see* Adhesions, peritoneum
  sciatic nerve — *see* Lesion, nerve, sciatic
  seminal vesicle N50.8
  shoulder (joint) — *see* Capsulitis, adhesive
  sigmoid flexure — *see* Adhesions, peritoneum
  spermatic cord (acquired) N50.8
    congenital Q55.4
  spinal canal G96.12
  stomach — *see* Adhesions, peritoneum
  subscapular — *see* Capsulitis, adhesive
  temporomandibular M26.61
  tendinitis (*see also* Tenosynovitis, specified type NEC)
    shoulder — *see* Capsulitis, adhesive
  testis N44.8
  tongue, congenital (to gum or roof of mouth) Q38.3
    acquired K14.8
  trachea J39.8
  tubo-ovarian N73.6
  tunica vaginalis N44.8

Adhesions, adhesive — *continued*
  uterus N73.6
    internal N85.6
    to abdominal wall N73.6
  vagina (chronic) N89.5
    postoperative N99.2
  vitreomacular H43.82- ☑
  vitreous H43.89
  vulva N90.89
Adiaspiromycosis B48.8
Adie (-Holmes) **pupil or syndrome** — *see* Anomaly,
    pupil, function, tonic pupil
Adiponecrosis neonatorum P83.8
Adiposis (*see also* Obesity)
  cerebralis E23.6
  dolorosa E88.2
Adiposity (*see also* Obesity)
  heart — *see* Degeneration, myocardial
  localized E65
Adiposogenital dystrophy E23.6
Adjustment
  disorder — *see* Disorder, adjustment
  implanted device — *see* Encounter (for), adjustment
    (of)
  prosthesis, external — *see* Fitting
  reaction — *see* Disorder, adjustment
Administration of tPA (rtPA) in a different facility within
    the last 24 hours prior to admission to current facil-
    ity Z92.82
Admission (for) (*see also* Encounter (for))
  adjustment (of)
    artificial
      arm Z44.00- ☑
        complete Z44.01- ☑
        partial Z44.02- ☑
      eye Z44.2 ☑
      leg Z44.10- ☑
        complete Z44.11- ☑
        partial Z44.12- ☑
    brain neuropacemaker Z46.2
      implanted Z45.42
    breast
      implant Z45.81 ☑
      prosthesis (external) Z44.3 ☑
    colostomy belt Z46.89
    contact lenses Z46.0
    cystostomy device Z46.6
    dental prosthesis Z46.3
    device NEC
      abdominal Z46.89
      implanted Z45.89
        cardiac Z45.09
          defibrillator (with synchronous cardiace
            pacemaker) Z45.02
          pacemaker Z45.018
            pulse generator Z45.010
        hearing device Z45.328
          bone conduction Z45.320
          cochlear Z45.321
        infusion pump Z45.1
        nervous system Z45.49
          CSF drainage Z45.41
          hearing device — *see* Admission, adjust-
            ment, device, implanted, hearing
            device
          neuropacemaker Z45.42
          visual substitution Z45.31
        specified NEC Z45.89
        vascular access Z45.2
        visual substitution Z45.31
      nervous system Z46.2
        implanted — *see* Admission, adjustment,
          device, implanted, nervous system
    orthodontic Z46.4
    prosthetic Z44.9
      arm — *see* Admission, adjustment, artificial,
        arm
      breast Z44.3 ☑
      dental Z46.3
      eye Z44.2 ☑
      leg — *see* Admission, adjustment, artificial,
        leg
      specified type NEC Z44.8

Admission — *continued*
  adjustment — *continued*
    device — *continued*
      substitution
        auditory Z46.2
          implanted — *see* Admission, adjust-
            ment, device, implanted, hearing
            device
        nervous system Z46.2
          implanted — *see* Admission, adjust-
            ment, device, implanted, nervous
            system
        visual Z46.2
          implanted Z45.31
      urinary Z46.6
    hearing aid Z46.1
      implanted — *see* Admission, adjustment, de-
        vice, implanted, hearing device
    ileostomy device Z46.89
    intestinal appliance or device NEC Z46.89
    neuropacemaker (brain) (peripheral nerve) (spinal
      cord) Z46.2
      implanted Z45.42
    orthodontic device Z46.4
    orthopedic (brace) (cast) (device) (shoes) Z46.89
    pacemaker
      cardiac Z45.018
        pulse generator Z45.010
      nervous system Z46.2
        implanted Z45.42
    portacath (port-a-cath) Z45.2
    prosthesis Z44.9
      arm — *see* Admission, adjustment, artificial,
        arm
      breast Z44.3 ☑
      dental Z46.3
      eye Z44.2 ☑
      leg — *see* Admission, adjustment, artificial, leg
      specified NEC Z44.8
    spectacles Z46.0
  aftercare (*see also* Aftercare) Z51.89
    postpartum
      immediately after delivery Z39.0
      routine follow-up Z39.2
    radiation therapy (antineoplastic) Z51.0
  attention to artificial opening (of) Z43.9
    artificial vagina Z43.7
    colostomy Z43.3
    cystostomy Z43.5
    enterostomy Z43.4
    gastrostomy Z43.1
    ileostomy Z43.2
    jejunostomy Z43.4
    nephrostomy Z43.6
    specified site NEC Z43.8
      intestinal tract Z43.4
      urinary tract Z43.6
    tracheostomy Z43.0
    ureterostomy Z43.6
    urethrostomy Z43.6
  breast augmentation or reduction Z41.1
  breast reconstruction following mastectomy Z42.1
  change of
    dressing (nonsurgical) Z48.00
    neuropacemaker device (brain) (peripheral nerve)
      (spinal cord) Z46.2
      implanted Z45.42
    surgical dressing Z48.01
  circumcision, ritual or routine (in absence of diagnosis)
    Z41.2
  clinical research investigation (control) (normal com-
    parison) (participant) Z00.6
  contraceptive management Z30.9
  cosmetic surgery NEC Z41.1
  counseling (*see also* Counseling)
    dietary Z71.3
    HIV Z71.7
    human immunodeficiency virus Z71.7
    nonattending third party Z71.0
    procreative management NEC Z31.69
  delivery, full-term, uncomplicated O80
    cesarean, without indication O82
  dietary surveillance and counseling Z71.3
  ear piercing Z41.3
  examination at health care facility (adult) (*see also*
    Examination) Z00.00
    with abnormal findings Z00.01

Admission — *continued*
  examination at health care facility (*see also* Examina-
    tion) — *continued*
    clinical research investigation (control) (normal
      comparison) (participant) Z00.6
    dental Z01.20
      with abnormal findings Z01.21
    donor (potential) Z00.5
    ear Z01.10
      with abnormal findings NEC Z01.118
    eye Z01.00
      with abnormal findings Z01.01
    general, specified reason NEC Z00.8
    hearing Z01.10
      with abnormal findings NEC Z01.118
    postpartum checkup Z39.2
    psychiatric (general) Z00.8
      requested by authority Z04.6
    vision Z01.00
      with abnormal findings Z01.01
  fitting (of)
    artificial
      arm — *see* Admission, adjustment, artificial,
        arm
      eye Z44.2 ☑
      leg — *see* Admission, adjustment, artificial, leg
    brain neuropacemaker Z46.2
      implanted Z45.42
    breast prosthesis (external) Z44.3 ☑
    colostomy belt Z46.89
    contact lenses Z46.0
    cystostomy device Z46.6
    dental prosthesis Z46.3
    dentures Z46.3
    device NEC
      abdominal Z46.89
      nervous system Z46.2
        implanted — *see* Admission, adjustment,
          device, implanted, nervous system
      orthodontic Z46.4
      prosthetic Z44.9
        breast Z44.3 ☑
        dental Z46.3
        eye Z44.2 ☑
      substitution
        auditory Z46.2
          implanted — *see* Admission, adjust-
            ment, device, implanted, hearing
            device
        nervous system Z46.2
          implanted — *see* Admission, adjust-
            ment, device, implanted, nervous
            system
        visual Z46.2
          implanted Z45.31
    hearing aid Z46.1
    ileostomy device Z46.89
    intestinal appliance or device NEC Z46.89
    neuropacemaker (brain) (peripheral nerve) (spinal
      cord) Z46.2
      implanted Z45.42
    orthodontic device Z46.4
    orthopedic device (brace) (cast) (shoes) Z46.89
    prosthesis Z44.9
      arm — *see* Admission, adjustment, artificial,
        arm
      breast Z44.3 ☑
      dental Z46.3
      eye Z44.2 ☑
      leg — *see* Admission, adjustment, artificial, leg
      specified type NEC Z44.8
    spectacles Z46.0
  follow-up examination Z09
  intrauterine device management Z30.431
    initial prescription Z30.014
  mental health evaluation Z00.8
    requested by authority Z04.6
  observation — *see* Observation
  Papanicolaou smear, cervix Z12.4
    for suspected malignant neoplasm Z12.4
  plastic and reconstructive surgery following medical
    procedure or healed injury NEC Z42.8
  plastic surgery, cosmetic NEC Z41.1
  postpartum observation
    immediately after delivery Z39.0
    routine follow-up Z39.2
  poststerilization (for restoration) Z31.0
    aftercare Z31.42

Admission — *continued*
  procreative management Z31.9
  prophylactic (measure)
    organ removal Z40.00
      breast Z40.01
      ovary Z40.02
      specified organ NEC Z40.09
      testes Z40.09
    vaccination Z23
  psychiatric examination (general) Z00.8
    requested by authority Z04.6
  radiation therapy (antineoplastic) Z51.0
  reconstructive surgery following medical procedure
      or healed injury NEC Z42.8
  removal of
    cystostomy catheter Z43.5
    drains Z48.03
    dressing (nonsurgical) Z48.00
    intrauterine contraceptive device Z30.432
    neuropacemaker (brain) (peripheral nerve) (spinal
        cord) Z46.2
      implanted Z45.42
    staples Z48.02
    surgical dressing Z48.01
    sutures Z48.02
    ureteral stent Z46.6
  respirator [ventilator] use during power failure Z99.12
  restoration of organ continuity (poststerilization) Z31.0
    aftercare Z31.42
  sensitivity test (*see also* Test, skin)
    allergy NEC Z01.82
    Mantoux Z11.1
  tuboplasty following previous sterilization Z31.0
    aftercare Z31.42
  vasoplasty following previous sterilization Z31.0
    aftercare Z31.42
  vision examination Z01.00
    with abnormal findings Z01.01
  waiting period for admission to other facility Z75.1
Adnexitis (suppurative) — *see* Salpingo-oophoritis
Adolescent X-linked adrenoleukodystrophy E71.521
Adrenal (gland) — *see* condition
Adrenalism, tuberculous A18.7
Adrenalitis, adrenitis E27.8
  autoimmune E27.1
  meningococcal, hemorrhagic A39.1
Adrenarche, premature E27.0
Adrenocortical syndrome — *see* Cushing's, syndrome
Adrenogenital syndrome E25.9
  acquired E25.8
  congenital E25.0
  salt loss E25.0
Adrenogenitalism, congenital E25.0
Adrenoleukodystrophy E71.529
  neonatal E71.511
  X-linked E71.529
    Addison only phenotype E71.528
    Addison-Schilder E71.528
    adolescent E71.521
    adrenomyeloneuropathy E71.522
    childhood cerebral E71.520
    other specified E71.528
Adrenomyeloneuropathy E71.522
Adventitious bursa — *see* Bursopathy, specified type
    NEC
Adverse effect — *see* Table of Drugs and Chemicals,
    categories T36-T50, with 6th character 5
Advice — *see* Counseling
Adynamia (episodica) (hereditary) (periodic) G72.3
Aeration lung imperfect, newborn — *see* Atelectasis
Aerobullosis T70.3 ☑
Aerocele — *see* Embolism, air
Aerodermectasia
  subcutaneous (traumatic) T79.7 ☑
Aerodontalgia T70.29 ☑
Aeroembolism T70.3 ☑
Aerogenes capsulatus infection A48.0
Aero-otitis media T70.0 ☑
Aerophagy, aerophagia (psychogenic) F45.8
Aerophobia F40.228
Aerosinusitis T70.1 ☑
Aerotitis T70.0 ☑
Affection — *see* Disease
Afibrinogenemia (*see also* Defect, coagulation) D68.8
  acquired D65
  congenital D68.2
  following ectopic or molar pregnancy O08.1

Afibrinogenemia — *continued*
  in abortion — *see* Abortion, by type, complicated by,
      afibrinogenemia
  puerperal O72.3
African
  sleeping sickness B56.9
  tick fever A68.1
  trypanosomiasis B56.9
    gambian B56.0
    rhodesian B56.1
Aftercare (*see also* Care) Z51.89
  following surgery (for) (on)
    amputation Z47.81
    attention to
      drains Z48.03
      dressings (nonsurgical) Z48.00
        surgical Z48.01
      sutures Z48.02
    circulatory system Z48.812
    delayed (planned) wound closure Z48.1
    digestive system Z48.815
    explantation of joint prosthesis (staged procedure)
      hip Z47.32
      knee Z47.33
      shoulder Z47.31
    genitourinary system Z48.816
    joint replacement Z47.1
    neoplasm Z48.3
    nervous system Z48.811
    oral cavity Z48.814
    organ transplant
      bone marrow Z48.290
      heart Z48.21
      heart-lung Z48.280
      kidney Z48.22
      liver Z48.23
      lung Z48.24
      multiple organs NEC Z48.288
      specified NEC Z48.298
    orthopedic NEC Z47.89
    planned wound closure Z48.1
    removal of internal fixation device Z47.2
    respiratory system Z48.813
    scoliosis Z47.82
    sense organs Z48.810
    skin and subcutaneous tissue Z48.817
    specified body system
      circulatory Z48.812
      digestive Z48.815
      genitourinary Z48.816
      nervous Z48.811
      oral cavity Z48.814
      respiratory Z48.813
      sense organs Z48.810
      skin and subcutaneous tissue Z48.817
      teeth Z48.814
    specified NEC Z48.89
    spinal Z48.89
    teeth Z48.814
  fracture — *code to* fracture with seventh character D
  involving
    removal of
      drains Z48.03
      dressings (nonsurgical) Z48.00
      staples Z48.02
      surgical dressings Z48.01
      sutures Z48.02
    neuropacemaker (brain) (peripheral nerve) (spinal
        cord) Z46.2
      implanted Z45.42
  orthopedic NEC Z47.89
  postprocedural — *see* Aftercare, following surgery
After-cataract — *see* Cataract, secondary
Agalactia (primary) O92.3
  elective, secondary or therapeutic O92.5
Agammaglobulinemia (acquired (secondary)) (nonfa-
    milial) D80.1
  with
    immunoglobulin-bearing B-lymphocytes D80.1
    lymphopenia D81.9
  autosomal recessive (Swiss type) D80.0
  Bruton's X-linked D80.0
  common variable (CVAgamma) D80.1
  congenital sex-linked D80.0
  hereditary D80.0
  lymphopenic D81.9
  Swiss type (autosomal recessive) D80.0

Agammaglobulinemia — *continued*
  X-linked (with growth hormone deficiency)(Bruton)
      D80.0
Aganglionosis (bowel) (colon) Q43.1
Age (old) — *see* Senility
Agenesis
  adrenal (gland) Q89.1
  alimentary tract (complete) (partial) NEC Q45.8
    upper Q40.8
  anus, anal (canal) Q42.3
    with fistula Q42.2
  aorta Q25.4
  appendix Q42.8
  arm (complete) Q71.0- ☑
    with hand present Q71.1- ☑
  artery (peripheral) Q27.9
    brain Q28.3
    coronary Q24.5
    pulmonary Q25.79
    specified NEC Q27.8
    umbilical Q27.0
  auditory (canal) (external) Q16.1
  auricle (ear) Q16.0
  bile duct or passage Q44.5
  bladder Q64.5
  bone Q79.9
  brain Q00.0
    part of Q04.3
  breast (with nipple present) Q83.8
    with absent nipple Q83.0
  bronchus Q32.4
  canaliculus lacrimalis Q10.4
  carpus — *see* Agenesis, hand
  cartilage Q79.9
  cecum Q42.8
  cerebellum Q04.3
  cervix Q51.5
  chin Q18.8
  cilia Q10.3
  circulatory system, part NOS Q28.9
  clavicle Q74.0
  clitoris Q52.6
  coccyx Q76.49
  colon Q42.9
    specified NEC Q42.8
  corpus callosum Q04.0
  cricoid cartilage Q31.8
  diaphragm (with hernia) Q79.1
  digestive organ(s) or tract (complete) (partial) NEC
      Q45.8
    upper Q40.8
  ductus arteriosus Q28.8
  duodenum Q41.0
  ear Q16.9
    auricle Q16.0
    lobe Q17.8
  ejaculatory duct Q55.4
  endocrine (gland) NEC Q89.2
  epiglottis Q31.8
  esophagus Q39.8
  eustachian tube Q16.2
  eye Q11.1
    adnexa Q15.8
  eyelid (fold) Q10.3
  face
    bones NEC Q75.8
    specified part NEC Q18.8
  fallopian tube Q50.6
  femur — *see* Defect, reduction, lower limb, longitudi-
      nal, femur
  fibula — *see* Defect, reduction, lower limb, longitudi-
      nal, fibula
  finger (complete) (partial) — *see* Agenesis, hand
  foot (and toes) (complete) (partial) Q72.3- ☑
  forearm (with hand present) — *see* Agenesis, arm,
      with hand present
    and hand Q71.2- ☑
  gallbladder Q44.0
  gastric Q40.2
  genitalia, genital (organ(s))
    female Q52.8
      external Q52.71
      internal NEC Q52.8
    male Q55.8
  glottis Q31.8
  hair Q84.0
  hand (and fingers) (complete) (partial) Q71.3- ☑

☑ **Additional Character Required — Refer to the Tabular List for Character Selection** ▽ **Subterms under main terms may continue to next column or page**

Agenesis — *continued*
  heart Q24.8
    valve NEC Q24.8
      pulmonary Q22.0
  hepatic Q44.7
  humerus — *see* Defect, reduction, upper limb
  hymen Q52.4
  ileum Q41.2
  incus Q16.3
  intestine (small) Q41.9
    large Q42.9
      specified NEC Q42.8
  iris (dilator fibers) Q13.1
  jaw M26.09
  jejunum Q41.1
  kidney(s) (partial) Q60.2
    bilateral Q60.1
    unilateral Q60.0
  labium (majus) (minus) Q52.71
  labyrinth, membranous Q16.5
  lacrimal apparatus Q10.4
  larynx Q31.8
  leg (complete) Q72.0- ☑
    with foot present Q72.1- ☑
    lower leg (with foot present) — *see* Agenesis, leg,
      with foot present
      and foot Q72.2- ☑
  lens Q12.3
  limb (complete) Q73.0
    lower — *see* Agenesis, leg
    upper — *see* Agenesis, arm
  lip Q38.0
  liver Q44.7
  lung (fissure) (lobe) (bilateral) (unilateral) Q33.3
  mandible, maxilla M26.09
  metacarpus — *see* Agenesis, hand
  metatarsus — *see* Agenesis, foot
  muscle Q79.8
    eyelid Q10.3
    ocular Q15.8
  musculoskeletal system NEC Q79.8
  nail(s) Q84.3
  neck, part Q18.8
  nerve Q07.8
  nervous system, part NEC Q07.8
  nipple Q83.2
  nose Q30.1
  nuclear Q07.8
  organ
    of Corti Q16.5
    or site not listed — *see* Anomaly, by site
  osseous meatus (ear) Q16.1
  ovary
    bilateral Q50.02
    unilateral Q50.01
  oviduct Q50.6
  pancreas Q45.0
  parathyroid (gland) Q89.2
  parotid gland(s) Q38.4
  patella Q74.1
  pelvic girdle (complete) (partial) Q74.2
  penis Q55.5
  pericardium Q24.8
  pituitary (gland) Q89.2
  prostate Q55.4
  punctum lacrimale Q10.4
  radioulnar — *see* Defect, reduction, upper limb
  radius — *see* Defect, reduction, upper limb, longitudi-
    nal, radius
  rectum Q42.1
    with fistula Q42.0
  renal Q60.2
    bilateral Q60.1
    unilateral Q60.0
  respiratory organ NEC Q34.8
  rib Q76.6
  roof of orbit Q75.8
  round ligament Q52.8
  sacrum Q76.49
  salivary gland Q38.4
  scapula Q74.0
  scrotum Q55.29
  seminal vesicles Q55.4
  septum
    atrial Q21.1
    between aorta and pulmonary artery Q21.4
    ventricular Q20.4
  shoulder girdle (complete) (partial) Q74.0

Agenesis — *continued*
  skull (bone) Q75.8
    with
      anencephaly Q00.0
      encephalocele — *see* Encephalocele
      hydrocephalus Q03.9
        with spina bifida — *see* Spina bifida, by site,
          with hydrocephalus
      microcephaly Q02
  spermatic cord Q55.4
  spinal cord Q06.0
  spine Q76.49
  spleen Q89.01
  sternum Q76.7
  stomach Q40.2
  submaxillary gland(s) (congenital) Q38.4
  tarsus — *see* Agenesis, foot
  tendon Q79.8
  testicle Q55.0
  thymus (gland) Q89.2
  thyroid (gland) E03.1
    cartilage Q31.8
  tibia — *see* Defect, reduction, lower limb, longitudinal,
    tibia
  tibiofibular — *see* Defect, reduction, lower limb,
    specified type NEC
  toe (and foot) (complete) (partial) — *see* Agenesis,
    foot
  tongue Q38.3
  trachea (cartilage) Q32.1
  ulna — *see* Defect, reduction, upper limb, longitudinal,
    ulna
  upper limb — *see* Agenesis, arm
  ureter Q62.4
  urethra Q64.5
  urinary tract NEC Q64.8
  uterus Q51.0
  uvula Q38.5
  vagina Q52.0
  vas deferens Q55.4
  vein(s) (peripheral) Q27.9
    brain Q28.3
    great NEC Q26.8
    portal Q26.5
  vena cava (inferior) (superior) Q26.8
  vermis of cerebellum Q04.3
  vertebra Q76.49
  vulva Q52.71
Ageusia R43.2
Agitated — *see* condition
Agitation R45.1
Aglossia (congenital) Q38.3
Aglossia-adactylia syndrome Q87.0
Aglycogenosis E74.00
Agnosia (body image) (other senses) (tactile) R48.1
  developmental F88
  verbal R48.1
    auditory R48.1
      developmental F80.2
    developmental F80.2
  visual (object) R48.3
Agoraphobia F40.00
  with panic disorder F40.01
  without panic disorder F40.02
Agrammatism R48.8
Agranulocytopenia — *see* Agranulocytosis
Agranulocytosis (chronic) (cyclical) (genetic) (infantile)
  (periodic) (pernicious) (*see also* Neutropenia) D70.9
  congenital D70.0
  cytoreductive cancer chemotherapy sequela D70.1
  drug-induced D70.2
    due to cytoreductive cancer chemotherapy D70.1
  due to infection D70.3
  secondary D70.4
    drug-induced D70.2
      due to cytoreductive cancer chemotherapy
        D70.1
Agraphia (absolute) R48.8
  with alexia R48.0
  developmental F81.81
Ague (dumb) — *see* Malaria
Agyria Q04.3
Ahumada-del Castillo syndrome E23.0
Aichomophobia F40.298
AIDS (related complex) B20
Ailment heart — *see* Disease, heart
Allurophobia F40.218
Ainhum (disease) L94.6

AIPHI (acute idiopathic pulmonary hemorrhage in infants
  (over 28 days old)) R04.81
Air
  anterior mediastinum J98.2
  compressed, disease T70.3 ☑
  conditioner lung or pneumonitis J67.7
  embolism (artery) (cerebral) (any site) T79.0 ☑
    with ectopic or molar pregnancy O08.2
    due to implanted device NEC — *see* Complications,
      by site and type, specified NEC
    following
      abortion — *see* Abortion by type, complicated
        by, embolism
      ectopic or molar pregnancy O08.2
      infusion, therapeutic injection or transfusion
        T80.0 ☑
    in pregnancy, childbirth or puerperium — *see*
      Embolism, obstetric
    traumatic T79.0 ☑
  hunger, psychogenic F45.8
  rarefied, effects of — *see* Effect, adverse, high altitude
  sickness T75.3 ☑
Airplane sickness T75.3 ☑
Akathisia (drug-induced) (treatment-induced) G25.71
  neuroleptic induced (acute) G25.71
Akinesia R29.898
Akinetic mutism R41.89
Akureyri's disease G93.3
Alactasia, congenital E73.0
Alagille's syndrome Q44.7
Alastrim B03
Albers-Schönberg syndrome Q78.2
Albert's syndrome — *see* Tendinitis, Achilles
Albinism, albino E70.30
  with hematologic abnormality E70.339
    Chédiak-Higashi syndrome E70.330
    Hermansky-Pudlak syndrome E70.331
    other specified E70.338
  I E70.320
  II E70.321
  ocular E70.319
    autosomal recessive E70.311
    other specified E70.318
    X-linked E70.310
  oculocutaneous E70.329
    other specified E70.328
    tyrosinase (ty) negative E70.320
    tyrosinase (ty) positive E70.321
  other specified E70.39
Albinismus E70.30
Albright (-McCune)(-Sternberg) syndrome Q78.1
Albuminous — *see* condition
Albuminuria, albuminuric (acute) (chronic) (subacute)
  (*see also* Proteinuria) R80.9
  complicating pregnancy — *see* Proteinuria, gestational
    with
      gestational hypertension — *see* Pre-eclampsia
      pre-existing hypertension — *see* Hypertension,
        complicating pregnancy, pre-existing,
        with, pre-eclampsia
    gestational — *see* Proteinuria, gestational
    with
      gestational hypertension — *see* Pre-eclampsia
      pre-existing hypertension — *see* Hypertension,
        complicating pregnancy, pre-existing,
        with, pre-eclampsia
  orthostatic R80.2
  postural R80.2
  pre-eclamptic — *see* Pre-eclampsia
  scarlatinal A38.8
Albuminurophobia F40.298
Alcaptonuria E70.29
Alcohol, alcoholic, alcohol-induced
  addiction (without remission) F10.20
    with remission F10.21
  amnestic disorder, persisting F10.96
    with dependence F10.26
  brain syndrome, chronic F10.97
    with dependence F10.27
  cardiopathy I42.6
  counseling and surveillance Z71.41
    family member Z71.42
  delirium (acute) (tremens) (withdrawal) F10.231
    with intoxication F10.921
    in
      abuse F10.121
      dependence F10.221

Alcohol, alcoholic, alcohol-induced — *continued*
- dementia F10.97
  - with dependence F10.27
- deterioration F10.97
  - with dependence F10.27
- hallucinosis (acute) F10.951
  - in
    - abuse F10.151
    - dependence F10.251
- insanity F10.959
- intoxication (acute) (without dependence) F10.129
  - with
    - delirium F10.121
    - dependence F10.229
      - with delirium F10.221
      - uncomplicated F10.220
    - uncomplicated F10.120
- jealousy F10.988
- Korsakoff's, Korsakov's, Korsakow's F10.26
- liver K70.9
  - acute — *see* Disease, liver, alcoholic, hepatitis
- mania (acute) (chronic) F10.959
- paranoia, paranoid (type) psychosis F10.950
- pellagra E52
- poisoning, accidental (acute) NEC — *see* Table of Drugs and Chemicals, alcohol, poisoning
- psychosis — *see* Psychosis, alcoholic
- withdrawal (without convulsions) F10.239
  - with delirium F10.231

Alcoholism (chronic) (without remission) F10.20
- with
  - psychosis — *see* Psychosis, alcoholic
  - remission F10.21
- Korsakov's F10.96
  - with dependence F10.26

Alder (-Reilly) **anomaly or syndrome** (leukocyte granulation) D72.0

Aldosteronism E26.9
- familial (type I) E26.02
- glucocorticoid-remediable E26.02
- primary (due to (bilateral) adrenal hyperplasia) E26.09
- primary NEC E26.09
- secondary E26.1
- specified NEC E26.89

Aldosteronoma D44.10

Aldrich (-Wiskott) **syndrome** (eczema-thrombocytopenia) D82.0

Alektorophobia F40.218

Aleppo boil B55.1

Aleukemic — *see* condition

Aleukia
- congenital D70.0
- hemorrhagica D61.9
  - congenital D61.09
- splenica D73.1

Alexia R48.0
- developmental F81.0
- secondary to organic lesion R48.0

Algoneurodystrophy M89.00
- ankle M89.07- ☑
- foot M89.07- ☑
- forearm M89.03- ☑
- hand M89.04- ☑
- lower leg M89.06- ☑
- multiple sites M89.0- ☑
- shoulder M89.01- ☑
- specified site NEC M89.08
- thigh M89.05- ☑
- upper arm M89.02- ☑

Algophobia F40.298

Alienation, mental — *see* Psychosis

Alkalemia E87.3

Alkalosis E87.3
- metabolic E87.3
  - with respiratory acidosis E87.4
- respiratory E87.3

Alkaptonuria E70.29

Allen-Masters syndrome N83.8

Allergy, allergic (reaction) (to) T78.40 ☑
- air-borne substance NEC (rhinitis) J30.89
- alveolitis (extrinsic) J67.9
  - due to
    - Aspergillus clavatus J67.4
    - Cryptostroma corticale J67.6
    - organisms (fungal, thermophilic actinomycete) growing in ventilation (air conditioning) systems J67.7

Allergy, allergic — *continued*
- alveolitis — *continued*
  - specified type NEC J67.8
- anaphylactic reaction or shock T78.2 ☑
- angioneurotic edema T78.3 ☑
- animal (dander) (epidermal) (hair) (rhinitis) J30.81
- bee sting (anaphylactic shock) — *see* Toxicity, venom, arthropod, bee
- biological — *see* Allergy, drug
- colitis K52.2
- dander (animal) (rhinitis) J30.81
- dandruff (rhinitis) J30.81
- dental restorative material (existing) K08.55
- dermatitis — *see* Dermatitis, contact, allergic
- diathesis — *see* History, allergy
- drug, medicament & biological (any) (external) (internal) T78.40 ☑
  - correct substance properly administered — *see* Table of Drugs and Chemicals, by drug, adverse effect
  - wrong substance given or taken NEC (by accident) — *see* Table of Drugs and Chemicals, by drug, poisoning
- due to pollen J30.1
- dust (house) (stock) (rhinitis) J30.89
  - with asthma — *see* Asthma, allergic extrinsic
- eczema — *see* Dermatitis, contact, allergic
- epidermal (animal) (rhinitis) J30.81
- feathers (rhinitis) J30.89
- food (any) (ingested) NEC T78.1 ☑
  - anaphylactic shock — *see* Shock, anaphylactic, due to food
  - dermatitis — *see* Dermatitis, due to, food
  - dietary counseling and surveillance Z71.3
  - in contact with skin L23.6
  - rhinitis J30.5
  - status (without reaction) Z91.018
    - eggs Z91.012
    - milk products Z91.011
    - peanuts Z91.010
    - seafood Z91.013
    - specified NEC Z91.018
- gastrointestinal K52.2
- grain J30.1
- grass (hay fever) (pollen) J30.1
  - asthma — *see* Asthma, allergic extrinsic
- hair (animal) (rhinitis) J30.81
- history (of) — *see* History, allergy
- horse serum — *see* Allergy, serum
- inhalant (rhinitis) J30.89
  - pollen J30.1
- kapok (rhinitis) J30.89
- medicine — *see* Allergy, drug
- milk protein K52.2
- nasal, seasonal due to pollen J30.1
- pneumonia J82
- pollen (any) (hay fever) J30.1
  - asthma — *see* Asthma, allergic extrinsic
- primrose J30.1
- primula J30.1
- purpura D69.0
- ragweed (hay fever) (pollen) J30.1
  - asthma — *see* Asthma, allergic extrinsic
- rose (pollen) J30.1
- seasonal NEC J30.2
- Senecio jacobae (pollen) J30.1
- serum (*see also* Reaction, serum) T80.69 ☑
  - anaphylactic shock T80.59 ☑
- shock (anaphylactic) T78.2 ☑
  - due to
    - administration of blood and blood products T80.51 ☑
    - adverse effect of correct medicinal substance properly administered T88.6 ☑
    - immunization T80.52 ☑
    - serum NEC T80.59 ☑
    - vaccination T80.52 ☑
- specific NEC T78.49 ☑
- tree (any) (hay fever) (pollen) J30.1
  - asthma — *see* Asthma, allergic extrinsic
- upper respiratory J30.9
- urticaria L50.0
- vaccine — *see* Allergy, serum
- wheat — *see* Allergy, food

Allescheriasis B48.2

Alligator skin disease Q80.9

Allocheiria, allochiria R20.8

Almeida's disease — *see* Paracoccidioidomycosis

Alopecia (hereditaria) (seborrheica) L65.9
- androgenic L64.9
  - drug-induced L64.0
  - specified NEC L64.8
- areata L63.9
  - ophiasis L63.2
  - specified NEC L63.8
  - totalis L63.0
  - universalis L63.1
- cicatricial L66.9
  - specified NEC L66.8
- circumscripta L63.9
- congenital, congenitalis Q84.0
- due to cytotoxic drugs NEC L65.8
- mucinosa L65.2
- postinfective NEC L65.8
- postpartum L65.0
- premature L64.8
- specific (syphilitic) A51.32
- specified NEC L65.8
- syphilitic (secondary) A51.32
- totalis (capitis) L63.0
- universalis (entire body) L63.1
- X-ray L58.1

Alpers' disease G31.81

Alpine sickness T70.29 ☑

Alport syndrome Q87.81

ALTE (apparent life threatening event) **in newborn and infant** R68.13

Alteration (of), **Altered**
- awareness, transient R40.4
- mental status R41.82
- pattern of family relationships affecting child Z62.898
- sensation
  - following
    - cerebrovascular disease I69.998
      - cerebral infarction I69.398
      - intracerebral hemorrhage I69.198
      - nontraumatic intracranial hemorrhage NEC I69.298
      - specified disease NEC I69.898
      - subarachnoid hemorrhage I69.098

Alternating — *see* condition

Altitude, high (effects) — *see* Effect, adverse, high altitude

Aluminosis (of lung) J63.0

Alveolitis
- allergic (extrinsic) — *see* Pneumonitis, hypersensitivity
  - due to
    - Aspergillus clavatus J67.4
    - Cryptostroma corticale J67.6
- fibrosing (cryptogenic) (idiopathic) J84.112
- jaw M27.3
- sicca dolorosa M27.3

Alveolus, alveolar — *see* condition

Alymphocytosis D72.810
- thymic (with immunodeficiency) D82.1

Alymphoplasia, thymic D82.1

Alzheimer's disease or sclerosis — *see* Disease, Alzheimer's

Amastia (with nipple present) Q83.8
- with absent nipple Q83.0

Amathophobia F40.228

Amaurosis (acquired) (congenital) (*see also* Blindness)
- fugax G45.3
- hysterical F44.6
- Leber's congenital H35.50
- uremic — *see* Uremia

Amaurotic idiocy (infantile) (juvenile) (late) E75.4

Amaxophobia F40.248

Amblyopia (congenital) (ex anopsia) (partial) (suppression) H53.00- ☑
- anisometropic — *see* Amblyopia, refractive
- deprivation H53.01- ☑
- hysterical F44.6
- nocturnal (*see also* Blindness, night)
  - vitamin A deficiency E50.5
- refractive H53.02- ☑
- strabismic H53.03- ☑
- tobacco H53.8
- toxic NEC H53.8
- uremic — *see* Uremia

Ameba, amebic (histolytica) (*see also* Amebiasis)
- abscess (liver) A06.4

Amebiasis A06.9
  with abscess — *see* Abscess, amebic
  acute A06.0
  chronic (intestine) A06.1
    with abscess — *see* Abscess, amebic
  cutaneous A06.7
  cutis A06.7
  cystitis A06.81
  genitourinary tract NEC A06.82
  hepatic — *see* Abscess, liver, amebic
  intestine A06.0
  nondysenteric colitis A06.2
  skin A06.7
  specified site NEC A06.89
Ameboma (of intestine) A06.3
Amelia Q73.0
  lower limb — *see* Agenesis, leg
  upper limb — *see* Agenesis, arm
Ameloblastoma (*see also* Cyst, calcifying odontogenic)
  long bones C40.9- ☑
    lower limb C40.2- ☑
    upper limb C40.0- ☑
  malignant C41.1
    jaw (bone) (lower) C41.1
      upper C41.0
  tibial C40.2- ☑
Amelogenesis imperfecta K00.5
  nonhereditaria (segmentalis) K00.4
Amenorrhea N91.2
  hyperhormonal E28.8
  primary N91.0
  secondary N91.1
Amentia — *see* Disability, intellectual
  Meynert's (nonalcoholic) F04
American
  leishmaniasis B55.2
  mountain tick fever A93.2
Ametropia — *see* Disorder, refraction
Amianthosis J61
Amimia R48.8
Amino-acid disorder E72.9
  anemia D53.0
Aminoacidopathy E72.9
Aminoaciduria E72.9
Amnesia R41.3
  anterograde R41.1
  auditory R48.8
  dissociative F44.0
  hysterical F44.0
  postictal in epilepsy — *see* Epilepsy
  psychogenic F44.0
  retrograde R41.2
  transient global G45.4
Amnes(t)ic syndrome (post-traumatic) F04
  induced by
    alcohol F10.96
      with dependence F10.26
    psychoactive NEC F19.96
      with
        abuse F19.16
        dependence F19.26
    sedative F13.96
      with dependence F13.26
Amnion, amniotic — *see* condition
Amnionitis — *see* Pregnancy, complicated by
Amok F68.8
Amoral traits F60.89
Ampulla
  lower esophagus K22.8
  phrenic K22.8
Amputation (*see also* Absence, by site, acquired)
  neuroma (postoperative) (traumatic) — *see* Complications, amputation stump, neuroma
  stump (surgical)
    abnormal, painful, or with complication (late) — *see* Complications, amputation stump
    healed or old NOS Z89.9
  traumatic (complete) (partial)
    arm (upper) (complete) S48.91- ☑
      at
        elbow S58.01- ☑
          partial S58.02- ☑
        shoulder joint (complete) S48.01- ☑
          partial S48.02- ☑
      between
        elbow and wrist (complete) S58.11- ☑
          partial S58.12- ☑

Amputation — *continued*
  traumatic — *continued*
    arm — *continued*
      between — *continued*
        shoulder and elbow (complete) S48.11- ☑
          partial S48.12- ☑
      partial S48.92- ☑
    breast (complete) S28.21- ☑
      partial S28.22- ☑
    clitoris (complete) S38.211 ☑
      partial S38.212 ☑
    ear (complete) S08.11- ☑
      partial S08.12- ☑
    finger (complete) (metacarpophalangeal) S68.11- ☑
      index S68.11- ☑
      little S68.11- ☑
      middle S68.11- ☑
      partial S68.12- ☑
        index S68.12- ☑
        little S68.12- ☑
        middle S68.12- ☑
        ring S68.12- ☑
      ring S68.11- ☑
      thumb — *see* Amputation, traumatic, thumb
      transphalangeal (complete) S68.61- ☑
        index S68.61- ☑
        little S68.61- ☑
        middle S68.61- ☑
        partial S68.62- ☑
          index S68.62- ☑
          little S68.62- ☑
          middle S68.62- ☑
          ring S68.62- ☑
        ring S68.61- ☑
    foot (complete) S98.91- ☑
      at ankle level S98.01- ☑
        partial S98.02- ☑
      midfoot S98.31- ☑
        partial S98.32- ☑
      partial S98.92- ☑
    forearm (complete) S58.91- ☑
      at elbow level (complete) S58.01- ☑
        partial S58.02- ☑
      between elbow and wrist (complete) S58.11- ☑
        partial S58.12- ☑
      partial S58.92- ☑
    genital organ(s) (external)
      female (complete) S38.211 ☑
        partial S38.212 ☑
      male
        penis (complete) S38.221 ☑
          partial S38.222 ☑
        scrotum (complete) S38.231 ☑
          partial S38.232 ☑
        testes (complete) S38.231 ☑
          partial S38.232 ☑
    hand (complete) (wrist level) S68.41- ☑
      finger(s) alone — *see* Amputation, traumatic, finger
      partial S68.42- ☑
      thumb alone — *see* Amputation, traumatic, thumb
      transmetacarpal (complete) S68.71- ☑
        partial S68.72- ☑
    head
      ear — *see* Amputation, traumatic, ear
      nose (partial) S08.812 ☑
        complete S08.811 ☑
      part S08.89 ☑
        scalp S08.0 ☑
    hip (and thigh) (complete) S78.91- ☑
      at hip joint (complete) S78.01- ☑
        partial S78.02- ☑
      between hip and knee (complete) S78.11- ☑
        partial S78.12- ☑
      partial S78.92- ☑
    labium (majus) (minus) (complete) S38.21- ☑
      partial S38.21- ☑
    leg (lower) S88.91- ☑
      at knee level S88.01- ☑
        partial S88.02- ☑
      between knee and ankle S88.11- ☑
        partial S88.12- ☑
      partial S88.92- ☑

Amputation — *continued*
  traumatic — *continued*
    nose (partial) S08.812 ☑
      complete S08.811 ☑
    penis (complete) S38.221 ☑
      partial S38.222 ☑
    scrotum (complete) S38.231 ☑
      partial S38.232 ☑
    shoulder — *see* Amputation, traumatic, arm
      at shoulder joint — *see* Amputation, traumatic, arm, at shoulder joint
    testes (complete) S38.231 ☑
      partial S38.232 ☑
    thigh — *see* Amputation, traumatic, hip
    thorax, part of S28.1
      breast — *see* Amputation, traumatic, breast
    thumb (complete) (metacarpophalangeal) S68.01- ☑
      partial S68.02- ☑
      transphalangeal (complete) S68.51- ☑
        partial S68.52- ☑
    toe (lesser) S98.13- ☑
      great S98.11- ☑
        partial S98.12- ☑
      more than one S98.21- ☑
        partial S98.22- ☑
      partial S98.14- ☑
    vulva (complete) S38.211 ☑
      partial S38.212 ☑
Amputee (bilateral) (old) Z89.9
Amsterdam dwarfism Q87.1
Amusia R48.8
  developmental F80.89
Amyelencephalus, amyelencephaly Q00.0
Amyelia Q06.0
Amygdalitis — *see* Tonsillitis
Amygdalolith J35.8
Amyloid heart (disease) E85.4 [I43]
Amyloidosis (generalized) (primary) E85.9
  with lung involvement E85.4 [J99]
  familial E85.2
  genetic E85.2
  heart E85.4 [I43]
  hemodialysis-associated E85.3
  liver E85.4 [K77]
  localized E85.4
  neuropathic heredofamilial E85.1
  non-neuropathic heredofamilial E85.0
  organ limited E85.4
  Portuguese E85.1
  pulmonary E85.4 [J99]
  secondary systemic E85.3
  skin (lichen) (macular) E85.4 [L99]
  specified NEC E85.8
  subglottic E85.4 [J99]
Amylopectinosis (brancher enzyme deficiency) E74.03
Amylophagia — *see* Pica
Amyoplasia congenita Q79.8
Amyotonia M62.89
  congenita G70.2
Amyotrophia, amyotrophy, amyotrophic G71.8
  congenita Q79.8
  diabetic — *see* Diabetes, amyotrophy
  lateral sclerosis G12.21
  neuralgic G54.5
  spinal progressive G12.21
Anacidity, gastric K31.83
  psychogenic F45.8
Anaerosis of newborn P28.89
Analbuminemia E88.09
Analgesia — *see* Anesthesia
Analphalipoproteinemia E78.6
Anaphylactic
  purpura D69.0
  shock or reaction — *see* Shock, anaphylactic
Anaphylactoid shock or reaction — *see* Shock, anaphylactic
Anaphylactoid syndrome of pregnancy O88.01- ☑
Anaphylaxis — *see* Shock, anaphylactic
Anaplasia cervix (*see also* Dysplasia, cervix) N87.9
Anaplasmosis, human A77.49
Anarthria R47.1
Anasarca R60.1
  cardiac — *see* Failure, heart, congestive
  lung J18.2
  newborn P83.2
  nutritional E43

Anasarca — *continued*
  pulmonary J18.2
  renal N04.9
Anastomosis
  aneurysmal — *see* Aneurysm
  arteriovenous ruptured brain I60.8
  intestinal K63.89
    complicated NEC K91.89
      involving urinary tract N99.89
  retinal and choroidal vessels (congenital) Q14.8
Anatomical narrow angle H40.03- ☑
Ancylostoma, ancylostomiasis (braziliense) (caninum) (ceylanicum) (duodenale) B76.0
  Necator americanus B76.1
Andersen's disease (glycogen storage) E74.09
Anderson-Fabry disease E75.21
Andes disease T70.29 ☑
Andrews' disease (bacterid) L08.89
Androblastoma
  benign
    specified site — *see* Neoplasm, benign, by site
    unspecified site
      female D27.9
      male D29.20
  malignant
    specified site — *see* Neoplasm, malignant, by site
    unspecified site
      female C56.9
      male C62.90
  specified site — *see* Neoplasm, uncertain behavior, by site
  tubular
    with lipid storage
      specified site — *see* Neoplasm, benign, by site
      unspecified site
        female D27.9
        male D29.20
    specified site — *see* Neoplasm, benign, by site
    unspecified site
      female D27.9
      male D29.20
  unspecified site
    female D39.10
    male D40.10
Androgen insensitivity syndrome (*see also* Syndrome, androgen insensitivity) E34.50
Androgen resistance syndrome (*see also* Syndrome, androgen insensitivity) E34.50
Android pelvis Q74.2
  with disproportion (fetopelvic) O33.3 ☑
    causing obstructed labor O65.3
Androphobia F40.290
Anectasis, pulmonary (newborn) — *see* Atelectasis
Anemia (essential) (general) (hemoglobin deficiency) (infantile) (primary) (profound) D64.9
  with (due to) (in)
    disorder of
      anaerobic glycolysis D55.2
      pentose phosphate pathway D55.1
    koilonychia D50.9
  achlorhydric D50.8
  achrestic D53.1
  Addison (-Biermer) (pernicious) D51.0
  agranulocytic — *see* Agranulocytosis
  amino-acid-deficiency D53.0
  aplastic D61.9
    congenital D61.09
    drug-induced D61.1
    due to
      drugs D61.1
      external agents NEC D61.2
      infection D61.2
      radiation D61.2
    idiopathic D61.3
    red cell (pure) D60.9
      chronic D60.0
      congenital D61.01
      specified type NEC D60.8
      transient D60.1
    specified type NEC D61.89
    toxic D61.2
  aregenerative
    congenital D61.09
  asiderotic D50.9
  atypical (primary) D64.9
  Baghdad spring D55.0
  Balantidium coli A07.0
  Biermer's (pernicious) D51.0

Anemia — *continued*
  blood loss (chronic) D50.0
    acute D62
  bothriocephalus B70.0 [D63.8]
  brickmaker's B76.9 [D63.8]
  cerebral I67.89
  childhood D58.9
  chlorotic D50.8
  chronic
    blood loss D50.0
    hemolytic D58.9
      idiopathic D59.9
    simple D53.9
  chronica congenita aregenerativa D61.09
  combined system disease NEC D51.0 [G32.0]
    due to dietary vitamin B12 deficiency D51.3 [G32.0]
  complicating Pregnancy, childbirth or puerperium — *see* Pregnancy, complicated by (management affected by), anemia
  congenital P61.4
    aplastic D61.09
    due to isoimmunization NOS P55.9
    dyserythropoietic, dyshematopoietic D64.4
    following fetal blood loss P61.3
    Heinz body D58.2
    hereditary hemolytic NOS D58.9
    pernicious D51.0
    spherocytic D58.0
  Cooley's (erythroblastic) D56.1
  cytogenic D51.0
  deficiency D53.9
    6-PGD D55.1
    2, 3 diphosphoglycurate mutase D55.2
    2, 3 PG D55.2
    6 phosphogluconate dehydrogenase D55.1
    amino-acid D53.0
    combined B12 and folate D53.1
    enzyme D55.9
      drug-induced (hemolytic) D59.2
      glucose-6-phosphate dehydrogenase (G6PD) D55.0
      glycolytic D55.2
      nucleotide metabolism D55.3
      related to hexose monophosphate (HMP) shunt pathway NEC D55.1
      specified type NEC D55.8
    erythrocytic glutathione D55.1
    folate D52.9
      dietary D52.0
      drug-induced D52.1
    folic acid D52.9
      dietary D52.0
      drug-induced D52.1
    G SH D55.1
    G6PD D55.0
    GGS-R D55.1
    glucose-6-phosphate dehydrogenase D55.0
    glutathione reductase D55.1
    glyceraldehyde phosphate dehydrogenase D55.2
    hexokinase D55.2
    iron D50.9
      secondary to blood loss (chronic) D50.0
    nutritional D53.9
      with
        poor iron absorption D50.8
        specified deficiency NEC D53.8
    phosphofructo-aldolase D55.2
    phosphoglycerate kinase D55.2
    PK D55.2
    protein D53.0
    pyruvate kinase D55.2
    transcobalamin II D51.2
    triose-phosphate isomerase D55.2
    vitamin B12 NOS D51.9
      dietary D51.3
      due to
        intrinsic factor deficiency D51.0
        selective vitamin B12 malabsorption with proteinuria D51.1
      pernicious D51.0
      specified type NEC D51.8
  Diamond-Blackfan (congenital hypoplastic) D61.01
  dibothriocephalus B70.0 [D63.8]
  dimorphic D53.1
  diphasic D53.1
  Diphyllobothrium (Dibothriocephalus) B70.0 [D63.8]
  due to (in) (with)
    antineoplastic chemotherapy D64.81

Anemia — *continued*
  due to — *continued*
    blood loss (chronic) D50.0
      acute D62
    chemotherapy, antineoplastic D64.81
    chronic disease classified elsewhere NEC D63.8
    chronic kidney disease D63.1
    deficiency
      amino-acid D53.0
      copper D53.8
      folate (folic acid) D52.9
        dietary D52.0
        drug-induced D52.1
      molybdenum D53.8
      protein D53.0
      zinc D53.8
    dietary vitamin B12 deficiency D51.3
    disorder of
      glutathione metabolism D55.1
      nucleotide metabolism D55.3
    drug — *see* Anemia, by type (*see also* Table of Drugs and Chemicals)
    end stage renal disease D63.1
    enzyme disorder D55.9
    fetal blood loss P61.3
    fish tapeworm (D.latum) infestation B70.0 [D63.8]
    hemorrhage (chronic) D50.0
      acute D62
    impaired absorption D50.9
    loss of blood (chronic) D50.0
      acute D62
    myxedema E03.9 [D63.8]
    Necator americanus B76.1 [D63.8]
    prematurity P61.2
    selective vitamin B12 malabsorption with proteinuria D51.1
    transcobalamin II deficiency D51.2
  Dyke-Young type (secondary) (symptomatic) D59.1
  dyserythropoietic (congenital) D64.4
  dyshematopoietic (congenital) D64.4
  Egyptian B76.9 [D63.8]
  elliptocytosis — *see* Elliptocytosis
  enzyme-deficiency, drug-induced D59.2
  epidemic (*see also* Ancylostomiasis) B76.9 [D63.8]
  erythroblastic
    familial D56.1
    newborn (*see also* Disease, hemolytic) P55.9
    of childhood D56.1
  erythrocytic glutathione deficiency D55.1
  erythropoietin-resistant anemia (EPO resistant anemia) D63.1
  Faber's (achlorhydric anemia) D50.9
  factitious (self-induced blood letting) D50.0
  familial erythroblastic D56.1
  Fanconi's (congenital pancytopenia) D61.09
  favism D55.0
  fish tapeworm (D. latum) infestation B70.0 [D63.8]
  folate (folic acid) deficiency D52.9
  glucose-6-phosphate dehydrogenase (G6PD) deficiency D55.0
  glutathione-reductase deficiency D55.1
  goat's milk D52.0
  granulocytic — *see* Agranulocytosis
  Heinz body, congenital D58.2
  hemolytic D58.9
    acquired D59.9
      with hemoglobinuria NEC D59.6
      autoimmune NEC D59.1
      infectious D59.4
      specified type NEC D59.8
      toxic D59.4
    acute D59.9
      due to enzyme deficiency specified type NEC D55.8
      Lederer's D59.1
    autoimmune D59.1
      drug-induced D59.0
    chronic D58.9
      idiopathic D59.9
    cold type (secondary) (symptomatic) D59.1
    congenital (spherocytic) — *see* Spherocytosis
    due to
      cardiac conditions D59.4
      drugs (nonautoimmune) D59.2
        autoimmune D59.0
      enzyme disorder D55.9
        drug-induced D59.2

Anemia — *continued*
  hemolytic — *continued*
    due to — *continued*
      presence of shunt or other internal prosthetic
          device D59.4
    familial D58.9
    hereditary D58.9
      due to enzyme disorder D55.9
        specified type NEC D55.8
      specified type NEC D58.8
    idiopathic (chronic) D59.9
    mechanical D59.4
    microangiopathic D59.4
    nonautoimmune D59.4
      drug-induced D59.2
    nonspherocytic
      congenital or hereditary NEC D55.8
        glucose-6-phosphate dehydrogenase defi-
            ciency D55.0
        pyruvate kinase deficiency D55.2
        type
            I D55.1
            II D55.2
        type
            I D55.1
            II D55.2
    secondary D59.4
      autoimmune D59.1
    specified (hereditary) type NEC D58.8
    Stransky-Regala type (*see also* Hemoglobinopathy)
        D58.8
    symptomatic D59.4
      autoimmune D59.1
    toxic D59.4
    warm type (secondary) (symptomatic) D59.1
  hemorrhagic (chronic) D50.0
    acute D62
  Herrick's D57.1
  hexokinase deficiency D55.2
  hookworm B76.9 [D63.8]
  hypochromic (idiopathic) (microcytic) (normoblastic)
      D50.9
    due to blood loss (chronic) D50.0
      acute D62
    familial sex-linked D64.0
    pyridoxine-responsive D64.3
    sideroblastic, sex-linked D64.0
  hypoplasia, red blood cells D61.9
    congenital or familial D61.01
  hypoplastic (idiopathic) D61.9
    congenital or familial (of childhood) D61.01
  hypoproliferative (refractive) D61.9
  idiopathic D64.9
    aplastic D61.3
    hemolytic, chronic D59.9
  in (due to) (with)
    chronic kidney disease D63.1
    end stage renal disease D63.1
    failure, kidney (renal) D63.1
    neoplastic disease (*see also* Neoplasm) D63.0
  intertropical (*see also* Ancylostomiasis) D63.8
  iron deficiency D50.9
    secondary to blood loss (chronic) D50.0
      acute D62
    specified type NEC D50.8
  Joseph-Diamond-Blackfan (congenital hypoplastic)
      D61.01
  Lederer's (hemolytic) D59.1
  leukoerythroblastic D61.82
  macrocytic D53.9
    nutritional D52.0
    tropical D52.8
  malarial (*see also* Malaria) B54 [D63.8]
  malignant (progressive) D51.0
  malnutrition D53.9
  marsh (*see also* Malaria) B54 [D63.8]
  Mediterranean (with other hemoglobinopathy) D56.9
  megaloblastic D53.1
    combined B12 and folate deficiency D53.1
    hereditary D51.1
    nutritional D52.0
    orotic aciduria D53.0
    refractory D53.1
    specified type NEC D53.1
  megalocytic D53.1
  microcytic (hypochromic) D50.9
    due to blood loss (chronic) D50.0
      acute D62

Anemia — *continued*
  microcytic — *continued*
    familial D56.8
  microdrepanocytosis D57.40
  microelliptopoikilocytic (Rietti-Greppi- Micheli) D56.9
  miner's B76.9 [D63.8]
  myelodysplastic D46.9
  myelofibrosis D75.81
  myelogenous D64.89
  myelopathic D64.89
  myelophthisic D61.82
  myeloproliferative D47.Z9 (*following* D47.4)
  newborn P61.4
    due to
      ABO (antibodies, isoimmunization, maternal/fe-
          tal incompatibility) P55.1
      Rh (antibodies, isoimmunization, maternal/fetal
          incompatibility) P55.0
    following fetal blood loss P61.3
    posthemorrhagic (fetal) P61.3
  nonspherocytic hemolytic — *see* Anemia, hemolytic,
      nonspherocytic
  normocytic (infectional) D64.9
    due to blood loss (chronic) D50.0
      acute D62
    myelophthisic D61.82
  nutritional (deficiency) D53.9
    with
      poor iron absorption D50.8
      specified deficiency NEC D53.8
    megaloblastic D52.0
  of prematurity P61.2
  orotaciduric (congenital) (hereditary) D53.0
  osteosclerotic D64.89
  ovalocytosis (hereditary) — *see* Elliptocytosis
  paludal (*see also* Malaria) B54 [D63.8]
  pernicious (congenital) (malignant) (progressive) D51.0
  pleochromic D64.89
    of sprue D52.8
  posthemorrhagic (chronic) D50.0
    acute D62
    newborn P61.3
  postoperative (postprocedural)
    due to (acute) blood loss D62
      chronic blood loss D50.0
    specified NEC D64.9
  postpartum O90.81
  pressure D64.89
  progressive D64.9
    malignant D51.0
    pernicious D51.0
  protein-deficiency D53.0
  pseudoleukemica infantum D64.89
  pure red cell D60.9
    congenital D61.01
  pyridoxine-responsive D64.3
  pyruvate kinase deficiency D55.2
  refractory D46.4
    with
      excess of blasts D46.20
        1 (RAEB 1) D46.21
        2 (RAEB 2) D46.22
        in transformation (RAEB T) — *see* Leukemia,
            acute myeloblastic
      hemochromatosis D46.1
      sideroblasts (ring) (RARS) D46.1
    without ring sideroblasts, so stated D46.0
    without sideroblasts without excess of blasts D46.0
    megaloblastic D53.1
    sideroblastic D46.1
    sideropenic D50.9
  Rietti-Greppi-Micheli D56.9
  scorbutic D53.2
  secondary to
    blood loss (chronic) D50.0
      acute D62
    hemorrhage (chronic) D50.0
      acute D62
  semiplastic D61.89
  sickle-cell — *see* Disease, sickle-cell
  sideroblastic D64.3
    hereditary D64.0
    hypochromic, sex-linked D64.0
    pyridoxine-responsive NEC D64.3
    refractory D46.1
    secondary (due to)
      disease D64.1
      drugs and toxins D64.2

Anemia — *continued*
  sideroblastic — *continued*
    specified type NEC D64.3
  sideropenic (refractory) D50.9
    due to blood loss (chronic) D50.0
      acute D62
  simple chronic D53.9
  specified type NEC D64.89
  spherocytic (hereditary) — *see* Spherocytosis
  splenic D64.89
  splenomegalic D64.89
  stomatocytosis D58.8
  syphilitic (acquired) (late) A52.79 [D63.8]
  target cell D64.89
  thalassemia D56.9
  thrombocytopenic — *see* Thrombocytopenia
  toxic D61.2
  tropical B76.9 [D63.8]
    macrocytic D52.8
  tuberculous A18.89 [D63.8]
  vegan D51.3
  vitamin
    B6-responsive D64.3
    B12 deficiency (dietary) pernicious D51.0
  von Jaksch's D64.89
  Witts' (achlorhydric anemia) D50.8
Anemophobia F40.228
Anencephalus, anencephaly Q00.0
Anergasia — *see* Psychosis, organic
Anesthesia, anesthetic R20.0
  complication or reaction NEC (*see also* Complications,
      anesthesia) T88.59 ☑
    due to
      correct substance properly administered — *see*
          Table of Drugs and Chemicals, by drug,
          adverse effect
      overdose or wrong substance given — *see* Ta-
          ble of Drugs and Chemicals, by drug,
          poisoning
  cornea H18.81- ☑
  dissociative F44.6
  functional (hysterical) F44.6
  hyperesthetic, thalamic G89.0
  hysterical F44.6
  local skin lesion R20.0
  sexual (psychogenic) F52.1
  shock (due to) T88.2 ☑
  skin R20.0
  testicular N50.9
Anetoderma (maculosum) (of) L90.8
  Jadassohn-Pellizzari L90.2
  Schweninger-Buzzi L90.1
Aneurin deficiency E51.9
Aneurysm (anastomotic) (artery) (cirsoid) (diffuse) (false)
      (fusiform) (multiple) (saccular) I72.9
  abdominal (aorta) I71.4
    ruptured I71.3
    syphilitic A52.01
  aorta, aortic (nonsyphilitic) I71.9
    abdominal I71.4
      ruptured I71.3
    arch I71.2
      ruptured I71.1
    arteriosclerotic I71.9
      ruptured I71.8
    ascending I71.2
      ruptured I71.1
    congenital Q25.4
    descending I71.9
      abdominal I71.4
        ruptured I71.3
      ruptured I71.8
      thoracic I71.2
        ruptured I71.1
    ruptured I71.8
    sinus, congenital Q25.4
    syphilitic A52.01
    thoracic I71.2
      ruptured I71.1
    thoracoabdominal I71.6
      ruptured I71.5
    thorax, thoracic (arch) I71.2
      ruptured I71.1
    transverse I71.2
      ruptured I71.1
  valve (heart) (*see also* Endocarditis, aortic) I35.8

▽ Subterms under main terms may continue to next column or page   ☑ Additional Character Required — Refer to the Tabular List for Character Selection   19

Anemia — Aneurysm

Aneurysm — *continued*
  arteriosclerotic I72.9
    cerebral I67.1
      ruptured — *see* Hemorrhage, intracranial, subarachnoid
  arteriovenous (congenital) (*see also* Malformation, arteriovenous)
    acquired I77.0
      brain I67.1
      coronary I25.41
      pulmonary I28.0
    brain Q28.2
      ruptured I60.8
    peripheral — *see* Malformation, arteriovenous, peripheral
    precerebral vessels Q28.0
    specified site NEC (*see also* Malformation, arteriovenous)
      acquired I77.0
  basal — *see* Aneurysm, brain
  berry (congenital) (nonruptured) I67.1
    ruptured I60.7
  brain I67.1
    arteriosclerotic I67.1
      ruptured — *see* Hemorrhage, intracranial, subarachnoid
    arteriovenous (congenital) (nonruptured) Q28.2
      acquired I67.1
        ruptured I60.8
      ruptured I60.8
    berry (congenital) (nonruptured) I67.1
      ruptured (*see also* Hemorrhage, intracranial, subarachnoid) I60.7
    congenital Q28.3
      ruptured I60.7
    meninges I67.1
      ruptured I60.8
    miliary (congenital) (nonruptured) I67.1
      ruptured (*see also* Hemorrhage, intracranial, subarachnoid) I60.7
    mycotic I33.0
    ruptured — *see* Hemorrhage, intracranial, subarachnoid
    syphilitic (hemorrhage) A52.05
  cardiac (false) (*see also* Aneurysm, heart) I25.3
  carotid artery (common) (external) I72.0
    internal (intracranial) I67.1
      extracranial portion I72.0
      ruptured into brain I60.0- ☑
      syphilitic A52.09
        intracranial A52.05
  cavernous sinus I67.1
    arteriovenous (congenital) (nonruptured) Q28.3
      ruptured I60.8
  celiac I72.8
  central nervous system, syphilitic A52.05
  cerebral — *see* Aneurysm, brain
  chest — *see* Aneurysm, thorax
  circle of Willis I67.1
    congenital Q28.3
      ruptured I60.6
    ruptured I60.6
  common iliac artery I72.3
  congenital (peripheral) Q27.8
    brain Q28.3
      ruptured I60.7
    coronary Q24.5
    digestive system Q27.8
    lower limb Q27.8
    pulmonary Q25.79
    retina Q14.1
    specified site NEC Q27.8
    upper limb Q27.8
  conjunctiva — *see* Abnormality, conjunctiva, vascular
  conus arteriosus — *see* Aneurysm, heart
  coronary (arteriosclerotic) (artery) I25.41
    arteriovenous, congenital Q24.5
    congenital Q24.5
    ruptured — *see* Infarct, myocardium
    syphilitic A52.06
    vein I25.89
  cylindroid (aorta) I71.9
    ruptured I71.8
    syphilitic A52.01
  ductus arteriosus Q25.0
  endocardial, infective (any valve) I33.0
  femoral (artery) (ruptured) I72.4
  gastroduodenal I72.8

Aneurysm — *continued*
  gastroepiploic I72.8
  heart (wall) (chronic or with a stated duration of over 4 weeks) I25.3
    valve — *see* Endocarditis
  hepatic I72.8
  iliac (common) (artery) (ruptured) I72.3
  infective I72.9
    endocardial (any valve) I33.0
  innominate (nonsyphilitic) I72.8
    syphilitic A52.09
  interauricular septum — *see* Aneurysm, heart
  interventricular septum — *see* Aneurysm, heart
  intrathoracic (nonsyphilitic) I71.2
    ruptured I71.1
    syphilitic A52.01
  lower limb I72.4
  lung (pulmonary artery) I28.1
  mediastinal (nonsyphilitic) I72.8
    syphilitic A52.09
  miliary (congenital) I67.1
    ruptured — *see* Hemorrhage, intracerebral, subarachnoid, intracranial
  mitral (heart) (valve) I34.8
  mural — *see* Aneurysm, heart
  mycotic I72.9
    endocardial (any valve) I33.0
    ruptured, brain — *see* Hemorrhage, intracerebral, subarachnoid
  myocardium — *see* Aneurysm, heart
  neck I72.0
  pancreaticoduodenal I72.8
  patent ductus arteriosus Q25.0
  peripheral NEC I72.8
    congenital Q27.8
      digestive system Q27.8
      lower limb Q27.8
      specified site NEC Q27.8
      upper limb Q27.8
  popliteal (artery) (ruptured) I72.4
  precerebral, congenital (nonruptured) Q28.1
  pulmonary I28.1
    arteriovenous Q25.72
      acquired I28.0
    syphilitic A52.09
    valve (heart) — *see* Endocarditis, pulmonary
  racemose (peripheral) I72.9
    congenital — *see* Aneurysm, congenital
  radial I72.1
  Rasmussen NEC A15.0
  renal (artery) I72.2
  retina (*see also* Disorder, retina, microaneurysms)
    congenital Q14.1
    diabetic — *see* Diabetes, microaneurysms, retinal
  sinus of Valsalva Q25.4
  specified NEC I72.8
  spinal (cord) I72.8
    syphilitic (hemorrhage) A52.09
  splenic I72.8
  subclavian (artery) (ruptured) I72.8
    syphilitic A52.09
  superior mesenteric I72.8
  syphilitic (aorta) A52.01
    central nervous system A52.05
    congenital (late) A50.54 [I79.0]
    spine, spinal A52.09
  thoracoabdominal (aorta) I71.6
    ruptured I71.5
    syphilitic A52.01
  thorax, thoracic (aorta) (arch) (nonsyphilitic) I71.2
    ruptured I71.1
    syphilitic A52.01
  traumatic (complication) (early), specified site — *see* Injury, blood vessel
  tricuspid (heart) (valve) I07.8
  ulnar I72.1
  upper limb (ruptured) I72.1
  valve, valvular — *see* Endocarditis
  venous (*see also* Varix) I86.8
    congenital Q27.8
      digestive system Q27.8
      lower limb Q27.8
      specified site NEC Q27.8
      upper limb Q27.8
  ventricle — *see* Aneurysm, heart
  visceral NEC I72.8
Angelman syndrome Q93.5
Anger R45.4

Angiectasis, angiectopia I99.8
Angiitis I77.6
  allergic granulomatous M30.1
  hypersensitivity M31.0
  necrotizing M31.9
    specified NEC M31.8
  nervous system, granulomatous I67.7
Angina (attack) (cardiac) (chest) (heart) (pectoris) (syndrome) (vasomotor) I20.9
  with
    atherosclerotic heart disease — *see* Arteriosclerosis, coronary (artery),
    documented spasm I20.1
  abdominal K55.1
  accelerated — *see* Angina, unstable
  agranulocytic — *see* Agranulocytosis
  angiospastic — *see* Angina, with documented spasm
  aphthous B08.5
  crescendo — *see* Angina, unstable
  croupous J05.0
  cruris I73.9
  de novo effort — *see* Angina, unstable
  diphtheritic, membranous A36.0
  equivalent I20.8
  exudative, chronic J37.0
  following acute myocardial infarction I23.7
  gangrenous diphtheritic A36.0
  intestinal K55.1
  Ludovici K12.2
  Ludwig's K12.2
  malignant diphtheritic A36.0
  membranous J05.0
    diphtheritic A36.0
    Vincent's A69.1
  mesenteric K55.1
  monocytic — *see* Mononucleosis, infectious
  of effort — *see* Angina, specified NEC
  phlegmonous J36
    diphtheritic A36.0
  post-infarctional I23.7
  pre-infarctional — *see* Angina, unstable
  Prinzmetal — *see* Angina, with documented spasm
  progressive — *see* Angina, unstable
  pseudomembranous A69.1
  pultaceous, diphtheritic A36.0
  spasm-induced — *see* Angina, with documented spasm
  specified NEC I20.8
  stable I20.9
  stenocardia — *see* Angina, specified NEC
  stridulous, diphtheritic A36.2
  tonsil J36
  trachealis J05.0
  unstable I20.0
  variant — *see* Angina, with documented spasm
  Vincent's A69.1
  worsening effort — *see* Angina, unstable
Angioblastoma — *see* Neoplasm, connective tissue, uncertain behavior
Angiocholecystitis — *see* Cholecystitis, acute
Angiocholitis (*see also* Cholecystitis, acute) K83.0
Angiodysgenesis spinalis G95.19
Angiodysplasia (cecum) (colon) K55.20
  with bleeding K55.21
  duodenum (and stomach) K31.819
    with bleeding K31.811
  stomach (and duodenum) K31.819
    with bleeding K31.811
Angioedema (allergic) (any site) (with urticaria) T78.3 ☑
  hereditary D84.1
Angioendothelioma — *see* Neoplasm, uncertain behavior, by site
  benign D18.00
    intra-abdominal D18.03
    intracranial D18.02
    skin D18.01
    specified site NEC D18.09
  bone — *see* Neoplasm, bone, malignant
  Ewing's — *see* Neoplasm, bone, malignant
Angioendotheliomatosis C85.8- ☑
Angiofibroma (*see also* Neoplasm, benign, by site)
  juvenile
    specified site — *see* Neoplasm, benign, by site
    unspecified site D10.6
Angiohemophilia (A) (B) D68.0
Angioid streaks (choroid) (macula) (retina) H35.33

Angiokeratoma — *see* Neoplasm, skin, benign
  corporis diffusum E75.21
Angioleiomyoma — *see* Neoplasm, connective tissue, benign
Angiolipoma (*see also* Lipoma)
  infiltrating — *see* Lipoma
Angioma (*see also* Hemangioma, by site)
  capillary I78.1
  hemorrhagicum hereditaria I78.0
  intra-abdominal D18.03
  intracranial D18.02
  malignant — *see* Neoplasm, connective tissue, malignant
  plexiform D18.00
    intra-abdominal D18.03
    intracranial D18.02
    skin D18.01
    specified site NEC D18.09
  senile I78.1
  serpiginosum L81.7
  skin D18.01
  specified site NEC D18.09
  spider I78.1
  stellate I78.1
  venous Q28.3
Angiomatosis Q82.8
  bacillary A79.89
  encephalotrigeminal Q85.8
  hemorrhagic familial I78.0
  hereditary familial I78.0
  liver K76.4
Angiomyolipoma — *see* Lipoma
Angiomyoliposarcoma — *see* Neoplasm, connective tissue, malignant
Angiomyoma — *see* Neoplasm, connective tissue, benign
Angiomyosarcoma — *see* Neoplasm, connective tissue, malignant
Angiomyxoma — *see* Neoplasm, connective tissue, uncertain behavior
Angioneurosis F45.8
Angioneurotic edema (allergic) (any site) (with urticaria) T78.3 ☑
  hereditary D84.1
Angiopathia, angiopathy I99.9
  cerebral I67.9
    amyloid E85.4 [I68.0]
  diabetic (peripheral) — *see* Diabetes, angiopathy
  peripheral I73.9
    diabetic — *see* Diabetes, angiopathy
    specified type NEC I73.89
  retinae syphilitica A52.05
  retinalis (juvenilis)
    diabetic — *see* Diabetes, retinopathy
    proliferative — *see* Retinopathy, proliferative
Angiosarcoma (*see also* Neoplasm, connective tissue, malignant)
  liver C22.3
Angiosclerosis — *see* Arteriosclerosis
Angiospasm (peripheral) (traumatic) (vessel) I73.9
  brachial plexus G54.0
  cerebral G45.9
  cervical plexus G54.2
  nerve
    arm — *see* Mononeuropathy, upper limb
      axillary G54.0
      median — *see* Lesion, nerve, median
      ulnar — *see* Lesion, nerve, ulnar
    axillary G54.0
    leg — *see* Mononeuropathy, lower limb
    median — *see* Lesion, nerve, median
    plantar — *see* Lesion, nerve, plantar
    ulnar — *see* Lesion, nerve, ulnar
Angiospastic disease or edema I73.9
Angiostrongyliasis
  due to
    Parastrongylus
      cantonensis B83.2
      costaricensis B81.3
    intestinal B81.3
Anguillulosis — *see* Strongyloidiasis
Angulation
  cecum — *see* Obstruction, intestine
  coccyx (acquired) (*see also* subcategory) M43.8 ☑
    congenital NEC Q76.49

Angulation — *continued*
  femur (acquired) (*see also* Deformity, limb, specified type NEC, thigh)
    congenital Q74.2
  intestine (large) (small) — *see* Obstruction, intestine
  sacrum (acquired) (*see also* subcategory) M43.8 ☑
    congenital NEC Q76.49
  sigmoid (flexure) — *see* Obstruction, intestine
  spine — *see* Dorsopathy, deforming, specified NEC
  tibia (acquired) (*see also* Deformity, limb, specified type NEC, lower leg)
    congenital Q74.2
  ureter N13.5
    with infection N13.6
  wrist (acquired) (*see also* Deformity, limb, specified type NEC, forearm)
    congenital Q74.0
Angulus infectiosus (lips) K13.0
Anhedonia R45.84
Anhidrosis L74.4
Anhydration, anhydremia E86.0
  with
    hypernatremia E87.0
    hyponatremia E87.1
Anhydremia E86.0
  with
    hypernatremia E87.0
    hyponatremia E87.1
Anidrosis L74.4
Aniridia (congenital) Q13.1
Anisakiasis (infection) (infestation) B81.0
Anisakis larvae infestation B81.0
Aniseikonia H52.32
Anisocoria (pupil) H57.02
  congenital Q13.2
Anisocytosis R71.8
Anisometropia (congenital) H52.31
Ankle — *see* condition
Ankyloblepharon (eyelid) (acquired) (*see also* Blepharophimosis)
  filiforme (adnatum) (congenital) Q10.3
  total Q10.3
Ankyloglossia Q38.1
Ankylosis (fibrous) (osseous) (joint) M24.60
  ankle M24.67- ☑
  arthrodesis status Z98.1
  cricoarytenoid (cartilage) (joint) (larynx) J38.7
  dental K03.5
  ear ossicles H74.31- ☑
  elbow M24.62- ☑
  foot M24.67- ☑
  hand M24.64- ☑
  hip M24.65- ☑
  incostapedial joint (infectional) — *see* Ankylosis, ear ossicles
  jaw (temporomandibular) M26.61
  knee M24.66- ☑
  lumbosacral (joint) M43.27
  postoperative (status) Z98.1
  produced by surgical fusion, status Z98.1
  sacro-iliac (joint) M43.28
  shoulder M24.61- ☑
  spine (joint) (*see also* Fusion, spine)
    spondylitic — *see* Spondylitis, ankylosing
  surgical Z98.1
  temporomandibular M26.61
  tooth, teeth (hard tissues) K03.5
  wrist M24.63- ☑
Ankylostoma — *see* Ancylostoma
Ankylostomiasis — *see* Ancylostomiasis
Ankylurethria — *see* Stricture, urethra
Annular (*see also* condition)
  detachment, cervix N88.8
  organ or site, congenital NEC — *see* Distortion
  pancreas (congenital) Q45.1
Anodontia (complete) (partial) (vera) K00.0
  acquired K08.10 ☑
Anomaly, anomalous (congenital) (unspecified type) Q89.9
  abdominal wall NEC Q79.59
  acoustic nerve Q07.8
  adrenal (gland) Q89.1
  Alder (-Reilly) (leukocyte granulation) D72.0
  alimentary tract Q45.9
    upper Q40.9

Anomaly, anomalous — *continued*
  alveolar M26.70
    hyperplasia M26.79
      mandibular M26.72
      maxillary M26.71
    hypoplasia M26.79
      mandibular M26.74
      maxillary M26.73
    ridge (process) M26.79
    specified NEC M26.79
  ankle (joint) Q74.2
  anus Q43.9
  aorta (arch) NEC Q25.4
    coarctation (preductal) (postductal) Q25.1
  aortic cusp or valve Q23.9
  appendix Q43.8
  apple peel syndrome Q41.1
  aqueduct of Sylvius Q03.0
    with spina bifida — *see* Spina bifida, with hydrocephalus
  arm Q74.0
  arteriovenous NEC
    coronary Q24.5
    gastrointestinal Q27.33
      acquired — *see* Angiodysplasia
  artery (peripheral) Q27.9
    basilar NEC Q28.1
    cerebral Q28.3
    coronary Q24.5
    digestive system Q27.8
    eye Q15.8
    great Q25.9
      specified NEC Q25.8
    lower limb Q27.8
    peripheral Q27.9
      specified NEC Q27.8
    pulmonary NEC Q25.79
    renal Q27.2
    retina Q14.1
    specified site NEC Q27.8
    subclavian Q27.8
    umbilical Q27.0
    upper limb Q27.8
    vertebral NEC Q28.1
  aryteno-epiglottic folds Q31.8
  atrial
    bands or folds Q20.8
    septa Q21.1
  atrioventricular
    excitation I45.6
    septum Q21.0
  auditory canal Q17.8
  auricle
    ear Q17.8
      causing impairment of hearing Q16.9
    heart Q20.8
  Axenfeld's Q15.0
  back Q89.9
  band
    atrial Q20.8
    heart Q24.8
    ventricular Q24.8
  Bartholin's duct Q38.4
  biliary duct or passage Q44.5
  bladder Q64.70
    absence Q64.5
    diverticulum Q64.6
    exstrophy Q64.10
      cloacal Q64.12
      extroversion Q64.19
      specified type NEC Q64.19
      supravesical fissure Q64.11
    neck obstruction Q64.31
    specified type NEC Q64.79
  bone Q79.9
    arm Q74.0
    face Q75.9
    leg Q74.2
    pelvic girdle Q74.2
    shoulder girdle Q74.0
    skull Q75.9
      with
        anencephaly Q00.0
        encephalocele — *see* Encephalocele
        hydrocephalus Q03.9
          with spina bifida — *see* Spina bifida, by site, with hydrocephalus
        microcephaly Q02

Anomaly, anomalous — *continued*
brain (multiple) Q04.9
  vessel Q28.3
breast Q83.9
broad ligament Q50.6
bronchus Q32.4
bulbus cordis Q21.9
bursa Q79.9
canal of Nuck Q52.4
canthus Q10.3
capillary Q27.9
cardiac Q24.9
  chambers Q20.9
    specified NEC Q20.8
  septal closure Q21.9
    specified NEC Q21.8
  valve NEC Q24.8
    pulmonary Q22.3
cardiovascular system Q28.8
carpus Q74.0
caruncle, lacrimal Q10.6
cascade stomach Q40.2
cauda equina Q06.3
cecum Q43.9
cerebral Q04.9
  vessels Q28.3
cervix Q51.9
Chédiak-Higashi (-Steinbrinck) (congenital gigantism of peroxidase granules) E70.330
cheek Q18.9
chest wall Q67.8
  bones Q76.9
chin Q18.9
chordae tendineae Q24.8
choroid Q14.3
  plexus Q07.8
chromosomes, chromosomal Q99.9
  D (1) — *see* condition, chromosome 13
  E (3) — *see* condition, chromosome 18
  G — *see* condition, chromosome 21
  sex
    female phenotype Q97.8
    gonadal dysgenesis (pure) Q99.1
    Klinefelter's Q98.4
    male phenotype Q98.9
    Turner's Q96.9
  specified NEC Q99.8
cilia Q10.3
circulatory system Q28.9
clavicle Q74.0
clitoris Q52.6
coccyx Q76.49
colon Q43.9
common duct Q44.5
communication
  coronary artery Q24.5
  left ventricle with right atrium Q21.0
concha (ear) Q17.3
connection
  portal vein Q26.5
  pulmonary venous Q26.4
    partial Q26.3
    total Q26.2
  renal artery with kidney Q27.2
cornea (shape) Q13.4
coronary artery or vein Q24.5
cranium — *see* Anomaly, skull
cricoid cartilage Q31.8
cystic duct Q44.5
dental
  alveolar — *see* Anomaly, alveolar
  arch relationship M26.20
    specified NEC M26.29
dentofacial M26.9
  alveolar — *see* Anomaly, alveolar
  dental arch relationship M26.20
    specified NEC M26.29
  functional M26.50
    specified NEC M26.59
  jaw size M26.00
    macrogenia M26.05
    mandibular
      hyperplasia M26.03
      hypoplasia M26.04
    maxillary
      hyperplasia M26.01
      hypoplasia M26.02
    microgenia M26.06

Anomaly, anomalous — *continued*
dentofacial — *continued*
  jaw size — *continued*
    specified type NEC M26.09
  jaw-cranial base relationship M26.10
    asymmetry M26.12
      maxillary M26.11
    specified type NEC M26.19
  malocclusion M26.4
    dental arch relationship NEC M26.29
    jaw size — *see* Anomaly, dentofacial, jaw size
    jaw-cranial base relationship — *see* Anomaly, dentofacial, jaw-cranial base relationship
  specified type NEC M26.89
  temporomandibular joint M26.60
    adhesions M26.61
    ankylosis M26.61
    arthralgia M26.62
    articular disc M26.63
    specified type NEC M26.69
  tooth position, fully erupted M26.30
    specified NEC M26.39
dermatoglyphic Q82.8
diaphragm (apertures) NEC Q79.1
digestive organ(s) or tract Q45.9
  lower Q43.9
  upper Q40.9
distance, interarch (excessive) (inadequate) M26.25
distribution, coronary artery Q24.5
ductus
  arteriosus Q25.0
  botalli Q25.0
duodenum Q43.9
dura (brain) Q04.9
  spinal cord Q06.9
ear (external) Q17.9
  causing impairment of hearing Q16.9
  inner Q16.5
  middle (causing impairment of hearing) Q16.4
    ossicles Q16.3
Ebstein's (heart) (tricuspid valve) Q22.5
ectodermal Q82.9
Eisenmenger's (ventricular septal defect) Q21.8
ejaculatory duct Q55.4
elbow Q74.0
endocrine gland NEC Q89.2
epididymis Q55.4
epiglottis Q31.8
esophagus Q39.9
eustachian tube Q17.8
eye Q15.9
  anterior segment Q13.9
    specified NEC Q13.89
  posterior segment Q14.9
    specified NEC Q14.8
  ptosis (eyelid) Q10.0
  specified NEC Q15.8
eyebrow Q18.8
eyelid Q10.3
  ptosis Q10.0
face Q18.9
  bone(s) Q75.9
fallopian tube Q50.6
fascia Q79.9
femur NEC Q74.2
fibula NEC Q74.2
finger Q74.0
fixation, intestine Q43.3
flexion (joint) NOS Q74.9
  hip or thigh Q65.89
foot NEC Q74.2
  varus (congenital) Q66.3
foramen
  Botalli Q21.1
  ovale Q21.1
forearm Q74.0
forehead Q75.8
form, teeth K00.2
fovea centralis Q14.1
frontal bone — *see* Anomaly, skull
gallbladder (position) (shape) (size) Q44.1
Gartner's duct Q52.4
gastrointestinal tract Q45.9
genitalia, genital organ(s) or system
  female Q52.9
    external Q52.70
    internal NOS Q52.9

Anomaly, anomalous — *continued*
genitalia, genital organ(s) or system — *continued*
  male Q55.9
    hydrocele P83.5
    specified NEC Q55.8
genitourinary NEC
  female Q52.9
  male Q55.9
Gerbode Q21.0
glottis Q31.8
granulation or granulocyte, genetic (constitutional) (leukocyte) D72.0
gum Q38.6
gyri Q07.9
hair Q84.2
hand Q74.0
hard tissue formation in pulp K04.3
head — *see* Anomaly, skull
heart Q24.9
  auricle Q20.8
  bands or folds Q24.8
  fibroelastosis cordis I42.4
  obstructive NEC Q22.6
  patent ductus arteriosus (Botalli) Q25.0
  septum Q21.9
    auricular Q21.1
    interatrial Q21.1
    interventricular Q21.0
      with pulmonary stenosis or atresia, dextra-position of aorta and hypertrophy of right ventricle Q21.3
    specified NEC Q21.8
    ventricular Q21.0
      with pulmonary stenosis or atresia, dextra-position of aorta and hypertrophy of right ventricle Q21.3
  tetralogy of Fallot Q21.3
  valve NEC Q24.8
    aortic
      bicuspid valve Q23.1
      insufficiency Q23.1
      stenosis Q23.0
        subaortic Q24.4
    mitral
      insufficiency Q23.3
      stenosis Q23.2
    pulmonary Q22.3
      atresia Q22.0
      insufficiency Q22.2
      stenosis Q22.1
        infundibular Q24.3
        subvalvular Q24.3
    tricuspid
      atresia Q22.4
      stenosis Q22.4
  ventricle Q20.8
heel NEC Q74.2
Hegglin's D72.0
hemianencephaly Q00.0
hemicephaly Q00.0
hemicrania Q00.0
hepatic duct Q44.5
hip NEC Q74.2
hourglass stomach Q40.2
humerus Q74.0
hydatid of Morgagni
  female Q50.5
  male (epididymal) Q55.4
    testicular Q55.29
hymen Q52.4
hypersegmentation of neutrophils, hereditary D72.0
hypophyseal Q89.2
ileocecal (coil) (valve) Q43.9
ileum Q43.9
ilium NEC Q74.2
integument Q84.9
  specified NEC Q84.8
interarch distance (excessive) (inadequate) M26.25
intervertebral cartilage or disc Q76.49
intestine (large) (small) Q43.9
  with anomalous adhesions, fixation or malrotation Q43.3
iris Q13.2
ischium NEC Q74.2
jaw — *see* Anomaly, dentofacial
  alveolar — *see* Anomaly, alveolar
jaw-cranial base relationship — *see* Anomaly, dentofacial, jaw-cranial base relationship

Anomaly, anomalous — *continued*
jejunum Q43.8
joint Q74.9
   specified NEC Q74.8
Jordan's D72.0
kidney(s) (calyx) (pelvis) Q63.9
   artery Q27.2
   specified NEC Q63.8
Klippel-Feil (brevicollis) Q76.1
knee Q74.1
labium (majus) (minus) Q52.70
labyrinth, membranous Q16.5
lacrimal apparatus or duct Q10.6
larynx, laryngeal (muscle) Q31.9
   web (bed) Q31.0
lens Q12.9
leukocytes, genetic D72.0
   granulation (constitutional) D72.0
lid (fold) Q10.3
ligament Q79.9
   broad Q50.6
   round Q52.8
limb Q74.9
   lower NEC Q74.2
      reduction deformity — *see* Defect, reduction,
         lower limb
   upper Q74.0
lip Q38.0
liver Q44.7
   duct Q44.5
lower limb NEC Q74.2
lumbosacral (joint) (region) Q76.49
   kyphosis — *see* Kyphosis, congenital
   lordosis — *see* Lordosis, congenital
lung (fissure) (lobe) Q33.9
mandible — *see* Anomaly, dentofacial
maxilla — *see* Anomaly, dentofacial
May (-Hegglin) D72.0
meatus urinarius NEC Q64.79
meningeal bands or folds Q07.9
   constriction of Q07.8
   spinal Q06.9
meninges Q07.9
   cerebral Q04.8
   spinal Q06.9
meningocele Q05.9
mesentery Q45.9
metacarpus Q74.0
metatarsus NEC Q74.2
middle ear Q16.4
   ossicles Q16.3
mitral (leaflets) (valve) Q23.9
   insufficiency Q23.3
   specified NEC Q23.8
   stenosis Q23.2
mouth Q38.6
Müllerian (*see also* Anomaly, by site)
   uterus NEC Q51.818
multiple NEC Q89.7
muscle Q79.9
   eyelid Q10.3
musculoskeletal system, except limbs Q79.9
myocardium Q24.8
nail Q84.6
narrowness, eyelid Q10.3
nasal sinus (wall) Q30.8
neck (any part) Q18.9
nerve Q07.9
   acoustic Q07.8
   optic Q07.8
nervous system (central) Q07.9
nipple Q83.9
nose, nasal (bones) (cartilage) (septum) (sinus) Q30.9
   specified NEC Q30.8
ocular muscle Q15.8
omphalomesenteric duct Q43.0
opening, pulmonary veins Q26.4
optic
   disc Q14.2
   nerve Q07.8
opticociliary vessels Q13.2
orbit (eye) Q10.7
organ Q89.9
   of Corti Q16.5
origin
   artery
      innominate Q25.8
      pulmonary Q25.79

Anomaly, anomalous — *continued*
origin — *continued*
   artery — *continued*
      renal Q27.2
      subclavian Q25.8
osseous meatus (ear) Q16.1
ovary Q50.39
oviduct Q50.6
palate (hard) (soft) NEC Q38.5
pancreas or pancreatic duct Q45.3
papillary muscles Q24.8
parathyroid gland Q89.2
paraurethral ducts Q64.79
parotid (gland) Q38.4
patella Q74.1
Pelger-Huët (hereditary hyposegmentation) D72.0
pelvic girdle NEC Q74.2
pelvis (bony) NEC Q74.2
   rachitic E64.3
penis (glans) Q55.69
pericardium Q24.8
peripheral vascular system Q27.9
Peter's Q13.4
pharynx Q38.8
pigmentation L81.9
   congenital Q82.8
pituitary (gland) Q89.2
pleural (folds) Q34.0
portal vein Q26.5
   connection Q26.5
position, tooth, teeth, fully erupted M26.30
   specified NEC M26.39
precerebral vessel Q28.1
prepuce Q55.69
prostate Q55.4
pulmonary Q33.9
   artery NEC Q25.79
   valve Q22.3
      atresia Q22.0
      insufficiency Q22.2
      specified type NEC Q22.3
      stenosis Q22.1
         infundibular Q24.3
         subvalvular Q24.3
   venous connection Q26.4
      partial Q26.3
      total Q26.2
pupil Q13.2
   function H57.00
      anisocoria H57.02
      Argyll Robertson pupil H57.01
      miosis H57.03
      mydriasis H57.04
      specified type NEC H57.09
      tonic pupil H57.05- ☑
pylorus Q40.3
radius Q74.0
rectum Q43.9
reduction (extremity) (limb)
   femur (longitudinal) — *see* Defect, reduction,
      lower limb, longitudinal, femur
   fibula (longitudinal) — *see* Defect, reduction, lower
      limb, longitudinal, fibula
   lower limb — *see* Defect, reduction, lower limb
   radius (longitudinal) — *see* Defect, reduction, up-
      per limb, longitudinal, radius
   tibia (longitudinal) — *see* Defect, reduction, lower
      limb, longitudinal, tibia
   ulna (longitudinal) — *see* Defect, reduction, upper
      limb, longitudinal, ulna
   upper limb — *see* Defect, reduction, upper limb
refraction — *see* Disorder, refraction
renal Q63.9
   artery Q27.2
   pelvis Q63.9
      specified NEC Q63.8
respiratory system Q34.9
   specified NEC Q34.8
retina Q14.1
rib Q76.6
   cervical Q76.5
Rieger's Q13.81
rotation — *see* Malrotation
   hip or thigh Q65.89
round ligament Q52.8
sacroiliac (joint) NEC Q74.2
sacrum NEC Q76.49
   kyphosis — *see* Kyphosis, congenital

Anomaly, anomalous — *continued*
sacrum — *continued*
   lordosis — *see* Lordosis, congenital
saddle nose, syphilitic A50.57
salivary duct or gland Q38.4
scapula Q74.0
scrotum — *see* Malformation, testis and scrotum
sebaceous gland Q82.9
seminal vesicles Q55.4
sense organs NEC Q07.8
sex chromosomes NEC (*see also* Anomaly, chromosomes)
   female phenotype Q97.8
   male phenotype Q98.9
shoulder (girdle) (joint) Q74.9
sigmoid (flexure) Q43.9
simian crease Q82.8
sinus of Valsalva Q25.4
skeleton generalized Q78.9
skin (appendage) Q82.9
skull Q75.9
   with
      anencephaly Q00.0
      encephalocele — *see* Encephalocele
      hydrocephalus Q03.9
         with spina bifida — *see* Spina bifida, by site,
            with hydrocephalus
      microcephaly Q02
specified organ or site NEC Q89.8
spermatic cord Q55.4
spine, spinal NEC Q76.49
   column NEC Q76.49
      kyphosis — *see* Kyphosis, congenital
      lordosis — *see* Lordosis, congenital
   cord Q06.9
   nerve root Q07.8
spleen Q89.09
   agenesis Q89.01
stenonian duct Q38.4
sternum NEC Q76.7
stomach Q40.3
submaxillary gland Q38.4
tarsus NEC Q74.2
tendon Q79.9
testis — *see* Malformation, testis and scrotum
thigh NEC Q74.2
thorax (wall) Q67.8
   bony Q76.9
throat Q38.8
thumb Q74.0
thymus gland Q89.2
thyroid (gland) Q89.2
   cartilage Q31.8
tibia NEC Q74.2
   saber A50.56
toe Q74.2
tongue Q38.3
tooth, teeth K00.9
   eruption K00.6
   position, fully erupted M26.30
   spacing, fully erupted M26.30
trachea (cartilage) Q32.1
tragus Q17.9
tricuspid (leaflet) (valve) Q22.9
   atresia or stenosis Q22.4
   Ebstein's Q22.5
Uhl's (hypoplasia of myocardium, right ventricle) Q24.8
ulna Q74.0
umbilical artery Q27.0
union
   cricoid cartilage and thyroid cartilage Q31.8
   thyroid cartilage and hyoid bone Q31.8
   trachea with larynx Q31.8
upper limb Q74.0
urachus Q64.4
ureter Q62.8
   obstructive NEC Q62.39
      cecoureterocele Q62.32
      orthotopic ureterocele Q62.31
urethra Q64.70
   absence Q64.5
   double Q64.74
   fistula to rectum Q64.73
   obstructive Q64.39
      stricture Q64.32
   prolapse Q64.71
   specified type NEC Q64.79
urinary tract Q64.9

Anomaly, anomalous — *continued*
uterus Q51.9
  with only one functioning horn Q51.4
uvula Q38.5
vagina Q52.4
valleculae Q31.8
valve (heart) NEC Q24.8
  coronary sinus Q24.5
  inferior vena cava Q24.8
  pulmonary Q22.3
  sinus coronario Q24.5
  venae cavae inferioris Q24.8
vas deferens Q55.4
vascular Q27.9
  brain Q28.3
  ring Q25.4
vein(s) (peripheral) Q27.9
  brain Q28.3
  cerebral Q28.3
  coronary Q24.5
  developmental Q28.3
  great Q26.9
    specified NEC Q26.8
vena cava (inferior) (superior) Q26.9
venous — *see* Anomaly, vein(s)
venous return Q26.8
ventricular
  bands or folds Q24.8
  septa Q21.0
vertebra Q76.49
  kyphosis — *see* Kyphosis, congenital
  lordosis — *see* Lordosis, congenital
vesicourethral orifice Q64.79
vessel(s) Q27.9
  optic papilla Q14.2
  precerebral Q28.1
vitelline duct Q43.0
vitreous body or humor Q14.0
vulva Q52.70
wrist (joint) Q74.0
Anomia R48.8
Anonychia (congenital) Q84.3
acquired L60.8
Anophthalmos, anophthalmus (congenital) (globe) Q11.1
acquired Z90.01
Anopia, anopsia H53.46- ☑
quadrant H53.46- ☑
Anorchia, anorchism, anorchidism Q55.0
Anorexia R63.0
hysterical F44.89
nervosa F50.00
  atypical F50.9
  binge-eating type F50.2
    with purging F50.02
  restricting type F50.01
Anorgasmy, psychogenic (female) F52.31
male F52.32
Anosmia R43.0
hysterical F44.6
postinfectional J39.8
Anosognosia R41.89
Anosteoplasia Q78.9
Anovulatory cycle N97.0
Anoxemia R09.02
newborn P84
Anoxia (pathological) R09.02
altitude T70.29 ☑
cerebral G93.1
  complicating
    anesthesia (general) (local) or other sedation T88.59 ☑
      in labor and delivery O74.3
      in pregnancy O29.21- ☑
      postpartum, puerperal O89.2
    delivery (cesarean) (instrumental) O75.4
  during a procedure G97.81
  newborn P84
  resulting from a procedure G97.82
due to
  drowning T75.1 ☑
  high altitude T70.29 ☑
heart — *see* Insufficiency, coronary
intrauterine P84
myocardial — *see* Insufficiency, coronary
newborn P84
spinal cord G95.11

Anoxia — *continued*
systemic (by suffocation) (low content in atmosphere) — *see* Asphyxia, traumatic
Anteflexion — *see* Anteversion
Antenatal
care (normal pregnancy) Z34.90
screening (encounter for) of mother Z36
Antepartum — *see* condition
Anterior — *see* condition
Antero-occlusion M26.220
Anteversion
cervix — *see* Anteversion, uterus
femur (neck), congenital Q65.89
uterus, uterine (cervix) (postinfectional) (postpartal, old) N85.4
  congenital Q51.818
  in pregnancy or childbirth — *see* Pregnancy, complicated by
Anthophobia F40.228
Anthracosilicosis J60
Anthracosis (lung) (occupational) J60
lingua K14.3
Anthrax A22.9
with pneumonia A22.1
cerebral A22.8
colitis A22.2
cutaneous A22.0
gastrointestinal A22.2
inhalation A22.1
intestinal A22.2
meningitis A22.8
pulmonary A22.1
respiratory A22.1
sepsis A22.7
specified manifestation NEC A22.8
Anthropoid pelvis Q74.2
with disproportion (fetopelvic) O33.0
Anthropophobia F40.10
generalized F40.11
Antibodies, maternal (blood group) — *see* Isoimmunization, affecting management of pregnancy
anti-D — *see* Isoimmunization, affecting management of pregnancy, Rh
newborn P55.0
Antibody
anticardiolipin R76.0
  with
    hemorrhagic disorder D68.312
    hypercoagulable state D68.61
antiphosphatidylglycerol R76.0
  with
    hemorrhagic disorder D68.312
    hypercoagulable state D68.61
antiphosphatidylinositol R76.0
  with
    hemorrhagic disorder D68.312
    hypercoagulable state D68.61
antiphosphatidylserine R76.0
  with
    hemorrhagic disorder D68.312
    hypercoagulable state D68.61
antipholipid R76.0
  with
    hemorrhagic disorder D68.312
    hypercoagulable state D68.61
Anticardiolipin syndrome D68.61
Anticoagulant, circulating (intrinsic) (*see also* Disorder, hemorrhagic) D68.318
drug-induced (extrinsic) (*see also* Disorder, hemorrhagic) D68.32
Antidiuretic hormone syndrome E22.2
Antimonial cholera — *see* Poisoning, antimony
Antiphospholipid
antibody
  with hemorrhagic disorder D68.312
  syndrome D68.61
Antisocial personality F60.2
Antithrombinemia — *see* Circulating anticoagulants
Antithromboplastinemia D68.318
Antithromboplastinogenemia D68.318
Antitoxin complication or reaction — *see* Complications, vaccination
Antlophobia F40.228
Antritis J32.0
maxilla J32.0
  acute J01.00
    recurrent J01.01

Antritis — *continued*
stomach K29.60
  with bleeding K29.61
Antrum, antral — *see* condition
Anuria R34
calculous (impacted) (recurrent) (*see also* Calculus, urinary) N20.9
following
  abortion — *see* Abortion by type complicated by, renal failure
  ectopic or molar pregnancy O08.4
newborn P96.0
postprocedural N99.0
postrenal N13.8
traumatic (following crushing) T79.5 ☑
Anus, anal — *see* condition
Anusitis K62.89
Anxiety F41.9
depression F40.8
episodic paroxysmal F41.0
generalized F41.1
hysteria F41.8
neurosis F41.1
panic type F41.0
reaction F41.1
separation, abnormal (of childhood) F93.0
specified NEC F41.8
state F41.1
Aorta, aortic — *see* condition
Aortectasia — *see* Ectasia, aorta
with aneurysm — *see* Aneurysm, aorta
Aortitis (nonsyphilitic) (calcific) I77.6
arteriosclerotic I70.0
Doehle-Heller A52.02
luetic A52.02
rheumatic — *see* Endocarditis, acute, rheumatic
specific (syphilitic) A52.02
syphilitic A52.02
  congenital A50.54 [I79.1]
Apathetic thyroid storm — *see* Thyrotoxicosis
Apathy R45.3
Apeirophobia F40.228
Apepsia K30
psychogenic F45.8
Aperistalsis, esophagus K22.0
Apertognathia M26.29
Apert's syndrome Q87.0
Aphagia R13.0
psychogenic F50.9
Aphakia (acquired) (postoperative) H27.0- ☑
congenital Q12.3
Aphasia (amnestic) (global) (nominal) (semantic) (syntactic) R47.01
acquired, with epilepsy (Landau-Kleffner syndrome) — *see* Epilepsy, specified NEC
auditory (developmental) F80.2
developmental (receptive type) F80.2
  expressive type F80.1
  Wernicke's F80.2
following
  cerebrovascular disease I69.920
    cerebral infarction I69.320
    intracerebral hemorrhage I69.120
    nontraumatic intracranial hemorrhage NEC I69.220
    specified disease NEC I69.820
    subarachnoid hemorrhage I69.020
primary progressive G31.01 [F02.80]
  with behavioral disturbance G31.01 [F02.81]
progressive isolated G31.01 [F02.80]
  with behavioral disturbance G31.01 [F02.81]
sensory F80.2
syphilis, tertiary A52.19
Wernicke's (developmental) F80.2
Aphonia (organic) R49.1
hysterical F44.4
psychogenic F44.4
Aphthae, aphthous (*see also* condition)
Bednar's K12.0
cachectic K14.0
epizootic B08.8
fever B08.8
oral (recurrent) K12.0
stomatitis (major) (minor) K12.0
thrush B37.0
ulcer (oral) (recurrent) K12.0
  genital organ(s) NEC
    female N76.6

  ☑ **Additional Character Required** — Refer to the Tabular List for Character Selection   ▽ **Subterms under main terms may continue to next column or page**

Aphthae, aphthous — *continued*
  ulcer — *continued*
    genital organ(s) — *continued*
      male N50.8
      larynx J38.7
Apical — *see* condition
Apiphobia F40.218
Aplasia (*see also* Agenesis)
  abdominal muscle syndrome Q79.4
  alveolar process (acquired) — *see* Anomaly, alveolar
    congenital Q38.6
  aorta (congenital) Q25.4
  axialis extracorticalis (congenita) E75.29
  bone marrow (myeloid) D61.9
    congenital D61.01
  brain Q00.0
    part of Q04.3
  bronchus Q32.4
  cementum K00.4
  cerebellum Q04.3
  cervix (congenital) Q51.5
  congenital pure red cell D61.01
  corpus callosum Q04.0
  cutis congenita Q84.8
  erythrocyte congenital D61.01
  extracortical axial E75.29
  eye Q11.1
  fovea centralis (congenital) Q14.1
  gallbladder, congenital Q44.0
  iris Q13.1
  labyrinth, membranous Q16.5
  limb (congenital) Q73.8
    lower — *see* Defect, reduction, lower limb
    upper — *see* Agenesis, arm
  lung, congenital (bilateral) (unilateral) Q33.3
  pancreas Q45.0
  parathyroid-thymic D82.1
  Pelizaeus-Merzbacher E75.29
  penis Q55.5
  prostate Q55.4
  red cell (with thymoma) D60.9
    acquired D60.9
      due to drugs D60.9
    adult D60.9
    chronic D60.0
    congenital D61.01
    constitutional D61.01
    due to drugs D60.9
    hereditary D61.01
    of infants D61.01
    primary D61.01
    pure D61.01
      due to drugs D60.9
    specified type NEC D60.8
    transient D60.1
  round ligament Q52.8
  skin Q84.8
  spermatic cord Q55.4
  spleen Q89.01
  testicle Q55.0
  thymic, with immunodeficiency D82.1
  thyroid (congenital) (with myxedema) E03.1
  uterus Q51.0
  ventral horn cell Q06.1
Apnea, apneic (of) (spells) R06.81
  newborn NEC P28.4
    obstructive P28.4
    sleep (central) (obstructive) (primary) P28.3
  prematurity P28.4
  sleep G47.30
    central (primary) G47.31
      in conditions classified elsewhere G47.37
    obstructive (adult) (pediatric) G47.33
    primary central G47.31
    specified NEC G47.39
Apneumatosis, newborn P28.0
Apocrine metaplasia (breast) — *see* Dysplasia, mammary, specified type NEC
Apophysitis (bone) (*see also* Osteochondropathy)
  calcaneus M92.8
  juvenile M92.9
Apoplectiform convulsions (cerebral ischemia) I67.82
Apoplexia, apoplexy, apoplectic
  adrenal A39.1
  heart (auricle) (ventricle) — *see* Infarct, myocardium
  heat T67.0 ☑
  hemorrhagic (stroke) — *see* Hemorrhage, intracranial

Apoplexia, apoplexy, apoplectic — *continued*
  meninges, hemorrhagic — *see* Hemorrhage, intracranial, subarachnoid
  uremic N18.9 [I68.8]
Appearance
  bizarre R46.1
  specified NEC R46.89
  very low level of personal hygiene R46.0
Appendage
  epididymal (organ of Morgagni) Q55.4
  intestine (epiploic) Q43.8
  preauricular Q17.0
  testicular (organ of Morgagni) Q55.29
Appendicitis (pneumococcal) (retrocecal) K37
  with
    perforation or rupture K35.2
    peritoneal abscess K35.3
    peritonitis NEC K35.3
      generalized (with perforation or rupture) K35.2
      localized (with perforation or rupture) K35.3
  acute (catarrhal) (fulminating) (gangrenous) (obstructive) (retrocecal) (suppurative) K35.80
    with
      peritoneal abscess K35.3
      peritonitis NEC K35.3
        generalized (with perforation or rupture) K35.2
        localized (with perforation or rupture) K35.3
    specified NEC K35.89
  amebic A06.89
  chronic (recurrent) K36
  exacerbation — *see* Appendicitis, acute
  gangrenous — *see* Appendicitis, acute
  healed (obliterative) K36
  interval K36
  neurogenic K36
  obstructive K36
  recurrent K36
  relapsing K36
  subacute (adhesive) K36
  subsiding K36
  suppurative — *see* Appendicitis, acute
  tuberculous A18.32
Appendicopathia oxyurica B80
Appendix, appendicular (*see also* condition)
  epididymis Q55.4
  Morgagni
    female Q50.5
    male (epididymal) Q55.4
      testicular Q55.29
  testis Q55.29
Appetite
  depraved — *see* Pica
  excessive R63.2
  lack or loss (*see also* Anorexia) R63.0
    nonorganic origin F50.8
    psychogenic F50.8
  perverted (hysterical) — *see* Pica
Apple peel syndrome Q41.1
Apprehension state F41.1
Apprehensiveness, abnormal F41.9
Approximal wear K03.0
Apraxia (classic) (ideational) (ideokinetic) (ideomotor) (motor) (verbal) R48.2
  following
    cerebrovascular disease I69.990
      cerebral infarction I69.390
      intracerebral hemorrhage I69.190
      nontraumatic intracranial hemorrhage NEC I69.290
      specified disease NEC I69.890
      subarachnoid hemorrhage I69.090
  oculomotor, congenital H51.8
Aptyalism K11.7
Apudoma — *see* Neoplasm, uncertain behavior, by site
Aqueous misdirection H40.83- ☑
Arabicum elephantiasis — *see* Infestation, filarial
Arachnitis — *see* Meningitis
Arachnodactyly — *see* Syndrome, Marfan's
Arachnoiditis (acute) (adhesive) (basal) (brain) (cerebrospinal) — *see* Meningitis
Arachnophobia F40.210
Arboencephalitis, Australian A83.4
Arborization block (heart) I45.5
ARC (AIDS-related complex) B20
Arches — *see* condition
Arcuate uterus Q51.810

Arcuatus uterus Q51.810
Arcus (cornea) senilis — *see* Degeneration, cornea, senile
Arc-welder's lung J63.4
Areflexia R29.2
Areola — *see* condition
Argentaffinoma (*see also* Neoplasm, uncertain behavior, by site)
  malignant — *see* Neoplasm, malignant, by site
  syndrome E34.0
Argininemia E72.21
Arginosuccinic aciduria E72.22
Argyll Robertson phenomenon, pupil or syndrome (syphilitic) A52.19
  atypical H57.09
  nonsyphilitic H57.09
Argyria, argyriasis
  conjunctival H11.13- ☑
  from drug or medicament — *see* Table of Drugs and Chemicals, by substance
Argyrosis, conjunctival H11.13- ☑
Arhinencephaly Q04.1
Ariboflavinosis E53.0
Arm — *see* condition
Arnold-Chiari disease, obstruction or syndrome (type II) Q07.00
  with
    hydrocephalus Q07.02
      with spina bifida Q07.03
    spina bifida Q07.01
      with hydrocephalus Q07.03
  type III — *see* Encephalocele
  type IV Q04.8
Aromatic amino-acid metabolism disorder E70.9
  specified NEC E70.8
Arousals, confusional G47.51
Arrest, arrested
  cardiac I46.9
    complicating
      abortion — *see* Abortion, by type, complicated by, cardiac arrest
      anesthesia (general) (local) or other sedation — *see* Table of Drugs and Chemicals, by drug
        in labor and delivery O74.2
        in pregnancy O29.11- ☑
          postpartum, puerperal O89.1
      delivery (cesarean) (instrumental) O75.4
    due to
      cardiac condition I46.2
      specified condition NEC I46.8
    intraoperative I97.71- ☑
    newborn P29.81
    postprocedural I97.12- ☑
      obstetric procedure O75.4
  cardiorespiratory — *see* Arrest, cardiac
  circulatory — *see* Arrest, cardiac
  deep transverse O64.0 ☑
  development or growth
    bone — *see* Disorder, bone, development or growth
    child R62.50
    tracheal rings Q32.1
  epiphyseal
    complete
      femur M89.15- ☑
      humerus M89.12- ☑
      tibia M89.16- ☑
      ulna M89.13- ☑
    forearm M89.13- ☑
      specified NEC M89.13- ☑
      ulna — *see* Arrest, epiphyseal, by type, ulna
    lower leg M89.16- ☑
      specified NEC M89.168
      tibia — *see* Arrest, epiphyseal, by type, tibia
    partial
      femur M89.15- ☑
      humerus M89.12- ☑
      tibia M89.16- ☑
      ulna M89.13- ☑
    specified NEC M89.18
  granulopoiesis — *see* Agranulocytosis
  growth plate — *see* Arrest, epiphyseal
  heart — *see* Arrest, cardiac
  legal, anxiety concerning Z65.3
  physeal — *see* Arrest, epiphyseal
  respiratory R09.2
    newborn P28.81

Arrest, arrested — continued
- sinus I45.5
- spermatogenesis (complete) — see Azoospermia
  - incomplete — see Oligospermia
- transverse (deep) O64.0 ☑

Arrhenoblastoma
- benign
  - specified site — see Neoplasm, benign, by site
  - unspecified site
    - female D27.9
    - male D29.20
- malignant
  - specified site — see Neoplasm, malignant, by site
  - unspecified site
    - female C56.9
    - male C62.90
- specified site — see Neoplasm, uncertain behavior, by site
- unspecified site
  - female D39.10
  - male D40.10

Arrhythmia (auricle) (cardiac) (juvenile) (nodal) (reflex) (sinus) (supraventricular) (transitory) (ventricle) I49.9
- block I45.9
- extrasystolic I49.49
- newborn
  - bradycardia P29.12
    - occurring before birth P03.819
      - before onset of labor P03.810
      - during labor P03.811
  - tachycardia P29.11
- psychogenic F45.8
- specified NEC I49.8
- vagal R55
- ventricular re-entry I47.0

Arrillaga-Ayerza syndrome (pulmonary sclerosis with pulmonary hypertension) I27.0

Arsenical pigmentation L81.8
- from drug or medicament — see Table of Drugs and Chemicals

Arsenism — see Poisoning, arsenic

Arterial — see condition

Arteriofibrosis — see Arteriosclerosis

Arteriolar sclerosis — see Arteriosclerosis

Arteriolith — see Arteriosclerosis

Arteriolitis I77.6
- necrotizing, kidney I77.5
- renal — see Hypertension, kidney

Arteriolosclerosis — see Arteriosclerosis

Arterionephrosclerosis — see Hypertension, kidney

Arteriopathy I77.9

Arteriosclerosis, arteriosclerotic (diffuse) (obliterans) (of) (senile) (with calcification) I70.90
- aorta I70.0
- arteries of extremities — see Arteriosclerosis, extremities
- brain I67.2
- bypass graft
  - coronary — see Arteriosclerosis, coronary, bypass graft
  - extremities — see Arteriosclerosis, extremities, bypass graft
- cardiac — see Disease, heart, ischemic, atherosclerotic
- cardiopathy — see Disease, heart, ischemic, atherosclerotic
- cardiorenal — see Hypertension, cardiorenal
- cardiovascular — see Disease, heart, ischemic, atherosclerotic
- carotid (see also Occlusion, artery, carotid) I65.2- ☑
- central nervous system I67.2
- cerebral I67.2
- cerebrovascular I67.2
- coronary (artery) I25.10
  - bypass graft I25.810
    - with
      - angina pectoris I25.709
        - with documented spasm I25.701
        - specified type NEC I25.708
        - unstable I25.700
      - ischemic chest pain I25.709
    - autologous artery I25.810
      - with
        - angina pectoris I25.729
          - with documented spasm I25.721
          - specified type I25.728
          - unstable I25.720
        - ischemic chest pain I25.729

Arteriosclerosis, arteriosclerotic — continued
- coronary — continued
  - bypass graft — continued
    - autologous vein I25.810
      - with
        - angina pectoris I25.719
          - with documented spasm I25.711
          - specified type I25.718
          - unstable I25.710
        - ischemic chest pain I25.719
    - nonautologous biological I25.810
      - with
        - angina pectoris I25.739
          - with documented spasm I25.731
          - specified type I25.738
          - unstable I25.730
        - ischemic chest pain I25.739
    - specified type NEC I25.810
      - with
        - angina pectoris I25.799
          - with documented spasm I25.791
          - specified type I25.798
          - unstable I25.790
        - ischemic chest pain I25.799
  - due to
    - calcified coronary lesion (severely) I25.84
    - lipid rich plaque I25.83
  - native vessel
    - with
      - angina pectoris I25.119
        - with documented spasm I25.111
        - specified type NEC I25.118
        - unstable I25.110
      - ischemic chest pain I25.119
  - transplanted heart I25.811
    - bypass graft I25.812
      - with
        - angina pectoris I25.769
          - with documented spasm I25.761
          - specified type I25.768
          - unstable I25.760
        - ischemic chest pain I25.769
    - native coronary artery I25.811
      - with
        - angina pectoris I25.759
          - with documented spasm I25.751
          - specified type I25.758
          - unstable I25.750
        - ischemic chest pain I25.759
- extremities (native arteries) I70.209
  - bypass graft I70.309
    - autologous vein graft I70.409
      - leg I70.409
        - with
          - gangrene (and intermittent claudication, rest pain and ulcer) I70.469
          - intermittent claudication I70.419
          - rest pain (and intermittent claudication) I70.429
        - bilateral I70.403
          - with
            - gangrene (and intermittent claudication, rest pain and ulcer) I70.463
            - intermittent claudication I70.463
            - rest pain (and intermittent claudication) I70.423
          - specified type NEC I70.493
        - left I70.402
          - with
            - gangrene (and intermittent claudication, rest pain and ulcer) I70.462
            - intermittent claudication I70.412
            - rest pain (and intermittent claudication) I70.422
            - ulceration (and intermittent claudication and rest pain) I70.449
              - ankle I70.443
              - calf I70.442
              - foot site NEC I70.445
              - heel I70.444
              - lower leg NEC I70.448
              - midfoot I70.444
              - thigh I70.441
          - specified type NEC I70.492

Arteriosclerosis, arteriosclerotic — continued
- extremities — continued
  - bypass graft — continued
    - autologous vein graft — continued
      - leg — continued
        - right I70.401
          - with
            - gangrene (and intermittent claudication, rest pain and ulcer) I70.461
            - intermittent claudication I70.411
            - rest pain (and intermittent claudication) I70.421
            - ulceration (and intermittent claudication and rest pain) I70.439
              - ankle I70.433
              - calf I70.432
              - foot site NEC I70.435
              - heel I70.434
              - lower leg NEC I70.438
              - midfoot I70.434
              - thigh I70.431
          - specified type NEC I70.491
        - specified type NEC I70.499
      - specified NEC I70.408
        - with
          - gangrene (and intermittent claudication, rest pain and ulcer) I70.468
          - intermittent claudication I70.418
          - rest pain (and intermittent claudication) I70.428
          - ulceration (and intermittent claudication and rest pain) I70.45
        - specified type NEC I70.498
  - leg I70.309
    - with
      - gangrene (and intermittent claudication, rest pain and ulcer) I70.369
      - intermittent claudication I70.319
      - rest pain (and intermittent claudication) I70.329
    - bilateral I70.303
      - with
        - gangrene (and intermittent claudication, rest pain and ulcer) I70.363
        - intermittent claudication I70.313
        - rest pain (and intermittent claudication) I70.323
      - specified type NEC I70.393
    - left I70.302
      - with
        - gangrene (and intermittent claudication, rest pain and ulcer) I70.362
        - intermittent claudication I70.312
        - rest pain (and intermittent claudication) I70.322
        - ulceration (and intermittent claudication and rest pain) I70.349
          - ankle I70.343
          - calf I70.342
          - foot site NEC I70.345
          - heel I70.344
          - lower leg NEC I70.348
          - midfoot I70.344
          - thigh I70.341
      - specified type NEC I70.392
    - right I70.301
      - with
        - gangrene (and intermittent claudication, rest pain and ulcer) I70.361
        - intermittent claudication I70.311
        - rest pain (and intermittent claudication) I70.321
        - ulceration (and intermittent claudication and rest pain I70.339
          - ankle I70.333
          - calf I70.332
          - foot site NEC I70.335
          - heel I70.334
          - lower leg NEC I70.338
          - midfoot I70.334
          - thigh I70.331
      - specified type NEC I70.391

Arteriosclerosis, arteriosclerotic — *continued*
  extremities — *continued*
    bypass graft — *continued*
      leg — *continued*
        specified type NEC I70.399
      nonautologous biological graft I70.509
        leg I70.509
          with
            gangrene (and intermittent claudication, rest pain and ulcer) I70.569
            intermittent claudication I70.519
            rest pain (and intermittent claudication) I70.529
          bilateral I70.503
            with
              gangrene (and intermittent claudication, rest pain and ulcer) I70.563
              intermittent claudication I70.513
              rest pain (and intermittent claudication) I70.523
            specified type NEC I70.593
          left I70.502
            with
              gangrene (and intermittent claudication, rest pain and ulcer) I70.562
              intermittent claudication I70.512
              rest pain (and intermittent claudication) I70.522
              ulceration (and intermittent claudication and rest pain) I70.549
                ankle I70.543
                calf I70.542
                foot site NEC I70.545
                heel I70.544
                lower leg NEC I70.548
                midfoot I70.544
                thigh I70.541
            specified type NEC I70.592
          right I70.501
            with
              gangrene (and intermittent claudication, rest pain and ulcer) I70.561
              intermittent claudication I70.511
              rest pain (and intermittent claudication) I70.521
              ulceration (and intermittent claudication and rest pain) I70.539
                ankle I70.533
                calf I70.532
                foot site NEC I70.535
                heel I70.534
                lower leg NEC I70.538
                midfoot I70.534
                thigh I70.531
            specified type NEC I70.591
        specified type NEC I70.599
      specified NEC I70.508
        with
          gangrene (and intermittent claudication, rest pain and ulcer) I70.568
          intermittent claudication I70.518
          rest pain (and intermittent claudication) I70.528
          ulceration (and intermittent claudication and rest pain) I70.55
        specified type NEC I70.598
      nonbiological graft I70.609
        leg I70.609
          with
            gangrene (and intermittent claudication, rest pain and ulcer) I70.669
            intermittent claudication I70.619
            rest pain (and intermittent claudication) I70.629
          bilateral I70.603
            with
              gangrene (and intermittent claudication, rest pain and ulcer) I70.663
              intermittent claudication I70.613

Arteriosclerosis, arteriosclerotic — *continued*
  extremities — *continued*
    bypass graft — *continued*
      nonbiological graft — *continued*
        leg — *continued*
          bilateral — *continued*
            with — *continued*
              rest pain (and intermittent claudication) I70.623
            specified type NEC I70.693
          left I70.602
            with
              gangrene (and intermittent claudication, rest pain and ulcer) I70.662
              intermittent claudication I70.612
              rest pain (and intermittent claudication) I70.622
              ulceration (and intermittent claudication and rest pain) I70.649
                ankle I70.643
                calf I70.642
                foot site NEC I70.645
                heel I70.644
                lower leg NEC I70.648
                midfoot I70.644
                thigh I70.641
            specified type NEC I70.692
          right I70.601
            with
              gangrene (and intermittent claudication, rest pain and ulcer) I70.661
              intermittent claudication I70.611
              rest pain (and intermittent claudication) I70.621
              ulceration (and intermittent claudication and rest pain) I70.639
                ankle I70.633
                calf I70.632
                foot site NEC I70.635
                heel I70.634
                lower leg NEC I70.638
                midfoot I70.634
                thigh I70.631
            specified type NEC I70.691
        specified type NEC I70.699
      specified NEC I70.608
        with
          gangrene (and intermittent claudication, rest pain and ulcer) I70.668
          intermittent claudication I70.618
          rest pain (and intermittent claudication) I70.628
          ulceration (and intermittent claudication and rest pain) I70.65
        specified type NEC I70.698
      specified graft NEC I70.709
        leg I70.709
          with
            gangrene (and intermittent claudication, rest pain and ulcer) I70.769
            intermittent claudication I70.719
            rest pain (and intermittent claudication) I70.729
          bilateral I70.703
            with
              gangrene (and intermittent claudication, rest pain and ulcer) I70.763
              intermittent claudication I70.713
              rest pain (and intermittent claudication) I70.723
            specified type NEC I70.793
          left I70.702
            with
              gangrene (and intermittent claudication, rest pain and ulcer) I70.762
              intermittent claudication I70.712
              rest pain (and intermittent claudication) I70.722

Arteriosclerosis, arteriosclerotic — *continued*
  extremities — *continued*
    bypass graft — *continued*
      specified graft — *continued*
        leg — *continued*
          left — *continued*
            with — *continued*
              ulceration (and intermittent claudication and rest pain) I70.749
                ankle I70.743
                calf I70.742
                foot site NEC I70.745
                heel I70.744
                lower leg NEC I70.748
                midfoot I70.744
                thigh I70.741
            specified type NEC I70.792
          right I70.701
            with
              gangrene (and intermittent claudication, rest pain and ulcer) I70.761
              intermittent claudication I70.711
              rest pain (and intermittent claudication) I70.721
              ulceration (and intermittent claudication and rest pain) I70.739
                ankle I70.733
                calf I70.732
                foot site NEC I70.735
                heel I70.734
                lower leg NEC I70.738
                midfoot I70.734
                thigh I70.731
            specified type NEC I70.791
        specified type NEC I70.799
      specified NEC I70.708
        with
          gangrene (and intermittent claudication, rest pain and ulcer) I70.768
          intermittent claudication I70.718
          rest pain (and intermittent claudication) I70.728
          ulceration (and intermittent claudication and rest pain) I70.75
        specified type NEC I70.798
    specified NEC I70.308
      with
        gangrene (and intermittent claudication, rest pain and ulcer) I70.368
        intermittent claudication I70.318
        rest pain (and intermittent claudication) I70.328
        ulceration (and intermittent claudication and rest pain) I70.35
      specifiec type NEC I70.398
    leg I70.209
      with
        gangrene (and intermittent claudication, rest pain and ulcer) I70.269
        intermittent claudication I70.219
        rest pain (and intermittent claudication) I70.229
      bilateral I70.203
        with
          gangrene (and intermittent claudication, rest pain and ulcer) I70.263
          intermittent claudication I70.213
          rest pain (and intermittent claudication) I70.223
        specified type NEC I70.293
      left I70.202
        with
          gangrene (and intermittent claudication, rest pain and ulcer) I70.262
          intermittent claudication I70.212
          rest pain (and intermittent claudication) I70.222
          ulceration (and intermittent claudication and rest pain) I70.249
            ankle I70.243
            calf I70.242
            foot site NEC I70.245
            heel I70.244
            lower leg NEC I70.248

Arteriosclerosis, arteriosclerotic — continued
  extremities — continued
    leg — continued
      left — continued
        with — continued
          ulceration — continued
            midfoot I70.244
            thigh I70.241
        specified type NEC I70.292
      right I70.201
        with
          gangrene (and intermittent claudication, rest pain and ulcer) I70.261
          intermittent claudication I70.211
          rest pain (and intermittent claudication) I70.221
          ulceration (and intermittent claudication and rest pain) I70.239
            ankle I70.233
            calf I70.232
            foot site NEC I70.235
            heel I70.234
            lower leg NEC I70.238
            midfoot I70.234
            thigh I70.231
        specified type NEC I70.291
    specified site NEC I70.208
      with
        gangrene (and intermittent claudication, rest pain and ulcer) I70.268
        intermittent claudication I70.218
        rest pain (and intermittent claudication) I70.228
        ulceration (and intermittent claudication and rest pain) I70.25
      specified type NEC I70.298
  generalized I70.91
  heart (disease) — see Arteriosclerosis, coronary (artery),
  kidney — see Hypertension, kidney
  medial — see Arteriosclerosis, extremities
  mesenteric (artery) K55.1
  Mönckeberg's — see Arteriosclerosis, extremities
  myocarditis I51.4
  peripheral (of extremities) — see Arteriosclerosis, extremities
  pulmonary (idiopathic) I27.0
  renal (arterioles) (see also Hypertension, kidney)
    artery I70.1
  retina (vascular) I70.8 [H35.0-] ☑
  specified artery NEC I70.8
  spinal (cord) G95.19
  vertebral (artery) I67.2
Arteriospasm I73.9
Arteriovenous — see condition
Arteritis I77.6
  allergic M31.0
  aorta (nonsyphilitic) I77.6
    syphilitic A52.02
  aortic arch M31.4
  brachiocephalic M31.4
  brain I67.7
    syphilitic A52.04
  cerebral I67.7
    in systemic lupus erythematosus M32.19
    listerial A32.89
    syphilitic A52.04
    tuberculous A18.89
  coronary (artery) I25.89
    rheumatic I01.8
      chronic I09.89
    syphilitic A52.06
  cranial (left) (right), giant cell M31.6
  deformans — see Arteriosclerosis
  giant cell NEC M31.6
    with polymyalgia rheumatica M31.5
  necrosing or necrotizing M31.9
    specified NEC M31.8
  nodosa M30.0
  obliterans — see Arteriosclerosis
  pulmonary I28.8
  rheumatic — see Fever, rheumatic
  senile — see Arteriosclerosis
  suppurative I77.2
  syphilitic (general) A52.09
    brain A52.04
    coronary A52.06

Arteritis — continued
  syphilitic — continued
    spinal A52.09
  temporal, giant cell M31.6
  young female aortic arch syndrome M31.4
Artery, arterial (see also condition)
  abscess I77.89
  single umbilical Q27.0
Arthralgia (allergic) (see also Pain, joint)
  in caisson disease T70.3 ☑
  temporomandibular M26.62
Arthritis, arthritic (acute) (chronic) (nonpyogenic) (subacute) M19.90
  allergic — see Arthritis, specified form NEC
  ankylosing (crippling) (spine) (see also Spondylitis, ankylosing)
    sites other than spine — see Arthritis, specified form NEC
  atrophic — see Osteoarthritis
    spine — see Spondylitis, ankylosing
  back — see Spondylopathy, inflammatory
  blennorrhagic (gonococcal) A54.42
  Charcot's — see Arthropathy, neuropathic
    diabetic — see Diabetes, arthropathy, neuropathic
    syringomyelic G95.0
  chylous (filarial) (see also category M01) B74.9
  climacteric (any site) NEC — see Arthritis, specified form NEC
  crystal (-induced) — see Arthritis, in, crystals
  deformans — see Osteoarthritis
  degenerative — see Osteoarthritis
  due to or associated with
    acromegaly E22.0
    brucellosis — see Brucellosis
    caisson disease T70.3 ☑
    diabetes — see Diabetes, arthropathy
    dracontiasis (see also category M01) B72
    enteritis NEC
      regional — see Enteritis, regional
    erysipelas (see also category M01) A46
    erythema
      epidemic A25.1
      nodosum L52
    filariasis NOS B74.9
    glanders A24.0
    helminthiasis (see also category M01) B83.9
    hemophilia D66 [M36.2]
    Henoch- (Schönlein) purpura D69.0 [M36.4]
    human parvovirus (see also category M01) B97.6
    infectious disease NEC M01 ☑
    leprosy (see also category M01) (see also Leprosy) A30.9
    Lyme disease A69.23
    mycobacteria (see also category M01) A31.8
    parasitic disease NEC (see also category M01) B89
    paratyphoid fever (see also category M01) (see also Fever, paratyphoid) A01.4
    rat bite fever (see also category M01) A25.1
    regional enteritis — see Enteritis, regional
    respiratory disorder NOS J98.9
    serum sickness (see also Reaction, serum) T80.69 ☑
    syringomyelia G95.0
    typhoid fever A01.04
  epidemic erythema A25.1
  febrile — see Fever, rheumatic
  gonococcal A54.42
  gouty (acute) — see Gout, idiopathic
  in (due to)
    acromegaly (see also subcategory M14.8-) E22.0
    amyloidosis (see also subcategory M14.8-) E85.4
    bacterial disease (see also subcategory M01) A49.9
    Behçet's syndrome M35.2
    caisson disease (see also subcategory M14.8-) T70.3 ☑
    coliform bacilli (Escherichia coli) — see Arthritis, in, pyogenic organism NEC
    crystals M11.9
      dicalcium phosphate — see Arthritis, in, crystals, specified type NEC
      hydroxyapatite M11.0- ☑
      pyrophosphate — see Arthritis, in, crystals, specified type NEC
      specified type NEC M11.80
        ankle M11.87- ☑
        elbow M11.82- ☑
        foot joint M11.87- ☑
        hand joint M11.84- ☑

Arthritis, arthritic — continued
  in — continued
    crystals — continued
      specified type — continued
        hip M11.85- ☑
        knee M11.86- ☑
        multiple sites M11.8- ☑
        shoulder M11.81- ☑
        vertebrae M11.88
        wrist M11.83- ☑
    dermatoarthritis, lipoid E78.81
    dracontiasis (dracunculiasis) (see also category M01) B72
    endocrine disorder NEC (see also subcategory M14.8-) E34.9
    enteritis, infectious NEC (see also category M01) A09
      specified organism NEC (see also category M01) A08.8
    erythema
      multiforme (see also subcategory M14.8-) L51.9
      nodosum (see also subcategory M14.8-) L52
    gout — see Gout, idiopathic
    helminthiasis NEC (see also category M01) B83.9
    hemochromatosis (see also subcategory M14.8-) E83.118
    hemoglobinopathy NEC D58.2 [M36.3]
    hemophilia NEC D66 [M36.2]
    Hemophilus influenzae M00.8- ☑ [B96.3]
    Henoch (-Schönlein) purpura D69.0 [M36.4]
    hyperparathyroidism NEC (see also subcategory M14.8-) E21.3
    hypersensitivity reaction NEC T78.49 ☑ [M36.4]
    hypogammaglobulinemia (see also subcategory M14.8-) D80.1
    hypothyroidism NEC (see also subcategory M14.8-) E03.9
    infection — see Arthritis, pyogenic or pyemic
      spine — see Spondylopathy, infective
    infectious disease NEC M01 ☑
    leprosy (see also category M01) A30.9
    leukemia NEC C95.9- ☑ [M36.1]
    lipoid dermatoarthritis E78.81
    Lyme disease A69.23
    Mediterranean fever, familial (see also subcategory M14.8-) E85.0
    Meningococcus A39.83
    metabolic disorder NEC (see also subcategory M14.8-) E88.9
    multiple myelomatosis C90.0- ☑ [M36.1]
    mumps B26.85
    mycosis NEC (see also category M01) B49
    myelomatosis (multiple) C90.0- ☑ [M36.1]
    neurological disorder NEC G98.0
    ochronosis (see also subcategory M14.8-) E70.29
    O'nyong-nyong (see also category M01) A92.1
    parasitic disease NEC (see also category M01) B89
    paratyphoid fever (see also category M01) A01.4
    Pseudomonas — see Arthritis, pyogenic, bacterial NEC
    psoriasis L40.50
    pyogenic organism NEC — see Arthritis, pyogenic, bacterial NEC
    Reiter's disease — see Reiter's disease
    respiratory disorder NEC (see also subcategory M14.8-) J98.9
    reticulosis, malignant (see also subcategory M14.8-) C86.0
    rubella B06.82
    Salmonella (arizonae) (cholerae-suis) (enteritidis) (typhimurium) A02.23
    sarcoidosis D86.86
    specified bacteria NEC — see Arthritis, pyogenic, bacterial NEC
    sporotrichosis B42.82
    syringomyelia G95.0
    thalassemia NEC D56.9 [M36.3]
    tuberculosis — see Tuberculosis, arthritis
    typhoid fever A01.04
    urethritis, Reiter's — see Reiter's disease
    viral disease NEC (see also category M01) B34.9
  infectious or infective (see also Arthritis, pyogenic or pyemic)
    spine — see Spondylopathy, infective
  juvenile M08.90
    with systemic onset — see Still's disease
    ankle M08.97- ☑

☑ **Additional Character Required — Refer to the Tabular List for Character Selection**   ▽ Subterms under main terms may continue to next column or page

Arthritis, arthritic — *continued*
  juvenile — *continued*
    elbow M08.92- ☑
    foot joint M08.97- ☑
    hand joint M08.94- ☑
    hip M08.95- ☑
    knee M08.96- ☑
    multiple site M08.99
    pauciarticular M08.40
      ankle M08.47- ☑
      elbow M08.42- ☑
      foot joint M08.47- ☑
      hand joint M08.44- ☑
      hip M08.45- ☑
      knee M08.46- ☑
      shoulder M08.41- ☑
      vertebrae M08.48
      wrist M08.43- ☑
    psoriatic L40.54
    rheumatoid — *see* Arthritis, rheumatoid, juvenile
    shoulder M08.91- ☑
    specified type NEC M08.80
      ankle M08.87- ☑
      elbow M08.82- ☑
      foot joint M08.87- ☑
      hand joint M08.84- ☑
      hip M08.85- ☑
      knee M08.86- ☑
      multiple site M08.89
      shoulder M08.81- ☑
      specified joint NEC M08.88
      vertebrae M08.88
      wrist M08.83- ☑
    wrist M08.93- ☑
  meaning osteoarthritis — *see* Osteoarthritis
  meningococcal A39.83
  menopausal (any site) NEC — *see* Arthritis, specified form NEC
  mutilans (psoriatic) L40.52
  mycotic NEC (*see also* category M01) B49
  neuropathic (Charcot) — *see* Arthropathy, neuropathic
    diabetic — *see* Diabetes, arthropathy, neuropathic
    nonsyphilitic NEC G98.0
    syringomyelic G95.0
  ochronotic (*see also* subcategory M14.8-) E70.29
  palindromic (any site) — *see* Rheumatism, palindromic
  pneumococcal M00.10
    ankle M00.17- ☑
    elbow M00.12- ☑
    foot joint — *see* Arthritis, pneumococcal, ankle
    hand joint M00.14- ☑
    hip M00.15- ☑
    knee M00.16- ☑
    multiple site M00.19
    shoulder M00.11- ☑
    vertebra M00.18
    wrist M00.13- ☑
  postdysenteric — *see* Arthropathy, postdysenteric
  postmeningococcal A39.84
  postrheumatic, chronic — *see* Arthropathy, postrheumatic, chronic
  primary progressive (*see also* Arthritis, specified form NEC)
    spine — *see* Spondylitis, ankylosing
  psoriatic L40.50
  purulent (any site except spine) — *see* Arthritis, pyogenic or pyemic
    spine — *see* Spondylopathy, infective
  pyogenic or pyemic (any site except spine) M00.9
    bacterial NEC M00.80
      ankle M00.87- ☑
      elbow M00.82- ☑
      foot joint — *see* Arthritis, pyogenic, bacterial NEC, ankle
      hand joint M00.84- ☑
      hip M00.85- ☑
      knee M00.86- ☑
      multiple site M00.89
      shoulder M00.81- ☑
      vertebra M00.88
      wrist M00.83- ☑
    pneumococcal — *see* Arthritis, pneumococcal
    spine — *see* Spondylopathy, infective
    staphylococcal — *see* Arthritis, staphylococcal
    streptococcal — *see* Arthritis, streptococcal NEC
      pneumococcal — *see* Arthritis, pneumococcal

Arthritis, arthritic — *continued*
  reactive — *see* Reiter's disease
  rheumatic (*see also* Arthritis, rheumatoid)
    acute or subacute — *see* Fever, rheumatic
  rheumatoid M06.9
    with
      carditis — *see* Rheumatoid, carditis
      endocarditis — *see* Rheumatoid, carditis
      heart involvement NEC — *see* Rheumatoid, carditis
      lung involvement — *see* Rheumatoid, lung
      myocarditis — *see* Rheumatoid, carditis
      myopathy — *see* Rheumatoid, myopathy
      pericarditis — *see* Rheumatoid, carditis
      polyneuropathy — *see* Rheumatoid, polyneuropathy
      rheumatoid factor — *see* Arthritis, rheumatoid, seropositive
      splenoadenomegaly and leukopenia — *see* Felty's syndrome
      vasculitis — *see* Rheumatoid, vasculitis
      visceral involvement NEC — *see* Rheumatoid, arthritis, with involvement of organs NEC
    juvenile (with or without rheumatoid factor) M08.00
      ankle M08.07- ☑
      elbow M08.02- ☑
      foot joint M08.07- ☑
      hand joint M08.04- ☑
      hip M08.05- ☑
      knee M08.06- ☑
      multiple site M08.09
      shoulder M08.01- ☑
      vertebra M08.08
      wrist M08.03- ☑
    seronegative M06.00
      ankle M06.07- ☑
      elbow M06.02- ☑
      foot joint M06.07- ☑
      hand joint M06.04- ☑
      hip M06.05- ☑
      knee M06.06- ☑
      multiple site M06.09
      shoulder M06.01- ☑
      vertebra M06.08
      wrist M06.03- ☑
    seropositive M05.9
      without organ involvement M05.70
        ankle M05.77- ☑
        elbow M05.72- ☑
        foot joint M05.77- ☑
        hand joint M05.74- ☑
        hip M05.75- ☑
        knee M05.76- ☑
        multiple sites M05.79
        shoulder M05.71- ☑
        vertebra — *see* Spondylitis, ankylosing
        wrist M05.73- ☑
      specified NEC M05.80
        ankle M05.87- ☑
        elbow M05.82- ☑
        foot joint M05.87- ☑
        hand joint M05.84- ☑
        hip M05.85- ☑
        knee M05.86- ☑
        multiple sites M05.89
        shoulder M05.81- ☑
        vertebra — *see* Spondylitis, ankylosing
        wrist M05.83- ☑
    specified type NEC M06.80
      ankle M06.87- ☑
      elbow M06.82- ☑
      foot joint M06.87- ☑
      hand joint M06.84- ☑
      hip M06.85- ☑
      knee M06.86- ☑
      multiple site M06.89
      shoulder M06.81- ☑
      vertebra M06.88
      wrist M06.83- ☑
    spine — *see* Spondylitis, ankylosing
  rubella B06.82
  scorbutic (*see also* subcategory M14.8-) E54
  senile or senescent — *see* Osteoarthritis

Arthritis, arthritic — *continued*
  septic (any site except spine) — *see* Arthritis, pyogenic or pyemic
    spine — *see* Spondylopathy, infective
  serum (nontherapeutic) (therapeutic) — *see* Arthropathy, postimmunization
  specified form NEC M13.80
    ankle M13.87- ☑
    elbow M13.82- ☑
    foot joint M13.87- ☑
    hand joint M13.84- ☑
    hip M13.85- ☑
    knee M13.86- ☑
    multiple site M13.89
    shoulder M13.81- ☑
    specified joint NEC M13.88
    wrist M13.83- ☑
  spine (*see also* Spondylopathy, inflammatory)
    infectious or infective NEC — *see* Spondylopathy, infective
    Marie-Strümpell — *see* Spondylitis, ankylosing
    pyogenic — *see* Spondylopathy, infective
    rheumatoid — *see* Spondylitis, ankylosing
    traumatic (old) — *see* Spondylopathy, traumatic
    tuberculous A18.01
  staphylococcal M00.00
    ankle M00.07- ☑
    elbow M00.02- ☑
    foot joint — *see* Arthritis, staphylococcal, ankle
    hand joint M00.04- ☑
    hip M00.05- ☑
    knee M00.06- ☑
    multiple site M00.09
    shoulder M00.01- ☑
    vertebra M00.08
    wrist M00.03- ☑
  streptococcal NEC M00.20
    ankle M00.27- ☑
    elbow M00.22- ☑
    foot joint — *see* Arthritis, streptococcal, ankle
    hand joint M00.24- ☑
    hip M00.25- ☑
    knee M00.26- ☑
    multiple site M00.29
    shoulder M00.21- ☑
    vertebra M00.28
    wrist M00.23- ☑
  suppurative — *see* Arthritis, pyogenic or pyemic
  syphilitic (late) A52.16
    congenital A50.55 [M12.80]
  syphilitica deformans (Charcot) A52.16
  temporomandibular M26.69
  toxic of menopause (any site) — *see* Arthritis, specified form NEC
  transient — *see* Arthropathy, specified form NEC
  traumatic (chronic) — *see* Arthropathy, traumatic
  tuberculous A18.02
    spine A18.01
  uratic — *see* Gout, idiopathic
  urethritica (Reiter's) — *see* Reiter's disease
  vertebral — *see* Spondylopathy, inflammatory
  villous (any site) — *see* Arthropathy, specified form NEC
Arthrocele — *see* Effusion, joint
Arthrodesis status Z98.1
Arthrodynia (*see also* Pain, joint)
Arthrodysplasia Q74.9
Arthrofibrosis, joint — *see* Ankylosis
Arthrogryposis (congenital) Q68.8
  multiplex congenita Q74.3
Arthrokatadysis M24.7
Arthropathy (*see also* Arthritis) M12.9
  Charcot's — *see* Arthropathy, neuropathic
    diabetic — *see* Diabetes, arthropathy, neuropathic
    syringomyelic G95.0
  cricoarytenoid J38.7
  crystal (-induced) — *see* Arthritis, in, crystals
  diabetic NEC — *see* Diabetes, arthropathy
  distal interphalangeal, psoriatic L40.51
  enteropathic M07.60
    ankle M07.67- ☑
    elbow M07.62- ☑
    foot joint M07.67- ☑
    hand joint M07.64- ☑
    hip M07.65- ☑
    knee M07.66- ☑

▽ Subterms under main terms may continue to next column or page   ☑ Additional Character Required — Refer to the Tabular List for Character Selection   29

Arthritis, arthritic — Arthropathy

Arthropathy — *continued*
 enteropathic — *continued*
  multiple site M07.69
  shoulder M07.61- ☑
  vertebra M07.68
  wrist M07.63- ☑
 following intestinal bypass M02.00
  ankle M02.07- ☑
  elbow M02.02- ☑
  foot joint M02.07- ☑
  hand joint M02.04- ☑
  hip M02.05- ☑
  knee M02.06- ☑
  multiple site M02.09
  shoulder M02.01- ☑
  vertebra M02.08
  wrist M02.03- ☑
 gouty (*see also* Gout, idiopathic)
  in (due to)
   Lesch-Nyhan syndrome E79.1 [M14.8-] ☑
   sickle-cell disorders D57- ☑ [M14.8-] ☑
 hemophilic NEC D66 [M36.2]
  in (due to)
   hyperparathyroidism NEC E21.3 [M14.8-] ☑
   metabolic disease NOS E88.9 [M14.8-] ☑
 in (due to)
  acromegaly E22.0 [M14.8-] ☑
  amyloidosis E85.4 [M14.8-] ☑
  blood disorder NOS D75.9 [M36.3]
  diabetes — *see* Diabetes, arthropathy
  endocrine disease NOS E34.9 [M14.8-] ☑
  erythema
   multiforme L51.9 [M14.8-] ☑
   nodosum L52 [M14.8-] ☑
  hemochromatosis E83.118 [M14.8-] ☑
  hemoglobinopathy NEC D58.2 [M36.3]
  hemophilia NEC D66 [M36.2]
  Henoch-Schönlein purpura D69.0 [M36.4]
  hyperthyroidism E05.90 [M14.8-] ☑
  hypothyroidism E03.9 [M14.8-] ☑
  infective endocarditis I33.0 [M12.80]
  leukemia NEC C95.9- ☑ [M36.1]
  malignant histiocytosis C96.A [M36.1]
  metabolic disease NOS E88.9 [M14.8-] ☑
  multiple myeloma C90.0- ☑ [M36.1]
  neoplastic disease NOS (*see also* Neoplasm)
    D49.9 [M36.1]
  nutritional deficiency (*see also* subcategory
    M14.8-) E63.9
  psoriasis NOS L40.50
  sarcoidosis D86.86
  syphilis (late) A52.77
   congenital A50.55 [M12.80]
  thyrotoxicosis (*see also* subcategory M14.8-) E05.90
  ulcerative colitis K51.90 [M07.60]
  viral hepatitis (postinfectious) NEC B19.9 [M12.80]
  Whipple's disease (*see also* subcategory M14.8-)
    K90.81
 Jaccoud — *see* Arthropathy, postrheumatic, chronic
 juvenile — *see* Arthritis, juvenile
  psoriatic L40.54
 mutilans (psoriatic) L40.52
 neuropathic (Charcot) M14.60
  ankle M14.67- ☑
  diabetic — *see* Diabetes, arthropathy, neuropathic
  elbow M14.62- ☑
  foot joint M14.67- ☑
  hand joint M14.64- ☑
  hip M14.65- ☑
  knee M14.66- ☑
  multiple site M14.69
  nonsyphilitic NEC G98.0
  shoulder M14.61- ☑
  syringomyelic G95.0
  vertebra M14.68
  wrist M14.63- ☑
 osteopulmonary — *see* Osteoarthropathy, hyper-
    trophic, specified NEC
 postdysenteric M02.10
  ankle M02.17- ☑
  elbow M02.12- ☑
  foot joint M02.17- ☑
  hand joint M02.14- ☑
  hip M02.15- ☑
  knee M02.16- ☑
  multiple site M02.19
  shoulder M02.11- ☑

Arthropathy — *continued*
 postdysenteric — *continued*
  vertebra M02.18
  wrist M02.13- ☑
 postimmunization M02.20
  ankle M02.27- ☑
  elbow M02.22- ☑
  foot joint M02.27- ☑
  hand joint M02.24- ☑
  hip M02.25- ☑
  knee M02.26- ☑
  multiple site M02.29
  shoulder M02.21- ☑
  vertebra M02.28
  wrist M02.23- ☑
 postinfectious NEC B99 ☑ [M12.80]
  in (due to)
   enteritis due to Yersinia enterocolitica
     A04.6 [M12.80]
   syphilis A52.77
   viral hepatitis NEC B19.9 [M12.80]
 postrheumatic, chronic (Jaccoud) M12.00
  ankle M12.07- ☑
  elbow M12.02- ☑
  foot joint M12.07- ☑
  hand joint M12.04- ☑
  hip M12.05- ☑
  knee M12.06- ☑
  multiple site M12.09
  shoulder M12.01- ☑
  specified joint NEC M12.08
  vertebrae M12.08
  wrist M12.03- ☑
 psoriatic NEC L40.59
  interphalangeal, distal L40.51
 reactive M02.9
  in (due to)
   infective endocarditis I33.0 [M02.9]
  specified type NEC M02.80
   ankle M02.87- ☑
   elbow M02.82- ☑
   foot joint M02.87- ☑
   hand joint M02.84- ☑
   hip M02.85- ☑
   knee M02.86- ☑
   multiple site M02.89
   shoulder M02.81- ☑
   vertebra M02.88
   wrist M02.83- ☑
 specified form NEC M12.80
  ankle M12.87- ☑
  elbow M12.82- ☑
  foot joint M12.87- ☑
  hand joint M12.84- ☑
  hip M12.85- ☑
  knee M12.86- ☑
  multiple site M12.89
  shoulder M12.81- ☑
  specified joint NEC M12.88
  vertebrae M12.88
  wrist M12.83- ☑
 syringomyelic G95.0
 tabes dorsalis A52.16
 tabetic A52.16
 transient — *see* Arthropathy, specified form NEC
 traumatic M12.50
  ankle M12.57- ☑
  elbow M12.52- ☑
  foot joint M12.57- ☑
  hand joint M12.54- ☑
  hip M12.55- ☑
  knee M12.56- ☑
  multiple site M12.59
  shoulder M12.51- ☑
  specified joint NEC M12.58
  vertebrae M12.58
  wrist M12.53- ☑
Arthropyosis — *see* Arthritis, pyogenic or pyemic
Arthrosis (deformans) (degenerative) (localized) (*see also*
  Osteoarthritis) M19.90
 spine — *see* Spondylosis
Arthus' phenomenon or reaction T78.41 ☑
 due to
  drug — *see* Table of Drugs and Chemicals, by drug
Articular — *see* condition
Articulation, reverse (teeth) M26.24

Artificial
 insemination complication — *see* Complications, arti-
    ficial, fertilization
 opening status (functioning) (without complication)
    Z93.9
  anus (colostomy) Z93.3
  colostomy Z93.3
  cystostomy Z93.50
   appendico-vesicostomy Z93.52
   cutaneous Z93.51
   specified NEC Z93.59
  enterostomy Z93.4
  gastrostomy Z93.1
  ileostomy Z93.2
  intestinal tract NEC Z93.4
  jejunostomy Z93.4
  nephrostomy Z93.6
  specified ostomy NEC Z93.8
  tracheostomy Z93.0
  ureterostomy Z93.6
  urethrostomy Z93.6
  urinary tract NEC Z93.6
  vagina Z93.8
 vagina status Z93.8
Arytenoid — *see* condition
Asbestosis (occupational) J61
Ascariasis B77.9
 with
  complications NEC B77.89
  intestinal complications B77.0
  pneumonia, pneumonitis B77.81
Ascaridosis, ascaridiasis — *see* Ascariasis
Ascaris (infection) (infestation) (lumbricoides) — *see*
  Ascariasis
Ascending — *see* condition
ASC-H (atypical squamous cells cannot exclude high
  grade squamous intraepithelial lesion on cytologic
  smear)
 anus R85.611
 cervix R87.611
 vagina R87.621
Aschoff's bodies — *see* Myocarditis, rheumatic
Ascites (abdominal) R18.8
 cardiac I50.9
 chylous (nonfilarial) I89.8
  filarial — *see* Infestation, filarial
 due to
  cirrhosis, alcoholic K70.31
  hepatitis
   alcoholic K70.11
   chronic active K71.51
  S. japonicum B65.2
 heart I50.9
 malignant R18.0
 pseudochylous R18.8
 syphilitic A52.74
 tuberculous A18.31
ASC-US (atypical squamous cells of undetermined significance on cytologic smear)
 anus R85.610
 cervix R87.610
 vagina R87.620
Aseptic — *see* condition
Asherman's syndrome N85.6
Asialia K11.7
Asiatic cholera — *see* Cholera
Asimultagnosia (simultanagnosia) R48.3
Askin's tumor — *see* Neoplasm, connective tissue, malignant
Asocial personality F60.2
Asomatognosia R41.4
Aspartylglucosaminuria E77.1
Asperger's disease or syndrome F84.5
Aspergilloma — *see* Aspergillosis
Aspergillosis (with pneumonia) B44.9
 bronchopulmonary, allergic B44.81
 disseminated B44.7
 generalized B44.7
 pulmonary NEC B44.1
  allergic B44.81
  invasive B44.0
 specified NEC B44.89
 tonsillar B44.2
Aspergillus (flavus) (fumigatus) (infection) (terreus) —
  see Aspergillosis
Aspermatogenesis — *see* Azoospermia
Aspermia (testis) — *see* Azoospermia

☑ **Additional Character Required** — Refer to the Tabular List for Character Selection   ▽ Subterms under main terms may continue to next column or page

Asphyxia, asphyxiation (by) R09.01
  antenatal P84
  birth P84
  bunny bag — *see* Asphyxia, due to, mechanical threat to breathing, trapped in bed clothes
  crushing S28.0 ☑
  drowning T75.1 ☑
  gas, fumes, or vapor — *see* Table of Drugs and Chemicals
  inhalation — *see* Inhalation
  intrauterine P84
  local I73.00
    with gangrene I73.01
  mucus (*see also* Foreign body, respiratory tract, causing asphyxia)
  newborn P84
  pathological R09.01
  postnatal P84
    mechanical — *see* Asphyxia, due to, mechanical threat to breathing
  prenatal P84
  reticularis R23.1
  strangulation — *see* Asphyxia, due to, mechanical threat to breathing
  submersion T75.1 ☑
  traumatic T71.9 ☑
    due to
      crushed chest S28.0 ☑
      foreign body (in) — *see* Foreign body, respiratory tract, causing asphyxia
      low oxygen content of ambient air T71.20 ☑
        due to
          being trapped in
            low oxygen environment T71.29 ☑
              in car trunk T71.221 ☑
                circumstances undetermined T71.224 ☑
                done with intent to harm by
                  another person T71.223 ☑
                  self T71.222 ☑
              in refrigerator T71.231 ☑
                circumstances undetermined T71.234 ☑
                done with intent to harm by
                  another person T71.233 ☑
                  self T71.232 ☑
            cave-in T71.21 ☑
      mechanical threat to breathing (accidental) T71.191 ☑
        circumstances undetermined T71.194 ☑
        done with intent to harm by
          another person T71.193 ☑
          self T71.192 ☑
        hanging T71.161 ☑
          circumstances undetermined T71.164 ☑
          done with intent to harm by
            another person T71.163 ☑
            self T71.162 ☑
        plastic bag T71.121 ☑
          circumstances undetermined T71.124 ☑
          done with intent to harm by
            another person T71.123 ☑
            self T71.122 ☑
        smothering
          in furniture T71.151 ☑
            circumstances undetermined T71.154 ☑
            done with intent to harm by
              another person T71.153 ☑
              self T71.152 ☑
          under
            another person's body T71.141 ☑
              circumstances undetermined T71.144 ☑
              done with intent to harm T71.143 ☑
            pillow T71.111 ☑
              circumstances undetermined T71.114 ☑
              done with intent to harm by
                another person T71.113 ☑
                self T71.112 ☑
        trapped in bed clothes T71.131 ☑
          circumstances undetermined T71.134 ☑
          done with intent to harm by
            another person T71.133 ☑
            self T71.132 ☑

Asphyxia, asphyxiation — *continued*
  vomiting, vomitus — *see* Foreign body, respiratory tract, causing asphyxia
Aspiration
  amniotic (clear) fluid (newborn) P24.10
    with
      pneumonia (pneumonitis) P24.11
      respiratory symptoms P24.11
  blood
    newborn (without respiratory symptoms) P24.20
      with
        pneumonia (pneumonitis) P24.21
        respiratory symptoms P24.21
      specified age NEC — *see* Foreign body, respiratory tract
  bronchitis J69.0
  food or foreign body (with asphyxiation) — *see* Asphyxia, food
  liquor (amnii) (newborn) P24.10
    with
      pneumonia (pneumonitis) P24.11
      respiratory symptoms P24.11
  meconium (newborn) (without respiratory symptoms) P24.00
    with
      pneumonia (pneumonitis) P24.01
      respiratory symptoms P24.01
  milk (newborn) (without respiratory symptoms) P24.30
    with
      pneumonia (pneumonitis) P24.31
      respiratory symptoms P24.31
    specified age NEC — *see* Foreign body, respiratory tract
  mucus (*see also* Foreign body, by site, causing asphyxia)
    newborn P24.10
      with
        pneumonia (pneumonitis) P24.11
        respiratory symptoms P24.11
  neonatal P24.9
    specific NEC (without respiratory symptoms) P24.80
      with
        pneumonia (pneumonitis) P24.81
        respiratory symptoms P24.81
  newborn P24.9
    specific NEC (without respiratory symptoms) P24.80
      with
        pneumonia (pneumonitis) P24.81
        respiratory symptoms P24.81
  pneumonia J69.0
  pneumonitis J69.0
  syndrome of newborn — *see* Aspiration, by substance, with pneumonia
  vernix caseosa (newborn) P24.80
    with
      pneumonia (pneumonitis) P24.81
      respiratory symptoms P24.81
  vomitus (*see also* Foreign body, respiratory tract)
    newborn (without respiratory symptoms) P24.30
      with
        pneumonia (pneumonitis) P24.31
        respiratory symptoms P24.31
Asplenia (congenital) Q89.01
  postsurgical Z90.81
Assam fever B55.0
Assault, sexual — *see* Maltreatment
Assmann's focus NEC A15.0
Astasia (-abasia) (hysterical) F44.4
Asteatosis cutis L85.3
Astereognosia, astereognosis R48.1
Asterixis R27.8
  in liver disease K71.3
Asteroid hyalitis — *see* Deposit, crystalline
Asthenia, asthenic R53.1
  cardiac (*see also* Failure, heart) I50.9
    psychogenic F45.8
  cardiovascular (*see also* Failure, heart) I50.9
    psychogenic F45.8
  heart (*see also* Failure, heart) I50.9
    psychogenic F45.8
  hysterical F44.4
  myocardial (*see also* Failure, heart) I50.9
    psychogenic F45.8
  nervous F48.8
  neurocirculatory F45.8
  neurotic F48.8
  psychogenic F48.8
  psychoneurotic F48.8

Asthenia, asthenic — *continued*
  psychophysiologic F48.8
  reaction (psychophysiologic) F48.8
  senile R54
Asthenopia (*see also* Discomfort, visual)
  hysterical F44.6
  psychogenic F44.6
Asthenospermia — *see* Abnormal, specimen, male genital organs
Asthma, asthmatic (bronchial) (catarrh) (spasmodic) J45.909
  with
    chronic obstructive bronchitis J44.9
      with
        acute lower respiratory infection J44.0
        exacerbation (acute) J44.1
    chronic obstructive pulmonary disease J44.9
      with
        acute lower respiratory infection J44.0
        exacerbation (acute) J44.1
    exacerbation (acute) J45.901
    hay fever — *see* Asthma, allergic extrinsic
    rhinitis, allergic — *see* Asthma, allergic extrinsic
    status asthmaticus J45.902
  allergic extrinsic J45.909
    with
      exacerbation (acute) J45.901
      status asthmaticus J45.902
  atopic — *see* Asthma, allergic extrinsic
  cardiac — *see* Failure, ventricular, left
  cardiobronchial I50.1
  childhood J45.909
    with
      exacerbation (acute) J45.901
      status asthmaticus J45.902
  chronic obstructive J44.9
    with
      acute lower respiratory infection J44.0
      exacerbation (acute) J44.1
  collier's J60
  cough variant J45.991
  detergent J69.8
  due to
    detergent J69.8
    inhalation of fumes J68.3
  eosinophilic J82
  extrinsic, allergic — *see* Asthma, allergic extrinsic
  grinder's J62.8
  hay — *see* Asthma, allergic extrinsic
  heart I50.1
  idiosyncratic — *see* Asthma, nonallergic
  intermittent (mild) J45.20
    with
      exacerbation (acute) J45.21
      status asthmaticus J45.22
  intrinsic, nonallergic — *see* Asthma, nonallergic
  Kopp's E32.8
  late-onset J45.909
    with
      exacerbation (acute) J45.901
      status asthmaticus J45.902
  mild intermittent J45.20
    with
      exacerbation (acute) J45.21
      status asthmaticus J45.22
  mild persistent J45.30
    with
      exacerbation (acute) J45.31
      status asthmaticus J45.32
  Millar's (laryngismus stridulus) J38.5
  miner's J60
  mixed J45.909
    with
      exacerbation (acute) J45.901
      status asthmaticus J45.902
  moderate persistent J45.40
    with
      exacerbation (acute) J45.41
      status asthmaticus J45.42
  nervous — *see* Asthma, nonallergic
  nonallergic (intrinsic) J45.909
    with
      exacerbation (acute) J45.901
      status asthmaticus J45.902
  persistent
    mild J45.30
      with
        exacerbation (acute) J45.31

Asphyxia, asphyxiation — Asthma, asthmatic

Asthma, asthmatic — continued
  persistent — continued
    mild — continued
      with — continued
        status asthmaticus J45.32
      moderate J45.40
        with
          exacerbation (acute) J45.41
          status asthmaticus J45.42
      severe J45.50
        with
          exacerbation (acute) J45.51
          status asthmaticus J45.52
  platinum J45.998
  pneumoconiotic NEC J64
  potter's J62.8
  predominantly allergic J45.909
  psychogenic F54
  pulmonary eosinophilic J82
  red cedar J67.8
  Rostan's I50.1
  sandblaster's J62.8
  sequoiosis J67.8
  severe persistent J45.50
    with
      exacerbation (acute) J45.51
      status asthmaticus J45.52
  specified NEC J45.998
  stonemason's J62.8
  thymic E32.8
  tuberculous — see Tuberculosis, pulmonary
  Wichmann's (laryngismus stridulus) J38.5
  wood J67.8
Astigmatism (compound) (congenital) H52.20- ☑
  irregular H52.21- ☑
  regular H52.22- ☑
Astraphobia F40.220
Astroblastoma
  specified site — see Neoplasm, malignant, by site
  unspecified site C71.9
Astrocytoma (cystic)
  anaplastic
    specified site — see Neoplasm, malignant, by site
    unspecified site C71.9
  fibrillary
    specified site — see Neoplasm, malignant, by site
    unspecified site C71.9
  fibrous
    specified site — see Neoplasm, malignant, by site
    unspecified site C71.9
  gemistocytic
    specified site — see Neoplasm, malignant, by site
    unspecified site C71.9
  juvenile
    specified site — see Neoplasm, malignant, by site
    unspecified site C71.9
  pilocytic
    specified site — see Neoplasm, malignant, by site
    unspecified site C71.9
  piloid
    specified site — see Neoplasm, malignant, by site
    unspecified site C71.9
  protoplasmic
    specified site — see Neoplasm, malignant, by site
    unspecified site C71.9
  specified site NEC — see Neoplasm, malignant, by site
  subependymal D43.2
    giant cell
      specified site — see Neoplasm, uncertain be-
        havior, by site
      unspecified site D43.2
    specified site — see Neoplasm, uncertain behavior,
      by site
    unspecified site D43.2
  unspecified site C71.9
Astroglioma
  specified site — see Neoplasm, malignant, by site
  unspecified site C71.9
Asymbolia R48.8
Asymmetry (see also Distortion)
  between native and reconstructed breast N65.1
  face Q67.0
  jaw (lower) — see Anomaly, dentofacial, jaw-cranial
    base relationship, asymmetry
Asynergia, asynergy R27.8
  ventricular I51.89
Asystole (heart) — see Arrest, cardiac

At risk
  for falling Z91.81
Ataxia, ataxy, ataxic R27.0
  acute R27.8
  brain (hereditary) G11.9
  cerebellar (hereditary) G11.9
    with defective DNA repair G11.3
    alcoholic G31.2
    early-onset G11.1
    in
      alcoholism G31.2
      myxedema E03.9 [G13.2]
      neoplastic disease (see also Neoplasm)
        D49.9 [G13.1]
      specified disease NEC G32.81
    late-onset (Marie's) G11.2
  cerebral (hereditary) G11.9
  congenital nonprogressive G11.0
  family, familial — see Ataxia, hereditary
  following
    cerebrovascular disease I69.993
      cerebral infarction I69.393
      intracerebral hemorrhage I69.193
      nontraumatic intracranial hemorrhage NEC
        I69.293
      specified disease NEC I69.893
      subarachnoid hemorrhage I69.093
  Friedreich's (heredofamilial) (cerebellar) (spinal) G11.1
  gait R26.0
    hysterical F44.4
  general R27.8
  gluten M35.9 [G32.81]
    with celiac disease K90.0 [G32.81]
  hereditary G11.9
    with neuropathy G60.2
    cerebellar — see Ataxia, cerebellar
    spastic G11.4
    specified NEC G11.8
    spinal (Friedreich's) G11.1
  heredofamilial — see Ataxia, hereditary
  Hunt's G11.1
  hysterical F44.4
  locomotor (progressive) (syphilitic) (partial) (spastic)
    A52.11
    diabetic — see Diabetes, ataxia
  Marie's (cerebellar) (heredofamilial) (late- onset) G11.2
  nonorganic origin F44.4
  nonprogressive, congenital G11.0
  psychogenic F44.4
  Roussy-Lévy G60.0
  Sanger-Brown's (hereditary) G11.2
  spastic hereditary G11.4
  spinal
    hereditary (Friedreich's) G11.1
    progressive (syphilitic) A52.11
  spinocerebellar, X-linked recessive G11.1
  telangiectasia (Louis-Bar) G11.3
Ataxia-telangiectasia (Louis-Bar) G11.3
Atelectasis (massive) (partial) (pressure) (pulmonary)
    J98.11
  newborn P28.10
    due to resorption P28.11
    partial P28.19
    primary P28.0
    secondary P28.19
  primary (newborn) P28.0
  tuberculous — see Tuberculosis, pulmonary
Atelocardia Q24.9
Atelomyelia Q06.1
Atheroembolism
  of
    extremities
      lower I75.02- ☑
      upper I75.01- ☑
    kidney I75.81
    specified NEC I75.89
Atheroma, atheromatous (see also Arteriosclerosis)
    I70.90
  aorta, aortic I70.0
    valve (see also Endocarditis, aortic) I35.8
  aorto-iliac I70.0
  artery — see Arteriosclerosis
  basilar (artery) I67.2
  carotid (artery) (common) (internal) I67.2
  cerebral (arteries) I67.2
  coronary (artery) I25.10
    with angina pectoris — see Arteriosclerosis, coro-
      nary (artery),

Atheroma, atheromatous — continued
  degeneration — see Arteriosclerosis
  heart, cardiac — see Disease, heart, ischemic,
    atherosclerotic
  mitral (valve) I34.8
  myocardium, myocardial — see Disease, heart, is-
    chemic, atherosclerotic
  pulmonary valve (heart) (see also Endocarditis, pul-
    monary) I37.8
  tricuspid (heart) (valve) I36.8
  valve, valvular — see Endocarditis
  vertebral (artery) I67.2
Atheromatosis — see Arteriosclerosis
Atherosclerosis (see also Arteriosclerosis)
  coronary
    artery I25.10
      with angina pectoris — see Arteriosclerosis,
        coronary (artery),
      due to
        calcified coronary lesion (severely) I25.84
        lipid rich plaque I25.83
    transplanted heart I25.811
      bypass graft I25.812
        with angina pectoris — see Arteriosclerosis,
          coronary (artery),
      native coronary artery I25.811
        with angina pectoris — see Arteriosclerosis,
          coronary (artery),
Athetosis (acquired) R25.8
  bilateral (congenital) G80.3
  congenital (bilateral) (double) G80.3
  double (congenital) G80.3
  unilateral R25.8
Athlete's
  foot B35.3
  heart I51.7
Athrepsia E41
Athyrea (acquired) (see also Hypothyroidism)
  congenital E03.1
Atonia, atony, atonic
  bladder (sphincter) (neurogenic) N31.2
  capillary I78.8
  cecum K59.8
    psychogenic F45.8
  colon — see Atony, intestine
  congenital P94.2
  esophagus K22.8
  intestine K59.8
    psychogenic F45.8
  stomach K31.89
    neurotic or psychogenic F45.8
  uterus (during labor) O62.2
    with hemorrhage (postpartum) O72.1
    postpartum (with hemorrhage) O72.1
      without hemorrhage O75.89
Atopy — see History, allergy
Atransferrinemia, congenital E88.09
Atresia, atretic
  alimentary organ or tract NEC Q45.8
    upper Q40.8
  ani, anus, anal (canal) Q42.3
    with fistula Q42.2
  aorta (arch) (ring) Q25.2
  aortic (orifice) (valve) Q23.0
    arch Q25.2
    congenital with hypoplasia of ascending aorta and
      defective development of left ventricle (with
      mitral stenosis) Q23.4
    in hypoplastic left heart syndrome Q23.4
  aqueduct of Sylvius Q03.0
    with spina bifida — see Spina bifida, with hydro-
      cephalus
  artery NEC Q27.8
    cerebral Q28.3
    coronary Q24.5
    digestive system Q27.8
    eye Q15.8
    lower limb Q27.8
    pulmonary Q25.5
    specified site NEC Q27.8
    umbilical Q27.0
    upper limb Q27.8
  auditory canal (external) Q16.1
  bile duct (common) (congenital) (hepatic) Q44.2
    acquired — see Obstruction, bile duct
  bladder (neck) Q64.39
    obstruction Q64.31
  bronchus Q32.4

☑ **Additional Character Required — Refer to the Tabular List for Character Selection**   ▽ **Subterms under main terms may continue to next column or page**

Atresia, atretic — *continued*
cecum Q42.8
cervix (acquired) N88.2
  congenital Q51.828
  in pregnancy or childbirth — *see* Anomaly, cervix,
    in pregnancy or childbirth
    causing obstructed labor O65.5
choana Q30.0
colon Q42.9
  specified NEC Q42.8
common duct Q44.2
cricoid cartilage Q31.8
cystic duct Q44.2
  acquired K82.8
    with obstruction K82.0
digestive organs NEC Q45.8
duodenum Q41.0
ear canal Q16.1
ejaculatory duct Q55.4
epiglottis Q31.8
esophagus Q39.0
  with tracheoesophageal fistula Q39.1
eustachian tube Q17.8
fallopian tube (congenital) Q50.6
  acquired N97.1
follicular cyst N83.0
foramen of
  Luschka Q03.1
    with spina bifida — *see* Spina bifida, with hy-
      drocephalus
  Magendie Q03.1
    with spina bifida — *see* Spina bifida, with hy-
      drocephalus
gallbladder Q44.1
genital organ
  external
    female Q52.79
    male Q55.8
  internal
    female Q52.8
    male Q55.8
glottis Q31.8
gullet Q39.0
  with tracheoesophageal fistula Q39.1
heart valve NEC Q24.8
  pulmonary Q22.0
  tricuspid Q22.4
hymen Q52.3
  acquired (postinfective) N89.6
ileum Q41.2
intestine (small) Q41.9
  large Q42.9
    specified NEC Q42.8
iris, filtration angle Q15.0
jejunum Q41.1
lacrimal apparatus Q10.4
larynx Q31.8
meatus urinarius Q64.33
mitral valve Q23.2
  in hypoplastic left heart syndrome Q23.4
nares (anterior) (posterior) Q30.0
nasopharynx Q34.8
nose, nostril Q30.0
  acquired J34.89
organ or site NEC Q89.8
osseous meatus (ear) Q16.1
oviduct (congenital) Q50.6
  acquired N97.1
parotid duct Q38.4
  acquired K11.8
pulmonary (artery) Q25.5
  valve Q22.0
pulmonic Q22.0
pupil Q13.2
rectum Q42.1
  with fistula Q42.0
salivary duct Q38.4
  acquired K11.8
sublingual duct Q38.4
  acquired K11.8
submandibular duct Q38.4
  acquired K11.8
submaxillary duct Q38.4
  acquired K11.8
thyroid cartilage Q31.8
trachea Q32.1
tricuspid valve Q22.4

Atresia, atretic — *continued*
ureter Q62.10
  pelvic junction Q62.11
  vesical orifice Q62.12
ureteropelvic junction Q62.11
ureterovesical orifice Q62.12
urethra (valvular) Q64.39
  stricture Q64.32
urinary tract NEC Q64.8
uterus Q51.818
  acquired N85.8
vagina (congenital) Q52.4
  acquired (postinfectional) (senile) N89.5
vas deferens Q55.3
vascular NEC Q27.8
  cerebral Q28.3
  digestive system Q27.8
  lower limb Q27.8
  specified site NEC Q27.8
  upper limb Q27.8
vein NEC Q27.8
  digestive system Q27.8
  great Q26.8
  lower limb Q27.8
  portal Q26.5
  pulmonary Q26.3
  specified site NEC Q27.8
  upper limb Q27.8
vena cava (inferior) (superior) Q26.8
vesicourethral orifice Q64.31
vulva Q52.79
  acquired N90.5
Atrichia, atrichosis — *see* Alopecia
Atrophia (*see also* Atrophy)
cutis senilis L90.8
  due to radiation L57.8
gyrata of choroid and retina H31.23
senilis R54
  dermatological L90.8
    due to radiation (nonionizing) (solar) L57.8
unguium L60.3
  congenita Q84.6
Atrophie blanche (en plaque) (de Milian) L95.0
Atrophoderma, atrophodermia (of) L90.9
diffusum (idiopathic) L90.4
maculatum L90.8
  et striatum L90.8
    due to syphilis A52.79
  syphilitic A51.39
neuriticum L90.8
Pasini and Pierini L90.3
pigmentosum Q82.1
reticulatum symmetricum faciei L66.4
senile L90.8
  due to radiation (nonionizing) (solar) L57.8
vermiculata (cheeks) L66.4
Atrophy, atrophic (of)
adrenal (capsule) (gland) E27.49
  primary (autoimmune) E27.1
alveolar process or ridge (edentulous) K08.20
anal sphincter (disuse) N81.84
appendix K38.8
arteriosclerotic — *see* Arteriosclerosis
bile duct (common) (hepatic) K83.8
bladder N32.89
  neurogenic N31.8
blanche (en plaque) (of Milian) L95.0
bone (senile) NEC (*see also* Disorder, bone, specified
  type NEC)
  due to
    tabes dorsalis (neurogenic) A52.11
brain (cortex) (progressive) G31.9
  frontotemporal circumscribed G31.01 [F02.80]
    with behavioral disturbance G31.01 [F02.81]
  senile NEC G31.1
breast N64.2
  obstetric — *see* Disorder, breast, specified type
    NEC
buccal cavity K13.79
cardiac — *see* Degeneration, myocardial
cartilage (infectional) (joint) — *see* Disorder, cartilage,
  specified NEC
cerebellar — *see* Atrophy, brain
cerebral — *see* Atrophy, brain
cervix (mucosa) (senile) (uteri) N88.8
  menopausal N95.8
Charcot-Marie-Tooth G60.0

Atrophy, atrophic — *continued*
choroid (central) (macular) (myopic) (retina) H31.10- ☑
  diffuse secondary H31.12- ☑
  gyrate H31.23
  senile H31.11- ☑
ciliary body — *see* Atrophy, iris
conjunctiva (senile) H11.89
corpus cavernosum N48.89
cortical — *see* Atrophy, brain
cystic duct K82.8
Déjérine-Thomas G23.8
disuse NEC — *see* Atrophy, muscle
Duchenne-Aran G12.21
ear H93.8- ☑
edentulous alveolar ridge K08.20
endometrium (senile) N85.8
  cervix N88.8
enteric K63.89
epididymis N50.8
eyeball — *see* Disorder, globe, degenerated condition,
  atrophy
eyelid (senile) — *see* Disorder, eyelid, degenerative
facial (skin) L90.9
fallopian tube (senile) N83.32
  with ovary N83.33
fascioscapulohumeral (Landouzy- Déjérine) G71.0
fatty, thymus (gland) E32.8
gallbladder K82.8
gastric K29.40
  with bleeding K29.41
gastrointestinal K63.89
glandular I89.8
globe H44.52- ☑
gum K06.0
hair L67.8
heart (brown) — *see* Degeneration, myocardial
hemifacial Q67.4
  Romberg G51.8
infantile E41
  paralysis, acute — *see* Poliomyelitis, paralytic
intestine K63.89
iris (essential) (progressive) H21.26- ☑
  specified NEC H21.29
kidney (senile) (terminal) (*see also* Sclerosis, renal)
  N26.1
  congenital or infantile Q60.5
    bilateral Q60.4
    unilateral Q60.3
  hydronephrotic — *see* Hydronephrosis
lacrimal gland (primary) H04.14- ☑
  secondary H04.15- ☑
Landouzy-Déjérine G71.0
laryngitis, infective J37.0
larynx J38.7
Leber's optic (hereditary) H47.22
lip K13.0
liver (yellow) K72.90
  with coma K72.91
  acute, subacute K72.00
    with coma K72.01
  chronic K72.10
    with coma K72.11
lung (senile) J98.4
macular (dermatological) L90.8
  syphilitic, skin A51.39
    striated A52.79
mandible (edentulous) K08.20
  minimal K08.21
  moderate K08.22
  severe K08.23
maxilla K08.20
  minimal K08.24
  moderate K08.25
  severe K08.26
muscle, muscular (diffuse) (general) (idiopathic) (primary) M62.50
  ankle M62.57- ☑
  Duchenne-Aran G12.21
  foot M62.57- ☑
  forearm M62.53- ☑
  hand M62.54- ☑
  infantile spinal G12.0
  lower leg M62.56- ☑
  multiple sites M62.59
  myelopathic — *see* Atrophy, muscle, spinal
  myotonic G71.11
  neuritic G58.9
  neuropathic (peroneal) (progressive) G60.0

Atrophy, atrophic — *continued*
  muscle, muscular — *continued*
    pelvic (disuse) N81.84
    peroneal G60.0
    progressive (bulbar) G12.21
      adult G12.1
      infantile (spinal) G12.0
      spinal G12.9
        adult G12.1
        infantile G12.0
    pseudohypertrophic G71.0
    shoulder region M62.51- ☑
    specified site NEC M62.58
    spinal G12.9
      adult form G12.1
      Aran-Duchenne G12.21
      childhood form, type II G12.1
      distal G12.1
      hereditary NEC G12.1
      infantile, type I (Werdnig-Hoffmann) G12.0
      juvenile form, type III (Kugelberg- Welander) G12.1
      progressive G12.21
      scapuloperoneal form G12.1
      specified NEC G12.8
    syphilitic A52.78
    thigh M62.55- ☑
    upper arm M62.52- ☑
  myocardium — *see* Degeneration, myocardial
  myometrium (senile) N85.8
    cervix N88.8
  myopathic NEC — *see* Atrophy, muscle
  myotonia G71.11
  nail L60.3
  nasopharynx J31.1
  nerve (*see also* Disorder, nerve)
    abducens — *see* Strabismus, paralytic, sixth nerve
    accessory G52.8
    acoustic or auditory H93.3 ☑
    cranial G52.9
      eighth (auditory) H93.3 ☑
      eleventh (accessory) G52.8
      fifth (trigeminal) G50.8
      first (olfactory) G52.0
      fourth (trochlear) — *see* Strabismus, paralytic, fourth nerve
      second (optic) H47.20
      sixth (abducens) — *see* Strabismus, paralytic, sixth nerve
      tenth (pneumogastric) (vagus) G52.2
      third (oculomotor) — *see* Strabismus, paralytic, third nerve
      twelfth (hypoglossal) G52.3
    hypoglossal G52.3
    oculomotor — *see* Strabismus, paralytic, third nerve
    olfactory G52.0
    optic (papillomacular bundle) H47.20
      syphilitic (late) A52.15
        congenital A50.44
    pneumogastric G52.2
    trigeminal G50.8
    trochlear — *see* Strabismus, paralytic, fourth nerve
    vagus (pneumogastric) G52.2
  neurogenic, bone, tabetic A52.11
  nutritional E41
  old age R54
  olivopontocerebellar G23.8
  optic (nerve) H47.20
    glaucomatous H47.23- ☑
    hereditary H47.22
    primary H47.21- ☑
    specified type NEC H47.29- ☑
    syphilitic (late) A52.15
      congenital A50.44
  orbit H05.31- ☑
  ovary (senile) N83.31
    with fallopian tube N83.33
  oviduct (senile) — *see* Atrophy, fallopian tube
  palsy, diffuse (progressive) G12.22
  pancreas (duct) (senile) K86.8
  parotid gland K11.0
  pelvic muscle N81.84
  penis N48.89
  pharynx J39.2
  pluriglandular E31.8
    autoimmune E31.0
  polyarthritis M15.9

Atrophy, atrophic — *continued*
  prostate N42.89
  pseudohypertrophic (muscle) G71.0
  renal (*see also* Sclerosis, renal) N26.1
  retina, retinal (postinfectional) H35.89
  rhinitis J31.0
  salivary gland K11.0
  scar L90.5
  sclerosis, lobar (of brain) G31.09 [F02.80]
    with behavioral disturbance G31.09 [F02.81]
  scrotum N50.8
  seminal vesicle N50.8
  senile R54
    due to radiation (nonionizing) (solar) L57.8
  skin (patches) (spots) L90.9
    degenerative (senile) L90.8
    due to radiation (nonionizing) (solar) L57.8
    senile L90.8
  spermatic cord N50.8
  spinal (acute) (cord) G95.89
    muscular — *see* Atrophy, muscle, spinal
    paralysis G12.20
      acute — *see* Poliomyelitis, paralytic
      meaning progressive muscular atrophy G12.21
  spine (column) — *see* Spondylopathy, specified NEC
  spleen (senile) D73.0
  stomach K29.40
    with bleeding K29.41
  striate (skin) L90.6
    syphilitic A52.79
  subcutaneous L90.9
  sublingual gland K11.0
  submandibular gland K11.0
  submaxillary gland K11.0
  Sudeck's — *see* Algoneurodystrophy
  suprarenal (capsule) (gland) E27.49
    primary E27.1
  systemic affecting central nervous system in
      myxedema E03.9 [G13.2]
      neoplastic disease (*see also* Neoplasm) D49.9 [G13.1]
      specified disease NEC G13.8
  tarso-orbital fascia, congenital Q10.3
  testis N50.0
  thenar, partial — *see* Syndrome, carpal tunnel
  thymus (fatty) E32.8
  thyroid (gland) (acquired) E03.4
    with cretinism E03.1
    congenital (with myxedema) E03.1
  tongue (senile) K14.8
    papillae K14.4
  trachea J39.8
  tunica vaginalis N50.8
  turbinate J34.89
  tympanic membrane (nonflaccid) H73.82- ☑
    flaccid H73.81- ☑
  upper respiratory tract J39.8
  uterus, uterine (senile) N85.8
    cervix N88.8
    due to radiation (intended effect) N85.8
      adverse effect or misadventure N99.89
  vagina (senile) N95.2
  vas deferens N50.8
  vascular I99.8
  vertebra (senile) — *see* Spondylopathy, specified NEC
  vulva (senile) N90.5
  Werdnig-Hoffmann G12.0
  yellow — *see* Failure, hepatic
Attack, attacks
  with alteration of consciousness (with automatisms) — *see* Epilepsy, localization-related, symptomatic, with complex partial seizures
  without alteration of consciousness — *see* Epilepsy, localization-related, symptomatic, with simple partial seizures
  Adams-Stokes I45.9
  akinetic — *see* Epilepsy, generalized, specified NEC
  angina — *see* Angina
  atonic — *see* Epilepsy, generalized, specified NEC
  benign shuddering G25.83
  cataleptic — *see* Catalepsy
  coronary — *see* Infarct, myocardium
  cyanotic, newborn P28.2
  drop NEC R55
  epileptic — *see* Epilepsy
  heart — *see* infarct, myocardium
  hysterical F44.9

Attack, attacks — *continued*
  jacksonian — *see* Epilepsy, localization-related, symptomatic, with simple partial seizures
  myocardium, myocardial — *see* Infarct, myocardium
  myoclonic — *see* Epilepsy, generalized, specified NEC
  panic F41.0
  psychomotor — *see* Epilepsy, localization-related, symptomatic, with complex partial seizures
  salaam — *see* Epilepsy, spasms
  schizophreniform, brief F23
  shuddering, benign G25.83
  Stokes-Adams I45.9
  syncope R55
  transient ischemic (TIA) G45.9
    specified NEC G45.8
  unconsciousness R55
    hysterical F44.89
  vasomotor R55
  vasovagal (paroxysmal) (idiopathic) R55
Attention (to)
  artificial
    opening (of) Z43.9
      digestive tract NEC Z43.4
        colon Z43.3
        ilium Z43.2
        stomach Z43.1
      specified NEC Z43.8
      trachea Z43.0
      urinary tract NEC Z43.6
        cystostomy Z43.5
        nephrostomy Z43.6
        ureterostomy Z43.6
        urethrostomy Z43.6
      vagina Z43.7
  colostomy Z43.3
  cystostomy Z43.5
  deficit disorder or syndrome F98.8
    with hyperactivity — *see* Disorder, attention-deficit hyperactivity
  gastrostomy Z43.1
  ileostomy Z43.2
  jejunostomy Z43.4
  nephrostomy Z43.6
  surgical dressings Z48.01
  sutures Z48.02
  tracheostomy Z43.0
  ureterostomy Z43.6
  urethrostomy Z43.6
Attrition
  gum K06.0
  tooth, teeth (excessive) (hard tissues) K03.0
Atypical, atypism (*see also* condition)
  cells (on cytolgocial smear) (endocervical) (endometrial) (glandular)
    cervix R87.619
    vagina R87.629
  cervical N87.9
  endometrium N85.9
    hyperplasia N85.00
  parenting situation Z62.9
Auditory — *see* condition
Aujeszky's disease B33.8
Aurantiasis, cutis E67.1
Auricle, auricular (*see also* condition)
  cervical Q18.2
Auriculotemporal syndrome G50.8
Austin Flint murmur (aortic insufficiency) I35.1
Australian
  Q fever A78
  X disease A83.4
Autism, autistic (childhood) (infantile) F84.0
  atypical F84.9
Autodigestion R68.89
Autoerythrocyte sensitization (syndrome) D69.2
Autographism L50.3
Autoimmune
  disease (systemic) M35.9
  inhibitors to clotting factors D68.311
  lymphoproliferative syndrome [ALPS] D89.82
  thyroiditis E06.3
Autointoxication R68.89
Automatism G93.89
  with temporal sclerosis G93.81
  epileptic — *see* Epilepsy, localization-related, symptomatic, with complex partial seizures
  paroxysmal, idiopathic — *see* Epilepsy, localization-related, symptomatic, with complex partial seizures

Autonomic, autonomous
　bladder (neurogenic) N31.2
　hysteria seizure F44.5
Autosensitivity, erythrocyte D69.2
Autosensitization, cutaneous L30.2
Autosome — *see* condition by chromosome involved
Autotopagnosia R48.1
Autotoxemia R68.89
Autumn — *see* condition
Avellis' syndrome G46.8
Aversion
　oral R63.3
　　newborn P92.- ☑
　　nonorganic origin F98.2 ☑
　sexual F52.1
Aviator's
　disease or sickness — *see* Effect, adverse, high altitude
　ear T70.0 ☑
Avitaminosis (multiple) (*see also* Deficiency, vitamin)
　　E56.9
　B E53.9
　　with
　　　beriberi E51.11
　　　pellagra E52
　　B2 E53.0
　　B6 E53.1
　　B12 E53.8
　　D E55.9
　　　with rickets E55.0
　　G E53.0
　　K E56.1
　　nicotinic acid E52
AVNRT (atrioventricular nodal re-entrant tachycardia)
　　I47.1
AVRT (atrioventricular nodal re-entrant tachycardia) I47.1
Avulsion (traumatic)
　blood vessel — *see* Injury, blood vessel
　bone — *see* Fracture, by site
　cartilage (*see also* Dislocation, by site)
　　symphyseal (inner), complicating delivery O71.6
　external site other than limb — *see* Wound, open, by
　　site
　eye S05.7- ☑
　head (intracranial)
　　external site NEC S08.89 ☑
　　scalp S08.0 ☑
　internal organ or site — *see* Injury, by site
　joint (*see also* Dislocation, by site)
　　capsule — *see* Sprain, by site
　kidney S37.06- ☑
　ligament — *see* Sprain, by site
　limb (*see also* Amputation, traumatic, by site)
　　skin and subcutaneous tissue — *see* Wound, open,
　　　by site
　muscle — *see* Injury, muscle
　nerve (root) — *see* Injury, nerve
　scalp S08.0 ☑
　skin and subcutaneous tissue — *see* Wound, open, by
　　site
　spleen S36.032 ☑
　symphyseal cartilage (inner), complicating delivery
　　O71.6
　tendon — *see* Injury, muscle
　tooth S03.2 ☑
Awareness of heart beat R00.2
Axenfeld's
　anomaly or syndrome Q15.0
　degeneration (calcareous) Q13.4
Axilla, axillary (*see also* condition)
　breast Q83.1
Axonotmesis — *see* Injury, nerve
Ayerza's disease or syndrome (pulmonary artery scle-
　　rosis with pulmonary hypertension) I27.0
Azoospermia (organic) N46.01
　due to
　　drug therapy N46.021
　　efferent duct obstruction N46.023
　　infection N46.022
　　radiation N46.024
　　specified cause NEC N46.029
　　systemic disease N46.025
Azotemia R79.89
　meaning uremia N19
Aztec ear Q17.3
Azygos
　continuation inferior vena cava Q26.8
　lobe (lung) Q33.1

B

Baastrup's disease — *see* Kissing spine
Babesiosis B60.0
Babington's disease (familial hemorrhagic telangiecta-
　　sia) I78.0
Babinski's syndrome A52.79
Baby
　crying constantly R68.11
　floppy (syndrome) P94.2
Bacillary — *see* condition
Bacilluria N39.0
Bacillus (*see also* Infection, bacillus)
　abortus infection A23.1
　anthracis infection A22.9
　coli infection (*see also* Escherichia coli) B96.20
　Flexner's A03.1
　mallei infection A24.0
　Shiga's A03.0
　suipestifer infection — *see* Infection, salmonella
Back — *see* condition
Backache (postural) M54.9
　sacroiliac M53.3
　specified NEC M54.89
Backflow — *see* Reflux
Backward reading (dyslexia) F81.0
Bacteremia R78.81
　with sepsis — *see* Sepsis
Bactericholia — *see* Cholecystitis, acute
Bacterid, bacteride (pustular) L40.3
Bacterium, bacteria, bacterial
　agent NEC, as cause of disease classified elsewhere
　　B96.89
　in blood — *see* Bacteremia
　in urine — *see* Bacteriuria
Bacteriuria, bacteruria N39.0
　asymptomatic N39.0
Bacteroides
　fragilis, as cause of disease classified elsewhere B96.6
Bad
　heart — *see* Disease, heart
　trip
　　due to drug abuse — *see* Abuse, drug, hallucino-
　　　gen
　　due to drug dependence — *see* Dependence, drug,
　　　hallucinogen
Baelz's disease (cheilitis glandularis apostematosa) K13.0
Baerensprung's disease (eczema marginatum) B35.6
Bagasse disease or pneumonitis J67.1
Bagassosis J67.1
Baker's cyst — *see* Cyst, Baker's
Bakwin-Krida syndrome (craniometaphyseal dysplasia)
　　Q78.5
Balancing side interference M26.56
Balanitis (circinata) (erosiva) (gangrenosa) (phagedenic)
　　(vulgaris) N48.1
　amebic A06.82
　candidal B37.42
　due to Haemophilus ducreyi A57
　gonococcal (acute) (chronic) A54.09
　xerotica obliterans N48.0
Balanoposthitis N47.6
　gonococcal (acute) (chronic) A54.09
　ulcerative (specific) A63.8
Balanorrhagia — *see* Balanitis
Balantidiasis, balantidiosis A07.0
Bald tongue K14.4
Baldness (*see also* Alopecia)
　male-pattern — *see* Alopecia, androgenic
Balkan grippe A78
Balloon disease — *see* Effect, adverse, high altitude
Balo's disease (concentric sclerosis) G37.5
Bamberger-Marie disease — *see* Osteoarthropathy,
　　hypertrophic, specified type NEC
Bancroft's filariasis B74.0
Band(s)
　adhesive — *see* Adhesions, peritoneum
　anomalous or congenital (*see also* Anomaly, by site)
　　heart (atrial) (ventricular) Q24.8
　　intestine Q43.3
　　omentum Q43.3
　cervix N88.1
　constricting, congenital Q79.8
　gallbladder (congenital) Q44.1
　intestinal (adhesive) — *see* Adhesions, peritoneum

Band(s) — *continued*
　obstructive
　　intestine K56.5
　　peritoneum K56.5
　periappendiceal, congenital Q43.3
　peritoneal (adhesive) — *see* Adhesions, peritoneum
　uterus N73.6
　　internal N85.6
　vagina N89.5
Bandemia D72.825
Bandl's ring (contraction), complicating delivery O62.4
Bangkok hemorrhagic fever A91
Bang's disease (brucella abortus) A23.1
Bankruptcy, anxiety concerning Z59.8
Bannister's disease T78.3 ☑
　hereditary D84.1
Banti's disease or syndrome (with cirrhosis) (with portal
　　hypertension) K76.6
Bar, median, prostate — *see* Enlargement, enlarged,
　　prostate
Barcoo disease or rot — *see* Ulcer, skin
Barlow's disease E54
Barodontalgia T70.29 ☑
Baron Münchausen syndrome — *see* Disorder, facti-
　　tious
Barosinusitis T70.1 ☑
Barotitis T70.0 ☑
Barotrauma T70.29 ☑
　odontalgia T70.29 ☑
　otitic T70.0 ☑
　sinus T70.1 ☑
Barraquer (-Simons) **disease or syndrome** (progressive
　　lipodystrophy) E88.1
Barré-Guillain disease or syndrome G61.0
Barrel chest M95.4
Barré-Liéou syndrome (posterior cervical sympathetic)
　　M53.0
Barrett's
　disease — *see* Barrett's, esophagus
　esophagus K22.70
　　with dysplasia K22.719
　　　high grade K22.711
　　　low grade K22.710
　　without dysplasia K22.70
　syndrome — *see* Barrett's, esophagus
　ulcer K22.10
　　with bleeding K22.11
　　without bleeding K22.10
Bársony (-Polgár) (-Teschendorf) **syndrome** (corkscrew
　　esophagus) K22.4
Barth syndrome E78.71
Bartholinitis (suppurating) N75.8
　gonococcal (acute) (chronic) (with abscess) A54.1
Bartonellosis A44.9
　cutaneous A44.1
　mucocutaneous A44.1
　specified NEC A44.8
　systemic A44.0
Barton's fracture S52.56- ☑
Bartter's syndrome E26.81
Basal — *see* condition
Basan's (hidrotic) ectodermal dysplasia Q82.4
Baseball finger — *see* Dislocation, finger
Basedow's disease (exophthalmic goiter) — *see* Hyper-
　　thyroidism, with, goiter
Basic — *see* condition
Basilar — *see* condition
Bason's (hidrotic) ectodermal dysplasia Q82.4
Basopenia — *see* Agranulocytosis
Basophilia D72.824
Basophilism (cortico-adrenal) (Cushing's) (pituitary)
　　E24.0
Bassen-Kornzweig disease or syndrome E78.6
Bat ear Q17.5
Bateman's
　disease B08.1
　purpura (senile) D69.2
Bathing cramp T75.1 ☑
Bathophobia F40.248
Batten (-Mayou) **disease** E75.4
　retina E75.4 [H36]
Batten-Steiner syndrome G71.11
Battered — *see* Maltreatment
Battey Mycobacterium infection A31.0
Battle exhaustion F43.0
Battledore placenta O43.19- ☑

Baumgarten-Cruveilhier cirrhosis, disease or syndrome K74.69
Bauxite fibrosis (of lung) J63.1
Bayle's disease (general paresis) A52.17
Bazin's disease (primary) (tuberculous) A18.4
Beach ear — *see* Swimmer's, ear
Beaded hair (congenital) Q84.1
Béal conjunctivitis or syndrome B30.2
Beard's disease (neurasthenia) F48.8
Beat(s)
   atrial, premature I49.1
   ectopic I49.49
   elbow — *see* Bursitis, elbow
   escaped, heart I49.49
   hand — *see* Bursitis, hand
   knee — *see* Bursitis, knee
   premature I49.40
     atrial I49.1
     auricular I49.1
     supraventricular I49.1
Beau's
   disease or syndrome — *see* Degeneration, myocardial
   lines (transverse furrows on fingernails) L60.4
Bechterev's syndrome — *see* Spondylitis, ankylosing
Becker's
   cardiomyopathy I42.8
   disease
     idiopathic mural endomyocardial disease I42.3
     myotonia congenita, recessive form G71.12
   dystrophy G71.0
   pigmented hairy nevus D22.5
Beck's syndrome (anterior spinal artery occlusion) I65.8
Beckwith-Wiedemann syndrome Q87.3
Bed confinement status Z74.01
Bed sore — *see* Ulcer, pressure, by site
Bedbug bite(s) — *see* Bite(s), by site, superficial, insect
Bedclothes, asphyxiation or suffocation by — *see* Asphyxia, traumatic, due to, mechanical, trapped
Bednar's
   aphthae K12.0
   tumor — *see* Neoplasm, malignant, by site
Bedridden Z74.01
Bedsore — *see* Ulcer, pressure, by site
Bedwetting — *see* Enuresis
Bee sting (with allergic or anaphylactic shock) — *see* Toxicity, venom, arthropod, bee
Beer drinker's heart (disease) I42.6
Begbie's disease (exophthalmic goiter) — *see* Hyperthyroidism, with, goiter
Behavior
   antisocial
     adult Z72.811
     child or adolescent Z72.810
   disorder, disturbance — *see* Disorder, conduct
   disruptive — *see* Disorder, conduct
   drug seeking Z72.89
   inexplicable R46.2
   marked evasiveness R46.5
   obsessive-compulsive R46.81
   overactivity R46.3
   poor responsiveness R46.4
   self-damaging (life-style) Z72.89
   sleep-incompatible Z72.821
   slowness R46.4
   specified NEC R46.89
   strange (and inexplicable) R46.2
   suspiciousness R46.5
   type A pattern Z73.1
   undue concern or preoccupation with stressful events R46.6
   verbosity and circumstantial detail obscuring reason for contact R46.7
Behçet's disease or syndrome M35.2
Behr's disease — *see* Degeneration, macula
Beigel's disease or morbus (white piedra) B36.2
Bejel A65
Bekhterev's syndrome — *see* Spondylitis, ankylosing
Belching — *see* Eructation
Bell's
   mania F30.8
   palsy, paralysis G51.0
     infant or newborn P11.3
   spasm G51.3
Bence Jones albuminuria or proteinuria NEC R80.3
Bends T70.3 ☑
Benedikt's paralysis or syndrome G46.3

Benign (*see also* condition)
   prostatic hyperplasia — *see* Hyperplasia, prostate
Bennett's fracture (displaced) S62.21- ☑
Benson's disease — *see* Deposit, crystalline
Bent
   back (hysterical) F44.4
   nose M95.0
     congenital Q67.4
Bereavement (uncomplicated) Z63.4
Bergeron's disease (hysterical chorea) F44.4
Berger's disease — *see* Nephropathy, IgA
Beriberi (dry) E51.11
   heart (disease) E51.12
   polyneuropathy E51.11
   wet E51.12
     involving circulatory system E51.11
Berlin's disease or edema (traumatic) S05.8X- ☑
Berlock (berloque) **dermatitis** L56.2
Bernard-Horner syndrome G90.2
Bernard-Soulier disease or thrombopathia D69.1
Bernhardt (-Roth) **disease** — *see* Mononeuropathy, lower limb, meralgia paresthetica
Bernheim's syndrome — *see* Failure, heart, congestive
Bertielliasis B71.8
Berylliosis (lung) J63.2
Besnier-Boeck (-Schaumann) **disease** — *see* Sarcoidosis
Besnier's
   lupus pernio D86.3
   prurigo L20.0
Bestiality F65.89
Best's disease H35.50
Betalipoproteinemia, broad or floating E78.2
Beta-mercaptolactate-cysteine disulfiduria E72.09
Betting and gambling Z72.6
   pathological (compulsive) F63.0
Bezoar T18.9 ☑
   intestine T18.3 ☑
   stomach T18.2 ☑
Bezold's abscess — *see* Mastoiditis, acute
Bianchi's syndrome R48.8
Bicornate or bicornis uterus Q51.3
   in pregnancy or childbirth O34.59- ☑
     causing obstructed labor O65.5
Bicuspid aortic valve Q23.1
Biedl-Bardet syndrome Q87.89
Bielschowsky (-Jansky) **disease** E75.4
Biermer's (pernicious) **anemia or disease** D51.0
Biett's disease L93.0
Bifid (congenital)
   apex, heart Q24.8
   clitoris Q52.6
   kidney Q63.8
   nose Q30.2
   patella Q74.1
   scrotum Q55.29
   toe NEC Q74.2
   tongue Q38.3
   ureter Q62.8
   uterus Q51.3
   uvula Q35.7
Biforis uterus (suprasimplex) Q51.3
Bifurcation (congenital)
   gallbladder Q44.1
   kidney pelvis Q63.8
   renal pelvis Q63.8
   rib Q76.6
   tongue, congenital Q38.3
   trachea Q32.1
   ureter Q62.8
   urethra Q64.74
   vertebra Q76.49
Big spleen syndrome D73.1
Bigeminal pulse R00.8
Bilateral — *see* condition
Bile
   duct — *see* condition
   pigments in urine R82.2
Bilharziasis (*see also* Schistosomiasis)
   chyluria B65.0
   cutaneous B65.3
   galacturia B65.0
   hematochyluria B65.0
   intestinal B65.1
   lipemia B65.9
   lipuria B65.0
   oriental B65.2
   piarhemia B65.9

Bilharziasis — *continued*
   pulmonary NOS B65.9 [J99]
     pneumonia B65.9 [J17]
   tropical hematuria B65.0
   vesical B65.0
Biliary — *see* condition
Bilirubin metabolism disorder E80.7
   specified NEC E80.6
Bilirubinemia, familial nonhemolytic E80.4
Bilirubinuria R82.2
Biliuria R82.2
Bilocular stomach K31.2
Binswanger's disease I67.3
Biparta, bipartite
   carpal scaphoid Q74.0
   patella Q74.1
   vagina Q52.10
Bird
   face Q75.8
   fancier's disease or lung J67.2
Birth
   complications in mother — *see* Delivery, complicated
   compression during NOS P15.9
   defect — *see* Anomaly
   immature (less than 37 completed weeks) — *see* Preterm, newborn
     extremely (less than 28 completed weeks) — *see* Immaturity, extreme
   inattention, at or after — *see* Maltreatment, child, neglect
   injury NOS P15.9
     basal ganglia P11.1
     brachial plexus NEC P14.3
     brain (compression) (pressure) P11.2
     central nervous system NOS P11.9
     cerebellum P11.1
     cerebral hemorrhage P10.1
     external genitalia P15.5
     eye P15.3
     face P15.4
     fracture
       bone P13.9
         specified NEC P13.8
       clavicle P13.4
       femur P13.2
       humerus P13.3
       long bone, except femur P13.3
       radius and ulna P13.3
       skull P13.0
       spine P11.5
       tibia and fibula P13 3
     intracranial P11.2
       laceration or hemorrhage P10.9
         specified NEC P10.8
     intraventricular hemorrhage P10.2
     laceration
       brain P10.1
       by scalpel P15.8
       peripheral nerve P14.9
     liver P15.0
     meninges
       brain P11.1
       spinal cord P11.5
     nerve
       brachial plexus P14.3
       cranial NEC (except facial) P11.4
       facial P11.3
       peripheral P14.9
       phrenic (paralysis) P14.2
     paralysis
       facial nerve P11.3
       spinal P11.5
     penis P15.5
     rupture
       spinal cord P11.5
     scalp P12.9
     scalpel wound P15.8
     scrotum P15.5
     skull NEC P13.1
       fracture P13.0
     specified type NEC P15.8
     spinal cord P11.5
     spine P11.5
     spleen P15.1
     sternomastoid (hematoma) P15.2
     subarachnoid hemorrhage P10.3
     subcutaneous fat necrosis P15.6
     subdural hemorrhage P10.0

Birth — *continued*
  injury — *continued*
    tentorial tear P10.4
    testes P15.5
    vulva P15.5
  lack of care, at or after — *see* Maltreatment, child, ne-
    glect
  neglect, at or after — *see* Maltreatment, child, neglect
  palsy or paralysis, newborn, NOS (birth injury) P14.9
  premature (infant) — *see* Preterm, newborn
  shock, newborn P96.89
  trauma — *see* Birth, injury
  weight
    4000 grams to 4499 grams P08.1
    4500 grams or more P08.0
    low (2499 grams or less) — *see* Low, birthweight
      extremely (999 grams or less) — *see* Low,
        birthweight, extreme
Birthmark Q82.5
Birt-Hogg-Dube syndrome Q87.89
Bisalbuminemia E88.09
Biskra's button B55.1
Bite(s) (animal) (human)
  abdomen, abdominal
    wall S31.159 ☑
      with penetration into peritoneal cavity
        S31.659 ☑
      epigastric region S31.152 ☑
        with penetration into peritoneal cavity
          S31.652 ☑
      left
        lower quadrant S31.154 ☑
          with penetration into peritoneal cavity
            S31.654 ☑
        upper quadrant S31.151 ☑
          with penetration into peritoneal cavity
            S31.651 ☑
      periumbilic region S31.155 ☑
        with penetration into peritoneal cavity
          S31.655 ☑
      right
        lower quadrant S31.153 ☑
          with penetration into peritoneal cavity
            S31.653 ☑
        upper quadrant S31.150 ☑
          with penetration into peritoneal cavity
            S31.650 ☑
      superficial NEC S30.871 ☑
        insect S30.861 ☑
  alveolar (process) — *see* Bite, oral cavity
  amphibian (venomous) — *see* Venom, bite, amphibian
  animal (*see also* Bite, by site)
    venomous — *see* Venom
  ankle S91.05- ☑
    superficial NEC S90.57- ☑
      insect S90.56- ☑
  antecubital space — *see* Bite, elbow
  anus S31.835 ☑
    superficial NEC S30.877 ☑
      insect S30.867 ☑
  arm (upper) S41.15- ☑
    lower — *see* Bite, forearm
    superficial NEC S40.87- ☑
      insect S40.86- ☑
  arthropod NEC — *see* Venom, bite, arthropod
  auditory canal (external) (meatus) — *see* Bite, ear
  auricle, ear — *see* Bite, ear
  axilla — *see* Bite, arm
  back (*see also* Bite, thorax, back)
    lower S31.050 ☑
      with penetration into retroperitoneal space
        S31.051 ☑
      superficial NEC S30.870 ☑
        insect S30.860 ☑
  bedbug — *see* Bite(s), by site, superficial, insect
  breast S21.05- ☑
    superficial NEC S20.17- ☑
      insect S20.16- ☑
  brow — *see* Bite, head, specified site NEC
  buttock S31.805 ☑
    left S31.825 ☑
    right S31.815 ☑
    superficial NEC S30.870 ☑
      insect S30.860 ☑
  calf — *see* Bite, leg
  canaliculus lacrimalis — *see* Bite, eyelid

Bite(s) — *continued*
  canthus, eye — *see* Bite, eyelid
  centipede — *see* Toxicity, venom, arthropod, cen-
    tipede
  cheek (external) S01.45- ☑
    internal — *see* Bite, oral cavity
    superficial NEC S00.87 ☑
      insect S00.86 ☑
  chest wall — *see* Bite, thorax
  chigger B88.0
  chin — *see* Bite, head, specified site NEC
  clitoris — *see* Bite, vulva
  costal region — *see* Bite, thorax
  digit(s)
    hand — *see* Bite, finger
    toe — *see* Bite, toe
  ear (canal) (external) S01.35- ☑
    superficial NEC S00.47- ☑
      insect S00.46- ☑
  elbow S51.05- ☑
    superficial NEC S50.37- ☑
      insect S50.36- ☑
  epididymis — *see* Bite, testis
  epigastric region — *see* Bite, abdomen
  epiglottis — *see* Bite, neck, specified site NEC
  esophagus, cervical S11.25 ☑
    superficial NEC S10.17 ☑
      insect S10.16 ☑
  eyebrow — *see* Bite, eyelid
  eyelid S01.15- ☑
    superficial NEC S00.27- ☑
      insect S00.26- ☑
  face NEC — *see* Bite, head, specified site NEC
  finger(s) S61.259 ☑
    with
      damage to nail S61.359 ☑
    index S61.258 ☑
      with
        damage to nail S61.358 ☑
      left S61.251 ☑
        with
          damage to nail S61.351 ☑
      right S61.250 ☑
        with
          damage to nail S61.350 ☑
      superficial NEC S60.478 ☑
        insect S60.46- ☑
    little S61.25- ☑
      with
        damage to nail S61.35- ☑
      superficial NEC S60.47- ☑
        insect S60.46- ☑
    middle S61.25- ☑
      with
        damage to nail S61.35- ☑
      superficial NEC S60.47- ☑
        insect S60.46- ☑
    ring S61.25- ☑
      with
        damage to nail S61.35- ☑
      superficial NEC S60.47- ☑
        insect S60.46- ☑
    superficial NEC S60.479 ☑
      insect S60.469 ☑
    thumb — *see* Bite, thumb
  flank — *see* Bite, abdomen, wall
  flea — *see* Bite, by site, superficial, insect
  foot (except toe(s) alone) S91.35- ☑
    superficial NEC S90.87- ☑
      insect S90.86- ☑
    toe — *see* Bite, toe
  forearm S51.85- ☑
    elbow only — *see* Bite, elbow
    superficial NEC S50.87- ☑
      insect S50.86- ☑
  forehead — *see* Bite, head, specified site NEC
  genital organs, external
    female S31.552 ☑
      superficial NEC S30.876 ☑
        insect S30.866 ☑
      vagina and vulva — *see* Bite, vulva
    male S31.551 ☑
      penis — *see* Bite, penis
      scrotum — *see* Bite, scrotum
      superficial NEC S30.875 ☑
        insect S30.865 ☑

Bite(s) — *continued*
  genital organs, external — *continued*
    male — *continued*
      testes — *see* Bite, testis
  groin — *see* Bite, abdomen, wall
  gum — *see* Bite, oral cavity
  hand S61.45- ☑
    finger — *see* Bite, finger
    superficial NEC S60.57- ☑
      insect S60.56- ☑
    thumb — *see* Bite, thumb
  head S01.95 ☑
    cheek — *see* Bite, cheek
    ear — *see* Bite, ear
    eyelid — *see* Bite, eyelid
    lip — *see* Bite, lip
    nose — *see* Bite, nose
    oral cavity — *see* Bite, oral cavity
    scalp — *see* Bite, scalp
    specified site NEC S01.85 ☑
      superficial NEC S00.87 ☑
        insect S00.86 ☑
    superficial NEC S00.97 ☑
      insect S00.96 ☑
    temporomandibular area — *see* Bite, cheek
  heel — *see* Bite, foot
  hip S71.05- ☑
    superficial NEC S70.27- ☑
      insect S70.26- ☑
  hymen S31.45 ☑
  hypochondrium — *see* Bite, abdomen, wall
  hypogastric region — *see* Bite, abdomen, wall
  inguinal region — *see* Bite, abdomen, wall
  insect — *see* Bite, by site, superficial, insect
  instep — *see* Bite, foot
  interscapular region — *see* Bite, thorax, back
  jaw — *see* Bite, head, specified site NEC
  knee S81.05- ☑
    superficial NEC S80.27- ☑
      insect S80.26- ☑
  labium (majus) (minus) — *see* Bite, vulva
  lacrimal duct — *see* Bite, eyelid
  larynx S11.015 ☑
    superficial NEC S10.17 ☑
      insect S10.16 ☑
  leg (lower) S81.85- ☑
    ankle — *see* Bite, ankle
    foot — *see* Bite, foot
    knee — *see* Bite, knee
    superficial NEC S80.87- ☑
      insect S80.86- ☑
    toe — *see* Bite, toe
    upper — *see* Bite, thigh
  lip S01.551 ☑
    superficial NEC S00.571 ☑
      insect S00.561 ☑
  lizard (venomous) — *see* Venom, bite, reptile
  loin — *see* Bite, abdomen, wall
  lower back — *see* Bite, back, lower
  lumbar region — *see* Bite, back, lower
  malar region — *see* Bite, head, specified site NEC
  mammary — *see* Bite, breast
  marine animals (venomous) — *see* Toxicity, venom,
    marine animal
  mastoid region — *see* Bite, head, specified site NEC
  mouth — *see* Bite, oral cavity
  nail
    finger — *see* Bite, finger
    toe — *see* Bite, toe
  nape — *see* Bite, neck, specified site NEC
  nasal (septum) (sinus) — *see* Bite, nose
  nasopharynx — *see* Bite, head, specified site NEC
  neck S11.95 ☑
    involving
      cervical esophagus — *see* Bite, esophagus,
        cervical
      larynx — *see* Bite, larynx
      pharynx — *see* Bite, pharynx
      thyroid gland S11.15 ☑
      trachea — *see* Bite, trachea
    specified site NEC S11.85 ☑
      superficial NEC S10.87 ☑
        insect S10.86 ☑
    superficial NEC S10.97 ☑
      insect S10.96 ☑

▽ Subterms under main terms may continue to next column or page   ☑ Additional Character Required — Refer to the Tabular List for Character Selection   **37**

Birth — Bite

Bite(s) — *continued*
- neck — *continued*
  - throat S11.85 ☑
    - superficial NEC S10.17 ☑
      - insect S10.16 ☑
- nose (septum) (sinus) S01.25 ☑
  - superficial NEC S00.37 ☑
    - insect S00.36 ☑
- occipital region — *see* Bite, scalp
- oral cavity S01.552 ☑
  - superficial NEC S00.572 ☑
    - insect S00.562 ☑
- orbital region — *see* Bite, eyelid
- palate — *see* Bite, oral cavity
- palm — *see* Bite, hand
- parietal region — *see* Bite, scalp
- pelvis S31.050 ☑
  - with penetration into retroperitoneal space S31.051 ☑
  - superficial NEC S30.870 ☑
    - insect S30.860 ☑
- penis S31.25 ☑
  - superficial NEC S30.872 ☑
    - insect S30.862 ☑
- perineum
  - female — *see* Bite, vulva
  - male — *see* Bite, pelvis
- periocular area (with or without lacrimal passages) — *see* Bite, eyelid
- phalanges
  - finger — *see* Bite, finger
  - toe — *see* Bite, toe
- pharynx S11.25 ☑
  - superficial NEC S10.17 ☑
    - insect S10.16 ☑
- pinna — *see* Bite, ear
- poisonous — *see* Venom
- popliteal space — *see* Bite, knee
- prepuce — *see* Bite, penis
- pubic region — *see* Bite, abdomen, wall
- rectovaginal septum — *see* Bite, vulva
- red bug B88.0
- reptile NEC (*see also* Venom, bite, reptile)
  - nonvenomous — *see* Bite, by site
  - snake — *see* Venom, bite, snake
- sacral region — *see* Bite, back, lower
- sacroiliac region — *see* Bite, back, lower
- salivary gland — *see* Bite, oral cavity
- scalp S01.05 ☑
  - superficial NEC S00.07 ☑
    - insect S00.06 ☑
- scapular region — *see* Bite, shoulder
- scrotum S31.35 ☑
  - superficial NEC S30.873 ☑
    - insect S30.863 ☑
- sea-snake (venomous) — *see* Toxicity, venom, snake, sea snake
- shin — *see* Bite, leg
- shoulder S41.05- ☑
  - superficial NEC S40.27- ☑
    - insect S40.26- ☑
- snake (*see also* Venom, bite, snake)
  - nonvenomous — *see* Bite, by site
- spermatic cord — *see* Bite, testis
- spider (venomous) — *see* Toxicity, venom, spider
  - nonvenomous — *see* Bite, by site, superficial, insect
- sternal region — *see* Bite, thorax, front
- submaxillary region — *see* Bite, head, specified site NEC
- submental region — *see* Bite, head, specified site NEC
- subungual
  - finger(s) — *see* Bite, finger
  - toe — *see* Bite, toe
- superficial — *see* Bite, by site, superficial
- supraclavicular fossa S11.85 ☑
- supraorbital — *see* Bite, head, specified site NEC
- temple, temporal region — *see* Bite, head, specified site NEC
- temporomandibular area — *see* Bite, cheek
- testis S31.35 ☑
  - superficial NEC S30.873 ☑
    - insect S30.863 ☑
- thigh S71.15- ☑
  - superficial NEC S70.37- ☑
    - insect S70.36- ☑

Bite(s) — *continued*
- thorax, thoracic (wall) S21.95 ☑
  - back S21.25- ☑
    - with penetration into thoracic cavity S21.45- ☑
  - breast — *see* Bite, breast
  - front S21.15- ☑
    - with penetration into thoracic cavity S21.35- ☑
  - superficial NEC S20.97 ☑
    - back S20.47- ☑
    - front S20.37- ☑
    - insect S20.96 ☑
      - back S20.46- ☑
      - front S20.36- ☑
- throat — *see* Bite, neck, throat
- thumb S61.05- ☑
  - with
    - damage to nail S61.15- ☑
  - superficial NEC S60.37- ☑
    - insect S60.36- ☑
- thyroid S11.15 ☑
  - superficial NEC S10.87 ☑
    - insect S10.86 ☑
- toe(s) S91.15- ☑
  - with
    - damage to nail S91.25- ☑
  - great S91.15- ☑
    - with
      - damage to nail S91.25- ☑
  - lesser S91.15- ☑
    - with
      - damage to nail S91.25- ☑
  - superficial NEC S90.47- ☑
    - great S90.47- ☑
    - insect S90.46- ☑
      - great S90.46- ☑
- tongue S01.552 ☑
- trachea S11.025 ☑
  - superficial NEC S10.17 ☑
    - insect S10.16 ☑
- tunica vaginalis — *see* Bite, testis
- tympanum, tympanic membrane — *see* Bite, ear
- umbilical region S31.155 ☑
- uvula — *see* Bite, oral cavity
- vagina — *see* Bite, vulva
- venomous — *see* Venom
- vocal cords S11.035 ☑
  - superficial NEC S10.17 ☑
    - insect S10.16 ☑
- vulva S31.45 ☑
  - superficial NEC S30.874 ☑
    - insect S30.864 ☑
- wrist S61.55- ☑
  - superficial NEC S60.87- ☑
    - insect S60.86- ☑

Biting, cheek or lip K13.1
Biventricular failure (heart) I50.9
Björck (-Thorson) **syndrome** (malignant carcinoid) E34.0
Black
- death A20.9
- eye S00.1- ☑
- hairy tongue K14.3
- heel (foot) S90.3- ☑
- lung (disease) J60
- palm (hand) S60.22- ☑

Blackfan-Diamond anemia or syndrome (congenital hypoplastic anemia) D61.01
Blackhead L70.0
Blackout R55
Bladder — *see* condition
Blast (air) (hydraulic) (immersion) (underwater)
- blindness S05.8X- ☑
- injury
  - abdomen or thorax — *see* Injury, by site
  - ear (acoustic nerve trauma) — *see* Injury, nerve, acoustic, specified type NEC
  - syndrome NEC T70.8 ☑
Blastoma — *see* Neoplasm, malignant, by site
- pulmonary — *see* Neoplasm, lung, malignant
Blastomycosis, blastomycotic B40.9
- Brazilian — *see* Paracoccidioidomycosis
- cutaneous B40.3
- disseminated B40.7
- European — *see* Cryptococcosis
- generalized B40.7
- keloidal B48.0
- North American B40.9

Blastomycosis, blastomycotic — *continued*
- primary pulmonary B40.0
- pulmonary B40.2
  - acute B40.0
  - chronic B40.1
- skin B40.3
- South American — *see* Paracoccidioidomycosis
- specified NEC B40.89
Bleb(s) R23.8
- emphysematous (lung) (solitary) J43.9
- endophthalmitis H59.43
- filtering (vitreous), after glaucoma surgery Z98.83
- inflammed (infected), postprocedural H59.40
  - stage 1 H59.41
  - stage 2 H59.42
  - stage 3 H59.43
- lung (ruptured) J43.9
  - congenital — *see* Atelectasis
  - newborn P25.8
- subpleural (emphysematous) J43.9
Blebitis, postprocedural H59.40
- stage 1 H59.41
- stage 2 H59.42
- stage 3 H59.43
Bleeder (familial) (hereditary) — *see* Hemophilia
Bleeding (*see also* Hemorrhage)
- anal K62.5
- anovulatory N97.0
- atonic, following delivery O72.1
- capillary I78.8
  - puerperal O72.2
- contact (postcoital) N93.0
- due to uterine subinvolution N85.3
- ear — *see* Otorrhagia
- excessive, associated with menopausal onset N92.4
- familial — *see* Defect, coagulation
- following intercourse N93.0
- gastrointestinal K92.2
- hemorrhoids — *see* Hemorrhoids
- intermenstrual (regular) N92.3
  - irregular N92.1
- intraoperative — *see* Complication, intraoperative, hemorrhage
- irregular N92.6
- menopausal N92.4
- newborn, intraventricular — *see* Newborn, affected by, hemorrhage, intraventricular
- nipple N64.59
- nose R04.0
- ovulation N92.3
- postclimacteric N95.0
- postcoital N93.0
- postmenopausal N95.0
- postoperative — *see* Complication, postprocedural, hemorrhage
- preclimacteric N92.4
- puberty (excessive, with onset of menstrual periods) N92.2
- rectum, rectal K62.5
  - newborn P54.2
- tendencies — *see* Defect, coagulation
- throat R04.1
- tooth socket (post-extraction) K91.840
- umbilical stump P51.9
- uterus, uterine NEC N93.9
  - climacteric N92.4
  - dysfunctional of functional N93.8
  - menopausal N92.4
  - preclimacteric or premenopausal N92.4
  - unrelated to menstrual cycle N93.9
- vagina, vaginal (abnormal) N93.9
  - dysfunctional or functional N93.8
  - newborn P54.6
- vicarious N94.89
Blennorrhagia, blennorrhagic — *see* Gonorrhea
Blennorrhea (acute) (chronic) (*see also* Gonorrhea)
- inclusion (neonatal) (newborn) P39.1
- lower genitourinary tract (gonococcal) A54.00
- neonatorum (gonococcal ophthalmia) A54.31
Blepharelosis — *see* Entropion
Blepharitis (angularis) (ciliaris) (eyelid) (marginal) (nonulcerative) H01.009
- herpes zoster B02.39
- left H01.006
  - lower H01.005
  - upper H01.004
- right H01.003
  - lower H01.002

☑ Additional Character Required — Refer to the Tabular List for Character Selection

� Subterms under main terms may continue to next column or page

Blepharitis — *continued*
  right — *continued*
    upper H01.001
    squamous H01.029
      left H01.026
        lower H01.025
        upper H01.024
      right H01.023
        lower H01.022
        upper H01.021
    ulcerative H01.019
      left H01.016
        lower H01.015
        upper H01.014
      right H01.013
        lower H01.012
        upper H01.011
Blepharochalasis H02.30
  congenital Q10.0
  left H02.36
    lower H02.35
    upper H02.34
  right H02.33
    lower H02.32
    upper H02.31
Blepharoclonus H02.59
Blepharoconjunctivitis H10.50- ☑
  angular H10.52- ☑
  contact H10.53- ☑
  ligneous H10.51- ☑
Blepharophimosis (eyelid) H02.529
  congenital Q10.3
  left H02.526
    lower H02.525
    upper H02.524
  right H02.523
    lower H02.522
    upper H02.521
Blepharoptosis H02.40- ☑
  congenital Q10.0
  mechanical H02.41- ☑
  myogenic H02.42- ☑
  neurogenic H02.43- ☑
  paralytic H02.43- ☑
Blepharopyorrhea, gonococcal A54.39
Blepharospasm G24.5
  drug induced G24.01
Blighted ovum O02.0
Blind (*see also* Blindness)
  bronchus (congenital) Q32.4
  loop syndrome K90.2
    congenital Q43.8
  sac, fallopian tube (congenital) Q50.6
  spot, enlarged — *see* Defect, visual field, localized, scotoma, blind spot area
  tract or tube, congenital NEC — *see* Atresia, by site
Blindness (acquired) (congenital) (both eyes) H54.0
  blast S05.8X- ☑
  color — *see* Deficiency, color vision
  concussion S05.8X- ☑
  cortical H47.619
    left brain H47.612
    right brain H47.611
  day H53.11
  due to injury (current episode) S05.9- ☑
    sequelae — *code to* injury with seventh character S
  eclipse (total) — *see* Retinopathy, solar
  emotional (hysterical) F44.6
  face H53.16
  hysterical F44.6
  legal (both eyes) (USA definition) H54.8
  mind R48.8
  night H53.60
    abnormal dark adaptation curve H53.61
    acquired H53.62
    congenital H53.63
    specified type NEC H53.69
    vitamin A deficiency E50.5
  one eye (other eye normal) H54.40
    left (normal vision on right) H54.42
      low vision on right H54.12
    low vision, other eye H54.10
    right (normal vision on left) H54.41
      low vision on left H54.11
  psychic R48.8
  river B73.01
  snow — *see* Photokeratitis

Blindness — *continued*
  sun, solar — *see* Retinopathy, solar
  transient — *see* Disturbance, vision, subjective, loss, transient
  traumatic (current episode) S05.9- ☑
  word (developmental) F81.0
    acquired R48.0
    secondary to organic lesion R48.0
Blister (nonthermal)
  abdominal wall S30.821 ☑
  alveolar process S00.522 ☑
  ankle S90.52- ☑
  antecubital space — *see* Blister, elbow
  anus S30.827 ☑
  arm (upper) S40.82- ☑
  auditory canal — *see* Blister, ear
  auricle — *see* Blister, ear
  axilla — *see* Blister, arm
  back, lower S30.820 ☑
  beetle dermatitis L24.89
  breast S20.12- ☑
  brow S00.82 ☑
  calf — *see* Blister, leg
  canthus — *see* Blister, eyelid
  cheek S00.82 ☑
    internal S00.522 ☑
  chest wall — *see* Blister, thorax
  chin S00.82 ☑
  costal region — *see* Blister, thorax
  digit(s)
    foot — *see* Blister, toe
    hand — *see* Blister, finger
  due to burn — *see* Burn, by site, second degree
  ear S00.42- ☑
  elbow S50.32- ☑
  epiglottis S10.12 ☑
  esophagus, cervical S10.12 ☑
  eyebrow — *see* Blister, eyelid
  eyelid S00.22- ☑
  face S00.82 ☑
  fever B00.1
  finger(s) S60.429 ☑
    index S60.42- ☑
    little S60.42- ☑
    middle S60.42- ☑
    ring S60.42- ☑
  foot (except toe(s) alone) S90.82- ☑
    toe — *see* Blister, toe
  forearm S50.82- ☑
    elbow only — *see* Blister, elbow
  forehead S00.82 ☑
  fracture — *omit code*
  genital organ
    female S30.826 ☑
    male S30.825 ☑
  gum S00.522 ☑
  hand S60.52- ☑
  head S00.92 ☑
    ear — *see* Blister, ear
    eyelid — *see* Blister, eyelid
    lip S00.521 ☑
    nose S00.32 ☑
    oral cavity S00.522 ☑
    scalp S00.02 ☑
    specified site NEC S00.82 ☑
  heel — *see* Blister, foot
  hip S70.22- ☑
  interscapular region S20.429 ☑
  jaw S00.82 ☑
  knee S80.22- ☑
  larynx S10.12 ☑
  leg (lower) S80.82- ☑
    knee — *see* Blister, knee
    upper — *see* Blister, thigh
  lip S00.521 ☑
  malar region S00.82 ☑
  mammary — *see* Blister, breast
  mastoid region S00.82 ☑
  mouth S00.522 ☑
  multiple, skin, nontraumatic R23.8
  nail
    finger — *see* Blister, finger
    toe — *see* Blister, toe
  nasal S00.32 ☑
  neck S10.92 ☑
    specified site NEC S10.82 ☑

Blister — *continued*
  neck — *continued*
    throat S10.12 ☑
  nose S00.32 ☑
  occipital region S00.02 ☑
  oral cavity S00.522 ☑
  orbital region — *see* Blister, eyelid
  palate S00.522 ☑
  palm — *see* Blister, hand
  parietal region S00.02 ☑
  pelvis S30.820 ☑
  penis S30.822 ☑
  periocular area — *see* Blister, eyelid
  phalanges
    finger — *see* Blister, finger
    toe — *see* Blister, toe
  pharynx S10.12 ☑
  pinna — *see* Blister, ear
  popliteal space — *see* Blister, knee
  scalp S00.02 ☑
  scapular region — *see* Blister, shoulder
  scrotum S30.823 ☑
  shin — *see* Blister, leg
  shoulder S40.22- ☑
  sternal region S20.329 ☑
  submaxillary region S00.82 ☑
  submental region S00.82 ☑
  subungual
    finger(s) — *see* Blister, finger
    toe(s) — *see* Blister, toe
  supraclavicular fossa S10.82 ☑
  supraorbital S00.82 ☑
  temple S00.82 ☑
  temporal region S00.82 ☑
  testis S30.823 ☑
  thermal — *see* Burn, second degree, by site
  thigh S70.32- ☑
  thorax, thoracic (wall) S20.92 ☑
    back S20.42- ☑
    front S20.32- ☑
  throat S10.12 ☑
  thumb S60.32- ☑
  toe(s) S90.42- ☑
    great S90.42- ☑
  tongue S00.522 ☑
  trachea S10.12 ☑
  tympanum, tympanic membrane — *see* Blister, ear
  upper arm — *see* Blister, arm (upper)
  uvula S00.522 ☑
  vagina S30.824 ☑
  vocal cords S10.12 ☑
  vulva S30.824 ☑
  wrist S60.82- ☑
Bloating R14.0
Bloch-Sulzberger disease or syndrome Q82.3
Block, blocked
  alveolocapillary J84.10
  arborization (heart) I45.5
  arrhythmic I45.9
  atrioventricular (incomplete) (partial) I44.30
    with atrioventricular dissociation I44.2
    complete I44.2
      congenital Q24.6
    congenital Q24.6
    first degree I44.0
    second degree (types I and II) I44.1
    specified NEC I44.39
    third degree I44.2
    types I and II I44.1
  auriculoventricular — *see* Block, atrioventricular
  bifascicular (cardiac) I45.2
  bundle-branch (complete) (false) (incomplete) I45.4
    bilateral I45.2
    left I44.7
      with right bundle branch block I45.2
      hemiblock I44.60
        anterior I44.4
        posterior I44.5
      incomplete I44.7
        with right bundle branch block I45.2
    right I45.10
      with
        left bundle branch block I45.2
        left fascicular block I45.2
      specified NEC I45.19
    Wilson's type I45.19
  cardiac I45.9

Block, blocked — *continued*
  conduction I45.9
    complete I44.2
  fascicular (left) I44.60
    anterior I44.4
    posterior I44.5
    right I45.0
    specified NEC I44.69
  foramen Magendie (acquired) G91.1
    congenital Q03.1
      with spina bifida — *see* Spina bifida, by site,
        with hydrocephalus
  heart I45.9
    bundle branch I45.4
      bilateral I45.2
    complete (atrioventricular) I44.2
    congenital Q24.6
    first degree (atrioventricular) I44.0
    second degree (atrioventricular) I44.1
    specified type NEC I45.5
    third degree (atrioventricular) I44.2
  hepatic vein I82.0
  intraventricular (nonspecific) I45.4
    bundle branch
      bilateral I45.2
  kidney N28.9
    postcystoscopic or postprocedural N99.0
  Mobitz (types I and II) I44.1
  myocardial — *see* Block, heart
  nodal I45.5
  organ or site, congenital NEC — *see* Atresia, by site
  portal (vein) I81
  second degree (types I and II) I44.1
  sinoatrial I45.5
  sinoauricular I45.5
  third degree I44.2
  trifascicular I45.3
  tubal N97.1
  vein NOS I82.90
  Wenckebach (types I and II) I44.1
Blockage — *see* Obstruction
Blocq's disease F44.4
Blood
  constituents, abnormal R78.9
  disease D75.9
  donor — *see* Donor, blood
  dyscrasia D75.9
    with
      abortion — *see* Abortion, by type, complicated
        by, hemorrhage
      ectopic pregnancy O08.1
      molar pregnancy O08.1
    following ectopic or molar pregnancy O08.1
    newborn P61.9
    puerperal, postpartum O72.3
  flukes NEC — *see* Schistosomiasis
  in
    feces K92.1
      occult R19.5
    urine — *see* Hematuria
  mole O02.0
  occult in feces R19.5
  pressure
    decreased, due to shock following injury T79.4 ☑
    examination only Z01.30
    fluctuating I99.8
    high — *see* Hypertension
      borderline R03.0
      incidental reading, without diagnosis of hyper-
        tension R03.0
    low (*see also* Hypotension)
      incidental reading, without diagnosis of hy-
        potension R03.1
  spitting — *see* Hemoptysis
  staining cornea — *see* Pigmentation, cornea, stromal
  transfusion
    reaction or complication — *see* Complications,
      transfusion
  type
    A (Rh positive) Z67.10
      Rh negative Z67.11
    AB (Rh positive) Z67.30
      Rh negative Z67.31
    B (Rh positive) Z67.20
      Rh negative Z67.21
    O (Rh positive) Z67.40
      Rh negative Z67.41
    Rh (positive) Z67.90

Blood — *continued*
  type — *continued*
    Rh (positive) Z67.90
      negative Z67.91
  vessel rupture — *see* Hemorrhage
  vomiting — *see* Hematemesis
Blood-forming organs, disease D75.9
Bloodgood's disease — *see* Mastopathy, cystic
Bloom (-Machacek)(-Torre) **syndrome** Q82.8
Blount's disease or osteochondrosis — *see* Osteochondrosis, juvenile, tibia
Blue
  baby Q24.9
  diaper syndrome E72.09
  dome cyst (breast) — *see* Cyst, breast
  dot cataract Q12.0
  nevus D22.9
  sclera Q13.5
    with fragility of bone and deafness Q78.0
  toe syndrome I75.02- ☑
Blueness — *see* Cyanosis
Blues, postpartal O90.6
  baby O90.6
Blurring, visual H53.8
Blushing (abnormal) (excessive) R23.2
BMI — *see* Body, mass index
Boarder, hospital NEC Z76.4
  accompanying sick person Z76.3
  healthy infant or child Z76.2
    foundling Z76.1
Bockhart's impetigo L01.02
Bodechtel-Guttman disease (subacute sclerosing panencephalitis) A81.1
Boder-Sedgwick syndrome (ataxia-telangiectasia)
  G11.3
Body, bodies
  Aschoff's — *see* Myocarditis, rheumatic
  asteroid, vitreous — *see* Deposit, crystalline
  cytoid (retina) — *see* Occlusion, artery, retina
  drusen (degenerative) (macula) (retinal) (*see also* De-
    generation, macula, drusen)
    optic disc — *see* Drusen, optic disc
  foreign — *see* Foreign body
  loose
    joint, except knee — *see* Loose, body, joint
      knee M23.4- ☑
    sheath, tendon — *see* Disorder, tendon, specified
      type NEC
  mass index (BMI)
    adult
      19 or less Z68.1
      20.0-20.9 Z68.20
      21.0-21.9 Z68.21
      22.0-22.9 Z68.22
      23.0-23.9 Z68.23
      24.0-24.9 Z68.24
      25.0-25.9 Z68.25
      26.0-26.9 Z68.26
      27.0-27.9 Z68.27
      28.0-28.9 Z68.28
      29.0-29.9 Z68.29
      30.0-30.9 Z68.30
      31.0-31.9 Z68.31
      32.0-32.9 Z68.32
      33.0-33.9 Z68.33
      34.0-34.9 Z68.34
      35.0-35.9 Z68.35
      36.0-36.9 Z68.36
      37.0-37.9 Z68.37
      38.0-38.9 Z68.38
      39.0-39.9 Z68.39
      40.0-44.9 Z68.41
      45.0-49.9 Z68.42
      50.0-59.9 Z68.43
      60.0-69.9 Z68.44
      70 and over Z68.45
    pediatric
      5th percentile to less than 85th percentile for
        age Z68.52
      85th percentile to less than 95th percentile for
        age Z68.53
      less than fifth percentile for age Z68.51
      greater than or equal to ninety-fifth percentile
        for age Z68.54
  Mooser's A75.2
  rice (*see also* Loose, body, joint)
    knee M23.4- ☑
  rocking F98.4

Boeck's
  disease or sarcoid — *see* Sarcoidosis
  lupoid (miliary) D86.3
Boerhaave's syndrome (spontaneous esophageal rup-
  ture) K22.3
Boggy
  cervix N88.8
  uterus N85.8
Boil (*see also* Furuncle, by site)
  Aleppo B55.1
  Baghdad B55.1
  Delhi B55.1
  lacrimal
    gland — *see* Dacryoadenitis
    passages (duct) (sac) — *see* Inflammation, lacrimal,
      passages, acute
  Natal B55.1
  orbit, orbital — *see* Abscess, orbit
  tropical B55.1
Bold hives — *see* Urticaria
Bombé, iris — *see* Membrane, pupillary
Bone — *see* condition
Bonnevie-Ullrich syndrome Q87.1
Bonnier's syndrome H81.8 ☑
Bonvale dam fever T73.3 ☑
Bony block of joint — *see* Ankylosis
BOOP (bronchiolitis obliterans organized pneumonia)
  J84.89
Borderline
  diabetes mellitus R73.09
  hypertension R03.0
  osteopenia M85.8- ☑
  pelvis, with obstruction during labor O65.1
  personality F60.3
Borna disease A83.9
Bornholm disease B33.0
Boston exanthem A88.0
Botalli, ductus (patent) (persistent) Q25.0
Bothriocephalus latus infestation B70.0
Botulism (foodborne intoxication) A05.1
  infant A48.51
  non-foodborne A48.52
  wound A48.52
Bouba — *see* Yaws
Bouchard's nodes (with arthropathy) M15.2
Bouffée délirante F23
Bouillaud's disease or syndrome (rheumatic heart
  disease) I01.9
Bourneville's disease Q85.1
Boutonniere deformity (finger) — *see* Deformity, finger,
  boutonniere
Bouveret (-Hoffmann) **syndrome** (paroxysmal tachycar-
  dia) I47.9
Bovine heart — *see* Hypertrophy, cardiac
Bowel — *see* condition
Bowen's
  dermatosis (precancerous) — *see* Neoplasm, skin, in
    situ
  disease — *see* Neoplasm, skin, in situ
  epithelioma — *see* Neoplasm, skin, in situ
  type
    epidermoid carcinoma-in-situ — *see* Neoplasm,
      skin, in situ
    intraepidermal squamous cell carcinoma — *see*
      Neoplasm, skin, in situ
Bowing
  femur (*see also* Deformity, limb, specified type NEC,
    thigh)
    congenital Q68.3
  fibula (*see also* Deformity, limb, specified type NEC,
    lower leg)
    congenital Q68.4
  forearm — *see* Deformity, limb, specified type NEC,
    forearm
  leg(s), long bones, congenital Q68.5
  radius — *see* Deformity, limb, specified type NEC,
    forearm
  tibia (*see also* Deformity, limb, specified type NEC,
    lower leg)
    congenital Q68.4
Bowleg(s) (acquired) M21.16- ☑
  congenital Q68.5
  rachitic E64.3
Boyd's dysentery A03.2
Brachial — *see* condition
Brachycardia R00.1
Brachycephaly Q75.0

☑ **Additional Character Required** — Refer to the Tabular List for Character Selection ▽ Subterms under main terms may continue to next column or page

Bradley's disease A08.19
Bradyarrhythmia, cardiac I49.8
Bradycardia (sinoatrial) (sinus) (vagal) R00.1
    neonatal P29.12
    reflex G90.09
    tachycardia syndrome I49.5
Bradykinesia R25.8
Bradypnea R06.89
Bradytachycardia I49.5
Brailsford's disease or osteochondrosis — *see* Osteochondrosis, juvenile, radius
Brain (*see also* condition)
    death G93.82
    syndrome — *see* Syndrome, brain
Branched-chain amino-acid disorder E71.2
Branchial — *see* condition
    cartilage, congenital Q18.2
Branchiogenic remnant (in neck) Q18.0
Brandt's syndrome (acrodermatitis enteropathica) E83.2
Brash (water) R12
Bravais-jacksonian epilepsy — *see* Epilepsy, localization-related, symptomatic, with simple partial seizures
Braxton Hicks contractions — *see* False, labor
Brazilian leishmaniasis B55.2
BRBPR K62.5
Break, retina (without detachment) H33.30- ☑
    with retinal detachment — *see* Detachment, retina
    horseshoe tear H33.31- ☑
    multiple H33.33- ☑
    round hole H33.32- ☑
Breakdown
    device, graft or implant (*see also* Complications, by site and type, mechanical) T85.618 ☑
        arterial graft NEC — *see* Complication, cardiovascular device, mechanical, vascular
        breast (implant) T85.41 ☑
        catheter NEC T85.618 ☑
            cystostomy T83.010 ☑
            dialysis (renal) T82.41 ☑
                intraperitoneal T85.611 ☑
            infusion NEC T82.514 ☑
                spinal (epidural) (subdural) T85.610 ☑
            urinary (indwelling) T83.018 ☑
        electronic (electrode) (pulse generator) (stimulator)
            bone T84.310 ☑
            cardiac T82.119 ☑
                electrode T82.110 ☑
                pulse generator T82.111 ☑
                specified type NEC T82.118 ☑
        nervous system — *see* Complication, prosthetic device, mechanical, electronic nervous system stimulator
        urinary — *see* Complication, genitourinary, device, urinary, mechanical
        fixation, internal (orthopedic) NEC — *see* Complication, fixation device, mechanical
        gastrointestinal — *see* Complications, prosthetic device, mechanical, gastrointestinal device
        genital NEC T83.418 ☑
            intrauterine contraceptive device T83.31 ☑
            penile prosthesis T83.410 ☑
        heart NEC — *see* Complication, cardiovascular device, mechanical
        joint prosthesis — *see* Complications..., joint prosthesis, internal, mechanical, by site
        ocular NEC — *see* Complications, prosthetic device, mechanical, ocular device
        orthopedic NEC — *see* Complication, orthopedic, device, mechanical
        specified NEC T85.618 ☑
        sutures, permanent T85.612 ☑
            used in bone repair — *see* Complications, fixation device, internal (orthopedic), mechanical
        urinary NEC (*see also* Complication, genitourinary, device, urinary, mechanical)
            graft T83.21 ☑
        vascular NEC — *see* Complication, cardiovascular device, mechanical
        ventricular intracranial shunt T85.01 ☑
    nervous F48.8
    perineum O90.1
    respirator J95.850
        specified NEC J95.859
    ventilator

Breakdown — *continued*
    ventilator J95.850
        specified NEC J95.859
Breast (*see also* condition)
    buds E30.1
        in newborn P96.89
    dense R92.2
    nodule N63
Breath
    foul R19.6
    holder, child R06.89
    holding spell R06.89
    shortness R06.02
Breathing
    labored — *see* Hyperventilation
    mouth R06.5
        causing malocclusion M26.5 ☑
    periodic R06.3
        high altitude G47.32
Breathlessness R06.81
Breda's disease — *see* Yaws
Breech presentation (mother) O32.1 ☑
    causing obstructed labor O64.1 ☑
    footling O32.8 ☑
        causing obstructed labor O64.8 ☑
    incomplete O32.8 ☑
        causing obstructed labor O64.8 ☑
Breisky's disease N90.4
Brennemann's syndrome I88.0
Brenner
    tumor (benign) D27.9
        borderline malignancy D39.1- ☑
        malignant C56 ☑
        proliferating D39.1- ☑
Bretonneau's disease or angina A36.0
Breus' mole O02.0
Brevicollis Q76.49
Brickmakers' anemia B76.9 [D63.8]
Bridge, myocardial Q24.5
Bright red blood per rectum (BRBPR) K62.5
Bright's disease (*see also* Nephritis)
    arteriosclerotic — *see* Hypertension, kidney
Brill (-Zinsser) **disease** (recrudescent typhus) A75.1
    flea-borne A75.2
    louse-borne A75.1
Brill-Symmers' disease C82.90
Brion-Kayser disease — *see* Fever, parathyroid
Briquet's disorder or syndrome F45.0
Brissaud's
    infantilism or dwarfism E23.0
    motor-verbal tic F95.2
Brittle
    bones disease Q78.0
    nails L60.3
        congenital Q84.6
Broad (*see also* condition)
    beta disease E78.2
    ligament laceration syndrome N83.8
Broad- or floating-betalipoproteinemia E78.2
Brock's syndrome (atelectasis due to enlarged lymph nodes) J98.19
Brocq-Duhring disease (dermatitis herpetiformis) L13.0
Brodie's abscess or disease M86.8X- ☑
Broken
    arches (*see also* Deformity, limb, flat foot)
    arm (meaning upper limb) — *see* Fracture, arm
    back — *see* Fracture, vertebra
    bone — *see* Fracture
    implant or internal device — *see* Complications, by site and type, mechanical
    leg (meaning lower limb) — *see* Fracture, leg
    nose S02.2 ☑
    tooth, teeth — *see* Fracture, tooth
Bromhidrosis, bromidrosis L75.0
Bromidism, bromism G92
    chronic (dependence) F13.20
    due to
        correct substance properly administered — *see* Table of Drugs and Chemicals, by drug, adverse effect
        overdose or wrong substance given or taken — *see* Table of Drugs and Chemicals, by drug, poisoning
Bromidrosiphobia F40.298
Bronchi, bronchial — *see* condition
Bronchiectasis (cylindrical) (diffuse) (fusiform) (localized) (saccular) J47.9

Bronchiectasis — *continued*
    with
        acute
            bronchitis J47.0
            lower respiratory infection J47.0
        exacerbation (acute) J47.1
    congenital Q33.4
    tuberculous NEC — *see* Tuberculosis, pulmonary
Bronchiolectasis — *see* Bronchiectasis
Bronchiolitis (acute) (infective) (subacute) J21.9
    with
        bronchospasm or obstruction J21.9
        influenza, flu or grippe — *see* Influenza, with, respiratory manifestations NEC
    chemical (chronic) J68.4
        acute J68.0
    chronic (fibrosing) (obliterative) J44.9
    due to
        external agent — *see* Bronchitis, acute, due to
        human metapneumovirus J21.1
        respiratory syncytial virus J21.0
        specified organism NEC J21.8
    fibrosa obliterans J44.9
    influenzal — *see* Influenza, with, respiratory manifestations NEC
    obliterans J42
        with organizing pneumonia (BOOP) J84.89
    obliterative (chronic) (subacute) J44.9
        due to chemicals, gases, fumes or vapors (inhalation) J68.4
        due to fumes or vapors J68.4
    respiratory, interstitial lung disease J84.115
Bronchitis (diffuse) (fibrinous) (hypostatic) (infective) (membranous) J40
    with
        influenza, flu or grippe — *see* Influenza, with, respiratory manifestations NEC
        obstruction (airway) (lung) J44.9
        tracheitis (l5 years of age and above) J40
            acute or subacute J20.9
            chronic J42
            under l5 years of age J20.9
    acute or subacute (with bronchospasm or obstruction) J20.9
        with
            bronchiectasis J47.0
            chronic obstructive pulmonary disease J44.0
        chemical (due to gases, fumes or vapors) J68.0
        due to
            fumes or vapors J68.0
            Haemophilus influenzae J20.1
            Mycoplasma pneumoniae J20.0
            radiation J70.0
            specified organism NEC J20.8
            Streptococcus J20.2
            virus
                coxsackie J20.3
                echovirus J20.7
                parainfluenzae J20.4
                respiratory syncytial J20.5
                rhinovirus J20.6
        viral NEC J20.8
    allergic (acute) J45.909
        with
            exacerbation (acute) J45.901
            status asthmaticus J45.902
    arachidic T17.528 ☑
    aspiration (due to fumes or vapors) J68.0
    asthmatic J45.9 ☑
        chronic J44.9
            with
                acute lower respiratory infection J44.0
                exacerbation (acute) J44.1
    capillary — *see* Pneumonia, broncho
    caseous (tuberculous) A15.5
    Castellani's A69.8
    catarrhal (l5 years of age and above) J40
        acute — *see* Bronchitis, acute
        chronic J41.0
        under l5 years of age J20.9
    chemical (acute) (subacute) J68.0
        chronic J68.4
        due to fumes or vapors J68.0
            chronic J68.4
    chronic J42
        with
            airways obstruction J44.9
            tracheitis (chronic) J42

Bronchitis — *continued*
  chronic — *continued*
    asthmatic (obstructive) J44.9
    catarrhal J41.0
    chemical (due to fumes or vapors) J68.4
    due to
      chemicals, gases, fumes or vapors (inhalation) J68.4
      radiation J70.1
      tobacco smoking J41.0
    emphysematous J44.9
    mucopurulent J41.1
    non-obstructive J41.0
    obliterans J44.9
    obstructive J44.9
    purulent J41.1
    simple J41.0
  croupous — *see* Bronchitis, acute
  due to gases, fumes or vapors (chemical) J68.0
  emphysematous (obstructive) J44.9
  exudative — *see* Bronchitis, acute
  fetid J41.1
  grippal — *see* Influenza, with, respiratory manifestations NEC
  in those under 15 years age — *see* Bronchitis, acute
    chronic — *see* Bronchitis, chronic
  influenzal — *see* Influenza, with, respiratory manifestations NEC
  mixed simple and mucopurulent J41.8
  moulder's J62.8
  mucopurulent (chronic) (recurrent) J41.1
    acute or subacute J20.9
    simple (mixed) J41.8
  obliterans (chronic) J44.9
  obstructive (chronic) (diffuse) J44.9
  pituitous J41.1
  pneumococcal, acute or subacute J20.2
  pseudomembranous, acute or subacute — *see* Bronchitis, acute
  purulent (chronic) (recurrent) J41.1
    acute or subacute — *see* Bronchitis, acute
  putrid J41.1
  senile (chronic) J42
  simple and mucopurulent (mixed) J41.8
  smokers' J41.0
  spirochetal NEC A69.8
  subacute — *see* Bronchitis, acute
  suppurative (chronic) J41.1
    acute or subacute — *see* Bronchitis, acute
  tuberculous A15.5
  under 15 years of age — *see* Bronchitis, acute
    chronic — *see* Bronchitis, chronic
  viral NEC, acute or subacute (*see also* Bronchitis, acute) J20.8
Bronchoalveolitis J18.0
Bronchoaspergillosis B44.1
Bronchocele meaning goiter E04.0
Broncholithiasis J98.09
  tuberculous NEC A15.5
Bronchomalacia J98.09
  congenital Q32.2
Bronchomycosis NOS B49 [J99]
  candidal B37.1
Bronchopleuropneumonia — *see* Pneumonia, broncho
Bronchopneumonia — *see* Pneumonia, broncho
Bronchopneumonitis — *see* Pneumonia, broncho
Bronchopulmonary — *see* condition
Bronchopulmonitis — *see* Pneumonia, broncho
Bronchorrhagia (see Hemoptysis)
Bronchorrhea J98.09
  acute J20.9
  chronic (infective) (purulent) J42
Bronchospasm (acute) J98.01
  with
    bronchiolitis, acute J21.9
    bronchitis, acute (conditions in J20) — *see* Bronchitis, acute
  due to external agent — *see* condition, respiratory, acute, due to
  exercise induced J45.990
Bronchospirochetosis A69.8
  Castellani A69.8
Bronchostenosis J98.09
Bronchus — *see* condition
Brontophobia F40.220
Bronze baby syndrome P83.8
Brooke's tumor — *see* Neoplasm, skin, benign

Brown enamel of teeth (hereditary) K00.5
Brown's sheath syndrome H50.61- ☑
Brown-Séquard disease, paralysis or syndrome G83.81
Bruce sepsis A23.0
Brucellosis (infection) A23.9
  abortus A23.1
  canis A23.3
  dermatitis A23.9
  melitensis A23.0
  mixed A23.8
  sepsis A23.9
    melitensis A23.0
    specified NEC A23.8
  suis A23.2
Bruck-de Lange disease Q87.1
Bruck's disease — *see* Deformity, limb
Brugsch's syndrome Q82.8
Bruise (skin surface intact) (*see also* Contusion)
  with
    open wound — *see* Wound, open
  internal organ — *see* Injury, by site
  newborn P54.5
  scalp, due to birth injury, newborn P12.3
  umbilical cord O69.5 ☑
Bruit (arterial) R09.89
  cardiac R01.1
Brush burn — *see* Abrasion, by site
Bruton's X-linked agammaglobulinemia D80.0
Bruxism
  psychogenic F45.8
  sleep related G47.63
Bubbly lung syndrome P27.0
Bubo I88.8
  blennorrhagic (gonococcal) A54.89
  chancroidal A57
  climatic A55
  due to Haemophilus ducreyi A57
  gonococcal A54.89
  indolent (nonspecific) I88.8
  inguinal (nonspecific) I88.8
    chancroidal A57
    climatic A55
    due to H. ducreyi A57
    infective I88.8
  scrofulous (tuberculous) A18.2
  soft chancre A57
  suppurating — *see* Lymphadenitis, acute
  syphilitic (primary) A51.0
    congenital A50.07
  tropical A55
  virulent (chancroidal) A57
Bubonic plague A20.0
Bubonocele — *see* Hernia, inguinal
Buccal — *see* condition
Buchanan's disease or osteochondrosis M91.0
Buchem's syndrome (hyperostosis corticalis) M85.2
Bucket-handle fracture or tear (semilunar cartilage) — *see* Tear, meniscus
Budd-Chiari syndrome (hepatic vein thrombosis) I82.0
Budgerigar fancier's disease or lung J67.2
Buds
  breast E30.1
    in newborn P96.89
Buerger's disease (thromboangiitis obliterans) I73.1
Bulbar — *see* condition
Bulbus cordis (left ventricle) (persistent) Q21.8
Bulimia (nervosa) F50.2
  atypical F50.9
  normal weight F50.9
Bulky
  stools R19.5
  uterus N85.2
Bulla (e) R23.8
  lung (emphysematous) (solitary) J43.9
    newborn P25.8
Bullet wound (*see also* Wound, open)
  fracture — *code as* Fracture, by site
  internal organ — *see* Injury, by site
Bundle
  branch block (complete) (false) (incomplete) — *see* Block, bundle-branch
  of His — *see* condition
Bunion — *see* Deformity, toe, hallux valgus
Buphthalmia, buphthalmos (congenital) Q15.0
Burdwan fever B55.0
Bürger-Grütz disease or syndrome E78.3

Buried
  penis (congenital) Q55.64
    acquired N48.83
  roots K08.3
Burke's syndrome K86.8
Burkitt
  cell leukemia C91.0- ☑
  lymphoma (malignant) C83.7- ☑
    small noncleaved, diffuse C83.7- ☑
    spleen C83.77
    undifferentiated C83.7- ☑
  tumor C83.7- ☑
  type
    acute lymphoblastic leukemia C91.0- ☑
    undifferentiated C83.7- ☑
Burn (electricity) (flame) (hot gas, liquid or hot object) (radiation) (steam) (thermal) T30.0
  abdomen, abdominal (muscle) (wall) T21.02 ☑
    first degree T21.12 ☑
    second degree T21.22 ☑
    third degree T21.32 ☑
  above elbow T22.039 ☑
    first degree T22.139 ☑
    left T22.032 ☑
      first degree T22.132 ☑
      second degree T22.232 ☑
      third degree T22.332 ☑
    right T22.031 ☑
      first degree T22.131 ☑
      second degree T22.231 ☑
      third degree T22.331 ☑
    second degree T22.239 ☑
    third degree T22.339 ☑
  acid (caustic) (external) (internal) — *see* Corrosion, by site
  alimentary tract NEC T28.2 ☑
    esophagus T28.1 ☑
    mouth T28.0 ☑
    pharynx T28.0 ☑
  alkaline (caustic) (external) (internal) — *see* Corrosion, by site
  ankle T25.019 ☑
    first degree T25.119 ☑
    left T25.012 ☑
      first degree T25.112 ☑
      second degree T25.212 ☑
      third degree T25.312 ☑
    multiple with foot — *see* Burn, lower, limb, multiple, ankle and foot
    right T25.011 ☑
      first degree T25.111 ☑
      second degree T25.211 ☑
      third degree T25.311 ☑
    second degree T25.219 ☑
    third degree T25.319 ☑
  anus — *see* Burn, buttock
  arm (lower) (upper) — *see* Burn, upper, limb
  axilla T22.049 ☑
    first degree T22.149 ☑
    left T22.042 ☑
      first degree T22.142 ☑
      second degree T22.242 ☑
      third degree T22.342 ☑
    right T22.041 ☑
      first degree T22.141 ☑
      second degree T22.241 ☑
      third degree T22.341 ☑
    second degree T22.249 ☑
    third degree T22.349 ☑
  back (lower) T21.04 ☑
    first degree T21.14 ☑
    second degree T21.24 ☑
    third degree T21.34 ☑
    upper T21.03 ☑
      first degree T21.13 ☑
      second degree T21.23 ☑
      third degree T21.33 ☑
  blisters — *code as* Burn, second degree, by site
  breast(s) — *see* Burn, chest wall
  buttock(s) T21.05 ☑
    first degree T21.15 ☑
    second degree T21.25 ☑
    third degree T21.35 ☑
  calf T24.039 ☑
    first degree T24.139 ☑

☑ **Additional Character Required — Refer to the Tabular List for Character Selection**   ▽ **Subterms under main terms may continue to next column or page**

Burn — *continued*
  calf — *continued*
    left T24.032 ☑
      first degree T24.132 ☑
      second degree T24.232 ☑
      third degree T24.332 ☑
    right T24.031 ☑
      first degree T24.131 ☑
      second degree T24.231 ☑
      third degree T24.331 ☑
    second degree T24.239 ☑
    third degree T24.339 ☑
  canthus (eye) — *see* Burn, eyelid
  caustic acid or alkaline — *see* Corrosion, by site
  cervix T28.3 ☑
  cheek T20.06 ☑
    first degree T20.16 ☑
    second degree T20.26 ☑
    third degree T20.36 ☑
  chemical (acids) (alkalines) (caustics) (external) (internal) — *see* Corrosion, by site
  chest wall T21.01 ☑
    first degree T21.11 ☑
    second degree T21.21 ☑
    third degree T21.31 ☑
  chin T20.03 ☑
    first degree T20.13 ☑
    second degree T20.23 ☑
    third degree T20.33 ☑
  colon T28.2 ☑
  conjunctiva (and cornea) — *see* Burn, cornea
  cornea (and conjunctiva) T26.1- ☑
    chemical — *see* Corrosion, cornea
  corrosion (external) (internal) — *see* Corrosion, by site
  deep necrosis of underlying tissue — *code as* Burn, third degree, by site
  dorsum of hand T23.069 ☑
    first degree T23.169 ☑
    left T23.062 ☑
      first degree T23.162 ☑
      second degree T23.262 ☑
      third degree T23.362 ☑
    right T23.061 ☑
      first degree T23.161 ☑
      second degree T23.261 ☑
      third degree T23.361 ☑
    second degree T23.269 ☑
    third degree T23.369 ☑
  due to ingested chemical agent — *see* Corrosion, by site
  ear (auricle) (external) (canal) T20.01 ☑
    first degree T20.11 ☑
    second degree T20.21 ☑
    third degree T20.31 ☑
  elbow T22.029 ☑
    first degree T22.129 ☑
    left T22.022 ☑
      first degree T22.122 ☑
      second degree T22.222 ☑
      third degree T22.322 ☑
    right T22.021 ☑
      first degree T22.121 ☑
      second degree T22.221 ☑
      third degree T22.321 ☑
    second degree T22.229 ☑
    third degree T22.329 ☑
  epidermal loss — *code as* Burn, second degree, by site
  erythema, erythematous — *code as* Burn, first degree, by site
  esophagus T28.1 ☑
  extent (percentage of body surface)
    less than 10 percent T31.0
    10-19 percent T31.10
      with 0-9 percent third degree burns T31.10
      with 10-19 percent third degree burns T31.11
    20-29 percent T31.20
      with 0-9 percent third degree burns T31.20
      with 10-19 percent third degree burns T31.21
      with 20-29 percent third degree burns T31.22
    30-39 percent T31.30
      with 0-9 percent third degree burns T31.30
      with 10-19 percent third degree burns T31.31
      with 20-29 percent third degree burns T31.32
      with 30-39 percent third degree burns T31.33
    40-49 percent T31.40
      with 0-9 percent third degree burns T31.40

Burn — *continued*
  extent — *continued*
    40-49 percent — *continued*
      with 10-19 percent third degree burns T31.41
      with 20-29 percent third degree burns T31.42
      with 30-39 percent third degree burns T31.43
      with 40-49 percent third degree burns T31.44
    50-59 percent T31.50
      with 0-9 percent third degree burns T31.50
      with 10-19 percent third degree burns T31.51
      with 20-29 percent third degree burns T31.52
      with 30-39 percent third degree burns T31.53
      with 40-49 percent third degree burns T31.54
      with 50-59 percent third degree burns T31.55
    60-69 percent T31.60
      with 0-9 percent third degree burns T31.60
      with 10-19 percent third degree burns T31.61
      with 20-29 percent third degree burns T31.62
      with 30-39 percent third degree burns T31.63
      with 40-49 percent third degree burns T31.64
      with 50-59 percent third degree burns T31.65
      with 60-69 percent third degree burns T31.66
    70-79 percent T31.70
      with 0-9 percent third degree burns T31.70
      with 10-19 percent third degree burns T31.71
      with 20-29 percent third degree burns T31.72
      with 30-39 percent third degree burns T31.73
      with 40-49 percent third degree burns T31.74
      with 50-59 percent third degree burns T31.75
      with 60-69 percent third degree burns T31.76
      with 70-79 percent third degree burns T31.77
    80-89 percent T31.80
      with 0-9 percent third degree burns T31.80
      with 10-19 percent third degree burns T31.81
      with 20-29 percent third degree burns T31.82
      with 30-39 percent third degree burns T31.83
      with 40-49 percent third degree burns T31.84
      with 50-59 percent third degree burns T31.85
      with 60-69 percent third degree burns T31.86
      with 70-79 percent third degree burns T31.87
      with 80-89 percent third degree burns T31.88
    90 percent or more T31.90
      with 0-9 percent third degree burns T31.90
      with 10-19 percent third degree burns T31.91
      with 20-29 percent third degree burns T31.92
      with 30-39 percent third degree burns T31.93
      with 40-49 percent third degree burns T31.94
      with 50-59 percent third degree burns T31.95
      with 60-69 percent third degree burns T31.96
      with 70-79 percent third degree burns T31.97
      with 80-89 percent third degree burns T31.98
      with 90 percent or more third degree burns T31.99
  extremity — *see* Burn, limb
  eye(s) and adnexa T26.4- ☑
    with resulting rupture and destruction of eyeball T26.2- ☑
    conjunctival sac — *see* Burn, cornea
    cornea — *see* Burn, cornea
    lid — *see* Burn, eyelid
    periocular area — *see* Burn, eyelid
    specified site NEC T26.3- ☑
  eyeball — *see* Burn, eye
  eyelid(s) T26.0- ☑
    chemical — *see* Corrosion, eyelid
  face — *see* Burn, head
  finger T23.029 ☑
    first degree T23.129 ☑
    left T23.022 ☑
      first degree T23.122 ☑
      second degree T23.222 ☑
      third degree T23.322 ☑
    multiple sites (without thumb) T23.039 ☑
      with thumb T23.049 ☑
        first degree T23.149 ☑
        left T23.042 ☑
          first degree T23.142 ☑
          second degree T23.242 ☑
          third degree T23.342 ☑
        right T23.041 ☑
          first degree T23.141 ☑
          second degree T23.241 ☑
          third degree T23.341 ☑
        second degree T23.249 ☑
        third degree T23.349 ☑
      first degree T23.139 ☑

Burn — *continued*
  finger — *continued*
    multiple sites — *continued*
      left T23.032 ☑
        first degree T23.132 ☑
        second degree T23.232 ☑
        third degree T23.332 ☑
      right T23.031 ☑
        first degree T23.131 ☑
        second degree T23.231 ☑
        third degree T23.331 ☑
      second degree T23.239 ☑
      third degree T23.339 ☑
    right T23.021 ☑
      first degree T23.121 ☑
      second degree T23.221 ☑
      third degree T23.321 ☑
    second degree T23.229 ☑
    third degree T23.329 ☑
  flank — *see* Burn, abdominal wall
  foot T25.029 ☑
    first degree T25.129 ☑
    left T25.022 ☑
      first degree T25.122 ☑
      second degree T25.222 ☑
      third degree T25.322 ☑
    multiple with ankle — *see* Burn, lower, limb, multiple, ankle and foot
    right T25.021 ☑
      first degree T25.121 ☑
      second degree T25.221 ☑
      third degree T25.321 ☑
    second degree T25.229 ☑
    third degree T25.329 ☑
  forearm T22.019 ☑
    first degree T22.119 ☑
    left T22.012 ☑
      first degree T22.112 ☑
      second degree T22.212 ☑
      third degree T22.312 ☑
    right T22.011 ☑
      first degree T22.111 ☑
      second degree T22.211 ☑
      third degree T22.311 ☑
    second degree T22.219 ☑
    third degree T22.319 ☑
  forehead T20.06 ☑
    first degree T20.16 ☑
    second degree T20.26 ☑
    third degree T20.36 ☑
  fourth degree — *code as* Burn, third degree, by site
  friction — *see* Burn, by site
  from swallowing caustic or corrosive substance NEC — *see* Corrosion, by site
  full thickness skin loss — *code as* Burn, third degree, by site
  gastrointestinal tract NEC T28.2 ☑
    from swallowing caustic or corrosive substance T28.7 ☑
  genital organs
    external
      female T21.07 ☑
        first degree T21.17 ☑
        second degree T21.27 ☑
        third degree T21.37 ☑
      male T21.06 ☑
        first degree T21.16 ☑
        second degree T21.26 ☑
        third degree T21.36 ☑
    internal T28.3 ☑
      from caustic or corrosive substance T28.8 ☑
  groin — *see* Burn, abdominal wall
  hand(s) T23.009 ☑
    back — *see* Burn, dorsum of hand
    finger — *see* Burn, finger
    first degree T23.109 ☑
    left T23.002 ☑
      first degree T23.102 ☑
      second degree T23.202 ☑
      third degree T23.302 ☑
    multiple sites with wrist T23.099 ☑
      first degree T23.199 ☑
      left T23.092 ☑
        first degree T23.192 ☑
        second degree T23.292 ☑
        third degree T23.392 ☑

Burn — *continued*
  hand(s) — *continued*
    multiple sites with wrist — *continued*
      right T23.091 ☑
        first degree T23.191 ☑
        second degree T23.291 ☑
        third degree T23.391 ☑
      second degree T23.299 ☑
      third degree T23.399 ☑
    palm — *see* Burn, palm
    right T23.001 ☑
      first degree T23.101 ☑
      second degree T23.201 ☑
      third degree T23.301 ☑
    second degree T23.209 ☑
    third degree T23.309 ☑
    thumb — *see* Burn, thumb
  head (and face) (and neck) T20.00 ☑
    cheek — *see* Burn, cheek
    chin — *see* Burn, chin
    ear — *see* Burn, ear
    eye(s) only — *see* Burn, eye
    first degree T20.10 ☑
    forehead — *see* Burn, forehead
    lip — *see* Burn, lip
    multiple sites T20.09 ☑
      first degree T20.19 ☑
      second degree T20.29 ☑
      third degree T20.39 ☑
    neck — *see* Burn, neck
    nose — *see* Burn, nose
    scalp — *see* Burn, scalp
    second degree T20.20 ☑
    third degree T20.30 ☑
  hip(s) — *see* Burn, lower, limb
  inhalation — *see* Burn, respiratory tract
    caustic or corrosive substance (fumes) — *see* Corrosion, respiratory tract
  internal organ(s) T28.40 ☑
    alimentary tract T28.2 ☑
      esophagus T28.1 ☑
    eardrum T28.41 ☑
    esophagus T28.1 ☑
    from caustic or corrosive substance (swallowing) NEC — *see* Corrosion, by site
    genitourinary T28.3 ☑
    mouth T28.0 ☑
    pharynx T28.0 ☑
    respiratory tract — *see* Burn, respiratory tract
    specified organ NEC T28.49 ☑
  interscapular region — *see* Burn, back, upper
  intestine (large) (small) T28.2 ☑
  knee T24.029 ☑
    first degree T24.129 ☑
    left T24.022 ☑
      first degree T24.122 ☑
      second degree T24.222 ☑
      third degree T24.322 ☑
    right T24.021 ☑
      first degree T24.121 ☑
      second degree T24.221 ☑
      third degree T24.321 ☑
    second degree T24.229 ☑
    third degree T24.329 ☑
  labium (majus) (minus) — *see* Burn, genital organs, external, female
  lacrimal apparatus, duct, gland or sac — *see* Burn, eye, specified site NEC
  larynx T27.0 ☑
    with lung T27.1 ☑
  leg(s) (lower) (upper) — *see* Burn, lower, limb
  lightning — *see* Burn, by site
  limb(s)
    lower (except ankle or foot alone) — *see* Burn, lower, limb
    upper — *see* Burn, upper limb
  lip(s) T20.02 ☑
    first degree T20.12 ☑
    second degree T20.22 ☑
    third degree T20.32 ☑
  lower
    back — *see* Burn, back
    limb T24.009 ☑
      ankle — *see* Burn, ankle
      calf — *see* Burn, calf
      first degree T24.109 ☑

Burn — *continued*
  lower — *continued*
    limb — *continued*
      foot — *see* Burn, foot
      hip — *see* Burn, thigh
      knee — *see* Burn, knee
      left T24.002 ☑
        first degree T24.102 ☑
        second degree T24.202 ☑
        third degree T24.302 ☑
      multiple sites, except ankle and foot T24.099 ☑
        ankle and foot T25.099 ☑
          first degree T25.199 ☑
          left T25.092 ☑
            first degree T25.192 ☑
            second degree T25.292 ☑
            third degree T25.392 ☑
          right T25.091 ☑
            first degree T25.191 ☑
            second degree T25.291 ☑
            third degree T25.391 ☑
          second degree T25.299 ☑
          third degree T25.399 ☑
        first degree T24.199 ☑
        left T24.092 ☑
          first degree T24.192 ☑
          second degree T24.292 ☑
          third degree T24.392 ☑
        right T24.091 ☑
          first degree T24.191 ☑
          second degree T24.291 ☑
          third degree T24.391 ☑
        second degree T24.299 ☑
        third degree T24.399 ☑
      right T24.001 ☑
        first degree T24.101 ☑
        second degree T24.201 ☑
        third degree T24.301 ☑
      second degree T24.209 ☑
      thigh — *see* Burn, thigh
      third degree T24.309 ☑
      toe — *see* Burn, toe
  lung (with larynx and trachea) T27.1 ☑
  mouth T28.0 ☑
  neck T20.07 ☑
    first degree T20.17 ☑
    second degree T20.27 ☑
    third degree T20.37 ☑
  nose (septum) T20.04 ☑
    first degree T20.14 ☑
    second degree T20.24 ☑
    third degree T20.34 ☑
  ocular adnexa — *see* Burn, eye
  orbit region — *see* Burn, eyelid
  palm T23.059 ☑
    first degree T23.159 ☑
    left T23.052 ☑
      first degree T23.152 ☑
      second degree T23.252 ☑
      third degree T23.352 ☑
    right T23.051 ☑
      first degree T23.151 ☑
      second degree T23.251 ☑
      third degree T23.351 ☑
    second degree T23.259 ☑
    third degree T23.359 ☑
  partial thickness — *code as* Burn, unspecified degree, by site
  pelvis — *see* Burn, trunk
  penis — *see* Burn, genital organs, external, male
  perineum
    female — *see* Burn, genital organs, external, female
    male — *see* Burn, genital organs, external, male
  periocular area — *see* Burn, eyelid
  pharynx T28.0 ☑
  rectum T28.2 ☑
  respiratory tract T27.3 ☑
    larynx — *see* Burn, larynx
    specified part NEC T27.2 ☑
    trachea — *see* Burn, trachea
  sac, lacrimal — *see* Burn, eye, specified site NEC
  scalp T20.05 ☑
    first degree T20.15 ☑
    second degree T20.25 ☑
    third degree T20.35 ☑

Burn — *continued*
  scapular region T22.069 ☑
    first degree T22.169 ☑
    left T22.062 ☑
      first degree T22.162 ☑
      second degree T22.262 ☑
      third degree T22.362 ☑
    right T22.061 ☑
      first degree T22.161 ☑
      second degree T22.261 ☑
      third degree T22.361 ☑
    second degree T22.269 ☑
    third degree T22.369 ☑
  sclera — *see* Burn, eye, specified site NEC
  scrotum — *see* Burn, genital organs, external, male
  shoulder T22.059 ☑
    first degree T22.159 ☑
    left T22.052 ☑
      first degree T22.152 ☑
      second degree T22.252 ☑
      third degree T22.352 ☑
    right T22.051 ☑
      first degree T22.151 ☑
      second degree T22.251 ☑
      third degree T22.351 ☑
    second degree T22.259 ☑
    third degree T22.359 ☑
  stomach T28.2 ☑
  temple — *see* Burn, head
  testis — *see* Burn, genital organs, external, male
  thigh T24.019 ☑
    first degree T24.119 ☑
    left T24.012 ☑
      first degree T24.112 ☑
      second degree T24.212 ☑
      third degree T24.312 ☑
    right T24.011 ☑
      first degree T24.111 ☑
      second degree T24.211 ☑
      third degree T24.311 ☑
    second degree T24.219 ☑
    third degree T24.319 ☑
  thorax (external) — *see* Burn, trunk
  throat (meaning pharynx) T28.0 ☑
  thumb(s) T23.019 ☑
    first degree T23.119 ☑
    left T23.012 ☑
      first degree T23.112 ☑
      second degree T23.212 ☑
      third degree T23.312 ☑
    multiple sites with fingers T23.049 ☑
      first degree T23.149 ☑
      left T23.042 ☑
        first degree T23.142 ☑
        second degree T23.242 ☑
        third degree T23.342 ☑
      right T23.041 ☑
        first degree T23.141 ☑
        second degree T23.241 ☑
        third degree T23.341 ☑
      second degree T23.249 ☑
      third degree T23.349 ☑
    right T23.011 ☑
      first degree T23.111 ☑
      second degree T23.211 ☑
      third degree T23.311 ☑
    second degree T23.219 ☑
    third degree T23.319 ☑
  toe T25.039 ☑
    first degree T25.139 ☑
    left T25.032 ☑
      first degree T25.132 ☑
      second degree T25.232 ☑
      third degree T25.332 ☑
    right T25.031 ☑
      first degree T25.131 ☑
      second degree T25.231 ☑
      third degree T25.331 ☑
    second degree T25.239 ☑
    third degree T25.339 ☑
  tongue T28.0 ☑
  tonsil(s) T28.0 ☑
  trachea T27.0 ☑
    with lung T27.1 ☑

Burn — *continued*
  trunk T21.00 ☑
    abdominal wall — *see* Burn, abdominal wall
    anus — *see* Burn, buttock
    axilla — *see* Burn, upper limb
    back — *see* Burn, back
    breast — *see* Burn, chest wall
    buttock — *see* Burn, buttock
    chest wall — *see* Burn, chest wall
    first degree T21.10 ☑
    flank — *see* Burn, abdominal wall
    genital
      female — *see* Burn, genital organs, external, female
      male — *see* Burn, genital organs, external, male
    groin — *see* Burn, abdominal wall
    interscapular region — *see* Burn, back, upper
    labia — *see* Burn, genital organs, external, female
    lower back — *see* Burn, back
    penis — *see* Burn, genital organs, external, male
    perineum
      female — *see* Burn, genital organs, external, female
      male — *see* Burn, genital organs, external, male
    scapula region — *see* Burn, scapular region
    scrotum — *see* Burn, genital organs, external, male
    second degree T21.20 ☑
    specified site NEC T21.09 ☑
      first degree T21.19 ☑
      second degree T21.29 ☑
      third degree T21.39 ☑
    testes — *see* Burn, genital organs, external, male
    third degree T21.30 ☑
    upper back — *see* Burn, back, upper
    vulva — *see* Burn, genital organs, external, female
  unspecified site with extent of body surface involved
    specified
      less than 10 per cent T31.0
      10-19 per cent (0-9 percent third degree) T31.10
        with 10-19 percent third degree T31.11
      20-29 per cent (0-9 percent third degree) T31.20
        with
          10-19 percent third degree T31.21
          20-29 percent third degree T31.22
      30-39 per cent (0-9 percent third degree) T31.30
        with
          10-19 percent third degree T31.31
          20-29 percent third degree T31.32
          30-39 percent third degree T31.33
      40-49 per cent (0-9 percent third degree) T31.40
        with
          10-19 percent third degree T31.41
          20-29 percent third degree T31.42
          30-39 percent third degree T31.43
          40-49 percent third degree T31.44
      50-59 per cent (0-9 percent third degree) T31.50
        with
          10-19 percent third degree T31.51
          20-29 percent third degree T31.52
          30-39 percent third degree T31.53
          40-49 percent third degree T31.54
          50-59 percent third degree T31.55
      60-69 per cent (0-9 percent third degree) T31.60
        with
          10-19 percent third degree T31.61
          20-29 percent third degree T31.62
          30-39 percent third degree T31.63
          40-49 percent third degree T31.64
          50-59 percent third degree T31.65
          60-69 percent third degree T31.66
      70-79 per cent (0-9 percent third degree) T31.70
        with
          10-19 percent third degree T31.71
          20-29 percent third degree T31.72
          30-39 percent third degree T31.73
          40-49 percent third degree T31.74
          50-59 percent third degree T31.75
          60-69 percent third degree T31.76
          70-79 percent third degree T31.77
      80-89 per cent (0-9 percent third degree) T31.80
        with
          10-19 percent third degree T31.81
          20-29 percent third degree T31.82
          30-39 percent third degree T31.83
          40-49 percent third degree T31.84
          50-59 percent third degree T31.85
          60-69 percent third degree T31.86
          70-79 percent third degree T31.87

Burn — *continued*
  unspecified site with extent of body surface involved
    specified — *continued*
      80-89 per cent — *continued*
        with — *continued*
          80-89 percent third degree T31.88
      90 per cent or more (0-9 percent third degree)
        T31.90
        with
          10-19 percent third degree T31.91
          20-29 percent third degree T31.92
          30-39 percent third degree T31.93
          40-49 percent third degree T31.94
          50-59 percent third degree T31.95
          60-69 percent third degree T31.96
          70-79 percent third degree T31.97
          80-89 percent third degree T31.98
          90-99 percent third degree T31.99
  upper limb T22.00 ☑
    above elbow — *see* Burn, above elbow
    axilla — *see* Burn, axilla
    elbow — *see* Burn, elbow
    first degree T22.10 ☑
    forearm — *see* Burn, forearm
    hand — *see* Burn, hand
    interscapular region — *see* Burn, back, upper
    multiple sites T22.099 ☑
      first degree T22.199 ☑
      left T22.092 ☑
        first degree T22.192 ☑
        second degree T22.292 ☑
        third degree T22.392 ☑
      right T22.091 ☑
        first degree T22.191 ☑
        second degree T22.291 ☑
        third degree T22.391 ☑
      second degree T22.299 ☑
      third degree T22.399 ☑
    scapular region — *see* Burn, scapular region
    second degree T22.20 ☑
    shoulder — *see* Burn, shoulder
    third degree T22.30 ☑
    wrist — *see* Burn, wrist
  uterus T28.3 ☑
  vagina T28.3 ☑
  vulva — *see* Burn, genital organs, external, female
  wrist T23.079 ☑
    first degree T23.179 ☑
    left T23.072 ☑
      first degree T23.172 ☑
      second degree T23.272 ☑
      third degree T23.372 ☑
    multiple sites with hand T23.099 ☑
      first degree T23.199 ☑
      left T23.092 ☑
        first degree T23.192 ☑
        second degree T23.292 ☑
        third degree T23.392 ☑
      right T23.091 ☑
        first degree T23.191 ☑
        second degree T23.291 ☑
        third degree T23.391 ☑
      second degree T23.299 ☑
      third degree T23.399 ☑
    right T23.071 ☑
      first degree T23.171 ☑
      second degree T23.271 ☑
      third degree T23.371 ☑
    second degree T23.279 ☑
    third degree T23.379 ☑
Burnett's syndrome E83.52
Burning
  feet syndrome E53.9
  sensation R20.8
  tongue K14.6
Burn-out (state) Z73.0
Burns' disease or osteochondrosis — *see* Osteochondrosis, juvenile, ulna
Bursa — *see* condition
Bursitis M71.9
  Achilles — *see* Tendinitis, Achilles
  adhesive — *see* Bursitis, specified NEC
  ankle — *see* Enthesopathy, lower limb, ankle, specified type NEC
  calcaneal — *see* Enthesopathy, foot, specified type NEC

Bursitis — *continued*
  collateral ligament, tibial — *see* Bursitis, tibial collateral
  due to use, overuse, pressure (*see also* Disorder, soft tissue, due to use, specified type NEC)
    specified NEC — *see* Disorder, soft tissue, due to use, specified NEC
  Duplay's M75.0 ☑
  elbow NEC M70.3- ☑
    olecranon M70.2- ☑
  finger — *see* Disorder, soft tissue, due to use, specified type NEC, hand
  foot — *see* Enthesopathy, foot, specified type NEC
  gonococcal A54.49
  gouty — *see* Gout, idiopathic
  hand M70.1- ☑
  hip NEC M70.7- ☑
    trochanteric M70.6- ☑
  infective NEC M71.10
    abscess — *see* Abscess, bursa
    ankle M71.17- ☑
    elbow M71.12- ☑
    foot M71.17- ☑
    hand M71.14- ☑
    hip M71.15- ☑
    knee M71.16- ☑
    multiple sites M71.19
    shoulder M71.11- ☑
    specified site NEC M71.18
    wrist M71.13- ☑
  ischial — *see* Bursitis, hip
  knee NEC M70.5- ☑
    prepatellar M70.4- ☑
  occupational NEC (*see also* Disorder, soft tissue, due to, use)
  olecranon — *see* Bursitis, elbow, olecranon
  pharyngeal J39.1
  popliteal — *see* Bursitis, knee
  prepatellar M70.4- ☑
  radiohumeral M77.8
  rheumatoid M06.20
    ankle M06.27- ☑
    elbow M06.22- ☑
    foot joint M06.27- ☑
    hand joint M06.24- ☑
    hip M06.25- ☑
    knee M06.26- ☑
    multiple site M06.29
    shoulder M06.21- ☑
    vertebra M06.28
    wrist M06.23- ☑
  scapulohumeral — *see* Bursitis, shoulder
  semimembranous muscle (knee) — *see* Bursitis, knee
  shoulder M75.5- ☑
    adhesive — *see* Capsulitis, adhesive
  specified NEC M71.50
    ankle M71.57- ☑
    due to use, overuse or pressure — *see* Disorder, soft tissue, due to, use
    elbow M71.52- ☑
    foot M71.57- ☑
    hand M71.54- ☑
    hip M71.55- ☑
    knee M71.56- ☑
    shoulder — *see* Bursitis, shoulder
    specified site NEC M71.58
    tibial collateral M76.4- ☑
    wrist M71.53- ☑
  subacromial — *see* Bursitis, shoulder
  subcoracoid — *see* Bursitis, shoulder
  subdeltoid — *see* Bursitis, shoulder
  syphilitic A52.78
  Thornwaldt, Tornwaldt J39.2
  tibial collateral — *see* Bursitis, tibial collateral
  toe — *see* Enthesopathy, foot, specified type NEC
  trochanteric (area) — *see* Bursitis, hip, trochanteric
  wrist — *see* Bursitis, hand
Bursopathy M71.9
  specified type NEC M71.80
    ankle M71.87- ☑
    elbow M71.82- ☑
    foot M71.87- ☑
    hand M71.84- ☑
    hip M71.85- ☑
    knee M71.86- ☑
    multiple sites M71.89
    shoulder M71.81- ☑

Subterms under main terms may continue to next column or page   ☑ Additional Character Required — Refer to the Tabular List for Character Selection   45

Burn — Bursopathy

Bursopathy — *continued*
  specified type — *continued*
    specified site NEC M71.88
    wrist M71.83- ☑
Burst stitches or sutures (complication of surgery)
  T81.31 ☑
  external operation wound T81.31 ☑
  internal operation wound T81.32 ☑
Buruli ulcer A31.1
Bury's disease L95.1
Buschke's
  disease B45.3
  scleredema — *see* Sclerosis, systemic
Busse-Buschke disease B45.3
Buttock — *see* condition
Button
  Biskra B55.1
  Delhi B55.1
  oriental B55.1
Buttonhole deformity (finger) — *see* Deformity, finger, boutonniere
Bwamba fever A92.8
Byssinosis J66.0
Bywaters' syndrome T79.5 ☑

C

Cachexia R64
  cancerous R64
  cardiac — *see* Disease, heart
  dehydration E86.0
    with
      hypernatremia E87.0
      hyponatremia E87.1
  due to malnutrition R64
  exophthalmic — *see* Hyperthyroidism
  heart — *see* Disease, heart
  hypophyseal E23.0
  hypopituitary E23.0
  lead — *see* Poisoning, lead
  malignant R64
  marsh — *see* Malaria
  nervous F48.8
  old age R54
  paludal — *see* Malaria
  pituitary E23.0
  renal N28.9
  saturnine — *see* Poisoning, lead
  senile R54
  Simmonds' E23.0
  splenica D73.0
  strumipriva E03.4
  tuberculous NEC — *see* Tuberculosis
Café, au lait spots L81.3
Caffey's syndrome Q78.8
Caisson disease T70.3 ☑
Cake kidney Q63.1
Caked breast (puerperal, postpartum) O92.79
Calabar swelling B74.3
Calcaneal spur — *see* Spur, bone, calcaneal
Calcaneo-apophysitis M92.8
Calcareous — *see* condition
Calcicosis J62.8
Calciferol (vitamin D) deficiency E55.9
  with rickets E55.0
Calcification
  adrenal (capsule) (gland) E27.49
    tuberculous E35 [B90.8]
  aorta I70.0
  artery (annular) — *see* Arteriosclerosis
  auricle (ear) — *see* Disorder, pinna, specified type NEC
  basal ganglia G23.8
  bladder N32.89
    due to Schistosoma hematobium B65.0
  brain (cortex) — *see* Calcification, cerebral
  bronchus J98.09
  bursa M71.40
    ankle M71.47- ☑
    elbow M71.42- ☑
    foot M71.47- ☑
    hand M71.44- ☑
    hip M71.45- ☑
    knee M71.46- ☑
    multiple sites M71.49
    shoulder M75.3- ☑
    specified site NEC M71.48
    wrist M71.43- ☑

Calcification — *continued*
  cardiac — *see* Degeneration, myocardial
  cerebral (cortex) G93.89
    artery I67.2
  cervix (uteri) N88.8
  choroid plexus G93.89
  conjunctiva — *see* Concretion, conjunctiva
  corpora cavernosa (penis) N48.89
  cortex (brain) — *see* Calcification, cerebral
  dental pulp (nodular) K04.2
  dentinal papilla K00.4
  fallopian tube N83.8
  falx cerebri G96.19
  gallbladder K82.8
  general E83.59
  heart (*see also* Degeneration, myocardial)
    valve — *see* Endocarditis
  idiopathic infantile arterial (IIAC) Q28.8
  intervertebral cartilage or disc (postinfective) — *see* Disorder, disc, specified NEC
  intracranial — *see* Calcification, cerebral
  joint — *see* Disorder, joint, specified type NEC
  kidney N28.89
    tuberculous N29 [B90.1]
  larynx (senile) J38.7
  lens — *see* Cataract, specified NEC
  lung (active) (postinfectional) J98.4
    tuberculous B90.9
  lymph gland or node (postinfectional) I89.8
    tuberculous (*see also* Tuberculosis, lymph gland) B90.8
  mammographic R92.1
  massive (paraplegic) — *see* Myositis, ossificans, in, quadriplegia
  medial — *see* Arteriosclerosis, extremities
  meninges (cerebral) (spinal) G96.19
  metastatic E83.59
  Mönckeberg's — *see* Arteriosclerosis, extremities
  muscle M61.9
    due to burns — *see* Myositis, ossificans, in, burns
    paralytic — *see* Myositis, ossificans, in, quadriplegia
    specified type NEC M61.40
      ankle M61.47- ☑
      foot M61.47- ☑
      forearm M61.43- ☑
      hand M61.44- ☑
      lower leg M61.46- ☑
      multiple sites M61.49
      pelvic region M61.45- ☑
      shoulder region M61.41- ☑
      specified site NEC M61.48
      thigh M61.45- ☑
      upper arm M61.42- ☑
  myocardium, myocardial — *see* Degeneration, myocardial
  ovary N83.8
  pancreas K86.8
  penis N48.89
  periarticular — *see* Disorder, joint, specified type NEC
  pericardium (*see also* Pericarditis) I31.1
  pineal gland E34.8
  pleura J94.8
    postinfectional J94.8
    tuberculous NEC B90.9
  pulpal (dental) (nodular) K04.2
  sclera H15.89
  spleen D73.89
  subcutaneous L94.2
  suprarenal (capsule) (gland) E27.49
  tendon (sheath) (*see also* Tenosynovitis, specified type NEC)
    with bursitis, synovitis or tenosynovitis — *see* Tendinitis, calcific
  trachea J39.8
  ureter N28.89
  uterus N85.8
  vitreous — *see* Deposit, crystalline
Calcified — *see* Calcification
Calcinosis (interstitial) (tumoral) (universalis) E83.59
  with Raynaud's phenomenon, esophageal dysfunction, sclerodactyly, telangiectasia (CREST syndrome) M34.1
  circumscripta (skin) L94.2
  cutis L94.2
Calciphylaxis (*see also* Calcification, by site) E83.59
Calcium
  deposits — *see* Calcification, by site

Calcium — *continued*
  metabolism disorder E83.50
  salts or soaps in vitreous — *see* Deposit, crystalline
Calciuria R82.99
Calculi — *see* Calculus
Calculosis, intrahepatic — *see* Calculus, bile duct
Calculus, calculi, calculous
  ampulla of Vater — *see* Calculus, bile duct
  anuria (impacted) (recurrent) (*see also* Calculus, urinary) N20.9
  appendix K38.1
  bile duct (common) (hepatic) K80.50
    with
      calculus of gallbladder — *see* Calculus, gallbladder and bile duct
      cholangitis K80.30
        with
          cholecystitis — *see* Calculus, bile duct, with cholecystitis
          obstruction K80.31
        acute K80.32
          with
            chronic cholangitis K80.36
              with obstruction K80.37
            obstruction K80.33
        chronic K80.34
          with
            acute cholangitis K80.36
              with obstruction K80.37
            obstruction K80.35
      cholecystitis (with cholangitis) K80.40
        with obstruction K80.41
        acute K80.42
          with
            chronic cholecystitis K80.46
              with obstruction K80.47
            obstruction K80.43
        chronic K80.44
          with
            acute cholecystitis K80.46
              with obstruction K80.47
            obstruction K80.45
      obstruction K80.51
  biliary (*see also* Calculus, gallbladder)
    specified NEC K80.80
      with obstruction K80.81
  bilirubin, multiple — *see* Calculus, gallbladder
  bladder (encysted) (impacted) (urinary) (diverticulum) N21.0
  bronchus J98.09
  calyx (kidney) (renal) — *see* Calculus, kidney
  cholesterol (pure) (solitary) — *see* Calculus, gallbladder
  common duct (bile) — *see* Calculus, bile duct
  conjunctiva — *see* Concretion, conjunctiva
  cystic N21.0
    duct — *see* Calculus, gallbladder
  dental (subgingival) (supragingival) K03.6
  diverticulum
    bladder N21.0
    kidney N20.0
  epididymis N50.8
  gallbladder K80.20
    with
      bile duct calculus — *see* Calculus, gallbladder and bile duct
      cholecystitis K80.10
        with obstruction K80.11
        acute K80.00
          with
            chronic cholecystitis K80.12
              with obstruction K80.13
            obstruction K80.01
        chronic K80.10
          with
            acute cholecystitis K80.12
              with obstruction K80.13
            obstruction K80.11
      specified NEC K80.18
        with obstruction K80.19
      obstruction K80.21
  gallbladder and bile duct K80.70
    with
      cholecystitis K80.60
        with obstruction K80.61
        acute K80.62
          with
            chronic cholecystitis K80.66
              with obstruction K80.67

☑ **Additional Character Required** — Refer to the Tabular List for Character Selection
▽ **Subterms under main terms may continue to next column or page**

Calculus, calculi, calculous — *continued*
  gallbladder and bile duct — *continued*
    with — *continued*
      cholecystitis — *continued*
        acute — *continued*
          with — *continued*
            obstruction K80.63
        chronic K80.64
          with
            acute cholecystitis K80.66
              with obstruction K80.67
            obstruction K80.65
      obstruction K80.71
  hepatic (duct) — *see* Calculus, bile duct
  ileal conduit N21.8
  intestinal (impaction) (obstruction) K56.49
  kidney (impacted) (multiple) (pelvis) (recurrent)
    (staghorn) N20.0
    with calculus, ureter N20.2
    congenital Q63.8
  lacrimal passages — *see* Dacryolith
  liver (impacted) — *see* Calculus, bile duct
  lung J98.4
  mammographic R92.1
  nephritic (impacted) (recurrent) — *see* Calculus, kidney
  nose J34.89
  pancreas (duct) K86.8
  parotid duct or gland K11.5
  pelvis, encysted — *see* Calculus, kidney
  prostate N42.0
  pulmonary J98.4
  pyelitis (impacted) (recurrent) N20.0
    with hydronephrosis N13.2
  pyelonephritis (impacted) (recurrent) N20 ☑
    with hydronephrosis N13.2
  renal (impacted) (recurrent) — *see* Calculus, kidney
  salivary (duct) (gland) K11.5
  seminal vesicle N50.8
  staghorn — *see* Calculus, kidney
  Stensen's duct K11.5
  stomach K31.89
  sublingual duct or gland K11.5
    congenital Q38.4
  submandibular duct, gland or region K11.5
  submaxillary duct, gland or region K11.5
  suburethral N21.8
  tonsil J35.8
  tooth, teeth (subgingival) (supragingival) K03.6
  tunica vaginalis N50.8
  ureter (impacted) (recurrent) N20.1
    with calculus, kidney N20.2
      with hydronephrosis N13.2
        with infection N13.6
  urethra (impacted) N21.1
  urinary (duct) (impacted) (passage) (tract) N20.9
    with hydronephrosis N13.2
      with infection N13.6
    in (due to)
    lower N21.9
      specified NEC N21.8
  vagina N89.8
  vesical (impacted) N21.0
  Wharton's duct K11.5
  xanthine E79.8 [N22]
Calicectasis N28.89
Caliectasis N28.89
California
  disease B38.9
  encephalitis A83.5
Caligo cornea — *see* Opacity, cornea, central
Callositas, callosity (infected) L84
Callus (infected) L84
  bone — *see* Osteophyte
  excessive, following fracture — *code as* Sequelae
    of fracture
Calorie deficiency or malnutrition (*see also* Malnutrition) E46
Calvé-Perthes disease — *see* Legg-Calvé-Perthes disease
Calvé's disease — *see* Osteochondrosis, juvenile, spine
Calvities — *see* Alopecia, androgenic
Cameroon fever — *see* Malaria
Camptocormia (hysterical) F44.4
Camurati-Engelmann syndrome Q78.3
Canal (*see also* condition)
  atrioventricular common Q21.2
Canaliculitis (lacrimal) (acute) (subacute) H04.33 ☑
  Actinomyces A42.89

Canaliculitis — *continued*
  chronic H04.42- ☑
Canavan's disease E75.29
Canceled procedure (surgical) Z53.9
  because of
    contraindication Z53.09
      smoking Z53.01
    left against medical advice (AMA) Z53.21
    patient's decision Z53.20
      for reasons of belief or group pressure Z53.1
      specified reason NEC Z53.29
    specified reason NEC Z53.8
Cancer (*see also* Neoplasm, by site, malignant)
  bile duct type liver C22.1
  blood — *see* Leukemia
  breast (*see also* Neoplasm, breast, malignant)
    C50.91- ☑
  hepatocellular C22.0
  lung (*see also* Neoplasm, lung, malignant) C34.90
  ovarian (*see also* Neoplasm ovary, malignant) C56.9
  unspecified site (primary) C80.1
Cancer (o)**phobia** F45.29
Cancerous — *see* Neoplasm, malignant, by site
Cancrum oris A69.0
Candidiasis, candidal B37.9
  balanitis B37.42
  bronchitis B37.1
  cheilitis B37.83
  congenital P37.5
  cystitis B37.41
  disseminated B37.7
  endocarditis B37.6
  enteritis B37.82
  esophagitis B37.81
  intertrigo B37.2
  lung B37.1
  meningitis B37.5
  mouth B37.0
  nails B37.2
  neonatal P37.5
  onychia B37.2
  oral B37.0
  osteomyelitis B37.89
  otitis externa B37.84
  paronychia B37.2
  perionyxis B37.2
  pneumonia B37.1
  proctitis B37.82
  pulmonary B37.1
  pyelonephritis B37.49
  sepsis B37.7
  skin B37.2
  specified site NEC B37.89
  stomatitis B37.0
  systemic B37.7
  urethritis B37.41
  urogenital site NEC B37.49
  vagina B37.3
  vulva B37.3
  vulvovaginitis B37.3
Candidid L30.2
Candidosis — *see* Candidiasis
Candiru infection or infestation B88.8
Canities (premature) L67.1
  congenital Q84.2
Canker (mouth) (sore) K12.0
  rash A38.9
Cannabinosis J66.2
Canton fever A75.9
Cantrell's syndrome Q87.89
Capillariasis (intestinal) B81.1
  hepatic B83.8
Capillary — *see* condition
Caplan's syndrome — *see* Rheumatoid, lung
Capsule — *see* condition
Capsulitis (joint) (*see also* Enthesopathy)
  adhesive (shoulder) M75.0- ☑
  hepatic K65.8
  labyrinthine — *see* Otosclerosis, specified NEC
  thyroid E06.9
Caput
  crepitus Q75.8
  medusae I86.8
  succedaneum P12.81
Car sickness T75.3 ☑
Carapata (disease) A68.0
Carate — *see* Pinta

Carbon lung J60
Carbuncle L02.93
  abdominal wall L02.231
  anus K61.0
  auditory canal, external — *see* Abscess, ear, external
  auricle ear — *see* Abscess, ear, external
  axilla L02.43- ☑
  back (any part) L02.232
  breast N61
  buttock L02.33
  cheek (external) L02.03
  chest wall L02.233
  chin L02.03
  corpus cavernosum N48.21
  ear (any part) (external) (middle) — *see* Abscess, ear,
    external
  external auditory canal — *see* Abscess, ear, external
  eyelid — *see* Abscess, eyelid
  face NEC L02.03
  femoral (region) — *see* Carbuncle, lower limb
  finger — *see* Carbuncle, hand
  flank L02.231
  foot L02.63- ☑
  forehead L02.03
  genital — *see* Abscess, genital
  gluteal (region) L02.33
  groin L02.234
  hand L02.53- ☑
  head NEC L02.831
  heel — *see* Carbuncle, foot
  hip — *see* Carbuncle, lower limb
  kidney — *see* Abscess, kidney
  knee — *see* Carbuncle, lower limb
  labium (majus) (minus) N76.4
  lacrimal
    gland — *see* Dacryoadenitis
    passages (duct) (sac) — *see* Inflammation, lacrimal,
      passages, acute
  leg — *see* Carbuncle, lower limb
  lower limb L02.43- ☑
  malignant A22.0
  navel L02.236
  neck L02.13
  nose (external) (septum) J34.0
  orbit, orbital — *see* Abscess, orbit
  palmar (space) — *see* Carbuncle, hand
  partes posteriores L02.33
  pectoral region L02.233
  penis N48.21
  perineum L02.235
  pinna — *see* Abscess, ear, external
  popliteal — *see* Carbuncle, lower limb
  scalp L02.831
  seminal vesicle N49.0
  shoulder — *see* Carbuncle, upper limb
  specified site NEC L02.838
  temple (region) L02.03
  thumb — *see* Carbuncle, hand
  toe — *see* Carbuncle, foot
  trunk L02.239
    abdominal wall L02.231
    back L02.232
    chest wall L02.233
    groin L02.234
    perineum L02.235
    umbilicus L02.236
  umbilicus L02.236
  upper limb L02.43- ☑
  urethra N34.0
  vulva N76.4
Carbunculus — *see* Carbuncle
Carcinoid (tumor) — *see* Tumor, carcinoid
Carcinoidosis E34.0
Carcinoma (malignant) (*see also* Neoplasm, by site, malignant)
  acidophil
    specified site — *see* Neoplasm, malignant, by site
    unspecified site C75.1
  acidophil-basophil, mixed
    specified site — *see* Neoplasm, malignant, by site
    unspecified site C75.1
  adnexal (skin) — *see* Neoplasm, skin, malignant
  adrenal cortical C74.0- ☑
  alveolar — *see* Neoplasm, lung, malignant
    cell — *see* Neoplasm, lung, malignant
  ameloblastic C41.1
    upper jaw (bone) C41.0

Index

Carcinoma — *continued*
apocrine
  breast — *see* Neoplasm, breast, malignant
  specified site NEC — *see* Neoplasm, skin, malignant
  unspecified site C44.99
basal cell (pigmented) (*see also* Neoplasm, skin, malignant) C44.91
  fibro-epithelial — *see* Neoplasm, skin, malignant
  morphea — *see* Neoplasm, skin, malignant
  multicentric — *see* Neoplasm, skin, malignant
basaloid
basal-squamous cell, mixed — *see* Neoplasm, skin, malignant
basophil
  specified site — *see* Neoplasm, malignant, by site
  unspecified site C75.1
basophil-acidophil, mixed
  specified site — *see* Neoplasm, malignant, by site
  unspecified site C75.1
basosquamous — *see* Neoplasm, skin, malignant
bile duct
  with hepatocellular, mixed C22.0
  liver C22.1
  specified site NEC — *see* Neoplasm, malignant, by site
  unspecified site C22.1
branchial or branchiogenic C10.4
bronchial or bronchiogenic — *see* Neoplasm, lung, malignant
bronchiolar — *see* Neoplasm, lung, malignant
bronchioloalveolar — *see* Neoplasm, lung, malignant
C cell
  specified site — *see* Neoplasm, malignant, by site
  unspecified site C73
ceruminous C44.29- ☑
cervix uteri
  in situ D06.9
    endocervix D06.0
    exocervix D06.1
    specified site NEC D06.7
chorionic
  specified site — *see* Neoplasm, malignant, by site
  unspecified site
    female C58
    male C62.90
chromophobe
  specified site — *see* Neoplasm, malignant, by site
  unspecified site C75.1
cloacogenic
  specified site — *see* Neoplasm, malignant, by site
  unspecified site C21.2
diffuse type
  specified site — *see* Neoplasm, malignant, by site
  unspecified site C16.9
duct (cell)
  with Paget's disease — *see* Neoplasm, breast, malignant
  infiltrating
    with lobular carcinoma (in situ)
      specified site — *see* Neoplasm, malignant, by site
      unspecified site (female) C50.91- ☑
        male C50.92- ☑
    specified site — *see* Neoplasm, malignant, by site
    unspecified site (female) C50.91- ☑
      male C50.92- ☑
ductal
  with lobular
    specified site — *see* Neoplasm, malignant, by site
    unspecified site (female) C50.91- ☑
      male C50.92- ☑
ductular, infiltrating
  specified site — *see* Neoplasm, malignant, by site
  unspecified site (female) C50.91- ☑
    male C50.92- ☑
embryonal
  liver C22.7
endometrioid
  specified site — *see* Neoplasm, malignant, by site
  unspecified site
    female C56.9
    male C61
eosinophil
  specified site — *see* Neoplasm, malignant, by site
  unspecified site C75.1

Carcinoma — *continued*
epidermoid (*see also* Neoplasm, skin, malignant)
  in situ, Bowen's type — *see* Neoplasm, skin, in situ
fibroepithelial, basal cell — *see* Neoplasm, skin, malignant
follicular
  with papillary (mixed) C73
  moderately differentiated C73
  pure follicle C73
  specified site — *see* Neoplasm, malignant, by site
  trabecular C73
  unspecified site C73
  well differentiated C73
generalized, with unspecified primary site C80.0
glycogen-rich — *see* Neoplasm, breast, malignant
granulosa cell C56- ☑
hepatic cell C22.0
hepatocellular C22.0
  with bile duct, mixed C22.0
  fibrolamellar C22.0
hepatocholangiolitic C22.0
Hurthle cell C73
in
  adenomatous
    polyposis coli C18.9
  pleomorphic adenoma — *see* Neoplasm, salivary glands, malignant
  situ — *see* Carcinoma-in-situ
infiltrating
  duct
    with lobular
      specified site — *see* Neoplasm, malignant, by site
      unspecified site (female) C50.91- ☑
        male C50.92- ☑
    with Paget's disease — *see* Neoplasm, breast, malignant
    specified site — *see* Neoplasm, malignant
    unspecified site (female) C50.91- ☑
      male C50.92- ☑
  ductular
    specified site — *see* Neoplasm, malignant
    unspecified site (female) C50.91- ☑
      male C50.92- ☑
  lobular
    specified site — *see* Neoplasm, malignant
    unspecified site (female) C50.91- ☑
      male C50.92- ☑
inflammatory
  specified site — *see* Neoplasm, malignant
  unspecified site (female) C50.91- ☑
    male C50.92- ☑
intestinal type
  specified site — *see* Neoplasm, malignant, by site
  unspecified site C16.9
intracystic
  noninfiltrating — *see* Neoplasm, in situ, by site
intraductal (noninfiltrating)
  with Paget's disease — *see* Neoplasm, breast, malignant
  breast D05.1- ☑
  papillary
    with invasion
      specified site — *see* Neoplasm, malignant, by site
      unspecified site (female) C50.91- ☑
        male C50.92- ☑
    breast D05.1- ☑
    specified site NEC — *see* Neoplasm, in situ, by site
    unspecified site (female) D05.1- ☑
  specified site NEC — *see* Neoplasm, in situ, by site
  unspecified site (female) D05.1- ☑
intraepidermal — *see* Neoplasm, in situ
  squamous cell, Bowen's type — *see* Neoplasm, skin, in situ
intraepithelial — *see* Neoplasm, in situ, by site
  squamous cell — *see* Neoplasm, in situ, by site
intraosseous C41.1
  upper jaw (bone) C41.0
islet cell
  with exocrine, mixed
    specified site — *see* Neoplasm, malignant, by site
    unspecified site C25.9
  pancreas C25.4

Carcinoma — *continued*
islet cell — *continued*
  specified site NEC — *see* Neoplasm, malignant, by site
  unspecified site C25.4
juvenile, breast — *see* Neoplasm, breast, malignant
large cell
  small cell
    specified site — *see* Neoplasm, malignant, by site
    unspecified site C34.90
Leydig cell (testis)
  specified site — *see* Neoplasm, malignant, by site
  unspecified site
    female C56.9
    male C62.90
lipid-rich (female) C50.91- ☑
  male C50.92- ☑
liver cell C22.0
liver NEC C22.7
lobular (infiltrating)
  with intraductal
    specified site — *see* Neoplasm, malignant, by site
    unspecified site (female) C50.91- ☑
      male C50.92- ☑
  noninfiltrating
    breast D05.0- ☑
    specified site NEC — *see* Neoplasm, in situ, by site
    unspecified site D05.0- ☑
  specified site — *see* Neoplasm, malignant, by site
  unspecified site (female) C50.91- ☑
    male C50.92- ☑
medullary
  with
    amyloid stroma
      specified site — *see* Neoplasm, malignant, by site
      unspecified site C73
    lymphoid stroma
      specified site — *see* Neoplasm, malignant, by site
      unspecified site (female) C50.91- ☑
        male C50.92- ☑
Merkel cell C4A.9 (*following* C43)
  anal margin C4A.51 (*following* C43)
  anal skin C4A.51 (*following* C43)
  canthus C4A.1- ☑ (*following* C43)
  ear and external auricular canal C4A.2- ☑ (*following* C43)
  external auricular canal C4A.2- ☑ (*following* C43)
  eyelid, including canthus C4A.1- ☑ (*following* C43)
  face C4A.30 (*following* C43)
    specified NEC C4A.39 (*following* C43)
  hip C4A.7- ☑ (*following* C43)
  lip C4A.0 (*following* C43)
  lower limb, including hip C4A.7- ☑ (*following* C43)
  neck C4A.4 (*following* C43)
  nodal presentation C7B.1 (*following* C75)
  nose C4A.31 (*following* C43)
  overlapping sites C4A.8 (*following* C43)
  perianal skin C4A.51 (*following* C43)
  scalp C4A.4 (*following* C43)
  secondary C7B.1 (*following* C75)
  shoulder C4A.6- ☑ (*following* C43)
  skin of breast C4A.52 (*following* C43)
  trunk NEC C4A.59 (*following* C43)
  upper limb, including shoulder C4A.6- ☑ (*following* C43)
  visceral metastatic C7B.1 (*following* C75)
metastatic — *see* Neoplasm, secondary, by site
metatypical — *see* Neoplasm, skin, malignant
morphea, basal cell — *see* Neoplasm, skin, malignant
mucoid
  cell
    specified site — *see* Neoplasm, malignant, by site
    unspecified site C75.1
neuroendocrine (*see also* Tumor, neuroendocrine)
  high grade, any site C7A.1 (*following* C75)
  poorly differentiated, any site C7A.1 (*following* C75)
nonencapsulated sclerosing C73
noninfiltrating
  intracystic — *see* Neoplasm, in situ, by site
  intraductal
    breast D05.1- ☑

☑ **Additional Character Required** — Refer to the Tabular List for Character Selection   **Subterms under main terms may continue to next column or page**

Carcinoma — *continued*
  noninfiltrating — *continued*
    intraductal — *continued*
      papillary
        breast D05.1- ☑
        specified site NEC — *see* Neoplasm, in situ, by site
        unspecified site D05.1- ☑
      specified site — *see* Neoplasm, in situ, by site
      unspecified site D05.1- ☑
    lobular
      breast D05.0- ☑
      specified site NEC — *see* Neoplasm, in situ, by site
      unspecified site (female) D05.0- ☑
  oat cell
    specified site — *see* Neoplasm, malignant, by site
    unspecified site C34.90
  odontogenic C41.1
    upper jaw (bone) C41.0
  papillary
    with follicular (mixed) C73
    follicular variant C73
    intraductal (noninfiltrating)
      with invasion
        specified site — *see* Neoplasm, malignant, by site
        unspecified site (female) C50.91- ☑
          male C50.92- ☑
      breast D05.1- ☑
      specified site NEC — *see* Neoplasm, in situ, by site
      unspecified site D05.1- ☑
    serous
      specified site — *see* Neoplasm, malignant, by site
      surface
        specified site — *see* Neoplasm, malignant, by site
        unspecified site C56.9
      unspecified site C56.9
  papillocystic
    specified site — *see* Neoplasm, malignant, by site
    unspecified site C56.9
  parafollicular cell
    specified site — *see* Neoplasm, malignant, by site
    unspecified site C73
  pilomatrix — *see* Neoplasm, skin, malignant
  pseudomucinous
    specified site — *see* Neoplasm, malignant, by site
    unspecified site C56.9
  renal cell C64- ☑
  Schmincke — *see* Neoplasm, nasopharynx, malignant
  Schneiderian
    specified site — *see* Neoplasm, malignant, by site
    unspecified site C30.0
  sebaceous — *see* Neoplasm, skin, malignant
  secondary (*see also* Neoplasm, secondary, by site)
    Merkel cell C7B.1 (*following* C75)
  secretory, breast — *see* Neoplasm, breast, malignant
  serous
    papillary
      specified site — *see* Neoplasm, malignant, by site
      unspecified site C56.9
    surface, papillary
      specified site — *see* Neoplasm, malignant, by site
      unspecified site C56.9
  Sertoli cell
    specified site — *see* Neoplasm, malignant, by site
    unspecified site C62.90
      female C56.9
      male C62.90
  skin appendage — *see* Neoplasm, skin, malignant
  small cell
    fusiform cell
      specified site — *see* Neoplasm, malignant, by site
      unspecified site C34.90
    intermediate cell
      specified site — *see* Neoplasm, malignant, by site
      unspecified site C34.90
    large cell
      specified site — *see* Neoplasm, malignant, by site

Carcinoma — *continued*
  small cell — *continued*
    large cell — *continued*
      unspecified site C34.90
    solid
      with amyloid stroma
        specified site — *see* Neoplasm, malignant, by site
        unspecified site C73
    microinvasive
      specified site — *see* Neoplasm, malignant, by site
      unspecified site C53.9
  sweat gland — *see* Neoplasm, skin, malignant
  theca cell C56.- ☑
  thymic C37
  unspecified site (primary) C80.1
  water-clear cell C75.0
Carcinoma-in-situ (*see also* Neoplasm, in situ, by site)
  breast NOS D05.9- ☑
    specified type NEC D05.8- ☑
  epidermoid (*see also* Neoplasm, in situ, by site)
    with questionable stromal invasion
      cervix D06.9
      specified site NEC — *see* Neoplasm, in situ, by site
      unspecified site D06.9
    Bowen's type — *see* Neoplasm, skin, in situ
  intraductal
    breast D05.1- ☑
    specified site NEC — *see* Neoplasm, in situ, by site
    unspecified site D05.1- ☑
  lobular
    with
      infiltrating duct
        breast (female) C50.91- ☑
          male C50.92- ☑
        specified site NEC — *see* Neoplasm, malignant
        unspecified site (female) C50.91- ☑
          male C50.92- ☑
      intraductal
        breast D05.8- ☑
        specified site NEC — *see* Neoplasm, in situ, by site
        unspecified site (female) D05.8- ☑
    breast D05.0- ☑
    specified site NEC — *see* Neoplasm, in situ, by site
    unspecified site D05.0- ☑
  squamous cell (*see also* Neoplasm, in situ, by site)
    with questionable stromal invasion
      cervix D06.9
      specified site NEC — *see* Neoplasm, in situ, by site
      unspecified site D06.9
Carcinomaphobia F45.29
Carcinomatosis C80.0
  peritonei C78.6
  unspecified site (primary) (secondary) C80.0
Carcinosarcoma — *see* Neoplasm, malignant, by site
  embryonal — *see* Neoplasm, malignant, by site
Cardia, cardial — *see* condition
Cardiac (*see also* condition)
  death, sudden — *see* Arrest, cardiac
  pacemaker
    in situ Z95.0
    management or adjustment Z45.018
  tamponade I31.4
Cardialgia — *see* Pain, precordial
Cardiectasis — *see* Hypertrophy, cardiac
Cardiochalasia K21.9
Cardiomalacia I51.5
Cardiomegalia glycogenica diffusa E74.02 [I43]
Cardiomegaly (*see also* Hypertrophy, cardiac)
  congenital Q24.8
  glycogen E74.02 [I43]
  idiopathic I51.7
Cardiomyoliposis I51.5
Cardiomyopathy (familial) (idiopathic) I42.9
  alcoholic I42.6
  amyloid E85.4 [I43]
  arteriosclerotic — *see* Disease, heart, ischemic, atherosclerotic
  beriberi E51.12
  cobalt-beer I42.6
  congenital I42.4
  congestive I42.0

Cardiomyopathy — *continued*
  constrictive NOS I42.5
  dilated I42.0
  due to
    alcohol I42.6
    beriberi E51.12
    cardiac glycogenosis E74.02 [I43]
    drugs I42.7
    external agents NEC I42.7
    Friedreich's ataxia G11.1
    myotonia atrophica G71.11 [I43]
    progressive muscular dystrophy G71.0
  glycogen storage E74.02 [I43]
  hypertensive — *see* Hypertension, heart
  hypertrophic (nonobstructive) I42.2
    obstructive I42.1
      congenital Q24.8
  in
    Chagas' disease (chronic) B57.2
      acute B57.0
    sarcoidosis D86.85
  ischemic I25.5
  metabolic E88.9 [I43]
    thyrotoxic E05.90 [I43]
      with thyroid storm E05.91 [I43]
  newborn I42.8
    congenital I42.4
  nutritional E63.9 [I43]
    beriberi E51.12
  obscure of Africa I42.8
  peripartum O90.3
  postpartum O90.3
  restrictive NEC I42.5
  rheumatic I09.0
  secondary I42.9
  stress induced I51.81
  takotsubo I51.81
  thyrotoxic E05.90 [I43]
    with thyroid storm E05.91 [I43]
  toxic NEC I42.7
  tuberculous A18.84
  viral B33.24
Cardionephritis — *see* Hypertension, cardiorenal
Cardionephropathy — *see* Hypertension, cardiorenal
Cardionephrosis — *see* Hypertension, cardiorenal
Cardiopathia nigra I27.0
Cardiopathy (*see also* Disease, heart) I51.9
  idiopathic I42.9
  mucopolysaccharidosis E76.3 [I52]
Cardiopericarditis — *see* Pericarditis
Cardiophobia F45.29
Cardiorenal — *see* condition
Cardiorrhexis — *see* Infarct, myocardium
Cardiosclerosis — *see* Disease, heart, ischemic, atherosclerotic
Cardiosis — *see* Disease, heart
Cardiospasm (esophagus) (reflex) (stomach) K22.0
  congenital Q39.5
    with megaesophagus Q39.5
Cardiostenosis — *see* Disease, heart
Cardiosymphysis I31.0
Cardiovascular — *see* condition
Carditis (acute) (bacterial) (chronic) (subacute) I51.89
  meningococcal A39.50
  rheumatic — *see* Disease, heart, rheumatic
  rheumatoid — *see* Rheumatoid, carditis
  viral B33.20
Care (of) (for) (following)
  child (routine) Z76.2
  family member (handicapped) (sick)
    creating problem for family Z63.6
    provided away from home for holiday relief Z75.5
    unavailable, due to
      absence (person rendering care) (sufferer) Z74.2
      inability (any reason) of person rendering care Z74.2
  foundling Z76.1
  holiday relief Z75.5
  improper — *see* Maltreatment
  lack of (at or after birth) (infant) — *see* Maltreatment, child, neglect
  lactating mother Z39.1
  palliative Z51.5
  postpartum
    immediately after delivery Z39.0
    routine follow-up Z39.2
  respite Z75.5

Index

Carcinoma — Care

Care — *continued*
unavailable, due to
absence of person rendering care Z74.2
inability (any reason) of person rendering care Z74.2
well-baby Z76.2
Caries
bone NEC A18.03
dental K02.9
arrested (coronal) (root) K02.3
chewing surface
limited to enamel K02.51
penetrating into dentin K02.52
penetrating into pulp K02.53
coronal surface
chewing surface
limited to enamel K02.51
penetrating into dentin K02.52
penetrating into pulp K02.53
pit and fissure surface
limited to enamel K02.51
penetrating into dentin K02.52
penetrating into pulp K02.53
smooth surface
limited to enamel K02.61
penetrating into dentin K02.62
penetrating into pulp K02.63
pit and fissure surface
limited to enamel K02.51
penetrating into dentin K02.52
penetrating into pulp K02.53
root K02.7
smooth surface
limited to enamel K02.61
penetrating into dentin K02.62
penetrating into pulp K02.63
external meatus — *see* Disorder, ear, external, specified type NEC
hip (tuberculous) A18.02
initial (tooth)
chewing surface K02.51
pit and fissure surface K02.51
smooth surface K02.61
knee (tuberculous) A18.02
labyrinth H83.8 ☑
limb NEC (tuberculous) A18.03
mastoid process (chronic) — *see* Mastoiditis, chronic
tuberculous A18.03
middle ear H74.8 ☑
nose (tuberculous) A18.03
orbit (tuberculous) A18.03
ossicles, ear — *see* Abnormal, ear ossicles
petrous bone — *see* Petrositis
root (dental) (tooth) K02.7
sacrum (tuberculous) A18.01
spine, spinal (column) (tuberculous) A18.01
syphilitic A52.77
congenital (early) A50.02 [M90.80]
tooth, teeth — *see* Caries, dental
tuberculous A18.03
vertebra (column) (tuberculous) A18.01
Carious teeth — *see* Caries, dental
Carneous mole O02.0
Carnitine insufficiency E71.40
Carotid body or sinus syndrome G90.01
Carotidynia G90.01
Carotinemia (dietary) E67.1
Carotinosis (cutis) (skin) E67.1
Carpal tunnel syndrome — *see* Syndrome, carpal tunnel
Carpenter's syndrome Q87.0
Carpopedal spasm — *see* Tetany
Carr-Barr-Plunkett syndrome Q97.1
Carrier (suspected) of
amebiasis Z22.1
bacterial disease NEC Z22.39
diphtheria Z22.2
intestinal infectious NEC Z22.1
typhoid Z22.0
meningococcal Z22.31
sexually transmitted Z22.4
specified NEC Z22.39
staphylococcal (Methicillin susceptible) Z22.321
Methicillin resistant Z22.322
streptococcal Z22.338
group B Z22.330
typhoid Z22.0
cholera Z22.1
diphtheria Z22.2

Carrier of — *continued*
gastrointestinal pathogens NEC Z22.1
genetic Z14.8
cystic fibrosis Z14.1
hemophilia A (asymptomatic) Z14.01
symptomatic Z14.02
gonorrhea Z22.4
HAA (hepatitis Australian-antigen) Z22.59
HB (c)(s)-AG Z22.51
hepatitis (viral) Z22.50
Australia-antigen (HAA) Z22.59
B surface antigen (HBsAg) Z22.51
with acute delta- (super)infection B17.0
C Z22.52
specified NEC Z22.59
human T-cell lymphotropic virus type-1 (HTLV-1) infection Z22.6
infectious organism Z22.9
specified NEC Z22.8
meningococci Z22.31
Salmonella typhosa Z22.0
serum hepatitis — *see* Carrier, hepatitis
staphylococci (Methicillin susceptible) Z22.321
Methicillin resistant Z22.322
streptococci Z22.338
group B Z22.330
syphilis Z22.4
typhoid Z22.0
venereal disease NEC Z22.4
Carrion's disease A44.0
Carter's relapsing fever (Asiatic) A68.1
Cartilage — *see* condition
Caruncle (inflamed)
conjunctiva (acute) — *see* Conjunctivitis, acute
labium (majus) (minus) N90.89
lacrimal — *see* Inflammation, lacrimal, passages
myrtiform N89.8
urethral (benign) N36.2
Cascade stomach K31.2
Caseation lymphatic gland (tuberculous) A18.2
Cassidy (-Scholte) syndrome (malignant carcinoid) E34.0
Castellani's disease A69.8
Castration, traumatic, male S38.231 ☑
Casts in urine R82.99
Cat
cry syndrome Q93.4
ear Q17.3
eye syndrome Q92.8
Catabolism, senile R54
Catalepsy (hysterical) F44.2
schizophrenic F20.2
Cataplexy (idiopathic) — *see* Narcolepsy
Cataract (cortical) (immature) (incipient) H26.9
with
neovascularization — *see* Cataract, complicated
age-related — *see* Cataract, senile
anterior
and posterior axial embryonal Q12.0
pyramidal Q12.0
associated with
galactosemia E74.21 [H28]
myotonic disorders G71.19 [H28]
blue Q12.0
central Q12.0
cerulean Q12.0
complicated H26.20
with
neovascularization H26.21- ☑
ocular disorder H26.22- ☑
glaucomatous flecks H26.23- ☑
congenital Q12.0
coraliform Q12.0
coronary Q12.0
crystalline Q12.0
diabetic — *see* Diabetes, cataract
drug-induced H26.3- ☑
due to
ocular disorder — *see* Cataract, complicated
radiation H26.8
electric H26.8
extraction status Z98.4- ☑
glass-blower's H26.8
heat ray H26.8
heterochromic — *see* Cataract, complicated
hypermature — *see* Cataract, senile, morgagnian type
in (due to)
chronic iridocyclitis — *see* Cataract, complicated

Cataract — *continued*
in — *continued*
diabetes — *see* Diabetes, cataract
endocrine disease E34.9 [H28]
eye disease — *see* Cataract, complicated
hypoparathyroidism E20.9 [H28]
malnutrition-dehydration E46 [H28]
metabolic disease E88.9 [H28]
myotonic disorders G71.19 [H28]
nutritional disease E63.9 [H28]
infantile — *see* Cataract, presenile
irradiational — *see* Cataract, specified NEC
juvenile — *see* Cataract, presenile
malnutrition-dehydration E46 [H28]
morgagnian — *see* Cataract, senile, morgagnian type
myotonic G71.19 [H28]
myxedema E03.9 [H28]
nuclear
embryonal Q12.0
sclerosis — *see* Cataract, senile, nuclear
presenile H26.00- ☑
combined forms H26.06- ☑
cortical H26.01- ☑
lamellar — *see* Cataract, presenile, cortical
nuclear H26.03- ☑
specified NEC H26.09
subcapsular polar (anterior) H26.04- ☑
posterior H26.05- ☑
zonular — *see* Cataract, presenile, cortical
secondary H26.40
Soemmering's ring H26.41- ☑
specified NEC H26.49- ☑
to eye disease — *see* Cataract, complicated
senile H25.9
brunescens — *see* Cataract, senile, nuclear
combined forms H25.81- ☑
coronary — *see* Cataract, senile, incipient
cortical H25.01- ☑
hypermature — *see* Cataract, senile, morgagnian type
incipient (mature) (total) H25.09- ☑
cortical — *see* Cataract, senile, cortical
subcapsular — *see* Cataract, senile, subcapsular
morgagnian type (hypermature) H25.2- ☑
nuclear (sclerosis) H25.1- ☑
polar subcapsular (anterior) (posterior) — *see* Cataract, senile, incipient
punctate — *see* Cataract, senile, incipient
specified NEC H25.89
subcapsular polar (anterior) H25.03- ☑
posterior H25.04- ☑
snowflake — *see* Diabetes, cataract
specified NEC H26.8
toxic — *see* Cataract, drug-induced
traumatic H26.10- ☑
localized H26.11- ☑
partially resolved H26.12- ☑
total H26.13- ☑
zonular (perinuclear) Q12.0
Cataracta (*see also* Cataract)
brunescens — *see* Cataract, senile, nuclear
centralis pulverulenta Q12.0
cerulea Q12.0
complicata — *see* Cataract, complicated
congenita Q12.0
coralliformis Q12.0
coronaria Q12.0
diabetic — *see* Diabetes, cataract
membranacea
accreta — *see* Cataract, secondary
congenita Q12.0
nigra — *see* Cataract, senile, nuclear
sunflower — *see* Cataract, complicated
Catarrh, catarrhal (acute) (febrile) (infectious) (inflammation) (*see also* condition) J00
bronchial — *see* Bronchitis
chest — *see* Bronchitis
chronic J31.0
due to congenital syphilis A50.03
enteric — *see* Enteritis
eustachian H68.009
fauces — *see* Pharyngitis
gastrointestinal — *see* Enteritis
gingivitis K05.00
nonplaque induced K05.01
plaque induced K05.00
hay — *see* Fever, hay

☑ Additional Character Required — Refer to the Tabular List for Character Selection ▽ Subterms under main terms may continue to next column or page

Catarrh, catarrhal — *continued*
  intestinal — *see* Enteritis
  larynx, chronic J37.0
  liver B15.9
    with hepatic coma B15.0
  lung — *see* Bronchitis
  middle ear, chronic — *see* Otitis, media, nonsuppurative, chronic, serous
  mouth K12.1
  nasal (chronic) — *see* Rhinitis
  nasobronchial J31.1
  nasopharyngeal (chronic) J31.1
    acute J00
  pulmonary — *see* Bronchitis
  spring (eye) (vernal) — *see* Conjunctivitis, acute, atopic
  summer (hay) — *see* Fever, hay
  throat J31.2
  tubotympanal (*see also* Otitis, media, nonsuppurative)
    chronic — *see* Otitis, media, nonsuppurative, chronic, serous
Catatonia (schizophrenic) F20.2
Catatonic
  disorder due to known physiologic condition F06.1
  schizophrenia F20.2
  stupor R40.1
Cat-scratch (*see also* Abrasion)
  disease or fever A28.1
Cauda equina — *see* condition
Cauliflower ear M95.1- ☑
Causalgia (upper limb) G56.4- ☑
  lower limb G57.7- ☑
Cause
  external, general effects T75.89 ☑
Caustic burn — *see* Corrosion, by site
Cavare's disease (familial periodic paralysis) G72.3
Cave-in, injury
  crushing (severe) — *see* Crush
  suffocation — *see* Asphyxia, traumatic, due to low oxygen, due to cave-in
Cavernitis (penis) N48.29
Cavernositis N48.29
Cavernous — *see* condition
Cavitation of lung (*see also* Tuberculosis, pulmonary)
  nontuberculous J98.4
Cavities, dental — *see* Caries, dental
Cavity
  lung — *see* Cavitation of lung
  optic papilla Q14.2
  pulmonary — *see* Cavitation of lung
Cavovarus foot, congenital Q66.1
Cavus foot (congenital) Q66.7
  acquired — *see* Deformity, limb, foot, specified NEC
Cazenave's disease L10.2
Cecitis K52.9
  with perforation, peritonitis, or rupture K65.8
Cecum — *see* condition
Celiac
  artery compression syndrome I77.4
  disease K90.0
  infantilism K90.0
Cell(s), **cellular** (*see also* condition)
  in urine R82.99
Cellulitis (diffuse) (phlegmonous) (septic) (suppurative) L03.90
  abdominal wall L03.311
  anaerobic A48.0
  ankle — *see* Cellulitis, lower limb
  anus K61.0
  arm — *see* Cellulitis, upper limb
  auricle (ear) — *see* Cellulitis, ear
  axilla L03.11- ☑
  back (any part) L03.312
  broad ligament
    acute N73.0
  buttock L03.317
  cervical (meaning neck) L03.221
  cervix (uteri) — *see* Cervicitis
  cheek (external) L03.211
    internal K12.2
  chest wall L03.313
  chronic L03.90
  clostridial A48.0
  corpus cavernosum N48.22
  digit
    finger — *see* Cellulitis, finger
    toe — *see* Cellulitis, toe

Cellulitis — *continued*
  Douglas' cul-de-sac or pouch
    acute N73.0
  drainage site (following operation) T81.4 ☑
  ear (external) H60.1- ☑
  eosinophilic (granulomatous) L98.3
  erysipelatous — *see* Erysipelas
  external auditory canal — *see* Cellulitis, ear
  eyelid — *see* Abscess, eyelid
  face NEC L03.211
  finger (intrathecal) (periosteal) (subcutaneous) (subcuticular) L03.01- ☑
  foot — *see* Cellulitis, lower limb
  gangrenous — *see* Gangrene
  genital organ NEC
    female (external) N76.4
    male N49.9
      multiple sites N49.8
      specified NEC N49.8
  gluteal (region) L03.317
  gonococcal A54.89
  groin L03.314
  hand — *see* Cellulitis, upper limb
  head NEC L03.811
    face (any part, except ear, eye and nose) L03.211
  heel — *see* Cellulitis, lower limb
  hip — *see* Cellulitis, lower limb
  jaw (region) L03.211
  knee — *see* Cellulitis, lower limb
  labium (majus) (minus) — *see* Vulvitis
  lacrimal passages — *see* Inflammation, lacrimal, passages
  larynx J38.7
  leg — *see* Cellulitis, lower limb
  lip K13.0
  lower limb L03.11- ☑
    toe — *see* Cellulitis, toe
  mouth (floor) K12.2
  multiple sites, so stated L03.90
  nasopharynx J39.1
  navel L03.316
    newborn P38.9
      with mild hemorrhage P38.1
      without hemorrhage P38.9
  neck (region) L03.221
  nose (septum) (external) J34.0
  orbit, orbital H05.01- ☑
  palate (soft) K12.2
  pectoral (region) L03.313
  pelvis, pelvic (chronic)
    female (*see also* Disease, pelvis, inflammatory) N73.2
      acute N73.0
    following ectopic or molar pregnancy O08.0
    male K65.0
  penis N48.22
  perineal, perineum L03.315
  perirectal K61.1
  peritonsillar J36
  periurethral N34.0
  periuterine (*see also* Disease, pelvis, inflammatory) N73.2
    acute N73.0
  pharynx J39.1
  rectum K61.1
  retroperitoneal K68.9
  round ligament
    acute N73.0
  scalp (any part) L03.811
  scrotum N49.2
  seminal vesicle N49.0
  shoulder — *see* Cellulitis, upper limb
  specified site NEC L03.818
  submandibular (region) (space) (triangle) K12.2
    gland K11.3
  submaxillary (region) K12.2
    gland K11.3
  thigh — *see* Cellulitis, lower limb
  thumb (intrathecal) (periosteal) (subcutaneous) (subcuticular) — *see* Cellulitis, finger
  toe (intrathecal) (periosteal) (subcutaneous) (subcuticular) L03.03- ☑
  tonsil J36
  trunk L03.319
    abdominal wall L03.311
    back (any part) L03.312
    buttock L03.317
    chest wall L03.313

Cellulitis — *continued*
  trunk — *continued*
    groin L03.314
    perineal, perineum L03.315
    umbilicus L03.316
    tuberculous (primary) A18.4
    umbilicus L03.316
    upper limb L03.11- ☑
      axilla — *see* Cellulitis, axilla
      finger — *see* Cellulitis, finger
      thumb — *see* Cellulitis, finger
  vaccinal T88.0 ☑
  vocal cord J38.3
  vulva — *see* Vulvitis
  wrist — *see* Cellulitis, upper limb
Cementoblastoma, benign — *see* Cyst, calcifying odontogenic
Cementoma — *see* Cyst, calcifying odontogenic
Cementoperiostitis — *see* Periodontitis
Cementosis K03.4
Central auditory processing disorder H93.25
Central pain syndrome G89.0
Cephalematocele, cephal (o)hematocele
  newborn P52.8
    birth injury P10.8
  traumatic — *see* Hematoma, brain
Cephalematoma, cephalhematoma (calcified)
  newborn (birth injury) P12.0
  traumatic — *see* Hematoma, brain
Cephalgia, cephalalgia (*see also* Headache)
  histamine G44.009
    intractable G44.001
    not intractable G44.009
  trigeminal autonomic (TAC) NEC G44.099
    intractable G44.091
    not intractable G44.099
Cephalic — *see* condition
Cephalitis — *see* Encephalitis
Cephalocele — *see* Encephalocele
Cephalomenia N94.89
Cephalopelvic — *see* condition
Cerclage (with cervical incompetence) in pregnancy — *see* Incompetence, cervix, in pregnancy
Cerebellitis — *see* Encephalitis
Cerebellum, cerebellar — *see* condition
Cerebral — *see* condition
Cerebritis — *see* Encephalitis
Cerebro-hepato-renal syndrome Q87.89
Cerebromalacia — *see* Softening, brain
  sequelae of cerebrovascular disease I69.398
Cerebroside lipidosis E75.22
Cerebrospasticity (congenital) G80.1
Cerebrospinal — *see* condition
Cerebrum — *see* condition
Ceroid-lipofuscinosis, neuronal E75.4
Cerumen (accumulation) (impacted) H61.2- ☑
Cervical (*see also* condition)
  auricle Q18.2
  dysplasia in pregnancy — *see* Abnormal, cervix, in pregnancy or childbirth
  erosion in pregnancy — *see* Abnormal, cervix, in pregnancy or childbirth
  fibrosis in pregnancy — *see* Abnormal, cervix, in pregnancy or childbirth
  fusion syndrome Q76.1
  rib Q76.5
  shortening (complicating pregnancy) O26.87- ☑
Cervicalgia M54.2
Cervicitis (acute) (chronic) (nonvenereal) (senile (atrophic)) (subacute) (with ulceration) N72
  with
    abortion — *see* Abortion, by type complicated by genital tract and pelvic infection
    ectopic pregnancy O08.0
    molar pregnancy O08.0
  chlamydial A56.09
  gonococcal A54.03
  herpesviral A60.03
  puerperal (postpartum) O86.11
  syphilitic A52.76
  trichomonal A59.09
  tuberculous A18.16
Cervicocolpitis (emphysematosa) (see also Cervicitis) N72
Cervix — *see* condition
Cesarean delivery, previous, affecting management of pregnancy O34.21

Céstan (-Chenais) paralysis or syndrome G46.3
Céstan-Raymond syndrome I65.8
Cestode infestation B71.9
  specified type NEC B71.8
Cestodiasis B71.9
Chabert's disease A22.9
Chacaleh E53.8
Chafing L30.4
Chagas' (-Mazza) disease (chronic) B57.2
  with
    cardiovascular involvement NEC B57.2
    digestive system involvement B57.30
      megacolon B57.32
      megaesophagus B57.31
      other specified B57.39
    megacolon B57.32
    megaesophagus B57.31
    myocarditis B57.2
    nervous system involvement B57.40
      meningitis B57.41
      meningoencephalitis B57.42
      other specified B57.49
    specified organ involvement NEC B57.5
  acute (with) B57.1
    cardiovascular NEC B57.0
    myocarditis B57.0
Chagres fever B50.9
Chairridden Z74.09
Chalasia (cardiac sphincter) K21.9
Chalazion H00.19
  left H00.16
    lower H00.15
    upper H00.14
  right H00.13
    lower H00.12
    upper H00.11
Chalcosis (see also Disorder, globe, degenerative, chalcosis)
  cornea — see Deposit, cornea
  crystalline lens — see Cataract, complicated
  retina H35.89
Chalicosis (pulmonum) J62.8
Chancre (any genital site) (hard) (hunterian) (mixed) (primary) (seronegative) (seropositive) (syphilitic) A51.0
  congenital A50.07
  conjunctiva NEC A51.2
  Ducrey's A57
  extragenital A51.2
  eyelid A51.2
  lip A51.2
  nipple A51.2
  Nisbet's A57
  of
    carate A67.0
    pinta A67.0
    yaws A66.0
  palate, soft A51.2
  phagedenic A57
  simple A57
  soft A57
    bubo A57
    palate A51.2
  urethra A51.0
  yaws A66.0
Chancroid (anus) (genital) (penis) (perineum) (rectum) (urethra) (vulva) A57
Chandler's disease (osteochondritis dissecans, hip) — see Osteochondritis, dissecans, hip
Change(s) (in) (of) (see also Removal)
  arteriosclerotic — see Arteriosclerosis
  bone (see also Disorder, bone)
    diabetic — see Diabetes, bone change
  bowel habit R19.4
  cardiorenal (vascular) — see Hypertension, cardiorenal
  cardiovascular — see Disease, cardiovascular
  circulatory I99.9
  cognitive (mild) (organic) R41.89
  color, tooth, teeth
    during formation K00.8
    posteruptive K03.7
  contraceptive device Z30.433
  corneal membrane H18.30
    Bowman's membrane fold or rupture H18.31- ☑
    Descemet's membrane
      fold H18.32- ☑
      rupture H18.33- ☑
  coronary — see Disease, heart, ischemic

Change(s) — continued
  degenerative, spine or vertebra — see Spondylosis
  dental pulp, regressive K04.2
  dressing (nonsurgical) Z48.00
    surgical Z48.01
  heart — see Disease, heart
  hip joint — see Derangement, joint, hip
  hyperplastic larynx J38.7
  hypertrophic
    nasal sinus J34.89
    turbinate, nasal J34.3
    upper respiratory tract J39.8
  indwelling catheter Z46.6
  inflammatory (see also Inflammation)
    sacroiliac M46.1
  job, anxiety concerning Z56.1
  joint — see Derangement, joint
  life — see Menopause
  mental status R41.82
  minimal (glomerular) (see also N00-N07 with fourth character .0) N05.0
  myocardium, myocardial — see Degeneration, myocardial
  of life — see Menopause
  pacemaker Z45.018
    pulse generator Z45.010
  personality (enduring) F68.8
    due to (secondary to)
      general medical condition F07.0
    secondary (nonspecific) F60.89
  regressive, dental pulp K04.2
  renal — see Disease, renal
  retina H35.9
    myopic H44.2- ☑
  sacroiliac joint M53.3
  senile (see also condition) R54
  sensory R20.8
  skin R23.9
    acute, due to ultraviolet radiation L56.9
      specified NEC L56.8
    chronic, due to nonionizing radiation L57.9
      specified NEC L57.8
    cyanosis R23.0
    flushing R23.2
    pallor R23.1
    petechiae R23.3
    specified change NEC R23.8
    swelling — see Mass, localized
    texture R23.4
  trophic
    arm — see Mononeuropathy, upper limb
    leg — see Mononeuropathy, lower limb
  vascular I99.9
  vasomotor I73.9
  voice R49.9
    psychogenic F44.4
    specified NEC R49.8
Changing sleep-work schedule, affecting sleep G47.26
Changuinola fever A93.1
Chapping skin T69.8 ☑
Charcot-Marie-Tooth disease, paralysis or syndrome G60.0
Charcot's
  arthropathy — see Arthropathy, neuropathic
  cirrhosis K74.3
  disease (tabetic arthropathy) A52.16
  joint (disease) (tabetic) A52.16
    diabetic — see Diabetes, with, arthropathy
    syringomyelic G95.0
  syndrome (intermittent claudication) I73.9
CHARGE association Q89.8
Charley-horse (quadriceps) M62.831
  traumatic (quadriceps) S76.11- ☑
Charlouis' disease — see Yaws
Cheadle's disease E54
Checking (of)
  cardiac pacemaker (battery) (electrode(s)) Z45.018
    pulse generator Z45.010
  intrauterine contraceptive device Z30.431
Check-up — see Examination
Chédiak-Higashi (-Steinbrinck) **syndrome** (congenital gigantism of peroxidase granules) E70.330
Cheek — see condition
Cheese itch B88.0
Cheese-washer's lung J67.8
Cheese-worker's lung J67.8

Cheilitis (acute) (angular) (catarrhal) (chronic) (exfoliative) (gangrenous) (glandular) (infectional) (suppurative) (ulcerative) (vesicular) K13.0
  actinic (due to sun) L56.8
    other than from sun L59.8
  candidal B37.83
Cheilodynia K13.0
Cheiloschisis — see Cleft, lip
Cheilosis (angular) K13.0
  with pellagra E52
  due to
    vitamin B2 (riboflavin) deficiency E53.0
Cheiromegaly M79.89
Cheiropompholyx L30.1
Cheloid — see Keloid
Chemical burn — see Corrosion, by site
Chemodectoma — see Paraganglioma, nonchromaffin
Chemosis, conjunctiva — see Edema, conjunctiva
Chemotherapy (session) (for)
  cancer Z51.11
  neoplasm Z51.11
Cherubism M27.8
Chest — see condition
Cheyne-Stokes breathing (respiration) R06.3
Chiari's
  disease or syndrome (hepatic vein thrombosis) I82.0
  malformation
    type I G93.5
    type II — see Spina bifida
  net Q24.8
Chicago disease B40.9
Chickenpox — see Varicella
Chiclero ulcer or sore B55.1
Chigger (infestation) B88.0
Chignon (disease) B36.8
  newborn (from vacuum extraction) (birth injury) P12.1
Chilaiditi's syndrome (subphrenic displacement, colon) Q43.3
Chilblain(s) (lupus) T69.1 ☑
Child
  custody dispute Z65.3
Childbirth — see Delivery
Childhood
  cerebral X-linked adrenoleukodystrophy E71.520
  period of rapid growth Z00.2
Chill(s) R68.83
  with fever R50.9
  without fever R68.83
  congestive in malarial regions B54
Chilomastigiasis A07.8
Chimera 46,XX/46,XY Q99.0
Chin — see condition
Chinese dysentery A03.9
Chionophobia F40.228
Chitral fever A93.1
Chlamydia, chlamydial A74.9
  cervicitis A56.09
  conjunctivitis A74.0
  cystitis A56.01
  endometritis A56.11
  epididymitis A56.19
  female
    pelvic inflammatory disease A56.11
    pelviperitonitis A56.11
  orchitis A56.19
  peritonitis A74.81
  pharyngitis A56.4
  proctitis A56.3
  psittaci (infection) A70
  salpingitis A56.11
  sexually-transmitted infection NEC A56.8
  specified NEC A74.89
  urethritis A56.01
  vulvovaginitis A56.02
Chlamydiosis — see Chlamydia
Chloasma (skin) (idiopathic) (symptomatic) L81.1
  eyelid H02.719
    hyperthyroid E05.90 [H02.719]
      with thyroid storm E05.91 [H02.719]
    left H02.716
      lower H02.715
      upper H02.714
    right H02.713
      lower H02.712
      upper H02.711
Chloroma C92.3- ☑

Céstan — Chloroma

Chlorosis D50.9
  Egyptian B76.9 [D63.8]
  miner's B76.9 [D63.8]
Chlorotic anemia D50.8
Chocolate cyst (ovary) N80.1
Choked
  disc or disk — *see* Papilledema
  on food, phlegm, or vomitus NOS — *see* Foreign body, by site
  while vomiting NOS — *see* Foreign body, by site
Chokes (resulting from bends) T70.3 ☑
Choking sensation R09.89
Cholangiectasis K83.8
Cholangiocarcinoma
  with hepatocellular carcinoma, combined C22.0
  liver C22.1
  specified site NEC — *see* Neoplasm, malignant, by site
  unspecified site C22.1
Cholangiohepatitis K83.8
  due to fluke infestation B66.1
Cholangiohepatoma C22.0
Cholangiolitis (acute) (chronic) (extrahepatic) (gangrenous) (intrahepatic) K83.0
  paratyphoidal — *see* Fever, paratyphoid
  typhoidal A01.09
Cholangioma D13.4
  malignant — *see* Cholangiocarcinoma
Cholangitis (ascending) (primary) (recurrent) (sclerosing) (secondary) (stenosing) (suppurative) K83.0
  with calculus, bile duct — *see* Calculus, bile duct, with cholangitis
  chronic nonsuppurative destructive K74.3
Cholecystectasia K82.8
Cholecystitis K81.9
  with
    calculus, stones in
      bile duct (common) (hepatic) — *see* Calculus, bile duct, with cholecystitis
      cystic duct — *see* Calculus, gallbladder, with cholecystitis
      gallbladder — *see* Calculus, gallbladder, with cholecystitis
      choledocholithiasis — *see* Calculus, bile duct, with cholecystitis
      cholelithiasis — *see* Calculus, gallbladder, with cholecystitis
    acute (emphysematous) (gangrenous) (suppurative) K81.0
      with
        calculus, stones in
          cystic duct — *see* Calculus, gallbladder, with cholecystitis, acute
          gallbladder — *see* Calculus, gallbladder, with cholecystitis, acute
          choledocholithiasis — *see* Calculus, bile duct, with cholecystitis, acute
          cholelithiasis — *see* Calculus, gallbladder, with cholecystitis, acute
        chronic cholecystitis K81.2
          with gallbladder calculus K80.12
            with obstruction K80.13
    chronic K81.1
      with acute cholecystitis K81.2
        with gallbladder calculus K80.12
          with obstruction K80.13
    emphysematous (acute) — *see* Cholecystitis, acute
    gangrenous — *see* Cholecystitis, acute
    paratyphoidal, current A01.4
    suppurative — *see* Cholecystitis, acute
    typhoidal A01.09
Cholecystolithiasis — *see* Calculus, gallbladder
Choledochitis (suppurative) K83.0
Choledocholith — *see* Calculus, bile duct
Choledocholithiasis (common duct) (hepatic duct) — *see* Calculus, bile duct
  cystic — *see* Calculus, gallbladder
  typhoidal A01.09
Cholelithiasis (cystic duct) (gallbladder) (impacted) (multiple) — *see* Calculus, gallbladder
  bile duct (common) (hepatic) — *see* Calculus, bile duct
  hepatic duct — *see* Calculus, bile duct
  specified NEC K80.80
    with obstruction K80.81
Cholemia (*see also* Jaundice)
  familial (simple) (congenital) E80.4
  Gilbert's E80.4
Choleperitoneum, choleperitonitis K65.3

Cholera (Asiatic) (epidemic) (malignant) A00.9
  antimonial — *see* Poisoning, antimony
  classical A00.0
  due to Vibrio cholerae 01 A00.9
    biovar cholerae A00.0
    biovar eltor A00.1
    el tor A00.1
  el tor A00.1
Cholerine — *see* Cholera
Cholestasis NEC K83.1
  with hepatocyte injury K71.0
  due to total parenteral nutrition (TPN) K76.89
  pure K71.0
Cholesteatoma (ear) (middle) (with reaction) H71.9- ☑
  attic H71.0- ☑
  external ear (canal) H60.4- ☑
  mastoid H71.2- ☑
  postmastoidectomy cavity (recurrent) — *see* Complications, postmastoidectomy, recurrent cholesteatoma
  recurrent (postmastoidectomy) — *see* Complications, postmastoidectomy, recurrent cholesteatoma
  tympanum H71.1- ☑
Cholesteatosis, diffuse H71.3- ☑
Cholesteremia E78.0
Cholesterin in vitreous — *see* Deposit, crystalline
Cholesterol
  deposit
    retina H35.89
    vitreous — *see* Deposit, crystalline
  elevated (high) E78.0
    with elevated (high) triglycerides E78.2
    screening for Z13.220
  imbibition of gallbladder K82.4
Cholesterolemia (essential) (familial) (hereditary) (pure) E78.0
Cholesterolosis, cholesterosis (gallbladder) K82.4
  cerebrotendinous E75.5
Cholocolic fistula K82.3
Choluria R82.2
Chondritis M94.8X9
  aurical H61.03- ☑
  costal (Tietze's) M94.0
  external ear H61.03- ☑
  patella, posttraumatic — *see* Chondromalacia, patella
  pinna H61.03- ☑
  purulent M94.8X- ☑
  tuberculous NEC A18.02
    intervertebral A18.01
Chondroblastoma (*see also* Neoplasm, bone, benign)
  malignant — *see* Neoplasm, bone, malignant
Chondrocalcinosis M11.20
  ankle M11.27- ☑
  elbow M11.22- ☑
  familial M11.10
    ankle M11.17- ☑
    elbow M11.12- ☑
    foot joint M11.17- ☑
    hand joint M11.14- ☑
    hip M11.15- ☑
    knee M11.16- ☑
    multiple site M11.19
    shoulder M11.11- ☑
    vertebrae M11.18
    wrist M11.13- ☑
  foot joint M11.27- ☑
  hand joint M11.24- ☑
  hip M11.25- ☑
  knee M11.26- ☑
  multiple site M11.29
  shoulder M11.21- ☑
  specified type NEC M11.20
    ankle M11.27- ☑
    elbow M11.22- ☑
    foot joint M11.27- ☑
    hand joint M11.24- ☑
    hip M11.25- ☑
    knee M11.26- ☑
    multiple site M11.29
    shoulder M11.21- ☑
    vertebrae M11.28
    wrist M11.23- ☑
  vertebrae M11.28
  wrist M11.23- ☑
Chondrodermatitis nodularis helicis or anthelicis — *see* Perichondritis, ear

Chondrodysplasia Q78.9
  with hemangioma Q78.4
  calcificans congenita Q77.3
  fetalis Q77.4
  metaphyseal (Jansen's) (McKusick's) (Schmid's) Q78.5
  punctata Q77.3
Chondrodystrophy, chondrodystrophia (familial) (fetalis) (hypoplastic) Q78.9
  calcificans congenita Q77.3
  myotonic (congenital) G71.13
  punctata Q77.3
Chondroectodermal dysplasia Q77.6
Chondrogenesis imperfecta Q77.4
Chondrolysis M94.35- ☑
Chondroma (*see also* Neoplasm, cartilage, benign)
  juxtacortical — *see* Neoplasm, bone, benign
  periosteal — *see* Neoplasm, bone, benign
Chondromalacia (systemic) M94.20
  acromioclavicular joint M94.21- ☑
  ankle M94.27- ☑
  elbow M94.22- ☑
  foot joint M94.27- ☑
  glenohumeral joint M94.21- ☑
  hand joint M94.24- ☑
  hip M94.25- ☑
  knee M94.26- ☑
    patella M22.4- ☑
  multiple sites M94.29
  patella M22.4- ☑
  rib M94.28
  sacroiliac joint M94.259
  shoulder M94.21- ☑
  sternoclavicular joint M94.21- ☑
  vertebral joint M94.28
  wrist M94.23- ☑
Chondromatosis (*see also* Neoplasm, cartilage, uncertain behavior)
  internal Q78.4
Chondromyxosarcoma — *see* Neoplasm, cartilage, malignant
Chondro-osteodysplasia (Morquio-Brailsford type) E76.219
Chondro-osteodystrophy E76.29
Chondro-osteoma — *see* Neoplasm, bone, benign
Chondropathia tuberosa M94.0
Chondrosarcoma — *see* Neoplasm, cartilage, malignant
  juxtacortical — *see* Neoplasm, bone, malignant
  mesenchymal — *see* Neoplasm, connective tissue, malignant
  myxoid — *see* Neoplasm, cartilage, malignant
Chordee (nonvenereal) N48.89
  congenital Q54.4
  gonococcal A54.09
Chorditis (fibrinous) (nodosa) (tuberosa) J38.2
Chordoma — *see* Neoplasm, vertebral (column), malignant
Chorea (chronic) (gravis) (posthemiplegic) (senile) (spasmodic) G25.5
  with
    heart involvement I02.0
      active or acute (conditions in I01-) I02.0
        rheumatic I02.0
          with valvular disorder I02.0
      rheumatic heart disease (chronic) (inactive)(quiescent) — *code to* rheumatic heart condition involved
  drug-induced G25.4
  habit F95.8
  hereditary G10
  Huntington's G10
  hysterical F44.4
  minor I02.9
    with heart involvement I02.0
  progressive G25.5
    hereditary G10
  rheumatic (chronic) I02.9
    with heart involvement I02.0
  Sydenham's I02.9
    with heart involvement — *see* Chorea, with rheumatic heart disease
    nonrheumatic G25.5
Choreoathetosis (paroxysmal) G25.5
Chorioadenoma (destruens) D39.2
Chorioamnionitis O41.12- ☑
Chorioangioma D26.7

Choriocarcinoma — *see* Neoplasm, malignant, by site
  combined with
      embryonal carcinoma — *see* Neoplasm, malignant,
        by site
      other germ cell elements — *see* Neoplasm, malig-
        nant, by site
      teratoma — *see* Neoplasm, malignant, by site
  specified site — *see* Neoplasm, malignant, by site
  unspecified site
    female C58
    male C62.90
Chorioencephalitis (acute) (lymphocytic) (serous) A87.2
Chorioepithelioma — *see* Choriocarcinoma
Choriomeningitis (acute) (lymphocytic) (serous) A87.2
Chorionepithelioma — *see* Choriocarcinoma
Chorioretinitis (*see also* Inflammation, chorioretinal)
  disseminated (*see also* Inflammation, chorioretinal,
    disseminated)
    in neurosyphilis A52.19
  Egyptian B76.9 [D63.8]
  focal (*see also* Inflammation, chorioretinal, focal)
  histoplasmic B39.9 [H32]
  in (due to)
    histoplasmosis B39.9 [H32]
    syphilis (secondary) A51.43
      late A52.71
    toxoplasmosis (acquired) B58.01
      congenital (active) P37.1 [H32]
    tuberculosis A18.53
  juxtapapillary, juxtapapillaris — *see* Inflammation,
    chorioretinal, focal, juxtapapillary
  leprous A30.9 [H32]
  miner's B76.9 [D63.8]
  progressive myopia (degeneration) H44.2- ☑
  syphilitic (secondary) A51.43
    congenital (early) A50.01 [H32]
      late A50.32
    late A52.71
  tuberculous A18.53
Chorioretinopathy, central serous H35.71- ☑
Choroid — *see* condition
Choroideremia H31.21
Choroiditis — *see* Chorioretinitis
Choroidopathy — *see* Disorder, choroid
Choroidoretinitis — *see* Chorioretinitis
Choroidoretinopathy, central serous — *see* Chori-
  oretinopathy, central serous
Christian-Weber disease M35.6
Christmas disease D67
Chromaffinoma (*see also* Neoplasm, benign, by site)
  malignant — *see* Neoplasm, malignant, by site
Chromatopsia — *see* Deficiency, color vision
Chromhidrosis, chromidrosis L75.1
Chromoblastomycosis — *see* Chromomycosis
Chromoconversion R82.91
Chromomycosis B43.9
  brain abscess B43.1
  cerebral B43.1
  cutaneous B43.0
  skin B43.0
  specified NEC B43.8
  subcutaneous abscess or cyst B43.2
Chromophytosis B36.0
Chromosome — *see* Anomaly, by chromosome involved
  D (1) — *see* Anomaly, chromosome 13
  E (3) — *see* Anomaly, chromosome 18
  G — *see* Anomaly, chromosome 21
Chromotrichomycosis B36.8
Chronic — *see* condition
  fracture — *see* Fracture, pathological
Churg-Strauss syndrome M30.1
Chyle cyst, mesentery I89.8
Chylocele (nonfilarial) I89.8
  filarial (*see also* Infestation, filarial) B74.9 [N51]
  tunica vaginalis N50.8
    filarial (*see also* Infestation, filarial) B74.9 [N51]
Chylomicronemia (fasting) (with hyperprebetalipopro-
  teinemia) E78.3
Chylopericardium I31.3
  acute I30.9
Chylothorax (nonfilarial) I89.8
  filarial (*see also* Infestation, filarial) B74.9 [J91.8]
Chylous — *see* condition
Chyluria (nonfilarial) R82.0
  due to
    bilharziasis B65.0

Chyluria — *continued*
  due to — *continued*
    Brugia (malayi) B74.1
      timori B74.2
    schistosomiasis (bilharziasis) B65.0
    Wuchereria (bancrofti) B74.0
  filarial — *see* Infestation, filarial
Cicatricial (deformity) — *see* Cicatrix
Cicatrix (adherent) (contracted) (painful) (vicious) (*see
  also* Scar) L90.5
  adenoid (and tonsil) J35.8
  alveolar process M26.79
  anus K62.89
  auricle — *see* Disorder, pinna, specified type NEC
  bile duct (common) (hepatic) K83.8
  bladder N32.89
  bone — *see* Disorder, bone, specified type NEC
  brain G93.89
  cervix (postoperative) (postpartal) N88.1
  common duct K83.8
  cornea H17.9
    tuberculous A18.59
  duodenum (bulb), obstructive K31.5
  esophagus K22.2
  eyelid — *see* Disorder, eyelid function
  hypopharynx J39.2
  lacrimal passages — *see* Obstruction, lacrimal
  larynx J38.7
  lung J98.4
  middle ear H74.8 ☑
  mouth K13.79
  muscle M62.89
    with contracture — *see* Contraction, muscle NEC
  nasopharynx J39.2
  palate (soft) K13.79
  penis N48.89
  pharynx J39.2
  prostate N42.89
  rectum K62.89
  retina — *see* Scar, chorioretinal
  semilunar cartilage — *see* Derangement, meniscus
  seminal vesicle N50.8
  skin L90.5
    infected L08.89
    postinfective L90.5
    tuberculous B90.8
  specified site NEC L90.5
  throat J39.2
  tongue K14.8
  tonsil (and adenoid) J35.8
  trachea J39.8
  tuberculous NEC B90.9
  urethra N36.8
  uterus N85.8
  vagina N89.8
    postoperative N99.2
  vocal cord J38.3
  wrist, constricting (annular) L90.5
CIDP (chronic inflammatory demyelinating polyneuropathy) G61.81
CIN — *see* Neoplasia, intraepithelial, cervix
Cinchonism — *see* Deafness, ototoxic
  correct substance properly administered — *see* Table
    of Drugs and Chemicals, by drug, adverse effect
  overdose or wrong substance given or taken — *see*
    Table of Drugs and Chemicals, by drug, poison-
    ing
Circle of Willis — *see* condition
Circular — *see* condition
Circulating anticoagulants (*see also* Disorder, hemorrhagic) D68.318
  due to drugs (*see also* Disorder, hemorrhagic) D68.32
  following childbirth O72.3
Circulation
  collateral, any site I99.8
  defective (lower extremity) I99.8
    congenital Q28.9
  embryonic Q28.9
  failure (peripheral) R57.9
    newborn P29.89
  fetal, persistent P29.3
  heart, incomplete Q28.9
Circulatory system — *see* condition
Circulus senilis (cornea) — *see* Degeneration, cornea,
  senile
Circumcision (in absence of medical indication) (ritual)
  (routine) Z41.2
Circumscribed — *see* condition

Circumvallate placenta O43.11- ☑
Cirrhosis, cirrhotic (hepatic) (liver) K74.60
  alcoholic K70.30
    with ascites K70.31
  atrophic — *see* Cirrhosis, liver
  Baumgarten-Cruveilhier K74.69
  biliary (cholangiolitic) (cholangitic) (hypertrophic)
    (obstructive) (pericholangiolitic) K74.5
    due to
      Clonorchiasis B66.1
      flukes B66.3
    primary K74.3
    secondary K74.4
  cardiac (of liver) K76.1
  Charcot's K74.3
  cholangiolitic, cholangitic, cholostatic (primary) K74.3
  congestive K76.1
  Cruveilhier-Baumgarten K74.69
  cryptogenic (liver) K74.69
  due to
    hepatolenticular degeneration E83.01
    Wilson's disease E83.01
    xanthomatosis E78.2
  fatty K76.0
    alcoholic K70.0
  Hanot's (hypertrophic) K74.3
  hepatic — *see* Cirrhosis, liver
  hypertrophic K74.3
  Indian childhood K74.69
  kidney — *see* Sclerosis, renal
  Laennec's K70.30
    with ascites K70.31
    alcoholic K70.30
      with ascites K70.31
    nonalcoholic K74.69
  liver K74.60
    alcoholic K70.30
      with ascites K70.31
      fatty K70.0
    congenital P78.81
    syphilitic A52.74
  lung (chronic) J84.10
  macronodular K74.69
    alcoholic K70.30
      with ascites K70.31
  micronodular K74.69
    alcoholic K70.30
      with ascites K70.31
  mixed type K74.69
  monolobular K74.3
  nephritis — *see* Sclerosis, renal
  nutritional K74.69
    alcoholic K70.30
      with ascites K70.31
  obstructive — *see* Cirrhosis, biliary
  ovarian N83.8
  pancreas (duct) K86.8
  pigmentary E83.110
  portal K74.69
    alcoholic K70.30
      with ascites K70.31
  postnecrotic K74.69
    alcoholic K70.30
      with ascites K70.31
  pulmonary J84.10
  renal — *see* Sclerosis, renal
  spleen D73.2
  stasis K76.1
  Todd's K74.3
  unilobar K74.3
  xanthomatous (biliary) K74.5
    due to xanthomatosis (familial) (metabolic) (prima-
      ry) E78.2
Cistern, subarachnoid R93.0
Citrullinemia E72.23
Citrullinuria E72.23
Civatte's disease or poikiloderma L57.3
Clam digger's itch B65.3
Clammy skin R23.1
Clap — *see* Gonorrhea
Clarke-Hadfield syndrome (pancreatic infantilism)
  K86.8
Clark's paralysis G80.9
Clastothrix L67.8
Claude Bernard-Horner syndrome G90.2
  traumatic — *see* Injury, nerve, cervical sympathetic
Claude's disease or syndrome G46.3
Claudicatio venosa intermittens I87.8

Claudication, intermittent I73.9
  cerebral (artery) G45.9
  spinal cord (arteriosclerotic) G95.19
    syphilitic A52.09
  venous (axillary) I87.8
Claustrophobia F40.240
Clavus (infected) L84
Clawfoot (congenital) Q66.89
  acquired — *see* Deformity, limb, clawfoot
Clawhand (acquired) (*see also* Deformity, limb, clawhand)
  congenital Q68.1
Clawtoe (congenital) Q66.89
  acquired — *see* Deformity, toe, specified NEC
Clay eating — *see* Pica
Cleansing of artificial opening — *see* Attention to, artificial, opening
Cleft (congenital) (*see also* Imperfect, closure)
  alveolar process M26.79
  branchial (cyst) (persistent) Q18.2
  cricoid cartilage, posterior Q31.8
  lip (unilateral) Q36.9
    with cleft palate Q37.9
      hard Q37.1
        with soft Q37.5
      soft Q37.3
        with hard Q37.5
      bilateral Q36.0
        with cleft palate Q37.8
          hard Q37.0
            with soft Q37.4
          soft Q37.2
            with hard Q37.4
    median Q36.1
  nose Q30.2
  palate Q35.9
    with cleft lip (unilateral) Q37.9
      bilateral Q37.8
    hard Q35.1
      with
        cleft lip (unilateral) Q37.1
          bilateral Q37.0
        soft Q35.5
          with cleft lip (unilateral) Q37.5
            bilateral Q37.4
    medial Q35.5
    soft Q35.3
      with
        cleft lip (unilateral) Q37.3
          bilateral Q37.2
        hard Q35.5
          with cleft lip (unilateral) Q37.5
            bilateral Q37.4
  penis Q55.69
  scrotum Q55.29
  thyroid cartilage Q31.8
  uvula Q35.7
Cleidocranial dysostosis Q74.0
Cleptomania F63.2
Clicking hip (newborn) R29.4
Climacteric (female) (*see also* Menopause)
  arthritis (any site) NEC — *see* Arthritis, specified form NEC
  depression (single episode) F32.8
  male (symptoms) (syndrome) NEC N50.8
  paranoid state F22
  polyarthritis NEC — *see* Arthritis, specified form NEC
  symptoms (female) N95.1
Clinical research investigation (clinical trial) (control subject) (normal comparison) (participant) Z00.6
Clitoris — *see* condition
Cloaca (persistent) Q43.7
Clonorchiasis, clonorchis infection (liver) B66.1
Clonus R25.8
Closed bite M26.29
Clostridium (C.) **perfringens, as cause of disease classified elsewhere** B96.7
Closure
  congenital, nose Q30.0
  cranial sutures, premature Q75.0
  defective or imperfect NEC — *see* Imperfect, closure
  fistula, delayed — *see* Fistula
  foramen ovale, imperfect Q21.1
  hymen N89.6
  interauricular septum, defective Q21.1
  interventricular septum, defective Q21.0
  lacrimal duct (*see also* Stenosis, lacrimal, duct)
    congenital Q10.5

Closure — *continued*
  nose (congenital) Q30.0
    acquired M95.0
  of artificial opening — *see* Attention to, artificial, opening
  vagina N89.5
  valve — *see* Endocarditis
  vulva N90.5
Clot (blood) (*see also* Embolism)
  artery (obstruction) (occlusion) — *see* Embolism
  bladder N32.89
  brain (intradural or extradural) — *see* Occlusion, artery, cerebral
  circulation I74.9
  heart (*see also* Infarct, myocardium)
    not resulting in infarction I24.0
  vein — *see* Thrombosis
Clouded state R40.1
  epileptic — *see* Epilepsy, specified NEC
  paroxysmal — *see* Epilepsy, specified NEC
Cloudy antrum, antra J32.0
Clouston's (hidrotic) **ectodermal dysplasia** Q82.4
Clubbed nail pachydermoperiostosis M89.40 [L62]
Clubbing of finger(s) (nails) R68.3
Clubfinger R68.3
  congenital Q68.1
Clubfoot (congenital) Q66.89
  acquired — *see* Deformity, limb, clubfoot
  equinovarus Q66.0
  paralytic — *see* Deformity, limb, clubfoot
Clubhand (congenital) (radial) Q71.4- ☑
  acquired — *see* Deformity, limb, clubhand
Clubnail R68.3
  congenital Q84.6
Clump, kidney Q63.1
Clumsiness, clumsy child syndrome F82
Cluttering F80.81
Clutton's joints A50.51 [M12.80]
Coagulation, intravascular (diffuse) (disseminated) (*see also* Defibrination syndrome)
  complicating abortion — *see* Abortion, by type, complicated by, intravascular coagulation
  following ectopic or molar pregnancy O08.1
Coagulopathy (*see also* Defect, coagulation)
  consumption D65
  intravascular D65
    newborn P60
Coalition
  calcaneo-scaphoid Q66.89
  tarsal Q66.89
Coalminer's
  elbow — *see* Bursitis, elbow, olecranon
  lung or pneumoconiosis J60
Coalworker's lung or pneumoconiosis J60
Coarctation
  aorta (preductal) (postductal) Q25.1
  pulmonary artery Q25.71
Coated tongue K14.3
Coats' disease (exudative retinopathy) — *see* Retinopathy, exudative
Cocainism — *see* Dependence, drug, cocaine
Coccidioidomycosis B38.9
  cutaneous B38.3
  disseminated B38.7
  generalized B38.7
  meninges B38.4
  prostate B38.81
  pulmonary B38.2
    acute B38.0
    chronic B38.1
  skin B38.3
  specified NEC B38.89
Coccidioidosis — *see* Coccidioidomycosis
Coccidiosis (intestinal) A07.3
Coccydynia, coccygodynia M53.3
Coccyx — *see* condition
Cochin-China diarrhea K90.1
Cocked up toe — *see* Deformity, toe, specified NEC
Cock's peculiar tumor L72.3
Codman's tumor — *see* Neoplasm, bone, benign
Coenurosis B71.8
Coffee-worker's lung J67.8
Cogan's syndrome H16.32- ☑
  oculomotor apraxia H51.8
Coitus, painful (female) N94.1
  male N53.12

Coitus, painful — *continued*
  psychogenic F52.6
Cold J00
  with influenza, flu, or grippe — *see* Influenza, with, respiratory manifestations NEC
  agglutinin disease or hemoglobinuria (chronic) D59.1
  bronchial — *see* Bronchitis
  chest — *see* Bronchitis
  common (head) J00
  effects of T69.9 ☑
    specified effect NEC T69.8 ☑
  excessive, effects of T69.9 ☑
    specified effect NEC T69.8 ☑
  exhaustion from T69.8 ☑
  exposure to T69.9 ☑
    specified effect NEC T69.8 ☑
  head J00
  injury syndrome (newborn) P80.0
  on lung — *see* Bronchitis
  rose J30.1
  sensitivity, auto-immune D59.1
  virus J00
Coldsore B00.1
Colibacillosis A49.8
  as the cause of other disease (*see also* Escherichia coli) B96.20
  generalized A41.50
Colic (bilious) (infantile) (intestinal) (recurrent) (spasmodic) R10.83
  abdomen R10.83
    psychogenic F45.8
  appendix, appendicular K38.8
  bile duct — *see* Calculus, bile duct
  biliary — *see* Calculus, bile duct
  common duct — *see* Calculus, bile duct
  cystic duct — *see* Calculus, gallbladder
  Devonshire NEC — *see* Poisoning, lead
  gallbladder — *see* Calculus, gallbladder
  gallstone — *see* Calculus, gallbladder
    gallbladder or cystic duct — *see* Calculus, gallbladder
  hepatic (duct) — *see* Calculus, bile duct
  hysterical F45.8
  kidney N23
  lead NEC — *see* Poisoning, lead
  mucous K58.9
    with diarrhea K58.0
    psychogenic F54
  nephritic N23
  painter's NEC — *see* Poisoning, lead
  pancreas K86.8
  psychogenic F45.8
  renal N23
  saturnine NEC — *see* Poisoning, lead
  ureter N23
  urethral N36.8
    due to calculus N21.1
  uterus NEC N94.89
    menstrual — *see* Dysmenorrhea
  worm NOS B83.9
Colicystitis — *see* Cystitis
Colitis (acute) (catarrhal) (chronic) (noninfective) (hemorrhagic) (*see also* Enteritis) K52.9
  allergic K52.2
  amebic (acute) (*see also* Amebiasis) A06.0
    nondysenteric A06.2
  anthrax A22.2
  bacillary — *see* Infection, Shigella
  balantidial A07.0
  Clostridium difficile A04.7
  coccidial A07.3
  collagenous K52.89
  cystica superficialis K52.89
  dietary counseling and surveillance (for) Z71.3
  dietetic K52.2
  drug-induced K52.1
  due to radiation K52.0
  eosinophilic K52.82
  food hypersensitivity K52.2
  giardial A07.1
  granulomatous — *see* Enteritis, regional, large intestine
  infectious — *see* Enteritis, infectious
  ischemic K55.9
    acute (fulminant) (subacute) K55.0
    chronic K55.1
    due to mesenteric artery insufficiency K55.1

Colitis — continued
 ischemic — continued
  fulminant (acute) K55.0
 left sided K51.50
  with
   abscess K51.514
   complication K51.519
    specified NEC K51.518
   fistula K51.513
   obstruction K51.512
   rectal bleeding K51.511
 lymphocytic K52.89
 membranous
  psychogenic F54
 microscopic (collagenous) (lymphocytic) K52.89
 mucous — see Syndrome, irritable, bowel
  psychogenic F54
 noninfective K52.9
  specified NEC K52.89
 polyposa — see Polyp, colon, inflammatory
 protozoal A07.9
 pseudomembranous A04.7
 pseudomucinous — see Syndrome, irritable, bowel
 regional — see Enteritis, regional, large intestine
 segmental — see Enteritis, regional, large intestine
 septic — see Enteritis, infectious
 spastic K58.9
  with diarrhea K58.0
  psychogenic F54
 staphylococcal A04.8
  foodborne A05.0
 subacute ischemic K55.0
 thromboulcerative K55.0
 toxic NEC K52.1
  due to Clostridium difficile A04.7
 transmural — see Enteritis, regional, large intestine
 trichomonal A07.8
 tuberculous (ulcerative) A18.32
 ulcerative (chronic) K51.90
  with
   complication K51.919
    abscess K51.914
    fistula K51.913
    obstruction K51.912
    rectal bleeding K51.911
    specified complication NEC K51.918
  enterocolitis — see Enterocolitis, ulcerative
  ileocolitis — see Ileocolitis, ulcerative
  mucosal proctocolitis — see Proctocolitis, mucosal
  proctitis — see Proctitis, ulcerative
  pseudopolyposis — see Polyp, colon, inflammatory
  psychogenic F54
  rectosigmoiditis — see Rectosigmoiditis, ulcerative
  specified type NEC K51.80
   with
    complication K51.819
     abscess K51.814
     fistula K51.813
     obstruction K51.812
     rectal bleeding K51.811
     specified complication NEC K51.818
Collagenosis, collagen disease (nonvascular) (vascular) M35.9
 cardiovascular I42.8
 reactive perforating L87.1
 specified NEC M35.8
Collapse R55
 adrenal E27.2
 cardiorespiratory R57.0
 cardiovascular R57.0
  newborn P29.89
 circulatory (peripheral) R57.9
  during or after labor and delivery O75.1
  following ectopic or molar pregnancy O08.3
  newborn P29.89
 during or
  after labor and delivery O75.1
  resulting from a procedure, not elsewhere classified T81.10 ☑
 external ear canal — see Stenosis, external ear canal
 general R55
 heart — see Disease, heart
 heat T67.1 ☑
 hysterical F44.89
 labyrinth, membranous (congenital) Q16.5

Collapse — continued
 lung (see also Atelectasis) J98.19
  pressure due to anesthesia (general) (local) or other sedation T88.2 ☑
   during labor and delivery O74.1
   in pregnancy O29.02- ☑
   postpartum, puerperal O89.09
 myocardial — see Disease, heart
 nervous F48.8
 neurocirculatory F45.8
 nose M95.0
 postoperative T81.10 ☑
 pulmonary (see also Atelectasis) J98.19
  newborn — see Atelectasis
 trachea J39.8
 tracheobronchial J98.09
 valvular — see Endocarditis
 vascular (peripheral) R57.9
  during or after labor and delivery O75.1
  following ectopic or molar pregnancy O08.3
  newborn P29.89
 vertebra M48.50-
  cervical region M48.52- ☑
  cervicothoracic region M48.53- ☑
  in (due to)
   metastasis — see Collapse, vertebra, in, specified disease NEC
   osteoporosis (see also Osteoporosis) M80.88 ☑
    cervical region M80.88 ☑
    cervicothoracic region M80.88 ☑
    lumbar region M80.88 ☑
    lumbosacral region M80.88 ☑
    multiple sites M80.88 ☑
    occipito-atlanto-axial region M80.88 ☑
    sacrococcygeal region M80.88 ☑
    thoracic region M80.88 ☑
    thoracolumbar region M80.88 ☑
   specified disease NEC M48.50- ☑
    cervical region M48.52- ☑
    cervicothoracic region M48.53- ☑
    lumbar region M48.56- ☑
    lumbosacral region M48.57- ☑
    occipito-atlanto-axial region M48.51- ☑
    sacrococcygeal region M48.58- ☑
    thoracic region M48.54- ☑
    thoracolumbar region M48.55- ☑
  lumbar region M48.56- ☑
  lumbosacral region M48.57- ☑
  occipito-atlanto-axial region M48.51- ☑
  sacrococcygeal region M48.58- ☑
  thoracic region M48.54- ☑
  thoracolumbar region M48.55- ☑
Collateral (see also condition)
 circulation (venous) I87.8
 dilation, veins I87.8
Colles' fracture S52.53- ☑
Collet (-Sicard) syndrome G52.7
Collier's asthma or lung J60
Collodion baby Q80.2
Colloid nodule (of thyroid) (cystic) E04.1
Coloboma (iris) Q13.0
 eyelid Q10.3
 fundus Q14.8
 lens Q12.2
 optic disc (congenital) Q14.2
  acquired H47.31- ☑
Coloenteritis — see Enteritis
Colon — see condition
Colonization
 MRSA (Methicillin resistant Staphylococcus aureus) Z22.322
 MSSA (Methicillin susceptible Staphylococcus aureus) Z22.321
 status — see Carrier (suspected) of
Coloptosis K63.4
Color blindness — see Deficiency, color vision
Colostomy
 attention to Z43.3
 fitting or adjustment Z46.89
 malfunctioning K94.03
 status Z93.3
Colpitis (acute) — see Vaginitis
Colpocele N81.5
Colpocystitis — see Vaginitis
Colpospasm N94.2
Column, spinal, vertebral — see condition

Coma R40.20
 with
  motor response (none) R40.231 ☑
   abnormal R40.233 ☑
   extension R40.232 ☑
   flexion withdrawal R40.234 ☑
   localizes pain R40.235 ☑
   obeys commands R40.236 ☑
  opening of eyes (never) R40.211 ☑
   in response to
    pain R40.212 ☑
    sound R40.213 ☑
   spontaneous R40.214 ☑
  verbal response (none) R40.221 ☑
   confused conversation R40.224 ☑
   inappropriate words R40.223 ☑
   incomprehensible words R40.222 ☑
   oriented R40.225 ☑
 eclamptic — see Eclampsia
 epileptic — see Epilepsy
 Glasgow, scale score — see Glasgow coma scale
 hepatic — see Failure, hepatic, by type, with coma
 hyperglycemic (diabetic) — see Diabetes, coma
 hyperosmolar (diabetic) — see Diabetes, coma
 hypoglycemic (diabetic) — see Diabetes, coma, hypoglycemic
  nondiabetic E15
 in diabetes — see Diabetes, coma
 insulin-induced — see Coma, hypoglycemic
 myxedematous E03.5
 newborn P91.5
 persistent vegetative state R40.3
 specified NEC, without documented Glasgow coma scale score, or with partial Glasgow coma scale score reported R40.244
Comatose — see Coma
Combat fatigue F43.0
Combined — see condition
Comedo, comedones (giant) L70.0
Comedocarcinoma (see also Neoplasm, breast, malignant)
 noninfiltrating
  breast D05.8- ☑
  specified site — see Neoplasm, in situ, by site
  unspecified site D05.8- ☑
Comedomastitis — see Ectasia, mammary duct
Comminuted fracture — code as Fracture, closed
Common
 arterial trunk Q20.0
 atrioventricular canal Q21.2
 atrium Q21.1
 cold (head) J00
 truncus (arteriosus) Q20.0
 variable immunodeficiency — see Immunodeficiency, common variable
 ventricle Q20.4
Commotio, commotion (current)
 brain — see Injury, intracranial, concussion
 cerebri — see Injury, intracranial, concussion
 retinae S05.8X- ☑
 spinal cord — see Injury, spinal cord, by region
 spinalis — see Injury, spinal cord, by region
Communication
 between
  base of aorta and pulmonary artery Q21.4
  left ventricle and right atrium Q20.5
  pericardial sac and pleural sac Q34.8
  pulmonary artery and pulmonary vein, congenital Q25.72
 congenital between uterus and digestive or urinary tract Q51.7
Compartment syndrome (deep) (posterior) (traumatic) T79.A0 ☑ (following T79.7)
 abdomen T79.A3 ☑ (following T79.7)
 lower extremity (hip, buttock, thigh, leg, foot, toes) T79.A2 ☑ (following T79.7)
 nontraumatic
  abdomen M79.A3 (following M79.7)
  lower extremity (hip, buttock, thigh, leg, foot, toes) M79.A2- ☑ (following M79.7)
  specified site NEC M79.A9 (following M79.7)
  upper extremity (shoulder, arm, forearm, wrist, hand, fingers) M79.A1- ☑ (following M79.7)
 specified site NEC T79.A9 ☑ (following T79.7)
 upper extremity (shoulder, arm, forearm, wrist, hand, fingers) T79.A1- ☑ (following T79.7)

☑ Additional Character Required — Refer to the Tabular List for Character Selection   ☝ Subterms under main terms may continue to next column or page

Compensation
  failure — *see* Disease, heart
  neurosis, psychoneurosis — *see* Disorder, factitious
Complaint (*see also* Disease)
  bowel, functional K59.9
    psychogenic F45.8
  intestine, functional K59.9
    psychogenic F45.8
  kidney — *see* Disease, renal
  miners' J60
Complete — *see* condition
Complex
  Addison-Schilder E71.528
  cardiorenal — *see* Hypertension, cardiorenal
  Costen's M26.69
  disseminated mycobacterium avium- intracellulare (DMAC) A31.2
  Eisenmenger's (ventricular septal defect) I27.89
  hypersexual F52.8
  jumped process, spine — *see* Dislocation, vertebra
  primary, tuberculous A15.7
  Schilder-Addison E71.528
  subluxation (vertebral) M99.19
    abdomen M99.19
    acromioclavicular M99.17
    cervical region M99.11
    cervicothoracic M99.11
    costochondral M99.18
    costovertebral M99.18
    head region M99.10
    hip M99.15
    lower extremity M99.16
    lumbar region M99.13
    lumbosacral M99.13
    occipitocervical M99.10
    pelvic region M99.15
    pubic M99.15
    rib cage M99.18
    sacral region M99.14
    sacrococcygeal M99.14
    sacroiliac M99.14
    specified NEC M99.19
    sternochondral M99.18
    sternoclavicular M99.17
    thoracic region M99.12
    thoracolumbar M99.12
    upper extremity M99.17
  Taussig-Bing (transposition, aorta and overriding pulmonary artery) Q20.1
Complication(s) (from) (of)
  accidental puncture or laceration during a procedure (of) — *see* Complications, intraoperative (intraprocedural), puncture or laceration
  amputation stump (surgical) (late) NEC T87.9
    dehiscence T87.81
    infection or inflammation T87.40
      lower limb T87.4- ☑
      upper limb T87.4- ☑
    necrosis T87.50
      lower limb T87.5- ☑
      upper limb T87.5- ☑
    neuroma T87.30
      lower limb T87.3- ☑
      upper limb T87.3- ☑
    specified type NEC T87.89
  anastomosis (and bypass) (*see also* Complications, prosthetic device or implant)
    intestinal (internal) NEC K91.89
      involving urinary tract N99.89
    urinary tract (involving intestinal tract) N99.89
    vascular — *see* Complications, cardiovascular device or implant
  anesthesia, anesthetic (*see also* Anesthesia, complication) T88.59 ☑
    brain, postpartum, puerperal O89.2
    cardiac
      in
        labor and delivery O74.2
        pregnancy O29.19- ☑
      postpartum, puerperal O89.1
    central nervous system
      in
        labor and delivery O74.3
        pregnancy O29.29- ☑
      postpartum, puerperal O89.2
    difficult or failed intubation T88.4 ☑
      in pregnancy O29.6- ☑

Complication(s) — *continued*
  anesthesia, anesthetic (*see also* Anesthesia, complication) — *continued*
    failed sedation (conscious) (moderate) during procedure T88.52 ☑
    hyperthermia, malignant T88.3 ☑
    hypothermia T88.51 ☑
    intubation failure T88.4 ☑
    malignant hyperthermia T88.3 ☑
    pulmonary
      in
        labor and delivery O74.1
        pregnancy NEC O29.09- ☑
      postpartum, puerperal O89.09
    shock T88.2 ☑
    spinal and epidural
      in
        labor and delivery NEC O74.6
          headache O74.5
        pregnancy NEC O29.5X- ☑
      postpartum, puerperal NEC O89.5
        headache O89.4
  anti-reflux device — *see* Complications, esophageal anti-reflux device
  aortic (bifurcation) graft — *see* Complications, graft, vascular
  aortocoronary (bypass) graft — *see* Complications, coronary artery (bypass) graft
  aortofemoral (bypass) graft — *see* Complications, extremity artery (bypass) graft
  arteriovenous
    fistula, surgically created T82.9 ☑
      embolism T82.818 ☑
      fibrosis T82.828 ☑
      hemorrhage T82.838 ☑
      infection or inflammation T82.7 ☑
      mechanical
        breakdown T82.510 ☑
        displacement T82.520 ☑
        leakage T82.530 ☑
        malposition T82.520 ☑
        obstruction T82.590 ☑
        perforation T82.590 ☑
        protrusion T82.590 ☑
      pain T82.848 ☑
      specified type NEC T82.898 ☑
      stenosis T82.858 ☑
      thrombosis T82.868 ☑
    shunt, surgically created T82.9 ☑
      embolism T82.818 ☑
      fibrosis T82.828 ☑
      hemorrhage T82.838 ☑
      infection or inflammation T82.7 ☑
      mechanical
        breakdown T82.511 ☑
        displacement T82.521 ☑
        leakage T82.531 ☑
        malposition T82.521 ☑
        obstruction T82.591 ☑
        perforation T82.591 ☑
        protrusion T82.591 ☑
      pain T82.848 ☑
      specified type NEC T82.898 ☑
      stenosis T82.858 ☑
      thrombosis T82.868 ☑
  arthroplasty — *see* Complications, joint prosthesis
  artificial
    fertilization or insemination N98.9
      attempted introduction (of)
        embryo in embryo transfer N98.3
        ovum following in vitro fertilization N98.2
      hyperstimulation of ovaries N98.1
      infection N98.0
      specified NEC N98.8
    heart T82.9 ☑
      embolism T82.817 ☑
      fibrosis T82.827 ☑
      hemorrhage T82.837 ☑
      infection or inflammation T82.7 ☑
      mechanical
        breakdown T82.512 ☑
        displacement T82.522 ☑
        leakage T82.532 ☑
        malposition T82.522 ☑
        obstruction T82.592 ☑
        perforation T82.592 ☑

Complication(s) — *continued*
  artificial — *continued*
    heart — *continued*
      mechanical — *continued*
        protrusion T82.592 ☑
      pain T82.847 ☑
      specified type NEC T82.897 ☑
      stenosis T82.857 ☑
      thrombosis T82.867 ☑
    opening
      cecostomy — *see* Complications, colostomy
      colostomy — *see* Complications, colostomy
      cystostomy — *see* Complications, cystostomy
      enterostomy — *see* Complications, enterostomy
      gastrostomy — *see* Complications, gastrostomy
      ileostomy — *see* Complications, enterostomy
      jejunostomy — *see* Complications, enterostomy
      nephrostomy — *see* Complications, stoma, urinary tract
      tracheostomy — *see* Complications, tracheostomy
      ureterostomy — *see* Complications, stoma, urinary tract
      urethrostomy — *see* Complications, stoma, urinary tract
  balloon implant or device
    gastrointestinal T85.9 ☑
      embolism T85.81 ☑
      fibrosis T85.82 ☑
      hemorrhage T85.83 ☑
      infection and inflammation T85.79 ☑
      pain T85.84 ☑
      specified type NEC T85.89 ☑
      stenosis T85.85 ☑
      thrombosis T85.86 ☑
    vascular (counterpulsation) T82.9 ☑
      embolism T82.818 ☑
      fibrosis T82.828 ☑
      hemorrhage T82.838 ☑
      infection or inflammation T82.7 ☑
      mechanical
        breakdown T82.513 ☑
        displacement T82.523 ☑
        leakage T82.533 ☑
        malposition T82.523 ☑
        obstruction T82.593 ☑
        perforation T82.593 ☑
        protrusion T82.593 ☑
      pain T82.848 ☑
      specified type NEC T82.898 ☑
      stenosis T82.858 ☑
      thrombosis T82.868 ☑
  bariatric procedure
    gastric band procedure K95.09
      infection K95.01
    specified procedure NEC K95.89
      infection K95.81
  bile duct implant (prosthetic) T85.9 ☑
    embolism T85.81 ☑
    fibrosis T85.82 ☑
    hemorrhage T85.83 ☑
    infection and inflammation T85.79 ☑
    mechanical
      breakdown T85.510 ☑
      displacement T85.520 ☑
      malfunction T85.510 ☑
      malposition T85.520 ☑
      obstruction T85.590 ☑
      perforation T85.590 ☑
      protrusion T85.590 ☑
      specified NEC T85.590 ☑
    pain T85.84 ☑
    specified type NEC T85.89 ☑
    stenosis T85.85 ☑
    thrombosis T85.86 ☑
  bladder device (auxiliary) — *see* Complications, genitourinary, device or implant, urinary system
  bleeding (postoperative) — *see* Complication, postoperative, hemorrhage
    intraoperative — *see* Complication, intraoperative, hemorrhage
  blood vessel graft — *see* Complications, graft, vascular
  bone
    device NEC T84.9 ☑
      embolism T84.81 ☑

Complication(s) — *continued*
  bone — *continued*
    device — *continued*
      fibrosis T84.82 ☑
      hemorrhage T84.83 ☑
      infection or inflammation T84.7 ☑
      mechanical
        breakdown T84.318 ☑
        displacement T84.328 ☑
        malposition T84.328 ☑
        obstruction T84.398 ☑
        perforation T84.398 ☑
        protrusion T84.398 ☑
      pain T84.84 ☑
      specified type NEC T84.89 ☑
      stenosis T84.85 ☑
      thrombosis T84.86 ☑
    graft — *see* Complications, graft, bone
    growth stimulator (electrode) — *see* Complications, electronic stimulator device, bone
    marrow transplant — *see* Complications, transplant, bone, marrow
  brain neurostimulator (electrode) — *see* Complications, electronic stimulator device, brain
  breast implant (prosthetic) T85.9 ☑
    capsular contracture T85.44 ☑
    embolism T85.81 ☑
    fibrosis T85.82 ☑
    hemorrhage T85.83 ☑
    infection and inflammation T85.79 ☑
    mechanical
      breakdown T85.41 ☑
      displacement T85.42 ☑
      leakage T85.43 ☑
      malposition T85.42 ☑
      obstruction T85.49 ☑
      perforation T85.49 ☑
      protrusion T85.49 ☑
      specified NEC T85.49 ☑
    pain T85.84 ☑
    specified type NEC T85.89 ☑
    stenosis T85.85 ☑
    thrombosis T85.86 ☑
  bypass (*see also* Complications, prosthetic device or implant)
    aortocoronary — *see* Complications, coronary artery (bypass) graft
    arterial (*see also* Complications, graft, vascular)
      extremity — *see* Complications, extremity artery (bypass) graft
  cardiac (*see also* Disease, heart)
    device, implant or graft T82.9 ☑
      embolism T82.817 ☑
      fibrosis T82.827 ☑
      hemorrhage T82.837 ☑
      infection or inflammation T82.7 ☑
        valve prosthesis T82.6 ☑
      mechanical
        breakdown T82.519 ☑
          specified device NEC T82.518 ☑
        displacement T82.529 ☑
          specified device NEC T82.528 ☑
        leakage T82.539 ☑
          specified device NEC T82.538 ☑
        malposition T82.529 ☑
          specified device NEC T82.528 ☑
        obstruction T82.599 ☑
          specified device NEC T82.598 ☑
        perforation T82.599 ☑
          specified device NEC T82.598 ☑
        protrusion T82.599 ☑
          specified device NEC T82.598 ☑
      pain T82.847 ☑
      specified type NEC T82.897 ☑
      stenosis T82.857 ☑
      thrombosis T82.867 ☑
  cardiovascular device, graft or implant T82.9 ☑
    aortic graft — *see* Complications, graft, vascular
    arteriovenous
      fistula, artificial — *see* Complication, arteriovenous, fistula, surgically created
      shunt — *see* Complication, arteriovenous, shunt, surgically created
    artificial heart — *see* Complication, artificial, heart
    balloon (counterpulsation) device — *see* Complication, balloon implant, vascular

Complication(s) — *continued*
  cardiovascular device, graft or implant — *continued*
    carotid artery graft — *see* Complications, graft, vascular
    coronary bypass graft — *see* Complication, coronary artery (bypass) graft
    dialysis catheter (vascular) — *see* Complication, catheter, dialysis
    electronic T82.9 ☑
      electrode T82.9 ☑
        embolism T82.817 ☑
        fibrosis T82.827 ☑
        hemorrhage T82.837 ☑
        infection T82.7 ☑
        mechanical
          breakdown T82.110 ☑
          displacement T82.120 ☑
          leakage T82.190 ☑
          obstruction T82.190 ☑
          perforation T82.190 ☑
          protrusion T82.190 ☑
          specified type NEC T82.190 ☑
        pain T82.847 ☑
        specified NEC T82.897 ☑
        stenosis T82.857 ☑
        thrombosis T82.867 ☑
      embolism T82.817 ☑
      fibrosis T82.827 ☑
      hemorrhage T82.837 ☑
      infection T82.7 ☑
      mechanical
        breakdown T82.119 ☑
        displacement T82.129 ☑
        leakage T82.199 ☑
        obstruction T82.199 ☑
        perforation T82.199 ☑
        protrusion T82.199 ☑
        specified type NEC T82.199 ☑
      pain T82.847 ☑
      pulse generator T82.9 ☑
        embolism T82.817 ☑
        fibrosis T82.827 ☑
        hemorrhage T82.837 ☑
        infection T82.7 ☑
        mechanical
          breakdown T82.111 ☑
          displacement T82.121 ☑
          leakage T82.191 ☑
          obstruction T82.191 ☑
          perforation T82.191 ☑
          protrusion T82.191 ☑
          specified type NEC T82.191 ☑
        pain T82.847 ☑
        specified NEC T82.897 ☑
        stenosis T82.857 ☑
        thrombosis T82.867 ☑
      specified condition NEC T82.897 ☑
      specified device NEC T82.9 ☑
        embolism T82.817 ☑
        fibrosis T82.827 ☑
        hemorrhage T82.837 ☑
        infection T82.7 ☑
        mechanical
          breakdown T82.118 ☑
          displacement T82.128 ☑
          leakage T82.198 ☑
          obstruction T82.198 ☑
          perforation T82.198 ☑
          protrusion T82.198 ☑
          specified type NEC T82.198 ☑
        pain T82.847 ☑
        specified NEC T82.897 ☑
        stenosis T82.857 ☑
        thrombosis T82.867 ☑
      stenosis T82.857 ☑
      thrombosis T82.867 ☑
    extremity artery graft — *see* Complication, extremity artery (bypass) graft
    femoral artery graft — *see* Complication, extremity artery (bypass) graft
    heart
      transplant — *see* Complication, transplant, heart
      valve — *see* Complication, prosthetic device, heart valve

Complication(s) — *continued*
  cardiovascular device, graft or implant — *continued*
    heart — *continued*
      valve — *see* Complication, prosthetic device, heart valve — *continued*
        graft — *see* Complication, heart, valve, graft
    heart-lung transplant — *see* Complication, transplant, heart, with lung
    infection or inflammation T82.7 ☑
    umbrella device — *see* Complication, umbrella device, vascular
    vascular graft (or anastomosis) — *see* Complication, graft, vascular
  carotid artery (bypass) graft — *see* Complications, graft, vascular
  catheter (device) NEC (*see also* Complications, prosthetic device or implant)
    cystostomy T83.9 ☑
      embolism T83.81 ☑
      fibrosis T83.82 ☑
      hemorrhage T83.83 ☑
      infection and inflammation T83.59 ☑
      mechanical
        breakdown T83.010 ☑
        displacement T83.020 ☑
        leakage T83.030 ☑
        malposition T83.020 ☑
        obstruction T83.090 ☑
        perforation T83.090 ☑
        protrusion T83.090 ☑
        specified NEC T83.090 ☑
      pain T83.84 ☑
      specified type NEC T83.89 ☑
      stenosis T83.85 ☑
      thrombosis T83.86 ☑
    dialysis (vascular) T82.9 ☑
      embolism T82.818 ☑
      fibrosis T82.828 ☑
      hemorrhage T82.838 ☑
      infection and inflammation T82.7 ☑
      intraperitoneal — *see* Complications, catheter, intraperitoneal
      mechanical
        breakdown T82.41 ☑
        displacement T82.42 ☑
        leakage T82.43 ☑
        malposition T82.42 ☑
        obstruction T82.49 ☑
        perforation T82.49 ☑
        protrusion T82.49 ☑
      pain T82.848 ☑
      specified type NEC T82.898 ☑
      stenosis T82.858 ☑
      thrombosis T82.868 ☑
    epidural infusion T85.9 ☑
      embolism T85.81 ☑
      fibrosis T85.82 ☑
      hemorrhage T85.83 ☑
      infection and inflammation T85.79 ☑
      mechanical
        breakdown T85.610 ☑
        displacement T85.620 ☑
        leakage T85.630 ☑
        malfunction T85.610 ☑
        malposition T85.620 ☑
        obstruction T85.690 ☑
        perforation T85.690 ☑
        protrusion T85.690 ☑
        specified NEC T85.690 ☑
      pain T85.84 ☑
      specified type NEC T85.89 ☑
      stenosis T85.85 ☑
      thrombosis T85.86 ☑
    intraperitoneal dialysis T85.9 ☑
      embolism T85.81 ☑
      fibrosis T85.82 ☑
      hemorrhage T85.83 ☑
      infection and inflammation T85.71 ☑
      mechanical
        breakdown T85.611 ☑
        displacement T85.621 ☑
        leakage T85.631 ☑
        malfunction T85.611 ☑
        malposition T85.621 ☑
        obstruction T85.691 ☑

Complication(s) — *continued*
  catheter (*see also* Complications, prosthetic device or
    implant) — *continued*
    intraperitoneal dialysis — *continued*
      mechanical — *continued*
        perforation T85.691 ☑
        protrusion T85.691 ☑
        specified NEC T85.691 ☑
      pain T85.84 ☑
      specified type NEC T85.89 ☑
      stenosis T85.85 ☑
      thrombosis T85.86 ☑
    intravenous infusion T82.9 ☑
      embolism T82.818 ☑
      fibrosis T82.828 ☑
      hemorrhage T82.838 ☑
      infection or inflammation T82.7 ☑
      mechanical
        breakdown T82.514 ☑
        displacement T82.524 ☑
        leakage T82.534 ☑
        malposition T82.524 ☑
        obstruction T82.594 ☑
        perforation T82.594 ☑
        protrusion T82.594 ☑
      pain T82.848 ☑
      specified type NEC T82.898 ☑
      stenosis T82.858 ☑
      thrombosis T82.868 ☑
    subdural infusion T85.9 ☑
      embolism T85.81 ☑
      fibrosis T85.82 ☑
      hemorrhage T85.83 ☑
      infection and inflammation T85.79 ☑
      mechanical
        breakdown T85.610 ☑
        displacement T85.620 ☑
        leakage T85.630 ☑
        malfunction T85.610 ☑
        malposition T85.620 ☑
        obstruction T85.690 ☑
        perforation T85.690 ☑
        protrusion T85.690 ☑
        specified NEC T85.690 ☑
      pain T85.84 ☑
      specified type NEC T85.89 ☑
      stenosis T85.85 ☑
      thrombosis T85.86 ☑
    urethral, indwelling T83.9 ☑
      displacement T83.028 ☑
      embolism T83.81 ☑
      fibrosis T83.82 ☑
      hemorrhage T83.83 ☑
      infection and inflammation T83.51 ☑
      leakage T83.038 ☑
      malposition T83.028 ☑
      mechanical
        breakdown T83.018 ☑
      obstruction (mechanical) T83.098 ☑
      pain T83.84 ☑
      perforation T83.098 ☑
      protrusion T83.098 ☑
      specified type NEC T83.098 ☑
      stenosis T83.85 ☑
      thrombosis T83.86 ☑
    urinary (indwelling) — *see* Complications, catheter,
      urethral, indwelling
  cecostomy (stoma) — *see* Complications, colostomy
  cesarean delivery wound NEC O90.89
    disruption O90.0
    hematoma O90.2
    infection (following delivery) O86.0
  chemotherapy (antineoplastic) NEC T88.7 ☑
  chin implant (prosthetic) — *see* Complication, pros-
    thetic device or implant, specified NEC
  circulatory system I99.8
    intraoperative I97.88
    postprocedural I97.89
      following cardiac surgery I97.19- ☑
        postcardiotomy syndrome I97.0
      hypertension I97.3
      lymphedema after mastectomy I97.2
      postcardiotomy syndrome I97.0
      specified NEC I97.89
  colostomy (stoma) K94.00
    hemorrhage K94.01

Complication(s) — *continued*
  colostomy — *continued*
    infection K94.02
    malfunction K94.03
    mechanical K94.03
    specified complication NEC K94.09
  contraceptive device, intrauterine — *see* Complica-
    tions, intrauterine, contraceptive device
  cord (umbilical) — *see* Complications, umbilical cord
  corneal graft — *see* Complications, graft, cornea
  coronary artery (bypass) graft T82.9 ☑
    atherosclerosis — *see* Arteriosclerosis, coronary
      (artery),
    embolism T82.818 ☑
    fibrosis T82.828 ☑
    hemorrhage T82.838 ☑
    infection and inflammation T82.7 ☑
    mechanical
      breakdown T82.211 ☑
      displacement T82.212 ☑
      leakage T82.213 ☑
      malposition T82.212 ☑
      obstruction T82.218 ☑
      perforation T82.218 ☑
      protrusion T82.218 ☑
      specified NEC T82.218 ☑
    pain T82.848 ☑
    specified type NEC T82.897 ☑
    stenosis T82.858 ☑
    thrombosis T82.868 ☑
  counterpulsation device (balloon), intra- aortic — *see*
    Complications, balloon implant, vascular
  cystostomy (stoma) N99.518
    catheter — *see* Complications, catheter, cystosto-
      my
    hemorrhage N99.510
    infection N99.511
    malfunction N99.512
    specified type NEC N99.518
  delivery (*see also* Complications, obstetric) O75.9
    procedure (instrumental) (manual) (surgical) O75.4
    specified NEC O75.89
  dialysis (peritoneal) (renal) (*see also* Complications,
    infusion)
    catheter (vascular) — *see* Complication, catheter,
      dialysis
      peritoneal, intraperitoneal — *see* Complica-
        tions, catheter, intraperitoneal
  dorsal column (spinal) neurostimulator — *see* Compli-
    cations, electronic stimulator device, spinal cord
  drug NEC T88.7 ☑
  ear procedure (*see also* Disorder, ear)
    intraoperative H95.88
      hematoma — *see* Complications, intraopera-
        tive, hemorrhage (hematoma) (of), ear
      hemorrhage — *see* Complications, intraopera-
        tive, hemorrhage (hematoma) (of), ear
      laceration — *see* Complications, intraoperative,
        puncture or laceration..., ear
      specified NEC H95.88
    postoperative H95.89
      external ear canal stenosis H95.81- ☑
      hematoma — *see* Complications, postprocedu-
        ral, hemorrhage (hematoma) (of), ear
      hemorrhage — *see* Complications, postproce-
        dural, hemorrhage (hematoma) (of), ear
      postmastoidectomy — *see* Complications,
        postmastoidectomy
      specified NEC H95.89
  ectopic pregnancy O08.9
    damage to pelvic organs O08.6
    embolism O08.2
    genital infection O08.0
    hemorrhage (delayed) (excessive) O08.1
    metabolic disorder O08.5
    renal failure O08.4
    shock O08.3
    specified type NEC O08.0
    venous complication NEC O08.7
  electronic stimulator device
    bladder (urinary) — *see* Complications, electronic
      stimulator device, urinary
    bone T84.9 ☑
      breakdown T84.310 ☑
      displacement T84.320 ☑
      embolism T84.81 ☑
      fibrosis T84.82 ☑

Complication(s) — *continued*
  electronic stimulator device — *continued*
    bone — *continued*
      hemorrhage T84.83 ☑
      infection or inflammation T84.7 ☑
      malfunction T84.310 ☑
      malposition T84.320 ☑
      mechanical NEC T84.390 ☑
      obstruction T84.390 ☑
      pain T84.84 ☑
      perforation T84.390 ☑
      protrusion T84.390 ☑
      specified type NEC T84.89 ☑
      stenosis T84.85 ☑
      thrombosis T84.86 ☑
    brain T85.9 ☑
      embolism T85.81 ☑
      fibrosis T85.82 ☑
      hemorrhage T85.83 ☑
      infection and inflammation T85.79 ☑
      mechanical
        breakdown T85.110 ☑
        displacement T85.120 ☑
        leakage T85.190 ☑
        malposition T85.120 ☑
        obstruction T85.190 ☑
        perforation T85.190 ☑
        protrusion T85.190 ☑
        specified NEC T85.190 ☑
      pain T85.84 ☑
      specified type NEC T85.89 ☑
      stenosis T85.85 ☑
      thrombosis T85.86 ☑
    cardiac (defibrillator) (pacemaker) — *see* Compli-
      cations, cardiovascular device or implant,
      electronic
    muscle T84.9 ☑
      breakdown T84.418 ☑
      displacement T84.428 ☑
      embolism T84.81 ☑
      fibrosis T84.82 ☑
      hemorrhage T84.83 ☑
      infection or inflammation T84.7 ☑
      mechanical NEC T84.498 ☑
      pain T84.84 ☑
      specified type NEC T84.89 ☑
      stenosis T84.85 ☑
      thrombosis T84.86 ☑
    nervous system T85.9 ☑
      brain — *see* Complications, electronic stimula-
        tor device, brain
      embolism T85.81 ☑
      fibrosis T85.82 ☑
      hemorrhage T85.83 ☑
      infection and inflammation T85.79 ☑
      mechanical
        breakdown T85.118 ☑
        displacement T85.128 ☑
        leakage T85.199 ☑
        malposition T85.128 ☑
        obstruction T85.199 ☑
        perforation T85.199 ☑
        protrusion T85.199 ☑
        specified NEC T85.199 ☑
      pain T85.84 ☑
      peripheral nerve — *see* Complications, electron-
        ic stimulator device, peripheral nerve
      specified type NEC T85.89 ☑
      spinal cord — *see* Complications, electronic
        stimulator device, spinal cord
      stenosis T85.85 ☑
      thrombosis T85.86 ☑
    peripheral nerve T85.9 ☑
      embolism T85.81 ☑
      fibrosis T85.82 ☑
      hemorrhage T85.83 ☑
      infection and inflammation T85.79 ☑
      mechanical
        breakdown T85.111 ☑
        displacement T85.121 ☑
        leakage T85.191 ☑
        malposition T85.121 ☑
        obstruction T85.191 ☑
        perforation T85.191 ☑
        protrusion T85.191 ☑
        specified NEC T85.191 ☑

Complication(s) — *continued*
  electronic stimulator device — *continued*
    peripheral nerve — *continued*
      pain T85.84
      specified type NEC T85.89 ☑
      stenosis T85.85 ☑
      thrombosis T85.86 ☑
    spinal cord T85.9 ☑
      embolism T85.81 ☑
      fibrosis T85.82 ☑
      hemorrhage T85.83 ☑
      infection and inflammation T85.79 ☑
      mechanical
        breakdown T85.112 ☑
        displacement T85.122 ☑
        leakage T85.192 ☑
        malposition T85.122 ☑
        obstruction T85.192 ☑
        perforation T85.192 ☑
        protrusion T85.192 ☑
        specified NEC T85.192 ☑
      pain T85.84 ☑
      specified type NEC T85.89 ☑
      stenosis T85.85 ☑
      thrombosis T85.86 ☑
    urinary T83.9 ☑
      embolism T83.81 ☑
      fibrosis T83.82 ☑
      hemorrhage T83.83 ☑
      infection and inflammation T83.59 ☑
      mechanical
        breakdown T83.110 ☑
        displacement T83.120 ☑
        malposition T83.120 ☑
        perforation T83.190 ☑
        protrusion T83.190 ☑
        specified NEC T83.190 ☑
      pain T83.84 ☑
      specified type NEC T83.89 ☑
      stenosis T83.85 ☑
      thrombosis T83.86 ☑
  electroshock therapy T88.9 ☑
    specified NEC T88.8 ☑
  endocrine E34.9
    postprocedural
      adrenal hypofunction E89.6
      hypoinsulinemia E89.1
      hypoparathyroidism E89.2
      hypopituitarism E89.3
      hypothyroidism E89.0
      ovarian failure E89.40
        asymptomatic E89.40
        symptomatic E89.41
      specified NEC E89.89
      testicular hypofunction E89.5
  endodontic treatment NEC M27.59
  enterostomy (stoma) K94.10
    hemorrhage K94.11
    infection K94.12
    malfunction K94.13
    mechanical K94.13
    specified complication NEC K94.19
  episiotomy, disruption O90.1
  esophageal anti-reflux device T85.9 ☑
    embolism T85.81 ☑
    fibrosis T85.82 ☑
    hemorrhage T85.83 ☑
    infection and inflammation T85.79 ☑
    mechanical
      breakdown T85.511 ☑
      displacement T85.521 ☑
      malfunction T85.511 ☑
      malposition T85.521 ☑
      obstruction T85.591 ☑
      perforation T85.591 ☑
      protrusion T85.591 ☑
      specified NEC T85.591 ☑
    pain T85.84 ☑
    specified type NEC T85.89 ☑
    stenosis T85.85 ☑
    thrombosis T85.86 ☑
  esophagostomy K94.30
    hemorrhage K94.31
    infection K94.32
    malfunction K94.33
    mechanical K94.33

Complication(s) — *continued*
  esophagostomy — *continued*
    specified complication NEC K94.39
  extracorporeal circulation T80.90 ☑
  extremity artery (bypass) graft T82.9 ☑
    arteriosclerosis — *see* Arteriosclerosis, extremities, bypass graft
    embolism T82.818 ☑
    fibrosis T82.828 ☑
    hemorrhage T82.838 ☑
    infection and inflammation T82.7 ☑
    mechanical
      breakdown T82.318 ☑
        femoral artery T82.312 ☑
      displacement T82.328 ☑
        femoral artery T82.322 ☑
      leakage T82.338 ☑
        femoral artery T82.332 ☑
      malposition T82.328 ☑
        femoral artery T82.322 ☑
      obstruction T82.398 ☑
        femoral artery T82.392 ☑
      perforation T82.398 ☑
        femoral artery T82.392 ☑
      protrusion T82.398 ☑
        femoral artery T82.392 ☑
    pain T82.848 ☑
    specified type NEC T82.898 ☑
    stenosis T82.858 ☑
    thrombosis T82.868 ☑
  eye H57.9
    corneal graft — *see* Complications, graft, cornea
    implant (prosthetic) T85.9 ☑
      embolism T85.81 ☑
      fibrosis T85.82 ☑
      hemorrhage T85.83 ☑
      infection and inflammation T85.79 ☑
      mechanical
        breakdown T85.318 ☑
        displacement T85.328 ☑
        leakage T85.398 ☑
        malposition T85.328 ☑
        obstruction T85.398 ☑
        perforation T85.398 ☑
        protrusion T85.398 ☑
        specified NEC T85.398 ☑
      pain T85.84 ☑
      specified type NEC T85.89 ☑
      stenosis T85.85 ☑
      thrombosis T85.86 ☑
    intraocular lens — *see* Complications, intraocular lens
    orbital prosthesis — *see* Complications, orbital prosthesis
  female genital N94.9
    device, implant or graft NEC — *see* Complications, genitourinary, device or implant, genital tract
  femoral artery (bypass) graft — *see* Complication, extremity artery (bypass) graft
  fixation device, internal (orthopedic) T84.9 ☑
    infection and inflammation T84.60 ☑
      arm T84.61- ☑
        humerus T84.61- ☑
        radius T84.61- ☑
        ulna T84.61- ☑
      leg T84.629 ☑
        femur T84.62- ☑
        fibula T84.62- ☑
        tibia T84.62- ☑
      specified site NEC T84.89 ☑
      spine T84.63 ☑
    mechanical
      breakdown
        limb T84.119 ☑
          carpal T84.210 ☑
          femur T84.11- ☑
          fibula T84.11- ☑
          humerus T84.11- ☑
          metacarpal T84.210 ☑
          metatarsal T84.213 ☑
          phalanx
            foot T84.213 ☑
            hand T84.210 ☑
          radius T84.11- ☑
          tarsal T84.213 ☑
          tibia T84.11- ☑

Complication(s) — *continued*
  fixation device, internal — *continued*
    mechanical — *continued*
      breakdown — *continued*
        limb — *continued*
          ulna T84.11- ☑
        specified bone NEC T84.218 ☑
        spine T84.216 ☑
      displacement
        limb T84.129 ☑
          carpal T84.220 ☑
          femur T84.12- ☑
          fibula T84.12- ☑
          humerus T84.12- ☑
          metacarpal T84.220 ☑
          metatarsal T84.223 ☑
          phalanx
            foot T84.223 ☑
            hand T84.220 ☑
          radius T84.12- ☑
          tarsal T84.223 ☑
          tibia T84.12- ☑
          ulna T84.12- ☑
        specified bone NEC T84.228 ☑
        spine T84.226 ☑
      malposition — *see* Complications, fixation device, internal, mechanical, displacement
      obstruction — *see* Complications, fixation device, internal, mechanical, specified type NEC
      perforation — *see* Complications, fixation device, internal, mechanical, specified type NEC
      protrusion — *see* Complications, fixation device, internal, mechanical, specified type NEC
      specified type NEC
        limb T84.199 ☑
          carpal T84.290 ☑
          femur T84.19- ☑
          fibula T84.19- ☑
          humerus T84.19- ☑
          metacarpal T84.290 ☑
          metatarsal T84.293 ☑
          phalanx
            foot T84.293 ☑
            hand T84.290 ☑
          radius T84.19- ☑
          tarsal T84.293 ☑
          tibia T84.19- ☑
          ulna T84.19- ☑
        specified bone NEC T84.298 ☑
        vertebra T84.296 ☑
    specified type NEC T84.89 ☑
      embolism T84.81 ☑
      fibrosis T84.82 ☑
      hemorrhage T84.83 ☑
      pain T84.84 ☑
      specified complication NEC T84.89 ☑
      stenosis T84.85 ☑
      thrombosis T84.86 ☑
  following
    acute myocardial infarction NEC I23.8
      aneurysm (false) (of cardiac wall) (of heart wall) (ruptured) I23.3
      angina I23.7
      atrial
        septal defect I23.1
        thrombosis I23.6
      cardiac wall rupture I23.3
      chordae tendinae rupture I23.4
      defect
        septal
          atrial (heart) I23.1
          ventricular (heart) I23.2
      hemopericardium I23.0
      papillary muscle rupture I23.5
      rupture
        cardiac wall I23.3
          with hemopericardium I23.0
        chordae tendineae I23.4
        papillary muscle I23.5
      specified NEC I23.8
      thrombosis
        atrium I23.6
        auricular appendage I23.6
        ventricle (heart) I23.6

Complication(s) — *continued*
  following — *continued*
    acute myocardial infarction — *continued*
      ventricular
        septal defect I23.2
        thrombosis I23.6
    ectopic or molar pregnancy O08.9
      cardiac arrest O08.81
      sepsis O08.82
      specified type NEC O08.89
      urinary tract infection O08.83
    termination of pregnancy — *see* Abortion
  gastrointestinal K92.9
    bile duct prosthesis — *see* Complications, bile duct
      implant
    esophageal anti-reflux device — *see* Complications,
      esophageal anti-reflux device
    postoperative
      colostomy — *see* Complications, colostomy
      dumping syndrome K91.1
      enterostomy — *see* Complications, enterosto-
        my
      gastrostomy — *see* Complications, gastrostomy
      malabsorption NEC K91.2
      obstruction K91.3
      postcholecystectomy syndrome K91.5
      specified NEC K91.89
      vomiting after GI surgery K91.0
    prosthetic device or implant
      bile duct prosthesis — *see* Complications, bile
        duct implant
      esophageal anti-reflux device — *see* Complica-
        tions, esophageal anti-reflux device
      specified type NEC
        embolism T85.81 ☑
        fibrosis T85.82 ☑
        hemorrhage T85.83 ☑
        mechanical
          breakdown T85.518 ☑
          displacement T85.528 ☑
          malfunction T85.518 ☑
          malposition T85.528 ☑
          obstruction T85.598 ☑
          perforation T85.598 ☑
          protrusion T85.598 ☑
          specified NEC T85.598 ☑
        pain T85.84 ☑
        specified complication NEC T85.89 ☑
        stenosis T85.85 ☑
        thrombosis T85.86 ☑
  gastrostomy (stoma) K94.20
    hemorrhage K94.21
    infection K94.22
    malfunction K94.23
    mechanical K94.23
    specified complication NEC K94.29
  genitourinary
    device or implant T83.9 ☑
      genital tract T83.9 ☑
        infection or inflammation T83.6 ☑
        intrauterine contraceptive device — *see*
          Complications, intrauterine, contra-
          ceptive device
        mechanical — *see* Complications, by device,
          mechanical
        mesh — *see* Complications, mesh
        penile prosthesis — *see* Complications,
          prosthetic device, penile
        specified type NEC T83.89 ☑
          embolism T83.81 ☑
          fibrosis T83.82 ☑
          hemorrhage T83.83 ☑
          pain T83.84 ☑
          specified complication NEC T83.89 ☑
          stenosis T83.85 ☑
          thrombosis T83.86 ☑
        vaginal mesh — *see* Complications, mesh
      urinary system T83.9 ☑
        cystostomy catheter — *see* Complication,
          catheter, cystostomy
        electronic stimulator — *see* Complications,
          electronic stimulator device, urinary
        indwelling urethral catheter — *see* Compli-
          cations, catheter, urethral, indwelling
        infection or inflammation T83.59 ☑
          indwelling urinary catheter T83.51 ☑

Complication(s) — *continued*
  genitourinary — *continued*
    device or implant — *continued*
      urinary system — *continued*
        kidney transplant — *see* Complication,
          transplant, kidney
        organ graft — *see* Complication, graft, uri-
          nary organ
        specified type NEC T83.89 ☑
          embolism T83.81 ☑
          fibrosis T83.82 ☑
          hemorrhage T83.83 ☑
          mechanical T83.198 ☑
            breakdown T83.118 ☑
            displacement T83.128 ☑
            malfunction T83.118 ☑
            malposition T83.128 ☑
            obstruction T83.198 ☑
            perforation T83.198 ☑
            protrusion T83.198 ☑
            specified NEC T83.198 ☑
          pain T83.84 ☑
          specified complication NEC T83.89 ☑
          stenosis T83.85 ☑
          thrombosis T83.86 ☑
        sphincter implant — *see* Complications,
          implant, urinary sphincter
    postprocedural
      pelvic peritoneal adhesions N99.4
      renal failure N99.0
      specified NEC N99.89
      stoma — *see* Complications, stoma, urinary
        tract
      urethral stricture — *see* Stricture, urethra,
        postprocedural
    vaginal
      adhesions N99.2
      vault prolapse N99.3
  graft (bypass) (patch) (*see also* Complications, prosthet-
      ic device or implant)
    aorta — *see* Complications, graft, vascular
    arterial — *see* Complication, graft, vascular
    bone T86.839
      failure T86.831
      infection T86.832
      mechanical T84.318 ☑
        breakdown T84.318 ☑
        displacement T84.328 ☑
        protrusion T84.398 ☑
        specified type NEC T84.398 ☑
      rejection T86.830
      specified type NEC T86.838
    carotid artery — *see* Complications, graft, vascular
    cornea T86.849
      failure T86.841
      infection T86.842
      mechanical T85.398 ☑
        breakdown T85.318 ☑
        displacement T85.328 ☑
        protrusion T85.398 ☑
        specified type NEC T85.398 ☑
      rejection T86.840
      retroprosthetic membrane T85.398 ☑
      specified type NEC T86.848
    femoral artery (bypass) — *see* Complication, ex-
      tremity artery (bypass) graft
    genital organ or tract — *see* Complications, geni-
      tourinary, device or implant, genital tract
    muscle T84.9 ☑
      breakdown T84.410 ☑
      displacement T84.420 ☑
      embolism T84.81 ☑
      fibrosis T84.82 ☑
      hemorrhage T84.83 ☑
      infection and inflammation T84.7 ☑
      mechanical NEC T84.490 ☑
      pain T84.84 ☑
      specified type NEC T84.89 ☑
      stenosis T84.85 ☑
      thrombosis T84.86 ☑
    nerve — *see* Complication, prosthetic device or
      implant, specified NEC
    skin — *see* Complications, prosthetic device or
      implant, skin graft
    tendon T84.9 ☑
      breakdown T84.410 ☑

Complication(s) — *continued*
  graft (*see also* Complications, prosthetic device or im-
      plant) — *continued*
    tendon — *continued*
      displacement T84.420 ☑
      embolism T84.81 ☑
      fibrosis T84.82 ☑
      hemorrhage T84.83 ☑
      infection and inflammation T84.7 ☑
      mechanical NEC T84.490 ☑
      pain T84.84 ☑
      specified type NEC T84.89 ☑
      stenosis T84.85 ☑
      thrombosis T84.86 ☑
    urinary organ T83.9 ☑
      embolism T83.81 ☑
      fibrosis T83.82 ☑
      hemorrhage T83.83 ☑
      infection and inflammation T83.59 ☑
        indwelling urinary catheter T83.51 ☑
      mechanical
        breakdown T83.21 ☑
        displacement T83.22 ☑
        leakage T83.23 ☑
        malposition T83.22 ☑
        obstruction T83.29 ☑
        perforation T83.29 ☑
        protrusion T83.29 ☑
        specified NEC T83.29 ☑
      pain T83.84 ☑
      specified type NEC T83.89 ☑
      stenosis T83.85 ☑
      thrombosis T83.86 ☑
    vascular T82.9 ☑
      embolism T82.818 ☑
      femoral artery — *see* Complication, extremity
        artery (bypass) graft
      fibrosis T82.828 ☑
      hemorrhage T82.838 ☑
      mechanical
        breakdown T82.319 ☑
          aorta (bifurcation) T82.310 ☑
          carotid artery T82.311 ☑
          specified vessel NEC T82.318 ☑
        displacement T82.329 ☑
          aorta (bifurcation) T82.320 ☑
          carotid artery T82.321 ☑
          specified vessel NEC T82.328 ☑
        leakage T82.339 ☑
          aorta (bifurcation) T82.330 ☑
          carotid artery T82.331 ☑
          specified vessel NEC T82.338 ☑
        malposition T82.329 ☑
          aorta (bifurcation) T82.320 ☑
          carotid artery T82.321 ☑
          specified vessel NEC T82.328 ☑
        obstruction T82.399 ☑
          aorta (bifurcation) T82.390 ☑
          carotid artery T82.391 ☑
          specified vessel NEC T82.398 ☑
        perforation T82.399 ☑
          aorta (bifurcation) T82.390 ☑
          carotid artery T82.391 ☑
          specified vessel NEC T82.398 ☑
        protrusion T82.399 ☑
          aorta (bifurcation) T82.390 ☑
          carotid artery T82.391 ☑
          specified vessel NEC T82.398 ☑
      pain T82.848 ☑
      specified complication NEC T82.898 ☑
      stenosis T82.858 ☑
      thrombosis T82.868 ☑
  heart I51.9
    assist device
      infection and inflammation T82.7 ☑
      following acute myocardial infarction — *see*
        Complications, following, acute myocardial
        infarction
      postoperative — *see* Complications, circulatory
        system
    transplant — *see* Complication, transplant, heart
      and lung(s) — *see* Complications, transplant,
        heart, with lung
    valve
      graft (biological) T82.9 ☑
        embolism T82.817 ☑

Complication(s) — *continued*
  heart — *continued*
    valve — *continued*
      graft — *continued*
        fibrosis T82.827 ☑
        hemorrhage T82.837 ☑
        infection and inflammation T82.7 ☑
        mechanical T82.228 ☑
          breakdown T82.221 ☑
          displacement T82.222 ☑
          leakage T82.223 ☑
          malposition T82.222 ☑
          obstruction T82.228 ☑
          perforation T82.228 ☑
          protrusion T82.228 ☑
        pain T82.847 ☑
        specified type NEC T82.897 ☑
        stenosis T82.857 ☑
        thrombosis T82.867 ☑
      prosthesis T82.9 ☑
        embolism T82.817 ☑
        fibrosis T82.827 ☑
        hemorrhage T82.837 ☑
        infection or inflammation T82.6 ☑
        mechanical T82.09 ☑
          breakdown T82.01 ☑
          displacement T82.02 ☑
          leakage T82.03 ☑
          malposition T82.02 ☑
          obstruction T82.09 ☑
          perforation T82.09 ☑
          protrusion T82.09 ☑
        pain T82.847 ☑
        specified type NEC T82.897 ☑
          mechanical T82.09 ☑
        stenosis T82.857 ☑
        thrombosis T82.867 ☑
  hematoma
    intraoperative — *see* Complication, intraoperative, hemorrhage
    postprocedural — *see* Complication, postprocedural, hemorrhage
  hemodialysis — *see* Complications, dialysis
  hemorrhage
    intraoperative — *see* Complication, intraoperative, hemorrhage
    postprocedural — *see* Complication, postprocedural, hemorrhage
  ileostomy (stoma) — *see* Complications, enterostomy
  immunization (procedure) — *see* Complications, vaccination
  implant (*see also* Complications, by site and type)
    urinary sphincter T83.9 ☑
      embolism T83.81 ☑
      fibrosis T83.82 ☑
      hemorrhage T83.83 ☑
      infection and inflammation T83.59 ☑
      mechanical
        breakdown T83.111 ☑
        displacement T83.121 ☑
        leakage T83.191 ☑
        malposition T83.121 ☑
        obstruction T83.191 ☑
        perforation T83.191 ☑
        protrusion T83.191 ☑
        specified NEC T83.191 ☑
      pain T83.84 ☑
      specified type NEC T83.89 ☑
      stenosis T83.85 ☑
      thrombosis T83.86 ☑
  infusion (procedure) T80.90 ☑
    air embolism T80.0 ☑
    blood — *see* Complications, transfusion
    catheter — *see* Complications, catheter
    infection T80.29 ☑
    pump — *see* Complications, cardiovascular, device or implant
    sepsis T80.29 ☑
    serum reaction (*see also* Reaction, serum) T80.69 ☑
      anaphylactic shock (*see also* Shock, anaphylactic) T80.59 ☑
    specified type NEC T80.89 ☑
  inhalation therapy NEC T81.81 ☑
  injection (procedure) T80.90 ☑
    drug reaction — *see* Reaction, drug
    infection T80.29 ☑

Complication(s) — *continued*
  injection — *continued*
    sepsis T80.29 ☑
    serum (prophylactic) (therapeutic) — *see* Complications, vaccination
    specified type NEC T80.89 ☑
    vaccine (any) — *see* Complications, vaccination
  inoculation (any) — *see* Complications, vaccination
  insulin pump
    infection and inflammation T85.72 ☑
    mechanical
      breakdown T85.614 ☑
      displacement T85.624 ☑
      leakage T85.633 ☑
      malposition T85.624 ☑
      obstruction T85.694 ☑
      perforation T85.694 ☑
      protrusion T85.694 ☑
      specified NEC T85.694 ☑
  intestinal pouch NEC K91.858
  intraocular lens (prosthetic) T85.9 ☑
    embolism T85.81 ☑
    fibrosis T85.82 ☑
    hemorrhage T85.83 ☑
    infection and inflammation T85.79 ☑
    mechanical
      breakdown T85.21 ☑
      displacement T85.22 ☑
      malposition T85.22 ☑
      obstruction T85.29 ☑
      perforation T85.29 ☑
      protrusion T85.29 ☑
      specified NEC T85.29 ☑
    pain T85.84 ☑
    specified type NEC T85.89 ☑
    stenosis T85.85 ☑
    thrombosis T85.86 ☑
  intraoperative (intraprocedural)
    cardiac arrest
      during cardiac surgery I97.710
      during other surgery I97.711
    cardiac functional disturbance NEC
      during cardiac surgery I97.790
      during other surgery I97.791
    hemorrhage (hematoma) (of)
      circulatory system organ or structure
        during cardiac bypass I97.411
        during cardiac catheterization I97.410
        during other circulatory system procedure I97.418
        during other procedure I97.42
      digestive system organ
        during procedure on digestive system K91.61
        during procedure on other organ K91.62
      ear
        during procedure on ear and mastoid process H95.21
        during procedure on other organ H95.22
      endocrine system organ or structure
        during procedure on endocrine system organ or structure E36.01
        during procedure on other organ E36.02
      eye and adnexa
        during ophthalmic procedure H59.11- ☑
        during other procedure H59.12- ☑
      genitourinary organ or structure
        during procedure on genitourinary organ or structure N99.61
        during procedure on other organ N99.62
      mastoid process
        during procedure on ear and mastoid process H95.21
        during procedure on other organ H95.22
      musculoskeletal structure
        during musculoskeletal surgery M96.810
        during non-orthopedic surgery M96.811
        during orthopedic surgery M96.810
      nervous system
        during a nervous system procedure G97.31
        during other procedure G97.32
      respiratory system
        during other procedure J95.62
        during procedure on respiratory system organ or structure J95.61
      skin and subcutaneous tissue
        during a dermatologic procedure L76.01

Complication(s) — *continued*
  intraoperative — *continued*
    hemorrhage — *continued*
      skin and subcutaneous tissue — *continued*
        during a procedure on other organ L76.02
      spleen
        during a procedure on other organ D78.02
        during a procedure on the spleen D78.01
    puncture or laceration (accidental) (unintentional) (of)
      brain
        during a nervous system procedure G97.48
        during other procedure G97.49
      circulatory system organ or structure
        during circulatory system procedure I97.51
        during other procedure I97.52
      digestive system
        during procedure on digestive system K91.71
        during procedure on other organ K91.72
      ear
        during procedure on ear and mastoid process H95.31
        during procedure on other organ H95.32
      endocrine system organ or structure
        during procedure on endocrine system organ or structure E36.11
        during procedure on other organ E36.12
      eye and adnexa
        during ophthalmic procedure H59.21- ☑
        during other procedure H59.22- ☑
      genitourinary organ or structure
        during procedure on genitourinary organ or structure N99.71
        during procedure on other organ N99.72
      mastoid process
        during procedure on ear and mastoid process H95.31
        during procedure on other organ H95.32
      musculoskeletal structure
        during musculoskeletal surgery M96.820
        during non-orthopedic surgery M96.821
        during orthopedic surgery M96.820
      nervous system
        during a nervous system procedure G97.48
        during other procedure G97.49
      respiratory system
        during other procedure J95.72
        during procedure on respiratory system organ or structure J95.71
      skin and subcutaneous tissue
        during a dermatologic procedure L76.11
        during a procedure on other organ L76.12
      spleen
        during a procedure on other organ D78.12
        during a procedure on the spleen D78.11
    specified NEC
      circulatory system I97.88
      digestive system K91.81
      ear H95.88
      endocrine system E36.8
      eye and adnexa H59.88
      genitourinary system N99.81
      mastoid process H95.88
      musculoskeletal structure M96.89
      nervous system G97.81
      respiratory system J95.88
      skin and subcutaneous tissue L76.81
      spleen D78.81
  intraperitoneal catheter (dialysis) (infusion) — *see* Complications, catheter, intraperitoneal
  intrauterine
    contraceptive device
      embolism T83.81 ☑
      fibrosis T83.82 ☑
      hemorrhage T83.83 ☑
      infection and inflammation T83.6 ☑
      mechanical
        breakdown T83.31 ☑
        displacement T83.32 ☑
        malposition T83.32 ☑
        obstruction T83.39 ☑
        perforation T83.39 ☑
        protrusion T83.39 ☑
        specified NEC T83.39 ☑
      pain T83.84 ☑
      specified type NEC T83.89 ☑
      stenosis T83.85 ☑

Complication(s) — *continued*
  intrauterine — *continued*
    contraceptive device — *continued*
      thrombosis T83.86 ☑
    procedure (fetal), to newborn P96.5
  jejunostomy (stoma) — *see* Complications, enterostomy
  joint prosthesis, internal T84.9 ☑
    breakage (fracture) T84.01- ☑
    dislocation T84.02- ☑
    fracture T84.01- ☑
    infection or inflammation T84.50 ☑
      hip T84.5- ☑
      knee T84.5- ☑
      specified joint NEC T84.59 ☑
    instability T84.02- ☑
    malposition — *see* Complications, joint prosthesis, mechanical, displacement
    mechanical
      breakage, broken T84.01- ☑
      dislocation T84.02- ☑
      fracture T84.01- ☑
      instability T84.02- ☑
      leakage — *see* Complications, joint prosthesis, mechanical, specified NEC
      loosening T84.039 ☑
        hip T84.03- ☑
        knee T84.03- ☑
        specified joint NEC T84.038 ☑
      obstruction — *see* Complications, joint prosthesis, mechanical, specified NEC
      perforation — *see* Complications, joint prosthesis, mechanical, specified NEC
      periprosthetic
        fracture T84.049 ☑
          hip T84.04- ☑
          knee T84.04- ☑
          other specified joint T84.048 ☑
        osteolysis T84.059 ☑
          hip T84.05- ☑
          knee T84.05- ☑
          other specified joint T84.058 ☑
      protrusion — *see* Complications, joint prosthesis, mechanical, specified NEC
      specified complication NEC T84.099 ☑
        hip T84.09- ☑
        knee T84.09- ☑
        other specified joint T84.098 ☑
      subluxation T84.02- ☑
      wear of articular bearing surface T84.069 ☑
        hip T84.06- ☑
        knee T84.06- ☑
        other specified joint T84.068 ☑
    specified joint NEC T84.89 ☑
      embolism T84.81 ☑
      fibrosis T84.82 ☑
      hemorrhage T84.83 ☑
      pain T84.84 ☑
      specified complication NEC T84.89 ☑
      stenosis T84.85 ☑
      thrombosis T84.86 ☑
      subluxation T84.02- ☑
  kidney transplant — *see* Complications, transplant, kidney
  labor O75.9
    specified NEC O75.89
  liver transplant (immune or nonimmune) — *see* Complications, transplant, liver
  lumbar puncture G97.1
    cerebrospinal fluid leak G97.0
    headache or reaction G97.1
  lung transplant — *see* Complications, transplant, lung
    and heart — *see* Complications, transplant, lung, with heart
  male genital N50.9
    device, implant or graft — *see* Complications, genitourinary, device or implant, genital tract
    postprocedural or postoperative — *see* Complications, genitourinary, postprocedural
      specified NEC N99.89
  mastoid (process) procedure
    intraoperative H95.88
      hematoma — *see* Complications, intraoperative, hemorrhage (hematoma) (of), mastoid process

Complication(s) — *continued*
  mastoid procedure — *continued*
    intraoperative — *continued*
      hemorrhage — *see* Complications, intraoperative, hemorrhage (hematoma) (of), mastoid process
      laceration — *see* Complications, intraoperative, puncture or laceration, mastoid process
      specified NEC H95.88
    postmastoidectomy — *see* Complications, postmastoidectomy
    postoperative H95.89
      external ear canal stenosis H95.81 ☑
      hematoma — *see* Complications, postprocedural, hemorrhage (hematoma) (of), mastoid process
      hemorrhage — *see* Complications, postprocedural, hemorrhage (hematoma) (of), mastoid process
      postmastoidectomy — *see* Complications, postmastoidectomy
      specified NEC H95.89
  mastoidectomy cavity — *see* Complications, postmastoidectomy
  mechanical — *see* Complications, by site and type, mechanical
  medical procedures (*see also* Complication(s), intraoperative) T88.9 ☑
  metabolic E88.9
    postoperative E89.89
      specified NEC E89.89
  molar pregnancy NOS O08.9
    damage to pelvic organs O08.6
    embolism O08.2
    genital infection O08.0
    hemorrhage (delayed) (excessive) O08.1
    metabolic disorder O08.5
    renal failure O08.4
    shock O08.3
    specified type NEC O08.0
    venous complication NEC O08.7
  musculoskeletal system (*see also* Complication, intraoperative (intraprocedural), by site)
    device, implant or graft NEC — *see* Complications, orthopedic, device or implant
    internal fixation (nail) (plate) (rod) — *see* Complications, fixation device, internal
    joint prosthesis — *see* Complications, joint prosthesis
    post radiation M96.89
      kyphosis M96.3
      scoliosis M96.5
      specified complication NEC M96.89
    postoperative (postprocedural) M96.89
      with osteoporosis — *see* Osteoporosis
      fracture following insertion of device — *see* Fracture, following insertion of orthopedic implant, joint prosthesis or bone plate
      joint instability after prosthesis removal M96.89
      lordosis M96.4
      postlaminectomy syndrome NEC M96.1
        kyphosis M96.3
      pseudarthrosis M96.0
      specified complication NEC M96.89
  nephrostomy (stoma) — *see* Complications, stoma, urinary tract, external NEC
  nervous system G98.8
    central G96.9
    device, implant or graft (*see also* Complication, prosthetic device or implant, specified NEC)
      electronic stimulator (electrode(s)) — *see* Complications, electronic stimulator device
      ventricular shunt — *see* Complications, ventricular shunt
    electronic stimulator (electrode(s)) — *see* Complications, electronic stimulator device
    postprocedural G97.82
      intracranial hypotension G97.2
      specified NEC G97.82
      spinal fluid leak G97.0
  newborn, due to intrauterine (fetal) procedure P96.5
  nonabsorbable (permanent) sutures — *see* Complication, sutures, permanent
  obstetric O75.9
    procedure (instrumental) (manual) (surgical)
      specified NEC O75.4
    specified NEC O75.89

Complication(s) — *continued*
  obstetric — *continued*
    surgical wound NEC O90.89
      hematoma O90.2
      infection O86.0
  ocular lens implant — *see* Complications, intraocular lens
  ophthalmologic
    postprocedural bleb — *see* Blebitis
  orbital prosthesis T85.9 ☑
    embolism T85.81 ☑
    fibrosis T85.82 ☑
    hemorrhage T85.83 ☑
    infection and inflammation T85.79 ☑
    mechanical
      breakdown T85.31- ☑
      displacement T85.32- ☑
      malposition T85.32- ☑
      obstruction T85.39- ☑
      perforation T85.39- ☑
      protrusion T85.39- ☑
      specified NEC T85.39- ☑
    pain T85.84 ☑
    specified type NEC T85.89 ☑
    stenosis T85.85 ☑
    thrombosis T85.86 ☑
  organ or tissue transplant (partial) (total) — *see* Complications, transplant
  orthopedic (*see also* Disorder, soft tissue)
    device or implant T84.9 ☑
      bone
        device or implant — *see* Complication, bone, device NEC
        graft — *see* Complication, graft, bone
      breakdown T84.418 ☑
      displacement T84.428 ☑
      electronic bone stimulator — *see* Complications, electronic stimulator device, bone
      embolism T84.81 ☑
      fibrosis T84.82 ☑
      fixation device — *see* Complication, fixation device, internal
      hemorrhage T84.83 ☑
      infection or inflammation T84.7 ☑
      joint prosthesis — *see* Complication, joint prosthesis, internal
      malfunction T84.418 ☑
      malposition T84.428 ☑
      mechanical NEC T84.498 ☑
      muscle graft — *see* Complications, graft, muscle
      obstruction T84.498 ☑
      pain T84.84 ☑
      perforation T84.498 ☑
      protrusion T84.498 ☑
      specified complication NEC T84.89 ☑
      stenosis T84.85 ☑
      tendon graft — *see* Complications, graft, tendon
      thrombosis T84.86 ☑
    fracture (following insertion of device) — *see* Fracture, following insertion of orthopedic implant, joint prosthesis or bone plate
    postprocedural M96.89
      fracture — *see* Fracture, following insertion of orthopedic implant, joint prosthesis or bone plate
      postlaminectomy syndrome NEC M96.1
        kyphosis M96.3
        lordosis M96.4
      postradiation
        kyphosis M96.2
        scoliosis M96.5
      pseudarthrosis post-fusion M96.0
      specified type NEC M96.89
  pacemaker (cardiac) — *see* Complications, cardiovascular device or implant, electronic
  pancreas transplant — *see* Complications, transplant, pancreas
  penile prosthesis (implant) — *see* Complications, prosthetic device, penile
  perfusion NEC T80.90 ☑
  perineal repair (obstetrical) NEC O90.89
    disruption O90.1
    hematoma O90.2
    infection (following delivery) O86.0
  phototherapy T88.9 ☑
    specified NEC T88.8 ☑

Complication(s) — *continued*
- postmastoidectomy NEC H95.19- ☑
  - cyst, mucosal H95.13- ☑
  - granulation H95.12- ☑
  - inflammation, chronic H95.11- ☑
  - recurrent cholesteatoma H95.0- ☑
- postoperative — *see* Complications, postprocedural
  - circulatory — *see* Complications, circulatory system
  - ear — *see* Complications, ear
  - endocrine — *see* Complications, endocrine
  - eye — *see* Complications, eye
  - lumbar puncture G97.1
    - cerebrospinal fluid leak G97.0
  - nervous system (central) (peripheral) — *see* Complications, nervous system
  - respiratory system — *see* Complications, respiratory system
- postprocedural (*see also* Complications, surgical procedure)
  - cardiac arrest
    - following cardiac surgery I97.120
    - following other surgery I97.121
  - cardiac functional disturbance NEC
    - following cardiac surgery I97.190
    - following other surgery I97.191
  - cardiac insufficiency
    - following cardiac surgery I97.110
    - following other surgery I97.111
  - chorioretinal scars following retinal surgery H59.81- ☑
  - following cataract surgery
    - cataract (lens) fragments H59.02- ☑
    - cystoid macular edema H59.03- ☑
    - specified NEC H59.09- ☑
    - vitreous (touch) syndrome H59.01- ☑
  - heart failure
    - following cardiac surgery I97.130
    - following other surgery I97.131
  - hemorrhage (hematoma) (of)
    - circulatory system organ or structure
      - following a cardiac bypass I97.611
      - following a cardiac catheterization I97.610
      - following other circulatory system procedure I97.618
      - following other procedure I97.62
    - digestive system
      - following procedure on digestive system K91.840
      - following procedure on other organ K91.841
    - ear
      - following other procedure H95.42
      - following procedure on ear and mastoid process H95.41
    - endocrine system
      - following endocrine system procedure E89.810
      - following other procedure E89.811
    - eye and adnexa
      - following ophthalmic procedure H59.31- ☑
      - following other procedure H59.32- ☑
    - genitourinary organ or structure
      - following procedure on genitourinary organ or structure N99.820
      - following procedure on other organ N99.821
    - mastoid process
      - following other procedure H95.42
      - following procedure on ear and mastoid process H95.41
    - musculoskeletal structure
      - following musculoskeletal surgery M96.830
      - following non-orthopedic surgery M96.831
      - following orthopedic surgery M96.830
    - nervous system
      - following a nervous system procedure G97.51
      - following other procedure G97.52
    - respiratory system
      - following a respiratory system procedure J95.830
      - following other procedure J95.831
    - skin and subcutaneous tissue
      - following a dermatologic procedure L76.21
      - following a procedure on other organ L76.22
    - spleen
      - following procedure on other organ D78.22
      - following procedure on the spleen D78.21

Complication(s) — *continued*
- postprocedural (*see also* Complications, surgical procedure) — *continued*
  - specified NEC
    - circulatory system I97.89
    - digestive K91.89
    - ear H95.89
    - endocrine E89.89
    - eye and adnexa H59.89
    - genitourinary N99.89
    - mastoid process H95.89
    - metabolic E89.89
    - musculoskeletal structure M96.89
    - nervous system G97.82
    - respiratory system J95.89
    - skin and subcutaneous tissue L76.82
    - spleen D78.89
- pregnancy NEC — *see* Pregnancy, complicated by
- prosthetic device or implant T85.9 ☑
  - bile duct — *see* Complications, bile duct implant
  - breast — *see* Complications, breast implant
  - cardiac and vascular NEC — *see* Complications, cardiovascular device or implant
  - corneal transplant — *see* Complications, graft, cornea
  - electronic nervous system stimulator — *see* Complications, electronic stimulator device
  - epidural infusion catheter — *see* Complications, catheter, epidural
  - esophageal anti-reflux device — *see* Complications, esophageal anti-reflux device
  - genital organ or tract — *see* Complications, genitourinary, device or implant, genital tract
  - heart valve — *see* Complications, heart, valve, prosthesis
  - infection or inflammation T85.79 ☑
    - intestine transplant T86.892
    - liver transplant T86.43
    - lung transplant T86.812
    - pancreas transplant T86.892
    - skin graft T86.822
  - intraocular lens — *see* Complications, intraocular lens
  - intraperitoneal (dialysis) catheter — *see* Complications, catheter, intraperitoneal
  - joint — *see* Complications, joint prosthesis, internal
  - mechanical NEC T85.698 ☑
    - dialysis catheter (vascular) (*see also* Complication, catheter, dialysis, mechanical)
      - peritoneal — *see* Complication, catheter, intraperitoneal, mechanical
    - gastrointestinal device T85.598 ☑
    - ocular device T85.398 ☑
    - subdural (infusion) catheter T85.690 ☑
    - suture, permanent T85.692 ☑
      - that for bone repair — *see* Complications, fixation device, internal (orthopedic), mechanical
    - ventricular shunt
      - breakdown T85.01 ☑
      - displacement T85.02 ☑
      - leakage T85.03 ☑
      - malposition T85.02 ☑
      - obstruction T85.09 ☑
      - perforation T85.09 ☑
      - protrusion T85.09 ☑
      - specified NEC T85.09 ☑
  - mesh
    - erosion (to surrounding organ or tissue) T83.718 ☑
      - vaginal (into pelvic floor muscles) T83.711 ☑
    - exposure (into surrounding organ or tissue) T83.728 ☑
      - vaginal (into vagina) (through vaginal wall) T83.721 ☑
  - orbital — *see* Complications, orbital prosthesis
  - penile T83.9 ☑
    - embolism T83.81 ☑
    - fibrosis T83.82 ☑
    - hemorrhage T83.83 ☑
    - infection and inflammation T83.6 ☑
    - mechanical
      - breakdown T83.410 ☑
      - displacement T83.420 ☑
      - leakage T83.490 ☑
      - malposition T83.420 ☑

Complication(s) — *continued*
- prosthetic device or implant — *continued*
  - penile — *continued*
    - mechanical — *continued*
      - obstruction T83.490 ☑
      - perforation T83.490 ☑
      - protrusion T83.490 ☑
      - specified NEC T83.490 ☑
    - pain T83.84 ☑
    - specified type NEC T83.89 ☑
    - stenosis T83.85 ☑
    - thrombosis T83.86 ☑
  - prosthetic materials NEC
    - erosion (to surrounding organ or tissue) T83.718 ☑
      - vaginal (into pelvic floor muscles) T83.711 ☑
    - exposure (into surrounding organ or tissue) T83.728 ☑
      - vaginal (into vagina) (through vaginal wall) T83.721 ☑
  - skin graft T86.829
    - artificial skin or decellularized allodermis
      - embolism T85.81 ☑
      - fibrosis T85.82 ☑
      - hemorrhage T85.83 ☑
      - infection and inflammation T85.79 ☑
      - mechanical
        - breakdown T85.613 ☑
        - displacement T85.623 ☑
        - malfunction T85.613 ☑
        - malposition T85.623 ☑
        - obstruction T85.693 ☑
        - perforation T85.693 ☑
        - protrusion T85.693 ☑
        - specified NEC T85.693 ☑
      - pain T85.84 ☑
      - specified type NEC T85.89 ☑
      - stenosis T85.85 ☑
      - thrombosis T85.86 ☑
    - failure T86.821
    - infection T86.822
    - rejection T86.820
    - specified NEC T86.828
  - specified NEC T85.9 ☑
    - embolism T85.81 ☑
    - fibrosis T85.82 ☑
    - hemorrhage T85.83 ☑
    - infection and inflammation T85.79 ☑
    - mechanical
      - breakdown T85.618 ☑
      - displacement T85.628 ☑
      - leakage T85.638 ☑
      - malfunction T85.618 ☑
      - malposition T85.628 ☑
      - obstruction T85.698 ☑
      - perforation T85.698 ☑
      - protrusion T85.698 ☑
      - specified NEC T85.698 ☑
    - pain T85.84 ☑
    - specified type NEC T85.89 ☑
    - stenosis T85.85 ☑
    - thrombosis T85.86 ☑
  - subdural infusion catheter — *see* Complications, catheter, subdural
  - sutures — *see* Complications, sutures
  - urinary organ or tract NEC — *see* Complications, genitourinary, device or implant, urinary system
  - vascular — *see* Complications, cardiovascular device or implant
  - ventricular shunt — *see* Complications, ventricular shunt (device)
- puerperium — *see* Puerperal
- puncture, spinal G97.1
  - cerebrospinal fluid leak G97.0
  - headache or reaction G97.1
- pyelogram N99.89
- radiation
  - kyphosis M96.2
  - scoliosis M96.5
- reattached
  - extremity (infection) (rejection)
    - lower T87.1X- ☑
    - upper T87.0X- ☑
  - specified body part NEC T87.2

Complication(s) — *continued*
- reconstructed breast
  - asymmetry between native and reconstructed breast N65.1
  - deformity N65.0
  - disproportion between native and reconstructed breast N65.1
  - excess tissue N65.0
  - misshapen N65.0
- reimplant NEC (*see also* Complications, prosthetic device or implant)
  - limb (infection) (rejection) — *see* Complications, reattached, extremity
  - organ (partial) (total) — *see* Complications, transplant
  - prosthetic device NEC — *see* Complications, prosthetic device
- renal N28.9
  - allograft — *see* Complications, transplant, kidney
  - dialysis — *see* Complications, dialysis
- respirator
  - mechancial J95.850
    - specified NEC J95.859
- respiratory system J98.9
  - device, implant or graft — *see* Complication, prosthetic device or implant, specified NEC
  - lung transplant — *see* Complications, prosthetic device or implant, lung transplant
  - postoperative J95.89
    - air leak J95.812
    - Mendelson's syndrome (chemical pneumonitis) J95.4
    - pneumothorax J95.811
    - pulmonary insufficiency (acute) (after nonthoracic surgery) J95.2
      - chronic J95.3
      - following thoracic surgery J95.1
    - respiratory failure (acute) J95.821
      - acute and chronic J95.822
    - specified NEC J95.89
    - subglottic stenosis J95.5
    - tracheostomy complication — *see* Complications, tracheostomy
  - therapy T81.89 ☑
- sedation during labor and delivery O74.9
  - cardiac O74.2
  - central nervous system O74.3
  - pulmonary NEC O74.1
- shunt (*see also* Complications, prosthetic device or implant)
  - arteriovenous — *see* Complications, arteriovenous, shunt
  - ventricular (communicating) — *see* Complications, ventricular shunt
- skin
  - graft T86.829
    - failure T86.821
    - infection T86.822
    - rejection T86.820
    - specified type NEC T86.828
- spinal
  - anesthesia — *see* Complications, anesthesia, spinal
  - catheter (epidural) (subdural) — *see* Complications, catheter
  - puncture or tap G97.1
    - cerebrospinal fluid leak G97.0
    - headache or reaction G97.1
- stent
  - bile duct — *see* Complications, bile duct prosthesis
  - urinary T83.9 ☑
    - embolism T83.81 ☑
    - fibrosis T83.82 ☑
    - hemorrhage T83.83 ☑
    - infection and inflammation T83.59 ☑
    - mechanical
      - breakdown T83.112 ☑
      - displacement T83.122 ☑
      - leakage T83.192 ☑
      - malposition T83.122 ☑
      - obstruction T83.192 ☑
      - perforation T83.192 ☑
      - protrusion T83.192 ☑
      - specified NEC T83.192 ☑
    - pain T83.84 ☑
    - specified type NEC T83.89 ☑
    - stenosis T83.85 ☑
    - thrombosis T83.86 ☑

Complication(s) — *continued*
- stoma
  - digestive tract
    - colostomy — *see* Complications, colostomy
    - enterostomy — *see* Complications, enterostomy
    - esophagostomy — *see* Complications, esophagostomy
    - gastrostomy — *see* Complications, gastrostomy
  - urinary tract N99.538
    - cystostomy — *see* Complications, cystostomy
    - external NOS N99.528
      - hemorrhage N99.520
      - infection N99.521
      - malfunction N99.522
      - specified type NEC N99.528
    - hemorrhage N99.530
    - infection N99.531
    - malfunction N99.532
    - specified type NEC N99.538
- stomach banding — *see* Complication(s), bariatric procedure
- stomach stapling — *see* Complication(s), bariatric procedure
- surgical material, nonabsorbable — *see* Complication, suture, permanent
- surgical procedure (on) T81.9 ☑
  - amputation stump (late) — *see* Complications, amputation stump
  - cardiac — *see* Complications, circulatory system
  - cholesteatoma, recurrent — *see* Complications, postmastoidectomy, recurrent cholesteatoma
  - circulatory (early) — *see* Complications, circulatory system
  - digestive system — *see* Complications, gastrointestinal
  - dumping syndrome (postgastrectomy) K91.1
  - ear — *see* Complications, ear
  - elephantiasis or lymphedema I97.89
    - postmastectomy I97.2
  - emphysema (surgical) T81.82 ☑
  - endocrine — *see* Complications, endocrine
  - eye — *see* Complications, eye
  - fistula (persistent postoperative) T81.83 ☑
  - foreign body inadvertently left in wound (sponge) (suture) (swab) — *see* Foreign body, accidentally left during a procedure
  - gastrointestinal — *see* Complications, gastrointestinal
  - genitourinary NEC N99.89
  - hematoma
    - intraoperative — *see* Complication, intraoperative, hemorrhage
    - postprocedural — *see* Complication, postprocedural, hemorrhage
  - hemorrhage
    - intraoperative — *see* Complication, intraoperative, hemorrhage
    - postprocedural — *see* Complication, postprocedural, hemorrhage
  - hepatic failure K91.82
  - hyperglycemia (postpancreatectomy) E89.1
  - hypoinsulinemia (postpancreatectomy) E89.1
  - hypoparathyroidism (postparathyroidectomy) E89.2
  - hypopituitarism (posthypophysectomy) E89.3
  - hypothyroidism (post-thyroidectomy) E89.0
  - intestinal obstruction K91.3
  - intracranial hypotension following ventricular shunting (ventriculostomy) G97.2
  - lymphedema I97.89
    - postmastectomy I97.2
  - malabsorption (postsurgical) NEC K91.2
    - osteoporosis — *see* Osteoporosis, postsurgical malabsorption
  - mastoidectomy cavity NEC — *see* Complications, postmastoidectomy
  - metabolic E89.89
    - specified NEC E89.89
  - musculoskeletal — *see* Complications, musculoskeletal system
  - nervous system (central) (peripheral) — *see* Complications, nervous system
  - ovarian failure E89.40
    - asymptomatic E89.40
    - symptomatic E89.41

Complication(s) — *continued*
- surgical procedure — *continued*
  - peripheral vascular — *see* Complications, surgical procedure, vascular
  - postcardiotomy syndrome I97.0
  - postcholecystectomy syndrome K91.5
  - postcommissurotomy syndrome I97.0
  - postgastrectomy dumping syndrome K91.1
  - postlaminectomy syndrome NEC M96.1
    - kyphosis M96.3
  - postmastectomy lymphedema syndrome I97.2
  - postmastoidectomy cholesteatoma — *see* Complications, postmastoidectomy, recurrent cholesteatoma
  - postvagotomy syndrome K91.1
  - postvalvulotomy syndrome I97.0
  - pulmonary insufficiency (acute) J95.2
    - chronic J95.3
    - following thoracic surgery J95.1
  - reattached body part — *see* Complications, reattached
  - respiratory — *see* Complications, respiratory system
  - shock (hypovolemic) T81.19 ☑
  - spleen (postoperative) D78.89
    - intraoperative D78.81
  - stitch abscess T81.4 ☑
  - subglottic stenosis (postsurgical) J95.5
  - testicular hypofunction E89.5
  - transplant — *see* Complications, organ or tissue transplant
  - urinary NEC N99.89
  - vaginal vault prolapse (posthysterectomy) N99.3
  - vascular (peripheral)
    - artery T81.719 ☑
      - mesenteric T81.710 ☑
      - renal T81.711 ☑
      - specified NEC T81.718 ☑
    - vein T81.72 ☑
  - wound infection T81.4 ☑
- suture, permanent (wire) NEC T85.9 ☑
  - with repair of bone — *see* Complications, fixation device, internal
  - embolism T85.81 ☑
  - fibrosis T85.82 ☑
  - hemorrhage T85.83 ☑
  - infection and inflammation T85.79 ☑
  - mechanical
    - breakdown T85.612 ☑
    - displacement T85.622 ☑
    - malfunction T85.612 ☑
    - malposition T85.622 ☑
    - obstruction T85.692 ☑
    - perforation T85.692 ☑
    - protrusion T85.692 ☑
    - specified NEC T85.692 ☑
  - pain T85.84 ☑
  - specified type NEC T85.89 ☑
  - stenosis T85.85 ☑
  - thrombosis T85.86 ☑
- tracheostomy J95.00
  - granuloma J95.09
  - hemorrhage J95.01
  - infection J95.02
  - malfunction J95.03
  - mechanical J95.03
  - obstruction J95.03
  - specified type NEC J95.09
  - tracheo-esophageal fistula J95.04
- transfusion (blood) (lymphocytes) (plasma) T80.92 ☑
  - air emblism T80.0 ☑
  - circulatory overload E87.71
  - febrile nonhemolytic transfusion reaction R50.84
  - hemochromatosis E83.111
  - hemolysis T80.89 ☑
  - hemolytic reaction (antigen unspecified) T80.919 ☑
  - incompatibility reaction (antigen unspecified) T80.919 ☑
    - ABO T80.30 ☑
      - delayed serologic (DSTR) T80.39 ☑
      - hemolytic transfusion reaction (HTR) (unspecified time after transfusion) T80.319 ☑
        - acute (AHTR) (less than 24 hours after transfusion) T80.310 ☑

Complication(s) — *continued*
 transfusion — *continued*
  incompatibility reaction — *continued*
   ABO — *continued*
    hemolytic transfusion reaction — *continued*
     delayed (DHTR) (24 hours or more after transfusion) T80.311 ☑
    specified NEC T80.39 ☑
   acute (antigen unspecified) T80.910 ☑
   delayed (antigen unspecified) T80.911 ☑
   delayed serologic (DSTR) T80.89 ☑
   non-ABO (minor antigens (Duffy) (Kell) (Kidd) (Lewis) (M) (N) (P) (S)) T80.A0 ☑ (*following* T80.4)
    delayed serologic (DSTR) T80.A9 ☑ (*following* T80.4)
    hemolytic transfusion reaction (HTR) (unspecified time after transfusion) T80.A19 ☑ (*following* T80.4)
     acute (AHTR) (less than 24 hours after transfusion) T80.A10 ☑ (*following* T80.4)
     delayed (DHTR) (24 hours or more after transfusion) T80.A11 ☑ (*following* T80.4)
    specified NEC T80.A9 ☑ (*following* T80.4)
   Rh (antigens (C) (c) (D) (E) (e)) (factor) T80.40 ☑
    delayed serologic (DSTR) T80.49 ☑
    hemolytic transfusion reaction (HTR) (unspecified time after transfusion) T80.419 ☑
     acute (AHTR) (less than 24 hours after transfusion) T80.410 ☑
     delayed (DHTR) (24 hours or more after transfusion) T80.411 ☑
    specified NEC T80.49 ☑
  infection T80.29 ☑
  reaction NEC T80.89 ☑
  sepsis T80.29 ☑
  shock T80.89 ☑
 transplant T86.90
  bone T86.839
   failure T86.831
   infection T86.832
   rejection T86.830
   specified type NEC T86.838
  bone marrow T86.00
   failure T86.02
   infection T86.03
   rejection T86.01
   specified type NEC T86.09
  cornea T86.849
   failure T86.841
   infection T86.842
   rejection T86.840
   specified type NEC T86.848
  failure T86.92
  heart T86.20
   with lung T86.30
   cardiac allograft vasculopathy T86.290
    failure T86.32
    infection T86.33
    rejection T86.31
    specified type NEC T86.39
   failure T86.22
   infection T86.23
   rejection T86.21
   specified type NEC T86.298
  infection T86.93
  intestine T86.859
   failure T86.851
   infection T86.852
   rejection T86.850
   specified type NEC T86.858
  kidney T86.10
   failure T86.12
   infection T86.13
   rejection T86.11
   specified type NEC T86.19
  liver T86.40
   failure T86.42
   infection T86.43
   rejection T86.41
   specified type NEC T86.49
  lung T86.819
   with heart T86.30
    failure T86.32

Complication(s) — *continued*
 transplant — *continued*
  lung — *continued*
   with heart — *continued*
    infection T86.33
    rejection T86.31
    specified type NEC T86.39
   failure T86.811
   infection T86.812
   rejection T86.810
   specified type NEC T86.818
  malignant neoplasm C80.2
  pancreas T86.899
   failure T86.891
   infection T86.892
   rejection T86.890
   specified type NEC T86.898
  peripheral blood stem cells T86.5
  post-transplant lymphoproliferative disorder (PTLD) D47.Z1 (*following* D47.4)
  rejection T86.91
  skin T86.829
   failure T86.821
   infection T86.822
   rejection T86.820
   specified type NEC T86.828
  specified
   tissue T86.899
    failure T86.891
    infection T86.892
    rejection T86.890
    specified type NEC T86.898
   type NEC T86.99
  stem cell (from peripheral blood) (from umbilical cord) T86.5
  umbilical cord stem cells T86.5
 trauma (early) T79.9 ☑
  specified NEC T79.8 ☑
 ultrasound therapy NEC T88.9 ☑
 umbilical cord NEC
  complicating delivery O69.9 ☑
   specified NEC O69.89 ☑
 umbrella device, vascular T82.9 ☑
  embolism T82.818 ☑
  fibrosis T82.828 ☑
  hemorrhage T82.838 ☑
  infection or inflammation T82.7 ☑
  mechanical
   breakdown T82.515 ☑
   displacement T82.525 ☑
   leakage T82.535 ☑
   malposition T82.525 ☑
   obstruction T82.595 ☑
   perforation T82.595 ☑
   protrusion T82.595 ☑
  pain T82.848 ☑
  specified type NEC T82.898 ☑
  stenosis T82.858 ☑
  thrombosis T82.868 ☑
 urethral catheter — *see* Complications, catheter, urethral, indwelling
 vaccination T88.1 ☑
  anaphylaxis NEC T80.52 ☑
  arthropathy — *see* Arthropathy, postimmunization
  cellulitis T88.0 ☑
  encephalitis or encephalomyelitis G04.02
  infection (general) (local) NEC T88.0 ☑
  meningitis G03.8
  myelitis G04.89
  protein sickness T80.62 ☑
  rash T88.1 ☑
  reaction (allergic) T88.1 ☑
   serum T80.62 ☑
  sepsis T88.0 ☑
  serum intoxication, sickness, rash, or other serum reaction NEC T80.62 ☑
   anaphylactic shock T80.52 ☑
  shock (allergic) (anaphylactic) T80.52 ☑
  vaccinia (generalized) (localized) T88.1 ☑
 vas deferens device or implant — *see* Complications, genitourinary, device or implant, genital tract
 vascular I99.9
  device or implant T82.9 ☑
   embolism T82.818 ☑
   fibrosis T82.828 ☑
   hemorrhage T82.838 ☑
   infection or inflammation T82.7 ☑

Complication(s) — *continued*
 vascular — *continued*
  device or implant — *continued*
   mechanical
    breakdown T82.519 ☑
     specified device NEC T82.518 ☑
    displacement T82.529 ☑
     specified device NEC T82.528 ☑
    leakage T82.539 ☑
     specified device NEC T82.538 ☑
    malposition T82.529 ☑
     specified device NEC T82.528 ☑
    obstruction T82.599 ☑
     specified device NEC T82.598 ☑
    perforation T82.599 ☑
     specified device NEC T82.598 ☑
    protrusion T82.599 ☑
     specified device NEC T82.598 ☑
   pain T82.848 ☑
   specified type NEC T82.898 ☑
   stenosis T82.858 ☑
   thrombosis T82.868 ☑
  dialysis catheter — *see* Complication, catheter, dialysis
  following infusion, therapeutic injection or transfusion T80.1 ☑
  graft T82.9 ☑
   embolism T82.818 ☑
   fibrosis T82.828 ☑
   hemorrhage T82.838 ☑
   mechanical
    breakdown T82.319 ☑
     aorta (bifurcation) T82.310 ☑
     carotid artery T82.311 ☑
     specified vessel NEC T82.318 ☑
    displacement T82.329 ☑
     aorta (bifurcation) T82.320 ☑
     carotid artery T82.321 ☑
     specified vessel NEC T82.328 ☑
    leakage T82.339 ☑
     aorta (bifurcation) T82.330 ☑
     carotid artery T82.331 ☑
     specified vessel NEC T82.338 ☑
    malposition T82.329 ☑
     aorta (bifurcation) T82.320 ☑
     carotid artery T82.321 ☑
     specified vessel NEC T82.328 ☑
    obstruction T82.399 ☑
     aorta (bifurcation) T82.390 ☑
     carotid artery T82.391 ☑
     specified vessel NEC T82.398 ☑
    perforation T82.399 ☑
     aorta (bifurcation) T82.390 ☑
     carotid artery T82.391 ☑
     specified vessel NEC T82.398 ☑
    protrusion T82.399 ☑
     aorta (bifurcation) T82.390 ☑
     carotid artery T82.391 ☑
     specified vessel NEC T82.398 ☑
   pain T82.848 ☑
   specified complication NEC T82.898 ☑
   stenosis T82.858 ☑
   thrombosis T82.868 ☑
  postoperative — *see* Complications, postoperative, circulatory
 vena cava device (filter) (sieve) (umbrella) — *see* Complications, umbrella device, vascular
 ventilation therapy NEC T81.81 ☑
 ventilator
  mechanical J95.850
   specified NEC J95.859
 ventricular (communicating) shunt (device) T85.9 ☑
  embolism T85.81 ☑
  fibrosis T85.82 ☑
  hemorrhage T85.83 ☑
  infection and inflammation T85.79 ☑
  mechanical
   breakdown T85.01 ☑
   displacement T85.02 ☑
   leakage T85.03 ☑
   malposition T85.02 ☑
   obstruction T85.09 ☑
   perforation T85.09 ☑
   protrusion T85.09 ☑
   specified NEC T85.09 ☑
  pain T85.84 ☑

⏀ Subterms under main terms may continue to next column or page   ☑ Additional Character Required — Refer to the Tabular List for Character Selection   67

Complication — Conjunctivitis

Conjunctivitis — continued
  acute — continued
    serous except viral H10.23- ☑
      viral — see Conjunctivitis, viral
    toxic H10.21- ☑
  adenoviral (acute) (follicular) B30.1
  allergic (acute) — see Conjunctivitis, acute, atopic
    chronic H10.45
      vernal H10.44
  anaphylactic — see Conjunctivitis, acute, atopic
  Apollo B30.3
  atopic (acute) — see Conjunctivitis, acute, atopic
  Béal's B30.2
  blennorrhagic (gonococcal) (neonatorum) A54.31
  chemical (acute) (see also Corrosion, cornea)
    H10.21- ☑
  chlamydial A74.0
    due to trachoma A71.1
    neonatal P39.1
  chronic (nodosa) (petrificans) (phlyctenular) H10.40- ☑
    allergic H10.45
      vernal H10.44
    follicular H10.43- ☑
    giant papillary H10.41- ☑
    simple H10.42- ☑
    vernal H10.44
  coxsackievirus 24 B30.3
  diphtheritic A36.86
  due to
    dust — see Conjunctivitis, acute, atopic
    filariasis B74.9
    mucocutaneous leishmaniasis B55.2
  enterovirus type 70 (hemorrhagic) B30.3
  epidemic (viral) B30.9
    hemorrhagic B30.3
  gonococcal (neonatorum) A54.31
  granular (trachomatous) A71.1
    sequelae (late effect) B94.0
  hemorrhagic (acute) (epidemic) B30.3
  herpes zoster B02.31
  in (due to)
    Acanthamoeba B60.12
    adenovirus (acute) (follicular) B30.1
    Chlamydia A74.0
    coxsackievirus 24 B30.3
    diphtheria A36.86
    enterovirus type 70 (hemorrhagic) B30.3
    filariasis B74.9
    gonococci A54.31
    herpes (simplex) virus B00.53
      zoster B02.31
    infectious disease NEC B99 ☑
    meningococci A39.89
    mucocutaneous leishmaniasis B55.2
    rosacea L71.9
    syphilis (late) A52.71
    zoster B02.31
  inclusion A74.0
  infantile P39.1
    gonococcal A54.31
  Koch-Weeks' — see Conjunctivitis, acute, mucopuru-
    lent
  light — see Conjunctivitis, acute, atopic
  ligneous — see Blepharoconjunctivitis, ligneous
  meningococcal A39.89
  mucopurulent — see Conjunctivitis, acute, mucopuru-
    lent
  neonatal P39.1
    gonococcal A54.31
  Newcastle B30.8
  of Béal B30.2
  parasitic
    filariasis B74.9
    mucocutaneous leishmaniasis B55.2
  Parinaud's H10.89
  petrificans H10.89
  rosacea L71.9
  specified NEC H10.89
  swimming-pool B30.1
  trachomatous A71.1
    acute A71.0
    sequelae (late effect) B94.0
  traumatic NEC H10.89
  tuberculous A18.59
  tularemic A21.1
  tularensis A21.1

Conjunctivitis — continued
  viral B30.9
    due to
      adenovirus B30.1
      enterovirus B30.3
    specified NEC B30.8
Conjunctivochalasis H11.82- ☑
Connective tissue — see condition
Conn's syndrome E26.01
Conradi (-Hunermann) **disease** Q77.3
Consanguinity Z84.3
  counseling Z71.89
Conscious simulation (of illness) Z76.5
Consecutive — see condition
Consolidation lung (base) — see Pneumonia, lobar
Constipation (atonic) (neurogenic) (simple) (spastic)
  K59.00
  drug-induced — see Table of Drugs and Chemicals
  outlet dysfunction K59.02
  psychogenic F45.8
  slow transit K59.01
  specified NEC K59.09
Constitutional (see also condition)
  substandard F60.7
Constitutionally substandard F60.7
Constriction (see also Stricture)
  auditory canal — see Stenosis, external ear canal
  bronchial J98.09
  duodenum K31.5
  esophagus K22.2
  external
    abdomen, abdominal (wall) S30.841 ☑
    alveolar process S00.542 ☑
    ankle S90.54- ☑
    antecubital space — see Constriction, external,
      forearm
    arm (upper) S40.84- ☑
    auricle — see Constriction, external, ear
    axilla — see Constriction, external, arm
    back, lower S30.840 ☑
    breast S20.14- ☑
    brow S00.84 ☑
    buttock S30.840 ☑
    calf — see Constriction, external, leg
    canthus — see Constriction, external, eyelid
    cheek S00.84 ☑
      internal S00.542 ☑
    chest wall — see Constriction, external, thorax
    chin S00.84 ☑
    clitoris S30.844 ☑
    costal region — see Constriction, external, thorax
    digit(s)
      foot — see Constriction, external, toe
      hand — see Constriction, external, finger
    ear S00.44- ☑
    elbow S50.34- ☑
    epididymis S30.843 ☑
    epigastric region S30.841 ☑
    esophagus, cervical S10.14 ☑
    eyebrow — see Constriction, external, eyelid
    eyelid S00.24- ☑
    face S00.84 ☑
    finger(s) S60.44- ☑
      index S60.44- ☑
      little S60.44- ☑
      middle S60.44- ☑
      ring S60.44- ☑
    flank S30.841 ☑
    foot (except toe(s) alone) S90.84- ☑
      toe — see Constriction, external, toe
    forearm S50.84- ☑
      elbow only — see Constriction, external, elbow
    forehead S00.84 ☑
    genital organs, external
      female S30.846 ☑
      male S30.845 ☑
    groin S30.841 ☑
    gum S00.542 ☑
    hand S60.54- ☑
    head S00.94 ☑
      ear — see Constriction, external, ear
      eyelid — see Constriction, external, eyelid
      lip S00.541 ☑
      nose S00.34 ☑
      oral cavity S00.542 ☑
      scalp S00.04 ☑

Constriction — continued
  external — continued
    head — continued
      specified site NEC S00.84 ☑
    heel — see Constriction, external, foot
    hip S70.24- ☑
    inguinal region S30.841 ☑
    interscapular region S20.449 ☑
    jaw S00.84 ☑
    knee S80.24- ☑
    labium (majus) (minus) S30.844 ☑
    larynx S10.14 ☑
    leg (lower) S80.84- ☑
      knee — see Constriction, external, knee
      upper — see Constriction, external, thigh
    lip S00.541 ☑
    lower back S30.840 ☑
    lumbar region S30.840 ☑
    malar region S00.84 ☑
    mammary — see Constriction, external, breast
    mastoid region S00.84 ☑
    mouth S00.542 ☑
    nail
      finger — see Constriction, external, finger
      toe — see Constriction, external, toe
    nasal S00.34 ☑
    neck S10.94 ☑
      specified site NEC S10.84 ☑
      throat S10.14 ☑
    nose S00.34 ☑
    occipital region S00.04 ☑
    oral cavity S00.542 ☑
    orbital region — see Constriction, external, eyelid
    palate S00.542 ☑
    palm — see Constriction, external, hand
    parietal region S00.04 ☑
    pelvis S30.840 ☑
    penis S30.842 ☑
    perineum
      female S30.844 ☑
      male S30.840 ☑
    periocular area — see Constriction, external, eyelid
    phalanges
      finger — see Constriction, external, finger
      toe — see Constriction, external, toe
    pharynx S10.14 ☑
    pinna — see Constriction, external, ear
    popliteal space — see Constriction, external, knee
    prepuce S30.842 ☑
    pubic region S30.840 ☑
    pudendum
      female S30.846 ☑
      male S30.845 ☑
    sacral region S30.840 ☑
    scalp S00.04 ☑
    scapular region — see Constriction, external,
      shoulder
    scrotum S30.843 ☑
    shin — see Constriction, external, leg
    shoulder S40.24- ☑
    sternal region S20.349 ☑
    submaxillary region S00.84 ☑
    submental region S00.84 ☑
    subungual
      finger(s) — see Constriction, external, finger
      toe(s) — see Constriction, external, toe
    supraclavicular fossa S10.84 ☑
    supraorbital S00.84 ☑
    temple S00.84 ☑
    temporal region S00.84 ☑
    testis S30.843 ☑
    thigh S70.34- ☑
    thorax, thoracic (wall) S20.94 ☑
      back S20.44- ☑
      front S20.34- ☑
    throat S10.14 ☑
    thumb S60.34- ☑
    toe(s) (lesser) S90.44- ☑
      great S90.44- ☑
    tongue S00.542 ☑
    trachea S10.14 ☑
    tunica vaginalis S30.843 ☑
    uvula S00.542 ☑
    vagina S30.844 ☑
    vulva S30.844 ☑
    wrist S60.84- ☑

☑ **Additional Character Required** — Refer to the Tabular List for Character Selection   ▨ **Subterms under main terms may continue to next column or page**

Constriction — *continued*
　gallbladder — *see* Obstruction, gallbladder
　intestine — *see* Obstruction, intestine
　larynx J38.6
　　congenital Q31.8
　　　specified NEC Q31.8
　　　subglottic Q31.1
　organ or site, congenital NEC — *see* Atresia, by site
　prepuce (acquired) (congenital) N47.1
　pylorus (adult hypertrophic) K31.1
　　congenital or infantile Q40.0
　　newborn Q40.0
　ring dystocia (uterus) O62.4
　spastic (*see also* Spasm)
　　ureter N13.5
　ureter N13.5
　　with infection N13.6
　urethra — *see* Stricture, urethra
　visual field (peripheral) (functional) — *see* Defect, visual field
Constrictive — *see* condition
Consultation
　without complaint or sickness Z71.9
　　feared complaint unfounded Z71.1
　　specified reason NEC Z71.89
　medical — *see* Counseling, medical
　religious Z71.81
　specified reason NEC Z71.89
　spiritual Z71.81
Consumption — *see* Tuberculosis
Contact (with) (*see also* Exposure (to))
　acariasis Z20.7
　AIDS virus Z20.6
　air pollution Z77.110
　algae and algae toxins Z77.121
　algae bloom Z77.121
　anthrax Z20.810
　aromatic amines Z77.020
　aromatic (hazardous) compounds NEC Z77.028
　aromatic dyes NOS Z77.028
　arsenic Z77.010
　asbestos Z77.090
　bacterial disease NEC Z20.818
　benzene Z77.021
　blue-green algae bloom Z77.121
　body fluids (potentially hazardous) Z77.21
　brown tide Z77.121
　chemicals (chiefly nonmedicinal) (hazardous) NEC Z77.098
　cholera Z20.09
　chromium compounds Z77.018
　communicable disease Z20.9
　　bacterial NEC Z20.818
　　specified NEC Z20.89
　　viral NEC Z20.828
　cyanobacteria bloom Z77.121
　dyes Z77.098
　Escherichia coli (E. coli) Z20.01
　fiberglass — *see* Table of Drugs and Chemicals, fiberglass
　German measles Z20.4
　gonorrhea Z20.2
　hazardous metals NEC Z77.018
　hazardous substances NEC Z77.29
　hazards in the physical environment NEC Z77.128
　hazards to health NEC Z77.9
　HIV Z20.6
　HTLV-III/LAV Z20.6
　human immunodeficiency virus (HIV) Z20.6
　infection Z20.9
　　specified NEC Z20.89
　infestation (parasitic) NEC Z20.7
　intestinal infectious disease NEC Z20.09
　　Escherichia coli (E. coli) Z20.01
　lead Z77.011
　meningococcus Z20.811
　mold (toxic) Z77.120
　nickel dust Z77.018
　noise Z77.122
　parasitic disease Z20.7
　pediculosis Z20.7
　pfiesteria piscicida Z77.121
　poliomyelitis Z20.89
　pollution
　　air Z77.110
　　environmental NEC Z77.118
　　soil Z77.112
　　water Z77.111

Contact — *continued*
　polycyclic aromatic hydrocarbons Z77.028
　rabies Z20.3
　radiation, naturally occurring NEC Z77.123
　radon Z77.123
　red tide (Florida) Z77.121
　rubella Z20.4
　sexually-transmitted disease Z20.2
　smallpox (laboratory) Z20.89
　syphilis Z20.2
　tuberculosis Z20.1
　uranium Z77.012
　varicella Z20.820
　venereal disease Z20.2
　viral disease NEC Z20.828
　viral hepatitis Z20.5
　water pollution Z77.111
Contamination, food — *see* Intoxication, foodborne
Contraception, contraceptive
　advice Z30.09
　counseling Z30.09
　device (intrauterine) (in situ) Z97.5
　　causing menorrhagia T83.83 ☑
　　checking Z30.431
　　complications — *see* Complications, intrauterine, contraceptive device
　　in place Z97.5
　　initial prescription Z30.014
　　reinsertion Z30.433
　　removal Z30.432
　　replacement Z30.433
　emergency (postcoital) Z30.012
　initial prescription Z30.019
　　injectable Z30.013
　　intrauterine device Z30.014
　　pills Z30.011
　　postcoital (emergency) Z30.012
　　specified type NEC Z30.018
　　subdermal implantable Z30.019
　maintenance Z30.40
　　examination Z30.8
　　injectable Z30.42
　　intrauterine device Z30.431
　　pills Z30.41
　　specified type NEC Z30.49
　　subdermal implantable Z30.49
　management Z30.9
　　specified NEC Z30.8
　postcoital (emergency) Z30.012
　prescription Z30.019
　　repeat Z30.40
　sterilization Z30.2
　surveillance (drug) — *see* Contraception, maintenance
Contraction(s), contracture, contracted
　Achilles tendon (*see also* Short, tendon, Achilles)
　　congenital Q66.89
　amputation stump (surgical) (flexion) (late) (next proximal joint) T87.89
　anus K59.8
　bile duct (common) (hepatic) K83.8
　bladder N32.89
　　neck or sphincter N32.0
　bowel, cecum, colon or intestine, any part — *see* Obstruction, intestine
　Braxton Hicks — *see* False, labor
　breast implant, capsular T85.44 ☑
　bronchial J98.09
　burn (old) — *see* Cicatrix
　cervix — *see* Stricture, cervix
　cicatricial — *see* Cicatrix
　conjunctiva, trachomatous, active A71.1
　　sequelae (late effect) B94.0
　Dupuytren's M72.0
　eyelid — *see* Disorder, eyelid function
　fascia (lata) (postural) M72.8
　　Dupuytren's M72.0
　　palmar M72.0
　　plantar M72.2
　finger NEC (*see also* Deformity, finger)
　　congenital Q68.1
　　joint — *see* Contraction, joint, hand
　flaccid — *see* Contraction, paralytic
　gallbladder K82.0
　heart valve — *see* Endocarditis
　hip — *see* Contraction, joint, hip
　hourglass
　　bladder N32.89
　　　congenital Q64.79

Contraction(s), contracture, contracted — *continued*
　hourglass — *continued*
　　gallbladder K82.0
　　　congenital Q44.1
　　stomach K31.89
　　　congenital Q40.2
　　　psychogenic F45.8
　　uterus (complicating delivery) O62.4
　hysterical F44.4
　internal os — *see* Stricture, cervix
　joint (abduction) (acquired) (adduction) (flexion) (rotation) M24.50
　　ankle M24.57- ☑
　　congenital NEC Q68.8
　　　hip Q65.89
　　elbow M24.52- ☑
　　foot joint M24.57- ☑
　　hand joint M24.54- ☑
　　hip M24.55- ☑
　　　congenital Q65.89
　　hysterical F44.4
　　knee M24.56- ☑
　　shoulder M24.51- ☑
　　wrist M24.53- ☑
　kidney (granular) (secondary) N26.9
　　congenital Q63.8
　　hydronephritic — *see* Hydronephrosis Page N26.2
　　pyelonephritic — *see* Pyelitis, chronic
　　tuberculous A18.11
　ligament (*see also* Disorder, ligament)
　　congenital Q79.8
　muscle (postinfective) (postural) NEC M62.40
　　with contracture of joint — *see* Contraction, joint
　　ankle M62.47- ☑
　　congenital Q79.8
　　　sternocleidomastoid Q68.0
　　extraocular — *see* Strabismus
　　eye (extrinsic) — *see* Strabismus
　　foot M62.47- ☑
　　forearm M62.43- ☑
　　hand M62.44- ☑
　　hysterical F44.4
　　ischemic (Volkmann's) T79.6 ☑
　　lower leg M62.46- ☑
　　multiple sites M62.49
　　pelvic region M62.45- ☑
　　posttraumatic — *see* Strabismus, paralytic
　　psychogenic F45.8
　　　conversion reaction F44.4
　　shoulder region M62.41- ☑
　　specified site NEC M62.48
　　thigh M62.45- ☑
　　upper arm M62.42- ☑
　neck — *see* Torticollis
　ocular muscle — *see* Strabismus
　organ or site, congenital NEC — *see* Atresia, by site
　outlet (pelvis) — *see* Contraction, pelvis
　palmar fascia M72.0
　paralytic
　　joint — *see* Contraction, joint
　　muscle (*see also* Contraction, muscle NEC)
　　　ocular — *see* Strabismus, paralytic
　pelvis (acquired) (general) M95.5
　　with disproportion (fetopelvic) O33.1
　　　causing obstructed labor O65.1
　　　inlet O33.2
　　　mid-cavity O33.3 ☑
　　　outlet O33.3 ☑
　plantar fascia M72.2
　premature
　　atrium I49.1
　　auriculoventricular I49.49
　　heart I49.49
　　junctional I49.2
　　supraventricular I49.1
　　ventricular I49.3
　prostate N42.89
　pylorus NEC (*see also* Pylorospasm)
　　psychogenic F45.8
　rectum, rectal (sphincter) K59.8
　ring (Bandl's) (complicating delivery) O62.4
　scar — *see* Cicatrix
　spine — *see* Dorsopathy, deforming
　sternocleidomastoid (muscle), congenital Q68.0

Contraction(s), contracture, contracted — *continued*

stomach K31.89
  hourglass K31.89
    congenital Q40.2
    psychogenic F45.8
  psychogenic F45.8
tendon (sheath) M62.40
  with contracture of joint — *see* Contraction, joint
  Achilles — *see* Short, tendon, Achilles
  ankle M62.47- ☑
    Achilles — *see* Short, tendon, Achilles
  foot M62.47- ☑
  forearm M62.43- ☑
  hand M62.44- ☑
  lower leg M62.46- ☑
  multiple sites M62.49
  neck M62.48
  pelvic region M62.45- ☑
  shoulder region M62.41- ☑
  specified site NEC M62.48
  thigh M62.45- ☑
  thorax M62.48
  trunk M62.48
  upper arm M62.42- ☑
toe — *see* Deformity, toe, specified NEC
ureterovesical orifice (postinfectional) N13.5
  with infection N13.6
urethra (*see also* Stricture, urethra)
  orifice N32.0
uterus N85.8
  abnormal NEC O62.9
  clonic (complicating delivery) O62.4
  dyscoordinate (complicating delivery) O62.4
  hourglass (complicating delivery) O62.4
  hypertonic O62.4
  hypotonic NEC O62.2
  inadequate
    primary O62.0
    secondary O62.1
  incoordinate (complicating delivery) O62.4
  poor O62.2
  tetanic (complicating delivery) O62.4
vagina (outlet) N89.5
vesical N32.89
  neck or urethral orifice N32.0
visual field — *see* Defect, visual field, generalized
Volkmann's (ischemic) T79.6

Contusion (skin surface intact) T14.8

abdomen, abdominal (muscle) (wall) S30.1 ☑
adnexa, eye NEC S05.8X- ☑
adrenal gland S37.812 ☑
alveolar process S00.532 ☑
ankle S90.0- ☑
antecubital space — *see* Contusion, forearm
anus S30.3 ☑
arm (upper) S40.02- ☑
  lower (with elbow) — *see* Contusion, forearm
auditory canal — *see* Contusion, ear
auricle — *see* Contusion, ear
axilla — *see* Contusion, arm, upper
back (*see also* Contusion, thorax, back)
  lower S30.0 ☑
bile duct S36.13 ☑
bladder S37.22 ☑
bone NEC T14.8
brain (diffuse) — *see* Injury, intracranial, diffuse
  focal — *see* Injury, intracranial, focal
brainstem S06.38- ☑
breast S20.0- ☑
broad ligament S37.892 ☑
brow S00.83 ☑
buttock S30.0 ☑
canthus, eye S00.1- ☑
cauda equina S34.3 ☑
cerebellar, traumatic S06.37- ☑
cerebral S06.33- ☑
  left side S06.32- ☑
  right side S06.31- ☑
cheek S00.83 ☑
  internal S00.532 ☑
chest (wall) — *see* Contusion, thorax
chin S00.83 ☑
clitoris S30.23 ☑
colon — *see* Injury, intestine, large, contusion
common bile duct S36.13 ☑

Contusion — *continued*

conjunctiva S05.1- ☑
  with foreign body (in conjunctival sac) — *see* Foreign body, conjunctival sac
conus medullaris (spine) S34.139 ☑
cornea — *see* Contusion, eyeball
  with foreign body — *see* Foreign body, cornea
corpus cavernosum S30.21 ☑
cortex (brain) (cerebral) — *see* Injury, intracranial, diffuse
  focal — *see* Injury, intracranial, focal
costal region — *see* Contusion, thorax
cystic duct S36.13 ☑
diaphragm S27.802 ☑
duodenum S36.420 ☑
ear S00.43- ☑
elbow S50.0- ☑
  with forearm — *see* Contusion, forearm
epididymis S30.22 ☑
epigastric region S30.1 ☑
epiglottis S10.0 ☑
esophagus (thoracic) S27.812 ☑
  cervical S10.0 ☑
eyeball S05.1- ☑
eyebrow S00.1- ☑
eyelid (and periocular area) S00.1- ☑
face NEC S00.83 ☑
fallopian tube S37.529 ☑
  bilateral S37.522 ☑
  unilateral S37.521 ☑
femoral triangle S30.1 ☑
finger(s) S60.00 ☑
  with damage to nail (matrix) S60.10 ☑
  index S60.02- ☑
    with damage to nail S60.12- ☑
  little S60.05- ☑
    with damage to nail S60.15- ☑
  middle S60.03- ☑
    with damage to nail S60.13- ☑
  ring S60.04- ☑
    with damage to nail S60.14- ☑
  thumb — *see* Contusion, thumb
flank S30.1 ☑
foot (except toe(s) alone) S90.3- ☑
  toe — *see* Contusion, toe
forearm S50.1- ☑
  elbow only — *see* Contusion, elbow
forehead S00.83 ☑
gallbladder S36.122 ☑
genital organs, external
  female S30.202 ☑
  male S30.201 ☑
globe (eye) — *see* Contusion, eyeball
groin S30.1 ☑
gum S00.532 ☑
hand S60.22- ☑
  finger(s) — *see* Contusion, finger
  wrist — *see* Contusion, wrist
head S00.93 ☑
  ear — *see* Contusion, ear
  eyelid — *see* Contusion, eyelid
  lip S00.531 ☑
  nose S00.33 ☑
  oral cavity S00.532 ☑
  scalp S00.03 ☑
  specified part NEC S00.83 ☑
heel — *see* Contusion, foot
hepatic duct S36.13 ☑
hip S70.0- ☑
ileum S36.428 ☑
iliac region S30.1 ☑
inguinal region S30.1 ☑
interscapular region S20.229 ☑
intra-abdominal organ S36.92 ☑
  colon — *see* Injury, intestine, large, contusion
  liver S36.112 ☑
  pancreas — *see* Contusion, pancreas
  rectum S36.62 ☑
  small intestine — *see* Injury, intestine, small, contusion
  specified organ NEC S36.892 ☑
  spleen — *see* Contusion, spleen
  stomach S36.32 ☑
iris (eye) — *see* Contusion, eyeball
jaw S00.83 ☑
jejunum S36.428 ☑

Contusion — *continued*

kidney S37.01- ☑
  major (greater than 2 cm) S37.02- ☑
  minor (less than 2 cm) S37.01- ☑
knee S80.0- ☑
labium (majus) (minus) S30.23 ☑
lacrimal apparatus, gland or sac S05.8X- ☑
larynx S10.0 ☑
leg (lower) S80.1- ☑
  knee — *see* Contusion, knee
lens — *see* Contusion, eyeball
lip S00.531 ☑
liver S36.112 ☑
lower back S30.0 ☑
lumbar region S30.0 ☑
lung S27.329 ☑
  bilateral S27.322 ☑
  unilateral S27.321 ☑
malar region S00.83 ☑
mastoid region S00.83 ☑
membrane, brain — *see* Injury, intracranial, diffuse
  focal — *see* Injury, intracranial, focal
mesentery S36.892 ☑
mesosalpinx S37.892 ☑
mouth S00.532 ☑
muscle — *see* Contusion, by site
nail
  finger — *see* Contusion, finger, with damage to nail
  toe — *see* Contusion, toe, with damage to nail
nasal S00.33 ☑
neck S10.93 ☑
  specified site NEC S10.83 ☑
  throat S10.0 ☑
nerve — *see* Injury, nerve
newborn P54.5
nose S00.33 ☑
occipital
  lobe (brain) — *see* Injury, intracranial, diffuse
    focal — *see* Injury, intracranial, focal
  region (scalp) S00.03 ☑
orbit (region) (tissues) S05.1- ☑
ovary S37.429 ☑
  bilateral S37.422 ☑
  unilateral S37.421 ☑
palate S00.532 ☑
pancreas S36.229 ☑
  body S36.221 ☑
  head S36.220 ☑
  tail S36.222 ☑
parietal
  lobe (brain) — *see* Injury, intracranial, diffuse
    focal — *see* Injury, intracranial, focal
  region (scalp) S00.03 ☑
pelvic organ S37.92 ☑
  adrenal gland S37.812 ☑
  bladder S37.22 ☑
  fallopian tube — *see* Contusion, fallopian tube
  kidney — *see* Contusion, kidney
  ovary — *see* Contusion, ovary
  prostate S37.822 ☑
  specified organ NEC S37.892 ☑
  ureter S37.12 ☑
  urethra S37.32 ☑
  uterus S37.62 ☑
pelvis S30.0 ☑
penis S30.21 ☑
perineum
  female S30.23 ☑
  male S30.0 ☑
periocular area S00.1- ☑
peritoneum S36.81 ☑
periurethral tissue — *see* Contusion, urethra
pharynx S10.0 ☑
pinna — *see* Contusion, ear
popliteal space — *see* Contusion, knee
prepuce S30.21 ☑
prostate S37.822 ☑
pubic region S30.1 ☑
pudendum
  female S30.202 ☑
  male S30.201 ☑
quadriceps femoris — *see* Contusion, thigh
rectum S36.62 ☑
retroperitoneum S36.892 ☑
round ligament S37.892 ☑

☑ Additional Character Required — Refer to the Tabular List for Character Selection

▽ Subterms under main terms may continue to next column or page

Index

Contraction(s), contracture, contracted — Contusion

Contusion — *continued*
  sacral region S30.0 ☑
  scalp S00.03 ☑
    due to birth injury P12.3
  scapular region — *see* Contusion, shoulder
  sclera — *see* Contusion, eyeball
  scrotum S30.22 ☑
  seminal vesicle S37.892 ☑
  shoulder S40.01- ☑
  skin NEC T14.8
  small intestine — *see* Injury, intestine, small, contusion
  spermatic cord S30.22 ☑
  spinal cord — *see* Injury, spinal cord, by region
    cauda equina S34.3 ☑
    conus medullaris S34.139 ☑
  spleen S36.029 ☑
    major S36.021 ☑
    minor S36.020 ☑
  sternal region S20.219 ☑
  stomach S36.32 ☑
  subconjunctival S05.1- ☑
  subcutaneous NEC T14.8
  submaxillary region S00.83 ☑
  submental region S00.83 ☑
  subperiosteal NEC T14.8
  subungual
    finger — *see* Contusion, finger, with damage to nail
    toe — *see* Contusion, toe, with damage to nail
  supraclavicular fossa S10.83 ☑
  supraorbital S00.83 ☑
  suprarenal gland S37.812 ☑
  temple (region) S00.83 ☑
  temporal
    lobe (brain) — *see* Injury, intracranial, diffuse
    focal — *see* Injury, intracranial, focal
    region S00.83 ☑
  testis S30.22 ☑
  thigh S70.1- ☑
  thorax (wall) S20.20 ☑
    back S20.22- ☑
    front S20.21- ☑
  throat S10.0 ☑
  thumb S60.01- ☑
    with damage to nail S60.11- ☑
  toe(s) (lesser) S90.12- ☑
    with damage to nail S90.22- ☑
    great S90.11- ☑
      with damage to nail S90.21- ☑
      specified type NEC S90.221 ☑
  tongue S00.532 ☑
  trachea (cervical) S10.0 ☑
    thoracic S27.52 ☑
  tunica vaginalis S30.22 ☑
  tympanum, tympanic membrane — *see* Contusion, ear
  ureter S37.12 ☑
  urethra S37.32 ☑
  urinary organ NEC S37.892 ☑
  uterus S37.62 ☑
  uvula S00.532 ☑
  vagina S30.23 ☑
  vas deferens S37.892 ☑
  vesical S37.22 ☑
  vocal cord(s) S10.0 ☑
  vulva S30.23 ☑
  wrist S60.21- ☑
Conus (congenital) (any type) Q14.8
  cornea — *see* Keratoconus
  medullaris syndrome G95.81
Conversion hysteria, neurosis or reaction F44.9
Converter, tuberculosis (test reaction) R76.11
Conviction (legal), **anxiety concerning** Z65.0
  with imprisonment Z65.1
Convulsions (idiopathic) (*see also* Seizure(s)) R56.9
  apoplectiform (cerebral ischemia) I67.82
  benign neonatal (familial) — *see* Epilepsy, generalized, idiopathic
  dissociative F44.5
  epileptic — *see* Epilepsy
  epileptiform, epileptoid — *see* Seizure, epileptiform
  ether (anesthetic) — *see* Table of Drugs and Chemicals, by drug
  febrile R56.00
    with status epilepticus G40.901

Convulsions — *continued*
  febrile — *continued*
    complex R56.01
      with status epilepticus G40.901
    simple R56.00
  hysterical F44.5
  infantile P90
    epilepsy — *see* Epilepsy
  jacksonian — *see* Epilepsy, localization-related, symptomatic, with simple partial seizures
  myoclonic G25.3
  neonatal, benign (familial) — *see* Epilepsy, generalized, idiopathic
  newborn P90
  obstetrical (nephritic) (uremic) — *see* Eclampsia
  paretic A52.17
  post traumatic R56.1
  psychomotor — *see* Epilepsy, localization-related, symptomatic, with complex partial seizures
  recurrent R56.9
  reflex R25.8
  scarlatinal A38.8
  tetanus, tetanic — *see* Tetanus
  thymic E32.8
Convulsive (*see also* Convulsions)
Cooley's anemia D56.1
Coolie itch B76.9
Cooper's
  disease — *see* Mastopathy, cystic
  hernia — *see* Hernia, abdomen, specified site NEC
Copra itch B88.0
Coprophagy F50.8
Coprophobia F40.298
Coproporphyria, hereditary E80.29
Cor
  biloculare Q20.8
  bovis, bovinum — *see* Hypertrophy, cardiac
  pulmonale (chronic) I27.81
    acute I26.09
  triatriatum, triatrium Q24.2
  triloculare Q20.8
    biatrium Q20.4
    biventriculare Q21.1
Corbus' disease (gangrenous balanitis) N48.1
Cord (*see also* condition)
  around neck (tightly) (with compression)
    complicating delivery O69.1 ☑
  bladder G95.89
    tabetic A52.19
Cordis ectopia Q24.8
Corditis (spermatic) N49.1
Corectopia Q13.2
Cori's disease (glycogen storage) E74.03
Corkhandler's disease or lung J67.3
Corkscrew esophagus K22.4
Corkworker's disease or lung J67.3
Corn (infected) L84
Cornea (*see also* condition)
  donor Z52.5
  plana Q13.4
Cornelia de Lange syndrome Q87.1
Cornu cutaneum L85.8
Cornual gestation or pregnancy O00.8
Coronary (artery) — *see* condition
Coronavirus, as cause of disease classified elsewhere B97.29
  SARS-associated B97.21
Corpora (*see also* condition)
  amylacea, prostate N42.89
  cavernosa — *see* condition
Corpulence — *see* Obesity
Corpus — *see* condition
Corrected transposition Q20.5
Corrosion (injury) (acid) (caustic) (chemical) (lime) (external) (internal) T30.4
  abdomen, abdominal (muscle) (wall) T21.42 ☑
    first degree T21.52 ☑
    second degree T21.62 ☑
    third degree T21.72 ☑
  above elbow T22.439 ☑
    first degree T22.539 ☑
    left T22.432 ☑
      first degree T22.532 ☑
      second degree T22.632 ☑
      third degree T22.732 ☑
    right T22.431 ☑
      first degree T22.531 ☑

Corrosion — *continued*
  above elbow — *continued*
    right — *continued*
      second degree T22.631 ☑
      third degree T22.731 ☑
    second degree T22.639 ☑
    third degree T22.739 ☑
  alimentary tract NEC T28.7 ☑
  ankle T25.419 ☑
    first degree T25.519 ☑
    left T25.412 ☑
      first degree T25.512 ☑
      second degree T25.612 ☑
      third degree T25.712 ☑
    multiple with foot — *see* Corrosion, lower, limb, multiple, ankle and foot
    right T25.411 ☑
      first degree T25.511 ☑
      second degree T25.611 ☑
      third degree T25.711 ☑
    second degree T25.619 ☑
    third degree T25.719 ☑
  anus — *see* Corrosion, buttock
  arm(s) (meaning upper limb(s)) — *see* Corrosion, upper limb
  axilla T22.449 ☑
    first degree T22.549 ☑
    left T22.442 ☑
      first degree T22.542 ☑
      second degree T22.642 ☑
      third degree T22.742 ☑
    right T22.441 ☑
      first degree T22.541 ☑
      second degree T22.641 ☑
      third degree T22.741 ☑
    second degree T22.649 ☑
    third degree T22.749 ☑
  back (lower) T21.44 ☑
    first degree T21.54 ☑
    second degree T21.64 ☑
    third degree T21.74 ☑
    upper T21.43 ☑
      first degree T21.53 ☑
      second degree T21.63 ☑
      third degree T21.73 ☑
  blisters — *code as* Corrosion, second degree, by site
  breast(s) — *see* Corrosion, chest wall
  buttock(s) T21.45 ☑
    first degree T21.55 ☑
    second degree T21.65 ☑
    third degree T21.75 ☑
  calf T24.439 ☑
    first degree T24.539 ☑
    left T24.432 ☑
      first degree T24.532 ☑
      second degree T24.632 ☑
      third degree T24.732 ☑
    right T24.431 ☑
      first degree T24.531 ☑
      second degree T24.631 ☑
      third degree T24.731 ☑
    second degree T24.639 ☑
    third degree T24.739 ☑
  canthus (eye) — *see* Corrosion, eyelid
  cervix T28.8 ☑
  cheek T20.46 ☑
    first degree T20.56 ☑
    second degree T20.66 ☑
    third degree T20.76 ☑
  chest wall T21.41 ☑
    first degree T21.51 ☑
    second degree T21.61 ☑
    third degree T21.71 ☑
  chin T20.43 ☑
    first degree T20.53 ☑
    second degree T20.63 ☑
    third degree T20.73 ☑
  colon T28.7 ☑
  conjunctiva (and cornea) — *see* Corrosion, cornea
  cornea (and conjunctiva) T26.6- ☑
  deep necrosis of underlying tissue — *code as* Corrosion, third degree, by site
  dorsum of hand T23.469 ☑
    first degree T23.569 ☑

Corrosion — *continued*
  dorsum of hand — *continued*
    left T23.462 ☑
      first degree T23.562 ☑
      second degree T23.662 ☑
      third degree T23.762 ☑
    right T23.461 ☑
      first degree T23.561 ☑
      second degree T23.661 ☑
      third degree T23.761 ☑
    second degree T23.669 ☑
    third degree T23.769 ☑
  ear (auricle) (external) (canal) T20.41 ☑
    drum T28.91 ☑
    first degree T20.51 ☑
    second degree T20.61 ☑
    third degree T20.71 ☑
  elbow T22.429 ☑
    first degree T22.529 ☑
    left T22.422 ☑
      first degree T22.522 ☑
      second degree T22.622 ☑
      third degree T22.722 ☑
    right T22.421 ☑
      first degree T22.521 ☑
      second degree T22.621 ☑
      third degree T22.721 ☑
    second degree T22.629 ☑
    third degree T22.729 ☑
  entire body — *see* Corrosion, multiple body regions
  epidermal loss — *code as* Corrosion, second degree, by site
  epiglottis T27.4 ☑
  erythema, erythematous — *code as* Corrosion, first degree, by site
  esophagus T28.6 ☑
  extent (percentage of body surface)
    less than 10 per cent T32.0
    10-19 per cent (0-9 percent third degree) T32.10
      with 10-19 percent third degree T32.11
    20-29 per cent (0-9 percent third degree) T32.20
      with
        10-19 percent third degree T32.21
        20-29 percent third degree T32.22
    30-39 per cent (0-9 percent third degree) T32.30
      with
        10-19 percent third degree T32.31
        20-29 percent third degree T32.32
        30-39 percent third degree T32.33
    40-49 per cent (0-9 percent third degree) T32.40
      with
        10-19 percent third degree T32.41
        20-29 percent third degree T32.42
        30-39 percent third degree T32.43
        40-49 percent third degree T32.44
    50-59 per cent (0-9 percent third degree) T32.50
      with
        10-19 percent third degree T32.51
        20-29 percent third degree T32.52
        30-39 percent third degree T32.53
        40-49 percent third degree T32.54
        50-59 percent third degree T32.55
    60-69 per cent (0-9 percent third degree) T32.60
      with
        10-19 percent third degree T32.61
        20-29 percent third degree T32.62
        30-39 percent third degree T32.63
        40-49 percent third degree T32.64
        50-59 percent third degree T32.65
        60-69 percent third degree T32.66
    70-79 per cent (0-9 percent third degree) T32.70
      with
        10-19 percent third degree T32.71
        20-29 percent third degree T32.72
        30-39 percent third degree T32.73
        40-49 percent third degree T32.74
        50-59 percent third degree T32.75
        60-69 percent third degree T32.76
        70-79 percent third degree T32.77
    80-89 per cent (0-9 percent third degree) T32.80
      with
        10-19 percent third degree T32.81
        20-29 percent third degree T32.82
        30-39 percent third degree T32.83
        40-49 percent third degree T32.84
        50-59 percent third degree T32.85
        60-69 percent third degree T32.86

  extent — *continued*
    80-89 per cent — *continued*
      with — *continued*
        70-79 percent third degree T32.87
        80-89 percent third degree T32.88
    90 per cent or more (0-9 percent third degree) T32.90
      with
        10-19 percent third degree T32.91
        20-29 percent third degree T32.92
        30-39 percent third degree T32.93
        40-49 percent third degree T32.94
        50-59 percent third degree T32.95
        60-69 percent third degree T32.96
        70-79 percent third degree T32.97
        80-89 percent third degree T32.98
        90-99 percent third degree T32.99
  extremity — *see* Corrosion, limb
  eye(s) and adnexa T26.9- ☑
    with resulting rupture and destruction of eyeball T26.7- ☑
    conjunctival sac — *see* Corrosion, cornea
    cornea — *see* Corrosion, cornea
    lid — *see* Corrosion, eyelid
    periocular area — *see* Corrosion eyelid
    specified site NEC T26.8- ☑
  eyeball — *see* Corrosion, eye
  eyelid(s) T26.5- ☑
  face — *see* Corrosion, head
  finger T23.429 ☑
    first degree T23.529 ☑
    left T23.422 ☑
      first degree T23.522 ☑
      second degree T23.622 ☑
      third degree T23.722 ☑
    multiple sites (without thumb) T23.439 ☑
      with thumb T23.449 ☑
        first degree T23.549 ☑
        left T23.442 ☑
          first degree T23.542 ☑
          second degree T23.642 ☑
          third degree T23.742 ☑
        right T23.441 ☑
          first degree T23.541 ☑
          second degree T23.641 ☑
          third degree T23.741 ☑
        second degree T23.649 ☑
        third degree T23.749 ☑
      first degree T23.539 ☑
      left T23.432 ☑
        first degree T23.532 ☑
        second degree T23.632 ☑
        third degree T23.732 ☑
      right T23.431 ☑
        first degree T23.531 ☑
        second degree T23.631 ☑
        third degree T23.731 ☑
      second degree T23.639 ☑
      third degree T23.739 ☑
    right T23.421 ☑
      first degree T23.521 ☑
      second degree T23.621 ☑
      third degree T23.721 ☑
    second degree T23.629 ☑
    third degree T23.729 ☑
  flank — *see* Corrosion, abdomen
  foot T25.429 ☑
    first degree T25.529 ☑
    left T25.422 ☑
      first degree T25.522 ☑
      second degree T25.622 ☑
      third degree T25.722 ☑
    multiple with ankle — *see* Corrosion, lower, limb, multiple, ankle and foot
    right T25.421 ☑
      first degree T25.521 ☑
      second degree T25.621 ☑
      third degree T25.721 ☑
    second degree T25.629 ☑
    third degree T25.729 ☑
  forearm T22.419 ☑
    first degree T22.519 ☑
    left T22.412 ☑
      first degree T22.512 ☑
      second degree T22.612 ☑

  forearm — *continued*
    left — *continued*
      third degree T22.712 ☑
    right T22.411 ☑
      first degree T22.511 ☑
      second degree T22.611 ☑
      third degree T22.711 ☑
    second degree T22.619 ☑
    third degree T22.719 ☑
  forehead T20.46 ☑
    first degree T20.56 ☑
    second degree T20.66 ☑
    third degree T20.76 ☑
  fourth degree — *code as* Corrosion, third degree, by site
  full thickness skin loss — *code as* Corrosion, third degree, by site
  gastrointestinal tract NEC T28.7 ☑
  genital organs
    external
      female T21.47 ☑
        first degree T21.57 ☑
        second degree T21.67 ☑
        third degree T21.77 ☑
      male T21.46 ☑
        first degree T21.56 ☑
        second degree T21.66 ☑
        third degree T21.76 ☑
    internal T28.8 ☑
  groin — *see* Corrosion, abdominal wall
  hand(s) T23.409 ☑
    back — *see* Corrosion, dorsum of hand
    finger — *see* Corrosion, finger
    first degree T23.509 ☑
    left T23.402 ☑
      first degree T23.502 ☑
      second degree T23.602 ☑
      third degree T23.702 ☑
    multiple sites with wrist T23.499 ☑
      first degree T23.599 ☑
      left T23.492 ☑
        first degree T23.592 ☑
        second degree T23.692 ☑
        third degree T23.792 ☑
      right T23.491 ☑
        first degree T23.591 ☑
        second degree T23.691 ☑
        third degree T23.791 ☑
      second degree T23.699 ☑
      third degree T23.799 ☑
    palm — *see* Corrosion, palm
    right T23.401 ☑
      first degree T23.501 ☑
      second degree T23.601 ☑
      third degree T23.701 ☑
    second degree T23.609 ☑
    third degree T23.709 ☑
    thumb — *see* Corrosion, thumb
  head (and face) (and neck) T20.40 ☑
    cheek — *see* Corrosion, cheek
    chin — *see* Corrosion, chin
    ear — *see* Corrosion, ear
    eye(s) only — *see* Corrosion, eye
    first degree T20.50 ☑
    forehead — *see* Corrosion, forehead
    lip — *see* Corrosion, lip
    multiple sites T20.49 ☑
      first degree T20.59 ☑
      second degree T20.69 ☑
      third degree T20.79 ☑
    neck — *see* Corrosion, neck
    nose — *see* Corrosion, nose
    scalp — *see* Corrosion, scalp
    second degree T20.60 ☑
    third degree T20.70 ☑
  hip(s) — *see* Corrosion, lower, limb
  inhalation — *see* Corrosion, respiratory tract
  internal organ(s) (*see also* Corrosion, by site) T28.90 ☑
    alimentary tract T28.7 ☑
      esophagus T28.6 ☑
    esophagus T28.6 ☑
    genitourinary T28.8 ☑
    mouth T28.5 ☑
    pharynx T28.5 ☑
    specified organ NEC T28.99 ☑

Corrosion — *continued*
  interscapular region — *see* Corrosion, back, upper
  intestine (large) (small) T28.7 ☑
  knee T24.429 ☑
    first degree T24.529 ☑
    left T24.422 ☑
      first degree T24.522 ☑
      second degree T24.622 ☑
      third degree T24.722 ☑
    right T24.421 ☑
      first degree T24.521 ☑
      second degree T24.621 ☑
      third degree T24.721 ☑
    second degree T24.629 ☑
    third degree T24.729 ☑
  labium (majus) (minus) — *see* Corrosion, genital organs, external, female
  lacrimal apparatus, duct, gland or sac — *see* Corrosion, eye, specified site NEC
  larynx T27.4 ☑
    with lung T27.5 ☑
  leg(s) (meaning lower limb(s)) — *see* Corrosion, lower limb
  limb(s)
    lower — *see* Corrosion, lower, limb
    upper — *see* Corrosion, upper limb
  lip(s) T20.42 ☑
    first degree T20.52 ☑
    second degree T20.62 ☑
    third degree T20.72 ☑
  lower
    back — *see* Corrosion, back
    limb T24.409 ☑
      ankle — *see* Corrosion, ankle
      calf — *see* Corrosion, calf
      first degree T24.509 ☑
      foot — *see* Corrosion, foot
      hip — *see* Corrosion, thigh
      knee — *see* Corrosion, knee
      left T24.402 ☑
        first degree T24.502 ☑
        second degree T24.602 ☑
        third degree T24.702 ☑
      multiple sites, except ankle and foot T24.499 ☑
        ankle and foot T25.499 ☑
          first degree T25.599 ☑
          left T25.492 ☑
            first degree T25.592 ☑
            second degree T25.692 ☑
            third degree T25.792 ☑
          right T25.491 ☑
            first degree T25.591 ☑
            second degree T25.691 ☑
            third degree T25.791 ☑
          second degree T25.699 ☑
          third degree T25.799 ☑
        first degree T24.599 ☑
        left T24.492 ☑
          first degree T24.592 ☑
          second degree T24.692 ☑
          third degree T24.792 ☑
        right T24.491 ☑
          first degree T24.591 ☑
          second degree T24.691 ☑
          third degree T24.791 ☑
        second degree T24.699 ☑
        thigh — *see* Corrosion, thigh
        third degree T24.709 ☑
      right T24.401 ☑
        first degree T24.501 ☑
        second degree T24.601 ☑
        third degree T24.701 ☑
      second degree T24.609 ☑
      thigh — *see* Corrosion, thigh
      third degree T24.709 ☑
  lung (with larynx and trachea) T27.5 ☑
  mouth T28.5 ☑
  neck T20.47 ☑
    first degree T20.57 ☑
    second degree T20.67 ☑
    third degree T20.77 ☑
  nose (septum) T20.44 ☑
    first degree T20.54 ☑
    second degree T20.64 ☑
    third degree T20.74 ☑
  ocular adnexa — *see* Corrosion, eye
  orbit region — *see* Corrosion, eyelid

Corrosion — *continued*
  palm T23.459 ☑
    first degree T23.559 ☑
    left T23.452 ☑
      first degree T23.552 ☑
      second degree T23.652 ☑
      third degree T23.752 ☑
    right T23.451 ☑
      first degree T23.551 ☑
      second degree T23.651 ☑
      third degree T23.751 ☑
    second degree T23.659 ☑
    third degree T23.759 ☑
  partial thickness — *code as* Corrosion, unspecified degree, by site
  pelvis — *see* Corrosion, trunk
  penis — *see* Corrosion, genital organs, external, male
  perineum
    female — *see* Corrosion, genital organs, external, female
    male — *see* Corrosion, genital organs, external, male
  periocular area — *see* Corrosion, eyelid
  pharynx T28.5 ☑
  rectum T28.7 ☑
  respiratory tract T27.7 ☑
    larynx — *see* Corrosion, larynx
    specified part NEC T27.6 ☑
    trachea — *see* Corrosion, larynx
  sac, lacrimal — *see* Corrosion, eye, specified site NEC
  scalp T20.45 ☑
    first degree T20.55 ☑
    second degree T20.65 ☑
    third degree T20.75 ☑
  scapular region T22.469 ☑
    first degree T22.569 ☑
    left T22.462 ☑
      first degree T22.562 ☑
      second degree T22.662 ☑
      third degree T22.762 ☑
    right T22.461 ☑
      first degree T22.561 ☑
      second degree T22.661 ☑
      third degree T22.761 ☑
    second degree T22.669 ☑
    third degree T22.769 ☑
  sclera — *see* Corrosion, eye, specified site NEC
  scrotum — *see* Corrosion, genital organs, external, male
  shoulder T22.459 ☑
    first degree T22.559 ☑
    left T22.452 ☑
      first degree T22.552 ☑
      second degree T22.652 ☑
      third degree T22.752 ☑
    right T22.451 ☑
      first degree T22.551 ☑
      second degree T22.651 ☑
      third degree T22.751 ☑
    second degree T22.659 ☑
    third degree T22.759 ☑
  stomach T28.7 ☑
  temple — *see* Corrosion, head
  testis — *see* Corrosion, genital organs, external, male
  thigh T24.419 ☑
    first degree T24.519 ☑
    left T24.412 ☑
      first degree T24.512 ☑
      second degree T24.612 ☑
      third degree T24.712 ☑
    right T24.411 ☑
      first degree T24.511 ☑
      second degree T24.611 ☑
      third degree T24.711 ☑
    second degree T24.619 ☑
    third degree T24.719 ☑
  thorax (external) — *see* Corrosion, trunk
  throat (meaning pharynx) T28.5 ☑
  thumb(s) T23.419 ☑
    first degree T23.519 ☑
    left T23.412 ☑
      first degree T23.512 ☑
      second degree T23.612 ☑
      third degree T23.712 ☑

Corrosion — *continued*
  thumb(s) — *continued*
    multiple sites with fingers T23.449 ☑
      first degree T23.549 ☑
      left T23.442 ☑
        first degree T23.542 ☑
        second degree T23.642 ☑
        third degree T23.742 ☑
      right T23.441 ☑
        first degree T23.541 ☑
        second degree T23.641 ☑
        third degree T23.741 ☑
      second degree T23.649 ☑
      third degree T23.749 ☑
    right T23.411 ☑
      first degree T23.511 ☑
      second degree T23.611 ☑
      third degree T23.711 ☑
    second degree T23.619 ☑
    third degree T23.719 ☑
  toe T25.439 ☑
    first degree T25.539 ☑
    left T25.432 ☑
      first degree T25.532 ☑
      second degree T25.632 ☑
      third degree T25.732 ☑
    right T25.431 ☑
      first degree T25.531 ☑
      second degree T25.631 ☑
      third degree T25.731 ☑
    second degree T25.639 ☑
    third degree T25.739 ☑
  tongue T28.5 ☑
  tonsil(s) T28.5 ☑
  total body — *see* Corrosion, multiple body regions
  trachea T27.4 ☑
    with lung T27.5 ☑
  trunk T21.40 ☑
    abdominal wall — *see* Corrosion, abdominal wall
    anus — *see* Corrosion, buttock
    axilla — *see* Corrosion, upper limb
    back — *see* Corrosion, back
    breast — *see* Corrosion, chest wall
    buttock — *see* Corrosion, buttock
    chest wall — *see* Corrosion, chest wall
    first degree T21.50 ☑
    flank — *see* Corrosion, abdominal wall
    genital
      female — *see* Corrosion, genital organs, external, female
      male — *see* Corrosion, genital organs, external, male
    groin — *see* Corrosion, abdominal wall
    interscapular region — *see* Corrosion, back, upper
    labia — *see* Corrosion, genital organs, external, female
    lower back — *see* Corrosion, back
    penis — *see* Corrosion, genital organs, external, male
    perineum
      female — *see* Corrosion, genital organs, external, female
      male — *see* Corrosion, genital organs, external, male
    scapular region — *see* Corrosion, upper limb
    scrotum — *see* Corrosion, genital organs, external, male
    second degree T21.60 ☑
    shoulder — *see* Corrosion, upper limb
    specified site NEC T21.49 ☑
      first degree T21.59 ☑
      second degree T21.69 ☑
      third degree T21.79 ☑
    testes — *see* Corrosion, genital organs, external, male
    third degree T21.70 ☑
    upper back — *see* Corrosion, back, upper
    vagina T28.8 ☑
    vulva — *see* Corrosion, genital organs, external, female
  unspecified site with extent of body surface involved specified
    less than 10 per cent T32.0
    10-19 per cent (0-9 percent third degree) T32.10
      with 10-19 percent third degree T32.11

Corrosion — *continued*
  unspecified site with extent of body surface involved
    specified — *continued*
      20-29 per cent (0-9 percent third degree) T32.20
        with
          10-19 percent third degree T32.21
          20-29 percent third degree T32.22
      30-39 per cent (0-9 percent third degree) T32.30
        with
          10-19 percent third degree T32.31
          20-29 percent third degree T32.32
          30-39 percent third degree T32.33
      40-49 per cent (0-9 percent third degree) T32.40
        with
          10-19 percent third degree T32.41
          20-29 percent third degree T32.42
          30-39 percent third degree T32.43
          40-49 percent third degree T32.44
      50-59 per cent (0-9 percent third degree) T32.50
        with
          10-19 percent third degree T32.51
          20-29 percent third degree T32.52
          30-39 percent third degree T32.53
          40-49 percent third degree T32.54
          50-59 percent third degree T32.55
      60-69 per cent (0-9 percent third degree) T32.60
        with
          10-19 percent third degree T32.61
          20-29 percent third degree T32.62
          30-39 percent third degree T32.63
          40-49 percent third degree T32.64
          50-59 percent third degree T32.65
          60-69 percent third degree T32.66
      70-79 per cent (0-9 percent third degree) T32.70
        with
          10-19 percent third degree T32.71
          20-29 percent third degree T32.72
          30-39 percent third degree T32.73
          40-49 percent third degree T32.74
          50-59 percent third degree T32.75
          60-69 percent third degree T32.76
          70-79 percent third degree T32.77
      80-89 per cent (0-9 percent third degree) T32.80
        with
          10-19 percent third degree T32.81
          20-29 percent third degree T32.82
          30-39 percent third degree T32.83
          40-49 percent third degree T32.84
          50-59 percent third degree T32.85
          60-69 percent third degree T32.86
          70-79 percent third degree T32.87
          80-89 percent third degree T32.88
      90 per cent or more (0-9 percent third degree)
        T32.90
        with
          10-19 percent third degree T32.91
          20-29 percent third degree T32.92
          30-39 percent third degree T32.93
          40-49 percent third degree T32.94
          50-59 percent third degree T32.95
          60-69 percent third degree T32.96
          70-79 percent third degree T32.97
          80-89 percent third degree T32.98
          90-99 percent third degree T32.99
  upper limb (axilla) (scapular region) T22.40 ☑
    above elbow — *see* Corrosion, above elbow
    axilla — *see* Corrosion, axilla
    elbow — *see* Corrosion, elbow
    first degree T22.50 ☑
    forearm — *see* Corrosion, forearm
    hand — *see* Corrosion, hand
    interscapular region — *see* Corrosion, back, upper
    multiple sites T22.499 ☑
      first degree T22.599 ☑
      left T22.492 ☑
        first degree T22.592 ☑
        second degree T22.692 ☑
        third degree T22.792 ☑
      right T22.491 ☑
        first degree T22.591 ☑
        second degree T22.691 ☑
        third degree T22.791 ☑
      second degree T22.699 ☑
      third degree T22.799 ☑
    scapular region — *see* Corrosion, scapular region
    second degree T22.60 ☑
    shoulder — *see* Corrosion, shoulder
    third degree T22.70 ☑

Corrosion — *continued*
  upper limb — *continued*
    wrist — *see* Corrosion, hand
  uterus T28.8 ☑
  vagina T28.8 ☑
  vulva — *see* Corrosion, genital organs, external, female
  wrist T23.479 ☑
    first degree T23.579 ☑
    left T23.472 ☑
      first degree T23.572 ☑
      second degree T23.672 ☑
      third degree T23.772 ☑
    multiple sites with hand T23.499 ☑
      first degree T23.599 ☑
      left T23.492 ☑
        first degree T23.592 ☑
        second degree T23.692 ☑
        third degree T23.792 ☑
      right T23.491 ☑
        first degree T23.591 ☑
        second degree T23.691 ☑
        third degree T23.791 ☑
      second degree T23.699 ☑
      third degree T23.799 ☑
    right T23.471 ☑
      first degree T23.571 ☑
      second degree T23.671 ☑
      third degree T23.771 ☑
    second degree T23.679 ☑
    third degree T23.779 ☑
Corrosive burn — *see* Corrosion
Corsican fever — *see* Malaria
Cortical — *see* condition
Cortico-adrenal — *see* condition
Coryza (acute) J00
  with grippe or influenza — *see* Influenza, with, respiratory manifestations NEC
  syphilitic
    congenital (chronic) A50.05
Costen's syndrome or complex M26.69
Costiveness — *see* Constipation
Costochondritis M94.0
Cot death R99
Cotard's syndrome F22
Cotia virus B08.8
Cotton wool spots (retinal) H35.81
Cotungo's disease — *see* Sciatica
Cough (affected) (chronic) (epidemic) (nervous) R05
  with hemorrhage — *see* Hemoptysis
  bronchial R05
    with grippe or influenza — *see* Influenza, with, respiratory manifestations NEC
  functional F45.8
  hysterical F45.8
  laryngeal, spasmodic R05
  psychogenic F45.8
  smokers' J41.0
  tea taster's B49
Counseling (for) Z71.9
  abuse NEC
    perpetrator Z69.82
    victim Z69.81
  alcohol abuser Z71.41
    family Z71.42
  child abuse
    nonparental
      perpetrator Z69.021
      victim Z69.020
    parental
      perpetrator Z69.011
      victim Z69.010
  consanguinity Z71.89
  contraceptive Z30.09
  dietary Z71.3
  drug abuser Z71.51
    family member Z71.52
  family Z71.89
  fertility preservation (prior to cancer therapy) (prior to removal of gonads) Z31.62
  for non-attending third party Z71.0
    related to sexual behavior or orientation Z70.2
  genetic NEC Z31.5
  health (advice) (education) (instruction) — *see* Counseling, medical
  human immunodeficiency virus (HIV) Z71.7
  impotence Z70.1
  insulin pump use Z46.81

Counseling — *continued*
  medical (for) Z71.9
    boarding school resident Z59.3
    consanguinity Z71.89
    feared complaint and no disease found Z71.1
    human immunodeficiency virus (HIV) Z71.7
    institutional resident Z59.3
    on behalf of another Z71.0
      related to sexual behavior or orientation Z70.2
    person living alone Z60.2
    specified reason NEC Z71.89
  natural family planning
    procreative Z31.61
    to avoid pregnancy Z30.02
  perpetrator (of)
    abuse NEC Z69.82
    child abuse
      non-parental Z69.021
      parental Z69.011
    rape NEC Z69.82
    spousal abuse Z69.12
  procreative NEC Z31.69
    fertility preservation (prior to cancer therapy) (prior to removal of gonads) Z31.62
    using natural family planning Z31.61
  promiscuity Z70.1
  rape victim Z69.81
  religious Z71.81
  sex, sexual (related to) Z70.9
    attitude(s) Z70.0
    behavior or orientation Z70.1
    combined concerns Z70.3
    non-responsiveness Z70.1
    on behalf of third party Z70.2
    specified reason NEC Z70.8
  specified reason NEC Z71.89
  spiritual Z71.81
  spousal abuse (perpetrator) Z69.12
    victim Z69.11
  substance abuse Z71.89
    alcohol Z71.41
    drug Z71.51
    tobacco Z71.6
  tobacco use Z71.6
  use (of)
    insulin pump Z46.81
  victim (of)
    abuse Z69.81
    child abuse
      by parent Z69.010
      non-parental Z69.020
    rape NEC Z69.81
Coupled rhythm R00.8
Couvelaire syndrome or uterus (complicating delivery) O45.8X- ☑
Cowperitis — *see* Urethritis
Cowper's gland — *see* condition
Cowpox B08.010
  due to vaccination T88.1 ☑
Coxa
  magna M91.4- ☑
  plana M91.2- ☑
  valga (acquired) (*see also* Deformity, limb, specified type NEC, thigh)
    congenital Q65.81
    sequelae (late effect) of rickets E64.3
  vara (acquired) (*see also* Deformity, limb, specified type NEC, thigh)
    congenital Q65.82
    sequelae (late effect) of rickets E64.3
Coxalgia, coxalgic (nontuberculous) (*see also* Pain, joint, hip)
  tuberculous A18.02
Coxitis — *see* Monoarthritis, hip
Coxsackie (virus) (infection) B34.1
  as cause of disease classified elsewhere B97.11
  carditis B33.20
  central nervous system NEC A88.8
  endocarditis B33.21
  enteritis A08.39
  meningitis (aseptic) A87.0
  myocarditis B33.22
  pericarditis B33.23
  pharyngitis B08.5
  pleurodynia B33.0
  specific disease NEC B33.8
Crabs, meaning pubic lice B85.3
Crack baby P04.41

Cracked nipple N64.0
  associated with
    lactation O92.13
    pregnancy O92.11- ☑
    puerperium O92.12
Cracked tooth K03.81
Cradle cap L21.0
Craft neurosis F48.8
Cramp(s) R25.2
  abdominal — *see* Pain, abdominal
  bathing T75.1 ☑
  colic R10.83
    psychogenic F45.8
  due to immersion T75.1 ☑
  fireman T67.2 ☑
  heat T67.2 ☑
  immersion T75.1 ☑
  intestinal — *see* Pain, abdominal
    psychogenic F45.8
  leg, sleep related G47.62
  limb (lower) (upper) NEC R25.2
    sleep related G47.62
  linotypist's F48.8
    organic G25.89
  muscle (limb) (general) R25.2
    due to immersion T75.1 ☑
    psychogenic F45.8
  occupational (hand) F48.8
    organic G25.89
  salt-depletion E87.1
  sleep related, leg G47.62
  stoker's T67.2 ☑
  swimmer's T75.1 ☑
  telegrapher's F48.8
    organic G25.89
  typist's F48.8
    organic G25.89
  uterus N94.89
    menstrual — *see* Dysmenorrhea
  writer's F48.8
    organic G25.89
Cranial — *see* condition
Craniocleidodysostosis Q74.0
Craniofenestria (skull) Q75.8
Craniolacunia (skull) Q75.8
Craniopagus Q89.4
Craniopathy, metabolic M85.2
Craniopharyngeal — *see* condition
Craniopharyngioma D44.4
Craniorachischisis (totalis) Q00.1
Cranioschisis Q75.8
Craniostenosis Q75.0
Craniosynostosis Q75.0
Craniotabes (cause unknown) M83.8
  neonatal P96.3
  rachitic E64.3
  syphilitic A50.56
Cranium — *see* condition
Craw-craw — *see* Onchocerciasis
Creaking joint — *see* Derangement, joint, specified type NEC
Creeping
  eruption B76.9
  palsy or paralysis G12.22
Crenated tongue K14.8
Creotoxism A05.9
Crepitus
  caput Q75.8
  joint — *see* Derangement, joint, specified type NEC
Crescent or conus choroid, congenital Q14.3
CREST syndrome M34.1
Cretin, cretinism (congenital) (endemic) (nongoitrous) (sporadic) E00.9
  pelvis
    with disproportion (fetopelvic) O33.0
      causing obstructed labor O65.0
  type
    hypothyroid E00.1
    mixed E00.2
    myxedematous E00.1
    neurological E00.0
Creutzfeldt-Jakob disease or syndrome (with dementia) A81.00
  familial A81.09
  iatrogenic A81.09
  specified NEC A81.09
  sporadic A81.09

Creutzfeldt-Jakob disease or syndrome — *continued*
  variant (vCJD) A81.01
Crib death R99
Cribriform hymen Q52.3
Cri-du-chat syndrome Q93.4
Crigler-Najjar disease or syndrome E80.5
Crime, victim of Z65.4
Crimean hemorrhagic fever A98.0
Criminalism F60.2
Crisis
  abdomen R10.0
  acute reaction F43.0
  addisonian E27.2
  adrenal (cortical) E27.2
  celiac K90.0
  Dietl's N13.8
  emotional (*see also* Disorder, adjustment)
    acute reaction to stress F43.0
    specific to childhood and adolescence F93.8
  glaucomatocyclitic — *see* Glaucoma, secondary, inflammation
  heart — *see* Failure, heart
  nitritoid I95.2
    correct substance properly administered — *see* Table of Drugs and Chemicals, by drug, adverse effect
    overdose or wrong substance given or taken — *see* Table of Drugs and Chemicals, by drug, poisoning
  oculogyric H51.8
    psychogenic F45.8
  Pel's (tabetic) A52.11
  psychosexual identity F64.2
  renal N28.0
  sickle-cell D57.00
    with
      acute chest syndrome D57.01
      splenic sequestration D57.02
  state (acute reaction) F43.0
  tabetic A52.11
  thyroid — *see* Thyrotoxicosis with thyroid storm
  thyrotoxic — *see* Thyrotoxicosis with thyroid storm
Crocq's disease (acrocyanosis) I73.89
Crohn's disease — *see* Enteritis, regional
Crooked septum, nasal J34.2
Cross syndrome E70.328
Crossbite (anterior) (posterior) M26.24
Cross-eye — *see* Strabismus, convergent concomitant
Croup, croupous (catarrhal) (infectious) (inflammatory) (nondiphtheritic) J05.0
  bronchial J20.9
  diphtheritic A36.2
  false J38.5
  spasmodic J38.5
    diphtheritic A36.2
  stridulous J38.5
    diphtheritic A36.2
Crouzon's disease Q75.1
Crowding, tooth, teeth, fully erupted M26.31
CRST syndrome M34.1
Cruchet's disease A85.8
Cruelty in children (*see also* Disorder, conduct)
Crural ulcer — *see* Ulcer, lower limb
Crush, crushed, crushing T14.8
  abdomen S38.1 ☑
  ankle S97.0- ☑
  arm (upper) (and shoulder) S47.- ☑
  axilla — *see* Crush, arm
  back, lower S38.1 ☑
  buttock S38.1 ☑
  cheek S07.0 ☑
  chest S28.0 ☑
  cranium S07.1 ☑
  ear S07.0 ☑
  elbow S57.0- ☑
  extremity
    lower
      ankle — *see* Crush, ankle
      below knee — *see* Crush, leg
      foot — *see* Crush, foot
      hip — *see* Crush, hip
      knee — *see* Crush, knee
      thigh — *see* Crush, thigh
      toe — *see* Crush, toe
    upper
      below elbow S67.9- ☑

Crush, crushed, crushing — *continued*
  extremity — *continued*
    upper — *continued*
      elbow — *see* Crush, elbow
      finger — *see* Crush, finger
      forearm — *see* Crush, forearm
      hand — *see* Crush, hand
      thumb — *see* Crush, thumb
      upper arm — *see* Crush, arm
      wrist — *see* Crush, wrist
  face S07.0 ☑
  finger(s) S67.1- ☑
    with hand (and wrist) — *see* Crush, hand, specified site NEC
    index S67.19- ☑
    little S67.19- ☑
    middle S67.19- ☑
    ring S67.19- ☑
    thumb — *see* Crush, thumb
  foot S97.8- ☑
    toe — *see* Crush, toe
  forearm S57.8- ☑
  genitalia, external
    female S38.002 ☑
      vagina S38.03 ☑
      vulva S38.03 ☑
    male S38.001 ☑
      penis S38.01 ☑
      scrotum S38.02 ☑
      testis S38.02 ☑
  hand (except fingers alone) S67.2- ☑
    with wrist S67.4- ☑
  head S07.9 ☑
    specified NEC S07.8 ☑
  heel — *see* Crush, foot
  hip S77.0- ☑
    with thigh S77.2- ☑
  internal organ (abdomen, chest, or pelvis) NEC T14.8
  knee S87.0- ☑
  labium (majus) (minus) S38.03 ☑
  larynx S17.0 ☑
  leg (lower) S87.8- ☑
    knee — *see* Crush, knee
  lip S07.0 ☑
  lower
    back S38.1 ☑
    leg — *see* Crush, leg
  neck S17.9 ☑
  nerve — *see* Injury, nerve
  nose S07.0 ☑
  pelvis S38.1 ☑
  penis S38.01 ☑
  scalp S07.8 ☑
  scapular region — *see* Crush, arm
  scrotum S38.02 ☑
  severe, unspecified site T14.8
  shoulder (and upper arm) — *see* Crush, arm
  skull S07.1 ☑
  syndrome (complication of trauma) T79.5 ☑
  testis S38.02 ☑
  thigh S77.1- ☑
    with hip S77.2- ☑
  throat S17.8 ☑
  thumb S67.0- ☑
    with hand (and wrist) — *see* Crush, hand, specified site NEC
  toe(s) S97.10- ☑
    great S97.11- ☑
    lesser S97.12- ☑
  trachea S17.0 ☑
  vagina S38.03 ☑
  vulva S38.03 ☑
  wrist S67.3- ☑
    with hand S67.4- ☑
Crusta lactea L21.0
Crusts R23.4
Crutch paralysis — *see* Injury, brachial plexus
Cruveilhier-Baumgarten cirrhosis, disease or syndrome K74.69
Cruveilhier's atrophy or disease G12.8
Crying (constant) (continuous) (excessive)
  child, adolescent, or adult R45.83
  infant (baby) (newborn) R68.11
Cryofibrinogenemia D89.2
Cryoglobulinemia (essential) (idiopathic) (mixed) (primary) (purpura) (secondary) (vasculitis) D89.1

Cryoglobulinemia — *continued*
   with lung involvement D89.1 [J99]
Cryptitis (anal) (rectal) K62.89
Cryptococcosis, cryptococcus (infection) (neoformans)
   B45.9
   bone B45.3
   cerebral B45.1
   cutaneous B45.2
   disseminated B45.7
   generalized B45.7
   meningitis B45.1
   meningocerebralis B45.1
   osseous B45.3
   pulmonary B45.0
   skin B45.2
   specified NEC B45.8
Cryptopapillitis (anus) K62.89
Cryptophthalmos Q11.2
   syndrome Q87.0
Cryptorchid, cryptorchism, cryptorchidism Q53.9
   bilateral Q53.20
     abdominal Q53.21
     perineal Q53.22
   unilateral Q53.10
     abdominal Q53.11
     perineal Q53.12
Cryptosporidiosis A07.2
   hepatobiliary B88.8
   respiratory B88.8
Cryptostromosis J67.6
Crystalluria R82.99
Cubitus
   congenital Q68.8
   valgus (acquired) M21.0- ☑
     congenital Q68.8
     sequelae (late effect) of rickets E64.3
   varus (acquired) M21.1- ☑
     congenital Q68.8
     sequelae (late effect) of rickets E64.3
Cultural deprivation or shock Z60.3
Curling esophagus K22.4
Curling's ulcer — *see* Ulcer, peptic, acute
Curschmann (-Batten) (-Steinert) **disease or syndrome**
   G71.11
Curse, Ondine's — *see* Apnea, sleep
Curvature
   organ or site, congenital NEC — *see* Distortion
   penis (lateral) Q55.61
   Pott's (spinal) A18.01
   radius, idiopathic, progressive (congenital) Q74.0
   spine (acquired) (angular) (idiopathic) (incorrect)
     (postural) — *see* Dorsopathy, deforming
     congenital Q67.5
     due to or associated with
       Charcot-Marie-Tooth disease (*see also* subcate-
         gory M49.8) G60.0
       osteitis
         deformans M88.88
         fibrosa cystica (*see also* subcategory M49.8)
           E21.0
       tuberculosis (Pott's curvature) A18.01
     sequelae (late effect) of rickets E64.3
     tuberculous A18.01
Cushingoid due to steroid therapy E24.2
   correct substance properly administered — *see* Table
     of Drugs and Chemicals, by drug, adverse effect
   overdose or wrong substance given or taken — *see*
     Table of Drugs and Chemicals, by drug, poison-
     ing
Cushing's
   syndrome or disease E24.9
     drug-induced E24.2
     iatrogenic E24.2
     pituitary-dependent E24.0
     specified NEC E24.8
   ulcer — *see* Ulcer, peptic, acute
Cusp, Carabelli — *omit code*
Cut (external) (*see also* Laceration)
   muscle — *see* Injury, muscle
Cutaneous (*see also* condition)
   hemorrhage R23.3
   larva migrans B76.9
Cutis (*see also* condition)
   hyperelastica Q82.8
     acquired L57.4
   laxa (hyperelastica) — *see* Dermatolysis
   marmorata R23.8

Cutis — *continued*
   osteosis L94.2
   pendula — *see* Dermatolysis
   rhomboidalis nuchae L57.2
   verticis gyrata Q82.8
     acquired L91.8
Cyanosis R23.0
   due to
     patent foramen botalli Q21.1
     persistent foramen ovale Q21.1
   enterogenous D74.8
   paroxysmal digital — *see* Raynaud's disease
     with gangrene I73.01
   retina, retinal H35.89
Cyanotic heart disease I24.9
   congenital Q24.9
Cycle
   anovulatory N97.0
   menstrual, irregular N92.6
Cyclencephaly Q04.9
Cyclical vomiting (*see also* Vomiting, cyclical) G43.A0
   (*following* G43.7)
   psychogenic F50.8
Cyclitis (*see also* Iridocyclitis) H20.9
   chronic — *see* Iridocyclitis, chronic
   Fuchs' heterochromic H20.81- ☑
   granulomatous — *see* Iridocyclitis, chronic
   lens-induced — *see* Iridocyclitis, lens-induced
   posterior H30.2- ☑
Cycloid personality F34.0
Cyclophoria H50.54
Cyclopia, cyclops Q87.0
Cyclopism Q87.0
Cyclosporiasis A07.4
Cyclothymia F34.0
Cyclothymic personality F34.0
Cyclotropia H50.41- ☑
Cylindroma (*see also* Neoplasm, malignant, by site)
   eccrine dermal — *see* Neoplasm, skin, benign
   skin — *see* Neoplasm, skin, benign
Cylindruria R82.99
Cynanche
   diphtheritic A36.2
   tonsillaris J36
Cynophobia F40.218
Cynorexia R63.2
Cyphosis — *see* Kyphosis
Cyprus fever — *see* Brucellosis
Cyst (colloid) (mucous) (simple) (retention)
   adenoid (infected) J35.8
   adrenal gland E27.8
     congenital Q89.1
   air, lung J98.4
   allantoic Q64.4
   alveolar process (jaw bone) M27.40
   amnion, amniotic O41.8X- ☑
   anterior
     chamber (eye) — *see* Cyst, iris
     nasopalatine K09.1
   antrum J34.1
   anus K62.89
   apical (tooth) (periodontal) K04.8
   appendix K38.8
   arachnoid, brain (acquired) G93.0
     congenital Q04.6
   arytenoid J38.7
   Baker's M71.2- ☑
     ruptured M66.0
     tuberculous A18.02
   Bartholin's gland N75.0
   bile duct (common) (hepatic) K83.5
   bladder (multiple) (trigone) N32.89
   blue dome (breast) — *see* Cyst, breast
   bone (local) NEC M85.60
     aneurysmal M85.50
       ankle M85.57- ☑
       foot M85.57- ☑
       forearm M85.53- ☑
       hand M85.54- ☑
       jaw M27.49
       lower leg M85.56- ☑
       multiple site M85.59
       neck M85.58
       rib M85.58
       shoulder M85.51- ☑
       skull M85.58
       specified site NEC M85.58

Cyst — *continued*
   bone — *continued*
     aneurysmal — *continued*
       thigh M85.55- ☑
       toe M85.57- ☑
       upper arm M85.52- ☑
       vertebra M85.58
     solitary M85.40
       ankle M85.47- ☑
       fibula M85.46- ☑
       foot M85.47- ☑
       hand M85.44- ☑
       humerus M85.42- ☑
       jaw M27.49
       neck M85.48
       pelvis M85.45- ☑
       radius M85.43- ☑
       rib M85.48
       shoulder M85.41- ☑
       skull M85.48
       specified site NEC M85.48
       tibia M85.46- ☑
       toe M85.47- ☑
       ulna M85.43- ☑
       vertebra M85.48
     specified type NEC M85.60
       ankle M85.67- ☑
       foot M85.67- ☑
       forearm M85.63- ☑
       hand M85.64- ☑
       jaw M27.40
         developmental (nonodontogenic) K09.1
         odontogenic K09.0
        latent M27.0
       lower leg M85.66- ☑
       multiple site M85.69
       neck M85.68
       rib M85.68
       shoulder M85.61- ☑
       skull M85.68
       specified site NEC M85.68
       thigh M85.65- ☑
       toe M85.67- ☑
       upper arm M85.62- ☑
       vertebra M85.68
   brain (acquired) G93.0
     congenital Q04.6
     hydatid B67.99 [G94]
     third ventricle (colloid), congenital Q04.6
   branchial (cleft) Q18.0
   branchiogenic Q18.0
   breast (benign) (blue dome) (pedunculated) (solitary)
     N60.0- ☑
     involution — *see* Dysplasia, mammary, specified
       type NEC
     sebaceous — *see* Dysplasia, mammary, specified
       type NEC
   broad ligament (benign) N83.8
   bronchogenic (mediastinal) (sequestration) J98.4
     congenital Q33.0
   buccal K09.8
   bulbourethral gland N36.8
   bursa, bursal NEC M71.30
     with rupture — *see* Rupture, synovium
     ankle M71.37- ☑
     elbow M71.32- ☑
     foot M71.37- ☑
     hand M71.34- ☑
     hip M71.35- ☑
     multiple sites M71.39
     pharyngeal J39.2
     popliteal space — *see* Cyst, Baker's
     shoulder M71.31- ☑
     specified site NEC M71.38
     wrist M71.33- ☑
   calcifying odontogenic D16.5
     upper jaw (bone) (maxilla) D16.4
   canal of Nuck (female) N94.89
     congenital Q52.4
   canthus — *see* Cyst, conjunctiva
   carcinomatous — *see* Neoplasm, malignant, by site
   cauda equina G95.89
   cavum septi pellucidi — *see* Cyst, brain
   celomic (pericardium) Q24.8
   cerebellopontine (angle) — *see* Cyst, brain
   cerebellum — *see* Cyst, brain
   cerebral — *see* Cyst, brain

☑ **Additional Character Required — Refer to the Tabular List for Character Selection**   ▽ **Subterms under main terms may continue to next column or page**

Cyst — *continued*
- cervical lateral Q18.1
- cervix NEC N88.8
  - embryonic Q51.6
  - nabothian N88.8
- chiasmal optic NEC — *see* Disorder, optic, chiasm
- chocolate (ovary) N80.1
- choledochus, congenital Q44.4
- chorion O41.8X- ☑
- choroid plexus G93.0
- ciliary body — *see* Cyst, iris
- clitoris N90.7
- colon K63.89
- common (bile) duct K83.5
- congenital NEC Q89.8
  - adrenal gland Q89.1
  - epiglottis Q31.8
  - esophagus Q39.8
  - fallopian tube Q50.4
  - kidney Q61.00
    - more than one (multiple) Q61.02
      - specified as polycystic Q61.3
        - adult type Q61.2
        - infantile type NEC Q61.19
          - collecting duct dilation Q61.11
    - solitary Q61.01
  - larynx Q31.8
  - liver Q44.6
  - lung Q33.0
  - mediastinum Q34.1
  - ovary Q50.1
  - oviduct Q50.4
  - periurethral (tissue) Q64.79
  - prepuce Q55.69
  - salivary gland (any) Q38.4
  - sublingual Q38.6
  - submaxillary gland Q38.6
  - thymus (gland) Q89.2
  - tongue Q38.3
  - ureterovesical orifice Q62.8
  - vulva Q52.79
- conjunctiva H11.44- ☑
- cornea H18.89- ☑
- corpora quadrigemina G93.0
- corpus
  - albicans N83.29
  - luteum (hemorrhagic) (ruptured) N83.1
- Cowper's gland (benign) (infected) N36.8
- cranial meninges G93.0
- craniobuccal pouch E23.6
- craniopharyngeal pouch E23.6
- cystic duct K82.8
- Cysticercus — *see* Cysticercosis
- Dandy-Walker Q03.1
  - with spina bifida — *see* Spina bifida
- dental (root) K04.8
  - developmental K09.0
  - eruption K09.0
  - primordial K09.0
- dentigerous (mandible) (maxilla) K09.0
- dermoid — *see* Neoplasm, benign, by site
  - with malignant transformation C56.- ☑
  - implantation
    - external area or site (skin) NEC L72.0
    - iris — *see* Cyst, iris, implantation
    - vagina N89.8
    - vulva N90.7
  - mouth K09.8
  - oral soft tissue K09.8
  - sacrococcygeal — *see* Cyst, pilonidal
- developmental K09.1
  - odontogenic K09.0
  - oral region (nonodontogenic) K09.1
  - ovary, ovarian Q50.1
- dura (cerebral) G93.0
  - spinal G96.19
- ear (external) Q18.1
- echinococcal — *see* Echinococcus
- embryonic
  - cervix uteri Q51.6
  - fallopian tube Q50.4
  - vagina Q51.6
- endometrium, endometrial (uterus) N85.8
  - ectopic — *see* Endometriosis
- enterogenous Q43.8
- epidermal, epidermoid (inclusion) (*see also* Cyst, skin) L72.0
  - mouth K09.8

Cyst — *continued*
- epidermal, epidermoid (*see also* Cyst, skin) — *continued*
  - oral soft tissue K09.8
- epididymis N50.3
- epiglottis J38.7
- epiphysis cerebri E34.8
- epithelial (inclusion) L72.0
- epoophoron Q50.5
- eruption K09.0
- esophagus K22.8
- ethmoid sinus J34.1
- external female genital organs NEC N90.7
- eyelid (sebaceous) H02.829
  - infected — *see* Hordeolum
  - left H02.826
    - lower H02.825
    - upper H02.824
  - right H02.823
    - lower H02.822
    - upper H02.821
- eye NEC H57.8
  - congenital Q15.8
- fallopian tube N83.8
  - congenital Q50.4
- fimbrial (twisted) Q50.4
- fissural (oral region) K09.1
- follicle (graafian) (hemorrhagic) N83.0
  - nabothian N88.8
- follicular (atretic) (hemorrhagic) (ovarian) N83.0
  - dentigerous K09.0
  - odontogenic K09.0
  - skin L72.9
    - specified NEC L72.8
- frontal sinus J34.1
- gallbladder K82.8
- ganglion — *see* Ganglion
- Gartner's duct Q52.4
- gingiva K09.0
- gland of Moll — *see* Cyst, eyelid
- globulomaxillary K09.1
- graafian follicle (hemorrhagic) N83.0
- granulosal lutein (hemorrhagic) N83.1
- hemangiomatous D18.00
  - intra-abdominal D18.03
  - intracranial D18.02
  - skin D18.01
  - specified site NEC D18.09
- hydatid (*see also* Echinococcus) B67.90
  - brain B67.99 [G94]
  - liver (*see also* Cyst, liver, hydatid) B67.8
  - lung NEC B67.99 [J99]
  - Morgagni
    - female Q50.5
    - male (epididymal) Q55.4
      - testicular Q55.29
  - specified site NEC B67.99
- hymen N89.8
  - embryonic Q52.4
- hypopharynx J39.2
- hypophysis, hypophyseal (duct) (recurrent) E23.6
  - cerebri E23.6
- implantation (dermoid)
  - external area or site (skin) NEC L72.0
  - iris — *see* Cyst, iris, implantation
  - vagina N89.8
  - vulva N90.7
- incisive canal K09.1
- inclusion (epidermal) (epithelial) (epidermoid) (squamous) L72.0
  - not of skin — *code under* Cyst, by site
- intestine (large) (small) K63.89
- intracranial — *see* Cyst, brain
- intraligamentous (*see also* Disorder, ligament)
  - knee — *see* Derangement, knee
- intrasellar E23.6
- iris H21.309
  - exudative H21.31- ☑
  - idiopathic H21.30- ☑
  - implantation H21.32- ☑
  - parasitic H21.33- ☑
  - pars plana (primary) H21.34- ☑
    - exudative H21.35- ☑
- jaw (bone) M27.40
  - aneurysmal M27.49
  - developmental (odontogenic) K09.0
  - fissural K09.1
  - hemorrhagic M27.49

Cyst — *continued*
- jaw — *continued*
  - traumatic M27.49
- joint NEC — *see* Disorder, joint, specified type NEC
- kidney (acquired) N28.1
  - calyceal — *see* Hydronephrosis
  - congenital Q61.00
    - more than one (multiple) Q61.02
      - specified as polycystic Q61.3
        - adult type (autosomal dominant) Q61.2
        - infantile type (autosomal recessive) NEC Q61.19
          - collecting duct dilation Q61.11
  - pyelogenic — *see* Hydronephrosis
  - simple N28.1
  - solitary (single) Q61.01
    - acquired N28.1
- labium (majus) (minus) N90.7
  - sebaceous N90.7
- lacrimal (*see also* Disorder, lacrimal system, specified NEC)
  - gland H04.13- ☑
  - passages or sac — *see* Disorder, lacrimal system, specified NEC
- larynx J38.7
- lateral periodontal K09.0
- lens H27.8
  - congenital Q12.8
- lip (gland) K13.0
- liver (idiopathic) (simple) K76.89
  - congenital Q44.6
  - hydatid B67.8
    - granulosus B67.0
    - multilocularis B67.5
- lung J98.4
  - congenital Q33.0
  - giant bullous J43.9
- lutein N83.1
- lymphangiomatous D18.1
- lymphoepithelial, oral soft tissue K09.8
- macula — *see* Degeneration, macula, hole
- malignant — *see* Neoplasm, malignant, by site
- mammary gland — *see* Cyst, breast
- mandible M27.40
  - dentigerous K09.0
  - radicular K04.8
- maxilla M27.40
  - dentigerous K09.0
  - radicular K04.8
- medial, face and neck Q18.8
- median
  - anterior maxillary K09.1
  - palatal K09.1
- mediastinum, congenital Q34.1
- meibomian (gland) — *see* Chalazion
  - infected — *see* Hordeolum
- membrane, brain G93.0
- meninges (cerebral) G93.0
  - spinal G96.19
- meniscus, knee — *see* Derangement, knee, meniscus, cystic
- mesentery, mesenteric K66.8
  - chyle I89.8
- mesonephric duct
  - female Q50.5
  - male Q55.4
- milk N64.89
- Morgagni (hydatid)
  - female Q50.5
  - male (epididymal) Q55.4
    - testicular Q55.29
- mouth K09.8
- Müllerian duct Q50.4
  - appendix testis Q55.29
  - cervix Q51.6
  - fallopian tube Q50.4
  - female Q50.4
  - male Q55.29
  - prostatic utricle Q55.4
  - vagina (embryonal) Q52.4
- multilocular (ovary) D39.10
  - benign — *see* Neoplasm, benign, by site
- myometrium N85.8
- nabothian (follicle) (ruptured) N88.8
- nasoalveolar K09.1
- nasolabial K09.1
- nasopalatine (anterior) (duct) K09.1
- nasopharynx J39.2

◁ **Subterms under main terms may continue to next column or page**   ☑ **Additional Character Required — Refer to the Tabular List for Character Selection**   **77**

Cyst — Cyst

Cyst — *continued*
- neoplastic — *see* Neoplasm, uncertain behavior, by site
  - benign — *see* Neoplasm, benign, by site
- nervous system NEC G96.8
- neuroenteric (congenital) Q06.8
- nipple — *see* Cyst, breast
- nose (turbinates) J34.1
  - sinus J34.1
- odontogenic, developmental K09.0
- omentum (lesser) K66.8
  - congenital Q45.8
- ora serrata — *see* Cyst, retina, ora serrata
- oral
  - region K09.9
    - developmental (nonodontogenic) K09.1
    - specified NEC K09.8
  - soft tissue K09.9
    - specified NEC K09.8
- orbit H05.81- ☑
- ovary, ovarian (twisted) N83.20
  - adherent N83.20
  - chocolate N80.1
  - corpus
    - albicans N83.29
    - luteum (hemorrhagic) N83.1
  - dermoid D27.9
  - developmental Q50.1
  - due to failure of involution NEC N83.20
  - endometrial N80.1
  - follicular (graafian) (hemorrhagic) N83.0
  - hemorrhagic N83.20
  - in pregnancy or childbirth O34.8- ☑
    - with obstructed labor O65.5
  - multilocular D39.10
  - pseudomucinous D27.9
  - retention N83.29
  - serous N83.20
  - specified NEC N83.29
  - theca lutein (hemorrhagic) N83.1
  - tuberculous A18.18
- oviduct N83.8
- palate (median) (fissural) K09.1
- palatine papilla (jaw) K09.1
- pancreas, pancreatic (hemorrhagic) (true) K86.2
  - congenital Q45.2
  - false K86.3
- paralabral
  - hip M24.85- ☑
  - shoulder S43.43- ☑
- paramesonephric duct Q50.4
  - female Q50.4
  - male Q55.29
- paranephric N28.1
- paraphysis, cerebri, congenital Q04.6
- parasitic B89
- parathyroid (gland) E21.4
- paratubal N83.8
- paraurethral duct N36.8
- paroophoron Q50.5
- parotid gland K11.6
- parovarian Q50.5
- pelvis, female N94.89
  - in pregnancy or childbirth O34.8- ☑
    - causing obstructed labor O65.5
- penis (sebaceous) N48.89
- periapical K04.8
- pericardial (congenital) Q24.8
  - acquired (secondary) I31.8
- pericoronal K09.0
- periodontal K04.8
  - lateral K09.0
- peripelvic (lymphatic) N28.1
- peritoneum K66.8
  - chylous I89.8
- periventricular, acquired, newborn P91.1
- pharynx (wall) J39.2
- pilar L72.11
- pilonidal (infected) (rectum) L05.91
  - with abscess L05.01
  - malignant C44.59- ☑
- pituitary (duct) (gland) E23.6
- placenta O43.19- ☑
- pleura J94.8
- popliteal — *see* Cyst, Baker's
- porencephalic Q04.6
  - acquired G93.0
- postanal (infected) — *see* Cyst, pilonidal

Cyst — *continued*
- postmastoidectomy cavity (mucosal) — *see* Complications, postmastoidectomy, cyst
- preauricular Q18.1
- prepuce N47.4
  - congenital Q55.69
- primordial (jaw) K09.0
- prostate N42.83
- pseudomucinous (ovary) D27.9
- pupillary, miotic H21.27- ☑
- radicular (residual) K04.8
- radiculodental K04.8
- ranular K11.8
- Rathke's pouch E23.6
- rectum (epithelium) (mucous) K62.89
- renal — *see* Cyst, kidney
- residual (radicular) K04.8
- retention (ovary) N83.29
  - salivary gland K11.6
- retina H33.19- ☑
  - ora serrata H33.11- ☑
  - parasitic H33.12- ☑
- retroperitoneal K68.9
- sacrococcygeal (dermoid) — *see* Cyst, pilonidal
- salivary gland or duct (mucous extravasation or retention) K11.6
- Sampson's N80.1
- sclera H15.89
- scrotum L72.9
  - sebaceous L72.3
- sebaceous (duct) (gland) L72.3
  - breast — *see* Dysplasia, mammary, specified type NEC
  - eyelid — *see* Cyst, eyelid
  - genital organ NEC
    - female N94.89
    - male N50.8
  - scrotum L72.3
- semilunar cartilage (knee) (multiple) — *see* Derangement, knee, meniscus, cystic
- seminal vesicle N50.8
- serous (ovary) N83.20
- sinus (accessory) (nasal) J34.1
- Skene's gland N36.8
- skin L72.9
  - breast — *see* Dysplasia, mammary, specified type NEC
  - epidermal, epidermoid L72.0
  - epithelial L72.0
  - eyelid — *see* Cyst, eyelid
  - genital organ NEC
    - female N90.7
    - male N50.8
  - inclusion L72.0
  - scrotum L72.9
  - sebaceous L72.3
  - sweat gland or duct L74.8
- solitary
  - bone — *see* Cyst, bone, solitary
  - jaw M27.40
  - kidney N28.1
- spermatic cord N50.8
- sphenoid sinus J34.1
- spinal meninges G96.19
- spleen NEC D73.4
  - congenital Q89.09
  - hydatid (*see also* Echinococcus) B67.99 [D77]
- Stafne's M27.0
- subarachnoid intrasellar R93.0
- subcutaneous, pheomycotic (chromomycotic) B43.2
- subdural (cerebral) G93.0
  - spinal cord G96.19
- sublingual gland K11.6
- submandibular gland K11.6
- submaxillary gland K11.6
- suburethral N36.8
- suprarenal gland E27.8
- suprasellar — *see* Cyst, brain
- sweat gland or duct L74.8
- synovial (*see also* Cyst, bursa)
  - ruptured — *see* Rupture, synovium
- tarsal — *see* Chalazion
- tendon (sheath) — *see* Disorder, tendon, specified type NEC
- testis N44.2
  - tunica albuginea N44.1
- theca lutein (ovary) N83.1
- Thornwaldt's J39.2

Cyst — *continued*
- thymus (gland) E32.8
- thyroglossal duct (infected) (persistent) Q89.2
- thyroid (gland) E04.1
- thyrolingual duct (infected) (persistent) Q89.2
- tongue K14.8
- tonsil J35.8
- tooth — *see* Cyst, dental
- Tornwaldt's J39.2
- trichilemmal (proliferating) L72.12
- trichodermal L72.12
- tubal (fallopian) N83.8
  - inflammatory — *see* Salpingitis, chronic
- tubo-ovarian N83.8
  - inflammatory N70.13
- tunica
  - albuginea testis N44.1
  - vaginalis N50.8
- turbinate (nose) J34.1
- Tyson's gland N48.89
- urachus, congenital Q64.4
- ureter N28.89
- ureterovesical orifice N28.89
- urethra, urethral (gland) N36.8
- uterine ligament N83.8
- uterus (body) (corpus) (recurrent) N85.8
  - embryonic Q51.818
    - cervix Q51.6
- vagina, vaginal (implantation) (inclusion) (squamous cell) (wall) N89.8
  - embryonic Q52.4
- vallecula, vallecular (epiglottis) J38.7
- vesical (orifice) N32.89
- vitreous body H43.89
- vulva (implantation) (inclusion) N90.7
  - congenital Q52.79
  - sebaceous gland N90.7
- vulvovaginal gland N90.7
- wolffian
  - female Q50.5
  - male Q55.4

Cystadenocarcinoma — *see* Neoplasm, malignant, by site
- bile duct C22.1
- endometrioid — *see* Neoplasm, malignant, by site
  - specified site — *see* Neoplasm, malignant, by site
  - unspecified site
    - female C56.9
    - male C61
- mucinous
  - papillary
    - specified site — *see* Neoplasm, malignant, by site
    - unspecified site C56.9
  - specified site — *see* Neoplasm, malignant, by site
  - unspecified site C56.9
- papillary
  - mucinous
    - specified site — *see* Neoplasm, malignant, by site
    - unspecified site C56.9
  - pseudomucinous
    - specified site — *see* Neoplasm, malignant, by site
    - unspecified site C56.9
  - serous
    - specified site — *see* Neoplasm, malignant, by site
    - unspecified site C56.9
  - specified site — *see* Neoplasm, malignant, by site
  - unspecified site C56.9
- pseudomucinous
  - papillary
    - specified site — *see* Neoplasm, malignant, by site
    - unspecified site C56.9
  - specified site — *see* Neoplasm, malignant, by site
  - unspecified site C56.9
- serous
  - papillary
    - specified site — *see* Neoplasm, malignant, by site
    - unspecified site C56.9
  - specified site — *see* Neoplasm, malignant, by site
  - unspecified site C56.9

Cystadenofibroma
- clear cell — *see* Neoplasm, benign, by site
- endometrioid D27.9

Cystadenofibroma — *continued*
  endometrioid D27.9
    borderline malignancy D39.1- ☑
    malignant C56.- ☑
  mucinous
    specified site — *see* Neoplasm, benign, by site
    unspecified site D27.9
  serous
    specified site — *see* Neoplasm, benign, by site
    unspecified site D27.9
  specified site — *see* Neoplasm, benign, by site
  unspecified site D27.9
Cystadenoma (*see also* Neoplasm, benign, by site)
  bile duct D13.4
  endometrioid — *see* Neoplasm, benign, by site
    borderline malignancy — *see* Neoplasm, uncertain
      behavior, by site
  malignant — *see* Neoplasm, malignant, by site
  mucinous
    borderline malignancy
      ovary C56.- ☑
      specified site NEC — *see* Neoplasm, uncertain
        behavior, by site
      unspecified site C56.9
    papillary
      borderline malignancy
        ovary C56.- ☑
        specified site NEC — *see* Neoplasm, uncer-
          tain behavior, by site
        unspecified site C56.9
      specified site — *see* Neoplasm, benign, by site
      unspecified site D27.9
    specified site — *see* Neoplasm, benign, by site
    unspecified site D27.9
  papillary
    borderline malignancy
      ovary C56.- ☑
      specified site NEC — *see* Neoplasm, uncertain
        behavior, by site
      unspecified site C56.9
    lymphomatosum
      specified site — *see* Neoplasm, benign, by site
      unspecified site D11.9
    mucinous
      borderline malignancy
        ovary C56.- ☑
        specified site NEC — *see* Neoplasm, uncer-
          tain behavior, by site
        unspecified site C56.9
      specified site — *see* Neoplasm, benign, by site
      unspecified site D27.9
    pseudomucinous
      borderline malignancy
        ovary C56.- ☑
        specified site NEC — *see* Neoplasm, uncer-
          tain behavior, by site
        unspecified site C56.9
      specified site — *see* Neoplasm, benign, by site
      unspecified site D27.9
    serous
      borderline malignancy
        ovary C56.- ☑
        specified site NEC — *see* Neoplasm, uncer-
          tain behavior, by site
        unspecified site C56.9
      specified site — *see* Neoplasm, benign, by site
      unspecified site D27.9
    specified site — *see* Neoplasm, benign, by site
    unspecified site D27.9
  pseudomucinous
    borderline malignancy
      ovary C56.- ☑
      specified site NEC — *see* Neoplasm, uncertain
        behavior, by site
      unspecified site C56.9
    papillary
      borderline malignancy
        ovary C56.- ☑
        specified site NEC — *see* Neoplasm, uncer-
          tain behavior, by site
        unspecified site C56.9
      specified site — *see* Neoplasm, benign, by site
      unspecified site D27.9
    specified site — *see* Neoplasm, benign, by site

Cystadenoma — *continued*
  pseudomucinous — *continued*
    unspecified site D27.9
  serous
    borderline malignancy
      ovary C56.- ☑
      specified site NEC — *see* Neoplasm, uncertain
        behavior, by site
      unspecified site C56.9
    papillary
      borderline malignancy
        ovary C56.- ☑
        specified site NEC — *see* Neoplasm, uncer-
          tain behavior, by site
        unspecified site C56.9
      specified site — *see* Neoplasm, benign, by site
      unspecified site D27.9
    specified site — *see* Neoplasm, benign, by site
    unspecified site D27.9
Cystathionine synthase deficiency E72.11
Cystathioninemia E72.19
Cystathioninuria E72.19
Cystic (*see also* condition)
  breast (chronic) — *see* Mastopathy, cystic
  corpora lutea (hemorrhagic) N83.1
  duct — *see* condition
  eyeball (congenital) Q11.0
  fibrosis — *see* Fibrosis, cystic
  kidney (congenital) Q61.9
    adult type Q61.2
    infantile type NEC Q61.19
      collecting duct dilatation Q61.11
    medullary Q61.5
  liver, congenital Q44.6
  lung disease J98.4
    congenital Q33.0
  mastitis, chronic — *see* Mastopathy, cystic
  medullary, kidney Q61.5
  meniscus — *see* Derangement, knee, meniscus, cystic
  ovary N83.20
Cysticercosis, cysticerciasis B69.9
  with
    epileptiform fits B69.0
    myositis B69.81
  brain B69.0
  central nervous system B69.0
  cerebral B69.0
  ocular B69.1
  specified NEC B69.89
Cysticercus cellulose infestation — *see* Cysticercosis
Cystinosis (malignant) E72.04
Cystinuria E72.01
Cystitis (exudative) (hemorrhagic) (septic) (suppurative)
    N30.90
  with
    fibrosis — *see* Cystitis, chronic, interstitial
    hematuria N30.91
    leukoplakia — *see* Cystitis, chronic, interstitial
    malakoplakia — *see* Cystitis, chronic, interstitial
    metaplasia — *see* Cystitis, chronic, interstitial
    prostatitis N41.3
  acute N30.00
    with hematuria N30.01
    of trigone N30.30
      with hematuria N30.31
  allergic — *see* Cystitis, specified type NEC
  amebic A06.81
  bilharzial B65.9 [N33]
  blennorrhagic (gonococcal) A54.01
  bullous — *see* Cystitis, specified type NEC
  calculus N21.0
  chlamydial A56.01
  chronic N30.20
    with hematuria N30.21
    interstitial N30.10
      with hematuria N30.11
    of trigone N30.30
      with hematuria N30.31
    specified NEC N30.20
      with hematuria N30.21
  cystic (a) — *see* Cystitis, specified type NEC
  diphtheritic A36.85
  echinococcal
    granulosus B67.39

Cystitis — *continued*
  echinococcal — *continued*
    multilocularis B67.69
  emphysematous — *see* Cystitis, specified type NEC
  encysted — *see* Cystitis, specified type NEC
  eosinophilic — *see* Cystitis, specified type NEC
  follicular — *see* Cystitis, of trigone
  gangrenous — *see* Cystitis, specified type NEC
  glandularis — *see* Cystitis, specified type NEC
  gonococcal A54.01
  incrusted — *see* Cystitis, specified type NEC
  interstitial (chronic) — *see* Cystitis, chronic, interstitial
  irradiation N30.40
    with hematuria N30.41
  irritation — *see* Cystitis, specified type NEC
  malignant — *see* Cystitis, specified type NEC
  of trigone N30.30
    with hematuria N30.31
  panmural — *see* Cystitis, chronic, interstitial
  polyposa — *see* Cystitis, specified type NEC
  prostatic N41.3
  puerperal (postpartum) O86.22
  radiation — *see* Cystitis, irradiation
  specified type NEC N30.80
    with hematuria N30.81
  subacute — *see* Cystitis, chronic
  submucous — *see* Cystitis, chronic, interstitial
  syphilitic (late) A52.76
  trichomonal A59.03
  tuberculous A18.12
  ulcerative — *see* Cystitis, chronic, interstitial
Cystocele (-urethrocele)
  female N81.10
    with prolapse of uterus — *see* Prolapse, uterus
    lateral N81.12
    midline N81.11
    paravaginal N81.12
  in pregnancy or childbirth O34.8- ☑
    causing obstructed labor O65.5
  male N32.89
Cystolithiasis N21.0
Cystoma (*see also* Neoplasm, benign, by site)
  endometrial, ovary N80.1
  mucinous
    specified site — *see* Neoplasm, benign, by site
    unspecified site D27.9
  serous
    specified site — *see* Neoplasm, benign, by site
    unspecified site D27.9
  simple (ovary) N83.29
Cystoplegia N31.2
Cystoptosis N32.89
Cystopyelitis — *see* Pyelonephritis
Cystorrhagia N32.89
Cystosarcoma phyllodes D48.6- ☑
  benign D24- ☑
  malignant — *see* Neoplasm, breast, malignant
Cystostomy
  attention to Z43.5
  complication — *see* Complications, cystostomy
  status Z93.50
    appendico-vesicostomy Z93.52
    cutaneous Z93.51
    specified NEC Z93.59
Cystourethritis — *see* Urethritis
Cystourethrocele (*see also* Cystocele)
  female N81.10
    with uterine prolapse — *see* Prolapse, uterus
    lateral N81.12
    midline N81.11
    paravaginal N81.12
  male N32.89
Cytomegalic inclusion disease
  congenital P35.1
Cytomegalovirus infection B25.9
Cytomycosis (reticuloendothelial) B39.4
Cytopenia D75.9
  refractory
    with multilineage dysplasia D46.A (*following* D46.2)
      and ring sideroblasts (RCMD RS) D46.B (*follow-*
        ing D46.2)
Czerny's disease (periodic hydrarthrosis of the knee) —
    see Effusion, joint, knee

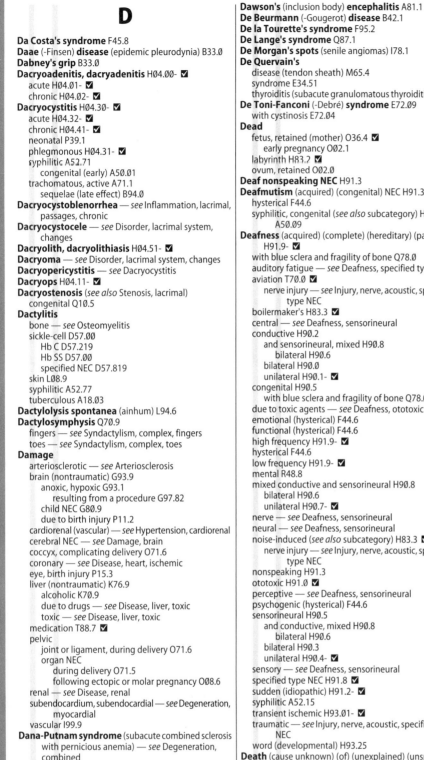

D

Da Costa's syndrome F45.8
Daae (-Finsen) **disease** (epidemic pleurodynia) B33.Ø
Dabney's grip B33.Ø
Dacryoadenitis, dacryadenitis HØ4.ØØ- ☑
  acute HØ4.Ø1- ☑
  chronic HØ4.Ø2- ☑
Dacryocystitis HØ4.3Ø- ☑
  acute HØ4.32- ☑
  chronic HØ4.41- ☑
  neonatal P39.1
  phlegmonous HØ4.31- ☑
  syphilitic A52.71
    congenital (early) A5Ø.Ø1
  trachomatous, active A71.1
    sequelae (late effect) B94.Ø
Dacryocystoblenorrhea — *see* Inflammation, lacrimal, passages, chronic
Dacryocystocele — *see* Disorder, lacrimal system, changes
Dacryolith, dacryolithiasis HØ4.51- ☑
Dacryoma — *see* Disorder, lacrimal system, changes
Dacryopericystitis — *see* Dacryocystitis
Dacryops HØ4.11- ☑
Dacryostenosis (*see also* Stenosis, lacrimal)
  congenital Q1Ø.5
Dactylitis
  bone — *see* Osteomyelitis
  sickle-cell D57.ØØ
    Hb C D57.219
    Hb SS D57.ØØ
    specified NEC D57.819
  skin LØ8.9
  syphilitic A52.77
  tuberculous A18.Ø3
Dactylolysis spontanea (ainhum) L94.6
Dactylosymphysis Q7Ø.9
  fingers — *see* Syndactylism, complex, fingers
  toes — *see* Syndactylism, complex, toes
Damage
  arteriosclerotic — *see* Arteriosclerosis
  brain (nontraumatic) G93.9
    anoxic, hypoxic G93.1
      resulting from a procedure G97.82
    child NEC G8Ø.9
    due to birth injury P11.2
  cardiorenal (vascular) — *see* Hypertension, cardiorenal
  cerebral NEC — *see* Damage, brain
  coccyx, complicating delivery O71.6
  coronary — *see* Disease, heart, ischemic
  eye, birth injury P15.3
  liver (nontraumatic) K76.9
    alcoholic K7Ø.9
    due to drugs — *see* Disease, liver, toxic
    toxic — *see* Disease, liver, toxic
  medication T88.7 ☑
  pelvic
    joint or ligament, during delivery O71.6
    organ NEC
      during delivery O71.5
      following ectopic or molar pregnancy OØ8.6
  renal — *see* Disease, renal
  subendocardium, subendocardial — *see* Degeneration, myocardial
  vascular I99.9
Dana-Putnam syndrome (subacute combined sclerosis with pernicious anemia) — *see* Degeneration, combined
Danbolt (-Cross) **syndrome** (acrodermatitis enteropathica) E83.2
Dandruff L21.Ø
Dandy-Walker syndrome QØ3.1
  with spina bifida — *see* Spina bifida
Danlos' syndrome Q79.6
Darier (-White) **disease** (congenital) Q82.8
  meaning erythema annulare centrifugum L53.1
Darier-Roussy sarcoid D86.3
Darling's disease or histoplasmosis B39.4
Darwin's tubercle Q17.8

Dawson's (inclusion body) **encephalitis** A81.1
De Beurmann (-Gougerot) **disease** B42.1
De la Tourette's syndrome F95.2
De Lange's syndrome Q87.1
De Morgan's spots (senile angiomas) I78.1
De Quervain's
  disease (tendon sheath) M65.4
  syndrome E34.51
  thyroiditis (subacute granulomatous thyroiditis) EØ6.1
De Toni-Fanconi (-Debré) **syndrome** E72.Ø9
  with cystinosis E72.Ø4
Dead
  fetus, retained (mother) O36.4 ☑
    early pregnancy OØ2.1
  labyrinth H83.2 ☑
  ovum, retained OØ2.Ø
Deaf nonspeaking NEC H91.3
Deafmutism (acquired) (congenital) NEC H91.3
  hysterical F44.6
  syphilitic, congenital (*see also* subcategory) H94.8 A5Ø.Ø9
Deafness (acquired) (complete) (hereditary) (partial) H91.9- ☑
  with blue sclera and fragility of bone Q78.Ø
  auditory fatigue — *see* Deafness, specified type NEC
  aviation T7Ø.Ø ☑
    nerve injury — *see* Injury, nerve, acoustic, specified type NEC
  boilermaker's H83.3 ☑
  central — *see* Deafness, sensorineural
  conductive H9Ø.2
    and sensorineural, mixed H9Ø.8
      bilateral H9Ø.6
    bilateral H9Ø.Ø
    unilateral H9Ø.1- ☑
  congenital H9Ø.5
    with blue sclera and fragility of bone Q78.Ø
  due to toxic agents — *see* Deafness, ototoxic
  emotional (hysterical) F44.6
  functional (hysterical) F44.6
  high frequency H91.9- ☑
  hysterical F44.6
  low frequency H91.9- ☑
  mental R48.8
  mixed conductive and sensorineural H9Ø.8
    bilateral H9Ø.6
    unilateral H9Ø.7- ☑
  nerve — *see* Deafness, sensorineural
  neural — *see* Deafness, sensorineural
  noise-induced (*see also* subcategory) H83.3 ☑
    nerve injury — *see* Injury, nerve, acoustic, specified type NEC
  nonspeaking H91.3
  ototoxic H91.Ø ☑
  perceptive — *see* Deafness, sensorineural
  psychogenic (hysterical) F44.6
  sensorineural H9Ø.5
    and conductive, mixed H9Ø.8
      bilateral H9Ø.6
    bilateral H9Ø.3
    unilateral H9Ø.4- ☑
  sensory — *see* Deafness, sensorineural
  specified type NEC H91.8 ☑
  sudden (idiopathic) H91.2- ☑
  syphilitic A52.15
  transient ischemic H93.Ø1- ☑
  traumatic — *see* Injury, nerve, acoustic, specified type NEC
  word (developmental) H93.25
Death (cause unknown) (of) (unexplained) (unspecified cause) R99
  brain G93.82
  cardiac (sudden) (with successful resuscitation) — *code to* underlying disease
    family history of Z82.41
    personal history of Z86.74
  family member (assumed) Z63.4
Debility (chronic) (general) (nervous) R53.81
  congenital or neonatal NOS P96.9
  nervous R53.81
  old age R54
  senile R54

Débove's disease (splenomegaly) R16.1
Decalcification
  bone — *see* Osteoporosis
  teeth KØ3.89
Decapsulation, kidney N28.89
Decay
  dental — *see* Caries, dental
  senile R54
  tooth, teeth — *see* Caries, dental
Deciduitis (acute)
  following ectopic or molar pregnancy OØ8.Ø
Decline (general) — *see* Debility
  cognitive, age-associated R41.81
Decompensation
  cardiac (acute) (chronic) — *see* Disease, heart
  cardiovascular — *see* Disease, cardiovascular
  heart — *see* Disease, heart
  hepatic — *see* Failure, hepatic
  myocardial (acute) (chronic) — *see* Disease, heart
  respiratory J98.8
Decompression sickness T7Ø.3 ☑
Decrease (d)
  absolute neutrophile count — *see* Neutropenia
  blood
    platelets — *see* Thrombocytopenia
    pressure RØ3.1
      due to shock following
        injury T79.4 ☑
        operation T81.19 ☑
  estrogen E28.39
    postablative E89.4Ø
      asymptomatic E89.4Ø
      symptomatic E89.41
  fragility of erythrocytes D58.8
  function
    lipase (pancreatic) K9Ø.3
    ovary in hypopituitarism E23.Ø
    parenchyma of pancreas K86.8
    pituitary (gland) (anterior) (lobe) E23.Ø
      posterior (lobe) E23.Ø
  functional activity R68.89
  glucose R73.Ø9
  hematocrit R71.Ø
  hemoglobin R71.Ø
  leukocytes D72.819
    specified NEC D72.818
  libido R68.82
  lymphocytes D72.81Ø
  platelets D69.6
  respiration, due to shock following injury T79.4 ☑
  sexual desire R68.82
  tear secretion NEC — *see* Syndrome, dry eye
  tolerance
    fat K9Ø.4
    glucose R73.Ø9
    pancreatic K9Ø.3
    salt and water E87.8
  vision NEC H54.7
  white blood cell count D72.819
    specified NEC D72.818
Decubitus (ulcer) — *see* Ulcer, pressure, by site
  cervix N86
Deepening acetabulum — *see* Derangement, joint, specified type NEC, hip
Defect, defective Q89.9
  3-beta-hydroxysteroid dehydrogenase E25.Ø
  11-hydroxylase E25.Ø
  21-hydroxylase E25.Ø
  abdominal wall, congenital Q79.59
  antibody immunodeficiency D8Ø.9
  aorticopulmonary septum Q21.4
  atrial septal (ostium secundum type) Q21.1
    following acute myocardial infarction (current complication) I23.1
    ostium primum type Q21.2
  atrioventricular
    canal Q21.2
    septum Q21.2
  auricular septal Q21.1
  bilirubin excretion NEC E8Ø.6
  biosynthesis, androgen (testicular) E29.1
  bulbar septum Q21.Ø

☑ **Additional Character Required — Refer to the Tabular List for Character Selection** ▽ **Subterms under main terms may continue to next column or page**

Defect, defective — *continued*
catalase E80.3
cell membrane receptor complex (CR3) D71
circulation I99.9
  congenital Q28.9
  newborn Q28.9
coagulation (factor) (*see also* Deficiency, factor) D68.9
  with
    ectopic pregnancy O08.1
    molar pregnancy O08.1
  acquired D68.4
  antepartum with hemorrhage — *see* Hemorrhage, antepartum, with coagulation defect
  due to
    liver disease D68.4
    vitamin K deficiency D68.4
  hereditary NEC D68.2
  intrapartum O67.0
  newborn, transient P61.6
  postpartum O72.3
  specified type NEC D68.8
complement system D84.1
conduction (heart) I45.9
  bone — *see* Deafness, conductive
congenital, organ or site not listed — *see* Anomaly, by site
coronary sinus Q21.1
cushion, endocardial Q21.2
degradation, glycoprotein E77.1
dental bridge, crown, fillings — *see* Defect, dental restoration
dental restoration K08.50
  specified NEC K08.59
dentin (hereditary) K00.5
Descemet's membrane, congenital Q13.89
developmental (*see also* Anomaly)
  cauda equina Q06.3
diaphragm
  with elevation, eventration or hernia — *see* Hernia, diaphragm
  congenital Q79.1
    with hernia Q79.0
    gross (with hernia) Q79.0
ectodermal, congenital Q82.9
Eisenmenger's Q21.8
enzyme
  catalase E80.3
  peroxidase E80.3
esophagus, congenital Q39.9
extensor retinaculum M62.89
fibrin polymerization D68.2
filling
  bladder R93.4
  kidney R93.4
  stomach R93.3
  ureter R93.4
Gerbode Q21.0
glycoprotein degradation E77.1
Hageman (factor) D68.2
hearing — *see* Deafness
high grade F70
interatrial septal Q21.1
interauricular septal Q21.1
interventricular septal Q21.0
  with dextroposition of aorta, pulmonary stenosis and hypertrophy of right ventricle Q21.3
  in tetralogy of Fallot Q21.3
learning (specific) — *see* Disorder, learning
lymphocyte function antigen-1 (LFA-1) D84.0
lysosomal enzyme, post-translational modification E77.0
major osseous M89.70
  ankle M89.77- ☑
  carpus M89.74- ☑
  clavicle M89.71- ☑
  femur M89.75- ☑
  fibula M89.76- ☑
  fingers M89.74- ☑
  foot M89.77- ☑
  forearm M89.73- ☑
  hand M89.74- ☑
  humerus M89.72- ☑
  lower leg M89.76- ☑
  metacarpus M89.74- ☑
  metatarsus M89.77- ☑
  multiple sites M89.79
  pelvic region M89.75- ☑
  pelvis M89.75- ☑

Defect, defective — *continued*
major osseous — *continued*
  radius M89.73- ☑
  scapula M89.71- ☑
  shoulder region M89.71- ☑
  specified NEC M89.78
  tarsus M89.77- ☑
  thigh M89.75- ☑
  tibia M89.76- ☑
  toes M89.77- ☑
  ulna M89.73- ☑
mental — *see* Disability, intellectual
modification, lysosomal enzymes, post-translational E77.0
obstructive, congenital
  renal pelvis Q62.39
  ureter Q62.39
    atresia — *see* Atresia, ureter
    cecoureterocele Q62.32
    megaureter Q62.2
    orthotopic ureterocele Q62.31
osseous, major M89.70
  ankle M89.77- ☑
  carpus M89.74- ☑
  clavicle M89.71- ☑
  femur M89.75- ☑
  fibula M89.76- ☑
  fingers M89.74- ☑
  foot M89.77- ☑
  forearm M89.73- ☑
  hand M89.74- ☑
  humerus M89.72- ☑
  lower leg M89.76- ☑
  metacarpus M89.74- ☑
  metatarsus M89.77- ☑
  multiple sites M89.9
  pelvic region M89.75- ☑
  pelvis M89.75- ☑
  radius M89.73- ☑
  scapula M89.71- ☑
  shoulder region M89.71- ☑
  specified NEC M89.78
  tarsus M89.77- ☑
  thigh M89.75- ☑
  tibia M89.76- ☑
  toes M89.77- ☑
  ulna M89.73- ☑
osteochondral NEC (*see also* Deformity) M95.8
ostium
  primum Q21.2
  secundum Q21.1
peroxidase E80.3
placental blood supply — *see* Insufficiency, placental
platelets, qualitative D69.1
  constitutional D68.0
postural NEC, spine — *see* Dorsopathy, deforming
reduction
  limb Q73.8
    lower Q72.9- ☑
      absence — *see* Agenesis, leg
        foot — *see* Agenesis, foot
      longitudinal
        femur Q72.4- ☑
        fibula Q72.6- ☑
        tibia Q72.5- ☑
      specified type NEC Q72.89- ☑
      split foot Q72.7- ☑
    specified type NEC Q73.8
    upper Q71.9- ☑
      absence — *see* Agenesis, arm
        forearm — *see* Agenesis, forearm
        hand — *see* Agenesis, hand
      lobster-claw hand Q71.6- ☑
      longitudinal
        radius Q71.4- ☑
        ulna Q71.5- ☑
      specified type NEC Q71.89- ☑
renal pelvis Q63.8
  obstructive Q62.39
respiratory system, congenital Q34.9
restoration, dental K08.50
  specified NEC K08.59
retinal nerve bundle fibers H35.89
septal (heart) NOS Q21.9
  acquired (atrial) (auricular) (ventricular) (old) I51.0

Defect, defective — *continued*
septal — *continued*
  atrial Q21.1
    concurrent with acute myocardial infarction — *see* Infarct, myocardium
    following acute myocardial infarction (current complication) I23.1
    ventricular (*see also* Defect, ventricular septal) Q21.0
  sinus venosus Q21.1
speech R47.9
  developmental F80.9
  specified NEC R47.89
Taussig-Bing (aortic transposition and overriding pulmonary artery) Q20.1
teeth, wedge K03.1
vascular (local) I99.9
  congenital Q27.9
ventricular septal Q21.0
  concurrent with acute myocardial infarction — *see* Infarct, myocardium
  following acute myocardial infarction (current complication) I23.2
  in tetralogy of Fallot Q21.3
vision NEC H54.7
visual field H53.40
  bilateral
    heteronymous H53.47
    homonymous H53.46- ☑
  generalized contraction H53.48- ☑
  localized
    arcuate H53.43- ☑
    scotoma (central area) H53.41- ☑
      blind spot area H53.42- ☑
    sector H53.43- ☑
    specified type NEC H53.45- ☑
voice R49.9
  specified NEC R49.8
wedge, tooth, teeth (abrasion) K03.1
Deferentitis N49.1
  gonorrheal (acute) (chronic) A54.23
Defibrination (syndrome) D65
  antepartum — *see* Hemorrhage, antepartum, with coagulation defect, disseminated intravascular coagulation
  following ectopic or molar pregnancy O08.1
  intrapartum O67.0
  newborn P60
  postpartum O72.3
Deficiency, deficient
  3-beta hydroxysteroid dehydrogenase E25.0
  5-alpha reductase (with male pseudohermaphroditism) E29.1
  11-hydroxylase E25.0
  21-hydroxylase E25.0
  abdominal muscle syndrome Q79.4
  AC globulin (congenital) (hereditary) D68.2
    acquired D68.4
  accelerator globulin (Ac G) (blood) D68.2
  acid phosphatase E83.39
  activating factor (blood) D68.2
  adenosine deaminase (ADA) D81.3
  aldolase (hereditary) E74.19
  alpha-1-antitrypsin E88.01
  amino-acids E72.9
  anemia — *see* Anemia
  aneurin E51.9
  antibody with
    hyperimmunoglobulinemia D80.6
    near-normal immunoglobins D80.6
  antidiuretic hormone E23.2
  anti-hemophilic
    factor (A) D66
      B D67
      C D68.1
    globulin (AHG) NEC D66
  antithrombin (antithrombin III) D68.59
  ascorbic acid E54
  attention (disorder) (syndrome) F98.8
    with hyperactivity — *see* Disorder, attention-deficit hyperactivity
  autoprothrombin
    C D68.2
    I D68.2
    II D67
  beta-glucuronidase E76.29
  biotin E53.8
  biotin-dependent carboxylase D81.819

Deficiency, deficient — *continued*
biotinidase D81.810
brancher enzyme (amylopectinosis) E74.03
C1 esterase inhibitor (C1-INH) D84.1
calciferol E55.9
   with
      adult osteomalacia M83.8
      rickets — *see* Rickets
calcium (dietary) E58
calorie, severe E43
   with marasmus E41
      and kwashiorkor E42
cardiac — *see* Insufficiency, myocardial
carnitine E71.40
   due to
      hemodialysis E71.43
      inborn errors of metabolism E71.42
      Valproic acid therapy E71.43
   iatrogenic E71.43
   muscle palmityltransferase E71.314
   primary E71.41
   secondary E71.448
carotene E50.9
central nervous system G96.8
ceruloplasmin (Wilson) E83.01
choline E53.8
Christmas factor D67
chromium E61.4
clotting (blood) (*see also* Deficiency, coagulation factor) D68.9
clotting factor NEC (hereditary) (*see also* Deficiency, factor) D68.2
coagulation NOS D68.9
   with
      ectopic pregnancy O08.1
      molar pregnancy O08.1
   acquired (any) D68.4
   antepartum hemorrhage — *see* Hemorrhage, antepartum, with coagulation defect
   clotting factor NEC (*see also* Deficiency, factor) D68.2
   due to
      hyperprothrombinemia D68.4
      liver disease D68.4
      vitamin K deficiency D68.4
   newborn, transient P61.6
   postpartum O72.3
   specified NEC D68.8
cognitive F09
color vision H53.50
   achromatopsia H53.51
   acquired H53.52
   deuteranomaly H53.53
   protanomaly H53.54
   specified type NEC H53.59
   tritanomaly H53.55
combined glucocorticoid and mineralocorticoid E27.49
contact factor D68.2
copper (nutritional) E61.0
corticoadrenal E27.40
   primary E27.1
craniofacial axis Q75.0
cyanocobalamin E53.8
debrancher enzyme (limit dextrinosis) E74.03
dehydrogenase
   long chain/very long chain acyl CoA E71.310
   medium chain acyl CoA E71.311
   short chain acyl CoA E71.312
diet E63.9
dihydropyrimidine dehydrogenase (DPD) E88.89
disaccharidase E73.9
edema — *see* Malnutrition, severe
endocrine E34.9
energy-supply — *see* Malnutrition
enzymes, circulating NEC E88.09
ergosterol E55.9
   with
      adult osteomalacia M83.8
      rickets — *see* Rickets
essential fatty acid (EFA) E63.0
factor (*see also* Deficiency, coagulation)
   Hageman D68.2
   I (congenital) (hereditary) D68.2
   II (congenital) (hereditary) D68.2
   IX (congenital) (functional) (hereditary) (with functional defect) D67
   multiple (congenital) D68.8
      acquired D68.4

Deficiency, deficient — *continued*
factor (*see also* Deficiency, coagulation) — *continued*
   V (congenital) (hereditary) D68.2
   VII (congenital) (hereditary) D68.2
   VIII (congenital) (functional) (hereditary) (with functional defect) D66
      with vascular defect D68.0
   X (congenital) (hereditary) D68.2
   XI (congenital) (hereditary) D68.1
   XII (congenital) (hereditary) D68.2
   XIII (congenital) (hereditary) D68.2
femoral, proximal focal (congenital) — *see* Defect, reduction, lower limb, longitudinal, femur
fibrinase D68.2
fibrinogen (congenital) (hereditary) D68.2
   acquired D65
fibrin-stabilizing factor (congenital) (hereditary) D68.2
   acquired D68.4
folate E53.8
folic acid E53.8
foreskin N47.3
fructokinase E74.11
fructose 1,6-diphosphatase E74.19
fructose-1-phosphate aldolase E74.19
galactokinase E74.29
galactose-1-phosphate uridyl transferase E74.29
gammaglobulin in blood D80.1
   hereditary D80.0
glass factor D68.2
glucocorticoid E27.49
   mineralocorticoid E27.49
glucose-6-phosphatase E74.01
glucose-6-phosphate dehydrogenase anemia D55.0
glucuronyl transferase E80.5
glycogen synthetase E74.09
gonadotropin (isolated) E23.0
growth hormone (idiopathic) (isolated) E23.0
Hageman factor D68.2
hemoglobin D64.9
hepatophosphorylase E74.09
homogentisate 1,2-dioxygenase E70.29
hormone
   anterior pituitary (partial) NEC E23.0
      growth E23.0
   growth (isolated) E23.0
   pituitary E23.0
   testicular E29.1
hypoxanthine- (guanine)-phosphoribosyltransferase (HG- PRT) (total H-PRT) E79.1
immunity D84.9
   cell-mediated D84.8
      with thrombocytopenia and eczema D82.0
   combined D81.9
   humoral D80.9
   IgA (secretory) D80.2
   IgG D80.3
   IgM D80.4
immuno — *see* Immunodeficiency
immunoglobulin, selective
   A (IgA) D80.2
   G (IgG) (subclasses) D80.3
   M (IgM) D80.4
inositol (B complex) E53.8
intrinsic
   factor (congenital) D51.0
   sphincter N36.42
      with urethral hypermobility N36.43
iodine E61.8
   congenital syndrome — *see* Syndrome, iodine-deficiency, congenital
iron E61.1
   anemia D50.9
kalium E87.6
kappa-light chain D80.8
labile factor (congenital) (hereditary) D68.2
   acquired D68.4
lacrimal fluid (acquired) (*see also* Syndrome, dry eye)
   congenital Q10.6
lactase
   congenital E73.0
   secondary E73.1
Laki-Lorand factor D68.2
lecithin cholesterol acyltransferase E78.6
lipocaic K86.8
lipoprotein (familial) (high density) E78.6
liver phosphorylase E74.09
lysosomal alpha-1, 4 glucosidase E74.02

Deficiency, deficient — *continued*
magnesium E61.2
major histocompatibility complex
   class I D81.6
   class II D81.7
manganese E61.3
menadione (vitamin K) E56.1
   newborn P53
mental (familial) (hereditary) — *see* Disability, intellectual
methylenetetrahydrofolate reductase (MTHFR) E72.12
mineralocorticoid E27.49
   with glucocorticoid E27.49
mineral NEC E61.8
molybdenum (nutritional) E61.5
moral F60.2
multiple nutrient elements E61.7
muscle
   carnitine (palmityltransferase) E71.314
   phosphofructokinase E74.09
myoadenylate deaminase E79.2
myocardial — *see* Insufficiency, myocardial
myophosphorylase E74.04
NADH diaphorase or reductase (congenital) D74.0
NADH-methemoglobin reductase (congenital) D74.0
natrium E87.1
niacin (amide) (-tryptophan) E52
nicotinamide E52
nicotinic acid E52
number of teeth — *see* Anodontia
nutrient element E61.9
   multiple E61.7
   specified NEC E61.8
nutrition, nutritional E63.9
   sequelae — *see* Sequelae, nutritional deficiency
   specified NEC E63.8
ornithine transcarbamylase E72.4
ovarian E28.39
oxygen — *see* Anoxia
pantothenic acid E53.8
parathyroid (gland) E20.9
perineum (female) N81.89
phenylalanine hydroxylase E70.1
phosphoenolpyruvate carboxykinase E74.4
phosphofructokinase E74.19
phosphomannomutase E74.8
phosphomannose isomerase E74.8
phosphomannosyl mutase E74.8
phosphorylase kinase, liver E74.09
pituitary hormone (isolated) E23.0
plasma thromboplastin
   antecedent (PTA) D68.1
   component (PTC) D67
platelet NEC D69.1
   constitutional D68.0
polyglandular E31.8
   autoimmune E31.0
potassium (K) E87.6
prepuce N47.3
proaccelerin (congenital) (hereditary) D68.2
   acquired D68.4
proconvertin factor (congenital) (hereditary) D68.2
   acquired D68.4
protein (*see also* Malnutrition) E46
   anemia D53.0
   C D68.59
   S D68.59
prothrombin (congenital) (hereditary) D68.2
   acquired D68.4
Prower factor D68.2
pseudocholinesterase E88.09
PTA (plasma thromboplastin antecedent) D68.1
PTC (plasma thromboplastin component) D67
purine nucleoside phosphorylase (PNP) D81.5
pyracin (alpha) (beta) E53.1
pyridoxal E53.1
pyridoxamine E53.1
pyridoxine (derivatives) E53.1
pyruvate
   carboxylase E74.4
   dehydrogenase E74.4
riboflavin (vitamin B2) E53.0
salt E87.1
secretion
   ovary E28.39
   salivary gland (any) K11.7
   urine R34
selenium (dietary) E59

☑ **Additional Character Required — Refer to the Tabular List for Character Selection** ▽ **Subterms under main terms may continue to next column or page**

Deficiency, deficient — *continued*
serum antitrypsin, familial E88.01
short stature homeobox gene (SHOX)
  with
    dyschondrosteosis Q78.8
    short stature (idiopathic) E34.3
    Turner's syndrome Q96.9
sodium (Na) E87.1
SPCA (factor VII) D68.2
sphincter, intrinsic N36.42
  with urethral hypermobility N36.43
stable factor (congenital) (hereditary) D68.2
  acquired D68.4
Stuart-Prower (factor X) D68.2
sucrase E74.39
sulfatase E75.29
sulfite oxidase E72.19
thiamin, thiaminic (chloride) E51.9
  beriberi (dry) E51.11
    wet E51.12
thrombokinase D68.2
  newborn P53
thyroid (gland) — *see* Hypothyroidism
tocopherol E56.0
tooth bud K00.0
transcobalamine II (anemia) D51.2
vanadium E61.6
vascular I99.9
vasopressin E23.2
viosterol — *see* Deficiency, calciferol
vitamin (multiple) NOS E56.9
  A E50.9
    with
      Bitot's spot (corneal) E50.1
      follicular keratosis E50.8
      keratomalacia E50.4
      manifestations NEC E50.8
      night blindness E50.5
      scar of cornea, xerophthalmic E50.6
      xeroderma E50.8
      xerophthalmia E50.7
      xerosis
        conjunctival E50.0
          and Bitot's spot E50.1
        cornea E50.2
          and ulceration E50.3
    sequelae E64.1
  B (complex) NOS E53.9
    with
      beriberi (dry) E51.11
        wet E51.12
      pellagra E52
  B1 NOS E51.9
    beriberi (dry) E51.11
      with circulatory system manifestations
        E51.11
      wet E51.12
  B2 (riboflavin) E53.0
  B6 E53.1
  B12 E53.8
  C E54
    sequelae E64.2
  D E55.9
    with
      adult osteomalacia M83.8
      rickets — *see* Rickets
      25-hydroxylase E83.32
  E E56.0
  folic acid E53.8
  G E53.0
  group B E53.9
    specified NEC E53.8
  H (biotin) E53.8
  K E56.1
    of newborn P53
  nicotinic E52
  P E56.8
  PP (pellagra-preventing) E52
  specified NEC E56.8
  thiamin E51.9
    beriberi — *see* Beriberi
zinc, dietary E60
Deficit (*see also* Deficiency)
attention and concentration R41.840
  disorder — *see* Attention, deficit
cognitive communication R41.841

Deficit — *continued*
cognitive NEC R41.89
  following
    cerebral infarction I69.31
    cerebrovascular disease I69.91
      specified disease NEC I69.81
    intracerebral hemorrhage I69.11
    nontraumatic intracranial hemorrhage NEC
      I69.21
    subarachnoid hemorrhage I69.01
concentration R41.840
executive function R41.844
frontal lobe R41.844
neurologic NEC R29.818
  ischemic
    reversible (RIND) I63.9
      prolonged (PRIND) I63.9
oxygen R09.02
prolonged reversible ischemic neurologic (PRIND) I63.9
psychomotor R41.843
visuospatial R41.842
Deflection
radius — *see* Deformity, limb, specified type NEC,
  forearm
septum (acquired) (nasal) (nose) J34.2
spine — *see* Curvature, spine
turbinate (nose) J34.2
Defluvium
capillorum — *see* Alopecia
ciliorum — *see* Madarosis
unguium L60.8
Deformity Q89.9
abdomen, congenital Q89.9
abdominal wall
  acquired M95.8
  congenital Q79.59
acquired (unspecified site) M95.9
adrenal gland Q89.1
alimentary tract, congenital Q45.9
  upper Q40.9
ankle (joint) (acquired) (*see also* Deformity, limb, lower
  leg)
  abduction — *see* Contraction, joint, ankle
  congenital Q68.8
  contraction — *see* Contraction, joint, ankle
  specified type NEC — *see* Deformity, limb, foot,
    specified NEC
anus (acquired) K62.89
  congenital Q43.9
aorta (arch) (congenital) Q25.4
  acquired I77.89
aortic
  arch, acquired I77.89
  cusp or valve (congenital) Q23.8
    acquired (*see also* Endocarditis, aortic) I35.8
arm (acquired) (upper) (*see also* Deformity, limb, upper
  arm)
  congenital Q68.8
  forearm — *see* Deformity, limb, forearm
artery (congenital) (peripheral) NOS Q27.9
  acquired I77.89
  coronary (acquired) I25.9
    congenital Q24.5
  umbilical Q27.0
atrial septal Q21.1
auditory canal (external) (congenital) (*see also* Malformation, ear, external)
  acquired — *see* Disorder, ear, external, specified
    type NEC
auricle
  ear (congenital) (*see also* Malformation, ear, exter-
    nal)
    acquired — *see* Disorder, pinna, deformity
back — *see* Dorsopathy, deforming
bile duct (common) (congenital) (hepatic) Q44.5
  acquired K83.8
biliary duct or passage (congenital) Q44.5
  acquired K83.8
bladder (neck) (trigone) (sphincter) (acquired) N32.89
  congenital Q64.79
bone (acquired) NOS M95.9
  congenital Q79.9
  turbinate M95.0
brain (congenital) Q04.9
  acquired G93.89
  reduction Q04.3
breast (acquired) N64.89
  congenital Q83.9

Deformity — *continued*
breast — *continued*
  reconstructed N65.0
bronchus (congenital) Q32.4
  acquired NEC J98.09
bursa, congenital Q79.9
canaliculi (lacrimalis) (acquired) (*see also* Disorder,
  lacrimal system, changes)
  congenital Q10.6
canthus, acquired — *see* Disorder, eyelid, specified
  type NEC
capillary (acquired) I78.8
cardiovascular system, congenital Q28.9
caruncle, lacrimal (acquired) (*see also* Disorder,
  lacrimal system, changes)
  congenital Q10.6
cascade, stomach K31.2
cecum (congenital) Q43.9
  acquired K63.89
cerebral, acquired G93.89
  congenital Q04.9
cervix (uterus) (acquired) NEC N88.8
  congenital Q51.9
cheek (acquired) M95.2
  congenital Q18.9
chest (acquired) (wall) M95.4
  congenital Q67.8
  sequelae (late effect) of rickets E64.3
chin (acquired) M95.2
  congenital Q18.9
choroid (congenital) Q14.3
  acquired H31.8
  plexus Q07.8
    acquired G96.19
cicatricial — *see* Cicatrix
cilia, acquired — *see* Disorder, eyelid, specified type
  NEC
clavicle (acquired) M95.8
  congenital Q68.8
clitoris (congenital) Q52.6
  acquired N90.89
clubfoot — *see* Clubfoot
coccyx (acquired) — *see* subcategory M43.8 ☑
colon (congenital) Q43.9
  acquired K63.89
concha (ear), congenital (*see also* Malformation, ear,
  external)
  acquired — *see* Disorder, pinna, deformity
cornea (acquired) H18.70
  congenital Q13.4
  descemetocele — *see* Descemetocele
  ectasia — *see* Ectasia, cornea
  specified NEC H18.79- ☑
  staphyloma — *see* Staphyloma, cornea
coronary artery (acquired) I25.9
  congenital Q24.5
cranium (acquired) — *see* Deformity, skull
cricoid cartilage (congenital) Q31.8
  acquired J38.7
cystic duct (congenital) Q44.5
  acquired K82.8
Dandy-Walker Q03.1
  with spina bifida — *see* Spina bifida
diaphragm (congenital) Q79.1
  acquired J98.6
digestive organ NOS Q45.9
ductus arteriosus Q25.0
duodenal bulb K31.89
duodenum (congenital) Q43.9
  acquired K31.89
dura — *see* Deformity, meninges
ear (acquired) (*see also* Disorder, pinna, deformity)
  congenital (external) Q17.9
    internal Q16.5
    middle Q16.4
      ossicles Q16.3
    ossicles Q16.3
ectodermal (congenital) NEC Q84.9
ejaculatory duct (congenital) Q55.4
  acquired N50.8
elbow (joint) (acquired) (*see also* Deformity, limb, upper arm)
  congenital Q68.8
  contraction — *see* Contraction, joint, elbow
endocrine gland NEC Q89.2
epididymis (congenital) Q55.4
  acquired N50.8

Deformity — *continued*
  epiglottis (congenital) Q31.8
    acquired J38.7
  esophagus (congenital) Q39.9
    acquired K22.8
  eustachian tube (congenital) NEC Q17.8
  eye, congenital Q15.9
  eyebrow (congenital) Q18.8
  eyelid (acquired) (*see also* Disorder, eyelid,
    specified type NEC)
    congenital Q10.3
  face (acquired) M95.2
    congenital Q18.9
  fallopian tube, acquired N83.8
  femur (acquired) — *see* Deformity, limb, specified type
    NEC, thigh
  fetal
    with fetopelvic disproportion O33.7
    causing obstructed labor O66.3
  finger (acquired) M20.00- ☑
    boutonniere M20.02- ☑
    congenital Q68.1
    flexion contracture — *see* Contraction, joint, hand
    mallet finger M20.01- ☑
    specified NEC M20.09- ☑
    swan-neck M20.03- ☑
  flexion (joint) (acquired) (*see also* Deformity, limb,
    flexion) M21.20
    congenital NOS Q74.9
      hip Q65.89
  foot (acquired) (*see also* Deformity, limb, lower leg)
    cavovarus (congenital) Q66.1
    congenital NOS Q66.9
      specified type NEC Q66.89
    specified type NEC — *see* Deformity, limb, foot,
      specified NEC
    valgus (congenital) Q66.6
      acquired — *see* Deformity, valgus, ankle
    varus (congenital) NEC Q66.3
      acquired — *see* Deformity, varus, ankle
  forearm (acquired) (*see also* Deformity, limb, forearm)
    congenital Q68.8
  forehead (acquired) M95.2
    congenital Q75.8
  frontal bone (acquired) M95.2
    congenital Q75.8
  gallbladder (congenital) Q44.1
    acquired K82.8
  gastrointestinal tract (congenital) NOS Q45.9
    acquired K63.89
  genitalia, genital organ(s) or system NEC
    female (congenital) Q52.9
      acquired N94.89
      external Q52.70
    male (congenital) Q55.9
      acquired N50.8
  globe (eye) (congenital) Q15.8
    acquired H44.89
  gum, acquired NEC K06.8
  hand (acquired) — *see* Deformity, limb, hand
    congenital Q68.1
  head (acquired) M95.2
    congenital Q75.8
  heart (congenital) Q24.9
    septum Q21.9
      auricular Q21.1
      ventricular Q21.0
    valve (congenital) NEC Q24.8
      acquired — *see* Endocarditis
  heel (acquired) — *see* Deformity, foot
  hepatic duct (congenital) Q44.5
    acquired K83.8
  hip (joint) (acquired) (*see also* Deformity, limb, thigh)
    congenital Q65.9
    due to (previous) juvenile osteochondrosis — *see*
      Coxa, plana
    flexion — *see* Contraction, joint, hip
  hourglass — *see* Contraction, hourglass
  humerus (acquired) M21.82- ☑
    congenital Q74.0
  hypophyseal (congenital) Q89.2
  ileocecal (coil) (valve) (acquired) K63.89
    congenital Q43.9
  ileum (congenital) Q43.9
    acquired K63.89
  ilium (acquired) M95.5
    congenital Q74.2
  integument (congenital) Q84.9

Deformity — *continued*
  intervertebral cartilage or disc (acquired) — *see* Disorder, disc, specified NEC
  intestine (large) (small) (congenital) NOS Q43.9
    acquired K63.89
  intrinsic minus or plus (hand) — *see* Deformity, limb, specified type NEC, forearm
  iris (acquired) H21.89
    congenital Q13.2
  ischium (acquired) M95.5
    congenital Q74.2
  jaw (acquired) (congenital) M26.9
  joint (acquired) NEC M21.90
    congenital Q68.8
    elbow M21.92- ☑
    hand M21.94- ☑
    hip M21.95- ☑
    knee M21.96- ☑
    shoulder M21.92- ☑
    wrist M21.93- ☑
  kidney(s) (calyx) (pelvis) (congenital) Q63.9
    acquired N28.89
    artery (congenital) Q27.2
      acquired I77.89
  Klippel-Feil (brevicollis) Q76.1
  knee (acquired) NEC (*see also* Deformity, limb, lower leg)
    congenital Q68.2
  labium (majus) (minus) (congenital) Q52.79
    acquired N90.89
  lacrimal passages or duct (congenital) NEC Q10.6
    acquired — *see* Disorder, lacrimal system, changes
  larynx (muscle) (congenital) Q31.8
    acquired J38.7
    web (glottic) Q31.0
  leg (upper) (acquired) NEC (*see also* Deformity, limb, thigh)
    congenital Q68.8
    lower leg — *see* Deformity, limb, lower leg
  lens (acquired) H27.8
    congenital Q12.9
  lid (fold) (acquired) (*see also* Disorder, eyelid, specified type NEC)
    congenital Q10.3
  ligament (acquired) — *see* Disorder, ligament
    congenital Q79.9
  limb (acquired) M21.90
    clawfoot M21.53- ☑
    clawhand M21.51- ☑
    clubfoot M21.54- ☑
    clubhand M21.52- ☑
    congenital, except reduction deformity Q74.9
    flat foot M21.4- ☑
    flexion M21.20
      ankle M21.27- ☑
      elbow M21.22- ☑
      finger M21.24- ☑
      hip M21.25- ☑
      knee M21.26- ☑
      shoulder M21.21- ☑
      toe M21.27- ☑
      wrist M21.23- ☑
    foot
      claw — *see* Deformity, limb, clawfoot
      club — *see* Deformity, limb, clubfoot
      drop M21.37- ☑
      flat — *see* Deformity, limb, flat foot
      specified NEC M21.6X- ☑
    forearm M21.93- ☑
    hand M21.94- ☑
    lower leg M21.96- ☑
    specified type NEC M21.80
      forearm M21.83- ☑
      lower leg M21.86- ☑
      thigh M21.85- ☑
      upper arm M21.82- ☑
    thigh M21.95- ☑
    unequal length M21.70
      short site is
        femur M21.75- ☑
        fibula M21.76- ☑
        humerus M21.72- ☑
        radius M21.73- ☑
        tibia M21.76- ☑
        ulna M21.73- ☑
    upper arm M21.92- ☑
    valgus — *see* Deformity, valgus

Deformity — *continued*
  limb — *continued*
    varus — *see* Deformity, varus
    wrist drop M21.33- ☑
  lip (acquired) NEC K13.0
    congenital Q38.0
  liver (congenital) Q44.7
    acquired K76.89
  lumbosacral (congenital) (joint) (region) Q76.49
    acquired — *see* subcategory M43.8 ☑
    kyphosis — *see* Kyphosis, congenital
    lordosis — *see* Lordosis, congenital
  lung (congenital) Q33.9
    acquired J98.4
  lymphatic system, congenital Q89.9
  Madelung's (radius) Q74.0
  mandible (acquired) (congenital) M26.9
  maxilla (acquired) (congenital) M26.9
  meninges or membrane (congenital) Q07.9
    cerebral Q04.8
      acquired G96.19
    spinal cord (congenital) G96.19
      acquired G96.19
  metacarpus (acquired) — *see* Deformity, limb, forearm
    congenital Q74.0
  metatarsus (acquired) — *see* Deformity, foot
    congenital Q66.9
  middle ear (congenital) Q16.4
    ossicles Q16.3
  mitral (leaflets) (valve) I05.8
    parachute Q23.2
    stenosis, congenital Q23.2
  mouth (acquired) K13.79
    congenital Q38.6
  multiple, congenital NEC Q89.7
  muscle (acquired) M62.89
    congenital Q79.9
      sternocleidomastoid Q68.0
  musculoskeletal system (acquired) M95.9
    congenital Q79.9
    specified NEC M95.8
  nail (acquired) L60.8
    congenital Q84.6
  nasal — *see* Deformity, nose
  neck (acquired) M95.3
    congenital Q18.9
      sternocleidomastoid Q68.0
  nervous system (congenital) Q07.9
  nipple (congenital) Q83.9
    acquired N64.89
  nose (acquired) (cartilage) M95.0
    bone (turbinate) M95.0
    congenital Q30.9
      bent or squashed Q67.4
    saddle M95.0
      syphilitic A50.57
    septum (acquired) J34.2
      congenital Q30.8
    sinus (wall) (congenital) Q30.8
      acquired M95.0
    syphilitic (congenital) A50.57
      late A52.73
  ocular muscle (congenital) Q10.3
    acquired — *see* Strabismus, mechanical
  opticociliary vessels (congenital) Q13.2
  orbit (eye) (acquired) H05.30
    atrophy — *see* Atrophy, orbit
    congenital Q10.7
    due to
      bone disease NEC H05.32- ☑
      trauma or surgery H05.33- ☑
    enlargement — *see* Enlargement, orbit
    exostosis — *see* Exostosis, orbit
  organ of Corti (congenital) Q16.5
  ovary (congenital) Q50.39
    acquired N83.8
  oviduct, acquired N83.8
  palate (congenital) Q38.5
    acquired M27.8
    cleft (congenital) — *see* Cleft, palate
  pancreas (congenital) Q45.3
    acquired K86.8
  parathyroid (gland) Q89.2
  parotid (gland) (congenital) Q38.4
    acquired K11.8
  patella (acquired) — *see* Disorder, patella, specified NEC

Deformity — *continued*
  pelvis, pelvic (acquired) (bony) M95.5
    with disproportion (fetopelvic) O33.0
      causing obstructed labor O65.0
    congenital Q74.2
    rachitic sequelae (late effect) E64.3
  penis (glans) (congenital) Q55.69
    acquired N48.89
  pericardium (congenital) Q24.8
    acquired — *see* Pericarditis
  pharynx (congenital) Q38.8
    acquired J39.2
  pinna, acquired (*see also* Disorder, pinna, deformity)
    congenital Q17.9
  pituitary (congenital) Q89.2
  posture — *see* Dorsopathy, deforming
  prepuce (congenital) Q55.69
    acquired N47.8
  prostate (congenital) Q55.4
    acquired N42.89
  pupil (congenital) Q13.2
    acquired — *see* Abnormality, pupillary
  pylorus (congenital) Q40.3
    acquired K31.89
  rachitic (acquired), old or healed E64.3
  radius (acquired) (*see also* Deformity, limb, forearm)
    congenital Q68.8
  rectum (congenital) Q43.9
    acquired K62.89
  reduction (extremity) (limb), congenital (*see also* condition and site) Q73.8
    brain Q04.3
    lower — *see* Defect, reduction, lower limb
    upper — *see* Defect, reduction, upper limb
  renal — *see* Deformity, kidney
  respiratory system (congenital) Q34.9
  rib (acquired) M95.4
    congenital Q76.6
    cervical Q76.5
  rotation (joint) (acquired) — *see* Deformity, limb, specified site NEC
    congenital Q74.9
    hip — *see* Deformity, limb, specified type NEC, thigh
      congenital Q65.89
  sacroiliac joint (congenital) — *see* subcategory Q74.2
    acquired — *see* subcategory M43.8 ☑
  sacrum (acquired) — *see* subcategory M43.8 ☑
  saddle
    back — *see* Lordosis
    nose M95.0
      syphilitic A50.57
  salivary gland or duct (congenital) Q38.4
    acquired K11.8
  scapula (acquired) M95.8
    congenital Q68.8
  scrotum (congenital) (*see also* Malformation, testis and scrotum)
    acquired N50.8
  seminal vesicles (congenital) Q55.4
    acquired N50.8
  septum, nasal (acquired) J34.2
  shoulder (joint) (acquired) — *see* Deformity, limb, upper arm
    congenital Q74.0
    contraction — *see* Contraction, joint, shoulder
  sigmoid (flexure) (congenital) Q43.9
    acquired K63.89
  skin (congenital) Q82.9
  skull (acquired) M95.2
    congenital Q75.8
      with
        anencephaly Q00.0
        encephalocele — *see* Encephalocele
        hydrocephalus Q03.9
          with spina bifida — *see* Spina bifida, by site, with hydrocephalus
        microcephaly Q02
  soft parts, organs or tissues (of pelvis)
    in pregnancy or childbirth NEC O34.8- ☑
      causing obstructed labor O65.5
  spermatic cord (congenital) Q55.4
    acquired N50.8
      torsion — *see* Torsion, spermatic cord
  spinal — *see* Dorsopathy, deforming
    column (acquired) — *see* Dorsopathy, deforming
    congenital Q67.5

Deformity — *continued*
  spinal — *see* Dorsopathy, deforming — *continued*
    cord (congenital) Q06.9
      acquired G95.89
      nerve root (congenital) Q07.9
  spine (acquired) (*see also* Dorsopathy, deforming)
    congenital Q67.5
    rachitic E64.3
    specified NEC — *see* Dorsopathy, deforming, specified NEC
  spleen
    acquired D73.89
    congenital Q89.09
  Sprengel's (congenital) Q74.0
  sternocleidomastoid (muscle), congenital Q68.0
  sternum (acquired) M95.4
    congenital NEC Q76.7
  stomach (congenital) Q40.3
    acquired K31.89
  submandibular gland (congenital) Q38.4
  submaxillary gland (congenital) Q38.4
    acquired K11.8
  talipes — *see* Talipes
  testis (congenital) (*see also* Malformation, testis and scrotum)
    acquired N44.8
      torsion — *see* Torsion, testis
  thigh (acquired) (*see also* Deformity, limb, thigh)
    congenital NEC Q68.8
  thorax (acquired) (wall) M95.4
    congenital Q67.8
    sequelae of rickets E64.3
  thumb (acquired) (*see also* Deformity, finger)
    congenital NEC Q68.1
  thymus (tissue) (congenital) Q89.2
  thyroid (gland) (congenital) Q89.2
    cartilage Q31.8
      acquired J38.7
  tibia (acquired) (*see also* Deformity, limb, specified type NEC, lower leg)
    congenital NEC Q68.8
    saber (syphilitic) A50.56
  toe (acquired) M20.6- ☑
    congenital Q66.9
    hallux rigidus M20.2- ☑
    hallux valgus M20.1- ☑
    hallux varus M20.3- ☑
    hammer toe M20.4- ☑
    specified NEC M20.5X- ☑
  tongue (congenital) Q38.3
    acquired K14.8
  tooth, teeth K00.2
  trachea (rings) (congenital) Q32.1
    acquired J39.8
  transverse aortic arch (congenital) Q25.4
  tricuspid (leaflets) (valve) I07.8
    atresia or stenosis Q22.4
    Ebstein's Q22.5
  trunk (acquired) M95.8
    congenital Q89.9
  ulna (acquired) (*see also* Deformity, limb, forearm)
    congenital NEC Q68.8
  urachus, congenital Q64.4
  ureter (opening) (congenital) Q62.8
    acquired N28.89
  urethra (congenital) Q64.79
    acquired N36.8
  urinary tract (congenital) Q64.9
    urachus Q64.4
  uterus (congenital) Q51.9
    acquired N85.8
  uvula (congenital) Q38.5
  vagina (acquired) N89.8
    congenital Q52.4
  valgus NEC M21.00
    ankle M21.07- ☑
    elbow M21.02- ☑
    hip M21.05- ☑
    knee M21.06- ☑
  valve, valvular (congenital) (heart) Q24.8
    acquired — *see* Endocarditis
  varus NEC M21.10
    ankle M21.17- ☑
    elbow M21.12- ☑
    hip M21.15 ☑
    knee M21.16- ☑
    tibia — *see* Osteochondrosis, juvenile, tibia

Deformity — *continued*
  vas deferens (congenital) Q55.4
    acquired N50.8
  vein (congenital) Q27.9
    great Q26.9
  vertebra — *see* Dorsopathy, deforming
  vertical talus (congenital) Q66.80
    left foot Q66.82
    right foot Q66.81
  vesicourethral orifice (acquired) N32.89
    congenital NEC Q64.79
  vessels of optic papilla (congenital) Q14.2
  visual field (contraction) — *see* Defect, visual field
  vitreous body, acquired H43.89
  vulva (congenital) Q52.79
    acquired N90.89
  wrist (joint) (acquired) (*see also* Deformity, limb, forearm)
    congenital Q68.8
    contraction — *see* Contraction, joint, wrist

Degeneration, degenerative
  adrenal (capsule) (fatty) (gland) (hyaline) (infectional) E27.8
  amyloid (*see also* Amyloidosis) E85.9
  anterior cornua, spinal cord G12.29
  anterior labral S43.49- ☑
  aorta, aortic I70.0
    fatty I77.89
  aortic valve (heart) — *see* Endocarditis, aortic
  arteriovascular — *see* Arteriosclerosis
  artery, arterial (atheromatous) (calcareous) (*see also* Arteriosclerosis)
    cerebral, amyloid E85.4 [I68.0]
    medial — *see* Arteriosclerosis, extremities
  articular cartilage NEC — *see* Derangement, joint, articular cartilage, by site
  atheromatous — *see* Arteriosclerosis
  basal nuclei or ganglia G23.9
    specified NEC G23.8
  bone NEC — *see* Disorder, bone, specified type NEC
  brachial plexus G54.0
  brain (cortical) (progressive) G31.9
    alcoholic G31.2
    arteriosclerotic I67.2
    childhood G31.9
      specified NEC G31.89
    cystic G31.89
      congenital Q04.6
    in
      alcoholism G31.2
      beriberi E51.2
      cerebrovascular disease I67.9
      congenital hydrocephalus Q03.9
        with spina bifida (*see also* Spina bifida)
      Fabry-Anderson disease E75.21
      Gaucher's disease E75.22
      Hunter's syndrome E76.1
      lipidosis
        cerebral E75.4
        generalized E75.6
      mucopolysaccharidosis — *see* Mucopolysaccharidosis
      myxedema E03.9 [G32.89]
      neoplastic disease (*see also* Neoplasm) D49.6 [G32.89]
      Niemann-Pick disease E75.249 [G32.89]
      sphingolipidosis E75.3 [G32.89]
      vitamin B12 deficiency E53.8 [G32.89]
    senile NEC G31.1
  breast N64.89
  Bruch's membrane — *see* Degeneration, choroid
  capillaries (fatty) I78.8
    amyloid E85.8 [I79.8]
  cardiac (*see also* Degeneration, myocardial)
    valve, valvular — *see* Endocarditis
  cardiorenal — *see* Hypertension, cardiorenal
  cardiovascular (*see also* Disease, cardiovascular)
    renal — *see* Hypertension, cardiorenal
  cerebellar NOS G31.9
    alcoholic G31.2
    primary (hereditary) (sporadic) G11.9
  cerebral — *see* Degeneration, brain
  cerebrovascular I67.9
    due to hypertension I67.4
  cervical plexus G54.2
  cervix N88.8
    due to radiation (intended effect) N88.8
      adverse effect or misadventure N99.89

Degeneration, degenerative — *continued*
- chamber angle H21.21- ☑
- changes, spine or vertebra — *see* Spondylosis
- chorioretinal (*see also* Degeneration, choroid)
  - hereditary H31.2Ø
- choroid (colloid) (drusen) H31.1Ø- ☑
  - atrophy — *see* Atrophy, choroidal
  - hereditary — *see* Dystrophy, choroidal, hereditary
- ciliary body H21.22- ☑
- cochlear — *see* subcategory H83.8 ☑
- combined (spinal cord) (subacute) E53.8 [G32.Ø]
  - with anemia (pernicious) D51.Ø [G32.Ø]
    - due to dietary vitamin B12 deficiency D51.3 [G32.Ø]
  - in (due to)
    - vitamin B12 deficiency E53.8 [G32.Ø]
      - anemia D51.9 [G32.Ø]
- conjunctiva H11.1Ø
  - concretions — *see* Concretion, conjunctiva
  - deposits — *see* Deposit, conjunctiva
  - pigmentations — *see* Pigmentation, conjunctiva
  - pinguecula — *see* Pinguecula
  - xerosis — *see* Xerosis, conjunctiva
- cornea H18.4Ø
  - calcerous H18.43
    - band keratopathy H18.42- ☑
  - familial, hereditary — *see* Dystrophy, cornea
  - hyaline (of old scars) H18.49
  - keratomalacia — *see* Keratomalacia
  - nodular H18.45- ☑
  - peripheral H18.46- ☑
  - senile H18.41- ☑
  - specified type NEC H18.49
- cortical (cerebellar) (parenchymatous) G31.89
  - alcoholic G31.2
  - diffuse, due to arteriopathy I67.2
- corticobasal G31.85
- cutis L98.8
  - amyloid E85.4 [L99]
- dental pulp KØ4.2
- disc disease — *see* Degeneration, intervertebral disc NEC
- dorsolateral (spinal cord) — *see* Degeneration, combined
- extrapyramidal G25.9
- eye, macular (*see also* Degeneration, macula)
  - congenital or hereditary — *see* Dystrophy, retina
- facet joints — *see* Spondylosis
- fatty
  - liver NEC K76.Ø
    - alcoholic K7Ø.Ø
- grey matter (brain) (Alpers') G31.81
- heart (*see also* Degeneration, myocardial)
  - amyloid E85.4 [I43]
  - atheromatous — *see* Disease, heart, ischemic, atherosclerotic
  - ischemic — *see* Disease, heart, ischemic
- hepatolenticular (Wilson's) E83.Ø1
- hepatorenal K76.7
- hyaline (diffuse) (generalized)
  - localized — *see* Degeneration, by site
- infrapatellar fat pad M79.4
- intervertebral disc NOS
  - with
    - myelopathy — *see* Disorder, disc, with, myelopathy
    - radiculitis or radiculopathy — *see* Disorder, disc, with, radiculopathy
  - cervical, cervicothoracic — *see* Disorder, disc, cervical, degeneration
    - with
      - myelopathy — *see* Disorder, disc, cervical, with myelopathy
      - neuritis, radiculitis or radiculopathy — *see* Disorder, disc, cervical, with neuritis
  - lumbar region M51.36
    - with
      - myelopathy M51.Ø6
      - neuritis, radiculitis, radiculopathy or sciatica M51.16
  - lumbosacral region M51.37
    - with
      - neuritis, radiculitis, radiculopathy or sciatica M51.17
  - sacrococcygeal region M53.3

Degeneration, degenerative — *continued*
- intervertebral disc — *continued*
  - thoracic region M51.34
    - with
      - myelopathy M51.Ø4
      - neuritis, radiculitis, radiculopathy M51.14
  - thoracolumbar region M51.35
    - with
      - myelopathy M51.Ø5
      - neuritis, radiculitis, radiculopathy M51.15
- intestine, amyloid E85.4
- iris (pigmentary) H21.23- ☑
- ischemic — *see* Ischemia
- joint disease — *see* Osteoarthritis
- kidney N28.89
  - amyloid E85.4 [N29]
  - cystic, congenital Q61.9
  - fatty N28.89
  - polycystic Q61.3
    - adult type (autosomal dominant) Q61.2
    - infantile type (autosomal recessive) NEC Q61.19
      - collecting duct dilatation Q61.11
- Kuhnt-Junius (*see also* Degeneration, macula) H35.32
- lens — *see* Cataract
- lenticular (familial) (progressive) (Wilson's) (with cirrhosis of liver) E83.Ø1
- liver (diffuse) NEC K76.89
  - amyloid E85.4 [K77]
  - cystic K76.89
    - congenital Q44.6
  - fatty NEC K76.Ø
    - alcoholic K7Ø.Ø
  - hypertrophic K76.89
  - parenchymatous, acute or subacute K72.ØØ
    - with coma K72.Ø1
  - pigmentary K76.89
  - toxic (acute) K71.9
- lung J98.4
- lymph gland I89.8
  - hyaline I89.8
- macula, macular (acquired) (age-related) (senile) H35.3Ø
  - angioid streaks H35.33
  - atrophic age-related H35.31
  - congenital or hereditary — *see* Dystrophy, retina
  - cystoid H35.35- ☑
  - drusen H35.36- ☑
  - exudative H35.32
  - hole H35.34- ☑
  - nonexudative H35.31
  - puckering H35.37- ☑
  - toxic H35.38- ☑
- membranous labyrinth, congenital (causing impairment of hearing) Q16.5
- meniscus — *see* Derangement, meniscus
- mitral — *see* Insufficiency, mitral
- Mönckeberg's — *see* Arteriosclerosis, extremities
- motor centers, senile G31.1
- multi-system G9Ø.3
- mural — *see* Degeneration, myocardial
- muscle (fatty) (fibrous) (hyaline) (progressive) M62.89
  - heart — *see* Degeneration, myocardial
- myelin, central nervous system G37.9
- myocardial, myocardium (fatty) (hyaline) (senile) I51.5
  - with rheumatic fever (conditions in IØØ) IØ9.Ø
    - active, acute or subacute IØ1.2
      - with chorea IØ2.Ø
    - inactive or quiescent (with chorea) IØ9.Ø
  - hypertensive — *see* Hypertension, heart
  - rheumatic — *see* Degeneration, myocardial, with rheumatic fever
  - syphilitic A52.Ø6
- nasal sinus (mucosa) J32.9
  - frontal J32.1
  - maxillary J32.Ø
- nerve — *see* Disorder, nerve
- nervous system G31.9
  - alcoholic G31.2
  - amyloid E85.4 [G99.8]
  - autonomic G9Ø.9
  - fatty G31.89
  - specified NEC G31.89
- nipple N64.89
- olivopontocerebellar (hereditary) (familial) G23.8
- osseous labyrinth — *see* subcategory H83.8 ☑
- ovary N83.8
  - cystic N83.2Ø
  - microcystic N83.2Ø

Degeneration, degenerative — *continued*
- pallidal pigmentary (progressive) G23.Ø
- pancreas K86.8
  - tuberculous A18.83
- penis N48.89
- pigmentary (diffuse) (general)
  - localized — *see* Degeneration, by site
  - pallidal (progressive) G23.Ø
- pineal gland E34.8
- pituitary (gland) E23.6
- popliteal fat pad M79.4
- posterolateral (spinal cord) — *see* Degeneration, combined
- pulmonary valve (heart) I37.8
- pulp (tooth) KØ4.2
- pupillary margin H21.24- ☑
- renal — *see* Degeneration, kidney
- retina H35.9
  - hereditary (cerebroretinal) (congenital) (juvenile) (macula) (peripheral) (pigmentary) — *see* Dystrophy, retina
  - Kuhnt-Junius (*see also* Degeneration, macula) H35.32
  - macula (cystic) (exudative) (hole) (nonexudative) (pseudohole) (senile) (toxic) — *see* Degeneration, macula
  - peripheral H35.4Ø
    - lattice H35.41- ☑
    - microcystoid H35.42- ☑
    - paving stone H35.43- ☑
    - secondary
      - pigmentary H35.45- ☑
      - vitreoretinal H35.46- ☑
    - senile reticular H35.44- ☑
  - pigmentary (primary) (*see also* Dystrophy, retina)
    - secondary — *see* Degeneration, retina, peripheral, secondary
  - posterior pole — *see* Degeneration, macula
- saccule, congenital (causing impairment of hearing) Q16.5
- senile R54
  - brain G31.1
  - cardiac, heart or myocardium — *see* Degeneration, myocardial
  - motor centers G31.1
  - vascular — *see* Arteriosclerosis
- sinus (cystic) (*see also* Sinusitis)
  - polypoid J33.1
- skin L98.8
  - amyloid E85.4 [L99]
  - colloid L98.8
- spinal (cord) G31.89
  - amyloid E85.4 [G32.89]
  - combined (subacute) — *see* Degeneration, combined
  - dorsolateral — *see* Degeneration, combined
  - familial NEC G31.89
  - fatty G31.89
  - funicular — *see* Degeneration, combined
  - posterolateral — *see* Degeneration, combined
  - subacute combined — *see* Degeneration, combined
  - tuberculous A17.81
- spleen D73.Ø
  - amyloid E85.4 [D77]
- stomach K31.89
- striatonigral G23.2
- suprarenal (capsule) (gland) E27.8
- synovial membrane (pulpy) — *see* Disorder, synovium, specified type NEC
- tapetoretinal — *see* Dystrophy, retina
- thymus (gland) E32.8
  - fatty E32.8
- thyroid (gland) EØ7.89
- tricuspid (heart) (valve) IØ7.9
- tuberculous NEC — *see* Tuberculosis
- turbinate J34.89
- uterus (cystic) N85.8
- vascular (senile) — *see* Arteriosclerosis
  - hypertensive — *see* Hypertension
- vitreoretinal, secondary — *see* Degeneration, retina, peripheral, secondary, vitreoretinal
- vitreous (body) H43.81- ☑
- Wallerian — *see* Disorder, nerve
- Wilson's hepatolenticular E83.Ø1

☑ Additional Character Required — Refer to the Tabular List for Character Selection ▽ Subterms under main terms may continue to next column or page

Deglutition
  paralysis R13.0
    hysterical F44.4
    pneumonia J69.0
Degos' disease I77.89
Dehiscence (of)
  amputation stump T87.81
  cesarean wound O90.0
  closure of
    cornea T81.31 ☑
    craniotomy T81.32 ☑
    fascia (muscular) (superficial) T81.32 ☑
    internal organ or tissue T81.32 ☑
    laceration (external) (internal) T81.33 ☑
    ligament T81.32 ☑
    mucosa T81.31 ☑
    muscle or muscle flap T81.32 ☑
    ribs or rib cage T81.32 ☑
    skin and subcutaneous tissue (full-thickness) (superficial) T81.31 ☑
    skull T81.32 ☑
    sternum (sternotomy) T81.32 ☑
    tendon T81.32 ☑
    traumatic laceration (external) (internal) T81.33 ☑
  episiotomy O90.1
  operation wound NEC T81.31 ☑
    external operation wound (superficial) T81.31 ☑
    internal operation wound (deep) T81.32 ☑
  perineal wound (postpartum) O90.1
  traumatic injury wound repair T81.33 ☑
  wound T81.30 ☑
    traumatic repair T81.33 ☑
Dehydration E86.0
  hypertonic E87.0
  hypotonic E87.1
  newborn P74.1
Déjérine-Roussy syndrome G89.0
Déjérine-Sottas disease or neuropathy (hypertrophic) G60.0
Déjérine-Thomas atrophy G23.8
Delay, delayed
  any plane in pelvis
    complicating delivery O66.9
  birth or delivery NOS O63.9
  closure, ductus arteriosus (Botalli) P29.3
  coagulation — see Defect, coagulation
  conduction (cardiac) (ventricular) I45.9
  delivery, second twin, triplet, etc O63.2
  development R62.50
    global F88
    intellectual (specific) F81.9
    language F80.9
      due to hearing loss F80.4
    learning F81.9
    pervasive F84.9
    physiological R62.50
      specified stage NEC R62.0
    reading F81.0
    sexual E30.0
    speech F80.9
      due to hearing loss F80.4
    spelling F81.81
  gastric emptying K30
  menarche E30.0
  menstruation (cause unknown) N91.0
  milestone R62.0
  passage of meconium (newborn) P76.0
  primary respiration P28.9
  puberty (constitutional) E30.0
  separation of umbilical cord P96.82
  sexual maturation, female E30.0
  sleep phase syndrome G47.21
  union, fracture — see Fracture, by site
  vaccination Z28.9
Deletion(s)
  autosome Q93.9
    identified by fluorescence in situ hybridization (FISH) Q93.89
    identified by in situ hybridization (ISH) Q93.89
  chromosome
    with complex rearrangements NEC Q93.7
    part of NEC Q93.5
    seen only at prometaphase Q93.89
    short arm
      22q11.2 Q93.81
      4 Q93.3
      5p Q93.4

Deletion(s) — continued
  chromosome — continued
    specified NEC Q93.89
    long arm chromosome 18 or 21 Q93.89
      with complex rearrangements NEC Q93.7
    microdeletions NEC Q93.88
Delhi boil or button B55.1
Delinquency (juvenile) (neurotic) F91.8
  group Z72.810
Delinquent immunization status Z28.3
Delirium, delirious (acute or subacute) (not alcohol- or drug-induced) (with dementia) R41.0
  alcoholic (acute) (tremens) (withdrawal) F10.921
    with intoxication F10.921
      in
        abuse F10.121
        dependence F10.221
  due to (secondary to)
    alcohol
      intoxication F10.921
        in
          abuse F10.121
          dependence F10.221
      withdrawal F10.231
    amphetamine intoxication F15.921
      in
        abuse F15.121
        dependence F15.221
    anxiolytic
      intoxication F13.921
        in
          abuse F13.121
          dependence F13.221
      withdrawal F13.231
    cannabis intoxication F12.921
      in
        abuse F12.121
        dependence F12.221
    cocaine intoxication (acute) F14.921
      in
        abuse F14.121
        dependence F14.221
    general medical condition F05
    hallucinogen intoxication F16.921
      in
        abuse F16.121
        dependence F16.221
    hypnotic
      intoxication F13.921
        in
          abuse F13.121
          dependence F13.221
      withdrawal F13.231
    inhalant intoxication (acute) F18.921
      in
        abuse F18.121
        dependence F18.221
    multiple etiologies F05
    opioid intoxication (acute) F11.921
      in
        abuse F11.121
        dependence F11.221
    phencyclidine intoxication (acute) F16.921
      in
        abuse F16.121
        dependence F16.221
    psychoactive substance NEC intoxication (acute) F19.921
      in
        abuse F19.121
        dependence F19.221
    sedative
      intoxication F13.921
        in
          abuse F13.121
          dependence F13.221
      withdrawal F13.231
    unknown etiology F05
  exhaustion F43.0
  hysterical F44.89
  postprocedural (postoperative) F05
  puerperal F05
  thyroid — see Thyrotoxicosis with thyroid storm
  traumatic — see Injury, intracranial
  tremens (alcohol-induced) F10.231
    sedative-induced F13.231
Delivery (childbirth) (labor)
  arrested active phase O62.1

Delivery — continued
  cesarean (for)
    without indication O82
    abnormal
      pelvis (bony) (deformity) (major) NEC with disproportion (fetopelvic) O33.0
        with obstructed labor O65.0
      presentation or position O32.9 ☑
    abruptio placentae (see also Abruptio placentae) O45.9-
    acromion presentation O32.2 ☑
    atony, uterus O62.2
    breech presentation O32.1 ☑
      incomplete O32.8 ☑
    brow presentation O32.3 ☑
    cephalopelvic disproportion O33.9
    cerclage O34.3-
    chin presentation O32.3 ☑
    cicatrix of cervix O34.4- ☑
    contracted pelvis (general)
      inlet O33.2
      outlet O33.3 ☑
    cord presentation or prolapse O69.0 ☑
    cystocele O34.8- ☑
    deformity (acquired) (congenital)
      pelvic organs or tissues NEC O34.8- ☑
      pelvis (bony) NEC O33.0
    disproportion NOS O33.9
    eclampsia — see Eclampsia
    face presentation O32.3 ☑
    failed
      forceps O66.5
      induction of labor O61.9
        instrumental O61.1
        mechanical O61.1
        medical O61.0
        specified NEC O61.8
        surgical O61.1
      trial of labor NOS O66.40
        following previous cesarean delivery O66.41
      vacuum extraction O66.5
      ventouse O66.5
    fetal-maternal hemorrhage O43.01- ☑
    hemorrhage (intrapartum) O67.9
      with coagulation defect O67.0
      specified cause NEC O67.8
    high head at term O32.4 ☑
    hydrocephalic fetus O33.6 ☑
    incarceration of uterus O34.51- ☑
    incoordinate uterine action O62.4
    increased size, fetus O33.5 ☑
    inertia, uterus O62.2
      primary O62.0
      secondary O62.1
    lateroversion, uterus O34.59- ☑
    mal lie O32.9 ☑
    malposition
      fetus O32.9 ☑
      pelvic organs or tissues NEC O34.8- ☑
      uterus NEC O34.59- ☑
    malpresentation NOS O32.9 ☑
    oblique presentation O32.2 ☑
    occurring after 37 completed weeks of gestation but before 39 completed weeks gestation due to (spontaneous) onset of labor O75.82
    oversize fetus O33.5 ☑
    pelvic tumor NEC O34.8- ☑
    placenta previa O44.1- ☑
      without hemorrhage O44.0- ☑
    placental insufficiency O36.51- ☑
    planned, occurring after 37 completed weeks of gestation but before 39 completed weeks gestation due to (spontaneous) onset of labor O75.82
    polyp, cervix O34.4- ☑
      causing obstructed labor O65.5
    poor dilatation, cervix O62.0
    pre-eclampsia O14.9- ☑
      mild O14.0- ☑
      moderate O14.0- ☑
      severe
        with hemolysis, elevated liver enzymes and low platelet count (HELLP) O14.2- ☑
    previous
      cesarean delivery O34.21
      surgery (to)
        cervix O34.4- ☑

Delivery — *continued*
  cesarean — *continued*
    previous — *continued*
      surgery — *continued*
        gynecological NEC O34.8- ☑
        rectum O34.7- ☑
        uterus O34.29
        vagina O34.6- ☑
    prolapse
      arm or hand O32.2 ☑
      uterus O34.52- ☑
    prolonged labor NOS O63.9
    rectocele O34.8- ☑
    retroversion
      uterus O34.53- ☑
    rigid
      cervix O34.4- ☑
      pelvic floor O34.8- ☑
      perineum O34.7- ☑
      vagina O34.6- ☑
      vulva O34.7- ☑
    sacculation, pregnant uterus O34.59- ☑
    scar(s)
      cervix O34.4- ☑
      cesarean delivery O34.21
      uterus O34.29
    Shirodkar suture in situ O34.3- ☑
    shoulder presentation O32.2 ☑
    stenosis or stricture, cervix O34.4- ☑
    streptococcus B carrier state O99.824
    transverse presentation or lie O32.2 ☑
    tumor, pelvic organs or tissues NEC O34.8- ☑
      cervix O34.4- ☑
    umbilical cord presentation or prolapse O69.0 ☑
  completely normal case O80
  complicated O75.9
    by
      abnormal, abnormality (of)
        forces of labor O62.9
          specified type NEC O62.8
        glucose O99.814
        uterine contractions NOS O62.9
      abruptio placentae (*see also* Abruptio placentae) O45.9- ☑
      abuse
        physical O9A.32 (*following* O99)
        psychological O9A.52 (*following* O99)
        sexual O9A.42 (*following* O99)
      adherent placenta O72.0
        without hemorrhage O73.0
      alcohol use O99.314
      anemia (pre-existing) O99.02
      anesthetic death O74.8
      annular detachment of cervix O71.3
      atony, uterus O62.2
      attempted vacuum extraction and forceps O66.5
      Bandl's ring O62.4
      bariatric surgery status O99.844
      biliary tract disorder O26.62
      bleeding — *see* Delivery, complicated by, hemorrhage
      blood disorder NEC O99.12
      cervical dystocia (hypotonic) O62.2
        primary O62.0
        secondary O62.1
      circulatory system disorder O99.42
      compression of cord (umbilical) NEC O69.2 ☑
      condition NEC O99.89
      contraction, contracted ring O62.4
      cord (umbilical)
        around neck
          with compression O69.1 ☑
          without compression O69.81 ☑
        bruising O69.5 ☑
        complication O69.9 ☑
          specified NEC O69.89 ☑
        compression NEC O69.2 ☑
        entanglement O69.2 ☑
          without compression O69.82 ☑
        hematoma O69.5 ☑
        presentation O69.0 ☑
        prolapse O69.0 ☑
        short O69.3 ☑
        thrombosis (vessels) O69.5 ☑
        vascular lesion O69.5 ☑
      Couvelaire uterus O45.8X- ☑

Delivery — *continued*
  complicated — *continued*
    by — *continued*
      damage to (injury to) NEC
        perineum O71.82
        periurethral tissue O71.82
        vulva O71.82
      delay following rupture of membranes (spontaneous) — *see* Pregnancy, complicated by, premature rupture of membranes
      depressed fetal heart tones O76
      diabetes O24.92
        gestational O24.429
          diet controlled O24.420
          insulin controlled O24.424
        pre-existing O24.32
          specified NEC O24.82
          type 1 O24.02
          type 2 O24.12
      diastasis recti (abdominis) O71.89
      dilatation
        bladder O66.8
        cervix incomplete, poor or slow O62.0
      disease NEC O99.89
      disruptio uteri — *see* Delivery, complicated by, rupture, uterus
      drug use O99.324
      dysfunction, uterus NOS O62.9
        hypertonic O62.4
        hypotonic O62.2
          primary O62.0
          secondary O62.1
        incoordinate O62.4
      eclampsia O15.1
      embolism (pulmonary) — *see* Embolism, obstetric
      endocrine, nutritional or metabolic disease NEC O99.284
      failed
        attempted vaginal birth after previous cesarean delivery O66.41
        induction of labor O61.9
          instrumental O61.1
          mechanical O61.1
          medical O61.0
          specified NEC O61.8
          surgical O61.1
        trial of labor O66.40
      female genital mutilation O65.5
      fetal
        abnormal acid-base balance O68
        acidemia O68
        acidosis O68
        alkalosis O68
        death, early O02.1
        deformity O66.3
        heart rate or rhythm (abnormal) (non-reassuring) O76
        hypoxia O77.8
        stress O77.9
          due to drug administration O77.1
          electrocardiographic evidence of O77.8
          specified NEC O77.8
          ultrasound evidence of O77.8
      fever during labor O75.2
      gastric banding status O99.844
      gastric bypass status O99.844
      gastrointestinal disease NEC O99.62
      gestational diabetes O24.429
        diet controlled O24.420
        insulin (and diet) controlled O24.424
      gonorrhea O98.22
      hematoma O71.7
        ischial spine O71.7
        pelvic O71.7
        vagina O71.7
        vulva or perineum O71.7
      hemorrhage (uterine) O67.9
        associated with
          afibrinogenemia O67.0
          coagulation defect O67.0
          hyperfibrinolysis O67.0
          hypofibrinogenemia O67.0
        due to
          low-lying placenta O44.1- ☑
          placenta previa O44.1- ☑

Delivery — *continued*
  complicated — *continued*
    by — *continued*
      hemorrhage — *continued*
        due to — *continued*
          premature separation of placenta (normally implanted) (*see also* Abruptio placentae) O45.9- ☑
          retained placenta O72.0
          uterine leiomyoma O67.8
        placenta NEC O67.8
        postpartum NEC (atonic) (immediate) O72.1
          with retained or trapped placenta O72.0
          delayed O72.2
          secondary O72.2
          third stage O72.0
      hourglass contraction, uterus O62.4
      hypertension, hypertensive (pre-existing) — *see* Hypertension, complicated by, childbirth (labor)
      hypotension O26.5- ☑
      incomplete dilatation (cervix) O62.0
      incoordinate uterus contractions O62.4
      inertia, uterus O62.2
        during latent phase of labor O62.0
        primary O62.0
        secondary O62.1
      infection (maternal) O98.92
        carrier state NEC O99.834
        gonorrhea O98.22
        human immunodeficiency virus (HIV) O98.72
        sexually transmitted NEC O98.32
        specified NEC O98.82
        syphilis O98.12
        tuberculosis O98.02
        viral hepatitis O98.42
        viral NEC O98.52
      injury (to mother) (*see also* Delivery, complicated, by, damage to) O71.9
        nonobstetric O9A.22 (*following* O99)
          caused by abuse — *see* Delivery, complicated by, abuse
      intrauterine fetal death, early O02.1
      inversion, uterus O71.2
      laceration (perineal) O70.9
        anus (sphincter) O70.4
          with third degree laceration O70.2
            with mucosa O70.3
          without third degree laceration O70.4
        bladder (urinary) O71.5
        bowel O71.5
        cervix (uteri) O71.3
        fourchette O70.0
        hymen O70.0
        labia O70.0
        pelvic
          floor O70.1
          organ NEC O71.5
        perineum, perineal O70.9
          first degree O70.0
          fourth degree O70.3
          muscles O70.1
          second degree O70.1
          skin O70.0
          slight O70.0
          third degree O70.2
        peritoneum (pelvic) O71.5
        rectovaginal (septum) (without perineal laceration) O71.4
          with perineum O70.2
            with anal or rectal mucosa O70.3
        specified NEC O71.89
        sphincter ani — *see* Delivery, complicated, by, laceration, anus (sphincter)
        urethra O71.5
        uterus O71.81
          before labor O71.81
        vagina, vaginal (deep) (high) (without perineal laceration) O71.4
          with perineum O70.0
          muscles, with perineum O70.1
        vulva O70.0
      liver disorder O26.62
      malignancy O9A.12 (*following* O99)
      malnutrition O25.2

☑ **Additional Character Required** — Refer to the Tabular List for Character Selection   ▽ **Subterms under main terms may continue to next column or page**

Delivery — *continued*
  complicated — *continued*
    by — *continued*
      malposition, malpresentation
        without obstruction (*see also* Delivery,
          complicated by, obstruction) O32.9 ☑
          breech O32.1 ☑
          compound O32.6 ☑
          face (brow) (chin) O32.3 ☑
          footling O32.8 ☑
          high head O32.4 ☑
          oblique O32.2 ☑
          specified NEC O32.8 ☑
          transverse O32.2 ☑
          unstable lie O32.0 ☑
      placenta (with hemorrhage) O44.1- ☑
        without hemorrhage O44.0- ☑
      uterus or cervix O65.5
    meconium in amniotic fluid O77.0
    mental disorder NEC O99.344
    metrorrhexis — *see* Delivery, complicated by,
      rupture, uterus
    nervous system disorder O99.354
    obesity (pre-existing) O99.214
    obesity surgery status O99.844
    obstetric trauma O71.9
      specified NEC O71.89
    obstructed labor
      due to
        breech (complete) (frank) presentation
          O64.1 ☑
          incomplete O64.8 ☑
        brow presenation O64.3 ☑
        buttock presentation O64.1 ☑
        chin presentation O64.2 ☑
        compound presentation O64.5 ☑
        contracted pelvis O65.1
        deep transverse arrest O64.0 ☑
        deformed pelvis O65.0
        dystocia (fetal) O66.9
          due to
            conjoined twins O66.3
            fetal
              abnormality NEC O66.3
              ascites O66.3
              hydrops O66.3
              meningomyelocele O66.3
              sacral teratoma O66.3
              tumor O66.3
            hydrocephalic fetus O66.3
          shoulder O66.0
        face presentation O64.2 ☑
        fetopelvic disproportion O65.4
        footling presentation O64.8 ☑
        impacted shoulders O66.0
        incomplete rotation of fetal head
          O64.0 ☑
        large fetus O66.2
        locked twins O66.1
        malposition O64.9 ☑
          specified NEC O64.8 ☑
        malpresentation O64.9 ☑
          specified NEC O64.8 ☑
        multiple fetuses NEC O66.6
        pelvic
          abnormality (maternal) O65.9
            organ O65.5
            specified NEC O65.8
          contraction
            inlet O65.2
            mid-cavity O65.3
            outlet O65.3
          persistent (position)
            occipitoiliac O64.0 ☑
            occipitoposterior O64.0 ☑
            occipitosacral O64.0 ☑
            occipitotransverse O64.0 ☑
          prolapsed arm O64.4 ☑
          shoulder presentation O64.4 ☑
        specified NEC O66.8
    pathological retraction ring, uterus O62.4
    penetration, pregnant uterus by instrument
      O71.1
    perforation — *see* Delivery, complicated by,
      laceration

Delivery — *continued*
  complicated — *continued*
    by — *continued*
      placenta, placental
        ablatio (*see also* Abruptio placentae)
          O45.9- ☑
        abnormality O43.9- ☑
          specified NEC O43.89- ☑
        abruptio (*see also* Abruptio placentae)
          O45.9- ☑
        accreta O43.21- ☑
        adherent (with hemorrhage) O72.0
          without hemorrhage O73.0
        detachment (premature) (*see also* Abruptio
          placentae) O45.9- ☑
        disorder O43.9- ☑
          specified NEC O43.89- ☑
        hemorrhage NEC O67.8
        increta O43.22- ☑
        low (implantation) O44.1- ☑
          without hemorrhage O44.0- ☑
        malformation O43.10- ☑
        malposition O44.1- ☑
          without hemorrhage O44.0- ☑
        percreta O43.23- ☑
        previa (central) (lateral) (low) (marginal)
          (partial) (total) O44.1- ☑
          without hemorrhage O44.0- ☑
        retained (with hemorrhage) O72.0
          without hemorrhage O73.0
        separation (premature) O45.9- ☑
          specified NEC O45.8X- ☑
        vicious insertion O44.1- ☑
      precipitate labor O62.3
      premature rupture, membranes (*see also* Preg-
        nancy, complicated by, premature rup-
        ture of membranes) O42.90
      prolapse
        arm or hand O32.2 ☑
        cord (umbilical) O69.0 ☑
        foot or leg O32.8 ☑
        uterus O34.52- ☑
      prolonged labor O63.9
        first stage O63.0
        second stage O63.1
      protozoal disease (maternal) O98.62
      respiratory disease NEC O99.52
      retained membranes or portions of placenta
        O72.2
        without hemorrhage O73.1
      retarded birth O63.9
      retention of secundines (with hemorrhage)
        O72.0
        without hemorrhage O73.0
        partial O72.2
          without hemorrhage O73.1
      rupture
        bladder (urinary) O71.5
        cervix O71.3
        pelvic organ NEC O71.5
        urethra O71.5
        uterus (during or after labor) O71.1
          before labor O71.0- ☑
      separation, pubic bone (symphysis pubis) O71.6
      shock O75.1
      shoulder presentation O64.4 ☑
      skin disorder NEC O99.72
      spasm, cervix O62.4
      stenosis or stricture, cervix O65.5
      streptococcus B carrier state O99.824
      subluxation of symphysis (pubis) O26.72
      syphilis (maternal) O98.12
      tear — *see* Delivery, complicated by, laceration
      tetanic uterus O62.4
      trauma (obstetrical) (*see also* Delivery, compli-
        cated, by, damage to) O71.9
        non-obstetric O9A.22 (*following* O99)
        periurethral O71.82
        specified NEC O71.89
      tuberculosis (maternal) O98.02
      tumor, pelvic organs or tissues NEC O65.5
      umbilical cord around neck
        with compression O69.1 ☑
        without compression O69.81 ☑
      uterine inertia O62.2
        during latent phase of labor O62.0
        primary O62.0

Delivery — *continued*
  complicated — *continued*
    by — *continued*
      uterine inertia — *continued*
        secondary O62.1
      vasa previa O69.4 ☑
      velamentous insertion of cord O43.12- ☑
    specified complication NEC O75.89
  delayed NOS O63.9
    following rupture of membranes
      artificial O75.5
    second twin, triplet, etc. O63.2
  forceps, low following failed vacuum extraction O66.5
  missed (at or near term) O36.4 ☑
  normal O80
  obstructed — *see* Delivery, complicated by, obstruc-
    tion
  precipitate O62.3
  preterm (*see also* Pregnancy, complicated by, preterm
    labor) O60.10 ☑
  spontaneous O80
  term pregnancy NOS O80
  uncomplicated O80
  vaginal, following previous cesarean delivery O34.21
Delusions (paranoid) — *see* Disorder, delusional
Dementia (degenerative (primary)) (old age) (persisting)
  F03.90
  with
    aggressive behavior F03.91
    behavioral disturbance F03.91
    combative behavior F03.91
    Lewy bodies G31.83 [F02.80]
      with behavioral disturbance G31.83 [F02.81]
    Parkinsonism G31.83 [F02.80]
      with behavioral disturbance G31.83 [F02.81]
    Parkinson's disease G20 [F02.80]
      with behavioral disturbance G20 [F02.81]
    violent behavior F03.91
  alcoholic F10.97
    with dependence F10.27
  Alzheimer's type — *see* Disease, Alzheimer's
  arteriosclerotic — *see* Dementia, vascular
  atypical, Alzheimer's type — *see* Disease, Alzheimer's,
    specified NEC
  congenital — *see* Disability, intellectual
  frontal (lobe) G31.09 [F02.80]
    with behavioral disturbance G31.09 [F02.81]
  frontotemporal G31.09 [F02.80]
    with behavioral disturbance G31.09 [F02.81]
    specified NEC G31.09 [F02.80]
      with behavioral disturbance G31.09 [F02.81]
  in (due to)
    with behavioral disturbance G31.83 [F02.81]
    alcohol F10.97
      with dependence F10.27
    Alzheimer's disease — *see* Disease, Alzheimer's
    arteriosclerotic brain disease — *see* Dementia,
      vascular
    cerebral lipidoses E75.- ☑ [F02.80]
      with behavioral disturbance E75.- ☑ [F02.81]
    Creutzfeldt-Jakob disease (*see also* Creutzfeldt-
      Jakob disease or syndrome (with dementia))
      A81.00
    epilepsy G40.- ☑ [F02.80]
      with behavioral disturbance G40.- ☑ [F02.81]
    hepatolenticular degeneration E83.01 [F02.80]
      with behavioral disturbance E83.01 [F02.81]
    human immunodeficiency virus (HIV) disease
      B20 [F02.80]
      with behavioral disturbance B20 [F02.81]
    Huntington's disease or chorea G10
    hypercalcemia E83.52 [F02.80]
      with behavioral disturbance E83.52 [F02.81]
    hypothyroidism, acquired E03.9 [F02.80]
      with behavioral disturbance E03.9 [F02.81]
      due to iodine deficiency E01.8 [F02.80]
        with behavioral disturbance E01.8 [F02.81]
    inhalants F18.97
      with dependence F18.27
    multiple
      etiologies F03
      sclerosis G35 [F02.80]
        with behavioral disturbance G35 [F02.81]
    neurosyphilis A52.17 [F02.80]
      with behavioral disturbance A52.17 [F02.81]
      juvenile A50.49 [F02.80]
        with behavioral disturbance A50.49 [F02.81]

Dementia — continued
in — continued
niacin deficiency E52 [F02.80]
with behavioral disturbance E52 [F02.81]
paralysis agitans G20 [F02.80]
with behavioral disturbance G20 [F02.81]
Parkinson's disease G20 [F02.80]
pellagra E52 [F02.80]
with behavioral disturbance E52 [F02.81]
Pick's G31.01 [F02.80]
with behavioral disturbance G31.01 [F02.81]
polyarteritis nodosa M30.0 [F02.80]
with behavioral disturbance M30.0 [F02.81]
psychoactive drug F19.97
with dependence F19.27
inhalants F18.97
with dependence F18.27
sedatives, hypnotics or anxiolytics F13.97
with dependence F13.27
sedatives, hypnotics or anxiolytics F13.97
with dependence F13.27
systemic lupus erythematosus M32.- ☑ [F02.80]
with behavioral disturbance M32.- ☑ [F02.81]
trypanosomiasis
African B56.9 [F02.80]
with behavioral disturbance B56.9 [F02.81]
unknown etiology F03 ☑
vitamin B12 deficiency E53.8 [F02.80]
with behavioral disturbance E53.8 [F02.81]
volatile solvents F18.97
with dependence F18.27
infantile, infantilis F84.3
Lewy body G31.83 [F02.80]
with behavioral disturbance G31.83 [F02.81]
multi-infarct — see Dementia, vascular
paralytica, paralytic (syphilitic) A52.17 [F02.80]
with behavioral disturbance A52.17 [F02.81]
juvenilis A50.45
paretic A52.17
praecox — see Schizophrenia
presenile F03 ☑
Alzheimer's type — see Disease, Alzheimer's, early onset
primary degenerative F03 ☑
progressive, syphilitic A52.17
senile F03 ☑
with acute confusional state F05
Alzheimer's type — see Disease, Alzheimer's, late onset
depressed or paranoid type F03 ☑
vascular (acute onset) (mixed) (multi-infarct) (subcortical) F01.50
with behavioral disturbance F01.51
Demineralization, bone — see Osteoporosis
Demodex folliculorum (infestation) B88.0
Demophobia F40.248
Demoralization R45.3
Demyelination, demyelinization
central nervous system G37.9
specified NEC G37.8
corpus callosum (central) G37.1
disseminated, acute G36.9
specified NEC G36.8
global G35
in optic neuritis G36.0
Dengue (classical) (fever) A90
hemorrhagic A91
sandfly A93.1
Dennie-Marfan syphilitic syndrome A50.45
Dens evaginatus, in dente or invaginatus K00.2
Dense breasts R92.2
Density
increased, bone (disseminated) (generalized) (spotted) — see Disorder, bone, density and structure, specified type NEC
lung (nodular) J98.4
Dental (see also condition)
examination Z01.20
with abnormal findings Z01.21
restoration
aesthetically inadequate or displeasing K08.56
defective K08.50
specified NEC K08.59
failure of marginal integrity K08.51
failure of periodontal anatomical integrity K08.54
Dentia praecox K00.6
Denticles (pulp) K04.2
Dentigerous cyst K09.0

Dentin
irregular (in pulp) K04.3
opalescent K00.5
secondary (in pulp) K04.3
sensitive K03.89
Dentinogenesis imperfecta K00.5
Dentinoma — see Cyst, calcifying odontogenic
Dentition (syndrome) K00.7
delayed K00.6
difficult K00.7
precocious K00.6
premature K00.6
retarded K00.6
Dependence (on) (syndrome) F19.20
with remission F19.21
alcohol (ethyl) (methyl) (without remission) F10.20
with
amnestic disorder, persisting F10.26
anxiety disorder F10.280
dementia, persisting F10.27
intoxication F10.229
with delirium F10.221
uncomplicated F10.220
mood disorder F10.24
psychotic disorder F10.259
with
delusions F10.250
hallucinations F10.251
remission F10.21
sexual dysfunction F10.281
sleep disorder F10.282
specified disorder NEC F10.288
withdrawal F10.239
with
delirium F10.231
perceptual disturbance F10.232
uncomplicated F10.230
counseling and surveillance Z71.41
amobarbital — see Dependence, drug, sedative
amphetamine(s) (type) — see Dependence, drug, stimulant NEC
amytal (sodium) — see Dependence, drug, sedative
analgesic NEC F55.8
anesthetic (agent) (gas) (general) (local) NEC — see Dependence, drug, psychoactive NEC
anxiolytic NEC — see Dependence, drug, sedative
barbital(s) — see Dependence, drug, sedative
barbiturate(s) (compounds) (drugs classifiable to T42) — see Dependence, drug, sedative
benzedrine — see Dependence, drug, stimulant NEC
bhang — see Dependence, drug, cannabis
bromide(s) NEC — see Dependence, drug, sedative
caffeine — see Dependence, drug, stimulant NEC
cannabis (sativa) (indica) (resin) (derivatives) (type) — see Dependence, drug, cannabis
chloral (betaine) (hydrate) — see Dependence, drug, sedative
chlordiazepoxide — see Dependence, drug, sedative
coca (leaf) (derivatives) — see Dependence, drug, cocaine
cocaine — see Dependence, drug, cocaine
codeine — see Dependence, drug, opioid
combinations of drugs F19.20
dagga — see Dependence, drug, cannabis
demerol — see Dependence, drug, opioid
dexamphetamine — see Dependence, drug, stimulant NEC
dexedrine — see Dependence, drug, stimulant NEC
dextromethorphan — see Dependence, drug, opioid
dextromoramide — see Dependence, drug, opioid
dextro-nor-pseudo-ephedrine — see Dependence, drug, stimulant NEC
dextrorphan — see Dependence, drug, opioid
diazepam — see Dependence, drug, sedative
dilaudid — see Dependence, drug, opioid
D-lysergic acid diethylamide — see Dependence, drug, hallucinogen
drug NEC F19.20
with sleep disorder F19.282
cannabis F12.20
with
anxiety disorder F12.280
intoxication F12.229
with
delirium F12.221
perceptual disturbance F12.222
uncomplicated F12.220

Dependence — continued
drug — continued
cannabis — continued
with — continued
other specified disorder F12.288
psychosis F12.259
delusions F12.250
hallucinations F12.251
unspecified disorder F12.29
in remission F12.21
cocaine F14.20
with
anxiety disorder F14.280
intoxication F14.229
with
delirium F14.221
perceptual disturbance F14.222
uncomplicated F14.220
mood disorder F14.24
other specified disorder F14.288
psychosis F14.259
delusions F14.250
hallucinations F14.251
sexual dysfunction F14.281
sleep disorder F14.282
unspecified disorder F14.29
withdrawal F14.23
in remission F14.21
withdrawal symptoms in newborn P96.1
counseling and surveillance Z71.51
hallucinogen F16.20
with
anxiety disorder F16.280
flashbacks F16.283
intoxication F16.229
with delirium F16.221
uncomplicated F16.220
mood disorder F16.24
other specified disorder F16.288
perception disorder, persisting F16.283
psychosis F16.259
delusions F16.250
hallucinations F16.251
unspecified disorder F16.29
in remission F16.21
in remission F19.21
inhalant F18.20
with
anxiety disorder F18.280
dementia, persisting F18.27
intoxication F18.229
with delirium F18.221
uncomplicated F18.220
mood disorder F18.24
other specified disorder F18.288
psychosis F18.259
delusions F18.250
hallucinations F18.251
unspecified disorder F18.29
in remission F18.21
nicotine F17.200
with disorder F17.209
remission F17.201
specified disorder NEC F17.208
withdrawal F17.203
chewing tobacco F17.220
with disorder F17.229
remission F17.221
specified disorder NEC F17.228
withdrawal F17.223
cigarettes F17.210
with disorder F17.219
remission F17.211
specified disorder NEC F17.218
withdrawal F17.213
specified product NEC F17.290
with disorder F17.299
remission F17.291
specified disorder NEC F17.298
withdrawal F17.293
opioid F11.20
with
intoxication F11.229
with
delirium F11.221
perceptual disturbance F11.222
uncomplicated F11.220
mood disorder F11.24

☑ **Additional Character Required** — Refer to the Tabular List for Character Selection   ▽ **Subterms under main terms may continue to next column or page**

Dependence — *continued*
  drug — *continued*
    opioid — *continued*
      with — *continued*
        other specified disorder F11.288
        psychosis F11.259
          delusions F11.250
          hallucinations F11.251
        sexual dysfunction F11.281
        sleep disorder F11.282
        unspecified disorder F11.29
        withdrawal F11.23
      in remission F11.21
    psychoactive NEC F19.20
      with
        amnestic disorder F19.26
        anxiety disorder F19.280
        dementia F19.27
        intoxication F19.229
          with
            delirium F19.221
            perceptual disturbance F19.222
          uncomplicated F19.220
        mood disorder F19.24
        other specified disorder F19.288
        psychosis F19.259
          delusions F19.250
          hallucinations F19.251
        sexual dysfunction F19.281
        sleep disorder F19.282
        unspecified disorder F19.29
        withdrawal F19.239
          with
            delirium F19.231
            perceptual disturbance F19.232
          uncomplicated F19.230
    sedative, hypnotic or anxiolytic F13.20
      with
        amnestic disorder F13.26
        anxiety disorder F13.280
        dementia, persisting F13.27
        intoxication F13.229
          with delirium F13.221
          uncomplicated F13.220
        mood disorder F13.24
        other specified disorder F13.288
        psychosis F13.259
          delusions F13.250
          hallucinations F13.251
        sexual dysfunction F13.281
        sleep disorder F13.282
        unspecified disorder F13.29
        withdrawal F13.239
          with
            delirium F13.231
            perceptual disturbance F13.232
          uncomplicated F13.230
      in remission F13.21
    stimulant NEC F15.20
      with
        anxiety disorder F15.280
        intoxication F15.229
          with
            delirium F15.221
            perceptual disturbance F15.222
          uncomplicated F15.220
        mood disorder F15.24
        other specified disorder F15.288
        psychosis F15.259
          delusions F15.250
          hallucinations F15.251
        sexual dysfunction F15.281
        sleep disorder F15.282
        unspecified disorder F15.29
        withdrawal F15.23
      in remission F15.21
  ethyl
    alcohol (without remission) F10.20
      with remission F10.21
    bromide — *see* Dependence, drug, sedative
    carbamate F19.20
    chloride F19.20
    morphine — *see* Dependence, drug, opioid
  ganja — *see* Dependence, drug, cannabis
  glue (airplane) (sniffing) — *see* Dependence, drug, inhalant
  glutethimide   *see* Dependence, drug, sedative

Dependence — *continued*
  hallucinogenics — *see* Dependence, drug, hallucinogen
  hashish — *see* Dependence, drug, cannabis
  hemp — *see* Dependence, drug, cannabis
  heroin (salt) (any) — *see* Dependence, drug, opioid
  hypnotic NEC — *see* Dependence, drug, sedative
  Indian hemp — *see* Dependence, drug, cannabis
  inhalants — *see* Dependence, drug, inhalant
  khat — *see* Dependence, drug, stimulant NEC
  laudanum — *see* Dependence, drug, opioid
  LSD (-25) (derivatives) — *see* Dependence, drug, hallucinogen
  luminal — *see* Dependence, drug, sedative
  lysergic acid — *see* Dependence, drug, hallucinogen
  maconha — *see* Dependence, drug, cannabis
  marihuana — *see* Dependence, drug, cannabis
  meprobamate — *see* Dependence, drug, sedative
  mescaline — *see* Dependence, drug, hallucinogen
  methadone — *see* Dependence, drug, opioid
  methamphetamine(s) — *see* Dependence, drug, stimulant NEC
  methaqualone — *see* Dependence, drug, sedative
  methyl
    alcohol (without remission) F10.20
      with remission F10.21
    bromide — *see* Dependence, drug, sedative
    morphine — *see* Dependence, drug, opioid
    phenidate — *see* Dependence, drug, stimulant NEC
    sulfonal — *see* Dependence, drug, sedative
  morphine (sulfate) (sulfite) (type) — *see* Dependence, drug, opioid
  narcotic (drug) NEC — *see* Dependence, drug, opioid
  nembutal — *see* Dependence, drug, sedative
  neraval — *see* Dependence, drug, sedative
  neravan — *see* Dependence, drug, sedative
  neurobarb — *see* Dependence, drug, sedative
  nicotine — *see* Dependence, drug, nicotine
  nitrous oxide F19.20
  nonbarbiturate sedatives and tranquilizers with similar effect — *see* Dependence, drug, sedative
  on
    artificial heart (fully implantable) (mechanical) Z95.812
    aspirator Z99.0
    care provider (because of) Z74.9
      impaired mobility Z74.09
      need for
        assistance with personal care Z74.1
        continuous supervision Z74.3
      no other household member able to render care Z74.2
      specified reason NEC Z74.8
    machine Z99.89
      enabling NEC Z99.89
      specified type NEC Z99.89
    renal dialysis (hemodialysis) (peritoneal) Z99.2
    respirator Z99.11
    ventilator Z99.11
    wheelchair Z99.3
  opiate — *see* Dependence, drug, opioid
  opioids — *see* Dependence, drug, opioid
  opium (alkaloids) (derivatives) (tincture) — *see* Dependence, drug, opioid
  oxygen (long-term) (supplemental) Z99.81
  paraldehyde — *see* Dependence, drug, sedative
  paregoric — *see* Dependence, drug, opioid
  PCP (phencyclidine) (*see also* Abuse, drug, hallucinogen) F16.20
  pentobarbital — *see* Dependence, drug, sedative
  pentobarbitone (sodium) — *see* Dependence, drug, sedative
  pentothal — *see* Dependence, drug, sedative
  peyote — *see* Dependence, drug, hallucinogen
  phencyclidine (PCP) (and related substances) (*see also* Abuse, drug, hallucinogen) F16.20
  phenmetrazine — *see* Dependence, drug, stimulant NEC
  phenobarbital — *see* Dependence, drug, sedative
  polysubstance F19.20
  psilocibin, psilocin, psilocyn, psilocyline — *see* Dependence, drug, hallucinogen
  psychostimulant NEC — *see* Dependence, drug, stimulant NEC
  secobarbital   *see* Dependence, drug, sedative
  seconal — *see* Dependence, drug, sedative

Dependence — *continued*
  sedative NEC — *see* Dependence, drug, sedative
  specified drug NEC — *see* Dependence, drug
  stimulant NEC — *see* Dependence, drug, stimulant NEC
  substance NEC — *see* Dependence, drug
  supplemental oxygen Z99.81
  tobacco — *see* Dependence, drug, nicotine
    counseling and surveillance Z71.6
  tranquilizer NEC — *see* Dependence, drug, sedative
  vitamin B6 E53.1
  volatile solvents — *see* Dependence, drug, inhalant
Dependency
  care-provider Z74.9
  passive F60.7
  reactions (persistent) F60.7
Depersonalization (in neurotic state) (neurotic) (syndrome) F48.1
Depletion
  extracellular fluid E86.9
  plasma E86.1
  potassium E87.6
    nephropathy N25.89
  salt or sodium E87.1
    causing heat exhaustion or prostration T67.4 ☑
    nephropathy N28.9
  volume NOS E86.9
Deployment (current) (military) status Z56.82
  in theater or in support of military war, peacekeeping and humanitarian operations Z56.82
  personal history of Z91.82
    military war, peacekeeping and humanitarian deployment (current or past conflict) Z91.82
  returned from Z91.82
Depolarization, premature I49.40
  atrial I49.1
  junctional I49.2
  specified NEC I49.49
  ventricular I49.3
Deposit
  bone in Boeck's sarcoid D86.89
  calcareous, calcium — *see* Calcification
  cholesterol
    retina H35.89
    vitreous (body) (humor) — *see* Deposit, crystalline
  conjunctiva H11.11- ☑
  cornea H18.00- ☑
    argentous H18.02- ☑
    due to metabolic disorder H18.03- ☑
    Kayser-Fleischer ring H18.04- ☑
    pigmentation — *see* Pigmentation, cornea
  crystalline, vitreous (body) (humor) H43.2- ☑
  hemosiderin in old scars of cornea — *see* Pigmentation, cornea, stromal
  metallic in lens — *see* Cataract, specified NEC
  skin R23.8
  tooth, teeth (betel) (black) (green) (materia alba) (orange) (tobacco) K03.6
  urate, kidney — *see* Calculus, kidney
Depraved appetite — *see* Pica
Depressed
  HDL cholesterol E78.6
Depression (acute) (mental) F32.9
  agitated (single episode) F32.2
  anaclitic — *see* Disorder, adjustment
  anxiety F41.8
    persistent F34.1
  arches (*see also* Deformity, limb, flat foot)
  atypical (single episode) F32.8
  basal metabolic rate R94.8
  bone marrow D75.89
  central nervous system R09.2
  cerebral R29.818
    newborn P91.4
  cerebrovascular I67.9
  chest wall M95.4
  climacteric (single episode) F32.8
  endogenous (without psychotic symptoms) F33.2
    with psychotic symptoms F33.3
  functional activity R68.89
  hysterical F44.89
  involutional (single episode) F32.8
  major F32.9
    with psychotic symptoms F32.3
    recurrent — *see* Disorder, depressive, recurrent
  manic-depressive — *see* Disorder, depressive, recurrent

▽ **Subterms under main terms may continue to next column or page**   ☑ **Additional Character Required — Refer to the Tabular List for Character Selection**   **91**

Dependence — Depression

Depression — *continued*
- masked (single episode) F32.8
- medullary G93.89
- menopausal (single episode) F32.8
- metatarsus — *see* Depression, arches
- monopolar F33.9
- nervous F34.1
- neurotic F34.1
- nose M95.0
- postnatal F53
- postpartum F53
- post-psychotic of schizophrenia F32.8
- post-schizophrenic F32.8
- psychogenic (reactive) (single episode) F32.9
- psychoneurotic F34.1
- psychotic (single episode) F32.3
  - recurrent F33.3
- reactive (psychogenic) (single episode) F32.9
  - psychotic (single episode) F32.3
- recurrent — *see* Disorder, depressive, recurrent
- respiratory center G93.89
- seasonal — *see* Disorder, depressive, recurrent
- senile F03 ✓
- severe, single episode F32.2
- situational F43.21
- skull Q67.4
- specified NEC (single episode) F32.8
- sternum M95.4
- visual field — *see* Defect, visual field
- vital (recurrent) (without psychotic symptoms) F33.2
  - with psychotic symptoms F33.3
  - single episode F32.2

Deprivation
- cultural Z60.3
- effects NOS T73.9 ✓
  - specified NEC T73.8 ✓
- emotional NEC Z65.8
  - affecting infant or child — *see* Maltreatment, child, psychological
- food T73.0 ✓
- protein — *see* Malnutrition
- sleep Z72.820
- social Z60.4
  - affecting infant or child — *see* Maltreatment, child, psychological
- specified NEC T73.8 ✓
- vitamins — *see* Deficiency, vitamin
- water T73.1 ✓

Derangement
- ankle (internal) — *see* Derangement, joint, ankle
- cartilage (articular) NEC — *see* Derangement, joint, articular cartilage, by site
  - recurrent — *see* Dislocation, recurrent
- cruciate ligament, anterior, current injury — *see* Sprain, knee, cruciate, anterior
- elbow (internal) — *see* Derangement, joint, elbow
- hip (joint) (internal) (old) — *see* Derangement, joint, hip
- joint (internal) M24.9
  - ankylosis — *see* Ankylosis
  - articular cartilage M24.10
    - ankle M24.17- ✓
    - elbow M24.12- ✓
    - foot M24.17- ✓
    - hand M24.14- ✓
    - hip M24.15- ✓
    - knee NEC M23.9- ✓
    - loose body — *see* Loose, body
    - shoulder M24.11- ✓
    - wrist M24.13- ✓
  - contracture — *see* Contraction, joint
  - current injury (*see also* Dislocation)
    - knee, meniscus or cartilage — *see* Tear, meniscus
  - dislocation
    - pathological — *see* Dislocation, pathological
    - recurrent — *see* Dislocation, recurrent
  - knee — *see* Derangement, knee
  - ligament — *see* Disorder, ligament
  - loose body — *see* Loose, body
  - recurrent — *see* Dislocation, recurrent
  - specified type NEC M24.80
    - ankle M24.87- ✓
    - elbow M24.82- ✓
    - foot joint M24.87- ✓
    - hand joint M24.84- ✓
    - hip M24.85- ✓

Derangement — *continued*
- joint — *continued*
  - specified type — *continued*
    - shoulder M24.81- ✓
    - wrist M24.83- ✓
  - temporomandibular M26.69
- knee (recurrent) M23.9- ✓
  - ligament disruption, spontaneous M23.60- ✓
    - anterior cruciate M23.61- ✓
    - capsular M23.67- ✓
    - instability, chronic M23.5- ✓
    - lateral collateral M23.64- ✓
    - medial collateral M23.63- ✓
    - posterior cruciate M23.62- ✓
  - loose body M23.4- ✓
  - meniscus M23.30- ✓
    - cystic M23.00- ✓
      - lateral M23.002
        - anterior horn M23.04- ✓
        - posterior horn M23.05- ✓
        - specified NEC M23.06- ✓
      - medial M23.005
        - anterior horn M23.01- ✓
        - posterior horn M23.02- ✓
        - specified NEC M23.03- ✓
    - degenerate — *see* Derangement, knee, meniscus, specified NEC
    - detached — *see* Derangement, knee, meniscus, specified NEC
    - due to old tear or injury M23.20- ✓
      - lateral M23.20- ✓
        - anterior horn M23.24- ✓
        - posterior horn M23.25- ✓
        - specified NEC M23.26- ✓
      - medial M23.20- ✓
        - anterior horn M23.21- ✓
        - posterior horn M23.22- ✓
        - specified NEC M23.23- ✓
    - retained — *see* Derangement, knee, meniscus, specified NEC
    - specified NEC M23.30- ✓
      - lateral M23.30- ✓
        - anterior horn M23.34- ✓
        - posterior horn M23.35- ✓
        - specified NEC M23.36- ✓
      - medial M23.30- ✓
        - anterior horn M23.31- ✓
        - posterior horn M23.32- ✓
        - specified NEC M23.33- ✓
    - old M23.8X- ✓
    - specified NEC — *see* subcategory M23.8 ✓
  - low back NEC — *see* Dorsopathy, specified NEC
  - meniscus — *see* Derangement, knee, meniscus
  - mental — *see* Psychosis
  - patella, specified NEC — *see* Disorder, patella, derangement NEC
  - semilunar cartilage (knee) — *see* Derangement, knee, meniscus, specified NEC
  - shoulder (internal) — *see* Derangement, joint, shoulder

Dercum's disease E88.2
Derealization (neurotic) F48.1
Dermal — *see* condition
Dermaphytid — *see* Dermatophytosis
Dermatitis (eczematous) L30.9
- ab igne L59.0
- acarine B88.0
- actinic (due to sun) L57.8
  - other than from sun L59.8
- allergic — *see* Dermatitis, contact, allergic
- ambustionis, due to burn or scald — *see* Burn
- amebic A06.7
- ammonia L22
- arsenical (ingested) L27.8
- artefacta L98.1
  - psychogenic F54
- atopic L20.9
  - psychogenic F54
  - specified NEC L20.89
- autoimmune progesterone L30.8
- berlock, berloque L56.2
- blastomycotic B40.3
- blister beetle L24.89
- bullous, bullosa L13.9
  - mucosynechial, atrophic L12.1
  - seasonal L30.8

Dermatitis — *continued*
- bullous, bullosa — *continued*
  - specified NEC L13.8
- calorica L59.0
  - due to burn or scald — *see* Burn
- caterpillar L24.89
- cercarial B65.3
- combustionis L59.0
  - due to burn or scald — *see* Burn
- congelationis T69.1 ✓
- contact (occupational) L25.9
  - allergic L23.9
    - due to
      - adhesives L23.1
      - cement L23.5
      - chemical products NEC L23.5
      - chromium L23.0
      - cosmetics L23.2
      - dander (cat) (dog) L23.81
      - drugs in contact with skin L23.3
      - dyes L23.4
      - food in contact with skin L23.6
      - hair (cat) (dog) L23.81
      - insecticide L23.5
      - metals L23.0
      - nickel L23.0
      - plants, non-food L23.7
      - plastic L23.5
      - rubber L23.5
      - specified agent NEC L23.89
  - due to
    - cement L25.3
    - chemical products NEC L25.3
    - cosmetics L25.0
    - dander (cat) (dog) L23.81
    - drugs in contact with skin L25.1
    - dyes L25.2
    - food in contact with skin L25.4
    - hair (cat) (dog) L23.81
    - plants, non-food L25.5
    - specified agent NEC L25.8
  - irritant L24.9
    - due to
      - cement L25.3
      - chemical products NEC L24.5
      - cosmetics L24.3
      - detergents L24.0
      - drugs in contact with skin L24.4
      - food in contact with skin L24.6
      - oils and greases L24.1
      - plants, non-food L24.7
      - solvents L24.2
      - specified agent NEC L24.89
- contusiformis L52
- diabetic — *see* E08-E13 with .620
- diaper L22
- diphtheritica A36.3
- dry skin L85.3
- due to
  - acetone (contact) (irritant) L24.2
  - acids (contact) (irritant) L24.5
  - adhesive(s) (allergic) (contact) (plaster) L23.1
    - irritant L24.5
  - alcohol (irritant) (skin contact) (substances in category T51) L24.2
    - taken internally L27.8
  - alkalis (contact) (irritant) L24.5
  - arsenic (ingested) L27.8
  - carbon disulfide (contact) (irritant) L24.2
  - caustics (contact) (irritant) L24.5
  - cement (contact) L25.3
  - cereal (ingested) L27.2
  - chemical(s) NEC L25.3
    - taken internally L27.8
  - chlorocompounds L24.2
  - chromium (contact) (irritant) L24.81
  - coffee (ingested) L27.2
  - cold weather L30.8
  - cosmetics (contact) L25.0
    - allergic L23.2
    - irritant L24.3
  - cyclohexanes L24.2
  - dander (cat) (dog) L23.81
  - Demodex species B88.0
  - Dermanyssus gallinae B88.0
  - detergents (contact) (irritant) L24.0
  - dichromate L24.81

Dermatitis — *continued*
  due to — *continued*
    drugs and medicaments (generalized) (internal use) L27.0
      external — *see* Dermatitis, due to, drugs, in contact with skin
      in contact with skin L25.1
        allergic L23.3
        irritant L24.4
      localized skin eruption L27.1
      specified substance — *see* Table of Drugs and Chemicals
    dyes (contact) L25.2
      allergic L23.4
      irritant L24.89
    epidermophytosis — *see* Dermatophytosis
    esters L24.2
    external irritant NEC L24.9
    fish (ingested) L27.2
    flour (ingested) L27.2
    food (ingested) L27.2
      in contact with skin L25.4
    fruit (ingested) L27.2
    furs (allergic) (contact) L23.81
    glues — *see* Dermatitis, due to, adhesives
    glycols L24.2
    greases NEC (contact) (irritant) L24.1
    hair (cat) (dog) L23.81
    hot
      objects and materials — *see* Burn
      weather or places L59.0
    hydrocarbons L24.2
    infrared rays L59.8
    ingestion, ingested substance L27.9
      chemical NEC L27.8
      drugs and medicaments — *see* Dermatitis, due to, drugs
      food L27.2
      specified NEC L27.8
    insecticide in contact with skin L24.5
    internal agent L27.9
      drugs and medicaments (generalized) — *see* Dermatitis, due to, drugs
      food L27.2
    irradiation — *see* Dermatitis, due to, radioactive substance
    ketones L24.2
    lacquer tree (allergic) (contact) L23.7
    light (sun) NEC L57.8
      acute L56.8
      other L59.8
    Liponyssoides sanguineus B88.0
    low temperature L30.8
    meat (ingested) L27.2
    metals, metal salts (contact) (irritant) L24.81
    milk (ingested) L27.2
    nickel (contact) (irritant) L24.81
    nylon (contact) (irritant) L24.5
    oils NEC (contact) (irritant) L24.1
    paint solvent (contact) (irritant) L24.2
    petroleum products (contact) (irritant) (substances in T52.0) L24.2
    plants NEC (contact) L25.5
      allergic L23.7
      irritant L24.7
    plasters (adhesive) (any) (allergic) (contact) L23.1
      irritant L24.5
    plastic (contact) L25.3
    preservatives (contact) — *see* Dermatitis, due to, chemical, in contact with skin
    primrose (allergic) (contact) L23.7
    primula (allergic) (contact) L23.7
    radiation L59.8
      nonionizing (chronic exposure) L57.8
      sun NEC L57.8
        acute L56.8
    radioactive substance L58.9
      acute L58.0
      chronic L58.1
    radium L58.9
      acute L58.0
      chronic L58.1
    ragweed (allergic) (contact) L23.7
    Rhus (allergic) (contact) (diversiloba) (radicans) (toxicodendron) (venenata) (verniciflua) L23.7
    rubber (contact) L24.5
    Senecio jacobaea (allergic) (contact) L23.7

Dermatitis — *continued*
  due to — *continued*
    solvents (contact) (irritant) (substances in category T52) L24.2
    specified agent NEC (contact) L25.8
      allergic L23.89
      irritant L24.89
    sunshine NEC L57.8
      acute L56.8
    tetrachlorethylene (contact) (irritant) L24.2
    toluene (contact) (irritant) L24.2
    turpentine (contact) L24.2
    ultraviolet rays (sun NEC) (chronic exposure) L57.8
      acute L56.8
    vaccine or vaccination L27.0
      specified substance — *see* Table of Drugs and Chemicals
    varicose veins — *see* Varix, leg, with, inflammation
    X-rays L58.9
      acute L58.0
      chronic L58.1
  dyshydrotic L30.1
  dysmenorrheica N94.6
  escharotica — *see* Burn
  exfoliative, exfoliativa (generalized) L26
    neonatorum L00
  eyelid (*see also* Dermatosis, eyelid)
    allergic H01.119
      left H01.116
        lower H01.115
        upper H01.114
      right H01.113
        lower H01.112
        upper H01.111
    contact — *see* Dermatitis, eyelid, allergic
    due to
      Demodex species B88.0
      herpes (zoster) B02.39
        simplex B00.59
    eczematous H01.139
      left H01.136
        lower H01.135
        upper H01.134
      right H01.133
        lower H01.132
        upper H01.131
  facta, factitia, factitial L98.1
    psychogenic F54
  flexural NEC L20.82
  friction L30.4
  fungus B36.9
    specified type NEC B36.8
  gangrenosa, gangrenous infantum L08.0
  harvest mite B88.0
  heat L59.0
  herpesviral, vesicular (ear) (lip) B00.1
  herpetiformis (bullous) (erythematous) (pustular) (vesicular) L13.0
    juvenile L12.2
    senile L12.0
  hiemalis L30.8
  hypostatic, hypostatica — *see* Varix, leg, with, inflammation
  infectious eczematoid L30.3
  infective L30.3
  irritant — *see* Dermatitis, contact, irritant
  Jacquet's (diaper dermatitis) L22
  Leptus B88.0
  lichenified NEC L28.0
  medicamentosa (generalized) (internal use) — *see* Dermatitis, due to drugs
  mite B88.0
  multiformis L13.0
    juvenile L12.2
  napkin L22
  neurotica L13.0
  nummular L30.0
  papillaris capillitii L73.0
  pellagrous E52
  perioral L71.0
  photocontact L56.2
  polymorpha dolorosa L13.0
  pruriginosa L13.0
  pruritic NEC L30.8
  psychogenic F54
  purulent L08.0
  pustular
    contagious B08.02

Dermatitis — *continued*
  pustular — *continued*
    subcorneal L13.1
  pyococcal L08.0
  pyogenica L08.0
  repens L40.2
  Ritter's (exfoliativa) L00
  Schamberg's L81.7
  schistosome B65.3
  seasonal bullous L30.8
  seborrheic L21.9
    infantile L21.1
    specified NEC L21.8
  sensitization NOS L23.9
  septic L08.0
  solare L57.8
  specified NEC L30.8
  stasis I87.2
    with varicose ulcer — *see* Varix, leg, with ulcer, with inflammation
    due to postthrombotic syndrome — *see* Syndrome, postthrombotic
  suppurative L08.0
  traumatic NEC L30.4
  trophoneurotica L13.0
  ultraviolet (sun) (chronic exposure) L57.8
    acute L56.8
  varicose — *see* Varix, leg, with, inflammation
  vegetans L10.1
  verrucosa B43.0
  vesicular, herpesviral B00.1

Dermatoarthritis, lipoid E78.81
Dermatochalasis, eyelid H02.839
  left H02.836
    lower H02.835
    upper H02.834
  right H02.833
    lower H02.832
    upper H02.831
Dermatofibroma (lenticulare) — *see* Neoplasm, skin, benign
  protuberans — *see* Neoplasm, skin, uncertain behavior
Dermatofibrosarcoma (pigmented) (protuberans) — *see* Neoplasm, skin, malignant
Dermatographia L50.3
Dermatolysis (exfoliativa) (congenital) Q82.8
  acquired L57.4
  eyelids — *see* Blepharochalasis
  palpebrarum — *see* Blepharochalasis
  senile L57.4
Dermatomegaly NEC Q82.8
Dermatomucosomyositis M33.10
  with
    myopathy M33.12
    respiratory involvement M33.11
    specified organ involvement NEC M33.19
Dermatomycosis B36.9
  furfuracea B36.0
  specified type NEC B36.8
Dermatomyositis (acute) (chronic) (*see also* Dermatopolymyositis)
  in (due to) neoplastic disease (*see also* Neoplasm) D49.9 [M36.0]
Dermatoneuritis of children — *see* Poisoning, mercury
Dermatophilosis A48.8
Dermatophytid L30.2
Dermatophytide — *see* Dermatophytosis
Dermatophytosis (epidermophyton) (infection) (Microsporum) (tinea) (Trichophyton) B35.9
  beard B35.0
  body B35.4
  capitis B35.0
  corporis B35.4
  deep-seated B35.8
  disseminated B35.8
  foot B35.3
  granulomatous B35.8
  groin B35.6
  hand B35.2
  nail B35.1
  perianal (area) B35.6
  scalp B35.0
  specified NEC B35.8
Dermatopolymyositis M33.90
  with
    myopathy M33.92
    respiratory involvement M33.91
    specified organ involvement NEC M33.99

Diabetes, diabetic — *continued*
 with — *continued*
  renal complication NEC E11.29
  renal tubular degeneration E11.29
  retinopathy E11.319
   with macular edema E11.311
   nonproliferative E11.329
    with macular edema E11.321
    mild E11.329
     with macular edema E11.321
    moderate E11.339
     with macular edema E11.331
    severe E11.349
     with macular edema E11.341
   proliferative E11.359
    with macular edema E11.351
  skin complication NEC E11.628
  skin ulcer NEC E11.622
 bronzed E83.110
 complicating pregnancy — *see* Pregnancy, complicated by, diabetes
 dietary counseling and surveillance Z71.3
 due to drug or chemical E09.9
  with
   amyotrophy E09.44
   arthropathy NEC E09.618
   autonomic (poly)neuropathy E09.43
   cataract E09.36
   Charcot's joints E09.610
   chronic kidney disease E09.22
   circulatory complication NEC E09.59
   complication E09.8
    specified NEC E09.69
   dermatitis E09.620
   foot ulcer E09.621
   gangrene E09.52
   gastroparesis E09.43
   glomerulonephrosis, intracapillary E09.21
   glomerulosclerosis, intercapillary E09.21
   hyperglycemia E09.65
   hyperosmolarity E09.00
    with coma E09.01
   hypoglycemia E09.649
    with coma E09.641
   ketoacidosis E09.10
    with coma E09.11
   kidney complications NEC E09.29
   Kimmelsteil-Wilson disease E09.21
   mononeuropathy E09.41
   myasthenia E09.44
   necrobiosis lipoidica E09.620
   nephropathy E09.21
   neuralgia E09.42
   neurologic complication NEC E09.49
   neuropathic arthropathy E09.610
   neuropathy E09.40
   ophthalmic complication NEC E09.39
   oral complication NEC E09.638
   periodontal disease E09.630
   peripheral angiopathy E09.51
    with gangrene E09.52
   polyneuropathy E09.42
   renal complication NEC E09.29
   renal tubular degeneration E09.29
   retinopathy E09.319
    with macular edema E09.311
    nonproliferative E09.329
     with macular edema E09.321
     mild E09.329
      with macular edema E09.321
     moderate E09.339
      with macular edema E09.331
     severe E09.349
      with macular edema E09.341
    proliferative E09.359
     with macular edema E09.351
   skin complication NEC E09.628
   skin ulcer NEC E09.622
 due to underlying condition E08.9
  with
   amyotrophy E08.44
   arthropathy NEC E08.618
   autonomic (poly)neuropathy E08.43
   cataract E08.36
   Charcot's joints E08.610
   chronic kidney disease E08.22
   circulatory complication NEC E08.59

Diabetes, diabetic — *continued*
 due to underlying condition — *continued*
  with — *continued*
   complication E08.8
    specified NEC E08.69
   dermatitis E08.620
   foot ulcer E08.621
   gangrene E08.52
   gastroparesis E08.43
   glomerulonephrosis, intracapillary E08.21
   glomerulosclerosis, intercapillary E08.21
   hyperglycemia E08.65
   hyperosmolarity E08.00
    with coma E08.01
   hypoglycemia E08.649
    with coma E08.641
   ketoacidosis E08.10
    with coma E08.11
   kidney complications NEC E08.29
   Kimmelsteil-WIlson disease E08.21
   mononeuropathy E08.41
   myasthenia E08.44
   necrobiosis lipoidica E08.620
   nephropathy E08.21
   neuralgia E08.42
   neurologic complication NEC E08.49
   neuropathic arthropathy E08.610
   neuropathy E08.40
   ophthalmic complication NEC E08.39
   oral complication NEC E08.638
   periodontal disease E08.630
   peripheral angiopathy E08.51
    with gangrene E08.52
   polyneuropathy E08.42
   renal complication NEC E08.29
   renal tubular degeneration E08.29
   retinopathy E08.319
    with macular edema E08.311
    nonproliferative E08.329
     with macular edema E08.321
     mild E08.329
      with macular edema E08.321
     moderate E08.339
      with macular edema E08.331
     severe E08.349
      with macular edema E08.341
    proliferative E08.359
     with macular edema E08.351
   skin complication NEC E08.628
   skin ulcer NEC E08.622
 gestational (in pregnancy) O24.419
  affecting newborn P70.0
  diet controlled O24.410
  in childbirth O24.429
   diet controlled O24.420
   insulin (and diet) controlled O24.424
  insulin (and diet) controlled O24.414
  puerperal O24.439
   diet controlled O24.430
   insulin (and diet) controlled O24.434
 hepatogenous E13.9
 inadequately controlled — *code to* Diabetes, by type, with hyperglycemia
 insipidus E23.2
  nephrogenic N25.1
  pituitary E23.2
  vasopressin resistant N25.1
 insulin dependent — *code to* type of diabetes
 juvenile-onset — *see* Diabetes, type 1
 ketosis-prone — *see* Diabetes, type 1
 latent R73.09
 neonatal (transient) P70.2
 non-insulin dependent — *code to* type of diabetes
 out of control — *code to* Diabetes, by type, with hyperglycemia
 phosphate E83.39
 poorly controlled — *code to* Diabetes, by type, with hyperglycemia
 postpancreatectomy — *see* Diabetes, specified type NEC
 postprocedural — *see* Diabetes, specified type NEC
 secondary diabetes mellitus NEC — *see* Diabetes, specified type NEC
 specified type NEC E13.9
  with
   amyotrophy E13.44
   arthropathy NEC E13.618
   autonomic (poly)neuropathy E13.43

Diabetes, diabetic — *continued*
 specified type — *continued*
  with — *continued*
   cataract E13.36
   Charcot's joints E13.610
   chronic kidney disease E13.22
   circulatory complication NEC E13.59
   complication E13.8
    specified NEC E13.69
   dermatitis E13.620
   foot ulcer E13.621
   gangrene E13.52
   gastroparesis E13.43
   glomerulonephrosis, intracapillary E13.21
   glomerulosclerosis, intercapillary E13.21
   hyperglycemia E13.65
   hyperosmolarity E13.00
    with coma E13.01
   hypoglycemia E13.649
    with coma E13.641
   ketoacidosis E13.10
    with coma E13.11
   kidney complications NEC E13.29
   Kimmelsteil-Wilson disease E13.21
   mononeuropathy E13.41
   myasthenia E13.44
   necrobiosis lipoidica E13.620
   nephropathy E13.21
   neuralgia E13.42
   neurologic complication NEC E13.49
   neuropathic arthropathy E13.610
   neuropathy E13.40
   ophthalmic complication NEC E13.39
   oral complication NEC E13.638
   periodontal disease E13.630
   peripheral angiopathy E13.51
    with gangrene E13.52
   polyneuropathy E13.42
   renal complication NEC E13.29
   renal tubular degeneration E13.29
   retinopathy E13.319
    with macular edema E13.311
    nonproliferative E13.329
     with macular edema E13.321
     mild E13.329
      with macular edema E13.321
     moderate E13.339
      with macular edema E13.331
     severe E13.349
      with macular edema E13.341
    proliferative E13.359
     with macular edema E13.351
   skin complication NEC E13.628
   skin ulcer NEC E13.622
 steroid-induced — *see* Diabetes, due to, drug or chemical
 type 1 E10.9
  with
   amyotrophy E10.44
   arthropathy NEC E10.618
   autonomic (poly)neuropathy E10.43
   cataract E10.36
   Charcot's joints E10.610
   chronic kidney disease E10.22
   circulatory complication NEC E10.59
   complication E10.8
    specified NEC E10.69
   dermatitis E10.620
   foot ulcer E10.621
   gangrene E10.52
   gastroparesis E10.43
   glomerulonephrosis, intracapillary E10.21
   glomerulosclerosis, intercapillary E10.21
   hyperglycemia E10.65
   hypoglycemia E10.649
    with coma E10.641
   ketoacidosis E10.10
    with coma E10.11
   kidney complications NEC E10.29
   Kimmelsteil-Wilson disease E10.21
   mononeuropathy E10.41
   myasthenia E10.44
   necrobiosis lipoidica E10.620
   nephropathy E10.21
   neuralgia E10.42
   neurologic complication NEC E10.49
   neuropathic arthropathy E10.610
   neuropathy E10.40

Diabetes, diabetic — continued
  type 1 — continued
    with — continued
      ophthalmic complication NEC E10.39
      oral complication NEC E10.638
      periodontal disease E10.630
      peripheral angiopathy E10.51
        with gangrene E10.52
      polyneuropathy E10.42
      renal complication NEC E10.29
      renal tubular degeneration E10.29
      retinopathy E10.319
        with macular edema E10.311
        nonproliferative E10.329
          with macular edema E10.321
          mild E10.329
            with macular edema E10.321
          moderate E10.339
            with macular edema E10.331
          severe E10.349
            with macular edema E10.341
        proliferative E10.359
          with macular edema E10.351
    skin complication NEC E10.628
    skin ulcer NEC E10.622
  type 2 E11.9
    with
      amyotrophy E11.44
      arthropathy NEC E11.618
      autonomic (poly)neuropathy E11.43
      cataract E11.36
      Charcot's joints E11.610
      chronic kidney disease E11.22
      circulatory complication NEC E11.59
      complication E11.8
        specified NEC E11.69
      dermatitis E11.620
      foot ulcer E11.621
      gangrene E11.52
      gastroparesis E11.43
      glomerulonephrosis, intracapillary E11.21
      glomerulosclerosis, intercapillary E11.21
      hyperglycemia E11.65
      hyperosmolarity E11.00
        with coma E11.01
      hypoglycemia E11.649
        with coma E11.641
      kidney complications NEC E11.29
      Kimmelstiel-Wilson disease E11.21
      mononeuropathy E11.41
      myasthenia E11.44
      necrobiosis lipoidica E11.620
      nephropathy E11.21
      neuralgia E11.42
      neurologic complication NEC E11.49
      neuropathic arthropathy E11.610
      neuropathy E11.40
      ophthalmic complication NEC E11.39
      oral complication NEC E11.638
      periodontal disease E11.630
      peripheral angiopathy E11.51
        with gangrene E11.52
      polyneuropathy E11.42
      renal complication NEC E11.29
      renal tubular degeneration E11.29
      retinopathy E11.319
        with macular edema E11.311
        nonproliferative E11.329
          with macular edema E11.321
          mild E11.329
            with macular edema E11.321
          moderate E11.339
            with macular edema E11.331
          severe E11.349
            with macular edema E11.341
        proliferative E11.359
          with macular edema E11.351
    skin complication NEC E11.628
    skin ulcer NEC E11.622
Diacyclothrombopathia D69.1
Diagnosis deferred R69
Dialysis (intermittent) (treatment)
  noncompliance (with) Z91.15
  renal (hemodialysis) (peritoneal), status Z99.2
  retina, retinal — see Detachment, retina, with retinal, dialysis
Diamond-Blackfan anemia (congenital hypoplastic) D61.01

Diamond-Gardener syndrome (autoerythrocyte sensitization) D69.2
Diaper rash L22
Diaphoresis (excessive) R61
Diaphragm — see condition
Diaphragmalgia R07.1
Diaphragmatitis, diaphragmitis J98.6
Diaphysial aclasis Q78.6
Diaphysitis — see Osteomyelitis, specified type NEC
Diarrhea, diarrheal (disease) (infantile) (inflammatory) R19.7
  achlorhydric K31.83
  allergic K52.2
  amebic (see also Amebiasis) A06.0
    with abscess — see Abscess, amebic
    acute A06.0
    chronic A06.1
    nondysenteric A06.2
  bacillary — see Dysentery, bacillary
  balantidial A07.0
  cachectic NEC K52.89
  Chilomastix A07.8
  choleriformis A00.1
  chronic (noninfectious) K52.9
  coccidial A07.3
  Cochin-China K90.1
    strongyloidiasis B78.0
  Dientamoeba A07.8
  dietetic K52.2
  drug-induced K52.1
  due to
    bacteria A04.9
      specified NEC A04.8
    Campylobacter A04.5
    Capillaria philippinensis B81.1
    Clostridium difficile A04.7
    Clostridium perfringens (C) (F) A04.8
    Cryptosporidium A07.2
    drugs K52.1
    Escherichia coli A04.4
      enteroaggregative A04.4
      enterohemorrhagic A04.3
      enteroinvasive A04.2
      enteropathogenic A04.0
      enterotoxigenic A04.1
      specified NEC A04.4
    food hypersensitivity K52.2
    Necator americanus B76.1
    S. japonicum B65.2
    specified organism NEC A08.8
      bacterial A04.8
      viral A08.39
    Staphylococcus A04.8
    Trichuris trichiuria B79
    virus — see Enteritis, viral
    Yersinia enterocolitica A04.6
  dysenteric A09
  endemic A09
  epidemic A09
  flagellate A07.9
  Flexner's (ulcerative) A03.1
  functional K59.1
    following gastrointestinal surgery K91.89
    psychogenic F45.8
  Giardia lamblia A07.1
  giardial A07.1
  hill K90.1
  infectious A09
  malarial — see Malaria
  mite B88.0
  mycotic NEC B49
  neonatal (noninfectious) P78.3
  nervous F45.8
  neurogenic K59.1
  noninfectious K52.9
  postgastrectomy K91.1
  postvagotomy K91.1
  protozoal A07.9
    specified NEC A07.8
  psychogenic F45.8
  specified
    bacterium NEC A04.8
    virus NEC A08.39
  strongyloidiasis B78.0
  toxic K52.1
  trichomonal A07.8
  tropical K90.1
  tuberculous A18.32

Diarrhea, diarrheal — continued
  viral — see Enteritis, viral
Diastasis
  cranial bones M84.88
    congenital NEC Q75.8
  joint (traumatic) — see Dislocation
  muscle M62.00
    ankle M62.07- ☑
    congenital Q79.8
    foot M62.07- ☑
    forearm M62.03- ☑
    hand M62.04- ☑
    lower leg M62.06- ☑
    pelvic region M62.05- ☑
    shoulder region M62.01- ☑
    specified site NEC M62.08
    thigh M62.05- ☑
    upper arm M62.02- ☑
  recti (abdomen)
    complicating delivery O71.89
    congenital Q79.59
Diastema, tooth, teeth, fully erupted M26.32
Diastematomyelia Q06.2
Diataxia, cerebral G80.4
Diathesis
  allergic — see History, allergy
  bleeding (familial) D69.9
  cystine (familial) E72.00
  gouty — see Gout
  hemorrhagic (familial) D69.9
    newborn NEC P53
  spasmophilic R29.0
Diaz's disease or osteochondrosis (juvenile) (talus) — see Osteochondrosis, juvenile, tarsus
Dibothriocephalus, dibothriocephaliasis (latus) (infection) (infestation) B70.0
  larval B70.1
Dicephalus, dicephaly Q89.4
Dichotomy, teeth K00.2
Dichromat, dichromatopsia (congenital) — see Deficiency, color vision
Dichuchwa A65
Dicrocoeliasis B66.2
Didelphia, didelphys — see Double uterus
Didymytis N45.1
  with orchitis N45.3
Dietary
  inadequacy or deficiency E63.9
  surveillance and counseling Z71.3
Dietl's crisis N13.8
Dieulafoy lesion (hemorrhagic)
  duodenum K31.82
  esophagus K22.8
  intestine (colon) K63.81
  stomach K31.82
Difficult, difficulty (in)
  acculturation Z60.3
  feeding R63.3
    newborn P92.9
      breast P92.5
      specified NEC P92.8
    nonorganic (infant or child) F98.29
  intubation, in anesthesia T88.4 ☑
  mechanical, gastroduodenal stoma K91.89
    causing obstruction K91.3
  reading (developmental) F81.0
    secondary to emotional disorders F93.9
  spelling (specific) F81.81
    with reading disorder F81.89
    due to inadequate teaching Z55.8
  swallowing — see Dysphagia
  walking R26.2
  work
    conditions NEC Z56.5
    schedule Z56.3
Diffuse — see condition
Digestive — see condition
Dihydropyrimidine dehydrogenase disease (DPD) E88.89
Diktyoma — see Neoplasm, malignant, by site
Dilaceration, tooth K00.4
Dilatation
  anus K59.8
    venule — see Hemorrhoids
  aorta (focal) (general) — see Ectasia, aorta
    with aneuysm — see Aneurysm, aorta
  artery — see Aneurysm

Dilatation — *continued*
  bladder (sphincter) N32.89
    congenital Q64.79
  blood vessel I99.8
  bronchial J47.9
    with
      exacerbation (acute) J47.1
      lower respiratory infection J47.0
  calyx (due to obstruction) — *see* Hydronephrosis
  capillaries I78.8
  cardiac (acute) (chronic) (*see also* Hypertrophy, cardiac)
    congenital Q24.8
      valve NEC Q24.8
        pulmonary Q22.3
    valve — *see* Endocarditis
  cavum septi pellucidi Q06.8
  cervix (uteri) (*see also* Incompetency, cervix)
    incomplete, poor, slow complicating delivery O62.0
  colon K59.3
    congenital Q43.1
    psychogenic F45.8
  common duct (acquired) K83.8
    congenital Q44.5
  cystic duct (acquired) K82.8
    congenital Q44.5
  duct, mammary — *see* Ectasia, mammary duct
  duodenum K59.8
  esophagus K22.8
    congenital Q39.5
    due to achalasia K22.0
  eustachian tube, congenital Q17.8
  gallbladder K82.8
  gastric — *see* Dilatation, stomach
  heart (acute) (chronic) (*see also* Hypertrophy, cardiac)
    congenital Q24.8
    valve — *see* Endocarditis
  ileum K59.8
    psychogenic F45.8
  jejunum K59.8
    psychogenic F45.8
  kidney (calyx) (collecting structures) (cystic)
    (parenchyma) (pelvis) (idiopathic) N28.89
  lacrimal passages or duct — *see* Disorder, lacrimal
    system, changes
  lymphatic vessel I89.0
  mammary duct — *see* Ectasia, mammary duct
  Meckel's diverticulum (congenital) Q43.0
    malignant — *see* Table of Neoplasms, small intestine, malignant
  myocardium (acute) (chronic) — *see* Hypertrophy, cardiac
  organ or site, congenital NEC — *see* Distortion
  pancreatic duct K86.8
  pericardium — *see* Pericarditis
  pharynx J39.2
  prostate N42.89
  pulmonary
    artery (idiopathic) I28.8
    valve, congenital Q22.3
  pupil H57.04
  rectum K59.3
  saccule, congenital Q16.5
  salivary gland (duct) K11.8
  sphincter ani K62.89
  stomach K31.89
    acute K31.0
    psychogenic F45.8
  submaxillary duct K11.8
  trachea, congenital Q32.1
  ureter (idiopathic) N28.82
    congenital Q62.2
    due to obstruction N13.4
  urethra (acquired) N36.8
  vasomotor I73.9
  vein I86.8
  ventricular, ventricle (acute) (chronic) (*see also* Hypertrophy, cardiac)
    cerebral, congenital Q04.8
  venule NEC I86.8
  vesical orifice N32.89
Dilated, dilation — *see* Dilatation
Diminished, diminution
  hearing (acuity) — *see* Deafness
  sense or sensation (cold) (heat) (tactile) (vibratory) R20.8
  vision NEC H54.7
  vital capacity R94.2
Diminuta taenia B71.0

Dimitri-Sturge-Weber disease Q85.8
Dimple
  parasacral, pilonidal or postanal — *see* Cyst, pilonidal
Dioctophyme renalis (infection) (infestation) B83.8
Dipetalonemiasis B74.4
Diphallus Q55.69
Diphtheria, diphtheritic (gangrenous) (hemorrhagic) A36.9
  carrier (suspected) Z22.2
  cutaneous A36.3
  faucial A36.0
  infection of wound A36.3
  laryngeal A36.2
  myocarditis A36.81
  nasal, anterior A36.89
  nasopharyngeal A36.1
  neurological complication A36.89
  pharyngeal A36.0
  specified site NEC A36.89
  tonsillar A36.0
Diphyllobothriasis (intestine) B70.0
  larval B70.1
Diplacusis H93.22- ☑
Diplegia (upper limbs) G83.0
  congenital (cerebral) G80.8
  facial G51.0
  lower limbs G82.20
  spastic G80.1
Diplococcus, diplococcal — *see* condition
Diplopia H53.2
Dipsomania F10.20
  with
    psychosis — *see* Psychosis, alcoholic
    remission F10.21
Dipylidiasis B71.1
Direction, teeth, abnormal, fully erupted M26.30
Dirofilariasis B74.8
Dirt-eating child F98.3
Disability, disabilities
  heart — *see* Disease, heart
  intellectual F79
    with
      autistic features F84.9
    mild (I.Q. 50-69) F70
    moderate (I.Q. 35-49) F71
    profound (I.Q. under 20) F73
    severe (I.Q. 20-34) F72
    specified level NEC F78
  knowledge acquisition F81.9
  learning F81.9
  limiting activities Z73.6
  spelling, specific F81.81
Disappearance of family member Z63.4
Disarticulation — *see* Amputation
  meaning traumatic amputation — *see* Amputation, traumatic
Discharge (from)
  abnormal finding in — *see* Abnormal, specimen
  breast (female) (male) N64.52
  diencephalic autonomic idiopathic — *see* Epilepsy, specified NEC
  ear (*see also* Otorrhea)
    blood — *see* Otorrhagia
  excessive urine R35.8
  nipple N64.52
  penile R36.9
  postnasal R09.82
  prison, anxiety concerning Z65.2
  urethral R36.9
    without blood R36.0
    hematospermia R36.1
  vaginal N89.8
Discitis, diskitis M46.40
  cervical region M46.42
  cervicothoracic region M46.43
  lumbar region M46.46
  lumbosacral region M46.47
  multiple sites M46.49
  occipito-atlanto-axial region M46.41
  pyogenic — *see* Infection, intervertebral disc, pyogenic
  sacrococcygeal region M46.48
  thoracic region M46.44
  thoracolumbar region M46.45
Discoid
  meniscus (congenital) Q68.6
  semilunar cartilage (congenital) — *see* Derangement, knee, meniscus, specified NEC

Discoloration
  nails L60.8
  teeth (posteruptive) K03.7
    during formation K00.8
Discomfort
  chest R07.89
  visual H53.14- ☑
Discontinuity, ossicles, ear H74.2- ☑
Discord (with)
  boss Z56.4
  classmates Z55.4
  counselor Z64.4
  employer Z56.4
  family Z63.8
  fellow employees Z56.4
  in-laws Z63.1
  landlord Z59.2
  lodgers Z59.2
  neighbors Z59.2
  probation officer Z64.4
  social worker Z64.4
  teachers Z55.4
  workmates Z56.4
Discordant connection
  atrioventricular (congenital) Q20.5
  ventriculoarterial Q20.3
Discrepancy
  centric occlusion maximum intercuspation M26.55
  leg length (acquired) — *see* Deformity, limb, unequal length
    congenital — *see* Defect, reduction, lower limb
  uterine size date O26.84- ☑
Discrimination
  ethnic Z60.5
  political Z60.5
  racial Z60.5
  religious Z60.5
  sex Z60.5
Disease, diseased (*see also* Syndrome)
  absorbent system I87.8
  acid-peptic K30
  Acosta's T70.29 ☑
  Adams-Stokes (-Morgagni) (syncope with heart block) I45.9
  Addison's anemia (pernicious) D51.0
  adenoids (and tonsils) J35.9
  adrenal (capsule) (cortex) (gland) (medullary) E27.9
    hyperfunction E27.0
    specified NEC E27.8
  ainhum L94.6
  airway
    obstructive, chronic J44.9
      due to
        cotton dust J66.0
        specific organic dusts NEC J66.8
    reactive — *see* Asthma
  akamushi (scrub typhus) A75.3
  Albers-Schönberg (marble bones) Q78.2
  Albert's — *see* Tendinitis, Achilles
  alimentary canal K63.9
  alligator-skin Q80.9
    acquired L85.0
  alpha heavy chain C88.3
  alpine T70.29 ☑
  altitude T70.20 ☑
  alveolar ridge
    edentulous K06.9
      specified NEC K06.8
  alveoli, teeth K08.9
  Alzheimer's G30.9 [F02.80]
    with behavioral disturbance G30.9 [F02.81]
    early onset G30.0 [F02.80]
      with behavioral disturbance G30.0 [F02.81]
    late onset G30.1 [F02.80]
      with behavioral disturbance G30.1 [F02.81]
    specified NEC G30.8 [F02.80]
      with behavioral disturbance G30.8 [F02.81]
  amyloid — *see* Amyloidosis
  Andersen's (glycogenosis IV) E74.09
  Andes T70.29 ☑
  Andrews' (bacterid) L08.89
  angiospastic I73.9
    cerebral G45.9
    vein I87.8
  anterior
    chamber H21.9
    horn cell G12.20

Disease, diseased — *continued*
- antiglomerular basement membrane (anti-GBM) antibody M31.0
  - tubulo-interstitial nephritis N12
- antral — *see* Sinusitis, maxillary
- anus K62.9
  - specified NEC K62.89
- aorta (nonsyphilitic) I77.9
  - syphilitic NEC A52.02
- aortic (heart) (valve) I35.9
  - rheumatic I06.9
- Apollo B30.3
- aponeuroses — *see* Enthesopathy
- appendix K38.9
  - specified NEC K38.8
- aqueous (chamber) H21.9
- Arnold-Chiari — *see* Arnold-Chiari disease
- arterial I77.9
  - occlusive — *see* Occlusion, by site
    - due to stricture or stenosis I77.1
- arteriocardiorenal — *see* Hypertension, cardiorenal
- arteriolar (generalized) (obliterative) I77.9
- arteriorenal — *see* Hypertension, kidney
- arteriosclerotic (*see also* Arteriosclerosis)
  - cardiovascular — *see* Disease, heart, ischemic, atherosclerotic
  - coronary (artery) — *see* Disease, heart, ischemic, atherosclerotic
  - heart — *see* Disease, heart, ischemic, atherosclerotic
- artery I77.9
  - cerebral I67.9
  - coronary I25.10
    - with angina pectoris — *see* Arteriosclerosis, coronary (artery)
- arthropod-borne NOS (viral) A94
  - specified type NEC A93.8
- atticoantral, chronic H66.20
  - left H66.22
    - with right H66.23
  - right H66.21
    - with left H66.23
- auditory canal — *see* Disorder, ear, external
- auricle, ear NEC — *see* Disorder, pinna
- Australian X A83.4
- autoimmune (systemic) NOS M35.9
  - hemolytic (cold type) (warm type) D59.1
    - drug-induced D59.0
  - thyroid E06.3
- aviator's — *see* Effect, adverse, high altitude
- Ayala's Q78.5
- Ayerza's (pulmonary artery sclerosis with pulmonary hypertension) I27.0
- Babington's (familial hemorrhagic telangiectasia) I78.0
- bacterial A49.9
  - specified NEC A48.8
  - zoonotic A28.9
    - specified type NEC A28.8
- Baelz's (cheilitis glandularis apostematosa) K13.0
- bagasse J67.1
- balloon — *see* Effect, adverse, high altitude
- Bang's (brucella abortus) A23.1
- Bannister's T78.3 ☑
- barometer makers' — *see* Poisoning, mercury
- Barraquer (-Simons') (progressive lipodystrophy) E88.1
- Barrett's — *see* Barrett's, esophagus
- Bartholin's gland N75.9
- basal ganglia G25.9
  - degenerative G23.9
    - specified NEC G23.8
  - specified NEC G25.89
- Basedow's (exophthalmic goiter) — *see* Hyperthyroidism, with, goiter (diffuse)
- Bateman's B08.1
- Batten-Steinert G71.11
- Battey A31.0
- Beard's (neurasthenia) F48.8
- Becker
  - idiopathic mural endomyocardial I42.3
  - myotonia congenita G71.12
- Begbie's (exophthalmic goiter) — *see* Hyperthyroidism, with, goiter (diffuse)
- behavioral, organic F07.9
- Beigel's (white piedra) B36.2
- Benson's — *see* Deposit, crystalline
- Bernard-Soulier (thrombopathy) D69.1
- Bernhardt (-Roth) — *see* Mononeuropathy, lower limb, meralgia paresthetica

Disease, diseased — *continued*
- Biermer's (pernicious anemia) D51.0
- bile duct (common) (hepatic) K83.9
  - with calculus, stones — *see* Calculus, bile duct
  - specified NEC K83.8
- biliary (tract) K83.9
  - specified NEC K83.8
- Billroth's — *see* Spina bifida
- bird fancier's J67.2
- black lung J60
- bladder N32.9
  - in (due to)
    - schistosomiasis (bilharziasis) B65.0 [N33]
  - specified NEC N32.89
- bleeder's D66
- blood D75.9
  - forming organs D75.9
  - vessel I99.9
- Bloodgood's — *see* Mastopathy, cystic
- Bodechtel-Guttmann (subacute sclerosing panencephalitis) A81.1
- bone (*see also* Disorder, bone)
  - aluminum M83.4
  - fibrocystic NEC
    - jaw M27.49
- bone-marrow D75.9
- Borna A83.9
- Bornholm (epidemic pleurodynia) B33.0
- Bouchard's (myopathic dilatation of the stomach) K31.0
- Bouillaud's (rheumatic heart disease) I01.9
- Bourneville (-Brissaud) (tuberous sclerosis) Q85.1
- Bouveret (-Hoffmann) (paroxysmal tachycardia) I47.9
- bowel K63.9
  - functional K59.9
    - psychogenic F45.8
- brain G93.9
  - arterial, artery I67.9
  - arteriosclerotic I67.2
  - congenital Q04.9
  - degenerative — *see* Degeneration, brain
  - inflammatory — *see* Encephalitis
  - organic G93.9
    - arteriosclerotic I67.2
  - parasitic NEC B71.9 [G94]
  - senile NEC G31.1
  - specified NEC G93.89
- breast (*see also* Disorder, breast) N64.9
  - cystic (chronic) — *see* Mastopathy, cystic
  - fibrocystic — *see* Mastopathy, cystic
  - Paget's
    - female, unspecified side C50.91- ☑
    - male, unspecified side C50.92- ☑
  - specified NEC N64.89
- Breda's — *see* Yaws
- Bretonneau's (diphtheritic malignant angina) A36.0
- Bright's — *see* Nephritis
  - arteriosclerotic — *see* Hypertension, kidney
- Brill's (recrudescent typhus) A75.1
- Brill-Zinsser (recrudescent typhus) A75.1
- Brion-Kayser — *see* Fever, paratyphoid
- broad
  - beta E78.2
  - ligament (noninflammatory) N83.9
    - inflammatory — *see* Disease, pelvis, inflammatory
    - specified NEC N83.8
- Brocq-Duhring (dermatitis herpetiformis) L13.0
- Brocq's
  - meaning
    - dermatitis herpetiformis L13.0
    - prurigo L28.2
- bronchopulmonary J98.4
- bronchus NEC J98.09
- bronze Addison's E27.1
  - tuberculous A18.7
- budgerigar fancier's J67.2
- Buerger's (thromboangiitis obliterans) I73.1
- bullous L13.9
  - chronic of childhood L12.2
  - specified NEC L13.8
- Bürger-Grütz (essential familial hyperlipemia) E78.3
- bursa — *see* Bursopathy
- caisson T70.3 ☑
- California — *see* Coccidioidomycosis
- capillaries I78.9
  - specified NEC I78.8
- Carapata A68.0

Disease, diseased — *continued*
- cardiac — *see* Disease, heart
- cardiopulmonary, chronic I27.9
- cardiorenal (hepatic) (hypertensive) (vascular) — *see* Hypertension, cardiorenal
- cardiovascular (atherosclerotic) I25.10
  - with angina pectoris — *see* Arteriosclerosis, coronary (artery),
  - congenital Q28.9
  - hypertensive — *see* Hypertension, heart
  - newborn P29.9
    - specified NEC P29.89
  - renal (hypertensive) — *see* Hypertension, cardiorenal
  - syphilitic (asymptomatic) A52.00
- cartilage — *see* Disorder, cartilage
- Castellani's A69.8
- cat-scratch A28.1
- Cavare's (familial periodic paralysis) G72.3
- cecum K63.9
- celiac (adult) (infantile) K90.0
- cellular tissue L98.9
- central core G71.2
- cerebellar, cerebellum — *see* Disease, brain
- cerebral (*see also* Disease, brain)
  - degenerative — *see* Degeneration, brain
- cerebrospinal G96.9
- cerebrovascular I67.9
  - acute I67.89
    - embolic I63.4- ☑
    - thrombotic I63.3- ☑
  - arteriosclerotic I67.2
  - specified NEC I67.89
- cervix (uteri) (noninflammatory) N88.9
  - inflammatory — *see* Cervicitis
  - specified NEC N88.8
- Chabert's A22.9
- Chandler's (osteochondritis dissecans, hip) — *see* Osteochondritis, dissecans, hip
- Charlouis — *see* Yaws
- Chédiak-Steinbrinck (-Higashi) (congenital gigantism of peroxidase granules) E70.330
- chest J98.9
- Chiari's (hepatic vein thrombosis) I82.0
- Chicago B40.9
- Chignon B36.8
- chigo, chigoe B88.1
- childhood granulomatous D71
- Chinese liver fluke B66.1
- chlamydial A74.9
  - specified NEC A74.89
- cholecystic K82.9
- choroid H31.9
  - specified NEC H31.8
- Christmas D67
- chronic bullous of childhood L12.2
- chylomicron retention E78.3
- ciliary body H21.9
  - specified NEC H21.89
- circulatory (system) NEC I99.8
  - newborn P29.9
  - syphilitic A52.00
    - congenital A50.54
- coagulation factor deficiency (congenital) — *see* Defect, coagulation
- coccidioidal — *see* Coccidioidomycosis
- cold
  - agglutinin or hemoglobinuria D59.1
    - paroxysmal D59.6
  - hemagglutinin (chronic) D59.1
- collagen NOS (nonvascular) (vascular) M35.9
  - specified NEC M35.8
- colon K63.9
  - functional K59.9
    - congenital Q43.2
  - ischemic K55.0
- combined system — *see* Degeneration, combined
- compressed air T70.3 ☑
- Concato's (pericardial polyserositis) A19.9
  - nontubercular I31.1
  - pleural — *see* Pleurisy, with effusion
- conjunctiva H11.9
  - chlamydial A74.0
  - specified NEC H11.89
  - viral B30.9
    - specified NEC B30.8

Disease, diseased — *continued*
- connective tissue, systemic (diffuse) M35.9
  - in (due to)
    - hypogammaglobulinemia D80.1 [M36.8]
    - ochronosis E70.29 [M36.8]
  - specified NEC M35.8
- Conor and Bruch's (boutonneuse fever) A77.1
- Cooper's — *see* Mastopathy, cystic
- Cori's (glycogenosis III) E74.03
- corkhandler's or corkworker's J67.3
- cornea H18.9
  - specified NEC H18.89- ☑
- coronary (artery) — *see* Disease, heart, ischemic, atherosclerotic
  - congenital Q24.5
  - ostial, syphilitic (aortic) (mitral) (pulmonary) A52.03
- corpus cavernosum N48.9
  - specified NEC N48.89
- Cotugno's — *see* Sciatica
- coxsackie (virus) NEC B34.1
- cranial nerve NOS G52.9
- Creutzfeldt-Jakob — *see* Creutzfeldt-Jakob disease or syndrome
- Crocq's (acrocyanosis) I73.89
- Crohn's — *see* Enteritis, regional
- Curschmann G71.11
- cystic
  - breast (chronic) — *see* Mastopathy, cystic
  - kidney, congenital Q61.9
  - liver, congenital Q44.6
  - lung J98.4
    - congenital Q33.0
- cytomegalic inclusion (generalized) B25.9
  - with pneumonia B25.0
  - congenital P35.1
- cytomegaloviral B25.9
  - specified NEC B25.8
- Czerny's (periodic hydrarthrosis of the knee) — *see* Effusion, joint, knee
- Daae (-Finsen) (epidemic pleurodynia) B33.0
- Darling's — *see* Histoplasmosis capsulati
- de Quervain's (tendon sheath) M65.4
  - thyroid (subacute granulomatous thyroiditis) E06.1
- Débove's (splenomegaly) R16.1
- deer fly — *see* Tularemia
- Degos' I77.89
- demyelinating, demyelinizating (nervous system) G37.9
  - multiple sclerosis G35
  - specified NEC G37.8
- dense deposit (*see also* N00-N07 with fourth character .6) N05.6
- deposition, hydroxyapatite — *see* Disease, hydroxyapatite deposition
- Devergie's (pityriasis rubra pilaris) L44.0
- Devic's G36.0
- diaphorase deficiency D74.0
- diaphragm J98.6
- diarrheal, infectious NEC A09
- digestive system K92.9
  - specified NEC K92.89
- disc, degenerative — *see* Degeneration, intervertebral disc
- discogenic (*see also* Displacement, intervertebral disc NEC)
  - with myelopathy — *see* Disorder, disc, with, myelopathy
- diverticular — *see* Diverticula
- Dubois (thymus) A50.59 [E35]
- Duchenne-Griesinger G71.0
- Duchenne's
  - muscular dystrophy G71.0
  - pseudohypertrophy, muscles G71.0
- ductless glands E34.9
- Duhring's (dermatitis herpetiformis) L13.0
- duodenum K31.9
  - specified NEC K31.89
- Dupré's (meningism) R29.1
- Dupuytren's (muscle contracture) M72.0
- Durand-Nicholas-Favre (climatic bubo) A55
- Duroziez's (congenital mitral stenosis) Q23.2
- ear — *see* Disorder, ear
- Eberth's — *see* Fever, typhoid
- Ebola (virus) A98.4
- Ebstein's heart Q22.5
- Echinococcus — *see* Echinococcus
- echovirus NEC B34.1
- Eddowes' (brittle bones and blue sclera) Q78.0

Disease, diseased — *continued*
- edentulous (alveolar) ridge K06.9
  - specified NEC K06.8
- Edsall's T67.2 ☑
- Eichstedt's (pityriasis versicolor) B36.0
- Ellis-van Creveld (chondroectodermal dysplasia) Q77.6
- end stage renal (ESRD) N18.6
  - due to hypertension I12.0
- endocrine glands or system NEC E34.9
- endomyocardial (eosinophilic) I42.3
- English (rickets) E55.0
- enteroviral, enterovirus NEC B34.1
  - central nervous system NEC A88.8
- epidemic B99.9
  - specified NEC B99.8
- epididymis N50.9
- Erb (-Landouzy) G71.0
- Erdheim-Chester (ECD) E88.89
- esophagus K22.9
  - functional K22.4
  - psychogenic F45.8
  - specified NEC K22.8
- Eulenburg's (congenital paramyotonia) G71.19
- eustachian tube — *see* Disorder, eustachian tube
- external
  - auditory canal — *see* Disorder, ear, external
  - ear — *see* Disorder, ear, external
- extrapyramidal G25.9
  - specified NEC G25.89
- eye H57.9
  - anterior chamber H21.9
  - inflammatory NEC H57.8
  - muscle (external) — *see* Strabismus
  - specified NEC H57.8
  - syphilitic — *see* Oculopathy, syphilitic
- eyeball H44.9
  - specified NEC H44.89
- eyelid — *see* Disorder, eyelid
  - specified NEC — *see* Disorder, eyelid, specified type NEC
- eyeworm of Africa B74.3
- facial nerve (seventh) G51.9
  - newborn (birth injury) P11.3
- Fahr (of brain) G23.8
- Fahr Volhard (of kidney) I12.- ☑
- fallopian tube (noninflammatory) N83.9
  - inflammatory — *see* Salpingo-oophoritis
  - specified NEC N83.8
- familial periodic paralysis G72.3
- Fanconi's (congenital pancytopenia) D61.09
- fascia NEC (*see also* Disorder, muscle)
  - inflammatory — *see* Myositis
  - specified NEC M62.89
- Fauchard's (periodontitis) — *see* Periodontitis
- Favre-Durand-Nicolas (climatic bubo) A55
- Fede's K14.0
- Feer's — *see* Poisoning, mercury
- female pelvic inflammatory (*see also* Disease, pelvis, inflammatory) N73.9
  - syphilitic (secondary) A51.42
  - tuberculous A18.17
- Fernels' (aortic aneurysm) I71.9
- fibrocaseous of lung — *see* Tuberculosis, pulmonary
- fibrocystic — *see* Fibrocystic disease
- Fiedler's (leptospiral jaundice) A27.0
- fifth B08.3
- file-cutter's — *see* Poisoning, lead
- fish-skin Q80.9
  - acquired L85.0
- Flajani (-Basedow) (exophthalmic goiter) — *see* Hyperthyroidism, with, goiter (diffuse)
- flax-dresser's J66.1
- fluke — *see* Infestation, fluke
- foot and mouth B08.8
- foot process N04.9
- Forbes' (glycogenosis III) E74.03
- Fordyce-Fox (apocrine miliaria) L75.2
- Fordyce's (ectopic sebaceous glands) (mouth) Q38.6
- Forestier's (rhizomelic pseudopolyarthritis) M35.3
  - meaning ankylosing hyperostosis — *see* Hyperostosis, ankylosing
- Fothergill's
  - neuralgia — *see* Neuralgia, trigeminal
  - scarlatina anginosa A38.9
- Fournier (gangrene) N49.3
  - female N76.89
- fourth B08.8
- Fox (-Fordyce) (apocrine miliaria) L75.2

Disease, diseased — *continued*
- Francis' — *see* Tularemia
- Franklin C88.2
- Frei's (climatic bubo) A55
- Friedreich's
  - combined systemic or ataxia G11.1
  - myoclonia G25.3
- frontal sinus — *see* Sinusitis, frontal
- fungus NEC B49
- Gaisböck's (polycythemia hypertonica) D75.1
- gallbladder K82.9
  - calculus — *see* Calculus, gallbladder
  - cholecystitis — *see* Cholecystitis
  - cholesterolosis K82.4
  - fistula — *see* Fistula, gallbladder
  - hydrops K82.1
  - obstruction — *see* Obstruction, gallbladder
  - perforation K82.2
  - specified NEC K82.8
- gamma heavy chain C88.2
- Gamna's (siderotic splenomegaly) D73.2
- Gamstorp's (adynamia episodica hereditaria) G72.3
- Gandy-Nanta (siderotic splenomegaly) D73.2
- ganister J62.8
- gastric — *see* Disease, stomach
- gastroesophageal reflux (GERD) K21.9
  - with esophagitis K21.0
- gastrointestinal (tract) K92.9
  - amyloid E85.4
  - functional K59.9
    - psychogenic F45.8
  - specified NEC K92.89
- Gee (-Herter) (-Heubner) (-Thaysen) (nontropical sprue) K90.0
- genital organs
  - female N94.9
  - male N50.9
- Gerhardt's (erythromelalgia) I73.81
- Gibert's (pityriasis rosea) L42
- Gierke's (glycogenosis I) E74.01
- Gilles de la Tourette's (motor-verbal tic) F95.2
- gingiva K06.9
  - specified NEC K06.8
- gland (lymph) I89.9
- Glanzmann's (hereditary hemorrhagic thrombasthenia) D69.1
- glass-blower's (cataract) — *see* Cataract, specified NEC
  - salivary gland hypertrophy K11.1
- Glisson's — *see* Rickets
- globe H44.9
  - specified NEC H44.89
- glomerular (*see also* Glomerulonephritis)
  - with edema — *see* Nephrosis
  - acute — *see* Nephritis, acute
  - chronic — *see* Nephritis, chronic
  - minimal change N05.0
  - rapidly progressive N01.9
- glycogen storage E74.00
  - Andersen's E74.09
  - Cori's E74.03
  - Forbes' E74.03
  - generalized E74.00
  - glucose-6-phosphatase deficiency E74.01
  - heart E74.02 [I43]
  - hepatorenal E74.09
  - Hers' E74.09
  - liver and kidney E74.09
  - McArdle's E74.04
  - muscle phosphofructokinase E74.09
  - myocardium E74.02 [I43]
  - Pompe's E74.02
  - Tauri's E74.09
  - type 0 E74.09
  - type I E74.01
  - type II E74.02
  - type III E74.03
  - type IV E74.09
  - type V E74.04
  - type VI-XI E74.09
  - Von Gierke's E74.01
- Goldstein's (familial hemorrhagic telangiectasia) I78.0
- gonococcal NOS A54.9
- graft-versus-host (GVH) D89.813
  - acute D89.810
  - acute on chronic D89.812
  - chronic D89.811
- grainhandler's J67.8
- granulomatous (childhood) (chronic) D71

▽ Subterms under main terms may continue to next column or page　　　☑ Additional Character Required — Refer to the Tabular List for Character Selection　　　**99**

Disease, diseased — *continued*
  Graves' (exophthalmic goiter) — *see* Hyperthyroidism, with, goiter (diffuse)
  Griesinger's — *see* Ancylostomiasis
  Grisel's M43.6
  Gruby's (tinea tonsurans) B35.0
  Guillain-Barré G61.0
  Guinon's (motor-verbal tic) F95.2
  gum K06.9
  gynecological N94.9
  H (Hartnup's) E72.02
  Haff — *see* Poisoning, mercury
  Hageman (congenital factor XII deficiency) D68.2
  hair (color) (shaft) L67.9
    follicles L73.9
      specified NEC L73.8
  Hamman's (spontaneous mediastinal emphysema) J98.2
  hand, foot and mouth B08.4
  Hansen's — *see* Leprosy
  Hantavirus, with pulmonary manifestations B33.4
    with renal manifestations A98.5
  Harada's H30.81- ☑
  Hartnup (pellagra-cerebellar ataxia-renal aminoaciduria) E72.02
  Hart's (pellagra-cerebellar ataxia-renal aminoaciduria) E72.02
  Hashimoto's (struma lymphomatosa) E06.3
  Hb — *see* Disease, hemoglobin
  heart (organic) I51.9
    with
      pulmonary edema (acute) (*see also* Failure, ventricular, left) I50.1
      rheumatic fever (conditions in I00)
        active I01.9
          with chorea I02.0
          specified NEC I01.8
        inactive or quiescent (with chorea) I09.9
          specified NEC I09.89
    amyloid E85.4 [I43]
    aortic (valve) I35.9
    arteriosclerotic or sclerotic (senile) — *see* Disease, heart, ischemic, atherosclerotic
    artery, arterial — *see* Disease, heart, ischemic, atherosclerotic
    beer drinkers' I42.6
    beriberi (wet) E51.12
    black I27.0
    congenital Q24.9
      cyanotic Q24.9
      specified NEC Q24.8
    coronary — *see* Disease, heart, ischemic
    cryptogenic I51.9
    fibroid — *see* Myocarditis
    functional I51.89
      psychogenic F45.8
    glycogen storage E74.02 [I43]
    gonococcal A54.83
    hypertensive — *see* Hypertension, heart
    hyperthyroid (*see also* Hyperthyroidism) E05.90 [I43]
      with thyroid storm E05.91 [I43]
    ischemic (chronic or with a stated duration of over 4 weeks) I25.9
      atherosclerotic (of) I25.10
        with angina pectoris — *see* Arteriosclerosis, coronary (artery)
        coronary artery bypass graft — *see* Arteriosclerosis, coronary (artery),
      cardiomyopathy I25.5
      diagnosed on ECG or other special investigation, but currently presenting no symptoms I25.6
      silent I25.6
      specified form NEC I25.89
    kyphoscoliotic I27.1
    meningococcal A39.50
      endocarditis A39.51
      myocarditis A39.52
      pericarditis A39.53
    mitral I05.9
      specified NEC I05.8
    muscular — *see* Degeneration, myocardial
    psychogenic (functional) F45.8
    pulmonary (chronic) I27.9
      in schistosomiasis B65.9 [I52]
      specified NEC I27.89

Disease, diseased — *continued*
  heart — *continued*
    rheumatic (chronic) (inactive) (old) (quiescent) (with chorea) I09.9
      active or acute I01.9
        with chorea (acute) (rheumatic) (Sydenham's) I02.0
      specified NEC I09.89
    senile — *see* Myocarditis
    syphilitic A52.06
      aortic A52.03
        aneurysm A52.01
      congenital A50.54 [I52]
    thyrotoxic (*see also* Thyrotoxicosis) E05.90 [I43]
      with thyroid storm E05.91 [I43]
    valve, valvular (obstructive) (regurgitant) (*see also* Endocarditis)
      congenital NEC Q24.8
        pulmonary Q22.3
    vascular — *see* Disease, cardiovascular
  heavy chain NEC C88.2
    alpha C88.3
    gamma C88.2
    mu C88.2
  Hebra's
    pityriasis
      maculata et circinata L42
      rubra pilaris L44.0
    prurigo L28.2
  hematopoietic organs D75.9
  hemoglobin or Hb
    abnormal (mixed) NEC D58.2
      with thalassemia D56.9
    AS genotype D57.3
    Bart's D56.0
    C (Hb-C) D58.2
      with other abnormal hemoglobin NEC D58.2
      elliptocytosis D58.1
      Hb-S D57.2- ☑
      sickle-cell D57.2- ☑
      thalassemia D56.8
    Constant Spring D58.2
    D (Hb-D) D58.2
    E (Hb-E) D58.2
    E-beta thalassemia D56.5
    elliptocytosis D58.1
    H (Hb-H) (thalassemia) D56.0
      with other abnormal hemoglobin NEC D56.9
      Constant Spring D56.0
    I thalassemia D56.9
    M D74.0
    S or SS D57.1
    SC D57.2- ☑
    SD D57.8- ☑
    SE D57.8- ☑
    spherocytosis D58.0
    unstable, hemolytic D58.2
  hemolytic (newborn) P55.9
    autoimmune (cold type) (warm type) D59.1
    drug-induced D59.0
    due to or with
      incompatibility
        ABO (blood group) P55.1
        blood (group) (Duffy) (K(ell)) (Kidd) (Lewis) (M) (S) NEC P55.8
        Rh (blood group) (factor) P55.0
          Rh negative mother P55.0
    specified type NEC P55.8
    unstable hemoglobin D58.2
  hemorrhagic D69.9
    newborn P53
  Henoch (-Schönlein) (purpura nervosa) D69.0
  hepatic — *see* Disease, liver
  hepatolenticular E83.01
  heredodegenerative NEC
    spinal cord G95.89
  herpesviral, disseminated B00.7
  Hers' (glycogenosis VI) E74.09
  Herter (-Gee) (-Heubner) (nontropical sprue) K90.0
  Heubner-Herter (nontropical sprue) K90.0
  high fetal gene or hemoglobin thalassemia D56.9
  Hildenbrand's — *see* Typhus
  hip (joint) M25.9
    congenital Q65.89
    suppurative M00.9
    tuberculous A18.02
  His (-Werner) (trench fever) A79.0

Disease, diseased — *continued*
  Hodgson's I71.2
    ruptured I71.1
  Holla — *see* Spherocytosis
  hookworm B76.9
    specified NEC B76.8
  host-versus-graft D89.813
    acute D89.810
    acute on chronic D89.812
    chronic D89.811
  human immunodeficiency virus (HIV) B20
  Huntington's G10
  Hutchinson's (cheiropompholyx) — *see* Hutchinson's disease
  hyaline (diffuse) (generalized)
    membrane (lung) (newborn) P22.0
      adult J80
  hydatid — *see* Echinococcus
  hydroxyapatite deposition M11.00
    ankle M11.07- ☑
    elbow M11.02- ☑
    foot joint M11.07- ☑
    hand joint M11.04- ☑
    hip M11.05- ☑
    knee M11.06- ☑
    multiple site M11.09
    shoulder M11.01- ☑
    vertebra M11.08
    wrist M11.03- ☑
  hyperkinetic — *see* Hyperkinesia
  hypertensive — *see* Hypertension
  hypophysis E23.7
  Iceland G93.3
  I-cell E77.0
  immune D89.9
  immunoproliferative (malignant) C88.9
    small intestinal C88.3
    specified NEC C88.8
  inclusion B25.9
    salivary gland B25.9
  infectious, infective B99.9
    congenital P37.9
      specified NEC P37.8
      viral P35.9
        specified type NEC P35.8
    specified NEC B99.8
  inflammatory
    penis N48.29
      abscess N48.21
      cellulitis N48.22
    prepuce N47.7
      balanoposthitis N47.6
    tubo-ovarian — *see* Salpingo-oophoritis
  intervertebral disc (*see also* Disorder, disc)
    with myelopathy — *see* Disorder, disc, with, myelopathy
    cervical, cervicothoracic — *see* Disorder, disc, cervical
      with
        myelopathy — *see* Disorder, disc, cervical, with myelopathy
        neuritis, radiculitis or radiculopathy — *see* Disorder, disc, cervical, with neuritis
        specified NEC — *see* Disorder, disc, cervical, specified type NEC
    lumbar (with)
      myelopathy M51.06
      neuritis, radiculitis, radiculopathy or sciatica M51.16
      specified NEC M51.86
    lumbosacral (with)
      neuritis, radiculitis, radiculopathy or sciatica M51.17
      specified NEC M51.87
    specified NEC — *see* Disorder, disc, specified NEC
    thoracic (with)
      myelopathy M51.04
      neuritis, radiculitis or radiculopathy M51.14
      specified NEC M51.84
    thoracolumbar (with)
      myelopathy M51.05
      neuritis, radiculitis or radiculopathy M51.15
      specified NEC M51.85
  intestine K63.9
    functional K59.9
      psychogenic F45.8
      specified NEC K59.8
    organic K63.9

Disease, diseased — *continued*
  intestine — *continued*
    protozoal A07.9
    specified NEC K63.89
  iris H21.9
    specified NEC H21.89
  iron metabolism or storage E83.10
  island (scrub typhus) A75.3
  itai-itai — *see* Poisoning, cadmium
  Jakob-Creutzfeldt — *see* Creutzfeldt-Jakob disease or syndrome
  jaw M27.9
    fibrocystic M27.49
    specified NEC M27.8
  jigger B88.1
  joint (*see also* Disorder, joint)
    Charcot's — *see* Arthropathy, neuropathic (Charcot)
    degenerative — *see* Osteoarthritis
      multiple M15.9
      spine — *see* Spondylosis
    hypertrophic — *see* Osteoarthritis
    sacroiliac M53.3
    specified NEC — *see* Disorder, joint, specified type NEC
    spine NEC — *see* Dorsopathy
    suppurative — *see* Arthritis, pyogenic or pyemic
  Jourdain's (acute gingivitis) K05.00
    nonplaque induced K05.01
    plaque induced K05.00
  Kaschin-Beck (endemic polyarthritis) M12.10
    ankle M12.17- ☑
    elbow M12.12- ☑
    foot joint M12.17- ☑
    hand joint M12.14- ☑
    hip M12.15- ☑
    knee M12.16- ☑
    multiple site M12.19
    shoulder M12.11- ☑
    vertebra M12.18
    wrist M12.13- ☑
  Katayama B65.2
  Kedani (scrub typhus) A75.3
  Keshan E59
  kidney (functional) (pelvis) N28.9
    chronic N18.9
      hypertensive — *see* Hypertension, kidney
      stage 1 N18.1
      stage 2 (mild) N18.2
      stage 3 (moderate) N18.3
      stage 4 (severe) N18.4
      stage 5 N18.5
    complicating pregnancy — *see* Pregnancy, complicated by, renal disease
    cystic (congenital) Q61.9
    fibrocystic (congenital) Q61.8
    hypertensive — *see* Hypertension, kidney
    in (due to)
      schistosomiasis (bilharziasis) B65.9 [N29]
    multicystic Q61.4
    polycystic Q61.3
      adult type Q61.2
      childhood type NEC Q61.19
        collecting duct dilatation Q61.11
  Kimmelstiel (-Wilson) (intercapillary polycystic (congenital) glomerulosclerosis) — *see* E08-E13 with .21
  Kinnier Wilson's (hepatolenticular degeneration) E83.01
  kissing — *see* Mononucleosis, infectious
  Klebs' (*see also* Glomerulonephritis) N05- ☑
  Klippel-Feil (brevicollis) Q76.1
  Köhler-Pellegrini-Stieda (calcification, knee joint) — *see* Bursitis, tibial collateral
  Kok Q89.8
  König's (osteochondritis dissecans) — *see* Osteochondritis, dissecans
  Korsakoff's (nonalcoholic) F04
    alcoholic F10.96
      with dependence F10.26
  Kostmann's (infantile genetic agranulocytosis) D70.0
  kuru A81.81
  Kyasanur Forest A98.2
  labyrinth, ear — *see* Disorder, ear, inner
  lacrimal system — *see* Disorder, lacrimal system
  Lafora's — *see* Epilepsy, generalized, idiopathic
  Lancereaux-Mathieu (leptospiral jaundice) A27.0
  Landry's G61.0

Disease, diseased — *continued*
  Larrey-Weil (leptospiral jaundice) A27.0
  larynx J38.7
  legionnaires' A48.1
    nonpneumonic A48.2
  Lenegre's I44.2
  lens H27.9
    specified NEC H27.8
  Lev's (acquired complete heart block) I44.2
  Lewy body (dementia) G31.83 [F02.80]
    with behavioral disturbance G31.83 [F02.81]
  Lichtheim's (subacute combined sclerosis with pernicious anemia) D51.0
  Lightwood's (renal tubular acidosis) N25.89
  Lignac's (cystinosis) E72.04
  lip K13.0
  lipid-storage E75.6
    specified NEC E75.5
  Lipschütz's N76.6
  liver (chronic) (organic) K76.9
    alcoholic (chronic) K70.9
      acute — *see* Disease, liver, alcoholic, hepatitis
      cirrhosis K70.30
        with ascites K70.31
      failure K70.40
        with coma K70.41
      fatty liver K70.0
      fibrosis K70.2
      hepatitis K70.10
        with ascites K70.11
      sclerosis K70.2
    cystic, congenital Q44.6
    drug-induced (idiosyncratic) (toxic) (predictable) (unpredictable) — *see* Disease, liver, toxic
    end stage K72.90
      due to hepatitis — *see* Hepatitis
    fatty, nonalcoholic (NAFLD) K76.0
      alcoholic K70.0
    fibrocystic (congenital) Q44.6
    fluke
      Chinese B66.1
      oriental B66.1
      sheep B66.3
    glycogen storage E74.09 [K77]
    in (due to)
      schistosomiasis (bilharziasis) B65.9 [K77]
    inflammatory K75.9
      alcoholic K70.1 ☑
      specified NEC K75.89
    polycystic (congenital) Q44.6
    toxic K71.9
      with
        cholestasis K71.0
        cirrhosis (liver) K71.7
        fibrosis (liver) K71.7
        focal nodular hyperplasia K71.8
        hepatic granuloma K71.8
        hepatic necrosis K71.10
          with coma K71.11
        hepatitis NEC K71.6
          acute K71.2
          chronic
            active K71.50
              with ascites K71.51
            lobular K71.4
            persistent K71.3
        lupoid K71.50
          with ascites K71.51
        peliosis hepatis K71.8
        veno-occlusive disease (VOD) of liver K71.8
    veno-occlusive K76.5
  Lobo's (keloid blastomycosis) B48.0
  Lobstein's (brittle bones and blue sclera) Q78.0
  Ludwig's (submaxillary cellulitis) K12.2
  lumbosacral region M53.87
  lung J98.4
    black J60
    congenital Q33.9
    cystic J98.4
      congenital Q33.0
    fibroid (chronic) — *see* Fibrosis, lung
    fluke B66.4
      oriental B66.4
    in
      amyloidosis E85.4 [J99]
      sarcoidosis D86.0
      Sjögren's syndrome M35.02

Disease, diseased — *continued*
  lung — *continued*
    in — *continued*
      systemic
        lupus erythematosus M32.13
        sclerosis M34.81
    interstitial J84.9
      of childhood, specified NEC J84.848
      respiratory bronchiolitis J84.115
      specified NEC J84.89
    obstructive (chronic) J44.9
      with
        acute
          bronchitis J44.0
          exacerbation NEC J44.1
          lower respiratory infection J44.0
        alveolitis, allergic J67.9
        asthma J44.9
        bronchiectasis J47.9
          with
            exacerbation (acute) J47.1
            lower respiratory infection J47.0
        bronchitis J44.9
          with
            exacerbation (acute) J44.1
            lower respiratory infection J44.0
        emphysema J44.9
        hypersensitivity pneumonitis J67.9
      decompensated J44.1
        with
          exacerbation (acute) J44.1
    polycystic J98.4
      congenital Q33.0
    rheumatoid (diffuse) (interstitial) — *see* Rheumatoid, lung
  Lutembacher's (atrial septal defect with mitral stenosis) Q21.1
  Lyme A69.20
  lymphatic (gland) (system) (channel) (vessel) I89.9
  lymphoproliferative D47.9
    specified NEC D47.Z9 (*following* D47.4)
    T-gamma D47.Z9 (*following* D47.4)
    X-linked D82.3
  Magitot's M27.2
  malarial — *see* Malaria
  malignant (*see also* Neoplasm, malignant, by site)
  Manson's B65.1
  maple bark J67.6
  maple-syrup-urine E71.0
  Marburg (virus) A98.3
  Marion's (bladder neck obstruction) N32.0
  Marsh's (exophthalmic goiter) — *see* Hyperthyroidism, with, goiter (diffuse)
  mastoid (process) — *see* Disorder, ear, middle
  Mathieu's (leptospiral jaundice) A27.0
  Maxcy's A75.2
  McArdle (-Schmid-Pearson) (glycogenosis V) E74.04
  mediastinum J98.5
  medullary center (idiopathic) (respiratory) G93.89
  Meige's (chronic hereditary edema) Q82.0
  meningococcal — *see* Infection, meningococcal
  mental F99
    organic F09
  mesenchymal M35.9
  mesenteric embolic K55.0
  metabolic, metabolism E88.9
    bilirubin E80.7
  metal-polisher's J62.8 .
  metastatic (*see also* Neoplasm, secondary, by site) C79.9
  microvascular - code to condition
  microvillus
    atrophy Q43.8
    inclusion (MVD) Q43.8
  middle ear — *see* Disorder, ear, middle
  Mikulicz' (dryness of mouth, absent or decreased lacrimation) K11.8
  Milroy's (chronic hereditary edema) Q82.0
  Minamata — *see* Poisoning, mercury
  minicore G71.2
  Minor's G95.19
  Minot's (hemorrhagic disease, newborn) P53
  Minot-von Willebrand-Jürgens (angiohemophilia) D68.0
  Mitchell's (erythromelalgia) I73.81
  mitral (valve) I05.9
    nonrheumatic I34.9
  mixed connective tissue M35.1

Disease, diseased — *continued*
- moldy hay J67.0
- Monge's T70.29 ☑
- Morgagni-Adams-Stokes (syncope with heart block) I45.9
- Morgagni's (syndrome) (hyperostosis frontalis interna) M85.2
- Morton's (with metatarsalgia) — *see* Lesion, nerve, plantar
- Morvan's G60.8
- motor neuron (bulbar) (familial) (mixed type) (spinal) G12.20
  - amyotrophic lateral sclerosis G12.21
  - progressive bulbar palsy G12.22
  - specified NEC G12.29
- moyamoya I67.5
- mu heavy chain disease C88.2
- multicore G71.2
- muscle (*see also* Disorder, muscle)
  - inflammatory — *see* Myositis
  - ocular (external) — *see* Strabismus
- musculoskeletal system, soft tissue — *see also* Disorder, soft tissue
  - specified NEC — *see* Disorder, soft tissue, specified type NEC
- mushroom workers' J67.5
- mycotic B49
- myelodysplastic, not classified C94.6
- myeloproliferative, not classified C94.6
  - chronic D47.1
- myocardium, myocardial (*see also* Degeneration, myocardial) I51.5
  - primary (idiopathic) I42.9
- myoneural G70.9
- Naegeli's D69.1
- nails L60.9
  - specified NEC L60.8
- Nairobi (sheep virus) A93.8
- nasal J34.9
- nemaline body G71.2
- nerve — *see* Disorder, nerve
- nervous system G98.8
  - autonomic G90.9
  - central G96.9
    - specified NEC G96.8
  - congenital Q07.9
  - parasympathetic G90.9
  - specified NEC G98.8
  - sympathetic G90.9
  - vegetative G90.9
- neuromuscular system G70.9
- Newcastle B30.8
- Nicolas (-Durand)-Favre (climatic bubo) A55
- nipple N64.9
  - Paget's C50.01- ☑
    - female C50.01- ☑
    - male C50.02- ☑
- Nishimoto (-Takeuchi) I67.5
- nonarthropod-borne NOS (viral) B34.9
  - enterovirus NEC B34.1
- nonautoimmune hemolytic D59.4
  - drug-induced D59.2
- Nonne-Milroy-Meige (chronic hereditary edema) Q82.0
- nose J34.9
- nucleus pulposus — *see* Disorder, disc
- nutritional E63.9
- oast-house-urine E72.19
  - ocular
    - herpesviral B00.50
    - zoster B02.30
- obliterative vascular I77.1
- Ohara's — *see* Tularemia
- Opitz's (congestive splenomegaly) D73.2
- Oppenheim-Urbach (necrobiosis lipoidica diabeticorum) — *see* E08-E13 with .620
- optic nerve NEC — *see* Disorder, nerve, optic
- orbit — *see* Disorder, orbit
- Oriental liver fluke B66.1
- Oriental lung fluke B66.4
- Ormond's N13.5
- Oropouche virus A93.0
- Osler-Rendu (familial hemorrhagic telangiectasia) I78.0
- osteofibrocystic E21.0
- Otto's M24.7
- outer ear — *see* Disorder, ear, external
- ovary (noninflammatory) N83.9
  - cystic N83.20
  - inflammatory — *see* Salpingo-oophoritis

Disease, diseased — *continued*
- ovary — *continued*
  - polycystic E28.2
  - specified NEC N83.8
- Owren's (congenital) — *see* Defect, coagulation
- pancreas K86.9
  - cystic K86.2
  - fibrocystic E84.9
  - specified NEC K86.8
- panvalvular I08.9
  - specified NEC I08.8
- parametrium (noninflammatory) N83.9
- parasitic B89
  - cerebral NEC B71.9 [G94]
  - intestinal NOS B82.9
  - mouth B37.0
  - skin NOS B88.9
  - specified type — *see* Infestation
  - tongue B37.0
- parathyroid (gland) E21.5
  - specified NEC E21.4
- Parkinson's G20
- parodontal K05.6
- Parrot's (syphilitic osteochondritis) A50.02
- Parry's (exophthalmic goiter) — *see* Hyperthyroidism, with, goiter (diffuse)
- Parson's (exophthalmic goiter) — *see* Hyperthyroidism, with, goiter (diffuse)
- Paxton's (white piedra) B36.2
- pearl-worker's — *see* Osteomyelitis, specified type NEC
- Pellegrini-Stieda (calcification, knee joint) — *see* Bursitis, tibial collateral
- pelvis, pelvic
  - female NOS N94.9
    - specified NEC N94.89
  - gonococcal (acute) (chronic) A54.24
  - inflammatory (female) N73.9
    - acute N73.0
    - chronic N73.1
    - specified NEC N73.8
    - syphilitic (secondary) A51.42
      - late A52.76
    - tuberculous A18.17
  - organ, female N94.9
  - peritoneum, female NEC N94.89
- penis N48.9
  - inflammatory N48.29
    - abscess N48.21
    - cellulitis N48.22
  - specified NEC N48.89
- periapical tissues NOS K04.90
- periodontal K05.6
  - specified NEC K05.5
- periosteum — *see* Disorder, bone, specified type NEC
- peripheral
  - arterial I73.9
  - autonomic nervous system G90.9
  - nerves — *see* Polyneuropathy
  - vascular NOS I73.9
- peritoneum K66.9
  - pelvic, female NEC N94.89
  - specified NEC K66.8
- persistent mucosal (middle ear) H66.20
  - left H66.22
    - with right H66.23
  - right H66.21
    - with left H66.23
- Petit's — *see* Hernia, abdomen, specified site NEC
- pharynx J39.2
  - specified NEC J39.2
- Phocas' — *see* Mastopathy, cystic
- photochromogenic (acid-fast bacilli) (pulmonary) A31.0
  - nonpulmonary A31.9
- Pick's G31.01 [F02.80]
  - with behavioral disturbance G31.01 [F02.81]
- pigeon fancier's J67.2
- pineal gland E34.8
- pink — *see* Poisoning, mercury
- Pinkus' (lichen nitidus) L44.1
- pinworm B80
- Piry virus A93.8
- pituitary (gland) E23.7
- pituitary-snuff-taker's J67.8
- pleura (cavity) J94.9
  - specified NEC J94.8
- pneumatic drill (hammer) T75.21 ☑

Disease, diseased — *continued*
- Pollitzer's (hidradenitis suppurativa) L73.2
- polycystic
  - kidney or renal Q61.3
    - adult type Q61.2
    - childhood type NEC Q61.19
      - collecting duct dilatation Q61.11
  - liver or hepatic Q44.6
  - lung or pulmonary J98.4
    - congenital Q33.0
  - ovary, ovaries E28.2
  - spleen Q89.09
- polyethylene T84.05- ☑
- Pompe's (glycogenosis II) E74.02
- Posadas-Wernicke B38.9
- Potain's (pulmonary edema) — *see* Edema, lung
- prepuce N47.8
  - inflammatory N47.7
    - balanoposthitis N47.6
- Pringle's (tuberous sclerosis) Q85.1
- prion, central nervous system A81.9
  - specified NEC A81.89
- prostate N42.9 (congenital) Q61.3
  - specified NEC N42.89
- protozoal B64
  - acanthamebiasis — *see* Acanthamebiasis
  - African trypanosomiasis — *see* African trypanosomiasis
  - babesiosis B60.0
  - Chagas disease — *see* Chagas disease
  - intestine, intestinal A07.9
  - leishmaniasis — *see* Leishmaniasis
  - malaria — *see* Malaria
  - naegleriasis B60.2
  - pneumocystosis B59
  - specified organism NEC B60.8
  - toxoplasmosis — *see* Toxoplasmosis
- pseudo-Hurler's E77.0
- psychiatric F99
- psychotic — *see* Psychosis
- Puente's (simple glandular cheilitis) K13.0
- puerperal (*see also* Puerperal) O90.89
- pulmonary (*see also* Disease, lung)
  - artery I28.9
  - chronic obstructive J44.9
    - with
      - acute bronchitis J44.0
        - exacerbation (acute) J44.1
      - lower respiratory infection (acute) J44.0
    - decompensated J44.1
      - with
        - exacerbation (acute) J44.1
  - heart I27.9
    - specified NEC I27.89
  - hypertensive (vascular) I27.0
  - valve I37.9
    - rheumatic I09.89
- pulp (dental) NOS K04.90
- pulseless M31.4
- Putnam's (subacute combined sclerosis with pernicious anemia) D51.0
- Pyle (-Cohn) (craniometaphyseal dysplasia) Q78.5
- ragpicker's or ragsorter's A22.1
- Raynaud's — *see* Raynaud's disease
- reactive airway — *see* Asthma
- Reclus' (cystic) — *see* Mastopathy, cystic
- rectum K62.9
  - specified NEC K62.89
- Refsum's (heredopathia atactica polyneuritiformis) G60.1
- renal (functional) (pelvis) (*see also* Disease, kidney) N28.9
  - with
    - edema — *see* Nephrosis
    - glomerular lesion — *see* Glomerulonephritis
      - with edema — *see* Nephrosis
    - interstitial nephritis N12
  - acute N28.9
  - chronic (*see also* Disease, kidney, chronic) N18.9
  - cystic, congenital Q61.9
  - diabetic — *see* E08-E13 with .22
  - end-stage (failure) N18.6
    - due to hypertension I12.0
  - fibrocystic (congenital) Q61.8
  - hypertensive — *see* Hypertension, kidney
  - lupus M32.14
  - phosphate-losing (tubular) N25.0

☑ Additional Character Required — Refer to the Tabular List for Character Selection   ▽ Subterms under main terms may continue to next column or page

Disease, diseased — *continued*
  renal (*see also* Disease, kidney) — *continued*
    polycystic (congenital) Q61.3
      adult type Q61.2
      childhood type NEC Q61.19
        collecting duct dilatation Q61.11
    rapidly progressive N01.9
    subacute N01.9
  Rendu-Osler-Weber (familial hemorrhagic telangiecta-sia) I78.0
  renovascular (arteriosclerotic) — *see* Hypertension, kidney
  respiratory (tract) J98.9
    acute or subacute NOS J06.9
      due to
        chemicals, gases, fumes or vapors (inhala-tion) J68.3
        external agent J70.9
          specified NEC J70.8
        radiation J70.0
        smoke inhalation J70.5
      noninfectious J39.8
    chronic NOS J98.9
      due to
        chemicals, gases, fumes or vapors J68.4
        external agent J70.9
          specified NEC J70.8
        radiation J70.1
      newborn P27.9
        specified NEC P27.8
    due to
      chemicals, gases, fumes or vapors J68.9
        acute or subacute NEC J68.3
        chronic J68.4
      external agent J70.9
        specified NEC J70.8
    newborn P28.9
      specified type NEC P28.89
    upper J39.9
      acute or subacute J06.9
      noninfectious NEC J39.8
      specified NEC J39.8
      streptococcal J06.9
  retina, retinal H35.9
    Batten's or Batten-Mayou E75.4 [H36]
    specified NEC H35.89
  rheumatoid — *see* Arthritis, rheumatoid
  rickettsial NOS A79.9
    specified type NEC A79.89
  Riga (-Fede) (cachectic aphthae) K14.0
  Riggs' (compound periodontitis) — *see* Periodontitis
  Ritter's L00
  Rivalta's (cervicofacial actinomycosis) A42.2
  Robles' (onchocerciasis) B73.01
  Roger's (congenital interventricular septal defect) Q21.0
  Rosenthal's (factor XI deficiency) D68.1
  Ross River B33.1
  Rossbach's (hyperchlorhydria) K30
  Rotes Quérol — *see* Hyperostosis, ankylosing
  Roth (-Bernhardt) — *see* Mononeuropathy, lower limb, meralgia paresthetica
  Runeberg's (progressive pernicious anemia) D51.0
  sacroiliac NEC M53.3
  salivary gland or duct K11.9
    inclusion B25.9
    specified NEC K11.8
    virus B25.9
  sandworm B76.9
  Schimmelbusch's — *see* Mastopathy, cystic
  Schmorl's — *see* Schmorl's disease or nodes
  Schönlein (-Henoch) (purpura rheumatica) D69.0
  Schottmüller's — *see* Fever, paratyphoid
  Schultz's (agranulocytosis) — *see* Agranulocytosis
  Schwalbe-Ziehen-Oppenheim G24.1
  Schwartz-Jampel G71.13
  sclera H15.9
    specified NEC H15.89
  scrofulous (tuberculous) A18.2
  scrotum N50.9
  sebaceous glands L73.9
  semilunar cartilage, cystic (*see also* Derangement, knee, meniscus, cystic)
  seminal vesicle N50.9
  serum NEC (*see also* Reaction, serum) T80.69 ☑
  sexually transmitted A64
    anogenital
      herpesviral infection — *see* Herpes, anogenital

Disease, diseased — *continued*
  sexually transmitted — *continued*
    anogenital — *continued*
      warts A63.0
    chancroid A57
    chlamydial infection — *see* Chlamydia
    gonorrhea — *see* Gonorrhea
    granuloma inguinale A58
    specified organism NEC A63.8
    syphilis — *see* Syphilis
    trichomoniasis — *see* Trichomoniasis
  Sézary C84.1- ☑
  shimamushi (scrub typhus) A75.3
  shipyard B30.0
  sickle-cell D57.1
    with crisis (vasoocclusive pain) D57.00
      with
        acute chest syndrome D57.01
        splenic sequestration D57.02
    elliptocytosis D57.8- ☑
    Hb-C D57.20
      with crisis (vasoocclusive pain) D57.219
        with
          acute chest syndrome D57.211
          splenic sequestration D57.212
      without crisis D57.20
    Hb-SD D57.80
      with crisis D57.819
        with
          acute chest syndrome D57.811
          splenic sequestration D57.812
    Hb-SE D57.80
      with crisis D57.819
        with
          acute chest syndrome D57.811
          splenic sequestration D57.812
    specified NEC D57.80
      with crisis D57.819
        with
          acute chest syndrome D57.811
          splenic sequestration D57.812
    spherocytosis D57.80
      with crisis D57.819
        with
          acute chest syndrome D57.811
          splenic sequestration D57.812
    thalassemia D57.40
      with crisis (vasoocclusive pain) D57.419
        with
          acute chest syndrome D57.411
          splenic sequestration D57.412
      without crisis D57.40
  silo-filler's J68.8
    bronchitis J68.0
    pneumonitis J68.0
    pulmonary edema J68.1
  simian B B00.4
  Simons' (progressive lipodystrophy) E88.1
  sin nombre virus B33.4
  sinus — *see* Sinusitis
  Sirkari's B55.0
  sixth B08.20
    due to human herpesvirus 6 B08.21
    due to human herpesvirus 7 B08.22
  skin L98.9
    due to metabolic disorder NEC E88.9 [L99]
    specified NEC L98.8
  slim (HIV) B20
  small vessel I73.9
  Sneddon-Wilkinson (subcorneal pustular dermatosis) L13.1
  South African creeping B88.0
  spinal (cord) G95.9
    congenital Q06.9
    specified NEC G95.89
  spine (*see also* Spondylopathy)
    joint — *see* Dorsopathy
    tuberculous A18.01
  spinocerebellar (hereditary) G11.9
    specified NEC G11.8
  spleen D73.9
    amyloid E85.4 [D77]
    organic D73.9
    polycystic Q89.09
    postinfectional D73.89
  sponge-diver's — *see* Toxicity, venom, marine animal, sea anemone
  Startle Q89.8

Disease, diseased — *continued*
  Steinert's G71.11
  Sticker's (erythema infectiosum) B08.3
  Stieda's (calcification, knee joint) — *see* Bursitis, tibial collateral
  Stokes' (exophthalmic goiter) — *see* Hyperthyroidism, with, goiter (diffuse)
  Stokes-Adams (syncope with heart block) I45.9
  stomach K31.9
    functional, psychogenic F45.8
    specified NEC K31.89
  stonemason's J62.8
  storage
    glycogen — *see* Disease, glycogen storage
    mucopolysaccharide — *see* Mucopolysaccharidosis
  striatopallidal system NEC G25.89
  Stuart-Prower (congenital factor X deficiency) D68.2
  Stuart's (congenital factor X deficiency) D68.2
  subcutaneous tissue — *see* Disease, skin
  supporting structures of teeth K08.9
    specified NEC K08.8
  suprarenal (capsule) (gland) E27.9
    hyperfunction E27.0
    specified NEC E27.8
  sweat glands L74.9
    specified NEC L74.8
  Sweeley-Klionsky E75.21
  Swift (-Feer) — *see* Poisoning, mercury
  swimming-pool granuloma A31.1
  Sylvest's (epidemic pleurodynia) B33.0
  sympathetic nervous system G90.9
  synovium — *see* Disorder, synovium
  syphilitic — *see* Syphilis
  systemic tissue mast cell C96.2
  tanapox (virus) B08.71
  Tangier E78.6
  Tarral-Besnier (pityriasis rubra pilaris) L44.0
  Tauri's E74.09
  tear duct — *see* Disorder, lacrimal system
  tendon, tendinous (*see also* Disorder, tendon)
    nodular — *see* Trigger finger
  terminal vessel I73.9
  testis N50.9
  thalassemia Hb-S — *see* Disease, sickle-cell, tha-lassemia
  Thaysen-Gee (nontropical sprue) K90.0
  Thomsen G71.12
  throat J39.2
    septic J02.0
  thromboembolic — *see* Embolism
  thymus (gland) E32.9
    specified NEC E32.8
  thyroid (gland) E07.9
    heart (*see also* Hyperthyroidism) E05.90 [I43]
      with thyroid storm E05.91 [I43]
    specified NEC E07.89
  Tietze's M94.0
  tongue K14.9
    specified NEC K14.8
  tonsils, tonsillar (and adenoids) J35.9
  tooth, teeth K08.9
    hard tissues K03.9
      specified NEC K03.89
    pulp NEC K04.99
    specified NEC K08.8
  Tourette's F95.2
  trachea NEC J39.8
  tricuspid I07.9
    nonrheumatic I36.9
  triglyceride-storage E75.5
  trophoblastic — *see* Mole, hydatidiform
  tsutsugamushi A75.3
  tube (fallopian) (noninflammatory) N83.9
    inflammatory — *see* Salpingitis
    specified NEC N83.8
  tuberculous NEC — *see* Tuberculosis
  tubo-ovarian (noninflammatory) N83.9
    inflammatory — *see* Salpingo-oophoritis
    specified NEC N83.8
  tubotympanic, chronic — *see* Otitis, media, suppura-tive, chronic, tubotympanic
  tubulo-interstitial N15.9
    specified NEC N15.8
  tympanum — *see* Disorder, tympanic membrane
  Uhl's Q24.8
  Underwood's (sclerema neonatorum) P83.0
  Unverricht (-Lundborg) — *see* Epilepsy, generalized, idiopathic

Index

Disease, diseased — Dislocation

Disease, diseased — *continued*
Urbach-Oppenheim (necrobiosis lipoidica diabetico-
      rum) — *see* E08-E13 with .620
ureter N28.9
   in (due to)
      schistosomiasis (bilharziasis) B65.0 [N29]
urethra N36.9
   specified NEC N36.8
urinary (tract) N39.9
   bladder N32.9
      specified NEC N32.89
   specified NEC N39.8
uterus (noninflammatory) N85.9
   infective — *see* Endometritis
   inflammatory — *see* Endometritis
   specified NEC N85.8
uveal tract (anterior) H21.9
   posterior H31.9
vagabond's B85.1
vagina, vaginal (noninflammatory) N89.9
   inflammatory NEC N76.89
   specified NEC N89.8
valve, valvular I38
   multiple I08.9
      specified NEC I08.8
van Creveld-von Gierke (glycogenosis I) E74.01
vas deferens N50.9
vascular I99.9
   arteriosclerotic — *see* Arteriosclerosis
   ciliary body NEC — *see* Disorder, iris, vascular
   hypertensive — *see* Hypertension
   iris NEC — *see* Disorder, iris, vascular
   obliterative I77.1
      peripheral I73.9
   occlusive I99.8
   peripheral (occlusive) I73.9
      in diabetes mellitus — *see* E08-E13 with .51
vasomotor I73.9
vasospastic I73.9
vein I87.9
venereal (*see also* Disease, sexually transmitted) A64
   chlamydial NEC A56.8
      anus A56.3
      genitourinary NOS A56.2
      pharynx A56.4
      rectum A56.3
   fifth A55
   sixth A55
   specified nature or type NEC A63.8
vertebra, vertebral (*see also* Spondylopathy)
   disc — *see* Disorder, disc
vibration — *see* Vibration, adverse effects
viral, virus (*see also* Disease, by type of virus) B34.9
   arbovirus NOS A94
   arthropod-borne NOS A94
   congenital P35.9
      specified NEC P35.8
   Hanta (with renal manifestations) (Dobrava) (Pu-
      umala) (Seoul) A98.5
      with pulmonary manifestations (Andes) (Bayou)
         (Bermejo) (Black Creek Canal) (Choclo)
         (Juquitiba) (Laguna negra) (Lechiguanas)
         (New York) (Oran) (Sin nombre) B33.4
   Hantaan (Korean hemorrhagic fever) A98.5
   human immunodeficiency (HIV) B20
   Kunjin A83.4
   nonarthropod-borne NOS B34.9
   Powassan A84.8
   Rocio (encephalitis) A83.6
   Sin nombre (Hantavirus) (cardio)-pulmonary syn-
      drome) B33.4
   Tahyna B33.8
   vesicular stomatitis A93.8
vitreous H43.9
   specified NEC H43.89
vocal cord J38.3
Volkmann's, acquired T79.6 ☑
von Eulenburg's (congenital paramyotonia) G71.19
von Gierke's (glycogenosis I) E74.01
von Graefe's — *see* Strabismus, paralytic, ophthalmo-
      plegia, progressive
von Willebrand (-Jürgens) (angiohemophilia) D68.0
Vrolik's (osteogenesis imperfecta) Q78.0
vulva (noninflammatory) N90.9
   inflammatory NEC N76.89
   specified NEC N90.89
Wallgren's (obstruction of splenic vein with collateral
      circulation) I87.8

Disease, diseased — *continued*
Wassilieff's (leptospiral jaundice) A27.0
wasting NEC R64
   due to malnutrition E41
Waterhouse-Friderichsen A39.1
Wegner's (syphilitic osteochondritis) A50.02
Weil's (leptospiral jaundice of lung) A27.0
Weir Mitchell's (erythromelalgia) I73.81
Werdnig-Hoffmann G12.0
Wermer's E31.21
Werner-His (trench fever) A79.0
Werner-Schultz (neutropenic splenomegaly) D73.81
Wernicke-Posadas B38.9
whipworm B79
white blood cells D72.9
   specified NEC D72.89
white matter R90.82
white-spot, meaning lichen sclerosus et atrophicus
      L90.0
   penis N48.0
   vulva N90.4
Wilkie's K55.1
Wilkinson-Sneddon (subcorneal pustular dermatosis)
      L13.1
Willis' — *see* Diabetes
Wilson's (hepatolenticular degeneration) E83.01
woolsorter's A22.1
yaba monkey tumor B08.72
yaba pox (virus) B08.72
zoonotic, bacterial A28.9
   specified type NEC A28.8
Disfigurement (due to scar) L90.5
Disgerminoma — *see* Dysgerminoma
DISH (diffuse idiopathic skeletal hyperostosis) — *see*
      Hyperostosis, ankylosing
Disinsertion, retina — *see* Detachment, retina
Dislocatable hip, congenital Q65.6
Dislocation (articular)
with fracture — *see* Fracture
   acromioclavicular (joint) S43.10- ☑
      with displacement
         100%-200% S43.12- ☑
         more than 200% S43.13- ☑
      inferior S43.14- ☑
      posterior S43.15- ☑
   ankle S93.0- ☑
   astragalus — *see* Dislocation, ankle
   atlantoaxial S13.121 ☑
   atlantooccipital S13.111 ☑
   atloidooccipital S13.111 ☑
   breast bone S23.29 ☑
   capsule, joint — *code by* site under Dislocation
   carpal (bone) — *see* Dislocation, wrist
   carpometacarpal (joint) NEC S63.05- ☑
      thumb S63.04- ☑
   cartilage (joint) — *code by* site under Dislocation
   cervical spine (vertebra) — *see* Dislocation, vertebra,
      cervical
   chronic — *see* Dislocation, recurrent
   clavicle — *see* Dislocation, acromioclavicular joint
   coccyx S33.2 ☑
   congenital NEC Q68.8
   coracoid — *see* Dislocation, shoulder
   costal cartilage S23.29 ☑
   costochondral S23.29 ☑
   cricoarytenoid articulation S13.29 ☑
   cricothyroid articulation S13.29 ☑
   dorsal vertebra — *see* Dislocation, vertebra, thoracic
   ear ossicle — *see* Discontinuity, ossicles, ear
   elbow S53.10- ☑
      congenital Q68.8
      pathological — *see* Dislocation, pathological NEC,
         elbow
      radial head alone — *see* Dislocation, radial head
      recurrent — *see* Dislocation, recurrent, elbow
      traumatic S53.10- ☑
         anterior S53.11- ☑
         lateral S53.14- ☑
         medial S53.13- ☑
         posterior S53.12- ☑
         specified type NEC S53.19- ☑
   eye, nontraumatic — *see* Luxation, globe
   eyeball, nontraumatic — *see* Luxation, globe
   femur
      distal end — *see* Dislocation, knee
      proximal end — *see* Dislocation, hip

Dislocation — *continued*
fibula
   distal end — *see* Dislocation, ankle
   proximal end — *see* Dislocation, knee
finger S63.25- ☑
   index S63.25- ☑
   interphalangeal S63.27- ☑
      distal S63.29- ☑
         index S63.29- ☑
         little S63.29- ☑
         middle S63.29- ☑
         ring S63.29- ☑
      index S63.27- ☑
      little S63.27- ☑
      middle S63.27- ☑
      proximal S63.28- ☑
         index S63.28- ☑
         little S63.28- ☑
         middle S63.28- ☑
         ring S63.28- ☑
      ring S63.27- ☑
   little S63.25- ☑
   metacarpophalangeal S63.26- ☑
      index S63.26- ☑
      little S63.26- ☑
      middle S63.26- ☑
      ring S63.26- ☑
   middle S63.25- ☑
   recurrent — *see* Dislocation, recurrent, finger
   ring S63.25- ☑
   thumb — *see* Dislocation, thumb
foot S93.30- ☑
   recurrent — *see* Dislocation, recurrent, foot
   specified site NEC S93.33- ☑
   tarsal joint S93.31- ☑
   tarsometatarsal joint S93.32- ☑
   toe — *see* Dislocation, toe
fracture — *see* Fracture
glenohumeral (joint) — *see* Dislocation, shoulder
glenoid — *see* Dislocation, shoulder
habitual — *see* Dislocation, recurrent
hip S73.00- ☑
   anterior S73.03- ☑
      obturator S73.02- ☑
   central S73.04- ☑
   congenital (total) Q65.2
      bilateral Q65.1
      partial Q65.5
         bilateral Q65.4
         unilateral Q65.3- ☑
      unilateral Q65.0- ☑
   developmental M24.85- ☑
   pathological — *see* Dislocation, pathological NEC,
      hip
   posterior S73.01- ☑
   recurrent — *see* Dislocation, recurrent, hip
humerus, proximal end — *see* Dislocation, shoulder
incomplete — *see* Subluxation, by site
incus — *see* Discontinuity, ossicles, ear
infracoracoid — *see* Dislocation, shoulder
innominate (pubic junction) (sacral junction) S33.39
   acetabulum — *see* Dislocation, hip
interphalangeal (joint(s))
   finger S63.279 ☑
      distal S63.29- ☑
         index S63.29- ☑
         little S63.29- ☑
         middle S63.29- ☑
         ring S63.29- ☑
      index S63.27- ☑
      little S63.27- ☑
      middle S63.27- ☑
      proximal S63.28- ☑
         index S63.28- ☑
         little S63.28- ☑
         middle S63.28- ☑
         ring S63.28- ☑
      ring S63.27- ☑
   foot or toe — *see* Dislocation, toe
   thumb S63.12- ☑
      distal joint S63.14- ☑
      proximal joint S63.13- ☑
jaw (cartilage) (meniscus) S03.0 ☑
joint prosthesis — *see* Complications, joint prosthesis,
      mechanical, displacement, by site
knee S83.106 ☑

☑ **Additional Character Required** — Refer to the Tabular List for Character Selection   ▽ **Subterms under main terms may continue to next column or page**

Dislocation — *continued*
- knee S83.106 ☑
  - cap — *see* Dislocation, patella
  - congenital Q68.2
  - old M23.8X-
  - patella — *see* Dislocation, patella
  - pathological — *see* Dislocation, pathological NEC, knee
  - proximal tibia
    - anteriorly S83.11-
    - laterally S83.14- ☑
    - medially S83.13- ☑
    - posteriorly S83.12- ☑
  - recurrent (*see also* Derangement, knee, specified NEC)
  - specified type NEC S83.19- ☑
- lacrimal gland H04.16- ☑
- lens (complete) H27.10
  - anterior H27.12-
  - congenital Q12.1
  - ocular implant — *see* Complications, intraocular lens
  - partial H27.11- ☑
  - posterior H27.13- ☑
  - traumatic S05.8X- ☑
- ligament — *code by* site under Dislocation
- lumbar (vertebra) — *see* Dislocation, vertebra, lumbar
- lumbosacral (vertebra) (*see also* Dislocation, vertebra, lumbar)
  - congenital Q76.49
- mandible S03.0 ☑
- meniscus (knee) — *see* Tear, meniscus
  - other sites - code by site under Dislocation
- metacarpal (bone)
  - distal end — *see* Dislocation, finger
  - proximal end S63.06- ☑
- metacarpophalangeal (joint)
  - finger S63.26- ☑
    - index S63.26- ☑
    - little S63.26- ☑
    - middle S63.26- ☑
    - ring S63.26- ☑
    - thumb S63.11- ☑
- metatarsal (bone) — *see* Dislocation, foot
- metatarsophalangeal (joint(s)) — *see* Dislocation, toe
- midcarpal (joint) S63.03- ☑
- midtarsal (joint) — *see* Dislocation, foot
- neck S13.20 ☑
  - specified site NEC S13.29 ☑
  - vertebra — *see* Dislocation, vertebra, cervical
- nose (septal cartilage) S03.1 ☑
- occipitoatloid S13.111 ☑
- old — *see* Derangement, joint, specified type NEC
- ossicles, ear — *see* Discontinuity, ossicles, ear
- partial — *see* Subluxation, by site
- patella S83.006 ☑
  - congenital Q74.1
  - lateral S83.01- ☑
  - recurrent (nontraumatic) M22.0- ☑
    - incomplete M22.1- ☑
  - specified type NEC S83.09- ☑
- pathological NEC M24.30
  - ankle M24.37- ☑
  - elbow M24.32- ☑
  - foot joint M24.37- ☑
  - hand joint M24.34- ☑
  - hip M24.35- ☑
  - knee M24.36- ☑
  - lumbosacral joint — *see* subcategory M53.2 ☑
  - pelvic region — *see* Dislocation, pathological, hip
  - sacroiliac — *see* subcategory M53.2 ☑
  - shoulder M24.31- ☑
  - wrist M24.33- ☑
- pelvis NEC S33.30 ☑
  - specified NEC S33.39 ☑
- phalanx
  - finger or hand — *see* Dislocation, finger
  - foot or toe — *see* Dislocation, toe
- prosthesis, internal — *see* Complications, prosthetic device, by site, mechanical
- radial head S53.006 ☑
  - anterior S53.01- ☑
  - posterior S53.02- ☑
  - specified type NEC S53.09- ☑
- radiocarpal (joint) S63.02- ☑
- radiohumeral (joint) — *see* Dislocation, radial head

Dislocation — *continued*
- radioulnar (joint)
  - distal S63.01- ☑
  - proximal — *see* Dislocation, elbow
- radius
  - distal end — *see* Dislocation, wrist
  - proximal end — *see* Dislocation, radial head
- recurrent M24.40
  - ankle M24.47- ☑
  - elbow M24.42- ☑
  - finger M24.44- ☑
  - foot joint M24.47- ☑
  - hand joint M24.44- ☑
  - hip M24.45- ☑
  - knee M24.46- ☑
    - patella — *see* Dislocation, patella, recurrent
  - patella — *see* Dislocation, patella, recurrent
  - sacroiliac — *see* subcategory M53.2 ☑
  - shoulder M24.41- ☑
  - toe M24.47- ☑
  - vertebra (*see also* subcategory) M43.5 ☑
    - atlantoaxial M43.4
      - with myelopathy M43.3
  - wrist M24.43- ☑
- rib (cartilage) S23.29 ☑
- sacrococcygeal S33.2 ☑
- sacroiliac (joint) (ligament) S33.2 ☑
  - congenital Q74.2
  - recurrent — *see* subcategory M53.2 ☑
- sacrum S33.2 ☑
- scaphoid (bone) (hand) (wrist) — *see* Dislocation, wrist
  - foot — *see* Dislocation, foot
- scapula — *see* Dislocation, shoulder, girdle, scapula
- semilunar cartilage, knee — *see* Tear, meniscus
- septal cartilage (nose) S03.1 ☑
- septum (nasal) (old) J34.2
- sesamoid bone — *code by* site under Dislocation
- shoulder (blade) (ligament) (joint) (traumatic) S43.006 ☑
  - acromioclavicular — *see* Dislocation, acromioclavicular
  - chronic — *see* Dislocation, recurrent, shoulder
  - congenital Q68.8
  - girdle S43.30- ☑
    - scapula S43.31- ☑
    - specified site NEC S43.39- ☑
  - humerus S43.00- ☑
    - anterior S43.01- ☑
    - inferior S43.03- ☑
    - posterior S43.02- ☑
  - pathological — *see* Dislocation, pathological NEC, shoulder
  - recurrent — *see* Dislocation, recurrent, shoulder
  - specified type NEC S43.08- ☑
- spine
  - cervical — *see* Dislocation, vertebra, cervical
  - congenital Q76.49
  - due to birth trauma P11.5
  - lumbar — *see* Dislocation, vertebra, lumbar
  - thoracic — *see* Dislocation, vertebra, thoracic
- spontaneous — *see* Dislocation, pathological
- sternoclavicular (joint) S43.206 ☑
  - anterior S43.21- ☑
  - posterior S43.22- ☑
- sternum S23.29 ☑
- subglenoid — *see* Dislocation, shoulder
- symphysis pubis S33.4 ☑
- talus — *see* Dislocation, ankle
- tarsal (bone(s)) (joint(s)) — *see* Dislocation, foot
- tarsometatarsal (joint(s)) — *see* Dislocation, foot
- temporomandibular (joint) S03.0 ☑
- thigh, proximal end — *see* Dislocation, hip
- thorax S23.20 ☑
  - specified site NEC S23.29 ☑
  - vertebra — *see* Dislocation, vertebra
- thumb S63.10- ☑
  - interphalangeal joint — *see* Dislocation, interphalangeal (joint), thumb
  - metacarpophalangeal joint — *see* Dislocation, metacarpophalangeal (joint), thumb
- thyroid cartilage S13.29 ☑
- tibia
  - distal end — *see* Dislocation, ankle
  - proximal end — *see* Dislocation, knee
- tibiofibular (joint)
  - distal — *see* Dislocation, ankle

Dislocation — *continued*
- tibiofibular — *continued*
  - superior — *see* Dislocation, knee
- toe(s) S93.106 ☑
  - great S93.10- ☑
    - interphalangeal joint S93.11- ☑
    - metatarsophalangeal joint S93.12- ☑
  - interphalangeal joint S93.119 ☑
  - lesser S93.106 ☑
    - interphalangeal joint S93.11- ☑
    - metatarsophalangeal joint S93.12- ☑
  - metatarsophalangeal joint S93.12- ☑
- tooth S03.2 ☑
- trachea S23.29 ☑
- ulna
  - distal end S63.07- ☑
  - proximal end — *see* Dislocation, elbow
- ulnohumeral (joint) — *see* Dislocation, elbow
- vertebra (articular process) (body) (traumatic)
  - cervical S13.101 ☑
    - atlantoaxial joint S13.121 ☑
    - atlantooccipital joint S13.111 ☑
    - atloidooccipital joint S13.111 ☑
    - joint between
      - C0 and C1 S13.111 ☑
      - C1 and C2 S13.121 ☑
      - C2 and C3 S13.131 ☑
      - C3 and C4 S13.141 ☑
      - C4 and C5 S13.151 ☑
      - C5 and C6 S13.161 ☑
      - C6 and C7 S13.171 ☑
      - C7 and T1 S13.181 ☑
    - occipitoatloid joint S13.111 ☑
  - congenital Q76.49
  - lumbar S33.101 ☑
    - joint between
      - L1 and L2 S33.111 ☑
      - L2 and L3 S33.121 ☑
      - L3 and L4 S33.131 ☑
      - L4 and L5 S33.141 ☑
  - nontraumatic — *see* Displacement, intervertebral disc
  - partial — *see* Subluxation, by site
  - recurrent NEC — *see* subcategory M43.5 ☑
  - thoracic S23.101 ☑
    - joint between
      - T1 and T2 S23.111 ☑
      - T2 and T3 S23.121 ☑
      - T3 and T4 S23.123 ☑
      - T4 and T5 S23.131 ☑
      - T5 and T6 S23.133 ☑
      - T6 and T7 S23.141 ☑
      - T7 and T8 S23.143 ☑
      - T8 and T9 S23.151 ☑
      - T9 and T10 S23.153 ☑
      - T10 and T11 S23.161 ☑
      - T11 and T12 S23.163 ☑
      - T12 and L1 S23.171 ☑
- wrist (carpal bone) S63.006 ☑
  - carpometacarpal joint — *see* Dislocation, carpometacarpal (joint)
  - distal radioulnar joint — *see* Dislocation, radioulnar (joint), distal
  - metacarpal bone, proximal — *see* Dislocation, metacarpal (bone), proximal end
  - midcarpal — *see* Dislocation, midcarpal (joint)
  - radiocarpal joint — *see* Dislocation, radiocarpal (joint)
  - recurrent — *see* Dislocation, recurrent, wrist
  - specified site NEC S63.09- ☑
  - ulna — *see* Dislocation, ulna, distal end
- xiphoid cartilage S23.29 ☑

Disorder (of) (*see also* Disease)
- acantholytic L11.9
  - specified NEC L11.8
- acute
  - psychotic — *see* Psychosis, acute
  - stress F43.0
- adjustment (grief) F43.20
  - with
    - anxiety F43.22
      - with depressed mood F43.23
    - conduct disturbance F43.24
      - with emotional disturbance F43.25
    - depressed mood F43.21
      - with anxiety F43.23

Disorder — continued
adjustment — continued
with — continued
other specified symptom F43.29
adrenal (capsule) (gland) (medullary) E27.9
specified NEC E27.8
adrenogenital E25.9
drug-induced E25.8
iatrogenic E25.8
idiopathic E25.8
adult personality (and behavior) F69
specified NEC F68.8
affective (mood) — see Disorder, mood
aggressive, unsocialized F91.1
alcohol-related F10.99
with
amnestic disorder, persisting F10.96
anxiety disorder F10.980
dementia, persisting F10.97
intoxication F10.929
with delirium F10.921
uncomplicated F10.920
mood disorder F10.94
other specified F10.988
psychotic disorder F10.959
with
delusions F10.950
hallucinations F10.951
sexual dysfunction F10.981
sleep disorder F10.982
allergic — see Allergy
alveolar NEC J84.09
amino-acid
cystathioninuria E72.19
cystinosis E72.04
cystinuria E72.01
glycinuria E72.09
homocystinuria E72.11
metabolism — see Disturbance, metabolism,
amino-acid
specified NEC E72.8
neonatal, transitory P74.8
renal transport NEC E72.09
transport NEC E72.09
amnesic, amnestic
alcohol-induced F10.96
with dependence F10.26
due to (secondary to) general medical condition
F04
psychoactive NEC-induced F19.96
with
abuse F19.16
dependence F19.26
sedative, hypnotic or anxiolytic-induced F13.96
with dependence F13.26
anaerobic glycolysis with anemia D55.2
anxiety F41.9
due to (secondary to)
alcohol F10.980
amphetamine F15.980
in
abuse F15.180
dependence F15.280
anxiolytic F13.980
in
abuse F13.180
dependence F13.280
caffeine F15.980
in
abuse F15.180
dependence F15.280
cannabis F12.980
in
abuse F12.180
dependence F12.280
cocaine F14.980
in
abuse F14.180
dependence F14.180
general medical condition F06.4
hallucinogen F16.980
in
abuse F16.180
dependence F16.280
hypnotic F13.980
in
abuse F13.180
dependence F13.280

Disorder — continued
anxiety — continued
due to — continued
inhalant F18.980
in
abuse F18.180
dependence F18.280
phencyclidine F16.980
in
abuse F16.180
dependence F16.280
psychoactive substance NEC F19.980
in
abuse F19.180
dependence F19.280
sedative F13.980
in
abuse F13.180
dependence F13.280
volatile solvents F18.980
in
abuse F18.180
dependence F18.280
generalized F41.1
mixed
with depression (mild) F41.8
specified NEC F41.3
organic F06.4
phobic F40.9
of childhood F40.8
specified NEC F41.8
aortic valve — see Endocarditis, aortic
aromatic amino-acid metabolism E70.9
specified NEC E70.8
arteriole NEC I77.89
artery NEC I77.89
articulation — see Disorder, joint
attachment (childhood)
disinhibited F94.2
reactive F94.1
attention-deficit hyperactivity (adolescent) (adult)
(child) F90.9
combined type F90.2
hyperactive type F90.1
inattentive type F90.0
specified type NEC F90.8
attention-deficit without hyperactivity (adolescent)
(adult) (child) F90.0
auditory processing (central) H93.25
autistic F84.0
autonomic nervous system G90.9
specified NEC G90.8
avoidant, child or adolescent F40.10
balance
acid-base E87.8
mixed E87.4
electrolyte E87.8
fluid NEC E87.8
behavioral (disruptive) — see Disorder, conduct
beta-amino-acid metabolism E72.8
bile acid and cholesterol metabolism E78.70
Barth syndrome E78.71
other specified E78.79
Smith-Lemli-Opitz syndrome E78.72
bilirubin excretion E80.6
binocular
movement H51.9
convergence
excess H51.12
insufficiency H51.11
internuclear ophthalmoplegia — see Ophthalmoplegia, internuclear
palsy of conjugate gaze H51.0
specified type NEC H51.8
vision NEC — see Disorder, vision, binocular
bipolar (I) F31.9
current episode
depressed F31.9
with psychotic features F31.5
without psychotic features F31.30
mild F31.31
moderate F31.32
severe (without psychotic features) F31.4
with psychotic features F31.5
hypomanic F31.0
manic F31.9
with psychotic features F31.2

Disorder — continued
bipolar — continued
current episode — continued
manic — continued
without psychotic features F31.10
mild F31.11
moderate F31.12
severe (without psychotic features)
F31.13
with psychotic features F31.2
mixed F31.60
mild F31.61
moderate F31.62
severe (without psychotic features) F31.63
with psychotic features F31.64
severe depression (without psychotic features)
F31.4
with psychotic features F31.5
in remission (currently) F31.70
in full remission
most recent episode
depressed F31.76
hypomanic F31.72
manic F31.74
mixed F31.78
in partial remission
most recent episode
depressed F31.75
hypomanic F31.71
manic F31.73
mixed F31.77
organic F06.30
single manic episode F30.9
mild F30.11
moderate F30.12
severe (without psychotic symptoms) F30.13
with psychotic symptoms F30.2
specified NEC F31.89
bipolar II F31.81
bladder N32.9
functional NEC N31.9
in schistosomiasis B65.0 [N33]
specified NEC N32.89
bleeding D68.9
blood D75.9
in congenital early syphilis A50.09 [D77]
body dysmorphic F45.22
bone M89.9
continuity M84.9
specified type NEC M84.80
ankle M84.87- ☑
fibula M84.86- ☑
foot M84.87- ☑
hand M84.84- ☑
humerus M84.82- ☑
neck M84.88
pelvis M84.859
radius M84.83- ☑
rib M84.88
shoulder M84.81- ☑
skull M84.88
thigh M84.85- ☑
tibia M84.86- ☑
ulna M84.83- ☑
vertebra M84.88
density and structure M85.9
cyst (see also Cyst, bone, specified type NEC)
aneurysmal — see Cyst, bone, aneurysmal
solitary — see Cyst, bone, solitary
diffuse idiopathic skeletal hyperostosis — see
Hyperostosis, ankylosing
fibrous dysplasia (monostotic) — see Dysplasia,
fibrous, bone
fluorosis — see Fluorosis, skeletal
hyperostosis of skull M85.2
osteitis condensans — see Osteitis, condensans
specified type NEC M85.8- ☑
ankle M85.87- ☑
foot M85.87- ☑
forearm M85.83- ☑
hand M85.84- ☑
lower leg M85.86- ☑
multiple sites M85.89
neck M85.88
rib M85.88
shoulder M85.81- ☑
skull M85.88
thigh M85.85- ☑

☑ **Additional Character Required** — Refer to the Tabular List for Character Selection   ⬥ Subterms under main terms may continue to next column or page

Disorder — *continued*
 bone — *continued*
  density and structure — *continued*
   specified type — *continued*
    upper arm M85.82- ☑
    vertebra M85.88
  development and growth NEC M89.20
   carpus M89.24- ☑
   clavicle M89.21- ☑
   femur M89.25- ☑
   fibula M89.26- ☑
   finger M89.24- ☑
   humerus M89.22- ☑
   ilium M89.259
   ischium M89.259
   metacarpus M89.24- ☑
   metatarsus M89.27- ☑
   multiple sites M89.29
   neck M89.28
   radius M89.23- ☑
   rib M89.28
   scapula M89.21- ☑
   skull M89.28
   tarsus M89.27- ☑
   tibia M89.26- ☑
   toe M89.27- ☑
   ulna M89.23- ☑
   vertebra M89.28
  specified type NEC M89.8X- ☑
 brachial plexus G54.0
 branched-chain amino-acid metabolism E71.2
  specified NEC E71.19
 breast N64.9
  agalactia — *see* Agalactia
  associated with
   lactation O92.70
    specified NEC O92.79
   pregnancy O92.20
    specified NEC O92.29
   puerperium O92.20
    specified NEC O92.29
  cracked nipple — *see* Cracked nipple
  galactorrhea — *see* Galactorrhea
  hypogalactia O92.4
  lactation disorder NEC O92.79
  mastitis — *see* Mastitis
  nipple infection — *see* Infection, nipple
  retracted nipple — *see* Retraction, nipple
  specified type NEC N64.89
 Briquet's F45.0
 bullous, in diseases classified elsewhere L14
 cannabis use
  due to drug abuse — *see* Abuse, drug, cannabis
  due to drug dependence — *see* Dependence, drug, cannabis
 carbohydrate
  absorption, intestinal NEC E74.39
  metabolism (congenital) E74.9
   specified NEC E74.8
 cardiac, functional I51.89
 carnitine metabolism E71.40
 cartilage M94.9
  articular NEC — *see* Derangement, joint, articular cartilage
  chondrocalcinosis — *see* Chondrocalcinosis
  specified type NEC M94.8X- ☑
   articular — *see* Derangement, joint, articular cartilage
   multiple sites M94.8X0
 catatonic
  due to (secondary to) known physiological condition F06.1
  organic F06.1
 central auditory processing H93.25
 cervical
  region NEC M53.82
  root (nerve) NEC G54.2
 character NOS F60.9
 childhood disintegrative NEC F84.3
 cholesterol and bile acid metabolism E78.70
  Barth syndrome E78.71
  other specified E78.79
  Smith-Lemli-Opitz syndrome E78.72
 choroid H31.9
  atrophy — *see* Atrophy, choroid
  degeneration — *see* Degeneration, choroid
  detachment — *see* Detachment, choroid

Disorder — *continued*
 choroid — *continued*
  dystrophy — *see* Dystrophy, choroid
  hemorrhage — *see* Hemorrhage, choroid
  rupture — *see* Rupture, choroid
  scar — *see* Scar, chorioretinal
  solar retinopathy — *see* Retinopathy, solar
  specified type NEC H31.8
 ciliary body — *see* Disorder, iris
  degeneration — *see* Degeneration, ciliary body
 coagulation (factor) (*see also* Defect, coagulation) D68.9
  newborn, transient P61.6
 coccyx NEC M53.3
 cognitive F09
  due to (secondary to) general medical condition F09
  persisting R41.89
   due to
    alcohol F10.97
     with dependence F10.27
    anxiolytics F13.97
     with dependence F13.27
    hypnotics F13.97
     with dependence F13.27
    sedatives F13.97
     with dependence F13.27
    specified substance NEC F19.97
     with
      abuse F19.17
      dependence F19.27
 communication F80.9
 conduct (childhood) F91.9
  adjustment reaction — *see* Disorder, adjustment
  adolescent onset type F91.2
  childhood onset type F91.1
  compulsive F63.9
  confined to family context F91.0
  depressive F91.8
  group type F91.2
  hyperkinetic — *see* Disorder, attention-deficit hyperactivity
  oppositional defiance F91.3
  socialized F91.2
  solitary aggressive type F91.1
  specified NEC F91.8
  unsocialized (aggressive) F91.1
 conduction, heart I45.9
 congenital glycosylation (CDG) E74.8
 conjunctiva H11.9
  infection — *see* Conjunctivitis
 connective tissue, localized L94.9
  specified NEC L94.8
 conversion — *see* Disorder, dissociative
 convulsive (secondary) — *see* Convulsions
 cornea H18.9
  deformity — *see* Deformity, cornea
  degeneration — *see* Degeneration, cornea
  deposits — *see* Deposit, cornea
  due to contact lens H18.82- ☑
   specified as edema — *see* Edema, cornea
  edema — *see* Edema, cornea
  keratitis — *see* Keratitis
  keratoconjunctivitis — *see* Keratoconjunctivitis
  membrane change — *see* Change, corneal membrane
  neovascularization — *see* Neovascularization, cornea
  scar — *see* Opacity, cornea
  specified type NEC H18.89- ☑
  ulcer — *see* Ulcer, cornea
 corpus cavernosum N48.9
 cranial nerve — *see* Disorder, nerve, cranial
 cyclothymic F34.0
 defiant oppositional F91.3
 delusional (persistent) (systematized) F22
  induced F24
 depersonalization F48.1
 depressive F32.9
  major F32.9
   with psychotic symptoms F32.3
   in remission (full) F32.5
    partial F32.4
   recurrent F33.9
   single episode F32.9
    mild F32.0
    moderate F32.1

Disorder — *continued*
 depressive — *continued*
  major — *continued*
   single episode — *continued*
    severe (without psychotic symptoms) F32.2
     with psychotic symptoms F32.3
   organic F06.31
   recurrent F33.9
    current episode
     mild F33.0
     moderate F33.1
     severe (without psychotic symptoms) F33.2
      with psychotic symptoms F33.3
    in remission F33.40
     full F33.42
     partial F33.41
    specified NEC F33.8
   single episode — *see* Episode, depressive
  developmental F89
   arithmetical skills F81.2
   coordination (motor) F82
   expressive writing F81.81
   language F80.9
    expressive F80.1
    mixed receptive and expressive F80.2
    receptive type F80.2
    specified NEC F80.89
   learning F81.9
    arithmetical F81.2
    reading F81.0
   mixed F88
   motor coordination or function F82
   pervasive F84.9
    specified NEC F84.8
   phonological F80.0
   reading F81.0
   scholastic skills (*see also* Disorder, learning)
    mixed F81.89
   specified NEC F88
   speech F80.9
    articulation F80.0
    specified NEC F80.89
   written expression F81.81
  diaphragm J98.6
  digestive (system) K92.9
   newborn P78.9
    specified NEC P78.89
   postprocedural — *see* Complication, gastrointestinal
   psychogenic F45.8
  disc (intervertebral) M51.9
   with
    myelopathy
     cervical region M50.00
     cervicothoracic region M50.03
     high cervical region M50.01
     lumbar region M51.06
     mid-cervical region M50.02
     sacrococcygeal region M53.3
     thoracic region M51.04
     thoracolumbar region M51.05
    radiculopathy
     cervical region M50.10
     cervicothoracic region M50.13
     high cervical region M50.11
     lumbar region M51.16
     lumbosacral region M51.17
     mid-cervical region M50.12
     sacrococcygeal region M53.3
     thoracic region M51.14
     thoracolumbar region M51.15
   cervical M50.90
    with
     myelopathy M50.00
      C2-C3 M50.01
      C3-C4 M50.01
      C4-C5 M50.02
      C5-C6 M50.02
      C6-C7 M50.02
      C7-T1 M50.03
      cervicothoracic region M50.03
      high cervical region M50.01
      mid-cervical region M50.02
     neuritis, radiculitis or radiculopathy M50.10
      C2-C3 M50.11
      C3-C4 M50.11
      C4-C5 M50.12
      C5-C6 M50.12

Disorder — *continued*
  disc — *continued*
    cervical — *continued*
      with — *continued*
        neuritis, radiculitis or radiculopathy — *continued*
          C6-C7 M50.12
          C7-T1 M50.13
          cervicothoracic region M50.13
          high cervical region M50.11
          mid-cervical region M50.12
        C2-C3 M50.91
        C3-C4 M50.91
        C4-C5 M50.92
        C5-C6 M50.92
        C6-C7 M50.92
        C7-T1 M50.93
        cervicothoracic region M50.93
        degeneration M50.30
          C2-C3 M50.31
          C3-C4 M50.31
          C4-C5 M50.32
          C5-C6 M50.32
          C6-C7 M50.32
          C7-T1 M50.33
          cervicothoracic region M50.33
          high cervical region M50.31
          mid-cervical region M50.32
        displacement M50.20
          C2-C3 M50.21
          C3-C4 M50.21
          C4-C5 M50.22
          C5-C6 M50.22
          C6-C7 M50.22
          C7-T1 M50.23
          cervicothoracic region M50.23
          high cervical region M50.21
          mid-cervical region M50.22
        high cervical region M50.91
        mid-cervical region M50.92
        specified type NEC M50.80
          C2-C3 M50.81
          C3-C4 M50.81
          C4-C5 M50.82
          C5-C6 M50.82
          C6-C7 M50.82
          C7-T1 M50.83
          cervicothoracic region M50.83
          high cervical region M50.81
          mid-cervical region M50.82
      specified NEC
        lumbar region M51.86
        lumbosacral region M51.87
        sacrococcygeal region M53.3
        thoracic region M51.84
        thoracolumbar region M51.85
  disinhibited attachment (childhood) F94.2
  disintegrative, childhood NEC F84.3
  disruptive behavior F98.9
  dissocial personality F60.2
  dissociative F44.9
    affecting
      motor function F44.4
        and sensation F44.7
      sensation F44.6
        and motor function F44.7
    brief reactive F43.0
    due to (secondary to) general medical condition F06.8
    mixed F44.7
    organic F06.8
    other specified NEC F44.89
  double heterozygous sickling — *see* Disease, sickle-cell
  dream anxiety F51.5
  drug induced hemorrhagic D68.32
  drug related F19.99
    abuse — *see* Abuse, drug
    dependence — *see* Dependence, drug
  dysmorphic body F45.1
  dysthymic F34.1
  ear H93.9- ☑
    bleeding — *see* Otorrhagia
    deafness — *see* Deafness
    degenerative H93.09- ☑
    discharge — *see* Otorrhea

Disorder — *continued*
  ear — *continued*
    external H61.9- ☑
      auditory canal stenosis — *see* Stenosis, external ear canal
      exostosis — *see* Exostosis, external ear canal
      impacted cerumen — *see* Impaction, cerumen
      otitis — *see* Otitis, externa
      perichondritis — *see* Perichondritis, ear
      pinna — *see* Disorder, pinna
      specified type NEC H61.89- ☑
    inner H83.9- ☑
      vestibular dysfunction — *see* Disorder, vestibular function
    middle H74.9- ☑
      adhesive H74.1- ☑
      ossicle — *see* Abnormal, ear ossicles
      polyp — *see* Polyp, ear (middle)
      specified NEC, in diseases classified elsewhere H75.8- ☑
    postprocedural — *see* Complications, ear, procedure
    specified NEC, in diseases classified elsewhere H94.8- ☑
  eating (adult) (psychogenic) F50.9
    anorexia — *see* Anorexia
    bulimia F50.2
    child F98.29
      pica F98.3
      rumination disorder F98.21
    pica F50.8
      childhood F98.3
  electrolyte (balance) NEC E87.8
    with
      abortion — *see* Abortion by type complicated by specified condition NEC
      ectopic pregnancy O08.5
      molar pregnancy O08.5
    acidosis (metabolic) (respiratory) E87.2
    alkalosis (metabolic) (respiratory) E87.3
  elimination, transepidermal L87.9
    specified NEC L87.8
  emotional (persistent) F34.9
    of childhood F93.9
      specified NEC F93.8
  endocrine E34.9
    postprocedural E89.89
    specified NEC E89.89
  erectile (male) (organic) (*see also* Dysfunction, sexual, male, erectile) N52.9
    nonorganic F52.21
  erythematous — *see* Erythema
  esophagus K22.9
    functional K22.4
    psychogenic F45.8
  eustachian tube H69.9- ☑
    infection — *see* Salpingitis, eustachian
    obstruction — *see* Obstruction, eustachian tube
    patulous — *see* Patulous, eustachian tube
    specified NEC H69.8- ☑
  extrapyramidal G25.9
    in diseases classified elsewhere — *see* category G26
    specified type NEC G25.89
  eye H57.9
    postprocedural — *see* Complication, postprocedural, eye
  eyelid H02.9
    cyst — *see* Cyst, eyelid
    degenerative H02.70
      chloasma — *see* Chloasma, eyelid
      madarosis — *see* Madarosis
      specified type NEC H02.79
      vitiligo — *see* Vitiligo, eyelid
      xanthelasma — *see* Xanthelasma
    dermatochalasis — *see* Dermatochalasis
    edema — *see* Edema, eyelid
    elephantiasis — *see* Elephantiasis, eyelid
    foreign body, retained — *see* Foreign body, retained, eyelid
    function H02.59
      abnormal innervation syndrome — *see* Syndrome, abnormal innervation
      blepharochalasis — *see* Blepharochalasis
      blepharoclonus — *see* Blepharoclonus
      blepharophimosis — *see* Blepharophimosis
      blepharoptosis — *see* Blepharoptosis

Disorder — *continued*
  eyelid — *continued*
    function — *continued*
      lagophthalmos — *see* Lagophthalmos
      lid retraction — *see* Retraction, lid
      hypertrichosis — *see* Hypertrichosis, eyelid
      specified type NEC H02.89
      vascular H02.879
        left H02.876
          lower H02.875
          upper H02.874
        right H02.873
          lower H02.872
          upper H02.871
  factitious F68.10
    with predominantly
      physical symptoms F68.12
        with psychological symptoms F68.13
      psychological symptoms F68.11
        with physical symptoms F68.13
  factor, coagulation — *see* Defect, coagulation
  fatty acid
    metabolism E71.30
      specified NEC E71.39
    oxidation
      LCAD E71.310
      MCAD E71.311
      SCAD E71.312
      specified deficiency NEC E71.318
  feeding (infant or child) (*see also* Disorder, eating) R63.3
  feigned (with obvious motivation) Z76.5
    without obvious motivation — *see* Disorder, factitious
  female
    hypoactive sexual desire F52.0
    orgasmic F52.31
    sexual arousal F52.22
  fibroblastic M72.9
    specified NEC M72.8
  fluency
    adult onset F98.5
    childhood onset F80.81
    following
      cerebral infarction I69.323
      cerebrovascular disease I69.923
        specified disease NEC I69.823
      intracerebral hemorrhage I69.123
      nontraumatic intracranial hemorrhage NEC I69.223
      subarachnoid hemorrhage I69.023
    in conditions classified elsewhere R47.82
  fluid balance E87.8
  follicular (skin) L73.9
    specified NEC L73.8
  fructose metabolism E74.10
    essential fructosuria E74.11
    fructokinase deficiency E74.11
    fructose-1, 6-diphosphatase deficiency E74.19
    hereditary fructose intolerance E74.12
    other specified E74.19
  functional polymorphonuclear neutrophils D71
  gallbladder, biliary tract and pancreas in diseases classified elsewhere K87
  gamma-glutamyl cycle E72.8
  gastric (functional) K31.9
    motility K30
    psychogenic F45.8
    secretion K30
  gastrointestinal (functional) NOS K92.9
    newborn P78.9
    psychogenic F45.8
  gender-identity or -role F64.9
    childhood F64.2
    effect on relationship F66
    of adolescence or adulthood (nontranssexual) F64.1
    specified NEC F64.8
    uncertainty F66
  genitourinary system
    female N94.9
    male N50.9
    psychogenic F45.8
  globe H44.9
    degenerated condition H44.50
      absolute glaucoma H44.51- ☑
      atrophy H44.52- ☑
      leucocoria H44.53- ☑
    degenerative H44.30

Disorder — *continued*
  globe — *continued*
    degenerative H44.30
      chalcosis H44.31- ☑
      myopia H44.2- ☑
      siderosis H44.32- ☑
      specified type NEC H44.39- ☑
    endophthalmitis — *see* Endophthalmitis
    foreign body, retained — *see* Foreign body, intraocular, old, retained
    hemophthalmos — *see* Hemophthalmos
    hypotony H44.40
      due to
        ocular fistula H44.42- ☑
        specified disorder NEC H44.43- ☑
      flat anterior chamber H44.41- ☑
      primary H44.44- ☑
    luxation — *see* Luxation, globe
    specified type NEC H44.89
  glomerular (in) N05.9
    amyloidosis E85.4 [N08]
    cryoglobulinemia D89.1 [N08]
    disseminated intravascular coagulation D65 [N08]
    Fabry's disease E75.21 [N08]
    familial lecithin cholesterol acyltransferase deficiency E78.6 [N08]
    Goodpasture's syndrome M31.0
    hemolytic-uremic syndrome D59.3
    Henoch (-Schönlein) purpura D69.0 [N08]
    malariae malaria B52.0
    microscopic polyangiitis M31.7 [N08]
    multiple myeloma C90.0- ☑ [N08]
    mumps B26.83
    schistosomiasis B65.9 [N08]
    sepsis NEC A41.- ☑ [N08]
      streptococcal A40.- ☑ [N08]
    sickle-cell disorders D57.- ☑ [N08]
    strongyloidiasis B78.9 [N08]
    subacute bacterial endocarditis I33.0 [N08]
    syphilis A52.75
    systemic lupus erythematosus M32.14
    thrombotic thrombocytopenic purpura M31.1 [N08]
    Waldenström macroglobulinemia C88.0 [N08]
    Wegener's granulomatosis M31.31
  gluconeogenesis E74.4
  glucosaminoglycan metabolism — *see* Disorder, metabolism, glucosaminoglycan
  glycine metabolism E72.50
    d-glycericacidemia E72.59
    hyperhydroxyprolinemia E72.59
    hyperoxaluria E72.53
    hyperprolinemia E72.59
    non-ketotic hyperglycinemia E72.51
    oxalosis E72.53
    oxaluria E72.53
    sarcosinemia E72.59
    trimethylaminuria E72.52
  glycoprotein metabolism E77.9
    specified NEC E77.8
  habit (and impulse) F63.9
    involving sexual behavior NEC F65.9
    specified NEC F63.89
  heart action I49.9
  hematological D75.9
    newborn (transient) P61.9
      specified NEC P61.8
  hematopoietic organs D75.9
  hemorrhagic NEC D69.9
    drug-induced D68.32
    due to
      extrinsic circulating anticoagulants D68.32
      increase in
        anti-IIa D68.32
        anti-Xa D68.32
      intrinsic
        circulating anticoagulants D68.318
        increase in
          anti-IXa D68.318
          antithrombin D68.318
          anti-VIIIa D68.318
          anti-XIa D68.318
    following childbirth O72.3
  hemostasis — *see* Defect, coagulation
  histidine metabolism E70.40
    histidinemia E70.41
    other specified E70.49

Disorder — *continued*
  hyperkinetic — *see* Disorder, attention-deficit hyperactivity
  hyperleucine-isoleucinemia E71.19
  hypervalinemia E71.19
  hypoactive sexual desire F52.0
  hypochondriacal F45.20
    body dysmorphic F45.22
    neurosis F45.21
    other specified F45.29
  identity
    dissociative F44.81
    of childhood F93.8
  immune mechanism (immunity) D89.9
    specified type NEC D89.89
  impaired renal tubular function N25.9
    specified NEC N25.89
  impulse (control) F63.9
  inflammatory
    pelvic, in diseases classified elsewhere — *see* category N74
    penis N48.29
      abscess N48.21
      cellulitis N48.22
  integument, newborn P83.9
    specified NEC P83.8
  intermittent explosive F63.81
  internal secretion pancreas — *see* Increased, secretion, pancreas, endocrine
  intestine, intestinal
    carbohydrate absorption NEC E74.39
      postoperative K91.2
    functional NEC K59.9
      postoperative K91.89
    psychogenic F45.8
    vascular K55.9
      chronic K55.1
      specified NEC K55.8
  intraoperative (intraprocedural) — *see* Complications, intraoperative
  involuntary emotional expression (IEED) F07.89
  iris H21.9
    adhesions — *see* Adhesions, iris
    atrophy — *see* Atrophy, iris
    chamber angle recession — *see* Recession, chamber angle
    cyst — *see* Cyst, iris
    degeneration — *see* Degeneration, iris
    in diseases classified elsewhere H22
    iridodialysis — *see* Iridodialysis
    iridoschisis — *see* Iridoschisis
    miotic pupillary cyst — *see* Cyst, pupillary
    pupillary
      abnormality — *see* Abnormality, pupillary
      membrane — *see* Membrane, pupillary
    specified type NEC H21.89
    vascular NEC H21.1X- ☑
  iron metabolism E83.10
    specified NEC E83.19
  isovaleric acidemia E71.110
  jaw, developmental M27.0
    temporomandibular — *see* Anomaly, dentofacial, temporomandibular joint
  joint M25.9
    derangement — *see* Derangement, joint
    effusion — *see* Effusion, joint
    fistula — *see* Fistula, joint
    hemarthrosis — *see* Hemarthrosis
    instability — *see* Instability, joint
    osteophyte — *see* Osteophyte
    pain — *see* Pain, joint
    psychogenic F45.8
    specified type NEC M25.80
      ankle M25.87- ☑
      elbow M25.82- ☑
      foot joint M25.87- ☑
      hand joint M25.84- ☑
      hip M25.85- ☑
      knee M25.86- ☑
      shoulder M25.81- ☑
      wrist M25.83- ☑
    stiffness — *see* Stiffness, joint
  ketone metabolism E71.32
  kidney N28.9
    functional (tubular) N25.9
    in
      schistosomiasis B65.9 [N29]

Disorder — *continued*
  kidney — *continued*
    tubular function N25.9
      specified NEC N25.89
  lacrimal system H04.9
    changes H04.69
      fistula — *see* Fistula, lacrimal
    gland H04.19
      atrophy — *see* Atrophy, lacrimal gland
      cyst — *see* Cyst, lacrimal, gland
      dacryops — *see* Dacryops
      dislocation — *see* Dislocation, lacrimal gland
      dry eye syndrome — *see* Syndrome, dry eye
      infection — *see* Dacryoadenitis
      granuloma — *see* Granuloma, lacrimal
      inflammation — *see* Inflammation, lacrimal
      obstruction — *see* Obstruction, lacrimal
      specified NEC H04.89
  lactation NEC O92.79
  language (developmental) F80.9
    expressive F80.1
    mixed receptive and expressive F80.2
    receptive F80.2
  late luteal phase dysphoric N94.89
  learning (specific) F81.9
    acalculia R48.8
    alexia R48.0
    mathematics F81.2
    reading F81.0
    specified NEC F81.89
    spelling F81.81
    written expression F81.81
  lens H27.9
    aphakia — *see* Aphakia
    cataract — *see* Cataract
    dislocation — *see* Dislocation, lens
    specified type NEC H27.8
  ligament M24.20
    ankle M24.27- ☑
    attachment, spine — *see* Enthesopathy, spinal
    elbow M24.22- ☑
    foot joint M24.27- ☑
    hand joint M24.24- ☑
    hip M24.25- ☑
    knee — *see* Derangement, knee, specified NEC
    shoulder M24.21- ☑
    vertebra M24.28
    wrist M24.23- ☑
  ligamentous attachments (*see also* Enthesopathy)
    spine — *see* Enthesopathy, spinal
  lipid
    metabolism, congenital E78.9
    storage E75.6
      specified NEC E75.5
  lipoprotein
    deficiency (familial) E78.6
    metabolism E78.9
      specified NEC E78.89
  liver K76.9
    malarial B54 [K77]
  low back (*see also* Dorsopathy, specified NEC)
  lumbosacral
    plexus G54.1
    root (nerve) NEC G54.4
  lung, interstitial, drug-induced J70.4
    acute J70.2
    chronic J70.3
  lymphoproliferative, post-transplant (PTLD) D47.Z1 (*following* D47.4)
  lysine and hydroxylysine metabolism E72.3
  male
    erectile (organic) (*see also* Dysfunction, sexual, male, erectile) N52.9
      nonorganic F52.21
    hypoactive sexual desire F52.0
    orgasmic F52.32
  manic F30.9
    organic F06.33
  mastoid (*see also* Disorder, ear, middle)
    postprocedural — *see* Complications, ear, procedure
  meniscus — *see* Derangement, knee, meniscus
  menopausal N95.9
    specified NEC N95.8
  menstrual N92.6
    psychogenic F45.8
    specified NEC N92.5

▽ Subterms under main terms may continue to next column or page   ☑ Additional Character Required — Refer to the Tabular List for Character Selection   109

Disorder — Disorder

Disorder — *continued*
  mental (or behavioral) (nonpsychotic) F99
    due to (secondary to)
      amphetamine
        due to drug abuse — *see* Abuse, drug,
            stimulant
        due to drug dependence — *see* Dependence, drug, stimulant
      brain disease, damage and dysfunction F09
      caffeine use
        due to drug abuse — *see* Abuse, drug,
            stimulant
        due to drug dependence — *see* Dependence, drug, stimulant
      cannabis use
        due to drug abuse — *see* Abuse, drug,
            cannabis
        due to drug dependence — *see* Dependence, drug, cannabis
      general medical condition F09
      sedative or hypnotic use
        due to drug abuse — *see* Abuse, drug,
            sedative
        due to drug dependence — *see* Dependence, drug, sedative
      tobacco (nicotine) use — *see* Dependence,
          drug, nicotine
    following organic brain damage F07.9
      frontal lobe syndrome F07.0
      personality change F07.0
      postconcussional syndrome F07.81
      specified NEC F07.89
    infancy, childhood or adolescence F98.9
    neurotic — *see* Neurosis
    organic or symptomatic F09
    presenile, psychotic F03 ☑
    problem NEC
    psychoneurotic — *see* Neurosis
    psychotic — *see* Psychosis
    puerperal F53
    senile, psychotic NEC F03 ☑
  metabolic, amino acid, transitory, newborn P74.8
  metabolism NOS E88.9
    amino-acid E72.9
      aromatic E70.9
        albinism — *see* Albinism
        histidine E70.40
          histidinemia E70.41
          other specified E70.49
        hyperphenylalaninemia E70.1
          classical phenylketonuria E70.0
        other specified E70.8
        tryptophan E70.5
        tyrosine E70.20
          hypertyrosinemia E70.21
          other specified E70.29
      branched chain E71.2
        3-methylglutaconic aciduria E71.111
        hyperleucine-isoleucinemia E71.19
        hypervalinemia E71.19
        isovaleric acidemia E71.110
        maple syrup urine disease E71.0
        methylmalonic acidemia E71.120
        organic aciduria NEC E71.118
        other specified E71.19
        proprionate NEC E71.128
        proprionic acidemia E71.121
      glycine E72.50
        d-glycericacidemia E72.59
        hyperhydroxyprolinemia E72.59
        hyperoxaluria E72.53
        hyperprolinemia E72.59
        non-ketotic hyperglycinemia E72.51
        other specified E72.59
        sarcosinemia E72.59
        trimethylaminuria E72.52
      hydroxylysine E72.3
      lysine E72.3
      ornithine E72.4
      other specified E72.8
        beta-amino acid E72.8
        gamma-glutamyl cycle E72.8
      straight-chain E72.8
      sulfur-bearing E72.10
        homocystinuria E72.11
        methylenetetrahydrofolate reductase deficiency E72.12
        other specified E72.19

Disorder — *continued*
  metabolism — *continued*
    bile acid and cholesterol metabolism E78.70
    bilirubin E80.7
      specified NEC E80.6
    calcium E83.50
      hypercalcemia E83.52
      hypocalcemia E83.51
      other specified E83.59
    carbohydrate E74.9
      specified NEC E74.8
    cholesterol and bile acid metabolism E78.70
    congenital E88.9
    copper E83.00
      specified type NEC E83.09
      Wilson's disease E83.01
    cystinuria E72.01
    fructose E74.10
    galactose E74.20
    glucosaminoglycan E76.9
      mucopolysaccharidosis — *see* Mucopolysaccharidosis
      specified NEC E76.8
    glutamine E72.8
    glycine E72.50
    glycogen storage (hepatorenal) E74.09
    glycoprotein E77.9
      specified NEC E77.8
    glycosaminoglycan E76.9
      specified NEC E76.8
    in labor and delivery O75.89
    iron E83.10
    isoleucine E71.19
    leucine E71.19
    lipoid E78.9
    lipoprotein E78.9
      specified NEC E78.89
    magnesium E83.40
      hypermagnesemia E83.41
      hypomagnesemia E83.42
      other specified E83.49
    mineral E83.9
      specified NEC E83.89
    mitochondrial E88.40
      MELAS syndrome E88.41
      MERRF syndrome (myoclonic epilepsy associated with ragged-red fibers) E88.42
      other specified E88.49
    ornithine E72.4
    phosphatases E83.30
    phosphorus E83.30
      acid phosphatase deficiency E83.39
      hypophosphatasia E83.39
      hypophosphatemia E83.39
        familial E83.31
      other specified E83.39
      pseudovitamin D deficiency E83.32
    plasma protein NEC E88.09
    porphyrin — *see* Porphyria
    postprocedural E89.89
      specified NEC E89.89
    purine E79.9
      specified NEC E79.8
    pyrimidine E79.9
      specified NEC E79.8
    pyruvate E74.4
    serine E72.8
    sodium E87.8
    specified NEC E88.89
    threonine E72.8
    valine E71.19
    zinc E83.2
  methylmalonic acidemia E71.120
  micturition NEC R39.19
    feeling of incomplete emptying R39.14
    hesitancy R39.11
    poor stream R39.12
    psychogenic F45.8
    split stream R39.13
    straining R39.16
    urgency R39.15
  mitochondrial metabolism E88.40
  mitral (valve) — *see* Endocarditis, mitral
  mixed
    anxiety and depressive F41.8
    of scholastic skills (developmental) F81.89
    receptive expressive language F80.2

Disorder — *continued*
  mood F39
    bipolar — *see* Disorder, bipolar
    depressive — *see* Disorder, depressive
    due to (secondary to)
      alcohol F10.94
      amphetamine F15.94
        in
          abuse F15.14
          dependence F15.24
      anxiolytic F13.94
        in
          abuse F13.14
          dependence F13.24
      cocaine F14.94
        in
          abuse F14.14
          dependence F14.24
      general medical condition F06.30
      hallucinogen F16.94
        in
          abuse F16.14
          dependence F16.24
      hypnotic F13.94
        in
          abuse F13.14
          dependence F13.24
      inhalant F18.94
        in
          abuse F18.14
          dependence F18.24
      opioid F11.94
        in
          abuse F11.14
          dependence F11.24
      phencyclidine (PCP) F16.94
        in
          abuse F16.14
          dependence F16.24
      physiological condition F06.30
        with
          depressive features F06.31
          major depressive-like episode F06.32
          manic features F06.33
          mixed features F06.34
      psychoactive substance NEC F19.94
        in
          abuse F19.14
          dependence F19.24
      sedative F13.94
        in
          abuse F13.14
          dependence F13.24
      volatile solvents F18.94
        in
          abuse F18.14
          dependence F18.24
    manic episode F30.9
      with psychotic symptoms F30.2
      without psychotic symptoms F30.10
        mild F30.11
        moderate F30.12
        severe F30.13
      in remission (full) F30.4
        partial F30.3
      specified type NEC F30.8
    organic F06.30
      right hemisphere F07.89
    persistent F34.9
      cyclothymia F34.0
      dysthymia F34.1
      specified type NEC F34.8
    recurrent F39
    right hemisphere organic F07.89
  movement G25.9
    drug-induced G25.70
      akathisia G25.71
      specified NEC G25.79
    hysterical F44.4
    in diseases classified elsewhere — *see* category
        G26
    periodic limb G47.61
      sleep related G47.61
    sleep related NEC G47.69
    specified NEC G25.89
    stereotyped F98.4
    treatment-induced G25.9
  multiple personality F44.81

Disorder — continued
  muscle M62.9
    attachment, spine — see Enthesopathy, spinal
    in trichinellosis — see Trichinellosis, with muscle
        disorder
    psychogenic F45.8
    specified type NEC M62.89
    tone, newborn P94.9
        specified NEC P94.8
  muscular
    attachments (see also Enthesopathy)
        spine — see Enthesopathy, spinal
    urethra N36.44
  musculoskeletal system, soft tissue — see Disorder,
        soft tissue
    postprocedural M96.89
    psychogenic F45.8
  myoneural G70.9
    due to lead G70.1
    specified NEC G70.89
    toxic G70.1
  myotonic NEC G71.19
  nail, in diseases classified elsewhere L62
  neck region NEC — see Dorsopathy, specified NEC
  nerve G58.9
    abducent NEC — see Strabismus, paralytic, sixth
        nerve
    accessory G52.8
    acoustic — see subcategory H93.3 ☑
    auditory — see subcategory H93.3 ☑
    auriculotemporal G50.8
    axillary G54.0
    cerebral — see Disorder, nerve, cranial
    cranial G52.9
        eighth — see subcategory H93.3 ☑
        eleventh G52.8
        fifth G50.9
        first G52.0
        fourth NEC — see Strabismus, paralytic, fourth
            nerve
        multiple G52.7
        ninth G52.1
        second NEC — see Disorder, nerve, optic
        seventh NEC G51.8
        sixth NEC — see Strabismus, paralytic, sixth
            nerve
        specified NEC G52.8
        tenth G52.2
        third NEC — see Strabismus, paralytic, third
            nerve
        twelfth G52.3
    entrapment — see Neuropathy, entrapment
    facial G51.9
        specified NEC G51.8
    femoral — see Lesion, nerve, femoral
    glossopharyngeal NEC G52.1
    hypoglossal G52.3
    intercostal G58.0
    lateral
        cutaneous of thigh — see Mononeuropathy,
            lower limb, meralgia paresthetica
        popliteal — see Lesion, nerve, popliteal
    lower limb — see Mononeuropathy, lower limb
    medial popliteal — see Lesion, nerve, popliteal,
        medial
    median NEC — see Lesion, nerve, median
    multiple G58.7
    oculomotor NEC — see Strabismus, paralytic, third
        nerve
    olfactory G52.0
    optic NEC H47.09- ☑
        hemorrhage into sheath — see Hemorrhage,
            optic nerve
        ischemic H47.01- ☑
    peroneal — see Lesion, nerve, popliteal
    phrenic G58.8
    plantar — see Lesion, nerve, plantar
    pneumogastric G52.2
    posterior tibial — see Syndrome, tarsal tunnel
    radial — see Lesion, nerve, radial
    recurrent laryngeal G52.2
    root G54.9
        cervical G54.2
        lumbosacral G54.1
        specified NEC G54.8
        thoracic G54.3
    sciatic NEC — see Lesion, nerve, sciatic

Disorder — continued
  nerve — continued
    specified NEC G58.8
        lower limb — see Mononeuropathy, lower limb,
            specified NEC
        upper limb — see Mononeuropathy, upper
            limb, specified NEC
    sympathetic G90.9
    tibial — see Lesion, nerve, popliteal, medial
    trigeminal G50.9
        specified NEC G50.8
    trochlear NEC — see Strabismus, paralytic, fourth
        nerve
    ulnar — see Lesion, nerve, ulnar
    upper limb — see Mononeuropathy, upper limb
    vagus G52.2
  nervous system G98.8
    autonomic (peripheral) G90.9
        specified NEC G90.8
    central G96.9
        specified NEC G96.8
    parasympathetic G90.9
    specified NEC G98.8
    sympathetic G90.9
    vegetative G90.9
  neurohypophysis NEC E23.3
  neurological NEC R29.818
  neuromuscular G70.9
    hereditary NEC G71.9
    specified NEC G70.89
    toxic G70.1
  neurotic F48.9
    specified NEC F48.8
  neutrophil, polymorphonuclear D71
  nicotine use — see Dependence, drug, nicotine
  nightmare F51.5
  nose J34.9
    specified NEC J34.89
  obsessive-compulsive F42
  odontogenesis NOS K00.9
  opioid use
    with
        opioid-induced psychotic disorder F11.959
            with
                delusions F11.950
                hallucinations F11.951
        due to drug abuse — see Abuse, drug, opioid
        due to drug dependence — see Dependence, drug,
            opioid
  oppositional defiant F91.3
  optic
    chiasm H47.49
        due to
            inflammatory disorder H47.41
            neoplasm H47.42
            vascular disorder H47.43
    disc H47.39- ☑
        coloboma — see Coloboma, optic disc
        drusen — see Drusen, optic disc
        pseudopapilledema — see Pseudopapilledema
    radiations — see Disorder, visual, pathway
    tracts — see Disorder, visual, pathway
  orbit H05.9
    cyst — see Cyst, orbit
    deformity — see Deformity, orbit
    edema — see Edema, orbit
    enophthalmos — see Enophthalmos
    exophthalmos — see Exophthalmos
    hemorrhage — see Hemorrhage, orbit
    inflammation — see Inflammation, orbit
    myopathy — see Myopathy, extraocular muscles
    retained foreign body — see Foreign body, orbit,
        old
    specified type NEC H05.89
  organic
    anxiety F06.4
    catatonic F06.1
    delusional F06.2
    dissociative F06.8
    emotionally labile (asthenic) F06.8
    mood (affective) F06.30
    schizophrenia-like F06.2
  orgasmic (female) F52.31
    male F52.32
  ornithine metabolism E72.4
  overanxious F41.1
    of childhood F93.8

Disorder — continued
  pain
    with related psychological factors F45.42
    exclusively related to psychological factors F45.41
  pancreatic internal secretion E16.9
    specified NEC E16.8
  panic F41.0
    with agoraphobia F40.01
  papulosquamous L44.9
    in diseases classified elsewhere L45
    specified NEC L44.8
  paranoid F22
    induced F24
    shared F24
  parathyroid (gland) E21.5
    specified NEC E21.4
  parietoalveolar NEC J84.09
  paroxysmal, mixed R56.9
  patella M22.9- ☑
    chondromalacia — see Chondromalacia, patella
    derangement NEC M22.3X- ☑
    recurrent
        dislocation — see Dislocation, patella, recurrent
        subluxation — see Dislocation, patella, recur-
            rent, incomplete
    specified NEC M22.8X- ☑
  patellofemoral M22.2X- ☑
  pentose phosphate pathway with anemia D55.1
  perception, due to hallucinogens F16.983
    in
        abuse F16.183
        dependence F16.283
  peripheral nervous system NEC G64
  peroxisomal E71.50
    biogenesis
        neonatal adrenoleukodystrophy E71.511
        specified disorder NEC E71.518
        Zellweger syndrome E71.510
    rhizomelic chondrodysplasia punctata E71.540
    specified form NEC E71.548
        group 1 E71.518
        group 2 E71.53
        group 3 E71.542
    X-linked adrenoleukodystrophy E71.529
        adolescent E71.521
        adrenomyeloneuropathy E71.522
        childhood E71.520
        specified form NEC E71.528
    Zellweger-like syndrome E71.541
  persistent
    (somatoform) pain F45.41
    affective (mood) F34.9
  personality (see also Personality) F60.9
    affective F34.0
    aggressive F60.3
    amoral F60.2
    anankastic F60.5
    antisocial F60.2
    anxious F60.6
    asocial F60.2
    asthenic F60.7
    avoidant F60.6
    borderline F60.3
    change (secondary) due to general medical condi-
        tion F07.0
    compulsive F60.5
    cyclothymic F34.0
    dependent (passive) F60.7
    depressive F34.1
    dissocial F60.2
    emotional instability F60.3
    expansive paranoid F60.0
    explosive F60.3
    following organic brain damage F07.9
    histrionic F60.4
    hyperthymic F34.0
    hypothymic F34.1
    hysterical F60.4
    immature F60.89
    inadequate F60.7
    labile F60.3
    mixed (nonspecific) F60.89
    moral deficiency F60.2
    narcissistic F60.81
    negativistic F60.89
    obsessional F60.5
    obsessive (-compulsive) F60.5
    organic F07.9

▽ Subterms under main terms may continue to next column or page   ☑ Additional Character Required — Refer to the Tabular List for Character Selection   111

Disorder — *continued*
personality (*see also* Personality) — *continued*
  overconscientious F60.5
  paranoid F60.0
  passive (-dependent) F60.7
  passive-aggressive F60.89
  pathological NEC F60.9
  pseudosocial F60.2
  psychopathic F60.2
  schizoid F60.1
  schizotypal F21
  self-defeating F60.7
  specified NEC F60.89
  type A F60.5
  unstable (emotional) F60.3
pervasive, developmental F84.9
phobic anxiety, childhood F40.8
phosphate-losing tubular N25.0
pigmentation L81.9
  choroid, congenital Q14.3
  diminished melanin formation L81.6
  iron L81.8
  specified NEC L81.8
pinna (noninfective) H61.10- ☑
  deformity, acquired H61.11- ☑
  hematoma H61.12- ☑
  perichondritis — *see* Perichondritis, ear
  specified type NEC H61.19- ☑
pituitary gland E23.7
  iatrogenic (postprocedural) E89.3
  specified NEC E23.6
platelets D69.1
plexus G54.9
  specified NEC G54.8
polymorphonuclear neutrophils D71
porphyrin metabolism — *see* Porphyria
postconcussional F07.81
posthallucinogen perception F16.983
  in
    abuse F16.183
    dependence F16.283
postmenopausal N95.9
  specified NEC N95.8
postprocedural (postoperative) — *see* Complications, postprocedural
post-transplant lymphoproliferative D47.Z1 (*following* D47.4)
post-traumatic stress (PTSD) F43.10
  acute F43.11
  chronic F43.12
premenstrual dysphoric (PMDD) N94.3
prepuce N47.8
propionic acidemia E71.121
prostate N42.9
  specified NEC N42.89
psychogenic NOS (*see also* condition) F45.9
  anxiety F41.8
  appetite F50.9
  asthenic F48.8
  cardiovascular (system) F45.8
  compulsive F42
  cutaneous F54
  depressive F32.9
  digestive (system) F45.8
  dysmenorrheic F45.8
  dyspneic F45.8
  endocrine (system) F54
  eye NEC F45.8
  feeding — *see* Disorder, eating
  functional NEC F45.8
  gastric F45.8
  gastrointestinal (system) F45.8
  genitourinary (system) F45.8
  heart (function) (rhythm) F45.8
  hyperventilatory F45.8
  hypochondriacal — *see* Disorder, hypochondriacal
  intestinal F45.8
  joint F45.8
  learning F81.9
  limb F45.8
  lymphatic (system) F45.8
  menstrual F45.8
  micturition F45.8
  monoplegic NEC F44.4
  motor F44.4
  muscle F45.8
  musculoskeletal F45.8
  neurocirculatory F45.8

Disorder — *continued*
psychogenic (*see also* condition) — *continued*
  obsessive F42
  occupational F48.8
  organ or part of body NEC F45.8
  paralytic NEC F44.4
  phobic F40.9
  physical NEC F45.8
  rectal F45.8
  respiratory (system) F45.8
  rheumatic F45.8
  sexual (function) F52.9
  skin (allergic) (eczematous) F54
  sleep F51.9
  specified part of body NEC F45.8
  stomach F45.8
psychological F99
  associated with
    disease classified elsewhere F54
    sexual
      development F66
      relationship F66
      uncertainty about gender identity F66
psychomotor NEC F44.4
  hysterical F44.4
psychoneurotic (*see also* Neurosis)
  mixed NEC F48.8
psychophysiologic — *see* Disorder, somatoform
psychosexual F65.9
  development F66
  identity of childhood F64.2
psychosomatic NOS — *see* Disorder, somatoform
  multiple F45.0
  undifferentiated F45.1
psychotic — *see* Psychosis
  transient (acute) F23
puberty E30.9
  specified NEC E30.8
pulmonary (valve) — *see* Endocarditis, pulmonary
purine metabolism E79.9
pyrimidine metabolism E79.9
pyruvate metabolism E74.4
reactive attachment (childhood) F94.1
reading R48.0
  developmental (specific) F81.0
receptive language F80.2
receptor, hormonal, peripheral (*see also* Syndrome, androgen insensitivity) E34.50
recurrent brief depressive F33.8
reflex R29.2
refraction H52.7
  aniseikonia H52.32
  anisometropia H52.31
  astigmatism — *see* Astigmatism
  hypermetropia — *see* Hypermetropia
  myopia — *see* Myopia
  presbyopia H52.4
  specified NEC H52.6
relationship F68.8
  due to sexual orientation F66
REM sleep behavior G47.52
renal function, impaired (tubular) N25.9
resonance R49.9
  specified NEC R49.8
respiratory function, impaired (*see also* Failure, respiration)
  postprocedural — *see* Complication, postoperative, respiratory system
  psychogenic F45.8
retina H35.9
  angioid streaks H35.33
  changes in vascular appearance H35.01- ☑
  degeneration — *see* Degeneration, retina
  dystrophy (hereditary) — *see* Dystrophy, retina
  edema H35.81
  hemorrhage — *see* Hemorrhage, retina
  ischemia H35.82
  macular degeneration — *see* Degeneration, macula
  microaneurysms H35.04- ☑
  microvascular abnormality NEC H35.09
  neovascularization — *see* Neovascularization, retina
  retinopathy — *see* Retinopathy
  separation of layers H35.70
    central serous chorioretinopathy H35.71- ☑
    pigment epithelium detachment (serous) H35.72- ☑
      hemorrhagic H35.73- ☑

Disorder — *continued*
retina — *continued*
  specified type NEC H35.89
  telangiectasis — *see* Telangiectasis, retina
  vasculitis — *see* Vasculitis, retina
retroperitoneal K68.9
right hemisphere organic affective F07.89
rumination (infant or child) F98.21
sacrum, sacrococcygeal NEC M53.3
schizoaffective F25.9
  bipolar type F25.0
  depressive type F25.1
  manic type F25.0
  mixed type F25.0
  specified NEC F25.8
schizoid of childhood F84.5
schizophreniform F20.81
  brief F23
schizotypal (personality) F21
secretion, thyrocalcitonin E07.0
seizure (*see also* Epilepsy) G40.909
  intractable G40.919
    with status epilepticus G40.911
semantic pragmatic F80.89
  with autism F84.0
sense of smell R43.1
  psychogenic F45.8
separation anxiety, of childhood F93.0
sexual
  arousal, female F52.22
  aversion F52.1
  function, psychogenic F52.9
  maturation F66
  nonorganic F52.9
  preference (*see also* Deviation, sexual) F65.9
    fetishistic transvestism F65.1
  relationship F66
shyness, of childhood and adolescence F40.10
sibling rivalry F93.8
sickle-cell (sickling) (homozygous) — *see* Disease, sickle-cell
  heterozygous D57.3
  specified type NEC D57.8- ☑
  trait D57.3
sinus (nasal) J34.9
  specified NEC J34.89
skin L98.9
  atrophic L90.9
    specified NEC L90.8
  granulomatous L92.9
    specified NEC L92.8
  hypertrophic L91.9
    specified NEC L91.8
  infiltrative NEC L98.6
  newborn P83.9
    specified NEC P83.8
  psychogenic (allergic) (eczematous) F54
sleep G47.9
  breathing-related — *see* Apnea, sleep
  circadian rhythm G47.20
    advance sleep phase type G47.22
    delayed sleep phase type G47.21
    due to
      alcohol
        abuse F10.182
        dependence F10.282
        use F10.982
      amphetamines
        abuse F15.182
        dependence F15.282
        use F15.982
      caffeine
        abuse F15.182
        dependence F15.282
        use F15.982
      cocaine
        abuse F14.182
        dependence F14.282
        use F14.982
      drug NEC
        abuse F19.182
        dependence F19.282
        use F19.982
      opioid
        abuse F11.182
        dependence F11.282
        use F11.982

☑ Additional Character Required — Refer to the Tabular List for Character Selection   ▽ Subterms under main terms may continue to next column or page

Disorder — *continued*
  sleep — *continued*
    circadian rhythm — *continued*
      due to — *continued*
        psychoactive substance NEC
          abuse F19.182
          dependence F19.282
          use F19.982
        sedative, hypnotic, or anxiolytic
          abuse F13.182
          dependence F13.282
          use F13.982
        stimulant NEC
          abuse F15.182
          dependence F15.282
          use F15.982
      free running type G47.24
      in conditions classified elsewhere G47.27
      irregular sleep wake type G47.23
      jet lag type G47.25
      shift work type G47.26
      specified NEC G47.29
    due to
      alcohol
        abuse F10.182
        dependence F10.282
        use F10.982
      amphetamine
        abuse F15.182
        dependence F15.282
        use F15.982
      anxiolytic
        abuse F13.182
        dependence F13.282
        use F13.982
      caffeine
        abuse F15.182
        dependence F15.282
        use F15.982
      cocaine
        abuse F14.182
        dependence F14.282
        use F14.982
      drug NEC
        abuse F19.182
        dependence F19.282
        use F19.982
      hypnotic
        abuse F13.182
        dependence F13.282
        use F13.982
      opioid
        abuse F11.182
        dependence F11.282
        use F11.982
      psychoactive substance NEC
        abuse F19.182
        dependence F19.282
        use F19.982
      sedative
        abuse F13.182
        dependence F13.282
        use F13.982
      stimulant NEC
        abuse F15.182
        dependence F15.282
        use F15.982
    emotional F51.9
    excessive somnolence — *see* Hypersomnia
    hypersomnia type — *see* Hypersomnia
    initiating or maintaining — *see* Insomnia
    nightmares F51.5
    nonorganic F51.9
      specified NEC F51.8
    parasomnia type G47.50
    specified NEC G47.8
    terrors F51.4
    walking F51.3
  sleep-wake pattern or schedule — *see* Disorder, sleep,
    circadian rhythm
  social
    anxiety of childhood F40.10
    functioning in childhood F94.9
      specified NEC F94.8
  soft tissue M79.9
    ankle M79.9
    due to use, overuse and pressure M70.90
      ankle M70.97- ☑

Disorder — *continued*
  soft tissue — *continued*
    due to use, overuse and pressure — *continued*
      bursitis — *see* Bursitis
      foot M70.97- ☑
      forearm M70.93- ☑
      hand M70.94- ☑
      lower leg M70.96- ☑
      multiple sites M70.99
      pelvic region M70.95- ☑
      shoulder region M70.91- ☑
      specified site NEC M70.98
      specified type NEC M70.80
        ankle M70.87- ☑
        foot M70.87- ☑
        forearm M70.83- ☑
        hand M70.84- ☑
        lower leg M70.86- ☑
        multiple sites M70.89
        pelvic region M70.85- ☑
        shoulder region M70.81- ☑
        specified site NEC M70.88
        thigh M70.85- ☑
        upper arm M70.82- ☑
      thigh M70.95- ☑
      upper arm M70.92- ☑
    foot M79.9
    forearm M79.9
    hand M79.9
    lower leg M79.9
    multiple sites M79.9
    occupational — *see* Disorder, soft tissue, due to
      use, overuse and pressure
    pelvic region M79.9
    shoulder region M79.9
    specified type NEC M79.89
    thigh M79.9
    upper arm M79.9
  somatization F45.0
  somatoform F45.9
    pain (persistent) F45.41
    somatization (multiple) (long-lasting) F45.0
    specified NEC F45.8
    undifferentiated F45.1
  somnolence, excessive — *see* Hypersomnia
  specific
    arithmetical F81.2
    developmental, of motor F82
    reading F81.0
    speech and language F80.9
    spelling F81.81
    written expression F81.81
  speech R47.9
    articulation (functional) (specific) F80.0
    developmental F80.9
    specified NEC R47.89
  spelling (specific) F81.81
  spine (*see also* Dorsopathy)
    ligamentous or muscular attachments, peripheral
      — *see* Enthesopathy, spinal
    specified NEC — *see* Dorsopathy, specified NEC
  stereotyped, habit or movement F98.4
  stomach (functional) — *see* Disorder, gastric
  stress F43.9
    post-traumatic F43.10
      acute F43.11
      chronic F43.12
  sulfur-bearing amino-acid metabolism E72.10
  sweat gland (eccrine) L74.9
    apocrine L75.9
      specified NEC L75.8
    specified NEC L74.8
  synovium M67.90
    acromioclavicular M67.91- ☑
    ankle M67.97- ☑
    elbow M67.92- ☑
    foot M67.97- ☑
    forearm M67.93- ☑
    hand M67.94- ☑
    hip M67.95- ☑
    knee M67.96- ☑
    multiple sites M67.99
    rupture — *see* Rupture, synovium
    shoulder M67.91- ☑
    specified type NEC M67.80
      acromioclavicular M67.81- ☑
      ankle M67.87- ☑

Disorder — *continued*
  synovium — *continued*
    specified type — *continued*
      elbow M67.82- ☑
      foot M67.87- ☑
      hand M67.84- ☑
      hip M67.85- ☑
      knee M67.86- ☑
      multiple sites M67.89
      wrist M67.83- ☑
    synovitis — *see* Synovitis
    upper arm M67.92- ☑
    wrist M67.93- ☑
  temperature regulation, newborn P81.9
    specified NEC P81.8
  temporomandibular joint — *see* Anomaly, dentofacial,
    temporomandibular joint
  tendon M67.90
    acromioclavicular M67.91- ☑
    ankle M67.97- ☑
    contracture — *see* Contracture, tendon
    elbow M67.92- ☑
    foot M67.97- ☑
    forearm M67.93- ☑
    hand M67.94- ☑
    hip M67.95- ☑
    knee M67.96- ☑
    multiple sites M67.99
    rupture — *see* Rupture, tendon
    shoulder M67.91- ☑
    specified type NEC M67.80
      acromioclavicular M67.81- ☑
      ankle M67.87- ☑
      elbow M67.82- ☑
      foot M67.87- ☑
      hand M67.84- ☑
      hip M67.85- ☑
      knee M67.86- ☑
      multiple sites M67.89
      trunk M67.88
      wrist M67.83- ☑
    synovitis — *see* Synovitis
    tendinitis — *see* Tendinitis
    tenosynovitis — *see* Tenosynovitis
    trunk M67.98
    upper arm M67.92- ☑
    wrist M67.93- ☑
  thoracic root (nerve) NEC G54.3
  thyrocalcitonin hypersecretion E07.0
  thyroid (gland) E07.9
    function NEC, neonatal, transitory P72.2
    iodine-deficiency related E01.8
    specified NEC E07.89
  tic — *see* Tic
  tooth K08.9
    development K00.9
      specified NEC K00.8
    eruption K00.6
  Tourette's F95.2
  trance and possession F44.89
  tricuspid (valve) — *see* Endocarditis, tricuspid
  tryptophan metabolism E70.5
  tubular, phosphate-losing N25.0
  tubulo-interstitial (in)
    brucellosis A23.9 [N16]
    cystinosis E72.04
    diphtheria A36.84
    glycogen storage disease E74.00 [N16]
    leukemia NEC C95.9- ☑ [N16]
    lymphoma NEC C85.9- ☑ [N16]
    mixed cryoglobulinemia D89.1 [N16]
    multiple myeloma C90.0- ☑ [N16]
    Salmonella infection A02.25
    sarcoidosis D86.84
    sepsis A41.9 [N16]
      streptococcal A40.9 [N16]
    systemic lupus erythematosus M32.15
    toxoplasmosis B58.83
    transplant rejection T86.91 [N16]
    Wilson's disease E83.01 [N16]
  tubulo-renal function, impaired N25.9
    specified NEC N25.89
  tympanic membrane H73.9- ☑
    atrophy — *see* Atrophy, tympanic membrane
    infection — *see* Myringitis
    perforation — *see* Perforation, tympanum
    specified NEC H73.89- ☑

▽ **Subterms under main terms may continue to next column or page**   ☑ **Additional Character Required — Refer to the Tabular List for Character Selection**   **113**

Disorder — Disorder

Disorder — *continued*
  unsocialized aggressive F91.1
  urea cycle metabolism E72.20
    argininemia E72.21
    arginosuccinic aciduria E72.22
    citrullinemia E72.23
    ornithine transcarbamylase deficiency E72.4
    other specified E72.29
  ureter (in) N28.9
    schistosomiasis B65.0 [N29]
    tuberculosis A18.11
  urethra N36.9
    specified NEC N36.8
  urinary system N39.9
    specified NEC N39.8
  valve, heart
    aortic — *see* Endocarditis, aortic
    mitral — *see* Endocarditis, mitral
    pulmonary — *see* Endocarditis, pulmonary
    rheumatic
      aortic — *see* Endocarditis, aortic, rheumatic
      mitral — *see* Endocarditis, mitral
      pulmonary — *see* Endocarditis, pulmonary,
        rheumatic
      tricuspid — *see* Endocarditis, tricuspid
    tricuspid — *see* Endocarditis, tricuspid
  vestibular function H81.9- ☑
    specified NEC — *see* subcategory H81.8 ☑
      in diseases classified elsewhere H82.- ☑
    vertigo — *see* Vertigo
  vision, binocular H53.30
    abnormal retinal correspondence H53.31
    diplopia H53.2
    fusion with defective stereopsis H53.32
    simultaneous perception H53.33
    suppression H53.34
  visual
    cortex
      blindness H47.619
        left brain H47.612
        right brain H47.611
      due to
        inflammatory disorder H47.629
          left brain H47.622
          right brain H47.621
        neoplasm H47.639
          left brain H47.632
          right brain H47.631
        vascular disorder H47.649
          left brain H47.642
          right brain H47.641
    pathway H47.9
      due to
        inflammatory disorder H47.51- ☑
        neoplasm H47.52- ☑
        vascular disorder H47.53- ☑
      optic chiasm — *see* Disorder, optic, chiasm
  vitreous body H43.9
    crystalline deposits — *see* Deposit, crystalline
    degeneration — *see* Degeneration, vitreous
    hemorrhage — *see* Hemorrhage, vitreous
    opacities — *see* Opacity, vitreous
    prolapse — *see* Prolapse, vitreous
    specified type NEC H43.89
  voice R49.9
    specified type NEC R49.8
  volatile solvent use
    due to drug abuse — *see* Abuse, drug, inhalant
    due to drug dependence — *see* Dependence, drug,
      inhalant
  white blood cells D72.9
    specified NEC D72.89
  withdrawing, child or adolescent F40.10
Disorientation R41.0
Displacement, displaced
  acquired traumatic of bone, cartilage, joint, tendon
    NEC — *see* Dislocation
  adrenal gland (congenital) Q89.1
  appendix, retrocecal (congenital) Q43.8
  auricle (congenital) Q17.4
  bladder (acquired) N32.89
    congenital Q64.19
  brachial plexus (congenital) Q07.8
  brain stem, caudal (congenital) Q04.8
  canaliculus (lacrimalis), congenital Q10.6
  cardia through esophageal hiatus (congenital) Q40.1
  cerebellum, caudal (congenital) Q04.8
  cervix — *see* Malposition, uterus

Displacement, displaced — *continued*
  colon (congenital) Q43.3
  device, implant or graft (*see also* Complications, by
    site and type, mechanical) T85.628 ☑
    arterial graft NEC — *see* Complication, cardiovas-
      cular device, mechanical, vascular
    breast (implant) T85.42 ☑
    catheter NEC T85.628 ☑
      dialysis (renal) T82.42 ☑
        intraperitoneal T85.621 ☑
      infusion NEC T82.524 ☑
        spinal (epidural) (subdural) T85.620 ☑
      urinary (indwelling) T83.028 ☑
        cystostomy T83.020 ☑
    electronic (electrode) (pulse generator) (stimulator)
      — *see* Complication, electronic stimulator
    fixation, internal (orthopedic) NEC — *see* Compli-
      cation, fixation device, mechanical
    gastrointestinal — *see* Complications, prosthetic
      device, mechanical, gastrointestinal device
    genital NEC T83.428 ☑
      intrauterine contraceptive device T83.32 ☑
      penile prosthesis T83.420 ☑
    heart NEC — *see* Complication, cardiovascular de-
      vice, mechanical
    joint prosthesis — *see* Complications, joint prosthe-
      sis, mechanical
    ocular — *see* Complications, prosthetic device,
      mechanical, ocular device
    orthopedic NEC — *see* Complication, orthopedic,
      device or graft, mechanical
    specified NEC T85.628 ☑
    urinary NEC (*see also* Complication, genitourinary,
      device, urinary, mechanical)
      graft T83.22 ☑
    vascular NEC — *see* Complication, cardiovascular
      device, mechanical
    ventricular intracranial shunt T85.02 ☑
  electronic stimulator
    bone T84.320 ☑
    cardiac — *see* Complications, cardiac device, elec-
      tronic
    nervous system — *see* Complication, prosthetic
      device, mechanical, electronic nervous sys-
      tem stimulator
    urinary — *see* Complications, electronic stimulator,
      urinary
  esophageal mucosa into cardia of stomach, congenital
    Q39.8
  esophagus (acquired) K22.8
    congenital Q39.8
  eyeball (acquired) (lateral) (old) — *see* Displacement,
    globe
    congenital Q15.8
    current — *see* Avulsion, eye
  fallopian tube (acquired) N83.4
    congenital Q50.6
    opening (congenital) Q50.6
  gallbladder (congenital) Q44.1
  gastric mucosa (congenital) Q40.2
  globe (acquired) (old) (lateral) H05.21- ☑
    current — *see* Avulsion, eye
  heart (congenital) Q24.8
    acquired I51.89
  hymen (upward) (congenital) Q52.4
  intervertebral disc NEC
    with myelopathy — *see* Disorder, disc, with,
      myelopathy
    cervical, cervicothoracic (with) M50.20
      myelopathy — *see* Disorder, disc, cervical, with
        myelopathy
      neuritis, radiculitis or radiculopathy — *see* Dis-
        order, disc, cervical, with neuritis
    due to trauma — *see* Dislocation, vertebra
    lumbar region M51.26
      with
        myelopathy M51.06
        neuritis, radiculitis, radiculopathy or sciatica
          M51.16
    lumbosacral region M51.27
      with
        neuritis, radiculitis, radiculopathy or sciatica
          M51.17
    sacrococcygeal region M53.3
    thoracic region M51.24
      with
        myelopathy M51.04

Displacement, displaced — *continued*
  intervertebral disc — *continued*
    thoracic region — *continued*
      with — *continued*
        neuritis, radiculitis, radiculopathy M51.14
    thoracolumbar region M51.25
      with
        myelopathy M51.05
        neuritis, radiculitis, radiculopathy M51.15
  intrauterine device T83.32 ☑
  kidney (acquired) N28.83
    congenital Q63.2
  lachrymal, lacrimal apparatus or duct (congenital)
    Q10.6
  lens, congenital Q12.1
  macula (congenital) Q14.1
  Meckel's diverticulum Q43.0
    malignant — *see* Table of Neoplasms, small intes-
      tine, malignant
  nail (congenital) Q84.6
    acquired L60.8
  opening of Wharton's duct in mouth Q38.4
  organ or site, congenital NEC — *see* Malposition,
    congenital
  ovary (acquired) N83.4
    congenital Q50.39
    free in peritoneal cavity (congenital) Q50.39
    into hernial sac N83.4
  oviduct (acquired) N83.4
    congenital Q50.6
  parathyroid (gland) E21.4
  parotid gland (congenital) Q38.4
  punctum lacrimale (congenital) Q10.6
  sacro-iliac (joint) (congenital) Q74.2
    current injury S33.2 ☑
    old — *see* subcategory M53.2 ☑
  salivary gland (any) (congenital) Q38.4
  spleen (congenital) Q89.09
  stomach, congenital Q40.2
  sublingual duct Q38.4
  tongue (downward) (congenital) Q38.3
  tooth, teeth, fully erupted M26.30
    horizontal M26.33
    vertical M26.34
  trachea (congenital) Q32.1
  ureter or ureteric opening or orifice (congenital)
    Q62.62
  uterine opening of oviducts or fallopian tubes Q50.6
  uterus, uterine — *see* Malposition, uterus
  ventricular septum Q21.0
    with rudimentary ventricle Q20.4
Disproportion
  between native and reconstructed breast N65.1
  fiber-type G71.2
Disruptio uteri — *see* Rupture, uterus
Disruption (of)
  ciliary body NEC H21.89
  closure of
    cornea T81.31 ☑
    craniotomy T81.32 ☑
    fascia (muscular) (superficial) T81.32 ☑
    internal organ or tissue T81.32 ☑
    laceration (external) (internal) T81.33 ☑
    ligament T81.32 ☑
    mucosa T81.31 ☑
    muscle or muscle flap T81.32 ☑
    ribs or rib cage T81.32 ☑
    skin and subcutaneous tissue (full-thickness) (su-
      perficial) T81.31 ☑
    skull T81.32 ☑
    sternum (sternotomy) T81.32 ☑
    tendon T81.32 ☑
    traumatic laceration (external) (internal) T81.33 ☑
  family Z63.8
    due to
      absence of family member due to military de-
        ployment Z63.31
      absence of family member NEC Z63.32
      alcoholism and drug addiction in family Z63.72
      bereavement Z63.4
      death (assumed) or disappearance of family
        member Z63.4
      divorce or separation Z63.5
      drug addiction in family Z63.72
      return of family member from military deploy-
        ment (current or past conflict) Z63.71
      stressful life events NEC Z63.79
  iris NEC H21.89

Disruption — *continued*
  ligament(s) (*see also* Sprain)
    knee
      current injury — *see* Dislocation, knee
      old (chronic) — *see* Derangement, knee, instability
      spontaneous NEC — *see* Derangement, knee, disruption ligament
    ossicular chain — *see* Discontinuity, ossicles, ear
  pelvic ring (stable) S32.810 ☑
    unstable S32.811 ☑
  traumatic injury wound repair T81.33 ☑
  wound T81.30 ☑
    episiotomy O90.1
    operation T81.31 ☑
      cesarean O90.0
      external operation wound (superficial) T81.31 ☑
      internal operation wound (deep) T81.32 ☑
    perineal (obstetric) O90.1
    traumatic injury repair T81.33 ☑
Dissatisfaction with
  employment Z56.9
  school environment Z55.4
Dissecting — *see* condition
Dissection
  aorta I71.00
    abdominal I71.02
    thoracic I71.01
    thoracoabdominal I71.03
  artery
    carotid I77.71
    cerebral (nonruptured) I67.0
      ruptured — *see* Hemorrhage, intracranial, subarachnoid
    coronary I25.42
    iliac I77.72
    renal I77.73
    specified NEC I77.79
    vertebral I77.74
  traumatic — *see* Wound, open, by site
  vascular I99.8
  wound — *see* Wound, open
Disseminated — *see* condition
Dissociation
  auriculoventricular or atrioventricular (AV) (any degree) (isorhythmic) I45.89
    with heart block I44.2
  interference I45.89
Dissociative reaction, state F44.9
Dissolution, vertebra — *see* Osteoporosis
Distension, distention
  abdomen R14.0
  bladder N32.89
  cecum K63.89
  colon K63.89
  gallbladder K82.8
  intestine K63.89
  kidney N28.89
  liver K76.89
  seminal vesicle N50.8
  stomach K31.89
    acute K31.0
    psychogenic F45.8
  ureter — *see* Dilatation, ureter
  uterus N85.8
Distoma hepaticum infestation B66.3
Distomiasis B66.9
  bile passages B66.3
  hemic B65.9
  hepatic B66.3
    due to Clonorchis sinensis B66.1
  intestinal B66.5
  liver B66.3
    due to Clonorchis sinensis B66.1
  lung B66.4
  pulmonary B66.4
Distomolar (fourth molar) K00.1
Disto-occlusion (Division I) (Division II) M26.212
Distortion(s) (congenital)
  adrenal (gland) Q89.1
  arm NEC Q68.8
  bile duct or passage Q44.5
  bladder Q64.79
  brain Q04.9
  cervix (uteri) Q51.9
  chest (wall) Q67.8

Distortion(s) — *continued*
  chest (wall) Q67.8
    bones Q76.8
  clavicle Q74.0
  clitoris Q52.6
  coccyx Q76.49
  common duct Q44.5
  coronary Q24.5
  cystic duct Q44.5
  ear (auricle) (external) Q17.3
    inner Q16.5
    middle Q16.4
      ossicles Q16.3
  endocrine NEC Q89.2
  eustachian tube Q17.8
  eye (adnexa) Q15.8
  face bone(s) NEC Q75.8
  fallopian tube Q50.6
  femur NEC Q68.8
  fibula NEC Q68.8
  finger(s) Q68.1
  foot Q66.9
  genitalia, genital organ(s)
    female Q52.8
      external Q52.79
      internal NEC Q52.8
  gyri Q04.8
  hand bone(s) Q68.1
  heart (auricle) (ventricle) Q24.8
    valve (cusp) Q24.8
  hepatic duct Q44.5
  humerus NEC Q68.8
  hymen Q52.4
  intrafamilial communications Z63.8
  jaw NEC M26.89
  labium (majus) (minus) Q52.79
  leg NEC Q68.8
  lens Q12.8
  liver Q44.7
  lumbar spine Q76.49
    with disproportion O33.8
      causing obstructed labor O65.0
  lumbosacral (joint) (region) Q76.49
    kyphosis — *see* Kyphosis, congenital
    lordosis — *see* Lordosis, congenital
  nerve Q07.8
  nose Q30.8
  organ
    of Corti Q16.5
    or site not listed — *see* Anomaly, by site
  ossicles, ear Q16.3
  oviduct Q50.6
  pancreas Q45.3
  parathyroid (gland) Q89.2
  pituitary (gland) Q89.2
  radius NEC Q68.8
  sacroiliac joint Q74.2
  sacrum Q76.49
  scapula Q74.0
  shoulder girdle Q74.0
  skull bone(s) NEC Q75.8
    with
      anencephalus Q00.0
      encephalocele — *see* Encephalocele
      hydrocephalus Q03.9
        with spina bifida — *see* Spina bifida, with hydrocephalus
      microcephaly Q02
  spinal cord Q06.8
  spine Q76.49
    kyphosis — *see* Kyphosis, congenital
    lordosis — *see* Lordosis, congenital
  spleen Q89.09
  sternum NEC Q76.7
  thorax (wall) Q67.8
    bony Q76.8
  thymus (gland) Q89.2
  thyroid (gland) Q89.2
  tibia NEC Q68.8
  toe(s) Q66.9
  tongue Q38.3
  trachea (cartilage) Q32.1
  ulna NEC Q68.8
  ureter Q62.8
  urethra Q64.79
    causing obstruction Q64.39
  uterus Q51.9
  vagina Q52.4

Distortion(s) — *continued*
  vertebra Q76.49
    kyphosis — *see* Kyphosis, congenital
    lordosis — *see* Lordosis, congenital
  visual (*see also* Disturbance, vision)
    shape and size H53.15
  vulva Q52.79
  wrist (bones) (joint) Q68.8
Distress
  abdomen — *see* Pain, abdominal
  acute respiratory (adult) (child) J80
  epigastric R10.13
  fetal P84
    complicating pregnancy — *see* Stress, fetal
  gastrointestinal (functional) K30
    psychogenic F45.8
  intestinal (functional) NOS K59.9
    psychogenic F45.8
  maternal, during labor and delivery O75.0
  respiratory R06.00
    adult J80
    child J80
    newborn P22.9
      specified NEC P22.8
    orthopnea R06.01
    psychogenic F45.8
    shortness of breath R06.02
    specified type NEC R06.09
Distribution vessel, atypical Q27.9
  coronary artery Q24.5
  precerebral Q28.1
Districhiasis L68.8
Disturbance(s) (*see also* Disease)
  absorption K90.9
    calcium E58
    carbohydrate K90.4
    fat K90.4
      pancreatic K90.3
    protein K90.4
    starch K90.4
    vitamin — *see* Deficiency, vitamin
  acid-base equilibrium E87.8
    mixed E87.4
  activity and attention (with hyperkinesis) — *see* Disorder, attention-deficit hyperactivity
  amino acid transport E72.00
  assimilation, food K90.9
  auditory nerve, except deafness — *see* subcategory H93.3 ☑
  behavior — *see* Disorder, conduct
  blood clotting (mechanism) (*see also* Defect, coagulation) D68.9
  cerebral
    nerve — *see* Disorder, nerve, cranial
    status, newborn P91.9
      specified NEC P91.8
  circulatory I99.9
  conduct (*see also* Disorder, conduct) F91.9
    adjustment reaction — *see* Disorder, adjustment
    compulsive F63.9
    disruptive F91.9
    hyperkinetic — *see* Disorder, attention-deficit hyperactivity
    socialized F91.2
    specified NEC F91.8
    unsocialized F91.1
  coordination R27.8
  cranial nerve — *see* Disorder, nerve, cranial
  deep sensibility — *see* Disturbance, sensation
  digestive K30
    psychogenic F45.8
  electrolyte (*see also* Imbalance, electrolyte)
    newborn, transitory P74.4
      hyperammonemia P74.6
      potassium balance P74.3
      sodium balance P74.2
      specified type NEC P74.4
  emotions specific to childhood and adolescence F93.9
    with
      anxiety and fearfulness NEC F93.8
      elective mutism F94.0
      oppositional disorder F91.3
      sensitivity (withdrawal) F40.10
      shyness F40.10
      social withdrawal F40.10
    involving relationship problems F93.8
    mixed F93.8
    specified NEC F93.8

Disturbance(s) — continued
  endocrine (gland) E34.9
    neonatal, transitory P72.9
      specified NEC P72.8
  equilibrium R42
  fructose metabolism E74.10
  gait — see Gait
    hysterical F44.4
    psychogenic F44.4
  gastrointestinal (functional) K30
    psychogenic F45.8
  habit, child F98.9
  hearing, except deafness and tinnitus — see Abnormal,
      auditory perception
  heart, functional (conditions in I44-I50)
    due to presence of (cardiac) prosthesis I97.19- ☑
    postoperative I97.89
      cardiac surgery I97.19- ☑
  hormones E34.9
  innervation uterus (parasympathetic) (sympathetic)
      N85.8
  keratinization NEC
    gingiva K05.10
      nonplaque induced K05.11
      plaque induced K05.10
    lip K13.0
    oral (mucosa) (soft tissue) K13.29
    tongue K13.29
  learning (specific) — see Disorder, learning
  memory — see Amnesia
    mild, following organic brain damage F06.8
  mental F99
    associated with diseases classified elsewhere F54
  metabolism E88.9
    with
      abortion — see Abortion, by type with other
          specified complication
      ectopic pregnancy O08.5
      molar pregnancy O08.5
    amino-acid E72.9
      aromatic E70.9
      branched-chain E71.2
      straight-chain E72.8
      sulfur-bearing E72.10
    ammonia E72.20
    arginine E72.21
    arginosuccinic acid E72.22
    carbohydrate E74.9
    cholesterol E78.9
    citrulline E72.23
    cystathionine E72.19
    general E88.9
    glutamine E72.8
    histidine E70.40
    homocystine E72.19
    hydroxylysine E72.3
    in labor or delivery O75.89
    iron E83.10
    lipoid E78.9
    lysine E72.3
    methionine E72.19
    neonatal, transitory P74.9
      calcium and magnesium P71.9
        specified type NEC P71.8
      carbohydrate metabolism P70.9
        specified type NEC P70.8
      specified NEC P74.8
    ornithine E72.4
    phosphate E83.39
    sodium NEC E87.8
    threonine E72.8
    tryptophan E70.5
    tyrosine E70.20
    urea cycle E72.20
  motor R29.2
  nervous, functional R45.0
  neuromuscular mechanism (eye), due to syphilis
      A52.15
  nutritional E63.9
    nail L60.3
  ocular motion H51.9
    psychogenic F45.8
  oculogyric H51.8
    psychogenic F45.8
  oculomotor H51.9
    psychogenic F45.8
  olfactory nerve R43.1
  optic nerve NEC — see Disorder, nerve, optic

Disturbance(s) — continued
  oral epithelium, including tongue NEC K13.29
  perceptual due to
    alcohol withdrawal F10.232
    amphetamine intoxication F15.922
      in
        abuse F15.122
        dependence F15.222
    anxiolytic withdrawal F13.232
    cannabis intoxication (acute) F12.922
      in
        abuse F12.122
        dependence F12.222
    cocaine intoxication (acute) F14.922
      in
        abuse F14.122
        dependence F14.222
    hypnotic withdrawal F13.232
    opioid intoxication (acute) F11.922
      in
        abuse F11.122
        dependence F11.222
    phencyclidine intoxication (acute) F19.922
      in
        abuse F19.122
        dependence F19.222
    sedative withdrawal F13.232
  personality (pattern) (trait) (see also Disorder, person-
      ality) F60.9
    following organic brain damage F07.9
  polyglandular E31.9
    specified NEC E31.8
  potassium balance, newborn P74.3
  psychogenic F45.9
  psychomotor F44.4
  psychophysical visual H53.16
  pupillary — see Anomaly, pupil, function
  reflex R29.2
  rhythm, heart I49.9
  salivary secretion K11.7
  sensation (cold) (heat) (localization) (tactile discrimi-
      nation) (texture) (vibratory) NEC R20.9
    hysterical F44.6
    skin R20.9
      anesthesia R20.0
      hyperesthesia R20.3
      hypoesthesia R20.1
      paresthesia R20.2
      specified type NEC R20.8
    smell R43.9
      and taste (mixed) R43.8
      anosmia R43.0
      parosmia R43.1
      specified NEC R43.8
    taste R43.9
      and smell (mixed) R43.8
      parageusia R43.2
      specified NEC R43.8
  sensory — see Disturbance, sensation
  situational (transient) (see also Disorder, adjustment)
    acute F43.0
  sleep G47.9
    nonorganic origin F51.9
  smell — see Disturbance, sensation, smell
  sociopathic F60.2
  sodium balance, newborn P74.2
  speech R47.9
    developmental F80.9
    specified NEC R47.89
  stomach (functional) K31.9
  sympathetic (nerve) G90.9
  taste — see Disturbance, sensation, taste
  temperature
    regulation, newborn P81.9
      specified NEC P81.8
    sense R20.8
      hysterical F44.6
  tooth
    eruption K00.6
    formation K00.4
    structure, hereditary NEC K00.5
  touch — see Disturbance, sensation
  vascular I99.9
    arteriosclerotic — see Arteriosclerosis
  vasomotor I73.9
  vasospastic I73.9
  vision, visual H53.9

Disturbance(s) — continued
  vision, visual — continued
    following
      cerebral infarction I69.398
      cerebrovascular disease I69.998
        specified NEC I69.898
      intracerebral hemorrhage I69.198
      nontraumatic intracranial hemorrhage NEC
          I69.298
      specified disease NEC I69.898
      subarachnoid hemorrhage I69.098
    psychophysical H53.16
    specified NEC H53.8
    subjective H53.10
      day blindness H53.11
      discomfort H53.14- ☑
      distortions of shape and size H53.15
      loss
        sudden H53.13- ☑
        transient H53.12- ☑
      specified type NEC H53.19
  voice R49.9
    psychogenic F44.4
    specified NEC R49.8
Diuresis R35.8
Diver's palsy, paralysis or squeeze T70.3 ☑
Diverticulitis (acute) K57.92
  bladder — see Cystitis
  ileum — see Diverticulitis, intestine, small
  intestine K57.92
    with
      abscess, perforation or peritonitis K57.80
        with bleeding K57.81
      bleeding K57.93
    congenital Q43.8
    large K57.32
      with
        abscess, perforation or peritonitis K57.20
          with bleeding K57.21
        bleeding K57.33
        small intestine K57.52
          with
            abscess, perforation or peritonitis
                K57.40
              with bleeding K57.41
            bleeding K57.53
    small K57.12
      with
        abscess, perforation or peritonitis K57.00
          with bleeding K57.01
        bleeding K57.13
        large intestine K57.52
          with
            abscess, perforation or peritonitis
                K57.40
              with bleeding K57.41
            bleeding K57.53
Diverticulosis K57.90
  with bleeding K57.91
  large intestine K57.30
    with
      bleeding K57.31
      small intestine K57.50
        with bleeding K57.51
  small intestine K57.10
    with
      bleeding K57.11
      large intestine K57.50
        with bleeding K57.51
Diverticulum, diverticula (multiple) K57.90
  appendix (noninflammatory) K38.2
  bladder (sphincter) N32.3
    congenital Q64.6
  bronchus (congenital) Q32.4
    acquired J98.09
  calyx, calyceal (kidney) N28.89
  cardia (stomach) K31.4
  cecum — see Diverticulosis, intestine, large
    congenital Q43.8
  colon — see Diverticulosis, intestine, large
    congenital Q43.8
  duodenum — see Diverticulosis, intestine, small
    congenital Q43.8
  epiphrenic (esophagus) K22.5
  esophagus (congenital) Q39.6
    acquired (epiphrenic) (pulsion) (traction) K22.5
  eustachian tube — see Disorder, eustachian tube,
      specified NEC

Diverticulum, diverticula — *continued*
  fallopian tube N83.8
  gastric K31.4
  heart (congenital) Q24.8
  ileum — *see* Diverticulosis, intestine, small
  jejunum — *see* Diverticulosis, intestine, small
  kidney (pelvis) (calyces) N28.89
    with calculus — *see* Calculus, kidney
  Meckel's (displaced) (hypertrophic) Q43.0
    malignant — *see* Table of Neoplasms, small intestine, malignant
  midthoracic K22.5
  organ or site, congenital NEC — *see* Distortion
  pericardium (congenital) (cyst) Q24.8
    acquired I31.8
  pharyngoesophageal (congenital) Q39.6
    acquired K22.5
  pharynx (congenital) Q38.7
  rectosigmoid — *see* Diverticulosis, intestine, large
    congenital Q43.8
  rectum — *see* Diverticulosis, intestine, large
  Rokitansky's K22.5
  seminal vesicle N50.8
  sigmoid — *see* Diverticulosis, intestine, large
    congenital Q43.8
  stomach (acquired) K31.4
    congenital Q40.2
  trachea (acquired) J39.8
  ureter (acquired) N28.89
    congenital Q62.8
  ureterovesical orifice N28.89
  urethra (acquired) N36.1
    congenital Q64.79
  ventricle, left (congenital) Q24.8
  vesical N32.3
    congenital Q64.6
  Zenker's (esophagus) K22.5

Division
  cervix uteri (acquired) N88.8
  glans penis Q55.69
  labia minora (congenital) Q52.79
  ligament (partial or complete) (current) (*see also* Sprain)
    with open wound — *see* Wound, open
  muscle (partial or complete) (current) (*see also* Injury, muscle)
    with open wound — *see* Wound, open
  nerve (traumatic) — *see* Injury, nerve
  spinal cord — *see* Injury, spinal cord, by region
  vein I87.8

Divorce, causing family disruption Z63.5
Dix-Hallpike neurolabyrinthitis — *see* Neuronitis, vestibular
Dizziness R42
  hysterical F44.89
  psychogenic F45.8
DMAC (disseminated mycobacterium avium- intracellulare complex) A31.2
DNR (do not resuscitate) Z66
Doan-Wiseman syndrome (primary splenic neutropenia) — *see* Agranulocytosis
Doehle-Heller aortitis A52.02
Dog bite — *see* Bite
Dohle body panmyelopathic syndrome D72.0
Dolichocephaly Q67.2
Dolichocolon Q43.8
Dolichostenomelia — *see* Syndrome, Marfan's
Donohue's syndrome E34.8
Donor (organ or tissue) Z52.9
  blood (whole) Z52.000
    autologous Z52.010
    specified component (lymphocytes) (platelets) NEC Z52.008
      autologous Z52.018
      specified donor NEC Z52.098
    specified donor NEC Z52.090
    stem cells Z52.001
      autologous Z52.011
      specified donor NEC Z52.091
  bone Z52.20
    autologous Z52.21
    marrow Z52.3
    specified type NEC Z52.29
  cornea Z52.5
  egg (Oocyte) Z52.819
    age 35 and over Z52.812
      anonymous recipient Z52.812
      designated recipient Z52.813

Donor — *continued*
  egg — *continued*
    under age 35 Z52.810
      anonymous recipient Z52.810
      designated recipient Z52.811
  kidney Z52.4
  liver Z52.6
  lung Z52.89
  lymphocyte — *see* Donor, blood, specified components NEC
  Oocyte — *see* Donor, egg
  platelets Z52.008
  potential, examination of Z00.5
  semen Z52.89
  skin Z52.10
    autologous Z52.11
    specified type NEC Z52.19
  specified organ or tissue NEC Z52.89
  sperm Z52.89
Donovanosis A58
Dorsalgia M54.9
  psychogenic F45.41
  specified NEC M54.89
Dorsopathy M53.9
  deforming M43.9
    specified NEC — *see* subcategory M43.8 ☑
  specified NEC M53.80
    cervical region M53.82
    cervicothoracic region M53.83
    lumbar region M53.86
    lumbosacral region M53.87
    occipito-atlanto-axial region M53.81
    sacrococcygeal region M53.88
    thoracic region M53.84
    thoracolumbar region M53.85
Double
  albumin E88.09
  aortic arch Q25.4
  auditory canal Q17.8
  auricle (heart) Q20.8
  bladder Q64.79
  cervix Q51.820
    with doubling of uterus (and vagina) Q51.10
      with obstruction Q51.11
  inlet ventricle Q20.4
  kidney with double pelvis (renal) Q63.0
  meatus urinarius Q64.75
  monster Q89.4
  outlet
    left ventricle Q20.2
    right ventricle Q20.1
  pelvis (renal) with double ureter Q62.5
  tongue Q38.3
  ureter (one or both sides) Q62.5
    with double pelvis (renal) Q62.5
  urethra Q64.74
  urinary meatus Q64.75
  uterus Q51.2
    with
      doubling of cervix (and vagina) Q51.10
        with obstruction Q51.11
    in pregnancy or childbirth O34.59- ☑
      causing obstructed labor O65.5
  vagina Q52.10
    with doubling of uterus (and cervix) Q51.10
      with obstruction Q51.11
  vision H53.2
  vulva Q52.79
Douglas' pouch, cul-de-sac — *see* condition
Down syndrome Q90.9
  meiotic nondisjunction Q90.0
  mitotic nondisjunction Q90.1
  mosaicism Q90.1
  translocation Q90.2
DPD (dihydropyrimidine dehydrogenase deficiency) E88.89
Dracontiasis B72
Dracunculiasis, dracunculosis B72
Dream state, hysterical F44.89
Drepanocytic anemia — *see* Disease, sickle-cell
Dresbach's syndrome (elliptocytosis) D58.1
Dreschlera (hawaiiensis) (infection) B43.8
Dressler's syndrome I24.1
Drift, ulnar — *see* Deformity, limb, specified type NEC, forearm

Drinking (alcohol)
  excessive, to excess NEC (without dependence) F10.10
    habitual (continual) (without remission) F10.20
      with remission F10.21
Drip, postnasal (chronic) R09.82
  due to
    allergic rhinitis — *see* Rhinitis, allergic
    common cold J00
    gastroesophageal reflux — *see* Reflux, gastroesophageal
    nasopharyngitis — *see* Nasopharyngitis
    other known condition — *code to* condition
    sinusitis — *see* Sinusitis
Droop
  facial R29.810
    cerebrovascular disease I69.992
      cerebral infarction I69.392
      intracerebral hemorrhage I69.192
      nontraumatic intracranial hemorrhage NEC I69.292
      specified disease NEC I69.892
      subarachnoid hemorrhage I69.092
Drop (in)
  attack NEC R55
  finger — *see* Deformity, finger
  foot — *see* Deformity, limb, foot, drop
  hematocrit (precipitous) R71.0
  hemoglobin R71.0
  toe — *see* Deformity, toe, specified NEC
  wrist — *see* Deformity, limb, wrist drop
Dropped heart beats I45.9
Dropsy, dropsical (*see also* Hydrops)
  abdomen R18.8
  brain — *see* Hydrocephalus
  cardiac, heart — *see* Failure, heart, congestive
  gangrenous — *see* Gangrene
  heart — *see* Failure, heart, congestive
  kidney — *see* Nephrosis
  lung — *see* Edema, lung
  newborn due to isoimmunization P56.0
  pericardium — *see* Pericarditis
Drowned, drowning (near) T75.1 ☑
Drowsiness R40.0
Drug
  abuse counseling and surveillance Z71.51
  addiction — *see* Dependence
  dependence — *see* Dependence
  habit — *see* Dependence
  harmful use — *see* Abuse, drug
  induced fever R50.2
  overdose — *see* Table of Drugs and Chemicals, by drug, poisoning
  poisoning — *see* Table of Drugs and Chemicals, by drug, poisoning
  resistant organism infection (*see also* Resistant, organism, to, drug) Z16.30
  therapy
    long term (current) (prophylactic) — *see* Therapy, drug long-term (current) (prophylactic)
    short term — *omit code*
  wrong substance given or taken in error — *see* Table of Drugs and Chemicals, by drug, poisoning
Drunkenness (without dependence) F10.129
  acute in alcoholism F10.229
  chronic (without remission) F10.20
    with remission F10.21
  pathological (without dependence) F10.129
    with dependence F10.229
  sleep F51.9
Drusen
  macula (degenerative) (retina) — *see* Degeneration, macula, drusen
  optic disc H47.32- ☑
Dry, dryness (*see also* condition)
  larynx J38.7
  mouth R68.2
    due to dehydration E86.0
  nose J34.89
  socket (teeth) M27.3
  throat J39.2
DSAP L56.5
Duane's syndrome H50.81- ☑
Dubin-Johnson disease or syndrome E80.6
Dubois' disease (thymus gland) A50.59 [E35]
Dubowitz' syndrome Q87.1
Duchenne-Aran muscular atrophy G12.21
Duchenne-Griesinger disease G71.0

Duchenne's
- disease or syndrome
  - motor neuron disease G12.22
  - muscular dystrophy G71.0
  - locomotor ataxia (syphilitic) A52.11
  - paralysis
    - birth injury P14.0
    - due to or associated with
      - motor neuron disease G12.22
      - muscular dystrophy G71.0

Ducrey's chancre A57
Duct, ductus — *see* condition
Duhring's disease (dermatitis herpetiformis) L13.0
Dullness, cardiac (decreased) (increased) R01.2
Dumb ague — *see* Malaria
Dumbness — *see* Aphasia
Dumdum fever B55.0
Dumping syndrome (postgastrectomy) K91.1
Duodenitis (nonspecific) (peptic) K29.80
- with bleeding K29.81

Duodenocholangitis — *see* Cholangitis
Duodenum, duodenal — *see* condition
Duplay's bursitis or periarthritis — *see* Tendinitis, calcific, shoulder
Duplication, duplex (*see also* Accessory)
- alimentary tract Q45.8
- anus Q43.4
- appendix (and cecum) Q43.4
- biliary duct (any) Q44.5
- bladder Q64.79
- cecum (and appendix) Q43.4
- cervix Q51.820
- chromosome NEC
  - with complex rearrangements NEC Q92.5
  - seen only at prometaphase Q92.8
- cystic duct Q44.5
- digestive organs Q45.8
- esophagus Q39.8
- frontonasal process Q75.8
- intestine (large) (small) Q43.4
- kidney Q63.0
- liver Q44.7
- pancreas Q45.3
- penis Q55.69
- respiratory organs NEC Q34.8
- salivary duct Q38.4
- spinal cord (incomplete) Q06.2
- stomach Q40.2

Dupré's disease (meningism) R29.1
Dupuytren's contraction or disease M72.0
Durand-Nicolas-Favre disease A55
Durotomy (inadvertent) (incidental) G97.41
Duroziez's disease (congenital mitral stenosis) Q23.2
Dutton's relapsing fever (West African) A68.1
Dwarfism E34.3
- achondroplastic Q77.4
- congenital E34.3
- constitutional E34.3
- hypochondroplastic Q77.4
- hypophyseal E23.0
- infantile E34.3
- Laron-type E34.3
- Lorain (-Levi) type E23.0
- metatropic Q77.8
- nephrotic-glycosuric (with hypophosphatemic rickets) E72.09
- nutritional E45
- pancreatic K86.8
- pituitary E23.0
- renal N25.0
- thanatophoric Q77.1

Dyke-Young anemia (secondary) (symptomatic) D59.1
Dysacusis — *see* Abnormal, auditory perception
Dysadrenocortism E27.9
- hyperfunction E27.0

Dysarthria R47.1
- following
  - cerebral infarction I69.322
  - cerebrovascular disease I69.922
    - specified disease NEC I69.822
  - intracerebral hemorrhage I69.122
  - nontraumatic intracranial hemorrhage NEC I69.222
  - subarachnoid hemorrhage I69.022

Dysautonomia (familial) G90.1
Dysbarism T70.3 ☑
Dysbasia R26.2
- angiosclerotica intermittens I73.9
- hysterical F44.4

Dysbasia — *continued*
- lordotica (progressiva) G24.1
- nonorganic origin F44.4
- psychogenic F44.4

Dysbetalipoproteinemia (familial) E78.2
Dyscalculia R48.8
- developmental F81.2

Dyschezia K59.00
Dyschondroplasia (with hemangiomata) Q78.4
Dyschromia (skin) L81.9
Dyscollagenosis M35.9
Dyscranio-pygo-phalangy Q87.0
Dyscrasia
- blood (with) D75.9
  - antepartum hemorrhage — *see* Hemorrhage, antepartum, with coagulation defect
  - intrapartum hemorrhage O67.0
  - newborn P61.9
    - specified type NEC P61.8
  - puerperal, postpartum O72.3
- polyglandular, pluriglandular E31.9

Dysendocrinism E34.9
Dysentery, dysenteric (catarrhal) (diarrhea) (epidemic) (hemorrhagic) (infectious) (sporadic) (tropical) A09
- abscess, liver A06.4
- amebic (*see also* Amebiasis) A06.0
  - with abscess — *see* Abscess, amebic
  - acute A06.0
  - chronic A06.1
- arthritis (*see also* category M01) A09
  - bacillary (*see also* category M01) A03.9
- bacillary A03.9
  - arthritis (*see also* category M01) A03.9
  - Boyd A03.2
  - Flexner A03.1
  - Schmitz (-Stutzer) A03.0
  - Shiga (-Kruse) A03.0
  - Shigella A03.9
    - boydii A03.2
    - dysenteriae A03.0
    - flexneri A03.1
    - group A A03.0
    - group B A03.1
    - group C A03.2
    - group D A03.3
    - sonnei A03.3
    - specified type NEC A03.8
  - Sonne A03.3
  - specified type NEC A03.8
- balantidial A07.0
- Balantidium coli A07.0
- Boyd's A03.2
- candidal B37.82
- Chilomastix A07.8
- Chinese A03.9
- coccidial A07.3
- Dientamoeba (fragilis) A07.8
- Embadomonas A07.8
- Entamoeba, entambic — *see* Dysentery, amebic
- Flexner-Boyd A03.2
- Flexner's A03.1
- Giardia lamblia A07.1
- Hiss-Russell A03.1
- Lamblia A07.1
- leishmanial B55.0
- malarial — *see* Malaria
- metazoal B82.0
- monilial B37.82
- protozoal A07.9
- Salmonella A02.0
- schistosomal B65.1
- Schmitz (-Stutzer) A03.0
- Shiga (-Kruse) A03.0
- Shigella NOS — *see* Dysentery, bacillary
- Sonne A03.3
- strongyloidiasis B78.0
- trichomonal A07.8
- viral (*see also* Enteritis, viral) A08.4

Dysequilibrium R42
Dysesthesia R20.8
- hysterical F44.6

Dysfibrinogenemia (congenital) D68.2
Dysfunction
- adrenal E27.9
  - hyperfunction E27.0
- autonomic
  - due to alcohol G31.2
  - somatoform F45.8

Dysfunction — *continued*
- bladder N31.9
  - neurogenic NOS — *see* Dysfunction, bladder, neuromuscular
  - neuromuscular NOS N31.9
    - atonic (motor) (sensory) N31.2
    - autonomous N31.2
    - flaccid N31.2
    - nonreflex N31.2
    - reflex N31.1
    - specified NEC N31.8
    - uninhibited N31.0
- bleeding, uterus N93.8
- cerebral G93.89
- colon K59.9
  - psychogenic F45.8
- colostomy K94.03
- cystic duct K82.8
- cystostomy (stoma) — *see* Complications, cystostomy
- ejaculatory N53.19
  - anejaculatory orgasm N53.13
  - painful N53.12
  - premature F52.4
  - retarded N53.11
- endocrine NOS E34.9
- endometrium N85.8
- enterostomy K94.13
- gallbladder K82.8
- gastrostomy (stoma) K94.23
- gland, glandular NOS E34.9
- heart I51.89
- hemoglobin D75.89
- hepatic K76.89
- hypophysis E23.7
- hypothalamic NEC E23.3
- ileostomy (stoma) K94.13
- jejunostomy (stoma) K94.13
- kidney — *see* Disease, renal
- labyrinthine — *see* subcategory H83.2 ☑
- left ventricular, following sudden emotional stress I51.81
- liver K76.89
- male — *see* Dysfunction, sexual, male
- orgasmic (female) F52.31
  - male F52.32
- ovary E28.9
  - specified NEC E28.8
- papillary muscle I51.89
- parathyroid E21.4
- physiological NEC R68.89
  - psychogenic F59
- pineal gland E34.8
- pituitary (gland) E23.3
- platelets D69.1
- polyglandular E31.9
  - specified NEC E31.8
- psychophysiologic F59
- psychosexual F52.9
  - with
    - dyspareunia F52.6
    - premature ejaculation F52.4
    - vaginismus F52.5
- pylorus K31.9
- rectum K59.9
  - psychogenic F45.8
- reflex (sympathetic) — *see* Syndrome, pain, complex regional I
- segmental — *see* Dysfunction, somatic
- senile R54
- sexual (due to) R37
  - alcohol F10.981
  - amphetamine F15.981
    - in
      - abuse F15.181
      - dependence F15.281
  - anxiolytic F13.981
    - in
      - abuse F13.181
      - dependence F13.281
  - cocaine F14.981
    - in
      - abuse F14.181
      - dependence F14.281
  - excessive sexual drive F52.8
  - failure of genital response (male) F52.21
    - female F52.22
  - female N94.9
    - aversion F52.1

Dysfunction — continued
  sexual — continued
    female — continued
      dyspareunia N94.1
        psychogenic F52.6
      frigidity F52.22
      nymphomania F52.8
      orgasmic F52.31
      psychogenic F52.9
        aversion F52.1
        dyspareunia F52.6
        frigidity F52.22
        nymphomania F52.8
        orgasmic F52.31
        vaginismus F52.5
      vaginismus N94.2
        psychogenic F52.5
    hypnotic F13.981
    in
      abuse F13.181
      dependence F13.281
    inhibited orgasm (female) F52.31
      male F52.32
    lack
      of sexual enjoyment F52.1
      or loss of sexual desire F52.0
    male N53.9
      anejaculatory orgasm N53.13
      ejaculatory N53.19
        painful N53.12
        premature F52.4
        retarded N53.11
      erectile N52.9
        drug induced N52.2
        due to
          disease classified elsewhere N52.1
          drug N52.2
        postoperative (postprocedural) N52.39
        following
          prostatectomy N52.34
            radical N52.31
          radical cystectomy N52.32
          urethral surgery N52.33
        psychogenic F52.21
        specified cause NEC N52.8
        vasculogenic
          arterial insufficiency N52.01
            with corporo-venous occlusive N52.03
          corporo-venous occlusive N52.02
            with arterial insufficiency N52.03
      impotence — see Dysfunction, sexual, male, erectile
      psychogenic F52.9
        aversion F52.1
        erectile F52.21
        orgasmic F52.32
        premature ejaculation F52.4
        satyriasis F52.8
        specified type NEC F52.8
      specified type NEC N53.8
    nonorganic F52.9
      specified NEC F52.8
    opioid F11.981
    in
      abuse F11.181
      dependence F11.281
    orgasmic dysfunction (female) F52.31
      male F52.32
    premature ejaculation F52.4
    psychoactive substances NEC F19.981
    in
      abuse F19.181
      dependence F19.281
    psychogenic F52.9
    sedative F13.981
    in
      abuse F13.181
      dependence F13.281
    sexual aversion F52.1
    vaginismus (nonorganic) (psychogenic) F52.5
  sinoatrial node I49.5
  somatic M99.09
    abdomen M99.09
    acromioclavicular M99.07
    cervical region M99.01
    cervicothoracic M99.01
    costochondral M99.08

Dysfunction — continued
  somatic — continued
    costovertebral M99.08
    head region M99.00
    hip M99.05
    lower extremity M99.06
    lumbar region M99.03
    lumbosacral M99.03
    occipitocervical M99.00
    pelvic region M99.05
    pubic M99.05
    rib cage M99.08
    sacral region M99.04
    sacrococcygeal M99.04
    sacroiliac M99.04
    specified NEC M99.09
    sternochondral M99.08
    sternoclavicular M99.07
    thoracic region M99.02
    thoracolumbar M99.02
    upper extremity M99.07
  somatoform autonomic F45.8
  stomach K31.89
    psychogenic F45.8
  suprarenal E27.9
    hyperfunction E27.0
  symbolic R48.9
    specified type NEC R48.8
  temporomandibular (joint) M26.69
    joint-pain syndrome M26.62
  testicular (endocrine) E29.9
    specified NEC E29.8
  thymus E32.9
  thyroid E07.9
  ureterostomy (stoma) — see Complications, stoma, urinary tract
  urethrostomy (stoma) — see Complications, stoma, urinary tract
  uterus, complicating delivery O62.9
    hypertonic O62.4
    hypotonic O62.2
      primary O62.0
      secondary O62.1
  ventricular I51.9
    with congestive heart failure I50.9
    left, reversible, following sudden emotional stress I51.81
Dysgenesis
  gonadal (due to chromosomal anomaly) Q96.9
    pure Q99.1
  renal Q60.5
    bilateral Q60.4
    unilateral Q60.3
  reticular D72.0
  tidal platelet D69.3
Dysgerminoma
  specified site — see Neoplasm, malignant, by site
  unspecified site
    female C56.9
    male C62.90
Dysgeusia R43.2
Dysgraphia R27.8
Dyshidrosis, dysidrosis L30.1
Dyskaryotic cervical smear R87.619
Dyskeratosis L85.8
  cervix — see Dysplasia, cervix
  congenital Q82.8
  uterus NEC N85.8
Dyskinesia G24.9
  biliary (cystic duct or gallbladder) K82.8
  drug induced
    orofacial G24.01
  esophagus K22.4
  hysterical F44.4
  intestinal K59.8
  nonorganic origin F44.4
  orofacial (idiopathic) G24.4
    drug induced G24.01
  psychogenic F44.4
  subacute, drug induced G24.01
  tardive G24.01
    neuroleptic induced G24.01
  trachea J39.8
  tracheobronchial J98.09
Dyslalia (developmental) F80.0
Dyslexia R48.0
  developmental F81.0

Dyslipidemia E78.5
  depressed HDL cholesterol E78.6
  elevated fasting triglycerides E78.1
Dysmaturity (see also Light for dates)
  pulmonary (newborn) (Wilson-Mikity) P27.0
Dysmenorrhea (essential) (exfoliative) N94.6
  congestive (syndrome) N94.6
  primary N94.4
  psychogenic F45.8
  secondary N94.5
Dysmetabolic syndrome X E88.81
Dysmetria R27.8
Dysmorphism (due to)
  alcohol Q86.0
  exogenous cause NEC Q86.8
  hydantoin Q86.1
  warfarin Q86.2
Dysmorphophobia (nondelusional) F45.22
  delusional F22
Dysnomia R47.01
Dysorexia R63.0
  psychogenic F50.8
Dysostosis
  cleidocranial, cleidocranialis Q74.0
  craniofacial Q75.1
  Fairbank's (idiopathic familial generalized osteophytosis) Q78.9
  mandibulofacial (incomplete) Q75.4
  multiplex E76.01
  oculomandibular Q75.5
Dyspareunia (female) N94.1
  male N53.12
  nonorganic F52.6
  psychogenic F52.6
  secondary N94.1
Dyspepsia R10.13
  atonic K30
  functional (allergic) (congenital) (gastrointestinal) (occupational) (reflex) K30
  intestinal K59.8
  nervous F45.8
  neurotic F45.8
  psychogenic F45.8
Dysphagia R13.10
  cervical R13.19
  following
    cerebral infarction I69.391
    cerebrovascular disease I69.991
      specified NEC I69.891
    intracerebral hemorrhage I69.191
    nontraumatic intracranial hemorrhage NEC I69.291
    specified disease NEC I69.891
    subarachnoid hemorrhage I69.091
  functional (hysterical) F45.8
  hysterical F45.8
  nervous (hysterical) F45.8
  neurogenic R13.19
  oral phase R13.11
  oropharyngeal phase R13.12
  pharyneal phase R13.13
  pharyngoesophageal phase R13.14
  psychogenic F45.8
  sideropenic D50.1
  spastica K22.4
  specified NEC R13.19
Dysphagocytosis, congenital D71
Dysphasia R47.02
  developmental
    expressive type F80.1
    receptive type F80.2
  following
    cerebrovascular disease I69.921
      cerebral infarction I69.321
      intracerebral hemorrhage I69.121
      nontraumatic intracranial hemorrhage NEC I69.221
      specified disease NEC I69.821
      subarachnoid hemorrhage I69.021
Dysphonia R49.0
  functional F44.4
  hysterical F44.4
  psychogenic F44.4
  spastica J38.3
Dysphoria, postpartal O90.6
Dyspituitarism E23.3
Dysplasia (see also Anomaly)
  acetabular, congenital Q65.89
  alveolar capillary, with vein misalignment J84.843

Dysplasia — continued
anus (histologically confirmed) (mild) (moderate) K62.82
  severe D01.3
arrhythmogenic right ventricular I42.8
arterial, fibromuscular I77.3
asphyxiating thoracic (congenital) Q77.2
brain Q07.9
bronchopulmonary, perinatal P27.1
cervix (uteri) N87.9
  mild N87.0
  moderate N87.1
  severe D06.9
chondroectodermal Q77.6
colon D12.6
craniometaphyseal Q78.5
dentinal K00.5
diaphyseal, progressive Q78.3
dystrophic Q77.5
ectodermal (anhidrotic) (congenital) (hereditary) Q82.4
  hydrotic Q82.8
epithelial, uterine cervix — see Dysplasia, cervix
eye (congenital) Q11.2
fibrous
  bone NEC (monostotic) M85.00
    ankle M85.07- ☑
    foot M85.07- ☑
    forearm M85.03- ☑
    hand M85.04- ☑
    lower leg M85.06- ☑
    multiple site M85.09
    neck M85.08
    rib M85.08
    shoulder M85.01- ☑
    skull M85.08
    specified site NEC M85.08
    thigh M85.05- ☑
    toe M85.07- ☑
    upper arm M85.02- ☑
    vertebra M85.08
  diaphyseal, progressive Q78.3
  jaw M27.8
  polyostotic Q78.1
florid osseous (see also Cyst, calcifying odontogenic)
high grade, focal D12.6
hip, congenital Q65.89
joint, congenital Q74.8
kidney Q61.4
  multicystic Q61.4
leg Q74.2
lung, congenital (not associated with short gestation) Q33.6
mammary (gland) (benign) N60.9- ☑
  cyst (solitary) — see Cyst, breast
  cystic — see Mastopathy, cystic
  duct ectasia — see Ectasia, mammary duct
  fibroadenosis — see Fibroadenosis, breast
  fibrosclerosis — see Fibrosclerosis, breast
  specified type NEC N60.8- ☑
metaphyseal (Jansen's) (McKusick's) (Schmid's) Q78.5
muscle Q79.8
oculodentodigital Q87.0
periapical (cemental) (cemento-osseous) — see Cyst, calcifying odontogenic
periosteum — see Disorder, bone, specified type NEC
polyostotic fibrous Q78.1
prostate (see also Neoplasia, intraepithelial, prostate) N42.3
  severe D07.5
renal Q61.4
  multicystic Q61.4
retinal, congenital Q14.1
right ventricular, arrhythmogenic I42.8
septo-optic Q04.4
skin L98.8
spinal cord Q06.1
spondyloepiphyseal Q77.7
thymic, with immunodeficiency D82.1
vagina N89.3
  mild N89.0
  moderate N89.1
  severe NEC D07.2
vulva N90.3
  mild N90.0
  moderate N90.1
  severe NEC D07.1

Dyspnea (nocturnal) (paroxysmal) R06.00
asthmatic (bronchial) J45.909
  with
    bronchitis J45.909
      with
        exacerbation (acute) J45.901
        status asthmaticus J45.902
      chronic J44.9
    exacerbation (acute) J45.901
    status asthmaticus J45.902
  cardiac — see Failure, ventricular, left
cardiac — see Failure, ventricular, left
functional F45.8
hyperventilation R06.4
hysterical F45.8
newborn P28.89
orthopnea R06.01
psychogenic F45.8
shortness of breath R06.02
specified type NEC R06.09
Dyspraxia R27.8
developmental (syndrome) F82
Dysproteinemia E88.09
Dysreflexia, autonomic G90.4
Dysrhythmia
cardiac I49.9
  newborn
    bradycardia P29.12
    occurring before birth P03.819
      before onset of labor P03.810
      during labor P03.811
    tachycardia P29.11
  postoperative I97.89
cerebral or cortical — see Epilepsy
Dyssomnia — see Disorder, sleep
Dyssynergia
biliary K83.8
bladder sphincter N36.44
cerebellaris myoclonica (Hunt's ataxia) G11.1
Dysthymia F34.1
Dysthyroidism E07.9
Dystocia O66.9
affecting newborn P03.1
cervical (hypotonic) O62.2
  affecting newborn P03.6
  primary O62.0
  secondary O62.1
contraction ring O62.4
fetal O66.9
  abnormality NEC O66.3
  conjoined twins O66.3
  oversize O66.2
maternal O66.9
positional O64.9 ☑
shoulder (girdle) O66.0
  causing obstructed labor O66.0
uterine NEC O62.4
Dystonia G24.9
deformans progressiva G24.1
drug induced NEC G24.09
  acute G24.02
  specified NEC G24.09
familial G24.1
idiopathic G24.1
  familial G24.1
  nonfamilial G24.2
  orofacial G24.4
lenticularis G24.1
musculorum deformans G24.1
neuroleptic induced (acute) G24.02
orofacial (idiopathic) G24.4
oromandibular G24.4
  due to drug G24.01
specified NEC G24.8
torsion (familial) (idiopathic) G24.1
  acquired G24.8
  genetic G24.1
  symptomatic (nonfamilial) G24.2
Dystonic movements R25.8
Dystrophy, dystrophia
adiposogenital E23.6
Becker's type G71.0
cervical sympathetic G90.2
choroid (hereditary) H31.20
  central areolar H31.22
  choroideremia H31.21
  gyrate atrophy H31.23
  specified type NEC H31.29

Dystrophy, dystrophia — continued
cornea (hereditary) H18.50
  endothelial H18.51
  epithelial H18.52
  granular H18.53
  lattice H18.54
  macular H18.55
  specified type NEC H18.59
Duchenne's type G71.0
due to malnutrition E45
Erb's G71.0
Fuchs' H18.51
Gower's muscular G71.0
hair L67.8
infantile neuraxonal G31.89
Landouzy-Déjérine G71.0
Leyden-Möbius G71.0
muscular G71.0
  benign (Becker type) G71.0
  congenital (hereditary) (progressive) (with specific morphological abnormalities of the muscle fiber) G71.0
    myotonic G71.11
  distal G71.0
  Duchenne type G71.0
  Emery-Dreifuss G71.0
  Erb type G71.0
  facioscapulohumeral G71.0
  Gower's G71.0
  hereditary (progressive) G71.0
  Landouzy-Déjérine type G71.0
  limb-girdle G71.0
  myotonic G71.11
  progressive (hereditary) G71.0
    Charcot-Marie (-Tooth) type G60.0
  pseudohypertrophic (infantile) G71.0
  severe (Duchenne type) G71.0
myocardium, myocardial — see Degeneration, myocardial
nail L60.3
  congenital Q84.6
nutritional E45
ocular G71.0
oculocerebrorenal E72.03
oculopharyngeal G71.0
ovarian N83.8
polyglandular E31.8
reflex (neuromuscular) (sympathetic) — see Syndrome, pain, complex regional I
retinal (hereditary) H35.50
  in
    lipid storage disorders E75.6 [H36]
    systemic lipidoses E75.6 [H36]
  involving
    pigment epithelium H35.54
    sensory area H35.53
  pigmentary H35.52
  vitreoretinal H35.51
Salzmann's nodular — see Degeneration, cornea, nodular
scapuloperoneal G71.0
skin NEC L98.8
sympathetic (reflex) — see Syndrome, pain, complex regional I
  cervical G90.2
tapetoretinal H35.54
thoracic, asphyxiating Q77.2
unguium L60.3
  congenital Q84.6
vitreoretinal H35.51
vulva N90.4
yellow (liver) — see Failure, hepatic
Dysuria R30.0
psychogenic F45.8

E

Eales' disease H35.06- ☑
Ear (see also condition)
piercing Z41.3
tropical B36.8
wax (impacted) H61.20
  left H61.22
    with right H61.23
  right H61.21
    with left H61.23
Earache — see subcategory H92.0 ☑
Early satiety R68.81

☑ **Additional Character Required — Refer to the Tabular List for Character Selection**

▽ **Subterms under main terms may continue to next column or page**

Eaton-Lambert syndrome — see Syndrome, Lambert-Eaton
Eberth's disease (typhoid fever) A01.00
Ebola virus disease A98.4
Ebstein's anomaly or syndrome (heart) Q22.5
Eccentro-osteochondrodysplasia E76.29
Ecchondroma — see Neoplasm, bone, benign
Ecchondrosis D48.0
Ecchymosis R58
  conjunctiva — see Hemorrhage, conjunctiva
  eye (traumatic) — see Contusion, eyeball
  eyelid (traumatic) — see Contusion, eyelid
  newborn P54.5
  spontaneous R23.3
  traumatic — see Contusion
Echinococciasis — see Echinococcus
Echinococcosis — see Echinococcus
Echinococcus (infection) B67.90
  granulosus B67.4
    bone B67.2
    liver B67.0
    lung B67.1
    multiple sites B67.32
    specified site NEC B67.39
    thyroid B67.31 [E35]
  liver NOS B67.8
    granulosus B67.0
    multilocularis B67.5
  lung NEC B67.99
    granulosus B67.1
    multilocularis B67.69
  multilocularis B67.7
    liver B67.5
    multiple sites B67.61
    specified site NEC B67.69
  specified site NEC B67.99
    granulosus B67.39
    multilocularis B67.69
  thyroid NEC B67.99
    granulosus B67.31 [E35]
    multilocularis B67.69 [E35]
Echinorhynchiasis B83.8
Echinostomiasis B66.8
Echolalia R48.8
Echovirus, as cause of disease classified elsewhere B97.12
Eclampsia, eclamptic (coma) (convulsions) (delirium) (with hypertension) NEC O15.9
  during labor and delivery O15.1
  postpartum O15.2
  pregnancy O15.0- ☑
  puerperal O15.2
Economic circumstances affecting care Z59.9
Economo's disease A85.8
Ectasia, ectasis
  annuloaortic I35.8
  aorta I77.819
    with aneurysm — see Aneurysm, aorta
    abdominal I77.811
    thoracic I77.810
    thoracoabdominal I77.812
  breast — see Ectasia, mammary duct
  capillary I78.8
  cornea H18.71- ☑
  gastric antral vascular (GAVE) K31.819
    with hemorrhage K31.811
    without hemorrhage K31.819
  mammary duct N60.4- ☑
  salivary gland (duct) K11.8
  sclera — see Sclerectasia
Ecthyma L08.0
  contagiosum B08.02
  gangrenosum L08.0
  infectiosum B08.02
Ectocardia Q24.8
Ectodermal dysplasia (anhidrotic) Q82.4
Ectodermosis erosiva pluriorificialis L51.1
Ectopic, ectopia (congenital)
  abdominal viscera Q45.8
    due to defect in anterior abdominal wall Q79.59
  ACTH syndrome E24.3
  adrenal gland Q89.1
  anus Q43.5
  atrial beats I49.1
  beats I49.49
    atrial I49.1
    ventricular I49.3

Ectopic, ectopia — continued
  bladder Q64.10
  bone and cartilage in lung Q33.5
  brain Q04.8
  breast tissue Q83.8
  cardiac Q24.8
  cerebral Q04.8
  cordis Q24.8
  endometrium — see Endometriosis
  gastric mucosa Q40.2
  gestation — see Pregnancy, by site
  heart Q24.8
  hormone secretion NEC E34.2
  kidney (crossed) (pelvis) Q63.2
  lens, lentis Q12.1
  mole — see Pregnancy, by site
  organ or site NEC — see Malposition, congenital
  pancreas Q45.3
  pregnancy — see Pregnancy, ectopic
  pupil — see Abnormality, pupillary
  renal Q63.2
  sebaceous glands of mouth Q38.6
  spleen Q89.09
  testis Q53.00
    bilateral Q53.02
    unilateral Q53.01
  thyroid Q89.2
  tissue in lung Q33.5
  ureter Q62.63
  ventricular beats I49.3
  vesicae Q64.10
Ectromelia Q73.8
  lower limb — see Defect, reduction, limb, lower, specified type NEC
  upper limb — see Defect, reduction, limb, upper, specified type NEC
Ectropion H02.109
  cervix N86
    with cervicitis N72
  congenital Q10.1
  eyelid (paralytic) H02.109
    cicatricial H02.119
      left H02.116
        lower H02.115
        upper H02.114
      right H02.113
        lower H02.112
        upper H02.111
    congenital Q10.1
    left H02.106
      lower H02.105
      upper H02.104
    mechanical H02.129
      left H02.126
        lower H02.125
        upper H02.124
      right H02.123
        lower H02.122
        upper H02.121
    right H02.103
      lower H02.102
      upper H02.101
    senile H02.139
      left H02.136
        lower H02.135
        upper H02.134
      right H02.133
        lower H02.132
        upper H02.131
    spastic H02.149
      left H02.146
        lower H02.145
        upper H02.144
      right H02.143
        lower H02.142
        upper H02.141
  iris H21.89
  lip (acquired) K13.0
    congenital Q38.0
  urethra N36.8
  uvea H21.89
Eczema (acute) (chronic) (erythematous) (fissum) (rubrum) (squamous) (see also Dermatitis) L30.9
  contact — see Dermatitis, contact
  dyshydrotic L30.1
  external ear — see Otitis, externa, acute, eczematoid
  flexural L20.82
  herpeticum B00.0

Eczema — continued
  hypertrophicum L28.0
  hypostatic — see Varix, leg, with, inflammation
  impetiginous L01.1
  infantile (due to any substance) L20.83
    intertriginous L21.1
    seborrheic L21.1
  intertriginous NEC L30.4
    infantile L21.1
  intrinsic (allergic) L20.84
  lichenified NEC L28.0
  marginatum (hebrae) B35.6
  pustular L30.3
  stasis — see Varix, leg, with, inflammation
  vaccination, vaccinatum T88.1 ☑
  varicose — see Varix, leg, with, inflammation
Eczematid L30.2
Eddowes (-Spurway) **syndrome** Q78.0
Edema, edematous (infectious) (pitting) (toxic) R60.9
  with nephritis — see Nephrosis
  allergic T78.3 ☑
  amputation stump (surgical) (sequelae) (late effect)) T87.89
  angioneurotic (allergic) (any site) (with urticaria) T78.3 ☑
    hereditary D84.1
  angiospastic I73.9
  Berlin's (traumatic) S05.8X- ☑
  brain (cytotoxic) (vasogenic) G93.6
    due to birth injury P11.0
    newborn (anoxia or hypoxia) P52.4
      birth injury P11.0
    traumatic — see Injury, intracranial, cerebral edema
  cardiac — see Failure, heart, congestive
  cardiovascular — see Failure, heart, congestive
  cerebral — see Edema, brain
  cerebrospinal — see Edema, brain
  cervix (uteri) (acute) N88.8
    puerperal, postpartum O90.89
  chronic hereditary Q82.0
  circumscribed, acute T78.3 ☑
    hereditary D84.1
  conjunctiva H11.42- ☑
  cornea H18.2- ☑
    idiopathic H18.22- ☑
    secondary H18.23- ☑
      due to contact lens H18.21- ☑
  due to
    lymphatic obstruction I89.0
    salt retention E87.0
  epiglottis — see Edema, glottis
  essential, acute T78.3 ☑
    hereditary D84.1
  extremities, lower — see Edema, legs
  eyelid NEC H02.849
    left H02.846
      lower H02.845
      upper H02.844
    right H02.843
      lower H02.842
      upper H02.841
  familial, hereditary Q82.0
  famine — see Malnutrition, severe
  generalized R60.1
  glottis, glottic, glottidis (obstructive) (passive) J38.4
    allergic T78.3 ☑
      hereditary D84.1
  heart — see Failure, heart, congestive
  heat T67.7 ☑
  hereditary Q82.0
  inanition — see Malnutrition, severe
  intracranial G93.6
  iris H21.89
  joint — see Effusion, joint
  larynx — see Edema, glottis
  legs R60.0
    due to venous obstruction I87.1
    hereditary Q82.0
  localized R60.0
    due to venous obstruction I87.1
  lower limbs — see Edema, legs
  lung J81.1
    with heart condition or failure — see Failure, ventricular, left
    acute J81.0
    chemical (acute) J68.1
      chronic J68.1

▽ Subterms under main terms may continue to next column or page   ☑ Additional Character Required — Refer to the Tabular List for Character Selection   121

Eaton-Lambert syndrome — Edema, edematous

Edema, edematous — *continued*
 lung — *continued*
  chronic J81.1
   due to
    chemicals, gases, fumes or vapors (inhalation) J68.1
    external agent J70.9
     specified NEC J70.8
    radiation J70.1
   due to
    chemicals, fumes or vapors (inhalation) J68.1
    external agent J70.9
     specified NEC J70.8
    high altitude T70.29 ☑
    near drowning T75.1 ☑
    radiation J70.0
  meaning failure, left ventricle I50.1
 lymphatic I89.0
  due to mastectomy I97.2
 macula H35.81
  cystoid, following cataract surgery — *see* Complications, postprocedural, following cataract surgery
  diabetic — *see* Diabetes, by type, with, retinopathy, with macular edema
 malignant — *see* Gangrene, gas
 Milroy's Q82.0
 nasopharynx J39.2
 newborn P83.30
  hydrops fetalis — *see* Hydrops, fetalis
  specified NEC P83.39
 nutritional (*see also* Malnutrition, severe)
  with dyspigmentation, skin and hair E40
 optic disc or nerve — *see* Papilledema
 orbit H05.22- ☑
 pancreas K86.8
 papilla, optic — *see* Papilledema
 penis N48.89
 periodic T78.3 ☑
  hereditary D84.1
 pharynx J39.2
 pulmonary — *see* Edema, lung
 Quincke's T78.3 ☑
  hereditary D84.1
 renal — *see* Nephrosis
 retina H35.81
  diabetic — *see* Diabetes, by type, with, retinopathy, with macular edema
 salt E87.0
 scrotum N50.8
 seminal vesicle N50.8
 spermatic cord N50.8
 spinal (cord) (vascular) (nontraumatic) G95.19
 starvation — *see* Malnutrition, severe
 stasis — *see* Hypertension, venous, (chronic)
 subglottic — *see* Edema, glottis
 supraglottic — *see* Edema, glottis
 testis N44.8
 tunica vaginalis N50.8
 vas deferens N50.8
 vulva (acute) N90.89
Edentulism — *see* Absence, teeth, acquired
Edsall's disease T67.2 ☑
Educational handicap Z55.9
 specified NEC Z55.8
Edward's syndrome — *see* Trisomy, 18
Effect(s) (of) (from) — *see* Effect, adverse NEC
Effect, adverse
 abnormal gravitational (G) forces or states T75.81 ☑
 abuse — *see* Maltreatment
 air pressure T70.9 ☑
  specified NEC T70.8 ☑
 altitude (high) — *see* Effect, adverse, high altitude
 anesthesia (*see also* Anesthesia) T88.59 ☑
  in labor and delivery O74.9
  in pregnancy NEC O29.3- ☑
  local, toxic
   in labor and delivery O74.4
   postpartum, puerperal O89.3
  postpartum, puerperal O89.9
  specified NEC T88.59 ☑
   in labor and delivery O74.8
   postpartum, puerperal O89.8
  spinal and epidural T88.59 ☑
   headache T88.59 ☑
    in labor and delivery O74.5
    postpartum, puerperal O89.4

Effect, adverse — *continued*
 anesthesia (*see also* Anesthesia) — *continued*
  spinal and epidural — *continued*
   specified NEC
    in labor and delivery O74.6
    postpartum, puerperal O89.5
 antitoxin — *see* Complications, vaccination
 atmospheric pressure T70.9 ☑
  due to explosion T70.8 ☑
  high T70.3 ☑
  low — *see* Effect, adverse, high altitude
  specified effect NEC T70.8 ☑
 biological, correct substance properly administered — *see* Effect, adverse, drug
 blood (derivatives) (serum) (transfusion) — *see* Complications, transfusion
 chemical substance — *see* Table of Drugs and Chemicals
 cold (temperature) (weather) T69.9 ☑
  chilblains T69.1 ☑
  frostbite — *see* Frostbite
  specified effect NEC T69.8 ☑
 drugs and medicaments T88.7 ☑
  specified drug — *see* Table of Drugs and Chemicals, by drug, adverse effect
  specified effect — *code to* condition
 electric current, electricity (shock) T75.4 ☑
  burn — *see* Burn
 exertion (excessive) T73.3 ☑
 exposure — *see* Exposure
 external cause NEC T75.89 ☑
 foodstuffs T78.1 ☑
  allergic reaction — *see* Allergy, food
   causing anaphylaxis — *see* Shock, anaphylactic, due to food
  noxious — *see* Poisoning, food, noxious
 gases, fumes, or vapors T59.9- ☑
  specified agent — *see* Table of Drugs and Chemicals
 glue (airplane) sniffing
  due to drug abuse — *see* Abuse, drug, inhalant
  due to drug dependence — *see* Dependence, drug, inhalant
 heat — *see* Heat
 high altitude NEC T70.29 ☑
  anoxia T70.29 ☑
  on
   ears T70.0 ☑
   sinuses T70.1 ☑
  polycythemia D75.1
 high pressure fluids T70.4 ☑
 hot weather — *see* Heat
 hunger T73.0 ☑
 immersion, foot — *see* Immersion
 immunization — *see* Complications, vaccination
 immunological agents — *see* Complications, vaccination
 infrared (radiation) (rays) NOS T66 ☑
  dermatitis or eczema L59.8
 infusion — *see* Complications, infusion
 lack of care of infants — *see* Maltreatment, child
 lightning — *see* Lightning
 medical care T88.9 ☑
  specified NEC T88.8 ☑
 medicinal substance, correct, properly administered — *see* Effect, adverse, drug
 motion T75.3 ☑
 noise, on inner ear — *see* subcategory H83.3 ☑
 overheated places — *see* Heat
 psychosocial, of work environment Z56.5
 radiation (diagnostic) (infrared) (natural source) (therapeutic) (ultraviolet) (X-ray) NOS T66 ☑
  dermatitis or eczema — *see* Dermatitis, due to, radiation
  fibrosis of lung J70.1
  pneumonitis J70.0
  pulmonary manifestations
   acute J70.0
   chronic J70.1
  skin L59.9
 radioactive substance NOS
  dermatitis or eczema — *see* Radiodermatitis
 reduced temperature T69.9 ☑
  immersion foot or hand — *see* Immersion
  specified effect NEC T69.8 ☑
 serum NEC (*see also* Reaction, serum) T80.69 ☑

Effect, adverse — *continued*
 specified NEC T78.8 ☑
  external cause NEC T75.89 ☑
 strangulation — *see* Asphyxia, traumatic
 submersion T75.1 ☑
 thirst T73.1 ☑
 toxic — *see* Toxicity
 transfusion — *see* Complications, transfusion
 ultraviolet (radiation) (rays) NOS T66 ☑
  burn — *see* Burn
  dermatitis or eczema — *see* Dermatitis, due to, ultraviolet rays
   acute L56.8
 vaccine (any) — *see* Complications, vaccination
 vibration — *see* Vibration, adverse effects
 water pressure NEC T70.9 ☑
  specified NEC T70.8 ☑
 weightlessness T75.82 ☑
 whole blood — *see* Complications, transfusion
 work environment Z56.5
Effects, late — *see* Sequelae
Effluvium
 anagen L65.1
 telogen L65.0
Effort syndrome (psychogenic) F45.8
Effusion
 amniotic fluid — *see* Pregnancy, complicated by, prematue rupture of membranes
 brain (serous) G93.6
 bronchial — *see* Bronchitis
 cerebral G93.6
 cerebrospinal (*see also* Meningitis)
  vessel G93.6
 chest — *see* Effusion, pleura
 chylous, chyliform (pleura) J94.0
 intracranial G93.6
 joint M25.40
  ankle M25.47- ☑
  elbow M25.42- ☑
  foot joint M25.47- ☑
  hand joint M25.44- ☑
  hip M25.45- ☑
  knee M25.46- ☑
  shoulder M25.41- ☑
  specified joint NEC M25.48
  wrist M25.43- ☑
 malignant pleural J91.0
 meninges — *see* Meningitis
 pericardium, pericardial (noninflammatory) I31.3
  acute — *see* Pericarditis, acute
 peritoneal (chronic) R18.8
 pleura, pleurisy, pleuritic, pleuropericardial J90
  chylous, chyliform J94.0
  due to systemic lupus erythematosis M32.13
  influenzal — *see* Influenza, with, respiratory manifestations NEC
  malignant J91.0
  newborn P28.89
  tuberculous NEC A15.6
   primary (progressive) A15.7
 spinal — *see* Meningitis
 thorax, thoracic — *see* Effusion, pleura
Egg shell nails L60.3
 congenital Q84.6
Egyptian splenomegaly B65.1
Ehlers-Danlos syndrome Q79.6
Ehrlichiosis A77.40
 due to
  E. chafeensis A77.41
  E. sennetsu A79.81
  specified organism NEC A77.49
Eichstedt's disease B36.0
Eisenmenger's
 complex or syndrome I27.89
 defect Q21.8
Ejaculation
 painful N53.12
 premature F52.4
 retarded N53.11
 retrograde N53.14
 semen, painful N53.12
  psychogenic F52.6
Ekbom's syndrome (restless legs) G25.81
Ekman's syndrome (brittle bones and blue sclera) Q78.0
Elastic skin Q82.8
 acquired L57.4

☑ **Additional Character Required — Refer to the Tabular List for Character Selection**   ▽ **Subterms under main terms may continue to next column or page**

Elastofibroma — see Neoplasm, connective tissue, benign
Elastoma (juvenile) Q82.8
    Miescher's L87.2
Elastomyofibrosis I42.4
Elastosis
    actinic, solar L57.8
    atrophicans (senile) L57.4
    perforans serpiginosa L87.2
    senilis L57.4
Elbow — see condition
Electric current, electricity, effects (concussion) (fatal) (nonfatal) (shock) T75.4 ☑
    burn — see Burn
Electric feet syndrome E53.8
Electrocution T75.4 ☑
    from electroshock gun (taser) T75.4 ☑
Electrolyte imbalance E87.8
    with
        abortion — see Abortion by type, complicated by, electrolyte imbalance
        ectopic pregnancy O08.5
        molar pregnancy O08.5
Elephantiasis (nonfilarial) I89.0
    arabicum — see Infestation, filarial
    bancroftian B74.0
    congenital (any site) (hereditary) Q82.0
    due to
        Brugia (malayi) B74.1
            timori B74.2
        mastectomy I97.2
        Wuchereria (bancrofti) B74.0
    eyelid H02.859
        left H02.856
            lower H02.855
            upper H02.854
        right H02.853
            lower H02.852
            upper H02.851
    filarial, filariensis — see Infestation, filarial
    glandular I89.0
    graecorum A30.9
    lymphangiectatic I89.0
    lymphatic vessel I89.0
        due to mastectomy I97.2
    scrotum (nonfilarial) I89.0
    streptococcal I89.0
    surgical I97.89
        postmastectomy I97.2
    telangiectodes I89.0
    vulva (nonfilarial) N90.89
Elevated, elevation
    antibody titer R76.0
    basal metabolic rate R94.8
    blood pressure (see also Hypertension)
        reading (incidental) (isolated) (nonspecific), no diagnosis of hypertension R03.0
    blood sugar R73.9
    body temperature (of unknown origin) R50.9
    cancer antigen 125 [CA 125] R97.1
    carcinoembryonic antigen [CEA] R97.0
    cholesterol E78.0
        with high triglycerides E78.2
    conjugate, eye H51.0
    C-reactive protein (CRP) R79.82
    diaphragm, congenital Q79.1
    erythrocyte sedimentation rate R70.0
    fasting glucose R73.01
    fasting triglycerides E78.1
    finding on laboratory examination — see Findings, abnormal, inconclusive, without diagnosis, by type of exam
    GFR (glomerular filtration rate) — see Findings, abnormal, inconclusive, without diagnosis, by type of exam
    glucose tolerance (oral) R73.02
    immunoglobulin level R76.8
    indoleacetic acid R82.5
    lactic acid dehydrogenase (LDH) level R74.0
    leukocytes D72.829
    lipoprotein a level E78.8 ☑
    liver function
        study R94.5
        test R79.89
            alkaline phosphatase R74.8
            aminotransferase R74.0
            bilirubin R17
            hepatic enzyme R74.8

Elevated, elevation — continued
    liver function — continued
        test — continued
            lactate dehydrogenase R74.0
    lymphocytes D72.820
    prostate specific antigen [PSA] R97.2
    Rh titer — see Complication(s), transfusion, incompatibility reaction, Rh (factor)
    scapula, congenital Q74.0
    sedimentation rate R70.0
    SGOT R74.0
    SGPT R74.0
    transaminase level R74.0
    triglycerides E78.1
        with high cholesterol E78.2
    tumor associated antigens [TAA] NEC R97.8
    tumor specific antigens [TSA] NEC R97.8
    urine level of
        17-ketosteroids R82.5
        catecholamine R82.5
        indoleacetic acid R82.5
        steroids R82.5
        vanillylmandelic acid (VMA) R82.5
    venous pressure I87.8
    white blood cell count D72.829
    specified NEC D72.828
Elliptocytosis (congenital) (hereditary) D58.1
    Hb C (disease) D58.1
    hemoglobin disease D58.1
    sickle-cell (disease) D57.8- ☑
        trait D57.3
Ellison-Zollinger syndrome E16.4
Ellis-van Creveld syndrome (chondroectodermal dysplasia) Q77.6
Elongated, elongation (congenital) (see also Distortion)
    bone Q79.9
    cervix (uteri) Q51.828
        acquired N88.4
        hypertrophic N88.4
    colon Q43.8
    common bile duct Q44.5
    cystic duct Q44.5
    frenulum, penis Q55.69
    labia minora (acquired) N90.6
    ligamentum patellae Q74.1
    petiolus (epiglottidis) Q31.8
    tooth, teeth K00.2
    uvula Q38.6
Eltor cholera A00.1
Emaciation (due to malnutrition) E41
Embadomoniasis A07.8
Embedded tooth, teeth K01.0
    root only K08.3
Embolic — see condition
Embolism (multiple) (paradoxical) I74.9
    air (any site) (traumatic) T79.0 ☑
        following
            abortion — see Abortion by type complicated by embolism
            ectopic pregnancy O08.2
            infusion, therapeutic injection or transfusion T80.0 ☑
            molar pregnancy O08.2
            procedure NEC
                artery T81.719 ☑
                    mesenteric T81.710 ☑
                    renal T81.711 ☑
                    specified NEC T81.718 ☑
                vein T81.72 ☑
        in pregnancy, childbirth or puerperium — see Embolism, obstetric
    amniotic fluid (pulmonary) (see also Embolism, obstetric)
        following
            abortion — see Abortion by type complicated by embolism
            ectopic pregnancy O08.2
            molar pregnancy O08.2
    aorta, aortic I74.10
        abdominal I74.09
            saddle I74.01
        bifurcation I74.09
        saddle I74.01
        thoracic I74.11
    artery I74.9
        auditory, internal I65.8
        basilar — see Occlusion, artery, basilar

Embolism — continued
    artery — continued
        carotid (common) (internal) — see Occlusion, artery, carotid
        cerebellar (anterior inferior) (posterior inferior) (superior) I66.3
        cerebral — see Occlusion, artery, cerebral
        choroidal (anterior) I66.8
        communicating posterior I66.8
        coronary (see also Infarct, myocardium)
            not resulting in infarction I24.0
        extremity I74.4
            lower I74.3
            upper I74.2
        hypophyseal I66.8
        iliac I74.5
        limb I74.4
            lower I74.3
            upper I74.2
        mesenteric (with gangrene) K55.0
        ophthalmic — see Occlusion, artery, retina
        peripheral I74.4
        pontine I66.8
        precerebral — see Occlusion, artery, precerebral
        pulmonary — see Embolism, pulmonary
        renal N28.0
        retinal — see Occlusion, artery, retina
        septic I76
        specified NEC I74.8
        vertebral — see Occlusion, artery, vertebral
    basilar (artery) I65.1
    blood clot
        following
            abortion — see Abortion by type complicated by embolism
            ectopic or molar pregnancy O08.2
        in pregnancy, childbirth or puerperium — see Embolism, obstetric
    brain (see also Occlusion, artery, cerebral)
        following
            abortion — see Abortion by type complicated by embolism
            ectopic or molar pregnancy O08.2
        puerperal, postpartum, childbirth — see Embolism, obstetric
    capillary I78.8
    cardiac (see also Infarct, myocardium)
        not resulting in infarction I24.0
    carotid (artery) (common) (internal) — see Occlusion, artery, carotid
    cavernous sinus (venous) — see Embolism, intracranial venous sinus
    cerebral — see Occlusion, artery, cerebral
    cholesterol — see Atheroembolism
    coronary (artery or vein) (systemic) — see Occlusion, coronary
    due to device, implant or graft (see also Complications, by site and type, specified NEC)
        arterial graft NEC T82.818 ☑
        breast (implant) T85.81 ☑
        catheter NEC T85.81 ☑
            dialysis (renal) T82.818 ☑
                intraperitoneal T85.81 ☑
            infusion NEC T82.818 ☑
                spinal (epidural) (subdural) T85.81 ☑
            urinary (indwelling) T83.81 ☑
        electronic (electrode) (pulse generator) (stimulator)
            bone T84.81 ☑
            cardiac T82.817 ☑
            nervous system (brain) (peripheral nerve) (spinal) T85.81 ☑
            urinary T83.81 ☑
        fixation, internal (orthopedic) NEC T84.81 ☑
        gastrointestinal (bile duct) (esophagus) T85.81 ☑
        genital NEC T83.81 ☑
        heart (graft) (valve) T82.817 ☑
        joint prosthesis T84.81 ☑
        ocular (corneal graft) (orbital implant) T85.81 ☑
        orthopedic (bone graft) NEC T86.838
        specified NEC T85.81 ☑
        urinary (graft) NEC T83.81 ☑
        vascular NEC T82.818 ☑
        ventricular intracranial shunt T85.81 ☑
    extremities
        lower — see Embolism, vein, lower extremity
            arterial I74.3
        upper I74.2

Embolism — *continued*
    eye H34.9
    fat (cerebral) (pulmonary) (systemic) T79.1 ☑
        complicating delivery — *see* Embolism, obstetric
        following
            abortion — *see* Abortion by type complicated
                by embolism
            ectopic or molar pregnancy O08.2
    following
        abortion — *see* Abortion by type complicated by
            embolism
        ectopic or molar pregnancy O08.2
        infusion, therapeutic injection or transfusion
            air T80.0 ☑
    heart (fatty) (*see also* Infarct, myocardium)
        not resulting in infarction I24.0
    hepatic (vein) I82.0
    in pregnancy, childbirth or puerperium — *see* Embolism, obstetric
    intestine (artery) (vein) (with gangrene) K55.0
    intracranial (*see also* Occlusion, artery, cerebral)
        venous sinus (any) G08
            nonpyogenic I67.6
    intraspinal venous sinuses or veins G08
        nonpyogenic G95.19
    kidney (artery) N28.0
    lateral sinus (venous) — *see* Embolism, intracranial,
        venous sinus
    leg — *see* Embolism, vein, lower extremity
        arterial I74.3
    longitudinal sinus (venous) — *see* Embolism, intracranial, venous sinus
    lung (massive) — *see* Embolism, pulmonary
    meninges I66.8
    mesenteric (artery) (vein) (with gangrene) K55.0
    obstetric (in) (pulmonary)
        childbirth O88.82
            air O88.02
            amniotic fluid O88.12
            blood clot O88.22
            fat O88.82
            pyemic O88.32
            septic O88.32
            specified type NEC O88.82
        pregnancy O88.81- ☑
            air O88.01- ☑
            amniotic fluid O88.11- ☑
            blood clot O88.21- ☑
            fat O88.81- ☑
            pyemic O88.31- ☑
            septic O88.31- ☑
            specified type NEC O88.81- ☑
        puerperal O88.83
            air O88.03
            amniotic fluid O88.13
            blood clot O88.23
            fat O88.83
            pyemic O88.33
            septic O88.33
            specified type NEC O88.83
    ophthalmic — *see* Occlusion, artery, retina
    penis N48.81
    peripheral artery NOS I74.4
    pituitary E23.6
    popliteal (artery) I74.3
    portal (vein) I81
    postoperative, postprocedural
        artery T81.719 ☑
            mesenteric T81.710 ☑
            renal T81.711 ☑
            specified NEC T81.718 ☑
        vein T81.72 ☑
    precerebral artery — *see* Occlusion, artery, precerebral
    puerperal — *see* Embolism, obstetric
    pulmonary (acute) (artery) (vein) I26.99
        with acute cor pulmonale I26.09
        chronic I27.82
        following
            abortion — *see* Abortion by type complicated
                by embolism
            ectopic or molar pregnancy O08.2
        healed or old Z86.711
        in pregnancy, childbirth or puerperium — *see*
            Embolism, obstetric
        personal history of Z86.711
        saddle I26.92
            with acute cor pulmonale I26.02

Embolism — *continued*
    pulmonary — *continued*
        septic I26.90
            with acute cor pulmonale I26.01
    pyemic (multiple) I76
        following
            abortion — *see* Abortion by type complicated
                by embolism
            ectopic or molar pregnancy O08.2
        Hemophilus influenzae A41.3
        pneumococcal A40.3
            with pneumonia J13
        puerperal, postpartum, childbirth (any organism)
            — *see* Embolism, obstetric
        specified organism NEC A41.89
        staphylococcal A41.2
        streptococcal A40.9
    renal (artery) N28.0
        vein I82.3
    retina, retinal — *see* Occlusion, artery, retina
    saddle
        abdominal aorta I74.01
        pulmonary artery I26.92
            with acute cor pulmonale I26.02
    septic (arterial) I76
        complicating abortion — *see* Abortion, by type,
            complicated by, embolism
    sinus — *see* Embolism, intracranial, venous sinus
    soap complicating abortion — *see* Abortion, by type,
        complicated by, embolism
    spinal cord G95.19
        pyogenic origin G06.1
    spleen, splenic (artery) I74.8
    upper extremity I74.2
    vein (acute) I82.90
        antecubital I82.61- ☑
            chronic I82.71- ☑
        axillary I82.A1- ☑ (*following* I82.7)
            chronic I82.A2- ☑ (*following* I82.7)
        basilic I82.61- ☑
            chronic I82.71- ☑
        brachial I82.62- ☑
            chronic I82.72- ☑
        brachiocephalic (innominate) I82.290
            chronic I82.291
        cephalic I82.61- ☑
            chronic I82.71- ☑
        chronic I82.91
        deep (DVT) I82.40- ☑
            calf I82.4Z- ☑
                chronic I82.5Z- ☑
            lower leg I82.4Z- ☑
                chronic I82.5Z- ☑
            thigh I82.4Y- ☑
                chronic I82.5Y- ☑
            upper leg I82.4Y ☑
                chronic I82.5Y-
        femoral I82.41- ☑
            chronic I82.51- ☑
        iliac (iliofemoral) I82.42- ☑
            chronic I82.52- ☑
        innominate I82.290
            chronic I82.291
        internal jugular I82.C1- ☑ (*following* I82.7)
            chronic I82.C2- ☑ (*following* I82.7)
        lower extremity
            deep I82.40- ☑
                chronic I82.50- ☑
                specified NEC I82.49- ☑
                    chronic NEC I82.59- ☑
            distal
                deep I82.4Z- ☑
            proximal
                deep I82.4Y- ☑
                    chronic I82.5Y- ☑
            superficial I82.81- ☑
        popliteal I82.43- ☑
            chronic I82.53- ☑
        radial I82.62- ☑
            chronic I82.72- ☑
        renal I82.3
        saphenous (greater) (lesser) I82.81- ☑
        specified NEC I82.890
            chronic NEC I82.891
        subclavian I82.B1- ☑ (*following* I82.7)
            chronic I82.B2- ☑ (*following* I82.7)

Embolism — *continued*
    vein — *continued*
        thoracic NEC I82.290
            chronic I82.291
        tibial I82.44- ☑
            chronic I82.54- ☑
        ulnar I82.62- ☑
            chronic I82.72- ☑
        upper extremity I82.60- ☑
            chronic I82.70- ☑
            deep I82.62- ☑
                chronic I82.72- ☑
            superficial I82.61- ☑
                chronic I82.71- ☑
        vena cava
            inferior (acute) I82.220
                chronic I82.221
            superior (acute) I82.210
                chronic I82.211
        venous sinus G08
        vessels of brain — *see* Occlusion, artery, cerebral
Embolus — *see* Embolism
Embryoma (*see also* Neoplasm, uncertain behavior, by
        site)
    benign — *see* Neoplasm, benign, by site
    kidney C64.- ☑
    liver C22.0
    malignant (*see also* Neoplasm, malignant, by site)
        kidney C64.- ☑
        liver C22.0
        testis C62.9- ☑
            descended (scrotal) C62.1- ☑
            undescended C62.0- ☑
    testis C62.9- ☑
        descended (scrotal) C62.1- ☑
        undescended C62.0- ☑
Embryonic
    circulation Q28.9
    heart Q28.9
    vas deferens Q55.4
Embryopathia NOS Q89.9
Embryotoxon Q13.4
Emesis — *see* Vomiting
Emotional lability R45.86
Emotionality, pathological F60.3
Emotogenic disease — *see* Disorder, psychogenic
Emphysema (atrophic) (bullous) (chronic) (interlobular)
        (lung) (obstructive) (pulmonary) (senile) (vesicular)
        J43.9
    cellular tissue (traumatic) T79.7 ☑
        surgical T81.82 ☑
    centrilobular J43.2
    compensatory J98.3
    congenital (interstitial) P25.0
    conjunctiva H11.89
    connective tissue (traumatic) T79.7 ☑
        surgical T81.82 ☑
    due to chemicals, gases, fumes or vapors J68.4
    eyelid(s) — *see* Disorder, eyelid, specified type NEC
        surgical T81.82 ☑
        traumatic T79.7 ☑
    interstitial J98.2
        congenital P25.0
        perinatal period P25.0
    laminated tissue T79.7 ☑
        surgical T81.82 ☑
    mediastinal J98.2
        newborn P25.2
    orbit, orbital — *see* Disorder, orbit, specified type NEC
    panacinar J43.1
    panlobular J43.1
    specified NEC J43.8
    subcutaneous (traumatic) T79.7 ☑
        nontraumatic J98.2
        postprocedural T81.82 ☑
        surgical T81.82 ☑
    surgical T81.82 ☑
    thymus (gland) (congenital) E32.8
    traumatic (subcutaneous) T79.7 ☑
    unilateral J43.0
Empty nest syndrome Z60.0
Empyema (acute) (chest) (double) (pleura) (supradi-
        aphragmatic) (thorax) J86.9
    with fistula J86.0
    accessory sinus (chronic) — *see* Sinusitis
    antrum (chronic) — *see* Sinusitis, maxillary
    brain (any part) — *see* Abscess, brain

Empyema — *continued*
   ethmoidal (chronic) (sinus) — *see* Sinusitis, ethmoidal
   extradural — *see* Abscess, extradural
   frontal (chronic) (sinus) — *see* Sinusitis, frontal
   gallbladder K81.0
   mastoid (process) (acute) — *see* Mastoiditis, acute
   maxilla, maxillary M27.2
      sinus (chronic) — *see* Sinusitis, maxillary
   nasal sinus (chronic) — *see* Sinusitis
   sinus (accessory) (chronic) (nasal) — *see* Sinusitis
   sphenoidal (sinus) (chronic) — *see* Sinusitis, sphenoidal
   subarachnoid — *see* Abscess, extradural
   subdural — *see* Abscess, subdural
   tuberculous A15.6
   ureter — *see* Ureteritis
   ventricular — *see* Abscess, brain
En coup de sabre lesion L94.1
Enamel pearls K00.2
Enameloma K00.2
Enanthema, viral B09
Encephalitis (chronic) (hemorrhagic) (idiopathic) (nonepidemic) (spurious) (subacute) G04.90
   acute (*see also* Encephalitis, viral) A86
      disseminated G04.00
         infectious G04.01
         noninfectious G04.81
         postimmunization (postvaccination) G04.02
         postinfectious G04.01
      inclusion body A85.8
      necrotizing hemorrhagic G04.30
         postimmunization G04.32
         postinfectious G04.31
         specified NEC G04.39
   arboviral, arbovirus NEC A85.2
   arthropod-borne NEC (viral) A85.2
   Australian A83.4
   California (virus) A83.5
   Central European (tick-borne) A84.1
   Czechoslovakian A84.1
   Dawson's (inclusion body) A81.1
   diffuse sclerosing A81.1
   disseminated, acute G04.00
   due to
      cat scratch disease A28.1
      human immunodeficiency virus (HIV) disease B20 [G05.3]
      malaria — *see* Malaria
      rickettsiosis — *see* Rickettsiosis
      smallpox inoculation G04.02
      typhus — *see* Typhus
   Eastern equine A83.2
   endemic (viral) A86
   epidemic NEC (viral) A86
   equine (acute) (infectious) (viral) A83.9
      Eastern A83.2
      Venezuelan A92.2
      Western A83.1
   Far Eastern (tick-borne) A84.0
   following vaccination or other immunization procedure G04.02
   herpes zoster B02.0
   herpesviral B00.4
      due to herpesvirus 6 B10.01
      due to herpesvirus 7 B10.09
      specified NEC B10.09
   Ilheus (virus) A83.8
   in (due to)
      actinomycosis A42.82
      adenovirus A85.1
      African trypanosomiasis B56.9 [G05.3]
      Chagas' disease (chronic) B57.42
      cytomegalovirus B25.8
      enterovirus A85.0
      herpes (simplex) virus B00.4
         due to herpesvirus 6 B10.01
         due to herpesvirus 7 B10.09
         specified NEC B10.09
      infectious disease NEC B99 ☑ [G05.3]
      influenza — *see* Influenza, with, encephalopathy
      listeriosis A32.12
      measles B05.0
      mumps B26.2
      naegleriasis B60.2
      parasitic disease NEC B89 [G05.3]
      poliovirus A80.9 [G05.3]
      rubella B06.01

Encephalitis — *continued*
   in — *continued*
      syphilis
         congenital A50.42
         late A52.14
      systemic lupus erythematosus M32.19
      toxoplasmosis (acquired) B58.2
         congenital P37.1
      tuberculosis A17.82
      zoster B02.0
   inclusion body A81.1
   infectious (acute) (virus) NEC A86
   Japanese (B type) A83.0
   La Crosse A83.5
   lead — *see* Poisoning, lead
   lethargica (acute) (infectious) A85.8
   louping ill A84.8
   lupus erythematosus, systemic M32.19
   lymphatica A87.2
   Mengo A85.8
   meningococcal A39.81
   Murray Valley A83.4
   otitic NEC H66.40 [G05.3]
   parasitic NOS B71.9
   periaxial G37.0
   periaxialis (concentrica) (diffuse) G37.5
   postchickenpox B01.11
   postexanthematous NEC B09
   postimmunization G04.02
   postinfectious NEC G04.01
   postmeasles B05.0
   postvaccinal G04.02
   postvaricella B01.11
   postviral NEC A86
   Powassan A84.8
   Rasmussen G04.81
   Rio Bravo A85.8
   Russian
      autumnal A83.0
      spring-summer (taiga) A84.0
   saturnine — *see* Poisoning, lead
   specified NEC G04.81
   St. Louis A83.3
   subacute sclerosing A81.1
   summer A83.0
   suppurative G04.81
   tick-borne A84.9
   Torula, torular (cryptococcal) B45.1
   toxic NEC G92
   trichinosis B75 [G05.3]
   type
      B A83.0
      C A83.3
   van Bogaert's A81.1
   Venezuelan equine A92.2
   Vienna A85.8
   viral, virus A86
      arthropod-borne NEC A85.2
         mosquito-borne A83.9
            Australian X disease A83.4
            California virus A83.5
            Eastern equine A83.2
            Japanese (B type) A83.0
            Murray Valley A83.4
            specified NEC A83.8
            St. Louis A83.3
            type B A83.0
            type C A83.3
            Western equine A83.1
         tick-borne A84.9
            biundulant A84.1
            central European A84.1
            Czechoslovakian A84.1
            diphasic meningoencephalitis A84.1
            Far Eastern A84.0
            Russian spring-summer (taiga) A84.0
            specified NEC A84.8
      specified type NEC A85.8
   Western equine A83.1
Encephalocele Q01.9
   frontal Q01.0
   nasofrontal Q01.1
   occipital Q01.2
   specified NEC Q01.8
Encephalocystocele — *see* Encephalocele
Encephaloduroarteriomyosynangiosis (EDAMS) I67.5
Encephalomalacia (brain) (cerebellar) (cerebral) — *see* Softening, brain

Encephalomeningitis — *see* Meningoencephalitis
Encephalomeningocele — *see* Encephalocele
Encephalomeningomyelitis — *see* Meningoencephalitis
Encephalomyelitis (*see also* Encephalitis) G04.90
   acute disseminated G04.00
      infectious G04.01
      noninfectious G04.81
      postimmunization G04.02
      postinfectious G04.01
   acute necrotizing hemorrhagic G04.30
      postimmunization G04.32
      postinfectious G04.31
      specified NEC G04.39
   benign myalgic G93.3
   equine A83.9
      Eastern A83.2
      Venezuelan A92.2
      Western A83.1
   in diseases classified elsewhere G05.3
   myalgic, benign G93.3
   postchickenpox B01.11
   postinfectious NEC G04.01
   postmeasles B05.0
   postvaccinal G04.02
   postvaricella B01.11
   rubella B06.01
   specified NEC G04.81
   Venezuelan equine A92.2
Encephalomyelocele — *see* Encephalocele
Encephalomyelomeningitis — *see* Meningoencephalitis
Encephalomyelopathy G96.9
Encephalomyeloradiculitis (acute) G61.0
Encephalomyeloradiculoneuritis (acute) (Guillain-Barré) G61.0
Encephalomyeloradiculopathy G96.9
Encephalopathia hyperbilirubinemica, newborn P57.9
   due to isoimmunization (conditions in P55) P57.0
Encephalopathy (acute) G93.40
   acute necrotizing hemorrhagic G04.30
      postimmunization G04.32
      postinfectious G04.31
      specified NEC G04.39
   alcoholic G31.2
   anoxic — *see* Damage, brain, anoxic
   arteriosclerotic I67.2
   centrolobar progressive (Schilder) G37.0
   congenital Q07.9
   degenerative, in specified disease NEC G32.89
   demyelinating callosal G37.1
   due to
      drugs (*see also* Table of Drugs and Chemicals) G92
   hepatic — *see* Failure, hepatic
   hyperbilirubinemic, newborn P57.9
      due to isoimmunization (conditions in P55) P57.0
   hypertensive I67.4
   hypoglycemic E16.2
   hypoxic — *see* Damage, brain, anoxic
   hypoxic ischemic P91.60
      mild P91.61
      moderate P91.62
      severe P91.63
   in (due to) (with)
      birth injury P11.1
      hyperinsulinism E16.1 [G94]
      influenza — *see* Influenza, with, encephalopathy
      lack of vitamin (*see also* Deficiency, vitamin) E56.9 [G32.89]
      neoplastic disease (*see also* Neoplasm) D49.9 [G13.1]
      serum (*see also* Reaction, serum) T80.69 ☑
      syphilis A52.17
      trauma (postconcussional) F07.81
         current injury — *see* Injury, intracranial
      vaccination G04.02
   lead — *see* Poisoning, lead
   metabolic G93.41
      drug induced G92
      toxic G92
   myoclonic, early, symptomatic — *see* Epilepsy, generalized, specified NEC
   necrotizing, subacute (Leigh) G31.82
   pellagrous E52 [G32.89]
   portosystemic — *see* Failure, hepatic
   postcontusional F07.81
      current injury — *see* Injury, intracranial, diffuse

◆ **Subterms under main terms may continue to next column or page**   ☑ **Additional Character Required** — Refer to the Tabular List for Character Selection   **125**

Empyema — Encephalopathy

Encephalopathy — continued
  posthypoglycemic (coma) E16.1 [G94]
  postradiation G93.89
  saturnine — see Poisoning, lead
  septic G93.41
  specified NEC G93.49
  spongiform, subacute (viral) A81.09
  toxic G92
    metabolic G92
  traumatic (postconcussional) F07.81
    current injury — see Injury, intracranial
  vitamin B deficiency NEC E53.9 [G32.89]
    vitamin B1 E51.2
  Wernicke's E51.2
Encephalorrhagia — see Hemorrhage, intracranial, intracerebral
Encephalosis, posttraumatic F07.81
Enchondroma (see also Neoplasm, bone, benign)
Enchondromatosis (cartilaginous) (multiple) Q78.4
Encopresis R15.9
  functional F98.1
  nonorganic origin F98.1
  psychogenic F98.1
Encounter (with health service) (for) Z76.89
  adjustment and management (of)
    breast implant Z45.81 ☑
    implanted device NEC Z45.89
    myringotomy device (stent) (tube) Z45.82
  administrative purpose only Z02.9
    examination for
      adoption Z02.82
      armed forces Z02.3
      disability determination Z02.71
      driving license Z02.4
      employment Z02.1
      insurance Z02.6
      medical certificate NEC Z02.79
      paternity testing Z02.81
      residential institution admission Z02.2
      school admission Z02.0
      sports Z02.5
    specified reason NEC Z02.89
  aftercare — see Aftercare
  antenatal screening Z36
  assisted reproductive fertility procedure cycle Z31.83
  blood typing Z01.83
    Rh typing Z01.83
  breast augmentation or reduction Z41.1
  breast implant exchange (different material) (different size) Z45.81 ☑
  breast reconstruction following mastectomy Z42.1
  check-up — see Examination
  chemotherapy for neoplasm Z51.11
  colonoscopy, screening Z12.11
  counseling — see Counseling
  delivery, full-term, uncomplicated O80
    cesarean, without indication O82
  ear piercing Z41.3
  examination — see Examination
  expectant parent(s) (adoptive) pre-birth pediatrician visit Z76.81
  fertility preservation procedure (prior to cancer therapy) (prior to removal of gonads) Z31.84
  fitting (of) — see Fitting (and adjustment) (of)
  genetic
    counseling Z31.5
    testing — see Test, genetic
  hearing conservation and treatment Z01.12
  immunotherapy for neoplasm Z51.12
  in vitro fertilization cycle Z31.83
  instruction (in)
    child care (postpartal) (prenatal) Z32.3
    childbirth Z32.2
    natural family planning
      procreative Z31.61
      to avoid pregnancy Z30.02
  insulin pump titration Z46.81
  joint prosthesis insertion following prior explantation of joint prosthesis (staged procedure)
    hip Z47.32
    knee Z47.33
    shoulder Z47.31
  laboratory (as part of a general medical examination) Z00.00
    with abnormal findings Z00.01
  mental health services (for)
    abuse NEC
      perpetrator Z69.82

Encounter — continued
  mental health services — continued
    abuse — continued
      victim Z69.81
    child abuse
      nonparental
        perpetrator Z69.021
        victim Z69.020
      parental
        perpetrator Z69.011
        victim Z69.010
    spousal or partner abuse
      perpetrator Z69.12
      victim Z69.11
  observation (for) (ruled out)
    exposure to (suspected)
      anthrax Z03.810
      biological agent NEC Z03.818
  pediatrician visit, by expectant parent(s) (adoptive) Z76.81
  plastic and reconstructive surgery following medical procedure or healed injury NEC Z42.8
  pregnancy
    supervision of — see Pregnancy, supervision of
    test Z32.00
      result negative Z32.02
      result positive Z32.01
  radiation therapy (antineoplastic) Z51.0
  radiological (as part of a general medical examination) Z00.00
    with abnormal findings Z00.01
  reconstructive surgery following medical procedure or healed injury NEC Z42.8
  removal (of) (see also Removal)
    artificial
      arm Z44.00- ☑
        complete Z44.01- ☑
        partial Z44.02- ☑
      eye Z44.2- ☑
      leg Z44.10- ☑
        complete Z44.11- ☑
        partial Z44.12- ☑
    breast implant Z45.81 ☑
      tissue expander (without synchronous insertion of permanent implant) Z45.81 ☑
    device Z46.9
      specified NEC Z46.89
    external
      fixation device — code to fracture with seventh character D
      prosthesis, prosthetic device Z44.9
        breast Z44.3- ☑
        specified NEC Z44.8
    implanted device NEC Z45.89
    insulin pump Z46.81
    internal fixation device Z47.2
    myringotomy device (stent) (tube) Z45.82
    nervous system device NEC Z46.2
      brain neuropacemaker Z46.2
      visual substitution device Z46.2
        implanted Z45.31
    non-vascular catheter Z46.82
    orthodontic device Z46.4
    stent
      ureteral Z46.6
    urinary device Z46.6
  repeat cervical smear to confirm findings of recent normal smear following initial abnormal smear Z01.42
  respirator [ventilator] use during power failure Z99.12
  Rh typing Z01.83
  screening — see Screening
  specified NEC Z76.89
  sterilization Z30.2
  suspected condition, ruled out
    amniotic cavity and membrane Z03.71
    cervical shortening Z03.75
    fetal anomaly Z03.73
    fetal growth Z03.74
    maternal and fetal conditions NEC Z03.79
    oligohydramnios Z03.71
    placental problem Z03.72
    polyhydramnios Z03.71
  suspected exposure (to), ruled out
    anthrax Z03.810
    biological agents NEC Z03.818
  termination of pregnancy, elective Z33.2
  testing — see Test

Encounter — continued
  therapeutic drug level monitoring Z51.81
  titration, insulin pump Z46.81
  to determine fetal viability of pregnancy O36.80 ☑
  training
    insulin pump Z46.81
  X-ray of chest (as part of a general medical examination) Z00.00
    with abnormal findings Z00.01
Encystment — see Cyst
Endarteritis (bacterial, subacute) (infective) I77.6
  brain I67.7
  cerebral or cerebrospinal I67.7
  deformans — see Arteriosclerosis
  embolic — see Embolism
  obliterans (see also Arteriosclerosis)
    pulmonary I28.8
  pulmonary I28.8
  retina — see Vasculitis, retina
  senile — see Arteriosclerosis
  syphilitic A52.09
    brain or cerebral A52.04
    congenital A50.54 [I79.8]
  tuberculous A18.89
Endemic — see condition
Endocarditis (chronic) (marantic) (nonbacterial) (thrombotic) (valvular) I38
  with rheumatic fever (conditions in I00)
    active — see Endocarditis, acute, rheumatic
    inactive or quiescent (with chorea) I09.1
  acute or subacute I33.9
    infective I33.0
      rheumatic (aortic) (mitral) (pulmonary) (tricuspid) I01.1
        with chorea (acute) (rheumatic) (Sydenham's) I02.0
  aortic (heart) (nonrheumatic) (valve) I35.8
    with
      mitral disease I08.0
        with tricuspid (valve) disease I08.3
        active or acute I01.1
          with chorea (acute) (rheumatic) (Sydenham's) I02.0
      rheumatic fever (conditions in I00)
        active — see Endocarditis, acute, rheumatic
        inactive or quiescent (with chorea) I06.9
      tricuspid (valve) disease I08.2
        with mitral (valve) disease I08.3
    acute or subacute I33.9
    arteriosclerotic I35.8
    rheumatic I06.9
      with mitral disease I08.0
        with tricuspid (valve) disease I08.3
        active or acute I01.1
          with chorea (acute) (rheumatic) (Sydenham's) I02.0
      active or acute I01.1
        with chorea (acute) (rheumatic) (Sydenham's) I02.0
      specified NEC I06.8
    specified cause NEC I35.8
    syphilitic A52.03
  arteriosclerotic I38
  atypical verrucous (Libman-Sacks) M32.11
  bacterial (acute) (any valve) (subacute) I33.0
  candidal B37.6
  congenital Q24.8
  constrictive I33.0
  Coxiella burnetii A78 [I39]
  Coxsackie B33.21
  due to
    prosthetic cardiac valve T82.6 ☑
    Q fever A78 [I39]
    Serratia marcescens I33.0
    typhoid (fever) A01.02
  gonococcal A54.83
  infectious or infective (acute) (any valve) (subacute) I33.0
  lenta (acute) (any valve) (subacute) I33.0
  Libman-Sacks M32.11
  listerial A32.82
  Löffler's I42.3
  malignant (acute) (any valve) (subacute) I33.0
  meningococcal A39.51
  mitral (chronic) (double) (fibroid) (heart) (inactive) (valve) (with chorea) I05.9
    with
      aortic (valve) disease I08.0

Endocarditis — continued
　mitral — continued
　　with — continued
　　　aortic disease — continued
　　　　with tricuspid (valve) disease I08.3
　　　　　active or acute I01.1
　　　　　　with chorea (acute) (rheumatic) (Syden-
　　　　　　　ham's) I02.0
　　　　rheumatic fever (conditions in I00)
　　　　　active — see Endocarditis, acute, rheumatic
　　　　　inactive or quiescent (with chorea) I05.9
　　　tricuspid (valve) disease I08.1
　　　　with aortic (valve) disease I08.3
　　active or acute I01.1
　　　with chorea (acute) (rheumatic) (Sydenham's)
　　　　I02.0
　　bacterial I33.0
　arteriosclerotic I34.8
　nonrheumatic I34.8
　　acute or subacute I33.9
　　specified NEC I05.8
　monilial B37.6
　multiple valves I08.9
　　specified disorders I08.8
　mycotic (acute) (any valve) (subacute) I33.0
　pneumococcal (acute) (any valve) (subacute) I33.0
　pulmonary (chronic) (heart) (valve) I37.8
　　with rheumatic fever (conditions in I00)
　　　active — see Endocarditis, acute, rheumatic
　　　inactive or quiescent (with chorea) I09.89
　　　　with aortic, mitral or tricuspid disease I08.8
　　acute or subacute I33.9
　　　rheumatic I01.1
　　　　with chorea (acute) (rheumatic) (Syden-
　　　　　ham's) I02.0
　　arteriosclerotic I37.8
　　congenital Q22.2
　　rheumatic (chronic) (inactive) (with chorea) I09.89
　　　active or acute I01.1
　　　　with chorea (acute) (rheumatic) (Syden-
　　　　　ham's) I02.0
　syphilitic A52.03
　purulent (acute) (any valve) (subacute) I33.0
　Q fever A78 [I39]
　rheumatic (chronic) (inactive) (with chorea) I09.1
　　active or acute (aortic) (mitral) (pulmonary) (tricus-
　　　pid) I01.1
　　　with chorea (acute) (rheumatic) (Sydenham's)
　　　　I02.0
　rheumatoid — see Rheumatoid, carditis
　septic (acute) (any valve) (subacute) I33.0
　streptococcal (acute) (any valve) (subacute) I33.0
　subacute — see Endocarditis, acute
　suppurative (acute) (any valve) (subacute) I33.0
　syphilitic A52.03
　toxic I33.9
　tricuspid (chronic) (heart) (inactive) (rheumatic) (valve)
　　(with chorea) I07.9
　　with
　　　aortic (valve) disease I08.2
　　　　mitral (valve) disease I08.3
　　　mitral (valve) disease I08.1
　　　　aortic (valve) disease I08.3
　　　rheumatic fever (conditions in I00)
　　　　active — see Endocarditis, acute, rheumatic
　　　　inactive or quiescent (with chorea) I07.8
　　active or acute I01.1
　　　with chorea (acute) (rheumatic) (Sydenham's)
　　　　I02.0
　　arteriosclerotic I36.8
　　nonrheumatic I36.8
　　　acute or subacute I33.9
　　specified cause, except rheumatic I36.8
　tuberculous — see Tuberculosis, endocarditis
　typhoid A01.02
　ulcerative (acute) (any valve) (subacute) I33.0
　vegetative (acute) (any valve) (subacute) I33.0
　verrucous (atypical) (nonbacterial) (nonrheumatic)
　　M32.11
Endocardium, endocardial (see also condition)
　cushion defect Q21.2
Endocervicitis (see also Cervicitis)
　due to intrauterine (contraceptive) device T83.6 ☑
　hyperplastic N72
Endocrine — see condition
Endocrinopathy, pluriglandular E31.9
Endodontic
　overfill M27.52

Endodontic — continued
　underfill M27.53
Endodontitis K04.0
Endomastoiditis — see Mastoiditis
Endometrioma N80.9
Endometriosis N80.9
　appendix N80.5
　bladder N80.8
　bowel N80.5
　broad ligament N80.3
　cervix N80.0
　colon N80.5
　cul-de-sac (Douglas') N80.3
　exocervix N80.0
　fallopian tube N80.2
　female genital organ NEC N80.8
　gallbladder N80.8
　in scar of skin N80.6
　internal N80.0
　intestine N80.5
　lung N80.8
　myometrium N80.0
　ovary N80.1
　parametrium N80.3
　pelvic peritoneum N80.3
　peritoneal (pelvic) N80.3
　rectovaginal septum N80.4
　rectum N80.5
　round ligament N80.3
　skin (scar) N80.6
　specified site NEC N80.8
　stromal D39.0
　umbilicus N80.8
　uterus (internal) N80.0
　vagina N80.4
　vulva N80.8
Endometritis (decidual) (nonspecific) (purulent) (senile)
　(atrophic) (suppurative) N71.9
　with ectopic pregnancy O08.0
　acute N71.0
　blenorrhagic (gonococcal) (acute) (chronic) A54.24
　cervix, cervical (with erosion or ectropion) (see also
　　Cervicitis)
　　hyperplastic N72
　chlamydial A56.11
　chronic N71.1
　following
　　abortion — see Abortion by type complicated by
　　　genital infection
　　ectopic or molar pregnancy O08.0
　gonococcal, gonorrheal (acute) (chronic) A54.24
　hyperplastic (see also Hyperplasia, endometrial) N85.00
　　cervix N72
　puerperal, postpartum, childbirth O86.12
　subacute N71.0
　tuberculous A18.17
Endometrium — see condition
Endomyocardiopathy, South African I42.3
Endomyocarditis — see Endocarditis
Endomyofibrosis I42.3
Endomyometritis — see Endometritis
Endopericarditis — see Endocarditis
Endoperineuritis — see Disorder, nerve
Endophlebitis — see Phlebitis
Endophthalmia — see Endophthalmitis, purulent
Endophthalmitis (acute) (infective) (metastatic) (suba-
　cute) H44.009
　bleb associated (see also Bleb, inflammed (infected),
　　postprocedural H59.4 ☑
　gonorrheal A54.39
　in (due to)
　　cysticercosis B69.1
　　onchocerciasis B73.01
　　toxocariasis B83.0
　panuveitis — see Panuveitis
　parasitic H44.12- ☑
　purulent H44.00- ☑
　　panophthalmitis — see Panophthalmitis
　　vitreous abscess H44.02- ☑
　specified NEC H44.19
　sympathetic — see Uveitis, sympathetic
Endosalpingioma D28.2
Endosalpingiosis N94.89
Endosteitis — see Osteomyelitis
Endothelioma, bone — see Neoplasm, bone, malignant
Endotheliosis (hemorrhagic infectional) D69.8
Endotoxemia — code to condition

Endotrachelitis — see Cervicitis
Engelmann (-Camurati) **syndrome** Q78.3
English disease — see Rickets
Engman's disease L30.3
Engorgement
　breast N64.59
　　newborn P83.4
　　puerperal, postpartum O92.79
　lung (passive) — see Edema, lung
　pulmonary (passive) — see Edema, lung
　stomach K31.89
　venous, retina — see Occlusion, retina, vein, engorge-
　　ment
Enlargement, enlarged (see also Hypertrophy)
　adenoids J35.2
　　with tonsils J35.3
　alveolar ridge K08.8
　　congenital — see Anomaly, alveolar
　apertures of diaphragm (congenital) Q79.1
　gingival K06.1
　heart, cardiac — see Hypertrophy, cardiac
　lacrimal gland, chronic H04.03- ☑
　liver — see Hypertrophy, liver
　lymph gland or node R59.9
　　generalized R59.1
　　localized R59.0
　orbit H05.34- ☑
　organ or site, congenital NEC — see Anomaly, by site
　parathyroid (gland) E21.0
　pituitary fossa R93.0
　prostate N40.0
　　with lower urinary tract symptoms (LUTS) N40.1
　　without lower urinary tract symtpoms (LUTS) N40.0
　sella turcica R93.0
　spleen — see Splenomegaly
　thymus (gland) (congenital) E32.0
　thyroid (gland) — see Goiter
　tongue K14.8
　tonsils J35.1
　　with adenoids J35.3
　uterus N85.2
Enophthalmos H05.40- ☑
　due to
　　orbital tissue atrophy H05.41- ☑
　　trauma or surgery H05.42- ☑
Enostosis M27.8
Entamebic, entamebiasis — see Amebiasis
Entanglement
　umbilical cord(s) O69.2 ☑
　　with compression O69.2 ☑
　　　without compression O69.82 ☑
　　around neck (with compression) O69.1 ☑
　　　without compression O69.81 ☑
　　of twins in monoamniotic sac O69.2 ☑
Enteralgia — see Pain, abdominal
Enteric — see condition
Enteritis (acute) (diarrheal) (hemorrhagic) (noninfective)
　(septic) K52.9
　adenovirus A08.2
　aertrycke infection A02.0
　allergic K52.2
　amebic (acute) A06.0
　　with abscess — see Abscess, amebic
　　chronic A06.1
　　　with abscess — see Abscess, amebic
　　　nondysenteric A06.2
　　nondysenteric A06.2
　astrovirus A08.32
　bacillary NOS A03.9
　bacterial A04.9
　　specified NEC A04.8
　calicivirus A08.31
　candidal B37.82
　Chilomastix A07.8
　choleriformis A00.1
　chronic (noninfectious) K52.9
　　ulcerative — see Colitis, ulcerative
　cicatrizing (chronic) — see Enteritis, regional, small
　　intestine
　Clostridium
　　botulinum (food poisoning) A05.1
　　difficile A04.7
　coccidial A07.3
　coxsackie virus A08.39
　dietetic K52.2
　drug-induced K52.1

Index

Enteritis — Enthesopathy

Enteritis — *continued*
due to
astrovirus A08.32
calicivirus A08.31
coxsackie virus A08.39
drugs K52.1
echovirus A08.39
enterovirus NEC A08.39
food hypersensitivity K52.2
infectious organism (bacterial) (viral) — *see* Enteritis, infectious
torovirus A08.39
Yersinia enterocolitica A04.6
echovirus A08.39
eltor A00.1
enterovirus NEC A08.39
eosinophilic K52.81
epidemic (infectious) A09
fulminant K55.0
gangrenous — *see* Enteritis, infectious
giardial A07.1
infectious NOS A09
due to
adenovirus A08.2
Aerobacter aerogenes A04.8
Arizona (bacillus) A02.0
bacteria NOS A04.9
specified NEC A04.8
Campylobacter A04.5
Clostridium difficile A04.7
Clostridium perfringens A04.8
Enterobacter aerogenes A04.8
enterovirus A08.39
Escherichia coli A04.4
enteroaggregative A04.4
enterohemorrhagic A04.3
enteroinvasive A04.2
enteropathogenic A04.0
enterotoxigenic A04.1
specified NEC A04.4
specified
bacteria NEC A04.8
virus NEC A08.39
Staphylococcus A04.8
virus NEC A08.4
specified type NEC A08.39
Yersinia enterocolitica A04.6
specified organism NEC A08.8
influenzal — *see* Influenza, with, digestive manifestations
ischemic K55.9
acute K55.0
chronic K55.1
microsporidial A07.8
mucomembranous, myxomembranous — *see* Syndrome, irritable bowel
mucous — *see* Syndrome, irritable bowel
necroticans A05.2
necrotizing of newborn — *see* Enterocolitis, necrotizing, in newborn
neurogenic — *see* Syndrome, irritable bowel
newborn necrotizing — *see* Enterocolitis, necrotizing, in newborn
noninfectious K52.9
norovirus A08.11
parasitic NEC B82.9
paratyphoid (fever) — *see* Fever, paratyphoid
protozoal A07.9
specified NEC A07.8
radiation K52.0
regional (of) K50.90
with
complication K50.919
abscess K50.914
fistula K50.913
intestinal obstruction K50.912
rectal bleeding K50.911
specified complication NEC K50.918
colon — *see* Enteritis, regional, large intestine
duodenum — *see* Enteritis, regional, small intestine
ileum — *see* Enteritis, regional, small intestine
jejunum — *see* Enteritis, regional, small intestine
large bowel — *see* Enteritis, regional, large intestine
large intestine (colon) (rectum) K50.10
with
complication K50.119
abscess K50.114

Enteritis — *continued*
regional — *continued*
large intestine — *continued*
with — *continued*
complication — *continued*
fistula K50.113
intestinal obstruction K50.112
rectal bleeding K50.111
small intestine (duodenum) (ileum) (jejunum) involvement K50.80
with
complication K50.819
abscess K50.814
fistula K50.813
intestinal obstruction K50.812
rectal bleeding K50.811
specified complication NEC K50.818
specified complication NEC K50.118
rectum — *see* Enteritis, regional, large intestine
small intestine (duodenum) (ileum) (jejunum) K50.00
with
complication K50.019
abscess K50.014
fistula K50.013
intestinal obstruction K50.012
large intestine (colon) (rectum) involvement K50.80
with
complication K50.819
abscess K50.814
fistula K50.813
intestinal obstruction K50.812
rectal bleeding K50.811
specified complication NEC K50.818
rectal bleeding K50.011
specified complication NEC K50.018
rotaviral A08.0
Salmonella, salmonellosis (arizonae) (cholerae-suis) (enteritidis) (typhimurium) A02.0
segmental — *see* Enteritis, regional
septic A09
Shigella — *see* Infection, Shigella
small round structured NEC A08.19
spasmodic, spastic — *see* Syndrome, irritable bowel
staphylococcal A04.8
due to food A05.0
torovirus A08.39
toxic NEC K52.1
due to Clostridium difficile A04.7
trichomonal A07.8
tuberculous A18.32
typhosa A01.00
ulcerative (chronic) — *see* Colitis, ulcerative
viral A08.4
adenovirus A08.2
enterovirus A08.39
Rotavirus A08.0
small round structured NEC A08.19
specified NEC A08.39
virus specified NEC A08.39
Enterobiasis B80
Enterobius vermicularis (infection) (infestation) B80
Enterocele (*see also* Hernia, abdomen)
pelvic, pelvis (acquired) (congenital) N81.5
vagina, vaginal (acquired) (congenital) NEC N81.5
Enterocolitis (*see also* Enteritis) K52.9
due to Clostridium difficile A04.7
fulminant ischemic K55.0
granulomatous — *see* Enteritis, regional
hemorrhagic (acute) K55.0
chronic K55.1
infectious NEC A09
ischemic K55.9
necrotizing
due to Clostridium difficile A04.7
in newborn P77.9
stage 1 (without pneumatosis, without perforation) P77.1
stage 2 (with pneumatosis, without perforation) P77.2
stage 3 (with pneumatosis, with perforation) P77.3
noninfectious K52.9
newborn — *see* Enterocolitis, necrotizing, in newborn

Enterocolitis — *continued*
pseudomembranous (newborn) A04.7
radiation K52.0
newborn — *see* Enterocolitis, necrotizing, in newborn
ulcerative (chronic) — *see* Pancolitis, ulcerative (chronic)
Enterogastritis — *see* Enteritis
Enteropathy K63.9
gluten-sensitive K90.0
hemorrhagic, terminal K55.0
protein-losing K90.4
Enteroperitonitis — *see* Peritonitis
Enteroptosis K63.4
Enterorrhagia K92.2
Enterospasm (*see also* Syndrome, irritable, bowel)
psychogenic F45.8
Enterostenosis (*see also* Obstruction, intestine) K56.69
Enterostomy
complication — *see* Complication, enterostomy
status Z93.4
Enterovirus, as cause of disease classified elsewhere B97.10
coxsackievirus B97.11
echovirus B97.12
other specified B97.19
Enthesopathy (peripheral) M77.9
Achilles tendinitis — *see* Tendinitis, Achilles
ankle and tarsus M77.9
specified type NEC — *see* Enthesopathy, foot, specified type NEC
anterior tibial syndrome M76.81- ☑
calcaneal spur — *see* Spur, bone, calcaneal
elbow region M77.8
lateral epicondylitis — *see* Epicondylitis, lateral
medial epicondylitis — *see* Epicondylitis, medial
foot NEC M77.9
metatarsalgia — *see* Metatarsalgia
specified type NEC M77.5- ☑
forearm M77.9
gluteal tendinitis — *see* Tendinitis, gluteal
hand M77.9
hip — *see* Enthesopathy, lower limb, specified type NEC
iliac crest spur — *see* Spur, bone, iliac crest
iliotibial band syndrome — *see* Syndrome, iliotibial band
knee — *see* Enthesopathy, lower limb, lower leg, specified type NEC
lateral epicondylitis — *see* Epicondylitis, lateral
lower limb (excluding foot) M76.9
Achilles tendinitis — *see* Tendinitis, Achilles
anterior tibial syndrome M76.81- ☑
gluteal tendinitis — *see* Tendinitis, gluteal
iliac crest spur — *see* Spur, bone, iliac crest
iliotibial band syndrome — *see* Syndrome, iliotibial band
patellar tendinitis — *see* Tendinitis, patellar
pelvic region — *see* Enthesopathy, lower limb, specified type NEC
peroneal tendinitis — *see* Tendinitis, peroneal
posterior tibial syndrome M76.82- ☑
psoas tendinitis — *see* Tendinitis, psoas
shoulder M77.9
specified type NEC M76.89- ☑
tibial collateral bursitis — *see* Bursitis, tibial collateral
medial epicondylitis — *see* Epicondylitis, medial
metatarsalgia — *see* Metatarsalgia
multiple sites M77.9
patellar tendinitis — *see* Tendinitis, patellar
pelvis M77.9
periarthritis of wrist — *see* Periarthritis, wrist
peroneal tendinitis — *see* Tendinitis, peroneal
posterior tibial syndrome M76.82- ☑
psoas tendinitis — *see* Tendinitis, psoas
shoulder region — *see* Lesion, shoulder
specified site NEC M77.9
specified type NEC M77.8
spinal M46.00
cervical region M46.02
cervicothoracic region M46.03
lumbar region M46.06
lumbosacral region M46.07
multiple sites M46.09
occipito-atlanto-axial region M46.01
sacrococcygeal region M46.08

Enthesopathy — *continued*
  spinal — *continued*
    thoracic region M46.04
    thoracolumbar region M46.05
  tibial collateral bursitis — *see* Bursitis, tibial collateral
  upper arm M77.9
  wrist and carpus NEC M77.8
    calcaneal spur — *see* Spur, bone, calcaneal
    periarthritis of wrist — *see* Periarthritis, wrist
Entomophobia F40.218
Entomophthoromycosis B46.8
Entrance, air into vein — *see* Embolism, air
Entrapment, nerve — *see* Neuropathy, entrapment
Entropion (eyelid) (paralytic) H02.009
  cicatricial H02.019
    left H02.016
      lower H02.015
      upper H02.014
    right H02.013
      lower H02.012
      upper H02.011
  congenital Q10.2
  left H02.006
    lower H02.005
    upper H02.004
  mechanical H02.029
    left H02.026
      lower H02.025
      upper H02.024
    right H02.023
      lower H02.022
      upper H02.021
  right H02.003
    lower H02.002
    upper H02.001
  senile H02.039
    left H02.036
      lower H02.035
      upper H02.034
    right H02.033
      lower H02.032
      upper H02.031
  spastic H02.049
    left H02.046
      lower H02.045
      upper H02.044
    right H02.043
      lower H02.042
      upper H02.041
Enucleated eye (traumatic, current) S05.7- ☑
Enuresis R32
  functional F98.0
  habit disturbance F98.0
  nocturnal N39.44
    psychogenic F98.0
  nonorganic origin F98.0
  psychogenic F98.0
Eosinopenia — *see* Agranulocytosis
Eosinophilia (allergic) (hereditary) (idiopathic) (secondary) D72.1
  with
    angiolymphoid hyperplasia (ALHE) D18.01
  infiltrative J82
  Löffler's J82
  peritoneal — *see* Peritonitis, eosinophilic
  pulmonary NEC J82
  tropical (pulmonary) J82
Eosinophilia-myalgia syndrome M35.8
Ependymitis (acute) (cerebral) (chronic) (granular) — *see* Encephalomyelitis
Ependymoblastoma
  specified site — *see* Neoplasm, malignant, by site
  unspecified site C71.9
Ependymoma (epithelial) (malignant)
  anaplastic
    specified site — *see* Neoplasm, malignant, by site
    unspecified site C71.9
  benign
    specified site — *see* Neoplasm, benign, by site
    unspecified site D33.2
  myxopapillary D43.2
    specified site — *see* Neoplasm, uncertain behavior, by site
    unspecified site D43.2
  papillary D43.2
    specified site — *see* Neoplasm, uncertain behavior, by site
    unspecified site D43.2

Ependymoma — *continued*
  specified site — *see* Neoplasm, malignant, by site
  unspecified site C71.9
Ependymopathy G93.89
Ephelis, ephelides L81.2
Epiblepharon (congenital) Q10.3
Epicanthus, epicanthic fold (eyelid) (congenital) Q10.3
Epicondylitis (elbow)
  lateral M77.1- ☑
  medial M77.0- ☑
Epicystitis — *see* Cystitis
Epidemic — *see* condition
Epidermidalization, cervix — *see* Dysplasia, cervix
Epidermis, epidermal — *see* condition
Epidermodysplasia verruciformis B07.8
Epidermolysis
  bullosa (congenital) Q81.9
    acquired L12.30
      drug-induced L12.31
      specified cause NEC L12.35
    dystrophica Q81.2
    letalis Q81.1
    simplex Q81.0
    specified NEC Q81.8
  necroticans combustiformis L51.2
    due to drug — *see* Table of Drugs and Chemicals, by drug
Epidermophytid — *see* Dermatophytosis
Epidermophytosis (infected) — *see* Dermatophytosis
Epididymis — *see* condition
Epididymitis (acute) (nonvenereal) (recurrent) (residual) N45.1
  with orchitis N45.3
  blennorrhagic (gonococcal) A54.23
  caseous (tuberculous) A18.15
  chlamydial A56.19
  filarial (*see also* Infestation, filarial) B74.9 [N51]
  gonococcal A54.23
  syphilitic A52.76
  tuberculous A18.15
Epididymo-orchitis (*see also* Epididymitis) N45.3
Epidural — *see* condition
Epigastrium, epigastric — *see* condition
Epigastrocele — *see* Hernia, ventral
Epiglottis — *see* condition
Epiglottitis, epiglottiditis (acute) J05.10
  with obstruction J05.11
  chronic J37.0
Epignathus Q89.4
Epilepsia partialis continua (*see also* Kozhevnikof's epilepsy) G40.1- ☑
Epilepsy, epileptic, epilepsia (attack) (cerebral) (convulsion) (fit) (seizure) G40.909

Note: the following terms are to be considered equivalent to intractable: pharmacoresistant (pharmacologically resistant), treatment resistant, refractory (medically) and poorly controlled

  with
    complex partial seizures — *see* Epilepsy, localization-related, symptomatic, with complex partial seizures
    grand mal seizures on awakening — *see* Epilepsy, generalized, specified NEC
    myoclonic absences — *see* Epilepsy, generalized, specified NEC
    myoclonic-astatic seizures — *see* Epilepsy, generalized, specified NEC
    simple partial seizures — *see* Epilepsy, localization-related, symptomatic, with simple partial seizures
  akinetic — *see* Epilepsy, generalized, specified NEC
  benign childhood with centrotemporal EEG spikes — *see* Epilepsy, localization-related, idiopathic
  benign myoclonic in infancy G40.80- ☑
  Bravais-jacksonian — *see* Epilepsy, localization-related, symptomatic, with simple partial seizures
  childhood
    with occipital EEG paroxysms — *see* Epilepsy, localization-related, idiopathic
    absence G40.A09 (*following* G40.3)
      intractable G40.A19 (*following* G40.3)
        with status epilepticus G40.A11 (*following* G40.3)
        without status epilepticus G40.A19 (*following* G40.3)

Epilepsy, epileptic, epilepsia — *continued*
  childhood — *continued*
    absence — *continued*
      not intractable G40.A09 (*following* G40.3)
        with status epilepticus G40.A01 (*following* G40.3)
        without status epilepticus G40.A09 (*following* G40.3)
  climacteric — *see* Epilepsy, specified NEC
  cysticercosis B69.0
  deterioration (mental) F06.8
  due to syphilis A52.19
  focal — *see* Epilepsy, localization-related, symptomatic, with simple partial seizures
  generalized
    idiopathic G40.309
      intractable G40.319
        with status epilepticus G40.311
        without status epilepticus G40.319
      not intractable G40.309
        with status epilepticus G40.301
        without status epilepticus G40.309
    specified NEC G40.409
      intractable G40.419
        with status epilepticus G40.411
        without status epilepticus G40.419
      not intractable G40.409
        with status epilepticus G40.401
        without status epilepticus G40.409
  impulsive petit mal — *see* Epilepsy, juvenile myoclonic
  intractable G40.919
    with status epilepticus G40.911
    without status epilepticus G40.919
  juvenile absence G40.A09 (*following* G40.3)
    intractable G40.A19 (*following* G40.3)
      with status epilepticus G40.A11 (*following* G40.3)
      without status epilepticus G40.A19 (*following* G40.3)
    not intractable G40.A09 (*following* G40.3)
      with status epilepticus G40.A01 (*following* G40.3)
      without status epilepticus G40.A09 (*following* G40.3)
  juvenile myoclonic G40.B09 (*following* G40.3)
    intractable G40.B19 (*following* G40.3)
      with status epilepticus G40.B11 (*following* G40.3)
      without status epilepticus G40.B19 (*following* G40.3)
    not intractable G40.B09 (*following* G40.3)
      with status epilepticus G40.B01 (*following* G40.3)
      without status epilepticus G40.B09 (*following* G40.3)
  localization-related (focal) (partial)
    idiopathic G40.009
      with seizures of localized onset G40.009
        intractable G40.019
          with status epilepticus G40.011
          without status epilepticus G40.019
        not intractable G40.009
          with status epilepticus G40.001
          without status epilepticus G40.009
    symptomatic
      with complex partial seizures G40.209
        intractable G40.219
          with status epilepticus G40.211
          without status epilepticus G40.219
        not intractable G40.209
          with status epilepticus G40.201
          without status epilepticus G40.209
      with simple partial seizures G40.109
        intractable G40.119
          with status epilepticus G40.111
          without status epilepticus G40.119
        not intractable G40.109
          with status epilepticus G40.101
          without status epilepticus G40.109
  myoclonus, myoclonic (progressive) — *see* Epilepsy, generalized, specified NEC
  not intractable G40.909
    with status epilepticus G40.901
    without status epilepticus G40.909
  on awakening — *see* Epilepsy, generalized, specified NEC
  parasitic NOS B71.9 [G94]

Epilepsy, epileptic, epilepsia — *continued*
- partialis continua (*see also* Kozhevnikof's epilepsy) G40.1- ☑
- peripheral — *see* Epilepsy, specified NEC
- procursiva — *see* Epilepsy, localization-related, symptomatic, with simple partial seizures
- progressive (familial) myoclonic — *see* Epilepsy, generalized, idiopathic
- reflex — *see* Epilepsy, specified NEC
- related to
  - alcohol G40.509
    - not intractable G40.509
      - with status epilepticus G40.501
      - without status epliepticus G40.509
  - drugs G40.509
    - not intractable G40.509
      - with status epilepticus G40.501
      - without status epliepticus G40.509
  - external causes G40.509
    - not intractable G40.509
      - with status epilepticus G40.501
      - without status epliepticus G40.509
  - hormonal changes G40.509
    - not intractable G40.509
      - with status epilepticus G40.501
      - without status epliepticus G40.509
  - sleep deprivation G40.509
    - not intractable G40.509
      - with status epilepticus G40.501
      - without status epliepticus G40.509
  - stress G40.509
    - not intractable G40.509
      - with status epilepticus G40.501
      - without status epliepticus G40.509
- somatomotor — *see* Epilepsy, localization-related, symptomatic, with simple partial seizures
- somatosensory — *see* Epilepsy, localization-related, symptomatic, with simple partial seizures
- spasms G40.822
  - intractable G40.824
    - with status epilepticus G40.823
    - without status epilepticus G40.824
  - not intractable G40.822
    - with status epilepticus G40.821
    - without status epilepticus G40.822
  - specified NEC G40.802
    - intractable G40.804
      - with status epilepticus G40.803
      - without status epilepticus G40.804
    - not intractable G40.802
      - with status epilepticus G40.801
      - without status epilepticus G40.802
- syndromes
  - generalized
    - idiopathic G40.309
      - intractable G40.319
        - with status epilepticus G40.311
        - without status epilepticus G40.319
      - not intractable G40.309
        - with status epilepticus G40.301
        - without status epilepticus G40.309
    - specified NEC G40.409
      - intractable G40.419
        - with status epilepticus G40.411
        - without status epilepticus G40.419
      - not intractable G40.409
        - with status epilepticus G40.401
        - without status epilepticus G40.409
  - localization-related (focal) (partial)
    - idiopathic G40.009
      - with seizures of localized onset G40.009
        - intractable G40.019
          - with status epilepticus G40.011
          - without status epilepticus G40.019
        - not intractable G40.009
          - with status epilepticus G40.001
          - without status epilepticus G40.009
    - symptomatic
      - with complex partial seizures G40.209
        - intractable G40.219
          - with status epilepticus G40.211
          - without status epilepticus G40.219
        - not intractable G40.209
          - with status epilepticus G40.201
          - without status epilepticus G40.209
      - with simple partial seizures G40.109
        - intractable G40.119
          - with status epilepticus G40.111

Epilepsy, epileptic, epilepsia — *continued*
- syndromes — *continued*
  - localization-related — *continued*
    - symptomatic — *continued*
      - with simple partial seizures — *continued*
        - intractable — *continued*
          - without status epilepticus G40.119
        - not intractable G40.109
          - with status epilepticus G40.101
          - without status epilepticus G40.109
    - specified NEC G40.802
      - intractable G40.804
        - with status epilepticus G40.803
        - without status epilepticus G40.804
      - not intractable G40.802
        - with status epilepticus G40.801
        - without status epilepticus G40.802
  - tonic (-clonic) — *see* Epilepsy, generalized, specified NEC
  - twilight F05
  - uncinate (gyrus) — *see* Epilepsy, localization-related, symptomatic, with complex partial seizures
  - Unverricht (-Lundborg) (familial myoclonic) — *see* Epilepsy, generalized, idiopathic
  - visceral — *see* Epilepsy, specified NEC
  - visual — *see* Epilepsy, specified NEC

Epiloia Q85.1
Epimenorrhea N92.0
Epipharyngitis — *see* Nasopharyngitis
Epiphora H04.20- ☑
- due to
  - excess lacrimation H04.21- ☑
  - insufficient drainage H04.22- ☑
Epiphyseal arrest — *see* Arrest, epiphyseal
Epiphyseolysis, epiphysiolysis — *see* Osteochondropathy
Epiphysitis (*see also* Osteochondropathy)
- juvenile M92.9
- syphilitic (congenital) A50.02
Epiplocele — *see* Hernia, abdomen
Epiploitis — *see* Peritonitis
Epiplosarcomphalocele — *see* Hernia, umbilicus
Episcleritis (suppurative) H15.10- ☑
- in (due to)
  - syphilis A52.71
  - tuberculosis A18.51
- nodular H15.12- ☑
- periodica fugax H15.11- ☑
  - angioneurotic — *see* Edema, angioneurotic
- syphilitic (late) A52.71
- tuberculous A18.51
Episode
- affective, mixed F39
- depersonalization (in neurotic state) F48.1
- depressive F32.9
  - major F32.9
    - mild F32.0
    - moderate F32.1
    - severe (without psychotic symptoms) F32.2
      - with psychotic symptoms F32.3
  - recurrent F33.9
    - brief F33.8
  - specified NEC F32.8
- hypomanic F30.8
- manic F30.9
  - with
    - psychotic symptoms F30.2
    - remission (full) F30.4
      - partial F30.3
  - without psychotic symptoms F30.10
    - mild F30.11
    - moderate F30.12
    - severe (without psychotic symptoms) F30.13
      - with psychotic symptoms F30.2
  - other specified F30.8
  - recurrent F31.89
- psychotic F23
  - organic F06.8
- schizophrenic (acute) NEC, brief F23
Epispadias (female) (male) Q64.0
Episplenitis D73.89
Epistaxis (multiple) R04.0
- hereditary I78.0
- vicarious menstruation N94.89
Epithelioma (malignant) (*see also* Neoplasm, malignant, by site)
- adenoides cysticum — *see* Neoplasm, skin, benign
- basal cell — *see* Neoplasm, skin, malignant

Epithelioma — *continued*
- benign — *see* Neoplasm, benign, by site
- Bowen's — *see* Neoplasm, skin, in situ
- calcifying, of Malherbe — *see* Neoplasm, skin, benign
- external site — *see* Neoplasm, skin, malignant
- intraepidermal, Jadassohn — *see* Neoplasm, skin, benign
- squamous cell — *see* Neoplasm, malignant, by site
Epitheliomatosis pigmented Q82.1
Epitheliopathy, multifocal placoid pigment H30.14- ☑
Epithelium, epithelial — *see* condition
Epituberculosis (with atelectasis) (allergic) A15.7
Eponychia Q84.6
Epstein's
- nephrosis or syndrome — *see* Nephrosis
- pearl K09.8
Epulis (gingiva) (fibrous) (giant cell) K06.8
Equinia A24.0
Equinovarus (congenital) (talipes) Q66.0
- acquired — *see* Deformity, limb, clubfoot
Equivalent
- convulsive (abdominal) — *see* Epilepsy, specified NEC
- epileptic (psychic) — *see* Epilepsy, localization-related, symptomatic, with complex partial seizures
Erb (-Duchenne) **paralysis** (birth injury) (newborn) P14.0
Erb-Goldflam disease or syndrome G70.00
- with exacerbation (acute) G70.01
- in crisis G70.01
Erb's
- disease G71.0
- palsy, paralysis (brachial) (birth) (newborn) P14.0
  - spinal (spastic) syphilitic A52.17
- pseudohypertrophic muscular dystrophy G71.0
Erdheim's syndrome (acromegalic macrospondylitis) E22.0
Erection, painful (persistent) — *see* Priapism
Ergosterol deficiency (vitamin D) E55.9
- with
  - adult osteomalacia M83.8
  - rickets — *see* Rickets
Ergotism (*see also* Poisoning, food, noxious, plant)
- from ergot used as drug (migraine therapy) — *see* Table of Drugs and Chemicals
Erosio interdigitalis blastomycetica B37.2
Erosion
- artery I77.2
  - without rupture I77.89
- bone — *see* Disorder, bone, density and structure, specified NEC
- bronchus J98.09
- cartilage (joint) — *see* Disorder, cartilage, specified type NEC
- cervix (uteri) (acquired) (chronic) (congenital) N86
  - with cervicitis N72
- cornea (nontraumatic) — *see* Ulcer, cornea
  - recurrent H18.83- ☑
  - traumatic — *see* Abrasion, cornea
- dental (idiopathic) (occupational) (due to diet, drugs or vomiting) K03.2
- duodenum, postpyloric — *see* Ulcer, duodenum
- esophagus K22.10
  - with bleeding K22.11
- gastric — *see* Ulcer, stomach
- gastrojejunal — *see* Ulcer, gastrojejunal
- implanted mesh — *see* Complications, mesh
- intestine K63.3
- lymphatic vessel I89.8
- pylorus, pyloric (ulcer) — *see* Ulcer, stomach
- spine, aneurysmal A52.09
- stomach — *see* Ulcer, stomach
- teeth (idiopathic) (occupational) (due to diet, drugs or vomiting) K03.2
- urethra N36.8
- uterus N85.8
Erotomania F52.8
Error
- metabolism, inborn — *see* Disorder, metabolism
- refractive — *see* Disorder, refraction
Eructation R14.2
- nervous or psychogenic F45.8
Eruption
- creeping B76.9
- drug (generalized) (taken internally) L27.0
  - fixed L27.1
  - in contact with skin — *see* Dermatitis, due to drugs
  - localized L27.1

Eruption — *continued*
  Hutchinson, summer L56.4
  Kaposi's varicelliform B00.0
  napkin L22
  polymorphous light (sun) L56.4
  recalcitrant pustular L13.8
  ringed R23.8
  skin (nonspecific) R21
    creeping (meaning hookworm) B76.9
    due to inoculation/vaccination (generalized) (*see also* Dermatitis, due to, vaccine) L27.0
      localized L27.1
    erysipeloid A26.0
    feigned L98.1
    Kaposi's varicelliform B00.0
    lichenoid L28.0
    meaning dermatitis — *see* Dermatitis
    toxic NEC L53.0
  tooth, teeth, abnormal (incomplete) (late) (premature) (sequence) K00.6
  vesicular R23.8
Erysipelas (gangrenous) (infantile) (newborn) (phlegmonous) (suppurative) A46
  external ear A46 [H62.40]
  puerperal, postpartum O86.89
Erysipeloid A26.9
  cutaneous (Rosenbach's) A26.0
  disseminated A26.8
  sepsis A26.7
  specified NEC A26.8
Erythema, erythematous (infectional) (inflammation) L53.9
  ab igne L59.0
  annulare (centrifugum) (rheumaticum) L53.1
  arthriticum epidemicum A25.1
  brucellum — *see* Brucellosis
  chronic figurate NEC L53.3
  chronicum migrans (Borrelia burgdorferi) A69.20
  diaper L22
  due to
    chemical NEC L53.0
      in contact with skin L24.5
    drug (internal use) — *see* Dermatitis, due to, drugs
  elevatum diutinum L95.1
  endemic E52
  epidemic, arthritic A25.1
  figuratum perstans L53.3
  gluteal L22
  heat — *code by site under* Burn, first degree
  ichthyosiforme congenitum bullous Q80.3
  in diseases classified elsewhere L54
  induratum (nontuberculous) L52
    tuberculous A18.4
  infectiosum B08.3
  intertrigo L30.4
  iris L51.9
  marginatum L53.2
    in (due to) acute rheumatic fever I00
  medicamentosum — *see* Dermatitis, due to, drugs
  migrans A26.0
    chronicum A69.20
    tongue K14.1
  multiforme (major) (minor) L51.9
    bullous, bullosum L51.1
    conjunctiva L51.1
    nonbullous L51.0
    pemphigoides L12.0
    specified NEC L51.8
  napkin L22
  neonatorum P83.8
    toxic P83.1
  nodosum L52
    tuberculous A18.4
  palmar L53.8
  pernio T69.1 ☑
  rash, newborn P83.8
  scarlatiniform (recurrent) (exfoliative) L53.8
  solare L55.0
  specified NEC L53.8
  toxic, toxicum NEC L53.0
    newborn P83.1
  tuberculous (primary) A18.4
Erythematous, erythematosus — *see* condition
Erythermalgia (primary) I73.81
Erythralgia I73.81
Erythrasma L08.1
Erythredema (polyneuropathy) — *see* Poisoning, mercury

Erythremia (acute) C94.0- ☑
  chronic D45
  secondary D75.1
Erythroblastopenia (*see also* Aplasia, red cell) D60.9
  congenital D61.01
Erythroblastophthisis D61.09
Erythroblastosis (fetalis) (newborn) P55.9
  due to
    ABO (antibodies) (incompatibility) (isoimmunization) P55.1
    Rh (antibodies) (incompatibility) (isoimmunization) P55.0
Erythrocyanosis (crurum) I73.89
Erythrocythemia — *see* Erythremia
Erythrocytosis (megalosplenic) (secondary) D75.1
  familial D75.0
  oval, hereditary — *see* Elliptocytosis
  secondary D75.1
  stress D75.1
Erythroderma (secondary) (*see also* Erythema) L53.9
  bullous ichthyosiform, congenital Q80.3
  desquamativum L21.1
  ichthyosiform, congenital (bullous) Q80.3
  neonatorum P83.8
  psoriaticum L40.8
Erythrodysesthesia, palmar plantar (PPE) L27.1
Erythrogenesis imperfecta D61.09
Erythroleukemia C94.0- ☑
Erythromelalgia I73.81
Erythrophagocytosis D75.89
Erythrophobia F40.298
Erythroplakia, oral epithelium, and tongue K13.29
Erythroplasia (Queyrat) D07.4
  specified site — *see* Neoplasm, skin, in situ
  unspecified site D07.4
Escherichia coli (E. coli), **as cause of disease classified elsewhere** B96.20
  non-O157 Shiga toxin-producing (with known O group) B96.22
  non-Shiga toxin-producing B96.29
  O157 B96.21
  O157 with confirmation of Shiga toxin when H antigen is unknown, or is not H7 B96.21
  O157:H- (nonmotile) with confirmation of Shiga toxin B96.21
  O157:H7 with or without confirmation of Shiga toxin-production B96.21
    specified NEC B96.22
  Shiga toxin-producing (with unspecified O group) (STEC) B96.23
  specified NEC B96.29
Esophagismus K22.4
Esophagitis (acute) (alkaline) (chemical) (chronic) (infectional) (necrotic) (peptic) (postoperative) K20.9
  candidal B37.81
  due to gastrointestinal reflux disease K21.0
  eosinophilic K20.0
  reflux K21.0
  specified NEC K20.8
  tuberculous A18.83
  ulcerative K22.10
    with bleeding K22.11
Esophagocele K22.5
Esophagomalacia K22.8
Esophagospasm K22.4
Esophagostenosis K22.2
Esophagostomiasis B81.8
Esophagotracheal — *see* condition
Esophagus — *see* condition
Esophoria H50.51
  convergence, excess H51.12
  divergence, insufficiency H51.8
Esotropia — *see* Strabismus, convergent concomitant
Espundia B55.2
Essential — *see* condition
Esthesioneuroblastoma C30.0
Esthesioneurocytoma C30.0
Esthesioneuroepithelioma C30.0
Esthiomene A55
Estivo-autumnal malaria (fever) B50.9
Estrangement (marital) Z63.5
  parent-child NEC Z62.890
Estriasis — *see* Myiasis
Ethanolism — *see* Alcoholism
Etherism — *see* Dependence, drug, inhalant
Ethmoid, ethmoidal — *see* condition

Ethmoiditis (chronic) (nonpurulent) (purulent) (*see also* Sinusitis, ethmoidal)
  influenzal — *see* Influenza, with, respiratory manifestations NEC
  Woakes' J33.1
Ethylism — *see* Alcoholism
Eulenburg's disease (congenital paramyotonia) G71.19
Eumycetoma B47.0
Eunuchoidism E29.1
  hypogonadotropic E23.0
European blastomycosis — *see* Cryptococcosis
Eustachian — *see* condition
Evaluation (for) (of)
  development state
    adolescent Z00.3
    period of
      delayed growth in childhood Z00.70
        with abnormal findings Z00.71
      rapid growth in childhood Z00.2
      puberty Z00.3
  growth and developmental state (period of rapid growth) Z00.2
  delayed growth Z00.70
    with abnormal findings Z00.71
  mental health (status) Z00.8
    requested by authority Z04.6
  period of
    delayed growth in childhood Z00.70
      with abnormal findings Z00.71
    rapid growth in childhood Z00.2
  suspected condition — *see* Observation
Evans syndrome D69.41
Event, apparent life threatening in newborn and infant (ALTE) R68.13
Eventration (*see also* Hernia, ventral)
  colon into chest — *see* Hernia, diaphragm
  diaphragm (congenital) Q79.1
Eversion
  bladder N32.89
  cervix (uteri) N86
    with cervicitis N72
  foot NEC (*see also* Deformity, valgus, ankle)
    congenital Q66.6
  punctum lacrimale (postinfectional) (senile) H04.52- ☑
  ureter (meatus) N28.89
  urethra (meatus) N36.8
  uterus N81.4
Evidence
  cytologic
    of malignancy on anal smear R85.614
    of malignancy on cervical smear R87.614
    of malignancy on vaginal smear R87.624
Evisceration
  birth injury P15.8
  traumatic NEC
    eye — *see* Enucleated eye
Evulsion — *see* Avulsion
Ewing's sarcoma or tumor — *see* Neoplasm, bone, malignant
Examination (for) (following) (general) (of) (routine) Z00.00
  with abnormal findings Z00.01
  abuse, physical (alleged), ruled out
    adult Z04.71
    child Z04.72
  adolescent (development state) Z00.3
  alleged rape or sexual assault (victim), ruled out
    adult Z04.41
    child Z04.42
  allergy Z01.82
  annual (adult) (periodic) (physical) Z00.00
    with abnormal findings Z00.01
    gynecological Z01.419
      with abnormal findings Z01.411
  antibody response Z01.84
  blood — *see* Examination, laboratory
  blood pressure Z01.30
    with abnormal findings Z01.31
  cancer staging — *see* Neoplasm, malignant, by site
  cervical Papanicolaou smear Z12.4
    as part of routine gynecological examination Z01.419
      with abnormal findings Z01.411
  child (over 28 days old) Z00.129
    with abnormal findings Z00.121
    under 28 days old — *see* Newborn, examination
  clinical research control or normal comparison (control) (participant) Z00.6

⛛ Subterms under main terms may continue to next column or page   ☑ Additional Character Required — Refer to the Tabular List for Character Selection

Examination — *continued*
  contraceptive (drug) maintenance (routine) Z30.8
    device (intrauterine) Z30.431
  dental Z01.20
    with abnormal findings Z01.21
  developmental — *see* Examination, child
  donor (potential) Z00.5
  ear Z01.10
    with abnormal findings NEC Z01.118
  eye Z01.00
    with abnormal findings Z01.01
  following
    accident NEC Z04.3
      transport Z04.1
      work Z04.2
    assault, alleged, ruled out
      adult Z04.71
      child Z04.72
    motor vehicle accident Z04.1
    treatment (for) Z09
      combined NEC Z09
        fracture Z09
        malignant neoplasm Z08
      malignant neoplasm Z08
      mental disorder Z09
      specified condition NEC Z09
  follow-up (routine) (following) Z09
    chemotherapy NEC Z09
      malignant neoplasm Z08
    fracture Z09
    malignant neoplasm Z08
    postpartum Z39.2
    psychotherapy Z09
    radiotherapy NEC Z09
      malignant neoplasm Z08
    surgery NEC Z09
      malignant neoplasm Z08
  gynecological Z01.419
    with abnormal findings Z01.411
    for contraceptive maintenance Z30.8
  health — *see* Examination, medical
  hearing Z01.10
    with abnormal findings NEC Z01.118
    following failed hearing screening Z01.110
  immunity status testing Z01.84
  laboratory (as part of a general medical examination)
      Z00.00
    with abnormal findings Z00.01
    preprocedural Z01.812
  lactating mother Z39.1
  medical (adult) (for) (of) Z00.00
    with abnormal findings Z00.01
    administrative purpose only Z02.9
      specified NEC Z02.89
    admission to
      armed forces Z02.3
      old age home Z02.2
      prison Z02.89
      residential institution Z02.2
      school Z02.0
        following illness or medical treatment Z02.0
      summer camp Z02.89
    adoption Z02.82
    blood alcohol or drug level Z02.83
    camp (summer) Z02.89
    clinical research, normal subject (control) (partici-
        pant) Z00.6
    control subject in clinical research (normal compar-
        ison) (participant) Z00.6
    donor (potential) Z00.5
    driving license Z02.4
    general (adult) Z00.00
      with abnormal findings Z00.01
    immigration Z02.89
    insurance purposes Z02.6
    marriage Z02.89
    medicolegal reasons NEC Z04.8
    naturalization Z02.89
    participation in sport Z02.5
    paternity testing Z02.81
    population survey Z00.8
    pre-employment Z02.1
    pre-operative — *see* Examination, pre-procedural
    pre-procedural
      cardiovascular Z01.810
      respiratory Z01.811
      specified NEC Z01.818

Examination — *continued*
  medical — *continued*
    preschool children
      for admission to school Z02.0
    prisoners
      for entrance into prison Z02.89
    recruitment for armed forces Z02.3
    specified NEC Z00.8
    sport competition Z02.5
  medicolegal reason NEC Z04.8
  newborn — *see* Newborn, examination
  pelvic (annual) (periodic) Z01.419
    with abnormal findings Z01.411
  period of rapid growth in childhood Z00.2
  periodic (adult) (annual) (routine) Z00.00
    with abnormal findings Z00.01
  physical (adult) (*see also* Examination, medical) Z00.00
    sports Z02.5
  postpartum
    immediately after delivery Z39.0
    routine follow-up Z39.2
  pre-chemotherapy (antineoplastic) Z01.818
  prenatal (normal pregnancy) (*see also* Pregnancy,
      normal) Z34.9- ☑
  pre-procedural (pre-operative)
    cardiovascular Z01.810
    laboratory Z01.812
    respiratory Z01.811
    specified NEC Z01.818
  prior to chemotherapy (antineoplastic) Z01.818
  psychiatric NEC Z00.8
    follow-up not needing further care Z09
    requested by authority Z04.6
  radiological (as part of a general medical examination)
      Z00.00
    with abnormal findings Z00.01
  repeat cervical smear to confirm findings of recent
      normal smear following initial abnormal smear
      Z01.42
  skin (hypersensitivity) Z01.82
  special (*see also* Examination, by type) Z01.89
    specified type NEC Z01.89
  specified type or reason NEC Z04.8
  teeth Z01.20
    with abnormal findings Z01.21
  urine — *see* Examination, laboratory
  vision Z01.00
    with abnormal findings Z01.01
Exanthem, exanthema (*see also* Rash)
  with enteroviral vesicular stomatitis B08.4
  Boston A88.0
  epidemic with meningitis A88.0 [G02]
  subitum B08.20
    due to human herpesvirus 6 B08.21
    due to human herpesvirus 7 B08.22
  viral, virus B09
    specified type NEC B08.8
Excess, excessive, excessively
  alcohol level in blood R78.0
  androgen (ovarian) E28.1
  attrition, tooth, teeth K03.0
  carotene, carotin (dietary) E67.1
  cold, effects of T69.9 ☑
    specified effect NEC T69.8 ☑
  convergence H51.12
  crying
    in child, adolescent, or adult R45.83
    in infant R68.11
  development, breast N62
  divergence H51.8
  drinking (alcohol) NEC (without dependence) F10.10
    habitual (continual) (without remission) F10.20
  eating R63.2
  estrogen E28.0
  fat (*see also* Obesity)
    in heart — *see* Degeneration, myocardial
    localized E65
  foreskin N47.8
  gas R14.0
  glucagon E16.3
  heat — *see* Heat
  intermaxillary vertical dimension of fully erupted teeth
      M26.37
  interocclusal distance of fully erupted teeth M26.37
  kalium E87.5
  large
    colon K59.3
      congenital Q43.8

Excess, excessive, excessively — *continued*
  large — *continued*
    infant P08.0
    organ or site, congenital NEC — *see* Anomaly, by
        site
  long
    organ or site, congenital NEC — *see* Anomaly, by
        site
  menstruation (with regular cycle) N92.0
    with irregular cycle N92.1
  napping Z72.821
  natrium E87.0
  number of teeth K00.1
  nutrient (dietary) NEC R63.2
  potassium (K) E87.5
  salivation K11.7
  secretion (*see also* Hypersecretion)
    milk O92.6
    sputum R09.3
    sweat R61
  sexual drive F52.8
  short
    organ or site, congenital NEC — *see* Anomaly, by
        site
    umbilical cord in labor or delivery O69.3 ☑
  skin, eyelid (acquired) — *see* Blepharochalasis
    congenital Q10.3
  sodium (Na) E87.0
  spacing of fully erupted teeth M26.32
  sputum R09.3
  sweating R61
  thirst R63.1
    due to deprivation of water T73.1 ☑
  tuberosity of jaw M26.07
  vitamin
    A (dietary) E67.0
      administered as drug (prolonged intake) — *see*
          Table of Drugs and Chemicals, vitamins,
          adverse effect
      overdose or wrong substance given or taken
          — *see* Table of Drugs and Chemicals, vi-
          tamins, poisoning
    D (dietary) E67.3
      administered as drug (prolonged intake) — *see*
          Table of Drugs and Chemicals, vitamins,
          adverse effect
      overdose or wrong substance given or taken
          — *see* Table of Drugs and Chemicals, vi-
          tamins, poisoning
  weight
    gain R63.5
    loss R63.4
Excitability, abnormal, under minor stress (personal-
    ity disorder) F60.3
Excitation
  anomalous atrioventricular I45.6
  psychogenic F30.8
  reactive (from emotional stress, psychological trauma)
      F30.8
Excitement
  hypomanic F30.8
  manic F30.9
  mental, reactive (from emotional stress, psychological
      trauma) F30.8
  state, reactive (from emotional stress, psychological
      trauma) F30.8
Excoriation (traumatic) (*see also* Abrasion)
  neurotic L98.1
Exfoliation
  due to erythematous conditions according to extent
      of body surface involved L49.0
    less than 10 percent of body surface L49.0
    10-19 percent of body surface L49.1
    20-29 percent of body surface L49.2
    30-39 percent of body surface L49.3
    40-49 percent of body surface L49.4
    50-59 percent of body surface L49.5
    60-69 percent of body surface L49.6
    70-79 percent of body surface L49.7
    80-89 percent of body surface L49.8
    90-99 percent of body surface L49.9
  teeth, due to systemic causes K08.0
Exfoliative — *see* condition
Exhaustion, exhaustive (physical NEC) R53.83
  battle F43.0
  cardiac — *see* Failure, heart
  delirium F43.0

Exhaustion, exhaustive — *continued*
due to
cold T69.8 ☑
excessive exertion T73.3 ☑
exposure T73.2 ☑
neurasthenia F48.8
heart — *see* Failure, heart
heat (*see also* Heat, exhaustion) T67.5 ☑
due to
salt depletion T67.4 ☑
water depletion T67.3 ☑
maternal, complicating delivery O75.81
mental F48.8
myocardium, myocardial — *see* Failure, heart
nervous F48.8
old age R54
psychogenic F48.8
psychosis F43.0
senile R54
vital NEC Z73.0
Exhibitionism F65.2
Exocervicitis — *see* Cervicitis
Exomphalos Q79.2
meaning hernia — *see* Hernia, umbilicus
Exophoria H50.52
convergence, insufficiency H51.11
divergence, excess H51.8
Exophthalmos H05.2- ☑
congenital Q15.8
constant NEC H05.24- ☑
displacement, globe — *see* Displacement, globe
due to thyrotoxicosis (hyperthyroidism) — *see* Hyperthyroidism, with, goiter (diffuse)
dysthyroid — *see* Hyperthyroidism, with, goiter (diffuse)
goiter — *see* Hyperthyroidism, with, goiter (diffuse)
intermittent NEC H05.25- ☑
malignant — *see* Hyperthyroidism, with, goiter (diffuse)
orbital
edema — *see* Edema, orbit
hemorrhage — *see* Hemorrhage, orbit
pulsating NEC H05.26- ☑
thyrotoxic, thyrotropic — *see* Hyperthyroidism, with, goiter (diffuse)
Exostosis (*see also* Disorder, bone)
cartilaginous — *see* Neoplasm, bone, benign
congenital (multiple) Q78.6
external ear canal H61.81- ☑
gonococcal A54.49
jaw (bone) M27.8
multiple, congenital Q78.6
orbit H05.35- ☑
osteocartilaginous — *see* Neoplasm, bone, benign
syphilitic A52.77
Exotropia — *see* Strabismus, divergent concomitant
Explanation of
investigation finding Z71.2
medication Z71.89
Exposure (to) (*see also* Contact, with) T75.89 ☑
acariasis Z20.7
AIDS virus Z20.6
air pollution Z77.110
algae and algae toxins Z77.121
algae bloom Z77.121
anthrax Z20.810
aromatic amines Z77.020
aromatic (hazardous) compounds NEC Z77.028
aromatic dyes NOS Z77.028
arsenic Z77.010
asbestos Z77.090
bacterial disease NEC Z20.818
benzene Z77.021
blue-green algae bloom Z77.121
body fluids (potentially hazardous) Z77.21
brown tide Z77.121
chemicals (chiefly nonmedicinal) (hazardous) NEC Z77.098
cholera Z20.09
chromium compounds Z77.018
cold, effects of T69.9 ☑
specified effect NEC T69.8 ☑
communicable disease Z20.9
bacterial NEC Z20.818
specified NEC Z20.89
viral NEC Z20.828
cyanobacteria bloom Z77.121

Exposure — *continued*
disaster Z65.5
discrimination Z60.5
dyes Z77.098
effects of T73.9 ☑
environmental tobacco smoke (acute) (chronic) Z77.22
Escherichia coli (E. coli) Z20.01
exhaustion due to T73.2 ☑
fiberglass — *see* Table of Drugs and Chemicals, fiberglass
German measles Z20.4
gonorrhea Z20.2
hazardous metals NEC Z77.018
hazardous substances NEC Z77.29
hazards in the physical environment NEC Z77.128
hazards to health NEC Z77.9
human immunodeficiency virus (HIV) Z20.6
human T-lymphotropic virus type-1 (HTLV-1) Z20.89
implanted
mesh — *see* Complications, mesh
prosthetic materials NEC — *see* Complications, prosthetic materials NEC
infestation (parasitic) NEC Z20.7
intestinal infectious disease NEC Z20.09
Escherichia coli (E. coli) Z20.01
lead Z77.011
meningococcus Z20.811
mold (toxic) Z77.120
nickel dust Z77.018
noise Z77.122
occupational
air contaminants NEC Z57.39
dust Z57.2
environmental tobacco smoke Z57.31
extreme temperature Z57.6
noise Z57.0
radiation Z57.1
risk factors Z57.9
specified NEC Z57.8
toxic agents (gases) (liquids) (solids) (vapors) in agriculture Z57.4
toxic agents (gases) (liquids) (solids) (vapors) in industry NEC Z57.5
vibration Z57.7
parasitic disease NEC Z20.7
pediculosis Z20.7
persecution Z60.5
pfiesteria piscicida Z77.121
poliomyelitis Z20.89
pollution
air Z77.110
environmental NEC Z77.118
soil Z77.112
water Z77.111
polycyclic aromatic hydrocarbons Z77.028
prenatal (drugs) (toxic chemicals) — *see* Newborn, affected by (suspected to be), noxious substances transmitted via placenta or breast milk
rabies Z20.3
radiation, naturally occurring NEC Z77.123
radon Z77.123
red tide (Florida) Z77.121
rubella Z20.4
second hand tobacco smoke (acute) (chronic) Z77.22
in the perinatal period P96.81
sexually-transmitted disease Z20.2
smallpox (laboratory) Z20.89
syphilis Z20.2
terrorism Z65.4
torture Z65.4
tuberculosis Z20.1
uranium Z77.012
varicella Z20.820
venereal disease Z20.2
viral disease NEC Z20.828
war Z65.5
water pollution Z77.111
Exsanguination — *see* Hemorrhage
Exstrophy
abdominal contents Q45.8
bladder Q64.10
cloacal Q64.12
specified type NEC Q64.19
supravesical fissure Q64.11
Extensive — *see* condition
Extra (*see also* Accessory)
marker chromosomes (normal individual) Q92.61
in abnormal individual Q92.62

Extra — *continued*
rib Q76.6
cervical Q76.5
Extrasystoles (supraventricular) I49.49
atrial I49.1
auricular I49.1
junctional I49.2
ventricular I49.3
Extrauterine gestation or pregnancy — *see* Pregnancy, by site
Extravasation
blood R58
chyle into mesentery I89.8
pelvicalyceal N13.8
pyelosinus N13.8
urine (from ureter) R39.0
vesicant agent
antineoplastic chemotherapy T80.810 ☑
other agent NEC T80.818 ☑
Extremity — *see* condition, limb
Extrophy — *see* Exstrophy
Extroversion
bladder Q64.19
uterus N81.4
complicating delivery O71.2
postpartal (old) N81.4
Extruded tooth (teeth) M26.34
Extrusion
breast implant (prosthetic) T85.42 ☑
eye implant (globe) (ball) T85.328 ☑
intervertebral disc — *see* Displacement, intervertebral disc
ocular lens implant (prosthetic) — *see* Complications, intraocular lens
vitreous — *see* Prolapse, vitreous
Exudate
pleural — *see* Effusion, pleura
retina H35.89
Exudative — *see* condition
Eye, eyeball, eyelid — *see* condition
Eyestrain — *see* Disturbance, vision, subjective
Eyeworm disease of Africa B74.3

F

Faber's syndrome (achlorhydric anemia) D50.9
Fabry (-Anderson) **disease** E75.21
Faciocephalalgia, autonomic (*see also* Neuropathy, peripheral, autonomic) G90.09
Factor(s)
psychic, associated with diseases classified elsewhere F54
psychological
affecting physical conditions F54
or behavioral
affecting general medical condition F54
associated with disorders or diseases classified elsewhere F54
Fahr disease (of brain) G23.8
Fahr Volhard disease (of kidney) I12.- ☑
Failure, failed
abortion — *see* Abortion, attempted
aortic (valve) I35.8
rheumatic I06.8
attempted abortion — *see* Abortion, attempted
biventricular I50.9
bone marrow — *see* Anemia, aplastic
cardiac — *see* Failure, heart
cardiorenal (chronic) I50.9
hypertensive I13.2
cardiorespiratory (*see also* Failure, heart) R09.2
cardiovascular (chronic) — *see* Failure, heart
cerebrovascular I67.9
cervical dilatation in labor O62.0
circulation, circulatory (peripheral) R57.9
newborn P29.89
compensation — *see* Disease, heart
compliance with medical treatment or regimen — *see* Noncompliance
congestive — *see* Failure, heart, congestive
dental implant (endosseous) M27.69
due to
failure of dental prosthesis M27.63
lack of attached gingiva M27.62
occlusal trauma (poor prosthetic design) M27.62
parafunctional habits M27.62

Failure, failed — *continued*
  dental implant — *continued*
    due to — *continued*
      periodontal infection (peri-implantitis) M27.62
      poor oral hygiene M27.62
    osseointegration M27.61
      due to
        complications of systemic disease M27.61
        poor bone quality M27.61
      iatrogenic M27.61
    post-osseointegration
      biological M27.62
      due to complications of systemic disease
        M27.62
      iatrogenic M27.62
      mechanical M27.63
    pre-integration M27.61
    pre-osseointegration M27.61
    specified NEC M27.69
  descent of head (at term) of pregnancy (mother)
    O32.4 ☑
  endosseous dental implant — *see* Failure, dental implant
  engagement of head (term of pregnancy) (mother)
    O32.4 ☑
  erection (penile) (*see also* Dysfunction, sexual, male,
    erectile) N52.9
    nonorgqanic F52.21
  examination(s), anxiety concerning Z55.2
  expansion terminal respiratory units (newborn) (primary) P28.0
  forceps NOS (with subsequent cesarean delivery) O66.5
  gain weight (child over 28 days old) R62.51
    adult R62.7
    newborn P92.6
  genital response (male) F52.21
    female F52.22
  heart (acute) (senile) (sudden) I50.9
    with
      acute pulmonary edema — *see* Failure, ventricular, left
      decompensation — *see* Failure, heart, congestive
      dilatation — *see* Disease, heart
    arteriosclerotic I70.90
    biventricular I50.9
    combined left-right sided I50.9
    compensated I50.9
    complicating
      anesthesia (general) (local) or other sedation
        in labor and delivery O74.2
        in pregnancy O29.12- ☑
        postpartum, puerperal O89.1
      delivery (cesarean) (instrumental) O75.4
    congestive (compensated) (decompensated) I50.9
      with rheumatic fever (conditions in I00)
        active I01.8
        inactive or quiescent (with chorea) I09.81
      newborn P29.0
      rheumatic (chronic) (inactive) (with chorea)
        I09.81
        active or acute I01.8
        with chorea I02.0
    decompensated I50.9
    degenerative — *see* Degeneration, myocardial
    diastolic (congestive) I50.30
      acute (congestive) I50.31
        and (on) chronic (congestive) I50.33
      chronic (congestive) I50.32
        and (on) acute (congestive) I50.33
      combined with systolic (congestive) I50.40
        acute (congestive) I50.41
          and (on) chronic (congestive) I50.43
        chronic (congestive) I50.42
          and (on) acute (congestive) I50.43
    due to presence of cardiac prosthesis I97.13- ☑
    following cardiac surgery I97.13- ☑
    high output NOS I50.9
    hypertensive — *see* Hypertension, heart
    left (ventricular) — *see* Failure, ventricular, left
    low output (syndrome) NOS I50.9
    newborn P29.0
    organic — *see* Disease, heart
    peripartum O90.3
    postprocedural I97.13- ☑
    rheumatic (chronic) (inactive) I09.9
    right (ventricular) (secondary to left heart failure)
      — *see* Failure, heart, congestive

Failure, failed — *continued*
  heart — *continued*
    systolic (congestive) I50.20
      acute (congestive) I50.21
        and (on) chronic (congestive) I50.23
      chronic (congestive) I50.22
        and (on) acute (congestive) I50.23
      combined with diastolic (congestive) I50.40
        acute (congestive) I50.41
          and (on) chronic (congestive) I50.43
        chronic (congestive) I50.42
          and (on) acute (congestive) I50.43
    thyrotoxic (*see also* Thyrotoxicosis) E05.90 [I43]
      with thyroid storm E05.91 [I43]
    valvular — *see* Endocarditis
  hepatic K72.90
    with coma K72.91
    acute or subacute K72.00
      with coma K72.01
      due to drugs K71.10
        with coma K71.11
      alcoholic (acute) (chronic) (subacute) K70.40
        with coma K70.41
    chronic K72.10
      with coma K72.11
      due to drugs (acute) (subacute) (chronic) K71.10
        with coma K71.11
    due to drugs (acute) (subacute) (chronic) K71.10
      with coma K71.11
    postprocedural K91.82
  hepatorenal K76.7
  induction (of labor) O61.9
    abortion — *see* Abortion, attempted
    by
      oxytocic drugs O61.0
      prostaglandins O61.0
    instrumental O61.1
    mechanical O61.1
    medical O61.0
    specified NEC O61.8
    surgical O61.1
  intubation during anesthesia T88.4 ☑
    in pregnancy O29.6- ☑
    labor and delivery O74.7
    postpartum, puerperal O89.6
  involution, thymus (gland) E32.0
  kidney (*see also* Disease, kidney, chronic) N19
    acute (*see also* Failure, renal, acute) N17.9
  lactation (complete) O92.3
    partial O92.4
  Leydig's cell, adult E29.1
  liver — *see* Failure, hepatic
  menstruation at puberty N91.0
  mitral I05.8
  myocardial, myocardium (*see also* Failure, heart) I50.9
    chronic (*see also* Failure, heart, congestive) I50.9
    congestive (*see also* Failure, heart, congestive) I50.9
  orgasm (female) (psychogenic) F52.31
    male F52.32
  ovarian (primary) E28.39
    iatrogenic E89.40
      asymptomatic E89.40
      symptomatic E89.41
    postprocedural (postablative) (postirradiation)
      (postsurgical) E89.40
      asymptomatic E89.40
      symptomatic E89.41
  ovulation causing infertility N97.0
  polyglandular, autoimmune E31.0
  prosthetic joint implant — *see* Complications, joint
    prosthesis, mechanical, breakdown, by site
  renal N19
    with
      tubular necrosis (acute) N17.0
    acute N17.9
      with
        cortical necrosis N17.1
        medullary necrosis N17.2
        tubular necrosis N17.0
      specified NEC N17.8
    chronic N18.9
      hypertensive — *see* Hypertension, kidney
    congenital P96.0
    end stage (chronic) N18.6
      due to hypertension I12.0
    following
      abortion — *see* Abortion by type complicated
        by specified condition NEC

Failure, failed — *continued*
  renal — *continued*
    following — *continued*
      crushing T79.5 ☑
      ectopic or molar pregnancy O08.4
      labor and delivery (acute) O90.4
    hypertensive — *see* Hypertension, kidney
    postprocedural N99.0
  respiration, respiratory J96.90
    with
      hypercapnia J96.92
      hypoxia J96.91
    acute J96.00
      with
        hypercapnia J96.02
        hypoxia J96.01
    acute and (on) chronic J96.20
      with
        hypercapnia J96.22
        hypoxia J96.21
    center G93.89
    chronic J96.10
      with
        hypercapnia J96.12
        hypoxia J96.11
    newborn P28.5
    postprocedural (acute) J95.821
      acute and chronic J95.822
  rotation
    cecum Q43.3
    colon Q43.3
    intestine Q43.3
    kidney Q63.2
  sedation (conscious) (moderate) during procedure
    T88.52 ☑
    history of Z92.83
  segmentation (*see also* Fusion)
    fingers — *see* Syndactylism, complex, fingers
    vertebra Q76.49
      with scoliosis Q76.3
  seminiferous tubule, adult E29.1
  senile (general) R54
  sexual arousal (male) F52.21
    female F52.22
  testicular endocrine function E29.1
  to thrive (child over 28 days old) R62.51
    adult R62.7
    newborn P92.6
  transplant T86.92
    bone T86.831
      marrow T86.02
    cornea T86.841
    heart T86.22
      with lung(s) T86.32
    intestine T86.851
    kidney T86.12
    liver T86.42
    lung(s) T86.811
      with heart T86.32
    pancreas T86.891
    skin (allograft) (autograft) T86.821
    specified organ or tissue NEC T86.891
    stem cell (peripheral blood) (umbilical cord) T86.5
  trial of labor (with subsequent cesarean delivery)
    O66.40
    following previous cesarean delivery O66.41
  tubal ligation N99.89
  urinary — *see* Disease, kidney, chronic
  vacuum extraction NOS (with subsequent cesarean
    delivery) O66.5
  vasectomy N99.89
  ventouse NOS (with subsequent cesarean delivery)
    O66.5
  ventricular (*see also* Failure, heart) I50.9
    left I50.1
      with rheumatic fever (conditions in I00)
        active I01.8
          with chorea I02.0
        inactive or quiescent (with chorea) I09.81
      rheumatic (chronic) (inactive) (with chorea)
        I09.81
        active or acute I01.8
          with chorea I02.0
    right (*see also* Failure, heart, congestive) I50.9
  vital centers, newborn P91.8
Fainting (fit) R55
Fallen arches — *see* Deformity, limb, flat foot

☑ **Additional Character Required — Refer to the Tabular List for Character Selection**   ⬦ **Subterms under main terms may continue to next column or page**

Falling, falls (repeated) R29.6
　any organ or part — see Prolapse
Fallopian
　insufflation Z31.41
　tube — see condition
Fallot's
　pentalogy Q21.8
　tetrad or tetralogy Q21.3
　triad or trilogy Q22.3
False (see also condition)
　croup J38.5
　joint — see Nonunion, fracture
　labor (pains) O47.9
　　at or after 37 completed weeks of gestation O47.1
　　before 37 completed weeks of gestation O47.0- ☑
　passage, urethra (prostatic) N36.5
　pregnancy F45.8
Family, familial (see also condition)
　disruption Z63.8
　　involving divorce or separation Z63.5
　Li-Fraumeni (syndrome) Z15.01
　planning advice Z30.09
　problem Z63.9
　　specified NEC Z63.8
　retinoblastoma C69.2- ☑
Famine (effects of) T73.0 ☑
　edema — see Malnutrition, severe
Fanconi (-de Toni)(-Debré) **syndrome** E72.09
　with cystinosis E72.04
Fanconi's anemia (congenital pancytopenia) D61.09
Farber's disease or syndrome E75.29
Farcy A24.0
Farmer's
　lung J67.0
　skin L57.8
Farsightedness — see Hypermetropia
Fascia — see condition
Fasciculation R25.3
Fasciitis M72.9
　diffuse (eosinophilic) M35.4
　infective M72.6
　　necrotizing M72.6
　necrotizing M72.6
　nodular M72.4
　perirenal (with ureteral obstruction) N13.5
　　with infection N13.6
　plantar M72.2
　specified NEC M72.8
　traumatic (old) M72.8
　　current — code by site under Sprain
Fascioliasis B66.3
Fasciolopsis, fasciolopsiasis (intestinal) B66.5
Fascioscapulohumeral myopathy G71.0
Fast pulse R00.0
Fat
　embolism — see Embolism, fat
　excessive (see also Obesity)
　　in heart — see Degeneration, myocardial
　in stool R19.5
　localized (pad) E65
　　heart — see Degeneration, myocardial
　　knee M79.4
　　retropatellar M79.4
　necrosis
　　breast N64.1
　　mesentery K65.4
　　omentum K65.4
　pad E65
　　knee M79.4
Fatigue R53.83
　auditory deafness — see Deafness
　chronic R53.82
　combat F43.0
　general R53.83
　　psychogenic F48.8
　heat (transient) T67.6 ☑
　muscle M62.89
　myocardium — see Failure, heart
　neoplasm-related R53.0
　nervous, neurosis F48.8
　operational F48.8
　psychogenic (general) F48.8
　senile R54
　voice R49.8
Fatness — see Obesity
Fatty (see also condition)
　apron E65

Fatty — continued
　degeneration — see Degeneration, fatty
　heart (enlarged) — see Degeneration, myocardial
　liver NEC K76.0
　　alcoholic K70.0
　　nonalcoholic K76.0
　necrosis — see Degeneration, fatty
Fauces — see condition
Fauchard's disease (periodontitis) — see Periodontitis
Faucitis J02.9
Favism (anemia) D55.0
Favus — see Dermatophytosis
Fazio-Londe disease or syndrome G12.1
Fear complex or reaction F40.9
Fear of — see Phobia
Feared complaint unfounded Z71.1
Febris, febrile (see also Fever)
　flava (see also Fever, yellow) A95.9
　melitensis A23.0
　pestis — see Plague
　recurrens — see Fever, relapsing
　rubra A38.9
Fecal
　incontinence R15.9
　smearing R15.1
　soiling R15.1
　urgency R15.2
Fecalith (impaction) K56.41
　appendix K38.1
　congenital P76.8
Fede's disease K14.0
Feeble rapid pulse due to shock following injury
　T79.4 ☑
Feeble-minded F70
Feeding
　difficulties R63.3
　problem R63.3
　　newborn P92.9
　　　specified NEC P92.8
　nonorganic (adult) — see Disorder, eating
Feeling (of)
　foreign body in throat R09.89
Feer's disease — see Poisoning, mercury
Feet — see condition
Feigned illness Z76.5
Feil-Klippel syndrome (brevicollis) Q76.1
Feinmesser's (hidrotic) **ectodermal dysplasia** Q82.4
Felinophobia F40.218
Felon (see also Cellulitis, digit)
　with lymphangitis — see Lymphangitis, acute, digit
Felty's syndrome M05.00
　ankle M05.07- ☑
　elbow M05.02- ☑
　foot joint M05.07- ☑
　hand joint M05.04- ☑
　hip M05.05- ☑
　knee M05.06- ☑
　multiple site M05.09
　shoulder M05.01- ☑
　vertebra — see Spondylitis, ankylosing
　wrist M05.03- ☑
Female genital cutting status — see Female genital
　mutilation status (FGM)
Female genital mutilation status (FGM) N90.810
　specified NEC N90.818
　type I (clitorectomy status) N90.811
　type II (clitorectomy with excision of labia minora status) N90.812
　type III (infibulation status) N90.813
　type IV N90.818
Femur, femoral — see condition
Fenestration, fenestrated (see also Imperfect, closure)
　aortico-pulmonary Q21.4
　cusps, heart valve NEC Q24.8
　　pulmonary Q22.3
　pulmonic cusps Q22.3
Fernell's disease (aortic aneurysm) I71.9
Fertile eunuch syndrome E23.0
Fetid
　breath R19.6
　sweat L75.0
Fetishism F65.0
　transvestic F65.1
Fetus, fetal (see also condition)
　alcohol syndrome (dysmorphic) Q86.0
　compressus O31.0- ☑
　hydantoin syndrome Q86.1

Fetus, fetal — continued
　lung tissue P28.0
　papyraceous O31.0- ☑
Fever (inanition) (of unknown origin) (persistent) (with chills) (with rigor) R50.9
　abortus A23.1
　Aden (dengue) A90
　African tick-borne A68.1
　American
　　mountain (tick) A93.2
　　spotted A77.0
　aphthous B08.8
　arbovirus, arboviral A94
　　hemorrhagic A94
　　specified NEC A93.8
　Argentinian hemorrhagic A96.0
　Assam B55.0
　Australian Q A78
　Bangkok hemorrhagic A91
　Barmah forest A92.8
　Bartonella A44.0
　bilious, hemoglobinuric B50.8
　blackwater B50.8
　blister B00.1
　Bolivian hemorrhagic A96.1
　Bonvale dam T73.3 ☑
　boutonneuse A77.1
　brain — see Encephalitis
　Brazilian purpuric A48.4
　breakbone A90
　Bullis A77.0
　Bunyamwera A92.8
　Burdwan B55.0
　Bwamba A92.8
　Cameroon — see Malaria
　Canton A75.9
　catarrhal (acute) J00
　　chronic J31.0
　cat-scratch A28.1
　Central Asian hemorrhagic A98.0
　cerebral — see Encephalitis
　cerebrospinal meningococcal A39.0
　Chagres B50.9
　Chandipura A92.8
　Changuinola A93.1
　Charcot's (biliary) (hepatic) (intermittent) — see Calculus, bile duct
　Chikungunya (viral) (hemorrhagic) A92.0
　Chitral A93.1
　Colombo — see Fever, paratyphoid
　Colorado tick (virus) A93.2
　congestive (remittent) — see Malaria
　Congo virus A98.0
　continued malarial B50.9
　Corsican — see Malaria
　Crimean-Congo hemorrhagic A98.0
　Cyprus — see Brucellosis
　dandy A90
　deer fly — see Tularemia
　dengue (virus) A90
　　hemorrhagic A91
　　sandfly A93.1
　desert B38.0
　drug induced R50.2
　due to
　　conditions classified elsewhere R50.81
　　heat T67.0 ☑
　enteric A01.00
　enteroviral exanthematous (Boston exanthem) A88.0
　ephemeral (of unknown origin) R50.9
　epidemic hemorrhagic A98.5
　erysipelatous — see Erysipelas
　estivo-autumnal (malarial) B50.9
　famine A75.0
　five day A79.0
　following delivery O86.4
　Fort Bragg A27.89
　gastroenteric A01.00
　gastromalarial — see Malaria
　Gibraltar — see Brucellosis
　glandular — see Mononucleosis, infectious
　Guama (viral) A92.8
　Haverhill A25.1
　hay (allergic) J30.1
　　with asthma (bronchial) J45.909
　　　with
　　　　exacerbation (acute) J45.901
　　　　status asthmaticus J45.902

Fever — *continued*

hay — *continued*
- due to
  - allergen other than pollen J30.89
  - pollen, any plant or tree J30.1
- heat (effects) T67.0 ☑
- hematuric, bilious B50.8
- hemoglobinuric (malarial) (bilious) B50.8
- hemorrhagic (arthropod-borne) NOS A94
  - with renal syndrome A98.5
  - arenaviral A96.9
    - specified NEC A96.8
  - Argentinian A96.0
  - Bangkok A91
  - Bolivian A96.1
  - Central Asian A98.0
  - Chikungunya A92.0
  - Crimean-Congo A98.0
  - dengue (virus) A91
  - epidemic A98.5
  - Junin (virus) A96.0
  - Korean A98.5
  - Kyasanur forest A98.2
  - Machupo (virus) A96.1
  - mite-borne A93.8
  - mosquito-borne A92.8
  - Omsk A98.1
  - Philippine A91
  - Russian A98.5
  - Singapore A91
  - Southeast Asia A91
  - Thailand A91
  - tick-borne NEC A93.8
  - viral A99
    - specified NEC A98.8
- hepatic — *see* Cholecystitis
- herpetic — *see* Herpes
- icterohemorrhagic A27.0
- Indiana A93.8
- infective B99.9
  - specified NEC B99.8
- intermittent (bilious) (*see also* Malaria)
  - of unknown origin R50.9
  - pernicious B50.9
- iodide R50.2
- Japanese river A75.3
- jungle (*see also* Malaria)
  - yellow A95.0
- Junin (virus) hemorrhagic A96.0
- Katayama B65.2
- kedani A75.3
- Kenya (tick) A77.1
- Kew Garden A79.1
- Korean hemorrhagic A98.5
- Lassa A96.2
- Lone Star A77.0
- Machupo (virus) hemorrhagic A96.1
- malaria, malarial — *see* Malaria
- Malta A23.9
- Marseilles A77.1
- marsh — *see* Malaria
- Mayaro (viral) A92.8
- Mediterranean (*see also* Brucellosis) A23.9
  - familial E85.0
  - tick A77.1
- meningeal — *see* Meningitis
- Meuse A79.0
- Mexican A75.2
- mianeh A68.1
- miasmatic — *see* Malaria
- mosquito-borne (viral) A92.9
  - hemorrhagic A92.8
- mountain (*see also* Brucellosis)
  - meaning Rocky Mountain spotted fever A77.0
  - tick (American) (Colorado) (viral) A93.2
- Mucambo (viral) A92.8
- mud A27.9
- Neapolitan — *see* Brucellosis
- neutropenic D70.9
- newborn P81.9
  - environmental P81.0
- Nine-Mile A78
- non-exanthematous tick A93.2
- North Asian tick-borne A77.2
- Omsk hemorrhagic A98.1
- O'nyong-nyong (viral) A92.1
- Oropouche (viral) A93.0
- Oroya A44.0

Fever — *continued*

- paludal — *see* Malaria
- Panama (malarial) B50.9
- Pappataci A93.1
- paratyphoid A01.4
  - A A01.1
  - B A01.2
  - C A01.3
- parrot A70
- periodic (Mediterranean) E85.0
- persistent (of unknown origin) R50.9
- petechial A39.0
- pharyngoconjunctival B30.2
- Philippine hemorrhagic A91
- phlebotomus A93.1
- Piry (virus) A93.8
- Pixuna (viral) A92.8
- Plasmodium ovale B53.0
- polioviral (nonparalytic) A80.4
- Pontiac A48.2
- postimmunization R50.83
- postoperative R50.82
  - due to infection T81.4 ☑
- posttransfusion R50.84
- postvaccination R50.83
- presenting with conditions classified elsewhere R50.81
- pretibial A27.89
- puerperal O86.4
- Q A78
- quadrilateral A78
- quartan (malaria) B52.9
- Queensland (coastal) (tick) A77.3
- quintan A79.0
- rabbit — *see* Tularemia
- rat-bite A25.9
  - due to
    - Spirillum A25.0
    - Streptobacillus moniliformis A25.1
- recurrent — *see* Fever, relapsing
- relapsing (Borrelia) A68.9
  - Carter's (Asiatic) A68.1
  - Dutton's (West African) A68.1
  - Koch's A68.9
  - louse-borne A68.0
  - Novy's
    - louse-borne A68.0
    - tick-borne A68.1
  - Obermeyer's (European) A68.0
  - tick-borne A68.1
- remittent (bilious) (congestive) (gastric) — *see* Malaria
- rheumatic (active) (acute) (chronic) (subacute) I00
  - with central nervous system involvement I02.9
  - active with heart involvement — *see* category I01 ☑
  - inactive or quiescent with
    - cardiac hypertrophy I09.89
    - carditis I09.9
    - endocarditis I09.1
      - aortic (valve) I06.9
        - with mitral (valve) disease I08.0
      - mitral (valve) I05.9
        - with aortic (valve) disease I08.0
      - pulmonary (valve) I09.89
      - tricuspid (valve) I07.8
    - heart disease NEC I09.89
    - heart failure (congestive) (conditions in I50.9) I09.81
    - left ventricular failure (conditions in I50.1) I09.81
    - myocarditis, myocardial degeneration (conditions in I51.4) I09.0
    - pancarditis I09.9
    - pericarditis I09.2
- Rift Valley (viral) A92.4
- Rocky Mountain spotted A77.0
- rose J30.1
- Ross River B33.1
- Russian hemorrhagic A98.5
- San Joaquin (Valley) B38.0
- sandfly A93.1
- Sao Paulo A77.0
- scarlet A38.9
- seven day (leptospirosis) (autumnal) (Japanese) A27.89
  - dengue A90
- shin-bone A79.0
- Singapore hemorrhagic A91
- solar A90
- Songo A98.5

Fever — *continued*

- sore B00.1
- South African tick-bite A68.1
- Southeast Asia hemorrhagic A91
- spinal — *see* Meningitis
- spirillary A25.0
- splenic — *see* Anthrax
- spotted A77.9
  - American A77.0
  - Brazilian A77.0
  - cerebrospinal meningitis A39.0
  - Colombian A77.0
  - due to Rickettsia
    - australis A77.3
    - conorii A77.1
    - rickettsii A77.0
    - sibirica A77.2
    - specified type NEC A77.8
  - Ehrlichiosis A77.40
    - due to
      - E. chafeensis A77.41
      - specified organism NEC A77.49
  - Rocky Mountain A77.0
- steroid R50.2
- streptobacillary A25.1
- subtertian B50.9
- Sumatran mite A75.3
- sun A90
- swamp A27.9
- swine A02.8
- sylvatic, yellow A95.0
- Tahyna B33.8
- tertian — *see* Malaria, tertian
- Thailand hemorrhagic A91
- thermic T67.0 ☑
- three-day A93.1
- tick
  - American mountain A93.2
  - Colorado A93.2
  - Kemerovo A93.8
  - Mediterranean A77.1
  - mountain A93.2
  - nonexanthematous A93.2
  - Quaranfil A93.8
- tick-bite NEC A93.8
- tick-borne (hemorrhagic) NEC A93.8
- trench A79.0
- tsutsugamushi A75.3
- typhogastric A01.00
- typhoid (abortive) (hemorrhagic) (intermittent) (malignant) A01.00
  - complicated by
    - arthritis A01.04
    - heart involvement A01.02
    - meningitis A01.01
    - osteomyelitis A01.05
    - pneumonia A01.03
    - specified NEC A01.09
- typhomalarial — *see* Malaria
- typhus — *see* Typhus (fever)
- undulant — *see* Brucellosis
- unknown origin R50.9
- uveoparotid D86.89
- valley B38.0
- Venezuelan equine A92.2
- vesicular stomatitis A93.8
- viral hemorrhagic — *see* Fever, hemorrhagic, by type of virus
- Volhynian A79.0
- Wesselsbron (viral) A92.8
- West
  - African B50.8
  - Nile (viral) A92.30
    - with
      - complications NEC A92.39
      - cranial nerve disorders A92.32
      - encephalitis A92.31
      - encephalomyelitis A92.31
      - neurologic manifestation NEC A92.32
      - optic neuritis A92.32
      - polyradiculitis A92.32
- Whitmore's — *see* Melioidosis
- Wolhynian A79.0
- worm B83.9
- yellow A95.9
  - jungle A95.0
  - sylvatic A95.0
  - urban A95.1

Fever — *continued*
  Zika (viral) A92.8
Fibrillation
  atrial or auricular (established) I48.91
    chronic I48.2
    paroxysmal I48.0
    permanent I48.2
    persistent I48.1
  cardiac I49.8
  heart I49.8
  muscular M62.89
  ventricular I49.01
Fibrin
  ball or bodies, pleural (sac) J94.1
  chamber, anterior (eye) (gelatinous exudate) — *see* Iridocyclitis, acute
Fibrinogenolysis — *see* Fibrinolysis
Fibrinogenopenia D68.8
  acquired D65
  congenital D68.2
Fibrinolysis (hemorrhagic) (acquired) D65
  antepartum hemorrhage — *see* Hemorrhage, antepartum, with coagulation defect
  following
    abortion — *see* Abortion by type complicated by hemorrhage
    ectopic or molar pregnancy O08.1
  intrapartum O67.0
  newborn, transient P60
  postpartum O72.3
Fibrinopenia (hereditary) D68.2
  acquired D68.4
Fibrinopurulent — *see* condition
Fibrinous — *see* condition
Fibroadenoma
  cellular intracanalicular D24- ☑
  giant D24- ☑
  intracanalicular
    cellular D24- ☑
    giant D24- ☑
    specified site — *see* Neoplasm, benign, by site
    unspecified site D24- ☑
  juvenile D24- ☑
  pericanalicular
    specified site — *see* Neoplasm, benign, by site
    unspecified site D24- ☑
  phyllodes D24- ☑
  prostate D29.1
  specified site NEC — *see* Neoplasm, benign, by site
  unspecified site D24- ☑
Fibroadenosis, breast (chronic) (cystic) (diffuse) (periodic) (segmental) N60.2- ☑
Fibroangioma (*see also* Neoplasm, benign, by site)
  juvenile
    specified site — *see* Neoplasm, benign, by site
    unspecified site D10.6
Fibrochondrosarcoma — *see* Neoplasm, cartilage, malignant
Fibrocystic
  disease (*see also* Fibrosis, cystic)
    breast — *see* Mastopathy, cystic
    jaw M27.49
    kidney (congenital) Q61.8
    liver Q44.6
    pancreas E84.9
  kidney (congenital) Q61.8
Fibrodysplasia ossificans progressiva — *see* Myositis, ossificans, progressiva
Fibroelastosis (cordis) (endocardial) (endomyocardial) I42.4
Fibroid (tumor) (*see also* Neoplasm, connective tissue, benign)
  disease, lung (chronic) — *see* Fibrosis, lung
  heart (disease) — *see* Myocarditis
  in pregnancy or childbirth O34.1- ☑
    causing obstructed labor O65.5
  induration, lung (chronic) — *see* Fibrosis, lung
  lung — *see* Fibrosis, lung
  pneumonia (chronic) — *see* Fibrosis, lung
  uterus D25.9
Fibrolipoma — *see* Lipoma
Fibroliposarcoma — *see* Neoplasm, connective tissue, malignant
Fibroma (*see also* Neoplasm, connective tissue, benign)
  ameloblastic — *see* Cyst, calcifying odontogenic
  bone (nonossifying) — *see* Disorder, bone, specified type NEC

Fibroma — *continued*
  bone — *see* Disorder, bone, specified type — *continued*
    ossifying — *see* Neoplasm, bone, benign
  cementifying — *see* Neoplasm, bone, benign
  chondromyxoid — *see* Neoplasm, bone, benign
  desmoplastic — *see* Neoplasm, connective tissue, uncertain behavior
  durum — *see* Neoplasm, connective tissue, benign
  fascial — *see* Neoplasm, connective tissue, benign
  invasive — *see* Neoplasm, connective tissue, uncertain behavior
  molle — *see* Lipoma
  myxoid — *see* Neoplasm, connective tissue, benign
  nasopharynx, nasopharyngeal (juvenile) D10.6
  nonosteogenic (nonossifying) — *see* Dysplasia, fibrous
  odontogenic (central) — *see* Cyst, calcifying odontogenic
  ossifying — *see* Neoplasm, bone, benign
  periosteal — *see* Neoplasm, bone, benign
  soft — *see* Lipoma
Fibromatosis M72.9
  abdominal — *see* Neoplasm, connective tissue, uncertain behavior
  aggressive — *see* Neoplasm, connective tissue, uncertain behavior
  congenital generalized — *see* Neoplasm, connective tissue, uncertain behavior
  Dupuytren's M72.0
  gingival K06.1
  palmar (fascial) M72.0
  plantar (fascial) M72.2
  pseudosarcomatous (proliferative) (subcutaneous) M72.4
  retroperitoneal D48.3
  specified NEC M72.8
Fibromyalgia M79.7
Fibromyoma (*see also* Neoplasm, connective tissue, benign)
  uterus (corpus) (*see also* Leiomyoma, uterus)
    in pregnancy or childbirth — *see* Fibroid, in pregnancy or childbirth
    causing obstructed labor O65.5
Fibromyositis M79.7
Fibromyxolipoma D17.9
Fibromyxoma — *see* Neoplasm, connective tissue, benign
Fibromyxosarcoma — *see* Neoplasm, connective tissue, malignant
Fibro-odontoma, ameloblastic — *see* Cyst, calcifying odontogenic
Fibro-osteoma — *see* Neoplasm, bone, benign
Fibroplasia, retrolental H35.17- ☑
Fibropurulent — *see* condition
Fibrosarcoma (*see also* Neoplasm, connective tissue, malignant)
  ameloblastic C41.1
    upper jaw (bone) C41.0
  congenital — *see* Neoplasm, connective tissue, malignant
  fascial — *see* Neoplasm, connective tissue, malignant
  infantile — *see* Neoplasm, connective tissue, malignant
  odontogenic C41.1
    upper jaw (bone) C41.0
  periosteal — *see* Neoplasm, bone, malignant
Fibrosclerosis
  breast N60.3- ☑
  multifocal M35.5
  penis (corpora cavernosa) N48.6
Fibrosis, fibrotic
  adrenal (gland) E27.8
  amnion O41.8X- ☑
  anal papillae K62.89
  arteriocapillary — *see* Arteriosclerosis
  bladder N32.89
    interstitial — *see* Cystitis, chronic, interstitial
    localized submucosal — *see* Cystitis, chronic, interstitial
    panmural — *see* Cystitis, chronic, interstitial
  breast — *see* Fibrosclerosis, breast
  capillary (*see also* Arteriosclerosis) I70.90
    lung (chronic) — *see* Fibrosis, lung
  cardiac — *see* Myocarditis
  cervix N88.8
  chorion O41.8X- ☑
  corpus cavernosum (sclerosing) N48.6

Fibrosis, fibrotic — *continued*
  cystic (of pancreas) E84.9
    with
      distal intestinal obstruction syndrome E84.19
      fecal impaction E84.19
      intestinal manifestations NEC E84.19
      pulmonary manifestations E84.0
      specified manifestations NEC E84.8
  due to device, implant or graft (*see also* Complications, by site and type, specified NEC) T85.82 ☑
    arterial graft NEC T82.828 ☑
    breast (implant) T85.82 ☑
    catheter NEC T85.82 ☑
      dialysis (renal) T82.828 ☑
        intraperitoneal T85.82 ☑
      infusion NEC T82.828 ☑
        spinal (epidural) (subdural) T85.82 ☑
      urinary (indwelling) T83.82 ☑
    electronic (electrode) (pulse generator) (stimulator)
      bone T84.82 ☑
      cardiac T82.827 ☑
      nervous system (brain) (peripheral nerve) (spinal) T85.82 ☑
      urinary T83.82 ☑
    fixation, internal (orthopedic) NEC T84.82 ☑
    gastrointestinal (bile duct) (esophagus) T85.82 ☑
    genital NEC T83.82 ☑
    heart NEC T82.827 ☑
    joint prosthesis T84.82 ☑
    ocular (corneal graft) (orbital implant) NEC T85.82 ☑
    orthopedic NEC T84.82 ☑
    specified NEC T85.82 ☑
    urinary NEC T83.82 ☑
    vascular NEC T82.828 ☑
    ventricular intracranial shunt T85.82 ☑
  ejaculatory duct N50.8
  endocardium — *see* Endocarditis
  endomyocardial (tropical) I42.3
  epididymis N50.8
  eye muscle — *see* Strabismus, mechanical
  heart — *see* Myocarditis
  hepatic — *see* Fibrosis, liver
  hepatolienal (portal hypertension) K76.6
  hepatosplenic (portal hypertension) K76.6
  infrapatellar fat pad M79.4
  intrascrotal N50.8
  kidney N26.9
  liver K74.0
    with sclerosis K74.2
    alcoholic K70.2
  lung (atrophic) (chronic) (confluent) (massive) (perialveolar) (peribronchial) J84.10
    with
      anthracosilicosis J60
      anthracosis J60
      asbestosis J61
      bagassosis J67.1
      bauxite J63.1
      berylliosis J63.2
      byssinosis J66.0
      calcicosis J62.8
      chalicosis J62.8
      dust reticulation J64
      farmer's lung J67.0
      ganister disease J62.8
      graphite J63.3
      pneumoconiosis NOS J64
      siderosis J63.4
      silicosis J62.8
    capillary J84.10
    congenital P27.8
    diffuse (idiopathic) J84.10
      chemicals, gases, fumes or vapors (inhalation) J68.4
      interstitial J84.10
        acute J84.114
      talc J62.0
    following radiation J70.1
    idiopathic J84.112
    postinflammatory J84.10
    silicotic J62.8
    tuberculous — *see* Tuberculosis, pulmonary
  lymphatic gland I89.8
  median bar — *see* Hyperplasia, prostate
  mediastinum (idiopathic) J98.5
  meninges G96.19

Fibrosis, fibrotic — *continued*
  myocardium, myocardial — *see* Myocarditis
  ovary N83.8
  oviduct N83.8
  pancreas K86.8
  penis NEC N48.6
  pericardium I31.0
  perineum, in pregnancy or childbirth O34.7- ☑
    causing obstructed labor O65.5
  pleura J94.1
  popliteal fat pad M79.4
  prostate (chronic) — *see* Hyperplasia, prostate
  pulmonary (*see also* Fibrosis, lung) J84.10
    congenital P27.8
    idiopathic J84.112
  rectal sphincter K62.89
  retroperitoneal, idiopathic (with ureteral obstruction) N13.5
    with infection N13.6
  sclerosing mesenteric (idiopathic) K65.4
  scrotum N50.8
  seminal vesicle N50.8
  senile R54
  skin L90.5
  spermatic cord N50.8
  spleen D73.89
    in schistosomiasis (bilharziasis) B65.9 [D77]
  subepidermal nodular — *see* Neoplasm, skin, benign
  submucous (oral) (tongue) K13.5
  testis N44.8
    chronic, due to syphilis A52.76
  thymus (gland) E32.8
  tongue, submucous K13.5
  tunica vaginalis N50.8
  uterus (non-neoplastic) N85.8
  vagina N89.8
  valve, heart — *see* Endocarditis
  vas deferens N50.8
  vein I87.8
Fibrositis (periarticular) M79.7
  nodular, chronic (Jaccoud's) (rheumatoid) — *see* Arthropathy, postrheumatic, chronic
Fibrothorax J94.1
Fibrotic — *see* Fibrosis
Fibrous — *see* condition
Fibroxanthoma (*see also* Neoplasm, connective tissue, benign)
  atypical — *see* Neoplasm, connective tissue, uncertain behavior
  malignant — *see* Neoplasm, connective tissue, malignant
Fibroxanthosarcoma — *see* Neoplasm, connective tissue, malignant
Fiedler's
  disease (icterohemorrhagic leptospirosis) A27.0
  myocarditis (acute) I40.1
Fifth disease B08.3
  venereal A55
Filaria, filarial, filariasis — *see* Infestation, filarial
Filatov's disease — *see* Mononucleosis, infectious
File-cutter's disease — *see* Poisoning, lead
Filling defect
  biliary tract R93.2
  bladder R93.4
  duodenum R93.3
  gallbladder R93.2
  gastrointestinal tract R93.3
  intestine R93.3
  kidney R93.4
  stomach R93.3
  ureter R93.4
Fimbrial cyst Q50.4
Financial problem affecting care NOS Z59.9
  bankruptcy Z59.8
  foreclosure on loan Z59.8
Findings, abnormal, inconclusive, without diagnosis
  (*see also* Abnormal)
  17-ketosteroids, elevated R82.5
  acetonuria R82.4
  alcohol in blood R78.0
  anisocytosis R71.8
  antenatal screening of mother O28.9
    biochemical O28.1
    chromosomal O28.5
    cytological O28.2
    genetic O28.5
    hematological O28.0
    radiological O28.4

Findings, abnormal, inconclusive, without diagnosis
  — *continued*
  antenatal screening of mother — *continued*
    specified NEC O28.8
    ultrasonic O28.3
  antibody titer, elevated R76.0
  anticardiolipin antibody R76.0
  antiphosphatidylglycerol antibody R76.0
  antiphosphatidylinositol antibody R76.0
  antiphosphatidylserine antibody R76.0
  antiphospholipid antibody R76.0
  bacteriuria N39.0
  bicarbonate E87.8
  bile in urine R82.2
  blood sugar R73.09
    high R73.9
    low (transient) E16.2
  body fluid or substance, specified NEC R88.8
  casts, urine R82.99
  catecholamines R82.5
  cells, urine R82.99
  chloride E87.8
  cholesterol E78.9
    high E78.0
      with high triglycerides E78.2
  chyluria R82.0
  cloudy
    dialysis effluent R88.0
    urine R82.90
  creatinine clearance R94.4
  crystals, urine R82.99
  culture
    blood R78.81
    positive — *see* Positive, culture
  echocardiogram R93.1
  electrolyte level, urinary R82.99
  function study NEC R94.8
    bladder R94.8
    endocrine NEC R94.7
      thyroid R94.6
    kidney R94.4
    liver R94.5
    pancreas R94.8
    placenta R94.8
    pulmonary R94.2
    spleen R94.8
  gallbladder, nonvisualization R93.2
  glucose (tolerance test) (non-fasting) R73.09
  glycosuria R81
  heart
    shadow R93.1
    sounds R01.2
  hematinuria R82.3
  hematocrit drop (precipitous) R71.0
  hemoglobinuria R82.3
  human papillomavirus (HPV) DNA test positive
    cervix
      high risk R87.810
      low risk R87.820
    vagina
      high risk R87.811
      low risk R87.821
  in blood (of substance not normally found in blood) R78.9
    addictive drug NEC R78.4
    alcohol (excessive level) R78.0
    cocaine R78.2
    hallucinogen R78.3
    heavy metals (abnormal level) R78.79
    lead R78.71
    lithium (abnormal level) R78.89
    opiate drug R78.1
    psychotropic drug R78.5
    specified substance NEC R78.89
    steroid agent R78.6
  indoleacetic acid, elevated R82.5
  ketonuria R82.4
  lactic acid dehydrogenase (LDH) R74.0
  liver function test R79.89
  mammogram NEC R92.8
    calcification (calculus) R92.1
    inconclusive result (due to dense breasts) R92.2
    microcalcification R92.0
  mediastinal shift R93.8
  melanin, urine R82.99
  myoglobinuria R82.1
  neonatal screening P09
  nonvisualization of gallbladder R93.2

Findings, abnormal, inconclusive, without diagnosis
  — *continued*
  odor of urine NOS R82.90
  Papanicolaou cervix R87.619
    non-atypical endometrial cells R87.618
  pneumoencephalogram R93.0
  poikilocytosis R71.8
  potassium (deficiency) E87.6
    excess E87.5
  PPD R76.11
  radiologic (X-ray) R93.8
    abdomen R93.5
    biliary tract R93.2
    breast R92.8
    gastrointestinal tract R93.3
    genitourinary organs R93.8
    head R93.0
    inconclusive due to excess body fat of patient R93.9
    intrathoracic organs NEC R93.1
    placenta R93.8
    retroperitoneum R93.5
    skin R93.8
    skull R93.0
    subcutaneous tissue R93.8
  red blood cell (count) (morphology) (sickling) (volume) R71.8
  scan NEC R94.8
    bladder R94.8
    bone R94.8
    kidney R94.4
    liver R93.2
    lung R94.2
    pancreas R94.8
    placental R94.8
    spleen R94.8
    thyroid R94.6
  sedimentation rate, elevated R70.0
  SGOT R74.0
  SGPT R74.0
  sodium (deficiency) E87.1
    excess E87.0
  specified body fluid NEC R88.8
  stress test R94.39
  thyroid (function) (metabolic rate) (scan) (uptake) R94.6
  transaminase (level) R74.0
  triglycerides E78.9
    high E78.1
      with high cholesterol E78.2
  tuberculin skin test (without active tuberculosis) R76.11
  urine R82.90
    acetone R82.4
    bacteria N39.0
    bile R82.2
    casts or cells R82.99
    chyle R82.0
    culture positive R82.7
    glucose R81
    hemoglobin R82.3
    ketone R82.4
    sugar R81
  vanillylmandelic acid (VMA), elevated R82.5
  vectorcardiogram (VCG) R94.39
  ventriculogram R93.0
  white blood cell (count) (differential) (morphology) D72.9
  xerography R92.8
Finger — *see* condition
Fire, Saint Anthony's — *see* Erysipelas
Fire-setting
  pathological (compulsive) F63.1
Fish hook stomach K31.89
Fishmeal-worker's lung J67.8
Fissure, fissured
  anus, anal K60.2
    acute K60.0
    chronic K60.1
    congenital Q43.8
  ear, lobule, congenital Q17.8
  epiglottis (congenital) Q31.8
  larynx J38.7
    congenital Q31.8
  lip K13.0
    congenital — *see* Cleft, lip
  nipple N64.0
    associated with
      lactation O92.13

Fissure, fissured — *continued*
  nipple — *continued*
    associated with — *continued*
      pregnancy O92.11- ☑
      puerperium O92.12
  nose Q30.2
  palate (congenital) — *see* Cleft, palate
  skin R23.4
  spine (congenital) (*see also* Spina bifida)
    with hydrocephalus — *see* Spina bifida, by site,
      with hydrocephalus
  tongue (acquired) K14.5
    congenital Q38.3
Fistula (cutaneous) L98.8
  abdomen (wall) K63.2
    bladder N32.2
    intestine NEC K63.2
    ureter N28.89
    uterus N82.5
  abdominorectal K63.2
  abdominosigmoidal K63.2
  abdominothoracic J86.0
  abdominouterine N82.5
    congenital Q51.7
  abdominovesical N32.2
  accessory sinuses — *see* Sinusitis
  actinomycotic — *see* Actinomycosis
  alveolar antrum — *see* Sinusitis, maxillary
  alveolar process K04.6
  anorectal K60.5
  antrobuccal — *see* Sinusitis, maxillary
  antrum — *see* Sinusitis, maxillary
  anus, anal (recurrent) (infectional) K60.3
    congenital Q43.6
      with absence, atresia and stenosis Q42.2
    tuberculous A18.32
  aorta-duodenal I77.2
  appendix, appendicular K38.3
  arteriovenous (acquired) (nonruptured) I77.0
    brain I67.1
      congenital Q28.2
        ruptured I60.8
      ruptured I60.8
    cerebral — *see* Fistula, arteriovenous, brain
    congenital (peripheral) (*see also* Malformation, ar-
      teriovenous)
      brain Q28.2
        ruptured I60.8
      coronary Q24.5
      pulmonary Q25.72
    coronary I25.41
      congenital Q24.5
    pulmonary I28.0
      congenital Q25.72
    surgically created (for dialysis) Z99.2
      complication — *see* Complication, arteriove-
        nous, fistula, surgically created
    traumatic — *see* Injury, blood vessel
  artery I77.2
  aural (mastoid) — *see* Mastoiditis, chronic
  auricle (*see also* Disorder, pinna, specified type NEC)
    congenital Q18.1
  Bartholin's gland N82.8
  bile duct (common) (hepatic) K83.3
    with calculus, stones — *see* Calculus, bile duct
  biliary (tract) — *see* Fistula, bile duct
  bladder (sphincter) NEC (*see also* Fistula, vesico-) N32.2
    into seminal vesicle N32.2
  bone (*see also* Disorder, bone, specified type NEC)
    with osteomyelitis, chronic — *see* Osteomyelitis,
      chronic, with draining sinus
  brain G93.89
    arteriovenous (acquired) I67.1
      congenital Q28.2
  branchial (cleft) Q18.0
  branchiogenous Q18.0
  breast N61
    puerperal, postpartum or gestational, due to mas-
      titis (purulent) — *see* Mastitis, obstetric, pu-
      rulent
  bronchial J86.0
  bronchocutaneous, bronchomediastinal, bronchopleu-
    ral, bronchopleuromediastinal (infective) J86.0
    tuberculous NEC A15.5
  bronchoesophageal J86.0
    congenital Q39.2
      with atresia of esophagus Q39.1
  bronchovisceral J86.0

Fistula — *continued*
  buccal cavity (infective) K12.2
  cecosigmoidal K63.2
  cecum K63.2
  cerebrospinal (fluid) G96.0
  cervical, lateral Q18.1
  cervicoaural Q18.1
  cervicosigmoidal N82.4
  cervicovesical N82.1
  cervix N82.8
  chest (wall) J86.0
  cholecystenteric — *see* Fistula, gallbladder
  cholecystocolic — *see* Fistula, gallbladder
  cholecystocolonic — *see* Fistula, gallbladder
  cholecystoduodenal — *see* Fistula, gallbladder
  cholecystogastric — *see* Fistula, gallbladder
  cholecystointestinal — *see* Fistula, gallbladder
  choledochoduodenal — *see* Fistula, bile duct
  cholocolic K82.3
  coccyx — *see* Sinus, pilonidal
  colon K63.2
  colostomy K94.09
  common duct — *see* Fistula, bile duct
  congenital, site not listed — *see* Anomaly, by site
  coronary, arteriovenous I25.41
    congenital Q24.5
  costal region J86.0
  cul-de-sac, Douglas' N82.8
  cystic duct (*see also* Fistula, gallbladder)
    congenital Q44.5
  dental K04.6
  diaphragm J86.0
  duodenum K31.6
  ear (external) (canal) — *see* Disorder, ear, external,
    specified type NEC
  enterocolic K63.2
  enterocutaneous K63.2
  enterouterine N82.4
    congenital Q51.7
  enterovaginal N82.4
    congenital Q52.2
    large intestine N82.3
    small intestine N82.2
  enterovesical N32.1
  epididymis N50.8
    tuberculous A18.15
  esophagobronchial J86.0
    congenital Q39.2
      with atresia of esophagus Q39.1
  esophagocutaneous K22.8
  esophagopleural-cutaneous J86.0
  esophagotracheal J86.0
    congenital Q39.2
      with atresia of esophagus Q39.1
  esophagus K22.8
    congenital Q39.2
      with atresia of esophagus Q39.1
  ethmoid — *see* Sinusitis, ethmoidal
  eyeball (cornea) (sclera) — *see* Disorder, globe, hy-
    potony
  eyelid H01.8
  fallopian tube, external N82.5
  fecal K63.2
    congenital Q43.6
  from periapical abscess K04.6
  frontal sinus — *see* Sinusitis, frontal
  gallbladder K82.3
    with calculus, cholelithiasis, stones — *see* Calculus,
      gallbladder
  gastric K31.6
  gastrocolic K31.6
    congenital Q40.2
    tuberculous A18.32
  gastroenterocolic K31.6
  gastroesophageal K31.6
  gastrojejunal K31.6
  gastrojejunocolic K31.6
  genital tract (female) N82.9
    specified NEC N82.8
    to intestine NEC N82.4
    to skin N82.5
  hepatic artery-portal vein, congenital Q26.6
  hepatopleural J86.0
  hepatopulmonary J86.0
  ileorectal or ileosigmoidal K63.2
  ileovaginal N82.2
  ileovesical N32.1
  ileum K63.2

Fistula — *continued*
  in ano K60.3
    tuberculous A18.32
  inner ear (labyrinth) — *see* subcategory H83.1 ☑
  intestine NEC K63.2
  intestinocolonic (abdominal) K63.2
  intestinoureteral N28.89
  intestinouterine N82.4
  intestinovaginal N82.4
    large intestine N82.3
    small intestine N82.2
  intestinovesical N32.1
  ischiorectal (fossa) K61.3
  jejunum K63.2
  joint M25.10
    ankle M25.17- ☑
    elbow M25.12- ☑
    foot joint M25.17- ☑
    hand joint M25.14- ☑
    hip M25.15- ☑
    knee M25.16- ☑
    shoulder M25.11- ☑
    specified joint NEC M25.18
    tuberculous — *see* Tuberculosis, joint
    vertebrae M25.18
    wrist M25.13- ☑
  kidney N28.89
  labium (majus) (minus) N82.8
  labyrinth — *see* subcategory H83.1 ☑
  lacrimal (gland) (sac) H04.61- ☑
  lacrimonasal duct — *see* Fistula, lacrimal
  laryngotracheal, congenital Q34.8
  larynx J38.7
  lip K13.0
    congenital Q38.0
  lumbar, tuberculous A18.01
  lung J86.0
  lymphatic I89.8
  mammary (gland) N61
  mastoid (process) (region) — *see* Mastoiditis, chronic
  maxillary J32.0
  medial, face and neck Q18.8
  mediastinal J86.0
  mediastinobronchial J86.0
  mediastinocutaneous J86.0
  middle ear — *see* subcategory H74.8 ☑
  mouth K12.2
  nasal J34.89
    sinus — *see* Sinusitis
  nasopharynx J39.2
  nipple N64.0
  nose J34.89
  oral (cutaneous) K12.2
    maxillary J32.0
    nasal (with cleft palate) — *see* Cleft, palate
  orbit, orbital — *see* Disorder, orbit, specified type NEC
  oroantral J32.0
  oviduct, external N82.5
  palate (hard) M27.8
  pancreatic K86.8
  pancreaticoduodenal K86.8
  parotid (gland) K11.4
    region K12.2
  penis N48.89
  perianal K60.3
  pericardium (pleura) (sac) — *see* Pericarditis
  pericecal K63.2
  perineorectal K60.4
  perineosigmoidal K63.2
  perineum, perineal (with urethral involvement) NEC
    N36.0
    tuberculous A18.13
    ureter N28.89
  perirectal K60.4
    tuberculous A18.32
  peritoneum K65.9
  pharyngoesophageal J39.2
  pharynx J39.2
    branchial cleft (congenital) Q18.0
  pilonidal (infected) (rectum) — *see* Sinus, pilonidal
  pleura, pleural, pleurocutaneous, pleuroperitoneal
    J86.0
    tuberculous NEC A15.6
  pleuropericardial I31.8
  portal vein-hepatic artery, congenital Q26.6
  postauricular H70.81- ☑
  postoperative, persistent I81.83 ☑
    specified site — *see* Fistula, by site

Fistula — *continued*
preauricular (congenital) Q18.1
prostate N42.89
pulmonary J86.0
arteriovenous I28.0
congenital Q25.72
tuberculous — *see* Tuberculosis, pulmonary
pulmonoperitoneal J86.0
rectolabial N82.4
rectosigmoid (intercommunicating) K63.2
rectoureteral N28.89
rectourethral N36.0
congenital Q64.73
rectouterine N82.4
congenital Q51.7
rectovaginal N82.3
congenital Q52.2
tuberculous A18.18
rectovesical N32.1
congenital Q64.79
rectovesicovaginal N82.3
rectovulval N82.4
congenital Q52.79
rectum (to skin) K60.4
congenital Q43.6
with absence, atresia and stenosis Q42.0
tuberculous A18.32
renal N28.89
retroauricular — *see* Fistula, postauricular
salivary duct or gland (any) K11.4
congenital Q38.4
scrotum (urinary) N50.8
tuberculous A18.15
semicircular canals — *see* subcategory H83.1 ☑
sigmoid K63.2
to bladder N32.1
sinus — *see* Sinusitis
skin L98.8
to genital tract (female) N82.5
splenocolic D73.89
stercoral K63.2
stomach K31.6
sublingual gland K11.4
submandibular gland K11.4
submaxillary (gland) K11.4
region K12.2
thoracic J86.0
duct I89.8
thoracoabdominal J86.0
thoracogastric J86.0
thoracointestinal J86.0
thorax J86.0
thyroglossal duct Q89.2
thyroid E07.89
trachea, congenital (external) (internal) Q32.1
tracheoesophageal J86.0
congenital Q39.2
with atresia of esophagus Q39.1
following tracheostomy J95.04
traumatic arteriovenous — *see* Injury, blood vessel, by site
tuberculous — *code by* site under Tuberculosis
typhoid A01.09
umbilicourinary Q64.8
urachus, congenital Q64.4
ureter (persistent) N28.89
ureteroabdominal N28.89
ureterorectal N28.89
ureterosigmoido-abdominal N28.89
ureterovaginal N82.1
ureterovesical N32.2
urethra N36.0
congenital Q64.79
tuberculous A18.13
urethroperineal N36.0
urethroperineovesical N32.2
urethrorectal N36.0
congenital Q64.73
urethroscrotal N50.8
urethrovaginal N82.1
urethrovesical N32.2
urinary (tract) (persistent) (recurrent) N36.0
uteroabdominal N82.5
congenital Q51.7
uteroenteric, uterointestinal N82.4
congenital Q51.7
uterorectal N82.4
congenital Q51.7

Fistula — *continued*
uteroureteric N82.1
uterourethral Q51.7
uterovaginal N82.8
uterovesical N82.1
congenital Q51.7
uterus N82.8
vagina (postpartal) (wall) N82.8
vaginocutaneous (postpartal) N82.5
vaginointestinal NEC N82.4
large intestine N82.3
small intestine N82.2
vaginoperineal N82.5
vasocutaneous, congenital Q55.7
vesical NEC N32.2
vesicoabdominal N32.2
vesicocervicovaginal N82.1
vesicocolic N32.1
vesicocutaneous N32.2
vesicoenteric N32.1
vesicointestinal N32.1
vesicometrorectal N82.4
vesicoperineal N32.2
vesicorectal N32.1
congenital Q64.79
vesicosigmoidal N32.1
vesicosigmoidovaginal N82.3
vesicoureteral N32.2
vesicoureterovaginal N82.1
vesicourethral N32.2
vesicourethrorectal N32.1
vesicouterine N82.1
congenital Q51.7
vesicovaginal N82.0
vulvorectal N82.4
congenital Q52.79
Fit R56.9
epileptic — *see* Epilepsy
fainting R55
hysterical F44.5
newborn P90
Fitting (and adjustment) (of)
artificial
arm — *see* Admission, adjustment, artificial, arm
breast Z44.3 ☑
eye Z44.2 ☑
leg — *see* Admission, adjustment, artificial, leg
automatic implantable cardiac defibrillator (with synchronous cardiac pacemaker) Z45.02
brain neuropacemaker Z46.2
implanted Z45.42
cardiac defibrillator — *see* Fitting (and adjustment) (of), automatic implantable cardiac defibrillator
catheter, non-vascular Z46.82
colostomy belt Z46.89
contact lenses Z46.0
cystostomy device Z46.6
defibrillator, cardiac — *see* Fitting (and adjustment) (of), automatic implantable cardiac defibrillator
dentures Z46.3
device NOS Z46.9
abdominal Z46.89
gastrointestinal NEC Z46.59
implanted NEC Z45.89
nervous system Z46.2
implanted — *see* Admission, adjustment, device, implanted, nervous system
orthodontic Z46.4
orthoptic Z46.0
orthotic Z46.89
prosthetic (external) Z44.9
breast Z44.3 ☑
dental Z46.3
eye Z44.2 ☑
specified NEC Z44.8
specified NEC Z46.89
substitution
auditory Z46.2
implanted — *see* Admission, adjustment, device, implanted, hearing device
nervous system Z46.2
implanted — *see* Admission, adjustment, device, implanted, nervous system
visual Z46.2
implanted Z45.31
urinary Z46.6
gastric lap band Z46.51
gastrointestinal appliance NEC Z46.59

Fitting — *continued*
glasses (reading) Z46.0
hearing aid Z46.1
ileostomy device Z46.89
insulin pump Z46.81
intestinal appliance NEC Z46.89
myringotomy device (stent) (tube) Z45.82
neuropacemaker Z46.2
implanted Z45.42
non-vascular catheter Z46.82
orthodontic device Z46.4
orthopedic device (brace) (cast) (corset) (shoes) Z46.89
pacemaker (cardiac) Z45.018
nervous system (brain) (peripheral nerve) (spinal cord) Z46.2
implanted Z45.42
pulse generator Z45.010
portacath (port-a-cath) Z45.2
prosthesis (external) Z44.9
arm — *see* Admission, adjustment, artificial, arm
breast Z44.3 ☑
dental Z46.3
eye Z44.2 ☑
leg — *see* Admission, adjustment, artificial, leg
specified NEC Z44.8
spectacles Z46.0
wheelchair Z46.89
Fitzhugh-Curtis syndrome
due to
Chlamydia trachomatis A74.81
Neisseria gonorrhorea (gonococcal peritonitis) A54.85
Fitz's syndrome (acute hemorrhagic pancreatitis) K85.8
Fixation
joint — *see* Ankylosis
larynx J38.7
stapes — *see* Ankylosis, ear ossicles
deafness — *see* Deafness, conductive
uterus (acquired) — *see* Malposition, uterus
vocal cord J38.3
Flabby ridge K06.8
Flaccid (*see also* condition)
palate, congenital Q38.5
Flail
chest S22.5 ☑
newborn (birth injury) P13.8
joint (paralytic) M25.20
ankle M25.27- ☑
elbow M25.22- ☑
foot joint M25.27- ☑
hand joint M25.24- ☑
hip M25.25- ☑
knee M25.26- ☑
shoulder M25.21- ☑
specified joint NEC M25.28
wrist M25.23- ☑
Flajani's disease — *see* Hyperthyroidism, with, goiter (diffuse)
Flap, liver K71.3
Flashbacks (residual to hallucinogen use) F16.283
Flat
chamber (eye) — *see* Disorder, globe, hypotony, flat anterior chamber
chest, congenital Q67.8
foot (acquired) (fixed type) (painful) (postural) (*see also* Deformity, limb, flat foot)
congenital (rigid) (spastic (everted)) Q66.5- ☑
rachitic sequelae (late effect) E64.3
organ or site, congenital NEC — *see* Anomaly, by site
pelvis M95.5
with disproportion (fetopelvic) O33.0
causing obstructed labor O65.0
congenital Q74.2
Flatau-Schilder disease G37.0
Flatback syndrome M40.30
lumbar region M40.36
lumbosacral region M40.37
thoracolumbar region M40.35
Flattening
head, femur M89.8X5
hip — *see* Coxa, plana
lip (congenital) Q18.8
nose (congenital) Q67.4
acquired M95.0
Flatulence R14.3
psychogenic F45.8
Flatus R14.3

☑ **Additional Character Required** — **Refer to the Tabular List for Character Selection**   ⩗ **Subterms under main terms may continue to next column or page**

Flatus — *continued*
   vaginalis N89.8
Flax-dresser's disease J66.1
Flea bite — *see* Injury, bite, by site, superficial, insect
Flecks, glaucomatous (subcapsular) — *see* Cataract, complicated
Fleischer (-Kayser) **ring** (cornea) H18.04- ☑
Fleshy mole O02.0
Flexibilitas cerea — *see* Catalepsy
Flexion
   amputation stump (surgical) T87.89
   cervix — *see* Malposition, uterus
   contracture, joint — *see* Contraction, joint
   deformity, joint (*see also* Deformity, limb, flexion) M21.20
      hip, congenital Q65.89
   uterus (*see also* Malposition, uterus)
      lateral — *see* Lateroversion, uterus
Flexner-Boyd dysentery A03.2
Flexner's dysentery A03.1
Flexure — *see* Flexion
Flint murmur (aortic insufficiency) I35.1
Floater, vitreous — *see* Opacity, vitreous
Floating
   cartilage (joint) (*see also* Loose, body, joint)
      knee — *see* Derangement, knee, loose body
   gallbladder, congenital Q44.1
   kidney N28.89
      congenital Q63.8
   spleen D73.89
Flooding N92.0
Floor — *see* condition
Floppy
   baby syndrome (nonspecific) P94.2
   iris syndrome (intraoperative) (IFIS) H21.81
   nonrheumatic mitral valve syndrome I34.1
Flu (*see also* Influenza)
   avian (*see also* Influenza, due to, identified novel influenza A virus) J09.X2
   bird (*see also* Influenza, due to, identified novel influenza A virus) J09.X2
   intestinal NEC A08.4
   swine (viruses that normally cause infections in pigs) (*see also* Influenza, due to, identified novel influenza A virus) J09.X2
Fluctuating blood pressure I99.8
Fluid
   abdomen R18.8
   chest J94.8
   heart — *see* Failure, heart, congestive
   joint — *see* Effusion, joint
   loss (acute) E86.9
      with
         hypernatremia E87.0
         hyponatremia E87.1
   lung — *see* Edema, lung
   overload E87.70
      specified NEC E87.79
   peritoneal cavity R18.8
   pleural cavity J94.8
   retention R60.9
Flukes NEC (*see also* Infestation, fluke)
   blood NEC — *see* Schistosomiasis
   liver B66.3
Fluor (vaginalis) N89.8
   trichomonal or due to Trichomonas (vaginalis) A59.00
Fluorosis
   dental K00.3
   skeletal M85.10
      ankle M85.17- ☑
      foot M85.17- ☑
      forearm M85.13- ☑
      hand M85.14- ☑
      lower leg M85.16- ☑
      multiple site M85.19
      neck M85.18
      rib M85.18
      shoulder M85.11- ☑
      skull M85.18
      specified site NEC M85.18
      thigh M85.15- ☑
      toe M85.17- ☑
      upper arm M85.12- ☑
      vertebra M85.18
Flush syndrome E34.0
Flushing R23.2
   menopausal N95.1

Flutter
   atrial or auricular I48.92
      atypical I48.4
      type I I48.3
      type II I48.4
      typical I48.3
   heart I49.8
      atrial or auricular I48.92
         atypical I48.4
         type I I48.3
         type II I48.4
         typical I48.3
      ventricular I49.02
   ventricular I49.02
FNHTR (febrile nonhemolytic transfusion reaction) R50.84
Fochier's abscess — *code by* site under Abscess
Focus, Assmann's — *see* Tuberculosis, pulmonary
Fogo selvagem L10.3
Foix-Alajouanine syndrome G95.19
Fold, folds (anomalous) (*see also* Anomaly, by site)
   Descemet's membrane — *see* Change, corneal membrane, Descemet's, fold
   epicanthic Q10.3
   heart Q24.8
Folie à deux F24
Follicle
   cervix (nabothian) (ruptured) N88.8
   graafian, ruptured, with hemorrhage N83.0
   nabothian N88.8
Follicular — *see* condition
Folliculitis (superficial) L73.9
   abscedens et suffodiens L66.3
   cyst N83.0
   decalvans L66.2
   deep — *see* Furuncle, by site
   gonococcal (acute) (chronic) A54.01
   keloid, keloidalis L73.0
   pustular L01.02
   ulerythematosa reticulata L66.4
Folliculome lipidique
   specified site — *see* Neoplasm, benign, by site
   unspecified site
      female D27.9
      male D29.20
Følling's disease E70.0
Follow-up — *see* Examination, follow-up
Fong's syndrome (hereditary osteo-onychodysplasia) Q78.5
Food
   allergy L27.2
   asphyxia (from aspiration or inhalation) — *see* Foreign body, by site
   choked on — *see* Foreign body, by site
   deprivation T73.0 ☑
      specified kind of food NEC E63.8
   intoxication — *see* Poisoning, food
   lack of T73.0 ☑
   poisoning — *see* Poisoning, food
   rejection NEC — *see* Disorder, eating
   strangulation or suffocation — *see* Foreign body, by site
   toxemia — *see* Poisoning, food
Foot — *see* condition
Foramen ovale (nonclosure) (patent) (persistent) Q21.1
Forbes' glycogen storage disease E74.03
Fordyce-Fox disease L75.2
Fordyce's disease (mouth) Q38.6
Forearm — *see* condition
Foreign body
   with
      laceration — *see* Laceration, by site, with foreign body
      puncture wound — *see* Puncture, by site, with foreign body
   accidentally left following a procedure T81.509 ☑
      aspiration T81.506 ☑
         resulting in
            adhesions T81.516 ☑
            obstruction T81.526 ☑
            perforation T81.536 ☑
            specified complication NEC T81.596 ☑
      cardiac catheterization T81.505 ☑
         resulting in
            acute reaction T81.60 ☑
               aseptic peritonitis T81.61 ☑
               specified NEC T81.69 ☑
            adhesions T81.515 ☑

Foreign body — *continued*
   accidentally left following a procedure — *continued*
      cardiac catheterization — *continued*
         resulting in — *continued*
            obstruction T81.525 ☑
            perforation T81.535 ☑
            specified complication NEC T81.595 ☑
      causing
         acute reaction T81.60 ☑
            aseptic peritonitis T81.61 ☑
            specified complication NEC T81.69 ☑
         adhesions T81.519 ☑
         aseptic peritonitis T81.61 ☑
         obstruction T81.529 ☑
         perforation T81.539 ☑
         specified complication NEC T81.599 ☑
      endoscopy T81.504 ☑
         resulting in
            adhesions T81.514 ☑
            obstruction T81.524 ☑
            perforation T81.534 ☑
            specified complication NEC T81.594 ☑
      immunization T81.503 ☑
         resulting in
            adhesions T81.513 ☑
            obstruction T81.523 ☑
            perforation T81.533 ☑
            specified complication NEC T81.593 ☑
      infusion T81.501 ☑
         resulting in
            adhesions T81.511 ☑
            obstruction T81.521 ☑
            perforation T81.531 ☑
            specified complication NEC T81.591 ☑
      injection T81.503 ☑
         resulting in
            adhesions T81.513 ☑
            obstruction T81.523 ☑
            perforation T81.533 ☑
            specified complication NEC T81.593 ☑
      kidney dialysis T81.502 ☑
         resulting in
            adhesions T81.512 ☑
            obstruction T81.522 ☑
            perforation T81.532 ☑
            specified complication NEC T81.592 ☑
      packing removal T81.507 ☑
         resulting in
            acute reaction T81.60 ☑
               aseptic peritonitis T81.61 ☑
               specified NEC T81.69 ☑
            adhesions T81.517 ☑
            obstruction T81.527 ☑
            perforation T81.537 ☑
            specified complication NEC T81.597 ☑
      puncture T81.506 ☑
         resulting in
            adhesions T81.516 ☑
            obstruction T81.526 ☑
            perforation T81.536 ☑
            specified complication NEC T81.596 ☑
      specified procedure NEC T81.508 ☑
         resulting in
            acute reaction T81.60 ☑
               aseptic peritonitis T81.61 ☑
               specified NEC T81.69 ☑
            adhesions T81.518 ☑
            obstruction T81.528 ☑
            perforation T81.538 ☑
            specified complication NEC T81.598 ☑
      surgical operation T81.500 ☑
         resulting in
            acute reaction T81.60 ☑
               aseptic peritonitis T81.61 ☑
               specified NEC T81.69 ☑
            adhesions T81.510 ☑
            obstruction T81.520 ☑
            perforation T81.530 ☑
            specified complication NEC T81.590 ☑
      transfusion T81.501 ☑
         resulting in
            adhesions T81.511 ☑
            obstruction T81.521 ☑
            perforation T81.531 ☑
            specified complication NEC T81.591 ☑

Foreign body — *continued*
- alimentary tract T18.9 ☑
  - anus T18.5 ☑
  - colon T18.4 ☑
  - esophagus — *see* Foreign body, esophagus
  - mouth T18.0 ☑
  - multiple sites T18.8 ☑
  - rectosigmoid (junction) T18.5 ☑
  - rectum T18.5 ☑
  - small intestine T18.3 ☑
  - specified site NEC T18.8 ☑
  - stomach T18.2 ☑
- anterior chamber (eye) S05.5- ☑
- auditory canal — *see* Foreign body, entering through orifice, ear
- bronchus T17.508 ☑
  - causing
    - asphyxiation T17.500 ☑
      - food (bone) (seed) T17.520 ☑
      - gastric contents (vomitus) T17.510 ☑
      - specified type NEC T17.590 ☑
    - injury NEC T17.508 ☑
      - food (bone) (seed) T17.528 ☑
      - gastric contents (vomitus) T17.518 ☑
      - specified type NEC T17.598 ☑
- canthus — *see* Foreign body, conjunctival sac
- ciliary body (eye) S05.5- ☑
- conjunctival sac T15.1- ☑
- cornea T15.0- ☑
- entering through orifice
  - accessory sinus T17.0 ☑
  - alimentary canal T18.9 ☑
    - multiple parts T18.8 ☑
    - specified part NEC T18.8 ☑
  - alveolar process T18.0 ☑
  - antrum (Highmore's) T17.0 ☑
  - anus T18.5 ☑
  - appendix T18.4 ☑
  - auditory canal — *see* Foreign body, entering through orifice, ear
  - auricle — *see* Foreign body, entering through orifice, ear
  - bladder T19.1 ☑
  - bronchioles — *see* Foreign body, respiratory tract, specified site NEC
  - bronchus (main) — *see* Foreign body, bronchus
  - buccal cavity T18.0 ☑
  - canthus (inner) — *see* Foreign body, conjunctival sac
  - cecum T18.4 ☑
  - cervix (canal) (uteri) T19.3 ☑
  - colon T18.4 ☑
  - conjunctival sac — *see* Foreign body, conjunctival sac
  - cornea — *see* Foreign body, cornea
  - digestive organ or tract NOS T18.9 ☑
    - multiple parts T18.8 ☑
    - specified part NEC T18.8 ☑
  - duodenum T18.3 ☑
  - ear (external) T16.- ☑
  - esophagus — *see* Foreign body, esophagus
  - eye (external) NOS T15.9- ☑
    - conjunctival sac — *see* Foreign body, conjunctival sac
    - cornea — *see* Foreign body, cornea
    - specified part NEC T15.8- ☑
  - eyeball (*see also* Foreign body, entering through orifice, eye, specified part NEC)
    - with penetrating wound — *see* Puncture, eyeball
  - eyelid (*see also* Foreign body, conjunctival sac) with
    - laceration — *see* Laceration, eyelid, with foreign body
    - puncture — *see* Puncture, eyelid, with foreign body
    - superficial injury — *see* Foreign body, superficial, eyelid
  - gastrointestinal tract T18.9 ☑
    - multiple parts T18.8 ☑
    - specified part NEC T18.8 ☑
  - genitourinary tract T19.9 ☑
    - multiple parts T19.8 ☑
    - specified part NEC T19.8 ☑
  - globe — *see* Foreign body, entering through orifice, eyeball

Foreign body — *continued*
- entering through orifice — *continued*
  - gum T18.0 ☑
  - Highmore's antrum T17.0 ☑
  - hypopharynx — *see* Foreign body, pharynx
  - ileum T18.3 ☑
  - intestine (small) T18.3 ☑
    - large T18.4 ☑
  - lacrimal apparatus (punctum) — *see* Foreign body, entering through orifice, eye, specified part NEC
  - large intestine T18.4 ☑
  - larynx — *see* Foreign body, larynx
  - lung — *see* Foreign body, respiratory tract, specified site NEC
  - maxillary sinus T17.0 ☑
  - mouth T18.0 ☑
  - nasal sinus T17.0 ☑
  - nasopharynx — *see* Foreign body, pharynx
  - nose (passage) T17.1 ☑
  - nostril T17.1 ☑
  - oral cavity T18.0 ☑
  - palate T18.0 ☑
  - penis T19.4 ☑
  - pharynx — *see* Foreign body, pharynx
  - piriform sinus — *see* Foreign body, pharynx
  - rectosigmoid (junction) T18.5 ☑
  - rectum T18.5 ☑
  - respiratory tract — *see* Foreign body, respiratory tract
  - sinus (accessory) (frontal) (maxillary) (nasal) T17.0 ☑
    - piriform — *see* Foreign body, pharynx
  - small intestine T18.3 ☑
  - stomach T18.2 ☑
  - suffocation by — *see* Foreign body, by site
  - tear ducts or glands — *see* Foreign body, entering through orifice, eye, specified part NEC
  - throat — *see* Foreign body, pharynx
  - tongue T18.0 ☑
  - tonsil, tonsillar (fossa) — *see* Foreign body, pharynx
  - trachea — *see* Foreign body, trachea
  - ureter T19.8 ☑
  - urethra T19.0 ☑
  - uterus (any part) T19.3 ☑
  - vagina T19.2 ☑
  - vulva T19.2 ☑
- esophagus T18.108 ☑
  - causing
    - injury NEC T18.108 ☑
      - food (bone) (seed) T18.128 ☑
      - gastric contents (vomitus) T18.118 ☑
      - specified type NEC T18.198 ☑
    - tracheal compression T18.100 ☑
      - food (bone) (seed) T18.120 ☑
      - gastric contents (vomitus) T18.110 ☑
      - specified type NEC T18.190 ☑
- felling of, in throat R09.89
- fragment — *see* Retained, foreign body fragments (type of)
- genitourinary tract T19.9 ☑
  - bladder T19.1 ☑
  - multiple parts T19.8 ☑
  - penis T19.4 ☑
  - specified site NEC T19.8 ☑
  - urethra T19.0 ☑
  - uterus T19.3 ☑
    - IUD Z97.5
  - vagina T19.2 ☑
    - contraceptive device Z97.5
  - vulva T19.2 ☑
- granuloma (old) (soft tissue) (*see also* Granuloma, foreign body)
  - skin L92.3
- in
  - laceration — *see* Laceration, by site, with foreign body
  - puncture wound — *see* Puncture, by site, with foreign body
  - soft tissue (residual) M79.5
- inadvertently left in operation wound — *see* Foreign body, accidentally left during a procedure
- ingestion, ingested NOS T18.9 ☑
- inhalation or inspiration — *see* Foreign body, by site
- internal organ, not entering through a natural orifice — code as specific injury with foreign body

Foreign body — *continued*
- intraocular S05.5- ☑
  - old, retained (nonmagnetic) H44.70- ☑
    - anterior chamber H44.71- ☑
    - ciliary body H44.72- ☑
    - iris H44.72- ☑
    - lens H44.73- ☑
    - magnetic H44.60- ☑
      - anterior chamber H44.61- ☑
      - ciliary body H44.62- ☑
      - iris H44.62- ☑
      - lens H44.63- ☑
      - posterior wall H44.64- ☑
      - specified site NEC H44.69- ☑
      - vitreous body H44.65- ☑
    - posterior wall H44.74- ☑
    - specified site NEC H44.79- ☑
    - vitreous body H44.75- ☑
  - iris — *see* Foreign body, intraocular
- lacrimal punctum — *see* Foreign body, entering through orifice, eye, specified part NEC
- larynx T17.308 ☑
  - causing
    - asphyxiation T17.300 ☑
      - food (bone) (seed) T17.320 ☑
      - gastric contents (vomitus) T17.310 ☑
      - specified type NEC T17.390 ☑
    - injury NEC T17.308 ☑
      - food (bone) (seed) T17.328 ☑
      - gastric contents (vomitus) T17.318 ☑
      - specified type NEC T17.398 ☑
- lens — *see* Foreign body, intraocular
- ocular muscle S05.4- ☑
  - old, retained — *see* Foreign body, orbit, old
- old or residual
  - soft tissue (residual) M79.5
- operation wound, left accidentally — *see* Foreign body, accidentally left during a procedure
- orbit S05.4- ☑
  - old, retained H05.5- ☑
- pharynx T17.208 ☑
  - causing
    - asphyxiation T17.200 ☑
      - food (bone) (seed) T17.220 ☑
      - gastric contents (vomitus) T17.210 ☑
      - specified type NEC T17.290 ☑
    - injury NEC T17.208 ☑
      - food (bone) (seed) T17.228 ☑
      - gastric contents (vomitus) T17.218 ☑
      - specified type NEC T17.298 ☑
- respiratory tract T17.908 ☑
  - bronchioles — *see* Foreign body, respiratory tract, specified site NEC
  - bronchus — *see* Foreign body, bronchus
  - causing
    - asphyxiation T17.900 ☑
      - food (bone) (seed) T17.920 ☑
      - gastric contents (vomitus) T17.910 ☑
      - specified type NEC T17.990 ☑
    - injury NEC T17.908 ☑
      - food (bone) (seed) T17.928 ☑
      - gastric contents (vomitus) T17.918 ☑
      - specified type NEC T17.998 ☑
  - larynx — *see* Foreign body, larynx
  - lung — *see* Foreign body, respiratory tract, specified site NEC
  - multiple parts — *see* Foreign body, respiratory tract, specified site NEC
  - nasal sinus T17.0 ☑
  - nasopharynx — *see* Foreign body, pharynx
  - nose T17.1 ☑
  - nostril T17.1 ☑
  - pharynx — *see* Foreign body, pharynx
  - specified site NEC T17.808 ☑
    - causing
      - asphyxiation T17.800 ☑
        - food (bone) (seed) T17.820 ☑
        - gastric contents (vomitus) T17.810 ☑
        - specified type NEC T17.890 ☑
      - injury NEC T17.808 ☑
        - food (bone) (seed) T17.828 ☑
        - gastric contents (vomitus) T17.818 ☑
        - specified type NEC T17.898 ☑
  - throat — *see* Foreign body, pharynx
  - trachea — *see* Foreign body, trachea

Foreign body — *continued*
  retained (old) (nonmagnetic) (in)
    anterior chamber (eye) — *see* Foreign body, intraocular, old, retained, anterior chamber
      magnetic — *see* Foreign body, intraocular, old, retained, magnetic, anterior chamber
    ciliary body — *see* Foreign body, intraocular, old, retained, ciliary body
      magnetic — *see* Foreign body, intraocular, old, retained, magnetic, ciliary body
    eyelid H02.819
      left H02.816
        lower H02.815
        upper H02.814
      right H02.813
        lower H02.812
        upper H02.811
    fragments — *see* Retained, foreign body fragments (type of)
    globe — *see* Foreign body, intraocular, old, retained
      magnetic — *see* Foreign body, intraocular, old, retained, magnetic
    intraocular — *see* Foreign body, intraocular, old, retained
      magnetic — *see* Foreign body, intraocular, old, retained, magnetic
    iris — *see* Foreign body, intraocular, old, retained, iris
      magnetic — *see* Foreign body, intraocular, old, retained, magnetic, iris
    lens — *see* Foreign body, intraocular, old, retained, lens
      magnetic — *see* Foreign body, intraocular, old, retained, magnetic, lens
    muscle — *see* Foreign body, retained, soft tissue
    orbit — *see* Foreign body, orbit, old
    posterior wall of globe — *see* Foreign body, intraocular, old, retained, posterior wall
      magnetic — *see* Foreign body, intraocular, old, retained, magnetic, posterior wall
    retrobulbar — *see* Foreign body, orbit, old, retrobulbar
    soft tissue M79.5
    vitreous — *see* Foreign body, intraocular, old, retained, vitreous body
      magnetic — *see* Foreign body, intraocular, old, retained, magnetic, vitreous body
  retina S05.5- ☑
  superficial, without open wound
    abdomen, abdominal (wall) S30.851 ☑
    alveolar process S00.552 ☑
    ankle S90.55- ☑
    antecubital space — *see* Foreign body, superficial, forearm
    anus S30.857 ☑
    arm (upper) S40.85- ☑
    auditory canal — *see* Foreign body, superficial, ear
    auricle — *see* Foreign body, superficial, ear
    axilla — *see* Foreign body, superficial, arm
    back, lower S30.850 ☑
    breast S20.15- ☑
    brow S00.85 ☑
    buttock S30.850 ☑
    calf — *see* Foreign body, superficial, leg
    canthus — *see* Foreign body, superficial, eyelid
    cheek S00.85 ☑
      internal S00.552 ☑
    chest wall — *see* Foreign body, superficial, thorax
    chin S00.85 ☑
    clitoris S30.854 ☑
    costal region — *see* Foreign body, superficial, thorax
    digit(s)
      foot — *see* Foreign body, superficial, toe
      hand — *see* Foreign body, superficial, finger
    ear S00.45- ☑
    elbow S50.35- ☑
    epididymis S30.853 ☑
    epigastric region S30.851 ☑
    epiglottis S10.15 ☑
    esophagus, cervical S10.15 ☑
    eyebrow — *see* Foreign body, superficial, eyelid
    eyelid S00.25- ☑
    face S00.85 ☑
    finger(s) S60.459 ☑
      index S60.45- ☑

Foreign body — *continued*
  superficial, without open wound — *continued*
    finger(s) — *continued*
      little S60.45- ☑
      middle S60.45- ☑
      ring S60.45- ☑
    flank S30.851 ☑
    foot (except toe(s) alone) S90.85- ☑
      toe — *see* Foreign body, superficial, toe
    forearm S50.85- ☑
      elbow only — *see* Foreign body, superficial, elbow
    forehead S00.85 ☑
    genital organs, external
      female S30.856 ☑
      male S30.855 ☑
    groin S30.851 ☑
    gum S00.552 ☑
    hand S60.55- ☑
    head S00.95 ☑
      ear — *see* Foreign body, superficial, ear
      eyelid — *see* Foreign body, superficial, eyelid
      lip S00.551 ☑
      nose S00.35 ☑
      oral cavity S00.552 ☑
      scalp S00.05 ☑
      specified site NEC S00.85 ☑
    heel — *see* Foreign body, superficial, foot
    hip S70.25- ☑
    inguinal region S30.851 ☑
    interscapular region S20.459 ☑
    jaw S00.85 ☑
    knee S80.25- ☑
    labium (majus) (minus) S30.854 ☑
    larynx S10.15 ☑
    leg (lower) S80.85- ☑
      knee — *see* Foreign body, superficial, knee
      upper — *see* Foreign body, superficial, thigh
    lip S00.551 ☑
    lower back S30.850 ☑
    lumbar region S30.850 ☑
    malar region S00.85 ☑
    mammary — *see* Foreign body, superficial, breast
    mastoid region S00.85 ☑
    mouth S00.552 ☑
    nail
      finger — *see* Foreign body, superficial, finger
      toe — *see* Foreign body, superficial, toe
    nape S10.85 ☑
    nasal S00.35 ☑
    neck S10.95 ☑
      specified site NEC S10.85 ☑
      throat S10.15 ☑
    nose S00.35 ☑
    occipital region S00.05 ☑
    oral cavity S00.552 ☑
    orbital region — *see* Foreign body, superficial, eyelid
    palate S00.552 ☑
    palm — *see* Foreign body, superficial, hand
    parietal region S00.05 ☑
    pelvis S30.850 ☑
    penis S30.852 ☑
    perineum
      female S30.854 ☑
      male S30.850 ☑
    periocular area — *see* Foreign body, superficial, eyelid
    phalanges
      finger — *see* Foreign body, superficial, finger
      toe — *see* Foreign body, superficial, toe
    pharynx S10.15 ☑
    pinna — *see* Foreign body, superficial, ear
    popliteal space — *see* Foreign body, superficial, knee
    prepuce S30.852 ☑
    pubic region S30.850 ☑
    pudendum
      female S30.856 ☑
      male S30.855 ☑
    sacral region S30.850 ☑
    scalp S00.05 ☑
    scapular region — *see* Foreign body, superficial, shoulder
    scrotum S30.853 ☑
    shin — *see* Foreign body, superficial, leg

Foreign body — *continued*
  superficial, without open wound — *continued*
    shoulder S40.25- ☑
    sternal region S20.359 ☑
    submaxillary region S00.85 ☑
    submental region S00.85 ☑
    subungual
      finger(s) — *see* Foreign body, superficial, finger
      toe(s) — *see* Foreign body, superficial, toe
    supraclavicular fossa S10.85 ☑
    supraorbital S00.85 ☑
    temple S00.85 ☑
    temporal region S00.85 ☑
    testis S30.853 ☑
    thigh S70.35- ☑
    thorax, thoracic (wall) S20.95 ☑
      back S20.45- ☑
      front S20.35- ☑
    throat S10.15 ☑
    thumb S60.35- ☑
    toe(s) (lesser) S90.456 ☑
      great S90.45- ☑
    tongue S00.552 ☑
    trachea S10.15 ☑
    tunica vaginalis S30.853 ☑
    tympanum, tympanic membrane — *see* Foreign body, superficial, ear
    uvula S00.552 ☑
    vagina S30.854 ☑
    vocal cords S10.15 ☑
    vulva S30.854 ☑
    wrist S60.85- ☑
  swallowed T18.9 ☑
  trachea T17.408 ☑
    causing
      asphyxiation T17.400 ☑
        food (bone) (seed) T17.420 ☑
        gastric contents (vomitus) T17.410 ☑
        specified type NEC T17.490 ☑
      injury NEC T17.408 ☑
        food (bone) (seed) T17.428 ☑
        gastric contents (vomitus) T17.418 ☑
        specified type NEC T17.498 ☑
  type of fragment — *see* Retained, foreign body fragments (type of)
  vitreous (humor) S05.5- ☑
Forestier's disease (rhizomelic pseudopolyarthritis) M35.3
  meaning ankylosing hyperostosis — *see* Hyperostosis, ankylosing
Formation
  hyalin in cornea — *see* Degeneration, cornea
  sequestrum in bone (due to infection) — *see* Osteomyelitis, chronic
  valve
    colon, congenital Q43.8
    ureter (congenital) Q62.39
Formication R20.2
Fort Bragg fever A27.89
Fossa (*see also* condition)
  pyriform — *see* condition
Foster-Kennedy syndrome H47.14- ☑
Fothergill's
  disease (trigeminal neuralgia) (*see also* Neuralgia, trigeminal)
  scarlatina anginosa A38.9
Foul breath R19.6
Foundling Z76.1
Fournier disease or gangrene N49.3
  female N76.89
Fourth
  cranial nerve — *see* condition
  molar K00.1
Foville's (peduncular) **disease or syndrome** G46.3
Fox (-Fordyce) disease (apocrine miliaria) L75.2
Fracture, burst — *see* Fracture, traumatic, by site
Fracture, chronic — *see* Fracture, pathological
Fracture, insufficiency — *see* Fracture, pathologic, by site
Fracture, pathological (pathologic) (*see also* Fracture, traumatic) M84.40 ☑
  ankle M84.47- ☑
  carpus M84.44- ☑
  clavicle M84.41- ☑
  dental implant M27.63

⬇ Subterms under main terms may continue to next column or page   ☑ Additional Character Required — Refer to the Tabular List for Character Selection   **143**

Foreign body — Fallen arches

Fracture, pathological — *continued*
  dental restorative material K08.539
    with loss of material K08.531
    without loss of material K08.530
  due to
    neoplastic disease NEC (*see also* Neoplasm)
      M84.50 ☑
      ankle M84.57- ☑
      carpus M84.54- ☑
      clavicle M84.51- ☑
      femur M84.55- ☑
      fibula M84.56- ☑
      finger M84.54- ☑
      hip M84.559 ☑
      humerus M84.52- ☑
      ilium M84.550 ☑
      ischium M84.550 ☑
      metacarpus M84.54- ☑
      metatarsus M84.57- ☑
      neck M84.58 ☑
      pelvis M84.550 ☑
      radius M84.53- ☑
      rib M84.58 ☑
      scapula M84.51- ☑
      skull M84.58 ☑
      specified site NEC M84.58 ☑
      tarsus M84.57- ☑
      tibia M84.56- ☑
      toe M84.57- ☑
      ulna M84.53- ☑
      vertebra M84.58 ☑
    osteoporosis M80.80 ☑
      disuse — *see* Osteoporosis, specified type NEC,
        with pathological fracture
      drug-induced — *see* Osteoporosis, drug in-
        duced, with pathological fracture
      idiopathic — *see* Osteoporosis, specified type
        NEC, with pathological fracture
      postmenopausal — *see* Osteoporosis, post-
        menopausal, with pathological fracture
      postoophorectomy — *see* Osteoporosis, pos-
        toophorectomy, with pathological frac-
        ture
      postsurgical malabsorption — *see* Osteoporo-
        sis, specified type NEC, with pathological
        fracture
      specified cause NEC — *see* Osteoporosis, spec-
        ified type NEC, with pathological fracture
  specified disease NEC M84.60 ☑
    ankle M84.67- ☑
    carpus M84.64- ☑
    clavicle M84.61- ☑
    femur M84.65- ☑
    fibula M84.66- ☑
    finger M84.64- ☑
    hip M84.65- ☑
    humerus M84.62- ☑
    ilium M84.650 ☑
    ischium M84.650 ☑
    metacarpus M84.64- ☑
    metatarsus M84.67- ☑
    neck M84.68 ☑
    radius M84.63- ☑
    rib M84.68 ☑
    scapula M84.61- ☑
    skull M84.68 ☑
    tarsus M84.67- ☑
    tibia M84.66- ☑
    toe M84.67- ☑
    ulna M84.63- ☑
    vertebra M84.68 ☑
  femur M84.45- ☑
  fibula M84.46- ☑
  finger M84.44- ☑
  hip M84.459 ☑
  humerus M84.42- ☑
  ilium M84.454 ☑
  ischium M84.454 ☑
  joint prosthesis — *see* Complications, joint prosthesis,
    mechanical, breakdown, by site
    periprosthetic — *see* Complications, joint prosthe-
      sis, mechanical, periprosthesis, fracture, by
      site
  metacarpus M84.44- ☑
  metatarsus M84.47- ☑
  neck M84.48 ☑

Fracture, pathological — *continued*
  pelvis M84.454 ☑
  radius M84.43- ☑
  restorative material (dental) K08.539
    with loss of material K08.531
    without loss of material K08.530
  rib M84.48 ☑
  scapula M84.41- ☑
  skull M84.48 ☑
  tarsus M84.47- ☑
  tibia M84.46- ☑
  toe M84.47- ☑
  ulna M84.43- ☑
  vertebra M84.48 ☑
Fracture, traumatic (abduction) (adduction) (separation)
  (*see also* Fracture, pathological) T14.8
  acetabulum S32.40- ☑
    column
      anterior (displaced) (iliopubic) S32.43- ☑
        nondisplaced S32.436 ☑
      posterior (displaced) (ilioischial) S32.443 ☑
        nondisplaced S32.44- ☑
    dome (displaced) S32.48- ☑
      nondisplaced S32.48 ☑
    specified NEC S32.49- ☑
    transverse (displaced) S32.45- ☑
      with associated posterior wall fracture (dis-
        placed) S32.46- ☑
        nondisplaced S32.46- ☑
      nondisplaced S32.45- ☑
    wall
      anterior (displaced) S32.41- ☑
        nondisplaced S32.41- ☑
      medial (displaced) S32.47- ☑
        nondisplaced S32.47- ☑
      posterior (displaced) S32.42- ☑
        with associated transverse fracture (dis-
          placed) S32.46- ☑
        nondisplaced S32.46- ☑
        nondisplaced S32.42- ☑
  acromion — *see* Fracture, scapula, acromial process
  ankle S82.899 ☑
    bimalleolar (displaced) S82.84- ☑
      nondisplaced S82.84- ☑
    lateral malleolus only (displaced) S82.6- ☑
      nondisplaced S82.6- ☑
    medial malleolus (displaced) S82.5- ☑
      associated with Maisonneuve's fracture — *see*
        Fracture, Maisonneuve's
      nondisplaced S82.5- ☑
    talus — *see* Fracture, tarsal, talus
    trimalleolar (displaced) S82.85- ☑
      nondisplaced S82.85- ☑
  arm (upper) (*see also* Fracture, humerus, shaft)
    humerus — *see* Fracture, humerus
    radius — *see* Fracture, radius
    ulna — *see* Fracture, ulna
  astragalus — *see* Fracture, tarsal, talus
  atlas — *see* Fracture, neck, cervical vertebra, first
  axis — *see* Fracture, neck, cervical vertebra, second
  back — *see* Fracture, vertebra
  Barton's — *see* Barton's fracture
  base of skull — *see* Fracture, skull, base
  basicervical (basal) (femoral) S72.0 ☑
  Bennett's — *see* Bennett's fracture
  bimalleolar — *see* Fracture, ankle, bimalleolar
  blow-out S02.3 ☑
  bone NEC T14.8
    birth injury P13.9
    following insertion of orthopedic implant, joint
      prosthesis or bone plate — *see* Fracture,
      following insertion of orthopedic implant,
      joint prosthesis or bone plate
    in (due to) neoplastic disease NEC — *see* Fracture,
      pathological, due to, neoplastic disease
    pathological (cause unknown) — *see* Fracture,
      pathological
  breast bone — *see* Fracture, sternum
  bucket handle (semilunar cartilage) — *see* Tear,
    meniscus
  burst — *see* Fracture, traumatic, by site
  calcaneus — *see* Fracture, tarsal, calcaneus
  carpal bone(s) S62.10- ☑
    capitate (displaced) S62.13- ☑
      nondisplaced S62.13- ☑
    cuneiform — *see* Fracture, carpal bone, triquetrum

Fracture, traumatic — *continued*
  carpal bone(s) — *continued*
    hamate (body) (displaced) S62.143 ☑
      hook process (displaced) S62.15- ☑
        nondisplaced S62.15- ☑
      nondisplaced S62.14- ☑
    larger multangular — *see* Fracture, carpal bones,
      trapezium
    lunate (displaced) S62.12- ☑
      nondisplaced S62.12- ☑
    navicular S62.00- ☑
      distal pole (displaced) S62.01- ☑
        nondisplaced S62.01- ☑
      middle third (displaced) S62.02- ☑
        nondisplaced S62.02- ☑
      proximal third (displaced) S62.03- ☑
        nondisplaced S62.03- ☑
      volar tuberosity — *see* Fracture, carpal bones,
        navicular, distal pole
    os magnum — *see* Fracture, carpal bones, capitate
    pisiform (displaced) S62.16- ☑
      nondisplaced S62.16- ☑
    semilunar — *see* Fracture, carpal bones, lunate
    smaller multangular — *see* Fracture, carpal bones,
      trapezoid
    trapezium (displaced) S62.17- ☑
      nondisplaced S62.17- ☑
    trapezoid (displaced) S62.18- ☑
      nondisplaced S62.18- ☑
    triquetrum (displaced) S62.11- ☑
      nondisplaced S62.11- ☑
    unciform — *see* Fracture, carpal bones, hamate
  cervical — *see* Fracture, vertebra, cervical
  clavicle S42.00- ☑
    acromial end (displaced) S42.03- ☑
      nondisplaced S42.03- ☑
    birth injury P13.4
    lateral end — *see* Fracture, clavicle, acromial end
    shaft (displaced) S42.02- ☑
      nondisplaced S42.02- ☑
    sternal end (anterior) (displaced) S42.01- ☑
      nondisplaced S42.01- ☑
      posterior S42.01- ☑
  coccyx S32.2 ☑
  collapsed — *see* Collapse, vertebra
  collar bone — *see* Fracture, clavicle
  Colles' — *see* Colles' fracture
  compression, not due to trauma — *see* Collapse, ver-
    tebra
  coronoid process — *see* Fracture, ulna, upper end,
    coronoid process
  corpus cavernosum penis S39.840 ☑
  costochondral cartilage S23.41 ☑
  costochondral, costosternal junction — *see* Fracture,
    rib
  cranium — *see* Fracture, skull
  cricoid cartilage S12.8 ☑
  cuboid (ankle) — *see* Fracture, tarsal, cuboid
  cuneiform
    foot — *see* Fracture, tarsal, cuneiform
    wrist — *see* Fracture, carpal, triquetrum
  delayed union — *see* Delay, union, fracture
  dental restorative material K08.539
    with loss of material K08.531
    without loss of material K08.530
  due to
    birth injury — *see* Birth, injury, fracture
    osteoporosis — *see* Osteoporosis, with fracture
  Dupuytren's — *see* Fracture, ankle, lateral malleolus
  elbow S42.40- ☑
  ethmoid (bone) (sinus) — *see* Fracture, skull, base
  face bone S02.92 ☑
  fatigue (*see also* Fracture, stress)
    vertebra M48.40 ☑
      cervical region M48.42 ☑
      cervicothoracic region M48.43 ☑
      lumbar region M48.46 ☑
      lumbosacral region M48.47 ☑
      occipito-atlanto-axial region M48.41 ☑
      sacrococcygeal region M48.48 ☑
      thoracic region M48.44 ☑
      thoracolumbar region M48.45 ☑
  femur, femoral S72.9- ☑
    basicervical (basal) S72.0 ☑
    birth injury P13.2
    capital epiphyseal S79.01- ☑

144

☑ **Additional Character Required** — Refer to the Tabular List for Character Selection   �𝕎 **Subterms under main terms may continue to next column or page**

Index

Fracture, pathological — Fracture, traumatic

Fracture, traumatic — *continued*
  femur, femoral — *continued*
    condyles, epicondyles — *see* Fracture, femur,
        lower end
    distal end — *see* Fracture, femur, lower end
    epiphysis
      head — *see* Fracture, femur, upper end, epiphysis
      lower — *see* Fracture, femur, lower end, epiphysis
      upper — *see* Fracture, femur, upper end, epiphysis
    following insertion of implant, prosthesis or plate
        M96.66- ✓
    head — *see* Fracture, femur, upper end, head
    intertrochanteric — *see* Fracture, femur,
        trochanteric
    intratrochanteric — *see* Fracture, femur,
        trochanteric
    lower end S72.40- ✓
      condyle (displaced) S72.41- ✓
        lateral (displaced) S72.42- ✓
          nondisplaced S72.42- ✓
        medial (displaced) S72.43- ✓
          nondisplaced S72.43- ✓
        nondisplaced S72.41- ✓
      epiphysis (displaced) S72.44- ✓
        nondisplaced S72.44- ✓
      physeal S79.10- ✓
        Salter-Harris
          Type I S79.11- ✓
          Type II S79.12- ✓
          Type III S79.13- ✓
          Type IV S79.14- ✓
          specified NEC S79.19- ✓
        specified NEC S72.49- ✓
      supracondylar (displaced) S72.45- ✓
        with intracondylar extension (displaced)
            S72.46- ✓
          nondisplaced S72.46- ✓
        nondisplaced S72.45- ✓
      torus S72.47- ✓
    neck — *see* Fracture, femur, upper end, neck
    pertrochanteric — *see* Fracture, femur,
        trochanteric
    shaft (lower third) (middle third) (upper third)
        S72.30- ✓
      comminuted (displaced) S72.35- ✓
        nondisplaced S72.35- ✓
      oblique (displaced) S72.33- ✓
        nondisplaced S72.33- ✓
      segmental (displaced) S72.36- ✓
        nondisplaced S72.36- ✓
      specified NEC S72.39- ✓
      spiral (displaced) S72.34- ✓
        nondisplaced S72.34- ✓
      transverse (displaced) S72.32- ✓
        nondisplaced S72.32- ✓
    specified site NEC — *see* subcategory S72.8 ✓
    subcapital (displaced) S72.01- ✓
    subtrochanteric (region) (section) (displaced)
        S72.2- ✓
      nondisplaced S72.2- ✓
    transcervical — *see* Fracture, femur, upper end,
        neck
    transtrochanteric — *see* Fracture, femur,
        trochanteric
    trochanteric S72.10- ✓
      apophyseal (displaced) S72.13- ✓
        nondisplaced S72.13- ✓
      greater trochanter (displaced) S72.11- ✓
        nondisplaced S72.11- ✓
      intertrochanteric (displaced) S72.14- ✓
        nondisplaced S72.14- ✓
      lesser trochanter (displaced) S72.12- ✓
        nondisplaced S72.12- ✓
    upper end S72.00- ✓
      apophyseal (displaced) S72.13- ✓
        nondisplaced S72.13- ✓
      cervicotrochanteric — *see* Fracture, femur, upper end, neck, base
      epiphysis (displaced) S72.02- ✓
        nondisplaced S72.02- ✓
      head S72.05- ✓
        articular (displaced) S72.06- ✓
          nondisplaced S72.06- ✓

Fracture, traumatic — *continued*
  femur, femoral — *continued*
    upper end — *continued*
      head — *continued*
        specified NEC S72.09- ✓
      intertrochanteric (displaced) S72.14- ✓
        nondisplaced S72.14- ✓
      intracapsular S72.01- ✓
      midcervical (displaced) S72.03- ✓
        nondisplaced S72.03- ✓
      neck S72.00- ✓
        base (displaced) S72.04- ✓
          nondisplaced S72.04- ✓
        specified NEC S72.09- ✓
      pertrochanteric — *see* Fracture, femur, upper
          end, trochanteric
      physeal S79.00- ✓
        Salter-Harris type I S79.01- ✓
        specified NEC S79.09- ✓
      subcapital (displaced) S72.01- ✓
      subtrochanteric (displaced) S72.2- ✓
        nondisplaced S72.2- ✓
      transcervical — *see* Fracture, femur, upper end,
          midcervical
      trochanteric S72.10- ✓
        greater (displaced) S72.11- ✓
          nondisplaced S72.11- ✓
        lesser (displaced) S72.12- ✓
          nondisplaced S72.12- ✓
  fibula (shaft) (styloid) S82.40- ✓
    comminuted (displaced) S82.45- ✓
      nondisplaced S82.45- ✓
    following insertion of implant, prosthesis or plate
        M96.67- ✓
    involving ankle or malleolus — *see* Fracture, fibula,
        lateral malleolus
    lateral malleolus (displaced) S82.6- ✓
      nondisplaced S82.6- ✓
    lower end
      physeal S89.30- ✓
        Salter-Harris
          Type I S89.31- ✓
          Type II S89.32- ✓
        specified NEC S89.39- ✓
      specified NEC S82.83- ✓
      torus S82.82- ✓
    oblique (displaced) S82.43- ✓
      nondisplaced S82.43- ✓
    segmental (displaced) S82.46- ✓
      nondisplaced S82.46- ✓
    specified NEC S82.49- ✓
    spiral (displaced) S82.44- ✓
      nondisplaced S82.44- ✓
    transverse (displaced) S82.42- ✓
      nondisplaced S82.42- ✓
    upper end
      physeal S89.20- ✓
        Salter-Harris
          Type I S89.21- ✓
          Type II S89.22- ✓
        specified NEC S89.29- ✓
      specified NEC S82.83- ✓
      torus S82.81- ✓
  finger (except thumb) S62.60- ✓
    distal phalanx (displaced) S62.63- ✓
      nondisplaced S62.66- ✓
    index S62.60- ✓
      distal phalanx (displaced) S62.63- ✓
        nondisplaced S62.66- ✓
      medial phalanx (displaced) S62.62- ✓
        nondisplaced S62.65- ✓
      proximal phalanx (displaced) S62.61- ✓
        nondisplaced S62.64- ✓
    little S62.60- ✓
      distal phalanx (displaced) S62.63- ✓
        nondisplaced S62.66- ✓
      medial phalanx (displaced) S62.62- ✓
        nondisplaced S62.65- ✓
      proximal phalanx (displaced) S62.61- ✓
        nondisplaced S62.64- ✓
    medial phalanx (displaced) S62.62- ✓
      nondisplaced S62.65- ✓
    middle S62.60- ✓
      distal phalanx (displaced) S62.63- ✓
        nondisplaced S62.66- ✓

Fracture, traumatic — *continued*
  finger — *continued*
    middle — *continued*
      medial phalanx (displaced) S62.62- ✓
        nondisplaced S62.65- ✓
      proximal phalanx (displaced) S62.61- ✓
        nondisplaced S62.64- ✓
    proximal phalanx (displaced) S62.61- ✓
      nondisplaced S62.64- ✓
    ring S62.60- ✓
      distal phalanx (displaced) S62.63- ✓
        nondisplaced S62.66- ✓
      medial phalanx (displaced) S62.62- ✓
        nondisplaced S62.65- ✓
      proximal phalanx (displaced) S62.61- ✓
        nondisplaced S62.64- ✓
    thumb — *see* Fracture, thumb
  following insertion (intraoperative) (postoperative) of
      orthopedic implant, joint prosthesis or bone
      plate M96.69
    femur M96.66- ✓
    fibula M96.67- ✓
    humerus M96.62- ✓
    pelvis M96.65
    radius M96.63- ✓
    specified bone NEC M96.69
    tibia M96.67- ✓
    ulna M96.63- ✓
  foot S92.90- ✓
    astragalus — *see* Fracture, tarsal, talus
    calcaneus — *see* Fracture, tarsal, calcaneus
    cuboid — *see* Fracture, tarsal, cuboid
    cuneiform — *see* Fracture, tarsal, cuneiform
    metatarsal — *see* Fracture, metatarsal
    navicular — *see* Fracture, tarsal, navicular
    talus — *see* Fracture, tarsal, talus
    tarsal — *see* Fracture, tarsal
    toe — *see* Fracture, toe
  forearm S52.9- ✓
    radius — *see* Fracture, radius
    ulna — *see* Fracture, ulna
  fossa (anterior) (middle) (posterior) S02.19 ✓
  frontal (bone) (skull) S02.0 ✓
    sinus S02.19 ✓
  glenoid (cavity) (scapula) — *see* Fracture, scapula,
      glenoid cavity
  greenstick — *see* Fracture, by site
  hallux — *see* Fracture, toe, great
  hand S62.9- ✓
    carpal — *see* Fracture, carpal bone
    finger (except thumb) — *see* Fracture, finger
    metacarpal — *see* Fracture, metacarpal
    navicular (scaphoid) (hand) — *see* Fracture, carpal
        bone, navicular
    thumb — *see* Fracture, thumb
  healed or old
    with complications — *code by* Nature of the complication
  heel bone — *see* Fracture, tarsal, calcaneus
  Hill-Sachs S42.29- ✓
  hip — *see* Fracture, femur, neck
  humerus S42.30- ✓
    anatomical neck — *see* Fracture, humerus, upper
        end
    articular process — *see* Fracture, humerus, lower
        end
    capitellum — *see* Fracture, humerus, lower end,
        condyle, lateral
    distal end — *see* Fracture, humerus, lower end
    epiphysis
      lower — *see* Fracture, humerus, lower end,
          physeal
      upper — *see* Fracture, humerus, upper end,
          physeal
    external condyle — *see* Fracture, humerus, lower
        end, condyle, lateral
    following insertion of implant, prosthesis or plate
        M96.62- ✓
    great tuberosity — *see* Fracture, humerus, upper
        end, greater tuberosity
    intercondylar — *see* Fracture, humerus, lower end
    internal epicondyle — *see* Fracture, humerus,
        lower end, epicondyle, medial
    lesser tuberosity — *see* Fracture, humerus, upper
        end, lesser tuberosity

Fracture, traumatic — *continued*
　humerus — *continued*
　　lower end S42.40- ☑
　　　condyle
　　　　lateral (displaced) S42.45- ☑
　　　　　nondisplaced S42.45- ☑
　　　　medial (displaced) S42.46- ☑
　　　　　nondisplaced S42.46- ☑
　　　epicondyle
　　　　lateral (displaced) S42.43- ☑
　　　　　nondisplaced S42.43- ☑
　　　　medial (displaced) S42.44- ☑
　　　　　incarcerated S42.44- ☑
　　　　　nondisplaced S42.44- ☑
　　　physeal S49.10- ☑
　　　　Salter-Harris
　　　　　Type I S49.11- ☑
　　　　　Type II S49.12- ☑
　　　　　Type III S49.13- ☑
　　　　　Type IV S49.14- ☑
　　　　specified NEC S49.19- ☑
　　　specified NEC (displaced) S42.49- ☑
　　　　nondisplaced S42.49- ☑
　　　supracondylar (simple) (displaced) S42.41- ☑
　　　　comminuted (displaced) S42.42- ☑
　　　　　nondisplaced S42.42- ☑
　　　　nondisplaced S42.41- ☑
　　　torus S42.48- ☑
　　　transcondylar (displaced) S42.47- ☑
　　　　nondisplaced S42.47- ☑
　　proximal end — *see* Fracture, humerus, upper end
　　shaft S42.30- ☑
　　　comminuted (displaced) S42.35- ☑
　　　　nondisplaced S42.35- ☑
　　　greenstick S42.31- ☑
　　　oblique (displaced) S42.33- ☑
　　　　nondisplaced S42.33- ☑
　　　segmental (displaced) S42.36- ☑
　　　　nondisplaced S42.36- ☑
　　　specified NEC S42.39- ☑
　　　spiral (displaced) S42.34- ☑
　　　　nondisplaced S42.34- ☑
　　　transverse (displaced) S42.32- ☑
　　　　nondisplaced S42.32- ☑
　　supracondylar — *see* Fracture, humerus, lower end
　　surgical neck — *see* Fracture, humerus, upper end, surgical neck
　　trochlea — *see* Fracture, humerus, lower end, condyle, medial
　　tuberosity — *see* Fracture, humerus, upper end
　　upper end S42.20- ☑
　　　anatomical neck — *see* Fracture, humerus, upper end, specified NEC
　　　articular head — *see* Fracture, humerus, upper end, specified NEC
　　　epiphysis — *see* Fracture, humerus, upper end, physeal
　　　greater tuberosity (displaced) S42.25- ☑
　　　　nondisplaced S42.25- ☑
　　　lesser tuberosity (displaced) S42.26- ☑
　　　　nondisplaced S42.26- ☑
　　　physeal S49.00- ☑
　　　　Salter-Harris
　　　　　Type I S49.01- ☑
　　　　　Type II S49.02- ☑
　　　　　Type III S49.03- ☑
　　　　　Type IV S49.04- ☑
　　　　specified NEC S49.09- ☑
　　　specified NEC (displaced) S42.29- ☑
　　　　nondisplaced S42.29- ☑
　　　surgical neck (displaced) S42.21- ☑
　　　　four-part S42.24- ☑
　　　　nondisplaced S42.21- ☑
　　　　three-part S42.23- ☑
　　　　two-part (displaced) S42.22- ☑
　　　　　nondisplaced S42.22- ☑
　　　torus S42.27- ☑
　　　transepiphyseal — *see* Fracture, humerus, upper end, physeal
　hyoid bone S12.8 ☑
　ilium S32.30- ☑
　　with disruption of pelvic ring — *see* Disruption, pelvic ring
　　avulsion (displaced) S32.31- ☑
　　　nondisplaced S32.31- ☑
　　specified NEC S32.39- ☑

Fracture, traumatic — *continued*
　impaction, impacted — *code as* Fracture, by site
　innominate bone — *see* Fracture, ilium
　instep — *see* Fracture, foot
　ischium S32.60- ☑
　　with disruption of pelvic ring — *see* Disruption, pelvic ring
　　avulsion (displaced) S32.61- ☑
　　　nondisplaced S32.61- ☑
　　specified NEC S32.69- ☑
　jaw (bone) (lower) — *see* Fracture, mandible
　　upper — *see* Fracture, maxilla
　joint prosthesis — *see* Complications, joint prosthesis, mechanical, breakdown, by site
　　periprosthetic — *see* Complications, joint prosthesis, mechanical, periprosthesis, fracture, by site
　knee cap — *see* Fracture, patella
　larynx S12.8 ☑
　late effects — *see* Sequelae, fracture
　leg (lower) S82.9- ☑
　　ankle — *see* Fracture, ankle
　　femur — *see* Fracture, femur
　　fibula — *see* Fracture, fibula
　　malleolus — *see* Fracture, ankle
　　patella — *see* Fracture, patella
　　specified site NEC S82.89- ☑
　　tibia — *see* Fracture, tibia
　lumbar spine — *see* Fracture, vertebra, lumbar
　lumbosacral spine S32.9
　Maisonneuve's (displaced) S82.86- ☑
　　nondisplaced S82.86- ☑
　malar bone (*see also* Fracture, maxilla) S02.400 ☑
　malleolus — *see* Fracture, ankle
　malunion — *see* Fracture, by site
　mandible (lower jaw (bone)) S02.609 ☑
　　alveolus S02.67 ☑
　　angle (of jaw) S02.65 ☑
　　body, unspecified S02.600 ☑
　　condylar process S02.61 ☑
　　coronoid process S02.63 ☑
　　ramus, unspecified S02.64 ☑
　　specified site NEC S02.69 ☑
　　subcondylar process S02.62 ☑
　　symphysis S02.66 ☑
　manubrium (sterni) S22.21 ☑
　　dissociation from sternum S22.23 ☑
　march — *see* Fracture, traumatic, stress, by site
　maxilla, maxillary (bone) (sinus) (superior) (upper jaw) S02.401 ☑
　　alveolus S02.42 ☑
　　inferior — *see* Fracture, mandible
　　LeFort I S02.411 ☑
　　LeFort II S02.412 ☑
　　LeFort III S02.413 ☑
　metacarpal S62.309 ☑
　　base (displaced) S62.319 ☑
　　　nondisplaced S62.349 ☑
　　fifth S62.30- ☑
　　　base (displaced) S62.31- ☑
　　　　nondisplaced S62.34- ☑
　　　neck (displaced) S62.33- ☑
　　　　nondisplaced S62.36- ☑
　　　shaft (displaced) S62.32- ☑
　　　　nondisplaced S62.35- ☑
　　　specified NEC S62.398 ☑
　　first S62.20- ☑
　　　base NEC (displaced) S62.23- ☑
　　　　nondisplaced S62.23- ☑
　　　Bennett's — *see* Bennett's fracture
　　　neck (displaced) S62.25- ☑
　　　　nondisplaced S62.25- ☑
　　　shaft (displaced) S62.24- ☑
　　　　nondisplaced S62.24- ☑
　　　specified NEC S62.29- ☑
　　fourth S62.30- ☑
　　　base (displaced) S62.31- ☑
　　　　nondisplaced S62.34- ☑
　　　neck (displaced) S62.33- ☑
　　　　nondisplaced S62.36- ☑
　　　shaft (displaced) S62.32- ☑
　　　　nondisplaced S62.35- ☑
　　　specified NEC S62.39- ☑
　　neck (displaced) S62.33- ☑
　　　nondisplaced S62.36- ☑
　　Rolando's — *see* Rolando's fracture

Fracture, traumatic — *continued*
　metacarpal — *continued*
　　second S62.30- ☑
　　　base (displaced) S62.31- ☑
　　　　nondisplaced S62.34- ☑
　　　neck (displaced) S62.33- ☑
　　　　nondisplaced S62.36- ☑
　　　shaft (displaced) S62.32- ☑
　　　　nondisplaced S62.35- ☑
　　　specified NEC S62.39- ☑
　　shaft (displaced) S62.32- ☑
　　　nondisplaced S62.35- ☑
　　specified NEC S62.399 ☑
　　third S62.30- ☑
　　　base (displaced) S62.31- ☑
　　　　nondisplaced S62.34- ☑
　　　neck (displaced) S62.33- ☑
　　　　nondisplaced S62.36- ☑
　　　shaft (displaced) S62.32- ☑
　　　　nondisplaced S62.35- ☑
　　　specified NEC S62.39- ☑
　metastatic — *see* Fracture, pathological, due to, neoplastic disease (*see also* Neoplasm)
　metatarsal bone S92.30- ☑
　　fifth (displaced) S92.35- ☑
　　　nondisplaced S92.35- ☑
　　first (displaced) S92.31- ☑
　　　nondisplaced S92.31- ☑
　　fourth (displaced) S92.34- ☑
　　　nondisplaced S92.34- ☑
　　second (displaced) S92.32- ☑
　　　nondisplaced S92.32- ☑
　　third (displaced) S92.33- ☑
　　　nondisplaced S92.33- ☑
　Monteggia's — *see* Monteggia's fracture
　multiple
　　hand (and wrist) NEC — *see* Fracture, by site
　　ribs — *see* Fracture, rib, multiple
　nasal (bone(s)) S02.2 ☑
　navicular (scaphoid) (foot) (*see also* Fracture, tarsal, navicular)
　　hand — *see* Fracture, carpal, navicular
　neck S12.9 ☑
　　cervical vertebra S12.9 ☑
　　　fifth (displaced) S12.400 ☑
　　　　nondisplaced S12.401 ☑
　　　　specified type NEC (displaced) S12.490 ☑
　　　　　nondisplaced S12.491 ☑
　　　first (displaced) S12.000 ☑
　　　　burst (stable) S12.01 ☑
　　　　　unstable S12.02 ☑
　　　　lateral mass (displaced) S12.040 ☑
　　　　　nondisplaced S12.041 ☑
　　　　nondisplaced S12.001 ☑
　　　　posterior arch (displaced) S12.030 ☑
　　　　　nondisplaced S12.031 ☑
　　　　specified type NEC (displaced) S12.090 ☑
　　　　　nondisplaced S12.091 ☑
　　　fourth (displaced) S12.300 ☑
　　　　nondisplaced S12.301 ☑
　　　　specified type NEC (displaced) S12.390 ☑
　　　　　nondisplaced S12.391 ☑
　　　second (displaced) S12.100 ☑
　　　　dens (anterior) (displaced) (type II) S12.110 ☑
　　　　　nondisplaced S12.112 ☑
　　　　　posterior S12.111 ☑
　　　　　specified type NEC (displaced) S12.120 ☑
　　　　　　nondisplaced S12.121 ☑
　　　　nondisplaced S12.101 ☑
　　　　specified type NEC (displaced) S12.190 ☑
　　　　　nondisplaced S12.191 ☑
　　　seventh (displaced) S12.600 ☑
　　　　nondisplaced S12.601 ☑
　　　　specified type NEC (displaced) S12.690 ☑
　　　　　displaced S12.691 ☑
　　　sixth (displaced) S12.500 ☑
　　　　nondisplaced S12.501 ☑
　　　　specified type NEC (displaced) S12.590 ☑
　　　　　displaced S12.591 ☑
　　　third (displaced) S12.200 ☑
　　　　nondisplaced S12.201 ☑
　　　　specified type NEC (displaced) S12.290 ☑
　　　　　displaced S12.291 ☑

Fracture, traumatic — *continued*
- neck — *continued*
  - hyoid bone S12.8 ☑
  - larynx S12.8 ☑
  - specified site NEC S12.8 ☑
  - thyroid cartilage S12.8 ☑
  - trachea S12.8 ☑
- neoplastic NEC — *see* Fracture, pathological, due to, neoplastic disease
- neural arch — *see* Fracture, vertebra
- newborn — *see* Birth, injury, fracture
- nontraumatic — *see* Fracture, pathological
- nonunion — *see* Nonunion, fracture
- nose, nasal (bone) (septum) S02.2 ☑
- occiput — *see* Fracture, skull, base, occiput
- odontoid process — *see* Fracture, neck, cervical vertebra, second
- olecranon (process) (ulna) — *see* Fracture, ulna, upper end, olecranon process
- orbit, orbital (bone) (region) S02.8 ☑
  - floor (blow-out) S02.3 ☑
  - roof S02.19 ☑
- os
  - calcis — *see* Fracture, tarsal, calcaneus
  - magnum — *see* Fracture, carpal, capitate
  - pubis — *see* Fracture, pubis
- palate S02.8 ☑
- parietal bone (skull) S02.0 ☑
- patella S82.00- ☑
  - comminuted (displaced) S82.04- ☑
    - nondisplaced S82.04- ☑
  - longitudinal (displaced) S82.02- ☑
    - nondisplaced S82.02- ☑
  - osteochondral (displaced) S82.01- ☑
    - nondisplaced S82.01- ☑
  - specified NEC S82.09- ☑
  - transverse (displaced) S82.03- ☑
    - nondisplaced S82.03- ☑
- pedicle (of vertebral arch) — *see* Fracture, vertebra
- pelvis, pelvic (bone) S32.9 ☑
  - acetabulum — *see* Fracture, acetabulum
  - circle — *see* Disruption, pelvic ring
  - following insertion of implant, prosthesis or plate M96.65
  - ilium — *see* Fracture, ilium
  - ischium — *see* Fracture, ischium
  - multiple
    - with disruption of pelvic ring (circle) — *see* Disruption, pelvic ring
    - without disruption of pelvic ring (circle) S32.82 ☑
  - pubis — *see* Fracture, pubis
  - sacrum — *see* Fracture, sacrum
  - specified site NEC S32.89 ☑
- phalanx
  - foot — *see* Fracture, toe
  - hand — *see* Fracture, finger
- pisiform — *see* Fracture, carpal, pisiform
- pond — *see* Fracture, skull
- prosthetic device, internal — *see* Complications, prosthetic device, by site, mechanical
- pubis S32.50- ☑
  - with disruption of pelvic ring — *see* Disruption, pelvic ring
  - specified site NEC S32.59- ☑
  - superior rim S32.51- ☑
- radius S52.9- ☑
  - distal end — *see* Fracture, radius, lower end
  - following insertion of implant, prosthesis or plate M96.63- ☑
  - head — *see* Fracture, radius, upper end, head
  - lower end S52.50- ☑
    - Barton's — *see* Barton's fracture
    - Colles' — *see* Colles' fracture
    - extraarticular NEC S52.55- ☑
    - intraarticular NEC S52.57- ☑
    - physeal S59.20- ☑
      - Salter-Harris
        - Type I S59.21- ☑
        - Type II S59.22- ☑
        - Type III S59.23- ☑
        - Type IV S59.24- ☑
        - specified NEC S59.29- ☑
    - Smith's — *see* Smith's fracture
    - specified NEC S52.59- ☑

Fracture, traumatic — *continued*
- radius — *continued*
  - lower end — *continued*
    - styloid process (displaced) S52.51- ☑
      - nondisplaced S52.51- ☑
    - torus S52.52- ☑
  - neck — *see* Fracture, radius, upper end
  - proximal end — *see* Fracture, radius, upper end
  - shaft S52.30- ☑
    - bent bone S52.38- ☑
    - comminuted (displaced) S52.35- ☑
      - nondisplaced S52.35- ☑
    - Galeazzi's — *see* Galeazzi's fracture
    - greenstick S52.31- ☑
    - oblique (displaced) S52.33- ☑
      - nondisplaced S52.33- ☑
    - segmental (displaced) S52.36- ☑
      - nondisplaced S52.36- ☑
    - specified NEC S52.39- ☑
    - spiral (displaced) S52.34- ☑
      - nondisplaced S52.34- ☑
    - transverse (displaced) S52.32- ☑
      - nondisplaced S52.32- ☑
  - upper end S52.10- ☑
    - head (displaced) S52.12- ☑
      - nondisplaced S52.12- ☑
    - neck (displaced) S52.13- ☑
      - nondisplaced S52.13- ☑
    - physeal S59.10- ☑
      - Salter-Harris
        - Type I S59.11- ☑
        - Type II S59.12- ☑
        - Type III S59.13- ☑
        - Type IV S59.14- ☑
        - specified NEC S59.19- ☑
    - specified NEC S52.18- ☑
    - torus S52.11- ☑
- ramus
  - inferior or superior, pubis — *see* Fracture, pubis
  - mandible — *see* Fracture, mandible
- restorative material (dental) K08.539
  - with loss of material K08.531
  - without loss of material K08.530
- rib S22.3- ☑
  - with flail chest — *see* Flail, chest
  - multiple S22.4- ☑
    - with flail chest — *see* Flail, chest
- root, tooth — *see* Fracture, tooth
- sacrum S32.10 ☑
  - specified NEC S32.19 ☑
  - Type
    - 1 S32.14 ☑
    - 2 S32.15 ☑
    - 3 S32.16 ☑
    - 4 S32.17 ☑
  - Zone
    - I S32.119 ☑
      - displaced (minimally) S32.111 ☑
        - severely S32.112 ☑
      - nondisplaced S32.110 ☑
    - II S32.129 ☑
      - displaced (minimally) S32.121 ☑
        - severely S32.122 ☑
      - nondisplaced S32.120 ☑
    - III S32.139 ☑
      - displaced (minimally) S32.131 ☑
        - severely S32.132 ☑
      - nondisplaced S32.130 ☑
- scaphoid (hand) (*see also* Fracture, carpal, navicular)
  - foot — *see* Fracture, tarsal, navicular
- scapula S42.10- ☑
  - acromial process (displaced) S42.12- ☑
    - nondisplaced S42.12- ☑
  - body (displaced) S42.11- ☑
    - nondisplaced S42.11- ☑
  - coracoid process (displaced) S42.13- ☑
    - nondisplaced S42.13- ☑
  - glenoid cavity (displaced) S42.14- ☑
    - nondisplaced S42.14- ☑
  - neck (displaced) S42.15- ☑
    - nondisplaced S42.15- ☑
  - specified NEC S42.19- ☑
- semilunar bone, wrist — *see* Fracture, carpal, lunate
- sequelae — *see* Sequelae, fracture
- sesamoid bone
  - hand — *see* Fracture, carpal

Fracture, traumatic — *continued*
- sesamoid bone — *continued*
  - other — *code by* site under Fracture
- shepherd's — *see* Fracture, tarsal, talus
- shoulder (girdle) S42.9- ☑
  - blade — *see* Fracture, scapula
- sinus (ethmoid) (frontal) S02.19 ☑
- skull S02.91 ☑
  - base S02.10 ☑
    - occiput S02.119 ☑
      - condyle S02.113 ☑
        - type I S02.110 ☑
        - type II S02.111 ☑
        - type III S02.112 ☑
        - specified NEC S02.118 ☑
      - specified NEC S02.19 ☑
  - birth injury P13.0
  - frontal bone S02.0 ☑
  - parietal bone S02.0 ☑
  - specified site NEC S02.8 ☑
  - temporal bone S02.19 ☑
  - vault S02.0 ☑
- Smith's — *see* Smith's fracture
- sphenoid (bone) (sinus) S02.19 ☑
- spine — *see* Fracture, vertebra
- spinous process — *see* Fracture, vertebra
- spontaneous (cause unknown) — *see* Fracture, pathological
- stave (of thumb) — *see* Fracture, metacarpal, first
- sternum S22.20 ☑
  - with flail chest — *see* Flail, chest
  - body S22.22 ☑
  - manubrium S22.21 ☑
  - xiphoid (process) S22.24 ☑
- stress M84.30 ☑
  - ankle M84.37- ☑
  - carpus M84.34- ☑
  - clavicle M84.31- ☑
  - femoral neck M84.359 ☑
  - femur M84.35- ☑
  - fibula M84.36- ☑
  - finger M84.34- ☑
  - hip M84.359 ☑
  - humerus M84.32- ☑
  - ilium M84.350 ☑
  - ischium M84.350 ☑
  - metacarpus M84.34- ☑
  - metatarsus M84.37- ☑
  - neck — *see* Fracture, fatigue, vertebra
  - pelvis M84.350 ☑
  - radius M84.33- ☑
  - rib M84.38 ☑
  - scapula M84.31- ☑
  - skull M84.38 ☑
  - tarsus M84.37- ☑
  - tibia M84.36- ☑
  - toe M84.37- ☑
  - ulna M84.33- ☑
  - vertebra — *see* Fracture, fatigue, vertebra
- supracondylar, elbow — *see* Fracture, humerus, lower end, supracondylar
- symphysis pubis — *see* Fracture, pubis
- talus (ankle bone) — *see* Fracture, tarsal, talus
- tarsal bone(s) S92.20- ☑
  - astragalus — *see* Fracture, tarsal, talus
  - calcaneus S92.00- ☑
    - anterior process (displaced) S92.02- ☑
      - nondisplaced S92.02- ☑
    - body (displaced) S92.01- ☑
      - nondisplaced S92.01- ☑
    - extraarticular NEC (displaced) S92.05- ☑
      - nondisplaced S92.05- ☑
    - intraarticular (displaced) S92.06- ☑
      - nondisplaced S92.06- ☑
    - tuberosity (displaced) S92.04- ☑
      - avulsion (displaced) S92.03- ☑
        - nondisplaced S92.03- ☑
      - nondisplaced S92.04- ☑
  - cuboid (displaced) S92.21- ☑
    - nondisplaced S92.21- ☑
  - cuneiform
    - intermediate (displaced) S92.23- ☑
      - nondisplaced S92.23- ☑
    - lateral (displaced) S92.22- ☑
      - nondisplaced S92.22- ☑

Fracture, traumatic — *continued*
   tarsal bone(s) — *continued*
     cuneiform — *continued*
      medial (displaced) S92.24- ☑
       nondisplaced S92.24- ☑
     navicular (displaced) S92.25- ☑
      nondisplaced S92.25- ☑
     scaphoid — *see* Fracture, tarsal, navicular
     talus S92.10- ☑
      avulsion (displaced) S92.15- ☑
       nondisplaced S92.15- ☑
      body (displaced) S92.12- ☑
       nondisplaced S92.12- ☑
      dome (displaced) S92.14- ☑
       nondisplaced S92.14- ☑
      head (displaced) S92.12- ☑
       nondisplaced S92.12- ☑
      lateral process (displaced) S92.14- ☑
       nondisplaced S92.14- ☑
      neck (displaced) S92.11- ☑
       nondisplaced S92.11- ☑
      posterior process (displaced) S92.13- ☑
       nondisplaced S92.13- ☑
      specified NEC S92.19- ☑
   temporal bone (styloid) S02.19 ☑
   thorax (bony) S22.9 ☑
    with flail chest — *see* Flail, chest
    rib S22.3- ☑
     multiple S22.4- ☑
      with flail chest — *see* Flail, chest
    sternum S22.20 ☑
     body S22.22 ☑
     manubrium S22.21 ☑
     xiphoid process S22.24 ☑
    vertebra (displaced) S22.009 ☑
     burst (stable) S22.001 ☑
      unstable S22.002 ☑
     eighth S22.069 ☑
      burst (stable) S22.061 ☑
       unstable S22.062 ☑
      specified type NEC S22.068 ☑
      wedge compression S22.060 ☑
     eleventh S22.089 ☑
      burst (stable) S22.081 ☑
       unstable S22.082 ☑
      specified type NEC S22.088 ☑
      wedge compression S22.080 ☑
     fifth S22.059 ☑
      burst (stable) S22.051 ☑
       unstable S22.052 ☑
      specified type NEC S22.058 ☑
      wedge compression S22.050 ☑
     first S22.019 ☑
      burst (stable) S22.011 ☑
       unstable S22.012 ☑
      specified type NEC S22.018 ☑
      wedge compression S22.010 ☑
     fourth S22.049 ☑
      burst (stable) S22.041 ☑
       unstable S22.042 ☑
      specified type NEC S22.048 ☑
      wedge compression S22.040 ☑
     ninth S22.079 ☑
      burst (stable) S22.071 ☑
       unstable S22.072 ☑
      specified type NEC S22.078 ☑
      wedge compression S22.070 ☑
     nondisplaced S22.001 ☑
     second S22.029 ☑
      burst (stable) S22.021 ☑
       unstable S22.022 ☑
      specified type NEC S22.028 ☑
      wedge compression S22.020 ☑
     seventh S22.069 ☑
      burst (stable) S22.061 ☑
       unstable S22.062 ☑
      specified type NEC S22.068 ☑
      wedge compression S22.060 ☑
     sixth S22.059 ☑
      burst (stable) S22.051 ☑
       unstable S22.052 ☑
      specified type NEC S22.058 ☑
      wedge compression S22.050 ☑
     specified type NEC S22.008 ☑

Fracture, traumatic — *continued*
   thorax — *continued*
    vertebra — *continued*
     tenth S22.079 ☑
      burst (stable) S22.071 ☑
       unstable S22.072 ☑
      specified type NEC S22.078 ☑
      wedge compression S22.070 ☑
     third S22.039 ☑
      burst (stable) S22.031 ☑
       unstable S22.032 ☑
      specified type NEC S22.038 ☑
      wedge compression S22.030 ☑
     twelfth S22.089 ☑
      burst (stable) S22.081 ☑
       unstable S22.082 ☑
      specified type NEC S22.088 ☑
      wedge compression S22.080 ☑
     wedge compression S22.000 ☑
   thumb S62.50- ☑
    distal phalanx (displaced) S62.52- ☑
     nondisplaced S62.52- ☑
    proximal phalanx (displaced) S62.51- ☑
     nondisplaced S62.51- ☑
   thyroid cartilage S12.8 ☑
   tibia (shaft) S82.20- ☑
    comminuted (displaced) S82.25- ☑
     nondisplaced S82.25- ☑
    condyles — *see* Fracture, tibia, upper end
    distal end — *see* Fracture, tibia, lower end
    epiphysis
     lower — *see* Fracture, tibia, lower end
     upper — *see* Fracture, tibia, upper end
    following insertion of implant, prosthesis or plate
     M96.67- ☑
    head (involving knee joint) — *see* Fracture, tibia, upper end
    intercondyloid eminence — *see* Fracture, tibia, upper end
    involving ankle or malleolus — *see* Fracture, ankle, medial malleolus
    lower end S82.30- ☑
     physeal S89.10- ☑
      Salter-Harris
       Type I S89.11- ☑
       Type II S89.12- ☑
       Type III S89.13- ☑
       Type IV S89.14- ☑
      specified NEC S89.19- ☑
     pilon (displaced) S82.87- ☑
      nondisplaced S82.87- ☑
     specified NEC S82.39- ☑
     torus S82.31- ☑
    malleolus — *see* Fracture, ankle, medial malleolus
    oblique (displaced) S82.23- ☑
     nondisplaced S82.23- ☑
    pilon — *see* Fracture, tibia, lower end, pilon
    proximal end — *see* Fracture, tibia, upper end
    segmental (displaced) S82.26- ☑
     nondisplaced S82.26- ☑
    specified NEC S82.29- ☑
    spine — *see* Fracture, tibia, upper end, spine
    spiral (displaced) S82.24- ☑
     nondisplaced S82.24- ☑
    transverse (displaced) S82.22- ☑
     nondisplaced S82.22- ☑
    tuberosity — *see* Fracture, tibia, upper end, tuberosity
    upper end S82.10- ☑
     bicondylar (displaced) S82.14- ☑
      nondisplaced S82.14- ☑
     lateral condyle (displaced) S82.12- ☑
      nondisplaced S82.12- ☑
     medial condyle (displaced) S82.13- ☑
      nondisplaced S82.13- ☑
     physeal S89.00- ☑
      Salter-Harris
       Type I S89.01- ☑
       Type II S89.02- ☑
       Type III S89.03- ☑
       Type IV S89.04- ☑
      specified NEC S89.09- ☑
     plateau — *see* Fracture, tibia, upper end, bicondylar
     specified NEC S82.19- ☑
     spine

Fracture, traumatic — *continued*
   tibia — *continued*
    upper end — *continued*
     spine (displaced) S82.11- ☑
      nondisplaced S82.11- ☑
     torus S82.16- ☑
     tuberosity (displaced) S82.15- ☑
      nondisplaced S82.15- ☑
   toe S92.91- ☑
    great (displaced) S92.40- ☑
     distal phalanx (displaced) S92.42- ☑
      nondisplaced S92.42- ☑
     nondisplaced S92.40- ☑
     proximal phalanx (displaced) S92.41- ☑
      nondisplaced S92.41- ☑
     specified NEC S92.49- ☑
    lesser (displaced) S92.50- ☑
     distal phalanx (displaced) S92.53- ☑
      nondisplaced S92.53- ☑
     medial phalanx (displaced) S92.52- ☑
      nondisplaced S92.52- ☑
     nondisplaced S92.50- ☑
     proximal phalanx (displaced) S92.51- ☑
      nondisplaced S92.51- ☑
     specified NEC S92.59- ☑
   tooth (root) S02.5 ☑
   trachea (cartilage) S12.8 ☑
   transverse process — *see* Fracture, vertebra
   trapezium or trapezoid bone — *see* Fracture, carpal
   trimalleolar — *see* Fracture, ankle, trimalleolar
   triquetrum (cuneiform of carpus) — *see* Fracture, carpal, triquetrum
   trochanter — *see* Fracture, femur, trochanteric
   tuberosity (external) — *code by* site under Fracture
   ulna (shaft) S52.20- ☑
    bent bone S52.28- ☑
    coronoid process — *see* Fracture, ulna, upper end, coronoid process
    distal end — *see* Fracture, ulna, lower end
    following insertion of implant, prosthesis or plate M96.63- ☑
    head S52.00- ☑
    lower end S52.60- ☑
     physeal S59.00- ☑
      Salter-Harris
       Type I S59.01- ☑
       Type II S59.02- ☑
       Type III S59.03- ☑
       Type IV S59.04- ☑
      specified NEC S59.09- ☑
     specified NEC S52.69- ☑
     styloid process (displaced) S52.61- ☑
      nondisplaced S52.61- ☑
     torus S52.62- ☑
    proximal end — *see* Fracture, ulna, upper end
    shaft S52.20- ☑
     comminuted (displaced) S52.25- ☑
      nondisplaced S52.25- ☑
     greenstick S52.21- ☑
     Monteggia's — *see* Monteggia's fracture
     oblique (displaced) S52.23- ☑
      nondisplaced S52.23- ☑
     segmental (displaced) S52.26- ☑
      nondisplaced S52.26- ☑
     specified NEC S52.29- ☑
     spiral (displaced) S52.24- ☑
      nondisplaced S52.24- ☑
     transverse (displaced) S52.22- ☑
      nondisplaced S52.22- ☑
    upper end S52.00- ☑
     coronoid process (displaced) S52.04- ☑
      nondisplaced S52.04- ☑
     olecranon process (displaced) S52.02- ☑
      with intraarticular extension S52.03- ☑
      nondisplaced S52.02- ☑
       with intraarticular extension S52.03- ☑
     specified NEC S52.09- ☑
     torus S52.01- ☑
   unciform — *see* Fracture, carpal, hamate
   vault of skull S02.0 ☑
   vertebra, vertebral (arch) (body) (column) (neural arch) (pedicle) (spinous process) (transverse process)
    atlas — *see* Fracture, neck, cervical vertebra, first
    axis — *see* Fracture, neck, cervical vertebra, second

Fracture, traumatic — *continued*
　vertebra, vertebral — *continued*
　　cervical (teardrop) S12.9 ☑
　　　axis — *see* Fracture, neck, cervical vertebra, second
　　　first (atlas) — *see* Fracture, neck, cervical vertebra, first
　　　second (axis) — *see* Fracture, neck, cervical vertebra, second
　　chronic M84.48 ☑
　　coccyx S32.2 ☑
　　dorsal — *see* Fracture, thorax, vertebra
　　lumbar S32.009 ☑
　　　burst (stable) S32.001 ☑
　　　　unstable S32.002 ☑
　　　fifth S32.059 ☑
　　　　burst (stable) S32.051 ☑
　　　　　unstable S32.052 ☑
　　　　specified type NEC S32.058 ☑
　　　　wedge compression S32.050 ☑
　　　first S32.019 ☑
　　　　burst (stable) S32.011 ☑
　　　　　unstable S32.012 ☑
　　　　specified type NEC S32.018 ☑
　　　　wedge compression S32.010 ☑
　　　fourth S32.049 ☑
　　　　burst (stable) S32.041 ☑
　　　　　unstable S32.042 ☑
　　　　specified type NEC S32.048 ☑
　　　　wedge compression S32.040 ☑
　　　second S32.029 ☑
　　　　burst (stable) S32.021 ☑
　　　　　unstable S32.022 ☑
　　　　specified type NEC S32.028 ☑
　　　　wedge compression S32.020 ☑
　　　specified type NEC S32.008 ☑
　　　third S32.039 ☑
　　　　burst (stable) S32.031 ☑
　　　　　unstable S32.032 ☑
　　　　specified type NEC S32.038 ☑
　　　　wedge compression S32.030 ☑
　　　wedge compression S32.000 ☑
　　metastatic — *see* Collapse, vertebra, in, specified disease NEC (*see also* Neoplasm)
　　newborn (birth injury) P11.5
　　sacrum S32.10 ☑
　　　specified NEC S32.19 ☑
　　　Type
　　　　1 S32.14 ☑
　　　　2 S32.15 ☑
　　　　3 S32.16 ☑
　　　　4 S32.17 ☑
　　　Zone
　　　　I S32.119 ☑
　　　　　displaced (minimally) S32.111 ☑
　　　　　　severely S32.112 ☑
　　　　　nondisplaced S32.110 ☑
　　　　II S32.129 ☑
　　　　　displaced (minimally) S32.121 ☑
　　　　　　severely S32.122 ☑
　　　　　nondisplaced S32.120 ☑
　　　　III S32.139 ☑
　　　　　displaced (minimally) S32.131 ☑
　　　　　　severely S32.132 ☑
　　　　　nondisplaced S32.130 ☑
　　thoracic — *see* Fracture, thorax, vertebra
　vertex S02.0 ☑
　vomer (bone) S02.2 ☑
　wrist S62.10- ☑
　　carpal — *see* Fracture, carpal bone
　　navicular (scaphoid) (hand) — *see* Fracture, carpal, navicular
　xiphisternum, xiphoid (process) S22.24 ☑
　zygoma S02.402 ☑
Fragile, fragility
　autosomal site Q95.5
　bone, congenital (with blue sclera) Q78.0
　capillary (hereditary) D69.8
　hair L67.8
　nails L60.3
　non-sex chromosome site Q95.5
　X chromosome Q99.2
Fragilitas
　crinium L67.8
　ossium (with blue sclerae) (hereditary) Q78.0
　unguium L60.3

Fragilitas — *continued*
　unguium L60.3
　　congenital Q84.6
Fragments, cataract (lens), **following cataract surgery** H59.02- ☑
　retained foreign body — *see* Retained, foreign body fragments (type of)
Frailty (frail) R54
　mental R41.81
Frambesia, frambesial (tropica) (*see also* Yaws)
　initial lesion or ulcer A66.0
　primary A66.0
Frambeside
　gummatous A66.4
　of early yaws A66.2
Frambesioma A66.1
Franceschetti-Klein (-Wildervanck) **disease or syndrome** Q75.4
Francis' disease — *see* Tularemia
Franklin disease C88.2
Frank's essential thrombocytopenia D69.3
Fraser's syndrome Q87.0
Freckle(s) L81.2
　malignant melanoma in — *see* Melanoma
　melanotic (Hutchinson's) — *see* Melanoma, in situ
　retinal D49.81
Frederickson's hyperlipoproteinemia, type
　I and V E78.3
　IIA E78.0
　IIB and III E78.2
　IV E78.1
Freeman Sheldon syndrome Q87.0
Freezing (*see also* Effect, adverse, cold) T69.9 ☑
Freiberg's disease (infraction of metatarsal head or osteochondrosis) — *see* Osteochondrosis, juvenile, metatarsus
Frei's disease A55
Fremitus, friction, cardiac R01.2
Frenum, frenulum
　external os Q51.828
　tongue (shortening) (congenital) Q38.1
Frequency micturition (nocturnal) R35.0
　psychogenic F45.8
Frey's syndrome
　auriculotemporal G50.8
　hyperhidrosis L74.52
Friction
　burn — *see* Burn, by site
　fremitus, cardiac R01.2
　precordial R01.2
　sounds, chest R09.89
Friderichsen-Waterhouse syndrome or disease A39.1
Friedländer's B (bacillus) **NEC** (*see also* condition) A49.8
Friedreich's
　ataxia G11.1
　combined systemic disease G11.1
　facial hemihypertrophy Q67.4
　sclerosis (cerebellum) (spinal cord) G11.1
Frigidity F52.22
Fröhlich's syndrome E23.6
Frontal (*see also* condition)
　lobe syndrome F07.0
Frostbite (superficial) T33.90 ☑
　with
　　partial thickness skin loss — *see* Frostbite (superficial), by site
　　tissue necrosis T34.90 ☑
　abdominal wall T33.3 ☑
　　with tissue necrosis T34.3 ☑
　ankle T33.81- ☑
　　with tissue necrosis T34.81- ☑
　arm T33.4- ☑
　　with tissue necrosis T34.4- ☑
　　finger(s) — *see* Frostbite, finger
　　hand — *see* Frostbite, hand
　　wrist — *see* Frostbite, wrist
　ear T33.01- ☑
　　with tissue necrosis T34.01- ☑
　face T33.09 ☑
　　with tissue necrosis T34.09 ☑
　finger T33.53- ☑
　　with tissue necrosis T34.53- ☑
　foot T33.82- ☑
　　with tissue necrosis T34.82- ☑
　hand T33.52- ☑
　　with tissue necrosis T34.52- ☑

Frostbite — *continued*
　head T33.09 ☑
　　with tissue necrosis T34.09 ☑
　　ear — *see* Frostbite, ear
　　nose — *see* Frostbite, nose
　hip (and thigh) T33.6- ☑
　　with tissue necrosis T34.6- ☑
　knee T33.7- ☑
　　with tissue necrosis T34.7- ☑
　leg T33.9- ☑
　　with tissue necrosis T34.9- ☑
　　ankle — *see* Frostbite, ankle
　　foot — *see* Frostbite, foot
　　knee — *see* Frostbite, knee
　　lower T33.7- ☑
　　　with tissue necrosis T34.7- ☑
　　thigh — *see* Frostbite, hip
　　toe — *see* Frostbite, toe
　limb
　　lower T33.99 ☑
　　　with tissue necrosis T34.99 ☑
　　upper — *see* Frostbite, arm
　neck T33.1 ☑
　　with tissue necrosis T34.1 ☑
　nose T33.02 ☑
　　with tissue necrosis T34.02 ☑
　pelvis T33.3 ☑
　　with tissue necrosis T34.3 ☑
　specified site NEC T33.99 ☑
　　with tissue necrosis T34.99 ☑
　thigh — *see* Frostbite, hip
　thorax T33.2 ☑
　　with tissue necrosis T34.2 ☑
　toes T33.83- ☑
　　with tissue necrosis T34.83- ☑
　trunk T33.99 ☑
　　with tissue necrosis T34.99 ☑
　wrist T33.51- ☑
　　with tissue necrosis T34.51- ☑
Frotteurism F65.81
Frozen (*see also* Effect, adverse, cold) T69.9 ☑
　pelvis (female) N94.89
　　male K66.8
　shoulder — *see* Capsulitis, adhesive
Fructokinase deficiency E74.11
Fructose 1,6 diphosphatase deficiency E74.19
Fructosemia (benign) (essential) E74.12
Fructosuria (benign) (essential) E74.11
Fuchs'
　black spot (myopic) H44.2- ☑
　dystrophy (corneal endothelium) H18.51
　heterochromic cyclitis — *see* Cyclitis, Fuchs' heterochromic
Fucosidosis E77.1
Fugue R68.89
　dissociative F44.1
　hysterical (dissociative) F44.1
　postictal in epilepsy — *see* Epilepsy
　reaction to exceptional stress (transient) F43.0
Fulminant, fulminating — *see* condition
Functional (*see also* condition)
　bleeding (uterus) N93.8
Functioning, intellectual, borderline R41.83
Fundus — *see* condition
Fungemia NOS B49
Fungus, fungous
　cerebral G93.89
　disease NOS B49
　infection — *see* Infection, fungus
Funiculitis (acute) (chronic) (endemic) N49.1
　gonococcal (acute) (chronic) A54.23
　tuberculous A18.15
Funnel
　breast (acquired) M95.4
　　congenital Q67.6
　　sequelae (late effect) of rickets E64.3
　chest (acquired) M95.4
　　congenital Q67.6
　　sequelae (late effect) of rickets E64.3
　pelvis (acquired) M95.5
　　with disproportion (fetopelvic) O33.3 ☑
　　　causing obstructed labor O65.3
　　congenital Q74.2
FUO (fever of unknown origin) R50.9
Furfur L21.0
　microsporon B36.0

Furrier's lung J67.8
Furrowed K14.5
  nail(s) (transverse) L60.4
    congenital Q84.6
  tongue K14.5
    congenital Q38.3
Furuncle L02.92
  abdominal wall L02.221
  ankle — *see* Furuncle, lower limb
  antecubital space — *see* Furuncle, upper limb
  anus K61.0
  arm — *see* Furuncle, upper limb
  auditory canal, external — *see* Abscess, ear, external
  auricle (ear) — *see* Abscess, ear, external
  axilla (region) L02.42- ☑
  back (any part) L02.222
  breast N61
  buttock L02.32
  cheek (external) L02.02
  chest wall L02.223
  chin L02.02
  corpus cavernosum N48.21
  ear, external — *see* Abscess, ear, external
  external auditory canal — *see* Abscess, ear, external
  eyelid — *see* Abscess, eyelid
  face L02.02
  femoral (region) — *see* Furuncle, lower limb
  finger — *see* Furuncle, hand
  flank L02.221
  foot L02.62- ☑
  forehead L02.02
  gluteal (region) L02.32
  groin L02.224
  hand L02.52- ☑
  head L02.821
    face L02.02
  hip — *see* Furuncle, lower limb
  kidney — *see* Abscess, kidney
  knee — *see* Furuncle, lower limb
  labium (majus) (minus) N76.4
  lacrimal
    gland — *see* Dacryoadenitis
    passages (duct) (sac) — *see* Inflammation, lacrimal,
      passages, acute
  leg (any part) — *see* Furuncle, lower limb
  lower limb L02.42- ☑
  malignant A22.0
  mouth K12.2
  navel L02.226

Furuncle — *continued*
  neck L02.12
  nose J34.0
  orbit, orbital — *see* Abscess, orbit
  palmar (space) — *see* Furuncle, hand
  partes posteriores L02.32
  pectoral region L02.223
  penis N48.21
  perineum L02.225
  pinna — *see* Abscess, ear, external
  popliteal — *see* Furuncle, lower limb
  prepatellar — *see* Furuncle, lower limb
  scalp L02.821
  seminal vesicle N49.0
  shoulder — *see* Furuncle, upper limb
  specified site NEC L02.828
  submandibular K12.2
  temple (region) L02.02
  thumb — *see* Furuncle, hand
  toe — *see* Furuncle, foot
  trunk L02.229
    abdominal wall L02.221
    back L02.222
    chest wall L02.223
    groin L02.224
    perineum L02.225
    umbilicus L02.226
  umbilicus L02.226
  upper limb L02.42- ☑
  vulva N76.4
Furunculosis — *see* Furuncle
Fused — *see* Fusion, fused
Fusion, fused (congenital)
  astragaloscaphoid Q74.2
  atria Q21.1
  auditory canal Q16.1
  auricles, heart Q21.1
  binocular with defective stereopsis H53.32
  bone Q79.8
  cervical spine M43.22
  choanal Q30.0
  commissure, mitral valve Q23.2
  cusps, heart valve NEC Q24.8
    mitral Q23.2
    pulmonary Q22.1
    tricuspid Q22.4
  ear ossicles Q16.3
  fingers Q70.0 ☑
  hymen Q52.3

Fusion, fused — *continued*
  joint (acquired) (*see also* Ankylosis)
    congenital Q74.8
  kidneys (incomplete) Q63.1
  labium (majus) (minus) Q52.5
  larynx and trachea Q34.8
  limb, congenital Q74.8
    lower Q74.2
    upper Q74.0
  lobes, lung Q33.8
  lumbosacral (acquired) M43.27
    arthrodesis status Z98.1
    congenital Q76.49
    postprocedural status Z98.1
  nares, nose, nasal, nostril(s) Q30.0
  organ or site not listed — *see* Anomaly, by site
  ossicles Q79.9
    auditory Q16.3
  pulmonic cusps Q22.1
  ribs Q76.6
  sacroiliac (joint) (acquired) M43.28
    arthrodesis status Z98.1
    congenital Q74.2
    postprocedural status Z98.1
  spine (acquired) NEC M43.20
    arthrodesis status Z98.1
    cervical region M43.22
    cervicothoracic region M43.23
    congenital Q76.49
    lumbar M43.26
    lumbosacral region M43.27
    occipito-atlanto-axial region M43.21
    postoperative status Z98.1
    sacrococcygeal region M43.28
    thoracic region M43.24
    thoracolumbar region M43.25
  sublingual duct with submaxillary duct at opening in
    mouth Q38.4
  testes Q55.1
  toes Q70.2- ☑
  tooth, teeth K00.2
  trachea and esophagus Q39.8
  twins Q89.4
  vagina Q52.4
  ventricles, heart Q21.0
  vertebra (arch) — *see* Fusion, spine
  vulva Q52.5
Fusospirillosis (mouth) (tongue) (tonsil) A69.1
Fussy baby R68.12

G

Gain in weight (abnormal) (excessive) (see also Weight, gain)
Gaisböck's disease (polycythemia hypertonica) D75.1
Gait abnormality R26.9
    ataxic R26.0
    falling R29.6
    hysterical (ataxic) (staggering) F44.4
    paralytic R26.1
    spastic R26.1
    specified type NEC R26.89
    staggering R26.0
    unsteadiness R26.81
    walking difficulty NEC R26.2
Galactocele (breast) N64.89
    puerperal, postpartum O92.79
Galactokinase deficiency E74.29
Galactophoritis N61
    gestational, puerperal, postpartum O91.2- ☑
Galactorrhea O92.6
    not associated with childbirth N64.3
Galactosemia (classic) (congenital) E74.21
Galactosuria E74.29
Galacturia R82.0
    schistosomiasis (bilharziasis) B65.0
Galeazzi's fracture S52.37- ☑
Galen's vein — see condition
Gall duct — see condition
Gallbladder (see also condition)
    acute K81.0
Gallop rhythm R00.8
Gallstone (colic) (cystic duct) (gallbladder) (impacted)
        (multiple) (see also Calculus, gallbladder)
    with
        cholecystitis — see Calculus, gallbladder, with
            cholecystitis
    bile duct (common) (hepatic) — see Calculus, bile duct
    causing intestinal obstruction K56.3
    specified NEC K80.80
        with obstruction K80.81
Gambling Z72.6
    pathological (compulsive) F63.0
Gammopathy (of undetermined significance [MGUS])
        D47.2
    associated with lymphoplasmacytic dyscrasia D47.2
    monoclonal D47.2
    polyclonal D89.0
Gamna's disease (siderotic splenomegaly) D73.1
Gamophobia F40.298
Gampsodactylia (congenital) Q66.7
Gamstorp's disease (adynamia episodica hereditaria)
        G72.3
Gandy-Nanta disease (siderotic splenomegaly) D73.1
Gang
    membership offenses Z72.810
Gangliocytoma D36.10
Ganglioglioma — see Neoplasm, uncertain behavior,
        by site
Ganglion (compound) (diffuse) (joint) (tendon (sheath))
        M67.40
    ankle M67.47- ☑
    foot M67.47- ☑
    forearm M67.43- ☑
    hand M67.44- ☑
    lower leg M67.46- ☑
    multiple sites M67.49
    of yaws (early) (late) A66.6
    pelvic region M67.45- ☑
    periosteal — see Periostitis
    shoulder region M67.41- ☑
    specified site NEC M67.48
    thigh region M67.45- ☑
    tuberculous A18.09
    upper arm M67.42- ☑
    wrist M67.43- ☑
Ganglioneuroblastoma — see Neoplasm, nerve, malig-
        nant

Ganglioneuroma D36.10
    malignant — see Neoplasm, nerve, malignant
Ganglioneuromatosis D36.10
Ganglionitis
    fifth nerve — see Neuralgia, trigeminal
    gasserian (postherpetic) (postzoster) B02.21
    geniculate G51.1
        newborn (birth injury) P11.3
        postherpetic, postzoster B02.21
    herpes zoster B02.21
    postherpetic geniculate B02.21
Gangliosidosis E75.10
    GM1 E75.19
    GM2 E75.00
        other specified E75.09
        Sandhoff disease E75.01
        Tay-Sachs disease E75.02
    GM3 E75.19
    mucolipidosis IV E75.11
Gangosa A66.5
Gangrene, gangrenous (connective tissue) (dropsical)
        (dry) (moist) (skin) (ulcer) (see also Necrosis) I96
    with diabetes (mellitus) — see Diabetes, gangrene
    abdomen (wall) I96
    alveolar M27.3
    appendix K35.80
        with
            perforation or rupture K35.2
            peritoneal abscess K35.3
            peritonitis NEC K35.3
                generalized (with perforation or rupture)
                    K35.2
                localized (with perforation or rupture) K35.3
    arteriosclerotic (general) (senile) — see Arteriosclero-
        sis, extremities, with, gangrene
    auricle I96
    Bacillus welchii A48.0
    bladder (infectious) — see Cystitis, specified type NEC
    bowel, cecum, or colon — see Gangrene, intestine
    Clostridium perfringens or welchii A48.0
    cornea H18.89- ☑
    corpora cavernosa N48.29
        noninfective N48.89
    cutaneous, spreading I96
    decubital — see Ulcer, pressure, by site
    diabetic (any site) — see Diabetes, gangrene
    emphysematous — see Gangrene, gas
    epidemic — see Poisoning, food, noxious, plant
    epididymis (infectional) N45.1
    erysipelas — see Erysipelas
    extremity (lower) (upper) I96
    Fournier N49.3
        female N76.89
    fusospirochetal A69.0
    gallbladder — see Cholecystitis, acute
    gas (bacillus) A48.0
        following
            abortion — see Abortion by type complicated
                by infection
            ectopic or molar pregnancy O08.0
    glossitis K14.0
    hernia — see Hernia, by site, with gangrene
    intestine, intestinal (hemorrhagic) (massive) K55.0
        with
            mesenteric embolism K55.0
            obstruction — see Obstruction, intestine
    laryngitis J04.0
    limb (lower) (upper) I96
    lung J85.0
        spirochetal A69.8
    lymphangitis I89.1
    Meleney's (synergistic) — see Ulcer, skin
    mesentery K55.0
        with
            embolism K55.0
            intestinal obstruction — see Obstruction, intes-
                tine
    mouth A69.0
    ovary — see Oophoritis
    pancreas K85.9
    penis N48.29
        noninfective N48.89

Gangrene, gangrenous — continued
    perineum I96
    pharynx (see also Pharyngitis)
        Vincent's A69.1
    presenile I73.1
    progressive synergistic — see Ulcer, skin
    pulmonary J85.0
    pulpal (dental) K04.1
    quinsy J36
    Raynaud's (symmetric gangrene) I73.01
    retropharyngeal J39.2
    scrotum N49.3
        noninfective N50.8
    senile (atherosclerotic) — see Arteriosclerosis, extrem-
        ities, with, gangrene
    spermatic cord N49.1
        noninfective N50.8
    spine I96
    spirochetal NEC A69.8
    spreading cutaneous I96
    stomatitis A69.0
    symmetrical I73.01
    testis (infectional) N45.2
        noninfective N44.8
    throat (see also Pharyngitis)
        diphtheritic A36.0
        Vincent's A69.1
    thyroid (gland) E07.89
    tooth (pulp) K04.1
    tuberculous NEC — see Tuberculosis
    tunica vaginalis N49.1
        noninfective N50.8
    umbilicus I96
    uterus — see Endometritis
    uvulitis K12.2
    vas deferens N49.1
        noninfective N50.8
    vulva N76.89
Ganister disease J62.8
Ganser's syndrome (hysterical) F44.89
Gardner-Diamond syndrome (autoerythrocyte sensiti-
        zation) D69.2
Gargoylism E76.01
Garré's disease, osteitis (sclerosing), osteomyelitis —
        see Osteomyelitis, specified type NEC
Garrod's pad, knuckle M72.1
Gartner's duct
    cyst Q52.4
    persistent Q50.6
Gas R14.3
    asphyxiation, inhalation, poisoning, suffocation NEC
        — see Table of Drugs and Chemicals
    excessive R14.0
    gangrene A48.0
        following
            abortion — see Abortion by type complicated
                by infection
            ectopic or molar pregnancy O08.0
    on stomach R14.0
    pains R14.1
Gastralgia (see also Pain, abdominal)
Gastrectasis K31.0
    psychogenic F45.8
Gastric — see condition
Gastrinoma
    malignant
        pancreas C25.4
        specified site NEC — see Neoplasm, malignant, by
            site
        unspecified site C25.4
    specified site — see Neoplasm, uncertain behavior
    unspecified site D37.9
Gastritis (simple) K29.70
    with bleeding K29.71
    acute (erosive) K29.00
        with bleeding K29.01
    alcoholic K29.20
        with bleeding K29.21
    allergic K29.60
        with bleeding K29.61
    atrophic (chronic) K29.40
        with bleeding K29.41

Gastritis — continued
  chronic (antral) (fundal) K29.5Ø
    with bleeding K29.51
    atrophic K29.4Ø
      with bleeding K29.41
    superficial K29.3Ø
      with bleeding K29.31
  dietary counseling and surveillance Z71.3
  due to diet deficiency E63.9
  eosinophilic K52.81
  giant hypertrophic K29.6Ø
    with bleeding K29.61
  granulomatous K29.6Ø
    with bleeding K29.61
  hypertrophic (mucosa) K29.6Ø
    with bleeding K29.61
  nervous F54
  spastic K29.6Ø
    with bleeding K29.61
  specified NEC K29.6Ø
    with bleeding K29.61
  superficial chronic K29.3Ø
    with bleeding K29.31
  tuberculous A18.83
  viral NEC A08.4
Gastrocarcinoma — see Neoplasm, malignant, stomach
Gastrocolic — see condition
Gastrodisciasis, gastrodiscoidiasis B66.8
Gastroduodenitis K29.9Ø
  with bleeding K29.91
  virus, viral A08.4
    specified type NEC A08.39
Gastrodynia — see Pain, abdominal
Gastroenteritis (acute) (chronic) (noninfectious) (see also Enteritis) K52.9
  allergic K52.2
  dietetic K52.2
  drug-induced K52.1
  due to
    Cryptosporidium A07.2
    drugs K52.1
    food poisoning — see Intoxication, foodborne
    radiation K52.Ø
  eosinophilic K52.81
  epidemic (infectious) A09
  food hypersensitivity K52.2
  infectious — see Enteritis, infectious
  influenzal — see Influenza, with gastroenteritis
  noninfectious K52.9
    specified NEC K52.89
  rotaviral A08.Ø
  Salmonella A02.Ø
  toxic K52.1
  viral NEC A08.4
    acute infectious A08.39
      type Norwalk A08.11
    infantile (acute) A08.39
    Norwalk agent A08.11
    rotaviral A08.Ø
    severe of infants A08.39
    specified type NEC A08.39
Gastroenteropathy (see also Gastroenteritis) K52.9
  acute, due to Norovirus A08.11
  acute, due to Norwalk agent A08.11
  infectious A09
Gastroenteroptosis K63.4
Gastroesophageal laceration- hemorrhage syndrome K22.6
Gastrointestinal — see condition
Gastrojejunal — see condition
Gastrojejunitis (see also Enteritis) K52.9
Gastrojejunocolic — see condition
Gastroliths K31.89
Gastromalacia K31.89
Gastroparalysis K31.84
  diabetic — see Diabetes, gastroparalysis
Gastroparesis K31.84
  diabetic — see Diabetes, by type, with gastroparesis
Gastropathy K31.9
  congestive portal K31.89
  erythematous K29.7Ø
  exudative K90.89
  portal hypertensive K31.89
Gastroptosis K31.89
Gastrorrhagia K92.2
  psychogenic F45.8
Gastroschisis (congenital) Q79.3

Gastrospasm (neurogenic) (reflex) K31.89
  neurotic F45.8
  psychogenic F45.8
Gastrostaxis — see Gastritis, with bleeding
Gastrostenosis K31.89
Gastrostomy
  attention to Z43.1
  status Z93.1
Gastrosuccorrhea (continuous) (intermittent) K31.89
  neurotic F45.8
  psychogenic F45.8
Gatophobia F4Ø.218
Gaucher's disease or splenomegaly (adult) (infantile) E75.22
Gee (-Herter)(-Thaysen) **disease** (nontropical sprue) K90.Ø
Gélineau's syndrome G47.419
  with cataplexy G47.411
Gemination, tooth, teeth KØØ.2
Gemistocytoma
  specified site — see Neoplasm, malignant, by site
  unspecified site C71.9
General, generalized — see condition
Genetic
  carrier (status)
    cystic fibrosis Z14.1
    hemophilia A (asymptomatic) Z14.Ø1
      symptomatic Z14.Ø2
    specified NEC Z14.8
  susceptibility to disease NEC Z15.89
    malignant neoplasm Z15.Ø9
      breast Z15.Ø1
      endometrium Z15.Ø4
      ovary Z15.Ø2
      prostate Z15.Ø3
      specified NEC Z15.Ø9
    multiple endocrine neoplasia Z15.81
Genital — see condition
Genito-anorectal syndrome A55
Genitourinary system — see condition
Genu
  congenital Q74.1
  extrorsum (acquired) (see also Deformity, varus, knee)
    congenital Q74.1
    sequelae (late effect) of rickets E64.3
  introrsum (acquired) (see also Deformity, valgus, knee)
    congenital Q74.1
    sequelae (late effect) of rickets E64.3
  rachitic (old) E64.3
  recurvatum (acquired) (see also Deformity, limb, specified type NEC, lower leg)
    congenital Q68.2
    sequelae (late effect) of rickets E64.3
  valgum (acquired) (knock-knee) M21.Ø6- ☑
    congenital Q74.1
    sequelae (late effect) of rickets E64.3
  varum (acquired) (bowleg) M21.16- ☑
    congenital Q74.1
    sequelae (late effect) of rickets E64.3
Geographic tongue K14.1
Geophagia — see Pica
Geotrichosis B48.3
  stomatitis B48.3
Gephyrophobia F4Ø.242
Gerbode defect Q21.Ø
GERD (gastroesophageal reflux disease) K21.9
Gerhardt's
  disease (erythromelalgia) I73.81
  syndrome (vocal cord paralysis) J38.ØØ
    bilateral J38.Ø2
    unilateral J38.Ø1
German measles (see also Rubella)
  exposure to Z20.4
Germinoblastoma (diffuse) C85.9- ☑
  follicular C82.9- ☑
Germinoma — see Neoplasm, malignant, by site
Gerontoxon — see Degeneration, cornea, senile
Gerstmann's syndrome R48.8
  developmental F81.2
Gerstmann-Sträussler-Scheinker syndrome (GSS) A81.82
Gestation (period) (see also Pregnancy)
  ectopic — see Pregnancy, by site
  multiple O30.9- ☑
    greater than quadruplets — see Pregnancy, multiple (gestation), specified NEC
    specified NEC — see Pregnancy, multiple (gestation), specified NEC

Gestational
  mammary abscess O91.11- ☑
  purulent mastitis O91.11- ☑
  subareolar abscess O91.11- ☑
Ghon tubercle, primary infection A15.7
Ghost
  teeth KØØ.4
  vessels (cornea) H16.41- ☑
Ghoul hand A66.3
Gianotti-Crosti disease L44.4
Giant
  cell
    epulis KØ6.8
    peripheral granuloma KØ6.8
  esophagus, congenital Q39.5
  kidney, congenital Q63.3
  urticaria T78.3 ☑
    hereditary D84.1
Giardiasis A07.1
Gibert's disease or pityriasis L42
Giddiness R42
  hysterical F44.89
  psychogenic F45.8
Gierke's disease (glycogenosis I) E74.Ø1
Gigantism (cerebral) (hypophyseal) (pituitary) E22.Ø
  constitutional E34.4
Gilbert's disease or syndrome E80.4
Gilchrist's disease B40.9
Gilford-Hutchinson disease E34.8
Gilles de la Tourette's disease or syndrome (motor-verbal tic) F95.2
Gingivitis KØ5.1Ø
  acute (catarrhal) KØ5.ØØ
    necrotizing A69.1
    nonplaque induced KØ5.Ø1
    plaque induced KØ5.ØØ
  chronic (desquamative) (hyperplastic) (simple marginal) (ulcerative) KØ5.1Ø
    nonplaque induced KØ5.11
    plaque induced KØ5.1Ø
  expulsiva — see Periodontitis
  necrotizing ulcerative (acute) A69.1
  pellagrous E52
    acute necrotizing A69.1
  Vincent's A69.1
Gingivoglossitis K14.Ø
Gingivopericementitis — see Periodontitis
Gingivosis — see Gingivitis, chronic
Gingivostomatitis KØ5.1Ø
  herpesviral BØØ.2
  necrotizing ulcerative (acute) A69.1
Gland, glandular — see condition
Glanders A24.Ø
Glanzmann (-Naegeli) **disease or thrombasthenia** D69.1
Glasgow coma scale
  total score
    3-8 R4Ø.243
    9-12 R4Ø.242
    13-15 R4Ø.241
Glass-blower's disease (cataract) — see Cataract, specified NEC
Glaucoma H4Ø.9
  with
    increased episcleral venous pressure H4Ø.81- ☑
    pseudoexfoliation of lens — see Glaucoma, open angle, primary, capsular
  absolute H44.51- ☑
  angle-closure (primary) H4Ø.20- ☑
    acute (attack) (crisis) H4Ø.21- ☑
    chronic H4Ø.22- ☑
    intermittent H4Ø.23- ☑
    residual stage H4Ø.24- ☑
  borderline H4Ø.ØØ- ☑
  capsular (with pseudoexfoliation of lens) — see Glaucoma, open angle, primary, capsular
  childhood Q15.Ø
  closed angle — see Glaucoma, angle-closure
  congenital Q15.Ø
  corticosteroid-induced — see Glaucoma, secondary, drugs
  hypersecretion H4Ø.82- ☑
  in (due to)
    amyloidosis E85.4 [H42]
    aniridia Q13.1 [H42]
    concussion of globe — see Glaucoma, secondary, trauma

Glaucoma — continued

  in — continued

    dislocation of lens — see Glaucoma, secondary

    disorder of lens NEC — see Glaucoma, secondary

    drugs — see Glaucoma, secondary, drugs

    endocrine disease NOS E34.9 [H42]

    eye

      inflammation — see Glaucoma, secondary, inflammation

      trauma — see Glaucoma, secondary, trauma

    hypermature cataract — see Glaucoma, secondary

    iridocyclitis — see Glaucoma, secondary, inflammation

    lens disorder — see Glaucoma, secondary

    Lowe's syndrome E72.03 [H42]

    metabolic disease NOS E88.9 [H42]

    ocular disorders NEC — see Glaucoma, secondary

    onchocerciasis B73.02

    pupillary block — see Glaucoma, secondary

    retinal vein occlusion — see Glaucoma, secondary

    Rieger's anomaly Q13.81 [H42]

    rubeosis of iris — see Glaucoma, secondary

    tumor of globe — see Glaucoma, secondary

  infantile Q15.0

  low tension — see Glaucoma, open angle, primary, low-tension

  malignant H40.83- ☑

  narrow angle — see Glaucoma, angle-closure

  newborn Q15.0

  noncongestive (chronic) — see Glaucoma, open angle

  nonobstructive — see Glaucoma, open angle

  obstructive (see also Glaucoma, angle-closure)

    due to lens changes — see Glaucoma, secondary

  open angle H40.10- ☑

    primary H40.11- ☑

      capsular (with pseudoexfoliation of lens) H40.14- ☑

      low-tension H40.12- ☑

      pigmentary H40.13- ☑

      residual stage H40.15- ☑

  phacolytic — see Glaucoma, secondary

  pigmentary — see Glaucoma, open angle, primary, pigmentary

  postinfectious — see Glaucoma, secondary, inflammation

  secondary (to) H40.5- ☑

    drugs H40.6- ☑

    inflammation H40.4- ☑

    trauma H40.3- ☑

  simple (chronic) H40.11 ☑

  simplex H40.11 ☑

  specified type NEC H40.89

  suspect H40.00- ☑

  syphilitic A52.71

  traumatic (see also Glaucoma, secondary, trauma)

    newborn (birth injury) P15.3

  tuberculous A18.59

Glaucomatous flecks (subcapsular) — see Cataract, complicated

Glazed tongue K14.4

Gleet (gonococcal) A54.01

Glénard's disease K63.4

Glioblastoma (multiforme)

  with sarcomatous component

    specified site — see Neoplasm, malignant, by site

    unspecified site C71.9

  giant cell

    specified site — see Neoplasm, malignant, by site

    unspecified site C71.9

  specified site — see Neoplasm, malignant, by site

  unspecified site C71.9

Glioma (malignant)

  astrocytic

    specified site — see Neoplasm, malignant, by site

    unspecified site C71.9

  mixed

    specified site — see Neoplasm, malignant, by site

    unspecified site C71.9

  nose Q30.8

  specified site NEC — see Neoplasm, malignant, by site

  subependymal D43.2

    specified site — see Neoplasm, uncertain behavior, by site

    unspecified site D43.2

  unspecified site C71.9

Gliomatosis cerebri C71.0

Glioneuroma — see Neoplasm, uncertain behavior, by site

Gliosarcoma

  specified site — see Neoplasm, malignant, by site

  unspecified site C71.9

Gliosis (cerebral) G93.89

  spinal G95.89

Glisson's disease — see Rickets

Globinuria R82.3

Globus (hystericus) F45.8

Glomangioma D18.00

  intra-abdominal D18.03

  intracranial D18.02

  skin D18.01

  specified site NEC D18.09

Glomangiomyoma D18.00

  intra-abdominal D18.03

  intracranial D18.02

  skin D18.01

  specified site NEC D18.09

Glomangiosarcoma — see Neoplasm, connective tissue, malignant

Glomerular

  disease in syphilis A52.75

  nephritis — see Glomerulonephritis

Glomerulitis — see Glomerulonephritis

Glomerulonephritis (see also Nephritis) N05.9

  with

    edema — see Nephrosis

    minimal change N05.0

    minor glomerular abnormality N05.0

  acute N00.9

  chronic N03.9

  crescentic (diffuse) NEC (see also N00-N07 with fourth character .7) N05.7

  dense deposit (see also N00-N07 with fourth character .6) N05.6

  diffuse

    crescentic (see also N00-N07 with fourth character .7) N05.7

    endocapillary proliferative (see also N00-N07 with fourth character .4) N05.4

    membranous (see also N00-N07 with fourth character .2) N05.2

    mesangial proliferative (see also N00-N07 with fourth character .3) N05.3

    mesangiocapillary (see also N00-N07 with fourth character .5) N05.5

    sclerosing N05.8

  endocapillary proliferative (diffuse) NEC (see also N00-N07 with fourth character .4) N05.4

  extracapillary NEC (see also N00-N07 with fourth character .7) N05.7

  focal (and segmental) (see also N00-N07 with fourth character .1) N05.1

  hypocomplementemic — see Glomerulonephritis, membranoproliferative

  IgA — see Nephropathy, IgA

  immune complex (circulating) NEC N05.8

  in (due to)

    amyloidosis E85.4 [N08]

    bilharziasis B65.9 [N08]

    cryoglobulinemia D89.1 [N08]

    defibrination syndrome D65 [N08]

    diabetes mellitus — see Diabetes, glomerulosclerosis

    disseminated intravascular coagulation D65 [N08]

    Fabry (-Anderson) disease E75.21 [N08]

    Goodpasture's syndrome M31.0

    hemolytic-uremic syndrome D59.3

    Henoch (-Schönlein) purpura D69.0 [N08]

    lecithin cholesterol acyltransferase deficiency E78.6 [N08]

    microscopic polyangiitis M31.7 [N08]

    multiple myeloma C90.0- ☑ [N08]

    Plasmodium malariae B52.0

    schistosomiasis B65.9 [N08]

    sepsis A41.9 [N08]

      streptococcal A40- ☑ [N08]

    sickle-cell disorders D57.- ☑ [N08]

    strongyloidiasis B78.9 [N08]

    subacute bacterial endocarditis I33.0 [N08]

    syphilis (late) congenital A50.59 [N08]

    systemic lupus erythematosus M32.14

    thrombotic thrombocytopenic purpura M31.1 [N08]

    typhoid fever A01.09

    Waldenström macroglobulinemia C88.0 [N08]

Glomerulonephritis — continued

  in — continued

    Wegener's granulomatosis M31.31

  latent or quiescent N03.9

  lobular, lobulonodular — see Glomerulonephritis, membranoproliferative

  membranoproliferative (diffuse)(type 1 or 3) (see also N00-N07 with fourth character .5) N05.5

    dense deposit (type 2) NEC (see also N00-N07 with fourth character .6) N05.6

  membranous (diffuse) NEC (see also N00-N07 with fourth character .2) N05.2

  mesangial

    IgA/IgG — see Nephropathy, IgA

    proliferative (diffuse) NEC (see also N00-N07 with fourth character .3) N05.3

  mesangiocapillary (diffuse) NEC (see also N00-N07 with fourth character .5) N05.5

  necrotic, necrotizing NEC (see also N00- N07 with fourth character .8) N05.8

  nodular — see Glomerulonephritis, membranoproliferative

  poststreptococcal NEC N05.9

    acute N00.9

    chronic N03.9

    rapidly progressive N01.9

  proliferative NEC (see also N00-N07 with fourth character .8) N05.8

    diffuse (lupus) M32.14

  rapidly progressive N01.9

  sclerosing, diffuse N05.8

  specified pathology NEC (see also N00- N07 with fourth character .8) N05.8

  subacute N01.9

Glomerulopathy — see Glomerulonephritis

Glomerulosclerosis (see also Sclerosis, renal)

  intercapillary (nodular) (with diabetes) — see Diabetes, glomerulosclerosis

  intracapillary — see Diabetes, glomerulosclerosis

Glossagra K14.6

Glossalgia K14.6

Glossitis (chronic superficial) (gangrenous) (Moeller's) K14.0

  areata exfoliativa K14.1

  atrophic K14.4

  benign migratory K14.1

  cortical superficial, sclerotic K14.0

  Hunter's D51.0

  interstitial, sclerous K14.0

  median rhomboid K14.2

  pellagrous E52

  superficial, chronic K14.0

Glossocele K14.8

Glossodynia K14.6

  exfoliativa K14.4

Glossoncus K14.8

Glossopathy K14.9

Glossophytia K14.3

Glossoplegia K14.8

Glossoptosis K14.8

Glossopyrosis K14.6

Glossotrichia K14.3

Glossy skin L90.8

Glottis — see condition

Glottitis (see also Laryngitis) J04.0

Glucagonoma

  pancreas

    benign D13.7

    malignant C25.4

    uncertain behavior D37.8

  specified site NEC

    benign — see Neoplasm, benign, by site

    malignant — see Neoplasm, malignant, by site

    uncertain behavior — see Neoplasm, uncertain behavior, by site

  unspecified site

    benign D13.7

    malignant C25.4

    uncertain behavior D37.8

Glucoglycinuria E72.51

Glucose-galactose malabsorption E74.39

Glue

  ear — see Otitis, media, nonsuppurative, chronic, mucoid

  sniffing (airplane) — see Abuse, drug, inhalant

    dependence — see Dependence, drug, inhalant

Glutaric aciduria E72.3

Index

Glycinemia — Gout, gouty

Glycinemia E72.51
Glycinuria (renal) (with ketosis) E72.09
Glycogen
   infiltration — *see* Disease, glycogen storage
   storage disease — *see* Disease, glycogen storage
Glycogenosis (diffuse) (generalized) (*see also* Disease,
   glycogen storage)
   cardiac E74.02 [143]
   diabetic, secondary — *see* Diabetes, glycogenosis,
      secondary
   pulmonary interstitial J84.842
Glycopenia E16.2
Glycosuria R81
   renal E74.8
Gnathostoma spinigerum (infection) (infestation),
   gnathostomiasis (wandering swelling) B83.1
Goiter (plunging) (substernal) E04.9
   with
      hyperthyroidism (recurrent) — *see* Hyperthy-
         roidism, with, goiter
      thyrotoxicosis — *see* Hyperthyroidism, with, goiter
   adenomatous — *see* Goiter, nodular
   cancerous C73
   congenital (nontoxic) E03.0
      diffuse E03.0
      parenchymatous E03.0
      transitory, with normal functioning P72.0
   cystic E04.2
      due to iodine-deficiency E01.1
   due to
      enzyme defect in synthesis of thyroid hormone
         E07.1
      iodine-deficiency (endemic) E01.2
   dyshormonogenetic (familial) E07.1
   endemic (iodine-deficiency) E01.2
      diffuse E01.0
      multinodular E01.1
   exophthalmic — *see* Hyperthyroidism, with, goiter
   iodine-deficiency (endemic) E01.2
      diffuse E01.0
      multinodular E01.1
      nodular E01.1
   lingual Q89.2
   lymphadenoid E06.3
   malignant C73
   multinodular (cystic) (nontoxic) E04.2
      toxic or with hyperthyroidism E05.20
         with thyroid storm E05.21
   neonatal NEC P72.0
   nodular (nontoxic) (due to) E04.9
      with
         hyperthyroidism E05.20
            with thyroid storm E05.21
         thyrotoxicosis E05.20
            with thyroid storm E05.21
      endemic E01.1
      iodine-deficiency E01.1
      sporadic E04.9
      toxic E05.20
         with thyroid storm E05.21
   nontoxic E04.9
      diffuse (colloid) E04.0
      multinodular E04.2
      simple E04.0
      specified NEC E04.8
      uninodular E04.1
   simple E04.0
   toxic — *see* Hyperthyroidism, with, goiter
   uninodular (nontoxic) E04.1
      toxic or with hyperthyroidism E05.10
         with thyroid storm E05.11
Goiter-deafness syndrome E07.1
Goldberg syndrome Q89.8
Goldberg-Maxwell syndrome E34.51
Goldblatt's hypertension or kidney I70.1
Goldenhar (-Gorlin) **syndrome** Q87.0
Goldflam-Erb disease or syndrome G70.00
   with exacerbation (acute) G70.01
   in crisis G70.01
Goldscheider's disease Q81.8
Goldstein's disease (familial hemorrhagic telangiectasia)
   I78.0
Golfer's elbow — *see* Epicondylitis, medial
Gonadoblastoma
   specified site — *see* Neoplasm, uncertain behavior,
      by site
   unspecified site
      female D39.10

Gonadoblastoma — *continued*
   unspecified site — *continued*
      male D40.10
Gonecystitis — *see* Vesiculitis
Gongylonemiasis B83.8
Goniosynechiae — *see* Adhesions, iris, goniosynechiae
Gonococcemia A54.86
Gonococcus, gonococcal (disease) (infection) (*see also*
   condition) A54.9
   anus A54.6
   bursa, bursitis A54.49
   conjunctiva, conjunctivitis (neonatorum) A54.31
   endocardium A54.83
   eye A54.30
      conjunctivitis A54.31
      iridocyclitis A54.32
      keratitis A54.33
      newborn A54.31
      other specified A54.39
   fallopian tubes (acute) (chronic) A54.24
   genitourinary (organ) (system) (tract) (acute)
      lower A54.00
         with abscess (accessory gland) (periurethral)
            A54.1
      upper (*see also* condition) A54.29
   heart A54.83
   iridocyclitis A54.32
   joint A54.42
   lymphatic (gland) (node) A54.89
   meninges, meningitis A54.81
   musculoskeletal A54.40
      arthritis A54.42
      osteomyelitis A54.43
      other specified A54.49
      spondylopathy A54.41
   pelviperitonitis A54.24
   pelvis (acute) (chronic) A54.24
   pharynx A54.5
   proctitis A54.6
   pyosalpinx (acute) (chronic) A54.24
   rectum A54.6
   skin A54.89
   specified site NEC A54.89
   tendon sheath A54.49
   throat A54.5
   urethra (acute) (chronic) A54.01
      with abscess (accessory gland) (periurethral) A54.1
   vulva (acute) (chronic) A54.02
Gonocytoma
   specified site — *see* Neoplasm, uncertain behavior,
      by site
   unspecified site
      female D39.10
      male D40.10
Gonorrhea (acute) (chronic) A54.9
   Bartholin's gland (acute) (chronic) (purulent) A54.02
      with abscess (accessory gland) (periurethral) A54.1
   bladder A54.01
   cervix A54.03
   conjunctiva, conjunctivitis (neonatorum) A54.31
   contact Z20.2
   Cowper's gland (with abscess) A54.1
   exposure to Z20.2
   fallopian tube (acute) (chronic) A54.24
   kidney (acute) (chronic) A54.21
   lower genitourinary tract A54.00
      with abscess (accessory gland) (periurethral) A54.1
   ovary (acute) (chronic) A54.24
   pelvis (acute) (chronic) A54.24
      female pelvic inflammatory disease A54.24
   penis A54.09
   prostate (acute) (chronic) A54.22
   seminal vesicle (acute) (chronic) A54.23
   specified site not listed (*see also* Gonococcus) A54.89
   spermatic cord (acute) (chronic) A54.23
   urethra A54.01
      with abscess (accessory gland) (periurethral) A54.1
   vagina A54.02
   vas deferens (acute) (chronic) A54.23
   vulva A54.02
Goodall's disease A08.19
Goodpasture's syndrome M31.0
Gopalan's syndrome (burning feet) E53.0
Gorlin-Chaudry-Moss syndrome Q87.0
Gottron's papules L94.4
Gougerot-Blum syndrome (pigmented purpuric
   lichenoid dermatitis) L81.7

Gougerot-Carteaud disease or syndrome (confluent
   reticulate papillomatosis) L83
Gougerot's syndrome (trisymptomatic) L81.7
Gouley's syndrome (constrictive pericarditis) I31.1
Goundou A66.6
Gout, chronic (*see also* Gout, gouty) M1A.9 ☑ (*following*
   M08)
   drug-induced M1A.20 ☑ (*following* M08)
      ankle M1A.27- ☑ (*following* M08)
      elbow M1A.22- ☑ (*following* M08)
      foot joint M1A.27- ☑ (*following* M08)
      hand joint M1A.24- ☑ (*following* M08)
      hip M1A.25- ☑ (*following* M08)
      knee M1A.26- ☑ (*following* M08)
      multiple site M1A.29- ☑ (*following* M08)
      shoulder M1A.21- ☑ (*following* M08)
      vertebrae M1A.28 ☑ (*following* M08)
      wrist M1A.23- ☑ (*following* M08)
   idiopathic M1A.00 ☑ (*following* M08)
      ankle M1A.07- ☑ (*following* M08)
      elbow M1A.02- ☑ (*following* M08)
      foot joint M1A.07- ☑ (*following* M08)
      hand joint M1A.04- ☑ (*following* M08)
      hip M1A.05- ☑ (*following* M08)
      knee M1A.06- ☑ (*following* M08)
      multiple site M1A.09 ☑ (*following* M08)
      shoulder M1A.01- ☑ (*following* M08)
      vertebrae M1A.08 ☑ (*following* M08)
      wrist M1A.03- ☑ (*following* M08)
   in (due to) renal impairment M1A.30 ☑ (*following*
      M08)
      ankle M1A.37- ☑ (*following* M08)
      elbow M1A.32- ☑ (*following* M08)
      foot joint M1A.37- ☑ (*following* M08)
      hand joint M1A.34- ☑ (*following* M08)
      hip M1A.35- ☑ (*following* M08)
      knee M1A.36- ☑ (*following* M08)
      multiple site M1A.39 ☑ (*following* M08)
      shoulder M1A.31- ☑ (*following* M08)
      vertebrae M1A.38 ☑ (*following* M08)
      wrist M1A.33- ☑ (*following* M08)
   lead-induced M1A.10 ☑ (*following* M08)
      ankle M1A.17- ☑ (*following* M08)
      elbow M1A.12- ☑ (*following* M08)
      foot joint M1A.17- ☑ (*following* M08)
      hand joint M1A.14- ☑ (*following* M08)
      hip M1A.15- ☑ (*following* M08)
      knee M1A.16- ☑ (*following* M08)
      multiple site M1A.19 ☑ (*following* M08)
      shoulder M1A.11- ☑ (*following* M08)
      vertebrae M1A.18 ☑ (*following* M08)
      wrist M1A.13- ☑ (*following* M08)
   primary — *see* Gout, chronic, idiopathic
   saturnine — *see* Gout, chronic, lead-induced
   secondary NEC M1A.40 ☑ (*following* M08)
      ankle M1A.47- ☑ (*following* M08)
      elbow M1A.42- ☑ (*following* M08)
      foot joint M1A.47- ☑ (*following* M08)
      hand joint M1A.44- ☑ (*following* M08)
      hip M1A.45- ☑ (*following* M08)
      knee M1A.46- ☑ (*following* M08)
      multiple site M1A.49 ☑ (*following* M08)
      shoulder M1A.41- ☑ (*following* M08)
      vertebrae M1A.48 ☑ (*following* M08)
      wrist M1A.43- ☑ (*following* M08)
   syphilitic (*see also* subcategory M14.8-) A52.77
   tophi M1A.9 ☑ (*following* M08)
Gout, gouty (acute) (attack) (flare) (*see also* Gout,
   chronic) M10.9
   drug-induced M10.20
      ankle M10.27- ☑
      elbow M10.22- ☑
      foot joint M10.27- ☑
      hand joint M10.24- ☑
      hip M10.25- ☑
      knee M10.26- ☑
      multiple site M10.29
      shoulder M10.21- ☑
      vertebrae M10.28
      wrist M10.23- ☑
   idiopathic M10.00
      ankle M10.07- ☑
      elbow M10.02- ☑
      foot joint M10.07- ☑
      hand joint M10.04- ☑
      hip M10.05- ☑

☑ **Additional Character Required** — Refer to the Tabular List for Character Selection   ▽ Subterms under main terms may continue to next column or page

Gout, gouty — *continued*
  idiopathic — *continued*
    knee M10.06- ☑
    multiple site M10.09
    shoulder M10.01- ☑
    vertebrae M10.08
    wrist M10.03- ☑
    in (due to) renal impairment M10.30
      ankle M10.37- ☑
      elbow M10.32- ☑
      foot joint M10.37- ☑
      hand joint M10.34- ☑
      hip M10.35- ☑
      knee M10.36- ☑
      multiple site M10.39
      shoulder M10.31- ☑
      vertebrae M10.38
      wrist M10.33- ☑
  lead-induced M10.10
    ankle M10.17- ☑
    elbow M10.12- ☑
    foot joint M10.17- ☑
    hand joint M10.14- ☑
    hip M10.15- ☑
    knee M10.16- ☑
    multiple site M10.19
    shoulder M10.11- ☑
    vertebrae M10.18
    wrist M10.13- ☑
  primary — *see* Gout, idiopathic
  saturnine — *see* Gout, lead-induced
  secondary NEC M10.40
    ankle M10.47- ☑
    elbow M10.42- ☑
    foot joint M10.47- ☑
    hand joint M10.44- ☑
    hip M10.45- ☑
    knee M10.46- ☑
    multiple site M10.49
    shoulder M10.41- ☑
    vertebrae M10.48
    wrist M10.43- ☑
  syphilitic (*see also* subcategory M14.8-) A52.77
  tophi — *see* Gout, chronic
Gower's
  muscular dystrophy G71.0
  syndrome (vasovagal attack) R55
Gradenigo's syndrome — *see* Otitis, media, suppurative, acute
Graefe's disease — *see* Strabismus, paralytic, ophthalmoplegia, progressive
Graft-versus-host disease D89.813
  acute D89.810
  acute on chronic D89.812
  chronic D89.811
Grain mite (itch) B88.0
Grainhandler's disease or lung J67.8
Grand mal — *see* Epilepsy, generalized, specified NEC
Grand multipara status only (not pregnant) Z64.1
  pregnant — *see* Pregnancy, complicated by, grand multiparity
Granite worker's lung J62.8
Granular (*see also* condition)
  inflammation, pharynx J31.2
  kidney (contracting) — *see* Sclerosis, renal
  liver K74.69
Granulation tissue (abnormal) (excessive) L92.9
  postmastoidectomy cavity — *see* Complications, postmastoidectomy, granulation
Granulocytopenia (primary) (malignant) — *see* Agranulocytosis
Granuloma L92.9
  abdomen K66.8
    from residual foreign body L92.3
    pyogenicum L98.0
  actinic L57.5
  annulare (perforating) L92.0
  apical K04.5
  aural — *see* Otitis, externa, specified NEC
  beryllium (skin) L92.3
  bone
    eosinophilic C96.6
    from residual foreign body — *see* Osteomyelitis, specified type NEC
    lung C96.6
  brain (any site) G06.0
    schistosomiasis B65.9 [G07]

Granuloma — *continued*
  canaliculus lacrimalis — *see* Granuloma, lacrimal
  candidal (cutaneous) B37.2
  cerebral (any site) G06.0
  coccidioidal (primary) (progressive) B38.7
    lung B38.1
    meninges B38.4
  colon K63.89
  conjunctiva H11.22- ☑
  dental K04.5
  ear, middle — *see* Cholesteatoma
  eosinophilic C96.6
    bone C96.6
    lung C96.6
    oral mucosa K13.4
    skin L92.2
  eyelid H01.8
  facial (e) L92.2
  foreign body (in soft tissue) NEC M60.20
    ankle M60.27- ☑
    foot M60.27- ☑
    forearm M60.23- ☑
    hand M60.24- ☑
    in operation wound — *see* Foreign body, accidentally left during a procedure
    lower leg M60.26- ☑
    pelvic region M60.25- ☑
    shoulder region M60.21- ☑
    skin L92.3
    specified site NEC M60.28
    subcutaneous tissue L92.3
    thigh M60.25- ☑
    upper arm M60.22- ☑
  gangraenescens M31.2
  genito-inguinale A58
  giant cell (central) (reparative) (jaw) M27.1
    gingiva (peripheral) K06.8
  gland (lymph) I88.8
  hepatic NEC K75.3
    in (due to)
      berylliosis J63.2 [K77]
      sarcoidosis D86.89
  Hodgkin C81.9 ☑
  ileum K63.89
  infectious B99.9
    specified NEC B99.8
  inguinale (Donovan) (venereal) A58
  intestine NEC K63.89
  intracranial (any site) G06.0
  intraspinal (any part) G06.1
  iridocyclitis — *see* Iridocyclitis, chronic
  jaw (bone) (central) M27.1
    reparative giant cell M27.1
  kidney (*see also* Infection, kidney) N15.8
  lacrimal H04.81- ☑
  larynx J38.7
  lethal midline (faciale(e)) M31.2
  liver NEC — *see* Granuloma, hepatic
  lung (infectious) (*see also* Fibrosis, lung)
    coccidioidal B38.1
    eosinophilic C96.6
  Majocchi's B35.8
  malignant (facial(e)) M31.2
  mandible (central) M27.1
  midline (lethal) M31.2
  monilial (cutaneous) B37.2
  nasal sinus — *see* Sinusitis
  operation wound T81.89 ☑
    foreign body — *see* Foreign body, accidentally left during a procedure
    stitch T81.89 ☑
    talc — *see* Foreign body, accidentally left during a procedure
  oral mucosa K13.4
  orbit, orbital H05.11- ☑
  paracoccidioidal B41.8
  penis, venereal A58
  periapical K04.5
  peritoneum K66.8
    due to ova of helminths NOS (*see also* Helminthiasis) B83.9 [K67]
  postmastoidectomy cavity — *see* Complications, postmastoidectomy, recurrent cholesteatoma
  prostate N42.89
  pudendi (ulcerating) A58
  pulp, internal (tooth) K03.3
  pyogenic, pyogenicum (of) (skin) L98.0
    gingiva K06.8

Granuloma — *continued*
  pyogenic, pyogenicum — *continued*
    maxillary alveolar ridge K04.5
    oral mucosa K13.4
  rectum K62.89
  reticulohistiocytic D76.3
  rubrum nasi L74.8
  Schistosoma — *see* Schistosomiasis
  septic (skin) L98.0
  silica (skin) L92.3
  sinus (accessory) (infective) (nasal) — *see* Sinusitis
  skin L92.9
    from residual foreign body L92.3
    pyogenicum L98.0
  spine
    syphilitic (epidural) A52.19
    tuberculous A18.01
  stitch (postoperative) T81.89 ☑
  suppurative (skin) L98.0
  swimming pool A31.1
  talc (*see also* Granuloma, foreign body)
    in operation wound — *see* Foreign body, accidentally left during a procedure
  telangiectaticum (skin) L98.0
  tracheostomy J95.09
  trichophyticum B35.8
  tropicum A66.4
  umbilicus L92.9
  urethra N36.8
  uveitis — *see* Iridocyclitis, chronic
  vagina A58
  venereum A58
  vocal cord J38.3
Granulomatosis L92.9
  lymphoid C83.8- ☑
  miliary (listerial) A32.89
  necrotizing, respiratory M31.30
  progressive septic D71
  specified NEC L92.8
  Wegener's M31.30
    with renal involvement M31.31
Granulomatous tissue (abnormal) (excessive) L92.9
Granulosis rubra nasi L74.8
Graphite fibrosis (of lung) J63.3
Graphospasm F48.8
  organic G25.89
Grating scapula M89.8X1
Gravel (urinary) — *see* Calculus, urinary
Graves' disease — *see* Hyperthyroidism, with, goiter
Gravis — *see* condition
Grawitz tumor C64.- ☑
Gray syndrome (newborn) P93.0
Grayness, hair (premature) L67.1
  congenital Q84.2
Green sickness D50.8
Greenfield's disease
  meaning
    concentric sclerosis (encephalitis periaxialis concentrica) G37.5
    metachromatic leukodystrophy E75.25
Greenstick fracture — code as Fracture, by site
Grey syndrome (newborn) P93.0
Grief F43.21
  prolonged F43.29
  reaction (*see also* Disorder, adjustment) F43.20
Griesinger's disease B76.9
Grinder's lung or pneumoconiosis J62.8
Grinding, teeth
  psychogenic F45.8
  sleep related G47.63
Grip
  Dabney's B33.0
  devil's B33.0
Grippe, grippal (*see also* Influenza)
  Balkan A78
  summer, of Italy A93.1
Grisel's disease M43.6
Groin — *see* condition
Grooved tongue K14.5
Ground itch B76.9
Grover's disease or syndrome L11.1
Growing pains, children R29.898
Growth (fungoid) (neoplastic) (new) (*see also* Neoplasm)
  adenoid (vegetative) J35.8
  benign — *see* Neoplasm, benign, by site
  malignant — *see* Neoplasm, malignant, by site
  rapid, childhood Z00.2

Growth — *continued*
secondary — *see* Neoplasm, secondary, by site
Gruby's disease B35.Ø
Gubler-Millard paralysis or syndrome G46.3
Guerin-Stern syndrome Q74.3
Guidance, insufficient anterior (occlusal) M26.54
Guillain-Barré disease or syndrome G61.Ø
sequelae G65.Ø
Guinea worms (infection) (infestation) B72
Guinon's disease (motor-verbal tic) F95.2
Gull's disease EØ3.4
Gum — *see* condition
Gumboil KØ4.7
with sinus KØ4.6
Gumma (syphilitic) A52.79
artery A52.Ø9
cerebral A52.Ø4
bone A52.77
of yaws (late) A66.6
brain A52.19
cauda equina A52.19
central nervous system A52.3
ciliary body A52.71
congenital A5Ø.59
eyelid A52.71
heart A52.Ø6
intracranial A52.19
iris A52.71
kidney A52.75
larynx A52.73
leptomeninges A52.19
liver A52.74
meninges A52.19
myocardium A52.Ø6
nasopharynx A52.73
neurosyphilitic A52.3
nose A52.73
orbit A52.71
palate (soft) A52.79
penis A52.76
pericardium A52.Ø6
pharynx A52.73
pituitary A52.79
scrofulous (tuberculous) A18.4
skin A52.79
specified site NEC A52.79
spinal cord A52.19
tongue A52.79
tonsil A52.73
trachea A52.73
tuberculous A18.4
ulcerative due to yaws A66.4
ureter A52.75
yaws A66.4
bone A66.6
Gunn's syndrome QØ7.8
Gunshot wound (*see also* Wound, open)
fracture — *code as* Fracture, by site
internal organs — *see* Injury, by site
Gynandrism Q56.Ø
Gynandroblastoma
specified site — *see* Neoplasm, uncertain behavior, by site
unspecified site
female D39.1Ø
male D4Ø.1Ø
Gynecological examination (periodic) (routine) ZØ1.419
with abnormal findings ZØ1.411
Gynecomastia N62
Gynephobia F4Ø.291
Gyrate scalp Q82.8

H

H (Hartnup's) **disease** E72.Ø2
Haas' disease or osteochondrosis (juvenile) (head of humerus) — *see* Osteochondrosis, juvenile, humerus
Habit, habituation
bad sleep Z72.821
chorea F95.8
disturbance, child F98.9
drug — *see* Dependence, drug
irregular sleep Z72.821
laxative F55.2
spasm — *see* Tic
tic — *see* Tic

Haemophilus (H.) **influenzae, as cause of disease classified elsewhere** B96.3
Haff disease — *see* Poisoning, mercury
Hageman's factor defect, deficiency or disease D68.2
Haglund's disease or osteochondrosis (juvenile) (os tibiale externum) — *see* Osteochondrosis, juvenile, tarsus
Hailey-Hailey disease Q82.8
Hair (*see also* condition)
plucking F63.3
in stereotyped movement disorder F98.4
tourniquet syndrome (*see also* Constriction, external, by site)
finger S6Ø.44- ☑
penis S3Ø.842 ☑
thumb S6Ø.34- ☑
toe S9Ø.44- ☑
Hairball in stomach T18.2 ☑
Hair-pulling, pathological (compulsive) F63.3
Hairy black tongue K14.3
Half vertebra Q76.49
Halitosis R19.6
Hallerman-Streiff syndrome Q87.Ø
Hallervorden-Spatz disease G23.Ø
Hallopeau's acrodermatitis or disease L4Ø.2
Hallucination R44.3
auditory R44.Ø
gustatory R44.2
olfactory R44.2
specified NEC R44.2
tactile R44.2
visual R44.1
Hallucinosis (chronic) F28
alcoholic (acute) F1Ø.951
in
abuse F1Ø.151
dependence F1Ø.251
drug-induced F19.951
cannabis F12.951
cocaine F14.951
hallucinogen F16.151
in
abuse F19.151
cannabis F12.151
cocaine F14.151
hallucinogen F16.151
inhalant F18.151
opioid F11.151
sedative, anxiolytic or hypnotic F13.151
stimulant NEC F15.151
dependence F19.251
cannabis F12.251
cocaine F14.251
hallucinogen F16.251
inhalant F18.251
opioid F11.251
sedative, anxiolytic or hypnotic F13.251
stimulant NEC F15.251
inhalant F18.951
opioid F11.951
sedative, anxiolytic or hypnotic F13.951
stimulant NEC F15.951
organic FØ6.Ø
Hallux
deformity (acquired) NEC M2Ø.5X- ☑
limitus M2Ø.5X- ☑
malleus (acquired) NEC M2Ø.3- ☑
rigidus (acquired) M2Ø.2- ☑
congenital Q74.2
sequelae (late effect) of rickets E64.3
valgus (acquired) M2Ø.1- ☑
congenital Q66.6
varus (acquired) M2Ø.3- ☑
congenital Q66.3
Halo, visual H53.19
Hamartoma, hamartoblastoma Q85.9
epithelial (gingival), odontogenic, central or peripheral — *see* Cyst, calcifying odontogenic
Hamartosis Q85.9
Hamman-Rich syndrome J84.114
Hammer toe (acquired) NEC (*see also* Deformity, toe, hammer toe)
congenital Q66.89
sequelae (late effect) of rickets E64.3
Hand — *see* condition
Hand-foot syndrome L27.1

Handicap, handicapped
educational Z55.9
specified NEC Z55.8
Hand-Schüller-Christian disease or syndrome C96.5
Hanging (asphyxia) (strangulation) (suffocation) — *see* Asphyxia, traumatic, due to mechanical threat
Hangnail (*see also* Cellulitis, digit)
with lymphangitis — *see* Lymphangitis, acute, digit
Hangover (alcohol) F1Ø.129
Hanhart's syndrome Q87.Ø
Hanot-Chauffard (-Troisier) **syndrome** E83.19
Hanot's cirrhosis or disease K74.3
Hansen's disease — *see* Leprosy
Hantaan virus disease (Korean hemorrhagic fever) A98.5
Hantavirus disease (with renal manifestations) (Dobrava) (Puumala) (Seoul) A98.5
with pulmonary manifestations (Andes) (Bayou) (Bermejo) (Black Creek Canal) (Choclo) (Juquitiba) (Laguna negra) (Lechiguanas) (New York) (Oran) (Sin nombre) B33.4
Happy puppet syndrome Q93.5
Harada's disease or syndrome H3Ø.81- ☑
Hardening
artery — *see* Arteriosclerosis
brain G93.89
Harelip (complete) (incomplete) — *see* Cleft, lip
Harlequin (newborn) Q8Ø.4
Harley's disease D59.6
Harmful use (of)
alcohol F1Ø.1Ø
anxiolytics — *see* Abuse, drug, sedative
cannabinoids — *see* Abuse, drug, cannabis
cocaine — *see* Abuse, drug, cocaine
drug — *see* Abuse, drug
hallucinogens — *see* Abuse, drug, hallucinogen
hypnotics — *see* Abuse, drug, sedative
opioids — *see* Abuse, drug, opioid
PCP (phencyclidine) — *see* Abuse, drug, hallucinogen
sedatives — *see* Abuse, drug, sedative
stimulants NEC — *see* Abuse, drug, stimulant
Harris' lines — *see* Arrest, epiphyseal
Hartnup's disease E72.Ø2
Harvester's lung J67.Ø
Harvesting ovum for in vitro fertilization Z31.83
Hashimoto's disease or thyroiditis EØ6.3
Hashitoxicosis (transient) EØ6.3
Hassal-Henle bodies or warts (cornea) H18.49
Haut mal — *see* Epilepsy, generalized, specified NEC
Haverhill fever A25.1
Hay fever (*see also* Fever, hay) J3Ø.1
Hayem-Widal syndrome D59.8
Haygarth's nodes M15.8
Haymaker's lung J67.Ø
Hb (abnormal)
Bart's disease D56.Ø
disease — *see* Disease, hemoglobin
trait — *see* Trait
Head — *see* condition
Headache R51
allergic NEC G44.89
associated with sexual activity G44.82
chronic daily R51
cluster G44.ØØ9
chronic G44.Ø29
intractable G44.Ø21
not intractable G44.Ø29
episodic G44.Ø19
intractable G44.Ø11
not intractable G44.Ø19
intractable G44.ØØ1
not intractable G44.ØØ9
cough (primary) G44.83
daily chronic R51
drug-induced NEC G44.4Ø
intractable G44.41
not intractable G44.4Ø
exertional (primary) G44.84
histamine G44.ØØ9
intractable G44.ØØ1
not intractable G44.ØØ9
hypnic G44.81
lumbar puncture G97.1
medication overuse G44.4Ø
intractable G44.41
not intractable G44.4Ø
menstrual — *see* Migraine, menstrual
migraine (type) (*see also* Migraine) G43.9Ø9

Headache — *continued*
  nasal septum R51
  neuralgiform, short lasting unilateral, with conjunctival
      injection and tearing (SUNCT) G44.059
    intractable G44.051
    not intractable G44.059
  new daily persistent (NDPH) G44.52
  orgasmic G44.82
  periodic syndromes in adults and children G43.C0
    (*following* G43.7)
    with refractory migraine G43.C1 (*following* G43.7)
    without refractory migraine G43.C0 (*following*
      G43.7)
    intractable G43.C1 (*following* G43.7)
    not intractable G43.C0 (*following* G43.7)
  postspinal puncture G97.1
  post-traumatic G44.309
    acute G44.319
      intractable G44.311
      not intractable G44.319
    chronic G44.329
      intractable G44.321
      not intractable G44.329
    intractable G44.301
    not intractable G44.309
  pre-menstrual — *see* Migraine, menstrual
  preorgasmic G44.82
  primary
    cough G44.83
    exertional G44.84
    stabbing G44.85
    thunderclap G44.53
  rebound G44.40
    intractable G44.41
    not intractable G44.40
  short lasting unilateral neuralgiform, with conjunctival
      injection and tearing (SUNCT) G44.059
    intractable G44.051
    not intractable G44.059
  specified syndrome NEC G44.89
  spinal and epidural anesthesia - induced T88.59 ☑
    in labor and delivery O74.5
    in pregnancy O29.4- ☑
    postpartum, puerperal O89.4
  spinal fluid loss (from puncture) G97.1
  stabbing (primary) G44.85
  tension (-type) G44.209
    chronic G44.229
      intractable G44.221
      not intractable G44.229
    episodic G44.219
      intractable G44.211
      not intractable G44.219
    intractable G44.201
    not intractable G44.209
  thunderclap (primary) G44.53
  vascular NEC G44.1
Healthy
  infant
    accompanying sick mother Z76.3
    receiving care Z76.2
  person accompanying sick person Z76.3
Hearing examination Z01.10
  with abnormal findings NEC Z01.118
  following failed hearing screening Z01.110
  for hearing conservation and treatment Z01.12
Heart — *see* condition
Heart beat
  abnormality R00.9
    specified NEC R00.8
  awareness R00.2
  rapid R00.0
  slow R00.1
Heartburn R12
  psychogenic F45.8
Heat (effects) T67.9 ☑
  apoplexy T67.0 ☑
  burn (*see also* Burn) L55.9
  collapse T67.1 ☑
  cramps T67.2 ☑
  dermatitis or eczema L59.0
  edema T67.7 ☑
  erythema — *code by site under* Burn, first degree
  excessive T67.9 ☑
    specified effect NEC T67.8 ☑
  exhaustion T67.5 ☑
    anhydrotic T67.3 ☑

Heat — *continued*
  exhaustion — *continued*
    due to
      salt (and water) depletion T67.4 ☑
      water depletion T67.3 ☑
        with salt depletion T67.4 ☑
  fatigue (transient) T67.6 ☑
  fever T67.0 ☑
  hyperpyrexia T67.0 ☑
  prickly L74.0
  prostration — *see* Heat, exhaustion
  pyrexia T67.0 ☑
  rash L74.0
  specified effect NEC T67.8 ☑
  stroke T67.0 ☑
  sunburn — *see* Sunburn
  syncope T67.1 ☑
Heavy-for-dates NEC (infant) (4000g to 4499g) P08.1
  exceptionally (4500g or more) P08.0
Hebephrenia, hebephrenic (schizophrenia) F20.1
Heberden's disease or nodes (with arthropathy) M15.1
Hebra's
  pityriasis L26
  prurigo L28.2
Heel — *see* condition
Heerfordt's disease D86.89
Hegglin's anomaly or syndrome D72.0
Heilmeyer-Schoner disease D45
Heine-Medin disease A80.9
Heinz body anemia, congenital D58.2
Heliophobia F40.228
Heller's disease or syndrome F84.3
HELLP syndrome (hemolysis, elevated liver enzymes
    and low platelet count) O14.2- ☑
Helminthiasis (*see also* Infestation, helminth)
  Ancylostoma B76.0
  intestinal B82.0
    mixed types (types classifiable to more than one
      of the titles B65.0-B81.3 and B81.8) B81.4
    specified type NEC B81.8
  mixed types (intestinal) (types classifiable to more
      than one of the titles B65.0-B81.3 and B81.8)
      B81.4
  Necator (americanus) B76.1
  specified type NEC B83.8
Heloma L84
Hemangioblastoma — *see* Neoplasm, connective tissue,
    uncertain behavior
  malignant — *see* Neoplasm, connective tissue, malig-
    nant
Hemangioendothelioma (*see also* Neoplasm, uncertain
    behavior, by site)
  benign D18.00
    intra-abdominal D18.03
    intracranial D18.02
    skin D18.01
    specified site NEC D18.09
  bone (diffuse) — *see* Neoplasm, bone, malignant
  epithelioid (*see also* Neoplasm, uncertain behavior,
    by site)
    malignant — *see* Neoplasm, malignant, by site
  malignant — *see* Neoplasm, connective tissue, malig-
    nant
Hemangiofibroma — *see* Neoplasm, benign, by site
Hemangiolipoma — *see* Lipoma
Hemangioma D18.00
  arteriovenous D18.00
    intra-abdominal D18.03
    intracranial D18.02
    skin D18.01
    specified site NEC D18.09
  capillary D18.00
    intra-abdominal D18.03
    intracranial D18.02
    skin D18.01
    specified site NEC D18.09
  cavernous D18.00
    intra-abdominal D18.03
    intracranial D18.02
    skin D18.01
    specified site NEC D18.09
  epithelioid D18.00
    intra-abdominal D18.03
    intracranial D18.02
    skin D18.01
    specified site NEC D18.09

Hemangioma — *continued*
  histiocytoid D18.00
    intra-abdominal D18.03
    intracranial D18.02
    skin D18.01
    specified site NEC D18.09
  infantile D18.00
    intra-abdominal D18.03
    intracranial D18.02
    skin D18.01
    specified site NEC D18.09
  intra-abdominal D18.03
  intracranial D18.02
  intramuscular D18.00
    intra-abdominal D18.03
    intracranial D18.02
    skin D18.01
    specified site NEC D18.09
  juvenile D18.00
  malignant — *see* Neoplasm,connective tissue, malig-
    nant
  plexiform D18.00
    intra-abdominal D18.03
    intracranial D18.02
    skin D18.01
    specified site NEC D18.09
  racemose D18.00
    intra-abdominal D18.03
    intracranial D18.02
    skin D18.01
    specified site NEC D18.09
  sclerosing — *see* Neoplasm, skin, benign
  simplex D18.00
    intra-abdominal D18.03
    intracranial D18.02
    skin D18.01
    specified site NEC D18.09
  skin D18.01
  specified site NEC D18.09
  venous D18.00
    intra-abdominal D18.03
    intracranial D18.02
    skin D18.01
    specified site NEC D18.09
  verrucous keratotic D18.00
    intra-abdominal D18.03
    intracranial D18.02
    skin D18.01
    specified site NEC D18.09
Hemangiomatosis (systemic) I78.8
  involving single site — *see* Hemangioma
Hemangiopericytoma (*see also* Neoplasm, connective
    tissue, uncertain behavior)
  benign — *see* Neoplasm, connective tissue, benign
  malignant — *see* Neoplasm, connective tissue, malig-
    nant
Hemangiosarcoma — *see* Neoplasm, connective tissue,
    malignant
Hemarthrosis (nontraumatic) M25.00
  ankle M25.07- ☑
  elbow M25.02- ☑
  foot joint M25.07- ☑
  hand joint M25.04- ☑
  hip M25.05- ☑
  in hemophilic arthropathy — *see* Arthropathy,
    hemophilic
  knee M25.06- ☑
  shoulder M25.01- ☑
  specified joint NEC M25.08
  traumatic — *see* Sprain, by site
  vertebrae M25.08
  wrist M25.03- ☑
Hematemesis K92.0
  with ulcer — *code by site under* Ulcer, with hemor-
    rhage K27.4
  newborn, neonatal P54.0
    due to swallowed maternal blood P78.2
Hematidrosis L74.8
Hematinuria (*see also* Hemoglobinuria)
  malarial B50.8
Hematobilia K83.8
Hematocele
  female NEC N94.89
    with ectopic pregnancy O00.9
    ovary N83.8
  male N50.1
Hematochezia (*see also* Melena) K92.1

Hematochyluria (see also Infestation, filarial)
   schistosomiasis (bilharziasis) B65.0
Hematocolpos (with hematometra or hematosalpinx)
   N89.7
Hematocornea — see Pigmentation, cornea, stromal
Hematogenous — see condition
Hematoma (traumatic) (skin surface intact) (see also
   Contusion)
   with
      injury of internal organs — see Injury, by site
      open wound — see Wound, open
   amputation stump (surgical) (late) T87.89
   aorta, dissecting I71.00
      abdominal I71.02
      thoracic I71.01
      thoracoabdominal I71.03
   aortic intramural — see Dissection, aorta
   arterial (complicating trauma) — see Injury, blood
      vessel, by site
   auricle — see Contusion, ear
      nontraumatic — see Disorder, pinna, hematoma
   birth injury NEC P15.8
   brain (traumatic)
      with
         cerebral laceration or contusion (diffuse) — see
            Injury, intracranial, diffuse
            focal — see Injury, intracranial, focal
      cerebellar, traumatic S06.37- ☑
      intracerebral, traumatic — see Injury, intracranial,
         intracerebral hemorrhage
      newborn NEC P52.4
         birth injury P10.1
      nontraumatic — see Hemorrhage, intracranial
      subarachnoid, arachnoid, traumatic — see Injury,
         intracranial, subarachnoid hemorrhage
      subdural, traumatic — see Injury, intracranial,
         subdural hemorrhage
   breast (nontraumatic) N64.89
   broad ligament (nontraumatic) N83.7
      traumatic S37.892 ☑
   cerebellar, traumatic S06.37- ☑
   cerebral — see Hematoma, brain
   cerebrum S06.36- ☑
      left S06.35- ☑
      right S06.34- ☑
   cesarean delivery wound O90.2
   complicating delivery (perineal) (pelvic) (vagina) (vul-
      va) O71.7
   corpus cavernosum (nontraumatic) N48.89
   epididymis (nontraumatic) N50.1
   epidural (traumatic) — see Injury, intracranial, epidural
      hemorrhage
      spinal — see Injury, spinal cord, by region
   episiotomy O90.2
   face, birth injury P15.4
   genital organ NEC (nontraumatic)
      female (nonobstetric) N94.89
         traumatic S30.202 ☑
      male N50.1
         traumatic S30.201 ☑
   internal organs — see Injury, by site
   intracerebral, traumatic — see Injury, intracranial, in-
      tracerebral hemorrhage
   intraoperative — see Complications, intraoperative,
      hemorrhage
   labia (nontraumatic) (nonobstetric) N90.89
   liver (subcapsular) (nontraumatic) K76.89
      birth injury P15.0
   mediastinum — see Injury, intrathoracic
   mesosalpinx (nontraumatic) N83.7
      traumatic S37.898 ☑
   muscle — code by site under Contusion
   nontraumatic
      muscle M79.81
      soft tissue M79.81
   obstetrical surgical wound O90.2
   orbit, orbital (nontraumatic) (see also Hemorrhage,
      orbit)
      traumatic — see Contusion, orbit
   pelvis (female) (nontraumatic) (nonobstetric) N94.89
      obstetric O71.7
      traumatic — see Injury, by site
   penis (nontraumatic) N48.89
      birth injury P15.5
   perianal (nontraumatic) K64.5
   perineal S30.23 ☑
      complicating delivery O71.7

Hematoma — continued
   perirenal — see Injury, kidney
   pinna — see Contusion, ear
      nontraumatic — see Disorder, pinna, hematoma
   placenta O43.89- ☑
   postoperative (postprocedural) — see Complication,
      postprocedural, hemorrhage
   retroperitoneal (nontraumatic) K66.1
      traumatic S36.892 ☑
   scrotum, superficial S30.22 ☑
      birth injury P15.5
   seminal vesicle (nontraumatic) N50.1
      traumatic S37.892 ☑
   spermatic cord (traumatic) S37.892 ☑
      nontraumatic N50.1
   spinal (cord) (meninges) (see also Injury, spinal cord,
      by region)
      newborn (birth injury) P11.5
   spleen D73.5
      intraoperative — see Complications, intraoperative,
         hemorrhage, spleen
      postprocedural (postoperative) — see Complica-
         tions, postprocedural, hemorrhage, spleen
   sternocleidomastoid, birth injury P15.2
   sternomastoid, birth injury P15.2
   subarachnoid (traumatic) — see Injury, intracranial,
      subarachnoid hemorrhage
      newborn P52.5
         due to birth injury P10.3
      nontraumatic — see Hemorrhage, intracranial,
         subarachnoid
   subdural (traumatic) — see Injury, intracranial, subdu-
      ral hemorrhage
      newborn (localized) P52.8
         birth injury P10.0
      nontraumatic — see Hemorrhage, intracranial,
         subdural
   superficial, newborn P54.5
   testis (nontraumatic) N50.1
      birth injury P15.5
   tunica vaginalis (nontraumatic) N50.1
   umbilical cord, complicating delivery O69.5 ☑
   uterine ligament (broad) (nontraumatic) N83.7
      traumatic S37.892 ☑
   vagina (ruptured) (nontraumatic) N89.8
      complicating delivery O71.7
   vas deferens (nontraumatic) N50.1
      traumatic S37.892 ☑
   vitreous — see Hemorrhage, vitreous
   vulva (nontraumatic) (nonobstetric) N90.89
      complicating delivery O71.7
      newborn (birth injury) P15.5
Hematometra N85.7
   with hematocolpos N89.7
Hematomyelia (central) G95.19
   newborn (birth injury) P11.5
   traumatic T14.8
Hematomyelitis G04.90
Hematoperitoneum — see Hemoperitoneum
Hematophobia F40.230
Hematopneumothorax (see Hemothorax)
Hematopoiesis, cyclic D70.4
Hematoporphyria — see Porphyria
Hematorachis, hematorrhachis G95.19
   newborn (birth injury) P11.5
Hematosalpinx N83.6
   with
      hematocolpos N89.7
      hematometra N85.7
         with hematocolpos N89.7
   infectional — see Salpingitis
Hematospermia R36.1
Hematothorax (see Hemothorax)
Hematuria R31.9
   benign (familial) (of childhood) (see also Hematuria,
      idiopathic)
      essential microscopic R31.1
   due to sulphonamide, sulfonamide — see Table of
      Drugs and Chemicals, by drug
   endemic (see also Schistosomiasis) B65.0
   gross R31.0
   idiopathic N02.9
      with glomerular lesion
         crescentic (diffuse) glomerulonephritis N02.7
         dense deposit disease N02.6
         endocapillary proliferative glomerulonephritis
            N02.4

Hematuria — continued
   idiopathic — continued
      with glomerular lesion — continued
         focal and segmental hyalinosis or sclerosis
            N02.1
         membranoproliferative (diffuse) N02.5
         membranous (diffuse) N02.2
         mesangial proliferative (diffuse) N02.3
         mesangiocapillary (diffuse) N02.5
         minor abnormality N02.0
         proliferative NEC N02.8
         specified pathology NEC N02.8
   intermittent — see Hematuria, idiopathic
   malarial B50.8
   microscopic NEC R31.2
      benign essential R31.1
   paroxysmal (see also Hematuria, idiopathic)
      nocturnal D59.5
   persistent — see Hematuria, idiopathic
   recurrent — see Hematuria, idiopathic
   tropical (see also Schistosomiasis) B65.0
   tuberculous A18.13
Hemeralopia (day blindness) H53.11
   vitamin A deficiency E50.5
Hemi-akinesia R41.4
Hemianalgesia R20.0
Hemianencephaly Q00.0
Hemianesthesia R20.0
Hemianopia, hemianopsia (heteronymous) H53.47
   homonymous H53.46- ☑
   syphilitic A52.71
Hemiathetosis R25.8
Hemiatrophy R68.89
   cerebellar G31.9
   face, facial, progressive (Romberg) G51.8
   tongue K14.8
Hemiballism (us) G25.5
Hemicardia Q24.8
Hemicephalus, hemicephaly Q00.0
Hemichorea G25.5
Hemicolitis, left — see Colitis, left sided
Hemicrania
   congenital malformation Q00.0
   continua G44.51
   meaning migraine (see also Migraine) G43.909
   paroxysmal G44.039
      chronic G44.049
         intractable G44.041
         not intractable G44.049
      episodic G44.039
         intractable G44.031
         not intractable G44.039
      intractable G44.031
      not intractable G44.039
Hemidystrophy — see Hemiatrophy
Hemiectromelia Q73.8
Hemihypalgesia R20.8
Hemihypesthesia R20.1
Hemi-inattention R41.4
Hemimelia Q73.8
   lower limb — see Defect, reduction, lower limb, spec-
      ified type NEC
   upper limb — see Defect, reduction, upper limb,
      specified type NEC
Hemiparalysis — see Hemiplegia
Hemiparesis — see Hemiplegia
Hemiparesthesia R20.2
Hemiparkinsonism G20
Hemiplegia G81.9- ☑
   alternans facialis G83.89
   ascending NEC G81.90
      spinal G95.89
   congenital (cerebral) G80.8
      spastic G80.2
   embolic (current episode) I63.4- ☑
   flaccid G81.0- ☑
   following
      cerebrovascular disease I69.959
         cerebral infarction I69.35- ☑
         intracerebral hemorrhage I69.15- ☑
         nontraumatic intracranial hemorrhage NEC
            I69.25- ☑
         specified disease NEC I69.85- ☑
         stroke NOS I69.35- ☑
         subarachnoid hemorrhage I69.05- ☑
   hysterical F44.4

   ☑ **Additional Character Required — Refer to the Tabular List for Character Selection**   ⩇ Subterms under main terms may continue to next column or page

Hemiplegia — *continued*
- newborn NEC P91.8
- birth injury P11.9
- spastic G81.1- ☑
- congenital G80.2
- thrombotic (current episode) I63.3 ☑

Hemisection, spinal cord — *see* Injury, spinal cord, by region

Hemispasm (facial) R25.2

Hemisporosis B48.8

Hemitremor R25.1

Hemivertebra Q76.49
- failure of segmentation with scoliosis Q76.3
- fusion with scoliosis Q76.3

Hemochromatosis E83.119
- with refractory anemia D46.1
- due to repeated red blood cell transfusion E83.111
- hereditary (primary) E83.110
- primary E83.110
- specified NEC E83.118

Hemoglobin (*see also* condition)
- abnormal (disease) — *see* Disease, hemoglobin
- AS genotype D57.3
- Constant Spring D58.2
- E-beta thalassemia D56.5
- fetal, hereditary persistence (HPFH) D56.4
- H Constant Spring D56.0
- low NOS D64.9
- S (Hb S), heterozygous D57.3

Hemoglobinemia D59.9
- due to blood transfusion T80.89 ☑
- paroxysmal D59.6
- nocturnal D59.5

Hemoglobinopathy (mixed) D58.2
- with thalassemia D56.8
- sickle-cell D57.1
- with thalassemia D57.40
- with crisis (vasoocclusive pain) D57.419
- with
- acute chest syndrome D57.411
- splenic sequestration D57.412
- without crisis D57.40

Hemoglobinuria R82.3
- with anemia, hemolytic, acquired (chronic) NEC D59.6
- cold (agglutinin) (paroxysmal) (with Raynaud's syndrome) D59.6
- due to exertion or hemolysis NEC D59.6
- intermittent D59.6
- malarial B50.8
- march D59.6
- nocturnal (paroxysmal) D59.5
- paroxysmal (cold) D59.6
- nocturnal D59.5

Hemolymphangioma D18.1

Hemolysis
- intravascular
- with
- abortion — *see* Abortion, by type, complicated by, hemorrhage
- ectopic or molar pregnancy O08.1
- hemorrhage
- antepartum — *see* Hemorrhage, antepartum, with coagulation defect
- intrapartum (*see also* Hemorrhage, complicating, delivery) O67.0
- postpartum O72.3
- neonatal (excessive) P58.9
- specified NEC P58.8

Hemolytic — *see* condition

Hemopericardium I31.2
- following acute myocardial infarction (current complication) I23.0
- newborn P54.8
- traumatic — *see* Injury, heart, with hemopericardium

Hemoperitoneum K66.1
- infectional K65.9
- traumatic S36.899 ☑
- with open wound — *see* Wound, open, with penetration into peritoneal cavity

Hemophilia (classical) (familial) (hereditary) D66
- A D66
- acquired D68.311
- autoimmune D68.311
- B D67
- C D68.1
- calcipriva (*see also* Defect, coagulation) D68.4
- nonfamilial (*see also* Defect, coagulation) D68.4
- secondary D68.311

Hemophilia — *continued*
- vascular D68.0

Hemophthalmos H44.81- ☑

Hemopneumothorax (*see also* Hemothorax)
- traumatic S27.2 ☑

Hemoptysis R04.2
- newborn P26.9
- tuberculous — *see* Tuberculosis, pulmonary

Hemorrhage, hemorrhagic (concealed) R58
- abdomen R58
- accidental antepartum — *see* Hemorrhage, antepartum
- acute idiopathic pulmonary, in infants R04.81
- adenoid J35.8
- adrenal (capsule) (gland) E27.49
- medulla E27.8
- newborn P54.4
- after delivery — *see* Hemorrhage, postpartum
- alveolar
- lung, newborn P26.8
- process K08.8
- alveolus K08.8
- amputation stump (surgical) T87.89
- anemia (chronic) D50.0
- acute D62
- antepartum (with) O46.90
- with coagulation defect O46.00- ☑
- afibrinogenemia O46.01- ☑
- disseminated intravascular coagulation O46.02- ☑
- hypofibrinogenemia O46.01- ☑
- specified defect NEC O46.09- ☑
- before 20 weeks gestation O20.9
- specified type NEC O20.8
- threatened abortion O20.0
- due to
- abruptio placenta (*see also* Abruptio placentae) O45.9- ☑
- leiomyoma, uterus — *see* Hemorrhage, antepartum, specified cause NEC
- placenta previa O44.1- ☑
- specified cause NEC — *see* subcategory O46.8X- ☑
- anus (sphincter) K62.5
- apoplexy (stroke) — *see* Hemorrhage, intracranial, intracerebral
- arachnoid — *see* Hemorrhage, intracranial, subarachnoid
- artery R58
- brain — *see* Hemorrhage, intracranial, intracerebral
- basilar (ganglion) I61.0
- bladder N32.89
- bowel K92.2
- newborn P54.3
- brain (miliary) (nontraumatic) — *see* Hemorrhage, intracranial, intracerebral
- due to
- birth injury P10.1
- syphilis A52.05
- epidural or extradural (traumatic) — *see* Injury, intracranial, epidural hemorrhage
- newborn P52.4
- birth injury P10.1
- subarachnoid — *see* Hemorrhage, intracranial, subarachnoid
- subdural — *see* Hemorrhage, intracranial, subdural
- brainstem (nontraumatic) I61.3
- traumatic S06.38- ☑
- breast N64.59
- bronchial tube — *see* Hemorrhage, lung
- bronchopulmonary — *see* Hemorrhage, lung
- bronchus — *see* Hemorrhage, lung
- bulbar I61.5
- capillary I78.8
- primary D69.8
- cecum K92.2
- cerebellar, cerebellum (nontraumatic) I61.4
- newborn P52.6
- traumatic S06.37- ☑
- cerebral, cerebrum (*see also* Hemorrhage, intracranial, intracerebral)
- lobe I61.1
- newborn (anoxic) P52.4
- birth injury P10.1
- cerebromeningeal I61.8
- cerebrospinal — *see* Hemorrhage, intracranial, intracerebral
- cervix (uteri) (stump) NEC N88.8

Hemorrhage, hemorrhagic — *continued*
- chamber, anterior (eye) — *see* Hyphema
- childbirth — *see* Hemorrhage, complicating, delivery
- choroid H31.30- ☑
- expulsive H31.31- ☑
- ciliary body — *see* Hyphema
- cochlea — *see* subcategory H83.8 ☑
- colon K92.2
- complicating
- abortion — *see* Abortion, by type, complicated by, hemorrhage
- delivery O67.9
- associated with coagulation defect (afibrinogenemia) (DIC) (hyperfibrinolysis) O67.0
- specified cause NEC O67.8
- surgical procedure — *see* Hemorrhage, intraoperative
- conjunctiva H11.3- ☑
- newborn P54.8
- cord, newborn (stump) P51.9
- corpus luteum (ruptured) cyst N83.1
- cortical (brain) I61.1
- cranial — *see* Hemorrhage, intracranial
- cutaneous R23.3
- due to autosensitivity, erythrocyte D69.2
- newborn P54.5
- delayed
- following ectopic or molar pregnancy O08.1
- postpartum O72.2
- diathesis (familial) D69.9
- disease D69.9
- newborn P53
- specified type NEC D69.8
- due to or associated with
- afibrinogenemia or other coagulation defect (conditions in categories D65- D69)
- antepartum — *see* Hemorrhage, antepartum, with coagulation defect
- intrapartum O67.0
- dental implant M27.61
- device, implant or graft (*see also* Complications, by site and type, specified NEC) T85.83 ☑
- arterial graft NEC T82.838 ☑
- breast T85.83 ☑
- catheter NEC T85.83 ☑
- dialysis (renal) T82.838 ☑
- intraperitoneal T85.83 ☑
- infusion NEC T82.838 ☑
- spinal (epidural) (subdural) T85.83 ☑
- urinary (indwelling) T83.83 ☑
- electronic (electrode) (pulse generator) (stimulator)
- bone T84.83 ☑
- cardiac T82.837 ☑
- nervous system (brain) (peripheral nerve) (spinal) T85.83 ☑
- urinary T83.83 ☑
- fixation, internal (orthopedic) NEC T84.83 ☑
- gastrointestinal (bile duct) (esophagus) T85.83 ☑
- genital NEC T83.83 ☑
- heart NEC T82.837 ☑
- joint prosthesis T84.83 ☑
- ocular (corneal graft) (orbital implant) NEC T85.83 ☑
- orthopedic NEC T84.83 ☑
- bone graft T86.838
- specified NEC T85.83 ☑
- urinary NEC T83.83 ☑
- vascular NEC T82.838 ☑
- ventricular intracranial shunt T85.83 ☑
- duodenum, duodenal K92.2
- ulcer — *see* Ulcer, duodenum, with hemorrhage
- dura mater — *see* Hemorrhage, intracranial, subdural
- endotracheal — *see* Hemorrhage, lung
- epicranial subaponeurotic (massive), birth injury P12.2
- epidural (traumatic) (*see also* Injury, intracranial, epidural hemorrhage)
- nontraumatic I62.1
- esophagus K22.8
- varix I85.01
- secondary I85.11
- excessive, following ectopic gestation (subsequent episode) O08.1
- extradural (traumatic) — *see* Injury, intracranial, epidural hemorrhage
- birth injury P10.8

Hemorrhage, hemorrhagic — *continued*
  extradural — *see* Injury, intracranial, epidural hemorrhage — *continued*
    newborn (anoxic) (nontraumatic) P52.8
    nontraumatic I62.1
  eye NEC H57.8
    fundus — *see* Hemorrhage, retina
    lid — *see* Disorder, eyelid, specified type NEC
  fallopian tube N83.6
  fibrinogenolysis — *see* Fibrinolysis
  fibrinolytic (acquired) — *see* Fibrinolysis
  from
    ear (nontraumatic) — *see* Otorrhagia
    tracheostomy stoma J95.01
  fundus, eye — *see* Hemorrhage, retina
  funis — *see* Hemorrhage, umbilicus, cord
  gastric — *see* Hemorrhage, stomach
  gastroenteric K92.2
    newborn P54.3
  gastrointestinal (tract) K92.2
    newborn P54.3
  genital organ, male N50.1
  genitourinary (tract) NOS R31.9
  gingiva K06.8
  globe (eye) — *see* Hemophthalmos
  graafian follicle cyst (ruptured) N83.0
  gum K06.8
  heart I51.89
  hypopharyngeal (throat) R04.1
  intermenstrual (regular) N92.3
    irregular N92.1
  internal (organs) NEC R58
    capsule I61.0
    ear — *see* subcategory H83.8 ☑
    newborn P54.8
  intestine K92.2
    newborn P54.3
  intra-abdominal R58
  intra-alveolar (lung), newborn P26.8
  intracerebral (nontraumatic) — *see* Hemorrhage, intracranial, intracerebral
  intracranial (nontraumatic) I62.9
    birth injury P10.9
    epidural, nontraumatic I62.1
    extradural, nontraumatic I62.1
    intracerebral (nontraumatic) (in) I61.9
      brain stem I61.3
      cerebellum I61.4
      hemisphere I61.2
        cortical (superficial) I61.1
        subcortical (deep) I61.0
      intraoperative
        during a nervous system procedure G97.31
        during other procedure G97.32
      intraventricular I61.5
      multiple localized I61.6
      newborn P52.4
        birth injury P10.1
      postprocedural
        following a nervous system procedure G97.51
        following other procedure G97.52
      specified NEC I61.8
      superficial I61.1
      traumatic (diffuse) — *see* Injury, intracranial, diffuse
        focal — *see* Injury, intracranial, focal
    newborn P52.9
      specified NEC P52.8
    subarachnoid (nontraumatic) (from) I60.9
      intracranial (cerebral) artery I60.7
        anterior communicating I60.2- ☑
        basilar I60.4
        carotid siphon and bifurcation I60.0- ☑
        communicating I60.7
          anterior I60.2- ☑
          posterior I60.3- ☑
        middle cerebral I60.1- ☑
        posterior communicating I60.3- ☑
        specified artery NEC I60.6
        vertebral I60.5- ☑
      newborn P52.5
        birth injury P10.3
      specified NEC I60.8
      traumatic S06.6X- ☑
    subdural (nontraumatic) I62.00
      acute I62.01
      birth injury P10.0

Hemorrhage, hemorrhagic — *continued*
  intracranial — *continued*
    subdural — *continued*
      chronic I62.03
      newborn (anoxic) (hypoxic) P52.8
        birth injury P10.0
      spinal G95.19
      subacute I62.02
      traumatic — *see* Injury, intracranial, subdural hemorrhage
    traumatic — *see* Injury, intracranial, focal brain injury
  intramedullary NEC G95.19
  intraocular — *see* Hemophthalmos
  intraoperative, intraprocedural — *see* Complication, hemorrhage (hematoma), intraoperative (intraprocedural), by site
  intrapartum — *see* Hemorrhage, complicating, delivery
  intrapelvic
    female N94.89
    male K66.1
  intraperitoneal K66.1
  intrapontine I61.3
  intraprocedural — *see* Complication, hemorrhage (hematoma), intraoperative (intraprocedural), by site
  intrauterine N85.7
    complicating delivery (*see also* Hemorrhage, complicating, delivery) O67.9
    postpartum — *see* Hemorrhage, postpartum
  intraventricular I61.5
    newborn (nontraumatic) (*see also* Newborn, affected by, hemorrhage) P52.3
      due to birth injury P10.2
      grade
        1 P52.0
        2 P52.1
        3 P52.21
        4 P52.22
  intravesical N32.89
  iris (postinfectional) (postinflammatory) (toxic) — *see* Hyphema
  joint (nontraumatic) — *see* Hemarthrosis
  kidney N28.89
  knee (joint) (nontraumatic) — *see* Hemarthrosis, knee
  labyrinth — *see* subcategory H83.8 ☑
  lenticular striate artery I61.0
  ligature, vessel — *see* Hemorrhage, postoperative
  liver K76.89
  lung R04.89
    newborn P26.9
      massive P26.1
      specified NEC P26.8
    tuberculous — *see* Tuberculosis, pulmonary
  massive umbilical, newborn P51.0
  mediastinum — *see* Hemorrhage, lung
  medulla I61.3
  membrane (brain) I60.8
    spinal cord — *see* Hemorrhage, spinal cord
  meninges, meningeal (brain) (middle) I60.8
    spinal cord — *see* Hemorrhage, spinal cord
  mesentery K66.1
  metritis — *see* Endometritis
  mouth K13.79
  mucous membrane NEC R58
    newborn P54.8
  muscle M62.89
  nail (subungual) L60.8
  nasal turbinate R04.0
    newborn P54.8
  navel, newborn P51.9
  newborn P54.9
    specified NEC P54.8
  nipple N64.59
  nose R04.0
    newborn P54.8
  omentum K66.1
  optic nerve (sheath) H47.02- ☑
  orbit, orbital H05.23- ☑
  ovary NEC N83.8
  oviduct N83.6
  pancreas K86.8
  parathyroid (gland) (spontaneous) E21.4
  parturition — *see* Hemorrhage, complicating, delivery
  penis N48.89
  pericardium, pericarditis I31.2
  peritoneum, peritoneal K66.1

Hemorrhage, hemorrhagic — *continued*
  peritonsillar tissue J35.8
    due to infection J36
  petechial R23.3
    due to autosensitivity, erythrocyte D69.2
  pituitary (gland) E23.6
  pleura — *see* Hemorrhage, lung
  polioencephalitis, superior E51.2
  polymyositis — *see* Polymyositis
  pons, pontine I61.3
  posterior fossa (nontraumatic) I61.8
    newborn P52.6
  postmenopausal N95.0
  postnasal R04.0
  postoperative — *see* Complications, postprocedural, hemorrhage, by site
  postpartum NEC (following delivery of placenta) O72.1
    delayed or secondary O72.2
    retained placenta O72.0
    third stage O72.0
  pregnancy — *see* Hemorrhage, antepartum
  preretinal — *see* Hemorrhage, retina
  prostate N42.1
  puerperal — *see* Hemorrhage, postpartum
    delayed or secondary O72.2
  pulmonary R04.89
    newborn P26.9
      massive P26.1
      specified NEC P26.8
    tuberculous — *see* Tuberculosis, pulmonary
  purpura (primary) D69.3
  rectum (sphincter) K62.5
    newborn P54.2
  recurring, following initial hemorrhage at time of injury T79.2 ☑
  renal N28.89
  respiratory passage or tract R04.9
    specified NEC R04.89
  retina, retinal (vessels) H35.6- ☑
    diabetic — *see* Diabetes, retinal, hemorrhage
  retroperitoneal R58
  scalp R58
  scrotum N50.1
  secondary (nontraumatic) R58
    following initial hemorrhage at time of injury T79.2 ☑
  seminal vesicle N50.1
  skin R23.3
    newborn P54.5
  slipped umbilical ligature P51.8
  spermatic cord N50.1
  spinal (cord) G95.19
    newborn (birth injury) P11.5
  spleen D73.5
    intraoperative — *see* Complications, intraoperative, hemorrhage, spleen
    postprocedural — *see* Complications, postprocedural, hemorrhage, spleen
  stomach K92.2
    newborn P54.3
    ulcer — *see* Ulcer, stomach, with hemorrhage
  subarachnoid (nontraumatic) — *see* Hemorrhage, intracranial, subarachnoid
  subconjunctival (*see also* Hemorrhage, conjunctiva)
    birth injury P15.3
  subcortical (brain) I61.0
  subcutaneous R23.3
  subdiaphragmatic R58
  subdural (acute) (nontraumatic) — *see* Hemorrhage, intracranial, subdural
  subependymal
    newborn P52.0
      with intraventricular extension P52.1
        and intracerebral extension P52.22
  subgaleal P12.1
  subhyaloid — *see* Hemorrhage, retina
  subperiosteal — *see* Disorder, bone, specified type NEC
  subretinal — *see* Hemorrhage, retina
  subtentorial — *see* Hemorrhage, intracranial, subdural
  subungual L60.8
  suprarenal (capsule) (gland) E27.49
    newborn P54.4
  tentorium (traumatic) NEC — *see* Hemorrhage, brain
    newborn (birth injury) P10.4
  testis N50.1
  third stage (postpartum) O72.0
  thorax — *see* Hemorrhage, lung

☑ **Additional Character Required** — Refer to the Tabular List for Character Selection   ▽ **Subterms under main terms may continue to next column or page**

Hemorrhage, hemorrhagic — *continued*
　throat R04.1
　thymus (gland) E32.8
　thyroid (cyst) (gland) E07.89
　tongue K14.8
　tonsil J35.8
　trachea — *see* Hemorrhage, lung
　tracheobronchial R04.89
　　newborn P26.0
　traumatic — *code to* specific injury
　　cerebellar — *see* Hemorrhage, brain
　　intracranial — *see* Hemorrhage, brain
　　recurring or secondary (following initial hemor-
　　　rhage at time of injury) T79.2 ☑
　tuberculous NEC (*see also* Tuberculosis, pulmonary)
　　A15.0
　tunica vaginalis N50.1
　ulcer — *code by* site under Ulcer, with hemorrhage
　　K27.4
　umbilicus, umbilical
　　cord
　　　after birth, newborn P51.9
　　　complicating delivery O69.5 ☑
　　newborn P51.9
　　　massive P51.0
　　　slipped ligature P51.8
　　stump P51.9
　urethra (idiopathic) N36.8
　uterus, uterine (abnormal) N93.9
　　climacteric N92.4
　　complicating delivery — *see* Hemorrhage, compli-
　　　cating, delivery
　　dysfunctional or functional N93.8
　　intermenstrual (regular) N92.3
　　　irregular N92.1
　　postmenopausal N95.0
　　postpartum — *see* Hemorrhage, postpartum
　　preclimacteric or premenopausal N92.4
　　prepubertal N93.8
　　pubertal N92.2
　vagina (abnormal) N93.9
　　newborn P54.6
　vas deferens N50.1
　vasa previa O69.4 ☑
　ventricular I61.5
　vesical N32.89
　viscera NEC R58
　　newborn P54.8
　vitreous (humor) (intraocular) H43.1- ☑
　vulva N90.89
Hemorrhoids (bleeding) (without mention of degree)
　K64.9
　1st degree (grade/stage I) (without prolapse outside
　　of anal canal) K64.0
　2nd degree (grade/stage II) (that prolapse with
　　straining but retract spontaneously) K64.1
　3rd degree (grade/stage III) (that prolapse with
　　straining and require manual replacement back
　　inside anal canal) K64.2
　4th degree (grade/stage IV) (with prolapsed tissue that
　　cannot be manually replaced) K64.3
　complicating
　　pregnancy O22.4 ☑
　　puerperium O87.2
　external K64.4
　　with
　　　thrombosis K64.5
　internal (without mention of degree) K64.8
　prolapsed K64.8
　skin tags
　　anus K64.4
　　residual K64.4
　specified NEC K64.8
　strangulated (*see also* Hemorrhoids, by degree) K64.8
　thrombosed (*see also* Hemorrhoids, by degree) K64.5
　ulcerated (*see also* Hemorrhoids, by degree) K64.8
Hemosalpinx N83.6
　with
　　hematocolpos N89.7
　　hematometra N85.7
　　　with hematocolpos N89.7
Hemosiderosis (dietary) E83.19
　pulmonary, idiopathic E83.1- ☑ [J84.03]
　transfusion T80.89 ☑
Hemothorax (bacterial) (nontuberculous) J94.2
　newborn P54.8
　traumatic S27.1 ☑
　　with pneumothorax S27.2 ☑

Hemothorax — *continued*
　tuberculous NEC A15.6
Henoch (-Schönlein) **disease or syndrome** (purpura)
　D69.0
Henpue, henpuye A66.6
Hepar lobatum (syphilitic) A52.74
Hepatalgia K76.89
Hepatitis K75.9
　acute B17.9
　　with coma K72.01
　　with hepatic failure — *see* Failure, hepatic
　　alcoholic — *see* Hepatitis, alcoholic
　　infectious B15.9
　　　with hepatic coma B15.0
　　viral B17.9
　alcoholic (acute) (chronic) K70.10
　　with ascites K70.11
　amebic — *see* Abscess, liver, amebic
　anicteric, (viral) — *see* Hepatitis, viral
　antigen-associated (HAA) — *see* Hepatitis, B
　Australia-antigen (positive) — *see* Hepatitis, B
　autoimmune K75.4
　B B19.10
　　with hepatic coma B19.11
　　acute B16.9
　　　with
　　　　delta-agent (coinfection) (without hepatic
　　　　　coma) B16.1
　　　　　with hepatic coma B16.0
　　　　hepatic coma (without delta-agent coinfec-
　　　　　tion) B16.2
　　chronic B18.1
　　　with delta-agent B18.0
　bacterial NEC K75.89
　C (viral) B19.20
　　with hepatic coma B19.21
　　acute B17.10
　　　with hepatic coma B17.11
　　chronic B18.2
　catarrhal (acute) B15.9
　　with hepatic coma B15.0
　cholangiolitic K75.89
　cholestatic K75.89
　chronic K73.9
　　active NEC K73.2
　　lobular NEC K73.1
　　persistent NEC K73.0
　　specified NEC K73.8
　cytomegaloviral B25.1
　due to ethanol (acute) (chronic) — *see* Hepatitis, alco-
　　holic
　epidemic B15.9
　　with hepatic coma B15.0
　fulminant NEC (viral) — *see* Hepatitis, viral
　granulomatous NEC K75.3
　herpesviral B00.81
　history of
　　B Z86.19
　　C Z86.19
　homologous serum — *see* Hepatitis, viral, type B
　in (due to)
　　mumps B26.81
　　toxoplasmosis (acquired) B58.1
　　　congenital (active) P37.1 [K77]
　infectious, infective (acute) (chronic) (subacute) B15.9
　　with hepatic coma B15.0
　inoculation — *see* Hepatitis, viral, type B
　interstitial (chronic) K74.69
　lupoid NEC K75.4
　malignant NEC (with hepatic failure) K72.90
　　with coma K72.91
　neonatal (idiopathic) (toxic) P59.29
　neonatal giant cell P59.29
　newborn P59.29
　postimmunization — *see* Hepatitis, viral, type B
　post-transfusion — *see* Hepatitis, viral, type B
　reactive, nonspecific K75.2
　serum — *see* Hepatitis, viral, type B
　specified type NEC
　　with hepatic failure — *see* Failure, hepatic
　syphilitic (late) A52.74
　　congenital (early) A50.08 [K77]
　　　late A50.59 [K77]
　　secondary A51.45
　toxic (*see also* Disease, liver, toxic) K71.6
　tuberculous A18.83
　viral, virus B19.9
　　with hepatic coma B19.0

Hepatitis — *continued*
　viral, virus — *continued*
　　acute B17.9
　　chronic B18.9
　　　specified NEC B18.8
　　　type
　　　　B B18.1
　　　　　with delta-agent B18.0
　　　　C B18.2
　　congenital P35.3
　　coxsackie B33.8 [K77]
　　cytomegalic inclusion B25.1
　　in remission, any type — *code to* Hepatitis, chronic,
　　　by type
　　non-A, non-B B17.8
　　specified type NEC (with or without coma) B17.8
　　type
　　　A B15.9
　　　　with hepatic coma B15.0
　　　B B19.10
　　　　with hepatic coma B19.11
　　　　acute B16.9
　　　　　with
　　　　　　delta-agent (coinfection) (without
　　　　　　　hepatic coma) B16.1
　　　　　　　with hepatic coma B16.0
　　　　　　hepatic coma (without delta-agent
　　　　　　　coinfection) B16.2
　　　　chronic B18.1
　　　　　with delta-agent B18.0
　　　C B19.20
　　　　with hepatic coma B19.21
　　　　acute B17.10
　　　　　with hepatic coma B17.11
　　　　chronic B18.2
　　　E B17.2
　　　non-A, non-B B17.8
Hepatization lung (acute) — *see* Pneumonia, lobar
Hepatoblastoma C22.2
Hepatocarcinoma C22.0
Hepatocholangiocarcinoma C22.0
Hepatocholangioma, benign D13.4
Hepatocholangitis K75.89
Hepatolenticular degeneration E83.01
Hepatoma (malignant) C22.0
　benign D13.4
　embryonal C22.0
Hepatomegaly (*see also* Hypertrophy, liver)
　with splenomegaly R16.2
　congenital Q44.7
　in mononucleosis
　　gammaherpesviral B27.09
　　infectious specified NEC B27.89
Hepatoptosis K76.89
Hepatorenal syndrome following labor and delivery
　O90.4
Hepatosis K76.89
Hepatosplenomegaly R16.2
　hyperlipemic (Bürger-Grütz type) E78.3 [K77]
Hereditary — *see* condition
Heredodegeneration, macular — *see* Dystrophy, retina
Heredopathia atactica polyneuritiformis G60.1
Heredosyphilis — *see* Syphilis, congenital
Herlitz' syndrome Q81.1
Hermansky-Pudlak syndrome E70.331
Hermaphrodite, hermaphroditism (true) Q56.0
　46,XX with streak gonads Q99.1
　46,XX/46,XY Q99.0
　46,XY with streak gonads Q99.1
　chimera 46,XX/46,XY Q99.0
Hernia, hernial (acquired) (recurrent) K46.9
　with
　　gangrene — *see* Hernia, by site, with, gangrene
　　incarceration — *see* Hernia, by site, with, obstruc-
　　　tion
　　irreducible — *see* Hernia, by site, with, obstruction
　　obstruction — *see* Hernia, by site, with, obstruction
　　strangulation — *see* Hernia, by site, with, obstruc-
　　　tion
　abdomen, abdominal K46.9
　　with
　　　gangrene (and obstruction) K46.1
　　　obstruction K46.0
　　femoral — *see* Hernia, femoral
　　incisional — *see* Hernia, incisional
　　inguinal — *see* Hernia, inguinal
　　specified site NEC K45.8

Hernia, hernial — *continued*
  abdomen, abdominal — *continued*
    specified site — *continued*
      with
        gangrene (and obstruction) K45.1
        obstruction K45.0
    umbilical — *see* Hernia, umbilical
    wall — *see* Hernia, ventral
  appendix — *see* Hernia, abdomen
  bladder (mucosa) (sphincter)
    congenital (female) (male) Q79.51
    female — *see* Cystocele
    male N32.89
  brain, congenital — *see* Encephalocele
  cartilage, vertebra — *see* Displacement, intervertebral disc
  cerebral, congenital (*see also* Encephalocele)
    endaural Q01.8
  ciliary body (traumatic) S05.2- ☑
  colon — *see* Hernia, abdomen
  Cooper's — *see* Hernia, abdomen, specified site NEC
  crural — *see* Hernia, femoral
  diaphragm, diaphragmatic K44.9
    with
      gangrene (and obstruction) K44.1
      obstruction K44.0
    congenital Q79.0
  direct (inguinal) — *see* Hernia, inguinal
  diverticulum, intestine — *see* Hernia, abdomen
  double (inguinal) — *see* Hernia, inguinal, bilateral
  due to adhesions (with obstruction) K56.5
  epigastric (*see also* Hernia, ventral) K43.9
  esophageal hiatus — *see* Hernia, hiatal
  external (inguinal) — *see* Hernia, inguinal
  fallopian tube N83.4
  fascia M62.89
  femoral K41.90
    with
      gangrene (and obstruction) K41.40
        not specified as recurrent K41.40
        recurrent K41.41
      obstruction K41.30
        not specified as recurrent K41.30
        recurrent K41.31
    bilateral K41.20
      with
        gangrene (and obstruction) K41.10
          not specified as recurrent K41.10
          recurrent K41.11
        obstruction K41.00
          not specified as recurrent K41.00
          recurrent K41.01
      not specified as recurrent K41.20
      recurrent K41.21
    not specified as recurrent K41.90
    recurrent K41.91
    unilateral K41.90
      with
        gangrene (and obstruction) K41.40
          not specified as recurrent K41.40
          recurrent K41.41
        obstruction K41.30
          not specified as recurrent K41.30
          recurrent K41.31
      not specified as recurrent K41.90
      recurrent K41.91
  foramen magnum G93.5
    congenital Q01.8
  funicular (umbilical) (*see also* Hernia, umbilicus)
    spermatic (cord) — *see* Hernia, inguinal
  gastrointestinal tract — *see* Hernia, abdomen
  Hesselbach's — *see* Hernia, femoral, specified site NEC
  hiatal (esophageal) (sliding) K44.9
    with
      gangrene (and obstruction) K44.1
      obstruction K44.0
    congenital Q40.1
  hypogastric — *see* Hernia, ventral
  incarcerated (*see also* Hernia, by site, with obstruction)
    with gangrene — *see* Hernia, by site, with gangrene
  incisional K43.2
    with
      gangrene (and obstruction) K43.1
      obstruction K43.0
  indirect (inguinal) — *see* Hernia, inguinal
  inguinal (direct) (external) (funicular) (indirect) (internal) (oblique) (scrotal) (sliding) K40.90

Hernia, hernial — *continued*
  inguinal — *continued*
    with
      gangrene (and obstruction) K40.40
        not specified as recurrent K40.40
        recurrent K40.41
      obstruction K40.30
        not specified as recurrent K40.30
        recurrent K40.31
    bilateral K40.20
      with
        gangrene (and obstruction) K40.10
          not specified as recurrent K40.10
          recurrent K40.11
        obstruction K40.00
          not specified as recurrent K40.00
          recurrent K40.01
      not specified as recurrent K40.20
      recurrent K40.21
    not specified as recurrent K40.90
    recurrent K40.91
    unilateral K40.90
      with
        gangrene (and obstruction) K40.40
          not specified as recurrent K40.40
          recurrent K40.41
        obstruction K40.30
          not specified as recurrent K40.30
          recurrent K40.31
      not specified as recurrent K40.90
      recurrent K40.91
  internal (*see also* Hernia, abdomen)
    inguinal — *see* Hernia, inguinal
  interstitial — *see* Hernia, abdomen
  intervertebral cartilage or disc — *see* Displacement, intervertebral disc
  intestine, intestinal — *see* Hernia, by site
  intra-abdominal — *see* Hernia, abdomen
  iris (traumatic) S05.2- ☑
  irreducible (*see also* Hernia, by site, with obstruction)
    with gangrene — *see* Hernia, by site, with gangrene
  ischiatic — *see* Hernia, abdomen, specified site NEC
  ischiorectal — *see* Hernia, abdomen, specified site NEC
  lens (traumatic) S05.2- ☑
  linea (alba) (semilunaris) — *see* Hernia, ventral
  Littre's — *see* Hernia, abdomen
  lumbar — *see* Hernia, abdomen, specified site NEC
  lung (subcutaneous) J98.4
  mediastinum J98.5
  mesenteric (internal) — *see* Hernia, abdomen
  midline — *see* Hernia, ventral
  muscle (sheath) M62.89
  nucleus pulposus — *see* Displacement, intervertebral disc
  oblique (inguinal) — *see* Hernia, inguinal
  obstructive (*see also* Hernia, by site, with obstruction)
    with gangrene — *see* Hernia, by site, with gangrene
  obturator — *see* Hernia, abdomen, specified site NEC
  omental — *see* Hernia, abdomen
  ovary N83.4
  oviduct N83.4
  paraesophageal (*see also* Hernia, diaphragm)
    congenital Q40.1
  parastomal K43.5
    with
      gangrene (and obstruction) K43.4
      obstruction K43.3
  paraumbilical — *see* Hernia, umbilicus
  perineal — *see* Hernia, abdomen, specified site NEC
  Petit's — *see* Hernia, abdomen, specified site NEC
  postoperative — *see* Hernia, incisional
  pregnant uterus — *see* Abnormal, uterus in pregnancy or childbirth
  prevesical N32.89
  properitoneal — *see* Hernia, abdomen, specified site NEC
  pudendal — *see* Hernia, abdomen, specified site NEC
  rectovaginal N81.6
  retroperitoneal — *see* Hernia, abdomen, specified site NEC
  Richter's — *see* Hernia, abdomen, with obstruction
  Rieux's, Riex's — *see* Hernia, abdomen, specified site NEC

Hernia, hernial — *continued*
  sac condition (adhesion) (dropsy) (inflammation) (laceration) (suppuration) — *code by site under* Hernia
  sciatic — *see* Hernia, abdomen, specified site NEC
  scrotum, scrotal — *see* Hernia, inguinal
  sliding (inguinal) (*see also* Hernia, inguinal)
    hiatus — *see* Hernia, hiatal
  spigelian — *see* Hernia, ventral
  spinal — *see* Spina bifida
  strangulated (*see also* Hernia, by site, with obstruction)
    with gangrene — *see* Hernia, by site, with gangrene
  subxiphoid — *see* Hernia, ventral
  supra-umbilicus — *see* Hernia, ventral
  tendon — *see* Disorder, tendon, specified type NEC
  Treitz's (fossa) — *see* Hernia, abdomen, specified site NEC
  tunica vaginalis Q55.29
  umbilicus, umbilical K42.9
    with
      gangrene (and obstruction) K42.1
      obstruction K42.0
  ureter N28.89
  urethra, congenital Q64.79
  urinary meatus, congenital Q64.79
  uterus N81.4
    pregnant — *see* Abnormal, uterus in pregnancy or childbirth
  vaginal (anterior) (wall) — *see* Cystocele
  Velpeau's — *see* Hernia, femoral
  ventral K43.9
    with
      gangrene (and obstruction) K43.7
      obstruction K43.6
    incisional K43.2
      with
        gangrene (and obstruction) K43.1
        obstruction K43.0
    recurrent — *see* Hernia, incisional
    specified NEC K43.9
      with
        gangrene (and obstruction) K43.7
        obstruction K43.6
  vesical
    congenital (female) (male) Q79.51
    female — *see* Cystocele
    male N32.89
  vitreous (into wound) S05.2- ☑
    into anterior chamber — *see* Prolapse, vitreous
Herniation (*see also* Hernia)
  brain (stem) G93.5
  cerebral G93.5
  mediastinum J98.5
  nucleus pulposus — *see* Displacement, intervertebral disc
Herpangina B08.5
Herpes, herpesvirus, herpetic B00.9
  anogenital A60.9
    perianal skin A60.1
    rectum A60.1
    urogenital tract A60.00
      cervix A60.03
      male genital organ NEC A60.02
      penis A60.01
      specified site NEC A60.09
      vagina A60.04
      vulva A60.04
  blepharitis (zoster) B02.39
    simplex B00.59
  circinatus B35.4
    bullosus L12.0
  conjunctivitis (simplex) B00.53
    zoster B02.31
  cornea B02.33
  encephalitis B00.4
    due to herpesvirus 6 B10.01
    due to herpesvirus 7 B10.09
    specified NEC B10.09
  eye (zoster) B02.30
    simplex B00.50
  eyelid (zoster) B02.39
    simplex B00.59
  facialis B00.1
  febrilis B00.1
  geniculate ganglionitis B02.21
  genital, genitalis A60.00
    female A60.09

Herpes, herpesvirus, herpetic — *continued*
  genital, genitalis — *continued*
    male A60.02
  gestational, gestationis O26.4- ☑
  gingivostomatitis B00.2
  human B00.9
    1 — *see* Herpes, simplex
    2 — *see* Herpes, simplex
    3 — *see* Varicella
    4 — *see* Mononucleosis, Epstein-Barr (virus)
    5 — *see* Disease, cytomegalic inclusion (generalized)
    6
      encephalitis B10.01
      specified NEC B10.81
    7
      encephalitis B10.09
      specified NEC B10.82
    8 B10.89
  infection NEC B10.89
    Kaposi's sarcoma associated B10.89
  iridocyclitis (simplex) B00.51
    zoster B02.32
  iris (vesicular erythema multiforme) L51.9
  iritis (simplex) B00.51
  Kaposi's sarcoma associated B10.89
  keratitis (simplex) (dendritic) (disciform) (interstitial) B00.52
    zoster (interstitial) B02.33
  keratoconjunctivitis (simplex) B00.52
    zoster B02.33
  labialis B00.1
  lip B00.1
  meningitis (simplex) B00.3
    zoster B02.1
  ophthalmicus (zoster) NEC B02.30
    simplex B00.50
  penis A60.01
  perianal skin A60.1
  pharyngitis, pharyngotonsillitis B00.2
  rectum A60.1
  scrotum A60.02
  sepsis B00.7
  simplex B00.9
    complicated NEC B00.89
    congenital P35.2
    conjunctivitis B00.53
    external ear B00.1
    eyelid B00.59
    hepatitis B00.81
    keratitis (interstitial) B00.52
    myeltis B00.82
    specified complication NEC B00.89
    visceral B00.89
  stomatitis B00.2
  tonsurans B35.0
  visceral B00.89
  vulva A60.04
  whitlow B00.89
  zoster (*see also* condition) B02.9
    auricularis B02.21
    complicated NEC B02.8
    conjunctivitis B02.31
    disseminated B02.7
    encephalitis B02.0
    eye (lid) B02.39
    geniculate ganglionitis B02.21
    keratitis (interstitial) B02.33
    meningitis B02.1
    myelitis B02.24
    neuritis, neuralgia B02.29
    ophthalmicus NEC B02.30
    oticus B02.21
    polyneuropathy B02.23
    specified complication NEC B02.8
    trigeminal neuralgia B02.22
Herpesvirus (human) — *see* Herpes
Herpetophobia F40.218
Herrick's anemia — *see* Disease, sickle-cell
Hers' disease E74.09
Herter-Gee syndrome K90.0
Herxheimer's reaction R68.89
Hesitancy
  of micturition R39.11
  urinary R39.11
Hesselbach's hernia — *see* Hernia, femoral, specified site NEC

Heterochromia (congenital) Q13.2
  cataract — *see* Cataract, complicated
  cyclitis (Fuchs) — *see* Cyclitis, Fuchs' heterochromic
  hair L67.1
  iritis — *see* Cyclitis, Fuchs' heterochromic
  retained metallic foreign body (nonmagnetic) — *see* Foreign body, intraocular, old, retained
    magnetic — *see* Foreign body, intraocular, old, retained, magnetic
  uveitis — *see* Cyclitis, Fuchs' heterochromic
Heterophoria — *see* Strabismus, heterophoria
Heterophyes, heterophyiasis (small intestine) B66.8
Heterotopia, heterotopic (*see also* Malposition, congenital)
  cerebralis Q04.8
Heterotropia — *see* Strabismus
Heubner-Herter disease K90.0
Hexadactylism Q69.9
HGSIL (cytology finding) (high grade squamous intraepithelial lesion on cytologic smear) (Pap smear finding)
  anus R85.613
  cervix R87.613
    biopsy (histology) finding — *code to* CIN II or CIN III
  vagina R87.623
    biopsy (histology) finding — *code to* VAIN II or VAIN III
Hibernoma — *see* Lipoma
Hiccup, hiccough R06.6
  epidemic B33.0
  psychogenic F45.8
Hidden penis (congenital) Q55.64
  acquired N48.83
Hidradenitis (axillaris) (suppurative) L73.2
Hidradenoma (nodular) (*see also* Neoplasm, skin, benign)
  clear cell — *see* Neoplasm, skin, benign
  papillary — *see* Neoplasm, skin, benign
Hidrocystoma — *see* Neoplasm, skin, benign
High
  altitude effects T70.20 ☑
    anoxia T70.29 ☑
    on
      ears T70.0 ☑
      sinuses T70.1 ☑
    polycythemia D75.1
  arch
    foot Q66.7
    palate, congenital Q38.5
  arterial tension — *see* Hypertension
  basal metabolic rate R94.8
  blood pressure (*see also* Hypertension)
    borderline R03.0
    reading (incidental) (isolated) (nonspecific), without diagnosis of hypertension R03.0
  cholesterol E78.0
    with high triglycerides E78.2
  diaphragm (congenital) Q79.1
  expressed emotional level within family Z63.8
  head at term O32.4 ☑
  palate, congenital Q38.5
  risk
    infant NEC Z76.2
    sexual behavior (heterosexual) Z72.51
      bisexual Z72.53
      homosexual Z72.52
  temperature (of unknown origin) R50.9
  thoracic rib Q76.6
  triglycerides E78.1
    with high cholesterol E78.2
Hildenbrand's disease A75.0
Hilum — *see* condition
Hip — *see* condition
Hippel's disease Q85.8
Hippophobia F40.218
Hippus H57.09
Hirschsprung's disease or megacolon Q43.1
Hirsutism, hirsuties L68.0
Hirudiniasis
  external B88.3
  internal B83.4
Hiss-Russell dysentery A03.1
Histidinemia, histidinuria E70.41
Histiocytoma (*see also* Neoplasm, skin, benign)
  fibrous (*see also* Neoplasm, skin, benign)
    atypical — *see* Neoplasm, connective tissue, uncertain behavior

Histiocytoma — *continued*
  fibrous (*see also* Neoplasm, skin, benign) — *continued*
    malignant — *see* Neoplasm, connective tissue, malignant
Histiocytosis D76.3
  acute differentiated progressive C96.0
  Langerhans' cell NEC C96.6
    multifocal X
      multisystemic (disseminated) C96.0
      unisystemic C96.5
    pulmonary, adult (adult PLCH) J84.82
    unifocal (X) C96.6
  lipid, lipoid D76.3
    essential E75.29
  malignant C96.A (*following* C96.6)
  mononuclear phagocytes NEC D76.1
    Langerhans' cells C96.6
  non-Langerhans cell D76.3
  polyostotic sclerosing D76.3
  sinus, with massive lymphadenopathy D76.3
  syndrome NEC D76.3
  X NEC C96.6
    acute (progressive) C96.0
    chronic C96.6
    multifocal C96.5
    multisystemic C96.0
    unifocal C96.6
Histoplasmosis B39.9
  with pneumonia NEC B39.2
  African B39.5
  American — *see* Histoplasmosis, capsulati
  capsulati B39.4
    disseminated B39.3
    generalized B39.3
    pulmonary B39.2
      acute B39.0
      chronic B39.1
  Darling's B39.4
  duboisii B39.5
  lung NEC B39.2
History
  family (of) (*see also* History, personal (of))
    alcohol abuse Z81.1
    allergy NEC Z84.89
    anemia Z83.2
    arthritis Z82.61
    asthma Z82.5
    blindness Z82.1
    cardiac death (sudden) Z82.41
    carrier of genetic disease Z84.81
    chromosomal anomaly Z82.79
    chronic
      disabling disease NEC Z82.8
      lower respiratory disease Z82.5
    colonic polyps Z83.71
    congenital malformations and deformations Z82.79
      polycystic kidney Z82.71
    consanguinity Z84.3
    deafness Z82.2
    diabetes mellitus Z83.3
    disability NEC Z82.8
    disease or disorder (of)
      allergic NEC Z84.89
      behavioral NEC Z81.8
      blood and blood-forming organs Z83.2
      cardiovascular NEC Z82.49
      chronic disabling NEC Z82.8
      digestive Z83.79
      ear NEC Z83.52
      endocrine NEC Z83.49
      eye NEC Z83.518
        glaucoma Z83.511
      genitourinary NEC Z84.2
      glaucoma Z83.511
      hematological Z83.2
      immune mechanism Z83.2
      infectious NEC Z83.1
      ischemic heart Z82.49
      kidney Z84.1
      mental NEC Z81.8
      metabolic Z83.49
      musculoskeletal NEC Z82.69
      neurological NEC Z82.0
      nutritional Z83.49
      parasitic NEC Z83.1
      psychiatric NEC Z81.8
      respiratory NEC Z83.6

History — *continued*
 family (*see also* History, personal) — *continued*
  disease or disorder — *continued*
   skin and subcutaneous tissue NEC Z84.0
   specified NEC Z84.89
  drug abuse NEC Z81.3
  epilepsy Z82.0
  genetic disease carrier Z84.81
  glaucoma Z83.511
  hearing loss Z82.2
  human immunodeficiency virus (HIV) infection
    Z83.0
  Huntington's chorea Z82.0
  intellectual disability Z81.0
  leukemia Z80.6
  malignant neoplasm (of) NOS Z80.9
   bladder Z80.52
   breast Z80.3
   bronchus Z80.1
   digestive organ Z80.0
   gastrointestinal tract Z80.0
   genital organ Z80.49
    ovary Z80.41
    prostate Z80.42
    specified organ NEC Z80.49
    testis Z80.43
   hematopoietic NEC Z80.7
   intrathoracic organ NEC Z80.2
   kidney Z80.51
   lung Z80.1
   lymphatic NEC Z80.7
   ovary Z80.41
   prostate Z80.42
   respiratory organ NEC Z80.2
   specified site NEC Z80.8
   testis Z80.43
   trachea Z80.1
   urinary organ or tract Z80.59
    bladder Z80.52
    kidney Z80.51
  mental
   disorder NEC Z81.8
  multiple endocrine neoplasia (MEN) syndrome
    Z83.41
  osteoporosis Z82.62
  polycystic kidney Z82.71
  polyps (colon) Z83.71
  psychiatric disorder Z81.8
  psychoactive substance abuse NEC Z81.3
  respiratory condition NEC Z83.6
   asthma and other lower respiratory conditions
    Z82.5
  self-harmful behavior Z81.8
  skin condition Z84.0
  specified condition NEC Z84.89
  stroke (cerebrovascular) Z82.3
  substance abuse NEC Z81.4
   alcohol Z81.1
   drug NEC Z81.3
   psychoactive NEC Z81.3
   tobacco Z81.2
  sudden cardiac death Z82.41
  tobacco abuse Z81.2
  violence, violent behavior Z81.8
  visual loss Z82.1
 personal (of) (*see also* History, family (of))
  abuse
   adult Z91.419
    physical and sexual Z91.410
    psychological Z91.411
   childhood Z62.819
    physical Z62.810
    psychological Z62.811
    sexual Z62.810
  alcohol dependence F10.21
  allergy (to) Z88.9
   analgesic agent NEC Z88.6
   anesthetic Z88.4
   antibiotic agent NEC Z88.1
   anti-infective agent NEC Z88.3
   contrast media Z91.041
   drugs, medicaments and biological substances
    Z88.9
    specified NEC Z88.8
   food Z91.018
    additives Z91.02
    eggs Z91.012
    milk products Z91.011

History — *continued*
 personal (*see also* History, family) — *continued*
  allergy — *continued*
   food — *continued*
    peanuts Z91.010
    seafood Z91.013
    specified food NEC Z91.018
   insect Z91.038
    bee Z91.030
   latex Z91.040
   medicinal agents Z88.9
    specified NEC Z88.8
   narcotic agent NEC Z88.5
   nonmedicinal agents Z91.048
   penicillin Z88.0
   serum Z88.7
   specified NEC Z91.09
   sulfonamides Z88.2
   vaccine Z88.7
  anaphylactic shock Z87.892
  anaphylaxis Z87.892
  behavioral disorders Z86.59
  benign carcinoid tumor Z86.012
  benign neoplasm Z86.018
   brain Z86.011
   carcinoid Z86.012
   colonic polyps Z86.010
  brain injury (traumatic) Z87.820
  breast implant removal Z98.86
  calculi, renal Z87.442
  cancer — *see* History, personal (of), malignant
    neoplasm (of)
  cardiac arrest (death), successfully resuscitated
    Z86.74
  cerebral infarction without residual deficit Z86.73
  cervical dysplasia Z87.410
  chemotherapy for neoplastic condition Z92.21
  childhood abuse — *see* History, personal (of),
    abuse
  cleft lip (corrected) Z87.730
  cleft palate (corrected) Z87.730
  collapsed vertebra (healed) Z87.311
   due to osteoporosis Z87.310
  combat and operational stress reaction Z86.51
  congenital malformation (corrected) Z87.798
   circulatory system (corrected) Z87.74
   digestive system (corrected) NEC Z87.738
   ear (corrected) Z87.720
   eye (corrected) Z87.721
   face and neck (corrected) Z87.790
   genitourinary system (corrected) NEC Z87.718
   heart (corrected) Z87.74
   integument (corrected) Z87.76
   limb(s) (corrected) Z87.76
   musculoskeletal system (corrected) Z87.76
   neck (corrected) Z87.790
   nervous system (corrected) NEC Z87.728
   respiratory system (corrected) Z87.75
   sense organs (corrected) NEC Z87.728
   specified NEC Z87.798
  contraception Z92.0
  deployment (military) Z91.82
  diabetic foot ulcer Z86.31
  disease or disorder (of) Z87.898
   anaphylaxis Z87.892
   blood and blood-forming organs Z86.2
   circulatory system Z86.79
    specified condition NEC Z86.79
   connective tissue Z87.39
   digestive system Z87.19
    colonic polyp Z86.010
    peptic ulcer disease Z87.11
    specified condition NEC Z87.19
   ear Z86.69
   endocrine Z86.39
    diabetic foot ulcer Z86.31
    gestational diabetes Z86.32
    specified type NEC Z86.39
   eye Z86.69
   genital (track) system NEC
    female Z87.42
    male Z87.438
   hematological Z86.2
   Hodgkin Z85.71
   immune mechanism Z86.2
   infectious Z86.19
    malaria Z86.13

History — *continued*
 personal (*see also* History, family) — *continued*
  disease or disorder — *continued*
   infectious — *continued*
    Methicillin resistant Staphylococcus aureus
     (MRSA) Z86.14
    poliomyelitis Z86.12
    specified NEC Z86.19
    tuberculosis Z86.11
   mental NEC Z86.59
   metabolic Z86.39
    diabetic foot ulcer Z86.31
    gestational diabetes Z86.32
    specified type NEC Z86.39
   musculoskeletal NEC Z87.39
   nervous system Z86.69
   nutritional Z86.39
   parasitic Z86.19
   respiratory system NEC Z87.09
   sense organs Z86.69
   skin Z87.2
   specified site or type NEC Z87.898
   subcutaneous tissue Z87.2
   trophoblastic Z87.59
   urinary system NEC Z87.448
  drug dependence — *see* Dependence, drug, by
    type, in remission
  drug therapy
   antineoplastic chemotherapy Z92.21
   estrogen Z92.23
   immunosupression Z92.25
   inhaled steroids Z92.240
   monoclonal drug Z92.22
   specified NEC Z92.29
   steroid Z92.241
   systemic steroids Z92.241
  dysplasia
   cervical Z87.410
   prostatic Z87.430
   vaginal Z87.411
   vulvar Z87.412
  embolism (venous) Z86.718
   pulmonary Z86.711
  encephalitis Z86.61
  estrogen therapy Z92.23
  extracorporeal membrane oxygenation (ECMO)
    Z92.81
  failed conscious sedation Z92.83
  failed moderate sedation Z92.83
  fall, falling Z91.81
  fracture (healed)
   fatigue Z87.312
   fragility Z87.310
   osteoporosis Z87.310
   pathological NEC Z87.311
   stress Z87.312
   traumatic Z87.81
  gestational diabetes Z86.32
  hepatitis
   B Z86.19
   C Z86.19
  Hodgkin disease Z85.71
  hyperthermia, malignant Z88.4
  hypospadias (corrected) Z87.710
  hysterectomy Z90.710
  immunosupression therapy Z92.25
  in situ neoplasm
   breast Z86.000
   cervix uteri Z86.001
   specified NEC Z86.008
  in utero procedure during pregnancy Z98.870
  in utero procedure while a fetus Z98.871
  infection NEC Z86.19
   central nervous system Z86.61
   Methicillin resistant Staphylococcus aureus
     (MRSA) Z86.14
   urinary (recurrent) (tract) Z87.440
  injury NEC Z87.828
  irradiation Z92.3
  kidney stones Z87.442
  leukemia Z85.6
  lymphoma (non-Hodgkin) Z85.72
  malignant melanoma (skin) Z85.820
  malignant neoplasm (of) Z85.9
   accessory sinuses Z85.22
   anus NEC Z85.048
    carcinoid Z85.040
   bladder Z85.51

History — *continued*
  personal (*see also* History, family) — *continued*
    malignant neoplasm — *continued*
      bone Z85.830
      brain Z85.841
      breast Z85.3
      bronchus NEC Z85.118
        carcinoid Z85.110
      carcinoid — *see* History, personal (of), malignant neoplasm, by site, carcinioid
      cervix Z85.41
      colon NEC Z85.038
        carcinoid Z85.030
      digestive organ Z85.00
        specified NEC Z85.09
      endocrine gland NEC Z85.858
      epididymis Z85.48
      esophagus Z85.01
      eye Z85.840
      gastrointestinal tract — *see* History, malignant neoplasm, digestive organ
      genital organ
        female Z85.40
          specified NEC Z85.44
        male Z85.45
          specified NEC Z85.49
      hematopoietic NEC Z85.79
      intrathoracic organ Z85.20
      kidney NEC Z85.528
        carcinoid Z85.520
      large intestine NEC Z85.038
        carcinoid Z85.030
      larynx Z85.21
      liver Z85.05
      lung NEC Z85.118
        carcinoid Z85.110
      mediastinum Z85.29
      Merkel cell Z85.821
      middle ear Z85.22
      nasal cavities Z85.22
      nervous system NEC Z85.848
      oral cavity Z85.819
        specified site NEC Z85.818
      ovary Z85.43
      pancreas Z85.07
      pelvis Z85.53
      pharynx Z85.819
        specified site NEC Z85.818
      pleura Z85.29
      prostate Z85.46
      rectosigmoid junction NEC Z85.048
        carcinoid Z85.040
      rectum NEC Z85.048
        carcinoid Z85.040
      respiratory organ Z85.20
      sinuses, accessory Z85.22
      skin NEC Z85.828
        melanoma Z85.820
        Merkel cell Z85.821
      small intestine NEC Z85.068
        carcinoid Z85.060
      soft tissue Z85.831
      specified site NEC Z85.89
      stomach NEC Z85.028
        carcinoid Z85.020
      testis Z85.47
      thymus NEC Z85.238
        carcinoid Z85.230
      thyroid Z85.850
      tongue Z85.810
      trachea Z85.12
      urinary organ or tract Z85.50
        specified NEC Z85.59
      uterus Z85.42
    maltreatment Z91.89
    medical treatment NEC Z92.89
    melanoma (malignant) (skin) Z85.820
    meningitis Z86.61
    mental disorder Z86.59
    Merkel cell carcinoma (skin) Z85.821
    Methicillin resistant Staphylococcus aureus (MRSA) Z86.14
    military deployment Z91.82
    military war, peacekeeping and humanitarian deployment (current or past conflict) Z91.82
    myocardial infarction (old) I25.2
    neglect (in)
      adult Z91.412

History — *continued*
  personal (*see also* History, family) — *continued*
    neglect — *continued*
      childhood Z62.812
    neoplasm
      benign Z86.018
        brain Z86.011
        colon polyp Z86.010
      in situ
        breast Z86.000
        cervix uteri Z86.001
        specified NEC Z86.008
      malignant — *see* History of, malignant neoplasm
      uncertain behavior Z86.03
    nephrotic syndrome Z87.441
    nicotine dependence Z87.891
    noncompliance with medical treatment or regimen — *see* Noncompliance
    nutritional deficiency Z86.39
    obstetric complications Z87.59
      childbirth Z87.59
      pregnancy Z87.59
      pre-term labor Z87.51
      puerperium Z87.59
    osteoporosis fractures Z87.31 ☑
    parasuicide (attempt) Z91.5
    physical trauma NEC Z87.828
      self-harm or suicide attempt Z91.5
    pneumonia (recurrent) Z87.01
    poisoning NEC Z91.89
      self-harm or suicide attempt Z91.5
    poor personal hygiene Z91.89
    preterm labor Z87.51
    procedure during pregnancy Z98.870
    procedure while a fetus Z98.871
    prolonged reversible ischemic neurologic deficit (PRIND) Z86.73
    prostatic dysplasia Z87.430
    psychological
      abuse
        adult Z91.411
        child Z62.811
      trauma, specified NEC Z91.49
    radiation therapy Z92.3
    removal
      implant
        breast Z98.86
    renal calculi Z87.442
    respiratory condition NEC Z87.09
    retained foreign body fully removed Z87.821
    risk factors NEC Z91.89
    self-harm Z91.5
    self-poisoning attempt Z91.5
    sex reassignment Z87.890
    sleep-wake cycle problem Z72.821
    specified NEC Z87.898
    steroid therapy (systemic) Z92.241
      inhaled Z92.240
    stroke without residual deficits Z86.73
    substance abuse NEC F10-F19 with fifth character 1
    sudden cardiac arrest Z86.74
    sudden cardiac death successfully resuscitated Z86.74
    suicide attempt Z91.5
    surgery NEC Z98.89
      sex reassignment Z87.890
      transplant — *see* Transplant
    thrombophlebitis Z86.72
    thrombosis (venous) Z86.718
      pulmonary Z86.711
    tobacco dependence Z87.891
    transient ischemic attack (TIA) without residual deficits Z86.73
    trauma (physical) NEC Z87.828
      psychological NEC Z91.49
      self-harm Z91.5
    traumatic brain injury Z87.820
    unhealthy sleep-wake cycle Z72.821
    urinary calculi Z87.442
    urinary (recurrent) (tract) infection(s) Z87.440
    vaginal dysplasia Z87.411
    venous thrombosis or embolism Z86.718
      pulmonary Z86.711
    vulvar dysplasia Z87.412
His-Werner disease A79.0

HIV (*see also* Human, immunodeficiency virus) B20
  laboratory evidence (nonconclusive) R75
  nonconclusive test (in infants) R75
  positive, seropositive Z21
Hives (bold) — *see* Urticaria
Hoarseness R49.0
Hobo Z59.0
Hodgkin disease — *see* Lymphoma, Hodgkin
Hodgson's disease I71.2
  ruptured I71.1
Hoffa-Kastert disease E88.89
Hoffa's disease E88.89
Hoffmann-Bouveret syndrome I47.9
Hoffmann's syndrome E03.9 [G73.7]
Hole (round)
  macula H35.34- ☑
  retina (without detachment) — *see* Break, retina, round hole
    with detachment — *see* Detachment, retina, with retinal, break
Holiday relief care Z75.5
Hollenhorst's plaque — *see* Occlusion, artery, retina
Hollow foot (congenital) Q66.7
  acquired — *see* Deformity, limb, foot, specified NEC
Holoprosencephaly Q04.2
Holt-Oram syndrome Q87.2
Homelessness Z59.0
Homesickness — *see* Disorder, adjustment
Homocystinemia, homocystinuria E72.11
Homogentisate 1,2-dioxygenase deficiency E70.29
Homologous serum hepatitis (prophylactic) (therapeutic) — *see* Hepatitis, viral, type B
Honeycomb lung J98.4
  congenital Q33.0
Hooded
  clitoris Q52.6
  penis Q55.69
Hookworm (anemia) (disease) (infection) (infestation) B76.9
  specified NEC B76.8
Hordeolum (eyelid) (externum) (recurrent) H00.019
  internum H00.029
    left H00.026
      lower H00.025
      upper H00.024
    right H00.023
      lower H00.022
      upper H00.021
  left H00.016
    lower H00.015
    upper H00.014
  right H00.013
    lower H00.012
    upper H00.011
Horn
  cutaneous L85.8
  nail L60.2
    congenital Q84.6
Horner (-Claude Bernard) **syndrome** G90.2
  traumatic — *see* Injury, nerve, cervical sympathetic
Horseshoe kidney (congenital) Q63.1
Horton's headache or neuralgia G44.099
  intractable G44.091
  not intractable G44.099
Hospital hopper syndrome — *see* Disorder, factitious
Hospitalism in children — *see* Disorder, adjustment
Hostility R45.5
  towards child Z62.3
Hot flashes
  menopausal N95.1
Hourglass (contracture) (*see also* Contraction, hourglass)
  stomach K31.89
    congenital Q40.2
    stricture K31.2
Household, housing circumstance affecting care Z59.9
  specified NEC Z59.8
Housemaid's knee — *see* Bursitis, prepatellar
Hudson (-Stähli) **line** (cornea) — *see* Pigmentation, cornea, anterior
Human
  bite (open wound) (*see also* Bite)
    intact skin surface — *see* Bite, superficial
  herpesvirus — *see* Herpes
  immunodeficiency virus (HIV) disease (infection) B20
    asymptomatic status Z21
    contact Z20.6

Human — *continued*
  immunodeficiency virus disease — *continued*
    counseling Z71.7
    dementia B20 [F02.80]
      with behavioral disturbance B20 [F02.81]
    exposure to Z20.6
    laboratory evidence R75
    type-2 (HIV 2) as cause of disease classified else-where B97.35
   papillomavirus (HPV)
    DNA test positive
      high risk
        cervix R87.810
        vagina R87.811
      low risk
        cervix R87.820
        vagina R87.821
    screening for Z11.51
   T-cell lymphotropic virus
    type-1 (HTLV-I) infection B33.3
      as cause of disease classified elsewhere B97.33
      carrier Z22.6
    type-2 (HTLV-II) as cause of disease classified else-where B97.34

Humidifier lung or pneumonitis J67.7
Humiliation (experience) **in childhood** Z62.898
Humpback (acquired) — *see* Kyphosis
Hunchback (acquired) — *see* Kyphosis
Hunger T73.0 ☑
  air, psychogenic F45.8
Hungry bone syndrome E83.81
Hunner's ulcer — *see* Cystitis, chronic, interstitial
Hunter's
  glossitis D51.0
  syndrome E76.1
Huntington's disease or chorea G10
  with dementia G10 [F02.80]
    with behavioral disturbance G10 [F02.81]
Hunt's
  disease or syndrome (herpetic geniculate ganglionitis) B02.21
    dyssynergia cerebellaris myoclonica G11.1
  neuralgia B02.21
Hurler (-Scheie) **disease or syndrome** E76.02
Hurst's disease G36.1
Hurthle cell
  adenocarcinoma C73
  adenoma D34
  carcinoma C73
  tumor D34
Hutchinson-Boeck disease or syndrome — *see* Sarcoidosis
Hutchinson-Gilford disease or syndrome E34.8
Hutchinson's
  disease, meaning
    angioma serpiginosum L81.7
    pompholyx (cheiropompholyx) L30.1
    prurigo estivalis L56.4
    summer eruption or summer prurigo L56.4
  melanotic freckle — *see* Melanoma, in situ
    malignant melanoma in — *see* Melanoma
  teeth or incisors (congenital syphilis) A50.52
  triad (congenital syphilis) A50.53
Hyalin plaque, sclera, senile H15.89
Hyaline membrane (disease) (lung) (pulmonary) (newborn) P22.0
Hyalinosis
  cutis (et mucosae) E78.89
  focal and segmental (glomerular) (*see also* N00-N07 with fourth character .1) N05.1
Hyalitis, hyalosis, asteroid (*see also* Deposit, crystalline)
  syphilitic (late) A52.71
Hydatid
  cyst or tumor — *see* Echinococcus
  mole — *see* Hydatidiform mole
  Morgagni
    female Q50.5
    male (epididymal) Q55.4
      testicular Q55.29
Hydatidiform mole (benign) (complicating pregnancy) (delivered) (undelivered) O01.9
  classical O01.0
  complete O01.0
  incomplete O01.1
  invasive D39.2
  malignant D39.2
  partial O01.1
Hydatidosis — *see* Echinococcus

Hydradenitis (axillaris) (suppurative) L73.2
Hydradenoma — *see* Hidradenoma
Hydramnios O40.- ☑
Hydramphaly, hydranencephaly Q04.3
  with spina bifida — *see* Spina bifida, with hydrocephalus
Hydrargyrism NEC — *see* Poisoning, mercury
Hydrarthrosis (*see also* Effusion, joint)
  gonococcal A54.42
  intermittent M12.40
    ankle M12.47- ☑
    elbow M12.42- ☑
    foot joint M12.47- ☑
    hand joint M12.44- ☑
    hip M12.45- ☑
    knee M12.46- ☑
    multiple site M12.49
    shoulder M12.41- ☑
    specified joint NEC M12.48
    wrist M12.43- ☑
  of yaws (early) (late) (*see also* subcategory M14.8-) A66.6
  syphilitic (late) A52.77
    congenital A50.55 [M12.80]
Hydremia D64.89
Hydrencephalocele (congenital) — *see* Encephalocele
Hydrencephalomeningocele (congenital) — *see* Encephalocele
Hydroa R23.8
  aestivale L56.4
  vacciniforme L56.4
Hydroadenitis (axillaris) (suppurative) L73.2
Hydrocalycosis — *see* Hydronephrosis
Hydrocele (spermatic cord) (testis) (tunica vaginalis) N43.3
  canal of Nuck N94.89
  communicating N43.2
    congenital P83.5
  congenital P83.5
  encysted N43.0
  female NEC N94.89
  infected N43.1
  newborn P83.5
  round ligament N94.89
  specified NEC N43.2
  spinalis — *see* Spina bifida
  vulva N90.89
Hydrocephalus (acquired) (external) (internal) (malignant) (recurrent) G91.9
  aqueduct Sylvius stricture Q03.0
  causing disproportion O33.6 ☑
    with obstructed labor O66.3
  communicating G91.0
  congenital (external) (internal) Q03.9
    with spina bifida Q05.4
      cervical Q05.0
      dorsal Q05.1
      lumbar Q05.2
      lumbosacral Q05.2
      sacral Q05.3
      thoracic Q05.1
      thoracolumbar Q05.1
    specified NEC Q03.8
  due to toxoplasmosis (congenital) P37.1
  foramen Magendie block (acquired) G91.1
    congenital (*see also* Hydrocephalus, congenital) Q03.1
  in (due to)
    infectious disease NEC B89 [G91.4]
    neoplastic disease NEC (*see also* Neoplasm) G91.4
    parasitic disease B89 [G91.4]
  newborn Q03.9
    with spina bifida — *see* Spina bifida, with hydrocephalus
  noncommunicating G91.1
  normal pressure G91.2
    secondary G91.0
  obstructive G91.1
  otitic G93.2
  post-traumatic NEC G91.3
  secondary G91.4
    post-traumatic G91.3
  specified NEC G91.8
  syphilitic, congenital A50.49
Hydrocolpos (congenital) N89.8
Hydrocystoma — *see* Neoplasm, skin, benign
Hydroencephalocele (congenital) — *see* Encephalocele

Hydroencephalomeningocele (congenital) — *see* Encephalocele
Hydrohematopneumothorax — *see* Hemothorax
Hydromeningitis — *see* Meningitis
Hydromeningocele (spinal) (*see also* Spina bifida)
  cranial — *see* Encephalocele
Hydrometra N85.8
Hydrometrocolpos N89.8
Hydromicrocephaly Q02
Hydromphalos (since birth) Q45.8
Hydromyelia Q06.4
Hydromyelocele — *see* Spina bifida
Hydronephrosis (atrophic) (early) (functionless) (intermittent) (primary) (secondary) NEC N13.30
  with
    infection N13.6
    obstruction (by) (of)
      renal calculus N13.2
        with infection N13.6
      ureteral NEC N13.1
        with infection N13.6
        calculus N13.2
          with infection N13.6
      ureteropelvic junction (congenital) Q62.0
        with infection N13.6
    ureteral stricture NEC N13.1
      with infection N13.6
  congenital Q62.0
  specified type NEC N13.39
  tuberculous A18.11
Hydropericarditis — *see* Pericarditis
Hydropericardium — *see* Pericarditis
Hydroperitoneum R18.8
Hydrophobia — *see* Rabies
Hydrophthalmos Q15.0
Hydropneumohemothorax — *see* Hemothorax
Hydropneumopericarditis — *see* Pericarditis
Hydropneumopericardium — *see* Pericarditis
Hydropneumothorax J94.8
  traumatic — *see* Injury, intrathoracic, lung
  tuberculous NEC A15.6
Hydrops R60.9
  abdominis R18.8
  articulorum intermittens — *see* Hydrarthrosis, intermittent
  cardiac — *see* Failure, heart, congestive
  causing obstructed labor O66.3
  endolymphatic H81.0- ☑
  fetal — *see* Pregnancy, complicated by, hydrops, fetalis
  fetalis P83.2
    due to
      ABO isoimmunization P56.0
      alpha thalassemia D56.0
      hemolytic disease P56.90
        specified NEC P56.99
      isoimmunization (ABO) (Rh) P56.0
      other specified nonhemolytic disease NEC P83.2
      Rh incompatibility P56.0
    during pregnancy — *see* Pregnancy, complicated by, hydrops, fetalis
  gallbladder K82.1
  joint — *see* Effusion, joint
  labyrinth H81.0- ☑
  newborn (idiopathic) P83.2
    due to
      ABO isoimmunization P56.0
      alpha thalassemia D56.0
      hemolytic disease P56.90
        specified NEC P56.99
      isoimmunization (ABO) (Rh) P56.0
      Rh incompatibility P56.0
  nutritional — *see* Malnutrition, severe
  pericardium — *see* Pericarditis
  pleura — *see* Hydrothorax
  spermatic cord — *see* Hydrocele
Hydropyonephrosis N13.6
Hydrorachis Q06.4
Hydrorrhea (nasal) J34.89
  pregnancy — *see* Rupture, membranes, premature
Hydrosadenitis (axillaris) (suppurative) L73.2
Hydrosalpinx (fallopian tube) (follicularis) N70.11
Hydrothorax (double) (pleura) J94.8
  chylous (nonfilarial) I89.8
    filarial (*see also* Infestation, filarial) B74.9 [J91.8]
  traumatic — *see* Injury, intrathoracic
  tuberculous NEC (non primary) A15.6

☑ **Additional Character Required** — Refer to the Tabular List for Character Selection   ▽ Subterms under main terms may continue to next column or page

Hydroureter (see also Hydronephrosis) N13.4
  with infection N13.6
  congenital Q62.39
Hydroureteronephrosis — see Hydronephrosis
Hydrourethra N36.8
Hydroxykynureninuria E70.8
Hydroxylysinemia E72.3
Hydroxyprolinemia E72.59
Hygiene, sleep
  abuse Z72.821
  inadequate Z72.821
  poor Z72.821
Hygroma (congenital) (cystic) D18.1
  praepatellare, prepatellar — see Bursitis, prepatellar
Hymen — see condition
Hymenolepis, hymenolepiasis (diminuta) (infection)
  (infestation) (nana) B71.0
Hypalgesia R20.8
Hyperacidity (gastric) K31.89
  psychogenic F45.8
Hyperactive, hyperactivity F90.9
  basal cell, uterine cervix — see Dysplasia, cervix
  bowel sounds R19.12
  cervix epithelial (basal) — see Dysplasia, cervix
  child F90.9
    attention deficit — see Disorder, attention-deficit
      hyperactivity
  detrusor muscle N32.81
  gastrointestinal K31.89
    psychogenic F45.8
  nasal mucous membrane J34.3
  stomach K31.89
  thyroid (gland) — see Hyperthyroidism
Hyperacusis H93.23- ☑
Hyperadrenalism E27.5
Hyperadrenocorticism E24.9
  congenital E25.0
  iatrogenic E24.2
    correct substance properly administered — see
      Table of Drugs and Chemicals, by drug, ad-
      verse effect
    overdose or wrong substance given or taken —
      see Table of Drugs and Chemicals, by drug,
      poisoning
  not associated with Cushing's syndrome E27.0
  pituitary-dependent E24.0
Hyperaldosteronism E26.9
  familial (type I) E26.02
  glucocorticoid-remediable E26.02
  primary (due to (bilateral) adrenal hyperplasia) E26.09
  primary NEC E26.09
  secondary E26.1
  specified NEC E26.89
Hyperalgesia R20.8
Hyperalimentation R63.2
  carotene, carotin E67.1
  specified NEC E67.8
  vitamin
    A E67.0
    D E67.3
Hyperaminoaciduria
  arginine E72.21
  cystine E72.01
  lysine E72.3
  ornithine E72.4
Hyperammonemia (congenital) E72.20
Hyperazotemia — see Uremia
Hyperbetalipoproteinemia (familial) E78.0
  with prebetalipoproteinemia E78.2
Hyperbilirubinemia
  constitutional E80.6
  familial conjugated E80.6
  neonatal (transient) — see Jaundice, newborn
Hypercalcemia, hypocalciuric, familial E83.52
Hypercalciuria, idiopathic E83.52
Hypercapnia R06.89
  newborn P84
Hypercarotenemia, hypercarotinemia (dietary) E67.1
Hypercementosis K03.4
Hyperchloremia E87.8
Hyperchlorhydria K31.89
  neurotic F45.8
  psychogenic F45.8
Hypercholesterinemia — see Hypercholesterolemia
Hypercholesterolemia (essential) (familial) (hereditary)
  (primary) (pure) E78.0
  with hyperglyceridemia, endogenous E78.2

Hypercholesterolemia — continued
  dietary counseling and surveillance Z71.3
Hyperchylia gastrica, psychogenic F45.8
Hyperchylomicronemia (familial) (primary) E78.3
  with hyperbetalipoproteinemia E78.3
Hypercoagulable (state) D68.59
  activated protein C resistance D68.51
  antithrombin (III) deficiency D68.59
  factor V Leiden mutation D68.51
  primary NEC D68.59
  protein C deficiency D68.59
  protein S deficiency D68.59
  prothrombin gene mutation D68.52
  secondary D68.69
  specified NEC D68.69
Hypercoagulation (state) D68.59
Hypercorticalism, pituitary-dependent E24.0
Hypercorticosolism — see Cushing's, syndrome
Hypercorticosteronism E24.2
  correct substance properly administered — see Table
    of Drugs and Chemicals, by drug, adverse effect
  overdose or wrong substance given or taken — see
    Table of Drugs and Chemicals, by drug, poison-
    ing
Hypercortisonism E24.2
  correct substance properly administered — see Table
    of Drugs and Chemicals, by drug, adverse effect
  overdose or wrong substance given or taken — see
    Table of Drugs and Chemicals, by drug, poison-
    ing
Hyperekplexia Q89.8
Hyperelectrolytemia E87.8
Hyperemesis R11.10
  with nausea R11.2
  gravidarum (mild) O21.0
    with
      carbohydrate depletion O21.1
      dehydration O21.1
      electrolyte imbalance O21.1
      metabolic disturbance O21.1
      severe (with metabolic disturbance) O21.1
  projectile R11.12
  psychogenic F45.8
Hyperemia (acute) (passive) R68.89
  anal mucosa K62.89
  bladder N32.89
  cerebral I67.89
  conjunctiva H11.43- ☑
  ear internal, acute — see subcategory H83.0 ☑
  enteric K59.8
  eye — see Hyperemia, conjunctiva
  eyelid (active) (passive) — see Disorder, eyelid, speci-
    fied type NEC
  intestine K59.8
  iris — see Disorder, iris, vascular
  kidney N28.89
  labyrinth — see subcategory H83.0 ☑
  liver (active) K76.89
  lung (passive) — see Edema, lung
  pulmonary (passive) — see Edema, lung
  renal N28.89
  retina H35.89
  stomach K31.89
Hyperesthesia (body surface) R20.3
  larynx (reflex) J38.7
    hysterical F44.89
  pharynx (reflex) J39.2
    hysterical F44.89
Hyperestrogenism (drug-induced) (iatrogenic) E28.0
Hyperexplexia Q89.8
Hyperfibrinolysis — see Fibrinolysis
Hyperfructosemia E74.19
Hyperfunction
  adrenal cortex, not associated with Cushing's syn-
    drome E27.0
  medulla E27.5
    adrenomedullary E27.5
  virilism E25.9
    congenital E25.0
  ovarian E28.8
  pancreas K86.8
  parathyroid (gland) E21.3
  pituitary (gland) (anterior) E22.9
    specified NEC E22.8
  polyglandular E31.1
  testicular E29.0

Hypergammaglobulinemia D89.2
  polyclonal D89.0
  Waldenström D89.0
Hypergastrinemia E16.4
Hyperglobulinemia R77.1
Hyperglycemia, hyperglycemic (transient) R73.9
  coma — see Diabetes, by type, with coma
  postpancreatectomy E89.1
Hyperglyceridemia (endogenous) (essential) (familial)
  (hereditary) (pure) E78.1
  mixed E78.3
Hyperglycinemia (non-ketotic) E72.51
Hypergonadism
  ovarian E28.8
  testicular (primary) (infantile) E29.0
Hyperheparinemia D68.32
Hyperhidrosis, hyperidrosis R61
  focal
    primary L74.519
      axilla L74.510
      face L74.511
      palms L74.512
      soles L74.513
    secondary L74.52
  generalized R61
  localized
    primary L74.519
      axilla L74.510
      face L74.511
      palms L74.512
      soles L74.513
    secondary L74.52
  psychogenic F45.8
  secondary R61
    focal L74.52
Hyperhistidinemia E70.41
Hyperhomocysteinemia E72.11
Hyperhydroxyprolinemia E72.59
Hyperinsulinism (functional) E16.1
  with
    coma (hypoglycemic) E15
    encephalopathy E16.1 [G94]
  ectopic E16.1
  therapeutic misadventure (from administration of in-
    sulin) — see subcategory T38.3 ☑
Hyperkalemia E87.5
Hyperkeratosis (see also Keratosis) L85.9
  cervix N88.0
  due to yaws (early) (late) (palmar or plantar) A66.3
  follicularis Q82.8
    penetrans (in cutem) L87.0
  palmoplantaris climacterica L85.1
  pinta A67.1
  senile (with pruritus) L57.0
  universalis congenita Q80.8
  vocal cord J38.3
  vulva N90.4
Hyperkinesia, hyperkinetic (disease) (reaction) (syndrome) (childhood) (adolescence) (see also Disorder,
  attention-deficit hyperactivity)
  heart I51.89
Hyperleucine-isoleucinemia E71.19
Hyperlipemia, hyperlipidemia E78.5
  combined E78.2
    familial E78.4
  group
    A E78.0
    B E78.1
    C E78.2
    D E78.3
  mixed E78.2
  specified NEC E78.4
Hyperlipidosis E75.6
  hereditary NEC E75.5
Hyperlipoproteinemia E78.5
  Fredrickson's type
    I E78.3
    IIa E78.0
    IIb E78.2
    III E78.2
    IV E78.1
    V E78.3
  low-density-lipoprotein-type (LDL) E78.0
  very-low-density-lipoprotein-type (VLDL) E78.1
Hyperlucent lung, unilateral J43.0
Hyperlysinemia E72.3
Hypermagnesemia E83.41
  neonatal P71.8

⚐ **Subterms under main terms may continue to next column or page**   ☑ **Additional Character Required** — Refer to the Tabular List for Character Selection

Hypermenorrhea N92.0
Hypermethioninemia E72.19
Hypermetropia (congenital) H52.0- ☑
Hypermobility, hypermotility
  cecum — *see* Syndrome, irritable bowel
  coccyx — *see* subcategory M53.2 ☑
  colon — *see* Syndrome, irritable bowel
    psychogenic F45.8
  ileum K58.9
  intestine (*see also* Syndrome, irritable bowel) K58.9
    psychogenic F45.8
  meniscus (knee) — *see* Derangement, knee, meniscus
  scapula — *see* Instability, joint, shoulder
  stomach K31.89
    psychogenic F45.8
  syndrome M35.7
  urethra N36.41
    with intrinsic sphincter deficiency N36.43
Hypernasality R49.21
Hypernatremia E87.0
Hypernephroma C64.- ☑
Hyperopia — *see* Hypermetropia
Hyperorexia nervosa F50.2
Hyperornithinemia E72.4
Hyperosmia R43.1
Hyperosmolality E87.0
Hyperostosis (monomelic) (*see also* Disorder, bone, density and structure, specified NEC)
  ankylosing (spine) M48.10
    cervical region M48.12
    cervicothoracic region M48.13
    lumbar region M48.16
    lumbosacral region M48.17
    multiple sites M48.19
    occipito-atlanto-axial region M48.11
    sacrococcygeal region M48.18
    thoracic region M48.14
    thoracolumbar region M48.15
  cortical (skull) M85.2
    infantile M89.8X- ☑
  frontal, internal of skull M85.2
  interna frontalis M85.2
  skeletal, diffuse idiopathic — *see* Hyperostosis, ankylosing
  skull M85.2
    congenital Q75.8
  vertebral, ankylosing — *see* Hyperostosis, ankylosing
Hyperovarism E28.8
Hyperoxaluria (primary) E72.53
Hyperparathyroidism E21.3
  primary E21.0
  secondary (renal) N25.81
    non-renal E21.1
  specified NEC E21.2
  tertiary E21.2
Hyperpathia R20.8
Hyperperistalsis R19.2
  psychogenic F45.8
Hyperpermeability, capillary I78.8
Hyperphagia R63.2
Hyperphenylalaninemia NEC E70.1
Hyperphoria (alternating) H50.53
Hyperphosphatemia E83.39
Hyperpiesis, hyperpiesia — *see* Hypertension
Hyperpigmentation (*see also* Pigmentation)
  melanin NEC L81.4
  postinflammatory L81.0
Hyperpinealism E34.8
Hyperpituitarism E22.9
Hyperplasia, hyperplastic
  adenoids J35.2
  adrenal (capsule) (cortex) (gland) E27.8
    with
      sexual precocity (male) E25.9
        congenital E25.0
      virilism, adrenal E25.9
        congenital E25.0
      virilization (female) E25.9
        congenital E25.0
    congenital E25.0
    salt-losing E25.0
  adrenomedullary E27.5
  angiolymphoid, eosinophilia (ALHE) D18.01
  appendix (lymphoid) K38.0
  artery, fibromuscular I77.3
  bone (*see also* Hypertrophy, bone)
    marrow D75.89

Hyperplasia, hyperplastic — *continued*
  breast (*see also* Hypertrophy, breast)
    ductal (atypical) N60.9- ☑
  C-cell, thyroid E07.0
  cementation (tooth) (teeth) K03.4
  cervical gland R59.0
  cervix (uteri) (basal cell) (endometrium) (polypoid) (*see also* Dysplasia, cervix)
    congenital Q51.828
  clitoris, congenital Q52.6
  denture K06.2
  endocervicitis N72
  endometrium, endometrial (adenomatous) (benign) (cystic) (glandular) (glandular-cystic) (polypoid) N85.00
    with atypia N85.02
    cervix — *see* Dysplasia, cervix
    complex (without atypia) N85.01
    simple (without atypia) N85.01
  epithelial L85.9
    focal, oral, including tongue K13.29
    nipple N62
    skin L85.9
    tongue K13.29
    vaginal wall N89.3
  erythroid D75.89
  fibromuscular of artery (carotid) (renal) I77.3
  genital
    female NEC N94.89
    male N50.8
  gingiva K06.1
  glandularis cystica uteri (interstitialis) (*see also* Hyperplasia, endometrial) N85.00
  gum K06.1
  hymen, congenital Q52.4
  irritative, edentulous (alveolar) K06.2
  jaw M26.09
    alveolar M26.79
    lower M26.03
      alveolar M26.72
    upper M26.01
      alveolar M26.71
  kidney (congenital) Q63.3
  labia N90.6
    epithelial N90.3
  liver (congenital) Q44.7
    nodular, focal K76.89
  lymph gland or node R59.9
  mandible, mandibular M26.03
    alveolar M26.72
    unilateral condylar M27.8
  maxilla, maxillary M26.01
    alveolar M26.71
  myometrium, myometrial N85.2
  neuroendocrine cell, of infancy J84.841
  nose
    lymphoid J34.89
    polypoid J33.9
  oral mucosa (irritative) K13.6
  organ or site, congenital NEC — *see* Anomaly, by site
  ovary N83.8
  palate, papillary (irritative) K13.6
  pancreatic islet cells E16.9
    alpha E16.8
      with excess
        gastrin E16.4
        glucagon E16.3
    beta E16.1
  parathyroid (gland) E21.0
  pharynx (lymphoid) J39.2
  prostate (adenofibromatous) (nodular) N40.0
    with lower urinary tract symptoms (LUTS) N40.1
    without lower urinary tract symtpoms (LUTS) N40.0
  renal artery I77.89
  reticulo-endothelial (cell) D75.89
  salivary gland (any) K11.1
  Schimmelbusch's — *see* Mastopathy, cystic
  suprarenal capsule (gland) E27.8
  thymus (gland) (persistent) E32.0
  thyroid (gland) — *see* Goiter
  tonsils (faucial) (infective) (lingual) (lymphoid) J35.1
    with adenoids J35.3
  unilateral condylar M27.8
  uterus, uterine N85.2
    endometrium (glandular) (*see also* Hyperplasia, endometrial) N85.00
  vulva N90.6
    epithelial N90.3

Hyperpnea — *see* Hyperventilation
Hyperpotassemia E87.5
Hyperprebetalipoproteinemia (familial) E78.1
Hyperprolactinemia E22.1
Hyperprolinemia (type I) (type II) E72.59
Hyperproteinemia E88.09
Hyperprothrombinemia, causing coagulation factor deficiency D68.4
Hyperpyrexia R50.9
  heat (effects) T67.0 ☑
  malignant, due to anesthetic T88.3 ☑
  rheumatic — *see* Fever, rheumatic
  unknown origin R50.9
Hyper-reflexia R29.2
Hypersalivation K11.7
Hypersecretion
  ACTH (not associated with Cushing's syndrome) E27.0
    pituitary E24.0
  adrenaline E27.5
  adrenomedullary E27.5
  androgen (testicular) E29.0
    ovarian (drug-induced) (iatrogenic) E28.1
  calcitonin E07.0
  catecholamine E27.5
  corticoadrenal E24.9
  cortisol E24.9
  epinephrine E27.5
  estrogen E28.0
  gastric K31.89
    psychogenic F45.8
  gastrin E16.4
  glucagon E16.3
  hormone(s)
    ACTH (not associated with Cushing's syndrome) E27.0
      pituitary E24.0
    antidiuretic E22.2
    growth E22.0
    intestinal NEC E34.1
    ovarian androgen E28.1
    pituitary E22.9
    testicular E29.0
    thyroid stimulating E05.80
      with thyroid storm E05.81
  insulin — *see* Hyperinsulinism
  lacrimal glands — *see* Epiphora
  medulloadrenal E27.5
  milk O92.6
  ovarian androgens E28.1
  salivary gland (any) K11.7
  thyrocalcitonin E07.0
  upper respiratory J39.8
Hypersegmentation, leukocytic, hereditary D72.0
Hypersensitive, hypersensitiveness, hypersensitivity (*see also* Allergy)
  carotid sinus G90.01
  colon — *see* Irritable, colon
  drug T88.7 ☑
  gastrointestinal K52.2
    psychogenic F45.8
  labyrinth — *see* subcategory H83.2 ☑
  pain R20.8
  pneumonitis — *see* Pneumonitis, allergic
  reaction T78.40 ☑
    upper respiratory tract NEC J39.3
Hypersomnia (organic) G47.10
  due to
    alcohol
      abuse F10.182
      dependence F10.282
      use F10.982
    amphetamines
      abuse F15.182
      dependence F15.282
      use F15.982
    caffeine
      abuse F15.182
      dependence F15.282
      use F15.982
    cocaine
      abuse F14.182
      dependence F14.282
      use F14.982
    drug NEC
      abuse F19.182
      dependence F19.282
      use F19.982
    medical condition G47.14

Hypersomnia — *continued*
  due to — *continued*
    mental disorder F51.13
    opioid
      abuse F11.182
      dependence F11.282
      use F11.982
    psychoactive substance NEC
      abuse F19.182
      dependence F19.282
      use F19.982
    sedative, hypnotic, or anxiolytic
      abuse F13.182
      dependence F13.282
      use F13.982
    stimulant NEC
      abuse F15.182
      dependence F15.282
      use F15.982
  idiopathic G47.11
    with long sleep time G47.11
    without long sleep time G47.12
  menstrual related G47.13
  nonorganic origin F51.11
    specified NEC F51.19
  not due to a substance or known physiological condition F51.11
    specified NEC F51.19
  primary F51.11
  recurrent G47.13
  specified NEC G47.19
Hypersplenia, hypersplenism D73.1
Hyperstimulation, ovaries (associated with induced ovulation) N98.1
Hypersusceptibility — *see* Allergy
Hypertelorism (ocular) (orbital) Q75.2
Hypertension, hypertensive (accelerated) (benign) (essential) (idiopathic) (malignant) (systemic) I10
  with
    heart involvement (conditions in I51.4 - I51.9 due to hypertension) — *see* Hypertension, heart
    kidney involvement — *see* Hypertension, kidney
  benign, intracranial G93.2
  borderline R03.0
  cardiorenal (disease) I13.10
    with heart failure I13.0
      with stage 1 through stage 4 chronic kidney disease I13.0
      with stage 5 or end stage renal disease I13.2
    without heart failure I13.10
      with stage 1 through stage 4 chronic kidney disease I13.10
      with stage 5 or end stage renal disease I13.11
  cardiovascular
    disease (arteriosclerotic) (sclerotic) — *see* Hypertension, heart
    renal (disease) — *see* Hypertension, cardiorenal
  chronic venous — *see* Hypertension, venous (chronic)
  complicating
    childbirth (labor) O10.92
      with
        heart disease O10.12
          with renal disease O10.32
        renal disease O10.22
          with heart disease O10.32
      essential O10.02
      secondary O10.42
    pregnancy O16.- ☑
      with edema (*see also* Pre-eclampsia) O14.9- ☑
      gestational (pregnancy induced) (transient) O13.- ☑
        (without proteinuria) O13.- ☑
        with proteinuria O14.9- ☑
          mild pre-eclampsia O14.0- ☑
          moderate pre-eclampsia O14.0- ☑
          severe pre-eclampsia O14.1- ☑
            with hemolysis, elevated liver enzymes and low platelet count (HELLP) O14.2- ☑
      pre-existing O10.91- ☑
        with
          heart disease O10.11- ☑
            with renal disease O10.31- ☑
          pre-eclampsia O11.- ☑
          renal disease O10.21- ☑
            with heart disease O10.31- ☑
        essential O10.01- ☑
        secondary O10.41- ☑

Hypertension, hypertensive — *continued*
  complicating — *continued*
    puerperium, pre-existing O10.93
      with
        heart disease O10.13
          with renal disease O10.33
        renal disease O10.23
          with heart disease O10.33
      essential O10.03
      pregnancy-induced O13.9
      secondary O10.43
  due to
    endocrine disorders I15.2
    pheochromocytoma I15.2
    renal disorders NEC I15.1
      arterial I15.0
    renovascular disorders I15.0
    specified disease NEC I15.8
  encephalopathy I67.4
  gestational (without significant proteinuria) (pregnancy-induced) (transient) O13.- ☑
    with significant proteinuria — *see* Pre-eclampsia
  Goldblatt's I70.1
  heart (disease) (conditions in I51.4-I51.9 due to hypertension) I11.9
    with
      heart failure (congestive) I11.0
      kidney disease (chronic) — *see* Hypertension, cardiorenal
  intracranial (benign) G93.2
  kidney I12.9
    with
      heart disease — *see* Hypertension, cardiorenal
      stage 1 through stage 4 chronic kidney disease I12.9
      stage 5 chronic kidney disease (CKD) or end stage renal disease (ESRD) I12.0
  lesser circulation I27.0
  newborn P29.2
    pulmonary (persistent) P29.3
  ocular H40.05- ☑
  pancreatic duct — *code to* underlying condition
    with chronic pancreatitis K86.1
  portal (due to chronic liver disease) (idiopathic) K76.6
    gastropathy K31.89
    in (due to) schistosomiasis (bilharziasis) B65.9 [K77]
  postoperative I97.3
  psychogenic F45.8
  pulmonary (artery) (secondary) NEC I27.2
    with
      cor pulmonale (chronic) I27.2
        acute I26.09
      right heart ventricular strain/failure I27.2
        acute I26.09
    of newborn (persistent) P29.3
    primary (idiopathic) I27.0
  renal — *see* Hypertension, kidney
  renovascular I15.0
  secondary NEC I15.9
    due to
      endocrine disorders I15.2
      pheochromocytoma I15.2
      renal disorders NEC I15.1
        arterial I15.0
      renovascular disorders I15.0
    specified NEC I15.8
  venous (chronic)
    due to
      deep vein thrombosis — *see* Syndrome, post-thrombotic
    idiopathic I87.309
      with
        inflammation I87.32- ☑
          with ulcer I87.33- ☑
        specified complication NEC I87.39- ☑
        ulcer I87.31- ☑
          with inflammation I87.33- ☑
        asymptomatic I87.30- ☑
Hypertensive urgency — *see* Hypertension
Hyperthecosis ovary E28.8
Hyperthermia (of unknown origin) (*see also* Hyperpyrexia)
  malignant, due to anesthesia T88.3 ☑
  newborn P81.9
    environmental P81.0
Hyperthyroid (recurrent) — *see* Hyperthyroidism

Hyperthyroidism (latent) (pre-adult) (recurrent) E05.90
  with
    goiter (diffuse) E05.00
      with thyroid storm E05.01
      nodular (multinodular) E05.20
        with thyroid storm E05.21
        uninodular E05.10
          with thyroid storm E05.11
    storm E05.91
  due to ectopic thyroid tissue E05.30
    with thyroid storm E05.31
  neonatal, transitory P72.1
  specified NEC E05.80
    with thyroid storm E05.81
Hypertony, hypertonia, hypertonicity
  bladder N31.8
  congenital P94.1
  stomach K31.89
    psychogenic F45.8
  uterus, uterine (contractions) (complicating delivery) O62.4
Hypertrichosis L68.9
  congenital Q84.2
  eyelid H02.869
    left H02.866
      lower H02.865
      upper H02.864
    right H02.863
      lower H02.862
      upper H02.861
  lanuginosa Q84.2
    acquired L68.1
  localized L68.2
  specified NEC L68.8
Hypertriglyceridemia, essential E78.1
Hypertrophy, hypertrophic
  adenofibromatous, prostate — *see* Enlargement, enlarged, prostate
  adenoids (infective) J35.2
    with tonsils J35.3
  adrenal cortex E27.8
  alveolar process or ridge — *see* Anomaly, alveolar
  anal papillae K62.89
  artery I77.89
    congenital NEC Q27.8
      digestive system Q27.8
      lower limb Q27.8
      specified site NEC Q27.8
      upper limb Q27.8
  auricular — *see* Hypertrophy, cardiac
  Bartholin's gland N75.8
  bile duct (common) (hepatic) K83.8
  bladder (sphincter) (trigone) N32.89
  bone M89.30
    carpus M89.34- ☑
    clavicle M89.31- ☑
    femur M89.35- ☑
    fibula M89.36- ☑
    finger M89.34- ☑
    humerus M89.32- ☑
    ilium M89.359
    ischium M89.359
    metacarpus M89.34- ☑
    metatarsus M89.37- ☑
    multiple sites M89.39
    neck M89.38
    radius M89.33- ☑
    rib M89.38
    scapula M89.31- ☑
    skull M89.38
    tarsus M89.37- ☑
    tibia M89.36- ☑
    toe M89.37- ☑
    ulna M89.33- ☑
    vertebra M89.38
  brain G93.89
  breast N62
    cystic — *see* Mastopathy, cystic
    newborn P83.4
    pubertal, massive N62
    puerperal, postpartum — *see* Disorder, breast, specified type NEC
    senile (parenchymatous) N62
  cardiac (chronic) (idiopathic) I51.7
    with rheumatic fever (conditions in I00)
      active I01.8
      inactive or quiescent (with chorea) I09.89
    congenital NEC Q24.8

Hypertrophy, hypertrophic — *continued*
  cardiac — *continued*
    fatty — *see* Degeneration, myocardial
    hypertensive — *see* Hypertension, heart
    rheumatic (with chorea) I09.89
      active or acute I01.8
        with chorea I02.0
    valve — *see* Endocarditis
  cartilage — *see* Disorder, cartilage, specified type NEC
  cecum — *see* Megacolon
  cervix (uteri) N88.8
    congenital Q51.828
    elongation N88.4
  clitoris (cirrhotic) N90.89
    congenital Q52.6
  colon (*see also* Megacolon)
    congenital Q43.2
  conjunctiva, lymphoid H11.89
  corpora cavernosa N48.89
  cystic duct K82.8
  duodenum K31.89
  endometrium (glandular) (*see also* Hyperplasia, endometrial) N85.00
    cervix N88.8
  epididymis N50.8
  esophageal hiatus (congenital) Q79.1
    with hernia — *see* Hernia, hiatal
  eyelid — *see* Disorder, eyelid, specified type NEC
  fat pad E65
    knee (infrapatellar) (popliteal) (prepatellar) (retropatellar) M79.4
  foot (congenital) Q74.2
  frenulum, frenum (tongue) K14.8
    lip K13.0
  gallbladder K82.8
  gastric mucosa K29.60
    with bleeding K29.61
  gland, glandular R59.9
    generalized R59.1
    localized R59.0
  gum (mucous membrane) K06.1
  heart (idiopathic) (*see also* Hypertrophy, cardiac)
    valve (*see also* Endocarditis) I38
  hemifacial Q67.4
  hepatic — *see* Hypertrophy, liver
  hiatus (esophageal) Q79.1
  hilus gland R59.0
  hymen, congenital Q52.4
  ileum K63.89
  intestine NEC K63.89
  jejunum K63.89
  kidney (compensatory) N28.81
    congenital Q63.3
  labium (majus) (minus) N90.6
  ligament — *see* Disorder, ligament
  lingual tonsil (infective) J35.1
    with adenoids J35.3
  lip K13.0
    congenital Q18.6
  liver R16.0
    acute K76.89
    cirrhotic — *see* Cirrhosis, liver
    congenital Q44.7
    fatty — *see* Fatty, liver
  lymph, lymphatic gland R59.9
    generalized R59.1
    localized R59.0
    tuberculous — *see* Tuberculosis, lymph gland
  mammary gland — *see* Hypertrophy, breast
  Meckel's diverticulum (congenital) Q43.0
    malignant — *see* Table of Neoplasms, small intestine, malignant
  median bar — *see* Hyperplasia, prostate
  meibomian gland — *see* Chalazion
  meniscus, knee, congenital Q74.1
  metatarsal head — *see* Hypertrophy, bone, metatarsus
  metatarsus — *see* Hypertrophy, bone, metatarsus
  mucous membrane
    alveolar ridge K06.2
    gum K06.1
    nose (turbinate) J34.3
  muscle M62.89
  muscular coat, artery I77.89
  myocardium (*see also* Hypertrophy, cardiac)
    idiopathic I42.2
  myometrium N85.2
  nail L60.2
    congenital Q84.5

Hypertrophy, hypertrophic — *continued*
  nasal J34.89
    alae J34.89
    bone J34.89
    cartilage J34.89
    mucous membrane (septum) J34.3
    sinus J34.89
    turbinate J34.3
  nasopharynx, lymphoid (infectional) (tissue) (wall) J35.2
  nipple N62
  organ or site, congenital NEC — *see* Anomaly, by site
  ovary N83.8
  palate (hard) M27.8
    soft K13.79
  pancreas, congenital Q45.3
  parathyroid (gland) E21.0
  parotid gland K11.1
  penis N48.89
  pharyngeal tonsil J35.2
  pharynx J39.2
    lymphoid (infectional) (tissue) (wall) J35.2
  pituitary (anterior) (fossa) (gland) E23.6
  prepuce (congenital) N47.8
    female N90.89
  prostate — *see* Enlargement, enlarged, prostate
    congenital Q55.4
  pseudomuscular G71.0
  pylorus (adult) (muscle) (sphincter) K31.1
    congenital or infantile Q40.0
  rectal, rectum (sphincter) K62.89
  rhinitis (turbinate) J31.0
  salivary gland (any) K11.1
    congenital Q38.4
  scaphoid (tarsal) — *see* Hypertrophy, bone, tarsus
  scar L91.0
  scrotum N50.8
  seminal vesicle N50.8
  sigmoid — *see* Megacolon
  skin L91.9
    specified NEC L91.8
  spermatic cord N50.8
  spleen — *see* Splenomegaly
  spondylitis — *see* Spondylosis
  stomach K31.89
  sublingual gland K11.1
  submandibular gland K11.1
  suprarenal cortex (gland) E27.8
  synovial NEC M67.20
    acromioclavicular M67.21- ☑
    ankle M67.27- ☑
    elbow M67.22- ☑
    foot M67.27- ☑
    hand M67.24- ☑
    hip M67.25- ☑
    knee M67.26- ☑
    multiple sites M67.29
    specified site NEC M67.28
    wrist M67.23- ☑
  tendon — *see* Disorder, tendon, specified type NEC
  testis N44.8
    congenital Q55.29
  thymic, thymus (gland) (congenital) E32.0
  thyroid (gland) — *see* Goiter
  toe (congenital) Q74.2
    acquired (*see also* Deformity, toe, specified NEC)
  tongue K14.8
    congenital Q38.2
    papillae (foliate) K14.3
  tonsils (faucial) (infective) (lingual) (lymphoid) J35.1
    with adenoids J35.3
  tunica vaginalis N50.8
  ureter N28.89
  urethra N36.8
  uterus N85.2
    neck (with elongation) N88.4
    puerperal O90.89
  uvula K13.79
  vagina N89.8
  vas deferens N50.8
  vein I87.8
  ventricle, ventricular (heart) (*see also* Hypertrophy, cardiac)
    congenital Q24.8
    in tetralogy of Fallot Q21.3
  verumontanum N36.8
  vocal cord J38.3

Hypertrophy, hypertrophic — *continued*
  vulva N90.6
    stasis (nonfilarial) N90.6
Hypertropia H50.2- ☑
Hypertyrosinemia E70.21
Hyperuricemia (asymptomatic) E79.0
Hypervalinemia E71.19
Hyperventilation (tetany) R06.4
  hysterical F45.8
  psychogenic F45.8
  syndrome F45.8
Hypervitaminosis (dietary) NEC E67.8
  A E67.0
    administered as drug (prolonged intake) — *see* Table of Drugs and Chemicals, vitamins, adverse effect
    overdose or wrong substance given or taken — *see* Table of Drugs and Chemicals, vitamins, poisoning
  B6 E67.2
  D E67.3
    administered as drug (prolonged intake) — *see* Table of Drugs and Chemicals, vitamins, adverse effect
    overdose or wrong substance given or taken — *see* Table of Drugs and Chemicals, vitamins, poisoning
  K E67.8
    administered as drug (prolonged intake) — *see* Table of Drugs and Chemicals, vitamins, adverse effect
    overdose or wrong substance given or taken — *see* Table of Drugs and Chemicals, vitamins, poisoning
Hypervolemia E87.70
  specified NEC E87.79
Hypesthesia R20.1
  cornea — *see* Anesthesia, cornea
Hyphema H21.0- ☑
  traumatic S05.1- ☑
Hypoacidity, gastric K31.89
  psychogenic F45.8
Hypoadrenalism, hypoadrenia E27.40
  primary E27.1
  tuberculous A18.7
Hypoadrenocorticism E27.40
  pituitary E23.0
  primary E27.1
Hypoalbuminemia E88.09
Hypoaldosteronism E27.40
Hypoalphalipoproteinemia E78.6
Hypobarism T70.29 ☑
Hypobaropathy T70.29 ☑
Hypobetalipoproteinemia (familial) E78.6
Hypocalcemia E83.51
  dietary E58
  neonatal P71.1
    due to cow's milk P71.0
  phosphate-loading (newborn) P71.1
Hypochloremia E87.8
Hypochlorhydria K31.89
  neurotic F45.8
  psychogenic F45.8
Hypochondria, hypochondriac, hypochondriasis (reaction) F45.21
  sleep F51.03
Hypochondrogenesis Q77.0
Hypochondroplasia Q77.4
Hypochromasia, blood cells D50.8
Hypodontia — *see* Anodontia
Hypoeosinophilia D72.89
Hypoesthesia R20.1
Hypofibrinogenemia D68.8
  acquired D65
  congenital (hereditary) D68.2
Hypofunction
  adrenocortical E27.40
    drug-induced E27.3
    postprocedural E89.6
    primary E27.1
  adrenomedullary, postprocedural E89.6
  cerebral R29.818
  corticoadrenal NEC E27.40
  intestinal K59.8
  labyrinth — *see* subcategory H83.2 ☑
  ovary E28.39
  pituitary (gland) (anterior) E23.0

Hypofunction — *continued*
  testicular E29.1
    postprocedural (postsurgical) (postirradiation) (iatrogenic) E89.5
Hypogalactia O92.4
Hypogammaglobulinemia (*see also* Agammaglobulinemia) D80.1
  hereditary D80.0
  nonfamilial D80.1
  transient, of infancy D80.7
Hypogenitalism (congenital) — *see* Hypogonadism
Hypoglossia Q38.3
Hypoglycemia (spontaneous) E16.2
  coma E15
    diabetic — *see* Diabetes, coma
  diabetic — *see* Diabetes, hypoglycemia
  dietary counseling and surveillance Z71.3
  drug-induced E16.0
    with coma (nondiabetic) E15
  due to insulin E16.0
    with coma (nondiabetic) E15
    therapeutic misadventure — *see* subcategory T38.3 ☑
  functional, nonhyperinsulinemic E16.1
  iatrogenic E16.0
    with coma (nondiabetic) E15
  in infant of diabetic mother P70.1
    gestational diabetes P70.0
  infantile E16.1
  leucine-induced E71.19
  neonatal (transitory) P70.4
    iatrogenic P70.3
  reactive (not drug-induced) E16.1
  transitory neonatal P70.4
Hypogonadism
  female E28.39
  hypogonadotropic E23.0
  male E29.1
  ovarian (primary) E28.39
  pituitary E23.0
  testicular (primary) E29.1
Hypohidrosis, hypoidrosis L74.4
Hypoinsulinemia, postprocedural E89.1
Hypokalemia E87.6
Hypoleukocytosis — *see* Agranulocytosis
Hypolipoproteinemia (alpha) (beta) E78.6
Hypomagnesemia E83.42
  neonatal P71.2
Hypomania, hypomanic reaction F30.8
Hypomenorrhea — *see* Oligomenorrhea
Hypometabolism R63.8
Hypomotility
  gastrointestinal (tract) K31.89
    psychogenic F45.8
  intestine K59.8
    psychogenic F45.8
  stomach K31.89
    psychogenic F45.8
Hyponasality R49.22
Hyponatremia E87.1
Hypo-osmolality E87.1
Hypo-ovarianism, hypo-ovarism E28.39
Hypoparathyroidism E20.9
  familial E20.8
  idiopathic E20.0
  neonatal, transitory P71.4
  postprocedural E89.2
  specified NEC E20.8
Hypoperfusion (in)
  newborn P96.89
Hypopharyngitis — *see* Laryngopharyngitis
Hypophoria H50.53
Hypophosphatemia, hypophosphatasia (acquired) (congenital) (renal) E83.39
  familial E83.31
Hypophyseal, hypophysis (*see also* condition)
  dwarfism E23.0
  gigantism E22.0
Hypopiesis — *see* Hypotension
Hypopinealism E34.8
Hypopituitarism (juvenile) E23.0
  drug-induced E23.1
  due to
    hypophysectomy E89.3
    radiotherapy E89.3
    iatrogenic NEC E23.1
    postirradiation E89.3

Hypopituitarism — *continued*
  postpartum E23.0
  postprocedural E89.3
Hypoplasia, hypoplastic
  adrenal (gland), congenital Q89.1
  alimentary tract, congenital Q45.8
    upper Q40.8
  anus, anal (canal) Q42.3
    with fistula Q42.2
  aorta, aortic Q25.4
    ascending, in hypoplastic left heart syndrome Q23.4
    valve Q23.1
      in hypoplastic left heart syndrome Q23.4
  areola, congenital Q83.8
  arm (congenital) — *see* Defect, reduction, upper limb
  artery (peripheral) Q27.8
    brain (congenital) Q28.3
    coronary Q24.5
    digestive system Q27.8
    lower limb Q27.8
    pulmonary Q25.79
      functional, unilateral J43.0
    retinal (congenital) Q14.1
    specified site NEC Q27.8
    umbilical Q27.0
    upper limb Q27.8
  auditory canal Q17.8
    causing impairment of hearing Q16.9
  biliary duct or passage Q44.5
  bone NOS Q79.9
    face Q75.8
    marrow D61.9
      megakaryocytic D69.49
    skull — *see* Hypoplasia, skull
  brain Q02
    gyri Q04.3
    part of Q04.3
  breast (areola) N64.82
  bronchus Q32.4
  cardiac Q24.8
  carpus — *see* Defect, reduction, upper limb, specified type NEC
  cartilage hair Q78.5
  cecum Q42.8
  cementum K00.4
  cephalic Q02
  cerebellum Q04.3
  cervix (uteri), congenital Q51.821
  clavicle (congenital) Q74.0
  coccyx Q76.49
  colon Q42.9
    specified NEC Q42.8
  corpus callosum Q04.0
  cricoid cartilage Q31.2
  digestive organ(s) or tract NEC Q45.8
    upper (congenital) Q40.8
  ear (auricle) (lobe) Q17.2
    middle Q16.4
  enamel of teeth (neonatal) (postnatal) (prenatal) K00.4
  endocrine (gland) NEC Q89.2
  endometrium N85.8
  epididymis (congenital) Q55.4
  epiglottis Q31.2
  erythroid, congenital D61.01
  esophagus (congenital) Q39.8
  eustachian tube Q17.8
  eye Q11.2
  eyelid (congenital) Q10.3
  face Q18.8
    bone(s) Q75.8
  femur (congenital) — *see* Defect, reduction, lower limb, specified type NEC
  fibula (congenital) — *see* Defect, reduction, lower limb, specified type NEC
  finger (congenital) — *see* Defect, reduction, upper limb, specified type NEC
  focal dermal Q82.8
  foot — *see* Defect, reduction, lower limb, specified type NEC
  gallbladder Q44.0
  genitalia, genital organ(s)
    female, congenital Q52.8
      external Q52.79
      internal NEC Q52.8
    in adiposogenital dystrophy E23.6
  glottis Q31.2
  hair Q84.2

Hypoplasia, hypoplastic — *continued*
  hand (congenital) — *see* Defect, reduction, upper limb, specified type NEC
  heart Q24.8
  humerus (congenital) — *see* Defect, reduction, upper limb, specified type NEC
  intestine (small) Q41.9
    large Q42.9
      specified NEC Q42.8
  jaw M26.09
    alveolar M26.79
    lower M26.04
      alveolar M26.74
    upper M26.02
      alveolar M26.73
  kidney(s) Q60.5
    bilateral Q60.4
    unilateral Q60.3
  labium (majus) (minus), congenital Q52.79
  larynx Q31.2
  left heart syndrome Q23.4
  leg (congenital) — *see* Defect, reduction, lower limb
  limb Q73.8
    lower (congenital) — *see* Defect, reduction, lower limb
    upper (congenital) — *see* Defect, reduction, upper limb
  liver Q44.7
  lung (lobe) (not associated with short gestation) Q33.6
    associated with immaturity, low birth weight, prematurity, or short gestation P28.0
  mammary (areola), congenital Q83.8
  mandible, mandibular M26.04
    alveolar M26.74
    unilateral condylar M27.8
  maxillary M26.02
    alveolar M26.73
  medullary D61.9
  megakaryocytic D69.49
  metacarpus — *see* Defect, reduction, upper limb, specified type NEC
  metatarsus — *see* Defect, reduction, lower limb, specified type NEC
  muscle Q79.8
  nail(s) Q84.6
  nose, nasal Q30.1
  optic nerve H47.03- ☑
  osseous meatus (ear) Q17.8
  ovary, congenital Q50.39
  pancreas Q45.0
  parathyroid (gland) Q89.2
  parotid gland Q38.4
  patella Q74.1
  pelvis, pelvic girdle Q74.2
  penis (congenital) Q55.62
  peripheral vascular system Q27.8
    digestive system Q27.8
    lower limb Q27.8
    specified site NEC Q27.8
    upper limb Q27.8
  pituitary (gland) (congenital) Q89.2
  pulmonary (not associated with short gestation) Q33.6
    artery, functional J43.0
    associated with short gestation P28.0
  radioulnar — *see* Defect, reduction, upper limb, specified type NEC
  radius — *see* Defect, reduction, upper limb
  rectum Q42.1
    with fistula Q42.0
  respiratory system NEC Q34.8
  rib Q76.6
  right heart syndrome Q22.6
  sacrum Q76.49
  scapula Q74.0
  scrotum Q55.1
  shoulder girdle Q74.0
  skin Q82.8
  skull (bone) Q75.8
    with
      anencephaly Q00.0
      encephalocele — *see* Encephalocele
      hydrocephalus Q03.9
        with spina bifida — *see* Spina bifida, by site, with hydrocephalus
      microcephaly Q02
  spinal (cord) (ventral horn cell) Q06.1
  spine Q76.49
  sternum Q76.7

Hypoplasia, hypoplastic — *continued*
  tarsus — *see* Defect, reduction, lower limb, specified
      type NEC
  testis Q55.1
  thymic, with immunodeficiency D82.1
  thymus (gland) Q89.2
      with immunodeficiency D82.1
  thyroid (gland) E03.1
      cartilage Q31.2
  tibiofibular (congenital) — *see* Defect, reduction,
      lower limb, specified type NEC
  toe — *see* Defect, reduction, lower limb, specified type
      NEC
  tongue Q38.3
  Turner's K00.4
  ulna (congenital) — *see* Defect, reduction, upper limb
  umbilical artery Q27.0
  unilateral condylar M27.8
  ureter Q62.8
  uterus, congenital Q51.811
  vagina Q52.4
  vascular NEC peripheral Q27.8
      brain Q28.3
      digestive system Q27.8
      lower limb Q27.8
      specified site NEC Q27.8
      upper limb Q27.8
  vein(s) (peripheral) Q27.8
      brain Q28.3
      digestive system Q27.8
      great Q26.8
      lower limb Q27.8
      specified site NEC Q27.8
      upper limb Q27.8
  vena cava (inferior) (superior) Q26.8
  vertebra Q76.49
  vulva, congenital Q52.79
  zonule (ciliary) Q12.8
Hypopotassemia E87.6
Hypoproconvertinemia, congenital (hereditary) D68.2
Hypoproteinemia E77.8
Hypoprothrombinemia (congenital) (hereditary) (idio-
      pathic) D68.2
  acquired D68.4
  newborn, transient P61.6
Hypoptyalism K11.7
Hypopyon (eye) (anterior chamber) — *see* Iridocyclitis,
      acute, hypopyon
Hypopyrexia R68.0
Hyporeflexia R29.2
Hyposecretion
  ACTH E23.0
  antidiuretic hormone E23.2
  ovary E28.39
  salivary gland (any) K11.7
  vasopressin E23.2
Hyposegmentation, leukocytic, hereditary D72.0
Hyposiderinemia D50.9
Hypospadias Q54.9
  balanic Q54.0
  coronal Q54.0
  glandular Q54.0
  penile Q54.1
  penoscrotal Q54.2
  perineal Q54.3
  specified NEC Q54.8
Hypospermatogenesis — *see* Oligospermia
Hyposplenism D73.0
Hypostasis pulmonary, passive — *see* Edema, lung
Hypostatic — *see* condition
Hyposthenuria N28.89
Hypotension (arterial) (constitutional) I95.9
  chronic I95.89
  drug-induced I95.2
  due to (of) hemodialysis I95.3
  iatrogenic I95.89
  idiopathic (permanent) I95.0
  intracranial, following ventricular shunting (ventricu-
      lostomy) G97.2
  intra-dialytic I95.3
  maternal, syndrome (following labor and delivery)
      O26.5- ☑
  neurogenic, orthostatic G90.3
  orthostatic (chronic) I95.1
      due to drugs I95.2
          neurogenic G90.3
  postoperative I95.81
  postural I95.1

Hypotension — *continued*
  specified NEC I95.89
Hypothermia (accidental) T68 ☑
  due to anesthesia, anesthetic T88.51 ☑
  low environmental temperature T68 ☑
  neonatal P80.9
      environmental (mild) NEC P80.8
      mild P80.8
      severe (chronic) (cold injury syndrome) P80.0
      specified NEC P80.8
  not associated with low environmental temperature
      R68.0
Hypothyroidism (acquired) E03.9
  congenital (without goiter) E03.1
      with goiter (diffuse) E03.0
  due to
      exogenous substance NEC E03.2
      iodine-deficiency, acquired E01.8
          subclinical E02
      irradiation therapy E89.0
      medicament NEC E03.2
      P-aminosalicylic acid (PAS) E03.2
      phenylbutazone E03.2
      resorcinol E03.2
      sulfonamide E03.2
      surgery E89.0
      thiourea group drugs E03.2
  iatrogenic NEC E03.2
  iodine-deficiency (acquired) E01.8
      congenital — *see* Syndrome, iodine- deficiency,
          congenital
      subclinical E02
  neonatal, transitory P72.2
  postinfectious E03.3
  postirradiation E89.0
  postprocedural E89.0
  postsurgical E89.0
  specified NEC E03.8
  subclinical, iodine-deficiency related E02
Hypotonia, hypotonicity, hypotony
  bladder N31.2
  congenital (benign) P94.2
  eye — *see* Disorder, globe, hypotony
Hypotrichosis — *see* Alopecia
Hypotropia H50.2- ☑
Hypoventilation R06.89
  congenital central alveolar G47.35
  sleep related
      idiopathic nonobstructive alveolar G47.34
      in conditions classified elsewhere G47.36
Hypovitaminosis — *see* Deficiency, vitamin
Hypovolemia E86.1
  surgical shock T81.19 ☑
  traumatic (shock) T79.4 ☑
Hypoxemia R09.02
  newborn P84
  sleep related, in conditions classified elsewhere G47.36
Hypoxia (*see also* Anoxia) R09.02
  cerebral, during a procedure NEC G97.81
      postprocedural NEC G97.82
  intrauterine P84
  myocardial — *see* Insufficiency, coronary
  newborn P84
  sleep-related G47.34
Hypsarhythmia — *see* Epilepsy, generalized, specified
      NEC
Hysteralgia, pregnant uterus O26.89- ☑
Hysteria, hysterical (conversion) (dissociative state)
      F44.9
  anxiety F41.8
  convulsions F44.5
  psychosis, acute F44.9
Hysteroepilepsy F44.5

I

Ichthyoparasitism due to Vandellia cirrhosa B88.8
Ichthyosis (congenital) Q80.9
  acquired L85.0
  fetalis Q80.4
  hystrix Q80.8
  lamellar Q80.2
  lingual K13.29
  palmaris and plantaris Q82.8
  simplex Q80.0
  vera Q80.8
  vulgaris Q80.0

Ichthyosis — *continued*
  X-linked Q80.1
Ichthyotoxism — *see* Poisoning, fish
  bacterial — *see* Intoxication, foodborne
Icteroanemia, hemolytic (acquired) D59.9
  congenital — *see* Spherocytosis
Icterus (*see also* Jaundice)
  conjunctiva R17
  gravis, newborn P55.0
  hematogenous (acquired) D59.9
  hemolytic (acquired) D59.9
      congenital — *see* Spherocytosis
  hemorrhagic (acute) (leptospiral) (spirochetal) A27.0
      newborn P53
  infectious B15.9
      with hepatic coma B15.0
      leptospiral A27.0
      spirochetal A27.0
  neonatorum — *see* Jaundice, newborn
  newborn P59.9
  spirochetal A27.0
Ictus solaris, solis T67.0 ☑
Id reaction (due to bacteria) L30.2
Ideation
  homicidal R45.850
  suicidal R45.851
Identity disorder (child) F64.9
  gender role F64.2
  psychosexual F64.2
Idioglossia F80.0
Idiopathic — *see* condition
Idiot, idiocy (congenital) F73
  amaurotic (Bielschowsky(-Jansky)) (family) (infantile
      (late) (juvenile (late)) (Vogt-Spielmeyer) E75.4
  microcephalic Q02
IgE asthma J45.909
IIAC (idiopathic infantile arterial calcification) Q28.8
Ileitis (chronic) (noninfectious) (*see also* Enteritis) K52.9
  backwash — *see* Pancolitis, ulcerative (chronic)
  infectious A09
  regional (ulcerative) — *see* Enteritis, regional, small
      intestine
  segmental — *see* Enteritis, regional
  terminal (ulcerative) — *see* Enteritis, regional, small
      intestine
Ileocolitis (*see also* Enteritis) K52.9
  infectious A09
  regional — *see* Enteritis, regional
Ileostomy
  attention to Z43.2
  malfunctioning K94.13
  status Z93.2
      with complication — *see* Complications, enteros-
          tomy
Ileotyphus — *see* Typhoid
Ileum — *see* condition
Ileus (bowel) (colon) (inhibitory) (intestine) K56.7
  adynamic K56.0
  due to gallstone (in intestine) K56.3
  duodenal (chronic) K31.5
  gallstone K56.3
  mechanical NEC K56.69
  meconium P76.0
      in cystic fibrosis E84.11
      meaning meconium plug (without cystic fibrosis)
          P76.0
  myxedema K59.8
  neurogenic K56.0
      Hirschsprung's disease or megacolon Q43.1
  newborn
      due to meconium P76.0
          in cystic fibrosis E84.11
          meaning meconium plug (without cystic fibro-
              sis) P76.0
      transitory P76.1
  obstructive K56.69
  paralytic K56.0
Iliac — *see* condition
Iliotibial band syndrome M76.3- ☑
Illiteracy Z55.0
Illness (*see also* Disease) R69
  manic-depressive — *see* Disorder, bipolar
Imbalance R26.89
  autonomic G90.8
  constituents of food intake E63.1
  electrolyte E87.8

☑ **Additional Character Required** — Refer to the Tabular List for Character Selection   ▽ **Subterms under main terms may continue to next column or page**

Imbalance — *continued*
  electrolyte — *continued*
    with
      abortion — *see* Abortion by type, complicated
        by, electrolyte imbalance
      molar pregnancy O08.5
    due to hyperemesis gravidarum O21.1
    following ectopic or molar pregnancy O08.5
    neonatal, transitory NEC P74.4
      potassium P74.3
      sodium P74.2
  endocrine E34.9
  eye muscle NOS H50.9
  hormone E34.9
  hysterical F44.4
  labyrinth — *see* subcategory H83.2 ☑
  posture R29.3
  protein-energy — *see* Malnutrition
  sympathetic G90.8
Imbecile, imbecility (I.Q. 35-49) F71
Imbedding, intrauterine device T83.39 ☑
Imbibition, cholesterol (gallbladder) K82.4
Imbrication, teeth,, fully erupted M26.30
Imerslund (-Gräsbeck) **syndrome** D51.1
Immature (*see also* Immaturity)
  birth (less than 37 completed weeks) — *see* Preterm,
    newborn
    extremely (less than 28 completed weeks) — *see*
      Immaturity, extreme
  personality F60.89
Immaturity (less than 37 completed weeks) (*see also*
  Preterm, newborn)
  extreme of newborn (less than 28 completed weeks
    of gestation) (less than 196 completed days of
    gestation) (unspecified weeks of gestation)
    P07.20
    gestational age
      less than 23 completed weeks P07.21
      23 completed weeks (23 weeks, 0 days through
        23 weeks, 6 days) P07.22
      24 completed weeks (24 weeks, 0 days through
        24 weeks, 6 days) P07.23
      25 completed weeks (25 weeks, 0 days through
        25 weeks, 6 days) P07.24
      26 completed weeks (26 weeks, 0 days through
        26 weeks, 6 days) P07.25
      27 completed weeks (27 weeks, 0 days through
        27 weeks, 6 days) P07.26
  fetus or infant light-for-dates — *see* Light-for-dates
  lung, newborn P28.0
  organ or site NEC — *see* Hypoplasia
  pulmonary, newborn P28.0
  reaction F60.89
  sexual (female) (male), after puberty E30.0
Immersion T75.1 ☑
  foot T69.02- ☑
  hand T69.01- ☑
Immobile, immobility
  complete, due to severe physical disability or frailty
    R53.2
  intestine K59.8
  syndrome (paraplegic) M62.3
Immune reconstitution (inflammatory) syndrome [IRIS]
  D89.3
Immunization (*see also* Vaccination)
  ABO — *see* Incompatibility, ABO
    in newborn P55.1
  complication — *see* Complications, vaccination
  encounter for Z23
  not done (not carried out) Z28.9
    because (of)
      acute illness of patient Z28.01
      allergy to vaccine (or component) Z28.04
      caregiver refusal Z28.82
      chronic illness of patient Z28.02
      contraindication NEC Z28.09
      group pressure Z28.1
      guardian refusal Z28.82
      immune compromised state of patient Z28.03
      parent refusal Z28.82
      patient had disease being vaccinated against
        Z28.81
      patient refusal Z28.21
      patient's belief Z28.1
      religious beliefs of patient Z28.1
      specified reason NEC Z28.89
        of patient Z28.29
      unspecified patient reason Z28.20

Immunization — *continued*
  Rh factor
    affecting management of pregnancy NEC
      O36.09- ☑
      anti-D antibody O36.01- ☑
    from transfusion — *see* Complication(s), transfu-
      sion, incompatibility reaction, Rh (factor)
Immunocytoma C83.0- ☑
Immunodeficiency D84.9
  with
    adenosine-deaminase deficiency D81.3
    antibody defects D80.9
      specified type NEC D80.8
    hyperimmunoglobulinemia D80.6
    increased immunoglobulin M (IgM) D80.5
    major defect D82.9
      specified type NEC D82.8
    partial albinism D82.8
    short-limbed stature D82.2
    thrombocytopenia and eczema D82.0
  antibody with
    hyperimmunoglobulinemia D80.6
    near-normal immunoglobulins D80.6
  autosomal recessive, Swiss type D80.0
  combined D81.9
    biotin-dependent carboxylase D81.819
      biotinidase D81.810
      holocarboxylase synthetase D81.818
      specified type NEC D81.818
    severe (SCID) D81.9
      with
        low or normal B-cell numbers D81.2
        low T- and B-cell numbers D81.1
        reticular dysgenesis D81.0
    specified type NEC D81.89
  common variable D83.9
    with
      abnormalities of B-cell numbers and function
        D83.0
      autoantibodies to B- or T-cells D83.2
      immunoregulatory T-cell disorders D83.1
    specified type NEC D83.8
  following hereditary defective response to Epstein-
    Barr virus (EBV) D82.3
  selective, immunoglobulin
    A (IgA) D80.2
    G (IgG) (subclasses) D80.3
    M (IgM) D80.4
  severe combined (SCID) D81.9
  specified type NEC D84.8
  X-linked, with increased IgM D80.5
Immunotherapy (encounter for)
  antineoplastic Z51.12
Impaction, impacted
  bowel, colon, rectum (*see also* Impaction, fecal) K56.49
    by gallstone K56.3
  calculus — *see* Calculus
  cerumen (ear) (external) H61.2- ☑
  cuspid — *see* Impaction, tooth
  dental (same or adjacent tooth) K01.1
  fecal, feces K56.41
  fracture — *see* Fracture, by site
  gallbladder — *see* Calculus, gallbladder
  gallstone(s) — *see* Calculus, gallbladder
    bile duct (common) (hepatic) — *see* Calculus, bile
      duct
    cystic duct — *see* Calculus, gallbladder
    in intestine, with obstruction (any part) K56.3
  intestine (calculous) NEC (*see also* Impaction, fecal)
    K56.49
    gallstone, with ileus K56.3
  intrauterine device (IUD) T83.39 ☑
  molar — *see* Impaction, tooth
  shoulder, causing obstructed labor O66.0
  tooth, teeth K01.1
  turbinate J34.89
Impaired, impairment (function)
  auditory discrimination — *see* Abnormal, auditory
    perception
  cognitive, mild, so stated G31.84
  dual sensory Z73.82
  fasting glucose R73.01
  glucose tolerance (oral) R73.02
  hearing — *see* Deafness
  heart — *see* Disease, heart
  kidney N28.9
    disorder resulting from N25.9
      specified NEC N25.89

Impaired, impairment — *continued*
  liver K72.90
    with coma K72.91
  mastication K08.8
  mild cognitive, so stated G31.84
  mobility
    ear ossicles — *see* Ankylosis, ear ossicles
    requiring care provider Z74.09
  myocardium, myocardial — *see* Insufficiency, myocar-
    dial
  rectal sphincter R19.8
  renal (acute) (chronic) N28.9
    disorder resulting from N25.9
      specified NEC N25.89
  vision NEC H54.7
    both eyes H54.3
Impediment, speech R47.9
  psychogenic (childhood) F98.8
  slurring R47.81
  specified NEC R47.89
Impending
  coronary syndrome I20.0
  delirium tremens F10.239
  myocardial infarction I20.0
Imperception auditory (acquired) (*see also* Deafness)
  congenital H93.25
Imperfect
  aeration, lung (newborn) NEC — *see* Atelectasis
  closure (congenital)
    alimentary tract NEC Q45.8
      lower Q43.8
      upper Q40.8
    atrioventricular ostium Q21.2
    atrium (secundum) Q21.1
    branchial cleft or sinus Q18.0
    choroid Q14.3
    cricoid cartilage Q31.8
    cusps, heart valve NEC Q24.8
      pulmonary Q22.3
    ductus
      arteriosus Q25.0
      Botalli Q25.0
    ear drum (causing impairment of hearing) Q16.4
    esophagus with communication to bronchus or
      trachea Q39.1
    eyelid Q10.3
    foramen
      botalli Q21.1
      ovale Q21.1
    genitalia, genital organ(s) or system
      female Q52.8
        external Q52.79
        internal NEC Q52.8
      male Q55.8
    glottis Q31.8
    interatrial ostium or septum Q21.1
    interauricular ostium or septum Q21.1
    interventricular ostium or septum Q21.0
    larynx Q31.8
    lip — *see* Cleft, lip
    nasal septum Q30.3
    nose Q30.2
    omphalomesenteric duct Q43.0
    optic nerve entry Q14.2
    organ or site not listed — *see* Anomaly, by site
    ostium
      interatrial Q21.1
      interauricular Q21.1
      interventricular Q21.0
    palate — *see* Cleft, palate
    preauricular sinus Q18.1
    retina Q14.1
    roof of orbit Q75.8
    sclera Q13.5
    septum
      aorticopulmonary Q21.4
      atrial (secundum) Q21.1
      between aorta and pulmonary artery Q21.4
      heart Q21.9
      interatrial (secundum) Q21.1
      interauricular (secundum) Q21.1
      interventricular Q21.0
        in tetralogy of Fallot Q21.3
      nasal Q30.3
      ventricular Q21.0
        with pulmonary stenosis or atresia, dextra-
          position of aorta, and hypertrophy of
          right ventricle Q21.3

Index

Imbalance — Imperfect

Imperfect — *continued*
  closure — *continued*
    septum — *continued*
      ventricular — *continued*
        in tetralogy of Fallot Q21.3
      skull Q75.0
        with
          anencephaly Q00.0
          encephalocele — *see* Encephalocele
          hydrocephalus Q03.9
            with spina bifida — *see* Spina bifida, by
              site, with hydrocephalus
          microcephaly Q02
    spine (with meningocele) — *see* Spina bifida
    trachea Q32.1
    tympanic membrane (causing impairment of
      hearing) Q16.4
    uterus Q51.818
    vitelline duct Q43.0
  erection — *see* Dysfunction, sexual, male, erectile
  fusion — *see* Imperfect, closure
  inflation, lung (newborn) — *see* Atelectasis
  posture R29.3
  rotation, intestine Q43.3
  septum, ventricular Q21.0
Imperfectly descended testis — *see* Cryptorchid
Imperforate (congenital) (*see also* Atresia)
  anus Q42.3
    with fistula Q42.2
  cervix (uteri) Q51.828
  esophagus Q39.0
    with tracheoesophageal fistula Q39.1
  hymen Q52.3
  jejunum Q41.1
  pharynx Q38.8
  rectum Q42.1
    with fistula Q42.0
  urethra Q64.39
  vagina Q52.4
Impervious (congenital) (*see also* Atresia)
  anus Q42.3
    with fistula Q42.2
  bile duct Q44.2
  esophagus Q39.0
    with tracheoesophageal fistula Q39.1
  intestine (small) Q41.9
    large Q42.9
      specified NEC Q42.8
  rectum Q42.1
    with fistula Q42.0
  ureter — *see* Atresia, ureter
  urethra Q64.39
Impetiginization of dermatoses L01.1
Impetigo (any organism) (any site) (circinate) (contagiosa) (simplex) (vulgaris) L01.00
  Bockhart's L01.02
  bullous, bullosa L01.03
  external ear L01.00 [H62.40]
  follicularis L01.02
  furfuracea L30.5
  herpetiformis L40.1
    nonobstetrical L40.1
  neonatorum L01.03
  nonbullous L01.01
  specified type NEC L01.09
  ulcerative L01.09
Impingement (on teeth)
  soft tissue
    anterior M26.81
    posterior M26.82
Implant, endometrial N80.9
Implantation
  anomalous — *see* Anomaly, by site
    ureter Q62.63
  cyst
    external area or site (skin) NEC L72.0
    iris — *see* Cyst, iris, implantation
    vagina N89.8
    vulva N90.7
  dermoid (cyst) — *see* Implantation, cyst
Impotence (sexual) N52.9
  counseling Z70.1
  organic origin (*see also* Dysfunction, sexual, male,
    erectile) N52.9
  psychogenic F52.21
Impression, basilar Q75.8
Imprisonment, anxiety concerning Z65.1
Improper care (child) (newborn) — *see* Maltreatment

Improperly tied umbilical cord (causing hemorrhage)
  P51.8
Impulsiveness (impulsive) R45.87
Inability to swallow — *see* Aphagia
Inaccessible, inaccessibility
  health care NEC Z75.3
    due to
      waiting period Z75.2
        for admission to facility elsewhere Z75.1
    other helping agencies Z75.4
Inactive — *see* condition
Inadequate, inadequacy
  aesthetics of dental restoration K08.56
  biologic, constitutional, functional, or social F60.7
  development
    child R62.50
    genitalia
      after puberty NEC E30.0
      congenital
        female Q52.8
          external Q52.79
          internal Q52.8
        male Q55.8
    lungs Q33.6
      associated with short gestation P28.0
    organ or site not listed — *see* Anomaly, by site
  diet (causing nutritional deficiency) E63.9
  eating habits Z72.4
  environment, household Z59.1
  family support Z63.8
  food (supply) NEC Z59.4
    hunger effects T73.0 ☑
  functional F60.7
  household care, due to
    family member
      handicapped or ill Z74.2
      on vacation Z75.5
      temporarily away from home Z74.2
    technical defects in home Z59.1
    temporary absence from home of person rendering
      care Z74.2
  housing (heating) (space) Z59.1
  income (financial) Z59.6
  intrafamilial communication Z63.8
  material resources Z59.9
  mental — *see* Disability, intellectual
  parental supervision or control of child Z62.0
  personality F60.7
  pulmonary
    function R06.89
      newborn P28.5
    ventilation, newborn P28.5
  sample of cytologic smear
    anus R85.615
    cervix R87.615
    vagina R87.625
  social F60.7
    insurance Z59.7
    skills NEC Z73.4
  supervision of child by parent Z62.0
  teaching affecting education Z55.8
  welfare support Z59.7
Inanition R64
  with edema — *see* Malnutrition, severe
  due to
    deprivation of food T73.0 ☑
    malnutrition — *see* Malnutrition
  fever R50.9
Inappropriate
  change in quantitative human chorionic gonadotropin
    (hCG) in early pregnancy O02.81
  diet or eating habits Z72.4
  level of quantitative human chorionic gonadotropin
    (hCG) for gestational age in early pregnancy
    O02.81
  secretion
    antidiuretic hormone (ADH) (excessive) E22.2
      deficiency E23.2
    pituitary (posterior) E22.2
Inattention at or after birth — *see* Neglect
Incarceration, incarcerated
  enterocele K46.0
    gangrenous K46.1
  epiplocele K46.0
    gangrenous K46.1
  exophthalmos K42.0
    gangrenous K42.1

Incarceration, incarcerated — *continued*
  hernia (*see also* Hernia, by site, with
    obstruction)
    with gangrene — *see* Hernia, by site, with gan-
      grene
  iris, in wound — *see* Injury, eye, laceration, with pro-
    lapse
  lens, in wound — *see* Injury, eye, laceration, with
    prolapse
  omphalocele K42.0
  prison, anxiety concerning Z65.1
  rupture — *see* Hernia, by site
  sarcoepiplocele K46.0
    gangrenous K46.1
  sarcoepiplomphalocele K42.0
    with gangrene K42.1
  uterus N85.8
    gravid O34.51- ☑
      causing obstructed labor O65.5
Incised wound
  external — *see* Laceration
  internal organs — *see* Injury, by site
Incision, incisional
  hernia K43.2
    with
      gangrene (and obstruction) K43.1
      obstruction K43.0
    surgical, complication — *see* Complications, surgical
      procedure
  traumatic
    external — *see* Laceration
    internal organs — *see* Injury, by site
Inclusion
  azurophilic leukocytic D72.0
  blennorrhea (neonatal) (newborn) P39.1
  gallbladder in liver (congenital) Q44.1
Incompatibility
  ABO
    affecting management of pregnancy O36.11- ☑
      anti-A sensitization O36.11- ☑
      anti-B sensitization O36.19- ☑
      specified NEC O36.19- ☑
    infusion or transfusion reaction — *see* Complica-
      tion(s), transfusion, incompatibility reaction,
      ABO
    newborn P55.1
  blood (group) (Duffy) (K(ell)) (Kidd) (Lewis) (M) (S) NEC
    affecting management of pregnancy O36.11- ☑
      anti-A sensitization O36.11- ☑
      anti-B sensitization O36.19- ☑
    infusion or transfusion reaction T80.89 ☑
    newborn P55.8
  divorce or estrangement Z63.5
  Rh (blood group) (factor) Z31.82
    affecting management of pregnancy NEC
      O36.09- ☑
      anti-D antibody O36.01- ☑
    infusion or transfusion reaction — *see* Complica-
      tion(s), transfusion, incompatibility reaction,
      Rh (factor)
    newborn P55.0
  rhesus — *see* Incompatibility, Rh
Incompetency, incompetent, incompetence
  annular
    aortic (valve) — *see* Insufficiency, aortic
    mitral (valve) I34.0
    pulmonary valve (heart) I37.1
  aortic (valve) — *see* Insufficiency, aortic
  cardiac valve — *see* Endocarditis
  cervix, cervical (os) N88.3
    in pregnancy O34.3- ☑
  chronotropic I45.89
    with
      autonomic dysfunction G90.8
      ischemic heart disease I25.89
      left ventricular dysfunction I51.89
      sinus node dysfunction I49.8
  esophagogastric (junction) (sphincter) K22.0
  mitral (valve) — *see* Insufficiency, mitral
  pelvic fundus N81.89
  pubocervical tissue N81.82
  pulmonary valve (heart) I37.1
    congenital Q22.3
  rectovaginal tissue N81.83
  tricuspid (annular) (valve) — *see* Insufficiency, tricuspid
  valvular — *see* Endocarditis
    congenital Q24.8

Incompetency, incompetent, incompetence — *continued*
  vein, venous (saphenous) (varicose) — *see* Varix, leg
Incomplete (*see also* condition)
  bladder, emptying R33.9
  defecation R15.0
  expansion lungs (newborn) NEC — *see* Atelectasis
  rotation, intestine Q43.3
Inconclusive
  diagnostic imaging due to excess body fat of patient R93.9
  findings on diagnostic imaging of breast NEC R92.8
  mammogram (due to dense breasts) R92.2
Incontinence R32
  anal sphincter R15.9
  feces R15.9
    nonorganic origin F98.1
  overflow N39.490
  psychogenic F45.8
  rectal R15.9
  reflex N39.498
  stress (female) (male) N39.3
    and urge N39.46
  urethral sphincter R32
  urge N39.41
    and stress (female) (male) N39.46
  urine (urinary) R32
    continuous N39.45
    due to cognitive impairment, or severe physical disability or immobility R39.81
    functional R39.81
    mixed (stress and urge) N39.46
    nocturnal N39.44
    nonorganic origin F98.0
    overflow N39.490
    post dribbling N39.43
    reflex N39.498
    specified NEC N39.498
    stress (female) (male) N39.3
      and urge N39.46
    total N39.498
    unaware N39.42
    urge N39.41
      and stress (female) (male) N39.46
Incontinentia pigmenti Q82.3
Incoordinate, incoordination
  esophageal-pharyngeal (newborn) — *see* Dysphagia
  muscular R27.8
  uterus (action) (contractions) (complicating delivery) O62.4
Increase, increased
  abnormal, in development R63.8
  androgens (ovarian) E28.1
  anticoagulants (antithrombin) (anti-VIIIa) (anti-IXa) (anti-Xa) (anti-XIa) — *see* Circulating anticoagulants
  cold sense R20.8
  estrogen E28.0
  function
    adrenal
      cortex — *see* Cushing's, syndrome
      medulla E27.5
    pituitary (gland) (anterior) (lobe) E22.9
      posterior E22.2
  heat sense R20.8
  intracranial pressure (benign) G93.2
  permeability, capillaries I78.8
  pressure, intracranial G93.2
  secretion
    gastrin E16.4
    glucagon E16.3
    pancreas, endocrine E16.9
      growth hormone-releasing hormone E16.8
      pancreatic polypeptide E16.8
      somatostatin E16.8
      vasoactive-intestinal polypeptide E16.8
  sphericity, lens Q12.4
  splenic activity D73.1
  venous pressure I87.8
    portal K76.6
Increta placenta O43.22- ☑
Incrustation, cornea, foreign body (lead)(zinc) — *see* Foreign body, cornea
Incyclophoria H50.54
Incyclotropia — *see* Cyclotropia
Indeterminate sex Q56.4
India rubber skin Q82.8

Indigestion (acid) (bilious) (functional) K30
  catarrhal K31.89
  due to decomposed food NOS A05.9
  nervous F45.8
  psychogenic F45.8
Indirect — *see* condition
Induratio penis plastica N48.6
Induration, indurated
  brain G93.89
  breast (fibrous) N64.51
    puerperal, postpartum O92.29
  broad ligament N83.8
  chancre
    anus A51.1
    congenital A50.07
    extragenital NEC A51.2
  corpora cavernosa (penis) (plastic) N48.6
  liver (chronic) K76.89
  lung (black) (chronic) (fibroid) (*see also* Fibrosis, lung) J84.10
    essential brown J84.03
  penile (plastic) N48.6
  phlebitic — *see* Phlebitis
  skin R23.4
Inebriety (without dependence) — *see* Alcohol, intoxication
Inefficiency, kidney N28.9
Inelasticity, skin R23.4
Inequality, leg (length) (acquired) (*see also* Deformity, limb, unequal length)
  congenital — *see* Defect, reduction, lower limb
  lower leg — *see* Deformity, limb, unequal length
Inertia
  bladder (neurogenic) N31.2
  stomach K31.89
    psychogenic F45.8
  uterus, uterine during labor O62.2
    during latent phase of labor O62.0
    primary O62.0
    secondary O62.1
  vesical (neurogenic) N31.2
Infancy, infantile, infantilism (*see also* condition)
  celiac K90.0
  genitalia, genitals (after puberty) E30.0
  Herter's (nontropical sprue) K90.0
  intestinal K90.0
  Lorain E23.0
  pancreatic K86.8
  pelvis M95.5
    with disproportion (fetopelvic) O33.1
      causing obstructed labor O65.1
  pituitary E23.0
  renal N25.0
  uterus — *see* Infantile, genitalia
Infant(s) (*see also* Infancy)
  excessive crying R68.11
  irritable child R68.12
  lack of care — *see* Neglect
  liveborn (singleton) Z38.2
    born in hospital Z38.00
      by cesarean Z38.01
    born outside hospital Z38.1
    multiple NEC Z38.8
      born in hospital Z38.68
        by cesarean Z38.69
      born outside hospital Z38.7
    quadruplet Z38.8
      born in hospital Z38.63
        by cesarean Z38.64
      born outside hospital Z38.7
    quintuplet Z38.8
      born in hospital Z38.65
        by cesarean Z38.66
      born outside hospital Z38.7
    triplet Z38.8
      born in hospital Z38.61
        by cesarean Z38.62
      born outside hospital Z38.7
    twin Z38.5
      born in hospital Z38.30
        by cesarean Z38.31
      born outside hospital Z38.4
  of diabetic mother (syndrome of) P70.1
    gestational diabetes P70.0
Infantile (*see also* condition)
  genitalia, genitals E30.0
  os, uterine E30.0
  penis E30.0

Infantile — *continued*
  testis E29.1
  uterus E30.0
Infantilism — *see* Infancy
Infarct, infarction
  adrenal (capsule) (gland) E27.49
  appendices epiploicae K55.0
  bowel K55.0
  brain (stem) — *see* Infarct, cerebral
  breast N64.89
  brewer's (kidney) N28.0
  cardiac — *see* Infarct, myocardium
  cerebellar — *see* Infarct, cerebral
  cerebral (*see also* Occlusion, artery cerebral or precerebral, with infarction) I63.9
    aborted I63.9
    cortical I63.9
    due to
      cerebral venous thrombosis, nonpyogenic I63.6
      embolism
        cerebral arteries I63.4- ☑
        precerebral arteries I63.1- ☑
      occlusion NEC
        cerebral arteries I63.5- ☑
        precerebral arteries I63.2- ☑
      stenosis NEC
        cerebral arteries I63.5- ☑
        precerebral arteries I63.2- ☑
      thrombosis
        cerebral artery I63.3- ☑
        precerebral artery I63.0- ☑
    intraoperative
      during cardiac surgery I97.810
      during other surgery I97.811
    postprocedural
      following cardiac surgery I97.820
      following other surgery I97.821
    specified NEC I63.8
  colon (acute) (agnogenic) (embolic) (hemorrhagic) (nonocclusive) (nonthrombotic) (occlusive) (segmental) (thrombotic) (with gangrene) K55.0
  coronary artery — *see* Infarct, myocardium
  embolic — *see* Embolism
  fallopian tube N83.8
  gallbladder K82.8
  heart — *see* Infarct, myocardium
  hepatic K76.3
  hypophysis (anterior lobe) E23.6
  impending (myocardium) I20.0
  intestine (acute) (agnogenic) (embolic) (hemorrhagic) (nonocclusive) (nonthrombotic) (occlusive) (thrombotic) (with gangrene) K55.0
  kidney N28.0
  liver K76.3
  lung (embolic) (thrombotic) — *see* Embolism, pulmonary
  lymph node I89.8
  mesentery, mesenteric (embolic) (thrombotic) (with gangrene) K55.0
  muscle (ischemic) M62.20
    ankle M62.27- ☑
    foot M62.27- ☑
    forearm M62.23- ☑
    hand M62.24- ☑
    lower leg M62.26- ☑
    pelvic region M62.25- ☑
    shoulder region M62.21- ☑
    specified site NEC M62.28
    thigh M62.25- ☑
    upper arm M62.22- ☑
  myocardium, myocardial (acute) (with stated duration of 4 weeks or less) I21.3
    diagnosed on ECG, but presenting no symptoms I25.2
    healed or old I25.2
    intraoperative
      during cardiac surgery I97.790
      during other surgery I97.791
    non-Q wave I21.4
    non-ST elevation (NSTEMI) I21.4
      subsequent I22.2
    nontransmural I21.4
    past (diagnosed on ECG or other investigation, but currently presenting no symptoms) I25.2
    postprocedural
      following cardiac surgery I97.190
      following other surgery I97.191
    Q wave (see also, Infarct, myocardium, by site) I21.3

Index — Infarct, infarction — Infection, infected, infective

Infarct, infarction — *continued*
myocardium, myocardial — *continued*
ST elevation (STEMI) I21.3
anterior (anteroapical) (anterolateral) (anteroseptal) (Q wave) (wall) I21.09
subsequent I22.0
inferior (diaphragmatic) (inferolateral) (inferoposterior) (wall) NEC I21.19
subsequent I22.1
inferoposterior transmural (Q wave) I21.11
involving
coronary artery of anterior wall NEC I21.09
coronary artery of inferior wall NEC I21.19
diagonal coronary artery I21.02
left anterior descending coronary artery I21.02
left circumflex coronary artery I21.21
left main coronary artery I21.01
oblique marginal coronary artery I21.21
right coronary artery I21.11
lateral (apical-lateral) (basal-lateral) (high) I21.29
subsequent I22.8
posterior (posterobasal) (posterolateral) (posteroseptal) (true) I21.29
subsequent I22.8
septal I21.29
subsequent I22.8
specified NEC I21.29
subsequent I22.8
subsequent I22.9
subsequent (recurrent) (reinfarction) I22.9
anterior (anteroapical) (anterolateral) (anteroseptal) (wall) I22.0
diaphragmatic (wall) I22.1
inferior (diaphragmatic) (inferolateral) (inferoposterior) (wall) I22.1
lateral (apical-lateral) (basal-lateral) (high) I22.8
non-ST elevation (NSTEMI) I22.2
posterior (posterobasal) (posterolateral) (posteroseptal) (true) I22.8
septal I22.8
specified NEC I22.8
ST elevation I22.9
anterior (anteroapical) (anterolateral) (anteroseptal) (wall) I22.0
inferior (diaphragmatic) (inferolateral) (inferoposterior) (wall) I22.1
specified NEC I22.8
subendocardial I22.2
transmural I22.9
anterior (anteroapical) (anterolateral) (anteroseptal) (wall) I22.0
diaphragmatic (wall) I22.1
inferior (diaphragmatic) (inferolateral) (inferoposterior) (wall) I22.1
lateral (apical-lateral) (basal-lateral) (high) I22.8
posterior (posterobasal) (posterolateral) (posteroseptal) (true) I22.8
specified NEC I22.8
syphilitic A52.06
transmural I21.3
anterior (anteroapical) (anterolateral) (anteroseptal) (Q wave) (wall) NEC I21.09
inferior (diaphragmatic) (inferolateral) (inferoposterior) (Q wave) (wall) NEC I21.19
inferoposterior (Q wave) I21.11
lateral (apical-lateral) (basal-lateral) (high) NEC I21.29
posterior (posterobasal) (posterolateral) (posteroseptal) (true) NEC I21.29
septal NEC I21.29
specified NEC I21.29
nontransmural I21.4
omentum K55.0
ovary N83.8
pancreas K86.8
papillary muscle — *see* Infarct, myocardium
parathyroid gland E21.4
pituitary (gland) E23.6
placenta O43.81- ☑
prostate N42.89
pulmonary (artery) (vein) (hemorrhagic) — *see* Embolism, pulmonary
renal (embolic) (thrombotic) N28.0
retina, retinal (artery) — *see* Occlusion, artery, retina
spinal (cord) (acute) (embolic) (nonembolic) G95.11

Infarct, infarction — *continued*
spleen D73.5
embolic or thrombotic I74.8
subendocardial (acute) (nontransmural) I21.4
suprarenal (capsule) (gland) E27.49
testis N50.1
thrombotic (*see also* Thrombosis)
artery, arterial — *see* Embolism
thyroid (gland) E07.89
ventricle (heart) — *see* Infarct, myocardium
Infecting — *see* condition
Infection, infected, infective (opportunistic) B99.9
with
drug resistant organism — *see* Resistance (to), drug (*see also* specific organism)
lymphangitis — *see* Lymphangitis
organ dysfunction (acute) R65.20
with septic shock R65.21
abscess (skin) — *code by* site under Abscess
Absidia — *see* Mucormycosis
Acanthamoeba — *see* Acanthamebiasis
Acanthocheilonema (perstans) (streptocerca) B74.4
accessory sinus (chronic) — *see* Sinusitis
achorion — *see* Dermatophytosis
acremonium falciforme B47.0
acromioclavicular M00.9
Actinobacillus (actinomycetem-comitans) A28.8
mallei A24.0
muris A25.1
Actinomadura B47.1
Actinomyces (israelii) (*see also* Actinomycosis) A42.9
Actinomycetales — *see* Actinomycosis
actinomycotic NOS — *see* Actinomycosis
adenoid (and tonsil) J03.90
chronic J35.02
adenovirus NEC
as cause of disease classified elsewhere B97.0
unspecified nature or site B34.0
aerogenes capsulatus A48.0
aertrycke — *see* Infection, salmonella
alimentary canal NOS — *see* Enteritis, infectious
Allescheria boydii B48.2
Alternaria B48.8
alveolus, alveolar (process) K04.7
Ameba, amebic (histolytica) — *see* Amebiasis
amniotic fluid, sac or cavity O41.10- ☑
chorioamnionitis O41.12- ☑
placentitis O41.14- ☑
amputation stump (surgical) — *see* Complication, amputation stump, infection
Ancylostoma (duodenalis) B76.0
Anisakiasis, Anisakis larvae B81.0
anthrax — *see* Anthrax
antrum (chronic) — *see* Sinusitis, maxillary
anus, anal (papillae) (sphincter) K62.89
arbovirus (arbor virus) A94
specified type NEC A93.8
artificial insemination N98.0
Ascaris lumbricoides — *see* Ascariasis
Ascomycetes B47.0
Aspergillus (flavus) (fumigatus) (terreus) — *see* Aspergillosis
atypical
acid-fast (bacilli) — *see* Mycobacterium, atypical
mycobacteria — *see* Mycobacterium, atypical
virus A81.9
specified type NEC A81.89
auditory meatus (external) — *see* Otitis, externa, infective
auricle (ear) — *see* Otitis, externa, infective
axillary gland (lymph) L04.2
Bacillus A49.9
abortus A23.1
anthracis — *see* Anthrax
Ducrey's (any location) A57
Flexner's A03.1
Friedländer's NEC A49.8
gas (gangrene) A48.0
mallei A24.0
melitensis A23.0
paratyphoid, paratyphosus A01.4
A A01.1
B A01.2
C A01.3
Shiga (-Kruse) A03.0
suipestifer — *see* Infection, salmonella
swimming pool A31.1

Infection, infected, infective — *continued*
Bacillus — *continued*
typhosa A01.00
welchii — *see* Gangrene, gas
bacterial NOS A49.9
as cause of disease classified elsewhere B96.89
Bacteroides fragilis [B. fragilis] B96.6
Clostridium perfringens [C. perfringens] B96.7
Enterobacter sakazakii B96.89
Enterococcus B95.2
Escherichia coli [E. coli] (*see also* Escherichia coli) B96.20
Helicobacter pylori [H.pylori] B96.81
Hemophilus influenzae [H. influenzae] B96.3
Klebsiella pneumoniae [K. pneumoniae] B96.1
Mycoplasma pneumoniae [M. pneumoniae] B96.0
Proteus (mirabilis) (morganii) B96.4
Pseudomonas (aeruginosa) (mallei) (pseudomallei) B96.5
Staphylococcus B95.8
aureus (methicillin susceptible) (MSSA) B95.61
methicillin resistant (MRSA) B95.62
specified NEC B95.7
Streptococcus B95.5
group A B95.0
group B B95.1
pneumoniae B95.3
specified NEC B95.4
Vibrio vulnificus B96.82
specified NEC A48.8
Bacterium
paratyphosum A01.4
A A01.1
B A01.2
C A01.3
typhosum A01.00
Bacteroides NEC A49.8
fragilis, as cause of disease classified elsewhere B96.6
Balantidium coli A07.0
Bartholin's gland N75.8
Basidiobolus B46.8
bile duct (common) (hepatic) — *see* Cholangitis
bladder — *see* Cystitis
Blastomyces, blastomycotic (*see also* Blastomycosis)
brasiliensis — *see* Paracoccidioidomycosis
dermatitidis — *see* Blastomycosis
European — *see* Cryptococcosis
Loboi B48.0
North American B40.9
South American — *see* Paracoccidioidomycosis
bleb, postprocedure — *see* Blebitis
bone — *see* Osteomyelitis
Bordetella — *see* Whooping cough
Borrelia bergdorfi A69.20
brain (*see also* Encephalitis) G04.90
membranes — *see* Meningitis
septic G06.0
meninges — *see* Meningitis, bacterial
branchial cyst Q18.0
breast — *see* Mastitis
bronchus — *see* Bronchitis
Brucella A23.9
abortus A23.1
canis A23.3
melitensis A23.0
mixed A23.8
specified NEC A23.8
suis A23.2
Brugia (malayi) B74.1
timori B74.2
bursa — *see* Bursitis, infective
buttocks (skin) L08.9
Campylobacter, intestinal A04.5
as cause of disease classified elsewhere B96.81
Candida (albicans) (tropicalis) — *see* Candidiasis
candiru B88.8
Capillaria (intestinal) B81.1
hepatica B83.8
philippinensis B81.1
cartilage — *see* Disorder, cartilage, specified type NEC
cat liver fluke B66.0
catheter-related bloodstream (CRBSI) T80.211 ☑
cellulitis — *code by* site under Cellulitis
central line-associated T80.219 ☑
bloodstream (CLABSI) T80.211 ☑

☑ Additional Character Required — Refer to the Tabular List for Character Selection   ▽ Subterms under main terms may continue to next column or page

Infection, infected, infective — *continued*
  central line-associated — *continued*
    specified NEC T80.218 ☑
  Cephalosporium falciforme B47.0
  cerebrospinal — *see* Meningitis
  cervical gland (lymph) L04.0
  cervix — *see* Cervicitis
  cesarean delivery wound (puerperal) O86.0
  cestodes — *see* Infestation, cestodes
  chest J22
  Chilomastix (intestinal) A07.8
  Chlamydia, chlamydial A74.9
    anus A56.3
    genitourinary tract A56.2
      lower A56.00
        specified NEC A56.19
    lymphogranuloma A55
    pharynx A56.4
    psittaci A70
    rectum A56.3
    sexually transmitted NEC A56.8
  cholera — *see* Cholera
  Cladosporium
    bantianum (brain abscess) B43.1
    carrionii B43.0
    castellanii B36.1
    trichoides (brain abscess) B43.1
    werneckii B36.1
  Clonorchis (sinensis) (liver) B66.1
  Clostridium NEC
    bifermentans A48.0
    botulinum (food poisoning) A05.1
      infant A48.51
      wound A48.52
    difficile
      as cause of disease classified elsewhere B96.89
      foodborne (disease) A04.7
      gas gangrene A48.0
      necrotizing enterocolitis A04.7
      sepsis A41.4
    gas-forming NEC A48.0
    histolyticum A48.0
    novyi, causing gas gangrene A48.0
    oedematiens A48.0
    perfringens
      as cause of disease classified elsewhere B96.7
      due to food A05.2
      foodborne (disease) A05.2
      gas gangrene A48.0
      sepsis A41.4
    septicum, causing gas gangrene A48.0
    sordellii, causing gas gangrene A48.0
    welchii
      as cause of disease classified elsewhere B96.7
      foodborne (disease) A05.2
      gas gangrene A48.0
      necrotizing enteritis A05.2
      sepsis A41.4
  Coccidioides (immitis) — *see* Coccidioidomycosis
  colon — *see* Enteritis, infectious
  colostomy K94.02
  common duct — *see* Cholangitis
  congenital P39.9
    Candida (albicans) P37.5
    cytomegalovirus P35.1
    hepatitis, viral P35.3
    herpes simplex P35.2
    infectious or parasitic disease P37.9
      specified NEC P37.8
    listeriosis (disseminated) P37.2
    malaria NEC P37.4
      falciparum P37.3
    Plasmodium falciparum P37.3
    poliomyelitis P35.8
    rubella P35.0
    skin P39.4
    toxoplasmosis (acute) (subacute) (chronic) P37.1
    tuberculosis P37.0
    urinary (tract) P39.3
    vaccinia P35.8
    virus P35.9
      specified type NEC P35.8
  Conidiobolus B46.8
  coronavirus NEC B34.2
    as cause of disease classified elsewhere B97.29
    severe acute respiratory syndrome (SARS associat-ed) B97.21
  corpus luteum — *see* Salpingo-oophoritis

Infection, infected, infective — *continued*
  Corynebacterium diphtheriae — *see* Diphtheria
  cotia virus B08.8
  Coxiella burnetii A78
  coxsackie — *see* Coxsackie
  Cryptococcus neoformans — *see* Cryptococcosis
  Cryptosporidium A07.2
  Cunninghamella — *see* Mucormycosis
  cyst — *see* Cyst
  cystic duct (*see also* Cholecystitis) K81.9
  Cysticercus cellulosae — *see* Cysticercosis
  cytomegalovirus, cytomegaloviral B25.9
    congenital P35.1
    maternal, maternal care for (suspected) damage to fetus O35.3 ☑
    mononucleosis B27.10
      with
        complication NEC B27.19
        meningitis B27.12
        polyneuropathy B27.11
  delta-agent (acute), in hepatitis B carrier B17.0
  dental (pulpal origin) K04.7
  Deuteromycetes B47.0
  Dicrocoelium dendriticum B66.2
  Dipetalonema (perstans) (streptocerca) B74.4
  diphtherial — *see* Diphtheria
  Diphyllobothrium (adult) (latum) (pacificum) B70.0
    larval B70.1
  Diplogonoporus (grandis) B71.8
  Dipylidium caninum B67.4
  Dirofilaria B74.8
  Dracunculus medinensis B72
  Drechslera (hawaiiensis) B43.8
  Ducrey Haemophilus (any location) A57
  due to or resulting from
    artificial insemination N98.0
    central venous catheter T80.219 ☑
      bloodstream T80.211 ☑
      exit or insertion site T80.212 ☑
      localized T80.212 ☑
      port or reservoir T80.212 ☑
      specified NEC T80.218 ☑
      tunnel T80.212 ☑
    device, implant or graft (*see also* Complications, by site and type, infection or inflammation) T85.79 ☑
      arterial graft NEC T82.7 ☑
      breast (implant) T85.79 ☑
      catheter NEC T85.79 ☑
        dialysis (renal) T82.7 ☑
          intraperitoneal T85.71 ☑
        infusion NEC T82.7 ☑
          spinal (epidural) (subdural) T85.79 ☑
        urinary (indwelling) T83.51 ☑
      electronic (electrode) (pulse generator) (stimulator)
        bone T84.7 ☑
        cardiac T82.7 ☑
        nervous system (brain) (peripheral nerve) (spinal) T85.79 ☑
        urinary T83.59 ☑
      fixation, internal (orthopedic) NEC — *see* Complication, fixation device, infection
      gastrointestinal (bile duct) (esophagus) T85.79 ☑
      genital NEC T83.6 ☑
      heart NEC T82.7 ☑
        valve (prosthesis) T82.6 ☑
          graft T82.7 ☑
      joint prosthesis — *see* Complication, joint prosthesis, infection
      ocular (corneal graft) (orbital implant) NEC T85.79 ☑
      orthopedic NEC T84.7 ☑
      specified NEC T85.79 ☑
      urinary NEC T83.59 ☑
      vascular NEC T82.7 ☑
      ventricular intracranial shunt T85.79 ☑
    Hickman catheter T80.219 ☑
      bloodstream T80.211 ☑
      localized T80.212 ☑
      specified NEC T80.218 ☑
    immunization or vaccination T88.0 ☑
    infusion, injection or transfusion NEC T80.29 ☑
    injury NEC — *code by* site under Wound, open

Infection, infected, infective — *continued*
  due to or resulting from — *continued*
    peripherally inserted central catheter (PICC) T80.219 ☑
      bloodstream T80.211 ☑
      localized T80.212 ☑
      specified NEC T80.218 ☑
    portacath (port-a-cath) T80.219 ☑
      bloodstream T80.211 ☑
      localized T80.212 ☑
      specified NEC T80.218 ☑
    surgery T81.4 ☑
    triple lumen catheter T80.219 ☑
      bloodstream T80.211 ☑
      localized T80.212 ☑
      specified NEC T80.218 ☑
    umbilical venous catheter T80.219 ☑
      bloodstream T80.211 ☑
      localized T80.212 ☑
      specified NEC T80.218 ☑
  during labor NEC O75.3
  ear (middle) (*see also* Otitis media)
    external — *see* Otitis, externa, infective
    inner — *see* subcategory H83.0 ☑
  Eberthella typhosa A01.00
  Echinococcus — *see* Echinococcus
  echovirus
    as cause of disease classified elsewhere B97.12
    unspecified nature or site B34.1
  endocardium I33.0
  endocervix — *see* Cervicitis
  Entamoeba — *see* Amebiasis
  enteric — *see* Enteritis, infectious
  Enterobacter sakazakii B96.89
  Enterobius vermicularis B80
  enterostomy K94.12
  enterovirus B34.1
    as cause of disease classified elsewhere B97.10
      coxsackievirus B97.11
      echovirus B97.12
      specified NEC B97.19
  Entomophthora B46.8
  Epidermophyton — *see* Dermatophytosis
  epididymis — *see* Epididymitis
  episiotomy (puerperal) O86.0
  Erysipelothrix (insidiosa) (rhusiopathiae) — *see* Erysipeloid
  erythema infectiosum B08.3
  Escherichia (E.) coli NEC A49.8
    as cause of disease classified elsewhere (*see also* Escherichia coli) B96.20
    congenital P39.8
      sepsis P36.4
    generalized A41.51
    intestinal — *see* Enteritis, infectious, due to, Escherichia coli
  ethmoidal (chronic) (sinus) — *see* Sinusitis, ethmoidal
  eustachian tube (ear) — *see* Salpingitis, eustachian
  external auditory canal (meatus) NEC — *see* Otitis, externa, infective
  eye (purulent) — *see* Endophthalmitis, purulent
  eyelid — *see* Inflammation, eyelid
  fallopian tube — *see* Salpingo-oophoritis
  Fasciola (gigantica) (hepatica) (indica) B66.3
  Fasciolopsis (buski) B66.5
  filarial — *see* Infestation, filarial
  finger (skin) L08.9
    nail L03.01- ☑
      fungus B35.1
  fish tapeworm B70.0
    larval B70.1
  flagellate, intestinal A07.9
  fluke — *see* Infestation, fluke
  focal
    teeth (pulpal origin) K04.7
    tonsils J35.01
  Fonsecaea (compactum) (pedrosoi) B43.0
  food — *see* Intoxication, foodborne
  foot (skin) L08.9
    dermatophytic fungus B35.3
  Francisella tularensis — *see* Tularemia
  frontal (sinus) (chronic) — *see* Sinusitis, frontal
  fungus NOS B49
    beard B35.0
    dermatophytic — *see* Dermatophytosis
    foot B35.3
    groin B35.6

Index

Infection, infected, infective — Infection, infected, infective

Infection, infected, infective

Infection, infected, infective — *continued*
fungus — *continued*
  hand B35.2
  nail B35.1
  pathogenic to compromised host only B48.8
  perianal (area) B35.6
  scalp B35.0
  skin B36.9
    foot B35.3
    hand B35.2
    toenails B35.1
  Fusarium B48.8
gallbladder — *see* Cholecystitis
gas bacillus — *see* Gangrene, gas
gastrointestinal — *see* Enteritis, infectious
generalized NEC — *see* Sepsis
genital organ or tract
  female — *see* Disease, pelvis, inflammatory
  male N49.9
    multiple sites N49.8
    specified NEC N49.8
Ghon tubercle, primary A15.7
Giardia lamblia A07.1
gingiva (chronic) K05.10
  acute K05.00
    nonplaque induced K05.01
    plaque induced K05.00
  nonplaque induced K05.11
  plaque induced K05.10
glanders A24.0
glenosporopsis B48.0
Gnathostoma (spinigerum) B83.1
Gongylonema B83.8
gonococcal — *see* Gonococcus
gram-negative bacilli NOS A49.9
guinea worm B72
gum (chronic) K05.10
  acute K05.00
    nonplaque induced K05.01
    plaque induced K05.00
  nonplaque induced K05.11
  plaque induced K05.10
Haemophilus — *see* Infection, Hemophilus
heart — *see* Carditis
Helicobacter pylori A04.8
  as cause of disease classified elsewhere B96.81
helminths B83.9
  intestinal B82.0
    mixed (types classifiable to more than one of
      the titles B65.0-B81.3 and B81.8) B81.4
    specified type NEC B81.8
  specified type NEC B83.8
Hemophilus
  aegyptius, systemic A48.4
  ducrey (any location) A57
  generalized A41.3
  influenzae NEC A49.2
    as cause of disease classified elsewhere B96.3
herpes (simplex) (*see also* Herpes)
  congenital P35.2
  disseminated B00.7
  zoster B02.9
herpesvirus, herpesviral — *see* Herpes
Heterophyes (heterophyes) B66.8
hip (joint) NEC M00.9
  due to internal joint prosthesis
    left T84.52 ☑
    right T84.51 ☑
  skin NEC L08.9
Histoplasma — *see* Histoplasmosis
  American B39.4
  capsulatum B39.4
hookworm B76.9
human
  papilloma virus A63.0
  T-cell lymphotropic virus type-1 (HTLV-1) B33.3
hydrocele N43.0
Hymenolepis B71.0
hypopharynx — *see* Pharyngitis
inguinal (lymph) glands L04.1
  due to soft chancre A57
intervertebral disc, pyogenic M46.30
  cervical region M46.32
  cervicothoracic region M46.33
  lumbar region M46.36
  lumbosacral region M46.37
  multiple sites M46.39
  occipito-atlanto-axial region M46.31

Infection, infected, infective — *continued*
intervertebral disc, pyogenic — *continued*
  sacrococcygeal region M46.38
  thoracic region M46.34
  thoracolumbar region M46.35
intestine, intestinal — *see* Enteritis, infectious
  specified NEC A08.8
intra-amniotic affecting newborn NEC P39.2
Isospora belli or hominis A07.3
Japanese B encephalitis A83.0
jaw (bone) (lower) (upper) M27.2
joint NEC M00.9
  due to internal joint prosthesis T84.50 ☑
kidney (cortex) (hematogenous) N15.9
  with calculus N20.0
    with hydronephrosis N13.6
  following ectopic gestation O08.83
  pelvis and ureter (cystic) N28.85
  puerperal (postpartum) O86.21
  specified NEC N15.8
Klebsiella (K.) pneumoniae NEC A49.8
  as cause of disease classified elsewhere B96.1
knee (joint) NEC M00.9
  due to internal joint prosthesis
    left T84.54 ☑
    right T84.53 ☑
  joint M00.9
  skin L08.9
Koch's — *see* Tuberculosis
labia (majora) (minora) (acute) — *see* Vulvitis
lacrimal
  gland — *see* Dacryoadenitis
  passages (duct) (sac) — *see* Inflammation, lacrimal,
    passages
lancet fluke B66.2
larynx NEC J38.7
leg (skin) NOS L08.9
Legionella pneumophila A48.1
  nonpneumonic A48.2
Leishmania (*see also* Leishmaniasis)
  aethiopica B55.1
  braziliensis B55.2
  chagasi B55.0
  donovani B55.0
  infantum B55.0
  major B55.1
  mexicana B55.1
  tropica B55.1
lentivirus, as cause of disease classified elsewhere
  B97.31
Leptosphaeria senegalensis B47.0
Leptospira interrogans A27.9
  autumnalis A27.89
  canicola A27.89
  hebdomadis A27.89
  icterohaemorrhagiae A27.0
  pomona A27.89
  specified type NEC A27.89
leptospirochetal NEC — *see* Leptospirosis
Listeria monocytogenes (*see also* Listeriosis)
  congenital P37.2
Loa loa B74.3
  with conjunctival infestation B74.3
  eyelid B74.3
Loboa loboi B48.0
local, skin (staphylococcal) (streptococcal) L08.9
  abscess — *code by* site under Abscess
  cellulitis — *code by* site under Cellulitis
  specified NEC L08.89
  ulcer — *see* Ulcer, skin
Loefflerella mallei A24.0
lung (*see also* Pneumonia) J18.9
  atypical Mycobacterium A31.0
  spirochetal A69.8
  tuberculous — *see* Tuberculosis, pulmonary
  virus — *see* Pneumonia, viral
lymph gland (*see also* Lymphadenitis, acute)
  mesenteric I88.0
lymphoid tissue, base of tongue or posterior pharynx,
  NEC (chronic) J35.03
Madurella (grisea) (mycetomii) B47.0
major
  following ectopic or molar pregnancy O08.0
  puerperal, postpartum, childbirth O85
Malassezia furfur B36.0
Malleomyces
  mallei A24.0
  pseudomallei (whitmori) — *see* Melioidosis

Infection, infected, infective — *continued*
mammary gland N61
Mansonella (ozzardi) (perstans) (streptocerca) B74.4
mastoid — *see* Mastoiditis
maxilla, maxillary M27.2
  sinus (chronic) — *see* Sinusitis, maxillary
mediastinum J98.5
Medina (worm) B72
meibomian cyst or gland — *see* Hordeolum
meninges — *see* Meningitis, bacterial
meningococcal (*see also* condition) A39.9
  adrenals A39.1
  brain A39.81
  cerebrospinal A39.0
  conjunctiva A39.89
  endocardium A39.51
  heart A39.50
    endocardium A39.51
    myocardium A39.52
    pericardium A39.53
  joint A39.83
  meninges A39.0
  meningococcemia A39.4
    acute A39.2
    chronic A39.3
  myocardium A39.52
  pericardium A39.53
  retrobulbar neuritis A39.82
  specified site NEC A39.89
mesenteric lymph nodes or glands NEC I88.0
Metagonimus B66.8
metatarsophalangeal M00.9
methicillin
  resistant Staphylococcus aureus (MRSA) A49.02
  susceptible Staphylococcus aureus (MSSA) A49.01
Microsporum, microsporic — *see* Dermatophytosis
mixed flora (bacterial) NEC A49.8
Monilia — *see* Candidiasis
Monosporium apiospermum B48.2
mouth, parasitic B37.0
Mucor — *see* Mucormycosis
muscle NEC — *see* Myositis, infective
mycelium NOS B49
mycetoma B47.9
  actinomycotic NEC B47.1
  mycotic NEC B47.0
Mycobacterium, mycobacterial — *see* Mycobacterium
Mycoplasma NEC A49.3
  pneumoniae, as cause of disease classified else-
    where B96.0
mycotic NOS B49
  pathogenic to compromised host only B48.8
  skin NOS B36.9
myocardium NEC I40.0
nail (chronic)
  with lymphangitis — *see* Lymphangitis, acute,
    digit
  finger L03.01- ☑
    fungus B35.1
  ingrowing L60.0
  toe L03.03- ☑
    fungus B35.1
nasal sinus (chronic) — *see* Sinusitis
nasopharynx — *see* Nasopharyngitis
navel L08.82
Necator americanus B76.1
Neisseria — *see* Gonococcus
Neotestudina rosatii B47.0
newborn P39.9
  intra-amniotic NEC P39.2
  skin P39.4
  specified type NEC P39.8
nipple N61
  associated with
    lactation O91.03
    pregnancy O91.01- ☑
    puerperium O91.02
Nocardia — *see* Nocardiosis
obstetrical surgical wound (puerperal) O86.0
Oesophagostomum (apiostomum) B81.8
Oestrus ovis — *see* Myiasis
Oidium albicans B37.9
Onchocerca (volvulus) — *see* Onchocerciasis
oncovirus, as cause of disease classified elsewhere
  B97.32
operation wound T81.4 ☑
Opisthorchis (felineus) (viverrini) B66.0
orbit, orbital — *see* Inflammation, orbit

☑ Additional Character Required — Refer to the Tabular List for Character Selection   🖑 Subterms under main terms may continue to next column or page

Infection, infected, infective — *continued*
  orthopoxvirus NEC B08.09
  ovary — *see* Salpingo-oophoritis
  Oxyuris vermicularis B80
  pancreas (acute) K85.9
    abscess — *see* Pancreatitis, acute
    specified NEC K85.8
  papillomavirus, as cause of disease classified elsewhere
      B97.7
  papovavirus NEC B34.4
  Paracoccidioides brasiliensis — *see* Paracoccidioidomy-
      cosis
  Paragonimus (westermani) B66.4
  parainfluenza virus B34.8
  parameningococcus NOS A39.9
  parapoxvirus B08.60
    specified NEC B08.69
  parasitic B89
  Parastrongylus
    cantonensis B83.2
    costaricensis B81.3
    paratyphoid A01.4
      Type A A01.1
      Type B A01.2
      Type C A01.3
  paraurethral ducts N34.2
  parotid gland — *see* Sialoadenitis
  parvovirus NEC B34.3
    as cause of disease classified elsewhere B97.6
  Pasteurella NEC A28.0
    multocida A28.0
    pestis — *see* Plague
    pseudotuberculosis A28.0
    septica (cat bite) (dog bite) A28.0
    tularensis — *see* Tularemia
  pelvic, female — *see* Disease, pelvis, inflammatory
  Penicillium (marneffei) B48.4
  penis (glans) (retention) NEC N48.29
  periapical K04.5
  peridental, periodontal K05.20
    generalized K05.22
    localized K05.21
  perinatal period P39.9
    specified type NEC P39.8
  perineal repair (puerperal) O86.0
  periorbital — *see* Inflammation, orbit
  perirectal K62.89
  perirenal — *see* Infection, kidney
  peritoneal — *see* Peritonitis
  periureteral N28.89
  Petriellidium boydii B48.2
  pharynx (*see also* Pharyngitis)
    coxsackievirus B08.5
    posterior, lymphoid (chronic) J35.03
  Phialophora
    gougerotii (subcutaneous abscess or cyst) B43.2
    jeanselmei (subcutaneous abscess or cyst) B43.2
    verrucosa (skin) B43.0
  Piedraia hortae B36.3
  pinta A67.9
    intermediate A67.1
    late A67.2
    mixed A67.3
    primary A67.0
  pinworm B80
  pityrosporum furfur B36.0
  pleuro-pneumonia-like organism (PPLO) NEC A49.3
    as cause of disease classified elsewhere B96.0
  pneumococcus, pneumococcal NEC A49.1
    as cause of disease classified elsewhere B95.3
    generalized (purulent) A40.3
      with pneumonia J13
  Pneumocystis carinii (pneumonia) B59
  Pneumocystis jiroveci (pneumonia) B59
  port or reservoir T80.212 ☑
  postoperative T81.4 ☑
  postoperative wound T81.4 ☑
  postprocedural T81.4 ☑
  postvaccinal T88.0 ☑
  prepuce NEC N47.7
    with penile inflammation N47.6
  prion — *see* Disease, prion, central nervous system
  prostate (capsule) — *see* Prostatitis
  Proteus (mirabilis) (morganii) (vulgaris) NEC A49.8
    as cause of disease classified elsewhere B96.4
  protozoal NEC B64
    intestinal A07.9
      specified NEC A07.8

Infection, infected, infective — *continued*
  protozoal — *continued*
    specified NEC B60.8
  Pseudoallescheria boydii B48.2
  Pseudomonas NEC A49.8
    as cause of disease classified elsewhere B96.5
    mallei A24.0
    pneumonia J15.1
    pseudomallei — *see* Melioidosis
  puerperal O86.4
    genitourinary tract NEC O86.89
    major or generalized O85
    minor O86.4
    specified NEC O86.89
  pulmonary — *see* Infection, lung
  purulent — *see* Abscess
  Pyrenochaeta romeroi B47.0
  Q fever A78
  rectum (sphincter) K62.89
  renal (*see also* Infection, kidney)
    pelvis and ureter (cystic) N28.85
  reovirus, as cause of disease classified elsewhere B97.5
  respiratory (tract) NEC J98.8
    acute J22
    chronic J98.8
    influenzal (upper) (acute) — *see* Influenza, with,
        respiratory manifestations NEC
    lower (acute) J22
      chronic — *see* Bronchitis, chronic
    rhinovirus J00
    syncytial virus, as cause of disease classified else-
        where B97.4
    upper (acute) NOS J06.9
      chronic J39.8
      streptococcal J06.9
      viral NOS J06.9
  resulting from
    presence of internal prosthesis, implant, graft —
        see Complications, by site and type, infection
  retortamoniasis A07.8
  retroperitoneal NEC K68.9
  retrovirus B33.3
    as cause of disease classified elsewhere B97.30
      human
        immunodeficiency, type 2 (HIV 2) B97.35
        T-cell lymphotropic
          type I (HTLV-I) B97.33
          type II (HTLV-II) B97.34
      lentivirus B97.31
      oncovirus B97.32
      specified NEC B97.39
  Rhinosporidium (seeberi) B48.1
  rhinovirus
    as cause of disease classified elsewhere B97.89
    unspecified nature or site B34.8
  Rhizopus — *see* Mucormycosis
  rickettsial NOS A79.9
  roundworm (large) NEC B82.0
    Ascariasis (*see also* Ascariasis) B77.9
  rubella — *see* Rubella
  Saccharomyces — *see* Candidiasis
  salivary duct or gland (any) — *see* Sialoadenitis
  Salmonella (aertrycke) (arizonae) (callinarum)
      (cholerae-suis) (enteritidis) (suipestifer) (ty-
      phimurium) A02.9
    with
      (gastro)enteritis A02.0
      sepsis A02.1
      specified manifestation NEC A02.8
    due to food (poisoning) A02.9
    hirschfeldii A01.3
    localized A02.20
      arthritis A02.23
      meningitis A02.21
      osteomyelitis A02.24
      pneumonia A02.22
      pyelonephritis A02.25
      specified NEC A02.29
    paratyphi A01.4
      A A01.1
      B A01.2
      C A01.3
    schottmuelleri A01.2
    typhi, typhosa — *see* Typhoid
  Sarcocystis A07.8
  scabies B86
  Schistosoma — *see* Infestation, Schistosoma
  scrotum (acute) NEC N49.2

Infection, infected, infective — *continued*
  seminal vesicle — *see* Vesiculitis
  septic
    localized, skin — *see* Abscess
  sheep liver fluke B66.3
  Shigella A03.9
    boydii A03.2
    dysenteriae A03.0
    flexneri A03.1
    group
      A A03.0
      B A03.1
      C A03.2
      D A03.3
    Schmitz (-Stutzer) A03.0
    schmitzii A03.0
    shigae A03.0
    sonnei A03.3
    specified NEC A03.8
  shoulder (joint) NEC M00.9
    due to internal joint prosthesis T84.59 ☑
    skin NEC L08.9
  sinus (accessory) (chronic) (nasal) (*see also* Sinusitis)
    pilonidal — *see* Sinus, pilonidal
    skin NEC L08.89
  Skene's duct or gland — *see* Urethritis
  skin (local) (staphylococcal) (streptococcal) L08.9
    abscess — *code by* site under Abscess
    cellulitis — *code by* site under Cellulitis
    due to fungus B36.9
      specified type NEC B36.8
    mycotic B36.9
      specified type NEC B36.8
    newborn P39.4
    ulcer — *see* Ulcer, skin
  slow virus A81.9
    specified NEC A81.89
  Sparganum (mansoni) (proliferum) (baxteri) B70.1
  specific (*see also* Syphilis)
    to perinatal period — *see* Infection, congenital
  specified NEC B99.8
  spermatic cord NEC N49.1
  sphenoidal (sinus) — *see* Sinusitis, sphenoidal
  spinal cord NOS (*see also* Myelitis) G04.91
    abscess G06.1
    meninges — *see* Meningitis
    streptococcal G04.89
  Spirillum A25.0
  spirochetal NOS A69.9
    lung A69.8
    specified NEC A69.8
  Spirometra larvae B70.1
  spleen D73.89
  Sporotrichum, Sporothrix (schenckii) — *see* Sporotri-
      chosis
  staphylococcal, unspecified site
    as cause of disease classified elsewhere B95.8
      aureus (methicillin susceptible) (MSSA) B95.61
        methicillin resistant (MRSA) B95.62
      specified NEC B95.7
    aureus (methicillin susceptible) (MSSA) A49.01
      methicillin resistant (MRSA) A49.02
    food poisoning A05.0
    generalized (purulent) A41.2
    pneumonia — *see* Pneumonia, staphylococcal
  Stellantchasmus falcatus B66.8
  streptobacillus moniliformis A25.1
  streptococcal NEC A49.1
    as cause of disease classified elsewhere B95.5
    B genitourinary complicating
      childbirth O98.82
      pregnancy O98.81- ☑
      puerperium O98.83
    congenital
      sepsis P36.10
        group B P36.0
        specified NEC P36.19
    generalized (purulent) A40.9
  Streptomyces B47.1
  Strongyloides (stercoralis) — *see* Strongyloidiasis
  stump (amputation) (surgical) — *see* Complication,
      amputation stump, infection
  subcutaneous tissue, local L08.9
  suipestifer — *see* Infection, salmonella
  swimming pool bacillus A31.1
  Taenia — *see* Infestation, Taenia
  Taeniarhynchus saginatus B68.1
  tapeworm — *see* Infestation, tapeworm

Infection, infected, infective — *continued*
- tendon (sheath) — *see* Tenosynovitis, infective NEC
- Ternidens diminutus B81.8
- testis — *see* Orchitis
- threadworm B80
- throat — *see* Pharyngitis
- thyroglossal duct K14.8
- toe (skin) L08.9
  - cellulitis L03.03- ☑
    - fungus B35.1
  - nail L03.03- ☑
    - fungus B35.1
- tongue NEC K14.0
  - parasitic B37.0
- tonsil (and adenoid) (faucial) (lingual) (pharyngeal) — *see* Tonsillitis
- tooth, teeth K04.7
  - periapical K04.7
  - peridental, periodontal K05.20
    - generalized K05.22
    - localized K05.21
  - pulp K04.0
  - socket M27.3
- TORCH — *see* Infection, congenital
  - without active infection P00.2
- Torula histolytica — *see* Cryptococcosis
- Toxocara (canis) (cati) (felis) B83.0
- Toxoplasma gondii — *see* Toxoplasma
- trachea, chronic J42
- trematode NEC — *see* Infestation, fluke
- trench fever A79.0
- Treponema pallidum — *see* Syphilis
- Trichinella (spiralis) B75
- Trichomonas A59.9
  - cervix A59.09
  - intestine A07.8
  - prostate A59.02
  - specified site NEC A59.8
  - urethra A59.03
  - urogenitalis A59.00
  - vagina A59.01
  - vulva A59.01
- Trichophyton, trichophytic — *see* Dermatophytosis
- Trichosporon (beigelii) cutaneum B36.2
- Trichostrongylus B81.2
- Trichuris (trichiura) B79
- Trombicula (irritans) B88.0
- Trypanosoma
  - brucei
    - gambiense B56.0
    - rhodesiense B56.1
  - cruzi — *see* Chagas' disease
- tubal — *see* Salpingo-oophoritis
- tuberculous NEC — *see* Tuberculosis
- tubo-ovarian — *see* Salpingo-oophoritis
- tunica vaginalis N49.1
- tunnel T80.212 ☑
- tympanic membrane NEC — *see* Myringitis
- typhoid (abortive) (ambulant) (bacillus) — *see* Typhoid
- typhus A75.9
  - flea-borne A75.2
  - mite-borne A75.3
  - recrudescent A75.1
  - tick-borne A77.9
    - African A77.1
    - North Asian A77.2
- umbilicus L08.82
- ureter N28.86
- urethra — *see* Urethritis
- urinary (tract) N39.0
  - bladder — *see* Cystitis
  - complicating
    - pregnancy O23.4- ☑
      - specified type NEC O23.3- ☑
  - kidney — *see* Infection, kidney
  - newborn P39.3
  - puerperal (postpartum) O86.20
  - tuberculous A18.13
  - urethra — *see* Urethritis
- uterus, uterine — *see* Endometritis
- vaccination T88.0 ☑
- vaccinia not from vaccination B08.011
- vagina (acute) — *see* Vaginitis
- varicella B01.9
- varicose veins — *see* Varix
- vas deferens NEC N49.1
- vesical — *see* Cystitis

Infection, infected, infective — *continued*
- Vibrio
  - cholerae A00.0
    - El Tor A00.1
  - parahaemolyticus (food poisoning) A05.3
  - vulnificus
    - as cause of disease classified elsewhere B96.82
    - foodborne intoxication A05.5
- Vincent's (gum) (mouth) (tonsil) A69.1
- virus, viral NOS B34.9
  - adenovirus
    - as cause of disease classified elsewhere B97.0
    - unspecified nature or site B34.0
  - arborvirus, arbovirus arthropod-borne A94
  - as cause of disease classified elsewhere B97.89
    - adenovirus B97.0
    - coronavirus B97.29
      - SARS-associated B97.21
    - coxsackievirus B97.11
    - echovirus B97.12
    - enterovirus B97.10
      - coxsackievirus B97.11
      - echovirus B97.12
      - specified NEC B97.19
    - human
      - immunodeficiency, type 2 (HIV 2) B97.35
      - metapneumovirus B97.81
      - T-cell lymphotropic,
        - type I (HTLV-I) B97.33
        - type II (HTLV-II) B97.34
    - papillomavirus B97.7
    - parvovirus B97.6
    - reovirus B97.5
    - respiratory syncytial B97.4
    - retrovirus B97.30
      - human
        - immunodeficiency, type 2 (HIV 2) B97.35
        - T-cell lymphotropic,
          - type I (HTLV-I) B97.33
          - type II (HTLV-II) B97.34
      - lentivirus B97.31
      - oncovirus B97.32
      - specified NEC B97.39
    - specified NEC B97.89
  - central nervous system A89
    - atypical A81.9
      - specified NEC A81.89
    - enterovirus NEC A88.8
      - meningitis A87.0
    - slow virus A81.9
      - specified NEC A81.89
    - specified NEC A88.8
  - chest J98.8
  - cotia B08.8
  - coxsackie (*see also* Infection, coxsackie) B34.1
    - as cause of disease classified elsewhere B97.11
  - ECHO
    - as cause of disease classified elsewhere B97.12
    - unspecified nature or site B34.1
  - encephalitis, tick-borne A84.9
  - enterovirus, as cause of disease classified elsewhere B97.10
    - coxsackievirus B97.11
    - echovirus B97.12
    - specified NEC B97.19
  - exanthem NOS B09
  - human metapneumovirus as cause of disease classified elsewhere B97.81
  - human papilloma as cause of disease classified elsewhere B97.7
  - intestine — *see* Enteritis, viral
  - respiratory syncytial
    - as cause of disease classified elsewhere B97.4
    - bronchopneumonia J12.1
    - common cold syndrome J00
    - nasopharyngitis (acute) J00
  - rhinovirus
    - as cause of disease classified elsewhere B97.89
    - unspecified nature or site B34.8
  - slow A81.9
    - specified NEC A81.89
  - specified type NEC B33.8
    - as cause of disease classified elsewhere B97.89
    - unspecified nature or site B34.8
  - unspecified nature or site B34.9
  - West Nile — *see* Virus, West Nile
- vulva (acute) — *see* Vulvitis
- West Nile — *see* Virus, West Nile

Infection, infected, infective — *continued*
- whipworm B79
- worms B83.9
  - specified type NEC B83.8
- Wuchereria (bancrofti) B74.0
  - malayi B74.1
- yatapoxvirus B08.70
  - specified NEC B08.79
- yeast (*see also* Candidiasis) B37.9
- yellow fever — *see* Fever, yellow
- Yersinia
  - enterocolitica (intestinal) A04.6
  - pestis — *see* Plague
  - pseudotuberculosis A28.2
- Zeis' gland — *see* Hordeolum
- zoonotic bacterial NOS A28.9
- Zopfia senegalensis B47.0

Infective, infectious — *see* condition

Infertility
- female N97.9
  - age-related N97.8
  - associated with
    - anovulation N97.0
    - cervical (mucus) disease or anomaly N88.3
    - congenital anomaly
      - cervix N88.3
      - fallopian tube N97.1
      - uterus N97.2
      - vagina N97.8
    - dysmucorrhea N88.3
    - fallopian tube disease or anomaly N97.1
    - pituitary-hypothalamic origin E23.0
    - specified origin NEC N97.8
    - Stein-Leventhal syndrome E28.2
    - uterine disease or anomaly N97.2
    - vaginal disease or anomaly N97.8
  - due to
    - cervical anomaly N88.3
    - fallopian tube anomaly N97.1
    - ovarian failure E28.39
    - Stein-Leventhal syndrome E28.2
    - uterine anomaly N97.2
    - vaginal anomaly N97.8
  - nonimplantation N97.2
  - origin
    - cervical N88.3
    - tubal (block) (occlusion) (stenosis) N97.1
    - uterine N97.2
    - vaginal N97.8
- male N46.9
  - azoospermia N46.01
    - extratesticular cause N46.029
      - drug therapy N46.021
      - efferent duct obstruction N46.023
      - infection N46.022
      - radiation N46.024
      - specified cause NEC N46.029
      - systemic disease N46.025
  - oligospermia N46.11
    - extratesticular cause N46.129
      - drug therapy N46.121
      - efferent duct obstruction N46.123
      - infection N46.122
      - radiation N46.124
      - specified cause NEC N46.129
      - systemic disease N46.125
  - specified type NEC N46.8

Infestation B88.9
- Acanthocheilonema (perstans) (streptocerca) B74.4
- Acariasis B88.0
  - demodex folliculorum B88.0
  - sarcoptes scabiei B86
  - trombiculae B88.0
- Agamofilaria streptocerca B74.4
- Ancylostoma, ankylostoma (braziliense) (caninum) (ceylanicum) (duodenale) B76.0
  - americanum B76.1
  - new world B76.1
- Anisakis larvae, anisakiasis B81.0
- arthropod NEC B88.2
- Ascaris lumbricoides — *see* Ascariasis
- Balantidium coli A07.0
- beef tapeworm B68.1
- Bothriocephalus (latus) B70.0
  - larval B70.1
- broad tapeworm B70.0
  - larval B70.1
- Brugia (malayi) B74.1

Infestation — *continued*
- Brugia (malayi) B74.1
  - timori B74.2
- candiru B88.8
- Capillaria
  - hepatica B83.8
  - philippinensis B81.1
- cat liver fluke B66.0
- cestodes B71.9
  - diphyllobothrium — *see* Infestation, diphyllobothrium
  - dipylidiasis B71.1
  - hymenolepiasis B71.0
  - specified type NEC B71.8
- chigger B88.0
- chigo, chigoe B88.1
- Clonorchis (sinensis) (liver) B66.1
- coccidial A07.3
- crab-lice B85.3
- Cysticercus cellulosae — *see* Cysticercosis
- Demodex (folliculorum) B88.0
- Dermanyssus gallinae B88.0
- Dermatobia (hominis) — *see* Myiasis
- Dibothriocephalus (latus) B70.0
  - larval B70.1
- Dicrocoelium dendriticum B66.2
- Diphyllobothrium (adult) (latum) (intestinal) (pacificum) B70.0
  - larval B70.1
- Diplogonoporus (grandis) B71.8
- Dipylidium caninum B67.4
- Distoma hepaticum B66.3
- dog tapeworm B67.4
- Dracunculus medinensis B72
- dragon worm B72
- dwarf tapeworm B71.0
- Echinococcus — *see* Echinococcus
- Echinostomum ilocanum B66.8
- Entamoeba (histolytica) — *see* Infection, Ameba
- Enterobius vermicularis B80
- eyelid
  - in (due to)
    - leishmaniasis B55.1
    - loiasis B74.3
    - onchocerciasis B73.09
    - phthiriasis B85.3
    - parasitic NOS B89
- eyeworm B74.3
- Fasciola (gigantica) (hepatica) (indica) B66.3
- Fasciolopsis (buski) (intestine) B66.5
- filarial B74.9
  - bancroftian B74.0
  - conjunctiva B74.9
  - due to
    - Acanthocheilonema (perstans) (streptocerca) B74.4
    - Brugia (malayi) B74.1
      - timori B74.2
    - Dracunculus medinensis B72
    - guinea worm B72
    - loa loa B74.3
    - Mansonella (ozzardi) (perstans) (streptocerca) B74.4
    - Onchocerca volvulus B73.00
      - eye B73.00
      - eyelid B73.09
    - Wuchereria (bancrofti) B74.0
  - Malayan B74.1
  - ozzardi B74.4
  - specified type NEC B74.8
- fish tapeworm B70.0
  - larval B70.1
- fluke B66.9
  - blood NOS — *see* Schistosomiasis
  - cat liver B66.0
  - intestinal B66.5
  - lancet B66.2
  - liver (sheep) B66.3
    - cat B66.0
    - Chinese B66.1
    - due to clonorchiasis B66.1
    - oriental B66.1
  - lung (oriental) B66.4
  - sheep liver B66.3
  - specified type NEC B66.8
- fly larvae — *see* Myiasis
- Gastrophilus (intestinalis) *see* Myiasis
- Gastrodiscoides hominis B66.8

Infestation — *continued*
- Giardia lamblia A07.1
- Gnathostoma (spinigerum) B83.1
- Gongylonema B83.8
- guinea worm B72
- helminth B83.9
  - angiostrongyliasis B83.2
    - intestinal B81.3
  - gnathostomiasis B83.1
  - hirudiniasis, internal B83.4
  - intestinal B82.0
    - angiostrongyliasis B81.3
    - anisakiasis B81.0
    - ascariasis — *see* Ascariasis
    - capillariasis B81.1
    - cysticercosis — *see* Cysticercosis
    - diphyllobothriasis — *see* Infestation, diphyllobothriasis
    - dracunculiasis B72
    - echinococcus — *see* Echinococcosis
    - enterobiasis B80
    - filariasis — *see* Infestation, filarial
    - fluke — *see* Infestation, fluke
    - hookworm — *see* Infestation, hookworm
    - mixed (types classifiable to more than one of the titles B65.0-B81.3 and B81.8) B81.4
    - onchocerciasis — *see* Onchocerciasis
    - schistosomiasis — *see* Infestation, schistosoma
    - specified
      - cestode NEC — *see* Infestation, cestode type NEC B81.8
    - strongyloidiasis — *see* Strongyloidiasis
    - taenia — *see* Infestation, taenia
    - trichinellosis B75
    - trichostrongyliasis B81.2
    - trichuriasis B79
  - specified type NEC B83.8
  - syngamiasis B83.3
  - visceral larva migrans B83.0
- Heterophyes (heterophyes) B66.8
- hookworm B76.9
  - ancylostomiasis B76.0
  - necatoriasis B76.1
  - specified type NEC B76.8
- Hymenolepis (diminuta) (nana) B71.0
- intestinal NEC B82.9
- leeches (aquatic) (land) — *see* Hirudiniasis
- Leishmania — *see* Leishmaniasis
- lice, louse — *see* Infestation, Pediculus
- Linguatula B88.8
- Liponyssoides sanguineus B88.0
- Loa loa B74.3
  - conjunctival B74.3
  - eyelid B74.3
- louse — *see* Infestation, Pediculus
- maggots — *see* Myiasis
- Mansonella (ozzardi) (perstans) (streptocerca) B74.4
- Medina (worm) B72
- Metagonimus (yokogawai) B66.8
- microfilaria streptocerca — *see* Onchocerciasis
  - eye B73.00
  - eyelid B73.09
- mites B88.9
  - scabic B86
- Monilia (albicans) — *see* Candidiasis
- mouth B37.0
- Necator americanus B76.1
- nematode NEC (intestinal) B82.0
  - Ancylostoma B76.0
  - conjunctiva NEC B83.9
  - Enterobius vermicularis B80
  - Gnathostoma spinigerum B83.1
  - physaloptera B80
  - specified NEC B81.8
  - trichostrongylus B81.2
  - trichuris (trichuria) B79
- Oesophagostomum (apiostomum) B81.8
- Oestrus ovis (*see also* Myiasis) B87.9
- Onchocerca (volvulus) — *see* Onchocerciasis
- Opisthorchis (felineus) (viverrini) B66.0
- orbit, parasitic NOS B89
- Oxyuris vermicularis B80
- Paragonimus (westermani) B66.4
- parasite, parasitic B89
  - eyelid B89
  - intestinal NOS B82.9
  - mouth B37.0
  - skin B88.9

Infestation — *continued*
- parasite, parasitic — *continued*
  - tongue B37.0
- Parastrongylus
  - cantonensis B83.2
  - costaricensis B81.3
- Pediculus B85.2
  - body B85.1
  - capitis (humanus) (any site) B85.0
  - corporis (humanus) (any site) B85.1
  - head B85.0
  - mixed (classifiable to more than one of the titles B85.0 - B85.3) B85.4
  - pubis (any site) B85.3
- Pentastoma B88.8
- Phthirus (pubis) (any site) B85.3
  - with any infestation classifiable to B85.0 - B85.2 B85.4
- pinworm B80
- pork tapeworm (adult) B68.0
- protozoal NEC B64
  - intestinal A07.9
    - specified NEC A07.8
  - specified NEC B60.8
- pubic, louse B85.3
- rat tapeworm B71.0
- red bug B88.0
- roundworm (large) NEC B82.0
  - Ascariasis (*see also* Ascariasis) B77.9
- sandflea B88.1
- Sarcoptes scabiei B86
- scabies B86
- Schistosoma B65.9
  - bovis B65.8
  - cercariae B65.3
  - haematobium B65.0
  - intercalatum B65.8
  - japonicum B65.2
  - mansoni B65.1
  - mattheei B65.8
  - mekongi B65.8
  - specified type NEC B65.8
  - spindale B65.8
- screw worms — *see* Myiasis
- skin NOS B88.9
- Sparganum (mansoni) (proliferum) (baxteri) B70.1
  - larval B70.1
- specified type NEC B88.8
- Spirometra larvae B70.1
- Stellantchasmus falcatus B66.8
- Strongyloides stercoralis — *see* Strongyloidiasis
- Taenia B68.9
  - diminuta B71.0
  - echinococcus — *see* Echinococcus
  - mediocanellata B68.1
  - nana B71.0
  - saginata B68.1
  - solium (intestinal form) B68.0
    - larval form — *see* Cysticercosis
- Taeniarhynchus saginatus B68.1
- tapeworm B71.9
  - beef B68.1
  - broad B70.0
    - larval B70.1
  - dog B67.4
  - dwarf B71.0
  - fish B70.0
    - larval B70.1
  - pork B68.0
  - rat B71.0
- Ternidens diminutus B81.8
- Tetranychus molestissimus B88.0
- threadworm B80
- tongue B37.0
- Toxocara (canis) (cati) (felis) B83.0
- trematode(s) NEC — *see* Infestation, fluke
- Trichinella (spiralis) B75
- Trichocephalus B79
- Trichomonas — *see* Trichomoniasis
- Trichostrongylus B81.2
- Trichuris (trichiura) B79
- Trombicula (irritans) B88.0
- Tunga penetrans B88.1
- Uncinaria americana B76.1
- Vandellia cirrhosa B88.8
- whipworm B79
- worms B83.9
  - intestinal B82.0

▽ Subterms under main terms may continue to next column or page   ☑ Additional Character Required — Refer to the Tabular List for Character Selection   **181**

Infestation — *continued*
  Wuchereria (bancrofti) B74.0
Infiltrate, infiltration
  amyloid (generalized) (localized) — *see* Amyloidosis
  calcareous NEC R89.7
    localized — *see* Degeneration, by site
  calcium salt R89.7
  cardiac
    fatty — *see* Degeneration, myocardial
    glycogenic E74.02 [I43]
  corneal — *see* Edema, cornea
  eyelid — *see* Inflammation, eyelid
  glycogen, glycogenic — *see* Disease, glycogen storage
  heart, cardiac
    fatty — *see* Degeneration, myocardial
    glycogenic E74.02 [I43]
  inflammatory in vitreous H43.89
  kidney N28.89
  leukemic — *see* Leukemia
  liver K76.89
    fatty — *see* Fatty, liver NEC
    glycogen (*see also* Disease, glycogen storage)
      E74.03 [K77]
  lung R91.8
    eosinophilic J82
  lymphatic (*see also* Leukemia, lymphatic) C91.9- ☑
    gland I88.9
  muscle, fatty M62.89
  myocardium, myocardial
    fatty — *see* Degeneration, myocardial
    glycogenic E74.02 [I43]
  on chest x-ray R91.8
  pulmonary R91.8
    with eosinophilia J82
  skin (lymphocytic) L98.6
  thymus (gland) (fatty) E32.8
  urine R39.0
  vesicant agent
    antineoplastic chemotherapy T80.810 ☑
    other agent NEC T80.818 ☑
  vitreous body H43.89
Infirmity R68.89
  senile R54
Inflammation, inflamed, inflammatory (with exudation)
  abducent (nerve) — *see* Strabismus, paralytic, sixth nerve
  accessory sinus (chronic) — *see* Sinusitis
  adrenal (gland) E27.8
  alveoli, teeth M27.3
    scorbutic E54
  anal canal, anus K62.89
  antrum (chronic) — *see* Sinusitis, maxillary
  appendix — *see* Appendicitis
  arachnoid — *see* Meningitis
  areola N61
    puerperal, postpartum or gestational — *see* Infection, nipple
  areolar tissue NOS L08.9
  artery — *see* Arteritis
  auditory meatus (external) — *see* Otitis, externa
  Bartholin's gland N75.8
  bile duct (common) (hepatic) or passage — *see* Cholangitis
  bladder — *see* Cystitis
  bone — *see* Osteomyelitis
  brain (*see also* Encephalitis)
    membrane — *see* Meningitis
  breast N61
    puerperal, postpartum, gestational — *see* Mastitis, obstetric
  broad ligament — *see* Disease, pelvis, inflammatory
  bronchi — *see* Bronchitis
  catarrhal J00
  cecum — *see* Appendicitis
  cerebral (*see also* Encephalitis)
    membrane — *see* Meningitis
  cerebrospinal
    meningococcal A39.0
  cervix (uteri) — *see* Cervicitis
  chest J98.8
  chorioretinal H30.9- ☑
    cyclitis — *see* Cyclitis
    disseminated H30.10- ☑
      generalized H30.13- ☑
      peripheral H30.12- ☑
      posterior pole H30.11- ☑

Inflammation, inflamed, inflammatory — *continued*
  chorioretinal — *continued*
    epitheliopathy — *see* Epitheliopathy
    focal H30.00- ☑
      juxtapapillary H30.01- ☑
      macular H30.04- ☑
      paramacular — *see* Inflammation, chorioretinal, focal, macular
      peripheral H30.03- ☑
      posterior pole H30.02- ☑
    specified type NEC H30.89- ☑
  choroid — *see* Inflammation, chorioretinal
  chronic, postmastoidectomy cavity — *see* Complications, postmastoidectomy, inflammation
  colon — *see* Enteritis
  connective tissue (diffuse) NEC — *see* Disorder, soft tissue, specified type NEC
  cornea — *see* Keratitis
  corpora cavernosa N48.29
  cranial nerve — *see* Disorder, nerve, cranial
  Douglas' cul-de-sac or pouch (chronic) N73.0
  due to device, implant or graft (*see also* Complications, by site and type, infection or inflammation)
    arterial graft T82.7 ☑
    breast (implant) T85.79 ☑
    catheter T85.79 ☑
      dialysis (renal) T82.7 ☑
        intraperitoneal T85.71 ☑
      infusion T82.7 ☑
        spinal (epidural) (subdural) T85.79 ☑
      urinary (indwelling) T83.51 ☑
    electronic (electrode) (pulse generator) (stimulator)
      bone T84.7 ☑
      cardiac T82.7 ☑
      nervous system (brain) (peripheral nerve) (spinal) T85.79 ☑
      urinary T83.59 ☑
    fixation, internal (orthopedic) NEC — *see* Complication, fixation device, infection
    gastrointestinal (bile duct) (esophagus) T85.79 ☑
    genital NEC T83.6 ☑
    heart NEC T82.7 ☑
      valve (prosthesis) T82.6 ☑
        graft T82.7 ☑
    joint prosthesis — *see* Complication, joint prosthesis, infection
    ocular (corneal graft) (orbital implant) NEC T85.79 ☑
    orthopedic NEC T84.7 ☑
    specified NEC T85.79 ☑
    urinary NEC T83.59 ☑
    vascular NEC T82.7 ☑
    ventricular intracranial shunt T85.79 ☑
  duodenum K29.80
    with bleeding K29.81
  dura mater — *see* Meningitis
  ear (middle) (*see also* Otitis, media)
    external — *see* Otitis, externa
    inner — *see* subcategory H83.0 ☑
  epididymis — *see* Epididymitis
  esophagus K20.9
  ethmoidal (sinus) (chronic) — *see* Sinusitis, ethmoidal
  eustachian tube (catarrhal) — *see* Salpingitis, eustachian
  eyelid H01.9
    abscess — *see* Abscess, eyelid
    blepharitis — *see* Blepharitis
    chalazion — *see* Chalazion
    dermatosis (noninfectious) — *see* Dermatosis, eyelid
    hordeolum — *see* Hordeolum
    specified NEC H01.8
  fallopian tube — *see* Salpingo-oophoritis
  fascia — *see* Myositis
  follicular, pharynx J31.2
  frontal (sinus) (chronic) — *see* Sinusitis, frontal
  gallbladder — *see* Cholecystitis
  gastric — *see* Gastritis
  gastrointestinal — *see* Enteritis
  genital organ (internal) (diffuse)
    female — *see* Disease, pelvis, inflammatory
    male N49.9
      multiple sites N49.8
      specified NEC N49.8
  gland (lymph) — *see* Lymphadenitis

Inflammation, inflamed, inflammatory — *continued*
  glottis — *see* Laryngitis
  granular, pharynx J31.2
  gum K05.10
    nonplaque induced K05.11
    plaque induced K05.10
  heart — *see* Carditis
  hepatic duct — *see* Cholangitis
  ileoanal (internal) pouch K91.850
  ileum (*see also* Enteritis)
    regional or terminal — *see* Enteritis, regional
  intestinal pouch K91.850
  intestine (any part) — *see* Enteritis
  jaw (acute) (bone) (chronic) (lower) (suppurative) (upper) M27.2
  joint NEC — *see* Arthritis
    sacroiliac M46.1
  kidney — *see* Nephritis
  knee (joint) M13.169
    tuberculous A18.02
  labium (majus) (minus) — *see* Vulvitis
  lacrimal
    gland — *see* Dacryoadenitis
    passages (duct) (sac) (*see also* Dacryocystitis)
      canaliculitis — *see* Canaliculitis, lacrimal
  larynx — *see* Laryngitis
  leg NOS L08.9
  lip K13.0
  liver (capsule) (*see also* Hepatitis)
    chronic K73.9
    suppurative K75.0
  lung (acute) (*see also* Pneumonia)
    chronic J98.4
  lymph gland or node — *see* Lymphadenitis
  lymphatic vessel — *see* Lymphangitis
  maxilla, maxillary M27.2
    sinus (chronic) — *see* Sinusitis, maxillary
  membranes of brain or spinal cord — *see* Meningitis
  meninges — *see* Meningitis
  mouth K12.1
  muscle — *see* Myositis
  myocardium — *see* Myocarditis
  nasal sinus (chronic) — *see* Sinusitis
  nasopharynx — *see* Nasopharyngitis
  navel L08.82
  nerve NEC — *see* Neuralgia
  nipple N61
    puerperal, postpartum or gestational — *see* Infection, nipple
  nose — *see* Rhinitis
  oculomotor (nerve) — *see* Strabismus, paralytic, third nerve
  optic nerve — *see* Neuritis, optic
  orbit (chronic) H05.10
    acute H05.00
      abscess — *see* Abscess, orbit
      cellulitis — *see* Cellulitis, orbit
      osteomyelitis — *see* Osteomyelitis, orbit
      periostitis — *see* Periostitis, orbital
      tenonitis — *see* Tenonitis, eye
    granuloma — *see* Granuloma, orbit
    myositis — *see* Myositis, orbital
  ovary — *see* Salpingo-oophoritis
  oviduct — *see* Salpingo-oophoritis
  pancreas (acute) — *see* Pancreatitis
  parametrium N73.0
  parotid region L08.9
  pelvis, female — *see* Disease, pelvis, inflammatory
  penis (corpora cavernosa) N48.29
  perianal K62.89
  pericardium — *see* Pericarditis
  perineum (female) (male) L08.9
  perirectal K62.89
  peritoneum — *see* Peritonitis
  periuterine — *see* Disease, pelvis, inflammatory
  perivesical — *see* Cystitis
  petrous bone (acute) (chronic) — *see* Petrositis
  pharynx (acute) — *see* Pharyngitis
  pia mater — *see* Meningitis
  pleura — *see* Pleurisy
  polyp, colon (*see also* Polyp, colon, inflammatory) K51.40
  prostate (*see also* Prostatitis)
    specified type NEC N41.8
  rectosigmoid — *see* Rectosigmoiditis
  rectum (*see also* Proctitis) K62.89

☑ Additional Character Required — Refer to the Tabular List for Character Selection   ⬇ Subterms under main terms may continue to next column or page

Inflammation, inflamed, inflammatory —
continued
  respiratory, upper (*see also* Infection, respiratory, upper) J06.9
    acute, due to radiation J70.0
    chronic, due to external agent — *see* condition, respiratory, chronic, due to
    due to
      chemicals, gases, fumes or vapors (inhalation) J68.2
      radiation J70.1
  retina — *see* Chorioretinitis
  retrocecal — *see* Appendicitis
  retroperitoneal — *see* Peritonitis
  salivary duct or gland (any) (suppurative) — *see* Sialoadenitis
  scorbutic, alveoli, teeth E54
  scrotum N49.2
  seminal vesicle — *see* Vesiculitis
  sigmoid — *see* Enteritis
  sinus — *see* Sinusitis
  Skene's duct or gland — *see* Urethritis
  skin L08.9
  spermatic cord N49.1
  sphenoidal (sinus) — *see* Sinusitis, sphenoidal
  spinal
    cord — *see* Encephalitis
    membrane — *see* Meningitis
    nerve — *see* Disorder, nerve
  spine — *see* Spondylopathy, inflammatory
  spleen (capsule) D73.89
  stomach — *see* Gastritis
  subcutaneous tissue L08.9
  suprarenal (gland) E27.8
  synovial — *see* Tenosynovitis
  tendon (sheath) NEC — *see* Tenosynovitis
  testis — *see* Orchitis
  throat (acute) — *see* Pharyngitis
  thymus (gland) E32.8
  thyroid (gland) — *see* Thyroiditis
  tongue K14.0
  tonsil — *see* Tonsillitis
  trachea — *see* Tracheitis
  trochlear (nerve) — *see* Strabismus, paralytic, fourth nerve
  tubal — *see* Salpingo-oophoritis
  tuberculous NEC — *see* Tuberculosis
  tubo-ovarian — *see* Salpingo-oophoritis
  tunica vaginalis N49.1
  tympanic membrane — *see* Tympanitis
  umbilicus, umbilical L08.82
  uterine ligament — *see* Disease, pelvis, inflammatory
  uterus (catarrhal) — *see* Endometritis
  uveal tract (anterior) NOS (*see also* Iridocyclitis)
    posterior — *see* Chorioretinitis
  vagina — *see* Vaginitis
  vas deferens N49.1
  vein (*see also* Phlebitis)
    intracranial or intraspinal (septic) G08
    thrombotic I80.9
      leg — *see* Phlebitis, leg
      lower extremity — *see* Phlebitis, leg
  vocal cord J38.3
  vulva — *see* Vulvitis
  Wharton's duct (suppurative) — *see* Sialoadenitis
Inflation, lung, imperfect (newborn) — *see* Atelectasis
Influenza (bronchial) (epidemic) (respiratory (upper)) (unidentified influenza virus) J11.1
  with
    digestive manifestations J11.2
    encephalopathy J11.81
    enteritis J11.2
    gastroenteritis J11.2
    gastrointestinal manifestations J11.2
    laryngitis J11.1
    myocarditis J11.82
    otitis media J11.83
    pharyngitis J11.1
    pneumonia J11.00
      specified type J11.08
    respiratory manifestations NEC J11.1
    specified manifestation NEC J11.89
  A/H5N1 (*see also* Influenza, due to, identified novel influenza A virus) J09.X2
  avian (*see also* Influenza, due to, identified novel influenza A virus) J09.X2

Influenza — *continued*
  bird (*see also* Influenza, due to, identified novel influenza A virus) J09.X2
  due to
    avian (*see also* Influenza, due to, identified novel influenza A virus) J09.X2
    identified influenza virus NEC J10.1
      with
        digestive manifestations J10.2
        encephalopathy J10.81
        enteritis J10.2
        gastroenteritis J10.2
        gastrointestinal manifestations J10.2
        laryngitis J10.1
        myocarditis J10.82
        otitis media J10.83
        pharyngitis J10.1
        pneumonia (unspecified type) J10.00
          with same identified influenza virus J10.01
          specified type NEC J10.08
        respiratory manifestations NEC J10.1
        specified manifestation NEC J10.89
    identified novel influenza A virus J09.X2
      with
        digestive manifestations J09.X3
        encephalopathy J09.X9
        enteritis J09.X3
        gastroenteritis J09.X3
        gastrointestinal manifestations J09.X3
        laryngitis J09.X2
        myocarditis J09.X9
        otitis media J09.X9
        pharyngitis J09.X2
        pneumonia J09.X1
        respiratory manifestations NEC J09.X2
        specified manifestation NEC J09.X9
        upper respiratory symptoms J09.X2
    novel (2009) H1N1 influenza (*see also* Influenza, due to, identified influenza virus NEC) J10.1
    novel influenza A/H1N1 (*see also* Influenza, due to, identified influenza virus NEC) J10.1
    of other animal origin, not bird or swine (*see also* Influenza, due to, identified novel influenza A virus) J09.X2
    swine (viruses that normally cause infections in pigs) (*see also* Influenza, due to, identified novel influenza A virus) J09.X2
Influenzal — *see* Influenza
Influenza-like disease — *see* Influenza
Infraction, Freiberg's (metatarsal head) — *see* Osteochondrosis, juvenile, metatarsus
Infraeruption of tooth (teeth) M26.34
Infusion complication, misadventure, or reaction — *see* Complications, infusion
Ingestion
  chemical — *see* Table of Drugs and Chemicals, by substance, poisoning
  drug or medicament
    correct substance properly administered — *see* Table of Drugs and Chemicals, by drug, adverse effect
    overdose or wrong substance given or taken — *see* Table of Drugs and Chemicals, by drug, poisoning
  foreign body — *see* Foreign body, alimentary tract
  tularemia A21.3
Ingrowing
  hair (beard) L73.1
  nail (finger) (toe) L60.0
Inguinal (*see also* condition)
  testicle Q53.9
    bilateral Q53.21
    unilateral Q53.11
Inhalation
  anthrax A22.1
  flame T27.3 ☑
  food or foreign body — *see* Foreign body, by site
  gases, fumes, or vapors NEC T59.9- ☑
    specified agent — *see* Table of Drugs and Chemicals, by substance
  liquid or vomitus — *see* Asphyxia
  meconium (newborn) P24.00
    with
      with respiratory symptoms P24.01
      pneumonia (pneumonitis) P24.01
  mucus — *see* Asphyxia, mucus

Inhalation — *continued*
  oil or gasoline (causing suffocation) — *see* Foreign body, by site
  smoke J70.5
    due to chemicals, gases, fumes and vapors J68.9
  steam — *see* Toxicity, vapors
  stomach contents or secretions — *see* Foreign body, by site
    due to anesthesia (general) (local) or other sedation T88.59
      in labor and delivery O74.0
      in pregnancy O29.01- ☑
      postpartum, puerperal O89.01
Inhibition, orgasm
  female F52.31
  male F52.32
Inhibitor, systemic lupus erythematosus (presence of) D68.62
Iniencephalus, iniencephaly Q00.2
Injection, traumatic jet (air) (industrial) (water) (paint or dye) T70.4 ☑
Injury (*see also* specified injury type) T14.90
  abdomen, abdominal S39.91
    blood vessel — *see* Injury, blood vessel, abdomen
    cavity — *see* Injury, intra-abdominal
    contusion S30.1 ☑
    internal — *see* Injury, intra-abdominal
    intra-abdominal organ — *see* Injury, intra-abdominal
    nerve — *see* Injury, nerve, abdomen
    open — *see* Wound, open, abdomen
    specified NEC S39.81 ☑
    superficial — *see* Injury, superficial, abdomen
  Achilles tendon S86.00- ☑
    laceration S86.02- ☑
    specified type NEC S86.09- ☑
    strain S86.01- ☑
  acoustic, resulting in deafness — *see* Injury, nerve, acoustic
  adrenal (gland) S37.819 ☑
    contusion S37.812 ☑
    laceration S37.813 ☑
    specified type NEC S37.818 ☑
  alveolar (process) S09.93 ☑
  ankle S99.91- ☑
    contusion — *see* Contusion, ankle
    dislocation — *see* Dislocation, ankle
    fracture — *see* Fracture, ankle
    nerve — *see* Injury, nerve, ankle
    open — *see* Wound, open, ankle
    specified type NEC S99.81- ☑
    sprain — *see* Sprain, ankle
    superficial — *see* Injury, superficial, ankle
  anterior chamber, eye — *see* Injury, eye, specified site NEC
  anus — *see* Injury, abdomen
  aorta (thoracic) S25.00 ☑
    abdominal S35.00 ☑
      laceration (minor) (superficial) S35.01 ☑
        major S35.02 ☑
      specified type NEC S35.09 ☑
    laceration (minor) (superficial) S25.01 ☑
      major S25.02 ☑
    specified type NEC S25.09 ☑
  arm (upper) S49.9- ☑
    blood vessel — *see* Injury, blood vessel, arm
    contusion — *see* Contusion, arm, upper
    fracture — *see* Fracture, humerus
    lower — *see* Injury, forearm
    muscle — *see* Injury, muscle, shoulder
    nerve — *see* Injury, nerve, arm
    open — *see* Wound, open, arm
    specified type NEC S49.8- ☑
    superficial — *see* Injury, superficial, arm
  artery (complicating trauma) (*see also* Injury, blood vessel, by site)
    cerebral or meningeal — *see* Injury, intracranial
  auditory canal (external) (meatus) S09.91 ☑
  auricle, auris, ear S09.91 ☑
  axilla — *see* Injury, shoulder
  back — *see* Injury, back, lower
  bile duct S36.13 ☑
  birth (*see also* Birth, injury) P15.9
  bladder (sphincter) S37.20 ☑
    at delivery O71.5
    contusion S37.22 ☑

Injury — continued
  bladder — continued
    laceration S37.23 ☑
    obstetrical trauma O71.5
    specified type NEC S37.29 ☑
  blast (air) (hydraulic) (immersion) (underwater) NEC
    T14.8
    acoustic nerve trauma — see Injury, nerve, acoustic
    bladder — see Injury, bladder
    brain — see Concussion
    colon — see Injury, intestine, large
    ear (primary) S09.31- ☑
      secondary S09.39- ☑
    generalized T70.8 ☑
    lung — see Injury, intrathoracic, lung
    multiple body organs T70.8 ☑
    peritoneum S36.81 ☑
    rectum S36.61 ☑
    retroperitoneum S36.898 ☑
    small intestine S36.419 ☑
      duodenum S36.410 ☑
      specified site NEC S36.418 ☑
    specified
      intra-abdominal organ NEC S36.898 ☑
      pelvic organ NEC S37.899 ☑
  blood vessel NEC T14.8
    abdomen S35.9 ☑
      aorta — see Injury, aorta, abdominal
      celiac artery — see Injury, blood vessel, celiac
        artery
      iliac vessel — see Injury, blood vessel, iliac
      laceration S35.91 ☑
      mesenteric vessel — see Injury, mesenteric
      portal vein — see Injury, blood vessel, portal
        vein
      renal vessel — see Injury, blood vessel, renal
      specified vessel NEC S35.8X- ☑
      splenic vessel — see Injury, blood vessel,
        splenic
      vena cava — see Injury, vena cava, inferior
    ankle — see Injury, blood vessel, foot
    aorta (abdominal) (thoracic) — see Injury, aorta
    arm (upper) NEC S45.90- ☑
      forearm — see Injury, blood vessel, forearm
      laceration S45.91- ☑
      specified
        site NEC S45.80- ☑
          laceration S45.81- ☑
          specified type NEC S45.89- ☑
        type NEC S45.99- ☑
      superficial vein S45.30- ☑
        laceration S45.31- ☑
        specified type NEC S45.39- ☑
    axillary
      artery S45.00- ☑
        laceration S45.01- ☑
        specified type NEC S45.09- ☑
      vein S45.20- ☑
        laceration S45.21- ☑
        specified type NEC S45.29- ☑
    azygos vein — see Injury, blood vessel, thoracic,
      specified site NEC
    brachial
      artery S45.10- ☑
        laceration S45.11- ☑
        specified type NEC S45.19- ☑
      vein S45.20- ☑
        laceration S45.219 ☑
        specified type NEC S45.29- ☑
    carotid artery (common) (external) (internal, ex-
      tracranial) S15.00- ☑
      internal, intracranial S06.8- ☑
      laceration (minor) (superficial) S15.01- ☑
        major S15.02- ☑
      specified type NEC S15.09- ☑
    celiac artery S35.219 ☑
      branch S35.299 ☑
        laceration (minor) (superficial) S35.291 ☑
          major S35.292 ☑
        specified NEC S35.298 ☑
      laceration (minor) (superficial) S35.211 ☑
        major S35.212 ☑
      specified type NEC S35.218 ☑
    cerebral — see Injury, intracranial
    deep plantar — see Injury, blood vessel, plantar
      artery

Injury — continued
  blood vessel — continued
    digital (hand) — see Injury, blood vessel, finger
    dorsal
      artery (foot) S95.00- ☑
        laceration S95.01- ☑
        specified type NEC S95.09- ☑
      vein (foot) S95.20- ☑
        laceration S95.21- ☑
        specified type NEC S95.29- ☑
    due to accidental laceration during procedure —
      see Laceration, accidental complicating
      surgery
    extremity — see Injury, blood vessel, limb
    femoral
      artery (common) (superficial) S75.00- ☑
        laceration (minor) (superficial) S75.01- ☑
          major S75.02- ☑
        specified type NEC S75.09- ☑
      vein (hip level) (thigh level) S75.10- ☑
        laceration (minor) (superficial) S75.11- ☑
          major S75.12- ☑
        specified type NEC S75.19- ☑
    finger S65.50- ☑
      index S65.50- ☑
        laceration S65.51- ☑
        specified type NEC S65.59- ☑
      laceration S65.51- ☑
      little S65.50- ☑
        laceration S65.51- ☑
        specified type NEC S65.59- ☑
      middle S65.50- ☑
        laceration S65.51- ☑
        specified type NEC S65.59- ☑
      specified type NEC S65.59- ☑
      thumb — see Injury, blood vessel, thumb
    foot S95.90- ☑
      dorsal
        artery — see Injury, blood vessel, dorsal,
          artery
        vein — see Injury, blood vessel, dorsal, vein
      laceration S95.91- ☑
      plantar artery — see Injury, blood vessel, plan-
        tar artery
      specified
        site NEC S95.80- ☑
          laceration S95.81- ☑
          specified type NEC S95.89- ☑
        specified type NEC S95.99- ☑
    forearm S55.90- ☑
      laceration S55.91- ☑
      radial artery — see Injury, blood vessel, radial
        artery
      specified
        site NEC S55.80- ☑
          laceration S55.81- ☑
          specified type NEC S55.89- ☑
        type NEC S55.99- ☑
      ulnar artery — see Injury, blood vessel, ulnar
        artery
      vein S55.20- ☑
        laceration S55.21- ☑
        specified type NEC S55.29- ☑
    gastric
      artery — see Injury, mesenteric, artery, branch
      vein — see Injury, blood vessel, abdomen
    gastroduodenal artery — see Injury, mesenteric,
      artery, branch
    greater saphenous vein (lower leg level) S85.30- ☑
      hip (and thigh) level S75.20- ☑
        laceration (minor) (superficial) S75.21- ☑
          major S75.22- ☑
        specified type NEC S75.29- ☑
      laceration S85.31- ☑
      specified type NEC S85.39- ☑
    hand (level) S65.90- ☑
      finger — see Injury, blood vessel, finger
      laceration S65.91- ☑
      palmar arch — see Injury, blood vessel, palmar
        arch
      radial artery — see Injury, blood vessel, radial
        artery, hand
      specified
        site NEC S65.80- ☑
          laceration S65.81- ☑
          specified type NEC S65.89- ☑

Injury — continued
  blood vessel — continued
    hand — continued
      specified — continued
        type NEC S65.99- ☑
      thumb — see Injury, blood vessel, thumb
      ulnar artery — see Injury, blood vessel, ulnar
        artery, hand
    head S09.0 ☑
      intracranial — see Injury, intracranial
      multiple S09.0 ☑
    hepatic
      artery — see Injury, mesenteric, artery
      vein — see Injury, vena cava, inferior
    hip S75.90- ☑
      femoral artery — see Injury, blood vessel,
        femoral, artery
      femoral vein — see Injury, blood vessel,
        femoral, vein
      greater saphenous vein — see Injury, blood
        vessel, greater saphenous, hip level
      laceration S75.91- ☑
      specified
        site NEC S75.80- ☑
          laceration S75.81- ☑
          specified type NEC S75.89- ☑
        type NEC S75.99- ☑
    hypogastric (artery) (vein) — see Injury, blood
      vessel, iliac
    iliac S35.5- ☑
      artery S35.51- ☑
      specified vessel NEC S35.5- ☑
      uterine vessel — see Injury, blood vessel, uter-
        ine
      vein S35.51- ☑
    innominate — see Injury, blood vessel, thoracic,
      innominate
    intercostal (artery) (vein) — see Injury, blood vessel,
      thoracic, intercostal
    jugular vein (external) S15.20- ☑
      internal S15.30- ☑
        laceration (minor) (superficial) S15.31- ☑
          major S15.32- ☑
        specified type NEC S15.39- ☑
      laceration (minor) (superficial) S15.21- ☑
        major S15.22- ☑
      specified type NEC S15.29- ☑
    leg (level) (lower) S85.90- ☑
      greater saphenous — see Injury, blood vessel,
        greater saphenous
      laceration S85.91- ☑
      lesser saphenous — see Injury, blood vessel,
        lesser saphenous
      peroneal artery — see Injury, blood vessel,
        peroneal artery
      popliteal
        artery — see Injury, blood vessel, popliteal,
          artery
        vein — see Injury, blood vessel, popliteal,
          vein
      specified
        site NEC S85.80- ☑
          laceration S85.81- ☑
          specified type NEC S85.89- ☑
        type NEC S85.99- ☑
      thigh — see Injury, blood vessel, hip
      tibial artery — see Injury, blood vessel, tibial
        artery
    lesser saphenous vein (lower leg level) S85.40- ☑
      laceration S85.41- ☑
      specified type NEC S85.49- ☑
    limb
      lower — see Injury, blood vessel, leg
      upper — see Injury, blood vessel, arm
    lower back — see Injury, blood vessel, abdomen
      specified NEC — see Injury, blood vessel, ab-
        domen, specified, site NEC
    mammary (artery) (vein) — see Injury, blood vessel,
      thoracic, specified site NEC
    mesenteric (inferior) (superior)
      artery — see Injury, mesenteric, artery
      vein — see Injury, blood vessel, mesenteric,
        vein
    neck S15.9 ☑
      specified site NEC S15.8 ☑
    ovarian (artery) (vein) — see subcategory S35.8 ☑

☑ Additional Character Required — Refer to the Tabular List for Character Selection   ▽ Subterms under main terms may continue to next column or page

Injury — *continued*
  blood vessel — *continued*
    palmar arch (superficial) S65.20- ☑
      deep S65.30- ☑
        laceration S65.31- ☑
        specified type NEC S65.39- ☑
      laceration S65.21- ☑
      specified type NEC S65.29- ☑
    pelvis — *see* Injury, blood vessel, abdomen
      specified NEC — *see* Injury, blood vessel, abdomen, specified, site NEC
    peroneal artery S85.20- ☑
      laceration S85.21- ☑
      specified type NEC S85.29- ☑
    plantar artery (deep) (foot) S95.10- ☑
      laceration S95.11- ☑
      specified type NEC S95.19- ☑
    popliteal
      artery S85.00- ☑
        laceration S85.01- ☑
        specified type NEC S85.09- ☑
      vein S85.50- ☑
        laceration S85.51- ☑
        specified type NEC S85.59- ☑
    portal vein S35.319 ☑
      laceration S35.311 ☑
      specified type NEC S35.318 ☑
    precerebral — *see* Injury, blood vessel, neck
    pulmonary (artery) (vein) — *see* Injury, blood vessel, thoracic, pulmonary
    radial artery (forearm level) S55.10- ☑
      hand and wrist (level) S65.10- ☑
        laceration S65.11- ☑
        specified type NEC S65.19- ☑
      laceration S55.11- ☑
      specified type NEC S55.19- ☑
    renal
      artery S35.40- ☑
        laceration S35.41- ☑
        specified NEC S35.49- ☑
      vein S35.40- ☑
        laceration S35.41- ☑
        specified NEC S35.49- ☑
    saphenous vein (greater) (lower leg level) — *see* Injury, blood vessel, greater saphenous
      hip and thigh level — *see* Injury, blood vessel, greater saphenous, hip level
      lesser — *see* Injury, blood vessel, lesser saphenous
    shoulder
      specified NEC — *see* Injury, blood vessel, arm, specified site NEC
      superficial vein — *see* Injury, blood vessel, arm, superficial vein
    specified NEC T14.8
    splenic
      artery — *see* Injury, blood vessel, celiac artery, branch
      vein S35.329 ☑
        laceration S35.321 ☑
        specified NEC S35.328 ☑
    subclavian — *see* Injury, blood vessel, thoracic, innominate
    thigh — *see* Injury, blood vessel, hip
    thoracic S25.90- ☑
      aorta S25.00- ☑
        laceration (minor) (superficial) S25.01 ☑
          major S25.02 ☑
        specified type NEC S25.09 ☑
      azygos vein — *see* Injury, blood vessel, thoracic, specified, site NEC
      innominate
        artery S25.10- ☑
          laceration (minor) (superficial) S25.11- ☑
            major S25.12- ☑
          specified type NEC S25.19- ☑
        vein S25.30- ☑
          laceration (minor) (superficial) S25.31- ☑
            major S25.32- ☑
          specified type NEC S25.39- ☑
      intercostal S25.50- ☑
        laceration S25.51- ☑
        specified type NEC S25.59- ☑
      laceration S25.91 ☑

Injury — *continued*
  blood vessel — *continued*
    thoracic — *continued*
      mammary vessel — *see* Injury, blood vessel, thoracic, specified, site NEC
      pulmonary S25.40- ☑
        laceration (minor) (superficial) S25.41- ☑
          major S25.42- ☑
        specified type NEC S25.49- ☑
      specified
        site NEC S25.80- ☑
          laceration S25.81 ☑
          specified type NEC S25.89 ☑
        type NEC S25.99 ☑
      subclavian — *see* Injury, blood vessel, thoracic, innominate
      vena cava (superior) S25.20 ☑
        laceration (minor) (superficial) S25.21 ☑
          major S25.22 ☑
        specified type NEC S25.29 ☑
    thumb S65.40- ☑
      laceration S65.41- ☑
      specified type NEC S65.49- ☑
    tibial artery S85.10- ☑
      anterior S85.13- ☑
        laceration S85.14- ☑
        specified injury NEC S85.15- ☑
      laceration S85.11- ☑
      posterior S85.16- ☑
        laceration S85.17- ☑
        specified injury NEC S85.18- ☑
      specified injury NEC S85.12- ☑
    ulnar artery (forearm level) S55.00- ☑
      hand and wrist (level) S65.00- ☑
        laceration S65.01- ☑
        specified type NEC S65.09- ☑
      laceration S55.01- ☑
      specified type NEC S55.09- ☑
    upper arm (level) — *see* Injury, blood vessel, arm
      superficial vein — *see* Injury, blood vessel, arm, superficial vein
    uterine S35.5- ☑
      artery S35.53- ☑
      vein S35.53- ☑
    vena cava — *see* Injury, vena cava
    vertebral artery S15.10- ☑
      laceration (minor) (superficial) S15.11- ☑
        major S15.12- ☑
      specified type NEC S15.19- ☑
    wrist (level) — *see* Injury, blood vessel, hand
  brachial plexus S14.3 ☑
    newborn P14.3
  brain (traumatic) S06.9- ☑
    diffuse (axonal) S06.2X- ☑
    focal S06.30- ☑
    traumatic — *see* category S06
  brainstem S06.38- ☑
  breast NOS S29.9 ☑
  broad ligament — *see* Injury, pelvic organ, specified site NEC
  bronchus, bronchi — *see* Injury, intrathoracic, bronchus
  brow S09.90 ☑
  buttock S39.92 ☑
  canthus, eye S05.90 ☑
  cardiac plexus — *see* Injury, nerve, thorax, sympathetic
  cauda equina S34.3 ☑
  cavernous sinus — *see* Injury, intracranial
  cecum — *see* Injury, colon
  celiac ganglion or plexus — *see* Injury, nerve, lumbosacral, sympathetic
  cerebellum — *see* Injury, intracranial
  cerebral — *see* Injury, intracranial
  cervix (uteri) — *see* Injury, uterus
  cheek (wall) S09.93 ☑
  chest — *see* Injury, thorax
  childbirth (newborn) (*see also* Birth, injury)
    maternal NEC O71.9
  chin S09.93 ☑
  choroid (eye) — *see* Injury, eye, specified site NEC
  clitoris S39.94 ☑
  coccyx (*see also* Injury, back, lower)
    complicating delivery O71.6
  colon — *see* Injury, intestine, large
  common bile duct — *see* Injury, liver
  conjunctiva (superficial) — *see* Injury, eye, conjunctiva

Injury — *continued*
  conus medullaris — *see* Injury, spinal, sacral
  cord
    spermatic (pelvic region) S37.898 ☑
      scrotal region S39.848
    spinal — *see* Injury, spinal cord, by region
  cornea — *see* Injury, eye, specified site NEC
    abrasion — *see* Injury, eye, cornea, abrasion
  cortex (cerebral) (*see also* Injury, intracranial)
    visual — *see* Injury, nerve, optic
  costal region NEC S29.9
  costochondral NEC S29.9 ☑
  cranial
    cavity — *see* Injury, intracranial
    nerve — *see* Injury, nerve, cranial
  crushing — *see* Crush
  cutaneous sensory nerve
  cystic duct — *see* Injury, liver
  deep tissue — *see* Contusion, by site
    meaning pressure ulcer — *see* Ulcer, pressure, unstageable, by site
  delivery (newborn) P15.9
    maternal NEC O71.9
  Descemet's membrane — *see* Injury, eyeball, penetrating
  diaphragm — *see* Injury, intrathoracic, diaphragm
  duodenum — *see* Injury, intestine, small, duodenum
  ear (auricle) (external) (canal) S09.91 ☑
    abrasion — *see* Abrasion, ear
    bite — *see* Bite, ear
    blister — *see* Blister, ear
    bruise — *see* Contusion, ear
    contusion — *see* Contusion, ear
    external constriction — *see* Constriction, external, ear
    hematoma — *see* Hematoma, ear
    inner — *see* Injury, ear, middle
    laceration — *see* Laceration, ear
    middle S09.30- ☑
      blast — *see* Injury, blast, ear
      specified NEC S09.39- ☑
    puncture — *see* Puncture, ear
    superficial — *see* Injury, superficial, ear
  eighth cranial nerve (acoustic or auditory) — *see* Injury, nerve, acoustic
  elbow S59.90- ☑
    contusion — *see* Contusion, elbow
    dislocation — *see* Dislocation, elbow
    fracture — *see* Fracture, ulna, upper end
    open — *see* Wound, open, elbow
    specified NEC S59.80- ☑
    sprain — *see* Sprain, elbow
    superficial — *see* Injury, superficial, elbow
  eleventh cranial nerve (accessory) — *see* Injury, nerve, accessory
  epididymis S39.94 ☑
  epigastric region S39.91 ☑
  epiglottis NEC S19.89 ☑
  esophageal plexus — *see* Injury, nerve, thorax, sympathetic
  esophagus (thoracic part) (*see also* Injury, intrathoracic, esophagus)
    cervical NEC S19.85 ☑
  eustachian tube S09.30 ☑
  eye S05.9- ☑
    avulsion S05.7- ☑
    ball — *see* Injury, eyeball
    conjunctiva S05.0- ☑
    cornea
      abrasion S05.0- ☑
      laceration S05.3- ☑
        with prolapse S05.2- ☑
    lacrimal apparatus S05.8X- ☑
    orbit penetration S05.4- ☑
    specified site NEC S05.8X- ☑
  eyeball S05.8X- ☑
    contusion S05.1- ☑
    penetrating S05.6- ☑
      with
        foreign body S05.5- ☑
        prolapse or loss of intraocular tissue S05.2- ☑
        without prolapse or loss of intraocular tissue S05.3- ☑
    specified type NEC S05.8- ☑
  eyebrow S09.93 ☑

Injury — continued
- eyelid S09.93 ☑
  - abrasion — see Abrasion, eyelid
  - contusion — see Contusion, eyelid
  - open — see Wound, open, eyelid
- face S09.93 ☑
- fallopian tube S37.509 ☑
  - bilateral S37.502 ☑
    - blast injury S37.512 ☑
    - contusion S37.522 ☑
    - laceration S37.532 ☑
    - specified type NEC S37.592 ☑
  - blast injury (primary) S37.519 ☑
    - bilateral S37.512 ☑
    - secondary — see Injury, fallopian tube, specified type NEC
    - unilateral S37.511 ☑
  - contusion S37.529 ☑
    - bilateral S37.522 ☑
    - unilateral S37.521 ☑
  - laceration S37.539 ☑
    - bilateral S37.532 ☑
    - unilateral S37.531 ☑
  - specified type NEC S37.599 ☑
    - bilateral S37.592 ☑
    - unilateral S37.591 ☑
  - unilateral S37.501 ☑
    - blast injury S37.511 ☑
    - contusion S37.521 ☑
    - laceration S37.531 ☑
    - specified type NEC S37.591 ☑
- fascia — see Injury, muscle
- fifth cranial nerve (trigeminal) — see Injury, nerve, trigeminal
- finger (nail) S69.9- ☑
  - blood vessel — see Injury, blood vessel, finger
  - contusion — see Contusion, finger
  - dislocation — see Dislocation, finger
  - fracture — see Fracture, finger
  - muscle — see Injury, muscle, finger
  - nerve — see Injury, nerve, digital, finger
  - open — see Wound, open, finger
  - specified NEC S69.8- ☑
  - sprain — see Sprain, finger
  - superficial — see Injury, superficial, finger
- first cranial nerve (olfactory) — see Injury, nerve, olfactory
- flank — see Injury, abdomen
- foot S99.92- ☑
  - blood vessel — see Injury, blood vessel, foot
  - contusion — see Contusion, foot
  - dislocation — see Dislocation, foot
  - fracture — see Fracture, foot
  - muscle — see Injury, muscle, foot
  - open — see Wound, open, foot
  - specified type NEC S99.82- ☑
  - sprain — see Sprain, foot
  - superficial — see Injury, superficial, foot
- forceps NOS P15.9
- forearm S59.91- ☑
  - blood vessel — see Injury, blood vessel, forearm
  - contusion — see Contusion, forearm
  - fracture — see Fracture, forearm
  - muscle — see Injury, muscle, forearm
  - nerve — see Injury, nerve, forearm
  - open — see Wound, open, forearm
  - specified NEC S59.81- ☑
  - superficial — see Injury, superficial, forearm
- forehead S09.90 ☑
- fourth cranial nerve (trochlear) — see Injury, nerve, trochlear
- gallbladder S36.129 ☑
  - contusion S36.122 ☑
  - laceration S36.123 ☑
  - specified NEC S36.128 ☑
- ganglion
  - celiac, coeliac — see Injury, nerve, lumbosacral, sympathetic
  - gasserian — see Injury, nerve, trigeminal
  - stellate — see Injury, nerve, thorax, sympathetic
  - thoracic sympathetic — see Injury, nerve, thorax, sympathetic
- gasserian ganglion — see Injury, nerve, trigeminal
- gastric artery — see Injury, blood vessel, celiac artery, branch

Injury — continued
- gastroduodenal artery — see Injury, blood vessel, celiac artery, branch
- gastrointestinal tract — see Injury, intra-abdominal
  - with open wound into abdominal cavity — see Wound, open, with penetration into peritoneal cavity
  - colon — see Injury, intestine, large
  - rectum — see Injury, intestine, large, rectum
    - with open wound into abdominal cavity S36.61 ☑
  - small intestine — see Injury, intestine, small
  - specified site NEC — see Injury, intra-abdominal, specified, site NEC
  - stomach — see Injury, stomach
- genital organ(s)
  - external S39.94 ☑
    - specified NEC S39.848 ☑
  - internal S37.90 ☑
    - fallopian tube — see Injury, fallopian tube
    - ovary — see Injury, ovary
    - prostate — see Injury, prostate
    - seminal vesicle — see Injury, pelvis, organ, specified site NEC
    - uterus — see Injury, uterus
    - vas deferens — see Injury, pelvis, organ, specified site NEC
  - obstetrical trauma O71.9
- gland
  - lacrimal laceration — see Injury, eye, specified site NEC
  - salivary S09.90 ☑
  - thyroid NEC S19.84 ☑
- globe (eye) S05.90 ☑
  - specified NEC S05.8X- ☑
- groin — see Injury, abdomen
- gum S09.90 ☑
- hand S69.9- ☑
  - blood vessel — see Injury, blood vessel, hand
  - contusion — see Contusion, hand
  - fracture — see Fracture, hand
  - muscle — see Injury, muscle, hand
  - nerve — see Injury, nerve, hand
  - open — see Wound, open, hand
  - specified NEC S69.8- ☑
  - sprain — see Sprain, hand
  - superficial — see Injury, superficial, hand
- head S09.90 ☑
  - with loss of consciousness S06.9- ☑
  - specified NEC S09.8 ☑
- heart S26.90 ☑
  - with hemopericardium S26.00 ☑
    - contusion S26.01 ☑
    - laceration (mild) S26.020 ☑
      - major S26.022 ☑
      - moderate S26.021 ☑
    - specified type NEC S26.09 ☑
  - without hemopericardium S26.10 ☑
    - contusion S26.11 ☑
    - laceration S26.12 ☑
    - specified type NEC S26.19 ☑
  - contusion S26.91 ☑
  - laceration S26.92 ☑
  - specified type NEC S26.99 ☑
- heel — see Injury, foot
- hepatic
  - artery — see Injury, blood vessel, celiac artery, branch
  - duct — see Injury, liver
  - vein — see Injury, vena cava, inferior
- hip S79.91- ☑
  - blood vessel — see Injury, blood vessel, hip
  - contusion — see Contusion, hip
  - dislocation — see Dislocation, hip
  - fracture — see Fracture, femur, neck
  - muscle — see Injury, muscle, hip
  - nerve — see Injury, nerve, hip
  - open — see Wound, open, hip
  - specified NEC S79.81- ☑
  - sprain — see Sprain, hip
  - superficial — see Injury, superficial, hip
- hymen S39.94 ☑
- hypogastric
  - blood vessel — see Injury, blood vessel, iliac
  - plexus — see Injury, nerve, lumbosacral, sympathetic

Injury — continued
- ileum — see Injury, intestine, small
- iliac region S39.91 ☑
- instrumental (during surgery) — see Laceration, accidental complicating surgery
  - birth injury — see Birth, injury
  - nonsurgical — see Injury, by site
- obstetrical O71.9
  - bladder O71.5
  - cervix O71.3
  - high vaginal O71.4
  - perineal NOS O70.9
  - urethra O71.5
  - uterus O71.5
    - with rupture or perforation O71.1
- internal T14.8
  - aorta — see Injury, aorta
  - bladder (sphincter) — see Injury, bladder
    - with
      - ectopic or molar pregnancy O08.6
      - following ectopic or molar pregnancy O08.6
      - obstetrical trauma O71.5
  - bronchus, bronchi — see Injury, intrathoracic, bronchus
  - cecum — see Injury, intestine, large
  - cervix (uteri) (see also Injury, uterus)
    - with ectopic or molar pregnancy O08.6
    - following ectopic or molar pregnancy O08.6
    - obstetrical trauma O71.3
  - chest — see Injury, intrathoracic
  - gastrointestinal tract — see Injury, intra-abdominal
  - heart — see Injury, heart
  - intestine NEC — see Injury, intestine
  - intrauterine — see Injury, uterus
  - mesentery — see Injury, intra-abdominal, specified, site NEC
  - pelvis, pelvic (organ) S37.90 ☑
    - following ectopic or molar pregnancy (subsequent episode) O08.6
    - obstetrical trauma NEC O71.5
      - rupture or perforation O71.1
    - specified NEC S39.83 ☑
  - rectum — see Injury, intestine, large, rectum
  - stomach — see Injury, stomach
  - ureter — see Injury, ureter
  - urethra (sphincter) following ectopic or molar pregnancy O08.6
  - uterus — see Injury, uterus
- interscapular area — see Injury, thorax
- intestine
  - large S36.509 ☑
    - ascending (right) S36.500 ☑
      - blast injury (primary) S36.510 ☑
        - secondary S36.590 ☑
      - contusion S36.520 ☑
      - laceration S36.530 ☑
      - specified type NEC S36.590 ☑
    - blast injury (primary) S36.519 ☑
      - ascending (right) S36.510 ☑
      - descending (left) S36.512 ☑
      - rectum S36.61 ☑
      - sigmoid S36.513 ☑
      - specified site NEC S36.518 ☑
      - transverse S36.511 ☑
    - contusion S36.529 ☑
      - ascending (right) S36.520 ☑
      - descending (left) S36.522 ☑
      - rectum S36.62 ☑
      - sigmoid S36.523 ☑
      - specified site NEC S36.528 ☑
      - transverse S36.521 ☑
    - descending (left) S36.502 ☑
      - blast injury (primary) S36.512 ☑
        - secondary S36.592 ☑
      - contusion S36.522 ☑
      - laceration S36.532 ☑
      - specified type NEC S36.592 ☑
    - laceration S36.539 ☑
      - ascending (right) S36.530 ☑
      - descending (left) S36.532 ☑
      - rectum S36.63 ☑
      - sigmoid S36.533 ☑
      - specified site NEC S36.538 ☑
      - transverse S36.531 ☑
    - rectum S36.60 ☑
      - blast injury (primary) S36.61 ☑

Injury — *continued*
  intestine — *continued*
    large — *continued*
      rectum — *continued*
        blast injury — *continued*
          secondary S36.69 ☑
        contusion S36.62 ☑
        laceration S36.63 ☑
        specified type NEC S36.69 ☑
      sigmoid S36.503 ☑
        blast injury (primary) S36.513 ☑
          secondary S36.593 ☑
        contusion S36.523 ☑
        laceration S36.533 ☑
        specified type NEC S36.593 ☑
      specified
        site NEC S36.508 ☑
          blast injury (primary) S36.518 ☑
            secondary S36.598 ☑
          contusion S36.528 ☑
          laceration S36.538 ☑
          specified type NEC S36.598 ☑
        type NEC S36.599 ☑
          ascending (right) S36.590 ☑
          descending (left) S36.592 ☑
          rectum S36.69 ☑
          sigmoid S36.593 ☑
          specified site NEC S36.598 ☑
          transverse S36.591 ☑
      transverse S36.501 ☑
        blast injury (primary) S36.511 ☑
          secondary S36.591 ☑
        contusion S36.521 ☑
        laceration S36.531 ☑
        specified type NEC S36.591 ☑
    small S36.409 ☑
      blast injury (primary) S36.419 ☑
        duodenum S36.410 ☑
        secondary S36.499 ☑
          duodenum S36.490 ☑
          specified site NEC S36.498 ☑
        specified site NEC S36.418 ☑
      contusion S36.429 ☑
        duodenum S36.420 ☑
        specified site NEC S36.428 ☑
      duodenum S36.400 ☑
        blast injury (primary) S36.410 ☑
          secondary S36.490 ☑
        contusion S36.420 ☑
        laceration S36.430 ☑
        specified NEC S36.490 ☑
      laceration S36.439 ☑
        duodenum S36.430 ☑
        specified site NEC S36.438 ☑
      specified
        site NEC S36.408 ☑
        type NEC S36.499 ☑
          duodenum S36.490 ☑
          specified site NEC S36.498 ☑
  intra-abdominal S36.90 ☑
    adrenal gland — *see* Injury, adrenal gland
    bladder — *see* Injury, bladder
    colon — *see* Injury, intestine, large
    contusion S36.92 ☑
    fallopian tube — *see* Injury, fallopian tube
    gallbladder — *see* Injury, gallbladder
    intestine — *see* Injury, intestine
    kidney — *see* Injury, kidney
    laceration S36.93 ☑
    liver — *see* Injury, liver
    ovary — *see* Injury, ovary
    pancreas — *see* Injury, pancreas
    pelvic NOS S37.90 ☑
    peritoneum — *see* Injury, intra-abdominal, specified, site NEC
    prostate — *see* Injury, prostate
    rectum — *see* Injury, intestine, large, rectum
    retroperitoneum — *see* Injury, intra-abdominal, specified, site NEC
    seminal vesicle — *see* Injury, pelvis, organ, specified site NEC
    small intestine — *see* Injury, intestine, small

Injury — *continued*
  intra-abdominal — *continued*
    specified
      pelvic S37.90 ☑
        specified
          site NEC S37.899 ☑
            specified type NEC S37.898 ☑
          type NEC S37.99 ☑
      site NEC S36.899 ☑
        contusion S36.892 ☑
        laceration S36.893 ☑
        specified type NEC S36.898 ☑
      type NEC S36.99 ☑
    spleen — *see* Injury, spleen
    stomach — *see* Injury, stomach
    ureter — *see* Injury, ureter
    urethra — *see* Injury, urethra
    uterus — *see* Injury, uterus
    vas deferens — *see* Injury, pelvis, organ, specified site NEC
  intracranial (traumatic) S06.9- ☑
    cerebellar hemorrhage, traumatic — *see* Injury, intracranial, focal
    cerebral edema, traumatic S06.1X- ☑
      diffuse S06.1X- ☑
      focal S06.1X- ☑
    diffuse (axonal) S06.2X- ☑
    epidural hemorrhage (traumatic) S06.4X- ☑
    focal brain injury S06.30- ☑
      contusion — *see* Contusion, cerebral
      laceration — *see* Laceration, cerebral
      intracerebral hemorrhage, traumatic S06.36- ☑
        left side S06.35- ☑
        right side S06.34- ☑
    subarachnoid hemorrhage, traumatic S06.6X- ☑
    subdural hemorrhage, traumatic S06.5X- ☑
  intraocular — *see* Injury, eyeball, penetrating
  intrathoracic S27.9 ☑
    bronchus S27.409 ☑
      bilateral S27.402 ☑
      blast injury (primary) S27.419 ☑
        bilateral S27.412 ☑
        secondary — *see* Injury, intrathoracic, bronchus, specified type NEC
        unilateral S27.411 ☑
      contusion S27.429 ☑
        bilateral S27.422 ☑
        unilateral S27.421 ☑
      laceration S27.439 ☑
        bilateral S27.432 ☑
        unilateral S27.431 ☑
      specified type NEC S27.499 ☑
        bilateral S27.492 ☑
        unilateral S27.491 ☑
      unilateral S27.401 ☑
    diaphragm S27.809 ☑
      contusion S27.802 ☑
      laceration S27.803 ☑
      specified type NEC S27.808 ☑
    esophagus (thoracic) S27.819 ☑
      contusion S27.812 ☑
      laceration S27.813 ☑
      specified type NEC S27.818 ☑
    heart — *see* Injury, heart
    hemopneumothorax S27.2 ☑
    hemothorax S27.1 ☑
    lung S27.309 ☑
      aspiration J69.0
      bilateral S27.302 ☑
      blast injury (primary) S27.319 ☑
        bilateral S27.312 ☑
        secondary — *see* Injury, intrathoracic, lung, specified type NEC
        unilateral S27.311 ☑
      contusion S27.329 ☑
        bilateral S27.322 ☑
        unilateral S27.321 ☑
      laceration S27.339 ☑
        bilateral S27.332 ☑
        unilateral S27.331 ☑
      specified type NEC S27.399 ☑
        bilateral S27.392 ☑
        unilateral S27.391 ☑
      unilateral S27.301 ☑
    pleura S27.60 ☑
      laceration S27.63 ☑

Injury — *continued*
  intrathoracic — *continued*
    pleura — *continued*
      specified type NEC S27.69 ☑
    pneumothorax S27.0 ☑
    specified organ NEC S27.899 ☑
      contusion S27.892 ☑
      laceration S27.893 ☑
      specified type NEC S27.898 ☑
      thoracic duct — *see* Injury, intrathoracic, specified organ NEC
      thymus gland — *see* Injury, intrathoracic, specified organ NEC
      trachea, thoracic S27.50 ☑
        blast (primary) S27.51 ☑
        contusion S27.52 ☑
        laceration S27.53 ☑
        specified type NEC S27.59 ☑
  iris — *see* Injury, eye, specified site NEC
    penetrating — *see* Injury, eyeball, penetrating
  jaw S09.93 ☑
  jejunum — *see* Injury, intestine, small
  joint NOS T14.8
    old or residual — *see* Disorder, joint, specified type NEC
  kidney S37.00- ☑
    acute (nontraumatic) N17.9
    contusion — *see* Contusion, kidney
    laceration — *see* Laceration, kidney
    specified NEC S37.09- ☑
  knee S89.9- ☑
    contusion — *see* Contusion, knee
    dislocation — *see* Dislocation, knee
    meniscus (lateral) (medial) — *see* Sprain, knee, specified site NEC
      old injury or tear — *see* Derangement, knee, meniscus, due to old injury
    open — *see* Wound, open, knee
    specified NEC S89.8- ☑
    sprain — *see* Sprain, knee
    superficial — *see* Injury, superficial, knee
  labium (majus) (minus) S39.94 ☑
  labyrinth, ear S09.30- ☑
  lacrimal apparatus, duct, gland, or sac — *see* Injury, eye, specified site NEC
  larynx NEC S19.81 ☑
  leg (lower) S89.9- ☑
    blood vessel — *see* Injury, blood vessel, leg
    contusion — *see* Contusion, leg
    fracture — *see* Fracture, leg
    muscle — *see* Injury, muscle, leg
    nerve — *see* Injury, nerve, leg
    open — *see* Wound, open, leg
    specified NEC S89.8- ☑
    superficial — *see* Injury, superficial, leg
  lens, eye — *see* Injury, eye, specified site NEC
    penetrating — *see* Injury, eyeball, penetrating
  limb NEC T14.8
  lip S09.93 ☑
  liver S36.119 ☑
    contusion S36.112 ☑
    laceration S36.113 ☑
      major (stellate) S36.116 ☑
      minor S36.114 ☑
      moderate S36.115 ☑
    specified NEC S36.118 ☑
  lower back S39.92 ☑
    specified NEC S39.82 ☑
  lumbar, lumbosacral (region) S39.92 ☑
    plexus — *see* Injury, lumbosacral plexus
  lumbosacral plexus S34.4 ☑
  lung (*see also* Injury, intrathoracic, lung)
    aspiration J69.0
    transfusion-related (TRALI) J95.84
  lymphatic thoracic duct — *see* Injury, intrathoracic, specified organ NEC
  malar region S09.93 ☑
  mastoid region S09.90 ☑
  maxilla S09.93 ☑
  mediastinum — *see* Injury, intrathoracic, specified organ NEC
  membrane, brain — *see* Injury, intracranial
  meningeal artery — *see* Injury, intracranial, subdural hemorrhage
  meninges (cerebral) — *see* Injury, intracranial

Injury — *continued*
  mesenteric
    artery
      branch S35.299 ✓
        laceration (minor) (superficial) S35.291 ✓
          major S35.292 ✓
        specified NEC S35.298 ✓
      inferior S35.239 ✓
        laceration (minor) (superficial) S35.231 ✓
          major S35.232 ✓
        specified NEC S35.238 ✓
      superior S35.229 ✓
        laceration (minor) (superficial) S35.221 ✓
          major S35.222 ✓
        specified NEC S35.228 ✓
    plexus (inferior) (superior) — *see* Injury, nerve,
      lumbosacral, sympathetic
    vein
      inferior S35.349 ✓
        laceration S35.341 ✓
        specified NEC S35.348 ✓
      superior S35.339 ✓
        laceration S35.331 ✓
        specified NEC S35.338 ✓
  mesentery — *see* Injury, intra-abdominal, specified
    site NEC
  mesosalpinx — *see* Injury, pelvic organ, specified site
    NEC
  middle ear S09.30- ✓
  midthoracic region NOS S29.9 ✓
  mouth S09.93 ✓
  multiple NOS T07
  muscle (and fascia) (and tendon)
    abdomen S39.001 ✓
      laceration S39.021 ✓
      specified type NEC S39.091 ✓
      strain S39.011 ✓
    abductor
      thumb, forearm level — *see* Injury, muscle,
        thumb, abductor
    adductor
      thigh S76.20- ✓
        laceration S76.22- ✓
        specified type NEC S76.29- ✓
        strain S76.21- ✓
    ankle — *see* Injury, muscle, foot
    anterior muscle group, at leg level (lower)
      S86.20- ✓
      laceration S86.22- ✓
      specified type NEC S86.29- ✓
      strain S86.21- ✓
    arm (upper) — *see* Injury, muscle, shoulder
    biceps (parts NEC) S46.20- ✓
      laceration S46.22- ✓
      long head S46.10- ✓
        laceration S46.12- ✓
        specified type NEC S46.19- ✓
        strain S46.11- ✓
      specified type NEC S46.29- ✓
      strain S46.21- ✓
    extensor
      finger(s) (other than thumb) — *see* Injury,
        muscle, finger by site, extensor
      forearm level, specified NEC — *see* Injury,
        muscle, forearm, extensor
      thumb — *see* Injury, muscle, thumb, extensor
      toe (large) (ankle level) (foot level) — *see* Injury,
        muscle, toe, extensor
    finger
      extensor (forearm level) S56.40- ✓
        hand level S66.309 ✓
          laceration S66.329 ✓
          specified type NEC S66.399 ✓
          strain S66.319 ✓
        laceration S56.429 ✓
        specified type NEC S56.499 ✓
        strain S56.419 ✓
      flexor (forearm level) S56.10- ✓
        hand level S66.109 ✓
          laceration S66.129 ✓
          specified type NEC S66.199 ✓
          strain S66.119 ✓
        laceration S56.129 ✓
        specified type NEC S56.199 ✓
        strain S56.119 ✓

Injury — *continued*
  muscle — *continued*
    finger — *continued*
      index
        extensor (forearm level)
          hand level S66.308 ✓
            laceration S66.32- ✓
            specified type NEC S66.39- ✓
            strain S66.31- ✓
          specified type NEC S56.492- ✓
        flexor (forearm level)
          hand level S66.108 ✓
            laceration S66.12- ✓
            specified type NEC S66.19- ✓
            strain S66.11- ✓
          specified type NEC S56.19- ✓
          strain S56.11- ✓
        intrinsic S66.50- ✓
          laceration S66.52- ✓
          specified type NEC S66.59- ✓
          strain S66.51- ✓
      intrinsic S66.509 ✓
        laceration S66.529 ✓
        specified type NEC S66.599 ✓
        strain S66.519 ✓
      little
        extensor (forearm level)
          hand level S66.30- ✓
            laceration S66.32- ✓
            specified type NEC S66.39- ✓
            strain S66.31- ✓
          laceration S56.42- ✓
          specified type NEC S56.49- ✓
          strain S56.41- ✓
        flexor (forearm level)
          hand level S66.10- ✓
            laceration S66.12- ✓
            specified type NEC S66.19- ✓
            strain S66.11- ✓
          laceration S56.12- ✓
          specified type NEC S56.19- ✓
          strain S56.11- ✓
        intrinsic S66.50- ✓
          laceration S66.52- ✓
          specified type NEC S66.59- ✓
          strain S66.51- ✓
      middle
        extensor (forearm level)
          hand level S66.30- ✓
            laceration S66.32- ✓
            specified type NEC S66.39- ✓
            strain S66.31- ✓
          laceration S56.42- ✓
          specified type NEC S56.49- ✓
          strain S56.41- ✓
        flexor (forearm level)
          hand level S66.10- ✓
            laceration S66.12- ✓
            specified type NEC S66.19- ✓
            strain S66.11- ✓
          laceration S56.12- ✓
          specified type NEC S56.19- ✓
          strain S56.11- ✓
        intrinsic S66.50- ✓
          laceration S66.52- ✓
          specified type NEC S66.59- ✓
          strain S66.51- ✓
      ring
        extensor (forearm level)
          hand level S66.30- ✓
            laceration S66.32- ✓
            specified type NEC S66.39- ✓
            strain S66.31- ✓
          laceration S56.42- ✓
          specified type NEC S56.49- ✓
          strain S56.41- ✓
        flexor (forearm level)
          hand level S66.10- ✓
            laceration S66.12- ✓
            specified type NEC S66.19- ✓
            strain S66.11- ✓
          laceration S56.12- ✓
          specified type NEC S56.19- ✓
          strain S56.11- ✓
        intrinsic S66.50- ✓
          laceration S66.52- ✓

Injury — *continued*
  muscle — *continued*
    finger — *continued*
      ring — *continued*
        intrinsic — *continued*
          specified type NEC S66.59- ✓
          strain S66.51- ✓
    flexor
      finger(s) (other than thumb) — *see* Injury,
        muscle, finger
      forearm level, specified NEC — *see* Injury,
        muscle, forearm, flexor
      thumb — *see* Injury, muscle, thumb, flexor
      toe (long) (ankle level) (foot level) — *see* Injury,
        muscle, toe, flexor
    foot S96.90- ✓
      intrinsic S96.20- ✓
        laceration S96.22- ✓
        specified type NEC S96.29- ✓
        strain S96.21- ✓
      laceration S96.92- ✓
      long extensor, toe — *see* Injury, muscle, toe,
        extensor
      long flexor, toe — *see* Injury, muscle, toe, flexor
      specified
        site NEC S96.80- ✓
          laceration S96.82- ✓
          specified type NEC S96.89- ✓
          strain S96.81- ✓
        type S96.99- ✓
      strain S96.91- ✓
    forearm (level) S56.90- ✓
      extensor S56.50- ✓
        laceration S56.52- ✓
        specified type NEC S56.59- ✓
        strain S56.51- ✓
      flexor S56.20- ✓
        laceration S56.22- ✓
        specified type NEC S56.29- ✓
        strain S56.21- ✓
      laceration S56.92- ✓
      specified S56.99- ✓
        site NEC S56.80- ✓
          laceration S56.82- ✓
          strain S56.81- ✓
          type NEC S56.89- ✓
      strain S56.91- ✓
    hand (level) S66.90- ✓
      laceration S66.92- ✓
      specified
        site NEC S66.80- ✓
          laceration S66.82- ✓
          specified type NEC S66.89- ✓
          strain S66.81- ✓
        type NEC S66.99- ✓
      strain S66.91- ✓
    head S09.10 ✓
      laceration S09.12 ✓
      specified type NEC S09.19 ✓
      strain S09.11 ✓
    hip NEC S76.00- ✓
      laceration S76.02- ✓
      specified type NEC S76.09- ✓
      strain S76.01- ✓
    intrinsic
      ankle and foot level — *see* Injury, muscle, foot,
        intrinsic
      finger (other than thumb) — *see* Injury, muscle,
        finger by site, intrinsic
      foot (level) — *see* Injury, muscle, foot, intrinsic
      thumb — *see* Injury, muscle, thumb, intrinsic
    leg (level) (lower) S86.90- ✓
      Achilles tendon — *see* Injury, Achilles tendon
      anterior muscle group — *see* Injury, muscle,
        anterior muscle group
      laceration S86.92- ✓
      peroneal muscle group — *see* Injury, muscle,
        peroneal muscle group
      posterior muscle group — *see* Injury, muscle,
        posterior muscle group, leg level
      specified
        site NEC S86.80- ✓
          laceration S86.82- ✓
          specified type NEC S86.89- ✓
          strain S86.81- ✓
        type NEC S86.99- ✓

Injury — *continued*
  muscle — *continued*
    leg — *continued*
      strain S86.91- ☑
    long
      extensor toe, at ankle and foot level — *see* Injury, muscle, toe, extensor
      flexor, toe, at ankle and foot level — *see* Injury, muscle, toe, flexor
      head, biceps — *see* Injury, muscle, biceps, long head
    lower back S39.002 ☑
      laceration S39.022 ☑
      specified type NEC S39.092 ☑
      strain S39.012 ☑
    neck (level) S16.9 ☑
      laceration S16.2 ☑
      specified type NEC S16.8 ☑
      strain S16.1 ☑
    pelvis S39.003 ☑
      laceration S39.023 ☑
      specified type NEC S39.093 ☑
      strain S39.013 ☑
    peroneal muscle group, at leg level (lower) S86.30- ☑
      laceration S86.32- ☑
      specified type NEC S86.39- ☑
      strain S86.31- ☑
    posterior muscle (group)
      leg level (lower) S86.10- ☑
        laceration S86.12- ☑
        specified type NEC S86.19- ☑
        strain S86.11- ☑
      thigh level S76.30- ☑
        laceration S76.32- ☑
        specified type NEC S76.39- ☑
        strain S76.31- ☑
    quadriceps (thigh) S76.10- ☑
      laceration S76.12- ☑
      specified type NEC S76.19- ☑
      strain S76.11- ☑
    shoulder S46.90- ☑
      laceration S46.92- ☑
      rotator cuff — *see* Injury, rotator cuff
      specified site NEC S46.80- ☑
        laceration S46.82- ☑
        specified type NEC S46.89- ☑
        strain S46.81- ☑
      specified type NEC S46.99- ☑
      strain S46.91- ☑
    thigh NEC (level) S76.90- ☑
      adductor — *see* Injury, muscle, adductor, thigh
      laceration S76.92- ☑
      posterior muscle (group) — *see* Injury, muscle, posterior muscle, thigh level
      quadriceps — *see* Injury, muscle, quadriceps
      specified
        site NEC S76.80- ☑
          laceration S76.82- ☑
          specified type NEC S76.89- ☑
          strain S76.81- ☑
        type NEC S76.99- ☑
      strain S76.91- ☑
    thorax (level) S29.009 ☑
      back wall S29.002 ☑
      front wall S29.001 ☑
      laceration S29.029 ☑
        back wall S29.022 ☑
        front wall S29.021 ☑
      specified type NEC S29.099 ☑
        back wall S29.092 ☑
        front wall S29.091 ☑
      strain S29.019 ☑
        back wall S29.012 ☑
        front wall S29.011 ☑
    thumb
      abductor (forearm level) S56.30- ☑
        laceration S56.32- ☑
        specified type NEC S56.39- ☑
        strain S56.31- ☑
      extensor (forearm level) S56.30- ☑
        hand level S66.20- ☑
          laceration S66.22- ☑
          specified type NEC S66.29- ☑
          strain S66.21- ☑
        laceration S56.32- ☑

Injury — *continued*
  muscle — *continued*
    thumb — *continued*
      extensor — *continued*
        specified type NEC S56.39- ☑
        strain S56.31- ☑
      flexor (forearm level) S56.00- ☑
        hand level S66.00- ☑
          laceration S66.02- ☑
          specified type NEC S66.09- ☑
          strain S66.01- ☑
        laceration S56.02- ☑
        specified type NEC S56.09- ☑
        strain S56.01- ☑
        wrist level — *see* Injury, muscle, thumb, flexor, hand level
      intrinsic S66.40- ☑
        laceration S66.42- ☑
        specified type NEC S66.49- ☑
        strain S66.41- ☑
    toe (*see also* Injury, muscle, foot)
      extensor, long S96.10- ☑
        laceration S96.12- ☑
        specified type NEC S96.19- ☑
        strain S96.11- ☑
      flexor, long S96.00- ☑
        laceration S96.02- ☑
        specified type NEC S96.09- ☑
        strain S96.01- ☑
    triceps S46.30- ☑
      laceration S46.32- ☑
      specified type NEC S46.39- ☑
      strain S46.31- ☑
    wrist (and hand) level — *see* Injury, muscle, hand
  musculocutaneous nerve — *see* Injury, nerve, musculocutaneous
  myocardium — *see* Injury, heart
  nape — *see* Injury, neck
  nasal (septum) (sinus) S09.92 ☑
  nasopharynx S09.92 ☑
  neck S19.9 ☑
    specified NEC S19.80 ☑
    specified site NEC S19.89 ☑
  nerve NEC T14.8
    abdomen S34.9 ☑
      peripheral S34.6 ☑
      specified site NEC S34.8 ☑
    abducens S04.4- ☑
      contusion S04.4- ☑
      laceration S04.4- ☑
      specified type NEC S04.4- ☑
    abducent — *see* Injury, nerve, abducens
    accessory S04.7- ☑
      contusion S04.7- ☑
      laceration S04.7- ☑
      specified type NEC S04.7- ☑
    acoustic S04.6- ☑
      contusion S04.6- ☑
      laceration S04.6- ☑
      specified type NEC S04.6- ☑
    ankle S94.9- ☑
      cutaneous sensory S94.3- ☑
      specified site NEC — *see* subcategory S94.8 ☑
    anterior crural, femoral — *see* Injury, nerve, femoral
    arm (upper) S44.9- ☑
      axillary — *see* Injury, nerve, axillary
      cutaneous — *see* Injury, nerve, cutaneous, arm
      median — *see* Injury, nerve, median, upper arm
      musculocutaneous — *see* Injury, nerve, musculocutaneous
      radial — *see* Injury, nerve, radial, upper arm
      specified site NEC — *see* subcategory S44.8 ☑
      ulnar — *see* Injury, nerve, ulnar, arm
    auditory — *see* Injury, nerve, acoustic
    axillary S44.3- ☑
    brachial plexus — *see* Injury, brachial plexus
    cervical sympathetic S14.5 ☑
    cranial S04.9 ☑
      contusion S04.9 ☑
      eighth (acoustic or auditory) — *see* Injury, nerve, acoustic
      eleventh (accessory) — *see* Injury, nerve, accessory
      fifth (trigeminal) — *see* Injury, nerve, trigeminal
      first (olfactory) — *see* Injury, nerve, olfactory
      fourth (trochlear) — *see* Injury, nerve, trochlear

Injury — *continued*
  nerve — *continued*
    cranial — *continued*
      laceration S04.9 ☑
      ninth (glossopharyngeal) — *see* Injury, nerve, glossopharyngeal
      second (optic) — *see* Injury, nerve, optic
      seventh (facial) — *see* Injury, nerve, facial
      sixth (abducent) — *see* Injury, nerve, abducens
      specified
        nerve NEC S04.89- ☑
          contusion S04.89- ☑
          laceration S04.89- ☑
          specified type NEC S04.89- ☑
        type NEC S04.9 ☑
      tenth (pneumogastric or vagus) — *see* Injury, nerve, vagus
      third (oculomotor) — *see* Injury, nerve, oculomotor
      twelfth (hypoglossal) — *see* Injury, nerve, hypoglossal
    cutaneous sensory
      ankle (level) S94.3- ☑
      arm (upper) (level) S44.5- ☑
      foot (level) — *see* Injury, nerve, cutaneous sensory, ankle
      forearm (level) S54.3- ☑
      hip (level) S74.2- ☑
      leg (lower level) S84.2- ☑
      shoulder (level) — *see* Injury, nerve, cutaneous sensory, arm
      thigh (level) — *see* Injury, nerve, cutaneous sensory, hip
    deep peroneal — *see* Injury, nerve, peroneal, foot
    digital
      finger S64.4- ☑
        index S64.49- ☑
        little S64.49- ☑
        middle S64.49- ☑
        ring S64.49- ☑
      thumb S64.3- ☑
      toe — *see* Injury, nerve, ankle, specified site NEC
    eighth cranial (acoustic or auditory) — *see* Injury, nerve, acoustic
    eleventh cranial (accessory) — *see* Injury, nerve, accessory
    facial S04.5- ☑
      contusion S04.5- ☑
      laceration S04.5- ☑
      newborn P11.3
      specified type NEC S04.5- ☑
    femoral (hip level) (thigh level) S74.1- ☑
    fifth cranial (trigeminal) — *see* Injury, nerve, trigeminal
    finger (digital) — *see* Injury, nerve, digital, finger
    first cranial (olfactory) — *see* Injury, nerve, olfactory
    foot S94.9- ☑
      cutaneous sensory S94.3- ☑
      deep peroneal S94.2- ☑
      lateral plantar S94.0- ☑
      medial plantar S94.1- ☑
      specified site NEC — *see* subcategory S94.8 ☑
    forearm (level) S54.9- ☑
      cutaneous sensory — *see* Injury, nerve, cutaneous sensory, forearm
      median — *see* Injury, nerve, median
      radial — *see* Injury, nerve, radial
      specified site NEC — *see* subcategory S54.8 ☑
      ulnar — *see* Injury, nerve, ulnar
    fourth cranial (trochlear) — *see* Injury, nerve, trochlear
    glossopharyngeal S04.89- ☑
      specified type NEC S04.89- ☑
    hand S64.9- ☑
      median — *see* Injury, nerve, median, hand
      radial — *see* Injury, nerve, radial, hand
      specified NEC — *see* subcategory S64.8 ☑
      ulnar — *see* Injury, nerve, ulnar, hand
    hip (level) S74.9- ☑
      cutaneous sensory — *see* Injury, nerve, cutaneous sensory, hip
      femoral — *see* Injury, nerve, femoral
      sciatic — *see* Injury, nerve, sciatic
      specified site NEC — *see* subcategory S74.8 ☑

▽ Subterms under main terms may continue to next column or page   ☑ Additional Character Required — Refer to the Tabular List for Character Selection   189

Injury — Injury

Injury — *continued*
  nerve — *continued*
    hypoglossal S04.89- ☑
      specified type NEC S04.89- ☑
    lateral plantar S94.0- ☑
    leg (lower) S84.9- ☑
      cutaneous sensory — *see* Injury, nerve, cutaneous sensory, leg
      peroneal — *see* Injury, nerve, peroneal
      specified site NEC — *see* subcategory S84.8 ☑
      tibial — *see* Injury, nerve, tibial
      upper — *see* Injury, nerve, thigh
    lower
      back — *see* Injury, nerve, abdomen, specified site NEC
        peripheral — *see* Injury, nerve, abdomen, peripheral
      limb — *see* Injury, nerve, leg
    lumbar plexus — *see* Injury, nerve, lumbosacral, sympathetic
    lumbar spinal — *see* Injury, nerve, spinal, lumbar
    lumbosacral
      plexus — *see* Injury, nerve, lumbosacral, sympathetic
      sympathetic S34.5 ☑
    medial plantar S94.1- ☑
    median (forearm level) S54.1- ☑
      hand (level) S64.1- ☑
      upper arm (level) S44.1- ☑
      wrist (level) — *see* Injury, nerve, median, hand
    musculocutaneous S44.4- ☑
    musculospiral (upper arm level) — *see* Injury, nerve, radial, upper arm
    neck S14.9 ☑
      peripheral S14.4 ☑
      specified site NEC S14.8 ☑
      sympathetic S14.5 ☑
    ninth cranial (glossopharyngeal) — *see* Injury, nerve, glossopharyngeal
    oculomotor S04.1- ☑
      contusion S04.1- ☑
      laceration S04.1- ☑
      specified type NEC S04.1- ☑
    olfactory S04.81- ☑
      specified type NEC S04.81- ☑
    optic S04.01- ☑
      contusion S04.01- ☑
      laceration S04.01- ☑
      specified type NEC S04.01- ☑
    pelvic girdle — *see* Injury, nerve, hip
    pelvis — *see* Injury, nerve, abdomen, specified site NEC
      peripheral — *see* Injury, nerve, abdomen, peripheral
    peripheral NEC T14.8
      abdomen — *see* Injury, nerve, abdomen, peripheral
      lower back — *see* Injury, nerve, abdomen, peripheral
      neck — *see* Injury, nerve, neck, peripheral
      pelvis — *see* Injury, nerve, abdomen, peripheral
      specified NEC T14.8
    peroneal (lower leg level) S84.1- ☑
      foot S94.2- ☑
    plexus
      brachial — *see* Injury, brachial plexus
      celiac, coeliac — *see* Injury, nerve, lumbosacral, sympathetic
      mesenteric, inferior — *see* Injury, nerve, lumbosacral, sympathetic
      sacral — *see* Injury, lumbosacral plexus
      spinal
        brachial — *see* Injury, brachial plexus
        lumbosacral — *see* Injury, lumbosacral plexus
    pneumogastric — *see* Injury, nerve, vagus
    radial (forearm level) S54.2- ☑
      hand (level) S64.2- ☑
      upper arm (level) S44.2- ☑
      wrist (level) — *see* Injury, nerve, radial, hand
    root — *see* Injury, nerve, spinal, root
    sacral plexus — *see* Injury, lumbosacral plexus
    sacral spinal — *see* Injury, nerve, spinal, sacral
    sciatic (hip level) (thigh level) S74.0- ☑
    second cranial (optic) — *see* Injury, nerve, optic
    seventh cranial (facial) — *see* Injury, nerve, facial

Injury — *continued*
  nerve — *continued*
    shoulder — *see* Injury, nerve, arm
    sixth cranial (abducent) — *see* Injury, nerve, abducens
    spinal
      plexus — *see* Injury, nerve, plexus, spinal
      root
        cervical S14.2 ☑
        dorsal S24.2 ☑
        lumbar S34.21 ☑
        sacral S34.22 ☑
        thoracic — *see* Injury, nerve, spinal, root, dorsal
    splanchnic — *see* Injury, nerve, lumbosacral, sympathetic
    sympathetic NEC — *see* Injury, nerve, lumbosacral, sympathetic
      cervical — *see* Injury, nerve, cervical sympathetic
    tenth cranial (pneumogastric or vagus) — *see* Injury, nerve, vagus
    thigh (level) — *see* Injury, nerve, hip
      cutaneous sensory — *see* Injury, nerve, cutaneous sensory, hip
      femoral — *see* Injury, nerve, femoral
      sciatic — *see* Injury, nerve, sciatic
      specified NEC — *see* Injury, nerve, hip
    third cranial (oculomotor) — *see* Injury, nerve, oculomotor
    thorax S24.9 ☑
      peripheral S24.3 ☑
      specified site NEC S24.8 ☑
      sympathetic S24.4 ☑
    thumb, digital — *see* Injury, nerve, digital, thumb
    tibial (lower leg level) (posterior) S84.0- ☑
    toe — *see* Injury, nerve, ankle
    trigeminal S04.3- ☑
      contusion S04.3- ☑
      laceration S04.3- ☑
      specified type NEC S04.3- ☑
    trochlear S04.2- ☑
      contusion S04.2- ☑
      laceration S04.2- ☑
      specified type NEC S04.2- ☑
    twelfth cranial (hypoglossal) — *see* Injury, nerve, hypoglossal
    ulnar (forearm level) S54.0- ☑
      arm (upper) (level) S44.0- ☑
      hand (level) S64.0- ☑
      wrist (level) — *see* Injury, nerve, ulnar, hand
    vagus S04.89- ☑
      specified type NEC S04.89- ☑
    wrist (level) — *see* Injury, nerve, hand
  ninth cranial nerve (glossopharyngeal) — *see* Injury, nerve, glossopharyngeal
  nose (septum) S09.92 ☑
  obstetrical O71.9
    specified NEC O71.89
  occipital (region) (scalp) S09.90 ☑
    lobe — *see* Injury, intracranial
  optic chiasm S04.02 ☑
  optic radiation S04.03- ☑
  optic tract and pathways S04.03- ☑
  orbit, orbital (region) — *see* Injury, eye
    penetrating (with foreign body) — *see* Injury, eye, orbit, penetrating
    specified NEC — *see* Injury, eye, specified site NEC
  ovary, ovarian S37.409 ☑
    bilateral S37.402 ☑
      contusion S37.422 ☑
      laceration S37.432 ☑
      specified type NEC S37.492 ☑
    blood vessel — *see* Injury, blood vessel, ovarian
    contusion S37.429 ☑
      bilateral S37.422 ☑
      unilateral S37.421 ☑
    laceration S37.439 ☑
      bilateral S37.432 ☑
      unilateral S37.431 ☑
    specified type NEC S37.499 ☑
      bilateral S37.492 ☑
      unilateral S37.491 ☑
    unilateral S37.401 ☑
      contusion S37.421 ☑
      laceration S37.431 ☑

Injury — *continued*
  ovary, ovarian — *continued*
    unilateral — *continued*
      specified type NEC S37.491 ☑
  palate (hard) (soft) S09.93 ☑
  pancreas S36.209 ☑
    body S36.201 ☑
      contusion S36.221 ☑
      laceration S36.231 ☑
        major S36.261 ☑
        minor S36.241 ☑
        moderate S36.251 ☑
      specified type NEC S36.291 ☑
    contusion S36.229 ☑
    head S36.200 ☑
      contusion S36.220 ☑
      laceration S36.230 ☑
        major S36.260 ☑
        minor S36.240 ☑
        moderate S36.250 ☑
      specified type NEC S36.290 ☑
    laceration S36.239 ☑
      major S36.269 ☑
      minor S36.249 ☑
      moderate S36.259 ☑
    specified type NEC S36.299 ☑
    tail S36.202 ☑
      contusion S36.222 ☑
      laceration S36.232 ☑
        major S36.262 ☑
        minor S36.242 ☑
        moderate S36.252 ☑
      specified type NEC S36.292 ☑
  parietal (region) (scalp) S09.90 ☑
    lobe — *see* Injury, intracranial
  patellar ligament (tendon) S76.10- ☑
    laceration S76.12- ☑
    specified NEC S76.19- ☑
    strain S76.11- ☑
  pelvis, pelvic (floor) S39.93 ☑
    complicating delivery O70.1
    joint or ligament, complicating delivery O71.6
    organ S37.90 ☑
      with ectopic or molar pregnancy O08.6
      complication of abortion — *see* Abortion
      contusion S37.92 ☑
      following ectopic or molar pregnancy O08.6
      laceration S37.93 ☑
      obstetrical trauma NEC O71.5
      specified
        site NEC S37.899 ☑
          contusion S37.892 ☑
          laceration S37.893 ☑
          specified type NEC S37.898 ☑
        type NEC S37.99 ☑
    specified NEC S39.83 ☑
  penis S39.94 ☑
  perineum S39.94 ☑
  peritoneum S36.81 ☑
    laceration S36.893 ☑
  periurethral tissue — *see* Injury, urethra
    complicating delivery O71.82
  phalanges
    foot — *see* Injury, foot
    hand — *see* Injury, hand
  pharynx NEC S19.85 ☑
  pleura — *see* Injury, intrathoracic, pleura
  plexus
    brachial — *see* Injury, brachial plexus
    cardiac — *see* Injury, nerve, thorax, sympathetic
    celiac, coeliac — *see* Injury, nerve, lumbosacral, sympathetic
    esophageal — *see* Injury, nerve, thorax, sympathetic
    hypogastric — *see* Injury, nerve, lumbosacral, sympathetic
    lumbar, lumbosacral — *see* Injury, lumbosacral plexus
    mesenteric — *see* Injury, nerve, lumbosacral, sympathetic
    pulmonary — *see* Injury, nerve, thorax, sympathetic
  postcardiac surgery (syndrome) I97.0
  prepuce S39.94 ☑
  prostate S37.829 ☑
    contusion S37.822 ☑

Injury — *continued*
  prostate — *continued*
    laceration S37.823 ☑
    specified type NEC S37.828 ☑
  pubic region S39.94 ☑
  pudendum S39.94 ☑
  pulmonary plexus — *see* Injury, nerve, thorax, sympa-
      thetic
  rectovaginal septum NEC S39.83 ☑
  rectum — *see* Injury, intestine, large, rectum
  retina — *see* Injury, eye, specified site NEC
    penetrating — *see* Injury, eyeball, penetrating
  retroperitoneal — *see* Injury, intra-abdominal, speci-
      fied site NEC
  rotator cuff (muscle(s)) (tendon(s)) S46.00- ☑
    laceration S46.02- ☑
    specified type NEC S46.09- ☑
    strain S46.01- ☑
  round ligament — *see* Injury, pelvic organ, specified
      site NEC
  sacral plexus — *see* Injury, lumbosacral plexus
  salivary duct or gland S09.93 ☑
  scalp S09.90 ☑
    newborn (birth injury) P12.9
      due to monitoring (electrode) (sampling inci-
          sion) P12.4
      specified NEC P12.89
        caput succedaneum P12.81
  scapular region — *see* Injury, shoulder
  sclera — *see* Injury, eye, specified site NEC
    penetrating — *see* Injury, eyeball, penetrating
  scrotum S39.94 ☑
  second cranial nerve (optic) — *see* Injury, nerve, optic
  seminal vesicle — *see* Injury, pelvic organ, specified
      site NEC
  seventh cranial nerve (facial) — *see* Injury, nerve, facial
  shoulder S49.9- ☑
    blood vessel — *see* Injury, blood vessel, arm
    contusion — *see* Contusion, shoulder
    dislocation — *see* Dislocation, shoulder
    fracture — *see* Fracture, shoulder
    muscle — *see* Injury, muscle, shoulder
    nerve — *see* Injury, nerve, shoulder
    open — *see* Wound, open, shoulder
    specified type NEC S49.8- ☑
    sprain — *see* Sprain, shoulder girdle
    superficial — *see* Injury, superficial, shoulder
  sinus
    cavernous — *see* Injury, intracranial
    nasal S09.92 ☑
  sixth cranial nerve (abducent) — *see* Injury, nerve,
      abducens
  skeleton, birth injury P13.9
    specified part NEC P13.8
  skin NEC T14.8
    surface intact — *see* Injury, superficial
  skull NEC S09.90 ☑
  specified NEC T14.8
  spermatic cord (pelvic region) S37.898 ☑
    scrotal region S39.848 ☑
  spinal (cord)
    cervical (neck) S14.109 ☑
      anterior cord syndrome S14.139 ☑
        C1 level S14.131 ☑
        C2 level S14.132 ☑
        C3 level S14.133 ☑
        C4 level S14.134 ☑
        C5 level S14.135 ☑
        C6 level S14.136 ☑
        C7 level S14.137 ☑
        C8 level S14.138 ☑
      Brown-Séquard syndrome S14.149 ☑
        C1 level S14.141 ☑
        C2 level S14.142 ☑
        C3 level S14.143 ☑
        C4 level S14.144 ☑
        C5 level S14.145 ☑
        C6 level S14.146 ☑
        C7 level S14.147 ☑
        C8 level S14.148 ☑
      C1 level S14.101 ☑
      C2 level S14.102 ☑
      C3 level S14.103 ☑
      C4 level S14.104 ☑
      C5 level S14.105 ☑
      C6 level S14.106 ☑

Injury — *continued*
  spinal — *continued*
    cervical –- *continued*
      C7 level S14.107 ☑
      C8 level S14.108 ☑
      central cord syndrome S14.129 ☑
        C1 level S14.121 ☑
        C2 level S14.122 ☑
        C3 level S14.123 ☑
        C4 level S14.124 ☑
        C5 level S14.125 ☑
        C6 level S14.126 ☑
        C7 level S14.127 ☑
        C8 level S14.128 ☑
      complete lesion S14.119 ☑
        C1 level S14.111 ☑
        C2 level S14.112 ☑
        C3 level S14.113 ☑
        C4 level S14.114 ☑
        C5 level S14.115 ☑
        C6 level S14.116 ☑
        C7 level S14.117 ☑
        C8 level S14.118 ☑
      concussion S14.0 ☑
      edema S14.0 ☑
      incomplete lesion specified NEC S14.159 ☑
        C1 level S14.151 ☑
        C2 level S14.152 ☑
        C3 level S14.153 ☑
        C4 level S14.154 ☑
        C5 level S14.155 ☑
        C6 level S14.156 ☑
        C7 level S14.157 ☑
        C8 level S14.158 ☑
      posterior cord syndrome S14.159 ☑
        C1 level S14.151 ☑
        C2 level S14.152 ☑
        C3 level S14.153 ☑
        C4 level S14.154 ☑
        C5 level S14.155 ☑
        C6 level S14.156 ☑
        C7 level S14.157 ☑
        C8 level S14.158 ☑
    dorsal — *see* Injury, spinal, thoracic
    lumbar S34.109 ☑
      complete lesion S34.119 ☑
        L1 level S34.111 ☑
        L2 level S34.112 ☑
        L3 level S34.113 ☑
        L4 level S34.114 ☑
        L5 level S34.115 ☑
      concussion S34.01 ☑
      edema S34.01 ☑
      incomplete lesion S34.129 ☑
        L1 level S34.121 ☑
        L2 level S34.122 ☑
        L3 level S34.123 ☑
        L4 level S34.124 ☑
        L5 level S34.125 ☑
      L1 level S34.101 ☑
      L2 level S34.102 ☑
      L3 level S34.103 ☑
      L4 level S34.104 ☑
      L5 level S34.105 ☑
    nerve root NEC
      cervical — *see* Injury, nerve, spinal, root, cervi-
          cal
      dorsal — *see* Injury, nerve, spinal, root, dorsal
      lumbar S34.21 ☑
      sacral S34.22 ☑
      thoracic — *see* Injury, nerve, spinal, root, dorsal
    plexus
      brachial — *see* Injury, brachial plexus
      lumbosacral — *see* Injury, lumbosacral plexus
    sacral S34.139 ☑
      complete lesion S34.131 ☑
      incomplete lesion S34.132 ☑
    thoracic S24.109 ☑
      anterior cord syndrome S24.139 ☑
        T1 level S24.131 ☑
        T2-T6 level S24.132 ☑
        T7-T10 level S24.133 ☑
        T11-T12 level S24.134 ☑
      Brown-Séquard syndrome S24.149 ☑
        T1 level S24.141 ☑

Injury — *continued*
  spinal — *continued*
    thoracic — *continued*
      Brown-Séquard syndrome — *continued*
        T2-T6 level S24.142 ☑
        T7-T10 level S24.143 ☑
        T11-T12 level S24.144 ☑
      complete lesion S24.119 ☑
        T1 level S24.111 ☑
        T2-T6 level S24.112 ☑
        T7-T10 level S24.113 ☑
        T11-T12 level S24.114 ☑
      concussion S24.0 ☑
      edema S24.0 ☑
      incomplete lesion specified NEC S24.159 ☑
        T1 level S24.151 ☑
        T2-T6 level S24.152 ☑
        T7-T10 level S24.153 ☑
        T11-T12 level S24.154 ☑
      posterior cord syndrome S24.159 ☑
        T1 level S24.151 ☑
        T2-T6 level S24.152 ☑
        T7-T10 level S24.153 ☑
        T11-T12 level S24.154 ☑
      T1 level S24.101 ☑
      T2-T6 level S24.102 ☑
      T7-T10 level S24.103 ☑
      T11-T12 level S24.104 ☑
  splanchnic nerve — *see* Injury, nerve, lumbosacral,
      sympathetic
  spleen S36.00 ☑
    contusion S36.029 ☑
      major S36.021 ☑
      minor S36.020 ☑
    laceration S36.039 ☑
      major (massive) (stellate) S36.032 ☑
      moderate S36.031 ☑
      superficial (capsular) (minor) S36.030 ☑
    specified type NEC S36.09 ☑
  splenic artery — *see* Injury, blood vessel, celiac artery,
      branch
  stellate ganglion — *see* Injury, nerve, thorax, sympa-
      thetic
  sternal region S29.9 ☑
  stomach S36.30 ☑
    contusion S36.32 ☑
    laceration S36.33 ☑
    specified type NEC S36.39 ☑
  subconjunctival — *see* Injury, eye, conjunctiva
  subcutaneous NEC T14.8
  submaxillary region S09.93 ☑
  submental region S09.93 ☑
  subungual
    fingers — *see* Injury, hand
    toes — *see* Injury, foot
  superficial NEC T14.8
    abdomen, abdominal (wall) S30.92 ☑
      abrasion S30.811 ☑
      bite S30.871 ☑
        insect S30.861 ☑
      contusion S30.1 ☑
      external constriction S30.841 ☑
      foreign body S30.851 ☑
    abrasion — *see* Abrasion, by site
    adnexa, eye NEC — *see* Injury, eye, specified site
        NEC
    alveolar process — *see* Injury, superficial, oral cav-
        ity
    ankle S90.91- ☑
      abrasion — *see* Abrasion, ankle
      bite — *see* Bite, ankle
      blister — *see* Blister, ankle
      contusion — *see* Contusion, ankle
      external constriction — *see* Constriction, exter-
          nal, ankle
      foreign body — *see* Foreign body, superficial,
          ankle
    anus S30.98 ☑
    arm (upper) S40.92- ☑
      abrasion — *see* Abrasion, arm
      bite — *see* Bite, superficial, arm
      blister — *see* Blister, arm (upper)
      contusion — *see* Contusion, arm
      external constriction — *see* Constriction, exter-
          nal, arm

Injury — *continued*
  superficial — *continued*
    arm — *continued*
      foreign body — *see* Foreign body, superficial, arm
    auditory canal (external) (meatus) — *see* Injury, superficial, ear
    auricle — *see* Injury, superficial, ear
    axilla — *see* Injury, superficial, arm
    back (*see also* Injury, superficial, thorax, back)
      lower S30.91 ☑
        abrasion S30.810 ☑
        contusion S30.0 ☑
        external constriction S30.840 ☑
        superficial
          bite NEC S30.870 ☑
            insect S30.860 ☑
          foreign body S30.850 ☑
    bite NEC — *see* Bite, superficial NEC, by site
    blister — *see* Blister, by site
    breast S20.10- ☑
      abrasion — *see* Abrasion, breast
      bite — *see* Bite, superficial, breast
      contusion — *see* Contusion, breast
      external constriction — *see* Constriction, external, breast
      foreign body — *see* Foreign body, superficial, breast
    brow — *see* Injury, superficial, head, specified NEC
    buttock S30.91 ☑
    calf — *see* Injury, superficial, leg
    canthus, eye — *see* Injury, superficial, periocular area
    cheek (external) — *see* Injury, superficial, head, specified NEC
      internal — *see* Injury, superficial, oral cavity
    chest wall — *see* Injury, superficial, thorax
    chin — *see* Injury, superficial, head NEC
    clitoris S30.95 ☑
    conjunctiva — *see* Injury, eye, conjunctiva
      with foreign body (in conjunctival sac) — *see* Foreign body, conjunctival sac
    contusion — *see* Contusion, by site
    costal region — *see* Injury, superficial, thorax
    digit(s)
      hand — *see* Injury, superficial, finger
    ear (auricle) (canal) (external) S00.40- ☑
      abrasion — *see* Abrasion, ear
      bite — *see* Bite, superficial, ear
      contusion — *see* Contusion, ear
      external constriction — *see* Constriction, external, ear
      foreign body — *see* Foreign body, superficial, ear
    elbow S50.90- ☑
      abrasion — *see* Abrasion, elbow
      bite — *see* Bite, superficial, elbow
      blister — *see* Blister, elbow
      contusion — *see* Contusion, elbow
      external constriction — *see* Constriction, external, elbow
      foreign body — *see* Foreign body, superficial, elbow
    epididymis S30.94 ☑
    epigastric region S30.92 ☑
    epiglottis — *see* Injury, superficial, throat
    esophagus
      cervical — *see* Injury, superficial, throat
    external constriction — *see* Constriction, external, by site
    extremity NEC T14.8
    eyeball NEC — *see* Injury, eye, specified site NEC
    eyebrow — *see* Injury, superficial, periocular area
    eyelid S00.20- ☑
      abrasion — *see* Abrasion, eyelid
      bite — *see* Bite, superficial, eyelid
      contusion — *see* Contusion, eyelid
      external constriction — *see* Constriction, external, eyelid
      foreign body — *see* Foreign body, superficial, eyelid
    face NEC — *see* Injury, superficial, head, specified NEC
    finger(s) S60.949 ☑
      abrasion — *see* Abrasion, finger
      bite — *see* Bite, superficial, finger

Injury — *continued*
  superficial — *continued*
    finger(s) — *continued*
      blister — *see* Blister, finger
      contusion — *see* Contusion, finger
      external constriction — *see* Constriction, external, finger
      foreign body — *see* Foreign body, superficial, finger
      index S60.94- ☑
      insect bite — *see* Bite, by site, superficial, insect
      little S60.94- ☑
      middle S60.94- ☑
      ring S60.94- ☑
    flank S30.92 ☑
    foot S90.92- ☑
      abrasion — *see* Abrasion, foot
      bite — *see* Bite, foot
      blister — *see* Blister, foot
      contusion — *see* Contusion, foot
      external constriction — *see* Constriction, external, foot
      foreign body — *see* Foreign body, superficial, foot
    forearm S50.91- ☑
      abrasion — *see* Abrasion, forearm
      bite — *see* Bite, forearm, superficial
      blister — *see* Blister, forearm
      contusion — *see* Contusion, forearm
      elbow only — *see* Injury, superficial, elbow
      external constriction — *see* Constriction, external, forearm
      foreign body — *see* Foreign body, superficial, forearm
    forehead — *see* Injury, superficial, head NEC
    foreign body — *see* Foreign body, superficial
    genital organs, external
      female S30.97 ☑
      male S30.96 ☑
    globe (eye) — *see* Injury, eye, specified site NEC
    groin S30.92 ☑
    gum — *see* Injury, superficial, oral cavity
    hand S60.92- ☑
      abrasion — *see* Abrasion, hand
      bite — *see* Bite, superficial, hand
      contusion — *see* Contusion, hand
      external constriction — *see* Constriction, external, hand
      foreign body — *see* Foreign body, superficial, hand
    head S00.90 ☑
      ear — *see* Injury, superficial, ear
      eyelid — *see* Injury, superficial, eyelid
      nose S00.30 ☑
      oral cavity S00.502 ☑
      scalp S00.00 ☑
      specified site NEC S00.80 ☑
    heel — *see* Injury, superficial, foot
    hip S70.91- ☑
      abrasion — *see* Abrasion, hip
      bite — *see* Bite, superficial, hip
      blister — *see* Blister, hip
      contusion — *see* Contusion, hip
      external constriction — *see* Constriction, external, hip
      foreign body — *see* Foreign body, superficial, hip
    iliac region — *see* Injury, superficial, abdomen
    inguinal region — *see* Injury, superficial, abdomen
    insect bite — *see* Bite, by site, superficial, insect
    interscapular region — *see* Injury, superficial, thorax, back
    jaw — *see* Injury, superficial, head, specified NEC
    knee S80.91- ☑
      abrasion — *see* Abrasion, knee
      bite — *see* Bite, superficial, knee
      blister — *see* Blister, knee
      contusion — *see* Contusion, knee
      external constriction — *see* Constriction, external, knee
      foreign body — *see* Foreign body, superficial, knee
    labium (majus) (minus) S30.95 ☑
    lacrimal (apparatus) (gland) (sac) — *see* Injury, eye, specified site NEC
    larynx — *see* Injury, superficial, throat

Injury — *continued*
  superficial — *continued*
    leg (lower) S80.92- ☑
      abrasion — *see* Abrasion, leg
      bite — *see* Bite, superficial, leg
      contusion — *see* Contusion, leg
      external constriction — *see* Constriction, external, leg
      foreign body — *see* Foreign body, superficial, leg
      knee — *see* Injury, superficial, knee
    limb NEC T14.8
    lip S00.501 ☑
    lower back S30.91 ☑
    lumbar region S30.91 ☑
    malar region — *see* Injury, superficial, head, specified NEC
    mammary — *see* Injury, superficial, breast
    mastoid region — *see* Injury, superficial, head, specified NEC
    mouth — *see* Injury, superficial, oral cavity
    muscle NEC T14.8
    nail NEC T14.8
      finger — *see* Injury, superficial, finger
      toe — *see* Injury, superficial, toe
    nasal (septum) — *see* Injury, superficial, nose
    neck S10.90 ☑
      specified site NEC S10.80 ☑
    nose (septum) S00.30 ☑
    occipital region — *see* Injury, superficial, scalp
    oral cavity S00.502 ☑
    orbital region — *see* Injury, superficial, periocular area
    palate — *see* Injury, superficial, oral cavity
    palm — *see* Injury, superficial, hand
    parietal region — *see* Injury, superficial, scalp
    pelvis S30.91 ☑
      girdle — *see* Injury, superficial, hip
    penis S30.93 ☑
    perineum
      female S30.95 ☑
      male S30.91 ☑
    periocular area S00.20- ☑
      abrasion — *see* Abrasion, eyelid
      bite — *see* Bite, superficial, eyelid
      contusion — *see* Contusion, eyelid
      external constriction — *see* Constriction, external, eyelid
      foreign body — *see* Foreign body, superficial, eyelid
    phalanges
      finger — *see* Injury, superficial, finger
      toe — *see* Injury, superficial, toe
    pharynx — *see* Injury, superficial, throat
    pinna — *see* Injury, superficial, ear
    popliteal space — *see* Injury, superficial, knee
    prepuce S30.93 ☑
    pubic region S30.91 ☑
    pudendum
      female S30.97 ☑
      male S30.96 ☑
    sacral region S30.91 ☑
    scalp S00.00 ☑
    scapular region — *see* Injury, superficial, shoulder
    sclera — *see* Injury, eye, specified site NEC
    scrotum S30.94 ☑
    shin — *see* Injury, superficial, leg
    shoulder S40.91- ☑
      abrasion — *see* Abrasion, shoulder
      bite — *see* Bite, superficial, shoulder
      blister — *see* Blister, shoulder
      contusion — *see* Contusion, shoulder
      external constriction — *see* Constriction, external, shoulder
      foreign body — *see* Foreign body, superficial, shoulder
    skin NEC T14.8
    sternal region — *see* Injury, superficial, thorax, front
    subconjunctival — *see* Injury, eye, specified site NEC
    subcutaneous NEC T14.8
    submaxillary region — *see* Injury, superficial, head, specified NEC
    submental region — *see* Injury, superficial, head, specified NEC

☑ **Additional Character Required** — Refer to the Tabular List for Character Selection   Subterms under main terms may continue to next column or page

Injury — *continued*
  superficial — *continued*
    subungual
      finger(s) — *see* Injury, superficial, finger
      toe(s) — *see* Injury, superficial, toe
    supraclavicular fossa — *see* Injury, superficial, neck
    supraorbital — *see* Injury, superficial, head, specified NEC
    temple — *see* Injury, superficial, head, specified NEC
    temporal region — *see* Injury, superficial, head, specified NEC
    testis S30.94 ☑
    thigh S70.92- ☑
      abrasion — *see* Abrasion, thigh
      bite — *see* Bite, superficial, thigh
      blister — *see* Blister, thigh
      contusion — *see* Contusion, thigh
      external constriction — *see* Constriction, external, thigh
      foreign body — *see* Foreign body, superficial, thigh
    thorax, thoracic (wall) S20.90 ☑
      abrasion — *see* Abrasion, thorax
      back S20.40- ☑
      bite — *see* Bite, thorax, superficial
      blister — *see* Blister, thorax
      contusion — *see* Contusion, thorax
      external constriction — *see* Constriction, external, thorax
      foreign body — *see* Foreign body, superficial, thorax
      front S20.30- ☑
    throat S10.10 ☑
      abrasion S10.11 ☑
      bite S10.17 ☑
        insect S10.16 ☑
      blister S10.12 ☑
      contusion S10.0 ☑
      external constriction S10.14 ☑
      foreign body S10.15 ☑
    thumb S60.93- ☑
      abrasion — *see* Abrasion, thumb
      bite — *see* Bite, superficial, thumb
      blister — *see* Blister, thumb
      contusion — *see* Contusion, thumb
      external constriction — *see* Constriction, external, thumb
      foreign body — *see* Foreign body, superficial, thumb
      insect bite — *see* Bite, by site, superficial, insect
      specified type NEC S60.39 ☑
    toe(s) S90.93- ☑
      abrasion — *see* Abrasion, toe
      bite — *see* Bite, toe
      blister — *see* Blister, toe
      contusion — *see* Contusion, toe
      external constriction — *see* Constriction, external, toe
      foreign body — *see* Foreign body, superficial, toe
      great S90.93- ☑
    tongue — *see* Injury, superficial, oral cavity
    tooth, teeth — *see* Injury, superficial, oral cavity
    trachea S10.10 ☑
    tunica vaginalis S30.94 ☑
    tympanum, tympanic membrane — *see* Injury, superficial, ear
    uvula — *see* Injury, superficial, oral cavity
    vagina S30.95 ☑
    vocal cords — *see* Injury, superficial, throat
    vulva S30.95 ☑
    wrist S60.91- ☑
  supraclavicular region — *see* Injury, neck
  supraorbital S09.93 ☑
  suprarenal gland (multiple) — *see* Injury, adrenal
  surgical complication (external or internal site) — *see* Laceration, accidental complicating surgery
  temple S09.90 ☑
  temporal region S09.90 ☑
  tendon (*see also* Injury, muscle, by site)
    abdomen — *see* Injury, muscle, abdomen
    Achilles — *see* Injury, Achilles tendon
    lower back — *see* Injury, muscle, lower back
    pelvic organs — *see* Injury, muscle, pelvis

Injury — *continued*
  tenth cranial nerve (pneumogastric or vagus) — *see* Injury, nerve, vagus
  testis S39.94 ☑
  thigh S79.92- ☑
    blood vessel — *see* Injury, blood vessel, hip
    contusion — *see* Contusion, thigh
    fracture — *see* Fracture, femur
    muscle — *see* Injury, muscle, thigh
    nerve — *see* Injury, nerve, thigh
    open — *see* Wound, open, thigh
    specified NEC S79.82- ☑
    superficial — *see* Injury, superficial, thigh
  third cranial nerve (oculomotor) — *see* Injury, nerve, oculomotor
  thorax, thoracic S29.9 ☑
    blood vessel — *see* Injury, blood vessel, thorax
    cavity — *see* Injury, intrathoracic
    dislocation — *see* Dislocation, thorax
    external (wall) S29.9 ☑
      contusion — *see* Contusion, thorax
      nerve — *see* Injury, nerve, thorax
      open — *see* Wound, open, thorax
      specified NEC S29.8 ☑
      sprain — *see* Sprain, thorax
      superficial — *see* Injury, superficial, thorax
    fracture — *see* Fracture, thorax
    internal — *see* Injury, intrathoracic
    intrathoracic organ — *see* Injury, intrathoracic
    sympathetic ganglion — *see* Injury, nerve, thorax, sympathetic
  throat (*see also* Injury, neck) S19.9 ☑
  thumb S69.9- ☑
    blood vessel — *see* Injury, blood vessel, thumb
    contusion — *see* Contusion, thumb
    dislocation — *see* Dislocation, thumb
    fracture — *see* Fracture, thumb
    muscle — *see* Injury, muscle, thumb
    nerve — *see* Injury, nerve, digital, thumb
    open — *see* Wound, open, thumb
    specified NEC S69.8- ☑
    sprain — *see* Sprain, thumb
    superficial — *see* Injury, superficial, thumb
  thymus (gland) — *see* Injury, intrathoracic, specified organ NEC
  thyroid (gland) NEC S19.84 ☑
  toe S99.92- ☑
    contusion — *see* Contusion, toe
    dislocation — *see* Dislocation, toe
    fracture — *see* Fracture, toe
    muscle — *see* Injury, muscle, toe
    open — *see* Wound, open, toe
    specified type NEC S99.82- ☑
    sprain — *see* Sprain, toe
    superficial — *see* Injury, superficial, toe
  tongue S09.93 ☑
  tonsil S09.93 ☑
  tooth S09.93 ☑
  trachea (cervical) NEC S19.82 ☑
    thoracic — *see* Injury, intrathoracic, trachea, thoracic
  transfusion-related acute lung (TRALI) J95.84
  tunica vaginalis S39.94 ☑
  twelfth cranial nerve (hypoglossal) — *see* Injury, nerve, hypoglossal
  ureter S37.10 ☑
    contusion S37.12 ☑
    laceration S37.13 ☑
    specified type NEC S37.19 ☑
  urethra (sphincter) S37.30 ☑
    at delivery O71.5
    contusion S37.32 ☑
    laceration S37.33 ☑
    specified type NEC S37.39 ☑
  urinary organ S37.90 ☑
    contusion S37.92 ☑
    laceration S37.93 ☑
    specified
      site NEC S37.899 ☑
        contusion S37.892 ☑
        laceration S37.893 ☑
        specified type NEC S37.898 ☑
      type NEC S37.99 ☑
  uterus, uterine S37.60 ☑
    with ectopic or molar pregnancy O08.6
    blood vessel — *see* Injury, blood vessel, iliac

Injury — *continued*
  uterus, uterine — *continued*
    contusion S37.62 ☑
    laceration S37.63 ☑
      cervix at delivery O71.3
    rupture associated with obstetrics — *see* Rupture, uterus
    specified type NEC S37.69 ☑
  uvula S09.93 ☑
  vagina S39.93 ☑
    abrasion S30.814 ☑
    bite S31.45 ☑
      insect S30.864 ☑
      superficial NEC S30.874 ☑
    contusion S30.23 ☑
    crush S38.03 ☑
    during delivery — *see* Laceration, vagina, during delivery
    external constriction S30.844 ☑
    insect bite S30.864 ☑
    laceration S31.41 ☑
      with foreign body S31.42 ☑
    open wound S31.40 ☑
    puncture S31.43 ☑
      with foreign body S31.44 ☑
    superficial S30.95 ☑
      foreign body S30.854 ☑
  vas deferens — *see* Injury, pelvic organ, specified site NEC
  vascular NEC T14.8
  vein — *see* Injury, blood vessel
  vena cava (superior) S25.20 ☑
    inferior S35.10 ☑
      laceration (minor) (superficial) S35.11 ☑
        major S35.12 ☑
      specified type NEC S35.19 ☑
    laceration (minor) (superficial) S25.21 ☑
      major S25.22 ☑
    specified type NEC S25.29 ☑
  vesical (sphincter) — *see* Injury, bladder
  visual cortex S04.04- ☑
  vitreous (humor) S05.90 ☑
    specified NEC S05.8X- ☑
  vocal cord NEC S19.83 ☑
  vulva S39.94 ☑
    abrasion S30.814 ☑
    bite S31.45 ☑
      insect S30.864 ☑
      superficial NEC S30.874 ☑
    contusion S30.23 ☑
    crush S38.03 ☑
    during delivery — *see* Laceration, perineum, female, during delivery
    external constriction S30.844 ☑
    insect bite S30.864 ☑
    laceration S31.41 ☑
      with foreign body S31.42 ☑
    open wound S31.40 ☑
    puncture S31.43 ☑
      with foreign body S31.44 ☑
    superficial S30.95 ☑
      foreign body S30.854 ☑
  whiplash (cervical spine) S13.4 ☑
  wrist S69.9- ☑
    blood vessel — *see* Injury, blood vessel, hand
    contusion — *see* Contusion, wrist
    dislocation — *see* Dislocation, wrist
    fracture — *see* Fracture, wrist
    muscle — *see* Injury, muscle, hand
    nerve — *see* Injury, nerve, hand
    open — *see* Wound, open, wrist
    specified NEC S69.8- ☑
    sprain — *see* Sprain, wrist
    superficial — *see* Injury, superficial, wrist
Inoculation (*see also* Vaccination)
  complication or reaction — *see* Complications, vaccination
Insanity, insane (*see also* Psychosis)
  adolescent — *see* Schizophrenia
  confusional F28
    acute or subacute F05
  delusional F22
  senile F03 ☑
Insect
  bite — *see* Bite, by site, superficial, insect

Insect — continued
  venomous, poisoning NEC (by) — see Venom, arthropod
Insensitivity
  adrenocorticotropin hormone (ACTH) E27.49
  androgen E34.50
    complete E34.51
    partial E34.52
Insertion
  cord (umbilical) lateral or velamentous O43.12- ☑
  intrauterine contraceptive device (encounter for) — see Intrauterine contraceptive device
Insolation (sunstroke) T67.0 ☑
Insomnia (organic) G47.00
  without objective findings F51.02
  adjustment F51.02
  adjustment disorder F51.02
  behavioral, of childhood Z73.819
    combined type Z73.812
    limit setting type Z73.811
    sleep-onset association type Z73.810
  childhood Z73.819
  chronic F51.04
    somatized tension F51.04
  conditioned F51.04
  due to
    alcohol
      abuse F10.182
      dependence F10.282
      use F10.982
    amphetamines
      abuse F15.182
      dependence F15.282
      use F15.982
    anxiety disorder F51.05
    caffeine
      abuse F15.182
      dependence F15.282
      use F15.982
    cocaine
      abuse F14.182
      dependence F14.282
      use F14.982
    depression F51.05
    drug NEC
      abuse F19.182
      dependence F19.282
      use F19.982
    medical condition G47.01
    mental disorder NEC F51.05
    opioid
      abuse F11.182
      dependence F11.282
      use F11.982
    psychoactive substance NEC
      abuse F19.182
      dependence F19.182
      use F19.982
    sedative, hypnotic, or anxiolytic
      abuse F13.182
      dependence F13.282
      use F13.982
    stimulant NEC
      abuse F15.182
      dependence F15.282
      use F15.982
  fatal familial (FFI) A81.83
  idiopathic F51.01
  learned F51.3
  nonorganic origin F51.01
  not due to a substance or known physiological condition F51.01
    specified NEC F51.09
  paradoxical F51.03
  primary F51.01
  psychiatric F51.05
  psychophysiologic F51.04
  related to psychopathology F51.05
  short-term F51.02
  specified NEC G47.09
  stress-related F51.02
  transient F51.02
Inspiration
  food or foreign body — see Foreign body, by site
  mucus — see Asphyxia, mucus
Inspissated bile syndrome (newborn) P59.1
Instability
  emotional (excessive) F60.3

Instability — continued
  joint (post-traumatic) M25.30
    ankle M25.37- ☑
    due to old ligament injury — see Disorder, ligament
    elbow M25.32- ☑
    flail — see Flail, joint
    foot M25.37- ☑
    hand M25.34- ☑
    hip M25.35- ☑
    knee M25.36- ☑
    lumbosacral — see subcategory M53.2 ☑
    prosthesis — see Complications, joint prosthesis, mechanical, displacement, by site
    sacroiliac — see subcategory M53.2 ☑
    secondary to
      old ligament injury — see Disorder, ligament
      removal of joint prosthesis M96.89
    shoulder (region) M25.31- ☑
    spine — see subcategory M53.2 ☑
    wrist M25.33- ☑
  knee (chronic) M23.5- ☑
  lumbosacral — see subcategory M53.2 ☑
  nervous F48.8
  personality (emotional) F60.3
  spine — see Instability, joint, spine
  vasomotor R55
Institutional syndrome (childhood) F94.2
Institutionalization, affecting child Z62.22
  disinhibited attachment F94.2
Insufficiency, insufficient
  accommodation, old age H52.4
  adrenal (gland) E27.40
    primary E27.1
  adrenocortical E27.40
    drug-induced E27.3
    iatrogenic E27.3
    primary E27.1
  anterior (occlusal) guidance M26.54
  anus K62.89
  aortic (valve) I35.1
    with
      mitral (valve) disease I08.0
        with tricuspid (valve) disease I08.3
      stenosis I35.2
      tricuspid (valve) disease I08.2
        with mitral (valve) disease I08.3
    congenital Q23.1
    rheumatic I06.1
      with
        mitral (valve) disease I08.0
          with tricuspid (valve) disease I08.3
        stenosis I06.2
          with mitral (valve) disease I08.0
            with tricuspid (valve) disease I08.3
        tricuspid (valve) disease I08.2
          with mitral (valve) disease I08.3
    specified cause NEC I35.1
    syphilitic A52.03
  arterial I77.1
    basilar G45.0
    carotid (hemispheric) G45.1
    cerebral I67.81
    coronary (acute or subacute) I24.8
    mesenteric K55.1
    peripheral I73.9
    precerebral (multiple) (bilateral) G45.2
    vertebral G45.0
  arteriovenous I99.8
  biliary K83.8
  cardiac (see also Insufficiency, myocardial)
    due to presence of (cardiac) prosthesis I97.11- ☑
    postprocedural I97.11- ☑
  cardiorenal, hypertensive I13.2
  cardiovascular — see Disease, cardiovascular
  cerebrovascular (acute) I67.81
    with transient focal neurological signs and symptoms G45.8
  circulatory NEC I99.8
    newborn P29.89
  convergence H51.11
  coronary (acute or subacute) I24.8
    chronic or with a stated duration of over 4 weeks I25.89
  corticoadrenal E27.40
    primary E27.1
  dietary E63.9
  divergence H51.8

Insufficiency, insufficient — continued
  food T73.0 ☑
  gastroesophageal K22.8
  gonadal
    ovary E28.39
    testis E29.1
  heart (see also Insufficiency, myocardial)
    newborn P29.0
    valve — see Endocarditis
  hepatic — see Failure, hepatic
  idiopathic autonomic G90.09
  interocclusal distance of fully erupted teeth (ridge) M26.36
  kidney N28.9
    acute N28.9
    chronic N18.9
  lacrimal (secretion) H04.12- ☑
    passages — see Stenosis, lacrimal
  liver — see Failure, hepatic
  lung — see Insufficiency, pulmonary
  mental (congenital) — see Disability, intellectual
  mesenteric K55.1
  mitral (valve) I34.0
    with
      aortic valve disease I08.0
        with tricuspid (valve) disease I08.3
      obstruction or stenosis I05.2
        with aortic valve disease I08.0
      tricuspid (valve) disease I08.1
        with aortic (valve) disease I08.3
    congenital Q23.3
    rheumatic I05.1
      with
        aortic valve disease I08.0
          with tricuspid (valve) disease I08.3
        obstruction or stenosis I05.2
          with aortic valve disease I08.0
            with tricuspid (valve) disease I08.3
        tricuspid (valve) disease I08.1
          with aortic (valve) disease I08.3
      active or acute I01.1
        with chorea, rheumatic (Sydenham's) I02.0
    specified cause, except rheumatic I34.0
  muscle (see also Disease, muscle)
    heart — see Insufficiency, myocardial
    ocular NEC H50.9
  myocardial, myocardium (with arteriosclerosis) I50.9
    with
      rheumatic fever (conditions in I00) I09.0
        active, acute or subacute I01.2
          with chorea I02.0
        inactive or quiescent (with chorea) I09.0
    congenital Q24.8
    hypertensive — see Hypertension, heart
    newborn P29.0
    rheumatic I09.0
      active, acute, or subacute I01.2
    syphilitic A52.06
  nourishment T73.0 ☑
  pancreatic K86.8
  parathyroid (gland) E20.9
  peripheral vascular (arterial) I73.9
  pituitary E23.0
  placental (mother) O36.51- ☑
  platelets D69.6
  prenatal care affecting management of pregnancy O09.3- ☑
  progressive pluriglandular E31.0
  pulmonary J98.4
    acute, following surgery (nonthoracic) J95.2
      thoracic J95.1
    chronic, following surgery J95.3
    following
      shock J98.4
      trauma J98.4
    newborn P28.5
    valve I37.1
      with stenosis I37.2
      congenital Q22.2
      rheumatic I09.89
        with aortic, mitral or tricuspid (valve) disease I08.8
  pyloric K31.89
  renal (acute) N28.9
    chronic N18.9
  respiratory R06.89
    newborn P28.5
  rotation — see Malrotation

Insufficiency, insufficient — *continued*
  sleep syndrome F51.12
  social insurance Z59.7
  suprarenal E27.40
    primary E27.1
  tarso-orbital fascia, congenital Q10.3
  testis E29.1
  thyroid (gland) (acquired) E03.9
    congenital E03.1
  tricuspid (valve) (rheumatic) I07.1
    with
      aortic (valve) disease I08.2
        with mitral (valve) disease I08.3
      mitral (valve) disease I08.1
        with aortic (valve) disease I08.3
      obstruction or stenosis I07.2
        with aortic (valve) disease I08.2
          with mitral (valve) disease I08.3
    congenital Q22.8
    nonrheumatic I36.1
      with stenosis I36.2
  urethral sphincter R32
  valve, valvular (heart) — *see* Endocarditis
    congenital Q24.8
  vascular I99.8
    intestine K55.9
      acute K55.0
      mesenteric K55.1
    peripheral I73.9
    renal — *see* Hypertension, kidney
  velopharyngeal
    acquired K13.79
    congenital Q38.8
  venous (chronic) (peripheral) I87.2
  ventricular — *see* Insufficiency, myocardial
  welfare support Z59.7
Insufflation, fallopian Z31.41
Insular — *see* condition
Insulinoma
  pancreas
    benign D13.7
    malignant C25.4
    uncertain behavior D37.8
  specified site
    benign — *see* Neoplasm, by site, benign
    malignant — *see* Neoplasm, by site, malignant
    uncertain behavior — *see* Neoplasm, by site, uncertain behavior
  unspecified site
    benign D13.7
    malignant C25.4
    uncertain behavior D37.8
Insuloma — *see* Insulinoma
Interference
  balancing side M26.56
  non-working side M26.56
Intermenstrual — *see* condition
Intermittent — *see* condition
Internal — *see* condition
Interrogation
  cardiac defibrillator (automatic) (implantable) Z45.02
  cardiac pacemaker Z45.018
  cardiac (event) (loop) recorder Z45.09
  infusion pump (implanted) (intrathecal) Z45.1
  neurostimulator Z46.2
Interruption
  bundle of His I44.30
  phase-shift, sleep cycle — *see* Disorder, sleep, circadian rhythm
  sleep phase-shift, or 24 hour sleep-wake cycle — *see* Disorder, sleep, circadian rhythm
Interstitial — *see* condition
Intertrigo L30.4
  labialis K13.0
Intervertebral disc — *see* condition
Intestine, intestinal — *see* condition
Intolerance
  carbohydrate K90.4
  disaccharide, hereditary E73.0
  fat NEC K90.4
    pancreatic K90.3
  food K90.4
    dietary counseling and surveillance Z71.3
  fructose E74.10
    hereditary E74.12
  glucose (-galactose) E74.39
  gluten K90.0

Intolerance — *continued*
  lactose E73.9
    specified NEC E73.8
  lysine E72.3
  milk NEC K90.4
    lactose E73.9
  protein K90.4
  starch NEC K90.4
  sucrose (-isomaltose) E74.31
Intoxicated NEC (without dependence) — *see* Alcohol, intoxication
Intoxication
  acid E87.2
  alcoholic (acute) (without dependence) — *see* Alcohol, intoxication
  alimentary canal K52.1
  amphetamine (without dependence) — *see* Abuse, drug, stimulant, with intoxication
    with dependence — *see* Dependence, drug, stimulant, with intoxication
  anxiolytic (acute) (without dependence) — *see* Abuse, drug, sedative, with intoxication
    with dependence — *see* Dependence, drug, sedative, with intoxication
  caffeine (acute) (without dependence) — *see* Abuse, drug, stimulant, with intoxication
    with dependence — *see* Dependence, drug, stimulant, with intoxication
  cannabinoids (acute) (without dependence) — *see* Abuse, drug, cannabis, with intoxication
    with dependence — *see* Dependence, drug, cannabis, with intoxication
  chemical — *see* Table of Drugs and Chemicals
    via placenta or breast milk — *see* - Absorption, chemical, through placenta
  cocaine (acute) (without dependence) — *see* Abuse, drug, cocaine, with intoxication
    with dependence — *see* Dependence, drug, cocaine, with intoxication
  drug
    acute (without dependence) — *see* Abuse, drug, by type with intoxication
      with dependence — *see* Dependence, drug, by type with intoxication
    addictive
      via placenta or breast milk — *see* Absorption, drug, addictive, through placenta
    newborn P93.8
      gray baby syndrome P93.0
    overdose or wrong substance given or taken — *see* Table of Drugs and Chemicals, by drug, poisoning
  enteric K52.1
  foodborne A05.9
    bacterial A05.9
    classical (Clostridium botulinum) A05.1
    due to
      Bacillus cereus A05.4
      bacterium A05.9
        specified NEC A05.8
      Clostridium
        botulinum A05.1
        perfringens A05.2
        welchii A05.2
      Salmonella A02.9
        with
          (gastro)enteritis A02.0
          localized infection(s) A02.20
            arthritis A02.23
            meningitis A02.21
            osteomyelitis A02.24
            pneumonia A02.22
            pyelonephritis A02.25
            specified NEC A02.29
          sepsis A02.1
          specified manifestation NEC A02.8
      Staphylococcus A05.0
      Vibrio
        parahaemolyticus A05.3
        vulnificus A05.5
    enterotoxin, staphylococcal A05.0
    noxious — *see* Poisoning, food, noxious
  gastrointestinal K52.1
  hallucinogenic (without dependence) — *see* Abuse, drug, hallucinogen, with intoxication
    with dependence — *see* Dependence, drug, hallucinogen, with intoxication

Intoxication — *continued*
  hypnotic (acute) (without dependence) — *see* Abuse, drug, sedative, with intoxication
    with dependence — *see* Dependence, drug, sedative, with intoxication
  inhalant (acute) (without dependence) — *see* Abuse, drug, inhalant, with intoxication
    with dependence — *see* Dependence, drug, inhalant, with intoxication
  meaning
    inebriation — *see* category F10 ☑
    poisoning — *see* Table of Drugs and Chemicals
  methyl alcohol (acute) (without dependence) — *see* Alcohol, intoxication
  opioid (acute) (without dependence) — *see* Abuse, drug, opioid, with intoxication
    with dependence — *see* Dependence, drug, opioid, with intoxication
  pathologic NEC (without dependence) — *see* Alcohol, intoxication
  phencyclidine (without dependence) — *see* Abuse, drug, psychoactive NEC, with intoxication
    with dependence — *see* Dependence, drug, psychoactive NEC, with intoxication
  potassium (K) E87.5
  psychoactive substance NEC (without dependence) — *see* Abuse, drug, psychoactive NEC, with intoxication
    with dependence — *see* Dependence, drug, psychoactive NEC, with intoxication
  sedative (acute) (without dependence) — *see* Abuse, drug, sedative, with intoxication
    with dependence — *see* Dependence, drug, sedative, with intoxication
  serum (*see also* Reaction, serum) T80.69 ☑
  uremic — *see* Uremia
  volatile solvents (acute) (without dependence) — *see* Abuse, drug, inhalant, with intoxication
    with dependence — *see* Dependence, drug, inhalant, with intoxication
  water E87.79
Intracranial — *see* condition
Intrahepatic gallbladder Q44.1
Intraligamentous — *see* condition
Intrathoracic (*see also* condition)
  kidney Q63.2
Intrauterine contraceptive device
  checking Z30.431
  in situ Z97.5
  insertion Z30.430
    immediately following removal Z30.433
  management Z30.431
  reinsertion Z30.433
  removal Z30.432
  replacement Z30.433
  retention in pregnancy O26.3- ☑
Intraventricular — *see* condition
Intrinsic deformity — *see* Deformity
Intubation, difficult or failed T88.4 ☑
Intumescence, lens (eye) (cataract) — *see* Cataract
Intussusception (bowel) (colon) (enteric) (ileocecal) (ileocolic) (intestine) (rectum) K56.1
  appendix K38.8
  congenital Q43.8
  ureter (with obstruction) N13.5
Invagination (bowel, colon, intestine or rectum) K56.1
Inversion
  albumin-globulin (A-G) ratio E88.09
  bladder N32.89
  cecum — *see* Intussusception
  cervix N88.8
  chromosome in normal individual Q95.1
  circadian rhythm — *see* Disorder, sleep, circadian rhythm
  nipple N64.59
    congenital Q83.8
    gestational — *see* Retraction, nipple
    puerperal, postpartum — *see* Retraction, nipple
  nyctohemeral rhythm — *see* Disorder, sleep, circadian rhythm
  optic papilla Q14.2
  organ or site, congenital NEC — *see* Anomaly, by site
  sleep rhythm — *see* Disorder, sleep, circadian rhythm
  testis (congenital) Q55.29
  uterus (chronic) (postinfectional) (postpartal, old) N85.5
    postpartum O71.2

Index

Insufficiency, insufficient — Inversion

Inversion — continued
  vagina (posthysterectomy) N99.3
  ventricular Q20.5
Investigation (see also Examination) Z04.9
  clinical research subject (control) (normal comparison)
    (participant) Z00.6
Involuntary movement, abnormal R25.9
Involution, involutional (see also condition)
  breast, cystic — see Dysplasia, mammary, specified
    type NEC
  depression (single episode) F32.8
    recurrent episode F33.9
  melancholia (recurrent episode) (single episode) F32.8
  ovary, senile — see Atrophy, ovary
  thymus failure E32.8
I.Q.
  under 20 F73
  20-34 F72
  35-49 F71
  50-69 F70
IRDS (type I) P22.0
  type II P22.1
Irideremia Q13.1
Iridis rubeosis — see Disorder, iris, vascular
Iridochoroiditis (panuveitis) — see Panuveitis
Iridocyclitis H20.9
  acute H20.0- ☑
    hypopyon H20.05- ☑
    primary H20.01- ☑
    recurrent H20.02- ☑
    secondary (noninfectious) H20.04- ☑
      infectious H20.03- ☑
  chronic H20.1- ☑
  due to allergy — see Iridocyclitis, acute, secondary
  endogenous — see Iridocyclitis, acute, primary
  Fuchs' — see Cyclitis, Fuchs' heterochromic
  gonococcal A54.32
  granulomatous — see Iridocyclitis, chronic
  herpes, herpetic (simplex) B00.51
    zoster B02.32
  hypopyon — see Iridocyclitis, acute, hypopyon
  in (due to)
    ankylosing spondylitis M45.9
    gonococcal infection A54.32
    herpes (simplex) virus B00.51
      zoster B02.32
    infectious disease NOS B99 ☑
    parasitic disease NOS B89 [H22]
    sarcoidosis D86.83
    syphilis A51.43
    tuberculosis A18.54
    zoster B02.32
  lens-induced H20.2- ☑
  nongranulomatous — see Iridocyclitis, acute
  recurrent — see Iridocyclitis, acute, recurrent
  rheumatic — see Iridocyclitis, chronic
  subacute — see Iridocyclitis, acute
  sympathetic — see Uveitis, sympathetic
  syphilitic (secondary) A51.43
  tuberculous (chronic) A18.54
  Vogt-Koyanagi H20.82- ☑
Iridocyclochoroiditis (panuveitis) — see Panuveitis
Iridodialysis H21.53- ☑
Iridodonesis H21.89
Iridoplegia (complete) (partial) (reflex) H57.09
Iridoschisis H21.25- ☑
Iris (see also condition)
  bombé — see Membrane, pupillary
Iritis (see also Iridocyclitis)
  chronic — see Iridocyclitis, chronic
  diabetic — see E08-E13 with .39
  due to
    herpes simplex B00.51
    leprosy A30.9 [H22]
  gonococcal A54.32
  gouty M10.9
  granulomatous — see Iridocyclitis, chronic
  lens induced — see Iridocyclitis, lens-induced
  papulosa (syphilitic) A52.71
  rheumatic — see Iridocyclitis, chronic
  syphilitic (secondary) A51.43
    congenital (early) A50.01
    late A52.71
  tuberculous A18.54
Iron — see condition
Iron-miner's lung J63.4
Irradiated enamel (tooth, teeth) K03.89

Irradiation effects, adverse T66 ☑
Irreducible, irreducibility — see condition
Irregular, irregularity
  action, heart I49.9
  alveolar process K08.8
  bleeding N92.6
  breathing R06.89
  contour of cornea (acquired) — see Deformity, cornea
    congenital Q13.4
  contour, reconstructed breast N65.0
  dentin (in pulp) K04.3
  eye movements H55.89
    nystagmus — see Nystagmus
    saccadic H55.81
  labor O62.2
  menstruation (cause unknown) N92.6
  periods N92.6
  prostate N42.9
  pupil — see Abnormality, pupillary
  reconstructed breast N65.0
  respiratory R06.89
  septum (nasal) J34.2
  shape, organ or site, congenital NEC — see Distortion
  sleep-wake pattern (rhythm) G47.23
Irritable, irritability R45.4
  bladder N32.89
  bowel (syndrome) K58.9
    with diarrhea K58.0
    psychogenic F45.8
  bronchial — see Bronchitis
  cerebral, in newborn P91.3
  colon K58.9
    with diarrhea K58.0
    psychogenic F45.8
  duodenum K59.8
  heart (psychogenic) F45.8
  hip — see Derangement, joint, specified type NEC, hip
  ileum K59.8
  infant R68.12
  jejunum K59.8
  rectum K59.8
  stomach K31.89
    psychogenic F45.8
  sympathetic G90.8
  urethra N36.8
Irritation
  anus K62.89
  axillary nerve G54.0
  bladder N32.89
  brachial plexus G54.0
  bronchial — see Bronchitis
  cervical plexus G54.2
  cervix — see Cervicitis
  choroid, sympathetic — see Endophthalmitis
  cranial nerve — see Disorder, nerve, cranial
  gastric K31.89
    psychogenic F45.8
  globe, sympathetic — see Uveitis, sympathetic
  labyrinth — see subcategory H83.2 ☑
  lumbosacral plexus G54.1
  meninges (traumatic) — see Injury, intracranial
    nontraumatic — see Meningismus
  nerve — see Disorder, nerve
  nervous R45.0
  penis N48.89
  perineum NEC L29.3
  peripheral autonomic nervous system G90.8
  peritoneum — see Peritonitis
  pharynx J39.2
  plantar nerve — see Lesion, nerve, plantar
  spinal (cord) (traumatic) (see also Injury, spinal cord,
    by region)
    nerve G58.9
      root NEC — see Radiculopathy
    nontraumatic — see Myelopathy
  stomach K31.89
    psychogenic F45.8
  sympathetic nerve NEC G90.8
  ulnar nerve — see Lesion, nerve, ulnar
  vagina N89.8
Ischemia, ischemic I99.8
  bowel (transient)
    acute K55.0
    chronic K55.1
    due to mesenteric artery insufficiency K55.1
  brain — see Ischemia, cerebral
  cardiac (see Disease, heart, ischemic)
  cardiomyopathy I25.5

Ischemia, ischemic — continued
  cerebral (chronic) (generalized) I67.82
    arteriosclerotic I67.2
    intermittent G45.9
    newborn P91.0
    recurrent focal G45.8
    transient G45.9
  colon chronic (due to mesenteric artery insufficiency)
    K55.1
  coronary — see Disease, heart, ischemic
  demand (coronary) (see also Angina) I24.8
  heart (chronic or with a stated duration of over 4
    weeks) I25.9
    acute or with a stated duration of 4 weeks or less
      I24.9
    subacute I24.9
  infarction, muscle — see Infarct, muscle
  intestine (large) (small) (transient) K55.9
    acute K55.0
    chronic K55.1
    due to mesenteric artery insufficiency K55.1
  kidney N28.0
  mesenteric, acute K55.0
  muscle, traumatic T79.6 ☑
  myocardium, myocardial (chronic or with a stated
    duration of over 4 weeks) I25.9
    acute, without myocardial infarction I24.0
    silent (asymptomatic) I25.6
    transient of newborn P29.4
  renal N28.0
  retina, retinal — see Occlusion, artery, retina
  small bowel
    acute K55.0
    chronic K55.1
    due to mesenteric artery insufficiency K55.1
  spinal cord G95.11
  subendocardial — see Insufficiency, coronary
  supply (coronary) (see also Angina) I25.9
    due to vasospasm I20.1
Ischial spine — see condition
Ischialgia — see Sciatica
Ischiopagus Q89.4
Ischium, ischial — see condition
Ischuria R34
Iselin's disease or osteochondrosis — see Osteochon-
    drosis, juvenile, metatarsus
Islands of
  parotid tissue in
    lymph nodes Q38.6
    neck structures Q38.6
  submaxillary glands in
    fascia Q38.6
    lymph nodes Q38.6
    neck muscles Q38.6
Islet cell tumor, pancreas D13.7
Isoimmunization NEC (see also Incompatibility)
  affecting management of pregnancy (ABO) (with hy-
    drops fetalis) O36.11-
    anti-A sensitization O36.11- ☑
    anti-B sensitization O36.19- ☑
    anti-c sensitization O36.09- ☑
    anti-C sensitization O36.09- ☑
    anti-E sensitization O36.09- ☑
    anti-e sensitization O36.09- ☑
    Rh NEC O36.09- ☑
      anti-D antibody O36.01- ☑
    specified NEC O36.19- ☑
  newborn P55.9
    with
      hydrops fetalis P56.0
      kernicterus P57.0
    ABO (blood groups) P55.1
    Rhesus (Rh) factor P55.0
    specified type NEC P55.8
Isolation, isolated
  dwelling Z59.8
  family Z63.79
  social Z60.4
Isoleucinosis E71.19
Isomerism atrial appendages (with asplenia or
    polysplenia) Q20.6
Isosporiasis, isosporosis A07.3
Isovaleric acidemia E71.110
Issue of
  medical certificate Z02.79
    for disability determination Z02.71

Issue of — *continued*
  repeat prescription (appliance) (glasses) (medicinal substance, medicament, medicine) Z76.Ø
    contraception — *see* Contraception
Itch, itching (*see also* Pruritus)
  baker's L23.6
  barber's B35.Ø
  bricklayer's L24.5
  cheese B88.Ø
  clam digger's B65.3
  coolie B76.9
  copra B88.Ø
  dew B76.9
  dhobi B35.6
  filarial — *see* Infestation, filarial
  grain B88.Ø
  grocer's B88.Ø
  ground B76.9
  harvest B88.Ø
  jock B35.6
  Malabar B35.5
    beard B35.Ø
    foot B35.3
    scalp B35.Ø
  meaning scabies B86
  Norwegian B86
  perianal L29.Ø
  poultrymen's B88.Ø
  sarcoptic B86
  scabies B86
  scrub B88.Ø
  straw B88.Ø
  swimmer's B65.3
  water B76.9
  winter L29.8
Ivemark's syndrome (asplenia with congenital heart disease) Q89.Ø1
Ivory bones Q78.2
Ixodiasis NEC B88.8

J

Jaccoud's syndrome — *see* Arthropathy, postrheumatic, chronic
Jackson's
  membrane Q43.3
  paralysis or syndrome G83.89
  veil Q43.3
Jacquet's dermatitis (diaper dermatitis) L22
Jadassohn-Pellizari's disease or anetoderma L9Ø.2
Jadassohn's
  blue nevus — *see* Nevus
  intraepidermal epithelioma — *see* Neoplasm, skin, benign
Jaffe-Lichtenstein (-Uehlinger) **syndrome** — *see* Dysplasia, fibrous, bone NEC
Jakob-Creutzfeldt disease or syndrome — *see* Creutzfeldt-Jakob disease or syndrome
Jaksch-Luzet disease D64.89
Jamaican
  neuropathy G92
  paraplegic tropical ataxic-spastic syndrome G92
Janet's disease F48.8
Janiceps Q89.4
Jansky-Bielschowsky amaurotic idiocy E75.4
Japanese
  B-type encephalitis A83.Ø
  river fever A75.3
Jaundice (yellow) R17
  acholuric (familial) (splenomegalic) (*see also* Spherocytosis)
    acquired D59.8
  breast-milk (inhibitor) P59.3
  catarrhal (acute) B15.9
    with hepatic coma B15.Ø
  cholestatic (benign) R17
  due to or associated with
    delayed conjugation P59.8
      associated with (due to) preterm delivery P59.Ø
    preterm delivery P59.Ø
  epidemic (catarrhal) B15.9
    with hepatic coma B15.Ø
    leptospiral A27.Ø
    spirochetal A27.Ø
  familial nonhemolytic (congenital) (Gilbert) E8Ø.4
    Crigler-Najjar E8Ø.5
  febrile (acute) B15.9
    with hepatic coma B15.Ø

Jaundice — *continued*
  febrile — *continued*
    leptospiral A27.Ø
    spirochetal A27.Ø
  hematogenous D59.9
  hemolytic (acquired) D59.9
    congenital — *see* Spherocytosis
  hemorrhagic (acute) (leptospiral) (spirochetal) A27.Ø
  infectious (acute) (subacute) B15.9
    with hepatic coma B15.Ø
    leptospiral A27.Ø
    spirochetal A27.Ø
  leptospiral (hemorrhagic) A27.Ø
  malignant (without coma) K72.9Ø
    with coma K72.91
  neonatal — *see* Jaundice, newborn
  newborn P59.9
    due to or associated with
      ABO
        antibodies P55.1
        incompatibility, maternal/fetal P55.1
        isoimmunization P55.1
      absence or deficiency of enzyme system for bilirubin conjugation (congenital) P59.8
      bleeding P58.1
      breast milk inhibitors to conjugation P59.3
        associated with preterm delivery P59.Ø
      bruising P58.Ø
      Crigler-Najjar syndrome E8Ø.5
      delayed conjugation P59.8
        associated with preterm delivery P59.Ø
      drugs or toxins
        given to newborn P58.42
        transmitted from mother P58.41
      excessive hemolysis P58.9
        due to
          bleeding P58.1
          bruising P58.Ø
          drugs or toxins
            given to newborn P58.42
            transmitted from mother P58.41
          infection P58.2
          polycythemia P58.3
          swallowed maternal blood P58.5
        specified type NEC P58.8
      galactosemia E74.21
      Gilbert syndrome E8Ø.4
      hemolytic disease P55.9
        ABO isoimmunization P55.1
        Rh isoimmunization P55.Ø
        specified NEC P55.8
      hepatocellular damage P59.2Ø
        specified NEC P59.29
      hereditary hemolytic anemia P58.8
      hypothyroidism, congenital EØ3.1
      incompatibility, maternal/fetal NOS P55.9
      infection P58.2
      inspissated bile syndrome P59.1
      isoimmunization NOS P55.9
      mucoviscidosis E84.9
      polycythemia P58.3
      preterm delivery P59.Ø
      Rh
        antibodies P55.Ø
        incompatibility, maternal/fetal P55.Ø
        isoimmunization P55.Ø
      specified cause NEC P59.8
      swallowed maternal blood P58.5
    spherocytosis (congenital) D58.Ø
  nonhemolytic congenital familial (Gilbert) E8Ø.4
  nuclear, newborn (*see also* Kernicterus of newborn) P57.9
  obstructive (*see also* Obstruction, bile duct) K83.1
  post-immunization — *see* Hepatitis, viral, type, B
  post-transfusion — *see* Hepatitis, viral, type, B
  regurgitation (*see also* Obstruction, bile duct) K83.1
  serum (homologous) (prophylactic) (therapeutic) — *see* Hepatitis, viral, type, B
  spirochetal (hemorrhagic) A27.Ø
  symptomatic R17
    newborn P59.9
Jaw — *see* condition
Jaw-winking phenomenon or syndrome QØ7.8
Jealousy
  alcoholic F1Ø.988
  childhood F93.8
  sibling F93.8
Jejunitis — *see* Enteritis

Jejunostomy status Z93.4
Jejunum, jejunal — *see* condition
Jensen's disease — *see* Inflammation, chorioretinal, focal, juxtapapillary
Jerks, myoclonic G25.3
Jervell-Lange-Nielsen syndrome I45.81
Jeune's disease Q77.2
Jigger disease B88.1
Job's syndrome (chronic granulomatous disease) D71
Joint (*see also* condition)
  mice — *see* Loose, body, joint
    knee M23.4- ☑
Jordan's anomaly or syndrome D72.Ø
Joseph-Diamond-Blackfan anemia (congenital hypoplastic) D61.Ø1
Jungle yellow fever A95.Ø
Jüngling's disease — *see* Sarcoidosis
Juvenile — *see* condition

K

Kahler's disease C9Ø.Ø- ☑
Kakke E51.11
Kala-azar B55.Ø
Kallmann's syndrome E23.Ø
Kanner's syndrome (autism) — *see* Psychosis, childhood
Kaposi's
  dermatosis (xeroderma pigmentosum) Q82.1
  lichen ruber L44.Ø
    acuminatus L44.Ø
  sarcoma
    colon C46.4
    connective tissue C46.1
    gastrointestinal organ C46.4
    lung C46.5- ☑
    lymph node (multiple) C46.3
    palate (hard) (soft) C46.2
    rectum C46.4
    skin (multiple sites) C46.Ø
    specified site NEC C46.7
    stomach C46.4
    unspecified site C46.9
  varicelliform eruption BØØ.Ø
    vaccinia T88.1 ☑
Kartagener's syndrome or triad (sinusitis, bronchiectasis, situs inversus) Q89.3
Karyotype
  with abnormality except iso (Xq) Q96.2
  45,X Q96.Ø
  46,X
    iso (Xq) Q96.1
  46,XX Q98.3
    with streak gonads Q5Ø.32
    hermaphrodite (true) Q99.1
    male Q98.3
  46,XY
    with streak gonads Q56.1
    female Q97.3
    hermaphrodite (true) Q99.1
  47,XXX Q97.Ø
  47,XXY Q98.Ø
  47,XYY Q98.5
Kaschin-Beck disease — *see* Disease, Kaschin-Beck
Katayama's disease or fever B65.2
Kawasaki's syndrome M3Ø.3
Kayser-Fleischer ring (cornea) (pseudosclerosis) H18.Ø4- ☑
Kaznelson's syndrome (congenital hypoplastic anemia) D61.Ø1
Kearns-Sayre syndrome H49.81- ☑
Kedani fever A75.3
Kelis L91.Ø
Kelly (-Patterson) **syndrome** (sideropenic dysphagia) D5Ø.1
Keloid, cheloid L91.Ø
  acne L73.Ø
  Addison's L94.Ø
  cornea — *see* Opacity, cornea
  Hawkin's L91.Ø
  scar L91.Ø
Keloma L91.Ø
Kenya fever A77.1
Keratectasia (*see also* Ectasia, cornea)
  congenital Q13.4
Keratinization of alveolar ridge mucosa
  excessive K13.23
  minimal K13.22

Keratinized residual ridge mucosa
  excessive K13.23
  minimal K13.22
Keratitis (nodular) (nonulcerative) (simple) (zonular) H16.9
  with ulceration (central) (marginal) (perforated) (ring) — see Ulcer, cornea
  actinic — see Photokeratitis
  arborescens (herpes simplex) B00.52
  areolar H16.11- ☑
  bullosa H16.8
  deep H16.309
    specified type NEC H16.399
  dendritic (a) (herpes simplex) B00.52
  disciform (is) (herpes simplex) B00.52
    varicella B01.81
  filamentary H16.12- ☑
  gonococcal (congenital or prenatal) A54.33
  herpes, herpetic (simplex) B00.52
    zoster B02.33
  in (due to)
    acanthamebiasis B60.13
    adenovirus B30.0
    exanthema (see also Exanthem) B09
    herpes (simplex) virus B00.52
    measles B05.81
    syphilis A50.31
    tuberculosis A18.52
    zoster B02.33
  interstitial (nonsyphilitic) H16.30- ☑
    diffuse H16.32- ☑
    herpes, herpetic (simplex) B00.52
      zoster B02.33
    sclerosing H16.33- ☑
    specified type NEC H16.39- ☑
    syphilitic (congenital) (late) A50.31
    tuberculous A18.52
  macular H16.11- ☑
  nummular H16.11- ☑
  oyster shuckers' H16.8
  parenchymatous — see Keratitis, interstitial
  petrificans H16.8
  postmeasles B05.81
  punctata
    leprosa A30.9 [H16.14-] ☑
    syphilitic (profunda) A50.31
  punctate H16.14- ☑
  purulent H16.8
  rosacea L71.8
  sclerosing H16.33- ☑
  specified type NEC H16.8
  stellate H16.11- ☑
  striate H16.11- ☑
  superficial H16.10- ☑
    with conjunctivitis — see Keratoconjunctivitis
    due to light — see Photokeratitis
  suppurative H16.8
  syphilitic (congenital) (prenatal) A50.31
  trachomatous A71.1
    sequelae B94.0
  tuberculous A18.52
  vesicular H16.8
  xerotic (see also Keratomalacia) H16.8
    vitamin A deficiency E50.4
Keratoacanthoma L85.8
Keratocele — see Descemetocele
Keratoconjunctivitis H16.20- ☑
  Acanthamoeba B60.13
  adenoviral B30.0
  epidemic B30.0
  exposure H16.21- ☑
  herpes, herpetic (simplex) B00.52
    zoster B02.33
  in exanthema (see also Exanthem) B09
  infectious B30.0
  lagophthalmic — see Keratoconjunctivitis, specified type NEC
  neurotrophic H16.23- ☑
  phlyctenular H16.25- ☑
  postmeasles B05.81
  shipyard B30.0
  sicca (Sjogren's) M35.0- ☑
    not Sjogren's H16.22- ☑
  specified type NEC H16.29- ☑
  tuberculous (phlyctenular) A18.52
  vernal H16.26- ☑
Keratoconus H18.60- ☑

Keratoconus H18.60- ☑
  congenital Q13.4
  stable H18.61- ☑
  unstable H18.62- ☑
Keratocyst (dental) (odontogenic) — see Cyst, calcifying odontogenic
Keratoderma, keratodermia (congenital) (palmaris et plantaris) (symmetrical) Q82.8
  acquired L85.1
    in diseases classified elsewhere L86
  climactericum L85.1
  gonococcal A54.89
  gonorrheal A54.89
  punctata L85.2
  Reiter's — see Reiter's disease
Keratodermatocele — see Descemetocele
Keratoglobus H18.79 ☑
  congenital Q15.8
    with glaucoma Q15.0
Keratohemia — see Pigmentation, cornea, stromal
Keratoiritis (see also Iridocyclitis)
  syphilitic A50.39
  tuberculous A18.54
Keratoma L57.0
  palmaris and plantaris hereditarium Q82.8
  senile L57.0
Keratomalacia H18.44- ☑
  vitamin A deficiency E50.4
Keratomegaly Q13.4
Keratomycosis B49
  nigrans, nigricans (palmaris) B36.1
Keratopathy H18.9
  band H18.42- ☑
  bullous (aphakic), following cataract surgery H59.01- ☑
  bullous H18.1- ☑
Keratoscleritis, tuberculous A18.52
Keratosis L57.0
  actinic L57.0
  arsenical L85.8
  congenital, specified NEC Q80.8
  female genital NEC N94.89
  follicularis Q82.8
    acquired L11.0
    congenita Q82.8
    et parafollicularis in cutem penetrans L87.0
    spinulosa (decalvans) Q82.8
    vitamin A deficiency E50.8
  gonococcal A54.89
  male genital (external) N50.8
  nigricans L83
  obturans, external ear (canal) — see Cholesteatoma, external ear
  palmaris et plantaris (inherited) (symmetrical) Q82.8
    acquired L85.1
  penile N48.89
  pharynx J39.2
  pilaris, acquired L85.8
  punctata (palmaris et plantaris) L85.2
  scrotal N50.8
  seborrheic L82.1
    inflamed L82.0
  senile L57.0
  solar L57.0
  tonsillaris J35.8
  vagina N89.4
  vegetans Q82.8
  vitamin A deficiency E50.8
  vocal cord J38.3
Kerato-uveitis — see Iridocyclitis
Kerion (celsi) B35.0
Kernicterus of newborn (not due to isoimmunization) P57.9
  due to isoimmunization (conditions in P55.0-P55.9) P57.0
  specified type NEC P57.8
Kerunoparalysis T75.09 ☑
Keshan disease E59
Ketoacidosis E87.2
  diabetic — see Diabetes, by type, with ketoacidosis
Ketonuria R82.4
Ketosis NEC E88.89
  diabetic — see Diabetes, by type, with with ketoacidosis
Kew Garden fever A79.1
Kidney — see condition

Kienböck's disease (see also Osteochondrosis, juvenile, hand, carpal lunate)
  adult M93.1
Kimmelstiel (-Wilson) **disease** — see Diabetes, Kimmelstiel (-Wilson) disease
Kink, kinking
  artery I77.1
  hair (acquired) L67.8
  ileum or intestine — see Obstruction, intestine
  Lane's — see Obstruction, intestine
  organ or site, congenital NEC — see Anomaly, by site
  ureter (pelvic junction) N13.5
    with
      hydronephrosis N13.1
        with infection N13.6
      pyelonephritis (chronic) N11.1
    congenital Q62.39
  vein(s) I87.8
    caval I87.1
    peripheral I87.1
Kinnier Wilson's disease (hepatolenticular degeneration) E83.01
Kissing spine M48.20
  cervical region M48.22
  cervicothoracic region M48.23
  lumbar region M48.26
  lumbosacral region M48.27
  occipito-atlanto-axial region M48.21
  thoracic region M48.24
  thoracolumbar region M48.25
Klatskin's tumor C22.1
Klauder's disease A26.8
Klebs' disease (see also Glomerulonephritis) N05- ☑
Klebsiella (K.) **pneumoniae, as cause of disease classified elsewhere** B96.1
Klein (e)-**Levin syndrome** G47.13
Kleptomania F63.2
Klinefelter's syndrome Q98.4
  karyotype 47,XXY Q98.0
  male with more than two X chromosomes Q98.1
Klippel-Feil deficiency, disease, or syndrome (brevicollis) Q76.1
Klippel's disease I67.2
Klippel-Trenaunay (-Weber) **syndrome** Q87.2
Klumpke (-Déjerine) **palsy, paralysis** (birth) (newborn) P14.1
Knee — see condition
Knock knee (acquired) M21.06- ☑
  congenital Q74.1
Knot(s)
  intestinal, syndrome (volvulus) K56.2
  surfer S89.8- ☑
  umbilical cord (true) O69.2 ☑
Knotting (of)
  hair L67.8
  intestine K56.2
Knuckle pad (Garrod's) M72.1
Koch's
  infection — see Tuberculosis
  relapsing fever A68.9
Koch-Weeks' conjunctivitis — see Conjunctivitis, acute, mucopurulent
Köebner's syndrome Q81.8
Köenig's disease (osteochondritis dissecans) — see Osteochondritis, dissecans
Köhler-Pellegrini-Steida disease or syndrome (calcification, knee joint) — see Bursitis, tibial collateral
Köhler's disease
  patellar — see Osteochondrosis, juvenile, patella
  tarsal navicular — see Osteochondrosis, juvenile, tarsus
Koilonychia L60.3
  congenital Q84.6
Kojevnikov's, epilepsy — see Kozhevnikof's epilepsy
Koplik's spots B05.9
Kopp's asthma E32.8
Korsakoff's (Wernicke) **disease, psychosis or syndrome** (alcoholic) F10.96
  with dependence F10.26
  drug-induced
    due to drug abuse — see Abuse, drug, by type, with amnestic disorder
    due to drug dependence — see Dependence, drug, by type, with amnestic disorder
  nonalcoholic F04
Korsakov's disease, psychosis or syndrome — see Korsakoff's disease

☑ **Additional Character Required** — Refer to the Tabular List for Character Selection   ☝ **Subterms under main terms may continue to next column or page**

Korsakow's disease, psychosis or syndrome — see Korsakoff's disease
Kostmann's disease or syndrome (infantile genetic agranulocytosis) — see Agranulocytosis
Kozhevnikof's epilepsy G40.109
  intractable G40.119
    with status epilepticus G40.111
    without status epilepticus G40.119
  not intractable G40.109
    with status epilepticus G40.101
    without status epilepticus G40.109
Krabbe's
  disease E75.23
  syndrome, congenital muscle hypoplasia Q79.8
Kraepelin-Morel disease — see Schizophrenia
Kraft-Weber-Dimitri disease Q85.8
Kraurosis
  ani K62.89
  penis N48.0
  vagina N89.8
  vulva N90.4
Kreotoxism A05.9
Krukenberg's
  spindle — see Pigmentation, cornea, posterior
  tumor C79.6- ☑
Kufs' disease E75.4
Kugelberg-Welander disease G12.1
Kuhnt-Junius degeneration (see also Degeneration, macula) H35.32
Kümmell's disease or spondylitis — see Spondylopathy, traumatic
Kupffer cell sarcoma C22.3
Kuru A81.81
Kussmaul's
  disease M30.0
  respiration E87.2
    in diabetic acidosis — see Diabetes, by type, with ketoacidosis
Kwashiorkor E40
  marasmic, marasmus type E42
Kyasanur Forest disease A98.2
Kyphoscoliosis, kyphoscoliotic (acquired) (see also Scoliosis) M41.9
  congenital Q67.5
  heart (disease) I27.1
  sequelae of rickets E64.3
  tuberculous A18.01
Kyphosis, kyphotic (acquired) M40.209
  cervical region M40.202
  cervicothoracic region M40.203
  congenital Q76.419
    cervical region Q76.412
    cervicothoracic region Q76.413
    occipito-atlanto-axial region Q76.411
    thoracic region Q76.414
    thoracolumbar region Q76.415
  Morquio-Brailsford type (spinal) (see also subcategory M49.8) E76.219
  postlaminectomy M96.3
  postradiation therapy M96.2
  postural (adolescent) M40.00
    cervicothoracic region M40.03
    thoracic region M40.04
    thoracolumbar region M40.05
  secondary NEC M40.10
    cervical region M40.12
    cervicothoracic region M40.13
    thoracic region M40.14
    thoracolumbar region M40.15
  sequelae of rickets E64.3
  specified type NEC M40.299
    cervical region M40.292
    cervicothoracic region M40.293
    thoracic region M40.294
    thoracolumbar region M40.295
  syphilitic, congenital A50.56
  thoracic region M40.204
  thoracolumbar region M40.205
  tuberculous A18.01
Kyrle disease L87.0

L

Labia, labium — see condition
Labile
  blood pressure R09.89
  vasomotor system I73.9

Labioglossal paralysis G12.29
Labium leporinum — see Cleft, lip
Labor — see Delivery
Labored breathing — see Hyperventilation
Labyrinthitis (circumscribed) (destructive) (diffuse) (inner ear) (latent) (purulent) (suppurative) (see also subcategory) H83.0 ☑
  syphilitic A52.79
Laceration
  with abortion — see Abortion, by type, complicated by laceration of pelvic organs
  abdomen, abdominal
    wall S31.119 ☑
      with
        foreign body S31.129 ☑
        penetration into peritoneal cavity S31.619 ☑
          with foreign body S31.629 ☑
      epigastric region S31.112 ☑
        with
          foreign body S31.122 ☑
          penetration into peritoneal cavity S31.612 ☑
            with foreign body S31.622 ☑
      left
        lower quadrant S31.114 ☑
          with
            foreign body S31.124 ☑
            penetration into peritoneal cavity S31.614 ☑
              with foreign body S31.624 ☑
        upper quadrant S31.111 ☑
          with
            foreign body S31.121 ☑
            penetration into peritoneal cavity S31.611 ☑
              with foreign body S31.621 ☑
      periumbilic region S31.115 ☑
        with
          foreign body S31.125 ☑
          penetration into peritoneal cavity S31.615 ☑
            with foreign body S31.625 ☑
      right
        lower quadrant S31.113 ☑
          with
            foreign body S31.123 ☑
            penetration into peritoneal cavity S31.613 ☑
              with foreign body S31.623 ☑
        upper quadrant S31.110 ☑
          with
            foreign body S31.120 ☑
            penetration into peritoneal cavity S31.610 ☑
              with foreign body S31.620 ☑
  accidental, complicating surgery — see Complications, surgical, accidental puncture or laceration
  Achilles tendon S86.02- ☑
  adrenal gland S37.813 ☑
  alveolar (process) — see Laceration, oral cavity
  ankle S91.01- ☑
    with
      foreign body S91.02- ☑
  antecubital space — see Laceration, elbow
  anus (sphincter) S31.831 ☑
    with
      ectopic or molar pregnancy O08.6
      foreign body S31.832 ☑
    complicating delivery — see Delivery, complicated, by, laceration, anus (sphincter)
    following ectopic or molar pregnancy O08.6
    nontraumatic, nonpuerperal — see Fissure, anus
  arm (upper) S41.11- ☑
    with foreign body S41.12- ☑
    lower — see Laceration, forearm
  auditory canal (external) (meatus) — see Laceration, ear
  auricle, ear — see Laceration, ear
  axilla — see Laceration, arm
  back (see also Laceration, thorax, back)
    lower S31.010 ☑
      with
        foreign body S31.020 ☑
        with penetration into retroperitoneal space S31.021 ☑

Laceration — continued
  back (see also Laceration, thorax, back) — continued
    lower — continued
      with — continued
        penetration into retroperitoneal space S31.011 ☑
  bile duct S36.13 ☑
  bladder S37.23 ☑
    with ectopic or molar pregnancy O08.6
    following ectopic or molar pregnancy O08.6
    obstetrical trauma O71.5
  blood vessel — see Injury, blood vessel
  bowel (see also Laceration, intestine)
    with ectopic or molar pregnancy O08.6
    complicating abortion — see Abortion, by type, complicated by, specified condition NEC
    following ectopic or molar pregnancy O08.6
    obstetrical trauma O71.5
  brain (any part) (cortex) (diffuse) (membrane) (see also Injury, intracranial, diffuse)
    during birth P10.8
      with hemorrhage P10.1
    focal — see Injury, intracranial, focal brain injury
  brainstem S06.38- ☑
  breast S21.01- ☑
    with foreign body S21.02- ☑
  broad ligament S37.893 ☑
    with ectopic or molar pregnancy O08.6
    following ectopic or molar pregnancy O08.6
    laceration syndrome N83.8
    obstetrical trauma O71.6
    syndrome (laceration) N83.8
  buttock S31.801 ☑
    with foreign body S31.802 ☑
    left S31.821 ☑
      with foreign body S31.822 ☑
    right S31.811 ☑
      with foreign body S31.812 ☑
  calf — see Laceration, leg
  canaliculus lacrimalis — see Laceration, eyelid
  canthus, eye — see Laceration, eyelid
  capsule, joint — see Sprain
  causing eversion of cervix uteri (old) N86
  central (perineal), complicating delivery O70.9
  cerebellum, traumatic S06.37- ☑
  cerebral S06.33- ☑
    during birth P10.8
      with hemorrhage P10.1
    left side S06.32- ☑
    right side S06.31- ☑
  cervix (uteri)
    with ectopic or molar pregnancy O08.6
    following ectopic or molar pregnancy O08.6
    nonpuerperal, nontraumatic N88.1
    obstetrical trauma (current) O71.3
    old (postpartal) N88.1
    traumatic S37.63 ☑
  cheek (external) S01.41- ☑
    with foreign body S01.42- ☑
    internal — see Laceration, oral cavity
  chest wall — see Laceration, thorax
  chin — see Laceration, head, specified site NEC
  chordae tendinae NEC I51.1
    concurrent with acute myocardial infarction — see Infarct, myocardium
    following acute myocardial infarction (current complication) I23.4
  clitoris — see Laceration, vulva
  colon — see Laceration, intestine, large, colon
  common bile duct S36.13 ☑
  cortex (cerebral) — see Injury, intracranial, diffuse
  costal region — see Laceration, thorax
  cystic duct S36.13 ☑
  diaphragm S27.803 ☑
  digit(s)
    foot — see Laceration, toe
    hand — see Laceration, finger
  duodenum S36.430 ☑
  ear (canal) (external) S01.31- ☑
    with foreign body S01.32- ☑
    drum S09.2- ☑
  elbow S51.01- ☑
    with
      foreign body S51.02- ☑
  epididymis — see Laceration, testis

Laceration — *continued*
- epigastric region — *see* Laceration, abdomen, wall, epigastric region
- esophagus K22.8
  - traumatic
    - cervical S11.21 ☑
      - with foreign body S11.22 ☑
    - thoracic S27.813 ☑
- eye (ball) S05.3- ☑
  - with prolapse or loss of intraocular tissue S05.2- ☑
  - penetrating S05.6- ☑
- eyebrow — *see* Laceration, eyelid
- eyelid S01.11- ☑
  - with foreign body S01.12- ☑
- face NEC — *see* Laceration, head, specified site NEC
- fallopian tube S37.539 ☑
  - bilateral S37.532 ☑
  - unilateral S37.531 ☑
- finger(s) S61.219 ☑
  - with
    - damage to nail S61.319 ☑
      - with
        - foreign body S61.329 ☑
    - foreign body S61.229 ☑
  - index S61.218 ☑
    - with
      - damage to nail S61.318 ☑
        - with
          - foreign body S61.328 ☑
      - foreign body S61.228 ☑
    - left S61.211 ☑
      - with
        - damage to nail S61.311 ☑
          - with
            - foreign body S61.321 ☑
        - foreign body S61.221 ☑
    - right S61.210 ☑
      - with
        - damage to nail S61.310 ☑
          - with
            - foreign body S61.320 ☑
        - foreign body S61.220 ☑
  - little S61.218 ☑
    - with
      - damage to nail S61.318 ☑
        - with
          - foreign body S61.328 ☑
      - foreign body S61.228 ☑
    - left S61.217 ☑
      - with
        - damage to nail S61.317 ☑
          - with
            - foreign body S61.327 ☑
        - foreign body S61.227 ☑
    - right S61.216 ☑
      - with
        - damage to nail S61.316 ☑
          - with
            - foreign body S61.326 ☑
        - foreign body S61.226 ☑
  - middle S61.218 ☑
    - with
      - damage to nail S61.318 ☑
        - with
          - foreign body S61.328 ☑
      - foreign body S61.228 ☑
    - left S61.213 ☑
      - with
        - damage to nail S61.313 ☑
          - with
            - foreign body S61.323 ☑
        - foreign body S61.223 ☑
    - right S61.212 ☑
      - with
        - damage to nail S61.312 ☑
          - with
            - foreign body S61.322 ☑
        - foreign body S61.222 ☑
  - ring S61.218 ☑
    - with
      - damage to nail S61.318 ☑
        - with
          - foreign body S61.328 ☑
      - foreign body S61.228 ☑

Laceration — *continued*
- finger(s) — *continued*
  - ring — *continued*
    - left S61.215 ☑
      - with
        - damage to nail S61.315 ☑
          - with
            - foreign body S61.325 ☑
        - foreign body S61.225 ☑
    - right S61.214 ☑
      - with
        - damage to nail S61.314 ☑
          - with
            - foreign body S61.324 ☑
        - foreign body S61.224 ☑
- flank S31.119 ☑
  - with foreign body S31.129 ☑
- foot (except toe(s) alone) S91.319 ☑
  - with foreign body S91.329 ☑
  - left S91.312 ☑
    - with foreign body S91.322 ☑
  - right S91.311 ☑
    - with foreign body S91.321 ☑
  - toe — *see* Laceration, toe
- forearm S51.819 ☑
  - with
    - foreign body S51.829 ☑
  - elbow only — *see* Laceration, elbow
  - left S51.812 ☑
    - with
      - foreign body S51.822 ☑
  - right S51.811 ☑
    - with
      - foreign body S51.821 ☑
- forehead S01.81 ☑
  - with foreign body S01.82 ☑
- fourchette O70.0
  - with ectopic or molar pregnancy O08.6
  - complicating delivery O70.0
  - following ectopic or molar pregnancy O08.6
- gallbladder S36.123 ☑
- genital organs, external
  - female S31.512 ☑
    - with foreign body S31.522 ☑
    - vagina — *see* Laceration, vagina
    - vulva — *see* Laceration, vulva
  - male S31.511 ☑
    - with foreign body S31.521 ☑
    - penis — *see* Laceration, penis
    - scrotum — *see* Laceration, scrotum
    - testis — *see* Laceration, testis
- groin — *see* Laceration, abdomen, wall
- gum — *see* Laceration, oral cavity
- hand S61.419 ☑
  - with
    - foreign body S61.429 ☑
  - finger — *see* Laceration, finger
  - left S61.412 ☑
    - with
      - foreign body S61.422 ☑
  - right S61.411 ☑
    - with
      - foreign body S61.421 ☑
  - thumb — *see* Laceration, thumb
- head S01.91 ☑
  - with foreign body S01.92 ☑
  - cheek — *see* Laceration, cheek
  - ear — *see* Laceration, ear
  - eyelid — *see* Laceration, eyelid
  - lip — *see* Laceration, lip
  - nose — *see* Laceration, nose
  - oral cavity — *see* Laceration, oral cavity
  - scalp S01.01 ☑
    - with foreign body S01.02 ☑
  - specified site NEC S01.81 ☑
    - with foreign body S01.82 ☑
  - temporomandibular area — *see* Laceration, cheek
- heart — *see* Injury, heart, laceration
- heel — *see* Laceration, foot
- hepatic duct S36.13 ☑
- hip S71.019 ☑
  - with foreign body S71.029 ☑
  - left S71.012 ☑
    - with foreign body S71.022 ☑
  - right S71.011 ☑
    - with foreign body S71.021 ☑

Laceration — *continued*
- hymen — *see* Laceration, vagina
- hypochondrium — *see* Laceration, abdomen, wall
- hypogastric region — *see* Laceration, abdomen, wall
- ileum S36.438 ☑
- inguinal region — *see* Laceration, abdomen, wall
- instep — *see* Laceration, foot
- internal organ — *see* Injury, by site
- interscapular region — *see* Laceration, thorax, back
- intestine
  - large
    - colon S36.539 ☑
      - ascending S36.530 ☑
      - descending S36.532 ☑
      - sigmoid S36.533 ☑
      - specified site NEC S36.538 ☑
    - rectum S36.63 ☑
    - transverse S36.531 ☑
  - small S36.439 ☑
    - duodenum S36.430 ☑
    - specified site NEC S36.438 ☑
- intra-abdominal organ S36.93 ☑
  - intestine — *see* Laceration, intestine
  - liver — *see* Laceration, liver
  - pancreas — *see* Laceration, pancreas
  - peritoneum S36.81 ☑
  - specified site NEC S36.893 ☑
  - spleen — *see* Laceration, spleen
  - stomach — *see* Laceration, stomach
- intracranial NEC (*see also* Injury, intracranial, diffuse)
  - birth injury P10.9
- jaw — *see* Laceration, head, specified site NEC
- jejunum S36.438 ☑
- joint capsule — *see* Sprain, by site
- kidney S37.03- ☑
  - major (greater than 3 cm) (massive) (stellate) S37.06- ☑
  - minor (less than 1 cm) S37.04- ☑
  - moderate (1 to 3 cm) S37.05- ☑
    - multiple S37.06- ☑
- knee S81.01- ☑
  - with foreign body S81.02- ☑
- labium (majus) (minus) — *see* Laceration, vulva
- lacrimal duct — *see* Laceration, eyelid
- large intestine — *see* Laceration, intestine, large
- larynx S11.011 ☑
  - with foreign body S11.012 ☑
- leg (lower) S81.819 ☑
  - with foreign body S81.829 ☑
  - foot — *see* Laceration, foot
  - knee — *see* Laceration, knee
  - left S81.812 ☑
    - with foreign body S81.822 ☑
  - right S81.811 ☑
    - with foreign body S81.821 ☑
  - upper — *see* Laceration, thigh
- ligament — *see* Sprain
- lip S01.511 ☑
  - with foreign body S01.521 ☑
- liver S36.113 ☑
  - major (stellate) S36.116 ☑
  - minor S36.114 ☑
  - moderate S36.115 ☑
- loin — *see* Laceration, abdomen, wall
- lower back — *see* Laceration, back, lower
- lumbar region — *see* Laceration, back, lower
- lung S27.339 ☑
  - bilateral S27.332 ☑
  - unilateral S27.331 ☑
- malar region — *see* Laceration, head, specified site NEC
- mammary — *see* Laceration, breast
- mastoid region — *see* Laceration, head, specified site NEC
- meninges — *see* Injury, intracranial, diffuse
- meniscus — *see* Tear, meniscus
- mesentery S36.893 ☑
- mesosalpinx S37.893 ☑
- mouth — *see* Laceration, oral cavity
- muscle — *see* Injury, muscle, by site, laceration
- nail
  - finger — *see* Laceration, finger, with damage to nail
  - toe — *see* Laceration, toe, with damage to nail
- nasal (septum) (sinus) — *see* Laceration, nose

Laceration — *continued*
  nasopharynx — *see* Laceration, head, specified site
    NEC
  neck S11.91 ☑
    with foreign body S11.92 ☑
    involving
      cervical esophagus S11.21 ☑
        with foreign body S11.22 ☑
      larynx — *see* Laceration, larynx
      pharynx — *see* Laceration, pharynx
      thyroid gland — *see* Laceration, thyroid gland
      trachea — *see* Laceration, trachea
    specified site NEC S11.81 ☑
      with foreign body S11.82 ☑
  nerve — *see* Injury, nerve
  nose (septum) (sinus) S01.21 ☑
    with foreign body S01.22 ☑
  ocular NOS S05.3- ☑
    adnexa NOS S01.11- ☑
  oral cavity S01.512 ☑
    with foreign body S01.522 ☑
  orbit (eye) — *see* Wound, open, ocular, orbit
  ovary S37.439 ☑
    bilateral S37.432 ☑
    unilateral S37.431 ☑
  palate — *see* Laceration, oral cavity
  palm — *see* Laceration, hand
  pancreas S36.239 ☑
  pelvic S31.010 ☑
    with
      foreign body S31.020 ☑
        penetration into retroperitoneal cavity
          S31.021 ☑
      penetration into retroperitoneal cavity
        S31.011 ☑
    floor (*see also* Laceration, back, lower)
      with ectopic or molar pregnancy O08.6
      complicating delivery O70.1
      following ectopic or molar pregnancy O08.6
      old (postpartal) N81.89
    organ S37.93 ☑
  penis S31.21 ☑
    with foreign body S31.22 ☑
  perineum
    female S31.41 ☑
      with
        ectopic or molar pregnancy O08.6
        foreign body S31.42 ☑
      during delivery O70.9
        first degree O70.0
        fourth degree O70.3
        second degree O70.1
        third degree O70.2
      old (postpartal) N81.89
      postpartal N81.89
      secondary (postpartal) O90.1
    male S31.119 ☑
      with foreign body S31.129 ☑
  periocular area (with or without lacrimal passages) —
    see Laceration, eyelid
  peritoneum S36.893 ☑
  periumbilic region — *see* Laceration, abdomen, wall,
    periumbilic
  periurethral tissue — *see* Laceration, urethra
  phalanges
    finger — *see* Laceration, finger
    toe — *see* Laceration, toe
  pharynx S11.21 ☑
    with foreign body S11.22 ☑
  pinna — *see* Laceration, ear
  popliteal space — *see* Laceration, knee
  prepuce — *see* Laceration, penis
  prostate S37.823 ☑
  pubic region S31.119 ☑
    with foreign body S31.129 ☑
  pudendum — *see* Laceration, genital organs, external
  rectovaginal septum — *see* Laceration, vagina
  rectum S36.63 ☑
  retroperitoneum S36.893 ☑
  round ligament S37.893 ☑
  sacral region — *see* Laceration, back, lower
  sacroiliac region — *see* Laceration, back, lower
  salivary gland — *see* Laceration, oral cavity
  scalp S01.01 ☑
    with foreign body S01.02 ☑
  scapular region — *see* Laceration, shoulder

Laceration — *continued*
  scrotum S31.31 ☑
    with foreign body S31.32 ☑
  seminal vesicle S37.893 ☑
  shin — *see* Laceration, leg
  shoulder S41.019 ☑
    with foreign body S41.029 ☑
    left S41.012 ☑
      with foreign body S41.022 ☑
    right S41.011 ☑
      with foreign body S41.021 ☑
  small intestine — *see* Laceration, intestine, small
  spermatic cord — *see* Laceration, testis
  spinal cord (meninges) (*see also* Injury, spinal cord, by
    region)
    due to injury at birth P11.5
    newborn (birth injury) P11.5
  spleen S36.039 ☑
    major (massive) (stellate) S36.032 ☑
    moderate S36.031 ☑
    superficial (minor) S36.030 ☑
  sternal region — *see* Laceration, thorax, front
  stomach S36.33 ☑
  submaxillary region — *see* Laceration, head, specified
    site NEC
  submental region — *see* Laceration, head, specified
    site NEC
  subungual
    finger(s) — *see* Laceration, finger, with damage to
      nail
    toe(s) — *see* Laceration, toe, with damage to nail
  suprarenal gland — *see* Laceration, adrenal gland
  temple, temporal region — *see* Laceration, head,
    specified site NEC
  temporomandibular area — *see* Laceration, cheek
  tendon — *see* Injury, muscle, by site, laceration
    Achilles S86.02- ☑
  tentorium cerebelli — *see* Injury, intracranial, diffuse
  testis S31.31 ☑
    with foreign body S31.32 ☑
  thigh S71.11- ☑
    with foreign body S71.12- ☑
  thorax, thoracic (wall) S21.91 ☑
    with foreign body S21.92 ☑
    back S21.22- ☑
      with penetration into thoracic cavity
        S21.42- ☑
    front S21.12- ☑
      with penetration into thoracic cavity
        S21.32- ☑
    back S21.21- ☑
      with
        foreign body S21.22- ☑
          with penetration into thoracic cavity
            S21.42- ☑
        penetration into thoracic cavity S21.41- ☑
    breast — *see* Laceration, breast
    front S21.11- ☑
      with
        foreign body S21.12- ☑
          with penetration into thoracic cavity
            S21.32- ☑
        penetration into thoracic cavity S21.31- ☑
  thumb S61.019 ☑
    with
      damage to nail S61.119 ☑
        with
          foreign body S61.129 ☑
      foreign body S61.029 ☑
    left S61.012 ☑
      with
        damage to nail S61.112 ☑
          with
            foreign body S61.122 ☑
        foreign body S61.022 ☑
    right S61.011 ☑
      with
        damage to nail S61.111 ☑
          with
            foreign body S61.121 ☑
        foreign body S61.021 ☑
  thyroid gland S11.11 ☑
    with foreign body S11.12 ☑

Laceration — *continued*
  toe(s) S91.119 ☑
    with
      damage to nail S91.219 ☑
        with
          foreign body S91.229 ☑
      foreign body S91.129 ☑
    great S91.113 ☑
      with
        damage to nail S91.213 ☑
          with
            foreign body S91.223 ☑
        foreign body S91.123 ☑
      left S91.112 ☑
        with
          damage to nail S91.212 ☑
            with
              foreign body S91.222 ☑
          foreign body S91.122 ☑
      right S91.111 ☑
        with
          damage to nail S91.211 ☑
            with
              foreign body S91.221 ☑
          foreign body S91.121 ☑
    lesser S91.116 ☑
      with
        damage to nail S91.216 ☑
          with
            foreign body S91.226 ☑
        foreign body S91.126 ☑
      left S91.115 ☑
        with
          damage to nail S91.215 ☑
            with
              foreign body S91.225 ☑
          foreign body S91.125 ☑
      right S91.114 ☑
        with
          damage to nail S91.214 ☑
            with
              foreign body S91.224 ☑
          foreign body S91.124 ☑
  tongue — *see* Laceration, oral cavity
  trachea S11.021 ☑
    with foreign body S11.022 ☑
  tunica vaginalis — *see* Laceration, testis
  tympanum, tympanic membrane — *see* Laceration,
    ear, drum
  umbilical region S31.115 ☑
    with foreign body S31.125 ☑
  ureter S37.13 ☑
  urethra S37.33 ☑
    with or following ectopic or molar pregnancy O08.6
    obstetrical trauma O71.5
  urinary organ NEC S37.893 ☑
  uterus S37.63 ☑
    with ectopic or molar pregnancy O08.6
    following ectopic or molar pregnancy O08.6
    nonpuerperal, nontraumatic N85.8
    obstetrical trauma NEC O71.81
    old (postpartal) N85.8
  uvula — *see* Laceration, oral cavity
  vagina S31.41 ☑
    with
      ectopic or molar pregnancy O08.6
      foreign body S31.42 ☑
    during delivery O71.4
      with perineal laceration — *see* Laceration, per-
        ineum, female, during delivery
    following ectopic or molar pregnancy O08.6
    nonpuerperal, nontraumatic N89.8
    old (postpartal) N89.8
  vas deferens S37.893 ☑
  vesical — *see* Laceration, bladder
  vocal cords S11.031 ☑
    with foreign body S11.032 ☑
  vulva S31.41 ☑
    with
      ectopic or molar pregnancy O08.6
      foreign body S31.42 ☑
    complicating delivery O70.0
    following ectopic or molar pregnancy O08.6
    nonpuerperal, nontraumatic N90.89
    old (postpartal) N90.89

Laceration — *continued*
  wrist S61.519 ☑
    with
      foreign body S61.529 ☑
    left S61.512 ☑
      with
        foreign body S61.522 ☑
    right S61.511 ☑
      with
        foreign body S61.521 ☑
Lack of
  achievement in school Z55.3
  adequate
    food Z59.4
    intermaxillary vertical dimension of fully erupted
        teeth M26.36
    sleep Z72.820
  appetite (see Anorexia) R63.0
  awareness R41.9
  care
    in home Z74.2
    of infant (at or after birth) T76.02 ☑
      confirmed T74.02 ☑
  cognitive functions R41.9
  coordination R27.9
    ataxia R27.0
    specified type NEC R27.8
  development (physiological) R62.50
    failure to thrive (child over 28 days old) R62.51
      adult R62.7
      newborn P92.6
    short stature R62.52
    specified type NEC R62.59
  energy R53.83
  financial resources Z59.6
  food T73.0 ☑
  growth R62.52
  heating Z59.1
  housing (permanent) (temporary) Z59.0
    adequate Z59.1
  learning experiences in childhood Z62.898
  leisure time (affecting life-style) Z73.2
  material resources Z59.9
  memory (see also Amnesia)
    mild, following organic brain damage F06.8
  ovulation N97.0
  parental supervision or control of child Z62.0
  person able to render necessary care Z74.2
  physical exercise Z72.3
  play experience in childhood Z62.898
  posterior occlusal support M26.57
  relaxation (affecting life-style) Z73.2
  sexual
    desire F52.0
    enjoyment F52.1
  shelter Z59.0
  sleep (adequate) Z72.820
  supervision of child by parent Z62.0
  support, posterior occlusal M26.57
  water T73.1 ☑
Lacrimal — *see* condition
Lacrimation, abnormal — *see* Epiphora
Lacrimonasal duct — *see* condition
Lactation, lactating (breast) (puerperal, postpartum)
  associated
    cracked nipple O92.13
    retracted nipple O92.03
  defective O92.4
  disorder NEC O92.79
  excessive O92.6
  failed (complete) O92.3
    partial O92.4
  mastitis NEC — *see* Mastitis, obstetric
  mother (care and/or examination) Z39.1
  nonpuerperal N64.3
Lacticemia, excessive E87.2
Lacunar skull Q75.8
Laennec's cirrhosis K74.69
  alcoholic K70.30
    with ascites K70.31
Lafora's disease — *see* Epilepsy, generalized, idiopathic
Lag, lid (nervous) — *see* Retraction, lid
Lagophthalmos (eyelid) (nervous) H02.209
  cicatricial H02.219
    left H02.216
      lower H02.215
      upper H02.214

Lagophthalmos — *continued*
  cicatricial — *continued*
    right H02.213
      lower H02.212
      upper H02.211
  keratoconjunctivitis — *see* Keratoconjunctivitis
  left H02.206
    lower H02.205
    upper H02.204
  mechanical H02.229
    left H02.226
      lower H02.225
      upper H02.224
    right H02.223
      lower H02.222
      upper H02.221
  paralytic H02.239
    left H02.236
      lower H02.235
      upper H02.234
    right H02.233
      lower H02.232
      upper H02.231
  right H02.203
    lower H02.202
    upper H02.201
Laki-Lorand factor deficiency — *see* Defect, coagulation, specified type NEC
Lalling F80.0
Lambert-Eaton syndrome — *see* Syndrome, Lambert-Eaton
Lambliasis, lambliosis A07.1
Landau-Kleffner syndrome — *see* Epilepsy, specified NEC
Landouzy-Déjérine dystrophy or facioscapulohumeral atrophy G71.0
Landouzy's disease (icterohemorrhagic leptospirosis) A27.0
Landry-Guillain-Barré, syndrome or paralysis G61.0
Landry's disease or paralysis G61.0
Lane's
  band Q43.3
  kink — *see* Obstruction, intestine
  syndrome K90.2
Langdon Down syndrome — *see* Trisomy, 21
Lapsed immunization schedule status Z28.3
Large
  baby (regardless of gestational age) (4000g to 4499g) P08.1
  ear, congenital Q17.1
  physiological cup Q14.2
  stature R68.89
Large-for-dates NEC (infant) (4000g to 4499g) P08.1
  affecting management of pregnancy O36.6- ☑
  exceptionally (4500g or more) P08.0
Larsen-Johansson disease orosteochondrosis — *see* Osteochondrosis, juvenile, patella
Larsen's syndrome (flattened facies and multiple congenital dislocations) Q74.8
Larva migrans
  cutaneous B76.9
    Ancylostoma B76.0
  visceral B83.0
Laryngeal — *see* condition
Laryngismus (stridulus) J38.5
  congenital P28.89
  diphtheritic A36.2
Laryngitis (acute) (edematous) (fibrinous) (infective) (infiltrative) (malignant) (membranous) (phlegmonous) (pneumococcal) (pseudomembranous) (septic) (subglottic) (suppurative) (ulcerative) J04.0
  with
    influenza, flu, or grippe — *see* Influenza, with, laryngitis
    tracheitis (acute) — *see* Laryngotracheitis
  atrophic J37.0
  catarrhal J37.0
  chronic J37.0
    with tracheitis (chronic) J37.1
  diphtheritic A36.2
  due to external agent — *see* Inflammation, respiratory, upper, due to
  H. influenzae J04.0
  Hemophilus influenzae J04.0
  hypertrophic J37.0
  influenzal — *see* Influenza, with, respiratory manifestations NEC
  obstructive J05.0

Laryngitis — *continued*
  sicca J37.0
  spasmodic J05.0
    acute J04.0
  streptococcal J04.0
  stridulous J05.0
  syphilitic (late) A52.73
    congenital A50.59 [J99]
      early A50.03 [J99]
  tuberculous A15.5
  Vincent's A69.1
Laryngocele (congenital) (ventricular) Q31.3
Laryngofissure J38.7
  congenital Q31.8
Laryngomalacia (congenital) Q31.5
Laryngopharyngitis (acute) J06.0
  chronic J37.0
  due to external agent — *see* Inflammation, respiratory, upper, due to
Laryngoplegia J38.00
  bilateral J38.02
  unilateral J38.01
Laryngoptosis J38.7
Laryngospasm J38.5
Laryngostenosis J38.6
Laryngotracheitis (acute) (Infectional) (infective) (viral) J04.2
  atrophic J37.1
  catarrhal J37.1
  chronic J37.1
  diphtheritic A36.2
  due to external agent — *see* Inflammation, respiratory, upper, due to
  Hemophilus influenzae J04.2
  hypertrophic J37.1
  influenzal — *see* Influenza, with, respiratory manifestations NEC
  pachydermic J38.7
  sicca J37.1
  spasmodic J38.5
    acute J05.0
  streptococcal J04.2
  stridulous J38.5
  syphilitic (late) A52.73
    congenital A50.59 [J99]
      early A50.03 [J99]
  tuberculous A15.5
  Vincent's A69.1
Laryngotracheobronchitis — *see* Bronchitis
Larynx, laryngeal — *see* condition
Lassa fever A96.2
Lassitude — *see* Weakness
Late
  talker R62.0
  walker R62.0
Late effect(s) — *see* Sequelae
Latent — *see* condition
Laterocession — *see* Lateroversion
Lateroflexion — *see* Lateroversion
Lateroversion
  cervix — *see* Lateroversion, uterus
  uterus, uterine (cervix) (postinfectional) (postpartal, old) N85.4
    congenital Q51.818
    in pregnancy or childbirth O34.59- ☑
Lathyrism — *see* Poisoning, food, noxious, plant
Launois' syndrome (pituitary gigantism) E22.0
Launois-Bensaude adenolipomatosis E88.89
Laurence-Moon (-Bardet)-**Biedl syndrome** Q87.89
Lax, laxity (see also Relaxation)
  ligament (ous) (see also Disorder, ligament)
    familial M35.7
    knee — *see* Derangement, knee
  skin (acquired) L57.4
    congenital Q82.8
Laxative habit F55.2
Lazy leukocyte syndrome D70.8
Lead miner's lung J63.6
Leak, leakage
  air NEC J93.82
    postprocedural J95.812
  amniotic fluid — *see* Rupture, membranes, premature
  blood (microscopic), fetal, into maternal circulation
    affecting management of pregnancy — *see* Pregnancy, complicated by
  cerebrospinal fluid G96.0
    from spinal (lumbar) puncture G97.0

Leak, leakage — *continued*
device, implant or graft (*see also* Complications, by site and type, mechanical)
arterial graft NEC — *see* Complication, cardiovascular device, mechanical, vascular
breast (implant) T85.43 ☑
catheter NEC T85.638 ☑
dialysis (renal) T82.43 ☑
intraperitoneal T85.631 ☑
infusion NEC T82.534 ☑
spinal (epidural) (subdural) T85.630 ☑
urinary, indwelling T83.038 ☑
cystostomy T83.030 ☑
gastrointestinal — *see* Complications, prosthetic device, mechanical, gastrointestinal device
genital NEC T83.498 ☑
penile prosthesis T83.490 ☑
heart NEC — *see* Complication, cardiovascular device, mechanical
joint prosthesis — *see* Complications, joint prosthesis, mechanical, specified NEC, by site
ocular NEC — *see* Complications, prosthetic device, mechanical, ocular device
orthopedic NEC — *see* Complication, orthopedic, device, mechanical
persistent air J93.82
specified NEC T85.638 ☑
urinary NEC (*see also* Complication, genitourinary, device, urinary, mechanical)
graft T83.23 ☑
vascular NEC — *see* Complication, cardiovascular device, mechanical
ventricular intracranial shunt T85.03 ☑
urine — *see* Incontinence
Leaky heart — *see* Endocarditis
Learning defect (specific) F81.9
Leather bottle stomach C16.9
Leber's
congenital amaurosis H35.50
optic atrophy (hereditary) H47.22
Lederer's anemia D59.1
Leeches (external) — *see* Hirudiniasis
Leg — *see* condition
Legg (-Calvé)-**Perthes disease, syndrome or osteochondrosis** M91.1- ☑
Legionellosis A48.1
nonpneumonic A48.2
Legionnaires'
disease A48.1
nonpneumonic A48.2
pneumonia A48.1
Leigh's disease G31.82
Leiner's disease L21.1
Leiofibromyoma — *see* Leiomyoma
Leiomyoblastoma — *see* Neoplasm, connective tissue, benign
Leiomyofibroma (*see also* Neoplasm, connective tissue, benign)
uterus (cervix) (corpus) D25.9
Leiomyoma (*see also* Neoplasm, connective tissue, benign)
bizarre — *see* Neoplasm, connective tissue, benign
cellular — *see* Neoplasm, connective tissue, benign
epithelioid — *see* Neoplasm, connective tissue, benign
uterus (cervix) (corpus) D25.9
intramural D25.1
submucous D25.0
subserosal D25.2
vascular — *see* Neoplasm, connective tissue, benign
Leiomyoma, leiomyomatosis (intravascular) — *see* Neoplasm, connective tissue, uncertain behavior
Leiomyosarcoma (*see also* Neoplasm, connective tissue, malignant)
epithelioid — *see* Neoplasm, connective tissue, malignant
myxoid — *see* Neoplasm, connective tissue, malignant
Leishmaniasis B55.9
American (mucocutaneous) B55.2
cutaneous B55.1
Asian Desert B55.1
Brazilian B55.2
cutaneous (any type) B55.1
dermal (*see also* Leishmaniasis, cutaneous)
post-kala-azar B55.0
eyelid B55.1
infantile B55.0
Mediterranean B55.0

Leishmaniasis — *continued*
mucocutaneous (American) (New World) B55.2
naso-oral B55.2
nasopharyngeal B55.2
old world B55.1
tegumentaria diffusa B55.1
visceral B55.0
Leishmanoid, dermal (*see also* Leishmaniasis, cutaneous)
post-kala-azar B55.0
Lenegre's disease I44.2
Lengthening, leg — *see* Deformity, limb, unequal length
Lennert's lymphoma — *see* Lymphoma, Lennert's
Lennox-Gastaut syndrome G40.812
intractable G40.814
with status epilepticus G40.813
without status epilepticus G40.814
not intractable G40.812
with status epilepticus G40.811
without status epilepticus G40.812
Lens — *see* condition
Lenticonus (anterior) (posterior) (congenital) Q12.8
Lenticular degeneration, progressive E83.01
Lentiglobus (posterior) (congenital) Q12.8
Lentigo (congenital) L81.4
maligna (*see also* Melanoma, in situ)
melanoma — *see* Melanoma
Lentivirus, as cause of disease classified elsewhere B97.31
Leontiasis
ossium M85.2
syphilitic (late) A52.78
congenital A50.59
Lepothrix A48.8
Lepra — *see* Leprosy
Leprechaunism E34.8
Leprosy A30.- ☑
with muscle disorder A30.9 [M63.80]
ankle A30.9 [M63.87-] ☑
foot A30.9 [M63.87-] ☑
forearm A30.9 [M63.83-] ☑
hand A30.9 [M63.84-] ☑
lower leg A30.9 [M63.86-] ☑
multiple sites A30.9 [M63.89]
pelvic region A30.9 [M63.85-] ☑
shoulder region A30.9 [M63.81-] ☑
specified site NEC A30.9 [M63.88]
thigh A30.9 [M63.85-] ☑
upper arm A30.9 [M63.82-] ☑
anesthetic A30.9
BB A30.3
BL A30.4
borderline (infiltrated) (neuritic) A30.3
lepromatous A30.4
tuberculoid A30.2
BT A30.2
dimorphous (infiltrated) (neuritic) A30.3
I A30.0
indeterminate (macular) (neuritic) A30.0
lepromatous (diffuse) (infiltrated) (macular) (neuritic) (nodular) A30.5
LL A30.5
macular (early) (neuritic) (simple) A30.9
maculoanesthetic A30.9
mixed A30.3
neural A30.9
nodular A30.5
primary neuritic A30.3
specified type NEC A30.8
TT A30.1
tuberculoid (major) (minor) A30.1
Leptocytosis, hereditary D56.9
Leptomeningitis (chronic) (circumscribed) (hemorrhagic) (nonsuppurative) — *see* Meningitis
Leptomeningopathy G96.19
Leptospiral — *see* condition
Leptospirochetal — *see* condition
Leptospirosis A27.9
canicola A27.89
due to Leptospira interrogans serovar icterohaemorrhagiae A27.0
icterohemorrhagica A27.0
pomona A27.89
Weil's disease A27.0
Leptus dermatitis B88.0
Leriche's syndrome (aortic bifurcation occlusion) I74.09
Leri's pleonosteosis Q78.8

Leri-Weill syndrome Q77.8
Lermoyez' syndrome — *see* Vertigo, peripheral NEC
Lesch-Nyhan syndrome E79.1
Leser-Trélat disease L82.1
inflamed L82.0
Lesion(s) (nontraumatic)
abducens nerve — *see* Strabismus, paralytic, sixth nerve
alveolar process K08.9
angiocentric immunoproliferative D47.Z9 (*following* D47.4)
anorectal K62.9
aortic (valve) I35.9
auditory nerve — *see* subcategory H93.3 ☑
basal ganglion G25.9
bile duct — *see* Disease, bile duct
biomechanical M99.9
specified type NEC M99.89
abdomen M99.89
acromioclavicular M99.87
cervical region M99.81
cervicothoracic M99.81
costochondral M99.88
costovertebral M99.88
head region M99.80
hip M99.85
lower extremity M99.86
lumbar region M99.83
lumbosacral M99.83
occipitocervical M99.80
pelvic region M99.85
pubic M99.85
rib cage M99.88
sacral region M99.84
sacrococcygeal M99.84
sacroiliac M99.84
specified NEC M99.89
sternochondral M99.88
sternoclavicular M99.87
thoracic region M99.82
thoracolumbar M99.82
upper extremity M99.87
bladder N32.9
bone — *see* Disorder, bone
brachial plexus G54.0
brain G93.9
congenital Q04.9
vascular I67.9
degenerative I67.9
hypertensive I67.4
buccal cavity K13.79
calcified — *see* Calcification
canthus — *see* Disorder, eyelid
carate — *see* Pinta, lesions
cardia K22.9
cardiac (*see also* Disease, heart) I51.9
congenital Q24.9
valvular — *see* Endocarditis
cauda equina G83.4
cecum K63.9
cerebral — *see* Lesion, brain
cerebrovascular I67.9
degenerative I67.9
hypertensive I67.4
cervical (nerve) root NEC G54.2
chiasmal — *see* Disorder, optic, chiasm
chorda tympani G51.8
coin, lung R91.1
colon K63.9
congenital — *see* Anomaly, by site
conjunctiva H11.9
conus medullaris — *see* Injury, conus medullaris
coronary artery — *see* Ischemia, heart
cranial nerve G52.9
eighth — *see* Disorder, ear
eleventh G52.9
fifth G50.9
first G52.0
fourth — *see* Strabismus, paralytic, fourth nerve
seventh G51.9
sixth — *see* Strabismus, paralytic, sixth nerve
tenth G52.2
twelfth G52.3
cystic — *see* Cyst
degenerative — *see* Degeneration
duodenum K31.9
edentulous (alveolar) ridge, associated with trauma, due to traumatic occlusion K06.2

Lesion(s) — *continued*
en coup de sabre L94.1
eyelid — *see* Disorder, eyelid
gasserian ganglion G50.8
gastric K31.9
gastroduodenal K31.9
gastrointestinal K63.9
gingiva, associated with trauma K06.2
glomerular
    focal and segmental (*see also* N00-N07 with fourth
             character .1) N05.1
    minimal change (*see also* N00-N07 with fourth
             character .0) N05.0
heart (organic) — *see* Disease, heart
hyperchromic, due to pinta (carate) A67.1
hyperkeratotic — *see* Hyperkeratosis
hypothalamic E23.7
ileocecal K63.9
ileum K63.9
iliohypogastric nerve G57.8- ☑
inflammatory — *see* Inflammation
intestine K63.9
intracerebral — *see* Lesion, brain
intrachiasmal (optic) — *see* Disorder, optic, chiasm
intracranial, space-occupying R90.0
joint — *see* Disorder, joint
    sacroiliac (old) M53.3
keratotic — *see* Keratosis
kidney — *see* Disease, renal
laryngeal nerve (recurrent) G52.2
lip K13.0
liver K76.9
lumbosacral
    plexus G54.1
    root (nerve) NEC G54.4
lung (coin) R91.1
maxillary sinus J32.0
mitral I05.9
Morel-Lavallée — *see* Hematoma, by site
motor cortex NEC G93.89
mouth K13.79
nerve G58.9
    femoral G57.2- ☑
    median G56.1- ☑
        carpal tunnel syndrome — *see* Syndrome,
            carpal tunnel
    plantar G57.6- ☑
    popliteal (lateral) G57.3- ☑
        medial G57.4- ☑
    radial G56.3- ☑
    sciatic G57.0- ☑
    spinal — *see* Injury, nerve, spinal
    ulnar G56.2- ☑
nervous system, congenital Q07.9
nonallopathic — *see* Lesion, biomechanical
nose (internal) J34.89
obstructive — *see* Obstruction
obturator nerve G57.8- ☑
oral mucosa K13.70
organ or site NEC — *see* Disease, by site
osteolytic — *see* Osteolysis
peptic K27.9
periodontal, due to traumatic occlusion K05.5
pharynx J39.2
pigment, pigmented (skin) L81.9
pinta — *see* Pinta, lesions
polypoid — *see* Polyp
prechiasmal (optic) — *see* Disorder, optic, chiasm
primary (*see also* Syphilis, primary) A51.0
    carate A67.0
    pinta A67.0
    yaws A66.0
pulmonary J98.4
    valve I37.9
pylorus K31.9
rectosigmoid K63.9
retina, retinal H35.9
sacroiliac (joint) (old) M53.3
salivary gland K11.9
    benign lymphoepithelial K11.8
saphenous nerve G57.8- ☑
sciatic nerve G57.0- ☑
secondary — *see* Syphilis, secondary
shoulder (region) M75.9- ☑
    specified NEC M75.8- ☑
sigmoid K63.9
sinus (accessory) (nasal) J34.89

Lesion(s) — *continued*
skin L98.9
    suppurative L08.0
SLAP S43.43- ☑
spinal cord G95.9
    congenital Q06.9
spleen D73.89
stomach K31.9
superior glenoid labrum S43.43- ☑
syphilitic — *see* Syphilis
tertiary — *see* Syphilis, tertiary
thoracic root (nerve) NEC G54.3
tonsillar fossa J35.9
tooth, teeth K08.9
    white spot
        chewing surface K02.51
        pit and fissure surface K02.51
        smooth surface K02.61
traumatic — *see* specific type of injury by site
tricuspid (valve) I07.9
    nonrheumatic I36.9
trigeminal nerve G50.9
ulcerated or ulcerative — *see* Ulcer, skin
uterus N85.9
vagus nerve G52.2
valvular — *see* Endocarditis
vascular I99.9
    affecting central nervous system I67.9
    following trauma NEC T14.8
    umbilical cord, complicating delivery O69.5 ☑
warty — *see* Verruca
white spot (tooth)
    chewing surface K02.51
    pit and fissure surface K02.51
    smooth surface K02.61
Lethargic — *see* condition
Lethargy R53.83
Letterer-Siwe's disease C96.0
Leukemia, leukemic C95.9- ☑
acute basophilic C94.8- ☑
acute bilineal C95.0- ☑
acute erythroid C94.0- ☑
acute lymphoblastic C91.0- ☑
acute megakaryoblastic C94.2- ☑
acute megakaryocytic C94.2- ☑
acute mixed lineage C95.0- ☑
acute monoblastic (monoblastic/monocytic) C93.0- ☑
acute monocytic (monoblastic/monocytic) C93.0- ☑
acute myeloblastic (minimal differentiation) (with
    maturation) C92.0- ☑
acute myeloid
    with
        11q23-abnormality C92.6- ☑
        dysplasia of remaining hematopoesis and/or
            myelodysplastic disease in its history
            C92.A- ☑ (*following* C92.6)
        multilineage dysplasia C92.A- ☑ (*following*
            C92.6)
        variation of MLL-gene C92.6- ☑
    M6 (a)(b) C94.0- ☑
    M7 C94.2- ☑
acute myelomonocytic C92.5- ☑
acute promyelocytic C92.4- ☑
adult T-cell (HTLV-1-associated) (acute variant)
    (chronic variant) (lymphomatoid variant)
    (smouldering variant) C91.5- ☑
aggressive NK-cell C94.8- ☑
AML (1/ETO) (M0) (M1) (M2) (without a FAB classifica-
    tion) C92.0- ☑
AML M3 C92.4- ☑
AML M4 (Eo with inv(16) or t(16;16)) C92.5- ☑
AML M5 C93.0- ☑
AML M5a C93.0- ☑
AML M5b C93.0- ☑
AML Me with t (15;17) and variants C92.4- ☑
atypical chronic myeloid, BCR/ABL-negative C92.2- ☑
biphenotypic acute C95.0- ☑
blast cell C95.0- ☑
Burkitt-type, mature B-cell C91.A- ☑ (*following* C91.6)
chronic lymphocytic, of B-cell type C91.1- ☑
chronic monocytic C93.1- ☑
chronic myelogenous (Philadelphia chromosome (Ph1)
    positive) (t(9;22)) (q34;q11) (with crisis of blast
    cells) C92.1- ☑
chronic myeloid, BCR/ABL-positive C92.1- ☑
    atypical, BCR/ABL-negative C92.2- ☑
chronic myelomonocytic C93.1- ☑

Leukemia, leukemic — *continued*
chronic neutrophilic D47.1
CMML (-1) (-2) (with eosinophilia) C93.1- ☑
granulocytic (*see also* Category C92) C92.9- ☑
hairy cell C91.4- ☑
juvenile myelomonocytic C93.3- ☑
lymphoid C91.9- ☑
    specified NEC C91.Z- ☑ (*following* C91.6)
mast cell C94.3- ☑
mature B-cell, Burkitt-type C91.A- ☑ (*following* C91.6)
monocytic (subacute) C93.9- ☑
    specified NEC C93.Z- ☑ (*following* C93.3)
myelogenous (*see also* Category C92) C92.9- ☑
myeloid C92.9- ☑
    specified NEC C92.Z- ☑ (*following* C92.6)
plasma cell C90.1- ☑
plasmacytic C90.1- ☑
prolymphocytic
    of B-cell type C91.3- ☑
    of T-cell type C91.6- ☑
specified NEC C94.8- ☑
stem cell, of unclear lineage C95.0- ☑
subacute lymphocytic C91.9- ☑
T-cell large granular lymphocytic C91.Z- ☑ (*following*
    C91.6)
unspecified cell type C95.9- ☑
    acute C95.0- ☑
    chronic C95.1- ☑
Leukemoid reaction (*see also* Reaction, leukemoid)
    D72.823
Leukoaraiosis (hypertensive) I67.81
Leukoariosis — *see* Leukoaraiosis
Leukocoria — *see* Disorder, globe, degenerated condi-
    tion, leucocoria
Leukocytopenia D72.819
Leukocytosis D72.829
    eosinophilic D72.1
Leukoderma, leukodermia NEC L81.5
    syphilitic A51.39
        late A52.79
Leukodystrophy E75.29
Leukoedema, oral epithelium K13.29
Leukoencephalitis G04.81
    acute (subacute) hemorrhagic G36.1
        postimmunization or postvaccinal G04.02
    postinfectious G04.01
    subacute sclerosing A81.1
    van Bogaert's (sclerosing) A81.1
Leukoencephalopathy (*see also* Encephalopathy)
    G93.49
    Binswanger's I67.3
    heroin vapor G92
    metachromatic E75.25
    multifocal (progressive) A81.2
    postimmunization and postvaccinal G04.02
    progressive multifocal A81.2
    reversible, posterior G93.6
    van Bogaert's (sclerosing) A81.1
    vascular, progressive I67.3
Leukoerythroblastosis D75.9
Leukokeratosis (*see also* Leukoplakia)
    mouth K13.21
    nicotina palati K13.24
    oral mucosa K13.21
    tongue K13.21
    vocal cord J38.3
Leukokraurosis vulva (e) N90.4
Leukoma (cornea) (*see also* Opacity, cornea)
    adherent H17.0- ☑
    interfering with central vision — *see* Opacity, cornea,
        central
Leukomalacia, cerebral, newborn P91.2
    periventricular P91.2
Leukomelanopathy, hereditary D72.0
Leukonychia (punctata) (striata) L60.8
    congenital Q84.4
Leukopathia unguium L60.8
    congenital Q84.4
Leukopenia D72.819
    basophilic D72.818
    chemotherapy (cancer) induced D70.1
    congenital D70.0
    cyclic D70.0
    drug induced NEC D70.2
        due to cytoreductive cancer chemotherapy D70.1
    eosinophilic D72.818
    familial D70.0

☑ **Additional Character Required** — **Refer to the Tabular List for Character Selection**   ▽ **Subterms under main terms may continue to next column or page**

Leukopenia — *continued*
  infantile genetic D70.0
  malignant D70.9
  periodic D70.0
  transitory neonatal P61.5
Leukopenic — *see* condition
Leukoplakia
  anus K62.89
  bladder (postinfectional) N32.89
  buccal K13.21
  cervix (uteri) N88.0
  esophagus K22.8
  gingiva K13.21
  hairy (oral mucosa) (tongue) K13.3
  kidney (pelvis) N28.89
  larynx J38.7
  lip K13.21
  mouth K13.21
  oral epithelium, including tongue (mucosa) K13.21
  palate K13.21
  pelvis (kidney) N28.89
  penis (infectional) N48.0
  rectum K62.89
  syphilitic (late) A52.79
  tongue K13.21
  ureter (postinfectional) N28.89
  urethra (postinfectional) N36.8
  uterus N85.8
  vagina N89.4
  vocal cord J38.3
  vulva N90.4
Leukorrhea N89.8
  due to Trichomonas (vaginalis) A59.00
  trichomonal A59.00
Leukosarcoma C85.9- ☑
Levocardia (isolated) Q24.1
  with situs inversus Q89.3
Levotransposition Q20.5
Lev's disease or syndrome (acquired complete heart
    block) I44.2
Levulosuria — *see* Fructosuria
Levurid L30.2
Lewy body (ies) (dementia) (disease) G31.83
Leyden-Moebius dystrophy G71.0
Leydig cell
  carcinoma
    specified site — *see* Neoplasm, malignant, by site
    unspecified site
      female C56.9
      male C62.9- ☑
  tumor
    benign
      specified site — *see* Neoplasm, benign, by site
      unspecified site
        female D27.- ☑
        male D29.2- ☑
    malignant
      specified site — *see* Neoplasm, malignant, by
          site
      unspecified site
        female C56.- ☑
        male C62.9- ☑
    specified site — *see* Neoplasm, uncertain behavior,
        by site
    unspecified site
      female D39.1- ☑
      male D40.1- ☑
Leydig-Sertoli cell tumor
  specified site — *see* Neoplasm, benign, by site
  unspecified site
    female D27.- ☑
    male D29.2- ☑
LGSIL (Low grade squamous intraepithelial lesion on cy-
    tologic smear of)
  anus R85.612
  cervix R87.612
  vagina R87.622
Liar, pathologic F60.2
Libido
  decreased R68.82
Libman-Sacks disease M32.11
Lice (infestation) B85.2
  body (Pediculus corporis) B85.1
  crab B85.3
  head (Pediculus capitis) B85.0
  mixed (classifiable to more than one of the titles B85.0-
      B85.3) B85.4

Lice — *continued*
  pubic (Phthirus pubis) B85.3
Lichen L28.0
  albus L90.0
    penis N48.0
    vulva N90.4
  amyloidosis E85.4 [L99]
  atrophicus L90.0
    penis N48.0
    vulva N90.4
  congenital Q82.8
  myxedematosus L98.5
  nitidus L44.1
  pilaris Q82.8
    acquired L85.8
  planopilaris L66.1
  planus (chronicus) L43.9
    annularis L43.8
    bullous L43.1
    follicular L66.1
    hypertrophic L43.0
    moniliformis L44.3
    of Wilson L43.9
    specified NEC L43.8
    subacute (active) L43.3
    tropicus L43.3
  ruber
    acuminatus L44.0
    moniliformis L44.3
    planus L43.9
  sclerosus (et atrophicus) L90.0
    penis N48.0
    vulva N90.4
  scrofulosus (primary) (tuberculous) A18.4
  simplex (chronicus) (circumscriptus) L28.0
  striatus L44.2
  urticatus L28.2
Lichenification L28.0
Lichenoides tuberculosis (primary) A18.4
Lichtheim's disease or syndrome — *see* Degeneration,
    combined
Lien migrans D73.89
Ligament — *see* condition
Light
  for gestational age — *see* Light for dates
  headedness R42
Light-for-dates (infant) P05.00
  with weight of
    1000-1249 grams P05.04
    1250-1499 grams P05.05
    1500-1749 grams P05.06
    1750-1999 grams P05.07
    2000-2499 grams P05.08
    499 grams or less P05.01
    500-749 grams P05.02
    750-999 grams P05.03
  affecting management of pregnancy O36.59- ☑
  and small-for-dates — *see* Small for dates
Lightning (effects) (stroke) (struck by) T75.00 ☑
  burn — *see* Burn
  foot E53.8
  shock T75.01 ☑
  specified effect NEC T75.09 ☑
Lightwood-Albright syndrome N25.89
Lightwood's disease or syndrome (renal tubular acido-
    sis) N25.89
Lignac (-de Toni) (-Fanconi) (-Debré) **disease or syn-
    drome** E72.09
  with cystinosis E72.04
Ligneous thyroiditis E06.5
Likoff's syndrome I20.8
Limb — *see* condition
Limbic epilepsy personality syndrome F07.0
Limitation, limited
  activities due to disability Z73.6
  cardiac reserve — *see* Disease, heart
  eye muscle duction, traumatic — *see* Strabismus,
      mechanical
  mandibular range of motion M26.52
Lindau (-von Hippel) **disease** Q85.8
Line(s)
  Beau's L60.4
  Harris' — *see* Arrest, epiphyseal
  Hudson's (cornea) — *see* Pigmentation, cornea, ante-
      rior
  Stähli's (cornea) — *see* Pigmentation, cornea, anterior
Linea corneae senilis — *see* Change, cornea, senile

Lingua
  geographica K14.1
  nigra (villosa) K14.3
  plicata K14.5
  tylosis K13.29
Lingual — *see* condition
Linguatulosis B88.8
Linitis (gastric) **plastica** C16.9
Lip — *see* condition
Lipedema — *see* Edema
Lipemia (*see also* Hyperlipidemia)
  retina, retinalis E78.3
Lipidosis E75.6
  cerebral (infantile) (juvenile) (late) E75.4
  cerebroretinal E75.4
  cerebroside E75.22
  cholesterol (cerebral) E75.5
  glycolipid E75.21
  hepatosplenomegalic E78.3
  sphingomyelin — *see* Niemann-Pick disease or syn-
      drome
  sulfatide E75.29
Lipoadenoma — *see* Neoplasm, benign, by site
Lipoblastoma — *see* Lipoma
Lipoblastomatosis — *see* Lipoma
Lipochondrodystrophy E76.01
Lipochrome histiocytosis (familial) D71
Lipodermatosclerosis — *see* Varix, leg, with, inflamma-
    tion
  ulcerated — *see* Varix, leg, with, ulcer, with inflamma-
      tion by site
Lipodystrophia progressiva E88.1
Lipodystrophy (progressive) E88.1
  insulin E88.1
  intestinal K90.81
  mesenteric K65.4
Lipofibroma — *see* Lipoma
Lipofuscinosis, neuronal (with ceroidosis) E75.4
Lipogranuloma, sclerosing L92.8
Lipogranulomatosis E78.89
Lipoid (*see also* condition)
  histiocytosis D76.3
    essential E75.29
  nephrosis N04.9
  proteinosis of Urbach E78.89
Lipoidemia — *see* Hyperlipidemia
Lipoidosis — *see* Lipidosis
Lipoma D17.9
  fetal D17.9
    fat cell D17.9
  infiltrating D17.9
  intramuscular D17.9
  pleomorphic D17.9
  site classification
    arms (skin) (subcutaneous) D17.2- ☑
    connective tissue D17.30
      intra-abdominal D17.5
      intrathoracic D17.4
      peritoneum D17.79
      retroperitoneum D17.79
      specified site NEC D17.39
      spermatic cord D17.6
    face (skin) (subcutaneous) D17.0
    genitourinary organ NEC D17.72
    head (skin) (subcutaneous) D17.0
    intra-abdominal D17.5
    intrathoracic D17.4
    kidney D17.71
    legs (skin) (subcutaneous) D17.2- ☑
    neck (skin) (subcutaneous) D17.0
    peritoneum D17.79
    retroperitoneum D17.79
    skin D17.30
      specified site NEC D17.39
    specified site NEC D17.79
    spermatic cord D17.6
    subcutaneous D17.30
      specified site NEC D17.39
    trunk (skin) (subcutaneous) D17.1
    unspecified D17.9
  spindle cell D17.9
Lipomatosis E88.2
  dolorosa (Dercum) E88.2
  fetal — *see* Lipoma
  Launois-Bensaude E88.89
Lipomyoma — *see* Lipoma
Lipomyxoma — *see* Lipoma

Lipomyxosarcoma — *see* Neoplasm, connective tissue, malignant
Lipoprotein metabolism disorder E78.9
Lipoproteinemia E78.5
 broad-beta E78.2
 floating-beta E78.2
 hyper-pre-beta E78.1
Liposarcoma (*see also* Neoplasm, connective tissue, malignant)
 dedifferentiated — *see* Neoplasm, connective tissue, malignant
 differentiated type — *see* Neoplasm, connective tissue, malignant
 embryonal — *see* Neoplasm, connective tissue, malignant
 mixed type — *see* Neoplasm, connective tissue, malignant
 myxoid — *see* Neoplasm, connective tissue, malignant
 pleomorphic — *see* Neoplasm, connective tissue, malignant
 round cell — *see* Neoplasm, connective tissue, malignant
 well differentiated type — *see* Neoplasm, connective tissue, malignant
Liposynovitis prepatellaris E88.89
Lipping, cervix N86
Lipschütz disease or ulcer N76.6
Lipuria R82.0
 schistosomiasis (bilharziasis) B65.0
Lisping F80.0
Lissauer's paralysis A52.17
Lissencephalia, lissencephaly Q04.3
Listeriosis, listerellosis A32.9
 congenital (disseminated) P37.2
 cutaneous A32.0
 neonatal, newborn (disseminated) P37.2
 oculoglandular A32.81
 specified NEC A32.89
Lithemia E79.0
Lithiasis — *see* Calculus
Lithosis J62.8
Lithuria R82.99
Litigation, anxiety concerning Z65.3
Little leaguer's elbow — *see* Epicondylitis, medial
Little's disease G80.9
Littre's
 gland — *see* condition
 hernia — *see* Hernia, abdomen
Littritis — *see* Urethritis
Livedo (annularis) (racemosa) (reticularis) R23.1
Liver — *see* condition
Living alone (problems with) Z60.2
 with handicapped person Z74.2
Lloyd's syndrome — *see* Adenomatosis, endocrine
Loa loa, loaiasis, loasis B74.3
Lobar — *see* condition
Lobomycosis B48.0
Lobo's disease B48.0
Lobotomy syndrome F07.0
Lobstein (-Ekman) **disease or syndrome** Q78.0
Lobster-claw hand Q71.6- ☑
Lobulation (congenital) (*see also* Anomaly, by site)
 kidney, Q63.1
 liver, abnormal Q44.7
 spleen Q89.09
Lobule, lobular — *see* condition
Local, localized — *see* condition
Locked twins causing obstructed labor O66.1
Locked-in state G83.5
Locking
 joint — *see* Derangement, joint, specified type NEC
 knee — *see* Derangement, knee
Lockjaw — *see* Tetanus
Löffler's
 endocarditis I42.3
 eosinophilia J82
 pneumonia J82
 syndrome (eosinophilic pneumonitis) J82
Loiasis (with conjunctival infestation) (eyelid) B74.3
Lone Star fever A77.0
Long
 labor O63.9
  first stage O63.0
  second stage O63.1
 QT syndrome I45.81
Longitudinal stripes or grooves, nails L60.8
 congenital Q84.6

Long-term (current) (prophylactic) **drug therapy** (use of)
 agents affecting estrogen receptors and estrogen levels NEC Z79.818
 anastrozole (Arimidex) Z79.811
 antibiotics Z79.2
  short-term use — *omit code*
 anticoagulants Z79.01
 anti-inflammatory, non-steroidal (NSAID) Z79.1
 antiplatelet Z79.02
 antithrombotics Z79.02
 aromatase inhibitors Z79.811
 aspirin Z79.82
 birth control pill or patch Z79.3
 bisphosphonates Z79.83
 contraceptive, oral Z79.3
 drug, specified NEC Z79.899
 estrogen receptor downregulators Z79.818
 Evista Z79.810
 exemestane (Aromasin) Z79.811
 Fareston Z79.810
 fulvestrant (Faslodex) Z79.818
 gonadotropin-releasing hormone (GnRH) agonist Z79.818
 goserelin acetate (Zoladex) Z79.818
 hormone replacement (postmenopausal) Z79.890
 insulin Z79.4
 letrozole (Femara) Z79.811
 leuprolide acetate (leuprorelin) (Lupron) Z79.818
 megestrol acetate (Megace) Z79.818
 methadone for pain management Z79.891
 Nolvadex Z79.810
 non-steroidal anti-inflammatories (NSAID) Z79.1
 opiate analgesic Z79.891
 oral contraceptive Z79.3
 raloxifene (Evista) Z79.810
 selective estrogen receptor modulators (SERMs) Z79.810
 steroids
  inhaled Z79.51
  systemic Z79.52
 tamoxifen (Nolvadex) Z79.810
 toremifene (Fareston) Z79.810
Loop
 intestine — *see* Volvulus
 vascular on papilla (optic) Q14.2
Loose (*see also* condition)
 body
  joint M24.00
   ankle M24.07- ☑
   elbow M24.02- ☑
   hand M24.04- ☑
   hip M24.05- ☑
   knee M23.4- ☑
   shoulder (region) M24.01- ☑
   specified site NEC M24.08
   toe M24.07- ☑
   vertebra M24.08
   wrist M24.03- ☑
  knee M23.4- ☑
  sheath, tendon — *see* Disorder, tendon, specified type NEC
 cartilage — *see* Loose, body, joint
 tooth, teeth K08.8
Loosening
 aseptic
  joint prosthesis — *see* Complications, joint prosthesis, mechanical, loosening, by site
 epiphysis — *see* Osteochondropathy
 mechanical
  joint prosthesis — *see* Complications, joint prosthesis, mechanical, loosening, by site
Looser-Milkman (-Debray) **syndrome** M83.8
Lop ear (deformity) Q17.3
Lorain (-Levi) **short stature syndrome** E23.0
Lordosis M40.50
 acquired — *see* Lordosis, specified type NEC
 congenital Q76.429
  lumbar region Q76.426
  lumbosacral region Q76.427
  sacral region Q76.428
  sacrococcygeal region Q76.428
  thoracolumbar region Q76.425
 lumbar region M40.56
 lumbosacral region M40.57
 postsurgical M96.4
 postural — *see* Lordosis, specified type NEC
 rachitic (late effect) (sequelae) E64.3

Lordosis — *continued*
 sequelae of rickets E64.3
 specified type NEC M40.40
  lumbar region M40.46
  lumbosacral region M40.47
  thoracolumbar region M40.45
 thoracolumbar region M40.55
 tuberculous A18.01
Loss (of)
 appetite (*see* Anorexia) R63.0
  hysterical F50.8
  nonorganic origin F50.8
  psychogenic F50.8
 blood — *see* Hemorrhage
 consciousness, transient R55
  traumatic — *see* Injury, intracranial
 control, sphincter, rectum R15.9
  nonorganic origin F98.1
 elasticity, skin R23.4
 family (member) in childhood Z62.898
 fluid (acute) E86.9
  with
   hypernatremia E87.0
   hyponatremia E87.1
 function of labyrinth — *see* subcategory H83.2 ☑
 hair, nonscarring — *see* Alopecia
 hearing (*see also* Deafness)
  central NOS H90.5
  neural NOS H90.5
  perceptive NOS H90.5
  sensorineural NOS H90.5
  sensory NOS H90.5
 height R29.890
 limb or member, traumatic, current — *see* Amputation, traumatic
 love relationship in childhood Z62.898
 memory (*see also* Amnesia)
  mild, following organic brain damage F06.8
 mind — *see* Psychosis
 occlusal vertical dimension of fully erupted teeth M26.37
 organ or part — *see* Absence, by site, acquired
 ossicles, ear (partial) H74.32- ☑
 parent in childhood Z63.4
 pregnancy, recurrent N96
  without current pregnancy N96
  care in current pregnancy O26.2- ☑
 recurrent pregnancy — *see* Loss, pregnancy, recurrent
 self-esteem, in childhood Z62.898
 sense of
  smell — *see* Disturbance, sensation, smell
  taste — *see* Disturbance, sensation, taste
  touch R20.8
 sensory R44.9
  dissociative F44.6
 sexual desire F52.0
 sight (acquired) (complete) (congenital) — *see* Blindness
 substance of
  bone — *see* Disorder, bone, density and structure, specified NEC
  cartilage — *see* Disorder, cartilage, specified type NEC
   auricle (ear) — *see* Disorder, pinna, specified type NEC
  vitreous (humor) H15.89
 tooth, teeth — *see* Absence, teeth, acquired
 vision, visual H54.7
  both eyes H54.3
  one eye H54.60
   left (normal vision on right) H54.62
   right (normal vision on left) H54.61
  specified as blindness — *see* Blindness
  subjective
   sudden H53.13- ☑
   transient H53.12- ☑
 vitreous — *see* Prolapse, vitreous
 voice — *see* Aphonia
 weight (abnormal) (cause unknown) R63.4
Louis-Bar syndrome (ataxia-telangiectasia) G11.3
Louping ill (encephalitis) A84.8
Louse, lousiness — *see* Lice
Low
 achiever, school Z55.3
 back syndrome M54.5
 basal metabolic rate R94.8
 birthweight (2499 grams or less) P07.10

Lymphangitis — continued
  acute — continued
    pectoral (region) L03.323
    perineal, perineum L03.325
    scalp (any part) L03.891
    shoulder — see Lymphangitis, acute, upper limb
    specified site NEC L03.898
    thigh — see Lymphangitis, acute, lower limb
    thumb (intrathecal) (periosteal) (subcutaneous)
        (subcuticular) — see Lymphangitis, acute,
        finger
    toe (intrathecal) (periosteal) (subcutaneous) (sub-
        cuticular) L03.04- ☑
    trunk L03.329
      abdominal wall L03.321
      back (any part) L03.322
      buttock L03.327
      chest wall L03.323
      groin L03.324
      perineal, perineum L03.325
      umbilicus L03.326
    umbilicus L03.326
    upper limb L03.12- ☑
      axilla — see Lymphangitis, acute, axilla
      finger — see Lymphangitis, acute, finger
      thumb — see Lymphangitis, acute, finger
    wrist — see Lymphangitis, acute, upper limb
  breast
    gestational — see Mastitis, obstetric
  chancroidal A57
  chronic (any site) I89.1
  due to
    Brugia (malayi) B74.1
      timori B74.2
    Wuchereria bancrofti B74.0
  following ectopic or molar pregnancy O08.89
  penis
    acute N48.29
    gonococcal (acute) (chronic) A54.09
  puerperal, postpartum, childbirth O86.89
  strumous, tuberculous A18.2
  subacute (any site) I89.1
  tuberculous — see Tuberculosis, lymph gland
Lymphatic (vessel) — see condition
Lymphatism E32.8
Lymphectasia I89.0
Lymphedema (acquired) (see also Elephantiasis)
  congenital Q82.0
  hereditary (chronic) (idiopathic) Q82.0
  postmastectomy I97.2
  praecox I89.0
  secondary I89.0
  surgical NEC I97.89
    postmastectomy (syndrome) I97.2
Lymphoblastic — see condition
Lymphoblastoma (diffuse) — see Lymphoma, lym-
    phoblastic (diffuse)
  giant follicular — see Lymphoma, lymphoblastic (dif-
    fuse)
  macrofollicular — see Lymphoma, lymphoblastic
    (diffuse)
Lymphocele I89.8
Lymphocytic
  chorioencephalitis (acute) (serous) A87.2
  choriomeningitis (acute) (serous) A87.2
  meningoencephalitis A87.2
Lymphocytoma, benign cutis L98.8
Lymphocytopenia D72.810
Lymphocytosis (symptomatic) D72.820
  infectious (acute) B33.8
Lymphoepithelioma — see Neoplasm, malignant, by
    site
Lymphogranuloma (malignant) (see also Lymphoma,
    Hodgkin)
  chlamydial A55
  inguinale A55
  venereum (any site) (chlamydial) (with stricture of
    rectum) A55
Lymphogranulomatosis (malignant) (see also Lym-
    phoma, Hodgkin)
  benign (Boeck's sarcoid) (Schaumann's) D86.1
Lymphohistiocytosis, hemophagocytic (familial) D76.1
Lymphoid — see condition
Lymphoma (of) (malignant) C85.90
  adult T-cell (HTLV-1-associated) (acute variant)
      (chronic variant) (lymphomatoid variant)
      (smouldering variant) C91.5- ☑

Lymphoma — continued
  anaplastic large cell
    ALK-negative C84.7- ☑
    ALK-positive C84.6- ☑
    CD30-positive C84.6- ☑
    primary cutaneous C86.6
  angioimmunoblastic T-cell C86.5
  BALT C88.4
  B-cell C85.1- ☑
  blastic NK-cell C86.4
  B-precursor C83.5- ☑
  bronchial-associated lymphoid tissue [BALT-lym-
    phoma] C88.4
  Burkitt (atypical) C83.7- ☑
  Burkitt-like C83.7- ☑
  centrocytic C83.1- ☑
  cutaneous follicle center C82.6- ☑
  cutaneous T-cell C84.A- ☑ (following C84.7)
  diffuse follicle center C82.5- ☑
  diffuse large cell C83.3- ☑
    anaplastic C83.3- ☑
    B-cell C83.3- ☑
    CD30-positive C83.3- ☑
    centroblastic C83.3- ☑
    immunoblastic C83.3- ☑
    plasmablastic C83.3- ☑
    subtype not specified C83.3- ☑
    T-cell rich C83.3- ☑
  enteropathy-type (associated) (intestinal) T-cell C86.2
  extranodal marginal zone B-cell lymphoma of mucosa-
      associated lymphoid tissue [MALT-lymphoma]
      C88.4
  extranodal NK/T-cell, nasal type C86.0
  follicular C82.9- ☑
    grade
      I C82.0- ☑
      II C82.1- ☑
      III C82.2- ☑
      IIIa C82.3- ☑
      IIIb C82.4- ☑
    specified NEC C82.8- ☑
  hepatosplenic T-cell (alpha-beta) (gamma-delta) C86.1
  histiocytic C96.9
    true C96.A (following C96.6)
  Hodgkin C81.9 ☑
    classical C81.7- ☑
      lymphocyte depleted C81.3- ☑
      lymphocyte-rich C81.4- ☑
      mixed cellularity C81.2- ☑
      nodular sclerosis C81.1- ☑
      specified NEC C81.7- ☑
    lymphocyte depleted classical C81.3- ☑
    lymphocyte-rich classical C81.4- ☑
    mixed cellularity classical C81.2- ☑
    nodular
      lymphocyte predominant C81.0- ☑
      sclerosis classical C81.1- ☑
  intravascular large B-cell C83.8- ☑
  Lennert's C84.4- ☑
  lymphoblastic (diffuse) C83.5- ☑
  lymphoblastic B-cell C83.5- ☑
  lymphoblastic T-cell C83.5- ☑
  lymphoepithelioid C84.4- ☑
  lymphoplasmacytic C83.0- ☑
    with IgM-production C88.0
  MALT C88.4
  mantle cell C83.1- ☑
  mature T-cell NEC C84.4- ☑
  mature T/NK-cell C84.9- ☑
    specified NEC C84.Z- ☑ (following C84.7)
  mediastinal (thymic) large B-cell C85.2- ☑
  Mediterranean C88.3
  mucosa-associated lymphoid tissue [MALT-lymphoma]
    C88.4
  NK/T cell C84.9- ☑
  nodal marginal zone C83.0- ☑
  non-follicular (diffuse) C83.9- ☑
    specified NEC C83.8- ☑
  non-Hodgkin (see also Lymphoma, by type) C85.9- ☑
    specified NEC C85.8- ☑
  non-leukemic variant of B-CLL C83.0- ☑
  peripheral T-cell, not classified C84.4- ☑
  primary cutaneous
    anaplastic large cell C86.6
    CD30-positive large T-cell C86.6
  primary effusion B-cell C83.8- ☑

Lymphoma — continued
  SALT C88.4
  skin-associated lymphoid tissue [SALT-lymphoma]
    C88.4
  small cell B-cell C83.0- ☑
  splenic marginal zone C83.0- ☑
  subcutaneous panniculitis-like T-cell C86.3
  T-precursor C83.5- ☑
  true histiocytic C96.A (following C96.6)
Lymphomatosis — see Lymphoma
Lymphopathia venereum, veneris A55
Lymphopenia D72.810
Lymphoplasmacytic leukemia — see Leukemia,
  chronic lymphocytic, B-cell type
Lymphoproliferation, X-linked disease D82.3
Lymphoreticulosis, benign (of inoculation) A28.1
Lymphorrhea I89.8
Lymphosarcoma (diffuse) (see also Lymphoma)
  C85.9- ☑
Lymphostasis I89.8
Lypemania — see Melancholia
Lysine and hydroxylysine metabolism disorder E72.3
Lyssa — see Rabies

M

Macacus ear Q17.3
Maceration, wet feet, tropical (syndrome) T69.02- ☑
MacLeod's syndrome J43.0
Macrocephalia, macrocephaly Q75.3
Macrocheilia, macrochilia (congenital) Q18.6
Macrocolon (see also Megacolon) Q43.1
Macrocornea Q15.8
  with glaucoma Q15.0
Macrocytic — see condition
Macrocytosis D75.89
Macrodactylia, macrodactylism (fingers) (thumbs)
  Q74.0
  toes Q74.2
Macrodontia K00.2
Macrogenia M26.05
Macrogenitosomia (adrenal) (male) (praecox) E25.9
  congenital E25.0
Macroglobulinemia (idiopathic) (primary) C88.0
  monoclonal (essential) D47.2
  Waldenström C88.0
Macroglossia (congenital) Q38.2
  acquired K14.8
Macrognathia, macrognathism (congenital)
  (mandibular) (maxillary) M26.09
Macrogyria (congenital) Q04.8
Macrohydrocephalus — see Hydrocephalus
Macromastia — see Hypertrophy, breast
Macrophthalmos Q11.3
  in congenital glaucoma Q15.0
Macropsia H53.15
Macrosigmoid K59.3
  congenital Q43.2
Macrospondylitis , acromegalic E22.0
Macrostomia (congenital) Q18.4
Macrotia (external ear) (congenital) Q17.1
Macula
  cornea, corneal — see Opacity, cornea
  degeneration (atrophic) (exudative) (senile) (see also
    Degeneration, macula)
    hereditary — see Dystrophy, retina
Maculae ceruleae B85.1
Maculopathy, toxic — see Degeneration, macula, toxic
Madarosis (eyelid) H02.729
  left H02.726
    lower H02.725
    upper H02.724
  right H02.723
    lower H02.722
    upper H02.721
Madelung's
  deformity (radius) Q74.0
  disease
    radial deformity Q74.0
    symmetrical lipomas, neck E88.89
Madness — see Psychosis
Madura
  foot B47.9
    actinomycotic B47.1
    mycotic B47.0
Maduromycosis B47.0
Maffucci's syndrome Q78.4

Magnesium metabolism disorder — *see* Disorder,
   metabolism, magnesium
Main en griffe (acquired) (*see also* Deformity, limb,
   clawhand)
   congenital Q74.0
Maintenance (encounter for)
   antineoplastic chemotherapy Z51.11
   antineoplastic radiation therapy Z51.0
   methadone F11.20
Majocchi's
   disease L81.7
   granuloma B35.8
Major — *see* condition
Mal de los pintos — *see* Pinta
Mal de mer T75.3 ☑
Malabar itch (any site) B35.5
Malabsorption K90.9
   calcium K90.89
   carbohydrate K90.4
   disaccharide E73.9
   fat K90.4
   galactose E74.20
   glucose (-galactose) E74.39
   intestinal K90.9
      specified NEC K90.89
   isomaltose E74.31
   lactose E73.9
   methionine E72.19
   monosaccharide E74.39
   postgastrectomy K91.2
   postsurgical K91.2
   protein K90.4
   starch K90.4
   sucrose E74.39
   syndrome K90.9
      postsurgical K91.2
Malacia, bone (adult) M83.9
   juvenile — *see* Rickets
Malacoplakia
   bladder N32.89
   pelvis (kidney) N28.89
   ureter N28.89
   urethra N36.8
Malacosteon, juvenile — *see* Rickets
Maladaptation — *see* Maladjustment
Maladie de Roger Q21.0
Maladjustment
   conjugal Z63.0
      involving divorce or estrangement Z63.5
   educational Z55.4
   family Z63.9
   marital Z63.0
      involving divorce or estrangement Z63.5
   occupational NEC Z56.89
   simple, adult — *see* Disorder, adjustment
   situational — *see* Disorder, adjustment
   social Z60.9
      due to
         acculturation difficulty Z60.3
         discrimination and persecution (perceived)
            Z60.5
         exclusion and isolation Z60.4
         life-cycle (phase of life) transition Z60.0
         rejection Z60.4
         specified reason NEC Z60.8
Malaise R53.81
Malakoplakia — *see* Malacoplakia
Malaria, malarial (fever) B54
   with
      blackwater fever B50.8
         hemoglobinuric (bilious) B50.8
      hemoglobinuria B50.8
   accidentally induced (therapeutically) — *code by* type
      under Malaria
   algid B50.9
   cerebral B50.0 [G94]
   clinically diagnosed (without parasitological confirma-
      tion) B54
   congenital NEC P37.4
      falciparum P37.3
   congestion, congestive B54
   continued (fever) B50.9
   estivo-autumnal B50.9
   falciparum B50.9
      with complications NEC B50.8
         cerebral B50.0 [G94]
      severe B50.8
   hemorrhagic B54

Malaria, malarial — *continued*
   malariae B52.9
      with
         complications NEC B52.8
         glomerular disorder B52.0
   malignant (tertian) — *see* Malaria, falciparum
   mixed infections — *code to* first listed type in B50-B53
   ovale B53.0
   parasitologically confirmed NEC B53.8
   pernicious, acute — *see* Malaria, falciparum
   Plasmodium (P.)
      falciparum NEC — *see* Malaria, falciparum
      malariae NEC B52.9
         with Plasmodium
            falciparum (and or vivax) — *see* Malaria,
               falciparum
            vivax (*see also* Malaria, vivax)
               and falciparum — *see* Malaria, falci-
                  parum
      ovale B53.0
         with Plasmodium malariae (*see also* Malaria,
            malariae)
            and vivax (*see also* Malaria, vivax)
               and falciparum — *see* Malaria, falci-
                  parum
      simian B53.1
         with Plasmodium malariae (*see also* Malaria,
            malariae)
            and vivax (*see also* Malaria, vivax)
               and falciparum — *see* Malaria, falci-
                  parum
      vivax NEC B51.9
         with Plasmodium falciparum — *see* Malaria,
            falciparum
   quartan — *see* Malaria, malariae
   quotidian — *see* Malaria, falciparum
   recurrent B54
   remittent B54
   specified type NEC (parasitologically confirmed) B53.8
   spleen B54
   subtertian (fever) — *see* Malaria, falciparum
   tertian (benign) (*see also* Malaria, vivax)
      malignant B50.9
   tropical B50.9
   typhoid B54
   vivax B51.9
      with
         complications NEC B51.8
         ruptured spleen B51.0
Malassez's disease (cystic) N50.8
Malassimilation K90.9
Maldescent, testis Q53.9
   bilateral Q53.20
      abdominal Q53.21
      perineal Q53.22
   unilateral Q53.10
      abdominal Q53.11
      perineal Q53.12
Maldevelopment (*see also* Anomaly)
   brain Q07.9
   colon Q43.9
   hip Q74.2
      congenital dislocation Q65.2
         bilateral Q65.1
         unilateral Q65.0- ☑
   mastoid process Q75.8
   middle ear Q16.4
      except ossicles Q16.4
      ossicles Q16.3
   ossicles Q16.3
   spine Q76.49
   toe Q74.2
Male type pelvis Q74.2
   with disproportion (fetopelvic) O33.3 ☑
      causing obstructed labor O65.3
Malformation (congenital) (*see also* Anomaly)
   adrenal gland Q89.1
   affecting multiple systems with skeletal changes NEC
      Q87.5
   alimentary tract Q45.9
      specified type NEC Q45.8
      upper Q40.9
         specified type NEC Q40.8
   aorta Q25.9
      atresia Q25.2
      coarctation (preductal) (postductal) Q25.1
      patent ductus arteriosus Q25.0
      specified type NEC Q25.4

Malformation — *continued*
   aorta — *continued*
      stenosis (supravalvular) Q25.3
   aortic valve Q23.9
      specified NEC Q23.8
   arteriovenous, aneurysmatic (congenital) Q27.30
      brain Q28.2
      cerebral Q28.2
      peripheral Q27.30
         digestive system Q27.33
         lower limb Q27.32
         other specified site Q27.39
         renal vessel Q27.34
         upper limb Q27.31
      precerebral vessels (nonruptured) Q28.0
   auricle
      ear (congenital) Q17.3
         acquired H61.119
            left H61.112
               with right H61.113
            right H61.111
               with left H61.113
   bile duct Q44.5
   bladder Q64.79
      aplasia Q64.5
      diverticulum Q64.6
      exstrophy — *see* Exstrophy, bladder
      neck obstruction Q64.31
   bone Q79.9
      face Q75.9
         specified type NEC Q75.8
      skull Q75.9
         specified type NEC Q75.8
   brain (multiple) Q04.9
      arteriovenous Q28.2
      specified type NEC Q04.8
   branchial cleft Q18.2
   breast Q83.9
      specified type NEC Q83.8
   broad ligament Q50.6
   bronchus Q32.4
   bursa Q79.9
   cardiac
      chambers Q20.9
         specified type NEC Q20.8
      septum Q21.9
         specified type NEC Q21.8
   cerebral Q04.9
      vessels Q28.3
   cervix uteri Q51.9
      specified type NEC Q51.828
   Chiari
      Type I G93.5
      Type II Q07.01
   choroid (congenital) Q14.3
      plexus Q07.8
   circulatory system Q28.9
   cochlea Q16.5
   cornea Q13.4
   coronary vessels Q24.5
   corpus callosum (congenital) Q04.0
   diaphragm Q79.1
   digestive system NEC, specified type NEC Q45.8
   dura Q07.9
      brain Q04.9
      spinal Q06.9
   ear Q17.9
      causing impairment of hearing Q16.9
      external Q17.9
         accessory auricle Q17.0
         causing impairment of hearing Q16.9
            absence of
               auditory canal Q16.1
               auricle Q16.0
         macrotia Q17.1
         microtia Q17.2
         misplacement Q17.4
         misshapen NEC Q17.3
         prominence Q17.5
         specified type NEC Q17.8
      inner Q16.5
      middle Q16.4
         absence of eustachian tube Q16.2
         ossicles (fusion) Q16.3
      ossicles Q16.3
      specified type NEC Q17.8
   epididymis Q55.4

Malformation — *continued*
esophagus Q39.9
specified type NEC Q39.8
eye Q15.9
lid Q10.3
specified NEC Q15.8
fallopian tube Q50.6
genital organ — *see* Anomaly, genitalia
great
artery Q25.9
aorta — *see* Malformation, aorta
pulmonary artery — *see* Malformation, pulmonary, artery
specified type NEC Q25.8
vein Q26.9
anomalous
portal venous connection Q26.5
pulmonary venous connection Q26.4
partial Q26.3
total Q26.2
persistent left superior vena cava Q26.1
portal vein-hepatic artery fistula Q26.6
specified type NEC Q26.8
vena cava stenosis, congenital Q26.0
gum Q38.6
hair Q84.2
heart Q24.9
specified type NEC Q24.8
integument Q84.9
specified type NEC Q84.8
internal ear Q16.5
intestine Q43.9
specified type NEC Q43.8
iris Q13.2
joint Q74.9
ankle Q74.2
lumbosacral Q76.49
sacroiliac Q74.2
specified type NEC Q74.8
kidney Q63.9
accessory Q63.0
giant Q63.3
horseshoe Q63.1
hydronephrosis Q62.0
malposition Q63.2
specified type NEC Q63.8
lacrimal apparatus Q10.6
lingual Q38.3
lip Q38.0
liver Q44.7
lung Q33.9
meninges or membrane (congenital) Q07.9
cerebral Q04.8
spinal (cord) Q06.9
middle ear Q16.4
ossicles Q16.3
mitral valve Q23.9
specified NEC Q23.8
Mondini's (congenital) (malformation, cochlea) Q16.5
mouth (congenital) Q38.6
multiple types NEC Q89.7
musculoskeletal system Q79.9
myocardium Q24.8
nail Q84.6
nervous system (central) Q07.9
nose Q30.9
specified type NEC Q30.8
optic disc Q14.2
orbit Q10.7
ovary Q50.39
palate Q38.5
parathyroid gland Q89.2
pelvic organs or tissues NEC
in pregnancy or childbirth O34.8- ☑
causing obstructed labor O65.5
penis Q55.69
aplasia Q55.5
curvature (lateral) Q55.61
hypoplasia Q55.62
pericardium Q24.8
peripheral vascular system Q27.9
specified type NEC Q27.8
pharynx Q38.8
precerebral vessels Q28.1
prostate Q55.4
pulmonary
arteriovenous Q25.72

Malformation — *continued*
pulmonary — *continued*
artery Q25.9
atresia Q25.5
specified type NEC Q25.79
stenosis Q25.6
valve Q22.3
renal artery Q27.2
respiratory system Q34.9
retina Q14.1
scrotum — *see* Malformation, testis and scrotum
seminal vesicles Q55.4
sense organs NEC Q07.9
skin Q82.9
specified NEC Q89.8
spinal
cord Q06.9
nerve root Q07.8
spine Q76.49
kyphosis — *see* Kyphosis, congenital
lordosis — *see* Lordosis, congenital
spleen Q89.09
stomach Q40.3
specified type NEC Q40.2
teeth, tooth K00.9
tendon Q79.9
testis and scrotum Q55.20
aplasia Q55.0
hypoplasia Q55.1
polyorchism Q55.21
retractile testis Q55.22
scrotal transposition Q55.23
specified NEC Q55.29
thorax, bony Q76.9
throat Q38.8
thyroid gland Q89.2
tongue (congenital) Q38.3
hypertrophy Q38.2
tie Q38.1
trachea Q32.1
tricuspid valve Q22.9
specified type NEC Q22.8
umbilical cord NEC (complicating delivery) O69.89 ☑
umbilicus Q89.9
ureter Q62.8
agenesis Q62.4
duplication Q62.5
malposition — *see* Malposition, congenital, ureter
obstructive defect — *see* Defect, obstructive, ureter
vesico-uretero-renal reflux Q62.7
urethra Q64.79
aplasia Q64.5
duplication Q64.74
posterior valves Q64.2
prolapse Q64.71
stricture Q64.32
urinary system Q64.9
uterus Q51.9
specified type NEC Q51.818
vagina Q52.4
vas deferens Q55.4
atresia Q55.3
vascular system, peripheral Q27.9
venous — *see* Anomaly, vein(s)
vulva Q52.70
Malfunction (*see also* Dysfunction)
cardiac electronic device T82.119 ☑
electrode T82.110 ☑
pulse generator T82.111 ☑
specified type NEC T82.118 ☑
catheter device NEC T85.618 ☑
cystostomy T83.010 ☑
dialysis (renal) (vascular) T82.41 ☑
intraperitoneal T85.611 ☑
infusion NEC T82.514 ☑
spinal (epidural) (subdural) T85.610 ☑
urinary, indwelling T83.018 ☑
colostomy K94.03
valve K94.03
cystostomy (stoma) N99.512
catheter T83.010 ☑
enteric stoma K94.13
enterostomy K94.13
esophagostomy K94.33
gastroenteric K31.89
gastrostomy K94.23
ileostomy K94.13
valve K94.13

Malfunction — *continued*
jejunostomy K94.13
pacemaker — *see* Malfunction, cardiac electronic device
prosthetic device, internal — *see* Complications, prosthetic device, by site, mechanical
tracheostomy J95.03
urinary device NEC — *see* Complication, genitourinary, device, urinary, mechanical
valve
colostomy K94.03
heart T82.09 ☑
ileostomy K94.13
vascular graft or shunt NEC — *see* Complication, cardiovascular device, mechanical, vascular
ventricular (communicating shunt) T85.01 ☑
Malherbe's tumor — *see* Neoplasm, skin, benign
Malibu disease L98.8
Malignancy (*see also* Neoplasm, malignant, by site)
unspecified site (primary) C80.1
Malignant — *see* condition
Malingerer, malingering Z76.5
Mallet finger (acquired) — *see* Deformity, finger, mallet finger
congenital Q74.0
sequelae of rickets E64.3
Malleus A24.0
Mallory's bodies R89.7
Mallory-Weiss syndrome K22.6
Malnutrition E46
degree
first E44.1
mild (protein) E44.1
moderate (protein) E44.0
second E44.0
severe (protein-energy) E43
intermediate form E42
with
kwashiorkor (and marasmus) E42
marasmus E41
third E43
following gastrointestinal surgery K91.2
intrauterine
light-for-dates — *see* Light for dates
small-for-dates — *see* Small for dates
lack of care, or neglect (child) (infant) T76.02 ☑
confirmed T74.02 ☑
malignant E40
protein E46
calorie E46
mild E44.1
moderate E44.0
severe E43
intermediate form E42
with
kwashiorkor (and marasmus) E42
marasmus E41
energy E46
mild E44.1
moderate E44.0
severe E43
intermediate form E42
with
kwashiorkor (and marasmus) E42
marasmus E41
severe (protein-energy) E43
with
kwashiorkor (and marasmus) E42
marasmus E41
Malocclusion (teeth) M26.4
Angle's M26.219
class I M26.211
class II M26.212
class III M26.213
due to
abnormal swallowing M26.59
mouth breathing M26.59
tongue, lip or finger habits M26.59
temporomandibular (joint) M26.69
Malposition
cervix — *see* Malposition, uterus
congenital
adrenal (gland) Q89.1
alimentary tract Q45.8
lower Q43.8
upper Q40.8
aorta Q25.4
appendix Q43.8

Malposition — *continued*
  congenital — *continued*
    arterial trunk Q20.0
    artery (peripheral) Q27.8
      coronary Q24.5
      digestive system Q27.8
      lower limb Q27.8
      pulmonary Q25.79
      specified site NEC Q27.8
      upper limb Q27.8
    auditory canal Q17.8
      causing impairment of hearing Q16.9
    auricle (ear) Q17.4
      causing impairment of hearing Q16.9
      cervical Q18.2
    biliary duct or passage Q44.5
    bladder (mucosa) — *see* Exstrophy, bladder
    brachial plexus Q07.8
    brain tissue Q04.8
    breast Q83.8
    bronchus Q32.4
    cecum Q43.8
    clavicle Q74.0
    colon Q43.8
    digestive organ or tract NEC Q45.8
      lower Q43.8
      upper Q40.8
    ear (auricle) (external) Q17.4
      ossicles Q16.3
    endocrine (gland) NEC Q89.2
    epiglottis Q31.8
    eustachian tube Q17.8
    eye Q15.8
    facial features Q18.8
    fallopian tube Q50.6
    finger(s) Q68.1
      supernumerary Q69.0
    foot Q66.9
    gallbladder Q44.1
    gastrointestinal tract Q45.8
    genitalia, genital organ(s) or tract
      female Q52.8
        external Q52.79
        internal NEC Q52.8
      male Q55.8
    glottis Q31.8
    hand Q68.1
    heart Q24.8
      dextrocardia Q24.0
        with complete transposition of viscera Q89.3
    hepatic duct Q44.5
    hip (joint) Q65.89
    intestine (large) (small) Q43.8
      with anomalous adhesions, fixation or malrotation Q43.3
    joint NEC Q68.8
    kidney Q63.2
    larynx Q31.8
    limb Q68.8
      lower Q68.8
      upper Q68.8
    liver Q44.7
    lung (lobe) Q33.8
    nail(s) Q84.6
    nerve Q07.8
    nervous system NEC Q07.8
    nose, nasal (septum) Q30.8
    organ or site not listed — *see* Anomaly, by site
    ovary Q50.39
    pancreas Q45.3
    parathyroid (gland) Q89.2
    patella Q74.1
    peripheral vascular system Q27.8
    pituitary (gland) Q89.2
    respiratory organ or system NEC Q34.8
    rib (cage) Q76.6
      supernumerary in cervical region Q76.5
    scapula Q74.0
    shoulder Q74.0
    spinal cord Q06.8
    spleen Q89.09
    sternum NEC Q76.7
    stomach Q40.2
    symphysis pubis Q74.2
    thymus (gland) Q89.2
    thyroid (gland) (tissue) Q89.2
      cartilage Q31.0

Malposition — *continued*
  congenital — *continued*
    toe(s) Q66.9
      supernumerary Q69.2
    tongue Q38.3
    trachea Q32.1
    ureter Q62.60
      deviation Q62.61
      displacement Q62.62
      ectopia Q62.63
      specified type NEC Q62.69
    uterus Q51.818
    vein(s) (peripheral) Q27.8
      great Q26.8
    vena cava (inferior) (superior) Q26.8
  device, implant or graft (*see also* Complications, by site and type, mechanical) T85.628 ☑
    arterial graft NEC — *see* Complication, cardiovascular device, mechanical, vascular
    breast (implant) T85.42 ☑
    catheter NEC T85.628 ☑
      cystostomy T83.020 ☑
      dialysis (renal) T82.42 ☑
        intraperitoneal T85.621 ☑
      infusion NEC T82.524 ☑
        spinal (epidural) (subdural) T85.620 ☑
      urinary, indwelling T83.028 ☑
    electronic (electrode) (pulse generator) (stimulator)
      bone T84.320 ☑
      cardiac T82.129 ☑
        electrode T82.120 ☑
        pulse generator T82.121 ☑
        specified type NEC T82.128 ☑
      nervous system — *see* Complication, prosthetic device, mechanical, electronic nervous system stimulator
      urinary — *see* Complication, genitourinary, device, urinary, mechanical
    fixation, internal (orthopedic) NEC — *see* Complication, fixation device, mechanical
    gastrointestinal — *see* Complications, prosthetic device, mechanical, gastrointestinal device
    genital NEC T83.428 ☑
      intrauterine contraceptive device T83.32 ☑
      penile prosthesis T83.420 ☑
    heart NEC — *see* Complication, cardiovascular device, mechanical
    joint prosthesis — *see* Complication, joint prosthesis, mechanical
    ocular NEC — *see* Complications, prosthetic device, mechanical, ocular device
    orthopedic NEC — *see* Complication, orthopedic, device, mechanical
    specified NEC T85.628 ☑
    urinary NEC (*see also* Complication, genitourinary, device, urinary, mechanical)
      graft T83.22 ☑
    vascular NEC — *see* Complication, cardiovascular device, mechanical
    ventricular intracranial shunt T85.02 ☑
  fetus — *see* Pregnancy, complicated by (management affected by), presentation, fetal
  gallbladder K82.8
  gastrointestinal tract, congenital Q45.8
  heart, congenital NEC Q24.8
  joint prosthesis — *see* Complications, joint prosthesis, mechanical, displacement, by site
  stomach K31.89
    congenital Q40.2
  tooth, teeth, fully erupted M26.30
  uterus (acute) (acquired) (adherent) (asymptomatic) (postinfectional) (postpartal, old) N85.4
    anteflexion or anteversion N85.4
      congenital Q51.818
    flexion N85.4
      lateral — *see* Lateroversion, uterus
    inversion N85.5
    lateral (flexion) (version) — *see* Lateroversion, uterus
      in pregnancy or childbirth — *see* subcategory O34.5 ☑
    retroflexion or retroversion — *see* Retroversion, uterus
Malposture R29.3
Malrotation
  cecum Q43.3
  colon Q43.3

Malrotation — *continued*
  intestine Q43.3
  kidney Q63.2
Malta fever — *see* Brucellosis
Maltreatment
  adult
    abandonment
      confirmed T74.01 ☑
      suspected T76.01 ☑
    confirmed T74.91 ☑
    history of Z91.419
    neglect
      confirmed T74.01 ☑
      suspected T76.01 ☑
    physical abuse
      confirmed T74.11 ☑
      suspected T76.11 ☑
    psychological abuse
      confirmed T74.31 ☑
      history of Z91.411
      suspected T76.31 ☑
    sexual abuse
      confirmed T74.21 ☑
      suspected T76.21 ☑
    suspected T76.91 ☑
  child
    abandonment
      confirmed T74.02 ☑
      suspected T76.02 ☑
    confirmed T74.92 ☑
    history of — *see* History, personal (of), abuse
    neglect
      confirmed T74.02 ☑
      history of — *see* History, personal (of), abuse
      suspected T76.02 ☑
    physical abuse
      confirmed T74.12 ☑
      history of — *see* History, personal (of), abuse
      suspected T76.12 ☑
    psychological abuse
      confirmed T74.32 ☑
      history of — *see* History, personal (of), abuse
      suspected T76.32 ☑
    sexual abuse
      confirmed T74.22 ☑
      history of — *see* History, personal (of), abuse
      suspected T76.22 ☑
    suspected T76.92 ☑
  personal history of Z91.89
Maltworker's lung J67.4
Malunion, fracture — *see* Fracture, by site
Mammillitis N61
  puerperal, postpartum O91.02
Mammitis — *see* Mastitis
Mammogram (examination) Z12.39
  routine Z12.31
Mammoplasia N62
Management (of)
  bone conduction hearing device (implanted) Z45.320
  cardiac pacemaker NEC Z45.018
  cerebrospinal fluid drainage device Z45.41
  cochlear device (implanted) Z45.321
  contraceptive Z30.9
    specified NEC Z30.8
  implanted device Z45.9
    specified NEC Z45.89
  infusion pump Z45.1
  procreative Z31.9
    male factor infertility in female Z31.81
    specified NEC Z31.89
  prosthesis (external) (*see also* Fitting) Z44.9
    implanted Z45.9
      specified NEC Z45.89
  renal dialysis catheter Z49.01
  vascular access device Z45.2
Mangled — *see* specified injury by site
Mania (monopolar) (*see also* Disorder, mood, manic episode)
  with psychotic symptoms F30.2
  without psychotic symptoms F30.10
    mild F30.11
    moderate F30.12
    severe F30.13
  Bell's F30.8
  chronic (recurrent) F31.89
  hysterical F44.09
  puerperal F30.8

Mania — *continued*
  recurrent F31.89
Manic-depressive insanity, psychosis, or syndrome
  — *see* Disorder, bipolar
Mannosidosis E77.1
Mansonelliasis, mansonellosis B74.4
Manson's
  disease B65.1
  schistosomiasis B65.1
Manual — *see* condition
Maple-bark-stripper's lung (disease) J67.6
Maple-syrup-urine disease E71.0
Marable's syndrome (celiac artery compression) I77.4
Marasmus E41
  due to malnutrition E41
  intestinal E41
  nutritional E41
  senile R54
  tuberculous NEC — *see* Tuberculosis
Marble
  bones Q78.2
  skin R23.8
Marburg virus disease A98.3
March
  fracture — *see* Fracture, traumatic, stress, by site
  hemoglobinuria D59.6
Marchesani (-Weill) **syndrome** Q87.0
Marchiafava (-Bignami) **syndrome or disease** G37.1
Marchiafava-Micheli syndrome D59.5
Marcus Gunn's syndrome Q07.8
Marfan's syndrome — *see* Syndrome, Marfan's
Marie-Bamberger disease — *see* Osteoarthropathy,
  hypertrophic, specified NEC
Marie-Charcot-Tooth neuropathic muscular atrophy
  G60.0
Marie's
  cerebellar ataxia (late-onset) G11.2
  disease or syndrome (acromegaly) E22.0
Marie-Strümpell arthritis, disease or spondylitis —
  see Spondylitis, ankylosing
Marion's disease (bladder neck obstruction) N32.0
Marital conflict Z63.0
Mark
  port wine Q82.5
  raspberry Q82.5
  strawberry Q82.5
  stretch L90.6
  tattoo L81.8
Marker heterochromatin — *see* Extra, marker chromo-
  somes
Maroteaux-Lamy syndrome (mild) (severe) E76.29
Marrow (bone)
  arrest D61.9
  poor function D75.89
Marseilles fever A77.1
Marsh fever — *see* Malaria
Marshall's (hidrotic) **ectodermal dysplasia** Q82.4
Marsh's disease (exophthalmic goiter) E05.00
  with storm E05.01
Masculinization (female) **with adrenal hyperplasia**
  E25.9
  congenital E25.0
Masculinovoblastoma D27.- ☑
Masochism (sexual) F65.51
Mason's lung J62.8
Mass
  abdominal R19.00
    epigastric R19.06
    generalized R19.07
    left lower quadrant R19.04
    left upper quadrant R19.02
    periumbilic R19.05
    right lower quadrant R19.03
    right upper quadrant R19.01
    specified site NEC R19.09
  breast N63
  chest R22.2
  cystic — *see* Cyst
  ear H93.8- ☑
  head R22.0
  intra-abdominal (diffuse) (generalized) — *see* Mass,
    abdominal
  kidney N28.89
  liver R16.0
  localized (skin) R22.9
    chest R22.2
    head R22.0

Mass — *continued*
  localized — *continued*
    limb
      lower R22.4- ☑
      upper R22.3- ☑
    neck R22.1
    trunk R22.2
  lung R91.8
  malignant — *see* Neoplasm, malignant, by site
  neck R22.1
  pelvic (diffuse) (generalized) — *see* Mass, abdominal
  specified organ NEC — *see* Disease, by site
  splenic R16.1
  substernal thyroid — *see* Goiter
  superficial (localized) R22.9
  umbilical (diffuse) (generalized) R19.09
Massive — *see* condition
Mast cell
  disease, systemic tissue D47.0
  leukemia C94.3- ☑
  sarcoma C96.2
  tumor D47.0
    malignant C96.2
Mastalgia N64.4
Masters-Allen syndrome N83.8
Mastitis (acute) (diffuse) (nonpuerperal) (subacute) N61
  chronic (cystic) — *see* Mastopathy, cystic
  cystic (Schimmelbusch's type) — *see* Mastopathy,
    cystic
  fibrocystic — *see* Mastopathy, cystic
  infective N61
    newborn P39.0
  interstitial, gestational or puerperal — *see* Mastitis,
    obstetric
  neonatal (noninfective) P83.4
    infective P39.0
  obstetric (interstitial) (nonpurulent)
    associated with
      lactation O91.23
      pregnancy O91.21- ☑
      puerperium O91.22
    purulent
      associated with
        lactation O91.13
        pregnancy O91.11- ☑
        puerperium O91.12
  periductal — *see* Ectasia, mammary duct
  phlegmonous — *see* Mastopathy, cystic
  plasma cell — *see* Ectasia, mammary duct
Mastocytoma D47.0
  malignant C96.2
Mastocytosis Q82.2
  aggressive systemic C96.2
  indolent systemic D47.0
  malignant C96.2
  systemic, associated with clonal hematopoetic non-
    mast-cell disease (SM-AHNMD) D47.0
Mastodynia N64.4
Mastoid — *see* condition
Mastoidalgia — *see* subcategory H92.0 ☑
Mastoiditis (coalescent) (hemorrhagic) (suppurative)
  H70.9- ☑
  acute, subacute H70.00- ☑
    complicated NEC H70.09- ☑
    subperiosteal H70.01- ☑
  chronic (necrotic) (recurrent) H70.1- ☑
  in (due to)
    infectious disease NEC B99 ☑ [H75.0-] ☑
    parasitic disease NEC B89 [H75.0-] ☑
    tuberculosis A18.03
  petrositis — *see* Petrositis
  postauricular fistula — *see* Fistula, postauricular
  specified NEC H70.89- ☑
  tuberculous A18.03
Mastopathy, mastopathia N64.9
  chronica cystica — *see* Mastopathy, cystic
  cystic (chronic) (diffuse) N60.1- ☑
    with epithelial proliferation N60.3- ☑
  diffuse cystic — *see* Mastopathy, cystic
  estrogenic, oestrogenica N64.89
  ovarian origin N64.89
Mastoplasia, mastoplastia N62
Masturbation (excessive) F98.8
Maternal care (for) — *see* Pregnancy (complicated by)
  (management affected by)
Matheiu's disease (leptospiral jaundice) A27.0

Mauclaire's disease or osteochondrosis — *see* Osteo-
  chondrosis, juvenile, hand, metacarpal
Maxcy's disease A75.2
Maxilla, maxillary — *see* condition
May (-Hegglin) **anomaly or syndrome** D72.0
McArdle (-Schmid)(-Pearson) **disease** (glycogen storage)
  E74.04
McCune-Albright syndrome Q78.1
McQuarrie's syndrome (idiopathic familial hypo-
  glycemia) E16.2
Meadow's syndrome Q86.1
Measles (black) (hemorrhagic) (suppressed) B05.9
  with
    complications NEC B05.89
    encephalitis B05.0
    intestinal complications B05.4
    keratitis (keratoconjunctivitis) B05.81
    meningitis B05.1
    otitis media B05.3
    pneumonia B05.2
  French — *see* Rubella
  German — *see* Rubella
  Liberty — *see* Rubella
Meatitis, urethral — *see* Urethritis
Meatus, meatal — *see* condition
Meat-wrappers' asthma J68.9
Meckel-Gruber syndrome Q61.9
Meckel's diverticulitis, diverticulum (displaced) (hypertrophic) Q43.0
  malignant — *see* Table of Neoplasms, small intestine,
    malignant
Meconium
  ileus, newborn P76.0
    in cystic fibrosis E84.11
    meaning meconium plug (without cystic fibrosis)
      P76.0
  obstruction, newborn P76.0
    due to fecaliths P76.0
    in mucoviscidosis E84.11
  peritonitis P78.0
  plug syndrome (newborn) NEC P76.0
Median (*see also* condition)
  arcuate ligament syndrome I77.4
  bar (prostate) (vesical orifice) — *see* Hyperplasia,
    prostate
  rhomboid glossitis K14.2
Mediastinal shift R93.8
Mediastinitis (acute) (chronic) J98.5
  syphilitic A52.73
  tuberculous A15.8
Mediastinopericarditis (*see also* Pericarditis)
  acute I30.9
  adhesive I31.0
  chronic I31.8
    rheumatic I09.2
Mediastinum, mediastinal — *see* condition
Medicine poisoning — *see* Table of Drugs and Chemicals, by drug, poisoning
Mediterranean
  fever — *see* Brucellosis
    familial E85.0
    tick A77.1
  kala-azar B55.0
  leishmaniasis B55.0
  tick fever A77.1
Medulla — *see* condition
Medullary cystic kidney Q61.5
Medullated fibers
  optic (nerve) Q14.8
  retina Q14.1
Medulloblastoma
  desmoplastic C71.6
  specified site — *see* Neoplasm, malignant, by site
  unspecified site C71.6
Medulloepithelioma (*see also* Neoplasm, malignant,
  by site)
  teratoid — *see* Neoplasm, malignant, by site
Medullomyoblastoma
  specified site — *see* Neoplasm, malignant, by site
  unspecified site C71.6
Meekeren-Ehlers-Danlos syndrome Q79.6
Megacolon (acquired) (functional) (not Hirschsprung's
  disease) (in) K59.3
  Chagas' disease B57.32
  congenital, congenitum (aganglionic) Q43.1
  Hirschsprung's (disease) Q43.1

Megacolon — *continued*
  toxic NEC K59.3
    due to Clostridium difficile A04.7
Megaesophagus (functional) K22.0
  congenital Q39.5
  in (due to) Chagas' disease B57.31
Megalencephaly Q04.5
Megalerythema (epidemic) B08.3
Megaloappendix Q43.8
Megalocephalus, megalocephaly NEC Q75.3
Megalocornea Q15.8
  with glaucoma Q15.0
Megalocytic anemia D53.1
Megalodactylia (fingers) (thumbs) (congenital) Q74.0
  toes Q74.2
Megaloduodenum Q43.8
Megaloesophagus (functional) K22.0
  congenital Q39.5
Megalogastria (acquired) K31.89
  congenital Q40.2
Megalophthalmos Q11.3
Megalopsia H53.15
Megalosplenia — *see* Splenomegaly
Megaloureter N28.82
  congenital Q62.2
Megarectum K62.89
Megasigmoid K59.3
  congenital Q43.2
Megaureter N28.82
  congenital Q62.2
Megavitamin-B6 syndrome E67.2
Megrim — *see* Migraine
Meibomian
  cyst, infected — *see* Hordeolum
  gland — *see* condition
  sty, stye — *see* Hordeolum
Meibomitis — *see* Hordeolum
Meige-Milroy disease (chronic hereditary edema) Q82.0
Meige's syndrome Q82.0
Melalgia, nutritional E53.8
Melancholia F32.9
  climacteric (single episode) F32.8
    recurrent episode F33.9
  hypochondriac F45.29
  intermittent (single episode) F32.8
    recurrent episode F33.9
  involutional (single episode) F32.8
    recurrent episode F33.9
  menopausal (single episode) F32.8
    recurrent episode F33.9
  puerperal F32.8
  reactive (emotional stress or trauma) F32.3
  recurrent F33.9
  senile F03 ☑
  stuporous (single episode) F32.8
    recurrent episode F33.9
Melanemia R79.89
Melanoameloblastoma — *see* Neoplasm, bone, benign
Melanoblastoma — *see* Melanoma
Melanocarcinoma — *see* Melanoma
Melanocytoma, eyeball D31.4- ☑
Melanocytosis, neurocutaneous Q82.8
Melanoderma, melanodermia L81.4
Melanodontia, infantile K03.89
Melanodontoclasia K03.89
Melanoepithelioma — *see* Melanoma
Melanoma (malignant) C43.9
  acral lentiginous, malignant — *see* Melanoma, skin, by site
  amelanotic — *see* Melanoma, skin, by site
  balloon cell — *see* Melanoma, skin, by site
  benign — *see* Nevus
  desmoplastic, malignant — *see* Melanoma, skin, by site
  epithelioid cell — *see* Melanoma, skin, by site
    with spindle cell, mixed — *see* Melanoma, skin, by site
  in
    giant pigmented nevus — *see* Melanoma, skin, by site
    Hutchinson's melanotic freckle — *see* Melanoma, skin, by site
    junctional nevus — *see* Melanoma, skin, by site
    precancerous melanosis — *see* Melanoma, skin, by site
  in situ D03.9
    abdominal wall D03.59

Melanoma — *continued*
  in situ — *continued*
    ala nasi D03.39
    ankle D03.7- ☑
    anus, anal (margin) (skin) D03.51
    arm D03.6- ☑
    auditory canal D03.2- ☑
    auricle (ear) D03.2- ☑
    auricular canal (external) D03.2- ☑
    axilla, axillary fold D03.59
    back D03.59
    breast D03.52
    brow D03.39
    buttock D03.59
    canthus (eye) D03.1- ☑
    cheek (external) D03.39
    chest wall D03.59
    chin D03.39
    choroid D03.8
    conjunctiva D03.8
    ear (external) D03.2- ☑
    external meatus (ear) D03.2- ☑
    eye D03.8
    eyebrow D03.39
    eyelid (lower) (upper) D03.1- ☑
    face D03.30
      specified NEC D03.39
    female genital organ (external) NEC D03.8
    finger D03.6- ☑
    flank D03.59
    foot D03.7- ☑
    forearm D03.6- ☑
    forehead D03.39
    foreskin D03.8
    gluteal region D03.59
    groin D03.59
    hand D03.6- ☑
    heel D03.7- ☑
    helix D03.2- ☑
    hip D03.7- ☑
    interscapular region D03.59
    iris D03.8
    jaw D03.39
    knee D03.7- ☑
    labium (majus) (minus) D03.8
    lacrimal gland D03.8
    leg D03.7- ☑
    lip (lower) (upper) D03.0
    lower limb NEC D03.7- ☑
    male genital organ (external) NEC D03.8
    nail D03.9
      finger D03.6- ☑
      toe D03.7- ☑
    neck D03.4
    nose (external) D03.39
    orbit D03.8
    penis D03.8
    perianal skin D03.51
    perineum D03.51
    pinna D03.2- ☑
    popliteal fossa or space D03.7- ☑
    prepuce D03.8
    pudendum D03.8
    retina D03.8
    retrobulbar D03.8
    scalp D03.4
    scrotum D03.8
    shoulder D03.6- ☑
    specified site NEC D03.8
    submammary fold D03.52
    temple D03.39
    thigh D03.7- ☑
    toe D03.7- ☑
    trunk NEC D03.59
    umbilicus D03.59
    upper limb NEC D03.6- ☑
    vulva D03.8
  juvenile — *see* Nevus
  malignant, of soft parts except skin — *see* Neoplasm, connective tissue, malignant
  metastatic
    breast C79.81
    genital organ C79.82
    specified site NEC C79.89
  neurotropic, malignant — *see* Melanoma, skin, by site
  nodular — *see* Melanoma, skin, by site
  regressing, malignant — *see* Melanoma, skin, by site

Melanoma — *continued*
  skin C43.9
    abdominal wall C43.59
    ala nasi C43.31
    ankle C43.7- ☑
    anus, anal (skin) C43.51
    arm C43.6- ☑
    auditory canal (external) C43.2- ☑
    auricle (ear) C43.2- ☑
    auricular canal (external) C43.2- ☑
    axilla, axillary fold C43.59
    back C43.59
    breast (female) (male) C43.52
    brow C43.39
    buttock C43.59
    canthus (eye) C43.1- ☑
    cheek (external) C43.39
    chest wall C43.59
    chin C43.39
    ear (external) C43.2- ☑
    elbow C43.6- ☑
    external meatus (ear) C43.2- ☑
    eyebrow C43.39
    eyelid (lower) (upper) C43.1- ☑
    face C43.30
      specified NEC C43.39
    female genital organ (external) NEC C51.9
    finger C43.6- ☑
    flank C43.59
    foot C43.7- ☑
    forearm C43.6- ☑
    forehead C43.39
    foreskin C60.0
    glabella C43.39
    gluteal region C43.59
    groin C43.59
    hand C43.6- ☑
    heel C43.7- ☑
    helix C43.2- ☑
    hip C43.7- ☑
    interscapular region C43.59
    jaw (external) C43.39
    knee C43.7- ☑
    labium C51.9
      majus C51.0
      minus C51.1
    leg C43.7- ☑
    lip (lower) (upper) C43.0
    lower limb NEC C43.7- ☑
    male genital organ (external) NEC C63.9
    nail
      finger C43.6- ☑
      toe C43.7- ☑
    nasolabial groove C43.39
    nates C43.59
    neck C43.4
    nose (external) C43.31
    overlapping site C43.8
    palpebra C43.1- ☑
    penis C60.9
    perianal skin C43.51
    perineum C43.51
    pinna C43.2- ☑
    popliteal fossa or space C43.7- ☑
    prepuce C60.0
    pudendum C51.9
    scalp C43.4
    scrotum C63.2
    shoulder C43.6- ☑
    skin NEC C43.9
    submammary fold C43.52
    temple C43.39
    thigh C43.7- ☑
    toe C43.7- ☑
    trunk NEC C43.59
    umbilicus C43.59
    upper limb NEC C43.6- ☑
    vulva C51.9
      overlapping sites C51.8
  spindle cell
    with epithelioid, mixed — *see* Melanoma, skin, by site
    type A C69.4- ☑
    type B C69.4- ☑
  superficial spreading — *see* Melanoma, skin, by site
Melanosarcoma (*see also* Melanoma)
  epithelioid cell — *see* Melanoma

Melanosis L81.4
  addisonian E27.1
    tuberculous A18.7
  adrenal E27.1
  colon K63.89
  conjunctiva — *see* Pigmentation, conjunctiva
    congenital Q13.89
  cornea (presenile) (senile) (*see also* Pigmentation,
    cornea)
    congenital Q13.4
  eye NEC H57.8
    congenital Q15.8
  lenticularis progressiva Q82.1
  liver K76.89
  precancerous (*see also* Melanoma, in situ)
    malignant melanoma in — *see* Melanoma
  Riehl's L81.4
  sclera H15.89
    congenital Q13.89
  suprarenal E27.1
  tar L81.4
  toxic L81.4
Melanuria R82.99
MELAS syndrome E88.41
Melasma L81.1
  adrenal (gland) E27.1
  suprarenal (gland) E27.1
Melena K92.1
  with ulcer — *code by* site under Ulcer, with hemor-
    rhage K27.4
  due to swallowed maternal blood P78.2
  newborn, neonatal P54.1
    due to swallowed maternal blood P78.2
Meleney's
  gangrene (cutaneous) — *see* Ulcer, skin
  ulcer (chronic undermining) — *see* Ulcer, skin
Melioidosis A24.9
  acute A24.1
  chronic A24.2
  fulminating A24.1
  pneumonia A24.1
  pulmonary (chronic) A24.2
    acute A24.1
    subacute A24.2
  sepsis A24.1
  specified NEC A24.3
  subacute A24.2
Melitensis, febris A23.0
Melkersson (-Rosenthal) **syndrome** G51.2
Mellitus, diabetes — *see* Diabetes
Melorheostosis (bone) — *see* Disorder, bone, density
  and structure, specified NEC
Meloschisis Q18.4
Melotia Q17.4
Membrana
  capsularis lentis posterior Q13.89
  epipapillaris Q14.2
Membranacea placenta O43.19- ☑
Membranaceous uterus N85.8
Membrane(s), membranous (*see also* condition)
  cyclitic — *see* Membrane, pupillary
  folds, congenital — *see* Web
  Jackson's Q43.3
  over face of newborn P28.9
  premature rupture — *see* Rupture, membranes, pre-
    mature
  pupillary H21.4- ☑
    persistent Q13.89
  retained (with hemorrhage) (complicating delivery)
    O72.2
    without hemorrhage O73.1
  secondary cataract — *see* Cataract, secondary
  unruptured (causing asphyxia) — *see* Asphyxia, new-
    born
  vitreous — *see* Opacity, vitreous, membranes and
    strands
Membranitis — *see* Chorioamnionitis
Memory disturbance, lack or loss (*see also* Amnesia)
  mild, following organic brain damage F06.8
Menadione deficiency E56.1
Menarche
  delayed E30.0
  precocious E30.1
Mendacity, pathologic F60.2
Mendelson's syndrome (due to anesthesia) J95.4
  in labor and delivery O74.0
  in pregnancy O29.01- ☑

Mendelson's syndrome — *continued*
  obstetric O74.0
  postpartum, puerperal O89.01
Ménétrier's disease or syndrome K29.60
  with bleeding K29.61
Ménière's disease, syndrome or vertigo H81.0- ☑
Meninges, meningeal — *see* condition
Meningioma (*see also* Neoplasm, meninges, benign)
  angioblastic — *see* Neoplasm, meninges, benign
  angiomatous — *see* Neoplasm, meninges, benign
  endotheliomatous — *see* Neoplasm, meninges, benign
  fibroblastic — *see* Neoplasm, meninges, benign
  fibrous — *see* Neoplasm, meninges, benign
  hemangioblastic — *see* Neoplasm, meninges, benign
  hemangiopericytic — *see* Neoplasm, meninges, be-
    nign
  malignant — *see* Neoplasm, meninges, malignant
  meningiothelial — *see* Neoplasm, meninges, benign
  meningotheliomatous — *see* Neoplasm, meninges,
    benign
  mixed — *see* Neoplasm, meninges, benign
  multiple — *see* Neoplasm, meninges, uncertain behav-
    ior
  papillary — *see* Neoplasm, meninges, uncertain behav-
    ior
  psammomatous — *see* Neoplasm, meninges, benign
  syncytial — *see* Neoplasm, meninges, benign
  transitional — *see* Neoplasm, meninges, benign
Meningiomatosis (diffuse) — *see* Neoplasm, meninges,
  uncertain behavior
Meningism — *see* Meningismus
Meningismus (infectional) (pneumococcal) R29.1
  due to serum or vaccine R29.1
  influenzal — *see* Influenza, with, manifestations NEC
Meningitis (basal) (basic) (brain) (cerebral) (cervical)
  (congestive) (diffuse) (hemorrhagic) (infantile)
  (membranous) (metastatic) (nonspecific) (pontine)
  (progressive) (simple) (spinal) (subacute) (sympathetic) (toxic) G03.9
  abacterial G03.0
  actinomycotic A42.81
  adenoviral A87.1
  arbovirus A87.8
  aseptic (acute) G03.0
  bacterial G00.9
    Escherichia coli (E. coli) G00.8
    Friedländer (bacillus) G00.8
    gram-negative G00.9
    H. influenzae G00.0
    Klebsiella G00.8
    pneumococcal G00.1
    specified organism NEC G00.8
    staphylococcal G00.3
    streptococcal (acute) G00.2
  benign recurrent (Mollaret) G03.2
  candidal B37.5
  caseous (tuberculous) A17.0
  cerebrospinal A39.0
  chronic NEC G03.1
  clear cerebrospinal fluid NEC G03.0
  coxsackievirus A87.0
  cryptococcal B45.1
  diplococcal (gram positive) A39.0
  echovirus A87.0
  enteroviral A87.0
  eosinophilic B83.2
  epidemic NEC A39.0
  Escherichia coli (E. coli) G00.8
  fibrinopurulent G00.9
    specified organism NEC G00.8
  Friedländer (bacillus) G00.8
  gonococcal A54.81
  gram-negative cocci G00.9
  gram-positive cocci G00.9
  H. influenzae G00.0
  Haemophilus (influenzae) G00.0
  in (due to)
    adenovirus A87.1
    African trypanosomiasis B56.9 [G02]
    anthrax A22.8
    bacterial disease NEC A48.8 [G01]
    Chagas' disease (chronic) B57.41
    chickenpox B01.0
    coccidioidomycosis B38.4
    Diplococcus pneumoniae G00.1
    enterovirus A87.0
    herpes (simplex) virus B00.3
      zoster B02.1

Meningitis — *continued*
  in — *continued*
    infectious mononucleosis B27.92
    leptospirosis A27.81
    Listeria monocytogenes A32.11
    Lyme disease A69.21
    measles B05.1
    mumps (virus) B26.1
    neurosyphilis (late) A52.13
    parasitic disease NEC B89 [G02]
    poliovirus A80.9 [G02]
    preventive immunization, inoculation or vaccina-
      tion G03.8
    rubella B06.02
    Salmonella infection A02.21
    specified cause NEC G03.8
    typhoid fever A01.01
    varicella B01.0
    viral disease NEC A87.8
    whooping cough A37.90
    zoster B02.1
  infectious G00.9
  influenzal (H. influenzae) G00.0
  Klebsiella G00.8
  leptospiral (aseptic) A27.81
  lymphocytic (acute) (benign) (serous) A87.2
  meningococcal A39.0
  Mima polymorpha G00.8
  Mollaret (benign recurrent) G03.2
  monilial B37.5
  mycotic NEC B49 [G02]
  Neisseria A39.0
  nonbacterial G03.0
  nonpyogenic NEC G03.0
  ossificans G96.19
  pneumococcal G00.1
  poliovirus A80.9 [G02]
  postmeasles B05.1
  purulent G00.9
    specified organism NEC G00.8
  pyogenic G00.9
    specified organism NEC G00.8
  Salmonella (arizonae) (Cholerae-Suis) (enteritidis) (ty-
    phimurium) A02.21
  septic G00.9
    specified organism NEC G00.8
  serosa circumscripta NEC G03.0
  serous NEC G93.2
  specified organism NEC G00.8
  sporotrichosis B42.81
  staphylococcal G00.3
  sterile G03.0
  streptococcal (acute) G00.2
  suppurative G00.9
    specified organism NEC G00.8
  syphilitic (late) (tertiary) A52.13
    acute A51.41
    congenital A50.41
    secondary A51.41
  Torula histolytica (cryptococcal) B45.1
  traumatic (complication of injury) T79.8 ☑
  tuberculous A17.0
  typhoid A01.01
  viral NEC A87.9
  Yersinia pestis A20.3
Meningocele (spinal) (*see also* Spina bifida)
  with hydrocephalus — *see* Spina bifida, by site, with
    hydrocephalus
  acquired (traumatic) G96.19
  cerebral — *see* Encephalocele
Meningocerebritis — *see* Meningoencephalitis
Meningococcemia A39.4
  acute A39.2
  chronic A39.3
Meningococcus, meningococcal (*see also* condition)
  A39.9
  adrenalitis, hemorrhagic A39.1
  carrier (suspected) of Z22.31
  meningitis (cerebrospinal) A39.0
Meningoencephalitis (*see also* Encephalitis) G04.90
  acute NEC (*see also* Encephalitis, viral) A86
  bacterial NEC G04.2
  California A83.5
  diphasic A84.1
  eosinophilic B83.2
  epidemic A39.81
  herpesviral, herpetic B00.4
    due to herpesvirus 6 B10.01

Meningoencephalitis — *continued*
  herpesviral, herpetic — *continued*
    due to herpesvirus 7 B10.09
    specified NEC B10.09
  in (due to)
    blastomycosis NEC B40.81
    diseases classified elsewhere G05.3
    free-living amebae B60.2
    H. influenzae G00.0
    Hemophilus influenzae (H .influenzae) G04.2
    herpes B00.4
      due to herpesvirus 6 B10.01
      due to herpesvirus 7 B10.09
      specified NEC B10.09
    Lyme disease A69.22
    mercury — *see* subcategory T56.1 ☑
    mumps B26.2
    Naegleria (amebae) (organisms) (fowleri) B60.2
    Parastrongylus cantonensis B83.2
    toxoplasmosis (acquired) B58.2
      congenital P37.1
  infectious (acute) (viral) A86
  influenzal (H. influenzae) G04.2
  Listeria monocytogenes A32.12
  lymphocytic (serous) A87.2
  mumps B26.2
  parasitic NEC B89 [G05.3]
  pneumococcal G00.1
  primary amebic B60.2
  specific (syphilitic) A52.14
  specified organism NEC G04.81
  staphylococcal G04.2
  streptococcal G04.2
  syphilitic A52.14
  toxic NEC G92
    due to mercury — *see* subcategory T56.1 ☑
  tuberculous A17.82
  virus NEC A86
Meningoencephalocele (*see also* Encephalocele)
  syphilitic A52.19
    congenital A50.49
Meningoencephalomyelitis (*see also* Meningoencephalitis)
  acute NEC (viral) A86
    disseminated G04.00
      postimmunization or postvaccination G04.02
      postinfectious G04.01
  due to
    actinomycosis A42.82
    Torula B45.1
    Toxoplasma or toxoplasmosis (acquired) B58.2
      congenital P37.1
  postimmunization or postvaccination G04.02
Meningoencephalomyelopathy G96.9
Meningoencephalopathy G96.9
Meningomyelitis (*see also* Meningoencephalitis)
  bacterial NEC G04.2
  blastomycotic NEC B40.81
  cryptococcal B45.1
  in diseases classified elsewhere G05.4
  meningococcal A39.81
  syphilitic A52.14
  tuberculous A17.82
Meningomyelocele (*see also* Spina bifida)
  syphilitic A52.19
Meningomyeloneuritis — *see* Meningoencephalitis
Meningoradiculitis — *see* Meningitis
Meningovascular — *see* condition
Menkes' disease or syndrome E83.09
  meaning maple-syrup-urine disease E71.0
Menometrorrhagia N92.1
Menopause, menopausal (asymptomatic) (state) Z78.0
  arthritis (any site) NEC — *see* Arthritis, specified form
    NEC
  bleeding N92.4
  depression (single episode) F32.8
    agitated (single episode) F32.2
      recurrent episode F33.9
    psychotic (single episode) F32.8
      recurrent episode F33.9
    recurrent episode F33.9
  melancholia (single episode) F32.8
    recurrent episode F33.9
  paranoid state F22
  premature E28.319
    asymptomatic E28.319
      postirradiation E89.40
      postsurgical E89.40

Menopause, menopausal — *continued*
  premature — *continued*
    symptomatic E28.310
      postirradiation E89.41
      postsurgical E89.41
  psychosis NEC F28
  symptomatic N95.1
  toxic polyarthritis NEC — *see* Arthritis, specified form
    NEC
Menorrhagia (primary) N92.0
  climacteric N92.4
    menopausal N92.4
  menopausal N92.4
  postclimacteric N95.0
  postmenopausal N95.0
  preclimacteric or premenopausal N92.4
  pubertal (menses retained) N92.2
Menostaxis N92.0
Menses, retention N94.89
Menstrual — *see* Menstruation
Menstruation
  absent — *see* Amenorrhea
  anovulatory N97.0
  cycle, irregular N92.6
  delayed N91.0
  disorder N93.9
    psychogenic F45.8
  during pregnancy O20.8
  excessive (with regular cycle) N92.0
    with irregular cycle N92.1
    at puberty N92.2
  frequent N92.0
  infrequent — *see* Oligomenorrhea
  irregular N92.6
    specified NEC N92.5
  latent N92.5
  membranous N92.5
  painful (*see also* Dysmenorrhea) N94.6
    primary N94.4
    psychogenic F45.8
    secondary N94.5
  passage of clots N92.0
  precocious E30.1
  protracted N92.5
  rare — *see* Oligomenorrhea
  retained N94.89
  retrograde N92.5
  scanty — *see* Oligomenorrhea
  suppression N94.89
  vicarious (nasal) N94.89
Mental (*see also* condition)
  deficiency — *see* Disability, intellectual
  deterioration — *see* Psychosis
  disorder — *see* Disorder, mental
  exhaustion F48.8
  insufficiency (congenital) — *see* Disability, intellectual
  observation without need for further medical care
    Z03.89
  retardation — *see* Disability, intellectual
  subnormality — *see* Disability, intellectuall
  upset — *see* Disorder, mental
Meralgia paresthetica G57.1- ☑
Mercurial — *see* condition
Mercurialism — *see* subcategory T56.1 ☑
Merkel cell tumor — *see* Carcinoma, Merkel cell
Merocele — *see* Hernia, femoral
Meromelia
  lower limb — *see* Defect, reduction, lower limb
    intercalary
      femur — *see* Defect, reduction, lower limb,
        specified type NEC
        tibiofibular (complete) (incomplete) — *see*
          Defect, reduction, lower limb
  upper limb — *see* Defect, reduction, upper limb
    intercalary, humeral, radioulnar — *see* Agenesis,
      arm, with hand present
MERRF syndrome (myoclonic epilepsy associated with
  ragged-red fiber) E88.42
Merzbacher-Pelizaeus disease E75.29
Mesaortitis — *see* Aortitis
Mesarteritis — *see* Arteritis
Mesencephalitis — *see* Encephalitis
Mesenchymoma (*see also* Neoplasm, connective tissue,
  uncertain behavior)
  benign — *see* Neoplasm, connective tissue, benign
  malignant — *see* Neoplasm, connective tissue, malig-
    nant

Mesenteritis
  retractile K65.4
  sclerosing K65.4
Mesentery, mesenteric — *see* condition
Mesiodens, mesiodentes K00.1
Mesio-occlusion M26.213
Mesocolon — *see* condition
Mesonephroma (malignant) — *see* Neoplasm, malig-
  nant, by site
  benign — *see* Neoplasm, benign, by site
Mesophlebitis — *see* Phlebitis
Mesostromal dysgenesis Q13.89
Mesothelioma (malignant) C45.9
  benign
    mesentery D19.1
    mesocolon D19.1
    omentum D19.1
    peritoneum D19.1
    pleura D19.0
    specified site NEC D19.7
    unspecified site D19.9
  biphasic C45.9
    benign
      mesentery D19.1
      mesocolon D19.1
      omentum D19.1
      peritoneum D19.1
      pleura D19.0
      specified site NEC D19.7
      unspecified site D19.9
  cystic D48.4
  epithelioid C45.9
    benign
      mesentery D19.1
      mesocolon D19.1
      omentum D19.1
      peritoneum D19.1
      pleura D19.0
      specified site NEC D19.7
      unspecified site D19.9
  fibrous C45.9
    benign
      mesentery D19.1
      mesocolon D19.1
      omentum D19.1
      peritoneum D19.1
      pleura D19.0
      specified site NEC D19.7
      unspecified site D19.9
  site classification
    liver C45.7
    lung C45.7
    mediastinum C45.7
    mesentery C45.1
    mesocolon C45.1
    omentum C45.1
    pericardium C45.2
    peritoneum C45.1
    pleura C45.0
      parietal C45.0
    retroperitoneum C45.7
    specified site NEC C45.7
    unspecified C45.9
Metabolic syndrome E88.81
Metagonimiasis B66.8
Metagonimus infestation (intestine) B66.8
Metal
  pigmentation L81.8
  polisher's disease J62.8
Metamorphopsia H53.15
Metaplasia
  apocrine (breast) — *see* Dysplasia, mammary, specified
    type NEC
  cervix (squamous) — *see* Dysplasia, cervix
  endometrium (squamous) (uterus) N85.8
  esophagus
  kidney (pelvis) (squamous) N28.89
  myelogenous D73.1
  myeloid (agnogenic) (megakaryocytic) D73.1
  spleen D73.1
  squamous cell, bladder N32.89
Metastasis, metastatic
  abscess — *see* Abscess
  calcification E83.59
  cancer
    from specified site — *see* Neoplasm, malignant,
      by site

Metastasis, metastatic — *continued*
cancer — *continued*
to specified site — *see* Neoplasm, secondary, by site
deposits (in) — *see* Neoplasm, secondary, by site
disease (*see also* Neoplasm, secondary, by site) C79.9
spread (to) — *see* Neoplasm, secondary, by site
Metastrongyliasis B83.8
Metatarsalgia M77.4- ☑
anterior G57.6- ☑
Morton's G57.6- ☑
Metatarsus, metatarsal (*see also* condition)
valgus (abductus), congenital Q66.6
varus (adductus) (congenital) Q66.2
Methadone use F11.20
Methemoglobinemia D74.9
acquired (with sulfhemoglobinemia) D74.8
congenital D74.0
enzymatic (congenital) D74.0
Hb M disease D74.0
hereditary D74.0
toxic D74.8
Methemoglobinuria — *see* Hemoglobinuria
Methioninemia E72.19
Methylmalonic acidemia E71.120
Metritis (catarrhal) (hemorrhagic) (septic) (suppurative)
(*see also* Endometritis)
cervical — *see* Cervicitis
Metropathia hemorrhagica N93.8
Metroperitonitis — *see* Peritonitis, pelvic, female
Metrorrhagia N92.1
climacteric N92.4
menopausal N92.4
postpartum NEC (atonic) (following delivery of placenta) O72.1
delayed or secondary O72.2
preclimacteric or premenopausal N92.4
psychogenic F45.8
Metrorrhexis — *see* Rupture, uterus
Metrosalpingitis N70.91
Metrostaxis N93.8
Metrovaginitis — *see* Endometritis
Meyer-Schwickerath and Weyers syndrome Q87.0
Meynert's amentia (nonalcoholic) F04
alcoholic F10.96
with dependence F10.26
Mibelli's disease (porokeratosis) Q82.8
Mice, joint — *see* Loose, body, joint
knee M23.4- ☑
Micrencephalon, micrencephaly Q02
Microalbuminuria R80.9
Microaneurysm, retinal (*see also* Disorder, retina, microaneurysms)
diabetic — *see* E08-E13 with .31
Microangiopathy (peripheral) I73.9
thrombotic M31.1
Microcalcifications, breast R92.0
Microcephalus, microcephalic, microcephaly Q02
due to toxoplasmosis (congenital) P37.1
Microcheilia Q18.7
Microcolon (congenital) Q43.8
Microcornea (congenital) Q13.4
Microcytic — *see* condition
Microdeletions NEC Q93.88
Microdontia K00.2
Microdrepanocytosis D57.40
with crisis (vasoocclusive pain) D57.419
with
acute chest syndrome D57.411
splenic sequestration D57.412
Microembolism
atherothrombotic — *see* Atheroembolism
retinal — *see* Occlusion, artery, retina
Microencephalon Q02
Microfilaria streptocerca infestation — *see* Onchocerciasis
Microgastria (congenital) Q40.2
Microgenia M26.06
Microgenitalia, congenital
female Q52.8
male Q55.8
Microglioma — *see* Lymphoma, non-Hodgkin, specified NEC
Microglossia (congenital) Q38.3
Micrognathia, micrognathism (congenital)
(mandibular) (maxillary) M26.09
Microgyria (congenital) Q04.3

Microinfarct of heart — *see* Insufficiency, coronary
Microlentia (congenital) Q12.8
Microlithiasis, alveolar, pulmonary J84.02
Micromastia N64.82
Micromyelia (congenital) Q06.8
Micropenis Q55.62
Microphakia (congenital) Q12.8
Microphthalmos, microphthalmia (congenital) Q11.2
due to toxoplasmosis P37.1
Micropsia H53.15
Microscopic polyangiitis (polyarteritis) M31.7
Microsporidiosis B60.8
intestinal A07.8
Microsporon furfur infestation B36.0
Microsporosis (*see also* Dermatophytosis)
nigra B36.1
Microstomia (congenital) Q18.5
Microtia (congenital) (external ear) Q17.2
Microtropia H50.40
Microvillus inclusion disease (MVD) (MVID) Q43.8
Micturition
disorder NEC R39.19
psychogenic F45.8
frequency R35.0
psychogenic F45.8
hesitancy R39.11
incomplete emptying R39.14
nocturnal R35.1
painful R30.9
dysuria R30.0
psychogenic F45.8
tenesmus R30.1
poor stream R39.12
split stream R39.13
straining R39.16
urgency R39.15
Mid plane — *see* condition
Middle
ear — *see* condition
lobe (right) syndrome J98.19
Miescher's elastoma L87.2
Mietens' syndrome Q87.2
Migraine (idiopathic) G43.909
with aura (acute-onset) (prolonged) (typical) (without headache) G43.109
with refractory migraine G43.119
with status migrainosus G43.111
without status migrainosus G43.119
without mention of refractory migraine G43.109
with status migrainosus G43.101
without status migrainosus G43.109
intractable G43.119
with status migrainosus G43.111
without status migrainosus G43.119
not intractable G43.109
with status migrainosus G43.101
without status migrainosus G43.109
persistent G43.509
with cerebral infarction G43.609
with refractory migraine G43.619
with status migrainosus G43.611
without status migrainosus G43.619
without refractory migraine G43.609
with status migrainosus G43.601
without status migrainosus G43.609
intractable G43.619
with status migrainosus G43.611
without status migrainosus G43.619
not intractable G43.609
with status migrainosus G43.601
without status migrainosus G43.609
without cerebral infarction G43.509
with refractory migraine G43.519
with status migrainosus G43.511
without status migrainosus G43.519
without refractory migraine G43.509
with status migrainosus G43.501
without status migrainosus G43.509
intractable G43.519
with status migrainosus G43.511
without status migrainosus G43.519
not intractable G43.509
with status migrainosus G43.501
without status migrainosus G43.509
with refractory migraine G43.919
with status migrainosus G43.911
without status migrainosus G43.919

Migraine — *continued*
without aura G43.009
with refractory migraine G43.019
with status migrainosus G43.011
without status migrainosus G43.019
without mention of refractory migraine G43.009
with status migrainosus G43.001
without status migrainosus G43.009
chronic G43.709
with refractory migraine G43.719
with status migrainosus G43.711
without status migrainosus G43.719
without refractory migraine G43.709
with status migrainosus G43.701
without status migrainosus G43.709
intractable
with status migrainosus G43.711
without status migrainosus G43.719
not intractable
with status migrainosus G43.701
without status migrainosus G43.709
intractable
with status migrainosus G43.011
without status migrainosus G43.019
not intractable
with status migrainosus G43.001
without status migrainosus G43.009
without refractory migraine G43.909
with status migrainosus G43.901
without status migrainosus G43.919
abdominal G43.D0 (*following* G43.7)
with refractory migraine G43.D1 (*following* G43.7)
without refractory migraine G43.D0 (*following* G43.7)
intractable G43.D1 (*following* G43.7)
not intractable G43.D0 (*following* G43.7)
basilar — *see* Migraine, with aura
classical — *see* Migraine, with aura
common — *see* Migraine, without aura
complicated G43.109
equivalents — *see* Migraine, with aura
familiar — *see* Migraine, hemiplegic
hemiplegic G43.409
with refractory migraine G43.419
with status migrainosus G43.411
without status migrainosus G43.419
without refractory migraine G43.409
with status migrainosus G43.401
without status migrainosus G43.409
intractable G43.419
with status migrainosus G43.411
without status migrainosus G43.419
not intractable G43.409
with status migrainosus G43.401
without status migrainosus G43.409
intractable G43.919
with status migrainosus G43.911
without status migrainosus G43.919
menstrual G43.829
with refractory migraine G43.839
with status migrainosus G43.831
without status migrainosus G43.839
without refractory migraine G43.829
with status migrainosus G43.821
without status migrainosus G43.829
intractable G43.839
with status migrainosus G43.831
without status migrainosus G43.839
not intractable 4G43.829
with status migrainosus G43.821
without status migrainosus G43.829
menstrually related — *see* Migraine, menstrual
not intractable G43.909
with status migrainosus G43.901
without status migrainosus G43.919
ophthalmoplegic G43.B0 (*following* G43.7)
with refractory migraine G43.B1 (*following* G43.7)
without refractory migraine G43.B0 (*following* G43.7)
intractable G43.B1 (*following* G43.7)
not intractable G43.B0 (*following* G43.7)
persistent aura (with, without) cerebral infarction — *see* Migraine, with aura, persistent
preceded or accompanied by transient focal neurological phenomena — *see* Migraine, with aura
pre-menstrual — *see* Migraine, menstrual
pure menstrual — *see* Migraine, menstrual
retinal — *see* Migraine, with aura

☑ **Additional Character Required — Refer to the Tabular List for Character Selection**   ▽ **Subterms under main terms may continue to next column or page**

Migraine — *continued*
  specified NEC G43.809
    intractable G43.819
      with status migrainosus G43.811
      without status migrainosus G43.819
    not intractable G43.809
      with status migrainosus G43.801
      without status migrainosus G43.809
  sporadic — *see* Migraine, hemiplegic
  transformed — *see* Migraine, without aura, chronic
  triggered seizures — *see* Migraine, with aura
Migrant, social Z59.0
Migration, anxiety concerning Z60.3
Migratory, migrating (*see also* condition)
  person Z59.0
  testis Q55.29
Mikity-Wilson disease or syndrome P27.0
Mikulicz' disease or syndrome K11.8
Miliaria L74.3
  alba L74.1
  apocrine L75.2
  crystallina L74.1
  profunda L74.2
  rubra L74.0
  tropicalis L74.2
Miliary — *see* condition
Milium L72.0
  colloid L57.8
Milk
  crust L21.0
  excessive secretion O92.6
  poisoning — *see* Poisoning, food, noxious
  retention O92.79
  sickness — *see* Poisoning, food, noxious
  spots I31.0
Milk-alkali disease or syndrome E83.52
Milk-leg (deep vessels) (nonpuerperal) — *see* Embolism, vein, lower extremity
  complicating pregnancy O22.3- ☑
  puerperal, postpartum, childbirth O87.1
Milkman's disease or syndrome M83.8
Milky urine — *see* Chyluria
Millard-Gubler (-Foville) **paralysis or syndrome** G46.3
Miliar's asthma J38.5
Miller Fisher syndrome G61.0
Milis' disease — *see* Hemiplegia
Millstone maker's pneumoconiosis J62.8
Milroy's disease (chronic hereditary edema) Q82.0
Minamata disease T26.1- ☑
Miners' asthma or lung J60
Minkowski-Chauffard syndrome — *see* Spherocytosis
Minor — *see* condition
Minor's disease (hematomyelia) G95.19
Minot's disease (hemorrhagic disease), newborn P53
Minot-von Willebrand-Jurgens disease or syndrome (angiohemophilia) D68.0
Minus (and plus) **hand** (intrinsic) — *see* Deformity, limb, specified type NEC, forearm
Miosis (pupil) H57.03
Mirizzi's syndrome (hepatic duct stenosis) K83.1
Mirror writing F81.0
Misadventure (of) (prophylactic) (therapeutic) (*see also* Complications) T88.9 ☑
  administration of insulin (by accident) — *see* subcategory T38.3
  infusion — *see* Complications, infusion
  local applications (of fomentations, plasters, etc.) T88.9 ☑
    burn or scald — *see* Burn
    specified NEC T88.8 ☑
  medical care (early) (late) T88.9 ☑
    adverse effect of drugs or chemicals — *see* Table of Drugs and Chemicals
    burn or scald — *see* Burn
    specified NEC T88.8 ☑
  specified NEC T88.8 ☑
  surgical procedure (early) (late) — *see* Complications, surgical procedure
  transfusion — *see* Complications, transfusion
  vaccination or other immunological procedure — *see* Complications, vaccination
Miscarriage O03.9
Misdirection, aqueous H40.83- ☑
Misperception, sleep state F51.02
Misplaced, misplacement
  ear Q17.4

Misplaced, misplacement — *continued*
  kidney (acquired) N28.89
    congenital Q63.2
  organ or site, congenital NEC — *see* Malposition, congenital
Missed
  abortion O02.1
  delivery O36.4 ☑
Missing — *see* Absence
Misuse of drugs F19.99
Mitchell's disease (erythromelalgia) I73.81
Mite(s) (infestation) B88.9
  diarrhea B88.0
  grain (itch) B88.0
  hair follicle (itch) B88.0
  in sputum B88.0
Mitral — *see* condition
Mittelschmerz N94.0
Mixed — *see* condition
MNGIE (Mitochondrial Neurogastrointestinal Encephalopathy) **syndrome** E88.49
Mobile, mobility
  cecum Q43.3
  excessive — *see* Hypermobility
  gallbladder, congenital Q44.1
  kidney N28.89
  organ or site, congenital NEC — *see* Malposition, congenital
Mobitz heart block (atrioventricular) I44.1
Moebius, Möbius
  disease (ophthalmoplegic migraine) — *see* Migraine, ophthalmoplegic
  syndrome Q87.0
    congenital oculofacial paralysis (with other anomalies) Q87.0
    ophthalmoplegic migraine — *see* Migraine, ophthalmoplegic
Moeller's glossitis K14.0
Mohr's syndrome (Types I and II) Q87.0
Mola destruens D39.2
Molar pregnancy O02.0
Molarization of premolars K00.2
Molding, head (during birth) — *omit code*
Mole (pigmented) (*see also* Nevus)
  blood O02.0
  Breus' O02.0
  cancerous — *see* Melanoma
  carneous O02.0
  destructive D39.2
  fleshy O02.0
  hydatid, hydatidiform (benign) (complicating pregnancy) (delivered) (undelivered) O01.9
    classical O01.0
    complete O01.0
    incomplete O01.1
    invasive D39.2
    malignant D39.2
    partial O01.1
  intrauterine O02.0
  invasive (hydatidiform) D39.2
  malignant
    meaning
      malignant hydatidiform mole D39.2
      melanoma — *see* Melanoma
  nonhydatidiform O02.0
  nonpigmented — *see* Nevus
  pregnancy NEC O02.0
  skin — *see* Nevus
  tubal O00.1
  vesicular — *see* Mole, hydatidiform
Molimen, molimina (menstrual) N94.3
Molluscum contagiosum (epitheliale) B08.1
Mönckeberg's arteriosclerosis, disease, or sclerosis — *see* Arteriosclerosis, extremities
Mondini's malformation (cochlea) Q16.5
Mondor's disease I80.8
Monge's disease T70.29 ☑
Monilethrix (congenital) Q84.1
Moniliasis (*see also* Candidiasis) B37.9
  neonatal P37.5
Monitoring (encounter for)
  therapeutic drug level Z51.81
Monkey malaria B53.1
Monkeypox B04
Monoarthritis M13.10
  ankle M13.17- ☑
  elbow M13.12- ☑

Monoarthritis — *continued*
  foot joint M13.17- ☑
  hand joint M13.14- ☑
  hip M13.15- ☑
  knee M13.16- ☑
  shoulder M13.11- ☑
  wrist M13.13- ☑
Monoblastic — *see* condition
Monochromat (ism), monochromatopsia (acquired) (congenital) H53.51
Monocytic — *see* condition
Monocytopenia D72.818
Monocytosis (symptomatic) D72.821
Monomania — *see* Psychosis
Mononeuritis G58.9
  cranial nerve — *see* Disorder, nerve, cranial
  femoral nerve G57.2- ☑
  lateral
    cutaneous nerve of thigh G57.1- ☑
    popliteal nerve G57.3- ☑
  lower limb G57.9- ☑
    specified nerve NEC G57.8- ☑
  medial popliteal nerve G57.4- ☑
  median nerve G56.1- ☑
  multiplex G58.7
  plantar nerve G57.6- ☑
  posterior tibial nerve G57.5- ☑
  radial nerve G56.3- ☑
  sciatic nerve G57.0- ☑
  specified NEC G58.8
  tibial nerve G57.4- ☑
  ulnar nerve G56.2- ☑
  upper limb G56.9- ☑
    specified nerve NEC G56.8- ☑
  vestibular — *see* subcategory H93.3 ☑
Mononeuropathy G58.9
  carpal tunnel syndrome — *see* Syndrome, carpal tunnel
  diabetic NEC — *see* E08-E13 with .41
  femoral nerve — *see* Lesion, nerve, femoral
  ilioinguinal nerve G57.8- ☑
  in diseases classified elsewhere — *see* category G59
  intercostal G58.0
  lower limb G57.9- ☑
    causalgia — *see* Causalgia, lower limb
    femoral nerve — *see* Lesion, nerve, femoral
    meralgia paresthetica G57.1- ☑
    plantar nerve — *see* Lesion, nerve, plantar
    popliteal nerve — *see* Lesion, nerve, popliteal
    sciatic nerve — *see* Lesion, nerve, sciatic
    specified NEC G57.8- ☑
    tarsal tunnel syndrome — *see* Syndrome, tarsal tunnel
  median nerve — *see* Lesion, nerve, median
  multiplex G58.7
  obturator nerve G57.8- ☑
  popliteal nerve — *see* Lesion, nerve, popliteal
  radial nerve — *see* Lesion, nerve, radial
  saphenous nerve G57.8- ☑
  specified NEC G58.8
  tarsal tunnel syndrome — *see* Syndrome, tarsal tunnel
  tuberculous A17.83
  ulnar nerve — *see* Lesion, nerve, ulnar
  upper limb G56.9- ☑
    carpal tunnel syndrome — *see* Syndrome, carpal tunnel
    causalgia — *see* Causalgia
    median nerve — *see* Lesion, nerve, median
    radial nerve — *see* Lesion, nerve, radial
    specified site NEC G56.8- ☑
    ulnar nerve — *see* Lesion, nerve, ulnar
Mononucleosis, infectious B27.90
  with
    complication NEC B27.99
    meningitis B27.92
    polyneuropathy B27.91
  cytomegaloviral B27.10
    with
      complication NEC B27.19
      meningitis B27.12
      polyneuropathy B27.11
  Epstein-Barr (virus) B27.00
    with
      complication NEC B27.09
      meningitis B27.02
      polyneuropathy B27.01

Index

Migraine — Mononucleosis, infectious

Mononucleosis, infectious — *continued*
  gammaherpesviral B27.00
    with
      complication NEC B27.09
      meningitis B27.02
      polyneuropathy B27.01
  specified NEC B27.80
    with
      complication NEC B27.89
      meningitis B27.82
      polyneuropathy B27.81
Monoplegia G83.3- ☑
  congenital (cerebral) G80.8
    spastic G80.1
  embolic (current episode) I63.4 ☑
  following
    cerebrovascular disease
      cerebral infarction
        lower limb I69.34- ☑
        upper limb I69.33- ☑
      intracerebral hemorrhage
        lower limb I69.14- ☑
        upper limb I69.13- ☑
      lower limb I69.94- ☑
      nontraumatic intracranial hemorrhage NEC
        lower limb I69.24- ☑
        upper limb I69.23- ☑
      specified disease NEC
        lower limb I69.84- ☑
        upper limb I69.83- ☑
      stroke NOS
        lower limb I69.34- ☑
        upper limb I69.33- ☑
      subarachnoid hemorrhage
        lower limb I69.04- ☑
        upper limb I69.03- ☑
      upper limb I69.93- ☑
  hysterical (transient) F44.4
  lower limb G83.1- ☑
  psychogenic (conversion reaction) F44.4
  thrombotic (current episode) I63.3 ☑
  transient R29.818
  upper limb G83.2- ☑
Monorchism, monorchidism Q55.0
Monosomy (*see also* Deletion, chromosome) Q93.9
  specified NEC Q93.89
  whole chromosome
    meiotic nondisjunction Q93.0
    mitotic nondisjunction Q93.1
    mosaicism Q93.1
  X Q96.9
Monster, monstrosity (single) Q89.7
  acephalic Q00.0
  twin Q89.4
Monteggia's fracture (-dislocation) S52.27- ☑
Mooren's ulcer (cornea) — *see* Ulcer, cornea, Mooren's
Moore's syndrome — *see* Epilepsy, specified NEC
Mooser-Neill reaction A75.2
Mooser's bodies A75.2
Morbidity not stated or unknown R69
Morbilli — *see* Measles
Morbus (*see also* Disease)
  angelicus, anglorum E55.0
  Beigel B36.2
  caducus — *see* Epilepsy
  celiacus K90.0
  comitialis — *see* Epilepsy
  cordis (*see also* Disease, heart) I51.9
    valvulorum — *see* Endocarditis
  coxae senilis M16.9
    tuberculous A18.02
  hemorrhagicus neonatorum P53
  maculosus neonatorum P54.5
Morel (-Stewart)(-Morgagni) **syndrome** M85.2
Morel-Kraepelin disease — *see* Schizophrenia
Morel-Moore syndrome M85.2
Morgagni's
  cyst, organ, hydatid, or appendage
    female Q50.5
    male (epididymal) Q55.4
      testicular Q55.29
  syndrome M85.2
Morgagni-Stewart-Morel syndrome M85.2
Morgagni-Stokes-Adams syndrome I45.9
Morgagni-Turner (-Albright) **syndrome** Q96.9
Moria F07.0
Moron (I.Q. 50-69) F70

Morphea L94.0
Morphinism (without remission) F11.20
  with remission F11.21
Morphinomania (without remission) F11.20
  with remission F11.21
Morquio (-Ullrich)(-Brailsford) **disease or syndrome** —
  see Mucopolysaccharidosis
Mortification (dry) (moist) — *see* Gangrene
Morton's metatarsalgia (neuralgia)(neuroma) (syn-
  drome) G57.6- ☑
Morvan's disease or syndrome G60.8
Mosaicism, mosaic (autosomal) (chromosomal)
  45,X/46,XX Q96.3
  45,X/other cell lines NEC with abnormal sex chromo-
    some Q96.4
  sex chromosome
    female Q97.8
    lines with various numbers of X chromosomes
      Q97.2
    male Q98.7
  XY Q96.3
Moschowitz' disease M31.1
Mother yaw A66.0
Motion sickness (from travel, any vehicle) (from round-
  abouts or swings) T75.3 ☑
Mottled, mottling, teeth (enamel) (endemic) (nonen-
  demic) K00.3
Mounier-Kuhn syndrome Q32.4
  with bronchiectasis J47.9
    exacerbation (acute) J47.1
    lower respiratory infection J47.0
  acquired J98.09
    with bronchiectasis J47.9
      with
        exacerbation (acute) J47.1
        lower respiratory infection J47.0
Mountain
  sickness T70.29 ☑
    with polycythemia , acquired (acute) D75.1
  tick fever A93.2
Mouse, joint — *see* Loose, body, joint
  knee M23.4- ☑
Mouth — *see* condition
Movable
  coccyx — *see* subcategory M53.2 ☑
  kidney N28.89
    congenital Q63.8
  spleen D73.89
Movements, dystonic R25.8
Moyamoya disease I67.5
MRSA (Methicillin resistant Staphylococcus aureus)
  infection A49.02
    as the cause of diseases classified elsewhere B95.62
  sepsis A41.02
MSSA (Methicillin susceptible Staphylococcus aureus)
  infection A49.01
    as the cause of diseases classified elsewhere B95.61
  sepsis A41.01
Mucha-Habermann disease L41.0
Mucinosis (cutaneous) (focal) (papular) (skin) L98.5
  oral K13.79
Mucocele
  appendix K38.8
  buccal cavity K13.79
  gallbladder K82.1
  lacrimal sac, chronic H04.43- ☑
  nasal sinus J34.1
  nose J34.1
  salivary gland (any) K11.6
  sinus (accessory) (nasal) J34.1
  turbinate (bone) (middle) (nasal) J34.1
  uterus N85.8
Mucolipidosis
  I E77.1
  II, III E77.0
  IV E75.11
Mucopolysaccharidosis E76.3
  beta-gluduronidase deficiency E76.29
  cardiopathy E76.3 [I52]
  Hunter's syndrome E76.1
  Hurler's syndrome E76.01
  Hurler-Scheie syndrome E76.02
  Maroteaux-Lamy syndrome E76.29
  Morquio syndrome E76.219
    A E76.210
    B E76.211
    classic E76.210

Mucopolysaccharidosis — *continued*
  Sanfilippo syndrome E76.22
  Scheie's syndrome E76.03
  specified NEC E76.29
  type
    I
      Hurler's syndrome E76.01
      Hurler-Scheie syndrome E76.02
      Scheie's syndrome E76.03
    II E76.1
    III E76.22
    IV E76.219
    IVA E76.210
    IVB E76.211
    VI E76.29
    VII E76.29
Mucormycosis B46.5
  cutaneous B46.3
  disseminated B46.4
  gastrointestinal B46.2
  generalized B46.4
  pulmonary B46.0
  rhinocerebral B46.1
  skin B46.3
  subcutaneous B46.3
Mucositis (ulcerative) K12.30
  due to drugs NEC K12.32
  gastrointestinal K92.81
  mouth (oral) (oropharyngeal) K12.30
    due to antineoplastic therapy K12.31
    due to drugs NEC K12.32
    due to radiation K12.33
    specified NEC K12.39
    viral K12.39
  nasal J34.81
  oral cavity — *see* Mucositis, mouth
  oral soft tissues — *see* Mucositis, mouth
  vagina and vulva N76.81
Mucositis necroticans agranulocytica — *see* Agranulocytosis
Mucous (*see also* condition)
  patches (syphilitic) A51.39
    congenital A50.07
Mucoviscidosis E84.9
  with meconium obstruction E84.11
Mucus
  asphyxia or suffocation — *see* Asphyxia, mucus
  in stool R19.5
  plug — *see* Asphyxia, mucus
Muguet B37.0
Mulberry molars (congenital syphilis) A50.52
Müllerian mixed tumor
  specified site — *see* Neoplasm, malignant, by site
  unspecified site C54.9
Multicystic kidney (development) Q61.4
Multiparity (grand) Z64.1
  affecting management of pregnancy, labor and deliv-
    ery (supervision only) O09.4- ☑
  requiring contraceptive management — *see* Contra-
    ception
Multipartita placenta O43.19- ☑
Multiple, multiplex (*see also* condition)
  digits (congenital) Q69.9
  endocrine neoplasia — *see* Neoplasia, endocrine,
    multiple (MEN)
  personality F44.81
Mumps B26.9
  arthritis B26.85
  complication NEC B26.89
  encephalitis B26.2
  hepatitis B26.81
  meningitis (aseptic) B26.1
  meningoencephalitis B26.2
  myocarditis B26.82
  oophoritis B26.89
  orchitis B26.0
  pancreatitis B26.3
  polyneuropathy B26.84
Mumu (*see also* Infestation, filarial) B74.9 [N51]
Münchausen's syndrome — *see* Disorder, factitious
Münchmeyer's syndrome — *see* Myositis, ossificans,
  progressiva
Mural — *see* condition
Murmur (cardiac) (heart) (organic) R01.1
  abdominal R19.15
  aortic (valve) — *see* Endocarditis, aortic
  benign R01.0
  diastolic — *see* Endocarditis

Murmur — *continued*
Flint I35.1
functional R01.0
Graham Steell I37.1
innocent R01.0
mitral (valve) — *see* Insufficiency, mitral
nonorganic R01.0
presystolic, mitral — *see* Insufficiency, mitral
pulmonic (valve) I37.8
systolic (valvular) — *see* Endocarditis
tricuspid (valve) I07.9
valvular — *see* Endocarditis
Murri's disease (intermittent hemoglobinuria) D59.6
Muscle, muscular (*see also* condition)
carnitine (palmityltransferase) deficiency E71.314
Musculoneuralgia — *see* Neuralgia
Mushrooming hip — *see* Derangement, joint, specified
NEC, hip
Mushroom-workers' (pickers') **disease or lung** J67.5
Mutation(s)
factor V Leiden D68.51
prothrombin gene D68.52
surfactant, of lung J84.83
Mutism (*see also* Aphasia)
deaf (acquired) (congenital) NEC H91.3
elective (adjustment reaction) (childhood) F94.0
hysterical F44.4
selective (childhood) F94.0
MVD (microvillus inclusion disease) Q43.8
MVID (microvillus inclusion disease) Q43.8
Myalgia M79.1
epidemic (cervical) B33.0
traumatic NEC T14.8
Myasthenia G70.9
congenital G70.2
cordis — *see* Failure, heart
developmental G70.2
gravis G70.00
with exacerbation (acute) G70.01
in crisis G70.01
neonatal, transient P94.0
pseudoparalytica G70.00
with exacerbation (acute) G70.01
in crisis G70.01
stomach, psychogenic F45.8
syndrome
in
diabetes mellitus — *see* E08-E13 with .44
neoplastic disease (*see also* Neoplasm)
D49.9 [G73.3]
pernicious anemia D51.0 [G73.3]
thyrotoxicosis E05.90 [G73.3]
with thyroid storm E05.91 [G73.3]
Myasthenic M62.81
Mycelium infection B49
Mycetismus — *see* Poisoning, food, noxious, mushroom
Mycetoma B47.9
actinomycotic B47.1
bone (mycotic) B47.9 [M90.80]
eumycotic B47.0
foot B47.9
actinomycotic B47.1
mycotic B47.0
madurae NEC B47.9
mycotic B47.0
maduromycotic B47.0
mycotic B47.0
nocardial B47.1
Mycobacteriosis — *see* Mycobacterium
Mycobacterium, mycobacterial (infection) A31.9
anonymous A31.9
atypical A31.9
cutaneous A31.1
pulmonary A31.0
tuberculous — *see* Tuberculosis, pulmonary
specified site NEC A31.8
avium (intracellulare complex) A31.0
balnei A31.1
Battey A31.0
chelonei A31.8
cutaneous A31.1
extrapulmonary systemic A31.8
fortuitum A31.8
intracellulare (Battey bacillus) A31.0
kakaferifu A31.8
kansasii (yellow bacillus) A31.0
kasongo A31.8
leprae (*see also* Leprosy) A30.9

Mycobacterium, mycobacterial — *continued*
luciflavum A31.1
marinum (M. balnei) A31.1
nonspecific — *see* Mycobacterium, atypical
pulmonary (atypical) A31.0
tuberculous — *see* Tuberculosis, pulmonary
scrofulaceum A31.8
simiae A31.8
systemic, extrapulmonary A31.8
szulgai A31.8
terrae A31.8
triviale A31.8
tuberculosis (human, bovine) — *see* Tuberculosis
ulcerans A31.1
xenopi A31.8
Mycoplasma (M.) **pneumoniae, as cause of disease
classified elsewhere** B96.0
Mycosis, mycotic B49
cutaneous NEC B36.9
ear B36.8
fungoides (extranodal) (solid organ) C84.0- ☑
mouth B37.0
nails B35.1
opportunistic B48.8
skin NEC B36.9
specified NEC B48.8
stomatitis B37.0
vagina, vaginitis (candidal) B37.3
Mydriasis (pupil) H57.04
Myelatelia Q06.1
Myelinolysis, pontine, central G37.2
Myelitis (acute) (ascending) (childhood) (chronic) (descending) (diffuse) (disseminated) (idiopathic)
(pressure) (progressive) (spinal cord) (subacute)
(*see also* Encephalitis) G04.91
herpes simplex B00.82
herpes zoster B02.24
in diseases classified elsewhere G05.4
necrotizing, subacute G37.4
optic neuritis in G36.0
postchickenpox B01.12
postherpetic B02.24
postimmunization G04.02
postinfectious NEC G04.89
postvaccinal G04.02
specified NEC G04.89
syphilitic (transverse) A52.14
toxic G92
transverse (in demyelinating diseases of central nervous system) G37.3
tuberculous A17.82
varicella B01.12
Myeloblastic — *see* condition
Myeloblastoma
granular cell (*see also* Neoplasm, connective tissue)
malignant — *see* Neoplasm, connective tissue,
malignant
tongue D10.1
Myelocele — *see* Spina bifida
Myelocystocele — *see* Spina bifida
Myelocytic — *see* condition
Myelodysplasia D46.9
specified NEC D46.Z (*following* D46.4)
spinal cord (congenital) Q06.1
Myelodysplastic syndrome D46.9
with
5q deletion D46.C (*following* D46.2)
isolated del (5q) chromosomal abnormality D46.C
(*following* D46.2)
specified NEC D46.Z (*following* D46.4)
Myeloencephalitis — *see* Encephalitis
Myelofibrosis D75.81
with myeloid metaplasia D47.4
acute C94.4- ☑
idiopathic (chronic) D47.4
primary D47.1
secondary D75.81
in myeloproliferative disease D47.4
Myelogenous — *see* condition
Myeloid — *see* condition
Myelokathexis D70.9
Myeloleukodystrophy E75.29
Myelolipoma — *see* Lipoma
Myeloma (multiple) C90.0- ☑
monostotic C90.3 ☑
plasma cell C90.0- ☑
plasma cell C90.0- ☑

Myeloma — *continued*
solitary (*see also* Plasmacytoma, solitary) C90.3- ☑
Myelomalacia G95.89
Myelomatosis C90.0- ☑
Myelomeningitis — *see* Meningoencephalitis
Myelomeningocele (spinal cord) — *see* Spina bifida
Myelo-osteo-musculodysplasia hereditaria Q79.8
Myelopathic
anemia D64.89
muscle atrophy — *see* Atrophy, muscle, spinal
pain syndrome G89.0
Myelopathy (spinal cord) G95.9
drug-induced G95.89
in (due to)
degeneration or displacement, intervertebral disc
NEC — *see* Disorder, disc, with, myelopathy
infection — *see* Encephalitis
intervertebral disc disorder (*see also* Disorder, disc,
with, myelopathy)
mercury — *see* subcategory T56.1 ☑
neoplastic disease (*see also* Neoplasm)
D49.9 [G99.2]
pernicious anemia D51.0 [G99.2]
spondylosis — *see* Spondylosis, with myelopathy
NEC
necrotic (subacute) (vascular) G95.19
radiation-induced G95.89
spondylogenic NEC — *see* Spondylosis, with
myelopathy NEC
toxic G95.89
transverse, acute G37.3
vascular G95.19
vitamin B12 E53.8 [G32.0]
Myelophthisis D61.82
Myeloradiculitis G04.91
Myeloradiculodysplasia (spinal) Q06.1
Myelosarcoma C92.3- ☑
Myelosclerosis D75.89
with myeloid metaplasia D47.4
disseminated, of nervous system G35
megakaryocytic D47.4
with myeloid metaplasia D47.4
Myelosis
acute C92.0- ☑
aleukemic C92.9- ☑
chronic D47.1
erythremic (acute) C94.0- ☑
megakaryocytic C94.2- ☑
nonleukemic D72.828
subacute C92.9- ☑
Myiasis (cavernous) B87.9
aural B87.4
creeping B87.0
cutaneous B87.0
dermal B87.0
ear (external) (middle) B87.4
eye B87.2
genitourinary B87.81
intestinal B87.82
laryngeal B87.3
nasopharyngeal B87.3
ocular B87.2
orbit B87.2
skin B87.0
specified site NEC B87.89
traumatic B87.1
wound B87.1
Myoadenoma, prostate — *see* Hyperplasia, prostate
Myoblastoma
granular cell (*see also* Neoplasm, connective tissue,
benign)
malignant — *see* Neoplasm, connective tissue,
malignant
tongue D10.1
Myocardial — *see* condition
Myocardiopathy (congestive) (constrictive) (familial)
(hypertrophic nonobstructive) (idiopathic) (infiltrative) (obstructive) (primary) (restrictive) (sporadic)
(*see also* Cardiomyopathy) I42.9
alcoholic I42.6
cobalt-beer I42.6
glycogen storage E74.02 [I43]
hypertrophic obstructive I42.1
in (due to)
beriberi E51.12
cardiac glycogenosis E74.02 [I43]
Friedreich's ataxia G11.1 [I43]

Myocardiopathy — *continued*
  in — *continued*
    myotonia atrophica G71.11 [I43]
    progressive muscular dystrophy G71.0 [I43]
  obscure (African) I42.8
  secondary I42.9
  thyrotoxic E05.90 [I43]
    with storm E05.91 [I43]
  toxic NEC I42.7
Myocarditis (with arteriosclerosis)(chronic)(fibroid) (interstitial) (old) (progressive) (senile) I51.4
  with
    rheumatic fever (conditions in I00) I09.0
      active — *see* Myocarditis, acute, rheumatic
      inactive or quiescent (with chorea) I09.0
  active I40.9
    rheumatic I01.2
      with chorea (acute) (rheumatic) (Sydenham's) I02.0
  acute or subacute (interstitial) I40.9
    due to
      streptococcus (beta-hemolytic) I01.2
    idiopathic I40.1
    rheumatic I01.2
      with chorea (acute) (rheumatic) (Sydenham's) I02.0
    specified NEC I40.8
  aseptic of newborn B33.22
  bacterial (acute) I40.0
  Coxsackie (virus) B33.22
  diphtheritic A36.81
  eosinophilic I40.1
  epidemic of newborn (Coxsackie) B33.22
  Fiedler's (acute) (isolated) I40.1
  giant cell (acute) (subacute) I40.1
  gonococcal A54.83
  granulomatous (idiopathic) (isolated) (nonspecific) I40.1
  hypertensive — *see* Hypertension, heart
  idiopathic (granulomatous) I40.1
  in (due to)
    diphtheria A36.81
    epidemic louse-borne typhus A75.0 [I41]
    Lyme disease A69.29
    sarcoidosis D86.85
    scarlet fever A38.1
    toxoplasmosis (acquired) B58.81
    typhoid A01.02
    typhus NEC A75.9 [I41]
  infective I40.0
  influenzal — *see* Influenza, with, myocarditis
  isolated (acute) I40.1
  meningococcal A39.52
  mumps B26.82
  nonrheumatic, active I40.9
  parenchymatous I40.9
  pneumococcal I40.0
  rheumatic (chronic) (inactive) (with chorea) I09.0
    active or acute I01.2
      with chorea (acute) (rheumatic) (Sydenham's) I02.0
  rheumatoid — *see* Rheumatoid, carditis
  septic I40.0
  staphylococcal I40.0
  suppurative I40.0
  syphilitic (chronic) A52.06
  toxic I40.8
    rheumatic — *see* Myocarditis, acute, rheumatic
  tuberculous A18.84
  typhoid A01.02
  valvular — *see* Endocarditis
  virus, viral I40.0
    of newborn (Coxsackie) B33.22
Myocardium, myocardial — *see* condition
Myocardosis — *see* Cardiomyopathy
Myoclonus, myoclonic, myoclonia (familial) (essential) (multifocal) (simplex) G25.3
  drug-induced G25.3
  epilepsy (*see also* Epilepsy, generalized, specified NEC) G40.4- ☑
    familial (progressive) G25.3
  epileptica G40.409
    with status epilepticus G40.401
  facial G51.3
  familial progressive G25.3
  Friedreich's G25.3
  jerks G25.3
  massive G25.3

Myoclonus, myoclonic, myoclonia — *continued*
  palatal G25.3
  pharyngeal G25.3
Myocytolysis I51.5
Myodiastasis — *see* Diastasis, muscle
Myoendocarditis — *see* Endocarditis
Myoepithelioma — *see* Neoplasm, benign, by site
Myofasciitis (acute) — *see* Myositis
Myofibroma (*see also* Neoplasm, connective tissue, benign)
  uterus (cervix) (corpus) — *see* Leiomyoma
Myofibromatosis D48.1
  infantile Q89.8
Myofibrosis M62.89
  heart — *see* Myocarditis
  scapulohumeral — *see* Lesion, shoulder, specified NEC
Myofibrositis M79.7
  scapulohumeral — *see* Lesion, shoulder, specified NEC
Myoglobulinuria, myoglobinuria (primary) R82.1
Myokymia, facial G51.4
Myolipoma — *see* Lipoma
Myoma (*see also* Neoplasm, connective tissue, benign)
  malignant — *see* Neoplasm, connective tissue, malignant
  prostate D29.1
  uterus (cervix) (corpus) — *see* Leiomyoma
Myomalacia M62.89
Myometritis — *see* Endometritis
Myometrium — *see* condition
Myonecrosis, clostridial A48.0
Myopathy G72.9
  acute
    necrotizing G72.81
    quadriplegic G72.81
  alcoholic G72.1
  benign congenital G71.2
  central core G71.2
  centronuclear G71.2
  congenital (benign) G71.2
  critical illness G72.81
  distal G71.0
  drug-induced G72.0
  endocrine NEC E34.9 [G73.7]
  extraocular muscles H05.82- ☑
  facioscapulohumeral G71.0
  hereditary G71.9
    specified NEC G71.8
  immune NEC G72.49
  in (due to)
    Addison's disease E27.1 [G73.7]
    alcohol G72.1
    amyloidosis E85.0 [G73.7]
    cretinism E00.9 [G73.7]
    Cushing's syndrome E24.9 [G73.7]
    drugs G72.0
    endocrine disease NEC E34.9 [G73.7]
    giant cell arteritis M31.6 [G73.7]
    glycogen storage disease E74.00 [G73.7]
    hyperadrenocorticism E24.9 [G73.7]
    hyperparathyroidism NEC E21.3 [G73.7]
    hypoparathyroidism E20.9 [G73.7]
    hypopituitarism E23.0 [G73.7]
    hypothyroidism E03.9 [G73.7]
    infectious disease NEC B99 ☑ [G73.7]
    lipid storage disease E75.6 [G73.7]
    metabolic disease NEC E88.9 [G73.7]
    myxedema E03.9 [G73.7]
    parasitic disease NEC B89 [G73.7]
    polyarteritis nodosa M30.0 [G73.7]
    rheumatoid arthritis — *see* Rheumatoid, myopathy
    sarcoidosis D86.87
    scleroderma M34.82
    sicca syndrome M35.03
    Sjögren's syndrome M35.03
    systemic lupus erythematosus M32.19
    thyrotoxicosis (hyperthyroidism) E05.90 [G73.7]
      with thyroid storm E05.91 [G73.7]
    toxic agent NEC G72.2
  inflammatory NEC G72.49
  intensive care (ICU) G72.81
  limb-girdle G71.0
  mitochondrial NEC G71.3
  myotubular G71.2
  myotonic, proximal (PROMM) G71.11
  nemaline G71.2
  ocular G71.0
  oculopharyngeal G71.0
  of critical illness G72.81

Myopathy — *continued*
  primary G71.9
    specified NEC G71.8
  progressive NEC G72.89
  proximal myotonic (PROMM) G71.11
  rod G71.2
  scapulohumeral G71.0
  specified NEC G72.89
  toxic G72.2
Myopericarditis (*see also* Pericarditis)
  chronic rheumatic I09.2
Myopia (axial) (congenital) H52.1- ☑
  degenerative (malignant) H44.2- ☑
  malignant H44.2- ☑
  pernicious H44.2- ☑
  progressive high (degenerative) H44.2- ☑
Myosarcoma — *see* Neoplasm, connective tissue, malignant
Myosis (pupil) H57.03
  stromal (endolymphatic) D39.0
Myositis M60.9
  clostridial A48.0
  due to posture — *see* Myositis, specified type NEC
  epidemic B33.0
  fibrosa or fibrous (chronic), Volkmann's T79.6 ☑
  foreign body granuloma — *see* Granuloma, foreign body
  in (due to)
    bilharziasis B65.9 [M63.8-] ☑
    cysticercosis B69.81
    leprosy A30.9 [M63.8-] ☑
    mycosis B49 [M63.8-] ☑
    sarcoidosis D86.87
    schistosomiasis B65.9 [M63.8-] ☑
    syphilis
      late A52.78
      secondary A51.49
    toxoplasmosis (acquired) B58.82
    trichinellosis B75 [M63.8-] ☑
    tuberculosis A18.09
  inclusion body [IBM] G72.41
  infective M60.009
    arm M60.002
      left M60.001
      right M60.000
    leg M60.005
      left M60.004
      right M60.003
    lower limb M60.005
      ankle M60.07- ☑
      foot M60.07- ☑
      lower leg M60.06- ☑
      thigh M60.05- ☑
      toe M60.07- ☑
    multiple sites M60.09
    specified site NEC M60.08
    upper limb M60.002
      finger M60.04- ☑
      forearm M60.03- ☑
      hand M60.04- ☑
      shoulder region M60.01- ☑
      upper arm M60.02- ☑
  interstitial M60.10
    ankle M60.17- ☑
    foot M60.17- ☑
    forearm M60.13- ☑
    hand M60.14- ☑
    lower leg M60.16- ☑
    multiple sites M60.19
    shoulder region M60.11- ☑
    specified site NEC M60.18
    thigh M60.15- ☑
    upper arm M60.12- ☑
  mycotic B49 [M63.8-] ☑
  orbital, chronic H05.12- ☑
  ossificans or ossifying (circumscripta) (*see also* Ossification, muscle, specified NEC)
    in (due to)
      burns M61.30
        ankle M61.37- ☑
        foot M61.37- ☑
        forearm M61.33- ☑
        hand M61.34- ☑
        lower leg M61.36- ☑
        multiple sites M61.39
        pelvic region M61.35- ☑
        shoulder region M61.31- ☑

Myositis — *continued*
  ossificans or ossifying (*see also* Ossification, muscle, specified) — *continued*
    in — *continued*
      burns — *continued*
        specified site NEC M61.38
        thigh M61.35- ☑
        upper arm M61.32- ☑
      quadriplegia or paraplegia M61.20
        ankle M61.27- ☑
        foot M61.27- ☑
        forearm M61.23- ☑
        hand M61.24- ☑
        lower leg M61.26- ☑
        multiple sites M61.29
        pelvic region M61.25- ☑
        shoulder region M61.21- ☑
        specified site NEC M61.28
        thigh M61.25- ☑
        upper arm M61.22- ☑
    progressiva M61.10
      ankle M61.17- ☑
      finger M61.14- ☑
      foot M61.17- ☑
      forearm M61.13- ☑
      hand M61.14- ☑
      lower leg M61.16- ☑
      multiple sites M61.19
      pelvic region M61.15- ☑
      shoulder region M61.11- ☑
      specified site NEC M61.18
      thigh M61.15- ☑
      toe M61.17- ☑
      upper arm M61.12- ☑
    traumatica M61.00
      ankle M61.07- ☑
      foot M61.07- ☑
      forearm M61.03- ☑
      hand M61.04- ☑

Myositis — *continued*
  ossificans or ossifying (*see also* Ossification, muscle, specified) — *continued*
    traumatica — *continued*
      lower leg M61.06- ☑
      multiple sites M61.09
      pelvic region M61.05- ☑
      shoulder region M61.01- ☑
      specified site NEC M61.08
      thigh M61.05- ☑
      upper arm M61.02- ☑
  purulent — *see* Myositis, infective
  specified type NEC M60.80
    ankle M60.87- ☑
    foot M60.87- ☑
    forearm M60.83- ☑
    hand M60.84- ☑
    lower leg M60.86- ☑
    multiple sites M60.89
    pelvic region M60.85- ☑
    shoulder region M60.81- ☑
    specified site NEC M60.88
    thigh M60.85- ☑
    upper arm M60.82- ☑
  suppurative — *see* Myositis, infective
  traumatic (old) — *see* Myositis, specified type NEC
Myospasia impulsiva F95.2
Myotonia (acquisita) (intermittens) M62.89
  atrophica G71.11
  chondrodystrophic G71.13
  congenita (acetazolamide responsive) (dominant) (recessive) G71.12
  drug-induced G71.14
  dystrophica G71.11
  fluctuans G71.19
  levior G71.12
  permanens G71.19
  symptomatic G71.19

Myotonic pupil — *see* Anomaly, pupil, function, tonic pupil
Myriapodiasis B88.2
Myringitis H73.2- ☑
  with otitis media — *see* Otitis, media
  acute H73.00- ☑
    bullous H73.01- ☑
    specified NEC H73.09- ☑
  bullous — *see* Myringitis, acute, bullous
  chronic H73.1- ☑
Mysophobia F40.228
Mytilotoxism — *see* Poisoning, fish
Myxadenitis labialis K13.0
Myxedema (adult) (idiocy) (infantile) (juvenile) (*see also* Hypothyroidism) E03.9
  circumscribed E05.90
    with storm E05.91
  coma E03.5
  congenital E00.1
  cutis L98.5
  localized (pretibial) E05.90
    with storm E05.91
  papular L98.5
Myxochondrosarcoma — *see* Neoplasm, cartilage, malignant
Myxofibroma — *see* Neoplasm, connective tissue, benign
  odontogenic — *see* Cyst, calcifying odontogenic
Myxofibrosarcoma — *see* Neoplasm, connective tissue, malignant
Myxolipoma D17.9
Myxoliposarcoma — *see* Neoplasm, connective tissue, malignant
Myxoma (*see also* Neoplasm, connective tissue, benign)
  nerve sheath — *see* Neoplasm, nerve, benign
  odontogenic — *see* Cyst, calcifying odontogenic
Myxosarcoma — *see* Neoplasm, connective tissue, malignant

N

Naegeli's
  disease Q82.8
  leukemia, monocytic C93.1- ☑
Naegleriasis (with meningoencephalitis) B60.2
Naffziger's syndrome G54.0
Naga sore — *see* Ulcer, skin
Nägele's pelvis M95.5
  with disproportion (fetopelvic) O33.0
    causing obstructed labor O65.0
Nail (*see also* condition)
  biting F98.8
  patella syndrome Q87.2
Nanism, nanosomia — *see* Dwarfism
Nanophyetiasis B66.8
Nanukayami A27.89
Napkin rash L22
Narcolepsy G47.419
  with cataplexy G47.411
  in conditions classified elsewhere G47.429
    with cataplexy G47.421
Narcosis R06.89
Narcotism — *see* Dependence
NARP (Neuropathy, Ataxia and Retinitis pigmentosa)
  syndrome E88.49
Narrow
  anterior chamber angle H40.03- ☑
  pelvis — *see* Contraction, pelvis
Narrowing (*see also* Stenosis)
  artery I77.1
    auditory, internal I65.8
    basilar — *see* Occlusion, artery, basilar
    carotid — *see* Occlusion, artery, carotid
    cerebellar — *see* Occlusion, artery, cerebellar
    cerebral — *see* Occlusion artery, cerebral
    choroidal — *see* Occlusion, artery, cerebral, speci-
      fied NEC
    communicating posterior — *see* Occlusion, artery,
      cerebral, specified NEC
    coronary (*see also* Disease, heart, ischemic,
      atherosclerotic)
      congenital Q24.5
        syphilitic A50.54 [I52]
      due to syphilis NEC A52.06
    hypophyseal — *see* Occlusion, artery, cerebral,
      specified NEC
    pontine — *see* Occlusion, artery, cerebral, specified
      NEC
    precerebral — *see* Occlusion, artery, precerebral
    vertebral — *see* Occlusion, artery, vertebral
  auditory canal (external) — *see* Stenosis, external ear
    canal
  eustachian tube — *see* Obstruction, eustachian tube
  eyelid — *see* Disorder, eyelid function
  larynx J38.6
  mesenteric artery K55.0
  palate M26.89
  palpebral fissure — *see* Disorder, eyelid function
  ureter N13.5
    with infection N13.6
  urethra — *see* Stricture, urethra
Narrowness, abnormal, eyelid Q10.3
Nasal — *see* condition
Nasolachrymal, nasolacrimal — *see* condition
Nasopharyngeal (*see also* condition)
  pituitary gland Q89.2
  torticollis M43.6
Nasopharyngitis (acute) (infective) (streptococcal)
  (subacute) J00
  chronic (suppurative) (ulcerative) J31.1
Nasopharynx, nasopharyngeal — *see* condition
Natal tooth, teeth K00.6
Nausea (without vomiting) R11.0
  with vomiting R11.2
  gravidarum — *see* Hyperemesis, gravidarum
  marina T75.3 ☑
  navalis T75.3 ☑
Navel — *see* condition
Neapolitan fever — *see* Brucellosis

Near drowning T75.1 ☑
Nearsightedness — *see* Myopia
Near-syncope R55
Nebula, cornea — *see* Opacity, cornea
Necator americanus infestation B76.1
Necatoriasis B76.1
Neck — *see* condition
Necrobiosis R68.89
  lipoidica NEC L92.1
    with diabetes — *see* E08-E13 with .620
Necrolysis, toxic epidermal L51.2
  due to drug
    correct substance properly administered — *see*
      Table of Drugs and Chemicals, by drug, ad-
      verse effect
    overdose or wrong substance given or taken —
      see Table of Drugs and Chemicals, by drug,
      poisoning
Necrophilia F65.89
Necrosis, necrotic (ischemic) (*see also* Gangrene)
  adrenal (capsule) (gland) E27.49
  amputation stump (surgical) (late) T87.50
    arm T87.5- ☑
    leg T87.5- ☑
  antrum J32.0
  aorta (hyaline) (*see also* Aneurysm, aorta)
    cystic medial — *see* Dissection, aorta
  artery I77.5
  bladder (aseptic) (sphincter) N32.89
  bone (*see also* Osteonecrosis) M87.9
    aseptic or avascular — *see* Osteonecrosis
      idiopathic M87.00
    ethmoid J32.2
    jaw M27.2
    tuberculous — *see* Tuberculosis, bone
  brain I67.89
  breast (aseptic) (fat) (segmental) N64.1
  bronchus J98.09
  central nervous system NEC I67.89
  cerebellar I67.89
  cerebral I67.89
  colon K55.0
  cornea H18.40
  cortical (acute) (renal) N17.1
  cystic medial (aorta) — *see* Dissection, aorta
  dental pulp K04.1
  esophagus K22.8
  ethmoid (bone) J32.2
  eyelid — *see* Disorder, eyelid, degenerative
  fat, fatty (generalized) (*see also* Disorder, soft tissue,
    specified type NEC)
    abdominal wall K65.4
    breast (aseptic) (segmental) N64.1
    localized — *see* Degeneration, by site, fatty
    mesentery K65.4
    omentum K65.4
    pancreas K86.8
    peritoneum K65.4
    skin (subcutaneous), newborn P83.0
    subcutaneous, due to birth injury P15.6
  gallbladder — *see* Cholecystitis, acute
  heart — *see* Infarct, myocardium
  hip, aseptic or avascular — *see* Osteonecrosis, by type,
    femur
  intestine (acute) (hemorrhagic) (massive) K55.0
  jaw M27.2
  kidney (bilateral) N28.0
    acute N17.9
    cortical (acute) (bilateral) N17.1
      with ectopic or molar pregnancy O08.4
    medullary (bilateral) (in acute renal failure) (papil-
      lary) N17.2
    papillary (bilateral) (in acute renal failure) N17.2
    tubular N17.0
      with ectopic or molar pregnancy O08.4
      complicating
        abortion — *see* Abortion, by type, compli-
          cated by, tubular necrosis
        ectopic or molar pregnancy O08.4
        pregnancy — *see* Pregnancy, complicated
          by, diseases of, specified type or sys-
          tem NEC

Necrosis, necrotic — *continued*
  kidney — *continued*
    tubular — *continued*
      following ectopic or molar pregnancy O08.4
      traumatic T79.5 ☑
  larynx J38.7
  liver (with hepatic failure) (cell) — *see* Failure, hepatic
    hemorrhagic, central K76.2
  lung J85.0
  lymphatic gland — *see* Lymphadenitis, acute
  mammary gland (fat) (segmental) N64.1
  mastoid (chronic) — *see* Mastoiditis, chronic
  medullary (acute) (renal) N17.2
  mesentery K55.0
    fat K65.4
  mitral valve — *see* Insufficiency, mitral
  myocardium, myocardial — *see* Infarct, myocardium
  nose J34.0
  omentum (with mesenteric infarction) K55.0
    fat K65.4
  orbit, orbital — *see* Osteomyelitis, orbit
  ossicles, ear — *see* Abnormal, ear ossicles
  ovary N70.92
  pancreas (aseptic) (duct) (fat) K86.8
    acute (infective) — *see* Pancreatitis, acute
    infective — *see* Pancreatitis, acute
  papillary (acute) (renal) N17.2
  perineum N90.89
  peritoneum (with mesenteric infarction) K55.0
    fat K65.4
  pharynx J02.9
    in granulocytopenia — *see* Neutropenia
      Vincent's A69.1
  phosphorus — *see* subcategory T54.2 ☑
  pituitary (gland) (postpartum) (Sheehan) E23.0
  pressure — *see* Ulcer, pressure, by site
  pulmonary J85.0
  pulp (dental) K04.1
  radiation — *see* Necrosis, by site
  radium — *see* Necrosis, by site
  renal — *see* Necrosis, kidney
  sclera H15.89
  scrotum N50.8
  skin or subcutaneous tissue NEC I96
  spine, spinal (column) (*see also* Osteonecrosis, by type,
    vertebra)
    cord G95.19
  spleen D73.5
  stomach K31.89
  stomatitis (ulcerative) A69.0
  subcutaneous fat, newborn P83.8
  subendocardial (acute) I21.4
    chronic I25.89
  suprarenal (capsule) (gland) E27.49
  testis N50.8
  thymus (gland) E32.8
  tonsil J35.8
  trachea J39.8
  tuberculous NEC — *see* Tuberculosis
  tubular (acute) (anoxic) (renal) (toxic) N17.0
    postprocedural N99.0
  vagina N89.8
  vertebra (*see also* Osteonecrosis, by type, vertebra)
    tuberculous A18.01
  vulva N90.89
  X-ray — *see* Necrosis, by site
Necrospermia — *see* Infertility, male
Need (for)
  care provider because of)
    assistance with personal care Z74.1
    continuous supervision required Z74.3
    impaired mobility Z74.09
    no other household member able to render care
      Z74.2
    specified reason NEC Z74.8
  immunization — *see* Vaccination
  vaccination — *see* Vaccination
Neglect
  adult
    confirmed T74.01 ☑
    history of Z91.412
    suspected T76.01 ☑

Naegeli's — Neglect

Index

222

☑ **Additional Character Required** — **Refer to the Tabular List for Character Selection**   ⬯ **Subterms under main terms may continue to next column or page**

Neglect — *continued*
  child (childhood)
    confirmed T74.02 ☑
    history of Z62.812
    suspected T76.02 ☑
  emotional, in childhood Z62.898
  hemispatial R41.4
  left-sided R41.4
  sensory R41.4
  visuospatial R41.4
Neisserian infection NEC — *see* Gonococcus
Nelaton's syndrome G60.8
Nelson's syndrome E24.1
Nematodiasis (intestinal) B82.0
  Ancylostoma B76.0
Neonatal (*see also* Newborn)
  acne L70.4
  bradycardia P29.12
  screening, abnormal findings on P09
  tachycardia P29.11
  tooth, teeth K00.6
Neonatorum — *see* condition
Neoplasia
  endocrine, multiple (MEN) E31.20
    type I E31.21
    type IIA E31.22
    type IIB E31.23
  intraepithelial (histologically confirmed)
    anal (AIN) (histologically confirmed) K62.82
      grade I K62.82
      grade II K62.82
      severe D01.3
    cervical glandular (histologically confirmed) D06.9
    cervix (uteri) (CIN) (histologically confirmed) N87.9
      glandular D06.9
      grade I N87.0
      grade II N87.1
      grade III (severe dysplasia) (*see also* Carcinoma, cervix uteri, in situ) D06.9
    prostate (histologically confirmed) (PIN I) (PIN II) N42.3
      grade I N42.3
      grade II N42.3
      severe D07.5
    vagina (histologically confirmed) (VAIN) N89.3
      grade I N89.0
      grade II N89.1
      grade III (severe dysplasia) D07.2
    vulva (histologically confirmed) (VIN) N90.3
      grade I N90.0
      grade II N90.1
      grade III (severe dysplasia) D07.1
Neoplasm, neoplastic (*see also* Table of Neoplasms)
  lipomatous, benign — *see* Lipoma
Neovascularization
  ciliary body — *see* Disorder, iris, vascular
  cornea H16.40- ☑
    deep H16.44- ☑
    ghost vessels — *see* Ghost, vessels
    localized H16.43- ☑
    pannus — *see* Pannus
  iris — *see* Disorder, iris, vascular
  retina H35.05- ☑
Nephralgia N23
Nephritis, nephritic (albuminuric) (azotemic) (congenital) (disseminated) (epithelial) (familial) (focal) (granulomatous) (hemorrhagic) (infantile) (nonsuppurative, excretory) (uremic) N05.9
  with
    dense deposit disease N05.6
    diffuse
      crescentic glomerulonephritis N05.7
      endocapillary proliferative glomerulonephritis N05.4
      membranous glomerulonephritis N05.2
      mesangial proliferative glomerulonephritis N05.3
      mesangiocapillary glomerulonephritis N05.5
    edema — *see* Nephrosis
    focal and segmental glomerular lesions N05.1
    foot process disease N04.9
    glomerular lesion
      diffuse sclerosing N05.8
      hypocomplementemic — *see* Nephritis, membranoproliferative
      IgA — *see* Nephropathy, IgA
      lobular, lobulonodular — *see* Nephritis, membranoproliferative

Nephritis, nephritic — *continued*
  with — *continued*
    glomerular lesion — *continued*
      nodular — *see* Nephritis, membranoproliferative
    lesion of
      glomerulonephritis, proliferative N05.8
      renal necrosis N05.9
    minor glomerular abnormality N05.0
    specified morphological changes NEC N05.8
  acute N00.9
    with
      dense deposit disease N00.6
      diffuse
        crescentic glomerulonephritis N00.7
        endocapillary proliferative glomerulonephritis N00.4
        membranous glomerulonephritis N00.2
        mesangial proliferative glomerulonephritis N00.3
        mesangiocapillary glomerulonephritis N00.5
      focal and segmental glomerular lesions N00.1
      minor glomerular abnormality N00.0
      specified morphological changes NEC N00.8
  amyloid E85.4 [N08]
  antiglomerular basement membrane (anti-GBM) antibody NEC
    in Goodpasture's syndrome M31.0
  antitubular basement membrane (tubulo-interstitial) NEC N12
    toxic — *see* Nephropathy, toxic
  arteriolar — *see* Hypertension, kidney
  arteriosclerotic — *see* Hypertension, kidney
  ascending — *see* Nephritis, tubulo-interstitial
  atrophic N03.9
  Balkan (endemic) N15.0
  calculous, calculus — *see* Calculus, kidney
  cardiac — *see* Hypertension, kidney
  cardiovascular — *see* Hypertension, kidney
  chronic N03.9
    with
      dense deposit disease N03.6
      diffuse
        crescentic glomerulonephritis N03.7
        endocapillary proliferative glomerulonephritis N03.4
        membranous glomerulonephritis N03.2
        mesangial proliferative glomerulonephritis N03.3
        mesangiocapillary glomerulonephritis N03.5
      focal and segmental glomerular lesions N03.1
      minor glomerular abnormality N03.0
      specified morphological changes NEC N03.8
    arteriosclerotic — *see* Hypertension, kidney
  cirrhotic N26.9
  complicating pregnancy O26.83- ☑
  croupous N00.9
  degenerative — *see* Nephrosis
  diffuse sclerosing N05.8
  due to
    diabetes mellitus — *see* E08-E13 with .21
    subacute bacterial endocarditis I33.0
    systemic lupus erythematosus (chronic) M32.14
    typhoid fever A01.09
  gonococcal (acute) (chronic) A54.21
  hypocomplementemic — *see* Nephritis, membranoproliferative
  IgA — *see* Nephropathy, IgA
  immune complex (circulating) NEC N05.8
  infective — *see* Nephritis, tubulo-interstitial
  interstitial — *see* Nephritis, tubulo-interstitial
  lead N14.3
  membranoproliferative (diffuse) (type 1 or 3) (*see also* N00-N07 with fourth character .5) N05.5
    type 2 (*see also* N00-N07 with fourth character .6) N05.6
  minimal change N05.0
  necrotic, necrotizing NEC (*see also* N00-N07 with fourth character .8) N05.8
  nephrotic — *see* Nephrosis
  nodular — *see* Nephritis, membranoproliferative
  polycystic Q61.3
    adult type Q61.2
    autosomal
      dominant Q61.2
      recessive NEC Q61.19
    childhood type NEC Q61.19
    infantile type NEC Q61.19

Nephritis, nephritic — *continued*
  poststreptococcal N05.9
    acute N00.9
    chronic N03.9
    rapidly progressive N01.9
  proliferative NEC (*see also* N00-N07 with fourth character .8) N05.8
  purulent — *see* Nephritis, tubulo-interstitial
  rapidly progressive N01.9
    with
      dense deposit disease N01.6
      diffuse
        crescentic glomerulonephritis N01.7
        endocapillary proliferative glomerulonephritis N01.4
        membranous glomerulonephritis N01.2
        mesangial proliferative glomerulonephritis N01.3
        mesangiocapillary glomerulonephritis N01.5
      focal and segmental glomerular lesions N01.1
      minor glomerular abnormality N01.0
      specified morphological changes NEC N01.8
  salt losing or wasting NEC N28.89
  saturnine N14.3
  sclerosing, diffuse N05.8
  septic — *see* Nephritis, tubulo-interstitial
  specified pathology NEC (*see also* N00-N07 with fourth character .8) N05.8
  subacute N01.9
  suppurative — *see* Nephritis, tubulo-interstitial
  syphilitic (late) A52.75
    congenital A50.59 [N08]
    early (secondary) A51.44
  toxic — *see* Nephropathy, toxic
  tubal, tubular — *see* Nephritis, tubulo-interstitial
  tuberculous A18.11
  tubulo-interstitial (in) N12
    acute (infectious) N10
    chronic (infectious) N11.9
      nonobstructive N11.8
        reflux-associated N11.0
      obstructive N11.1
      specified NEC N11.8
    due to
      brucellosis A23.9 [N16]
      cryoglobulinemia D89.1 [N16]
      glycogen storage disease E74.00 [N16]
    Sjögren's syndrome M35.04
  vascular — *see* Hypertension, kidney
  war N00.9
Nephroblastoma (epithelial) (mesenchymal) C64- ☑
Nephrocalcinosis E83.59 [N29]
Nephrocystitis, pustular — *see* Nephritis, tubulo-interstitial
Nephrolithiasis (congenital) (pelvis) (recurrent) (*see also* Calculus, kidney)
Nephroma C64- ☑
  mesoblastic D41.0- ☑
Nephronephritis — *see* Nephrosis
Nephronophthisis Q61.5
Nephropathia epidemica A98.5
Nephropathy (*see also* Nephritis) N28.9
  with
    edema — *see* Nephrosis
    glomerular lesion — *see* Glomerulonephritis
  amyloid, hereditary E85.0
  analgesic N14.0
    with medullary necrosis, acute N17.2
  Balkan (endemic) N15.0
  chemical — *see* Nephropathy, toxic
  diabetic — *see* E08-E13 with .21
  drug-induced N14.2
    specified NEC N14.1
  focal and segmental hyalinosis or sclerosis N02.1
  heavy metal-induced N14.3
  hereditary NEC N07.9
    with
      dense deposit disease N07.6
      diffuse
        crescentic glomerulonephritis N07.7
        endocapillary proliferative glomerulonephritis N07.4
        membranous glomerulonephritis N07.2
        mesangial proliferative glomerulonephritis N07.3
        mesangiocapillary glomerulonephritis N07.5
      focal and segmental glomerular lesions N07.1
      minor glomerular abnormality N07.0

Nephropathy — *continued*
 hereditary — *continued*
  with — *continued*
   specified morphological changes NEC N07.8
 hypercalcemic N25.89
 hypertensive — *see* Hypertension, kidney
 hypokalemic (vacuolar) N25.89
 IgA N02.8
  with glomerular lesion N02.9
   focal and segmental hyalinosis or sclerosis N02.1
   membranoproliferative (diffuse) N02.5
   membranous (diffuse) N02.2
   mesangial proliferative (diffuse) N02.3
   mesangiocapillary (diffuse) N02.5
   proliferative NEC N02.8
   specified pathology NEC N02.8
 lead N14.3
 membranoproliferative (diffuse) N02.5
 membranous (diffuse) N02.2
 mesangial (IgA/IgG) — *see* Nephropathy, IgA
  proliferative (diffuse) N02.3
 mesangiocapillary (diffuse) N02.5
 obstructive N13.8
 phenacetin N17.2
 phosphate-losing N25.0
 potassium depletion N25.89
 pregnancy-related O26.83- ☑
 proliferative NEC (*see also* N00-N07 with fourth character .8) N05.8
 protein-losing N25.89
 saturnine N14.3
 sickle-cell D57.- ☑ [N08]
 toxic NEC N14.4
  due to
   drugs N14.2
    analgesic N14.0
    specified NEC N14.1
   heavy metals N14.3
 vasomotor N17.0
 water-losing N25.89
Nephroptosis N28.83
Nephropyosis — *see* Abscess, kidney
Nephrorrhagia N28.89
Nephrosclerosis (arteriolar)(arteriosclerotic) (chronic) (hyaline) (*see also* Hypertension, kidney)
 hyperplastic — *see* Hypertension, kidney
 senile N26.9
Nephrosis, nephrotic (Epstein's) (syndrome) (congenital) N04.9
 with
  foot process disease N04.9
  glomerular lesion N04.1
  hypocomplementemic N04.5
 acute N04.9
 anoxic — *see* Nephrosis, tubular
 chemical — *see* Nephrosis, tubular
 cholemic K76.7
 diabetic — *see* E08-E13 with .21
 Finnish type (congenital) Q89.8
 hemoglobin N10
 hemoglobinuric — *see* Nephrosis, tubular
 in
  amyloidosis E85.4 [N08]
  diabetes mellitus — *see* E08-E13 with .21
  epidemic hemorrhagic fever A98.5
  malaria (malariae) B52.0
 ischemic — *see* Nephrosis, tubular
 lipoid N04.9
 lower nephron — *see* Nephrosis, tubular
 malarial (malariae) B52.0
 minimal change N04.0
 myoglobin N10
 necrotizing — *see* Nephrosis, tubular
 osmotic (sucrose) N25.89
 radiation N04.9
 syphilitic (late) A52.75
 toxic — *see* Nephrosis, tubular
 tubular (acute) N17.0
  postprocedural N99.0
  radiation N04.9
Nephrosonephritis, hemorrhagic (endemic) A98.5
Nephrostomy
 attention to Z43.6
 status Z93.6
Nerve (*see also* condition)
 injury — *see* Injury, nerve, by body site
Nerves R45.0

Nervous (*see also* condition) R45.0
 heart F45.8
 stomach F45.8
 tension R45.0
Nervousness R45.0
Nesidioblastoma
 pancreas D13.7
 specified site NEC — *see* Neoplasm, benign, by site
 unspecified site D13.7
Nettleship's syndrome Q82.2
Neumann's disease or syndrome L10.1
Neuralgia, neuralgic (acute) M79.2
 accessory (nerve) G52.8
 acoustic (nerve) — *see* subcategory H93.3 ☑
 auditory (nerve) — *see* subcategory H93.3 ☑
 ciliary G44.009
  intractable G44.001
  not intractable G44.009
 cranial
  nerve (*see also* Disorder, nerve, cranial)
   fifth or trigeminal — *see* Neuralgia, trigeminal
  postherpetic, postzoster B02.29
 ear — *see* subcategory H92.0 ☑
 facialis vera G51.1
 Fothergill's — *see* Neuralgia, trigeminal
 glossopharyngeal (nerve) G52.1
 Horton's G44.099
  intractable G44.091
  not intractable G44.099
 Hunt's B02.21
 hypoglossal (nerve) G52.3
 infraorbital — *see* Neuralgia, trigeminal
 malarial — *see* Malaria
 migrainous G44.009
  intractable G44.001
  not intractable G44.009
 Morton's G57.6- ☑
 nerve, cranial — *see* Disorder, nerve, cranial
 nose G52.0
 occipital M54.81
 olfactory G52.0
 penis N48.9
 perineum R10.2
 postherpetic NEC B02.29
  trigeminal B02.22
 pubic region R10.2
 scrotum R10.2
 Sluder's G44.89
 specified nerve NEC G58.8
 spermatic cord R10.2
 sphenopalatine (ganglion) G90.09
 trifacial — *see* Neuralgia, trigeminal
 trigeminal G50.0
  postherpetic, postzoster B02.22
 vagus (nerve) G52.2
 writer's F48.8
  organic G25.89
Neurapraxia — *see* Injury, nerve
Neurasthenia F48.8
 cardiac F45.8
 gastric F45.8
 heart F45.8
Neurilemmoma (*see also* Neoplasm, nerve, benign)
 acoustic (nerve) D33.3
 malignant (*see also* Neoplasm, nerve, malignant)
  acoustic (nerve) C72.4- ☑
Neurilemmosarcoma — *see* Neoplasm, nerve, malignant
Neurinoma — *see* Neoplasm, nerve, benign
Neurinomatosis — *see* Neoplasm, nerve, uncertain behavior
Neuritis (rheumatoid) M79.2
 abducens (nerve) — *see* Strabismus, paralytic, sixth nerve
 accessory (nerve) G52.8
 acoustic (nerve) (*see also* subcategory) H93.3 ☑
  in (due to)
   infectious disease NEC B99 ☑ [H94.0-] ☑
   parasitic disease NEC B89 [H94.0-] ☑
   syphilitic A52.15
 alcoholic G62.1
  with psychosis — *see* Psychosis, alcoholic
 amyloid, any site E85.4 [G63]
 auditory (nerve) — *see* subcategory H93.3 ☑
 brachial — *see* Radiculopathy
  due to displacement, intervertebral disc — *see* Disorder, disc, cervical, with neuritis

Neuritis — *continued*
 cranial nerve
  due to Lyme disease A69.22
  eighth or acoustic or auditory — *see* subcategory H93.3 ☑
  eleventh or accessory G52.8
  fifth or trigeminal G51.0
  first or olfactory G52.0
  fourth or trochlear — *see* Strabismus, paralytic, fourth nerve
  second or optic — *see* Neuritis, optic
  seventh or facial G51.8
   newborn (birth injury) P11.3
  sixth or abducent — *see* Strabismus, paralytic, sixth nerve
  tenth or vagus G52.2
  third or oculomotor — *see* Strabismus, paralytic, third nerve
  twelfth or hypoglossal G52.3
 Déjérine-Sottas G60.0
 diabetic (mononeuropathy) — *see* E08-E13 with .41
  polyneuropathy — *see* E08-E13 with .42
 due to
  beriberi E51.11
  displacement, prolapse or rupture, intervertebral disc — *see* Disorder, disc, with, radiculopathy
  herniation, nucleus pulposus M51.9 [G55]
 endemic E51.11
 facial G51.8
  newborn (birth injury) P11.3
 general — *see* Polyneuropathy
 geniculate ganglion G51.1
  due to herpes (zoster) B02.21
 gouty M10.00 [G63]
 hypoglossal (nerve) G52.3
 ilioinguinal (nerve) G57.9- ☑
 infectious (multiple) NEC G61.0
 interstitial hypertrophic progressive G60.0
 lumbar M54.16
 lumbosacral M54.17
 multiple (*see also* Polyneuropathy)
  endemic E51.11
  infective, acute G61.0
 multiplex endemica E51.11
 nerve root — *see* Radiculopathy
 oculomotor (nerve) — *see* Strabismus, paralytic, third nerve
 olfactory nerve G52.0
 optic (nerve) (hereditary) (sympathetic) H46.9
  with demyelination G36.0
  in myelitis G36.0
  nutritional H46.2
  papillitis — *see* Papillitis, optic
  retrobulbar H46.1- ☑
  specified type NEC H46.8
  toxic H46.3
 peripheral (nerve) G62.9
  multiple — *see* Polyneuropathy
  single — *see* Mononeuritis
 pneumogastric (nerve) G52.2
 postherpetic, postzoster B02.29
 progressive hypertrophic interstitial G60.0
 retrobulbar (*see also* Neuritis, optic, retrobulbar)
  in (due to)
   late syphilis A52.15
   meningococcal infection A39.82
  meningococcal A39.82
  syphilitic A52.15
 sciatic (nerve) (*see also* Sciatica)
  due to displacement of intervertebral disc — *see* Disorder, disc, with, radiculopathy
 serum (*see also* Reaction, serum) T80.69 ☑
 shoulder-girdle G54.5
 specified nerve NEC G58.8
 spinal (nerve) root — *see* Radiculopathy
 syphilitic A52.15
 thenar (median) G56.1- ☑
 thoracic M54.14
 toxic NEC G62.2
 trochlear (nerve) — *see* Strabismus, paralytic, fourth nerve
 vagus (nerve) G52.2
Neuroastrocytoma — *see* Neoplasm, uncertain behavior, by site
Neuroavitaminosis E56.9 [G99.8]
Neuroblastoma
 olfactory C30.0
 specified site — *see* Neoplasm, malignant, by site

Neuroblastoma — *continued*
  unspecified site C74.90
Neurochorioretinitis — *see* Chorioretinitis
Neurocirculatory asthenia F45.8
Neurocysticercosis B69.0
Neurocytoma — *see* Neoplasm, benign, by site
Neurodermatitis (circumscribed) (circumscripta) (local) L28.0
  atopic L20.81
  diffuse (Brocq) L20.81
  disseminated L20.81
Neuroencephalomyelopathy, optic G36.0
Neuroepithelioma (*see also* Neoplasm, malignant, by site)
  olfactory C30.0
Neurofibroma (*see also* Neoplasm, nerve, benign)
  melanotic — *see* Neoplasm, nerve, benign
  multiple — *see* Neurofibromatosis
  plexiform — *see* Neoplasm, nerve, benign
Neurofibromatosis (multiple) (nonmalignant) Q85.00
  acoustic Q85.02
  malignant — *see* Neoplasm, nerve, malignant
  specified NEC Q85.09
  type 1 (von Recklinghausen) Q85.01
  type 2 Q85.02
Neurofibrosarcoma — *see* Neoplasm, nerve, malignant
Neurogenic (*see also* condition)
  bladder (*see also* Dysfunction, bladder, neuromuscular) N31.9
    cauda equina syndrome G83.4
  bowel NEC K59.2
  heart F45.8
Neuroglioma — *see* Neoplasm, uncertain behavior, by site
Neurolabyrinthitis (of Dix and Hallpike) — *see* Neuronitis, vestibular
Neurolathyrism — *see* Poisoning, food, noxious, plant
Neuroleprosy A30.9
Neuroma (*see also* Neoplasm, nerve, benign)
  acoustic (nerve) D33.3
  amputation (stump) (traumatic) (surgical complication) (late) T87.3- ☑
    arm T87.3- ☑
    leg T87.3- ☑
  digital (toe) G57.6- ☑
  interdigital (toe) G58.8
    lower limb G57.8- ☑
    upper limb G56.8- ☑
  intermetatarsal G57.8- ☑
  Morton's G57.6- ☑
  nonneoplastic
    arm G56.9- ☑
    leg G57.9- ☑
    lower extremity G57.9- ☑
    upper extremity G56.9- ☑
  optic (nerve) D33.3
  plantar G57.6- ☑
  plexiform — *see* Neoplasm, nerve, benign
  surgical (nonneoplastic)
    arm G56.9- ☑
    leg G57.9- ☑
    lower extremity G57.9- ☑
    upper extremity G56.9- ☑
Neuromyalgia — *see* Neuralgia
Neuromyasthenia (epidemic) (postinfectious) G93.3
Neuromyelitis G36.9
  ascending G61.0
  optica G36.0
Neuromyopathy G70.9
  paraneoplastic D49.9 [G13.0]
Neuromyotonia (Isaacs) G71.19
Neuronevus — *see* Nevus
Neuronitis G58.9
  ascending (acute) G57.2- ☑
  vestibular H81.2- ☑
Neuroparalytic — *see* condition
Neuropathy, neuropathic G62.9
  acute motor G62.81
  alcoholic G62.1
    with psychosis — *see* Psychosis, alcoholic
  arm G56.9- ☑
  autonomic, peripheral — *see* Neuropathy, peripheral, autonomic
  axillary G56.9- ☑
  bladder N31.9
    atonic (motor) (sensory) N31.2
    autonomous N31.2

Neuropathy, neuropathic — *continued*
  bladder — *continued*
    flaccid N31.2
    nonreflex N31.2
    reflex N31.1
    uninhibited N31.0
  brachial plexus G54.0
  cervical plexus G54.2
  chronic
    progressive segmentally demyelinating G62.89
    relapsing demyelinating G62.89
  Déjérine-Sottas G60.0
  diabetic — *see* E08-E13 with .40
    mononeuropathy — *see* E08-E13 with .41
    polyneuropathy — *see* E08-E13 with .42
  entrapment G58.9
    iliohypogastric nerve G57.8- ☑
    ilioinguinal nerve G57.8- ☑
    lateral cutaneous nerve of thigh G57.1- ☑
    median nerve G56.0- ☑
    obturator nerve G57.8- ☑
    peroneal nerve G57.3- ☑
    posterior tibial nerve G57.5- ☑
    saphenous nerve G57.8- ☑
    ulnar nerve G56.2- ☑
  facial nerve G51.9
  hereditary G60.9
    motor and sensory (types I-IV) G60.0
    sensory G60.8
    specified NEC G60.8
  hypertrophic G60.0
    Charcot-Marie-Tooth G60.0
    Déjérine-Sottas G60.0
    interstitial progressive G60.0
    of infancy G60.0
    Refsum G60.1
  idiopathic G60.9
    progressive G60.3
    specified NEC G60.8
  in association with hereditary ataxia G60.2
  intercostal G58.0
  ischemic — *see* Disorder, nerve
  Jamaica (ginger) G62.2
  leg NEC G57.9- ☑
  lower extremity G57.9- ☑
  lumbar plexus G54.1
  median nerve G56.1- ☑
  motor and sensory (*see also* Polyneuropathy)
    hereditary (types I-IV) G60.0
  multiple (acute) (chronic) — *see* Polyneuropathy
  optic (nerve) (*see also* Neuritis, optic)
    ischemic H47.01- ☑
  paraneoplastic (sensorial) (Denny Brown) D49.9 [G13.0]
  peripheral (nerve) (*see also* Polyneuropathy) G62.9
    autonomic G90.9
      idiopathic G90.09
      in (due to)
        amyloidosis E85.4 [G99.0]
        diabetes mellitus — *see* E08-E13 with .43
        endocrine disease NEC E34.9 [G99.0]
        gout M10.00 [G99.0]
        hyperthyroidism E05.90 [G99.0]
          with thyroid storm E05.91 [G99.0]
        metabolic disease NEC E88.9 [G99.0]
    idiopathic G60.9
      progressive G60.3
    in (due to)
      antitetanus serum G62.0
      arsenic G62.2
      drugs NEC G62.0
      lead G62.2
      organophosphate compounds G62.2
      toxic agent NEC G62.2
  plantar nerves G57.6- ☑
  progressive
    hypertrophic interstitial G60.0
    inflammatory G62.81
  radicular NEC — *see* Radiculopathy
  sacral plexus G54.1
  sciatic G57.0- ☑
  serum G61.1
  toxic NEC G62.2
  trigeminal sensory G50.8
  ulnar nerve G56.2- ☑
  uremic N18.9 [G63]
  vitamin B12 E53.8 [G63]
    with anemia (pernicious) D51.0 [G63]
      due to dietary deficiency D51.3 [G63]

Neurophthisis (*see also* Disorder, nerve)
  peripheral, diabetic — *see* E08-E13 with .42
Neuroretinitis — *see* Chorioretinitis
Neuroretinopathy, hereditary optic H47.22
Neurosarcoma — *see* Neoplasm, nerve, malignant
Neurosclerosis — *see* Disorder, nerve
Neurosis, neurotic F48.9
  anankastic F42
  anxiety (state) F41.1
    panic type F41.0
  asthenic F48.8
  bladder F45.8
  cardiac (reflex) F45.8
  cardiovascular F45.8
  character F60.9
  colon F45.8
  compensation F68.1 ☑
  compulsive, compulsion F42
  conversion F44.9
  craft F48.8
  cutaneous F45.8
  depersonalization F48.1
  depressive (reaction) (type) F34.1
  environmental F48.8
  excoriation L98.1
  fatigue F48.8
  functional — *see* Disorder, somatoform
  gastric F45.8
  gastrointestinal F45.8
  heart F45.8
  hypochondriacal F45.21
  hysterical F44.9
  incoordination F45.8
    larynx F45.8
    vocal cord F45.8
  intestine F45.8
  larynx (sensory) F45.8
    hysterical F44.4
  mixed NEC F48.8
  musculoskeletal F45.8
  obsessional F48.8
  obsessive-compulsive F42
  occupational F48.8
  ocular NEC F45.8
  organ — *see* Disorder, somatoform
  pharynx F45.8
  phobic F40.9
  posttraumatic (situational) F43.10
    acute F43.11
    chronic F43.12
  psychasthenic (type) F48.8
  railroad F48.8
  rectum F45.8
  respiratory F45.8
  rumination F45.8
  sexual F65.9
  situational F48.8
  social F40.10
    generalized F40.11
  specified type NEC F48.8
  state F48.9
    with depersonalization episode F48.1
  stomach F45.8
  traumatic F43.10
    acute F43.11
    chronic F43.12
  vasomotor F45.8
  visceral F45.8
  war F48.8
Neurospongioblastosis diffusa Q85.1
Neurosyphilis (arrested) (early) (gumma) (late) (latent) (recurrent) (relapse) A52.3
  with ataxia (cerebellar) (locomotor) (spastic) (spinal) A52.19
  aneurysm (cerebral) A52.05
  arachnoid (adhesive) A52.13
  arteritis (any artery) (cerebral) A52.04
  asymptomatic A52.2
  congenital A50.40
  dura (mater) A52.13
  general paresis A52.17
  hemorrhagic A52.05
  juvenile (asymptomatic) (meningeal) A50.40
  leptomeninges (aseptic) A52.13
  meningeal, meninges (adhesive) A52.13
  meningitis A52.13
  meningovascular (diffuse) A52.13
  optic atrophy A52.15

Neurosyphilis — *continued*
  parenchymatous (degenerative) A52.19
  paresis, paretic A52.17
    juvenile A50.45
  remission in (sustained) A52.3
  serological (without symptoms) A52.2
  specified nature or site NEC A52.19
  tabes, tabetic (dorsalis) A52.11
    juvenile A50.45
  taboparesis A52.17
    juvenile A50.45
  thrombosis (cerebral) A52.05
  vascular (cerebral) NEC A52.05
Neurothekeoma — *see* Neoplasm, nerve, benign
Neurotic — *see* Neurosis
Neurotoxemia — *see* Toxemia
Neuroclusion M26.211
Neutropenia, neutropenic (chronic) (genetic) (idiopath-
    ic) (immune) (infantile) (malignant) (pernicious)
    (splenic) D70.9
  congenital (primary) D70.0
  cyclic D70.4
  cytoreductive cancer chemotherapy sequela D70.1
  drug-induced D70.2
    due to cytoreductive cancer chemotherapy D70.1
  due to infection D70.3
  fever D70.9
  neonatal, transitory (isoimmune) (maternal transfer)
    P61.5
  periodic D70.4
  secondary (cyclic) (periodic) (splenic) D70.4
    drug-induced D70.2
      due to cytoreductive cancer chemotherapy
        D70.1
  toxic D70.8
Neutrophilia, hereditary giant D72.0
Nevocarcinoma — *see* Melanoma
Nevus D22.9
  achromic — *see* Neoplasm, skin, benign
  amelanotic — *see* Neoplasm, skin, benign
  angiomatousD18.00
    intra-abdominal D18.03
    intracranial D18.02
    skin D18.01
    specified site NEC D18.09
  araneus I78.1
  balloon cell — *see* Neoplasm, skin, benign
  bathing trunk D48.5
  blue — *see* Neoplasm, skin, benign
    cellular — *see* Neoplasm, skin, benign
    giant — *see* Neoplasm, skin, benign
    Jadassohn's — *see* Neoplasm, skin, benign
    malignant — *see* Melanoma
  capillary D18.00
    intra-abdominal D18.03
    intracranial D18.02
    skin D18.01
    specified site NEC D18.09
  cavernous D18.00
    intra-abdominal D18.03
    intracranial D18.02
    skin D18.01
    specified site NEC D18.09
  cellular — *see* Neoplasm, skin, benign
    blue — *see* Neoplasm, skin, benign
  choroid D31.3- ☑
  comedonicus Q82.5
  conjunctiva D31.0- ☑
  dermal — *see* Neoplasm, skin, benign
    with epidermal nevus — *see* Neoplasm, skin, be-
      nign
  dysplastic — *see* Neoplasm, skin, benign
  eye D31.9- ☑
  flammeus Q82.5
  hemangiomatous D18.00
    intra-abdominal D18.03
    intracranial D18.02
    skin D18.01
    specified site NEC D18.09
  iris D31.4- ☑
  lacrimal gland D31.5- ☑
  lymphatic D18.1
  magnocellular
    specified site — *see* Neoplasm, benign, by site
    unspecified site D31.40
  malignant — *see* Melanoma
  meaning hemangioma D18.00
    intra-abdominal D18.03

Nevus — *continued*
  meaning hemangioma — *continued*
    intracranial D18.02
    skin D18.01
    specified site NEC D18.09
  mouth (mucosa) D10.30
    specified site NEC D10.39
    white sponge Q38.6
  multiplex Q85.1
  non-neoplastic I78.1
  oral mucosa D10.30
    specified site NEC D10.39
    white sponge Q38.6
  orbit D31.6- ☑
  pigmented
    giant (*see also* Neoplasm, skin, uncertain behavior)
      D48.5
      malignant melanoma in — *see* Melanoma
  portwine Q82.5
  retina D31.2- ☑
  retrobulbar D31.6- ☑
  sanguineous Q82.5
  senile I78.1
  skin D22.9
    abdominal wall D22.5
    ala nasi D22.39
    ankle D22.7- ☑
    anus, anal D22.5
    arm D22.6- ☑
    auditory canal (external) D22.2- ☑
    auricle (ear) D22.2- ☑
    auricular canal (external) D22.2- ☑
    axilla, axillary fold D22.5
    back D22.5
    breast D22.5
    brow D22.39
    buttock D22.5
    canthus (eye) D22.1- ☑
    cheek (external) D22.39
    chest wall D22.5
    chin D22.39
    ear (external) D22.2- ☑
    external meatus (ear) D22.2- ☑
    eyebrow D22.39
    eyelid (lower) (upper) D22.1- ☑
    face D22.30
      specified NEC D22.39
    female genital organ (external) NEC D28.0
    finger D22.6- ☑
    flank D22.5
    foot D22.7- ☑
    forearm D22.6- ☑
    forehead D22.39
    foreskin D29.0
    genital organ (external) NEC
      female D28.0
      male D29.9
    gluteal region D22.5
    groin D22.5
    hand D22.6- ☑
    heel D22.7- ☑
    helix D22.2- ☑
    hip D22.7- ☑
    interscapular region D22.5
    jaw D22.39
    knee D22.7- ☑
    labium (majus) (minus) D28.0
    leg D22.7- ☑
    lip (lower) (upper) D22.0
    lower limb D22.7- ☑
    male genital organ (external) D29.9
    nail D22.9
      finger D22.6- ☑
      toe D22.7- ☑
    nasolabial groove D22.39
    nates D22.5
    neck D22.4
    nose (external) D22.39
    palpebra D22.1- ☑
    penis D29.0
    perianal skin D22.5
    perineum D22.5
    pinna D22.2- ☑
    popliteal fossa or space D22.7- ☑
    prepuce D29.0
    pudendum D28.0
    scalp D22.4

Nevus — *continued*
  skin — *continued*
    scrotum D29.4
    shoulder D22.6- ☑
    submammary fold D22.5
    temple D22.39
    thigh D22.7- ☑
    toe D22.7- ☑
    trunk NEC D22.5
    umbilicus D22.5
    upper limb D22.6- ☑
    vulva D28.0
  specified site NEC — *see* Neoplasm, by site, benign
  spider I78.1
  stellar I78.1
  strawberry Q82.5
  Sutton's — *see* Neoplasm, skin, benign
  unius lateris Q82.5
  Unna's Q82.5
  vascular Q82.5
  verrucous Q82.5
Newborn (infant) (liveborn) (singleton) Z38.2
  abstinence syndrome P96.1
  acne L70.4
  affected by (suspected to be)
    abnormalities of membranes P02.9
      specified NEC P02.8
    abruptio placenta P02.1
    amino-acid metabolic disorder, transitory P74.8
    amniocentesis (while in utero) P00.6
    amnionitis P02.7
    apparent life threatening event (ALTE) R68.13
    bleeding (into)
      cerebral cortex P52.22
      germinal matrix P52.0
      ventricles P52.1
    breech delivery P03.0
    cardiac arrest P29.81
    cardiomyopathy I42.8
      congenital I42.4
    cerebral ischemia P91.0
    Cesarean delivery P03.4
    chemotherapy agents P04.1
    chorioamnionitis P02.7
    cocaine (crack) P04.41
    complications of labor and delivery P03.9
      specified NEC P03.89
    compression of umbilical cord NEC P02.5
    contracted pelvis P03.1
    delivery P03.9
      Cesarean P03.4
      forceps P03.2
      vacuum extractor P03.3
    entanglement (knot) in umbilical cord P02.5
    environmental chemicals P04.6
    fetal (intrauterine)
      growth retardation P05.9
      malnutrition not light or small for gestational
        age P05.2
    forceps delivery P03.2
    heart rate abnormalities
      bradycardia P29.12
        intrauterine P03.819
          before onset of labor P03.810
          during labor P03.811
      tachycardia P29.11
    hemorrhage (antepartum) P02.1
      cerebellar (nontraumatic) P52.6
      intracerebral (nontraumatic) P52.4
      intracranial (nontraumatic) P52.9
        specified NEC P52.8
      intraventricular (nontraumatic) P52.3
        grade 1 P52.0
        grade 2 P52.1
        grade 3 P52.21
        grade 4 P52.22
      posterior fossa (nontraumatic) P52.6
      subarachnoid (nontraumatic) P52.5
      subependymal P52.0
        with intracerebral extension P52.22
        with intraventricular extension P52.1
          with enlargment of ventricles P52.21
        without intraventricular extension P52.0
    hypoxic ischemic encephalopathy [HIE] P91.60
      mild P91.61
      moderate P91.62
      severe P91.63
    induction of labor P03.89

Index

Neurosyphilis — Newborn

Newborn — *continued*
  affected by — *continued*
    intestinal perforation P78.0
    intrauterine (fetal) blood loss P50.9
      due to (from)
        cut end of co-twin cord P50.5
        hemorrhage into
          co-twin P50.3
            maternal circulation P50.4
          placenta P50.2
        ruptured cord blood P50.1
        vasa previa P50.0
      specified NEC P50.8
    intrauterine (fetal) hemorrhage P50.9
    intrauterine (in utero) procedure P96.5
    malpresentation (malposition) NEC P03.1
    maternal (complication of) (use of)
      alcohol P04.3
      analgesia (maternal) P04.0
      anesthesia (maternal) P04.0
      blood loss P02.1
      circulatory disease P00.3
      condition P00.9
        specified NEC P00.89
      delivery P03.9
        Cesarean P03.4
        forceps P03.2
        vacuum extractor P03.3
      diabetes mellitus (pre-existing) P70.1
      disorder P00.9
        specified NEC P00.89
      drugs (addictive) (illegal) NEC P04.49
      ectopic pregnancy P01.4
      gestational diabetes P70.0
      hemorrhage P02.1
      hypertensive disorder P00.0
      incompetent cervix P01.0
      infectious disease P00.2
      injury P00.5
      labor and delivery P03.9
      malpresentation before labor P01.7
      maternal death P01.6
      medical procedure P00.7
      medication P04.1
      multiple pregnancy P01.5
      nutritional disorder P00.4
      oligohydramnios P01.2
      parasitic disease P00.2
      periodontal disease P00.81
      placenta previa P02.0
      polyhydramnios P01.3
      precipitate delivery P03.5
      pregnancy P01.9
        specified P01.8
      premature rupture of membranes P01.1
      renal disease P00.1
      respiratory disease P00.3
      surgical procedure P00.6
      urinary tract disease P00.1
      uterine contraction (abnormal) P03.6
    meconium peritonitis P78.0
    medication (legal) (maternal use) (prescribed) P04.1
    membrane abnormalities P02.9
      specified NEC P02.8
    membranitis P02.7
    methamphetamine(s) P04.49
    mixed metabolic and respiratory acidosis P84
    neonatal abstinence syndrome P96.1
    noxious substances transmitted via placenta or
      breast milk P04.9
      specified NEC P04.8
    nutritional supplements P04.5
    placenta previa P02.0
    placental
      abnormality (functional) (morphological)
        P02.20
        specified NEC P02.29
      dysfunction P02.29
      infarction P02.29
      insufficiency P02.29
      separation NEC P02.1
      transfusion syndromes P02.3
    placentitis P02.7
    precipitate delivery P03.5
    prolapsed cord P02.4
    respiratory arrest P28.81
    slow intrauterine growth P05.9
    tobacco P04.2

Newborn — *continued*
  affected by — *continued*
    twin to twin transplacental transfusion P02.3
    umbilical cord (tightly) around neck P02.5
    umbilical cord condition P02.60
      short cord P02.69
      specified NEC P02.69
    uterine contractions (abnormal) P03.6
    vasa previa P02.69
      from intrauterine blood loss P50.0
  apnea P28.3
    obstructive P28.4
    primary P28.3
    specified P28.4
  born in hospital Z38.00
    by cesarean Z38.01
  born outside hospital Z38.1
  breast buds P96.89
  breast engorgement P83.4
  check-up — *see* Newborn, examination
  convulsion P90
  dehydration P74.1
  examination
    8 to 28 days old Z00.111
    under 8 days old Z00.110
  fever P81.9
    environmentally-induced P81.0
  hyperbilirubinemia P59.9
    of prematurity P59.0
  hypernatremia P74.2
  hyponatremia P74.2
  infection P39.9
    candidal P37.5
    specified NEC P39.8
    urinary tract P39.3
  jaundice P59.8
    due to
      breast milk inhibitor P59.3
      hepatocellular damage P59.20
        specified NEC P59.29
      preterm delivery P59.0
    of prematurity P59.0
    specified NEC P59.8
  late metabolic acidosis P74.0
  mastitis P39.0
    infective P39.0
    noninfective P83.4
  multiple born NEC Z38.8
    born in hospital Z38.68
      by cesarean Z38.69
    born outside hospital Z38.7
  omphalitis P38.9
    with mild hemorrhage P38.1
    without hemorrhage P38.9
  post-term P08.21
  prolonged gestation (over 42 completed weeks)
    P08.22
  quadruplet Z38.8
    born in hospital Z38.63
      by cesarean Z38.64
    born outside hospital Z38.7
  quintuplet Z38.8
    born in hospital Z38.65
      by cesarean Z38.66
    born outside hospital Z38.7
  seizure P90
  sepsis (congenital) P36.9
    due to
      anaerobes NEC P36.5
      Escherichia coli P36.4
      Staphylococcus P36.30
        aureus P36.2
        specified NEC P36.39
      Streptococcus P36.10
        group B P36.0
        specified NEC P36.19
      specified NEC P36.8
  triplet Z38.8
    born in hospital Z38.61
      by cesarean Z38.62
    born outside hospital Z38.7
  twin Z38.5
    born in hospital Z38.30
      by cesarean Z38.31
    born outside hospital Z38.4
  vomiting P92.09
    bilious P92.01
  weight check Z00.111

Newcastle conjunctivitis or disease B30.8
Nezelof's syndrome (pure alymphocytosis) D81.4
Niacin (amide) **deficiency** E52
Nicolas (-Durand)-**Favre disease** A55
Nicotine — *see* Tobacco
Nicotinic acid deficiency E52
Niemann-Pick disease or syndrome E75.249
  specified NEC E75.248
  type
    A E75.240
    B E75.241
    C E75.242
    D E75.243
Night
  blindness — *see* Blindness, night
  sweats R61
  terrors (child) F51.4
Nightmares (REM sleep type) F51.5
Nipple — *see* condition
Nisbet's chancre A57
Nishimoto (-Takeuchi) **disease** I67.5
Nitritoid crisis or reaction — *see* Crisis, nitritoid
Nitrosohemoglobinemia D74.8
Njovera A65
Nocardiosis, nocardiasis A43.9
  cutaneous A43.1
  lung A43.0
  pneumonia A43.0
  pulmonary A43.0
  specified site NEC A43.8
Nocturia R35.1
  psychogenic F45.8
Nocturnal — *see* condition
Nodal rhythm I49.8
Node(s) (*see also* Nodule)
  Bouchard's (with arthropathy) M15.2
  Haygarth's M15.8
  Heberden's (with arthropathy) M15.1
  larynx J38.7
  lymph — *see* condition
  milker's B08.03
  Osler's I33.0
  Schmorl's — *see* Schmorl's disease
  singer's J38.2
  teacher's J38.2
  tuberculous — *see* Tuberculosis, lymph gland
  vocal cord J38.2
Nodule(s), **nodular**
  actinomycotic — *see* Actinomycosis
  breast NEC N63
  colloid (cystic), thyroid E04.1
  cutaneous — *see* Swelling, localized
  endometrial (stromal) D26.1
  Haygarth's M15.8
  inflammatory — *see* Inflammation
  juxta-articular
    syphilitic A52.77
    yaws A66.7
  larynx J38.7
  lung, solitary (subsegmental branch of the bronchial
    tree) R91.1
    multiple R91.8
  milker's B08.03
  prostate N40.2
    with lower urinary tract symptoms (LUTS) N40.3
    without lower urinary tract symtpoms (LUTS) N40.2
  pulmonary, solitary (subsegmental branch of the
    bronchial tree) R91.1
  retrocardiac R09.89
  rheumatoid M06.30
    ankle M06.37- ☑
    elbow M06.32- ☑
    foot joint M06.37- ☑
    hand joint M06.34- ☑
    hip M06.35- ☑
    knee M06.36- ☑
    multiple site M06.39
    shoulder M06.31- ☑
    vertebra M06.38
    wrist M06.33- ☑
  scrotum (inflammatory) N49.2
  singer's J38.2
  solitary, lung (subsegmental branch of the bronchial
    tree) R91.1
    multiple R91.8
  subcutaneous — *see* Swelling, localized
  teacher's J38.2

Nodule(s), nodular — *continued*
  thyroid (cold) (gland) (nontoxic) E04.1
    with thyrotoxicosis E05.20
      with thyroid storm E05.21
      toxic or with hyperthyroidism E05.20
        with thyroid storm E05.21
    vocal cord J38.2
Noma (gangrenous) (hospital) (infective) A69.0
  auricle I96
  mouth A69.0
  pudendi N76.89
  vulvae N76.89
Nomad, nomadism Z59.0
Nonautoimmune hemolytic anemia D59.4
  drug-induced D59.2
Nonclosure (*see also* Imperfect, closure)
  ductus arteriosus (Botallo's) Q25.0
  foramen
    botalli Q21.1
    ovale Q21.1
Noncompliance Z91.19
  with
    dialysis Z91.15
    dietary regimen Z91.11
    medical treatment Z91.19
    medication regimen NEC Z91.14
      underdosing (*see also* Table of Drugs and
        Chemicals, categories T36-T50, with final
        character 6) Z91.14
      intentional NEC Z91.128
        due to financial hardship of patient
          Z91.120
      unintentional NEC Z91.138
        due to patient's age related debility
          Z91.130
    renal dialysis Z91.15
Nondescent (congenital) (*see also* Malposition, congen-
    ital)
  cecum Q43.3
  colon Q43.3
  testicle Q53.9
    bilateral Q53.20
      abdominal Q53.21
      perineal Q53.22
    unilateral Q53.10
      abdominal Q53.11
      perineal Q53.12
Nondevelopment
  brain Q02
    part of Q04.3
  heart Q24.8
  organ or site, congenital NEC — *see* Hypoplasia
Nonengagement
  head NEC O32.4 ☑
    in labor, causing obstructed labor O64.8 ☑
Nonexanthematous tick fever A93.2
Nonexpansion, lung (newborn) P28.0
Nonfunctioning
  cystic duct (*see also* Disease, gallbladder) K82.8
  gallbladder (*see also* Disease, gallbladder) K82.8
  kidney N28.9
  labyrinth — *see* subcategory H83.2 ☑
Non-Hodgkin lymphoma NEC — *see* Lymphoma, non-
    Hodgkin
Nonimplantation, ovum N97.2
Noninsufflation, fallopian tube N97.1
Non-ketotic hyperglycinemia E72.51
Nonne-Milroy syndrome Q82.0
Nonovulation N97.0
Nonpatent fallopian tube N97.1
Nonpneumatization, lung NEC P28.0
Nonrotation — *see* Malrotation
Nonsecretion, urine — *see* Anuria
Nonunion
  fracture — *see* Fracture, by site
  organ or site, congenital NEC — *see* Imperfect, closure
  symphysis pubis, congenital Q74.2
Nonvisualization, gallbladder R93.2
Nonvital, nonvitalized tooth K04.99
Non-working side interference M26.56
Noonan's syndrome Q87.1
Normocytic anemia (infectional) due to blood loss
    (chronic) D50.0
  acute D62
Norrie's disease (congenital) Q15.8
North American blastomycosis B40.9
Norwegian itch B86

Nose, nasal — *see* condition
Nosebleed R04.0
Nose-picking F98.8
Nosomania F45.21
Nosophobia F45.22
Nostalgia F43.20
Notch of iris Q13.2
Notching nose, congenital (tip) Q30.2
Nothnagel's
  syndrome — *see* Strabismus, paralytic, third nerve
  vasomotor acroparesthesia I73.89
Novy's relapsing fever A68.9
  louse-borne A68.0
  tick-borne A68.1
Noxious
  foodstuffs, poisoning by — *see* Poisoning, food, nox-
    ious, plant
  substances transmitted through placenta or breast
    milk P04.9
Nucleus pulposus — *see* condition
Numbness R20.0
Nuns' knee — *see* Bursitis, prepatellar
Nursemaid's elbow S53.03- ☑
Nutcracker esophagus K22.4
Nutmeg liver K76.1
Nutrient element deficiency E61.9
  specified NEC E61.8
Nutrition deficient or insufficient (*see also* Malnutri-
    tion) E46
  due to
    insufficient food T73.0 ☑
    lack of
      care (child) T76.02 ☑
        adult T76.01 ☑
      food T73.0 ☑
Nutritional stunting E45
Nyctalopia (night blindness) — *see* Blindness, night
Nycturia R35.1
  psychogenic F45.8
Nymphomania F52.8
Nystagmus H55.00
  benign paroxysmal — *see* Vertigo, benign paroxysmal
  central positional H81.4- ☑
  congenital H55.01
  dissociated H55.04
  latent H55.02
  miners' H55.09
  positional
    benign paroxysmal H81.4- ☑
    central H81.4- ☑
  specified form NEC H55.09
  visual deprivation H55.03

O

Obermeyer's relapsing fever (European) A68.0
Obesity E66.9
  with alveolar hyperventilation E66.2
  adrenal E27.8
  complicating
    childbirth O99.214
    pregnancy O99.21- ☑
    puerperium O99.215
  constitutional E66.8
  dietary counseling and surveillance Z71.3
  drug-induced E66.1
  due to
    drug E66.1
    excess calories E66.09
      morbid E66.01
      severe E66.01
  endocrine E66.8
  endogenous E66.8
  familial E66.8
  glandular E66.8
  hypothyroid — *see* Hypothyroidism
  morbid E66.01
    with alveolar hypoventilation E66.2
    due to excess calories E66.01
  nutritional E66.09
  pituitary E23.6
  severe E66.01
  specified type NEC E66.8
Oblique — *see* condition
Obliteration
  appendix (lumen) K38.8
  artery I77.1

Obliteration — *continued*
  bile duct (noncalculous) K83.1
  common duct (noncalculous) K83.1
  cystic duct — *see* Obstruction, gallbladder
  disease, arteriolar I77.1
  endometrium N85.8
  eye, anterior chamber — *see* Disorder, globe, hy-
    potony
  fallopian tube N97.1
  lymphatic vessel I89.0
    due to mastectomy I97.2
  organ or site, congenital NEC — *see* Atresia, by site
  ureter N13.5
    with infection N13.6
  urethra — *see* Stricture, urethra
  vein I87.8
  vestibule (oral) K08.8
Observation (following) (for) (without need for further
    medical care) Z04.9
  accident NEC Z04.3
    at work Z04.2
    transport Z04.1
  adverse effect of drug Z03.6
  alleged rape or sexual assault (victim), ruled out
    adult Z04.41
    child Z04.42
  criminal assault Z04.8
  development state
    adolescent Z00.3
      period of rapid growth in childhood Z00.2
      puberty Z00.3
  disease, specified NEC Z03.89
  following work accident Z04.2
  growth and development state — *see* Observation,
    development state
  injuries (accidental) NEC (*see also* Observation, acci-
    dent)
  newborn (for suspected condition, ruled out) — *see*
    Newborn, affected by (suspected to be), mater-
    nal (complication of) (use of)
  postpartum
    immediately after delivery Z39.0
    routine follow-up Z39.2
  pregnancy (normal) (without complication) Z34.9- ☑
    high risk O09.9- ☑
  suicide attempt, alleged NEC Z03.89
    self-poisoning Z03.6
  suspected, ruled out (*see also* Suspected condition,
    ruled out)
    abuse, physical
      adult Z04.71
      child Z04.72
    accident at work Z04.2
    adult battering victim Z04.71
    child battering victim Z04.72
    condition NEC Z03.89
      newborn — *see* Newborn, affected by (suspect-
        ed to be), maternal (complication of) (use
        of)
    drug poisoning or adverse effect Z03.6
    exposure (to)
      anthrax Z03.810
      biological agent NEC Z03.818
    inflicted injury NEC Z04.8
    suicide attempt, alleged Z03.89
      self-poisoning Z03.6
    toxic effects from ingested substance (drug) (poi-
      son) Z03.6
  toxic effects from ingested substance (drug) (poison)
    Z03.6
Obsession, obsessional state F42
Obsessive-compulsive neurosis or reaction F42
Obstetric embolism, septic — *see* Embolism, obstetric,
    septic
Obstetrical trauma (complicating delivery) O71.9
  with or following ectopic or molar pregnancy O08.6
  specified type NEC O71.89
Obstipation — *see* Constipation
Obstruction, obstructed, obstructive
  airway J98.8
    with
      allergic alveolitis J67.9
      asthma J45.909
        with
          exacerbation (acute) J45.901
          status asthmaticus J45.902
      bronchiectasis J47.9

☑ **Additional Character Required — Refer to the Tabular List for Character Selection**   🐦 **Subterms under main terms may continue to next column or page**

Obstruction, obstructed, obstructive — *continued*
  airway — *continued*
    with
      bronchiectasis — *continued*
        with — *continued*
          exacerbation (acute) J47.1
          lower respiratory infection J47.0
      bronchitis (chronic) J44.9
      emphysema J43.9
    chronic J44.9
      with
        allergic alveolitis — *see* Pneumonitis, hyper-
          sensitivity
        bronchiectasis J47.9
          with
            exacerbation (acute) J47.1
            lower respiratory infection J47.0
    due to
      foreign body — *see* Foreign body, by site,
        causing asphyxia
      inhalation of fumes or vapors J68.9
      laryngospasm J38.5
  ampulla of Vater K83.1
  aortic (heart) (valve) — *see* Stenosis, aortic
  aortoiliac I74.09
  aqueduct of Sylvius G91.1
    congenital Q03.0
      with spina bifida — *see* Spina bifida, by site,
        with hydrocephalus
  Arnold-Chiari — *see* Arnold-Chiari disease
  artery (*see also* Embolism, artery) I74.9
    basilar (complete) (partial) — *see* Occlusion, artery,
      basilar
    carotid (complete) (partial) — *see* Occlusion, artery,
      carotid
    cerebellar — *see* Occlusion, artery, cerebellar
    cerebral (anterior) (middle) (posterior) — *see* Oc-
      clusion, artery, cerebral
    precerebral — *see* Occlusion, artery, precerebral
    renal N28.0
    retinal NEC — *see* Occlusion, artery, retina
    vertebral (complete) (partial) — *see* Occlusion,
      artery, vertebral
  band (intestinal) K56.69
  bile duct or passage (common) (hepatic) (noncalcu-
    lous) K83.1
    with calculus K80.51
    congenital (causing jaundice) Q44.3
  biliary (duct) (tract) K83.1
    gallbladder K82.0
  bladder-neck (acquired) N32.0
    congenital Q64.31
    due to hyperplasia (hypertrophy) of prostate —
      see Hyperplasia, prostate
  bowel — *see* Obstruction, intestine
  bronchus J98.09
  canal, ear — *see* Stenosis, external ear canal
  cardia K22.2
  caval veins (inferior) (superior) I87.1
  cecum — *see* Obstruction, intestine
  circulatory I99.8
  colon — *see* Obstruction, intestine
  common duct (noncalculous) K83.1
  coronary (artery) — *see* Occlusion, coronary
  cystic duct (*see also* Obstruction, gallbladder)
    with calculus K80.21
  device, implant or graft (*see also* Complications, by
    site and type, mechanical) T85.698 ☑
    arterial graft NEC — *see* Complication, cardiovas-
      cular device, mechanical, vascular
    catheter NEC T85.628 ☑
      cystostomy T83.090 ☑
      dialysis (renal) T82.49 ☑
        intraperitoneal T85.691 ☑
      infusion NEC T82.594 ☑
        spinal (epidural) (subdural) T85.690 ☑
      urinary, indwelling T83.098 ☑
    due to infection T85.79 ☑
    gastrointestinal — *see* Complications, prosthetic
      device, mechanical, gastrointestinal device
    genital NEC T83.498 ☑
      intrauterine contraceptive device T83.39 ☑
      penile prosthesis T83.490 ☑
    heart NEC — *see* Complication, cardiovascular de-
      vice, mechanical
    joint prosthesis — *see* Complications, joint prosthe-
      sis, mechanical, specified NEC, by site

Obstruction, obstructed, obstructive — *continued*
  device, implant or graft (*see also* Complications, by site
    and type, mechanical) — *continued*
    orthopedic NEC — *see* Complication, orthopedic,
      device, mechanical
    specified NEC T85.628 ☑
    urinary NEC (*see also* Complication, genitourinary,
      device, urinary, mechanical)
      graft T83.29 ☑
    vascular NEC — *see* Complication, cardiovascular
      device, mechanical
    ventricular intracranial shunt T85.09 ☑
  due to foreign body accidentally left in operative
    wound T81.529 ☑
  duodenum K31.5
  ejaculatory duct N50.8
  esophagus K22.2
  eustachian tube (complete) (partial) H68.10- ☑
    cartilagenous (extrinsic) H68.13- ☑
      intrinsic H68.12- ☑
    osseous H68.11- ☑
  fallopian tube (bilateral) N97.1
  fecal K56.41
    with hernia — *see* Hernia, by site, with obstruction
  foramen of Monro (congenital) Q03.8
    with spina bifida — *see* Spina bifida, by site, with
      hydrocephalus
  foreign body — *see* Foreign body
  gallbladder K82.0
    with calculus, stones K80.21
    congenital Q44.1
  gastric outlet K31.1
  gastrointestinal —- *see* Obstruction, intestine
  hepatic K76.89
    duct (noncalculous) K83.1
  ileum — *see* Obstruction, intestine
  iliofemoral (artery) I74.5
  intestine K56.60
    with
      adhesions (intestinal) (peritoneal) K56.5
    adynamic K56.0
    by gallstone K56.3
    congenital (small) Q41.9
      large Q42.9
        specified part NEC Q42.8
    neurogenic K56.0
      Hirschsprung's disease or megacolon Q43.1
    newborn P76.9
      due to
        fecaliths P76.8
        inspissated milk P76.2
        meconium (plug) P76.0
          in mucoviscidosis E84.11
      specified NEC P76.8
    postoperative K91.3
    reflex K56.0
    specified NEC K56.69
    volvulus K56.2
  intracardiac ball valve prosthesis T82.09 ☑
  jejunum — *see* Obstruction, intestine
  joint prosthesis — *see* Complications, joint prosthesis,
    mechanical, specified NEC, by site
  kidney (calices) N28.89
  labor — *see* Delivery
  lacrimal (passages) (duct)
    by
      dacryolith — *see* Dacryolith
      stenosis — *see* Stenosis, lacrimal
    congenital Q10.5
    neonatal H04.53- ☑
  lacrimonasal duct — *see* Obstruction, lacrimal
  lacteal, with steatorrhea K90.2
  laryngitis — *see* Laryngitis
  larynx NEC J38.6
    congenital Q31.8
  lung J98.4
    disease, chronic J44.9
  lymphatic I89.0
  meconium (plug)
    newborn P76.0
      due to fecaliths P76.0
      in mucoviscidosis E84.11
  mitral — *see* Stenosis, mitral
  nasal J34.89
  nasolacrimal duct (*see also* Obstruction, lacrimal)
    congenital Q10.5
  nasopharynx J39.2
  nose J34.89

Obstruction, obstructed, obstructive — *continued*
  organ or site, congenital NEC — *see* Atresia, by site
  pancreatic duct K86.8
  parotid duct or gland K11.8
  pelviureteral junction N13.5
    congenital Q62.39
  pharynx J39.2
  portal (circulation) (vein) I81
  prostate (*see also* Hyperplasia, prostate)
    valve (urinary) N32.0
  pulmonary valve (heart) I37.0
  pyelonephritis (chronic) N11.1
  pylorus
    adult K31.1
    congenital or infantile Q40.0
  rectosigmoid — *see* Obstruction, intestine
  rectum K62.4
  renal N28.89
    outflow N13.8
    pelvis, congenital Q62.39
  respiratory J98.8
    chronic J44.9
  retinal (vessels) H34.9
  salivary duct (any) K11.8
    with calculus K11.5
  sigmoid — *see* Obstruction, intestine
  sinus (accessory) (nasal) J34.89
  Stensen's duct K11.8
  stomach NEC K31.89
    acute K31.0
    congenital Q40.2
    due to pylorospasm K31.3
  submandibular duct K11.8
  submaxillary gland K11.8
    with calculus K11.5
  thoracic duct I89.0
  thrombotic — *see* Thrombosis
  trachea J39.8
  tracheostomy airway J95.03
  tricuspid (valve) — *see* Stenosis, tricuspid
  upper respiratory, congenital Q34.8
  ureter (functional) (pelvic junction) NEC N13.5
    with
      hydronephrosis N13.1
        with infection N13.6
      pyelonephritis (chronic) N11.1
    congenital Q62.39
    due to calculus — *see* Calculus, ureter
  urethra NEC N36.8
    congenital Q64.39
  urinary (moderate) N13.9
    due to hyperplasia (hypertrophy) of prostate —
      see Hyperplasia, prostate
    organ or tract (lower) N13.9
    prostatic valve N32.0
    specified NEC N13.8
  uropathy N13.9
  uterus N85.8
  vagina N89.5
  valvular — *see* Endocarditis
  vein, venous I87.1
    caval (inferior) (superior) I87.1
    thrombotic — *see* Thrombosis
  vena cava (inferior) (superior) I87.1
  vesical NEC N32.0
  vesicourethral orifice N32.0
    congenital Q64.31
  vessel NEC I99.8
Obturator — *see* condition
Occlusal wear, teeth K03.0
Occlusio pupillae — *see* Membrane, pupillary
Occlusion, occluded
  anus K62.4
    congenital Q42.3
      with fistula Q42.2
  aortoiliac (chronic) I74.09
  aqueduct of Sylvius G91.1
    congenital Q03.0
      with spina bifida — *see* Spina bifida, by site,
        with hydrocephalus
  artery (*see also* Embolism, artery) I74.9
    auditory, internal I65.8
    basilar I65.1
      with
        infarction I63.22
          due to
            embolism I63.12
            thrombosis I63.02

Occlusion, occluded — *continued*
  artery (*see also* Embolism, artery) — *continued*
    brain or cerebral I66.9
      with infarction (due to) I63.5 ☑
        embolism I63.4 ☑
        thrombosis I63.3 ☑
    carotid I65.2- ☑
      with
        infarction I63.23- ☑
          due to
            embolism I63.13- ☑
            thrombosis I63.03- ☑
    cerebellar (anterior inferior) (posterior inferior)
        (superior) I66.3
      with infarction I63.54- ☑
        due to
          embolism I63.44- ☑
          thrombosis I63.34- ☑
    cerebral I66.9
      with infarction I63.50
        due to
          embolism I63.40
            specified NEC I63.49
          thrombosis I63.30
            specified NEC I63.39
      anterior I66.1- ☑
        with infarction I63.52- ☑
          due to
            embolism I63.42- ☑
            thrombosis I63.32- ☑
      middle I66.0- ☑
        with infarction I63.51- ☑
          due to
            embolism I63.41- ☑
            thrombosis I63.31- ☑
      posterior I66.2- ☑
        with infarction I63.53- ☑
          due to
            embolism I63.43- ☑
            thrombosis I63.33- ☑
      specified NEC I66.8
        with infarction I63.59
          due to
            embolism I63.4 ☑
            thrombosis I63.3 ☑
    choroidal (anterior) — *see* Occlusion, artery, pre-
        cerebral, specified NEC
    communicating posterior — *see* Occlusion, artery,
        cerebral, specified NEC
    complete
      coronary I25.82
      extremities I70.92
    coronary (acute) (thrombotic) (without myocardial
        infarction) I24.0
      with myocardial infarction — *see* Infarction,
        myocardium
      chronic total I25.82
      complete I25.82
      healed or old I25.2
      total (chronic) I25.82
    hypophyseal — *see* Occlusion, artery, precerebral,
        specified NEC
    iliac I74.5
    lower extremities due to stenosis or stricture I77.1
    mesenteric (embolic) (thrombotic) K55.0
    perforating — *see* Occlusion, artery, cerebral,
        specified NEC
    peripheral I77.9
      thrombotic or embolic I74.4
    pontine — *see* Occlusion, artery, cerebral, specified
        NEC
    precerebral I65.9
      with infarction I63.20
        due to
          embolism I63.10
            specified NEC I63.19
          thrombosis I63.00
            specified NEC I63.09
        specified NEC I63.29
      basilar — *see* Occlusion, artery, basilar
      carotid — *see* Occlusion, artery, carotid
      puerperal O88.23
      specified NEC I65.8
        with infarction I63.29
          due to
            embolism I63.19
            thrombosis I63.00

Occlusion, occluded — *continued*
  artery (*see also* Embolism, artery) — *continued*
    precerebral — *continued*
      vertebral — *see* Occlusion, artery, vertebral
    renal N28.0
    retinal
      branch H34.23- ☑
      central H34.1- ☑
      partial H34.21- ☑
      transient H34.0- ☑
    spinal — *see* Occlusion, artery, precerebral, verte-
        bral
    total (chronic)
      coronary I25.82
      extremities I70.92
    vertebral I65.0- ☑
      with
        infarction I63.21- ☑
          due to
            embolism I63.11- ☑
            thrombosis I63.01- ☑
  basilar artery — *see* Occlusion, artery, basilar
  bile duct (common) (hepatic) (noncalculous) K83.1
  bowel — *see* Obstruction, intestine
  carotid (artery) (common) (internal) — *see* Occlusion,
      artery, carotid
  centric (of teeth) M26.59
    maximum intercuspation discrepancy M26.55
  cerebellar (artery) — *see* Occlusion, artery, cerebellar
  cerebral (artery) — *see* Occlusion, artery, cerebral
  cerebrovascular (*see also* Occlusion, artery, cerebral)
    with infarction I63.5 ☑
  cervical canal — *see* Stricture, cervix
  cervix (uteri) — *see* Stricture, cervix
  choanal Q30.0
  choroidal (artery) — *see* Occlusion, artery, precerebral,
      specified NEC
  colon — *see* Obstruction, intestine
  communicating posterior artery — *see* Occlusion,
      artery, precerebral, specified NEC
  coronary (artery) (vein) (thrombotic) (*see also* Infarct,
      myocardium)
    chronic total I25.82
    healed or old I25.2
    not resulting in infarction I24.0
    total (chronic) I25.82
  cystic duct — *see* Obstruction, gallbladder
  embolic — *see* Embolism
  fallopian tube N97.1
    congenital Q50.6
  gallbladder (*see also* Obstruction, gallbladder)
    congenital (causing jaundice) Q44.1
  gingiva, traumatic K06.2
  hymen N89.6
    congenital Q52.3
  hypophyseal (artery) — *see* Occlusion, artery, precere-
      bral, specified NEC
  iliac artery I74.5
  intestine — *see* Obstruction, intestine
  lacrimal passages — *see* Obstruction, lacrimal
  lung J98.4
  lymph or lymphatic channel I89.0
  mammary duct N64.89
  mesenteric artery (embolic) (thrombotic) K55.0
  nose J34.89
    congenital Q30.0
  organ or site, congenital NEC — *see* Atresia, by site
  oviduct N97.1
    congenital Q50.6
  peripheral arteries
    due to stricture or stenosis I77.1
    upper extremity I74.2
  pontine (artery) — *see* Occlusion, artery, precerebral,
      specified NEC
  posterior lingual, of mandibular teeth M26.29
  precerebral artery — *see* Occlusion, artery, precerebral
  punctum lacrimale — *see* Obstruction, lacrimal
  pupil — *see* Membrane, pupillary
  pylorus, adult (*see also* Stricture, pylorus) K31.1
  renal artery N28.0
  retina, retinal
    artery — *see* Occlusion, artery, retinal
    vein (central) H34.81- ☑
      engorgement H34.82- ☑
      tributary H34.83- ☑
    vessels H34.9

Occlusion, occluded — *continued*
  spinal artery — *see* Occlusion, artery, precerebral,
      vertebral
  teeth (mandibular) (posterior lingual) M26.29
  thoracic duct I89.0
  thrombotic — *see* Thrombosis, artery
  traumatic
    edentulous (alveolar) ridge K06.2
    gingiva K06.2
    periodontal K05.5
  tubal N97.1
  ureter (complete) (partial) N13.5
    congenital Q62.10
  ureteropelvic junction N13.5
    congenital Q62.11
  ureterovesical orifice N13.5
    congenital Q62.12
  urethra — *see* Stricture, urethra
  uterus N85.8
  vagina N89.5
  vascular NEC I99.8
  vein — *see* Thrombosis
    retinal — *see* Occlusion, retinal, vein
  vena cava (inferior) (superior) — *see* Embolism, vena
      cava
  ventricle (brain) NEC G91.1
  vertebral (artery) — *see* Occlusion, artery, vertebral
  vessel (blood) I99.8
  vulva N90.5
Occult
  blood in feces (stools) R19.5
Occupational
  problems NEC Z56.89
Ochlophobia — *see* Agoraphobia
Ochronosis (endogenous) E70.29
Ocular muscle — *see* condition
Oculogyric crisis or disturbance H51.8
  psychogenic F45.8
Oculomotor syndrome H51.9
Oculopathy
  syphilitic NEC A52.71
    congenital
      early A50.01
      late A50.30
    early (secondary) A51.43
    late A52.71
Oddi's sphincter spasm K83.4
Odontalgia K08.8
Odontoameloblastoma — *see* Cyst, calcifying odonto-
    genic
Odontoclasia K03.89
Odontodysplasia, regional K00.4
Odontogenesis imperfecta K00.5
Odontoma (ameloblastic) (complex) (compound) (fi-
    broameloblastic) — *see* Cyst, calcifying odontogenic
Odontomyelitis (closed) (open) K04.0
Odontorrhagia K08.8
Odontosarcoma, ameloblastic C41.1
  upper jaw (bone) C41.0
Oestriasis — *see* Myiasis
Oguchi's disease H53.63
Ohara's disease — *see* Tularemia
Oidiomycosis — *see* Candidiasis
Oidium albicans infection — *see* Candidiasis
Old age (without mention of debility) R54
  dementia F03 ☑
Old (previous) **myocardial infarction** I25.2
Olfactory — *see* condition
Oligemia — *see* Anemia
Oligoastrocytoma
  specified site — *see* Neoplasm, malignant, by site
  unspecified site C71.9
Oligocythemia D64.9
Oligodendroblastoma
  specified site — *see* Neoplasm, malignant
  unspecified site C71.9
Oligodendroglioma
  anaplastic type
    specified site — *see* Neoplasm, malignant, by site
    unspecified site C71.9
  specified site — *see* Neoplasm, malignant, by site
  unspecified site C71.9
Oligodontia — *see* Anodontia
Oligoencephalon Q02
Oligohidrosis L74.4
Oligohydramnios O41.0- ☑
Oligohydrosis L74.4

☑ **Additional Character Required — Refer to the Tabular List for Character Selection**   ▽ Subterms under main terms may continue to next column or page

Ossification — *continued*
  myocardium, myocardial — *see* Degeneration, myocardial
  penis N48.89
  periarticular — *see* Disorder, joint, specified type NEC
  pinna — *see* Disorder, pinna, specified type NEC
  rider's bone — *see* Ossification, muscle, specified NEC
  sclera H15.89
  subperiosteal, post-traumatic M89.8X- ☑
  tendon — *see* Disorder, tendon, specified type NEC
  trachea J39.8
  tympanic membrane — *see* Disorder, tympanic membrane, specified NEC
  vitreous (humor) — *see* Deposit, crystalline
Osteitis (*see also* Osteomyelitis)
  alveolar M27.3
  condensans M85.30
    ankle M85.37- ☑
    foot M85.37- ☑
    forearm M85.33- ☑
    hand M85.34- ☑
    lower leg M85.36- ☑
    multiple site M85.39
    neck M85.38
    rib M85.38
    shoulder M85.31- ☑
    skull M85.38
    specified site NEC M85.38
    thigh M85.35- ☑
    toe M85.37- ☑
    upper arm M85.32- ☑
    vertebra M85.38
  deformans M88.9
    in (due to)
      malignant neoplasm of bone C41.9 [M90.60]
      neoplastic disease (*see also* Neoplasm) D49.9 [M90.60]
        carpus D49.9 [M90.64-] ☑
        clavicle D49.9 [M90.61-] ☑
        femur D49.9 [M90.65-] ☑
        fibula D49.9 [M90.66-] ☑
        finger D49.9 [M90.64-] ☑
        humerus D49.9 [M90.62-] ☑
        ilium D49.9 [M90.65-] ☑
        ischium D49.9 [M90.65-] ☑
        metacarpus D49.9 [M90.64-] ☑
        metatarsus D49.9 [M90.67-] ☑
        multiple sites D49.9 [M90.69]
        neck D49.9 [M90.68]
        radius D49.9 [M90.63-] ☑
        rib D49.9 [M90.68]
        scapula D49.9 [M90.61-] ☑
        skull D49.9 [M90.68]
        tarsus D49.9 [M90.67-] ☑
        tibia D49.9 [M90.66-] ☑
        toe D49.9 [M90.67-] ☑
        ulna D49.9 [M90.63-] ☑
        vertebra D49.9 [M90.68]
    skull M88.0
    specified NEC — *see* Paget's disease, bone, by site
    vertebra M88.1
  due to yaws A66.6
  fibrosa NEC — *see* Cyst, bone, by site
    circumscripta — *see* Dysplasia, fibrous, bone NEC
    cystica (generalisata) E21.0
    disseminata Q78.1
    osteoplastica E21.0
  fragilitans Q78.0
  Garr's (sclerosing) — *see* Osteomyelitis, specified type NEC
  jaw (acute) (chronic) (lower) (suppurative) (upper) M27.2
  parathyroid E21.0
  petrous bone (acute) (chronic) — *see* Petrositis
  sclerotic, nonsuppurative –– *see* Osteomyelitis, specified type NEC
  tuberculosa A18.09
    cystica D86.89
    multiplex cystoides D86.89
Osteoarthritis M19.90
  ankle M19.07- ☑
  elbow M19.02- ☑
  foot joint M19.07- ☑
  generalized M15.9
    erosive M15.4
    primary M15.0
    specified NEC M15.8

Osteoarthritis — *continued*
  hand joint M19.04- ☑
    first carpometacarpal joint M18.9
  hip M16.1- ☑
    bilateral M16.0
    due to hip dysplasia (unilateral) M16.3- ☑
      bilateral M16.2
  interphalangeal
    distal (Heberden) M15.1
    proximal (Bouchard) M15.2
  knee M17.9
    bilateral M17.0
  post-traumatic NEC M19.92
    ankle M19.17- ☑
    elbow M19.12- ☑
    foot joint M19.17- ☑
    hand joint M19.14- ☑
      first carpometacarpal joint M18.3- ☑
        bilateral M18.2
    hip M16.5- ☑
      bilateral M16.4
    knee M17.3- ☑
      bilateral M17.2
    shoulder M19.11- ☑
    wrist M19.13- ☑
  primary M19.91
    ankle M19.07- ☑
    elbow M19.02- ☑
    foot joint M19.07- ☑
    hand joint M19.04- ☑
      first carpometacarpal joint M18.1- ☑
        bilateral M18.0
    hip M16.1- ☑
      bilateral M16.0
    knee M17.1- ☑
      bilateral M17.0
    shoulder M19.01- ☑
    spine — *see* Spondylosis
    wrist M19.03- ☑
  secondary M19.93
    ankle M19.27- ☑
    elbow M19.22- ☑
    foot joint M19.27- ☑
    hand joint M19.24- ☑
      first carpometacarpal joint M18.5- ☑
        bilateral M18.4
    hip M16.7
      bilateral M16.6
    knee M17.5
      bilateral M17.4
    multiple M15.3
    shoulder M19.21- ☑
    spine — *see* Spondylosis
    wrist M19.23- ☑
  shoulder M19.01- ☑
  spine — *see* Spondylosis
  wrist M19.03- ☑
Osteoarthropathy (hypertrophic) M19.90
  ankle — *see* Osteoarthritis, primary, ankle
  elbow — *see* Osteoarthritis, primary, elbow
  foot joint — *see* Osteoarthritis, primary, foot
  hand joint — *see* Osteoarthritis, primary, hand joint
  knee joint — *see* Osteoarthritis, primary, knee
  multiple site — *see* Osteoarthritis, primary, multiple joint
  pulmonary (*see also* Osteoarthropathy, specified type NEC)
    hypertrophic — *see* Osteoarthropathy, hypertrophic, specified type NEC
  secondary — *see* Osteoarthropathy, specified type NEC
  secondary hypertrophic — *see* Osteoarthropathy, specified type NEC
  shoulder — *see* Osteoarthritis, primary, shoulder
  specified joint NEC — *see* Osteoarthritis, primary, specified joint NEC
  specified type NEC M89.40
    carpus M89.44- ☑
    clavicle M89.41- ☑
    femur M89.45- ☑
    fibula M89.46- ☑
    finger M89.44- ☑
    humerus M89.42- ☑
    ilium M89.459
    ischium M89.459
    metacarpus M89.44- ☑

Osteoarthropathy — *continued*
  specified type — *continued*
    metatarsus M89.47- ☑
    multiple sites M89.49
    neck M89.48
    radius M89.43- ☑
    rib M89.48
    scapula M89.41- ☑
    skull M89.48
    tarsus M89.47- ☑
    tibia M89.46- ☑
    toe M89.47- ☑
    ulna M89.43- ☑
    vertebra M89.48
  spine — *see* Spondylosis
  wrist — *see* Osteoarthritis, primary, wrist
Osteoarthrosis (degenerative) (hypertrophic) (joint) (*see also* Osteoarthritis)
  deformans alkaptonurica E70.29 [M36.8]
  erosive M15.4
  generalized M15.9
    primary M15.0
  polyarticular M15.9
  spine — *see* Spondylosis
Osteoblastoma — *see* Neoplasm, bone, benign
  aggressive — *see* Neoplasm, bone, uncertain behavior
Osteochondritis (*see also* Osteochondropathy, by site)
  Brailsford's — *see* Osteochondrosis, juvenile, radius
  dissecans M93.20
    ankle M93.27- ☑
    elbow M93.22- ☑
    foot M93.27- ☑
    hand M93.24- ☑
    hip M93.25- ☑
    knee M93.26- ☑
    multiple sites M93.29
    shoulder joint M93.21- ☑
    specified site NEC M93.28
    wrist M93.23- ☑
  juvenile M92.9
    patellar — *see* Osteochondrosis, juvenile, patella
  syphilitic (congenital) (early) A50.02 [M90.80]
    ankle A50.02 [M90.87-] ☑
    elbow A50.02 [M90.82-] ☑
    foot A50.02 [M90.87-] ☑
    forearm A50.02 [M90.83-] ☑
    hand A50.02 [M90.84-] ☑
    hip A50.02 [M90.85-] ☑
    knee A50.02 [M90.86-] ☑
    multiple sites A50.02 [M90.89]
    shoulder joint A50.02 [M90.81-] ☑
    specified site NEC A50.02 [M90.88]
Osteochondroarthrosis deformans endemica — *see* Disease, Kaschin-Beck
Osteochondrodysplasia Q78.9
  with defects of growth of tubular bones and spine Q77.9
    specified NEC Q77.8
  specified NEC Q78.8
Osteochondrodystrophy E78.9
Osteochondrolysis — *see* Osteochondritis, dissecans
Osteochondroma — *see* Neoplasm, bone, benign
Osteochondromatosis D48.0
  syndrome Q78.4
Osteochondromyxosarcoma — *see* Neoplasm, bone, malignant
Osteochondropathy M93.90
  ankle M93.97- ☑
  elbow M93.92- ☑
  foot M93.97- ☑
  hand M93.94- ☑
  hip M93.95- ☑
  Kienböck's disease of adults M93.1
  knee M93.96- ☑
  multiple joints M93.99
  osteochondritis dissecans — *see* Osteochondritis, dissecans
  osteochondrosis — *see* Osteochondrosis
  shoulder region M93.91- ☑
  slipped upper femoral epiphysis — *see* Slipped, epiphysis, upper femoral
  specified joint NEC M93.98
  specified type NEC M93.80
    ankle M93.87- ☑
    elbow M93.82- ☑
    foot M93.87- ☑

☑ Additional Character Required — Refer to the Tabular List for Character Selection   🐦 Subterms under main terms may continue to next column or page

Osteochondropathy — *continued*
　specified type — *continued*
　　hand M93.84- ☑
　　hip M93.85- ☑
　　knee M93.86- ☑
　　multiple joints M93.89
　　shoulder region M93.81- ☑
　　specified joint NEC M93.88
　　wrist M93.83- ☑
　syphilitic, congenital
　　early A50.02 [M90.80]
　　late A50.56 [M90.80]
　wrist M93.93- ☑
Osteochondrosarcoma — *see* Neoplasm, bone, malignant
Osteochondrosis (*see also* Osteochondropathy, by site)
　acetabulum (juvenile) M91.0
　adult — *see* Osteochondropathy, specified type NEC, by site
　astragalus (juvenile) — *see* Osteochondrosis, juvenile, tarsus
　Blount's — *see* Osteochondrosis, juvenile, tibia
　Buchanan's M91.0
　Burns' — *see* Osteochondrosis, juvenile, ulna
　calcaneus (juvenile) — *see* Osteochondrosis, juvenile, tarsus
　capitular epiphysis (femur) (juvenile) — *see* Legg-Calvé-Perthes disease
　carpal (juvenile) (lunate) (scaphoid) — *see* Osteochondrosis, juvenile, hand, carpal lunate
　　adult M93.1
　coxae juvenilis — *see* Legg-Calvé-Perthes disease
　deformans juvenilis, coxae — *see* Legg-Calvé-Perthes disease
　Diaz's — *see* Osteochondrosis, juvenile, tarsus
　dissecans (knee) (shoulder) — *see* Osteochondritis, dissecans
　femoral capital epiphysis (juvenile) — *see* Legg-Calvé-Perthes disease
　femur (head), juvenile — *see* Legg-Calvé-Perthes disease
　fibula (juvenile) — *see* Osteochondrosis, juvenile, fibula
　foot NEC (juvenile) M92.8
　Freiberg's — *see* Osteochondrosis, juvenile, metatarsus
　Haas' (juvenile) — *see* Osteochondrosis, juvenile, humerus
　Haglund's — *see* Osteochondrosis, juvenile, tarsus
　hip (juvenile) — *see* Legg-Calvé-Perthes disease
　humerus (capitulum) (head) (juvenile) — *see* Osteochondrosis, juvenile, humerus
　ilium, iliac crest (juvenile) M91.0
　ischiopubic synchondrosis M91.0
　Iselin's — *see* Osteochondrosis, juvenile, metatarsus
　juvenile, juvenilis M92.9
　　after congenital dislocation of hip reduction — *see* Osteochondrosis, juvenile, hip, specified NEC
　　arm — *see* Osteochondrosis, juvenile, upper limb NEC
　　capitular epiphysis (femur) — *see* Legg-Calvé-Perthes disease
　　clavicle, sternal epiphysis — *see* Osteochondrosis, juvenile, upper limb NEC
　　coxae — *see* Legg-Calvé-Perthes disease
　　deformans M92.9
　　fibula M92.5- ☑
　　foot NEC M92.8
　　hand M92.20- ☑
　　　carpal lunate M92.21- ☑
　　　metacarpal head M92.22- ☑
　　　specified site NEC M92.29- ☑
　　head of femur — *see* Legg-Calvé-Perthes disease
　　hip and pelvis M91.9- ☑
　　　coxa plana — *see* Coxa, plana
　　　femoral head — *see* Legg-Calvé-Perthes disease
　　　pelvis M91.0
　　　pseudocoxalgia — *see* Pseudocoxalgia
　　　specified NEC M91.8- ☑
　　humerus M92.0- ☑
　　limb
　　　lower NEC M92.8
　　　upper NEC — *see* Osteochondrosis, juvenile, upper limb NEC
　　medial cuneiform bone — *see* Osteochondrosis, juvenile, tarsus
　　metatarsus M92.7- ☑
　　patella M92.4- ☑

Osteochondrosis — *continued*
　juvenile, juvenilis — *continued*
　　radius M92.1- ☑
　　specified site NEC M92.8
　　spine M42.00
　　　cervical region M42.02
　　　cervicothoracic region M42.03
　　　lumbar region M42.06
　　　lumbosacral region M42.07
　　　multiple sites M42.09
　　　occipito-atlanto-axial region M42.01
　　　sacrococcygeal region M42.08
　　　thoracic region M42.04
　　　thoracolumbar region M42.05
　　tarsus M92.6- ☑
　　tibia M92.5- ☑
　　ulna M92.1- ☑
　　upper limb NEC M92.3- ☑
　　vertebra (body) (epiphyseal plates) (Calvé's) (Scheuermann's) — *see* Osteochondrosis, juvenile, spine
　Kienböck's — *see* Osteochondrosis, juvenile, hand, carpal lunate
　　adult M93.1
　Köhler's
　　patellar — *see* Osteochondrosis, juvenile, patella
　　tarsal navicular — *see* Osteochondrosis, juvenile, tarsus
　Legg-Perthes (-Calvé)(-Waldenström) — *see* Legg-Calvé-Perthes disease
　limb
　　lower NEC (juvenile) M92.8
　　upper NEC (juvenile) — *see* Osteochondrosis, juvenile, upper limb NEC
　lunate bone (carpal) (juvenile) (*see also* Osteochondrosis, juvenile, hand, carpal lunate)
　　adult M93.1
　Mauclaire's — *see* Osteochondrosis, juvenile, hand, metacarpal
　metacarpal (head) (juvenile) — *see* Osteochondrosis, juvenile, hand, metacarpal
　metatarsus (fifth) (head) (juvenile) (second) — *see* Osteochondrosis, juvenile, metatarsus
　navicular (juvenile) — *see* Osteochondrosis, juvenile, tarsus
　os
　　calcis (juvenile) — *see* Osteochondrosis, juvenile, tarsus
　　tibiale externum (juvenile) — *see* Osteochondrosis, juvenile, tarsus
　Osgood-Schlatter — *see* Osteochondrosis, juvenile, tibia
　Panner's — *see* Osteochondrosis, juvenile, humerus
　patellar center (juvenile) (primary) (secondary) — *see* Osteochondrosis, juvenile, patella
　pelvis (juvenile) M91.0
　Pierson's M91.0
　radius (head) (juvenile) — *see* Osteochondrosis, juvenile, radius
　Scheuermann's — *see* Osteochondrosis, juvenile, spine
　Sever's — *see* Osteochondrosis, juvenile, tarsus
　Sinding-Larsen — *see* Osteochondrosis, juvenile, patella
　spine M42.9
　　adult M42.10
　　　cervical region M42.12
　　　cervicothoracic region M42.13
　　　lumbar region M42.16
　　　lumbosacral region M42.17
　　　multiple sites M42.19
　　　occipito-atlanto-axial region M42.11
　　　sacrococcygeal region M42.18
　　　thoracic region M42.14
　　　thoracolumbar region M42.15
　　juvenile — *see* Osteochondrosis, juvenile, spine
　symphysis pubis (juvenile) M91.0
　syphilitic (congenital) A50.02
　talus (juvenile) — *see* Osteochondrosis, juvenile, tarsus
　tarsus (navicular) (juvenile) — *see* Osteochondrosis, juvenile, tarsus
　tibia (proximal) (tubercle) (juvenile) — *see* Osteochondrosis, juvenile, tibia
　tuberculous — *see* Tuberculosis, bone
　ulna (lower) (juvenile) — *see* Osteochondrosis, juvenile, ulna
　van Neck's M91.0
　vertebral — *see* Osteochondrosis, spine

Osteoclastoma D48.0
　malignant — *see* Neoplasm, bone, malignant
Osteodynia — *see* Disorder, bone, specified type NEC
Osteodystrophy Q78.9
　azotemic N25.0
　congenital Q78.9
　parathyroid, secondary E21.1
　renal N25.0
Osteofibroma — *see* Neoplasm, bone, benign
Osteofibrosarcoma — *see* Neoplasm, bone, malignant
Osteogenesis imperfecta Q78.0
Osteogenic — *see* condition
Osteolysis M89.50
　carpus M89.54- ☑
　clavicle M89.51- ☑
　femur M89.55- ☑
　fibula M89.56- ☑
　finger M89.54- ☑
　humerus M89.52- ☑
　ilium M89.559
　ischium M89.559
　joint prosthesis (periprosthetic) — *see* Complications, joint prosthesis, mechanical, periprosthetic, osteolysis, by site
　metacarpus M89.54- ☑
　metatarsus M89.57- ☑
　multiple sites M89.59
　neck M89.58
　periprosthetic — *see* Complications, joint prosthesis, mechanical, periprosthetic, osteolysis, by site
　radius M89.53- ☑
　rib M89.58
　scapula M89.51- ☑
　skull M89.58
　tarsus M89.57- ☑
　tibia M89.56- ☑
　toe M89.57- ☑
　ulna M89.53- ☑
　vertebra M89.58
Osteoma (*see also* Neoplasm, bone, benign)
　osteoid (*see also* Neoplasm, bone, benign)
　　giant — *see* Neoplasm, bone, benign
Osteomalacia M83.9
　adult M83.9
　　drug-induced NEC M83.5
　　due to
　　　malabsorption (postsurgical) M83.2
　　　malnutrition M83.3
　　specified NEC M83.8
　aluminium-induced M83.4
　infantile — *see* Rickets
　juvenile — *see* Rickets
　oncogenic E83.89
　pelvis M83.8
　puerperal M83.0
　senile M83.1
　vitamin-D-resistant in adults E83.31 [M90.8-] ☑
　　carpus E83.31 [M90.84-] ☑
　　clavicle E83.31 [M90.81-] ☑
　　femur E83.31 [M90.85-] ☑
　　fibula E83.31 [M90.86-] ☑
　　finger E83.31 [M90.84-] ☑
　　humerus E83.31 [M90.82-] ☑
　　ilium E83.31 [M90.859]
　　ischium E83.31 [M90.859]
　　metacarpus E83.31 [M90.84-] ☑
　　metatarsus E83.31 [M90.87-] ☑
　　multiple sites E83.31 [M90.89]
　　neck E83.31 [M90.88]
　　radius E83.31 [M90.83-] ☑
　　rib E83.31 [M90.88]
　　scapula E83.31 [M90.819]
　　skull E83.31 [M90.88]
　　tarsus E83.31 [M90.879]
　　tibia E83.31 [M90.869]
　　toe E83.31 [M90.879]
　　ulna E83.31 [M90.839]
　　vertebra E83.31 [M90.88]
Osteomyelitis (general) (infective) (localized) (neonatal) (purulent) (septic) (staphylococcal) (streptococcal) (suppurative) (with periostitis) M86.9
　acute M86.10
　　carpus M86.14- ☑
　　clavicle M86.11- ☑
　　femur M86.15- ☑
　　fibula M86.16 ☑
　　finger M86.14- ☑

Osteomyelitis — *continued*
  acute — *continued*
    hematogenous M86.00
      carpus M86.04- ☑
      clavicle M86.01- ☑
      femur M86.05- ☑
      fibula M86.06- ☑
      finger M86.04- ☑
      humerus M86.02- ☑
      ilium M86.059
      ischium M86.059
      mandible M27.2
      metacarpus M86.04- ☑
      metatarsus M86.07- ☑
      multiple sites M86.09
      neck M86.08
      orbit H05.02- ☑
      petrous bone — *see* Petrositis
      radius M86.03- ☑
      rib M86.08
      scapula M86.01- ☑
      skull M86.08
      tarsus M86.07- ☑
      tibia M86.06- ☑
      toe M86.07- ☑
      ulna M86.03- ☑
      vertebra — *see* Osteomyelitis, vertebra
    humerus M86.12- ☑
    ilium M86.159
    ischium M86.159
    mandible M27.2
    metacarpus M86.14- ☑
    metatarsus M86.17- ☑
    multiple sites M86.19
    neck M86.18
    orbit H05.02- ☑
    petrous bone — *see* Petrositis
    radius M86.13- ☑
    rib M86.18
    scapula M86.11- ☑
    skull M86.18
    tarsus M86.17- ☑
    tibia M86.16- ☑
    toe M86.17- ☑
    ulna M86.13- ☑
    vertebra — *see* Osteomyelitis, vertebra
  chronic (or old) M86.60
    with draining sinus M86.40
      carpus M86.44- ☑
      clavicle M86.41- ☑
      femur M86.45- ☑
      fibula M86.46- ☑
      finger M86.44- ☑
      humerus M86.42- ☑
      ilium M86.459
      ischium M86.459
      mandible M27.2
      metacarpus M86.44- ☑
      metatarsus M86.47- ☑
      multiple sites M86.49
      neck M86.48
      orbit H05.02- ☑
      petrous bone — *see* Petrositis
      radius M86.43- ☑
      rib M86.48
      scapula M86.41- ☑
      skull M86.48
      tarsus M86.47- ☑
      tibia M86.46- ☑
      toe M86.47- ☑
      ulna M86.43- ☑
      vertebra — *see* Osteomyelitis, vertebra
    carpus M86.64- ☑
    clavicle M86.61- ☑
    femur M86.65- ☑
    fibula M86.66- ☑
    finger M86.64- ☑
    hematogenous NEC M86.50
      carpus M86.54- ☑
      clavicle M86.51- ☑
      femur M86.55- ☑
      fibula M86.56- ☑
      finger M86.54- ☑
      humerus M86.52- ☑
      ilium M86.559
      ischium M86.559

Osteomyelitis — *continued*
  chronic — *continued*
    hematogenous — *continued*
      mandible M27.2
      metacarpus M86.54- ☑
      metatarsus M86.57- ☑
      multifocal M86.30
        carpus M86.34- ☑
        clavicle M86.31- ☑
        femur M86.35- ☑
        fibula M86.36- ☑
        finger M86.34- ☑
        humerus M86.32- ☑
        ilium M86.359
        ischium M86.359
        metacarpus M86.34- ☑
        metatarsus M86.37- ☑
        multiple sites M86.39
        neck M86.38
        radius M86.33- ☑
        rib M86.38
        scapula M86.31- ☑
        skull M86.38
        tarsus M86.37- ☑
        tibia M86.36- ☑
        toe M86.37- ☑
        ulna M86.33- ☑
        vertebra — *see* Osteomyelitis, vertebra
      multiple sites M86.59
      neck M86.58
      orbit H05.02- ☑
      petrous bone — *see* Petrositis
      radius M86.53- ☑
      rib M86.58
      scapula M86.51- ☑
      skull M86.58
      tarsus M86.57- ☑
      tibia M86.56- ☑
      toe M86.57- ☑
      ulna M86.53- ☑
      vertebra — *see* Osteomyelitis, vertebra
    humerus M86.62- ☑
    ilium M86.659
    ischium M86.659
    mandible M27.2
    metacarpus M86.64- ☑
    metatarsus M86.67- ☑
    multifocal — *see* Osteomyelitis, chronic, hematogenous, multifocal
    multiple sites M86.69
    neck M86.68
    orbit H05.02- ☑
    petrous bone — *see* Petrositis
    radius M86.63- ☑
    rib M86.68
    scapula M86.61- ☑
    skull M86.68
    tarsus M86.67- ☑
    tibia M86.66- ☑
    toe M86.67- ☑
    ulna M86.63- ☑
    vertebra — *see* Osteomyelitis, vertebra
  echinococcal B67.2
  Garr's — *see* Osteomyelitis, specified type NEC
  jaw (acute) (chronic) (lower) (neonatal) (suppurative) (upper) M27.2
  nonsuppurating — *see* Osteomyelitis, specified type NEC
  orbit H05.02- ☑
  petrous bone — *see* Petrositis
  Salmonella (arizonae) (cholerae-suis) (enteritidis) (typhimurium) A02.24
  sclerosing, nonsuppurative — *see* Osteomyelitis, specified type NEC
  specified type NEC (*see also* subcategory) M86.8X- ☑
    mandible M27.2
    orbit H05.02- ☑
    petrous bone — *see* Petrositis
    vertebra — *see* Osteomyelitis, vertebra
  subacute M86.20
    carpus M86.24- ☑
    clavicle M86.21- ☑
    femur M86.25- ☑
    fibula M86.26- ☑
    finger M86.24- ☑
    humerus M86.22- ☑

Osteomyelitis — *continued*
  subacute — *continued*
    mandible M27.2
    metacarpus M86.24- ☑
    metatarsus M86.27- ☑
    multiple sites M86.29
    neck M86.28
    orbit H05.02- ☑
    petrous bone — *see* Petrositis
    radius M86.23- ☑
    rib M86.28
    scapula M86.21- ☑
    skull M86.28
    tarsus M86.27- ☑
    tibia M86.26- ☑
    toe M86.27- ☑
    ulna M86.23- ☑
    vertebra — *see* Osteomyelitis, vertebra
  syphilitic A52.77
    congenital (early) A50.02 [M90.80]
  tuberculous — *see* Tuberculosis, bone
  typhoid A01.05
  vertebra M46.20
    cervical region M46.22
    cervicothoracic region M46.23
    lumbar region M46.26
    lumbosacral region M46.27
    occipito-atlanto-axial region M46.21
    sacrococcygeal region M46.28
    thoracic region M46.24
    thoracolumbar region M46.25
Osteomyelofibrosis D75.89
Osteomyelosclerosis D75.89
Osteonecrosis M87.9
  due to
    drugs — *see* Osteonecrosis, secondary, due to, drugs
    trauma — *see* Osteonecrosis, secondary, due to, trauma
  idiopathic aseptic M87.00
    ankle M87.07- ☑
    carpus M87.03- ☑
    clavicle M87.01- ☑
    femur M87.05- ☑
    fibula M87.06- ☑
    finger M87.04- ☑
    humerus M87.02- ☑
    ilium M87.050
    ischium M87.050
    metacarpus M87.04- ☑
    metatarsus M87.07- ☑
    multiple sites M87.09
    neck M87.08
    pelvis M87.050
    radius M87.03- ☑
    rib M87.08
    scapula M87.01- ☑
    skull M87.08
    tarsus M87.07- ☑
    tibia M87.06- ☑
    toe M87.07- ☑
    ulna M87.03- ☑
    vertebra M87.08
  secondary NEC M87.30
    carpus M87.33- ☑
    clavicle M87.31- ☑
    due to
      drugs M87.10
        carpus M87.13- ☑
        clavicle M87.11- ☑
        femur M87.15- ☑
        fibula M87.16- ☑
        finger M87.14- ☑
        humerus M87.12- ☑
        ilium M87.159
        ischium M87.159
        jaw M87.180
        metacarpus M87.14- ☑
        metatarsus M87.17- ☑
        multiple sites M87.19
        neck M87.18
        radius M87.13- ☑
        rib M87.18
        scapula M87.11- ☑
        skull M87.18
        tarsus M87.17- ☑
        tibia M87.16- ☑

☑ Additional Character Required — Refer to the Tabular List for Character Selection

▽ Subterms under main terms may continue to next column or page

Osteonecrosis — *continued*
  secondary — *continued*
    due to — *continued*
      drugs — *continued*
        toe M87.17- ✓
        ulna M87.13- ✓
        vertebra M87.18 ✓
      hemoglobinopathy NEC D58.2 [M90.50]
        carpus D58.2 [M90.54-] ✓
        clavicle D58.2 [M90.51-] ✓
        femur D58.2 [M90.55-] ✓
        fibula D58.2 [M90.56-] ✓
        finger D58.2 [M90.54-] ✓
        humerus D58.2 [M90.52-] ✓
        ilium D58.2 [M90.55-] ✓
        ischium D58.2 [M90.55-] ✓
        metacarpus D58.2 [M90.54-] ✓
        metatarsus D58.2 [M90.57-] ✓
        multiple sites D58.2 [M90.58]
        neck D58.2 [M90.58]
        radius D58.2 [M90.53-] ✓
        rib D58.2 [M90.58]
        scapula D58.2 [M90.51-] ✓
        skull D58.2 [M90.58]
        tarsus D58.2 [M90.57-] ✓
        tibia D58.2 [M90.56-] ✓
        toe D58.2 [M90.57-] ✓
        ulna D58.2 [M90.53-] ✓
        vertebra D58.2 [M90.58]
      trauma (previous) M87.20
        carpus M87.23- ✓
        clavicle M87.21- ✓
        femur M87.25- ✓
        fibula M87.26- ✓
        finger M87.24- ✓
        humerus M87.22- ✓
        ilium M87.25- ✓
        ischium M87.25- ✓
        metacarpus M87.24- ✓
        metatarsus M87.27- ✓
        multiple sites M87.29
        neck M87.28
        radius M87.23- ✓
        rib M87.28
        scapula M87.21- ✓
        skull M87.28
        tarsus M87.27- ✓
        tibia M87.26- ✓
        toe M87.27- ✓
        ulna M87.23- ✓
        vertebra M87.28
  femur M87.35- ✓
  fibula M87.36- ✓
  finger M87.34- ✓
  humerus M87.32- ✓
  ilium M87.350
  in
    caisson disease T70.3 ✓ [M90.50]
      carpus T70.3 ✓ [M90.54-] ✓
      clavicle T70.3 ✓ [M90.51-] ✓
      femur T70.3 ✓ [M90.55-] ✓
      fibula T70.3 ✓ [M90.56-] ✓
      finger T70.3 ✓ [M90.54-] ✓
      humerus T70.3 ✓ [M90.52-] ✓
      ilium T70.3 ✓ [M90.55-] ✓
      ischium T70.3 ✓ [M90.55-] ✓
      metacarpus T70.3 ✓ [M90.54-] ✓
      metatarsus T70.3 ✓ [M90.57-] ✓
      multiple sites T70.3 ✓ [M90.59]
      neck T70.3 ✓ [M90.58]
      radius T70.3 ✓ [M90.53-] ✓
      rib T70.3 ✓ [M90.58]
      scapula T70.3 ✓ [M90.51-] ✓
      skull T70.3 ✓ [M90.58]
      tarsus T70.3 ✓ [M90.57-] ✓
      tibia T70.3 ✓ [M90.56-] ✓
      toe T70.3 ✓ [M90.57-] ✓
      ulna T70.3 ✓ [M90.53-] ✓
      vertebra T70.3 ✓ [M90.58]
  ischium M87.350
  metacarpus M87.34- ✓
  metatarsus M87.37- ✓
  multiple site M87.39
  neck M87.38
  radius M87.33- ✓
  rib M87.38

Osteonecrosis — *continued*
  secondary — *continued*
    scapula M87.319
    skull M87.38
    tarsus M87.379
    tibia M87.366
    toe M87.379
    ulna M87.33- ✓
    vertebra M87.38
    specified type NEC M87.80
      carpus M87.83- ✓
      clavicle M87.81- ✓
      femur M87.85- ✓
      fibula M87.86- ✓
      finger M87.84- ✓
      humerus M87.82- ✓
      ilium M87.85- ✓
      ischium M87.85- ✓
      metacarpus M87.84- ✓
      metatarsus M87.87- ✓
      multiple sites M87.89
      neck M87.88
      radius M87.83- ✓
      rib M87.88
      scapula M87.81- ✓
      skull M87.88
      tarsus M87.87- ✓
      tibia M87.86- ✓
      toe M87.87- ✓
      ulna M87.83- ✓
      vertebra M87.88
Osteo-onycho-arthro-dysplasia Q79.8
Osteo-onychodysplasia, hereditary Q79.8
Osteopathia condensans disseminata Q78.8
Osteopathy (*see also* Osteomyelitis, Osteonecrosis, Osteoporosis)
  after poliomyelitis M89.60
    carpus M89.64- ✓
    clavicle M89.61- ✓
    femur M89.65- ✓
    fibula M89.66- ✓
    finger M89.64- ✓
    humerus M89.62- ✓
    ilium M89.659
    ischium M89.659
    metacarpus M89.64- ✓
    metatarsus M89.67- ✓
    multiple sites M89.69
    neck M89.68
    radius M89.63- ✓
    rib M89.68
    scapula M89.61- ✓
    skull M89.68
    tarsus M89.67- ✓
    tibia M89.66- ✓
    toe M89.67- ✓
    ulna M89.63- ✓
    vertebra M89.68
  in (due to)
    renal osteodystrophy N25.0
    specified diseases classified elsewhere — *see* subcategory M90.8 ✓
Osteopenia M85.8- ✓
  borderline M85.8- ✓
Osteoperiostitis — *see* Osteomyelitis, specified type NEC
Osteopetrosis (familial) Q78.2
Osteophyte M25.70
  ankle M25.77- ✓
  elbow M25.72- ✓
  foot joint M25.77- ✓
  hand joint M25.74- ✓
  hip M25.75- ✓
  knee M25.76- ✓
  shoulder M25.71- ✓
  spine M25.78
  vertebrae M25.78
  wrist M25.73- ✓
Osteopoikilosis Q78.8
Osteoporosis (female) (male) M81.0
  with current pathological fracture M80.00 ✓
  age-related M81.0
    with current pathologic fracture M80.00 ✓
      carpus M80.04- ✓
      clavicle M80.01- ✓
      fibula M80.06- ✓

Osteoporosis — *continued*
  age-related — *continued*
    with current pathologic fracture — *continued*
      finger M80.04- ✓
      humerus M80.02- ✓
      ilium M80.05- ✓
      ischium M80.05- ✓
      metacarpus M80.04- ✓
      metatarsus M80.07- ✓
      pelvis M80.05- ✓
      radius M80.03- ✓
      scapula M80.01- ✓
      tarsus M80.07- ✓
      tibia M80.06- ✓
      toe M80.07- ✓
      ulna M80.03- ✓
      vertebra M80.08 ✓
  disuse M81.8
    with current pathological fracture M80.80 ✓
      carpus M80.84- ✓
      clavicle M80.81- ✓
      fibula M80.86- ✓
      finger M80.84- ✓
      humerus M80.82- ✓
      ilium M80.85- ✓
      ischium M80.85- ✓
      metacarpus M80.84- ✓
      metatarsus M80.87- ✓
      pelvis M80.85- ✓
      radius M80.83- ✓
      scapula M80.81- ✓
      tarsus M80.87- ✓
      tibia M80.86- ✓
      toe M80.87- ✓
      ulna M80.83- ✓
      vertebra M80.88 ✓
  drug-induced — *see* Osteoporosis, specified type NEC
  idiopathic — *see* Osteoporosis, specified type NEC
  involutional — *see* Osteoporosis, age-related
  Lequesne M81.6
  localized M81.6
  postmenopausal M81.0
    with pathological fracture M80.00 ✓
      carpus M80.04- ✓
      clavicle M80.01- ✓
      fibula M80.06- ✓
      finger M80.04- ✓
      humerus M80.02- ✓
      ilium M80.05- ✓
      ischium M80.05- ✓
      metacarpus M80.04- ✓
      metatarsus M80.07- ✓
      pelvis M80.05- ✓
      radius M80.03- ✓
      scapula M80.01- ✓
      tarsus M80.07- ✓
      tibia M80.06- ✓
      toe M80.07- ✓
      ulna M80.03- ✓
      vertebra M80.08 ✓
  postoophorectomy — *see* Osteoporosis, specified type NEC
  postsurgical malabsorption — *see* Osteoporosis, specified type NEC
  post-traumatic — *see* Osteoporosis, specified type NEC
  senile — *see* Osteoporosis, age-related
  specified type NEC M81.8
    with pathological fracture M80.80 ✓
      carpus M80.84- ✓
      clavicle M80.81- ✓
      fibula M80.86- ✓
      finger M80.84- ✓
      humerus M80.82- ✓
      ilium M80.85- ✓
      ischium M80.85- ✓
      metacarpus M80.84- ✓
      metatarsus M80.87- ✓
      pelvis M80.85- ✓
      radius M80.83- ✓
      scapula M80.81- ✓
      tarsus M80.87- ✓
      tibia M80.86- ✓
      toe M80.87- ✓
      ulna M80.83- ✓
      vertebra M80.88 ✓

Osteopsathyrosis (idiopathica) Q78.0
Osteoradionecrosis, jaw (acute) (chronic) (lower) (suppurative) (upper) M27.2
Osteosarcoma (any form) — see Neoplasm, bone, malignant
Osteosclerosis Q78.2
  acquired M85.8- ☑
  congenita Q77.4
  fragilitas (generalisata) Q78.2
  myelofibrosis D75.81
Osteosclerotic anemia D64.89
Osteosis
  cutis L94.2
  renal fibrocystic N25.0
Österreicher-Turner syndrome Q87.2
Ostium
  atrioventriculare commune Q21.2
  primum (arteriosum) (defect) (persistent) Q21.2
  secundum (arteriosum) (defect) (patent) (persistent) Q21.1
Ostrum-Furst syndrome Q75.8
Otalgia H92.0 ☑
Otitis (acute) H66.90
  with effusion (see also Otitis, media, nonsuppurative)
    purulent — see Otitis, media, suppurative
  adhesive — see subcategory H74.1 ☑
  chronic (see also Otitis, media, chronic)
    with effusion (see also Otitis, media, nonsuppurative, chronic)
  externa H60.9- ☑
    abscess — see Abscess, ear, external
    acute (noninfective) H60.50- ☑
      actinic H60.51- ☑
      chemical H60.52- ☑
      contact H60.53- ☑
      eczematoid H60.54- ☑
      infective — see Otitis, externa, infective
      reactive H60.55- ☑
      specified NEC H60.59- ☑
    cellulitis — see Cellulitis, ear
    chronic H60.6- ☑
    diffuse — see Otitis, externa, infective, diffuse
    hemorrhagic — see Otitis, externa, infective, hemorrhagic
    in (due to)
      aspergillosis B44.89
      candidiasis B37.84
      erysipelas A46 [H62.40]
      herpes (simplex) virus infection B00.1
        zoster B02.8
      impetigo L01.00 [H62.40]
      infectious disease NEC B99 ☑ [H62.4-] ☑
      mycosis NEC B36.9 [H62.40]
      parasitic disease NEC B89 [H62.40]
      viral disease NEC B34.9 [H62.40]
      zoster B02.8
    infective NEC H60.39- ☑
      abscess — see Abscess, ear, external
      cellulitis — see Cellulitis, ear
      diffuse H60.31- ☑
      hemorrhagic H60.32- ☑
      swimmer's ear — see Swimmer's, ear
    malignant H60.2- ☑
    mycotic B36.9 [H62.40]
    necrotizing — see Otitis, externa, malignant
    Pseudomonas aeruginosa — see Otitis, externa, malignant
    reactive — see Otitis, externa, acute, reactive
    specified NEC — see subcategory H60.8 ☑
    tropical B36.8
  insidiosa — see Otosclerosis
  interna H83.0 ☑
  media (hemorrhagic) (staphylococcal) (streptococcal) H66.9-
    with effusion (nonpurulent) — see Otitis, media, nonsuppurative
    acute, subacute H66.90
      allergic — see Otitis, media, nonsuppurative, acute, allergic
      exudative — see Otitis, media, nonsuppurative, acute
      mucoid — see Otitis, media, nonsuppurative, acute
      necrotizing (see also Otitis, media, suppurative, acute)
        in
          measles B05.3

Otitis — continued
  media — continued
    acute, subacute — continued
      necrotizing (see also Otitis, media, suppurative, acute) — continued
        in — continued
          scarlet fever A38.0
      nonsuppurative NEC — see Otitis, media, nonsuppurative, acute
      purulent — see Otitis, media, suppurative, acute
      sanguinous — see Otitis, media, nonsuppurative, acute
      secretory — see Otitis, media, nonsuppurative, acute, serous
      seromucinous — see Otitis, media, nonsuppurative, acute
      serous — see Otitis, media, nonsuppurative, acute, serous
      suppurative — see Otitis, media, suppurative, acute
    allergic — see Otitis, media, nonsuppurative
    catarrhal — see Otitis, media, nonsuppurative
    chronic H66.90
      with effusion (nonpurulent) — see Otitis, media, nonsuppurative, chronic
      allergic — see Otitis, media, nonsuppurative, chronic, allergic
      benign suppurative — see Otitis, media, suppurative, chronic, tubotympanic
      catarrhal — see Otitis, media, nonsuppurative, chronic, serous
      exudative — see Otitis, media, nonsuppurative, chronic
      mucinous — see Otitis, media, nonsuppurative, chronic, mucoid
      mucoid — see Otitis, media, nonsuppurative, chronic, mucoid
      nonsuppurative NEC — see Otitis, media, nonsuppurative, chronic
      purulent — see Otitis, media, suppurative, chronic
      secretory — see Otitis, media, nonsuppurative, chronic, mucoid
      seromucinous — see Otitis, media, nonsuppurative, chronic
      serous — see Otitis, media, nonsuppurative, chronic, serous
      suppurative — see Otitis, media, suppurative, chronic
      transudative — see Otitis, media, nonsuppurative, chronic, mucoid
    exudative — see Otitis, media, nonsuppurative
    in (due to) (with)
      influenza — see Influenza, with, otitis media
      measles B05.3
      scarlet fever A38.0
      tuberculosis A18.6
      viral disease NEC B34.- [H67.-] ☑
    mucoid — see Otitis, media, nonsuppurative
    nonsuppurative H65.9- ☑
      acute or subacute NEC H65.19- ☑
        allergic H65.11- ☑
          recurrent H65.11- ☑
        recurrent H65.19- ☑
        secretory — see Otitis, media, nonsuppurative, serous
        serous H65.0- ☑
          recurrent H65.0- ☑
      chronic H65.49- ☑
        allergic H65.41- ☑
        mucoid H65.3- ☑
        serous H65.2- ☑
    postmeasles B05.3
    purulent — see Otitis, media, suppurative
    secretory — see Otitis, media, nonsuppurative
    seromucinous — see Otitis, media, nonsuppurative
    serous — see Otitis, media, nonsuppurative
    suppurative H66.4- ☑
      acute H66.00- ☑
        with rupture of ear drum H66.01- ☑
        recurrent H66.00- ☑
          with rupture of ear drum H66.01- ☑
      chronic (see also subcategory) H66.3 ☑
        atticoantral H66.2- ☑
        benign — see Otitis, media, suppurative, chronic, tubotympanic

Otitis — continued
  media — continued
    suppurative — continued
      chronic (see also subcategory) — continued
        tubotympanic H66.1- ☑
    transudative — see Otitis, media, nonsuppurative
    tuberculous A18.6
Otocephaly Q18.2
Otolith syndrome — see subcategory H81.8 ☑
Otomycosis (diffuse) NEC B36.9 [H62.40]
  in
    aspergillosis B44.89
    candidiasis B37.84
    moniliasis B37.84
Otoporosis — see Otosclerosis
Otorrhagia (nontraumatic) H92.2- ☑
  traumatic — code by Type of injury
Otorrhea H92.1- ☑
  cerebrospinal G96.0
Otosclerosis (general) H80.9- ☑
  cochlear (endosteal) H80.2- ☑
  involving
    otic capsule — see Otosclerosis, cochlear
    oval window
      nonobliterative H80.0- ☑
      obliterative H80.1- ☑
    round window — see Otosclerosis, cochlear
  nonobliterative — see Otosclerosis, involving, oval window, nonobliterative
  obliterative — see Otosclerosis, involving, oval window, obliterative
  specified NEC H80.8- ☑
Otospongiosis — see Otosclerosis
Otto's disease or pelvis M24.7
Outcome of delivery Z37.9
  multiple births Z37.9
    all liveborn Z37.50
      quadruplets Z37.52
      quintuplets Z37.53
      sextuplets Z37.54
      specified number NEC Z37.59
      triplets Z37.51
    all stillborn Z37.7
    some liveborn Z37.60
      quadruplets Z37.62
      quintuplets Z37.63
      sextuplets Z37.64
      specified number NEC Z37.69
      triplets Z37.61
  single NEC Z37.9
    liveborn Z37.0
    stillborn Z37.1
  twins NEC Z37.9
    both liveborn Z37.2
    both stillborn Z37.4
    one liveborn, one stillborn Z37.3
Outlet — see condition
Ovalocytosis (congenital) (hereditary) — see Elliptocytosis
Ovarian — see Condition
Ovariocele N83.4
Ovaritis (cystic) — see Oophoritis
Ovary, ovarian (see also condition)
  resistant syndrome E28.39
  vein syndrome N13.8
Overactive (see also Hyperfunction)
  adrenal cortex NEC E27.0
  bladder N32.81
  hypothalamus E23.3
  thyroid — see Hyperthyroidism
Overactivity R46.3
  child — see Disorder, attention-deficit hyperactivity
Overbite (deep) (excessive) (horizontal) (vertical) M26.29
Overbreathing — see Hyperventilation
Overconscientious personality F60.5
Overdevelopment — see Hypertrophy
Overdistension — see Distension
Overdose, overdosage (drug) — see Table of Drugs and Chemicals, by drug, poisoning
Overeating R63.2
  nonorganic origin F50.8
  psychogenic F50.8
Overexertion (effects) (exhaustion) T73.3 ☑
Overexposure (effects) T73.9 ☑
  exhaustion T73.2 ☑
Overfeeding — see Overeating
  newborn P92.4

☑ Additional Character Required — Refer to the Tabular List for Character Selection   ▼ Subterms under main terms may continue to next column or page

Overfill, endodontic M27.52
Overgrowth, bone — *see* Hypertrophy, bone
Overhanging of dental restorative material (unrepairable) K08.52
Overheated (places) (effects) — *see* Heat
Overjet (excessive horizontal) M26.23
Overlaid, overlying (suffocation) — *see* Asphyxia, traumatic, due to mechanical threat
Overlap, excessive horizontal (teeth) M26.23
Overlapping toe (acquired) (*see also* Deformity, toe, specified NEC)
   congenital (fifth toe) Q66.89
Overload
   circulatory, due to transfusion (blood) (blood components) (TACO) E87.71
   fluid E87.70
      due to transfusion (blood) (blood components) E87.71
      specified NEC E87.79
   iron, due to repeated red blood cell transfusions E83.111
   potassium (K) E87.5
   sodium (Na) E87.0
Overnutrition — *see* Hyperalimentation
Overproduction (*see also* Hypersecretion)
   ACTH E27.0
   catecholamine E27.5
   growth hormone E22.0
Overprotection, child by parent Z62.1
Overriding
   aorta Q25.4
   finger (acquired) — *see* Deformity, finger
      congenital Q68.1
   toe (acquired) (*see also* Deformity, toe, specified NEC)
      congenital Q66.89
Overstrained R53.83
   heart — *see* Hypertrophy, cardiac
Overuse, muscle NEC M70.8- ☑
Overweight E66.3
Overworked R53.83
Oviduct — *see* condition
Ovotestis Q56.0
Ovulation (cycle)
   failure or lack of N97.0
   pain N94.0
Ovum — *see* condition
Owren's disease or syndrome (parahemophilia) D68.2
Ox heart — *see* Hypertrophy, cardiac
Oxalosis E72.53
Oxaluria E72.53
Oxycephaly, oxycephalic Q75.0
   syphilitic, congenital A50.02
Oxyuriasis B80
Oxyuris vermicularis (infestation) B80
Ozena J31.0

P

Pachyderma, pachydermia L85.9
   larynx (verrucosa) J38.7
Pachydermatocele (congenital) Q82.8
Pachydermoperiostosis (*see also* Osteoarthropathy, hypertrophic, specified type NEC)
   clubbed nail M89.40 [L62]
Pachygyria Q04.3
Pachymeningitis (adhesive) (basal) (brain) (cervical) (chronic)(circumscribed) (external) (fibrous) (hemorrhagic) (hypertrophic) (internal) (purulent) (spinal) (suppurative) — *see* Meningitis
Pachyonychia (congenital) Q84.5
Pacinian tumor — *see* Neoplasm, skin, benign
Pad, knuckle or Garrod's M72.1
Paget's disease
   with infiltrating duct carcinoma — *see* Neoplasm, breast, malignant
   bone M88.9
      carpus M88.84- ☑
      clavicle M88.81- ☑
      femur M88.85- ☑
      fibula M88.86- ☑
      finger M88.84- ☑
      humerus M88.82- ☑
      ilium M88.85- ☑
      in neoplastic disease — *see* Osteitis, deformans, in neoplastic disease
      ischium M88.85- ☑
      metacarpus M88.84- ☑

Paget's disease — *continued*
   bone — *continued*
      metatarsus M88.87- ☑
      multiple sites M88.89
      neck M88.88
      radius M88.83- ☑
      rib M88.88
      scapula M88.81- ☑
      skull M88.0
      tarsus M88.87- ☑
      tibia M88.86- ☑
      toe M88.87- ☑
      ulna M88.83- ☑
      vertebra M88.88
   breast (female) C50.01- ☑
      male C50.02- ☑
   extramammary (*see also* Neoplasm, skin, malignant)
      anus C21.0
      margin C44.590
      skin C44.590
   intraductal carcinoma — *see* Neoplasm, breast, malignant
   malignant — *see* Neoplasm, skin, malignant
      breast (female) C50.01- ☑
      male C50.02- ☑
      unspecified site (female) C50.01- ☑
      male C50.02- ☑
   mammary — *see* Paget's disease, breast
   nipple — *see* Paget's disease, breast
   osteitis deformans — *see* Paget's disease, bone
Paget-Schroetter syndrome I82.890
Pain(s) (*see also* Painful) R52
   abdominal R10.9
      colic R10.83
      generalized R10.84
         with acute abdomen R10.0
      lower R10.30
         left quadrant R10.32
         pelvic or perineal R10.2
         periumbilical R10.33
         right quadrant R10.31
      rebound — *see* Tenderness, abdominal, rebound
      severe with abdominal rigidity R10.0
      tenderness — *see* Tenderness, abdominal
      upper R10.10
         epigastric R10.13
         left quadrant R10.12
         right quadrant R10.11
   acute R52
      due to trauma G89.11
      neoplasm related G89.3
      postprocedural NEC G89.18
      post-thoracotomy G89.12
      specified by site — *code to* Pain, by site
   adnexa (uteri) R10.2
   anginoid — *see* Pain, precordial
   anus K62.89
   arm — *see* Pain, limb, upper
   axillary (axilla) M79.62- ☑
   back (postural) M54.9
   bladder R39.89
      associated with micturition — *see* Micturition, painful
   bone — *see* Disorder, bone, specified type NEC
   breast N64.4
   broad ligament R10.2
   cancer associated (acute) (chronic) G89.3
   cecum — *see* Pain, abdominal
   cervicobrachial M53.1
   chest (central) R07.9
      anterior wall R07.89
      atypical R07.89
      ischemic I20.9
      musculoskeletal R07.89
      non-cardiac R07.89
      on breathing R07.1
      pleurodynia R07.81
      precordial R07.2
      wall (anterior) R07.89
   chronic G89.29
      associated with significant psychosocial dysfunction G89.4
      due to trauma G89.21
      neoplasm related G89.3
      postoperative NEC G89.28
      postprocedural NEC G89.28
      post-thoracotomy G89.22

Pain(s) — *continued*
   chronic — *continued*
      specified NEC G89.29
   coccyx M53.3
   colon — *see* Pain, abdominal
   coronary — *see* Angina
   costochondral R07.1
   diaphragm R07.1
   due to cancer G89.3
   due to device, implant or graft (*see also* Complications, by site and type, specified NEC) T85.84 ☑
      arterial graft NEC T82.848 ☑
      breast (implant) T85.84 ☑
      catheter NEC T85.84 ☑
         dialysis (renal) T82.848 ☑
            intraperitoneal T85.84 ☑
         infusion NEC T82.848 ☑
            spinal (epidural) (subdural) T85.84 ☑
         urinary (indwelling) T83.84 ☑
      electronic (electrode) (pulse generator) (stimulator)
         bone T84.84 ☑
         cardiac T82.847 ☑
         nervous system (brain) (peripheral nerve) (spinal) T85.84 ☑
         urinary T83.84 ☑
      fixation, internal (orthopedic) NEC T84.84 ☑
      gastrointestinal (bile duct) (esophagus) T85.84 ☑
      genital NEC T83.84 ☑
      heart NEC T82.847 ☑
      infusion NEC T85.84 ☑
      joint prosthesis T84.84 ☑
      ocular (corneal graft) (orbital implant) NEC T85.84 ☑
      orthopedic NEC T84.84 ☑
      specified NEC T85.84 ☑
      urinary NEC T83.84 ☑
      vascular NEC T82.848 ☑
      ventricular intracranial shunt T85.84 ☑
   due to malignancy (primary) (secondary) G89.3
   ear — *see* subcategory H92.0 ☑
   epigastric, epigastrium R10.13
   eye — *see* Pain, ocular
   face, facial R51
      atypical G50.1
   female genital organs NEC N94.89
   finger — *see* Pain, limb, upper
   flank — *see* Pain, abdominal
   foot — *see* Pain, limb, lower
   gallbladder K82.9
   gas (intestinal) R14.1
   gastric — *see* Pain, abdominal
   generalized NOS R52
   genital organ
      female N94.89
      male N50.8
   groin — *see* Pain, abdominal, lower
   hand — *see* Pain, limb, upper
   head — *see* Headache
   heart — *see* Pain, precordial
   infra-orbital — *see* Neuralgia, trigeminal
   intercostal R07.82
   intermenstrual N94.0
   jaw R68.84
   joint M25.50
      ankle M25.57- ☑
      elbow M25.52- ☑
      finger M79.64- ☑
      foot M79.67- ☑
      hand M79.64- ☑
      hip M25.55- ☑
      knee M25.56- ☑
      shoulder M25.51- ☑
      toe M79.67- ☑
      wrist M25.53- ☑
   kidney N23
   laryngeal R07.0
   leg — *see* Pain, limb, lower
   limb M79.609
      lower M79.60- ☑
         foot M79.67- ☑
         lower leg M79.66- ☑
         thigh M79.65- ☑
         toe M79.67- ☑
      upper M79.60- ☑
         axilla M79.62- ☑
         finger M79.64- ☑

Panic (attack) (state) F41.0
  reaction to exceptional stress (transient) F43.0
Panmyelopathy, familial, constitutional D61.09
Panmyelophthisis D61.82
  congenital D61.09
Panmyelosis (acute) (with myelofibrosis) C94.4- ☑
Panner's disease — see Osteochondrosis, juvenile, humerus
Panneuritis endemica E51.11
Panniculitis (nodular) (nonsuppurative) M79.3
  back M54.00
    cervical region M54.02
    cervicothoracic region M54.03
    lumbar region M54.06
    lumbosacral region M54.07
    multiple sites M54.09
    occipito-atlanto-axial region M54.01
    sacrococcygeal region M54.08
    thoracic region M54.04
    thoracolumbar region M54.05
  lupus L93.2
  mesenteric K65.4
  neck M54.02
    cervicothoracic region M54.03
    occipito-atlanto-axial region M54.01
  relapsing M35.6
Panniculus adiposus (abdominal) E65
Pannus (allergic) (cornea) (degenerativus) (keratic) H16.42- ☑
  abdominal (symptomatic) E65
  trachomatosus, trachomatous (active) A71.1
Panophthalmitis H44.01- ☑
Pansinusitis (chronic) (hyperplastic) (nonpurulent) (purulent) J32.4
  acute J01.40
    recurrent J01.41
  tuberculous A15.8
Panuveitis (sympathetic) H44.11- ☑
Panvalvular disease I08.9
  specified NEC I08.8
Papanicolaou smear, cervix Z12.4
  as part of routine gynecological examination Z01.419
    with abnormal findings Z01.411
  for suspected neoplasm Z12.4
  nonspecific abnormal finding R87.619
  routine Z01.419
    with abnormal findings Z01.411
Papilledema (choked disc) H47.10
  associated with
    decreased ocular pressure H47.12
    increased intracranial pressure H47.11
    retinal disorder H47.13
  Foster-Kennedy syndrome H47.14- ☑
Papillitis H46.00
  anus K62.89
  chronic lingual K14.4
  necrotizing, kidney N17.2
  optic H46.0- ☑
  rectum K62.89
  renal, necrotizing N17.2
  tongue K14.0
Papilloma (see also Neoplasm, benign, by site)
  acuminatum (female) (male) (anogenital) A63.0
  benign pinta (primary) A67.0
  bladder (urinary) (transitional cell) D41.4
  choroid plexus (lateral ventricle) (third ventricle) D33.0
    anaplastic C71.5
    fourth ventricle D33.1
    malignant C71.5
  renal pelvis (transitional cell) D41.1- ☑
    benign D30.1- ☑
  Schneiderian
    specified site — see Neoplasm, benign, by site
    unspecified site D14.0
  serous surface
    borderline malignancy
      specified site — see Neoplasm, uncertain behavior, by site
      unspecified site D39.10
    specified site — see Neoplasm, benign, by site
    unspecified site D27.9
  transitional (cell)
    bladder (urinary) D41.4
    inverted type — see Neoplasm, uncertain behavior, by site
    renal pelvis D41.1- ☑
    ureter D41.2- ☑

Papilloma — continued
  ureter (transitional cell) D41.2- ☑
    benign D30.2- ☑
  urothelial — see Neoplasm, uncertain behavior, by site
  villous — see Neoplasm, uncertain behavior, by site
    adenocarcinoma in — see Neoplasm, malignant, by site
    in situ — see Neoplasm, in situ
  yaws, plantar or palmar A66.1
Papillomata, multiple, of yaws A66.1
Papillomatosis (see also Neoplasm, benign, by site)
  confluent and reticulated L83
  cystic, breast — see Mastopathy, cystic
  ductal, breast — see Mastopathy, cystic
  intraductal (diffuse) — see Neoplasm, benign, by site
  subareolar duct D24- ☑
Papillomavirus, as cause of disease classified elsewhere B97.7
Papillon-Léage and Psaume syndrome Q87.0
Papule(s) R23.8
  carate (primary) A67.0
  fibrous, of nose D22.39
  Gottron's L94.4
  pinta (primary) A67.0
Papulosis
  lymphomatoid C86.6
  malignant I77.89
Papyraceous fetus O31.0- ☑
Para-albuminemia E88.09
Paracephalus Q89.7
Parachute mitral valve Q23.2
Paracoccidioidomycosis B41.9
  disseminated B41.7
  generalized B41.7
  mucocutaneous-lymphangitic B41.8
  pulmonary B41.0
  specified NEC B41.8
  visceral B41.8
Paradentosis K05.4
Paraffinoma T88.8 ☑
Paraganglioma D44.7
  adrenal D35.0- ☑
    malignant C74.1- ☑
  aortic body D44.7
    malignant C75.5
  carotid body D44.6
    malignant C75.4
  chromaffin (see also Neoplasm, benign, by site)
    malignant — see Neoplasm, malignant, by site
  extra-adrenal D44.7
    malignant C75.5
      specified site — see Neoplasm, malignant, by site
      unspecified site C75.5
    specified site — see Neoplasm, uncertain behavior, by site
    unspecified site D44.7
  gangliocytic D13.2
    specified site — see Neoplasm, benign, by site
    unspecified site D13.2
  glomus jugulare D44.7
    malignant C75.5
  jugular D44.7
  malignant C75.5
    specified site — see Neoplasm, malignant, by site
    unspecified site C75.5
  nonchromaffin D44.7
    malignant C75.5
      specified site — see Neoplasm, malignant, by site
      unspecified site C75.5
    specified site — see Neoplasm, uncertain behavior, by site
    unspecified site D44.7
  parasympathetic D44.7
    specified site — see Neoplasm, uncertain behavior, by site
    unspecified site D44.7
  specified site — see Neoplasm, uncertain behavior, by site
  sympathetic D44.7
    specified site — see Neoplasm, uncertain behavior, by site
    unspecified site D44.7
  unspecified site D44.7

Parageusia R43.2
  psychogenic F45.8
Paragonimiasis B66.4
Paragranuloma, Hodgkin — see Lymphoma, Hodgkin, classical, specified NEC
Parahemophilia (see also Defect, coagulation) D68.2
Parakeratosis R23.4
  variegata L41.0
Paralysis, paralytic (complete) (incomplete) G83.9
  with
    syphilis A52.17
  abducens, abducent (nerve) — see Strabismus, paralytic, sixth nerve
  abductor, lower extremity G57.9- ☑
  accessory nerve G52.8
  accommodation (see also Paresis, of accommodation)
    hysterical F44.89
  acoustic nerve (except Deafness) H93.3 ☑
  agitans (see also Parkinsonism) G20
    arteriosclerotic G21.4
  alternating (oculomotor) G83.89
  amyotrophic G12.21
  ankle G57.9- ☑
  anus (sphincter) K62.89
  arm — see Monoplegia, upper limb
  ascending (spinal), acute G61.0
  association G12.29
  asthenic bulbar G70.00
    with exacerbation (acute) G70.01
    in crisis G70.01
  ataxic (hereditary) G11.9
    general (syphilitic) A52.17
  atrophic G58.9
    infantile, acute — see Poliomyelitis, paralytic
    progressive G12.22
    spinal (acute) — see Poliomyelitis, paralytic
  axillary G54.0
  Babinski-Nageotte's G83.89
  Bell's G51.0
    newborn P11.3
  Benedikt's G46.3
  birth injury P14.9
    spinal cord P11.5
  bladder (neurogenic) (sphincter) N31.2
  bowel, colon or intestine K56.0
  brachial plexus G54.0
    birth injury P14.3
    newborn (birth injury) P14.3
  brain G83.9
    diplegia G83.0
    triplegia G83.89
  bronchial J98.09
  Brown-Séquard G83.81
  bulbar (chronic) (progressive) G12.22
    infantile — see Poliomyelitis, paralytic
    poliomyelitic — see Poliomyelitis, paralytic
    pseudo G12.29
  bulbospinal G70.00
    with exacerbation (acute) G70.01
    in crisis G70.01
  cardiac (see also Failure, heart) I50.9
  cerebrocerebellar, diplegic G80.1
  cervical
    plexus G54.2
    sympathetic G90.09
  Cèstan-Chenais G46.3
  Charcot-Marie-Tooth type G60.0
  Clark's G80.9
  colon K56.0
  compressed air T70.3 ☑
  compression
    arm G56.9- ☑
    leg G57.9- ☑
    lower extremity G57.9- ☑
    upper extremity G56.9- ☑
  congenital (cerebral) — see Palsy, cerebral
  conjugate movement (gaze) (of eye) H51.0
    cortical (nuclear) (supranuclear) H51.0
  cordis — see Failure, heart
  cranial or cerebral nerve G52.9
  creeping G12.22
  crossed leg G83.89
  crutch — see Injury, brachial plexus
  deglutition R13.0
    hysterical F44.4
  dementia A52.17
  descending (spinal) NEC G12.29

Paralysis, paralytic — *continued*
- diaphragm (flaccid) J98.6
  - due to accidental dissection of phrenic nerve during procedure — *see* Puncture, accidental complicating surgery
- digestive organs NEC K59.8
- diplegic — *see* Diplegia
- divergence (nuclear) H51.8
- diver's T70.3 ☑
- Duchenne's
  - birth injury P14.0
  - due to or associated with
    - motor neuron disease G12.22
    - muscular dystrophy G71.0
  - due to intracranial or spinal birth injury — *see* Palsy, cerebral
- embolic (current episode) I63.4 ☑
- Erb (-Duchenne) (birth) (newborn) P14.0
- Erb's syphilitic spastic spinal A52.17
- esophagus K22.8
- eye muscle (extrinsic) H49.9
  - intrinsic (*see also* Paresis, of accommodation)
- facial (nerve) G51.0
  - birth injury P11.3
  - congenital P11.3
  - following operation NEC — *see* Puncture, accidental complicating surgery
  - newborn (birth injury) P11.3
- familial (recurrent) (periodic) G72.3
  - spastic G11.4
- fauces J39.2
- finger G56.9- ☑
- gait R26.1
- gastric nerve (nondiabetic) G52.2
- gaze, conjugate H51.0
- general (progressive) (syphilitic) A52.17
  - juvenile A50.45
- glottis J38.00
  - bilateral J38.02
  - unilateral J38.01
- gluteal G54.1
- Gubler (-Millard) G46.3
- hand — *see* Monoplegia, upper limb
- heart — *see* Arrest, cardiac
- hemiplegic — *see* Hemiplegia
- hyperkalemic periodic (familial) G72.3
- hypoglossal (nerve) G52.3
- hypokalemic periodic G72.3
- hysterical F44.4
- ileus K56.0
- infantile (*see also* Poliomyelitis, paralytic) A80.30
  - bulbar — *see* Poliomyelitis, paralytic
  - cerebral — *see* Palsy, cerebral
  - spastic — *see* Palsy, cerebral, spastic
- infective — *see* Poliomyelitis, paralytic
- inferior nuclear G83.9
- internuclear — *see* Ophthalmoplegia, internuclear
- intestine K56.0
- iris H57.09
  - due to diphtheria (toxin) A36.89
- ischemic, Volkmann's (complicating trauma) T79.6 ☑
- Jackson's G83.89
- jake — *see* Poisoning, food, noxious, plant
- Jamaica ginger (jake) G62.2
- juvenile general A50.45
- Klumpke (-Déjérine) (birth) (newborn) P14.1
- labioglossal (laryngeal) (pharyngeal) G12.29
- Landry's G61.0
- laryngeal nerve (recurrent) (superior) (unilateral) J38.00
  - bilateral J38.02
  - unilateral J38.01
- larynx J38.00
  - bilateral J38.02
  - due to diphtheria (toxin) A36.2
  - unilateral J38.01
- lateral G12.21
- lead T56.0 ☑
- left side — *see* Hemiplegia
- leg G83.1- ☑
  - both — *see* Paraplegia
  - crossed G83.89
  - hysterical F44.4
  - psychogenic F44.4
  - transient or transitory R29.818
    - traumatic NEC — *see* Injury, nerve, leg
- levator palpebrae superioris — *see* Blepharoptosis, paralytic
- limb — *see* Monoplegia

Paralysis, paralytic — *continued*
- lip K13.0
- Lissauer's A52.17
- lower limb — *see* Monoplegia, lower limb
  - both — *see* Paraplegia
- lung J98.4
- median nerve G56.1- ☑
- medullary (tegmental) G83.89
- mesencephalic NEC G83.89
  - tegmental G83.89
- middle alternating G83.89
- Millard-Gubler-Foville G46.3
- monoplegic — *see* Monoplegia
- motor G83.9
- muscle, muscular NEC G72.89
  - due to nerve lesion G58.9
  - eye (extrinsic) H49.9
    - intrinsic (*see also* Paresis, of accommodation)
    - oblique — *see* Strabismus, paralytic, fourth nerve
  - iris sphincter H21.9
  - ischemic (Volkmann's) (complicating trauma) T79.6
  - progressive G12.21
  - pseudohypertrophic G71.0
- musculocutaneous nerve G56.9- ☑
- musculospiral G56.9- ☑
- nerve (*see also* Disorder, nerve)
  - abducent — *see* Strabismus, paralytic, sixth nerve
  - accessory G52.8
  - auditory (except Deafness) H93.3 ☑
  - birth injury P14.9
  - cranial or cerebral G52.9
  - facial G51.0
    - birth injury P11.3
    - congenital P11.3
    - newborn (birth injury) P11.3
  - fourth or trochlear — *see* Strabismus, paralytic, fourth nerve
  - newborn (birth injury) P14.9
  - oculomotor — *see* Strabismus, paralytic, third nerve
  - phrenic (birth injury) P14.2
  - radial G56.3- ☑
  - seventh or facial G51.0
    - newborn (birth injury) P11.3
  - sixth or abducent — *see* Strabismus, paralytic, sixth nerve
  - syphilitic A52.15
  - third or oculomotor — *see* Strabismus, paralytic, third nerve
  - trigeminal G50.9
  - trochlear — *see* Strabismus, paralytic, fourth nerve
  - ulnar G56.2- ☑
- normokalemic periodic G72.3
- ocular H49.9
  - alternating G83.89
- oculofacial, congenital (Moebius) Q87.0
- oculomotor (external bilateral) (nerve) — *see* Strabismus, paralytic, third nerve
- palate (soft) K13.79
- paratrigeminal G50.9
- periodic (familial) (hyperkalemic) (hypokalemic) (myotonic) (normokalemic) (potassium sensitive) (secondary) G72.3
- peripheral autonomic nervous system — *see* Neuropathy, peripheral, autonomic
- peroneal (nerve) G57.3- ☑
- pharynx J39.2
- phrenic nerve G56.8- ☑
- plantar nerve(s) G57.6- ☑
- pneumogastric nerve G52.2
- poliomyelitis (current) — *see* Poliomyelitis, paralytic
- popliteal nerve G57.3- ☑
- postepileptic transitory G83.84
- progressive (atrophic) (bulbar) (spinal) G12.22
  - general A52.17
  - infantile acute — *see* Poliomyelitis, paralytic
  - supranuclear G23.1
- pseudobulbar G12.29
- pseudohypertrophic (muscle) G71.0
- psychogenic F44.4
- quadriceps G57.9- ☑
- quadriplegic — *see* Tetraplegia
- radial nerve G56.3- ☑
- rectus muscle (eye) H49.9
- recurrent isolated sleep G47.53

Paralysis, paralytic — *continued*
- respiratory (muscle) (system) (tract) R06.81
  - center NEC G93.89
  - congenital P28.89
  - newborn P28.89
- right side — *see* Hemiplegia
- saturnine T56.0 ☑
- sciatic nerve G57.0- ☑
- senile G83.9
- shaking — *see* Parkinsonism
- shoulder G56.9- ☑
- sleep, recurrent isolated G47.53
- spastic G83.9
  - cerebral — *see* Palsy, cerebral, spastic
  - congenital (cerebral) — *see* Palsy, cerebral, spastic
  - familial G11.4
  - hereditary G11.4
  - quadriplegic G80.0
  - syphilitic (spinal) A52.17
- sphincter, bladder — *see* Paralysis, bladder
- spinal (cord) G83.9
  - accessory nerve G52.8
  - acute — *see* Poliomyelitis, paralytic
  - ascending acute G61.0
  - atrophic (acute) (*see also* Poliomyelitis, paralytic)
    - spastic, syphilitic A52.17
  - congenital NEC — *see* Palsy, cerebral
  - hereditary G95.89
  - infantile — *see* Poliomyelitis, paralytic
  - progressive G12.21
  - sequelae NEC G83.89
- sternomastoid G52.8
- stomach K31.84
  - diabetic — *see* Diabetes, by type, with gastroparesis
  - nerve G52.2
    - diabetic — *see* Diabetes, by type, with gastroparesis
- stroke — *see* Infarct, brain
- subcapsularis G56.8- ☑
- supranuclear (progressive) G23.1
- sympathetic G90.8
  - cervical G90.09
  - nervous system — *see* Neuropathy, peripheral, autonomic
- syndrome G83.9
  - specified NEC G83.89
- syphilitic spastic spinal (Erb's) A52.17
- thigh G57.9- ☑
- throat J39.2
  - diphtheritic A36.0
  - muscle J39.2
- thrombotic (current episode) I63.3 ☑
- thumb G56.9- ☑
- tick — *see* Toxicity, venom, arthropod, specified NEC
- Todd's (postepileptic transitory paralysis) G83.84
- toe G57.6- ☑
- tongue K14.8
- transient R29.5
  - arm or leg NEC R29.818
    - traumatic NEC — *see* Injury, nerve
- trapezius G52.8
- traumatic, transient NEC — *see* Injury, nerve
- trembling — *see* Parkinsonism
- triceps brachii G56.9- ☑
- trigeminal nerve G50.9
- trochlear (nerve) — *see* Strabismus, paralytic, fourth nerve
- ulnar nerve G56.2- ☑
- upper limb — *see* Monoplegia, upper limb
- uremic N18.9 [G99.8]
- uveoparotitic D86.89
- uvula K13.79
  - postdiphtheritic A36.0
- vagus nerve G52.2
- vasomotor NEC G90.8
- velum palati K13.79
- vesical — *see* Paralysis, bladder
- vestibular nerve (except Vertigo) H93.3 ☑
- vocal cords J38.00
  - bilateral J38.02
  - unilateral J38.01
- Volkmann's (complicating trauma) T79.6 ☑
- wasting G12.29
- Weber's G46.3
- wrist G56.9- ☑

Paramedial urethrovesical orifice Q64.79

Paramenia N92.6
Parametritis (*see also* Disease, pelvis, inflammatory)
  N73.2
  acute N73.0
  complicating abortion — *see* Abortion, by type, complicated by, parametritis
Parametrium, parametric — *see* condition
Paramnesia — *see* Amnesia
Paramolar K00.1
Paramyloidosis E85.8
Paramyoclonus multiplex G25.3
Paramyotonia (congenita) G71.19
Parangi — *see* Yaws
Paranoia (querulans) F22
  senile F03 ☑
Paranoid
  dementia (senile) F03 ☑
    praecox — *see* Schizophrenia
  personality F60.0
  psychosis (climacteric) (involutional) (menopausal)
    F22
    psychogenic (acute) F23
    senile F03 ☑
  reaction (acute) F23
    chronic F22
  schizophrenia F20.0
  state (climacteric) (involutional) (menopausal) (simple)
    F22
    senile F03 ☑
  tendencies F60.0
  traits F60.0
  trends F60.0
  type, psychopathic personality F60.0
Paraparesis — *see* Paraplegia
Paraphasia R47.02
Paraphilia F65.9
Paraphimosis (congenital) N47.2
  chancroidal A57
Paraphrenia, paraphrenic (late) F22
  schizophrenia F20.0
Paraplegia (lower) G82.20
  ataxic — *see* Degeneration, combined, spinal cord
  complete G82.21
  congenital (cerebral) G80.8
    spastic G80.1
  familial spastic G11.4
  functional (hysterical) F44.4
  hereditary, spastic G11.4
  hysterical F44.4
  incomplete G82.22
  Pott's A18.01
  psychogenic F44.4
  spastic
    Erb's spinal, syphilitic A52.17
    hereditary G11.4
    tropical G04.1
  syphilitic (spastic) A52.17
  tropical spastic G04.1
Parapoxvirus B08.60
  specified NEC B08.69
Paraproteinemia D89.2
  benign (familial) D89.2
  monoclonal D47.2
  secondary to malignant disease D47.2
Parapsoriasis L41.9
  en plaques L41.4
  guttata L41.1
  large plaque L41.4
  retiform, retiformis L41.5
  small plaque L41.3
  specified NEC L41.8
  varioliformis (acuta) L41.0
Parasitic (*see also* condition)
  disease NEC B89
  stomatitis B37.0
  sycosis (beard) (scalp) B35.0
  twin Q89.4
Parasitism B89
  intestinal B82.9
  skin B88.9
  specified — *see* Infestation
Parasitophobia F40.218
Parasomnia G47.50
  due to
    alcohol
      abuse F10.182
      dependence F10.282

Parasomnia — *continued*
  due to — *continued*
    alcohol — *continued*
      use F10.982
    amphetamines
      abuse F15.182
      dependence F15.282
      use F15.982
    caffeine
      abuse F15.182
      dependence F15.282
      use F15.982
    cocaine
      abuse F14.182
      dependence F14.282
      use F14.982
    drug NEC
      abuse F19.182
      dependence F19.282
      use F19.982
    opioid
      abuse F11.182
      dependence F11.282
      use F11.982
    psychoactive substance NEC
      abuse F19.182
      dependence F19.282
      use F19.982
    sedative, hypnotic, or anxiolytic
      abuse F13.182
      dependence F13.282
      use F13.982
    stimulant NEC
      abuse F15.182
      dependence F15.282
      use F15.982
  in conditions classified elsewhere G47.54
  nonorganic origin F51.8
  organic G47.50
  specified NEC G47.59
Paraspadias Q54.9
Paraspasmus facialis G51.8
Parasuicide (attempt)
  history of (personal) Z91.5
    in family Z81.8
Parathyroid gland — *see* condition
Parathyroid tetany E20.9
Paratrachoma A74.0
Paratyphilitis — *see* Appendicitis
Paratyphoid (fever) — *see* Fever, paratyphoid
Paratyphus — *see* Fever, paratyphoid
Paraurethral duct Q64.79
  nonorganic origin F51.5
Paraurethritis (*see also* Urethritis)
  gonococcal (acute) (chronic) (with abscess) A54.1
Paravaccinia NEC B08.04
Paravaginitis — *see* Vaginitis
Parencephalitis (*see also* Encephalitis)
  sequelae G09
Parent-child conflict — *see* Conflict, parent-child
  estrangement NEC Z62.890
Paresis (*see also* Paralysis)
  accommodation — *see* Paresis, of accommodation
  Bernhardt's G57.1- ☑
  bladder (sphincter) (*see also* Paralysis, bladder)
    tabetic A52.17
  bowel, colon or intestine K56.0
  extrinsic muscle, eye H49.9
  general (progressive) (syphilitic) A52.17
    juvenile A50.45
  heart — *see* Failure, heart
  insane (syphilitic) A52.17
  juvenile (general) A50.45
  of accommodation H52.52- ☑
  peripheral progressive (idiopathic) G60.3
  pseudohypertrophic G71.0
  senile G83.9
  syphilitic (general) A52.17
    congenital A50.45
  vesical NEC N31.2
Paresthesia (*see also* Disturbance, sensation)
  Bernhardt G57.1- ☑
Paretic — *see* condition
Parinaud's
  conjunctivitis H10.89
  oculoglandular syndrome H10.89
  ophthalmoplegia H49.88- ☑

Parkinsonism (idiopathic) (primary) G20
  with neurogenic orthostatic hypotension (symptomatic) G90.3
  arteriosclerotic G21.4
  dementia G31.83 [F02.80]
    with behavioral disturbance G31.83 [F02.81]
  due to
    drugs NEC G21.19
      neuroleptic G21.11
  neuroleptic induced G21.11
  postencephalitic G21.3
  secondary G21.9
    due to
      arteriosclerosis G21.4
      drugs NEC G21.19
        neuroleptic G21.11
      encephalitis G21.3
      external agents NEC G21.2
      syphilis A52.19
    specified NEC G21.8
  syphilitic A52.19
  treatment-induced NEC G21.19
  vascular G21.4
Parkinson's disease, syndrome or tremor — *see* Parkinsonism
Parodontitis — *see* Periodontitis
Parodontosis K05.4
Paronychia (*see also* Cellulitis, digit)
  with lymphangitis — *see* Lymphangitis, acute, digit
  candidal (chronic) B37.2
  tuberculous (primary) A18.4
Parorexia (psychogenic) F50.8
Parosmia R43.1
  psychogenic F45.8
Parotid gland — *see* condition
Parotitis, parotiditis (allergic)(nonspecific toxic) (purulent) (septic) (suppurative) (*see also* Sialoadenitis)
  epidemic — *see* Mumps
  infectious — *see* Mumps
  postoperative K91.89
  surgical K91.89
Parrot fever A70
Parrot's disease (early congenital syphilitic pseudoparalysis) A50.02
Parry-Romberg syndrome G51.8
Parry's disease or syndrome E05.00
  with thyroid storm E05.01
Pars planitis — *see* Cyclitis
Parsonage (-Aldren)-Turner syndrome G54.5
Parson's disease (exophthalmic goiter) E05.00
  with thyroid storm E05.01
Particolored infant Q82.8
Parturition — *see* Delivery
Parulis K04.7
  with sinus K04.6
Parvovirus, as cause of disease classified elsewhere B97.6
Pasini and Pierini's atrophoderma L90.3
Passage
  false, urethra N36.5
  meconium (newborn) during delivery P03.82
  of sounds or bougies — *see* Attention to, artificial, opening
Passive — *see* condition
  smoking Z77.22
Pasteurella septica A28.0
Pasteurellosis — *see* Infection, Pasteurella
PAT (paroxysmal atrial tachycardia) I47.1
Patau's syndrome — *see* Trisomy, 13
Patches
  mucous (syphilitic) A51.39
    congenital A50.07
  smokers' (mouth) K13.24
Patellar — *see* condition
Patent (*see also* Imperfect, closure)
  canal of Nuck Q52.4
  cervix N88.3
  ductus arteriosus or Botallo's Q25.0
  foramen
    botalli Q21.1
    ovale Q21.1
  interauricular septum Q21.1
  interventricular septum Q21.0
  omphalomesenteric duct Q43.0
  os (uteri) — *see* Patent, cervix
  ostium secundum Q21.1
  urachus Q64.4

Patent — *continued*
vitelline duct Q43.0
Paterson (-Brown)(-Kelly) **syndrome or web** D50.1
Pathologic, pathological (*see also* condition)
asphyxia R09.01
fire-setting F63.1
gambling F63.0
ovum O02.0
resorption, tooth K03.3
stealing F63.2
Pathology (of) — *see* Disease
periradicular, associated with previous endodontic
treatment NEC M27.59
Pattern, sleep-wake, irregular G47.23
Patulous (*see also* Imperfect, closure (congenital))
alimentary tract Q45.8
lower Q43.8
upper Q40.8
eustachian tube H69.0- ☑
Pause, sinoatrial I49.5
Paxton's disease B36.2
Pearl(s)
enamel K00.2
Epstein's K09.8
Pearl-worker's disease — *see* Osteomyelitis, specified
type NEC
Pectenosis K62.4
Pectoral — *see* condition
Pectus
carinatum (congenital) Q67.7
acquired M95.4
rachitic sequelae (late effect) E64.3
excavatum (congenital) Q67.6
acquired M95.4
rachitic sequelae (late effect) E64.3
recurvatum (congenital) Q67.6
Pedatrophia E41
Pederosis F65.4
Pediculosis (infestation) B85.2
capitis (head-louse) (any site) B85.0
corporis (body-louse) (any site) B85.1
eyelid B85.0
mixed (classifiable to more than one of the titles B85.0-
B85.3) B85.4
pubis (pubic louse) (any site) B85.3
vestimenti B85.1
vulvae B85.3
Pediculus (infestation) — *see* Pediculosis
Pedophilia F65.4
Peg-shaped teeth K00.2
Pelade — *see* Alopecia, areata
Pelger-Huët anomaly or syndrome D72.0
Peliosis (rheumatica) D69.0
hepatis K76.4
with toxic liver disease K71.8
Pelizaeus-Merzbacher disease E75.29
Pellagra (alcoholic) (with polyneuropathy) E52
Pellagra-cerebellar-ataxia-renal aminoaciduria
syndrome E72.02
Pellegrini (-Stieda) **disease or syndrome** — *see* Bursitis,
tibial collateral
Pellizzi's syndrome E34.8
Pel's crisis A52.11
Pelvic (*see also* condition)
examination (periodic) (routine) Z01.419
with abnormal findings Z01.411
kidney, congenital Q63.2
Pelviolithiasis — *see* Calculus, kidney
Pelviperitonitis (*see also* Peritonitis, pelvic)
gonococcal A54.24
puerperal O85
Pelvis — *see* condition or type
Pemphigoid L12.9
benign, mucous membrane L12.1
bullous L12.0
cicatricial L12.1
juvenile L12.2
ocular L12.1
specified NEC L12.8
Pemphigus L10.9
benign familial (chronic) Q82.8
Brazilian L10.3
circinatus L13.0
conjunctiva L12.1
drug-induced L10.5
erythematosus L10.4
foliaceous L10.2

Pemphigus — *continued*
gangrenous — *see* Gangrene
neonatorum L01.03
ocular L12.1
paraneoplastic L10.81
specified NEC L10.89
syphilitic (congenital) A50.06
vegetans L10.1
vulgaris L10.0
wildfire L10.3
Pendred's syndrome E07.1
Pendulous
abdomen, in pregnancy — *see* Pregnancy, complicated by, abnormal, pelvic organs or tissues NEC
breast N64.89
Penetrating wound (*see also* Puncture)
with internal injury — *see* Injury, by site
eyeball — *see* Puncture, eyeball
orbit (with or without foreign body) — *see* Puncture,
orbit
uterus by instrument with or following ectopic or
molar pregnancy O08.6
Penicillosis B48.4
Penis — *see* condition
Penitis N48.29
Pentalogy of Fallot Q21.8
Pentasomy X syndrome Q97.1
Pentosuria (essential) E74.8
Percreta placenta - O43.23 ☑
Peregrinating patient — *see* Disorder, factitious
Perforation, perforated (nontraumatic) (of)
accidental during procedure (blood vessel) (nerve)
(organ) — *see* Complication, accidental puncture or laceration
antrum — *see* Sinusitis, maxillary
appendix K35.2
atrial septum, multiple Q21.1
attic, ear — *see* Perforation, tympanum, attic
bile duct (common) (hepatic) K83.2
cystic K82.2
bladder (urinary)
with or following ectopic or molar pregnancy O08.6
obstetrical trauma O71.5
traumatic S37.29 ☑
at delivery O71.5
bowel K63.1
with or following ectopic or molar pregnancy O08.6
newborn P78.0
obstetrical trauma O71.5
traumatic — *see* Laceration, intestine
broad ligament N83.8
with or following ectopic or molar pregnancy O08.6
obstetrical trauma O71.6
by
device, implant or graft (*see also* Complications,
by site and type, mechanical) T85.628 ☑
arterial graft NEC — *see* Complication, cardiovascular device, mechanical, vascular
breast (implant) T85.49 ☑
catheter NEC T85.698 ☑
cystostomy T83.090 ☑
dialysis (renal) T82.49 ☑
intraperitoneal T85.691 ☑
infusion NEC T82.594 ☑
spinal (epidural) (subdural) T85.690 ☑
electronic (electrode) (pulse generator) (stimulator)
bone T84.390 ☑
cardiac T82.199 ☑
electrode T82.190 ☑
pulse generator T82.191 ☑
specified type NEC T82.198 ☑
nervous system — *see* Complication, prosthetic device, mechanical, electronic
nervous system stimulator
urinary — *see* Complication, genitourinary,
device, urinary, mechanical
fixation, internal (orthopedic) NEC — *see*
Complication, fixation device, mechanical
gastrointestinal — *see* Complications, prosthetic device, mechanical, gastrointestinal
device
genital NEC T83.498 ☑
intrauterine contraceptive device T83.39 ☑
penile prosthesis T83.490 ☑
heart NEC — *see* Complication, cardiovascular
device, mechanical

Perforation, perforated — *continued*
by — *continued*
device, implant or graft (*see also* Complications, by
site and type, mechanical) — *continued*
joint prosthesis — *see* Complications, joint
prosthesis, mechanical, specified NEC, by
site
ocular NEC — *see* Complications, prosthetic
device, mechanical, ocular device
orthopedic NEC — *see* Complication, orthopedic, device, mechanical
specified NEC T85.628 ☑
urinary, indwelling T83.098 ☑
urinary NEC (*see also* Complication, genitourinary, device, urinary, mechanical)
graft T83.29 ☑
vascular NEC — *see* Complication, cardiovascular device, mechanical
ventricular intracranial shunt T85.09 ☑
foreign body left accidentally in operative wound
T81.539 ☑
instrument (any) during a procedure, accidental
— *see* Puncture, accidental complicating
surgery
cecum K35.2
cervix (uteri) N88.8
with or following ectopic or molar pregnancy O08.6
obstetrical trauma O71.3
colon K63.1
newborn P78.0
obstetrical trauma O71.5
traumatic — *see* Laceration, intestine, large
common duct (bile) K83.2
cornea (due to ulceration) — *see* Ulcer, cornea, perforated
cystic duct K82.2
diverticulum (intestine) K57.80
with bleeding K57.81
large intestine K57.20
with
bleeding K57.21
small intestine K57.40
with bleeding K57.41
small intestine K57.00
with
bleeding K57.01
large intestine K57.40
with bleeding K57.41
ear drum — *see* Perforation, tympanum
esophagus K22.3
ethmoidal sinus — *see* Sinusitis, ethmoidal
frontal sinus — *see* Sinusitis, frontal
gallbladder K82.2
heart valve — *see* Endocarditis
ileum K63.1
newborn P78.0
obstetrical trauma O71.5
traumatic — *see* Laceration, intestine, small
instrumental, surgical (accidental) (blood vessel)
(nerve) (organ) — *see* Puncture, accidental
complicating surgery
intestine NEC K63.1
with ectopic or molar pregnancy O08.6
newborn P78.0
obstetrical trauma O71.5
traumatic — *see* Laceration, intestine
ulcerative NEC K63.1
newborn P78.0
jejunum, jejunal K63.1
obstetrical trauma O71.5
traumatic — *see* Laceration, intestine, small
ulcer — *see* Ulcer, gastrojejunal, with perforation
joint prosthesis — *see* Complications, joint prosthesis,
mechanical, specified NEC, by site
mastoid (antrum) (cell) — *see* Disorder, mastoid,
specified NEC
maxillary sinus — *see* Sinusitis, maxillary
membrana tympani — *see* Perforation, tympanum
nasal
septum J34.89
congenital Q30.3
syphilitic A52.73
sinus J34.89
congenital Q30.8
due to sinusitis — *see* Sinusitis
palate (*see also* Cleft, palate) Q35.9
syphilitic A52.79

☑ **Additional Character Required** — Refer to the Tabular List for Character Selection   ▽ **Subterms under main terms may continue to next column or page**

Perforation, perforated — *continued*
  palatine vault (*see also* Cleft, palate, hard) Q35.1
    syphilitic A52.79
      congenital A50.59
  pars flaccida (ear drum) — *see* Perforation, tympanum, attic
  pelvic
    floor S31.030 ☑
      with
        ectopic or molar pregnancy O08.6
        penetration into retroperitoneal space S31.031 ☑
        retained foreign body S31.040 ☑
          with penetration into retroperitoneal space S31.041 ☑
      following ectopic or molar pregnancy O08.6
      obstetrical trauma O70.1
    organ S37.99 ☑
      adrenal gland S37.818 ☑
      bladder — *see* Perforation, bladder
      fallopian tube S37.599 ☑
        bilateral S37.592 ☑
        unilateral S37.591 ☑
      kidney S37.09- ☑
      obstetrical trauma O71.5
      ovary S37.499 ☑
        bilateral S37.492 ☑
        unilateral S37.491 ☑
      prostate S37.828 ☑
      specified organ NEC S37.898 ☑
      ureter — *see* Perforation, ureter
      urethra — *see* Perforation, urethra
      uterus — *see* Perforation, uterus
  perineum — *see* Laceration, perineum
  pharynx J39.2
  rectum K63.1
    newborn P78.0
    obstetrical trauma O71.5
    traumatic S36.63 ☑
  root canal space due to endodontic treatment M27.51
  sigmoid K63.1
    newborn P78.0
    obstetrical trauma O71.5
    traumatic S36.533 ☑
  sinus (accessory) (chronic) (nasal) J34.89
  sphenoidal sinus — *see* Sinusitis, sphenoidal
  surgical (accidental) (by instrument) (blood vessel) (nerve) (organ) — *see* Puncture, accidental complicating surgery
  traumatic
    external — *see* Puncture
    eye — *see* Puncture, eyeball
    internal organ — *see* Injury, by site
  tympanum, tympanic (membrane) (persistent post-traumatic) (postinflammatory) H72.9- ☑
    attic H72.1- ☑
      multiple — *see* Perforation, tympanum, multiple
      total — *see* Perforation, tympanum, total
    central H72.0- ☑
      multiple — *see* Perforation, tympanum, multiple
      total — *see* Perforation, tympanum, total
    marginal NEC — *see* subcategory H72.2 ☑
    multiple H72.81- ☑
    pars flaccida — *see* Perforation, tympanum, attic
    total H72.82- ☑
    traumatic, current episode S09.2- ☑
  typhoid, gastrointestinal — *see* Typhoid
  ulcer — *see* Ulcer, by site, with perforation
  ureter N28.89
    traumatic S37.19 ☑
  urethra N36.8
    with ectopic or molar pregnancy O08.6
    following ectopic or molar pregnancy O08.6
    obstetrical trauma O71.5
    traumatic S37.39 ☑
      at delivery O71.5
  uterus
    with ectopic or molar pregnancy O08.6
    by intrauterine contraceptive device T83.39 ☑
    following ectopic or molar pregnancy O08.6
    obstetrical trauma O71.1
    traumatic S37.69 ☑
      obstetric O71.1
  uvula K13.79
    syphilitic A52.79

Perforation, perforated — *continued*
  vagina O71.4
    obstetrical trauma O71.4
    other trauma — *see* Puncture, vagina
Periadenitis mucosa necrotica recurrens K12.0
Periappendicitis (acute) — *see* Appendicitis
Periarteritis nodosa (disseminated) (infectious) (necrotizing) M30.0
Periarthritis (joint) (*see also* Enthesopathy)
  Duplay's M75.0-
  gonococcal A54.42
  humeroscapularis — *see* Capsulitis, adhesive
  scapulohumeral — *see* Capsulitis, adhesive
  shoulder — *see* Capsulitis, adhesive
  wrist M77.2- ☑
Periarthrosis (angioneural) — *see* Enthesopathy
Pericapsulitis, adhesive (shoulder) — *see* Capsulitis, adhesive
Pericarditis (with decompensation) (with effusion) I31.9
  with rheumatic fever (conditions in I00)
    active — *see* Pericarditis, rheumatic
    inactive or quiescent I09.2
  acute (hemorrhagic) (nonrheumatic) (Sicca) I30.9
    with chorea (acute) (rheumatic) (Sydenham's) I02.0
    benign I30.8
    nonspecific I30.0
    rheumatic I01.0
      with chorea (acute) (Sydenham's) I02.0
  adhesive or adherent (chronic) (external) (internal) I31.0
    acute — *see* Pericarditis, acute
    rheumatic I09.2
  bacterial (acute) (subacute) (with serous or seropurulent effusion) I30.1
  calcareous I31.1
  cholesterol (chronic) I31.8
    acute I30.9
  chronic (nonrheumatic) I31.9
    rheumatic I09.2
  constrictive (chronic) I31.1
  coxsackie B33.23
  fibrinocaseous (tuberculous) A18.84
  fibrinopurulent I30.1
  fibrinous I30.8
  fibrous I31.0
  gonococcal A54.83
  idiopathic I30.0
  in systemic lupus erythematosus M32.12
  infective I30.1
  meningococcal A39.53
  neoplastic (chronic) I31.8
    acute I30.9
  obliterans, obliterating I31.0
  plastic I31.0
  pneumococcal I30.1
  postinfarction I24.1
  purulent I30.1
  rheumatic (active) (acute) (with effusion) (with pneumonia) I01.0
    with chorea (acute) (rheumatic) (Sydenham's) I02.0
    chronic or inactive (with chorea) I09.2
  rheumatoid — *see* Rheumatoid, carditis
  septic I30.1
  serofibrinous I30.8
  staphylococcal I30.1
  streptococcal I30.1
  suppurative I30.1
  syphilitic A52.06
  tuberculous A18.84
  uremic N18.9 [I32]
  viral I30.1
Pericardium, pericardial — *see* condition
Pericellulitis — *see* Cellulitis
Pericementitis (chronic) (suppurative) (*see also* Periodontitis)
  acute K05.20
    generalized K05.22
    localized K05.21
Perichondritis
  auricle — *see* Perichondritis, ear
  bronchus J98.09
  ear (external) H61.00- ☑
    acute H61.01- ☑
    chronic H61.02- ☑
  external auditory canal — *see* Perichondritis, ear
  larynx J38.7
    syphilitic A52.73
    typhoid A01.09

Perichondritis — *continued*
  nose J34.89
  pinna — *see* Perichondritis, ear
  trachea J39.8
Periclasia K05.4
Pericoronitis — *see* Periodontitis
Pericystitis N30.90
  with hematuria N30.91
Peridiverticulitis (intestine) K57.92
  cecum — *see* Diverticulitis, intestine, large
  colon — *see* Diverticulitis, intestine, large
  duodenum — *see* Diverticulitis, intestine, small
  intestine — *see* Diverticulitis, intestine
  jejunum — *see* Diverticulitis, intestine, small
  rectosigmoid — *see* Diverticulitis, intestine, large
  rectum — *see* Diverticulitis, intestine, large
  sigmoid — *see* Diverticulitis, intestine, large
Periendocarditis — *see* Endocarditis
Periepididymitis N45.1
Perifolliculitis L01.02
  abscedens, caput, scalp L66.3
  capitis, abscedens (et suffodiens) L66.3
  superficial pustular L01.02
Perihepatitis K65.8
Perilabyrinthitis (acute) — *see* subcategory H83.0 ☑
Perimeningitis — *see* Meningitis
Perimetritis — *see* Endometritis
Perimetrosalpingitis — *see* Salpingo-oophoritis
Perineocele N81.81
Perinephric, perinephritic — *see* condition
Perinephritis (*see also* Infection, kidney)
  purulent — *see* Abscess, kidney
Perineum, perineal — *see* condition
Perineuritis NEC — *see* Neuralgia
Periodic — *see* condition
Periodontitis (chronic) (complex) (compound) (local) (simplex) K05.30
  acute K05.20
    generalized K05.22
    localized K05.21
  apical K04.5
    acute (pulpal origin) K04.4
  generalized K05.32
  localized K05.31
Periodontoclasia K05.4
Periodontosis (juvenile) K05.4
Periods (*see also* Menstruation)
  heavy N92.0
  irregular N92.6
  shortened intervals (irregular) N92.1
Perionychia (*see also* Cellulitis, digit)
  with lymphangitis — *see* Lymphangitis, acute, digit
Perioophoritis — *see* Salpingo-oophoritis
Periorchitis N45.2
Periosteum, periosteal — *see* condition
Periostitis (albuminosa) (circumscribed) (diffuse) (infective) (monomelic) (*see also* Osteomyelitis)
  alveolar M27.3
  alveolodental M27.3
  dental M27.3
  gonorrheal A54.43
  jaw (lower) (upper) M27.2
  orbit H05.03- ☑
  syphilitic A52.77
    congenital (early) A50.02 [M90.80]
    secondary A51.46
  tuberculous — *see* Tuberculosis, bone
  yaws (hypertrophic) (early) (late) A66.6 [M90.80]
Periostosis (hyperplastic) (*see also* Disorder, bone, specified type NEC)
  with osteomyelitis — *see* Osteomyelitis, specified type NEC
Peripartum
  cardiomyopathy O90.3
Periphlebitis — *see* Phlebitis
Periproctitis K62.89
Periprostatitis — *see* Prostatitis
Perirectal — *see* condition
Perirenal — *see* condition
Perisalpingitis — *see* Salpingo-oophoritis
Perisplenitis (infectional) D73.89
Peristalsis, visible or reversed R19.2
Peritendinitis — *see* Enthesopathy
Peritoneum, peritoneal — *see* condition
Peritonitis (adhesive) (bacterial) (fibrinous) (hemorrhagic) (idiopathic) (localized) (perforative) (primary) (with adhesions) (with effusion) K65.9

Peritonitis — continued
  with or following
    abscess K65.1
    appendicitis K35.2
      with perforation or rupture K35.2
      generalized K35.2
      localized K35.3
    diverticular disease (intestine) K57.80
      with bleeding K57.81
      ectopic or molar pregnancy O08.0
      large intestine K57.20
        with
          bleeding K57.21
          small intestine K57.40
            with bleeding K57.41
      small intestine K57.00
        with
          bleeding K57.01
          large intestine K57.40
            with bleeding K57.41
  acute (generalized) K65.0
  aseptic T81.61 ☑
  bile, biliary K65.3
  chemical T81.61 ☑
  chlamydial A74.81
  chronic proliferative K65.8
  complicating abortion — see Abortion, by type, complicated by, pelvic peritonitis
  congenital P78.1
  diaphragmatic K65.0
  diffuse K65.0
  diphtheritic A36.89
  disseminated K65.0
  due to
    bile K65.3
    foreign
      body or object accidentally left during a procedure (instrument) (sponge) (swab) T81.599 ☑
      substance accidentally left during a procedure (chemical) (powder) (talc) T81.61 ☑
    talc T81.61 ☑
    urine K65.8
  eosinophilic K65.8
    acute K65.0
  fibrocaseous (tuberculous) A18.31
  fibropurulent K65.0
  following ectopic or molar pregnancy O08.0
  general (ized) K65.0
  gonococcal A54.85
  meconium (newborn) P78.0
  neonatal P78.1
    meconium P78.0
  pancreatic K65.0
  paroxysmal, familial E85.0
    benign E85.0
  pelvic
    female N73.5
      acute N73.3
      chronic N73.4
        with adhesions N73.6
    male K65.0
  periodic, familial E85.0
  proliferative, chronic K65.8
  puerperal, postpartum, childbirth O85
  purulent K65.0
  septic K65.0
  specified NEC K65.8
  spontaneous bacterial K65.2
  subdiaphragmatic K65.0
  subphrenic K65.0
  suppurative K65.0
  syphilitic A52.74
    congenital (early) A50.08 [K67]
  talc T81.61 ☑
  tuberculous A18.31
  urine K65.8
Peritonsillar — see condition
Peritonsillitis J36
Perityphlitis K37
Periurethral — see condition
Periurethritis (gangrenous) — see Urethritis
Periuterine — see condition
Perivaginitis — see Vaginitis
Perivasculitis, retinal H35.06- ☑
Perivasitis (chronic) N49.1
Perivesiculitis (seminal) — see Vesiculitis

Perlèche NEC K13.0
  due to
    candidiasis B37.83
    moniliasis B37.83
    riboflavin deficiency E53.0
    vitamin B2 (riboflavin) deficiency E53.0
Pernicious — see condition
Pernio, perniosis T69.1 ☑
Perpetrator (of abuse) — see Index to External Causes of Injury, Perpetrator
Persecution
  delusion F22
  social Z60.5
Perseveration (tonic) R48.8
Persistence, persistent (congenital)
  anal membrane Q42.3
    with fistula Q42.2
  arteria stapedia Q16.3
  atrioventricular canal Q21.2
  branchial cleft Q18.0
  bulbus cordis in left ventricle Q21.8
  canal of Cloquet Q14.0
  capsule (opaque) Q12.8
  cilioretinal artery or vein Q14.8
  cloaca Q43.7
  communication — see Fistula, congenital
  convolutions
    aortic arch Q25.4
    fallopian tube Q50.6
    oviduct Q50.6
    uterine tube Q50.6
  double aortic arch Q25.4
  ductus arteriosus (Botalli) Q25.0
  fetal
    circulation P29.3
    form of cervix (uteri) Q51.828
    hemoglobin, hereditary (HPFH) D56.4
  foramen
    Botalli Q21.1
    ovale Q21.1
  Gartner's duct Q52.4
  hemoglobin, fetal (hereditary) (HPFH) D56.4
  hyaloid
    artery (generally incomplete) Q14.0
    system Q14.8
  hymen, in pregnancy or childbirth — see Pregnancy, complicated by, abnormal, vulva
  lanugo Q84.2
  left
    posterior cardinal vein Q26.8
    root with right arch of aorta Q25.4
    superior vena cava Q26.1
  Meckel's diverticulum Q43.0
    malignant — see Table of Neoplasms, small intestine, malignant
  mucosal disease (middle ear) — see Otitis, media, suppurative, chronic, tubotympanic
  nail(s), anomalous Q84.6
  omphalomesenteric duct Q43.0
  organ or site not listed — see Anomaly, by site
  ostium
    atrioventriculare commune Q21.2
    primum Q21.2
    secundum Q21.1
  ovarian rests in fallopian tube Q50.6
  pancreatic tissue in intestinal tract Q43.8
  primary (deciduous)
    teeth K00.6
    vitreous hyperplasia Q14.0
  pupillary membrane Q13.89
  rhesus (Rh) titer — see Complication(s), transfusion, incompatibility reaction, Rh (factor)
  right aortic arch Q25.4
  sinus
    urogenitalis
      female Q52.8
      male Q55.8
    venosus with imperfect incorporation in right auricle Q26.8
  thymus (gland) (hyperplasia) E32.0
  thyroglossal duct Q89.2
  thyrolingual duct Q89.2
  truncus arteriosus or communis Q20.0
  tunica vasculosa lentis Q12.2
  umbilical sinus Q64.4
  urachus Q64.4
  vitelline duct Q43.0

Person (with)
  admitted for clinical research, as a control subject (normal comparison) (participant) Z00.6
  awaiting admission to adequate facility elsewhere Z75.1
  concern (normal) about sick person in family Z63.6
  consulting on behalf of another Z71.0
  feigning illness Z76.5
  living (in)
    without
      adequate housing (heating) (space) Z59.1
      housing (permanent) (temporary) Z59.0
      person able to render necessary care Z74.2
      shelter Z59.1
    alone Z60.2
    boarding school Z59.3
    residential institution Z59.3
  on waiting list Z75.1
  sick or handicapped in family Z63.6
Personality (disorder) F60.9
  accentuation of traits (type A pattern) Z73.1
  affective F34.0
  aggressive F60.3
  amoral F60.2
  anacastic, anankastic F60.5
  antisocial F60.2
  anxious F60.6
  asocial F60.2
  asthenic F60.7
  avoidant F60.6
  borderline F60.3
  change due to organic condition (enduring) F07.0
  compulsive F60.5
  cycloid F34.0
  cyclothymic F34.0
  dependent F60.7
  depressive F34.1
  dissocial F60.2
  dual F44.81
  eccentric F60.89
  emotionally unstable F60.3
  expansive paranoid F60.0
  explosive F60.3
  fanatic F60.0
  haltlose type F60.89
  histrionic F60.4
  hyperthymic F34.0
  hypothymic F34.1
  hysterical F60.4
  immature F60.89
  inadequate F60.7
  labile (emotional) F60.3
  mixed (nonspecific) F60.81
  morally defective F60.2
  multiple F44.81
  narcissistic F60.81
  obsessional F60.5
  obsessive (-compulsive) F60.5
  organic F07.0
  overconscientious F60.5
  paranoid F60.0
  passive (-dependent) F60.7
  passive-aggressive F60.89
  pathologic F60.9
  pattern defect or disturbance F60.9
  pseudopsychopathic (organic) F07.0
  pseudoretarded (organic) F07.0
  psychoinfantile F60.4
  psychoneurotic NEC F60.89
  psychopathic F60.2
  querulant F60.0
  sadistic F60.89
  schizoid F60.1
  self-defeating F60.7
  sensitive paranoid F60.0
  sociopathic (amoral) (antisocial) (asocial) (dissocial) F60.2
  specified NEC F60.89
  type A Z73.1
  unstable (emotional) F60.3
Perthes' disease — see Legg-Calvé-Perthes disease
Pertussis (see also Whooping cough) A37.90
Perversion, perverted
  appetite F50.8
    psychogenic F50.8
  function
    pituitary gland E23.2
      posterior lobe E22.2

Perversion, perverted — *continued*
  sense of smell and taste R43.8
    psychogenic F45.8
  sexual — *see* Deviation, sexual
Pervious, congenital (*see also* Imperfect, closure)
  ductus arteriosus Q25.0
Pes (congenital) (*see also* Talipes)
  acquired (*see also* Deformity, limb, foot, specified NEC)
    planus — *see* Deformity, limb, flat foot
  adductus Q66.89
  cavus Q66.7
  deformity NEC, acquired — *see* Deformity, limb, foot, specified NEC
  planus (acquired) (any degree) (*see also* Deformity, limb, flat foot)
    rachitic sequelae (late effect) E64.3
  valgus Q66.6
Pest, pestis — *see* Plague
Petechia, petechiae R23.3
  newborn P54.5
Petechial typhus A75.9
Peter's anomaly Q13.4
Petit mal seizure — *see* Epilepsy, generalized, specified NEC
Petit's hernia — *see* Hernia, abdomen, specified site NEC
Petrellidosis B48.2
Petrositis H70.20- ☑
  acute H70.21- ☑
  chronic H70.22- ☑
Peutz-Jeghers disease or syndrome Q85.8
Peyronie's disease N48.6
Pfeiffer's disease — *see* Mononucleosis, infectious
Phagedena (dry) (moist) (sloughing) (*see also* Gangrene)
  geometric L88
  penis N48.29
  tropical — *see* Ulcer, skin
  vulva N76.6
Phagedenic — *see* condition
Phakoma H35.89
Phakomatosis (*see also* specific eponymous syndromes) Q85.9
  Bourneville's Q85.1
  specified NEC Q85.8
Phantom limb syndrome (without pain) G54.7
  with pain G54.6
Pharyngeal pouch syndrome D82.1
Pharyngitis (acute) (catarrhal) (gangrenous) (infective) (malignant) (membranous) (phlegmonous) (pseudomembranous) (simple) (subacute) (suppurative) (ulcerative) (viral) J02.9
  with influenza, flu, or grippe — *see* Influenza, with, pharyngitis
  aphthous B08.5
  atrophic J31.2
  chlamydial A56.4
  chronic (atrophic) (granular) (hypertrophic) J31.2
  coxsackievirus B08.5
  diphtheritic A36.0
  enteroviral vesicular B08.5
  follicular (chronic) J31.2
  fusospirochetal A69.1
  gonococcal A54.5
  granular (chronic) J31.2
  herpesviral B00.2
  hypertrophic J31.2
  infectional, chronic J31.2
  influenzal — *see* Influenza, with, respiratory manifestations NEC
  lymphonodular, acute (enteroviral) B08.8
  pneumococcal J02.8
  purulent J02.9
  putrid J02.9
  septic J02.0
  sicca J31.2
  specified organism NEC J02.8
  staphylococcal J02.8
  streptococcal J02.0
  syphilitic, congenital (early) A50.03
  tuberculous A15.8
  vesicular, enteroviral B08.5
  viral NEC J02.8
Pharyngoconjunctivitis, viral B30.2
Pharyngolaryngitis (acute) J06.0
  chronic J37.0
Pharyngoplegia J39.2
Pharyngotonsillitis, herpesviral B00.2

Pharyngotracheitis, chronic J42
Pharynx, pharyngeal — *see* condition
Phenomenon
  Arthus' — *see* Arthus' phenomenon
  jaw-winking Q07.8
  lupus erythematosus (LE) cell M32.9
  Raynaud's (secondary) I73.00
    with gangrene I73.01
  vasomotor R55
  vasospastic I73.9
  vasovagal R55
  Wenckebach's I44.1
Phenylketonuria E70.1
  classical E70.0
  maternal E70.1
Pheochromoblastoma
  specified site — *see* Neoplasm, malignant, by site
  unspecified site C74.10
Pheochromocytoma
  malignant
    specified site — *see* Neoplasm, malignant, by site
    unspecified site C74.10
  specified site — *see* Neoplasm, benign, by site
  unspecified site D35.00
Pheohyphomycosis — *see* Chromomycosis
Pheomycosis — *see* Chromomycosis
Phimosis (congenital) (due to infection) N47.1
  chancroidal A57
Phlebectasia (*see also* Varix)
  congenital Q27.4
Phlebitis (infective) (pyemic) (septic) (suppurative) I80.9
  antepartum — *see* Thrombophlebitis, antepartum
  blue — *see* Phlebitis, leg, deep
  breast, superficial I80.8
  cavernous (venous) sinus — *see* Phlebitis, intracranial (venous) sinus
  cerebral (venous) sinus — *see* Phlebitis, intracranial (venous) sinus
  chest wall, superficial I80.8
  cranial (venous) sinus — *see* Phlebitis, intracranial (venous) sinus
  deep (vessels) — *see* Phlebitis, leg, deep
  due to implanted device — *see* Complications, by site and type, specified NEC
  during or resulting from a procedure T81.72 ☑
  femoral vein (superficial) I80.1- ☑
  femoropopliteal vein I80.0- ☑
  gestational — *see* Phlebopathy, gestational
  hepatic veins I80.8
  iliofemoral — *see* Phlebitis, femoral vein
  intracranial (venous) sinus (any) G08
    nonpyogenic I67.6
  intraspinal venous sinuses and veins G08
    nonpyogenic G95.19
  lateral (venous) sinus — *see* Phlebitis, intracranial (venous) sinus
  leg I80.3
    antepartum — *see* Thrombophlebitis, antepartum
    deep (vessels) NEC I80.20- ☑
      iliac I80.21- ☑
      popliteal vein I80.22- ☑
      specified vessel NEC I80.29- ☑
      tibial vein I80.23- ☑
    femoral vein (superficial) I80.1- ☑
    superficial (vessels) I80.0- ☑
  longitudinal sinus — *see* Phlebitis, intracranial (venous) sinus
  lower limb — *see* Phlebitis, leg
  migrans, migrating (superficial) I82.1
  pelvic
    with ectopic or molar pregnancy O08.0
    following ectopic or molar pregnancy O08.0
    puerperal, postpartum O87.1
  popliteal vein — *see* Phlebitis, leg, deep, popliteal
  portal (vein) K75.1
  postoperative T81.72 ☑
  pregnancy — *see* Thrombophlebitis, antepartum
  puerperal, postpartum, childbirth O87.0
    deep O87.1
    pelvic O87.1
    superficial O87.0
  retina — *see* Vasculitis, retina
  saphenous (accessory) (great) (long) (small) — *see* Phlebitis, leg, superficial
  sinus (meninges) — *see* Phlebitis, intracranial (venous) sinus
  specified site NEC I80.8

Phlebitis — *continued*
  syphilitic A52.09
  tibial vein — *see* Phlebitis, leg, deep, tibial
  ulcerative I80.9
    leg — *see* Phlebitis, leg
  umbilicus I80.8
  uterus (septic) — *see* Endometritis
  varicose (leg) (lower limb) — *see* Varix, leg, with, inflammation
Phlebofibrosis I87.8
Phleboliths I87.8
Phlebopathy,
  gestational O22.9- ☑
  puerperal O87.9
Phlebosclerosis I87.8
Phlebothrombosis (*see also* Thrombosis)
  antepartum — *see* Thrombophlebitis, antepartum
  pregnancy — *see* Thrombophlebitis, antepartum
  puerperal — *see* Thrombophlebitis, puerperal
Phlebotomus fever A93.1
Phlegmasia
  alba dolens O87.1
    nonpuerperal — *see* Phlebitis, femoral vein
  cerulea dolens — *see* Phlebitis, leg, deep
Phlegmon — *see* Abscess
Phlegmonous — *see* condition
Phlyctenulosis (allergic) (keratoconjunctivitis) (nontuberculous) (*see also* Keratoconjunctivitis)
  cornea — *see* Keratoconjunctivitis
  tuberculous A18.52
Phobia, phobic F40.9
  animal F40.218
    spiders F40.210
  examination F40.298
  reaction F40.9
  simple F40.298
  social F40.10
    generalized F40.11
  specific (isolated) F40.298
    animal F40.218
      spiders F40.210
    blood F40.230
    injection F40.231
    injury F40.233
    men F40.290
    natural environment F40.228
      thunderstorms F40.220
    situational F40.248
      bridges F40.242
      closed in spaces F40.240
      flying F40.243
      heights F40.241
    specified focus NEC F40.298
    transfusion F40.231
    women F40.291
  specified NEC F40.8
    medical care NEC F40.232
  state F40.9
Phocas' disease — *see* Mastopathy, cystic
Phocomelia Q73.1
  lower limb — *see* Agenesis, leg, with foot present
  upper limb — *see* Agenesis, arm, with hand present
Phoria H50.50
Phosphate-losing tubular disorder N25.0
Phosphatemia E83.39
Phosphaturia E83.39
Photodermatitis (sun) L56.8
  chronic L57.8
  due to drug L56.8
  light other than sun L59.8
Photokeratitis H16.13- ☑
Photophobia H53.14- ☑
Photophthalmia — *see* Photokeratitis
Photopsia H53.19
Photoretinitis — *see* Retinopathy, solar
Photosensitivity, photosensitization (sun) skin L56.8
  light other than sun L59.8
Phrenitis — *see* Encephalitis
Phrynoderma (vitamin A deficiency) E50.8
Phthiriasis (pubis) B85.3
  with any infestation classifiable to B85.0-B85.2 B85.4
Phthirus infestation — *see* Phthiriasis
Phthisis (*see also* Tuberculosis)
  bulbi (infectional) — *see* Disorder, globe, degenerated condition, atrophy
  eyeball (due to infection) — *see* Disorder, globe, degenerated condition, atrophy

Index

Phycomycosis — Pneumocephalus

Phycomycosis — *see* Zygomycosis
Physalopteriasis B81.8
Physical restraint status Z78.1
Phytobezoar T18.9 ☑
  intestine T18.3 ☑
  stomach T18.2 ☑
Pian — *see* Yaws
Pianoma A66.1
Pica F50.8
  in adults F50.8
  infant or child F98.3
Picking, nose F98.8
Pick-Niemann disease — *see* Niemann-Pick disease or
  syndrome
Pick's
  cerebral atrophy G31.01 [F02.80]
    with behavioral disturbance G31.01 [F02.81]
  disease or syndrome (brain) G31.01 [F02.80]
    with behavioral disturbance G31.01 [F02.81]
Pickwickian syndrome E66.2
Piebaldism E70.39
Piedra (beard) (scalp) B36.8
  black B36.3
  white B36.2
Pierre Robin deformity or syndrome Q87.0
Pierson's disease or osteochondrosis M91.0
Pig-bel A05.2
Pigeon
  breast or chest (acquired) M95.4
    congenital Q67.7
    rachitic sequelae (late effect) E64.3
  breeder's disease or lung J67.2
  fancier's disease or lung J67.2
  toe — *see* Deformity, toe, specified NEC
Pigmentation (abnormal) (anomaly) L81.9
  conjunctiva H11.13- ☑
  cornea (anterior) H18.01- ☑
    posterior H18.05- ☑
    stromal H18.06- ☑
  diminished melanin formation NEC L81.6
  iron L81.8
  lids, congenital Q82.8
  limbus corneae — *see* Pigmentation, cornea
  metals L81.8
  optic papilla, congenital Q14.2
  retina, congenital (grouped) (nevoid) Q14.1
  scrotum, congenital Q82.8
  tattoo L81.8
Piles (*see also* Hemorrhoids) K64.9
Pili
  annulati or torti (congenital) Q84.1
  incarnati L73.1
Pill roller hand (intrinsic) — *see* Parkinsonism
Pilomatrixoma — *see* Neoplasm, skin, benign
  malignant — *see* Neoplasm, skin, malignant
Pilonidal — *see* condition
Pimple R23.8
Pinched nerve — *see* Neuropathy, entrapment
Pindborg tumor — *see* Cyst, calcifying odontogenic
Pineal body or gland — *see* condition
Pinealoblastoma C75.3
Pinealoma D44.5
  malignant C75.3
Pineoblastoma C75.3
Pineocytoma D44.5
Pinguecula H11.15- ☑
Pingueculitis H10.81- ☑
Pinhole meatus (*see also* Stricture, urethra) N35.9
Pink
  disease — *see* subcategory T56.1 ☑
  eye — *see* Conjunctivitis, acute, mucopurulent
Pinkus' disease (lichen nitidus) L44.1
Pinpoint
  meatus — *see* Stricture, urethra
  os (uteri) — *see* Stricture, cervix
Pins and needles R20.2
Pinta A67.9
  cardiovascular lesions A67.2
  chancre (primary) A67.0
  erythematous plaques A67.1
  hyperchromic lesions A67.1
  hyperkeratosis A67.1
  lesions A67.9
    cardiovascular A67.2
    hyperchromic A67.1
    intermediate A67.1
    late A67.2

Pinta — *continued*
  lesions — *continued*
    mixed A67.3
    primary A67.0
    skin (achromic) (cicatricial) (dyschromic) A67.2
      hyperchromic A67.1
      mixed (achromic and hyperchromic) A67.3
  papule (primary) A67.0
  skin lesions (achromic) (cicatricial) (dyschromic) A67.2
    hyperchromic A67.1
    mixed (achromic and hyperchromic) A67.3
  vitiligo A67.2
Pintids A67.1
Pinworm (disease) (infection) (infestation) B80
Piroplasmosis B60.0
Pistol wound — *see* Gunshot wound
Pitchers' elbow — *see* Derangement, joint, specified
  type NEC, elbow
Pithecoid pelvis Q74.2
  with disproportion (fetopelvic) O33.0
    causing obstructed labor O65.0
Pithiatism F48.8
Pitted — *see* Pitting
Pitting (*see also* Edema) R60.9
  lip R60.0
  nail L60.8
  teeth K00.4
Pituitary gland — *see* condition
Pituitary-snuff-taker's disease J67.8
Pityriasis (capitis) L21.0
  alba L30.5
  circinata (et maculata) L42
  furfuracea L21.0
  Hebra's L26
  lichenoides L41.0
    chronica L41.1
    et varioliformis (acuta) L41.0
  maculata (et circinata) L30.5
  nigra B36.1
  pilaris, Hebra's L44.0
  rosea L42
  rotunda L44.8
  rubra (Hebra) pilaris L44.0
  simplex L30.5
  specified type NEC L30.5
  streptogenes L30.5
  versicolor (scrotal) B36.0
Placenta, placental — *see* Pregnancy, complicated by
  (care of) (management affected by), specified condition
Placentitis O41.14- ☑
Plagiocephaly Q67.3
Plague A20.9
  abortive A20.8
  ambulatory A20.8
  asymptomatic A20.8
  bubonic A20.0
  cellulocutaneous A20.1
  cutaneobubonic A20.1
  lymphatic gland A20.0
  meningitis A20.3
  pharyngeal A20.8
  pneumonic (primary) (secondary) A20.2
  pulmonary, pulmonic A20.2
  septicemic A20.7
  tonsillar A20.8
    septicemic A20.7
Planning, family
  contraception Z30.9
  procreation Z31.69
Plaque(s)
  artery, arterial — *see* Arteriosclerosis
  calcareous — *see* Calcification
  coronary, lipid rich I25.83
  epicardial I31.8
  erythematous, of pinta A67.1
  Hollenhorst's — *see* Occlusion, artery, retina
  lipid rich, coronary I25.83
  pleural (without asbestos) J92.9
    with asbestos J92.0
  tongue K13.29
Plasmacytoma C90.3- ☑
  extramedullary C90.2- ☑
  medullary C90.0- ☑
  solitary C90.3- ☑
Plasmacytopenia D72.818
Plasmacytosis D72.822
Plaster ulcer — *see* Ulcer, pressure, by site

Plateau iris syndrome (post-iridectomy) (postprocedu-
  ral) (without glaucoma) H21.82
  with glaucoma H40.22- ☑
Platybasia Q75.8
Platyonychia (congenital) Q84.6
  acquired L60.8
Platypelloid pelvis M95.5
  with disproportion (fetopelvic) O33.0
    causing obstructed labor O65.0
  congenital Q74.2
Platyspondylisis Q76.49
Plaut (-Vincent) **disease** (*see also* Vincent's) A69.1
Plethora R23.2
  newborn P61.1
Pleura, pleural — *see* condition
Pleuralgia R07.81
Pleurisy (acute) (adhesive) (chronic) (costal) (diaphragmatic) (double) (dry) (fibrinous) (fibrous) (interlobar)
  (latent) (plastic) (primary) (residual) (sicca) (sterile)
  (subacute) (unresolved) R09.1
  with
    adherent pleura J86.0
    effusion J90
      chylous, chyliform J94.0
      tuberculous (non primary) A15.6
        primary (progressive) A15.7
    tuberculosis — *see* Pleurisy, tuberculous (non pri-
      mary)
  encysted — *see* Pleurisy, with effusion
  exudative — *see* Pleurisy, with effusion
  fibrinopurulent, fibropurulent — *see* Pyothorax
  hemorrhagic — *see* Hemothorax
  pneumococcal J90
  purulent — *see* Pyothorax
  septic — *see* Pyothorax
  serofibrinous — *see* Pleurisy, with effusion
  seropurulent — *see* Pyothorax
  serous — *see* Pleurisy, with effusion
  staphylococcal J86.9
  streptococcal J90
  suppurative — *see* Pyothorax
  traumatic (post) (current) — *see* Injury, intrathoracic,
    pleura
  tuberculous (with effusion) (non primary) A15.6
    primary (progressive) A15.7
Pleuritis sicca — *see* Pleurisy
Pleurobronchopneumonia — *see* Pneumonia, broncho-
Pleurodynia R07.81
  epidemic B33.0
  viral B33.0
Pleuropericarditis (*see also* Pericarditis)
  acute I30.9
Pleuropneumonia (acute) (bilateral) (double) (septic)
  (*see also* Pneumonia) J18.8
  chronic — *see* Fibrosis, lung
Pleuro-pneumonia-like-organism (PPLO), as cause of
  disease classified elsewhere B96.0
Pleurorrhea — *see* Pleurisy, with effusion
Plexitis, brachial G54.0
Plica
  polonica B85.0
  syndrome, knee M67.5- ☑
  tonsil J35.8
Plicated tongue K14.5
Plug
  bronchus NEC J98.09
  meconium (newborn) NEC syndrome P76.0
  mucus — *see* Asphyxia, mucus
Plumbism — *see* subcategory T56.0 ☑
Plummer's disease E05.20
  with thyroid storm E05.21
Plummer-Vinson syndrome D50.1
Pluricarential syndrome of infancy E40
Plus (and minus) **hand** (intrinsic) — *see* Deformity, limb,
  specified type NEC, forearm
Pneumathemia — *see* Air, embolism
Pneumatic hammer (drill) syndrome T75.21 ☑
Pneumatocele (lung) J98.4
  intracranial G93.89
  tension J44.9
Pneumatosis
  cystoides intestinalis K63.89
  intestinalis K63.89
  peritonei K66.8
Pneumaturia R39.89
Pneumoblastoma — *see* Neoplasm, lung, malignant
Pneumocephalus G93.89

Pneumococcemia A40.3
Pneumococcus, pneumococcal — *see* condition
Pneumoconiosis (due to) (inhalation of) J64
  with tuberculosis (any type in A15) J65
  aluminum J63.0
  asbestos J61
  bagasse, bagassosis J67.1
  bauxite J63.1
  beryllium J63.2
  coal miners' (simple) J60
  coalworkers' (simple) J60
  collier's J60
  cotton dust J66.0
  diatomite (diatomaceous earth) J62.8
  dust
    inorganic NEC J63.6
    lime J62.8
    marble J62.8
    organic NEC J66.8
  fumes or vapors (from silo) J68.9
  graphite J63.3
  grinder's J62.8
  kaolin J62.8
  mica J62.8
  millstone maker's J62.8
  mineral fibers NEC J61
  miner's J60
  moldy hay J67.0
  potter's J62.8
  rheumatoid — *see* Rheumatoid, lung
  sandblaster's J62.8
  silica, silicate NEC J62.8
    with carbon J60
  stonemason's J62.8
  talc (dust) J62.0
Pneumocystis carinii pneumonia B59
Pneumocystis jiroveci (pneumonia) B59
Pneumocystosis (with pneumonia) B59
Pneumohemopericardium I31.2
Pneumohemothorax J94.2
  traumatic S27.2 ☑
Pneumohydropericardium — *see* Pericarditis
Pneumohydrothorax — *see* Hydrothorax
Pneumomediastinum J98.2
  congenital or perinatal P25.2
Pneumomycosis B49 [J99]
Pneumonia (acute) (double) (migratory) (purulent)
  (septic) (unresolved) J18.9
  with
    influenza — *see* Influenza, with, pneumonia
    lung abscess J85.1
      due to specified organism — *see* Pneumonia,
        in (due to)
  adenoviral J12.0
  adynamic J18.2
  alba A50.04
  allergic (eosinophilic) J82
  alveolar — *see* Pneumonia, lobar
  anaerobes J15.8
  anthrax A22.1
  apex, apical — *see* Pneumonia, lobar
  Ascaris B77.81
  aspiration J69.0
    due to
      aspiration of microorganisms
        bacterial J15.9
        viral J12.9
      food (regurgitated) J69.0
      gastric secretions J69.0
      milk (regurgitated) J69.0
      oils, essences J69.1
      solids, liquids NEC J69.8
      vomitus J69.0
    newborn P24.81
      amniotic fluid (clear) P24.11
      blood P24.21
      food (regurgitated) P24.31
      liquor (amnii) P24.11
      meconium P24.01
      milk P24.31
      mucus P24.11
      specified NEC P24.81
      stomach contents P24.31
    postprocedural J95.4
  atypical NEC J18.9
  bacillus J15.9
    specified NEC J15.8

Pneumonia — *continued*
  bacterial J15.9
    specified NEC J15.8
  Bacteroides (fragilis) (oralis) (melaninogenicus) J15.8
  basal, basic, basilar — *see* Pneumonia, by type
  bronchiolitis obliterans organized (BOOP) J84.89
  broncho-, bronchial (confluent) (croupous) (diffuse)
    (disseminated) (hemorrhagic) (involving lobes)
    (lobar) (terminal) J18.0
    allergic (eosinophilic) J82
    aspiration — *see* Pneumonia, aspiration
    bacterial J15.9
      specified NEC J15.8
    chronic — *see* Fibrosis, lung
    diplococcal J13
    Eaton's agent J15.7
    Escherichia coli (E. coli) J15.5
    Friedländer's bacillus J15.0
    Hemophilus influenzae J14
    hypostatic J18.2
    inhalation (*see also* Pneumonia, aspiration)
      due to fumes or vapors (chemical) J68.0
      of oils or essences J69.1
    Klebsiella (pneumoniae) J15.0
    lipid, lipoid J69.1
      endogenous J84.89
    Mycoplasma (pneumoniae) J15.7
    pleuro-pneumonia-like-organisms (PPLO) J15.7
    pneumococcal J13
    Proteus J15.6
    Pseudomonas J15.1
    Serratia marcescens J15.6
    specified organism NEC J16.8
    staphylococcal — *see* Pneumonia, staphylococcal
    streptococcal NEC J15.4
      group B J15.3
      pneumoniae J13
    viral, virus — *see* Pneumonia, viral
  Butyrivibrio (fibriosolvens) J15.8
  Candida B37.1
  caseous — *see* Tuberculosis, pulmonary
  catarrhal — *see* Pneumonia, broncho
  chlamydial J16.0
    congenital P23.1
  cholesterol J84.89
  cirrhotic (chronic) — *see* Fibrosis, lung
  Clostridium (haemolyticum) (novyi) J15.8
  confluent — *see* Pneumonia, broncho
  congenital (infective) P23.9
    due to
      bacterium NEC P23.6
      Chlamydia P23.1
      Escherichia coli P23.4
      Haemophilus influenzae P23.6
      infective organism NEC P23.8
      Klebsiella pneumoniae P23.6
      Mycoplasma P23.6
      Pseudomonas P23.5
      Staphylococcus P23.2
      Streptococcus (except group B) P23.6
        group B P23.3
      viral agent P23.0
    specified NEC P23.8
  croupous — *see* Pneumonia, lobar
  cryptogenic organizing J84.116
  cytomegalic inclusion B25.0
  cytomegaloviral B25.0
  deglutition — *see* Pneumonia, aspiration
  desquamative interstitial J84.117
  diffuse — *see* Pneumonia, broncho
  diplococcal, diplococcus (broncho-) (lobar) J13
  disseminated (focal) — *see* Pneumonia, broncho
  Eaton's agent J15.7
  embolic, embolism — *see* Embolism, pulmonary
  Enterobacter J15.6
  eosinophilic J82
  Escherichia coli (E. coli) J15.5
  Eubacterium J15.8
  fibrinous — *see* Pneumonia, lobar
  fibroid, fibrous (chronic) — *see* Fibrosis, lung
  Friedländer's bacillus J15.0
  Fusobacterium (nucleatum) J15.8
  gangrenous J85.0
  giant cell (measles) B05.2
  gonococcal A54.84
  gram-negative bacteria NEC J15.6
    anaerobic J15.8
  Hemophilus influenzae (broncho) (lobar) J14

Pneumonia — *continued*
  human metapneumovirus J12.3
  hypostatic (broncho) (lobar) J18.2
  in (due to)
    actinomycosis A42.0
    adenovirus J12.0
    anthrax A22.1
    ascariasis B77.81
    aspergillosis B44.9
    Bacillus anthracis A22.1
    Bacterium anitratum J15.6
    candidiasis B37.1
    chickenpox B01.2
    Chlamydia J16.0
      neonatal P23.1
    coccidioidomycosis B38.2
      acute B38.0
      chronic B38.1
    cytomegalovirus disease B25.0
    Diplococcus (pneumoniae) J13
    Eaton's agent J15.7
    Enterobacter J15.6
    Escherichia coli (E. coli) J15.5
    Friedländer's bacillus J15.0
    fumes and vapors (chemical) (inhalation) J68.0
    gonorrhea A54.84
    Hemophilus influenzae (H. influenzae) J14
    Herellea J15.6
    histoplasmosis B39.2
      acute B39.0
      chronic B39.1
    human metapneumovirus J12.3
    Klebsiella (pneumoniae) J15.0
    measles B05.2
    Mycoplasma (pneumoniae) J15.7
    nocardiosis, nocardiasis A43.0
    ornithosis A70
    parainfluenza virus J12.2
    pleuro-pneumonia-like-organism (PPLO) J15.7
    pneumococcus J13
    pneumocystosis (Pneumocystis carinii) (Pneumo-
      cystis jiroveci) B59
    Proteus J15.6
    Pseudomonas NEC J15.1
      pseudomallei A24.1
    psittacosis A70
    Q fever A78
    respiratory syncytial virus J12.1
    rheumatic fever I00 [J17]
    rubella B06.81
    Salmonella (infection) A02.22
      typhi A01.03
    schistosomiasis B65.9 [J17]
    Serratia marcescens J15.6
    specified
      bacterium NEC J15.8
      organism NEC J16.8
    spirochetal NEC A69.8
    Staphylococcus J15.20
      aureus (methicillin susceptible) (MSSA) J15.211
        methicillin resistant (MRSA) J15.212
      specified NEC J15.29
    Streptococcus J15.4
      group B J15.3
      pneumoniae J13
      specified NEC J15.4
    toxoplasmosis B58.3
    tularemia A21.2
    typhoid (fever) A01.03
    varicella B01.2
    virus — *see* Pneumonia, viral
    whooping cough A37.91
      due to
        Bordetella parapertussis A37.11
        Bordetella pertussis A37.01
        specified NEC A37.81
    Yersinia pestis A20.2
  inhalation of food or vomit — *see* Pneumonia, aspira-
    tion
  interstitial J84.9
    chronic J84.111
    desquamative J84.117
    due to
      collagen vascular disease J84.17
      known underlying cause J84.17
    idiopathic NOS J84.111
    in disease classified elsewhere J84.17

Pneumonia — *continued*
 interstitial — *continued*
  lymphocytic (due to collagen vascular disease) (in diseases classified elsewhere) J84.17
  lymphoid J84.2
  non-specific J84.89
   due to
    collagen vascular disease J84.17
    known underlying cause J84.17
   idiopathic J84.113
   in diseases classified elsewhere J84.17
  plasma cell B59
  pseudomonas J15.1
  usual J84.112
   due to collagen vascular disease J84.17
   idiopathic J84.112
   in diseases classified elsewhere J84.17
 Klebsiella (pneumoniae) J15.0
 lipid, lipoid (exogenous) J69.1
  endogenous J84.89
 lobar (disseminated) (double) (interstitial) J18.1
  bacterial J15.9
   specified NEC J15.8
  chronic — *see* Fibrosis, lung
  Escherichia coli (E. coli) J15.5
  Friedländer's bacillus J15.0
  Hemophilus influenzae J14
  hypostatic J18.2
  Klebsiella (pneumoniae) J15.0
  pneumococcal J13
  Proteus J15.6
  Pseudomonas J15.1
  specified organism NEC J16.8
  staphylococcal — *see* Pneumonia, staphylococcal
  streptococcal NEC J15.4
  Streptococcus pneumoniae J13
  viral, virus — *see* Pneumonia, viral
 lobular — *see* Pneumonia, broncho
 Löffler's J82
 lymphoid interstitial J84.2
 massive — *see* Pneumonia, lobar
 meconium P24.01
 MSSA (methicillin susceptible Staphylococcus aureus) J15.211
 multilobar — *see* Pneumonia, by type
 Mycoplasma (pneumoniae) J15.7
 necrotic J85.0
 neonatal P23.9
  aspiration — *see* Aspiration, by substance, with pneumonia
 nitrogen dioxide J68.9
 organizing J84.89
  due to
   collagen vascular disease J84.17
   known underlying cause J84.17
  in diseases classified elsewhere J84.17
 orthostatic J18.2
 parainfluenza virus J12.2
 parenchymatous — *see* Fibrosis, lung
 passive J18.2
 patchy — *see* Pneumonia, broncho
 Peptococcus J15.8
 Peptostreptococcus J15.8
 plasma cell (of infants) B59
 pleurolobar — *see* Pneumonia, lobar
 pleuro-pneumonia-like organism (PPLO) J15.7
 pneumococcal (broncho) (lobar) J13
 Pneumocystis (carinii) (jiroveci) B59
 postinfectional NEC B99 ☑ [J17]
 postmeasles B05.2
 Proteus J15.6
 Pseudomonas J15.1
 psittacosis A70
 radiation J70.0
 respiratory syncytial virus J12.1
 resulting from a procedure J95.89
 rheumatic I00 [J17]
 Salmonella (arizonae) (cholerae-suis) (enteritidis) (typhimurium) A02.22
  typhi A01.03
  typhoid fever A01.03
 SARS-associated coronavirus J12.81
 segmented, segmental — *see* Pneumonia, broncho-
 Serratia marcescens J15.6
 specified NEC J18.8
  bacterium NEC J15.8
  organism NEC J16.8
  virus NEC J12.89

Pneumonia — *continued*
 spirochetal NEC A69.8
 staphylococcal (broncho) (lobar) J15.20
  aureus (methicillin susceptible) (MSSA) J15.211
   methicillin resistant (MRSA) J15.212
  specified NEC J15.29
 static, stasis J18.2
 streptococcal NEC (broncho) (lobar) J15.4
  group
   A J15.4
   B J15.3
   specified NEC J15.4
 Streptococcus pneumoniae J13
 syphilitic, congenital (early) A50.04
 traumatic (complication) (early) (secondary) T79.8 ☑
 tuberculous (any) — *see* Tuberculosis, pulmonary
 tularemic A21.2
 varicella B01.2
 Veillonella J15.8
 ventilator associated J95.851
 viral, virus (broncho) (interstitial) (lobar) J12.9
  adenoviral J12.0
  congenital P23.0
  human metapneumovirus J12.3
  parainfluenza J12.2
  respiratory syncytial J12.1
  SARS-associated coronavirus J12.81
  specified NEC J12.89
 white (congenital) A50.04
Pneumonic — *see* condition
Pneumonitis (acute) (primary) (*see also* Pneumonia)
 air-conditioner J67.7
 allergic (due to) J67.9
  organic dust NEC J67.8
  red cedar dust J67.8
  sequoiosis J67.8
  wood dust J67.8
 aspiration J69.0
  due to
   anesthesia J95.4
    during
     labor and delivery O74.0
     pregnancy O29.01- ☑
     puerperium O89.01
   fumes or gases J68.0
  obstetric O74.0
 chemical (due to gases, fumes or vapors) (inhalation) J68.0
  due to anesthesia J95.4
 cholesterol J84.89
 chronic — *see* Fibrosis, lung
 congenital rubella P35.0
 crack (cocaine) J68.0
 due to
  beryllium J68.0
  cadmium J68.0
  crack (cocaine) J68.0
  detergent J69.8
  fluorocarbon-polymer J68.0
  food, vomit (aspiration) J69.0
  fumes or vapors J68.0
  gases, fumes or vapors (inhalation) J68.0
  inhalation
   blood J69.8
   essences J69.1
   food (regurgitated), milk, vomit J69.0
   oils, essences J69.1
   saliva J69.0
   solids, liquids NEC J69.8
  manganese J68.0
  nitrogen dioxide J68.0
  oils, essences J69.1
  solids, liquids NEC J69.8
  toxoplasmosis (acquired) B58.3
   congenital P37.1
  vanadium J68.0
  ventilator J95.851
 eosinophilic J82
 hypersensitivity J67.9
  air conditioner lung J67.7
  bagassosis J67.1
  bird fancier's lung J67.2
  farmer's lung J67.0
  maltworker's lung J67.4
  maple bark-stripper's lung J67.6
  mushroom worker's lung J67.5
  specified organic dust NEC J67.8
  suberosis J67.3

Pneumonitis — *continued*
 interstitial (chronic) J84.89
  acute J84.114
  lymphoid J84.2
  non-specific J84.89
   idiopathic J84.113
 lymphoid, interstitial J84.2
 meconium P24.01
 postanesthetic J95.4
  correct substance properly administered — *see* Table of Drugs and Chemicals, by drug, adverse effect
  in labor and delivery O74.0
  in pregnancy O29.01- ☑
   obstetric O74.0
  overdose or wrong substance given or taken (by accident) — *see* Table of Drugs and Chemicals, by drug, poisoning
  postpartum, puerperal O89.01
 postoperative J95.4
  obstetric O74.0
 radiation J70.0
 rubella, congenital P35.0
 ventilation (air-conditioning) J67.7
 ventilator associated J95.851
 wood-dust J67.8
Pneumonoconiosis — *see* Pneumoconiosis
Pneumoparotid K11.8
Pneumopathy NEC J98.4
 alveolar J84.09
 due to organic dust NEC J66.8
 parietoalveolar J84.09
Pneumopericarditis (*see also* Pericarditis)
 acute I30.9
Pneumopericardium (*see also* Pericarditis)
 congenital P25.3
 newborn P25.3
 traumatic (post) — *see* Injury, heart
Pneumophagia (psychogenic) F45.8
Pneumopleurisy, pneumopleuritis (*see also* Pneumonia) J18.8
Pneumopyopericardium I30.1
Pneumopyothorax — *see* Pyopneumothorax
 with fistula J86.0
Pneumorrhagia (*see also* Hemorrhage, lung)
 tuberculous — *see* Tuberculosis, pulmonary
Pneumothorax NOS J93.9
 acute J93.83
 chronic J93.81
 congenital P25.1
 perinatal period P25.1
 postprocedural J95.811
 specified NEC J93.83
 spontaneous NOS J93.83
  newborn P25.1
  primary J93.11
  secondary J93.12
  tension J93.0
 tense valvular, infectional J93.0
 tension (spontaneous) J93.0
 traumatic S27.0 ☑
  with hemothorax S27.2 ☑
 tuberculous — *see* Tuberculosis, pulmonary
Podagra (*see also* Gout) M10.9
Podencephalus Q01.9
Poikilocytosis R71.8
Poikiloderma L81.6
 Civatte's L57.3
 congenital Q82.8
 vasculare atrophicans L94.5
Poikilodermatomyositis M33.10
 with
  myopathy M33.12
  respiratory involvement M33.11
  specified organ involvement NEC M33.19
Pointed ear (congenital) Q17.3
Poison ivy, oak, sumac or other plant dermatitis (allergic) (contact) L23.7
Poisoning (acute) (*see also* Table of Drugs and Chemicals)
 algae and toxins T65.82- ☑
 Bacillus B (aertrycke) (cholerae (suis)) (paratyphosus) (suipestifer) A02.9
  botulinus A05.1
 bacterial toxins A05.9
 berries, noxious — *see* Poisoning, food, noxious, berries
 botulism A05.1
 ciguatera fish T61.0- ☑

Poisoning — *continued*
  Clostridium botulinum A05.1
  death-cap (Amanita phalloides) (Amanita verna) —
    see Poisoning, food, noxious, mushrooms
  drug — *see* Table of Drugs and Chemicals, by drug,
    poisoning
  epidemic, fish (noxious) — *see* Poisoning, seafood
    bacterial A05.9
  fava bean D55.0
  fish (noxious) T61.9- ☑
    bacterial — *see* Intoxication, foodborne, by agent
    ciguatera fish — *see* Poisoning, ciguatera fish
    scombroid fish — *see* Poisoning, scombroid fish
    specified type NEC T61.77- ☑
  food (acute) (diseased) (infected) (noxious) NEC
    T62.9-
    bacterial — *see* Intoxication, foodborne, by agent
    due to
      Bacillus (aertrycke) (choleraesuis) (paratypho-
        sus) (suipestifer) A02.9
        botulinus A05.1
      Clostridium (perfringens) (Welchii) A05.2
      salmonella (aertrycke) (callinarum) (choleraesu-
        is) (enteritidis) (paratyphi) (suipestifer)
        A02.9
        with
          gastroenteritis A02.0
          sepsis A02.1
      staphylococcus A05.0
      Vibrio
        parahaemolyticus A05.3
        vulnificus A05.5
    noxious or naturally toxic T62.9- ☑
      berries — *see* subcategory T62.1 ☑
      fish — *see* Poisoning, seafood
      mushrooms — *see* subcategory T62.0X ☑
      plants NEC — *see* subcategory T62.2X ☑
      seafood — *see* Poisoning, seafood
      specified NEC — *see* subcategory T62.8X ☑
  ichthyotoxism — *see* Poisoning, seafood
  kreotoxism, food A05.9
  latex T65.81- ☑
  lead T56.0- ☑
  mushroom — *see* Poisoning, food, noxious, mushroom
  mussels (*see also* Poisoning, shellfish)
    bacterial — *see* Intoxication, foodborne, by agent
  nicotine (tobacco) T65.2- ☑
  noxious foodstuffs — *see* Poisoning, food, noxious
  plants, noxious — *see* Poisoning, food, noxious, plants
    NEC
  ptomaine — *see* Poisoning, food
  radiation J70.0
  Salmonella (arizonae) (cholerae-suis) (enteritidis) (ty-
    phimurium) A02.9
  scombroid fish T61.1- ☑
  seafood (noxious) T61.9- ☑
    bacterial — *see* Intoxication, foodborne, by agent
    fish — *see* Poisoning, fish
    shellfish — *see* Poisoning, shellfish
    specified NEC — *see* subcategory T61.8X ☑
  shellfish (amnesic) (azaspiracid) (diarrheic) (neurotoxic)
    (noxious) (paralytic) T61.78- ☑
    bacterial — *see* Intoxication, foodborne, by agent
    ciguatera mollusk — *see* Poisoning, ciguatera fish
  specified substance NEC T65.891 ☑
  Staphylococcus, food A05.0
  tobacco (nicotine) T65.2- ☑
  water E87.79
Poker spine — *see* Spondylitis, ankylosing
Poland syndrome Q79.8
Polioencephalitis (acute) (bulbar) A80.9
  inferior G12.22
  influenzal — *see* Influenza, with, encephalopathy
  superior hemorrhagic (acute) (Wernicke's) E51.2
  Wernicke's E51.2
Polioencephalomyelitis (acute) (anterior) A80.9
  with beriberi E51.2
Polioencephalopathy, superior hemorrhagic E51.2
  with
    beriberi E51.11
    pellagra E52
Poliomeningoencephalitis — *see* Meningoencephalitis
Poliomyelitis (acute) (anterior) (epidemic) A80.9
  with paralysis (bulbar) — *see* Poliomyelitis, paralytic
  abortive A80.4
  ascending (progressive) — *see* Poliomyelitis, paralytic
  bulbar (paralytic) — *see* Poliomyelitis, paralytic

Poliomyelitis — *continued*
  congenital P35.8
  nonepidemic A80.9
  nonparalytic A80.4
  paralytic A80.30
    specified NEC A80.39
    vaccine-associated A80.0
    wild virus
      imported A80.1
      indigenous A80.2
  spinal, acute A80.9
Poliosis (eyebrow) (eyelashes) L67.1
  circumscripta, acquired L67.1
Pollakiuria R35.0
  psychogenic F45.8
Pollinosis J30.1
Pollitzer's disease L73.2
Polyadenitis (*see also* Lymphadenitis)
  malignant A20.0
Polyalgia M79.89
Polyangiitis M30.0
  microscopic M31.7
  overlap syndrome M30.8
Polyarteritis
  microscopic M31.7
  nodosa M30.0
    with lung involvement M30.1
    juvenile M30.2
    related condition NEC M30.8
Polyarthralgia — *see* Pain, joint
Polyarthritis, polyarthropathy (*see also* Arthritis) M13.0
  due to or associated with other specified conditions
    — *see* Arthritis
  epidemic (Australian) (with exanthema) B33.1
  infective — *see* Arthritis, pyogenic or pyemic
  inflammatory M06.4
  juvenile (chronic) (seronegative) M08.3
  migratory — *see* Fever, rheumatic
  rheumatic, acute — *see* Fever, rheumatic
Polyarthrosis M15.9
  post-traumatic M15.3
  primary M15.0
  specified NEC M15.8
Polycarential syndrome of infancy E40
Polychondritis (atrophic) (chronic) (*see also* Disorder,
  cartilage, specified type NEC)
  relapsing M94.1
Polycoria Q13.2
Polycystic (disease)
  degeneration, kidney Q61.3
    autosomal dominant (adult type) Q61.2
    autosomal recessive (infantile type) NEC Q61.19
  kidney Q61.3
    autosomal
      dominant Q61.2
      recessive NEC Q61.19
    autosomal dominant (adult type) Q61.2
    autosomal recessive (childhood type) NEC Q61.19
    infantile type NEC Q61.19
  liver Q44.6
  lung J98.4
    congenital Q33.0
  ovary, ovaries E28.2
  spleen Q89.09
Polycythemia (secondary) D75.1
  acquired D75.1
  benign (familial) D75.0
  due to
    donor twin P61.1
    erythropoietin D75.1
    fall in plasma volume D75.1
    high altitude D75.1
    maternal-fetal transfusion P61.1
    stress D75.1
  emotional D75.1
  erythropoietin D75.1
  familial (benign) D75.0
  Gaisböck's (hypertonica) D75.1
  high altitude D75.1
  hypertonica D75.1
  hypoxemic D75.1
  neonatorum P61.1
  nephrogenous D75.1
  relative D75.1
  secondary D75.1
  spurious D75.1
  stress D75.1
  vera D45

Polycytosis cryptogenica D75.1
Polydactylism, polydactyly Q69.9
  toes Q69.2
Polydipsia R63.1
Polydystrophy, pseudo-Hurler E77.0
Polyembryoma — *see* Neoplasm, malignant, by site
Polyglandular
  deficiency E31.0
  dyscrasia E31.9
  dysfunction E31.9
  syndrome E31.8
Polyhydramnios O40.- ☑
Polymastia Q83.1
Polymenorrhea N92.0
Polymyalgia M35.3
  arteritica, giant cell M31.5
  rheumatica M35.3
    with giant cell arteritis M31.5
Polymyositis (acute) (chronic) (hemorrhagic) M33.20
  with
    myopathy M33.22
    respiratory involvement M33.21
    skin involvement — *see* Dermatopolymyositis
    specified organ involvement NEC M33.29
  ossificans (generalisata) (progressiva) — *see* Myositis,
    ossificans, progressiva
Polyneuritis, polyneuritic (*see also* Polyneuropathy)
  acute (post-)infective G61.0
  alcoholic G62.1
  cranialis G52.7
  demyelinating, chronic inflammatory (CIDP) G61.81
  diabetic — *see* Diabetes, polyneuropathy
  diphtheritic A36.83
  due to lack of vitamin NEC E56.9 [G63]
  endemic E51.11
  erythredema — *see* subcategory T56.1 ☑
  febrile, acute G61.0
  hereditary ataxic G60.1
  idiopathic, acute G61.0
  infective (acute) G61.0
  inflammatory, chronic demyelinating (CIDP) G61.81
  nutritional E63.9 [G63]
  postinfective (acute) G61.0
  specified NEC G62.89
Polyneuropathy (peripheral) G62.9
  alcoholic G62.1
  amyloid (Portuguese) E85.1 [G63]
  arsenical G62.2
  critical illness G62.81
  demyelinating, chronic inflammatory (CIDP) G61.81
  diabetic — *see* Diabetes, polyneuropathy
  drug-induced G62.0
  hereditary G60.9
    specified NEC G60.8
  idiopathic G60.9
    progressive G60.3
  in (due to)
    alcohol G62.1
      sequelae G65.2
    amyloidosis, familial (Portuguese) E85.1 [G63]
    antitetanus serum G61.1
    arsenic G62.2
      sequelae G65.2
    avitaminosis NEC E56.9 [G63]
    beriberi E51.11
    collagen vascular disease NEC M35.9 [G63]
    deficiency (of)
      B (-complex) vitamins E53.9 [G63]
      vitamin B6 E53.1 [G63]
    diabetes — *see* Diabetes, polyneuropathy
    diphtheria A36.83
    drug or medicament G62.0
      correct substance properly administered — *see*
        Table of Drugs and Chemicals, by drug,
        adverse effect
      overdose or wrong substance given or taken
        — *see* Table of Drugs and Chemicals, by
        drug, poisoning
    endocrine disease NEC E34.9 [G63]
    herpes zoster B02.23
    hypoglycemia E16.2 [G63]
    infectious
      disease NEC B99 ☑ [G63]
      mononucleosis B27.91
    lack of vitamin NEC E56.9 [G63]
    lead G62.2
      sequelae G65.2
    leprosy A30.9 [G63]

Polyneuropathy — *continued*
  in — *continued*
    Lyme disease A69.22
    metabolic disease NEC E88.9 [G63]
    microscopic polyangiitis M31.7 [G63]
    mumps B26.84
    neoplastic disease (*see also* Neoplasm) D49.9 [G63]
    nutritional deficiency NEC E63.9 [G63]
    organophosphate compounds G62.2
      sequelae G65.2
    parasitic disease NEC B89 [G63]
    pellagra E52 [G63]
    polyarteritis nodosa M30.0
    porphyria E80.20 [G63]
    radiation G62.82
    rheumatoid arthritis — *see* Rheumatoid, polyneu-
      ropathy
    sarcoidosis D86.89
    serum G61.1
    syphilis (late) A52.15
      congenital A50.43
    systemic
      connective tissue disorder M35.9 [G63]
      lupus erythematosus M32.19
    toxic agent NEC G62.2
      sequelae G65.2
    triorthocresyl phosphate G62.2
      sequelae G65.2
    tuberculosis A17.89
    uremia N18.9 [G63]
    vitamin B12 deficiency E53.8 [G63]
      with anemia (pernicious) D51.0 [G63]
        due to dietary deficiency D51.3 [G63]
    zoster B02.23
  inflammatory G61.9
    chronic demyelinating (CIDP) G61.81
    sequelae G65.1
    specified NEC G61.89
  lead G62.2
    sequelae G65.2
  nutritional NEC E63.9 [G63]
  postherpetic (zoster) B02.23
  progressive G60.3
  radiation-induced G62.82
  sensory (hereditary) (idiopathic) G60.8
  specified NEC G62.89
  syphilitic (late) A52.15
    congenital A50.43
Polyopia H53.8
Polyorchism, polyorchidism Q55.21
Polyosteoarthritis (*see also* Osteoarthritis, generalized)
  M15.9
  post-traumatic M15.3
  specified NEC M15.8
Polyostotic fibrous dysplasia Q78.1
Polyotia Q17.0
Polyp, polypus
  accessory sinus J33.8
  adenocarcinoma in — *see* Neoplasm, malignant, by
    site
  adenocarcinoma in situ in — *see* Neoplasm, in situ, by
    site
  adenoid tissue J33.0
  adenomatous (*see also* Neoplasm, benign, by site)
    adenocarcinoma in — *see* Neoplasm, malignant,
      by site
    adenocarcinoma in situ in — *see* Neoplasm, in situ,
      by site
    carcinoma in — *see* Neoplasm, malignant, by site
    carcinoma in situ in — *see* Neoplasm, in situ, by
      site
    multiple — *see* Neoplasm, benign
      adenocarcinoma in — *see* Neoplasm, malig-
        nant, by site
      adenocarcinoma in situ in — *see* Neoplasm, in
        situ, by site
  antrum J33.8
  anus, anal (canal) K62.0
  Bartholin's gland N84.3
  bladder D41.4
  carcinoma in — *see* Neoplasm, malignant, by site
  carcinoma in situ in — *see* Neoplasm, in situ, by site
  cecum D12.0
  cervix (uteri) N84.1
    in pregnancy or childbirth — *see* Pregnancy,
      complicated by, abnormal, cervix
    mucous N84.1
    nonneoplastic N84.1

Polyp, polypus — *continued*
  choanal J33.0
  cholesterol K82.4
  clitoris N84.3
  colon K63.5
    adenomatous D12.6
    ascending D12.2
    cecum D12.0
    descending D12.4
    inflammatory K51.40
      with
        abscess K51.414
        complication K51.419
          specified NEC K51.418
        fistula K51.413
        intestinal obstruction K51.412
        rectal bleeding K51.411
    sigmoid D12.5
    transverse D12.3
  corpus uteri N84.0
  dental K04.0
  duodenum K31.7
  ear (middle) H74.4- ☑
  endometrium N84.0
  ethmoidal (sinus) J33.8
  fallopian tube N84.8
  female genital tract N84.9
    specified NEC N84.8
  frontal (sinus) J33.8
  gallbladder K82.4
  gingiva, gum K06.8
  labia, labium (majus) (minus) N84.3
  larynx (mucous) J38.1
    adenomatous D14.1
  malignant –– *see* Neoplasm, malignant, by site
  maxillary (sinus) J33.8
  middle ear — *see* Polyp, ear (middle)
  myometrium N84.0
  nares
    anterior J33.9
    posterior J33.0
  nasal (mucous) J33.9
    cavity J33.0
    septum J33.0
  nasopharyngeal J33.0
  nose (mucous) J33.9
  oviduct N84.8
  pharynx J39.2
  placenta O90.89
  prostate — *see* Enlargement, enlarged, prostate
  pudenda, pudendum N84.3
  pulpal (dental) K04.0
  rectum (nonadenomatous) K62.1
    adenomatous — *see* Polyp, adenomatous
  septum (nasal) J33.0
  sinus (accessory) (ethmoidal) (frontal) (maxillary)
    (sphenoidal) J33.8
  sphenoidal (sinus) J33.8
  stomach K31.7
    adenomatous D13.1
  tube, fallopian N84.8
  turbinate, mucous membrane J33.8
  umbilical, newborn P83.6
  ureter N28.89
  urethra N36.2
  uterus (body) (corpus) (mucous) N84.0
    cervix N84.1
    in pregnancy or childbirth — *see* Pregnancy,
      complicated by, tumor, uterus
  vagina N84.2
  vocal cord (mucous) J38.1
  vulva N84.3
Polyphagia R63.2
Polyphagia R63.2
Polyploidy Q92.7
Polypoid — *see* condition
Polyposis (*see also* Polyp)
  coli (adenomatous) D12.6
    adenocarcinoma in C18.9
    adenocarcinoma in situ in — *see* Neoplasm, in situ,
      by site
    carcinoma in C18.9
  colon (adenomatous) D12.6
  familial D12.6
    adenocarcinoma in situ in — *see* Neoplasm, in situ,
      by site
  intestinal (adenomatous) D12.6
  malignant lymphomatous C83.1- ☑

Polyposis — *continued*
  multiple, adenomatous (*see also* Neoplasm, benign)
    D36.9
Polyradiculitis — *see* Polyneuropathy
Polyradiculoneuropathy (acute) (postinfective) (seg-
  mentally demyelinating) G61.0
Polyserositis
  due to pericarditis I31.1
  pericardial I31.1
  periodic, familial E85.0
  tuberculous A19.9
    acute A19.1
    chronic A19.8
Polysplenia syndrome Q89.09
Polysyndactyly (*see also* Syndactylism, syndactyly) Q70.4
Polytrichia L68.3
Polyunguia Q84.6
Polyuria R35.8
  nocturnal R35.1
  psychogenic F45.8
Pompe's disease (glycogen storage) E74.02
Pompholyx L30.1
Poncet's disease (tuberculous rheumatism) A18.09
Pond fracture — *see* Fracture, skull
Ponos B55.0
Pons, pontine — *see* condition
Poor
  aesthetic of existing restoration of tooth K08.56
  contractions, labor O62.2
  gingival margin to tooth restoration K08.51
  personal hygiene R46.0
  prenatal care, affecting management of pregnancy
    — *see* Pregnancy, complicated by, insufficient,
    prenatal care
  sucking reflex (newborn) R29.2
  urinary stream R39.12
  vision NEC H54.7
Poradenitis, nostras inguinalis or venerea A55
Porencephaly (congenital) (developmental) (true) Q04.6
  acquired G93.0
  nondevelopmental G93.0
  traumatic (post) F07.89
Porocephaliasis B88.8
Porokeratosis Q82.8
Poroma, eccrine — *see* Neoplasm, skin, benign
Porphyria (South African) E80.20
  acquired E80.20
  acute intermittent (hepatic) (Swedish) E80.21
  cutanea tarda (hereditary) (symptomatic) E80.1
  due to drugs E80.20
    correct substance properly administered — *see*
      Table of Drugs and Chemicals, by drug, ad-
      verse effect
    overdose or wrong substance given or taken —
      see Table of Drugs and Chemicals, by drug,
      poisoning
  erythropoietic (congenital) (hereditary) E80.0
  hepatocutaneous type E80.1
  secondary E80.20
  toxic NEC E80.20
  variegata E80.20
Porphyrinuria — *see* Porphyria
Porphyruria — *see* Porphyria
Port wine nevus, mark, or stain Q82.5
Portal — *see* condition
Posadas-Wernicke disease B38.9
Positive
  culture (nonspecific)
    blood R78.81
    bronchial washings R84.5
    cerebrospinal fluid R83.5
    cervix uteri R87.5
    nasal secretions R84.5
    nipple discharge R89.5
    nose R84.5
      staphylococcus (Methicillin susceptible) Z22.321
        Methicillin resistant Z22.322
    peritoneal fluid R85.5
    pleural fluid R84.5
    prostatic secretions R86.5
    saliva R85.5
    seminal fluid R86.5
    sputum R84.5
    synovial fluid R89.5
    throat scrapings R84.5
    urine R82.7
    vagina R87.5
    vulva R87.5

☑ **Additional Character Required** — Refer to the Tabular List for Character Selection   🐦 Subterms under main terms may continue to next column or page

Positive — *continued*
  culture — *continued*
    wound secretions R89.5
  PPD (skin test) R76.11
  serology for syphilis A53.0
    with signs or symptoms — *code as* Syphilis, by site
      and stage
    false R76.8
  skin test, tuberculin (without active tuberculosis)
    R76.11
  test, human immunodeficiency virus (HIV) R75
  VDRL A53.0
    with signs or symptoms — *code by* site and stage
      under Syphilis A53.9
  Wassermann reaction A53.0
Postcardiotomy syndrome I97.0
Postcaval ureter Q62.62
Postcholecystectomy syndrome K91.5
Postclimacteric bleeding N95.0
Postcommissurotomy syndrome I97.0
Postconcussional syndrome F07.81
Postcontusional syndrome F07.81
Postcricoid region — *see* condition
Post-dates (40-42 weeks) (pregnancy) (mother) O48.0
  more than 42 weeks gestation O48.1
Postencephalitic syndrome F07.89
Posterior — *see* condition
Posterolateral sclerosis (spinal cord) — *see* Degeneration, combined
Postexanthematous — *see* condition
Postfebrile — *see* condition
Postgastrectomy dumping syndrome K91.1
Posthemiplegic chorea — *see* Monoplegia
Posthemorrhagic anemia (chronic) D50.0
  acute D62
  newborn P61.3
Postherpetic neuralgia (zoster) B02.29
  trigeminal B02.22
Posthitis N47.7
Postimmunization complication or reaction — *see* Complications, vaccination
Postinfectious — *see* condition
Postlaminectomy syndrome NEC M96.1
Postleukotomy syndrome F07.0
Postmastectomy lymphedema (syndrome) I97.2
Postmaturity, postmature (over 42 weeks)
  maternal (over 42 weeks gestation) O48.1
  newborn P08.22
Postmeasles complication NEC (*see also* condition) B05.89
Postmenopausal
  endometrium (atrophic) N95.8
    suppurative (*see also* Endometritis) N71.9
  osteoporosis — *see* Osteoporosis, postmenopausal
Postnasal drip R09.82
  due to
    allergic rhinitis — *see* Rhinitis, allergic
    common cold J00
    gastroesophageal reflux — *see* Reflux, gastroesophageal
    nasopharyngitis — *see* Nasopharyngitis
    other known condition — *code to* condition
    sinusitis — *see* Sinusitis
Postnatal — *see* condition
Postoperative (postprocedural) — *see* Complication, postoperative
  pneumothorax, therapeutic Z98.3
  state NEC Z98.89
Postpancreatectomy hyperglycemia E89.1
Postpartum — *see* Puerperal
Postphlebitic syndrome — *see* Syndrome, postthrombotic
Postpolio (myelitic) **syndrome** G14
Postpoliomyelitic (*see also* condition)
  osteopathy — *see* Osteopathy, after poliomyelitis
Postprocedural (*see also* Postoperative)
  hypoinsulinemia E89.1
Postschizophrenic depression F32.8
Postsurgery status (*see also* Status (post))
  pneumothorax, therapeutic Z98.3
Post-term (40-42 weeks) (pregnancy) (mother) O48.0
  infant P08.21
  more than 42 weeks gestation (mother) O48.1
Post-traumatic brain syndrome, nonpsychotic F07.81
Post-typhoid abscess A01.09
Postures, hysterical F44.2

Postvaccinal reaction or complication — *see* Complications, vaccination
Postvalvulotomy syndrome I97.0
Potain's
  disease (pulmonary edema) — *see* Edema, lung
  syndrome (gastrectasis with dyspepsia) K31.0
Potter's
  asthma J62.8
  facies Q60.6
  lung J62.8
  syndrome (with renal agenesis) Q60.6
Pott's
  curvature (spinal) A18.01
  disease or paraplegia A18.01
  spinal curvature A18.01
  tumor, puffy — *see* Osteomyelitis, specified type NEC
Pouch
  bronchus Q32.4
  Douglas' — *see* condition
  esophagus, esophageal, congenital Q39.6
    acquired K22.5
  gastric K31.4
  Hartmann's K82.8
  pharynx, pharyngeal (congenital) Q38.7
Pouchitis K91.850
Poultrymen's itch B88.0
Poverty NEC Z59.6
  extreme Z59.5
Poxvirus NEC B08.8
Prader-Willi syndrome Q87.1
Preauricular appendage or tag Q17.0
Prebetalipoproteinemia (acquired) (essential) (familial) (hereditary) (primary) (secondary) E78.1
  with chylomicronemia E78.3
Precipitate labor or delivery O62.3
Preclimacteric bleeding (menorrhagia) N92.4
Precocious
  adrenarche E30.1
  menarche E30.1
  menstruation E30.1
  pubarche E30.1
  puberty E30.1
    central E22.8
  sexual development NEC E30.1
  thelarche E30.8
Precocity, sexual (constitutional) (cryptogenic) (female) (idiopathic) (male) E30.1
  with adrenal hyperplasia E25.9
    congenital E25.0
Precordial pain R07.2
Predeciduous teeth K00.2
Prediabetes, prediabetic R73.09
  complicating
    pregnancy — *see* Pregnancy, complicated by, diseases of, specified type or system NEC
    puerperium O99.89
Predislocation status of hip at birth Q65.6
Pre-eclampsia O14.9- ☑
  with pre-existing hypertension — *see* Hypertension, complicating pregnancy, pre-existing, with, preeclampsia
  mild O14.0- ☑
  moderate O14.0- ☑
  severe O14.1- ☑
    with hemolysis, elevated liver enzymes and low platelet count (HELLP) O14.2- ☑
Pre-eruptive color change, teeth, tooth K00.8
Pre-excitation atrioventricular conduction I45.6
Preglaucoma H40.00- ☑
Pregnancy (single) (uterine) (*see also* Delivery and Puerperal)

Note: The Tabular must be reviewed for assignment of appropriate seventh character for multiple gestation codes in Chapter 15

Note: The Tabular must be reviewed for assignment of the appropriate character indicating the trimester of the pregnancy

  abdominal (ectopic) O00.0
    with viable fetus O36.7- ☑
  ampullar O00.1
  biochemical O02.81
  broad ligament O00.8
  cervical O00.8
  chemical O02.81

Pregnancy — *continued*
  complicated by (care of) (management affected by)
    abnormal, abnormality
      cervix O34.4- ☑
        causing obstructed labor O65.5
      cord (umbilical) O69.9 ☑
      findings on antenatal screening of mother O28.9
        biochemical O28.1
        chromosomal O28.5
        cytological O28.2
        genetic O28.5
        hematological O28.0
        radiological O28.4
        specified NEC O28.8
        ultrasonic O28.3
      glucose (tolerance) NEC O99.810
      pelvic organs O34.9- ☑
        specified NEC O34.8- ☑
          causing obstructed labor O65.5
      pelvis (bony) (major) NEC O33.0
      perineum O34.7- ☑
      position
        placenta O44.1- ☑
          without hemorrhage O44.0- ☑
        uterus O34.59- ☑
      uterus O34.59- ☑
        causing obstructed labor O65.5
        congenital O34.0- ☑
      vagina O34.6- ☑
        causing obstructed labor O65.5
      vulva O34.7- ☑
        causing obstructed labor O65.5
    abruptio placentae — *see* Abruptio placentae
    abscess or cellulitis
      bladder O23.1- ☑
      breast O91.11- ☑
      genital organ or tract O23.9- ☑
    abuse
      physical O9A.31 ☑ (*following* O99)
      psychological O9A.51 ☑ (*following* O99)
      sexual O9A.41 ☑ (*following* O99)
    adverse effect anesthesia O29.9- ☑
      aspiration pneumonitis O29.01- ☑
      cardiac arrest O29.11- ☑
      cardiac complication NEC O29.19- ☑
      cardiac failure O29.12- ☑
      central nervous system complication NEC O29.29- ☑
      cerebral anoxia O29.21- ☑
      failed or difficult intubation O29.6- ☑
      inhalation of stomach contents or secretions NOS O29.01- ☑
      local, toxic reaction O29.3X- ☑
      Mendelson's syndrome O29.01- ☑
      pressure collapse of lung O29.02- ☑
      pulmonary complications NEC O29.09- ☑
      specified NEC O29.8X- ☑
      spinal and epidural type NEC O29.5X ☑
        induced headache O29.4- ☑
    albuminuria O12.1- ☑
    alcohol use O99.31- ☑
    amnionitis O41.12- ☑
    anaphylactoid syndrome of pregnancy O88.01- ☑
    anemia (conditions in D50-D64) (pre-existing) O99.01- ☑
      complicating the puerperium O99.03
    antepartum hemorrhage O46.9- ☑
      with coagulation defect — *see* Hemorrhage, antepartum, with coagulation defect
      specified NEC O46.8X- ☑
    appendicitis O99.61- ☑
    atrophy (yellow) (acute) liver (subacute) O26.61- ☑
    bariatric surgery status O99.84- ☑
    bicornis or bicornuate uterus O34.59- ☑
    biliary tract problems O26.61- ☑
    breech presentation O32.1 ☑
    cardiovascular diseases (conditions in I00-I09, I20-I52, I70-I99) O99.41- ☑
    cerebrovascular disorders (conditions in I60-I69) O99.41- ☑
    cervical shortening O26.87- ☑
    cervicitis O23.51- ☑
    chloasma (gravidarum) O26.89- ☑
    cholecystitis O99.61- ☑
    cholestasis (intrahepatic) O26.61- ☑

Pregnancy — *continued*
    complicated by — *continued*
        chorioamnionitis O41.12- ☑
        circulatory system disorder (conditions in I00-I09, I20-I99, O99.41-)
        compound presentation O32.6 ☑
        conjoined twins O30.02- ☑
        connective system disorders (conditions in M00-M99) O99.89
        contracted pelvis (general) O33.1
            inlet O33.2
            outlet O33.3 ☑
        convulsions (eclamptic) (uremic) (*see also* Eclampsia) O15.9
        cracked nipple O92.11- ☑
        cystitis O23.1- ☑
        cystocele O34.8- ☑
        death of fetus (near term) O36.4 ☑
            early pregnancy O02.1
            of one fetus or more in multiple gestation O31.2- ☑
        deciduitis O41.14- ☑
        decreased fetal movement O36.81- ☑
        dental problems O99.61- ☑
        diabetes (mellitus) O24.91- ☑
            gestational (pregnancy induced) — *see* Diabetes, gestational
            pre-existing O24.31- ☑
                specified NEC O24.81- ☑
                type 1 O24.01- ☑
                type 2 O24.11- ☑
        digestive system disorders (conditions in K00-K93) O99.61- ☑
        diseases of — *see* Pregnancy, complicated by, specified body system disease
            biliary tract O26.61- ☑
            blood NEC (conditions in D65-D77) O99.11- ☑
            liver O26.61- ☑
            specified NEC O99.89
        disorders of — *see* Pregnancy, complicated by, specified body system disorder
            amniotic fluid and membranes O41.9- ☑
                specified NEC O41.8X- ☑
            biliary tract O26.61- ☑
            ear and mastoid process (conditions in H60-H95) O99.89
            eye and adnexa (conditions in H00-H59) O99.89
            liver O26.61- ☑
            skin (conditions in L00-L99) O99.71- ☑
            specified NEC O99.89
        displacement, uterus NEC O34.59- ☑
            causing obstructed labor O65.5
        disproportion (due to) O33.9
            fetal deformities NEC O33.7
            generally contracted pelvis O33.1
            hydrocephalic fetus O33.6 ☑
            inlet contraction of pelvis O33.2
            mixed maternal and fetal origin O33.4 ☑
            specified NEC O33.8
        double uterus O34.59- ☑
            causing obstructed labor O65.5
        drug use (conditions in F11-F19) O99.32- ☑
        eclampsia, eclamptic (coma) (convulsions) (delirium) (nephritis) (uremia) (*see also* Eclampsia) O15.- ☑
        ectopic pregnancy — *see* Pregnancy, ectopic
        edema O12.0- ☑
            with
                gestational hypertension, mild (*see also* Pre-eclampsia) O14.0- ☑
                proteinuria O12.2- ☑
        effusion, amniotic fluid — *see* Pregnancy, complicated by, premature rupture of membranes
        elderly
            multigravida O09.52- ☑
            primigravida O09.51- ☑
        embolism (*see also* Embolism, obstetric, pregnancy) O88.- ☑
        endocrine diseases NEC O99.28- ☑
        endometritis O86.12
        excessive weight gain O26.0- ☑
        exhaustion O26.81- ☑
            during labor and delivery O75.81
        face presentation O32.3 ☑
        failed induction of labor O61.9
            instrumental O61.1
            mechanical O61.1

Pregnancy — *continued*
    complicated by — *continued*
        failed induction of labor — *continued*
            medical O61.0
            specified NEC O61.8
            surgical O61.1
        failed or difficult intubation for anesthesia O29.6- ☑
        false labor (pains) O47.9
            at or after 37 completed weeks of pregnancy O47.1
            before 37 completed weeks of pregnancy O47.0- ☑
        fatigue O26.81- ☑
            during labor and delivery O75.81
        fatty metamorphosis of liver O26.61- ☑
        female genital mutilation O34.8- ☑ [N90.81-] ☑
        fetal (maternal care for)
            abnormality or damage O35.9 ☑
                acid-base balance O68
                specified type NEC O35.8 ☑
            acidemia O68
            acidosis O68
            alkalosis O68
            anemia and thrombocytopenia O36.82- ☑
            anencephaly O35.0 ☑
            chromosomal abnormality (conditions in Q90-Q99) O35.1 ☑
            conjoined twins O30.02- ☑
            damage from
                amniocentesis O35.7 ☑
                biopsy procedures O35.7 ☑
                drug addiction O35.5 ☑
                hematological investigation O35.7 ☑
                intrauterine contraceptive device O35.7 ☑
                maternal
                    alcohol addiction O35.4 ☑
                    cytomegalovirus infection O35.3 ☑
                    disease NEC O35.8 ☑
                    drug addiction O35.5 ☑
                    listeriosis O35.8 ☑
                    rubella O35.3 ☑
                    toxoplasmosis O35.8 ☑
                    viral infection O35.3 ☑
                medical procedure NEC O35.7 ☑
                radiation O35.6 ☑
            death (near term) O36.4 ☑
               early pregnancy O02.1
            decreased movement O36.81- ☑
            disproportion due to deformity (fetal) O33.7
            excessive growth (large for dates) O36.6- ☑
            growth retardation O36.59- ☑
               light for dates O36.59- ☑
               small for dates O36.59- ☑
            heart rate irregularity (bradycardia) (decelerations) (tachycardia) O76
            hereditary disease O35.2 ☑
            hydrocephalus O35.0 ☑
            intrauterine death O36.4 ☑
            poor growth O36.59- ☑
               light for dates O36.59- ☑
               small for dates O36.59- ☑
            problem O36.9- ☑
               specified NEC O36.89- ☑
            reduction (elective) O31.3- ☑
            selective termination O31.3- ☑
            spina bifida O35.0 ☑
            thrombocytopenia O36.82- ☑
        fibroid (tumor) (uterus) O34.1- ☑
        fissure of nipple O92.11- ☑
        gallstones O99.61- ☑
        gastric banding status O99.84- ☑
        gastric bypass status O99.84- ☑
        genital herpes (asymptomatic) (history of) (inactive) O98.51- ☑
        genital tract infection O23.9- ☑
        glomerular diseases (conditions in N00-N07) O26.83- ☑
            with hypertension, pre-existing — *see* Hypertension, complicating, pregnancy, pre-existing, with, renal disease
        gonorrhea O98.21- ☑
        grand multiparity O09.4 ☑
        habitual aborter — *see* Pregnancy, complicated by, recurrent pregnancy loss

Pregnancy — *continued*
    complicated by — *continued*
        HELLP syndrome (hemolysis, elevated liver enzymes and low platelet count) O14.2- ☑
        hemorrhage
            antepartum — *see* Hemorrhage, antepartum
            before 20 completed weeks gestation O20.9
               specified NEC O20.8
            due to premature separation, placenta (*see also* Abruptio placentae) O45.9- ☑
            early O20.9
               specified NEC O20.8
            threatened abortion O20.0
        hemorrhoids O22.4- ☑
        hepatitis (viral) O98.41- ☑
        herniation of uterus O34.59- ☑
        high
            head at term O32.4 ☑
            risk — *see* Supervision (of) (for), high-risk
        history of in utero procedure during previous pregnancy O09.82- ☑
        HIV O98.71- ☑
        human immunodeficiency virus (HIV) disease O98.71- ☑
        hydatidiform mole (*see also* Mole, hydatidiform) O01.9
        hydramnios O40.- ☑
        hydrocephalic fetus (disproportion) O33.6 ☑
        hydrops
            amnii O40.- ☑
            fetalis O36.2- ☑
               associated with isoimmunization (*see also* Pregnancy, complicated by, isoimmunization) O36.11- ☑
        hydrorrhea O42.90
        hyperemesis (gravidarum) (mild) (*see also* Hyperemesis, gravidarum) O21.0
        hypertension — *see* Hypertension, complicating pregnancy
        hypertensive
            heart and renal disease, pre-existing — *see* Hypertension, complicating, pregnancy, pre-existing, with, heart disease, with renal disease
            heart disease, pre-existing — *see* Hypertension, complicating, pregnancy, pre-existing, with, heart disease
            renal disease, pre-existing — *see* Hypertension, complicating, pregnancy, pre-existing, with, renal disease
        hypotension O26.5- ☑
        immune disorders NEC (conditions in D80-D89) O99.11- ☑
        incarceration, uterus O34.51- ☑
        incompetent cervix O34.3- ☑
        inconclusive fetal viability O36.80 ☑
        infection(s) O98.91- ☑
            amniotic fluid or sac O41.10- ☑
            bladder O23.1- ☑
            carrier state NEC O99.830
               streptococcus B O99.820
            genital organ or tract O23.9- ☑
               specified NEC O23.59- ☑
            genitourinary tract O23.9- ☑
            gonorrhea O98.21- ☑
            hepatitis (viral) O98.41- ☑
            HIV O98.71- ☑
            human immunodeficiency virus (HIV) O98.71- ☑
            kidney O23.0- ☑
            nipple O91.01- ☑
            parasitic disease O98.91- ☑
               specified NEC O98.81- ☑
            protozoal disease O98.61- ☑
            sexually transmitted NEC O98.31- ☑
            specified type NEC O98.81- ☑
            syphilis O98.11- ☑
            tuberculosis O98.01- ☑
            urethra O23.2- ☑
            urinary (tract) O23.4- ☑
               specified NEC O23.3- ☑
            viral disease O98.51- ☑
        injury or poisoning (conditions in S00-T88) O9A.21- ☑ (*following* O99)
            due to abuse
               physical O9A.31- ☑ (*following* O99)

☑ Additional Character Required — Refer to the Tabular List for Character Selection   ▽ Subterms under main terms may continue to next column or page

Pregnancy — *continued*
  complicated by — *continued*
    injury or poisoning — *continued*
      due to abuse — *continued*
        psychological O9A.51- ☑ (*following* O99)
        sexual O9A.41- ☑ (*following* O99)
    insufficient
      prenatal care O09.3- ☑
      weight gain O26.1- ☑
    insulin resistance O26.89 ☑
    intrauterine fetal death (near term) O36.4 ☑
      early pregnancy O02.1
      multiple gestation (one fetus or more)
        O31.2- ☑
    isoimmunization O36.11- ☑
      anti-A sensitization O36.11- ☑
      anti-B sensitization O36.19- ☑
      Rh O36.09- ☑
        anti-D antibody O36.01- ☑
      specified NEC O36.19- ☑
    laceration of uterus NEC O71.81
    malformation
      placenta, placental (vessel) O43.10- ☑
        specified NEC O43.19- ☑
      uterus (congenital) O34.0- ☑
    malnutrition (conditions in E40-E46) O25.1- ☑
    maternal hypotension syndrome O26.5- ☑
    mental disorders (conditions in F01-F09, F20-F99)
      O99.34- ☑
      alcohol use O99.31- ☑
      drug use O99.32- ☑
      smoking O99.33- ☑
    mentum presentation O32.3
    metabolic disorders O99.28- ☑
    missed
      abortion O02.1
      delivery O36.4
    multiple gestations O30.9- ☑
      conjoined twins O30.02- ☑
      quadruplet — *see* Pregnancy, quadruplet
      specified complication NEC O31.8X- ☑
      specified number of multiples NEC — *see*
        Pregnancy, multiple (gestation), specified
        NEC
      triplet — *see* Pregnancy, triplet
      twin — *see* Pregnancy, twin
    musculoskeletal condition (conditions is M00-M99)
      O99.89
    necrosis, liver (conditions in K72) O26.61- ☑
    neoplasm
      benign
        cervix O34.4- ☑
        corpus uteri O34.1- ☑
        uterus O34.1- ☑
      malignant O9A.11- ☑ (*following* O99)
    nephropathy NEC O26.83- ☑
    nervous system condition (conditions in G00-G99)
      O99.35- ☑
    nutritional diseases NEC O99.28- ☑
    obesity (pre-existing) O99.21- ☑
    obesity surgery status O99.84- ☑
    oblique lie or presentation O32.2 ☑
    older mother — *see* Pregnancy, complicated by,
      elderly
    oligohydramnios O41.0- ☑
      with premature rupture of membranes (*see also*
        Pregnancy, complicated by, premature
        rupture of membranes) O42.- ☑
    onset (spontaneous) of labor after 37 completed
      weeks of gestation but before 39 completed
      weeks gestation, with delivery by (planned)
      cesarean section O75.82
    oophoritis O23.52- ☑
    overdose, drug (*see also* Table of Drugs and
      Chemicals, by drug, poisoning) O9A.21- ☑
      (*following* O99)
    oversize fetus O33.5 ☑
    papyraceous fetus O31.0- ☑
    pelvic inflammatory disease O99.89
    periodontal disease O99.61- ☑
    peripheral neuritis O26.82- ☑
    peritoneal (pelvic) adhesions O99.89
    phlebitis O22.9- ☑
    phlebopathy O22.9- ☑
    phlebothrombosis (superficial) O22.2- ☑
      deep O22.3- ☑

Pregnancy — *continued*
  complicated by — *continued*
    placenta accreta O43.21- ☑
    placenta increta O43.22- ☑
    placenta percreta O43.23- ☑
    placenta previa O44.1- ☑
      without hemorrhage O44.0- ☑
    placental disorder O43.9- ☑
      specified NEC O43.89- ☑
    placental dysfunction O43.89- ☑
    placental infarction O43.81- ☑
    placental insufficiency O36.51- ☑
    placental transfusion syndromes
      fetomaternal O43.01- ☑
      fetus to fetus O43.02- ☑
      maternofetal O43.01- ☑
    placentitis O41.14- ☑
    pneumonia O99.51- ☑
    poisoning (*see also* Table of Drugs and Chemicals)
      O9A.21 ☑ (*following* O99)
    polyhydramnios O40- ☑
    polymorphic eruption of pregnancy O26.86
    poor obstetric history NEC O09.29- ☑
    postmaturity (post-term) (40 to 42 weeks) O48.0
      more than 42 completed weeks gestation
        (prolonged) O48.1
    pre-eclampsia O14.9- ☑
      mild O14.0- ☑
      moderate O14.0- ☑
      severe O14.1- ☑
        with hemolysis, elevated liver enzymes and
          low platelet count (HELLP) O14.2- ☑
    premature labor — *see* Pregnancy, complicated
      by, preterm labor
    premature rupture of membranes O42.90
      with onset of labor
        after 24 hours O42.10
          after 37 weeks gestation O42.12
          pre-term (before 37 completed weeks
            of gestation) O42.11- ☑
        within 24 hours O42.00
          after 37 weeks gestation O42.02
          pre-term (before 37 completed weeks
            of gestation) O42.01- ☑
      after 37 weeks gestation O42.92
      full-term O42.92
      pre-term (before 37 completed weeks of gesta-
        tion) O42.91- ☑
    premature separation of placenta (*see also* Abrup-
      tio placentae) O45.9- ☑
    presentation, fetal — *see* Delivery, complicated
      by, malposition
    preterm delivery O60.10 ☑
    preterm labor
      with delivery O60.10 ☑
        preterm O60.10 ☑
        term O60.20 ☑
      without delivery O60.00
        second trimester O60.02
        third trimester O60.03
      second trimester
        with preterm delivery
          second trimester O60.12 ☑
          third trimester O60.13 ☑
        with term delivery O60.22 ☑
        without delivery O60.02
      third trimester
        with term delivery O60.23 ☑
        with third trimester preterm delivery
          O60.14 ☑
        without delivery O60.03
    previous history of — *see* Pregnancy, supervision
      of, high-risk
    prolapse, uterus O34.52- ☑
    proteinuria (gestational) O12.1- ☑
      with edema O12.2- ☑
    pruritic urticarial papules and plaques of pregnancy
      (PUPPP) O26.86
    pruritus (neurogenic) O26.89- ☑
    psychosis or psychoneurosis (puerperal) F53
    ptyalism O26.89- ☑
    PUPPP (pruritic urticarial papules and plaques of
      pregnancy) O26.86
    pyelitis O23.0- ☑
    recurrent pregnancy loss O26.2- ☑

Pregnancy — *continued*
  complicated by — *continued*
    renal disease or failure NEC O26.83- ☑
      with secondary hypertension, pre-existing —
        see Hypertension, complicating, pregnan-
        cy, pre-existing, secondary
      hypertensive, pre-existing — *see* Hypertension,
        complicating, pregnancy, pre-existing,
        with, renal disease
    respiratory condition (conditions in J00-J99)
      O99.51- ☑
    retained, retention
      dead ovum O02.0
      intrauterine contraceptive device O26.3- ☑
    retroversion, uterus O34.53- ☑
    Rh immunization, incompatibility or sensitization
      NEC O36.09- ☑
      anti-D antibody O36.01- ☑
    rupture
      amnion (premature) (*see also* Pregnancy, com-
        plicated by, premature rupture of mem-
        branes) O42- ☑
      membranes (premature) (*see also* Pregnancy,
        complicated by, premature rupture of
        membranes) O42- ☑
      uterus (during labor) O71.1
        before onset of labor O71.0- ☑
    salivation (excessive) O26.89- ☑
    salpingitis O23.52- ☑
    salpingo-oophoritis O23.52- ☑
    sepsis (conditions in A40, A41) O98.81- ☑
    size date discrepancy (uterine) O26.84- ☑
    skin condition (conditions in L00-L99) O99.71- ☑
    smoking (tobacco) O99.33- ☑
    social problem O09.7- ☑
    specified condition NEC O26.89- ☑
    spotting O26.85- ☑
    streptococcus B carrier state O99.820
    subluxation of symphysis (pubis) O26.71- ☑
    syphilis (conditions in A50-A53) O98.11- ☑
    threatened
      abortion O20.0
      labor O47.9
        at or after 37 completed weeks of gestation
          O47.1
        before 37 completed weeks of gestation
          O47.0- ☑
    thrombophlebitis (superficial) O22.2- ☑
    thrombosis O22.9- ☑
      cerebral venous O22.5- ☑
      cerebrovenous sinus O22.5- ☑
      deep O22.3- ☑
    torsion of uterus O34.59- ☑
    toxemia O14.9- ☑
    transverse lie or presentation O32.2 ☑
    tuberculosis (conditions in A15-A19) O98.01- ☑
    tumor (benign)
      cervix O34.4- ☑
      malignant O9A.11- ☑ (*following* O99)
      uterus O34.1- ☑
    unstable lie O32.0 ☑
    upper respiratory infection O99.51- ☑
    urethritis O23.2- ☑
    uterine size date discrepancy O26.84- ☑
    vaginitis or vulvitis O23.59- ☑
    varicose veins (lower extremities) O22.0- ☑
      genitals O22.1- ☑
      legs O22.0- ☑
      perineal O22.1- ☑
      vaginal or vulval O22.1- ☑
    venereal disease NEC (conditions in A63.8)
      O98.31- ☑
    venous disorders O22.9- ☑
      specified NEC O22.8X- ☑
    very young mother — *see* Pregnancy, complicated
      by, young mother
    viral diseases (conditions in A80-B09, B25-B34)
      O98.51- ☑
    vomiting O21.9
      due to diseases classified elsewhere O21.8
      hyperemesis gravidarum (mild) (*see also* Hyper-
        emesis, gravidarum) O21.0
      late (occurring after 20 weeks of gestation)
        O21.2
    young mother
      multigravida O09.62- ☑

Index

Pregnancy — Pregnancy

Pregnancy — *continued*
  complicated by — *continued*
    young mother — *continued*
      primigravida O09.61- ☑
  complicated NOS O26.9- ☑
  concealed O09.3- ☑
  continuing following
    elective fetal reduction of one or more fetus
      O31.3- ☑
    intrauterine death of one or more fetus O31.2- ☑
    spontaneous abortion of one or more fetus
      O31.1- ☑
  cornual O00.8
  ectopic (ruptured) O00.9
    abdominal O00.0
      with viable fetus O36.7- ☑
    cervical O00.8
    complicated (by) O08.9
      afibrinogenemia O08.1
      cardiac arrest O08.81
      chemical damage of pelvic organ(s) O08.6
      circulatory collapse O08.3
      defibrination syndrome O08.1
      electrolyte imbalance O08.5
      embolism (amniotic fluid) (blood clot) (pul-
        monary) (septic) O08.2
      endometritis O08.0
      genital tract and pelvic infection O08.0
      hemorrhage (delayed) (excessive) O08.1
      infection
        genital tract or pelvic O08.0
        kidney O08.83
        urinary tract O08.3
      intravascular coagulation O08.1
      laceration of pelvic organ(s) O08.6
      metabolic disorder O08.5
      oliguria O08.4
      oophoritis O08.0
      parametritis O08.0
      pelvic peritonitis O08.0
      perforation of pelvic organ(s) O08.6
      renal failure or shutdown O08.4
      salpingitis or salpingo-oophoritis O08.0
      sepsis O08.82
      shock O08.83
        septic O08.82
      specified condition NEC O08.89
      tubular necrosis (renal) O08.4
      uremia O08.4
      urinary infection O08.83
      venous complication NEC O08.7
        embolism O08.2
    cornual O00.8
    intraligamentous O00.8
    mural O00.8
    ovarian O00.2
    specified site NEC O00.8
    tubal (ruptured) O00.1
  examination (normal) Z34.9- ☑
    first Z34.0- ☑
    high-risk — *see* Pregnancy, supervision of, high-
      risk
    specified Z34.8- ☑
  extrauterine — *see* Pregnancy, ectopic
  fallopian O00.1
  false F45.8
  hidden O09.3- ☑
  high-risk — *see* Pregnancy, supervision of, high-risk
  incidental finding Z33.1
  interstitial O00.8
  intraligamentous O00.8
  intramural O00.8
  intraperitoneal O00.0
  isthmian O00.1
  mesometric (mural) O00.8
  molar NEC O02.0
    complicated (by) O08.9
      afibrinogenemia O08.1
      cardiac arrest O08.81
      chemical damage of pelvic organ(s) O08.6
      circulatory collapse O08.3
      defibrination syndrome O08.1
      electrolyte imbalance O08.5
      embolism (amniotic fluid) (blood clot) (pul-
        monary) (septic) O08.2
      endometritis O08.0
      genital tract and pelvic infection O08.0
      hemorrhage (delayed) (excessive) O08.1

Pregnancy — *continued*
  molar — *continued*
    complicated — *continued*
      infection
        genital tract or pelvic O08.0
        kidney O08.83
        urinary tract O08.83
      intravascular coagulation O08.1
      laceration of pelvic organ(s) O08.6
      metabolic disorder O08.5
      oliguria O08.4
      oophoritis O08.0
      parametritis O08.0
      pelvic peritonitis O08.0
      perforation of pelvic organ(s) O08.6
      renal failure or shutdown O08.4
      salpingitis or salpingo-oophoritis O08.0
      sepsis O08.82
      shock O08.3
        septic O08.82
      specified condition NEC O08.89
      tubular necrosis (renal) O08.4
      uremia O08.4
      urinary infection O08.83
      venous complication NEC O08.7
        embolism O08.2
    hydatidiform (*see also* Mole, hydatidiform) O01.9
  multiple (gestation) O30.9- ☑
    greater than quadruplets — *see* Pregnancy, multi-
      ple (gestation), specified NEC
    specified NEC O30.80- ☑
      with
        two or more monoamniotic fetuses
          O30.82- ☑
        two or more monochorionic fetuses
          O30.81- ☑
      two or more monoamniotic fetuses O30.82- ☑
      two or more monochorionic fetuses O30.81- ☑
      unable to determine number of placenta and
        number of amniotic sacs O30.89- ☑
      unspecified number of placenta and unspeci-
        fied number of amniotic sacs O30.80- ☑
  mural O00.8
  normal (supervision of) Z34.9- ☑
    first Z34.0- ☑
    high-risk — *see* Pregnancy, supervision of, high-
      risk
    specified Z34.8- ☑
  ovarian O00.2
  postmature (40 to 42 weeks) O48.0
    more than 42 weeks gestation O48.1
  post-term (40 to 42 weeks) O48.0
  prenatal care only Z34.9- ☑
    first Z34.0- ☑
    high-risk — *see* Pregnancy, supervision of, high-
      risk
    specified Z34.8- ☑
  prolonged (more than 42 weeks gestation) O48.1
  quadruplet O30.20- ☑
    with
      two or more monoamniotic fetuses O30.22- ☑
      two or more monochorionic fetuses O30.21- ☑
    two or more monoamniotic fetuses O30.22- ☑
    two or more monochorionic fetuses O30.21- ☑
    unable to determine number of placenta and
      number of amniotic sacs O30.29- ☑
    unspecified number of placenta and unspecified
      number of amniotic sacs O30.20- ☑
  quintuplet — *see* Pregnancy, multiple (gestation),
    specified NEC
  sextuplet — *see* Pregnancy, multiple (gestation),
    specified NEC
  supervision of
    concealed pregnancy O09.3- ☑
    elderly mother
      multigravida O09.52- ☑
      primigravida O09.51- ☑
    hidden pregnancy O09.3- ☑
    high-risk O09.9- ☑
      due to (history of)
        ectopic pregnancy O09.1- ☑
        elderly — *see* Pregnancy, supervision, elder-
          ly mother
        grand multiparity O09.4 ☑
        in utero procedure during previous pregnan-
          cy O09.82- ☑
        in vitro fertilization O09.81- ☑

Pregnancy — *continued*
  supervision of — *continued*
    high-risk — *continued*
      due to — *continued*
        infertility O09.0- ☑
        insufficient prenatal care O09.3- ☑
        molar pregnancy O09.1- ☑
        multiple previous pregnancies O09.4- ☑
        older mother — *see* Pregnancy, supervision
          of, elderly mother
        poor reproductive or obstetric history NEC
          O09.29- ☑
        pre-term labor O09.21- ☑
        previous
          neonatal death O09.29- ☑
        social problems O09.7- ☑
        specified NEC O09.89- ☑
        very young mother — *see* Pregnancy, super-
          vision, young mother
      resulting from in vitro fertilization O09.81- ☑
    normal Z34.9- ☑
      first Z34.0- ☑
      specified NEC Z34.8- ☑
    young mother
      multigravida O09.62- ☑
      primigravida O09.61- ☑
  triplet O30.10- ☑
    with
      two or more monoamniotic fetuses O30.12- ☑
      two or more monochrorionic fetuses O30.11- ☑
    two or more monoamniotic fetuses O30.12- ☑
    two or more monochrorionic fetuses O30.11- ☑
    unable to determine number of placenta and
      number of amniotic sacs O30.19- ☑
    unspecified number of placenta and unspecified
      number of amniotic sacs O30.10- ☑
  tubal (with abortion) (with rupture) O00.1
  twin O30.00- ☑
    conjoined O30.02- ☑
    dichorionic/diamniotic (two placenta, two amniotic
      sacs) O30.04- ☑
    monochorionic/diamniotic (one placenta, two
      amniotic sacs) O30.03- ☑
    monochorionic/monoamniotic (one placenta, one
      amniotic sac) O30.01- ☑
    unable to determine number of placenta and
      number of amniotic sacs O30.09- ☑
    unspecified number of placenta and unspecified
      number of amniotic sacs O30.00- ☑
  unwanted Z64.0
  weeks of gestation
    8 weeks Z3A.08 (*following* Z36)
    9 weeks Z3A.09 (*following* Z36)
    10 weeks Z3A.10 (*following* Z36)
    11 weeks Z3A.11 (*following* Z36)
    12 weeks Z3A.12 (*following* Z36)
    13 weeks Z3A.13 (*following* Z36)
    14 weeks Z3A.14 (*following* Z36)
    15 weeks Z3A.15 (*following* Z36)
    16 weeks Z3A.16 (*following* Z36)
    17 weeks Z3A.17 (*following* Z36)
    18 weeks Z3A.18 (*following* Z36)
    19 weeks Z3A.19 (*following* Z36)
    20 weeks Z3A.20 (*following* Z36)
    21 weeks Z3A.21 (*following* Z36)
    22 weeks Z3A.22 (*following* Z36)
    23 weeks Z3A.23 (*following* Z36)
    24 weeks Z3A.24 (*following* Z36)
    25 weeks Z3A.25 (*following* Z36)
    26 weeks Z3A.26 (*following* Z36)
    27 weeks Z3A.27 (*following* Z36)
    28 weeks Z3A.28 (*following* Z36)
    29 weeks Z3A.29 (*following* Z36)
    30 weeks Z3A.30 (*following* Z36)
    31 weeks Z3A.31 (*following* Z36)
    32 weeks Z3A.32 (*following* Z36)
    33 weeks Z3A.33 (*following* Z36)
    34 weeks Z3A.34 (*following* Z36)
    35 weeks Z3A.35 (*following* Z36)
    36 weeks Z3A.36 (*following* Z36)
    37 weeks Z3A.37 (*following* Z36)
    38 weeks Z3A.38 (*following* Z36)
    39 weeks Z3A.39 (*following* Z36)
    40 weeks Z3A.40 (*following* Z36)
    41 weeks Z3A.41 (*following* Z36)
    42 weeks Z3A.42 (*following* Z36)

☑ **Additional Character Required** — Refer to the Tabular List for Character Selection   ▽ **Subterms under main terms may continue to next column or page**

Pregnancy — *continued*
  weeks of gestation — *continued*
    greater than 42 weeks Z3A.49 (*following* Z36)
    less than 8 weeks Z3A.01 (*following* Z36)
    not specified Z3A.00 (*following* Z36)
Preiser's disease — *see* Osteonecrosis, secondary, due to, trauma, metacarpus
Pre-kwashiorkor — *see* Malnutrition, severe
Preleukemia (syndrome) D46.9
Preluxation, hip, congenital Q65.6
Premature (*see also* condition)
  adrenarche E27.0
  aging E34.8
  beats I49.40
    atrial I49.1
    auricular I49.1
    supraventricular I49.1
  birth NEC — *see* Preterm, newborn
  closure, foramen ovale Q21.8
  contraction
    atrial I49.1
    atrioventricular I49.2
    auricular I49.1
    auriculoventricular I49.49
    heart (extrasystole) I49.49
    junctional I49.2
    ventricular I49.3
  delivery (*see also* Pregnancy, complicated by, preterm labor) O60.10 ☑
  ejaculation F52.4
  infant NEC — *see* Preterm, newborn
    light-for-dates — *see* Light for dates
  labor — *see* Pregnancy, complicated by, preterm labor
  lungs P28.0
  menopause E28.319
    asymptomatic E28.319
    symptomatic E28.310
  newborn
    less than 37 completed weeks — *see* Preterm, newborn
    extreme (less than 28 completed weeks) — *see* Immaturity, extreme
  puberty E30.1
  rupture membranes or amnion — *see* Pregnancy, complicated by, premature rupture of membranes
  senility E34.8
  thelarche E30.8
  ventricular systole I49.3
Prematurity NEC (less than 37 completed weeks) — *see* Preterm, newborn
  extreme (less than 28 completed weeks) — *see* Immaturity, extreme
Premenstrual
  dysphoric disorder (PMDD) N94.3
  tension (syndrome) N94.3
Premolarization, cuspids K00.2
Prenatal
  care, normal pregnancy — *see* Pregnancy, normal
  screening of mother Z36
  teeth K00.6
Preparatory care for subsequent treatment NEC
  for dialysis Z49.01
    peritoneal Z49.02
Prepartum — *see* condition
Preponderance, left or right ventricular I51.7
Prepuce — *see* condition
PRES (posterior reversible encephalopathy syndrome) I67.83
Presbycardia R54
Presbycusis, presbyacusia H91.1- ☑
Presbyesophagus K22.8
Presbyophrenia F03 ☑
Presbyopia H52.4
Prescription of contraceptives (initial) Z30.019
  emergency (postcoital) Z30.012
  implantable subdermal Z30.019
  injectable Z30.013
  intrauterine contraceptive device Z30.014
  pills Z30.011
  postcoital (emergency) Z30.012
  repeat Z30.40
    implantable subdermal Z30.49
    injectable Z30.42
    pills Z30.41
    specified type NEC Z30.49
  specified type NEC Z30.018

Presence (of)
  ankle-joint implant (functional) (prosthesis) Z96.66- ☑
  aortocoronary (bypass) graft Z95.1
  arterial-venous shunt (dialysis) Z99.2
  artificial
    eye (globe) Z97.0
    heart (fully implantable) (mechanical) Z95.812
      valve Z95.2
    larynx Z96.3
    lens (intraocular) Z96.1
    limb (complete) (partial) Z97.1- ☑
      arm Z97.1- ☑
        bilateral Z97.15
      leg Z97.1- ☑
        bilateral Z97.16
  audiological implant (functional) Z96.29
  bladder implant (functional) Z96.0
  bone
    conduction hearing device Z96.29
    implant (functional) NEC Z96.7
    joint (prosthesis) — *see* Presence, joint implant
  cardiac
    defibrillator (functional) (with synchronous cardiac pacemaker) Z95.810
    implant or graft Z95.9
      specified type NEC Z95.818
    pacemaker Z95.0
  cerebrospinal fluid drainage device Z98.2
  cochlear implant (functional) Z96.21
  contact lens (es) Z97.3
  coronary artery graft or prosthesis Z95.5
  CSF shunt Z98.2
  dental prosthesis device Z97.2
  dentures Z97.2
  device (external) NEC Z97.8
    cardiac NEC Z95.818
    heart assist Z95.811
    implanted (functional) Z96.9
      specified NEC Z96.89
    prosthetic Z97.8
  ear implant Z96.20
    cochlear implant Z96.21
    myringotomy tube Z96.22
    specified type NEC Z96.29
  elbow-joint implant (functional) (prosthesis) Z96.62- ☑
  endocrine implant (functional) NEC Z96.49
  eustachian tube stent or device (functional) Z96.29
  external hearing-aid or device Z97.4
  finger-joint implant (functional) (prosthetic) Z96.69- ☑
  functional implant Z96.9
    specified NEC Z96.89
  graft
    cardiac NEC Z95.818
    vascular NEC Z95.828
  hearing-aid or device (external) Z97.4
    implant (bone) (cochlear) (functional) Z96.21
  heart assist device Z95.811
  heart valve implant (functional) Z95.2
    prosthetic Z95.2
    specified type NEC Z95.4
    xenogenic Z95.3
  hip-joint implant (functional) (prosthesis) Z96.64- ☑
  implanted device (artificial) (functional) (prosthetic) Z96.9
    automatic cardiac defibrillator (with synchronous cardiac pacemaker) Z95.810
    cardiac pacemaker Z95.0
    cochlear Z96.21
    dental Z96.5
    heart Z95.812
    heart valve Z95.2
      prosthetic Z95.2
      specified NEC Z95.4
      xenogenic Z95.3
    insulin pump Z96.41
    intraocular lens Z96.1
    joint Z96.60
      ankle Z96.66- ☑
      elbow Z96.62- ☑
      finger Z96.69- ☑
      hip Z96.64- ☑
      knee Z96.65- ☑
      shoulder Z96.61- ☑
      specified NEC Z96.698
      wrist Z96.63- ☑
    larynx Z96.3
    myringotomy tube Z96.22

Presence — *continued*
  implanted device — *continued*
    otological Z96.20
      cochlear Z96.21
      eustachian stent Z96.29
      myringotomy Z96.22
      specified NEC Z96.29
      stapes Z96.29
    skin Z96.81
    skull plate Z96.7
    specified NEC Z96.89
    urogenital Z96.0
  insulin pump (functional) Z96.41
  intestinal bypass or anastomosis Z98.0
  intraocular lens (functional) Z96.1
  intrauterine contraceptive device (IUD) Z97.5
  intravascular implant (functional) (prosthetic) NEC Z95.9
    coronary artery Z95.5
    defibrillator (with synchronous cardiac pacemaker) Z95.810
    peripheral vessel (with angioplasty) Z95.820
  joint implant (prosthetic) (any) Z96.60
    ankle — *see* Presence, ankle joint implant
    elbow — *see* Presence, elbow joint implant
    finger — *see* Presence, finger joint implant
    hip — *see* Presence, hip joint implant
    knee — *see* Presence, knee joint implant
    shoulder — *see* Presence, shoulder joint implant
    specified joint NEC Z96.698
    wrist — *see* Presence, wrist joint implant
  knee-joint implant (functional) (prosthesis) Z96.65- ☑
  laryngeal implant (functional) Z96.3
  mandibular implant (dental) Z96.5
  myringotomy tube(s) Z96.22
  orthopedic-joint implant (prosthetic) (any) — *see* Presence, joint implant
  otological implant (functional) Z96.29
  shoulder-joint implant (functional) (prosthesis) Z96.61- ☑
  skull-plate implant Z96.7
  spectacles Z97.3
  stapes implant (functional) Z96.29
  systemic lupus erythematosus [SLE] inhibitor D68.62
  tendon implant (functional) (graft) Z96.7
  tooth root(s) implant Z96.5
  ureteral stent Z96.0
  urethral stent Z96.0
  urogenital implant (functional) Z96.0
  vascular implant or device Z95.9
    access port device Z95.828
    specified type NEC Z95.828
  wrist-joint implant (functional) (prosthesis) Z96.63- ☑
Presenile (*see also* condition)
  dementia F03 ☑
  premature aging E34.8
Presentation, fetal — *see* Delivery, complicated by, malposition
Prespondylolisthesis (congenital) Q76.2
Pressure
  area, skin — *see* Ulcer, pressure, by site
  brachial plexus G54.0
  brain G93.5
    injury at birth NEC P11.1
  cerebral — *see* Pressure, brain
  chest R07.89
  cone, tentorial G93.5
  hyposystolic (*see also* Hypotension)
    incidental reading, without diagnosis of hypotension R03.1
  increased
    intracranial (benign) G93.2
      injury at birth P11.0
    intraocular H40.05- ☑
  lumbosacral plexus G54.1
  mediastinum J98.5
  necrosis (chronic) — *see* Ulcer, pressure, by site
  parental, inappropriate (excessive) Z62.6
  sore (chronic) — *see* Ulcer, pressure, by site
  spinal cord G95.20
  ulcer (chronic) — *see* Ulcer, pressure, by site
  venous, increased I87.8
Pre-syncope R55
Preterm
  delivery (*see also* Pregnancy, complicated by, preterm labor) O60.10 ☑
  labor — *see* Pregnancy, complicated by, preterm labor

Preterm — *continued*
  newborn (infant) P07.30
    gestational age
      28 completed weeks (28 weeks, 0 days through
        28 weeks, 6 days) P07.31
      29 completed weeks (29 weeks, 0 days through
        29 weeks, 6 days) P07.32
      30 completed weeks (30 weeks, 0 days through
        30 weeks, 6 days) P07.33
      31 completed weeks (31 weeks, 0 days through
        31 weeks, 6 days) P07.34
      32 completed weeks (32 weeks, 0 days through
        32 weeks, 6 days) P07.35
      33 completed weeks (33 weeks, 0 days through
        33 weeks, 6 days) P07.36
      34 completed weeks (34 weeks, 0 days through
        34 weeks, 6 days) P07.37
      35 completed weeks (35 weeks, 0 days through
        35 weeks, 6 days) P07.38
      36 completed weeks (36 weeks, 0 days through
        36 weeks, 6 days) P07.39
Previa
  placenta (low) (marginal) (partial) (total) (with hemor-
    rhage) O44.1- ☑
    without hemorrhage O44.0- ☑
  vasa O69.4 ☑
Priapism N48.30
  due to
    disease classified elsewhere N48.32
    drug N48.33
    specified cause NEC N48.39
    trauma N48.31
Prickling sensation (skin) R20.2
Prickly heat L74.0
Primary — *see* condition
Primigravida
  elderly, affecting management of pregnancy, labor
    and delivery (supervision only) — *see* Pregnan-
    cy, complicated by, elderly, primigravida
  older, affecting management of pregnancy, labor and
    delivery (supervision only) — *see* Pregnancy,
    complicated by, elderly, primigravida
  very young, affecting management of pregnancy, labor
    and delivery (supervision only) — *see* Pregnan-
    cy, complicated by, young mother, primigravida
Primipara
  elderly, affecting management of pregnancy, labor
    and delivery (supervision only) — *see* Pregnan-
    cy, complicated by, elderly, primigravida
  older, affecting management of pregnancy, labor and
    delivery (supervision only) — *see* Pregnancy,
    complicated by, elderly, primigravida
  very young, affecting management of pregnancy, labor
    and delivery (supervision only) — *see* Pregnan-
    cy, complicated by, young mother, primigravida
Primus varus (bilateral) Q66.2
PRIND (Prolonged reversible ischemic neurologic deficit)
  I63.9
Pringle's disease (tuberous sclerosis) Q85.1
Prinzmetal angina I20.1
Prizefighter ear — *see* Cauliflower ear
Problem (with) (related to)
  academic Z55.8
  acculturation Z60.3
  adjustment (to)
    change of job Z56.1
    life-cycle transition Z60.0
    pension Z60.0
    retirement Z60.0
  adopted child Z62.821
  alcoholism in family Z63.72
  atypical parenting situation Z62.9
  bankruptcy Z59.8
  behavioral (adult) F69
    drug seeking Z72.89
  birth of sibling affecting child Z62.898
  care (of)
    provider dependency Z74.9
      specified NEC Z74.8
    sick or handicapped person in family or household
      Z63.6
  child
    abuse (affecting the child) — *see* Maltreatment,
      child
    custody or support proceedings Z65.3
    in care of non-parental family member Z62.21
    in foster care Z62.21
    in welfare custody Z62.21

Problem — *continued*
  child — *continued*
    living in orphanage or group home Z62.22
  child-rearing Z62.9
    specified NEC Z62.898
  communication (developmental) F80.9
  conflict or discord (with)
    boss Z56.4
    classmates Z55.4
    counselor Z64.4
    employer Z56.4
    family Z63.9
      specified NEC Z63.8
    probation officer Z64.4
    social worker Z64.4
    teachers Z55.4
    workmates Z56.4
  conviction in legal proceedings Z65.0
    with imprisonment Z65.1
  counselor Z64.4
  creditors Z59.8
  digestive K92.9
  drug addict in family Z63.72
  ear — *see* Disorder, ear
  economic Z59.9
    affecting care Z59.9
    specified NEC Z59.8
  education Z55.9
    specified NEC Z55.8
  employment Z56.9
    change of job Z56.1
    discord Z56.4
    environment Z56.5
    sexual harassment Z56.81
    specified NEC Z56.89
    stressful schedule Z56.3
    stress NEC Z56.6
    threat of job loss Z56.2
    unemployment Z56.0
  enuresis, child F98.0
  eye H57.9
  failed examinations (school) Z55.2
  falling Z91.81
  family (*see also* Disruption, family) Z63.9
    specified NEC Z63.8
  feeding (elderly) (infant) R63.3
    newborn P92.9
      breast P92.5
      overfeeding P92.4
      slow P92.2
      specified NEC P92.8
      underfeeding P92.3
    nonorganic F50.8
  finance Z59.9
    specified NEC Z59.8
  foreclosure on loan Z59.8
  foster child Z62.822
  frightening experience(s) in childhood Z62.898
  genital NEC
    female N94.9
    male N50.9
  health care Z75.9
    specified NEC Z75.8
  hearing — *see* Deafness
  homelessness Z59.0
  housing Z59.9
    inadequate Z59.1
    isolated Z59.8
    specified NEC Z59.8
  identity (of childhood) F93.8
  illegitimate pregnancy (unwanted) Z64.0
  illiteracy Z55.0
  impaired mobility Z74.09
  imprisonment or incarceration Z65.1
  inadequate teaching affecting education Z55.8
  inappropriate (excessive) parental pressure Z62.6
  influencing health status NEC Z78.9
  in-law Z63.1
  institutionalization, affecting child Z62.22
  intrafamilial communication Z63.8
  jealousy, child F93.8
  landlord Z59.2
  language (developmental) F80.9
  learning (developmental) F81.9
  legal Z65.3
    conviction without imprisonment Z65.0
    imprisonment Z65.1
    release from prison Z65.2

Problem — *continued*
  life-management Z73.9
    specified NEC Z73.89
  life-style Z72.9
    gambling Z72.6
    high-risk sexual behavior (heterosexual) Z72.51
      bisexual Z72.53
      homosexual Z72.52
    inappropriate eating habits Z72.4
    self-damaging behavior NEC Z72.89
    specified NEC Z72.89
    tobacco use Z72.0
  literacy Z55.9
    low level Z55.0
    specified NEC Z55.8
  living alone Z60.2
  lodgers Z59.2
  loss of love relationship in childhood Z62.898
  marital Z63.0
    involving
      divorce Z63.5
      estrangement Z63.5
      gender identity F66
  mastication K08.8
  medical
    care, within family Z63.6
    facilities Z75.9
      specified NEC Z75.8
  mental F48.9
  multiparity Z64.1
  negative life events in childhood Z62.9
    altered pattern of family relationships Z62.898
    frightening experience Z62.898
    loss of
      love relationship Z62.898
      self-esteem Z62.898
    physical abuse (alleged) — *see* Maltreatment, child
    removal from home Z62.29
    specified event NEC Z62.898
  neighbor Z59.2
  neurological NEC R29.818
  new step-parent affecting child Z62.898
  none (feared complaint unfounded) Z71.1
  occupational NEC Z56.89
  parent-child — *see* Conflict, parent-child
  personal hygiene Z91.89
  personality F69
  phase-of-life transition, adjustment Z60.0
  presence of sick or disabled person in family or
    household Z63.79
    needing care Z63.6
  primary support group (family) Z63.9
    specified NEC Z63.8
  probation officer Z64.4
  psychiatric F99
  psychosexual (development) F66
  psychosocial Z65.9
    specified NEC Z65.8
  relationship Z63.9
    childhood F93.8
  release from prison Z65.2
  removal from home affecting child Z62.29
  seeking and accepting known hazardous and harmful
    behavioral or psychological interventions Z65.8
    chemical, nutritional or physical interventions Z65.8
  sexual function (nonorganic) F52.9
  sight H54.7
  sleep disorder, child F51.9
  smell — *see* Disturbance, sensation, smell
  social
    environment Z60.9
      specified NEC Z60.8
    exclusion and rejection Z60.4
    worker Z64.4
  speech R47.9
    developmental F80.9
    specified NEC R47.89
  swallowing — *see* Dysphagia
  taste — *see* Disturbance, sensation, taste
  tic, child F95.0
  underachievement in school Z55.3
  unemployment Z56.0
    threatened Z56.2
  unwanted pregnancy Z64.0
  upbringing Z62.9
    specified NEC Z62.898
  urinary N39.9
  voice production R47.89

Problem — *continued*
  work schedule (stressful) Z56.3
Procedure (surgical)
  for purpose other than remedying health state Z41.9
    specified NEC Z41.8
  not done Z53.9
    because of
      administrative reasons Z53.8
      contraindication Z53.09
        smoking Z53.01
      patient's decision Z53.20
        for reasons of belief or group pressure Z53.1
        left against medical advice (AMA) Z53.21
        specified reason NEC Z53.29
      specified reason NEC Z53.8
Procidentia (uteri) N81.3
Proctalgia K62.89
  fugax K59.4
  spasmodic K59.4
Proctitis K62.89
  amebic (acute) A06.0
  chlamydial A56.3
  gonococcal A54.6
  granulomatous — *see* Enteritis, regional, large intestine
  herpetic A60.1
  radiation K62.7
  tuberculous A18.32
  ulcerative (chronic) K51.20
    with
      complication K51.219
        abscess K51.214
        fistula K51.213
        obstruction K51.212
        rectal bleeding K51.211
        specified NEC K51.218
Proctocele
  female (without uterine prolapse) N81.6
    with uterine prolapse N81.2
      complete N81.3
  male K62.3
Proctocolitis, mucosal — *see* Rectosigmoiditis, ulcerative
Proctoptosis K62.3
Proctorrhagia K62.5
Proctosigmoiditis K63.89
  ulcerative (chronic) — *see* Rectosigmoiditis, ulcerative
Proctospasm K59.4
  psychogenic F45.8
Profichet's disease — *see* Disorder, soft tissue, specified type NEC
Progeria E34.8
Prognathism (mandibular) (maxillary) M26.19
Progonoma (melanotic) — *see* Neoplasm, benign, by site
Progressive — *see* condition
Prolactinoma
  specified site — *see* Neoplasm, benign, by site
  unspecified site D35.2
Prolapse, prolapsed
  anus, anal (canal) (sphincter) K62.2
  arm or hand O32.2 ☑
    causing obstructed labor O64.4 ☑
  bladder (mucosa) (sphincter) (acquired)
    congenital Q79.4
    female — *see* Cystocele
    male N32.89
  breast implant (prosthetic) T85.49 ☑
  cecostomy K94.09
  cecum K63.4
  cervix, cervical (hypertrophied) N81.2
    anterior lip, obstructing labor O65.5
    congenital Q51.828
    postpartal, old N81.2
    stump N81.85
  ciliary body (traumatic) — *see* Laceration, eye(ball), with prolapse or loss of interocular tissue
  colon (pedunculated) K63.4
  colostomy K94.09
  disc (intervertebral) — *see* Displacement, intervertebral disc
  eye implant (orbital) T85.398 ☑
    lens (ocular) — *see* Complications, intraocular lens
  fallopian tube N83.4
  gastric (mucosa) K31.89
  genital, female N81.9
    specified NEC N81.89
  globe, nontraumatic — *see* Luxation, globe

Prolapse, prolapsed — *continued*
  ileostomy bud K94.19
  intervertebral disc — *see* Displacement, intervertebral disc
  intestine (small) K63.4
  iris (traumatic) — *see* Laceration, eye(ball), with prolapse or loss of interocular tissue
    nontraumatic H21.89
  kidney N28.83
    congenital Q63.2
  laryngeal muscles or ventricle J38.7
  liver K76.89
  meatus urinarius N36.8
  mitral (valve) I34.1
  ocular lens implant — *see* Complications, intraocular lens
  organ or site, congenital NEC — *see* Malposition, congenital
  ovary N83.4
  pelvic floor, female N81.89
  perineum, female N81.89
  rectum (mucosa) (sphincter) K62.3
    due to trichuris trichuria B79
  spleen D73.89
  stomach K31.89
  umbilical cord
    complicating delivery O69.0 ☑
  urachus, congenital Q64.4
  ureter N28.89
    with obstruction N13.5
      with infection N13.6
  ureterovesical orifice N28.89
  urethra (acquired) (infected) (mucosa) N36.8
    congenital Q64.71
  urinary meatus N36.8
    congenital Q64.72
  uterovaginal N81.4
    complete N81.3
    incomplete N81.2
  uterus (with prolapse of vagina) N81.4
    complete N81.3
    congenital Q51.818
    first degree N81.2
    in pregnancy or childbirth — *see* Pregnancy, complicated by, abnormal, uterus
    incomplete N81.2
    postpartal (old) N81.4
    second degree N81.2
    third degree N81.3
  uveal (traumatic) — *see* Laceration, eye(ball), with prolapse or loss of interocular tissue
  vagina (anterior) (wall) — *see* Cystocele
    with prolapse of uterus N81.4
      complete N81.3
      incomplete N81.2
    posterior wall N81.6
    posthysterectomy N99.3
  vitreous (humor) H43.0- ☑
    in wound — *see* Laceration, eye(ball), with prolapse or loss of interocular tissue
  womb — *see* Prolapse, uterus
Prolapsus, female N81.9
  specified NEC N81.89
Proliferation(s)
  primary cutaneous CD30-positive large T-cell C86.6
Proliferative — *see* condition
Prolonged, prolongation (of)
  bleeding (time) (idiopathic) R79.1
  coagulation (time) R79.1
  gestation (over 42 completed weeks)
    mother O48.1
    newborn P08.22
  interval I44.0
  labor O63.9
    first stage O63.0
    second stage O63.1
  partial thromboplastin time (PTT) R79.1
  pregnancy (more than 42 weeks gestation) O48.1
  prothrombin time R79.1
  QT interval I45.81
  uterine contractions in labor O62.4
Prominence, prominent
  auricle (congenital) (ear) Q17.5
  ischial spine or sacral promontory
    with disproportion (fetopelvic) O33.0
      causing obstructed labor O65.0
  nose (congenital) acquired M95.0
Promiscuity — *see* High, risk, sexual behavior

Pronation
  ankle — *see* Deformity, limb, foot, specified NEC
  foot (*see also* Deformity, limb, foot, specified NEC)
    congenital Q74.2
Prophylactic
  administration of
    antibiotics, long-term Z79.2
      short-term use — *omit code*
    drug (*see also* Long-term (current) drug therapy (use of)) Z79.899
  medication Z79.899
  organ removal (for neoplasia management) Z40.00
    breast Z40.01
    ovary Z40.02
    specified site NEC Z40.09
  surgery Z40.9
    for risk factors related to malignant neoplasm — *see* Prophylactic, organ removal
    specified NEC Z40.8
  vaccination Z23
Propionic acidemia E71.121
Proptosis (ocular) (*see also* Exophthalmos)
  thyroid — *see* Hyperthyroidism, with goiter
Prosecution, anxiety concerning Z65.3
Prosopagnosia R48.3
Prostadynia N42.81
Prostate, prostatic — *see* condition
Prostatism — *see* Hyperplasia, prostate
Prostatitis (congestive) (suppurative) (with cystitis) N41.9
  acute N41.0
  cavitary N41.8
  chronic N41.1
  diverticular N41.8
  due to Trichomonas (vaginalis) A59.02
  fibrous N41.1
  gonococcal (acute) (chronic) A54.22
  granulomatous N41.4
  hypertrophic N41.1
  subacute N41.1
  trichomonal A59.02
  tuberculous A18.14
Prostatocystitis N41.3
Prostatorrhea N42.89
Prostatosis N42.82
Prostration R53.83
  heat (*see also* Heat, exhaustion)
    anhydrotic T67.3 ☑
    due to
      salt (and water) depletion T67.4 ☑
      water depletion T67.3 ☑
  nervous F48.8
  senile R54
Protanomaly (anomalous trichromat) H53.54
Protanopia (complete) (incomplete) H53.54
Protection (against) (from) — *see* Prophylactic
Protein
  deficiency NEC — *see* Malnutrition
  malnutrition — *see* Malnutrition
  sickness (*see also* Reaction, serum) T80.69 ☑
Proteinemia R77.9
Proteinosis
  alveolar (pulmonary) J84.01
  lipid or lipoid (of Urbach) E78.89
Proteinuria R80.9
  Bence Jones R80.3
  complicating pregnancy — *see* Proteinuria, gestational
  gestational O12.1- ☑
    with edema O12.2- ☑
  idiopathic R80.0
  isolated R80.0
    with glomerular lesion N06.9
      dense deposit disease N06.6
      diffuse
        crescentic glomerulonephritis N06.7
        endocapillary proliferative glomerulonephritis N06.4
        mesangiocapillary glomerulonephritis N06.5
      focal and segmental hyalinosis or sclerosis N06.1
      membranous (diffuse) N06.2
      mesangial proliferative (diffuse) N06.3
      minimal change N06.0
      specified pathology NEC N06.8
  orthostatic R80.2
    with glomerular lesion — *see* Proteinuria, isolated, with glomerular lesion

▽ Subterms under main terms may continue to next column or page   ☑ Additional Character Required — Refer to the Tabular List for Character Selection   257

Problem — Proteinuria

Proteinuria — continued
persistent R80.1
with glomerular lesion — see Proteinuria, isolated, with glomerular lesion
postural R80.2
with glomerular lesion — see Proteinuria, isolated, with glomerular lesion
pre-eclamptic — see Pre-eclampsia
specified type NEC R80.8
Proteolysis, pathologic D65
Proteus (mirabilis) (morganii), **as cause of disease classified elsewhere** B96.4
Prothrombin gene mutation D68.52
Protoporphyria, erythropoietic E80.0
Protozoal (see also condition)
disease B64
specified NEC B60.8
Protrusion, protrusio
acetabuli M24.7
acetabulum (into pelvis) M24.7
device, implant or graft (see also Complications, by site and type, mechanical) T85.698 ☑
arterial graft NEC — see Complication, cardiovascular device, mechanical, vascular
breast (implant) T85.49 ☑
catheter NEC T85.698 ☑
cystostomy T83.090 ☑
dialysis (renal) T82.49 ☑
intraperitoneal T85.691 ☑
infusion NEC T82.594 ☑
spinal (epidural) (subdural) T85.690 ☑
urinary, indwelling T83.098 ☑
electronic (electrode) (pulse generator) (stimulator)
bone T84.390 ☑
nervous system — see Complication, prosthetic device, mechanical, electronic nervous system stimulator
fixation, internal (orthopedic) NEC — see Complication, fixation device, mechanical
gastrointestinal — see Complications, prosthetic device, mechanical, gastrointestinal device
genital NEC T83.498 ☑
intrauterine contraceptive device T83.39 ☑
penile prosthesis T83.490 ☑
heart NEC — see Complication, cardiovascular device, mechanical
joint prosthesis — see Complications, joint prosthesis, mechanical, specified NEC, by site
ocular NEC — see Complications, prosthetic device, mechanical, ocular device
orthopedic NEC — see Complication, orthopedic, device, mechanical
specified NEC T85.628 ☑
urinary NEC (see also Complication, genitourinary, device, urinary, mechanical)
graft T83.29 ☑
vascular NEC — see Complication, cardiovascular device, mechanical
ventricular intracranial shunt T85.09 ☑
intervertebral disc — see Displacement, intervertebral disc
joint prosthesis — see Complications, joint prosthesis, mechanical, specified NEC, by site
nucleus pulposus — see Displacement, intervertebral disc
Prune belly (syndrome) Q79.4
Prurigo (ferox) (gravis) (Hebrae) (Hebra's) (mitis) (simplex) L28.2
Besnier's L20.0
estivalis L56.4
nodularis L28.1
psychogenic F45.8
Pruritus, pruritic (essential) L29.9
ani, anus L29.0
psychogenic F45.8
anogenital L29.3
psychogenic F45.8
due to onchocerca volvulus B73.1
gravidarum — see Pregnancy, complicated by, specified pregnancy-related condition NEC
hiemalis L29.8
neurogenic (any site) F45.8
perianal L29.0
psychogenic (any site) F45.8
scroti, scrotum L29.1
psychogenic F45.8
senile, senilis L29.8

Pruritus, pruritic — continued
specified NEC L29.8
psychogenic F45.8
Trichomonas A59.9
vulva, vulvae L29.2
psychogenic F45.8
Pseudarthrosis, pseudoarthrosis (bone) — see Nonunion, fracture
clavicle, congenital Q74.0
joint, following fusion or arthrodesis M96.0
Pseudoaneurysm — see Aneurysm
Pseudoangina (pectoris) — see Angina
Pseudoangioma I81
Pseudoarteriosus Q28.8
Pseudoarthrosis — see Pseudarthrosis
Pseudobulbar affect (PBA) F48.8
Pseudochromhidrosis L67.8
Pseudocirrhosis, liver, pericardial I31.1
Pseudocowpox B08.03
Pseudocoxalgia M91.3- ☑
Pseudocroup J38.5
Pseudo-Cushing's syndrome, alcohol-induced E24.4
Pseudocyesis F45.8
Pseudocyst
lung J98.4
pancreas K86.3
retina — see Cyst, retina
Pseudoelephantiasis neuroarthritica Q82.0
Pseudoexfoliation, capsule (lens) — see Cataract, specified NEC
Pseudofolliculitis barbae L73.1
Pseudoglioma H44.89
Pseudohemophilia (Bernuth's) (hereditary) (type B) D68.0
Type A D69.8
vascular D69.8
Pseudohermaphroditism Q56.3
adrenal E25.8
female Q56.2
with adrenocortical disorder E25.8
without adrenocortical disorder Q56.2
adrenal, congenital E25.0
male Q56.1
with
5-alpha-reductase deficiency E29.1
adrenocortical disorder E25.8
androgen resistance E34.51
cleft scrotum Q56.1
feminizing testis E34.51
without gonadal disorder Q56.1
adrenal E25.8
Pseudo-Hurler's polydystrophy E77.0
Pseudohydrocephalus G93.2
Pseudohypertrophic muscular dystrophy (Erb's) G71.0
Pseudohypertrophy, muscle G71.0
Pseudohypoparathyroidism E20.1
Pseudoinsomnia F51.03
Pseudoleukemia, infantile D64.89
Pseudomembranous — see condition
Pseudomeningocele (cerebral) (infective) (post-traumatic) G96.19
postprocedural (spinal) G97.82
Pseudomenses (newborn) P54.6
Pseudomenstruation (newborn) P54.6
Pseudomonas
aeruginosa, as cause of disease classified elsewhere B96.5
mallei infection A24.0
as cause of disease classified elsewhere B96.5
pseudomallei, as cause of disease classified elsewhere B96.5
Pseudomyotonia G71.19
Pseudomyxoma peritonei C78.6
Pseudoneuritis, optic (nerve) (disc) (papilla), **congenital** Q14.2
Pseudo-obstruction intestine (acute) (chronic) (idiopathic) (intermittent secondary) (primary) K59.8
Pseudopapilledema H47.33- ☑
congenital Q14.2
Pseudoparalysis
arm or leg R29.818
atonic, congenital P94.2
Pseudopelade L66.0
Pseudophakia Z96.1
Pseudopolyarthritis, rhizomelic M35.3
Pseudopolycythemia D75.1
Pseudopseudohypoparathyroidism E20.1

Pseudopterygium H11.81- ☑
Pseudoptosis (eyelid) — see Blepharochalasis
Pseudopuberty, precocious
female heterosexual E25.8
male isosexual E25.8
Pseudorickets (renal) N25.0
Pseudorubella B08.20
Pseudosclerema, newborn P83.8
Pseudosclerosis (brain)
Jakob's — see Creutzfeldt-Jakob disease or syndrome
of Westphal (Strümpell) E83.01
spastic — see Creutzfeldt-Jakob disease or syndrome
Pseudotetanus — see Convulsions
Pseudotetany R29.0
hysterical F44.5
Pseudotruncus arteriosus Q25.4
Pseudotuberculosis A28.2
enterocolitis A04.8
pasteurella (infection) A28.0
Pseudotumor
cerebri G93.2
orbital H05.11 ☑
Pseudoxanthoma elasticum Q82.8
Psilosis (sprue) (tropical) K90.1
nontropical K90.0
Psittacosis A70
Psoitis M60.88
Psoriasis L40.9
arthropathic L40.50
arthritis mutilans L40.52
distal interphalangeal L40.51
juvenile L40.54
other specified L40.59
spondylitis L40.53
buccal K13.29
flexural L40.8
guttate L40.4
mouth K13.29
nummular L40.0
plaque L40.0
psychogenic F54
pustular (generalized) L40.1
palmaris et plantaris L40.3
specified NEC L40.8
vulgaris L40.0
Psychasthenia F48.8
Psychiatric disorder or problem F99
Psychogenic (see also condition)
factors associated with physical conditions F54
Psychological and behavioral factors affecting medical condition F59
Psychoneurosis, psychoneurotic (see also Neurosis)
anxiety (state) F41.1
depersonalization F48.1
hypochondriacal F45.21
hysteria F44.9
neurasthenic F48.8
personality NEC F60.89
Psychopathy, psychopathic
affectionless F94.2
autistic F84.5
constitution, post-traumatic F07.81
personality — see Disorder, personality
sexual — see Deviation, sexual
state F60.2
Psychosexual identity disorder of childhood F64.2
Psychosis, psychotic F29
acute (transient) F23
hysterical F44.9
affective — see Disorder, mood
alcoholic F10.959
with
abuse F10.159
anxiety disorder F10.980
with
abuse F10.180
dependence F10.280
delirium tremens F10.231
delusions F10.950
with
abuse F10.150
dependence F10.250
dementia F10.97
with dependence F10.27
dependence F10.259

☑ **Additional Character Required** — Refer to the Tabular List for Character Selection   ▽ Subterms under main terms may continue to next column or page

Psychosis, psychotic — *continued*
  alcoholic — *continued*
    with — *continued*
      hallucinosis F10.951
        with
          abuse F10.151
          dependence F10.251
      mood disorder F10.94
        with
          abuse F10.14
          dependence F10.24
      paranoia F10.950
        with
          abuse F10.150
          dependence F10.250
      persisting amnesia F10.96
        with dependence F10.26
    amnestic confabulatory F10.96
      with dependence F10.26
    delirium tremens F10.231
    Korsakoff's, Korsakov's, Korsakow's F10.26
    paranoid type F10.950
      with
        abuse F10.150
        dependence F10.250
  anergastic — *see* Psychosis, organic
  arteriosclerotic (simple type) (uncomplicated) F01.50
    with behavioral disturbance F01.51
  childhood F84.0
    atypical F84.8
  climacteric — *see* Psychosis, involutional
  confusional F29
    acute or subacute F05
    reactive F23
  cycloid F23
  depressive — *see* Disorder, depressive
  disintegrative (childhood) F84.3
  drug-induced — *see* F11-F19 with .X59
    paranoid and hallucinatory states — *see* F11-F19
      with .X50 or .X51
  due to or associated with
    addiction, drug — *see* F11-F19 with .X59
    dependence
      alcohol F10.259
      drug — *see* F11-F19 with .X59
    epilepsy F06.8
    Huntington's chorea F06.8
    ischemia, cerebrovascular (generalized) F06.8
    multiple sclerosis F06.8
    physical disease F06.8
    presenile dementia F03 ☑
    senile dementia F03 ☑
    vascular disease (arteriosclerotic) (cerebral) F01.50
      with behavioral disturbance F01.51
  epileptic F06.8
  episode F23
    due to or associated with physical condition F06.8
  exhaustive F43.0
  hallucinatory, chronic F28
  hypomanic F30.8
  hysterical (acute) F44.9
  induced F24
  infantile F84.0
    atypical F84.8
  infective (acute) (subacute) F05
  involutional F28
    depressive — *see* Disorder, depressive
    melancholic — *see* Disorder, depressive
    paranoid (state) F22
  Korsakoff's, Korsakov's, Korsakow's (nonalcoholic) F04
    alcoholic F10.96
      in dependence F10.26
    induced by other psychoactive substance — *see*
      categories F11-F19 with .X5X
  mania, manic (single episode) F30.2
    recurrent type F31.89
  manic-depressive — *see* Disorder, mood
  menopausal — *see* Psychosis, involutional
  mixed schizophrenic and affective F25.8
  multi-infarct (cerebrovascular) F01.50
    with behavioral disturbance F01.51
  nonorganic F29
    specified NEC F28
  organic F09
    due to or associated with
      arteriosclerosis (cerebral) — *see* Psychosis, arte-
        riosclerotic

Psychosis, psychotic — *continued*
  organic — *continued*
    due to or associated with — *continued*
      cerebrovascular disease, arteriosclerotic — *see*
        Psychosis, arteriosclerotic
      childbirth — *see* Psychosis, puerperal
      Creutzfeldt-Jakob disease or syndrome — *see*
        Creutzfeldt-Jakob disease or syndrome
      dependence, alcohol F10.259
      disease
        alcoholic liver F10.259
        brain, arteriosclerotic — *see* Psychosis, arte-
          riosclerotic
        cerebrovascular F01.50
          with behavioral disturbance F01.51
        Creutzfeldt-Jakob — *see* Creutzfeldt-Jakob
          disease or syndrome
        endocrine or metabolic F06.8
          acute or subacute F05
        liver, alcoholic F10.259
      epilepsy transient (acute) F05
      infection
        brain (intracranial) F06.8
          acute or subacute F05
      intoxication
        alcoholic (acute) F10.259
        drug F11-F19 with .X59
      ischemia, cerebrovascular (generalized) — *see*
        Psychosis, arteriosclerotic
      puerperium — *see* Psychosis, puerperal
      trauma, brain (birth) (from electric current)
        (surgical) F06.8
        acute or subacute F05
    infective F06.8
      acute or subacute F05
    post-traumatic F06.8
      acute or subacute F05
  paranoiac F22
  paranoid (climacteric) (involutional) (menopausal) F22
    psychogenic (acute) F23
    schizophrenic F20.0
    senile F03 ☑
  postpartum F53
  presbyophrenic (type) F03 ☑
  presenile F03 ☑
  psychogenic (paranoid) F23
    depressive F32.3
  puerperal F53
    specified type — *see* Psychosis, by type
  reactive (brief) (transient) (emotional stress) (psycho-
      logical trauma) F23
    depressive F32.3
      recurrent F33.3
    excitative type F30.8
  schizoaffective F25.9
    depressive type F25.1
    manic type F25.0
  schizophrenia, schizophrenic — *see* Schizophrenia
  schizophrenia-like, in epilepsy F06.2
  schizophreniform F20.81
    affective type F25.9
    brief F23
    confusional type F23
    depressive type F25.1
    manic type F25.0
    mixed type F25.0
  senile NEC F03 ☑
    depressed or paranoid type F03 ☑
    simple deterioration F03 ☑
    specified type — *code to* condition
  shared F24
  situational (reactive) F23
  symbiotic (childhood) F84.3
  symptomatic F09
Psychosomatic — *see* Disorder, psychosomatic
Psychosyndrome, organic F07.9
**Psychotic episode due to or associated with physical
  condition** F06.8
Pterygium (eye) H11.00- ☑
  amyloid H11.01- ☑
  central H11.02- ☑
  colli Q18.3
  double H11.03- ☑
  peripheral
    progressive H11.05- ☑
    stationary H11.04- ☑
  recurrent H11.06- ☑

Ptilosis (eyelid) — *see* Madarosis
Ptomaine (poisoning) — *see* Poisoning, food
Ptosis (*see also* Blepharoptosis)
  adiposa (false) — *see* Blepharoptosis
  breast N64.81
  cecum K63.4
  colon K63.4
  congenital (eyelid) Q10.0
    specified site NEC — *see* Anomaly, by site
  eyelid — *see* Blepharoptosis
    congenital Q10.0
  gastric K31.89
  intestine K63.4
  kidney N28.83
  liver K76.89
  renal N28.83
  splanchnic K63.4
  spleen D73.89
  stomach K31.89
  viscera K63.4
PTP D69.51
Ptyalism (periodic) K11.7
  hysterical F45.8
  pregnancy — *see* Pregnancy, complicated by, specified
    pregnancy-related condition NEC
  psychogenic F45.8
Ptyalolithiasis K11.5
Pubarche, precocious E30.1
Pubertas praecox E30.1
Puberty (development state) Z00.3
  bleeding (excessive) N92.2
  delayed E30.0
  precocious (constitutional) (cryptogenic) (idiopathic)
      E30.1
    central E22.8
    due to
      ovarian hyperfunction E28.1
        estrogen E28.0
      testicular hyperfunction E29.0
  premature E30.1
    due to
      adrenal cortical hyperfunction E25.8
      pineal tumor E34.8
      pituitary (anterior) hyperfunction E22.8
Puckering, macula — *see* Degeneration, macula, puckering
Pudenda, pudendum — *see* condition
Puente's disease (simple glandular cheilitis) K13.0
Puerperal, puerperium (complicated by, complications)
  abnormal glucose (tolerance test) O99.815
  abscess
    areola O91.02
      associated with lactation O91.03
    Bartholin's gland O86.19
    breast O91.12
      associated with lactation O91.13
    cervix (uteri) O86.11
    genital organ NEC O86.19
    kidney O86.21
    mammary O91.12
      associated with lactation O91.13
    nipple O91.02
      associated with lactation O91.03
    peritoneum O85
    subareolar O91.12
      associated with lactation O91.13
    urinary tract — *see* Puerperal, infection, urinary
    uterus O86.12
    vagina (wall) O86.13
    vaginorectal O86.13
    vulvovaginal gland O86.13
  adnexitis O86.19
  afibrinogenemia, or other coagulation defect O72.3
  albuminuria (acute) (subacute) — *see* Proteinuria,
    gestational
  alcohol use O99.315
  anemia O90.81
    pre-existing (pre-pregnancy) O99.03
  anesthetic death O89.8
  apoplexy O99.43
  bariatric surgery status O99.845
  blood disorder NEC O99.13
  blood dyscrasia O72.3
  cardiomyopathy O90.3
  cerebrovascular disorder (conditions in I60-I69) O99.43
  cervicitis O86.11
  circulatory system disorder O99.43
  coagulopathy (any) O72.3

Puerperal, puerperium — *continued*
complications O90.9
  specified NEC O90.89
convulsions — *see* Eclampsia
cystitis O86.22
cystopyelitis O86.29
delirium NEC F05
diabetes O24.93
  gestational — *see* Puerperal, gestational diabetes
  pre-existing O24.33
    specified NEC O24.83
    type 1 O24.03
    type 2 O24.13
digestive system disorder O99.63
disease O90.9
  breast NEC O92.29
  cerebrovascular (acute) O99.43
  nonobstetric NEC O99.89
  tubo-ovarian O86.19
  Valsuani's O99.03
disorder O90.9
  biliary tract O26.63
  lactation O92.70
  liver O26.63
  nonobstetric NEC O99.89
disruption
  cesarean wound O90.0
  episiotomy wound O90.1
  perineal laceration wound O90.1
drug use O99.325
eclampsia (with pre-existing hypertension) O15.2
embolism (pulmonary) (blood clot) — *see* Embolism, obstetric, puerperal
endocrine, nutritional or metabolic disease NEC O99.285
endophlebitis — *see* Puerperal, phlebitis
endotrachelitis O86.11
failure
  lactation (complete) O92.3
    partial O92.4
  renal, acute O90.4
fever (of unknown origin) O86.4
  septic O85
fissure, nipple O92.12
  associated with lactation O92.13
fistula
  breast (due to mastitis) O91.12
    associated with lactation O91.13
  nipple O91.02
    associated with lactation O91.03
galactophoritis O91.22
  associated with lactation O91.23
galactorrhea O92.6
gastric banding status O99.845
gastric bypass status O99.845
gastrointestinal disease NEC O99.63
gestational diabetes O24.439
  diet controlled O24.430
  insulin (and diet) controlled O24.434
gonorrhea O98.23
hematoma, subdural O99.43
hemiplegia, cerebral O99.355
  due to cerbrovascular disorder O99.43
hemorrhage O72.1
  brain O99.43
  bulbar O99.43
  cerebellar O99.43
  cerebral O99.43
  cortical O99.43
  delayed or secondary O72.2
  extradural O99.43
  internal capsule O99.43
  intracranial O99.43
  intrapontine O99.43
  meningeal O99.43
  pontine O99.43
  retained placenta O72.0
  subarachnoid O99.43
  subcortical O99.43
  subdural O99.43
  third stage O72.0
  uterine, delayed O72.2
  ventricular O99.43
hemorrhoids O87.2
hepatorenal syndrome O90.4
hypertension — *see* Hypertension, complicating, puerperium
hypertrophy, breast O92.29

Puerperal, puerperium — *continued*
induration breast (fibrous) O92.29
infection O86.4
  cervix O86.11
  generalized O85
  genital tract NEC O86.19
    obstetric surgical wound O86.0
  kidney (bacillus coli) O86.21
  maternal O98.93
    carrier state NEC O99.835
    gonorrhea O98.23
    human immunodeficiency virus (HIV) O98.73
    protozoal O98.63
    sexually transmitted NEC O98.33
    specified NEC O98.83
    streptococcus B carrier state O99.825
    syphilis O98.13
    tuberculosis O98.03
    viral hepatitis O98.43
    viral NEC O98.53
  nipple O91.02
    associated with lactation O91.03
  peritoneum O85
  renal O86.21
  specified NEC O86.89
  urinary (asymptomatic) (tract) NEC O86.20
    bladder O86.22
    kidney O86.21
    specified site NEC O86.29
    urethra O86.22
  vagina O86.13
  vein — *see* Puerperal, phlebitis
ischemia, cerebral O99.43
lymphangitis O86.89
  breast O91.22
    associated with lactation O91.23
malignancy O9A.13 (*following* O99)
malnutrition O25.3
mammillitis O91.02
  associated with lactation O91.03
mammitis O91.22
  associated with lactation O91.23
mania F30.8
mastitis O91.22
  associated with lactation O91.23
  purulent O91.12
    associated with lactation O91.13
melancholia — *see* Disorder, depressive
mental disorder NEC O99.345
metroperitonitis O85
metrorrhagia — *see* Hemorrhage, postpartum
metrosalpingitis O86.19
metrovaginitis O86.13
milk leg O87.1
monoplegia, cerebral O99.43
mood disturbance O90.6
necrosis, liver (acute) (subacute) (conditions in subcategory K72.0) O26.63
  with renal failure O90.4
nervous system disorder O99.355
obesity (pre-existing prior to pregnancy) O99.215
obesity surgery status O99.845
occlusion, precerebral artery O99.43
paralysis
  bladder (sphincter) O90.89
  cerebral O99.43
paralytic stroke O99.43
parametritis O85
paravaginitis O86.13
pelviperitonitis O85
perimetritis O86.12
perimetrosalpingitis O86.19
perinephritis O86.21
periphlebitis — *see* Puerperal phlebitis
peritoneal infection O85
peritonitis (pelvic) O85
perivaginitis O86.13
phlebitis O87.0
  deep O87.1
  pelvic O87.1
  superficial O87.0
phlebothrombosis, deep O87.1
phlegmasia alba dolens O87.1
placental polyp O90.89
pneumonia, embolic — *see* Embolism, obstetric, puerperal
pre-eclampsia — *see* Pre-eclampsia
psychosis F53

Puerperal, puerperium — *continued*
pyelitis O86.21
pyelocystitis O86.29
pyelonephritis O86.21
pyelonephrosis O86.21
pyemia O85
pyocystitis O86.29
pyohemia O85
pyometra O86.12
pyonephritis O86.21
pyosalpingitis O86.19
pyrexia (of unknown origin) O86.4
renal
  disease NEC O90.89
  failure O90.4
respiratory disease NEC O99.53
retention
  decidua — *see* Retention, decidua
  placenta O72.0
  secundines — *see* Retention, secundines
retrated nipple O92.02
salpingo-ovaritis O86.19
salpingoperitonitis O85
secondary perineal tear O90.1
sepsis (pelvic) O85
sepsis O85
septic thrombophlebitis O86.81
skin disorder NEC O99.73
specified condition NEC O99.89
stroke O99.43
subinvolution (uterus) O90.89
subluxation of symphysis (pubis) O26.73
suppuration — *see* Puerperal, abscess
tetanus A34
thelitis O91.02
  associated with lactation O91.03
thrombocytopenia O72.3
thrombophlebitis (superficial) O87.0
  deep O87.1
  pelvic O87.1
  septic O86.81
thrombosis (venous) — *see* Thrombosis, puerperal
thyroiditis O90.5
toxemia (eclamptic) (pre-eclamptic) (with convulsions) O15.2
trauma, non-obstetric O9A.23 (*following* O99)
  caused by abuse (physical) (suspected) O9A.33 (*following* O99)
    confirmed O9A.33 (*following* O99)
    psychological (suspected) O9A.53 (*following* O99)
      confirmed O9A.53 (*following* O99)
    sexual (suspected) O9A.43 (*following* O99)
      confirmed O9A.43 (*following* O99)
uremia (due to renal failure) O90.4
urethritis O86.22
vaginitis O86.13
varicose veins (legs) O87.4
  vulva or perineum O87.8
venous O87.9
vulvitis O86.19
vulvovaginitis O86.13
white leg O87.1
Puerperium — *see* Puerperal
Pulmolithiasis J98.4
Pulmonary — *see* condition
Pulpitis (acute) (anachoretic) (chronic) (hyperplastic) (irreversible) (putrescent) (reversible) (suppurative) (ulcerative) K04.0
Pulpless tooth K04.99
Pulse
alternating R00.8
bigeminal R00.8
fast R00.0
feeble, rapid due to shock following injury T79.4 ☑
rapid R00.0
weak R09.89
Pulsus alternans or trigeminus R00.8
Punch drunk F07.81
Punctum lacrimale occlusion — *see* Obstruction, lacrimal
Puncture
abdomen, abdominal
  wall S31.139 ☑
    with
      foreign body S31.149 ☑

Puncture — *continued*
  abdomen, abdominal — *continued*
    wall — *continued*
      with — *continued*
        penetration into peritoneal cavity S31.639 ☑
          with foreign body S31.649 ☑
        epigastric region S31.132 ☑
          with
            foreign body S31.142 ☑
            penetration into peritoneal cavity S31.632 ☑
              with foreign body S31.642 ☑
        left
          lower quadrant S31.134 ☑
            with
              foreign body S31.144 ☑
              penetration into peritoneal cavity S31.634 ☑
                with foreign body S31.644 ☑
          upper quadrant S31.131 ☑
            with
              foreign body S31.141 ☑
              penetration into peritoneal cavity S31.631 ☑
                with foreign body S31.641 ☑
        periumbilic region S31.135 ☑
          with
            foreign body S31.145 ☑
            penetration into peritoneal cavity S31.635 ☑
              with foreign body S31.645 ☑
        right
          lower quadrant S31.133 ☑
            with
              foreign body S31.143 ☑
              penetration into peritoneal cavity S31.633 ☑
                with foreign body S31.643 ☑
          upper quadrant S31.130 ☑
            with
              foreign body S31.140 ☑
              penetration into peritoneal cavity S31.630 ☑
                with foreign body S31.640 ☑
  accidental, complicating surgery — *see* Complication, accidental puncture or laceration
  alveolar (process) — *see* Puncture, oral cavity
  ankle S91.039 ☑
    with
      foreign body S91.049 ☑
    left S91.032 ☑
      with
        foreign body S91.042 ☑
    right S91.031 ☑
      with
        foreign body S91.041 ☑
  anus S31.833 ☑
    with foreign body S31.834 ☑
  arm (upper) S41.139 ☑
    with foreign body S41.149 ☑
    left S41.132 ☑
      with foreign body S41.142 ☑
    lower — *see* Puncture, forearm
    right S41.131 ☑
      with foreign body S41.141 ☑
  auditory canal (external) (meatus) — *see* Puncture, ear
  auricle, ear — *see* Puncture, ear
  axilla — *see* Puncture, arm
  back (*see also* Puncture, thorax, back)
    lower S31.030 ☑
      with
        foreign body S31.040 ☑
          with penetration into retroperitoneal space S31.041 ☑
        penetration into retroperitoneal space S31.031 ☑
  bladder (traumatic) S37.29 ☑
    nontraumatic N32.89
  breast S21.039 ☑
    with foreign body S21.049 ☑
    left S21.032 ☑
      with foreign body S21.042 ☑
    right S21.031 ☑
      with foreign body S21.041 ☑

Puncture — *continued*
  buttock S31.803 ☑
    with foreign body S31.804 ☑
    left S31.823 ☑
      with foreign body S31.824 ☑
    right S31.813 ☑
      with foreign body S31.814 ☑
  by
    device, implant or graft — *see* Complications, by site and type, mechanical
    foreign body left accidentally in operative wound T81.539 ☑
    instrument (any) during a procedure, accidental — *see* Puncture, accidental complicating surgery
  calf — *see* Puncture, leg
  canaliculus lacrimalis — *see* Puncture, eyelid
  canthus, eye — *see* Puncture, eyelid
  cervical esophagus S11.23 ☑
    with foreign body S11.24 ☑
  cheek (external) S01.439 ☑
    with foreign body S01.449 ☑
    internal — *see* Puncture, oral cavity
    left S01.432 ☑
      with foreign body S01.442 ☑
    right S01.431 ☑
      with foreign body S01.441 ☑
  chest wall — *see* Puncture, thorax
  chin — *see* Puncture, head, specified site NEC
  clitoris — *see* Puncture, vulva
  costal region — *see* Puncture, thorax
  digit(s)
    foot — *see* Puncture, toe
    hand — *see* Puncture, finger
  ear (canal) (external) S01.339 ☑
    with foreign body S01.349 ☑
    drum S09.2- ☑
    left S01.332 ☑
      with foreign body S01.342 ☑
    right S01.331 ☑
      with foreign body S01.341 ☑
  elbow S51.039 ☑
    with
      foreign body S51.049 ☑
    left S51.032 ☑
      with
        foreign body S51.042 ☑
    right S51.031 ☑
      with
        foreign body S51.041 ☑
  epididymis — *see* Puncture, testis
  epigastric region — *see* Puncture, abdomen, wall, epigastric
  epiglottis S11.83 ☑
    with foreign body S11.84 ☑
  esophagus
    cervical S11.23 ☑
      with foreign body S11.24 ☑
    thoracic S27.818 ☑
  eyeball S05.6- ☑
    with foreign body S05.5- ☑
  eyebrow — *see* Puncture, eyelid
  eyelid S01.13- ☑
    with foreign body S01.14- ☑
    left S01.132 ☑
      with foreign body S01.142 ☑
    right S01.131 ☑
      with foreign body S01.141 ☑
  face NEC — *see* Puncture, head, specified site NEC
  finger(s) S61.239 ☑
    with
      damage to nail S61.339 ☑
        with
          foreign body S61.349 ☑
      foreign body S61.249 ☑
    index S61.238 ☑
      with
        damage to nail S61.338 ☑
          with
            foreign body S61.348 ☑
        foreign body S61.248 ☑
      left S61.231 ☑
        with
          damage to nail S61.331 ☑
            with
              foreign body S61.341 ☑

Puncture — *continued*
  finger(s) — *continued*
    index — *continued*
      left — *continued*
        with — *continued*
          foreign body S61.241 ☑
      right S61.230 ☑
        with
          damage to nail S61.330 ☑
            with
              foreign body S61.340 ☑
          foreign body S61.240 ☑
    little S61.238 ☑
      with
        damage to nail S61.338 ☑
          with
            foreign body S61.348 ☑
        foreign body S61.248 ☑
      left S61.237 ☑
        with
          damage to nail S61.337 ☑
            with
              foreign body S61.347 ☑
          foreign body S61.247 ☑
      right S61.236 ☑
        with
          damage to nail S61.336 ☑
            with
              foreign body S61.346 ☑
          foreign body S61.246 ☑
    middle S61.238 ☑
      with
        damage to nail S61.338 ☑
          with
            foreign body S61.348 ☑
        foreign body S61.248 ☑
      left S61.233 ☑
        with
          damage to nail S61.333 ☑
            with
              foreign body S61.343 ☑
          foreign body S61.243 ☑
      right S61.232 ☑
        with
          damage to nail S61.332 ☑
            with
              foreign body S61.342 ☑
          foreign body S61.242 ☑
    ring S61.238 ☑
      with
        damage to nail S61.338 ☑
          with
            foreign body S61.348 ☑
        foreign body S61.248 ☑
      left S61.235 ☑
        with
          damage to nail S61.335 ☑
            with
              foreign body S61.345 ☑
          foreign body S61.245 ☑
      right S61.234 ☑
        with
          damage to nail S61.334 ☑
            with
              foreign body S61.344 ☑
          foreign body S61.244 ☑
  flank S31.139 ☑
    with foreign body S31.149 ☑
  foot (except toe(s) alone) S91.339 ☑
    with foreign body S91.349 ☑
    left S91.332 ☑
      with foreign body S91.342 ☑
    right S91.331 ☑
      with foreign body S91.341 ☑
    toe — *see* Puncture, toe
  forearm S51.839 ☑
    with
      foreign body S51.849 ☑
    elbow only — *see* Puncture, elbow
    left S51.832 ☑
      with
        foreign body S51.842 ☑
    right S51.831 ☑
      with
        foreign body S51.841 ☑
  forehead — *see* Puncture, head, specified site NEC

Puncture — *continued*
  genital organs, external
    female S31.532 ☑
      with foreign body S31.542 ☑
      vagina — *see* Puncture, vagina
      vulva — *see* Puncture, vulva
    male S31.531 ☑
      with foreign body S31.541 ☑
      penis — *see* Puncture, penis
      scrotum — *see* Puncture, scrotum
      testis — *see* Puncture, testis
  groin — *see* Puncture, abdomen, wall
  gum — *see* Puncture, oral cavity
  hand S61.439 ☑
    with
      foreign body S61.449 ☑
    finger — *see* Puncture, finger
    left S61.432 ☑
      with
        foreign body S61.442 ☑
    right S61.431 ☑
      with
        foreign body S61.441 ☑
    thumb — *see* Puncture, thumb
  head S01.93 ☑
    with foreign body S01.94 ☑
    cheek — *see* Puncture, cheek
    ear — *see* Puncture, ear
    eyelid — *see* Puncture, eyelid
    lip — *see* Puncture, oral cavity
    nose — *see* Puncture, nose
    oral cavity — *see* Puncture, oral cavity
    scalp S01.03 ☑
      with foreign body S01.04 ☑
    specified site NEC S01.83 ☑
      with foreign body S01.84 ☑
    temporomandibular area — *see* Puncture, cheek
  heart S26.99 ☑
    with hemopericardium S26.09 ☑
    without hemopericardium S26.19 ☑
  heel — *see* Puncture, foot
  hip S71.039 ☑
    with foreign body S71.049 ☑
    left S71.032 ☑
      with foreign body S71.042 ☑
    right S71.031 ☑
      with foreign body S71.041 ☑
  hymen — *see* Puncture, vagina
  hypochondrium — *see* Puncture, abdomen, wall
  hypogastric region — *see* Puncture, abdomen, wall
  inguinal region — *see* Puncture, abdomen, wall
  instep — *see* Puncture, foot
  internal organs — *see* Injury, by site
  interscapular region — *see* Puncture, thorax, back
  intestine
    large
      colon S36.599 ☑
        ascending S36.590 ☑
        descending S36.592 ☑
        sigmoid S36.593 ☑
        specified site NEC S36.598 ☑
        transverse S36.591 ☑
      rectum S36.69 ☑
    small S36.499 ☑
      duodenum S36.490 ☑
      specified site NEC S36.498 ☑
  intra-abdominal organ S36.99 ☑
    gallbladder S36.128 ☑
    intestine — *see* Puncture, intestine
    liver S36.118 ☑
    pancreas — *see* Puncture, pancreas
    peritoneum S36.81 ☑
    specified site NEC S36.898 ☑
    spleen S36.09 ☑
    stomach S36.39 ☑
  jaw — *see* Puncture, head, specified site NEC
  knee S81.039 ☑
    with foreign body S81.049 ☑
    left S81.032 ☑
      with foreign body S81.042 ☑
    right S81.031 ☑
      with foreign body S81.041 ☑
  labium (majus) (minus) — *see* Puncture, vulva
  lacrimal duct — *see* Puncture, eyelid
  larynx S11.013 ☑
    with foreign body S11.014 ☑

Puncture — *continued*
  leg (lower) S81.839 ☑
    with foreign body S81.849 ☑
    foot — *see* Puncture, foot
    knee — *see* Puncture, knee
    left S81.832 ☑
      with foreign body S81.842 ☑
    right S81.831 ☑
      with foreign body S81.841 ☑
    upper — *see* Puncture, thigh
  lip S01.531 ☑
    with foreign body S01.541 ☑
  loin — *see* Puncture, abdomen, wall
  lower back — *see* Puncture, back, lower
  lumbar region — *see* Puncture, back, lower
  malar region — *see* Puncture, head, specified site NEC
  mammary — *see* Puncture, breast
  mastoid region — *see* Puncture, head, specified site NEC
  mouth — *see* Puncture, oral cavity
  nail
    finger — *see* Puncture, finger, with damage to nail
    toe — *see* Puncture, toe, with damage to nail
  nasal (septum) (sinus) — *see* Puncture, nose
  nasopharynx — *see* Puncture, head, specified site NEC
  neck S11.93 ☑
    with foreign body S11.94 ☑
    involving
      cervical esophagus — *see* Puncture, cervical esophagus
      larynx — *see* Puncture, larynx
      pharynx — *see* Puncture, pharynx
      thyroid gland — *see* Puncture, thyroid gland
      trachea — *see* Puncture, trachea
    specified site NEC S11.83 ☑
      with foreign body S11.84 ☑
  nose (septum) (sinus) S01.23 ☑
    with foreign body S01.24 ☑
  ocular — *see* Puncture, eyeball
  oral cavity S01.532 ☑
    with foreign body S01.542 ☑
  orbit S05.4- ☑
  palate — *see* Puncture, oral cavity
  palm — *see* Puncture, hand
  pancreas S36.299 ☑
    body S36.291 ☑
    head S36.290 ☑
    tail S36.292 ☑
  pelvis — *see* Puncture, back, lower
  penis S31.23 ☑
    with foreign body S31.24 ☑
  perineum
    female S31.43 ☑
      with foreign body S31.44 ☑
    male S31.139 ☑
      with foreign body S31.149 ☑
  periocular area (with or without lacrimal passages) — *see* Puncture, eyelid
  phalanges
    finger — *see* Puncture, finger
    toe — *see* Puncture, toe
  pharynx S11.23 ☑
    with foreign body S11.24 ☑
  pinna — *see* Puncture, ear
  popliteal space — *see* Puncture, knee
  prepuce — *see* Puncture, penis
  pubic region S31.139 ☑
    with foreign body S31.149 ☑
  pudendum — *see* Puncture, genital organs, external
  rectovaginal septum — *see* Puncture, vagina
  sacral region — *see* Puncture, back, lower
  sacroiliac region — *see* Puncture, back, lower
  salivary gland — *see* Puncture, oral cavity
  scalp S01.03 ☑
    with foreign body S01.04 ☑
  scapular region — *see* Puncture, shoulder
  scrotum S31.33 ☑
    with foreign body S31.34 ☑
  shin — *see* Puncture, leg
  shoulder S41.039 ☑
    with foreign body S41.049 ☑
    left S41.032 ☑
      with foreign body S41.042 ☑
    right S41.031 ☑
      with foreign body S41.041 ☑
  spermatic cord — *see* Puncture, testis

Puncture — *continued*
  sternal region — *see* Puncture, thorax, front
  submaxillary region — *see* Puncture, head, specified site NEC
  submental region — *see* Puncture, head, specified site NEC
  subungual
    finger(s) — *see* Puncture, finger, with damage to nail
    toe — *see* Puncture, toe, with damage to nail
  supraclavicular fossa — *see* Puncture, neck, specified site NEC
  temple, temporal region — *see* Puncture, head, specified site NEC
  temporomandibular area — *see* Puncture, cheek
  testis S31.33 ☑
    with foreign body S31.34 ☑
  thigh S71.139 ☑
    with foreign body S71.149 ☑
    left S71.132 ☑
      with foreign body S71.142 ☑
    right S71.131 ☑
      with foreign body S71.141 ☑
  thorax, thoracic (wall) S21.93 ☑
    with foreign body S21.94 ☑
    back S21.23- ☑
      with
        foreign body S21.24- ☑
          with penetration S21.44 ☑
        penetration S21.43 ☑
    breast — *see* Puncture, breast
    front S21.13- ☑
      with
        foreign body S21.14- ☑
          with penetration S21.34 ☑
        penetration S21.33 ☑
  throat — *see* Puncture, neck
  thumb S61.039 ☑
    with
      damage to nail S61.139 ☑
        with
          foreign body S61.149 ☑
      foreign body S61.049 ☑
    left S61.032 ☑
      with
        damage to nail S61.132 ☑
          with
            foreign body S61.142 ☑
        foreign body S61.042 ☑
    right S61.031 ☑
      with
        damage to nail S61.131 ☑
          with
            foreign body S61.141 ☑
        foreign body S61.041 ☑
  thyroid gland S11.13 ☑
    with foreign body S11.14 ☑
  toe(s) S91.139 ☑
    with
      damage to nail S91.239 ☑
        with
          foreign body S91.249 ☑
      foreign body S91.149 ☑
    great S91.133 ☑
      with
        damage to nail S91.233 ☑
          with
            foreign body S91.243 ☑
        foreign body S91.143 ☑
      left S91.132 ☑
        with
          damage to nail S91.232 ☑
            with
              foreign body S91.242 ☑
          foreign body S91.142 ☑
      right S91.131 ☑
        with
          damage to nail S91.231 ☑
            with
              foreign body S91.241 ☑
          foreign body S91.141 ☑
    lesser S91.136 ☑
      with
        damage to nail S91.236 ☑
          with
            foreign body S91.246 ☑

☑ **Additional Character Required — Refer to the Tabular List for Character Selection**   ▽ **Subterms under main terms may continue to next column or page**

Puncture — *continued*
  toe(s) — *continued*
    lesser — *continued*
      with — *continued*
        foreign body S91.146 ☑
        left S91.135 ☑
          with
            damage to nail S91.235 ☑
              with
                foreign body S91.245 ☑
            foreign body S91.145 ☑
        right S91.134 ☑
          with
            damage to nail S91.234 ☑
              with
                foreign body S91.244 ☑
            foreign body S91.144 ☑
  tongue — *see* Puncture, oral cavity
  trachea S11.023 ☑
    with foreign body S11.024 ☑
  tunica vaginalis — *see* Puncture, testis
  tympanum, tympanic membrane S09.2- ☑
  umbilical region S31.135 ☑
    with foreign body S31.145 ☑
  uvula — *see* Puncture, oral cavity
  vagina S31.43 ☑
    with foreign body S31.44 ☑
  vocal cords S11.033 ☑
    with foreign body S11.034 ☑
  vulva S31.43 ☑
    with foreign body S31.44 ☑
  wrist S61.539 ☑
    with
      foreign body S61.549 ☑
    left S61.532 ☑
      with
        foreign body S61.542 ☑
    right S61.531 ☑
      with
        foreign body S61.541 ☑
PUO (pyrexia of unknown origin) R50.9
Pupillary membrane (persistent) Q13.89
Pupillotonia — *see* Anomaly, pupil, function, tonic pupil
Purpura D69.2
  abdominal D69.0
  allergic D69.0
  anaphylactoid D69.0
  annularis telangiectodes L81.7
  arthritic D69.0
  autoerythrocyte sensitization D69.2
  autoimmune D69.0
  bacterial D69.0
  Bateman's (senile) D69.2
  capillary fragility (hereditary) (idiopathic) D69.8
  cryoglobulinemic D89.1
  Devil's pinches D69.2
  fibrinolytic — *see* Fibrinolysis
  fulminans, fulminous D65
  gangrenous D65
  hemorrhagic, hemorrhagica D69.3
    not due to thrombocytopenia D69.0
  Henoch (-Schönlein) (allergic) D69.0
  hypergammaglobulinemic (benign) (Waldenström)
    D89.0
  idiopathic (thrombocytopenic) D69.3
    nonthrombocytopenic D69.0
  immune thrombocytopenic D69.3
  infectious D69.0
  malignant D69.0
  neonatorum P54.5
  nervosa D69.0
  newborn P54.5
  nonthrombocytopenic D69.2
    hemorrhagic D69.0
    idiopathic D69.0
  nonthrombopenic D69.2
  peliosis rheumatica D69.0
  posttransfusion (post-transfusion) (from (fresh) whole
    blood or blood products) D69.51
  primary D69.49
  red cell membrane sensitivity D69.2
  rheumatica D69.0
  Schönlein (-Henoch) (allergic) D69.0
  scorbutic E54 [D77]
  senile D69.2
  simplex D69.2
  symptomatica D69.0

Purpura — *continued*
  telangiectasia annularis L81.7
  thrombocytopenic D69.49
    congenital D69.42
    hemorrhagic D69.3
    hereditary D69.42
    idiopathic D69.3
    immune D69.3
    neonatal, transitory P61.0
    thrombotic M31.1
  thrombohemolytic — *see* Fibrinolysis
  thrombolytic — *see* Fibrinolysis
  thrombopenic D69.49
  thrombotic, thrombocytopenic M31.1
  toxic D69.0
  vascular D69.0
  visceral symptoms D69.0
Purpuric spots R23.3
Purulent — *see* condition
Pus
  in
    stool R19.5
    urine N39.0
  tube (rupture) — *see* Salpingo-oophoritis
Pustular rash L08.0
Pustule (nonmalignant) L08.9
  malignant A22.0
Pustulosis palmaris et plantaris L40.3
Putnam (-Dana) **disease or syndrome** — *see* Degeneration, combined
Putrescent pulp (dental) K04.1
Pyarthritis, pyarthrosis — *see* Arthritis, pyogenic or pyemic
  tuberculous — *see* Tuberculosis, joint
Pyelectasis — *see* Hydronephrosis
Pyelitis (congenital) (uremic) (*see also* Pyelonephritis)
  with
    calculus — *see* category N20 ☑
      with hydronephrosis N13.2
    contracted kidney N11.9
  acute N10
  chronic N11.9
    with calculus — *see* category N20 ☑
      with hydronephrosis N13.2
  cystica N28.84
  puerperal (postpartum) O86.21
  tuberculous A18.11
Pyelocystitis — *see* Pyelonephritis
Pyelonephritis (*see also* Nephritis, tubulo-interstitial)
  with
    calculus — *see* category N20 ☑
      with hydronephrosis N13.2
    contracted kidney N11.9
  acute N10
  calculous — *see* category N20 ☑
    with hydronephrosis N13.2
  chronic N11.9
    with calculus — *see* category N20 ☑
      with hydronephrosis N13.2
    associated with ureteral obstruction or stricture
      N11.1
    nonobstructive N11.8
      with reflux (vesicoureteral) N11.0
    obstructive N11.1
    specified NEC N11.8
  in (due to)
    brucellosis A23.9 [N16]
    cryoglobulinemia (mixed) D89.1 [N16]
    cystinosis E72.04
    diphtheria A36.84
    glycogen storage disease E74.09 [N16]
    leukemia NEC C95.9- ☑ [N16]
    lymphoma NEC C85.90 [N16]
    multiple myeloma C90.0- ☑ [N16]
    obstruction N11.1
    Salmonella infection A02.25
    sarcoidosis D86.84
    sepsis A41.9 [N16]
    Sjögren's disease M35.04
    toxoplasmosis B58.83
    transplant rejection T86.91 [N16]
    Wilson's disease E83.01 [N16]
  nonobstructive N12
    with reflux (vesicoureteral) N11.0
    chronic N11.8
  syphilitic A52.75
Pyelonephrosis (obstructive) N11.1
  chronic N11.9

Pyelophlebitis I80.8
Pyeloureteritis cystica N28.85
Pyemia, pyemic (fever) (infection) (purulent) (*see also* Sepsis)
  joint — *see* Arthritis, pyogenic or pyemic
  liver K75.1
  pneumococcal A40.3
  portal K75.1
  postvaccinal T88.0 ☑
  puerperal, postpartum, childbirth O85
  specified organism NEC A41.89
  tuberculous — *see* Tuberculosis, miliary
Pygopagus Q89.4
Pyknoepilepsy (idiopathic) — *see* Pyknolepsy
Pyknolepsy G40.A09 (*following* G40.3)
  intractable G40.A19 (*following* G40.3)
    with status epilepticus G40.A11 (*following* G40.3)
    without status epilepticus G40.A19 (*following* G40.3)
  not intractable G40.A09 (*following* G40.3)
    with status epilepticus G40.A01 (*following* G40.3)
    without status epilepticus G40.A09 (*following* G40.3)
Pylephlebitis K75.1
Pyle's syndrome Q78.5
Pylethrombophlebitis K75.1
Pylethrombosis K75.1
Pyloritis K29.90
  with bleeding K29.91
Pylorospasm (reflex) **NEC** K31.3
  congenital or infantile Q40.0
  neurotic F45.8
  newborn Q40.0
  psychogenic F45.8
Pylorus, pyloric — *see* condition
Pyoarthrosis — *see* Arthritis, pyogenic or pyemic
Pyocele
  mastoid — *see* Mastoiditis, acute
  sinus (accessory) — *see* Sinusitis
  turbinate (bone) J32.9
  urethra (*see also* Urethritis) N34.0
Pyocolpos — *see* Vaginitis
Pyocystitis N30.80
  with hematuria N30.81
Pyoderma, pyodermia L08.0
  gangrenosum L88
  newborn P39.4
  phagedenic L88
  vegetans L08.81
Pyodermatitis L08.0
  vegetans L08.81
Pyogenic — *see* condition
Pyohydronephrosis N13.6
Pyometra, pyometrium, pyometritis — *see* Endometritis
Pyomyositis (tropical) — *see* Myositis, infective
Pyonephritis N12
Pyonephrosis N13.6
  tuberculous A18.11
Pyo-oophoritis — *see* Salpingo-oophoritis
Pyo-ovarium — *see* Salpingo-oophoritis
Pyopericarditis, pyopericardium I30.1
Pyophlebitis — *see* Phlebitis
Pyopneumopericardium I30.1
Pyopneumothorax (infective) J86.9
  with fistula J86.0
  tuberculous NEC A15.6
Pyosalpinx, pyosalpingitis (*see also* Salpingo-oophoritis)
Pyothorax J86.9
  with fistula J86.0
  tuberculous NEC A15.6
Pyoureter N28.89
  tuberculous A18.11
Pyramidopallidonigral syndrome G20
Pyrexia (of unknown origin) R50.9
  atmospheric T67.0 ☑
  during labor NEC O75.2
  heat T67.0 ☑
  newborn P81.9
    environmentally-induced P81.0
  persistent R50.9
  puerperal O86.4
Pyroglobulinemia NEC E88.09
Pyromania F63.1
Pyrosis R12
Pyuria (bacterial) N39.0

Q

Q fever A78
  with pneumonia A78
Quadricuspid aortic valve Q23.8
Quadrilateral fever A78
Quadriparesis — *see* Quadriplegia
  meaning muscle weakness M62.81
Quadriplegia G82.50
  complete
      C1-C4 level G82.51
      C5-C7 level G82.53
  congenital (cerebral) (spinal) G80.8
      spastic G80.0
  embolic (current episode) I63.4 ☑
  functional R53.2
  incomplete
      C1-C4 level G82.52
      C5-C7 level G82.54
  thrombotic (current episode) I63.3 ☑
  traumatic — *code to* injury with seventh character S
      current episode — *see* Injury, spinal (cord), cervical
Quadruplet, pregnancy — *see* Pregnancy, quadruplet
Quarrelsomeness F60.3
Queensland fever A77.3
Quervain's disease M65.4
  thyroid E06.1
Queyrat's erythroplasia D07.4
  penis D07.4
  specified site — *see* Neoplasm, skin, in situ
  unspecified site D07.4
Quincke's disease or edema T78.3 ☑
  hereditary D84.1
Quinsy (gangrenous) J36
Quintan fever A79.0
Quintuplet, pregnancy — *see* Pregnancy, quintuplet

R

Rabbit fever — *see* Tularemia
Rabies A82.9
  contact Z20.3
  exposure to Z20.3
  inoculation reaction — *see* Complications, vaccination
  sylvatic A82.0
  urban A82.1
Rachischisis — *see* Spina bifida
Rachitic (*see also* condition)
  deformities of spine (late effect) (sequelae) E64.3
  pelvis (late effect) (sequelae) E64.3
      with disproportion (fetopelvic) O33.0
          causing obstructed labor O65.0
Rachitis, rachitism (acute) (tarda) (*see also* Rickets)
  renalis N25.0
  sequelae E64.3
Radial nerve — *see* condition
Radiation
  burn — *see* Burn
  effects NOS T66 ☑
  sickness NOS T66 ☑
  therapy, encounter for Z51.0
Radiculitis (pressure) (vertebrogenic) — *see* Radiculopathy
Radiculomyelitis (*see also* Encephalitis)
  toxic, due to
      Clostridium tetani A35
      Corynebacterium diphtheriae A36.82
Radiculopathy M54.10
  cervical region M54.12
  cervicothoracic region M54.13
  due to
      disc disorder
          C3 M50.11
          C4 M50.11
          C5 M50.12
          C6 M50.12
          C7 M50.12
          C8 M50.13
      displacement of intervertebral disc — *see* Disorder, disc, with, radiculopathy
  leg M54.1- ☑
  lumbar region M54.16
  lumbosacral region M54.17
  occipito-atlanto-axial region M54.11
  postherpetic B02.29
  sacrococcygeal region M54.18

Radiculopathy — *continued*
  syphilitic A52.11
  thoracic region (with visceral pain) M54.14
  thoracolumbar region M54.15
Radiodermal burns (acute, chronic, or occupational) — *see* Burn
Radiodermatitis L58.9
  acute L58.0
  chronic L58.1
Radiotherapy session Z51.0
Rage, meaning rabies — *see* Rabies
Ragpicker's disease A22.1
Ragsorter's disease A22.1
Raillietiniasis B71.8
Railroad neurosis F48.8
Railway spine F48.8
Raised (*see also* Elevated)
  antibody titer R76.0
Rake teeth, tooth M26.39
Rales R09.89
Ramifying renal pelvis Q63.8
Ramsay-Hunt disease or syndrome (*see also* Hunt's disease) B02.21
  meaning dyssynergia cerebellaris myoclonica G11.1
Ranula K11.6
  congenital Q38.4
Rape
  adult
      confirmed T74.21 ☑
      suspected T76.21 ☑
  alleged, observation or examination, ruled out
      adult Z04.41
      child Z04.42
  child
      confirmed T74.22 ☑
      suspected T76.22 ☑
Rapid
  feeble pulse, due to shock, following injury T79.4 ☑
  heart (beat) R00.0
      psychogenic F45.8
  second stage (delivery) O62.3
  time-zone change syndrome — *see* Disorder, sleep, circadian rhythm, psychogenic
Rarefaction, bone — *see* Disorder, bone, density and structure, specified NEC
Rash (toxic) R21
  canker A38.9
  diaper L22
  drug (internal use) L27.0
      contact (*see also* Dermatitis, due to, drugs, external) L25.1
  following immunization T88.1 ☑
  food — *see* Dermatitis, due to, food
  heat L74.0
  napkin (psoriasiform) L22
  nettle — *see* Urticaria
  pustular L08.0
  rose R21
      epidemic B06.9
  scarlet A38.9
  serum (*see also* Reaction, serum) T80.69 ☑
  wandering tongue K14.1
Rasmussen aneurysm — *see* Tuberculosis, pulmonary
Rasmussen encephalitis G04.81
Rat-bite fever A25.9
  due to Streptobacillus moniliformis A25.1
  spirochetal (morsus muris) A25.0
Rathke's pouch tumor D44.3
Raymond (-Céstan) **syndrome** I65.8
Raynaud's disease, phenomenon or syndrome (secondary) I73.00
  with gangrene (symmetric) I73.01
RDS (newborn) (type I) P22.0
  type II P22.1
Reaction (*see also* Disorder)
  adaptation — *see* Disorder, adjustment
  adjustment (anxiety) (conduct disorder) (depressiveness) (distress) — *see* Disorder, adjustment
      with
          mutism, elective (child) (adolescent) F94.0
  adverse
      food (any) (ingested) NEC T78.1 ☑
          anaphylactic — *see* Shock, anaphylactic, due to food
  affective — *see* Disorder, mood
  allergic — *see* Allergy
  anaphylactic — *see* Shock, anaphylactic

Reaction — *continued*
  anaphylactoid — *see* Shock, anaphylactic
  anesthesia — *see* Anesthesia, complication
  antitoxin (prophylactic) (therapeutic) — *see* Complications, vaccination
  anxiety F41.1
  Arthus — *see* Arthus' phenomenon
  asthenic F48.8
  combat and operational stress F43.0
  compulsive F42
  conversion F44.9
  crisis, acute F43.0
  deoxyribonuclease (DNA) (DNase) hypersensitivity D69.2
  depressive (single episode) F32.9
      affective (single episode) F31.4
          recurrent episode F33.9
      neurotic F34.1
      psychoneurotic F34.1
      psychotic F32.3
      recurrent — *see* Disorder, depressive, recurrent
  dissociative F44.9
  drug NEC T88.7 ☑
      addictive — *see* Dependence, drug
          transmitted via placenta or breast milk — *see* Absorption, drug, addictive, through placenta
      allergic — *see* Allergy, drug
      lichenoid L43.2
      newborn P93.8
          gray baby syndrome P93.0
      overdose or poisoning (by accident) — *see* Table of Drugs and Chemicals, by drug, poisoning
      photoallergic L56.1
      phototoxic L56.0
      withdrawal — *see* Dependence, by drug, with, withdrawal
          infant of dependent mother P96.1
          newborn P96.1
      wrong substance given or taken (by accident) — *see* Table of Drugs and Chemicals, by drug, poisoning
  fear F40.9
      child (abnormal) F93.8
  febrile nonhemolytic transfusion (FNHTR) R50.84
  fluid loss, cerebrospinal G97.1
  foreign
      body NEC — *see* Granuloma, foreign body
          in operative wound (inadvertently left) — *see* Foreign body, accidentally left during a procedure
      substance accidentally left during a procedure (chemical) (powder) (talc) T81.60 ☑
          aseptic peritonitis T81.61 ☑
          body or object (instrument) (sponge) (swab) — *see* Foreign body, accidentally left during a procedure
          specified reaction NEC T81.69 ☑
  grief — *see* Disorder, adjustment
  Herxheimer's R68.89
  hyperkinetic — *see* Hyperkinesia
  hypochondriacal F45.20
  hypoglycemic, due to insulin E16.0
      with coma (diabetic) — *see* Diabetes, coma nondiabetic E15
      therapeutic misadventure — *see* subcategory T38.3
  hypomanic F30.8
  hysterical F44.9
  immunization — *see* Complications, vaccination
  incompatibility
      ABO blood group (infusion) (transfusion) — *see* Complication(s), transfusion, incompatibility reaction, ABO
          delayed serologic T80.39 ☑
      minor blood group (Duffy) (E) (K(ell)) (Kidd) (Lewis) (M) (N) (P) (S) T80.89 ☑
      Rh (factor) (infusion) (transfusion) — *see* Complication(s), transfusion, incompatibility reaction, Rh (factor)
  inflammatory — *see* Infection
  infusion — *see* Complications, infusion
  inoculation (immune serum) — *see* Complications, vaccination
  insulin T38.3- ☑
  involutional psychotic — *see* Disorder, depressive

☑ **Additional Character Required** — Refer to the Tabular List for Character Selection   ⚠ **Subterms under main terms may continue to next column or page**

Reaction — *continued*
  leukemoid D72.823
    basophilic D72.823
    lymphocytic D72.823
    monocytic D72.823
    myelocytic D72.823
    neutrophilic D72.823
  LSD (acute)
    due to drug abuse — *see* Abuse, drug, hallucinogen
    due to drug dependence — *see* Dependence, drug, hallucinogen
  lumbar puncture G97.1
  manic-depressive — *see* Disorder, bipolar
  neurasthenic F48.8
  neurogenic — *see* Neurosis
  neurotic F48.9
  neurotic-depressive F34.1
  nitritoid — *see* Crisis, nitritoid
  nonspecific
    to
      cell mediated immunity measurement of gamma interferon antigen response without active tuberculosis R76.12
      QuantiFERON-TB test (QFT) without active tuberculosis R76.12
      tuberculin test (*see also* Reaction, tuberculin skin test) R76.11
  obsessive-compulsive F42
  organic, acute or subacute — *see* Delirium
  paranoid (acute) F23
    chronic F22
    senile F03 ☑
  passive dependency F60.7
  phobic F40.9
  post-traumatic stress, uncomplicated Z73.3
  psychogenic F99
  psychoneurotic (*see also* Neurosis)
    compulsive F42
    depersonalization F48.1
    depressive F34.1
    hypochondriacal F45.20
    neurasthenic F48.8
    obsessive F42
  psychophysiologic — *see* Disorder, somatoform
  psychosomatic — *see* Disorder, somatoform
  psychotic — *see* Psychosis
  scarlet fever toxin — *see* Complications, vaccination
  schizophrenic F23
    acute (brief) (undifferentiated) F23
    latent F21
    undifferentiated (acute) (brief) F23
  serological for syphilis — *see* Serology for syphilis
  serum T80.69 ☑
    anaphylactic (immediate) (*see also* Shock, anaphylactic) T80.59 ☑
    specified reaction NEC
      due to
        administration of blood and blood products T80.61 ☑
        immunization T80.62 ☑
        serum specified NEC T80.69 ☑
        vaccination T80.62 ☑
  situational — *see* Disorder, adjustment
  somatization — *see* Disorder, somatoform
  spinal puncture G97.1
  stress (severe) F43.9
    acute (agitation) ("daze") (disorientation) (disturbance of consciousness) (flight reaction) (fugue) F43.0
    specified NEC F43.8
  surgical procedure — *see* Complications, surgical procedure
  tetanus antitoxin — *see* Complications, vaccination
  toxic, to local anesthesia T81.89 ☑
    in labor and delivery O74.4
    in pregnancy O29.3X- ☑
    postpartum, puerperal O89.3
  toxin-antitoxin — *see* Complications, vaccination
  transfusion (blood) (bone marrow) (lymphocytes) (allergic) — *see* Complications, transfusion
  tuberculin skin test, abnormal R76.11
  vaccination (any) — *see* Complications, vaccination
  withdrawing, child or adolescent F93.8
Reactive airway disease — *see* Asthma
Reactive depression — *see* Reaction, depressive

Rearrangement
  chromosomal
    balanced (in) Q95.9
      abnormal individual (autosomal) Q95.2
        non-sex (autosomal) chromosomes Q95.2
        sex/non-sex chromosomes Q95.3
      specified NEC Q95.8
Recalcitrant patient — *see* Noncompliance
Recanalization, thrombus — *see* Thrombosis
Recession, receding
  chamber angle (eye) H21.55- ☑
  chin M26.09
  gingival (generalized) (localized) (postinfective) (postoperative) K06.0
Recklinghausen disease Q85.01
  bones E21.0
Reclus' disease (cystic) — *see* Mastopathy, cystic
Recrudescent typhus (fever) A75.1
Recruitment, auditory H93.21- ☑
Rectalgia K62.89
Rectitis K62.89
Rectocele
  female (without uterine prolapse) N81.6
    with uterine prolapse N81.4
      incomplete N81.2
  in pregnancy — *see* Pregnancy, complicated by, abnormal, pelvic organs or tissues NEC
  male K62.3
Rectosigmoid junction — *see* condition
Rectosigmoiditis K63.89
  ulcerative (chronic) K51.30
    with
      complication K51.319
        abscess K51.314
        fistula K51.313
        obstruction K51.312
        rectal bleeding K51.311
        specified NEC K51.318
Rectourethral — *see* condition
Rectovaginal — *see* condition
Rectovesical — *see* condition
Rectum, rectal — *see* condition
Recurrent — *see* condition
  pregnancy loss — *see* Loss (of), pregnancy, recurrent
Red bugs B88.0
Red tide (*see also* Table of Drugs and Chemicals) T65.82- ☑
Red-cedar lung or pneumonitis J67.8
Reduced
  mobility Z74.09
  ventilatory or vital capacity R94.2
Redundant, redundancy
  anus (congenital) Q43.8
  clitoris N90.89
  colon (congenital) Q43.8
  foreskin (congenital) N47.8
  intestine (congenital) Q43.8
  labia N90.6
  organ or site, congenital NEC — *see* Accessory
  panniculus (abdominal) E65
  prepuce (congenital) N47.8
  pylorus K31.89
  rectum (congenital) Q43.8
  scrotum N50.8
  sigmoid (congenital) Q43.8
  skin (of face) L57.4
    eyelids — *see* Blepharochalasis
  stomach K31.89
Reduplication — *see* Duplication
Reflex R29.2
  hyperactive gag J39.2
  pupillary, abnormal — *see* Anomaly, pupil, function
  vasoconstriction I73.9
  vasovagal R55
Reflux K21.9
  acid K21.9
  esophageal K21.9
    with esophagitis K21.0
    newborn P78.83
  gastroesophageal K21.9
    with esophagitis K21.0
  mitral — *see* Insufficiency, mitral
  ureteral — *see* Reflux, vesicoureteral

Reflux — *continued*
  vesicoureteral (with scarring) N13.70
    with
      nephropathy N13.729
        with hydroureter N13.739
          bilateral N13.732
          unilateral N13.731
        without hydroureter N13.729
          bilateral N13.722
          unilateral N13.721
        bilateral N13.722
        unilateral N13.721
      pyelonephritis (chronic) N11.0
    without nephropathy N13.71
    congenital Q62.7
Reforming, artificial openings — *see* Attention to, artificial, opening
Refractive error — *see* Disorder, refraction
Refsum's disease or syndrome G60.1
Refusal of
  food, psychogenic F50.8
  treatment (because of) Z53.20
    left against medical advice (AMA) Z53.21
    patient's decision NEC Z53.29
    reasons of belief or group pressure Z53.1
Regional — *see* condition
Regurgitation R11.10
  aortic (valve) — *see* Insufficiency, aortic
  food (*see also* Vomiting)
    with reswallowing — *see* Rumination
    newborn P92.1
  gastric contents — *see* Vomiting
  heart — *see* Endocarditis
  mitral (valve) — *see* Insufficiency, mitral
    congenital Q23.3
  myocardial — *see* Endocarditis
  pulmonary (valve) (heart) I37.1
    congenital Q22.2
    syphilitic A52.03
  tricuspid — *see* Insufficiency, tricuspid
  valve, valvular — *see* Endocarditis
    congenital Q24.8
  vesicoureteral — *see* Reflux, vesicoureteral
Reichmann's disease or syndrome K31.89
Reifenstein syndrome E34.52
Reinsertion, contraceptive device Z30.433
Reiter's disease, syndrome, or urethritis M02.30
  ankle M02.37- ☑
  elbow M02.32- ☑
  foot joint M02.37- ☑
  hand joint M02.34- ☑
  hip M02.35- ☑
  knee M02.36- ☑
  multiple site M02.39
  shoulder M02.31- ☑
  vertebra M02.38
  wrist M02.33- ☑
Rejection
  food, psychogenic F50.8
  transplant T86.91
    bone T86.830
      marrow T86.01
    cornea T86.840
    heart T86.21
      with lung(s) T86.31
    intestine T86.850
    kidney T86.11
    liver T86.41
    lung(s) T86.810
      with heart T86.31
    organ (immune or nonimmune cause) T86.91
    pancreas T86.890
    skin (allograft) (autograft) T86.820
    specified NEC T86.890
    stem cell (peripheral blood) (umbilical cord) T86.5
Relapsing fever A68.9
  Carter's (Asiatic) A68.1
  Dutton's (West African) A68.1
  Koch's A68.9
  louse-borne (epidemic) A68.0
  Novy's (American) A68.1
  Obermeyers's (European) A68.0
  Spirillum A68.9
  tick-borne (endemic) A68.1
Relationship
  occlusal
    open anterior M26.220

Relationship — *continued*
  occlusal — *continued*
    open posterior M26.221
Relaxation
  anus (sphincter) K62.89
    psychogenic F45.8
  arch (foot) (see also Deformity, limb, flat foot)
  back ligaments — *see* Instability, joint, spine
  bladder (sphincter) N31.2
  cardioesophageal K21.9
  cervix — *see* Incompetency, cervix
  diaphragm J98.6
  joint (capsule) (ligament) (paralytic) — *see* Flail, joint
    congenital NEC Q74.8
  lumbosacral (joint) — *see* subcategory M53.2 ☑
  pelvic floor N81.89
  perineum N81.89
  posture R29.3
  rectum (sphincter) K62.89
  sacroiliac (joint) — *see* subcategory M53.2 ☑
  scrotum N50.8
  urethra (sphincter) N36.44
  vesical N31.2
Release from prison, anxiety concerning Z65.2
Remains
  canal of Cloquet Q14.0
  capsule (opaque) Q14.8
Remittent fever (malarial) B54
Remnant
  canal of Cloquet Q14.0
  capsule (opaque) Q14.8
  cervix, cervical stump (acquired) (postoperative) N88.8
  cystic duct, postcholecystectomy K91.5
  fingernail L60.8
    congenital Q84.6
  meniscus, knee — *see* Derangement, knee, meniscus,
    specified NEC
  thyroglossal duct Q89.2
  tonsil J35.8
    infected (chronic) J35.01
  urachus Q64.4
Removal (from) (of)
  artificial
    arm Z44.00- ☑
      complete Z44.01- ☑
      partial Z44.02- ☑
    eye Z44.2- ☑
    leg Z44.10- ☑
      complete Z44.11- ☑
      partial Z44.12- ☑
  breast implant Z45.81 ☑
  cardiac pulse generator (battery) (end-of-life) Z45.010
  catheter (urinary) (indwelling) Z46.6
    from artificial opening — *see* Attention to, artificial,
      opening
    non-vascular Z46.82
    vascular NEC Z45.2
  device Z46.9
    contraceptive Z30.432
    implanted NEC Z45.89
    specified NEC Z46.89
  drains Z48.03
  dressing (nonsurgical) Z48.00
    surgical Z48.01
  external
    fixation device — *code to* fracture with seventh
      character D
    prosthesis, prosthetic device Z44.9
      breast Z44.3- ☑
      specified NEC Z44.8
  home in childhood (to foster home or institution)
    Z62.29
  ileostomy Z43.2
  insulin pump Z46.81
  myringotomy device (stent) (tube) Z45.82
  nervous system device NEC Z46.2
    brain neuropacemaker Z46.2
    visual substitution device Z46.2
      implanted Z45.31
  non-vascular catheter Z46.82
  organ, prophylactic (for neoplasia management) —
    see Prophylactic, organ removal
  orthodontic device Z46.4
  staples Z48.02
  stent
    ureteral Z46.6
  suture Z48.02
  urinary device Z46.6

Removal — *continued*
  vascular access device or catheter Z45.2
Ren
  arcuatus Q63.1
  mobile, mobilis N28.89
    congenital Q63.8
  unguliformis Q63.1
Renal — *see* condition
Rendu-Osler-Weber disease or syndrome I78.0
Reninoma D41.0- ☑
Renon-Delille syndrome E23.3
Reovirus, as cause of disease classified elsewhere
  B97.5
Repeated falls NEC R29.6
Replaced chromosome by dicentric ring Q93.2
Replacement by artificial or mechanical device or
    prosthesis of
  bladder Z96.0
  blood vessel NEC Z95.828
  bone NEC Z96.7
  cochlea Z96.21
  coronary artery Z95.5
  eustachian tube Z96.29
  eye globe Z97.0
  heart Z95.812
    valve Z95.2
      prosthetic Z95.2
      specified NEC Z95.4
      xenogenic Z95.3
  intestine Z96.89
  joint Z96.60
    hip — *see* Presence, hip joint implant
    knee — *see* Presence, knee joint implant
    specified site NEC Z96.698
  larynx Z96.3
  lens Z96.1
  limb(s) — *see* Presence, artificial, limb
  mandible NEC (for tooth root implant(s)) Z96.5
  organ NEC Z96.89
  peripheral vessel NEC Z95.828
  stapes Z96.29
  teeth Z97.2
  tendon Z96.7
  tissue NEC Z96.89
  tooth root(s) Z96.5
  vessel NEC Z95.828
    coronary (artery) Z95.5
Request for expert evidence Z04.8
Reserve, decreased or low
  cardiac — *see* Disease, heart
  kidney N28.89
Residual (see also condition)
  ovary syndrome N99.83
  state, schizophrenic F20.5
  urine R39.19
Resistance, resistant (to)
  activated protein C D68.51
  complicating pregnancy O26.89 ☑
  insulin E88.81
  organism(s)
    to
      drug
        aminoglycosides Z16.29
        amoxicillin Z16.11
        ampicillin Z16.11
        antibiotic(s) Z16.20
          multiple Z16.24
          specified NEC Z16.29
        antifungal Z16.32
        antimicrobial (single) Z16.30
          multiple Z16.35
          specified NEC Z16.39
        antimycbacterial (single) Z16.341
          multiple Z16.342
        antiparasitic Z16.31
        antiviral Z16.33
        beta lactam antibiotics Z16.10
          specified NEC Z16.19
        cephalosporins Z16.19
        extended beta lactamase (ESBL) Z16.12
        fluoroquinolones Z16.23
        macrolides Z16.29
        methicillin — *see* MRSA
        multiple drugs (MDRO)
          antibiotics Z16.24
        penicillins Z16.11
        quinine (and related compounds) Z16.31
        quinolones Z16.23

Resistance, resistant — *continued*
  organism(s) — *continued*
    to — *continued*
      drug — *continued*
        sulfonamides Z16.29
        tetracyclines Z16.29
        tuberculostatics (single) Z16.341
          multiple Z16.342
        vancomycin Z16.21
          related antibiotics Z16.22
    thyroid hormone E07.89
Resorption
  dental (roots) K03.3
    alveoli M26.79
  teeth (external) (internal) (pathological) (roots) K03.3
Respiration
  Cheyne-Stokes R06.3
  decreased due to shock, following injury T79.4 ☑
  disorder of, psychogenic F45.8
  insufficient, or poor R06.89
    newborn P28.5
  painful R07.1
  sighing, psychogenic F45.8
Respiratory (see also condition)
  distress syndrome (newborn) (type I) P22.0
    type II P22.1
  syncytial virus, as cause of disease classified elsewhere
    B97.4
Respite care Z75.5
Response (drug)
  photoallergic L56.1
  phototoxic L56.0
Restless legs (syndrome) G25.81
Restlessness R45.1
Restoration (of)
  dental
    aesthetically inadequate or displeasing K08.56
    defective K08.50
      specified NEC K08.59
    failure of marginal integrity K08.51
    failure of periodontal anatomical intergrity K08.54
  organ continuity from previous sterilization (tuboplas-
    ty) (vasoplasty) Z31.0
    aftercare Z31.42
  tooth (existing)
    contours biologically incompatible with oral health
      K08.54
    open margins K08.51
    overhanging K08.52
    poor aesthetic K08.56
    poor gingival margins K08.51
  unsatisfactory, of tooth K08.50
    specified NEC K08.59
Restorative material (dental)
  allergy to K08.55
  fractured K08.539
    with loss of material K08.531
    without loss of material K08.530
  unrepairable overhanging of K08.52
Restriction of housing space Z59.1
Rests, ovarian, in fallopian tube Q50.6
Restzustand (schizophrenic) F20.5
Retained (see also Retention)
  cholelithiasis following cholecystectomy K91.86
  foreign body fragments (type of) Z18.9
    acrylics Z18.2
    animal quill(s) or spines Z18.31
    cement Z18.83
    concrete Z18.83
    crystalline Z18.83
    depleted isotope Z18.09
    depleted uranium Z18.01
    diethylhexylphthalates Z18.2
    glass Z18.81
    isocyanate Z18.2
    magnetic metal Z18.11
    metal Z18.10
    nonmagnectic metal Z18.12
    nontherapeutic radioactive Z18.09
    organic NEC Z18.39
    plastic Z18.2
    quill(s) (animal) Z18.31
    radioactive (nontherapeutic) NEC Z18.09
    specified NEC Z18.89
    spine(s) (animal) Z18.31
    stone Z18.83
    tooth (teeth) Z18.32
    wood Z18.33

☑ **Additional Character Required** — Refer to the Tabular List for Character Selection   ▽ **Subterms under main terms may continue to next column or page**

Retained — *continued*
  fragments (type of) Z18.9
    acrylics Z18.2
    animal quill(s) or spines Z18.31
    cement Z18.83
    concrete Z18.83
    crystalline Z18.83
    depleted isotope Z18.09
    depleted uranium Z18.01
    diethylhexylphthalates Z18.2
    glass Z18.81
    isocyanate Z18.2
    magnetic metal Z18.11
    metal Z18.10
    nonmagnectic metal Z18.12
    nontherapeutic radioactive Z18.09
    organic NEC Z18.39
    plastic Z18.2
    quill(s) (animal) Z18.31
    radioactive (nontherapeutic) NEC Z18.09
    specified NEC Z18.89
    spine(s) (animal) Z18.31
    stone Z18.83
    tooth (teeth) Z18.32
    wood Z18.33
  gallstones, following cholecystectomy K91.86
Retardation
  development, developmental, specific — *see* Disorder,
      developmental
  endochondral bone growth — *see* Disorder, bone,
      development or growth
  growth R62.50
    due to malnutrition E45
  mental — *see* Disability, intellectual
  motor function, specific F82
  physical (child) R62.52
    due to malnutrition E45
  reading (specific) F81.0
  spelling (specific) (without reading disorder) F81.81
Retching — *see* Vomiting
Retention (*see also* Retained)
  bladder — *see* Retention, urine
  carbon dioxide E87.2
  cholelithiasis following cholecystectomy K91.86
  cyst — *see* Cyst
  dead
    fetus (at or near term) (mother) O36.4 ☑
      early fetal death O02.1
    ovum O02.0
  decidua (fragments) (following delivery) (with hemor-
      rhage) O72.2
    without hemorrhage O73.1
  deciduous tooth K00.6
  dental root K08.3
  fecal — *see* Constipation
  fetus
    dead O36.4 ☑
      early O02.1
  fluid R60.9
  foreign body (*see also* Foreign body, retained)
    current trauma — *code as* Foreign body, by site or
        type
  gallstones, following cholecystectomy K91.86
  gastric K31.89
  intrauterine contraceptive device, in pregnancy — *see*
      Pregnancy, complicated by, retention, intrauter-
      ine device
  membranes (complicating delivery) (with hemorrhage)
      O72.2
    with abortion — *see* Abortion, by type
    without hemorrhage O73.1
  meniscus — *see* Derangement, meniscus
  menses N94.89
  milk (puerperal, postpartum) O92.79
  nitrogen, extrarenal R39.2
  ovary syndrome N99.83
  placenta (total) (with hemorrhage) O72.0
    without hemorrhage O73.0
    portions or fragments (with hemorrhage) O72.2
      without hemorrhage O73.1
  products of conception
    early pregnancy (dead fetus) O02.1
    following
      delivery (with hemorrhage) O72.2
        without hemorrhage O73.1
  secundines (following delivery) (with hemorrhage)
      O72.0
    without hemorrhage O73.0

Retention — *continued*
  secundines — *continued*
    complicating puerperium (delayed hemorrhage)
        O72.2
    partial O72.2
      without hemorrhage O73.1
  smegma, clitoris N90.89
  urine R33.9
    drug-induced R33.0
    due to hyperplasia (hypertrophy) of prostate —
        see Hyperplasia, prostate
    organic R33.8
      drug-induced R33.0
    psychogenic F45.8
    specified NEC R33.8
  water (in tissues) — *see* Edema
Reticulation, dust — *see* Pneumoconiosis
Reticulocytosis R70.1
Reticuloendotheliosis
  acute infantile C96.0
  leukemic C91.4- ☑
  malignant C96.9
  nonlipid C96.0
Reticulohistiocytoma (giant-cell) D76.3
Reticuloid, actinic L57.1
Reticulosis (skin)
  acute of infancy C96.0
  hemophagocytic, familial D76.1
  histiocytic medullary C96.9
  lipomelanotic I89.8
  malignant (midline) C86.0
  nonlipid C96.0
  polymorphic C83.8- ☑
  Sézary — *see* Sézary disease
Retina, retinal (*see also* condition)
  dark area D49.81
Retinitis (*see also* Inflammation, chorioretinal)
  albuminurica N18.9 [H32]
  diabetic — *see* Diabetes, retinitis
  disciformis — *see* Degeneration, macula
  focal — *see* Inflammation, chorioretinal, focal
  gravidarum — *see* Pregnancy, complicated by, speci-
      fied pregnancy-related condition NEC
  juxtapapillaris — *see* Inflammation, chorioretinal, focal,
      juxtapapillary
  luetic — *see* Retinitis, syphilitic
  pigmentosa H35.52
  proliferans — *see* Disorder, globe, degenerative,
      specified type NEC
  proliferating — *see* Disorder, globe, degenerative,
      specified type NEC
  renal N18.9 [H32]
  syphilitic (early) (secondary) A51.43
    central, recurrent A52.71
    congenital (early) A50.01 [H32]
    late A52.71
  tuberculous A18.53
Retinoblastoma C69.2- ☑
  differentiated C69.2- ☑
  undifferentiated C69.2- ☑
Retinochoroiditis (*see also* Inflammation, chorioretinal)
  disseminated — *see* Inflammation, chorioretinal, dis-
      seminated
    syphilitic A52.71
  focal — *see* Inflammation, chorioretinal
  juxtapapillaris — *see* Inflammation, chorioretinal, focal,
      juxtapapillary
Retinopathy (background) H35.00
  arteriosclerotic I70.8 [H35.0-] ☑
  atherosclerotic I70.8 [H35.0-] ☑
  central serous — *see* Chorioretinopathy, central serous
  Coats H35.02- ☑
  diabetic — *see* Diabetes, retinopathy
  exudative H35.02- ☑
  hypertensive H35.03- ☑
  in (due to)
    diabetes — *see* Diabetes, retinopathy
    sickle-cell disorders D57.- ☑ [H36]
  of prematurity H35.10- ☑
    stage 0 H35.11- ☑
    stage 1 H35.12- ☑
    stage 2 H35.13- ☑
    stage 3 H35.14- ☑
    stage 4 H35.15- ☑
    stage 5 H35.16- ☑
  pigmentary, congenital — *see* Dystrophy, retina

Retinopathy — *continued*
  proliferative NEC H35.2- ☑
    diabetic — *see* Diabetes, retinopathy, proliferative
    sickle-cell D57.- ☑ [H36]
  solar H31.02- ☑
Retinoschisis H33.10- ☑
  congenital Q14.1
  specified type NEC H33.19- ☑
Retortamoniasis A07.8
Retractile testis Q55.22
Retraction
  cervix — *see* Retroversion, uterus
  drum (membrane) — *see* Disorder, tympanic mem-
      brane, specified NEC
  finger — *see* Deformity, finger
  lid H02.539
    left H02.536
      lower H02.535
      upper H02.534
    right H02.533
      lower H02.532
      upper H02.531
  lung J98.4
  mediastinum J98.5
  nipple N64.53
    associated with
      lactation O92.03
      pregnancy O92.01- ☑
      puerperium O92.02
    congenital Q83.8
  palmar fascia M72.0
  pleura — *see* Pleurisy
  ring, uterus (Bandl's) (pathological) O62.4
  sternum (congenital) Q76.7
    acquired M95.4
  uterus — *see* Retroversion, uterus
  valve (heart) — *see* Endocarditis
Retrobulbar — *see* condition
Retrocecal — *see* condition
Retrocession — *see* Retroversion
Retrodisplacement — *see* Retroversion
Retroflection, retroflexion — *see* Retroversion
Retrognathia, retrognathism (mandibular) (maxillary)
    M26.19
Retrograde menstruation N92.5
Retroperineal — *see* condition
Retroperitoneal — *see* condition
Retroperitonitis K68.9
Retropharyngeal — *see* condition
Retroplacental — *see* condition
Retroposition — *see* Retroversion
Retroprosthetic membrane T85.398 ☑
Retrosternal thyroid (congenital) Q89.2
Retroversion, retroverted
  cervix — *see* Retroversion, uterus
  female NEC — *see* Retroversion, uterus
  iris H21.89
  testis (congenital) Q55.29
  uterus (acquired) (acute) (any degree) (asymptomatic)
      (cervix) (postinfectional) (postpartal, old) N85.4
    congenital Q51.818
    in pregnancy O34.53- ☑
Retrovirus, as cause of disease classified elsewhere
    B97.30
  human
    immunodeficiency, type 2 (HIV 2) B97.35
    T-cell lymphotropic
      type I (HTLV-I) B97.33
      type II (HTLV-II) B97.34
  lentivirus B97.31
  oncovirus B97.32
  specified NEC B97.39
Retrusion, premaxilla (developmental) M26.09
Rett's disease or syndrome F84.2
Reverse peristalsis R19.2
Reye's syndrome G93.7
Rh (factor)
  hemolytic disease (newborn) P55.0
  incompatibility, immunization or sensitization
    affecting management of pregnancy NEC
        O36.09- ☑
      anti-D antibody O36.01- ☑
    newborn P55.0
    transfusion reaction — *see* Complication(s), trans-
        fusion, incompatibility reaction, Rh (factor)
  negative mother affecting newborn P55.0

Rh — *continued*
  titer elevated — *see* Complication(s), transfusion, incompatibility reaction, Rh (factor)
  transfusion reaction — *see* Complication(s), transfusion, incompatibility reaction, Rh (factor)
Rhabdomyolysis (idiopathic) NEC M62.82
  traumatic T79.6 ☑
Rhabdomyoma (*see also* Neoplasm, connective tissue, benign)
  adult — *see* Neoplasm, connective tissue, benign
  fetal — *see* Neoplasm, connective tissue, benign
  glycogenic — *see* Neoplasm, connective tissue, benign
Rhabdomyosarcoma (any type) — *see* Neoplasm, connective tissue, malignant
Rhabdosarcoma — *see* Rhabdomyosarcoma
Rhesus (factor) **incompatibility** — *see* Rh, incompatibility
Rheumatic (acute) (subacute) (chronic)
  adherent pericardium I09.2
  coronary arteritis I01.9
  degeneration, myocardium I09.0
  fever (acute) — *see* Fever, rheumatic
  heart — *see* Disease, heart, rheumatic
  myocardial degeneration — *see* Degeneration, myocardium
  myocarditis (chronic) (inactive) (with chorea) I09.0
    with chorea (acute) (rheumatic) (Sydenham's) I02.0
    active or acute I01.2
  pancarditis, acute I01.8
    with chorea (acute (rheumatic) Sydenham's) I02.0
  pericarditis (active) (acute) (with effusion) (with pneumonia) I01.0
    with chorea (acute) (rheumatic) (Sydenham's) I02.0
    chronic or inactive I09.2
  pneumonia I00 [J17]
  torticollis M43.6
  typhoid fever A01.09
Rheumatism (articular) (neuralgic) (nonarticular) M79.0
  gout — *see* Arthritis, rheumatoid
  intercostal, meaning Tietze's disease M94.0
  palindromic (any site) M12.30
    ankle M12.37- ☑
    elbow M12.32- ☑
    foot joint M12.37- ☑
    hand joint M12.34- ☑
    hip M12.35- ☑
    knee M12.36- ☑
    multiple site M12.39
    shoulder M12.31- ☑
    specified joint NEC M12.38
    vertebrae M12.38
    wrist M12.33- ☑
  sciatic M54.4- ☑
Rheumatoid (*see also* condition)
  arthritis (*see also* Arthritis, rheumatoid)
    with involvement of organs NEC M05.60
      ankle M05.67- ☑
      elbow M05.62- ☑
      foot joint M05.67- ☑
      hand joint M05.64- ☑
      hip M05.65- ☑
      knee M05.66- ☑
      multiple site M05.69
      shoulder M05.61- ☑
      vertebra — *see* Spondylitis, ankylosing
      wrist M05.63- ☑
    seronegative — *see* Arthritis, rheumatoid, seronegative
    seropositive — *see* Arthritis, rheumatoid, seropositive
  carditis M05.30
    ankle M05.37- ☑
    elbow M05.32- ☑
    foot joint M05.37- ☑
    hand joint M05.34- ☑
    hip M05.35- ☑
    knee M05.36- ☑
    multiple site M05.39
    shoulder M05.31- ☑
    vertebra — *see* Spondylitis, ankylosing
    wrist M05.33- ☑
  endocarditis — *see* Rheumatoid, carditis
  lung (disease) M05.10
    ankle M05.17- ☑
    elbow M05.12- ☑
    foot joint M05.17- ☑
    hand joint M05.14- ☑

Rheumatoid — *continued*
  lung — *continued*
    hip M05.15- ☑
    knee M05.16- ☑
    multiple site M05.19
    shoulder M05.11- ☑
    vertebra — *see* Spondylitis, ankylosing
    wrist M05.13- ☑
  myocarditis — *see* Rheumatoid, carditis
  myopathy M05.40
    ankle M05.47- ☑
    elbow M05.42- ☑
    foot joint M05.47- ☑
    hand joint M05.44- ☑
    hip M05.45- ☑
    knee M05.46- ☑
    multiple site M05.49
    shoulder M05.41- ☑
    vertebra — *see* Spondylitis, ankylosing
    wrist M05.43- ☑
  pericarditis — *see* Rheumatoid, carditis
  polyarthritis — *see* Arthritis, rheumatoid
  polyneuropathy M05.50
    ankle M05.57- ☑
    elbow M05.52- ☑
    foot joint M05.57- ☑
    hand joint M05.54- ☑
    hip M05.55- ☑
    knee M05.56- ☑
    multiple site M05.59
    shoulder M05.51- ☑
    vertebra — *see* Spondylitis, ankylosing
    wrist M05.53- ☑
  vasculitis M05.20
    ankle M05.27- ☑
    elbow M05.22- ☑
    foot joint M05.27- ☑
    hand joint M05.24- ☑
    hip M05.25- ☑
    knee M05.26- ☑
    multiple site M05.29
    shoulder M05.21- ☑
    vertebra — *see* Spondylitis, ankylosing
    wrist M05.23- ☑
Rhinitis (atrophic) (catarrhal) (chronic) (croupous) (fibrinous) (granulomatous) (hyperplastic) (hypertrophic) (membranous) (obstructive) (purulent) (suppurative) (ulcerative) J31.0
  with
    sore throat — *see* Nasopharyngitis
  acute J00
  allergic J30.9
    with asthma J45.909
      with
        exacerbation (acute) J45.901
        status asthmaticus J45.902
    due to
      food J30.5
      pollen J30.1
    nonseasonal J30.89
    perennial J30.89
    seasonal NEC J30.2
    specified NEC J30.89
  infective J00
  pneumococcal J00
  syphilitic A52.73
    congenital A50.05 [J99]
  tuberculous A15.8
  vasomotor J30.0
Rhinoantritis (chronic) — *see* Sinusitis, maxillary
Rhinodacryolith — *see* Dacryolith
Rhinolith (nasal sinus) J34.89
Rhinomegaly J34.89
Rhinopharyngitis (acute) (subacute) (*see also* Nasopharyngitis)
  chronic J31.1
  destructive ulcerating A66.5
  mutilans A66.5
Rhinophyma L71.1
Rhinorrhea J34.89
  cerebrospinal (fluid) G96.0
  paroxysmal — *see* Rhinitis, allergic
  spasmodic — *see* Rhinitis, allergic
Rhinosalpingitis — *see* Salpingitis, eustachian
Rhinoscleroma A48.8
Rhinosporidiosis B48.1
Rhinovirus infection NEC B34.8

Rhizomelic chondrodysplasia punctata E71.540
Rhythm
  atrioventricular nodal I49.8
  disorder I49.9
    coronary sinus I49.8
    ectopic I49.8
    nodal I49.8
  escape I49.9
  heart, abnormal I49.9
  idioventricular I44.2
  nodal I49.8
  sleep, inversion G47.2- ☑
    nonorganic origin — *see* Disorder, sleep, circadian rhythm, psychogenic
Rhytidosis facialis L98.8
Rib (*see also* condition)
  cervical Q76.5
Riboflavin deficiency E53.0
Rice bodies (*see also* Loose, body, joint)
  knee M23.4- ☑
Richter syndrome — *see* Leukemia, chronic lymphocytic, B-cell type
Richter's hernia — *see* Hernia, abdomen, with obstruction
Ricinism — *see* Poisoning, food, noxious, plant
Rickets (active) (acute) (adolescent) (chest wall) (congenital) (current) (infantile) (intestinal) E55.0
  adult — *see* Osteomalacia
  celiac K90.0
  hypophosphatemic with nephrotic-glycosuric dwarfism E72.09
  inactive E64.3
  kidney N25.0
  renal N25.0
  sequelae, any E64.3
  vitamin-D-resistant E83.31 [M90.80]
Rickettsial disease A79.9
  specified type NEC A79.89
Rickettsialpox (Rickettsia akari) A79.1
Rickettsiosis A79.9
  due to
    Ehrlichia sennetsu A79.81
    Rickettsia akari (rickettsialpox) A79.1
  specified type NEC A79.89
  tick-borne A77.9
  vesicular A79.1
Rider's bone — *see* Ossification, muscle, specified NEC
Ridge, alveolus (*see also* condition)
  flabby K06.8
Ridged ear, congenital Q17.3
Riedel's
  lobe, liver Q44.7
  struma, thyroiditis or disease E06.5
Rieger's anomaly or syndrome Q13.81
Riehl's melanosis L81.4
Rietti-Greppi-Micheli anemia D56.9
Rieux's hernia — *see* Hernia, abdomen, specified site NEC
Riga (-Fede) **disease** K14.0
Riggs' disease — *see* Periodontitis
Right middle lobe syndrome J98.11
Rigid, rigidity (*see also* condition)
  abdominal R19.30
    with severe abdominal pain R10.0
    epigastric R19.36
    generalized R19.37
    left lower quadrant R19.34
    left upper quadrant R19.32
    periumbilic R19.35
    right lower quadrant R19.33
    right upper quadrant R19.31
  articular, multiple, congenital Q68.8
  cervix (uteri) in pregnancy — *see* Pregnancy, complicated by, abnormal, cervix
  hymen (acquired) (congenital) N89.6
  nuchal R29.1
  pelvic floor in pregnancy — *see* Pregnancy, complicated by, abnormal, pelvic organs or tissues NEC
  perineum or vulva in pregnancy — *see* Pregnancy, complicated by, abnormal, vulva
  spine — *see* Dorsopathy, specified NEC
  vagina in pregnancy — *see* Pregnancy, complicated by, abnormal, vagina
Rigors R68.89
  with fever R50.9
Riley-Day syndrome G90.1
RIND (reversible ischemic neurologic deficit) I63.9

268 ☑ Additional Character Required — Refer to the Tabular List for Character Selection   Subterms under main terms may continue to next column or page

Rh — RIND

Ring(s)
  aorta (vascular) Q25.4
  Bandl's O62.4
  contraction, complicating delivery O62.4
  esophageal, lower (muscular) K22.2
  Fleischer's (cornea) H18.04- ☑
  hymenal, tight (acquired) (congenital) N89.6
  Kayser-Fleischer (cornea) H18.04- ☑
  retraction, uterus, pathological O62.4
  Schatzki's (esophagus) (lower) K22.2
    congenital Q39.3
  Soemmering's — *see* Cataract, secondary
  vascular (congenital) Q25.8
    aorta Q25.4
Ringed hair (congenital) Q84.1
Ringworm B35.9
  beard B35.0
  black dot B35.0
  body B35.4
  Burmese B35.5
  corporeal B35.4
  foot B35.3
  groin B35.6
  hand B35.2
  honeycomb B35.0
  nails B35.1
  perianal (area) B35.6
  scalp B35.0
  specified NEC B35.8
  Tokelau B35.5
Rise, venous pressure I87.8
Risk, suicidal
  meaning personal history of attempted suicide Z91.5
  meaning suicidal ideation — *see* Ideation, suicidal
Ritter's disease L00
Rivalry, sibling Z62.891
Rivalta's disease A42.2
River blindness B73.01
Robert's pelvis Q74.2
  with disproportion (fetopelvic) O33.0
    causing obstructed labor O65.0
Robin (-Pierre) **syndrome** Q87.0
Robinow-Silvermann-Smith syndrome Q87.1
Robinson's (hidrotic) **ectodermal dysplasia or syndrome** Q82.4
Robles' disease B73.01
Rocky Mountain (spotted) **fever** A77.0
Roetheln — *see* Rubella
Roger's disease Q21.0
Rokitansky-Aschoff sinuses (gallbladder) K82.8
Rolando's fracture (displaced) S62.22- ☑
  nondisplaced- S62.22- ☑
Romano-Ward (prolonged QT interval) **syndrome** I45.81
Romberg's disease or syndrome G51.8
Roof, mouth — *see* condition
Rosacea L71.9
  acne L71.9
  keratitis L71.8
  specified NEC L71.8
Rosary, rachitic E55.0
Rose
  cold J30.1
  fever J30.1
  rash R21
    epidemic B06.9
Rosenbach's erysipeloid A26.0
Rosenthal's disease or syndrome D68.1
Roseola B09
  infantum B08.20
    due to human herpesvirus 6 B08.21
    due to human herpesvirus 7 B08.22
Ross River disease or fever B33.1
Rossbach's disease K31.89
  psychogenic F45.8
Rostan's asthma (cardiac) — *see* Failure, ventricular, left
Rotation
  anomalous, incomplete or insufficient, intestine Q43.3
  cecum (congenital) Q43.3
  colon (congenital) Q43.3
  spine, incomplete or insufficient — *see* Dorsopathy, deforming, specified NEC
  tooth, teeth, fully erupted M26.35
  vertebra, incomplete or insufficient — *see* Dorsopathy, deforming, specified NEC
Rotes Quérol disease or syndrome — *see* Hyperostosis, ankylosing

Roth (-Bernhardt) **disease or syndrome** — *see* Meralgia paraesthetica
Rothmund (-Thomson) **syndrome** Q82.8
Rotor's disease or syndrome E80.6
Round
  back (with wedging of vertebrae) — *see* Kyphosis
    sequelae (late effect) of rickets E64.3
  worms (large) (infestation) NEC B82.0
    Ascariasis (*see also* Ascariasis) B77.9
Roussy-Lévy syndrome G60.0
Rubella (German measles) B06.9
  complication NEC B06.09
    neurological B06.00
  congenital P35.0
  contact Z20.4
  exposure to Z20.4
  maternal
    care for (suspected) damage to fetus O35.3 ☑
    manifest rubella in infant P35.0
    suspected damage to fetus affecting management of pregnancy O35.3 ☑
  specified complications NEC B06.89
Rubeola (meaning measles) — *see* Measles
  meaning rubella — *see* Rubella
Rubeosis, iris — *see* Disorder, iris, vascular
Rubinstein-Taybi syndrome Q87.2
Rudimentary (congenital) (*see also* Agenesis)
  arm — *see* Defect, reduction, upper limb
  bone Q79.9
  cervix uteri Q51.828
  eye Q11.2
  lobule of ear Q17.3
  patella Q74.1
  respiratory organs in thoracopagus Q89.4
  tracheal bronchus Q32.4
  uterus Q51.818
    in male Q56.1
  vagina Q52.0
Ruled out condition — *see* Observation, suspected
Rumination R11.10
  with nausea R11.2
  disorder of infancy F98.21
  neurotic F42
  newborn P92.1
  obsessional F42
  psychogenic F42
Runeberg's disease D51.0
Runny nose R09.89
Rupia (syphilitic) A51.39
  congenital A50.06
  tertiary A52.79
Rupture, ruptured
  abscess (spontaneous) — *code by site under* Abscess
  aneurysm — *see* Aneurysm
  anus (sphincter) — *see* Laceration, anus
  aorta, aortic I71.8
    abdominal I71.3
    arch I71.1
    ascending I71.1
    descending I71.8
      abdominal I71.3
      thoracic I71.1
    syphilitic A52.01
    thoracoabdominal I71.5
    thorax, thoracic I71.1
    transverse I71.1
    traumatic — *see* Injury, aorta, laceration, major
    valve or cusp (*see also* Endocarditis, aortic) I35.8
  appendix (with peritonitis) K35.2
  arteriovenous fistula, brain I60.8
  artery I77.2
    brain — *see* Hemorrhage, intracranial, intracerebral
    coronary — *see* Infarct, myocardium
    heart — *see* Infarct, myocardium
    pulmonary I28.8
    traumatic (complication) — *see* Injury, blood vessel
  bile duct (common) (hepatic) K83.2
    cystic K82.2
  bladder (sphincter) (nontraumatic) (spontaneous) N32.89
    following ectopic or molar pregnancy O08.6
    obstetrical trauma O71.5
    traumatic S37.29 ☑
  blood vessel (*see also* Hemorrhage)
    brain — *see* Hemorrhage, intracranial, intracerebral
    heart — *see* Infarct, myocardium

Rupture, ruptured — *continued*
  blood vessel (*see also* Hemorrhage) — *continued*
    traumatic (complication) — *see* Injury, blood vessel, laceration, major, by site
  bone — *see* Fracture
  bowel (nontraumatic) K63.1
  brain
    aneurysm (congenital) (*see also* Hemorrhage, intracranial, subarachnoid)
      syphilitic A52.05
    hemorrhagic — *see* Hemorrhage, intracranial, intracerebral
  capillaries I78.8
  cardiac (auricle) (ventricle) (wall) I23.3
    with hemopericardium I23.0
    infectional I40.9
    traumatic — *see* Injury, heart
  cartilage (articular) (current) (*see also* Sprain)
    knee S83.3- ☑
    semilunar — *see* Tear, meniscus
  cecum (with peritonitis) K65.0
    with peritoneal abscess K35.3
    traumatic S36.598 ☑
  celiac artery, traumatic — *see* Injury, blood vessel, celiac artery, laceration, major
  cerebral aneurysm (congenital) (*see* Hemorrhage, intracranial, subarachnoid)
  cervix (uteri)
    with ectopic or molar pregnancy O08.6
    following ectopic or molar pregnancy O08.6
    obstetrical trauma O71.3
    traumatic S37.69 ☑
  chordae tendineae NEC I51.1
    concurrent with acute myocardial infarction — *see* Infarct, myocardium
    following acute myocardial infarction (current complication) I23.4
  choroid (direct) (indirect) (traumatic) H31.32- ☑
  circle of Willis I60.6
  colon (nontraumatic) K63.1
    traumatic — *see* Injury, intestine, large
  cornea (traumatic) — *see* Injury, eye, laceration
  coronary (artery) (thrombotic) — *see* Infarct, myocardium
  corpus luteum (infected) (ovary) N83.1
  cyst — *see* Cyst
  cystic duct K82.2
  Descemet's membrane — *see* Change, corneal membrane, Descemet's, rupture
    traumatic — *see* Injury, eye, laceration
  diaphragm, traumatic — *see* Injury, intrathoracic, diaphragm
  disc — *see* Rupture, intervertebral disc
  diverticulum (intestine) K57.80
    with bleeding K57.81
    bladder N32.3
    large intestine K57.20
      with
        bleeding K57.21
        small intestine K57.40
          with bleeding K57.41
    small intestine K57.00
      with
        bleeding K57.01
        large intestine K57.40
          with bleeding K57.41
  duodenal stump K31.89
  ear drum (nontraumatic) (*see also* Perforation, tympanum)
    traumatic S09.2- ☑
    due to blast injury — *see* Injury, blast, ear
  esophagus K22.3
  eye (without prolapse or loss of intraocular tissue) — *see* Injury, eye, laceration
  fallopian tube NEC (nonobstetric) (nontraumatic) N83.8
    due to pregnancy O00.1
  fontanel P13.1
  gallbladder K82.2
    traumatic S36.128 ☑
  gastric (*see also* Rupture, stomach)
    vessel K92.2
  globe (eye) (traumatic) — *see* Injury, eye, laceration
  graafian follicle (hematoma) N83.0
  heart — *see* Rupture, cardiac
  hymen (nontraumatic) (nonintentional) N89.8
  internal organ, traumatic — *see* Injury, by site

Rupture, ruptured — *continued*
- intervertebral disc — *see* Displacement, intervertebral disc
  - traumatic — *see* Rupture, traumatic, intervertebral disc
- intestine NEC (nontraumatic) K63.1
  - traumatic — *see* Injury, intestine
- iris (*see also* Abnormality, pupillary)
  - traumatic — *see* Injury, eye, laceration
- joint capsule, traumatic — *see* Sprain
- kidney (traumatic) S37.06- ☑
  - birth injury P15.8
  - nontraumatic N28.89
- lacrimal duct (traumatic) –-- *see* Injury, eye, specified site NEC
- lens (cataract) (traumatic) — *see* Cataract, traumatic
- ligament, traumatic — *see* Rupture, traumatic, ligament, by site
- liver S36.116 ☑
  - birth injury P15.0
- lymphatic vessel I89.8
- marginal sinus (placental) (with hemorrhage) — *see* Hemorrhage, antepartum, specified cause NEC
- membrana tympani (nontraumatic) — *see* Perforation, tympanum
- membranes (spontaneous)
  - artificial
    - delayed delivery following O75.5
  - delayed delivery following — *see* Pregnancy, complicated by, premature rupture of membranes
- meningeal artery I60.8
- meniscus (knee) (*see also* Tear, meniscus)
  - old — *see* Derangement, meniscus
  - site other than knee — *code as* Sprain
- mesenteric artery, traumatic — *see* Injury, mesenteric, artery, laceration, major
- mesentery (nontraumatic) K66.8
  - traumatic — *see* Injury, intra-abdominal, specified, site NEC
- mitral (valve) I34.8
- muscle (traumatic) (*see also* Strain)
  - diastasis — *see* Diastasis, muscle
  - nontraumatic M62.10
    - ankle M62.17- ☑
    - foot M62.17- ☑
    - forearm M62.13- ☑
    - hand M62.14- ☑
    - lower leg M62.16- ☑
    - pelvic region M62.15- ☑
    - shoulder region M62.11- ☑
    - specified site NEC M62.18
    - thigh M62.15- ☑
    - upper arm M62.12- ☑
  - traumatic — *see* Strain, by site
- musculotendinous junction NEC, nontraumatic — *see* Rupture, tendon, spontaneous
- mycotic aneurysm causing cerebral hemorrhage — *see* Hemorrhage, intracranial, subarachnoid
- myocardium, myocardial — *see* Rupture, cardiac
  - traumatic — *see* Injury, heart
- nontraumatic, meaning hernia — *see* Hernia
- obstructed — *see* Hernia, by site, obstructed
- operation wound — *see* Disruption, wound, operation
- ovary, ovarian N83.8
  - corpus luteum cyst N83.1
  - follicle (graafian) N83.0
- oviduct (nonobstetric) (nontraumatic) N83.8
  - due to pregnancy O00.1
- pancreas (nontraumatic) K86.8
  - traumatic S36.299 ☑
- papillary muscle NEC I51.2
  - following acute myocardial infarction (current complication) I23.5
- pelvic
  - floor, complicating delivery O70.1
  - organ NEC, obstetrical trauma O71.5
- perineum (nonobstetric) (nontraumatic) N90.89
  - complicating delivery — *see* Delivery, complicated, by, laceration, anus (sphincter)
- postoperative wound — *see* Disruption, wound, operation
- prostate (traumatic) S37.828 ☑
- pulmonary
  - artery I28.8
  - valve (heart) I37.8
  - vein I28.8

Rupture, ruptured — *continued*
- pulmonary — *continued*
  - vessel I28.8
- pus tube — *see* Salpingitis
- pyosalpinx — *see* Salpingitis
- rectum (nontraumatic) K63.1
  - traumatic S36.69 ☑
- retina, retinal (traumatic) (without detachment) (*see also* Break, retina)
  - with detachment — *see* Detachment, retina, with retinal, break
- rotator cuff (nontraumatic) M75.10- ☑
  - complete M75.12- ☑
  - incomplete M75.11- ☑
- sclera — *see* Injury, eye, laceration
- sigmoid (nontraumatic) K63.1
  - traumatic S36.593 ☑
- spinal cord (*see also* Injury, spinal cord, by region)
  - due to injury at birth P11.5
  - newborn (birth injury) P11.5
- spleen (traumatic) S36.09 ☑
  - birth injury P15.1
  - congenital (birth injury) P15.1
  - due to P. vivax malaria B51.0
  - nontraumatic D73.5
  - spontaneous D73.5
- splenic vein R58
  - traumatic — *see* Injury, blood vessel, splenic vein
- stomach (nontraumatic) (spontaneous) K31.89
  - traumatic S36.39 ☑
- supraspinatus (complete) (incomplete) (nontraumatic) — *see* Tear, rotator cuff
- symphysis pubis
  - obstetric O71.6
  - traumatic S33.4 ☑
- synovium (cyst) M66.10
  - ankle M66.17- ☑
  - elbow M66.12- ☑
  - finger M66.14- ☑
  - foot M66.17- ☑
  - forearm M66.13- ☑
  - hand M66.14- ☑
  - pelvic region M66.15- ☑
  - shoulder region M66.11- ☑
  - specified site NEC M66.18
  - thigh M66.15- ☑
  - toe M66.17- ☑
  - upper arm M66.12- ☑
  - wrist M66.13- ☑
- tendon (traumatic) — *see* Strain
  - nontraumatic (spontaneous) M66.9
    - ankle M66.87- ☑
    - extensor M66.20
      - ankle M66.27- ☑
      - foot M66.27- ☑
      - forearm M66.23- ☑
      - hand M66.24- ☑
      - lower leg M66.26- ☑
      - multiple sites M66.29
      - pelvic region M66.25- ☑
      - shoulder region M66.21- ☑
      - specified site NEC M66.28
      - thigh M66.25- ☑
      - upper arm M66.22- ☑
    - flexor M66.30
      - ankle M66.37- ☑
      - foot M66.37- ☑
      - forearm M66.33- ☑
      - hand M66.34- ☑
      - lower leg M66.36- ☑
      - multiple sites M66.39
      - pelvic region M66.35- ☑
      - shoulder region M66.31- ☑
      - specified site NEC M66.38
      - thigh M66.35- ☑
      - upper arm M66.32- ☑
    - foot M66.87- ☑
    - forearm M66.83- ☑
    - hand M66.84- ☑
    - lower leg M66.86- ☑
    - multiple sites M66.89
    - pelvic region M66.85- ☑
    - shoulder region M66.81- ☑
    - specified
      - site NEC M66.88
      - tendon M66.80

Rupture, ruptured — *continued*
- tendon — *see* Strain — *continued*
  - nontraumatic — *continued*
    - thigh M66.85- ☑
    - upper arm M66.82- ☑
- thoracic duct I89.8
- tonsil J35.8
- traumatic
  - aorta — *see* Injury, aorta, laceration, major
  - diaphragm — *see* Injury, intrathoracic, diaphragm
  - external site — *see* Wound, open, by site
  - eye — *see* Injury, eye, laceration
  - internal organ — *see* Injury, by site
  - intervertebral disc
    - cervical S13.0 ☑
    - lumbar S33.0 ☑
    - thoracic S23.0 ☑
  - kidney S37.06- ☑
  - ligament (*see also* Sprain)
    - ankle — *see* Sprain, ankle
    - carpus — *see* Rupture, traumatic, ligament, wrist
    - collateral (hand) — *see* Rupture, traumatic, ligament, finger, collateral
    - finger (metacarpophalangeal) (interphalangeal) S63.40- ☑
      - collateral S63.41- ☑
        - index S63.41- ☑
        - little S63.41- ☑
        - middle S63.41- ☑
        - ring S63.41- ☑
      - index S63.40- ☑
      - little S63.40- ☑
      - middle S63.40- ☑
      - palmar S63.42- ☑
        - index S63.42- ☑
        - little S63.42- ☑
        - middle S63.42- ☑
        - ring S63.42- ☑
      - ring S63.40- ☑
      - specified site NEC S63.499 ☑
        - index S63.49- ☑
        - little S63.49- ☑
        - middle S63.49- ☑
        - ring S63.49- ☑
      - volar plate S63.43- ☑
        - index S63.43- ☑
        - little S63.43- ☑
        - middle S63.43- ☑
        - ring S63.43- ☑
    - foot — *see* Sprain, foot
    - radial collateral S53.2- ☑
    - radiocarpal — *see* Rupture, traumatic, ligament, wrist, radiocarpal
    - ulnar collateral S53.3- ☑
    - ulnocarpal — *see* Rupture, traumatic, ligament, wrist, ulnocarpal
    - wrist S63.30- ☑
      - collateral S63.31- ☑
      - radiocarpal S63.32- ☑
      - specified site NEC S63.39- ☑
      - ulnocarpal (palmar) S63.33- ☑
  - liver S36.116 ☑
  - membrana tympani — *see* Rupture, ear drum, traumatic
  - muscle or tendon — *see* Strain
  - myocardium — *see* Injury, heart
  - pancreas S36.299 ☑
  - rectum S36.69 ☑
  - sigmoid S36.593 ☑
  - spleen S36.09 ☑
  - stomach S36.39 ☑
  - symphysis pubis S33.4 ☑
  - tympanum, tympanic (membrane) — *see* Rupture, ear drum, traumatic
  - ureter S37.19 ☑
  - uterus S37.69 ☑
  - vagina — *see* Injury, vagina
  - vena cava — *see* Injury, vena cava, laceration, major
- tricuspid (heart) (valve) I07.8
- tube, tubal (nonobstetric) (nontraumatic) N83.8
  - abscess — *see* Salpingitis
  - due to pregnancy O00.1

☑ **Additional Character Required** — Refer to the Tabular List for Character Selection   ◥ **Subterms under main terms may continue to next column or page**

Rupture, ruptured — *continued*
  tympanum, tympanic (membrane) (nontraumatic)
    (*see also* Perforation, tympanic membrane)
    H72.9- ☑
    traumatic — *see* Rupture, ear drum, traumatic
  umbilical cord, complicating delivery O69.89 ☑
  ureter (traumatic) S37.19 ☑
    nontraumatic N28.89
  urethra (nontraumatic) N36.8
    with ectopic or molar pregnancy O08.6
    following ectopic or molar pregnancy O08.6
    obstetrical trauma O71.5
    traumatic S37.39 ☑
  uterosacral ligament (nonobstetric) (nontraumatic)
    N83.8
  uterus (traumatic) S37.69 ☑
    before labor O71.0- ☑
    during or after labor O71.1
    nonpuerperal, nontraumatic N85.8
    pregnant (during labor) O71.1
      before labor O71.0- ☑
  vagina — *see* Injury, vagina
  valve, valvular (heart) — *see* Endocarditis
  varicose vein — *see* Varix
  varix — *see* Varix
  vena cava R58
    traumatic — *see* Injury, vena cava, laceration, major
  vesical (urinary) N32.89
  vessel (blood) R58
    pulmonary I28.8
    traumatic — *see* Injury, blood vessel
  viscus R19.8
  vulva complicating delivery O70.0
Russell-Silver syndrome Q87.1
Russian spring-summer type encephalitis A84.0
Rust's disease (tuberculous cervical spondylitis) A18.01
Ruvalcaba-Myhre-Smith syndrome E71.440
Rytand-Lipsitch syndrome I44.2

S

Saber, sabre shin or tibia (syphilitic) A50.56 [M90.8-] ☑
Sac lacrimal — *see* condition
Saccharomyces infection B37.9
Saccharopinuria E72.3
Saccular — *see* condition
Sacculation
  aorta (nonsyphilitic) — *see* Aneurysm, aorta
  bladder N32.3
  intralaryngeal (congenital) (ventricular) Q31.3
  larynx (congenital) (ventricular) Q31.3
  organ or site, congenital — *see* Distortion
  pregnant uterus — *see* Pregnancy, complicated by,
    abnormal, uterus
  ureter N28.89
  urethra N36.1
  vesical N32.3
Sachs' amaurotic familial idiocy or disease E75.02
Sachs-Tay disease E75.02
Sacks-Libman disease M32.11
Sacralgia M53.3
Sacralization Q76.49
Sacrodynia M53.3
Sacroiliac joint — *see* condition
Sacroiliitis NEC M46.1
Sacrum — *see* condition
Saddle
  back — *see* Lordosis
  embolus
    abdominal aorta I74.01
    pulmonary artery I26.92
      with acute cor pulmonale I26.02
  injury — *code to* condition
  nose M95.0
    due to syphilis A50.57
Sadism (sexual) F65.52
Sadness, postpartal O90.6
Sadomasochism F65.50
Saemisch's ulcer (cornea) — *see* Ulcer, cornea, central
Sahib disease B55.0
Sailors' skin L57.8
Saint
  Anthony's fire — *see* Erysipelas
  triad — *see* Hernia, diaphragm
  Vitus' dance — *see* Chorea, Sydenham's
Salaam
  attack(s) — *see* Epilepsy, spasms

Salaam — *continued*
  tic R25.8
Salicylism
  abuse F55.8
  overdose or wrong substance given — *see* Table of
    Drugs and Chemicals, by drug, poisoning
Salivary duct or gland — *see* condition
Salivation, excessive K11.7
Salmonella — *see* Infection, Salmonella
Salmonellosis A02.0
Salpingitis (catarrhal) (fallopian tube) (nodular) (pseud-
  ofollicular) (purulent) (septic) N70.91
  with oophoritis N70.93
  acute N70.01
    with oophoritis N70.03
  chlamydial A56.11
  chronic N70.11
    with oophoritis N70.13
  complicating abortion — *see* Abortion, by type, com-
    plicated by, salpingitis
  ear — *see* Salpingitis, eustachian
  eustachian (tube) H68.00- ☑
    acute H68.01- ☑
    chronic H68.02- ☑
  follicularis N70.11
    with oophoritis N70.13
  gonococcal (acute) (chronic) A54.24
  interstitial, chronic N70.11
    with oophoritis N70.13
  isthmica nodosa N70.11
    with oophoritis N70.13
  specific (gonococcal) (acute) (chronic) A54.24
  tuberculous (acute) (chronic) A18.17
  venereal (gonococcal) (acute) (chronic) A54.24
Salpingocele N83.4
Salpingo-oophoritis (catarrhal) (purulent) (ruptured)
  (septic) (suppurative) N70.93
  acute N70.03
    with ectopic or molar pregnancy O08.0
    following ectopic or molar pregnancy O08.0
    gonococcal A54.24
  chronic N70.13
  following ectopic or molar pregnancy O08.0
  gonococcal (acute) (chronic) A54.24
  puerperal O86.19
  specific (gonococcal) (acute) (chronic) A54.24
  subacute N70.03
  tuberculous (acute) (chronic) A18.17
  venereal (gonococcal) (acute) (chronic) A54.24
Salpingo-ovaritis — *see* Salpingo-oophoritis
Salpingoperitonitis — *see* Salpingo-oophoritis
Salzmann's nodular dystrophy — *see* Degeneration,
  cornea, nodular
Sampson's cyst or tumor N80.1
San Joaquin (Valley) **fever** B38.0
Sandblaster's asthma, lung or pneumoconiosis J62.8
Sander's disease (paranoia) F22
Sandfly fever A93.1
Sandhoff's disease E75.01
Sanfilippo (Type B) (Type C) (Type D) **syndrome** E76.22
Sanger-Brown ataxia G11.2
Sao Paulo fever or typhus A77.0
Saponification, mesenteric K65.8
Sarcocele (benign)
  syphilitic A52.76
    congenital A50.59
Sarcocystosis A07.8
Sarcoepiplocele — *see* Hernia
Sarcoepiplomphalocele Q79.2
Sarcoid (*see also* Sarcoidosis)
  arthropathy D86.86
  Boeck's D86.9
  Darier-Roussy D86.3
  iridocyclitis D86.83
  meningitis D86.81
  myocarditis D86.85
  myositis D86.87
  pyelonephritis D86.84
  Spiegler-Fendt L08.89
Sarcoidosis D86.9
  with
    cranial nerve palsies D86.82
    hepatic granuloma D86.89
    polyarthritis D86.86
    tubulo-interstitial nephropathy D86.84
    combined sites NEC D86.89

Sarcoidosis — *continued*
  lung D86.0
    and lymph nodes D86.2
  lymph nodes D86.1
    and lung D86.2
  meninges D86.81
  skin D86.3
  specified type NEC D86.89
Sarcoma (of) (*see also* Neoplasm, connective tissue, malignant)
  alveolar soft part — *see* Neoplasm, connective tissue,
    malignant
  ameloblastic C41.1
    upper jaw (bone) C41.0
  botryoid — *see* Neoplasm, connective tissue, malig-
    nant
  botryoides — *see* Neoplasm, connective tissue, malig-
    nant
  cerebellar C71.6
    circumscribed (arachnoidal) C71.6
  circumscribed (arachnoidal) cerebellar C71.6
  clear cell (*see also* Neoplasm, connective tissue, malig-
    nant)
    kidney C64.- ☑
  dendritic cells (accessory cells) C96.4
  embryonal — *see* Neoplasm, connective tissue, malig-
    nant
  endometrial (stromal) C54.1
    isthmus C54.0
  epithelioid (cell) — *see* Neoplasm, connective tissue,
    malignant
  Ewing's — *see* Neoplasm, bone, malignant
  follicular dendritic cell C96.4
  germinoblastic (diffuse) — *see* Lymphoma, diffuse
    large cell
    follicular — *see* Lymphoma, follicular, specified
      NEC
  giant cell (except of bone) (*see also* Neoplasm, connec-
    tive tissue, malignant)
    bone — *see* Neoplasm, bone, malignant
  glomoid — *see* Neoplasm, connective tissue, malig-
    nant
  granulocytic C92.3- ☑
  hemangioendothelial — *see* Neoplasm, connective
    tissue, malignant
  hemorrhagic, multiple — *see* Sarcoma, Kaposi's
  histiocytic C96.A (*following* C96.6)
  Hodgkin — *see* Lymphoma, Hodgkin
  immunoblastic (diffuse) — *see* Lymphoma, diffuse
    large cell
  interdigitating dendritic cell C96.4
  Kaposi's
    colon C46.4
    connective tissue C46.1
    gastrointestinal organ C46.4
    lung C46.5- ☑
    lymph node(s) C46.3
    palate (hard) (soft) C46.2
    rectum C46.4
    skin C46.0
    specified site NEC C46.7
    stomach C46.4
    unspecified site C46.9
  Kupffer cell C22.3
  Langerhans cell C96.4
  leptomeningeal — *see* Neoplasm, meninges, malig-
    nant
  liver NEC C22.4
  lymphangioendothelial — *see* Neoplasm, connective
    tissue, malignant
  lymphoblastic — *see* Lymphoma, lymphoblastic (dif-
    fuse)
  lymphocytic — *see* Lymphoma, small cell B-cell
  mast cell C96.2
  melanotic — *see* Melanoma
  meningeal — *see* Neoplasm, meninges, malignant
  meningothelial — *see* Neoplasm, meninges, malignant
  mesenchymal (*see also* Neoplasm, connective tissue,
    malignant)
    mixed — *see* Neoplasm, connective tissue, malig-
      nant
  mesothelial — *see* Mesothelioma
  monstrocellular
    specified site — *see* Neoplasm, malignant, by site
    unspecified site C71.9
  myeloid C92.3- ☑
  neurogenic — *see* Neoplasm, nerve, malignant

Sarcoma — *continued*
odontogenic C41.1
upper jaw (bone) C41.0
osteoblastic — *see* Neoplasm, bone, malignant
osteogenic (*see also* Neoplasm, bone, malignant)
juxtacortical — *see* Neoplasm, bone, malignant
periosteal — *see* Neoplasm, bone, malignant
periosteal (*see also* Neoplasm, bone, malignant)
osteogenic — *see* Neoplasm, bone, malignant
pleomorphic cell — *see* Neoplasm, connective tissue, malignant
reticulum cell (diffuse) — *see* Lymphoma, diffuse large cell
nodular — *see* Lymphoma, follicular
pleomorphic cell type — *see* Lymphoma, diffuse large cell
rhabdoid — *see* Neoplasm, malignant, by site
round cell — *see* Neoplasm, connective tissue, malignant
small cell — *see* Neoplasm, connective tissue, malignant
soft tissue — *see* Neoplasm, connective tissue, malignant
spindle cell — *see* Neoplasm, connective tissue, malignant
stromal (endometrial) C54.1
isthmus C54.0
synovial (*see also* Neoplasm, connective tissue, malignant)
biphasic — *see* Neoplasm, connective tissue, malignant
epithelioid cell — *see* Neoplasm, connective tissue, malignant
spindle cell — *see* Neoplasm, connective tissue, malignant
Sarcomatosis
meningeal — *see* Neoplasm, meninges, malignant
specified site NEC — *see* Neoplasm, connective tissue, malignant
unspecified site C80.1
Sarcosinemia E72.59
Sarcosporidiosis (intestinal) A07.8
Satiety, early R68.81
Saturnine — *see* condition
Saturnism
overdose or wrong substance given or taken — *see* Table of Drugs and Chemicals, by drug, poisoning
Satyriasis F52.8
Sauriasis — *see* Ichthyosis
SBE (subacute bacterial endocarditis) I33.0
Scabies (any site) B86
Scabs R23.4
Scaglietti-Dagnini syndrome E22.0
Scald — *see* Burn
Scalenus anticus (anterior) **syndrome** G54.0
Scales R23.4
Scaling, skin R23.4
Scalp — *see* condition
Scapegoating affecting child Z62.3
Scaphocephaly Q75.0
Scapulalgia M89.8X1
Scapulohumeral myopathy G71.0
Scar, scarring (*see also* Cicatrix) L90.5
adherent L90.5
atrophic L90.5
cervix
in pregnancy or childbirth — *see* Pregnancy, complicated by, abnormal cervix
cheloid L91.0
chorioretinal H31.00- ☑
posterior pole macula H31.01- ☑
postsurgical H59.81- ☑
solar retinopathy H31.02- ☑
specified type NEC H31.09- ☑
choroid — *see* Scar, chorioretinal
conjunctiva H11.24- ☑
cornea H17.9
xerophthalmic (*see also* Opacity, cornea)
vitamin A deficiency E50.6
duodenum, obstructive K31.5
hypertrophic L91.0
keloid L91.0
labia N90.89
lung (base) J98.4
macula — *see* Scar, chorioretinal, posterior pole
muscle M62.89

Scar, scarring — *continued*
myocardium, myocardial I25.2
painful L90.5
posterior pole (eye) — *see* Scar, chorioretinal, posterior pole
retina — *see* Scar, chorioretinal
trachea J39.8
uterus N85.8
in pregnancy O34.29
vagina N89.8
postoperative N99.2
vulva N90.89
Scarabiasis B88.2
Scarlatina (anginosa) (maligna) (ulcerosa) A38.9
myocarditis (acute) A38.1
old — *see* Myocarditis
otitis media A38.0
Scarlet fever (albuminuria) (angina) A38.9
Schamberg's disease (progressive pigmentary dermatosis) L81.7
Schatzki's ring (acquired) (esophagus) (lower) K22.2
congenital Q39.3
Schaufenster krankheit I20.8
Schaumann's
benign lymphogranulomatosis D86.1
disease or syndrome — *see* Sarcoidosis
Scheie's syndrome E76.03
Schenck's disease B42.1
Scheuermann's disease or osteochondrosis — *see* Osteochondrosis, juvenile, spine
Schilder (-Flatau) **disease** G37.0
Schilling-type monocytic leukemia C93.0- ☑
Schimmelbusch's disease, cystic mastitis, or hyperplasia — *see* Mastopathy, cystic
Schistosoma infestation — *see* Infestation, Schistosoma
Schistosomiasis B65.9
with muscle disorder B65.9 [M63.80]
ankle B65.9 [M63.87-] ☑
foot B65.9 [M63.87-] ☑
forearm B65.9 [M63.83-] ☑
hand B65.9 [M63.84-] ☑
lower leg B65.9 [M63.86-] ☑
multiple sites B65.9 [M63.89]
pelvic region B65.9 [M63.85-] ☑
shoulder region B65.9 [M63.81-] ☑
specified site NEC B65.9 [M63.88]
thigh B65.9 [M63.85-] ☑
upper arm B65.9 [M63.82-] ☑
Asiatic B65.2
bladder B65.0
chestermani B65.8
colon B65.1
cutaneous B65.3
due to
S. haematobium B65.0
S. japonicum B65.2
S. mansoni B65.1
S. mattheii B65.8
Eastern B65.2
genitourinary tract B65.0
intestinal B65.1
lung NEC B65.9 [J99]
pneumonia B65.9 [J17]
Manson's (intestinal) B65.1
oriental B65.2
pulmonary NEC B65.9 [J99]
pneumonia B65.9
Schistosoma
haematobium B65.0
japonicum B65.2
mansoni B65.1
specified type NEC B65.8
urinary B65.0
vesical B65.0
Schizencephaly Q04.6
Schizoaffective psychosis F25.9
Schizodontia K00.2
Schizoid personality F60.1
Schizophrenia, schizophrenic F20.9
acute (brief) (undifferentiated) F23
atypical (form) F20.3
borderline F21
catalepsy F20.2
catatonic (type) (excited) (withdrawn) F20.2
cenesthopathic, cenesthesiopathic F20.89
childhood type F84.5
chronic undifferentiated F20.5

Schizophrenia, schizophrenic — *continued*
cyclic F25.0
disorganized (type) F20.1
flexibilitas cerea F20.2
hebephrenic (type) F20.1
incipient F21
latent F21
negative type F20.5
paranoid (type) F20.0
paraphrenic F20.0
post-psychotic depression F32.8
prepsychotic F21
prodromal F21
pseudoneurotic F21
pseudopsychopathic F21
reaction F23
residual (state) (type) F20.5
restzustand F20.5
schizoaffective (type) — *see* Psychosis, schizoaffective
simple (type) F20.89
simplex F20.89
specified type NEC F20.89
stupor F20.2
syndrome of childhood F84.5
undifferentiated (type) F20.3
chronic F20.5
Schizothymia (persistent) F60.1
Schlatter-Osgood disease or osteochondrosis — *see* Osteochondrosis, juvenile, tibia
Schlatter's tibia — *see* Osteochondrosis, juvenile, tibia
Schmidt's syndrome (polyglandular, autoimmune) E31.0
Schmincke's carcinoma or tumor — *see* Neoplasm, nasopharynx, malignant
Schmitz (-Stutzer) **dysentery** A03.0
Schmorl's disease or nodes
lumbar region M51.46
lumbosacral region M51.47
sacrococcygeal region M53.3
thoracic region M51.44
thoracolumbar region M51.45
Schneiderian
papilloma — *see* Neoplasm, nasopharynx, benign
specified site — *see* Neoplasm, benign, by site
unspecified site D14.0
specified site — *see* Neoplasm, malignant, by site
unspecified site C30.0
Scholte's syndrome (malignant carcinoid) E34.0
Scholz (-Bielchowsky-Henneberg) **disease or syndrome** E75.25
Schönlein (-Henoch) disease or purpura (primary) (rheumatic) D69.0
Schottmuller's disease A01.4
Schroeder's syndrome (endocrine hypertensive) E27.0
Schüller-Christian disease or syndrome C96.5
Schultze's type acroparesthesia, simple I73.89
Schultz's disease or syndrome — *see* Agranulocytosis
Schwalbe-Ziehen-Oppenheim disease G24.1
Schwannoma (*see also* Neoplasm, nerve, benign)
malignant (*see also* Neoplasm, nerve, malignant)
with rhabdomyoblastic differentiation — *see* Neoplasm, nerve, malignant
melanocytic — *see* Neoplasm, nerve, benign
pigmented — *see* Neoplasm, nerve, benign
Schwannomatosis Q85.03
Schwartz (-Jampel) **syndrome** G71.13
Schwartz-Bartter syndrome E22.2
Schweniger-Buzzi anetoderma L90.1
Sciatic — *see* condition
Sciatica (infective)
with lumbago M54.4- ☑
due to intervertebral disc disorder — *see* Disorder, disc, with, radiculopathy
due to displacement of intervertebral disc (with lumbago) — *see* Disorder, disc, with, radiculopathy
wallet M54.3- ☑
Scimitar syndrome Q26.8
Sclera — *see* condition
Sclerectasia H15.84- ☑
Scleredema
adultorum — *see* Sclerosis, systemic
Buschke's — *see* Sclerosis, systemic
newborn P83.0
Sclerema (adiposum) (edematosum) (neonatorum) (newborn) P83.0
adultorum — *see* Sclerosis, systemic
Scleriasis — *see* Scleroderma

☑ **Additional Character Required — Refer to the Tabular List for Character Selection**   ⸰ **Subterms under main terms may continue to next column or page**

Scleritis H15.00- ☑
with corneal involvement H15.04- ☑
anterior H15.01- ☑
brawny H15.02- ☑
in (due to) zoster B02.34
posterior H15.03- ☑
specified type NEC H15.09- ☑
syphilitic A52.71
tuberculous (nodular) A18.51
Sclerochoroiditis H31.8
Scleroconjunctivitis — *see* Scleritis
Sclerocystic ovary syndrome E28.2
Sclerodactyly, sclerodactylia L94.3
Scleroderma, sclerodermia (acrosclerotic) (diffuse)
(generalized) (progressive) (pulmonary) (*see also*
Sclerosis, systemic) M34.9
circumscribed L94.0
linear L94.1
localized L94.0
newborn P83.8
systemic M34.9
Sclerokeratitis H16.8
tuberculous A18.52
Scleroma nasi A48.8
Scleromalacia (perforans) H15.05- ☑
Scleromyxedema L98.5
Sclérose en plaques G35
Sclerosis, sclerotic
adrenal (gland) E27.8
Alzheimer's — *see* Disease, Alzheimer's
amyotrophic (lateral) G12.21
aorta, aortic I70.0
valve — *see* Endocarditis, aortic
artery, arterial, arteriolar, arteriovascular — *see* Arteriosclerosis
ascending multiple G35
brain (generalized) (lobular) G37.9
artery, arterial I67.2
diffuse G37.0
disseminated G35
insular G35
Krabbe's E75.23
miliary G35
multiple G35
presenile (Alzheimer's) — *see* Disease, Alzheimer's, early onset
senile (arteriosclerotic) I67.2
stem, multiple G35
tuberous Q85.1
bulbar, multiple G35
bundle of His I44.39
cardiac — *see* Disease, heart, ischemic, atherosclerotic
cardiorenal — *see* Hypertension, cardiorenal
cardiovascular (*see also* Disease, cardiovascular)
renal — *see* Hypertension, cardiorenal
cerebellar — *see* Sclerosis, brain
cerebral — *see* Sclerosis, brain
cerebrospinal (disseminated) (multiple) G35
cerebrovascular I67.2
choroid — *see* Degeneration, choroid
combined (spinal cord) (*see also* Degeneration, combined)
multiple G35
concentric (Balo) G37.5
cornea — *see* Opacity, cornea
coronary (artery) I25.10
with angina pectoris — *see* Arteriosclerosis, coronary (artery),
corpus cavernosum
female N90.89
male N48.6
diffuse (brain) (spinal cord) G37.0
disseminated G35
dorsal G35
dorsolateral (spinal cord) — *see* Degeneration, combined
endometrium N85.5
extrapyramidal G25.9
eye, nuclear (senile) — *see* Cataract, senile, nuclear
focal and segmental (glomerular) (*see also* N00-N07
with fourth character .1) N05.1
Friedreich's (spinal cord) G11.1
funicular (spermatic cord) N50.8
general (vascular) — *see* Arteriosclerosis
gland (lymphatic) I89.8
hepatic K74.1
alcoholic K70.2

Sclerosis, sclerotic — *continued*
hereditary
cerebellar G11.9
spinal (Friedreich's ataxia) G11.1
hippocampal G93.81
insular G35
kidney — *see* Sclerosis, renal
larynx J38.7
lateral (amyotrophic) (descending) (primary) (spinal)
G12.21
lens, senile nuclear — *see* Cataract, senile, nuclear
liver K74.1
with fibrosis K74.2
alcoholic K70.2
alcoholic K70.2
cardiac K76.1
lung — *see* Fibrosis, lung
mastoid — *see* Mastoiditis, chronic
mesial temporal G93.81
mitral I05.8
Mönckeberg's (medial) — *see* Arteriosclerosis, extremities
multiple (brain stem) (cerebral) (generalized) (spinal cord) G35
myocardium, myocardial — *see* Disease, heart, ischemic, atherosclerotic
nuclear (senile), eye — *see* Cataract, senile, nuclear
ovary N83.8
pancreas K86.8
penis N48.6
peripheral arteries — *see* Arteriosclerosis, extremities
plaques G35
pluriglandular E31.8
polyglandular E31.8
posterolateral (spinal cord) — *see* Degeneration, combined
presenile (Alzheimer's) — *see* Disease, Alzheimer's, early onset
primary, lateral G12.29
progressive, systemic M34.0
pulmonary — *see* Fibrosis, lung
artery I27.0
valve (heart) — *see* Endocarditis, pulmonary
renal N26.9
with
cystine storage disease E72.09
hypertensive heart disease (conditions in I11) — *see* Hypertension, cardiorenal
arteriolar (hyaline) (hyperplastic) — *see* Hypertension, kidney
retina (senile) (vascular) H35.00
senile (vascular) — *see* Arteriosclerosis
spinal (cord) (progressive) G95.89
ascending G61.0
combined (*see also* Degeneration, combined)
multiple G35
syphilitic A52.11
disseminated G35
dorsolateral — *see* Degeneration, combined
hereditary (Friedreich's) (mixed form) G11.1
lateral (amyotrophic) G12.21
multiple G35
posterior (syphilitic) A52.11
stomach K31.89
subendocardial, congenital I42.4
systemic M34.9
with
lung involvement M34.81
myopathy M34.82
polyneuropathy M34.83
drug-induced M34.2
due to chemicals NEC M34.2
progressive M34.0
specified NEC M34.89
temporal (mesial) G93.81
tricuspid (heart) (valve) I07.8
tuberous (brain) Q85.1
tympanic membrane — *see* Disorder, tympanic membrane, specified NEC
valve, valvular (heart) — *see* Endocarditis
vascular — *see* Arteriosclerosis
vein I87.8
Scoliosis (acquired) (postural) M41.9
adolescent (idiopathic) — *see* Scoliosis, idiopathic, juvenile
congenital Q67.5
due to bony malformation Q76.3
failure of segmentation (hemivertebra) Q76.3

Scoliosis — *continued*
congenital — *continued*
hemivertebra fusion Q76.3
postural Q67.5
idiopathic M41.20
adolescent M41.129
cervical region M41.122
cervicothoracic region M41.123
lumbar region M41.126
lumbosacral region M41.127
thoracic region M41.124
thoracolumbar region M41.125
cervical region M41.22
cervicothoracic region M41.23
infantile M41.00
cervical region M41.02
cervicothoracic region M41.03
lumbar region M41.06
lumbosacral region M41.07
sacrococcygeal region M41.08
thoracic region M41.04
thoracolumbar region M41.05
juvenile M41.119
cervical region M41.112
cervicothoracic region M41.113
lumbar region M41.116
lumbosacral region M41.117
thoracic region M41.114
thoracolumbar region M41.115
lumbar region M41.26
lumbosacral region M41.27
thoracic region M41.24
thoracolumbar region M41.25
neuromuscular M41.40
cervical region M41.42
cervicothoracic region M41.43
lumbar region M41.46
lumbosacral region M41.47
occipito-atlanto-axial region M41.41
thoracic region M41.44
thoracolumbar region M41.45
paralytic — *see* Scoliosis, neuromuscular
postradiation therapy M96.5
rachitic (late effect or sequelae) E64.3 [M49.80]
cervical region E64.3 [M49.82]
cervicothoracic region E64.3 [M49.83]
lumbar region E64.3 [M49.86]
lumbosacral region E64.3 [M49.87]
multiple sites E64.3 [M49.89]
occipito-atlanto-axial region E64.3 [M49.81]
sacrococcygeal region E64.3 [M49.88]
thoracic region E64.3 [M49.84]
thoracolumbar region E64.3 [M49.85]
sciatic M54.4- ☑
secondary (to) NEC M41.50
cerebral palsy, Friedreich's ataxia, poliomyelitis, neuromuscular disorders — *see* Scoliosis, neuromuscular
cervical region M41.52
cervicothoracic region M41.53
lumbar region M41.56
lumbosacral region M41.57
thoracic region M41.54
thoracolumbar region M41.55
specified form NEC M41.80
cervical region M41.82
cervicothoracic region M41.83
lumbar region M41.86
lumbosacral region M41.87
thoracic region M41.84
thoracolumbar region M41.85
thoracogenic M41.30
thoracic region M41.34
thoracolumbar region M41.35
tuberculous A18.01
Scoliotic pelvis
with disproportion (fetopelvic) O33.0
causing obstructed labor O65.0
Scorbutus, scorbutic (*see also* Scurvy)
anemia D53.2
Scotoma (arcuate) (Bjerrum) (central) (ring) (*see also* Defect, visual field, localized, scotoma)
scintillating H53.19
Scratch — *see* Abrasion
Scratchy throat R09.89
Screening (for) Z13.9
alcoholism Z13.89
anemia Z13.0

▽ **Subterms under main terms may continue to next column or page**			☑ **Additional Character Required — Refer to the Tabular List for Character Selection**			**273**

Scleritis — Screening

Screening — *continued*
anomaly, congenital Z13.89
antenatal, of mother Z36
arterial hypertension Z13.6
arthropod-borne viral disease NEC Z11.59
bacteriuria, asymptomatic Z13.89
behavioral disorder Z13.89
brain injury, traumatic Z13.850
bronchitis, chronic Z13.83
brucellosis Z11.2
cardiovascular disorder Z13.6
cataract Z13.5
chlamydial diseases Z11.8
cholera Z11.0
chromosomal abnormalities (nonprocreative) NEC
Z13.79
colonoscopy Z12.11
congenital
dislocation of hip Z13.89
eye disorder Z13.5
malformation or deformation Z13.89
contamination NEC Z13.88
cystic fibrosis Z13.228
dengue fever Z11.59
dental disorder Z13.84
depression Z13.89
developmental handicap Z13.4
in early childhood Z13.4
diabetes mellitus Z13.1
diphtheria Z11.2
disability, intellectual Z13.4
disease or disorder Z13.9
bacterial NEC Z11.2
intestinal infectious Z11.0
respiratory tuberculosis Z11.1
blood or blood-forming organ Z13.0
cardiovascular Z13.6
Chagas' Z11.6
chlamydial Z11.8
dental Z13.89
developmental Z13.4
digestive tract NEC Z13.818
lower GI Z13.811
upper GI Z13.810
ear Z13.5
endocrine Z13.29
eye Z13.5
genitourinary Z13.89
heart Z13.6
human immunodeficiency virus (HIV) infection
Z11.4
immunity Z13.0
infection
intestinal Z11.0
specified NEC Z11.6
infectious Z11.9
mental Z13.89
metabolic Z13.228
neurological Z13.89
nutritional Z13.21
metabolic Z13.228
lipoid disorders Z13.220
protozoal Z11.6
intestinal Z11.0
respiratory Z13.83
rheumatic Z13.828
rickettsial Z11.8
sexually-transmitted NEC Z11.3
human immunodeficiency virus (HIV) Z11.4
sickle-cell (trait) Z13.0
skin Z13.89
specified NEC Z13.89
spirochetal Z11.8
thyroid Z13.29
vascular Z13.6
venereal Z11.3
viral NEC Z11.59
human immunodeficiency virus (HIV) Z11.4
intestinal Z11.0
elevated titer Z13.89
emphysema Z13.83
encephalitis, viral (mosquito- or tick-borne) Z11.59
exposure to contaminants (toxic) Z13.88
fever
dengue Z11.59
hemorrhagic Z11.59
yellow Z11.59
filariasis Z11.6

Screening — *continued*
galactosemia Z13.228
gastrointestinal condition Z13.818
genetic (nonprocreative) - for procreative management — *see* Testing, genetic, for procreative
management
disease carrier status (nonprocreative) Z13.71
specified NEC (nonprocreative) Z13.79
genitourinary condition Z13.89
glaucoma Z13.5
gonorrhea Z11.3
gout Z13.89
helminthiasis (intestinal) Z11.6
hematopoietic malignancy Z12.89
hemoglobinopathies NEC Z13.0
hemorrhagic fever Z11.59
Hodgkin disease Z12.89
human immunodeficiency virus (HIV) Z11.4
human papillomavirus Z11.51
hypertension Z13.6
immunity disorders Z13.0
infection
mycotic Z11.8
parasitic Z11.8
ingestion of radioactive substance Z13.88
intellectual disability Z13.4
intestinal
helminthiasis Z11.6
infectious disease Z11.0
leishmaniasis Z11.6
leprosy Z11.2
leptospirosis Z11.8
leukemia Z12.89
lymphoma Z12.89
malaria Z11.6
malnutrition Z13.29
metabolic Z13.228
nutritional Z13.21
measles Z11.59
mental disorder Z13.89
metabolic errors, inborn Z13.228
multiphasic Z13.89
musculoskeletal disorder Z13.828
osteoporosis Z13.820
mycoses Z11.8
myocardial infarction (acute) Z13.6
neoplasm (malignant) (of) Z12.9
bladder Z12.6
blood Z12.89
breast Z12.39
routine mammogram Z12.31
cervix Z12.4
colon Z12.11
genitourinary organs NEC Z12.79
bladder Z12.6
cervix Z12.4
ovary Z12.73
prostate Z12.5
testis Z12.71
vagina Z12.72
hematopoietic system Z12.89
intestinal tract Z12.10
colon Z12.11
rectum Z12.12
small intestine Z12.13
lung Z12.2
lymph (glands) Z12.89
nervous system Z12.82
oral cavity Z12.81
prostate Z12.5
rectum Z12.12
respiratory organs Z12.2
skin Z12.83
small intestine Z12.13
specified site NEC Z12.89
stomach Z12.0
nephropathy Z13.89
nervous system disorders NEC Z13.858
neurological condition Z13.89
osteoporosis Z13.820
parasitic infestation Z11.9
specified NEC Z11.8
phenylketonuria Z13.228
plague Z11.2
poisoning (chemical) (heavy metal) Z13.88
poliomyelitis Z11.59
postnatal, chromosomal abnormalities Z13.89
prenatal, of mother Z36

Screening — *continued*
protozoal disease Z11.6
intestinal Z11.0
pulmonary tuberculosis Z11.1
radiation exposure Z13.88
respiratory condition Z13.83
respiratory tuberculosis Z11.1
rheumatoid arthritis Z13.828
rubella Z11.59
schistosomiasis Z11.6
sexually-transmitted disease NEC Z11.3
human immunodeficiency virus (HIV) Z11.4
sickle-cell disease or trait Z13.0
skin condition Z13.89
sleeping sickness Z11.6
special Z13.9
specified NEC Z13.89
syphilis Z11.3
tetanus Z11.2
trachoma Z11.8
traumatic brain injury Z13.850
trypanosomiasis Z11.6
tuberculosis, respiratory Z11.1
venereal disease Z11.3
viral encephalitis (mosquito- or tick-borne) Z11.59
whooping cough Z11.2
worms, intestinal Z11.6
yaws Z11.8
yellow fever Z11.59
Scrofula, scrofulosis (tuberculosis of cervical lymph
glands) A18.2
Scrofulide (primary) (tuberculous) A18.4
Scrofuloderma, scrofulodermia (any site) (primary)
A18.4
Scrofulosus lichen (primary) (tuberculous) A18.4
Scrofulous — *see* condition
Scrotal tongue K14.5
Scrotum — *see* condition
Scurvy, scorbutic E54
anemia D53.2
gum E54
infantile E54
rickets E55.0 [M90.80]
Sealpox B08.62
Seasickness T75.3 ☑
Seatworm (infection) (infestation) B80
Sebaceous (*see also* condition)
cyst — *see* Cyst, sebaceous
Seborrhea, seborrheic L21.9
capillitii R23.8
capitis L21.0
dermatitis L21.9
infantile L21.1
eczema L21.9
infantile L21.1
sicca L21.0
Seckel's syndrome Q87.1
Seclusion, pupil — *see* Membrane, pupillary
Second hand tobacco smoke exposure (acute)
(chronic) Z77.22
in the perinatal period P96.81
Secondary
dentin (in pulp) K04.3
neoplasm, secondaries — *see* Table of Neoplasms,
secondary
Secretion
antidiuretic hormone, inappropriate E22.2
catecholamine, by pheochromocytoma E27.5
hormone
antidiuretic, inappropriate (syndrome) E22.2
by
carcinoid tumor E34.0
pheochromocytoma E27.5
ectopic NEC E34.2
urinary
excessive R35.8
suppression R34
Section
nerve, traumatic — *see* Injury, nerve
Segmentation, incomplete (congenital) (*see also* Fusion)
bone NEC Q78.8
lumbosacral (joint) (vertebra) Q76.49
Seitelberger's syndrome (infantile neuraxonal dystrophy) G31.89
Seizure(s) (*see also* Convulsions) R56.9
akinetic — *see* Epilepsy, generalized, specified NEC
atonic — *see* Epilepsy, generalized, specified NEC

☑ **Additional Character Required — Refer to the Tabular List for Character Selection** ▽ Subterms under main terms may continue to next column or page

Seizure(s) — *continued*
  autonomic (hysterical) F44.5
  convulsive — *see* Convulsions
  cortical (focal) (motor) — *see* Epilepsy, localization-related, symptomatic, with simple partial seizures
  disorder (*see also* Epilepsy) G40.909
  due to stroke — *see* Sequelae (of), disease, cerebrovascular, by type, specified NEC
  epileptic — *see* Epilepsy
  febrile (simple) R56.00
    with status epilepticus G40.901
    complex (atypical) (complicated) R56.01
      with status epilepticus G40.901
  grand mal G40.409
    intractable G40.419
      with status epilepticus G40.411
      without status epilepticus G40.419
    not intractable G40.409
      with status epilepticus G40.401
      without status epilepticus G40.409
  heart — *see* Disease, heart
  hysterical F44.5
  intractable G40.919
    with status epilepticus G40.911
  Jacksonian (focal) (motor type) (sensory type) — *see* Epilepsy, localization-related, symptomatic, with simple partial seizures
  newborn P90
  nonspecific epileptic
    atonic — *see* Epilepsy, generalized, specified NEC
    clonic — *see* Epilepsy, generalized, specified NEC
    myoclonic — *see* Epilepsy, generalized, specified NEC
    tonic — *see* Epilepsy, generalized, specified NEC
    tonic-clonic — *see* Epilepsy, generalized, specified NEC
  partial, developing into secondarily generalized seizures
    complex — *see* Epilepsy, localization-related, symptomatic, with complex partial seizures
    simple — *see* Epilepsy, localization-related, symptomatic, with simple partial seizures
  petit mal G40.409
    intractable G40.419
      with status epilepticus G40.411
      without status epilepticus G40.419
    not intractable G40.409
      with status epilepticus G40.401
      without status epilepticus G40.409
  post traumatic R56.1
  recurrent G40.909
  specified NEC G40.89
  uncinate — *see* Epilepsy, localization-related, symptomatic, with complex partial seizures
Selenium deficiency, dietary E59
Self-damaging behavior (life-style) Z72.89
Self-harm (attempted)
  history (personal) Z91.5
    in family Z81.8
Self-mutilation (attempted)
  history (personal) Z91.5
    in family Z81.8
Self-poisoning
  history (personal) Z91.5
    in family Z81.8
  observation following (alleged) attempt Z03.6
Semicoma R40.1
Seminal vesiculitis N49.0
Seminoma C62.9-
  specified site — *see* Neoplasm, malignant, by site
Senear-Usher disease or syndrome L10.4
Senectus R54
Senescence (without mention of psychosis) R54
Senile, senility (*see also* condition) R41.81
  with
    acute confusional state F05
    mental changes NOS F03 ☑
    psychosis NEC — *see* Psychosis, senile
  asthenia R54
  cervix (atrophic) N88.8
  debility R54
  endometrium (atrophic) N85.8
  fallopian tube (atrophic) — *see* Atrophy, fallopian tube
  heart (failure) R54
  ovary (atrophic) — *see* Atrophy, ovary
  premature E34.8

Senile, senility — *continued*
  vagina, vaginitis (atrophic) N95.2
  wart L82.1
Sensation
  burning (skin) R20.8
    tongue K14.6
  loss of R20.8
  prickling (skin) R20.2
  tingling (skin) R20.2
Sense loss
  smell — *see* Disturbance, sensation, smell
  taste — *see* Disturbance, sensation, taste
  touch R20.8
Sensibility disturbance (cortical) (deep) (vibratory) R20.9
Sensitive, sensitivity (*see also* Allergy)
  carotid sinus G90.01
  child (excessive) F93.8
  cold, autoimmune D59.1
  dentin K03.89
  latex Z91.040
  methemoglobin D74.8
  tuberculin, without clinical or radiological symptoms R76.11
  visual
    glare H53.71
    impaired contrast H53.72
Sensitiver Beziehungswahn F22
Sensitization, auto-erythrocytic D69.2
Separation
  anxiety, abnormal (of childhood) F93.0
  apophysis, traumatic — *code as* Fracture, by site
  choroid — *see* Detachment, choroid
  epiphysis, epiphyseal
    nontraumatic (*see also* Osteochondropathy, specified type NEC)
      upper femoral — *see* Slipped, epiphysis, upper femoral
    traumatic — *code as* Fracture, by site
  fracture — *see* Fracture
  infundibulum cardiac from right ventricle by a partition Q24.3
  joint (traumatic) (current) — *code by* site under Dislocation
  pubic bone, obstetrical trauma O71.6
  retina, retinal — *see* Detachment, retina
  symphysis pubis, obstetrical trauma O71.6
  tracheal ring, incomplete, congenital Q32.1
Sepsis (generalized) (unspecified organism) A41.9
  with
    organ dysfunction (acute) (multiple) R65.20
      with septic shock R65.21
  actinomycotic A42.7
  adrenal hemorrhage syndrome (meningococcal) A39.1
  anaerobic A41.4
  Bacillus anthracis A22.7
  Brucella (*see also* Brucellosis) A23.9
  candidal B37.7
  cryptogenic A41.9
  due to device, implant or graft T85.79 ☑
    arterial graft NEC T82.7 ☑
    breast (implant) T85.79 ☑
    catheter NEC T85.79 ☑
      dialysis (renal) T82.7 ☑
        intraperitoneal T85.71 ☑
      infusion NEC T82.7 ☑
        spinal (epidural) (subdural) T85.79 ☑
      urinary (indwelling) T83.51 ☑
    ectopic or molar pregnancy O08.82
    electronic (electrode) (pulse generator) (stimulator)
      bone T84.7 ☑
      cardiac T82.7 ☑
      nervous system (brain) (peripheral nerve) (spinal) T85.79 ☑
      urinary T83.59 ☑
    fixation, internal (orthopedic) — *see* Complication, fixation device, infection
    gastrointestinal (bile duct) (esophagus) T85.79 ☑
    genital T83.6 ☑
    heart NEC T82.7 ☑
      valve (prosthesis) T82.6 ☑
        graft T82.7 ☑
    joint prosthesis — *see* Complication, joint prosthesis, infection
    ocular (corneal graft) (orbital implant) T85.79 ☑
    orthopedic NEC T84.7 ☑

Sepsis — *continued*
  due to device, implant or graft — *continued*
    orthopedic — *continued*
      fixation device, internal — *see* Complication, fixation device, infection
    specified NEC T85.79 ☑
    vascular T82.7 ☑
    ventricular intracranial shunt T85.79 ☑
  during labor O75.3
  Enterococcus A41.81
  Erysipelothrix (rhusiopathiae) (erysipeloid) A26.7
  Escherichia coli (E. coli) A41.5 ☑
  extraintestinal yersiniosis A28.2
  following
    abortion (subsequent episode) O08.0
      current episode — *see* Abortion
    ectopic or molar pregnancy O08.82
    immunization T88.0 ☑
    infusion, therapeutic injection or transfusion NEC T80.29 ☑
  gangrenous A41.9
  gonococcal A54.86
  Gram-negative (organism) A41.5 ☑
    anaerobic A41.4
  Haemophilus influenzae A41.3
  herpesviral B00.7
  intra-abdominal K65.1
  intraocular — *see* Endophthalmitis, purulent
  Listeria monocytogenes A32.7
  localized — *code to* specific localized infection
    in operation wound T81.4 ☑
    skin — *see* Abscess
  malleus A24.0
  melioidosis A24.1
  meningeal — *see* Meningitis
  meningococcal A39.4
    acute A39.2
    chronic A39.3
  MSSA (Methicillin susceptible Staphylococcus aureus) A41.01
  newborn P36.9
    due to
      anaerobes NEC P36.5
      Escherichia coli P36.4
      Staphylococcus P36.30
        aureus P36.2
        specified NEC P36.39
      Streptococcus P36.10
        group B P36.0
        specified NEC P36.19
      specified NEC P36.8
  Pasteurella multocida A28.0
  pelvic, puerperal, postpartum, childbirth O85
  pneumococcal A40.3
  postprocedural T81.4 ☑
  puerperal, postpartum, childbirth (pelvic) O85
  Salmonella (arizonae) (cholerae-suis) (enteritidis) (typhimurium) A02.1
  severe R65.20
    with septic shock R65.21
  Shigella (*see also* Dysentery, bacillary) A03.9
  skin, localized — *see* Abscess
  specified organism NEC A41.89
  Staphylococcus, staphylococcal A41.2
    aureus (methicillin susceptible) (MSSA) A41.01
      methicillin resistant (MRSA) A41.02
    coagulase-negative A41.1
    specified NEC A41.1
  Streptococcus, streptococcal A40.9
    agalactiae A40.1
    group
      A A40.0
      B A40.1
      D A41.81
    neonatal P36.10
      group B P36.0
      specified NEC P36.19
    pneumoniae A40.3
    pyogenes A40.0
    specified NEC A40.8
  tracheostomy stoma J95.02
  tularemic A21.7
  umbilical, umbilical cord (newborn) — *see* Sepsis, newborn
  Yersinia pestis A20.7
Septate — *see* Septum

Septic — see condition
  arm — see Cellulitis, upper limb
    with lymphangitis — see Lymphangitis, acute, upper limb
  embolus — see Embolism
  finger — see Cellulitis, digit
    with lymphangitis — see Lymphangitis, acute, digit
  foot — see Cellulitis, lower limb
    with lymphangitis — see Lymphangitis, acute, lower limb
  gallbladder (acute) K81.0
  hand — see Cellulitis, upper limb
    with lymphangitis — see Lymphangitis, acute, upper limb
  joint — see Arthritis, pyogenic or pyemic
  leg — see Cellulitis, lower limb
    with lymphangitis — see Lymphangitis, acute, lower limb
  nail (see also Cellulitis, digit)
    with lymphangitis — see Lymphangitis, acute, digit
  sore (see also Abscess)
    throat J02.0
      streptococcal J02.0
  spleen (acute) D73.89
  teeth, tooth (pulpal origin) K04.4
  throat — see Pharyngitis
  thrombus — see Thrombosis
  toe — see Cellulitis, digit
    with lymphangitis — see Lymphangitis, acute, digit
  tonsils, chronic J35.01
    with adenoiditis J35.03
  uterus — see Endometritis
Septicemia A41.9
  meaning sepsis — see Sepsis
Septum, septate (congenital) (see also Anomaly, by site)
  anal Q42.3
    with fistula Q42.2
  aqueduct of Sylvius Q03.0
    with spina bifida — see Spina bifida, by site, with hydrocephalus
  uterus (complete) (partial) Q51.2
  vagina Q52.10
    in pregnancy — see Pregnancy, complicated by, abnormal vagina
      causing obstructed labor O65.5
    longitudinal (with or without obstruction) Q52.12
    transverse Q52.11
Sequelae (of) (see also condition)
  abscess, intracranial or intraspinal (conditions in G06) G09
  amputation — code to injury with seventh character S
  burn and corrosion — code to injury with seventh character S
  calcium deficiency E64.8
  cerebrovascular disease — see Sequelae, disease, cerebrovascular
  childbirth O94
  contusion — code to injury with seventh character S
  corrosion — see Sequelae, burn and corrosion
  crushing injury — code to injury with seventh character S
  disease
    cerebrovascular I69.90
      alteration of sensation I69.998
      aphasia I69.920
      apraxia I69.990
      ataxia I69.993
      cognitive deficits I69.91
      disturbance of vision I69.998
      dysarthria I69.922
      dysphagia I69.991
      dysphasia I69.921
      facial droop I69.992
      facial weakness I69.992
      fluency disorder I69.923
      hemiplegia I69.95- ☑
      hemorrhage
        intracerebral — see Sequelae, hemorrhage, intracerebral
        intracranial, nontraumatic NEC — see Sequelae, hemorrhage, intracranial, nontraumatic

Sequelae — continued
  disease — continued
    cerebrovascular — continued
      hemorrhage — continued
        subarachnoid — see Sequelae, hemorrhage, subarachnoid
      language deficit I69.928
      monoplegia
        lower limb I69.84- ☑
        upper limb I69.93- ☑
      paralytic syndrome I69.96- ☑
      specified effect NEC I69.998
      specified type NEC I69.80
        alteration of sensation I69.898
        aphasia I69.820
        apraxia I69.890
        ataxia I69.893
        cognitive deficits I69.81
        disturbance of vision I69.898
        dysarthria I69.822
        dysphagia I69.891
        dysphasia I69.821
        facial droop I69.892
        facial weakness I69.892
        fluency disorder I69.823
        hemiplegia I69.85- ☑
        language deficit I69.828
        monoplegia
          lower limb I69.84- ☑
          upper limb I69.83- ☑
        paralytic syndrome I69.86- ☑
        specified effect NEC I69.898
      speech deficit I69.928
        speech deficit I69.828
      stroke NOS — see Sequelae, stroke NOS
  dislocation — code to injury with seventh character S
  encephalitis or encephalomyelitis (conditions in G04) G09
    in infectious disease NEC B94.8
    viral B94.1
  external cause — code to injury with seventh character S
  foreign body entering natural orifice — code to injury with seventh character S
  fracture — code to injury with seventh character S
  frostbite — code to injury with seventh character S
  Hansen's disease B92
  hemorrhage
    intracerebral I69.10
      alteration of sensation I69.198
      aphasia I69.120
      apraxia I69.190
      ataxia I69.193
      cognitive deficits I69.11
      disturbance of vision I69.198
      dysarthria I69.122
      dysphagia I69.191
      dysphasia I69.121
      facial droop I69.192
      facial weakness I69.192
      fluency disorder I69.123
      hemiplegia I69.15- ☑
      language deficit NEC I69.128
      monoplegia
        lower limb I69.14- ☑
        upper limb I69.13- ☑
      paralytic syndrome I69.16- ☑
      specified effect NEC I69.198
      speech deficit NEC I69.128
    intracranial, nontraumatic NEC I69.20
      alteration of sensation I69.298
      aphasia I69.220
      apraxia I69.290
      ataxia I69.293
      cognitive deficits I69.21
      disturbance of vision I69.298
      dysarthria I69.222
      dysphagia I69.291
      dysphasia I69.221
      facial droop I69.292
      facial weakness I69.292
      fluency disorder I69.223
      hemiplegia I69.25- ☑
      language deficit NEC I69.228
      monoplegia
        lower limb I69.24- ☑
        upper limb I69.23- ☑
      paralytic syndrome I69.26- ☑

Sequelae — continued
  hemorrhage — continued
    intracranial, nontraumatic — continued
      specified effect NEC I69.298
      speech deficit NEC I69.228
    subarachnoid I69.00
      alteration of sensation I69.098
      aphasia I69.020
      apraxia I69.090
      ataxia I69.093
      cognitive deficits I69.01
      disturbance of vision I69.098
      dysarthria I69.022
      dysphagia I69.091
      dysphasia I69.021
      facial droop I69.092
      facial weakness I69.092
      fluency disorder I69.023
      hemiplegia I69.05- ☑
      language deficit NEC I69.028
      monoplegia
        lower limb I69.04- ☑
        upper limb I69.03- ☑
      paralytic syndrome I69.06- ☑
      specified effect NEC I69.098
      speech deficit NEC I69.028
  hepatitis, viral B94.2
  hyperalimentation E68
  infarction
    cerebral I69.30
      alteration of sensation I69.398
      aphasia I69.320
      apraxia I69.390
      ataxia I69.393
      cognitive deficits I69.31
      disturbance of vision I69.398
      dysarthria I69.322
      dysphagia I69.391
      dysphasia I69.321
      facial droop I69.392
      facial weakness I69.392
      fluency disorder I69.323
      hemiplegia I69.35- ☑
      language deficit NEC I69.328
      monoplegia
        lower limb I69.34- ☑
        upper limb I69.33- ☑
      paralytic syndrome I69.36- ☑
      specified effect NEC I69.398
      speech deficit NEC I69.328
  infection, pyogenic, intracranial or intraspinal G09
  infectious disease B94.9
    specified NEC B94.8
  injury — code to injury with seventh character S
  leprosy B92
  meningitis
    bacterial (conditions in G00) G09
    other or unspecified cause (conditions in G03) G09
  muscle (and tendon) injury — code to injury with seventh character S
  myelitis — see Sequelae, encephalitis
  niacin deficiency E64.8
  nutritional deficiency E64.9
    specified NEC E64.8
  obstetrical condition O94
  parasitic disease B94.9
  phlebitis or thrombophlebitis of intracranial or intraspinal venous sinuses and veins (conditions in G08) G09
  poisoning — code to poisoning with seventh character S
    nonmedicinal substance — see Sequelae, toxic effect, nonmedicinal substance
  poliomyelitis (acute) B91
  pregnancy O94
  protein-energy malnutrition E64.0
  puerperium O94
  rickets E64.3
  selenium deficiency E64.8
  sprain and strain — code to injury with seventh character S
  stroke NOS I69.30
    alteration in sensation I69.398
    aphasia I69.320
    apraxia I69.390
    ataxia I69.393
    cognitive deficits I69.31
    disturbance of vision I69.398

Sequelae — *continued*
  stroke — *continued*
    dysarthria I69.322
    dysphagia I69.391
    dysphasia I69.321
    facial droop I69.392
    facial weakness I69.392
    hemiplegia I69.35- ☑
    language deficit NEC I69.328
    monoplegia
      lower limb I69.34- ☑
      upper limb I69.33- ☑
    paralytic syndrome I69.36- ☑
    specified effect NEC I69.398
    speech deficit NEC I69.328
  tendon and muscle injury — *code to* injury with seventh character S
  thiamine deficiency E64.8
  trachoma B94.0
  tuberculosis B90.9
    bones and joints B90.2
    central nervous system B90.0
    genitourinary B90.1
    pulmonary (respiratory) B90.9
    specified organs NEC B90.8
  viral
    encephalitis B94.1
    hepatitis B94.2
  vitamin deficiency NEC E64.8
    A E64.1
    B E64.8
    C E64.2
  wound, open — *code to* injury with seventh character S

Sequestration (*see also* Sequestrum)
  lung, congenital Q33.2

Sequestrum
  bone — *see* Osteomyelitis, chronic
  dental M27.2
  jaw bone M27.2
  orbit — *see* Osteomyelitis, orbit
  sinus (accessory) (nasal) — *see* Sinusitis

Sequoiosis lung or pneumonitis J67.8

Serology for syphilis
  doubtful
    with signs or symptoms — *code by* site and stage under Syphilis
    follow-up of latent syphilis — *see* Syphilis, latent
  negative, with signs or symptoms — *code by* site and stage under Syphilis
  positive A53.0
    with signs or symptoms — *code by* site and stage under Syphilis
  reactivated A53.0

Seroma (*see also* Hematoma)
  traumatic, secondary and recurrent T79.2 ☑

Seropurulent — *see* condition

Serositis, multiple K65.8
  pericardial I31.1
  peritoneal K65.8

Serous — *see* condition

Sertoli cell
  adenoma
    specified site — *see* Neoplasm, benign, by site
    unspecified site
      female D27.9
      male D29.20
  carcinoma
    specified site — *see* Neoplasm, malignant, by site
    unspecified site (male) C62.9- ☑
      female C56.9
  tumor
    with lipid storage
      specified site — *see* Neoplasm, benign, by site
      unspecified site
        female D27.9
        male D29.20
    specified site — *see* Neoplasm, benign, by site
    unspecified site
      female D27.9
      male D29.20

Sertoli-Leydig cell tumor — *see* Neoplasm, benign, by site
  specified site — *see* Neoplasm, benign, by site
  unspecified site
    female D27.9
    male D29.20

Serum
  allergy, allergic reaction (*see also* Reaction, serum) T80.69 ☑
    shock (*see also* Shock, anaphylactic) T80.59 ☑
  arthritis (*see also* Reaction, serum) T80.69 ☑
  complication or reaction NEC (*see also* Reaction, serum) T80.69 ☑
  disease NEC (*see also* Reaction, serum) T80.69 ☑
  hepatitis (*see also* Hepatitis, viral, type B)
    carrier (suspected) of Z22.51
  intoxication (*see also* Reaction, serum) T80.69 ☑
  neuritis (*see also* Reaction, serum) T80.69 ☑
  neuropathy G61.1
  poisoning NEC (*see also* Reaction, serum) T80.69 ☑
  rash NEC (*see also* Reaction, serum) T80.69 ☑
  reaction NEC (*see also* Reaction, serum) T80.69 ☑
  sickness NEC (*see also* Reaction, serum) T80.69 ☑
  urticaria (*see also* Reaction, serum) T80.69 ☑

Sesamoiditis M25.8- ☑

Severe sepsis R65.20
  with septic shock R65.21

Sever's disease or osteochondrosis — *see* Osteochondrosis, juvenile, tarsus

Sex
  chromosome mosaics Q97.8
    lines with various numbers of X chromosomes Q97.2
  education Z70.8
  reassignment surgery status Z87.890

Sextuplet pregnancy — *see* Pregnancy, sextuplet

Sexual
  function, disorder of (psychogenic) F52.9
  immaturity (female) (male) E30.0
  impotence (psychogenic) organic origin NEC — *see* Dysfunction, sexual, male
  precocity (constitutional) (cryptogenic)(female) (idiopathic) (male) E30.1

Sexuality, pathologic — *see* Deviation, sexual

Sézary disease C84.1- ☑

Shadow, lung R91.8

Shaking palsy or paralysis — *see* Parkinsonism

Shallowness, acetabulum — *see* Derangement, joint, specified type NEC, hip

Shaver's disease J63.1

Sheath (tendon) — *see* condition

Sheathing, retinal vessels H35.01- ☑

Shedding
  nail L60.8
  premature, primary (deciduous) teeth K00.6

Sheehan's disease or syndrome E23.0

Shelf, rectal K62.89

Shell teeth K00.5

Shellshock (current) F43.0
  lasting state — *see* Disorder, post-traumatic stress

Shield kidney Q63.1

Shift
  auditory threshold (temporary) H93.24- ☑
  mediastinal R93.8

Shifting sleep-work schedule (affecting sleep) G47.26

Shiga (-Kruse) **dysentery** A03.0

Shiga's bacillus A03.0

Shigella (dysentery) — *see* Dysentery, bacillary

Shigellosis A03.9
  Group A A03.0
  Group B A03.1
  Group C A03.2
  Group D A03.3

Shin splints S86.89- ☑

Shingles — *see* Herpes, zoster

Shipyard disease or eye B30.0

Shirodkar suture, in pregnancy — *see* Pregnancy, complicated by, incompetent cervix

Shock R57.9
  with ectopic or molar pregnancy O08.3
  adrenal (cortical) (Addisonian) E27.2
  adverse food reaction (anaphylactic) — *see* Shock, anaphylactic, due to food
  allergic — *see* Shock, anaphylactic
  anaphylactic T78.2 ☑
    chemical — *see* Table of Drugs and Chemicals
    due to drug or medicinal substance
      correct substance properly administered T88.6 ☑
      overdose or wrong substance given or taken (by accident) — *see* Table of Drugs and Chemicals, by drug, poisoning

Shock — *continued*
  anaphylactic — *continued*
    due to food (nonpoisonous) T78.00 ☑
      additives T78.06 ☑
      dairy products T78.07 ☑
      eggs T78.08 ☑
      fish T78.03 ☑
        shellfish T78.02 ☑
      fruit T78.04 ☑
      milk T78.07 ☑
      nuts T78.05 ☑
        peanuts T78.01 ☑
      peanuts T78.01 ☑
      seeds T78.05 ☑
      specified type NEC T78.09 ☑
      vegetable T78.04 ☑
    following sting(s) — *see* Venom
    immunization T80.52 ☑
    serum T80.59 ☑
      blood and blood products T80.51 ☑
      immunization T80.52 ☑
      specified NEC T80.59 ☑
      vaccination T80.52 ☑
  anaphylactoid — *see* Shock, anaphylactic
  anesthetic
    correct substance properly administered T88.2 ☑
    overdose or wrong substance given or taken — *see* Table of Drugs and Chemicals, by drug, poisoning
    specified anesthetic — *see* Table of Drugs and Chemicals, by drug, poisoning
  cardiogenic R57.0
  chemical substance — *see* Table of Drugs and Chemicals
  complicating ectopic or molar pregnancy O08.3
  culture — *see* Disorder, adjustment
  drug
    due to correct substance properly administered T88.6 ☑
    overdose or wrong substance given or taken (by accident) — *see* Table of Drugs and Chemicals, by drug, poisoning
  during or after labor and delivery O75.1
  electric T75.4 ☑
    (taser) T75.4 ☑
  endotoxic R65.21
    postprocedural (during or resulting from a procedure, not elsewhere classified) T81.12 ☑
  following
    ectopic or molar pregnancy O08.3
    injury (immediate) (delayed) T79.4 ☑
    labor and delivery O75.1
  food (anaphylactic) — *see* Shock, anaphylactic, due to food
  from electroshock gun (taser) T75.4 ☑
  gram-negative R65.21
    postprocedural (during or resulting from a procedure, not elsewhere classified) T81.12 ☑
  hematologic R57.8
  hemorrhagic
    surgery (intraoperative) (postoperative) T81.19 ☑
    trauma T79.4 ☑
  hypovolemic R57.1
    surgical T81.19 ☑
    traumatic T79.4 ☑
  insulin E15
    therapeutic misadventure — *see* subcategory T38.3 ☑
  kidney N17.0
    traumatic (following crushing) T79.5 ☑
  lightning T75.01 ☑
  lung J80
  obstetric O75.1
    with ectopic or molar pregnancy O08.3
    following ectopic or molar pregnancy O08.3
  pleural (surgical) T81.19 ☑
    due to trauma T79.4 ☑
  postprocedural (postoperative) T81.10 ☑
    with ectopic or molar pregnancy O08.3
    cardiogenic T81.11 ☑
    endotoxic T81.12 ☑
    following ectopic or molar pregnancy O08.3
    gram-negative T81.12 ☑
    hypovolemic T81.19 ☑
    septic T81.12 ☑
    specified type NEC T81.19 ☑

Shock — *continued*
  psychic F43.Ø
  septic (due to severe sepsis) R65.21
  specified NEC R57.8
  surgical T81.1Ø ☑
  taser gun (taser) T75.4 ☑
  therapeutic misadventure NEC T81.1Ø ☑
  thyroxin
    overdose or wrong substance given or taken —
        see Table of Drugs and Chemicals, by drug,
        poisoning
  toxic, syndrome A48.3
  transfusion — *see* Complications, transfusion
  traumatic (immediate) (delayed) T79.4 ☑
Shoemaker's chest M95.4
Short, shortening, shortness
  arm (acquired) (*see also* Deformity, limb, unequal
        length)
    congenital Q71.81- ☑
    forearm — *see* Deformity, limb, unequal length
  bowel syndrome K91.2
  breath RØ6.Ø2
  cervical (complicating pregnancy) O26.87- ☑
    non-gravid uterus N88.3
  common bile duct, congenital Q44.5
  cord (umbilical), complicating delivery O69.3 ☑
  cystic duct, congenital Q44.5
  esophagus (congenital) Q39.8
  femur (acquired) — *see* Deformity, limb, unequal
        length, femur
    congenital — *see* Defect, reduction, lower limb,
        longitudinal, femur
  frenum, frenulum, linguae (congenital) Q38.1
  hip (acquired) (*see also* Deformity, limb, unequal
        length)
    congenital Q65.89
  leg (acquired) (*see also* Deformity, limb, unequal
        length)
    congenital Q72.81- ☑
    lower leg (*see also* Deformity, limb, unequal length)
  limbed stature, with immunodeficiency D82.2
  lower limb (acquired) (*see also* Deformity, limb, un-
        equal length)
    congenital Q72.81- ☑
  organ or site, congenital NEC — *see* Distortion
  palate, congenital Q38.5
  radius (acquired) (*see also* Deformity, limb, unequal
        length)
    congenital — *see* Defect, reduction, upper limb,
        longitudinal, radius
  rib syndrome Q77.2
  stature (child) (hereditary) (idiopathic) NEC R62.52
    constitutional E34.3
    due to endocrine disorder E34.3
    Laron-type E34.3
  tendon (*see also* Contraction, tendon)
    with contracture of joint — *see* Contraction, joint
    Achilles (acquired) M67.Ø- ☑
        congenital Q66.89
    congenital Q79.8
  thigh (acquired) (*see also* Deformity, limb, unequal
        length, femur)
    congenital — *see* Defect, reduction, lower limb,
        longitudinal, femur
  tibialis anterior (tendon) — *see* Contraction, tendon
  umbilical cord
    complicating delivery O69.3 ☑
  upper limb, congenital — *see* Defect, reduction, upper
        limb, specified type NEC
  urethra N36.8
  uvula, congenital Q38.5
  vagina (congenital) Q52.4
Shortsightedness — *see* Myopia
Shoshin (acute fulminating beriberi) E51.11
Shoulder — *see* condition
Shovel-shaped incisors KØØ.2
Shower, thromboembolic — *see* Embolism
Shunt
  arterial-venous (dialysis) Z99.2
  arteriovenous, pulmonary (acquired) I28.Ø
    congenital Q25.72
  cerebral ventricle (communicating) in situ Z98.2
  surgical, prosthetic, with complications — *see* Compli-
        cations, cardiovascular, device or implant
Shutdown, renal N28.9
Shy-Drager syndrome G9Ø.3

Sialadenitis, sialadenosis (any gland) (chronic) (period-
        ic) (suppurative) — *see* Sialoadenitis
Sialectasia K11.8
Sialidosis E77.1
Sialitis, silitis (any gland) (chronic) (suppurative) — *see*
        Sialoadenitis
Sialoadenitis (any gland) (periodic) (suppurative) K11.2Ø
  acute K11.21
    recurrent K11.22
  chronic K11.23
Sialoadenopathy K11.9
Sialoangitis — *see* Sialoadenitis
Sialodochitis (fibrinosa) — *see* Sialoadenitis
Sialodocholithiasis K11.5
Sialolithiasis K11.5
Sialometaplasia, necrotizing K11.8
Sialorrhea (*see also* Ptyalism)
  periodic — *see* Sialoadenitis
Sialosis K11.7
Siamese twin Q89.4
Sibling rivalry Z62.891
Sicard's syndrome G52.7
Sicca syndrome M35.ØØ
  with
    keratoconjunctivitis M35.Ø1
    lung involvement M35.Ø2
    myopathy M35.Ø3
    renal tubulo-interstitial disorders M35.Ø4
  specified organ involvement NEC M35.Ø9
Sick R69
  or handicapped person in family Z63.79
    needing care at home Z63.6
  sinus (syndrome) I49.5
Sick-euthyroid syndrome EØ7.81
Sickle-cell
  anemia — *see* Disease, sickle-cell
  trait D57.3
Sicklemia (*see also* Disease, sickle-cell)
  trait D57.3
Sickness
  air (travel) T75.3 ☑
  airplane T75.3 ☑
  alpine T70.29 ☑
  altitude T70.2Ø ☑
  Andes T70.29 ☑
  aviator's T70.29 ☑
  balloon T70.29 ☑
  car T75.3 ☑
  compressed air T70.3 ☑
  decompression T70.3 ☑
  green D5Ø.8
  milk — *see* Poisoning, food, noxious
  motion T75.3 ☑
  mountain T70.29 ☑
    acute D75.1
  protein (*see also* Reaction, serum) T80.69 ☑
  radiation T66 ☑
  roundabout (motion) T75.3 ☑
  sea T75.3 ☑
  serum NEC (*see also* Reaction, serum) T80.69 ☑
  sleeping (African) B56.9
    by Trypanosoma B56.9
      brucei
        gambiense B56.Ø
        rhodesiense B56.1
    East African B56.1
    Gambian B56.Ø
    Rhodesian B56.1
    West African B56.Ø
  swing (motion) T75.3 ☑
  train (railway) (travel) T75.3 ☑
  travel (any vehicle) T75.3 ☑
Sideropenia — *see* Anemia, iron deficiency
Siderosilicosis J62.8
Siderosis (lung) J63.4
  eye (globe) — *see* Disorder, globe, degenerative,
        siderosis
Siemens' syndrome (ectodermal dysplasia) Q82.8
Sighing RØ6.89
  psychogenic F45.8
Sigmoid (*see also* condition)
  flexure — *see* condition
  kidney Q63.1
Sigmoiditis (*see also* Enteritis) K52.9
  infectious AØ9
  noninfectious K52.9
Silfversköld's syndrome Q78.9

Silicosiderosis J62.8
Silicosis, silicotic (simple) (complicated) J62.8
  with tuberculosis J65
Silicotuberculosis J65
Silo-fillers' disease J68.8
  bronchitis J68.Ø
  pneumonitis J68.Ø
  pulmonary edema J68.1
Silver's syndrome Q87.1
Simian malaria B53.1
Simmonds' cachexia or disease E23.Ø
Simons' disease or syndrome (progressive lipodystro-
        phy) E88.1
Simple, simplex — *see* condition
Simulation, conscious (of illness) Z76.5
Simultanagnosia (asimultagnosia) R48.3
Sin Nombre virus disease (Hantavirus) (cardio)-pul-
        monary syndrome) B33.4
Sinding-Larsen disease or osteochondrosis — *see*
        Osteochondrosis, juvenile, patella
Singapore hemorrhagic fever A91
Singer's node or nodule J38.2
Single
  atrium Q21.2
  coronary artery Q24.5
  umbilical artery Q27.Ø
  ventricle Q2Ø.4
Singultus RØ6.6
  epidemicus B33.Ø
Sinus (*see also* Fistula)
  abdominal K63.89
  arrest I45.5
  arrhythmia I49.8
  bradycardia RØØ.1
  branchial cleft (internal) (external) Q18.Ø
  coccygeal — *see* Sinus, pilonidal
  dental KØ4.6
  dermal (congenital) QØ6.8
    with abscess QØ6.8
    coccygeal, pilonidal — *see* Sinus, coccygeal
  infected, skin NEC LØ8.89
  marginal, ruptured or bleeding — *see* Hemorrhage,
        antepartum, specified cause NEC
  medial, face and neck Q18.8
  pause I45.5
  pericranii QØ1.9
  pilonidal (infected) (rectum) LØ5.92
    with abscess LØ5.Ø2
  preauricular Q18.1
  rectovaginal N82.3
  Rokitansky-Aschoff (gallbladder) K82.8
  sacrococcygeal (dermoid) (infected) — *see* Sinus, pi-
        lonidal
  tachycardia RØØ.Ø
    paroxysmal I47.1
  tarsi syndrome M25.57- ☑
  testis N5Ø.8
  tract (postinfective) — *see* Fistula
  urachus Q64.4
Sinusitis (accessory) (chronic) (hyperplastic) (nasal)
        (nonpurulent) (purulent) J32.9
  acute JØ1.9Ø
    ethmoidal JØ1.2Ø
      recurrent JØ1.21
    frontal JØ1.1Ø
      recurrent JØ1.11
    involving more than one sinus, other than pansi-
        nusitis JØ1.8Ø
      recurrent JØ1.81
    maxillary JØ1.ØØ
      recurrent JØ1.Ø1
    pansinusitis JØ1.4Ø
      recurrent JØ1.41
    recurrent JØ1.91
    specified NEC JØ1.8Ø
      recurrent JØ1.81
    sphenoidal JØ1.3Ø
      recurrent JØ1.31
  allergic — *see* Rhinitis, allergic
  due to high altitude T70.1 ☑
  ethmoidal J32.2
    acute JØ1.2Ø
      recurrent JØ1.21
  frontal J32.1
    acute JØ1.1Ø
      recurrent JØ1.11
  influenzal — *see* Influenza, with, respiratory manifes-
        tations NEC

☑ Additional Character Required — Refer to the Tabular List for Character Selection   ▽ Subterms under main terms may continue to next column or page

Sinusitis — *continued*
  involving more than one sinus but not pansinusitis J32.8
    acute J01.80
      recurrent J01.81
  maxillary J32.0
    acute J01.00
      recurrent J01.01
  sphenoidal J32.3
    acute J01.30
      recurrent J01.31
  tuberculous, any sinus A15.8
Sinusitis-bronchiectasis-situs inversus (syndrome) (triad) Q89.3
Sipple's syndrome E31.22
Sirenomelia (syndrome) Q87.2
Siriasis T67.0 ☑
Sirkari's disease B55.0
Siti A65
Situation, psychiatric F99
Situational
  disturbance (transient) — *see* Disorder, adjustment
    acute F43.0
  maladjustment — *see* Disorder, adjustment
  reaction — *see* Disorder, adjustment
    acute F43.0
Situs inversus or transversus (abdominalis) (thoracis) Q89.3
Sixth disease B08.20
  due to human herpesvirus 6 B08.21
  due to human herpesvirus 7 B08.22
Sjögren-Larsson syndrome Q87.1
Sjögren's syndrome or disease — *see* Sicca syndrome
Skeletal — *see* condition
Skene's gland — *see* condition
Skenitis — *see* Urethritis
Skerljevo A65
Skevas-Zerfus disease — *see* Toxicity, venom, marine animal, sea anemone
Skin (*see also* condition)
  clammy R23.1
  donor — *see* Donor, skin
  hidebound M35.9
Slate-dressers' or slate-miners' lung J62.8
Sleep
  apnea — *see* Apnea, sleep
  deprivation Z72.820
  disorder or disturbance G47.9
    child F51.9
    nonorganic origin F51.9
    specified NEC G47.8
  disturbance G47.9
    nonorganic origin F51.9
  drunkenness F51.9
  rhythm inversion G47.2- ☑
  terrors F51.4
  walking F51.3
    hysterical F44.89
Sleep hygiene
  abuse Z72.821
  inadequate Z72.821
  poor Z72.821
Sleeping sickness — *see* Sickness, sleeping
Sleeplessness — *see* Insomnia
  menopausal N95.1
Sleep-wake schedule disorder G47.20
Slim disease (in HIV infection) B20
Slipped, slipping
  epiphysis (traumatic) (*see also* Osteochondropathy, specified type NEC)
    capital femoral (traumatic)
      acute (on chronic) S79.01- ☑
    current traumatic — *code as* Fracture, by site
    upper femoral (nontraumatic) M93.00- ☑
      acute M93.01- ☑
        on chronic M93.03- ☑
      chronic M93.02- ☑
  intervertebral disc — *see* Displacement, intervertebral disc
  ligature, umbilical P51.8
  patella — *see* Disorder, patella, derangement NEC
  rib M89.8X8
  sacroiliac joint — *see* subcategory M53.2 ☑
  tendon — *see* Disorder, tendon
  ulnar nerve, nontraumatic — *see* Lesion, nerve, ulnar
  vertebra NEC — *see* Spondylolisthesis
Slocumb's syndrome E27.0

Sloughing (multiple) (phagedena) (skin) (*see also* Gangrene)
  abscess — *see* Abscess
  appendix K38.8
  fascia — *see* Disorder, soft tissue, specified type NEC
  scrotum N50.8
  tendon — *see* Disorder, tendon
  transplanted organ — *see* Rejection, transplant
  ulcer — *see* Ulcer, skin
Slow
  feeding, newborn P92.2
  flow syndrome, coronary I20.8
  heart (beat) R00.1
Slowing, urinary stream R39.19
Sluder's neuralgia (syndrome) G44.89
Slurred, slurring speech R47.81
Small (ness)
  for gestational age — *see* Small for dates
  introitus, vagina N89.6
  kidney (unknown cause) N27.9
    bilateral N27.1
    unilateral N27.0
  ovary (congenital) Q50.39
  pelvis
    with disproportion (fetopelvic) O33.1
      causing obstructed labor O65.1
  uterus N85.8
  white kidney N03.9
Small-and-light-for-dates — *see* Small for dates
Small-for-dates (infant) P05.10
  with weight of
    1000-1249 grams P05.14
    1250-1499 grams P05.15
    1500-1749 grams P05.16
    1750-1999 grams P05.17
    2000-2499 grams P05.18
    499 grams or less P05.11
    500-749 grams P05.12
    750-999 grams P05.13
Smallpox B03
Smearing, fecal R15.1
Smith-Lemli-Opitz syndrome E78.72
Smith's fracture S52.54- ☑
Smoker — *see* Dependence, drug, nicotine
Smoker's
  bronchitis J41.0
  cough J41.0
  palate K13.24
  throat J31.2
  tongue K13.24
Smoking
  passive Z77.22
Smothering spells R06.81
Snaggle teeth, tooth M26.39
Snapping
  finger — *see* Trigger finger
  hip — *see* Derangement, joint, specified type NEC, hip
    involving the iliotiblial band M76.3- ☑
  knee — *see* Derangement, knee
    involving the iliotiblial band M76.3- ☑
Sneddon-Wilkinson disease or syndrome (sub-corneal pustular dermatosis) L13.1
Sneezing (intractable) R06.7
Sniffing
  cocaine
    abuse — *see* Abuse, drug, cocaine
    dependence — *see* Dependence, drug, cocaine
  gasoline
    abuse — *see* Abuse, drug, inhalant
    dependence — *see* Dependence, drug, inhalant
  glue (airplane)
    abuse — *see* Abuse, drug, inhalant
    drug dependence — *see* Dependence, drug, inhalant
Sniffles
  newborn P28.89
Snoring R06.83
Snow blindness — *see* Photokeratitis
Snuffles (non-syphilitic) R06.5
  newborn P28.89
  syphilitic (infant) A50.05 [J99]
Social
  exclusion Z60.4
    due to discrimination or persecution (perceived) Z60.5
  migrant Z59.0
    acculturation difficulty Z60.3

Social — *continued*
  rejection Z60.4
    due to discrimination or persecution Z60.5
  role conflict NEC Z73.5
  skills inadequacy NEC Z73.4
  transplantation Z60.3
Sodoku A25.0
Soemmerring's ring — *see* Cataract, secondary
Soft (*see also* condition)
  nails L60.3
Softening
  bone — *see* Osteomalacia
  brain (necrotic) (progressive) G93.89
    congenital Q04.8
    embolic I63.4 ☑
    hemorrhagic — *see* Hemorrhage, intracranial, intracerebral
    occlusive I63.5 ☑
    thrombotic I63.3 ☑
  cartilage M94.2- ☑
    patella M22.4- ☑
  cerebellar — *see* Softening, brain
  cerebral — *see* Softening, brain
  cerebrospinal — *see* Softening, brain
  myocardial, heart — *see* Degeneration, myocardial
  spinal cord G95.89
  stomach K31.89
Soldier's
  heart F45.8
  patches I31.0
Solitary
  cyst, kidney N28.1
  kidney, congenital Q60.0
Solvent abuse — *see* Abuse, drug, inhalant
  dependence — *see* Dependence, drug, inhalant
Somatization reaction, somatic reaction — *see* Disorder, somatoform
Somnambulism F51.3
  hysterical F44.89
Somnolence R40.0
  nonorganic origin F51.11
Sonne dysentery A03.3
Soor B37.0
Sore
  bed — *see* Ulcer, pressure, by site
  chiclero B55.1
  Delhi B55.1
  desert — *see* Ulcer, skin
  eye H57.1- ☑
  Lahore B55.1
  mouth K13.79
    canker K12.0
  muscle M79.1
  Naga — *see* Ulcer, skin
  of skin — *see* Ulcer, skin
  oriental B55.1
  pressure — *see* Ulcer, pressure, by site
  skin L98.9
  soft A57
  throat (acute) (*see also* Pharyngitis)
    with influenza, flu, or grippe — *see* Influenza, with, respiratory manifestations NEC
    chronic J31.2
    coxsackie (virus) B08.5
    diphtheritic A36.0
    herpesviral B00.2
    influenzal — *see* Influenza, with, respiratory manifestations NEC
    septic J02.0
    streptococcal (ulcerative) J02.0
    viral NEC J02.8
      coxsackie B08.5
  tropical — *see* Ulcer, skin
  veldt — *see* Ulcer, skin
Soto's syndrome (cerebral gigantism) Q87.3
South African cardiomyopathy syndrome I42.8
Southeast Asian hemorrhagic fever A91
Spacing
  abnormal, tooth, teeth, fully erupted M26.30
  excessive, tooth, fully erupted M26.32
Spade-like hand (congenital) Q68.1
Spading nail L60.8
  congenital Q84.6
Spanish collar N47.1
Sparganosis B70.1
Spasm(s), spastic, spasticity (*see also* condition) R25.2
  accommodation — *see* Spasm, of accommodation

Spasm(s), spastic, spasticity — *continued*
ampulla of Vater K83.4
anus, ani (sphincter) (reflex) K59.4
   psychogenic F45.8
artery I73.9
   cerebral G45.9
Bell's G51.3
bladder (sphincter, external or internal) N32.89
   psychogenic F45.8
bronchus, bronchiole J98.01
cardia K22.0
cardiac I20.1
carpopedal — *see* Tetany
cerebral (arteries) (vascular) G45.9
cervix, complicating delivery O62.4
ciliary body (of accommodation) — *see* Spasm, of accommodation
colon K58.9
   with diarrhea K58.0
   psychogenic F45.8
common duct K83.8
compulsive — *see* Tic
conjugate H51.8
coronary (artery) I20.1
diaphragm (reflex) R06.6
   epidemic B33.0
   psychogenic F45.8
duodenum K59.8
epidemic diaphragmatic (transient) B33.0
esophagus (diffuse) K22.4
   psychogenic F45.8
facial G51.3
fallopian tube N83.8
gastrointestinal (tract) K31.89
   psychogenic F45.8
glottis J38.5
   hysterical F44.4
   psychogenic F45.8
      conversion reaction F44.4
   reflex through recurrent laryngeal nerve J38.5
habit — *see* Tic
heart I20.1
hemifacial (clonic) G51.3
hourglass — *see* Contraction, hourglass
hysterical F44.4
infantile — *see* Epilepsy, spasms
inferior oblique, eye H51.8
intestinal (*see also* Syndrome, irritable bowel) K58.9
   psychogenic F45.8
larynx, laryngeal J38.5
   hysterical F44.4
   psychogenic F45.8
      conversion reaction F44.4
levator palpebrae superioris — *see* Disorder, eyelid function
muscle NEC M62.838
   back M62.830
nerve, trigeminal G51.0
nervous F45.8
nodding F98.4
occupational F48.8
oculogyric H51.8
   psychogenic F45.8
of accommodation H52.53- ☑
ophthalmic artery — *see* Occlusion, artery, retina
perineal, female N94.89
peroneo-extensor (*see also* Deformity, limb, flat foot)
pharynx (reflex) J39.2
   hysterical F45.8
   psychogenic F45.8
psychogenic F45.8
pylorus NEC K31.3
   adult hypertrophic K31.89
   congenital or infantile Q40.0
   psychogenic F45.8
rectum (sphincter) K59.4
   psychogenic F45.8
retinal (artery) — *see* Occlusion, artery, retina
sigmoid (*see also* Syndrome, irritable bowel) K58.9
   psychogenic F45.8
sphincter of Oddi K83.4
stomach K31.89
   neurotic F45.8
throat J39.2
   hysterical F45.8
   psychogenic F45.8
tic F95.9
   chronic F95.1

Spasm(s), spastic, spasticity — *continued*
tic — *continued*
   transient of childhood F95.0
tongue K14.8
torsion (progressive) G24.1
trigeminal nerve — *see* Neuralgia, trigeminal
ureter N13.5
urethra (sphincter) N35.9
uterus N85.8
   complicating labor O62.4
vagina N94.2
   psychogenic F52.5
vascular I73.9
vasomotor I73.9
vein NEC I87.8
viscera — *see* Pain, abdominal
Spasmodic — *see* condition
Spasmophilia — *see* Tetany
Spasmus nutans F98.4
Spastic, spasticity (*see also* Spasm)
   child (cerebral) (congenital) (paralysis) G80.1
Speaker's throat R49.8
Specific, specified — *see* condition
Speech
   defect, disorder, disturbance, impediment R47.9
      psychogenic, in childhood and adolescence F98.8
      slurring R47.81
      specified NEC R47.89
Spencer's disease A08.19
Spens' syndrome (syncope with heart block) I45.9
Sperm counts (fertility testing) Z31.41
   postvasectomy Z30.8
   reversal Z31.42
Spermatic cord — *see* condition
Spermatocele N43.40
   congenital Q55.4
   multiple N43.42
   single N43.41
Spermatocystitis N49.0
Spermatocytoma C62.9- ☑
   specified site — *see* Neoplasm, malignant, by site
Spermatorrhea N50.8
Sphacelus — *see* Gangrene
Sphenoidal — *see* condition
Sphenoiditis (chronic) — *see* Sinusitis, sphenoidal
Sphenopalatine ganglion neuralgia G90.09
Sphericity, increased, lens (congenital) Q12.4
Spherocytosis (congenital) (familial) (hereditary) D58.0
   hemoglobin disease D58.0
   sickle-cell (disease) D57.8- ☑
Spherophakia Q12.4
Sphincter — *see* condition
Sphincteritis, sphincter of Oddi — *see* Cholangitis
Sphingolipidosis E75.3
   specified NEC E75.29
Sphingomyelinosis E75.3
Spicule tooth K00.2
Spider
   bite — *see* Toxicity, venom, spider
   fingers — *see* Syndrome, Marfan's
   nevus I78.1
   toes — *see* Syndrome, Marfan's
   vascular I78.1
Spiegler-Fendt
   benign lymphocytoma L98.8
   sarcoid L08.89
Spielmeyer-Vogt disease E75.4
Spina bifida (aperta) Q05.9
   with hydrocephalus NEC Q05.4
   cervical Q05.5
      with hydrocephalus Q05.0
   dorsal Q05.6
      with hydrocephalus Q05.1
   lumbar Q05.7
      with hydrocephalus Q05.2
   lumbosacral Q05.7
      with hydrocephalus Q05.2
   occulta Q76.0
   sacral Q05.8
      with hydrocephalus Q05.3
   thoracic Q05.6
      with hydrocephalus Q05.1
   thoracolumbar Q05.6
      with hydrocephalus Q05.1
Spindle, Krukenberg's — *see* Pigmentation, cornea, posterior
Spine, spinal — *see* condition

Spiradenoma (eccrine) — *see* Neoplasm, skin, benign
Spirillosis A25.0
Spirillum
   minus A25.0
   obermeieri infection A68.0
Spirochetal — *see* condition
Spirochetosis A69.9
   arthritic, arthritica A69.9
   bronchopulmonary A69.8
   icterohemorrhagic A27.0
   lung A69.8
Spirometrosis B70.1
Spitting blood — *see* Hemoptysis
Splanchnoptosis K63.4
Spleen, splenic — *see* condition
Splenectasis — *see* Splenomegaly
Splenitis (interstitial) (malignant) (nonspecific) D73.89
   malarial (*see also* Malaria) B54 [D77]
   tuberculous A18.85
Splenocele D73.89
Splenomegaly, splenomegalia (Bengal) (cryptogenic) (idiopathic) (tropical) R16.1
   with hepatomegaly R16.2
   cirrhotic D73.2
   congenital Q89.09
   congestive, chronic D73.2
   Egyptian B65.1
   Gaucher's E75.22
   malarial (*see also* Malaria) B54 [D77]
   neutropenic D73.81
   Niemann-Pick — *see* Niemann-Pick disease or syndrome
   sideritic D73.2
   syphilitic A52.79
      congenital (early) A50.08 [D77]
Splenopathy D73.9
Splenoptosis D73.89
Splenosis D73.89
Splinter — *see* Foreign body, superficial, by site
Split, splitting
   foot Q72.7- ☑
   heart sounds R01.2
   lip, congenital — *see* Cleft, lip
   nails L60.3
   urinary stream R39.13
Spondylarthrosis — *see* Spondylosis
Spondylitis (chronic) (*see also* Spondylopathy, inflammatory)
   ankylopoietica — *see* Spondylitis, ankylosing
   ankylosing (chronic) M45.9
      with lung involvement M45.9 [J99]
      cervical region M45.2
      cervicothoracic region M45.3
      juvenile M08.1
      lumbar region M45.6
      lumbosacral region M45.7
      multiple sites M45.0
      occipito-atlanto-axial region M45.1
      sacrococcygeal region M45.8
      thoracic region M45.4
      thoracolumbar region M45.5
   atrophic (ligamentous) — *see* Spondylitis, ankylosing
   deformans (chronic) — *see* Spondylosis
   gonococcal A54.41
   gouty M10.08
   in (due to)
      brucellosis A23.9 [M49.80]
         cervical region A23.9 [M49.82]
         cervicothoracic region A23.9 [M49.83]
         lumbar region A23.9 [M49.86]
         lumbosacral region A23.9 [M49.87]
         multiple sites A23.9 [M49.89]
         occipito-atlanto-axial region A23.9 [M49.81]
         sacrococcygeal region A23.9 [M49.88]
         thoracic region A23.9 [M49.84]
         thoracolumbar region A23.9 [M49.85]
      enterobacteria (*see also* subcategory M49.8) A04.9
      tuberculosis A18.01
   infectious NEC — *see* Spondylopathy, infective
   juvenile ankylosing (chronic) M08.1
   Kümmell's — *see* Spondylopathy, traumatic
   Marie-Strümpell — *see* Spondylitis, ankylosing
   muscularis — *see* Spondylopathy, specified NEC
   psoriatic L40.53
   rheumatoid — *see* Spondylitis, ankylosing
   rhizomelica — *see* Spondylitis, ankylosing
   sacroiliac NEC M46.1

☑ **Additional Character Required** — Refer to the Tabular List for Character Selection   ⩗ Subterms under main terms may continue to next column or page

Spondylitis — *continued*
  senescent, senile — *see* Spondylosis
  traumatic (chronic) or post-traumatic — *see* Spondylopathy, traumatic
  tuberculous A18.01
  typhosa A01.05
Spondylolisthesis (acquired) (degenerative) M43.10
  with disproportion (fetopelvic) O33.0
    causing obstructed labor O65.0
  cervical region M43.12
  cervicothoracic region M43.13
  congenital Q76.2
  lumbar region M43.16
  lumbosacral region M43.17
  multiple sites M43.19
  occipito-atlanto-axial region M43.11
  sacrococcygeal region M43.18
  thoracic region M43.14
  thoracolumbar region M43.15
  traumatic (old) M43.10
    acute
      fifth cervical (displaced) S12.430 ☑
        nondisplaced S12.431 ☑
        specified type NEC (displaced) S12.450 ☑
          nondisplaced S12.451 ☑
          type III S12.44 ☑
      fourth cervical (displaced) S12.330 ☑
        nondisplaced S12.331 ☑
        specified type NEC (displaced) S12.350 ☑
          nondisplaced S12.351 ☑
          type III S12.34 ☑
      second cervical (displaced) S12.130 ☑
        nondisplaced S12.131 ☑
        specified type NEC (displaced) S12.150 ☑
          nondisplaced S12.151 ☑
          type III S12.14 ☑
      seventh cervical (displaced) S12.630 ☑
        nondisplaced S12.631 ☑
        specified type NEC (displaced) S12.650 ☑
          nondisplaced S12.651 ☑
          type III S12.64 ☑
      sixth cervical (displaced) S12.530 ☑
        nondisplaced S12.531 ☑
        specified type NEC (displaced) S12.550 ☑
          nondisplaced S12.551 ☑
          type III S12.54 ☑
      third cervical (displaced) S12.230 ☑
        nondisplaced S12.231 ☑
        specified type NEC (displaced) S12.250 ☑
          nondisplaced S12.251 ☑
          type III S12.24 ☑
Spondylolysis (acquired) M43.00
  cervical region M43.02
  cervicothoracic region M43.03
  congenital Q76.2
  lumbar region M43.06
  lumbosacral region M43.07
    with disproportion (fetopelvic) O33.0
      causing obstructed labor O65.8
  multiple sites M43.09
  occipito-atlanto-axial region M43.01
  sacrococcygeal region M43.08
  thoracic region M43.04
  thoracolumbar region M43.05
Spondylopathy M48.9
  infective NEC M46.50
    cervical region M46.52
    cervicothoracic region M46.53
    lumbar region M46.56
    lumbosacral region M46.57
    multiple sites M46.59
    occipito-atlanto-axial region M46.51
    sacrococcygeal region M46.58
    thoracic region M46.54
    thoracolumbar region M46.55
  inflammatory M46.90
    cervical region M46.92
    cervicothoracic region M46.93
    lumbar region M46.96
    lumbosacral region M46.97
    multiple sites M46.99
    occipito-atlanto-axial region M46.91
    sacrococcygeal region M46.98
    specified type NEC M46.80
      cervical region M46.82
      cervicothoracic region M46.83
      lumbar region M46.86

Spondylopathy — *continued*
  inflammatory — *continued*
    specified type — *continued*
      lumbosacral region M46.87
      multiple sites M46.89
      occipito-atlanto-axial region M46.81
      sacrococcygeal region M46.88
      thoracic region M46.84
      thoracolumbar region M46.85
    thoracic region M46.94
    thoracolumbar region M46.95
  neuropathic, in
    syringomyelia and syringobulbia G95.0
    tabes dorsalis A52.11
  specified NEC — *see* subcategory M48.8 ☑
  traumatic M48.30
    cervical region M48.32
    cervicothoracic region M48.33
    lumbar region M48.36
    lumbosacral region M48.37
    occipito-atlanto-axial region M48.31
    sacrococcygeal region M48.38
    thoracic region M48.34
    thoracolumbar region M48.35
Spondylosis M47.9
  with
    disproportion (fetopelvic) O33.0
      causing obstructed labor O65.0
    myelopathy NEC M47.10
      cervical region M47.12
      cervicothoracic region M47.13
      lumbar region M47.16
      occipito-atlanto-axial region M47.11
      thoracic region M47.14
      thoracolumbar region M47.15
    radiculopathy M47.20
      cervical region M47.22
      cervicothoracic region M47.23
      lumbar region M47.26
      lumbosacral region M47.27
      occipito-atlanto-axial region M47.21
      sacrococcygeal region M47.28
      thoracic region M47.24
      thoracolumbar region M47.25
  without myelopathy or radiculopathy M47.819
    cervical region M47.812
    cervicothoracic region M47.813
    lumbar region M47.816
    lumbosacral region M47.817
    occipito-atlanto-axial region M47.811
    sacrococcygeal region M47.818
    thoracic region M47.814
    thoracolumbar region M47.815
  specified NEC M47.899
    cervical region M47.892
    cervicothoracic region M47.893
    lumbar region M47.896
    lumbosacral region M47.897
    occipito-atlanto-axial region M47.891
    sacrococcygeal region M47.898
    thoracic region M47.894
    thoracolumbar region M47.895
  traumatic — *see* Spondylopathy, traumatic
Sponge
  inadvertently left in operation wound — *see* Foreign body, accidentally left during a procedure
  kidney (medullary) Q61.5
Sponge-diver's disease — *see* Toxicity, venom, marine animal, sea anemone
Spongioblastoma (any type) — *see* Neoplasm, malignant, by site
  specified site — *see* Neoplasm, malignant, by site
  unspecified site C71.9
Spongioneuroblastoma — *see* Neoplasm, malignant, by site
Spontaneous (*see also* condition)
  fracture (cause unknown) — *see* Fracture, pathological
Spoon nail L60.3
  congenital Q84.6
Sporadic — *see* condition
Sporothrix schenckii infection — *see* Sporotrichosis
Sporotrichosis B42.9
  arthritis B42.82
  disseminated B42.7
  generalized B42.7
  lymphocutaneous (fixed) (progressive) B42.1
  pulmonary B42.0
  specified NEC B42.89

Spots, spotting (in) (of)
  Bitot's (*see also* Pigmentation, conjunctiva)
    in the young child E50.1
    vitamin A deficiency E50.1
  café, au lait L81.3
  Cayenne pepper I78.1
  cotton wool, retina — *see* Occlusion, artery, retina
  de Morgan's (senile angiomas) I78.1
  Fuchs' black (myopic) H44.2- ☑
  intermenstrual (regular) N92.0
    irregular N92.1
  Koplik's B05.9
  liver L81.4
  pregnancy O26.85- ☑
  purpuric R23.3
  ruby I78.1
Spotted fever — *see* Fever, spotted N92.3
Sprain (joint) (ligament)
  acromioclavicular joint or ligament S43.5- ☑
  ankle S93.40- ☑
    calcaneofibular ligament S93.41- ☑
    deltoid ligament S93.42- ☑
    internal collateral ligament — *see* Sprain, ankle, specified ligament NEC
    specified ligament NEC S93.49- ☑
    talofibular ligament — *see* Sprain, ankle, specified ligament NEC
    tibiofibular ligament S93.43- ☑
  anterior longitudinal, cervical S13.4 ☑
  atlas, atlanto-axial, atlanto-occipital S13.4 ☑
  breast bone — *see* Sprain, sternum
  calcaneofibular — *see* Sprain, ankle
  carpal — *see* Sprain, wrist
  carpometacarpal — *see* Sprain, hand, specified site NEC
  cartilage
    costal S23.41 ☑
    semilunar (knee) — *see* Sprain, knee, specified site NEC
      with current tear — *see* Tear, meniscus
    thyroid region S13.5 ☑
    xiphoid — *see* Sprain, sternum
  cervical, cervicodorsal, cervicothoracic S13.4 ☑
  chondrosternal S23.421 ☑
  coracoclavicular S43.8- ☑
  coracohumeral S43.41- ☑
  coronary, knee — *see* Sprain, knee, specified site NEC
  costal cartilage S23.41 ☑
  cricoarytenoid articulation or ligament S13.5 ☑
  cricothyroid articulation S13.5 ☑
  cruciate, knee — *see* Sprain, knee, cruciate
  deltoid, ankle — *see* Sprain, ankle
  dorsal (spine) S23.3 ☑
  elbow S53.40- ☑
    radial collateral ligament S53.43- ☑
    radiohumeral S53.41- ☑
    rupture
      radial collateral ligament — *see* Rupture, traumatic, ligament, radial collateral
      ulnar collateral ligament — *see* Rupture, traumatic, ligament, ulnar collateral
    specified type NEC S53.49- ☑
    ulnar collateral ligament S53.44- ☑
    ulnohumeral S53.42- ☑
  femur, head — *see* Sprain, hip
  fibular collateral, knee — *see* Sprain, knee, collateral
  fibulocalcaneal — *see* Sprain, ankle
  finger(s) S63.61- ☑
    index S63.61- ☑
    interphalangeal (joint) S63.63- ☑
      index S63.63- ☑
      little S63.63- ☑
      middle S63.63- ☑
      ring S63.63- ☑
    little S63.61- ☑
    metacarpophalangeal (joint) S63.65- ☑
    middle S63.61- ☑
    ring S63.61- ☑
    specified site NEC S63.69- ☑
      index S63.69- ☑
      little S63.69- ☑
      middle S63.69- ☑
      ring S63.69- ☑
  foot S93.60- ☑
    specified ligament NEC S93.69- ☑
    tarsal ligament S93.61- ☑

Sprain — continued
  foot — continued
    tarsometatarsal ligament S93.62- ☑
    toe — see Sprain, toe
  hand S63.9- ☑
    finger — see Sprain, finger
    specified site NEC — see subcategory S63.8 ☑
    thumb — see Sprain, thumb
  head S03.9 ☑
  hip S73.10- ☑
    iliofemoral ligament S73.11- ☑
    ischiocapsular (ligament) S73.12- ☑
    specified NEC S73.19- ☑
  iliofemoral — see Sprain, hip
  innominate
    acetabulum — see Sprain, hip
    sacral junction S33.6 ☑
  internal
    collateral, ankle — see Sprain, ankle
    semilunar cartilage — see Sprain, knee, specified site NEC
  interphalangeal
    finger — see Sprain, finger, interphalangeal (joint)
    toe — see Sprain, toe, interphalangeal joint
  ischiocapsular — see Sprain, hip
  ischiofemoral — see Sprain, hip
  jaw (articular disc) (cartilage) (meniscus) S03.4 ☑
    old M26.69
  knee S83.9- ☑
    collateral ligament S83.40- ☑
      lateral (fibular) S83.42- ☑
      medial (tibial) S83.41- ☑
    cruciate ligament S83.50- ☑
      anterior S83.51- ☑
      posterior S83.52- ☑
    lateral (fibular) collateral ligament S83.42- ☑
    medial (tibial) collateral ligament S83.41- ☑
    patellar ligament S76.11- ☑
    specified site NEC S83.8X- ☑
    superior tibiofibular joint (ligament) S83.6- ☑
  lateral collateral, knee — see Sprain, knee, collateral
  lumbar (spine) S33.5 ☑
  lumbosacral S33.9 ☑
  mandible (articular disc) S03.4 ☑
    old M26.69
  medial collateral, knee — see Sprain, knee, collateral
  meniscus
    jaw S03.4 ☑
      old M26.69
    knee — see Sprain, knee, specified site NEC
      with current tear — see Tear, meniscus
        old — see Derangement, knee, meniscus, due to old tear
    mandible S03.4 ☑
      old M26.69
  metacarpal (distal) (proximal) — see Sprain, hand, specified site NEC
  metacarpophalangeal — see Sprain, finger, metacarpophalangeal (joint)
  metatarsophalangeal — see Sprain, toe, metatarsophalangeal joint
  midcarpal — see Sprain, hand, specified site NEC
  midtarsal — see Sprain, foot, specified site NEC
  neck S13.9 ☑
    anterior longitudinal cervical ligament S13.4 ☑
    atlanto-axial joint S13.4 ☑
    atlanto-occipital joint S13.4 ☑
    cervical spine S13.4 ☑
    cricoarytenoid ligament S13.5 ☑
    cricothyroid ligament S13.5 ☑
    specified site NEC S13.8 ☑
    thyroid region (cartilage) S13.5 ☑
  nose S03.8 ☑
  orbicular, hip — see Sprain, hip
  patella — see Sprain, knee, specified site NEC
  patellar ligament S76.11- ☑
  pelvis NEC S33.8 ☑
  phalanx
    finger — see Sprain, finger
    toe — see Sprain, toe
  pubofemoral — see Sprain, hip
  radiocarpal — see Sprain, wrist
  radiohumeral — see Sprain, elbow
  radius, collateral — see Rupture, traumatic, ligament, radial collateral
  rib (cage) S23.41 ☑

Sprain — continued
  rotator cuff (capsule) S43.42- ☑
  sacroiliac (region)
    chronic or old — see subcategory M53.2
    joint S33.6 ☑
  scaphoid (hand) — see Sprain, hand, specified site NEC
  scapula (r) — see Sprain, shoulder girdle, specified site NEC
  semilunar cartilage (knee) — see Sprain, knee, specified site NEC
    with current tear — see Tear, meniscus
      old — see Derangement, knee, meniscus, due to old tear
  shoulder joint S43.40- ☑
    acromioclavicular joint (ligament) — see Sprain, acromioclavicular joint
    blade — see Sprain, shoulder, girdle, specified site NEC
    coracoclavicular joint (ligament) — see Sprain, coracoclavicular joint
    coracohumeral ligament — see Sprain, coracohumeral joint
    girdle S43.9- ☑
      specified site NEC S43.8- ☑
    rotator cuff — see Sprain, rotator cuff
    specified site NEC S43.49- ☑
    sternoclavicular joint (ligament) — see Sprain, sternoclavicular joint
  spine
    cervical S13.4 ☑
    lumbar S33.5 ☑
    thoracic S23.3 ☑
  sternoclavicular joint S43.6- ☑
  sternum S23.429 ☑
    chondrosternal joint S23.421 ☑
    specified site NEC S23.428 ☑
    sternoclavicular (joint) (ligament) S23.420 ☑
  symphysis
    jaw S03.4 ☑
      old M26.69
    mandibular S03.4 ☑
      old M26.69
  talofibular — see Sprain, ankle
  tarsal — see Sprain, foot, specified site NEC
  tarsometatarsal — see Sprain, foot, specified site NEC
  temporomandibular S03.4 ☑
    old M26.69
  thorax S23.9 ☑
    ribs S23.41 ☑
    specified site NEC S23.8 ☑
    spine S23.3 ☑
    sternum — see Sprain, sternum
  thumb S63.60- ☑
    interphalangeal (joint) S63.62- ☑
    metacarpophalangeal (joint) S63.64- ☑
    specified site NEC S63.68- ☑
  thyroid cartilage or region S13.5 ☑
  tibia (proximal end) — see Sprain, knee, specified site NEC
  tibial collateral, knee — see Sprain, knee, collateral
  tibiofibular
    distal — see Sprain, ankle
    superior — see Sprain, knee, specified site NEC
  toe(s) S93.50- ☑
    great S93.50- ☑
    interphalangeal joint S93.51- ☑
      great S93.51- ☑
      lesser S93.51- ☑
    lesser S93.50- ☑
    metatarsophalangeal joint S93.52- ☑
      great S93.52- ☑
      lesser S93.52- ☑
  ulna, collateral — see Rupture, traumatic, ligament, ulnar collateral
  ulnohumeral — see Sprain, elbow
  wrist S63.50- ☑
    carpal S63.51- ☑
    radiocarpal S63.52- ☑
    specified site NEC S63.59- ☑
  xiphoid cartilage — see Sprain, sternum
Sprengel's deformity (congenital) Q74.0
Sprue (tropical) K90.1
  celiac K90.0
  idiopathic K90.0
  meaning thrush B37.0

Sprue — continued
  nontropical K90.0
Spur, bone (see also Enthesopathy)
  calcaneal M77.3- ☑
  iliac crest M76.2- ☑
  nose (septum) J34.89
Spurway's syndrome Q78.0
Sputum
  abnormal (amount) (color) (odor) (purulent) R09.3
  blood-stained R04.2
  excessive (cause unknown) R09.3
Squamous (see also condition)
  epithelium in
    cervical canal (congenital) Q51.828
    uterine mucosa (congenital) Q51.818
Squashed nose M95.0
  congenital Q67.4
Squeeze, diver's T70.3 ☑
Squint (see also Strabismus)
  accommodative — see Strabismus, convergent concomitant
St. Hubert's disease A82.9
Stab (see also Laceration)
  internal organs — see Injury, by site
Stafne's cyst or cavity M27.0
Staggering gait R26.0
  hysterical F44.4
Staghorn calculus — see Calculus, kidney
Stähli's line (cornea) (pigment) — see Pigmentation, cornea, anterior
Stain, staining
  meconium (newborn) P96.83
  port wine Q82.5
  tooth, teeth (hard tissues) (extrinsic) K03.6
    due to
      accretions K03.6
      deposits (betel) (black) (green) (materia alba) (orange) (soft) (tobacco) K03.6
      metals (copper) (silver) K03.7
      nicotine K03.6
      pulpal bleeding K03.7
      tobacco K03.6
    intrinsic K00.8
Stammering (see also Disorder, fluency) F80.81
Standstill
  auricular I45.5
  cardiac — see Arrest, cardiac
  sinoatrial I45.5
  ventricular — see Arrest, cardiac
Stannosis J63.5
Stanton's disease — see Melioidosis
Staphylitis (acute) (catarrhal) (chronic) (gangrenous) (membranous) (suppurative) (ulcerative) K12.2
Staphylococcal scalded skin syndrome L00
Staphylococcemia A41.2
Staphylococcus, staphylococcal (see also condition)
  as cause of disease classified elsewhere B95.8
    aureus (methicillin susceptible) (MSSA) B95.61
      methicillin resistant (MRSA) B95.62
    specified NEC, as cause of disease classified elsewhere B95.7
Staphyloma (sclera)
  cornea H18.72- ☑
  equatorial H15.81- ☑
  localized (anterior) H15.82- ☑
  posticum H15.83- ☑
  ring H15.85- ☑
Stargardt's disease — see Dystrophy, retina
Starvation (inanition) (due to lack of food) T73.0 ☑
  edema — see Malnutrition, severe
Stasis
  bile (noncalculous) K83.1
  bronchus J98.09
    with infection — see Bronchitis
  cardiac — see Failure, heart, congestive
  cecum K59.8
  colon K59.8
  dermatitis — see Varix, leg, with, inflammation
  duodenal K31.5
  eczema — see Varix, leg, with, inflammation
  edema — see Hypertension, venous (chronic), idiopathic
  foot T69.0- ☑
  ileocecal coil K59.8
  ileum K59.8
  intestinal K59.8
  jejunum K59.8

☑ Additional Character Required — Refer to the Tabular List for Character Selection   Subterms under main terms may continue to next column or page

Stasis — *continued*
  kidney N19
  liver (cirrhotic) K76.1
  lymphatic I89.8
  pneumonia J18.2
  pulmonary — *see* Edema, lung
  rectal K59.8
  renal N19
    tubular N17.0
  ulcer — *see* Varix, leg, with, ulcer
    without varicose veins I87.2
  urine — *see* Retention, urine
  venous I87.8
State (of)
  affective and paranoid, mixed, organic psychotic F06.8
  agitated R45.1
    acute reaction to stress F43.0
  anxiety (neurotic) F41.1
  apprehension F41.1
  burn-out Z73.0
  climacteric, female Z78.0
    symptomatic N95.1
  compulsive F42
    mixed with obsessional thoughts F42
  confusional (psychogenic) F44.89
    acute (*see also* Delirium)
      with
        arteriosclerotic dementia F01.50
          with behavioral disturbance F01.51
        senility or dementia F05
      alcoholic F10.231
    epileptic F05
    reactive (from emotional stress, psychological trauma) F44.89
    subacute — *see* Delirium
  convulsive — *see* Convulsions
  crisis F43.0
  depressive F32.9
    neurotic F34.1
  dissociative F44.9
  emotional shock (stress) R45.7
  hypercoagulation — *see* Hypercoagulable
  locked-in G83.5
  menopausal Z78.0
    symptomatic N95.1
  neurotic F48.9
    with depersonalization F48.1
  obsessional F42
  oneiroid (schizophrenia-like) F23
  organic
    hallucinatory (nonalcoholic) F06.0
    paranoid (-hallucinatory) F06.2
  panic F41.0
  paranoid F22
    climacteric F22
    involutional F22
    menopausal F22
    organic F06.2
    senile F03 ☑
    simple F22
  persistent vegetative R40.3
  phobic F40.9
  postleukotomy F07.0
  pregnant, incidental Z33.1
  psychogenic, twilight F44.89
  psychopathic (constitutional) F60.2
  psychotic, organic (*see also* Psychosis, organic)
    mixed paranoid and affective F06.8
    senile or presenile F03 ☑
    transient NEC F06.8
      with
        depression F06.31
        hallucinations F06.0
  residual schizophrenic F20.5
  restlessness R45.1
  stress (emotional) R45.7
  tension (mental) F48.9
    specified NEC F48.8
  transient organic psychotic NEC F06.8
    depressive type F06.31
    hallucinatory type F06.30
  twilight
    epileptic F05
    psychogenic F44.89
  vegetative, persistent R40.3
  vital exhaustion Z73.0
  withdrawal, — *see* Withdrawal, state

Status (post) (*see also* Presence (of))
  absence, epileptic — *see* Epilepsy, by type, with status epilepticus
  administration of tPA (rtPA) in a different facility within the last 24 hours prior to admission to current facility Z92.82
  adrenalectomy (unilateral) (bilateral) E89.6
  anastomosis Z98.0
  anginosus I20.9
  angioplasty (peripheral) Z98.62
    with implant Z95.820
    coronary artery Z98.61
      with implant Z95.5
  aortocoronary bypass Z95.1
  arthrodesis Z98.1
  artificial opening (of) Z93.9
    gastrointestinal tract Z93.4
    specified NEC Z93.8
    urinary tract Z93.6
    vagina Z93.8
  asthmaticus — *see* Asthma, by type, with status asthmaticus
  awaiting organ transplant Z76.82
  bariatric surgery Z98.84
  bed confinement Z74.01
  bleb, filtering (vitreous), after glaucoma surgery Z98.83
  breast implant Z98.82
    removal Z98.86
  cataract extraction Z98.4- ☑
  cholecystectomy Z90.49
  clitorectomy N90.811
    with excision of labia minora N90.812
  colectomy (complete) (partial) Z90.49
  colonization — *see* Carrier (suspected) of
  colostomy Z93.3
  convulsivus idiopathicus — *see* Epilepsy, by type, with status epilepticus
  coronary artery angioplasty — *see* Status, angioplasty, coronary artery
  cystectomy (urinary bladder) Z90.6
  cystostomy Z93.50
    appendico-vesicostomy Z93.52
    cutaneous Z93.51
    specified NEC Z93.59
  delinquent immunization Z28.3
  dental Z98.818
    crown Z98.811
    fillings Z98.811
    restoration Z98.811
    sealant Z98.810
    specified NEC Z98.818
  deployment (current) (military) Z56.82
  dialysis (hemodialysis) (peritoneal) Z99.2
  do not resuscitate (DNR) Z66
  donor — *see* Donor
  embedded fragments — *see* Retained, foreign body fragments (type of)
  embedded splinter — *see* Retained, foreign body fragments (type of)
  enterostomy Z93.4
  epileptic, epilepticus (*see also* Epilepsy, by type, with status epilepticus) G40.901
  estrogen receptor
    negative Z17.1
    positive Z17.0
  female genital cutting — *see* Female genital mutilation status
  female genital mutilation — *see* Female genital mutilation status
  filtering (vitreous) bleb after glaucoma surgery Z98.83
  gastrectomy (complete) (partial) Z90.3
  gastric banding Z98.84
  gastric bypass for obesity Z98.84
  gastrostomy Z93.1
  human immunodeficiency virus (HIV) infection, asymptomatic Z21
  hysterectomy (complete) (total) Z90.710
    partial (with remaining cervial stump) Z90.711
  ileostomy Z93.2
  implant
    breast Z98.82
  infibulation N90.813
  intestinal bypass Z98.0
  jejunostomy Z93.4
  lapsed immunization schedule Z28.3
  laryngectomy Z90.02
  lymphaticus E32.8
  marmoratus G80.3

Status — *continued*
  mastectomy (unilateral) (bilateral) Z90.1- ☑
  military deployment status (current) Z56.82
    in theater or in support of military war, peacekeeping and humanitarian operations Z56.82
  nephrectomy (unilateral) (bilateral) Z90.5
  nephrostomy Z93.6
  obesity surgery Z98.84
  oophorectomy
    bilateral Z90.722
    unilateral Z90.721
  organ replacement
    by artificial or mechanical device or prosthesis of
      artery Z95.828
      bladder Z96.0
      blood vessel Z95.828
      breast Z97.8
      eye globe Z97.0
      heart Z95.812
        valve Z95.2
      intestine Z97.8
      joint Z96.60
        hip — *see* Presence, hip joint implant
        knee — *see* Presence, knee joint implant
        specified site NEC Z96.698
      kidney Z97.8
      larynx Z96.3
      lens Z96.1
      limbs — *see* Presence, artificial, limb
      liver Z97.8
      lung Z97.8
      pancreas Z97.8
    by organ transplant (heterologous)(homologous) — *see* Transplant
  pacemaker
    brain Z96.89
    cardiac Z95.0
    specified NEC Z96.89
  pancreatectomy Z90.410
    complete Z90.410
    partial Z90.411
    total Z90.410
  physical restraint Z78.1
  pneumonectomy (complete) (partial) Z90.2
  pneumothorax, therapeutic Z98.3
  postcommotio cerebri F07.81
  postoperative (postprocedural) NEC Z98.89
    breast implant Z98.82
    dental Z98.818
      crown Z98.811
      fillings Z98.811
      restoration Z98.811
      sealant Z98.810
      specified NEC Z98.818
    pneumothorax, therapeutic Z98.3
  postpartum (routine follow-up) Z39.2
    care immediately after delivery Z39.0
  postsurgical (postprocedural) NEC Z98.89
    pneumothorax, therapeutic Z98.3
  pregnancy, incidental Z33.1
  prosthesis coronary angioplasty Z95.5
  pseudophakia Z96.1
  renal dialysis (hemodialysis) (peritoneal) Z99.2
  retained foreign body — *see* Retained, foreign body fragments (type of)
  reversed jejunal transposition (for bypass) Z98.0
  salpingo-oophorectomy
    bilateral Z90.722
    unilateral Z90.721
  sex reassignment surgery status Z87.890
  shunt
    arteriovenous (for dialysis) Z99.2
    cerebrospinal fluid Z98.2
    ventricular (communicating) (for drainage) Z98.2
  splenectomy Z90.81
  thymicolymphaticus E32.8
  thymicus E32.8
  thymolymphaticus E32.8
  thyroidectomy (hypothyroidism) E89.0
  tooth (teeth) extraction (*see also* Absence, teeth, acquired) K08.409
  tPA (rtPA) administration in a different facility within the last 24 hours prior to admission to current facility Z92.82
  tracheostomy Z93.0
  transplant — *see* Transplant
    organ removed Z98.85
  tubal ligation Z98.51

▽ Subterms under main terms may continue to next column or page   ☑ Additional Character Required — Refer to the Tabular List for Character Selection   283

Stasis — Status

Status — *continued*
  underimmunization Z28.3
  ureterostomy Z93.6
  urethrostomy Z93.6
  vagina, artificial Z93.8
  vasectomy Z98.52
  wheelchair confinement Z99.3
Stealing
  child problem F91.8
    in company with others Z72.810
  pathological (compulsive) F63.2
Steam burn — *see* Burn
Steatocystoma multiplex L72.2
Steatohepatitis (nonalcoholic) (NASH) K75.81
Steatoma L72.3
  eyelid (cystic) — *see* Dermatosis, eyelid
    infected — *see* Hordeolum
Steatorrhea (chronic) K90.4
  with lacteal obstruction K90.2
  idiopathic (adult) (infantile) K90.0
  pancreatic K90.3
  primary K90.0
  tropical K90.1
Steatosis E88.89
  heart — *see* Degeneration, myocardial
  kidney N28.89
  liver NEC K76.0
Steele-Richardson-Olszewski disease or syndrome
  G23.1
Steinbrocker's syndrome G90.8
Steinert's disease G71.11
Stein-Leventhal syndrome E28.2
Stein's syndrome E28.2
STEMI (*see also* Infarct, myocardium, ST elevation) I21.3
Stenocardia I20.8
Stenocephaly Q75.8
Stenosis, stenotic (cicatricial) (*see also* Stricture)
  ampulla of Vater K83.1
  anus, anal (canal) (sphincter) K62.4
    and rectum K62.4
    congenital Q42.3
      with fistula Q42.2
  aorta (ascending) (supraventricular) (congenital) Q25.3
    arteriosclerotic I70.0
    calcified I70.0
  aortic (valve) I35.0
    with insufficiency I35.2
    congenital Q23.0
    rheumatic I06.0
      with
        incompetency, insufficiency or regurgitation
          I06.2
          with mitral (valve) disease I08.0
            with tricuspid (valve) disease I08.3
        mitral (valve) disease I08.0
          with tricuspid (valve) disease I08.3
        tricuspid (valve) disease I08.2
          with mitral (valve) disease I08.3
    specified cause NEC I35.8
    syphilitic A52.03
  aqueduct of Sylvius (congenital) Q03.0
    with spina bifida — *see* Spina bifida, by site, with
      hydrocephalus
    acquired G91.1
  artery NEC (*see also* Arteriosclerosis) I77.1
    celiac I77.4
    cerebral — *see* Occlusion, artery, cerebral
    extremities — *see* Arteriosclerosis, extremities
    precerebral — *see* Occlusion, artery, precerebral
    pulmonary (congenital) Q25.6
      acquired I28.8
    renal I70.1
  bile duct (common) (hepatic) K83.1
    congenital Q44.3
  bladder-neck (acquired) N32.0
    congenital Q64.31
  brain G93.89
  bronchus J98.09
    congenital Q32.3
    syphilitic A52.72
  cardia (stomach) K22.2
    congenital Q39.3
  cardiovascular — *see* Disease, cardiovascular
  caudal M48.08
  cervix, cervical (canal) N88.2
    congenital Q51.828
    in pregnancy or childbirth — *see* Pregnancy,
      complicated by, abnormal cervix

Stenosis, stenotic — *continued*
  colon (*see also* Obstruction, intestine)
    congenital Q42.9
      specified NEC Q42.8
  colostomy K94.03
  common (bile) duct K83.1
    congenital Q44.3
  coronary (artery) — *see* Disease, heart, ischemic,
    atherosclerotic
  cystic duct — *see* Obstruction, gallbladder
  due to presence of device, implant or graft (*see also*
    Complications, by site and type, specified NEC)
    T85.85 ☑
    arterial graft NEC T82.858 ☑
    breast (implant) T85.85 ☑
    catheter T85.85 ☑
      dialysis (renal) T82.858 ☑
        intraperitoneal T85.85 ☑
      infusion NEC T82.858 ☑
        spinal (epidural) (subdural) T85.85 ☑
      urinary (indwelling) T83.85 ☑
    fixation, internal (orthopedic) NEC T84.85 ☑
    gastrointestinal (bile duct) (esophagus) T85.85 ☑
    genital NEC T83.85 ☑
    heart NEC T82.857 ☑
    joint prosthesis T84.85 ☑
    ocular (corneal graft) (orbital implant) NEC
      T85.85 ☑
    orthopedic NEC T84.85 ☑
    specified NEC T85.85 ☑
    urinary NEC T83.85 ☑
    vascular NEC T82.858 ☑
    ventricular intracranial shunt T85.85 ☑
  duodenum K31.5
    congenital Q41.0
  ejaculatory duct NEC N50.8
  endocervical os — *see* Stenosis, cervix
  enterostomy K94.13
  esophagus K22.2
    congenital Q39.3
    syphilitic A52.79
      congenital A50.59 [K23]
  eustachian tube — *see* Obstruction, eustachian tube
  external ear canal (acquired) H61.30- ☑
    congenital Q16.1
    due to
      inflammation H61.32- ☑
      trauma H61.31- ☑
    postprocedural H95.81- ☑
    specified cause NEC H61.39- ☑
  gallbladder — *see* Obstruction, gallbladder
  glottis J38.6
  heart valve (congenital) Q24.8
    aortic Q23.0
    mitral Q23.2
    pulmonary Q22.1
    tricuspid Q22.4
  hepatic duct K83.1
  hymen N89.6
  hypertrophic subaortic (idiopathic) I42.1
  ileum K56.69
    congenital Q41.2
  infundibulum cardia Q24.3
  intervertebral foramina (*see also* Lesion, biomechani-
    cal, specified NEC)
    connective tissue M99.79
      abdomen M99.79
      cervical region M99.71
      cervicothoracic M99.71
      head region M99.70
      lumbar region M99.73
      lumbosacral M99.73
      occipitocervical M99.70
      sacral region M99.74
      sacrococcygeal M99.74
      sacroiliac M99.74
      specified NEC M99.79
      thoracic region M99.72
      thoracolumbar M99.72
    disc M99.79
      abdomen M99.79
      cervical region M99.71
      cervicothoracic M99.71
      head region M99.70
      lower extremity M99.76
      lumbar region M99.73
      lumbosacral M99.73

Stenosis, stenotic — *continued*
  intervertebral foramina (*see also* Lesion, biomechanical,
    specified) — *continued*
    disc — *continued*
      occipitocervical M99.70
      pelvic M99.75
      rib cage M99.78
      sacral region M99.74
      sacrococcygeal M99.74
      sacroiliac M99.74
      specified NEC M99.79
      thoracic region M99.72
      thoracolumbar M99.72
      upper extremity M99.77
    osseous M99.69
      abdomen M99.69
      cervical region M99.61
      cervicothoracic M99.61
      head region M99.60
      lower extremity M99.66
      lumbar region M99.63
      lumbosacral M99.63
      occipitocervical M99.60
      pelvic M99.65
      rib cage M99.68
      sacral region M99.64
      sacrococcygeal M99.64
      sacroiliac M99.64
      specified NEC M99.69
      thoracic region M99.62
      thoracolumbar M99.62
      upper extremity M99.67
    subluxation — *see* Stenosis, intervertebral forami-
      na, osseous
  intestine (*see also* Obstruction, intestine)
    congenital (small) Q41.9
      large Q42.9
        specified NEC Q42.8
      specified NEC Q41.8
  jejunum K56.69
    congenital Q41.1
  lacrimal (passage)
    canaliculi H04.54- ☑
    congenital Q10.5
    duct H04.55- ☑
    punctum H04.56- ☑
    sac H04.57- ☑
  lacrimonasal duct — *see* Stenosis, lacrimal, duct
    congenital Q10.5
  larynx J38.6
    congenital NEC Q31.8
      subglottic Q31.1
    syphilitic A52.73
      congenital A50.59 [J99]
  mitral (chronic) (inactive) (valve) I05.0
    with
      aortic valve disease I08.0
      incompetency, insufficiency or regurgitation
        I05.2
    active or acute I01.1
      with rheumatic or Sydenham's chorea I02.0
    congenital Q23.2
    specified cause, except rheumatic I34.2
    syphilitic A52.03
  myocardium, myocardial (*see also* Degeneration, my-
    ocardial)
    hypertrophic subaortic (idiopathic) I42.1
  nares (anterior) (posterior) J34.89
    congenital Q30.0
  nasal duct (*see also* Stenosis, lacrimal, duct)
    congenital Q10.5
  nasolacrimal duct (*see also* Stenosis, lacrimal, duct)
    congenital Q10.5
  neural canal (*see also* Lesion, biomechanical, specified
    NEC)
    connective tissue M99.49
      abdomen M99.49
      cervical region M99.41
      cervicothoracic M99.41
      head region M99.40
      lower extremity M99.46
      lumbar region M99.43
      lumbosacral M99.43
      occipitocervical M99.40
      pelvic M99.45
      rib cage M99.48
      sacral region M99.44
      sacrococcygeal M99.44

☑ **Additional Character Required** — Refer to the Tabular List for Character Selection   ▽ Subterms under main terms may continue to next column or page

Stenosis, stenotic — continued
  neural canal (see also Lesion, biomechanical, specified)
    — continued
    connective tissue — continued
      sacroiliac M99.44
      specified NEC M99.49
      thoracic region M99.42
      thoracolumbar M99.42
      upper extremity M99.47
    intervertebral disc M99.59
      abdomen M99.59
      cervical region M99.51
      cervicothoracic M99.51
      head region M99.50
      lower extremity M99.56
      lumbar region M99.53
      lumbosacral M99.53
      occipitocervical M99.50
      pelvic M99.55
      rib cage M99.58
      sacral region M99.54
      sacrococcygeal M99.54
      sacroiliac M99.54
      specified NEC M99.59
      thoracic region M99.52
      thoracolumbar M99.52
      upper extremity M99.57
    osseous M99.39
      abdomen M99.39
      cervical region M99.31
      cervicothoracic M99.31
      head region M99.30
      lower extremity M99.36
      lumbar region M99.33
      lumbosacral M99.33
      occipitocervical M99.30
      pelvic M99.35
      rib cage M99.38
      sacral region M99.34
      sacrococcygeal M99.34
      sacroiliac M99.34
      specified NEC M99.39
      thoracic region M99.32
      thoracolumbar M99.32
      upper extremity M99.37
    subluxation M99.29
      cervical region M99.21
      cervicothoracic M99.21
      head region M99.20
      lower extremity M99.26
      lumbar region M99.23
      lumbosacral M99.23
      occipitocervical M99.20
      pelvic M99.25
      rib cage M99.28
      sacral region M99.24
      sacrococcygeal M99.24
      sacroiliac M99.24
      specified NEC M99.29
      thoracic region M99.22
      thoracolumbar M99.22
      upper extremity M99.27
  organ or site, congenital NEC — see Atresia, by site
  papilla of Vater K83.1
  pulmonary (artery) (congenital) Q25.6
    with ventricular septal defect, transposition of
      aorta, and hypertrophy of right ventricle
      Q21.3
    acquired I28.8
    in tetralogy of Fallot Q21.3
    infundibular Q24.3
    subvalvular Q24.3
    supravalvular Q25.6
    valve I37.0
      with insufficiency I37.2
      congenital Q22.1
      rheumatic I09.89
        with aortic, mitral or tricuspid (valve) disease
          I08.8
    vein, acquired I28.8
    vessel NEC I28.8
  pulmonic (congenital) Q22.1
    infundibular Q24.3
    subvalvular Q24.3
  pylorus (hypertrophic) (acquired) K31.1
    adult K31.1
    congenital Q40.0
    infantile Q40.0

Stenosis, stenotic — continued
  rectum (sphincter) — see Stricture, rectum
  renal artery I70.1
    congenital Q27.1
  salivary duct (any) K11.8
  sphincter of Oddi K83.1
  spinal M48.00
    cervical region M48.02
    cervicothoracic region M48.03
    lumbar region M48.06
    lumbosacral region M48.07
    occipito-atlanto-axial region M48.01
    sacrococcygeal region M48.08
    thoracic region M48.04
    thoracolumbar region M48.05
  stomach, hourglass K31.2
  subaortic (congenital) Q24.4
    hypertrophic (idiopathic) I42.1
  subglottic J38.6
    congenital Q31.1
    postprocedural J95.5
  trachea J39.8
    congenital Q32.1
    syphilitic A52.73
    tuberculous NEC A15.5
  tracheostomy J95.03
  tricuspid (valve) I07.0
    with
      aortic (valve) disease I08.2
      incompetency, insufficiency or regurgitation
        I07.2
        with aortic (valve) disease I08.2
          with mitral (valve) disease I08.3
      mitral (valve) disease I08.1
        with aortic (valve) disease I08.3
    congenital Q22.4
    nonrheumatic I36.0
      with insufficiency I36.2
  tubal N97.1
  ureter — see Atresia, ureter
  ureteropelvic junction, congenital Q62.11
  ureterovesical orifice, congenital Q62.12
  urethra (valve) (see also Stricture, urethra)
    congenital Q64.32
  urinary meatus, congenital Q64.33
  vagina N89.5
    congenital Q52.4
    in pregnancy — see Pregnancy, complicated by,
      abnormal vagina
      causing obstructed labor O65.5
  valve (cardiac) (heart) (see also Endocarditis) I38
    congenital Q24.8
      aortic Q23.0
      mitral Q23.2
      pulmonary Q22.1
      tricuspid Q22.4
  vena cava (inferior) (superior) I87.1
    congenital Q26.0
  vesicourethral orifice Q64.31
  vulva N90.5
Stent jail T82.897 ☑
Stercolith (impaction) K56.41
  appendix K38.1
Stercoraceous, stercoral ulcer K63.3
  anus or rectum K62.6
Stereotypies NEC F98.4
Sterility — see Infertility
Sterilization — see Encounter (for), sterilization
Sternalgia — see Angina
Sternopagus Q89.4
Sternum bifidum Q76.7
Steroid
  effects (adverse) (adrenocortical) (iatrogenic)
    cushingoid E24.2
      correct substance properly administered — see
        Table of Drugs and Chemicals, by drug,
        adverse effect
      overdose or wrong substance given or taken
        — see Table of Drugs and Chemicals, by
        drug, poisoning
    diabetes — see subcategory E09 ☑
      correct substance properly administered — see
        Table of Drugs and Chemicals, by drug,
        adverse effect
      overdose or wrong substance given or taken
        — see Table of Drugs and Chemicals, by
        drug, poisoning
    fever R50.2

Steroid — continued
  effects — continued
    insufficiency E27.3
      correct substance properly administered — see
        Table of Drugs and Chemicals, by drug,
        adverse effect
      overdose or wrong substance given or taken
        — see Table of Drugs and Chemicals, by
        drug, poisoning
  responder H40.04- ☑
Stevens-Johnson disease or syndrome L51.1
  toxic epidermal necrolysis overlap L51.3
Stewart-Morel syndrome M85.2
Sticker's disease B08.3
Sticky eye — see Conjunctivitis, acute, mucopurulent
Stieda's disease — see Bursitis, tibial collateral
Stiff neck — see Torticollis
Stiff-man syndrome G25.82
Stiffness, joint NEC M25.60
  ankle M25.67- ☑
  ankylosis — see Ankylosis, joint
  contracture — see Contraction, joint
  elbow M25.62- ☑
  foot M25.67- ☑
  hand M25.64- ☑
  hip M25.65- ☑
  knee M25.66- ☑
  shoulder M25.61- ☑
  wrist M25.63- ☑
Stigmata congenital syphilis A50.59
Stillbirth P95
Still-Felty syndrome — see Felty's syndrome
Still's disease or syndrome (juvenile) M08.20
  adult-onset M06.1
  ankle M08.27- ☑
  elbow M08.22- ☑
  foot joint M08.27- ☑
  hand joint M08.24- ☑
  hip M08.25- ☑
  knee M08.26- ☑
  multiple site M08.29
  shoulder M08.21- ☑
  vertebra M08.28
  wrist M08.23- ☑
Stimulation, ovary E28.1
Sting (venomous) (with allergic or anaphylactic shock)
    — see Table of Drugs and Chemicals, by animal or
    substance, poisoning
Stippled epiphyses Q78.8
Stitch
  abscess T81.4 ☑
  burst (in operation wound) — see Disruption, wound,
    operation
Stokes' disease E05.00
  with thyroid storm E05.01
Stokes-Adams disease or syndrome I45.9
Stokvis (-Talma) **disease** D74.8
Stoma malfunction
  colostomy K94.03
  enterostomy K94.13
  gastrostomy K94.23
  ileostomy K94.13
  tracheostomy J95.03
Stomach — see condition
Stomatitis (denture) (ulcerative) K12.1
  angular K13.0
    due to dietary or vitamin deficiency E53.0
  aphthous K12.0
  bovine B08.61
  candidal B37.0
  catarrhal K12.1
  diphtheritic A36.89
  due to
    dietary deficiency E53.0
    thrush B37.0
    vitamin deficiency
      B group NEC E53.9
      B2 (riboflavin) E53.0
  epidemic B08.8
  epizootic B08.8
  follicular K12.1
  gangrenous A69.0
  Geotrichum B48.3
  herpesviral, herpetic B00.2
  herpetiformis K12.0
  malignant K12.1
  membranous acute K12.1

Stomatitis — *continued*
 monilial B37.0
 mycotic B37.0
 necrotizing ulcerative A69.0
 parasitic B37.0
 septic K12.1
 spirochetal A69.1
 suppurative (acute) K12.2
 ulceromembranous A69.1
 vesicular K12.1
  with exanthem (enteroviral) B08.4
  virus disease A93.8
 Vincent's A69.1
Stomatocytosis D58.8
Stomatomycosis B37.0
Stomatorrhagia K13.79
Stone(s) (*see also* Calculus)
 bladder (diverticulum) N21.0
 cystine E72.09
 heart syndrome I50.1
 kidney N20.0
 prostate N42.0
 pulpal (dental) K04.2
 renal N20.0
 salivary gland or duct (any) K11.5
 urethra (impacted) N21.1
 urinary (duct) (impacted) (passage) N20.9
  bladder (diverticulum) N21.0
  lower tract N21.9
  specified NEC N21.8
 xanthine E79.8 [N22]
Stonecutter's lung J62.8
Stonemason's asthma, disease, lung or pneumoco-niosis J62.8
Stoppage
 heart — *see* Arrest, cardiac
 urine — *see* Retention, urine
Storm, thyroid — *see* Thyrotoxicosis
Strabismus (congenital) (nonparalytic) H50.9
 concomitant H50.40
  convergent — *see* Strabismus, convergent concomitant
  divergent — *see* Strabismus, divergent concomitant
 convergent concomitant H50.00
  accommodative component H50.43
  alternating H50.05
   with
    A pattern H50.06
    specified nonconcomitances NEC H50.08
    V pattern H50.07
  monocular H50.01- ☑
   with
    A pattern H50.02- ☑
    specified nonconcomitances NEC H50.04- ☑
    V pattern H50.03- ☑
   intermittent H50.31- ☑
    alternating H50.32
 cyclotropia H50.1- ☑
 divergent concomitant H50.10
  alternating H50.15
   with
    A pattern H50.16
    specified noncomitances NEC H50.18
    V pattern H50.17
  monocular H50.11- ☑
   with
    A pattern H50.12- ☑
    specified noncomitances NEC H50.14- ☑
    V pattern H50.13- ☑
   intermittent H50.33 ☑
    alternating H50.34
 Duane's syndrome H50.81- ☑
 due to adhesions, scars H50.69
 heterophoria H50.50
  alternating H50.55
  cyclophoria H50.54
  esophoria H50.51
  exophoria H50.52
  vertical H50.53
 heterotropia H50.40
  intermittent H50.30
 hypertropia H50.2- ☑
 hypotropia — *see* Hypertropia
 latent H50.50
 mechanical H50.60
  Brown's sheath syndrome H50.61- ☑

Strabismus — *continued*
 mechanical — *continued*
  specified type NEC H50.69
 monofixation syndrome H50.42
 paralytic H49.9
  abducens nerve H49.2- ☑
  fourth nerve H49.1- ☑
  Kearns-Sayre syndrome H49.81- ☑
  ophthalmoplegia (external)
   progressive H49.4- ☑
    with pigmentary retinopathy H49.81- ☑
   total H49.3- ☑
  sixth nerve H49.2- ☑
  specified type NEC H49.88- ☑
  third nerve H49.0- ☑
  trochlear nerve H49.1- ☑
 specified type NEC H50.89
 vertical H50.2- ☑
Strain
 back S39.012 ☑
 cervical S16.1 ☑
 eye NEC — *see* Disturbance, vision, subjective
 heart — *see* Disease, heart
 low back S39.012 ☑
 mental NOS Z73.3
  work-related Z56.6
 muscle (tendon) — *see* Injury, muscle, by site, strain
 neck S16.1 ☑
 physical NOS Z73.3
  work-related Z56.6
 postural (*see also* Disorder, soft tissue, due to use)
 psychological NEC Z73.3
 tendon — *see* Injury, muscle, by site, strain
Straining, on urination R39.16
Strand, vitreous — *see* Opacity, vitreous, membranes and strands
Strangulation, strangulated (*see also* Asphyxia, traumatic)
 appendix K38.8
 bladder-neck N32.0
 bowel or colon K56.2
 food or foreign body — *see* Foreign body, by site
 hemorrhoids — *see* Hemorrhoids, with complication
 hernia (*see also* Hernia, by site, with obstruction)
  with gangrene — *see* Hernia, by site, with gangrene
 intestine (large) (small) K56.2
  with hernia (*see also* Hernia, by site, with obstruction)
   with gangrene — *see* Hernia, by site, with gangrene
 mesentery K56.2
 mucus — *see* Asphyxia, mucus
 omentum K56.2
 organ or site, congenital NEC — *see* Atresia, by site
 ovary — *see* Torsion, ovary
 penis N48.89
  foreign body T19.4 ☑
 rupture — *see* Hernia, by site, with obstruction
 stomach due to hernia (*see also* Hernia, by site, with obstruction)
  with gangrene — *see* Hernia, by site, with gangrene
 vesicourethral orifice N32.0
Strangury R30.0
Straw itch B88.0
Strawberry
 gallbladder K82.4
 mark Q82.5
 tongue (red) (white) K14.3
Streak(s)
 macula, angioid H35.33
 ovarian Q50.32
Strephosymbolia F81.0
 secondary to organic lesion R48.8
Streptobacillary fever A25.1
Streptobacillosis A25.1
Streptobacillus moniliformis A25.1
Streptococcus, streptococcal (*see also* condition)
 as cause of disease classified elsewhere B95.5
 group
  A, as cause of disease classified elsewhere B95.0
  B, as cause of disease classified elsewhere B95.1
  D, as cause of disease classified elsewhere B95.2
  pneumoniae, as cause of disease classified elsewhere B95.3

Streptococcus, streptococcal — *continued*
 specified NEC, as cause of disease classified elsewhere B95.4
Streptomycosis B47.1
Streptotrichosis A48.8
Stress F43.9
 family — *see* Disruption, family
 fetal P84
  complicating pregnancy O77.9
   due to drug administration O77.1
 mental NEC Z73.3
  work-related Z56.6
 physical NEC Z73.3
  work-related Z56.6
 polycythemia D75.1
 reaction (*see also* Reaction, stress) F43.9
 work schedule Z56.3
Stretching, nerve — *see* Injury, nerve
Striae albicantes, atrophicae or distensae (cutis) L90.6
Stricture (*see also* Stenosis)
 ampulla of Vater K83.1
 anus (sphincter) K62.4
  congenital Q42.3
   with fistula Q42.2
  infantile Q42.3
   with fistula Q42.2
 aorta (ascending) (congenital) Q25.3
  arteriosclerotic I70.0
  calcified I70.0
  supravalvular, congenital Q25.3
 aortic (valve) — *see* Stenosis, aortic
 aqueduct of Sylvius (congenital) Q03.0
  with spina bifida — *see* Spina bifida, by site, with hydrocephalus
  acquired G91.1
 artery I77.1
  basilar — *see* Occlusion, artery, basilar
  carotid — *see* Occlusion, artery, carotid
  celiac I77.4
  congenital (peripheral) Q27.8
   cerebral Q28.3
   coronary Q24.5
   digestive system Q27.8
   lower limb Q27.8
   retinal Q14.1
   specified site NEC Q27.8
   umbilical Q27.0
   upper limb Q27.8
  coronary — *see* Disease, heart, ischemic, atherosclerotic
   congenital Q24.5
  precerebral — *see* Occlusion, artery, precerebral
  pulmonary (congenital) Q25.6
   acquired I28.8
  renal I70.1
  vertebral — *see* Occlusion, artery, vertebral
 auditory canal (external) (congenital)
  acquired — *see* Stenosis, external ear canal
 bile duct (common) (hepatic) K83.1
  congenital Q44.3
  postoperative K91.89
 bladder N32.89
  neck N32.0
 bowel — *see* Obstruction, intestine
 brain G93.89
 bronchus J98.09
  congenital Q32.3
  syphilitic A52.72
 cardia (stomach) K22.2
  congenital Q39.3
 cardiac (*see also* Disease, heart)
  orifice (stomach) K22.2
 cecum — *see* Obstruction, intestine
 cervix, cervical (canal) N88.2
  congenital Q51.828
  in pregnancy — *see* Pregnancy, complicated by, abnormal cervix
   causing obstructed labor O65.5
 colon (*see also* Obstruction, intestine)
  congenital Q42.9
   specified NEC Q42.8
 colostomy K94.03
 common (bile) duct K83.1
 coronary (artery) — *see* Disease, heart, ischemic, atherosclerotic
 cystic duct — *see* Obstruction, gallbladder
 digestive organs NEC, congenital Q45.8

☑ **Additional Character Required** — Refer to the Tabular List for Character Selection   ▽ **Subterms under main terms may continue to next column or page**

Stricture — *continued*
  duodenum K31.5
    congenital Q41.0
  ear canal (external) (congenital) Q16.1
    acquired — *see* Stricture, auditory canal, acquired
  ejaculatory duct N50.8
  enterostomy K94.13
  esophagus K22.2
    congenital Q39.3
    syphilitic A52.79
      congenital A50.59 [K23]
  eustachian tube (*see also* Obstruction, eustachian tube)
    congenital Q17.8
  fallopian tube N97.1
    gonococcal A54.24
    tuberculous A18.17
  gallbladder — *see* Obstruction, gallbladder
  glottis J38.6
  heart (*see also* Disease, heart)
    valve (*see also* Endocarditis) I38
      aortic Q23.0
      mitral Q23.4
      pulmonary Q22.1
      tricuspid Q22.4
  hepatic duct K83.1
  hourglass, of stomach K31.2
  hymen N89.6
  hypopharynx J39.2
  ileum K56.69
    congenital Q41.2
  intestine (*see also* Obstruction, intestine)
    congenital (small) Q41.9
      large Q42.9
        specified NEC Q42.8
      specified NEC Q41.8
    ischemic K55.1
  jejunum K56.69
    congenital Q41.1
  lacrimal passages (*see also* Stenosis, lacrimal)
    congenital Q10.5
  larynx J38.6
    congenital NEC Q31.8
      subglottic Q31.1
    syphilitic A52.73
      congenital A50.59 [J99]
  meatus
    ear (congenital) Q16.1
      acquired — *see* Stricture, auditory canal, acquired
      osseous (ear) (congenital) Q16.1
        acquired — *see* Stricture, auditory canal, acquired
    urinarius (*see also* Stricture, urethra)
      congenital Q64.33
  mitral (valve) — *see* Stenosis, mitral
  myocardium, myocardial I51.5
    hypertrophic subaortic (idiopathic) I42.1
  nares (anterior) (posterior) J34.89
    congenital Q30.0
  nasal duct (*see also* Stenosis, lacrimal, duct)
    congenital Q10.5
  nasolacrimal duct (*see also* Stenosis, lacrimal, duct)
    congenital Q10.5
  nasopharynx J39.2
    syphilitic A52.73
  nose J34.89
    congenital Q30.0
    syphilitic A52.73
      congenital A50.59 [J99]
  organ or site, congenital NEC — *see* Atresia, by site
  os uteri — *see* Stricture, cervix
  osseous meatus (ear) (congenital) Q16.1
    acquired — *see* Stricture, auditory canal, acquired
  oviduct — *see* Stricture, fallopian tube
  pelviureteric junction (congenital) Q62.11
  penis, by foreign body T19.4 ☑
  pharynx J39.2
  prostate N42.89
  pulmonary, pulmonic
    artery (congenital) Q25.6
      acquired I28.8
      noncongenital I28.8
    infundibulum (congenital) Q24.3
    valve I37.0
      congenital Q22.1
    vein, acquired I28.8

Stricture — *continued*
  pulmonary, pulmonic — *continued*
    vessel NEC I28.8
  punctum lacrimale (*see also* Stenosis, lacrimal, punctum)
    congenital Q10.5
  pylorus (hypertrophic) K31.1
    adult K31.1
    congenital Q40.0
    infantile Q40.0
  rectosigmoid K56.69
  rectum (sphincter) K62.4
    congenital Q42.1
      with fistula Q42.0
    due to
      chlamydial lymphogranuloma A55
      irradiation K91.89
      lymphogranuloma venereum A55
    gonococcal A54.6
    inflammatory (chlamydial) A55
    syphilitic A52.74
    tuberculous A18.32
  renal artery I70.1
    congenital Q27.1
  salivary duct or gland (any) K11.8
  sigmoid (flexure) — *see* Obstruction, intestine
  spermatic cord N50.8
  stoma (following) (of)
    colostomy K94.03
    enterostomy K94.13
    gastrostomy K94.23
    ileostomy K94.13
    tracheostomy J95.03
  stomach K31.89
    congenital Q40.2
    hourglass K31.2
  subaortic Q24.4
    hypertrophic (acquired) (idiopathic) I42.1
  subglottic J38.6
  syphilitic NEC A52.79
  trachea J39.8
    congenital Q32.1
    syphilitic A52.73
    tuberculous NEC A15.5
  tracheostomy J95.03
  tricuspid (valve) — *see* Stenosis, tricuspid
  tunica vaginalis N50.8
  ureter (postoperative) N13.5
    with
      hydronephrosis N13.1
        with infection N13.6
      pyelonephritis (chronic) N11.1
    congenital — *see* Atresia, ureter
    tuberculous A18.11
  ureteropelvic junction (congenital) Q62.11
  ureterovesical orifice N13.5
    with infection N13.6
  urethra (organic) (spasmodic) N35.9
    associated with schistosomiasis B65.0 [N37]
    congenital Q64.39
      valvular (posterior) Q64.2
    due to
      infection — *see* Stricture, urethra, postinfective
      trauma — *see* Stricture, urethra, post-traumatic
    gonococcal, gonorrheal A54.01
    infective NEC — *see* Stricture, urethra, postinfective
    late effect (sequelae) of injury — *see* Stricture, urethra, post-traumatic
    postcatheterization — *see* Stricture, urethra, postprocedural
    postinfective NEC
      female N35.12
      male N35.119
        anterior urethra N35.114
        bulbous urethra N35.112
        meatal N35.111
        membranous urethra N35.113
    postobstetric N35.021
    postoperative — *see* Stricture, urethra, postprocedural
    postprocedural
      female N99.12
      male N99.114
        anterior urethra N99.113
        bulbous urethra N99.111
        meatal N99.110
        membranous urethra N99.112

Stricture — *continued*
  urethra — *continued*
    post-traumatic
      female N35.028
        due to childbirth N35.021
      male N35.014
        anterior urethra N35.013
        bulbous urethra N35.011
        meatal N35.010
        membranous urethra N35.012
    sequela (late effect) of
      childbirth N35.021
      injury — *see* Stricture, urethra, post-traumatic
    specified cause NEC N35.8
    syphilitic A52.76
    traumatic — *see* Stricture, urethra, post-traumatic
    valvular (posterior), congenital Q64.2
  urinary meatus — *see* Stricture, urethra
  uterus, uterine (synechiae) N85.6
    os (external) (internal) — *see* Stricture, cervix
  vagina (outlet) — *see* Stenosis, vagina
  valve (cardiac) (heart) (*see also* Endocarditis)
    congenital
      aortic Q23.0
      mitral Q23.2
      pulmonary Q22.1
      tricuspid Q22.4
  vas deferens N50.8
    congenital Q55.4
  vein I87.1
  vena cava (inferior) (superior) NEC I87.1
    congenital Q26.0
  vesicourethral orifice N32.0
    congenital Q64.31
  vulva (acquired) N90.5
Stridor R06.1
  congenital (larynx) P28.89
Stridulous — *see* condition
Stroke (apoplectic) (brain) (embolic) (ischemic) (paralytic) (thrombotic) I63.9
  epileptic — *see* Epilepsy
  heat T67.0 ☑
  in evolution I63.9
  intraoperative
    during cardiac surgery I97.810
    during other surgery I97.811
  lightning — *see* Lightning
  meaning
    cerebral hemorrhage — *code to* Hemorrhage, intracranial
    cerebral infarction — *code to* Infarction, cerebral
  postprocedural
    following cardiac surgery I97.820
    following other surgery I97.821
  unspecified (NOS) I63.9
Stromatosis, endometrial D39.0
Strongyloidiasis, strongyloidosis B78.9
  cutaneous B78.1
  disseminated B78.7
  intestinal B78.0
Strophulus pruriginosus L28.2
Struck by lightning — *see* Lightning
Struma (*see also* Goiter)
  Hashimoto E06.3
  lymphomatosa E06.3
  nodosa (simplex) E04.9
    endemic E01.2
      multinodular E01.1
    multinodular E04.2
      iodine-deficiency related E01.1
    toxic or with hyperthyroidism E05.20
      with thyroid storm E05.21
      multinodular E05.20
        with thyroid storm E05.21
      uninodular E05.10
        with thyroid storm E05.11
    toxicosa E05.20
      with thyroid storm E05.21
      multinodular E05.20
        with thyroid storm E05.21
      uninodular E05.10
        with thyroid storm E05.11
    uninodular E04.1
  ovarii D27.- ☑
  Riedel's E06.5
Strumipriva cachexia E03.4
Strümpell-Marie spine — *see* Spondylitis, ankylosing
Strümpell-Westphal pseudosclerosis E83.01

Stuart deficiency disease (factor X) D68.2
Stuart-Prower factor deficiency (factor X) D68.2
Student's elbow — *see* Bursitis, elbow, olecranon
Stump — *see* Amputation
Stunting, nutritional E45
Stupor (catatonic) R40.1
　depressive F32.8
　dissociative F44.2
　manic F30.2
　manic-depressive F31.89
　psychogenic (anergic) F44.2
　reaction to exceptional stress (transient) F43.0
Sturge (-Weber) (-Dimitri) (-Kalischer) **disease or syn-
　drome** Q85.8
Stuttering F80.81
　adult onset F98.5
　childhood onset F80.81
　following cerebrovascular disease — *see* Disorder,
　　fluency. following cerebrovascular disease
　in conditions classified elsewhere R47.82
Sty, stye (external) (internal) (meibomian) (zeisian) —
　　see Hordeolum
Subacidity, gastric K31.89
　psychogenic F45.8
Subacute — *see* condition
Subarachnoid — *see* condition
Subcortical — *see* condition
Subcostal syndrome, nerve compression — *see*
　　Mononeuropathy, upper limb, specified site NEC
Subcutaneous, subcuticular — *see* condition
Subdural — *see* condition
Subendocardium — *see* condition
Subependymoma
　specified site — *see* Neoplasm, uncertain behavior,
　　by site
　unspecified site D43.2
Suberosis J67.3
Subglossitis — *see* Glossitis
Subhemophilia D66
Subinvolution
　breast (postlactational) (postpuerperal) N64.89
　puerperal O90.89
　uterus (chronic) (nonpuerperal) N85.3
　　puerperal O90.89
Sublingual — *see* condition
Sublinguitis — *see* Sialoadenitis
Subluxatable hip Q65.6
Subluxation (*see also* Dislocation)
　acromioclavicular S43.11- ☑
　ankle S93.0- ☑
　atlantoaxial, recurrent M43.4
　　with myelopathy M43.3
　carpometacarpal (joint) NEC S63.05- ☑
　　thumb S63.04- ☑
　complex, vertebral — *see* Complex, subluxation
　congenital (*see also* Malposition, congenital)
　　hip — *see* Dislocation, hip, congenital, partial
　　joint (excluding hip)
　　　lower limb Q68.8
　　　shoulder Q68.8
　　　upper limb Q68.8
　elbow (traumatic) S53.10- ☑
　　anterior S53.11- ☑
　　lateral S53.14- ☑
　　medial S53.13- ☑
　　posterior S53.12- ☑
　　specified type NEC S53.19- ☑
　finger S63.20- ☑
　　index S63.20- ☑
　　interphalangeal S63.22- ☑
　　　distal S63.24- ☑
　　　　index S63.24- ☑
　　　　little S63.24- ☑
　　　　middle S63.24- ☑
　　　　ring S63.24- ☑
　　　index S63.22- ☑
　　　little S63.22- ☑
　　　middle S63.22- ☑
　　　proximal S63.23- ☑
　　　　index S63.23- ☑
　　　　little S63.23- ☑
　　　　middle S63.23- ☑
　　　　ring S63.23- ☑
　　　ring S63.22- ☑
　　little S63.20- ☑

Subluxation — *continued*
　finger — *continued*
　　metacarpophalangeal S63.21- ☑
　　　index S63.21- ☑
　　　little S63.21- ☑
　　　middle S63.21- ☑
　　　ring S63.21- ☑
　　middle S63.20- ☑
　　ring S63.20- ☑
　foot S93.30- ☑
　　specified site NEC S93.33- ☑
　　tarsal joint S93.31- ☑
　　tarsometatarsal joint S93.32- ☑
　　toe — *see* Subluxation, toe
　hip S73.00- ☑
　　anterior S73.03- ☑
　　obturator S73.02- ☑
　　central S73.04- ☑
　　posterior S73.01- ☑
　interphalangeal (joint)
　　finger S63.22- ☑
　　　distal joint S63.24- ☑
　　　　index S63.24- ☑
　　　　little S63.24- ☑
　　　　middle S63.24- ☑
　　　　ring S63.24- ☑
　　　index S63.22- ☑
　　　little S63.22- ☑
　　　middle S63.22- ☑
　　　proximal joint S63.23- ☑
　　　　index S63.23- ☑
　　　　little S63.23- ☑
　　　　middle S63.23- ☑
　　　　ring S63.23- ☑
　　　ring S63.22- ☑
　　thumb S63.12- ☑
　　　distal joint S63.14- ☑
　　　proximal joint S63.13- ☑
　　toe S93.13- ☑
　　　great S93.13- ☑
　　　lesser S93.13- ☑
　joint prosthesis — *see* Complications, joint prosthesis,
　　mechanical, displacement, by site
　knee S83.10- ☑
　　cap — *see* Subluxation, patella
　　patella — *see* Subluxation, patella
　　proximal tibia
　　　anteriorly S83.11- ☑
　　　laterally S83.14- ☑
　　　medially S83.13- ☑
　　　posteriorly S83.12- ☑
　　specified type NEC S83.19- ☑
　lens — *see* Dislocation, lens, partial
　ligament, traumatic — *see* Sprain, by site
　metacarpal (bone)
　　proximal end S63.06- ☑
　metacarpophalangeal (joint)
　　finger S63.21- ☑
　　　index S63.21- ☑
　　　little S63.21- ☑
　　　middle S63.21- ☑
　　　ring S63.21- ☑
　　thumb S63.11- ☑
　metatarsophalangeal joint S93.14- ☑
　　great toe S93.14- ☑
　　lesser toe S93.14- ☑
　midcarpal (joint) S63.03- ☑
　patella S83.00- ☑
　　lateral S83.01- ☑
　　recurrent (nontraumatic) — *see* Dislocation,
　　　patella, recurrent, incomplete
　　specified type NEC S83.09- ☑
　pathological — *see* Dislocation, pathological
　radial head S53.00- ☑
　　anterior S53.01- ☑
　　nursemaid's elbow S53.03- ☑
　　posterior S53.02- ☑
　　specified type NEC S53.09- ☑
　radiocarpal (joint) S63.02- ☑
　radioulnar (joint)
　　distal S63.01- ☑
　　proximal — *see* Subluxation, elbow
　shoulder
　　congenital Q68.8
　　girdle S43.30- ☑
　　　scapula S43.31- ☑

Subluxation — *continued*
　shoulder — *continued*
　　girdle — *continued*
　　　specified site NEC S43.39- ☑
　　traumatic S43.00- ☑
　　　anterior S43.01- ☑
　　　inferior S43.03- ☑
　　　posterior S43.02- ☑
　　　specified type NEC S43.08- ☑
　sternoclavicular (joint) S43.20- ☑
　　anterior S43.21- ☑
　　posterior S43.22- ☑
　symphysis (pubis)
　thumb S63.103 ☑
　　interphalangeal joint — *see* Subluxation, interpha-
　　　langeal (joint), thumb
　　metacarpophalangeal joint — *see* Subluxation,
　　　metacarpophalangeal (joint), thumb
　toe(s) S93.10- ☑
　　great S93.10- ☑
　　　interphalangeal joint S93.13- ☑
　　　metatarsophalangeal joint S93.14- ☑
　　interphalangeal joint S93.13- ☑
　　lesser S93.10- ☑
　　　interphalangeal joint S93.13- ☑
　　　metatarsophalangeal joint S93.14- ☑
　　metatarsophalangeal joint S93.149 ☑
　ulna
　　distal end S63.07- ☑
　　proximal end — *see* Subluxation, elbow
　ulnohumeral joint — *see* Subluxation, elbow
　vertebral
　　recurrent NEC — *see* subcategory M43.5 ☑
　　traumatic
　　　cervical S13.100 ☑
　　　　atlantoaxial joint S13.120 ☑
　　　　atlantooccipital joint S13.110 ☑
　　　　atloidooccipital joint S13.110 ☑
　　　　joint between
　　　　　C0 and C1 S13.110 ☑
　　　　　C1 and C2 S13.120 ☑
　　　　　C2 and C3 S13.130 ☑
　　　　　C3 and C4 S13.140 ☑
　　　　　C4 and C5 S13.150 ☑
　　　　　C5 and C6 S13.160 ☑
　　　　　C6 and C7 S13.170 ☑
　　　　　C7 and T1 S13.180 ☑
　　　　occipitoatloid joint S13.110 ☑
　　　lumbar S33.100 ☑
　　　　joint between
　　　　　L1 and L2 S33.110 ☑
　　　　　L2 and L3 S33.120 ☑
　　　　　L3 and L4 S33.130 ☑
　　　　　L4 and L5 S33.140 ☑
　　　thoracic S23.100 ☑
　　　　joint between
　　　　　T1 and T2 S23.110 ☑
　　　　　T2 and T3 S23.120 ☑
　　　　　T3 and T4 S23.122 ☑
　　　　　T4 and T5 S23.130 ☑
　　　　　T5 and T6 S23.132 ☑
　　　　　T6 and T7 S23.140 ☑
　　　　　T7 and T8 S23.142 ☑
　　　　　T8 and T9 S23.150 ☑
　　　　　T9 and T10 S23.152 ☑
　　　　　T10 and T11 S23.160 ☑
　　　　　T11 and T12 S23.162 ☑
　　　　　T12 and L1 S23.170 ☑
　wrist (carpal bone) S63.00- ☑
　　carpometacarpal joint — *see* Subluxation, car-
　　　pometacarpal (joint)
　　distal radioulnar joint — *see* Subluxation, radioul-
　　　nar (joint), distal
　　metacarpal bone, proximal — *see* Subluxation,
　　　metacarpal (bone), proximal end
　　midcarpal — *see* Subluxation, midcarpal (joint)
　　radiocarpal joint — *see* Subluxation, radiocarpal
　　　(joint)
　　recurrent — *see* Dislocation, recurrent, wrist
　　specified site NEC S63.09- ☑
　　ulna — *see* Subluxation, ulna, distal end
Submaxillary — *see* condition
Submersion (fatal) (nonfatal) T75.1 ☑
Submucous — *see* condition
Subnormal, subnormality
　accommodation (old age) H52.4

　☑ **Additional Character Required — Refer to the Tabular List for Character Selection**　　▽ **Subterms under main terms may continue to next column or page**

Subnormal, subnormality — *continued*
mental — *see* Disability, intellectual
    temperature (accidental) T68 ☑
Subphrenic — *see* condition
Subscapular nerve — *see* condition
Subseptus uterus Q51.2
Subsiding appendicitis K36
Substernal thyroid E04.9
    congenital Q89.2
Substitution disorder F44.9
Subtentorial — *see* condition
Subthyroidism (acquired) (*see also* Hypothyroidism)
    congenital E03.1
Succenturiate placenta O43.19- ☑
Sucking thumb, child (excessive) F98.8
Sudamen, sudamina L74.1
Sudanese kala-azar B55.0
Sudden
hearing loss — *see* Deafness, sudden
heart failure — *see* Failure, heart
Sudeck's atrophy, disease, or syndrome — *see* Algoneurodystrophy
Suffocation — *see* Asphyxia, traumatic
Sugar
blood
    high (transient) R73.9
    low (transient) E16.2
in urine R81
Suicide, suicidal (attempted) T14.91
by poisoning — *see* Table of Drugs and Chemicals
history of (personal) Z91.5
    in family Z81.8
ideation — *see* Ideation, suicidal
risk
    meaning personal history of attempted suicide Z91.5
    meaning suicidal ideation — *see* Ideation, suicidal
tendencies
    meaning personal history of attempted suicide Z91.5
    meaning suicidal ideation — *see* Ideation, suicidal
trauma — *see* nature of injury by site
Suipestifer infection — *see* Infection, salmonella
Sulfhemoglobinemia, sulphemoglobinemia (acquired) (with methemoglobinemia) D74.8
Sumatran mite fever A75.3
Summer — *see* condition
Sunburn L55.9
first degree L55.0
second degree L55.1
third degree L55.2
SUNCT (short lasting unilateral neuralgiform headache with conjunctival injection and tearing) G44.059
intractable G44.051
not intractable G44.059
Sunken acetabulum — *see* Derangement, joint, specified type NEC, hip
Sunstroke T67.0 ☑
Superfecundation — *see* Pregnancy, multiple
Superfetation — *see* Pregnancy, multiple
Superinvolution (uterus) N85.8
Supernumerary (congenital)
aortic cusps Q23.8
auditory ossicles Q16.3
bone Q79.8
breast Q83.1
carpal bones Q74.0
cusps, heart valve NEC Q24.8
    aortic Q23.8
    mitral Q23.2
    pulmonary Q22.3
digit(s) Q69.9
ear (lobule) Q17.0
fallopian tube Q50.6
finger Q69.0
hymen Q52.4
kidney Q63.0
lacrimonasal duct Q10.6
lobule (ear) Q17.0
mitral cusps Q23.2
muscle Q79.8
nipple(s) Q83.3
organ or site not listed — *see* Accessory
ossicles, auditory Q16.3
ovary Q50.31
oviduct Q50.6
pulmonary, pulmonic cusps Q22.3

Supernumerary — *continued*
rib Q76.6
    cervical or first (syndrome) Q76.5
roots (of teeth) K00.2
spleen Q89.09
tarsal bones Q74.2
teeth K00.1
testis Q55.29
thumb Q69.1
toe Q69.2
uterus Q51.2
vagina Q52.1 ☑
vertebra Q76.49
Supervision (of)
contraceptive — *see* Prescription, contraceptives
dietary (for) Z71.3
    allergy (food) Z71.3
    colitis Z71.3
    diabetes mellitus Z71.3
    food allergy or intolerance Z71.3
    gastritis Z71.3
    hypercholesterolemia Z71.3
    hypoglycemia Z71.3
    intolerance (food) Z71.3
    obesity Z71.3
    specified NEC Z71.3
healthy infant or child Z76.2
    foundling Z76.1
high-risk pregnancy — *see* Pregnancy, complicated by, high, risk
lactation Z39.1
pregnancy — *see* Pregnancy, supervision of
Supplemental teeth K00.1
Suppression
binocular vision H53.34
lactation O92.5
menstruation N94.89
ovarian secretion E28.39
renal N28.9
urine, urinary secretion R34
Suppuration, suppurative (*see also* condition)
accessory sinus (chronic) — *see* Sinusitis
adrenal gland
antrum (chronic) — *see* Sinusitis, maxillary
bladder — *see* Cystitis
brain G06.0
    sequelae G09
breast N61
    puerperal, postpartum or gestational — *see* Mastitis, obstetric, purulent
dental periosteum M27.3
ear (middle) (*see also* Otitis, media)
    external NEC — *see* Otitis, externa, infective
    internal — *see* subcategory H83.0 ☑
ethmoidal (chronic) (sinus) — *see* Sinusitis, ethmoidal
fallopian tube — *see* Salpingo-oophoritis
frontal (chronic) (sinus) — *see* Sinusitis, frontal
gallbladder (acute) K81.0
gum K05.20
    generalized K05.22
    localized K05.21
intracranial G06.0
joint — *see* Arthritis, pyogenic or pyemic
labyrinthine — *see* subcategory H83.0 ☑
lung — *see* Abscess, lung
mammary gland N61
    puerperal, postpartum O91.12
        associated with lactation O91.13
maxilla, maxillary M27.2
    sinus (chronic) — *see* Sinusitis, maxillary
muscle — *see* Myositis, infective
nasal sinus (chronic) — *see* Sinusitis
pancreas, acute K85.8
parotid gland — *see* Sialoadenitis
pelvis, pelvic
    female — *see* Disease, pelvis, inflammatory
    male K65.0
pericranial — *see* Osteomyelitis
salivary duct or gland (any) — *see* Sialoadenitis
sinus (accessory) (chronic) (nasal) — *see* Sinusitis
sphenoidal sinus (chronic) — *see* Sinusitis, sphenoidal
thymus (gland) E32.1
thyroid (gland) E06.0
tonsil — *see* Tonsillitis
uterus — *see* Endometritis
Supraeruption of tooth (teeth) M26.34

Supraglottitis J04.30
with obstruction J04.31
Suprarenal (gland) — *see* condition
Suprascapular nerve — *see* condition
Suprasellar — *see* condition
Surfer's knots or nodules S89.8- ☑
Surgical
emphysema T81.82 ☑
procedures, complication or misadventure — *see* Complications, surgical procedures
shock T81.10 ☑
Surveillance (of) (for) (*see also* Observation)
alcohol abuse Z71.41
contraceptive — *see* Prescription, contraceptives
dietary Z71.3
drug abuse Z71.51
Susceptibility to disease, genetic Z15.89
malignant neoplasm Z15.09
    breast Z15.01
    endometrium Z15.04
    ovary Z15.02
    prostate Z15.03
    specified NEC Z15.09
multiple endocrine neoplasia Z15.81
Suspected condition, ruled out (*see also* Observation, suspected)
amniotic cavity and membrane Z03.71
cervical shortening Z03.75
fetal anomaly Z03.73
fetal growth Z03.74
maternal and fetal conditions NEC Z03.79
oligohydramnios Z03.71
placental problem Z03.72
polyhydramnios Z03.71
Suspended uterus
in pregnancy or childbirth — *see* Pregnancy, complicated by, abnormal uterus
Sutton's nevus D22.9
Suture
burst (in operation wound) T81.31 ☑
    external operation wound T81.31 ☑
    internal operation wound T81.32 ☑
inadvertently left in operation wound — *see* Foreign body, accidentally left during a procedure
removal Z48.02
Swab inadvertently left in operation wound — *see* Foreign body, accidentally left during a procedure
Swallowed, swallowing
difficulty — *see* Dysphagia
foreign body — *see* Foreign body, alimentary tract
Swan-neck deformity (finger) — *see* Deformity, finger, swan-neck
Swearing, compulsive F42
in Gilles de la Tourette's syndrome F95.2
Sweat, sweats
fetid L75.0
night R61
Sweating, excessive R61
Sweeley-Klionsky disease E75.21
Sweet's disease or dermatosis L98.2
Swelling (of) R60.9
abdomen, abdominal (not referable to any particular organ) — *see* Mass, abdominal
ankle — *see* Effusion, joint, ankle
arm M79.89
    forearm M79.89
breast N63
Calabar B74.3
cervical gland R59.0
chest, localized R22.2
ear H93.8- ☑
extremity (lower) (upper) — *see* Disorder, soft tissue, specified type NEC
finger M79.89
foot M79.89
glands R59.9
    generalized R59.1
    localized R59.0
hand M79.89
head (localized) R22.0
inflammatory — *see* Inflammation
intra-abdominal — *see* Mass, abdominal
joint — *see* Effusion, joint
leg M79.89
    lower M79.89
limb — *see* Disorder, soft tissue, specified type NEC

Swelling — *continued*
  localized (skin) R22.9
    chest R22.2
    head R22.0
    limb
      lower — *see* Mass, localized, limb, lower
      upper — *see* Mass, localized, limb, upper
    neck R22.1
    trunk R22.2
  neck (localized) R22.1
  pelvic — *see* Mass, abdominal
  scrotum N50.8
  splenic — *see* Splenomegaly
  testis N50.8
  toe M79.89
  umbilical R19.09
  wandering, due to Gnathostoma (spinigerum) B83.1
  white — *see* Tuberculosis, arthritis
Swift (-Feer) **disease**
  overdose or wrong substance given or taken — *see* Table of Drugs and Chemicals, by drug, poisoning
Swimmer's
  cramp T75.1 ☑
  ear H60.33- ☑
  itch B65.3
Swimming in the head R42
Swollen — *see* Swelling
Swyer syndrome Q99.1
Sycosis L73.8
  barbae (not parasitic) L73.8
  contagiosa (mycotic) B35.0
  lupoides L73.8
  mycotic B35.0
  parasitic B35.0
  vulgaris L73.8
Sydenham's chorea — *see* Chorea, Sydenham's
Sylvatic yellow fever A95.0
Sylvest's disease B33.0
Symblepharon H11.23- ☑
  congenital Q10.3
Symond's syndrome G93.2
Sympathetic — *see* condition
Sympatheticotonia G90.8
Sympathicoblastoma
  specified site — *see* Neoplasm, malignant, by site
  unspecified site C74.90
Sympathogonioma — *see* Sympathicoblastoma
Symphalangy (fingers) (toes) Q70.9
Symptoms NEC R68.89
  breast NEC N64.59
  development NEC R63.8
  factitious, self-induced — *see* Disorder, factitious
  genital organs, female R10.2
  involving
    abdomen NEC R19.8
    appearance NEC R46.89
    awareness R41.9
      altered mental status R41.82
      amnesia — *see* Amnesia
      borderline intellectual functioning R41.83
      coma — *see* Coma
      disorientation R41.0
      neurologic neglect syndrome R41.4
      senile cognitive decline R41.81
      specified symptom NEC R41.89
    behavior NEC R46.89
    cardiovascular system NEC R09.89
    chest NEC R09.89
    circulatory system NEC R09.89
    cognitive functions R41.9
      altered mental status R41.82
      amnesia — *see* Amnesia
      borderline intellectual functioning R41.83
      coma — *see* Coma
      disorientation R41.0
      neurologic neglect syndrome R41.4
      senile cognitive decline R41.81
      specified symptom NEC R41.89
    development NEC R62.50
    digestive system NEC R19.8
    emotional state NEC R45.89
      emotional lability R45.86
    food and fluid intake R63.8
    general perceptions and sensations R44.9
      specified NEC R44.8
    musculoskeletal system R29.91

Symptoms — *continued*
  involving — *continued*
    musculoskeletal system R29.91
      specified NEC R29.898
    nervous system R29.90
      specified NEC R29.818
    pelvis NEC R19.8
    respiratory system NEC R09.89
    skin and integument R23.9
    urinary system R39.9
  menopausal N95.1
  metabolism NEC R63.8
  neurotic F48.8
  of infancy R68.19
  pelvis NEC, female R10.2
  skin and integument NEC R23.9
  subcutaneous tissue NEC R23.9
Sympus Q74.2
Syncephalus Q89.4
Synchondrosis
  abnormal (congenital) Q78.8
  ischiopubic M91.0
Synchysis (scintillans) (senile) (vitreous body) H43.89
Syncope (near) (pre-) R55
  anginosa I20.8
  bradycardia R00.1
  cardiac R55
  carotid sinus G90.01
  due to spinal (lumbar) puncture G97.1
  heart R55
  heat T67.1 ☑
  laryngeal R05
  psychogenic F48.8
  tussive R05
  vasoconstriction R55
  vasodepressor R55
  vasomotor R55
  vasovagal R55
Syndactylism, syndactyly Q70.9
  complex (with synostosis)
    fingers Q70.0- ☑
    toes Q70.2- ☑
  simple (without synostosis)
    fingers Q70.1- ☑
    toes Q70.3- ☑
Syndrome (*see also* Disease)
  48,XXXX Q97.1
  49,XXXXX Q97.1
  5q minus NOS D46.C (*following* D46.2)
  abdominal
    acute R10.0
    muscle deficiency Q79.4
  abnormal innervation H02.519
    left H02.516
      lower H02.515
      upper H02.514
    right H02.513
      lower H02.512
      upper H02.511
  abstinence, neonatal P96.1
  acid pulmonary aspiration, obstetric O74.0
  acquired immunodeficiency — *see* Human, immunodeficiency virus (HIV) disease
  acute abdominal R10.0
  acute respiratory distress (adult) (child) J80
  Adair-Dighton Q78.0
  Adams-Stokes (-Morgagni) I45.9
  adiposogenital E23.6
  adrenal
    hemorrhage (meningococcal) A39.1
    meningococcic A39.1
  adrenocortical — *see* Cushing's, syndrome
  adrenogenital E25.9
    congenital, associated with enzyme deficiency E25.0
  afferent loop NEC K91.89
  Alagille's Q44.7
  alcohol withdrawal (without convulsions) — *see* Dependence, alcohol, with, withdrawal
  Alder's D72.0
  Aldrich (-Wiskott) D82.0
  alien hand R41.4
  Alport Q87.81
  alveolar hypoventilation E66.2
  alveolocapillary block J84.10
  amnesic, amnestic (confabulatory) (due to) — *see* Disorder, amnesic
  amyostatic (Wilson's disease) E83.01

Syndrome — *continued*
  androgen insensitivity E34.50
    complete E34.51
    partial E34.52
  androgen resistance (*see also* Syndrome, androgen insensitivity) E34.50
  Angelman Q93.5
  anginal — *see* Angina
  ankyloglossia superior Q38.1
  anterior
    chest wall R07.89
    cord G83.82
    spinal artery G95.19
      compression M47.019
        cervical region M47.012
        cervicothoracic region M47.013
        lumbar region M47.016
        occipito-atlanto-axial region M47.011
        thoracic region M47.014
        thoracolumbar region M47.015
    tibial M76.81- ☑
  antibody deficiency D80.9
    agammaglobulinemic D80.1
      hereditary D80.0
    congenital D80.0
    hypogammaglobulinemic D80.1
      hereditary D80.0
  anticardiolipin (-antibody) D68.61
  antiphospholipid (-antibody) D68.61
  aortic
    arch M31.4
    bifurcation I74.09
  aortomesenteric duodenum occlusion K31.5
  apical ballooning (transient left ventricular) I51.81
  arcuate ligament I77.4
  argentaffin, argintaffinoma E34.0
  Arnold-Chiari — *see* Arnold-Chiari disease
  Arrillaga-Ayerza I27.0
  Asherman's N85.6
  aspiration, of newborn — *see* Aspiration, by substance, with pneumonia
    meconium P24.01
  ataxia-telangiectasia G11.3
  auriculotemporal G50.8
  autoerythrocyte sensitization (Gardner-Diamond) D69.2
  autoimmune lymphoproliferative [ALPS] D89.82
  autoimmune polyglandular E31.0
  autosomal — *see* Abnormal, autosomes
  Avellis' G46.8
  Ayerza (-Arrillaga) I27.0
  Babinski-Nageotte G83.89
  Bakwin-Krida Q79.8
  bare lymphocyte D81.6
  Barré-Guillain G61.0
  Barré-Liéou M53.0
  Barrett's — *see* Barrett's, esophagus
  Barsony-Polgar K22.4
  Bársony-Teschendorf K22.4
  Barth E78.71
  Bartter's E26.81
  basal cell nevus Q87.89
  Basedow's E05.00
    with thyroid storm E05.01
  basilar artery G45.0
  Batten-Steinert G71.11
  battered
    baby or child — *see* Maltreatment, child, physical abuse
    spouse — *see* Maltreatment, adult, physical abuse
  Beals Q87.40
  Beau's I51.5
  Beck's I65.8
  Benedikt's G46.3
  Béquez César (-Steinbrinck-Chédiak-Higashi) E70.330
  Bernhardt-Roth — *see* Meralgia paresthetica
  Bernheim's I50.9
  big spleen D73.1
  bilateral polycystic ovarian E28.2
  Bing-Horton's — *see* Horton's headache
  Birt-Hogg-Dube syndrome Q87.89
  Björck (-Thorsen) E34.0
  black
    lung J60
    widow spider bite — *see* Toxicity, venom, spider, black widow
  Blackfan-Diamond D61.01

☑ **Additional Character Required** — Refer to the Tabular List for Character Selection   ⬇ Subterms under main terms may continue to next column or page

Syndrome — *continued*
- blind loop K90.2
  - congenital Q43.8
  - postsurgical K91.2
- blue sclera Q78.0
- blue toe I75.02- ☑
- Boder-Sedgewick G11.3
- Boerhaave's K22.3
- Borjeson Forssman Lehmann Q89.8
- Bouillaud's I01.9
- Bourneville (-Pringle) Q85.1
- Bouveret (-Hoffman) I47.9
- brachial plexus G54.0
- bradycardia-tachycardia I49.5
- brain (nonpsychotic) F09
  - with psychosis, psychotic reaction F09
  - acute or subacute — *see* Delirium
  - congenital — *see* Disability, intellectual
  - organic F09
    - post-traumatic (nonpsychotic) F07.81
      - psychotic F09
  - personality change F07.0
  - postcontusional F07.81
  - post-traumatic, nonpsychotic F07.81
  - psycho-organic F09
  - psychotic F06.8
- brain stem stroke G46.3
- Brandt's (acrodermatitis enteropathica) E83.2
- broad ligament laceration N83.8
- Brock's J98.11
- bronze baby P83.8
- Brown-Sequard G83.81
- bubbly lung P27.0
- Buchem's M85.2
- Budd-Chiari I82.0
- bulbar (progressive) G12.22
- Bürger-Grütz E78.3
- Burke's K86.8
- Burnett's (milk-alkali) E83.52
- burning feet E53.9
- Bywaters' T79.5 ☑
- Call-Fleming I67.841
- carbohydrate-deficient glycoprotein (CDGS) E77.8
- carcinogenic thrombophlebitis I82.1
- carcinoid E34.0
- cardiac asthma I50.1
- cardiacos negros I27.0
- cardiofaciocutaneous Q87.89
- cardiopulmonary-obesity E66.2
- cardiorenal — *see* Hypertension, cardiorenal
- cardiorespiratory distress (idiopathic), newborn P22.0
- cardiovascular renal — *see* Hypertension, cardiorenal
- carotid
  - artery (hemispheric) (internal) G45.1
  - body G90.01
  - sinus G90.01
- carpal tunnel G56.0- ☑
- Cassidy (-Scholte) E34.0
- cat cry Q93.4
- cat eye Q92.8
- cauda equina G83.4
- causalgia — *see* Causalgia
- celiac K90.0
  - artery compression I77.4
  - axis I77.4
- central pain G89.0
- cerebellar
  - hereditary G11.9
  - stroke G46.4
- cerebellomedullary malformation — *see* Spina bifida
- cerebral
  - artery
    - anterior G46.1
    - middle G46.0
    - posterior G46.2
  - gigantism E22.0
- cervical (root) M53.1
  - disc — *see* Disorder, disc, cervical, with neuritis
  - fusion Q76.1
  - posterior, sympathicus M53.0
  - rib Q76.5
  - sympathetic paralysis G90.2
- cervicobrachial (diffuse) M53.1
- cervicocranial M53.0
- cervicodorsal outlet G54.2
- cervicothoracic outlet G54.0
- Céstan (-Raymond) I65.8

Syndrome — *continued*
- Charcot's (angina cruris) (intermittent claudication) I73.9
- Charcot-Weiss-Baker G90.09
- CHARGE Q89.8
- Chédiak-Higashi (-Steinbrinck) E70.330
- chest wall R07.1
- Chiari's (hepatic vein thrombosis) I82.0
- Chilaiditi's Q43.3
- child maltreatment — *see* Maltreatment, child
- chondrocostal junction M94.0
- chondroectodermal dysplasia Q77.6
- chromosome 4 short arm deletion Q93.3
- chromosome 5 short arm deletion Q93.4
- chronic
  - pain G89.4
    - personality F68.8
- Clarke-Hadfield K86.8
- Clerambault's automatism G93.89
- Clouston's (hidrotic ectodermal dysplasia) Q82.4
- clumsiness, clumsy child F82
- cluster headache G44.009
  - intractable G44.001
  - not intractable G44.009
- Coffin-Lowry Q89.8
- cold injury (newborn) P80.0
- combined immunity deficiency D81.9
- compartment (deep) (posterior) (traumatic) T79.A0 ☑ (*following* T79.7)
  - abdomen T79.A3 ☑ (*following* T79.7)
  - lower extremity (hip, buttock, thigh, leg, foot, toes) T79.A2 ☑ (*following* T79.7)
  - nontraumatic
    - abdomen M79.A3 (*following* M79.7)
    - lower extremity (hip, buttock, thigh, leg, foot, toes) M79.A2- ☑ (*following* M79.7)
    - specified site NEC M79.A9 (*following* M79.7)
    - upper extremity (shoulder, arm, forearm, wrist, hand, fingers) M79.A1- ☑ (*following* M79.7)
  - postprocedural — *see* Syndrome, compartment, nontraumatic
  - specified site NEC T79.A9 ☑ (*following* T79.7)
  - upper extremity (shoulder, arm, forearm, wrist, hand, fingers) T79.A1 ☑ (*following* T79.7)
- complex regional pain — *see* Syndrome, pain, complex regional
- compression T79.5 ☑
  - anterior spinal — *see* Syndrome, anterior, spinal artery, compression
  - cauda equina G83.4
  - celiac artery I77.4
  - vertebral artery M47.029
    - cervical region M47.022
    - occipito-atlanto-axial region M47.021
- concussion F07.81
- congenital
  - affecting multiple systems NEC Q87.89
  - central alveolar hypoventilation G47.35
  - facial diplegia Q87.0
  - muscular hypertrophy-cerebral Q87.89
  - oculo-auriculovertebral Q87.0
  - oculofacial diplegia (Moebius) Q87.0
  - rubella (manifest) P35.0
- congestion-fibrosis (pelvic), female N94.89
- congestive dysmenorrhea N94.6
- connective tissue M35.9
  - overlap NEC M35.1
- Conn's E26.01
- conus medullaris G95.81
- cord
  - anterior G83.82
  - posterior G83.83
- coronary
  - acute NEC I24.9
  - insufficiency or intermediate I20.0
  - slow flow I20.8
- Costen's (complex) M26.69
- costochondral junction M94.0
- costoclavicular G54.0
- costovertebral E22.0
- Cowden Q85.8
- craniovertebral M53.0
- Creutzfeldt-Jakob — *see* Creutzfeldt-Jakob disease or syndrome
- crib death R99
- cricopharyngeal — *see* Dysphagia
- cri-du-chat Q93.4

Syndrome — *continued*
- croup J05.0
- CRPS I — *see* Syndrome, pain, complex regional I
- crush T79.5 ☑
- cryptophthalmos Q87.0
- cubital tunnel — *see* Lesion, nerve, ulnar
- Curschmann (-Batten) (-Steinert) G71.11
- Cushing's E24.9
  - alcohol-induced E24.4
  - drug-induced E24.2
  - due to
    - alcohol
    - drugs E24.2
    - ectopic ACTH E24.3
    - overproduction of pituitary ACTH E24.0
  - overdose or wrong substance given or taken — *see* Table of Drugs and Chemicals, by drug, poisoning
  - pituitary-dependent E24.0
  - specified type NEC E24.8
- cystic duct stump K91.5
- Dana-Putnam D51.0
- Danbolt (-Cross) (acrodermatitis enteropathica) E83.2
- Dandy-Walker Q03.1
  - with spina bifida Q07.01
- Danlos' Q79.8
- De Quervain E34.51
- de Toni-Fanconi (-Debré) E72.09
  - with cystinosis E72.04
- defibrination (*see also* Fibrinolysis)
  - with
    - antepartum hemorrhage — *see* Hemorrhage, antepartum, with coagulation defect
    - intrapartum hemorrhage — *see* Hemorrhage, complicating, delivery
  - newborn P60
  - postpartum O72.3
- Degos' I77.89
- Déjérine-Roussy G89.0
- delayed sleep phase G47.21
- demyelinating G37.9
- dependence — *see* F10-F19 with fourth character .2
- depersonalization (-derealization) F48.1
- di George's D82.1
- diabetes mellitus in newborn infant P70.2
- diabetes mellitus-hypertension-nephrosis — *see* Diabetes, nephrosis
- diabetes-nephrosis — *see* Diabetes, nephrosis
- diabetic amyotrophy — *see* Diabetes, amyotrophy
- Diamond-Blackfan D61.01
- Diamond-Gardener D69.2
- DIC (diffuse or disseminated intravascular coagulopathy) D65
- Dighton's Q78.0
- disequilibrium E87.8
- Döhle body-panmyelopathic D72.0
- dorsolateral medullary G46.4
- double athetosis G80.3
- Down (*see also* Down syndrome) Q90.9
- Dresbach's (elliptocytosis) D58.1
- Dressler's (postmyocardial infarction) I24.1
  - postcardiotomy I97.0
- drug withdrawal, infant of dependent mother P96.1
- dry eye H04.12- ☑
- due to abnormality
  - chromosomal Q99.9
  - sex
    - female phenotype Q97.9
    - male phenotype Q98.9
  - specified NEC Q99.8
- dumping (postgastrectomy) K91.1
  - nonsurgical K31.89
- Dupré's (meningism) R29.1
- dysmetabolic X E88.81
- dyspraxia, developmental F82
- Eagle-Barrett Q79.4
- Eaton-Lambert — *see* Syndrome, Lambert-Eaton
- Ebstein's Q22.5
- ectopic ACTH E24.3
- eczema-thrombocytopenia D82.0
- Eddowes' Q78.0
- effort (psychogenic) F45.8
- Ehlers-Danlos Q79.6
- Eisenmenger's I27.89
- Ekman's Q78.0
- electric feet E53.8
- Ellis van Creveld Q77.6
- empty nest Z60.0

▽ Subterms under main terms may continue to next column or page   ☑ Additional Character Required — Refer to the Tabular List for Character Selection   291

Syndrome — *continued*
- endocrine-hypertensive E27.Ø
- entrapment — *see* Neuropathy, entrapment
- eosinophilia-myalgia M35.8
- epileptic (*see also* Epilepsy, by type)
  - absence G4Ø.AØ9 (*following* G4Ø.3)
    - intractable G4Ø.A19 (*following* G4Ø.3)
      - with status epilepticus G4Ø.A11 (*following* G4Ø.3)
      - without status epilepticus G4Ø.A19 (*following* G4Ø.3)
    - not intractable G4Ø.AØ9 (*following* G4Ø.3)
      - with status epilepticus G4Ø.AØ1 (*following* G4Ø.3)
      - without status epilepticus G4Ø.AØ9 (*following* G4Ø.3)
- Erdheim-Chester (ECD) E88.89
- Erdheim's E22.Ø
- erythrocyte fragmentation D59.4
- Evans D69.41
- exhaustion F48.8
- extrapyramidal G25.9
  - specified NEC G25.89
- eye retraction — *see* Strabismus
- eyelid-malar-mandible Q87.Ø
- Faber's D5Ø.9
- facial pain, paroxysmal G5Ø.Ø
- Fallot's Q21.3
- familial eczema-thrombocytopenia (Wiskott-Aldrich) D82.Ø
- Fanconi (-de Toni) (-Debré) E72.Ø9
  - with cystinosis E72.Ø4
- Fanconi's (anemia) (congenital pancytopenia) D61.Ø9
- fatigue
  - chronic R53.82
  - psychogenic F48.8
- faulty bowel habit K59.3
- Feil-Klippel (brevicollis) Q76.1
- Felty's — *see* Felty's syndrome
- fertile eunuch E23.Ø
- fetal
  - alcohol (dysmorphic) Q86.Ø
  - hydantoin Q86.1
- Fiedler's I4Ø.1
- first arch Q87.Ø
- fish odor E72.8
- Fisher's G61.Ø
- Fitzhugh-Curtis
  - due to
    - Chlamydia trachomatis A74.81
    - Neisseria gonorrhorea (gonococcal peritonitis) A54.85
- Fitz's K85.8
- Flajani (-Basedow) EØ5.ØØ
  - with thyroid storm EØ5.Ø1
- flatback — *see* Flatback syndrome
- floppy
  - baby P94.2
  - iris (intraoeprative) (IFIS) H21.81
  - mitral valve I34.1
- flush E34.Ø
- Foix-Alajouanine G95.19
- Fong's Q79.8
- foramen magnum G93.5
- Foster-Kennedy H47.14- ☑
- Foville's (peduncular) G46.3
- fragile X Q99.2
- Franceschetti Q75.4
- Frey's
  - auriculotemporal G5Ø.8
  - hyperhidrosis L74.52
- Friderichsen-Waterhouse A39.1
- Froin's G95.89
- frontal lobe FØ7.Ø
- Fukuhara E88.49
- functional
  - bowel K59.9
  - prepubertal castrate E29.1
- Gaisböck's D75.1
- ganglion (basal ganglia brain) G25.9
  - geniculi G51.1
- Gardner-Diamond D69.2
- gastroesophageal
  - junction K22.Ø
  - laceration-hemorrhage K22.6
- gastrojejunal loop obstruction K91.89
- Gee-Herter-Heubner K9Ø.Ø

Syndrome — *continued*
- Gelineau's G47.419
  - with cataplexy G47.411
- genito-anorectal A55
- Gerstmann-Sträussler-Scheinker (GSS) A81.82
- Gianotti-Crosti L44.4
- giant platelet (Bernard-Soulier) D69.1
- Gilles de la Tourette's F95.2
- goiter-deafness EØ7.1
- Goldberg Q89.8
- Goldberg-Maxwell E34.51
- Good's D83.8
- Gopalan' (burning feet) E53.8
- Gorlin's Q87.89
- Gougerot-Blum L81.7
- Gouley's I31.1
- Gower's R55
- gray or grey (newborn) P93.Ø
  - platelet D69.1
- Gubler-Millard G46.3
- Guillain-Barré (-Strohl) G61.Ø
- gustatory sweating G5Ø.8
- Hadfield-Clarke K86.8
- hair tourniquet — *see* Constriction, external, by site
- Hamman's J98.19
- hand-foot L27.1
- hand-shoulder G9Ø.8
- hantavirus (cardio)-pulmonary (HPS) (HCPS) B33.4
- happy puppet Q93.5
- Harada's H3Ø.81- ☑
- Hayem-Faber D5Ø.9
- headache NEC G44.89
  - complicated NEC G44.59
- Heberden's I2Ø.8
- Hedinger's E34.Ø
- Hegglin's D72.Ø
- HELLP (hemolysis, elevated liver enzymes and low platelet count) O14.2- ☑
- hemolytic-uremic D59.3
- hemophagocytic, infection-associated D76.2
- Henoch-Schönlein D69.Ø
- hepatic flexure K59.8
- hepatopulmonary K76.81
- hepatorenal K76.7
  - following delivery O9Ø.4
  - postoperative or postprocedural K91.83
  - postpartum, puerperal O9Ø.4
- hepatourologic K76.7
- Herter (-Gee) (nontropical sprue) K9Ø.Ø
- Heubner-Herter K9Ø.Ø
- Heyd's K76.7
- Hilger's G9Ø.Ø9
- histamine-like (fish poisoning) — *see* Poisoning, fish
- histiocytic D76.3
- histiocytosis NEC D76.3
- HIV infection, acute B2Ø
- Hoffmann-Werdnig G12.Ø
- Hollander-Simons E88.1
- Hoppe-Goldflam G7Ø.ØØ
  - with exacerbation (acute) G7Ø.Ø1
  - in crisis G7Ø.Ø1
- Horner's G9Ø.2
- hungry bone E83.81
- hunterian glossitis D51.Ø
- Hutchinson's triad A5Ø.53
- hyperabduction G54.Ø
- hyperammonemia-hyperornithinemia-homocitrulline-mia E72.4
- hypereosinophilic (idiopathic) D72.1
- hyperimmunoglobulin E (IgE) D82.4
- hyperkalemic E87.5
- hyperkinetic — *see* Hyperkinesia
- hypermobility M35.7
- hypernatremia E87.Ø
- hyperosmolarity E87.Ø
- hyperperfusion G97.82
- hypersplenic D73.1
- hypertransfusion, newborn P61.1
- hyperventilation F45.8
- hyperviscosity (of serum)
  - polycythemic D75.1
  - sclerothymic D58.8
- hypoglycemic (familial) (neonatal) E16.2
- hypokalemic E87.6
- hyponatremic E87.1
- hypopituitarism E23.Ø
- hypoplastic left-heart Q23.4
- hypopotassemia E87.6

Syndrome — *continued*
- hyposmolality E87.1
- hypotension, maternal O26.5- ☑
- hypothenar hammer I73.89
- ICF (intravascular coagulation-fibrinolysis) D65
- idiopathic
  - cardiorespiratory distress, newborn P22.Ø
  - nephrotic (infantile) NØ4.9
- iliotibial band M76.3- ☑
- immobility, immobilization (paraplegic) M62.3
- immune reconstitution D89.3
- immune reconstitution inflammatory [IRIS] D89.3
- immunity deficiency, combined D81.9
- immunodeficiency
  - acquired — *see* Human, immunodeficiency virus (HIV) disease
  - combined D81.9
- impending coronary I2Ø.Ø
- impingement, shoulder M75.4- ☑
- inappropriate secretion of antidiuretic hormone E22.2
- infant
  - gestational diabetes P7Ø.Ø
  - of diabetic mother P7Ø.1
- infantilism (pituitary) E23.Ø
- inferior vena cava I87.1
- inspissated bile (newborn) P59.1
- institutional (childhood) F94.2
- insufficient sleep F51.12
- intermediate coronary (artery) I2Ø.Ø
- interspinous ligament — *see* Spondylopathy, specified NEC
- intestinal
  - carcinoid E34.Ø
  - knot K56.2
- intravascular coagulation-fibrinolysis (ICF) D65
- iodine-deficiency, congenital EØØ.9
  - type
    - mixed EØØ.2
    - myxedematous EØØ.1
    - neurological EØØ.Ø
- IRDS (idiopathic respiratory distress, newborn) P22.Ø
- irritable
  - bowel K58.9
    - with diarrhea K58.Ø
    - psychogenic F45.8
  - heart (psychogenic) F45.8
  - weakness F48.8
- ischemic bowel (transient) K55.9
  - chronic K55.1
  - due to mesenteric artery insufficiency K55.1
- IVC (intravascular coagulopathy) D65
- Ivemark's Q89.Ø1
- Jaccoud's — *see* Arthropathy, postrheumatic, chronic
- Jackson's G83.89
- Jakob-Creutzfeldt — *see* Creutzfeldt-Jakob disease or syndrome
- jaw-winking QØ7.8
- Jervell-Lange-Nielsen I45.81
- jet lag G47.25
- Job's D71
- Joseph-Diamond-Blackfan D61.Ø1
- jugular foramen G52.7
- Kabuki Q89.8
- Kanner's (autism) F84.Ø
- Kartagener's Q89.3
- Kelly's D5Ø.1
- Kimmelstiel-Wilson — *see* Diabetes, specified type, with Kimmelstiel-Wilson disease
- Klein (e)-Levine G47.13
- Klippel-Feil (brevicollis) Q76.1
- Köhler-Pellegrini-Steida — *see* Bursitis, tibial collateral
- König's K59.8
- Korsakoff (-Wernicke) (nonalcoholic) FØ4
  - alcoholic F1Ø.26
- Kostmann's D7Ø.Ø
- Krabbe's congenital muscle hypoplasia Q79.8
- labyrinthine — *see* subcategory H83.2 ☑
- lacunar NEC G46.7
- Lambert-Eaton G7Ø.8Ø
  - in
    - neoplastic disease G73.1
    - specified disease NEC G7Ø.81
- Landau-Kleffner — *see* Epilepsy, specified NEC
- Larsen's Q74.8
- lateral
  - cutaneous nerve of thigh G57.1- ☑
  - medullary G46.4
- Launois' E22.Ø

☑ Additional Character Required — Refer to the Tabular List for Character Selection   ▽ Subterms under main terms may continue to next column or page

Syndrome — continued
lazy
  leukocyte D70.8
  posture M62.3
Lemiere I80.8
Lennox-Gastaut G40.812
  intractable G40.814
    with status epilepticus G40.813
    without status epilepticus G40.814
  not intractable G40.812
    with status epilepticus G40.811
    without status epilepticus G40.812
lenticular, progressive E83.01
Leopold-Levi's E05.90
Lev's I44.2
Lichtheim's D51.0
Li-Fraumeni Z15.01
Lightwood's N25.89
Lignac (de Toni) (-Fanconi) (-Debré) E72.09
  with cystinosis E72.04
Likoff's I20.8
limbic epilepsy personality F07.0
liver-kidney K76.7
lobotomy F07.0
Loffler's J82
long arm 18 or 21 deletion Q93.89
long QT I45.81
Louis-Barré G11.3
low
  atmospheric pressure T70.29 ☑
  back M54.5
  output (cardiac) I50.9
lower radicular, newborn (birth injury) P14.8
Luetscher's (dehydration) E86.0
Lupus anticoagulant D68.62
Lutembacher's Q21.1
macrophage activation D76.1
  due to infection D76.2
magnesium-deficiency R29.0
Mal de Debarquement R42
malabsorption K90.9
  postsurgical K91.2
malformation, congenital, due to
  alcohol Q86.0
  exogenous cause NEC Q86.8
  hydantoin Q86.1
  warfarin Q86.2
malignant
  carcinoid E34.0
  neuroleptic G21.0
Mallory-Weiss K22.6
mandibulofacial dysostosis Q75.4
manic-depressive — see Disorder, bipolar, affective
maple-syrup-urine E71.0
Marable's I77.4
Marfan's Q87.40
  with
    cardiovascular manifestations Q87.418
      aortic dilation Q87.410
    ocular manifestations Q87.42
    skeletal manifestations Q87.43
Marie's (acromegaly) E22.0
maternal hypotension — see Syndrome, hypotension, maternal
May (-Hegglin) D72.0
McArdle (-Schmidt) (-Pearson) E74.04
McQuarrie's E16.2
meconium plug (newborn) P76.0
median arcuate ligament I77.4
Meekeren-Ehlers-Danlos Q79.6
megavitamin-B6 E67.2
Meige G24.4
MELAS E88.41
Mendelson's O74.0
MERRF (myoclonic epilepsy associated with ragged-red fibers) E88.42
mesenteric
  artery (superior) K55.1
  vascular insufficiency K55.1
metabolic E88.81
metastatic carcinoid E34.0
micrognathia-glossoptosis Q87.0
midbrain NEC G93.89
middle lobe (lung) J98.19
middle radicular G54.0
migraine (see also Migraine) G43.909
Mikulicz' K11.8
milk-alkali E83.52

Syndrome — continued
Millard-Gubler G46.3
Miller-Dieker Q93.88
Miller-Fisher G61.0
Minkowski-Chauffard D58.0
Mirizzi's K83.1
MNGIE (Mitochondrial Neurogastrointestinal Encephalopathy) E88.49
Möbius, ophthalmoplegic migraine — see Migraine, ophthalmoplegic
monofixation H50.42
Morel-Moore M85.2
Morel-Morgagni M85.2
Morgagni (-Morel) (-Stewart) M85.2
Morgagni-Adams-Stokes I45.9
Mounier-Kuhn Q32.4
  with bronchiectasis J47.9
    with
      exacerbation (acute) J47.1
      lower respiratory infection J47.0
  acquired J98.09
    with bronchiectasis J47.9
      with
        exacerbation (acute) J47.1
        lower respiratory infection J47.0
mucocutaneous lymph node (acute febrile) (MCLS) M30.3
multiple endocrine neoplasia (MEN) — see Neoplasia, endocrine, multiple (MEN)
multiple operations — see Disorder, factitious
myasthenic G70.9
  in
    diabetes mellitus — see Diabetes, amyotrophy
    endocrine disease NEC E34.9 [G73.3]
    neoplastic disease (see also Neoplasm) D49.9 [G73.3]
    thyrotoxicosis (hyperthyroidism) E05.90 [G73.3]
      with thyroid storm E05.91 [G73.3]
myelodysplastic D46.9
  with
    5q deletion D46.C (following D46.2)
    isolated del (5q) chromosomal abnormality D46.C (following D46.2)
  lesions, low grade D46.20
  specified NEC D46.Z (following D46.4)
myelopathic pain G89.0
myeloproliferative (chronic) D47.1
myofascial pain M79.1
Naffziger's G54.0
nail patella Q87.2
NARP (Neuropathy, Ataxia and Retinitis pigmentosa) E88.49
neonatal abstinence P96.1
nephritic (see also Nephritis)
  with edema — see Nephrosis
  acute N00.9
  chronic N03.9
  rapidly progressive N01.9
nephrotic (congenital) (see also Nephrosis) N04.9
  with
    dense deposit disease N04.6
    diffuse
      crescentic glomerulonephritis N04.7
      endocapillary proliferative glomerulonephritis N04.4
      membranous glomerulonephritis N04.2
      mesangial proliferative glomerulonephritis N04.3
      mesangiocapillary glomerulonephritis N04.5
    focal and segmental glomerular lesions N04.1
    minor glomerular abnormality N04.0
    specified morphological changes NEC N04.8
  diabetic — see Diabetes, nephrosis
neurologic neglect R41.4
Nezelof's D81.4
Nonne-Milroy-Meige Q82.0
Nothnagel's vasomotor acroparesthesia I73.89
oculomotor H51.9
ophthalmoplegia-cerebellar ataxia — see Strabismus, paralytic, third nerve
oral-facial-digital Q87.0
organic
  affective F06.30
  amnesic (not alcohol- or drug-induced) F04
  brain F09
  depressive F06.31
  hallucinosis F06.0
  personality F07.0

Syndrome — continued
Ormond's N13.5
oro-facial-digital Q87.0
os trigonum Q68.8
Osler-Weber-Rendu I78.0
osteoporosis-osteomalacia M83.8
Osterreicher-Turner Q79.8
otolith — see subcategory H81.8 ☑
oto-palatal-digital Q87.0
outlet (thoracic) G54.0
ovary
  polycystic E28.2
  resistant E28.39
  sclerocystic E28.2
Owren's D68.2
Paget-Schroetter I82.890
pain (see also Pain)
  complex regional I G90.50
    lower limb G90.52- ☑
    specified site NEC G90.59
    upper limb G90.51- ☑
  complex regional II — see Causalgia
painful
  bruising D69.2
  feet E53.8
  prostate N42.81
paralysis agitans — see Parkinsonism
paralytic G83.9
  specified NEC G83.89
Parinaud's H51.0
parkinsonian — see Parkinsonism
Parkinson's — see Parkinsonism
paroxysmal facial pain G50.0
Parry's E05.00
  with thyroid storm E05.01
Parsonage (-Aldren)-Turner G54.5
patella clunk M25.86- ☑
Paterson (-Brown) (-Kelly) D50.1
pectoral girdle I77.89
pectoralis minor I77.89
Pelger-Huet D72.0
pellagra-cerebellar ataxia-renal aminoaciduria E72.02
pellagroid E52
Pellegrini-Stieda — see Bursitis, tibial collateral
pelvic congestion-fibrosis, female N94.89
penta X Q97.1
peptic ulcer — see Ulcer, peptic
perabduction I77.89
periodic headache, in adults and children — see Headache, periodic syndromes in adults and children
periurethral fibrosis N13.5
phantom limb (without pain) G54.7
  with pain G54.6
pharyngeal pouch D82.1
Pick's (heart) (liver) I31.1
Pickwickian E66.2
PIE (pulmonary infiltration with eosinophilia) J82
pigmentary pallidal degeneration (progressive) G23.0
pineal E34.8
pituitary E22.0
placental transfusion — see Pregnancy, complicated by, placental transfusion syndromes
plantar fascia M72.2
plateau iris (post-iridectomy) (postprocedural) H21.82
Plummer-Vinson D50.1
pluricarential of infancy E40
plurideficiency E40
pluriglandular (compensatory) E31.8
  autoimmune E31.0
pneumatic hammer T75.21 ☑
polyangiitis overlap M30.8
polycarential of infancy E40
polyglandular E31.8
  autoimmune E31.0
polysplenia Q89.09
pontine NEC G93.89
popliteal
  artery entrapment I77.89
  web Q87.89
post chemoembolization — code to associated conditions
postcardiac injury
  postcardiotomy I97.0
  postmyocardial infarction I24.1
postcardiotomy I97.0
postcholecystectomy K91.5
postcommissurotomy I97.0

Syndrome — *continued*
  postconcussional F07.81
  postcontusional F07.81
  postencephalitic F07.89
  posterior
    cervical sympathetic M53.0
    cord G83.83
    fossa compression G93.5
    reversible encephalopathy (PRES) I67.83
  postgastrectomy (dumping) K91.1
  postgastric surgery K91.1
  postinfarction I24.1
  postlaminectomy NEC M96.1
  postleukotomy F07.0
  postmastectomy lymphedema I97.2
  postmyocardial infarction I24.1
  postoperative NEC T81.9 ☑
    blind loop K90.2
  postpartum panhypopituitary (Sheehan) E23.0
  postpolio (myelitic) G14
  postthrombotic I87.009
    with
      inflammation I87.02- ☑
        with ulcer I87.03- ☑
      specified complication NEC I87.09- ☑
      ulcer I87.01- ☑
        with inflammation I87.03- ☑
    asymptomatic I87.00- ☑
  postvagotomy K91.1
  postvalvulotomy I97.0
  postviral NEC G93.3
    fatigue G93.3
  Potain's K31.0
  potassium intoxication E87.5
  precerebral artery (multiple) (bilateral) G45.2
  preinfarction I20.0
  preleukemic D46.9
  premature senility E34.8
  premenstrual dysphoric N94.3
  premenstrual tension N94.3
  Prinzmetal-Massumi R07.1
  prune belly Q79.4
  pseudo -Turner's Q87.1
  pseudocarpal tunnel (sublimis) — *see* Syndrome,
    carpal tunnel
  pseudoparalytica G70.00
    with exacerbation (acute) G70.01
    in crisis G70.01
  psycho-organic (nonpsychotic severity) F07.9
    acute or subacute F05
    depressive type F06.31
    hallucinatory type F06.0
    nonpsychotic severity F07.0
    specified NEC F07.89
  pulmonary
    arteriosclerosis I27.0
    dysmaturity (Wilson-Mikity) P27.0
    hypoperfusion (idiopathic) P22.0
    renal (hemorrhagic) (Goodpasture's) M31.0
  pure
    motor lacunar G46.5
    sensory lacunar G46.6
  Putnam-Dana D51.0
  pyramidopallidonigral G20
  pyriformis — *see* Lesion, nerve, sciatic
  QT interval prolongation I45.81
  radicular NEC — *see* Radiculopathy
    upper limbs, newborn (birth injury) P14.3
  rapid time-zone change G47.25
  Rasmussen G04.81
  Raymond (-Céstan) I65.8
  Raynaud's I73.00
    with gangrene I73.01
  RDS (respiratory distress syndrome, newborn) P22.0
  reactive airways dysfunction J68.3
  Refsum's G60.1
  Reifenstein E34.52
  renal glomerulohyalinosis-diabetic — *see* Diabetes,
    nephrosis
  Rendu-Osler-Weber I78.0
  residual ovary N99.83
  resistant ovary E28.39
  respiratory
    distress
      acute J80
        adult J80
        child J80

Syndrome — *continued*
  respiratory — *continued*
    distress — *continued*
      newborn (idiopathic) (type I) P22.0
        type II P22.1
  restless legs G25.81
  retinoblastoma (familial) C69.2 ☑
  retroperitoneal fibrosis N13.5
  retroviral seroconversion (acute) Z21
  Reye's G93.7
  Richter — *see* Leukemia, chronic lymphocytic, B-cell
    type
  Ridley's I50.1
  right
    heart, hypoplastic Q22.6
    ventricular obstruction — *see* Failure, heart, con-
      gestive
  Romano-Ward (prolonged QT interval) I45.81
  rotator cuff, shoulder (*see also* Tear, rotator cuff)
    M75.10- ☑
  Rotes Quérol — *see* Hyperostosis, ankylosing
  Roth — *see* Meralgia paresthetica
  rubella (congenital) P35.0
  Ruvalcaba-Myhre-Smith E71.440
  Rytand-Lipsitch I44.2
  salt
    depletion E87.1
      due to heat NEC T67.8 ☑
        causing heat exhaustion or prostration
          T67.4 ☑
    low E87.1
  salt-losing N28.89
  Scaglietti-Dagnini E22.0
  scalenus anticus (anterior) G54.0
  scapulocostal — *see* Mononeuropathy, upper limb,
    specified site NEC
  scapuloperoneal G71.0
  schizophrenic, of childhood NEC F84.5
  Schnitzler D47.2
  Scholte's E34.0
  Schroeder's E27.0
  Schüller-Christian C96.5
  Schwachman's — *see* Syndrome, Shwachman's
  Schwartz (-Jampel) G71.13
  Schwartz-Bartter E22.2
  scimitar Q26.8
  sclerocystic ovary E28.2
  Seitelberger's G31.89
  septicemic adrenal hemorrhage A39.1
  seroconversion, retroviral (acute) Z21
  serous meningitis G93.2
  severe acute respiratory (SARS) J12.81
  shaken infant T74.4 ☑
  shock (traumatic) T79.4 ☑
    kidney N17.0
      following crush injury T79.5 ☑
    toxic A48.3
  shock-lung J80
  Shone's — *code to* specific anomalies
  short
    bowel K91.2
    rib Q77.2
  shoulder-hand — *see* Algoneurodystrophy
  Shwachman's D70.4
  sicca — *see* Sicca syndrome
  sick
    cell E87.1
    sinus I49.5
  sick-euthyroid E07.81
  sideropenic D50.1
  Siemens' ectodermal dysplasia Q82.4
  Silfversköld's Q78.9
  Simons' E88.1
  sinus tarsi M25.57- ☑
  sinusitis-bronchiectasis-situs inversus Q89.3
  Sipple's E31.22
  sirenomelia Q87.2
  Slocumb's E27.0
  slow flow, coronary I20.8
  Sluder's G44.89
  Smith-Magenis Q93.88
  Sneddon-Wilkinson L13.1
  Sotos' E22.0
  South African cardiomyopathy I42.8
  spasmodic
    upward movement, eyes H51.8
    winking F95.8
  Spen's I45.9

Syndrome — *continued*
  splenic
    agenesis Q89.01
    flexure K59.8
    neutropenia D73.81
  Spurway's Q78.0
  staphylococcal scalded skin L00
  Stein-Leventhal E28.2
  Stein's E28.2
  Stevens-Johnson syndrome L51.1
    toxic epidermal necrolysis overlap L51.3
  Stewart-Morel M85.2
  Stickler Q89.8
  stiff baby Q89.8
  stiff man G25.82
  Still-Felty — *see* Felty's syndrome
  Stokes (-Adams) I45.9
  stone heart I50.1
  straight back, congenital Q76.49
  subclavian steal G45.8
  subcoracoid-pectoralis minor G54.0
  subcostal nerve compression I77.89
  subphrenic interposition Q43.3
  superior
    cerebellar artery I63.8
    mesenteric artery K55.1
    semi-circular canal dehiscence H83.8X- ☑
    vena cava I87.1
  supine hypotensive (maternal) — *see* Syndrome, hy-
    potension, maternal
  suprarenal cortical E27.0
  supraspinatus (*see also* Tear, rotator cuff) M75.10- ☑
  Susac G93.49
  swallowed blood P78.2
  sweat retention L74.0
  Swyer Q99.1
  Symond's G93.2
  sympathetic
    cervical paralysis G90.2
    pelvic, female N94.89
  systemic inflammatory response (SIRS), of non-infec-
    tious origin (without organ dysfunction) R65.10
    with acute organ dysfunction R65.11
  tachycardia-bradycardia I49.5
  takotsubo I51.81
  TAR (thrombocytopenia with absent radius) Q87.2
  tarsal tunnel G57.5- ☑
  teething K00.7
  tegmental G93.89
  telangiectasic-pigmentation-cataract Q82.8
  temporal pyramidal apex — *see* Otitis, media, suppu-
    rative, acute
  temporomandibular joint-pain-dysfunction M26.62
  Terry's H44.2- ☑
  testicular feminization (*see also* Syndrome, androgen
    insensitivity) E34.51
  thalamic pain (hyperesthetic) G89.0
  thoracic outlet (compression) G54.0
  Thorson-Björck E34.0
  thrombocytopenia with absent radius (TAR) Q87.2
  thyroid-adrenocortical insufficiency E31.0
  tibial
    anterior M76.81- ☑
    posterior M76.82- ☑
  Tietze's M94.0
  time-zone (rapid) G47.25
  Toni-Fanconi E72.09
    with cystinosis E72.04
  Touraine's Q79.8
  tourniquet — *see* Constriction, external, by site
  toxic shock A48.3
  transient left ventricular apical ballooning I51.81
  traumatic vasospastic T75.22 ☑
  Treacher Collins Q75.4
  triple X, female Q97.0
  trisomy Q92.9
    13 Q91.7
      meiotic nondisjunction Q91.4
      mitotic nondisjunction Q91.5
      mosaicism Q91.5
      translocation Q91.6
    18 Q91.3
      meiotic nondisjunction Q91.0
      mitotic nondisjunction Q91.1
      mosaicism Q91.1
      translocation Q91.2
    20 (q)(p) Q92.8

☑ **Additional Character Required** — Refer to the Tabular List for Character Selection   ⬇ **Subterms under main terms may continue to next column or page**

Syndrome — *continued*
trisomy — *continued*
  21 Q90.9
    meiotic nondisjunction Q90.0
    mitotic nondisjunction Q90.1
    mosaicism Q90.1
    translocation Q90.2
  22 Q92.8
tropical wet feet T69.0- ☑
Trousseau's I82.1
tumor lysis (following antineoplastic chemotherapy) (spontaneous) NEC E88.3
Twiddler's (due to)
  automatic implantable defibrillator T82.198 ☑
  cardiac pacemaker T82.198 ☑
Unverricht (-Lundborg) — *see* Epilepsy, generalized, idiopathic
upward gaze H51.8
uremia, chronic (*see also* Disease, kidney, chronic) N18.9
urethral N34.3
urethro-oculo-articular — *see* Reiter's disease
urohepatic K76.7
vago-hypoglossal G52.7
van Buchem's M85.2
van der Hoeve's Q78.0
vascular NEC in cerebrovascular disease G46.8
vasoconstriction, reversible cerebrovascular I67.841
vasomotor I73.9
vasospastic (traumatic) T75.22 ☑
vasovagal R55
VATER Q87.2
velo-cardio-facial Q93.81
vena cava (inferior) (superior) (obstruction) I87.1
vertebral
  artery G45.0
    compression — *see* Syndrome, anterior, spinal artery, compression
    steal G45.0
vertebro-basilar artery G45.0
vertebrogenic (pain) M54.89
vertiginous — *see* Disorder, vestibular function
Vinson-Plummer D50.1
virus B34.9
visceral larva migrans B83.0
visual disorientation H53.8
vitamin B6 deficiency E53.1
vitreal corneal H59.01- ☑
vitreous (touch) H59.01- ☑
Vogt-Koyanagi H20.82- ☑
Volkmann's T79.6 ☑
von Schroetter's I82.890
von Willebrand (-Jürgen) D68.0
Waldenström-Kjellberg D50.1
Wallenberg's G46.3
water retention E87.79
Waterhouse (-Friderichsen) A39.1
Weber-Gubler G46.3
Weber-Leyden G46.3
Weber's G46.3
Wegener's M31.30
  with
    kidney involvement M31.31
    lung involvement M31.30
      with kidney involvement M31.31
Weingarten's (tropical eosinophilia) J82
Weiss-Baker G90.09
Werdnig-Hoffman G12.0
Wermer's E31.21
Werner's E34.8
Wernicke-Korsakoff (nonalcoholic) F04
  alcoholic F10.26
Westphal-Strümpell E83.01
West's — *see* Epilepsy, spasms
wet
  feet (maceration) (tropical) T69.0- ☑
  lung, newborn P22.1
whiplash S13.4 ☑
whistling face Q87.0
Wilkie's K55.1
Wilkinson-Sneddon L13.1
Willebrand (-Jürgens) D68.0
Wilson's (hepatolenticular degeneration) E83.01
Wiskott-Aldrich D82.0
withdrawal — *see* Withdrawal, state
  drug
    infant of dependent mother P96.1
    therapeutic use, newborn P96.2

Syndrome — *continued*
Woakes' (ethmoiditis) J33.1
Wright's (hyperabduction) I77.89
X I20.9
XXXX Q97.1
XXXXX Q97.1
XXXXY Q98.1
XXY Q98.0
yellow nail L60.5
Zahorsky's B08.5
Zellweger syndrome E71.510
Zellweger-like syndrome E71.541
Synechia (anterior) (iris) (posterior) (pupil) (*see also* Adhesions, iris)
  intra-uterine (traumatic) N85.6
Synesthesia R20.8
Syngamiasis, syngamosis B83.3
Synodontia K00.2
Synorchidism, synorchism Q55.1
Synostosis (congenital) Q78.8
  astragalo-scaphoid Q74.2
  radioulnar Q74.0
Synovial sarcoma — *see* Neoplasm, connective tissue, malignant
Synovioma (malignant) (*see also* Neoplasm, connective tissue, malignant)
  benign — *see* Neoplasm, connective tissue, benign
Synoviosarcoma — *see* Neoplasm, connective tissue, malignant
Synovitis (*see also* Tenosynovitis)
  crepitant
    hand M70.0- ☑
    wrist M70.03- ☑
  gonococcal A54.49
  gouty — *see* Gout, idiopathic
  in (due to)
    crystals M65.8- ☑
    gonorrhea A54.49
    syphilis (late) A52.78
    use, overuse, pressure — *see* Disorder, soft tissue, due to use
  infective NEC — *see* Tenosynovitis, infective NEC
  specified NEC — *see* Tenosynovitis, specified type NEC
  syphilitic A52.78
    congenital (early) A50.02
  toxic — *see* Synovitis, transient
  transient M67.3- ☑
    ankle M67.37- ☑
    elbow M67.32- ☑
    foot joint M67.37- ☑
    hand joint M67.34- ☑
    hip M67.35- ☑
    knee M67.36- ☑
    multiple site M67.39
    pelvic region M67.35- ☑
    shoulder M67.31- ☑
    specified joint NEC M67.38
    wrist M67.33- ☑
  traumatic, current — *see* Sprain
  tuberculous — *see* Tuberculosis, synovitis
  villonodular (pigmented) M12.2- ☑
    ankle M12.27- ☑
    elbow M12.22- ☑
    foot joint M12.27- ☑
    hand joint M12.24- ☑
    hip M12.25- ☑
    knee M12.26- ☑
    multiple site M12.29
    pelvic region M12.25- ☑
    shoulder M12.21- ☑
    specified joint NEC M12.28
    vertebrae M12.28
    wrist M12.23- ☑
Syphilid A51.39
  congenital A50.06
  newborn A50.06
  tubercular (late) A52.79
Syphilis, syphilitic (acquired) A53.9
  abdomen (late) A52.79
  acoustic nerve A52.15
  adenopathy (secondary) A51.49
  adrenal (gland) (with cortical hypofunction) A52.79
  age under 2 years NOS (*see also* Syphilis, congenital, early)
    acquired A51.9
  alopecia (secondary) A51.32
  anemia (late) A52.79 [D63.8]

Syphilis, syphilitic — *continued*
aneurysm (aorta) (ruptured) A52.01
  central nervous system A52.05
  congenital A50.54 [I79.0]
anus (late) A52.74
  primary A51.1
  secondary A51.39
aorta (arch) (abdominal) (thoracic) A52.02
  aneurysm A52.01
aortic (insufficiency) (regurgitation) (stenosis) A52.03
  aneurysm A52.01
arachnoid (adhesive) (cerebral) (spinal) A52.13
asymptomatic — *see* Syphilis, latent
ataxia (locomotor) A52.11
atrophoderma maculatum A51.39
auricular fibrillation A52.06
bladder (late) A52.76
bone A52.77
  secondary A51.46
brain A52.17
breast (late) A52.79
bronchus (late) A52.72
bubo (primary) A51.0
bulbar palsy A52.19
bursa (late) A52.78
cardiac decompensation A52.06
cardiovascular A52.00
central nervous system (late) (recurrent) (relapse) (tertiary) A52.3
  with
    ataxia A52.11
    general paralysis A52.17
      juvenile A50.45
    paresis (general) A52.17
      juvenile A50.45
    tabes (dorsalis) A52.11
      juvenile A50.45
    taboparesis A52.17
      juvenile A50.45
  aneurysm A52.05
  congenital A50.40
  juvenile A50.40
  remission in (sustained) A52.3
  serology doubtful, negative, or positive A52.3
  specified nature or site NEC A52.19
  vascular A52.05
cerebral A52.17
  meningovascular A52.13
  nerves (multiple palsies) A52.15
  sclerosis A52.17
  thrombosis A52.05
cerebrospinal (tabetic type) A52.12
cerebrovascular A52.05
cervix (late) A52.76
chancre (multiple) A51.0
  extragenital A51.2
  Rollet's A51.0
Charcot's joint A52.16
chorioretinitis A51.43
  congenital A50.01
  late A52.71
  prenatal A50.01
choroiditis — *see* Syphilitic chorioretinitis
choroidoretinitis — *see* Syphilitic chorioretinitis
ciliary body (secondary) A51.43
  late A52.71
colon (late) A52.74
combined spinal sclerosis A52.11
condyloma (latum) A51.31
congenital A50.9
  with
    paresis (general) A50.45
    tabes (dorsalis) A50.45
    taboparesis A50.45
  early, or less than 2 years after birth NEC A50.2
    with manifestations — *see* Syphilis, congenital, early, symptomatic
    latent (without manifestations) A50.1
      negative spinal fluid test A50.1
      serology positive A50.1
    symptomatic A50.09
      cutaneous A50.06
      mucocutaneous A50.07
      oculopathy A50.01
      osteochondropathy A50.02
      pharyngitis A50.03
      pneumonia A50.04
      rhinitis A50.05

Syphilis, syphilitic — *continued*
  congenital — *continued*
    early, or less than 2 years after birth — *continued*
      symptomatic — *continued*
        visceral A50.08
    chorioretinitis, choroiditis A50.01 [H32]
    interstitial keratitis A50.31
    juvenile neurosyphilis A50.45
    late, or 2 years or more after birth NEC A50.7
      chorioretinitis, choroiditis A50.32
      interstitial keratitis A50.31
      juvenile neurosyphilis A50.45
      latent (without manifestations) A50.6
        negative spinal fluid test A50.6
        serology positive A50.6
      symptomatic or with manifestations NEC A50.59
        arthropathy A50.55
        cardiovascular A50.54
        Clutton's joints A50.51
        Hutchinson's teeth A50.52
        Hutchinson's triad A50.53
        osteochondropathy A50.56
        saddle nose A50.57
  conjugal A53.9
    tabes A52.11
  conjunctiva (late) A52.71
  contact Z20.2
  cord bladder A52.19
  cornea, late A52.71
  coronary (artery) (sclerosis) A52.06
  coryza, congenital A50.05
  cranial nerve A52.15
    multiple palsies A52.15
  cutaneous — *see* Syphilis, skin
  dacryocystitis (late) A52.71
  degeneration, spinal cord A52.12
  dementia paralytica A52.17
    juvenilis A50.45
  destruction of bone A52.77
  dilatation, aorta A52.01
  due to blood transfusion A53.9
  dura mater A52.13
  ear A52.79
    inner A52.79
      nerve (eighth) A52.15
      neurorecurrence A52.15
  early A51.9
    cardiovascular A52.00
    central nervous system A52.3
    latent (without manifestations) (less than 2 years after infection) A51.5
      negative spinal fluid test A51.5
      serological relapse after treatment A51.5
      serology positive A51.5
    relapse (treated, untreated) A51.9
    skin A51.39
    symptomatic A51.9
      extragenital chancre A51.2
      primary, except extragenital chancre A51.0
      secondary (*see also* Syphilis, secondary) A51.39
        relapse (treated, untreated) A51.49
    ulcer A51.39
  eighth nerve (neuritis) A52.15
  endemic A65
  endocarditis A52.03
    aortic A52.03
    pulmonary A52.03
  epididymis (late) A52.76
  epiglottis (late) A52.73
  epiphysitis (congenital) (early) A50.02
  episcleritis (late) A52.71
  esophagus A52.79
  eustachian tube A52.73
  exposure to Z20.2
  eye A52.71
  eyelid (late) (with gumma) A52.71
  fallopian tube (late) A52.76
  fracture A52.77
  gallbladder (late) A52.74
  gastric (polyposis) (late) A52.74
  general A53.9
    paralysis A52.17
      juvenile A50.45
  genital (primary) A51.0
  glaucoma A52.71

Syphilis, syphilitic — *continued*
  gumma NEC A52.79
    cardiovascular system A52.00
    central nervous system A52.3
    congenital A50.59
  heart (block) (decompensation) (disease) (failure) A52.06 [I52]
    valve NEC A52.03
  hemianesthesia A52.19
  hemianopsia A52.71
  hemiparesis A52.17
  hemiplegia A52.17
  hepatic artery A52.09
  hepatis A52.74
  hepatomegaly, congenital A50.08
  hereditaria tarda — *see* Syphilis, congenital, late
  hereditary — *see* Syphilis, congenital
  Hutchinson's teeth A50.52
  hyalitis A52.71
  inactive — *see* Syphilis, latent
  infantum — *see* Syphilis, congenital
  inherited — *see* Syphilis, congenital
  internal ear A52.79
  intestine (late) A52.74
  iris, iritis (secondary) A51.43
    late A52.71
  joint (late) A52.77
  keratitis (congenital) (interstitial) (late) A50.31
  kidney (late) A52.75
  lacrimal passages (late) A52.71
  larynx (late) A52.73
  late A52.9
    cardiovascular A52.00
    central nervous system A52.3
    kidney A52.75
    latent or 2 years or more after infection (without manifestations) A52.8
      negative spinal fluid test A52.8
      serology positive A52.8
    paresis A52.17
    specified site NEC A52.79
    symptomatic or with manifestations A52.79
    tabes A52.11
  latent A53.0
    with signs or symptoms — *code by* site and stage under Syphilis
    early, or less than 2 years after infection A51.5
    central nervous system A52.2
    date of infection unspecified A53.0
    follow-up of latent syphilis A53.0
      date of infection unspecified A53.0
      late, or 2 years or more after infection A52.8
    late, or 2 years or more after infection A52.8
    positive serology (only finding) A53.0
      early, or less than 2 years after infection A51.5
      date of infection unspecified A53.0
      late, or 2 years or more after infection A52.8
  lens (late) A52.71
  leukoderma A51.39
    late A52.79
  lienitis A52.79
  lip A51.39
    chancre (primary) A51.2
    late A52.79
  Lissauer's paralysis A52.17
  liver A52.74
  locomotor ataxia A52.11
  lung A52.72
  lymph gland (early) (secondary) A51.49
    late A52.79
  lymphadenitis (secondary) A51.49
  macular atrophy of skin A51.39
    striated A52.79
  mediastinum (late) A52.73
  meninges (adhesive) (brain) (spinal cord) A52.13
  meningitis A52.13
    acute (secondary) A51.41
    congenital A50.41
  meningoencephalitis A52.14
  meningovascular A52.13
    congenital A50.41
  mesarteritis A52.09
    brain A52.04
  middle ear A52.77
  mitral stenosis A52.03
  monoplegia A52.17
  mouth (secondary) A51.39
    late A52.79

Syphilis, syphilitic — *continued*
  mucocutaneous (secondary) A51.39
    late A52.79
  mucous
    membrane (secondary) A51.39
      late A52.79
    patches A51.39
      congenital A50.07
  mulberry molars A50.52
  muscle A52.78
  myocardium A52.06
  nasal sinus (late) A52.73
  neonatorum — *see* Syphilis, congenital
  nephrotic syndrome (secondary) A51.44
  nerve palsy (any cranial nerve) A52.15
    multiple A52.15
  nervous system, central A52.3
  neuritis A52.15
    acoustic A52.15
  neurorecidive of retina A52.19
  neuroretinitis A52.19
  newborn — *see* Syphilis, congenital
  nodular superficial (late) A52.79
  nonvenereal A65
  nose (late) A52.73
    saddle back deformity A50.57
  occlusive arterial disease A52.09
  oculopathy A52.71
  ophthalmic (late) A52.71
  optic nerve (atrophy) (neuritis) (papilla) A52.15
  orbit (late) A52.71
  organic A53.9
  osseous (late) A52.77
  osteochondritis (congenital) (early) A50.02 [M90.80]
  osteoporosis A52.77
  ovary (late) A52.76
  oviduct (late) A52.76
  palate (late) A52.79
  pancreas (late) A52.74
  paralysis A52.17
    general A52.17
      juvenile A50.45
  paresis (general) A52.17
    juvenile A50.45
  paresthesia A52.19
  Parkinson's disease or syndrome A52.19
  paroxysmal tachycardia A52.06
  pemphigus (congenital) A50.06
  penis (chancre) A51.0
    late A52.76
  pericardium A52.06
  perichondritis, larynx (late) A52.73
  periosteum (late) A52.77
    congenital (early) A50.02 [M90.80]
    early (secondary) A51.46
  peripheral nerve A52.79
  petrous bone (late) A52.77
  pharynx (late) A52.73
    secondary A51.39
  pituitary (gland) A52.79
  pleura (late) A52.73
  pneumonia, white A50.04
  pontine lesion A52.17
  portal vein A52.09
  primary A51.0
    anal A51.1
    and secondary — *see* Syphilis, secondary
    central nervous system A52.3
    extragenital chancre NEC A51.2
      fingers A51.2
      genital A51.0
      lip A51.2
      specified site NEC A51.2
      tonsils A51.2
  prostate (late) A52.76
  ptosis (eyelid) A52.71
  pulmonary (late) A52.72
    artery A52.09
  pyelonephritis (late) A52.75
  recently acquired, symptomatic A51.9
  rectum (late) A52.74
  respiratory tract (late) A52.73
  retina, late A52.71
  retrobulbar neuritis A52.15
  salpingitis A52.76
  sclera (late) A52.71
  sclerosis
    cerebral A52.17

☑ **Additional Character Required — Refer to the Tabular List for Character Selection**   ▽ **Subterms under main terms may continue to next column or page**

Syphilis, syphilitic — *continued*
  sclerosis — *continued*
    coronary A52.06
    multiple A52.11
  scotoma (central) A52.71
  scrotum (late) A52.76
  secondary (and primary) A51.49
    adenopathy A51.49
    anus A51.39
    bone A51.46
    chorioretinitis, choroiditis A51.43
    hepatitis A51.45
    liver A51.45
    lymphadenitis A51.49
    meningitis (acute) A51.41
    mouth A51.39
    mucous membranes A51.39
    periosteum, periostitis A51.46
    pharynx A51.39
    relapse (treated, untreated) A51.49
    skin A51.39
    specified form NEC A51.49
    tonsil A51.39
    ulcer A51.39
    viscera NEC A51.49
    vulva A51.39
  seminal vesicle (late) A52.76
  seronegative with signs or symptoms — *code by* site
    and stage under Syphilis
  seropositive
    with signs or symptoms — *code by* site and stage
      under Syphilis
    follow-up of latent syphilis — *see* Syphilis, latent
    only finding — *see* Syphilis, latent
  seventh nerve (paralysis) A52.15
  sinus, sinusitis (late) A52.73
  skeletal system A52.77
  skin (with ulceration) (early) (secondary) A51.39
    late or tertiary A52.79
  small intestine A52.74
  spastic spinal paralysis A52.17
  spermatic cord (late) A52.76
  spinal (cord) A52.12

Syphilis, syphilitic — *continued*
  spleen A52.79
  splenomegaly A52.79
  spondylitis A52.77
  staphyloma A52.71
  stigmata (congenital) A50.59
  stomach A52.74
  synovium A52.78
  tabes dorsalis (late) A52.11
    juvenile A50.45
  tabetic type A52.11
    juvenile A50.45
  taboparesis A52.17
    juvenile A50.45
  tachycardia A52.06
  tendon (late) A52.78
  tertiary A52.9
    with symptoms NEC A52.79
    cardiovascular A52.00
    central nervous system A52.3
    multiple NEC A52.79
    specified site NEC A52.79
  testis A52.76
  thorax A52.73
  throat A52.73
  thymus (gland) (late) A52.79
  thyroid (late) A52.79
  tongue (late) A52.79
  tonsil (lingual) (late) A52.73
    primary A51.2
    secondary A51.39
  trachea (late) A52.73
  tunica vaginalis (late) A52.76
  ulcer (any site) (early) (secondary) A51.39
    late A52.79
    perforating A52.79
      foot A52.11
  urethra (late) A52.76
  urogenital (late) A52.76
  uterus (late) A52.76
  uveal tract (secondary) A51.43
    late A52.71

Syphilis, syphilitic — *continued*
  uveitis (secondary) A51.43
    late A52.71
  uvula (late) (perforated) A52.79
  vagina A51.0
    late A52.76
  valvulitis NEC A52.03
  vascular A52.00
    brain (cerebral) A52.05
  ventriculi A52.74
  vesicae urinariae (late) A52.76
  viscera (abdominal) (late) A52.74
    secondary A51.49
  vitreous (opacities) (late) A52.71
    hemorrhage A52.71
  vulva A51.0
    late A52.76
    secondary A51.39
Syphiloma A52.79
  cardiovascular system A52.00
  central nervous system A52.3
  circulatory system A52.00
  congenital A50.59
Syphilophobia F45.29
Syringadenoma (*see also* Neoplasm, skin, benign)
  papillary — *see* Neoplasm, skin, benign
Syringobulbia G95.0
Syringocystadenoma — *see* Neoplasm, skin, benign
  papillary — *see* Neoplasm, skin, benign
Syringoma (*see also* Neoplasm, skin, benign)
  chondroid — *see* Neoplasm, skin, benign
Syringomyelia G95.0
Syringomyelitis — *see* Encephalitis
Syringomyelocele — *see* Spina bifida
Syringopontia G95.0
System, systemic (*see also* condition)
  disease, combined — *see* Degeneration, combined
  inflammatory response syndrome (SIRS) of non-infec-
    tious origin (without organ dysfunction) R65.10
    with acute organ dysfunction R65.11
  lupus erythematosus M32.9
    inhibitor present D68.62

T

Tabacism, tabacosis, tabagism (*see also* Poisoning, tobacco)
  meaning dependence (without remission) F17.200
    with
      disorder F17.299
        remission F17.211
        specified disorder NEC F17.298
        withdrawal F17.203
Tabardillo A75.9
  flea-borne A75.2
  louse-borne A75.0
Tabes, tabetic A52.10
  with
    central nervous system syphilis A52.10
    Charcot's joint A52.16
    cord bladder A52.19
    crisis, viscera (any) A52.19
    paralysis, general A52.17
    paresis (general) A52.17
    perforating ulcer (foot) A52.19
  arthropathy (Charcot) A52.16
  bladder A52.19
  bone A52.11
  cerebrospinal A52.12
  congenital A50.45
  conjugal A52.10
  dorsalis A52.11
    juvenile A50.49
  juvenile A50.49
  latent A52.19
  mesenterica A18.39
  paralysis, insane, general A52.17
  spasmodic A52.17
  syphilis (cerebrospinal) A52.12
Taboparalysis A52.17
Taboparesis (remission) A52.17
  juvenile A50.45
TAC (trigeminal autonomic cephalgia) **NEC** G44.099
  intractable G44.091
  not intractable G44.099
Tache noir S60.22-
Tachyalimentation K91.2
Tachyarrhythmia, tachyrhythmia — *see* Tachycardia
Tachycardia R00.0
  atrial (paroxysmal) I47.1
  auricular I47.1
  AV nodal re-entry (re-entrant) I47.1
  junctional (paroxysmal) I47.1
  newborn P29.11
  nodal (paroxysmal) I47.1
  non-paroxysmal AV nodal I45.89
  paroxysmal (sustained) (nonsustained) I47.9
    with sinus bradycardia I49.5
    atrial (PAT) I47.1
    atrioventricular (AV) (re-entrant) I47.1
      psychogenic F54
    junctional I47.1
      ectopic I47.1
    nodal I47.1
    psychogenic (atrial) (supraventricular) (ventricular) F54
    supraventricular (sustained) I47.1
      psychogenic F54
    ventricular I47.2
      psychogenic F54
  psychogenic F45.8
  sick sinus I49.5
  sinoauricular NOS R00.0
    paroxysmal I47.1
  sinus [sinusal] NOS R00.0
    paroxysmal I47.1
  supraventricular I47.1
  ventricular (paroxysmal) (sustained) I47.2
    psychogenic F54
Tachygastria K31.89
Tachypnea R06.82
  hysterical F45.8
  newborn (idiopathic) (transitory) P22.1
  psychogenic F45.8
  transitory, of newborn P22.1

TACO (transfusion associated circulatory overload) E87.71
Taenia (infection) (infestation) B68.9
  diminuta B71.0
  echinococcal infestation B67.90
  mediocanellata B68.1
  nana B71.0
  saginata B68.1
  solium (intestinal form) B68.0
    larval form — *see* Cysticercosis
Taeniasis (intestine) — *see* Taenia
Tag (hypertrophied skin) (infected) L91.8
  adenoid J35.8
  anus K64.4
  hemorrhoidal K64.4
  hymen N89.8
  perineal N90.89
  preauricular Q17.0
  sentinel K64.4
  skin L91.8
    accessory (congenital) Q82.8
    anus K64.4
    congenital Q82.8
    preauricular Q17.0
  tonsil J35.8
  urethra, urethral N36.8
  vulva N90.89
Tahyna fever B33.8
Takahara's disease E80.3
Takayasu's disease or syndrome M31.4
Talcosis (pulmonary) J62.0
Talipes (congenital) Q66.89
  acquired, planus — *see* Deformity, limb, flat foot
  asymmetric Q66.89
  calcaneovalgus Q66.4
  calcaneovarus Q66.1
  calcaneus Q66.89
  cavus Q66.7
  equinovalgus Q66.6
  equinovarus Q66.0
  equinus Q66.89
  percavus Q66.7
  planovalgus Q66.6
  planus (acquired) (any degree) (*see also* Deformity, limb, flat foot)
    congenital Q66.5-
    due to rickets (sequelae) E64.3
  valgus Q66.6
  varus Q66.3
Tall stature, constitutional E34.4
Talma's disease M62.89
Talon noir S90.3-
  hand S60.22-
  heel S90.3-
  toe S90.1-
Tamponade, heart I31.4
Tanapox (virus disease) B08.71
Tangier disease E78.6
Tantrum, child problem F91.8
Tapeworm (infection) (infestation) — *see* Infestation, tapeworm
Tapia's syndrome G52.7
TAR (thrombocytopenia with absent radius) **syndrome** Q87.2
Tarral-Besnier disease L44.0
Tarsal tunnel syndrome — *see* Syndrome, tarsal tunnel
Tarsalgia — *see* Pain, limb, lower
Tarsitis (eyelid) H01.8
  syphilitic A52.71
  tuberculous A18.4
Tartar (teeth) (dental calculus) K03.6
Tattoo (mark) L81.8
Tauri's disease E74.09
Taurodontism K00.2
Taussig-Bing syndrome Q20.1
Taybi's syndrome Q87.2
Tay-Sachs amaurotic familial idiocy or disease E75.02
TBI (traumatic brain injury) — *see* category S06
Teacher's node or nodule J38.2
Tear, torn (traumatic) (*see also* Laceration)
  with abortion — *see* Abortion
  annular fibrosis M51.35
  anus, anal (sphincter) S31.831

Tear, torn — *continued*
  anus, anal — *continued*
    complicating delivery
      with third degree perineal laceration O70.2
        with mucosa O70.3
      without third degree perineal laceration O70.4
    nontraumatic (healed) (old) K62.81
  articular cartilage, old — *see* Derangement, joint, articular cartilage, by site
  bladder
    with ectopic or molar pregnancy O08.6
    following ectopic or molar pregnancy O08.6
    obstetrical O71.5
    traumatic — *see* Injury, bladder
  bowel
    with ectopic or molar pregnancy O08.6
    following ectopic or molar pregnancy O08.6
    obstetrical trauma O71.5
  broad ligament
    with ectopic or molar pregnancy O08.6
    following ectopic or molar pregnancy O08.6
    obstetrical trauma O71.6
  bucket handle (knee) (meniscus) — *see* Tear, meniscus
  capsule, joint — *see* Sprain
  cartilage (*see also* Sprain)
    articular, old — *see* Derangement, joint, articular cartilage, by site
  cervix
    with ectopic or molar pregnancy O08.6
    following ectopic or molar pregnancy O08.6
    obstetrical trauma (current) O71.3
    old N88.1
    traumatic — *see* Injury, uterus
  dural G97.41
    nontraumatic G96.11
  internal organ — *see* Injury, by site
  knee cartilage
    articular (current) S83.3-
    old — *see* Derangement, knee, meniscus, due to old tear
  ligament — *see* Sprain
  meniscus (knee) (current injury) S83.209
    bucket-handle S83.20-
    lateral
      bucket-handle S83.25-
      complex S83.27-
      peripheral S83.26-
      specified type NEC S83.28-
    medial
      bucket-handle S83.21-
      complex S83.23-
      peripheral S83.22-
      specified type NEC S83.24-
    old — *see* Derangement, knee, meniscus, due to old tear
    site other than knee — *code as* Sprain
    specified type NEC S83.20-
  muscle — *see* Strain
  pelvic
    floor, complicating delivery O70.1
    organ NEC, obstetrical trauma O71.5
      with ectopic or molar pregnancy O08.6
      following ectopic or molar pregnancy O08.6
  perineal, secondary O90.1
  periurethral tissue, obstetrical trauma O71.82
    with ectopic or molar pregnancy O08.6
    following ectopic or molar pregnancy O08.6
  rectovaginal septum — *see* Laceration, vagina
  retina, retinal (without detachment) (horseshoe) (*see also* Break, retina, horseshoe)
    with detachment — *see* Detachment, retina, with retinal, break
  rotator cuff (nontraumatic) M75.10-
    complete M75.12-
    incomplete M75.11-
    traumatic S46.01-
      capsule S43.42-
  semilunar cartilage, knee — *see* Tear, meniscus
  supraspinatus (complete) (incomplete) (nontraumatic) (*see also* Tear, rotator cuff) M75.10-
  tendon — *see* Strain
  tentorial, at birth P10.4

Tear, torn — *continued*
 umbilical cord
  complicating delivery O69.89 ☑
 urethra
  with ectopic or molar pregnancy O08.6
  following ectopic or molar pregnancy O08.6
  obstetrical trauma O71.5
 uterus — *see* Injury, uterus
 vagina — *see* Laceration, vagina
 vessel, from catheter — *see* Puncture, accidental complicating surgery
 vulva, complicating delivery O70.0
Tear-stone — *see* Dacryolith
Teeth (*see also* condition)
 grinding
  psychogenic F45.8
  sleep related G47.63
Teething (syndrome) K00.7
Telangiectasia, telangiectasis (verrucous) I78.1
 ataxic (cerebellar) (Louis-Bar) G11.3
 familial I78.0
 hemorrhagic, hereditary (congenital) (senile) I78.0
 hereditary, hemorrhagic (congenital) (senile) I78.0
 juxtafoveal H35.07-
 macular H35.07- ☑
 parafoveal H35.07- ☑
 retinal (idiopathic) (juxtafoveal) (macular) (parafoveal) H35.07- ☑
 spider I78.1
Telephone scatologia F65.89
Telescoped bowel or intestine K56.1
 congenital Q43.8
Temperature
 body, high (of unknown origin) R50.9
 cold, trauma from T69.9 ☑
  newborn P80.0
  specified effect NEC T69.8 ☑
Temple — *see* condition
Temporal — *see* condition
Temporomandibular joint pain-dysfunction syndrome M26.62
Temporosphenoidal — *see* condition
Tendency
 bleeding — *see* Defect, coagulation
 suicide
  meaning personal history of attempted suicide Z91.5
  meaning suicidal ideation — *see* Ideation, suicidal
 to fall R29.6
Tenderness, abdominal R10.819
 epigastric R10.816
 generalized R10.817
 left lower quadrant R10.814
 left upper quadrant R10.812
 periumbilic R10.815
 rebound R10.829
  epigastric R10.826
  generalized R10.827
  left lower quadrant R10.824
  left upper quadrant R10.822
  periumbilic R10.825
  right lower quadrant R10.823
  right upper quadrant R10.821
 right lower quadrant R10.813
 right upper quadrant R10.811
Tendinitis, tendonitis (*see also* Enthesopathy)
 Achilles M76.6- ☑
 adhesive — *see* Tenosynovitis, specified type NEC
  shoulder — *see* Capsulitis, adhesive
 bicipital M75.2- ☑
 calcific M65.2- ☑
  ankle M65.27- ☑
  foot M65.27- ☑
  forearm M65.23- ☑
  hand M65.24- ☑
  lower leg M65.26- ☑
  multiple sites M65.29
  pelvic region M65.25- ☑
  shoulder M75.3- ☑
  specified site NEC M65.28
  thigh M65.25- ☑
  upper arm M65.22- ☑
 due to use, overuse, pressure (*see also* Disorder, soft tissue, due to use)
  specified NEC — *see* Disorder, soft tissue, due to use, specified NEC
 gluteal M76.0- ☑

Tendinitis, tendonitis — *continued*
 patellar M76.5- ☑
 peroneal M76.7- ☑
 psoas M76.1- ☑
 tibial (posterior) M76.82- ☑
  anterior M76.81- ☑
 trochanteric — *see* Bursitis, hip, trochanteric
Tendon — *see* condition
Tendosynovitis — *see* Tenosynovitis
Tenesmus (rectal) R19.8
 vesical R30.1
Tennis elbow — *see* Epicondylitis, lateral
Tenonitis (*see also* Tenosynovitis)
 eye (capsule) H05.04- ☑
Tenontosynovitis — *see* Tenosynovitis
Tenontothecitis — *see* Tenosynovitis
Tenophyte — *see* Disorder, synovium, specified type NEC
Tenosynovitis (*see also* Synovitis) M65.9
 adhesive — *see* Tenosynovitis, specified type NEC
  shoulder — *see* Capsulitis, adhesive
 bicipital (calcifying) — *see* Tendinitis, bicipital
 gonococcal A54.49
 in (due to)
  crystals M65.8- ☑
  gonorrhea A54.49
  syphilis (late) A52.78
  use, overuse, pressure (*see also* Disorder, soft tissue, due to use)
   specified NEC — *see* Disorder, soft tissue, due to use, specified NEC
 infective NEC M65.1- ☑
  ankle M65.17- ☑
  foot M65.17- ☑
  forearm M65.13- ☑
  hand M65.14- ☑
  lower leg M65.16- ☑
  multiple sites M65.19
  pelvic region M65.15- ☑
  shoulder region M65.11- ☑
  specified site NEC M65.18
  thigh M65.15- ☑
  upper arm M65.12- ☑
 radial styloid M65.4
 shoulder region M65.81- ☑
  adhesive — *see* Capsulitis, adhesive
 specified type NEC M65.88
  ankle M65.87- ☑
  foot M65.87- ☑
  forearm M65.83- ☑
  hand M65.84- ☑
  lower leg M65.86- ☑
  multiple sites M65.89
  pelvic region M65.85- ☑
  shoulder region M65.81- ☑
  specified site NEC M65.88
  thigh M65.85- ☑
  upper arm M65.82- ☑
 tuberculous — *see* Tuberculosis, tenosynovitis
Tenovaginitis — *see* Tenosynovitis
Tension
 arterial, high (*see also* Hypertension)
  without diagnosis of hypertension R03.0
 headache G44.209
  intractable G44.201
  not intractable G44.209
 nervous R45.0
 pneumothorax J93.0
 premenstrual N94.3
 state (mental) F48.9
Tentorium — *see* condition
Teratencephalus Q89.8
Teratism Q89.7
Teratoblastoma (malignant) — *see* Neoplasm, malignant, by site
Teratocarcinoma (*see also* Neoplasm, malignant, by site)
 liver C22.7
Teratoma (solid) (*see also* Neoplasm, uncertain behavior, by site)
 with embryonal carcinoma, mixed — *see* Neoplasm, malignant, by site
 with malignant transformation — *see* Neoplasm, malignant, by site
 adult (cystic) — *see* Neoplasm, benign, by site
 benign — *see* Neoplasm, benign, by site

Teratoma — *continued*
 combined with choriocarcinoma — *see* Neoplasm, malignant, by site
 cystic (adult) — *see* Neoplasm, benign, by site
 differentiated — *see* Neoplasm, benign, by site
 embryonal (*see also* Neoplasm, malignant, by site)
  liver C22.7
 immature — *see* Neoplasm, malignant, by site
 liver C22.7
  adult, benign, cystic, differentiated type or mature D13.4
 malignant (*see also* Neoplasm, malignant, by site)
  anaplastic — *see* Neoplasm, malignant, by site
  intermediate — *see* Neoplasm, malignant, by site
   specified site — *see* Neoplasm, malignant, by site
  unspecified site C62.90
  undifferentiated — *see* Neoplasm, malignant, by site
 mature — *see* Neoplasm, uncertain behavior, by site
  malignant — *see* Neoplasm, by site, malignant, by site
 ovary D27.- ☑
  embryonal, immature or malignant C56- ☑
 solid — *see* Neoplasm, uncertain behavior, by site
 testis C62.9- ☑
  adult, benign, cystic, differentiated type or mature D29.2- ☑
  scrotal C62.1- ☑
  undescended C62.0- ☑
Termination
 anomalous (*see also* Malposition, congenital)
  right pulmonary vein Q26.3
 pregnancy, elective Z33.2
Ternidens diminutus infestation B81.8
Ternidensiasis B81.8
Terror(s) night (child) F51.4
Terrorism, victim of Z65.4
Terry's syndrome H44.2- ☑
Tertiary — *see* condition
Test, tests, testing (for)
 adequacy (for dialysis)
  hemodialysis Z49.31
  peritoneal Z49.32
 blood pressure Z01.30
  abnormal reading — *see* Blood, pressure
 blood typing Z01.83
  Rh typing Z01.83
 blood-alcohol Z04.8
  positive — *see* Findings, abnormal, in blood
 blood-drug Z04.8
  positive — *see* Findings, abnormal, in blood
 cardiac pulse generator (battery) Z45.010
 fertility Z31.41
 genetic
  disease carrier status for procreative management
   female Z31.430
   male Z31.440
  male partner of patient with recurrent pregnancy loss Z31.441
  procreative management NEC
   female Z31.438
   male Z31.448
 hearing Z01.10
  with abnormal findings NEC Z01.118
 HIV (human immunodeficiency virus)
  nonconclusive (in infants) R75
  positive Z21
  seropositive Z21
 immunity status Z01.84
 intelligence NEC Z01.89
 laboratory (as part of a general medical examination) Z00.00
  with abnormal finding Z00.01
  for medicolegal reason NEC Z04.8
 male partner of patient with recurrent pregnancy loss Z31.441
 Mantoux (for tuberculosis) Z11.1
  abnormal result R76.11
 pregnancy, positive first pregnancy — *see* Pregnancy, normal, first
 procreative Z31.49
  fertility Z31.41
 skin, diagnostic
  allergy Z01.82
   special screening examination — *see* Screening, by name of disease

▽ **Subterms under main terms may continue to next column or page**   ☑ **Additional Character Required — Refer to the Tabular List for Character Selection**

299

Tear, torn — Test, tests, testing

Test, tests, testing — continued
  skin, diagnostic — continued
    Mantoux Z11.1
    tuberculin Z11.1
  specified NEC Z01.89
  tuberculin Z11.1
    abnormal result R76.11
  vision Z01.00
    with abnormal findings Z01.01
  Wassermann Z11.3
    positive — see Serology for syphilis, positive
Testicle, testicular, testis (see also condition)
  feminization syndrome (see also Syndrome, androgen
    insensitivity) E34.51
  migrans Q55.29
Tetanus, tetanic (cephalic) (convulsions) A35
  with
    abortion A34
    ectopic or molar pregnancy O08.0
  following ectopic or molar pregnancy O08.0
  inoculation reaction (due to serum) — see Complica-
    tions, vaccination
  neonatorum A33
  obstetrical A34
  puerperal, postpartum, childbirth A34
Tetany (due to) R29.0
  alkalosis E87.3
  associated with rickets E55.0
  convulsions R29.0
    hysterical F44.5
  functional (hysterical) F44.5
  hyperkinetic R29.0
    hysterical F44.5
  hyperpnea R06.4
    hysterical F44.5
    psychogenic F45.8
  hyperventilation (see also Hyperventilation) R06.4
    hysterical F44.5
  neonatal (without calcium or magnesium deficiency)
    P71.3
  parathyroid (gland) E20.9
  parathyroprival E89.2
  post- (para)thyroidectomy E89.2
  postoperative E89.2
  pseudotetany R29.0
  psychogenic (conversion reaction) F44.5
Tetralogy of Fallot Q21.3
Tetraplegia (chronic) (see also Quadriplegia) G82.50
Thailand hemorrhagic fever A91
Thalassanemia — see Thalassemia
Thalassemia (anemia) (disease) D56.9
  with other hemoglobinopathy D56.8
  alpha (major) (severe) (triple gene defect) D56.0
    minor D56.3
    silent carrier D56.3
    trait D56.3
  beta (severe) D56.1
    homozygous D56.1
    major D56.1
    minor D56.3
    trait D56.3
  delta-beta (homozygous) D56.2
    minor D56.3
    trait D56.3
  dominant D56.8
  hemoglobin
    C D56.8
    E-beta D56.5
  intermedia D56.1
  major D56.1
  minor D56.3
  mixed D56.8
  sickle-cell — see Disease, sickle-cell, thalassemia
  specified type NEC D56.8
  trait D56.3
  variants D56.8
Thanatophoric dwarfism or short stature Q77.1
Thaysen-Gee disease (nontropical sprue) K90.0
Thaysen's disease K90.0
Thecoma D27- ☑
  luteinized D27- ☑
  malignant C56- ☑
Thelarche, premature E30.8
Thelaziasis B83.8
Thelitis N61
  puerperal, postpartum or gestational — see Infection,
    nipple
Therapeutic — see condition

Therapy
  drug, long-term (current) (prophylactic)
    agents affecting estrogen receptors and estrogen
      levels NEC Z79.818
    anastrozole (Arimidex) Z79.811
    antibiotics Z79.2
      short-term use — omit code
    anticoagulants Z79.01
    anti-inflammatory Z79.1
    antiplatelet Z79.02
    antithrombotics Z79.02
    aromatase inhibitors Z79.811
    aspirin Z79.82
    birth control pill or patch Z79.3
    bisphosphonates Z79.83
    contraceptive, oral Z79.3
    drug, specified NEC Z79.899
    estrogen receptor downregulators Z79.818
    Evista Z79.810
    exemestane (Aromasin) Z79.811
    Fareston Z79.810
    fulvestrant (Faslodex) Z79.818
    gonadotropin-releasing hormone (GnRH) agonist
      Z79.818
    goserelin acetate (Zoladex) Z79.818
    hormone replacement (postmenopausal) Z79.890
    insulin Z79.4
    letrozole (Femara) Z79.811
    leuprolide acetate (leuprorelin) (Lupron) Z79.818
    megestrol acetate (Megace) Z79.818
    methadone
      for pain management Z79.891
      maintenance therapy F11.20
    Nolvadex Z79.810
    opiate analgesic Z79.891
    oral contraceptive Z79.3
    raloxifene (Evista) Z79.810
    selective estrogen receptor modulators (SERMs)
      Z79.810
    short term — omit code
    steroids
      inhaled Z79.51
      systemic Z79.52
    tamoxifen (Nolvadex) Z79.810
    toremifene (Fareston) Z79.810
Thermic — see condition
Thermography (abnormal) (see also Abnormal, diagnostic imaging) R93.8
  breast R92.8
Thermoplegia T67.0 ☑
Thesaurismosis, glycogen — see Disease, glycogen
  storage
Thiamin deficiency E51.9
  specified NEC E51.8
Thiaminic deficiency with beriberi E51.11
Thibierge-Weissenbach syndrome — see Sclerosis,
  systemic
Thickening
  bone — see Hypertrophy, bone
  breast N64.59
  endometrium R93.8
  epidermal L85.9
    specified NEC L85.8
  hymen N89.6
  larynx J38.7
  nail L60.2
    congenital Q84.5
  periosteal — see Hypertrophy, bone
  pleura J92.9
    with asbestos J92.0
  skin R23.4
  subepiglottic J38.7
  tongue K14.8
  valve, heart — see Endocarditis
Thigh — see condition
Thinning vertebra — see Spondylopathy, specified NEC
Thirst, excessive R63.1
  due to deprivation of water T73.1 ☑
Thomsen disease G71.12
Thoracic (see also condition)
  kidney Q63.2
  outlet syndrome G54.0
Thoracogastroschisis (congenital) Q79.8
Thoracopagus Q89.4
Thorax — see condition
Thorn's syndrome N28.89
Thorson-Björck syndrome E34.0
Threadworm (infection) (infestation) B80

Threatened
  abortion O20.0
    with subsequent abortion O03.9
  job loss, anxiety concerning Z56.2
  labor (without delivery) O47.9
    after 37 completed weeks of gestation O47.1
    before 37 completed weeks of gestation O47.0- ☑
  loss of job, anxiety concerning Z56.2
  miscarriage O20.0
  unemployment, anxiety concerning Z56.2
Three-day fever A93.1
Threshers' lung J67.0
Thrix annulata (congenital) Q84.1
Throat — see condition
Thrombasthenia (Glanzmann) (hemorrhagic) (heredi-
  tary) D69.1
Thromboangiitis I73.1
  obliterans (general) I73.1
    cerebral I67.89
    vessels
      brain I67.89
      spinal cord I67.89
Thromboarteritis — see Arteritis
Thromboasthenia (Glanzmann) (hemorrhagic) (hereditary) D69.1
Thrombocytasthenia (Glanzmann) D69.1
Thrombocythemia (essential) (hemorrhagic) (idiopathic)
  (primary) D47.3
Thrombocytopathy (dystrophic) (granulopenic) D69.1
Thrombocytopenia, thrombocytopenic D69.6
  with absent radius (TAR) Q87.2
  congenital D69.42
  dilutional D69.59
  due to
    (massive) blood transfusion D69.59
    drugs D69.59
    extracorporeal circulation of blood D69.59
    platelet alloimmunization D69.59
  essential D69.3
  heparin induced (HIT) D75.82
  hereditary D69.42
  idiopathic D69.3
  neonatal, transitory P61.0
    due to
      exchange transfusion P61.0
      idiopathic maternal thrombocytopenia P61.0
      isoimmunization P61.0
  primary NEC D69.49
    idiopathic D69.3
  puerperal, postpartum O72.3
  secondary D69.59
  transient neonatal P61.0
Thrombocytosis, essential D47.3
  primary D47.3
Thromboembolism — see Embolism
Thrombopathy (Bernard-Soulier) D69.1
  constitutional D68.0
  Willebrand-Jurgens D68.0
Thrombopenia — see Thrombocytopenia
Thrombophilia D68.59
  primary NEC D68.59
  secondary NEC D68.69
  specified NEC D68.69
Thrombophlebitis I80.9
  antepartum O22.2- ☑
    deep O22.3- ☑
    superficial O22.2- ☑
  cavernous (venous) sinus G08
    complicating pregnancy O22.5- ☑
    nonpyogenic I67.6
  cerebral (sinus) (vein) G08
    nonpyogenic I67.6
    sequelae G09
  due to implanted device — see Complications, by site
    and type, specified NEC
  during or resulting from a procedure NEC T81.72 ☑
  femoral vein (superficial) I80.1- ☑
  femoropopliteal vein I80.0- ☑
  hepatic (vein) I80.8
  idiopathic, recurrent I82.1
  iliofemoral I80.1- ☑
  intracranial venous sinus (any) G08
    nonpyogenic I67.6
    sequelae G09
  intraspinal venous sinuses and veins G08
    nonpyogenic G95.19
  lateral (venous) sinus G08
    nonpyogenic I67.6

Thrombophlebitis — *continued*
leg I80.299
 superficial I80.0- ☑
longitudinal (venous) sinus G08
 nonpyogenic I67.6
lower extremity I80.299
migrans, migrating I82.1
pelvic
 with ectopic or molar pregnancy O08.0
 following ectopic or molar pregnancy O08.0
 puerperal O87.1
popliteal vein — *see* Phlebitis, leg, deep, popliteal
portal (vein) K75.1
postoperative T81.72 ☑
pregnancy — *see* Thrombophlebitis, antepartum
puerperal, postpartum, childbirth O87.0
 deep O87.1
 pelvic O87.1
 septic O86.81
 superficial O87.0
saphenous (greater) (lesser) I80.0- ☑
sinus (intracranial) G08
 nonpyogenic I67.6
specified site NEC I80.8
tibial vein I80.23- ☑

Thrombosis, thrombotic (bland) (multiple) (progressive)
 (silent) (vessel) I82.90
anal K64.5
antepartum — *see* Thrombophlebitis, antepartum
aorta, aortic I74.10
 abdominal I74.09
  saddle I74.01
 bifurcation I74.09
 saddle I74.01
 specified site NEC I74.19
 terminal I74.09
 thoracic I74.11
 valve — *see* Endocarditis, aortic
apoplexy I63.3 ☑
artery, arteries (postinfectional) I74.9
 auditory, internal — *see* Occlusion, artery, precerebral, specified NEC
 basilar — *see* Occlusion, artery, basilar
 carotid (common) (internal) — *see* Occlusion, artery, carotid
 cerebellar (anterior inferior) (posterior inferior) (superior) — *see* Occlusion, artery, cerebellar
 cerebral — *see* Occlusion, artery, cerebral
 choroidal (anterior) — *see* Occlusion, artery, cerebral, specified NEC
 communicating, posterior — *see* Occlusion, artery, cerebral, specified NEC
 coronary (*see also* Infarct, myocardium)
  not resulting in infarction I24.0
 hepatic I74.8
 hypophyseal — *see* Occlusion, artery, cerebral, specified NEC
 iliac I74.5
 limb I74.4
  lower I74.3
  upper I74.2
 meningeal, anterior or posterior — *see* Occlusion, artery, cerebral, specified NEC
 mesenteric (with gangrene) K55.0
 ophthalmic — *see* Occlusion, artery, retina
 pontine — *see* Occlusion, artery, cerebral, specified NEC
 precerebral — *see* Occlusion, artery, precerebral
 pulmonary (iatrogenic) — *see* Embolism, pulmonary
 renal N28.0
 retinal — *see* Occlusion, artery, retina
 spinal, anterior or posterior G95.11
 traumatic NEC T14.8
 vertebral — *see* Occlusion, artery, vertebral
atrium, auricular (*see also* Infarct, myocardium)
 following acute myocardial infarction (current complication) I23.6
 not resulting in infarction I24.0
basilar (artery) — *see* Occlusion, artery, basilar
brain (artery) (stem) (*see also* Occlusion, artery, cerebral)
 due to syphilis A52.05
 puerperal O99.43
 sinus — *see* Thrombosis, intracranial venous sinus
capillary I78.8

Thrombosis, thrombotic — *continued*
cardiac (*see also* Infarct, myocardium)
 not resulting in infarction I24.0
 valve — *see* Endocarditis
carotid (artery) (common) (internal) — *see* Occlusion, artery, carotid
cavernous (venous) sinus — *see* Thrombosis, intracranial venous sinus
cerebellar artery (anterior inferior) (posterior inferior) (superior) I66.3
cerebral (artery) — *see* Occlusion, artery, cerebral
cerebrovenous sinus (*see also* Thrombosis, intracranial venous sinus)
 puerperium O87.3
chronic I82.91
coronary (artery) (vein) (*see also* Infarct, myocardium)
 not resulting in infarction I24.0
corpus cavernosum N48.89
cortical I66.9
deep — *see* Embolism, vein, lower extremity
due to device, implant or graft (*see also* Complications, by site and type, specified NEC) T85.86 ☑
 arterial graft NEC T82.868 ☑
 breast (implant) T85.86 ☑
 catheter NEC T85.86 ☑
  dialysis (renal) T82.868 ☑
   intraperitoneal T85.86 ☑
  infusion NEC T82.868 ☑
   spinal (epidural) (subdural) T85.86 ☑
  urinary (indwelling) T83.86 ☑
 electronic (electrode) (pulse generator) (stimulator)
  bone T84.86 ☑
  cardiac T82.867 ☑
  nervous system (brain) (peripheral nerve) (spinal) T85.86 ☑
  urinary T83.86 ☑
 fixation, internal (orthopedic) NEC T84.86 ☑
 gastrointestinal (bile duct) (esophagus) T85.86 ☑
 genital NEC T83.86 ☑
 heart T82.867 ☑
 joint prosthesis T84.86 ☑
 ocular (corneal graft) (orbital implant) NEC T85.86 ☑
 orthopedic NEC T84.86 ☑
 specified NEC T85.86 ☑
 urinary NEC T83.86 ☑
 vascular NEC T82.868 ☑
 ventricular intracranial shunt T85.86 ☑
during the puerperium — *see* Thrombosis, puerperal
endocardial (*see also* Infarct, myocardium)
 not resulting in infarction I24.0
eye — *see* Occlusion, retina
genital organ
 female NEC N94.89
  pregnancy — *see* Thrombophlebitis, antepartum
 male N50.1
gestational — *see* Phlebopathy, gestational
heart (chamber) (*see also* Infarct, myocardium)
 not resulting in infarction I24.0
hepatic (vein) I82.0
 artery I74.8
history (of) Z86.718
intestine (with gangrene) K55.0
intracardiac NEC (apical) (atrial) (auricular) (ventricular) (old) I51.3
intracranial (arterial) I66.9
 venous sinus (any) G08
  nonpyogenic origin I67.6
  puerperium O87.3
intramural (*see also* Infarct, myocardium)
 not resulting in infarction I24.0
intraspinal venous sinuses and veins G08
 nonpyogenic G95.19
kidney (artery) N28.0
lateral (venous) sinus — *see* Thrombosis, intracranial venous sinus
leg — *see* Thrombosis, vein, lower extremity
 arterial I74.3
liver (venous) I82.0
 artery I74.8
 portal vein I81
longitudinal (venous) sinus — *see* Thrombosis, intracranial venous sinus
lower limb — *see* Thrombosis, vein, lower extremity
lung (iatrogenic) (postoperative) — *see* Embolism, pulmonary

Thrombosis, thrombotic — *continued*
meninges (brain) (arterial) I66.8
mesenteric (artery) (with gangrene) K55.0
 vein (inferior) (superior) I81
mitral I34.8
mural (*see also* Infarct, myocardium)
 due to syphilis A52.06
 not resulting in infarction I24.0
omentum (with gangrene) K55.0
ophthalmic — *see* Occlusion, retina
pampiniform plexus (male) N50.1
parietal (*see also* Infarct, myocardium)
 not resulting in infarction I24.0
penis, superficial vein N48.81
perianal venous K64.5
peripheral arteries I74.4
 upper I74.2
personal history (of) Z86.718
portal I81
 due to syphilis A52.09
precerebral artery — *see* Occlusion, artery, precerebral
puerperal, postpartum O87.0
 brain (artery) O99.43
  venous (sinus) O87.3
 cardiac O99.43
 cerebral (artery) O99.43
  venous (sinus) O87.3
 superficial O87.0
pulmonary (artery) (iatrogenic) (postoperative) (vein) — *see* Embolism, pulmonary
renal (artery) N28.0
 vein I82.3
resulting from presence of device, implant or graft — *see* Complications, by site and type, specified NEC
retina, retinal — *see* Occlusion, retina
scrotum N50.1
seminal vesicle N50.1
sigmoid (venous) sinus — *see* Thrombosis, intracranial venous sinus
sinus, intracranial (any) — *see* Thrombosis, intracranial venous sinus
specified site NEC I82.890
 chronic I82.891
spermatic cord N50.1
spinal cord (arterial) G95.11
 due to syphilis A52.09
 pyogenic origin G06.1
spleen, splenic D73.5
 artery I74.8
testis N50.1
traumatic NEC T14.8
tricuspid I07.8
tumor — *see* Neoplasm, unspecified behavior, by site
tunica vaginalis N50.1
umbilical cord (vessels), complicating delivery O69.5 ☑
vas deferens N50.1
vein (acute) I82.90
 antecubital I82.61- ☑
  chronic I82.71- ☑
 axillary I82.A1- ☑ (*following* I82.7)
  chronic I82.A2- ☑ (*following* I82.7)
 basilic I82.61- ☑
  chronic I82.71- ☑
 brachial I82.62- ☑
  chronic I82.72- ☑
 brachiocephalic (innominate) I82.290
  chronic I82.291
 cephalic I82.61- ☑
  chronic I82.71- ☑
 cerebral, nonpyogenic I67.6
 chronic I82.91
 deep (DVT) I82.40- ☑
  calf I82.4Z- ☑
   chronic I82.5Z- ☑
  lower leg I82.4Z- ☑
   chronic I82.5Z- ☑
  thigh I82.4Y- ☑
   chronic I82.5Y- ☑
  upper leg I82.4Y ☑
   chronic I82.5y--
 femoral I82.41- ☑
  chronic I82.51- ☑
 iliac (iliofemoral) I82.42- ☑
  chronic I82.52- ☑
 innominate I82.290
  chronic I82.291

Index (left margin)

Thrombosis, thrombotic — Tommaselli's disease (left margin)

Thrombosis, thrombotic — *continued*
  vein — *continued*
    internal jugular I82.C1- ☑ (*following* I82.7)
      chronic I82.C2- ☑ (*following* I82.7)
    lower extremity
      deep I82.40- ☑
        chronic I82.50- ☑
        specified NEC I82.49- ☑
          chronic NEC I82.59- ☑
      distal
        deep I82.4Z- ☑
      proximal
        deep I82.4Y- ☑
          chronic I82.5Y- ☑
      superficial I82.81- ☑
    perianal K64.5
    popliteal I82.43- ☑
      chronic I82.53- ☑
    radial I82.62- ☑
      chronic I82.72- ☑
    renal I82.3
    saphenous (greater) (lesser) I82.81- ☑
    specified NEC I82.890
      chronic NEC I82.891
    subclavian I82.B1- ☑ (*following* I82.7)
      chronic I82.B2- ☑ (*following* I82.7)
    thoracic NEC I82.290
      chronic I82.291
    tibial I82.44- ☑
      chronic I82.54- ☑
    ulnar I82.62- ☑
      chronic I82.72- ☑
    upper extremity I82.60- ☑
      chronic I82.70- ☑
      deep I82.62- ☑
        chronic I82.72- ☑
      superficial I82.61- ☑
        chronic I82.71- ☑
  vena cava
    inferior I82.220
      chronic I82.221
    superior I82.210
      chronic I82.211
  venous, perianal K64.5
  ventricle (*see also* Infarct, myocardium)
    following acute myocardial infarction (current complication) I23.6
    not resulting in infarction I24.0
Thrombus — *see* Thrombosis
Thrush (*see also* Candidiasis)
  newborn P37.5
  oral B37.0
  vaginal B37.3
Thumb (*see also* condition)
  sucking (child problem) F98.8
Thymitis E32.8
Thymoma (benign) D15.0
  malignant C37
Thymus, thymic (gland) — *see* condition
Thyrocele — *see* Goiter
Thyroglossal (*see also* condition)
  cyst Q89.2
  duct, persistent Q89.2
Thyroid (gland) (body) (*see also* condition)
  hormone resistance E07.89
  lingual Q89.2
  nodule (cystic) (nontoxic) (single) E04.1
Thyroiditis E06.9
  acute (nonsuppurative) (pyogenic) (suppurative) E06.0
  autoimmune E06.3
  chronic (nonspecific) (sclerosing) E06.5
    with thyrotoxicosis, transient E06.2
    fibrous E06.5
    lymphadenoid E06.3
    lymphocytic E06.3
    lymphoid E06.3
  de Quervain's E06.1
  drug-induced E06.4
  fibrous (chronic) E06.5
  giant-cell (follicular) E06.1
  granulomatous (de Quervain) (subacute) E06.1
  Hashimoto's (struma lymphomatosa) E06.3
  iatrogenic E06.4
  ligneous E06.5
  lymphocytic (chronic) E06.3
  lymphoid E06.3
  lymphomatous E06.3

Thyroiditis — *continued*
  nonsuppurative E06.1
  postpartum, puerperal O90.5
  pseudotuberculous E06.1
  pyogenic E06.0
  radiation E06.4
  Riedel's E06.5
  subacute (granulomatous) E06.1
  suppurative E06.0
  tuberculous A18.81
  viral E06.1
  woody E06.5
Thyrolingual duct, persistent Q89.2
Thyromegaly E01.0
Thyrotoxic
  crisis — *see* Thyrotoxicosis
  heart disease or failure (*see also* Thyrotoxicosis) E05.90 [I43]
    with thyroid storm E05.91 [I43]
  storm — *see* Thyrotoxicosis
Thyrotoxicosis (recurrent) E05.90
  with
    goiter (diffuse) E05.00
      with thyroid storm E05.01
      adenomatous uninodular E05.10
        with thyroid storm E05.11
      multinodular E05.20
        with thyroid storm E05.21
      nodular E05.20
        with thyroid storm E05.21
      uninodular E05.10
        with thyroid storm E05.11
    infiltrative
      dermopathy E05.00
        with thyroid storm E05.01
      ophthalmopathy E05.00
        with thyroid storm E05.01
    single thyroid nodule E05.10
      with thyroid storm E05.11
    thyroid storm E05.91
  due to
    ectopic thyroid nodule or tissue E05.30
      with thyroid storm E05.31
    ingestion of (excessive) thyroid material E05.40
      with thyroid storm E05.41
    overproduction of thyroid-stimulating hormone E05.80
      with thyroid storm E05.81
    specified cause NEC E05.80
      with thyroid storm E05.81
  factitia E05.40
    with thyroid storm E05.41
  heart E05.90 [I43]
    with thyroid storm E05.91 [I43]
    failure E05.90 [I43]
  neonatal (transient) P72.1
  transient with chronic thyroiditis E06.2
Tibia vara — *see* Osteochondrosis, juvenile, tibia
Tic (disorder) F95.9
  breathing F95.8
  child problem F95.0
  compulsive F95.1
  de la Tourette F95.2
  degenerative (generalized) (localized) G25.69
    facial G25.69
  disorder
    chronic
      motor F95.1
      vocal F95.1
    combined vocal and multiple motor F95.2
    transient F95.0
  douloureux G50.0
    atypical G50.1
    postherpetic, postzoster B02.22
  drug-induced G25.61
  eyelid F95.8
  habit F95.9
    chronic F95.1
    transient of childhood F95.0
  lid, transient of childhood F95.0
  motor-verbal F95.2
  occupational F48.8
  orbicularis F95.8
    transient of childhood F95.0
  organic origin G25.69
  postchoreic G25.69
  psychogenic, compulsive F95.1
  salaam R25.8

Tic — *continued*
  spasm (motor or vocal) F95.9
    chronic F95.1
    transient of childhood F95.0
  specified NEC F95.8
Tick-borne — *see* condition
Tietze's disease or syndrome M94.0
Tight, tightness
  anus K62.89
  chest R07.89
  fascia (lata) M62.89
  foreskin (congenital) N47.1
  hymen, hymenal ring N89.6
  introitus (acquired) (congenital) N89.6
  rectal sphincter K62.89
  tendon — *see* Short, tendon
  urethral sphincter N35.9
Tilting vertebra — *see* Dorsopathy, deforming, specified NEC
Timidity, child F93.8
Tinea (intersecta) (tarsi) B35.9
  amiantacea L44.8
  asbestina B35.0
  barbae B35.0
  beard B35.0
  black dot B35.0
  blanca B36.2
  capitis B35.0
  corporis B35.4
  cruris B35.6
  flava B36.0
  foot B35.3
  furfuracea B36.0
  imbricata (Tokelau) B35.5
  kerion B35.0
  manuum B35.2
  microsporic — *see* Dermatophytosis
  nigra B36.1
  nodosa — *see* Piedra
  pedis B35.3
  scalp B35.0
  specified site NEC B35.8
  sycosis B35.0
  tonsurans B35.0
  trichophytic — *see* Dermatophytosis
  unguium B35.1
  versicolor B36.0
Tingling sensation (skin) R20.2
Tin-miner's lung J63.5
Tinnitus (audible) (aurium) (subjective) — *see* subcategory H93.1 ☑
Tipped tooth (teeth) M26.33
Tipping
  pelvis M95.5
    with disproportion (fetopelvic) O33.0
      causing obstructed labor O65.0
  tooth (teeth), fully erupted M26.33
Tiredness R53.83
Tissue — *see* condition
Tobacco (nicotine)
  dependence — *see* Dependence, drug, nicotine
  harmful use Z72.0
  heart — *see* Tobacco, toxic effect
  maternal use, affecting newborn P04.2
  toxic effect — *see* Table of Drugs and Chemicals, by substance, poisoning
    chewing tobacco — *see* Table of Drugs and Chemicals, by substance, poisoning
    cigarettes — *see* Table of Drugs and Chemicals, by substance, poisoning
  use Z72.0
    complicating
      childbirth O99.334
      pregnancy O99.33- ☑
      puerperium O99.335
    counseling and surveillance Z71.6
  withdrawal state — *see* Dependence, drug, nicotine
Tocopherol deficiency E56.0
Todd's
  cirrhosis K74.3
  paralysis (postepileptic) (transitory) G83.84
Toe — *see* condition
Toilet, artificial opening — *see* Attention to, artificial, opening
Tokelau (ringworm) B35.5
Tollwut — *see* Rabies
Tommaselli's disease R31.9

Tommaselli's disease — *continued*
  correct substance properly administered — *see* Table of Drugs and Chemicals, by drug, adverse effect
  overdose or wrong substance given or taken — *see* Table of Drugs and Chemicals, by drug, poisoning
Tongue (*see also* condition)
  tie Q38.1
Tonic pupil — *see* Anomaly, pupil, function, tonic pupil
Toni-Fanconi syndrome (cystinosis) E72.09
  with cystinosis E72.04
Tonsil — *see* condition
Tonsillitis (acute) (catarrhal) (croupous) (follicular) (gangrenous) (infective) (lacunar) (lingual) (malignant) (membranous) (parenchymatous) (phlegmonous) (pseudomembranous) (purulent) (septic) (subacute) (suppurative) (toxic) (ulcerative) (vesicular) (viral) J03.90
  chronic J35.01
    with adenoiditis J35.03
  diphtheritic A36.0
  hypertrophic J35.01
    with adenoiditis J35.03
  recurrent J03.91
  specified organism NEC J03.80
    recurrent J03.81
  staphylococcal J03.80
    recurrent J03.81
  streptococcal J03.00
    recurrent J03.01
  tuberculous A15.8
  Vincent's A69.1
Tooth, teeth — *see* condition
Toothache K08.8
Topagnosis R20.8
Tophi — *see* Gout, chronic
TORCH infection — *see* Infection, congenital
  without active infection P00.2
Torn — *see* Tear
Tornwaldt's cyst or disease J39.2
Torsion
  accessory tube — *see* Torsion, fallopian tube
  adnexa (female) — *see* Torsion, fallopian tube
  aorta, acquired I77.1
  appendix epididymis N44.04
  appendix testis N44.03
  bile duct (common) (hepatic) K83.8
    congenital Q44.5
  bowel, colon or intestine K56.2
  cervix — *see* Malposition, uterus
  cystic duct K82.8
  dystonia — *see* Dystonia, torsion
  epididymis (appendix) N44.04
  fallopian tube N83.52
    with ovary N83.53
  gallbladder K82.8
    congenital Q44.1
  hydatid of Morgagni
    female N83.52
    male N44.03
  kidney (pedicle) (leading to infarction) N28.0
  Meckel's diverticulum (congenital) Q43.0
    malignant — *see* Table of Neoplasms, small intestine, malignant
  mesentery K56.2
  omentum K56.2
  organ or site, congenital NEC — *see* Anomaly, by site
  ovary (pedicle) N83.51
    with fallopian tube N83.53
    congenital Q50.2
  oviduct — *see* Torsion, fallopian tube
  penis (acquired) N48.82
    congenital Q55.63
  spasm — *see* Dystonia, torsion
  spermatic cord N44.02
    extravaginal N44.01
    intravaginal N44.02
  spleen D73.5
  testis, testicle N44.00
    appendix N44.03
  tibia — *see* Deformity, limb, specified type NEC, lower leg
  uterus — *see* Malposition, uterus
Torticollis (intermittent) (spastic) M43.6
  congenital (sternomastoid) Q68.0
  due to birth injury P15.8
  hysterical F44.4
  ocular R29.891

Torticollis — *continued*
  psychogenic F45.8
    conversion reaction F44.4
  rheumatic M43.6
  rheumatoid M06.88
  spasmodic G24.3
  traumatic, current S13.4 ☑
Tortipelvis G24.1
Tortuous
  artery I77.1
  organ or site, congenital NEC — *see* Distortion
  retinal vessel, congenital Q14.1
  ureter N13.8
  urethra N36.8
  vein — *see* Varix
Torture, victim of Z65.4
Torula, torular (histolytica) (infection) — *see* Cryptococcosis
Torulosis — *see* Cryptococcosis
Torus (mandibularis) (palatinus) M27.0
  fracture — *see* Fracture, by site, torus
Touraine's syndrome Q79.8
Tourette's syndrome F95.2
Tourniquet syndrome — *see* Constriction, external, by site
Tower skull Q75.0
  with exophthalmos Q87.0
Toxemia R68.89
  bacterial — *see* Sepsis
  burn — *see* Burn
  eclamptic (with pre-existing hypertension) — *see* Eclampsia
  erysipelatous — *see* Erysipelas
  fatigue R68.89
  food — *see* Poisoning, food
  gastrointestinal K52.1
  intestinal K52.1
  kidney — *see* Uremia
  malarial — *see* Malaria
  myocardial — *see* Myocarditis, toxic
  of pregnancy — *see* Pre-eclampsia
  pre-eclamptic — *see* Pre-eclampsia
  small intestine K52.1
  staphylococcal, due to food A05.0
  stasis R68.89
  uremic — *see* Uremia
  urinary — *see* Uremia
Toxemica cerebropathia psychica (nonalcoholic) F04
  alcoholic — *see* Alcohol, amnestic disorder
Toxic (poisoning) (*see also* condition) T65.91 ☑
  effect — *see* Table of Drugs and Chemicals, by substance, poisoning
  shock syndrome A48.3
  thyroid (gland) — *see* Thyrotoxicosis
Toxicemia — *see* Toxemia
Toxicity — *see* Table of Drugs and Chemicals, by substance, poisoning
  fava bean D55.0
  food, noxious — *see* Poisoning, food
  from drug or nonmedicinal substance — *see* Table of Drugs and Chemicals, by drug
Toxicosis (*see also* Toxemia)
  capillary, hemorrhagic D69.0
Toxinfection, gastrointestinal K52.1
Toxocariasis B83.0
Toxoplasma, toxoplasmosis (acquired) B58.9
  with
    hepatitis B58.1
    meningoencephalitis B58.2
    ocular involvement B58.00
    other organ involvement B58.89
    pneumonia, pneumonitis B58.3
  congenital (acute) (subacute) (chronic) P37.1
  maternal, manifest toxoplasmosis in infant (acute) (subacute) (chronic) P37.1
tPA (rtPA) administration in a different facility within the last 24 hours prior to admission to current facility Z92.82
Trabeculation, bladder N32.89
Trachea — *see* condition
Tracheitis (catarrhal) (infantile) (membranous) (plastic) (septal) (suppurative) (viral) J04.10
  with
    bronchitis (15 years of age and above) J40
      acute or subacute — *see* Bronchitis, acute
      chronic J42
      tuberculous NEC A15.5

Tracheitis — *continued*
  with — *continued*
    bronchitis — *continued*
      under 15 years of age J20.9
    laryngitis (acute) J04.2
      chronic J37.1
      tuberculous NEC A15.5
  acute J04.10
    with obstruction J04.11
  chronic J42
    with
      bronchitis (chronic) J42
      laryngitis (chronic) J37.1
  diphtheritic (membranous) A36.89
  due to external agent — *see* Inflammation, respiratory, upper, due to
  syphilitic A52.73
  tuberculous A15.5
Trachelitis (nonvenereal) — *see* Cervicitis
Tracheobronchial — *see* condition
Tracheobronchitis (15 years of age and above) (*see also* Bronchitis)
  due to
    Bordetella bronchiseptica A37.80
      with pneumonia A37.81
    Francisella tularensis A21.8
Tracheobronchomegaly Q32.4
  with bronchiectasis J47.9
    with
      exacerbation (acute) J47.1
      lower respiratory infection J47.0
  acquired J98.09
    with bronchiectasis J47.9
      with
        exacerbation (acute) J47.1
        lower respiratory infection J47.0
Tracheobronchopneumonitis — *see* Pneumonia, broncho-
Tracheocele (external) (internal) J39.8
  congenital Q32.1
Tracheomalacia J39.8
  congenital Q32.0
Tracheopharyngitis (acute) J06.9
  chronic J42
  due to external agent — *see* Inflammation, respiratory, upper, due to
Tracheostenosis J39.8
Tracheostomy
  complication — *see* Complication, tracheostomy
  status Z93.0
    attention to Z43.0
    malfunctioning J95.03
Trachoma, trachomatous A71.9
  active (stage) A71.1
  contraction of conjunctiva A71.1
  dubium A71.0
  healed or sequelae B94.0
  initial (stage) A71.0
  pannus A71.1
  Türck's J37.0
Traction, vitreomacular H43.82- ☑
Train sickness T75.3 ☑
Trait(s)
  Hb-S D57.3
  hemoglobin
    abnormal NEC D58.2
      with thalassemia D56.3
    C — *see* Disease, hemoglobin C
    S (Hb-S) D57.3
  Lepore D56.3
  personality, accentuated Z73.1
  sickle-cell D57.3
    with elliptocytosis or spherocytosis D57.3
  type A personality Z73.1
Tramp Z59.0
Trance R41.89
  hysterical F44.89
Transaminasemia R74.0
Transection
  abdomen (partial) S38.3 ☑
  aorta (incomplete) (*see also* Injury, aorta)
    complete — *see* Injury, aorta, laceration, major
  carotid artery (incomplete) (*see also* Injury, blood vessel, carotid, laceration)
    complete — *see* Injury, blood vessel, carotid, laceration, major
  celiac artery (incomplete) S35.211 ☑

Transection — continued
  celiac artery — continued
    branch (incomplete) S35.291 ☑
      complete S35.292 ☑
    complete S35.212 ☑
  innominate
    artery (incomplete) (see also Injury, blood vessel,
      thoracic, innominate, artery, laceration)
      complete — see Injury, blood vessel, thoracic,
        innominate, artery, laceration, major
    vein (incomplete) (see also Injury, blood vessel,
      thoracic, innominate, vein, laceration)
      complete — see Injury, blood vessel, thoracic,
        innominate, vein, laceration, major
  jugular vein (external) (incomplete) (see also Injury,
    blood vessel, jugular vein, laceration)
    complete — see Injury, blood vessel, jugular vein,
      laceration, major
    internal (incomplete) (see also Injury, blood vessel,
      jugular vein, internal, laceration)
      complete — see Injury, blood vessel, jugular
        vein, internal, laceration, major
  mesenteric artery (incomplete) (see also Injury,
    mesenteric, artery, laceration)
    complete — see Injury, mesenteric artery, lacera-
      tion, major
  pulmonary vessel (incomplete) (see also Injury, blood
    vessel, thoracic, pulmonary, laceration)
    complete — see Injury, blood vessel, thoracic,
      pulmonary, laceration, major
  subclavian — see Transection, innominate
  vena cava (incomplete) (see also Injury, vena cava)
    complete — see Injury, vena cava, laceration, major
  vertebral artery (incomplete) (see also Injury, blood
    vessel, vertebral, laceration)
    complete — see Injury, blood vessel, vertebral,
      laceration, major
Transfusion
  associated (red blood cell) hemochromatosis E83.111
  blood
    ABO incompatible — see Complication(s), transfu-
      sion, incompatibility reaction, ABO
    minor blood group (Duffy) (E) (K(ell)) (Kidd) (Lewis)
      (M) (N) (P) (S) T80.89 ☑
    reaction or complication — see Complications,
      transfusion
  fetomaternal (mother) — see Pregnancy, complicated
    by, placenta, transfusion syndrome
  maternofetal (mother) — see Pregnancy, complicated
    by, placenta, transfusion syndrome
  placental (syndrome) (mother) — see Pregnancy,
    complicated by, placenta, transfusion syndrome
  reaction (adverse) — see Complications, transfusion
  related acute lung injury (TRALI) J95.84
  twin-to-twin — see Pregnancy, complicated by, pla-
    centa, transfusion syndrome, fetus to fetus
Transient (meaning homeless) (see also condition) Z59.0
Translocation
  balanced autosomal Q95.9
    in normal individual Q95.0
  chromosomes NEC Q99.8
    balanced and insertion in normal individual Q95.0
  Down syndrome Q90.2
  trisomy
    13 Q91.6
    18 Q91.2
    21 Q90.2
Translucency, iris — see Degeneration, iris
Transmission of chemical substances through the
  placenta — see Absorption, chemical, through
  placenta
Transparency, lung, unilateral J43.0
Transplant (ed) (status) Z94.9
  awaiting organ Z76.82
  bone Z94.6
    marrow Z94.81
  candidate Z76.82
  complication — see Complication, transplant
  cornea Z94.7
  heart Z94.1
    and lung(s) Z94.3
    valve Z95.2
      prosthetic Z95.2
      specified NEC Z95.4
      xenogenic Z95.3
  intestine Z94.82
  kidney Z94.0

Transplant — continued
  liver Z94.4
  lung(s) Z94.2
    and heart Z94.3
  organ (failure) (infection) (rejection) Z94.9
    removal status Z98.85
  pancreas Z94.83
  skin Z94.5
  social Z60.3
  specified organ or tissue NEC Z94.89
  stem cells Z94.84
  tissue Z94.9
Transplants, ovarian, endometrial N80.1
Transposed — see Transposition
Transposition (congenital) (see also Malposition, congenital)
  abdominal viscera Q89.3
  aorta (dextra) Q20.3
  appendix Q43.8
  colon Q43.8
  corrected Q20.5
  great vessels (complete) (partial) Q20.3
  heart Q24.0
    with complete transposition of viscera Q89.3
  intestine (large) (small) Q43.8
  reversed jejunal (for bypass) (status) Z98.0
  scrotum Q55.23
  stomach Q40.2
    with general transposition of viscera Q89.3
  tooth, teeth, fully erupted M26.30
  vessels, great (complete) (partial) Q20.3
  viscera (abdominal) (thoracic) Q89.3
Transsexualism F64.1
Transverse (see also condition)
  arrest (deep), in labor O64.0 ☑
  lie (mother) O32.2 ☑
    causing obstructed labor O64.8 ☑
Transvestism, transvestitism (dual-role) F64.1
  fetishistic F65.1
Trapped placenta (with hemorrhage) O72.0
  without hemorrhage O73.0
Trauma, traumatism (see also Injury)
  acoustic — see subcategory H83.3 ☑
  birth — see Birth, injury
  complicating ectopic or molar pregnancy O08.6
  during delivery O71.9
  following ectopic or molar pregnancy O08.6
  obstetric O71.9
    specified NEC O71.89
Traumatic (see also condition)
  brain injury — see category S06 ☑
Treacher Collins syndrome Q75.4
Treitz's hernia — see Hernia, abdomen, specified site
  NEC
Trematode infestation — see Infestation, fluke
Trematodiasis — see Infestation, fluke
Trembling paralysis — see Parkinsonism
Tremor(s) R25.1
  drug induced G25.1
  essential (benign) G25.0
  familial G25.0
  hereditary G25.0
  hysterical F44.4
  intention G25.2
  medication induced postural G25.1
  mercurial — see subcategory T56.1 ☑
  Parkinson's — see Parkinsonism
  psychogenic (conversion reaction) F44.4
  senilis R54
  specified type NEC G25.2
Trench
  fever A79.0
  foot — see Immersion, foot
  mouth A69.1
Treponema pallidum infection — see Syphilis
Treponematosis
  due to
    T. pallidum — see Syphilis
    T. pertenue — see Yaws
Triad
  Hutchinson's (congenital syphilis) A50.53
  Kartagener's Q89.3
  Saint's — see Hernia, diaphragm
Trichiasis (eyelid) H02.059
  with entropion — see Entropion
  left H02.056
    lower H02.055

Trichiasis — continued
  left — continued
    upper H02.054
  right H02.053
    lower H02.052
    upper H02.051
Trichinella spiralis (infection) (infestation) B75
Trichinellosis, trichiniasis, trichinelliasis, trichinosis
  B75
  with muscle disorder B75 [M63.80]
    ankle B75 [M63.87-] ☑
    foot B75 [M63.87-] ☑
    forearm B75 [M63.83-] ☑
    hand B75 [M63.84-] ☑
    lower leg B75 [M63.86-] ☑
    multiple sites B75 [M63.89]
    pelvic region B75 [M63.85-] ☑
    shoulder region B75 [M63.81-] ☑
    specified site NEC B75 [M63.88]
    thigh B75 [M63.85-] ☑
    upper arm B75 [M63.82-] ☑
Trichobezoar T18.9 ☑
  intestine T18.3 ☑
  stomach T18.2 ☑
Trichocephaliasis, trichocephalosis B79
Trichocephalus infestation B79
Trichoclasis L67.8
Trichoepithelioma (see also Neoplasm, skin, benign)
  malignant — see Neoplasm, skin, malignant
Trichofolliculoma — see Neoplasm, skin, benign
Tricholemmoma — see Neoplasm, skin, benign
Trichomoniasis A59.9
  bladder A59.03
  cervix A59.09
  intestinal A07.8
  prostate A59.02
  seminal vesicles A59.09
  specified site NEC A59.8
  urethra A59.03
  urogenitalis A59.00
  vagina A59.01
  vulva A59.01
Trichomycosis
  axillaris A48.8
  nodosa, nodularis B36.8
Trichonodosis L67.8
Trichophytid, trichophyton infection — see Dermato-
  phytosis
Trichophytobezoar T18.9 ☑
  intestine T18.3 ☑
  stomach T18.2 ☑
Trichophytosis — see Dermatophytosis
Trichoptilosis L67.8
Trichorrhexis (nodosa) (invaginata) L67.0
Trichosis axillaris A48.8
Trichosporosis nodosa B36.2
Trichostasis spinulosa (congenital) Q84.1
Trichostrongyliasis, trichostrongylosis (small intes-
  tine) B81.2
Trichostrongylus infection B81.2
Trichotillomania F63.3
Trichromat, trichromatopsia, anomalous (congenital)
  H53.55
Trichuriasis B79
Trichuris trichiura (infection) (infestation) (any site) B79
Tricuspid (valve) — see condition
Trifid (see also Accessory)
  kidney (pelvis) Q63.8
  tongue Q38.3
Trigeminal neuralgia — see Neuralgia, trigeminal
Trigeminy R00.8
Trigger finger (acquired) M65.30
  congenital Q74.0
  index finger M65.32- ☑
  little finger M65.35- ☑
  middle finger M65.33- ☑
  ring finger M65.34- ☑
  thumb M65.31- ☑
Trigonitis (bladder) (chronic) (pseudomembranous)
  N30.30
  with hematuria N30.31
Trigonocephaly Q75.0
Trilocular heart — see Cor triloculare
Trimethylaminuria E72.52
Tripartite placenta O43.19- ☑
Triphalangeal thumb Q74.0

☑ Additional Character Required — Refer to the Tabular List for Character Selection   ▽ Subterms under main terms may continue to next column or page

Triple (see also Accessory)
  kidneys Q63.0
  uteri Q51.818
  X, female Q97.0
Triplegia G83.89
  congenital G80.8
Triplet (newborn) (see also Newborn, triplet)
  complicating pregnancy — see Pregnancy, triplet
Triplication — see Accessory
Triploidy Q92.7
Trismus R25.2
  neonatorum A33
  newborn A33
Trisomy (syndrome) Q92.9
  13 (partial) Q91.7
    meiotic nondisjunction Q91.4
    mitotic nondisjunction Q91.5
    mosaicism Q91.5
    translocation Q91.6
  18 (partial) Q91.3
    meiotic nondisjunction Q91.0
    mitotic nondisjunction Q91.1
    mosaicism Q91.1
    translocation Q91.2
  20 Q92.8
  21 (partial) Q90.9
    meiotic nondisjunction Q90.0
    mitotic nondisjunction Q90.1
    mosaicism Q90.1
    translocation Q90.2
  22 Q92.8
  autosomes Q92.9
  chromosome specified NEC Q92.8
    partial Q92.2
      due to unbalanced translocation Q92.5
    specified NEC Q92.8
    whole (nonsex chromosome)
      meiotic nondisjunction Q92.0
      mitotic nondisjunction Q92.1
      mosaicism Q92.1
  due to
    dicentrics — see Extra, marker chromosomes
    extra rings — see Extra, marker chromosomes
    isochromosomes — see Extra, marker chromo-
      somes
  specified NEC Q92.8
  whole chromosome Q92.9
    meiotic nondisjunction Q92.0
    mitotic nondisjunction Q92.1
    mosaicism Q92.1
    partial Q92.9
    specified NEC Q92.8
Tritanomaly, tritanopia H53.55
Trombiculosis, trombiculiasis, trombidiosis B88.0
Trophedema (congenital) (hereditary) Q82.0
Trophoblastic disease (see also Mole, hydatidiform)
  O01.9
Tropholymphedema Q82.0
Trophoneurosis NEC G96.8
  disseminated M34.9
Tropical — see condition
Trouble (see also Disease)
  heart — see Disease, heart
  kidney — see Disease, renal
  nervous R45.0
  sinus — see Sinusitis
Trousseau's syndrome (thrombophlebitis migrans) I82.1
Truancy, childhood
  from school Z72.810
Truncus
  arteriosus (persistent) Q20.0
  communis Q20.0
Trunk — see condition
Trypanosomiasis
  African B56.9
    by Trypanosoma brucei
      gambiense B56.0
      rhodesiense B56.1
  American — see Chagas' disease
  Brazilian — see Chagas' disease
  by Trypanosoma
    brucei gambiense B56.0
    brucei rhodesiense B56.1
    cruzi — see Chagas' disease
  gambiensis, Gambian B56.0
  rhodesiensis, Rhodesian B56.1
  South American — see Chagas' disease
  where

Trypanosomiasis — continued
  where — continued
    African trypanosomiasis is prevalent B56.9
    Chagas' disease is prevalent B57.2
T-shaped incisors K00.2
Tsutsugamushi (disease) (fever) A75.3
Tube, tubal, tubular — see condition
Tubercle (see also Tuberculosis)
  brain, solitary A17.81
  Darwin's Q17.8
  Ghon, primary infection A15.7
Tuberculid, tuberculide (indurating, subcutaneous)
  (lichenoid) (miliary) (papulonecrotic) (primary) (skin)
  A18.4
Tuberculoma (see also Tuberculosis)
  brain A17.81
  meninges (cerebral) (spinal) A17.1
  spinal cord A17.81
Tuberculosis, tubercular, tuberculous (calcification)
  (calcified) (caseous) (chromogenic acid-fast bacilli)
  (degeneration) (fibrocaseous) (fistula) (interstitial)
  (isolated circumscribed lesions) (necrosis)
  (parenchymatous) (ulcerative) A15.9
  with pneumoconiosis (any condition in J60-J64) J65
  abdomen (lymph gland) A18.39
  abscess (respiratory) A15.9
    bone A18.03
      hip A18.02
      knee A18.02
      sacrum A18.01
      specified site NEC A18.03
      spinal A18.01
      vertebra A18.01
    brain A17.81
    breast A18.89
    Cowper's gland A18.15
    dura (mater) (cerebral) (spinal) A17.81
    epidural (cerebral) (spinal) A17.81
    female pelvis A18.17
    frontal sinus A15.8
    genital organs NEC A18.10
    genitourinary A18.10
    gland (lymphatic) — see Tuberculosis, lymph gland
    hip A18.02
    intestine A18.32
    ischiorectal A18.32
    joint NEC A18.02
      hip A18.02
      knee A18.02
      specified NEC A18.02
      vertebral A18.01
    kidney A18.11
    knee A18.02
    latent R76.11
    lumbar (spine) A18.01
    lung — see Tuberculosis, pulmonary
    meninges (cerebral) (spinal) A17.0
    muscle A18.09
    perianal (fistula) A18.32
    perinephritic A18.11
    perirectal A18.32
    rectum A18.32
    retropharyngeal A15.8
    sacrum A18.01
    scrofulous A18.2
    scrotum A18.15
    skin (primary) A18.4
    spinal cord A17.81
    spine or vertebra (column) A18.01
    subdiaphragmatic A18.31
    testis A18.15
    urinary A18.13
    uterus A18.17
  accessory sinus — see Tuberculosis, sinus
  Addison's disease A18.7
  adenitis — see Tuberculosis, lymph gland
  adenoids A15.8
  adenopathy — see Tuberculosis, lymph gland
  adherent pericardium A18.84
  adnexa (uteri) A18.17
  adrenal (capsule) (gland) A18.7
  alimentary canal A18.32
  anemia A18.89
  ankle (joint) (bone) A18.02
  anus A18.32
  apex, apical — see Tuberculosis, pulmonary
  appendicitis, appendix A18.32
  arachnoid A17.0

Tuberculosis, tubercular, tuberculous — continued
  artery, arteritis A18.89
    cerebral A18.89
  arthritis (chronic) (synovial) A18.02
    spine or vertebra (column) A18.01
  articular — see Tuberculosis, joint
  ascites A18.31
  asthma — see Tuberculosis, pulmonary
  axilla, axillary (gland) A18.2
  bladder A18.12
  bone A18.03
    hip A18.02
    knee A18.02
    limb NEC A18.03
    sacrum A18.01
    spine or vertebral column A18.01
  bowel (miliary) A18.32
  brain A17.81
  breast A18.89
  broad ligament A18.17
  bronchi, bronchial, bronchus A15.5
    ectasia, ectasis (bronchiectasis) — see Tuberculosis,
      pulmonary
    fistula A15.5
      primary (progressive) A15.7
    gland or node A15.4
      primary (progressive) A15.7
    lymph gland or node A15.4
      primary (progressive) A15.7
  bronchiectasis — see Tuberculosis, pulmonary
  bronchitis A15.5
  bronchopleural A15.6
  bronchopneumonia, bronchopneumonic — see Tuber-
    culosis, pulmonary
  bronchorrhagia A15.5
  bronchotracheal A15.5
  bronze disease A18.7
  buccal cavity A18.83
  bulbourethral gland A18.15
  bursa A18.09
  cachexia A15.9
  cardiomyopathy A18.84
  caries — see Tuberculosis, bone
  cartilage A18.02
    intervertebral A18.01
  catarrhal — see Tuberculosis, respiratory
  cecum A18.32
  cellulitis (primary) A18.4
  cerebellum A17.81
  cerebral, cerebrum A17.81
  cerebrospinal A17.81
    meninges A17.0
  cervical (lymph gland or node) A18.2
  cervicitis, cervix (uteri) A18.16
  chest — see Tuberculosis, respiratory
  chorioretinitis A18.53
  choroid, choroiditis A18.53
  ciliary body A18.54
  colitis A18.32
  collier's J65
  colliquativa (primary) A18.4
  colon A18.32
  complex, primary A15.7
  congenital P37.0
  conjunctiva A18.59
  connective tissue (systemic) A18.89
  contact Z20.1
  cornea (ulcer) A18.52
  Cowper's gland A18.15
  coxae A18.02
  coxalgia A18.02
  cul-de-sac of Douglas A18.17
  curvature, spine A18.01
  cutis (colliquativa) (primary) A18.4
  cyst, ovary A18.18
  cystitis A18.12
  dactylitis A18.03
  diarrhea A18.32
  diffuse — see Tuberculosis, miliary
  digestive tract A18.32
  disseminated — see Tuberculosis, miliary
  duodenum A18.32
  dura (mater) (cerebral) (spinal) A17.0
    abscess (cerebral) (spinal) A17.81
  dysentery A18.32
  ear (inner) (middle) A18.6
    bone A18.03
    external (primary) A18.4

⏷ **Subterms under main terms may continue to next column or page**   ☑ **Additional Character Required — Refer to the Tabular List for Character Selection**

Tuberculosis, tubercular, tuberculous — *continued*

ear — *continued*
   skin (primary) A18.4
elbow A18.02
emphysema — *see* Tuberculosis, pulmonary
empyema A15.6
encephalitis A17.82
endarteritis A18.89
endocarditis A18.84
   aortic A18.84
   mitral A18.84
   pulmonary A18.84
   tricuspid A18.84
endocrine glands NEC A18.82
endometrium A18.17
enteric, enterica, enteritis A18.32
enterocolitis A18.32
epididymis, epididymitis A18.15
epidural abscess (cerebral) (spinal) A17.81
epiglottis A15.5
episcleritis A18.51
erythema (induratum) (nodosum) (primary) A18.4
esophagus A18.83
eustachian tube A18.6
exposure (to) Z20.1
exudative — *see* Tuberculosis, pulmonary
eye A18.50
eyelid (primary) (lupus) A18.4
fallopian tube (acute) (chronic) A18.17
fascia A18.09
fauces A15.8
female pelvic inflammatory disease A18.17
finger A18.03
first infection A15.7
gallbladder A18.83
ganglion A18.09
gastritis A18.83
gastrocolic fistula A18.32
gastroenteritis A18.32
gastrointestinal tract A18.32
general, generalized — *see* Tuberculosis, miliary
genital organs A18.10
genitourinary A18.10
genu A18.02
glandula suprarenalis A18.7
glandular, general A18.2
glottis A15.5
grinder's J65
gum A18.83
hand A18.03
heart A18.84
hematogenous — *see* Tuberculosis, miliary
hemoptysis — *see* Tuberculosis, pulmonary
hemorrhage NEC — *see* Tuberculosis, pulmonary
hemothorax A15.6
hepatitis A18.83
hilar lymph nodes A15.4
   primary (progressive) A15.7
hip (joint) (disease) (bone) A18.02
hydropneumothorax A15.6
hydrothorax A15.6
hypoadrenalism A18.7
hypopharynx A15.8
ileocecal (hyperplastic) A18.32
ileocolitis A18.32
ileum A18.32
iliac spine (superior) A18.03
immunological findings only A15.7
indurativa (primary) A18.4
infantile A15.7
infection A15.9
   without clinical manifestations A15.7
infraclavicular gland A18.2
inguinal gland A18.2
inguinalis A18.2
intestine (any part) A18.32
iridocyclitis A18.54
iris, iritis A18.54
ischiorectal A18.32
jaw A18.03
jejunum A18.32
joint A18.02
   vertebral A18.01
keratitis (interstitial) A18.52
keratoconjunctivitis A18.52
kidney A18.11
knee (joint) A18.02
kyphosis, kyphoscoliosis A18.01

Tuberculosis, tubercular, tuberculous — *continued*

laryngitis A15.5
larynx A15.5
latent R76.11
leptomeninges, leptomeningitis (cerebral) (spinal) A17.0
lichenoides (primary) A18.4
linguae A18.83
lip A18.83
liver A18.83
lordosis A18.01
lung — *see* Tuberculosis, pulmonary
lupus vulgaris A18.4
lymph gland or node (peripheral) A18.2
   abdomen A18.39
   bronchial A15.4
     primary (progressive) A15.7
   cervical A18.2
   hilar A15.4
     primary (progressive) A15.7
   intrathoracic A15.4
     primary (progressive) A15.7
   mediastinal A15.4
     primary (progressive) A15.7
   mesenteric A18.39
   retroperitoneal A18.39
   tracheobronchial A15.4
     primary (progressive) A15.7
lymphadenitis — *see* Tuberculosis, lymph gland
lymphangitis — *see* Tuberculosis, lymph gland
lymphatic (gland) (vessel) — *see* Tuberculosis, lymph gland
mammary gland A18.89
marasmus A15.9
mastoiditis A18.03
mediastinal lymph gland or node A15.4
   primary (progressive) A15.7
mediastinitis A15.8
   primary (progressive) A15.7
mediastinum A15.8
   primary (progressive) A15.7
medulla A17.81
melanosis, Addisonian A18.7
meninges, meningitis (basilar) (cerebral) (cerebrospinal) (spinal) A17.0
meningoencephalitis A17.82
mesentery, mesenteric (gland or node) A18.39
miliary A19.9
   acute A19.2
     multiple sites A19.1
     single specified site A19.0
   chronic A19.8
   specified NEC A19.8
millstone makers' J65
miner's J65
molder's J65
mouth A18.83
multiple A19.9
   acute A19.1
   chronic A19.8
muscle A18.09
myelitis A17.82
myocardium, myocarditis A18.84
nasal (passage) (sinus) A15.8
nasopharynx A15.8
neck gland A18.2
nephritis A18.11
nerve (mononeuropathy) A17.83
nervous system A17.9
nose (septum) A15.8
ocular A18.50
omentum A18.31
oophoritis (acute) (chronic) A18.17
optic (nerve trunk) (papilla) A18.59
orbit A18.59
orchitis A18.15
organ, specified NEC A18.89
osseous — *see* Tuberculosis, bone
osteitis — *see* Tuberculosis, bone
osteomyelitis — *see* Tuberculosis, bone
otitis media A18.6
ovary, ovaritis (acute) (chronic) A18.17
oviduct (acute) (chronic) A18.17
pachymeningitis A17.0
palate (soft) A18.83
pancreas A18.83
papulonecrotic (a) (primary) A18.4
parathyroid glands A18.82

Tuberculosis, tubercular, tuberculous — *continued*

paronychia (primary) A18.4
parotid gland or region A18.83
pelvis (bony) A18.03
penis A18.15
peribronchitis A15.5
pericardium, pericarditis A18.84
perichondritis, larynx A15.5
periostitis — *see* Tuberculosis, bone
perirectal fistula A18.32
peritoneum NEC A18.31
peritonitis A18.31
pharynx, pharyngitis A15.8
phlyctenulosis (keratoconjunctivitis) A18.52
phthisis NEC — *see* Tuberculosis, pulmonary
pituitary gland A18.82
pleura, pleural, pleurisy, pleuritis (fibrinous) (obliterative) (purulent) (simple plastic) (with effusion) A15.6
   primary (progressive) A15.7
pneumonia, pneumonic — *see* Tuberculosis, pulmonary
pneumothorax (spontaneous) (tense valvular) — *see* Tuberculosis, pulmonary
polyneuropathy A17.89
polyserositis A19.9
   acute A19.1
   chronic A19.8
potter's J65
prepuce A18.15
primary (complex) A15.7
proctitis A18.32
prostate, prostatitis A18.14
pulmonalis — *see* Tuberculosis, pulmonary
pulmonary (cavitated) (fibrotic) (infiltrative) (nodular) A15.0
   childhood type or first infection A15.7
   primary (complex) A15.7
pyelitis A18.11
pyelonephritis A18.11
pyemia — *see* Tuberculosis, miliary
pyonephrosis A18.11
pyopneumothorax A15.6
pyothorax A15.6
rectum (fistula) (with abscess) A18.32
reinfection stage — *see* Tuberculosis, pulmonary
renal A18.11
renis A18.11
respiratory A15.9
   primary A15.7
   specified site NEC A15.8
retina, retinitis A18.53
retroperitoneal (lymph gland or node) A18.39
rheumatism NEC A18.09
rhinitis A15.8
sacroiliac (joint) A18.01
sacrum A18.01
salivary gland A18.83
salpingitis (acute) (chronic) A18.17
sandblaster's J65
sclera A18.51
scoliosis A18.01
scrofulous A18.2
scrotum A18.15
seminal tract or vesicle A18.15
senile A15.9
septic — *see* Tuberculosis, miliary
shoulder (joint) A18.02
   blade A18.03
sigmoid A18.32
sinus (any nasal) A15.8
   bone A18.03
   epididymis A18.15
skeletal NEC A18.03
skin (any site) (primary) A18.4
small intestine A18.32
soft palate A18.83
spermatic cord A18.15
spine, spinal (column) A18.01
   cord A17.81
   medulla A17.81
   membrane A17.0
   meninges A17.0
spleen, splenitis A18.85
spondylitis A18.01
sternoclavicular joint A18.02
stomach A18.83
stonemason's J65

Ulcer, ulcerated, ulcerating, ulceration, ulcerative

— *continued*
gum K06.8
gumma, due to yaws A66.4
heel — *see* Ulcer, lower limb
hemorrhoid (*see also* Hemorrhoids, by degree) K64.8
Hunner's — *see* Cystitis, interstitial
hypopharynx J39.2
hypopyon (chronic) (subacute) — *see* Ulcer, cornea,
  with hypopyon
hypostaticum — *see* Ulcer, varicose
ileum — *see* Ulcer, intestine
intestine, intestinal K63.3
  with perforation K63.1
  amebic A06.1
  duodenal — *see* Ulcer, duodenum
  granulocytopenic (with hemorrhage) — *see* Neu-
    tropenia
  marginal — *see* Ulcer, gastrojejunal
  perforating K63.1
    newborn P78.0
  primary, small intestine K63.3
  rectum K62.6
  stercoraceous, stercoral K63.3
  tuberculous A18.32
  typhoid (fever) — *see* Typhoid
  varicose I86.8
jejunum, jejunal — *see* Ulcer, gastrojejunal
keratitis — *see* Ulcer, cornea
knee — *see* Ulcer, lower limb
labium (majus) (minus) N76.6
laryngitis — *see* Laryngitis
larynx (aphthous) (contact) J38.7
  diphtheritic A36.2
leg — *see* Ulcer, lower limb
lip K13.0
Lipschütz's N76.6
lower limb (atrophic) (chronic) (neurogenic) (perforat-
    ing) (pyogenic) (trophic) (tropical) L97.909
  with
    bone necrosis L97.904
    exposed fat layer L97.902
    muscle necrosis L97.903
    skin breakdown only L97.901
  ankle L97.309
    with
      bone necrosis L97.304
      exposed fat layer L97.302
      muscle necrosis L97.303
      skin breakdown only L97.301
    left L97.329
      with
        bone necrosis L97.324
        exposed fat layer L97.322
        muscle necrosis L97.323
        skin breakdown only L97.321
    right L97.319
      with
        bone necrosis L97.314
        exposed fat layer L97.312
        muscle necrosis L97.313
        skin breakdown only L97.311
  calf L97.209
    with
      bone necrosis L97.204
      exposed fat layer L97.202
      muscle necrosis L97.203
      skin breakdown only L97.201
    left L97.229
      with
        bone necrosis L97.224
        exposed fat layer L97.222
        muscle necrosis L97.223
        skin breakdown only L97.221
    right L97.219
      with
        bone necrosis L97.214
        exposed fat layer L97.212
        muscle necrosis L97.213
        skin breakdown only L97.211
  decubitus — *see* Ulcer, pressure, by site
  foot specified NEC L97.509
    with
      bone necrosis L97.504
      exposed fat layer L97.502
      muscle necrosis L97.503
      skin breakdown only L97.501
    left L97.529

Ulcer, ulcerated, ulcerating, ulceration, ulcerative

— *continued*
lower limb — *continued*
  foot specified — *continued*
    left — *continued*
      with
        bone necrosis L97.524
        exposed fat layer L97.522
        muscle necrosis L97.523
        skin breakdown only L97.521
    right L97.519
      with
        bone necrosis L97.514
        exposed fat layer L97.512
        muscle necrosis L97.513
        skin breakdown only L97.511
  heel L97.409
    with
      bone necrosis L97.404
      exposed fat layer L97.402
      muscle necrosis L97.403
      skin breakdown only L97.401
    left L97.429
      with
        bone necrosis L97.424
        exposed fat layer L97.422
        muscle necrosis L97.423
        skin breakdown only L97.421
    right L97.419
      with
        bone necrosis L97.414
        exposed fat layer L97.412
        muscle necrosis L97.413
        skin breakdown only L97.411
  left L97.929
    with
      bone necrosis L97.924
      exposed fat layer L97.922
      muscle necrosis L97.923
      skin breakdown only L97.921
  leprous A30.1
  lower leg NOS L97.909
    with
      bone necrosis L97.904
      exposed fat layer L97.902
      muscle necrosis L97.903
      skin breakdown only L97.901
    left L97.929
      with
        bone necrosis L97.924
        exposed fat layer L97.922
        muscle necrosis L97.923
        skin breakdown only L97.921
    right L97.919
      with
        bone necrosis L97.914
        exposed fat layer L97.912
        muscle necrosis L97.913
        skin breakdown only L97.911
  specified site NEC L97.809
    with
      bone necrosis L97.804
      exposed fat layer L97.802
      muscle necrosis L97.803
      skin breakdown only L97.801
    left L97.829
      with
        bone necrosis L97.824
        exposed fat layer L97.822
        muscle necrosis L97.823
        skin breakdown only L97.821
    right L97.819
      with
        bone necrosis L97.814
        exposed fat layer L97.812
        muscle necrosis L97.813
        skin breakdown only L97.811
  midfoot L97.409
    with
      bone necrosis L97.404
      exposed fat layer L97.402
      muscle necrosis L97.403
      skin breakdown only L97.401
    left L97.429
      with
        bone necrosis L97.424
        exposed fat layer L97.422
        muscle necrosis L97.423

Ulcer, ulcerated, ulcerating, ulceration, ulcerative

— *continued*
lower limb — *continued*
  midfoot — *continued*
    left — *continued*
      with — *continued*
        skin breakdown only L97.421
    right L97.419
      with
        bone necrosis L97.414
        exposed fat layer L97.412
        muscle necrosis L97.413
        skin breakdown only L97.411
  right L97.919
    with
      bone necrosis L97.914
      exposed fat layer L97.912
      muscle necrosis L97.913
      skin breakdown only L97.911
  syphilitic A52.19
  thigh L97.109
    with
      bone necrosis L97.104
      exposed fat layer L97.102
      muscle necrosis L97.103
      skin breakdown only L97.101
    left L97.129
      with
        bone necrosis L97.124
        exposed fat layer L97.122
        muscle necrosis L97.123
        skin breakdown only L97.121
    right L97.119
      with
        bone necrosis L97.114
        exposed fat layer L97.112
        muscle necrosis L97.113
        skin breakdown only L97.111
  toe L97.509
    with
      bone necrosis L97.504
      exposed fat layer L97.502
      muscle necrosis L97.503
      skin breakdown only L97.501
    left L97.529
      with
        bone necrosis L97.524
        exposed fat layer L97.522
        muscle necrosis L97.523
        skin breakdown only L97.521
    right L97.519
      with
        bone necrosis L97.514
        exposed fat layer L97.512
        muscle necrosis L97.513
        skin breakdown only L97.511
  varicose — *see* Varix, leg, with, ulcer
luetic — *see* Ulcer, syphilitic
lung J98.4
  tuberculous — *see* Tuberculosis, pulmonary
malignant — *see* Neoplasm, malignant, by site
marginal NEC — *see* Ulcer, gastrojejunal
meatus (urinarius) N34.2
Meckel's diverticulum Q43.0
  malignant — *see* Table of Neoplasms, small intes-
    tine, malignant
Meleney's (chronic undermining) — *see* Ulcer, skin
Mooren's (cornea) — *see* Ulcer, cornea, Mooren's
mycobacterial (skin) A31.1
nasopharynx J39.2
neck, uterus N86
neurogenic NEC — *see* Ulcer, skin
nose, nasal (passage) (infective) (septum) J34.0
  skin — *see* Ulcer, skin
  spirochetal A69.8
  varicose (bleeding) I86.8
oral mucosa (traumatic) K12.1
palate (soft) K12.1
penis (chronic) N48.5
peptic (site unspecified) K27.9
  with
    hemorrhage K27.4
      and perforation K27.6
    perforation K27.5
  acute K27.3
    with
      hemorrhage K27.0
        and perforation K27.2

Ulcer, ulcerated, ulcerating, ulceration, ulcerative
— *continued*
　peptic — *continued*
　　acute — *continued*
　　　with — *continued*
　　　　perforation K27.1
　　chronic K27.7
　　　with
　　　　hemorrhage K27.4
　　　　　and perforation K27.6
　　　　perforation K27.5
　　esophagus K22.10
　　　with bleeding K22.11
　　newborn P78.82
　　perforating K27.5
　skin — *see* Ulcer, skin
　peritonsillar J35.8
　phagedenic (tropical) — *see* Ulcer, skin
　pharynx J39.2
　phlebitis — *see* Phlebitis
　plaster — *see* Ulcer, pressure, by site
　popliteal space — *see* Ulcer, lower limb
　postpyloric — *see* Ulcer, duodenum
　prepuce N47.7
　prepyloric — *see* Ulcer, stomach
　pressure (pressure area) L89.9- ☑
　　ankle L89.5- ☑
　　back L89.1- ☑
　　buttock L89.3- ☑
　　coccyx L89.15- ☑
　　contiguous site of back, buttock, hip L89.4- ☑
　　elbow L89.0- ☑
　　face L89.81- ☑
　　head L89.81- ☑
　　heel L89.6- ☑
　　hip L89.2- ☑
　　sacral region (tailbone) L89.15- ☑
　　specified site NEC L89.89- ☑
　　stage 1 (healing) (pre-ulcer skin changes limited to persistent focal edema)
　　　ankle L89.5- ☑
　　　back L89.1- ☑
　　　buttock L89.3- ☑
　　　coccyx L89.15- ☑
　　　contiguous site of back, buttock, hip L89.4- ☑
　　　elbow L89.0- ☑
　　　face L89.81- ☑
　　　head L89.81- ☑
　　　heel L89.6- ☑
　　　hip L89.2- ☑
　　　sacral region (tailbone) L89.15- ☑
　　　specified site NEC L89.89- ☑
　　stage 2 (healing) (abrasion, blister, partial thickness skin loss involving epidermis and/or dermis)
　　　ankle L89.5- ☑
　　　back L89.1- ☑
　　　buttock L89.3- ☑
　　　coccyx L89.15- ☑
　　　contiguous site of back, buttock, hip L89.4- ☑
　　　elbow L89.0- ☑
　　　face L89.81- ☑
　　　head L89.81- ☑
　　　heel L89.6- ☑
　　　hip L89.2- ☑
　　　sacral region (tailbone) L89.15- ☑
　　　specified site NEC L89.89- ☑
　　stage 3 (healing) (full thickness skin loss involving damage or necrosis of subcutaneous tissue)
　　　ankle L89.5- ☑
　　　back L89.1- ☑
　　　buttock L89.3- ☑
　　　coccyx L89.15- ☑
　　　contiguous site of back, buttock, hip L89.4- ☑
　　　elbow L89.0- ☑
　　　face L89.81- ☑
　　　head L89.81- ☑
　　　heel L89.6- ☑
　　　hip L89.2- ☑
　　　sacral region (tailbone) L89.15- ☑
　　　specified site NEC L89.89- ☑
　　stage 4 (healing) (necrosis of soft tissues through to underlying muscle, tendon, or bone)
　　　ankle L89.5- ☑
　　　back L89.1- ☑
　　　buttock L89.3- ☑
　　　coccyx L89.15- ☑

Ulcer, ulcerated, ulcerating, ulceration, ulcerative
— *continued*
　pressure — *continued*
　　stage 4 — *continued*
　　　contiguous site of back, buttock, hip L89.4- ☑
　　　elbow L89.0- ☑
　　　face L89.81- ☑
　　　head L89.81- ☑
　　　heel L89.6- ☑
　　　hip L89.2- ☑
　　　sacral region (tailbone) L89.15- ☑
　　　specified site NEC L89.89- ☑
　　unspecified stage
　　　ankle L89.5- ☑
　　　back L89.1- ☑
　　　buttock L89.3- ☑
　　　coccyx L89.15- ☑
　　　contiguous site of back, buttock, hip L89.4- ☑
　　　elbow L89.0- ☑
　　　face L89.81- ☑
　　　head L89.81- ☑
　　　heel L89.6- ☑
　　　hip L89.2- ☑
　　　sacral region (tailbone) L89.15- ☑
　　　specified site NEC L89.89- ☑
　　unstageable
　　　ankle L89.5- ☑
　　　back L89.1- ☑
　　　buttock L89.3- ☑
　　　coccyx L89.15- ☑
　　　contiguous site of back, buttock, hip L89.4- ☑
　　　elbow L89.0- ☑
　　　face L89.81- ☑
　　　head L89.81- ☑
　　　heel L89.6- ☑
　　　hip L89.2- ☑
　　　sacral region (tailbone) L89.15- ☑
　　　specified site NEC L89.89- ☑
　primary of intestine K63.3
　　with perforation K63.1
　prostate N41.9
　pyloric — *see* Ulcer, stomach
　rectosigmoid K63.3
　　with perforation K63.1
　rectum (sphincter) (solitary) K62.6
　　stercoraceous, stercoral K62.6
　retina — *see* Inflammation, chorioretinal
　rodent (*see also* Neoplasm, skin, malignant)
　sclera — *see* Scleritis
　scrofulous (tuberculous) A18.2
　scrotum N50.8
　　tuberculous A18.15
　　varicose I86.1
　seminal vesicle N50.8
　sigmoid — *see* Ulcer, intestine
　skin (atrophic) (chronic) (neurogenic) (non-healing) (perforating) (pyogenic) (trophic) (tropical) L98.499
　　with gangrene — *see* Gangrene
　　amebic A06.7
　　back — *see* Ulcer, back
　　buttock — *see* Ulcer, buttock
　　decubitus — *see* Ulcer, pressure
　　lower limb — *see* Ulcer, lower limb
　　mycobacterial A31.1
　　specified site NEC L98.499
　　　with
　　　　bone necrosis L98.494
　　　　exposed fat layer L98.492
　　　　muscle necrosis L98.493
　　　　skin breakdown only L98.491
　　tuberculous (primary) A18.4
　　varicose — *see* Ulcer, varicose
　sloughing — *see* Ulcer, skin
　solitary, anus or rectum (sphincter) K62.6
　sore throat J02.9
　　streptococcal J02.0
　spermatic cord N50.8
　spine (tuberculous) A18.01
　stasis (venous) — *see* Varix, leg, with, ulcer
　　without varicose veins I87.2
　stercoraceous, stercoral K63.3
　　with perforation K63.1
　　anus or rectum K62.6
　stoma, stomal — *see* Ulcer, gastrojejunal
　stomach (eroded) (peptic) (round) K25.9
　　with

Ulcer, ulcerated, ulcerating, ulceration, ulcerative
— *continued*
　stomach — *continued*
　　with — *continued*
　　　hemorrhage K25.4
　　　　and perforation K25.6
　　　perforation K25.5
　　acute K25.3
　　　with
　　　　hemorrhage K25.0
　　　　　and perforation K25.2
　　　　perforation K25.1
　　chronic K25.7
　　　with
　　　　hemorrhage K25.4
　　　　　and perforation K25.6
　　　　perforation K25.5
　stomal — *see* Ulcer, gastrojejunal
　stomatitis K12.1
　stress — *see* Ulcer, peptic
　strumous (tuberculous) A18.2
　submucosal, bladder — *see* Cystitis, interstitial
　syphilitic (any site) (early) (secondary) A51.39
　　late A52.79
　　　perforating A52.79
　　　　foot A52.11
　testis N50.8
　thigh — *see* Ulcer, lower limb
　throat J39.2
　　diphtheritic A36.0
　toe — *see* Ulcer, lower limb
　tongue (traumatic) K14.0
　tonsil J35.8
　　diphtheritic A36.0
　trachea J39.8
　trophic — *see* Ulcer, skin
　tropical — *see* Ulcer, skin
　tuberculous — *see* Tuberculosis, ulcer
　tunica vaginalis N50.8
　turbinate J34.89
　typhoid (perforating) — *see* Typhoid
　unspecified site — *see* Ulcer, skin
　urethra (meatus) — *see* Urethritis
　uterus N85.8
　　cervix N86
　　　with cervicitis N72
　　neck N86
　　　with cervicitis N72
　vagina N76.5
　　in Behçet's disease M35.2 [N77.0]
　　pessary N89.8
　valve, heart I33.0
　varicose (lower limb, any part) (*see also* Varix, leg, with, ulcer)
　　broad ligament I86.2
　　esophagus — *see* Varix, esophagus
　　inflamed or infected — *see* Varix, leg, with ulcer, with inflammation
　　nasal septum I86.8
　　perineum I86.3
　　scrotum I86.1
　　specified site NEC I86.8
　　sublingual I86.0
　　vulva I86.3
　vas deferens N50.8
　vulva (acute) (infectional) N76.6
　　in (due to)
　　　Behçet's disease M35.2 [N77.0]
　　　herpesviral (herpes simplex) infection A60.04
　　　tuberculosis A18.18
　vulvobuccal, recurring N76.6
　X-ray L58.1
　yaws A66.4

Ulcerosa scarlatina A38.8

Ulcus (*see also* Ulcer)
　cutis tuberculosum A18.4
　duodeni — *see* Ulcer, duodenum
　durum (syphilitic) A51.0
　　extragenital A51.2
　gastrojejunale — *see* Ulcer, gastrojejunal
　hypostaticum — *see* Ulcer, varicose
　molle (cutis) (skin) A57
　serpens corneae — *see* Ulcer, cornea, central
　ventriculi — *see* Ulcer, stomach

Ulegyria Q04.8

Ulerythema
　ophryogenes, congenital Q84.2
　sycosiforme L73.8

Ullrich (-Bonnevie)(-Turner) **syndrome** Q87.1
Ullrich-Feichtiger syndrome Q87.0
Ulnar — *see* condition
Ulorrhagia, ulorrhea K06.8
Umbilicus, umbilical — *see* condition
Unacceptable
  contours of tooth K08.54
  morphology of tooth K08.54
Unavailability (of)
  bed at medical facility Z75.1
  health service-related agencies Z75.4
  medical facilities (at) Z75.3
    due to
      investigation by social service agency Z75.2
      lack of services at home Z75.0
      remoteness from facility Z75.3
      waiting list Z75.1
    home Z75.0
    outpatient clinic Z75.3
  schooling Z55.1
  social service agencies Z75.4
Uncinaria americana infestation B76.1
Uncinariasis B76.9
Uncongenial work Z56.5
Unconscious (ness) — *see* Coma
Under observation — *see* Observation
Underachievement in school Z55.3
Underdevelopment (*see also* Undeveloped)
  nose Q30.1
  sexual E30.0
Underdosing (*see also* Table of Drugs and Chemicals,
    categories T36-T50, with final character 6) Z91.14
  intentional NEC Z91.128
    due to financial hardship of patient Z91.120
  unintentional NEC Z91.138
    due to patient's age related debility Z91.130
Underfeeding, newborn P92.3
Underfill, endodontic M27.53
Underimmunization status Z28.3
Undernourishment — *see* Malnutrition
Undernutrition — *see* Malnutrition
Underweight R63.6
  for gestational age — *see* Light for dates
Underwood's disease P83.0
Undescended (*see also* Malposition, congenital)
  cecum Q43.3
  colon Q43.3
  testicle — *see* Cryptorchid
Undeveloped, undevelopment (*see also* Hypoplasia)
  brain (congenital) Q02
  cerebral (congenital) Q02
  heart Q24.8
  lung Q33.6
  testis E29.1
  uterus E30.0
Undiagnosed (disease) R69
Undulant fever — *see* Brucellosis
Unemployment, anxiety concerning Z56.0
  threatened Z56.2
Unequal length (acquired) (limb) (*see also* Deformity,
    limb, unequal length)
  leg (*see also* Deformity, limb, unequal length)
    congenital Q72.9- ☑
Unextracted dental root K08.3
Unguis incarnatus L60.0
Unhappiness R45.2
Unicornate uterus Q51.4
Unilateral (*see also* condition)
  development, breast N64.89
  organ or site, congenital NEC — *see* Agenesis, by site
Unilocular heart Q20.8
Union, abnormal (*see also* Fusion)
  larynx and trachea Q34.8
Universal mesentery Q43.3
Unrepairable overhanging of dental restorative
    materials K08.52
Unsatisfactory
  restoration of tooth K08.50
    specified NEC K08.59
  sample of cytologic smear
    anus R85.615
    cervix R87.615
    vagina R87.625
  surroundings Z59.1
  work Z56.5
Unsoundness of mind — *see* Psychosis

Unstable
  back NEC — *see* Instability, joint, spine
  hip (congenital) Q65.6
    acquired — *see* Derangement, joint, specified type
      NEC, hip
  joint — *see* Instability, joint
    secondary to removal of joint prosthesis M96.89
  lie (mother) O32.0 ☑
  lumbosacral joint (congenital)
    acquired — *see* subcategory M53.2 ☑
  sacroiliac — *see* subcategory M53.2 ☑
  spine NEC — *see* Instability, joint, spine
Unsteadiness on feet R26.81
Untruthfulness, child problem F91.8
Unverricht (-Lundborg) **disease or epilepsy** — *see*
    Epilepsy, generalized, idiopathic
Unwanted pregnancy Z64.0
Upbringing, institutional Z62.22
  away from parents NEC Z62.29
  in care of non-parental family member Z62.21
  in foster care Z62.21
  in orphanage or group home Z62.22
  in welfare custody Z62.21
Upper respiratory — *see* condition
Upset
  gastric K30
  gastrointestinal K30
    psychogenic F45.8
  intestinal (large) (small) K59.9
    psychogenic F45.8
  menstruation N93.9
  mental F48.9
  stomach K30
    psychogenic F45.8
Urachus (*see also* condition)
  patent or persistent Q64.4
Urbach-Oppenheim disease (necrobiosis lipoidica dia-
    beticorum) — *see* E08-E13 with .620
Urbach's lipoid proteinosis E78.89
Urbach-Wiethe disease E78.89
Urban yellow fever A95.1
Urea
  blood, high — *see* Uremia
  cycle metabolism disorder — *see* Disorder, urea cycle
    metabolism
Uremia, uremic N19
  with
    ectopic or molar pregnancy O08.4
    polyneuropathy N18.9 [G63]
  chronic (*see also* Disease, kidney, chronic) N18.9
    due to hypertension — *see* Hypertensive, kidney
  complicating
    ectopic or molar pregnancy O08.4
  congenital P96.0
  extrarenal R39.2
  following ectopic or molar pregnancy O08.4
  newborn P96.0
  prerenal R39.2
Ureter, ureteral — *see* condition
Ureteralgia N23
Ureterectasis — *see* Hydroureter
Ureteritis N28.89
  cystica N28.86
  due to calculus N20.1
    with calculus, kidney N20.2
      with hydronephrosis N13.2
  gonococcal (acute) (chronic) A54.21
  nonspecific N28.89
Ureterocele N28.89
  congenital (orthotopic) Q62.31
  ectopic Q62.32
Ureterolith, ureterolithiasis — *see* Calculus, ureter
Ureterostomy
  attention to Z43.6
  status Z93.6
Urethra, urethral — *see* condition
Urethralgia R39.89
Urethritis (anterior) (posterior) N34.2
  calculous N21.1
  candidal B37.41
  chlamydial A56.01
  diplococcal (gonococcal) A54.01
    with abscess (accessory gland) (periurethral) A54.1
  gonococcal A54.01
    with abscess (accessory gland) (periurethral) A54.1
  nongonococcal N34.1
    Reiter's — *see* Reiter's disease

Urethritis — *continued*
  nonspecific N34.1
  nonvenereal N34.1
  postmenopausal N34.2
  puerperal O86.22
  Reiter's — *see* Reiter's disease
  specified NEC N34.2
  trichomonal or due to Trichomonas (vaginalis) A59.03
Urethrocele N81.0
  with
    cystocele — *see* Cystocele
    prolapse of uterus — *see* Prolapse, uterus
Urethrolithiasis (with colic or infection) N21.1
Urethrorectal — *see* condition
Urethrorrhagia N36.8
Urethrorrhea R36.9
Urethrostomy
  attention to Z43.6
  status Z93.6
Urethrotrigonitis — *see* Trigonitis
Urethrovaginal — *see* condition
Urgency
  fecal R15.2
  hypertensive — *see* Hypertension
  urinary N39.41
Urhidrosis, uridrosis L74.8
Uric acid in blood (increased) E79.0
Uricacidemia (asymptomatic) E79.0
Uricemia (asymptomatic) E79.0
Uricosuria R82.99
Urinary — *see* condition
Urination
  frequent R35.0
  painful R30.9
Urine
  blood in — *see* Hematuria
  discharge, excessive R35.8
  enuresis, nonorganic origin F98.0
  extravasation R39.0
  frequency R35.0
  incontinence R32
    nonorganic origin F98.0
  intermittent stream R39.19
  pus in N39.0
  retention or stasis R33.9
    organic R33.8
      drug-induced R33.0
    psychogenic F45.8
  secretion
    deficient R34
    excessive R35.8
    frequency R35.0
  stream
    intermittent R39.19
    slowing R39.19
    splitting R39.13
    weak R39.12
Urinemia — *see* Uremia
Urinoma, urethra N36.8
Uroarthritis, infectious (Reiter's) — *see* Reiter's disease
Urodialysis R34
Urolithiasis — *see* Calculus, urinary
Uronephrosis — *see* Hydronephrosis
Uropathy N39.9
  obstructive N13.9
    specified NEC N13.8
  reflux N13.9
    specified NEC N13.8
  vesicoureteral reflux-associated — *see* Reflux, vesi-
    coureteral
Urosepsis — *code to* condition
Urticaria L50.9
  with angioneurotic edema T78.3 ☑
    hereditary D84.1
  allergic L50.0
  cholinergic L50.5
  chronic L50.8
  cold, familial L50.2
  contact L50.6
  dermatographic L50.3
  due to
    cold or heat L50.2
    drugs L50.0
    food L50.0
    inhalants L50.0
    plants L50.6
    serum (*see also* Reaction, serum) T80.69 ☑

Urticaria — *continued*
  factitial L50.3
  giant T78.3 ☑
    hereditary D84.1
  gigantea T78.3 ☑
  idiopathic L50.1
  larynx T78.3 ☑
    hereditary D84.1
  neonatorum P83.8
  nonallergic L50.9
  papulosa (Hebra) L28.2
  pigmentosa Q82.2
  recurrent periodic L50.8
  serum (*see also* Reaction, serum) T80.69 ☑
  solar L56.3
  specified type NEC L50.8
  thermal (cold) (heat) L50.2
  vibratory L50.4
  xanthelasmoidea Q82.2
Use (of)
  alcohol F10.99
    with sleep disorder F10.982
    harmful — *see* Abuse, alcohol
  amphetamines — *see* Use, stimulant NEC
  caffeine — *see* Use, stimulant NEC
  cannabis F12.90
    with
      anxiety disorder F12.980
      intoxication F12.929
        with
          delirium F12.921
          perceptual disturbance F12.922
        uncomplicated F12.920
      other specified disorder F12.988
      psychosis F12.959
        delusions F12.950
        hallucinations F12.951
      unspecified disorder F12.99
  cocaine F14.90
    with
      anxiety disorder F14.980
      intoxication F14.929
        with
          delirium F14.921
          perceptual disturbance F14.922
        uncomplicated F14.920
      other specified disorder F14.988
      psychosis F14.959
        delusions F14.950
        hallucinations F14.951
      sexual dysfunction F14.981
      sleep disorder F14.982
      unspecified disorder F14.99
    harmful — *see* Abuse, drug, cocaine
  drug(s) NEC F19.90
    with sleep disorder F19.982
    harmful — *see* Abuse, drug, by type
  hallucinogen NEC F16.90
    with
      anxiety disorder F16.980
      intoxication F16.929
        with
          delirium F16.921
        uncomplicated F16.920
      mood disorder F16.94
      other specified disorder F16.988
      perception disorder (flashbacks) F16.983
      psychosis F16.959
        delusions F16.950
        hallucinations F16.951
      unspecified disorder F16.99
    harmful — *see* Abuse, drug, hallucinogen NEC
  inhalants F18.90
    with
      anxiety disorder F18.980
      intoxication F18.929
        with delirium F18.921
        uncomplicated F18.920
      mood disorder F18.94
      other specified disorder F18.988
      persisting dementia F18.97
      psychosis F18.959
        delusions F18.950
        hallucinations F18.951
      unspecified disorder F18.99
    harmful — *see* Abuse, drug, inhalant
    methadone F11.20

Use — *continued*
  nonprescribed drugs F19.90
    harmful — *see* Abuse, non-psychoactive substance
  opioid F11.90
    with
      disorder F11.99
        mood F11.94
        sleep F11.982
        specified type NEC F11.988
      intoxication F11.929
        with
          delirium F11.921
          perceptual disturbance F11.922
        uncomplicated F11.920
      withdrawal F11.93
    harmful — *see* Abuse, drug, opioid
  patent medicines F19.90
    harmful — *see* Abuse, non-psychoactive substance
  psychoactive drug NEC F19.90
    with
      anxiety disorder F19.980
      intoxication F19.929
        with
          delirium F19.921
          perceptual disturbance F19.922
        uncomplicated F19.920
      mood disorder F19.94
      other specified disorder F19.988
      persisting
        amnestic disorder F19.96
        dementia F19.97
      psychosis F19.959
        delusions F19.950
        hallucinations F19.951
      sexual dysfunction F19.981
      sleep disorder F19.982
      unspecified disorder F19.99
      withdrawal F19.939
        with
          delirium F19.931
          perceptual disturbance F19.932
        uncomplicated F19.930
    harmful — *see* Abuse, drug NEC, psychoactive NEC
  sedative, hypnotic, or anxiolytic F13.90
    with
      anxiety disorder F13.980
      intoxication F13.929
        with
          delirium F13.921
        uncomplicated F13.920
      other specified disorder F13.988
      persisting
        amnestic disorder F13.96
        dementia F13.97
      psychosis F13.959
        delusions F13.950
        hallucinations F13.951
      sexual dysfunction F13.981
      sleep disorder F13.982
      unspecified disorder F13.99
    harmful — *see* Abuse, drug, sedative, hypnotic, or anxiolytic
  stimulant NEC F15.90
    with
      anxiety disorder F15.980
      intoxication F15.929
        with
          delirium F15.921
          perceptual disturbance F15.922
        uncomplicated F15.920
      mood disorder F15.94
      other specified disorder F15.988
      psychosis F15.959
        delusions F15.950
        hallucinations F15.951
      sexual dysfunction F15.981
      sleep disorder F15.982
      unspecified disorder F15.99
      withdrawal F15.93
    harmful — *see* Abuse, drug, stimulant NEC
  tobacco Z72.0
    with dependence — *see* Dependence, drug, nicotine
  volatile solvents (*see also* Use, inhalant) F18.90
    harmful — *see* Abuse, drug, inhalant
Usher-Senear disease or syndrome L10.4
Uta B55.1
Uteromegaly N85.2

Uterovaginal — *see* condition
Uterovesical — *see* condition
Uveal — *see* condition
Uveitis (anterior) (*see also* Iridocyclitis)
  acute — *see* Iridocyclitis, acute
  chronic — *see* Iridocyclitis, chronic
  due to toxoplasmosis (acquired) B58.09
    congenital P37.1
  granulomatous — *see* Iridocyclitis, chronic
  heterochromic — *see* Cyclitis, Fuchs' heterochromic
  lens-induced — *see* Iridocyclitis, lens-induced
  posterior — *see* Chorioretinitis
  sympathetic H44.13- ☑
  syphilitic (secondary) A51.43
    congenital (early) A50.01
    late A52.71
  tuberculous A18.54
Uveoencephalitis — *see* Inflammation, chorioretinal
Uveokeratitis — *see* Iridocyclitis
Uveoparotitis D86.89
Uvula — *see* condition
Uvulitis (acute) (catarrhal) (chronic) (membranous) (suppurative) (ulcerative) K12.2

V

Vaccination (prophylactic)
  complication or reaction — *see* Complications, vaccination
  delayed Z28.9
  encounter for Z23
  not done — *see* Immunization, not done, because (of)
Vaccinia (generalized) (localized) T88.1 ☑
  without vaccination B08.011
  congenital P35.8
Vacuum, in sinus (accessory) (nasal) J34.89
Vagabond, vagabondage Z59.0
Vagabond's disease B85.1
Vagina, vaginal — *see* condition
Vaginalitis (tunica) (testis) N49.1
Vaginismus (reflex) N94.2
  functional F52.5
  nonorganic F52.5
  psychogenic F52.5
  secondary N94.2
Vaginitis (acute) (circumscribed) (diffuse) (emphysematous) (nonvenereal) (ulcerative) N76.0
  with ectopic or molar pregnancy O08.0
  amebic A06.82
  atrophic, postmenopausal N95.2
  bacterial N76.0
  blennorrhagic (gonococcal) A54.02
  candidal B37.3
  chlamydial A56.02
  chronic N76.1
  due to Trichomonas (vaginalis) A59.01
  following ectopic or molar pregnancy O08.0
  gonococcal A54.02
    with abscess (accessory gland) (periurethral) A54.1
  granuloma A58
  in (due to)
    candidiasis B37.3
    herpesviral (herpes simplex) infection A60.04
    pinworm infection B80 [N77.1]
  monilial B37.3
  mycotic (candidal) B37.3
  postmenopausal atrophic N95.2
  puerperal (postpartum) O86.13
  senile (atrophic) N95.2
  subacute or chronic N76.1
  syphilitic (early) A51.0
    late A52.76
  trichomonal A59.01
  tuberculous A18.18
Vaginosis — *see* Vaginitis
Vagotonia G52.2
Vagrancy Z59.0
VAIN — *see* Neoplasia, intraepithelial, vagina
Vallecula — *see* condition
Valley fever B38.0
Valsuani's disease — *see* Anemia, obstetric
Valve, valvular (formation) (*see also* condition)
  cerebral ventricle (communicating) in situ Z98.2
  cervix, internal os Q51.828
  congenital NEC — *see* Atresia, by site
  ureter (pelvic junction) (vesical orifice) Q62.39
  urethra (congenital) (posterior) Q64.2

Valvulitis (chronic) — *see* Endocarditis
Valvulopathy — *see* Endocarditis
Van Bogaert's leukoencephalopathy (sclerosing) (subacute) A81.1
Van Bogaert-Scherer-Epstein disease or syndrome E75.5
Van Buchem's syndrome M85.2
Van Creveld-von Gierke disease E74.01
Van der Hoeve (-de Kleyn) **syndrome** Q78.0
Van der Woude's syndrome Q38.0
Van Neck's disease or osteochondrosis M91.0
Vanishing lung J44.9
Vapor asphyxia or suffocation T59.9 ☑
   specified agent — *see* Table of Drugs and Chemicals
Variance, lethal ball, prosthetic heart valve T82.09 ☑
Variants, thalassemic D56.8
Variations in hair color L67.1
Varicella B01.9
  with
    complications NEC B01.89
    encephalitis B01.11
    encephalomyelitis B01.11
    meningitis B01.0
    myelitis B01.12
    pneumonia B01.2
  congenital P35.8
Varices — *see* Varix
Varicocele (scrotum) (thrombosed) I86.1
  ovary I86.2
  perineum I86.3
  spermatic cord (ulcerated) I86.1
Varicose
  aneurysm (ruptured) I77.0
  dermatitis — *see* Varix, leg, with, inflammation
  eczema — *see* Varix, leg, with, inflammation
  phlebitis — *see* Varix, with, inflammation
  tumor — *see* Varix
  ulcer (lower limb, any part) (*see also* Varix, leg, with, ulcer)
    anus (*see also* Hemorrhoids) K64.8
    esophagus — *see* Varix, esophagus
    inflamed or infected — *see* Varix, leg, with ulcer, with inflammation
    nasal septum I86.8
    perineum I86.3
    scrotum I86.1
    specified site NEC I86.8
  vein — *see* Varix
  vessel — *see* Varix, leg
Varicosis, varicosities, varicosity — *see* Varix
Variola (major) (minor) B03
Varioloid B03
Varix (lower limb) (ruptured) I83.90
  with
    edema I83.899
    inflammation I83.10
      with ulcer (venous) I83.209
    pain I83.819
    specified complication NEC I83.899
    stasis dermatitis I83.10
      with ulcer (venous) I83.209
    swelling I83.899
    ulcer I83.009
      with inflammation I83.209
  aneurysmal I77.0
  asymptomatic I83.9- ☑
  bladder I86.2
  broad ligament I86.2
  complicating
    childbirth (lower extremity) O87.4
      anus or rectum O87.2
      genital (vagina, vulva or perineum) O87.8
    pregnancy (lower extremity) O22.0- ☑
      anus or rectum O22.4- ☑
      genital (vagina, vulva or perineum) O22.1- ☑
    puerperium (lower extremity) O87.4
      anus or rectum O87.2
      genital (vagina, vulva, perineum) O87.8
  congenital (any site) Q27.8
  esophagus (idiopathic) (primary) (ulcerated) I85.00
    bleeding I85.01
    congenital Q27.8
    in (due to)
      alcoholic liver disease I85.10
        bleeding I85.11
      cirrhosis of liver I85.10
        bleeding I85.11

Varix — *continued*
  esophagus — *continued*
    in — *continued*
      portal hypertension I85.10
        bleeding I85.11
      schistosomiasis I85.10
        bleeding I85.11
      toxic liver disease I85.10
        bleeding I85.11
    secondary I85.10
      bleeding I85.11
  gastric I86.4
  inflamed or infected I83.10
    ulcerated I83.209
  labia (majora) I86.3
  leg (asymptomatic) I83.90
    with
      edema I83.899
      inflammation I83.10
        with ulcer — *see* Varix, leg, with, ulcer, with inflammation by site
      pain I83.819
      specified complication NEC I83.899
      swelling I83.899
      ulcer I83.009
        with inflammation I83.209
        ankle I83.003
          with inflammation I83.203
        calf I83.002
          with inflammation I83.202
        foot NEC I83.005
          with inflammation I83.205
        heel I83.004
          with inflammation I83.204
        lower leg NEC I83.008
          with inflammation I83.208
        midfoot I83.004
          with inflammation I83.204
        thigh I83.001
          with inflammation I83.201
    bilateral (asymptomatic) I83.93
      with
        edema I83.893
        pain I83.813
        specified complication NEC I83.893
        swelling I83.893
        ulcer I83.009
          with inflammation I83.209
    left (asymptomatic) I83.92
      with
        edema I83.892
        inflammation I83.12
          with ulcer — *see* Varix, leg, with, ulcer, with inflammation by site
        pain I83.812
        specified complication NEC I83.892
        swelling I83.892
        ulcer I83.029
          with inflammation I83.229
          ankle I83.023
            with inflammation I83.223
          calf I83.022
            with inflammation I83.222
          foot NEC I83.025
            with inflammation I83.225
          heel I83.024
            with inflammation I83.224
          lower leg NEC I83.028
            with inflammation I83.228
          midfoot I83.024
            with inflammation I83.224
          thigh I83.021
            with inflammation I83.221
    right (asymptomatic) I83.91
      with
        edema I83.891
        inflammation I83.11
          with ulcer — *see* Varix, leg, with, ulcer, with inflammation by site
        pain I83.811
        specified complication NEC I83.891
        swelling I83.891
        ulcer I83.019
          with inflammation I83.219
          ankle I83.013
            with inflammation I83.213
          calf I83.012
            with inflammation I83.212

Varix — *continued*
  leg — *continued*
    right — *continued*
      with — *continued*
        ulcer — *continued*
          foot NEC I83.015
            with inflammation I83.215
          heel I83.014
            with inflammation I83.214
          lower leg NEC I83.018
            with inflammation I83.218
          midfoot I83.014
            with inflammation I83.214
          thigh I83.011
            with inflammation I83.211
  nasal septum I86.8
  orbit I86.8
    congenital Q27.8
  ovary I86.2
  papillary I78.1
  pelvis I86.2
  perineum I86.3
  pharynx I86.8
  placenta O43.89- ☑
  renal papilla I86.8
  retina H35.09
  scrotum (ulcerated) I86.1
  sigmoid colon I86.8
  specified site NEC I86.8
  spinal (cord) (vessels) I86.8
  spleen, splenic (vein) (with phlebolith) I86.8
  stomach I86.4
  sublingual I86.0
  ulcerated I83.009
    inflamed or infected I83.209
  uterine ligament I86.2
  vagina I86.8
  vocal cord I86.8
  vulva I86.3
Vas deferens — *see* condition
Vas deferentitis N49.1
Vasa previa O69.4 ☑
  hemorrhage from, affecting newborn P50.0
Vascular (*see also* condition)
  loop on optic papilla Q14.2
  spasm I73.9
  spider I78.1
Vascularization, cornea — *see* Neovascularization, cornea
Vasculitis I77.6
  allergic D69.0
  cryoglobulinemic D89.1
  disseminated I77.6
  hypocomplementemic M31.8
  kidney I77.89
  livedoid L95.0
  nodular L95.8
  retina H35.06- ☑
  rheumatic — *see* Fever, rheumatic
  rheumatoid — *see* Rheumatoid, vasculitis
  skin (limited to) L95.9
    specified NEC L95.8
Vasculopathy, necrotizing M31.9
  cardiac allograft T86.290
  specified NEC M31.8
Vasitis (nodosa) N49.1
  tuberculous A18.15
Vasodilation I73.9
Vasomotor — *see* condition
Vasoplasty, after previous sterilization Z31.0
  aftercare Z31.42
Vasospasm (vasoconstriction) I73.9
  cerebral (cerebrovascular) (artery) I67.848
    reversible I67.841
  coronary I20.1
  nerve
    arm — *see* Mononeuropathy, upper limb
    brachial plexus G54.0
    cervical plexus G54.2
    leg — *see* Mononeuropathy, lower limb
    peripheral NOS I73.9
  retina (artery) — *see* Occlusion, artery, retina
Vasospastic — *see* condition
Vasovagal attack (paroxysmal) R55
  psychogenic F45.8
VATER syndrome Q87.2
Vater's ampulla — *see* condition

Vegetation, vegetative
  adenoid (nasal fossa) J35.8
  endocarditis (acute) (any valve) (subacute) I33.0
  heart (mycotic) (valve) I33.0
Veil
  Jackson's Q43.3
Vein, venous — *see* condition
Veldt sore — *see* Ulcer, skin
Velpeau's hernia — *see* Hernia, femoral
Venereal
  bubo A55
  disease A64
  granuloma inguinale A58
  lymphogranuloma (Durand-Nicolas-Favre) A55
Venofibrosis I87.8
Venom, venomous — *see* Table of Drugs and Chemicals, by animal or substance, poisoning
Venous — *see* condition
Ventilator lung, newborn P27.8
Ventral — *see* condition
Ventricle, ventricular (*see also* condition)
  escape I49.3
  inversion Q20.5
Ventriculitis (cerebral) (*see also* Encephalitis) G04.90
Ventriculostomy status Z98.2
Vernet's syndrome G52.7
Verneuil's disease (syphilitic bursitis) A52.78
Verruca (due to HPV) (filiformis) (simplex) (viral) (vulgaris) B07.9
  acuminata A63.0
  necrogenica (primary) (tuberculosa) A18.4
  plana B07.8
  plantaris B07.0
  seborrheica L82.1
    inflamed L82.0
  senile (seborrheic) L82.1
    inflamed L82.0
  tuberculosa (primary) A18.4
  venereal A63.0
Verrucosities — *see* Verruca
Verruga peruana, peruviana A44.1
Version
  with extraction
  cervix — *see* Malposition, uterus
  uterus (postinfectional) (postpartal, old) — *see* Malposition, uterus
Vertebra, vertebral — *see* condition
Vertical talus (congenital) Q66.80
  left foot Q66.82
  right foot Q66.81
Vertigo R42
  auditory — *see* Vertigo, aural
  aural H81.31- ☑
  benign paroxysmal (positional) H81.1- ☑
  central (origin) H81.4- ☑
  cerebral H81.4- ☑
  Dix and Hallpike (epidemic) — *see* Neuronitis, vestibular
  due to infrasound T75.23 ☑
  epidemic A88.1
    Dix and Hallpike — *see* Neuronitis, vestibular
    Pedersen's — *see* Neuronitis, vestibular
    vestibular neuronitis — *see* Neuronitis, vestibular
  hysterical F44.89
  infrasound T75.23 ☑
  labyrinthine — *see* subcategory H81.0 ☑
  laryngeal R05
  malignant positional H81.4- ☑
  Ménière's — *see* subcategory H81.0 ☑
  menopausal N95.1
  otogenic — *see* Vertigo, aural
  paroxysmal positional, benign — *see* Vertigo, benign paroxysmal
  Pedersen's (epidemic) — *see* Neuronitis, vestibular
  peripheral NEC H81.39- ☑
  positional
    benign paroxysmal — *see* Vertigo, benign paroxysmal
    malignant H81.4- ☑
Very-low-density-lipoprotein-type (VLDL) **hyperlipoproteinemia** E78.1
Vesania — *see* Psychosis
Vesical — *see* condition
Vesicle
  cutaneous R23.8
  seminal — *see* condition
  skin R23.8

Vesicocolic — *see* condition
Vesicoperineal — *see* condition
Vesicorectal — *see* condition
Vesicourethrorectal — *see* condition
Vesicovaginal — *see* condition
Vesicular — *see* condition
Vesiculitis (seminal) N49.0
  amebic A06.82
  gonorrheal (acute) (chronic) A54.23
  trichomonal A59.09
  tuberculous A18.15
Vestibulitis (ear) (*see also* subcategory) H83.0 ☑
  nose (external) J34.89
  vulvar N94.810
Vestibulopathy , acute peripheral (recurrent) — *see* Neuronitis, vestibular
Vestige, vestigial (*see also* Persistence)
  branchial Q18.0
  structures in vitreous Q14.0
Vibration
  adverse effects T75.20 ☑
    pneumatic hammer syndrome T75.21 ☑
    specified effect NEC T75.29 ☑
    vasospastic syndrome T75.22 ☑
    vertigo from infrasound T75.23 ☑
  exposure (occupational) Z57.7
  vertigo T75.23 ☑
Vibriosis A28.9
Victim (of)
  crime Z65.4
  disaster Z65.5
  terrorism Z65.4
  torture Z65.4
  war Z65.5
Vidal's disease L28.0
Villaret's syndrome G52.7
Villous — *see* condition
VIN — *see* Neoplasia, intraepithelial, vulva
Vincent's infection (angina) (gingivitis) A69.1
  stomatitis NEC A69.1
Vinson-Plummer syndrome D50.1
Violence, physical R45.6
Viosterol deficiency — *see* Deficiency, calciferol
Vipoma — *see* Neoplasm, malignant, by site
Viremia B34.9
Virilism (adrenal) E25.9
  congenital E25.0
Virilization (female) (suprarenal) E25.9
  congenital E25.0
  isosexual E28.2
Virulent bubo A57
Virus, viral (*see also* condition)
  as cause of disease classified elsewhere B97.89
  cytomegalovirus B25.9
  human immunodeficiency (HIV) — *see* Human, immunodeficiency virus (HIV) disease
  infection — *see* Infection, virus
  specified NEC B34.8
  swine influenza (viruses that normally cause infections in pigs) (*see also* Influenza, due to, identified novel influenza A virus) J09.X2
  West Nile (fever) A92.30
    with
      complications NEC A92.39
      cranial nerve disorders A92.32
      encephalitis A92.31
      encephalomyelitis A92.31
      neurologic manifestation NEC A92.32
      optic neuritis A92.32
      polyradiculitis A92.32
Viscera, visceral — *see* condition
Visceroptosis K63.4
Visible peristalsis R19.2
Vision, visual
  binocular, suppression H53.34
  blurred, blurring H53.8
    hysterical F44.6
  defect, defective NEC H54.7
  disorientation (syndrome) H53.8
  disturbance H53.9
    hysterical F44.6
  double H53.2
  examination Z01.00
    with abnormal findings Z01.01
  field, limitation (defect) — *see* Defect, visual field
  hallucinations R44.1
  halos H53.19

Vision, visual — *continued*
  loss — *see* Loss, vision
    sudden — *see* Disturbance, vision, subjective, loss, sudden
  low (both eyes) — *see* Low, vision
  perception, simultaneous without fusion H53.33
Vitality, lack or want of R53.83
  newborn P96.89
Vitamin deficiency — *see* Deficiency, vitamin
Vitelline duct, persistent Q43.0
Vitiligo L80
  eyelid H02.739
    left H02.736
      lower H02.735
      upper H02.734
    right H02.733
      lower H02.732
      upper H02.731
  pinta A67.2
  vulva N90.89
Vitreal corneal syndrome H59.01- ☑
Vitreoretinopathy, proliferative (*see also* Retinopathy, proliferative)
  with retinal detachment — *see* Detachment, retina, traction
Vitreous (*see also* condition)
  touch syndrome — *see* Complication, postprocedural, following cataract surgery
Vocal cord — *see* condition
Vogt-Koyanagi syndrome H20.82- ☑
Vogt's disease or syndrome G80.3
Vogt-Spielmeyer amaurotic idiocy or disease E75.4
Voice
  change R49.9
    specified NEC R49.8
  loss — *see* Aphonia
Volhynian fever A79.0
Volkmann's ischemic contracture or paralysis (complicating trauma) T79.6 ☑
Volvulus (bowel) (colon) (duodenum) (intestine) K56.2
  with perforation K56.2
  congenital Q43.8
  fallopian tube — *see* Torsion, fallopian tube
  oviduct — *see* Torsion, fallopian tube
  stomach (due to absence of gastrocolic ligament) K31.89
Vomiting R11.10
  with nausea R11.2
  without nausea R11.11
  asphyxia — *see* Foreign body, by site, causing asphyxia, gastric contents
  bilious (cause unknown) R11.14
    following gastro-intestinal surgery K91.0
    in newborn P92.01
  blood — *see* Hematemesis
  causing asphyxia, choking, or suffocation — *see* Foreign body, by site
  cyclical G43.A0 (*following* G43.7)
    with refractory migraine G43.A1 (*following* G43.7)
    without refractory migraine G43.A0 (*following* G43.7)
    intractable G43.A1 (*following* G43.7)
    not intractable G43.A0 (*following* G43.7)
    psychogenic F50.8
  fecal mater R11.13
  following gastrointestinal surgery K91.0
    psychogenic F50.8
  functional K31.89
  hysterical F50.8
  nervous F50.8
  neurotic F50.8
  newborn NEC P92.09
    bilious P92.01
  periodic R11.10
    psychogenic F50.8
  projectile R11.12
  psychogenic F50.8
  uremic — *see* Uremia
Vomito negro — *see* Fever, yellow
Von Bezold's abscess — *see* Mastoiditis, acute
Von Economo-Cruchet disease A85.8
Von Eulenburg's disease G71.19
Von Gierke's disease E74.01
Von Hippel (-Lindau) **disease or syndrome** Q85.8
Von Jaksch's anemia or disease D64.89

Von Recklinghausen
  disease (neurofibromatosis) Q85.01
    bones E21.0
Von Schroetter's syndrome I82.890
Von Willebrand (-Jurgens)(-Minot) **disease or syndrome** D68.0
Von Zumbusch's disease L40.1
Voyeurism F65.3
Vrolik's disease Q78.0
Vulva — *see* condition
Vulvismus N94.2
Vulvitis (acute) (allergic) (atrophic) (hypertrophic) (intertriginous) (senile) N76.2
  with ectopic or molar pregnancy O08.0
  adhesive, congenital Q52.79
  blennorrhagic (gonococcal) A54.02
  candidal B37.3
  chlamydial A56.02
  due to Haemophilus ducreyi A57
  following ectopic or molar pregnancy O08.0
  gonococcal A54.02
    with abscess (accessory gland) (periurethral) A54.1
  herpesviral A60.04
  leukoplakic N90.4
  monilial B37.3
  puerperal (postpartum) O86.19
  subacute or chronic N76.3
  syphilitic (early) A51.0
    late A52.76
  trichomonal A59.01
  tuberculous A18.18
Vulvodynia N94.819
  specified NEC N94.818
Vulvorectal — *see* condition
Vulvovaginitis (acute) — *see* Vaginitis

W

Waiting list, person on Z75.1
  for organ transplant Z76.82
  undergoing social agency investigation Z75.2
Waldenström
  hypergammaglobulinemia D89.0
  syndrome or macroglobulinemia C88.0
Waldenström-Kjellberg syndrome D50.1
Walking
  difficulty R26.2
    psychogenic F44.4
  sleep F51.3
    hysterical F44.89
Wall, abdominal — *see* condition
Wallenberg's disease or syndrome G46.3
Wallgren's disease I87.8
Wandering
  gallbladder, congenital Q44.1
  in diseases classified elsewhere Z91.83
  kidney, congenital Q63.8
  organ or site, congenital NEC — *see* Malposition, congenital, by site
  pacemaker (heart) I49.8
  spleen D73.89
War neurosis F48.8
Wart (due to HPV) (filiform) (infectious) (viral) B07.9
  anogenital region (venereal) A63.0
  common B07.8
  external genital organs (venereal) A63.0
  flat B07.8
  Hassal-Henle's (of cornea) H18.49
  Peruvian A44.1
  plantar B07.0
  prosector (tuberculous) A18.4
  seborrheic L82.1
    inflamed L82.0
  senile (seborrheic) L82.1
    inflamed L82.0
  tuberculous A18.4
  venereal A63.0
Warthin's tumor — *see* Neoplasm, salivary gland, benign
Wassilieff's disease A27.0
Wasting
  disease R64
    due to malnutrition E41
  extreme (due to malnutrition) E41
  muscle NEC — *see* Atrophy, muscle
Water
  clefts (senile cataract) — *see* Cataract, senile, incipient
  deprivation of T73.1 ☑

Water — *continued*
  intoxication E87.79
  itch B76.9
  lack of T73.1 ☑
  loading E87.70
  on
    brain — *see* Hydrocephalus
    chest J94.8
  poisoning E87.79
Waterbrash R12
Waterhouse (-Friderichsen) **syndrome or disease** (meningococcal) A39.1
Water-losing nephritis N25.89
Watermelon stomach K31.819
  with hemorrhage K31.811
  without hemorrhage K31.819
Watsoniasis B66.8
Wax in ear — *see* Impaction, cerumen
Weak, weakening, weakness (generalized) R53.1
  arches (acquired) (*see also* Deformity, limb, flat foot) R53.1
  bladder (sphincter) R32
  facial R29.810
    following
      cerebrovascular disease I69.992
        cerebral infarction I69.392
        intracerebral hemorrhage I69.192
        nontraumatic intracranial hemorrhage NEC I69.292
        specified disease NEC I69.892
        stroke I69.392
        subarachnoid hemorrhage I69.092
  foot (double) — *see* Weak, arches
  heart, cardiac — *see* Failure, heart
  mind F70
  muscle M62.81
  myocardium — *see* Failure, heart
  newborn P96.89
  pelvic fundus N81.89
  pubocervical tissue N81.82
  rectovaginal tissue N81.83
  senile R54
  urinary stream R39.12
  valvular — *see* Endocarditis
Wear, worn (with normal or routine use)
  articular bearing surface of internal joint prosthesis — *see* Complications, joint prosthesis, mechanical, wear of articular bearing surfaces, by site
  device, implant or graft — *see* Complications, by site, mechanical complication
  tooth, teeth (approximal) (hard tissues) (interproximal) (occlusal) K03.0
Weather, weathered
  effects of
    cold T69.9 ☑
      specified effect NEC T69.8 ☑
    hot — *see* Heat
  skin L57.8
Weaver's syndrome Q87.3
Web, webbed (congenital)
  duodenal Q43.8
  esophagus Q39.4
  fingers Q70.1- ☑
  larynx (glottic) (subglottic) Q31.0
  neck (pterygium colli) Q18.3
  Paterson-Kelly D50.1
  popliteal syndrome Q87.89
  toes Q70.3- ☑
Weber-Christian disease M35.6
Weber-Cockayne syndrome (epidermolysis bullosa) Q81.8
Weber-Gubler syndrome G46.3
Weber-Leyden syndrome G46.3
Weber-Osler syndrome I78.0
Weber's paralysis or syndrome G46.3
Wedge-shaped or wedging vertebra — *see* Collapse, vertebra NEC
Wegener's granulomatosis or syndrome M31.30
  with
    kidney involvement M31.31
    lung involvement M31.30
      with kidney involvement M31.31
Wegner's disease A50.02
Weight
  1000-2499 grams at birth (low) — *see* Low, birthweight
  999 grams or less at birth (extremely low) — *see* Low, birthweight, extreme

Weight — *continued*
  gain (abnormal) (excessive) R63.5
    in pregnancy — *see* Pregnancy, complicated by, excessive weight gain
    low — *see* Pregnancy, complicated by, insufficient, weight gain
  loss (abnormal) (cause unknown) R63.4
Weightlessness (effect of) T75.82 ☑
Weil (I)**-Marchesani syndrome** Q87.1
Weil's disease A27.0
Weingarten's syndrome J82
Weir Mitchell's disease I73.81
Weiss-Baker syndrome G90.09
Wells' disease L98.3
Wen — *see* Cyst, sebaceous
Wenckebach's block or phenomenon I44.1
Werdnig-Hoffmann syndrome (muscular atrophy) G12.0
Werlhof's disease D69.3
Wermer's disease or syndrome E31.21
Werner-His disease A79.0
Werner's disease or syndrome E34.8
Wernicke-Korsakoff's syndrome or psychosis (alcoholic) F10.96
  with dependence F10.26
  drug-induced
    due to drug abuse — *see* Abuse, drug, by type, with amnestic disorder
    due to drug dependence — *see* Dependence, drug, by type, with amnestic disorder
  nonalcoholic F04
Wernicke-Posadas disease B38.9
Wernicke's
  developmental aphasia F80.2
  disease or syndrome E51.2
  encephalopathy E51.2
  polioencephalitis, superior E51.2
West African fever B50.8
Westphal-Strümpell syndrome E83.01
West's syndrome — *see* Epilepsy, spasms
Wet
  feet, tropical (maceration) (syndrome) — *see* Immersion, foot
  lung (syndrome), newborn P22.1
Wharton's duct — *see* condition
Wheal — *see* Urticaria
Wheezing R06.2
Whiplash injury S13.4 ☑
Whipple's disease (*see also* subcategory M14.8-) K90.81
Whipworm (disease) (infection) (infestation) B79
Whistling face Q87.0
White (*see also* condition)
  kidney, small N03.9
  leg, puerperal, postpartum, childbirth O87.1
  mouth B37.0
  patches of mouth K13.29
  spot lesions, teeth
    chewing surface K02.51
    pit and fissure surface K02.51
    smooth surface K02.61
Whitehead L70.0
Whitlow (*see also* Cellulitis, digit)
  with lymphangitis — *see* Lymphangitis, acute, digit
  herpesviral B00.89
Whitmore's disease or fever — *see* Melioidosis
Whooping cough A37.90
  with pneumonia A37.91
    due to Bordetella
      bronchiseptica A37.81
      parapertussis A37.11
      pertussis A37.01
    specified organism NEC A37.81
  due to
    Bordetella
      bronchiseptica A37.80
        with pneumonia A37.81
      parapertussis A37.10
        with pneumonia A37.11
      pertussis A37.00
        with pneumonia A37.01
    specified NEC A37.80
      with pneumonia A37.81
Wichman's asthma J38.5
Wide cranial sutures, newborn P96.3
Widening aorta — *see* Ectasia, aorta
  with aneurysm — *see* Aneurysm, aorta
Wilkie's disease or syndrome K55.1

Wilkinson-Sneddon disease or syndrome L13.1
Willebrand (-Jürgens) **thrombopathy** D68.0
Willige-Hunt disease or syndrome G23.1
Wilms' tumor C64- ☑
Wilson-Mikity syndrome P27.0
Wilson's
  disease or syndrome E83.01
  hepatolenticular degeneration E83.01
  lichen ruber L43.9
Window (*see also* Imperfect, closure)
  aorticopulmonary Q21.4
Winter — *see* condition
Wiskott-Aldrich syndrome D82.0
Withdrawal state (*see also* Dependence, drug by type,
    with withdrawal)
  newborn
    correct therapeutic substance properly adminis-
      tered P96.2
    infant of dependent mother P96.1
    therapeutic substance, neonatal P96.2
Witts' anemia D50.8
Witzelsucht F07.0
Woakes' ethmoiditis or syndrome J33.1
Wolff-Hirschorn syndrome Q93.3
Wolff-Parkinson-White syndrome I45.6
Wolhynian fever A79.0
Wolman's disease E75.5
Wood lung or pneumonitis J67.8
Woolly, wooly hair (congenital) (nevus) Q84.1
Woolsorter's disease A22.1
Word
  blindness (congenital) (developmental) F81.0
  deafness (congenital) (developmental) H93.25
Worm(s) (infection) (infestation) (*see also* Infestation,
    helminth)
  guinea B72
  in intestine NEC B82.0
Worm-eaten soles A66.3
Worn out — *see* Exhaustion
  cardiac
    defibrillator (with synchronous cardiace pacemak-
      er) Z45.02
    pacemaker
      battery Z45.010
      lead Z45.018
  device, implant or graft — *see* Complications, by site,
    mechanical
Worried well Z71.1
Worries R45.82
Wound, open
  abdomen, abdominal
    wall S31.109 ☑
      with penetration into peritoneal cavity
        S31.609 ☑
      bite — *see* Bite, abdomen, wall
      epigastric region S31.102 ☑
        with penetration into peritoneal cavity
          S31.602 ☑
        bite — *see* Bite, abdomen, wall, epigastric
          region
        laceration — *see* Laceration, abdomen, wall,
          epigastric region
        puncture — *see* Puncture, abdomen, wall,
          epigastric region
      laceration — *see* Laceration, abdomen, wall
      left
        lower quadrant S31.104 ☑
          with penetration into peritoneal cavity
            S31.604 ☑
          bite — *see* Bite, abdomen, wall, left,
            lower quadrant
          laceration — *see* Laceration, abdomen,
            wall, left, lower quadrant
          puncture — *see* Puncture, abdomen,
            wall, left, lower quadrant
        upper quadrant S31.101 ☑
          with penetration into peritoneal cavity
            S31.601 ☑
          bite — *see* Bite, abdomen, wall, left, up-
            per quadrant
          laceration — *see* Laceration, abdomen,
            wall, left, upper quadrant
          puncture — *see* Puncture, abdomen,
            wall, left, upper quadrant
      periumbilic region S31.105 ☑
        with penetration into peritoneal cavity
          S31.605 ☑

Wound, open — *continued*
  abdomen, abdominal — *continued*
    wall — *continued*
      periumbilic region — *continued*
        bite — *see* Bite, abdomen, wall, periumbilic
          region
        laceration — *see* Laceration, abdomen, wall,
          periumbilic region
        puncture — *see* Puncture, abdomen, wall,
          periumbilic region
      puncture — *see* Puncture, abdomen, wall
      right
        lower quadrant S31.103 ☑
          with penetration into peritoneal cavity
            S31.603 ☑
          bite — *see* Bite, abdomen, wall, right,
            lower quadrant
          laceration — *see* Laceration, abdomen,
            wall, right, lower quadrant
          puncture — *see* Puncture, abdomen,
            wall, right, lower quadrant
        upper quadrant S31.100 ☑
          with penetration into peritoneal cavity
            S31.600 ☑
          bite — *see* Bite, abdomen, wall, right,
            upper quadrant
          laceration — *see* Laceration, abdomen,
            wall, right, upper quadrant
          puncture — *see* Puncture, abdomen,
            wall, right, upper quadrant
    alveolar (process) — *see* Wound, open, oral cavity
    ankle S91.00- ☑
      bite — *see* Bite, ankle
      laceration — *see* Laceration, ankle
      puncture — *see* Puncture, ankle
    antecubital space — *see* Wound, open, elbow
    anterior chamber, eye — *see* Wound, open, ocular
    anus S31.839 ☑
      bite S31.835 ☑
      laceration — *see* Laceration, anus
      puncture — *see* Puncture, anus
    arm (upper) S41.10- ☑
      with amputation — *see* Amputation, traumatic,
        arm
      bite — *see* Bite, arm
      forearm — *see* Wound, open, forearm
      laceration — *see* Laceration, arm
      puncture — *see* Puncture, arm
    auditory canal (external) (meatus) — *see* Wound, open,
      ear
    auricle, ear — *see* Wound, open, ear
    axilla — *see* Wound, open, arm
    back (*see also* Wound, open, thorax, back)
      lower S31.000 ☑
        with penetration into retroperitoneal space
          S31.001 ☑
        bite — *see* Bite, back, lower
        laceration — *see* Laceration, back, lower
        puncture — *see* Puncture, back, lower
    bite — *see* Bite
    blood vessel — *see* Injury, blood vessel
    breast S21.00- ☑
      with amputation — *see* Amputation, traumatic,
        breast
      bite — *see* Bite, breast
      laceration — *see* Laceration, breast
      puncture — *see* Puncture, breast
    buttock S31.809 ☑
      bite — *see* Bite, buttock
      laceration — *see* Laceration, buttock
      left S31.829 ☑
      puncture — *see* Puncture, buttock
      right S31.819 ☑
    calf — *see* Wound, open, leg
    canaliculus lacrimalis — *see* Wound, open, eyelid
    canthus, eye — *see* Wound, open, eyelid
    cervical esophagus S11.20 ☑
      bite S11.25 ☑
      laceration — *see* Laceration, esophagus, traumatic,
        cervical
      puncture — *see* Puncture, cervical esophagus
    cheek (external) S01.40- ☑
      bite — *see* Bite, cheek
      internal — *see* Wound, open, oral cavity
      laceration — *see* Laceration, cheek
      puncture — *see* Puncture, cheek

Wound, open — *continued*
  chest wall — *see* Wound, open, thorax
  chin — *see* Wound, open, head, specified site NEC
  choroid — *see* Wound, open, ocular
  ciliary body (eye) — *see* Wound, open, ocular
  clitoris S31.40 ☑
    with amputation — *see* Amputation, traumatic,
      clitoris
    bite S31.45 ☑
    laceration — *see* Laceration, vulva
    puncture — *see* Puncture, vulva
  conjunctiva — *see* Wound, open, ocular
  cornea — *see* Wound, open, ocular
  costal region — *see* Wound, open, thorax
  Descemet's membrane — *see* Wound, open, ocular
  digit(s)
    foot — *see* Wound, open, toe
    hand — *see* Wound, open, finger
  ear (canal) (external) S01.30- ☑
    with amputation — *see* Amputation, traumatic,
      ear
    bite — *see* Bite, ear
    drum S09.2- ☑
    laceration — *see* Laceration, ear
    puncture — *see* Puncture, ear
  elbow S51.00- ☑
    bite — *see* Bite, elbow
    laceration — *see* Laceration, elbow
    puncture — *see* Puncture, elbow
  epididymis — *see* Wound, open, testis
  epigastric region S31.102 ☑
    with penetration into peritoneal cavity S31.602 ☑
    bite — *see* Bite, abdomen, wall, epigastric region
    laceration — *see* Laceration, abdomen, wall, epi-
      gastric region
    puncture — *see* Puncture, abdomen, wall, epigas-
      tric region
  epiglottis — *see* Wound, open, neck, specified site
    NEC
  esophagus (thoracic) S27.819 ☑
    cervical — *see* Wound, open, cervical esophagus
    laceration S27.813 ☑
    specified type NEC S27.818 ☑
  eye — *see* Wound, open, ocular
  eyeball — *see* Wound, open, ocular
  eyebrow — *see* Wound, open, eyelid
  eyelid S01.10- ☑
    bite — *see* Bite, eyelid
    laceration — *see* Laceration, eyelid
    puncture — *see* Puncture, eyelid
  face NEC — *see* Wound, open, head, specified site NEC
  finger(s) S61.209 ☑
    with
      amputation — *see* Amputation, traumatic, fin-
        ger
      damage to nail S61.309 ☑
    bite — *see* Bite, finger
    index S61.208 ☑
      with
        damage to nail S61.308 ☑
      left S61.201 ☑
        with
          damage to nail S61.301 ☑
      right S61.200 ☑
        with
          damage to nail S61.300 ☑
    laceration — *see* Laceration, finger
    little S61.208 ☑
      with
        damage to nail S61.308 ☑
      left S61.207 ☑
        with damage to nail S61.307 ☑
      right S61.206 ☑
        with damage to nail S61.306 ☑
    middle S61.208 ☑
      with
        damage to nail S61.308 ☑
      left S61.203 ☑
        with damage to nail S61.303 ☑
      right S61.202 ☑
        with damage to nail S61.302 ☑
    puncture — *see* Puncture, finger
    ring S61.208 ☑
      with
        damage to nail S61.308 ☑

Wound, open — *continued*
  finger(s) — *continued*
    ring — *continued*
      left S61.205 ☑
        with damage to nail S61.305 ☑
      right S61.204 ☑
        with damage to nail S61.304 ☑
  flank — *see* Wound, open, abdomen, wall
  foot (except toe(s) alone) S91.30- ☑
    with amputation — *see* Amputation, traumatic, foot
    bite — *see* Bite, foot
    laceration — *see* Laceration, foot
    puncture — *see* Puncture, foot
    toe — *see* Wound, open, toe
  forearm S51.80- ☑
    with
      amputation — *see* Amputation, traumatic, forearm
    bite — *see* Bite, forearm
    elbow only — *see* Wound, open, elbow
    laceration — *see* Laceration, forearm
    puncture — *see* Puncture, forearm
  forehead — *see* Wound, open, head, specified site NEC
  genital organs, external
    with amputation — *see* Amputation, traumatic, genital organs
    bite — *see* Bite, genital organ
    female S31.502 ☑
      vagina S31.40 ☑
      vulva S31.40 ☑
    laceration — *see* Laceration, genital organ
    male S31.501 ☑
      penis S31.20 ☑
      scrotum S31.30 ☑
      testes S31.30 ☑
    puncture — *see* Puncture, genital organ
  globe (eye) — *see* Wound, open, ocular
  groin — *see* Wound, open, abdomen, wall
  gum — *see* Wound, open, oral cavity
  hand S61.40- ☑
    with
      amputation — *see* Amputation, traumatic, hand
    bite — *see* Bite, hand
    finger(s) — *see* Wound, open, finger
    laceration — *see* Laceration, hand
    puncture — *see* Puncture, hand
    thumb — *see* Wound, open, thumb
  head S01.90 ☑
    bite — *see* Bite, head
    cheek — *see* Wound, open, cheek
    ear — *see* Wound, open, ear
    eyelid — *see* Wound, open, eyelid
    laceration — *see* Laceration, head
    lip — *see* Wound, open, lip
    nose S01.20 ☑
    oral cavity — *see* Wound, open, oral cavity
    puncture — *see* Puncture, head
    scalp — *see* Wound, open, scalp
    specified site NEC S01.80 ☑
    temporomandibular area — *see* Wound, open, cheek
  heel — *see* Wound, open, foot
  hip S71.00- ☑
    with amputation — *see* Amputation, traumatic, hip
    bite — *see* Bite, hip
    laceration — *see* Laceration, hip
    puncture — *see* Puncture, hip
  hymen S31.40 ☑
    bite — *see* Bite, vulva
    laceration — *see* Laceration, vagina
    puncture — *see* Puncture, vagina
  hypochondrium S31.109 ☑
    bite — *see* Bite, hypochondrium
    laceration — *see* Laceration, hypochondrium
    puncture — *see* Puncture, hypochondrium
  hypogastric region S31.109 ☑
    bite — *see* Bite, hypogastric region
    laceration — *see* Laceration, hypogastric region
    puncture — *see* Puncture, hypogastric region
  iliac (region) — *see* Wound, open, inguinal region
  inguinal region S31.109 ☑
    bite — *see* Bite, abdomen, wall, lower quadrant
    laceration — *see* Laceration, inguinal region

Wound, open — *continued*
  inguinal region — *continued*
    puncture — *see* Puncture, inguinal region
  instep — *see* Wound, open, foot
  interscapular region — *see* Wound, open, thorax, back
  intraocular — *see* Wound, open, ocular
  iris — *see* Wound, open, ocular
  jaw — *see* Wound, open, head, specified site NEC
  knee S81.00- ☑
    bite — *see* Bite, knee
    laceration — *see* Laceration, knee
    puncture — *see* Puncture, knee
  labium (majus) (minus) — *see* Wound, open, vulva
  laceration — *see* Laceration, by site
  lacrimal duct — *see* Wound, open, eyelid
  larynx S11.019 ☑
    bite — *see* Bite, larynx
    laceration — *see* Laceration, larynx
    puncture — *see* Puncture, larynx
  left
    lower quadrant S31.104 ☑
      with penetration into peritoneal cavity S31.604 ☑
      bite — *see* Bite, abdomen, wall, left, lower quadrant
      laceration — *see* Laceration, abdomen, wall, left, lower quadrant
      puncture — *see* Puncture, abdomen, wall, left, lower quadrant
    upper quadrant S31.101 ☑
      with penetration into peritoneal cavity S31.601 ☑
      bite — *see* Bite, abdomen, wall, left, upper quadrant
      laceration — *see* Laceration, abdomen, wall, left, upper quadrant
      puncture — *see* Puncture, abdomen, wall, left, upper quadrant
  leg (lower) S81.80- ☑
    with amputation — *see* Amputation, traumatic, leg
    ankle — *see* Wound, open, ankle
    bite — *see* Bite, leg
    foot — *see* Wound, open, foot
    knee — *see* Wound, open, knee
    laceration — *see* Laceration, leg
    puncture — *see* Puncture, leg
    toe — *see* Wound, open, toe
    upper — *see* Wound, open, thigh
  lip S01.501 ☑
    bite — *see* Bite, lip
    laceration — *see* Laceration, lip
    puncture — *see* Puncture, lip
  loin S31.109 ☑
    bite — *see* Bite, abdomen, wall
    laceration — *see* Laceration, loin
    puncture — *see* Puncture, loin
  lower back — *see* Wound, open, back, lower
  lumbar region — *see* Wound, open, back, lower
  malar region — *see* Wound, open, head, specified site NEC
  mammary — *see* Wound, open, breast
  mastoid region — *see* Wound, open, head, specified site NEC
  mouth — *see* Wound, open, oral cavity
  nail
    finger — *see* Wound, open, finger, with damage to nail
    toe — *see* Wound, open, toe, with damage to nail
  nape (neck) — *see* Wound, open, neck
  nasal (septum) (sinus) — *see* Wound, open, nose
  nasopharynx — *see* Wound, open, head, specified site NEC
  neck S11.90 ☑
    bite — *see* Bite, neck
    involving
      cervical esophagus S11.20 ☑
      larynx — *see* Wound, open, larynx
      pharynx S11.20 ☑
      thyroid S11.10 ☑
      trachea (cervical) S11.029 ☑
        bite — *see* Bite, trachea
        laceration S11.021 ☑
          with foreign body S11.022 ☑
        puncture S11.023 ☑
          with foreign body S11.024 ☑

Wound, open — *continued*
  neck — *continued*
    laceration — *see* Laceration, neck
    puncture — *see* Puncture, neck
    specified site NEC S11.80 ☑
      specified type NEC S11.89 ☑
  nose (septum) (sinus) S01.20 ☑
    with amputation — *see* Amputation, traumatic, nose
    bite — *see* Bite, nose
    laceration — *see* Laceration, nose
    puncture — *see* Puncture, nose
  ocular S05.90 ☑
    avulsion (traumatic enucleation) S05.7- ☑
    eyeball S05.6- ☑
      with foreign body S05.5- ☑
    eyelid — *see* Wound, open, eyelid
    laceration and rupture S05.3- ☑
      with prolapse or loss of intraocular tissue S05.2- ☑
    orbit (penetrating) (with or without foreign body) S05.4- ☑
    periocular area — *see* Wound, open, eyelid
    specified NEC S05.8X- ☑
  oral cavity S01.502 ☑
    bite S01.552 ☑
    laceration — *see* Laceration, oral cavity
    puncture — *see* Puncture, oral cavity
  orbit — *see* Wound, open, ocular, orbit
  palate — *see* Wound, open, oral cavity
  palm — *see* Wound, open, hand
  pelvis, pelvic (*see also* Wound, open, back, lower)
    girdle — *see* Wound, open, hip
  penetrating — *see* Puncture, by site
  penis S31.20 ☑
    with amputation — *see* Amputation, traumatic, penis
    bite S31.25 ☑
    laceration — *see* Laceration, penis
    puncture — *see* Puncture, penis
  perineum
    bite — *see* Bite, perineum
    female S31.502 ☑
    laceration — *see* Laceration, perineum
    male S31.501 ☑
    puncture — *see* Puncture, perineum
  periocular area (with or without lacrimal passages) — *see* Wound, open, eyelid
  periumbilic region S31.105 ☑
    with penetration into peritoneal cavity S31.605 ☑
    bite — *see* Bite, abdomen, wall, periumbilic region
    laceration — *see* Laceration, abdomen, wall, periumbilic region
    puncture — *see* Puncture, abdomen, wall, periumbilic region
  phalanges
    finger — *see* Wound, open, finger
    toe — *see* Wound, open, toe
  pharynx S11.20 ☑
  pinna — *see* Wound, open, ear
  popliteal space — *see* Wound, open, knee
  prepuce — *see* Wound, open, penis
  pubic region — *see* Wound, open, back, lower
  pudendum — *see* Wound, open, genital organs, external
  puncture wound — *see* Puncture
  rectovaginal septum — *see* Wound, open, vagina
  right
    lower quadrant S31.103 ☑
      with penetration into peritoneal cavity S31.603 ☑
      bite — *see* Bite, abdomen, wall, right, lower quadrant
      laceration — *see* Laceration, abdomen, wall, right, lower quadrant
      puncture — *see* Puncture, abdomen, wall, right, lower quadrant
    upper quadrant S31.100 ☑
      with penetration into peritoneal cavity S31.600 ☑
      bite — *see* Bite, abdomen, wall, right, upper quadrant
      laceration — *see* Laceration, abdomen, wall, right, upper quadrant
      puncture — *see* Puncture, abdomen, wall, right, upper quadrant

Yaws — *continued*
gummatous — *continued*
periostitis A66.6
hydrarthrosis (*see also* subcategory M14.8-) A66.6
hyperkeratosis (early) (late) A66.3
initial lesions A66.0
joint lesions (*see also* subcategory M14.8-) A66.6
juxta-articular nodules A66.7
late nodular (ulcerated) A66.4
latent (without clinical manifestations) (with positive
serology) A66.8
mother A66.0
mucosal A66.7
multiple papillomata A66.1
nodular, late (ulcerated) A66.4
osteitis A66.6
papilloma, plantar or palmar A66.1
periostitis (hypertrophic) A66.6

Yaws — *continued*
specified NEC A66.7
ulcers A66.4
wet crab A66.1
Yeast infection (*see also* Candidiasis) B37.9
Yellow
atrophy (liver) — *see* Failure, hepatic
fever — *see* Fever, yellow
jack — *see* Fever, yellow
jaundice — *see* Jaundice
nail syndrome L60.5
Yersiniosis (*see also* Infection, Yersinia) A28.9
extraintestinal A28.2
intestinal A04.6

Z

Zahorsky's syndrome (herpangina) B08.5

Zellweger's syndrome Q87.89
Zenker's diverticulum (esophagus) K22.5
Ziehen-Oppenheim disease G24.1
Zieve's syndrome K70.0
Zinc
deficiency, dietary E60
metabolism disorder E83.2
Zollinger-Ellison syndrome E16.4
Zona — *see* Herpes, zoster
Zoophobia F40.218
Zoster (herpes) — *see* Herpes, zoster
Zygomycosis B46.9
specified NEC B46.8
Zymotic — *see* condition

☑ **Additional Character Required — Refer to the Tabular List for Character Selection**   ▽ **Subterms under main terms may continue to next column or page**

ICD-10-CM Neoplasm Table

Note: The list below gives the code number for neoplasms by anatomical site. For each site there are six possible code numbers according to whether the neoplasm in question is malignant, benign, in situ, of uncertain behavior, or of unspecified nature. The description of the neoplasm will often indicate which of the six columns is appropriate; e.g., malignant melanoma of skin, benign fibroadenoma of breast, carcinoma in situ of cervix uteri. Where such descriptors are not present, the remainder of the Index should be consulted where guidance is given to the appropriate column for each morphological (histological) variety listed; e.g., Mesonephroma – see Neoplasm, malignant; Embryoma (see also Neoplasm, uncertain behavior); Disease, Bowen's – see Neoplasm, skin, in situ. However, the guidance in the Index can be overridden if one of the descriptors mentioned above is present; e.g., malignant adenoma of colon is coded to C18.9 and not to D12.6 as the adjective "malignant" overrides the Index entry "Adenoma (see also Neoplasm, benign)." Codes listed with a dash -, following the code have a required 5th character for laterality. The tabular list must be reviewed for the complete code.

	Malignant Primary	Malignant Secondary	Ca in situ	Benign	Uncertain	Unspecified Behavior
Neoplasm, neoplastic	C80.1	C79.9	D09.9	D36.9	D48.9	D49.9
abdomen, abdominal	C76.2	C79.8-✓	D09.8	D36.7	D48.7	D49.89
cavity	C76.2	C79.8-✓	D09.8	D36.7	D48.7	D49.89
organ	C76.2	C79.8-✓	D09.8	D36.7	D48.7	D49.89
viscera	C76.2	C79.8-✓	D09.8	D36.7	D48.7	D49.89
wall — *see also* Neoplasm, abdomen, wall, skin	C44.509	C79.2	D04.5	D23.5	D48.5	D49.2
connective tissue	C49.4	C79.8-✓	—	D21.4	D48.1	D49.2
skin	C44.509	—	—	—	—	—
basal cell carcinoma	C44.519	—	—	—	—	—
specified type NEC	C44.599	—	—	—	—	—
squamous cell carcinoma	C44.529	—	—	—	—	—
abdominopelvic	C76.8	C79.8-✓	—	D36.7	D48.7	D49.89
accessory sinus — *see* Neoplasm, sinus						
acoustic nerve	C72.4-✓	C79.49	—	D33.3	D43.3	D49.7
adenoid (pharynx) (tissue)	C11.1	C79.89	D00.08	D10.6	D37.05	D49.0
adipose tissue — *see also* Neoplasm, connective tissue	C49.4	C79.89	—	D21.9	D48.1	D49.2
adnexa (uterine)	C57.4	C79.89	D07.39	D28.7	D39.8	D49.5
adrenal	C74.9-✓	C79.7-✓	D09.3	D35.0-✓	D44.1-✓	D49.7
capsule	C74.9-✓	C79.7-✓	D09.3	D35.0-✓	D44.1-✓	D49.7
cortex	C74.0-✓	C79.7-✓	D09.3	D35.0-✓	D44.1-✓	D49.7
gland	C74.9-✓	C79.7-✓	D09.3	D35.0-✓	D44.1-✓	D49.7
medulla	C74.1-✓	C79.7-✓	D09.3	D35.0-✓	D44.1-✓	D49.7
ala nasi (external) — *see also* Neoplasm, skin, nose	C44.301	C79.2	D04.39	D23.39	D48.5	D49.2
alimentary canal or tract NEC	C26.9	C78.80	D01.9	D13.9	D37.9	D49.0
alveolar	C03.9	C79.89	D00.03	D10.39	D37.09	D49.0
mucosa	C03.9	C79.89	D00.03	D10.39	D37.09	D49.0
lower	C03.1	C79.89	D00.03	D10.39	D37.09	D49.0
upper	C03.0	C79.89	D00.03	D10.39	D37.09	D49.0
ridge or process	C41.1	C79.51	—	D16.5	D48.0	D49.2
carcinoma	C03.9	C79.8-✓	—	—	—	—
lower	C03.1	C79.8-✓	—	—	—	—
upper	C03.0	C79.8-✓	—	—	—	—
lower	C41.1	C79.51	—	D16.5	D48.0	D49.2
mucosa	C03.9	C79.89	D00.03	D10.39	D37.09	D49.0
lower	C03.1	C79.89	D00.03	D10.39	D37.09	D49.0
upper	C03.0	C79.89	D00.03	D10.39	D37.09	D49.0
upper	C41.0	C79.51	—	D16.4	D48.0	D49.2
sulcus	C06.1	C79.89	D00.02	D10.39	D37.09	D49.0
alveolus	C03.9	C79.89	D00.03	D10.39	D37.09	D49.0
lower	C03.1	C79.89	D00.03	D10.39	D37.09	D49.0
upper	C03.0	C79.89	D00.03	D10.39	D37.09	D49.0
ampulla of Vater	C24.1	C78.89	D01.5	D13.5	D37.6	D49.0
ankle NEC	C76.5-✓	C79.89	D04.7-✓	D36.7	D48.7	D49.89

	Malignant Primary	Malignant Secondary	Ca in situ	Benign	Uncertain	Unspecified Behavior
Neoplasm, neoplastic — *continued*						
anorectum, anorectal (junction)	C21.8	C78.5	D01.3	D12.9	D37.8	D49.0
antecubital fossa or space	C76.4-✓	C79.89	D04.6-✓	D36.7	D48.7	D49.89
antrum (Highmore) (maxillary)	C31.0	C78.39	D02.3	D14.0	D38.5	D49.1
pyloric	C16.3	C78.89	D00.2	D13.1	D37.1	D49.0
tympanicum	C30.1	C78.39	D02.3	D14.0	D38.5	D49.1
anus, anal	C21.0	C78.5	D01.3	D12.9	D37.8	D49.0
canal	C21.1	C78.5	D01.3	D12.9	D37.8	D49.0
cloacogenic zone	C21.2	C78.5	D01.3	D12.9	D37.8	D49.0
margin — *see also* Neoplasm, anus, skin	C44.500	C79.2	D04.5	D23.5	D48.5	D49.2
overlapping lesion with rectosigmoid junction or rectum	C21.8	—	—	—	—	—
skin	C44.500	C79.2	D04.5	D23.5	D48.5	D49.2
basal cell carcinoma	C44.510	—	—	—	—	—
specified type NEC	C44.590	—	—	—	—	—
squamous cell carcinoma	C44.520	—	—	—	—	—
sphincter	C21.1	C78.5	D01.3	D12.9	D37.8	D49.0
aorta (thoracic)	C49.3	C79.89	—	D21.3	D48.1	D49.2
abdominal	C49.4	C79.89	—	D21.4	D48.1	D49.2
aortic body	C75.5	C79.89	—	D35.6	D44.7	D49.7
aponeurosis	C49.9	C79.89	—	D21.9	D48.1	D49.2
palmar	C49.1-✓	C79.89	—	D21.1-✓	D48.1	D49.2
plantar	C49.2-✓	C79.89	—	D21.2-✓	D48.1	D49.2
appendix	C18.1	C78.5	D01.0	D12.1	D37.3	D49.0
arachnoid	C70.9	C79.49	—	D32.9	D42.9	D49.7
cerebral	C70.0	C79.32	—	D32.0	D42.0	D49.7
spinal	C70.1	C79.49	—	D32.1	D42.1	D49.7
areola	C50.0-✓	C79.81	D05-✓	D24-✓	D48.6-✓	D49.3
arm NEC	C76.4-✓	C79.89	D04.6-✓	D36.7	D48.7	D49.89
artery — *see* Neoplasm, connective tissue						
aryepiglottic fold	C13.1	C79.89	D00.08	D10.7	D37.05	D49.0
hypopharyngeal aspect	C13.1	C79.89	D00.08	D10.7	D37.05	D49.0
laryngeal aspect	C32.1	C78.39	D02.0	D14.1	D38.0	D49.1
marginal zone	C13.1	C79.89	D00.08	D10.7	D37.05	D49.0
arytenoid (cartilage)	C32.3	C78.39	D02.0	D14.1	D38.0	D49.1
fold — *see* Neoplasm, aryepiglottic						
associated with transplanted organ	C80.2	—	—	—	—	—
atlas	C41.2	C79.51	—	D16.6	D48.0	D49.2
atrium, cardiac	C38.0	C79.89	—	D15.1	D48.7	D49.89
auditory						
canal (external) (skin) A81	C44.20-✓	C79.2	D04.2-✓	D23.2-✓	D48.5	D49.2
internal	C30.1	C78.39	D02.3	D14.0	D38.5	D49.1
nerve	C72.4-✓	C79.49	—	D33.3	D43.3	D49.7
tube	C30.1	C78.39	D02.3	D14.0	D38.5	D49.1
opening	C11.2	C79.89	D00.08	D10.6	D37.05	D49.0
auricle, ear — *see also* Neoplasm, skin, ear	C44.20-✓	C79.2	D04.2-✓	D23.2-✓	D48.5	D49.2
auricular canal (external) — *see also* Neoplasm, skin, ear	C44.20-✓	C79.2	D04.2-✓	D23.2-✓	D48.5	D49.2
internal	C30.1	C78.39	D02.3	D14.0	D38.5	D49.2
autonomic nerve or nervous system NEC (see Neoplasm, nerve, peripheral)						
axilla, axillary	C76.1	C79.89	D09.8	D36.7	D48.7	D49.89
fold — *see also* Neoplasm, skin, trunk	C44.509	C79.2	D04.5	D23.5	D48.5	D49.2
back NEC	C76.8	C79.89	D04.5	D36.7	D48.7	D49.89

Neoplasm Table

Neoplasm, Bartholin's gland — Neoplasm, brain NEC

Neoplasm, neoplastic — *continued*	Malignant Primary	Malignant Secondary	Ca in situ	Benign	Uncertain	Unspecified Behavior
Bartholin's gland	C51.0	C79.82	D07.1	D28.0	D39.8	D49.5
basal ganglia	C71.0	C79.31	—	D33.0	D43.0	D49.6
basis pedunculi	C71.7	C79.31	—	D33.1	D43.1	D49.6
bile or biliary (tract)	C24.9	C78.89	D01.5	D13.5	D37.6	D49.0
canaliculi (biliferi) (intrahepatic)	C22.1	C78.7	D01.5	D13.4	D37.6	D49.0
canals, interlobular	C22.1	C78.89	D01.5	D13.4	D37.6	D49.0
duct or passage (common) (cystic) (extrahepatic)	C24.0	C78.89	D01.5	D13.5	D37.6	D49.0
interlobular	C22.1	C78.89	D01.5	D13.4	D37.6	D49.0
intrahepatic	C22.1	C78.7	D01.5	D13.4	D37.6	D49.0
and extrahepatic	C24.8	C78.89	D01.5	D13.5	D37.6	D49.0
bladder (urinary)	C67.9	C79.11	D09.0	D30.3	D41.4	D49.4
dome	C67.1	C79.11	D09.0	D30.3	D41.4	D49.4
neck	C67.5	C79.11	D09.0	D30.3	D41.4	D49.4
orifice	C67.9	C79.11	D09.0	D30.3	D41.4	D49.4
ureteric	C67.6	C79.11	D09.0	D30.3	D41.4	D49.4
urethral	C67.5	C79.11	D09.0	D30.3	D41.4	D49.4
overlapping lesion	C67.8	—	—	—	—	—
sphincter	C67.8	C79.11	D09.0	D30.3	D41.4	D49.4
trigone	C67.0	C79.11	D09.0	D30.3	D41.4	D49.4
urachus	C67.7	C79.11	D09.0	D30.3	D41.4	D49.4
wall	C67.9	C79.11	D09.0	D30.3	D41.4	D49.4
anterior	C67.3	C79.11	D09.0	D30.3	D41.4	D49.4
lateral	C67.2	C79.11	D09.0	D30.3	D41.4	D49.4
posterior	C67.4	C79.11	D09.0	D30.3	D41.4	D49.4
blood vessel — *see* Neoplasm, connective tissue						
bone (periosteum)	C41.9	C79.51	—	D16.9	D48.0	D49.2
acetabulum	C41.4	C79.51	—	D16.8	D48.0	D49.2
ankle	C40.3-☑	C79.51	—	D16.3-☑	—	—
arm NEC	C40.0-☑	C79.51	—	D16.0-☑	—	—
astragalus	C40.3-☑	C79.51	—	D16.3-☑	—	—
atlas	C41.2	C79.51	—	D16.6	D48.0	D49.2
axis	C41.2	C79.51	—	D16.6	D48.0	D49.2
back NEC	C41.2	C79.51	—	D16.6	D48.0	D49.2
calcaneus	C40.3-☑	C79.51	—	D16.3-☑	—	—
calvarium	C41.0	C79.51	—	D16.4	D48.0	D49.2
carpus (any)	C40.1-☑	C79.51	—	D16.1-☑	—	—
cartilage NEC	C41.9	C79.51	—	D16.9	D48.0	D49.2
clavicle	C41.3	C79.51	—	D16.7	D48.0	D49.2
clivus	C41.0	C79.51	—	D16.4	D48.0	D49.2
coccygeal vertebra	C41.4	C79.51	—	D16.8	D48.0	D49.2
coccyx	C41.4	C79.51	—	D16.8	D48.0	D49.2
costal cartilage	C41.3	C79.51	—	D16.7	D48.0	D49.2
costovertebral joint	C41.3	C79.51	—	D16.7	D48.0	D49.2
cranial	C41.0	C79.51	—	D16.4	D48.0	D49.2
cuboid	C40.3-☑	C79.51	—	D16.3-☑	—	—
cuneiform	C41.9	C79.51	—	D16.9	D48.0	D49.2
elbow	C40.0-☑	C79.51	—	D16.0-☑	—	—
ethmoid (labyrinth)	C41.0	C79.51	—	D16.4	D48.0	D49.2
face	C41.0	C79.51	—	D16.4	D48.0	D49.2
femur (any part)	C40.2-☑	C79.51	—	D16.2-☑	—	—
fibula (any part)	C40.2-☑	C79.51	—	D16.2-☑	—	—
finger (any)	C40.1-☑	C79.51	—	D16.1-☑	—	—
foot	C40.3-☑	C79.51	—	D16.3-☑	—	—
forearm	C40.0-☑	C79.51	—	D16.0-☑	—	—
frontal	C41.0	C79.51	—	D16.4	D48.0	D49.2
hand	C40.1-☑	C79.51	—	D16.1-☑	—	—
heel	C40.3-☑	C79.51	—	D16.3-☑	—	—
hip	C41.4	C79.51	—	D16.8	D48.0	D49.2
humerus (any part)	C40.0-☑	C79.51	—	D16.0-☑	—	—
hyoid	C41.0	C79.51	—	D16.4	D48.0	D49.2
ilium	C41.4	C79.51	—	D16.8	D48.0	D49.2
innominate	C41.4	C79.51	—	D16.8	D48.0	D49.2
intervertebral cartilage or disc	C41.2	C79.51	—	D16.6	D48.0	D49.2
ischium	C41.4	C79.51	—	D16.8	D48.0	D49.2
jaw (lower)	C41.1	C79.51	—	D16.5	D48.0	D49.2
knee	C40.2-☑	C79.51	—	D16.2-☑	—	—
leg NEC	C40.2-☑	C79.51	—	D16.2-☑	—	—
limb NEC	C40.9-☑	C79.51	—	D16.9	—	—

Neoplasm, neoplastic — *continued*	Malignant Primary	Malignant Secondary	Ca in situ	Benign	Uncertain	Unspecified Behavior
bone — *continued*						
limb — *continued*						
lower (long bones)	C40.2-☑	C79.51	—	D16.2-☑	—	—
short bones	C40.3-☑	C79.51	—	D16.3-☑	—	—
upper (long bones)	C40.0-☑	C79.51	—	D16.0-☑	—	—
short bones	C40.1-☑	C79.51	—	D16.1-☑	—	—
malar	C41.0	C79.51	—	D16.4	D48.0	D49.2
mandible	C41.1	C79.51	—	D16.5	D48.0	D49.2
marrow NEC (any bone)	C96.9	C79.52	—	—	D47.9	D49.89
mastoid	C41.0	C79.51	—	D16.4	D48.0	D49.2
maxilla, maxillary (superior)	C41.0	C79.51	—	D16.4	D48.0	D49.2
inferior	C41.1	C79.51	—	D16.5	D48.0	D49.2
metacarpus (any)	C40.1-☑	C79.51	—	D16.1-☑	—	—
metatarsus (any)	C40.3-☑	C79.51	—	D16.3-☑	—	—
navicular ankle	C40.3-☑	C79.51	—	—	—	—
hand	C40.1-☑	C79.51	—	—	—	—
nose, nasal	C41.0	C79.51	—	D16.4	D48.0	D49.2
occipital	C41.0	C79.51	—	D16.4	D48.0	D49.2
orbit	C41.0	C79.51	—	D16.4	D48.0	D49.2
overlapping sites	C40.8-☑	—	—	—	—	—
parietal	C41.0	C79.51	—	D16.4	D48.0	D49.2
patella	C40.2-☑	C79.51	—	—	—	—
pelvic	C41.4	C79.51	—	D16.8	D48.0	D49.2
phalanges foot	C40.3-☑	C79.51	—	—	—	—
hand	C40.1-☑	C79.51	—	—	—	—
pubic	C41.4	C79.51	—	D16.8	D48.0	D49.2
radius (any part)	C40.0-☑	C79.51	—	D16.0-☑	—	—
rib	C41.3	C79.51	—	D16.7	D48.0	D49.2
sacral vertebra	C41.4	C79.51	—	D16.8	D48.0	D49.2
sacrum	C41.4	C79.51	—	D16.8	D48.0	D49.2
scaphoid of ankle	C40.3-☑	C79.51	—	—	—	—
of hand	C40.1-☑	C79.51	—	—	—	—
scapula (any part)	C40.0-☑	C79.51	—	D16.0-☑	—	—
sella turcica	C41.0	C79.51	—	D16.4	D48.0	D49.2
shoulder	C40.0-☑	C79.51	—	D16.0-☑	—	—
skull	C41.0	C79.51	—	D16.4	D48.0	D49.2
sphenoid	C41.0	C79.51	—	D16.4	D48.0	D49.2
spine, spinal (column)	C41.2	C79.51	—	D16.6	D48.0	D49.2
coccyx	C41.4	C79.51	—	D16.8	D48.0	D49.2
sacrum	C41.4	C79.51	—	D16.8	D48.0	D49.2
sternum	C41.3	C79.51	—	D16.7	D48.0	D49.2
tarsus (any)	C40.3-☑	C79.51	—	—	—	—
temporal	C41.0	C79.51	—	D16.4	D48.0	D49.2
thumb	C40.1-☑	C79.51	—	—	—	—
tibia (any part)	C40.2-☑	C79.51	—	—	—	—
toe (any)	C40.3-☑	C79.51	—	—	—	—
trapezium	C40.1-☑	C79.51	—	—	—	—
trapezoid	C40.1-☑	C79.51	—	—	—	—
turbinate	C41.0	C79.51	—	D16.4	D48.0	D49.2
ulna (any part)	C40.0-☑	C79.51	—	D16.0-☑	—	—
unciform	C40.1-☑	C79.51	—	—	—	—
vertebra (column)	C41.2	C79.51	—	D16.6	D48.0	D49.2
coccyx	C41.4	C79.51	—	D16.8	D48.0	D49.2
sacrum	C41.4	C79.51	—	D16.8	D48.0	D49.2
vomer	C41.0	C79.51	—	D16.4	D48.0	D49.2
wrist	C40.1-☑	C79.51	—	—	—	—
xiphoid process	C41.3	C79.51	—	D16.7	D48.0	D49.2
zygomatic	C41.0	C79.51	—	D16.4	D48.0	D49.2
book-leaf (mouth) — *ventral surface of tongue and floor of mouth*	C06.89	C79.89	D00.00	D10.39	D37.09	D49.0
bowel — *see* Neoplasm, intestine						
brachial plexus	C47.1-☑	C79.89	—	D36.12	D48.2	D49.2
brain NEC	C71.9	C79.31	—	D33.2	D43.2	D49.6
basal ganglia	C71.0	C79.31	—	D33.0	D43.0	D49.6
cerebellopontine angle	C71.6	C79.31	—	D33.1	D43.1	D49.6
cerebellum NOS	C71.6	C79.31	—	D33.1	D43.1	D49.6
cerebrum	C71.0	C79.31	—	D33.0	D43.0	D49.6

☑ Additional Character Required — Refer to the Tabular List for Character Selection   ▽ Subterms under main terms may continue to next column or page

	Malignant Primary	Malignant Secondary	Ca in situ	Benign	Uncertain	Unspecified Behavior
Neoplasm, neoplastic — *continued*						
brain — *continued*						
choroid plexus	C71.7	C79.31	—	D33.1	D43.1	D49.6
corpus callosum	C71.8	C79.31	—	D33.2	D43.2	D49.6
corpus striatum	C71.0	C79.31	—	D33.0	D43.0	D49.6
cortex (cerebral)	C71.0	C79.31	—	D33.0	D43.0	D49.6
frontal lobe	C71.1	C79.31	—	D33.0	D43.0	D49.6
globus pallidus	C71.0	C79.31	—	D33.0	D43.0	D49.6
hippocampus	C71.2	C79.31	—	D33.0	D43.0	D49.6
hypothalamus	C71.0	C79.31	—	D33.0	D43.0	D49.6
internal capsule	C71.0	C79.31	—	D33.0	D43.0	D49.6
medulla oblongata	C71.7	C79.31	—	D33.1	D43.1	D49.6
meninges	C70.0	C79.32	—	D32.0	D42.0	D49.7
midbrain	C71.7	C79.31	—	D33.1	D43.1	D49.6
occipital lobe	C71.4	C79.31	—	D33.0	D43.0	D49.6
overlapping lesion	C71.8	C79.31	—	—	—	—
parietal lobe	C71.3	C79.31	—	D33.0	D43.0	D49.6
peduncle	C71.7	C79.31	—	D33.1	D43.1	D49.6
pons	C71.7	C79.31	—	D33.1	D43.1	D49.6
stem	C71.7	C79.31	—	D33.1	D43.1	D49.6
tapetum	C71.8	C79.31	—	D33.2	D43.2	D49.6
temporal lobe	C71.2	C79.31	—	D33.0	D43.0	D49.6
thalamus	C71.0	C79.31	—	D33.0	D43.0	D49.6
uncus	C71.2	C79.31	—	D33.0	D43.0	D49.6
ventricle (floor)	C71.5	C79.31	—	D33.0	D43.0	D49.6
fourth	C71.7	C79.31	—	D33.1	D43.1	D49.6
branchial (cleft) (cyst) (vestiges)	C10.4	C79.89	D00.08	D10.5	D37.05	D49.0
breast (connective tissue) (glandular tissue) (soft parts)	C50.9-☑	C79.81	D05.-☑	D24.-☑	D48.6-☑	D49.3
areola	C50.0-☑	C79.81	D05.-☑	D24.-☑	D48.6-☑	D49.3
axillary tail	C50.6-☑	C79.81	D05.-☑	D24.-☑	D48.6-☑	D49.3
central portion	C50.1-☑	C79.81	D05.-☑	D24.-☑	D48.6-☑	D49.3
inner	C50.8-☑	C79.81	D05.-☑	D24.-☑	D48.6-☑	D49.3
lower	C50.8-☑	C79.81	D05.-☑	D24.-☑	D48.6-☑	D49.3
lower-inner quadrant	C50.3-☑	C79.81	D05.-☑	D24.-☑	D48.6-☑	D49.3
lower-outer quadrant	C50.5-☑	C79.81	D05.-☑	D24.-☑	D48.6-☑	D49.3
mastectomy site (skin) — *see also* Neoplasm, breast, skin	C44.501	C79.2		—	—	—
specified as breast tissue	C50.8-☑	C79.81	—	—	—	—
midline	C50.8-☑	C79.81	D05.-☑	D24.-☑	D48.6-☑	D49.3
nipple	C50.0-☑	C79.81	D05.-☑	D24.-☑	D48.6-☑	D49.3
outer	C50.8-☑	C79.81	D05.-☑	D24.-☑	D48.6-☑	D49.3
overlapping lesion	C50.8-☑	—	—	—	—	—
skin	C44.501	C79.2	D04.5	D23.5	D48.5	D49.2
basal cell carcinoma	C44.511			—	—	—
specified type NEC	C44.591			—	—	—
squamous cell carcinoma	C44.521			—	—	—
tail (axillary)	C50.6-☑	C79.81	D05.-☑	D24.-☑	D48.6-☑	D49.3
upper	C50.8-☑	C79.81	D05.-☑	D24.-☑	D48.6-☑	D49.3
upper-inner quadrant	C50.2-☑	C79.81	D05.-☑	D24.-☑	D48.6-☑	D49.3
upper-outer quadrant	C50.4-☑	C79.81	D05.-☑	D24.-☑	D48.6-☑	D49.3
broad ligament	C57.1-☑	C79.82	D07.39	D28.2	D39.8	D49.5
bronchiogenic, bronchogenic (lung)	C34.9-☑	C78.0-☑	D02.2-☑	D14.3-☑	D38.1	D49.1
bronchiole	C34.9-☑	C78.0-☑	D02.2-☑	D14.3-☑	D38.1	D49.1
bronchus	C34.9-☑	C78.0-☑	D02.2-☑	D14.3-☑	D38.1	D49.1
carina	C34.0-☑	C78.0-☑	D02.2-☑	D14.3-☑	D38.1	D49.1
lower lobe of lung	C34.3-☑	C78.0-☑	D02.2-☑	D14.3-☑	D38.1	D49.1
main	C34.0-☑	C78.0-☑	D02.2-☑	D14.3-☑	D38.1	D49.1
middle lobe of lung	C34.2	C78.0-☑	D02.21	D14.31	D38.1	D49.1
overlapping lesion	C34.8-☑	—	—	—	—	—
upper lobe of lung	C34.1-☑	C78.0-☑	D02.2-☑	D14.3-☑	D38.1	D49.1
brow	C44.309	C79.2	D04.39	D23.39	D48.5	D49.2
basal cell carcinoma	C44.319	—	—	—	—	—
specified type NEC	C44.399	—	—	—	—	—

	Malignant Primary	Malignant Secondary	Ca in situ	Benign	Uncertain	Unspecified Behavior
Neoplasm, neoplastic — *continued*						
brow — *continued*						
squamous cell carcinoma	C44.329	—	—	—	—	—
buccal (cavity)	C06.9	C79.89	D00.00	D10.39	D37.09	D49.0
commissure	C06.0	C79.89	D00.02	D10.39	D37.09	D49.0
groove (lower) (upper)	C06.1	C79.89	D00.02	D10.39	D37.09	D49.0
mucosa	C06.0	C79.89	D00.02	D10.39	D37.09	D49.0
sulcus (lower) (upper)	C06.1	C79.89	D00.02	D10.39	D37.09	D49.0
bulbourethral gland	C68.0	C79.19	D09.19	D30.4	D41.3	D49.5
bursa — *see* Neoplasm, connective tissue						
buttock NEC	C76.3	C79.89	D04.5	D36.7	D48.7	D49.89
calf	C76.5-☑	C79.89	D04.7-☑	D36.7	D48.7	D49.89
calvarium	C41.0	C79.51		D16.4	D48.0	D49.2
calyx, renal	C65.-☑	C79.0-☑	D09.19	D30.1-☑	D41.1-☑	D49.5
canal						
anal	C21.1	C78.5	D01.3	D12.9	D37.8	D49.0
auditory (external) — *see also* Neoplasm, skin, ear	C44.20-☑	C79.2	D04.2-☑	D23.2-☑	D48.5	D49.2
auricular (external) — *see also* Neoplasm, skin, ear	C44.20-☑	C79.2	D04.2-☑	D23.2-☑	D48.5	D49.2
canaliculi, biliary (biliferi) (intrahepatic)	C22.1	C78.7	D01.5	D13.4	D37.6	D49.0
canthus (eye) (inner) (outer)	C44.10-☑	C79.2	D04.1-☑	D23.1-☑	D48.5	D49.2
basal cell carcinoma	C44.11-☑	—	—	—	—	—
specified type NEC	C44.19-☑	—	—	—	—	—
squamous cell carcinoma	C44.12-☑	—	—	—	—	—
capillary — *see* Neoplasm, connective tissue						
caput coli	C18.0	C78.5	D01.0	D12.0	D37.4	D49.0
carcinoid — *see* Tumor, carcinoid						
cardia (gastric)	C16.0	C78.89	D00.2	D13.1	D37.1	D49.0
cardiac orifice (stomach)	C16.0	C78.89	D00.2	D13.1	D37.1	D49.0
cardio-esophageal junction	C16.0	C78.89	D00.2	D13.1	D37.1	D49.0
cardio-esophagus	C16.0	C78.89	D00.2	D13.1	D37.1	D49.0
carina (bronchus)	C34.0-☑	C78.0-☑	D02.2-☑	D14.3-☑	D38.1	D49.1
carotid (artery)	C49.0	C79.89	—	D21.0	D48.1	D49.2
body	C75.4	C79.89	—	D35.5	D44.6	D49.7
carpus (any bone)	C40.1-☑	C79.51	—	D16.1-☑	—	—
cartilage (articular) (joint) NEC — *see also* Neoplasm, bone	C41.9	C79.51	—	D16.9	D48.0	D49.2
arytenoid	C32.3	C78.39	D02.0	D14.1	D38.0	D49.1
auricular	C49.0	C79.89	—	D21.0	D48.1	D49.2
bronchi	C34.0-☑	C78.39	—	D14.3-☑	D38.1	D49.1
costal	C41.3	C79.51	—	D16.7	D48.0	D49.2
cricoid	C32.3	C78.39	D02.0	D14.1	D38.0	D49.1
cuneiform	C32.3	C78.39	D02.0	D14.1	D38.0	D49.1
ear (external)	C49.0	C79.89	—	D21.0	D48.1	D49.2
ensiform	C41.3	C79.51	—	D16.7	D48.0	D49.2
epiglottis	C32.1	C78.39	D02.0	D14.1	D38.0	D49.1
anterior surface	C10.1	C79.89	D00.08	D10.5	D37.05	D49.0
eyelid	C49.0	C79.89	—	D21.0	D48.1	D49.2
intervertebral	C41.2	C79.51	—	D16.6	D48.0	D49.2
larynx, laryngeal	C32.3	C78.39	D02.0	D14.1	D38.0	D49.1
nose, nasal	C30.0	C78.39	D02.3	D14.0	D38.5	D49.1
pinna	C49.0	C79.89	—	D21.0	D48.1	D49.2
rib	C41.3	C79.51	—	D16.7	D48.0	D49.2
semilunar (knee)	C40.2-☑	C79.51	—	D16.2-☑	D48.0	D49.2
thyroid	C32.3	C78.39	D02.0	D14.1	D38.0	D49.1
trachea	C33	C78.39	D02.1	D14.2	D38.1	D49.1
cauda equina	C72.1	C79.49	—	D33.4	D43.4	D49.7
cavity						
buccal	C06.9	C79.89	D00.00	D10.30	D37.09	D49.0
nasal	C30.0	C78.39	D02.3	D14.0	D38.5	D49.1
oral	C06.9	C79.89	D00.00	D10.30	D37.09	D49.0
peritoneal	C48.2	C78.6		D20.1	D48.4	D49.0
tympanic	C30.1	C78.39	D02.3	D14.0	D38.5	D49.1
cecum	C18.0	C78.5	D01.0	D12.0	D37.4	D49.0

	Malignant Primary	Malignant Secondary	Ca in situ	Benign	Uncertain	Unspecified Behavior
Neoplasm, neoplastic —						
continued						
central nervous						
system	C72.9	C79.40	—	—	—	—
cerebellopontine						
(angle)	C71.6	C79.31	—	D33.1	D43.1	D49.6
cerebellum,						
cerebellar	C71.6	C79.31	—	D33.1	D43.1	D49.6
cerebrum, cerebral						
(cortex) (hemisphere)						
(white matter)	C71.0	C79.31	—	D33.0	D43.0	D49.6
meninges	C70.0	C79.32	—	D32.0	D42.0	D49.7
peduncle	C71.7	C79.31	—	D33.1	D43.1	D49.6
ventricle	C71.5	C79.31	—	D33.0	D43.0	D49.6
fourth	C71.7	C79.31	—	D33.1	D43.1	D49.6
cervical region	C76.0	C79.89	D09.8	D36.7	D48.7	D49.89
cervix (cervical) (uteri)						
(uterus)	C53.9	C79.82	D06.9	D26.0	D39.0	D49.5
canal	C53.0	C79.82	D06.0	D26.0	D39.0	D49.5
endocervix (canal)						
(gland)	C53.0	C79.82	D06.0	D26.0	D39.0	D49.5
exocervix	C53.1	C79.82	D06.1	D26.0	D39.0	D49.5
external os	C53.1	C79.82	D06.1	D26.0	D39.0	D49.5
internal os	C53.0	C79.82	D06.0	D26.0	D39.0	D49.5
nabothian gland	C53.0	C79.82	D06.0	D26.0	D39.0	D49.5
overlapping lesion	C53.8	—	—	—	—	—
squamocolumnar						
junction	C53.8	C79.82	D06.7	D26.0	D39.0	D49.5
stump	C53.8	C79.82	D06.7	D26.0	D39.0	D49.5
cheek	C76.0	C79.89	D09.8	D36.7	D48.7	D49.89
external	C44.309	C79.2	D04.39	D23.39	D48.5	D49.2
basal cell						
carcinoma	C44.319	—	—	—	—	—
specified type						
NEC	C44.399	—	—	—	—	—
squamous cell						
carcinoma	C44.329	—	—	—	—	—
inner aspect	C06.0	C79.89	D00.02	D10.39	D37.09	D49.0
internal	C06.0	C79.89	D00.02	D10.39	D37.09	D49.0
mucosa	C06.0	C79.89	D00.02	D10.39	D37.09	D49.0
chest (wall) NEC	C76.1	C79.89	D09.8	D36.7	D48.7	D49.89
chiasma opticum	C72.3-☑	C79.49	—	D33.3	D43.3	D49.7
chin	C44.309	C79.2	D04.39	D23.39	D48.5	D49.2
basal cell						
carcinoma	C44.319	—	—	—	—	—
specified type NEC	C44.399	—	—	—	—	—
squamous cell						
carcinoma	C44.329	—	—	—	—	—
choana	C11.3	C79.89	D00.08	D10.6	D37.05	D49.0
cholangiole	C22.1	C78.89	D01.5	D13.4	D37.6	D49.0
choledochal duct	C24.0	C78.89	D01.5	D13.5	D37.6	D49.0
choroid	C69.3-☑	C79.49	D09.2-☑	D31.3-☑	D48.7	D49.81
plexus	C71.5	C79.31	—	D33.0	D43.0	D49.6
ciliary body	C69.4-☑	C79.49	D09.2-☑	D31.4-☑	D48.7	D49.89
clavicle	C41.3	C79.51	—	D16.7	D48.0	D49.2
clitoris	C51.2	C79.82	D07.1	D28.0	D39.8	D49.5
clivus	C41.0	C79.51	—	D16.4	D48.0	D49.2
cloacogenic zone	C21.2	C78.5	D01.3	D12.9	D37.8	D49.0
coccygeal						
body or glomus	C49.5	C79.89	—	D21.5	D48.1	D49.2
vertebra	C41.4	C79.51	—	D16.8	D48.0	D49.2
coccyx	C41.4	C79.51	—	D16.8	D48.0	D49.2
colon — *see also*						
Neoplasm, intestine,						
large	C18.9	C78.5	—	—	—	—
with rectum	C19	C78.5	D01.1	D12.7	D37.5	D49.0
columnella — *see also*						
Neoplasm, skin,						
face	C44.390	C79.2	D04.39	D23.39	D48.5	D49.2
column, spinal — *see*						
Neoplasm, spine						
commissure						
labial, lip	C00.6	C79.89	D00.01	D10.39	D37.01	D49.0
laryngeal	C32.0	C78.39	D02.0	D14.1	D38.0	D49.1
common (bile) duct	C24.0	C78.89	D01.5	D13.5	D37.6	D49.0
concha — *see also*						
Neoplasm, skin,						
ear	C44.20-☑	C79.2	D04.2-☑	D23.2-☑	D48.5	D49.2
nose	C30.0	C78.39	D02.3	D14.0	D38.5	D49.1
conjunctiva	C69.0-☑	C79.49	D09.2-☑	D31.0-☑	D48.7	D49.89

	Malignant Primary	Malignant Secondary	Ca in situ	Benign	Uncertain	Unspecified Behavior
Neoplasm, neoplastic —						
continued						
connective tissue						
NEC	C49.9	C79.89	—	D21.9	D48.1	D49.2

Note: For neoplasms of connective tissue (blood vessel, bursa, fascia, ligament, muscle, peripheral nerves, sympathetic and parasympathetic nerves and ganglia, synovia, tendon, etc.) or of morphological types that indicate connective tissue, code according to the list under "Neoplasm, connective tissue". For sites that do not appear in this list, code to neoplasm of that site; e.g., fibrosarcoma, pancreas (C25.9)

Note: Morphological types that indicate connective tissue appear in their proper place in the alphabetic index with the instruction "see Neoplasm, connective tissue ...."

	Malignant Primary	Malignant Secondary	Ca in situ	Benign	Uncertain	Unspecified Behavior
abdomen	C49.4	C79.89	—	D21.4	D48.1	D49.2
abdominal wall	C49.4	C79.89	—	D21.4	D48.1	D49.2
ankle	C49.2-☑	C79.89	—	D21.2-☑	D48.1	D49.2
antecubital fossa or						
space	C49.1-☑	C79.89	—	D21.1-☑	D48.1	D49.2
arm	C49.1-☑	C79.89	—	D21.1-☑	D48.1	D49.2
auricle (ear)	C49.0	C79.89	—	D21.0	D48.1	D49.2
axilla	C49.3	C79.89	—	D21.3	D48.1	D49.2
back	C49.6	C79.89	—	D21.6	D48.1	D49.2
breast — *see* Neoplasm,						
breast						
buttock	C49.5	C79.89	—	D21.5	D48.1	D49.2
calf	C49.2-☑	C79.89	—	D21.2-☑	D48.1	D49.2
cervical region	C49.0	C79.89	—	D21.0	D48.1	D49.2
cheek	C49.0	C79.89	—	D21.0	D48.1	D49.2
chest (wall)	C49.3	C79.89	—	D21.3	D48.1	D49.2
chin	C49.0	C79.89	—	D21.0	D48.1	D49.2
diaphragm	C49.3	C79.89	—	D21.3	D48.1	D49.2
ear (external)	C49.0	C79.89	—	D21.0	D48.1	D49.2
elbow	C49.1-☑	C79.89	—	D21.1-☑	D48.1	D49.2
extrarectal	C49.5	C79.89	—	D21.5	D48.1	D49.2
extremity	C49.9	C79.89	—	D21.9	D48.1	D49.2
lower	C49.2-☑	C79.89	—	D21.2-☑	D48.1	D49.2
upper	C49.1-☑	C79.89	—	D21.1-☑	D48.1	D49.2
eyelid	C49.0	C79.89	—	D21.0	D48.1	D49.2
face	C49.0	C79.89	—	D21.0	D48.1	D49.2
finger	C49.1-☑	C79.89	—	D21.1-☑	D48.1	D49.2
flank	C49.6	C79.89	—	D21.6	D48.1	D49.2
foot	C49.2-☑	C79.89	—	D21.2-☑	D48.1	D49.2
forearm	C49.1-☑	C79.89	—	D21.1-☑	D48.1	D49.2
forehead	C49.0	C79.89	—	D21.0	D48.1	D49.2
gastric	C49.4	C79.89	—	D21.4	D48.1	D49.2
gastrointestinal	C49.4	C79.89	—	D21.4	D48.1	D49.2
gluteal region	C49.5	C79.89	—	D21.5	D48.1	D49.2
great vessels NEC	C49.3	C79.89	—	D21.3	D48.1	D49.2
groin	C49.5	C79.89	—	D21.5	D48.1	D49.2
hand	C49.1-☑	C79.89	—	D21.1-☑	D48.1	D49.2
head	C49.0	C79.89	—	D21.0	D48.1	D49.2
heel	C49.2-☑	C79.89	—	D21.2-☑	D48.1	D49.2
hip	C49.2-☑	C79.89	—	D21.2-☑	D48.1	D49.2
hypochondrium	C49.4	C79.89	—	D21.4	D48.1	D49.2
iliopsoas muscle	C49.5	C79.89	—	D21.5	D48.1	D49.2
infraclavicular						
region	C49.3	C79.89	—	D21.3	D48.1	D49.2
inguinal (canal)						
(region)	C49.5	C79.89	—	D21.5	D48.1	D49.2
intestinal	C49.4	C79.89	—	D21.4	D48.1	D49.2
intrathoracic	C49.3	C79.89	—	D21.3	D48.1	D49.2
ischiorectal fossa	C49.5	C79.89	—	D21.5	D48.1	D49.2
jaw	C03.9	C79.89	D00.03	D10.39	D48.1	D49.0
knee	C49.2-☑	C79.89	—	D21.2-☑	D48.1	D49.2
leg	C49.2-☑	C79.89	—	D21.2-☑	D48.1	D49.2
limb NEC	C49.9	C79.89	—	D21.9	D48.1	D49.2
lower	C49.2-☑	C79.89	—	D21.2-☑	D48.1	D49.2
upper	C49.1-☑	C79.89	—	D21.1-☑	D48.1	D49.2
nates	C49.5	C79.89	—	D21.5	D48.1	D49.2
neck	C49.0	C79.89	—	D21.0	D48.1	D49.2
orbit	C69.6-☑	C79.49	D09.2-☑	D31.6-☑	D48.1	D49.89
overlapping lesion	C49.8	—	—	—	—	—
pararectal	C49.5	C79.89	—	D21.5	D48.1	D49.2
para-urethral	C49.5	C79.89	—	D21.5	D48.1	D49.2
paravaginal	C49.5	C79.89	—	D21.5	D48.1	D49.2
pelvis (floor)	C49.5	C79.89	—	D21.5	D48.1	D49.2
pelvo-abdominal	C49.8	C79.89	—	D21.6	D48.1	D49.2
perineum	C49.5	C79.89	—	D21.5	D48.1	D49.2
perirectal (tissue)	C49.5	C79.89	—	D21.5	D48.1	D49.2

☑ **Additional Character Required — Refer to the Tabular List for Character Selection**   ▽ **Subterms under main terms may continue to next column or page**

Neoplasm, neoplastic —	Malignant Primary	Malignant Secondary	Ca in situ	Benign	Uncertain	Unspecified Behavior
continued						
connective tissue —						
continued						
periurethral						
(tissue)	C49.5	C79.89	—	D21.5	D48.1	D49.2
popliteal fossa or						
space	C49.2-☑	C79.89	—	D21.2-☑	D48.1	D49.2
presacral	C49.5	C79.89	—	D21.5	D48.1	D49.2
psoas muscle	C49.4	C79.89	—	D21.4	D48.1	D49.2
pterygoid fossa	C49.0	C79.89	—	D21.0	D48.1	D49.2
rectovaginal septum or						
wall	C49.5	C79.89	—	D21.5	D48.1	D49.2
rectovesical	C49.5	C79.89	—	D21.5	D48.1	D49.2
retroperitoneum	C48.0	C78.6	—	D20.0	D48.3	D49.0
sacrococcygeal						
region	C49.5	C79.89	—	D21.5	D48.1	D49.2
scalp	C49.0	C79.89	—	D21.0	D48.1	D49.2
scapular region	C49.3	C79.89	—	D21.3	D48.1	D49.2
shoulder	C49.1-☑	C79.89	—	D21.1-☑	D48.1	D49.2
skin (dermis) NEC — *see*						
also Neoplasm, skin,						
by site	C44.90	C79.2	D04.9	D23.9	D48.5	D49.2
stomach	C49.4	C79.89	—	D21.4	D48.1	D49.2
submental	C49.0	C79.89	—	D21.0	D48.1	D49.2
supraclavicular						
region	C49.0	C79.89	—	D21.0	D48.1	D49.2
temple	C49.0	C79.89	—	D21.0	D48.1	D49.2
temporal region	C49.0	C79.89	—	D21.0	D48.1	D49.2
thigh	C49.2-☑	C79.89	—	D21.2-☑	D48.1	D49.2
thoracic (duct)						
(wall)	C49.3	C79.89	—	D21.3	D48.1	D49.2
thorax	C49.3	C79.89	—	D21.3	D48.1	D49.2
thumb	C49.1-☑	C79.89	—	D21.1-☑	D48.1	D49.2
toe	C49.2-☑	C79.89	—	D21.2-☑	D48.1	D49.2
trunk	C49.6	C79.89	—	D21.6	D48.1	D49.2
umbilicus	C49.4	C79.89	—	D21.4	D48.1	D49.2
vesicorectal	C49.5	C79.89	—	D21.5	D48.1	D49.2
wrist	C49.1-☑	C79.89	—	D21.1-☑	D48.1	D49.2
conus medullaris	C72.0	C79.49	—	D33.4	D43.4	D49.7
cord (true) (vocal)	C32.0	C78.39	D02.0	D14.1	D38.0	D49.1
false	C32.1	C78.39	D02.0	D14.1	D38.0	D49.1
spermatic	C63.1-☑	C79.82	D07.69	D29.8	D40.8	D49.5
spinal (cervical)						
(lumbar)						
(thoracic)	C72.0	C79.49	—	D33.4	D43.4	D49.7
cornea (limbus)	C69.1-☑	C79.49	D09.2-☑	D31.1-☑	D48.7	D49.89
corpus						
albicans	C56.-☑	C79.6-☑	D07.39	D27.-☑	D39.1-☑	D49.5
callosum, brain	C71.0	C79.31	—	D33.2	D43.2	D49.6
cavernosum	C60.2	C79.82	D07.4	D29.0	D40.8	D49.5
gastric	C16.2	C78.89	D00.2	D13.1	D37.1	D49.0
overlapping sites	C54.8	—	—	—	—	—
penis	C60.2	C79.82	D07.4	D29.0	D40.8	D49.5
striatum,						
cerebrum	C71.0	C79.31	—	D33.0	D43.0	D49.6
uteri	C54.9	C79.82	D07.0	D26.1	D39.0	D49.5
isthmus	C54.0	C79.82	D07.0	D26.1	D39.0	D49.5
cortex						
adrenal	C74.0-☑	C79.7-☑	D09.3	D35.0-☑	D44.1-☑	D49.7
cerebral	C71.0	C79.31	—	D33.0	D43.0	D49.6
costal cartilage	C41.3	C79.51	—	D16.7	D48.0	D49.2
costovertebral joint	C41.3	C79.51	—	D16.7	D48.0	D49.2
Cowper's gland	C68.0	C79.19	D09.19	D30.4	D41.3	D49.5
cranial (fossa, any)	C71.9	C79.31	—	D33.2	D43.2	D49.6
meninges	C70.0	C79.32	—	D32.0	D42.0	D49.7
nerve	C72.50	C79.49	—	D33.3	D43.3	D49.7
specified NEC	C72.59	C79.49	—	D33.3	D43.3	D49.7
craniobuccal pouch	C75.2	C79.89	D09.3	D35.2	D44.3	D49.7
craniopharyngeal (duct)						
(pouch)	C75.2	C79.89	D09.3	D35.3	D44.4	D49.7
cricoid	C13.0	C79.89	D00.08	D10.7	D37.05	D49.0
cartilage	C32.3	C78.39	D02.0	D14.1	D38.0	D49.1
cricopharynx	C13.0	C79.89	D00.08	D10.7	D37.05	D49.0
crypt of Morgagni	C21.8	C78.5	D01.3	D12.9	D37.8	D49.0
crystalline lens	C69.4-☑	C79.49	D09.2-☑	D31.4-☑	D48.7	D49.89
cul-de-sac						
(Douglas')	C48.1	C78.6	—	D20.1	D48.4	D49.0
cuneiform cartilage	C32.3	C78.39	D02.0	D14.1	D38.0	D49.1
cutaneous — *see*						
Neoplasm, skin						
cutis — *see* Neoplasm,						
skin						

Neoplasm, neoplastic —	Malignant Primary	Malignant Secondary	Ca in situ	Benign	Uncertain	Unspecified Behavior
continued						
cystic (bile) duct						
(common)	C24.0	C78.89	D01.5	D13.5	D37.6	D49.0
dermis — *see* Neoplasm,						
skin						
diaphragm	C49.3	C79.89	—	D21.3	D48.1	D49.2
digestive organs, system,						
tube, or tract						
NEC	C26.9	C78.89	D01.9	D13.9	D37.9	D49.0
disc, intervertebral	C41.2	C79.51	—	D16.6	D48.0	D49.2
disease, generalized	C80.0	—	—	—	—	—
disseminated	C80.0	—	—	—	—	—
Douglas' cul-de-sac or						
pouch	C48.1	C78.6	—	D20.1	D48.4	D49.0
duodenojejunal						
junction	C17.8	C78.4	D01.49	D13.39	D37.2	D49.0
duodenum	C17.0	C78.4	D01.49	D13.2	D37.2	D49.0
dura (cranial)						
(mater)	C70.9	C79.49	—	D32.9	D42.9	D49.7
cerebral	C70.0	C79.32	—	D32.0	D42.0	D49.7
spinal	C70.1	C79.49	—	D32.1	D42.1	D49.7
ear (external) — *see also*						
Neoplasm, skin,						
ear	C44.20-☑	C79.2	D04.2-☑	D23.2-☑	D48.5	D49.2
auricle or auris — *see*						
also Neoplasm, skin,						
ear	C44.20-☑	C79.2	D04.2-☑	D23.2-☑	D48.5	D49.2
canal, external — *see*						
also Neoplasm, skin,						
ear	C44.20-☑	C79.2	D04.2-☑	D23.2-☑	D48.5	D49.2
cartilage	C49.0	C79.89	—	D21.0	D48.1	D49.2
external meatus — *see*						
also Neoplasm, skin,						
ear	C44.20-☑	C79.2	D04.2-☑	D23.2-☑	D48.5	D49.2
inner	C30.1	C78.39	D02.3	D14.0	D38.5	D49.1
lobule — *see also*						
Neoplasm, skin,						
ear	C44.20-☑	C79.2	D04.2-☑	D23.2-☑	D48.5	D49.2
middle	C30.1	C78.39	D02.3	D14.0	D38.5	D49.1
overlapping lesion with						
accessory						
sinuses	C31.8	—	—	—	—	—
skin	C44.20-☑	C79.2	D04.2-☑	D23.2-☑	D48.5	D49.2
basal cell						
carcinoma	C44.21-☑	—	—	—	—	—
specified type						
NEC	C44.29-☑	—	—	—	—	—
squamous cell						
carcinoma	C44.22-☑	—	—	—	—	—
earlobe	C44.20-☑	C79.2	D04.2-☑	D23.2-☑	D48.5	D49.2
basal cell						
carcinoma	C44.21-☑	—	—	—	—	—
specified type NEC	C44.29-☑	—	—	—	—	—
squamous cell						
carcinoma	C44.22-☑	—	—	—	—	—
ejaculatory duct	C63.7	C79.82	D07.69	D29.8	D40.8	D49.5
elbow NEC	C76.4-☑	C79.89	D04.6-☑	D36.7	D48.7	D49.89
endocardium	C38.0	C79.89	—	D15.1	D48.7	D49.89
endocervix (canal)						
(gland)	C53.0	C79.82	D06.0	D26.0	D39.0	D49.5
endocrine gland						
NEC	C75.9	C79.89	D09.3	D35.9	D44.9	D49.7
pluriglandular	C75.8	C79.89	D09.3	D35.7	D44.9	D49.7
endometrium (gland)						
(stroma)	C54.1	C79.82	D07.0	D26.1	D39.0	D49.5
ensiform cartilage	C41.3	C79.51	—	D16.7	D48.0	D49.2
enteric — *see* Neoplasm,						
intestine						
ependyma (brain)	C71.5	C79.31	—	D33.0	D43.0	D49.6
fourth ventricle	C71.7	C79.31	—	D33.1	D43.1	D49.6
epicardium	C38.0	C79.89	—	D15.1	D48.7	D49.89
epididymis	C63.0-☑	C79.82	D07.69	D29.3-☑	D40.8	D49.5
epidural	C72.9	C79.49	—	D33.9	D43.9	D49.7
epiglottis	C32.1	C78.39	D02.0	D14.1	D38.0	D49.1
anterior aspect or						
surface	C10.1	C79.89	D00.08	D10.5	D37.05	D49.0
cartilage	C32.3	C78.39	D02.0	D14.1	D38.0	D49.1
free border						
(margin)	C10.1	C79.89	D00.08	D10.5	D37.05	D49.0
junctional region	C10.8	C79.89	D00.08	D10.5	D37.05	D49.0
posterior (laryngeal)						
surface	C32.1	C78.39	D02.0	D14.1	D38.0	D49.1

☟ **Subterms under main terms may continue to next column or page**   ☑ **Additional Character Required — Refer to the Tabular List for Character Selection**

Neoplasm Table

Neoplasm, epiglottis — Neoplasm, gland, glandular

Neoplasm, neoplastic — continued	Malignant Primary	Malignant Secondary	Ca in situ	Benign	Uncertain	Unspecified Behavior
epiglottis — continued						
suprahyoid portion	C32.1	C78.39	D02.0	D14.1	D38.0	D49.1
esophagogastric junction	C16.0	C78.89	D00.2	D13.1	D37.1	D49.0
esophagus	C15.9	C78.89	D00.1	D13.0	D37.8	D49.0
abdominal	C15.5	C78.89	D00.1	D13.0	D37.8	D49.0
cervical	C15.3	C78.89	D00.1	D13.0	D37.8	D49.0
distal (third)	C15.5	C78.89	D00.1	D13.0	D37.8	D49.0
lower (third)	C15.5	C78.89	D00.1	D13.0	D37.8	D49.0
middle (third)	C15.4	C78.89	D00.1	D13.0	D37.8	D49.0
overlapping lesion	C15.8	—	—	—	—	—
proximal (third)	C15.3	C78.89	D00.1	D13.0	D37.8	D49.0
thoracic	C15.4	C78.89	D00.1	D13.0	D37.8	D49.0
upper (third)	C15.3	C78.89	D00.1	D13.0	D37.8	D49.0
ethmoid (sinus)	C31.1	C78.39	D02.3	D14.0	D38.5	D49.1
bone or labyrinth	C41.0	C79.51	—	D16.4	D48.0	D49.2
eustachian tube	C30.1	C78.39	D02.3	D14.0	D38.5	D49.1
exocervix	C53.1	C79.82	D06.1	D26.0	D39.0	D49.5
external						
meatus (ear) — see also Neoplasm, skin, ear	C44.20-☑	C79.2	D04.2-☑	D23.2-☑	D48.5	D49.2
os, cervix uteri	C53.1	C79.82	D06.1	D26.0	D39.0	D49.5
extradural	C72.9	C79.49	—	D33.9	D43.9	D49.7
extrahepatic (bile) duct	C24.0	C78.89	D01.5	D13.5	D37.6	D49.0
overlapping lesion with gallbladder	C24.8	—	—	—	—	—
extraocular muscle	C69.6-☑	C79.49	D09.2-☑	D31.6-☑	D48.7	D49.89
extrarectal	C76.3	C79.89	D09.8	D36.7	D48.7	D49.89
extremity	C76.8	C79.89	D04.8	D36.7	D48.7	D49.89
lower	C76.5-☑	C79.89	D04.7-☑	D36.7	D48.7	D49.89
upper	C76.4-☑	C79.89	D04.6-☑	D36.7	D48.7	D49.89
eyeball	C69.9-☑	C79.49	D09.2-☑	D31.9-☑	D48.7	D49.89
eyebrow	C44.309	C79.2	D04.39	D23.39	D48.5	D49.2
basal cell carcinoma	C44.319	—	—	—	—	—
specified type NEC	C44.399	—	—	—	—	—
squamous cell carcinoma	C44.329	—	—	—	—	—
eyelid (lower) (skin) (upper)	C44.10-☑	—	—	—	—	—
basal cell carcinoma	C44.11-☑	—	—	—	—	—
cartilage	C49.0	C79.89	—	D21.0	D48.1	D49.2
specified type NEC	C44.19-☑	—	—	—	—	—
squamous cell carcinoma	C44.12-☑	—	—	—	—	—
eye NEC	C69.9-☑	C79.49	D09.2-☑	D31.9-☑	D48.7	D49.89
overlapping sites	C69.8-☑	—	—	—	—	—
face NEC	C76.0	C79.89	D04.39	D36.7	D48.7	D49.89
fallopian tube (accessory)	C57.0-☑	C79.82	D07.39	D28.2	D39.8	D49.5
falx (cerebella) (cerebri)	C70.0	C79.32	—	D32.0	D42.0	D49.7
fascia — see also Neoplasm, connective tissue						
palmar	C49.1-☑	C79.89	—	D21.1-☑	D48.1	D49.2
plantar	C49.2-☑	C79.89	—	D21.2-☑	D48.1	D49.2
fatty tissue — see Neoplasm, connective tissue						
fauces, faucial NEC	C10.9	C79.89	D00.08	D10.5	D37.05	D49.0
pillars	C09.1	C79.89	D00.08	D10.5	D37.05	D49.0
tonsil	C09.9	C79.89	D00.08	D10.4	D37.05	D49.0
femur (any part)	C40.2-☑	—	—	D16.2-☑	—	—
fetal membrane	C58	C79.82	D07.0	D26.7	D39.2	D49.5
fibrous tissue — see Neoplasm, connective tissue						
fibula (any part)	C40.2-☑	C79.51	—	D16.2-☑	—	—
filum terminale	C72.0	C79.49	—	D33.4	D43.4	D49.7
finger NEC	C76.4-☑	C79.89	D04.6-☑	D36.7	D48.7	D49.89
flank NEC	C76.8	C79.89	D04.5	D36.7	D48.7	D49.89
follicle, nabothian	C53.0	C79.82	D06.0	D26.0	D39.0	D49.5
foot NEC	C76.5-☑	C79.89	D04.7-☑	D36.7	D48.7	D49.89
forearm NEC	C76.4-☑	C79.89	D04.6-☑	D36.7	D48.7	D49.89
forehead (skin)	C44.309	C79.2	D04.39	D23.39	D48.5	D49.2

Neoplasm, neoplastic — continued	Malignant Primary	Malignant Secondary	Ca in situ	Benign	Uncertain	Unspecified Behavior
forehead — continued						
basal cell carcinoma	C44.319	—	—	—	—	—
specified type NEC	C44.399	—	—	—	—	—
squamous cell carcinoma	C44.329	—	—	—	—	—
foreskin	C60.0	C79.82	D07.4	D29.0	D40.8	D49.5
fornix						
pharyngeal	C11.3	C79.89	D00.08	D10.6	D37.05	D49.0
vagina	C52	C79.82	D07.2	D28.1	D39.8	D49.5
fossa (of)						
anterior (cranial)	C71.9	C79.31	—	D33.2	D43.2	D49.6
cranial	C71.9	C79.31	—	D33.2	D43.2	D49.6
ischiorectal	C76.3	C79.89	D09.8	D36.7	D48.7	D49.89
middle (cranial)	C71.9	C79.31	—	D33.2	D43.2	D49.6
piriform	C12	C79.89	D00.08	D10.7	D37.05	D49.0
pituitary	C75.1	C79.89	D09.3	D35.2	D44.3	D49.7
posterior (cranial)	C71.9	C79.31	—	D33.2	D43.2	D49.6
pterygoid	C49.0	C79.89	—	D21.0	D48.1	D49.2
pyriform	C12	C79.89	D00.08	D10.7	D37.05	D49.0
Rosenmuller	C11.2	C79.89	D00.08	D10.6	D37.05	D49.0
tonsillar	C09.0	C79.89	D00.08	D10.5	D37.05	D49.0
fourchette	C51.9	C79.82	D07.1	D28.0	D39.8	D49.5
frenulum						
labii — see Neoplasm, lip, internal						
linguae	C02.2	C79.89	D00.07	D10.1	D37.02	D49.0
frontal						
bone	C41.0	C79.51	—	D16.4	D48.0	D49.2
lobe, brain	C71.1	C79.31	—	D33.0	D43.0	D49.6
pole	C71.1	C79.31	—	D33.0	D43.0	D49.6
sinus	C31.2	C78.39	D02.3	D14.0	D38.5	D49.1
fundus						
stomach	C16.1	C78.89	D00.2	D13.1	D37.1	D49.0
uterus	C54.3	C79.82	D07.0	D26.1	D39.0	D49.5
gallbladder	C23	C78.89	D01.5	D13.5	D37.6	D49.0
overlapping lesion with extrahepatic bile ducts	C24.8	—	—	—	—	—
gall duct (extrahepatic)	C24.0	C78.89	D01.5	D13.5	D37.6	D49.0
intrahepatic	C22.1	C78.7	D01.5	D13.4	D37.6	D49.0
ganglia — see also Neoplasm, nerve, peripheral	C47.9	C79.89	—	D36.10	D48.2	D49.2
basal	C71.0	C79.31	—	D33.0	D43.0	D49.6
cranial nerve	C72.50	C79.49	—	D33.3	D43.3	D49.7
Gartner's duct	C52	C79.82	D07.2	D28.1	D39.8	D49.5
gastric — see Neoplasm, stomach						
gastrocolic	C26.9	C78.89	D01.9	D13.9	D37.9	D49.0
gastroesophageal junction	C16.0	C78.89	D00.2	D13.1	D37.1	D49.0
gastrointestinal (tract) NEC	C26.9	C78.89	D01.9	D13.9	D37.9	D49.0
generalized	C80.0	—	—	—	—	—
genital organ or tract						
female NEC	C57.9	C79.82	D07.30	D28.9	D39.9	D49.5
overlapping lesion	C57.8	—	—	—	—	—
specified site NEC	C57.7	C79.82	D07.39	D28.7	D39.8	D49.5
male NEC	C63.9	C79.82	D07.60	D29.9	D40.9	D49.5
overlapping lesion	C63.8	—	—	—	—	—
specified site NEC	C63.7	C79.82	D07.69	D29.8	D40.8	D49.5
genitourinary tract						
female	C57.9	C79.82	D07.30	D28.9	D39.9	D49.5
male	C63.9	C79.82	D07.60	D29.9	D40.9	D49.5
gingiva (alveolar) (marginal)	C03.9	C79.89	D00.03	D10.39	D37.09	D49.0
lower	C03.1	C79.89	D00.03	D10.39	D37.09	D49.0
mandibular	C03.1	C79.89	D00.03	D10.39	D37.09	D49.0
maxillary	C03.0	C79.89	D00.03	D10.39	D37.09	D49.0
upper	C03.0	C79.89	D00.03	D10.39	D37.09	D49.0
gland, glandular (lymphatic) (system) — see also Neoplasm, lymph gland						
endocrine NEC	C75.9	C79.89	D09.3	D35.9	D44.9	D49.7

☑ **Additional Character Required** — Refer to the Tabular List for Character Selection ⬙ Subterms under main terms may continue to next column or page

	Malignant Primary	Malignant Secondary	Ca in situ	Benign	Uncertain	Unspecified Behavior
Neoplasm, neoplastic — *continued*						
gland, glandular — *see also* Neoplasm, lymph gland — *continued*						
salivary — *see* Neoplasm, salivary gland						
glans penis	C60.1	C79.82	D07.4	D29.0	D40.8	D49.5
globus pallidus	C71.0	C79.31	—	D33.0	D43.0	D49.6
glomus						
coccygeal	C49.5	C79.89	—	D21.5	D48.1	D49.2
jugularis	C75.5	C79.89	—	D35.6	D44.7	D49.7
glosso-epiglottic fold(s)	C10.1	C79.89	D00.08	D10.5	D37.05	D49.0
glossopalatine fold	C09.1	C79.89	D00.08	D10.5	D37.05	D49.0
glossopharyngeal sulcus	C09.0	C79.89	D00.08	D10.5	D37.05	D49.0
glottis	C32.0	C78.39	D02.0	D14.1	D38.0	D49.1
gluteal region	C76.3	C79.89	D04.5	D36.7	D48.7	D49.89
great vessels NEC	C49.3	C79.89	—	D21.3	D48.1	D49.2
groin NEC	C76.3	C79.89	D04.5	D36.7	D48.7	D49.89
gum	C03.9	C79.89	D00.03	D10.39	D37.09	D49.0
lower	C03.1	C79.89	D00.03	D10.39	D37.09	D49.0
upper	C03.0	C79.89	D00.03	D10.39	D37.09	D49.0
hand NEC	C76.4-☑	C79.89	D04.6-☑	D36.7	D48.7	D49.89
head NEC	C76.0	C79.89	D04.4	D36.7	D48.7	D49.89
heart	C38.0	C79.89	—	D15.1	D48.7	D49.89
heel NEC	C76.5-☑	C79.89	D04.7-☑	D36.7	D48.7	D49.89
helix — *see also* Neoplasm, skin, ear	C44.20-☑	C79.2	D04.2-☑	D23.2-☑	D48.5	D49.2
hematopoietic, hemopoietic tissue NEC	C96.9	—	—	—	—	—
specified NEC	C96.Z	—	—	—	—	—
hemisphere, cerebral	C71.0	C79.31	—	D33.0	D43.0	D49.6
hemorrhoidal zone	C21.1	C78.5	D01.3	D12.9	D37.8	D49.0
hepatic — *see also* Index to disease, by histology	C22.9	C78.7	D01.5	D13.4	D37.6	D49.0
duct (bile)	C24.0	C78.89	D01.5	D13.5	D37.6	D49.0
flexure (colon)	C18.3	C78.5	D01.0	D12.3	D37.4	D49.0
primary	C22.8	C78.7	D01.5	D13.4	D37.6	D49.0
hepatobiliary	C24.9	C78.89	D01.5	D13.5	D37.6	D49.0
hepatoblastoma	C22.2	C78.7	D01.5	D13.4	D37.6	D49.0
hepatoma	C22.0	C78.7	D01.5	D13.4	D37.6	D49.0
hilus of lung	C34.0-☑	C78.0-☑	D02.2-☑	D14.3-☑	D38.1	D49.1
hippocampus, brain	C71.2	C79.31	—	D33.0	D43.0	D49.6
hip NEC	C76.5-☑	C79.89	D04.7-☑	D36.7	D48.7	D49.89
humerus (any part)	C40.0-☑	C79.51	—	D16.0-☑	—	—
hymen	C52	C79.82	D07.2	D28.1	D39.8	D49.5
hypopharynx, hypopharyngeal NEC	C13.9	C79.89	D00.08	D10.7	D37.05	D49.0
overlapping lesion	C13.8	—	—	—	—	—
postcricoid region	C13.0	C79.89	D00.08	D10.7	D37.05	D49.0
posterior wall	C13.2	C79.89	D00.08	D10.7	D37.05	D49.0
pyriform fossa (sinus)	C12	C79.89	D00.08	D10.7	D37.05	D49.0
hypophysis	C75.1	C79.89	D09.3	D35.2	D44.3	D49.7
hypothalamus	C71.0	C79.31	—	D33.0	D43.0	D49.6
ileocecum, ileocecal (coil) (junction) (valve)	C18.0	C78.5	D01.0	D12.0	D37.4	D49.0
ileum	C17.2	C78.4	D01.49	D13.39	D37.2	D49.0
ilium	C41.4	C79.51	—	D16.8	D48.0	D49.2
immunoproliferative NEC	C88.9	—	—	—	—	—
infraclavicular (region)	C76.1	C79.89	D04.5	D36.7	D48.7	D49.89
inguinal (region)	C76.3	C79.89	D04.5	D36.7	D48.7	D49.89
insula	C71.0	C79.31	—	D33.0	D43.0	D49.6
insular tissue (pancreas)	C25.4	C78.89	D01.7	D13.7	D37.8	D49.0
brain	C71.0	C79.31	—	D33.0	D43.0	D49.6
interarytenoid fold	C13.1	C78.39	D00.08	D10.7	D37.05	D49.0
hypopharyngeal aspect	C13.1	C79.89	D00.08	D10.7	D37.05	D49.0
laryngeal aspect	C32.1	C78.39	D02.0	D14.1	D38.0	D49.1
marginal zone	C13.1	C79.89	D00.08	D10.7	D37.05	D49.0
interdental papillae	C03.9	C79.89	D00.03	D10.39	D37.09	D49.0

	Malignant Primary	Malignant Secondary	Ca in situ	Benign	Uncertain	Unspecified Behavior
Neoplasm, neoplastic — *continued*						
interdental papillae — *continued*						
lower	C03.1	C79.89	D00.03	D10.39	D37.09	D49.0
upper	C03.0	C79.89	D00.03	D10.39	D37.09	D49.0
internal						
capsule	C71.0	C79.31	—	D33.0	D43.0	D49.6
os (cervix)	C53.0	C79.82	D06.0	D26.0	D39.0	D49.5
intervertebral cartilage or disc	C41.2	C79.51	—	D16.6	D48.0	D49.2
intestine, intestinal	C26.0	C78.80	D01.40	D13.9	D37.8	D49.0
large	C18.9	C78.5	D01.0	D12.6	D37.4	D49.0
appendix	C18.1	C78.5	D01.0	D12.1	D37.3	D49.0
caput coli	C18.0	C78.5	D01.0	D12.0	D37.4	D49.0
cecum	C18.0	C78.5	D01.0	D12.0	D37.4	D49.0
colon	C18.9	C78.5	D01.0	D12.6	D37.4	D49.0
and rectum	C19	C78.5	D01.1	D12.7	D37.5	D49.0
ascending	C18.2	C78.5	D01.0	D12.2	D37.4	D49.0
caput	C18.0	C78.5	D01.0	D12.0	D37.4	D49.0
descending	C18.6	C78.5	D01.0	D12.4	D37.4	D49.0
distal	C18.6	C78.5	D01.0	D12.4	D37.4	D49.0
left	C18.6	C78.5	D01.0	D12.4	D37.4	D49.0
overlapping lesion	C18.8	—	—	—	—	—
pelvic	C18.7	C78.5	D01.0	D12.5	D37.4	D49.0
right	C18.2	C78.5	D01.0	D12.2	D37.4	D49.0
sigmoid (flexure)	C18.7	C78.5	D01.0	D12.5	D37.4	D49.0
transverse	C18.4	C78.5	D01.0	D12.3	D37.4	D49.0
hepatic flexure	C18.3	C78.5	D01.0	D12.3	D37.4	D49.0
ileocecum, ileocecal (coil) (valve)	C18.0	C78.5	D01.0	D12.0	D37.4	D49.0
overlapping lesion	C18.8	—	—	—	—	—
sigmoid flexure (lower) (upper)	C18.7	C78.5	D01.0	D12.5	D37.4	D49.0
splenic flexure	C18.5	C78.5	D01.0	D12.3	D37.4	D49.0
small	C17.9	C78.4	D01.40	D13.30	D37.2	D49.0
duodenum	C17.0	C78.4	D01.49	D13.2	D37.2	D49.0
ileum	C17.2	C78.4	D01.49	D13.39	D37.2	D49.0
jejunum	C17.1	C78.4	D01.49	D13.39	D37.2	D49.0
overlapping lesion	C17.8	—	—	—	—	—
tract NEC	C26.0	C78.89	D01.40	D13.9	D37.8	D49.0
intra-abdominal	C76.2	C79.89	D09.8	D36.7	D48.7	D49.89
intracranial NEC	C71.9	C79.31	—	D33.2	D43.2	D49.6
intrahepatic (bile) duct	C22.1	C78.7	D01.5	D13.4	D37.6	D49.0
intraocular	C69.9-☑	C79.49	D09.2-☑	D31.9-☑	D48.7	D49.89
intraorbital	C69.6-☑	C79.49	D09.2-☑	D31.6-☑	D48.7	D49.89
intrasellar	C75.1	C79.89	D09.3	D35.2	D44.3	D49.7
intrathoracic (cavity) (organs)	C76.1	C79.89	D09.8	D15.9	D48.7	D49.89
specified NEC	C76.1	C79.89	D09.8	D15.7	—	—
iris	C69.4-☑	C79.49	D09.2-☑	D31.4-☑	D48.7	D49.89
ischiorectal (fossa)	C76.3	C79.89	D09.8	D36.7	D48.7	D49.89
ischium	C41.4	C79.51	—	D16.8	D48.0	D49.2
island of Reil	C71.0	C79.31	—	D33.0	D43.0	D49.6
islands or islets of Langerhans	C25.4	C78.89	D01.7	D13.7	D37.8	D49.0
isthmus uteri	C54.0	C79.82	D07.0	D26.1	D39.0	D49.5
jaw	C76.0	C79.89	D09.8	D36.7	D48.7	D49.89
bone	C41.1	C79.51	—	D16.5	D48.0	D49.2
lower	C41.1	C79.51	—	D16.5	—	—
upper	C41.0	C79.51	—	D16.4	—	—
carcinoma (any type) (lower) (upper)	C76.0	C79.89	—	—	—	—
skin — *see also* Neoplasm, skin, face	C44.309	C79.2	D04.39	D23.39	D48.5	D49.2
soft tissues	C03.9	C79.89	D00.03	D10.39	D37.09	D49.0
lower	C03.1	C79.89	D00.03	D10.39	D37.09	D49.0
upper	C03.0	C79.89	D00.03	D10.39	D37.09	D49.0
jejunum	C17.1	C78.4	D01.49	D13.39	D37.2	D49.0
joint NEC — *see also* Neoplasm, bone	C41.9	C79.51	—	D16.9	D48.0	D49.2
acromioclavicular	C40.0-☑	C79.51	—	D16.0-☑	—	—

Neoplasm Table

Neoplasm, joint NEC — Neoplasm, lung

	Malignant Primary	Malignant Secondary	Ca in situ	Benign	Uncertain	Unspecified Behavior
Neoplasm, neoplastic — *continued*						
joint — *see also* Neoplasm, bone — *continued*						
bursa or synovial membrane — *see* Neoplasm, connective tissue						
costovertebral	C41.3	C79.51	—	D16.7	D48.0	D49.2
sternocostal	C41.3	C79.51	—	D16.7	D48.0	D49.2
temporomandibular	C41.1	C79.51	—	D16.5	D48.0	D49.2
junction						
anorectal	C21.8	C78.5	D01.3	D12.9	D37.8	D49.0
cardioesophageal	C16.0	C78.89	D00.2	D13.1	D37.1	D49.0
esophagogastric	C16.0	C78.89	D00.2	D13.1	D37.1	D49.0
gastroesophageal	C16.0	C78.89	D00.2	D13.1	D37.1	D49.0
hard and soft palate	C05.9	C79.89	D00.00	D10.39	D37.09	D49.0
ileocecal	C18.0	C78.5	D01.0	D12.0	D37.4	D49.0
pelvirectal	C19	C78.5	D01.1	D12.7	D37.5	D49.0
pelviureteric	C65.-☑	C79.0-☑	D09.19	D30.1-☑	D41.1-☑	D49.5
rectosigmoid	C19	C78.5	D01.1	D12.7	D37.5	D49.0
squamocolumnar, of cervix	C53.8	C79.82	D06.7	D26.0	D39.0	D49.5
Kaposi's sarcoma — *see* Kaposi's, sarcoma						
kidney (parenchymal)	C64.-☑	C79.0-☑	D09.19	D30.0-☑	D41.0-☑	D49.5
calyx	C65.-☑	C79.0-☑	D09.19	D30.1-☑	D41.1-☑	D49.5
hilus	C65.-☑	C79.0-☑	D09.19	D30.1-☑	D41.1-☑	D49.5
pelvis	C65.-☑	C79.0-☑	D09.19	D30.1-☑	D41.1-☑	D49.5
knee NEC	C76.5-☑	C79.89	D04.7-☑	D36.7	D48.7	D49.89
labia (skin)	C51.9	C79.82	D07.1	D28.0	D39.8	D49.5
majora	C51.0	C79.82	D07.1	D28.0	D39.8	D49.5
minora	C51.1	C79.82	D07.1	D28.0	D39.8	D49.5
labial — *see also* Neoplasm, lip	C00.9	C79.89	D00.01	D10.0	D37.01	D49.0
sulcus (lower) (upper)	C06.1	C79.89	D00.02	D10.39	D37.09	D49.0
labium (skin)	C51.9	C79.82	D07.1	D28.0	D39.8	D49.5
majus	C51.0	C79.82	D07.1	D28.0	D39.8	D49.5
minus	C51.1	C79.82	D07.1	D28.0	D39.8	D49.5
lacrimal						
canaliculi	C69.5-☑	C79.49	D09.2-☑	D31.5-☑	D48.7	D49.89
duct (nasal)	C69.5-☑	C79.49	D09.2-☑	D31.5-☑	D48.7	D49.89
gland	C69.5-☑	C79.49	D09.2-☑	D31.5-☑	D48.7	D49.89
punctum	C69.5-☑	C79.49	D09.2-☑	D31.5-☑	D48.7	D49.89
sac	C69.5-☑	C79.49	D09.2-☑	D31.5-☑	D48.7	D49.89
Langerhans, islands or islets	C25.4	C78.89	D01.7	D13.7	D37.8	D49.0
laryngopharynx	C13.9	C79.89	D00.08	D10.7	D37.05	D49.0
larynx, laryngeal NEC	C32.9	C78.39	D02.0	D14.1	D38.0	D49.1
aryepiglottic fold	C32.1	C78.39	D02.0	D14.1	D38.0	D49.1
cartilage (arytenoid) (cricoid) (cuneiform) (thyroid)	C32.3	C78.39	D02.0	D14.1	D38.0	D49.1
commissure (anterior) (posterior)	C32.0	C78.39	D02.0	D14.1	D38.0	D49.1
extrinsic NEC	C32.1	C78.39	D02.0	D14.1	D38.0	D49.1
meaning hypopharynx	C13.9	C79.89	D00.08	D10.7	D37.05	D49.0
interarytenoid fold	C32.1	C78.39	D02.0	D14.1	D38.0	D49.1
intrinsic	C32.0	C78.39	D02.0	D14.1	D38.0	D49.1
overlapping lesion	C32.8	—	—	—	—	—
ventricular band	C32.1	C78.39	D02.0	D14.1	D38.0	D49.1
leg NEC	C76.5-☑	C79.89	D04.7-☑	D36.7	D48.7	D49.89
lens, crystalline	C69.4-☑	C79.49	D09.2-☑	D31.4-☑	D48.7	D49.89
lid (lower) (upper)	C44.10-☑	C79.2	D04.1-☑	D23.1-☑	D48.5	D49.2
basal cell carcinoma	C44.11-☑	—	—	—	—	—
specified type NEC	C44.19-☑	—	—	—	—	—
squamous cell carcinoma	C44.12-☑	—	—	—	—	—
ligament — *see also* Neoplasm, connective tissue						

	Malignant Primary	Malignant Secondary	Ca in situ	Benign	Uncertain	Unspecified Behavior
Neoplasm, neoplastic — *continued*						
ligament — *see also* Neoplasm, connective tissue — *continued*						
broad	C57.1-☑	C79.82	D07.39	D28.2	D39.8	D49.5
Mackenrodt's	C57.7	C79.82	D07.39	D28.7	D39.8	D49.5
non-uterine — *see* Neoplasm, connective tissue						
round	C57.2-☑	C79.82	—	D28.2	D39.8	D49.5
sacro-uterine	C57.3	C79.82	—	D28.2	D39.8	D49.5
uterine	C57.3	C79.82	—	D28.2	D39.8	D49.5
utero-ovarian	C57.7	C79.82	D07.39	D28.2	D39.8	D49.5
uterosacral	C57.3	C79.82	—	D28.2	D39.8	D49.5
limb	C76.8	C79.89	D04.8	D36.7	D48.7	D49.89
lower	C76.5-☑	C79.89	D04.7-☑	D36.7	D48.7	D49.89
upper	C76.4-☑	C79.89	D04.6-☑	D36.7	D48.7	D49.89
limbus of cornea	C69.1-☑	C79.49	D09.2-☑	D31.1-☑	D48.7	D49.89
lingual NEC — *see also* Neoplasm, tongue	C02.9	C79.89	D00.07	D10.1	D37.02	D49.0
lingula, lung	C34.1-☑	C78.0-☑	D02.2-☑	D14.3-☑	D38.1	D49.1
lip	C00.9	C79.89	D00.01	D10.0	D37.01	D49.0
buccal aspect — *see* Neoplasm, lip, internal						
commissure	C00.6	C79.89	D00.01	D10.0	D37.01	D49.0
external	C00.2	C79.89	D00.01	D10.0	D37.01	D49.0
lower	C00.1	C79.89	D00.01	D10.0	D37.01	D49.0
upper	C00.0	C79.89	D00.01	D10.0	D37.01	D49.0
frenulum — *see* Neoplasm, lip, internal						
inner aspect — *see* Neoplasm, lip, internal						
internal	C00.5	C79.89	D00.01	D10.0	D37.01	D49.0
lower	C00.4	C79.89	D00.01	D10.0	D37.01	D49.0
upper	C00.3	C79.89	D00.01	D10.0	D37.01	D49.0
lipstick area	C00.2	C79.89	D00.01	D10.0	D37.01	D49.0
lower	C00.1	C79.89	D00.01	D10.0	D37.01	D49.0
upper	C00.0	C79.89	D00.01	D10.0	D37.01	D49.0
lower	C00.1	C79.89	D00.01	D10.0	D37.01	D49.0
internal	C00.4	C79.89	D00.01	D10.0	D37.01	D49.0
mucosa — *see* Neoplasm, lip, internal						
oral aspect — *see* Neoplasm, lip, internal						
overlapping lesion	C00.8	—	—	—	—	—
with oral cavity or pharynx	C14.8	—	—	—	—	—
skin (commissure) (lower) (upper)	C44.00	C79.2	D04.0	D23.0	D48.5	D49.2
basal cell carcinoma	C44.01	—	—	—	—	—
specified type NEC	C44.09	—	—	—	—	—
squamous cell carcinoma	C44.02	—	—	—	—	—
upper	C00.0	C79.89	D00.01	D10.0	D37.01	D49.0
internal	C00.3	C79.89	D00.01	D10.0	D37.01	D49.0
vermilion border	C00.2	C79.89	D00.01	D10.0	D37.01	D49.0
lower	C00.1	C79.89	D00.01	D10.0	D37.01	D49.0
upper	C00.0	C79.89	D00.01	D10.0	D37.01	D49.0
lipomatous — *see* Lipoma, by site						
liver — *see also* Index to disease, by histology	C22.9	C78.7	D01.5	D13.4	D37.6	D49.0
primary	C22.8	C78.7	D01.5	D13.4	D37.6	D49.0
lumbosacral plexus	C47.5	C79.89	—	D36.16	D48.2	D49.2
lung	C34.9-☑	C78.0-☑	D02.2-☑	D14.3-☑	D38.1	D49.1
azygos lobe	C34.1-☑	C78.0-☑	D02.2-☑	D14.3-☑	D38.1	D49.1
carina	C34.0-☑	C78.0-☑	D02.2-☑	D14.3-☑	D38.1	D49.1
hilus	C34.0-☑	C78.0-☑	D02.2-☑	D14.3-☑	D38.1	D49.1
lingula	C34.1-☑	C78.0-☑	D02.2-☑	D14.3-☑	D38.1	D49.1
lobe NEC	C34.9-☑	C78.0-☑	D02.2-☑	D14.3-☑	D38.1	D49.1
lower lobe	C34.3-☑	C78.0-☑	D02.2-☑	D14.3-☑	D38.1	D49.1

☑ **Additional Character Required** — Refer to the Tabular List for Character Selection   ▽ Subterms under main terms may continue to next column or page

Neoplasm, neoplastic — *continued*	Malignant Primary	Malignant Secondary	Ca in situ	Benign	Uncertain	Unspecified Behavior
lung — *continued*						
main bronchus	C34.0-☑	C78.0-☑	D02.2-☑	D14.3-☑	D38.1	D49.1
mesothelioma — *see* Mesothelioma						
middle lobe	C34.2	C78.0-☑	D02.21	D14.31	D38.1	D49.1
overlapping lesion	C34.8-☑	—	—	—	—	—
upper lobe	C34.1-☑	C78.0-☑	D02.2-☑	D14.3-☑	D38.1	D49.1
lymph, lymphatic channel						
NEC	C49.9	C79.89	—	D21.9	D48.1	D49.2
gland (secondary)	—	C77.9	—	D36.0	D48.7	D49.89
abdominal	—	C77.2	—	D36.0	D48.7	D49.89
aortic	—	C77.2	—	D36.0	D48.7	D49.89
arm	—	C77.3	—	D36.0	D48.7	D49.89
auricular (anterior) (posterior)	—	C77.0	—	D36.0	D48.7	D49.89
axilla, axillary	—	C77.3	—	D36.0	D48.7	D49.89
brachial	—	C77.3	—	D36.0	D48.7	D49.89
bronchial	—	C77.1	—	D36.0	D48.7	D49.89
bronchopulmonary	—	C77.1	—	D36.0	D48.7	D49.89
celiac	—	C77.2	—	D36.0	D48.7	D49.89
cervical	—	C77.0	—	D36.0	D48.7	D49.89
cervicofacial	—	C77.0	—	D36.0	D48.7	D49.89
Cloquet	—	C77.4	—	D36.0	D48.7	D49.89
colic	—	C77.2	—	D36.0	D48.7	D49.89
common duct	—	C77.2	—	D36.0	D48.7	D49.89
cubital	—	C77.3	—	D36.0	D48.7	D49.89
diaphragmatic	—	C77.1	—	D36.0	D48.7	D49.89
epigastric, inferior	—	C77.1	—	D36.0	D48.7	D49.89
epitrochlear	—	C77.3	—	D36.0	D48.7	D49.89
esophageal	—	C77.1	—	D36.0	D48.7	D49.89
face	—	C77.0	—	D36.0	D48.7	D49.89
femoral	—	C77.4	—	D36.0	D48.7	D49.89
gastric	—	C77.2	—	D36.0	D48.7	D49.89
groin	—	C77.4	—	D36.0	D48.7	D49.89
head	—	C77.0	—	D36.0	D48.7	D49.89
hepatic	—	C77.2	—	D36.0	D48.7	D49.89
hilar (pulmonary)	—	C77.1	—	D36.0	D48.7	D49.89
splenic	—	C77.2	—	D36.0	D48.7	D49.89
hypogastric	—	C77.5	—	D36.0	D48.7	D49.89
ileocolic	—	C77.2	—	D36.0	D48.7	D49.89
iliac	—	C77.5	—	D36.0	D48.7	D49.89
infraclavicular	—	C77.3	—	D36.0	D48.7	D49.89
inguina, inguinal	—	C77.4	—	D36.0	D48.7	D49.89
innominate	—	C77.1	—	D36.0	D48.7	D49.89
intercostal	—	C77.1	—	D36.0	D48.7	D49.89
intestinal	—	C77.2	—	D36.0	D48.7	D49.89
intrabdominal	—	C77.2	—	D36.0	D48.7	D49.89
intrapelvic	—	C77.5	—	D36.0	D48.7	D49.89
intrathoracic	—	C77.1	—	D36.0	D48.7	D49.89
jugular	—	C77.0	—	D36.0	D48.7	D49.89
leg	—	C77.4	—	D36.0	D48.7	D49.89
limb						
lower	—	C77.4	—	D36.0	D48.7	D49.89
upper	—	C77.3	—	D36.0	D48.7	D49.89
lower limb	—	C77.4	—	D36.0	D48.7	D49.89
lumbar	—	C77.2	—	D36.0	D48.7	D49.89
mandibular	—	C77.0	—	D36.0	D48.7	D49.89
mediastinal	—	C77.1	—	D36.0	D48.7	D49.89
mesenteric (inferior) (superior)	—	C77.2	—	D36.0	D48.7	D49.89
midcolic	—	C77.2	—	D36.0	D48.7	D49.89
multiple sites in categories C77.0-C77.5	—	C77.8	—	D36.0	D48.7	D49.89
neck	—	C77.0	—	D36.0	D48.7	D49.89
obturator	—	C77.5	—	D36.0	D48.7	D49.89
occipital	—	C77.0	—	D36.0	D48.7	D49.89
pancreatic	—	C77.2	—	D36.0	D48.7	D49.89
para-aortic	—	C77.2	—	D36.0	D48.7	D49.89
paracervical	—	C77.5	—	D36.0	D48.7	D49.89
parametrial	—	C77.5	—	D36.0	D48.7	D49.89
parasternal	—	C77.1	—	D36.0	D48.7	D49.89
parotid	—	C77.0	—	D36.0	D48.7	D49.89
pectoral	—	C77.3	—	D36.0	D48.7	D49.89
pelvic	—	C77.5	—	D36.0	D48.7	D49.89
peri-aortic	—	C77.2	—	D36.0	D48.7	D49.89
peripancreatic	—	C77.2	—	D36.0	D48.7	D49.89
popliteal	—	C77.1	—	D36.0	D48.7	D49.89
porta hepatis	—	C77.2	—	D36.0	D48.7	D49.89

Neoplasm, neoplastic — *continued*	Malignant Primary	Malignant Secondary	Ca in situ	Benign	Uncertain	Unspecified Behavior
lymph, lymphatic channel — *continued*						
gland — *continued*						
portal	—	C77.2	—	D36.0	D48.7	D49.89
preauricular	—	C77.0	—	D36.0	D48.7	D49.89
prelaryngeal	—	C77.0	—	D36.0	D48.7	D49.89
presymphysial	—	C77.5	—	D36.0	D48.7	D49.89
pretracheal	—	C77.0	—	D36.0	D48.7	D49.89
primary (any site) NEC	C96.9	—	—	—	—	—
pulmonary (hiler)	—	C77.1	—	D36.0	D48.7	D49.89
pyloric	—	C77.2	—	D36.0	D48.7	D49.89
retroperitoneal	—	C77.2	—	D36.0	D48.7	D49.89
retropharyngeal	—	C77.0	—	D36.0	D48.7	D49.89
Rosenmuller's	—	C77.4	—	D36.0	D48.7	D49.89
sacral	—	C77.5	—	D36.0	D48.7	D49.89
scalene	—	C77.0	—	D36.0	D48.7	D49.89
site NEC	—	C77.9	—	D36.0	D48.7	D49.89
splenic (hilar)	—	C77.2	—	D36.0	D48.7	D49.89
subclavicular	—	C77.3	—	D36.0	D48.7	D49.89
subinguinal	—	C77.4	—	D36.0	D48.7	D49.89
sublingual	—	C77.0	—	D36.0	D48.7	D49.89
submandibular	—	C77.0	—	D36.0	D48.7	D49.89
submaxillary	—	C77.0	—	D36.0	D48.7	D49.89
submental	—	C77.0	—	D36.0	D48.7	D49.89
subscapular	—	C77.3	—	D36.0	D48.7	D49.89
supraclavicular	—	C77.0	—	D36.0	D48.7	D49.89
thoracic	—	C77.1	—	D36.0	D48.7	D49.89
tibial	—	C77.4	—	D36.0	D48.7	D49.89
tracheal	—	C77.1	—	D36.0	D48.7	D49.89
tracheobronchial	—	C77.1	—	D36.0	D48.7	D49.89
upper limb	—	C77.3	—	D36.0	D48.7	D49.89
Virchow's	—	C77.0	—	D36.0	D48.7	D49.89
node — *see also* Neoplasm, lymph gland						
primary NEC	C96.9	—	—	—	—	—
vessel — *see also* Neoplasm, connective tissue	C49.9	C79.89	—	D21.9	D48.1	D49.2
Mackenrodt's ligament	C57.7	C79.82	D07.39	D28.7	D39.8	D49.5
malar	C41.0	C79.51	—	D16.4	D48.0	D49.2
region — *see* Neoplasm, cheek						
mammary gland — *see* Neoplasm, breast						
mandible	C41.1	C79.51	—	D16.5	D48.0	D49.2
alveolar						
mucosa (carcinoma)	C03.1	C79.89	D00.03	D10.39	D37.09	D49.0
ridge or process	C41.1	C79.51	—	D16.5	D48.0	D49.2
marrow (bone) NEC	C96.9	C79.52	—	—	D47.9	D49.89
mastectomy site (skin) — *see also* Neoplasm, breast, skin	C44.501	C79.2	—	—	—	D49.2
specified as breast tissue	C50.8-☑	C79.81	—	—	—	—
mastoid (air cells) (antrum) (cavity)	C30.1	C78.39	D02.3	D14.0	D38.5	D49.1
bone or process	C41.0	C79.51	—	D16.4	D48.0	D49.2
maxilla, maxillary (superior)	C41.0	C79.51	—	D16.4	D48.0	D49.2
alveolar						
mucosa	C03.0	C79.89	D00.03	D10.39	D37.09	D49.0
ridge or process (carcinoma)	C41.0	C79.51	—	D16.4	D48.0	D49.2
antrum	C31.0	C78.39	D02.3	D14.0	D38.5	D49.1
carcinoma	C03.0	C79.51	—	—	—	—
inferior — *see* Neoplasm, mandible						
sinus	C31.0	C78.39	D02.3	D14.0	D38.5	D49.1
meatus external (ear) — *see also* Neoplasm, skin, ear	C44.20-☑	C79.2	D04.2-☑	D23.2-☑	D48.5	D49.2
Meckel diverticulum, malignant	C17.3	C78.4	D01.49	D13.39	D37.2	D49.0

▽ Subterms under main terms may continue to next column or page　　　☑ Additional Character Required — Refer to the Tabular List for Character Selection

Neoplasm Table

	Malignant Primary	Malignant Secondary	Ca in situ	Benign	Uncertain	Unspecified Behavior
Neoplasm, neoplastic — *continued*						
mediastinum,						
mediastinal	C38.3	C78.1	—	D15.2	D38.3	D49.89
anterior	C38.1	C78.1	—	D15.2	D38.3	D49.89
posterior	C38.2	C78.1	—	D15.2	D38.3	D49.89
medulla						
adrenal	C74.1-☑	C79.7-☑	D09.3	D35.0-☑	D44.1-☑	D49.7
oblongata	C71.7	C79.31		D33.1	D43.1	D49.6
meibomian gland	C44.10-☑	C79.2	D04.1-☑	D23.1-☑	D48.5	D49.2
basal cell carcinoma	C44.11-☑	—	—	—	—	—
specified type NEC	C44.19-☑	—	—	—	—	—
squamous cell carcinoma	C44.12-☑	—	—	—	—	—
melanoma — *see* Melanoma						
meninges	C70.9	C79.49	—	D32.9	D42.9	D49.7
brain	C70.0	C79.32	—	D32.0	D42.0	D49.7
cerebral	C70.0	C79.32	—	D32.0	D42.0	D49.7
crainial	C70.0	C79.32	—	D32.0	D42.0	D49.7
intracranial	C70.0	C79.32	—	D32.0	D42.0	D49.7
spinal (cord)	C70.1	C79.49	—	D32.1	D42.1	D49.7
meniscus, knee joint (lateral) (medial)	C40.2-☑	C79.51	—	D16.2-☑	D48.0	D49.2
Merkel cell — *see* Carcinoma, Merkel cell						
mesentery, mesenteric	C48.1	C78.6	—	D20.1	D48.4	D49.0
mesoappendix	C48.1	C78.6	—	D20.1	D48.4	D49.0
mesocolon	C48.1	C78.6	—	D20.1	D48.4	D49.0
mesopharynx — *see* Neoplasm, oropharynx						
mesosalpinx	C57.1-☑	C79.82	D07.39	D28.2	D39.8	D49.5
mesothelial tissue — *see* Mesothelioma						
mesothelioma — *see* Mesothelioma						
mesovarium	C57.1-☑	C79.82	D07.39	D28.2	D39.8	D49.5
metacarpus (any bone)	C40.1-☑	C79.51	—	D16.1-☑	—	—
metastatic NEC — *see also* Neoplasm, by site, secondary	—	C79.9	—	—	—	—
metatarsus (any bone)	C40.3-☑	C79.51	—	D16.3-☑	—	—
midbrain	C71.7	C79.31	—	D33.1	D43.1	D49.6
milk duct — *see* Neoplasm, breast						
mons						
pubis	C51.9	C79.82	D07.1	D28.0	D39.8	D49.5
veneris	C51.9	C79.82	D07.1	D28.0	D39.8	D49.5
motor tract	C72.9	C79.49	—	D33.9	D43.9	D49.7
brain	C71.9	C79.31	—	D33.2	D43.2	D49.6
cauda equina	C72.1	C79.49	—	D33.4	D43.4	D49.7
spinal	C72.0	C79.49	—	D33.4	D43.4	D49.7
mouth	C06.9	C79.89	D00.00	D10.30	D37.09	D49.0
book-leaf	C06.89	C79.89	—	—	—	—
floor	C04.9	C79.89	D00.06	D10.2	D37.09	D49.0
anterior portion	C04.0	C79.89	D00.06	D10.2	D37.09	D49.0
lateral portion	C04.1	C79.89	D00.06	D10.2	D37.09	D49.0
overlapping lesion	C04.8	—	—	—	—	—
overlapping NEC	C06.80	—	—	—	—	—
roof	C05.9	C79.89	D00.00	D10.39	D37.09	D49.0
specified part NEC	C06.89	C79.89	D00.00	D10.39	D37.09	D49.0
vestibule	C06.1	C79.89	D00.00	D10.39	D37.09	D49.0
mucosa						
alveolar (ridge or process)	C03.9	C79.89	D00.03	D10.39	D37.09	D49.0
lower	C03.1	C79.89	D00.03	D10.39	D37.09	D49.0
upper	C03.0	C79.89	D00.03	D10.39	D37.09	D49.0
buccal	C06.0	C79.89	D00.02	D10.39	D37.09	D49.0
cheek	C06.0	C79.89	D00.02	D10.39	D37.09	D49.0
lip — *see* Neoplasm, lip, internal						
nasal	C30.0	C78.39	D02.3	D14.0	D38.5	D49.1
oral	C06.0	C79.89	D00.02	D10.39	D37.09	D49.0
Mullerian duct						
female	C57.7	C79.82	D07.39	D28.7	D39.8	D49.5
male	C63.7	C79.82	D07.69	D29.8	D40.8	D49.5
Neoplasm, neoplastic — *continued*						
muscle — *see also* Neoplasm, connective tissue						
extraocular	C69.6-☑	C79.49	D09.2-☑	D31.6-☑	D48.7	D49.89
myocardium	C38.0	C79.89	—	D15.1	D48.7	D49.89
myometrium	C54.2	C79.82	D07.0	D26.1	D39.0	D49.5
myopericardium	C38.0	C79.89	—	D15.1	D48.7	D49.89
nabothian gland (follicle)	C53.0	C79.82	D06.0	D26.0	D39.0	D49.5
nail — *see also* Neoplasm, skin, limb	C44.90	C79.2	D04.9	D23.9	D48.5	D49.2
finger — *see also* Neoplasm, skin, limb, upper	C44.60-☑	C79.2	D04.6-☑	D23.6-☑	D48.5	D49.2
toe — *see also* Neoplasm, skin, limb, lower	C44.70-☑	C79.2	D04.7-☑	D23.7-☑	D48.5	D49.2
nares, naris (anterior) (posterior)	C30.0	C78.39	D02.3	D14.0	D38.5	D49.1
nasal — *see* Neoplasm, nose						
nasolabial groove — *see also* Neoplasm, skin, face	C44.309	C79.2	D04.39	D23.39	D48.5	D49.2
nasolacrimal duct	C69.5-☑	C79.49	D09.2-☑	D31.5-☑	D48.7	D49.89
nasopharynx, nasopharyngeal	C11.9	C79.89	D00.08	D10.6	D37.05	D49.0
floor	C11.3	C79.89	D00.08	D10.6	D37.05	D49.0
overlapping lesion	C11.8	—	—	—	—	—
roof	C11.0	C79.89	D00.08	D10.6	D37.05	D49.0
wall	C11.9	C79.89	D00.08	D10.6	D37.05	D49.0
anterior	C11.3	C79.89	D00.08	D10.6	D37.05	D49.0
lateral	C11.2	C79.89	D00.08	D10.6	D37.05	D49.0
posterior	C11.1	C79.89	D00.08	D10.6	D37.05	D49.0
superior	C11.0	C79.89	D00.08	D10.6	D37.05	D49.0
nates — *see also* Neoplasm, skin, trunk	C44.509	C79.2	D04.5	D23.5	D48.5	D49.2
neck NEC	C76.0	C79.89	D09.8	D36.7	D48.7	D49.89
skin	C44.40	—	—	—	—	—
basal cell carcinoma	C44.41	—	—	—	—	—
specified type NEC	C44.49	—	—	—	—	—
squamous cell carcinoma	C44.42	—	—	—	—	—
nerve (ganglion)	C47.9	C79.89	—	D36.10	D48.2	D49.2
abducens	C72.59	C79.49	—	D33.3	D43.3	D49.7
accessory (spinal)	C72.59	C79.49	—	D33.3	D43.3	D49.7
acoustic	C72.4-☑	C79.49	—	D33.3	D43.3	D49.7
auditory	C72.4-☑	C79.49	—	D33.3	D43.3	D49.7
autonomic NEC — *see also* Neoplasm, nerve, peripheral	C47.9	C79.89	—	D36.10	D48.2	D49.2
brachial	C47.1-☑	C79.89	—	D36.12	D48.2	D49.2
cranial	C72.50	C79.49	—	D33.3	D43.3	D49.7
specified NEC	C72.59	C79.49	—	D33.3	D43.3	D49.7
facial	C72.59	C79.49	—	D33.3	D43.3	D49.7
femoral	C47.2-☑	C79.89	—	D36.13	D48.2	D49.2
ganglion NEC — *see also* Neoplasm, nerve, peripheral	C47.9	C79.89	—	D36.10	D48.2	D49.2
glossopharyngeal	C72.59	C79.49	—	D33.3	D43.3	D49.7
hypoglossal	C72.59	C79.49	—	D33.3	D43.3	D49.7
intercostal	C47.3	C79.89	—	D36.14	D48.2	D49.2
lumbar	C47.6	C79.89	—	D36.17	D48.2	D49.2
median	C47.1-☑	C79.89	—	D36.12	D48.2	D49.2
obturator	C47.2-☑	C79.89	—	D36.13	D48.2	D49.2
oculomotor	C72.59	C79.49	—	D33.3	D43.3	D49.7
olfactory	C72.2-☑	C79.49	—	D33.3	D43.3	D49.7
optic	C72.3-☑	C79.49	—	D33.3	D43.3	D49.7
parasympathetic NEC	C47.9	C79.89	—	D36.10	D48.2	D49.2
peripheral NEC	C47.9	C79.89	—	D36.10	D48.2	D49.2
abdomen	C47.4	C79.89	—	D36.15	D48.2	D49.2
abdominal wall	C47.4	C79.89	—	D36.15	D48.2	D49.2
ankle	C47.2-☑	C79.89	—	D36.13	D48.2	D49.2

☑ Additional Character Required — Refer to the Tabular List for Character Selection   Subterms under main terms may continue to next column or page

Neoplasm, neoplastic — continued
nerve — continued
  peripheral — continued

	Malignant Primary	Malignant Secondary	Ca in situ	Benign	Uncertain	Unspecified Behavior
antecubital fossa or space	C47.1-☑	C79.89	—	D36.12	D48.2	D49.2
arm	C47.1-☑	C79.89	—	D36.12	D48.2	D49.2
auricle (ear)	C47.0	C79.89	—	D36.11	D48.2	D49.2
axilla	C47.3	C79.89	—	D36.12	D48.2	D49.2
back	C47.6	C79.89	—	D36.17	D48.2	D49.2
buttock	C47.5	C79.89	—	D36.16	D48.2	D49.2
calf	C47.2-☑	C79.89	—	D36.13	D48.2	D49.2
cervical region	C47.0	C79.89	—	D36.11	D48.2	D49.2
cheek	C47.0	C79.89	—	D36.11	D48.2	D49.2
chest (wall)	C47.3	C79.89	—	D36.14	D48.2	D49.2
chin	C47.0	C79.89	—	D36.11	D48.2	D49.2
ear (external)	C47.0	C79.89	—	D36.11	D48.2	D49.2
elbow	C47.1-☑	C79.89	—	D36.12	D48.2	D49.2
extrarectal	C47.5	C79.89	—	D36.16	D48.2	D49.2
extremity	C47.9	C79.89	—	D36.10	D48.2	D49.2
lower	C47.2-☑	C79.89	—	D36.13	D48.2	D49.2
upper	C47.1-☑	C79.89	—	D36.12	D48.2	D49.2
eyelid	C47.0	C79.89	—	D36.11	D48.2	D49.2
face	C47.0	C79.89	—	D36.11	D48.2	D49.2
finger	C47.1-☑	C79.89	—	D36.12	D48.2	D49.2
flank	C47.6	C79.89	—	D36.17	D48.2	D49.2
foot	C47.2-☑	C79.89	—	D36.13	D48.2	D49.2
forearm	C47.1-☑	C79.89	—	D36.12	D48.2	D49.2
forehead	C47.0	C79.89	—	D36.11	D48.2	D49.2
gluteal region	C47.5	C79.89	—	D36.16	D48.2	D49.2
groin	C47.5	C79.89	—	D36.16	D48.2	D49.2
hand	C47.1-☑	C79.89	—	D36.12	D48.2	D49.2
head	C47.0	C79.89	—	D36.11	D48.2	D49.2
heel	C47.2-☑	C79.89	—	D36.13	D48.2	D49.2
hip	C47.2-☑	C79.89	—	D36.13	D48.2	D49.2
infraclavicular region	C47.3	C79.89	—	D36.14	D48.2	D49.2
inguinal (canal) (region)	C47.5	C79.89	—	D36.16	D48.2	D49.2
intrathoracic	C47.3	C79.89	—	D36.14	D48.2	D49.2
ischiorectal fossa	C47.5	C79.89	—	D36.16	D48.2	D49.2
knee	C47.2-☑	C79.89	—	D36.13	D48.2	D49.2
leg	C47.2-☑	C79.89	—	D36.13	D48.2	D49.2
limb NEC	C47.9	C79.89	—	D36.10	D48.2	D49.2
lower	C47.2-☑	C79.89	—	D36.13	D48.2	D49.2
upper	C47.1-☑	C79.89	—	D36.12	D48.2	D49.2
nates	C47.5	C79.89	—	D36.16	D48.2	D49.2
neck	C47.0	C79.89	—	D36.11	D48.2	D49.2
orbit	C69.6-☑	C79.49	—	D31.6-☑	D48.7	D49.2
pararectal	C47.5	C79.89	—	D36.16	D48.2	D49.2
paraurethral	C47.5	C79.89	—	D36.16	D48.2	D49.2
paravaginal	C47.5	C79.89	—	D36.16	D48.2	D49.2
pelvis (floor)	C47.5	C79.89	—	D36.16	D48.2	D49.2
pelvoabdominal	C47.8	C79.89	—	D36.17	D48.2	D49.2
perineum	C47.5	C79.89	—	D36.16	D48.2	D49.2
perirectal (tissue)	C47.5	C79.89	—	D36.16	D48.2	D49.2
periurethral (tissue)	C47.5	C79.89	—	D36.16	D48.2	D49.2
popliteal fossa or space	C47.2-☑	C79.89	—	D36.13	D48.2	D49.2
presacral	C47.5	C79.89	—	D36.16	D48.2	D49.2
pterygoid fossa	C47.0	C79.89	—	D36.11	D48.2	D49.2
rectovaginal septum or wall	C47.5	C79.89	—	D36.16	D48.2	D49.2
rectovesical	C47.5	C79.89	—	D36.16	D48.2	D49.2
sacrococcygeal region	C47.5	C79.89	—	D36.16	D48.2	D49.2
scalp	C47.0	C79.89	—	D36.11	D48.2	D49.2
scapular region	C47.3	C79.89	—	D36.14	D48.2	D49.2
shoulder	C47.1-☑	C79.89	—	D36.12	D48.2	D49.2
submental	C47.0	C79.89	—	D36.11	D48.2	D49.2
supraclavicular region	C47.0	C79.89	—	D36.11	D48.2	D49.2
temple	C47.0	C79.89	—	D36.11	D48.2	D49.2
temporal region	C47.0	C79.89	—	D36.11	D48.2	D49.2
thigh	C47.2-☑	C79.89	—	D36.13	D48.2	D49.2
thoracic (duct) (wall)	C47.3	C79.89	—	D36.14	D48.2	D49.2
thorax	C47.3	C79.89	—	D36.14	D48.2	D49.2
thumb	C47.1-☑	C79.89	—	D36.12	D48.2	D49.2

Neoplasm, neoplastic — continued
nerve — continued
  peripheral — continued

	Malignant Primary	Malignant Secondary	Ca in situ	Benign	Uncertain	Unspecified Behavior
toe	C47.2-☑	C79.89	—	D36.13	D48.2	D49.2
trunk	C47.6	C79.89	—	D36.17	D48.2	D49.2
umbilicus	C47.4	C79.89	—	D36.15	D48.2	D49.2
vesicorectal	C47.5	C79.89	—	D36.16	D48.2	D49.2
wrist	C47.1-☑	C79.89	—	D36.12	D48.2	D49.2
radial	C47.1-☑	C79.89	—	D36.12	D48.2	D49.2
sacral	C47.5	C79.89	—	D36.16	D48.2	D49.2
sciatic	C47.2-☑	C79.89	—	D36.13	D48.2	D49.2
spinal NEC	C47.9	C79.89	—	D36.10	D48.2	D49.2
accessory	C72.59	C79.49	—	D33.3	D43.3	D49.7
sympathetic NEC — see also Neoplasm, nerve, peripheral	C47.9	C79.89	—	D36.10	D48.2	D49.2
trigeminal	C72.59	C79.49	—	D33.3	D43.3	D49.7
trochlear	C72.59	C79.49	—	D33.3	D43.3	D49.7
ulnar	C47.1-☑	C79.89	—	D36.12	D48.2	D49.2
vagus	C72.59	C79.49	—	D33.3	D43.3	D49.7
nervous system (central)	C72.9	C79.40	—	D33.9	D43.9	D49.7
autonomic — see Neoplasm, nerve, peripheral						
parasympathetic — see Neoplasm, nerve, peripheral						
specified site NEC	—	C79.49	—	D33.7	D43.8	—
sympathetic — see Neoplasm, nerve, peripheral						
nevus — see Nevus						
nipple	C50.0-☑	C79.81	D05.-☑	D24.-☑	—	—
nose, nasal	C76.0	C79.89	D09.8	D36.7	D48.7	D49.89
ala (external) (nasi) — see also Neoplasm, nose, skin	C44.301	C79.2	D04.39	D23.39	D48.5	D49.2
bone	C41.0	C79.51	—	D16.4	D48.0	D49.2
cartilage	C30.0	C78.39	D02.3	D14.0	D38.5	D49.1
cavity	C30.0	C78.39	D02.3	D14.0	D38.5	D49.1
choana	C11.3	C79.89	D00.08	D10.6	D37.05	D49.0
external (skin) — see also Neoplasm, nose, skin	C44.301	C79.2	D04.39	D23.39	D48.5	D49.2
fossa	C30.0	C78.39	D02.3	D14.0	D38.5	D49.1
internal	C30.0	C78.39	D02.3	D14.0	D38.5	D49.1
mucosa	C30.0	C78.39	D02.3	D14.0	D38.5	D49.1
septum	C30.0	C78.39	D02.3	D14.0	D38.5	D49.1
posterior margin	C11.3	C79.89	D00.08	D10.6	D37.05	D49.0
sinus — see Neoplasm, sinus						
skin	C44.301	C79.2	D04.39	D23.39	D48.5	D49.2
basal cell carcinoma	C44.311	—	—	—	—	—
specified type NEC	C44.391	—	—	—	—	—
squamous cell carcinoma	C44.321	—	—	—	—	—
turbinate (mucosa)	C30.0	C78.39	D02.3	D14.0	D38.5	D49.1
bone	C41.0	C79.51	—	D16.4	D48.0	D49.2
vestibule	C30.0	C78.39	D02.3	D14.0	D38.5	D49.1
nostril	C30.0	C78.39	D02.3	D14.0	D38.5	D49.1
nucleus pulposus	C41.2	C79.51	—	D16.6	D48.0	D49.2
occipital						
bone	C41.0	C79.51	—	D16.4	D48.0	D49.2
lobe or pole, brain	C71.4	C79.31	—	D33.0	D43.0	D49.6
odontogenic — see Neoplasm, jaw bone						
olfactory nerve or bulb	C72.2-☑	C79.49	—	D33.3	D43.3	D49.7
olive (brain)	C71.7	C79.31	—	D33.1	D43.1	D49.6
omentum	C48.1	C78.6	—	D20.1	D48.4	D49.0
operculum (brain)	C71.0	C79.31	—	D33.0	D43.0	D49.6
optic nerve, chiasm, or tract	C72.3-☑	C79.49	—	D33.3	D43.3	D49.7
oral (cavity)	C06.9	C79.89	D00.00	D10.30	D37.09	D49.0
ill-defined	C14.8	C79.89	D00.00	D10.30	D37.09	D49.0
mucosa	C06.0	C79.89	D00.02	D10.39	D37.09	D49.0

	Malignant Primary	Malignant Secondary	Ca in situ	Benign	Uncertain	Unspecified Behavior
Neoplasm, neoplastic — *continued*						
orbit	C69.6-☑	C79.49	D09.2-☑	D31.6-☑	D48.7	D49.89
autonomic nerve	C69.6-☑	C79.49	—	D31.6-☑	D48.7	D49.2
bone	C41.0	C79.51	—	D16.4	D48.7	D49.2
eye	C69.6-☑	C79.49	D09.2-☑	D31.6-☑	D48.7	D49.89
peripheral nerves	C69.6-☑	C79.49	—	D31.6-☑	D48.7	D49.2
soft parts	C69.6-☑	C79.49	D09.2-☑	D31.6-☑	D48.7	D49.89
organ of Zuckerkandl	C75.5	C79.89	—	D35.6	D44.7	D49.7
oropharynx	C10.9	C79.89	D00.08	D10.5	D37.05	D49.0
branchial cleft (vestige)	C10.4	C79.89	D00.08	D10.5	D37.05	D49.0
junctional region	C10.8	C79.89	D00.08	D10.5	D37.05	D49.0
lateral wall	C10.2	C79.89	D00.08	D10.5	D37.05	D49.0
overlapping lesion	C10.8	—	—	—	—	—
pillars or fauces	C09.1	C79.89	D00.08	D10.5	D37.05	D49.0
posterior wall	C10.3	C79.89	D00.08	D10.5	D37.05	D49.0
vallecula	C10.0	C79.89	D00.08	D10.5	D37.05	D49.0
os						
external	C53.1	C79.82	D06.1	D26.0	D39.0	D49.5
internal	C53.0	C79.82	D06.0	D26.0	D39.0	D49.5
ovary	C56.-☑	C79.6-☑	D07.39	D27.-☑	D39.1-☑	D49.5
oviduct	C57.0-☑	C79.82	D07.39	D28.2	D39.8	D49.5
palate	C05.9	C79.89	D00.00	D10.39	D37.09	D49.0
hard	C05.0	C79.89	D00.05	D10.39	D37.09	D49.0
junction of hard and soft palate	C05.9	C79.89	D00.00	D10.39	D37.09	D49.0
overlapping lesions	C05.8	—	—	—	—	—
soft	C05.1	C79.89	D00.04	D10.39	D37.09	D49.0
nasopharyngeal surface	C11.3	C79.89	D00.08	D10.6	D37.05	D49.0
posterior surface	C11.3	C79.89	D00.08	D10.6	D37.05	D49.0
superior surface	C11.3	C79.89	D00.08	D10.6	D37.05	D49.0
palatoglossal arch	C09.1	C79.89	D00.00	D10.5	D37.09	D49.0
palatopharyngeal arch	C09.1	C79.89	D00.00	D10.5	D37.09	D49.0
pallium	C71.0	C79.31	—	D33.0	D43.0	D49.6
palpebra	C44.10-☑	C79.2	D04.1-☑	D23.1-☑	D48.5	D49.2
basal cell carcinoma	C44.11-☑	—	—	—	—	—
specified type NEC	C44.19-☑	—	—	—	—	—
squamous cell carcinoma	C44.12-☑	—	—	—	—	—
pancreas	C25.9	C78.89	D01.7	D13.6	D37.8	D49.0
body	C25.1	C78.89	D01.7	D13.6	D37.8	D49.0
duct (of Santorini) (of Wirsung)	C25.3	C78.89	D01.7	D13.6	D37.8	D49.0
ectopic tissue	C25.7	C78.89	—	D13.6	D37.8	D49.0
head	C25.0	C78.89	D01.7	D13.6	D37.8	D49.0
islet cells	C25.4	C78.89	D01.7	D13.7	D37.8	D49.0
neck	C25.7	C78.89	D01.7	D13.6	D37.8	D49.0
overlapping lesion	C25.8	—	—	—	—	—
tail	C25.2	C78.89	D01.7	D13.6	D37.8	D49.0
para-aortic body	C75.5	C79.89	—	D35.6	D44.7	D49.7
paraganglion NEC	C75.5	C79.89	—	D35.6	D44.7	D49.7
parametrium	C57.3	C79.82	—	D28.2	D39.8	D49.5
paranephric	C48.0	C78.6	—	D20.0	D48.3	D49.0
pararectal	C76.3	C79.89	—	D36.7	D48.7	D49.89
parasagittal (region)	C76.0	C79.89	D09.8	D36.7	D48.7	D49.89
parasellar	C72.9	C79.49	—	D33.9	D43.8	D49.7
parathyroid (gland)	C75.0	C79.89	D09.3	D35.1	D44.2	D49.7
paraurethral	C76.3	C79.89	—	D36.7	D48.7	D49.89
gland	C68.1	C79.19	D09.19	D30.8	D41.8	D49.5
paravaginal	C76.3	C79.89	—	D36.7	D48.7	D49.89
parenchyma, kidney	C64.-☑	C79.0-☑	D09.19	D30.0-☑	D41.0-☑	D49.5
parietal						
bone	C41.0	C79.51	—	D16.4	D48.0	D49.2
lobe, brain	C71.3	C79.31	—	D33.0	D43.0	D49.6
paroophoron	C57.1-☑	C79.82	D07.39	D28.2	D39.8	D49.5
parotid (duct) (gland)	C07	C79.89	D00.00	D11.0	D37.030	D49.0
parovarium	C57.1-☑	C79.82	D07.39	D28.2	D39.8	D49.5
patella	C40.20	C79.51	—	—	—	—
peduncle, cerebral	C71.7	C79.31	—	D33.1	D43.1	D49.6
pelvirectal junction	C19	C78.5	D01.1	D12.7	D37.5	D49.0
pelvis, pelvic	C76.3	C79.89	D09.8	D36.7	D48.7	D49.89
bone	C41.4	C79.51	—	D16.8	D48.0	D49.2
floor	C76.3	C79.89	D09.8	D36.7	D48.7	D49.89
renal	C65.-☑	C79.0-☑	D09.19	D30.1-☑	D41.1-☑	D49.5
viscera	C76.3	C79.89	D09.8	D36.7	D48.7	D49.89

	Malignant Primary	Malignant Secondary	Ca in situ	Benign	Uncertain	Unspecified Behavior
Neoplasm, neoplastic — *continued*						
pelvis, pelvic — *continued*						
wall	C76.3	C79.89	D09.8	D36.7	D48.7	D49.89
pelvo-abdominal	C76.8	C79.89	D09.8	D36.7	D48.7	D49.89
penis	C60.9	C79.82	D07.4	D29.0	D40.8	D49.5
body	C60.2	C79.82	D07.4	D29.0	D40.8	D49.5
corpus (cavernosum)	C60.2	C79.82	D07.4	D29.0	D40.8	D49.5
glans	C60.1	C79.82	D07.4	D29.0	D40.8	D49.5
overlapping sites	C60.8	—	—	—	—	—
skin NEC	C60.9	C79.82	D07.4	D29.0	D40.8	D49.5
periadrenal (tissue)	C48.0	C78.6	—	D20.0	D48.3	D49.0
perianal (skin) — *see also Neoplasm, anus, skin*	C44.500	C79.2	D04.5	D23.5	D48.5	D49.2
pericardium	C38.0	C79.89	—	D15.1	D48.7	D49.89
perinephric	C48.0	C78.6	—	D20.0	D48.3	D49.0
perineum	C76.3	C79.89	D09.8	D36.7	D48.7	D49.89
periodontal tissue NEC	C03.9	C79.89	D00.03	D10.39	D37.09	D49.0
periosteum — *see Neoplasm, bone*						
peripancreatic	C48.0	C78.6	—	D20.0	D48.3	D49.0
peripheral nerve NEC	C47.9	C79.89	—	D36.10	D48.2	D49.2
perirectal (tissue)	C76.3	C79.89	—	D36.7	D48.7	D49.89
perirenal (tissue)	C48.0	C78.6	—	D20.0	D48.3	D49.0
peritoneum, peritoneal (cavity)	C48.2	C78.6	—	D20.1	D48.4	D49.0
benign mesothelial tissue — *see Mesothelioma, benign*						
overlapping lesion with digestive organs	C48.8	—	—	—	—	—
	C26.9	—	—	—	—	—
parietal	C48.1	C78.6	—	D20.1	D48.4	D49.0
pelvic	C48.1	C78.6	—	D20.1	D48.4	D49.0
specified part NEC	C48.1	C78.6	—	D20.1	D48.4	D49.0
peritonsillar (tissue)	C76.0	C79.89	D09.8	D36.7	D48.7	D49.89
periurethral tissue	C76.3	C79.89	—	D36.7	D48.7	D49.89
phalanges						
foot	C40.3-☑	C79.51	—	D16.3-☑	—	—
hand	C40.1-☑	C79.51	—	D16.1-☑	—	—
pharynx, pharyngeal	C14.0	C79.89	D00.08	D10.9	D37.05	D49.0
bursa	C11.1	C79.89	D00.08	D10.6	D37.05	D49.0
fornix	C11.3	C79.89	D00.08	D10.6	D37.05	D49.0
recess	C11.2	C79.89	D00.08	D10.6	D37.05	D49.0
region	C14.0	C79.89	D00.08	D10.9	D37.05	D49.0
tonsil	C11.1	C79.89	D00.08	D10.6	D37.05	D49.0
wall (lateral) (posterior)	C14.0	C79.89	D00.08	D10.9	D37.05	D49.0
pia mater	C70.9	C79.40	—	D32.9	D42.9	D49.7
cerebral	C70.0	C79.32	—	D32.0	D42.0	D49.7
cranial	C70.0	C79.32	—	D32.0	D42.0	D49.7
spinal	C70.1	C79.49	—	D32.1	D42.1	D49.7
pillars of fauces	C09.1	C79.89	D00.08	D10.5	D37.05	D49.0
pineal (body) (gland)	C75.3	C79.89	D09.3	D35.4	D44.5	D49.7
pinna (ear) NEC — *see also Neoplasm, skin, ear*	C44.20-☑	C79.2	D04.2-☑	D23.2-☑	D48.5	D49.2
piriform fossa or sinus	C12	C79.89	D00.08	D10.7	D37.05	D49.0
pituitary (body) (fossa) (gland) (lobe)	C75.1	C79.89	D09.3	D35.2	D44.3	D49.7
placenta	C58	C79.82	D07.0	D26.7	D39.2	D49.5
pleura, pleural (cavity)	C38.4	C78.2	—	D19.0	D38.2	D49.1
overlapping lesion with heart or mediastinum	C38.8	—	—	—	—	—
parietal	C38.4	C78.2	—	D19.0	D38.2	D49.1
visceral	C38.4	C78.2	—	D19.0	D38.2	D49.1
plexus						
brachial	C47.1-☑	C79.89	—	D36.12	D48.2	D49.2
cervical	C47.0	C79.89	—	D36.11	D48.2	D49.2
choroid	C71.5	C79.31	—	D33.0	D43.0	D49.6
lumbosacral	C47.5	C79.89	—	D36.16	D48.2	D49.2
sacral	C47.5	C79.89	—	D36.16	D48.2	D49.2
pluriendocrine	C75.8	C79.89	D09.3	D35.7	D44.9	D49.7

☑ **Additional Character Required — Refer to the Tabular List for Character Selection**   ▽ **Subterms under main terms may continue to next column or page**

Neoplasm Table

Neoplasm, neoplastic — continued

	Malignant Primary	Malignant Secondary	Ca in situ	Benign	Uncertain	Unspecified Behavior
pole						
frontal	C71.1	C79.31	—	D33.0	D43.0	D49.6
occipital	C71.4	C79.31	—	D33.0	D43.0	D49.6
pons (varolii)	C71.7	C79.31	—	D33.1	D43.1	D49.6
popliteal fossa or space	C76.5-☑	C79.89	D04.7-☑	D36.7	D48.7	D49.89
postcricoid (region)	C13.0	C79.89	D00.08	D10.7	D37.05	D49.0
posterior fossa (cranial)	C71.9	C79.31	—	D33.2	D43.2	D49.6
postnasal space	C11.9	C79.89	D00.08	D10.6	D37.05	D49.0
prepuce	C60.0	C79.82	D07.4	D29.0	D40.8	D49.5
prepylorus	C16.4	C78.89	D00.2	D13.1	D37.1	D49.0
presacral (region)	C76.3	C79.89	—	D36.7	D48.7	D49.89
prostate (gland)	C61	C79.82	D07.5	D29.1	D40.0	D49.5
utricle	C68.0	C79.19	D09.19	D30.4	D41.3	D49.5
pterygoid fossa	C49.0	C79.89	—	D21.0	D48.1	D49.2
pubic bone	C41.4	C79.51	—	D16.8	D48.0	D49.2
pudenda, pudendum (female)	C51.9	C79.82	D07.1	D28.0	D39.8	D49.5
pulmonary — see also Neoplasm, lung	C34.9-☑	C78.0-☑	D02.2-☑	D14.3-☑	D38.1	D49.1
putamen	C71.0	C79.31	—	D33.0	D43.0	D49.6
pyloric						
antrum	C16.3	C78.89	D00.2	D13.1	D37.1	D49.0
canal	C16.4	C78.89	D00.2	D13.1	D37.1	D49.0
pylorus	C16.4	C78.89	D00.2	D13.1	D37.1	D49.0
pyramid (brain)	C71.7	C79.31	—	D33.1	D43.1	D49.6
pyriform fossa or sinus	C12	C79.89	D00.08	D10.7	D37.05	D49.0
radius (any part)	C40.0-☑	C79.51	—	D16.0-☑	—	—
Rathke's pouch	C75.1	C79.89	D09.3	D35.2	D44.3	D49.7
rectosigmoid (junction)	C19	C78.5	D01.1	D12.7	D37.5	D49.0
overlapping lesion with anus or rectum	C21.8	—	—	—	—	—
rectouterine pouch	C48.1	C78.6	—	D20.1	D48.4	D49.0
rectovaginal septum or wall	C76.3	C79.89	D09.8	D36.7	D48.7	D49.89
rectovesical septum	C76.3	C79.89	D09.8	D36.7	D48.7	D49.89
rectum (ampulla)	C20	C78.5	D01.2	D12.8	D37.5	D49.0
and colon	C19	C78.5	D01.1	D12.7	D37.5	D49.0
overlapping lesion with anus or rectosigmoid junction	C21.8	—	—	—	—	—
renal	C64.-☑	C79.0-☑	D09.19	D30.0-☑	D41.0-☑	D49.5
calyx	C65.-☑	C79.0-☑	D09.19	D30.1-☑	D41.1-☑	D49.5
hilus	C65.-☑	C79.0-☑	D09.19	D30.1-☑	D41.1-☑	D49.5
parenchyma	C64.-☑	C79.0-☑	D09.19	D30.0-☑	D41.0-☑	D49.5
pelvis	C65.-☑	C79.0-☑	D09.19	D30.1-☑	D41.1-☑	D49.5
respiratory						
organs or system NEC	C39.9	C78.30	D02.4	D14.4	D38.6	D49.1
tract NEC	C39.9	C78.30	D02.4	D14.4	D38.5	D49.1
upper	C39.0	C78.30	D02.4	D14.4	D38.5	D49.1
retina	C69.2-☑	C79.49	D09.2-☑	D31.2-☑	D48.7	D49.81
retrobulbar	C69.6-☑	C79.49	—	D31.6-☑	D48.7	D49.89
retrocecal	C48.0	C78.6	—	D20.0	D48.3	D49.0
retromolar (area) (triangle) (trigone)	C06.2	C79.89	D00.00	D10.39	D37.09	D49.0
retro-orbital	C76.0	C79.89	D09.8	D36.7	D48.7	D49.89
retroperitoneal (space) (tissue)	C48.0	C78.6	—	D20.0	D48.3	D49.0
retroperitoneum	C48.0	C78.6	—	D20.0	D48.3	D49.0
retropharyngeal	C14.0	C79.89	D00.08	D10.9	D37.05	D49.0
retrovesical (septum)	C76.3	C79.89	D09.8	D36.7	D48.7	D49.89
rhinencephalon	C71.0	C79.31	—	D33.0	D43.0	D49.6
rib	C41.3	C79.51	—	D16.7	D48.0	D49.2
Rosenmuller's fossa	C11.2	C79.89	D00.08	D10.6	D37.05	D49.0
round ligament	C57.2☑	C79.82	—	D28.2	D39.8	D49.5
sacrococcyx, sacrococcygeal	C41.4	C79.51	—	D16.8	D48.0	D49.2
region	C76.3	C79.89	D09.8	D36.7	D48.7	D49.89
sacrouterine ligament	C57.3	C79.82	—	D28.2	D39.8	D49.5
sacrum, sacral (vertebra)	C41.4	C79.51	—	D16.8	D48.0	D49.2

Neoplasm, neoplastic — continued

	Malignant Primary	Malignant Secondary	Ca in situ	Benign	Uncertain	Unspecified Behavior
salivary gland or duct (major)	C08.9	C79.89	D00.00	D11.9	D37.039	D49.0
minor NEC	C06.9	C79.89	D00.00	D10.39	D37.04	D49.0
overlapping lesion	C08.9	—	—	—	—	—
parotid	C07	C79.89	D00.00	D11.0	D37.030	D49.0
pluriglandular	C08.9	C79.89	D00.00	D11.9	D37.039	D49.0
sublingual	C08.1	C79.89	D00.00	D11.7	D37.031	D49.0
submandibular	C08.0	C79.89	D00.00	D11.7	D37.032	D49.0
submaxillary	C08.0	C79.89	D00.00	D11.7	D37.032	D49.0
salpinx (uterine)	C57.0-☑	C79.82	D07.39	D28.2	D39.8	D49.5
Santorini's duct	C25.3	C78.89	D01.7	D13.6	D37.8	D49.0
scalp	C44.40	C79.2	D04.4	D23.4	D48.5	D49.2
basal cell carcinoma	C44.41	—	—	—	—	—
specified type NEC	C44.49	—	—	—	—	—
squamous cell carcinoma	C44.42	—	—	—	—	—
scapula (any part)	C40.0-☑	C79.51	—	D16.0-☑	—	—
scapular region	C76.1	C79.89	D09.8	D36.7	D48.7	D49.89
scar NEC — see also Neoplasm, skin, by site	C44.90	C79.2	D04.9	D23.9	D48.5	D49.2
sciatic nerve	C47.2-☑	C79.89	—	D36.13	D48.2	D49.2
sclera	C69.4-☑	C79.49	D09.2-☑	D31.4-☑	D48.7	D49.89
scrotum (skin)	C63.2	C79.82	D07.61	D29.4	D40.8	D49.5
sebaceous gland — see Neoplasm, skin						
sella turcica	C75.1	C79.89	D09.3	D35.2	D44.3	D49.7
bone	C41.0	C79.51	—	D16.4	D48.0	D49.2
semilunar cartilage (knee)	C40.2-☑	C79.51	—	D16.2-☑	D48.0	D49.2
seminal vesicle	C63.7	C79.82	D07.69	D29.8	D40.8	D49.5
septum						
nasal	C30.0	C78.39	D02.3	D14.0	D38.5	D49.1
posterior margin	C11.3	C79.89	D00.08	D10.6	D37.05	D49.0
rectovaginal	C76.3	C79.89	D09.8	D36.7	D48.7	D49.89
rectovesical	C76.3	C79.89	D09.8	D36.7	D48.7	D49.89
urethrovaginal	C57.9	C79.82	D07.30	D28.9	D39.9	D49.5
vesicovaginal	C57.9	C79.82	D07.30	D28.9	D39.9	D49.5
shoulder NEC	C76.4-☑	C79.89	D04.6-☑	D36.7	D48.7	D49.89
sigmoid flexure (lower) (upper)	C18.7	C78.5	D01.0	D12.5	D37.4	D49.0
sinus (accessory)	C31.9	C78.39	D02.3	D14.0	D38.5	D49.1
bone (any)	C41.0	C79.51	—	D16.4	D48.0	D49.2
ethmoidal	C31.1	C78.39	D02.3	D14.0	D38.5	D49.1
frontal	C31.2	C78.39	D02.3	D14.0	D38.5	D49.1
maxillary	C31.0	C78.39	D02.3	D14.0	D38.5	D49.1
nasal, paranasal NEC	C31.9	C78.39	D02.3	D14.0	D38.5	D49.1
overlapping lesion	C31.8	—	—	—	—	—
pyriform	C12	C79.89	D00.08	D10.7	D37.05	D49.0
sphenoid	C31.3	C78.39	D02.3	D14.0	D38.5	D49.1
skeleton, skeletal NEC	C41.9	C79.51	—	D16.9	D48.0	D49.2
Skene's gland	C68.1	C79.19	D09.19	D30.8	D41.8	D49.5
skin NOS	C44.90	C79.2	D04.9	D23.9	D48.5	D49.2
abdominal wall	C44.509	C79.2	D04.5	D23.5	D48.5	D49.2
basal cell carcinoma	C44.519	—	—	—	—	—
specified type NEC	C44.599	—	—	—	—	—
squamous cell carcinoma	C44.529	—	—	—	—	—
ala nasi — see also Neoplasm, nose, skin	C44.301	C79.2	D04.39	D23.39	D48.5	D49.2
ankle — see also Neoplasm, skin, limb, lower	C44.70-☑	C79.2	D04.7-☑	D23.7-☑	D48.5	D49.2
antecubital space — see also Neoplasm, skin, limb, upper	C44.60-☑	C79.2	D04.6-☑	D23.6-☑	D48.5	D49.2
anus	C44.500	C79.2	D04.5	D23.5	D48.5	D49.2
basal cell carcinoma	C44.510	—	—	—	—	—
specified type NEC	C44.590	—	—	—	—	—
squamous cell carcinoma	C44.520	—				

Neoplasm Table

Neoplasm, neoplastic — continued
skin — continued

	Malignant Primary	Malignant Secondary	Ca in situ	Benign	Uncertain	Unspecified Behavior
arm — see also Neoplasm, skin, limb, upper	C44.60-✓	C79.2	D04.6-✓	D23.6-✓	D48.5	D49.2
auditory canal (external) — see also Neoplasm, skin, ear	C44.20-✓	C79.2	D04.2-✓	D23.2-✓	D48.5	D49.2
auricle (ear) — see also Neoplasm, skin, ear	C44.20-✓	C79.2	D04.2-✓	D23.2-✓	D48.5	D49.2
auricular canal (external) — see also Neoplasm, skin, ear	C44.20-✓	C79.2	D04.2-✓	D23.2-✓	D48.5	D49.2
axilla, axillary fold — see also Neoplasm, skin, trunk	C44.509	C79.2	D04.5	D23.5	D48.5	D49.2
back — see also Neoplasm, skin, trunk	C44.509	C79.2	D04.5	D23.5	D48.5	D49.2
basal cell carcinoma	C44.91	—	—	—	—	—
breast	C44.501	C79.2	D04.5	D23.5	D48.5	D49.2
basal cell carcinoma	C44.511	—	—	—	—	—
specified type NEC	C44.591	—	—	—	—	—
squamous cell carcinoma	C44.521	—	—	—	—	—
brow — see also Neoplasm, skin, face	C44.309	C79.2	D04.39	D23.39	D48.5	D49.2
buttock — see also Neoplasm, skin, trunk	C44.509	C79.2	D04.5	D23.5	D48.5	D49.2
calf — see also Neoplasm, skin, limb, lower	C44.70-✓	C79.2	D04.7-✓	D23.7-✓	D48.5	D49.2
canthus (eye) (inner) (outer)	C44.10-✓	C79.2	D04.1-✓	D23.1-✓	D48.5	D49.2
basal cell carcinoma	C44.11-✓	—	—	—	—	—
specified type NEC	C44.19-✓	—	—	—	—	—
squamous cell carcinoma	C44.12-✓	—	—	—	—	—
cervical region — see also Neoplasm, skin, neck	C44.40	C79.2	D04.4	D23.4	D48.5	D49.2
cheek (external) — see also Neoplasm, skin, face	C44.309	C79.2	D04.39	D23.39	D48.5	D49.2
chest (wall) — see also Neoplasm, skin, trunk	C44.509	C79.2	D04.5	D23.5	D48.5	D49.2
chin — see also Neoplasm, skin, face	C44.309	C79.2	D04.39	D23.39	D48.5	D49.2
clavicular area — see also Neoplasm, skin, trunk	C44.509	C79.2	D04.5	D23.5	D48.5	D49.2
clitoris	C51.2	C79.82	D07.1	D28.0	D39.8	D49.5
columnella — see also Neoplasm, skin, face	C44.309	C79.2	D04.39	D23.39	D48.5	D49.2
concha — see also Neoplasm, skin, ear	C44.20-✓	C79.2	D04.2-✓	D23.2-✓	D48.5	D49.2
ear (external)	C44.20-✓	C79.2	D04.2-✓	D23.2-✓	D48.5	D49.2
basal cell carcinoma	C44.21-✓	—	—	—	—	—
specified type NEC	C44.29-✓	—	—	—	—	—
squamous cell carcinoma	C44.22-✓	—	—	—	—	—
elbow — see also Neoplasm, skin, limb, upper	C44.60-✓	C79.2	D04.6-✓	D23.6-✓	D48.5	D49.2

Neoplasm, neoplastic — continued
skin — continued

	Malignant Primary	Malignant Secondary	Ca in situ	Benign	Uncertain	Unspecified Behavior
eyebrow — see also Neoplasm, skin, face	C44.309	C79.2	D04.39	D23.39	D48.5	D49.2
eyelid	C44.10-✓	C79.2	D04.1-✓	D23.1-✓	D48.5	D49.2
basal cell carcinoma	C44.11-✓	—	—	—	—	—
specified type NEC	C44.19-✓	—	—	—	—	—
squamous cell carcinoma	C44.12-✓	—	—	—	—	—
face NOS	C44.300	C79.2	D04.30	D23.30	D48.5	D49.2
basal cell carcinoma	C44.310	—	—	—	—	—
specified type NEC	C44.390	—	—	—	—	—
squamous cell carcinoma	C44.320	—	—	—	—	—
female genital organs (external)	C51.9	C79.82	D07.1	D28.0	D39.8	D49.5
clitoris	C51.2	C79.82	D07.1	D28.0	D39.8	D49.5
labium NEC	C51.9	C79.82	D07.1	D28.0	D39.8	D49.5
majus	C51.0	C79.82	D07.1	D28.0	D39.8	D49.5
minus	C51.1	C79.82	D07.1	D28.0	D39.8	D49.5
pudendum	C51.9	C79.82	D07.1	D28.0	D39.8	D49.5
vulva	C51.9	C79.82	D07.1	D28.0	D39.8	D49.5
finger — see also Neoplasm, skin, limb, upper	C44.60-✓	C79.2	D04.6-✓	D23.6-✓	D48.5	D49.2
flank — see also Neoplasm, skin, trunk	C44.509	C79.2	D04.5	D23.5	D48.5	D49.2
foot — see also Neoplasm, skin, limb, lower	C44.70-✓	C79.2	D04.7-✓	D23.7-✓	D48.5	D49.2
forearm — see also Neoplasm, skin, limb, upper	C44.60-✓	C79.2	D04.6-✓	D23.6-✓	D48.5	D49.2
forehead — see also Neoplasm, skin, face	C44.309	C79.2	D04.39	D23.39	D48.5	D49.2
glabella — see also Neoplasm, skin, face	C44.309	C79.2	D04.39	D23.39	D48.5	D49.2
gluteal region — see also Neoplasm, skin, trunk	C44.509	C79.2	D04.5	D23.5	D48.5	D49.2
groin — see also Neoplasm, skin, trunk	C44.509	C79.2	D04.5	D23.5	D48.5	D49.2
hand — see also Neoplasm, skin, limb, upper	C44.60-✓	C79.2	D04.6-✓	D23.6-✓	D48.5	D49.2
head NEC — see also Neoplasm, skin, scalp	C44.40	C79.2	D04.4	D23.4	D48.5	D49.2
heel — see also Neoplasm, skin, limb, lower	C44.70-✓	C79.2	D04.7-✓	D23.7-✓	D48.5	D49.2
helix — see also Neoplasm, skin, ear	C44.20-✓	C79.2	D04.2-✓	D23.2-✓	D48.5	D49.2
hip — see also Neoplasm, skin, limb, lower	C44.70-✓	C79.2	D04.7-✓	D23.7-✓	D48.5	D49.2
infraclavicular region — see also Neoplasm, skin, trunk	C44.509	C79.2	D04.5	D23.5	D48.5	D49.2
inguinal region — see also Neoplasm, skin, trunk	C44.509	C79.2	D04.5	D23.5	D48.5	D49.2
jaw — see also Neoplasm, skin, face	C44.309	C79.2	D04.39	D23.39	D48.5	D49.2
Kaposi's sarcoma — see Kaposi's, sarcoma, skin						
knee — see also Neoplasm, skin, limb, lower	C44.70-✓	C79.2	D04.7-✓	D23.7-✓	D48.5	D49.2

✓ Additional Character Required — Refer to the Tabular List for Character Selection   Subterms under main terms may continue to next column or page

Neoplasm, neoplastic — continued / skin — continued

	Malignant Primary	Malignant Secondary	Ca in situ	Benign	Uncertain	Unspecified Behavior
labia						
majora	C51.0	C79.82	D07.1	D28.0	D39.8	D49.5
minora	C51.1	C79.82	D07.1	D28.0	D39.8	D49.5
leg — see also Neoplasm, skin, limb, lower	C44.70-☑	C79.2	D04.7-☑	D23.7-☑	D48.5	D49.2
lid (lower) (upper)	C44.10-☑	C79.2	D04.1-☑	D23.1-☑	D48.5	D49.2
basal cell carcinoma	C44.11-☑	—	—	—	—	—
specified type NEC	C44.19-☑	—	—	—	—	—
squamous cell carcinoma	C44.12-☑	—	—	—	—	—
limb NEC	C44.90	C79.2	D04.9	D23.9	D48.5	D49.2
basal cell carcinoma	C44.91	—	—	—	—	—
lower	C44.70-☑	C79.2	D04.7-☑	D23.7-☑	D48.5	D49.2
basal cell carcinoma	C44.71-☑	—	—	—	—	—
specified type NEC	C44.79-☑	—	—	—	—	—
squamous cell carcinoma	C44.72-☑	—	—	—	—	—
upper	C44.60-☑	C79.2	D04.6-☑	D23.6-☑	D48.5	D49.2
basal cell carcinoma	C44.61-☑	—	—	—	—	—
specified type NEC	C44.69-☑	—	—	—	—	—
squamous cell carcinoma	C44.62-☑	—	—	—	—	—
lip (lower) (upper)	C44.00	C79.2	D04.0	D23.0	D48.5	D49.2
basal cell carcinoma	C44.01	—	—	—	—	—
specified type NEC	C44.09	—	—	—	—	—
squamous cell carcinoma	C44.02	—	—	—	—	—
male genital organs	C63.9	C79.82	D07.60	D29.9	D40.8	D49.5
penis	C60.9	C79.82	D07.4	D29.0	D40.8	D49.5
prepuce	C60.0	C79.82	D07.4	D29.0	D40.8	D49.5
scrotum	C63.2	C79.82	D07.61	D29.4	D40.8	D49.5
mastectomy site (skin) — see also Neoplasm, skin, breast	C44.501	C79.2				
specified as breast tissue	C50.8-☑	C79.81				
meatus, acoustic (external) — see also Neoplasm, skin, ear	C44.20-☑	C79.2	D04.2-☑	D23.2-☑	D48.5	D49.2
melanotic — see Melanoma						
Merkel cell — see Carcinoma, Merkel cell						
nates — see also Neoplasm, skin, trunk	C44.509	C79.2	D04.5	D23.5	D48.5	D49.2
neck	C44.40	C79.2	D04.4	D23.4	D48.5	D49.2
basal cell carcinoma	C44.41	—	—	—	—	—
specified type NEC	C44.49	—	—	—	—	—
squamous cell carcinoma	C44.42	—	—	—	—	—
nevus — see Nevus, skin						
nose (external) — see also Neoplasm, nose, skin	C44.301	C79.2	D04.39	D23.39	D48.5	D49.2
overlapping lesion	C44.80	—	—	—	—	—
basal cell carcinoma	C44.81	—	—	—	—	—
specified type NEC	C44.89	—	—	—	—	—
squamous cell carcinoma	C44.82	—	—	—	—	—

Neoplasm, neoplastic — continued / skin — continued

	Malignant Primary	Malignant Secondary	Ca in situ	Benign	Uncertain	Unspecified Behavior
palm — see also Neoplasm, skin, limb, upper	C44.60-☑	C79.2	D04.6-☑	D23.6-☑	D48.5	D49.2
palpebra	C44.10-☑	C79.2	D04.1-☑	D23.1-☑	D48.5	D49.2
basal cell carcinoma	C44.11-☑	—	—	—	—	—
specified type NEC	C44.19-☑	—	—	—	—	—
squamous cell carcinoma	C44.12-☑	—	—	—	—	—
penis NEC	C60.9	C79.82	D07.4	D29.0	D40.8	D49.5
perianal — see also Neoplasm, skin, anus	C44.500	C79.2	D04.5	D23.5	D48.5	D49.2
perineum — see also Neoplasm, skin, anus	C44.500	C79.2	D04.5	D23.5	D48.5	D49.2
pinna — see also Neoplasm, skin, ear	C44.20-☑	C79.2	D04.2-☑	D23.2-☑	D48.5	D49.2
plantar — see also Neoplasm, skin, limb, lower	C44.70-☑	C79.2	D04.7-☑	D23.7-☑	D48.5	D49.2
popliteal fossa or space — see also Neoplasm, skin, limb, lower	C44.70-☑	C79.2	D04.7-☑	D23.7-☑	D48.5	D49.2
prepuce	C60.0	C79.82	D07.4	D29.0	D40.8	D49.5
pubes — see also Neoplasm, skin, trunk	C44.509	C79.2	D04.5	D23.5	D48.5	D49.2
sacrococcygeal region — see also Neoplasm, skin, trunk	C44.509	C79.2	D04.5	D23.5	D48.5	D49.2
scalp	C44.40	C79.2	D04.4	D23.4	D48.5	D49.2
basal cell carcinoma	C44.41	—	—	—	—	—
specified type NEC	C44.49	—	—	—	—	—
squamous cell carcinoma	C44.42	—	—	—	—	—
scapular region — see also Neoplasm, skin, trunk	C44.509	C79.2	D04.5	D23.5	D48.5	D49.2
scrotum	C63.2	C79.82	D07.61	D29.4	D40.8	D49.5
shoulder — see also Neoplasm, skin, limb, upper	C44.60-☑	C79.2	D04.6-☑	D23.6-☑	D48.5	D49.2
sole (foot) — see also Neoplasm, skin, limb, lower	C44.70-☑	C79.2	D04.7-☑	D23.7-☑	D48.5	D49.2
specified sites NEC	C44.80	C79.2	D04.8	D23.9	D48.5	D49.2
basal cell carcinoma	C44.81	—	—	—	—	—
specified type NEC	C44.89	—	—	—	—	—
squamous cell carcinoma	C44.82	—	—	—	—	—
specified type NEC	C44.99	—	—	—	—	—
squamous cell carcinoma	C44.92	—	—	—	—	—
submammary fold — see also Neoplasm, skin, trunk	C44.509	C79.2	D04.5	D23.5	D48.5	D49.2
supraclavicular region — see also Neoplasm, skin, neck	C44.40	C79.2	D04.4	D23.4	D48.5	D49.2
temple — see also Neoplasm, skin, face	C44.309	C79.2	D04.39	D23.39	D48.5	D49.2
thigh — see also Neoplasm, skin, limb, lower	C44.70-☑	C79.2	D04.7-☑	D23.7-☑	D48.5	D49.2
thoracic wall — see also Neoplasm, skin, trunk	C44.509	C79.2	D04.5	D23.5	D48.5	D49.2

Neoplasm Table

Neoplasm, skin NOS — Neoplasm, skin NOS

Neoplasm Table

Neoplasm, skin NOS — Neoplasm, thyroglossal duct

Neoplasm, neoplastic —	Malignant Primary	Malignant Secondary	Ca in situ	Benign	Uncertain	Unspecified Behavior
continued						
skin — continued						
thumb — see also						
Neoplasm, skin, limb, upper	C44.60-✓	C79.2	D04.6-✓	D23.6-✓	D48.5	D49.2
toe — see also						
Neoplasm, skin, limb, lower	C44.70-✓	C79.2	D04.7-✓	D23.7-✓	D48.5	D49.2
tragus — see also						
Neoplasm, skin, ear	C44.20-✓	C79.2	D04.2-✓	D23.2-✓	D48.5	D49.2
trunk	C44.509	C79.2	D04.5	D23.5	D48.5	D49.2
basal cell carcinoma	C44.519	—	—	—	—	—
specified type NEC	C44.599	—	—	—	—	—
squamous cell carcinoma	C44.529	—	—	—	—	—
umbilicus — see also						
Neoplasm, skin, trunk	C44.509	C79.2	D04.5	D23.5	D48.5	D49.2
vulva	C51.9	C79.82	D07.1	D28.0	D39.8	D49.5
overlapping lesion	C51.8	—	—	—	—	—
wrist — see also						
Neoplasm, skin, limb, upper	C44.60-✓	C79.2	D04.6-✓	D23.6-✓	D48.5	D49.2
skull	C41.0	C79.51	—	D16.4	D48.0	D49.2
soft parts or tissues — see Neoplasm, connective tissue						
specified site NEC	C76.8	C79.89	D09.8	D36.7	D48.7	D49.89
spermatic cord	C63.1-✓	C79.82	D07.69	D29.8	D40.8	D49.5
sphenoid	C31.3	C78.39	D02.3	D14.0	D38.5	D49.1
bone	C41.0	C79.51	—	D16.4	D48.0	D49.2
sinus	C31.3	C78.39	D02.3	D14.0	D38.5	D49.1
sphincter						
anal	C21.1	C78.5	D01.3	D12.9	D37.8	D49.0
of Oddi	C24.0	C78.89	D01.5	D13.5	D37.6	D49.0
spine, spinal (column)	C41.2	C79.51	—	D16.6	D48.0	D49.2
bulb	C71.7	C79.31	—	D33.1	D43.1	D49.6
coccyx	C41.4	C79.51	—	D16.8	D48.0	D49.2
cord (cervical) (lumbar) (sacral) (thoracic)	C72.0	C79.49	—	D33.4	D43.4	D49.7
dura mater	C70.1	C79.49	—	D32.1	D42.1	D49.7
lumbosacral	C41.2	C79.51	—	D16.6	D48.0	D49.2
marrow NEC	C96.9	C79.52	—	—	D47.9	D49.89
membrane	C70.1	C79.49	—	D32.1	D42.1	D49.7
meninges	C70.1	C79.49	—	D32.1	D42.1	D49.7
nerve (root)	C47.9	C79.89	—	D36.10	D48.2	D49.2
pia mater	C70.1	C79.49	—	D32.1	D42.1	D49.7
root	C47.9	C79.89	—	D36.10	D48.2	D49.2
sacrum	C41.4	C79.51	—	D16.8	D48.0	D49.2
spleen, splenic NEC	C26.1	C78.89	D01.7	D13.9	D37.8	D49.0
flexure (colon)	C18.5	C78.5	D01.0	D12.3	D37.4	D49.0
stem, brain	C71.7	C79.31	—	D33.1	D43.1	D49.6
Stensen's duct	C07	C79.89	D00.00	D11.0	D37.030	D49.0
sternum	C41.3	C79.51	—	D16.7	D48.0	D49.2
stomach	C16.9	C78.89	D00.2	D13.1	D37.1	D49.0
antrum (pyloric)	C16.3	C78.89	D00.2	D13.1	D37.1	D49.0
body	C16.2	C78.89	D00.2	D13.1	D37.1	D49.0
cardia	C16.0	C78.89	D00.2	D13.1	D37.1	D49.0
cardiac orifice	C16.0	C78.89	D00.2	D13.1	D37.1	D49.0
corpus	C16.2	C78.89	D00.2	D13.1	D37.1	D49.0
fundus	C16.1	C78.89	D00.2	D13.1	D37.1	D49.0
greater curvature NEC	C16.6	C78.89	D00.2	D13.1	D37.1	D49.0
lesser curvature NEC	C16.5	C78.89	D00.2	D13.1	D37.1	D49.0
overlapping lesion	C16.8	—	—	—	—	—
prepylorus	C16.4	C78.89	D00.2	D13.1	D37.1	D49.0
pylorus	C16.4	C78.89	D00.2	D13.1	D37.1	D49.0
wall NEC	C16.9	C78.89	D00.2	D13.1	D37.1	D49.0
anterior NEC	C16.8	C78.89	D00.2	D13.1	D37.1	D49.0
posterior NEC	C16.8	C78.89	D00.2	D13.1	D37.1	D49.0
stroma, endometrial	C54.1	C79.82	D07.0	D26.1	D39.0	D49.5
stump, cervical	C53.8	C79.82	D06.7	D26.0	D39.0	D49.5

Neoplasm, neoplastic —	Malignant Primary	Malignant Secondary	Ca in situ	Benign	Uncertain	Unspecified Behavior
continued						
subcutaneous (nodule) (tissue) NEC — see Neoplasm, connective tissue						
subdural	C70.9	C79.32	—	D32.9	D42.9	D49.7
subglottis, subglottic	C32.2	C78.39	D02.0	D14.1	D38.0	D49.1
sublingual	C04.9	C79.89	D00.06	D10.2	D37.09	D49.0
gland or duct	C08.1	C79.89	D00.00	D11.7	D37.031	D49.0
submandibular gland	C08.0	C79.89	D00.00	D11.7	D37.032	D49.0
submaxillary gland or duct	C08.0	C79.89	D00.00	D11.7	D37.032	D49.0
submental	C76.0	C79.89	D09.8	D36.7	D48.7	D49.89
subpleural	C34.9-✓	C78.0-✓	D02.2-✓	D14.3-✓	D38.1	D49.1
substernal	C38.1	C78.1	—	D15.2	D38.3	D49.89
sudoriferous, sudoriparous gland, site unspecified	C44.90	C79.2	D04.9	D23.9	D48.5	D49.2
specified site — see Neoplasm, skin						
supraclavicular region	C76.0	C79.89	D09.8	D36.7	D48.7	D49.89
supraglottis	C32.1	C78.39	D02.0	D14.1	D38.0	D49.1
suprarenal	C74.9-✓	C79.7-✓	D09.3	D35.0-✓	D44.1-✓	D49.7
capsule	C74.9-✓	C79.7-✓	D09.3	D35.0-✓	D44.1-✓	D49.7
cortex	C74.0-✓	C79.7-✓	D09.3	D35.0-✓	D44.1-✓	D49.7
gland	C74.9-✓	C79.7-✓	D09.3	D35.0-✓	D44.1-✓	D49.7
medulla	C74.1-✓	C79.7-✓	D09.3	D35.0-✓	D44.1-✓	D49.7
suprasellar (region)	C71.9	C79.31	—	D33.2	D43.2	D49.6
supratentorial (brain) NEC	C71.0	C79.31	—	D33.0	D43.0	D49.6
sweat gland (apocrine) (eccrine), site unspecified	C44.90	C79.2	D04.9	D23.9	D48.5	D49.2
specified site — see Neoplasm, skin						
sympathetic nerve or nervous system NEC	C47.9	C79.89	—	D36.10	D48.2	D49.2
symphysis pubis	C41.4	C79.51	—	D16.8	D48.0	D49.2
synovial membrane — see Neoplasm, connective tissue						
tapetum, brain	C71.8	C79.31	—	D33.2	D43.2	D49.6
tarsus (any bone)	C40.3-✓	C79.51	—	D16.3-✓	—	—
temple (skin) — see also Neoplasm, skin, face	C44.309	C79.2	D04.39	D23.39	D48.5	D49.2
temporal						
bone	C41.0	C79.51	—	D16.4	D48.0	D49.2
lobe or pole	C71.2	C79.31	—	D33.0	D43.0	D49.6
region	C76.0	C79.89	D09.8	D36.7	D48.7	D49.89
skin — see also Neoplasm, skin, face	C44.309	C79.2	D04.39	D23.39	D48.5	D49.2
tendon (sheath) — see Neoplasm, connective tissue						
tentorium (cerebelli)	C70.0	C79.32	—	D32.0	D42.0	D49.7
testis, testes	C62.9-✓	C79.82	D07.69	D29.2-✓	D40.1-✓	D49.5
descended	C62.1-✓	C79.82	D07.69	D29.2-✓	D40.1-✓	D49.5
ectopic	C62.0-✓	C79.82	D07.69	D29.2-✓	D40.1-✓	D49.5
retained	C62.0-✓	C79.82	D07.69	D29.2-✓	D40.1-✓	D49.5
scrotal	C62.1-✓	C79.82	D07.69	D29.2-✓	D40.1-✓	D49.5
undescended	C62.0-✓	C79.82	D07.69	D29.2-✓	D40.1-✓	D49.5
unspecified whether descended or undescended	C62.9-✓	C79.82	D07.69	D29.2-✓	D40.1-✓	D49.5
thalamus	C71.0	C79.31	—	D33.0	D43.0	D49.6
thigh NEC	C76.5-✓	C79.89	D04.7-✓	D36.7	D48.7	D49.89
thorax, thoracic (cavity) (organs NEC)	C76.1	C79.89	D09.8	D36.7	D48.7	D49.89
duct	C49.3	C79.89	—	D21.3	D48.1	D49.2
wall NEC	C76.1	C79.89	D09.8	D36.7	D48.7	D49.89
throat	C14.0	C79.89	D00.08	D10.9	D37.05	D49.0
thumb NEC	C76.4-✓	C79.89	D04.6-✓	D36.7	D48.7	D49.89
thymus (gland)	C37	C79.89	D09.3	D15.0	D38.4	D49.89
thyroglossal duct	C73	C79.89	D09.3	D34	D44.0	D49.7

✓ Additional Character Required — Refer to the Tabular List for Character Selection ▽ Subterms under main terms may continue to next column or page

Neoplasm Table

Neoplasm, thyroid — Neoplasm, Wharton's duct

Neoplasm, neoplastic — continued	Malignant Primary	Malignant Secondary	Ca in situ	Benign	Uncertain	Unspecified Behavior
thyroid (gland)	C73	C79.89	D09.3	D34	D44.0	D49.7
cartilage	C32.3	C78.39	D02.0	D14.1	D38.0	D49.1
tibia (any part)	C40.2-☑	C79.51	—	D16.2-☑	—	—
toe NEC	C76.5-☑	C79.89	D04.7-☑	D36.7	D48.7	D49.89
tongue	C02.9	C79.89	D00.07	D10.1	D37.02	D49.0
anterior (two-thirds) NEC	C02.3	C79.89	D00.07	D10.1	D37.02	D49.0
dorsal surface	C02.0	C79.89	D00.07	D10.1	D37.02	D49.0
ventral surface	C02.2	C79.89	D00.07	D10.1	D37.02	D49.0
base (dorsal surface)	C01	C79.89	D00.07	D10.1	D37.02	D49.0
border (lateral)	C02.1	C79.89	D00.07	D10.1	D37.02	D49.0
dorsal surface NEC	C02.0	C79.89	D00.07	D10.1	D37.02	D49.0
fixed part NEC	C01	C79.89	D00.07	D10.1	D37.02	D49.0
foreamen cecum	C02.0	C79.89	D00.07	D10.1	D37.02	D49.0
frenulum linguae	C02.2	C79.89	D00.07	D10.1	D37.02	D49.0
junctional zone	C02.8	C79.89	D00.07	D10.1	D37.02	D49.0
margin (lateral)	C02.1	C79.89	D00.07	D10.1	D37.02	D49.0
midline NEC	C02.0	C79.89	D00.07	D10.1	D37.02	D49.0
mobile part NEC	C02.3	C79.89	D00.07	D10.1	D37.02	D49.0
overlapping lesion	C02.8	—	—	—	—	—
posterior (third)	C01	C79.89	D00.07	D10.1	D37.02	D49.0
root	C01	C79.89	D00.07	D10.1	D37.02	D49.0
surface (dorsal)	C02.0	C79.89	D00.07	D10.1	D37.02	D49.0
base	C01	C79.89	D00.07	D10.1	D37.02	D49.0
ventral	C02.2	C79.89	D00.07	D10.1	D37.02	D49.0
tip	C02.1	C79.89	D00.07	D10.1	D37.02	D49.0
tonsil	C02.4	C79.89	D00.07	D10.1	D37.02	D49.0
tonsil	C09.9	C79.89	D00.08	D10.4	D37.05	D49.0
fauces, faucial	C09.9	C79.89	D00.08	D10.4	D37.05	D49.0
lingual	C02.4	C79.89	D00.07	D10.1	D37.02	D49.0
overlapping sites	C09.8	—	—	—	—	—
palatine	C09.9	C79.89	D00.08	D10.4	D37.05	D49.0
pharyngeal	C11.1	C79.89	D00.08	D10.6	D37.05	D49.0
pillar (anterior) (posterior)	C09.1	C79.89	D00.08	D10.5	D37.05	D49.0
tonsillar fossa	C09.0	C79.89	D00.08	D10.5	D37.05	D49.0
tooth socket NEC	C03.9	C79.89	D00.03	D10.39	D37.09	D49.0
trachea (cartilage) (mucosa)	C33	C78.39	D02.1	D14.2	D38.1	D49.1
overlapping lesion with bronchus or lung	C34.8-☑	—	—	—	—	—
tracheobronchial	C34.8-☑	C78.39	D02.1	D14.2	D38.1	D49.1
overlapping lesion with lung	C34.8-☑	—	—	—	—	—
tragus — see also Neoplasm, skin, ear	C44.20-☑	C79.2	D04.2-☑	D23.2-☑	D48.5	D49.2
trunk NEC	C76.8	C79.89	D04.5	D36.7	D48.7	D49.89
tubo-ovarian	C57.8	C79.82	D07.39	D28.7	D39.8	D49.5
tunica vaginalis	C63.7	C79.82	D07.69	D29.8	D40.8	D49.5
turbinate (bone)	C41.0	C79.51	—	D16.4	D48.0	D49.2
nasal	C30.0	C78.39	D02.3	D14.0	D38.5	D49.1
tympanic cavity	C30.1	C78.39	D02.3	D14.0	D38.5	D49.1
ulna (any part)	C40.0-☑	C79.51	—	D16.0-☑	—	—
umbilicus, umbilical — see also Neoplasm, skin, trunk	C44.509	C79.2	D04.5	D23.5	D48.5	D49.2
uncus, brain	C71.2	C79.31	—	D33.0	D43.0	D49.6
unknown site or unspecified	C80.1	C79.9	D09.9	D36.9	D48.9	D49.9
urachus	C67.7	C79.11	D09.0	D30.3	D41.4	D49.4
ureter-bladder (junction)	C67.6	C79.11	D09.0	D30.3	D41.4	D49.4
ureter, ureteral	C66.-☑	C79.19	D09.19	D30.2-☑	D41.2-☑	D49.5
orifice (bladder)	C67.6	C79.11	D09.0	D30.3	D41.4	D49.4
urethra, urethral (gland)	C68.0	C79.19	D09.19	D30.4	D41.3	D49.5
orifice, internal	C67.5	C79.11	D09.0	D30.3	D41.4	D49.4
urethrovaginal (septum)	C57.9	C79.82	D07.30	D28.9	D39.8	D49.5
urinary organ or system	C68.9	C79.10	D09.10	D30.9	D41.9	D49.5
bladder — see Neoplasm, bladder						
overlapping lesion	C68.8	—	—	—	—	—
specified sites NEC	C68.8	C79.19	D09.19	D30.8	D41.8	D49.5
utero-ovarian	C57.8	C79.82	D07.39	D28.7	D39.8	D49.5
ligament	C57.1-☑	C79.82	D07.30	D28.2	D39.8	D49.5
uterosacral ligament	C57.3	C79.82	—	D28.2	D39.8	D49.5

Neoplasm, neoplastic — continued	Malignant Primary	Malignant Secondary	Ca in situ	Benign	Uncertain	Unspecified Behavior
uterus, uteri, uterine	C55	C79.82	D07.0	D26.9	D39.0	D49.5
adnexa NEC	C57.4	C79.82	D07.39	D28.7	D39.8	D49.5
body	C54.9	C79.82	D07.0	D26.1	D39.0	D49.5
cervix	C53.9	C79.82	D06.9	D26.0	D39.0	D49.5
cornu	C54.9	C79.82	D07.0	D26.1	D39.0	D49.5
corpus	C54.9	C79.82	D07.0	D26.1	D39.0	D49.5
endocervix (canal) (gland)	C53.0	C79.82	D06.0	D26.0	D39.0	D49.5
endometrium	C54.1	C79.82	D07.0	D26.1	D39.0	D49.5
exocervix	C53.1	C79.82	D06.1	D26.0	D39.0	D49.5
external os	C53.1	C79.82	D06.1	D26.0	D39.0	D49.5
fundus	C54.3	C79.82	D07.0	D26.1	D39.0	D49.5
internal os	C53.0	C79.82	D06.0	D26.0	D39.0	D49.5
isthmus	C54.0	C79.82	D07.0	D26.1	D39.0	D49.5
ligament	C57.3	C79.82	—	D28.2	D39.8	D49.5
broad	C57.1-☑	C79.82	D07.39	D28.2	D39.8	D49.5
round	C57.2-☑	C79.82	—	D28.2	D39.8	D49.5
lower segment	C54.0	C79.82	D07.0	D26.1	D39.0	D49.5
myometrium	C54.2	C79.82	D07.0	D26.1	D39.0	D49.5
overlapping sites	C54.8	—	—	—	—	—
squamocolumnar junction	C53.8	C79.82	D06.7	D26.0	D39.0	D49.5
tube	C57.0-☑	C79.82	D07.39	D28.2	D39.8	D49.5
utricle, prostatic	C68.0	C79.19	D09.19	D30.4	D41.3	D49.5
uveal tract	C69.4-☑	C79.49	D09.2-☑	D31.4-☑	D48.7	D49.89
uvula	C05.2	C79.89	D00.04	D10.39	D37.09	D49.0
vagina, vaginal (fornix) (vault) (wall)	C52	C79.82	D07.2	D28.1	D39.8	D49.5
vaginovesical	C57.9	C79.82	D07.30	D28.9	D39.9	D49.5
septum	C57.9	C79.82	D07.30	D28.9	D39.9	D49.5
vallecula (epiglottis)	C10.0	C79.89	D00.08	D10.5	D37.05	D49.0
vascular — see Neoplasm, connective tissue						
vas deferens	C63.1-☑	C79.82	D07.69	D29.8	D40.8	D49.5
Vater's ampulla	C24.1	C78.89	D01.5	D13.5	D37.6	D49.0
vein, venous — see Neoplasm, connective tissue						
vena cava (abdominal) (inferior)	C49.4	C79.89	—	D21.4	D48.1	D49.2
superior	C49.3	C79.89	—	D21.3	D48.1	D49.2
ventricle (cerebral) (floor) (lateral) (third)	C71.5	C79.31	—	D33.0	D43.0	D49.6
cardiac (left) (right)	C38.0	C79.89	—	D15.1	D48.7	D49.89
fourth	C71.7	C79.31	—	D33.1	D43.1	D49.6
ventricular band of larynx	C32.1	C78.39	D02.0	D14.1	D38.0	D49.1
ventriculus — see Neoplasm, stomach						
vermillion border — see Neoplasm, lip						
vermis, cerebellum	C71.6	C79.31	—	D33.1	D43.1	D49.6
vertebra (column)	C41.2	C79.51	—	D16.6	D48.0	D49.2
coccyx	C41.4	C79.51	—	D16.8	D48.0	D49.2
marrow NEC	C96.9	C79.52	—	—	D47.9	D49.89
sacrum	C41.4	C79.51	—	D16.8	D48.0	D49.2
vesical — see Neoplasm, bladder						
vesicle, seminal	C63.7	C79.82	D07.69	D29.8	D40.8	D49.5
vesicocervical tissue	C57.9	C79.82	D07.30	D28.9	D39.9	D49.5
vesicorectal	C76.3	C79.82	D09.8	D36.7	D48.7	D49.89
vesicovaginal	C57.9	C79.82	D07.30	D28.9	D39.8	D49.5
septum	C57.9	C79.82	D07.30	D28.9	D39.8	D49.5
vessel (blood) — see Neoplasm, connective tissue						
vestibular gland, greater	C51.0	C79.82	D07.1	D28.0	D39.8	D49.5
vestibule						
mouth	C06.1	C79.89	D00.00	D10.39	D37.09	D49.0
nose	C30.0	C78.39	D02.3	D14.0	D38.5	D49.1
Virchow's gland	C77.0	C77.0	—	D36.0	D48.7	D49.89
viscera NEC	C76.8	C79.89	D09.8	D36.7	D48.7	D49.89
vocal cords (true)	C32.0	C78.39	D02.0	D14.1	D38.0	D49.1
false	C32.1	C78.39	D02.0	D14.1	D38.0	D49.1
vomer	C41.0	C79.51	—	D16.4	D48.0	D49.2
vulva	C51.9	C79.82	D07.1	D28	D39.8	D49.5
vulvovaginal gland	C51.0	C79.82	D07.1	D28.0	D39.8	D49.5
Waldeyer's ring	C14.2	C79.89	D00.08	D10.9	D37.05	D49.0
Wharton's duct	C08.0	C79.89	D00.00	D11.7	D37.032	D49.0

Neoplasm Table

Neoplasm, neoplastic —	Malignant Primary	Malignant Secondary	Ca in situ	Benign	Uncertain	Unspecified Behavior
continued						
white matter (central)						
(cerebral)	C71.0	C79.31	—	D33.0	D43.0	D49.6
windpipe	C33	C78.39	D02.1	D14.2	D38.1	D49.1
Wirsung's duct	C25.3	C78.89	D01.7	D13.6	D37.8	D49.0
wolffian (body) (duct)						
female	C57.7	C79.82	D07.39	D28.7	D39.8	D49.5
male	C63.7	C79.82	D07.69	D29.8	D40.8	D49.5
womb — *see* Neoplasm, uterus						
wrist NEC	C76.4-☑	C79.89	D04.6-☑	D36.7	D48.7	D49.89
xiphoid process	C41.3	C79.51	—	D16.7	D48.0	D49.2
Zuckerkandl organ	C75.5	C79.89	—	D35.6	D44.7	D49.7

☑ Additional Character Required — Refer to the Tabular List for Character Selection   ▽ Subterms under main terms may continue to next column or page

ICD-10-CM Table of Drugs and Chemicals

Substance	Poisoning, Accidental (unintentional)	Poisoning, Intentional Self-harm	Poisoning, Assault	Poisoning, Undetermined	Adverse Effect	Under-dosing
14-Hydroxydihydromorphinone	T40.2X1	T40.2X2	T40.2X3	T40.2X4	T40.2X5	T40.2X6
1-Propanol	T51.3X1	T51.3X2	T51.3X3	T51.3X4	—	—
2,3,7,8-Tetrachlorodibenzo-p-dioxin	T53.7X1	T53.7X2	T53.7X3	T53.7X4	—	—
2,4,5-T (trichlorophenoxyacetic acid)	T60.1X1	T60.1X2	T60.1X3	T60.1X4	—	—
2,4,5-Trichlorophenoxyacetic acid	T60.3X1	T60.3X2	T60.3X3	T60.3X4	—	—
2,4-D (dichlorophenoxyacetic acid)	T60.3X1	T60.3X2	T60.3X3	T60.3X4	—	—
2,4-Toluene diisocyanate	T65.0X1	T65.0X2	T65.0X3	T65.0X4	—	—
2-Deoxy-5-fluorouridine	T45.1X1	T45.1X2	T45.1X3	T45.1X4	T45.1X5	T45.1X6
2-Ethoxyethanol	T52.3X1	T52.3X2	T52.3X3	T52.3X4	—	—
2-Methoxyethanol	T52.3X1	T52.3X2	T52.3X3	T52.3X4	—	—
2-Propanol	T51.2X1	T51.2X2	T51.2X3	T51.2X4	—	—
4-Aminobutyric acid	T43.8X1	T43.8X2	T43.8X3	T43.8X4	T43.8X5	T43.8X6
4-Aminophenol derivatives	T39.1X1	T39.1X2	T39.1X3	T39.1X4	T39.1X5	T39.1X6
5-Deoxy-5-fluorouridine	T45.1X1	T45.1X2	T45.1X3	T45.1X4	T45.1X5	T45.1X6
5-Methoxypsoralen (5-MOP)	T50.991	T50.992	T50.993	T50.994	T50.995	T50.996
8-Aminoquinoline drugs	T37.2X1	T37.2X2	T37.2X3	T37.2X4	T37.2X5	T37.2X6
8-Methoxypsoralen (8-MOP)	T50.991	T50.992	T50.993	T50.994	T50.995	T50.996
ABOB	T37.5X1	T37.5X2	T37.5X3	T37.5X4	T37.5X5	T37.5X6
Abrine	T62.2X1	T62.2X2	T62.2X3	T62.2X4	—	—
Abrus (seed)	T62.2X1	T62.2X2	T62.2X3	T62.2X4	—	—
Absinthe	T51.0X1	T51.0X2	T51.0X3	T51.0X4	—	—
beverage	T51.0X1	T51.0X2	T51.0X3	T51.0X4	—	—
Acaricide	T60.8X1	T60.8X2	T60.8X3	T60.8X4	—	—
Acebutolol	T44.7X1	T44.7X2	T44.7X3	T44.7X4	T44.7X5	T44.7X6
Acecarbromal	T42.6X1	T42.6X2	T42.6X3	T42.6X4	T42.6X5	T42.6X6
Aceclidine	T44.1X1	T44.1X2	T44.1X3	T44.1X4	T44.1X5	T44.1X6
Acedapsone	T37.0X1	T37.0X2	T37.0X3	T37.0X4	T37.0X5	T37.0X6
Acefylline piperazine	T48.6X1	T48.6X2	T48.6X3	T48.6X4	T48.6X5	T48.6X6
Acemorphan	T40.2X1	T40.2X2	T40.2X3	T40.2X4	T40.2X5	T40.2X6
Acenocoumarin	T45.511	T45.512	T45.513	T45.514	T45.515	T45.516
Acenocoumarol	T45.511	T45.512	T45.513	T45.514	T45.515	T45.516
Acepifylline	T48.6X1	T48.6X2	T48.6X3	T48.6X4	T48.6X5	T48.6X6
Acepromazine	T43.3X1	T43.3X2	T43.3X3	T43.3X4	T43.3X5	T43.3X6
Acesulfamethoxypyridazine	T37.0X1	T37.0X2	T37.0X3	T37.0X4	T37.0X5	T37.0X6
Acetal	T52.8X1	T52.8X2	T52.8X3	T52.8X4	—	—
Acetaldehyde (vapor)	T52.8X1	T52.8X2	T52.8X3	T52.8X4	—	—
liquid	T65.891	T65.892	T65.893	T65.894	—	—
Acetaminophen	T39.1X1	T39.1X2	T39.1X3	T39.1X4	T39.1X5	T39.1X6
Acetaminosalol	T39.1X1	T39.1X2	T39.1X3	T39.1X4	T39.1X5	T39.1X6
Acetanilide	T39.1X1	T39.1X2	T39.1X3	T39.1X4	T39.1X5	T39.1X6
Acetarsol	T37.3X1	T37.3X2	T37.3X3	T37.3X4	T37.3X5	T37.3X6
Acetazolamide	T50.2X1	T50.2X2	T50.2X3	T50.2X4	T50.2X5	T50.2X6
Acetiamine	T45.2X1	T45.2X2	T45.2X3	T45.2X4	T45.2X5	T45.2X6
Acetic						
acid	T54.2X1	T54.2X2	T54.2X3	T54.2X4	—	—
with sodium acetate (ointment)	T49.3X1	T49.3X2	T49.3X3	T49.3X4	T49.3X5	T49.3X6
ester (solvent)(vapor)	T52.8X1	T52.8X2	T52.8X3	T52.8X4	—	—
irrigating solution	T50.3X1	T50.3X2	T50.3X3	T50.3X4	T50.3X5	T50.3X6
medicinal (lotion)	T49.2X1	T49.2X2	T49.2X3	T49.2X4	T49.2X5	T49.2X6
anhydride	T65.891	T65.892	T65.893	T65.894	—	—
ether (vapor)	T52.8X1	T52.8X2	T52.8X3	T52.8X4	—	—
Acetohexamide	T38.3X1	T38.3X2	T38.3X3	T38.3X4	T38.3X5	T38.3X6
Acetohydroxamic acid	T50.991	T50.992	T50.993	T50.994	T50.995	T50.996
Acetomenaphthone	T45.7X1	T45.7X2	T45.7X3	T45.7X4	T45.7X5	T45.7X6
Acetomorphine	T40.1X1	T40.1X2	T40.1X3	T40.1X4	—	—
Acetone (oils)	T52.4X1	T52.4X2	T52.4X3	T52.4X4	—	—
chlorinated	T52.4X1	T52.4X2	T52.4X3	T52.4X4	—	—
vapor	T52.4X1	T52.4X2	T52.4X3	T52.4X4	—	—
Acetonitrile	T52.8X1	T52.8X2	T52.8X3	T52.8X4	—	—
Acetophenazine	T43.3X1	T43.3X2	T43.3X3	T43.3X4	T43.3X5	T43.3X6
Acetophenetedin	T39.1X1	T39.1X2	T39.1X3	T39.1X4	T39.1X5	T39.1X6
Acetophenone	T52.4X1	T52.4X2	T52.4X3	T52.4X4	—	—
Acetorphine	T40.2X1	T40.2X2	T40.2X3	T40.2X4	—	—
Acetosulfone (sodium)	T37.1X1	T37.1X2	T37.1X3	T37.1X4	T37.1X5	T37.1X6
Acetrizoate (sodium)	T50.8X1	T50.8X2	T50.8X3	T50.8X4	T50.8X5	T50.8X6
Acetrizoic acid	T50.8X1	T50.8X2	T50.8X3	T50.8X4	T50.8X5	T50.8X6
Acetyl						
bromide	T53.6X1	T53.6X2	T53.6X3	T53.6X4	—	—
chloride	T53.6X1	T53.6X2	T53.6X3	T53.6X4	—	—
Acetylcarbromal	T42.6X1	T42.6X2	T42.6X3	T42.6X4	T42.6X5	T42.6X6
Acetylcholine						
chloride	T44.1X1	T44.1X2	T44.1X3	T44.1X4	T44.1X5	T44.1X6
derivative	T44.1X1	T44.1X2	T44.1X3	T44.1X4	T44.1X5	T44.1X6
Acetylcysteine	T48.4X1	T48.4X2	T48.4X3	T48.4X4	T48.4X5	T48.4X6
Acetyldigitoxin	T46.0X1	T46.0X2	T46.0X3	T46.0X4	T46.0X5	T46.0X6
Acetyldigoxin	T46.0X1	T46.0X2	T46.0X3	T46.0X4	T46.0X5	T46.0X6
Acetyldihydrocodeine	T40.2X1	T40.2X2	T40.2X3	T40.2X4	—	—
Acetyldihydrocodeinone	T40.2X1	T40.2X2	T40.2X3	T40.2X4	—	—
Acetylene (gas)	T59.891	T59.892	T59.893	T59.894	—	—
dichloride	T53.6X1	T53.6X2	T53.6X3	T53.6X4	—	—
incomplete combustion of	T58.11	T58.12	T58.13	T58.14	—	—
industrial	T59.891	T59.892	T59.893	T59.894	—	—
tetrachloride	T53.6X1	T53.6X2	T53.6X3	T53.6X4	—	—
vapor	T53.6X1	T53.6X2	T53.6X3	T53.6X4	—	—
Acetylpheneturide	T42.6X1	T42.6X2	T42.6X3	T42.6X4	T42.6X5	T42.6X6
Acetylphenylhydrazine	T39.8X1	T39.8X2	T39.8X3	T39.8X4	T39.8X5	T39.8X6
Acetylsalicylic acid (salts)	T39.011	T39.012	T39.013	T39.014	T39.015	T39.016
enteric coated	T39.011	T39.012	T39.013	T39.014	T39.015	T39.016
Acetylsulfamethoxypyridazine	T37.0X1	T37.0X2	T37.0X3	T37.0X4	T37.0X5	T37.0X6
Achromycin	T36.4X1	T36.4X2	T36.4X3	T36.4X4	T36.4X5	T36.4X6
ophthalmic preparation	T49.5X1	T49.5X2	T49.5X3	T49.5X4	T49.5X5	T49.5X6
topical NEC	T49.0X1	T49.0X2	T49.0X3	T49.0X4	T49.0X5	T49.0X6
Aciclovir	T37.5X1	T37.5X2	T37.5X3	T37.5X4	T37.5X5	T37.5X6
Acidifying agent NEC	T50.901	T50.902	T50.903	T50.904	T50.905	T50.906
Acid (corrosive) NEC	T54.2X1	T54.2X2	T54.2X3	T54.2X4	—	—
Acipimox	T46.6X1	T46.6X2	T46.6X3	T46.6X4	T46.6X5	T46.6X6
Acitretin	T50.991	T50.992	T50.993	T50.994	T50.995	T50.996
Aclarubicin	T45.1X1	T45.1X2	T45.1X3	T45.1X4	T45.1X5	T45.1X6
Aclatonium napadisilate	T48.1X1	T48.1X2	T48.1X3	T48.1X4	T48.1X5	T48.1X6
Aconite (wild)	T46.991	T46.992	T46.993	T46.994	T46.995	T46.996
Aconitine	T46.991	T46.992	T46.993	T46.994	T46.995	T46.996
Aconitum ferox	T46.991	T46.992	T46.993	T46.994	T46.995	T46.996
Acridine	T65.6X1	T65.6X2	T65.6X3	T65.6X4	—	—
vapor	T59.891	T59.892	T59.893	T59.894	—	—
Acriflavine	T37.91	T37.92	T37.93	T37.94	T37.95	T37.96
Acriflavinium chloride	T49.0X1	T49.0X2	T49.0X3	T49.0X4	T49.0X5	T49.0X6
Acrinol	T49.0X1	T49.0X2	T49.0X3	T49.0X4	T49.0X5	T49.0X6
Acrisorcin	T49.0X1	T49.0X2	T49.0X3	T49.0X4	T49.0X5	T49.0X6
Acrivastine	T45.0X1	T45.0X2	T45.0X3	T45.0X4	T45.0X5	T45.0X6
Acrolein (gas)	T59.891	T59.892	T59.893	T59.894	—	—
liquid	T54.1X1	T54.1X2	T54.1X3	T54.1X4	—	—
Acrylamide	T65.891	T65.892	T65.893	T65.894	—	—
Acrylic resin	T49.3X1	T49.3X2	T49.3X3	T49.3X4	T49.3X5	T49.3X6
Acrylonitrile	T65.891	T65.892	T65.893	T65.894	—	—
Actaea spicata	T62.2X1	T62.2X2	T62.2X3	T62.2X4	—	—
berry	T62.1X1	T62.1X2	T62.1X3	T62.1X4	—	—
Acterol	T37.3X1	T37.3X2	T37.3X3	T37.3X4	T37.3X5	T37.3X6
ACTH	T38.811	T38.812	T38.813	T38.814	T38.815	T38.816
Actinomycin C	T45.1X1	T45.1X2	T45.1X3	T45.1X4	T45.1X5	T45.1X6
Actinomycin D	T45.1X1	T45.1X2	T45.1X3	T45.1X4	T45.1X5	T45.1X6
Activated charcoal — see also Charcoal, medicinal	T47.6X1	T47.6X2	T47.6X3	T47.6X4	T47.6X5	T47.6X6
Acyclovir	T37.5X1	T37.5X2	T37.5X3	T37.5X4	T37.5X5	T37.5X6
Adenine	T45.2X1	T45.2X2	T45.2X3	T45.2X4	T45.2X5	T45.2X6
arabinoside	T37.5X1	T37.5X2	T37.5X3	T37.5X4	T37.5X5	T37.5X6
Adenosine (phosphate)	T46.2X1	T46.2X2	T46.2X3	T46.2X4	T46.2X5	T46.2X6
ADH	T38.891	T38.892	T38.893	T38.894	T38.895	T38.896
Adhesive NEC	T65.891	T65.892	T65.893	T65.894	—	—
Adicillin	T36.0X1	T36.0X2	T36.0X3	T36.0X4	T36.0X5	T36.0X6
Adiphenine	T44.3X1	T44.3X2	T44.3X3	T44.3X4	T44.3X5	T44.3X6
Adipiodone	T50.8X1	T50.8X2	T50.8X3	T50.8X4	T50.8X5	T50.8X6
Adjunct, pharmaceutical	T50.901	T50.902	T50.903	T50.904	T50.905	T50.906
Adrenal (extract, cortex or medulla) (glucocorticoids) (hormones) (mineralocorticoids)	T38.0X1	T38.0X2	T38.0X3	T38.0X4	T38.0X5	T38.0X6
ENT agent	T49.6X1	T49.6X2	T49.6X3	T49.6X4	T49.6X5	T49.6X6
ophthalmic preparation	T49.5X1	T49.5X2	T49.5X3	T49.5X4	T49.5X5	T49.5X6
topical NEC	T49.0X1	T49.0X2	T49.0X3	T49.0X4	T49.0X5	T49.0X6
Adrenalin — see Adrenaline						
Adrenaline	T44.5X1	T44.5X2	T44.5X3	T44.5X4	T44.5X5	T44.5X6
Adrenergic NEC	T44.901	T44.902	T44.903	T44.904	T44.905	T44.906
blocking agent NEC	T44.8X1	T44.8X2	T44.8X3	T44.8X4	T44.8X5	T44.8X6
beta, heart	T44.7X1	T44.7X2	T44.7X3	T44.7X4	T44.7X5	T44.7X6
specified NEC	T44.991	T44.992	T44.993	T44.994	T44.995	T44.996
Adrenochrome						
derivative	T46.991	T46.992	T46.993	T46.994	T46.995	T46.996

Table of Drugs and Chemicals

Adrenochrome — Aluminium, aluminum

Substance	Poisoning, Accidental (unintentional)	Poisoning, Intentional Self-harm	Poisoning, Assault	Poisoning, Undetermined	Adverse Effect	Under-dosing
Adrenochrome — continued						
(mono) semicarbazone	T46.991	T46.992	T46.993	T46.994	T46.995	T46.996
Adrenocorticotrophic hormone	T38.811	T38.812	T38.813	T38.814	T38.815	T38.816
Adrenocorticotrophin	T38.811	T38.812	T38.813	T38.814	T38.815	T38.816
Adriamycin	T45.1X1	T45.1X2	T45.1X3	T45.1X4	T45.1X5	T45.1X6
Aerosol spray NEC	T65.91	T65.92	T65.93	T65.94	—	—
Aerosporin	T36.8X1	T36.8X2	T36.8X3	T36.8X4	T36.8X5	T36.8X6
ENT agent	T49.6X1	T49.6X2	T49.6X3	T49.6X4	T49.6X5	T49.6X6
ophthalmic preparation	T49.5X1	T49.5X2	T49.5X3	T49.5X4	T49.5X5	T49.5X6
topical NEC	T49.0X1	T49.0X2	T49.0X3	T49.0X4	T49.0X5	T49.0X6
Aethusa cynapium	T62.2X1	T62.2X2	T62.2X3	T62.2X4	—	—
Afghanistan black	T40.7X1	T40.7X2	T40.7X3	T40.7X4	T40.7X5	T40.7X6
Aflatoxin	T64.01	T64.02	T64.03	T64.04	—	—
Afloqualone	T42.8X1	T42.8X2	T42.8X3	T42.8X4	T42.8X5	T42.8X6
African boxwood	T62.2X1	T62.2X2	T62.2X3	T62.2X4	—	—
Agar	T47.4X1	T47.4X2	T47.4X3	T47.4X4	T47.4X5	T47.4X6
Agonist						
predominantly						
alpha-adrenoreceptor	T44.4X1	T44.4X2	T44.4X3	T44.4X4	T44.4X5	T44.4X6
beta-adrenoreceptor	T44.5X1	T44.5X2	T44.5X3	T44.5X4	T44.5X5	T44.5X6
Agricultural agent NEC	T65.91	T65.92	T65.93	T65.94	—	—
Agrypnal	T42.3X1	T42.3X2	T42.3X3	T42.3X4	T42.3X5	T42.3X6
AHLG	T50.Z11	T50.Z12	T50.Z13	T50.Z14	T50.Z15	T50.Z16
Air contaminant(s), source/type NOS	T65.91	T65.92	T65.93	T65.94	—	—
Ajmaline	T46.2X1	T46.2X2	T46.2X3	T46.2X4	T46.2X5	T46.2X6
Akee	T62.1X1	T62.1X2	T62.1X3	T62.1X4	—	—
Akrinol	T49.0X1	T49.0X2	T49.0X3	T49.0X4	T49.0X5	T49.0X6
Akritoin	T37.8X1	T37.8X2	T37.8X3	T37.8X4	T37.8X5	T37.8X6
Alacepril	T46.4X1	T46.4X2	T46.4X3	T46.4X4	T46.4X5	T46.4X6
Alantolactone	T37.4X1	T37.4X2	T37.4X3	T37.4X4	T37.4X5	T37.4X6
Albamycin	T36.8X1	T36.8X2	T36.8X3	T36.8X4	T36.8X5	T36.8X6
Albendazole	T37.4X1	T37.4X2	T37.4X3	T37.4X4	T37.4X5	T37.4X6
Albumin						
bovine	T45.8X1	T45.8X2	T45.8X3	T45.8X4	T45.8X5	T45.8X6
human serum	T45.8X1	T45.8X2	T45.8X3	T45.8X4	T45.8X5	T45.8X6
salt-poor	T45.8X1	T45.8X2	T45.8X3	T45.8X4	T45.8X5	T45.8X6
normal human serum	T45.8X1	T45.8X2	T45.8X3	T45.8X4	T45.8X5	T45.8X6
Albuterol	T48.6X1	T48.6X2	T48.6X3	T48.6X4	T48.6X5	T48.6X6
Albutoin	T42.0X1	T42.0X2	T42.0X3	T42.0X4	T42.0X5	T42.0X6
Alclometasone	T49.0X1	T49.0X2	T49.0X3	T49.0X4	T49.0X5	T49.0X6
Alcohol	T51.91	T51.92	T51.93	T51.94	—	—
absolute	T51.0X1	T51.0X2	T51.0X3	T51.0X4	—	—
beverage	T51.0X1	T51.0X2	T51.0X3	T51.0X4	—	—
allyl	T51.8X1	T51.8X2	T51.8X3	T51.8X4	—	—
amyl	T51.3X1	T51.3X2	T51.3X3	T51.3X4	—	—
antifreeze	T51.1X1	T51.1X2	T51.1X3	T51.1X4	—	—
beverage	T51.0X1	T51.0X2	T51.0X3	T51.0X4	—	—
butyl	T51.3X1	T51.3X2	T51.3X3	T51.3X4	—	—
dehydrated	T51.0X1	T51.0X2	T51.0X3	T51.0X4	—	—
beverage	T51.0X1	T51.0X2	T51.0X3	T51.0X4	—	—
denatured	T51.0X1	T51.0X2	T51.0X3	T51.0X4	—	—
deterrent NEC	T50.6X1	T50.6X2	T50.6X3	T50.6X4	T50.6X5	T50.6X6
diagnostic (gastric function)	T50.8X1	T50.8X2	T50.8X3	T50.8X4	T50.8X5	T50.8X6
ethyl	T51.0X1	T51.0X2	T51.0X3	T51.0X4	—	—
beverage	T51.0X1	T51.0X2	T51.0X3	T51.0X4	—	—
grain	T51.0X1	T51.0X2	T51.0X3	T51.0X4	—	—
beverage	T51.0X1	T51.0X2	T51.0X3	T51.0X4	—	—
industrial	T51.0X1	T51.0X2	T51.0X3	T51.0X4	—	—
isopropyl	T51.2X1	T51.2X2	T51.2X3	T51.2X4	—	—
methyl	T51.1X1	T51.1X2	T51.1X3	T51.1X4	—	—
preparation for consumption	T51.0X1	T51.0X2	T51.0X3	T51.0X4	—	—
propyl	T51.3X1	T51.3X2	T51.3X3	T51.3X4	—	—
secondary	T51.2X1	T51.2X2	T51.2X3	T51.2X4	—	—
radiator	T51.1X1	T51.1X2	T51.1X3	T51.1X4	—	—
rubbing	T51.2X1	T51.2X2	T51.2X3	T51.2X4	—	—
specified type NEC	T51.8X1	T51.8X2	T51.8X3	T51.8X4	—	—
surgical	T51.0X1	T51.0X2	T51.0X3	T51.0X4	—	—
vapor (from any type of Alcohol)	T59.891	T59.892	T59.893	T59.894	—	—
wood	T51.1X1	T51.1X2	T51.1X3	T51.1X4	—	—
Alcuronium (chloride)	T48.1X1	T48.1X2	T48.1X3	T48.1X4	T48.1X5	T48.1X6
Aldactone	T50.0X1	T50.0X2	T50.0X3	T50.0X4	T50.0X5	T50.0X6
Aldesulfone sodium	T37.1X1	T37.1X2	T37.1X3	T37.1X4	T37.1X5	T37.1X6
Aldicarb	T60.0X1	T60.0X2	T60.0X3	T60.0X4	—	—
Aldomet	T46.5X1	T46.5X2	T46.5X3	T46.5X4	T46.5X5	T46.5X6
Aldosterone	T50.0X1	T50.0X2	T50.0X3	T50.0X4	T50.0X5	T50.0X6
Aldrin (dust)	T60.1X1	T60.1X2	T60.1X3	T60.1X4	—	—
Aleve — see Naproxen						
Alexitol sodium	T47.1X1	T47.1X2	T47.1X3	T47.1X4	T47.1X5	T47.1X6
Alfacalcidol	T45.2X1	T45.2X2	T45.2X3	T45.2X4	T45.2X5	T45.2X6
Alfadolone	T41.1X1	T41.1X2	T41.1X3	T41.1X4	T41.1X5	T41.1X6
Alfaxalone	T41.1X1	T41.1X2	T41.1X3	T41.1X4	T41.1X5	T41.1X6
Alfentanil	T40.4X1	T40.4X2	T40.4X3	T40.4X4	T40.4X5	T40.4X6
Alfuzosin (hydrochloride)	T44.8X1	T44.8X2	T44.8X3	T44.8X4	T44.8X5	T44.8X6
Algae (harmful) (toxin)	T65.821	T65.822	T65.823	T65.824	—	—
Algeldrate	T47.1X1	T47.1X2	T47.1X3	T47.1X4	T47.1X5	T47.1X6
Algin	T47.8X1	T47.8X2	T47.8X3	T47.8X4	T47.8X5	T47.8X6
Alglucerase	T45.3X1	T45.3X2	T45.3X3	T45.3X4	T45.3X5	T45.3X6
Alidase	T45.3X1	T45.3X2	T45.3X3	T45.3X4	T45.3X5	T45.3X6
Alimemazine	T43.3X1	T43.3X2	T43.3X3	T43.3X4	T43.3X5	T43.3X6
Aliphatic thiocyanates	T65.0X1	T65.0X2	T65.0X3	T65.0X4	—	—
Alizapride	T45.0X1	T45.0X2	T45.0X3	T45.0X4	T45.0X5	T45.0X6
Alkali (caustic)	T54.3X1	T54.3X2	T54.3X3	T54.3X4	—	—
Alkaline antiseptic solution (aromatic)	T49.6X1	T49.6X2	T49.6X3	T49.6X4	T49.6X5	T49.6X6
Alkalinizing agents (medicinal)	T50.901	T50.902	T50.903	T50.904	T50.905	T50.906
Alkalizing agent NEC	T50.901	T50.902	T50.903	T50.904	T50.905	T50.906
Alka-seltzer	T39.011	T39.012	T39.013	T39.014	T39.015	T39.016
Alkavervir	T46.5X1	T46.5X2	T46.5X3	T46.5X4	T46.5X5	T46.5X6
Alkonium (bromide)	T49.0X1	T49.0X2	T49.0X3	T49.0X4	T49.0X5	T49.0X6
Alkylating drug NEC	T45.1X1	T45.1X2	T45.1X3	T45.1X4	T45.1X5	T45.1X6
antimyeloproliferative	T45.1X1	T45.1X2	T45.1X3	T45.1X4	T45.1X5	T45.1X6
lymphatic	T45.1X1	T45.1X2	T45.1X3	T45.1X4	T45.1X5	T45.1X6
Alkylisocyanate	T65.0X1	T65.0X2	T65.0X3	T65.0X4	—	—
Allantoin	T49.4X1	T49.4X2	T49.4X3	T49.4X4	T49.4X5	T49.4X6
Allegron	T43.011	T43.012	T43.013	T43.014	T43.015	T43.016
Allethrin	T49.0X1	T49.0X2	T49.0X3	T49.0X4	T49.0X5	T49.0X6
Allobarbital	T42.3X1	T42.3X2	T42.3X3	T42.3X4	T42.3X5	T42.3X6
Allopurinol	T50.4X1	T50.4X2	T50.4X3	T50.4X4	T50.4X5	T50.4X6
Allyl						
alcohol	T51.8X1	T51.8X2	T51.8X3	T51.8X4	—	—
disulfide	T46.6X1	T46.6X2	T46.6X3	T46.6X4	T46.6X5	T46.6X6
Allylestrenol	T38.5X1	T38.5X2	T38.5X3	T38.5X4	T38.5X5	T38.5X6
Allylisopropylacetylurea	T42.6X1	T42.6X2	T42.6X3	T42.6X4	T42.6X5	T42.6X6
Allylisopropylmalonylurea	T42.3X1	T42.3X2	T42.3X3	T42.3X4	T42.3X5	T42.3X6
Allylthiourea	T49.3X1	T49.3X2	T49.3X3	T49.3X4	T49.3X5	T49.3X6
Allyltribromide	T42.6X1	T42.6X2	T42.6X3	T42.6X4	T42.6X5	T42.6X6
Allypropymal	T42.3X1	T42.3X2	T42.3X3	T42.3X4	T42.3X5	T42.3X6
Almagate	T47.1X1	T47.1X2	T47.1X3	T47.1X4	T47.1X5	T47.1X6
Almasilate	T47.1X1	T47.1X2	T47.1X3	T47.1X4	T47.1X5	T47.1X6
Almitrine	T50.7X1	T50.7X2	T50.7X3	T50.7X4	T50.7X5	T50.7X6
Aloes	T47.2X1	T47.2X2	T47.2X3	T47.2X4	T47.2X5	T47.2X6
Aloglutamol	T47.1X1	T47.1X2	T47.1X3	T47.1X4	T47.1X5	T47.1X6
Aloin	T47.2X1	T47.2X2	T47.2X3	T47.2X4	T47.2X5	T47.2X6
Aloxidone	T42.2X1	T42.2X2	T42.2X3	T42.2X4	T42.2X5	T42.2X6
Alpha						
acetyldigoxin	T46.0X1	T46.0X2	T46.0X3	T46.0X4	T46.0X5	T46.0X6
adrenergic blocking drug	T44.6X1	T44.6X2	T44.6X3	T44.6X4	T44.6X5	T44.6X6
amylase	T45.3X1	T45.3X2	T45.3X3	T45.3X4	T45.3X5	T45.3X6
tocoferol (acetate)	T45.2X1	T45.2X2	T45.2X3	T45.2X4	T45.2X5	T45.2X6
tocopherol	T45.2X1	T45.2X2	T45.2X3	T45.2X4	T45.2X5	T45.2X6
Alphadolone	T41.1X1	T41.1X2	T41.1X3	T41.1X4	T41.1X5	T41.1X6
Alphaprodine	T40.4X1	T40.4X2	T40.4X3	T40.4X4	T40.4X5	T40.4X6
Alphaxalone	T41.1X1	T41.1X2	T41.1X3	T41.1X4	T41.1X5	T41.1X6
Alprazolam	T42.4X1	T42.4X2	T42.4X3	T42.4X4	T42.4X5	T42.4X6
Alprenolol	T44.7X1	T44.7X2	T44.7X3	T44.7X4	T44.7X5	T44.7X6
Alprostadil	T46.7X1	T46.7X2	T46.7X3	T46.7X4	T46.7X5	T46.7X6
Alsactide	T38.811	T38.812	T38.813	T38.814	T38.815	T38.816
Alseroxylon	T46.5X1	T46.5X2	T46.5X3	T46.5X4	T46.5X5	T46.5X6
Alteplase	T45.611	T45.612	T45.613	T45.614	T45.615	T45.616
Altizide	T50.2X1	T50.2X2	T50.2X3	T50.2X4	T50.2X5	T50.2X6
Altretamine	T45.1X1	T45.1X2	T45.1X3	T45.1X4	T45.1X5	T45.1X6
Alum (medicinal)	T49.4X1	T49.4X2	T49.4X3	T49.4X4	T49.4X5	T49.4X6
nonmedicinal (ammonium) (potassium)	T56.891	T56.892	T56.893	T56.894	—	—
Aluminium, aluminum						
acetate	T49.2X1	T49.2X2	T49.2X3	T49.2X4	T49.2X5	T49.2X6
solution	T49.0X1	T49.0X2	T49.0X3	T49.0X4	T49.0X5	T49.0X6
aspirin	T39.011	T39.012	T39.013	T39.014	T39.015	T39.016
bis (acetylsalicylate)	T39.011	T39.012	T39.013	T39.014	T39.015	T39.016
carbonate (gel, basic)	T47.1X1	T47.1X2	T47.1X3	T47.1X4	T47.1X5	T47.1X6
chlorhydroxide-complex	T47.1X1	T47.1X2	T47.1X3	T47.1X4	T47.1X5	T47.1X6
chloride	T49.2X1	T49.2X2	T49.2X3	T49.2X4	T49.2X5	T49.2X6
clofibrate	T46.6X1	T46.6X2	T46.6X3	T46.6X4	T46.6X5	T46.6X6
diacetate	T49.2X1	T49.2X2	T49.2X3	T49.2X4	T49.2X5	T49.2X6
glycinate	T47.1X1	T47.1X2	T47.1X3	T47.1X4	T47.1X5	T47.1X6
hydroxide (gel)	T47.1X1	T47.1X2	T47.1X3	T47.1X4	T47.1X5	T47.1X6
hydroxide-magnesium carb. gel	T47.1X1	T47.1X2	T47.1X3	T47.1X4	T47.1X5	T47.1X6
magnesium silicate	T47.1X1	T47.1X2	T47.1X3	T47.1X4	T47.1X5	T47.1X6
nicotinate	T46.7X1	T46.7X2	T46.7X3	T46.7X4	T46.7X5	T46.7X6

Substance	Poisoning, Accidental (unintentional)	Poisoning, Intentional Self-harm	Poisoning, Assault	Poisoning, Undetermined	Adverse Effect	Under-dosing
Aluminium, aluminum — *continued*						
ointment (surgical) (topical)	T49.3X1	T49.3X2	T49.3X3	T49.3X4	T49.3X5	T49.3X6
phosphate	T47.1X1	T47.1X2	T47.1X3	T47.1X4	T47.1X5	T47.1X6
salicylate	T39.091	T39.092	T39.093	T39.094	T39.095	T39.096
silicate	T47.1X1	T47.1X2	T47.1X3	T47.1X4	T47.1X5	T47.1X6
sodium silicate	T47.1X1	T47.1X2	T47.1X3	T47.1X4	T47.1X5	T47.1X6
subacetate	T49.2X1	T49.2X2	T49.2X3	T49.2X4	T49.2X5	T49.2X6
sulfate	T49.0X1	T49.0X2	T49.0X3	T49.0X4	T49.0X5	T49.0X6
tannate	T47.6X1	T47.6X2	T47.6X3	T47.6X4	T47.6X5	T47.6X6
topical NEC	T49.3X1	T49.3X2	T49.3X3	T49.3X4	T49.3X5	T49.3X6
Alurate	T42.3X1	T42.3X2	T42.3X3	T42.3X4	T42.3X5	T42.3X6
Alverine	T44.3X1	T44.3X2	T44.3X3	T44.3X4	T44.3X5	T44.3X6
Alvodine	T40.2X1	T40.2X2	T40.2X3	T40.2X4	T40.2X5	T40.2X6
Amanita phalloides	T62.0X1	T62.0X2	T62.0X3	T62.0X4	—	—
Amanitine	T62.0X1	T62.0X2	T62.0X3	T62.0X4	—	—
Amantadine	T42.8X1	T42.8X2	T42.8X3	T42.8X4	T42.8X5	T42.8X6
Ambazone	T49.6X1	T49.6X2	T49.6X3	T49.6X4	T49.6X5	T49.6X6
Ambenonium (chloride)	T44.0X1	T44.0X2	T44.0X3	T44.0X4	T44.0X5	T44.0X6
Ambroxol	T48.4X1	T48.4X2	T48.4X3	T48.4X4	T48.4X5	T48.4X6
Ambuphylline	T48.6X1	T48.6X2	T48.6X3	T48.6X4	T48.6X5	T48.6X6
Ambutonium bromide	T44.3X1	T44.3X2	T44.3X3	T44.3X4	T44.3X5	T44.3X6
Amcinonide	T49.0X1	T49.0X2	T49.0X3	T49.0X4	T49.0X5	T49.0X6
Amdinocilline	T36.0X1	T36.0X2	T36.0X3	T36.0X4	T36.0X5	T36.0X6
Ametazole	T50.8X1	T50.8X2	T50.8X3	T50.8X4	T50.8X5	T50.8X6
Amethocaine	T41.3X1	T41.3X2	T41.3X3	T41.3X4	T41.3X5	T41.3X6
regional	T41.3X1	T41.3X2	T41.3X3	T41.3X4	T41.3X5	T41.3X6
spinal	T41.3X1	T41.3X2	T41.3X3	T41.3X4	T41.3X5	T41.3X6
Amethopterin	T45.1X1	T45.1X2	T45.1X3	T45.1X4	T45.1X5	T45.1X6
Amezinium metilsulfate	T44.991	T44.992	T44.993	T44.994	T44.995	T44.996
Amfebutamone	T43.291	T43.292	T43.293	T43.294	T43.295	T43.296
Amfepramone	T50.5X1	T50.5X2	T50.5X3	T50.5X4	T50.5X5	T50.5X6
Amfetamine	T43.621	T43.622	T43.623	T43.624	T43.625	T43.626
Amfetaminil	T43.621	T43.622	T43.623	T43.624	T43.625	T43.626
Amfomycin	T36.8X1	T36.8X2	T36.8X3	T36.8X4	T36.8X5	T36.8X6
Amidefrine mesilate	T48.5X1	T48.5X2	T48.5X3	T48.5X4	T48.5X5	T48.5X6
Amidone	T40.3X1	T40.3X2	T40.3X3	T40.3X4	T40.3X5	T40.3X6
Amidopyrine	T39.2X1	T39.2X2	T39.2X3	T39.2X4	T39.2X5	T39.2X6
Amidotrizoate	T50.8X1	T50.8X2	T50.8X3	T50.8X4	T50.8X5	T50.8X6
Amiflamine	T43.1X1	T43.1X2	T43.1X3	T43.1X4	T43.1X5	T43.1X6
Amikacin	T36.5X1	T36.5X2	T36.5X3	T36.5X4	T36.5X5	T36.5X6
Amikhelline	T46.3X1	T46.3X2	T46.3X3	T46.3X4	T46.3X5	T46.3X6
Amiloride	T50.2X1	T50.2X2	T50.2X3	T50.2X4	T50.2X5	T50.2X6
Aminacrine	T49.0X1	T49.0X2	T49.0X3	T49.0X4	T49.0X5	T49.0X6
Amineptine	T43.011	T43.012	T43.013	T43.014	T43.015	T43.016
Aminitrozole	T37.3X1	T37.3X2	T37.3X3	T37.3X4	T37.3X5	T37.3X6
Aminoacetic acid (derivatives)	T50.3X1	T50.3X2	T50.3X3	T50.3X4	T50.3X5	T50.3X6
Amino acids	T50.3X1	T50.3X2	T50.3X3	T50.3X4	T50.3X5	T50.3X6
Aminoacridine	T49.0X1	T49.0X2	T49.0X3	T49.0X4	T49.0X5	T49.0X6
Aminobenzoic acid (-p)	T49.3X1	T49.3X2	T49.3X3	T49.3X4	T49.3X5	T49.3X6
Aminocaproic acid	T45.621	T45.622	T45.623	T45.624	T45.625	T45.626
Aminoethylisothiourium	T45.8X1	T45.8X2	T45.8X3	T45.8X4	T45.8X5	T45.8X6
Aminofenazone	T39.2X1	T39.2X2	T39.2X3	T39.2X4	T39.2X5	T39.2X6
Aminoglutethimide	T45.1X1	T45.1X2	T45.1X3	T45.1X4	T45.1X5	T45.1X6
Aminohippuric acid	T50.8X1	T50.8X2	T50.8X3	T50.8X4	T50.8X5	T50.8X6
Aminomethylbenzoic acid	T45.691	T45.692	T45.693	T45.694	T45.695	T45.696
Aminometradine	T50.2X1	T50.2X2	T50.2X3	T50.2X4	T50.2X5	T50.2X6
Aminopentamide	T44.3X1	T44.3X2	T44.3X3	T44.3X4	T44.3X5	T44.3X6
Aminophenazone	T39.2X1	T39.2X2	T39.2X3	T39.2X4	T39.2X5	T39.2X6
Aminophenol	T54.0X1	T54.0X2	T54.0X3	T54.0X4	—	—
Aminophenylpyridone	T43.591	T43.592	T43.593	T43.594	T43.595	T43.596
Aminophylline	T48.6X1	T48.6X2	T48.6X3	T48.6X4	T48.6X5	T48.6X6
Aminopterin sodium	T45.1X1	T45.1X2	T45.1X3	T45.1X4	T45.1X5	T45.1X6
Aminopyrine	T39.2X1	T39.2X2	T39.2X3	T39.2X4	T39.2X5	T39.2X6
Aminorex	T50.5X1	T50.5X2	T50.5X3	T50.5X4	T50.5X5	T50.5X6
Aminosalicylic acid	T37.1X1	T37.1X2	T37.1X3	T37.1X4	T37.1X5	T37.1X6
Aminosalylum	T37.1X1	T37.1X2	T37.1X3	T37.1X4	T37.1X5	T37.1X6
Amiodarone	T46.2X1	T46.2X2	T46.2X3	T46.2X4	T46.2X5	T46.2X6
Amiphenazole	T50.7X1	T50.7X2	T50.7X3	T50.7X4	T50.7X5	T50.7X6
Amiquinsin	T46.5X1	T46.5X2	T46.5X3	T46.5X4	T46.5X5	T46.5X6
Amisometradine	T50.2X1	T50.2X2	T50.2X3	T50.2X4	T50.2X5	T50.2X6
Amisulpride	T43.591	T43.592	T43.593	T43.594	T43.595	T43.596
Amitriptyline	T43.011	T43.012	T43.013	T43.014	T43.015	T43.016
Amitriptylinoxide	T43.011	T43.012	T43.013	T43.014	T43.015	T43.016
Amlexanox	T48.6X1	T48.6X2	T48.6X3	T48.6X4	T48.6X5	T48.6X6
Ammonia (fumes) (gas) (vapor)	T59.891	T59.892	T59.893	T59.894	—	—
aromatic spirit	T48.991	T48.992	T48.993	T48.994	T48.995	T48.996
liquid (household)	T54.3X1	T54.3X2	T54.3X3	T54.3X4	—	—
Ammoniated mercury	T49.0X1	T49.0X2	T49.0X3	T49.0X4	T49.0X5	T49.0X6
Ammonium						
acid tartrate	T49.5X1	T49.5X2	T49.5X3	T49.5X4	T49.5X5	T49.5X6

Substance	Poisoning, Accidental (unintentional)	Poisoning, Intentional Self-harm	Poisoning, Assault	Poisoning, Undetermined	Adverse Effect	Under-dosing
Ammonium — *continued*						
bromide	T42.6X1	T42.6X2	T42.6X3	T42.6X4	T42.6X5	T42.6X6
carbonate	T54.3X1	T54.3X2	T54.3X3	T54.3X4	—	—
chloride	T50.991	T50.992	T50.993	T50.994	T50.995	T50.996
expectorant	T48.4X1	T48.4X2	T48.4X3	T48.4X4	T48.4X5	T48.4X6
compounds (household) NEC	T54.3X1	T54.3X2	T54.3X3	T54.3X4	—	—
fumes (any usage)	T59.891	T59.892	T59.893	T59.894	—	—
industrial	T54.3X1	T54.3X2	T54.3X3	T54.3X4	—	—
ichthyosulronate	T49.4X1	T49.4X2	T49.4X3	T49.4X4	T49.4X5	T49.4X6
mandelate	T37.91	T37.92	T37.93	T37.94	T37.95	T37.96
sulfamate	T60.3X1	T60.3X2	T60.3X3	T60.3X4	—	—
sulfonate resin	T47.8X1	T47.8X2	T47.8X3	T47.8X4	T47.8X5	T47.8X6
Amobarbital (sodium)	T42.3X1	T42.3X2	T42.3X3	T42.3X4	T42.3X5	T42.3X6
Amodiaquine	T37.2X1	T37.2X2	T37.2X3	T37.2X4	T37.2X5	T37.2X6
Amopyroquin (e)	T37.2X1	T37.2X2	T37.2X3	T37.2X4	T37.2X5	T37.2X6
Amoxapine	T43.011	T43.012	T43.013	T43.014	T43.015	T43.016
Amoxicillin	T36.0X1	T36.0X2	T36.0X3	T36.0X4	T36.0X5	T36.0X6
Amperozide	T43.591	T43.592	T43.593	T43.594	T43.595	T43.596
Amphenidone	T43.591	T43.592	T43.593	T43.594	T43.595	T43.596
Amphetamine NEC	T43.621	T43.622	T43.623	T43.624	T43.625	T43.626
Amphomycin	T36.8X1	T36.8X2	T36.8X3	T36.8X4	T36.8X5	T36.8X6
Amphotalide	T37.4X1	T37.4X2	T37.4X3	T37.4X4	T37.4X5	T37.4X6
Amphotericin B	T36.7X1	T36.7X2	T36.7X3	T36.7X4	T36.7X5	T36.7X6
topical	T49.0X1	T49.0X2	T49.0X3	T49.0X4	T49.0X5	T49.0X6
Ampicillin	T36.0X1	T36.0X2	T36.0X3	T36.0X4	T36.0X5	T36.0X6
Amprotropine	T44.3X1	T44.3X2	T44.3X3	T44.3X4	T44.3X5	T44.3X6
Amsacrine	T45.1X1	T45.1X2	T45.1X3	T45.1X4	T45.1X5	T45.1X6
Amygdaline	T62.2X1	T62.2X2	T62.2X3	T62.2X4	—	—
Amyl						
acetate	T52.8X1	T52.8X2	T52.8X3	T52.8X4	—	—
vapor	T59.891	T59.892	T59.893	T59.894	—	—
alcohol	T51.3X1	T51.3X2	T51.3X3	T51.3X4	—	—
chloride	T53.6X1	T53.6X2	T53.6X3	T53.6X4	—	—
formate	T52.8X1	T52.8X2	T52.8X3	T52.8X4	—	—
nitrite	T46.3X1	T46.3X2	T46.3X3	T46.3X4	T46.3X5	T46.3X6
propionate	T65.891	T65.892	T65.893	T65.894	—	—
Amylase	T47.5X1	T47.5X2	T47.5X3	T47.5X4	T47.5X5	T47.5X6
Amyleine, regional	T41.3X1	T41.3X2	T41.3X3	T41.3X4	T41.3X5	T41.3X6
Amylene						
dichloride	T53.6X1	T53.6X2	T53.6X3	T53.6X4	—	—
hydrate	T51.3X1	T51.3X2	T51.3X3	T51.3X4	—	—
Amylmetacresol	T49.6X1	T49.6X2	T49.6X3	T49.6X4	T49.6X5	T49.6X6
Amylobarbitone	T42.3X1	T42.3X2	T42.3X3	T42.3X4	T42.3X5	T42.3X6
Amylocaine, regional	T41.3X1	T41.3X2	T41.3X3	T41.3X4	T41.3X5	T41.3X6
infiltration (subcutaneous)	T41.3X1	T41.3X2	T41.3X3	T41.3X4	T41.3X5	T41.3X6
nerve block (peripheral) (plexus)	T41.3X1	T41.3X2	T41.3X3	T41.3X4	T41.3X5	T41.3X6
spinal	T41.3X1	T41.3X2	T41.3X3	T41.3X4	T41.3X5	T41.3X6
topical (surface)	T41.3X1	T41.3X2	T41.3X3	T41.3X4	T41.3X5	T41.3X6
Amylopectin	T47.6X1	T47.6X2	T47.6X3	T47.6X4	T47.6X5	T47.6X6
Amytal (sodium)	T42.3X1	T42.3X2	T42.3X3	T42.3X4	T42.3X5	T42.3X6
Anabolic steroid	T38.7X1	T38.7X2	T38.7X3	T38.7X4	T38.7X5	T38.7X6
Analeptic NEC	T50.7X1	T50.7X2	T50.7X3	T50.7X4	T50.7X5	T50.7X6
Analgesic	T39.91	T39.92	T39.93	T39.94	T39.95	T39.96
anti-inflammatory NEC	T39.91	T39.92	T39.93	T39.94	T39.95	T39.96
propionic acid derivative	T39.311	T39.312	T39.313	T39.314	T39.315	T39.316
antirheumatic NEC	T39.4X1	T39.4X2	T39.4X3	T39.4X4	T39.4X5	T39.4X6
aromatic NEC	T39.1X1	T39.1X2	T39.1X3	T39.1X4	T39.1X5	T39.1X6
narcotic NEC	T40.601	T40.602	T40.603	T40.604	T40.605	T40.606
combination	T40.601	T40.602	T40.603	T40.604	T40.605	T40.606
obstetric	T40.601	T40.602	T40.603	T40.604	T40.605	T40.606
non-narcotic NEC	T39.91	T39.92	T39.93	T39.94	T39.95	T39.96
combination	T39.91	T39.92	T39.93	T39.94	T39.95	T39.96
pyrazole	T39.2X1	T39.2X2	T39.2X3	T39.2X4	T39.2X5	T39.2X6
specified NEC	T39.8X1	T39.8X2	T39.8X3	T39.8X4	T39.8X5	T39.8X6
Analgin	T39.2X1	T39.2X2	T39.2X3	T39.2X4	T39.2X5	T39.2X6
Anamirta cocculus	T62.1X1	T62.1X2	T62.1X3	T62.1X4	—	—
Ancillin	T36.0X1	T36.0X2	T36.0X3	T36.0X4	T36.0X5	T36.0X6
Ancrod	T45.691	T45.692	T45.693	T45.694	T45.695	T45.696
Androgen	T38.7X1	T38.7X2	T38.7X3	T38.7X4	T38.7X5	T38.7X6
Androgen-estrogen mixture	T38.7X1	T38.7X2	T38.7X3	T38.7X4	T38.7X5	T38.7X6
Androstalone	T38.7X1	T38.7X2	T38.7X3	T38.7X4	T38.7X5	T38.7X6
Androstanolone	T38.7X1	T38.7X2	T38.7X3	T38.7X4	T38.7X5	T38.7X6
Androsterone	T38.7X1	T38.7X2	T38.7X3	T38.7X4	T38.7X5	T38.7X6
Anemone pulsatilla	T62.2X1	T62.2X2	T62.2X3	T62.2X4	—	—
Anesthesia						
caudal	T41.3X1	T41.3X2	T41.3X3	T41.3X4	T41.3X5	T41.3X6
endotracheal	T41.0X1	T41.0X2	T41.0X3	T41.0X4	T41.0X5	T41.0X6
epidural	T41.3X1	T41.3X2	T41.3X3	T41.3X4	T41.3X5	T41.3X6
inhalation	T41.0X1	T41.0X2	T41.0X3	T41.0X4	T41.0X5	T41.0X6
local	T41.3X1	T41.3X2	T41.3X3	T41.3X4	T41.3X5	T41.3X6

Table of Drugs and Chemicals

Anesthesia — Antifreeze

Substance	Poisoning, Accidental (unintentional)	Poisoning, Intentional Self-harm	Poisoning, Assault	Poisoning, Undetermined	Adverse Effect	Under-dosing
Anesthesia — continued						
mucosal	T41.3X1	T41.3X2	T41.3X3	T41.3X4	T41.3X5	T41.3X6
muscle relaxation	T48.1X1	T48.1X2	T48.1X3	T48.1X4	T48.1X5	T48.1X6
nerve blocking	T41.3X1	T41.3X2	T41.3X3	T41.3X4	T41.3X5	T41.3X6
plexus blocking	T41.3X1	T41.3X2	T41.3X3	T41.3X4	T41.3X5	T41.3X6
potentiated	T41.201	T41.202	T41.203	T41.204	T41.205	T41.206
rectal	T41.201	T41.202	T41.203	T41.204	T41.205	T41.206
general	T41.201	T41.202	T41.203	T41.204	T41.205	T41.206
local	T41.3X1	T41.3X2	T41.3X3	T41.3X4	T41.3X5	T41.3X6
regional	T41.3X1	T41.3X2	T41.3X3	T41.3X4	T41.3X5	T41.3X6
surface	T41.3X1	T41.3X2	T41.3X3	T41.3X4	T41.3X5	T41.3X6
Anesthetic NEC — see also	T41.41	T41.42	T41.43	T41.44	T41.45	T41.46
Anesthesia						
with muscle relaxant	T41.201	T41.202	T41.203	T41.204	T41.205	T41.206
general	T41.201	T41.202	T41.203	T41.204	T41.205	T41.206
local	T41.3X1	T41.3X2	T41.3X3	T41.3X4	T41.3X5	T41.3X6
gaseous NEC	T41.0X1	T41.0X2	T41.0X3	T41.0X4	T41.0X5	T41.0X6
general NEC	T41.201	T41.202	T41.203	T41.204	T41.205	T41.206
halogenated hydrocarbon derivatives NEC	T41.0X1	T41.0X2	T41.0X3	T41.0X4	T41.0X5	T41.0X6
infiltration NEC	T41.3X1	T41.3X2	T41.3X3	T41.3X4	T41.3X5	T41.3X6
intravenous NEC	T41.1X1	T41.1X2	T41.1X3	T41.1X4	T41.1X5	T41.1X6
local NEC	T41.3X1	T41.3X2	T41.3X3	T41.3X4	T41.3X5	T41.3X6
rectal	T41.201	T41.202	T41.203	T41.204	T41.205	T41.206
general	T41.201	T41.202	T41.203	T41.204	T41.205	T41.206
local	T41.3X1	T41.3X2	T41.3X3	T41.3X4	T41.3X5	T41.3X6
regional NEC	T41.3X1	T41.3X2	T41.3X3	T41.3X4	T41.3X5	T41.3X6
spinal NEC	T41.3X1	T41.3X2	T41.3X3	T41.3X4	T41.3X5	T41.3X6
thiobarbiturate	T41.1X1	T41.1X2	T41.1X3	T41.1X4	T41.1X5	T41.1X6
topical	T41.3X1	T41.3X2	T41.3X3	T41.3X4	T41.3X5	T41.3X6
Aneurine	T45.2X1	T45.2X2	T45.2X3	T45.2X4	T45.2X5	T45.2X6
Angio-Conray	T50.8X1	T50.8X2	T50.8X3	T50.8X4	T50.8X5	T50.8X6
Angiotensin	T44.5X1	T44.5X2	T44.5X3	T44.5X4	T44.5X5	T44.5X6
Angiotensinamide	T44.991	T44.992	T44.993	T44.994	T44.995	T44.996
Anhydrohydroxy-progesterone	T38.5X1	T38.5X2	T38.5X3	T38.5X4	T38.5X5	T38.5X6
Anhydron	T50.2X1	T50.2X2	T50.2X3	T50.2X4	T50.2X5	T50.2X6
Anileridine	T40.4X1	T40.4X2	T40.4X3	T40.4X4	T40.4X5	T40.4X6
Aniline (dye) (liquid)	T65.3X1	T65.3X2	T65.3X3	T65.3X4	—	—
analgesic	T39.1X1	T39.1X2	T39.1X3	T39.1X4	T39.1X5	T39.1X6
derivatives, therapeutic NEC	T39.1X1	T39.1X2	T39.1X3	T39.1X4	T39.1X5	T39.1X6
vapor	T65.3X1	T65.3X2	T65.3X3	T65.3X4	—	—
Aniscoropine	T44.3X1	T44.3X2	T44.3X3	T44.3X4	T44.3X5	T44.3X6
Anise oil	T47.5X1	T47.5X2	T47.5X3	T47.5X4	T47.5X5	T47.5X6
Anisidine	T65.3X1	T65.3X2	T65.3X3	T65.3X4	—	—
Anisindione	T45.511	T45.512	T45.513	T45.514	T45.515	T45.516
Anisotropine methyl-bromide	T44.3X1	T44.3X2	T44.3X3	T44.3X4	T44.3X5	T44.3X6
Anistreplase	T45.611	T45.612	T45.613	T45.614	T45.615	T45.616
Anorexiant (central)	T50.5X1	T50.5X2	T50.5X3	T50.5X4	T50.5X5	T50.5X6
Anorexic agents	T50.5X1	T50.5X2	T50.5X3	T50.5X4	T50.5X5	T50.5X6
Ansamycin	T36.6X1	T36.6X2	T36.6X3	T36.6X4	T36.6X5	T36.6X6
Ant (bite) (sting)	T63.421	T63.422	T63.423	T63.424	—	—
Antabuse	T50.6X1	T50.6X2	T50.6X3	T50.6X4	T50.6X5	T50.6X6
Antacid NEC	T47.1X1	T47.1X2	T47.1X3	T47.1X4	T47.1X5	T47.1X6
Antagonist						
Aldosterone	T50.0X1	T50.0X2	T50.0X3	T50.0X4	T50.0X5	T50.0X6
alpha-adrenoreceptor	T44.6X1	T44.6X2	T44.6X3	T44.6X4	T44.6X5	T44.6X6
anticoagulant	T45.7X1	T45.7X2	T45.7X3	T45.7X4	T45.7X5	T45.7X6
beta-adrenoreceptor	T44.7X1	T44.7X2	T44.7X3	T44.7X4	T44.7X5	T44.7X6
extrapyramidal NEC	T44.3X1	T44.3X2	T44.3X3	T44.3X4	T44.3X5	T44.3X6
folic acid	T45.1X1	T45.1X2	T45.1X3	T45.1X4	T45.1X5	T45.1X6
H2 receptor	T47.0X1	T47.0X2	T47.0X3	T47.0X4	T47.0X5	T47.0X6
heavy metal	T45.8X1	T45.8X2	T45.8X3	T45.8X4	T45.8X5	T45.8X6
narcotic analgesic	T50.7X1	T50.7X2	T50.7X3	T50.7X4	T50.7X5	T50.7X6
opiate	T50.7X1	T50.7X2	T50.7X3	T50.7X4	T50.7X5	T50.7X6
pyrimidine	T45.1X1	T45.1X2	T45.1X3	T45.1X4	T45.1X5	T45.1X6
serotonin	T46.5X1	T46.5X2	T46.5X3	T46.5X4	T46.5X5	T46.5X6
Antazolin (e)	T45.0X1	T45.0X2	T45.0X3	T45.0X4	T45.0X5	T45.0X6
Anterior pituitary hormone NEC	T38.811	T38.812	T38.813	T38.814	T38.815	T38.816
Anthelmintic NEC	T37.4X1	T37.4X2	T37.4X3	T37.4X4	T37.4X5	T37.4X6
Anthiolimine	T37.4X1	T37.4X2	T37.4X3	T37.4X4	T37.4X5	T37.4X6
Anthralin	T49.4X1	T49.4X2	T49.4X3	T49.4X4	T49.4X5	T49.4X6
Anthramycin	T45.1X1	T45.1X2	T45.1X3	T45.1X4	T45.1X5	T45.1X6
Antiadrenergic NEC	T44.8X1	T44.8X2	T44.8X3	T44.8X4	T44.8X5	T44.8X6
Antiallergic NEC	T45.0X1	T45.0X2	T45.0X3	T45.0X4	T45.0X5	T45.0X6
Antiandrogen NEC	T38.6X1	T38.6X2	T38.6X3	T38.6X4	T38.6X5	T38.6X6
Anti-anemic (drug) (preparation)	T45.8X1	T45.8X2	T45.8X3	T45.8X4	T45.8X5	T45.8X6
Antianxiety drug NEC	T43.501	T43.502	T43.503	T43.504	T43.505	T43.506
Antiaris toxicaria	T65.891	T65.892	T65.893	T65.894	—	—
Antiarteriosclerotic drug	T46.6X1	T46.6X2	T46.6X3	T46.6X4	T46.6X5	T46.6X6

Substance	Poisoning, Accidental (unintentional)	Poisoning, Intentional Self-harm	Poisoning, Assault	Poisoning, Undetermined	Adverse Effect	Under-dosing
Antiasthmatic drug NEC	T48.6X1	T48.6X2	T48.6X3	T48.6X4	T48.6X5	T48.6X6
Antibiotic NEC	T36.91	T36.92	T36.93	T36.94	T36.95	T36.96
aminoglycoside	T36.5X1	T36.5X2	T36.5X3	T36.5X4	T36.5X5	T36.5X6
anticancer	T45.1X1	T45.1X2	T45.1X3	T45.1X4	T45.1X5	T45.1X6
antifungal	T36.7X1	T36.7X2	T36.7X3	T36.7X4	T36.7X5	T36.7X6
antimycobacterial	T36.5X1	T36.5X2	T36.5X3	T36.5X4	T36.5X5	T36.5X6
antineoplastic	T45.1X1	T45.1X2	T45.1X3	T45.1X4	T45.1X5	T45.1X6
b-lactam NEC	T36.1X1	T36.1X2	T36.1X3	T36.1X4	T36.1X5	T36.1X6
cephalosporin (group)	T36.1X1	T36.1X2	T36.1X3	T36.1X4	T36.1X5	T36.1X6
chloramphenicol (group)	T36.2X1	T36.2X2	T36.2X3	T36.2X4	T36.2X5	T36.2X6
ENT	T49.6X1	T49.6X2	T49.6X3	T49.6X4	T49.6X5	T49.6X6
eye	T49.5X1	T49.5X2	T49.5X3	T49.5X4	T49.5X5	T49.5X6
fungicidal (local)	T49.0X1	T49.0X2	T49.0X3	T49.0X4	T49.0X5	T49.0X6
intestinal	T36.8X1	T36.8X2	T36.8X3	T36.8X4	T36.8X5	T36.8X6
local	T49.0X1	T49.0X2	T49.0X3	T49.0X4	T49.0X5	T49.0X6
macrolides	T36.3X1	T36.3X2	T36.3X3	T36.3X4	T36.3X5	T36.3X6
polypeptide	T36.8X1	T36.8X2	T36.8X3	T36.8X4	T36.8X5	T36.8X6
specified NEC	T36.8X1	T36.8X2	T36.8X3	T36.8X4	T36.8X5	T36.8X6
tetracycline (group)	T36.4X1	T36.4X2	T36.4X3	T36.4X4	T36.4X5	T36.4X6
throat	T49.6X1	T49.6X2	T49.6X3	T49.6X4	T49.6X5	T49.6X6
Anticancer agents NEC	T45.1X1	T45.1X2	T45.1X3	T45.1X4	T45.1X5	T45.1X6
Anticholesterolemic drug NEC	T46.6X1	T46.6X2	T46.6X3	T46.6X4	T46.6X5	T46.6X6
Anticholinergic NEC	T44.3X1	T44.3X2	T44.3X3	T44.3X4	T44.3X5	T44.3X6
Anticholinesterase	T44.0X1	T44.0X2	T44.0X3	T44.0X4	T44.0X5	T44.0X6
organophosphorus	T44.0X1	T44.0X2	T44.0X3	T44.0X4	T44.0X5	T44.0X6
insecticide	T60.0X1	T60.0X2	T60.0X3	T60.0X4	—	—
nerve gas	T59.891	T59.892	T59.893	T59.894	—	—
reversible	T44.0X1	T44.0X2	T44.0X3	T44.0X4	T44.0X5	T44.0X6
ophthalmological	T49.5X1	T49.5X2	T49.5X3	T49.5X4	T49.5X5	T49.5X6
Anticoagulant NEC	T45.511	T45.512	T45.513	T45.514	T45.515	T45.516
Antagonist	T45.7X1	T45.7X2	T45.7X3	T45.7X4	T45.7X5	T45.7X6
Anti-common-cold drug NEC	T48.5X1	T48.5X2	T48.5X3	T48.5X4	T48.5X5	T48.5X6
Anticonvulsant	T42.71	T42.72	T42.73	T42.74	T42.75	T42.76
barbiturate	T42.3X1	T42.3X2	T42.3X3	T42.3X4	T42.3X5	T42.3X6
combination (with barbiturate)	T42.3X1	T42.3X2	T42.3X3	T42.3X4	T42.3X5	T42.3X6
hydantoin	T42.0X1	T42.0X2	T42.0X3	T42.0X4	T42.0X5	T42.0X6
hypnotic NEC	T42.6X1	T42.6X2	T42.6X3	T42.6X4	T42.6X5	T42.6X6
oxazolidinedione	T42.2X1	T42.2X2	T42.2X3	T42.2X4	T42.2X5	T42.2X6
pyrimidinedione	T42.6X1	T42.6X2	T42.6X3	T42.6X4	T42.6X5	T42.6X6
specified NEC	T42.6X1	T42.6X2	T42.6X3	T42.6X4	T42.6X5	T42.6X6
succinimide	T42.2X1	T42.2X2	T42.2X3	T42.2X4	T42.2X5	T42.2X6
Antidepressant	T43.201	T43.202	T43.203	T43.204	T43.205	T43.206
monoamine oxidase inhibitor	T43.1X1	T43.1X2	T43.1X3	T43.1X4	T43.1X5	T43.1X6
selective serotonin norepinephrine reuptake inhibitor	T43.211	T43.212	T43.213	T43.214	T43.215	T43.216
selective serotonin reuptake inhibitor	T43.221	T43.222	T43.223	T43.224	T43.225	T43.226
specified NEC	T43.291	T43.292	T43.293	T43.294	T43.295	T43.296
tetracyclic	T43.021	T43.022	T43.023	T43.024	T43.025	T43.026
triazolopyridine	T43.211	T43.212	T43.213	T43.214	T43.215	T43.216
tricyclic	T43.011	T43.012	T43.013	T43.014	T43.015	T43.016
Antidiabetic NEC	T38.3X1	T38.3X2	T38.3X3	T38.3X4	T38.3X5	T38.3X6
biguanide	T38.3X1	T38.3X2	T38.3X3	T38.3X4	T38.3X5	T38.3X6
and sulfonyl combined	T38.3X1	T38.3X2	T38.3X3	T38.3X4	T38.3X5	T38.3X6
combined	T38.3X1	T38.3X2	T38.3X3	T38.3X4	T38.3X5	T38.3X6
sulfonylurea	T38.3X1	T38.3X2	T38.3X3	T38.3X4	T38.3X5	T38.3X6
Antidiarrheal drug NEC	T47.6X1	T47.6X2	T47.6X3	T47.6X4	T47.6X5	T47.6X6
absorbent	T47.6X1	T47.6X2	T47.6X3	T47.6X4	T47.6X5	T47.6X6
Anti-D immunoglobulin (human)	T50.Z11	T50.Z12	T50.Z13	T50.Z14	T50.Z15	T50.Z16
Antidiphtheria serum	T50.Z11	T50.Z12	T50.Z13	T50.Z14	T50.Z15	T50.Z16
Antidiuretic hormone	T38.891	T38.892	T38.893	T38.894	T38.895	T38.896
Antidote NEC	T50.6X1	T50.6X2	T50.6X3	T50.6X4	T50.6X5	T50.6X6
heavy metal	T45.8X1	T45.8X2	T45.8X3	T45.8X4	T45.8X5	T45.8X6
Antidysrhythmic NEC	T46.2X1	T46.2X2	T46.2X3	T46.2X4	T46.2X5	T46.2X6
Antiemetic drug	T45.0X1	T45.0X2	T45.0X3	T45.0X4	T45.0X5	T45.0X6
Antiepilepsy agent	T42.71	T42.72	T42.73	T42.74	T42.75	T42.76
combination	T42.5X1	T42.5X2	T42.5X3	T42.5X4	T42.5X5	T42.5X6
mixed	T42.5X1	T42.5X2	T42.5X3	T42.5X4	T42.5X5	T42.5X6
specified, NEC	T42.6X1	T42.6X2	T42.6X3	T42.6X4	T42.6X5	T42.6X6
Antiestrogen NEC	T38.6X1	T38.6X2	T38.6X3	T38.6X4	T38.6X5	T38.6X6
Antifertility pill	T38.4X1	T38.4X2	T38.4X3	T38.4X4	T38.4X5	T38.4X6
Antifibrinolytic drug	T45.621	T45.622	T45.623	T45.624	T45.625	T45.626
Antifilarial drug	T37.4X1	T37.4X2	T37.4X3	T37.4X4	T37.4X5	T37.4X6
Antiflatulent	T47.5X1	T47.5X2	T47.5X3	T47.5X4	T47.5X5	T47.5X6
Antifreeze	T65.91	T65.92	T65.93	T65.94	—	—
alcohol	T51.1X1	T51.1X2	T51.1X3	T51.1X4	—	—
ethylene glycol	T51.8X1	T51.8X2	T51.8X3	T51.8X4	—	—

Substance	Poisoning, Accidental (unintentional)	Poisoning, Intentional Self-harm	Poisoning, Assault	Poisoning, Undetermined	Adverse Effect	Under-dosing
Antifungal						
antibiotic (systemic)	T36.7X1	T36.7X2	T36.7X3	T36.7X4	T36.7X5	T36.7X6
anti-infective NEC	T37.91	T37.92	T37.93	T37.94	T37.95	T37.96
disinfectant, local	T49.0X1	T49.0X2	T49.0X3	T49.0X4	T49.0X5	T49.0X6
nonmedicinal (spray)	T60.3X1	T60.3X2	T60.3X3	T60.3X4	—	—
topical	T49.0X1	T49.0X2	T49.0X3	T49.0X4	T49.0X5	T49.0X6
Anti-gastric-secretion drug NEC	T47.1X1	T47.1X2	T47.1X3	T47.1X4	T47.1X5	T47.1X6
Antigonadotrophin NEC	T38.6X1	T38.6X2	T38.6X3	T38.6X4	T38.6X5	T38.6X6
Antihallucinogen	T43.501	T43.502	T43.503	T43.504	T43.505	T43.506
Antihelmintics	T37.4X1	T37.4X2	T37.4X3	T37.4X4	T37.4X5	T37.4X6
Antihemophilic						
factor	T45.8X1	T45.8X2	T45.8X3	T45.8X4	T45.8X5	T45.8X6
fraction	T45.8X1	T45.8X2	T45.8X3	T45.8X4	T45.8X5	T45.8X6
globulin concentrate	T45.7X1	T45.7X2	T45.7X3	T45.7X4	T45.7X5	T45.7X6
human plasma	T45.8X1	T45.8X2	T45.8X3	T45.8X4	T45.8X5	T45.8X6
plasma, dried	T45.7X1	T45.7X2	T45.7X3	T45.7X4	T45.7X5	T45.7X6
Antihemorrhoidal preparation	T49.2X1	T49.2X2	T49.2X3	T49.2X4	T49.2X5	T49.2X6
Antiheparin drug	T45.7X1	T45.7X2	T45.7X3	T45.7X4	T45.7X5	T45.7X6
Antihistamine	T45.0X1	T45.0X2	T45.0X3	T45.0X4	T45.0X5	T45.0X6
Antihookworm drug	T37.4X1	T37.4X2	T37.4X3	T37.4X4	T37.4X5	T37.4X6
Anti-human lymphocytic globulin	T50.Z11	T50.Z12	T50.Z13	T50.Z14	T50.Z15	T50.Z16
Antihyperlipidemic drug	T46.6X1	T46.6X2	T46.6X3	T46.6X4	T46.6X5	T46.6X6
Antihypertensive drug NEC	T46.5X1	T46.5X2	T46.5X3	T46.5X4	T46.5X5	T46.5X6
Anti-infective NEC	T37.91	T37.92	T37.93	T37.94	T37.95	T37.96
anthelmintic	T37.4X1	T37.4X2	T37.4X3	T37.4X4	T37.4X5	T37.4X6
antibiotics	T36.91	T36.92	T36.93	T36.94	T36.95	T36.96
specified NEC	T36.8X1	T36.8X2	T36.8X3	T36.8X4	T36.8X5	T36.8X6
antimalarial	T37.2X1	T37.2X2	T37.2X3	T37.2X4	T37.2X5	T37.2X6
antimycobacterial NEC	T37.1X1	T37.1X2	T37.1X3	T37.1X4	T37.1X5	T37.1X6
antibiotics	T36.5X1	T36.5X2	T36.5X3	T36.5X4	T36.5X5	T36.5X6
antiprotozoal NEC	T37.3X1	T37.3X2	T37.3X3	T37.3X4	T37.3X5	T37.3X6
blood	T37.2X1	T37.2X2	T37.2X3	T37.2X4	T37.2X5	T37.2X6
antiviral	T37.5X1	T37.5X2	T37.5X3	T37.5X4	T37.5X5	T37.5X6
arsenical	T37.8X1	T37.8X2	T37.8X3	T37.8X4	T37.8X5	T37.8X6
bismuth, local	T49.0X1	T49.0X2	T49.0X3	T49.0X4	T49.0X5	T49.0X6
ENT	T49.6X1	T49.6X2	T49.6X3	T49.6X4	T49.6X5	T49.6X6
eye NEC	T49.5X1	T49.5X2	T49.5X3	T49.5X4	T49.5X5	T49.5X6
heavy metals NEC	T37.8X1	T37.8X2	T37.8X3	T37.8X4	T37.8X5	T37.8X6
local NEC	T49.0X1	T49.0X2	T49.0X3	T49.0X4	T49.0X5	T49.0X6
specified NEC	T49.0X1	T49.0X2	T49.0X3	T49.0X4	T49.0X5	T49.0X6
mixed	T37.91	T37.92	T37.93	T37.94	T37.95	T37.96
ophthalmic preparation	T49.5X1	T49.5X2	T49.5X3	T49.5X4	T49.5X5	T49.5X6
topical NEC	T49.0X1	T49.0X2	T49.0X3	T49.0X4	T49.0X5	T49.0X6
Anti-inflammatory drug NEC	T39.391	T39.392	T39.393	T39.394	T39.395	T39.396
local	T49.0X1	T49.0X2	T49.0X3	T49.0X4	T49.0X5	T49.0X6
nonsteroidal NEC	T39.391	T39.392	T39.393	T39.394	T39.395	T39.396
propionic acid derivative	T39.311	T39.312	T39.313	T39.314	T39.315	T39.316
specified NEC	T39.391	T39.392	T39.393	T39.394	T39.395	T39.396
Antikaluretic	T50.3X1	T50.3X2	T50.3X3	T50.3X4	T50.3X5	T50.3X6
Antiknock (tetraethyl lead)	T56.0X1	T56.0X2	T56.0X3	T56.0X4	—	—
Antilipemic drug NEC	T46.6X1	T46.6X2	T46.6X3	T46.6X4	T46.6X5	T46.6X6
Antimalarial	T37.2X1	T37.2X2	T37.2X3	T37.2X4	T37.2X5	T37.2X6
prophylactic NEC	T37.2X1	T37.2X2	T37.2X3	T37.2X4	T37.2X5	T37.2X6
pyrimidine derivative	T37.2X1	T37.2X2	T37.2X3	T37.2X4	T37.2X5	T37.2X6
Antimetabolite	T45.1X1	T45.1X2	T45.1X3	T45.1X4	T45.1X5	T45.1X6
Antimitotic agent	T45.1X1	T45.1X2	T45.1X3	T45.1X4	T45.1X5	T45.1X6
Antimony (compounds) (vapor) NEC	T56.891	T56.892	T56.893	T56.894	—	—
anti-infectives	T37.8X1	T37.8X2	T37.8X3	T37.8X4	T37.8X5	T37.8X6
dimercaptosuccinate	T37.3X1	T37.3X2	T37.3X3	T37.3X4	T37.3X5	T37.3X6
hydride	T56.891	T56.892	T56.893	T56.894	—	—
pesticide (vapor)	T60.8X1	T60.8X2	T60.8X3	T60.8X4	—	—
potassium (sodium) tartrate	T37.8X1	T37.8X2	T37.8X3	T37.8X4	T37.8X5	T37.8X6
sodium dimercaptosuccinate	T37.3X1	T37.3X2	T37.3X3	T37.3X4	T37.3X5	T37.3X6
tartrated	T37.8X1	T37.8X2	T37.8X3	T37.8X4	T37.8X5	T37.8X6
Antimuscarinic NEC	T44.3X1	T44.3X2	T44.3X3	T44.3X4	T44.3X5	T44.3X6
Antimycobacterial drug NEC	T37.1X1	T37.1X2	T37.1X3	T37.1X4	T37.1X5	T37.1X6
antibiotics	T36.5X1	T36.5X2	T36.5X3	T36.5X4	T36.5X5	T36.5X6
combination	T37.1X1	T37.1X2	T37.1X3	T37.1X4	T37.1X5	T37.1X6
Antinausea drug	T45.0X1	T45.0X2	T45.0X3	T45.0X4	T45.0X5	T45.0X6
Antinematode drug	T37.4X1	T37.4X2	T37.4X3	T37.4X4	T37.4X5	T37.4X6
Antineoplastic NEC	T45.1X1	T45.1X2	T45.1X3	T45.1X4	T45.1X5	T45.1X6
alkaloidal	T45.1X1	T45.1X2	T45.1X3	T45.1X4	T45.1X5	T45.1X6
antibiotics	T45.1X1	T45.1X2	T45.1X3	T45.1X4	T45.1X5	T45.1X6
combination	T45.1X1	T45.1X2	T45.1X3	T45.1X4	T45.1X5	T45.1X6
estrogen	T38.5X1	T38.5X2	T38.5X3	T38.5X4	T38.5X5	T38.5X6

Substance	Poisoning, Accidental (unintentional)	Poisoning, Intentional Self-harm	Poisoning, Assault	Poisoning, Undetermined	Adverse Effect	Under-dosing
Antineoplastic — *continued*						
steroid	T38.7X1	T38.7X2	T38.7X3	T38.7X4	T38.7X5	T38.7X6
Antiparasitic drug (systemic)	T37.91	T37.92	T37.93	T37.94	T37.95	T37.96
local	T49.0X1	T49.0X2	T49.0X3	T49.0X4	T49.0X5	T49.0X6
specified NEC	T37.8X1	T37.8X2	T37.8X3	T37.8X4	T37.8X5	T37.8X6
Antiparkinsonism drug NEC	T42.8X1	T42.8X2	T42.8X3	T42.8X4	T42.8X5	T42.8X6
Antiperspirant NEC	T49.2X1	T49.2X2	T49.2X3	T49.2X4	T49.2X5	T49.2X6
Antiphlogistic NEC	T39.4X1	T39.4X2	T39.4X3	T39.4X4	T39.4X5	T39.4X6
Antiplatyhelmintic drug	T37.4X1	T37.4X2	T37.4X3	T37.4X4	T37.4X5	T37.4X6
Antiprotozoal drug NEC	T37.3X1	T37.3X2	T37.3X3	T37.3X4	T37.3X5	T37.3X6
blood	T37.2X1	T37.2X2	T37.2X3	T37.2X4	T37.2X5	T37.2X6
local	T49.0X1	T49.0X2	T49.0X3	T49.0X4	T49.0X5	T49.0X6
Antipruritic drug NEC	T49.1X1	T49.1X2	T49.1X3	T49.1X4	T49.1X5	T49.1X6
Antipsychotic drug	T43.501	T43.502	T43.503	T43.504	T43.505	T43.506
specified NEC	T43.591	T43.592	T43.593	T43.594	T43.595	T43.596
Antipyretic	T39.91	T39.92	T39.93	T39.94	T39.95	T39.96
specified NEC	T39.8X1	T39.8X2	T39.8X3	T39.8X4	T39.8X5	T39.8X6
Antipyrine	T39.2X1	T39.2X2	T39.2X3	T39.2X4	T39.2X5	T39.2X6
Antirabies hyperimmune serum	T50.Z11	T50.Z12	T50.Z13	T50.Z14	T50.Z15	T50.Z16
Antirheumatic NEC	T39.4X1	T39.4X2	T39.4X3	T39.4X4	T39.4X5	T39.4X6
Antirigidity drug NEC	T42.8X1	T42.8X2	T42.8X3	T42.8X4	T42.8X5	T42.8X6
Antischistosomal drug	T37.4X1	T37.4X2	T37.4X3	T37.4X4	T37.4X5	T37.4X6
Antiscorpion sera	T50.Z11	T50.Z12	T50.Z13	T50.Z14	T50.Z15	T50.Z16
Antiseborrheics	T49.4X1	T49.4X2	T49.4X3	T49.4X4	T49.4X5	T49.4X6
Antiseptics (external) (medicinal)	T49.0X1	T49.0X2	T49.0X3	T49.0X4	T49.0X5	T49.0X6
Antistine	T45.0X1	T45.0X2	T45.0X3	T45.0X4	T45.0X5	T45.0X6
Antitapeworm drug	T37.4X1	T37.4X2	T37.4X3	T37.4X4	T37.4X5	T37.4X6
Antitetanus immunoglobulin	T50.Z11	T50.Z12	T50.Z13	T50.Z14	T50.Z15	T50.Z16
Antithyroid drug NEC	T38.2X1	T38.2X2	T38.2X3	T38.2X4	T38.2X5	T38.2X6
Antitoxin	T50.Z11	T50.Z12	T50.Z13	T50.Z14	T50.Z15	T50.Z16
diphtheria	T50.Z11	T50.Z12	T50.Z13	T50.Z14	T50.Z15	T50.Z16
gas gangrene	T50.Z11	T50.Z12	T50.Z13	T50.Z14	T50.Z15	T50.Z16
tetanus	T50.Z11	T50.Z12	T50.Z13	T50.Z14	T50.Z15	T50.Z16
Antitrichomonal drug	T37.3X1	T37.3X2	T37.3X3	T37.3X4	T37.3X5	T37.3X6
Antituberculars	T37.1X1	T37.1X2	T37.1X3	T37.1X4	T37.1X5	T37.1X6
antibiotics	T36.5X1	T36.5X2	T36.5X3	T36.5X4	T36.5X5	T36.5X6
Antitussive NEC	T48.3X1	T48.3X2	T48.3X3	T48.3X4	T48.3X5	T48.3X6
codeine mixture	T40.2X1	T40.2X2	T40.2X3	T40.2X4	T40.2X5	T40.2X6
opiate	T40.2X1	T40.2X2	T40.2X3	T40.2X4	T40.2X5	T40.2X6
Antivaricose drug	T46.8X1	T46.8X2	T46.8X3	T46.8X4	T46.8X5	T46.8X6
Antivenin, antivenom (sera)	T50.Z11	T50.Z12	T50.Z13	T50.Z14	T50.Z15	T50.Z16
crotaline	T50.Z11	T50.Z12	T50.Z13	T50.Z14	T50.Z15	T50.Z16
spider bite	T50.Z11	T50.Z12	T50.Z13	T50.Z14	T50.Z15	T50.Z16
Antivertigo drug	T45.0X1	T45.0X2	T45.0X3	T45.0X4	T45.0X5	T45.0X6
Antiviral drug NEC	T37.5X1	T37.5X2	T37.5X3	T37.5X4	T37.5X5	T37.5X6
eye	T49.5X1	T49.5X2	T49.5X3	T49.5X4	T49.5X5	T49.5X6
Antiwhipworm drug	T37.4X1	T37.4X2	T37.4X3	T37.4X4	T37.4X5	T37.4X6
Ant poison — *see* Insecticide						
Antrol — *see also* by specific chemical substance	T60.91	T60.92	T60.93	T60.94	—	—
fungicide	T60.91	T60.92	T60.93	T60.94	—	—
ANTU (alpha naphthylthiourea)	T60.4X1	T60.4X2	T60.4X3	T60.4X4	—	—
Apalcillin	T36.0X1	T36.0X2	T36.0X3	T36.0X4	T36.0X5	T36.0X6
APC	T48.5X1	T48.5X2	T48.5X3	T48.5X4	T48.5X5	T48.5X6
Aplonidine	T44.4X1	T44.4X2	T44.4X3	T44.4X4	T44.4X5	T44.4X6
Apomorphine	T47.7X1	T47.7X2	T47.7X3	T47.7X4	T47.7X5	T47.7X6
Appetite depressants, central	T50.5X1	T50.5X2	T50.5X3	T50.5X4	T50.5X5	T50.5X6
Apraclonidine (hydrochloride)	T44.4X1	T44.4X2	T44.4X3	T44.4X4	T44.4X5	T44.4X6
Apresoline	T46.5X1	T46.5X2	T46.5X3	T46.5X4	T46.5X5	T46.5X6
Aprindine	T46.2X1	T46.2X2	T46.2X3	T46.2X4	T46.2X5	T46.2X6
Aprobarbital	T42.3X1	T42.3X2	T42.3X3	T42.3X4	T42.3X5	T42.3X6
Apronalide	T42.6X1	T42.6X2	T42.6X3	T42.6X4	T42.6X5	T42.6X6
Aprotinin	T45.621	T45.622	T45.623	T45.624	T45.625	T45.626
Aptocaine	T41.3X1	T41.3X2	T41.3X3	T41.3X4	T41.3X5	T41.3X6
Aqua fortis	T54.2X1	T54.2X2	T54.2X3	T54.2X4	—	—
Ara-A	T37.5X1	T37.5X2	T37.5X3	T37.5X4	T37.5X5	T37.5X6
Ara-C	T45.1X1	T45.1X2	T45.1X3	T45.1X4	T45.1X5	T45.1X6
Arachis oil	T49.3X1	T49.3X2	T49.3X3	T49.3X4	T49.3X5	T49.3X6
cathartic	T47.4X1	T47.4X2	T47.4X3	T47.4X4	T47.4X5	T47.4X6
Aralen	T37.2X1	T37.2X2	T37.2X3	T37.2X4	T37.2X5	T37.2X6
Arecoline	T44.1X1	T44.1X2	T44.1X3	T44.1X4	T44.1X5	T44.1X6
Arginine	T50.991	T50.992	T50.993	T50.994	T50.995	T50.996
glutamate	T50.991	T50.992	T50.993	T50.994	T50.995	T50.996
Argyrol	T49.0X1	T49.0X2	T49.0X3	T49.0X4	T49.0X5	T49.0X6
ENT agent	T49.6X1	T49.6X2	T49.6X3	T49.6X4	T49.6X5	T49.6X6

Substance	Poisoning, Accidental (unintentional)	Poisoning, Intentional Self-harm	Poisoning, Assault	Poisoning, Undetermined	Adverse Effect	Under-dosing
Argyrol — continued						
ophthalmic preparation	T49.5X1	T49.5X2	T49.5X3	T49.5X4	T49.5X5	T49.5X6
Aristocort	T38.0X1	T38.0X2	T38.0X3	T38.0X4	T38.0X5	T38.0X6
ENT agent	T49.6X1	T49.6X2	T49.6X3	T49.6X4	T49.6X5	T49.6X6
ophthalmic preparation	T49.5X1	T49.5X2	T49.5X3	T49.5X4	T49.5X5	T49.5X6
topical NEC	T49.0X1	T49.0X2	T49.0X3	T49.0X4	T49.0X5	T49.0X6
Aromatics, corrosive	T54.1X1	T54.1X2	T54.1X3	T54.1X4	—	—
disinfectants	T54.1X1	T54.1X2	T54.1X3	T54.1X4	—	—
Arsenate of lead	T57.0X1	T57.0X2	T57.0X3	T57.0X4	—	—
herbicide	T57.0X1	T57.0X2	T57.0X3	T57.0X4	—	—
Arsenic, arsenicals (compounds) (dust) (vapor) **NEC**	T57.0X1	T57.0X2	T57.0X3	T57.0X4	—	—
anti-infectives	T37.8X1	T37.8X2	T37.8X3	T37.8X4	T37.8X5	T37.8X6
pesticide (dust) (fumes)	T57.0X1	T57.0X2	T57.0X3	T57.0X4	—	—
Arsine (gas)	T57.0X1	T57.0X2	T57.0X3	T57.0X4	—	—
Arsphenamine (silver)	T37.8X1	T37.8X2	T37.8X3	T37.8X4	T37.8X5	T37.8X6
Arsthinol	T37.3X1	T37.3X2	T37.3X3	T37.3X4	T37.3X5	T37.3X6
Artane	T44.3X1	T44.3X2	T44.3X3	T44.3X4	T44.3X5	T44.3X6
Arthropod (venomous) **NEC**	T63.481	T63.482	T63.483	T63.484	—	—
Articaine	T41.3X1	T41.3X2	T41.3X3	T41.3X4	T41.3X5	T41.3X6
Asbestos	T57.8X1	T57.8X2	T57.8X3	T57.8X4	—	—
Ascaridole	T37.4X1	T37.4X2	T37.4X3	T37.4X4	T37.4X5	T37.4X6
Ascorbic acid	T45.2X1	T45.2X2	T45.2X3	T45.2X4	T45.2X5	T45.2X6
Asiaticoside	T49.0X1	T49.0X2	T49.0X3	T49.0X4	T49.0X5	T49.0X6
Asparaginase	T45.1X1	T45.1X2	T45.1X3	T45.1X4	T45.1X5	T45.1X6
Aspidium (oleoresin)	T37.4X1	T37.4X2	T37.4X3	T37.4X4	T37.4X5	T37.4X6
Aspirin (aluminum) (soluble)	T39.011	T39.012	T39.013	T39.014	T39.015	T39.016
Aspoxicillin	T36.0X1	T36.0X2	T36.0X3	T36.0X4	T36.0X5	T36.0X6
Astemizole	T45.0X1	T45.0X2	T45.0X3	T45.0X4	T45.0X5	T45.0X6
Astringent (local)	T49.2X1	T49.2X2	T49.2X3	T49.2X4	T49.2X5	T49.2X6
specified NEC	T49.2X1	T49.2X2	T49.2X3	T49.2X4	T49.2X5	T49.2X6
Astromicin	T36.5X1	T36.5X2	T36.5X3	T36.5X4	T36.5X5	T36.5X6
Ataractic drug NEC	T43.501	T43.502	T43.503	T43.504	T43.505	T43.506
Atenolol	T44.7X1	T44.7X2	T44.7X3	T44.7X4	T44.7X5	T44.7X6
Atonia drug, intestinal	T47.4X1	T47.4X2	T47.4X3	T47.4X4	T47.4X5	T47.4X6
Atophan	T50.4X1	T50.4X2	T50.4X3	T50.4X4	T50.4X5	T50.4X6
Atracurium besilate	T48.1X1	T48.1X2	T48.1X3	T48.1X4	T48.1X5	T48.1X6
Atropine	T44.3X1	T44.3X2	T44.3X3	T44.3X4	T44.3X5	T44.3X6
derivative	T44.3X1	T44.3X2	T44.3X3	T44.3X4	T44.3X5	T44.3X6
methonitrate	T44.3X1	T44.3X2	T44.3X3	T44.3X4	T44.3X5	T44.3X6
Attapulgite	T47.6X1	T47.6X2	T47.6X3	T47.6X4	T47.6X5	T47.6X6
Auramine	T65.891	T65.892	T65.893	T65.894	—	—
dye	T65.6X1	T65.6X2	T65.6X3	T65.6X4	—	—
fungicide	T60.3X1	T60.3X2	T60.3X3	T60.3X4	—	—
Auranofin	T39.4X1	T39.4X2	T39.4X3	T39.4X4	T39.4X5	T39.4X6
Aurantiin	T46.991	T46.992	T46.993	T46.994	T46.995	T46.996
Aureomycin	T36.4X1	T36.4X2	T36.4X3	T36.4X4	T36.4X5	T36.4X6
ophthalmic preparation	T49.5X1	T49.5X2	T49.5X3	T49.5X4	T49.5X5	T49.5X6
topical NEC	T49.0X1	T49.0X2	T49.0X3	T49.0X4	T49.0X5	T49.0X6
Aurothioglucose	T39.4X1	T39.4X2	T39.4X3	T39.4X4	T39.4X5	T39.4X6
Aurothioglycanide	T39.4X1	T39.4X2	T39.4X3	T39.4X4	T39.4X5	T39.4X6
Aurothiomalate sodium	T39.4X1	T39.4X2	T39.4X3	T39.4X4	T39.4X5	T39.4X6
Aurotioprol	T39.4X1	T39.4X2	T39.4X3	T39.4X4	T39.4X5	T39.4X6
Automobile fuel	T52.0X1	T52.0X2	T52.0X3	T52.0X4	—	—
Autonomic nervous system agent NEC	T44.901	T44.902	T44.903	T44.904	T44.905	T44.906
Avlosulfon	T37.1X1	T37.1X2	T37.1X3	T37.1X4	T37.1X5	T37.1X6
Avomine	T42.6X1	T42.6X2	T42.6X3	T42.6X4	T42.6X5	T42.6X6
Axerophthol	T45.2X1	T45.2X2	T45.2X3	T45.2X4	T45.2X5	T45.2X6
Azacitidine	T45.1X1	T45.1X2	T45.1X3	T45.1X4	T45.1X5	T45.1X6
Azacyclonol	T43.591	T43.592	T43.593	T43.594	T43.595	T43.596
Azadirachta	T60.2X1	T60.2X2	T60.2X3	T60.2X4	—	—
Azanidazole	T37.3X1	T37.3X2	T37.3X3	T37.3X4	T37.3X5	T37.3X6
Azapetine	T46.7X1	T46.7X2	T46.7X3	T46.7X4	T46.7X5	T46.7X6
Azapropazone	T39.2X1	T39.2X2	T39.2X3	T39.2X4	T39.2X5	T39.2X6
Azaribine	T45.1X1	T45.1X2	T45.1X3	T45.1X4	T45.1X5	T45.1X6
Azaserine	T45.1X1	T45.1X2	T45.1X3	T45.1X4	T45.1X5	T45.1X6
Azatadine	T45.0X1	T45.0X2	T45.0X3	T45.0X4	T45.0X5	T45.0X6
Azatepa	T45.1X1	T45.1X2	T45.1X3	T45.1X4	T45.1X5	T45.1X6
Azathioprine	T45.1X1	T45.1X2	T45.1X3	T45.1X4	T45.1X5	T45.1X6
Azelaic acid	T49.0X1	T49.0X2	T49.0X3	T49.0X4	T49.0X5	T49.0X6
Azelastine	T45.0X1	T45.0X2	T45.0X3	T45.0X4	T45.0X5	T45.0X6
Azidocillin	T36.0X1	T36.0X2	T36.0X3	T36.0X4	T36.0X5	T36.0X6
Azidothymidine	T37.5X1	T37.5X2	T37.5X3	T37.5X4	T37.5X5	T37.5X6
Azinphos (ethyl) (methyl)	T60.0X1	T60.0X2	T60.0X3	T60.0X4	—	—
Aziridine (chelating)	T54.1X1	T54.1X2	T54.1X3	T54.1X4	—	—
Azithromycin	T36.3X1	T36.3X2	T36.3X3	T36.3X4	T36.3X5	T36.3X6
Azlocillin	T36.0X1	T36.0X2	T36.0X3	T36.0X4	T36.0X5	T36.0X6
Azobenzene smoke	T65.3X1	T65.3X2	T65.3X3	T65.3X4	—	—
acaricide	T60.8X1	T60.8X2	T60.8X3	T60.8X4	—	—
Azosulfamide	T37.0X1	T37.0X2	T37.0X3	T37.0X4	T37.0X5	T37.0X6
AZT	T37.5X1	T37.5X2	T37.5X3	T37.5X4	T37.5X5	T37.5X6
Aztreonam	T36.1X1	T36.1X2	T36.1X3	T36.1X4	T36.1X5	T36.1X6

Substance	Poisoning, Accidental (unintentional)	Poisoning, Intentional Self-harm	Poisoning, Assault	Poisoning, Undetermined	Adverse Effect	Under-dosing
Azulfidine	T37.0X1	T37.0X2	T37.0X3	T37.0X4	T37.0X5	T37.0X6
Azuresin	T50.8X1	T50.8X2	T50.8X3	T50.8X4	T50.8X5	T50.8X6
b-acetyldigoxin	T46.0X1	T46.0X2	T46.0X3	T46.0X4	T46.0X5	T46.0X6
P-Acetamidophenol	T39.1X1	T39.1X2	T39.1X3	T39.1X4	T39.1X5	T39.1X6
Bacampicillin	T36.0X1	T36.0X2	T36.0X3	T36.0X4	T36.0X5	T36.0X6
Bacillus						
lactobacillus	T47.8X1	T47.8X2	T47.8X3	T47.8X4	T47.8X5	T47.8X6
subtilis	T47.6X1	T47.6X2	T47.6X3	T47.6X4	T47.6X5	T47.6X6
Bacimycin	T49.0X1	T49.0X2	T49.0X3	T49.0X4	T49.0X5	T49.0X6
ophthalmic preparation	T49.5X1	T49.5X2	T49.5X3	T49.5X4	T49.5X5	T49.5X6
Bacitracin zinc	T49.0X1	T49.0X2	T49.0X3	T49.0X4	T49.0X5	T49.0X6
with neomycin	T49.0X1	T49.0X2	T49.0X3	T49.0X4	T49.0X5	T49.0X6
ENT agent	T49.6X1	T49.6X2	T49.6X3	T49.6X4	T49.6X5	T49.6X6
ophthalmic preparation	T49.5X1	T49.5X2	T49.5X3	T49.5X4	T49.5X5	T49.5X6
topical NEC	T49.0X1	T49.0X2	T49.0X3	T49.0X4	T49.0X5	T49.0X6
Baclofen	T42.8X1	T42.8X2	T42.8X3	T42.8X4	T42.8X5	T42.8X6
Baking soda	T50.991	T50.992	T50.993	T50.994	T50.995	T50.996
BAL	T45.8X1	T45.8X2	T45.8X3	T45.8X4	T45.8X5	T45.8X6
Bambuterol	T48.6X1	T48.6X2	T48.6X3	T48.6X4	T48.6X5	T48.6X6
Bamethan (sulfate)	T46.7X1	T46.7X2	T46.7X3	T46.7X4	T46.7X5	T46.7X6
Bamifylline	T48.6X1	T48.6X2	T48.6X3	T48.6X4	T48.6X5	T48.6X6
Bamipine	T45.0X1	T45.0X2	T45.0X3	T45.0X4	T45.0X5	T45.0X6
Baneberry — see Actaea spicata						
Banewort — see Belladonna						
Barbenyl	T42.3X1	T42.3X2	T42.3X3	T42.3X4	T42.3X5	T42.3X6
Barbexaclone	T42.6X1	T42.6X2	T42.6X3	T42.6X4	T42.6X5	T42.6X6
Barbital	T42.3X1	T42.3X2	T42.3X3	T42.3X4	T42.3X5	T42.3X6
sodium	T42.3X1	T42.3X2	T42.3X3	T42.3X4	T42.3X5	T42.3X6
Barbitone	T42.3X1	T42.3X2	T42.3X3	T42.3X4	T42.3X5	T42.3X6
Barbiturate NEC	T42.3X1	T42.3X2	T42.3X3	T42.3X4	T42.3X5	T42.3X6
with tranquilizer	T42.3X1	T42.3X2	T42.3X3	T42.3X4	T42.3X5	T42.3X6
anesthetic (intravenous)	T41.1X1	T41.1X2	T41.1X3	T41.1X4	T41.1X5	T41.1X6
Barium (carbonate) (chloride) (sulfite)	T57.8X1	T57.8X2	T57.8X3	T57.8X4	—	—
diagnostic agent	T50.8X1	T50.8X2	T50.8X3	T50.8X4	T50.8X5	T50.8X6
pesticide	T60.4X1	T60.4X2	T60.4X3	T60.4X4	—	—
rodenticide	T60.4X1	T60.4X2	T60.4X3	T60.4X4	—	—
sulfate (medicinal)	T50.8X1	T50.8X2	T50.8X3	T50.8X4	T50.8X5	T50.8X6
Barrier cream	T49.3X1	T49.3X2	T49.3X3	T49.3X4	T49.3X5	T49.3X6
Basic fuchsin	T49.0X1	T49.0X2	T49.0X3	T49.0X4	T49.0X5	T49.0X6
Battery acid or fluid	T54.2X1	T54.2X2	T54.2X3	T54.2X4	—	—
Bay rum	T51.8X1	T51.8X2	T51.8X3	T51.8X4	—	—
b-benzalbutyramide	T46.6X1	T46.6X2	T46.6X3	T46.6X4	T46.6X5	T46.6X6
BCG (vaccine)	T50.A91	T50.A92	T50.A93	T50.A94	T50.A95	T50.A96
BCNU	T45.1X1	T45.1X2	T45.1X3	T45.1X4	T45.1X5	T45.1X6
Bearsfoot	T62.2X1	T62.2X2	T62.2X3	T62.2X4	—	—
Beclamide	T42.6X1	T42.6X2	T42.6X3	T42.6X4	T42.6X5	T42.6X6
Beclomethasone	T44.5X1	T44.5X2	T44.5X3	T44.5X4	T44.5X5	T44.5X6
Bee (sting) (venom)	T63.441	T63.442	T63.443	T63.444	—	—
Befunolol	T49.5X1	T49.5X2	T49.5X3	T49.5X4	T49.5X5	T49.5X6
Bekanamycin	T36.5X1	T36.5X2	T36.5X3	T36.5X4	T36.5X5	T36.5X6
Belladonna — see also Nightshade						
alkaloids	T44.3X1	T44.3X2	T44.3X3	T44.3X4	T44.3X5	T44.3X6
extract	T44.3X1	T44.3X2	T44.3X3	T44.3X4	T44.3X5	T44.3X6
herb	T44.3X1	T44.3X2	T44.3X3	T44.3X4	T44.3X5	T44.3X6
Bemegride	T50.7X1	T50.7X2	T50.7X3	T50.7X4	T50.7X5	T50.7X6
Benactyzine	T44.3X1	T44.3X2	T44.3X3	T44.3X4	T44.3X5	T44.3X6
Benadryl	T45.0X1	T45.0X2	T45.0X3	T45.0X4	T45.0X5	T45.0X6
Benaprizine	T44.3X1	T44.3X2	T44.3X3	T44.3X4	T44.3X5	T44.3X6
Benazepril	T46.4X1	T46.4X2	T46.4X3	T46.4X4	T46.4X5	T46.4X6
Bencyclane	T46.7X1	T46.7X2	T46.7X3	T46.7X4	T46.7X5	T46.7X6
Bendazol	T46.3X1	T46.3X2	T46.3X3	T46.3X4	T46.3X5	T46.3X6
Bendrofluazide	T50.2X1	T50.2X2	T50.2X3	T50.2X4	T50.2X5	T50.2X6
Bendroflumethiazide	T50.2X1	T50.2X2	T50.2X3	T50.2X4	T50.2X5	T50.2X6
Benemid	T50.4X1	T50.4X2	T50.4X3	T50.4X4	T50.4X5	T50.4X6
Benethamine penicillin	T36.0X1	T36.0X2	T36.0X3	T36.0X4	T36.0X5	T36.0X6
Benexate	T47.1X1	T47.1X2	T47.1X3	T47.1X4	T47.1X5	T47.1X6
Benfluorex	T46.6X1	T46.6X2	T46.6X3	T46.6X4	T46.6X5	T46.6X6
Benfotiamine	T45.2X1	T45.2X2	T45.2X3	T45.2X4	T45.2X5	T45.2X6
Benisone	T49.0X1	T49.0X2	T49.0X3	T49.0X4	T49.0X5	T49.0X6
Benomyl	T60.0X1	T60.0X2	T60.0X3	T60.0X4	—	—
Benoquin	T49.8X1	T49.8X2	T49.8X3	T49.8X4	T49.8X5	T49.8X6
Benoxinate	T41.3X1	T41.3X2	T41.3X3	T41.3X4	T41.3X5	T41.3X6
Benperidol	T43.4X1	T43.4X2	T43.4X3	T43.4X4	T43.4X5	T43.4X6
Benproperine	T48.3X1	T48.3X2	T48.3X3	T48.3X4	T48.3X5	T48.3X6
Benserazide	T42.8X1	T42.8X2	T42.8X3	T42.8X4	T42.8X5	T42.8X6
Bentazepam	T42.4X1	T42.4X2	T42.4X3	T42.4X4	T42.4X5	T42.4X6
Bentiromide	T50.8X1	T50.8X2	T50.8X3	T50.8X4	T50.8X5	T50.8X6
Bentonite	T49.3X1	T49.3X2	T49.3X3	T49.3X4	T49.3X5	T49.3X6
Benzalbutyramide	T46.6X1	T46.6X2	T46.6X3	T46.6X4	T46.6X5	T46.6X6
Benzalkonium (chloride)	T49.0X1	T49.0X2	T49.0X3	T49.0X4	T49.0X5	T49.0X6
ophthalmic preparation	T49.5X1	T49.5X2	T49.5X3	T49.5X4	T49.5X5	T49.5X6

Additional Character May Be Required — Refer to the Tabular List for Character Selection   ▽ **Subterms under main terms may continue to next column or page**

Substance	Poisoning, Accidental (unintentional)	Poisoning, Intentional Self-harm	Poisoning, Assault	Poisoning, Undetermined	Adverse Effect	Under-dosing
Benzamidosalicylate (calcium)	T37.1X1	T37.1X2	T37.1X3	T37.1X4	T37.1X5	T37.1X6
Benzamine	T41.3X1	T41.3X2	T41.3X3	T41.3X4	T41.3X5	T41.3X6
lactate	T49.1X1	T49.1X2	T49.1X3	T49.1X4	T49.1X5	T49.1X6
Benzamphetamine	T50.5X1	T50.5X2	T50.5X3	T50.5X4	T50.5X5	T50.5X6
Benzapril hydrochloride	T46.5X1	T46.5X2	T46.5X3	T46.5X4	T46.5X5	T46.5X6
Benzathine benzylpenicillin	T36.0X1	T36.0X2	T36.0X3	T36.0X4	T36.0X5	T36.0X6
Benzathine penicillin	T36.0X1	T36.0X2	T36.0X3	T36.0X4	T36.0X5	T36.0X6
Benzatropine	T42.8X1	T42.8X2	T42.8X3	T42.8X4	T42.8X5	T42.8X6
Benzbromarone	T50.4X1	T50.4X2	T50.4X3	T50.4X4	T50.4X5	T50.4X6
Benzcarbimine	T45.1X1	T45.1X2	T45.1X3	T45.1X4	T45.1X5	T45.1X6
Benzedrex	T44.991	T44.992	T44.993	T44.994	T44.995	T44.996
Benzedrine (amphetamine)	T43.621	T43.622	T43.623	T43.624	T43.625	T43.626
Benzenamine	T65.3X1	T65.3X2	T65.3X3	T65.3X4	—	—
Benzene	T52.1X1	T52.1X2	T52.1X3	T52.1X4	—	—
homologues (acetyl) (dimethyl) (methyl) (solvent)	T52.2X1	T52.2X2	T52.2X3	T52.2X4	—	—
Benzethonium (chloride)	T49.0X1	T49.0X2	T49.0X3	T49.0X4	T49.0X5	T49.0X6
Benzfetamine	T50.5X1	T50.5X2	T50.5X3	T50.5X4	T50.5X5	T50.5X6
Benzhexol	T44.3X1	T44.3X2	T44.3X3	T44.3X4	T44.3X5	T44.3X6
Benzhydramine (chloride)	T45.0X1	T45.0X2	T45.0X3	T45.0X4	T45.0X5	T45.0X6
Benzidine	T65.891	T65.892	T65.893	T65.894	—	—
Benzilonium bromide	T44.3X1	T44.3X2	T44.3X3	T44.3X4	T44.3X5	T44.3X6
Benzimidazole	T60.3X1	T60.3X2	T60.3X3	T60.3X4	—	—
Benzin (e) — see Ligroin						
Benziodarone	T46.3X1	T46.3X2	T46.3X3	T46.3X4	T46.3X5	T46.3X6
Benznidazole	T37.3X1	T37.3X2	T37.3X3	T37.3X4	T37.3X5	T37.3X6
Benzocaine	T41.3X1	T41.3X2	T41.3X3	T41.3X4	T41.3X5	T41.3X6
Benzodiapin	T42.4X1	T42.4X2	T42.4X3	T42.4X4	T42.4X5	T42.4X6
Benzodiazepine NEC	T42.4X1	T42.4X2	T42.4X3	T42.4X4	T42.4X5	T42.4X6
Benzoic acid	T49.0X1	T49.0X2	T49.0X3	T49.0X4	T49.0X5	T49.0X6
with salicylic acid	T49.0X1	T49.0X2	T49.0X3	T49.0X4	T49.0X5	T49.0X6
Benzoin (tincture)	T48.5X1	T48.5X2	T48.5X3	T48.5X4	T48.5X5	T48.5X6
Benzol (benzene)	T52.1X1	T52.1X2	T52.1X3	T52.1X4	—	—
vapor	T52.0X1	T52.0X2	T52.0X3	T52.0X4	—	—
Benzomorphan	T40.2X1	T40.2X2	T40.2X3	T40.2X4	T40.2X5	T40.2X6
Benzonatate	T48.3X1	T48.3X2	T48.3X3	T48.3X4	T48.3X5	T48.3X6
Benzophenones	T49.3X1	T49.3X2	T49.3X3	T49.3X4	T49.3X5	T49.3X6
Benzopyrone	T46.991	T46.992	T46.993	T46.994	T46.995	T46.996
Benzothiadiazides	T50.2X1	T50.2X2	T50.2X3	T50.2X4	T50.2X5	T50.2X6
Benzoxonium chloride	T49.0X1	T49.0X2	T49.0X3	T49.0X4	T49.0X5	T49.0X6
Benzoylpas calcium	T37.1X1	T37.1X2	T37.1X3	T37.1X4	T37.1X5	T37.1X6
Benzoyl peroxide	T49.0X1	T49.0X2	T49.0X3	T49.0X4	T49.0X5	T49.0X6
Benzperidin	T43.591	T43.592	T43.593	T43.594	T43.595	T43.596
Benzperidol	T43.591	T43.592	T43.593	T43.594	T43.595	T43.596
Benzphetamine	T50.5X1	T50.5X2	T50.5X3	T50.5X4	T50.5X5	T50.5X6
Benzpyrinium bromide	T44.1X1	T44.1X2	T44.1X3	T44.1X4	T44.1X5	T44.1X6
Benzquinamide	T45.0X1	T45.0X2	T45.0X3	T45.0X4	T45.0X5	T45.0X6
Benzthiazide	T50.2X1	T50.2X2	T50.2X3	T50.2X4	T50.2X5	T50.2X6
Benztropine						
anticholinergic	T44.3X1	T44.3X2	T44.3X3	T44.3X4	T44.3X5	T44.3X6
antiparkinson	T42.8X1	T42.8X2	T42.8X3	T42.8X4	T42.8X5	T42.8X6
Benzydamine	T49.0X1	T49.0X2	T49.0X3	T49.0X4	T49.0X5	T49.0X6
Benzyl						
acetate	T52.8X1	T52.8X2	T52.8X3	T52.8X4	—	—
alcohol	T49.0X1	T49.0X2	T49.0X3	T49.0X4	T49.0X5	T49.0X6
benzoate	T49.0X1	T49.0X2	T49.0X3	T49.0X4	T49.0X5	T49.0X6
Benzoic acid	T49.0X1	T49.0X2	T49.0X3	T49.0X4	T49.0X5	T49.0X6
morphine	T40.2X1	T40.2X2	T40.2X3	T40.2X4	—	—
nicotinate	T46.6X1	T46.6X2	T46.6X3	T46.6X4	T46.6X5	T46.6X6
penicillin	T36.0X1	T36.0X2	T36.0X3	T36.0X4	T36.0X5	T36.0X6
Benzylhydrochlorthiazide	T50.2X1	T50.2X2	T50.2X3	T50.2X4	T50.2X5	T50.2X6
Benzylpenicillin	T36.0X1	T36.0X2	T36.0X3	T36.0X4	T36.0X5	T36.0X6
Benzylthiouracil	T38.2X1	T38.2X2	T38.2X3	T38.2X4	T38.2X5	T38.2X6
Bephenium	T37.4X1	T37.4X2	T37.4X3	T37.4X4	T37.4X5	T37.4X6
hydroxynaphthoate						
Bepridil	T46.1X1	T46.1X2	T46.1X3	T46.1X4	T46.1X5	T46.1X6
Bergamot oil	T65.891	T65.892	T65.893	T65.894	—	—
Bergapten	T50.991	T50.992	T50.993	T50.994	T50.995	T50.996
Berries, poisonous	T62.1X1	T62.1X2	T62.1X3	T62.1X4	—	—
Beryllium (compounds)	T56.7X1	T56.7X2	T56.7X3	T56.7X4	—	—
beta adrenergic blocking agent, heart	T44.7X1	T44.7X2	T44.7X3	T44.7X4	T44.7X5	T44.7X6
Betacarotene	T45.2X1	T45.2X2	T45.2X3	T45.2X4	T45.2X5	T45.2X6
Beta-Chlor	T42.6X1	T42.6X2	T42.6X3	T42.6X4	T42.6X5	T42.6X6
Betahistine	T46.7X1	T46.7X2	T46.7X3	T46.7X4	T46.7X5	T46.7X6
Betaine	T47.5X1	T47.5X2	T47.5X3	T47.5X4	T47.5X5	T47.5X6
Betamethasone	T49.0X1	T49.0X2	T49.0X3	T49.0X4	T49.0X5	T49.0X6
topical	T49.0X1	T49.0X2	T49.0X3	T49.0X4	T49.0X5	T49.0X6
Betamicin	T36.8X1	T36.8X2	T36.8X3	T36.8X4	T36.8X5	T36.8X6
Betanidine	T46.5X1	T46.5X2	T46.5X3	T46.5X4	T46.5X5	T46.5X6
Betaxolol	T44.7X1	T44.7X2	T44.7X3	T44.7X4	T44.7X5	T44.7X6

Substance	Poisoning, Accidental (unintentional)	Poisoning, Intentional Self-harm	Poisoning, Assault	Poisoning, Undetermined	Adverse Effect	Under-dosing
Betazole	T50.8X1	T50.8X2	T50.8X3	T50.8X4	T50.8X5	T50.8X6
Bethanechol	T44.1X1	T44.1X2	T44.1X3	T44.1X4	T44.1X5	T44.1X6
chloride	T44.1X1	T44.1X2	T44.1X3	T44.1X4	T44.1X5	T44.1X6
Bethanidine	T46.5X1	T46.5X2	T46.5X3	T46.5X4	T46.5X5	T46.5X6
Betoxycaine	T41.3X1	T41.3X2	T41.3X3	T41.3X4	T41.3X5	T41.3X6
Betula oil	T49.3X1	T49.3X2	T49.3X3	T49.3X4	T49.3X5	T49.3X6
Bevantolol	T44.7X1	T44.7X2	T44.7X3	T44.7X4	T44.7X5	T44.7X6
Bevonium metilsulfate	T44.3X1	T44.3X2	T44.3X3	T44.3X4	T44.3X5	T44.3X6
Bezafibrate	T46.6X1	T46.6X2	T46.6X3	T46.6X4	T46.6X5	T46.6X6
Bezitramide	T40.4X1	T40.4X2	T40.4X3	T40.4X4	T40.4X5	T40.4X6
BHA	T50.991	T50.992	T50.993	T50.994	T50.995	T50.996
Bhang	T40.7X1	T40.7X2	T40.7X3	T40.7X4	T40.7X5	T40.7X6
BHC (medicinal)	T49.0X1	T49.0X2	T49.0X3	T49.0X4	T49.0X5	T49.0X6
nonmedicinal (vapor)	T53.6X1	T53.6X2	T53.6X3	T53.6X4	—	—
Bialamicol	T37.3X1	T37.3X2	T37.3X3	T37.3X4	T37.3X5	T37.3X6
Bibenzonium bromide	T48.3X1	T48.3X2	T48.3X3	T48.3X4	T48.3X5	T48.3X6
Bibrocathol	T49.5X1	T49.5X2	T49.5X3	T49.5X4	T49.5X5	T49.5X6
Bichloride of mercury — see Mercury, chloride						
Bichromates (calcium) (potassium)(sodium) (crystals)	T57.8X1	T57.8X2	T57.8X3	T57.8X4		
fumes	T56.2X1	T56.2X2	T56.2X3	T56.2X4	—	—
Biclotymol	T49.6X1	T49.6X2	T49.6X3	T49.6X4	T49.6X5	T49.6X6
Bicucculine	T50.7X1	T50.7X2	T50.7X3	T50.7X4	T50.7X5	T50.7X6
Bifemelane	T43.291	T43.292	T43.293	T43.294	T43.295	T43.296
Biguanide derivatives, oral	T38.3X1	T38.3X2	T38.3X3	T38.3X4	T38.3X5	T38.3X6
Bile salts	T47.5X1	T47.5X2	T47.5X3	T47.5X4	T47.5X5	T47.5X6
Biligrafin	T50.8X1	T50.8X2	T50.8X3	T50.8X4	T50.8X5	T50.8X6
Bilopaque	T50.8X1	T50.8X2	T50.8X3	T50.8X4	T50.8X5	T50.8X6
Binifibrate	T46.6X1	T46.6X2	T46.6X3	T46.6X4	T46.6X5	T46.6X6
Binitrobenzol	T65.3X1	T65.3X2	T65.3X3	T65.3X4	—	—
Bioflavonoid(s)	T46.991	T46.992	T46.993	T46.994	T46.995	T46.996
Biological substance NEC	T50.901	T50.902	T50.903	T50.904	T50.905	T50.906
Biotin	T45.2X1	T45.2X2	T45.2X3	T45.2X4	T45.2X5	T45.2X6
Biperiden	T44.3X1	T44.3X2	T44.3X3	T44.3X4	T44.3X5	T44.3X6
Bisacodyl	T47.2X1	T47.2X2	T47.2X3	T47.2X4	T47.2X5	T47.2X6
Bisbentiamine	T45.2X1	T45.2X2	T45.2X3	T45.2X4	T45.2X5	T45.2X6
Bisbutiamine	T45.2X1	T45.2X2	T45.2X3	T45.2X4	T45.2X5	T45.2X6
Bisdequalinium (salts) (diacetate)	T49.6X1	T49.6X2	T49.6X3	T49.6X4	T49.6X5	T49.6X6
Bishydroxycoumarin	T45.511	T45.512	T45.513	T45.514	T45.515	T45.516
Bismarsen	T37.8X1	T37.8X2	T37.8X3	T37.8X4	T37.8X5	T37.8X6
Bismuth salts	T47.6X1	T47.6X2	T47.6X3	T47.6X4	T47.6X5	T47.6X6
aluminate	T47.1X1	T47.1X2	T47.1X3	T47.1X4	T47.1X5	T47.1X6
anti-infectives	T37.8X1	T37.8X2	T37.8X3	T37.8X4	T37.8X5	T37.8X6
formic iodide	T49.0X1	T49.0X2	T49.0X3	T49.0X4	T49.0X5	T49.0X6
glycolylarsenate	T49.0X1	T49.0X2	T49.0X3	T49.0X4	T49.0X5	T49.0X6
nonmedicinal (compounds) NEC	T65.91	T65.92	T65.93	T65.94	—	—
subcarbonate	T47.6X1	T47.6X2	T47.6X3	T47.6X4	T47.6X5	T47.6X6
subsalicylate	T37.8X1	T37.8X2	T37.8X3	T37.8X4	T37.8X5	T37.8X6
sulfarsphenamine	T37.8X1	T37.8X2	T37.8X3	T37.8X4	T37.8X5	T37.8X6
Bisoprolol	T44.7X1	T44.7X2	T44.7X3	T44.7X4	T44.7X5	T44.7X6
Bisoxatin	T47.2X1	T47.2X2	T47.2X3	T47.2X4	T47.2X5	T47.2X6
Bisulepin (hydrochloride)	T45.0X1	T45.0X2	T45.0X3	T45.0X4	T45.0X5	T45.0X6
Bithionol	T37.8X1	T37.8X2	T37.8X3	T37.8X4	T37.8X5	T37.8X6
anthelminthic	T37.4X1	T37.4X2	T37.4X3	T37.4X4	T37.4X5	T37.4X6
Bitolterol	T48.6X1	T48.6X2	T48.6X3	T48.6X4	T48.6X5	T48.6X6
Bitoscanate	T37.4X1	T37.4X2	T37.4X3	T37.4X4	T37.4X5	T37.4X6
Bitter almond oil	T62.8X1	T62.8X2	T62.8X3	T62.8X4	—	—
Bittersweet	T62.2X1	T62.2X2	T62.2X3	T62.2X4	—	—
Black						
flag	T60.91	T60.92	T60.93	T60.94	—	—
henbane	T62.2X1	T62.2X2	T62.2X3	T62.2X4	—	—
leaf (40)	T60.91	T60.92	T60.93	T60.94	—	—
widow spider (bite)	T63.311	T63.312	T63.313	T63.314	—	—
antivenin	T50.Z11	T50.Z12	T50.Z13	T50.Z14	T50.Z15	T50.Z16
Blast furnace gas (carbon monoxide from)	T58.8X1	T58.8X2	T58.8X3	T58.8X4	—	—
Bleach	T54.91	T54.92	T54.93	T54.94	—	—
Bleaching agent (medicinal)	T49.4X1	T49.4X2	T49.4X3	T49.4X4	T49.4X5	T49.4X6
Bleomycin	T45.1X1	T45.1X2	T45.1X3	T45.1X4	T45.1X5	T45.1X6
Blockain	T41.3X1	T41.3X2	T41.3X3	T41.3X4	T41.3X5	T41.3X6
infiltration (subcutaneous)	T41.3X1	T41.3X2	T41.3X3	T41.3X4	T41.3X5	T41.3X6
nerve block (peripheral) (plexus)	T41.3X1	T41.3X2	T41.3X3	T41.3X4	T41.3X5	T41.3X6
topical (surface)	T41.3X1	T41.3X2	T41.3X3	T41.3X4	T41.3X5	T41.3X6
Blockers, calcium channel	T46.1X1	T46.1X2	T46.1X3	T46.1X4	T46.1X5	T46.1X6
Blood (derivatives) (natural) (plasma) (whole)	T45.8X1	T45.8X2	T45.8X3	T45.8X4	T45.8X5	T45.8X6
dried	T45.8X1	T45.8X2	T45.0X3	T45.0X4	T45.0X5	T45.0X6
drug affecting NEC	T45.91	T45.92	T45.93	T45.94	T45.95	T45.96

Benzamidosalicylate — Blood

Table of Drugs and Chemicals

Substance	Poisoning, Accidental (unintentional)	Poisoning, Intentional Self-harm	Poisoning, Assault	Poisoning, Undetermined	Adverse Effect	Under-dosing
Blood — continued						
expander NEC	T45.8X1	T45.8X2	T45.8X3	T45.8X4	T45.8X5	T45.8X6
fraction NEC	T45.8X1	T45.8X2	T45.8X3	T45.8X4	T45.8X5	T45.8X6
substitute (macromolecular)	T45.8X1	T45.8X2	T45.8X3	T45.8X4	T45.8X5	T45.8X6
Blue velvet	T40.2X1	T40.2X2	T40.2X3	T40.2X4	—	—
Bone meal	T62.8X1	T62.8X2	T62.8X3	T62.8X4	—	—
Bonine	T45.0X1	T45.0X2	T45.0X3	T45.0X4	T45.0X5	T45.0X6
Bopindolol	T44.7X1	T44.7X2	T44.7X3	T44.7X4	T44.7X5	T44.7X6
Boracic acid	T49.0X1	T49.0X2	T49.0X3	T49.0X4	T49.0X5	T49.0X6
ENT agent	T49.6X1	T49.6X2	T49.6X3	T49.6X4	T49.6X5	T49.6X6
ophthalmic preparation	T49.5X1	T49.5X2	T49.5X3	T49.5X4	T49.5X5	T49.5X6
Borane complex	T57.8X1	T57.8X2	T57.8X3	T57.8X4	—	—
Borate(s)	T57.8X1	T57.8X2	T57.8X3	T57.8X4	—	—
buffer	T50.991	T50.992	T50.993	T50.994	T50.995	T50.996
cleanser	T54.91	T54.92	T54.93	T54.94	—	—
sodium	T57.8X1	T57.8X2	T57.8X3	T57.8X4	—	—
Borax (cleanser)	T54.91	T54.92	T54.93	T54.94	—	—
Bordeaux mixture	T60.3X1	T60.3X2	T60.3X3	T60.3X4	—	—
Boric acid	T49.0X1	T49.0X2	T49.0X3	T49.0X4	T49.0X5	T49.0X6
ENT agent	T49.6X1	T49.6X2	T49.6X3	T49.6X4	T49.6X5	T49.6X6
ophthalmic preparation	T49.5X1	T49.5X2	T49.5X3	T49.5X4	T49.5X5	T49.5X6
Bornaprine	T44.3X1	T44.3X2	T44.3X3	T44.3X4	T44.3X5	T44.3X6
Boron	T57.8X1	T57.8X2	T57.8X3	T57.8X4	—	—
hydride NEC	T57.8X1	T57.8X2	T57.8X3	T57.8X4	—	—
fumes or gas	T57.8X1	T57.8X2	T57.8X3	T57.8X4	—	—
trifluoride	T59.891	T59.892	T59.893	T59.894	—	—
Botox	T48.291	T48.292	T48.293	T48.294	T48.295	T48.296
Botulinus anti-toxin (type A, B)	T50.Z11	T50.Z12	T50.Z13	T50.Z14	T50.Z15	T50.Z16
Brake fluid vapor	T59.891	T59.892	T59.893	T59.894	—	—
Brallobarbital	T42.3X1	T42.3X2	T42.3X3	T42.3X4	T42.3X5	T42.3X6
Bran (wheat)	T47.4X1	T47.4X2	T47.4X3	T47.4X4	T47.4X5	T47.4X6
Brass (fumes)	T56.891	T56.892	T56.893	T56.894	—	—
Brasso	T52.0X1	T52.0X2	T52.0X3	T52.0X4	—	—
Bretylium tosilate	T46.2X1	T46.2X2	T46.2X3	T46.2X4	T46.2X5	T46.2X6
Brevital (sodium)	T41.1X1	T41.1X2	T41.1X3	T41.1X4	T41.1X5	T41.1X6
Brinase	T45.3X1	T45.3X2	T45.3X3	T45.3X4	T45.3X5	T45.3X6
British antilewisite	T45.8X1	T45.8X2	T45.8X3	T45.8X4	T45.8X5	T45.8X6
Brodifacoum	T60.4X1	T60.4X2	T60.4X3	T60.4X4	—	—
Bromal (hydrate)	T42.6X1	T42.6X2	T42.6X3	T42.6X4	T42.6X5	T42.6X6
Bromazepam	T42.4X1	T42.4X2	T42.4X3	T42.4X4	T42.4X5	T42.4X6
Bromazine	T45.0X1	T45.0X2	T45.0X3	T45.0X4	T45.0X5	T45.0X6
Brombenzylcyanide	T59.3X1	T59.3X2	T59.3X3	T59.3X4	—	—
Bromelains	T45.3X1	T45.3X2	T45.3X3	T45.3X4	T45.3X5	T45.3X6
Bromethalin	T60.4X1	T60.4X2	T60.4X3	T60.4X4	—	—
Bromhexine	T48.4X1	T48.4X2	T48.4X3	T48.4X4	T48.4X5	T48.4X6
Bromide salts	T42.6X1	T42.6X2	T42.6X3	T42.6X4	T42.6X5	T42.6X6
Bromindione	T45.511	T45.512	T45.513	T45.514	T45.515	T45.516
Bromine						
compounds (medicinal)	T42.6X1	T42.6X2	T42.6X3	T42.6X4	T42.6X5	T42.6X6
sedative	T42.6X1	T42.6X2	T42.6X3	T42.6X4	T42.6X5	T42.6X6
vapor	T59.891	T59.892	T59.893	T59.894	—	—
Bromisoval	T42.6X1	T42.6X2	T42.6X3	T42.6X4	T42.6X5	T42.6X6
Bromisovalum	T42.6X1	T42.6X2	T42.6X3	T42.6X4	T42.6X5	T42.6X6
Bromobenzylcyanide	T59.3X1	T59.3X2	T59.3X3	T59.3X4	—	—
Bromochlorosalicylani-lide	T49.0X1	T49.0X2	T49.0X3	T49.0X4	—	T49.0X6
Bromocriptine	T42.8X1	T42.8X2	T42.8X3	T42.8X4	T42.8X5	T42.8X6
Bromodiphenhydramine	T45.0X1	T45.0X2	T45.0X3	T45.0X4	T45.0X5	T45.0X6
Bromoform	T42.6X1	T42.6X2	T42.6X3	T42.6X4	T42.6X5	T42.6X6
Bromophenol blue reagent	T50.991	T50.992	T50.993	T50.994	T50.995	T50.996
Bromopride	T47.8X1	T47.8X2	T47.8X3	T47.8X4	T47.8X5	T47.8X6
Bromosalicylchloranitide	T49.0X1	T49.0X2	T49.0X3	T49.0X4	T49.0X5	T49.0X6
Bromosalicylhydroxamic acid	T37.1X1	T37.1X2	T37.1X3	T37.1X4	T37.1X5	T37.1X6
Bromo-seltzer	T39.1X1	T39.1X2	T39.1X3	T39.1X4	T39.1X5	T39.1X6
Bromoxynil	T60.3X1	T60.3X2	T60.3X3	T60.3X4	—	—
Bromperidol	T43.4X1	T43.4X2	T43.4X3	T43.4X4	T43.4X5	T43.4X6
Brompheniramine	T45.0X1	T45.0X2	T45.0X3	T45.0X4	T45.0X5	T45.0X6
Bromsulphthalein	T50.8X1	T50.8X2	T50.8X3	T50.8X4	T50.8X5	T50.8X6
Bromural	T42.6X1	T42.6X2	T42.6X3	T42.6X4	T42.6X5	T42.6X6
Bromvaletone	T42.6X1	T42.6X2	T42.6X3	T42.6X4	T42.6X5	T42.6X6
Bronchodilator NEC	T48.6X1	T48.6X2	T48.6X3	T48.6X4	T48.6X5	T48.6X6
Brotizolam	T42.4X1	T42.4X2	T42.4X3	T42.4X4	T42.4X5	T42.4X6
Brovincamine	T46.7X1	T46.7X2	T46.7X3	T46.7X4	T46.7X5	T46.7X6
Brown recluse spider (bite) (venom)	T63.331	T63.332	T63.333	T63.334	—	—
Brown spider (bite) (venom)	T63.391	T63.392	T63.393	T63.394	—	—
Broxaterol	T48.6X1	T48.6X2	T48.6X3	T48.6X4	T48.6X5	T48.6X6
Broxuridine	T45.1X1	T45.1X2	T45.1X3	T45.1X4	T45.1X5	T45.1X6
Broxyquinoline	T37.8X1	T37.8X2	T37.8X3	T37.8X4	T37.8X5	T37.8X6
Bruceine	T48.291	T48.292	T48.293	T48.294	T48.295	T48.296
Brucia	T62.2X1	T62.2X2	T62.2X3	T62.2X4	—	—

Substance	Poisoning, Accidental (unintentional)	Poisoning, Intentional Self-harm	Poisoning, Assault	Poisoning, Undetermined	Adverse Effect	Under-dosing
Brucine	T65.1X1	T65.1X2	T65.1X3	T65.1X4	—	—
Brunswick green — see Copper						
Bruten — see Ibuprofen						
Bryonia	T47.2X1	T47.2X2	T47.2X3	T47.2X4	T47.2X5	T47.2X6
Buclizine	T45.0X1	T45.0X2	T45.0X3	T45.0X4	T45.0X5	T45.0X6
Buclosamide	T49.0X1	T49.0X2	T49.0X3	T49.0X4	T49.0X5	T49.0X6
Budesonide	T44.5X1	T44.5X2	T44.5X3	T44.5X4	T44.5X5	T44.5X6
Budralazine	T46.5X1	T46.5X2	T46.5X3	T46.5X4	T46.5X5	T46.5X6
Bufferin	T39.011	T39.012	T39.013	T39.014	T39.015	T39.016
Buflomedil	T46.7X1	T46.7X2	T46.7X3	T46.7X4	T46.7X5	T46.7X6
Buformin	T38.3X1	T38.3X2	T38.3X3	T38.3X4	T38.3X5	T38.3X6
Bufotenine	T40.991	T40.992	T40.993	T40.994	—	—
Bufrolin	T48.6X1	T48.6X2	T48.6X3	T48.6X4	T48.6X5	T48.6X6
Bufylline	T48.6X1	T48.6X2	T48.6X3	T48.6X4	T48.6X5	T48.6X6
Bulk filler	T50.5X1	T50.5X2	T50.5X3	T50.5X4	T50.5X5	T50.5X6
cathartic	T47.4X1	T47.4X2	T47.4X3	T47.4X4	T47.4X5	T47.4X6
Bumetanide	T50.1X1	T50.1X2	T50.1X3	T50.1X4	T50.1X5	T50.1X6
Bunaftine	T46.2X1	T46.2X2	T46.2X3	T46.2X4	T46.2X5	T46.2X6
Bunamiodyl	T50.8X1	T50.8X2	T50.8X3	T50.8X4	T50.8X5	T50.8X6
Bunazosin	T44.6X1	T44.6X2	T44.6X3	T44.6X4	T44.6X5	T44.6X6
Bunitrolol	T44.7X1	T44.7X2	T44.7X3	T44.7X4	T44.7X5	T44.7X6
Buphenine	T46.7X1	T46.7X2	T46.7X3	T46.7X4	T46.7X5	T46.7X6
Bupivacaine	T41.3X1	T41.3X2	T41.3X3	T41.3X4	T41.3X5	T41.3X6
infiltration (subcutaneous)	T41.3X1	T41.3X2	T41.3X3	T41.3X4	T41.3X5	T41.3X6
nerve block (peripheral) (plexus)	T41.3X1	T41.3X2	T41.3X3	T41.3X4	T41.3X5	T41.3X6
spinal	T41.3X1	T41.3X2	T41.3X3	T41.3X4	T41.3X5	T41.3X6
Bupranolol	T44.7X1	T44.7X2	T44.7X3	T44.7X4	T44.7X5	T44.7X6
Buprenorphine	T40.4X1	T40.4X2	T40.4X3	T40.4X4	T40.4X5	T40.4X6
Bupropion	T43.291	T43.292	T43.293	T43.294	T43.295	T43.296
Burimamide	T47.1X1	T47.1X2	T47.1X3	T47.1X4	T47.1X5	T47.1X6
Buserelin	T38.891	T38.892	T38.893	T38.894	T38.895	T38.896
Buspirone	T43.591	T43.592	T43.593	T43.594	T43.595	T43.596
Busulfan, busulphan	T45.1X1	T45.1X2	T45.1X3	T45.1X4	T45.1X5	T45.1X6
Butabarbital (sodium)	T42.3X1	T42.3X2	T42.3X3	T42.3X4	T42.3X5	T42.3X6
Butabarbitone	T42.3X1	T42.3X2	T42.3X3	T42.3X4	T42.3X5	T42.3X6
Butabarpal	T42.3X1	T42.3X2	T42.3X3	T42.3X4	T42.3X5	T42.3X6
Butacaine	T41.3X1	T41.3X2	T41.3X3	T41.3X4	T41.3X5	T41.3X6
Butalamine	T46.7X1	T46.7X2	T46.7X3	T46.7X4	T46.7X5	T46.7X6
Butalbital	T42.3X1	T42.3X2	T42.3X3	T42.3X4	T42.3X5	T42.3X6
Butallylonal	T42.3X1	T42.3X2	T42.3X3	T42.3X4	T42.3X5	T42.3X6
Butamben	T41.3X1	T41.3X2	T41.3X3	T41.3X4	T41.3X5	T41.3X6
Butamirate	T48.3X1	T48.3X2	T48.3X3	T48.3X4	T48.3X5	T48.3X6
Butane (distributed in mobile container)	T59.891	T59.892	T59.893	T59.894	—	—
distributed through pipes	T59.891	T59.892	T59.893	T59.894	—	—
incomplete combustion	T58.11	T58.12	T58.13	T58.14	—	—
Butanilicaine	T41.3X1	T41.3X2	T41.3X3	T41.3X4	T41.3X5	T41.3X6
Butanol	T51.3X1	T51.3X2	T51.3X3	T51.3X4	—	—
Butanone, 2-butanone	T52.4X1	T52.4X2	T52.4X3	T52.4X4	—	—
Butantrone	T49.4X1	T49.4X2	T49.4X3	T49.4X4	T49.4X5	T49.4X6
Butaperazine	T43.3X1	T43.3X2	T43.3X3	T43.3X4	T43.3X5	T43.3X6
Butazolidin	T39.2X1	T39.2X2	T39.2X3	T39.2X4	T39.2X5	T39.2X6
Butetamate	T48.6X1	T48.6X2	T48.6X3	T48.6X4	T48.6X5	T48.6X6
Butethal	T42.3X1	T42.3X2	T42.3X3	T42.3X4	T42.3X5	T42.3X6
Butethamate	T44.3X1	T44.3X2	T44.3X3	T44.3X4	T44.3X5	T44.3X6
Buthalitone (sodium)	T41.1X1	T41.1X2	T41.1X3	T41.1X4	T41.1X5	T41.1X6
Butisol (sodium)	T42.3X1	T42.3X2	T42.3X3	T42.3X4	T42.3X5	T42.3X6
Butizide	T50.2X1	T50.2X2	T50.2X3	T50.2X4	T50.2X5	T50.2X6
Butobarbital	T42.3X1	T42.3X2	T42.3X3	T42.3X4	T42.3X5	T42.3X6
sodium	T42.3X1	T42.3X2	T42.3X3	T42.3X4	T42.3X5	T42.3X6
Butobarbitone	T42.3X1	T42.3X2	T42.3X3	T42.3X4	T42.3X5	T42.3X6
Butoconazole (nitrate)	T49.0X1	T49.0X2	T49.0X3	T49.0X4	T49.0X5	T49.0X6
Butorphanol	T40.4X1	T40.4X2	T40.4X3	T40.4X4	T40.4X5	T40.4X6
Butriptyline	T43.011	T43.012	T43.013	T43.014	T43.015	T43.016
Butropium bromide	T44.3X1	T44.3X2	T44.3X3	T44.3X4	T44.3X5	T44.3X6
Buttercups	T62.2X1	T62.2X2	T62.2X3	T62.2X4	—	—
Butter of antimony — see Antimony						
Butyl						
acetate (secondary)	T52.8X1	T52.8X2	T52.8X3	T52.8X4	—	—
alcohol	T51.3X1	T51.3X2	T51.3X3	T51.3X4	—	—
aminobenzoate	T41.3X1	T41.3X2	T41.3X3	T41.3X4	T41.3X5	T41.3X6
butyrate	T52.8X1	T52.8X2	T52.8X3	T52.8X4	—	—
carbinol	T51.3X1	T51.3X2	T51.3X3	T51.3X4	—	—
carbitol	T52.3X1	T52.3X2	T52.3X3	T52.3X4	—	—
cellosolve	T52.3X1	T52.3X2	T52.3X3	T52.3X4	—	—
chloral (hydrate)	T42.6X1	T42.6X2	T42.6X3	T42.6X4	T42.6X5	T42.6X6
formate	T52.8X1	T52.8X2	T52.8X3	T52.8X4	—	—
lactate	T52.8X1	T52.8X2	T52.8X3	T52.8X4	—	—
propionate	T52.8X1	T52.8X2	T52.8X3	T52.8X4	—	—
scopolamine bromide	T44.3X1	T44.3X2	T44.3X3	T44.3X4	T44.3X5	T44.3X6
thiobarbital sodium	T41.1X1	T41.1X2	T41.1X3	T41.1X4	T41.1X5	T41.1X6

Blood — Butyl

Substance	Poisoning, Accidental (unintentional)	Poisoning, Intentional Self-harm	Poisoning, Assault	Poisoning, Undetermined	Adverse Effect	Under-dosing
Butylated hydroxyanisole	T50.991	T50.992	T50.993	T50.994	T50.995	T50.996
Butylchloral hydrate	T42.6X1	T42.6X2	T42.6X3	T42.6X4	T42.6X5	T42.6X6
Butyltoluene	T52.2X1	T52.2X2	T52.2X3	T52.2X4	—	—
Butyn	T41.3X1	T41.3X2	T41.3X3	T41.3X4	T41.3X5	T41.3X6
Butyrophenone (-based tranquilizers)	T43.4X1	T43.4X2	T43.4X3	T43.4X4	T43.4X5	T43.4X6
Cabergoline	T42.8X1	T42.8X2	T42.8X3	T42.8X4	T42.8X5	T42.8X6
Cacodyl, cacodylic acid	T57.0X1	T57.0X2	T57.0X3	T57.0X4	—	—
Cactinomycin	T45.1X1	T45.1X2	T45.1X3	T45.1X4	T45.1X5	T45.1X6
Cade oil	T49.4X1	T49.4X2	T49.4X3	T49.4X4	T49.4X5	T49.4X6
Cadexomer iodine	T49.0X1	T49.0X2	T49.0X3	T49.0X4	T49.0X5	T49.0X6
Cadmium (chloride) (fumes) (oxide)	T56.3X1	T56.3X2	T56.3X3	T56.3X4	—	—
sulfide (medicinal) NEC	T49.4X1	T49.4X2	T49.4X3	T49.4X4	T49.4X5	T49.4X6
Cadralazine	T46.5X1	T46.5X2	T46.5X3	T46.5X4	T46.5X5	T46.5X6
Caffeine	T43.611	T43.612	T43.613	T43.614	T43.615	T43.616
Calabar bean	T62.2X1	T62.2X2	T62.2X3	T62.2X4	—	—
Caladium seguinum	T62.2X1	T62.2X2	T62.2X3	T62.2X4	—	—
Calamine (lotion)	T49.3X1	T49.3X2	T49.3X3	T49.3X4	T49.3X5	T49.3X6
Calcifediol	T45.2X1	T45.2X2	T45.2X3	T45.2X4	T45.2X5	T45.2X6
Calciferol	T45.2X1	T45.2X2	T45.2X3	T45.2X4	T45.2X5	T45.2X6
Calcitonin	T50.991	T50.992	T50.993	T50.994	T50.995	T50.996
Calcitriol	T45.2X1	T45.2X2	T45.2X3	T45.2X4	T45.2X5	T45.2X6
Calcium	T50.3X1	T50.3X2	T50.3X3	T50.3X4	T50.3X5	T50.3X6
actylsalicylate	T39.011	T39.012	T39.013	T39.014	T39.015	T39.016
benzamidosalicylate	T37.1X1	T37.1X2	T37.1X3	T37.1X4	T37.1X5	T37.1X6
bromide	T42.6X1	T42.6X2	T42.6X3	T42.6X4	T42.6X5	T42.6X6
bromolactobionate	T42.6X1	T42.6X2	T42.6X3	T42.6X4	T42.6X5	T42.6X6
carbaspirin	T39.011	T39.012	T39.013	T39.014	T39.015	T39.016
carbimide	T50.6X1	T50.6X2	T50.6X3	T50.6X4	T50.6X5	T50.6X6
carbonate	T47.1X1	T47.1X2	T47.1X3	T47.1X4	T47.1X5	T47.1X6
chloride	T50.991	T50.992	T50.993	T50.994	T50.995	T50.996
anhydrous	T50.991	T50.992	T50.993	T50.994	T50.995	T50.996
cyanide	T57.8X1	T57.8X2	T57.8X3	T57.8X4	—	—
dioctyl sulfosuccinate	T47.4X1	T47.4X2	T47.4X3	T47.4X4	T47.4X5	T47.4X6
disodium edathamil	T45.8X1	T45.8X2	T45.8X3	T45.8X4	T45.8X5	T45.8X6
disodium edetate	T45.8X1	T45.8X2	T45.8X3	T45.8X4	T45.8X5	T45.8X6
dobesilate	T46.991	T46.992	T46.993	T46.994	T46.995	T46.996
EDTA	T45.8X1	T45.8X2	T45.8X3	T45.8X4	T45.8X5	T45.8X6
ferrous citrate	T45.4X1	T45.4X2	T45.4X3	T45.4X4	T45.4X5	T45.4X6
folinate	T45.8X1	T45.8X2	T45.8X3	T45.8X4	T45.8X5	T45.8X6
glubionate	T50.3X1	T50.3X2	T50.3X3	T50.3X4	T50.3X5	T50.3X6
gluconate	T50.3X1	T50.3X2	T50.3X3	T50.3X4	T50.3X5	T50.3X6
gluconogalactogluconate	T50.3X1	T50.3X2	T50.3X3	T50.3X4	T50.3X5	T50.3X6
hydrate, hydroxide	T54.3X1	T54.3X2	T54.3X3	T54.3X4	—	—
hypochlorite	T54.3X1	T54.3X2	T54.3X3	T54.3X4	—	—
iodide	T48.4X1	T48.4X2	T48.4X3	T48.4X4	T48.4X5	T48.4X6
ipodate	T50.8X1	T50.8X2	T50.8X3	T50.8X4	T50.8X5	T50.8X6
lactate	T50.3X1	T50.3X2	T50.3X3	T50.3X4	T50.3X5	T50.3X6
leucovorin	T45.8X1	T45.8X2	T45.8X3	T45.8X4	T45.8X5	T45.8X6
mandelate	T37.91	T37.92	T37.93	T37.94	T37.95	T37.96
oxide	T54.3X1	T54.3X2	T54.3X3	T54.3X4	—	—
pantothenate	T45.2X1	T45.2X2	T45.2X3	T45.2X4	T45.2X5	T45.2X6
phosphate	T50.3X1	T50.3X2	T50.3X3	T50.3X4	T50.3X5	T50.3X6
salicylate	T39.091	T39.092	T39.093	T39.094	T39.095	T39.096
salts	T50.3X1	T50.3X2	T50.3X3	T50.3X4	T50.3X5	T50.3X6
Calculus-dissolving drug	T50.991	T50.992	T50.993	T50.994	T50.995	T50.996
Calomel	T49.0X1	T49.0X2	T49.0X3	T49.0X4	T49.0X5	T49.0X6
Caloric agent	T50.3X1	T50.3X2	T50.3X3	T50.3X4	T50.3X5	T50.3X6
Calusterone	T38.7X1	T38.7X2	T38.7X3	T38.7X4	T38.7X5	T38.7X6
Camazepam	T42.4X1	T42.4X2	T42.4X3	T42.4X4	T42.4X5	T42.4X6
Camomile	T49.0X1	T49.0X2	T49.0X3	T49.0X4	T49.0X5	T49.0X6
Camoquin	T37.2X1	T37.2X2	T37.2X3	T37.2X4	T37.2X5	T37.2X6
Camphor						
insecticide	T60.2X1	T60.2X2	T60.2X3	T60.2X4	—	—
medicinal	T49.8X1	T49.8X2	T49.8X3	T49.8X4	T49.8X5	T49.8X6
Camylofin	T44.3X1	T44.3X2	T44.3X3	T44.3X4	T44.3X5	T44.3X6
Cancer chemotherapy drug regimen	T45.1X1	T45.1X2	T45.1X3	T45.1X4	T45.1X5	T45.1X6
Candeptin	T49.0X1	T49.0X2	T49.0X3	T49.0X4	T49.0X5	T49.0X6
Candicidin	T49.0X1	T49.0X2	T49.0X3	T49.0X4	T49.0X5	T49.0X6
Cannabinol	T40.7X1	T40.7X2	T40.7X3	T40.7X4	T40.7X5	T40.7X6
Cannabis (derivatives)	T40.7X1	T40.7X2	T40.7X3	T40.7X4	T40.7X5	T40.7X6
Canned heat	T51.1X1	T51.1X2	T51.1X3	T51.1X4	—	—
Canrenoic acid	T50.0X1	T50.0X2	T50.0X3	T50.0X4	T50.0X5	T50.0X6
Canrenone	T50.0X1	T50.0X2	T50.0X3	T50.0X4	T50.0X5	T50.0X6
Cantharides, cantharidin, cantharis	T49.8X1	T49.8X2	T49.8X3	T49.8X4	T49.8X5	T49.8X6
Canthaxanthin	T50.991	T50.992	T50.993	T50.994	T50.995	T50.996
Capillary-active drug NEC	T46.901	T46.902	T46.903	T46.904	T46.905	T46.906
Capreomycin	T36.8X1	T36.8X2	T36.8X3	T36.8X4	T36.8X5	T36.8X6
Capsicum	T49.4X1	T49.4X2	T49.4X3	T49.4X4	T49.4X5	T49.4X6
Captafol	T60.3X1	T60.3X2	T60.3X3	T60.3X4	—	—
Captan	T60.3X1	T60.3X2	T60.3X3	T60.3X4	—	—
Captodiame, captodiamine	T43.591	T43.592	T43.593	T43.594	T43.595	T43.596
Captopril	T46.4X1	T46.4X2	T46.4X3	T46.4X4	T46.4X5	T46.4X6
Caramiphen	T44.3X1	T44.3X2	T44.3X3	T44.3X4	T44.3X5	T44.3X6
Carazolol	T44.7X1	T44.7X2	T44.7X3	T44.7X4	T44.7X5	T44.7X6
Carbachol	T44.1X1	T44.1X2	T44.1X3	T44.1X4	T44.1X5	T44.1X6
Carbacrylamine (resin)	T50.3X1	T50.3X2	T50.3X3	T50.3X4	T50.3X5	T50.3X6
Carbamate (insecticide)	T60.0X1	T60.0X2	T60.0X3	T60.0X4	—	—
Carbamate (sedative)	T42.6X1	T42.6X2	T42.6X3	T42.6X4	T42.6X5	T42.6X6
herbicide	T60.0X1	T60.0X2	T60.0X3	T60.0X4	—	—
insecticide	T60.0X1	T60.0X2	T60.0X3	T60.0X4	—	—
Carbamazepine	T42.1X1	T42.1X2	T42.1X3	T42.1X4	T42.1X5	T42.1X6
Carbamide	T47.3X1	T47.3X2	T47.3X3	T47.3X4	T47.3X5	T47.3X6
peroxide	T49.0X1	T49.0X2	T49.0X3	T49.0X4	T49.0X5	T49.0X6
topical	T49.8X1	T49.8X2	T49.8X3	T49.8X4	T49.8X5	T49.8X6
Carbamylcholine chloride	T44.1X1	T44.1X2	T44.1X3	T44.1X4	T44.1X5	T44.1X6
Carbaril	T60.0X1	T60.0X2	T60.0X3	T60.0X4	—	—
Carbarsone	T37.3X1	T37.3X2	T37.3X3	T37.3X4	T37.3X5	T37.3X6
Carbaryl	T60.0X1	T60.0X2	T60.0X3	T60.0X4	—	—
Carbaspirin	T39.011	T39.012	T39.013	T39.014	T39.015	T39.016
Carbazochrome (salicylate) (sodium sulfonate)	T49.4X1	T49.4X2	T49.4X3	T49.4X4	T49.4X5	T49.4X6
Carbenicillin	T36.0X1	T36.0X2	T36.0X3	T36.0X4	T36.0X5	T36.0X6
Carbenoxolone	T47.1X1	T47.1X2	T47.1X3	T47.1X4	T47.1X5	T47.1X6
Carbetapentane	T48.3X1	T48.3X2	T48.3X3	T48.3X4	T48.3X5	T48.3X6
Carbethyl salicylate	T39.091	T39.092	T39.093	T39.094	T39.095	T39.096
Carbidopa (with levodopa)	T42.8X1	T42.8X2	T42.8X3	T42.8X4	T42.8X5	T42.8X6
Carbimazole	T38.2X1	T38.2X2	T38.2X3	T38.2X4	T38.2X5	T38.2X6
Carbinol	T51.1X1	T51.1X2	T51.1X3	T51.1X4	—	—
Carbinoxamine	T45.0X1	T45.0X2	T45.0X3	T45.0X4	T45.0X5	T45.0X6
Carbiphene	T39.8X1	T39.8X2	T39.8X3	T39.8X4	T39.8X5	T39.8X6
Carbitol	T52.3X1	T52.3X2	T52.3X3	T52.3X4	—	—
Carbocaine	T41.3X1	T41.3X2	T41.3X3	T41.3X4	T41.3X5	T41.3X6
infiltration (subcutaneous)	T41.3X1	T41.3X2	T41.3X3	T41.3X4	T41.3X5	T41.3X6
nerve block (peripheral) (plexus)	T41.3X1	T41.3X2	T41.3X3	T41.3X4	T41.3X5	T41.3X6
topical (surface)	T41.3X1	T41.3X2	T41.3X3	T41.3X4	T41.3X5	T41.3X6
Carbocisteine	T48.4X1	T48.4X2	T48.4X3	T48.4X4	T48.4X5	T48.4X6
Carbocromen	T46.3X1	T46.3X2	T46.3X3	T46.3X4	T46.3X5	T46.3X6
Carbol fuchsin	T49.0X1	T49.0X2	T49.0X3	T49.0X4	T49.0X5	T49.0X6
Carbolic acid — see also Phenol	T54.0X1	T54.0X2	T54.0X3	T54.0X4	—	—
Carbolonium (bromide)	T48.1X1	T48.1X2	T48.1X3	T48.1X4	T48.1X5	T48.1X6
Carbo medicinalis	T47.6X1	T47.6X2	T47.6X3	T47.6X4	T47.6X5	T47.6X6
Carbomycin	T36.8X1	T36.8X2	T36.8X3	T36.8X4	T36.8X5	T36.8X6
Carbon						
bisulfide (liquid)	T65.4X1	T65.4X2	T65.4X3	T65.4X4	—	—
vapor	T65.4X1	T65.4X2	T65.4X3	T65.4X4	—	—
dioxide (gas)	T59.7X1	T59.7X2	T59.7X3	T59.7X4	—	—
medicinal	T41.5X1	T41.5X2	T41.5X3	T41.5X4	T41.5X5	T41.5X6
nonmedicinal	T59.7X1	T59.7X2	T59.7X3	T59.7X4	—	—
snow	T49.4X1	T49.4X2	T49.4X3	T49.4X4	T49.4X5	T49.4X6
disulfide (liquid)	T65.4X1	T65.4X2	T65.4X3	T65.4X4	—	—
vapor	T65.4X1	T65.4X2	T65.4X3	T65.4X4	—	—
monoxide (from incomplete combustion)	T58.91	T58.92	T58.93	T58.94	—	—
blast furnace gas	T58.8X1	T58.8X2	T58.8X3	T58.8X4	—	—
butane (distributed in mobile container)	T58.11	T58.12	T58.13	T58.14	—	—
distributed through pipes	T58.11	T58.12	T58.13	T58.14	—	—
charcoal fumes	T58.2X1	T58.2X2	T58.2X3	T58.2X4	—	—
coal	T58.2X1	T58.2X2	T58.2X3	T58.2X4	—	—
coke (in domestic stoves, fireplaces)	T58.2X1	T58.2X2	T58.2X3	T58.2X4	—	—
exhaust gas (motor) not in transit	T58.01	T58.02	T58.03	T58.04	—	—
combustion engine, any not in watercraft	T58.01	T58.02	T58.03	T58.04	—	—
farm tractor, not in transit	T58.01	T58.02	T58.03	T58.04	—	—
gas engine	T58.01	T58.02	T58.03	T58.04	—	—
motor pump	T58.01	T58.02	T58.03	T58.04	—	—
motor vehicle, not in transit	T58.01	T58.02	T58.03	T58.04	—	—
fuel (in domestic use)	T58.2X1	T58.2X2	T58.2X3	T58.2X4	—	—
gas (piped)	T58.11	T58.12	T58.13	T58.14	—	—
in mobile container	T58.11	T58.12	T58.13	T58.14	—	—
piped (natural)	T58.11	T58.12	T58.13	T58.14	—	—
utility	T58.11	T58.12	T58.13	T58.14	—	—
in mobile container	T58.11	T58.12	T58.13	T58.14	—	—
gas (piped)	T58.11	T58.12	T58.13	T58.14	—	—
illuminating gas	T58.11	T58.12	T58.13	T58.14	—	—

Table of Drugs and Chemicals

Carbon — Central nervous system

Substance	Poisoning, Accidental (unintentional)	Poisoning, Intentional Self-harm	Poisoning, Assault	Poisoning, Undetermined	Adverse Effect	Under-dosing
Carbon — continued						
monoxide — continued						
industrial fuels or gases, any	T58.8X1	T58.8X2	T58.8X3	T58.8X4	—	—
kerosene (in domestic stoves, fireplaces)	T58.2X1	T58.2X2	T58.2X3	T58.2X4	—	—
kiln gas or vapor	T58.8X1	T58.8X2	T58.8X3	T58.8X4	—	—
motor exhaust gas, not in transit	T58.01	T58.02	T58.03	T58.04	—	—
piped gas (manufactured) (natural)	T58.11	T58.12	T58.13	T58.14	—	—
producer gas	T58.8X1	T58.8X2	T58.8X3	T58.8X4	—	—
propane (distributed in mobile container)	T58.11	T58.12	T58.13	T58.14	—	—
distributed through pipes	T58.11	T58.12	T58.13	T58.14	—	—
solid (in domestic stoves, fireplaces)	T58.2X1	T58.2X2	T58.2X3	T58.2X4	—	—
specified source NEC	T58.8X1	T58.8X2	T58.8X3	T58.8X4	—	—
stove gas	T58.11	T58.12	T58.13	T58.14	—	—
piped	T58.11	T58.12	T58.13	T58.14	—	—
utility gas	T58.11	T58.12	T58.13	T58.14	—	—
piped	T58.11	T58.12	T58.13	T58.14	—	—
water gas	T58.11	T58.12	T58.13	T58.14	—	—
wood (in domestic stoves, fireplaces)	T58.2X1	T58.2X2	T58.2X3	T58.2X4	—	—
tetrachloride (vapor) NEC	T53.0X1	T53.0X2	T53.0X3	T53.0X4	—	—
liquid (cleansing agent) NEC	T53.0X1	T53.0X2	T53.0X3	T53.0X4	—	—
solvent	T53.0X1	T53.0X2	T53.0X3	T53.0X4	—	—
Carbonic acid gas	T59.7X1	T59.7X2	T59.7X3	T59.7X4	—	—
anhydrase inhibitor NEC	T50.2X1	T50.2X2	T50.2X3	T50.2X4	T50.2X5	T50.2X6
Carbophenothion	T60.0X1	T60.0X2	T60.0X3	T60.0X4	—	—
Carboplatin	T45.1X1	T45.1X2	T45.1X3	T45.1X4	T45.1X5	T45.1X6
Carboprost	T48.0X1	T48.0X2	T48.0X3	T48.0X4	T48.0X5	T48.0X6
Carboquone	T45.1X1	T45.1X2	T45.1X3	T45.1X4	T45.1X5	T45.1X6
Carbowax	T49.3X1	T49.3X2	T49.3X3	T49.3X4	T49.3X5	T49.3X6
Carboxymethylcellulose	T47.4X1	T47.4X2	T47.4X3	T47.4X4	T47.4X5	T47.4X6
Carbrital	T42.3X1	T42.3X2	T42.3X3	T42.3X4	T42.3X5	T42.3X6
Carbromal	T42.6X1	T42.6X2	T42.6X3	T42.6X4	T42.6X5	T42.6X6
Carbutamide	T38.3X1	T38.3X2	T38.3X3	T38.3X4	T38.3X5	T38.3X6
Carbuterol	T48.6X1	T48.6X2	T48.6X3	T48.6X4	T48.6X5	T48.6X6
Cardiac						
depressants	T46.2X1	T46.2X2	T46.2X3	T46.2X4	T46.2X5	T46.2X6
rhythm regulator	T46.2X1	T46.2X2	T46.2X3	T46.2X4	T46.2X5	T46.2X6
specified NEC	T46.2X1	T46.2X2	T46.2X3	T46.2X4	T46.2X5	T46.2X6
Cardiografin	T50.8X1	T50.8X2	T50.8X3	T50.8X4	T50.8X5	T50.8X6
Cardiogreen	T50.8X1	T50.8X2	T50.8X3	T50.8X4	T50.8X5	T50.8X6
Cardiotonic (glycoside) **NEC**	T46.0X1	T46.0X2	T46.0X3	T46.0X4	T46.0X5	T46.0X6
Cardiovascular drug NEC	T46.901	T46.902	T46.903	T46.904	T46.905	T46.906
Cardrase	T50.2X1	T50.2X2	T50.2X3	T50.2X4	T50.2X5	T50.2X6
Carfecillin	T36.0X1	T36.0X2	T36.0X3	T36.0X4	T36.0X5	T36.0X6
Carfenazine	T43.3X1	T43.3X2	T43.3X3	T43.3X4	T43.3X5	T43.3X6
Carfusin	T49.0X1	T49.0X2	T49.0X3	T49.0X4	T49.0X5	T49.0X6
Carindacillin	T36.0X1	T36.0X2	T36.0X3	T36.0X4	T36.0X5	T36.0X6
Carisoprodol	T42.8X1	T42.8X2	T42.8X3	T42.8X4	T42.8X5	T42.8X6
Carmellose	T47.4X1	T47.4X2	T47.4X3	T47.4X4	T47.4X5	T47.4X6
Carminative	T47.5X1	T47.5X2	T47.5X3	T47.5X4	T47.5X5	T47.5X6
Carmofur	T45.1X1	T45.1X2	T45.1X3	T45.1X4	T45.1X5	T45.1X6
Carmustine	T45.1X1	T45.1X2	T45.1X3	T45.1X4	T45.1X5	T45.1X6
Carotene	T45.2X1	T45.2X2	T45.2X3	T45.2X4	T45.2X5	T45.2X6
Carphenazine	T43.3X1	T43.3X2	T43.3X3	T43.3X4	T43.3X5	T43.3X6
Carpipramine	T42.4X1	T42.4X2	T42.4X3	T42.4X4	T42.4X5	T42.4X6
Carprofen	T39.311	T39.312	T39.313	T39.314	T39.315	T39.316
Carpronium chloride	T44.3X1	T44.3X2	T44.3X3	T44.3X4	T44.3X5	T44.3X6
Carrageenan	T47.8X1	T47.8X2	T47.8X3	T47.8X4	T47.8X5	T47.8X6
Carteolol	T44.7X1	T44.7X2	T44.7X3	T44.7X4	T44.7X5	T44.7X6
Carter's Little Pills	T47.2X1	T47.2X2	T47.2X3	T47.2X4	T47.2X5	T47.2X6
Cascara (sagrada)	T47.2X1	T47.2X2	T47.2X3	T47.2X4	T47.2X5	T47.2X6
Cassava	T62.2X1	T62.2X2	T62.2X3	T62.2X4	—	—
Castellani's paint	T49.0X1	T49.0X2	T49.0X3	T49.0X4	T49.0X5	T49.0X6
Castor						
bean	T62.2X1	T62.2X2	T62.2X3	T62.2X4	—	—
oil	T47.2X1	T47.2X2	T47.2X3	T47.2X4	T47.2X5	T47.2X6
Catalase	T45.3X1	T45.3X2	T45.3X3	T45.3X4	T45.3X5	T45.3X6
Caterpillar (sting)	T63.431	T63.432	T63.433	T63.434	—	—
Catha (edulis) (tea)	T43.691	T43.692	T43.693	T43.694	—	—
Cathartic NEC	T47.4X1	T47.4X2	T47.4X3	T47.4X4	T47.4X5	T47.4X6
anthacene derivative	T47.2X1	T47.2X2	T47.2X3	T47.2X4	T47.2X5	T47.2X6
bulk	T47.4X1	T47.4X2	T47.4X3	T47.4X4	T47.4X5	T47.4X6
contact	T47.2X1	T47.2X2	T47.2X3	T47.2X4	T47.2X5	T47.2X6
emollient NEC	T47.4X1	T47.4X2	T47.4X3	T47.4X4	T47.4X5	T47.4X6
irritant NEC	T47.2X1	T47.2X2	T47.2X3	T47.2X4	T47.2X5	T47.2X6

Substance	Poisoning, Accidental (unintentional)	Poisoning, Intentional Self-harm	Poisoning, Assault	Poisoning, Undetermined	Adverse Effect	Under-dosing
Cathartic — continued						
mucilage	T47.4X1	T47.4X2	T47.4X3	T47.4X4	T47.4X5	T47.4X6
saline	T47.3X1	T47.3X2	T47.3X3	T47.3X4	T47.3X5	T47.3X6
vegetable	T47.2X1	T47.2X2	T47.2X3	T47.2X4	T47.2X5	T47.2X6
Cathine	T50.5X1	T50.5X2	T50.5X3	T50.5X4	T50.5X5	T50.5X6
Cathomycin	T36.8X1	T36.8X2	T36.8X3	T36.8X4	T36.8X5	T36.8X6
Cation exchange resin	T50.3X1	T50.3X2	T50.3X3	T50.3X4	T50.3X5	T50.3X6
Caustic(s) NEC	T54.91	T54.92	T54.93	T54.94	—	—
alkali	T54.3X1	T54.3X2	T54.3X3	T54.3X4	—	—
hydroxide	T54.3X1	T54.3X2	T54.3X3	T54.3X4	—	—
potash	T54.3X1	T54.3X2	T54.3X3	T54.3X4	—	—
soda	T54.3X1	T54.3X2	T54.3X3	T54.3X4	—	—
specified NEC	T54.91	T54.92	T54.93	T54.94	—	—
Ceepryn	T49.0X1	T49.0X2	T49.0X3	T49.0X4	T49.0X5	T49.0X6
ENT agent	T49.6X1	T49.6X2	T49.6X3	T49.6X4	T49.6X5	T49.6X6
lozenges	T49.6X1	T49.6X2	T49.6X3	T49.6X4	T49.6X5	T49.6X6
Cefacetrile	T36.1X1	T36.1X2	T36.1X3	T36.1X4	T36.1X5	T36.1X6
Cefaclor	T36.1X1	T36.1X2	T36.1X3	T36.1X4	T36.1X5	T36.1X6
Cefadroxil	T36.1X1	T36.1X2	T36.1X3	T36.1X4	T36.1X5	T36.1X6
Cefalexin	T36.1X1	T36.1X2	T36.1X3	T36.1X4	T36.1X5	T36.1X6
Cefaloglycin	T36.1X1	T36.1X2	T36.1X3	T36.1X4	T36.1X5	T36.1X6
Cefaloridine	T36.1X1	T36.1X2	T36.1X3	T36.1X4	T36.1X5	T36.1X6
Cefalosporins	T36.1X1	T36.1X2	T36.1X3	T36.1X4	T36.1X5	T36.1X6
Cefalotin	T36.1X1	T36.1X2	T36.1X3	T36.1X4	T36.1X5	T36.1X6
Cefamandole	T36.1X1	T36.1X2	T36.1X3	T36.1X4	T36.1X5	T36.1X6
Cefamycin antibiotic	T36.1X1	T36.1X2	T36.1X3	T36.1X4	T36.1X5	T36.1X6
Cefapirin	T36.1X1	T36.1X2	T36.1X3	T36.1X4	T36.1X5	T36.1X6
Cefatrizine	T36.1X1	T36.1X2	T36.1X3	T36.1X4	T36.1X5	T36.1X6
Cefazedone	T36.1X1	T36.1X2	T36.1X3	T36.1X4	T36.1X5	T36.1X6
Cefazolin	T36.1X1	T36.1X2	T36.1X3	T36.1X4	T36.1X5	T36.1X6
Cefbuperazone	T36.1X1	T36.1X2	T36.1X3	T36.1X4	T36.1X5	T36.1X6
Cefetamet	T36.1X1	T36.1X2	T36.1X3	T36.1X4	T36.1X5	T36.1X6
Cefixime	T36.1X1	T36.1X2	T36.1X3	T36.1X4	T36.1X5	T36.1X6
Cefmenoxime	T36.1X1	T36.1X2	T36.1X3	T36.1X4	T36.1X5	T36.1X6
Cefmetazole	T36.1X1	T36.1X2	T36.1X3	T36.1X4	T36.1X5	T36.1X6
Cefminox	T36.1X1	T36.1X2	T36.1X3	T36.1X4	T36.1X5	T36.1X6
Cefonicid	T36.1X1	T36.1X2	T36.1X3	T36.1X4	T36.1X5	T36.1X6
Cefoperazone	T36.1X1	T36.1X2	T36.1X3	T36.1X4	T36.1X5	T36.1X6
Ceforanide	T36.1X1	T36.1X2	T36.1X3	T36.1X4	T36.1X5	T36.1X6
Cefotaxime	T36.1X1	T36.1X2	T36.1X3	T36.1X4	T36.1X5	T36.1X6
Cefotetan	T36.1X1	T36.1X2	T36.1X3	T36.1X4	T36.1X5	T36.1X6
Cefotiam	T36.1X1	T36.1X2	T36.1X3	T36.1X4	T36.1X5	T36.1X6
Cefoxitin	T36.1X1	T36.1X2	T36.1X3	T36.1X4	T36.1X5	T36.1X6
Cefpimizole	T36.1X1	T36.1X2	T36.1X3	T36.1X4	T36.1X5	T36.1X6
Cefpiramide	T36.1X1	T36.1X2	T36.1X3	T36.1X4	T36.1X5	T36.1X6
Cefradine	T36.1X1	T36.1X2	T36.1X3	T36.1X4	T36.1X5	T36.1X6
Cefroxadine	T36.1X1	T36.1X2	T36.1X3	T36.1X4	T36.1X5	T36.1X6
Cefsulodin	T36.1X1	T36.1X2	T36.1X3	T36.1X4	T36.1X5	T36.1X6
Ceftazidime	T36.1X1	T36.1X2	T36.1X3	T36.1X4	T36.1X5	T36.1X6
Cefteram	T36.1X1	T36.1X2	T36.1X3	T36.1X4	T36.1X5	T36.1X6
Ceftezole	T36.1X1	T36.1X2	T36.1X3	T36.1X4	T36.1X5	T36.1X6
Ceftizoxime	T36.1X1	T36.1X2	T36.1X3	T36.1X4	T36.1X5	T36.1X6
Ceftriaxone	T36.1X1	T36.1X2	T36.1X3	T36.1X4	T36.1X5	T36.1X6
Cefuroxime	T36.1X1	T36.1X2	T36.1X3	T36.1X4	T36.1X5	T36.1X6
Cefuzonam	T36.1X1	T36.1X2	T36.1X3	T36.1X4	T36.1X5	T36.1X6
Celestone	T38.0X1	T38.0X2	T38.0X3	T38.0X4	T38.0X5	T38.0X6
topical	T49.0X1	T49.0X2	T49.0X3	T49.0X4	T49.0X5	T49.0X6
Celiprolol	T44.7X1	T44.7X2	T44.7X3	T44.7X4	T44.7X5	T44.7X6
Cellosolve	T52.91	T52.92	T52.93	T52.94	—	—
Cell stimulants and proliferants	T49.8X1	T49.8X2	T49.8X3	T49.8X4	T49.8X5	T49.8X6
Cellulose						
cathartic	T47.4X1	T47.4X2	T47.4X3	T47.4X4	T47.4X5	T47.4X6
hydroxyethyl	T47.4X1	T47.4X2	T47.4X3	T47.4X4	T47.4X5	T47.4X6
nitrates (topical)	T49.3X1	T49.3X2	T49.3X3	T49.3X4	T49.3X5	T49.3X6
oxidized	T49.4X1	T49.4X2	T49.4X3	T49.4X4	T49.4X5	T49.4X6
Centipede (bite)	T63.411	T63.412	T63.413	T63.414	—	—
Central nervous system						
depressants	T42.71	T42.72	T42.73	T42.74	T42.75	T42.76
anesthetic (general) NEC	T41.201	T41.202	T41.203	T41.204	T41.205	T41.206
gases NEC	T41.0X1	T41.0X2	T41.0X3	T41.0X4	T41.0X5	T41.0X6
intravenous	T41.1X1	T41.1X2	T41.1X3	T41.1X4	T41.1X5	T41.1X6
barbiturates	T42.3X1	T42.3X2	T42.3X3	T42.3X4	T42.3X5	T42.3X6
benzodiazepines	T42.4X1	T42.4X2	T42.4X3	T42.4X4	T42.4X5	T42.4X6
bromides	T42.6X1	T42.6X2	T42.6X3	T42.6X4	T42.6X5	T42.6X6
cannabis sativa	T40.7X1	T40.7X2	T40.7X3	T40.7X4	T40.7X5	T40.7X6
chloral hydrate	T42.6X1	T42.6X2	T42.6X3	T42.6X4	T42.6X5	T42.6X6
ethanol	T51.0X1	T51.0X2	T51.0X3	T51.0X4	—	—
hallucinogenics	T40.901	T40.902	T40.903	T40.904	T40.905	T40.906
hypnotics	T42.71	T42.72	T42.73	T42.74	T42.75	T42.76
specified NEC	T42.6X1	T42.6X2	T42.6X3	T42.6X4	T42.6X5	T42.6X6
muscle relaxants	T42.8X1	T42.8X2	T42.8X3	T42.8X4	T42.8X5	T42.8X6
paraldehyde	T42.6X1	T42.6X2	T42.6X3	T42.6X4	T42.6X5	T42.6X6

Additional Character May Be Required — Refer to the Tabular List for Character Selection ▽ Subterms under main terms may continue to next column or page

Substance	Poisoning, Accidental (unintentional)	Poisoning, Intentional Self-harm	Poisoning, Assault	Poisoning, Undetermined	Adverse Effect	Under-dosing
Central nervous system —						
continued						
depressants — *continued*						
sedatives;	T42.71	T42.72	T42.73	T42.74	T42.75	T42.76
sedative-hypnotics						
mixed NEC	T42.6X1	T42.6X2	T42.6X3	T42.6X4	T42.6X5	T42.6X6
specified NEC	T42.6X1	T42.6X2	T42.6X3	T42.6X4	T42.6X5	T42.6X6
muscle-tone depressants	T42.8X1	T42.8X2	T42.8X3	T42.8X4	T42.8X5	T42.8X6
stimulants	T43.601	T43.602	T43.603	T43.604	T43.605	T43.606
amphetamines	T43.621	T43.622	T43.623	T43.624	T43.625	T43.626
analeptics	T50.7X1	T50.7X2	T50.7X3	T50.7X4	T50.7X5	T50.7X6
antidepressants	T43.201	T43.202	T43.203	T43.204	T43.205	T43.206
opiate antagonists	T50.7X1	T50.7X2	T50.7X3	T50.7X4	T50.7X5	T50.7X6
specified NEC	T43.691	T43.692	T43.693	T43.694	T43.695	T43.696
Cephalexin	T36.1X1	T36.1X2	T36.1X3	T36.1X4	T36.1X5	T36.1X6
Cephaloglycin	T36.1X1	T36.1X2	T36.1X3	T36.1X4	T36.1X5	T36.1X6
Cephaloridine	T36.1X1	T36.1X2	T36.1X3	T36.1X4	T36.1X5	T36.1X6
Cephalosporins	T36.1X1	T36.1X2	T36.1X3	T36.1X4	T36.1X5	T36.1X6
N (adicillin)	T36.0X1	T36.0X2	T36.0X3	T36.0X4	T36.0X5	T36.0X6
Cephalothin	T36.1X1	T36.1X2	T36.1X3	T36.1X4	T36.1X5	T36.1X6
Cephalotin	T36.1X1	T36.1X2	T36.1X3	T36.1X4	T36.1X5	T36.1X6
Cephradine	T36.1X1	T36.1X2	T36.1X3	T36.1X4	T36.1X5	T36.1X6
Cerbera (odallam)	T62.2X1	T62.2X2	T62.2X3	T62.2X4	—	—
Cerberin	T46.0X1	T46.0X2	T46.0X3	T46.0X4	T46.0X5	T46.0X6
Cerebral stimulants	T43.601	T43.602	T43.603	T43.604	T43.605	T43.606
psychotherapeutic	T43.601	T43.602	T43.603	T43.604	T43.605	T43.606
specified NEC	T43.691	T43.692	T43.693	T43.694	T43.695	T43.696
Cerium oxalate	T45.0X1	T45.0X2	T45.0X3	T45.0X4	T45.0X5	T45.0X6
Cerous oxalate	T45.0X1	T45.0X2	T45.0X3	T45.0X4	T45.0X5	T45.0X6
Ceruletide	T50.8X1	T50.8X2	T50.8X3	T50.8X4	T50.8X5	T50.8X6
Cetalkonium (chloride)	T49.0X1	T49.0X2	T49.0X3	T49.0X4	T49.0X5	T49.0X6
Cethexonium chloride	T49.0X1	T49.0X2	T49.0X3	T49.0X4	T49.0X5	T49.0X6
Cetiedil	T46.7X1	T46.7X2	T46.7X3	T46.7X4	T46.7X5	T46.7X6
Cetirizine	T45.0X1	T45.0X2	T45.0X3	T45.0X4	T45.0X5	T45.0X6
Cetomacrogol	T50.991	T50.992	T50.993	T50.994	T50.995	T50.996
Cetotiamine	T45.2X1	T45.2X2	T45.2X3	T45.2X4	T45.2X5	T45.2X6
Cetoxime	T45.0X1	T45.0X2	T45.0X3	T45.0X4	T45.0X5	T45.0X6
Cetraxate	T47.1X1	T47.1X2	T47.1X4	T47.1X4	T47.1X5	T47.1X6
Cetrimide	T49.0X1	T49.0X2	T49.0X3	T49.0X4	T49.0X5	T49.0X6
Cetrimonium (bromide)	T49.0X1	T49.0X2	T49.0X3	T49.0X4	T49.0X5	T49.0X6
Cetylpyridinium chloride	T49.0X1	T49.0X2	T49.0X3	T49.0X4	T49.0X5	T49.0X6
ENT agent	T49.6X1	T49.6X2	T49.6X3	T49.6X4	T49.6X5	T49.6X6
lozenges	T49.6X1	T49.6X2	T49.6X3	T49.6X4	T49.6X5	T49.6X6
Cevadilla — *see* Sabadilla						
Cevitamic acid	T45.2X1	T45.2X2	T45.2X3	T45.2X4	T45.2X5	T45.2X6
Chalk, precipitated	T47.1X1	T47.1X2	T47.1X3	T47.1X4	T47.1X5	T47.1X6
Chamomile	T49.0X1	T49.0X2	T49.0X3	T49.0X4	T49.0X5	T49.0X6
Ch'an su	T46.0X1	T46.0X2	T46.0X3	T46.0X4	T46.0X5	T46.0X6
Charcoal	T47.6X1	T47.6X2	T47.6X3	T47.6X4	T47.6X5	T47.6X6
activated — *see also* Charcoal,	T47.6X1	T47.6X2	T47.6X3	T47.6X4	T47.6X5	T47.6X6
medicinal						
fumes (Carbon monoxide)	T58.2X1	T58.2X2	T58.2X3	T58.2X4	—	—
industrial	T58.8X1	T58.8X2	T58.8X3	T58.8X4	—	—
medicinal (activated)	T47.6X1	T47.6X2	T47.6X3	T47.6X4	T47.6X5	T47.6X6
antidiarrheal	T47.6X1	T47.6X2	T47.6X3	T47.6X4	T47.6X5	T47.6X6
poison control	T47.8X1	T47.8X2	T47.8X3	T47.8X4	T47.8X5	T47.8X6
specified use other than for	T47.8X1	T47.8X2	T47.8X3	T47.8X4	T47.8X5	T47.8X6
diarrhea						
topical	T49.8X1	T49.8X2	T49.8X3	T49.8X4	T49.8X5	T49.8X6
Chaulmosulfone	T37.1X1	T37.1X2	T37.1X3	T37.1X4	T37.1X5	T37.1X6
Chelating agent NEC	T50.6X1	T50.6X2	T50.6X3	T50.6X4	T50.6X5	T50.6X6
Chelidonium majus	T62.2X1	T62.2X2	T62.2X3	T62.2X4	—	—
Chemical substance NEC	T65.91	T65.92	T65.93	T65.94	—	—
Chenodeoxycholic acid	T47.5X1	T47.5X2	T47.5X3	T47.5X4	T47.5X5	T47.5X6
Chenodiol	T47.5X1	T47.5X2	T47.5X3	T47.5X4	T47.5X5	T47.5X6
Chenopodium	T37.4X1	T37.4X2	T37.4X3	T37.4X4	T37.4X5	T37.4X6
Cherry laurel	T62.2X1	T62.2X2	T62.2X3	T62.2X4	—	—
Chinidin (e)	T46.2X1	T46.2X2	T46.2X3	T46.2X4	T46.2X5	T46.2X6
Chiniofon	T37.8X1	T37.8X2	T37.8X3	T37.8X4	T37.8X5	T37.8X6
Chlophedianol	T48.3X1	T48.3X2	T48.3X3	T48.3X4	T48.3X5	T48.3X6
Chloral	T42.6X1	T42.6X2	T42.6X3	T42.6X4	T42.6X5	T42.6X6
derivative	T42.6X1	T42.6X2	T42.6X3	T42.6X4	T42.6X5	T42.6X6
hydrate	T42.6X1	T42.6X2	T42.6X3	T42.6X4	T42.6X5	T42.6X6
Chloralamide	T42.6X1	T42.6X2	T42.6X3	T42.6X4	T42.6X5	T42.6X6
Chloralodol	T42.6X1	T42.6X2	T42.6X3	T42.6X4	T42.6X5	T42.6X6
Chloralose	T60.4X1	T60.4X2	T60.4X3	T60.4X4	—	—
Chlorambucil	T45.1X1	T45.1X2	T45.1X3	T45.1X4	T45.1X5	T45.1X6
Chloramine	T57.8X1	T57.8X2	T57.8X3	T57.8X4	—	—
T	T49.0X1	T49.0X2	T49.0X3	T49.0X4	T49.0X5	T49.0X6
topical	T49.0X1	T49.0X2	T49.0X3	T49.0X4	T49.0X5	T49.0X6
Chloramphenicol	T36.2X1	T36.2X2	T36.2X3	T36.2X4	T36.2X5	T36.2X6
ENT agent	T49.6X1	T49.6X2	T49.6X3	T49.6X4	T49.6X5	T49.6X6
ophthalmic preparation	T49.5X1	T49.5X2	T49.5X3	T49.5X4	T49.5X5	T49.5X6

Substance	Poisoning, Accidental (unintentional)	Poisoning, Intentional Self-harm	Poisoning, Assault	Poisoning, Undetermined	Adverse Effect	Under-dosing
Chloramphenicol — *continued*						
topical NEC	T49.0X1	T49.0X2	T49.0X3	T49.0X4	T49.0X5	T49.0X6
Chlorate (potassium) (sodium)	T60.3X1	T60.3X2	T60.3X3	T60.3X4	—	—
NEC						
herbicide	T60.3X1	T60.3X2	T60.3X3	T60.3X4	—	—
Chlorazanil	T50.2X1	T50.2X2	T50.2X3	T50.2X4	T50.2X5	T50.2X6
Chlorbenzene, chlorbenzol	T53.7X1	T53.7X2	T53.7X3	T53.7X4	—	—
Chlorbenzoxamine	T44.3X1	T44.3X2	T44.3X3	T44.3X4	T44.3X5	T44.3X6
Chlorbutol	T42.6X1	T42.6X2	T42.6X3	T42.6X4	T42.6X5	T42.6X6
Chlorcyclizine	T45.0X1	T45.0X2	T45.0X3	T45.0X4	T45.0X5	T45.0X6
Chlordan (e) (dust)	T60.1X1	T60.1X2	T60.1X3	T60.1X4	—	—
Chlordantoin	T49.0X1	T49.0X2	T49.0X3	T49.0X4	T49.0X5	T49.0X6
Chlordiazepoxide	T42.4X1	T42.4X2	T42.4X3	T42.4X4	T42.4X5	T42.4X6
Chlordiethyl benzamide	T49.3X1	T49.3X2	T49.3X3	T49.3X4	T49.3X5	T49.3X6
Chloresium	T49.8X1	T49.8X2	T49.8X3	T49.8X4	T49.8X5	T49.8X6
Chlorethiazol	T42.6X1	T42.6X2	T42.6X3	T42.6X4	T42.6X5	T42.6X6
Chlorethyl — *see* Ethyl chloride						
Chloretone	T42.6X1	T42.6X2	T42.6X3	T42.6X4	T42.6X5	T42.6X6
Chlorex	T53.6X1	T53.6X2	T53.6X3	T53.6X4	—	—
insecticide	T60.1X1	T60.1X2	T60.1X3	T60.1X4	—	—
Chlorfenvinphos	T60.0X1	T60.0X2	T60.0X3	T60.0X4	—	—
Chlorhexadol	T42.6X1	T42.6X2	T42.6X3	T42.6X4	T42.6X5	T42.6X6
Chlorhexamide	T45.1X1	T45.1X2	T45.1X3	T45.1X4	T45.1X5	T45.1X6
Chlorhexidine	T49.0X1	T49.0X2	T49.0X3	T49.0X4	T49.0X5	T49.0X6
Chlorhydroxyquinolin	T49.0X1	T49.0X2	T49.0X3	T49.0X4	T49.0X5	T49.0X6
Chloride of lime (bleach)	T54.3X1	T54.3X2	T54.3X3	T54.3X4	—	—
Chlorimipramine	T43.011	T43.012	T43.013	T43.014	T43.015	T43.016
Chlorinated						
camphene	T53.6X1	T53.6X2	T53.6X3	T53.6X4	—	—
diphenyl	T53.7X1	T53.7X2	T53.7X3	T53.7X4	—	—
hydrocarbons NEC	T53.91	T53.92	T53.93	T53.94	—	—
solvents	T53.91	T53.92	T53.93	T53.94	—	—
lime (bleach)	T54.3X1	T54.3X2	T54.3X3	T54.3X4	—	—
and boric acid solution	T49.0X1	T49.0X2	T49.0X3	T49.0X4	T49.0X5	T49.0X6
naphthalene (insecticide)	T60.1X1	T60.1X2	T60.1X3	T60.1X4	—	—
industrial (non-pesticide)	T53.7X1	T53.7X2	T53.7X3	T53.7X4	—	—
pesticide NEC	T60.8X1	T60.8X2	T60.8X3	T60.8X4	—	—
soda — *see also* sodium						
hypochlorite						
solution	T49.0X1	T49.0X2	T49.0X3	T49.0X4	T49.0X5	T49.0X6
Chlorine (fumes) (gas)	T59.4X1	T59.4X2	T59.4X3	T59.4X4	—	—
bleach	T54.3X1	T54.3X2	T54.3X3	T54.3X4	—	—
compound gas NEC	T59.4X1	T59.4X2	T59.4X3	T59.4X4	—	—
disinfectant	T59.4X1	T59.4X2	T59.4X3	T59.4X4	—	—
releasing agents NEC	T59.4X1	T59.4X2	T59.4X3	T59.4X4	—	—
Chlorisondamine chloride	T46.991	T46.992	T46.993	T46.994	T46.995	T46.996
Chlormadinone	T38.5X1	T38.5X2	T38.5X3	T38.5X4	T38.5X5	T38.5X6
Chlormephos	T60.0X1	T60.0X2	T60.0X3	T60.0X4	—	—
Chlormerodrin	T50.2X1	T50.2X2	T50.2X3	T50.2X4	T50.2X5	T50.2X6
Chlormethiazole	T42.6X1	T42.6X2	T42.6X3	T42.6X4	T42.6X5	T42.6X6
Chlormethine	T45.1X1	T45.1X2	T45.1X3	T45.1X4	T45.1X5	T45.1X6
Chlormethylenecycline	T36.4X1	T36.4X2	T36.4X3	T36.4X4	T36.4X5	T36.4X6
Chlormezanone	T42.6X1	T42.6X2	T42.6X3	T42.6X4	T42.6X5	T42.6X6
Chloroacetic acid	T60.3X1	T60.3X2	T60.3X3	T60.3X4	—	—
Chloroacetone	T59.3X1	T59.3X2	T59.3X3	T59.3X4	—	—
Chloroacetophenone	T59.3X1	T59.3X2	T59.3X3	T59.3X4	—	—
Chloroaniline	T53.7X1	T53.7X2	T53.7X3	T53.7X4	—	—
Chlorobenzene, chlorobenzol	T53.7X1	T53.7X2	T53.7X3	T53.7X4	—	—
Chlorobromomethane (fire extinguisher)	T53.6X1	T53.6X2	T53.6X3	T53.6X4	—	—
Chlorobutanol	T49.0X1	T49.0X2	T49.0X3	T49.0X4	T49.0X5	T49.0X6
Chlorocresol	T49.0X1	T49.0X2	T49.0X3	T49.0X4	T49.0X5	T49.0X6
Chlorodehydromethyltestosterone	T38.7X1	T38.7X2	T38.7X3	T38.7X4	T38.7X5	T38.7X6
Chlorodinitrobenzene	T53.7X1	T53.7X2	T53.7X3	T53.7X4	—	—
dust or vapor	T53.7X1	T53.7X2	T53.7X3	T53.7X4	—	—
Chlorodiphenyl	T53.7X1	T53.7X2	T53.7X3	T53.7X4	—	—
Chloroethane — *see* Ethyl chloride						
Chloroethylene	T53.6X1	T53.6X2	T53.6X3	T53.6X4	—	—
Chlorofluorocarbons	T53.5X1	T53.5X2	T53.5X3	T53.5X4	—	—
Chloroform (fumes) (vapor)	T53.1X1	T53.1X2	T53.1X3	T53.1X4	—	—
anesthetic	T41.0X1	T41.0X2	T41.0X3	T41.0X4	T41.0X5	T41.0X6
solvent	T53.1X1	T53.1X2	T53.1X3	T53.1X4	—	—
water, concentrated	T41.0X1	T41.0X2	T41.0X3	T41.0X4	T41.0X5	T41.0X6
Chloroguanide	T37.2X1	T37.2X2	T37.2X3	T37.2X4	T37.2X5	T37.2X6
Chloromycetin	T36.2X1	T36.2X2	T36.2X3	T36.2X4	T36.2X5	T36.2X6
ENT agent	T49.6X1	T49.6X2	T49.6X3	T49.6X4	T49.6X5	T49.6X6
ophthalmic preparation	T49.5X1	T49.5X2	T49.5X3	T49.5X4	T49.5X5	T49.5X6
otic solution	T49.6X1	T49.6X2	T49.6X3	T49.6X4	T49.6X5	T49.6X6
topical NEC	T49.0X1	T49.0X2	T49.0X3	T49.0X4	T49.0X5	T49.0X6
Chloronitrobenzene	T53.7X1	T53.7X2	T53.7X3	T53.7X4	—	—
dust or vapor	T53.7X1	T53.7X2	T53.7X3	T53.7X4	—	—

Substance	Poisoning, Accidental (unintentional)	Poisoning, Intentional Self-harm	Poisoning, Assault	Poisoning, Undetermined	Adverse Effect	Under-dosing
Chlorophacinone	T60.4X1	T60.4X2	T60.4X3	T60.4X4	—	—
Chlorophenol	T53.7X1	T53.7X2	T53.7X3	T53.7X4	—	—
Chlorophenothane	T60.1X1	T60.1X2	T60.1X3	T60.1X4	—	—
Chlorophyll	T50.991	T50.992	T50.993	T50.994	T50.995	T50.996
Chloropicrin (fumes)	T53.6X1	T53.6X2	T53.6X3	T53.6X4	—	—
fumigant	T60.8X1	T60.8X2	T60.8X3	T60.8X4	—	—
fungicide	T60.3X1	T60.3X2	T60.3X3	T60.3X4	—	—
pesticide	T60.8X1	T60.8X2	T60.8X3	T60.8X4	—	—
Chloroprocaine	T41.3X1	T41.3X2	T41.3X3	T41.3X4	T41.3X5	T41.3X6
infiltration (subcutaneous)	T41.3X1	T41.3X2	T41.3X3	T41.3X4	T41.3X5	T41.3X6
nerve block (peripheral) (plexus)	T41.3X1	T41.3X2	T41.3X3	T41.3X4	T41.3X5	T41.3X6
spinal	T41.3X1	T41.3X2	T41.3X3	T41.3X4	T41.3X5	T41.3X6
Chloroptic	T49.5X1	T49.5X2	T49.5X3	T49.5X4	T49.5X5	T49.5X6
Chloropurine	T45.1X1	T45.1X2	T45.1X3	T45.1X4	T45.1X5	T45.1X6
Chloropyramine	T45.0X1	T45.0X2	T45.0X3	T45.0X4	T45.0X5	T45.0X6
Chloropyrifos	T60.0X1	T60.0X2	T60.0X3	T60.0X4	—	—
Chloropyrilene	T45.0X1	T45.0X2	T45.0X3	T45.0X4	T45.0X5	T45.0X6
Chloroquine	T37.2X1	T37.2X2	T37.2X3	T37.2X4	T37.2X5	T37.2X6
Chlorothalonil	T60.3X1	T60.3X2	T60.3X3	T60.3X4	—	—
Chlorothen	T45.0X1	T45.0X2	T45.0X3	T45.0X4	T45.0X5	T45.0X6
Chlorothiazide	T50.2X1	T50.2X2	T50.2X3	T50.2X4	T50.2X5	T50.2X6
Chlorothymol	T49.4X1	T49.4X2	T49.4X3	T49.4X4	T49.4X5	T49.4X6
Chlorotrianisene	T38.5X1	T38.5X2	T38.5X3	T38.5X4	T38.5X5	T38.5X6
Chlorovinyldichloroarsine, not in war	T57.0X1	T57.0X2	T57.0X3	T57.0X4	—	—
Chloroxine	T49.4X1	T49.4X2	T49.4X3	T49.4X4	T49.4X5	T49.4X6
Chloroxylenol	T49.0X1	T49.0X2	T49.0X3	T49.0X4	T49.0X5	T49.0X6
Chlorphenamine	T45.0X1	T45.0X2	T45.0X3	T45.0X4	T45.0X5	T45.0X6
Chlorphenesin	T42.8X1	T42.8X2	T42.8X3	T42.8X4	T42.8X5	T42.8X6
topical (antifungal)	T49.0X1	T49.0X2	T49.0X3	T49.0X4	T49.0X5	T49.0X6
Chlorpheniramine	T45.0X1	T45.0X2	T45.0X3	T45.0X4	T45.0X5	T45.0X6
Chlorphenoxamine	T45.0X1	T45.0X2	T45.0X3	T45.0X4	T45.0X5	T45.0X6
Chlorphentermine	T50.5X1	T50.5X2	T50.5X3	T50.5X4	T50.5X5	T50.5X6
Chlorprocaine — see Chloroprocaine						
Chlorproguanil	T37.2X1	T37.2X2	T37.2X3	T37.2X4	T37.2X5	T37.2X6
Chlorpromazine	T43.3X1	T43.3X2	T43.3X3	T43.3X4	T43.3X5	T43.3X6
Chlorpropamide	T38.3X1	T38.3X2	T38.3X3	T38.3X4	T38.3X5	T38.3X6
Chlorprothixene	T43.4X1	T43.4X2	T43.4X3	T43.4X4	T43.4X5	T43.4X6
Chlorquinaldol	T49.0X1	T49.0X2	T49.0X3	T49.0X4	T49.0X5	T49.0X6
Chlorquinol	T49.0X1	T49.0X2	T49.0X3	T49.0X4	T49.0X5	T49.0X6
Chlortalidone	T50.2X1	T50.2X2	T50.2X3	T50.2X4	T50.2X5	T50.2X6
Chlortetracycline	T36.4X1	T36.4X2	T36.4X3	T36.4X4	T36.4X5	T36.4X6
Chlorthalidone	T50.2X1	T50.2X2	T50.2X3	T50.2X4	T50.2X5	T50.2X6
Chlorthion	T60.0X1	T60.0X2	T60.0X3	T60.0X4	—	—
Chlorthiophos	T60.0X1	T60.0X2	T60.0X3	T60.0X4	—	—
Chlortrianisene	T38.5X1	T38.5X2	T38.5X3	T38.5X4	T38.5X5	T38.5X6
Chlor-Trimeton	T45.0X1	T45.0X2	T45.0X3	T45.0X4	T45.0X5	T45.0X6
Chlorzoxazone	T42.8X1	T42.8X2	T42.8X3	T42.8X4	T42.8X5	T42.8X6
Choke damp	T59.7X1	T59.7X2	T59.7X3	T59.7X4	—	—
Cholagogues	T47.5X1	T47.5X2	T47.5X3	T47.5X4	T47.5X5	T47.5X6
Cholebrine	T50.8X1	T50.8X2	T50.8X3	T50.8X4	T50.8X5	T50.8X6
Cholecalciferol	T45.2X1	T45.2X2	T45.2X3	T45.2X4	T45.2X5	T45.2X6
Cholecystokinin	T50.8X1	T50.8X2	T50.8X3	T50.8X4	T50.8X5	T50.8X6
Cholera vaccine	T50.A91	T50.A92	T50.A93	T50.A94	T50.A95	T50.A96
Choleretic	T47.5X1	T47.5X2	T47.5X3	T47.5X4	T47.5X5	T47.5X6
Cholesterol-lowering agents	T46.6X1	T46.6X2	T46.6X3	T46.6X4	T46.6X5	T46.6X6
Cholestyramine (resin)	T46.6X1	T46.6X2	T46.6X3	T46.6X4	T46.6X5	T46.6X6
Cholic acid	T47.5X1	T47.5X2	T47.5X3	T47.5X4	T47.5X5	T47.5X6
Choline	T48.6X1	T48.6X2	T48.6X3	T48.6X4	T48.6X5	T48.6X6
chloride	T50.991	T50.992	T50.993	T50.994	T50.995	T50.996
dihydrogen citrate	T50.991	T50.992	T50.993	T50.994	T50.995	T50.996
salicylate	T39.091	T39.092	T39.093	T39.094	T39.095	T39.096
theophyllinate	T48.6X1	T48.6X2	T48.6X3	T48.6X4	T48.6X5	T48.6X6
Cholinergic (drug) NEC	T44.1X1	T44.1X2	T44.1X3	T44.1X4	T44.1X5	T44.1X6
muscle tone enhancer	T44.1X1	T44.1X2	T44.1X3	T44.1X4	T44.1X5	T44.1X6
organophosphorus	T44.0X1	T44.0X2	T44.0X3	T44.0X4	T44.0X5	T44.0X6
insecticide	T60.0X1	T60.0X2	T60.0X3	T60.0X4	—	—
nerve gas	T59.891	T59.892	T59.893	T59.894	—	—
trimethyl ammonium propanediol	T44.1X1	T44.1X2	T44.1X3	T44.1X4	T44.1X5	T44.1X6
Cholinesterase reactivator	T50.6X1	T50.6X2	T50.6X3	T50.6X4	T50.6X5	T50.6X6
Cholografin	T50.8X1	T50.8X2	T50.8X3	T50.8X4	T50.8X5	T50.8X6
Chorionic gonadotropin	T38.891	T38.892	T38.893	T38.894	T38.895	T38.896
Chromate	T56.2X1	T56.2X2	T56.2X3	T56.2X4	—	—
dust or mist	T56.2X1	T56.2X2	T56.2X3	T56.2X4	—	—
lead — see also lead	T56.0X1	T56.0X2	T56.0X3	T56.0X4	—	—
paint	T56.0X1	T56.0X2	T56.0X3	T56.0X4	—	—
Chromic						
acid	T56.2X1	T56.2X2	T56.2X3	T56.2X4	—	—
dust or mist	T56.2X1	T56.2X2	T56.2X3	T56.2X4	—	—

Substance	Poisoning, Accidental (unintentional)	Poisoning, Intentional Self-harm	Poisoning, Assault	Poisoning, Undetermined	Adverse Effect	Under-dosing
Chromic — continued						
phosphate 32P	T45.1X1	T45.1X2	T45.1X3	T45.1X4	T45.1X5	T45.1X6
Chromium	T56.2X1	T56.2X2	T56.2X3	T56.2X4	—	—
compounds — see Chromate						
sesquioxide	T50.8X1	T50.8X2	T50.8X3	T50.8X4	T50.8X5	T50.8X6
Chromomycin A3	T45.1X1	T45.1X2	T45.1X3	T45.1X4	T45.1X5	T45.1X6
Chromonar	T46.3X1	T46.3X2	T46.3X3	T46.3X4	T46.3X5	T46.3X6
Chromyl chloride	T56.2X1	T56.2X2	T56.2X3	T56.2X4	—	—
Chrysarobin	T49.4X1	T49.4X2	T49.4X3	T49.4X4	T49.4X5	T49.4X6
Chrysazin	T47.2X1	T47.2X2	T47.2X3	T47.2X4	T47.2X5	T47.2X6
Chymar	T45.3X1	T45.3X2	T45.3X3	T45.3X4	T45.3X5	T45.3X6
ophthalmic preparation	T49.5X1	T49.5X2	T49.5X3	T49.5X4	T49.5X5	T49.5X6
Chymopapain	T45.3X1	T45.3X2	T45.3X3	T45.3X4	T45.3X5	T45.3X6
Chymotrypsin	T45.3X1	T45.3X2	T45.3X3	T45.3X4	T45.3X5	T45.3X6
ophthalmic preparation	T49.5X1	T49.5X2	T49.5X3	T49.5X4	T49.5X5	T49.5X6
Cianidanol	T50.991	T50.992	T50.993	T50.994	T50.995	T50.996
Cianopramine	T43.011	T43.012	T43.013	T43.014	T43.015	T43.016
Cibenzoline	T46.2X1	T46.2X2	T46.2X3	T46.2X4	T46.2X5	T46.2X6
Ciclacillin	T36.0X1	T36.0X2	T36.0X3	T36.0X4	T36.0X5	T36.0X6
Ciclobarbital — see Hexobarbital						
Ciclonicate	T46.7X1	T46.7X2	T46.7X3	T46.7X4	T46.7X5	T46.7X6
Ciclopirox (olamine)	T49.0X1	T49.0X2	T49.0X3	T49.0X4	T49.0X5	T49.0X6
Ciclosporin	T45.1X1	T45.1X2	T45.1X3	T45.1X4	T45.1X5	T45.1X6
Cicuta maculata or virosa	T62.2X1	T62.2X2	T62.2X3	T62.2X4	—	—
Cicutoxin	T62.2X1	T62.2X2	T62.2X3	T62.2X4	—	—
Cigarette lighter fluid	T52.0X1	T52.0X2	T52.0X3	T52.0X4	—	—
Cigarettes (tobacco)	T65.221	T65.222	T65.223	T65.224	—	—
Ciguatoxin	T61.01	T61.02	T61.03	T61.04	—	—
Cilazapril	T46.4X1	T46.4X2	T46.4X3	T46.4X4	T46.4X5	T46.4X6
Cimetidine	T47.0X1	T47.0X2	T47.0X3	T47.0X4	T47.0X5	T47.0X6
Cimetropium bromide	T44.3X1	T44.3X2	T44.3X3	T44.3X4	T44.3X5	T44.3X6
Cinchocaine	T41.3X1	T41.3X2	T41.3X3	T41.3X4	T41.3X5	T41.3X6
topical (surface)	T41.3X1	T41.3X2	T41.3X3	T41.3X4	T41.3X5	T41.3X6
Cinchona	T37.2X1	T37.2X2	T37.2X3	T37.2X4	T37.2X5	T37.2X6
Cinchonine alkaloids	T37.2X1	T37.2X2	T37.2X3	T37.2X4	T37.2X5	T37.2X6
Cinchophen	T50.4X1	T50.4X2	T50.4X3	T50.4X4	T50.4X5	T50.4X6
Cinepazide	T46.7X1	T46.7X2	T46.7X3	T46.7X4	T46.7X5	T46.7X6
Cinnamedrine	T48.5X1	T48.5X2	T48.5X3	T48.5X4	T48.5X5	T48.5X6
Cinnarizine	T45.0X1	T45.0X2	T45.0X3	T45.0X4	T45.0X5	T45.0X6
Cinoxacin	T37.8X1	T37.8X2	T37.8X3	T37.8X4	T37.8X5	T37.8X6
Ciprofibrate	T46.6X1	T46.6X2	T46.6X3	T46.6X4	T46.6X5	T46.6X6
Ciprofloxacin	T36.8X1	T36.8X2	T36.8X3	T36.8X4	T36.8X5	T36.8X6
Cisapride	T47.8X1	T47.8X2	T47.8X3	T47.8X4	T47.8X5	T47.8X6
Cisplatin	T45.1X1	T45.1X2	T45.1X3	T45.1X4	T45.1X5	T45.1X6
Citalopram	T43.221	T43.222	T43.223	T43.224	T43.225	T43.226
Citanest	T41.3X1	T41.3X2	T41.3X3	T41.3X4	T41.3X5	T41.3X6
infiltration (subcutaneous)	T41.3X1	T41.3X2	T41.3X3	T41.3X4	T41.3X5	T41.3X6
nerve block (peripheral) (plexus)	T41.3X1	T41.3X2	T41.3X3	T41.3X4	T41.3X5	T41.3X6
Citric acid	T47.5X1	T47.5X2	T47.5X3	T47.5X4	T47.5X5	T47.5X6
Citrovorum (factor)	T45.8X1	T45.8X2	T45.8X3	T45.8X4	T45.8X5	T45.8X6
Claviceps purpurea	T62.2X1	T62.2X2	T62.2X3	T62.2X4	—	—
Clavulanic acid	T36.1X1	T36.1X2	T36.1X3	T36.1X4	T36.1X5	T36.1X6
Cleaner, cleansing agent, type not specified	T65.891	T65.892	T65.893	T65.894	—	—
of paint or varnish	T52.91	T52.92	T52.93	T52.94	—	—
specified type NEC	T65.891	T65.892	T65.893	T65.894	—	—
Clebopride	T47.8X1	T47.8X2	T47.8X3	T47.8X4	T47.8X5	T47.8X6
Clefamide	T37.3X1	T37.3X2	T37.3X3	T37.3X4	T37.3X5	T37.3X6
Clemastine	T45.0X1	T45.0X2	T45.0X3	T45.0X4	T45.0X5	T45.0X6
Clematis vitalba	T62.2X1	T62.2X2	T62.2X3	T62.2X4	—	—
Clemizole	T45.0X1	T45.0X2	T45.0X3	T45.0X4	T45.0X5	T45.0X6
penicillin	T36.0X1	T36.0X2	T36.0X3	T36.0X4	T36.0X5	T36.0X6
Clenbuterol	T48.6X1	T48.6X2	T48.6X3	T48.6X4	T48.6X5	T48.6X6
Clidinium bromide	T44.3X1	T44.3X2	T44.3X3	T44.3X4	T44.3X5	T44.3X6
Clindamycin	T36.8X1	T36.8X2	T36.8X3	T36.8X4	T36.8X5	T36.8X6
Clinofibrate	T46.6X1	T46.6X2	T46.6X3	T46.6X4	T46.6X5	T46.6X6
Clioquinol	T37.8X1	T37.8X2	T37.8X3	T37.8X4	T37.8X5	T37.8X6
Cliradon	T40.2X1	T40.2X2	T40.2X3	T40.2X4	—	—
Clobazam	T42.4X1	T42.4X2	T42.4X3	T42.4X4	T42.4X5	T42.4X6
Clobenzorex	T50.5X1	T50.5X2	T50.5X3	T50.5X4	T50.5X5	T50.5X6
Clobetasol	T49.0X1	T49.0X2	T49.0X3	T49.0X4	T49.0X5	T49.0X6
Clobetasone	T49.0X1	T49.0X2	T49.0X3	T49.0X4	T49.0X5	T49.0X6
Clobutinol	T48.3X1	T48.3X2	T48.3X3	T48.3X4	T48.3X5	T48.3X6
Clocortolone	T38.0X1	T38.0X2	T38.0X3	T38.0X4	T38.0X5	T38.0X6
Clodantoin	T49.0X1	T49.0X2	T49.0X3	T49.0X4	T49.0X5	T49.0X6
Clodronic acid	T50.991	T50.992	T50.993	T50.994	T50.995	T50.996
Clofazimine	T37.1X1	T37.1X2	T37.1X3	T37.1X4	T37.1X5	T37.1X6
Clofedanol	T48.3X1	T48.3X2	T48.3X3	T48.3X4	T48.3X5	T48.3X6
Clofenamide	T50.2X1	T50.2X2	T50.2X3	T50.2X4	T50.2X5	T50.2X6
Clofenotane	T49.0X1	T49.0X2	T49.0X3	T49.0X4	T49.0X5	T49.0X6
Clofezone	T39.2X1	T39.2X2	T39.2X3	T39.2X4	T39.2X5	T39.2X6
Clofibrate	T46.6X1	T46.6X2	T46.6X3	T46.6X4	T46.6X5	T46.6X6

Additional Character May Be Required — Refer to the Tabular List for Character Selection   ▽ Subterms under main terms may continue to next column or page

Substance	Poisoning, Accidental (unintentional)	Poisoning, Intentional Self-harm	Poisoning, Assault	Poisoning, Undetermined	Adverse Effect	Under-dosing
Clofibride	T46.6X1	T46.6X2	T46.6X3	T46.6X4	T46.6X5	T46.6X6
Cloforex	T50.5X1	T50.5X2	T50.5X3	T50.5X4	T50.5X5	T50.5X6
Clomethiazole	T42.6X1	T42.6X2	T42.6X3	T42.6X4	T42.6X5	T42.6X6
Clometocillin	T36.0X1	T36.0X2	T36.0X3	T36.0X4	T36.0X5	T36.0X6
Clomifene	T38.5X1	T38.5X2	T38.5X3	T38.5X4	T38.5X5	T38.5X6
Clomiphene	T38.5X1	T38.5X2	T38.5X3	T38.5X4	T38.5X5	T38.5X6
Clomipramine	T43.011	T43.012	T43.013	T43.014	T43.015	T43.016
Clomocycline	T36.4X1	T36.4X2	T36.4X3	T36.4X4	T36.4X5	T36.4X6
Clonazepam	T42.4X1	T42.4X2	T42.4X3	T42.4X4	T42.4X5	T42.4X6
Clonidine	T46.5X1	T46.5X2	T46.5X3	T46.5X4	T46.5X5	T46.5X6
Clonixin	T39.8X1	T39.8X2	T39.8X3	T39.8X4	T39.8X5	T39.8X6
Clopamide	T50.2X1	T50.2X2	T50.2X3	T50.2X4	T50.2X5	T50.2X6
Clopenthixol	T43.4X1	T43.4X2	T43.4X3	T43.4X4	T43.4X5	T43.4X6
Cloperastine	T48.3X1	T48.3X2	T48.3X3	T48.3X4	T48.3X5	T48.3X6
Clophedianol	T48.3X1	T48.3X2	T48.3X3	T48.3X4	T48.3X5	T48.3X6
Cloponone	T36.2X1	T36.2X2	T36.2X3	T36.2X4	T36.2X5	T36.2X6
Cloprednol	T38.0X1	T38.0X2	T38.0X3	T38.0X4	T38.0X5	T38.0X6
Cloral betaine	T42.6X1	T42.6X2	T42.6X3	T42.6X4	T42.6X5	T42.6X6
Cloramfenicol	T36.2X1	T36.2X2	T36.2X3	T36.2X4	T36.2X5	T36.2X6
Clorazepate (dipotassium)	T42.4X1	T42.4X2	T42.4X3	T42.4X4	T42.4X5	T42.4X6
Clorexolone	T50.2X1	T50.2X2	T50.2X3	T50.2X4	T50.2X5	T50.2X6
Clorfenamine	T45.0X1	T45.0X2	T45.0X3	T45.0X4	T45.0X5	T45.0X6
Clorgiline	T43.1X1	T43.1X2	T43.1X3	T43.1X4	T43.1X5	T43.1X6
Clorotepine	T44.3X1	T44.3X2	T44.3X3	T44.3X4	T44.3X5	T44.3X6
Clorox (bleach)	T54.91	T54.92	T54.93	T54.94	—	—
Clorprenaline	T48.6X1	T48.6X2	T48.6X3	T48.6X4	T48.6X5	T48.6X6
Clortermine	T50.5X1	T50.5X2	T50.5X3	T50.5X4	T50.5X5	T50.5X6
Clotiapine	T43.591	T43.592	T43.593	T43.594	T43.595	T43.596
Clotiazepam	T42.4X1	T42.4X2	T42.4X3	T42.4X4	T42.4X5	T42.4X6
Clotibric acid	T46.6X1	T46.6X2	T46.6X3	T46.6X4	T46.6X5	T46.6X6
Clotrimazole	T49.0X1	T49.0X2	T49.0X3	T49.0X4	T49.0X5	T49.0X6
Cloxacillin	T36.0X1	T36.0X2	T36.0X3	T36.0X4	T36.0X5	T36.0X6
Cloxazolam	T42.4X1	T42.4X2	T42.4X3	T42.4X4	T42.4X5	T42.4X6
Cloxiquine	T49.0X1	T49.0X2	T49.0X3	T49.0X4	T49.0X5	T49.0X6
Clozapine	T42.4X1	T42.4X2	T42.4X3	T42.4X4	T42.4X5	T42.4X6
Coagulant NEC	T45.7X1	T45.7X2	T45.7X3	T45.7X4	T45.7X5	T45.7X6
Coal (carbon monoxide from) — see also Carbon, monoxide, coal	T58.2X1	T58.2X2	T58.2X3	T58.2X4	—	—
oil — see Kerosene						
tar	T49.1X1	T49.1X2	T49.1X3	T49.1X4	T49.1X5	T49.1X6
fumes	T59.891	T59.892	T59.893	T59.894		
medicinal (ointment)	T49.4X1	T49.4X2	T49.4X3	T49.4X4	T49.4X5	T49.4X6
analgesics NEC	T39.2X1	T39.2X2	T39.2X3	T39.2X4	T39.2X5	T39.2X6
naphtha (solvent)	T52.0X1	T52.0X2	T52.0X3	T52.0X4		
Cobalamine	T45.2X1	T45.2X2	T45.2X3	T45.2X4	T45.2X5	T45.2X6
Cobalt (nonmedicinal) (fumes) (industrial)	T56.891	T56.892	T56.893	T56.894	—	—
medicinal (trace) (chloride)	T45.8X1	T45.8X2	T45.8X3	T45.8X4	T45.8X5	T45.8X6
Cobra (venom)	T63.041	T63.042	T63.043	T63.044	—	—
Coca (leaf)	T40.5X1	T40.5X2	T40.5X3	T40.5X4	T40.5X5	T40.5X6
Cocaine	T40.5X1	T40.5X2	T40.5X3	T40.5X4	T40.5X5	T40.5X6
topical anesthetic	T41.3X1	T41.3X2	T41.3X3	T41.3X4	T41.3X5	T41.3X6
Cocarboxylase	T45.3X1	T45.3X2	T45.3X3	T45.3X4	T45.3X5	T45.3X6
Coccidioidin	T50.8X1	T50.8X2	T50.8X3	T50.8X4	T50.8X5	T50.8X6
Cocculus indicus	T62.1X1	T62.1X2	T62.1X3	T62.1X4	—	—
Cochineal	T65.6X1	T65.6X2	T65.6X3	T65.6X4	—	—
medicinal products	T50.991	T50.992	T50.993	T50.994	T50.995	T50.996
Codeine	T40.2X1	T40.2X2	T40.2X3	T40.2X4	T40.2X5	T40.2X6
Cod-liver oil	T45.2X1	T45.2X2	T45.2X3	T45.2X4	T45.2X5	T45.2X6
Coenzyme A	T50.991	T50.992	T50.993	T50.994	T50.995	T50.996
Coffee	T62.8X1	T62.8X2	T62.8X3	T62.8X4	—	—
Cogalactoisomerase	T50.991	T50.992	T50.993	T50.994	T50.995	T50.996
Cogentin	T44.3X1	T44.3X2	T44.3X3	T44.3X4	T44.3X5	T44.3X6
Coke fumes or gas (carbon monoxide)	T58.2X1	T58.2X2	T58.2X3	T58.2X4	—	—
industrial use	T58.8X1	T58.8X2	T58.8X3	T58.8X4	—	—
Colace	T47.4X1	T47.4X2	T47.4X3	T47.4X4	T47.4X5	T47.4X6
Colaspase	T45.1X1	T45.1X2	T45.1X3	T45.1X4	T45.1X5	T45.1X6
Colchicine	T50.4X1	T50.4X2	T50.4X3	T50.4X4	T50.4X5	T50.4X6
Colchicum	T62.2X1	T62.2X2	T62.2X3	T62.2X4	—	—
Cold cream	T49.3X1	T49.3X2	T49.3X3	T49.3X4	T49.3X5	T49.3X6
Colecalciferol	T45.2X1	T45.2X2	T45.2X3	T45.2X4	T45.2X5	T45.2X6
Colestipol	T46.6X1	T46.6X2	T46.6X3	T46.6X4	T46.6X5	T46.6X6
Colestyramine	T46.6X1	T46.6X2	T46.6X3	T46.6X4	T46.6X5	T46.6X6
Colimycin	T36.8X1	T36.8X2	T36.8X3	T36.8X4	T36.8X5	T36.8X6
Colistimethate	T36.8X1	T36.8X2	T36.8X3	T36.8X4	T36.8X5	T36.8X6
Colistin	T36.8X1	T36.8X2	T36.8X3	T36.8X4	T36.8X5	T36.8X6
sulfate (eye preparation)	T49.5X1	T49.5X2	T49.5X3	T49.5X4	T49.5X5	T49.5X6
Collagen	T50.991	T50.992	T50.993	T50.994	T50.995	T50.996
Collagenase	T49.4X1	T49.4X2	T49.4X3	T49.4X4	T49.4X5	T49.4X6
Collodion	T49.3X1	T49.3X2	T49.3X3	T49.3X4	T49.3X5	T49.3X6
Colocynth	T47.2X1	T47.2X2	T47.2X3	T47.2X4	T47.2X5	T47.2X6

Substance	Poisoning, Accidental (unintentional)	Poisoning, Intentional Self-harm	Poisoning, Assault	Poisoning, Undetermined	Adverse Effect	Under-dosing
Colophony adhesive	T49.3X1	T49.3X2	T49.3X3	T49.3X4	T49.3X5	T49.3X6
Colorant — see also Dye	T50.991	T50.992	T50.993	T50.994	T50.995	T50.996
Coloring matter — see Dye(s)						
Combustion gas (after combustion) — see Carbon, monoxide						
prior to combustion	T59.891	T59.892	T59.893	T59.894	—	—
Compazine	T43.3X1	T43.3X2	T43.3X3	T43.3X4	T43.3X5	T43.3X6
Compound						
1080 (sodium fluoroacetate)	T60.4X1	T60.4X2	T60.4X3	T60.4X4		
269 (endrin)	T60.1X1	T60.1X2	T60.1X3	T60.1X4		
3422 (parathion)	T60.0X1	T60.0X2	T60.0X3	T60.0X4		
3911 (phorate)	T60.0X1	T60.0X2	T60.0X3	T60.0X4		
3956 (toxaphene)	T60.1X1	T60.1X2	T60.1X3	T60.1X4		
4049 (malathion)	T60.0X1	T60.0X2	T60.0X3	T60.0X4		
4069 (malathion)	T60.0X1	T60.0X2	T60.0X3	T60.0X4		
4124 (dicapthon)	T60.0X1	T60.0X2	T60.0X3	T60.0X4		
42 (warfarin)	T60.4X1	T60.4X2	T60.4X3	T60.4X4		
497 (dieldrin)	T60.1X1	T60.1X2	T60.1X3	T60.1X4		
E (cortisone)	T38.0X1	T38.0X2	T38.0X3	T38.0X4	T38.0X5	T38.0X6
F (hydrocortisone)	T38.0X1	T38.0X2	T38.0X3	T38.0X4	T38.0X5	T38.0X6
Congener, anabolic	T38.7X1	T38.7X2	T38.7X3	T38.7X4	T38.7X5	T38.7X6
Congo red	T50.8X1	T50.8X2	T50.8X3	T50.8X4	T50.8X5	T50.8X6
Coniine, conine	T62.2X1	T62.2X2	T62.2X3	T62.2X4	—	—
Conium (maculatum)	T62.2X1	T62.2X2	T62.2X3	T62.2X4	—	—
Conjugated estrogenic substances	T38.5X1	T38.5X2	T38.5X3	T38.5X4	T38.5X5	T38.5X6
Contac	T48.5X1	T48.5X2	T48.5X3	T48.5X4	T48.5X5	T48.5X6
Contact lens solution	T49.5X1	T49.5X2	T49.5X3	T49.5X4	T49.5X5	T49.5X6
Contraceptive (oral)	T38.4X1	T38.4X2	T38.4X3	T38.4X4	T38.4X5	T38.4X6
vaginal	T49.8X1	T49.8X2	T49.8X3	T49.8X4	T49.8X5	T49.8X6
Contrast medium, radiography	T50.8X1	T50.8X2	T50.8X3	T50.8X4	T50.8X5	T50.8X6
Convallaria glycosides	T46.0X1	T46.0X2	T46.0X3	T46.0X4	T46.0X5	T46.0X6
Convallaria majalis	T62.2X1	T62.2X2	T62.2X3	T62.2X4	—	—
berry	T62.1X1	T62.1X2	T62.1X3	T62.1X4	—	—
Copperhead snake (bite) (venom)	T63.061	T63.062	T63.063	T63.064	—	—
Copper (dust) (fumes) (nonmedicinal) NEC	T56.4X1	T56.4X2	T56.4X3	T56.4X4		
arsenate, arsenite	T57.0X1	T57.0X2	T57.0X3	T57.0X4	—	—
insecticide	T60.2X1	T60.2X2	T60.2X3	T60.2X4	—	—
emetic	T47.7X1	T47.7X2	T47.7X3	T47.7X4	T47.7X5	T47.7X6
fungicide	T60.3X1	T60.3X2	T60.3X3	T60.3X4	—	—
gluconate	T49.0X1	T49.0X2	T49.0X3	T49.0X4	T49.0X5	T49.0X6
insecticide	T60.2X1	T60.2X2	T60.2X3	T60.2X4	—	—
medicinal (trace)	T45.8X1	T45.8X2	T45.8X3	T45.8X4	T45.8X5	T45.8X6
oleate	T49.0X1	T49.0X2	T49.0X3	T49.0X4	T49.0X5	T49.0X6
sulfate	T56.4X1	T56.4X2	T56.4X3	T56.4X4		
cupric	T56.4X1	T56.4X2	T56.4X3	T56.4X4		
fungicide	T60.3X1	T60.3X2	T60.3X3	T60.3X4		
medicinal						
ear	T49.6X1	T49.6X2	T49.6X3	T49.6X4	T49.6X5	T49.6X6
emetic	T47.7X1	T47.7X2	T47.7X3	T47.7X4	T47.7X5	T47.7X6
eye	T49.5X1	T49.5X2	T49.5X3	T49.5X4	T49.5X5	T49.5X6
cuprous	T56.4X1	T56.4X2	T56.4X3	T56.4X4		
fungicide	T60.3X1	T60.3X2	T60.3X3	T60.3X4		
medicinal						
ear	T49.6X1	T49.6X2	T49.6X3	T49.6X4	T49.6X5	T49.6X6
emetic	T47.7X1	T47.7X2	T47.7X3	T47.7X4	T47.7X5	T47.7X6
eye	T49.5X1	T49.5X2	T49.5X3	T49.5X4	T49.5X5	T49.5X6
Coral (sting)	T63.691	T63.692	T63.693	T63.694	—	—
snake (bite) (venom)	T63.021	T63.022	T63.023	T63.024	—	—
Corbadrine	T49.6X1	T49.6X2	T49.6X3	T49.6X4	T49.6X5	T49.6X6
Cordite	T65.891	T65.892	T65.893	T65.894	—	—
vapor	T59.891	T59.892	T59.893	T59.894	—	—
Cordran	T49.0X1	T49.0X2	T49.0X3	T49.0X4	T49.0X5	T49.0X6
Corn cures	T49.4X1	T49.4X2	T49.4X3	T49.4X4	T49.4X5	T49.4X6
Cornhusker's lotion	T49.3X1	T49.3X2	T49.3X3	T49.3X4	T49.3X5	T49.3X6
Corn starch	T49.3X1	T49.3X2	T49.3X3	T49.3X4	T49.3X5	T49.3X6
Coronary vasodilator NEC	T46.3X1	T46.3X2	T46.3X3	T46.3X4	T46.3X5	T46.3X6
Corrosive NEC	T54.91	T54.92	T54.93	T54.94	—	—
acid NEC	T54.2X1	T54.2X2	T54.2X3	T54.2X4	—	—
aromatics	T54.1X1	T54.1X2	T54.1X3	T54.1X4	—	—
disinfectant	T54.1X1	T54.1X2	T54.1X3	T54.1X4	—	—
fumes NEC	T54.91	T54.92	T54.93	T54.94	—	—
specified NEC	T54.91	T54.92	T54.93	T54.94	—	—
sublimate	T56.1X1	T56.1X2	T56.1X3	T56.1X4	—	—
Cortate	T38.0X1	T38.0X2	T38.0X3	T38.0X4	T38.0X5	T38.0X6
Cort-Dome	T38.0X1	T38.0X2	T38.0X3	T38.0X4	T38.0X5	T38.0X6
ENT agent	T49.6X1	T49.6X2	T49.6X3	T49.6X4	T49.6X5	T49.6X6
ophthalmic preparation	T49.5X1	T49.5X2	T49.5X3	T49.5X4	T49.5X5	T49.5X6

Table of Drugs and Chemicals

Clofibride — Cort-Dome

Table of Drugs and Chemicals

Substance	Poisoning, Accidental (unintentional)	Poisoning, Intentional Self-harm	Poisoning, Assault	Poisoning, Undetermined	Adverse Effect	Under-dosing
Cort-Dome — *continued*						
topical NEC	T49.0X1	T49.0X2	T49.0X3	T49.0X4	T49.0X5	T49.0X6
Cortef	T38.0X1	T38.0X2	T38.0X3	T38.0X4	T38.0X5	T38.0X6
ENT agent	T49.6X1	T49.6X2	T49.6X3	T49.6X4	T49.6X5	T49.6X6
ophthalmic preparation	T49.5X1	T49.5X2	T49.5X3	T49.5X4	T49.5X5	T49.5X6
topical NEC	T49.0X1	T49.0X2	T49.0X3	T49.0X4	T49.0X5	T49.0X6
Corticosteroid	T38.0X1	T38.0X2	T38.0X3	T38.0X4	T38.0X5	T38.0X6
ENT agent	T49.6X1	T49.6X2	T49.6X3	T49.6X4	T49.6X5	T49.6X6
mineral	T50.0X1	T50.0X2	T50.0X3	T50.0X4	T50.0X5	T50.0X6
ophthalmic	T49.5X1	T49.5X2	T49.5X3	T49.5X4	T49.5X5	T49.5X6
topical NEC	T49.0X1	T49.0X2	T49.0X3	T49.0X4	T49.0X5	T49.0X6
Corticotropin	T38.811	T38.812	T38.813	T38.814	T38.815	T38.816
Cortisol	T49.0X1	T49.0X2	T49.0X3	T49.0X4	T49.0X5	T49.0X6
ENT agent	T49.6X1	T49.6X2	T49.6X3	T49.6X4	T49.6X5	T49.6X6
ophthalmic preparation	T49.5X1	T49.5X2	T49.5X3	T49.5X4	T49.5X5	T49.5X6
topical NEC	T49.0X1	T49.0X2	T49.0X3	T49.0X4	T49.0X5	T49.0X6
Cortisone (acetate)	T38.0X1	T38.0X2	T38.0X3	T38.0X4	T38.0X5	T38.0X6
ENT agent	T49.6X1	T49.6X2	T49.6X3	T49.6X4	T49.6X5	T49.6X6
ophthalmic preparation	T49.5X1	T49.5X2	T49.5X3	T49.5X4	T49.5X5	T49.5X6
topical NEC	T49.0X1	T49.0X2	T49.0X3	T49.0X4	T49.0X5	T49.0X6
Cortivazol	T38.0X1	T38.0X2	T38.0X3	T38.0X4	T38.0X5	T38.0X6
Cortogen	T38.0X1	T38.0X2	T38.0X3	T38.0X4	T38.0X5	T38.0X6
ENT agent	T49.6X1	T49.6X2	T49.6X3	T49.6X4	T49.6X5	T49.6X6
ophthalmic preparation	T49.5X1	T49.5X2	T49.5X3	T49.5X4	T49.5X5	T49.5X6
Cortone	T38.0X1	T38.0X2	T38.0X3	T38.0X4	T38.0X5	T38.0X6
ENT agent	T49.6X1	T49.6X2	T49.6X3	T49.6X4	T49.6X5	T49.6X6
ophthalmic preparation	T49.5X1	T49.5X2	T49.5X3	T49.5X4	T49.5X5	T49.5X6
Cortril	T38.0X1	T38.0X2	T38.0X3	T38.0X4	T38.0X5	T38.0X6
ENT agent	T49.6X1	T49.6X2	T49.6X3	T49.6X4	T49.6X5	T49.6X6
ophthalmic preparation	T49.5X1	T49.5X2	T49.5X3	T49.5X4	T49.5X5	T49.5X6
topical NEC	T49.0X1	T49.0X2	T49.0X3	T49.0X4	T49.0X5	T49.0X6
Corynebacterium parvum	T45.1X1	T45.1X2	T45.1X3	T45.1X4	T45.1X5	T45.1X6
Cosmetic preparation	T49.8X1	T49.8X2	T49.8X3	T49.8X4	T49.8X5	T49.8X6
Cosmetics	T49.8X1	T49.8X2	T49.8X3	T49.8X4	T49.8X5	T49.8X6
Cosyntropin	T38.811	T38.812	T38.813	T38.814	T38.815	T38.816
Cotarnine	T45.7X1	T45.7X2	T45.7X3	T45.7X4	T45.7X5	T45.7X6
Co-trimoxazole	T36.8X1	T36.8X2	T36.8X3	T36.8X4	T36.8X5	T36.8X6
Cottonseed oil	T49.3X1	T49.3X2	T49.3X3	T49.3X4	T49.3X5	T49.3X6
Cough mixture (syrup)	T48.4X1	T48.4X2	T48.4X3	T48.4X4	T48.4X5	T48.4X6
containing opiates	T40.2X1	T40.2X2	T40.2X3	T40.2X4	T40.2X5	T40.2X6
expectorants	T48.4X1	T48.4X2	T48.4X3	T48.4X4	T48.4X5	T48.4X6
Coumadin	T45.511	T45.512	T45.513	T45.514	T45.515	T45.516
rodenticide	T60.4X1	T60.4X2	T60.4X3	T60.4X4	—	—
Coumaphos	T60.0X1	T60.0X2	T60.0X3	T60.0X4	—	—
Coumarin	T45.511	T45.512	T45.513	T45.514	T45.515	T45.516
Coumetarol	T45.511	T45.512	T45.513	T45.514	T45.515	T45.516
Cowbane	T62.2X1	T62.2X2	T62.2X3	T62.2X4	—	—
Cozyme	T45.2X1	T45.2X2	T45.2X3	T45.2X4	T45.2X5	T45.2X6
Crack	T40.5X1	T40.5X2	T40.5X3	T40.5X4	—	—
Crataegus extract	T46.0X1	T46.0X2	T46.0X3	T46.0X4	T46.0X5	T46.0X6
Creolin	T54.1X1	T54.1X2	T54.1X3	T54.1X4	—	—
disinfectant	T54.1X1	T54.1X2	T54.1X3	T54.1X4	—	—
Creosol (compound)	T49.0X1	T49.0X2	T49.0X3	T49.0X4	T49.0X5	T49.0X6
Creosote (coal tar)	T49.0X1	T49.0X2	T49.0X3	T49.0X4	T49.0X5	T49.0X6
(beechwood)						
medicinal (expectorant)	T48.4X1	T48.4X2	T48.4X3	T48.4X4	T48.4X5	T48.4X6
syrup	T48.4X1	T48.4X2	T48.4X3	T48.4X4	T48.4X5	T48.4X6
Cresol(s)	T49.0X1	T49.0X2	T49.0X3	T49.0X4	T49.0X5	T49.0X6
and soap solution	T49.0X1	T49.0X2	T49.0X3	T49.0X4	T49.0X5	T49.0X6
Cresyl acetate	T49.0X1	T49.0X2	T49.0X3	T49.0X4	T49.0X5	T49.0X6
Cresylic acid	T49.0X1	T49.0X2	T49.0X3	T49.0X4	T49.0X5	T49.0X6
Crimidine	T60.4X1	T60.4X2	T60.4X3	T60.4X4	—	—
Croconazole	T37.8X1	T37.8X2	T37.8X3	T37.8X4	T37.8X5	T37.8X6
Cromoglicic acid	T48.6X1	T48.6X2	T48.6X3	T48.6X4	T48.6X5	T48.6X6
Cromolyn	T48.6X1	T48.6X2	T48.6X3	T48.6X4	T48.6X5	T48.6X6
Cromonar	T46.3X1	T46.3X2	T46.3X3	T46.3X4	T46.3X5	T46.3X6
Cropropamide	T39.8X1	T39.8X2	T39.8X3	T39.8X4	T39.8X5	T39.8X6
with crotethamide	T50.7X1	T50.7X2	T50.7X3	T50.7X4	T50.7X5	T50.7X6
Crotamiton	T49.0X1	T49.0X2	T49.0X3	T49.0X4	T49.0X5	T49.0X6
Crotethamide	T39.8X1	T39.8X2	T39.8X3	T39.8X4	T39.8X5	T39.8X6
with cropropamide	T50.7X1	T50.7X2	T50.7X3	T50.7X4	T50.7X5	T50.7X6
Croton (oil)	T47.2X1	T47.2X2	T47.2X3	T47.2X4	T47.2X5	T47.2X6
chloral	T42.6X1	T42.6X2	T42.6X3	T42.6X4	T42.6X5	T42.6X6
Crude oil	T52.0X1	T52.0X2	T52.0X3	T52.0X4	—	—
Cryogenine	T39.8X1	T39.8X2	T39.8X3	T39.8X4	T39.8X5	T39.8X6
Cryolite (vapor)	T60.1X1	T60.1X2	T60.1X3	T60.1X4	—	—
insecticide	T60.1X1	T60.1X2	T60.1X3	T60.1X4	—	—
Cryptenamine (tannates)	T46.5X1	T46.5X2	T46.5X3	T46.5X4	T46.5X5	T46.5X6
Crystal violet	T49.0X1	T49.0X2	T49.0X3	T49.0X4	T49.0X5	T49.0X6
Cuckoopint	T62.2X1	T62.2X2	T62.2X3	T62.2X4	—	—
Cumetharol	T45.511	T45.512	T45.513	T45.514	T45.515	T45.516
Cupric						
acetate	T60.3X1	T60.3X2	T60.3X3	T60.3X4	—	—
Cupric — *continued*						
acetoarsenite	T57.0X1	T57.0X2	T57.0X3	T57.0X4	—	—
arsenate	T57.0X1	T57.0X2	T57.0X3	T57.0X4	—	—
gluconate	T49.0X1	T49.0X2	T49.0X3	T49.0X4	T49.0X5	T49.0X6
oleate	T49.0X1	T49.0X2	T49.0X3	T49.0X4	T49.0X5	T49.0X6
sulfate	T56.4X1	T56.4X2	T56.4X3	T56.4X4	—	—
Cuprous sulfate — *see also*	T56.4X1	T56.4X2	T56.4X3	T56.4X4	—	—
Copper sulfate						
Curare, curarine	T48.1X1	T48.1X2	T48.1X3	T48.1X4	T48.1X5	T48.1X6
Cyamemazine	T43.3X1	T43.3X2	T43.3X3	T43.3X4	T43.3X5	T43.3X6
Cyamopsis tetragonoloba	T46.6X1	T46.6X2	T46.6X3	T46.6X4	T46.6X5	T46.6X6
Cyanacetyl hydrazide	T37.1X1	T37.1X2	T37.1X3	T37.1X4	T37.1X5	T37.1X6
Cyanic acid (gas)	T59.891	T59.892	T59.893	T59.894	—	—
Cyanide(s) (compounds)	T65.0X1	T65.0X2	T65.0X3	T65.0X4	—	—
(potassium) (sodium)						
NEC						
dust or gas (inhalation) NEC	T57.3X1	T57.3X2	T57.3X3	T57.3X4	—	—
fumigant	T65.0X1	T65.0X2	T65.0X3	T65.0X4	—	—
hydrogen	T57.3X1	T57.3X2	T57.3X3	T57.3X4	—	—
mercuric — *see* Mercury						
pesticide (dust) (fumes)	T65.0X1	T65.0X2	T65.0X3	T65.0X4	—	—
Cyanoacrylate adhesive	T49.3X1	T49.3X2	T49.3X3	T49.3X4	T49.3X5	T49.3X6
Cyanocobalamin	T45.8X1	T45.8X2	T45.8X3	T45.8X4	T45.8X5	T45.8X6
Cyanogen (chloride) (gas)	T59.891	T59.892	T59.893	T59.894	—	—
NEC						
Cyclacillin	T36.0X1	T36.0X2	T36.0X3	T36.0X4	T36.0X5	T36.0X6
Cyclaine	T41.3X1	T41.3X2	T41.3X3	T41.3X4	T41.3X5	T41.3X6
Cyclamate	T50.991	T50.992	T50.993	T50.994	T50.995	T50.996
Cyclamen europaeum	T62.2X1	T62.2X2	T62.2X3	T62.2X4	—	—
Cyclandelate	T46.7X1	T46.7X2	T46.7X3	T46.7X4	T46.7X5	T46.7X6
Cyclazocine	T50.7X1	T50.7X2	T50.7X3	T50.7X4	T50.7X5	T50.7X6
Cyclizine	T45.0X1	T45.0X2	T45.0X3	T45.0X4	T45.0X5	T45.0X6
Cyclobarbital	T42.3X1	T42.3X2	T42.3X3	T42.3X4	T42.3X5	T42.3X6
Cyclobarbitone	T42.3X1	T42.3X2	T42.3X3	T42.3X4	T42.3X5	T42.3X6
Cyclobenzaprine	T48.1X1	T48.1X2	T48.1X3	T48.1X4	T48.1X5	T48.1X6
Cyclodrine	T44.3X1	T44.3X2	T44.3X3	T44.3X4	T44.3X5	T44.3X6
Cycloguanil embonate	T37.2X1	T37.2X2	T37.2X3	T37.2X4	T37.2X5	T37.2X6
Cyclohexane	T52.8X1	T52.8X2	T52.8X3	T52.8X4	—	—
Cyclohexanol	T51.8X1	T51.8X2	T51.8X3	T51.8X4	—	—
Cyclohexanone	T52.4X1	T52.4X2	T52.4X3	T52.4X4	—	—
Cycloheximide	T60.3X1	T60.3X2	T60.3X3	T60.3X4	—	—
Cyclohexyl acetate	T52.8X1	T52.8X2	T52.8X3	T52.8X4	—	—
Cycloleucin	T45.1X1	T45.1X2	T45.1X3	T45.1X4	T45.1X5	T45.1X6
Cyclomethycaine	T41.3X1	T41.3X2	T41.3X3	T41.3X4	T41.3X5	T41.3X6
Cyclopentamine	T44.4X1	T44.4X2	T44.4X3	T44.4X4	T44.4X5	T44.4X6
Cyclopenthiazide	T50.2X1	T50.2X2	T50.2X3	T50.2X4	T50.2X5	T50.2X6
Cyclopentolate	T44.3X1	T44.3X2	T44.3X3	T44.3X4	T44.3X5	T44.3X6
Cyclophosphamide	T45.1X1	T45.1X2	T45.1X3	T45.1X4	T45.1X5	T45.1X6
Cycloplegic drug	T49.5X1	T49.5X2	T49.5X3	T49.5X4	T49.5X5	T49.5X6
Cyclopropane	T41.291	T41.292	T41.293	T41.294	T41.295	T41.296
Cyclopyrabital	T39.8X1	T39.8X2	T39.8X3	T39.8X4	T39.8X5	T39.8X6
Cycloserine	T37.1X1	T37.1X2	T37.1X3	T37.1X4	T37.1X5	T37.1X6
Cyclosporin	T45.1X1	T45.1X2	T45.1X3	T45.1X4	T45.1X5	T45.1X6
Cyclothiazide	T50.2X1	T50.2X2	T50.2X3	T50.2X4	T50.2X5	T50.2X6
Cycrimine	T44.3X1	T44.3X2	T44.3X3	T44.3X4	T44.3X5	T44.3X6
Cyhalothrin	T60.1X1	T60.1X2	T60.1X3	T60.1X4	—	—
Cymarin	T46.0X1	T46.0X2	T46.0X3	T46.0X4	T46.0X5	T46.0X6
Cypermethrin	T60.1X1	T60.1X2	T60.1X3	T60.1X4	—	—
Cyphenothrin	T60.2X1	T60.2X2	T60.2X3	T60.2X4	—	—
Cyproheptadine	T45.0X1	T45.0X2	T45.0X3	T45.0X4	T45.0X5	T45.0X6
Cyproterone	T38.6X1	T38.6X2	T38.6X3	T38.6X4	T38.6X5	T38.6X6
Cysteamine	T50.6X1	T50.6X2	T50.6X3	T50.6X4	T50.6X5	T50.6X6
Cytarabine	T45.1X1	T45.1X2	T45.1X3	T45.1X4	T45.1X5	T45.1X6
Cytisus						
laburnum	T62.2X1	T62.2X2	T62.2X3	T62.2X4	—	—
scoparius	T62.2X1	T62.2X2	T62.2X3	T62.2X4	—	—
Cytochrome C	T47.5X1	T47.5X2	T47.5X3	T47.5X4	T47.5X5	T47.5X6
Cytomel	T38.1X1	T38.1X2	T38.1X3	T38.1X4	T38.1X5	T38.1X6
Cytosine arabinoside	T45.1X1	T45.1X2	T45.1X3	T45.1X4	T45.1X5	T45.1X6
Cytoxan	T45.1X1	T45.1X2	T45.1X3	T45.1X4	T45.1X5	T45.1X6
Cytozyme	T45.7X1	T45.7X2	T45.7X3	T45.7X4	T45.7X5	T45.7X6
S-Carboxymethylcysteine	T48.4X1	T48.4X2	T48.4X3	T48.4X4	T48.4X5	T48.4X6
Dacarbazine	T45.1X1	T45.1X2	T45.1X3	T45.1X4	T45.1X5	T45.1X6
Dactinomycin	T45.1X1	T45.1X2	T45.1X3	T45.1X4	T45.1X5	T45.1X6
DADPS	T37.1X1	T37.1X2	T37.1X3	T37.1X4	T37.1X5	T37.1X6
Dakin's solution	T49.0X1	T49.0X2	T49.0X3	T49.0X4	T49.0X5	T49.0X6
Dalapon (sodium)	T60.3X1	T60.3X2	T60.3X3	T60.3X4	—	—
Dalmane	T42.4X1	T42.4X2	T42.4X3	T42.4X4	T42.4X5	T42.4X6
Danazol	T38.6X1	T38.6X2	T38.6X3	T38.6X4	T38.6X5	T38.6X6
Danilone	T45.511	T45.512	T45.513	T45.514	T45.515	T45.516
Danthron	T47.2X1	T47.2X2	T47.2X3	T47.2X4	T47.2X5	T47.2X6
Dantrolene	T42.8X1	T42.8X2	T42.8X3	T42.8X4	T42.8X5	T42.8X6
Dantron	T47.2X1	T47.2X2	T47.2X3	T47.2X4	T47.2X5	T47.2X6

Additional Character May Be Required — Refer to the Tabular List for Character Selection ▽ Subterms under main terms may continue to next column or page

Cort-Dome — Dantron

Substance	Poisoning, Accidental (unintentional)	Poisoning, Intentional Self-harm	Poisoning, Assault	Poisoning, Undetermined	Adverse Effect	Under-dosing
Daphne (gnidium) (mezereum)	T62.2X1	T62.2X2	T62.2X3	T62.2X4	—	—
berry	T62.1X1	T62.1X2	T62.1X3	T62.1X4	—	—
Dapsone	T37.1X1	T37.1X2	T37.1X3	T37.1X4	T37.1X5	T37.1X6
Daraprim	T37.2X1	T37.2X2	T37.2X3	T37.2X4	T37.2X5	T37.2X6
Darnel	T62.2X1	T62.2X2	T62.2X3	T62.2X4	—	—
Darvon	T39.8X1	T39.8X2	T39.8X3	T39.8X4	T39.8X5	T39.8X6
Daunomycin	T45.1X1	T45.1X2	T45.1X3	T45.1X4	T45.1X5	T45.1X6
Daunorubicin	T45.1X1	T45.1X2	T45.1X3	T45.1X4	T45.1X5	T45.1X6
DBI	T38.3X1	T38.3X2	T38.3X3	T38.3X4	T38.3X5	T38.3X6
D-Con	T60.91	T60.92	T60.93	T60.94	—	—
insecticide	T60.2X1	T60.2X2	T60.2X3	T60.2X4	—	—
rodenticide	T60.4X1	T60.4X2	T60.4X3	T60.4X4	—	—
DDAVP	T38.891	T38.892	T38.893	T38.894	T38.895	T38.896
DDE (bis(chlorophenyl)-dichloroethylene)	T60.2X1	T60.2X2	T60.2X3	T60.2X4	—	—
DDS	T37.1X1	T37.1X2	T37.1X3	T37.1X4	T37.1X5	T37.1X6
DDT (dust)	T60.1X1	T60.1X2	T60.1X3	T60.1X4	—	—
Deadly nightshade — *see also* Belladonna	T62.2X1	T62.2X2	T62.2X3	T62.2X4	—	—
berry	T62.1X1	T62.1X2	T62.1X3	T62.1X4	—	—
Deamino-D-arginine vasopressin	T38.891	T38.892	T38.893	T38.894	T38.895	T38.896
Deanol (aceglumate)	T50.991	T50.992	T50.993	T50.994	T50.995	T50.996
Debrisoquine	T46.5X1	T46.5X2	T46.5X3	T46.5X4	T46.5X5	T46.5X6
Decaborane	T57.8X1	T57.8X2	T57.8X3	T57.8X4	—	—
fumes	T59.891	T59.892	T59.893	T59.894	—	—
Decadron	T38.0X1	T38.0X2	T38.0X3	T38.0X4	T38.0X5	T38.0X6
ENT agent	T49.6X1	T49.6X2	T49.6X3	T49.6X4	T49.6X5	T49.6X6
ophthalmic preparation	T49.5X1	T49.5X2	T49.5X3	T49.5X4	T49.5X5	T49.5X6
topical NEC	T49.0X1	T49.0X2	T49.0X3	T49.0X4	T49.0X5	T49.0X6
Decahydronaphthalene	T52.8X1	T52.8X2	T52.8X3	T52.8X4	—	—
Decalin	T52.8X1	T52.8X2	T52.8X3	T52.8X4	—	—
Decamethonium (bromide)	T48.1X1	T48.1X2	T48.1X3	T48.1X4	T48.1X5	T48.1X6
Decholin	T47.5X1	T47.5X2	T47.5X3	T47.5X4	T47.5X5	T47.5X6
Declomycin	T36.4X1	T36.4X2	T36.4X3	T36.4X4	T36.4X5	T36.4X6
Decongestant, nasal (mucosa)	T48.5X1	T48.5X2	T48.5X3	T48.5X4	T48.5X5	T48.5X6
combination	T48.5X1	T48.5X2	T48.5X3	T48.5X4	T48.5X5	T48.5X6
Deet	T60.8X1	T60.8X2	T60.8X3	T60.8X4	—	—
Deferoxamine	T45.8X1	T45.8X2	T45.8X3	T45.8X4	T45.8X5	T45.8X6
Deflazacort	T38.0X1	T38.0X2	T38.0X3	T38.0X4	T38.0X5	T38.0X6
Deglycyrrhizinized extract of licorice	T48.4X1	T48.4X2	T48.4X3	T48.4X4	T48.4X5	T48.4X6
Dehydrocholic acid	T47.5X1	T47.5X2	T47.5X3	T47.5X4	T47.5X5	T47.5X6
Dehydroemetine	T37.3X1	T37.3X2	T37.3X3	T37.3X4	T37.3X5	T37.3X6
Dekalin	T52.8X1	T52.8X2	T52.8X3	T52.8X4	—	—
Delalutin	T38.5X1	T38.5X2	T38.5X3	T38.5X4	T38.5X5	T38.5X6
Delorazepam	T42.4X1	T42.4X2	T42.4X3	T42.4X4	T42.4X5	T42.4X6
Delphinium	T62.2X1	T62.2X2	T62.2X3	T62.2X4	—	—
Deltamethrin	T60.1X1	T60.1X2	T60.1X3	T60.1X4	—	—
Deltasone	T38.0X1	T38.0X2	T38.0X3	T38.0X4	T38.0X5	T38.0X6
Deltra	T38.0X1	T38.0X2	T38.0X3	T38.0X4	T38.0X5	T38.0X6
Delvinal	T42.3X1	T42.3X2	T42.3X3	T42.3X4	T42.3X5	T42.3X6
Demecarium (bromide)	T49.5X1	T49.5X2	T49.5X3	T49.5X4	T49.5X5	T49.5X6
Demeclocycline	T36.4X1	T36.4X2	T36.4X3	T36.4X4	T36.4X5	T36.4X6
Demecolcine	T45.1X1	T45.1X2	T45.1X3	T45.1X4	T45.1X5	T45.1X6
Demegestone	T38.5X1	T38.5X2	T38.5X3	T38.5X4	T38.5X5	T38.5X6
Demelanizing agents	T49.8X1	T49.8X2	T49.8X3	T49.8X4	T49.8X5	T49.8X6
Demephion -O and -S	T60.0X1	T60.0X2	T60.0X3	T60.0X4	—	—
Demerol	T40.2X1	T40.2X2	T40.2X3	T40.2X4	T40.2X5	T40.2X6
Demethylchlortetracycline	T36.4X1	T36.4X2	T36.4X3	T36.4X4	T36.4X5	T36.4X6
Demethyltetracycline	T36.4X1	T36.4X2	T36.4X3	T36.4X4	T36.4X5	T36.4X6
Demeton -O and -S	T60.0X1	T60.0X2	T60.0X3	T60.0X4	—	—
Demulcent (external)	T49.3X1	T49.3X2	T49.3X3	T49.3X4	T49.3X5	T49.3X6
specified NEC	T49.3X1	T49.3X2	T49.3X3	T49.3X4	T49.3X5	T49.3X6
Demulen	T38.4X1	T38.4X2	T38.4X3	T38.4X4	T38.4X5	T38.4X6
Denatured alcohol	T51.0X1	T51.0X2	T51.0X3	T51.0X4	—	—
Dendrid	T49.5X1	T49.5X2	T49.5X3	T49.5X4	T49.5X5	T49.5X6
Dental drug, topical application NEC	T49.7X1	T49.7X2	T49.7X3	T49.7X4	T49.7X5	T49.7X6
Dentifrice	T49.7X1	T49.7X2	T49.7X3	T49.7X4	T49.7X5	T49.7X6
Deodorant spray (feminine hygiene)	T49.8X1	T49.8X2	T49.8X3	T49.8X4	T49.8X5	T49.8X6
Deoxycortone	T50.0X1	T50.0X2	T50.0X3	T50.0X4	T50.0X5	T50.0X6
Deoxyribonuclease (pancreatic)	T45.3X1	T45.3X2	T45.3X3	T45.3X4	T45.3X5	T45.3X6
Depilatory	T49.4X1	T49.4X2	T49.4X3	T49.4X4	T49.4X5	T49.4X6
Deprenalin	T42.8X1	T42.8X2	T42.8X3	T42.8X4	T42.8X5	T42.8X6
Deprenyl	T42.8X1	T42.8X2	T42.8X3	T42.8X4	T42.8X5	T42.8X6
Depressant						
appetite (central)	T50.5X1	T50.5X2	T50.5X3	T50.5X4	T50.5X5	T50.5X6
cardiac	T46.2X1	T46.2X2	T46.2X3	T46.2X4	T46.2X5	T46.2X6

Substance	Poisoning, Accidental (unintentional)	Poisoning, Intentional Self-harm	Poisoning, Assault	Poisoning, Undetermined	Adverse Effect	Under-dosing
Depressant — *continued* central nervous system (anesthetic) — *see also* Central nervous system, depressants	T42.71	T42.72	T42.73	T42.74	T42.75	T42.76
general anesthetic	T41.201	T41.202	T41.203	T41.204	T41.205	T41.206
muscle tone	T42.8X1	T42.8X2	T42.8X3	T42.8X4	T42.8X5	T42.8X6
muscle tone, central	T42.8X1	T42.8X2	T42.8X3	T42.8X4	T42.8X5	T42.8X6
psychotherapeutic	T43.501	T43.502	T43.503	T43.504	T43.505	T43.506
Depressant, appetite	T50.5X1	T50.5X2	T50.5X3	T50.5X4	T50.5X5	T50.5X6
Deptropine	T45.0X1	T45.0X2	T45.0X3	T45.0X4	T45.0X5	T45.0X6
Dequalinium (chloride)	T49.0X1	T49.0X2	T49.0X3	T49.0X4	T49.0X5	T49.0X6
Derris root	T60.2X1	T60.2X2	T60.2X3	T60.2X4	—	—
Deserpidine	T46.5X1	T46.5X2	T46.5X3	T46.5X4	T46.5X5	T46.5X6
Desferrioxamine	T45.8X1	T45.8X2	T45.8X3	T45.8X4	T45.8X5	T45.8X6
Desipramine	T43.011	T43.012	T43.013	T43.014	T43.015	T43.016
Deslanoside	T46.0X1	T46.0X2	T46.0X3	T46.0X4	T46.0X5	T46.0X6
Desloughing agent	T49.4X1	T49.4X2	T49.4X3	T49.4X4	T49.4X5	T49.4X6
Desmethylimipramine	T43.011	T43.012	T43.013	T43.014	T43.015	T43.016
Desmopressin	T38.891	T38.892	T38.893	T38.894	T38.895	T38.896
Desocodeine	T40.2X1	T40.2X2	T40.2X3	T40.2X4	T40.2X5	T40.2X6
Desogestrel	T38.5X1	T38.5X2	T38.5X3	T38.5X4	T38.5X5	T38.5X6
Desomorphine	T40.2X1	T40.2X2	T40.2X3	T40.2X4	—	—
Desonide	T49.0X1	T49.0X2	T49.0X3	T49.0X4	T49.0X5	T49.0X6
Desoximetasone	T49.0X1	T49.0X2	T49.0X3	T49.0X4	T49.0X5	T49.0X6
Desoxycorticosteroid	T50.0X1	T50.0X2	T50.0X3	T50.0X4	T50.0X5	T50.0X6
Desoxycortone	T50.0X1	T50.0X2	T50.0X3	T50.0X4	T50.0X5	T50.0X6
Desoxyephedrine	T43.621	T43.622	T43.623	T43.624	T43.625	T43.626
Detaxtran	T46.6X1	T46.6X2	T46.6X3	T46.6X4	T46.6X5	T46.6X6
Detergent	T49.2X1	T49.2X2	T49.2X3	T49.2X4	T49.2X5	T49.2X6
external medication	T49.2X1	T49.2X2	T49.2X3	T49.2X4	T49.2X5	T49.2X6
local	T49.2X1	T49.2X2	T49.2X3	T49.2X4	T49.2X5	T49.2X6
medicinal	T49.2X1	T49.2X2	T49.2X3	T49.2X4	T49.2X5	T49.2X6
nonmedicinal	T55.1X1	T55.1X2	T55.1X3	T55.1X4	—	—
specified NEC	T55.1X1	T55.1X2	T55.1X3	T55.1X4	—	—
Deterrent, alcohol	T50.6X1	T50.6X2	T50.6X3	T50.6X4	T50.6X5	T50.6X6
Detoxifying agent	T50.6X1	T50.6X2	T50.6X3	T50.6X4	T50.6X5	T50.6X6
Detrothyronine	T38.1X1	T38.1X2	T38.1X3	T38.1X4	T38.1X5	T38.1X6
Dettol (external medication)	T49.0X1	T49.0X2	T49.0X3	T49.0X4	T49.0X5	T49.0X6
Dexamethasone	T38.0X1	T38.0X2	T38.0X3	T38.0X4	T38.0X5	T38.0X6
ENT agent	T49.6X1	T49.6X2	T49.6X3	T49.6X4	T49.6X5	T49.6X6
ophthalmic preparation	T49.5X1	T49.5X2	T49.5X3	T49.5X4	T49.5X5	T49.5X6
topical NEC	T49.0X1	T49.0X2	T49.0X3	T49.0X4	T49.0X5	T49.0X6
Dexamfetamine	T43.621	T43.622	T43.623	T43.624	T43.625	T43.626
Dexamphetamine	T43.621	T43.622	T43.623	T43.624	T43.625	T43.626
Dexbrompheniramine	T45.0X1	T45.0X2	T45.0X3	T45.0X4	T45.0X5	T45.0X6
Dexchlorpheniramine	T45.0X1	T45.0X2	T45.0X3	T45.0X4	T45.0X5	T45.0X6
Dexedrine	T43.621	T43.622	T43.623	T43.624	T43.625	T43.626
Dexetimide	T44.3X1	T44.3X2	T44.3X3	T44.3X4	T44.3X5	T44.3X6
Dexfenfluramine	T50.5X1	T50.5X2	T50.5X3	T50.5X4	T50.5X5	T50.5X6
Dexpanthenol	T45.2X1	T45.2X2	T45.2X3	T45.2X4	T45.2X5	T45.2X6
Dextran (40) (70) (150)	T45.8X1	T45.8X2	T45.8X3	T45.8X4	T45.8X5	T45.8X6
Dextriferron	T45.4X1	T45.4X2	T45.4X3	T45.4X4	T45.4X5	T45.4X6
Dextroamphetamine	T43.621	T43.622	T43.623	T43.624	T43.625	T43.626
Dextro calcium pantothenate	T45.2X1	T45.2X2	T45.2X3	T45.2X4	T45.2X5	T45.2X6
Dextromethorphan	T48.3X1	T48.3X2	T48.3X3	T48.3X4	T48.3X5	T48.3X6
Dextromoramide	T40.4X1	T40.4X2	T40.4X3	T40.4X4	—	—
topical	T49.8X1	T49.8X2	T49.8X3	T49.8X4	T49.8X5	T49.8X6
Dextro pantothenyl alcohol	T45.2X1	T45.2X2	T45.2X3	T45.2X4	T45.2X5	T45.2X6
Dextropropoxyphene	T40.4X1	T40.4X2	T40.4X3	T40.4X4	T40.4X5	T40.4X6
Dextrorphan	T40.2X1	T40.2X2	T40.2X3	T40.2X4	T40.2X5	T40.2X6
Dextrose	T50.3X1	T50.3X2	T50.3X3	T50.3X4	T50.3X5	T50.3X6
concentrated solution, intravenous	T46.8X1	T46.8X2	T46.8X3	T46.8X4	T46.8X5	T46.8X6
Dextrothyroxin	T38.1X1	T38.1X2	T38.1X3	T38.1X4	T38.1X5	T38.1X6
Dextrothyroxine sodium	T38.1X1	T38.1X2	T38.1X3	T38.1X4	T38.1X5	T38.1X6
DFP	T44.0X1	T44.0X2	T44.0X3	T44.0X4	T44.0X5	T44.0X6
DHE	T37.3X1	T37.3X2	T37.3X3	T37.3X4	T37.3X5	T37.3X6
45	T46.5X1	T46.5X2	T46.5X3	T46.5X4	T46.5X5	T46.5X6
Diabinese	T38.3X1	T38.3X2	T38.3X3	T38.3X4	T38.3X5	T38.3X6
Diacetone alcohol	T52.4X1	T52.4X2	T52.4X3	T52.4X4	—	—
Diacetyl monoxime	T50.991	T50.992	T50.993	T50.994	—	—
Diacetylmorphine	T40.1X1	T40.1X2	T40.1X3	T40.1X4	—	—
Diachylon plaster	T49.4X1	T49.4X2	T49.4X3	T49.4X4	T49.4X5	T49.4X6
Diaethylstilboestrolum	T38.5X1	T38.5X2	T38.5X3	T38.5X4	T38.5X5	T38.5X6
Diagnostic agent NEC	T50.8X1	T50.8X2	T50.8X3	T50.8X4	T50.8X5	T50.8X6
Dial (soap)	T49.2X1	T49.2X2	T49.2X3	T49.2X4	T49.2X5	T49.2X6
sedative	T42.3X1	T42.3X2	T42.3X3	T42.3X4	T42.3X5	T42.3X6
Dialkyl carbonate	T52.91	T52.92	T52.93	T52.94	—	—
Diallylbarbituric acid	T42.3X1	T42.3X2	T42.3X3	T42.3X4	T42.3X5	T42.3X6
Diallymal	T42.3X1	T42.3X2	T42.3X3	T42.3X4	T42.3X5	T42.3X6

▽ Subterms under main terms may continue to next column or page   Additional Character May Be Required — Refer to the Tabular List for Character Selection   353

Daphne — Diallymal

Substance	Poisoning, Accidental (unintentional)	Poisoning, Intentional Self-harm	Poisoning, Assault	Poisoning, Undetermined	Adverse Effect	Under-dosing
Dialysis solution (intraperitoneal)	T50.3X1	T50.3X2	T50.3X3	T50.3X4	T50.3X5	T50.3X6
Diaminodiphenylsulfone	T37.1X1	T37.1X2	T37.1X3	T37.1X4	T37.1X5	T37.1X6
Diamorphine	T40.1X1	T40.1X2	T40.1X3	T40.1X4	—	—
Diamox	T50.2X1	T50.2X2	T50.2X3	T50.2X4	T50.2X5	T50.2X6
Diamthazole	T49.0X1	T49.0X2	T49.0X3	T49.0X4	T49.0X5	T49.0X6
Dianthone	T47.2X1	T47.2X2	T47.2X3	T47.2X4	T47.2X5	T47.2X6
Diaphenylsulfone	T37.0X1	T37.0X2	T37.0X3	T37.0X4	T37.0X5	T37.0X6
Diasone (sodium)	T37.1X1	T37.1X2	T37.1X3	T37.1X4	T37.1X5	T37.1X6
Diastase	T47.5X1	T47.5X2	T47.5X3	T47.5X4	T47.5X5	T47.5X6
Diatrizoate	T50.8X1	T50.8X2	T50.8X3	T50.8X4	T50.8X5	T50.8X6
Diazepam	T42.4X1	T42.4X2	T42.4X3	T42.4X4	T42.4X5	T42.4X6
Diazinon	T60.0X1	T60.0X2	T60.0X3	T60.0X4	—	—
Diazomethane (gas)	T59.891	T59.892	T59.893	T59.894	—	—
Diazoxide	T46.5X1	T46.5X2	T46.5X3	T46.5X4	T46.5X5	T46.5X6
Dibekacin	T36.5X1	T36.5X2	T36.5X3	T36.5X4	T36.5X5	T36.5X6
Dibenamine	T44.6X1	T44.6X2	T44.6X3	T44.6X4	T44.6X5	T44.6X6
Dibenzepin	T43.011	T43.012	T43.013	T43.014	T43.015	T43.016
Dibenzheptropine	T45.0X1	T45.0X2	T45.0X3	T45.0X4	T45.0X5	T45.0X6
Dibenzyline	T44.6X1	T44.6X2	T44.6X3	T44.6X4	T44.6X5	T44.6X6
Diborane (gas)	T59.891	T59.892	T59.893	T59.894	—	—
Dibromochloropropane	T60.8X1	T60.8X2	T60.8X3	T60.8X4	—	—
Dibromodulcitol	T45.1X1	T45.1X2	T45.1X3	T45.1X4	T45.1X5	T45.1X6
Dibromoethane	T53.6X1	T53.6X2	T53.6X3	T53.6X4	—	—
Dibromomannitol	T45.1X1	T45.1X2	T45.1X3	T45.1X4	T45.1X5	T45.1X6
Dibromopropamidine isethionate	T49.0X1	T49.0X2	T49.0X3	T49.0X4	T49.0X5	T49.0X6
Dibrompropamidine	T49.0X1	T49.0X2	T49.0X3	T49.0X4	T49.0X5	T49.0X6
Dibucaine	T41.3X1	T41.3X2	T41.3X3	T41.3X4	T41.3X5	T41.3X6
topical (surface)	T41.3X1	T41.3X2	T41.3X3	T41.3X4	T41.3X5	T41.3X6
Dibunate sodium	T48.3X1	T48.3X2	T48.3X3	T48.3X4	T48.3X5	T48.3X6
Dibutoline sulfate	T44.3X1	T44.3X2	T44.3X3	T44.3X4	T44.3X5	T44.3X6
Dicamba	T60.3X1	T60.3X2	T60.3X3	T60.3X4	—	—
Dicapthon	T60.0X1	T60.0X2	T60.0X3	T60.0X4	—	—
Dichlobenil	T60.3X1	T60.3X2	T60.3X3	T60.3X4	—	—
Dichlone	T60.3X1	T60.3X2	T60.3X3	T60.3X4	—	—
Dichloralphenozone	T42.6X1	T42.6X2	T42.6X3	T42.6X4	T42.6X5	T42.6X6
Dichlorbenzidine	T65.3X1	T65.3X2	T65.3X3	T65.3X4	—	—
Dichlorhydrin	T52.8X1	T52.8X2	T52.8X3	T52.8X4	—	—
Dichlorhydroxyquinoline	T37.8X1	T37.8X2	T37.8X3	T37.8X4	T37.8X5	T37.8X6
Dichlorobenzene	T53.7X1	T53.7X2	T53.7X3	T53.7X4	—	—
Dichlorobenzyl alcohol	T49.6X1	T49.6X2	T49.6X3	T49.6X4	T49.6X5	T49.6X6
Dichlorodifluoromethane	T53.5X1	T53.5X2	T53.5X3	T53.5X4	—	—
Dichloroethane	T52.8X1	T52.8X2	T52.8X3	T52.8X4	—	—
Dichloroethylene	T53.6X1	T53.6X2	T53.6X3	T53.6X4	—	—
Dichloroethyl sulfide, not in war	T59.891	T59.892	T59.893	T59.894	—	—
Dichloroformoxine, not in war	T59.891	T59.892	T59.893	T59.894		
Dichlorohydrin, alpha-dichlorohydrin	T52.8X1	T52.8X2	T52.8X3	T52.8X4	—	—
Dichloromethane (solvent)	T53.4X1	T53.4X2	T53.4X3	T53.4X4	—	—
vapor	T53.4X1	T53.4X2	T53.4X3	T53.4X4	—	—
Dichloronaphthoquinone	T60.3X1	T60.3X2	T60.3X3	T60.3X4	—	—
Dichlorophen	T37.4X1	T37.4X2	T37.4X3	T37.4X4	T37.4X5	T37.4X6
Dichloropropene	T60.3X1	T60.3X2	T60.3X3	T60.3X4	—	—
Dichloropropionic acid	T60.3X1	T60.3X2	T60.3X3	T60.3X4	—	—
Dichlorphenamide	T50.2X1	T50.2X2	T50.2X3	T50.2X4	T50.2X5	T50.2X6
Dichlorvos	T60.0X1	T60.0X2	T60.0X3	T60.0X4	—	—
Diclofenac	T39.391	T39.392	T39.393	T39.394	T39.395	T39.396
Diclofenamide	T50.2X1	T50.2X2	T50.2X3	T50.2X4	T50.2X5	T50.2X6
Diclofensine	T43.291	T43.292	T43.293	T43.294	T43.295	T43.296
Diclonixine	T39.8X1	T39.8X2	T39.8X3	T39.8X4	T39.8X5	T39.8X6
Dicloxacillin	T36.0X1	T36.0X2	T36.0X3	T36.0X4	T36.0X5	T36.0X6
Dicophane	T49.0X1	T49.0X2	T49.0X3	T49.0X4	T49.0X5	T49.0X6
Dicoumarol, dicoumarin, dicumarol	T45.511	T45.512	T45.513	T45.514	T45.515	T45.516
Dicrotophos	T60.0X1	T60.0X2	T60.0X3	T60.0X4	—	—
Dicyanogen (gas)	T65.0X1	T65.0X2	T65.0X3	T65.0X4	—	—
Dicyclomine	T44.3X1	T44.3X2	T44.3X3	T44.3X4	T44.3X5	T44.3X6
Dicycloverine	T44.3X1	T44.3X2	T44.3X3	T44.3X4	T44.3X5	T44.3X6
Dideoxycytidine	T37.5X1	T37.5X2	T37.5X3	T37.5X4	T37.5X5	T37.5X6
Dideoxyinosine	T37.5X1	T37.5X2	T37.5X3	T37.5X4	T37.5X5	T37.5X6
Dieldrin (vapor)	T60.1X1	T60.1X2	T60.1X3	T60.1X4	—	—
Diemal	T42.3X1	T42.3X2	T42.3X3	T42.3X4	T42.3X5	T42.3X6
Dienestrol	T38.5X1	T38.5X2	T38.5X3	T38.5X4	T38.5X5	T38.5X6
Dienoestrol	T38.5X1	T38.5X2	T38.5X3	T38.5X4	T38.5X5	T38.5X6
Dietetic drug NEC	T50.901	T50.902	T50.903	T50.904	T50.905	T50.906
Diethazine	T42.8X1	T42.8X2	T42.8X3	T42.8X4	T42.8X5	T42.8X6
Diethyl						
barbituric acid	T42.3X1	T42.3X2	T42.3X3	T42.3X4	T42.3X5	T42.3X6
carbamazine	T37.4X1	T37.4X2	T37.4X3	T37.4X4	T37.4X5	T37.4X6
carbinol	T51.3X1	T51.3X2	T51.3X3	T51.3X4	—	—

Substance	Poisoning, Accidental (unintentional)	Poisoning, Intentional Self-harm	Poisoning, Assault	Poisoning, Undetermined	Adverse Effect	Under-dosing
Diethyl — continued						
carbonate	T52.8X1	T52.8X2	T52.8X3	T52.8X4	—	—
ether (vapor) — see also ether	T41.0X1	T41.0X2	T41.0X3	T41.0X4	T41.0X5	T41.0X6
oxide	T52.8X1	T52.8X2	T52.8X3	T52.8X4	—	—
propion	T50.5X1	T50.5X2	T50.5X3	T50.5X4	T50.5X5	T50.5X6
stilbestrol	T38.5X1	T38.5X2	T38.5X3	T38.5X4	T38.5X5	T38.5X6
toluamide (nonmedicinal)	T60.8X1	T60.8X2	T60.8X3	T60.8X4	—	—
medicinal	T49.3X1	T49.3X2	T49.3X3	T49.3X4	T49.3X5	T49.3X6
Diethylcarbamazine	T37.4X1	T37.4X2	T37.4X3	T37.4X4	T37.4X5	T37.4X6
Diethylene						
dioxide	T52.8X1	T52.8X2	T52.8X3	T52.8X4	—	—
glycol (monoacetate) (monobutyl ether) (monoethyl ether)	T52.3X1	T52.3X2	T52.3X3	T52.3X4	—	—
Diethylhexylphthalate	T65.891	T65.892	T65.893	T65.894	—	—
Diethylpropion	T50.5X1	T50.5X2	T50.5X3	T50.5X4	T50.5X5	T50.5X6
Diethylstilbestrol	T38.5X1	T38.5X2	T38.5X3	T38.5X4	T38.5X5	T38.5X6
Diethylstilboestrol	T38.5X1	T38.5X2	T38.5X3	T38.5X4	T38.5X5	T38.5X6
Diethylsulfone-diethylmethane	T42.6X1	T42.6X2	T42.6X3	T42.6X4	T42.6X5	T42.6X6
Diethyltoluamide	T49.0X1	T49.0X2	T49.0X3	T49.0X4	T49.0X5	T49.0X6
Diethyltryptamine (DET)	T40.991	T40.992	T40.993	T40.994	—	—
Difebarbamate	T42.3X1	T42.3X2	T42.3X3	T42.3X4	T42.3X5	T42.3X6
Difencloxazine	T40.2X1	T40.2X2	T40.2X3	T40.2X4	T40.2X5	T40.2X6
Difenidol	T45.0X1	T45.0X2	T45.0X3	T45.0X4	T45.0X5	T45.0X6
Difenoxin	T47.6X1	T47.6X2	T47.6X3	T47.6X4	T47.6X5	T47.6X6
Difetarsone	T37.3X1	T37.3X2	T37.3X3	T37.3X4	T37.3X5	T37.3X6
Diffusin	T45.3X1	T45.3X2	T45.3X3	T45.3X4	T45.3X5	T45.3X6
Diflorasone	T49.0X1	T49.0X2	T49.0X3	T49.0X4	T49.0X5	T49.0X6
Diflos	T44.0X1	T44.0X2	T44.0X3	T44.0X4	T44.0X5	T44.0X6
Diflubenzuron	T60.1X1	T60.1X2	T60.1X3	T60.1X4	—	—
Diflucortolone	T49.0X1	T49.0X2	T49.0X3	T49.0X4	T49.0X5	T49.0X6
Diflunisal	T39.091	T39.092	T39.093	T39.094	T39.095	T39.096
Difluoromethyldopa	T42.8X1	T42.8X2	T42.8X3	T42.8X4	T42.8X5	T42.8X6
Difluorophate	T44.0X1	T44.0X2	T44.0X3	T44.0X4	T44.0X5	T44.0X6
Digestant NEC	T47.5X1	T47.5X2	T47.5X3	T47.5X4	T47.5X5	T47.5X6
Digitalin (e)	T46.0X1	T46.0X2	T46.0X3	T46.0X4	T46.0X5	T46.0X6
Digitalis (leaf)(glycoside)	T46.0X1	T46.0X2	T46.0X3	T46.0X4	T46.0X5	T46.0X6
lanata	T46.0X1	T46.0X2	T46.0X3	T46.0X4	T46.0X5	T46.0X6
purpurea	T46.0X1	T46.0X2	T46.0X3	T46.0X4	T46.0X5	T46.0X6
Digitoxin	T46.0X1	T46.0X2	T46.0X3	T46.0X4	T46.0X5	T46.0X6
Digitoxose	T46.0X1	T46.0X2	T46.0X3	T46.0X4	T46.0X5	T46.0X6
Digoxin	T46.0X1	T46.0X2	T46.0X3	T46.0X4	T46.0X5	T46.0X6
Digoxine	T46.0X1	T46.0X2	T46.0X3	T46.0X4	T46.0X5	T46.0X6
Dihydralazine	T46.5X1	T46.5X2	T46.5X3	T46.5X4	T46.5X5	T46.5X6
Dihydrazine	T46.5X1	T46.5X2	T46.5X3	T46.5X4	T46.5X5	T46.5X6
Dihydrocodeine	T40.2X1	T40.2X2	T40.2X3	T40.2X4	T40.2X5	T40.2X6
Dihydrocodeinone	T40.2X1	T40.2X2	T40.2X3	T40.2X4	T40.2X5	T40.2X6
Dihydroergocornine	T46.7X1	T46.7X2	T46.7X3	T46.7X4	T46.7X5	T46.7X6
Dihydroergocristine (mesilate)	T46.7X1	T46.7X2	T46.7X3	T46.7X4	T46.7X5	T46.7X6
Dihydroergokryptine	T46.7X1	T46.7X2	T46.7X3	T46.7X4	T46.7X5	T46.7X6
Dihydroergotamine	T46.5X1	T46.5X2	T46.5X3	T46.5X4	T46.5X5	T46.5X6
Dihydroergotoxine	T46.7X1	T46.7X2	T46.7X3	T46.7X4	T46.7X5	T46.7X6
mesilate	T46.7X1	T46.7X2	T46.7X3	T46.7X4	T46.7X5	T46.7X6
Dihydrohydroxycodeinone	T40.2X1	T40.2X2	T40.2X3	T40.2X4	T40.2X5	T40.2X6
Dihydrohydroxymorphinone	T40.2X1	T40.2X2	T40.2X3	T40.2X4	T40.2X5	T40.2X6
Dihydroisocodeine	T40.2X1	T40.2X2	T40.2X3	T40.2X4	T40.2X5	T40.2X6
Dihydromorphine	T40.2X1	T40.2X2	T40.2X3	T40.2X4	—	—
Dihydromorphinone	T40.2X1	T40.2X2	T40.2X3	T40.2X4	T40.2X5	T40.2X6
Dihydrostreptomycin	T36.5X1	T36.5X2	T36.5X3	T36.5X4	T36.5X5	T36.5X6
Dihydrotachysterol	T45.2X1	T45.2X2	T45.2X3	T45.2X4	T45.2X5	T45.2X6
Dihydroxyaluminum aminoacetate	T47.1X1	T47.1X2	T47.1X3	T47.1X4	T47.1X5	T47.1X6
Dihydroxyaluminum sodium carbonate	T47.1X1	T47.1X2	T47.1X3	T47.1X4	T47.1X5	T47.1X6
Dihydroxyanthraquinone	T47.2X1	T47.2X2	T47.2X3	T47.2X4	T47.2X5	T47.2X6
Dihydroxycodeinone	T40.2X1	T40.2X2	T40.2X3	T40.2X4	T40.2X5	T40.2X6
Dihydroxypropyl theophylline	T50.2X1	T50.2X2	T50.2X3	T50.2X4	T50.2X5	T50.2X6
Diiodohydroxyquin	T37.8X1	T37.8X2	T37.8X3	T37.8X4	T37.8X5	T37.8X6
topical	T49.0X1	T49.0X2	T49.0X3	T49.0X4	T49.0X5	T49.0X6
Diiodohydroxyquinoline	T37.8X1	T37.8X2	T37.8X3	T37.8X4	T37.8X5	T37.8X6
Diiodotyrosine	T38.2X1	T38.2X2	T38.2X3	T38.2X4	T38.2X5	T38.2X6
Diisopromine	T44.3X1	T44.3X2	T44.3X3	T44.3X4	T44.3X5	T44.3X6
Diisopropylamine	T46.3X1	T46.3X2	T46.3X3	T46.3X4	T46.3X5	T46.3X6
Diisopropylfluorophosphonate	T44.0X1	T44.0X2	T44.0X3	T44.0X4	T44.0X5	T44.0X6
Dilantin	T42.0X1	T42.0X2	T42.0X3	T42.0X4	T42.0X5	T42.0X6
Dilaudid	T40.2X1	T40.2X2	T40.2X3	T40.2X4	T40.2X5	T40.2X6
Dilazep	T46.3X1	T46.3X2	T46.3X3	T46.3X4	T46.3X5	T46.3X6
Dill	T47.5X1	T47.5X2	T47.5X3	T47.5X4	T47.5X5	T47.5X6
Diloxanide	T37.3X1	T37.3X2	T37.3X3	T37.3X4	T37.3X5	T37.3X6
Diltiazem	T46.1X1	T46.1X2	T46.1X3	T46.1X4	T46.1X5	T46.1X6

Additional Character May Be Required — Refer to the Tabular List for Character Selection

▽ Subterms under main terms may continue to next column or page

Substance	Poisoning, Accidental (unintentional)	Poisoning, Intentional Self-harm	Poisoning, Assault	Poisoning, Undetermined	Adverse Effect	Under-dosing
Dimazole	T49.0X1	T49.0X2	T49.0X3	T49.0X4	T49.0X5	T49.0X6
Dimefline	T50.7X1	T50.7X2	T50.7X3	T50.7X4	T50.7X5	T50.7X6
Dimefox	T60.0X1	T60.0X2	T60.0X3	T60.0X4	—	—
Dimemorfan	T48.3X1	T48.3X2	T48.3X3	T48.3X4	T48.3X5	T48.3X6
Dimenhydrinate	T45.0X1	T45.0X2	T45.0X3	T45.0X4	T45.0X5	T45.0X6
Dimercaprol (British anti-lewisite)	T45.8X1	T45.8X2	T45.8X3	T45.8X4	T45.8X5	T45.8X6
Dimercaptopropanol	T45.8X1	T45.8X2	T45.8X3	T45.8X4	T45.8X5	T45.8X6
Dimestrol	T38.5X1	T38.5X2	T38.5X3	T38.5X4	T38.5X5	T38.5X6
Dimetane	T45.0X1	T45.0X2	T45.0X3	T45.0X4	T45.0X5	T45.0X6
Dimethicone	T47.1X1	T47.1X2	T47.1X3	T47.1X4	T47.1X5	T47.1X6
Dimethindene	T45.0X1	T45.0X2	T45.0X3	T45.0X4	T45.0X5	T45.0X6
Dimethisoquin	T49.1X1	T49.1X2	T49.1X3	T49.1X4	T49.1X5	T49.1X6
Dimethisterone	T38.5X1	T38.5X2	T38.5X3	T38.5X4	T38.5X5	T38.5X6
Dimethoate	T60.0X1	T60.0X2	T60.0X3	T60.0X4	—	—
Dimethocaine	T41.3X1	T41.3X2	T41.3X3	T41.3X4	T41.3X5	T41.3X6
Dimethoxanate	T48.3X1	T48.3X2	T48.3X3	T48.3X4	T48.3X5	T48.3X6
Dimethyl						
arsine, arsinic acid	T57.0X1	T57.0X2	T57.0X3	T57.0X4	—	—
carbinol	T51.2X1	T51.2X2	T51.2X3	T51.2X4	—	—
carbonate	T52.8X1	T52.8X2	T52.8X3	T52.8X4	—	—
diguanide	T38.3X1	T38.3X2	T38.3X3	T38.3X4	T38.3X5	T38.3X6
ketone	T52.4X1	T52.4X2	T52.4X3	T52.4X4	—	—
vapor	T52.4X1	T52.4X2	T52.4X3	T52.4X4	—	—
meperidine	T40.2X1	T40.2X2	T40.2X3	T40.2X4	T40.2X5	T40.2X6
parathion	T60.0X1	T60.0X2	T60.0X3	T60.0X4	—	—
phthlate	T49.3X1	T49.3X2	T49.3X3	T49.3X4	T49.3X5	T49.3X6
polysiloxane	T47.8X1	T47.8X2	T47.8X3	T47.8X4	T47.8X5	T47.8X6
sulfate (fumes)	T59.891	T59.892	T59.893	T59.894	—	—
liquid	T65.891	T65.892	T65.893	T65.894	—	—
sulfoxide (nonmedicinal)	T52.8X1	T52.8X2	T52.8X3	T52.8X4	—	—
medicinal	T49.4X1	T49.4X2	T49.4X3	T49.4X4	T49.4X5	T49.4X6
tryptamine	T40.991	T40.992	T40.993	T40.994	—	—
tubocurarine	T48.1X1	T48.1X2	T48.1X3	T48.1X4	T48.1X5	T48.1X6
Dimethylamine sulfate	T49.4X1	T49.4X2	T49.4X3	T49.4X4	T49.4X5	T49.4X6
Dimethylformamide	T52.8X1	T52.8X2	T52.8X3	T52.8X4	—	—
Dimethyltubocurarinium chloride	T48.1X1	T48.1X2	T48.1X3	T48.1X4	T48.1X5	T48.1X6
Dimeticone	T47.1X1	T47.1X2	T47.1X3	T47.1X4	T47.1X5	T47.1X6
Dimetilan	T60.0X1	T60.0X2	T60.0X3	T60.0X4	—	—
Dimetindene	T45.0X1	T45.0X2	T45.0X3	T45.0X4	T45.0X5	T45.0X6
Dimetotiazine	T43.3X1	T43.3X2	T43.3X3	T43.3X4	T43.3X5	T43.3X6
Dimorpholamine	T50.7X1	T50.7X2	T50.7X3	T50.7X4	T50.7X5	T50.7X6
Dimoxyline	T46.3X1	T46.3X2	T46.3X3	T46.3X4	—	—
Dinitrobenzene	T65.3X1	T65.3X2	T65.3X3	T65.3X4	—	—
vapor	T59.891	T59.892	T59.893	T59.894	—	—
Dinitrobenzol	T65.3X1	T65.3X2	T65.3X3	T65.3X4	—	—
vapor	T59.891	T59.892	T59.893	T59.894	—	—
Dinitrobutylphenol	T65.3X1	T65.3X2	T65.3X3	T65.3X4	—	—
Dinitro (-ortho-)cresol (pesticide) (spray)	T65.3X1	T65.3X2	T65.3X3	T65.3X4	—	—
Dinitrocyclohexylphenol	T65.3X1	T65.3X2	T65.3X3	T65.3X4	—	—
Dinitrophenol	T65.3X1	T65.3X2	T65.3X3	T65.3X4	—	—
Dinoprost	T48.0X1	T48.0X2	T48.0X3	T48.0X4	T48.0X5	T48.0X6
Dinoprostone	T48.0X1	T48.0X2	T48.0X3	T48.0X4	T48.0X5	T48.0X6
Dinoseb	T60.3X1	T60.3X2	T60.3X3	T60.3X4	—	—
Dioctyl sulfosuccinate (calcium) (sodium)	T47.4X1	T47.4X2	T47.4X3	T47.4X4	T47.4X5	T47.4X6
Diodone	T50.8X1	T50.8X2	T50.8X3	T50.8X4	T50.8X5	T50.8X6
Diodoquin	T37.8X1	T37.8X2	T37.8X3	T37.8X4	T37.8X5	T37.8X6
Dionin	T40.2X1	T40.2X2	T40.2X3	T40.2X4	T40.2X5	T40.2X6
Diosmin	T46.991	T46.992	T46.993	T46.994	T46.995	T46.996
Dioxane	T52.8X1	T52.8X2	T52.8X3	T52.8X4	—	—
Dioxathion	T60.0X1	T60.0X2	T60.0X3	T60.0X4	—	—
Dioxin	T53.7X1	T53.7X2	T53.7X3	T53.7X4	—	—
Dioxopromethazine	T43.3X1	T43.3X2	T43.3X3	T43.3X4	T43.3X5	T43.3X6
Dioxyline	T46.3X1	T46.3X2	T46.3X3	T46.3X4	T46.3X5	T46.3X6
Dipentene	T52.8X1	T52.8X2	T52.8X3	T52.8X4	—	—
Diperodon	T41.3X1	T41.3X2	T41.3X3	T41.3X4	T41.3X5	T41.3X6
Diphacinone	T60.4X1	T60.4X2	T60.4X3	T60.4X4	—	—
Diphemanil	T44.3X1	T44.3X2	T44.3X3	T44.3X4	T44.3X5	T44.3X6
metilsulfate	T44.3X1	T44.3X2	T44.3X3	T44.3X4	T44.3X5	T44.3X6
Diphenadione	T45.511	T45.512	T45.513	T45.514	T45.515	T45.516
rodenticide	T60.4X1	T60.4X2	T60.4X3	T60.4X4	—	—
Diphenhydramine	T45.0X1	T45.0X2	T45.0X3	T45.0X4	T45.0X5	T45.0X6
Diphenidol	T45.0X1	T45.0X2	T45.0X3	T45.0X4	T45.0X5	T45.0X6
Diphenoxylate	T47.6X1	T47.6X2	T47.6X3	T47.6X4	T47.6X5	T47.6X6
Diphenylamine	T65.3X1	T65.3X2	T65.3X3	T65.3X4	—	—
Diphenylbutazone	T39.2X1	T39.2X2	T39.2X3	T39.2X4	T39.2X5	T39.2X6
Diphenylchloroarsine, not in war	T57.0X1	T57.0X2	T57.0X3	T57.0X4	—	—
Diphenylhydantoin	T42.0X1	T42.0X2	T42.0X3	T42.0X4	T42.0X5	T42.0X6
Diphenylmethane dye	T52.1X1	T52.1X2	T52.1X3	T52.1X4	—	—

Substance	Poisoning, Accidental (unintentional)	Poisoning, Intentional Self-harm	Poisoning, Assault	Poisoning, Undetermined	Adverse Effect	Under-dosing
Diphenylpyraline	T45.0X1	T45.0X2	T45.0X3	T45.0X4	T45.0X5	T45.0X6
Diphtheria						
antitoxin	T50.Z11	T50.Z12	T50.Z13	T50.Z14	T50.Z15	T50.Z16
toxoid	T50.A91	T50.A92	T50.A93	T50.A94	T50.A95	T50.A96
with tetanus toxoid	T50.A21	T50.A22	T50.A23	T50.A24	T50.A25	T50.A26
with pertussis component	T50.A11	T50.A12	T50.A13	T50.A14	T50.A15	T50.A16
vaccine	T50.A91	T50.A92	T50.A93	T50.A94	T50.A95	T50.A96
combination						
without pertussis	T50.A21	T50.A22	T50.A23	T50.A24	T50.A25	T50.A26
including pertussis	T50.A11	T50.A12	T50.A13	T50.A14	T50.A15	T50.A16
Diphylline	T50.2X1	T50.2X2	T50.2X3	T50.2X4	T50.2X5	T50.2X6
Dipipanone	T40.4X1	T40.4X2	T40.4X3	T40.4X4	—	—
Dipivefrine	T49.5X1	T49.5X2	T49.5X3	T49.5X4	T49.5X5	T49.5X6
Diplovax	T50.B91	T50.B92	T50.B93	T50.B94	T50.B95	T50.B96
Diprophylline	T50.2X1	T50.2X2	T50.2X3	T50.2X4	T50.2X5	T50.2X6
Dipropyline	T48.291	T48.292	T48.293	T48.294	T48.295	T48.296
Dipyridamole	T46.3X1	T46.3X2	T46.3X3	T46.3X4	T46.3X5	T46.3X6
Dipyrone	T39.2X1	T39.2X2	T39.2X3	T39.2X4	T39.2X5	T39.2X6
Diquat (dibromide)	T60.3X1	T60.3X2	T60.3X3	T60.3X4	—	—
Disinfectant	T65.891	T65.892	T65.893	T65.894	—	—
alkaline	T54.3X1	T54.3X2	T54.3X3	T54.3X4	—	—
aromatic	T54.1X1	T54.1X2	T54.1X3	T54.1X4	—	—
intestinal	T37.8X1	T37.8X2	T37.8X3	T37.8X4	T37.8X5	T37.8X6
Disipal	T42.8X1	T42.8X2	T42.8X3	T42.8X4	T42.8X5	T42.8X6
Disodium edetate	T50.6X1	T50.6X2	T50.6X3	T50.6X4	T50.6X5	T50.6X6
Disoprofol	T41.291	T41.292	T41.293	T41.294	T41.295	T41.296
Disopyramide	T46.2X1	T46.2X2	T46.2X3	T46.2X4	T46.2X5	T46.2X6
Distigmine (bromide)	T44.0X1	T44.0X2	T44.0X3	T44.0X4	T44.0X5	T44.0X6
Disulfamide	T50.2X1	T50.2X2	T50.2X3	T50.2X4	T50.2X5	T50.2X6
Disulfanilamide	T37.0X1	T37.0X2	T37.0X3	T37.0X4	T37.0X5	T37.0X6
Disulfiram	T50.6X1	T50.6X2	T50.6X3	T50.6X4	T50.6X5	T50.6X6
Disulfoton	T60.0X1	T60.0X2	T60.0X3	T60.0X4	—	—
Dithiazanine iodide	T37.4X1	T37.4X2	T37.4X3	T37.4X4	T37.4X5	T37.4X6
Dithiocarbamate	T60.0X1	T60.0X2	T60.0X3	T60.0X4	—	—
Dithranol	T49.4X1	T49.4X2	T49.4X3	T49.4X4	T49.4X5	T49.4X6
Diucardin	T50.2X1	T50.2X2	T50.2X3	T50.2X4	T50.2X5	T50.2X6
Diupres	T50.2X1	T50.2X2	T50.2X3	T50.2X4	T50.2X5	T50.2X6
Diuretic NEC	T50.2X1	T50.2X2	T50.2X3	T50.2X4	T50.2X5	T50.2X6
benzothiadiazine	T50.2X1	T50.2X2	T50.2X3	T50.2X4	T50.2X5	T50.2X6
carbonic acid anhydrase inhibitors	T50.2X1	T50.2X2	T50.2X3	T50.2X4	T50.2X5	T50.2X6
furfuryl NEC	T50.2X1	T50.2X2	T50.2X3	T50.2X4	T50.2X5	T50.2X6
loop (high-ceiling)	T50.1X1	T50.1X2	T50.1X3	T50.1X4	T50.1X5	T50.1X6
mercurial NEC	T50.2X1	T50.2X2	T50.2X3	T50.2X4	T50.2X5	T50.2X6
osmotic	T50.2X1	T50.2X2	T50.2X3	T50.2X4	T50.2X5	T50.2X6
purine NEC	T50.2X1	T50.2X2	T50.2X3	T50.2X4	T50.2X5	T50.2X6
saluretic NEC	T50.2X1	T50.2X2	T50.2X3	T50.2X4	T50.2X5	T50.2X6
sulfonamide	T50.2X1	T50.2X2	T50.2X3	T50.2X4	T50.2X5	T50.2X6
thiazide NEC	T50.2X1	T50.2X2	T50.2X3	T50.2X4	T50.2X5	T50.2X6
xanthine	T50.2X1	T50.2X2	T50.2X3	T50.2X4	T50.2X5	T50.2X6
Diurgin	T50.2X1	T50.2X2	T50.2X3	T50.2X4	T50.2X5	T50.2X6
Diuril	T50.2X1	T50.2X2	T50.2X3	T50.2X4	T50.2X5	T50.2X6
Diuron	T60.3X1	T60.3X2	T60.3X3	T60.3X4	—	—
Divalproex	T42.6X1	T42.6X2	T42.6X3	T42.6X4	T42.6X5	T42.6X6
Divinyl ether	T41.0X1	T41.0X2	T41.0X3	T41.0X4	T41.0X5	T41.0X6
Dixanthogen	T49.0X1	T49.0X2	T49.0X3	T49.0X4	T49.0X5	T49.0X6
Dixyrazine	T43.3X1	T43.3X2	T43.3X3	T43.3X4	T43.3X5	T43.3X6
D-lysergic acid diethylamide	T40.8X1	T40.8X2	T40.8X3	T40.8X4	—	—
DMCT	T36.4X1	T36.4X2	T36.4X3	T36.4X4	T36.4X5	T36.4X6
DMSO — see Dimethyl sulfoxide						
DNBP	T60.3X1	T60.3X2	T60.3X3	T60.3X4	—	—
DNOC	T65.3X1	T65.3X2	T65.3X3	T65.3X4	—	—
Dobutamine	T44.5X1	T44.5X2	T44.5X3	T44.5X4	T44.5X5	T44.5X6
DOCA	T38.0X1	T38.0X2	T38.0X3	T38.0X4	T38.0X5	T38.0X6
Docusate sodium	T47.4X1	T47.4X2	T47.4X3	T47.4X4	T47.4X5	T47.4X6
Dodicin	T49.0X1	T49.0X2	T49.0X3	T49.0X4	T49.0X5	T49.0X6
Dofamium chloride	T49.0X1	T49.0X2	T49.0X3	T49.0X4	T49.0X5	T49.0X6
Dolophine	T40.3X1	T40.3X2	T40.3X3	T40.3X4	T40.3X5	T40.3X6
Doloxene	T39.8X1	T39.8X2	T39.8X3	T39.8X4	T39.8X5	T39.8X6
Domestic gas (after combustion) — see Gas, utility						
prior to combustion	T59.891	T59.892	T59.893	T59.894	—	—
Domiodol	T48.4X1	T48.4X2	T48.4X3	T48.4X4	T48.4X5	T48.4X6
Domiphen (bromide)	T49.0X1	T49.0X2	T49.0X3	T49.0X4	T49.0X5	T49.0X6
Domperidone	T45.0X1	T45.0X2	T45.0X3	T45.0X4	T45.0X5	T45.0X6
Dopa	T42.8X1	T42.8X2	T42.8X3	T42.8X4	T42.8X5	T42.8X6
Dopamine	T44.991	T44.992	T44.993	T44.994	T44.995	T44.996
Doriden	T42.6X1	T42.6X2	T42.6X3	T42.6X4	T42.6X5	T42.6X6
Dormiral	T42.3X1	T42.3X2	T42.3X3	T42.3X4	T42.3X5	T42.3X6
Dormison	T42.6X1	T42.6X2	T42.6X3	T42.6X4	T42.6X5	T42.6X6
Dornase	T48.4X1	T48.4X2	T48.4X3	T48.4X4	T48.4X5	T48.4X6

Table of Drugs and Chemicals

Substance	Poisoning, Accidental (unintentional)	Poisoning, Intentional Self-harm	Poisoning, Assault	Poisoning, Undetermined	Adverse Effect	Under-dosing
Dorsacaine	T41.3X1	T41.3X2	T41.3X3	T41.3X4	T41.3X5	T41.3X6
Dosulepin	T43.011	T43.012	T43.013	T43.014	T43.015	T43.016
Dothiepin	T43.011	T43.012	T43.013	T43.014	T43.015	T43.016
Doxantrazole	T48.6X1	T48.6X2	T48.6X3	T48.6X4	T48.6X5	T48.6X6
Doxapram	T50.7X1	T50.7X2	T50.7X3	T50.7X4	T50.7X5	T50.7X6
Doxazosin	T44.6X1	T44.6X2	T44.6X3	T44.6X4	T44.6X5	T44.6X6
Doxepin	T43.011	T43.012	T43.013	T43.014	T43.015	T43.016
Doxifluridine	T45.1X1	T45.1X2	T45.1X3	T45.1X4	T45.1X5	T45.1X6
Doxorubicin	T45.1X1	T45.1X2	T45.1X3	T45.1X4	T45.1X5	T45.1X6
Doxycycline	T36.4X1	T36.4X2	T36.4X3	T36.4X4	T36.4X5	T36.4X6
Doxylamine	T45.0X1	T45.0X2	T45.0X3	T45.0X4	T45.0X5	T45.0X6
Dramamine	T45.0X1	T45.0X2	T45.0X3	T45.0X4	T45.0X5	T45.0X6
Drano (drain cleaner)	T54.3X1	T54.3X2	T54.3X3	T54.3X4	—	—
Dressing, live pulp	T49.7X1	T49.7X2	T49.7X3	T49.7X4	T49.7X5	T49.7X6
Drocode	T40.2X1	T40.2X2	T40.2X3	T40.2X4	T40.2X5	T40.2X6
Dromoran	T40.2X1	T40.2X2	T40.2X3	T40.2X4	T40.2X5	T40.2X6
Dromostanolone	T38.7X1	T38.7X2	T38.7X3	T38.7X4	T38.7X5	T38.7X6
Dronabinol	T40.7X1	T40.7X2	T40.7X3	T40.7X4	T40.7X5	T40.7X6
Droperidol	T43.591	T43.592	T43.593	T43.594	T43.595	T43.596
Dropropizine	T48.3X1	T48.3X2	T48.3X3	T48.3X4	T48.3X5	T48.3X6
Drostanolone	T38.7X1	T38.7X2	T38.7X3	T38.7X4	T38.7X5	T38.7X6
Drotaverine	T44.3X1	T44.3X2	T44.3X3	T44.3X4	T44.3X5	T44.3X6
Drotrecogin alfa	T45.511	T45.512	T45.513	T45.514	T45.515	T45.516
Drug NEC	T50.901	T50.902	T50.903	T50.904	T50.905	T50.906
specified NEC	T50.991	T50.992	T50.993	T50.994	T50.995	T50.996
DTIC	T45.1X1	T45.1X2	T45.1X3	T45.1X4	T45.1X5	T45.1X6
Duboisine	T44.3X1	T44.3X2	T44.3X3	T44.3X4	T44.3X5	T44.3X6
Dulcolax	T47.2X1	T47.2X2	T47.2X3	T47.2X4	T47.2X5	T47.2X6
Duponol (C) (EP)	T49.2X1	T49.2X2	T49.2X3	T49.2X4	T49.2X5	T49.2X6
Durabolin	T38.7X1	T38.7X2	T38.7X3	T38.7X4	T38.7X5	T38.7X6
Dyclone	T41.3X1	T41.3X2	T41.3X3	T41.3X4	T41.3X5	T41.3X6
Dyclonine	T41.3X1	T41.3X2	T41.3X3	T41.3X4	T41.3X5	T41.3X6
Dydrogesterone	T38.5X1	T38.5X2	T38.5X3	T38.5X4	T38.5X5	T38.5X6
Dye NEC	T65.6X1	T65.6X2	T65.6X3	T65.6X4	—	—
antiseptic	T49.0X1	T49.0X2	T49.0X3	T49.0X4	T49.0X5	T49.0X6
diagnostic agents	T50.8X1	T50.8X2	T50.8X3	T50.8X4	T50.8X5	T50.8X6
pharmaceutical NEC	T50.901	T50.902	T50.903	T50.904	T50.905	T50.906
Dyflos	T44.0X1	T44.0X2	T44.0X3	T44.0X4	T44.0X5	T44.0X6
Dymelor	T38.3X1	T38.3X2	T38.3X3	T38.3X4	T38.3X5	T38.3X6
Dynamite	T65.3X1	T65.3X2	T65.3X3	T65.3X4	—	—
fumes	T59.891	T59.892	T59.893	T59.894	—	—
Dyphylline	T44.3X1	T44.3X2	T44.3X3	T44.3X4	T44.3X5	T44.3X6
b-eucaine	T49.1X1	T49.1X2	T49.1X3	T49.1X4	T49.1X5	T49.1X6
Ear drug NEC	T49.6X1	T49.6X2	T49.6X3	T49.6X4	T49.6X5	T49.6X6
Ear preparations	T49.6X1	T49.6X2	T49.6X3	T49.6X4	T49.6X5	T49.6X6
Echothiophate, echothiopate, ecothiopate	T49.5X1	T49.5X2	T49.5X3	T49.5X4	T49.5X5	T49.5X6
Econazole	T49.0X1	T49.0X2	T49.0X3	T49.0X4	T49.0X5	T49.0X6
Ecothiopate iodide	T49.5X1	T49.5X2	T49.5X3	T49.5X4	T49.5X5	T49.5X6
Ecstasy	T43.621	T43.622	T43.623	T43.624	T43.625	T43.626
Ectylurea	T42.6X1	T42.6X2	T42.6X3	T42.6X4	T42.6X5	T42.6X6
Edathamil disodium	T45.8X1	T45.8X2	T45.8X3	T45.8X4	T45.8X5	T45.8X6
Edecrin	T50.1X1	T50.1X2	T50.1X3	T50.1X4	T50.1X5	T50.1X6
Edetate, disodium (calcium)	T45.8X1	T45.8X2	T45.8X3	T45.8X4	T45.8X5	T45.8X6
Edoxudine	T49.5X1	T49.5X2	T49.5X3	T49.5X4	T49.5X5	T49.5X6
Edrophonium	T44.0X1	T44.0X2	T44.0X3	T44.0X4	T44.0X5	T44.0X6
chloride	T44.0X1	T44.0X2	T44.0X3	T44.0X4	T44.0X5	T44.0X6
EDTA	T50.6X1	T50.6X2	T50.6X3	T50.6X4	T50.6X5	T50.6X6
Eflornithine	T37.2X1	T37.2X2	T37.2X3	T37.2X4	T37.2X5	T37.2X6
Efloxate	T46.3X1	T46.3X2	T46.3X3	T46.3X4	T46.3X5	T46.3X6
Elase	T49.8X1	T49.8X2	T49.8X3	T49.8X4	T49.8X5	T49.8X6
Elastase	T47.5X1	T47.5X2	T47.5X3	T47.5X4	T47.5X5	T47.5X6
Elaterium	T47.2X1	T47.2X2	T47.2X3	T47.2X4	T47.2X5	T47.2X6
Elcatonin	T50.991	T50.992	T50.993	T50.994	T50.995	T50.996
Elder	T62.2X1	T62.2X2	T62.2X3	T62.2X4	—	—
berry, (unripe)	T62.1X1	T62.1X2	T62.1X3	T62.1X4	—	—
Electrolyte balance drug	T50.3X1	T50.3X2	T50.3X3	T50.3X4	T50.3X5	T50.3X6
Electrolytes NEC	T50.3X1	T50.3X2	T50.3X3	T50.3X4	T50.3X5	T50.3X6
Electrolytic agent NEC	T50.3X1	T50.3X2	T50.3X3	T50.3X4	T50.3X5	T50.3X6
Elemental diet	T50.901	T50.902	T50.903	T50.904	T50.905	T50.906
Elliptinium acetate	T45.1X1	T45.1X2	T45.1X3	T45.1X4	T45.1X5	T45.1X6
Embramine	T45.0X1	T45.0X2	T45.0X3	T45.0X4	T45.0X5	T45.0X6
Emepronium (salts)	T44.3X1	T44.3X2	T44.3X3	T44.3X4	T44.3X5	T44.3X6
bromide	T44.3X1	T44.3X2	T44.3X3	T44.3X4	T44.3X5	T44.3X6
Emetic NEC	T47.7X1	T47.7X2	T47.7X3	T47.7X4	T47.7X5	T47.7X6
Emetine	T37.3X1	T37.3X2	T37.3X3	T37.3X4	T37.3X5	T37.3X6
Emollient NEC	T49.3X1	T49.3X2	T49.3X3	T49.3X4	T49.3X5	T49.3X6
Emorfazone	T39.8X1	T39.8X2	T39.8X3	T39.8X4	T39.8X5	T39.8X6
Emylcamate	T43.591	T43.592	T43.593	T43.594	T43.595	T43.596
Enalapril	T46.4X1	T46.4X2	T46.4X3	T46.4X4	T46.4X5	T46.4X6
Enalaprilat	T46.4X1	T46.4X2	T46.4X3	T46.4X4	T46.4X5	T46.4X6
Encainide	T46.2X1	T46.2X2	T46.2X3	T46.2X4	T46.2X5	T46.2X6
Endocaine	T41.3X1	T41.3X2	T41.3X3	T41.3X4	T41.3X5	T41.3X6

Substance	Poisoning, Accidental (unintentional)	Poisoning, Intentional Self-harm	Poisoning, Assault	Poisoning, Undetermined	Adverse Effect	Under-dosing
Endosulfan	T60.2X1	T60.2X2	T60.2X3	T60.2X4	—	—
Endothall	T60.3X1	T60.3X2	T60.3X3	T60.3X4	—	—
Endralazine	T46.5X1	T46.5X2	T46.5X3	T46.5X4	T46.5X5	T46.5X6
Endrin	T60.1X1	T60.1X2	T60.1X3	T60.1X4	—	—
Enflurane	T41.0X1	T41.0X2	T41.0X3	T41.0X4	T41.0X5	T41.0X6
Enhexymal	T42.3X1	T42.3X2	T42.3X3	T42.3X4	T42.3X5	T42.3X6
Enocitabine	T45.1X1	T45.1X2	T45.1X3	T45.1X4	T45.1X5	T45.1X6
Enovid	T38.4X1	T38.4X2	T38.4X3	T38.4X4	T38.4X5	T38.4X6
Enoxacin	T36.8X1	T36.8X2	T36.8X3	T36.8X4	T36.8X5	T36.8X6
Enoxaparin (sodium)	T45.511	T45.512	T45.513	T45.514	T45.515	T45.515
Enpiprazole	T43.591	T43.592	T43.593	T43.594	T43.595	T43.596
Enprofylline	T48.6X1	T48.6X2	T48.6X3	T48.6X4	T48.6X5	T48.6X6
Enprostil	T47.1X1	T47.1X2	T47.1X3	T47.1X4	T47.1X5	T47.1X6
Enterogastrone	T38.891	T38.892	T38.893	T38.894	T38.895	T38.896
ENT preparations (anti-infectives)	T49.6X1	T49.6X2	T49.6X3	T49.6X4	T49.6X5	T49.6X6
Enviomycin	T36.8X1	T36.8X2	T36.8X3	T36.8X4	T36.8X5	T36.8X6
Enzodase	T45.3X1	T45.3X2	T45.3X3	T45.3X4	T45.3X5	T45.3X6
Enzyme NEC	T45.3X1	T45.3X2	T45.3X3	T45.3X4	T45.3X5	T45.3X6
depolymerizing	T49.8X1	T49.8X2	T49.8X3	T49.8X4	T49.8X5	T49.8X6
fibrolytic	T45.3X1	T45.3X2	T45.3X3	T45.3X4	T45.3X5	T45.3X6
gastric	T47.5X1	T47.5X2	T47.5X3	T47.5X4	T47.5X5	T47.5X6
intestinal	T47.5X1	T47.5X2	T47.5X3	T47.5X4	T47.5X5	T47.5X6
local action	T49.4X1	T49.4X2	T49.4X3	T49.4X4	T49.4X5	T49.4X6
proteolytic	T49.4X1	T49.4X2	T49.4X3	T49.4X4	T49.4X5	T49.4X6
thrombolytic	T45.3X1	T45.3X2	T45.3X3	T45.3X4	T45.3X5	T45.3X6
EPAB	T41.3X1	T41.3X2	T41.3X3	T41.3X4	T41.3X5	T41.3X6
Epanutin	T42.0X1	T42.0X2	T42.0X3	T42.0X4	T42.0X5	T42.0X6
Ephedra	T44.991	T44.992	T44.993	T44.994	T44.995	T44.996
Ephedrine	T44.991	T44.992	T44.993	T44.994	T44.995	T44.996
Epichlorhydrin, epichlorohydrin	T52.8X1	T52.8X2	T52.8X3	T52.8X4	—	—
Epicillin	T36.0X1	T36.0X2	T36.0X3	T36.0X4	T36.0X5	T36.0X6
Epiestriol	T38.5X1	T38.5X2	T38.5X3	T38.5X4	T38.5X5	T38.5X6
Epilim — see Sodium valproate						
Epimestrol	T38.5X1	T38.5X2	T38.5X3	T38.5X4	T38.5X5	T38.5X6
Epinephrine	T44.5X1	T44.5X2	T44.5X3	T44.5X4	T44.5X5	T44.5X6
Epirubicin	T45.1X1	T45.1X2	T45.1X3	T45.1X4	T45.1X5	T45.1X6
Epitiostanol	T38.7X1	T38.7X2	T38.7X3	T38.7X4	T38.7X5	T38.7X6
Epitizide	T50.2X1	T50.2X2	T50.2X3	T50.2X4	T50.2X5	T50.2X6
EPN	T60.0X1	T60.0X2	T60.0X3	T60.0X4	—	—
EPO	T45.8X1	T45.8X2	T45.8X3	T45.8X4	T45.8X5	T45.8X6
Epoetin alpha	T45.8X1	T45.8X2	T45.8X3	T45.8X4	T45.8X5	T45.8X6
Epomediol	T50.991	T50.992	T50.993	T50.994	T50.995	T50.996
Epoprostenol	T45.521	T45.522	T45.523	T45.524	T45.525	T45.526
Epoxy resin	T65.891	T65.892	T65.893	T65.894	—	—
Eprazinone	T48.4X1	T48.4X2	T48.4X3	T48.4X4	T48.4X5	T48.4X6
Epsilon aminocaproic acid	T45.621	T45.622	T45.623	T45.624	T45.625	T45.626
Epsom salt	T47.3X1	T47.3X2	T47.3X3	T47.3X4	T47.3X5	T47.3X6
Eptazocine	T40.4X1	T40.4X2	T40.4X3	T40.4X4	T40.4X5	T40.4X6
Equanil	T43.591	T43.592	T43.593	T43.594	T43.595	T43.596
Equisetum	T62.2X1	T62.2X2	T62.2X3	T62.2X4	—	—
diuretic	T50.2X1	T50.2X2	T50.2X3	T50.2X4	T50.2X5	T50.2X6
Ergobasine	T48.0X1	T48.0X2	T48.0X3	T48.0X4	T48.0X5	T48.0X6
Ergocalciferol	T45.2X1	T45.2X2	T45.2X3	T45.2X4	T45.2X5	T45.2X6
Ergoloid mesylates	T46.7X1	T46.7X2	T46.7X3	T46.7X4	T46.7X5	T46.7X6
Ergometrine	T48.0X1	T48.0X2	T48.0X3	T48.0X4	T48.0X5	T48.0X6
Ergonovine	T48.0X1	T48.0X2	T48.0X3	T48.0X4	T48.0X5	T48.0X6
Ergotamine	T46.5X1	T46.5X2	T46.5X3	T46.5X4	T46.5X5	T46.5X6
Ergotocine	T48.0X1	T48.0X2	T48.0X3	T48.0X4	T48.0X5	T48.0X6
Ergotrate	T48.0X1	T48.0X2	T48.0X3	T48.0X4	T48.0X5	T48.0X6
Ergot NEC	T64.81	T64.82	T64.83	T64.84	—	—
derivative	T48.0X1	T48.0X2	T48.0X3	T48.0X4	T48.0X5	T48.0X6
medicinal (alkaloids)	T48.0X1	T48.0X2	T48.0X3	T48.0X4	T48.0X5	T48.0X6
prepared	T48.0X1	T48.0X2	T48.0X3	T48.0X4	T48.0X5	T48.0X6
Eritrityl tetranitrate	T46.3X1	T46.3X2	T46.3X3	T46.3X4	T46.3X5	T46.3X6
Erythrityl tetranitrate	T46.3X1	T46.3X2	T46.3X3	T46.3X4	T46.3X5	T46.3X6
Erythrol tetranitrate	T46.3X1	T46.3X2	T46.3X3	T46.3X4	T46.3X5	T46.3X6
Erythromycin (salts)	T36.3X1	T36.3X2	T36.3X3	T36.3X4	T36.3X5	T36.3X6
ophthalmic preparation	T49.5X1	T49.5X2	T49.5X3	T49.5X4	T49.5X5	T49.5X6
topical NEC	T49.0X1	T49.0X2	T49.0X3	T49.0X4	T49.0X5	T49.0X6
Erythropoietin	T45.8X1	T45.8X2	T45.8X3	T45.8X4	T45.8X5	T45.8X6
human	T45.8X1	T45.8X2	T45.8X3	T45.8X4	T45.8X5	T45.8X6
Escin	T46.991	T46.992	T46.993	T46.994	T46.995	T46.996
Esculin	T45.2X1	T45.2X2	T45.2X3	T45.2X4	T45.2X5	T45.2X6
Esculoside	T45.2X1	T45.2X2	T45.2X3	T45.2X4	T45.2X5	T45.2X6
ESDT (ether-soluble tar distillate)	T49.1X1	T49.1X2	T49.1X3	T49.1X4	T49.1X5	T49.1X6
Eserine	T49.5X1	T49.5X2	T49.5X3	T49.5X4	T49.5X5	T49.5X6
Esflurbiprofen	T39.311	T39.312	T39.313	T39.314	T39.315	T39.316
Eskabarb	T42.3X1	T42.3X2	T42.3X3	T42.3X4	T42.3X5	T42.3X6
Eskalith	T43.8X1	T43.8X2	T43.8X3	T43.8X4	T43.8X5	T43.8X6
Esmolol	T44.7X1	T44.7X2	T44.7X3	T44.7X4	T44.7X5	T44.7X6

Additional Character May Be Required — Refer to the Tabular List for Character Selection   ▽ Subterms under main terms may continue to next column or page

Dorsacaine — Esmolol

Substance	Poisoning, Accidental (unintentional)	Poisoning, Intentional Self-harm	Poisoning, Assault	Poisoning, Undetermined	Adverse Effect	Underdosing
Estanozolol	T38.7X1	T38.7X2	T38.7X3	T38.7X4	T38.7X5	T38.7X6
Estazolam	T42.4X1	T42.4X2	T42.4X3	T42.4X4	T42.4X5	T42.4X6
Estradiol	T38.5X1	T38.5X2	T38.5X3	T38.5X4	T38.5X5	T38.5X6
with testosterone	T38.7X1	T38.7X2	T38.7X3	T38.7X4	T38.7X5	T38.7X6
benzoate	T38.5X1	T38.5X2	T38.5X3	T38.5X4	T38.5X5	T38.5X6
Estramustine	T45.1X1	T45.1X2	T45.1X3	T45.1X4	T45.1X5	T45.1X6
Estriol	T38.5X1	T38.5X2	T38.5X3	T38.5X4	T38.5X5	T38.5X6
Estrogen	T38.5X1	T38.5X2	T38.5X3	T38.5X4	T38.5X5	T38.5X6
with progesterone	T38.5X1	T38.5X2	T38.5X3	T38.5X4	T38.5X5	T38.5X6
conjugated	T38.5X1	T38.5X2	T38.5X3	T38.5X4	T38.5X5	T38.5X6
Estrone	T38.5X1	T38.5X2	T38.5X3	T38.5X4	T38.5X5	T38.5X6
Estropipate	T38.5X1	T38.5X2	T38.5X3	T38.5X4	T38.5X5	T38.5X6
Etacrynate sodium	T50.1X1	T50.1X2	T50.1X3	T50.1X4	T50.1X5	T50.1X6
Etacrynic acid	T50.1X1	T50.1X2	T50.1X3	T50.1X4	T50.1X5	T50.1X6
Etafedrine	T48.6X1	T48.6X2	T48.6X3	T48.6X4	T48.6X5	T48.6X6
Etafenone	T46.3X1	T46.3X2	T46.3X3	T46.3X4	T46.3X5	T46.3X6
Etambutol	T37.1X1	T37.1X2	T37.1X3	T37.1X4	T37.1X5	T37.1X6
Etamiphyllin	T48.6X1	T48.6X2	T48.6X3	T48.6X4	T48.6X5	T48.6X6
Etamivan	T50.7X1	T50.7X2	T50.7X3	T50.7X4	T50.7X5	T50.7X6
Etamsylate	T45.7X1	T45.7X2	T45.7X3	T45.7X4	T45.7X5	T45.7X6
Etebenecid	T50.4X1	T50.4X2	T50.4X3	T50.4X4	T50.4X5	T50.4X6
Ethacridine	T49.0X1	T49.0X2	T49.0X3	T49.0X4	T49.0X5	T49.0X6
Ethacrynic acid	T50.1X1	T50.1X2	T50.1X3	T50.1X4	T50.1X5	T50.1X6
Ethadione	T42.2X1	T42.2X2	T42.2X3	T42.2X4	T42.2X5	T42.2X6
Ethambutol	T37.1X1	T37.1X2	T37.1X3	T37.1X4	T37.1X5	T37.1X6
Ethamide	T50.2X1	T50.2X2	T50.2X3	T50.2X4	T50.2X5	T50.2X6
Ethamivan	T50.7X1	T50.7X2	T50.7X3	T50.7X4	T50.7X5	T50.7X6
Ethamsylate	T45.7X1	T45.7X2	T45.7X3	T45.7X4	T45.7X5	T45.7X6
Ethanol	T51.0X1	T51.0X2	T51.0X3	T51.0X4	—	—
beverage	T51.0X1	T51.0X2	T51.0X3	T51.0X4	—	—
Ethanolamine oleate	T46.8X1	T46.8X2	T46.8X3	T46.8X4	T46.8X5	T46.8X6
Ethaverine	T44.3X1	T44.3X2	T44.3X3	T44.3X4	T44.3X5	T44.3X6
Ethchlorvynol	T42.6X1	T42.6X2	T42.6X3	T42.6X4	T42.6X5	T42.6X6
Ethebenecid	T50.4X1	T50.4X2	T50.4X3	T50.4X4	T50.4X5	T50.4X6
Ether (vapor)	T41.0X1	T41.0X2	T41.0X3	T41.0X4	T41.0X5	T41.0X6
anesthetic	T41.0X1	T41.0X2	T41.0X3	T41.0X4	T41.0X5	T41.0X6
divinyl	T41.0X1	T41.0X2	T41.0X3	T41.0X4	T41.0X5	T41.0X6
ethyl (medicinal)	T41.0X1	T41.0X2	T41.0X3	T41.0X4	T41.0X5	T41.0X6
nonmedicinal	T52.8X1	T52.8X2	T52.8X3	T52.8X4	—	—
petroleum — see Ligroin						
solvent	T52.8X1	T52.8X2	T52.8X3	T52.8X4	—	—
Ethiazide	T50.2X1	T50.2X2	T50.2X3	T50.2X4	T50.2X5	T50.2X6
Ethidium chloride (vapor)	T59.891	T59.892	T59.893	T59.894		
Ethinamate	T42.6X1	T42.6X2	T42.6X3	T42.6X4	T42.6X5	T42.6X6
Ethinylestradiol, ethinyloestradiol	T38.5X1	T38.5X2	T38.5X3	T38.5X4	T38.5X5	T38.5X6
with						
levonorgestrel	T38.4X1	T38.4X2	T38.4X3	T38.4X4	T38.4X5	T38.4X6
norethisterone	T38.4X1	T38.4X2	T38.4X3	T38.4X4	T38.4X5	T38.4X6
Ethiodized oil (131 I)	T50.8X1	T50.8X2	T50.8X3	T50.8X4	T50.8X5	T50.8X6
Ethion	T60.0X1	T60.0X2	T60.0X3	T60.0X4	—	—
Ethionamide	T37.1X1	T37.1X2	T37.1X3	T37.1X4	T37.1X5	T37.1X6
Ethioniamide	T37.1X1	T37.1X2	T37.1X3	T37.1X4	T37.1X5	T37.1X6
Ethisterone	T38.5X1	T38.5X2	T38.5X3	T38.5X4	T38.5X5	T38.5X6
Ethobral	T42.3X1	T42.3X2	T42.3X3	T42.3X4	T42.3X5	T42.3X6
Ethocaine (infiltration)	T41.3X1	T41.3X2	T41.3X3	T41.3X4	T41.3X5	T41.3X6
(topical)	T41.3X1	T41.3X2	T41.3X3	T41.3X4	T41.3X5	T41.3X6
nerve block (peripheral) (plexus)	T41.3X1	T41.3X2	T41.3X3	T41.3X4	T41.3X5	T41.3X6
spinal	T41.3X1	T41.3X2	T41.3X3	T41.3X4	T41.3X5	T41.3X6
Ethoheptazine	T40.4X1	T40.4X2	T40.4X3	T40.4X4	T40.4X5	T40.4X6
Ethopropazine	T44.3X1	T44.3X2	T44.3X3	T44.3X4	T44.3X5	T44.3X6
Ethosuximide	T42.2X1	T42.2X2	T42.2X3	T42.2X4	T42.2X5	T42.2X6
Ethotoin	T42.0X1	T42.0X2	T42.0X3	T42.0X4	T42.0X5	T42.0X6
Ethoxazene	T37.91	T37.92	T37.93	T37.94	T37.95	T37.96
Ethoxazorutoside	T46.991	T46.992	T46.993	T46.994	T46.995	T46.996
Ethoxzolamide	T50.2X1	T50.2X2	T50.2X3	T50.2X4	T50.2X5	T50.2X6
Ethyl						
acetate	T52.8X1	T52.8X2	T52.8X3	T52.8X4	—	—
alcohol	T51.0X1	T51.0X2	T51.0X3	T51.0X4	—	—
beverage	T51.0X1	T51.0X2	T51.0X3	T51.0X4	—	—
aldehyde (vapor)	T59.891	T59.892	T59.893	T59.894	—	—
liquid	T52.8X1	T52.8X2	T52.8X3	T52.8X4	—	—
aminobenzoate	T41.3X1	T41.3X2	T41.3X3	T41.3X4	T41.3X5	T41.3X6
aminophenothiazine	T43.3X1	T43.3X2	T43.3X3	T43.3X4	T43.3X5	T43.3X6
benzoate	T52.8X1	T52.8X2	T52.8X3	T52.8X4	—	—
biscoumacetate	T45.511	T45.512	T45.513	T45.514	T45.515	T45.516
bromide (anesthetic)	T41.0X1	T41.0X2	T41.0X3	T41.0X4	T41.0X5	T41.0X6
carbamate	T45.1X1	T45.1X2	T45.1X3	T45.1X4	T45.1X5	T45.1X6
carbinol	T51.3X1	T51.3X2	T51.3X3	T51.3X4	—	—
carbonate	T52.8X1	T52.8X2	T52.8X3	T52.8X4	—	—
chaulmoograte	T37.1X1	T37.1X2	T37.1X3	T37.1X4	T37.1X5	T37.1X6
chloride (anesthetic)	T41.0X1	T41.0X2	T41.0X3	T41.0X4	T41.0X5	T41.0X6

Substance	Poisoning, Accidental (unintentional)	Poisoning, Intentional Self-harm	Poisoning, Assault	Poisoning, Undetermined	Adverse Effect	Underdosing
Ethyl — continued						
chloride — continued						
anesthetic (local)	T41.3X1	T41.3X2	T41.3X3	T41.3X4	T41.3X5	T41.3X6
inhaled	T41.0X1	T41.0X2	T41.0X3	T41.0X4	T41.0X5	T41.0X6
local	T49.4X1	T49.4X2	T49.4X3	T49.4X4	T49.4X5	T49.4X6
solvent	T53.6X1	T53.6X2	T53.6X3	T53.6X4	—	—
dibunate	T48.3X1	T48.3X2	T48.3X3	T48.3X4	T48.3X5	T48.3X6
dichloroarsine (vapor)	T57.0X1	T57.0X2	T57.0X3	T57.0X4	—	—
estranol	T38.7X1	T38.7X2	T38.7X3	T38.7X4	T38.7X5	T38.7X6
ether — see also ether						
formate NEC (solvent)	T52.0X1	T52.0X2	T52.0X3	T52.0X4	—	—
fumarate	T49.4X1	T49.4X2	T49.4X3	T49.4X4	T49.4X5	T49.4X6
hydroxyisobutyrate NEC (solvent)	T52.8X1	T52.8X2	T52.8X3	T52.8X4	—	—
iodoacetate	T59.3X1	T59.3X2	T59.3X3	T59.3X4		
lactate NEC (solvent)	T52.8X1	T52.8X2	T52.8X3	T52.8X4	—	—
loflazepate	T42.4X1	T42.4X2	T42.4X3	T42.4X4	T42.4X5	T42.4X6
mercuric chloride	T56.1X1	T56.1X2	T56.1X3	T56.1X4	—	—
methylcarbinol	T51.8X1	T51.8X2	T51.8X3	T51.8X4	—	—
morphine	T40.2X1	T40.2X2	T40.2X3	T40.2X4	T40.2X5	T40.2X6
noradrenaline	T48.6X1	T48.6X2	T48.6X3	T48.6X4	T48.6X5	T48.6X6
oxybutyrate NEC (solvent)	T52.8X1	T52.8X2	T52.8X3	T52.8X4	—	—
Ethylene (gas)	T59.891	T59.892	T59.893	T59.894		
anesthetic (general)	T41.0X1	T41.0X2	T41.0X3	T41.0X4	T41.0X5	T41.0X6
chlorohydrin	T52.8X1	T52.8X2	T52.8X3	T52.8X4		
vapor	T53.6X1	T53.6X2	T53.6X3	T53.6X4		
dichloride	T52.8X1	T52.8X2	T52.8X3	T52.8X4		
vapor	T53.6X1	T53.6X2	T53.6X3	T53.6X4		
dinitrate	T52.3X1	T52.3X2	T52.3X3	T52.3X4		
glycol(s)	T52.8X1	T52.8X2	T52.8X3	T52.8X4		
dinitrate	T52.3X1	T52.3X2	T52.3X3	T52.3X4		
monobutyl ether	T52.3X1	T52.3X2	T52.3X3	T52.3X4		
imine	T54.1X1	T54.1X2	T54.1X3	T54.1X4		
oxide (fumigant) (nonmedicinal)	T59.891	T59.892	T59.893	T59.894		
medicinal	T49.0X1	T49.0X2	T49.0X3	T49.0X4	T49.0X5	T49.0X6
Ethylenediaminetetra-acetic acid	T50.6X1	T50.6X2	T50.6X3	T50.6X4	T50.6X5	T50.6X6
Ethylenediamine theophylline	T48.6X1	T48.6X2	T48.6X3	T48.6X4	T48.6X5	T48.6X6
Ethylenedinitrilotetra-acetate	T50.6X1	T50.6X2	T50.6X3	T50.6X4	T50.6X5	T50.6X6
Ethylestrenol	T38.7X1	T38.7X2	T38.7X3	T38.7X4	T38.7X5	T38.7X6
Ethylhydroxycellulose	T47.4X1	T47.4X2	T47.4X3	T47.4X4	T47.4X5	T47.4X6
Ethylidene						
chloride NEC	T53.6X1	T53.6X2	T53.6X3	T53.6X4	—	—
diacetate	T60.3X1	T60.3X2	T60.3X3	T60.3X4	—	—
dicoumarin	T45.511	T45.512	T45.513	T45.514	T45.515	T45.516
dicoumarol	T45.511	T45.512	T45.513	T45.514	T45.515	T45.516
diethyl ether	T52.0X1	T52.0X2	T52.0X3	T52.0X4	—	—
Ethylmorphine	T40.2X1	T40.2X2	T40.2X3	T40.2X4	T40.2X5	T40.2X6
Ethylnorepinephrine	T48.6X1	T48.6X2	T48.6X3	T48.6X4	T48.6X5	T48.6X6
Ethylparachlorophen-oxyisobutyrate	T46.6X1	T46.6X2	T46.6X3	T46.6X4	T46.6X5	T46.6X6
Ethynodiol	T38.4X1	T38.4X2	T38.4X3	T38.4X4	T38.4X5	T38.4X6
with mestranol diacetate	T38.4X1	T38.4X2	T38.4X3	T38.4X4	T38.4X5	T38.4X6
Etidocaine	T41.3X1	T41.3X2	T41.3X3	T41.3X4	T41.3X5	T41.3X6
infiltration (subcutaneous)	T41.3X1	T41.3X2	T41.3X3	T41.3X4	T41.3X5	T41.3X6
nerve (peripheral) (plexus)	T41.3X1	T41.3X2	T41.3X3	T41.3X4	T41.3X5	T41.3X6
Etidronate	T50.991	T50.992	T50.993	T50.994	T50.995	T50.996
Etidronic acid (disodium salt)	T50.991	T50.992	T50.993	T50.994	T50.995	T50.996
Etifoxine	T42.6X1	T42.6X2	T42.6X3	T42.6X4	T42.6X5	T42.6X6
Etilefrine	T44.4X1	T44.4X2	T44.4X3	T44.4X4	T44.4X5	T44.4X6
Etilfen	T42.3X1	T42.3X2	T42.3X3	T42.3X4	T42.3X5	T42.3X6
Etinodiol	T38.4X1	T38.4X2	T38.4X3	T38.4X4	T38.4X5	T38.4X6
Etiroxate	T46.6X1	T46.6X2	T46.6X3	T46.6X4	T46.6X5	T46.6X6
Etizolam	T42.4X1	T42.4X2	T42.4X3	T42.4X4	T42.4X5	T42.4X6
Etodolac	T39.391	T39.392	T39.393	T39.394	T39.395	T39.396
Etofamide	T37.3X1	T37.3X2	T37.3X3	T37.3X4	T37.3X5	T37.3X6
Etofibrate	T46.6X1	T46.6X2	T46.6X3	T46.6X4	T46.6X5	T46.6X6
Etofylline	T46.7X1	T46.7X2	T46.7X3	T46.7X4	T46.7X5	T46.7X6
clofibrate	T46.6X1	T46.6X2	T46.6X3	T46.6X4	T46.6X5	T46.6X6
Etoglucid	T45.1X1	T45.1X2	T45.1X3	T45.1X4	T45.1X5	T45.1X6
Etomidate	T41.1X1	T41.1X2	T41.1X3	T41.1X4	T41.1X5	T41.1X6
Etomide	T39.8X1	T39.8X2	T39.8X3	T39.8X4	T39.8X5	T39.8X6
Etomidoline	T44.3X1	T44.3X2	T44.3X3	T44.3X4	T44.3X5	T44.3X6
Etoposide	T45.1X1	T45.1X2	T45.1X3	T45.1X4	T45.1X5	T45.1X6
Etorphine	T40.2X1	T40.2X2	T40.2X3	T40.2X4	T40.2X5	T40.2X6
Etoval	T42.3X1	T42.3X2	T42.3X3	T42.3X4	T42.3X5	T42.3X6
Etozolin	T50.1X1	T50.1X2	T50.1X3	T50.1X4	T50.1X5	T50.1X6
Etretinate	T50.991	T50.992	T50.993	T50.994	T50.995	T50.996
Etryptamine	T43.691	T43.692	T43.693	T43.694	T43.695	T43.696
Etybenzatropine	T44.3X1	T44.3X2	T44.3X3	T44.3X4	T44.3X5	T44.3X6

▽ **Subterms under main terms may continue to next column or page** Additional Character May Be Required — Refer to the Tabular List for Character Selection **357**

Estanozolol — Etybenzatropine

Substance	Poisoning, Accidental (unintentional)	Poisoning, Intentional Self-harm	Poisoning, Assault	Poisoning, Undetermined	Adverse Effect	Under-dosing
Etynodiol	T38.4X1	T38.4X2	T38.4X3	T38.4X4	T38.4X5	T38.4X6
Eucaine	T41.3X1	T41.3X2	T41.3X3	T41.3X4	T41.3X5	T41.3X6
Eucalyptus oil	T49.7X1	T49.7X2	T49.7X3	T49.7X4	T49.7X5	T49.7X6
Eucatropine	T49.5X1	T49.5X2	T49.5X3	T49.5X4	T49.5X5	T49.5X6
Eucodal	T40.2X1	T40.2X2	T40.2X3	T40.2X4	T40.2X5	T40.2X6
Euneryl	T42.3X1	T42.3X2	T42.3X3	T42.3X4	T42.3X5	T42.3X6
Euphthalmine	T44.3X1	T44.3X2	T44.3X3	T44.3X4	T44.3X5	T44.3X6
Eurax	T49.0X1	T49.0X2	T49.0X3	T49.0X4	T49.0X5	T49.0X6
Euresol	T49.4X1	T49.4X2	T49.4X3	T49.4X4	T49.4X5	T49.4X6
Euthroid	T38.1X1	T38.1X2	T38.1X3	T38.1X4	T38.1X5	T38.1X6
Evans blue	T50.8X1	T50.8X2	T50.8X3	T50.8X4	T50.8X5	T50.8X6
Evipal	T42.3X1	T42.3X2	T42.3X3	T42.3X4	T42.3X5	T42.3X6
sodium	T41.1X1	T41.1X2	T41.1X3	T41.1X4	T41.1X5	T41.1X6
Evipan	T42.3X1	T42.3X2	T42.3X3	T42.3X4	T42.3X5	T42.3X6
sodium	T41.1X1	T41.1X2	T41.1X3	T41.1X4	T41.1X5	T41.1X6
Exalamide	T49.0X1	T49.0X2	T49.0X3	T49.0X4	T49.0X5	T49.0X6
Exalgin	T39.1X1	T39.1X2	T39.1X3	T39.1X4	T39.1X5	T39.1X6
Excipients, pharmaceutical	T50.901	T50.902	T50.903	T50.904	T50.905	T50.906
Exhaust gas (engine) (motor vehicle)	T58.01	T58.02	T58.03	T58.04	—	—
Ex-Lax (phenolphthalein)	T47.2X1	T47.2X2	T47.2X3	T47.2X4	T47.2X5	T47.2X6
Expectorant NEC	T48.4X1	T48.4X2	T48.4X3	T48.4X4	T48.4X5	T48.4X6
Extended insulin zinc suspension	T38.3X1	T38.3X2	T38.3X3	T38.3X4	T38.3X5	T38.3X6
External medications (skin) (mucous membrane)	T49.91	T49.92	T49.93	T49.94	T49.95	T49.96
dental agent	T49.7X1	T49.7X2	T49.7X3	T49.7X4	T49.7X5	T49.7X6
ENT agent	T49.6X1	T49.6X2	T49.6X3	T49.6X4	T49.6X5	T49.6X6
ophthalmic preparation	T49.5X1	T49.5X2	T49.5X3	T49.5X4	T49.5X5	T49.5X6
specified NEC	T49.8X1	T49.8X2	T49.8X3	T49.8X4	T49.8X5	T49.8X6
Extrapyramidal antagonist NEC	T44.3X1	T44.3X2	T44.3X3	T44.3X4	T44.3X5	T44.3X6
Eye agents (anti-infective)	T49.5X1	T49.5X2	T49.5X3	T49.5X4	T49.5X5	T49.5X6
Eye drug NEC	T49.5X1	T49.5X2	T49.5X3	T49.5X4	T49.5X5	T49.5X6
FAC (fluorouracil + doxorubicin + cyclophosphamide)	T45.1X1	T45.1X2	T45.1X3	T45.1X4	T45.1X5	T45.1X6
Factor						
I (fibrinogen)	T45.8X1	T45.8X2	T45.8X3	T45.8X4	T45.8X5	T45.8X6
III (thromboplastin)	T45.8X1	T45.8X2	T45.8X3	T45.8X4	T45.8X5	T45.8X6
IX complex	T45.7X1	T45.7X2	T45.7X3	T45.7X4	T45.7X5	T45.7X6
human	T45.8X1	T45.8X2	T45.8X3	T45.8X4	T45.8X5	T45.8X6
VIII (antihemophilic Factor) (concentrate)	T45.8X1	T45.8X2	T45.8X3	T45.8X4	T45.8X5	T45.8X6
Famotidine	T47.0X1	T47.0X2	T47.0X3	T47.0X4	T47.0X5	T47.0X6
Fat suspension, intravenous	T50.991	T50.992	T50.993	T50.994	T50.995	T50.996
Fazadinium bromide	T48.1X1	T48.1X2	T48.1X3	T48.1X4	T48.1X5	T48.1X6
Febarbamate	T42.3X1	T42.3X2	T42.3X3	T42.3X4	T42.3X5	T42.3X6
Fecal softener	T47.4X1	T47.4X2	T47.4X3	T47.4X4	T47.4X5	T47.4X6
Fedrilate	T48.3X1	T48.3X2	T48.3X3	T48.3X4	T48.3X5	T48.3X6
Felodipine	T46.1X1	T46.1X2	T46.1X3	T46.1X4	T46.1X5	T46.1X6
Felypressin	T38.891	T38.892	T38.893	T38.894	T38.895	T38.896
Femoxetine	T43.221	T43.222	T43.223	T43.224	T43.225	T43.226
Fenalcomine	T46.3X1	T46.3X2	T46.3X3	T46.3X4	T46.3X5	T46.3X6
Fenamisal	T37.1X1	T37.1X2	T37.1X3	T37.1X4	T37.1X5	T37.1X6
Fenazone	T39.2X1	T39.2X2	T39.2X3	T39.2X4	T39.2X5	T39.2X6
Fenbendazole	T37.4X1	T37.4X2	T37.4X3	T37.4X4	T37.4X5	T37.4X6
Fenbutrazate	T50.5X1	T50.5X2	T50.5X3	T50.5X4	T50.5X5	T50.5X6
Fencamfamine	T43.691	T43.692	T43.693	T43.694	T43.695	T43.696
Fendiline	T46.1X1	T46.1X2	T46.1X3	T46.1X4	T46.1X5	T46.1X6
Fenetylline	T43.691	T43.692	T43.693	T43.694	T43.695	T43.696
Fenflumizole	T39.391	T39.392	T39.393	T39.394	T39.395	T39.396
Fenfluramine	T50.5X1	T50.5X2	T50.5X3	T50.5X4	T50.5X5	T50.5X6
Fenobarbital	T42.3X1	T42.3X2	T42.3X3	T42.3X4	T42.3X5	T42.3X6
Fenofibrate	T46.6X1	T46.6X2	T46.6X3	T46.6X4	T46.6X5	T46.6X6
Fenoprofen	T39.311	T39.312	T39.313	T39.314	T39.315	T39.316
Fenoterol	T48.6X1	T48.6X2	T48.6X3	T48.6X4	T48.6X5	T48.6X6
Fenoverine	T44.3X1	T44.3X2	T44.3X3	T44.3X4	T44.3X5	T44.3X6
Fenoxazoline	T48.5X1	T48.5X2	T48.5X3	T48.5X4	T48.5X5	T48.5X6
Fenproporex	T50.5X1	T50.5X2	T50.5X3	T50.5X4	T50.5X5	T50.5X6
Fenquizone	T50.2X1	T50.2X2	T50.2X3	T50.2X4	T50.2X5	T50.2X6
Fentanyl	T40.4X1	T40.4X2	T40.4X3	T40.4X4	T40.4X5	T40.4X6
Fentazin	T43.3X1	T43.3X2	T43.3X3	T43.3X4	T43.3X5	T43.3X6
Fenthion	T60.0X1	T60.0X2	T60.0X3	T60.0X4	—	—
Fenticlor	T49.0X1	T49.0X2	T49.0X3	T49.0X4	T49.0X5	T49.0X6
Fenylbutazone	T39.2X1	T39.2X2	T39.2X3	T39.2X4	T39.2X5	T39.2X6
Feprazone	T39.2X1	T39.2X2	T39.2X3	T39.2X4	T39.2X5	T39.2X6
Fer de lance (bite) (venom)	T63.061	T63.062	T63.063	T63.064	—	—
Ferric — see also Iron						
chloride	T45.4X1	T45.4X2	T45.4X3	T45.4X4	T45.4X5	T45.4X6
citrate	T45.4X1	T45.4X2	T45.4X3	T45.4X4	T45.4X5	T45.4X6
hydroxide						
colloidal	T45.4X1	T45.4X2	T45.4X3	T45.4X4	T45.4X5	T45.4X6

Substance	Poisoning, Accidental (unintentional)	Poisoning, Intentional Self-harm	Poisoning, Assault	Poisoning, Undetermined	Adverse Effect	Under-dosing
Ferric — see also Iron — continued						
hydroxide — continued						
polymaltose	T45.4X1	T45.4X2	T45.4X3	T45.4X4	T45.4X5	T45.4X6
pyrophosphate	T45.4X1	T45.4X2	T45.4X3	T45.4X4	T45.4X5	T45.4X6
Ferritin	T45.4X1	T45.4X2	T45.4X3	T45.4X4	T45.4X5	T45.4X6
Ferrocholinate	T45.4X1	T45.4X2	T45.4X3	T45.4X4	T45.4X5	T45.4X6
Ferrodextrane	T45.4X1	T45.4X2	T45.4X3	T45.4X4	T45.4X5	T45.4X6
Ferropolimaler	T45.4X1	T45.4X2	T45.4X3	T45.4X4	T45.4X5	T45.4X6
Ferrous — see also Iron						
phosphate	T45.4X1	T45.4X2	T45.4X3	T45.4X4	T45.4X5	T45.4X6
salt	T45.4X1	T45.4X2	T45.4X3	T45.4X4	T45.4X5	T45.4X6
with folic acid	T45.4X1	T45.4X2	T45.4X3	T45.4X4	T45.4X5	T45.4X6
Ferrous fumarate, gluconate, lactate, salt NEC, sulfate (medicinal)	T45.4X1	T45.4X2	T45.4X3	T45.4X4	T45.4X5	T45.4X6
Ferrovanadium (fumes)	T59.891	T59.892	T59.893	T59.894	—	—
Ferrum — see Iron						
Fertilizers NEC	T65.891	T65.892	T65.893	T65.894	—	—
with herbicide mixture	T60.3X1	T60.3X2	T60.3X3	T60.3X4	—	—
Fetoxilate	T47.6X1	T47.6X2	T47.6X3	T47.6X4	T47.6X5	T47.6X6
Fiber, dietary	T47.4X1	T47.4X2	T47.4X3	T47.4X4	T47.4X5	T47.4X6
Fiberglass	T65.831	T65.832	T65.833	T65.834	—	—
Fibrinogen (human)	T45.8X1	T45.8X2	T45.8X3	T45.8X4	T45.8X5	T45.8X6
Fibrinolysin (human)	T45.691	T45.692	T45.693	T45.694	T45.695	T45.696
Fibrinolysis						
affecting drug	T45.601	T45.602	T45.603	T45.604	T45.605	T45.606
inhibitor NEC	T45.621	T45.622	T45.623	T45.624	T45.625	T45.626
Fibrinolytic drug	T45.611	T45.612	T45.613	T45.614	T45.615	T45.616
Filix mas	T37.4X1	T37.4X2	T37.4X3	T37.4X4	T37.4X5	T37.4X6
Filtering cream	T49.3X1	T49.3X2	T49.3X3	T49.3X4	T49.3X5	T49.3X6
Fiorinal	T39.011	T39.012	T39.013	T39.014	T39.015	T39.016
Firedamp	T59.891	T59.892	T59.893	T59.894	—	—
Fish, noxious, nonbacterial	T61.91	T61.92	T61.93	T61.94	—	—
ciguatera	T61.01	T61.02	T61.03	T61.04	—	—
scombroid	T61.11	T61.12	T61.13	T61.14	—	—
shell	T61.781	T61.782	T61.783	T61.784	—	—
specified NEC	T61.771	T61.772	T61.773	T61.774	—	—
Flagyl	T37.3X1	T37.3X2	T37.3X3	T37.3X4	T37.3X5	T37.3X6
Flavine adenine dinucleotide	T45.2X1	T45.2X2	T45.2X3	T45.2X4	T45.2X5	T45.2X6
Flavodic acid	T46.991	T46.992	T46.993	T46.994	T46.995	T46.996
Flavoxate	T44.3X1	T44.3X2	T44.3X3	T44.3X4	T44.3X5	T44.3X6
Flaxedil	T48.1X1	T48.1X2	T48.1X3	T48.1X4	T48.1X5	T48.1X6
Flaxseed (medicinal)	T49.3X1	T49.3X2	T49.3X3	T49.3X4	T49.3X5	T49.3X6
Flecainide	T46.2X1	T46.2X2	T46.2X3	T46.2X4	T46.2X5	T46.2X6
Fleroxacin	T36.8X1	T36.8X2	T36.8X3	T36.8X4	T36.8X5	T36.8X6
Floctafenine	T39.8X1	T39.8X2	T39.8X3	T39.8X4	T39.8X5	T39.8X6
Flomax	T44.6X1	T44.6X2	T44.6X3	T44.6X4	T44.6X5	T44.6X6
Flomoxef	T36.1X1	T36.1X2	T36.1X3	T36.1X4	T36.1X5	T36.1X6
Flopropione	T44.3X1	T44.3X2	T44.3X3	T44.3X4	T44.3X5	T44.3X6
Florantyrone	T47.5X1	T47.5X2	T47.5X3	T47.5X4	T47.5X5	T47.5X6
Floraquin	T37.8X1	T37.8X2	T37.8X3	T37.8X4	T37.8X5	T37.8X6
Florinef	T38.0X1	T38.0X2	T38.0X3	T38.0X4	T38.0X5	T38.0X6
ENT agent	T49.6X1	T49.6X2	T49.6X3	T49.6X4	T49.6X5	T49.6X6
ophthalmic preparation	T49.5X1	T49.5X2	T49.5X3	T49.5X4	T49.5X5	T49.5X6
topical NEC	T49.0X1	T49.0X2	T49.0X3	T49.0X4	T49.0X5	T49.0X6
Flowers of sulfur	T49.4X1	T49.4X2	T49.4X3	T49.4X4	T49.4X5	T49.4X6
Floxuridine	T45.1X1	T45.1X2	T45.1X3	T45.1X4	T45.1X5	T45.1X6
Fluanisone	T43.4X1	T43.4X2	T43.4X3	T43.4X4	T43.4X5	T43.4X6
Flubendazole	T37.4X1	T37.4X2	T37.4X3	T37.4X4	T37.4X5	T37.4X6
Fluclorolone acetonide	T49.0X1	T49.0X2	T49.0X3	T49.0X4	T49.0X5	T49.0X6
Flucloxacillin	T36.0X1	T36.0X2	T36.0X3	T36.0X4	T36.0X5	T36.0X6
Fluconazole	T37.8X1	T37.8X2	T37.8X3	T37.8X4	T37.8X5	T37.8X6
Flucytosine	T37.8X1	T37.8X2	T37.8X3	T37.8X4	T37.8X5	T37.8X6
Fludeoxyglucose (18F)	T50.8X1	T50.8X2	T50.8X3	T50.8X4	T50.8X5	T50.8X6
Fludiazepam	T42.4X1	T42.4X2	T42.4X3	T42.4X4	T42.4X5	T42.4X6
Fludrocortisone	T50.0X1	T50.0X2	T50.0X3	T50.0X4	T50.0X5	T50.0X6
ENT agent	T49.6X1	T49.6X2	T49.6X3	T49.6X4	T49.6X5	T49.6X6
ophthalmic preparation	T49.5X1	T49.5X2	T49.5X3	T49.5X4	T49.5X5	T49.5X6
topical NEC	T49.0X1	T49.0X2	T49.0X3	T49.0X4	T49.0X5	T49.0X6
Fludroxycortide	T49.0X1	T49.0X2	T49.0X3	T49.0X4	T49.0X5	T49.0X6
Flufenamic acid	T39.391	T39.392	T39.393	T39.394	T39.395	T39.396
Fluindione	T45.511	T45.512	T45.513	T45.514	T45.515	T45.516
Flumequine	T37.8X1	T37.8X2	T37.8X3	T37.8X4	T37.8X5	T37.8X6
Flumethasone	T49.0X1	T49.0X2	T49.0X3	T49.0X4	T49.0X5	T49.0X6
Flumethiazide	T50.2X1	T50.2X2	T50.2X3	T50.2X4	T50.2X5	T50.2X6
Flumidin	T37.5X1	T37.5X2	T37.5X3	T37.5X4	T37.5X5	T37.5X6
Flunarizine	T46.7X1	T46.7X2	T46.7X3	T46.7X4	T46.7X5	T46.7X6
Flunidazole	T37.8X1	T37.8X2	T37.8X3	T37.8X4	T37.8X5	T37.8X6
Flunisolide	T48.6X1	T48.6X2	T48.6X3	T48.6X4	T48.6X5	T48.6X6
Flunitrazepam	T42.4X1	T42.4X2	T42.4X3	T42.4X4	T42.4X5	T42.4X6
Fluocinolone (acetonide)	T49.0X1	T49.0X2	T49.0X3	T49.0X4	T49.0X5	T49.0X6
Fluocinonide	T49.0X1	T49.0X2	T49.0X3	T49.0X4	T49.0X5	T49.0X6

358

Additional Character May Be Required — Refer to the Tabular List for Character Selection   ▽ Subterms under main terms may continue to next column or page

Substance	Poisoning, Accidental (unintentional)	Poisoning, Intentional Self-harm	Poisoning, Assault	Poisoning, Undetermined	Adverse Effect	Under-dosing
Fluocortin (butyl)	T49.0X1	T49.0X2	T49.0X3	T49.0X4	T49.0X5	T49.0X6
Fluocortolone	T49.0X1	T49.0X2	T49.0X3	T49.0X4	T49.0X5	T49.0X6
Fluohydrocortisone	T38.0X1	T38.0X2	T38.0X3	T38.0X4	T38.0X5	T38.0X6
ENT agent	T49.6X1	T49.6X2	T49.6X3	T49.6X4	T49.6X5	T49.6X6
ophthalmic preparation	T49.5X1	T49.5X2	T49.5X3	T49.5X4	T49.5X5	T49.5X6
topical NEC	T49.0X1	T49.0X2	T49.0X3	T49.0X4	T49.0X5	T49.0X6
Fluonid	T49.0X1	T49.0X2	T49.0X3	T49.0X4	T49.0X5	T49.0X6
Fluopromazine	T43.3X1	T43.3X2	T43.3X3	T43.3X4	T43.3X5	T43.3X6
Fluoracetate	T60.8X1	T60.8X2	T60.8X3	T60.8X4	—	—
Fluorescein	T50.8X1	T50.8X2	T50.8X3	T50.8X4	T50.8X5	T50.8X6
Fluorhydrocortisone	T50.0X1	T50.0X2	T50.0X3	T50.0X4	T50.0X5	T50.0X6
Fluoride (nonmedicinal) (pesticide) (sodium) **NEC**	T60.8X1	T60.8X2	T60.8X3	T60.8X4	—	—
hydrogen — *see* Hydrofluoric acid						
medicinal NEC	T50.991	T50.992	T50.993	T50.994	T50.995	T50.996
dental use	T49.7X1	T49.7X2	T49.7X3	T49.7X4	T49.7X5	T49.7X6
not pesticide NEC	T54.91	T54.92	T54.93	T54.94	—	—
stannous	T49.7X1	T49.7X2	T49.7X3	T49.7X4	T49.7X5	T49.7X6
Fluorinated corticosteroids	T38.0X1	T38.0X2	T38.0X3	T38.0X4	T38.0X5	T38.0X6
Fluorine (gas)	T59.5X1	T59.5X2	T59.5X3	T59.5X4	—	—
salt — *see* Fluoride(s)						
Fluoristan	T49.7X1	T49.7X2	T49.7X3	T49.7X4	T49.7X5	T49.7X6
Fluormetholone	T49.0X1	T49.0X2	T49.0X3	T49.0X4	T49.0X5	T49.0X6
Fluoroacetate	T60.8X1	T60.8X2	T60.8X3	T60.8X4	—	—
Fluorocarbon monomer	T53.6X1	T53.6X2	T53.6X3	T53.6X4	—	—
Fluorocytosine	T37.8X1	T37.8X2	T37.8X3	T37.8X4	T37.8X5	T37.8X6
Fluorodeoxyuridine	T45.1X1	T45.1X2	T45.1X3	T45.1X4	T45.1X5	T45.1X6
Fluorometholone	T49.0X1	T49.0X2	T49.0X3	T49.0X4	T49.0X5	T49.0X6
ophthalmic preparation	T49.5X1	T49.5X2	T49.5X3	T49.5X4	T49.5X5	T49.5X6
Fluorophosphate insecticide	T60.0X1	T60.0X2	T60.0X3	T60.0X4	—	—
Fluorosol	T46.3X1	T46.3X2	T46.3X3	T46.3X4	T46.3X5	T46.3X6
Fluorouracil	T45.1X1	T45.1X2	T45.1X3	T45.1X4	T45.1X5	T45.1X6
Fluorphenylalanine	T49.5X1	T49.5X2	T49.5X3	T49.5X4	T49.5X5	T49.5X6
Fluothane	T41.0X1	T41.0X2	T41.0X3	T41.0X4	T41.0X5	T41.0X6
Fluoxetine	T43.221	T43.222	T43.223	T43.224	T43.225	T43.226
Fluoxymesterone	T38.7X1	T38.7X2	T38.7X3	T38.7X4	T38.7X5	T38.7X6
Flupenthixol	T43.4X1	T43.4X2	T43.4X3	T43.4X4	T43.4X5	T43.4X6
Flupentixol	T43.4X1	T43.4X2	T43.4X3	T43.4X4	T43.4X5	T43.4X6
Fluphenazine	T43.3X1	T43.3X2	T43.3X3	T43.3X4	T43.3X5	T43.3X6
Fluprednidene	T49.0X1	T49.0X2	T49.0X3	T49.0X4	T49.0X5	T49.0X6
Fluprednisolone	T38.0X1	T38.0X2	T38.0X3	T38.0X4	T38.0X5	T38.0X6
Fluradoline	T39.8X1	T39.8X2	T39.8X3	T39.8X4	T39.8X5	T39.8X6
Flurandrenolide	T49.0X1	T49.0X2	T49.0X3	T49.0X4	T49.0X5	T49.0X6
Flurandrenolone	T49.0X1	T49.0X2	T49.0X3	T49.0X4	T49.0X5	T49.0X6
Flurazepam	T42.4X1	T42.4X2	T42.4X3	T42.4X4	T42.4X5	T42.4X6
Flurbiprofen	T39.311	T39.312	T39.313	T39.314	T39.315	T39.316
Flurobate	T49.0X1	T49.0X2	T49.0X3	T49.0X4	T49.0X5	T49.0X6
Fluroxene	T41.0X1	T41.0X2	T41.0X3	T41.0X4	T41.0X5	T41.0X6
Fluspirilene	T43.591	T43.592	T43.593	T43.594	T43.595	T43.596
Flutamide	T38.6X1	T38.6X2	T38.6X3	T38.6X4	T38.6X5	T38.6X6
Flutazolam	T42.4X1	T42.4X2	T42.4X3	T42.4X4	T42.4X5	T42.4X6
Fluticasone propionate	T49.1X1	T49.1X2	T49.1X3	T49.1X4	T49.1X5	T49.1X6
Flutoprazepam	T42.4X1	T42.4X2	T42.4X3	T42.4X4	T42.4X5	T42.4X6
Flutropium bromide	T48.6X1	T48.6X2	T48.6X3	T48.6X4	T48.6X5	T48.6X6
Fluvoxamine	T43.221	T43.222	T43.223	T43.224	T43.225	T43.226
Folacin	T45.8X1	T45.8X2	T45.8X3	T45.8X4	T45.8X5	T45.8X6
Folic acid	T45.8X1	T45.8X2	T45.8X3	T45.8X4	T45.8X5	T45.8X6
with ferrous salt	T45.2X1	T45.2X2	T45.2X3	T45.2X4	T45.2X5	T45.2X6
antagonist	T45.1X1	T45.1X2	T45.1X3	T45.1X4	T45.1X5	T45.1X6
Folinic acid	T45.8X1	T45.8X2	T45.8X3	T45.8X4	T45.8X5	T45.8X6
Folium stramoniae	T48.6X1	T48.6X2	T48.6X3	T48.6X4	T48.6X5	T48.6X6
Follicle-stimulating hormone, human	T38.811	T38.812	T38.813	T38.814	T38.815	T38.816
Folpet	T60.3X1	T60.3X2	T60.3X3	T60.3X4	—	—
Fominoben	T48.3X1	T48.3X2	T48.3X3	T48.3X4	T48.3X5	T48.3X6
Food, foodstuffs, noxious, nonbacterial, NEC	T62.91	T62.92	T62.93	T62.94	—	—
berries	T62.1X1	T62.1X2	T62.1X3	T62.1X4	—	—
fish — *see also* Fish	T61.91	T61.92	T61.93	T61.94	—	—
mushrooms	T62.0X1	T62.0X2	T62.0X3	T62.0X4	—	—
plants	T62.2X1	T62.2X2	T62.2X3	T62.2X4	—	—
seafood	T61.91	T61.92	T61.93	T61.94	—	—
specified NEC	T61.8X1	T61.8X2	T61.8X3	T61.8X4	—	—
seeds	T62.2X1	T62.2X2	T62.2X3	T62.2X4	—	—
shellfish	T61.781	T61.782	T61.783	T61.784	—	—
specified NEC	T62.8X1	T62.8X2	T62.8X3	T62.8X4	—	—
Fool's parsley	T62.2X1	T62.2X2	T62.2X3	T62.2X4	—	—
Formaldehyde (solution), gas or vapor	T59.2X1	T59.2X2	T59.2X3	T59.2X4	—	—
fungicide	T60.3X1	T60.3X2	T60.3X3	T60.3X4	—	—
Formalin	T59.2X1	T59.2X2	T59.2X3	T59.2X4	—	—
fungicide	T60.3X1	T60.3X2	T60.3X3	T60.3X4	—	—
vapor	T59.2X1	T59.2X2	T59.2X3	T59.2X4	—	—
Formic acid	T54.2X1	T54.2X2	T54.2X3	T54.2X4	—	—
vapor	T59.891	T59.892	T59.893	T59.894	—	—
Foscarnet sodium	T37.5X1	T37.5X2	T37.5X3	T37.5X4	T37.5X5	T37.5X6
Fosfestrol	T38.5X1	T38.5X2	T38.5X3	T38.5X4	T38.5X5	T38.5X6
Fosfomycin	T36.8X1	T36.8X2	T36.8X3	T36.8X4	T36.8X5	T36.8X6
Fosfonet sodium	T37.5X1	T37.5X2	T37.5X3	T37.5X4	T37.5X5	T37.5X6
Fosinopril	T46.4X1	T46.4X2	T46.4X3	T46.4X4	T46.4X5	T46.4X6
sodium	T46.4X1	T46.4X2	T46.4X3	T46.4X4	T46.4X5	T46.4X6
Fowler's solution	T57.0X1	T57.0X2	T57.0X3	T57.0X4	—	—
Foxglove	T62.2X1	T62.2X2	T62.2X3	T62.2X4	—	—
Framycetin	T36.5X1	T36.5X2	T36.5X3	T36.5X4	T36.5X5	T36.5X6
Frangula	T47.2X1	T47.2X2	T47.2X3	T47.2X4	T47.2X5	T47.2X6
extract	T47.2X1	T47.2X2	T47.2X3	T47.2X4	T47.2X5	T47.2X6
Frei antigen	T50.8X1	T50.8X2	T50.8X3	T50.8X4	T50.8X5	T50.8X6
Freon	T53.5X1	T53.5X2	T53.5X3	T53.5X4	—	—
Fructose	T50.3X1	T50.3X2	T50.3X3	T50.3X4	T50.3X5	T50.3X6
Frusemide	T50.1X1	T50.1X2	T50.1X3	T50.1X4	T50.1X5	T50.1X6
FSH	T38.811	T38.812	T38.813	T38.814	T38.815	T38.816
Ftorafur	T45.1X1	T45.1X2	T45.1X3	T45.1X4	T45.1X5	T45.1X6
Fuel						
automobile	T52.0X1	T52.0X2	T52.0X3	T52.0X4	—	—
exhaust gas, not in transit	T58.01	T58.02	T58.03	T58.04	—	—
vapor NEC	T52.0X1	T52.0X2	T52.0X3	T52.0X4	—	—
gas (domestic use) — *see also* Carbon, monoxide, fuel, utility	T59.891	T59.892	T59.893	T59.894	—	—
utility	T59.891	T59.892	T59.893	T59.894	—	—
incomplete combustion of — *see* Carbon, monoxide, fuel, utility						
in mobile container	T59.891	T59.892	T59.893	T59.894	—	—
piped (natural)	T59.891	T59.892	T59.893	T59.894	—	—
industrial, incomplete combustion	T58.8X1	T58.8X2	T58.8X3	T58.8X4	—	—
Fugillin	T36.8X1	T36.8X2	T36.8X3	T36.8X4	T36.8X5	T36.8X6
Fulminate of mercury	T56.1X1	T56.1X2	T56.1X3	T56.1X4	—	—
Fulvicin	T36.7X1	T36.7X2	T36.7X3	T36.7X4	T36.7X5	T36.7X6
Fumadil	T36.8X1	T36.8X2	T36.8X3	T36.8X4	T36.8X5	T36.8X6
Fumagillin	T36.8X1	T36.8X2	T36.8X3	T36.8X4	T36.8X5	T36.8X6
Fumaric acid	T49.4X1	T49.4X2	T49.4X3	T49.4X4	T49.4X5	T49.4X6
Fumes (from)	T59.91	T59.92	T59.93	T59.94	—	—
carbon monoxide — *see* Carbon, monoxide						
charcoal (domestic use) — *see* Charcoal, fumes						
chloroform — *see* Chloroform						
coke (in domestic stoves, fireplaces) — *see* Coke fumes						
corrosive NEC	T54.91	T54.92	T54.93	T54.94	—	—
ether — *see* ether						
freons	T53.5X1	T53.5X2	T53.5X3	T53.5X4	—	—
hydrocarbons	T59.891	T59.892	T59.893	T59.894	—	—
petroleum (liquefied)	T59.891	T59.892	T59.893	T59.894	—	—
distributed through pipes (pure or mixed with air)	T59.891	T59.892	T59.893	T59.894	—	—
lead — *see* lead						
metal — *see* Metals, or the specified metal						
nitrogen dioxide	T59.0X1	T59.0X2	T59.0X3	T59.0X4	—	—
pesticides — *see* Pesticides						
petroleum (liquefied)	T59.891	T59.892	T59.893	T59.894	—	—
distributed through pipes (pure or mixed with air)	T59.891	T59.892	T59.893	T59.894	—	—
polyester	T59.891	T59.892	T59.893	T59.894	—	—
specified source NEC — *see also* substance specified	T59.891	T59.892	T59.893	T59.894	—	—
sulfur dioxide	T59.1X1	T59.1X2	T59.1X3	T59.1X4	—	—
Fumigant NEC	T60.91	T60.92	T60.93	T60.94	—	—
Fungicide NEC (nonmedicinal)	T60.3X1	T60.3X2	T60.3X3	T60.3X4	—	—
Fungi, noxious, used as food	T62.0X1	T62.0X2	T62.0X3	T62.0X4	—	—
Fungizone	T36.7X1	T36.7X2	T36.7X3	T36.7X4	T36.7X5	T36.7X6
topical	T49.0X1	T49.0X2	T49.0X3	T49.0X4	T49.0X5	T49.0X6
Furacin	T49.0X1	T49.0X2	T49.0X3	T49.0X4	T49.0X5	T49.0X6
Furadantin	T37.91	T37.92	T37.93	T37.94	T37.95	T37.96
Furazolidone	T37.8X1	T37.8X2	T37.8X3	T37.8X4	T37.8X5	T37.8X6

Substance	Poisoning, Accidental (unintentional)	Poisoning, Intentional Self-harm	Poisoning, Assault	Poisoning, Undetermined	Adverse Effect	Under-dosing
Furazolium chloride	T49.0X1	T49.0X2	T49.0X3	T49.0X4	T49.0X5	T49.0X6
Furfural	T52.8X1	T52.8X2	T52.8X3	T52.8X4	—	—
Furnace (coal burning) (domestic), gas from	T58.2X1	T58.2X2	T58.2X3	T58.2X4	—	—
industrial	T58.8X1	T58.8X2	T58.8X3	T58.8X4	—	—
Furniture polish	T65.891	T65.892	T65.893	T65.894	—	—
Furosemide	T50.1X1	T50.1X2	T50.1X3	T50.1X4	T50.1X5	T50.1X6
Furoxone	T37.91	T37.92	T37.93	T37.94	T37.95	T37.96
Fursultiamine	T45.2X1	T45.2X2	T45.2X3	T45.2X4	T45.2X5	T45.2X6
Fusafungine	T36.8X1	T36.8X2	T36.8X3	T36.8X4	T36.8X5	T36.8X6
Fusel oil (any) (amyl) (butyl) (propyl), vapor	T51.3X1	T51.3X2	T51.3X3	T51.3X4	—	—
Fusidate (ethanolamine) (sodium)	T36.8X1	T36.8X2	T36.8X3	T36.8X4	T36.8X5	T36.8X6
Fusidic acid	T36.8X1	T36.8X2	T36.8X3	T36.8X4	T36.8X5	T36.8X6
Fytic acid, nonasodium	T50.6X1	T50.6X2	T50.6X3	T50.6X4	T50.6X5	T50.6X6
b-Galactosidase	T47.5X1	T47.5X2	T47.5X3	T47.5X4	T47.5X5	T47.5X6
GABA	T43.8X1	T43.8X2	T43.8X3	T43.8X4	T43.8X5	T43.8X6
Gadopentetic acid	T50.8X1	T50.8X2	T50.8X3	T50.8X4	T50.8X5	T50.8X6
Galactose	T50.3X1	T50.3X2	T50.3X3	T50.3X4	T50.3X5	T50.3X6
Galantamine	T44.0X1	T44.0X2	T44.0X3	T44.0X4	T44.0X5	T44.0X6
Gallamine (triethiodide)	T48.1X1	T48.1X2	T48.1X3	T48.1X4	T48.1X5	T48.1X6
Gallium citrate	T50.991	T50.992	T50.993	T50.994	T50.995	T50.996
Gallopamil	T46.1X1	T46.1X2	T46.1X3	T46.1X4	T46.1X5	T46.1X6
Gamboge	T47.2X1	T47.2X2	T47.2X3	T47.2X4	T47.2X5	T47.2X6
Gamimune	T50.Z11	T50.Z12	T50.Z13	T50.Z14	T50.Z15	T50.Z16
Gamma-aminobutyric acid	T43.8X1	T43.8X2	T43.8X3	T43.8X4	T43.8X5	T43.8X6
Gamma-benzene hexachloride (medicinal)	T49.0X1	T49.0X2	T49.0X3	T49.0X4	T49.0X5	T49.0X6
nonmedicinal, vapor	T53.6X1	T53.6X2	T53.6X3	T53.6X4	—	—
Gamma-BHC (medicinal) — see also Gamma-benzene hexachloride	T49.0X1	T49.0X2	T49.0X3	T49.0X4	T49.0X5	T49.0X6
Gamma globulin	T50.Z11	T50.Z12	T50.Z13	T50.Z14	T50.Z15	T50.Z16
Gamulin	T50.Z11	T50.Z12	T50.Z13	T50.Z14	T50.Z15	T50.Z16
Ganciclovir (sodium)	T37.5X1	T37.5X2	T37.5X3	T37.5X4	T37.5X5	T37.5X6
Ganglionic blocking drug NEC	T44.2X1	T44.2X2	T44.2X3	T44.2X4	T44.2X5	T44.2X6
specified NEC	T44.2X1	T44.2X2	T44.2X3	T44.2X4	T44.2X5	T44.2X6
Ganja	T40.7X1	T40.7X2	T40.7X3	T40.7X4	T40.7X5	T40.7X6
Garamycin	T36.5X1	T36.5X2	T36.5X3	T36.5X4	T36.5X5	T36.5X6
ophthalmic preparation	T49.5X1	T49.5X2	T49.5X3	T49.5X4	T49.5X5	T49.5X6
topical NEC	T49.0X1	T49.0X2	T49.0X3	T49.0X4	T49.0X5	T49.0X6
Gardenal	T42.3X1	T42.3X2	T42.3X3	T42.3X4	T42.3X5	T42.3X6
Gardepanyl	T42.3X1	T42.3X2	T42.3X3	T42.3X4	T42.3X5	T42.3X6
Gas	T59.91	T59.92	T59.93	T59.94	—	—
acetylene	T59.891	T59.892	T59.893	T59.894	—	—
incomplete combustion of	T58.11	T58.12	T58.13	T58.14	—	—
air contaminants, source or type not specified	T59.91	T59.92	T59.93	T59.94	—	—
anesthetic	T41.0X1	T41.0X2	T41.0X3	T41.0X4	T41.0X5	T41.0X6
blast furnace	T58.8X1	T58.8X2	T58.8X3	T58.8X4	—	—
butane — see butane						
carbon monoxide — see Carbon, monoxide						
chlorine	T59.4X1	T59.4X2	T59.4X3	T59.4X4	—	—
coal	T58.2X1	T58.2X2	T58.2X3	T58.2X4	—	—
cyanide	T57.3X1	T57.3X2	T57.3X3	T57.3X4	—	—
dicyanogen	T65.0X1	T65.0X2	T65.0X3	T65.0X4	—	—
domestic — see Domestic gas						
exhaust	T58.01	T58.02	T58.03	T58.04	—	—
from utility (for cooking, heating, or lighting) (after combustion) — see Carbon, monoxide, fuel, utility						
prior to combustion	T59.891	T59.892	T59.893	T59.894	—	—
from wood- or coal-burning stove or fireplace	T58.2X1	T58.2X2	T58.2X3	T58.2X4	—	—
fuel (domestic use) (after combustion) — see also Carbon, monoxide, fuel						
industrial use	T58.8X1	T58.8X2	T58.8X3	T58.8X4	—	—
prior to combustion	T59.891	T59.892	T59.893	T59.894	—	—
utility	T59.891	T59.892	T59.893	T59.894	—	—
incomplete combustion of — see Carbon, monoxide, fuel, utility						
in mobile container	T59.891	T59.892	T59.893	T59.894	—	—
piped (natural)	T59.891	T59.892	T59.893	T59.894	—	—
garage	T58.01	T58.02	T58.03	T58.04	—	—

Substance	Poisoning, Accidental (unintentional)	Poisoning, Intentional Self-harm	Poisoning, Assault	Poisoning, Undetermined	Adverse Effect	Under-dosing
Gas — continued						
hydrocarbon NEC	T59.891	T59.892	T59.893	T59.894	—	—
incomplete combustion of — see Carbon, monoxide, fuel, utility						
liquefied — see butane						
piped	T59.891	T59.892	T59.893	T59.894	—	—
hydrocyanic acid	T65.0X1	T65.0X2	T65.0X3	T65.0X4	—	—
illuminating (after combustion)	T58.11	T58.12	T58.13	T58.14	—	—
prior to combustion	T59.891	T59.892	T59.893	T59.894	—	—
incomplete combustion, any — see Carbon, monoxide						
kiln	T58.8X1	T58.8X2	T58.8X3	T58.8X4	—	—
lacrimogenic	T59.3X1	T59.3X2	T59.3X3	T59.3X4	—	—
liquefied petroleum — see butane						
marsh	T59.891	T59.892	T59.893	T59.894	—	—
motor exhaust, not in transit	T58.01	T58.02	T58.03	T58.04	—	—
mustard, not in war	T59.891	T59.892	T59.893	T59.894	—	—
natural	T59.891	T59.892	T59.893	T59.894	—	—
nerve, not in war	T59.91	T59.92	T59.93	T59.94	—	—
oil	T52.0X1	T52.0X2	T52.0X3	T52.0X4	—	—
petroleum (liquefied) (distributed in mobile containers)	T59.891	T59.892	T59.893	T59.894	—	—
piped (pure or mixed with air)	T59.891	T59.892	T59.893	T59.894	—	—
piped (manufactured) (natural) NEC	T59.891	T59.892	T59.893	T59.894	—	—
producer	T58.8X1	T58.8X2	T58.8X3	T58.8X4	—	—
propane — see propane						
refrigerant (chlorofluoro-carbon)	T53.5X1	T53.5X2	T53.5X3	T53.5X4	—	—
not chlorofluoro-carbon	T59.891	T59.892	T59.893	T59.894	—	—
sewer	T59.91	T59.92	T59.93	T59.94	—	—
specified source NEC	T59.91	T59.92	T59.93	T59.94	—	—
stove (after combustion)	T58.11	T58.12	T58.13	T58.14	—	—
prior to combustion	T59.891	T59.892	T59.893	T59.894	—	—
tear	T59.3X1	T59.3X2	T59.3X3	T59.3X4	—	—
therapeutic	T41.5X1	T41.5X2	T41.5X3	T41.5X4	T41.5X5	T41.5X6
utility (for cooking, heating, or lighting) (piped) NEC	T59.891	T59.892	T59.893	T59.894	—	—
incomplete combustion of — see Carbon, monoxide, fuel, utility						
in mobile container	T59.891	T59.892	T59.893	T59.894	—	—
piped (natural)	T59.891	T59.892	T59.893	T59.894	—	—
water	T58.11	T58.12	T58.13	T58.14	—	—
incomplete combustion of — see Carbon, monoxide, fuel, utility						
Gaseous substance — see Gas						
Gasoline	T52.0X1	T52.0X2	T52.0X3	T52.0X4	—	—
vapor	T52.0X1	T52.0X2	T52.0X3	T52.0X4	—	—
Gastric enzymes	T47.5X1	T47.5X2	T47.5X3	T47.5X4	T47.5X5	T47.5X6
Gastrografin	T50.8X1	T50.8X2	T50.8X3	T50.8X4	T50.8X5	T50.8X6
Gastrointestinal drug	T47.91	T47.92	T47.93	T47.94	T47.95	T47.96
biological	T47.8X1	T47.8X2	T47.8X3	T47.8X4	T47.8X5	T47.8X6
specified NEC	T47.8X1	T47.8X2	T47.8X3	T47.8X4	T47.8X5	T47.8X6
Gaultheria procumbens	T62.2X1	T62.2X2	T62.2X3	T62.2X4	—	—
Gefarnate	T44.3X1	T44.3X2	T44.3X3	T44.3X4	T44.3X5	T44.3X6
Gelatin (intravenous)	T45.8X1	T45.8X2	T45.8X3	T45.8X4	T45.8X5	T45.8X6
absorbable (sponge)	T45.7X1	T45.7X2	T45.7X3	T45.7X4	T45.7X5	T45.7X6
Gelfilm	T49.8X1	T49.8X2	T49.8X3	T49.8X4	T49.8X5	T49.8X6
Gelfoam	T45.7X1	T45.7X2	T45.7X3	T45.7X4	T45.7X5	T45.7X6
Gelsemine	T50.991	T50.992	T50.993	T50.994	T50.995	T50.996
Gelsemium (sempervirens)	T62.2X1	T62.2X2	T62.2X3	T62.2X4	—	—
Gemeprost	T48.0X1	T48.0X2	T48.0X3	T48.0X4	T48.0X5	T48.0X6
Gemfibrozil	T46.6X1	T46.6X2	T46.6X3	T46.6X4	T46.6X5	T46.6X6
Gemonil	T42.3X1	T42.3X2	T42.3X3	T42.3X4	T42.3X5	T42.3X6
Gentamicin	T36.5X1	T36.5X2	T36.5X3	T36.5X4	T36.5X5	T36.5X6
ophthalmic preparation	T49.5X1	T49.5X2	T49.5X3	T49.5X4	T49.5X5	T49.5X6
topical NEC	T49.0X1	T49.0X2	T49.0X3	T49.0X4	T49.0X5	T49.0X6
Gentian	T47.5X1	T47.5X2	T47.5X3	T47.5X4	T47.5X5	T47.5X6
violet	T49.0X1	T49.0X2	T49.0X3	T49.0X4	T49.0X5	T49.0X6
Gepefrine	T44.4X1	T44.4X2	T44.4X3	T44.4X4	T44.4X5	T44.4X6
Gestonorone caproate	T38.5X1	T38.5X2	T38.5X3	T38.5X4	T38.5X5	T38.5X6
Gexane	T49.0X1	T49.0X2	T49.0X3	T49.0X4	T49.0X5	T49.0X6
Gila monster (venom)	T63.111	T63.112	T63.113	T63.114	—	—
Ginger	T47.5X1	T47.5X2	T47.5X3	T47.5X4	T47.5X5	T47.5X6
Jamaica — see Jamaica, ginger						

Substance	Poisoning, Accidental (unintentional)	Poisoning, Intentional Self-harm	Poisoning, Assault	Poisoning, Undetermined	Adverse Effect	Under-dosing
Gitalin	T46.0X1	T46.0X2	T46.0X3	T46.0X4	T46.0X5	T46.0X6
amorphous	T46.0X1	T46.0X2	T46.0X3	T46.0X4	T46.0X5	T46.0X6
Gitaloxin	T46.0X1	T46.0X2	T46.0X3	T46.0X4	T46.0X5	T46.0X6
Gitoxin	T46.0X1	T46.0X2	T46.0X3	T46.0X4	T46.0X5	T46.0X6
Glafenine	T39.8X1	T39.8X2	T39.8X3	T39.8X4	T39.8X5	T39.8X6
Glandular extract (medicinal) **NEC**	T50.Z91	T50.Z92	T50.Z93	T50.Z94	T50.Z95	T50.Z96
Glaucarubin	T37.3X1	T37.3X2	T37.3X3	T37.3X4	T37.3X5	T37.3X6
Glibenclamide	T38.3X1	T38.3X2	T38.3X3	T38.3X4	T38.3X5	T38.3X6
Glibornuride	T38.3X1	T38.3X2	T38.3X3	T38.3X4	T38.3X5	T38.3X6
Gliclazide	T38.3X1	T38.3X2	T38.3X3	T38.3X4	T38.3X5	T38.3X6
Glimidine	T38.3X1	T38.3X2	T38.3X3	T38.3X4	T38.3X5	T38.3X6
Glipizide	T38.3X1	T38.3X2	T38.3X3	T38.3X4	T38.3X5	T38.3X6
Gliquidone	T38.3X1	T38.3X2	T38.3X3	T38.3X4	T38.3X5	T38.3X6
Glisolamide	T38.3X1	T38.3X2	T38.3X3	T38.3X4	T38.3X5	T38.3X6
Glisoxepide	T38.3X1	T38.3X2	T38.3X3	T38.3X4	T38.3X5	T38.3X6
Globin zinc insulin	T38.3X1	T38.3X2	T38.3X3	T38.3X4	T38.3X5	T38.3X6
Globulin						
antilymphocytic	T50.Z11	T50.Z12	T50.Z13	T50.Z14	T50.Z15	T50.Z16
antirhesus	T50.Z11	T50.Z12	T50.Z13	T50.Z14	T50.Z15	T50.Z16
antivenin	T50.Z11	T50.Z12	T50.Z13	T50.Z14	T50.Z15	T50.Z16
antiviral	T50.Z11	T50.Z12	T50.Z13	T50.Z14	T50.Z15	T50.Z16
Glucagon	T38.3X1	T38.3X2	T38.3X3	T38.3X4	T38.3X5	T38.3X6
Glucocorticoids	T38.0X1	T38.0X2	T38.0X3	T38.0X4	T38.0X5	T38.0X6
Glucocorticosteroid	T38.0X1	T38.0X2	T38.0X3	T38.0X4	T38.0X5	T38.0X6
Gluconic acid	T50.991	T50.992	T50.993	T50.994	T50.995	T50.996
Glucosamine sulfate	T39.4X1	T39.4X2	T39.4X3	T39.4X4	T39.4X5	T39.4X6
Glucose	T50.3X1	T50.3X2	T50.3X3	T50.3X4	T50.3X5	T50.3X6
with sodium chloride	T50.3X1	T50.3X2	T50.3X3	T50.3X4	T50.3X5	T50.3X6
Glucosulfone sodium	T37.1X1	T37.1X2	T37.1X3	T37.1X4	T37.1X5	T37.1X6
Glucurolactone	T47.8X1	T47.8X2	T47.8X3	T47.8X4	T47.8X5	T47.8X6
Glue NEC	T52.8X1	T52.8X2	T52.8X3	T52.8X4	—	—
Glutamic acid	T47.5X1	T47.5X2	T47.5X3	T47.5X4	T47.5X5	T47.5X6
Glutaral (medicinal)	T49.0X1	T49.0X2	T49.0X3	T49.0X4	T49.0X5	T49.0X6
nonmedicinal	T65.891	T65.892	T65.893	T65.894	—	—
Glutaraldehyde (nonmedicinal)	T65.891	T65.892	T65.893	T65.894	—	—
medicinal	T49.0X1	T49.0X2	T49.0X3	T49.0X4	T49.0X5	T49.0X6
Glutathione	T50.6X1	T50.6X2	T50.6X3	T50.6X4	T50.6X5	T50.6X6
Glutethimide	T42.6X1	T42.6X2	T42.6X3	T42.6X4	T42.6X5	T42.6X6
Glyburide	T38.3X1	T38.3X2	T38.3X3	T38.3X4	T38.3X5	T38.3X6
Glycerin	T47.4X1	T47.4X2	T47.4X3	T47.4X4	T47.4X5	T47.4X6
Glycerol	T47.4X1	T47.4X2	T47.4X3	T47.4X4	T47.4X5	T47.4X6
borax	T49.6X1	T49.6X2	T49.6X3	T49.6X4	T49.6X5	T49.6X6
intravenous	T50.3X1	T50.3X2	T50.3X3	T50.3X4	T50.3X5	T50.3X6
iodinated	T48.4X1	T48.4X2	T48.4X3	T48.4X4	T48.4X5	T48.4X6
Glycerophosphate	T50.991	T50.992	T50.993	T50.994	T50.995	T50.996
Glyceryl						
gualacolate	T48.4X1	T48.4X2	T48.4X3	T48.4X4	T48.4X5	T48.4X6
nitrate	T46.3X1	T46.3X2	T46.3X3	T46.3X4	T46.3X5	T46.3X6
triacetate (topical)	T49.0X1	T49.0X2	T49.0X3	T49.0X4	T49.0X5	T49.0X6
trinitrate	T46.3X1	T46.3X2	T46.3X3	T46.3X4	T46.3X5	T46.3X6
Glycine	T50.3X1	T50.3X2	T50.3X3	T50.3X4	T50.3X5	T50.3X6
Glyclopyramide	T38.3X1	T38.3X2	T38.3X3	T38.3X4	T38.3X5	T38.3X6
Glycobiarsol	T37.3X1	T37.3X2	T37.3X3	T37.3X4	T37.3X5	T37.3X6
Glycols (ether)	T52.3X1	T52.3X2	T52.3X3	T52.3X4	—	—
Glyconiazide	T37.1X1	T37.1X2	T37.1X3	T37.1X4	T37.1X5	T37.1X6
Glycopyrrolate	T44.3X1	T44.3X2	T44.3X3	T44.3X4	T44.3X5	T44.3X6
Glycopyrronium	T44.3X1	T44.3X2	T44.3X3	T44.3X4	T44.3X5	T44.3X6
bromide	T44.3X1	T44.3X2	T44.3X3	T44.3X4	T44.3X5	T44.3X6
Glycoside, cardiac (stimulant)	T46.0X1	T46.0X2	T46.0X3	T46.0X4	T46.0X5	T46.0X6
Glycyclamide	T38.3X1	T38.3X2	T38.3X3	T38.3X4	T38.3X5	T38.3X6
Glycyrrhiza extract	T48.4X1	T48.4X2	T48.4X3	T48.4X4	T48.4X5	T48.4X6
Glycyrrhizic acid	T48.4X1	T48.4X2	T48.4X3	T48.4X4	T48.4X5	T48.4X6
Glycyrrhizinate potassium	T48.4X1	T48.4X2	T48.4X3	T48.4X4	T48.4X5	T48.4X6
Glymidine sodium	T38.3X1	T38.3X2	T38.3X3	T38.3X4	T38.3X5	T38.3X6
Glyphosate	T60.3X1	T60.3X2	T60.3X3	T60.3X4	—	—
Glyphylline	T48.6X1	T48.6X2	T48.6X3	T48.6X4	T48.6X5	T48.6X6
Gold						
colloidal (l98Au)	T45.1X1	T45.1X2	T45.1X3	T45.1X4	T45.1X5	T45.1X6
salts	T39.4X1	T39.4X2	T39.4X3	T39.4X4	T39.4X5	T39.4X6
Golden sulfide of antimony	T56.891	T56.892	T56.893	T56.894	—	—
Goldylocks	T62.2X1	T62.2X2	T62.2X3	T62.2X4	—	—
Gonadal tissue extract	T38.901	T38.902	T38.903	T38.904	T38.905	T38.906
female	T38.5X1	T38.5X2	T38.5X3	T38.5X4	T38.5X5	T38.5X6
male	T38.7X1	T38.7X2	T38.7X3	T38.7X4	T38.7X5	T38.7X6
Gonadorelin	T38.891	T38.892	T38.893	T38.894	T38.895	T38.896
Gonadotropin	T38.891	T38.892	T38.893	T38.894	T38.895	T38.896
chorionic	T38.891	T38.892	T38.893	T38.894	T38.895	T38.896
pituitary	T38.811	T38.812	T38.813	T38.814	T38.815	T38.816
Goserelin	T45.1X1	T45.1X2	T45.1X3	T45.1X4	T45.1X5	T45.1X6
Grain alcohol	T51.0X1	T51.0X2	T51.0X3	T51.0X4	—	—
Gramicidin	T49.0X1	T49.0X2	T49.0X3	T49.0X4	T49.0X5	T49.0X6
Granisetron	T45.0X1	T45.0X2	T45.0X3	T45.0X4	T45.0X5	T45.0X6
Gratiola officinalis	T62.2X1	T62.2X2	T62.2X3	T62.2X4	—	—
Grease	T65.891	T65.892	T65.893	T65.894	—	—
Green hellebore	T62.2X1	T62.2X2	T62.2X3	T62.2X4	—	—
Green soap	T49.2X1	T49.2X2	T49.2X3	T49.2X4	T49.2X5	T49.2X6
Grifulvin	T36.7X1	T36.7X2	T36.7X3	T36.7X4	T36.7X5	T36.7X6
Griseofulvin	T36.7X1	T36.7X2	T36.7X3	T36.7X4	T36.7X5	T36.7X6
Growth hormone	T38.811	T38.812	T38.813	T38.814	T38.815	T38.816
Guaiacol derivatives	T48.4X1	T48.4X2	T48.4X3	T48.4X4	T48.4X5	T48.4X6
Guaiac reagent	T50.991	T50.992	T50.993	T50.994	T50.995	T50.996
Guaifenesin	T48.4X1	T48.4X2	T48.4X3	T48.4X4	T48.4X5	T48.4X6
Guaimesal	T48.4X1	T48.4X2	T48.4X3	T48.4X4	T48.4X5	T48.4X6
Guaiphenesin	T48.4X1	T48.4X2	T48.4X3	T48.4X4	T48.4X5	T48.4X6
Guamecycline	T36.4X1	T36.4X2	T36.4X3	T36.4X4	T36.4X5	T36.4X6
Guanabenz	T46.5X1	T46.5X2	T46.5X3	T46.5X4	T46.5X5	T46.5X6
Guanacline	T46.5X1	T46.5X2	T46.5X3	T46.5X4	T46.5X5	T46.5X6
Guanadrel	T46.5X1	T46.5X2	T46.5X3	T46.5X4	T46.5X5	T46.5X6
Guanatol	T37.2X1	T37.2X2	T37.2X3	T37.2X4	T37.2X5	T37.2X6
Guanethidine	T46.5X1	T46.5X2	T46.5X3	T46.5X4	T46.5X5	T46.5X6
Guanfacine	T46.5X1	T46.5X2	T46.5X3	T46.5X4	T46.5X5	T46.5X6
Guano	T65.891	T65.892	T65.893	T65.894	—	—
Guanochlor	T46.5X1	T46.5X2	T46.5X3	T46.5X4	T46.5X5	T46.5X6
Guanoclor	T46.5X1	T46.5X2	T46.5X3	T46.5X4	T46.5X5	T46.5X6
Guanoctine	T46.5X1	T46.5X2	T46.5X3	T46.5X4	T46.5X5	T46.5X6
Guanoxabenz	T46.5X1	T46.5X2	T46.5X3	T46.5X4	T46.5X5	T46.5X6
Guanoxan	T46.5X1	T46.5X2	T46.5X3	T46.5X4	T46.5X5	T46.5X6
Guar gum (medicinal)	T46.6X1	T46.6X2	T46.6X3	T46.6X4	T46.6X5	T46.6X6
Hachimycin	T36.7X1	T36.7X2	T36.7X3	T36.7X4	T36.7X5	T36.7X6
Hair						
dye	T49.4X1	T49.4X2	T49.4X3	T49.4X4	T49.4X5	T49.4X6
preparation NEC	T49.4X1	T49.4X2	T49.4X3	T49.4X4	T49.4X5	T49.4X6
Halazepam	T42.4X1	T42.4X2	T42.4X3	T42.4X4	T42.4X5	T42.4X6
Halcinolone	T49.0X1	T49.0X2	T49.0X3	T49.0X4	T49.0X5	T49.0X6
Halcinonide	T49.0X1	T49.0X2	T49.0X3	T49.0X4	T49.0X5	T49.0X6
Halethazole	T49.0X1	T49.0X2	T49.0X3	T49.0X4	T49.0X5	T49.0X6
Hallucinogen NEC	T40.901	T40.902	T40.903	T40.904	T40.905	T40.906
Halofantrine	T37.2X1	T37.2X2	T37.2X3	T37.2X4	T37.2X5	T37.2X6
Halofenate	T46.6X1	T46.6X2	T46.6X3	T46.6X4	T46.6X5	T46.6X6
Halometasone	T49.0X1	T49.0X2	T49.0X3	T49.0X4	T49.0X5	T49.0X6
Haloperidol	T43.4X1	T43.4X2	T43.4X3	T43.4X4	T43.4X5	T43.4X6
Haloprogin	T49.0X1	T49.0X2	T49.0X3	T49.0X4	T49.0X5	T49.0X6
Halotex	T49.0X1	T49.0X2	T49.0X3	T49.0X4		
Halothane	T41.0X1	T41.0X2	T41.0X3	T41.0X4	T41.0X5	T41.0X6
Haloxazolam	T42.4X1	T42.4X2	T42.4X3	T42.4X4	T42.4X5	T42.4X6
Halquinols	T49.0X1	T49.0X2	T49.0X3	T49.0X4	T49.0X5	T49.0X6
Hamamelis	T49.2X1	T49.2X2	T49.2X3	T49.2X4	T49.2X5	T49.2X6
Haptendextran	T45.8X1	T45.8X2	T45.8X3	T45.8X4	T45.8X5	T45.8X6
Harmonyl	T46.5X1	T46.5X2	T46.5X3	T46.5X4	T46.5X5	T46.5X6
Hartmann's solution	T50.3X1	T50.3X2	T50.3X3	T50.3X4	T50.3X5	T50.3X6
Hashish	T40.7X1	T40.7X2	T40.7X3	T40.7X4	T40.7X5	T40.7X6
Hawaiian Woodrose seeds	T40.991	T40.992	T40.993	T40.994	—	—
HCB	T60.3X1	T60.3X2	T60.3X3	T60.3X4	—	—
HCH	T53.6X1	T53.6X2	T53.6X3	T53.6X4	—	—
medicinal	T49.0X1	T49.0X2	T49.0X3	T49.0X4	T49.0X5	T49.0X6
HCN	T57.3X1	T57.3X2	T57.3X3	T57.3X4	—	—
Headache cures, drugs, powders NEC	T50.901	T50.902	T50.903	T50.904	T50.905	T50.906
Heavenly Blue (morning glory)	T40.991	T40.992	T40.993	T40.994	—	—
Heavy metal antidote	T45.8X1	T45.8X2	T45.8X3	T45.8X4	T45.8X5	T45.8X6
Hedaquinium	T49.0X1	T49.0X2	T49.0X3	T49.0X4	T49.0X5	T49.0X6
Hedge hyssop	T62.2X1	T62.2X2	T62.2X3	T62.2X4	—	—
Heet	T49.8X1	T49.8X2	T49.8X3	T49.8X4	T49.8X5	T49.8X6
Helenin	T37.4X1	T37.4X2	T37.4X3	T37.4X4	T37.4X5	T37.4X6
Helium (nonmedicinal) **NEC**	T59.891	T59.892	T59.893	T59.894	—	—
medicinal	T48.991	T48.992	T48.993	T48.994	T48.995	T48.996
Hellebore (black) (green) (white)	T62.2X1	T62.2X2	T62.2X3	T62.2X4	—	—
Hematin	T45.8X1	T45.8X2	T45.8X3	T45.8X4	T45.8X5	T45.8X6
Hematinic preparation	T45.8X1	T45.8X2	T45.8X3	T45.8X4	T45.8X5	T45.8X6
Hematological agent	T45.91	T45.92	T45.93	T45.94	T45.95	T45.96
specified NEC	T45.8X1	T45.8X2	T45.8X3	T45.8X4	T45.8X5	T45.8X6
Hemlock	T62.2X1	T62.2X2	T62.2X3	T62.2X4	—	—
Hemostatic	T45.621	T45.622	T45.623	T45.624	T45.625	T45.626
drug, systemic	T45.621	T45.622	T45.623	T45.624	T45.625	T45.626
Hemostyptic	T49.4X1	T49.4X2	T49.4X3	T49.4X4	T49.4X5	T49.4X6
Henbane	T62.2X1	T62.2X2	T62.2X3	T62.2X4	—	—
Heparin (sodium)	T45.511	T45.512	T45.513	T45.514	T45.515	T45.516
action reverser	T45.7X1	T45.7X2	T45.7X3	T45.7X4	T45.7X5	T45.7X6
Heparin-fraction	T45.511	T45.512	T45.513	T45.514	T45.515	T45.516
Heparinoid (systemic)	T45.511	T45.512	T45.513	T45.514	T45.515	T45.516

Table of Drugs and Chemicals

Hepatic secretion stimulant — Hydrogen

Substance	Poisoning, Accidental (unintentional)	Poisoning, Intentional Self-harm	Poisoning, Assault	Poisoning, Undetermined	Adverse Effect	Under-dosing
Hepatic secretion stimulant	T47.8X1	T47.8X2	T47.8X3	T47.8X4	T47.8X5	T47.8X6
Hepatitis B						
immune globulin	T50.Z11	T50.Z12	T50.Z13	T50.Z14	T50.Z15	T50.Z16
vaccine	T50.B91	T50.B92	T50.B93	T50.B94	T50.B95	T50.B96
Hepronicate	T46.7X1	T46.7X2	T46.7X3	T46.7X4	T46.7X5	T46.7X6
Heptabarb	T42.3X1	T42.3X2	T42.3X3	T42.3X4	T42.3X5	T42.3X6
Heptabarbital	T42.3X1	T42.3X2	T42.3X3	T42.3X4	T42.3X5	T42.3X6
Heptabarbitone	T42.3X1	T42.3X2	T42.3X3	T42.3X4	T42.3X5	T42.3X6
Heptachlor	T60.1X1	T60.1X2	T60.1X3	T60.1X4	—	—
Heptalgin	T40.2X1	T40.2X2	T40.2X3	T40.2X4	T40.2X5	T40.2X6
Heptaminol	T46.3X1	T46.3X2	T46.3X3	T46.3X4	T46.3X5	T46.3X6
Herbicide NEC	T60.3X1	T60.3X2	T60.3X3	T60.3X4	—	—
Heroin	T40.1X1	T40.1X2	T40.1X3	T40.1X4	—	—
Herplex	T49.5X1	T49.5X2	T49.5X3	T49.5X4	T49.5X5	T49.5X6
HES	T45.8X1	T45.8X2	T45.8X3	T45.8X4	T45.8X5	T45.8X6
Hesperidin	T46.991	T46.992	T46.993	T46.994	T46.995	T46.996
Hetacillin	T36.0X1	T36.0X2	T36.0X3	T36.0X4	T36.0X5	T36.0X6
Hetastarch	T45.8X1	T45.8X2	T45.8X3	T45.8X4	T45.8X5	T45.8X6
HETP	T60.0X1	T60.0X2	T60.0X3	T60.0X4	—	—
Hexachlorobenzene (vapor)	T60.3X1	T60.3X2	T60.3X3	T60.3X4	—	—
Hexachlorocyclohexane	T53.6X1	T53.6X2	T53.6X3	T53.6X4	—	—
Hexachlorophene	T49.0X1	T49.0X2	T49.0X3	T49.0X4	T49.0X5	T49.0X6
Hexadiline	T46.3X1	T46.3X2	T46.3X3	T46.3X4	T46.3X5	T46.3X6
Hexadimethrine (bromide)	T45.7X1	T45.7X2	T45.7X3	T45.7X4	T45.7X5	T45.7X6
Hexadylamine	T46.3X1	T46.3X2	T46.3X3	T46.3X4	T46.3X5	T46.3X6
Hexaethyl tetraphosphate	T60.0X1	T60.0X2	T60.0X3	T60.0X4	—	—
Hexafluorenium bromide	T48.1X1	T48.1X2	T48.1X3	T48.1X4	T48.1X5	T48.1X6
Hexafluronium (bromide)	T48.1X1	T48.1X2	T48.1X3	T48.1X4	T48.1X5	T48.1X6
Hexa-germ	T49.2X1	T49.2X2	T49.2X3	T49.2X4	T49.2X5	T49.2X6
Hexahydrobenzol	T52.8X1	T52.8X2	T52.8X3	T52.8X4	—	—
Hexahydrocresol(s)	T51.8X1	T51.8X2	T51.8X3	T51.8X4	—	—
arsenide	T57.0X1	T57.0X2	T57.0X3	T57.0X4	—	—
arseniurated	T57.0X1	T57.0X2	T57.0X3	T57.0X4	—	—
cyanide	T57.3X1	T57.3X2	T57.3X3	T57.3X4	—	—
gas	T59.891	T59.892	T59.893	T59.894	—	—
Fluoride (liquid)	T57.8X1	T57.8X2	T57.8X3	T57.8X4	—	—
vapor	T59.891	T59.892	T59.893	T59.894	—	—
phophorated	T60.0X1	T60.0X2	T60.0X3	T60.0X4	—	—
sulfate	T57.8X1	T57.8X2	T57.8X3	T57.8X4	—	—
sulfide (gas)	T59.6X1	T59.6X2	T59.6X3	T59.6X4	—	—
arseniurated	T57.0X1	T57.0X2	T57.0X3	T57.0X4	—	—
sulfurated	T57.8X1	T57.8X2	T57.8X3	T57.8X4	—	—
Hexahydrophenol	T51.8X1	T51.8X2	T51.8X3	T51.8X4	—	—
Hexalen	T51.8X1	T51.8X2	T51.8X3	T51.8X4	—	—
Hexamethonium bromide	T44.2X1	T44.2X2	T44.2X3	T44.2X4	T44.2X5	T44.2X6
Hexamethylene	T52.8X1	T52.8X2	T52.8X3	T52.8X4	—	—
Hexamethylmelamine	T45.1X1	T45.1X2	T45.1X3	T45.1X4	T45.1X5	T45.1X6
Hexamidine	T49.0X1	T49.0X2	T49.0X3	T49.0X4	T49.0X5	T49.0X6
Hexamine (mandelate)	T37.8X1	T37.8X2	T37.8X3	T37.8X4	T37.8X5	T37.8X6
Hexanone, 2-hexanone	T52.4X1	T52.4X2	T52.4X3	T52.4X4	—	—
Hexanuorenium	T48.1X1	T48.1X2	T48.1X3	T48.1X4	T48.1X5	T48.1X6
Hexapropymate	T42.6X1	T42.6X2	T42.6X3	T42.6X4	T42.6X5	T42.6X6
Hexasonium iodide	T44.3X1	T44.3X2	T44.3X3	T44.3X4	T44.3X5	T44.3X6
Hexcarbacholine bromide	T48.1X1	T48.1X2	T48.1X3	T48.1X4	T48.1X5	T48.1X6
Hexemal	T42.3X1	T42.3X2	T42.3X3	T42.3X4	T42.3X5	T42.3X6
Hexestrol	T38.5X1	T38.5X2	T38.5X3	T38.5X4	T38.5X5	T38.5X6
Hexethal (sodium)	T42.3X1	T42.3X2	T42.3X3	T42.3X4	T42.3X5	T42.3X6
Hexetidine	T37.8X1	T37.8X2	T37.8X3	T37.8X4	T37.8X5	T37.8X6
Hexobarbital	T42.3X1	T42.3X2	T42.3X3	T42.3X4	T42.3X5	T42.3X6
rectal	T41.291	T41.292	T41.293	T41.294	T41.295	T41.296
sodium	T41.1X1	T41.1X2	T41.1X3	T41.1X4	T41.1X5	T41.1X6
Hexobendine	T46.3X1	T46.3X2	T46.3X3	T46.3X4	T46.3X5	T46.3X6
Hexocyclium	T44.3X1	T44.3X2	T44.3X3	T44.3X4	T44.3X5	T44.3X6
metilsulfate	T44.3X1	T44.3X2	T44.3X3	T44.3X4	T44.3X5	T44.3X6
Hexoestrol	T38.5X1	T38.5X2	T38.5X3	T38.5X4	T38.5X5	T38.5X6
Hexone	T52.4X1	T52.4X2	T52.4X3	T52.4X4	—	—
Hexoprenaline	T48.6X1	T48.6X2	T48.6X3	T48.6X4	T48.6X5	T48.6X6
Hexylcaine	T41.3X1	T41.3X2	T41.3X3	T41.3X4	T41.3X5	T41.3X6
Hexylresorcinol	T52.2X1	T52.2X2	T52.2X3	T52.2X4	—	—
HGH (human growth hormone)	T38.811	T38.812	T38.813	T38.814	T38.815	T38.816
Hinkle's pills	T47.2X1	T47.2X2	T47.2X3	T47.2X4	T47.2X5	T47.2X6
Histalog	T50.8X1	T50.8X2	T50.8X3	T50.8X4	T50.8X5	T50.8X6
Histamine (phosphate)	T50.8X1	T50.8X2	T50.8X3	T50.8X4	T50.8X5	T50.8X6
Histoplasmin	T50.8X1	T50.8X2	T50.8X3	T50.8X4	T50.8X5	T50.8X6
Holly berries	T62.2X1	T62.2X2	T62.2X3	T62.2X4	—	—
Homatropine	T44.3X1	T44.3X2	T44.3X3	T44.3X4	T44.3X5	T44.3X6
methylbromide	T44.3X1	T44.3X2	T44.3X3	T44.3X4	T44.3X5	T44.3X6
Homochlorcyclizine	T45.0X1	T45.0X2	T45.0X3	T45.0X4	T45.0X5	T45.0X6
Homosalate	T49.3X1	T49.3X2	T49.3X3	T49.3X4	T49.3X5	T49.3X6
Homo-tet	T50.Z11	T50.Z12	T50.Z13	T50.Z14	T50.Z15	T50.Z16

Substance	Poisoning, Accidental (unintentional)	Poisoning, Intentional Self-harm	Poisoning, Assault	Poisoning, Undetermined	Adverse Effect	Under-dosing
Hormone	T38.801	T38.802	T38.803	T38.804	T38.805	T38.806
adrenal cortical steroids	T38.0X1	T38.0X2	T38.0X3	T38.0X4	T38.0X5	T38.0X6
androgenic	T38.7X1	T38.7X2	T38.7X3	T38.7X4	T38.7X5	T38.7X6
anterior pituitary NEC	T38.811	T38.812	T38.813	T38.814	T38.815	T38.816
antidiabetic agents	T38.3X1	T38.3X2	T38.3X3	T38.3X4	T38.3X5	T38.3X6
antidiuretic	T38.891	T38.892	T38.893	T38.894	T38.895	T38.896
cancer therapy	T45.1X1	T45.1X2	T45.1X3	T45.1X4	T45.1X5	T45.1X6
follicle stimulating	T38.811	T38.812	T38.813	T38.814	T38.815	T38.816
gonadotropic	T38.891	T38.892	T38.893	T38.894	T38.895	T38.896
pituitary	T38.811	T38.812	T38.813	T38.814	T38.815	T38.816
growth	T38.811	T38.812	T38.813	T38.814	T38.815	T38.816
luteinizing	T38.811	T38.812	T38.813	T38.814	T38.815	T38.816
ovarian	T38.5X1	T38.5X2	T38.5X3	T38.5X4	T38.5X5	T38.5X6
oxytocic	T48.0X1	T48.0X2	T48.0X3	T48.0X4	T48.0X5	T48.0X6
parathyroid (derivatives)	T50.991	T50.992	T50.993	T50.994	T50.995	T50.996
pituitary (posterior) NEC	T38.891	T38.892	T38.893	T38.894	T38.895	T38.896
anterior	T38.811	T38.812	T38.813	T38.814	T38.815	T38.816
specified, NEC	T38.891	T38.892	T38.893	T38.894	T38.895	T38.896
thyroid	T38.1X1	T38.1X2	T38.1X3	T38.1X4	T38.1X5	T38.1X6
Hornet (sting)	T63.451	T63.452	T63.453	T63.454	—	—
Horse anti-human lymphocytic serum	T50.Z11	T50.Z12	T50.Z13	T50.Z14	T50.Z15	T50.Z16
Horticulture agent NEC	T65.91	T65.92	T65.93	T65.94	—	—
with pesticide	T60.91	T60.92	T60.93	T60.94	—	—
Human						
albumin	T45.8X1	T45.8X2	T45.8X3	T45.8X4	T45.8X5	T45.8X6
growth hormone (HGH)	T38.811	T38.812	T38.813	T38.814	T38.815	T38.816
immune serum	T50.Z11	T50.Z12	T50.Z13	T50.Z14	T50.Z15	T50.Z16
Hyaluronidase	T45.3X1	T45.3X2	T45.3X3	T45.3X4	T45.3X5	T45.3X6
Hyazyme	T45.3X1	T45.3X2	T45.3X3	T45.3X4	T45.3X5	T45.3X6
Hycodan	T40.2X1	T40.2X2	T40.2X3	T40.2X4	T40.2X5	T40.2X6
Hydantoin derivative NEC	T42.0X1	T42.0X2	T42.0X3	T42.0X4	T42.0X5	T42.0X6
Hydeltra	T38.0X1	T38.0X2	T38.0X3	T38.0X4	T38.0X5	T38.0X6
Hydergine	T44.6X1	T44.6X2	T44.6X3	T44.6X4	T44.6X5	T44.6X6
Hydrabamine penicillin	T36.0X1	T36.0X2	T36.0X3	T36.0X4	T36.0X5	T36.0X6
Hydralazine	T46.5X1	T46.5X2	T46.5X3	T46.5X4	T46.5X5	T46.5X6
Hydrargaphen	T49.0X1	T49.0X2	T49.0X3	T49.0X4	T49.0X5	T49.0X6
Hydrargyri aminochloridum	T49.0X1	T49.0X2	T49.0X3	T49.0X4	T49.0X5	T49.0X6
Hydrastine	T48.291	T48.292	T48.293	T48.294	T48.295	T48.296
Hydrazine	T54.1X1	T54.1X2	T54.1X3	T54.1X4	—	—
monoamine oxidase inhibitors	T43.1X1	T43.1X2	T43.1X3	T43.1X4	T43.1X5	T43.1X6
Hydrazoic acid, azides	T54.2X1	T54.2X2	T54.2X3	T54.2X4	—	—
Hydriodic acid	T48.4X1	T48.4X2	T48.4X3	T48.4X4	T48.4X5	T48.4X6
Hydrocarbon gas	T59.891	T59.892	T59.893	T59.894	—	—
incomplete combustion of — see Carbon, monoxide, fuel, utility						
liquefied (mobile container)	T59.891	T59.892	T59.893	T59.894	—	—
piped (natural)	T59.891	T59.892	T59.893	T59.894	—	—
Hydrochloric acid (liquid)	T54.2X1	T54.2X2	T54.2X3	T54.2X4	—	—
medicinal (digestant)	T47.5X1	T47.5X2	T47.5X3	T47.5X4	T47.5X5	T47.5X6
vapor	T59.891	T59.892	T59.893	T59.894	—	—
Hydrochlorothiazide	T50.2X1	T50.2X2	T50.2X3	T50.2X4	T50.2X5	T50.2X6
Hydrocodone	T40.2X1	T40.2X2	T40.2X3	T40.2X4	T40.2X5	T40.2X6
Hydrocortisone (derivatives)	T49.0X1	T49.0X2	T49.0X3	T49.0X4	T49.0X5	T49.0X6
aceponate	T49.0X1	T49.0X2	T49.0X3	T49.0X4	T49.0X5	T49.0X6
ENT agent	T49.6X1	T49.6X2	T49.6X3	T49.6X4	T49.6X5	T49.6X6
ophthalmic preparation	T49.5X1	T49.5X2	T49.5X3	T49.5X4	T49.5X5	T49.5X6
topical NEC	T49.0X1	T49.0X2	T49.0X3	T49.0X4	T49.0X5	T49.0X6
Hydrocortone	T38.0X1	T38.0X2	T38.0X3	T38.0X4	T38.0X5	T38.0X6
ENT agent	T49.6X1	T49.6X2	T49.6X3	T49.6X4	T49.6X5	T49.6X6
ophthalmic preparation	T49.5X1	T49.5X2	T49.5X3	T49.5X4	T49.5X5	T49.5X6
topical NEC	T49.0X1	T49.0X2	T49.0X3	T49.0X4	T49.0X5	T49.0X6
Hydrocyanic acid (liquid)	T57.3X1	T57.3X2	T57.3X3	T57.3X4	—	—
gas	T65.0X1	T65.0X2	T65.0X3	T65.0X4	—	—
Hydroflumethiazide	T50.2X1	T50.2X2	T50.2X3	T50.2X4	T50.2X5	T50.2X6
Hydrofluoric acid (liquid)	T54.2X1	T54.2X2	T54.2X3	T54.2X4	—	—
vapor	T59.891	T59.892	T59.893	T59.894	—	—
Hydrogen	T59.891	T59.892	T59.893	T59.894	—	—
arsenide	T57.0X1	T57.0X2	T57.0X3	T57.0X4	—	—
arseniureted	T57.0X1	T57.0X2	T57.0X3	T57.0X4	—	—
chloride	T57.8X1	T57.8X2	T57.8X3	T57.8X4	—	—
cyanide (salts)	T57.3X1	T57.3X2	T57.3X3	T57.3X4	—	—
gas	T57.3X1	T57.3X2	T57.3X3	T57.3X4	—	—
Fluoride	T59.5X1	T59.5X2	T59.5X3	T59.5X4	—	—
vapor	T59.5X1	T59.5X2	T59.5X3	T59.5X4	—	—
peroxide	T49.0X1	T49.0X2	T49.0X3	T49.0X4	T49.0X5	T49.0X6
phosphureted	T57.1X1	T57.1X2	T57.1X3	T57.1X4	—	—
sulfide	T59.6X1	T59.6X2	T59.6X3	T59.6X4	—	—
arseniureted	T57.0X1	T57.0X2	T57.0X3	T57.0X4	—	—
sulfureted	T59.6X1	T59.6X2	T59.6X3	T59.6X4	—	—

Substance	Poisoning, Accidental (unintentional)	Poisoning, Intentional Self-harm	Poisoning, Assault	Poisoning, Undetermined	Adverse Effect	Under-dosing
Hydromethylpyridine	T46.7X1	T46.7X2	T46.7X3	T46.7X4	T46.7X5	T46.7X6
Hydromorphinol	T40.2X1	T40.2X2	T40.2X3	T40.2X4	—	—
Hydromorphinone	T40.2X1	T40.2X2	T40.2X3	T40.2X4	T40.2X5	T40.2X6
Hydromorphone	T40.2X1	T40.2X2	T40.2X3	T40.2X4	T40.2X5	T40.2X6
Hydromox	T50.2X1	T50.2X2	T50.2X3	T50.2X4	T50.2X5	T50.2X6
Hydrophilic lotion	T49.3X1	T49.3X2	T49.3X3	T49.3X4	T49.3X5	T49.3X6
Hydroquinidine	T46.2X1	T46.2X2	T46.2X3	T46.2X4	T46.2X5	T46.2X6
Hydroquinone	T52.2X1	T52.2X2	T52.2X3	T52.2X4	—	—
vapor	T59.891	T59.892	T59.893	T59.894	—	—
Hydrosulfuric acid (gas)	T59.6X1	T59.6X2	T59.6X3	T59.6X4	—	—
Hydrotalcite	T47.1X1	T47.1X2	T47.1X3	T47.1X4	T47.1X5	T47.1X6
Hydrous wool fat	T49.3X1	T49.3X2	T49.3X3	T49.3X4	T49.3X5	T49.3X6
Hydroxide, caustic	T54.3X1	T54.3X2	T54.3X3	T54.3X4	—	—
Hydroxocobalamin	T45.8X1	T45.8X2	T45.8X3	T45.8X4	T45.8X5	T45.8X6
Hydroxyamphetamine	T49.5X1	T49.5X2	T49.5X3	T49.5X4	T49.5X5	T49.5X6
Hydroxycarbamide	T45.1X1	T45.1X2	T45.1X3	T45.1X4	T45.1X5	T45.1X6
Hydroxychloroquine	T37.8X1	T37.8X2	T37.8X3	T37.8X4	T37.8X5	T37.8X6
Hydroxydihydrocodeinone	T40.2X1	T40.2X2	T40.2X3	T40.2X4	T40.2X5	T40.2X6
Hydroxyestrone	T38.5X1	T38.5X2	T38.5X3	T38.5X4	T38.5X5	T38.5X6
Hydroxyethyl starch	T45.8X1	T45.8X2	T45.8X3	T45.8X4	T45.8X5	T45.8X6
Hydroxymethylpentanone	T52.4X1	T52.4X2	T52.4X3	T52.4X4	—	—
Hydroxyphenamate	T43.591	T43.592	T43.593	T43.594	T43.595	T43.596
Hydroxyphenylbutazone	T39.2X1	T39.2X2	T39.2X3	T39.2X4	T39.2X5	T39.2X6
Hydroxyprogesterone	T38.5X1	T38.5X2	T38.5X3	T38.5X4	T38.5X5	T38.5X6
caproate	T38.5X1	T38.5X2	T38.5X3	T38.5X4	T38.5X5	T38.5X6
Hydroxyquinoline (derivatives) NEC	T37.8X1	T37.8X2	T37.8X3	T37.8X4	T37.8X5	T37.8X6
Hydroxystilbamidine	T37.3X1	T37.3X2	T37.3X3	T37.3X4	T37.3X5	T37.3X6
Hydroxytoluene (nonmedicinal)	T54.0X1	T54.0X2	T54.0X3	T54.0X4	—	—
medicinal	T49.0X1	T49.0X2	T49.0X3	T49.0X4	T49.0X5	T49.0X6
Hydroxyurea	T45.1X1	T45.1X2	T45.1X3	T45.1X4	T45.1X5	T45.1X6
Hydroxyzine	T43.591	T43.592	T43.593	T43.594	T43.595	T43.596
Hyoscine	T44.3X1	T44.3X2	T44.3X3	T44.3X4	T44.3X5	T44.3X6
Hyoscyamine	T44.3X1	T44.3X2	T44.3X3	T44.3X4	T44.3X5	T44.3X6
Hyoscyamus	T44.3X1	T44.3X2	T44.3X3	T44.3X4	T44.3X5	T44.3X6
dry extract	T44.3X1	T44.3X2	T44.3X3	T44.3X4	T44.3X5	T44.3X6
Hypaque	T50.8X1	T50.8X2	T50.8X3	T50.8X4	T50.8X5	T50.8X6
Hypertussis	T50.Z11	T50.Z12	T50.Z13	T50.Z14	T50.Z15	T50.Z16
Hypnotic	T42.71	T42.72	T42.73	T42.74	T42.75	T42.76
anticonvulsant	T42.71	T42.72	T42.73	T42.74	T42.75	T42.76
specified NEC	T42.6X1	T42.6X2	T42.6X3	T42.6X4	T42.6X5	T42.6X6
Hypochlorite	T49.0X1	T49.0X2	T49.0X3	T49.0X4	T49.0X5	T49.0X6
Hypophysis, posterior	T38.891	T38.892	T38.893	T38.894	T38.895	T38.896
Hypotensive NEC	T46.5X1	T46.5X2	T46.5X3	T46.5X4	T46.5X5	T46.5X6
Hypromellose	T49.5X1	T49.5X2	T49.5X3	T49.5X4	T49.5X5	T49.5X6
Ibacitabine	T37.5X1	T37.5X2	T37.5X3	T37.5X4	T37.5X5	T37.5X6
Ibopamine	T44.991	T44.992	T44.993	T44.994	T44.995	T44.996
Ibufenac	T39.311	T39.312	T39.313	T39.314	T39.315	T39.316
Ibuprofen	T39.311	T39.312	T39.313	T39.314	T39.315	T39.316
Ibuproxam	T39.311	T39.312	T39.313	T39.314	T39.315	T39.316
Ibuterol	T48.6X1	T48.6X2	T48.6X3	T48.6X4	T48.6X5	T48.6X6
Ichthammol	T49.0X1	T49.0X2	T49.0X3	T49.0X4	T49.0X5	T49.0X6
Ichthyol	T49.4X1	T49.4X2	T49.4X3	T49.4X4	T49.4X5	T49.4X6
Idarubicin	T45.1X1	T45.1X2	T45.1X3	T45.1X4	T45.1X5	T45.1X6
Idrocilamide	T42.8X1	T42.8X2	T42.8X3	T42.8X4	T42.8X5	T42.8X6
Ifenprodil	T46.7X1	T46.7X2	T46.7X3	T46.7X4	T46.7X5	T46.7X6
Ifosfamide	T45.1X1	T45.1X2	T45.1X3	T45.1X4	T45.1X5	T45.1X6
Iletin	T38.3X1	T38.3X2	T38.3X3	T38.3X4	T38.3X5	T38.3X6
Ilex	T62.2X1	T62.2X2	T62.2X3	T62.2X4	—	—
Illuminating gas (after combustion)	T58.11	T58.12	T58.13	T58.14	—	—
prior to combustion	T59.891	T59.892	T59.893	T59.894	—	—
Ilopan	T45.2X1	T45.2X2	T45.2X3	T45.2X4	T45.2X5	T45.2X6
Iloprost	T46.7X1	T46.7X2	T46.7X3	T46.7X4	T46.7X5	T46.7X6
Ilotycin	T36.3X1	T36.3X2	T36.3X3	T36.3X4	T36.3X5	T36.3X6
ophthalmic preparation	T49.5X1	T49.5X2	T49.5X3	T49.5X4	T49.5X5	T49.5X6
topical NEC	T49.0X1	T49.0X2	T49.0X3	T49.0X4	T49.0X5	T49.0X6
Imidazole-4-carboxamide	T45.1X1	T45.1X2	T45.1X3	T45.1X4	T45.1X5	T45.1X6
Iminostilbene	T42.1X1	T42.1X2	T42.1X3	T42.1X4	T42.1X5	T42.1X6
Imipenem	T36.0X1	T36.0X2	T36.0X3	T36.0X4	T36.0X5	T36.0X6
Imipramine	T43.011	T43.012	T43.013	T43.014	T43.015	T43.016
Immu-G	T50.Z11	T50.Z12	T50.Z13	T50.Z14	T50.Z15	T50.Z16
Immuglobin	T50.Z11	T50.Z12	T50.Z13	T50.Z14	T50.Z15	T50.Z16
Immune						
globulin	T50.Z11	T50.Z12	T50.Z13	T50.Z14	T50.Z15	T50.Z16
serum globulin	T50.Z11	T50.Z12	T50.Z13	T50.Z14	T50.Z15	T50.Z16
Immunoglobin human (intravenous) (normal)	T50.Z11	T50.Z12	T50.Z13	T50.Z14	T50.Z15	T50.Z16
unmodified	T50.Z11	T50.Z12	T50.Z13	T50.Z14	T50.Z15	T50.Z16
Immunosuppressive drug	T45.1X1	T45.1X2	T45.1X3	T45.1X4	T45.1X5	T45.1X6
Immu-tetanus	T50.Z11	T50.Z12	T50.Z13	T50.Z14	T50.Z15	T50.Z16
Indalpine	T43.221	T43.222	T43.223	T43.224	T43.225	T43.226
Indanazoline	T48.5X1	T48.5X2	T48.5X3	T48.5X4	T48.5X5	T48.5X6
Indandione (derivatives)	T45.511	T45.512	T45.513	T45.514	T45.515	T45.516
Indapamide	T46.5X1	T46.5X2	T46.5X3	T46.5X4	T46.5X5	T46.5X6
Indendione (derivatives)	T45.511	T45.512	T45.513	T45.514	T45.515	T45.516
Indenolol	T44.7X1	T44.7X2	T44.7X3	T44.7X4	T44.7X5	T44.7X6
Inderal	T44.7X1	T44.7X2	T44.7X3	T44.7X4	T44.7X5	T44.7X6
Indian						
hemp	T40.7X1	T40.7X2	T40.7X3	T40.7X4	T40.7X5	T40.7X6
tobacco	T62.2X1	T62.2X2	T62.2X3	T62.2X4	—	—
Indigo carmine	T50.8X1	T50.8X2	T50.8X3	T50.8X4	T50.8X5	T50.8X6
Indobufen	T45.521	T45.522	T45.523	T45.524	T45.525	T45.526
Indocin	T39.2X1	T39.2X2	T39.2X3	T39.2X4	T39.2X5	T39.2X6
Indocyanine green	T50.8X1	T50.8X2	T50.8X3	T50.8X4	T50.8X5	T50.8X6
Indometacin	T39.391	T39.392	T39.393	T39.394	T39.395	T39.396
Indomethacin	T39.391	T39.392	T39.393	T39.394	T39.395	T39.396
farnesil	T39.4X1	T39.4X2	T39.4X3	T39.4X4	T39.4X5	T39.4X6
Indoramin	T44.6X1	T44.6X2	T44.6X3	T44.6X4	T44.6X5	T44.6X6
Industrial						
alcohol	T51.0X1	T51.0X2	T51.0X3	T51.0X4	—	—
fumes	T59.891	T59.892	T59.893	T59.894	—	—
solvents (fumes) (vapors)	T52.91	T52.92	T52.93	T52.94	—	—
Influenza vaccine	T50.B91	T50.B92	T50.B93	T50.B94	T50.B95	T50.B96
Ingested substance NEC	T65.91	T65.92	T65.93	T65.94	—	—
INH	T37.1X1	T37.1X2	T37.1X3	T37.1X4	T37.1X5	T37.1X6
Inhalation, gas (noxious) — see Gas						
Inhibitor						
angiotensin-converting enzyme	T46.4X1	T46.4X2	T46.4X3	T46.4X4	T46.4X5	T46.4X6
carbonic anhydrase	T50.2X1	T50.2X2	T50.2X3	T50.2X4	T50.2X5	T50.2X6
fibrinolysis	T45.621	T45.622	T45.623	T45.624	T45.625	T45.626
monoamine oxidase NEC	T43.1X1	T43.1X2	T43.1X3	T43.1X4	T43.1X5	T43.1X6
hydrazine	T43.1X1	T43.1X2	T43.1X3	T43.1X4	T43.1X5	T43.1X6
postsynaptic	T43.8X1	T43.8X2	T43.8X3	T43.8X4	T43.8X5	T43.8X6
prothrombin synthesis	T45.511	T45.512	T45.513	T45.514	T45.515	T45.516
Ink	T65.891	T65.892	T65.893	T65.894	—	—
Inorganic substance NEC	T57.91	T57.92	T57.93	T57.94	—	—
Inosine pranobex	T37.5X1	T37.5X2	T37.5X3	T37.5X4	T37.5X5	T37.5X6
Inositol	T50.991	T50.992	T50.993	T50.994	T50.995	T50.996
nicotinate	T46.7X1	T46.7X2	T46.7X3	T46.7X4	T46.7X5	T46.7X6
Inproquone	T45.1X1	T45.1X2	T45.1X3	T45.1X4	T45.1X5	T45.1X6
Insecticide NEC	T60.91	T60.92	T60.93	T60.94	—	—
carbamate	T60.0X1	T60.0X2	T60.0X3	T60.0X4	—	—
chlorinated	T60.1X1	T60.1X2	T60.1X3	T60.1X4	—	—
mixed	T60.91	T60.92	T60.93	T60.94	—	—
organochlorine	T60.1X1	T60.1X2	T60.1X3	T60.1X4	—	—
organophosphorus	T60.0X1	T60.0X2	T60.0X3	T60.0X4	—	—
Insect (sting), venomous	T63.481	T63.482	T63.483	T63.484	—	—
ant	T63.421	T63.422	T63.423	T63.424	—	—
bee	T63.441	T63.442	T63.443	T63.444	—	—
caterpillar	T63.431	T63.432	T63.433	T63.434	—	—
hornet	T63.451	T63.452	T63.453	T63.454	—	—
wasp	T63.461	T63.462	T63.463	T63.464	—	—
Insular tissue extract	T38.3X1	T38.3X2	T38.3X3	T38.3X4	T38.3X5	T38.3X6
Insulin (amorphous) (globin) (isophane) (Lente) (NPH) (Semilente) (Ultralente)	T38.3X1	T38.3X2	T38.3X3	T38.3X4	T38.3X5	T38.3X6
defalan	T38.3X1	T38.3X2	T38.3X3	T38.3X4	T38.3X5	T38.3X6
human	T38.3X1	T38.3X2	T38.3X3	T38.3X4	T38.3X5	T38.3X6
injection, soluble	T38.3X1	T38.3X2	T38.3X3	T38.3X4	T38.3X5	T38.3X6
biphasic	T38.3X1	T38.3X2	T38.3X3	T38.3X4	T38.3X5	T38.3X6
intermediate acting	T38.3X1	T38.3X2	T38.3X3	T38.3X4	T38.3X5	T38.3X6
protamine zinc	T38.3X1	T38.3X2	T38.3X3	T38.3X4	T38.3X5	T38.3X6
slow acting	T38.3X1	T38.3X2	T38.3X3	T38.3X4	T38.3X5	T38.3X6
zinc						
protamine injection	T38.3X1	T38.3X2	T38.3X3	T38.3X4	T38.3X5	T38.3X6
suspension (amorphous) (crystalline)	T38.3X1	T38.3X2	T38.3X3	T38.3X4	T38.3X5	T38.3X6
Interferon (alpha) (beta) (gamma)	T37.5X1	T37.5X2	T37.5X3	T37.5X4	T37.5X5	T37.5X6
Intestinal motility control drug	T47.6X1	T47.6X2	T47.6X3	T47.6X4	T47.6X5	T47.6X6
biological	T47.8X1	T47.8X2	T47.8X3	T47.8X4	T47.8X5	T47.8X6
Intranarcon	T41.1X1	T41.1X2	T41.1X3	T41.1X4	T41.1X5	T41.1X6
Intravenous						
amino acids	T50.991	T50.992	T50.993	T50.994	T50.995	T50.996
fat suspension	T50.991	T50.992	T50.993	T50.994	T50.995	T50.996
Inulin	T50.8X1	T50.8X2	T50.8X3	T50.8X4	T50.8X5	T50.8X6
Invert sugar	T50.3X1	T50.3X2	T50.3X3	T50.3X4	T50.3X5	T50.3X6
Inza — see Naproxen						
Iobenzamic acid	T50.8X1	T50.8X2	T50.8X3	T50.8X4	T50.8X5	T50.8X6
Iocetamic acid	T50.8X1	T50.8X2	T50.8X3	T50.8X4	T50.8X5	T50.8X6
Iocetamic acid	T50.8X1	T50.8X2	T50.8X3	T50.8X4	T50.8X5	T50.8X6

Substance	Poisoning, Accidental (unintentional)	Poisoning, Intentional Self-harm	Poisoning, Assault	Poisoning, Undetermined	Adverse Effect	Under-dosing
Iodamide	T50.8X1	T50.8X2	T50.8X3	T50.8X4	T50.8X5	T50.8X6
Iodide NEC — *see also* Iodine	T49.0X1	T49.0X2	T49.0X3	T49.0X4	T49.0X5	T49.0X6
mercury (ointment)	T49.0X1	T49.0X2	T49.0X3	T49.0X4	T49.0X5	T49.0X6
methylate	T49.0X1	T49.0X2	T49.0X3	T49.0X4	T49.0X5	T49.0X6
potassium (expectorant) NEC	T48.4X1	T48.4X2	T48.4X3	T48.4X4	T48.4X5	T48.4X6
Iodinated						
contrast medium	T50.8X1	T50.8X2	T50.8X3	T50.8X4	T50.8X5	T50.8X6
glycerol	T48.4X1	T48.4X2	T48.4X3	T48.4X4	T48.4X5	T48.4X6
human serum albumin (131I)	T50.8X1	T50.8X2	T50.8X3	T50.8X4	T50.8X5	T50.8X6
Iodine (antiseptic, external) (tincture) **NEC**	T49.0X1	T49.0X2	T49.0X3	T49.0X4	T49.0X5	T49.0X6
125 — *see also* Radiation sickness, and Exposure to radioactivce isotopes	T50.8X1	T50.8X2	T50.8X3	T50.8X4		T50.8X6
therapeutic	T50.991	T50.992	T50.993	T50.994	T50.995	T50.996
131 — *see also* Radiation sickness, and Exposure to radioactivce isotopes	T50.8X1	T50.8X2	T50.8X3	T50.8X4	T50.8X5	T50.8X6
therapeutic	T38.2X1	T38.2X2	T38.2X3	T38.2X4	T38.2X5	T38.2X6
diagnostic	T50.8X1	T50.8X2	T50.8X3	T50.8X4	T50.8X5	T50.8X6
for thyroid conditions (antithyroid)	T38.2X1	T38.2X2	T38.2X3	T38.2X4	T38.2X5	T38.2X6
solution	T49.0X1	T49.0X2	T49.0X3	T49.0X4	T49.0X5	T49.0X6
vapor	T59.891	T59.892	T59.893	T59.894	—	—
Iodipamide	T50.8X1	T50.8X2	T50.8X3	T50.8X4	T50.8X5	T50.8X6
Iodized (poppy seed) oil	T50.8X1	T50.8X2	T50.8X3	T50.8X4	T50.8X5	T50.8X6
Iodobismitol	T37.8X1	T37.8X2	T37.8X3	T37.8X4	T37.8X5	T37.8X6
Iodochlorhydroxyquin	T37.8X1	T37.8X2	T37.8X3	T37.8X4	T37.8X5	T37.8X6
topical	T49.0X1	T49.0X2	T49.0X3	T49.0X4	T49.0X5	T49.0X6
Iodochlorhydroxyquinoline	T37.8X1	T37.8X2	T37.8X3	T37.8X4	T37.8X5	T37.8X6
Iodocholesterol (131I)	T50.8X1	T50.8X2	T50.8X3	T50.8X4	T50.8X5	T50.8X6
Iodoform	T49.0X1	T49.0X2	T49.0X3	T49.0X4	T49.0X5	T49.0X6
Iodohippuric acid	T50.8X1	T50.8X2	T50.8X3	T50.8X4	T50.8X5	T50.8X6
Iodopanoic acid	T50.8X1	T50.8X2	T50.8X3	T50.8X4	T50.8X5	T50.8X6
Iodophthalein (sodium)	T50.8X1	T50.8X2	T50.8X3	T50.8X4	T50.8X5	T50.8X6
Iodopyracet	T50.8X1	T50.8X2	T50.8X3	T50.8X4	T50.8X5	T50.8X6
Iodoquinol	T37.8X1	T37.8X2	T37.8X3	T37.8X4	T37.8X5	T37.8X6
Iodoxamic acid	T50.8X1	T50.8X2	T50.8X3	T50.8X4	T50.8X5	T50.8X6
Iofendylate	T50.8X1	T50.8X2	T50.8X3	T50.8X4	T50.8X5	T50.8X6
Ioglycamic acid	T50.8X1	T50.8X2	T50.8X3	T50.8X4	T50.8X5	T50.8X6
Iohexol	T50.8X1	T50.8X2	T50.8X3	T50.8X4	T50.8X5	T50.8X6
Ion exchange resin						
anion	T47.8X1	T47.8X2	T47.8X3	T47.8X4	T47.8X5	T47.8X6
cation	T50.3X1	T50.3X2	T50.3X3	T50.3X4	T50.3X5	T50.3X6
cholestyramine	T46.6X1	T46.6X2	T46.6X3	T46.6X4	T46.6X5	T46.6X6
intestinal	T47.8X1	T47.8X2	T47.8X3	T47.8X4	T47.8X5	T47.8X6
Iopamidol	T50.8X1	T50.8X2	T50.8X3	T50.8X4	T50.8X5	T50.8X6
Iopanoic acid	T50.8X1	T50.8X2	T50.8X3	T50.8X4	T50.8X5	T50.8X6
Iophenoic acid	T50.8X1	T50.8X2	T50.8X3	T50.8X4	T50.8X5	T50.8X6
Iopodate, sodium	T50.8X1	T50.8X2	T50.8X3	T50.8X4	T50.8X5	T50.8X6
Iopodic acid	T50.8X1	T50.8X2	T50.8X3	T50.8X4	T50.8X5	T50.8X6
Iopromide	T50.8X1	T50.8X2	T50.8X3	T50.8X4	T50.8X5	T50.8X6
Iopydol	T50.8X1	T50.8X2	T50.8X3	T50.8X4	T50.8X5	T50.8X6
Iotalamic acid	T50.8X1	T50.8X2	T50.8X3	T50.8X4	T50.8X5	T50.8X6
Iothalamate	T50.8X1	T50.8X2	T50.8X3	T50.8X4	T50.8X5	T50.8X6
Iothiouracil	T38.2X1	T38.2X2	T38.2X3	T38.2X4	T38.2X5	T38.2X6
Iotrol	T50.8X1	T50.8X2	T50.8X3	T50.8X4	T50.8X5	T50.8X6
Iotrolan	T50.8X1	T50.8X2	T50.8X3	T50.8X4	T50.8X5	T50.8X6
Iotroxate	T50.8X1	T50.8X2	T50.8X3	T50.8X4	T50.8X5	T50.8X6
Iotroxic acid	T50.8X1	T50.8X2	T50.8X3	T50.8X4	T50.8X5	T50.8X6
Ioversol	T50.8X1	T50.8X2	T50.8X3	T50.8X4	T50.8X5	T50.8X6
Ioxaglate	T50.8X1	T50.8X2	T50.8X3	T50.8X4	T50.8X5	T50.8X6
Ioxaglic acid	T50.8X1	T50.8X2	T50.8X3	T50.8X4	T50.8X5	T50.8X6
Ioxitalamic acid	T50.8X1	T50.8X2	T50.8X3	T50.8X4	T50.8X5	T50.8X6
Ipecac	T47.7X1	T47.7X2	T47.7X3	T47.7X4	T47.7X5	T47.7X6
Ipecacuanha	T48.4X1	T48.4X2	T48.4X3	T48.4X4	T48.4X5	T48.4X6
Ipodate, calcium	T50.8X1	T50.8X2	T50.8X3	T50.8X4	T50.8X5	T50.8X6
Ipral	T42.3X1	T42.3X2	T42.3X3	T42.3X4	T42.3X5	T42.3X6
Ipratropium (bromide)	T48.6X1	T48.6X2	T48.6X3	T48.6X4	T48.6X5	T48.6X6
Ipriflavone	T46.3X1	T46.3X2	T46.3X3	T46.3X4	T46.3X5	T46.3X6
Iprindole	T43.011	T43.012	T43.013	T43.014	T43.015	T43.016
Iproclozide	T43.1X1	T43.1X2	T43.1X3	T43.1X4	T43.1X5	T43.1X6
Iprofenin	T50.8X1	T50.8X2	T50.8X3	T50.8X4	T50.8X5	T50.8X6
Iproheptine	T49.2X1	T49.2X2	T49.2X3	T49.2X4	T49.2X5	T49.2X6
Iproniazid	T43.1X1	T43.1X2	T43.1X3	T43.1X4	T43.1X5	T43.1X6
Iproplatin	T45.1X1	T45.1X2	T45.1X3	T45.1X4	T45.1X5	T45.1X6
Iproveratril	T46.1X1	T46.1X2	T46.1X3	T46.1X4	T46.1X5	T46.1X6
Iron (compounds) (medicinal) **NEC**	T45.4X1	T45.4X2	T45.4X3	T45.4X4	T45.4X5	T45.4X6
ammonium	T45.4X1	T45.4X2	T45.4X3	T45.4X4	T45.4X5	T45.4X6
dextran injection	T45.4X1	T45.4X2	T45.4X3	T45.4X4	T45.4X5	T45.4X6
Iron (compounds) (medicinal) **NEC** — *continued*						
nonmedicinal	T56.891	T56.892	T56.893	T56.894	—	—
salts	T45.4X1	T45.4X2	T45.4X3	T45.4X4	T45.4X5	T45.4X6
sorbitex	T45.4X1	T45.4X2	T45.4X3	T45.4X4	T45.4X5	T45.4X6
sorbitol citric acid complex	T45.4X1	T45.4X2	T45.4X3	T45.4X4	T45.4X5	T45.4X6
Irrigating fluid (vaginal)	T49.8X1	T49.8X2	T49.8X3	T49.8X4	T49.8X5	T49.8X6
eye	T49.5X1	T49.5X2	T49.5X3	T49.5X4	T49.5X5	T49.5X6
Isepamicin	T36.5X1	T36.5X2	T36.5X3	T36.5X4	T36.5X5	T36.5X6
Isoaminile (citrate)	T48.3X1	T48.3X2	T48.3X3	T48.3X4	T48.3X5	T48.3X6
Isoamyl nitrite	T46.3X1	T46.3X2	T46.3X3	T46.3X4	T46.3X5	T46.3X6
Isobenzan	T60.1X1	T60.1X2	T60.1X3	T60.1X4	—	—
Isobutyl acetate	T52.8X1	T52.8X2	T52.8X3	T52.8X4	—	—
Isocarboxazid	T43.1X1	T43.1X2	T43.1X3	T43.1X4	T43.1X5	T43.1X6
Isoconazole	T49.0X1	T49.0X2	T49.0X3	T49.0X4	T49.0X5	T49.0X6
Isocyanate	T65.0X1	T65.0X2	T65.0X3	T65.0X4	—	—
Isoephedrine	T44.991	T44.992	T44.993	T44.994	T44.995	T44.996
Isoetarine	T48.6X1	T48.6X2	T48.6X3	T48.6X4	T48.6X5	T48.6X6
Isoethadione	T42.2X1	T42.2X2	T42.2X3	T42.2X4	T42.2X5	T42.2X6
Isoetharine	T44.5X1	T44.5X2	T44.5X3	T44.5X4	T44.5X5	T44.5X6
Isoflurane	T41.0X1	T41.0X2	T41.0X3	T41.0X4	T41.0X5	T41.0X6
Isoflurophate	T44.0X1	T44.0X2	T44.0X3	T44.0X4	T44.0X5	T44.0X6
Isomaltose, ferric complex	T45.4X1	T45.4X2	T45.4X3	T45.4X4	T45.4X5	T45.4X6
Isometheptene	T44.3X1	T44.3X2	T44.3X3	T44.3X4	T44.3X5	T44.3X6
Isoniazid	T37.1X1	T37.1X2	T37.1X3	T37.1X4	T37.1X5	T37.1X6
with						
rifampicin	T36.6X1	T36.6X2	T36.6X3	T36.6X4	T36.6X5	T36.6X6
thioacetazone	T37.1X1	T37.1X2	T37.1X3	T37.1X4	T37.1X5	T37.1X6
Isonicotinic acid hydrazide	T37.1X1	T37.1X2	T37.1X3	T37.1X4	T37.1X5	T37.1X6
Isonipecaine	T40.4X1	T40.4X2	T40.4X3	T40.4X4	T40.4X5	T40.4X6
Isopentaquine	T37.2X1	T37.2X2	T37.2X3	T37.2X4	T37.2X5	T37.2X6
Isophane insulin	T38.3X1	T38.3X2	T38.3X3	T38.3X4	T38.3X5	T38.3X6
Isophorone	T65.891	T65.892	T65.893	T65.894	—	—
Isophosphamide	T45.1X1	T45.1X2	T45.1X3	T45.1X4	T45.1X5	T45.1X6
Isopregnenone	T38.5X1	T38.5X2	T38.5X3	T38.5X4	T38.5X5	T38.5X6
Isoprenaline	T48.6X1	T48.6X2	T48.6X3	T48.6X4	T48.6X5	T48.6X6
Isopromethazine	T43.3X1	T43.3X2	T43.3X3	T43.3X4	T43.3X5	T43.3X6
Isopropamide	T44.3X1	T44.3X2	T44.3X3	T44.3X4	T44.3X5	T44.3X6
iodide	T44.3X1	T44.3X2	T44.3X3	T44.3X4	T44.3X5	T44.3X6
Isopropanol	T51.2X1	T51.2X2	T51.2X3	T51.2X4		
Isopropyl						
acetate	T52.8X1	T52.8X2	T52.8X3	T52.8X4	—	—
alcohol	T51.2X1	T51.2X2	T51.2X3	T51.2X4	—	—
medicinal	T49.4X1	T49.4X2	T49.4X3	T49.4X4	T49.4X5	T49.4X6
ether	T52.8X1	T52.8X2	T52.8X3	T52.8X4	—	—
Isopropylaminophenazone	T39.2X1	T39.2X2	T39.2X3	T39.2X4	T39.2X5	T39.2X6
Isoproterenol	T48.6X1	T48.6X2	T48.6X3	T48.6X4	T48.6X5	T48.6X6
Isosorbide dinitrate	T46.3X1	T46.3X2	T46.3X3	T46.3X4	T46.3X5	T46.3X6
Isothipendyl	T45.0X1	T45.0X2	T45.0X3	T45.0X4	T45.0X5	T45.0X6
Isotretinoin	T50.991	T50.992	T50.993	T50.994	T50.995	T50.996
Isoxazolyl penicillin	T36.0X1	T36.0X2	T36.0X3	T36.0X4	T36.0X5	T36.0X6
Isoxicam	T39.391	T39.392	T39.393	T39.394	T39.395	T39.396
Isoxsuprine	T46.7X1	T46.7X2	T46.7X3	T46.7X4	T46.7X5	T46.7X6
Ispagula	T47.4X1	T47.4X2	T47.4X3	T47.4X4	T47.4X5	T47.4X6
husk	T47.4X1	T47.4X2	T47.4X3	T47.4X4	T47.4X5	T47.4X6
Isradipine	T46.1X1	T46.1X2	T46.1X3	T46.1X4	T46.1X5	T46.1X6
l-thyroxine sodium	T38.1X1	T38.1X2	T38.1X3	T38.1X4	T38.1X5	T38.1X6
Itraconazole	T37.8X1	T37.8X2	T37.8X3	T37.8X4	T37.8X5	T37.8X6
Itramin tosilate	T46.3X1	T46.3X2	T46.3X3	T46.3X4	T46.3X5	T46.3X6
Ivermectin	T37.4X1	T37.4X2	T37.4X3	T37.4X4	T37.4X5	T37.4X6
Izoniazid	T37.1X1	T37.1X2	T37.1X3	T37.1X4	T37.1X5	T37.1X6
with thioacetazone	T37.1X1	T37.1X2	T37.1X3	T37.1X4	T37.1X5	T37.1X6
Jalap	T47.2X1	T47.2X2	T47.2X3	T47.2X4	T47.2X5	T47.2X6
Jamaica						
dogwood (bark)	T39.8X1	T39.8X2	T39.8X3	T39.8X4	T39.8X5	T39.8X6
ginger	T65.891	T65.892	T65.893	T65.894	—	—
root	T62.2X1	T62.2X2	T62.2X3	T62.2X4	—	—
Jatropha	T62.2X1	T62.2X2	T62.2X3	T62.2X4	—	—
curcas	T62.2X1	T62.2X2	T62.2X3	T62.2X4	—	—
Jectofer	T45.4X1	T45.4X2	T45.4X3	T45.4X4	T45.4X5	T45.4X6
Jellyfish (sting)	T63.621	T63.622	T63.623	T63.624	—	—
Jequirity (bean)	T62.2X1	T62.2X2	T62.2X3	T62.2X4	—	—
Jimson weed (stramonium)	T62.2X1	T62.2X2	T62.2X3	T62.2X4	—	—
seeds	T62.2X1	T62.2X2	T62.2X3	T62.2X4	—	—
Josamycin	T36.3X1	T36.3X2	T36.3X3	T36.3X4	T36.3X5	T36.3X6
Juniper tar	T49.1X1	T49.1X2	T49.1X3	T49.1X4	T49.1X5	T49.1X6
Kallidinogenase	T46.7X1	T46.7X2	T46.7X3	T46.7X4	T46.7X5	T46.7X6
Kallikrein	T46.7X1	T46.7X2	T46.7X3	T46.7X4	T46.7X5	T46.7X6
Kanamycin	T36.5X1	T36.5X2	T36.5X3	T36.5X4	T36.5X5	T36.5X6
Kantrex	T36.5X1	T36.5X2	T36.5X3	T36.5X4	T36.5X5	T36.5X6
Kaolin	T47.6X1	T47.6X2	T47.6X3	T47.6X4	T47.6X5	T47.6X6
light	T47.6X1	T47.6X2	T47.6X3	T47.6X4	T47.6X5	T47.6X6
Karaya (gum)	T47.4X1	T47.4X2	T47.4X3	T47.4X4	T47.4X5	T47.4X6

Substance	Poisoning, Accidental (unintentional)	Poisoning, Intentional Self-harm	Poisoning, Assault	Poisoning, Undetermined	Adverse Effect	Under-dosing
Kebuzone	T39.2X1	T39.2X2	T39.2X3	T39.2X4	T39.2X5	T39.2X6
Kelevan	T60.1X1	T60.1X2	T60.1X3	T60.1X4	—	—
Kemithal	T41.1X1	T41.1X2	T41.1X3	T41.1X4	T41.1X5	T41.1X6
Kenacort	T38.0X1	T38.0X2	T38.0X3	T38.0X4	T38.0X5	T38.0X6
Keratolytic drug NEC	T49.4X1	T49.4X2	T49.4X3	T49.4X4	T49.4X5	T49.4X6
anthracene	T49.4X1	T49.4X2	T49.4X3	T49.4X4	T49.4X5	T49.4X6
Keratoplastic NEC	T49.4X1	T49.4X2	T49.4X3	T49.4X4	T49.4X5	T49.4X6
Kerosene, kerosine (fuel) (solvent) **NEC**	T52.0X1	T52.0X2	T52.0X3	T52.0X4	—	—
insecticide	T52.0X1	T52.0X2	T52.0X3	T52.0X4	—	—
vapor	T52.0X1	T52.0X2	T52.0X3	T52.0X4	—	—
Ketamine	T41.291	T41.292	T41.293	T41.294	T41.295	T41.296
Ketazolam	T42.4X1	T42.4X2	T42.4X3	T42.4X4	T42.4X5	T42.4X6
Ketazon	T39.2X1	T39.2X2	T39.2X3	T39.2X4	T39.2X5	T39.2X6
Ketobemidone	T40.4X1	T40.4X2	T40.4X3	T40.4X4	—	—
Ketoconazole	T49.0X1	T49.0X2	T49.0X3	T49.0X4	T49.0X5	T49.0X6
Ketols	T52.4X1	T52.4X2	T52.4X3	T52.4X4	—	—
Ketone oils	T52.4X1	T52.4X2	T52.4X3	T52.4X4	—	—
Ketoprofen	T39.311	T39.312	T39.313	T39.314	T39.315	T39.316
Ketorolac	T39.8X1	T39.8X2	T39.8X3	T39.8X4	T39.8X5	T39.8X6
Ketotifen	T45.0X1	T45.0X2	T45.0X3	T45.0X4	T45.0X5	T45.0X6
Khat	T43.691	T43.692	T43.693	T43.694	—	—
Khellin	T46.3X1	T46.3X2	T46.3X3	T46.3X4	T46.3X5	T46.3X6
Khelloside	T46.3X1	T46.3X2	T46.3X3	T46.3X4	T46.3X5	T46.3X6
Kiln gas or vapor (carbon monoxide)	T58.8X1	T58.8X2	T58.8X3	T58.8X4	—	—
Kitasamycin	T36.3X1	T36.3X2	T36.3X3	T36.3X4	T36.3X5	T36.3X6
Konsyl	T47.4X1	T47.4X2	T47.4X3	T47.4X4	T47.4X5	T47.4X6
Kosam seed	T62.2X1	T62.2X2	T62.2X3	T62.2X4	—	—
Krait (venom)	T63.091	T63.092	T63.093	T63.094	—	—
Kwell (insecticide)	T60.1X1	T60.1X2	T60.1X3	T60.1X4	—	—
anti-infective (topical)	T49.0X1	T49.0X2	T49.0X3	T49.0X4	T49.0X5	T49.0X6
Labetalol	T44.8X1	T44.8X2	T44.8X3	T44.8X4	T44.8X5	T44.8X6
Laburnum (seeds)	T62.2X1	T62.2X2	T62.2X3	T62.2X4	—	—
leaves	T62.2X1	T62.2X2	T62.2X3	T62.2X4	—	—
Lachesine	T49.5X1	T49.5X2	T49.5X3	T49.5X4	T49.5X5	T49.5X6
Lacidipine	T46.5X1	T46.5X2	T46.5X3	T46.5X4	T46.5X5	T46.5X6
Lacquer	T65.6X1	T65.6X2	T65.6X3	T65.6X4	—	—
Lacrimogenic gas	T59.3X1	T59.3X2	T59.3X3	T59.3X4	—	—
Lactated potassic saline	T50.3X1	T50.3X2	T50.3X3	T50.3X4	T50.3X5	T50.3X6
Lactic acid	T49.8X1	T49.8X2	T49.8X3	T49.8X4	T49.8X5	T49.8X6
Lactobacillus						
acidophilus	T47.6X1	T47.6X2	T47.6X3	T47.6X4	T47.6X5	T47.6X6
compound	T47.6X1	T47.6X2	T47.6X3	T47.6X4	T47.6X5	T47.6X6
bifidus, lyophilized	T47.6X1	T47.6X2	T47.6X3	T47.6X4	T47.6X5	T47.6X6
bulgaricus	T47.6X1	T47.6X2	T47.6X3	T47.6X4	T47.6X5	T47.6X6
sporogenes	T47.6X1	T47.6X2	T47.6X3	T47.6X4	T47.6X5	T47.6X6
Lactoflavin	T45.2X1	T45.2X2	T45.2X3	T45.2X4	T45.2X5	T45.2X6
Lactose (as excipient)	T50.901	T50.902	T50.903	T50.904	T50.905	T50.906
Lactuca (virosa) (extract)	T42.6X1	T42.6X2	T42.6X3	T42.6X4	T42.6X5	T42.6X6
Lactucarium	T42.6X1	T42.6X2	T42.6X3	T42.6X4	T42.6X5	T42.6X6
Lactulose	T47.3X1	T47.3X2	T47.3X3	T47.3X4	T47.3X5	T47.3X6
Laevo — see Levo-						
Lanatosides	T46.0X1	T46.0X2	T46.0X3	T46.0X4	T46.0X5	T46.0X6
Lanolin	T49.3X1	T49.3X2	T49.3X3	T49.3X4	T49.3X5	T49.3X6
Largactil	T43.3X1	T43.3X2	T43.3X3	T43.3X4	T43.3X5	T43.3X6
Larkspur	T62.2X1	T62.2X2	T62.2X3	T62.2X4	—	—
Laroxyl	T43.011	T43.012	T43.013	T43.014	T43.015	T43.016
Lasix	T50.1X1	T50.1X2	T50.1X3	T50.1X4	T50.1X5	T50.1X6
Lassar's paste	T49.4X1	T49.4X2	T49.4X3	T49.4X4	T49.4X5	T49.4X6
Latamoxef	T36.1X1	T36.1X2	T36.1X3	T36.1X4	T36.1X5	T36.1X6
Latex	T65.811	T65.812	T65.813	T65.814	—	—
Lathyrus (seed)	T62.2X1	T62.2X2	T62.2X3	T62.2X4	—	—
Laudanum	T40.0X1	T40.0X2	T40.0X3	T40.0X4	T40.0X5	T40.0X6
Laudexium	T48.1X1	T48.1X2	T48.1X3	T48.1X4	T48.1X5	T48.1X6
Laughing gas	T41.0X1	T41.0X2	T41.0X3	T41.0X4	T41.0X5	T41.0X6
Laurel, black or cherry	T62.2X1	T62.2X2	T62.2X3	T62.2X4	—	—
Laurolinium	T49.0X1	T49.0X2	T49.0X3	T49.0X4	T49.0X5	T49.0X6
Lauryl sulfoacetate	T49.2X1	T49.2X2	T49.2X3	T49.2X4	T49.2X5	T49.2X6
Laxative NEC	T47.4X1	T47.4X2	T47.4X3	T47.4X4	T47.4X5	T47.4X6
osmotic	T47.3X1	T47.3X2	T47.3X3	T47.3X4	T47.3X5	T47.3X6
saline	T47.3X1	T47.3X2	T47.3X3	T47.3X4	T47.3X5	T47.3X6
stimulant	T47.2X1	T47.2X2	T47.2X3	T47.2X4	T47.2X5	T47.2X6
L-dopa	T42.8X1	T42.8X2	T42.8X3	T42.8X4	T42.8X5	T42.8X6
Lead (dust) (fumes) (vapor)	T56.0X1	T56.0X2	T56.0X3	T56.0X4	—	—
NEC						
acetate	T49.2X1	T49.2X2	T49.2X3	T49.2X4	T49.2X5	T49.2X6
alkyl (fuel additive)	T56.0X1	T56.0X2	T56.0X3	T56.0X4	—	—
anti-infectives	T37.8X1	T37.8X2	T37.8X3	T37.8X4	T37.8X5	T37.8X6
antiknock compound (tetraethyl)	T56.0X1	T56.0X2	T56.0X3	T56.0X4	—	—

Substance	Poisoning, Accidental (unintentional)	Poisoning, Intentional Self-harm	Poisoning, Assault	Poisoning, Undetermined	Adverse Effect	Under-dosing
Lead (dust) (fumes) (vapor) **NEC**						
— continued						
arsenate, arsenite (dust)(herbicide) (insecticide) (vapor)	T57.0X1	T57.0X2	T57.0X3	T57.0X4	—	—
carbonate	T56.0X1	T56.0X2	T56.0X3	T56.0X4	—	—
paint	T56.0X1	T56.0X2	T56.0X3	T56.0X4	—	—
chromate	T56.0X1	T56.0X2	T56.0X3	T56.0X4	—	—
paint	T56.0X1	T56.0X2	T56.0X3	T56.0X4	—	—
dioxide	T56.0X1	T56.0X2	T56.0X3	T56.0X4	—	—
inorganic	T56.0X1	T56.0X2	T56.0X3	T56.0X4	—	—
iodide	T56.0X1	T56.0X2	T56.0X3	T56.0X4	—	—
pigment (paint)	T56.0X1	T56.0X2	T56.0X3	T56.0X4	—	—
monoxide (dust)	T56.0X1	T56.0X2	T56.0X3	T56.0X4	—	—
paint	T56.0X1	T56.0X2	T56.0X3	T56.0X4	—	—
organic	T56.0X1	T56.0X2	T56.0X3	T56.0X4	—	—
oxide	T56.0X1	T56.0X2	T56.0X3	T56.0X4	—	—
paint	T56.0X1	T56.0X2	T56.0X3	T56.0X4	—	—
paint	T56.0X1	T56.0X2	T56.0X3	T56.0X4	—	—
salts	T56.0X1	T56.0X2	T56.0X3	T56.0X4	—	—
specified compound NEC	T56.0X1	T56.0X2	T56.0X3	T56.0X4	—	—
tetra-ethyl	T56.0X1	T56.0X2	T56.0X3	T56.0X4	—	—
Lebanese red	T40.7X1	T40.7X2	T40.7X3	T40.7X4	T40.7X5	T40.7X6
Lefetamine	T39.8X1	T39.8X2	T39.8X3	T39.8X4	T39.8X5	T39.8X6
Lenperone	T43.4X1	T43.4X2	T43.4X3	T43.4X4	T43.4X5	T43.4X6
Lente lietin (insulin)	T38.3X1	T38.3X2	T38.3X3	T38.3X4	T38.3X5	T38.3X6
Leptazol	T50.7X1	T50.7X2	T50.7X3	T50.7X4	T50.7X5	T50.7X6
Leptophos	T60.0X1	T60.0X2	T60.0X3	T60.0X4	—	—
Leritine	T40.2X1	T40.2X2	T40.2X3	T40.2X4	T40.2X5	T40.2X6
Letosteine	T48.4X1	T48.4X2	T48.4X3	T48.4X4	T48.4X5	T48.4X6
Letter	T38.1X1	T38.1X2	T38.1X3	T38.1X4	T38.1X5	T38.1X6
Lettuce opium	T42.6X1	T42.6X2	T42.6X3	T42.6X4	T42.6X5	T42.6X6
Leucinocaine	T41.3X1	T41.3X2	T41.3X3	T41.3X4	T41.3X5	T41.3X6
Leucocianidol	T46.991	T46.992	T46.993	T46.994	T46.995	T46.996
Leucovorin (factor)	T45.8X1	T45.8X2	T45.8X3	T45.8X4	T45.8X5	T45.8X6
Leukeran	T45.1X1	T45.1X2	T45.1X3	T45.1X4	T45.1X5	T45.1X6
Leuprolide	T38.891	T38.892	T38.893	T38.894	T38.895	T38.896
Levalbuterol	T48.6X1	T48.6X2	T48.6X3	T48.6X4	T48.6X5	T48.6X6
Levallorphan	T50.7X1	T50.7X2	T50.7X3	T50.7X4	T50.7X5	T50.7X6
Levamisole	T37.4X1	T37.4X2	T37.4X3	T37.4X4	T37.4X5	T37.4X6
Levanil	T42.6X1	T42.6X2	T42.6X3	T42.6X4	T42.6X5	T42.6X6
Levarterenol	T44.4X1	T44.4X2	T44.4X3	T44.4X4	T44.4X5	T44.4X6
Levdropropizine	T48.3X1	T48.3X2	T48.3X3	T48.3X4	T48.3X5	T48.3X6
Levobunolol	T49.5X1	T49.5X2	T49.5X3	T49.5X4	T49.5X5	T49.5X6
Levocabastine (hydrochloride)	T45.0X1	T45.0X2	T45.0X3	T45.0X4	T45.0X5	T45.0X6
Levocarnitine	T50.991	T50.992	T50.993	T50.994	T50.995	T50.996
Levodopa	T42.8X1	T42.8X2	T42.8X3	T42.8X4	T42.8X5	T42.8X6
with carbidopa	T42.8X1	T42.8X2	T42.8X3	T42.8X4	T42.8X5	T42.8X6
Levo-dromoran	T40.2X1	T40.2X2	T40.2X3	T40.2X4	T40.2X5	T40.2X6
Levoglutamide	T50.991	T50.992	T50.993	T50.994	T50.995	T50.996
Levoid	T38.1X1	T38.1X2	T38.1X3	T38.1X4	T38.1X5	T38.1X6
Levo-isomethadone	T40.3X1	T40.3X2	T40.3X3	T40.3X4	T40.3X5	T40.3X6
Levomepromazine	T43.3X1	T43.3X2	T43.3X3	T43.3X4	T43.3X5	T43.3X6
Levonordefrin	T49.6X1	T49.6X2	T49.6X3	T49.6X4	T49.6X5	T49.6X6
Levonorgestrel	T38.4X1	T38.4X2	T38.4X3	T38.4X4	T38.4X5	T38.4X6
with ethinylestradiol	T38.5X1	T38.5X2	T38.5X3	T38.5X4	T38.5X5	T38.5X6
Levopromazine	T43.3X1	T43.3X2	T43.3X3	T43.3X4	T43.3X5	T43.3X6
Levoprome	T42.6X1	T42.6X2	T42.6X3	T42.6X4	T42.6X5	T42.6X6
Levopropoxyphene	T40.4X1	T40.4X2	T40.4X3	T40.4X4	T40.4X5	T40.4X6
Levopropylhexedrine	T50.5X1	T50.5X2	T50.5X3	T50.5X4	T50.5X5	T50.5X6
Levoproxyphylline	T48.6X1	T48.6X2	T48.6X3	T48.6X4	T48.6X5	T48.6X6
Levorphanol	T40.4X1	T40.4X2	T40.4X3	T40.4X4	T40.4X5	T40.4X6
Levothyroxine	T38.1X1	T38.1X2	T38.1X3	T38.1X4	T38.1X5	T38.1X6
sodium	T38.1X1	T38.1X2	T38.1X3	T38.1X4	T38.1X5	T38.1X6
Levsin	T44.3X1	T44.3X2	T44.3X3	T44.3X4	T44.3X5	T44.3X6
Levulose	T50.3X1	T50.3X2	T50.3X3	T50.3X4	T50.3X5	T50.3X6
Lewisite (gas), not in war	T57.0X1	T57.0X2	T57.0X3	T57.0X4	—	—
Librium	T42.4X1	T42.4X2	T42.4X3	T42.4X4	T42.4X5	T42.4X6
Lidex	T49.0X1	T49.0X2	T49.0X3	T49.0X4	T49.0X5	T49.0X6
Lidocaine	T41.3X1	T41.3X2	T41.3X3	T41.3X4	T41.3X5	T41.3X6
regional	T41.3X1	T41.3X2	T41.3X3	T41.3X4	T41.3X5	T41.3X6
spinal	T41.3X1	T41.3X2	T41.3X3	T41.3X4	T41.3X5	T41.3X6
Lidofenin	T50.8X1	T50.8X2	T50.8X3	T50.8X4	T50.8X5	T50.8X6
Lidoflazine	T46.1X1	T46.1X2	T46.1X3	T46.1X4	T46.1X5	T46.1X6
Lighter fluid	T52.0X1	T52.0X2	T52.0X3	T52.0X4	—	—
Lignin hemicellulose	T47.6X1	T47.6X2	T47.6X3	T47.6X4	T47.6X5	T47.6X6
Lignocaine	T41.3X1	T41.3X2	T41.3X3	T41.3X4	T41.3X5	T41.3X6
regional	T41.3X1	T41.3X2	T41.3X3	T41.3X4	T41.3X5	T41.3X6
spinal	T41.3X1	T41.3X2	T41.3X3	T41.3X4	T41.3X5	T41.3X6
Ligroin (e) (solvent)	T52.0X1	T52.0X2	T52.0X3	T52.0X4	—	—
vapor	T59.891	T59.892	T59.893	T59.894	—	—
Ligustrum vulgare	T62.2X1	T62.2X2	T62.2X3	T62.2X4	—	—

Table of Drugs and Chemicals

Lily of the valley — Mecoprop

Substance	Poisoning, Accidental (unintentional)	Poisoning, Intentional Self-harm	Poisoning, Assault	Poisoning, Undetermined	Adverse Effect	Under-dosing
Lily of the valley	T62.2X1	T62.2X2	T62.2X3	T62.2X4	—	—
Lime (chloride)	T54.3X1	T54.3X2	T54.3X3	T54.3X4	—	—
Limonene	T52.8X1	T52.8X2	T52.8X3	T52.8X4	—	—
Lincomycin	T36.8X1	T36.8X2	T36.8X3	T36.8X4	T36.8X5	T36.8X6
Lindane (insecticide) (nonmedicinal) (vapor)	T53.6X1	T53.6X2	T53.6X3	T53.6X4	—	—
medicinal	T49.0X1	T49.0X2	T49.0X3	T49.0X4	T49.0X5	T49.0X6
Liniments NEC	T49.91	T49.92	T49.93	T49.94	T49.95	T49.96
Linoleic acid	T46.6X1	T46.6X2	T46.6X3	T46.6X4	T46.6X5	T46.6X6
Linolenic acid	T46.6X1	T46.6X2	T46.6X3	T46.6X4	T46.6X5	T46.6X6
Linseed	T47.4X1	T47.4X2	T47.4X3	T47.4X4	T47.4X5	T47.4X6
Liothyronine	T38.1X1	T38.1X2	T38.1X3	T38.1X4	T38.1X5	T38.1X6
Liotrix	T38.1X1	T38.1X2	T38.1X3	T38.1X4	T38.1X5	T38.1X6
Lipancreatin	T47.5X1	T47.5X2	T47.5X3	T47.5X4	T47.5X5	T47.5X6
Lipo-alprostadil	T46.7X1	T46.7X2	T46.7X3	T46.7X4	T46.7X5	T46.7X6
Lipo-Lutin	T38.5X1	T38.5X2	T38.5X3	T38.5X4	T38.5X5	T38.5X6
Lipotropic drug NEC	T50.901	T50.902	T50.903	T50.904	T50.905	T50.906
Liquefied petroleum gases	T59.891	T59.892	T59.893	T59.894	—	—
piped (pure or mixed with air)	T59.891	T59.892	T59.893	T59.894	—	—
Liquid						
paraffin	T47.4X1	T47.4X2	T47.4X3	T47.4X4	T47.4X5	T47.4X6
petrolatum	T47.4X1	T47.4X2	T47.4X3	T47.4X4	T47.4X5	T47.4X6
topical	T49.3X1	T49.3X2	T49.3X3	T49.3X4	T49.3X5	T49.3X6
specified NEC	T65.891	T65.892	T65.893	T65.894	—	—
substance	T65.91	T65.92	T65.93	T65.94	—	—
Liquor creosolis compositus	T65.891	T65.892	T65.893	T65.894	—	—
Liquorice	T48.4X1	T48.4X2	T48.4X3	T48.4X4	T48.4X5	T48.4X6
extract	T47.8X1	T47.8X2	T47.8X3	T47.8X4	T47.8X5	T47.8X6
Lisinopril	T46.4X1	T46.4X2	T46.4X3	T46.4X4	T46.4X5	T46.4X6
Lisuride	T42.8X1	T42.8X2	T42.8X3	T42.8X4	T42.8X5	T42.8X6
Lithane	T43.8X1	T43.8X2	T43.8X3	T43.8X4	T43.8X5	T43.8X6
Lithium	T56.891	T56.892	T56.893	T56.894	—	—
gluconate	T43.591	T43.592	T43.593	T43.594	T43.595	T43.596
salts (carbonate)	T43.591	T43.592	T43.593	T43.594	T43.595	T43.596
Lithonate	T43.8X1	T43.8X2	T43.8X3	T43.8X4	T43.8X5	T43.8X6
Liver						
extract	T45.8X1	T45.8X2	T45.8X3	T45.8X4	T45.8X5	T45.8X6
for parenteral use	T45.8X1	T45.8X2	T45.8X3	T45.8X4	T45.8X5	T45.8X6
fraction 1	T45.8X1	T45.8X2	T45.8X3	T45.8X4	T45.8X5	T45.8X6
hydrolysate	T45.8X1	T45.8X2	T45.8X3	T45.8X4	T45.8X5	T45.8X6
Lizard (bite) (venom)	T63.121	T63.122	T63.123	T63.124		
LMD	T45.8X1	T45.8X2	T45.8X3	T45.8X4	T45.8X5	T45.8X6
Lobelia	T62.2X1	T62.2X2	T62.2X3	T62.2X4	—	—
Lobeline	T50.7X1	T50.7X2	T50.7X3	T50.7X4	T50.7X5	T50.7X6
Local action drug NEC	T49.8X1	T49.8X2	T49.8X3	T49.8X4	T49.8X5	T49.8X6
Locorten	T49.0X1	T49.0X2	T49.0X3	T49.0X4	T49.0X5	T49.0X6
Lofepramine	T43.011	T43.012	T43.013	T43.014	T43.015	T43.016
Lolium temulentum	T62.2X1	T62.2X2	T62.2X3	T62.2X4	—	—
Lomotil	T47.6X1	T47.6X2	T47.6X3	T47.6X4	T47.6X5	T47.6X6
Lomustine	T45.1X1	T45.1X2	T45.1X3	T45.1X4	T45.1X5	T45.1X6
Lonidamine	T45.1X1	T45.1X2	T45.1X3	T45.1X4	T45.1X5	T45.1X6
Loperamide	T47.6X1	T47.6X2	T47.6X3	T47.6X4	T47.6X5	T47.6X6
Loprazolam	T42.4X1	T42.4X2	T42.4X3	T42.4X4	T42.4X5	T42.4X6
Lorajmine	T46.2X1	T46.2X2	T46.2X3	T46.2X4	T46.2X5	T46.2X6
Loratidine	T45.0X1	T45.0X2	T45.0X3	T45.0X4	T45.0X5	T45.0X6
Lorazepam	T42.4X1	T42.4X2	T42.4X3	T42.4X4	T42.4X5	T42.4X6
Lorcainide	T46.2X1	T46.2X2	T46.2X3	T46.2X4	T46.2X5	T46.2X6
Lormetazepam	T42.4X1	T42.4X2	T42.4X3	T42.4X4	T42.4X5	T42.4X6
Lotions NEC	T49.91	T49.92	T49.93	T49.94	T49.95	T49.96
Lotusate	T42.3X1	T42.3X2	T42.3X3	T42.3X4	T42.3X5	T42.3X6
Lovastatin	T46.6X1	T46.6X2	T46.6X3	T46.6X4	T46.6X5	T46.6X6
Lowila	T49.2X1	T49.2X2	T49.2X3	T49.2X4	T49.2X5	T49.2X6
Loxapine	T43.591	T43.592	T43.593	T43.594	T43.595	T43.596
Lozenges (throat)	T49.6X1	T49.6X2	T49.6X3	T49.6X4	T49.6X5	T49.6X6
LSD	T40.8X1	T40.8X2	T40.8X3	T40.8X4		
L-Tryptophan — see amino acid						
Lubricant, eye	T49.5X1	T49.5X2	T49.5X3	T49.5X4	T49.5X5	T49.5X6
Lubricating oil NEC	T52.0X1	T52.0X2	T52.0X3	T52.0X4	—	—
Lucanthone	T37.4X1	T37.4X2	T37.4X3	T37.4X4	T37.4X5	T37.4X6
Luminal	T42.3X1	T42.3X2	T42.3X3	T42.3X4	T42.3X5	T42.3X6
Lung irritant (gas) NEC	T59.91	T59.92	T59.93	T59.94		
Luteinizing hormone	T38.811	T38.812	T38.813	T38.814	T38.815	T38.816
Lutocylol	T38.5X1	T38.5X2	T38.5X3	T38.5X4	T38.5X5	T38.5X6
Lutromone	T38.5X1	T38.5X2	T38.5X3	T38.5X4	T38.5X5	T38.5X6
Lututrin	T48.291	T48.292	T48.293	T48.294	T48.295	T48.296
Lye (concentrated)	T54.3X1	T54.3X2	T54.3X3	T54.3X4	—	—
Lygranum (skin test)	T50.8X1	T50.8X2	T50.8X3	T50.8X4	T50.8X5	T50.8X6
Lymecycline	T36.4X1	T36.4X2	T36.4X3	T36.4X4	T36.4X5	T36.4X6
Lymphogranuloma venereum antigen	T50.8X1	T50.8X2	T50.8X3	T50.8X4	T50.8X5	T50.8X6
Lynestrenol	T38.4X1	T38.4X2	T38.4X3	T38.4X4	T38.4X5	T38.4X6

Substance	Poisoning, Accidental (unintentional)	Poisoning, Intentional Self-harm	Poisoning, Assault	Poisoning, Undetermined	Adverse Effect	Under-dosing
Lyovac Sodium Edecrin	T50.1X1	T50.1X2	T50.1X3	T50.1X4	T50.1X5	T50.1X6
Lypressin	T38.891	T38.892	T38.893	T38.894	T38.895	T38.896
Lysergic acid diethylamide	T40.8X1	T40.8X2	T40.8X3	T40.8X4	—	—
Lysergide	T40.8X1	T40.8X2	T40.8X3	T40.8X4	—	—
Lysine vasopressin	T38.891	T38.892	T38.893	T38.894	T38.895	T38.896
Lysol	T54.1X1	T54.1X2	T54.1X3	T54.1X4	—	—
Lysozyme	T49.0X1	T49.0X2	T49.0X3	T49.0X4	T49.0X5	T49.0X6
Lytta (vitatta)	T49.8X1	T49.8X2	T49.8X3	T49.8X4	T49.8X5	T49.8X6
Mace	T59.3X1	T59.3X2	T59.3X3	T59.3X4	—	—
Macrogol	T50.991	T50.992	T50.993	T50.994	T50.995	T50.996
Macrolide						
anabolic drug	T38.7X1	T38.7X2	T38.7X3	T38.7X4	T38.7X5	T38.7X6
antibiotic	T36.3X1	T36.3X2	T36.3X3	T36.3X4	T36.3X5	T36.3X6
Mafenide	T49.0X1	T49.0X2	T49.0X3	T49.0X4	T49.0X5	T49.0X6
Magaldrate	T47.1X1	T47.1X2	T47.1X3	T47.1X4	T47.1X5	T47.1X6
Magic mushroom	T40.991	T40.992	T40.993	T40.994	—	—
Magnamycin	T36.8X1	T36.8X2	T36.8X3	T36.8X4	T36.8X5	T36.8X6
Magnesia magma	T47.1X1	T47.1X2	T47.1X3	T47.1X4	T47.1X5	T47.1X6
Magnesium NEC	T56.891	T56.892	T56.893	T56.894	—	—
carbonate	T47.1X1	T47.1X2	T47.1X3	T47.1X4	T47.1X5	T47.1X6
citrate	T47.4X1	T47.4X2	T47.4X3	T47.4X4	T47.4X5	T47.4X6
hydroxide	T47.1X1	T47.1X2	T47.1X3	T47.1X4	T47.1X5	T47.1X6
oxide	T47.1X1	T47.1X2	T47.1X3	T47.1X4	T47.1X5	T47.1X6
peroxide	T49.0X1	T49.0X2	T49.0X3	T49.0X4	T49.0X5	T49.0X6
salicylate	T39.091	T39.092	T39.093	T39.094	T39.095	T39.096
silicofluoride	T50.3X1	T50.3X2	T50.3X3	T50.3X4	T50.3X5	T50.3X6
sulfate	T47.4X1	T47.4X2	T47.4X3	T47.4X4	T47.4X5	T47.4X6
thiosulfate	T45.0X1	T45.0X2	T45.0X3	T45.0X4	T45.0X5	T45.0X6
trisilicate	T47.1X1	T47.1X2	T47.1X3	T47.1X4	T47.1X5	T47.1X6
Malathion (medicinal)	T49.0X1	T49.0X2	T49.0X3	T49.0X4	T49.0X5	T49.0X6
insecticide	T60.0X1	T60.0X2	T60.0X3	T60.0X4	—	—
Male fern extract	T37.4X1	T37.4X2	T37.4X3	T37.4X4	T37.4X5	T37.4X6
M-AMSA	T45.1X1	T45.1X2	T45.1X3	T45.1X4	T45.1X5	T45.1X6
Mandelic acid	T37.8X1	T37.8X2	T37.8X3	T37.8X4	T37.8X5	T37.8X6
Manganese (dioxide) (salts)	T57.2X1	T57.2X2	T57.2X3	T57.2X4	—	—
medicinal	T50.991	T50.992	T50.993	T50.994	T50.995	T50.996
Mannitol	T47.3X1	T47.3X2	T47.3X3	T47.3X4	T47.3X5	T47.3X6
hexanitrate	T46.3X1	T46.3X2	T46.3X3	T46.3X4	T46.3X5	T46.3X6
Mannomustine	T45.1X1	T45.1X2	T45.1X3	T45.1X4	T45.1X5	T45.1X6
MAO inhibitors	T43.1X1	T43.1X2	T43.1X3	T43.1X4	T43.1X5	T43.1X6
Mapharsen	T37.8X1	T37.8X2	T37.8X3	T37.8X4	T37.8X5	T37.8X6
Maphenide	T49.0X1	T49.0X2	T49.0X3	T49.0X4	T49.0X5	T49.0X6
Maprotiline	T43.021	T43.022	T43.023	T43.024	T43.025	T43.026
Marcaine	T41.3X1	T41.3X2	T41.3X3	T41.3X4	T41.3X5	T41.3X6
infiltration (subcutaneous)	T41.3X1	T41.3X2	T41.3X3	T41.3X4	T41.3X5	T41.3X6
nerve block (peripheral) (plexus)	T41.3X1	T41.3X2	T41.3X3	T41.3X4	T41.3X5	T41.3X6
Marezine	T45.0X1	T45.0X2	T45.0X3	T45.0X4	T45.0X5	T45.0X6
Marihuana	T40.7X1	T40.7X2	T40.7X3	T40.7X4	T40.7X5	T40.7X6
Marijuana	T40.7X1	T40.7X2	T40.7X3	T40.7X4	T40.7X5	T40.7X6
Marine (sting)	T63.691	T63.692	T63.693	T63.694	—	—
animals (sting)	T63.691	T63.692	T63.693	T63.694	—	—
plants (sting)	T63.711	T63.712	T63.713	T63.714	—	—
Marplan	T43.1X1	T43.1X2	T43.1X3	T43.1X4	T43.1X5	T43.1X6
Marsh gas	T59.891	T59.892	T59.893	T59.894	—	—
Marsilid	T43.1X1	T43.1X2	T43.1X3	T43.1X4	T43.1X5	T43.1X6
Matulane	T45.1X1	T45.1X2	T45.1X3	T45.1X4	T45.1X5	T45.1X6
Mazindol	T50.5X1	T50.5X2	T50.5X3	T50.5X4	T50.5X5	T50.5X6
MCPA	T60.3X1	T60.3X2	T60.3X3	T60.3X4	—	—
MDMA	T43.621	T43.622	T43.623	T43.624	T43.625	T43.626
Meadow saffron	T62.2X1	T62.2X2	T62.2X3	T62.2X4	—	—
Measles virus vaccine (attenuated)	T50.B91	T50.B92	T50.B93	T50.B94	T50.B95	T50.B96
Meat, noxious	T62.8X1	T62.8X2	T62.8X3	T62.8X4	—	—
Meballymal	T42.3X1	T42.3X2	T42.3X3	T42.3X4	T42.3X5	T42.3X6
Mebanazine	T43.1X1	T43.1X2	T43.1X3	T43.1X4	T43.1X5	T43.1X6
Mebaral	T42.3X1	T42.3X2	T42.3X3	T42.3X4	T42.3X5	T42.3X6
Mebendazole	T37.4X1	T37.4X2	T37.4X3	T37.4X4	T37.4X5	T37.4X6
Mebeverine	T44.3X1	T44.3X2	T44.3X3	T44.3X4	T44.3X5	T44.3X6
Mebhydrolin	T45.0X1	T45.0X2	T45.0X3	T45.0X4	T45.0X5	T45.0X6
Mebumal	T42.3X1	T42.3X2	T42.3X3	T42.3X4	T42.3X5	T42.3X6
Mebutamate	T43.591	T43.592	T43.593	T43.594	T43.595	T43.596
Mecamylamine	T44.2X1	T44.2X2	T44.2X3	T44.2X4	T44.2X5	T44.2X6
Mechlorethamine	T45.1X1	T45.1X2	T45.1X3	T45.1X4	T45.1X5	T45.1X6
Mecillinam	T36.0X1	T36.0X2	T36.0X3	T36.0X4	T36.0X5	T36.0X6
Meclizine (hydrochloride)	T45.0X1	T45.0X2	T45.0X3	T45.0X4	T45.0X5	T45.0X6
Meclocycline	T36.4X1	T36.4X2	T36.4X3	T36.4X4	T36.4X5	T36.4X6
Meclofenamate	T39.391	T39.392	T39.393	T39.394	T39.395	T39.396
Meclofenamic acid	T39.391	T39.392	T39.393	T39.394	T39.395	T39.396
Meclofenoxate	T43.691	T43.692	T43.693	T43.694	ICD.695	T43.696
Meclozine	T45.0X1	T45.0X2	T45.0X3	T45.0X4	T45.0X5	T45.0X6
Mecobalamin	T45.8X1	T45.8X2	T45.8X3	T45.8X4	T45.8X5	T45.8X6
Mecoprop	T60.3X1	T60.3X2	T60.3X3	T60.3X4	—	—

Additional Character May Be Required — Refer to the Tabular List for Character Selection   ▽ Subterms under main terms may continue to next column or page

Table of Drugs and Chemicals

Substance	Poisoning, Accidental (unintentional)	Poisoning, Intentional Self-harm	Poisoning, Assault	Poisoning, Undetermined	Adverse Effect	Under-dosing
Mecrilate	T49.3X1	T49.3X2	T49.3X3	T49.3X4	T49.3X5	T49.3X6
Mecysteine	T48.4X1	T48.4X2	T48.4X3	T48.4X4	T48.4X5	T48.4X6
Medazepam	T42.4X1	T42.4X2	T42.4X3	T42.4X4	T42.4X5	T42.4X6
Medicament NEC	T50.901	T50.902	T50.903	T50.904	T50.905	T50.906
Medinal	T42.3X1	T42.3X2	T42.3X3	T42.3X4	T42.3X5	T42.3X6
Medomin	T42.3X1	T42.3X2	T42.3X3	T42.3X4	T42.3X5	T42.3X6
Medrogestone	T38.5X1	T38.5X2	T38.5X3	T38.5X4	T38.5X5	T38.5X6
Medroxalol	T44.8X1	T44.8X2	T44.8X3	T44.8X4	T44.8X5	T44.8X6
Medroxyprogesterone acetate (depot)	T38.5X1	T38.5X2	T38.5X3	T38.5X4	T38.5X5	T38.5X6
Medrysone	T49.0X1	T49.0X2	T49.0X3	T49.0X4	T49.0X5	T49.0X6
Mefenamic acid	T39.391	T39.392	T39.393	T39.394	T39.395	T39.396
Mefenorex	T50.5X1	T50.5X2	T50.5X3	T50.5X4	T50.5X5	T50.5X6
Mefloquine	T37.2X1	T37.2X2	T37.2X3	T37.2X4	T37.2X5	T37.2X6
Mefruside	T50.2X1	T50.2X2	T50.2X3	T50.2X4	T50.2X5	T50.2X6
Megahallucinogen	T40.901	T40.902	T40.903	T40.904	T40.905	T40.906
Megestrol	T38.5X1	T38.5X2	T38.5X3	T38.5X4	T38.5X5	T38.5X6
Meglumine						
antimoniate	T37.8X1	T37.8X2	T37.8X3	T37.8X4	T37.8X5	T37.8X6
diatrizoate	T50.8X1	T50.8X2	T50.8X3	T50.8X4	T50.8X5	T50.8X6
iodipamide	T50.8X1	T50.8X2	T50.8X3	T50.8X4	T50.8X5	T50.8X6
iotroxate	T50.8X1	T50.8X2	T50.8X3	T50.8X4	T50.8X5	T50.8X6
MEK (methyl ethyl ketone)	T52.4X1	T52.4X2	T52.4X3	T52.4X4		
Meladinin	T49.3X1	T49.3X2	T49.3X3	T49.3X4	T49.3X5	T49.3X6
Meladrazine	T44.3X1	T44.3X2	T44.3X3	T44.3X4	T44.3X5	T44.3X6
Melaleuca alternifolia oil	T49.0X1	T49.0X2	T49.0X3	T49.0X4	T49.0X5	T49.0X6
Melanizing agents	T49.3X1	T49.3X2	T49.3X3	T49.3X4	T49.3X5	T49.3X6
Melanocyte-stimulating hormone	T38.891	T38.892	T38.893	T38.894	T38.895	T38.896
Melarsonyl potassium	T37.3X1	T37.3X2	T37.3X3	T37.3X4	T37.3X5	T37.3X6
Melarsoprol	T37.3X1	T37.3X2	T37.3X3	T37.3X4	T37.3X5	T37.3X6
Melia azedarach	T62.2X1	T62.2X2	T62.2X3	T62.2X4	—	—
Melitracen	T43.011	T43.012	T43.013	T43.014	T43.015	T43.016
Mellaril	T43.3X1	T43.3X2	T43.3X3	T43.3X4	T43.3X5	T43.3X6
Meloxine	T49.3X1	T49.3X2	T49.3X3	T49.3X4	T49.3X5	T49.3X6
Melperone	T43.4X1	T43.4X2	T43.4X3	T43.4X4	T43.4X5	T43.4X6
Melphalan	T45.1X1	T45.1X2	T45.1X3	T45.1X4	T45.1X5	T45.1X6
Memantine	T43.8X1	T43.8X2	T43.8X3	T43.8X4	T43.8X5	T43.8X6
Menadiol	T45.7X1	T45.7X2	T45.7X3	T45.7X4	T45.7X5	T45.7X6
sodium sulfate	T45.7X1	T45.7X2	T45.7X3	T45.7X4	T45.7X5	T45.7X6
Menadione	T45.7X1	T45.7X2	T45.7X3	T45.7X4	T45.7X5	T45.7X6
sodium bisulfite	T45.7X1	T45.7X2	T45.7X3	T45.7X4	T45.7X5	T45.7X6
Menaphthone	T45.7X1	T45.7X2	T45.7X3	T45.7X4	T45.7X5	T45.7X6
Menaquinone	T45.7X1	T45.7X2	T45.7X3	T45.7X4	T45.7X5	T45.7X6
Menatetrenone	T45.7X1	T45.7X2	T45.7X3	T45.7X4	T45.7X5	T45.7X6
Meningococcal vaccine	T50.A91	T50.A92	T50.A93	T50.A94	T50.A95	T50.A96
Menningovax (-AC) (-C)	T50.A91	T50.A92	T50.A93	T50.A94	T50.A95	T50.A96
Menotropins	T38.811	T38.812	T38.813	T38.814	T38.815	T38.816
Menthol	T48.5X1	T48.5X2	T48.5X3	T48.5X4	T48.5X5	T48.5X6
Mepacrine	T37.2X1	T37.2X2	T37.2X3	T37.2X4	T37.2X5	T37.2X6
Meparfynol	T42.6X1	T42.6X2	T42.6X3	T42.6X4	T42.6X5	T42.6X6
Mepartricin	T36.7X1	T36.7X2	T36.7X3	T36.7X4	T36.7X5	T36.7X6
Mepazine	T43.3X1	T43.3X2	T43.3X3	T43.3X4	T43.3X5	T43.3X6
Mepenzolate	T44.3X1	T44.3X2	T44.3X3	T44.3X4	T44.3X5	T44.3X6
bromide	T44.3X1	T44.3X2	T44.3X3	T44.3X4	T44.3X5	T44.3X6
Meperidine	T40.4X1	T40.4X2	T40.4X3	T40.4X4	T40.4X5	T40.4X6
Mephebarbital	T42.3X1	T42.3X2	T42.3X3	T42.3X4	T42.3X5	T42.3X6
Mephenamin (e)	T42.8X1	T42.8X2	T42.8X3	T42.8X4	T42.8X5	T42.8X6
Mephenesin	T42.8X1	T42.8X2	T42.8X3	T42.8X4	T42.8X5	T42.8X6
Mephenhydramine	T45.0X1	T45.0X2	T45.0X3	T45.0X4	T45.0X5	T45.0X6
Mephenoxalone	T42.8X1	T42.8X2	T42.8X3	T42.8X4	T42.8X5	T42.8X6
Mephentermine	T44.991	T44.992	T44.993	T44.994	T44.995	T44.996
Mephenytoin	T42.0X1	T42.0X2	T42.0X3	T42.0X4	T42.0X5	T42.0X6
with phenobarbital	T42.3X1	T42.3X2	T42.3X3	T42.3X4	T42.3X5	T42.3X6
Mephobarbital	T42.3X1	T42.3X2	T42.3X3	T42.3X4	T42.3X5	T42.3X6
Mephosfolan	T60.0X1	T60.0X2	T60.0X3	T60.0X4	—	—
Mepindolol	T44.7X1	T44.7X2	T44.7X3	T44.7X4	T44.7X5	T44.7X6
Mepiperphenidol	T44.3X1	T44.3X2	T44.3X3	T44.3X4	T44.3X5	T44.3X6
Mepitiostane	T38.7X1	T38.7X2	T38.7X3	T38.7X4	T38.7X5	T38.7X6
Mepivacaine	T41.3X1	T41.3X2	T41.3X3	T41.3X4	T41.3X5	T41.3X6
epidural	T41.3X1	T41.3X2	T41.3X3	T41.3X4	T41.3X5	T41.3X6
Meprednisone	T38.0X1	T38.0X2	T38.0X3	T38.0X4	T38.0X5	T38.0X6
Meprobam	T43.591	T43.592	T43.593	T43.594	T43.595	T43.596
Meprobamate	T43.591	T43.592	T43.593	T43.594	T43.595	T43.596
Meproscillarin	T46.0X1	T46.0X2	T46.0X3	T46.0X4	T46.0X5	T46.0X6
Meprylcaine	T41.3X1	T41.3X2	T41.3X3	T41.3X4	T41.3X5	T41.3X6
Meptazinol	T39.8X1	T39.8X2	T39.8X3	T39.8X4	T39.8X5	T39.8X6
Mepyramine	T45.0X1	T45.0X2	T45.0X3	T45.0X4	T45.0X5	T45.0X6
Mequitazine	T43.3X1	T43.3X2	T43.3X3	T43.3X4	T43.3X5	T43.3X6
Meralluride	T50.2X1	T50.2X2	T50.2X3	T50.2X4	T50.2X5	T50.2X6
Merbaphen	T50.2X1	T50.2X2	T50.2X3	T50.2X4	T50.2X5	T50.2X6
Merbromin	T49.0X1	T49.0X2	T49.0X3	T49.0X4	T49.0X5	T49.0X6

Substance	Poisoning, Accidental (unintentional)	Poisoning, Intentional Self-harm	Poisoning, Assault	Poisoning, Undetermined	Adverse Effect	Under-dosing
Mercaptobenzothiazole salts	T49.0X1	T49.0X2	T49.0X3	T49.0X4	T49.0X5	T49.0X6
Mercaptomerin	T50.2X1	T50.2X2	T50.2X3	T50.2X4	T50.2X5	T50.2X6
Mercaptopurine	T45.1X1	T45.1X2	T45.1X3	T45.1X4	T45.1X5	T45.1X6
Mercumatilin	T50.2X1	T50.2X2	T50.2X3	T50.2X4	T50.2X5	T50.2X6
Mercuramide	T50.2X1	T50.2X2	T50.2X3	T50.2X4	T50.2X5	T50.2X6
Mercurochrome	T49.0X1	T49.0X2	T49.0X3	T49.0X4	T49.0X5	T49.0X6
Mercurophylline	T50.2X1	T50.2X2	T50.2X3	T50.2X4	T50.2X5	T50.2X6
Mercury, mercurial, mercuric, mercurous (compounds) (cyanide) (fumes) (nonmedicinal) (vapor) NEC	T56.1X1	T56.1X2	T56.1X3	T56.1X4	—	—
ammoniated	T49.0X1	T49.0X2	T49.0X3	T49.0X4	T49.0X5	T49.0X6
anti-infective						
local	T49.0X1	T49.0X2	T49.0X3	T49.0X4	T49.0X5	T49.0X6
systemic	T37.8X1	T37.8X2	T37.8X3	T37.8X4	T37.8X5	T37.8X6
topical	T49.0X1	T49.0X2	T49.0X3	T49.0X4	T49.0X5	T49.0X6
chloride (ammoniated)	T49.0X1	T49.0X2	T49.0X3	T49.0X4	T49.0X5	T49.0X6
fungicide	T56.1X1	T56.1X2	T56.1X3	T56.1X4	—	—
diuretic NEC	T50.2X1	T50.2X2	T50.2X3	T50.2X4	T50.2X5	T50.2X6
fungicide	T56.1X1	T56.1X2	T56.1X3	T56.1X4	—	—
organic (fungicide)	T56.1X1	T56.1X2	T56.1X3	T56.1X4	—	—
oxide, yellow	T49.0X1	T49.0X2	T49.0X3	T49.0X4	T49.0X5	T49.0X6
Mersalyl	T50.2X1	T50.2X2	T50.2X3	T50.2X4	T50.2X5	T50.2X6
Merthiolate	T49.0X1	T49.0X2	T49.0X3	T49.0X4	T49.0X5	T49.0X6
ophthalmic preparation	T49.5X1	T49.5X2	T49.5X3	T49.5X4	T49.5X5	T49.5X6
Meruvax	T50.B91	T50.B92	T50.B93	T50.B94	T50.B95	T50.B96
Mesalazine	T47.8X1	T47.8X2	T47.8X3	T47.8X4	T47.8X5	T47.8X6
Mescal buttons	T40.991	T40.992	T40.993	T40.994	—	—
Mescaline	T40.991	T40.992	T40.993	T40.994	—	—
Mesna	T48.4X1	T48.4X2	T48.4X3	T48.4X4	T48.4X5	T48.4X6
Mesoglycan	T46.6X1	T46.6X2	T46.6X3	T46.6X4	T46.6X5	T46.6X6
Mesoridazine	T43.3X1	T43.3X2	T43.3X3	T43.3X4	T43.3X5	T43.3X6
Mestanolone	T38.7X1	T38.7X2	T38.7X3	T38.7X4	T38.7X5	T38.7X6
Mesterolone	T38.7X1	T38.7X2	T38.7X3	T38.7X4	T38.7X5	T38.7X6
Mestranol	T38.5X1	T38.5X2	T38.5X3	T38.5X4	T38.5X5	T38.5X6
Mesulergine	T42.8X1	T42.8X2	T42.8X3	T42.8X4	T42.8X5	T42.8X6
Mesulfen	T49.0X1	T49.0X2	T49.0X3	T49.0X4	T49.0X5	T49.0X6
Mesuximide	T42.2X1	T42.2X2	T42.2X3	T42.2X4	T42.2X5	T42.2X6
Metabutethamine	T41.3X1	T41.3X2	T41.3X3	T41.3X4	T41.3X5	T41.3X6
Metactesylacetate	T49.0X1	T49.0X2	T49.0X3	T49.0X4	T49.0X5	T49.0X6
Metacycline	T36.4X1	T36.4X2	T36.4X3	T36.4X4	T36.4X5	T36.4X6
Metaldehyde (snail killer) NEC	T60.8X1	T60.8X2	T60.8X3	T60.8X4		
Metals (heavy) (nonmedicinal)	T56.91	T56.92	T56.93	T56.94	—	—
dust, fumes, or vapor NEC	T56.91	T56.92	T56.93	T56.94	—	—
light NEC	T56.91	T56.92	T56.93	T56.94	—	—
dust, fumes, or vapor NEC	T56.891	T56.892	T56.893	T56.894	—	—
specified NEC	T56.891	T56.892	T56.893	T56.894	—	—
thallium	T56.811	T56.812	T56.813	T56.814	—	—
Metamfetamine	T43.621	T43.622	T43.623	T43.624	T43.625	T43.626
Metamizole sodium	T39.2X1	T39.2X2	T39.2X3	T39.2X4	T39.2X5	T39.2X6
Metampicillin	T36.0X1	T36.0X2	T36.0X3	T36.0X4	T36.0X5	T36.0X6
Metamucil	T47.4X1	T47.4X2	T47.4X3	T47.4X4	T47.4X5	T47.4X6
Metandienone	T38.7X1	T38.7X2	T38.7X3	T38.7X4	T38.7X5	T38.7X6
Metandrostenolone	T38.7X1	T38.7X2	T38.7X3	T38.7X4	T38.7X5	T38.7X6
Metaphen	T49.0X1	T49.0X2	T49.0X3	T49.0X4	T49.0X5	T49.0X6
Metaphos	T60.0X1	T60.0X2	T60.0X3	T60.0X4	—	—
Metapramine	T43.011	T43.012	T43.013	T43.014	T43.015	T43.016
Metaproterenol	T48.291	T48.292	T48.293	T48.294	T48.295	T48.296
Metaraminol	T44.4X1	T44.4X2	T44.4X3	T44.4X4	T44.4X5	T44.4X6
Metaxalone	T42.8X1	T42.8X2	T42.8X3	T42.8X4	T42.8X5	T42.8X6
Metenolone	T38.7X1	T38.7X2	T38.7X3	T38.7X4	T38.7X5	T38.7X6
Metergoline	T42.8X1	T42.8X2	T42.8X3	T42.8X4	T42.8X5	T42.8X6
Metescufylline	T46.991	T46.992	T46.993	T46.994	T46.995	T46.996
Metetoin	T42.0X1	T42.0X2	T42.0X3	T42.0X4	T42.0X5	T42.0X6
Metformin	T38.3X1	T38.3X2	T38.3X3	T38.3X4	T38.3X5	T38.3X6
Methacholine	T44.1X1	T44.1X2	T44.1X3	T44.1X4	T44.1X5	T44.1X6
Methacycline	T36.4X1	T36.4X2	T36.4X3	T36.4X4	T36.4X5	T36.4X6
Methadone	T40.3X1	T40.3X2	T40.3X3	T40.3X4	T40.3X5	T40.3X6
Methallenestril	T38.5X1	T38.5X2	T38.5X3	T38.5X4	T38.5X5	T38.5X6
Methallenoestril	T38.5X1	T38.5X2	T38.5X3	T38.5X4	T38.5X5	T38.5X6
Methamphetamine	T43.621	T43.622	T43.623	T43.624	T43.625	T43.626
Methampyrone	T39.2X1	T39.2X2	T39.2X3	T39.2X4	T39.2X5	T39.2X6
Methandienone	T38.7X1	T38.7X2	T38.7X3	T38.7X4	T38.7X5	T38.7X6
Methandriol	T38.7X1	T38.7X2	T38.7X3	T38.7X4	T38.7X5	T38.7X6
Methandrostenolone	T38.7X1	T38.7X2	T38.7X3	T38.7X4	T38.7X5	T38.7X6
Methane	T59.891	T59.892	T59.893	T59.894	—	—
Methanethiol	T59.891	T59.892	T59.893	T59.894	—	—
Methaniazide	T37.1X1	T37.1X2	T37.1X3	T37.1X4	T37.1X5	T37.1X6
Methanol (vapor)	T51.1X1	T51.1X2	T51.1X3	T51.1X4		

Substance	Poisoning, Accidental (unintentional)	Poisoning, Intentional Self-harm	Poisoning, Assault	Poisoning, Undetermined	Adverse Effect	Underdosing
Methantheline	T44.3X1	T44.3X2	T44.3X3	T44.3X4	T44.3X5	T44.3X6
Methanthelinium bromide	T44.3X1	T44.3X2	T44.3X3	T44.3X4	T44.3X5	T44.3X6
Methaphenilene	T45.0X1	T45.0X2	T45.0X3	T45.0X4	T45.0X5	T45.0X6
Methapyrilene	T45.0X1	T45.0X2	T45.0X3	T45.0X4	T45.0X5	T45.0X6
Methaqualone (compound)	T42.6X1	T42.6X2	T42.6X3	T42.6X4	T42.6X5	T42.6X6
Metharbital	T42.3X1	T42.3X2	T42.3X3	T42.3X4	T42.3X5	T42.3X6
Methazolamide	T50.2X1	T50.2X2	T50.2X3	T50.2X4	T50.2X5	T50.2X6
Methdilazine	T43.3X1	T43.3X2	T43.3X3	T43.3X4	T43.3X5	T43.3X6
Methedrine	T43.621	T43.622	T43.623	T43.624	T43.625	T43.626
Methenamine (mandelate)	T37.8X1	T37.8X2	T37.8X3	T37.8X4	T37.8X5	T37.8X6
Methenolone	T38.7X1	T38.7X2	T38.7X3	T38.7X4	T38.7X5	T38.7X6
Methergine	T48.0X1	T48.0X2	T48.0X3	T48.0X4	T48.0X5	T48.0X6
Methetoin	T42.0X1	T42.0X2	T42.0X3	T42.0X4	T42.0X5	T42.0X6
Methiacil	T38.2X1	T38.2X2	T38.2X3	T38.2X4	T38.2X5	T38.2X6
Methicillin	T36.0X1	T36.0X2	T36.0X3	T36.0X4	T36.0X5	T36.0X6
Methimazole	T38.2X1	T38.2X2	T38.2X3	T38.2X4	T38.2X5	T38.2X6
Methiodal sodium	T50.8X1	T50.8X2	T50.8X3	T50.8X4	T50.8X5	T50.8X6
Methionine	T50.991	T50.992	T50.993	T50.994	T50.995	T50.996
Methisazone	T37.5X1	T37.5X2	T37.5X3	T37.5X4	T37.5X5	T37.5X6
Methisoprinol	T37.5X1	T37.5X2	T37.5X3	T37.5X4	T37.5X5	T37.5X6
Methitural	T42.3X1	T42.3X2	T42.3X3	T42.3X4	T42.3X5	T42.3X6
Methixene	T44.3X1	T44.3X2	T44.3X3	T44.3X4	T44.3X5	T44.3X6
Methobarbital, methobarbitone	T42.3X1	T42.3X2	T42.3X3	T42.3X4	T42.3X5	T42.3X6
Methocarbamol	T42.8X1	T42.8X2	T42.8X3	T42.8X4	T42.8X5	T42.8X6
skeletal muscle relaxant	T48.1X1	T48.1X2	T48.1X3	T48.1X4	T48.1X5	T48.1X6
Methohexital	T41.1X1	T41.1X2	T41.1X3	T41.1X4	T41.1X5	T41.1X6
Methohexitone	T41.1X1	T41.1X2	T41.1X3	T41.1X4	T41.1X5	T41.1X6
Methoin	T42.0X1	T42.0X2	T42.0X3	T42.0X4	T42.0X5	T42.0X6
Methopholine	T39.8X1	T39.8X2	T39.8X3	T39.8X4	T39.8X5	T39.8X6
Methopromazine	T43.3X1	T43.3X2	T43.3X3	T43.3X4	T43.3X5	T43.3X6
Methorate	T48.3X1	T48.3X2	T48.3X3	T48.3X4	T48.3X5	T48.3X6
Methoserpidine	T46.5X1	T46.5X2	T46.5X3	T46.5X4	T46.5X5	T46.5X6
Methotrexate	T45.1X1	T45.1X2	T45.1X3	T45.1X4	T45.1X5	T45.1X6
Methotrimeprazine	T43.3X1	T43.3X2	T43.3X3	T43.3X4	T43.3X5	T43.3X6
Methoxa-Dome	T49.3X1	T49.3X2	T49.3X3	T49.3X4	T49.3X5	T49.3X6
Methoxamine	T44.4X1	T44.4X2	T44.4X3	T44.4X4	T44.4X5	T44.4X6
Methoxsalen	T50.991	T50.992	T50.993	T50.994	T50.995	T50.996
Methoxyaniline	T65.3X1	T65.3X2	T65.3X3	T65.3X4	—	—
Methoxybenzyl penicillin	T36.0X1	T36.0X2	T36.0X3	T36.0X4	—	T36.0X6
Methoxychlor	T53.7X1	T53.7X2	T53.7X3	T53.7X4	—	—
Methoxy-DDT	T53.7X1	T53.7X2	T53.7X3	T53.7X4	—	—
Methoxyflurane	T41.0X1	T41.0X2	T41.0X3	T41.0X4	T41.0X5	T41.0X6
Methoxyphenamine	T48.6X1	T48.6X2	T48.6X3	T48.6X4	T48.6X5	T48.6X6
Methoxypromazine	T43.3X1	T43.3X2	T43.3X3	T43.3X4	T43.3X5	T43.3X6
Methscopolamine bromide	T44.3X1	T44.3X2	T44.3X3	T44.3X4	T44.3X5	T44.3X6
Methsuximide	T42.2X1	T42.2X2	T42.2X3	T42.2X4	T42.2X5	T42.2X6
Methyclothiazide	T50.2X1	T50.2X2	T50.2X3	T50.2X4	T50.2X5	T50.2X6
Methyl						
acetate	T52.4X1	T52.4X2	T52.4X3	T52.4X4	—	—
acetone	T52.4X1	T52.4X2	T52.4X3	T52.4X4	—	—
acrylate	T65.891	T65.892	T65.893	T65.894	—	—
alcohol	T51.1X1	T51.1X2	T51.1X3	T51.1X4	—	—
aminophenol	T65.3X1	T65.3X2	T65.3X3	T65.3X4	—	—
amphetamine	T43.621	T43.622	T43.623	T43.624	T43.625	T43.626
androstanolone	T38.7X1	T38.7X2	T38.7X3	T38.7X4	T38.7X5	T38.7X6
atropine	T44.3X1	T44.3X2	T44.3X3	T44.3X4	T44.3X5	T44.3X6
benzene	T52.2X1	T52.2X2	T52.2X3	T52.2X4	—	—
benzoate	T52.8X1	T52.8X2	T52.8X3	T52.8X4	—	—
benzol	T52.2X1	T52.2X2	T52.2X3	T52.2X4	—	—
bromide (gas)	T59.891	T59.892	T59.893	T59.894	—	—
fumigant	T60.8X1	T60.8X2	T60.8X3	T60.8X4	—	—
butanol	T51.3X1	T51.3X2	T51.3X3	T51.3X4	—	—
carbinol	T51.1X1	T51.1X2	T51.1X3	T51.1X4	—	—
carbonate	T52.8X1	T52.8X2	T52.8X3	T52.8X4	—	—
CCNU	T45.1X1	T45.1X2	T45.1X3	T45.1X4	T45.1X5	T45.1X6
cellosolve	T52.91	T52.92	T52.93	T52.94	—	—
cellulose	T47.4X1	T47.4X2	T47.4X3	T47.4X4	T47.4X5	T47.4X6
chloride (gas)	T59.891	T59.892	T59.893	T59.894	—	—
chloroformate	T59.3X1	T59.3X2	T59.3X3	T59.3X4	—	—
cyclohexane	T52.8X1	T52.8X2	T52.8X3	T52.8X4	—	—
cyclohexanol	T51.8X1	T51.8X2	T51.8X3	T51.8X4	—	—
cyclohexanone	T52.8X1	T52.8X2	T52.8X3	T52.8X4	—	—
cyclohexyl acetate	T52.8X1	T52.8X2	T52.8X3	T52.8X4	—	—
demeton	T60.0X1	T60.0X2	T60.0X3	T60.0X4	—	—
dihydromorphinone	T40.2X1	T40.2X2	T40.2X3	T40.2X4	T40.2X5	T40.2X6
ergometrine	T48.0X1	T48.0X2	T48.0X3	T48.0X4	T48.0X5	T48.0X6
ergonovine	T48.0X1	T48.0X2	T48.0X3	T48.0X4	T48.0X5	T48.0X6
ethyl ketone	T52.4X1	T52.4X2	T52.4X3	T52.4X4	—	—
glucamine antimonate	T37.8X1	T37.8X2	T37.8X3	T37.8X4	T37.8X5	T37.8X6
hydrazine	T65.891	T65.892	T65.893	T65.894	—	—
iodide	T65.891	T65.892	T65.893	T65.894	—	—
isobutyl ketone	T52.4X1	T52.4X2	T52.4X3	T52.4X4	—	—
Methyl — continued						
isothiocyanate	T60.3X1	T60.3X2	T60.3X3	T60.3X4	—	—
mercaptan	T59.891	T59.892	T59.893	T59.894	—	—
morphine NEC	T40.2X1	T40.2X2	T40.2X3	T40.2X4	T40.2X5	T40.2X6
nicotinate	T49.4X1	T49.4X2	T49.4X3	T49.4X4	T49.4X5	T49.4X6
paraben	T49.0X1	T49.0X2	T49.0X3	T49.0X4	T49.0X5	T49.0X6
parafynol	T42.6X1	T42.6X2	T42.6X3	T42.6X4	T42.6X5	T42.6X6
parathion	T60.0X1	T60.0X2	T60.0X3	T60.0X4	—	—
peridol	T43.4X1	T43.4X2	T43.4X3	T43.4X4	T43.4X5	T43.4X6
phenidate	T43.631	T43.632	T43.633	T43.634	T43.635	T43.636
prednisolone	T38.0X1	T38.0X2	T38.0X3	T38.0X4	T38.0X5	T38.0X6
ENT agent	T49.6X1	T49.6X2	T49.6X3	T49.6X4	T49.6X5	T49.6X6
ophthalmic preparation	T49.5X1	T49.5X2	T49.5X3	T49.5X4	T49.5X5	T49.5X6
topical NEC	T49.0X1	T49.0X2	T49.0X3	T49.0X4	T49.0X5	T49.0X6
propylcarbinol	T51.3X1	T51.3X2	T51.3X3	T51.3X4	—	—
rosaniline NEC	T49.0X1	T49.0X2	T49.0X3	T49.0X4	T49.0X5	T49.0X6
salicylate	T49.2X1	T49.2X2	T49.2X3	T49.2X4	T49.2X5	T49.2X6
sulfate (fumes)	T59.891	T59.892	T59.893	T59.894	—	—
liquid	T52.8X1	T52.8X2	T52.8X3	T52.8X4	—	—
sulfonal	T42.6X1	T42.6X2	T42.6X3	T42.6X4	T42.6X5	T42.6X6
testosterone	T38.7X1	T38.7X2	T38.7X3	T38.7X4	T38.7X5	T38.7X6
thiouracil	T38.2X1	T38.2X2	T38.2X3	T38.2X4	T38.2X5	T38.2X6
Methylamphetamine	T43.621	T43.622	T43.623	T43.624	T43.625	T43.626
Methylated spirit	T51.1X1	T51.1X2	T51.1X3	T51.1X4	—	—
Methylatropine nitrate	T44.3X1	T44.3X2	T44.3X3	T44.3X4	T44.3X5	T44.3X6
Methylbenactyzium bromide	T44.3X1	T44.3X2	T44.3X3	T44.3X4	T44.3X5	T44.3X6
Methylbenzethonium chloride	T49.0X1	T49.0X2	T49.0X3	T49.0X4	T49.0X5	T49.0X6
Methylcellulose	T47.4X1	T47.4X2	T47.4X3	T47.4X4	T47.4X5	T47.4X6
laxative	T47.4X1	T47.4X2	T47.4X3	T47.4X4	T47.4X5	T47.4X6
Methylchlorophenoxyacetic acid	T60.3X1	T60.3X2	T60.3X3	T60.3X4	—	—
Methyldopa	T46.5X1	T46.5X2	T46.5X3	T46.5X4	T46.5X5	T46.5X6
Methyldopate	T46.5X1	T46.5X2	T46.5X3	T46.5X4	T46.5X5	T46.5X6
Methylene						
blue	T50.6X1	T50.6X2	T50.6X3	T50.6X4	T50.6X5	T50.6X6
chloride or dichloride (solvent) NEC	T53.4X1	T53.4X2	T53.4X3	T53.4X4	—	—
Methylenedioxyamphetamine	T43.621	T43.622	T43.623	T43.624	T43.625	T43.626
Methylenedioxymethamphetamine	T43.621	T43.622	T43.623	T43.624	T43.625	T43.626
Methylergometrine	T48.0X1	T48.0X2	T48.0X3	T48.0X4	T48.0X5	T48.0X6
Methylergonovine	T48.0X1	T48.0X2	T48.0X3	T48.0X4	T48.0X5	T48.0X6
Methylestrenolone	T38.5X1	T38.5X2	T38.5X3	T38.5X4	T38.5X5	T38.5X6
Methylethyl cellulose	T50.991	T50.992	T50.993	T50.994	T50.995	T50.996
Methylhexabital	T42.3X1	T42.3X2	T42.3X3	T42.3X4	T42.3X5	T42.3X6
Methylmorphine	T40.2X1	T40.2X2	T40.2X3	T40.2X4	T40.2X5	T40.2X6
Methylparaben (ophthalmic)	T49.5X1	T49.5X2	T49.5X3	T49.5X4	T49.5X5	T49.5X6
Methylparafynol	T42.6X1	T42.6X2	T42.6X3	T42.6X4	T42.6X5	T42.6X6
Methylpentynol, methylpenthynol	T42.6X1	T42.6X2	T42.6X3	T42.6X4	T42.6X5	T42.6X6
Methylphenidate	T43.631	T43.632	T43.633	T43.634	T43.635	T43.636
Methylphenobarbital	T42.3X1	T42.3X2	T42.3X3	T42.3X4	T42.3X5	T42.3X6
Methylpolysiloxane	T47.1X1	T47.1X2	T47.1X3	T47.1X4	T47.1X5	T47.1X6
Methylprednisolone — see Methyl, prednisolone						
Methylrosaniline	T49.0X1	T49.0X2	T49.0X3	T49.0X4	T49.0X5	T49.0X6
Methylrosanilinium chloride	T49.0X1	T49.0X2	T49.0X3	T49.0X4	T49.0X5	T49.0X6
Methyltestosterone	T38.7X1	T38.7X2	T38.7X3	T38.7X4	T38.7X5	T38.7X6
Methylthionine chloride	T50.6X1	T50.6X2	T50.6X3	T50.6X4	T50.6X5	T50.6X6
Methylthioninium chloride	T50.6X1	T50.6X2	T50.6X3	T50.6X4	T50.6X5	T50.6X6
Methylthiouracil	T38.2X1	T38.2X2	T38.2X3	T38.2X4	T38.2X5	T38.2X6
Methyprylon	T42.6X1	T42.6X2	T42.6X3	T42.6X4	T42.6X5	T42.6X6
Methysergide	T46.5X1	T46.5X2	T46.5X3	T46.5X4	T46.5X5	T46.5X6
Metiamide	T47.1X1	T47.1X2	T47.1X3	T47.1X4	T47.1X5	T47.1X6
Meticillin	T36.0X1	T36.0X2	T36.0X3	T36.0X4	T36.0X5	T36.0X6
Meticrane	T50.2X1	T50.2X2	T50.2X3	T50.2X4	T50.2X5	T50.2X6
Metildigoxin	T46.0X1	T46.0X2	T46.0X3	T46.0X4	T46.0X5	T46.0X6
Metipranolol	T49.5X1	T49.5X2	T49.5X3	T49.5X4	T49.5X5	T49.5X6
Metirosine	T46.5X1	T46.5X2	T46.5X3	T46.5X4	T46.5X5	T46.5X6
Metisazone	T37.5X1	T37.5X2	T37.5X3	T37.5X4	T37.5X5	T37.5X6
Metixene	T44.3X1	T44.3X2	T44.3X3	T44.3X4	T44.3X5	T44.3X6
Metizoline	T48.5X1	T48.5X2	T48.5X3	T48.5X4	T48.5X5	T48.5X6
Metoclopramide	T45.0X1	T45.0X2	T45.0X3	T45.0X4	T45.0X5	T45.0X6
Metofenazate	T43.3X1	T43.3X2	T43.3X3	T43.3X4	T43.3X5	T43.3X6
Metofoline	T39.8X1	T39.8X2	T39.8X3	T39.8X4	T39.8X5	T39.8X6
Metolazone	T50.2X1	T50.2X2	T50.2X3	T50.2X4	T50.2X5	T50.2X6
Metopon	T40.2X1	T40.2X2	T40.2X3	T40.2X4	T40.2X5	T40.2X6
Metopine	T45.1X1	T45.1X2	T45.1X3	T45.1X4	T45.1X5	T45.1X6
Metoprolol	T44.7X1	T44.7X2	T44.7X3	T44.7X4	T44.7X5	T44.7X6
Metrifonate	T60.0X1	T60.0X2	T60.0X3	T60.0X4	—	—

Substance	Poisoning, Accidental (unintentional)	Poisoning, Intentional Self-harm	Poisoning, Assault	Poisoning, Undetermined	Adverse Effect	Under-dosing
Metrizamide	T50.8X1	T50.8X2	T50.8X3	T50.8X4	T50.8X5	T50.8X6
Metrizoic acid	T50.8X1	T50.8X2	T50.8X3	T50.8X4	T50.8X5	T50.8X6
Metronidazole	T37.8X1	T37.8X2	T37.8X3	T37.8X4	T37.8X5	T37.8X6
Metycaine	T41.3X1	T41.3X2	T41.3X3	T41.3X4	T41.3X5	T41.3X6
infiltration (subcutaneous)	T41.3X1	T41.3X2	T41.3X3	T41.3X4	T41.3X5	T41.3X6
nerve block (peripheral) (plexus)	T41.3X1	T41.3X2	T41.3X3	T41.3X4	T41.3X5	T41.3X6
topical (surface)	T41.3X1	T41.3X2	T41.3X3	T41.3X4	T41.3X5	T41.3X6
Metyrapone	T50.8X1	T50.8X2	T50.8X3	T50.8X4	T50.8X5	T50.8X6
Mevinphos	T60.0X1	T60.0X2	T60.0X3	T60.0X4	—	—
Mexazolam	T42.4X1	T42.4X2	T42.4X3	T42.4X4	T42.4X5	T42.4X6
Mexenone	T49.3X1	T49.3X2	T49.3X3	T49.3X4	T49.3X5	T49.3X6
Mexiletine	T46.2X1	T46.2X2	T46.2X3	T46.2X4	T46.2X5	T46.2X6
Mezereon	T62.2X1	T62.2X2	T62.2X3	T62.2X4	—	—
berries	T62.1X1	T62.1X2	T62.1X3	T62.1X4	—	—
Mezlocillin	T36.0X1	T36.0X2	T36.0X3	T36.0X4	T36.0X5	T36.0X6
Mianserin	T43.021	T43.022	T43.023	T43.024	T43.025	T43.026
Micatin	T49.0X1	T49.0X2	T49.0X3	T49.0X4	T49.0X5	T49.0X6
Miconazole	T49.0X1	T49.0X2	T49.0X3	T49.0X4	T49.0X5	T49.0X6
Micronomicin	T36.5X1	T36.5X2	T36.5X3	T36.5X4	T36.5X5	T36.5X6
Midazolam	T42.4X1	T42.4X2	T42.4X3	T42.4X4	T42.4X5	T42.4X6
Midecamycin	T36.3X1	T36.3X2	T36.3X3	T36.3X4	T36.3X5	T36.3X6
Mifepristone	T38.6X1	T38.6X2	T38.6X3	T38.6X4	T38.6X5	T38.6X6
Milk of magnesia	T47.1X1	T47.1X2	T47.1X3	T47.1X4	T47.1X5	T47.1X6
Millipede (tropical) (venomous)	T63.411	T63.412	T63.413	T63.414	—	—
Miltown	T43.591	T43.592	T43.593	T43.594	T43.595	T43.596
Milverine	T44.3X1	T44.3X2	T44.3X3	T44.3X4	T44.3X5	T44.3X6
Minaprine	T43.291	T43.292	T43.293	T43.294	T43.295	T43.296
Minaxolone	T41.291	T41.292	T41.293	T41.294	T41.295	T41.296
Mineral						
acids	T54.2X1	T54.2X2	T54.2X3	T54.2X4	—	—
oil (laxative)(medicinal)	T47.4X1	T47.4X2	T47.4X3	T47.4X4	T47.4X5	T47.4X6
emulsion	T47.2X1	T47.2X2	T47.2X3	T47.2X4	T47.2X5	T47.2X6
nonmedicinal	T52.0X1	T52.0X2	T52.0X3	T52.0X4	—	—
topical	T49.3X1	T49.3X2	T49.3X3	T49.3X4	T49.3X5	T49.3X6
salt NEC	T50.3X1	T50.3X2	T50.3X3	T50.3X4	T50.3X5	T50.3X6
spirits	T52.0X1	T52.0X2	T52.0X3	T52.0X4	—	—
Mineralocorticosteroid	T50.0X1	T50.0X2	T50.0X3	T50.0X4	T50.0X5	T50.0X6
Minocycline	T36.4X1	T36.4X2	T36.4X3	T36.4X4	T36.4X5	T36.4X6
Minoxidil	T46.7X1	T46.7X2	T46.7X3	T46.7X4	T46.7X5	T46.7X6
Miokamycin	T36.3X1	T36.3X2	T36.3X3	T36.3X4	T36.3X5	T36.3X6
Miotic drug	T49.5X1	T49.5X2	T49.5X3	T49.5X4	T49.5X5	T49.5X6
Mipafox	T60.0X1	T60.0X2	T60.0X3	T60.0X4	—	—
Mirex	T60.1X1	T60.1X2	T60.1X3	T60.1X4	—	—
Mirtazapine	T43.021	T43.022	T43.023	T43.024	T43.025	T43.026
Misonidazole	T37.3X1	T37.3X2	T37.3X3	T37.3X4	T37.3X5	T37.3X6
Misoprostol	T47.1X1	T47.1X2	T47.1X3	T47.1X4	T47.1X5	T47.1X6
Mithramycin	T45.1X1	T45.1X2	T45.1X3	T45.1X4	T45.1X5	T45.1X6
Mitobronitol	T45.1X1	T45.1X2	T45.1X3	T45.1X4	T45.1X5	T45.1X6
Mitoguazone	T45.1X1	T45.1X2	T45.1X3	T45.1X4	T45.1X5	T45.1X6
Mitolactol	T45.1X1	T45.1X2	T45.1X3	T45.1X4	T45.1X5	T45.1X6
Mitomycin	T45.1X1	T45.1X2	T45.1X3	T45.1X4	T45.1X5	T45.1X6
Mitopodozide	T45.1X1	T45.1X2	T45.1X3	T45.1X4	T45.1X5	T45.1X6
Mitotane	T45.1X1	T45.1X2	T45.1X3	T45.1X4	T45.1X5	T45.1X6
Mitoxantrone	T45.1X1	T45.1X2	T45.1X3	T45.1X4	T45.1X5	T45.1X6
Mivacurium chloride	T48.1X1	T48.1X2	T48.1X3	T48.1X4	T48.1X5	T48.1X6
Miyari bacteria	T47.6X1	T47.6X2	T47.6X3	T47.6X4	T47.6X5	T47.6X6
Moclobemide	T43.1X1	T43.1X2	T43.1X3	T43.1X4	T43.1X5	T43.1X6
Moderil	T46.5X1	T46.5X2	T46.5X3	T46.5X4	T46.5X5	T46.5X6
Mofebutazone	T39.2X1	T39.2X2	T39.2X3	T39.2X4	T39.2X5	T39.2X6
Mogadon — see Nitrazepam						
Molindone	T43.591	T43.592	T43.593	T43.594	T43.595	T43.596
Molsidomine	T46.3X1	T46.3X2	T46.3X3	T46.3X4	T46.3X5	T46.3X6
Mometasone	T49.0X1	T49.0X2	T49.0X3	T49.0X4	T49.0X5	T49.0X6
Monistat	T49.0X1	T49.0X2	T49.0X3	T49.0X4	T49.0X5	T49.0X6
Monkshood	T62.2X1	T62.2X2	T62.2X3	T62.2X4	—	—
Monoamine oxidase inhibitor NEC	T43.1X1	T43.1X2	T43.1X3	T43.1X4	T43.1X5	T43.1X6
hydrazine	T43.1X1	T43.1X2	T43.1X3	T43.1X4	T43.1X5	T43.1X6
Monobenzone	T49.4X1	T49.4X2	T49.4X3	T49.4X4	T49.4X5	T49.4X6
Monochloroacetic acid	T60.3X1	T60.3X2	T60.3X3	T60.3X4	—	—
Monochlorobenzene	T53.7X1	T53.7X2	T53.7X3	T53.7X4	—	—
Monoethanolamine	T46.8X1	T46.8X2	T46.8X3	T46.8X4	T46.8X5	T46.8X6
oleate	T46.8X1	T46.8X2	T46.8X3	T46.8X4	T46.8X5	T46.8X6
Monooctanoin	T50.991	T50.992	T50.993	T50.994	T50.995	T50.996
Monophenylbutazone	T39.2X1	T39.2X2	T39.2X3	T39.2X4	T39.2X5	T39.2X6
Monosodium glutamate	T65.891	T65.892	T65.893	T65.894	—	—
Monosulfiram	T49.0X1	T49.0X2	T49.0X3	T49.0X4	T49.0X5	T49.0X6
Monoxide, carbon — see Carbon, monoxide						
Monoxidine hydrochloride	T46.1X1	T46.1X2	T46.1X3	T46.1X4	T46.1X5	T46.1X6
Monuron	T60.3X1	T60.3X2	T60.3X3	T60.3X4	—	—

Substance	Poisoning, Accidental (unintentional)	Poisoning, Intentional Self-harm	Poisoning, Assault	Poisoning, Undetermined	Adverse Effect	Under-dosing
Moperone	T43.4X1	T43.4X2	T43.4X3	T43.4X4	T43.4X5	T43.4X6
Mopidamol	T45.1X1	T45.1X2	T45.1X3	T45.1X4	T45.1X5	T45.1X6
MOPP (mechloreth-amine + vincristine + prednisone + procarba-zine)	T45.1X1	T45.1X2	T45.1X3	T45.1X4	T45.1X5	T45.1X6
Morfin	T40.2X1	T40.2X2	T40.2X3	T40.2X4	T40.2X5	T40.2X6
Morinamide	T37.1X1	T37.1X2	T37.1X3	T37.1X4	T37.1X5	T37.1X6
Morning glory seeds	T40.991	T40.992	T40.993	T40.994	—	—
Moroxydine	T37.5X1	T37.5X2	T37.5X3	T37.5X4	T37.5X5	T37.5X6
Morphazinamide	T37.1X1	T37.1X2	T37.1X3	T37.1X4	T37.1X5	T37.1X6
Morphine	T40.2X1	T40.2X2	T40.2X3	T40.2X4	T40.2X5	T40.2X6
antagonist	T50.7X1	T50.7X2	T50.7X3	T50.7X4	T50.7X5	T50.7X6
Morpholinylethylmorphine	T40.2X1	T40.2X2	T40.2X3	T40.2X4		
Morsuximide	T42.2X1	T42.2X2	T42.2X3	T42.2X4	T42.2X5	T42.2X6
Mosapramine	T43.591	T43.592	T43.593	T43.594	T43.595	T43.596
Moth balls — see also Pesticides	T60.2X1	T60.2X2	T60.2X3	T60.2X4		
naphthalene	T60.2X1	T60.2X2	T60.2X3	T60.2X4		
paradichlorobenzene	T60.1X1	T60.1X2	T60.1X3	T60.1X4		
Motor exhaust gas	T58.01	T58.02	T58.03	T58.04		
Mouthwash (antiseptic) (zinc chloride)	T49.6X1	T49.6X2	T49.6X3	T49.6X4	T49.6X5	T49.6X6
Moxastine	T45.0X1	T45.0X2	T45.0X3	T45.0X4	T45.0X5	T45.0X6
Moxaverine	T44.3X1	T44.3X2	T44.3X3	T44.3X4	T44.3X5	T44.3X6
Moxisylyte	T46.7X1	T46.7X2	T46.7X3	T46.7X4	T46.7X5	T46.7X6
Mucilage, plant	T47.4X1	T47.4X2	T47.4X3	T47.4X4	T47.4X5	T47.4X6
Mucolytic drug	T48.4X1	T48.4X2	T48.4X3	T48.4X4	T48.4X5	T48.4X6
Mucomyst	T48.4X1	T48.4X2	T48.4X3	T48.4X4	T48.4X5	T48.4X6
Mucous membrane agents (external)	T49.91	T49.92	T49.93	T49.94	T49.95	T49.96
specified NEC	T49.8X1	T49.8X2	T49.8X3	T49.8X4	T49.8X5	T49.8X6
Mumps						
immune globulin (human)	T50.Z11	T50.Z12	T50.Z13	T50.Z14	T50.Z15	T50.Z16
skin test antigen	T50.8X1	T50.8X2	T50.8X3	T50.8X4	T50.8X5	T50.8X6
vaccine	T50.B91	T50.B92	T50.B93	T50.B94	T50.B95	T50.B96
Mumpsvax	T50.B91	T50.B92	T50.B93	T50.B94	T50.B95	T50.B96
Mupirocin	T49.0X1	T49.0X2	T49.0X3	T49.0X4	T49.0X5	T49.0X6
Muriatic acid — see Hydrochloric acid						
Muromonab-CD3	T45.1X1	T45.1X2	T45.1X3	T45.1X4	T45.1X5	T45.1X6
Muscle-action drug NEC	T48.201	T48.202	T48.203	T48.204	T48.205	T48.206
Muscle affecting agents NEC	T48.201	T48.202	T48.203	T48.204	T48.205	T48.206
oxytocic	T48.0X1	T48.0X2	T48.0X3	T48.0X4	T48.0X5	T48.0X6
relaxants	T48.201	T48.202	T48.203	T48.204	T48.205	T48.206
central nervous system	T42.8X1	T42.8X2	T42.8X3	T42.8X4	T42.8X5	T42.8X6
skeletal	T48.1X1	T48.1X2	T48.1X3	T48.1X4	T48.1X5	T48.1X6
smooth	T44.3X1	T44.3X2	T44.3X3	T44.3X4	T44.3X5	T44.3X6
Muscle relaxant — see Relaxant, muscle						
Muscle-tone depressant, central NEC	T42.8X1	T42.8X2	T42.8X3	T42.8X4	T42.8X5	T42.8X6
specified NEC	T42.8X1	T42.8X2	T42.8X3	T42.8X4	T42.8X5	T42.8X6
Mushroom, noxious	T62.0X1	T62.0X2	T62.0X3	T62.0X4	—	—
Mussel, noxious	T61.781	T61.782	T61.783	T61.784	—	—
Mustard (emetic)	T47.7X1	T47.7X2	T47.7X3	T47.7X4	T47.7X5	T47.7X6
black	T47.7X1	T47.7X2	T47.7X3	T47.7X4	T47.7X5	T47.7X6
gas, not in war	T59.91	T59.92	T59.93	T59.94	—	—
nitrogen	T45.1X1	T45.1X2	T45.1X3	T45.1X4	T45.1X5	T45.1X6
Mustine	T45.1X1	T45.1X2	T45.1X3	T45.1X4	T45.1X5	T45.1X6
M-vac	T45.1X1	T45.1X2	T45.1X3	T45.1X4	T45.1X5	T45.1X6
Mycifradin	T36.5X1	T36.5X2	T36.5X3	T36.5X4	T36.5X5	T36.5X6
topical	T49.0X1	T49.0X2	T49.0X3	T49.0X4	T49.0X5	T49.0X6
Mycitracin	T36.8X1	T36.8X2	T36.8X3	T36.8X4	T36.8X5	T36.8X6
ophthalmic preparation	T49.5X1	T49.5X2	T49.5X3	T49.5X4	T49.5X5	T49.5X6
Mycostatin	T36.7X1	T36.7X2	T36.7X3	T36.7X4	T36.7X5	T36.7X6
topical	T49.0X1	T49.0X2	T49.0X3	T49.0X4	T49.0X5	T49.0X6
Mycotoxins	T64.81	T64.82	T64.83	T64.84	—	—
aflatoxin	T64.01	T64.02	T64.03	T64.04	—	—
specified NEC	T64.81	T64.82	T64.83	T64.84	—	—
Mydriacyl	T44.3X1	T44.3X2	T44.3X3	T44.3X4	T44.3X5	T44.3X6
Mydriatic drug	T49.5X1	T49.5X2	T49.5X3	T49.5X4	T49.5X5	T49.5X6
Myelobromal	T45.1X1	T45.1X2	T45.1X3	T45.1X4	T45.1X5	T45.1X6
Myleran	T45.1X1	T45.1X2	T45.1X3	T45.1X4	T45.1X5	T45.1X6
Myochrysin (e)	T39.2X1	T39.2X2	T39.2X3	T39.2X4	T39.2X5	T39.2X6
Myoneural blocking agents	T48.1X1	T48.1X2	T48.1X3	T48.1X4	T48.1X5	T48.1X6
Myralact	T49.0X1	T49.0X2	T49.0X3	T49.0X4	T49.0X5	T49.0X6
Myristica fragrans	T62.2X1	T62.2X2	T62.2X3	T62.2X4	—	—
Myristicin	T65.891	T65.892	T65.893	T65.894	—	—
Mysoline	T42.3X1	T42.3X2	T42.3X3	T42.3X4	T42.3X5	T42.3X6
Nabilone	T40.7X1	T40.7X2	T40.7X3	T40.7X4	T40.7X5	T40.7X6
Nabumetone	T39.391	T39.392	T39.393	T39.394	T39.395	T39.396
Nadolol	T44.7X1	T44.7X2	T44.7X3	T44.7X4	T44.7X5	T44.7X6

▽ **Subterms under main terms may continue to next column or page** Additional Character May Be Required — Refer to the Tabular List for Character Selection 369

Metrizamide — Nadolol

Substance	Poisoning, Accidental (unintentional)	Poisoning, Intentional Self-harm	Poisoning, Assault	Poisoning, Undetermined	Adverse Effect	Under-dosing
Nafcillin	T36.0X1	T36.0X2	T36.0X3	T36.0X4	T36.0X5	T36.0X6
Nafoxidine	T38.6X1	T38.6X2	T38.6X3	T38.6X4	T38.6X5	T38.6X6
Naftazone	T46.991	T46.992	T46.993	T46.994	T46.995	T46.996
Naftidrofuryl (oxalate)	T46.7X1	T46.7X2	T46.7X3	T46.7X4	T46.7X5	T46.7X6
Naftifine	T49.0X1	T49.0X2	T49.0X3	T49.0X4	T49.0X5	T49.0X6
Nail polish remover	T52.91	T52.92	T52.93	T52.94		
Nalbuphine	T40.4X1	T40.4X2	T40.4X3	T40.4X4	T40.4X5	T40.4X6
Naled	T60.0X1	T60.0X2	T60.0X3	T60.0X4	—	
Nalidixic acid	T37.8X1	T37.8X2	T37.8X3	T37.8X4	T37.8X5	T37.8X6
Nalorphine	T50.7X1	T50.7X2	T50.7X3	T50.7X4	T50.7X5	T50.7X6
Naloxone	T50.7X1	T50.7X2	T50.7X3	T50.7X4	T50.7X5	T50.7X6
Naltrexone	T50.7X1	T50.7X2	T50.7X3	T50.7X4	T50.7X5	T50.7X6
Namenda	T43.8X1	T43.8X2	T43.8X3	T43.8X4	T43.8X5	T43.8X6
Nandrolone	T38.7X1	T38.7X2	T38.7X3	T38.7X4	T38.7X5	T38.7X6
Naphazoline	T48.5X1	T48.5X2	T48.5X3	T48.5X4	T48.5X5	T48.5X6
Naphtha (painters') (petroleum)	T52.0X1	T52.0X2	T52.0X3	T52.0X4	—	
solvent	T52.0X1	T52.0X2	T52.0X3	T52.0X4	—	
vapor	T52.0X1	T52.0X2	T52.0X3	T52.0X4	—	
Naphthalene (non-chlorinated)	T60.2X1	T60.2X2	T60.2X3	T60.2X4	—	
chlorinated	T60.1X1	T60.1X2	T60.1X3	T60.1X4	—	
vapor	T60.1X1	T60.1X2	T60.1X3	T60.1X4	—	
insecticide or moth repellent	T60.2X1	T60.2X2	T60.2X3	T60.2X4	—	
chlorinated	T60.1X1	T60.1X2	T60.1X3	T60.1X4	—	
vapor	T60.2X1	T60.2X2	T60.2X3	T60.2X4	—	
chlorinated	T60.1X1	T60.1X2	T60.1X3	T60.1X4	—	
Naphthol	T65.891	T65.892	T65.893	T65.894	—	
Naphthylamine	T65.891	T65.892	T65.893	T65.894	—	
Naphthylthiourea (ANTU)	T60.4X1	T60.4X2	T60.4X3	T60.4X4	—	
Naprosyn — *see* Naproxen						
Naproxen	T39.311	T39.312	T39.313	T39.314	T39.315	T39.316
Narcotic (drug)	T40.601	T40.602	T40.603	T40.604	T40.605	T40.606
analgesic NEC	T40.601	T40.602	T40.603	T40.604	T40.605	T40.606
antagonist	T50.7X1	T50.7X2	T50.7X3	T50.7X4	T50.7X5	T50.7X6
specified NEC	T40.691	T40.692	T40.693	T40.694	T40.695	T40.696
synthetic	T40.4X1	T40.4X2	T40.4X3	T40.4X4	T40.4X5	T40.4X6
Narcotine	T48.3X1	T48.3X2	T48.3X3	T48.3X4	T48.3X5	T48.3X6
Nardil	T43.1X1	T43.1X2	T43.1X3	T43.1X4	T43.1X5	T43.1X6
Nasal drug NEC	T49.6X1	T49.6X2	T49.6X3	T49.6X4	T49.6X5	T49.6X6
Natamycin	T49.0X1	T49.0X2	T49.0X3	T49.0X4	T49.0X5	T49.0X6
Natrium cyanide — *see* Cyanide(s)						
Natural						
blood (product)	T45.8X1	T45.8X2	T45.8X3	T45.8X4	T45.8X5	T45.8X6
gas (piped)	T59.891	T59.892	T59.893	T59.894	—	
incomplete combustion	T58.11	T58.12	T58.13	T58.14		
Nealbarbital	T42.3X1	T42.3X2	T42.3X3	T42.3X4	T42.3X5	T42.3X6
Nectadon	T48.3X1	T48.3X2	T48.3X3	T48.3X4	T48.3X5	T48.3X6
Nedocromil	T48.6X1	T48.6X2	T48.6X3	T48.6X4	T48.6X5	T48.6X6
Nefopam	T39.8X1	T39.8X2	T39.8X3	T39.8X4	T39.8X5	T39.8X6
Nematocyst (sting)	T63.691	T63.692	T63.693	T63.694		
Nembutal	T42.3X1	T42.3X2	T42.3X3	T42.3X4	T42.3X5	T42.3X6
Nemonapride	T43.591	T43.592	T43.593	T43.594	T43.595	T43.596
Neoarsphenamine	T37.8X1	T37.8X2	T37.8X3	T37.8X4	T37.8X5	T37.8X6
Neocinchophen	T50.4X1	T50.4X2	T50.4X3	T50.4X4	T50.4X5	T50.4X6
Neomycin (derivatives)	T36.5X1	T36.5X2	T36.5X3	T36.5X4	T36.5X5	T36.5X6
with						
bacitracin	T49.0X1	T49.0X2	T49.0X3	T49.0X4	T49.0X5	T49.0X6
neostigmine	T44.0X1	T44.0X2	T44.0X3	T44.0X4	T44.0X5	T44.0X6
ENT agent	T49.6X1	T49.6X2	T49.6X3	T49.6X4	T49.6X5	T49.6X6
ophthalmic preparation	T49.5X1	T49.5X2	T49.5X3	T49.5X4	T49.5X5	T49.5X6
topical NEC	T49.0X1	T49.0X2	T49.0X3	T49.0X4	T49.0X5	T49.0X6
Neonal	T42.3X1	T42.3X2	T42.3X3	T42.3X4	T42.3X5	T42.3X6
Neoprontosil	T37.0X1	T37.0X2	T37.0X3	T37.0X4	T37.0X5	T37.0X6
Neosalvarsan	T37.8X1	T37.8X2	T37.8X3	T37.8X4	T37.8X5	T37.8X6
Neosilversalvarsan	T37.8X1	T37.8X2	T37.8X3	T37.8X4	T37.8X5	T37.8X6
Neosporin	T36.8X1	T36.8X2	T36.8X3	T36.8X4	T36.8X5	T36.8X6
ENT agent	T49.6X1	T49.6X2	T49.6X3	T49.6X4	T49.6X5	T49.6X6
opthalmic preparation	T49.5X1	T49.5X2	T49.5X3	T49.5X4	T49.5X5	T49.5X6
topical NEC	T49.0X1	T49.0X2	T49.0X3	T49.0X4	T49.0X5	T49.0X6
Neostigmine bromide	T44.0X1	T44.0X2	T44.0X3	T44.0X4	T44.0X5	T44.0X6
Neraval	T42.3X1	T42.3X2	T42.3X3	T42.3X4	T42.3X5	T42.3X6
Neravan	T42.3X1	T42.3X2	T42.3X3	T42.3X4	T42.3X5	T42.3X6
Nerium oleander	T62.2X1	T62.2X2	T62.2X3	T62.2X4	—	—
Nerve gas, not in war	T59.91	T59.92	T59.93	T59.94	—	—
Nesacaine	T41.3X1	T41.3X2	T41.3X3	T41.3X4	T41.3X5	T41.3X6
infiltration (subcutaneous)	T41.3X1	T41.3X2	T41.3X3	T41.3X4	T41.3X5	T41.3X6
nerve block (peripheral) (plexus)	T41.3X1	T41.3X2	T41.3X3	T41.3X4	T41.3X5	T41.3X6
Netilmicin	T36.5X1	T36.5X2	T36.5X3	T36.5X4	T36.5X5	T36.5X6
Neurobarb	T42.3X1	T42.3X2	T42.3X3	T42.3X4	T42.3X5	T42.3X6
Neuroleptic drug NEC	T43.501	T43.502	T43.503	T43.504	T43.505	T43.506
Neuromuscular blocking drug	T48.1X1	T48.1X2	T48.1X3	T48.1X4	T48.1X5	T48.1X6
Neutral insulin injection	T38.3X1	T38.3X2	T38.3X3	T38.3X4	T38.3X5	T38.3X6
Neutral spirits	T51.0X1	T51.0X2	T51.0X3	T51.0X4	—	
beverage	T51.0X1	T51.0X2	T51.0X3	T51.0X4	—	
Niacin	T46.7X1	T46.7X2	T46.7X3	T46.7X4	T46.7X5	T46.7X6
Niacinamide	T45.2X1	T45.2X2	T45.2X3	T45.2X4	T45.2X5	T45.2X6
Nialamide	T43.1X1	T43.1X2	T43.1X3	T43.1X4	T43.1X5	T43.1X6
Niaprazine	T42.6X1	T42.6X2	T42.6X3	T42.6X4	T42.6X5	T42.6X6
Nicametate	T46.7X1	T46.7X2	T46.7X3	T46.7X4	T46.7X5	T46.7X6
Nicardipine	T46.1X1	T46.1X2	T46.1X3	T46.1X4	T46.1X5	T46.1X6
Nicergoline	T46.7X1	T46.7X2	T46.7X3	T46.7X4	T46.7X5	T46.7X6
Nickel (carbonyl) (tetra-carbonyl) (fumes) (vapor)	T56.891	T56.892	T56.893	T56.894	—	
Nickelocene	T56.891	T56.892	T56.893	T56.894	—	—
Niclosamide	T37.4X1	T37.4X2	T37.4X3	T37.4X4	T37.4X5	T37.4X6
Nicofuranose	T46.7X1	T46.7X2	T46.7X3	T46.7X4	T46.7X5	T46.7X6
Nicomorphine	T40.2X1	T40.2X2	T40.2X3	T40.2X4	—	
Nicorandil	T46.3X1	T46.3X2	T46.3X3	T46.3X4	T46.3X5	T46.3X6
Nicotiana (plant)	T62.2X1	T62.2X2	T62.2X3	T62.2X4		
Nicotinamide	T45.2X1	T45.2X2	T45.2X3	T45.2X4	T45.2X5	T45.2X6
Nicotine (insecticide) (spray) (sulfate) NEC	T60.2X1	T60.2X2	T60.2X3	T60.2X4	—	
from tobacco	T65.291	T65.292	T65.293	T65.294	—	
cigarettes	T65.221	T65.222	T65.223	T65.224	—	
not insecticide	T65.291	T65.292	T65.293	T65.294		
Nicotinic acid	T46.7X1	T46.7X2	T46.7X3	T46.7X4	T46.7X5	T46.7X6
Nicotinyl alcohol	T46.7X1	T46.7X2	T46.7X3	T46.7X4	T46.7X5	T46.7X6
Nicoumalone	T45.511	T45.512	T45.513	T45.514	T45.515	T45.516
Nifedipine	T46.1X1	T46.1X2	T46.1X3	T46.1X4	T46.1X5	T46.1X6
Nifenazone	T39.2X1	T39.2X2	T39.2X3	T39.2X4	T39.2X5	T39.2X6
Nifuraldezone	T37.91	T37.92	T37.93	T37.94	T37.95	T37.96
Nifuratel	T37.8X1	T37.8X2	T37.8X3	T37.8X4	T37.8X5	T37.8X6
Nifurtimox	T37.3X1	T37.3X2	T37.3X3	T37.3X4	T37.3X5	T37.3X6
Nifurtoinol	T37.8X1	T37.8X2	T37.8X3	T37.8X4	T37.8X5	T37.8X6
Nightshade, deadly (solanum) — *see also* Belladonna	T62.2X1	T62.2X2	T62.2X3	T62.2X4		
berry	T62.1X1	T62.1X2	T62.1X3	T62.1X4		
Nikethamide	T50.7X1	T50.7X2	T50.7X3	T50.7X4	T50.7X5	T50.7X6
Nilstat	T36.7X1	T36.7X2	T36.7X3	T36.7X4	T36.7X5	T36.7X6
topical	T49.0X1	T49.0X2	T49.0X3	T49.0X4	T49.0X5	T49.0X6
Nilutamide	T38.6X1	T38.6X2	T38.6X3	T38.6X4	T38.6X5	T38.6X6
Nimesulide	T39.391	T39.392	T39.393	T39.394	T39.395	T39.396
Nimetazepam	T42.4X1	T42.4X2	T42.4X3	T42.4X4	T42.4X5	T42.4X6
Nimodipine	T46.1X1	T46.1X2	T46.1X3	T46.1X4	T46.1X5	T46.1X6
Nimorazole	T37.3X1	T37.3X2	T37.3X3	T37.3X4	T37.3X5	T37.3X6
Nimustine	T45.1X1	T45.1X2	T45.1X3	T45.1X4	T45.1X5	T45.1X6
Niridazole	T37.4X1	T37.4X2	T37.4X3	T37.4X4	T37.4X5	T37.4X6
Nisentil	T40.2X1	T40.2X2	T40.2X3	T40.2X4	T40.2X5	T40.2X6
Nisoldipine	T46.1X1	T46.1X2	T46.1X3	T46.1X4	T46.1X5	T46.1X6
Nitramine	T65.3X1	T65.3X2	T65.3X3	T65.3X4	—	—
Nitrate, organic	T46.3X1	T46.3X2	T46.3X3	T46.3X4	T46.3X5	T46.3X6
Nitrazepam	T42.4X1	T42.4X2	T42.4X3	T42.4X4	T42.4X5	T42.4X6
Nitrefazole	T50.6X1	T50.6X2	T50.6X3	T50.6X4	T50.6X5	T50.6X6
Nitrendipine	T46.1X1	T46.1X2	T46.1X3	T46.1X4	T46.1X5	T46.1X6
Nitric						
acid (liquid)	T54.2X1	T54.2X2	T54.2X3	T54.2X4	—	
vapor	T59.891	T59.892	T59.893	T59.894	—	
oxide (gas)	T59.0X1	T59.0X2	T59.0X3	T59.0X4	—	
Nitrimidazine	T37.3X1	T37.3X2	T37.3X3	T37.3X4	T37.3X5	T37.3X6
Nitrite, amyl (medicinal) (vapor)	T46.3X1	T46.3X2	T46.3X3	T46.3X4	T46.3X5	T46.3X6
Nitroaniline	T65.3X1	T65.3X2	T65.3X3	T65.3X4	—	
vapor	T59.891	T59.892	T59.893	T59.894	—	
Nitrobenzene, nitrobenzol	T65.3X1	T65.3X2	T65.3X3	T65.3X4	—	
vapor	T65.3X1	T65.3X2	T65.3X3	T65.3X4	—	
Nitrocellulose	T65.891	T65.892	T65.893	T65.894	—	
lacquer	T65.891	T65.892	T65.893	T65.894	—	
Nitrodiphenyl	T65.3X1	T65.3X2	T65.3X3	T65.3X4	—	
Nitrofural	T49.0X1	T49.0X2	T49.0X3	T49.0X4	T49.0X5	T49.0X6
Nitrofurantoin	T37.8X1	T37.8X2	T37.8X3	T37.8X4	T37.8X5	T37.8X6
Nitrofurazone	T49.0X1	T49.0X2	T49.0X3	T49.0X4	T49.0X5	T49.0X6
Nitrogen	T59.0X1	T59.0X2	T59.0X3	T59.0X4	—	
mustard	T45.1X1	T45.1X2	T45.1X3	T45.1X4	T45.1X5	T45.1X6
Nitroglycerin, nitroglycerol (medicinal)	T46.3X1	T46.3X2	T46.3X3	T46.3X4	T46.3X5	T46.3X6
nonmedicinal	T65.5X1	T65.5X2	T65.5X3	T65.5X4	—	
fumes	T65.5X1	T65.5X2	T65.5X3	T65.5X4	—	
Nitroglycol	T52.3X1	T52.3X2	T52.3X3	T52.3X4	—	
Nitrohydrochloric acid	T54.2X1	T54.2X2	T54.2X3	T54.2X4	—	
Nitromersol	T49.0X1	T49.0X2	T49.0X3	T49.0X4	T49.0X5	T49.0X6
Nitronaphthalene	T65.891	T65.892	T65.893	T65.894		

Additional Character May Be Required — Refer to the Tabular List for Character Selection   ▽ Subterms under main terms may continue to next column or page

Substance	Poisoning, Accidental (unintentional)	Poisoning, Intentional Self-harm	Poisoning, Assault	Poisoning, Undetermined	Adverse Effect	Under-dosing
Nitrophenol	T54.0X1	T54.0X2	T54.0X3	T54.0X4	—	—
Nitropropane	T52.8X1	T52.8X2	T52.8X3	T52.8X4	—	—
Nitroprusside	T46.5X1	T46.5X2	T46.5X3	T46.5X4	T46.5X5	T46.5X6
Nitrosodimethylamine	T65.3X1	T65.3X2	T65.3X3	T65.3X4	—	—
Nitrothiazol	T37.4X1	T37.4X2	T37.4X3	T37.4X4	T37.4X5	T37.4X6
Nitrotoluene, nitrotoluol	T65.3X1	T65.3X2	T65.3X3	T65.3X4	—	—
vapor	T65.3X1	T65.3X2	T65.3X3	T65.3X4	—	—
Nitrous						
acid (liquid)	T54.2X1	T54.2X2	T54.2X3	T54.2X4	—	—
fumes	T59.891	T59.892	T59.893	T59.894	—	—
ether spirit	T46.3X1	T46.3X2	T46.3X3	T46.3X4	T46.3X5	T46.3X6
oxide	T41.0X1	T41.0X2	T41.0X3	T41.0X4	T41.0X5	T41.0X6
Nitroxoline	T37.8X1	T37.8X2	T37.8X3	T37.8X4	T37.8X5	T37.8X6
Nitrozone	T49.0X1	T49.0X2	T49.0X3	T49.0X4	T49.0X5	T49.0X6
Nizatidine	T47.0X1	T47.0X2	T47.0X3	T47.0X4	T47.0X5	T47.0X6
Nizofenone	T43.8X1	T43.8X2	T43.8X3	T43.8X4	T43.8X5	T43.8X6
Noctec	T42.6X1	T42.6X2	T42.6X3	T42.6X4	T42.6X5	T42.6X6
Noludar	T42.6X1	T42.6X2	T42.6X3	T42.6X4	T42.6X5	T42.6X6
Nomegestrol	T38.5X1	T38.5X2	T38.5X3	T38.5X4	T38.5X5	T38.5X6
Nomifensine	T43.291	T43.292	T43.293	T43.294	T43.295	T43.296
Nonoxinol	T49.8X1	T49.8X2	T49.8X3	T49.8X4	T49.8X5	T49.8X6
Nonylphenoxy (polyethoxyethanol)	T49.8X1	T49.8X2	T49.8X3	T49.8X4	T49.8X5	T49.8X6
Noptil	T42.3X1	T42.3X2	T42.3X3	T42.3X4	T42.3X5	T42.3X6
Noradrenaline	T44.4X1	T44.4X2	T44.4X3	T44.4X4	T44.4X5	T44.4X6
Noramidopyrine	T39.2X1	T39.2X2	T39.2X3	T39.2X4	T39.2X5	T39.2X6
methanesulfonate sodium	T39.2X1	T39.2X2	T39.2X3	T39.2X4	T39.2X5	T39.2X6
Norbormide	T60.4X1	T60.4X2	T60.4X3	T60.4X4	—	—
Nordazepam	T42.4X1	T42.4X2	T42.4X3	T42.4X4	T42.4X5	T42.4X6
Norepinephrine	T44.4X1	T44.4X2	T44.4X3	T44.4X4	T44.4X5	T44.4X6
Norethandrolone	T38.7X1	T38.7X2	T38.7X3	T38.7X4	T38.7X5	T38.7X6
Norethindrone	T38.4X1	T38.4X2	T38.4X3	T38.4X4	T38.4X5	T38.4X6
Norethisterone (acetate) (enantate)	T38.4X1	T38.4X2	T38.4X3	T38.4X4	T38.4X5	T38.4X6
with ethinylestradiol	T38.5X1	T38.5X2	T38.5X3	T38.5X4	T38.5X5	T38.5X6
Noretynodrel	T38.5X1	T38.5X2	T38.5X3	T38.5X4	T38.5X5	T38.5X6
Norfenefrine	T44.4X1	T44.4X2	T44.4X3	T44.4X4	T44.4X5	T44.4X6
Norfloxacin	T36.8X1	T36.8X2	T36.8X3	T36.8X4	T36.8X5	T36.8X6
Norgestrel	T38.4X1	T38.4X2	T38.4X3	T38.4X4	T38.4X5	T38.4X6
Norgestrienone	T38.4X1	T38.4X2	T38.4X3	T38.4X4	T38.4X5	T38.4X6
Norlestrin	T38.4X1	T38.4X2	T38.4X3	T38.4X4	T38.4X5	T38.4X6
Norlutin	T38.4X1	T38.4X2	T38.4X3	T38.4X4	T38.4X5	T38.4X6
Normal serum albumin (human), salt-poor	T45.8X1	T45.8X2	T45.8X3	T45.8X4	T45.8X5	T45.8X6
Normethandrone	T38.5X1	T38.5X2	T38.5X3	T38.5X4	T38.5X5	T38.5X6
Normison — see Benzodiazepines						
Normorphine	T40.2X1	T40.2X2	T40.2X3	T40.2X4	—	—
Norpseudoephedrine	T50.5X1	T50.5X2	T50.5X3	T50.5X4	T50.5X5	T50.5X6
Nortestosterone (furanpropionate)	T38.7X1	T38.7X2	T38.7X3	T38.7X4	T38.7X5	T38.7X6
Nortriptyline	T43.011	T43.012	T43.013	T43.014	T43.015	T43.016
Noscapine	T48.3X1	T48.3X2	T48.3X3	T48.3X4	T48.3X5	T48.3X6
Nose preparations	T49.6X1	T49.6X2	T49.6X3	T49.6X4	T49.6X5	T49.6X6
Novobiocin	T36.5X1	T36.5X2	T36.5X3	T36.5X4	T36.5X5	T36.5X6
Novocain (infiltration) (topical)	T41.3X1	T41.3X2	T41.3X3	T41.3X4	T41.3X5	T41.3X6
nerve block (peripheral) (plexus)	T41.3X1	T41.3X2	T41.3X3	T41.3X4	T41.3X5	T41.3X6
spinal	T41.3X1	T41.3X2	T41.3X3	T41.3X4	T41.3X5	T41.3X6
Noxious foodstuff	T62.91	T62.92	T62.93	T62.94	—	—
specified NEC	T62.8X1	T62.8X2	T62.8X3	T62.8X4	—	—
Noxiptiline	T43.011	T43.012	T43.013	T43.014	T43.015	T43.016
Noxytiolin	T49.0X1	T49.0X2	T49.0X3	T49.0X4	T49.0X5	T49.0X6
NPH Iletin (insulin)	T38.3X1	T38.3X2	T38.3X3	T38.3X4	T38.3X5	T38.3X6
Numorphan	T40.2X1	T40.2X2	T40.2X3	T40.2X4	T40.2X5	T40.2X6
Nunol	T42.3X1	T42.3X2	T42.3X3	T42.3X4	T42.3X5	T42.3X6
Nupercaine (spinal anesthetic)	T41.3X1	T41.3X2	T41.3X3	T41.3X4	T41.3X5	T41.3X6
topical (surface)	T41.3X1	T41.3X2	T41.3X3	T41.3X4	T41.3X5	T41.3X6
Nutmeg oil (liniment)	T49.3X1	T49.3X2	T49.3X3	T49.3X4	T49.3X5	T49.3X6
Nutritional supplement	T50.901	T50.902	T50.903	T50.904	T50.905	T50.906
Nux vomica	T65.1X1	T65.1X2	T65.1X3	T65.1X4	—	—
Nydrazid	T37.1X1	T37.1X2	T37.1X3	T37.1X4	T37.1X5	T37.1X6
Nylidrin	T46.7X1	T46.7X2	T46.7X3	T46.7X4	T46.7X5	T46.7X6
Nystatin	T36.7X1	T36.7X2	T36.7X3	T36.7X4	T36.7X5	T36.7X6
topical	T49.0X1	T49.0X2	T49.0X3	T49.0X4	T49.0X5	T49.0X6
Nytol	T45.0X1	T45.0X2	T45.0X3	T45.0X4	T45.0X5	T45.0X6
Obidoxime chloride	T50.6X1	T50.6X2	T50.6X3	T50.6X4	T50.6X5	T50.6X6
Octafonium (chloride)	T49.3X1	T49.3X2	T49.3X3	T49.3X4	T49.3X5	T49.3X6
Octamethyl pyrophosphoramide	T60.0X1	T60.0X2	T60.0X3	T60.0X4	—	—
Octanoin	T50.991	T50.992	T50.993	T50.994	T50.995	T50.996
Octatropine methylbromide	T44.3X1	T44.3X2	T44.3X3	T44.3X4	T44.3X5	T44.3X6
Octotiamine	T45.2X1	T45.2X2	T45.2X3	T45.2X4	T45.2X5	T45.2X6
Octoxinol (9)	T49.8X1	T49.8X2	T49.8X3	T49.8X4	T49.8X5	T49.8X6
Octreotide	T38.991	T38.992	T38.993	T38.994	T38.995	T38.996
Octyl nitrite	T46.3X1	T46.3X2	T46.3X3	T46.3X4	T46.3X5	T46.3X6
Oestradiol	T38.5X1	T38.5X2	T38.5X3	T38.5X4	T38.5X5	T38.5X6
Oestriol	T38.5X1	T38.5X2	T38.5X3	T38.5X4	T38.5X5	T38.5X6
Oestrogen	T38.5X1	T38.5X2	T38.5X3	T38.5X4	T38.5X5	T38.5X6
Oestrone	T38.5X1	T38.5X2	T38.5X3	T38.5X4	T38.5X5	T38.5X6
Ofloxacin	T36.8X1	T36.8X2	T36.8X3	T36.8X4	T36.8X5	T36.8X6
Oil (of)	T65.891	T65.892	T65.893	T65.894	—	—
bitter almond	T62.8X1	T62.8X2	T62.8X3	T62.8X4	—	—
cloves	T49.7X1	T49.7X2	T49.7X3	T49.7X4	T49.7X5	T49.7X6
colors	T65.6X1	T65.6X2	T65.6X3	T65.6X4	—	—
fumes	T59.891	T59.892	T59.893	T59.894	—	—
lubricating	T52.0X1	T52.0X2	T52.0X3	T52.0X4	—	—
Niobe	T52.8X1	T52.8X2	T52.8X3	T52.8X4	—	—
vitriol (liquid)	T54.2X1	T54.2X2	T54.2X3	T54.2X4	—	—
fumes	T54.2X1	T54.2X2	T54.2X3	T54.2X4	—	—
wintergreen (bitter) NEC	T49.3X1	T49.3X2	T49.3X3	T49.3X4	T49.3X5	T49.3X6
Oily preparation (for skin)	T49.3X1	T49.3X2	T49.3X3	T49.3X4	T49.3X5	T49.3X6
Ointment NEC	T49.3X1	T49.3X2	T49.3X3	T49.3X4	T49.3X5	T49.3X6
Olanzapine	T43.591	T43.592	T43.593	T43.594	T43.595	T43.596
Oleander	T62.2X1	T62.2X2	T62.2X3	T62.2X4	—	—
Oleandomycin	T36.3X1	T36.3X2	T36.3X3	T36.3X4	T36.3X5	T36.3X6
Oleandrin	T46.0X1	T46.0X2	T46.0X3	T46.0X4	T46.0X5	T46.0X6
Oleic acid	T46.6X1	T46.6X2	T46.6X3	T46.6X4	T46.6X5	T46.6X6
Oleovitamin A	T45.2X1	T45.2X2	T45.2X3	T45.2X4	T45.2X5	T45.2X6
Oleum ricini	T47.2X1	T47.2X2	T47.2X3	T47.2X4	T47.2X5	T47.2X6
Olive oil (medicinal) **NEC**	T47.4X1	T47.4X2	T47.4X3	T47.4X4	T47.4X5	T47.4X6
Olivomycin	T45.1X1	T45.1X2	T45.1X3	T45.1X4	T45.1X5	T45.1X6
Olsalazine	T47.8X1	T47.8X2	T47.8X3	T47.8X4	T47.8X5	T47.8X6
Omeprazole	T47.1X1	T47.1X2	T47.1X3	T47.1X4	T47.1X5	T47.1X6
OMPA	T60.0X1	T60.0X2	T60.0X3	T60.0X4	—	—
Oncovin	T45.1X1	T45.1X2	T45.1X3	T45.1X4	—	T45.1X6
Ondansetron	T45.0X1	T45.0X2	T45.0X3	T45.0X4	T45.0X5	T45.0X6
Ophthaine	T41.3X1	T41.3X2	T41.3X3	T41.3X4	T41.3X5	T41.3X6
Ophthetic	T41.3X1	T41.3X2	T41.3X3	T41.3X4	T41.3X5	T41.3X6
Opiate NEC	T40.601	T40.602	T40.603	T40.604	T40.605	T40.606
antagonists	T50.7X1	T50.7X2	T50.7X3	T50.7X4	T50.7X5	T50.7X6
Opioid NEC	T40.2X1	T40.2X2	T40.2X3	T40.2X4	T40.2X5	T40.2X6
Opipramol	T43.011	T43.012	T43.013	T43.014	T43.015	T43.016
Opium alkaloids (total)	T40.0X1	T40.0X2	T40.0X3	T40.0X4	T40.0X5	T40.0X6
standardized powdered	T40.0X1	T40.0X2	T40.0X3	T40.0X4	T40.0X5	T40.0X6
tincture (camphorated)	T40.0X1	T40.0X2	T40.0X3	T40.0X4	T40.0X5	T40.0X6
Oracon	T38.4X1	T38.4X2	T38.4X3	T38.4X4	T38.4X5	T38.4X6
Oragrafin	T50.8X1	T50.8X2	T50.8X3	T50.8X4	T50.8X5	T50.8X6
Oral contraceptives	T38.4X1	T38.4X2	T38.4X3	T38.4X4	T38.4X5	T38.4X6
Oral rehydration salts	T50.3X1	T50.3X2	T50.3X3	T50.3X4	T50.3X5	T50.3X6
Orazamide	T50.991	T50.992	T50.993	T50.994	T50.995	T50.996
Orciprenaline	T48.291	T48.292	T48.293	T48.294	T48.295	T48.296
Organidin	T48.4X1	T48.4X2	T48.4X3	T48.4X4	T48.4X5	T48.4X6
Organonitrate NEC	T46.3X1	T46.3X2	T46.3X3	T46.3X4	T46.3X5	T46.3X6
Organophosphates	T60.0X1	T60.0X2	T60.0X3	T60.0X4	—	—
Orimune	T50.B91	T50.B92	T50.B93	T50.B94	T50.B95	T50.B96
Orinase	T38.3X1	T38.3X2	T38.3X3	T38.3X4	T38.3X5	T38.3X6
Ormeloxifene	T38.6X1	T38.6X2	T38.6X3	T38.6X4	T38.6X5	T38.6X6
Ornidazole	T37.3X1	T37.3X2	T37.3X3	T37.3X4	T37.3X5	T37.3X6
Ornithine aspartate	T50.991	T50.992	T50.993	T50.994	T50.995	T50.996
Ornoprostil	T47.1X1	T47.1X2	T47.1X3	T47.1X4	T47.1X5	T47.1X6
Orphenadrine (hydrochloride)	T42.8X1	T42.8X2	T42.8X3	T42.8X4	T42.8X5	T42.8X6
Ortal (sodium)	T42.3X1	T42.3X2	T42.3X3	T42.3X4	T42.3X5	T42.3X6
Orthoboric acid	T49.0X1	T49.0X2	T49.0X3	T49.0X4	T49.0X5	T49.0X6
ENT agent	T49.6X1	T49.6X2	T49.6X3	T49.6X4	T49.6X5	T49.6X6
ophthalmic preparation	T49.5X1	T49.5X2	T49.5X3	T49.5X4	T49.5X5	T49.5X6
Orthocaine	T41.3X1	T41.3X2	T41.3X3	T41.3X4	T41.3X5	T41.3X6
Orthodichlorobenzene	T53.7X1	T53.7X2	T53.7X3	T53.7X4	—	—
Ortho-Novum	T38.4X1	T38.4X2	T38.4X3	T38.4X4	T38.4X5	T38.4X6
Orthotolidine (reagent)	T54.2X1	T54.2X2	T54.2X3	T54.2X4	—	—
Osmic acid (liquid)	T54.2X1	T54.2X2	T54.2X3	T54.2X4	—	—
fumes	T54.2X1	T54.2X2	T54.2X3	T54.2X4	—	—
Osmotic diuretics	T50.2X1	T50.2X2	T50.2X3	T50.2X4	T50.2X5	T50.2X6
Otilonium bromide	T44.3X1	T44.3X2	T44.3X3	T44.3X4	T44.3X5	T44.3X6
Otorhinolaryngological drug NEC	T49.6X1	T49.6X2	T49.6X3	T49.6X4	T49.6X5	T49.6X6
Ouabain (e)	T46.0X1	T46.0X2	T46.0X3	T46.0X4	T46.0X5	T46.0X6
Ovarian						
hormone	T38.5X1	T38.5X2	T38.5X3	T38.5X4	T38.5X5	T38.5X6
stimulant	T38.5X1	T38.5X2	T38.5X3	T38.5X4	T38.5X5	T38.5X6
Ovral	T38.4X1	T38.4X2	T38.4X3	T38.4X4	T38.4X5	T38.4X6
Ovulen	T38.4X1	T38.4X2	T38.4X3	T38.4X4	T38.4X5	T38.4X6

▽ Subterms under main terms may continue to next column or page   Additional Character May Be Required — Refer to the Tabular List for Character Selection   371

Nitrophenol — Ovulen

Substance	Poisoning, Accidental (unintentional)	Poisoning, Intentional Self-harm	Poisoning, Assault	Poisoning, Undetermined	Adverse Effect	Under-dosing
Oxacillin	T36.0X1	T36.0X2	T36.0X3	T36.0X4	T36.0X5	T36.0X6
Oxalic acid	T54.2X1	T54.2X2	T54.2X3	T54.2X4		
ammonium salt	T50.991	T50.992	T50.993	T50.994	T50.995	T50.996
Oxamniquine	T37.4X1	T37.4X2	T37.4X3	T37.4X4	T37.4X5	T37.4X6
Oxanamide	T43.591	T43.592	T43.593	T43.594	T43.595	T43.596
Oxandrolone	T38.7X1	T38.7X2	T38.7X3	T38.7X4	T38.7X5	T38.7X6
Oxantel	T37.4X1	T37.4X2	T37.4X3	T37.4X4	T37.4X5	T37.4X6
Oxapium iodide	T44.3X1	T44.3X2	T44.3X3	T44.3X4	T44.3X5	T44.3X6
Oxaprotiline	T43.021	T43.022	T43.023	T43.024	T43.025	T43.026
Oxaprozin	T39.311	T39.312	T39.313	T39.314	T39.315	T39.316
Oxatomide	T45.0X1	T45.0X2	T45.0X3	T45.0X4	T45.0X5	T45.0X6
Oxazepam	T42.4X1	T42.4X2	T42.4X3	T42.4X4	T42.4X5	T42.4X6
Oxazimedrine	T50.5X1	T50.5X2	T50.5X3	T50.5X4	T50.5X5	T50.5X6
Oxazolam	T42.4X1	T42.4X2	T42.4X3	T42.4X4	T42.4X5	T42.4X6
Oxazolidine derivatives	T42.2X1	T42.2X2	T42.2X3	T42.2X4	T42.2X5	T42.2X6
Oxazolidinedione (derivative)	T42.2X1	T42.2X2	T42.2X3	T42.2X4	T42.2X5	T42.2X6
Ox bile extract	T47.5X1	T47.5X2	T47.5X3	T47.5X4	T47.5X5	T47.5X6
Oxcarbazepine	T42.1X1	T42.1X2	T42.1X3	T42.1X4	T42.1X5	T42.1X6
Oxedrine	T44.4X1	T44.4X2	T44.4X3	T44.4X4	T44.4X5	T44.4X6
Oxeladin (citrate)	T48.3X1	T48.3X2	T48.3X3	T48.3X4	T48.3X5	T48.3X6
Oxendolone	T38.5X1	T38.5X2	T38.5X3	T38.5X4	T38.5X5	T38.5X6
Oxetacaine	T41.3X1	T41.3X2	T41.3X3	T41.3X4	T41.3X5	T41.3X6
Oxethazine	T41.3X1	T41.3X2	T41.3X3	T41.3X4	T41.3X5	T41.3X6
Oxetorone	T39.8X1	T39.8X2	T39.8X3	T39.8X4	T39.8X5	T39.8X6
Oxiconazole	T49.0X1	T49.0X2	T49.0X3	T49.0X4	T49.0X5	T49.0X6
Oxidizing agent NEC	T54.91	T54.92	T54.93	T54.94		
Oxipurinol	T50.4X1	T50.4X2	T50.4X3	T50.4X4	T50.4X5	T50.4X6
Oxitriptan	T43.291	T43.292	T43.293	T43.294	T43.295	T43.296
Oxitropium bromide	T48.6X1	T48.6X2	T48.6X3	T48.6X4	T48.6X5	T48.6X6
Oxodipine	T46.1X1	T46.1X2	T46.1X3	T46.1X4	T46.1X5	T46.1X6
Oxolamine	T48.3X1	T48.3X2	T48.3X3	T48.3X4	T48.3X5	T48.3X6
Oxolinic acid	T37.8X1	T37.8X2	T37.8X3	T37.8X4	T37.8X5	T37.8X6
Oxomemazine	T43.3X1	T43.3X2	T43.3X3	T43.3X4	T43.3X5	T43.3X6
Oxophenarsine	T37.3X1	T37.3X2	T37.3X3	T37.3X4	T37.3X5	T37.3X6
Oxprenolol	T44.7X1	T44.7X2	T44.7X3	T44.7X4	T44.7X5	T44.7X6
Oxsoralen	T49.3X1	T49.3X2	T49.3X3	T49.3X4	T49.3X5	T49.3X6
Oxtriphylline	T48.6X1	T48.6X2	T48.6X3	T48.6X4	T48.6X5	T48.6X6
Oxybate sodium	T41.291	T41.292	T41.293	T41.294	T41.295	T41.296
Oxybuprocaine	T41.3X1	T41.3X2	T41.3X3	T41.3X4	T41.3X5	T41.3X6
Oxybutynin	T44.3X1	T44.3X2	T44.3X3	T44.3X4	T44.3X5	T44.3X6
Oxychlorosene	T49.0X1	T49.0X2	T49.0X3	T49.0X4	T49.0X5	T49.0X6
Oxycodone	T40.2X1	T40.2X2	T40.2X3	T40.2X4	T40.2X5	T40.2X6
Oxyfedrine	T46.3X1	T46.3X2	T46.3X3	T46.3X4	T46.3X5	T46.3X6
Oxygen	T41.5X1	T41.5X2	T41.5X3	T41.5X4	T41.5X5	T41.5X6
Oxylone	T49.0X1	T49.0X2	T49.0X3	T49.0X4	T49.0X5	T49.0X6
ophthalmic preparation	T49.5X1	T49.5X2	T49.5X3	T49.5X4	T49.5X5	T49.5X6
Oxymesterone	T38.7X1	T38.7X2	T38.7X3	T38.7X4	T38.7X5	T38.7X6
Oxymetazoline	T48.5X1	T48.5X2	T48.5X3	T48.5X4	T48.5X5	T48.5X6
Oxymetholone	T38.7X1	T38.7X2	T38.7X3	T38.7X4	T38.7X5	T38.7X6
Oxymorphone	T40.2X1	T40.2X2	T40.2X3	T40.2X4	T40.2X5	T40.2X6
Oxypertine	T43.591	T43.592	T43.593	T43.594	T43.595	T43.596
Oxyphenbutazone	T39.2X1	T39.2X2	T39.2X3	T39.2X4	T39.2X5	T39.2X6
Oxyphencyclimine	T44.3X1	T44.3X2	T44.3X3	T44.3X4	T44.3X5	T44.3X6
Oxyphenisatine	T47.2X1	T47.2X2	T47.2X3	T47.2X4	T47.2X5	T47.2X6
Oxyphenonium bromide	T44.3X1	T44.3X2	T44.3X3	T44.3X4	T44.3X5	T44.3X6
Oxypolygelatin	T45.8X1	T45.8X2	T45.8X3	T45.8X4	T45.8X5	T45.8X6
Oxyquinoline (derivatives)	T37.8X1	T37.8X2	T37.8X3	T37.8X4	T37.8X5	T37.8X6
Oxytetracycline	T36.4X1	T36.4X2	T36.4X3	T36.4X4	T36.4X5	T36.4X6
Oxytocic drug NEC	T48.0X1	T48.0X2	T48.0X3	T48.0X4	T48.0X5	T48.0X6
Oxytocin (synthetic)	T48.0X1	T48.0X2	T48.0X3	T48.0X4	T48.0X5	T48.0X6
Ozone	T59.891	T59.892	T59.893	T59.894	—	—
PABA	T49.3X1	T49.3X2	T49.3X3	T49.3X4	T49.3X5	T49.3X6
Packed red cells	T45.8X1	T45.8X2	T45.8X3	T45.8X4	T45.8X5	T45.8X6
Padimate	T49.3X1	T49.3X2	T49.3X3	T49.3X4	T49.3X5	T49.3X6
Paint NEC	T65.6X1	T65.6X2	T65.6X3	T65.6X4	—	—
cleaner	T52.91	T52.92	T52.93	T52.94	—	—
fumes NEC	T59.891	T59.892	T59.893	T59.894	—	—
lead (fumes)	T56.0X1	T56.0X2	T56.0X3	T56.0X4	—	—
solvent NEC	T52.8X1	T52.8X2	T52.8X3	T52.8X4	—	—
stripper	T52.8X1	T52.8X2	T52.8X3	T52.8X4	—	—
Palfium	T40.2X1	T40.2X2	T40.2X3	T40.2X4	—	—
Palm kernel oil	T50.991	T50.992	T50.993	T50.994	T50.995	T50.996
Paludrine	T37.2X1	T37.2X2	T37.2X3	T37.2X4	T37.2X5	T37.2X6
PAM (pralidoxime)	T50.6X1	T50.6X2	T50.6X3	T50.6X4	T50.6X5	T50.6X6
Pamaquine (naphthoute)	T37.2X1	T37.2X2	T37.2X3	T37.2X4	T37.2X5	T37.2X6
Panadol	T39.1X1	T39.1X2	T39.1X3	T39.1X4	T39.1X5	T39.1X6
Pancreatic						
digestive secretion stimulant	T47.8X1	T47.8X2	T47.8X3	T47.8X4	T47.8X5	T47.8X6
dornase	T45.3X1	T45.3X2	T45.3X3	T45.3X4	T45.3X5	T45.3X6
Pancreatin	T47.5X1	T47.5X2	T47.5X3	T47.5X4	T47.5X5	T47.5X6
Pancrelipase	T47.5X1	T47.5X2	T47.5X3	T47.5X4	T47.5X5	T47.5X6

Substance	Poisoning, Accidental (unintentional)	Poisoning, Intentional Self-harm	Poisoning, Assault	Poisoning, Undetermined	Adverse Effect	Under-dosing
Pancuronium (bromide)	T48.1X1	T48.1X2	T48.1X3	T48.1X4	T48.1X5	T48.1X6
Pangamic acid	T45.2X1	T45.2X2	T45.2X3	T45.2X4	T45.2X5	T45.2X6
Panthenol	T45.2X1	T45.2X2	T45.2X3	T45.2X4	T45.2X5	T45.2X6
topical	T49.8X1	T49.8X2	T49.8X3	T49.8X4	T49.8X5	T49.8X6
Pantopon	T40.0X1	T40.0X2	T40.0X3	T40.0X4	T40.0X5	T40.0X6
Pantothenic acid	T45.2X1	T45.2X2	T45.2X3	T45.2X4	T45.2X5	T45.2X6
Panwarfin	T45.511	T45.512	T45.513	T45.514	T45.515	T45.516
Papain	T47.5X1	T47.5X2	T47.5X3	T47.5X4	T47.5X5	T47.5X6
digestant	T47.5X1	T47.5X2	T47.5X3	T47.5X4	T47.5X5	T47.5X6
Papaveretum	T40.0X1	T40.0X2	T40.0X3	T40.0X4	T40.0X5	T40.0X6
Papaverine	T44.3X1	T44.3X2	T44.3X3	T44.3X4	T44.3X5	T44.3X6
Para-acetamidophenol	T39.1X1	T39.1X2	T39.1X3	T39.1X4	T39.1X5	T39.1X6
Para-aminobenzoic acid	T49.3X1	T49.3X2	T49.3X3	T49.3X4	T49.3X5	T49.3X6
Para-aminophenol derivatives	T39.1X1	T39.1X2	T39.1X3	T39.1X4	T39.1X5	T39.1X6
Para-aminosalicylic acid	T37.1X1	T37.1X2	T37.1X3	T37.1X4	T37.1X5	T37.1X6
Paracetaldehyde	T42.6X1	T42.6X2	T42.6X3	T42.6X4	T42.6X5	T42.6X6
Paracetamol	T39.1X1	T39.1X2	T39.1X3	T39.1X4	T39.1X5	T39.1X6
Parachlorophenol (camphorated)	T49.0X1	T49.0X2	T49.0X3	T49.0X4	T49.0X5	T49.0X6
Paracodin	T40.2X1	T40.2X2	T40.2X3	T40.2X4	T40.2X5	T40.2X6
Paradione	T42.2X1	T42.2X2	T42.2X3	T42.2X4	T42.2X5	T42.2X6
Paraffin(s) (wax)	T52.0X1	T52.0X2	T52.0X3	T52.0X4		
liquid (medicinal)	T47.4X1	T47.4X2	T47.4X3	T47.4X4	T47.4X5	T47.4X6
nonmedicinal	T52.0X1	T52.0X2	T52.0X3	T52.0X4	—	—
Paraformaldehyde	T60.3X1	T60.3X2	T60.3X3	T60.3X4	—	—
Paraldehyde	T42.6X1	T42.6X2	T42.6X3	T42.6X4	T42.6X5	T42.6X6
Paramethadione	T42.2X1	T42.2X2	T42.2X3	T42.2X4	T42.2X5	T42.2X6
Paramethasone	T38.0X1	T38.0X2	T38.0X3	T38.0X4	T38.0X5	T38.0X6
acetate	T49.0X1	T49.0X2	T49.0X3	T49.0X4	T49.0X5	T49.0X6
Paraoxon	T60.0X1	T60.0X2	T60.0X3	T60.0X4	—	—
Paraquat	T60.3X1	T60.3X2	T60.3X3	T60.3X4	—	—
Parasympatholytic NEC	T44.3X1	T44.3X2	T44.3X3	T44.3X4	T44.3X5	T44.3X6
Parasympathomimetic drug NEC	T44.1X1	T44.1X2	T44.1X3	T44.1X4	T44.1X5	T44.1X6
Parathion	T60.0X1	T60.0X2	T60.0X3	T60.0X4	—	—
Parathormone	T50.991	T50.992	T50.993	T50.994	T50.995	T50.996
Parathyroid extract	T50.991	T50.992	T50.993	T50.994	T50.995	T50.996
Paratyphoid vaccine	T50.A91	T50.A92	T50.A93	T50.A94	T50.A95	T50.A96
Paredrine	T44.4X1	T44.4X2	T44.4X3	T44.4X4	T44.4X5	T44.4X6
Paregoric	T40.0X1	T40.0X2	T40.0X3	T40.0X4	T40.0X5	T40.0X6
Pargyline	T46.5X1	T46.5X2	T46.5X3	T46.5X4	T46.5X5	T46.5X6
Paris green	T57.0X1	T57.0X2	T57.0X3	T57.0X4	—	—
insecticide	T57.0X1	T57.0X2	T57.0X3	T57.0X4	—	—
Parnate	T43.1X1	T43.1X2	T43.1X3	T43.1X4	T43.1X5	T43.1X6
Paromomycin	T36.5X1	T36.5X2	T36.5X3	T36.5X4	T36.5X5	T36.5X6
Paroxypropione	T45.1X1	T45.1X2	T45.1X3	T45.1X4	T45.1X5	T45.1X6
Parzone	T40.2X1	T40.2X2	T40.2X3	T40.2X4	T40.2X5	T40.2X6
PAS	T37.1X1	T37.1X2	T37.1X3	T37.1X4	T37.1X5	T37.1X6
Pasiniazid	T37.1X1	T37.1X2	T37.1X3	T37.1X4	T37.1X5	T37.1X6
PBB (polybrominated biphenyls)	T65.891	T65.892	T65.893	T65.894	—	—
PCB	T65.891	T65.892	T65.893	T65.894	—	—
PCP						
meaning pentachlorophenol	T60.1X1	T60.1X2	T60.1X3	T60.1X4	—	—
fungicide	T60.3X1	T60.3X2	T60.3X3	T60.3X4	—	—
herbicide	T60.3X1	T60.3X2	T60.3X3	T60.3X4	—	—
insecticide	T60.1X1	T60.1X2	T60.1X3	T60.1X4	—	—
meaning phencyclidine	T40.991	T40.992	T40.993	T40.994	—	—
Peach kernel oil (emulsion)	T47.4X1	T47.4X2	T47.4X3	T47.4X4	T47.4X5	T47.4X6
Peanut oil (emulsion) NEC	T47.4X1	T47.4X2	T47.4X3	T47.4X4	T47.4X5	T47.4X6
topical	T49.3X1	T49.3X2	T49.3X3	T49.3X4	T49.3X5	T49.3X6
Pearly Gates (morning glory seeds)	T40.991	T40.992	T40.993	T40.994		
Pecazine	T43.3X1	T43.3X2	T43.3X3	T43.3X4	T43.3X5	T43.3X6
Pectin	T47.6X1	T47.6X2	T47.6X3	T47.6X4	T47.6X5	T47.6X6
Pefloxacin	T37.8X1	T37.8X2	T37.8X3	T37.8X4	T37.8X5	T37.8X6
Pegademase, bovine	T50.Z91	T50.Z92	T50.Z93	T50.Z94	T50.Z95	T50.Z96
Pelletierine tannate	T37.4X1	T37.4X2	T37.4X3	T37.4X4	T37.4X5	T37.4X6
Pemirolast (potassium)	T48.6X1	T48.6X2	T48.6X3	T48.6X4	T48.6X5	T48.6X6
Pemoline	T50.7X1	T50.7X2	T50.7X3	T50.7X4	T50.7X5	T50.7X6
Pempidine	T44.2X1	T44.2X2	T44.2X3	T44.2X4	T44.2X5	T44.2X6
Penamecillin	T36.0X1	T36.0X2	T36.0X3	T36.0X4	T36.0X5	T36.0X6
Penbutolol	T44.7X1	T44.7X2	T44.7X3	T44.7X4	T44.7X5	T44.7X6
Penethamate	T36.0X1	T36.0X2	T36.0X3	T36.0X4	T36.0X5	T36.0X6
Penfluridol	T43.591	T43.592	T43.593	T43.594	T43.595	T43.596
Penflutizide	T50.2X1	T50.2X2	T50.2X3	T50.2X4	T50.2X5	T50.2X6
Pengitoxin	T46.0X1	T46.0X2	T46.0X3	T46.0X4	T46.0X5	T46.0X6
Penicillamine	T50.6X1	T50.6X2	T50.6X3	T50.6X4	T50.6X5	T50.6X6
Penicillin (any)	T36.0X1	T36.0X2	T36.0X3	T36.0X4	T36.0X5	T36.0X6
Penicillinase	T45.3X1	T45.3X2	T45.3X3	T45.3X4	T45.3X5	T45.3X6
Penicilloyl polylysine	T50.8X1	T50.8X2	T50.8X3	T50.8X4	T50.8X5	T50.8X6

Substance	Poisoning, Accidental (unintentional)	Poisoning, Intentional Self-harm	Poisoning, Assault	Poisoning, Undetermined	Adverse Effect	Under-dosing
Penimepicycline	T36.4X1	T36.4X2	T36.4X3	T36.4X4	T36.4X5	T36.4X6
Pentachloroethane	T53.6X1	T53.6X2	T53.6X3	T53.6X4	—	—
Pentachloronaphthalene	T53.7X1	T53.7X2	T53.7X3	T53.7X4	—	—
Pentachlorophenol	T60.1X1	T60.1X2	T60.1X3	T60.1X4	—	—
(pesticide)						
fungicide	T60.3X1	T60.3X2	T60.3X3	T60.3X4	—	—
herbicide	T60.3X1	T60.3X2	T60.3X3	T60.3X4	—	—
insecticide	T60.1X1	T60.1X2	T60.1X3	T60.1X4	—	—
Pentaerythritol	T46.3X1	T46.3X2	T46.3X3	T46.3X4	T46.3X5	T46.3X6
chloral	T42.6X1	T42.6X2	T42.6X3	T42.6X4	T42.6X5	T42.6X6
tetranitrate NEC	T46.3X1	T46.3X2	T46.3X3	T46.3X4	T46.3X5	T46.3X6
Pentaerythrityl	T46.3X1	T46.3X2	T46.3X3	T46.3X4	T46.3X5	T46.3X6
tetranitrate						
Pentagastrin	T50.8X1	T50.8X2	T50.8X3	T50.8X4	T50.8X5	T50.8X6
Pentalin	T53.6X1	T53.6X2	T53.6X3	T53.6X4	—	—
Pentamethonium bromide	T44.2X1	T44.2X2	T44.2X3	T44.2X4	T44.2X5	T44.2X6
Pentamidine	T37.3X1	T37.3X2	T37.3X3	T37.3X4	T37.3X5	T37.3X6
Pentanol	T51.3X1	T51.3X2	T51.3X3	T51.3X4	—	—
Pentapyrrolinium	T44.2X1	T44.2X2	T44.2X3	T44.2X4	T44.2X5	T44.2X6
(bitartrate)						
Pentaquine	T37.2X1	T37.2X2	T37.2X3	T37.2X4	T37.2X5	T37.2X6
Pentazocine	T40.4X1	T40.4X2	T40.4X3	T40.4X4	T40.4X5	T40.4X6
Pentetrazole	T50.7X1	T50.7X2	T50.7X3	T50.7X4	T50.7X5	T50.7X6
Penthienate bromide	T44.3X1	T44.3X2	T44.3X3	T44.3X4	T44.3X5	T44.3X6
Pentifylline	T46.7X1	T46.7X2	T46.7X3	T46.7X4	T46.7X5	T46.7X6
Pentobarbital	T42.3X1	T42.3X2	T42.3X3	T42.3X4	T42.3X5	T42.3X6
sodium	T42.3X1	T42.3X2	T42.3X3	T42.3X4	T42.3X5	T42.3X6
Pentobarbitone	T42.3X1	T42.3X2	T42.3X3	T42.3X4	T42.3X5	T42.3X6
Pentolonium tartrate	T44.2X1	T44.2X2	T44.2X3	T44.2X4	T44.2X5	T44.2X6
Pentosan polysulfate	T39.8X1	T39.8X2	T39.8X3	T39.8X4	T39.8X5	T39.8X6
(sodium)						
Pentostatin	T45.1X1	T45.1X2	T45.1X3	T45.1X4	T45.1X5	T45.1X6
Pentothal	T41.1X1	T41.1X2	T41.1X3	T41.1X4	T41.1X5	T41.1X6
Pentoxifylline	T46.7X1	T46.7X2	T46.7X3	T46.7X4	T46.7X5	T46.7X6
Pentoxyverine	T48.3X1	T48.3X2	T48.3X3	T48.3X4	T48.3X5	T48.3X6
Pentrinat	T46.3X1	T46.3X2	T46.3X3	T46.3X4	T46.3X5	T46.3X6
Pentylenetetrazole	T50.7X1	T50.7X2	T50.7X3	T50.7X4	T50.7X5	T50.7X6
Pentylsalicylamide	T37.1X1	T37.1X2	T37.1X3	T37.1X4	T37.1X5	T37.1X6
Pentymal	T42.3X1	T42.3X2	T42.3X3	T42.3X4	T42.3X5	T42.3X6
Peplomycin	T45.1X1	T45.1X2	T45.1X3	T45.1X4	T45.1X5	T45.1X6
Peppermint (oil)	T47.5X1	T47.5X2	T47.5X3	T47.5X4	T47.5X5	T47.5X6
Pepsin	T47.5X1	T47.5X2	T47.5X3	T47.5X4	T47.5X5	T47.5X6
digestant	T47.5X1	T47.5X2	T47.5X3	T47.5X4	T47.5X5	T47.5X6
Pepstatin	T47.1X1	T47.1X2	T47.1X3	T47.1X4	T47.1X5	T47.1X6
Peptavlon	T50.8X1	T50.8X2	T50.8X3	T50.8X4	T50.8X5	T50.8X6
Perazine	T43.3X1	T43.3X2	T43.3X3	T43.3X4	T43.3X5	T43.3X6
Percaine (spinal)	T41.3X1	T41.3X2	T41.3X3	T41.3X4	T41.3X5	T41.3X6
topical (surface)	T41.3X1	T41.3X2	T41.3X3	T41.3X4	T41.3X5	T41.3X6
Perchloroethylene	T53.3X1	T53.3X2	T53.3X3	T53.3X4	—	—
medicinal	T37.4X1	T37.4X2	T37.4X3	T37.4X4	T37.4X5	T37.4X6
vapor	T53.3X1	T53.3X2	T53.3X3	T53.3X4	—	—
Percodan	T40.2X1	T40.2X2	T40.2X3	T40.2X4	T40.2X5	T40.2X6
Percogesic — see also	T45.0X1	T45.0X2	T45.0X3	T45.0X4	T45.0X5	T45.0X6
acetaminophen						
Percorten	T38.0X1	T38.0X2	T38.0X3	T38.0X4	T38.0X5	T38.0X6
Pergolide	T42.8X1	T42.8X2	T42.8X3	T42.8X4	T42.8X5	T42.8X6
Pergonal	T38.811	T38.812	T38.813	T38.814	T38.815	T38.816
Perhexilene	T46.3X1	T46.3X2	T46.3X3	T46.3X4	T46.3X5	T46.3X6
Perhexiline (maleate)	T46.3X1	T46.3X2	T46.3X3	T46.3X4	T46.3X5	T46.3X6
Periactin	T45.0X1	T45.0X2	T45.0X3	T45.0X4	T45.0X5	T45.0X6
Periciazine	T43.3X1	T43.3X2	T43.3X3	T43.3X4	T43.3X5	T43.3X6
Periclor	T42.6X1	T42.6X2	T42.6X3	T42.6X4	T42.6X5	T42.6X6
Perindopril	T46.4X1	T46.4X2	T46.4X3	T46.4X4	T46.4X5	T46.4X6
Perisoxal	T39.8X1	T39.8X2	T39.8X3	T39.8X4	T39.8X5	T39.8X6
Peritoneal dialysis solution	T50.3X1	T50.3X2	T50.3X3	T50.3X4	T50.3X5	T50.3X6
Peritrate	T46.3X1	T46.3X2	T46.3X3	T46.3X4	T46.3X5	T46.3X6
Perlapine	T42.4X1	T42.4X2	T42.4X3	T42.4X4	T42.4X5	T42.4X6
Permanganate	T65.891	T65.892	T65.893	T65.894	—	—
Permethrin	T60.1X1	T60.1X2	T60.1X3	T60.1X4	—	—
Pernocton	T42.3X1	T42.3X2	T42.3X3	T42.3X4	T42.3X5	T42.3X6
Pernoston	T42.3X1	T42.3X2	T42.3X3	T42.3X4	T42.3X5	T42.3X6
Peronine	T40.2X1	T40.2X2	T40.2X3	T40.2X4	—	—
Perphenazine	T43.3X1	T43.3X2	T43.3X3	T43.3X4	T43.3X5	T43.3X6
Pertofrane	T43.011	T43.012	T43.013	T43.014	T43.015	T43.016
Pertussis						
immune serum (human)	T50.Z11	T50.Z12	T50.Z13	T50.Z14	T50.Z15	T50.Z16
vaccine (with diphtheria toxoid)	T50.A11	T50.A12	T50.A13	T50.A14	T50.A15	T50.A16
(with tetanus toxoid)						
Peruvian balsam	T49.0X1	T49.0X2	T49.0X3	T49.0X4	T49.0X5	T49.0X6
Peruvoside	T46.0X1	T46.0X2	T46.0X3	T46.0X4	T46.0X5	T46.0X6
Pesticide (dust) (fumes) (vapor)	T60.91	T60.92	T60.93	T60.94	—	—
NEC						
arsenic	T57.0X1	T57.0X2	T57.0X3	T57.0X4	—	—
Pesticide (dust) (fumes) (vapor)						
NEC — continued						
chlorinated	T60.1X1	T60.1X2	T60.1X3	T60.1X4	—	—
cyanide	T65.0X1	T65.0X2	T65.0X3	T65.0X4	—	—
kerosene	T52.0X1	T52.0X2	T52.0X3	T52.0X4	—	—
mixture (of compounds)	T60.91	T60.92	T60.93	T60.94		
naphthalene	T60.2X1	T60.2X2	T60.2X3	T60.2X4	—	—
organochlorine	T60.1X1	T60.1X2	T60.1X3	T60.1X4	—	—
(compounds)						
petroleum (distillate) (products) NEC	T60.8X1	T60.8X2	T60.8X3	T60.8X4	—	—
specified ingredient NEC	T60.8X1	T60.8X2	T60.8X3	T60.8X4	—	—
strychnine	T65.1X1	T65.1X2	T65.1X3	T65.1X4	—	—
thallium	T60.4X1	T60.4X2	T60.4X3	T60.4X4	—	—
Pethidine	T40.4X1	T40.4X2	T40.4X3	T40.4X4	T40.4X5	T40.4X6
Petrichloral	T42.6X1	T42.6X2	T42.6X3	T42.6X4	T42.6X5	T42.6X6
Petrol	T52.0X1	T52.0X2	T52.0X3	T52.0X4	—	—
vapor	T52.0X1	T52.0X2	T52.0X3	T52.0X4	—	—
Petrolatum	T49.3X1	T49.3X2	T49.3X3	T49.3X4	T49.3X5	T49.3X6
hydrophilic	T49.3X1	T49.3X2	T49.3X3	T49.3X4	T49.3X5	T49.3X6
liquid	T47.4X1	T47.4X2	T47.4X3	T47.4X4	T47.4X5	T47.4X6
topical	T49.3X1	T49.3X2	T49.3X3	T49.3X4	T49.3X5	T49.3X6
nonmedicinal	T52.0X1	T52.0X2	T52.0X3	T52.0X4	—	—
red veterinary	T49.3X1	T49.3X2	T49.3X3	T49.3X4	T49.3X5	T49.3X6
white	T49.3X1	T49.3X2	T49.3X3	T49.3X4	T49.3X5	T49.3X6
Petroleum (products) NEC	T52.0X1	T52.0X2	T52.0X3	T52.0X4	—	—
benzine(s) — see Ligroin						
ether — see Ligroin						
jelly — see Petrolatum						
naphtha — see Ligroin						
pesticide	T60.8X1	T60.8X2	T60.8X3	T60.8X4	—	—
solids	T52.0X1	T52.0X2	T52.0X3	T52.0X4	—	—
solvents	T52.0X1	T52.0X2	T52.0X3	T52.0X4	—	—
vapor	T52.0X1	T52.0X2	T52.0X3	T52.0X4	—	—
Peyote	T40.991	T40.992	T40.993	T40.994		
Phanodorm, phanodorn	T42.3X1	T42.3X2	T42.3X3	T42.3X4	T42.3X5	T42.3X6
Phanquinone	T37.3X1	T37.3X2	T37.3X3	T37.3X4	T37.3X5	T37.3X6
Phanquone	T37.3X1	T37.3X2	T37.3X3	T37.3X4	T37.3X5	T37.3X6
Pharmaceutical						
adjunct NEC	T50.901	T50.902	T50.903	T50.904	T50.905	T50.906
excipient NEC	T50.901	T50.902	T50.903	T50.904	T50.905	T50.906
sweetener	T50.901	T50.902	T50.903	T50.904	T50.905	T50.906
viscous agent	T50.901	T50.902	T50.903	T50.904	T50.905	T50.906
Phemitone	T42.3X1	T42.3X2	T42.3X3	T42.3X4	T42.3X5	T42.3X6
Phenacaine	T41.3X1	T41.3X2	T41.3X3	T41.3X4	T41.3X5	T41.3X6
Phenacemide	T42.6X1	T42.6X2	T42.6X3	T42.6X4	T42.6X5	T42.6X6
Phenacetin	T39.1X1	T39.1X2	T39.1X3	T39.1X4	T39.1X5	T39.1X6
Phenadoxone	T40.2X1	T40.2X2	T40.2X3	T40.2X4		
Phenaglycodol	T43.591	T43.592	T43.593	T43.594	T43.595	T43.596
Phenantoin	T42.0X1	T42.0X2	T42.0X3	T42.0X4	T42.0X5	T42.0X6
Phenaphthazine reagent	T50.991	T50.992	T50.993	T50.994	T50.995	T50.996
Phenazocine	T40.4X1	T40.4X2	T40.4X3	T40.4X4	T40.4X5	T40.4X6
Phenazone	T39.2X1	T39.2X2	T39.2X3	T39.2X4	T39.2X5	T39.2X6
Phenazopyridine	T39.8X1	T39.8X2	T39.8X3	T39.8X4	T39.8X5	T39.8X6
Phenbenicillin	T36.0X1	T36.0X2	T36.0X3	T36.0X4	T36.0X5	T36.0X6
Phenbutrazate	T50.5X1	T50.5X2	T50.5X3	T50.5X4	T50.5X5	T50.5X6
Phencyclidine	T40.991	T40.992	T40.993	T40.994	T40.995	T40.996
Phendimetrazine	T50.5X1	T50.5X2	T50.5X3	T50.5X4	T50.5X5	T50.5X6
Phenelzine	T43.1X1	T43.1X2	T43.1X3	T43.1X4	T43.1X5	T43.1X6
Phenemal	T42.3X1	T42.3X2	T42.3X3	T42.3X4	T42.3X5	T42.3X6
Phenergan	T42.6X1	T42.6X2	T42.6X3	T42.6X4	T42.6X5	T42.6X6
Pheneticillin	T36.0X1	T36.0X2	T36.0X3	T36.0X4	T36.0X5	T36.0X6
Pheneturide	T42.6X1	T42.6X2	T42.6X3	T42.6X4	T42.6X5	T42.6X6
Phenformin	T38.3X1	T38.3X2	T38.3X3	T38.3X4	T38.3X5	T38.3X6
Phenglutarimide	T44.3X1	T44.3X2	T44.3X3	T44.3X4	T44.3X5	T44.3X6
Phenicarbazide	T39.8X1	T39.8X2	T39.8X3	T39.8X4	T39.8X5	T39.8X6
Phenindamine	T45.0X1	T45.0X2	T45.0X3	T45.0X4	T45.0X5	T45.0X6
Phenindione	T45.511	T45.511	T45.511	T45.514	T45.515	T45.516
Pheniprazine	T43.1X1	T43.1X2	T43.1X3	T43.1X4	T43.1X5	T43.1X6
Pheniramine	T45.0X1	T45.0X2	T45.0X3	T45.0X4	T45.0X5	T45.0X6
Phenisatin	T47.2X1	T47.2X2	T47.2X3	T47.2X4	T47.2X5	T47.2X6
Phenmetrazine	T50.5X1	T50.5X2	T50.5X3	T50.5X4	T50.5X5	T50.5X6
Phenobal	T42.3X1	T42.3X2	T42.3X3	T42.3X4	T42.3X5	T42.3X6
Phenobarbital	T42.3X1	T42.3X2	T42.3X3	T42.3X4	T42.3X5	T42.3X6
with						
mephenytoin	T42.3X1	T42.3X2	T42.3X3	T42.3X4	T42.3X5	T42.3X6
phenytoin	T42.3X1	T42.3X2	T42.3X3	T42.3X4	T42.3X5	T42.3X6
sodium	T42.3X1	T42.3X2	T42.3X3	T42.3X4	T42.3X5	T42.3X6
Phenobarbitone	T42.3X1	T42.3X2	T42.3X3	T42.3X4	T42.3X5	T42.3X6
Phenobutiodil	T50.8X1	T50.8X2	T50.8X3	T50.8X4	T50.8X5	T50.8X6
Phenoctide	T49.0X1	T49.0X2	T49.0X3	T49.0X4	T49.0X5	T49.0X6
Phenol	T49.0X1	T49.0X2	T49.0X3	T49.0X4	T49.0X5	T49.0X6
disinfectant	T54.0X1	T54.0X2	T54.0X3	T54.0X4		

Table of Drugs and Chemicals

Substance	Poisoning, Accidental (unintentional)	Poisoning, Intentional Self-harm	Poisoning, Assault	Poisoning, Undetermined	Adverse Effect	Under-dosing
Phenol — *continued*						
in oil injection	T46.8X1	T46.8X2	T46.8X3	T46.8X4	T46.8X5	T46.8X6
medicinal	T49.1X1	T49.1X2	T49.1X3	T49.1X4	T49.1X5	T49.1X6
nonmedicinal NEC	T54.0X1	T54.0X2	T54.0X3	T54.0X4	—	—
pesticide	T60.8X1	T60.8X2	T60.8X3	T60.8X4	—	—
red	T50.8X1	T50.8X2	T50.8X3	T50.8X4	T50.8X5	T50.8X6
Phenolic preparation	T49.1X1	T49.1X2	T49.1X3	T49.1X4	T49.1X5	T49.1X6
Phenolphthalein	T47.2X1	T47.2X2	T47.2X3	T47.2X4	T47.2X5	T47.2X6
Phenolsulfonphthalein	T50.8X1	T50.8X2	T50.8X3	T50.8X4	T50.8X5	T50.8X6
Phenomorphan	T40.2X1	T40.2X2	T40.2X3	T40.2X4	—	—
Phenonyl	T42.3X1	T42.3X2	T42.3X3	T42.3X4	T42.3X5	T42.3X6
Phenoperidine	T40.4X1	T40.4X2	T40.4X3	T40.4X4	—	—
Phenopyrazone	T46.991	T46.992	T46.993	T46.994	T46.995	T46.996
Phenoquin	T50.4X1	T50.4X2	T50.4X3	T50.4X4	T50.4X5	T50.4X6
Phenothiazine (psychotropic) NEC	T43.3X1	T43.3X2	T43.3X3	T43.3X4	T43.3X5	T43.3X6
insecticide	T60.2X1	T60.2X2	T60.2X3	T60.2X4	—	—
Phenothrin	T49.0X1	T49.0X2	T49.0X3	T49.0X4	T49.0X5	T49.0X6
Phenoxybenzamine	T46.7X1	T46.7X2	T46.7X3	T46.7X4	T46.7X5	T46.7X6
Phenoxyethanol	T49.0X1	T49.0X2	T49.0X3	T49.0X4	T49.0X5	T49.0X6
Phenoxymethyl penicillin	T36.0X1	T36.0X2	T36.0X3	T36.0X4	T36.0X5	T36.0X6
Phenprobamate	T42.8X1	T42.8X2	T42.8X3	T42.8X4	T42.8X5	T42.8X6
Phenprocoumon	T45.511	T45.512	T45.513	T45.514	T45.515	T45.516
Phensuximide	T42.2X1	T42.2X2	T42.2X3	T42.2X4	T42.2X5	T42.2X6
Phentermine	T50.5X1	T50.5X2	T50.5X3	T50.5X4	T50.5X5	T50.5X6
Phenthicillin	T36.0X1	T36.0X2	T36.0X3	T36.0X4	T36.0X5	T36.0X6
Phentolamine	T46.7X1	T46.7X2	T46.7X3	T46.7X4	T46.7X5	T46.7X6
Phenyl						
butazone	T39.2X1	T39.2X2	T39.2X3	T39.2X4	T39.2X5	T39.2X6
enediamine	T65.3X1	T65.3X2	T65.3X3	T65.3X4	—	—
hydrazine	T65.3X1	T65.3X2	T65.3X3	T65.3X4	—	—
antineoplastic	T45.1X1	T45.1X2	T45.1X3	T45.1X4	T45.1X5	T45.1X6
mercuric compounds — *see* Mercury						
salicylate	T49.3X1	T49.3X2	T49.3X3	T49.3X4	T49.3X5	T49.3X6
Phenylalanine mustard	T45.1X1	T45.1X2	T45.1X3	T45.1X4	T45.1X5	T45.1X6
Phenylbutazone	T39.2X1	T39.2X2	T39.2X3	T39.2X4	T39.2X5	T39.2X6
Phenylenediamine	T65.3X1	T65.3X2	T65.3X3	T65.3X4	—	—
Phenylephrine	T44.4X1	T44.4X2	T44.4X3	T44.4X4	T44.4X5	T44.4X6
Phenylethylbiguanide	T38.3X1	T38.3X2	T38.3X3	T38.3X4	T38.3X5	T38.3X6
Phenylmercuric						
acetate	T49.0X1	T49.0X2	T49.0X3	T49.0X4	T49.0X5	T49.0X6
borate	T49.0X1	T49.0X2	T49.0X3	T49.0X4	T49.0X5	T49.0X6
nitrate	T49.0X1	T49.0X2	T49.0X3	T49.0X4	T49.0X5	T49.0X6
Phenylmethylbarbitone	T42.3X1	T42.3X2	T42.3X3	T42.3X4	T42.3X5	T42.3X6
Phenylpropanol	T47.5X1	T47.5X2	T47.5X3	T47.5X4	T47.5X5	T47.5X6
Phenylpropanolamine	T44.991	T44.992	T44.993	T44.994	T44.995	T44.996
Phenylsulfthion	T60.0X1	T60.0X2	T60.0X3	T60.0X4	—	—
Phenyltoloxamine	T45.0X1	T45.0X2	T45.0X3	T45.0X4	T45.0X5	T45.0X6
Phenyramidol, phenyramidon	T39.8X1	T39.8X2	T39.8X3	T39.8X4	T39.8X5	T39.8X6
Phenytoin	T42.0X1	T42.0X2	T42.0X3	T42.0X4	T42.0X5	T42.0X6
with Phenobarbital	T42.3X1	T42.3X2	T42.3X3	T42.3X4	T42.3X5	T42.3X6
pHisoHex	T49.2X1	T49.2X2	T49.2X3	T49.2X4	T49.2X5	T49.2X6
Pholcodine	T48.3X1	T48.3X2	T48.3X3	T48.3X4	T48.3X5	T48.3X6
Pholedrine	T46.991	T46.992	T46.993	T46.994	T46.995	T46.996
Phorate	T60.0X1	T60.0X2	T60.0X3	T60.0X4	—	—
Phosdrin	T60.0X1	T60.0X2	T60.0X3	T60.0X4	—	—
Phosfolan	T60.0X1	T60.0X2	T60.0X3	T60.0X4	—	—
Phosgene (gas)	T59.891	T59.892	T59.893	T59.894	—	—
Phosphamidon	T60.0X1	T60.0X2	T60.0X3	T60.0X4	—	—
Phosphate	T65.891	T65.892	T65.893	T65.894	—	—
laxative	T47.4X1	T47.4X2	T47.4X3	T47.4X4	T47.4X5	T47.4X6
organic	T60.0X1	T60.0X2	T60.0X3	T60.0X4	—	—
solvent	T52.91	T52.92	T52.93	T52.94	—	—
tricresyl	T65.891	T65.892	T65.893	T65.894	—	—
Phosphine	T57.1X1	T57.1X2	T57.1X3	T57.1X4	—	—
fumigant	T57.1X1	T57.1X2	T57.1X3	T57.1X4	—	—
Phospholine	T49.5X1	T49.5X2	T49.5X3	T49.5X4	T49.5X5	T49.5X6
Phosphoric acid	T54.2X1	T54.2X2	T54.2X3	T54.2X4	—	—
Phosphorus (compound) NEC	T57.1X1	T57.1X2	T57.1X3	T57.1X4	—	—
pesticide	T60.0X1	T60.0X2	T60.0X3	T60.0X4	—	—
Phthalates	T65.891	T65.892	T65.893	T65.894	—	—
Phthalic anhydride	I65.891	T65.892	T65.893	T65.894	—	—
Phthalimidoglutarimide	T42.6X1	T42.6X2	T42.6X3	T42.6X4	T42.6X5	T42.6X6
Phthalylsulfathiazole	T37.0X1	T37.0X2	T37.0X3	T37.0X4	T37.0X5	T37.0X6
Phylloquinone	T45.7X1	T45.7X2	T45.7X3	T45.7X4	T45.7X5	T45.7X6
Physeptone	T40.3X1	T40.3X2	T40.3X3	T40.3X4	T40.3X5	T40.3X6
Physostigma venenosum	T62.2X1	T62.2X2	T62.2X3	T62.2X4	—	—
Physostigmine	T49.5X1	T49.5X2	T49.5X3	T49.5X4	T49.5X5	T49.5X6
Phytolacca decandra	T62.2X1	T62.2X2	T62.2X3	T62.2X4	—	—
berries	T62.1X1	T62.1X2	T62.1X3	T62.1X4	—	—

Substance	Poisoning, Accidental (unintentional)	Poisoning, Intentional Self-harm	Poisoning, Assault	Poisoning, Undetermined	Adverse Effect	Under-dosing
Phytomenadione	T45.7X1	T45.7X2	T45.7X3	T45.7X4	T45.7X5	T45.7X6
Phytonadione	T45.7X1	T45.7X2	T45.7X3	T45.7X4	T45.7X5	T45.7X6
Picoperine	T48.3X1	T48.3X2	T48.3X3	T48.3X4	T48.3X5	T48.3X6
Picosulfate (sodium)	T47.2X1	T47.2X2	T47.2X3	T47.2X4	T47.2X5	T47.2X6
Picric (acid)	T54.2X1	T54.2X2	T54.2X3	T54.2X4	—	—
Picrotoxin	T50.7X1	T50.7X2	T50.7X3	T50.7X4	T50.7X5	T50.7X6
Piketoprofen	T49.0X1	T49.0X2	T49.0X3	T49.0X4	T49.0X5	T49.0X6
Pilocarpine	T44.1X1	T44.1X2	T44.1X3	T44.1X4	T44.1X5	T44.1X6
Pilocarpus (jaborandi) extract	T44.1X1	T44.1X2	T44.1X3	T44.1X4	T44.1X5	T44.1X6
Pilsicainide (hydrochloride)	T46.2X1	T46.2X2	T46.2X3	T46.2X4	T46.2X5	T46.2X6
Pimaricin	T36.7X1	T36.7X2	T36.7X3	T36.7X4	T36.7X5	T36.7X6
Pimeclone	T50.7X1	T50.7X2	T50.7X3	T50.7X4	T50.7X5	T50.7X6
Pimelic ketone	T52.8X1	T52.8X2	T52.8X3	T52.8X4	—	—
Pimethixene	T45.0X1	T45.0X2	T45.0X3	T45.0X4	T45.0X5	T45.0X6
Piminodine	T40.2X1	T40.2X2	T40.2X3	T40.2X4	T40.2X5	T40.2X6
Pimozide	T43.591	T43.592	T43.593	T43.594	T43.595	T43.596
Pinacidil	T46.5X1	T46.5X2	T46.5X3	T46.5X4	T46.5X5	T46.5X6
Pinaverium bromide	T44.3X1	T44.3X2	T44.3X3	T44.3X4	T44.3X5	T44.3X6
Pinazepam	T42.4X1	T42.4X2	T42.4X3	T42.4X4	T42.4X5	T42.4X6
Pindolol	T44.7X1	T44.7X2	T44.7X3	T44.7X4	T44.7X5	T44.7X6
Pindone	T60.4X1	T60.4X2	T60.4X3	T60.4X4	—	—
Pine oil (disinfectant)	T65.891	T65.892	T65.893	T65.894	—	—
Pinkroot	T37.4X1	T37.4X2	T37.4X3	T37.4X4	T37.4X5	T37.4X6
Pipadone	T40.2X1	T40.2X2	T40.2X3	T40.2X4	—	—
Pipamazine	T45.0X1	T45.0X2	T45.0X3	T45.0X4	T45.0X5	T45.0X6
Pipamperone	T43.4X1	T43.4X2	T43.4X3	T43.4X4	T43.4X5	T43.4X6
Pipazetate	T48.3X1	T48.3X2	T48.3X3	T48.3X4	T48.3X5	T48.3X6
Pipemidic acid	T37.8X1	T37.8X2	T37.8X3	T37.8X4	T37.8X5	T37.8X6
Pipenzolate bromide	T44.3X1	T44.3X2	T44.3X3	T44.3X4	T44.3X5	T44.3X6
Piperacetazine	T43.3X1	T43.3X2	T43.3X3	T43.3X4	T43.3X5	T43.3X6
Piperacillin	T36.0X1	T36.0X2	T36.0X3	T36.0X4	T36.0X5	T36.0X6
Piperazine	T37.4X1	T37.4X2	T37.4X3	T37.4X4	T37.4X5	T37.4X6
estrone sulfate	T38.5X1	T38.5X2	T38.5X3	T38.5X4	T38.5X5	T38.5X6
Piper cubeba	T62.2X1	T62.2X2	T62.2X3	T62.2X4	—	—
Piperidione	T48.3X1	T48.3X2	T48.3X3	T48.3X4	T48.3X5	T48.3X6
Piperidolate	T44.3X1	T44.3X2	T44.3X3	T44.3X4	T44.3X5	T44.3X6
Piperocaine						
infiltration (subcutaneous)	T41.3X1	T41.3X2	T41.3X3	T41.3X4	T41.3X5	T41.3X6
nerve block (peripheral) (plexus)	T41.3X1	T41.3X2	T41.3X3	T41.3X4	T41.3X5	T41.3X6
topical (surface)	T41.3X1	T41.3X2	T41.3X3	T41.3X4	T41.3X5	T41.3X6
Piperonyl butoxide	T60.8X1	T60.8X2	T60.8X3	T60.8X4	—	—
Pipethanate	T44.3X1	T44.3X2	T44.3X3	T44.3X4	T44.3X5	T44.3X6
Pipobroman	T45.1X1	T45.1X2	T45.1X3	T45.1X4	T45.1X5	T45.1X6
Pipotiazine	T43.3X1	T43.3X2	T43.3X3	T43.3X4	T43.3X5	T43.3X6
Pipoxizine	T45.0X1	T45.0X2	T45.0X3	T45.0X4	T45.0X5	T45.0X6
Pipradrol	T43.691	T43.692	T43.693	T43.694	T43.695	T43.696
Piprinhydrinate	T45.0X1	T45.0X2	T45.0X3	T45.0X4	T45.0X5	T45.0X6
Pirarubicin	T45.1X1	T45.1X2	T45.1X3	T45.1X4	T45.1X5	T45.1X6
Pirazinamide	T37.1X1	T37.1X2	T37.1X3	T37.1X4	T37.1X5	T37.1X6
Pirbuterol	T48.6X1	T48.6X2	T48.6X3	T48.6X4	T48.6X5	T48.6X6
Pirenzepine	T47.1X1	T47.1X2	T47.1X3	T47.1X4	T47.1X5	T47.1X6
Piretanide	T50.1X1	T50.1X2	T50.1X3	T50.1X4	T50.1X5	T50.1X6
Piribedil	T42.8X1	T42.8X2	T42.8X3	T42.8X4	T42.8X5	T42.8X6
Piridoxilate	T46.3X1	T46.3X2	T46.3X3	T46.3X4	T46.3X5	T46.3X6
Piritramide	T40.4X1	T40.4X2	T40.4X3	T40.4X4	—	—
Piromidic acid	T37.8X1	T37.8X2	T37.8X3	T37.8X4	T37.8X5	T37.8X6
Piroxicam	T39.391	T39.392	T39.393	T39.394	T39.395	T39.396
beta-cyclodextrin complex	T39.8X1	T39.8X2	T39.8X3	T39.8X4	T39.8X5	T39.8X6
Pirozadil	T46.6X1	T46.6X2	T46.6X3	T46.6X4	T46.6X5	T46.6X6
Piscidia (bark) (erythrina)	T39.8X1	T39.8X2	T39.8X3	T39.8X4	T39.8X5	T39.8X6
Pitch	T65.891	T65.892	T65.893	T65.894	—	—
Pitkin's solution	T41.3X1	T41.3X2	T41.3X3	T41.3X4	T41.3X5	T41.3X6
Pitocin	T48.0X1	T48.0X2	T48.0X3	T48.0X4	T48.0X5	T48.0X6
Pitressin (tannate)	T38.891	T38.892	T38.893	T38.894	T38.895	T38.896
Pituitary extracts (posterior)	T38.891	T38.892	T38.893	T38.894	T38.895	T38.896
anterior	T38.811	T38.812	T38.813	T38.814	T38.815	T38.816
Pituitrin	T38.891	T38.892	T38.893	T38.894	T38.895	T38.896
Pivampicillin	T36.0X1	T36.0X2	T36.0X3	T36.0X4	T36.0X5	T36.0X6
Pivmecillinam	T36.0X1	T36.0X2	T36.0X3	T36.0X4	T36.0X5	T36.0X6
Placental hormone	T38.891	T38.892	T38.893	T38.894	T38.895	T38.896
Placidyl	T42.6X1	T42.6X2	T42.6X3	T42.6X4	T42.6X5	T42.6X6
Plague vaccine	T50.A91	T50.A92	T50.A93	T50.A94	T50.A95	T50.A96
Plant						
food or fertilizer NEC	T65.891	T65.892	T65.893	T65.894	—	—
containing herbicide	T60.3X1	T60.3X2	T60.3X3	T60.3X4	—	—
noxious, used as food	T62.2X1	T62.2X2	T62.2X3	T62.2X4	—	—
berries	T62.1X1	T62.1X2	T62.1X3	T62.1X4	—	—
seeds	T62.2X1	T62.2X2	T62.2X3	T62.2X4	—	—
specified type NEC	T62.2X1	T62.2X2	T62.2X3	T62.2X4	—	—
Plasma	T45.8X1	T45.8X2	T45.8X3	T45.8X4	T45.8X5	T45.8X6
expander NEC	T45.8X1	T45.8X2	T45.8X3	T45.8X4	T45.8X5	T45.8X6

Additional Character May Be Required — Refer to the Tabular List for Character Selection

▽ Subterms under main terms may continue to next column or page

Phenol — Plasma

Substance	Poisoning, Accidental (unintentional)	Poisoning, Intentional Self-harm	Poisoning, Assault	Poisoning, Undetermined	Adverse Effect	Under-dosing
Plasma — *continued*						
protein fraction (human)	T45.8X1	T45.8X2	T45.8X3	T45.8X4	T45.8X5	T45.8X6
Plasmanate	T45.8X1	T45.8X2	T45.8X3	T45.8X4	T45.8X5	T45.8X6
Plasminogen (tissue)	T45.611	T45.612	T45.613	T45.614	T45.615	T45.616
activator						
Plaster dressing	T49.3X1	T49.3X2	T49.3X3	T49.3X4	T49.3X5	T49.3X6
Plastic dressing	T49.3X1	T49.3X2	T49.3X3	T49.3X4	T49.3X5	T49.3X6
Plegicil	T43.3X1	T43.3X2	T43.3X3	T43.3X4	T43.3X5	T43.3X6
Plicamycin	T45.1X1	T45.1X2	T45.1X3	T45.1X4	T45.1X5	T45.1X6
Podophyllotoxin	T49.8X1	T49.8X2	T49.8X3	T49.8X4	T49.8X5	T49.8X6
Podophyllum (resin)	T49.4X1	T49.4X2	T49.4X3	T49.4X4	T49.4X5	T49.4X6
Poisonous berries	T62.1X1	T62.1X2	T62.1X3	T62.1X4	—	—
Poison NEC	T65.91	T65.92	T65.93	T65.94	—	—
Pokeweed (any part)	T62.2X1	T62.2X2	T62.2X3	T62.2X4	—	—
Poldine metilsulfate	T44.3X1	T44.3X2	T44.3X3	T44.3X4	T44.3X5	T44.3X6
Polidexide (sulfate)	T46.6X1	T46.6X2	T46.6X3	T46.6X4	T46.6X5	T46.6X6
Polidocanol	T46.8X1	T46.8X2	T46.8X3	T46.8X4	T46.8X5	T46.8X6
Poliomyelitis vaccine	T50.B91	T50.B92	T50.B93	T50.B94	T50.B95	T50.B96
Polish (car) (floor) (furniture)	T65.891	T65.892	T65.893	T65.894	—	—
(metal) (porcelain) (silver)						
abrasive	T65.891	T65.892	T65.893	T65.894	—	—
porcelain	T65.891	T65.892	T65.893	T65.894	—	—
Poloxalkol	T47.4X1	T47.4X2	T47.4X3	T47.4X4	T47.4X5	T47.4X6
Poloxamer	T47.4X1	T47.4X2	T47.4X3	T47.4X4	T47.4X5	T47.4X6
Polyaminostyrene resins	T50.3X1	T50.3X2	T50.3X3	T50.3X4	T50.3X5	T50.3X6
Polycarbophil	T47.4X1	T47.4X2	T47.4X3	T47.4X4	T47.4X5	T47.4X6
Polychlorinated biphenyl	T65.891	T65.892	T65.893	T65.894	—	—
Polycycline	T36.4X1	T36.4X2	T36.4X3	T36.4X4	T36.4X5	T36.4X6
Polyester fumes	T59.891	T59.892	T59.893	T59.894	—	—
Polyester resin hardener	T52.91	T52.92	T52.93	T52.94	—	—
fumes	T59.891	T59.892	T59.893	T59.894	—	—
Polyestradiol phosphate	T38.5X1	T38.5X2	T38.5X3	T38.5X4	T38.5X5	T38.5X6
Polyethanolamine alkyl sulfate	T49.2X1	T49.2X2	T49.2X3	T49.2X4	T49.2X5	T49.2X6
Polyethylene adhesive	T49.3X1	T49.3X2	T49.3X3	T49.3X4	T49.3X5	T49.3X6
Polyferose	T45.4X1	T45.4X2	T45.4X3	T45.4X4	T45.4X5	T45.4X6
Polygeline	T45.8X1	T45.8X2	T45.8X3	T45.8X4	T45.8X5	T45.8X6
Polymyxin	T36.8X1	T36.8X2	T36.8X3	T36.8X4	T36.8X5	T36.8X6
B	T36.8X1	T36.8X2	T36.8X3	T36.8X4	T36.8X5	T36.8X6
ENT agent	T49.6X1	T49.6X2	T49.6X3	T49.6X4	T49.6X5	T49.6X6
ophthalmic preparation	T49.5X1	T49.5X2	T49.5X3	T49.5X4	T49.5X5	T49.5X6
topical NEC	T49.0X1	T49.0X2	T49.0X3	T49.0X4	T49.0X5	T49.0X6
E sulfate (eye preparation)	T49.5X1	T49.5X2	T49.5X3	T49.5X4	T49.5X5	T49.5X6
Polynoxylin	T49.0X1	T49.0X2	T49.0X3	T49.0X4	T49.0X5	T49.0X6
Polyoestradiol phosphate	T38.5X1	T38.5X2	T38.5X3	T38.5X4	T38.5X5	T38.5X6
Polyoxymethyleneurea	T49.0X1	T49.0X2	T49.0X3	T49.0X4	T49.0X5	T49.0X6
Polysilane	T47.8X1	T47.8X2	T47.8X3	T47.8X4	T47.8X5	T47.8X6
Polytetrafluoroethylene (inhaled)	T59.891	T59.892	T59.893	T59.894	—	—
Polythiazide	T50.2X1	T50.2X2	T50.2X3	T50.2X4	T50.2X5	T50.2X6
Polyvidone	T45.8X1	T45.8X2	T45.8X3	T45.8X4	T45.8X5	T45.8X6
Polyvinylpyrrolidone	T45.8X1	T45.8X2	T45.8X3	T45.8X4	T45.8X5	T45.8X6
Pontocaine (hydrochloride) (infiltration) (topical)	T41.3X1	T41.3X2	T41.3X3	T41.3X4	T41.3X5	T41.3X6
nerve block (peripheral) (plexus)	T41.3X1	T41.3X2	T41.3X3	T41.3X4	T41.3X5	T41.3X6
spinal	T41.3X1	T41.3X2	T41.3X3	T41.3X4	T41.3X5	T41.3X6
Porfiromycin	T45.1X1	T45.1X2	T45.1X3	T45.1X4	T45.1X5	T45.1X6
Posterior pituitary hormone NEC	T38.891	T38.892	T38.893	T38.894	T38.895	T38.896
Pot	T40.7X1	T40.7X2	T40.7X3	T40.7X4	T40.7X5	T40.7X6
Potash (caustic)	T54.3X1	T54.3X2	T54.3X3	T54.3X4	—	—
Potassic saline injection (lactated)	T50.3X1	T50.3X2	T50.3X3	T50.3X4	T50.3X5	T50.3X6
Potassium-removing resin	T50.3X1	T50.3X2	T50.3X3	T50.3X4	T50.3X5	T50.3X6
Potassium-retaining drug	T50.3X1	T50.3X2	T50.3X3	T50.3X4	T50.3X5	T50.3X6
Potassium (salts) NEC	T50.3X1	T50.3X2	T50.3X3	T50.3X4	T50.3X5	T50.3X6
aminobenzoate	T45.8X1	T45.8X2	T45.8X3	T45.8X4	T45.8X5	T45.8X6
aminosalicylate	T37.1X1	T37.1X2	T37.1X3	T37.1X4	T37.1X5	T37.1X6
antimony ' tartrate'	T37.8X1	T37.8X2	T37.8X3	T37.8X4	T37.8X5	T37.8X6
arsenite (solution)	T57.0X1	T57.0X2	T57.0X3	T57.0X4	—	—
bichromate	T56.2X1	T56.2X2	T56.2X3	T56.2X4	—	—
bisulfate	T47.3X1	T47.3X2	T47.3X3	T47.3X4	T47.3X5	T47.3X6
bromide	T42.6X1	T42.6X2	T42.6X3	T42.6X4	T42.6X5	T42.6X6
canrenoate	T50.0X1	T50.0X2	T50.0X3	T50.0X4	T50.0X5	T50.0X6
carbonate	T54.3X1	T54.3X2	T54.3X3	T54.3X4	—	—
chlorate NEC	T65.891	T65.892	T65.893	T65.894	—	—
chloride	T50.3X1	T50.3X2	T50.3X3	T50.3X4	T50.3X5	T50.3X6
citrate	T50.991	T50.992	T50.993	T50.994	T50.995	T50.996
cyanide	T65.0X1	T65.0X2	T65.0X3	T65.0X4	—	—
ferric hexacyanoferrate (medicinal)	T50.6X1	T50.6X2	T50.6X3	T50.6X4	T50.6X5	T50.6X6
nonmedicinal	T65.891	T65.892	T65.893	T65.894	—	—

Substance	Poisoning, Accidental (unintentional)	Poisoning, Intentional Self-harm	Poisoning, Assault	Poisoning, Undetermined	Adverse Effect	Under-dosing
Potassium (salts) NEC — *continued*						
Fluoride	T57.8X1	T57.8X2	T57.8X3	T57.8X4	—	—
glucaldrate	T47.1X1	T47.1X2	T47.1X3	T47.1X4	T47.1X5	T47.1X6
hydroxide	T54.3X1	T54.3X2	T54.3X3	T54.3X4	—	—
iodate	T49.0X1	T49.0X2	T49.0X3	T49.0X4	T49.0X5	T49.0X6
iodide	T48.4X1	T48.4X2	T48.4X3	T48.4X4	T48.4X5	T48.4X6
nitrate	T57.8X1	T57.8X2	T57.8X3	T57.8X4	—	—
oxalate	T65.891	T65.892	T65.893	T65.894	—	—
perchlorate (nonmedicinal) NEC	T65.891	T65.892	T65.893	T65.894	—	—
antithyroid	T38.2X1	T38.2X2	T38.2X3	T38.2X4	T38.2X5	T38.2X6
medicinal	T38.2X1	T38.2X2	T38.2X3	T38.2X4	T38.2X5	T38.2X6
Permanganate (nonmedicinal)	T65.891	T65.892	T65.893	T65.894	—	—
medicinal	T49.0X1	T49.0X2	T49.0X3	T49.0X4	T49.0X5	T49.0X6
sulfate	T47.2X1	T47.2X2	T47.2X3	T47.2X4	T47.2X5	T47.2X6
Povidone	T45.8X1	T45.8X2	T45.8X3	T45.8X4	T45.8X5	T45.8X6
iodine	T49.0X1	T49.0X2	T49.0X3	T49.0X4	T49.0X5	T49.0X6
Practolol	T44.7X1	T44.7X2	T44.7X3	T44.7X4	T44.7X5	T44.7X6
Prajmalium bitartrate	T46.2X1	T46.2X2	T46.2X3	T46.2X4	T46.2X5	T46.2X6
Pralidoxime (iodide)	T50.6X1	T50.6X2	T50.6X3	T50.6X4	T50.6X5	T50.6X6
chloride	T50.6X1	T50.6X2	T50.6X3	T50.6X4	T50.6X5	T50.6X6
Pramiverine	T44.3X1	T44.3X2	T44.3X3	T44.3X4	T44.3X5	T44.3X6
Pramocaine	T49.1X1	T49.1X2	T49.1X3	T49.1X4	T49.1X5	T49.1X6
Pramoxine	T49.1X1	T49.1X2	T49.1X3	T49.1X4	T49.1X5	T49.1X6
Prasterone	T38.7X1	T38.7X2	T38.7X3	T38.7X4	T38.7X5	T38.7X6
Pravastatin	T46.6X1	T46.6X2	T46.6X3	T46.6X4	T46.6X5	T46.6X6
Prazepam	T42.4X1	T42.4X2	T42.4X3	T42.4X4	T42.4X5	T42.4X6
Praziquantel	T37.4X1	T37.4X2	T37.4X3	T37.4X4	T37.4X5	T37.4X6
Prazitone	T43.291	T43.292	T43.293	T43.294	T43.295	T43.296
Prazosin	T44.6X1	T44.6X2	T44.6X3	T44.6X4	T44.6X5	T44.6X6
Prednicarbate	T49.0X1	T49.0X2	T49.0X3	T49.0X4	T49.0X5	T49.0X6
Prednimustine	T45.1X1	T45.1X2	T45.1X3	T45.1X4	T45.1X5	T45.1X6
Prednisolone	T38.0X1	T38.0X2	T38.0X3	T38.0X4	T38.0X5	T38.0X6
ENT agent	T49.6X1	T49.6X2	T49.6X3	T49.6X4	T49.6X5	T49.6X6
ophthalmic preparation	T49.5X1	T49.5X2	T49.5X3	T49.5X4	T49.5X5	T49.5X6
steaglate	T49.0X1	T49.0X2	T49.0X3	T49.0X4	T49.0X5	T49.0X6
topical NEC	T49.0X1	T49.0X2	T49.0X3	T49.0X4	T49.0X5	T49.0X6
Prednisone	T38.0X1	T38.0X2	T38.0X3	T38.0X4	T38.0X5	T38.0X6
Prednylidene	T38.0X1	T38.0X2	T38.0X3	T38.0X4	T38.0X5	T38.0X6
Pregnandiol	T38.5X1	T38.5X2	T38.5X3	T38.5X4	T38.5X5	T38.5X6
Pregneninolone	T38.5X1	T38.5X2	T38.5X3	T38.5X4	T38.5X5	T38.5X6
Preludin	T43.691	T43.692	T43.693	T43.694	T43.695	T43.696
Premarin	T38.5X1	T38.5X2	T38.5X3	T38.5X4	T38.5X5	T38.5X6
Premedication anesthetic	T41.201	T41.202	T41.203	T41.204	T41.205	T41.206
Prenalterol	T44.5X1	T44.5X2	T44.5X3	T44.5X4	T44.5X5	T44.5X6
Prenoxdiazine	T48.3X1	T48.3X2	T48.3X3	T48.3X4	T48.3X5	T48.3X6
Prenylamine	T46.3X1	T46.3X2	T46.3X3	T46.3X4	T46.3X5	T46.3X6
Preparation H	T49.8X1	T49.8X2	T49.8X3	T49.8X4	T49.8X5	T49.8X6
Preparation, local	T49.4X1	T49.4X2	T49.4X3	T49.4X4	T49.4X5	T49.4X6
Preservative (nonmedicinal)	T65.891	T65.892	T65.893	T65.894	—	—
medicinal	T50.901	T50.902	T50.903	T50.904	T50.905	T50.906
wood	T60.91	T60.92	T60.93	T60.94	—	—
Prethcamide	T50.7X1	T50.7X2	T50.7X3	T50.7X4	T50.7X5	T50.7X6
Pride of China	T62.2X1	T62.2X2	T62.2X3	T62.2X4	—	—
Pridinol	T44.3X1	T44.3X2	T44.3X3	T44.3X4	T44.3X5	T44.3X6
Prifinium bromide	T44.3X1	T44.3X2	T44.3X3	T44.3X4	T44.3X5	T44.3X6
Prilocaine	T41.3X1	T41.3X2	T41.3X3	T41.3X4	T41.3X5	T41.3X6
infiltration (subcutaneous)	T41.3X1	T41.3X2	T41.3X3	T41.3X4	T41.3X5	T41.3X6
nerve block (peripheral) (plexus)	T41.3X1	T41.3X2	T41.3X3	T41.3X4	T41.3X5	T41.3X6
regional	T41.3X1	T41.3X2	T41.3X3	T41.3X4	T41.3X5	T41.3X6
Primaquine	T37.2X1	T37.2X2	T37.2X3	T37.2X4	T37.2X5	T37.2X6
Primidone	T42.6X1	T42.6X2	T42.6X3	T42.6X4	T42.6X5	T42.6X6
Primula (veris)	T62.2X1	T62.2X2	T62.2X3	T62.2X4	—	—
Prinadol	T40.2X1	T40.2X2	T40.2X3	T40.2X4	T40.2X5	T40.2X6
Priscol, Priscoline	T44.6X1	T44.6X2	T44.6X3	T44.6X4	T44.6X5	T44.6X6
Pristinamycin	T36.3X1	T36.3X2	T36.3X3	T36.3X4	T36.3X5	T36.3X6
Privet	T62.2X1	T62.2X2	T62.2X3	T62.2X4	—	—
berries	T62.1X1	T62.1X2	T62.1X3	T62.1X4	—	—
Privine	T44.4X1	T44.4X2	T44.4X3	T44.4X4	T44.4X5	T44.4X6
Pro-Banthine	T44.3X1	T44.3X2	T44.3X3	T44.3X4	T44.3X5	T44.3X6
Probarbital	T42.3X1	T42.3X2	T42.3X3	T42.3X4	T42.3X5	T42.3X6
Probenecid	T50.4X1	T50.4X2	T50.4X3	T50.4X4	T50.4X5	T50.4X6
Probucol	T46.6X1	T46.6X2	T46.6X3	T46.6X4	T46.6X5	T46.6X6
Procainamide	T46.2X1	T46.2X2	T46.2X3	T46.2X4	T46.2X5	T46.2X6
Procaine	T41.3X1	T41.3X2	T41.3X3	T41.3X4	T41.3X5	T41.3X6
benzylpenicillin	T36.0X1	T36.0X2	T36.0X3	T36.0X4	T36.0X5	T36.0X6
nerve block (periphreal) (plexus)	T41.3X1	T41.3X2	T41.3X3	T41.3X4	T41.3X5	T41.3X6
penicillin G	T36.0X1	T36.0X2	T36.0X3	T36.0X4	T36.0X5	T36.0X6
regional	T41.3X1	T41.3X2	T41.3X3	T41.3X4	T41.3X5	T41.3X6

Substance	Poisoning, Accidental (unintentional)	Poisoning, Intentional Self-harm	Poisoning, Assault	Poisoning, Undetermined	Adverse Effect	Under-dosing
Procaine — *continued*						
spinal	T41.3X1	T41.3X2	T41.3X3	T41.3X4	T41.3X5	T41.3X6
Procalmidol	T43.591	T43.592	T43.593	T43.594	T43.595	T43.596
Procarbazine	T45.1X1	T45.1X2	T45.1X3	T45.1X4	T45.1X5	T45.1X6
Procaterol	T44.5X1	T44.5X2	T44.5X3	T44.5X4	T44.5X5	T44.5X6
Prochlorperazine	T43.3X1	T43.3X2	T43.3X3	T43.3X4	T43.3X5	T43.3X6
Procyclidine	T44.3X1	T44.3X2	T44.3X3	T44.3X4	T44.3X5	T44.3X6
Producer gas	T58.8X1	T58.8X2	T58.8X3	T58.8X4	—	—
Profadol	T40.4X1	T40.4X2	T40.4X3	T40.4X4	T40.4X5	T40.4X6
Profenamine	T44.3X1	T44.3X2	T44.3X3	T44.3X4	T44.3X5	T44.3X6
Profenil	T44.3X1	T44.3X2	T44.3X3	T44.3X4	T44.3X5	T44.3X6
Proflavine	T49.0X1	T49.0X2	T49.0X3	T49.0X4	T49.0X5	T49.0X6
Progabide	T42.6X1	T42.6X2	T42.6X3	T42.6X4	T42.6X5	T42.6X6
Progesterone	T38.5X1	T38.5X2	T38.5X3	T38.5X4	T38.5X5	T38.5X6
Progestin	T38.5X1	T38.5X2	T38.5X3	T38.5X4	T38.5X5	T38.5X6
oral contraceptive	T38.4X1	T38.4X2	T38.4X3	T38.4X4	T38.4X5	T38.4X6
Progestogen NEC	T38.5X1	T38.5X2	T38.5X3	T38.5X4	T38.5X5	T38.5X6
Progestone	T38.5X1	T38.5X2	T38.5X3	T38.5X4	T38.5X5	T38.5X6
Proglumide	T47.1X1	T47.1X2	T47.1X3	T47.1X4	T47.1X5	T47.1X6
Proguanil	T37.2X1	T37.2X2	T37.2X3	T37.2X4	T37.2X5	T37.2X6
Prolactin	T38.811	T38.812	T38.813	T38.814	T38.815	T38.816
Prolintane	T43.691	T43.692	T43.693	T43.694	T43.695	T43.696
Proloid	T38.1X1	T38.1X2	T38.1X3	T38.1X4	T38.1X5	T38.1X6
Proluton	T38.5X1	T38.5X2	T38.5X3	T38.5X4	T38.5X5	T38.5X6
Promacetin	T37.1X1	T37.1X2	T37.1X3	T37.1X4	T37.1X5	T37.1X6
Promazine	T43.3X1	T43.3X2	T43.3X3	T43.3X4	T43.3X5	T43.3X6
Promedol	T40.2X1	T40.2X2	T40.2X3	T40.2X4	—	—
Promegestone	T38.5X1	T38.5X2	T38.5X3	T38.5X4	T38.5X5	T38.5X6
Promethazine (teoclate)	T43.3X1	T43.3X2	T43.3X3	T43.3X4	T43.3X5	T43.3X6
Promin	T37.1X1	T37.1X2	T37.1X3	T37.1X4	T37.1X5	T37.1X6
Pronase	T45.3X1	T45.3X2	T45.3X3	T45.3X4	T45.3X5	T45.3X6
Pronestyl (hydrochloride)	T46.2X1	T46.2X2	T46.2X3	T46.2X4	T46.2X5	T46.2X6
Pronetalol	T44.7X1	T44.7X2	T44.7X3	T44.7X4	T44.7X5	T44.7X6
Prontosil	T37.0X1	T37.0X2	T37.0X3	T37.0X4	T37.0X5	T37.0X6
Propachlor	T60.3X1	T60.3X2	T60.3X3	T60.3X4	—	—
Propafenone	T46.2X1	T46.2X2	T46.2X3	T46.2X4	T46.2X5	T46.2X6
Propallylonal	T42.3X1	T42.3X2	T42.3X3	T42.3X4	T42.3X5	T42.3X6
Propamidine	T49.0X1	T49.0X2	T49.0X3	T49.0X4	T49.0X5	T49.0X6
Propane (distributed in mobile container)	T59.891	T59.892	T59.893	T59.894	—	—
distributed through pipes	T59.891	T59.892	T59.893	T59.894	—	—
incomplete combustion	T58.11	T58.12	T58.13	T58.14	—	—
Propanidid	T41.291	T41.292	T41.293	T41.294	T41.295	T41.296
Propanil	T60.3X1	T60.3X2	T60.3X3	T60.3X4	—	—
Propantheline	T44.3X1	T44.3X2	T44.3X3	T44.3X4	T44.3X5	T44.3X6
bromide	T44.3X1	T44.3X2	T44.3X3	T44.3X4	T44.3X5	T44.3X6
Proparacaine	T41.3X1	T41.3X2	T41.3X3	T41.3X4	T41.3X5	T41.3X6
Propatylnitrate	T46.3X1	T46.3X2	T46.3X3	T46.3X4	T46.3X5	T46.3X6
Propicillin	T36.0X1	T36.0X2	T36.0X3	T36.0X4	T36.0X5	T36.0X6
Propiolactone	T49.0X1	T49.0X2	T49.0X3	T49.0X4	T49.0X5	T49.0X6
Propiomazine	T45.0X1	T45.0X2	T45.0X3	T45.0X4	T45.0X5	T45.0X6
Propionaidehyde (medicinal)	T42.6X1	T42.6X2	T42.6X3	T42.6X4	T42.6X5	T42.6X6
Propionate (calcium) (sodium)	T49.0X1	T49.0X2	T49.0X3	T49.0X4	T49.0X5	T49.0X6
Propion gel	T49.0X1	T49.0X2	T49.0X3	T49.0X4	T49.0X5	T49.0X6
Propitocaine	T41.3X1	T41.3X2	T41.3X3	T41.3X4	T41.3X5	T41.3X6
infiltration (subcutaneous)	T41.3X1	T41.3X2	T41.3X3	T41.3X4	T41.3X5	T41.3X6
nerve block (peripheral) (plexus)	T41.3X1	T41.3X2	T41.3X3	T41.3X4	T41.3X5	T41.3X6
Propofol	T41.291	T41.292	T41.293	T41.294	T41.295	T41.296
Propoxur	T60.0X1	T60.0X2	T60.0X3	T60.0X4	—	—
Propoxycaine	T41.3X1	T41.3X2	T41.3X3	T41.3X4	T41.3X5	T41.3X6
infiltration (subcutaneous)	T41.3X1	T41.3X2	T41.3X3	T41.3X4	T41.3X5	T41.3X6
nerve block (peripheral) (plexus)	T41.3X1	T41.3X2	T41.3X3	T41.3X4	T41.3X5	T41.3X6
topical (surface)	T41.3X1	T41.3X2	T41.3X3	T41.3X4	T41.3X5	T41.3X6
Propoxyphene	T40.4X1	T40.4X2	T40.4X3	T40.4X4	T40.4X5	T40.4X6
Propranolol	T44.7X1	T44.7X2	T44.7X3	T44.7X4	T44.7X5	T44.7X6
Propyl						
alcohol	T51.3X1	T51.3X2	T51.3X3	T51.3X4	—	—
carbinol	T51.3X1	T51.3X2	T51.3X3	T51.3X4	—	—
hexadrine	T44.4X1	T44.4X2	T44.4X3	T44.4X4	T44.4X5	T44.4X6
iodone	T50.8X1	T50.8X2	T50.8X3	T50.8X4	T50.8X5	T50.8X6
thiouracil	T38.2X1	T38.2X2	T38.2X3	T38.2X4	T38.2X5	T38.2X6
Propylaminophenothiazine	T43.3X1	T43.3X2	T43.3X3	T43.3X4	T43.3X5	T43.3X6
Propylene	T59.891	T59.892	T59.893	T59.894	—	—
Propylhexedrine	T48.5X1	T48.5X2	T48.5X3	T48.5X4	T48.5X5	T48.5X6
Propyliodone	T50.8X1	T50.8X2	T50.8X3	T50.8X4	T50.8X5	T50.8X6
Propylparaben (ophthalmic)	T49.5X1	T49.5X2	T49.5X3	T49.5X4	T49.5X5	T49.5X6
Propylthiouracil	T38.2X1	T38.2X2	T38.2X3	T38.2X4	T38.2X5	T38.2X6
Propyphenazone	T39.2X1	T39.2X2	T39.2X3	T39.2X4	T39.2X5	T39.2X6
Proquazone	T39.391	T39.392	T39.393	T39.394	T39.395	T39.396

Substance	Poisoning, Accidental (unintentional)	Poisoning, Intentional Self-harm	Poisoning, Assault	Poisoning, Undetermined	Adverse Effect	Under-dosing
Proscillaridin	T46.0X1	T46.0X2	T46.0X3	T46.0X4	T46.0X5	T46.0X6
Prostacyclin	T45.521	T45.522	T45.523	T45.524	T45.525	T45.526
Prostaglandin (I2)	T45.521	T45.522	T45.523	T45.524	T45.525	T45.526
E1	T46.7X1	T46.7X2	T46.7X3	T46.7X4	T46.7X5	T46.7X6
E2	T48.0X1	T48.0X2	T48.0X3	T48.0X4	T48.0X5	T48.0X6
F2 alpha	T48.0X1	T48.0X2	T48.0X3	T48.0X4	T48.0X5	T48.0X6
Prostigmin	T44.0X1	T44.0X2	T44.0X3	T44.0X4	T44.0X5	T44.0X6
Prosultiamine	T45.2X1	T45.2X2	T45.2X3	T45.2X4	T45.2X5	T45.2X6
Protamine sulfate	T45.7X1	T45.7X2	T45.7X3	T45.7X4	T45.7X5	T45.7X6
zinc insulin	T38.3X1	T38.3X2	T38.3X3	T38.3X4	T38.3X5	T38.3X6
Protease	T47.5X1	T47.5X2	T47.5X3	T47.5X4	T47.5X5	T47.5X6
Protectant, skin NEC	T49.3X1	T49.3X2	T49.3X3	T49.3X4	T49.3X5	T49.3X6
Protein hydrolysate	T50.991	T50.992	T50.993	T50.994	T50.995	T50.996
Prothiaden — *see* Dothiepin hydrochloride						
Prothionamide	T37.1X1	T37.1X2	T37.1X3	T37.1X4	T37.1X5	T37.1X6
Prothipendyl	T43.591	T43.592	T43.593	T43.594	T43.595	T43.596
Prothoate	T60.0X1	T60.0X2	T60.0X3	T60.0X4	—	—
Prothrombin						
activator	T45.7X1	T45.7X2	T45.7X3	T45.7X4	T45.7X5	T45.7X6
synthesis inhibitor	T45.511	T45.512	T45.513	T45.514	T45.515	T45.516
Protionamide	T37.1X1	T37.1X2	T37.1X3	T37.1X4	T37.1X5	T37.1X6
Protirelin	T38.891	T38.892	T38.893	T38.894	T38.895	T38.896
Protokylol	T48.6X1	T48.6X2	T48.6X3	T48.6X4	T48.6X5	T48.6X6
Protopam	T50.6X1	T50.6X2	T50.6X3	T50.6X4	T50.6X5	T50.6X6
Protoveratrine(s) (A) (B)	T46.5X1	T46.5X2	T46.5X3	T46.5X4	T46.5X5	T46.5X6
Protriptyline	T43.011	T43.012	T43.013	T43.014	T43.015	T43.016
Provera	T38.5X1	T38.5X2	T38.5X3	T38.5X4	T38.5X5	T38.5X6
Provitamin A	T45.2X1	T45.2X2	T45.2X3	T45.2X4	T45.2X5	T45.2X6
Proxibarbal	T42.3X1	T42.3X2	T42.3X3	T42.3X4	T42.3X5	T42.3X6
Proxymetacaine	T41.3X1	T41.3X2	T41.3X3	T41.3X4	T41.3X5	T41.3X6
Proxyphylline	T48.6X1	T48.6X2	T48.6X3	T48.6X4	T48.6X5	T48.6X6
Prozac — *see* Fluoxetine hydrochloride						
Prunus						
laurocerasus	T62.2X1	T62.2X2	T62.2X3	T62.2X4	—	—
virginiana	T62.2X1	T62.2X2	T62.2X3	T62.2X4	—	—
Prussian blue						
commercial	T65.891	T65.892	T65.893	T65.894	—	—
therapeutic	T50.6X1	T50.6X2	T50.6X3	T50.6X4	T50.6X5	T50.6X6
Prussic acid	T65.0X1	T65.0X2	T65.0X3	T65.0X4	—	—
vapor	T57.3X1	T57.3X2	T57.3X3	T57.3X4	—	—
Pseudoephedrine	T44.991	T44.992	T44.993	T44.994	T44.995	T44.996
Psilocin	T40.991	T40.992	T40.993	T40.994	—	—
Psilocybin	T40.991	T40.992	T40.993	T40.994	—	—
Psilocybine	T40.991	T40.992	T40.993	T40.994	—	—
Psoralene (nonmedicinal)	T65.891	T65.892	T65.893	T65.894	—	—
Psoralens (medicinal)	T50.991	T50.992	T50.993	T50.994	T50.995	T50.996
PSP (phenolsulfonphthalein)	T50.8X1	T50.8X2	T50.8X3	T50.8X4	T50.8X5	T50.8X6
Psychodysleptic drug NEC	T40.901	T40.902	T40.903	T40.904	T40.905	T40.906
Psychostimulant	T43.601	T43.602	T43.603	T43.604	T43.605	T43.606
amphetamine	T43.621	T43.622	T43.623	T43.624	T43.625	T43.626
caffeine	T43.611	T43.612	T43.613	T43.614	T43.615	T43.616
methylphenidate	T43.631	T43.632	T43.633	T43.634	T43.635	T43.636
specified NEC	T43.691	T43.692	T43.693	T43.694	T43.695	T43.696
Psychotherapeutic drug NEC	T43.91	T43.92	T43.93	T43.94	T43.95	T43.96
antidepressants — *see also* Antidepressant	T43.201	T43.202	T43.203	T43.204	T43.205	T43.206
specified NEC	T43.8X1	T43.8X2	T43.8X3	T43.8X4	T43.8X5	T43.8X6
tranquilizers NEC	T43.501	T43.502	T43.503	T43.504	T43.505	T43.506
Psychotomimetic agents	T40.901	T40.902	T40.903	T40.904	T40.905	T40.906
Psychotropic drug NEC	T43.91	T43.92	T43.93	T43.94	T43.95	T43.96
specified NEC	T43.8X1	T43.8X2	T43.8X3	T43.8X4	T43.8X5	T43.8X6
Psyllium hydrophilic mucilloid	T47.4X1	T47.4X2	T47.4X3	T47.4X4	T47.4X5	T47.4X6
Pteroylglutamic acid	T45.8X1	T45.8X2	T45.8X3	T45.8X4	T45.8X5	T45.8X6
Pteroyltriglutamate	T45.1X1	T45.1X2	T45.1X3	T45.1X4	T45.1X5	T45.1X6
PTFE — *see* Polytetrafluoroethylene						
Pulp						
devitalizing paste	T49.7X1	T49.7X2	T49.7X3	T49.7X4	T49.7X5	T49.7X6
dressing	T49.7X1	T49.7X2	T49.7X3	T49.7X4	T49.7X5	T49.7X6
Pulsatilla	T62.2X1	T62.2X2	T62.2X3	T62.2X4	—	—
Pumpkin seed extract	T37.4X1	T37.4X2	T37.4X3	T37.4X4	T37.4X5	T37.4X6
Purex (bleach)	T54.91	T54.92	T54.93	T54.94	—	—
Purgative NEC — *see also* Cathartic	T47.4X1	T47.4X2	T47.4X3	T47.4X4	T47.4X5	T47.4X6
Purine analogue (antineoplastic)	T45.1X1	T45.1X2	T45.1X3	T45.1X4	T45.1X5	T45.1X6
Purine diuretics	T50.2X1	T50.2X2	T50.2X3	T50.2X4	T50.2X5	T50.2X6
Purinethol	T45.1X1	T45.1X2	T45.1X3	T45.1X4	T45.1X5	T45.1X6
PVP	T45.8X1	T45.8X2	T45.8X3	T45.8X4	T45.8X5	T45.8X6

Substance	Poisoning, Accidental (unintentional)	Poisoning, Intentional Self-harm	Poisoning, Assault	Poisoning, Undetermined	Adverse Effect	Under-dosing
Pyrabital	T39.8X1	T39.8X2	T39.8X3	T39.8X4	T39.8X5	T39.8X6
Pyramidon	T39.2X1	T39.2X2	T39.2X3	T39.2X4	T39.2X5	T39.2X6
Pyrantel	T37.4X1	T37.4X2	T37.4X3	T37.4X4	T37.4X5	T37.4X6
Pyrathiazine	T45.0X1	T45.0X2	T45.0X3	T45.0X4	T45.0X5	T45.0X6
Pyrazinamide	T37.1X1	T37.1X2	T37.1X3	T37.1X4	T37.1X5	T37.1X6
Pyrazinoic acid (amide)	T37.1X1	T37.1X2	T37.1X3	T37.1X4	T37.1X5	T37.1X6
Pyrazole (derivatives)	T39.2X1	T39.2X2	T39.2X3	T39.2X4	T39.2X5	T39.2X6
Pyrazolone analgesic NEC	T39.2X1	T39.2X2	T39.2X3	T39.2X4	T39.2X5	T39.2X6
Pyrethrin, pyrethrum (nonmedicinal)	T60.2X1	T60.2X2	T60.2X3	T60.2X4	—	—
Pyrethrum extract	T49.0X1	T49.0X2	T49.0X3	T49.0X4	T49.0X5	T49.0X6
Pyribenzamine	T45.0X1	T45.0X2	T45.0X3	T45.0X4	T45.0X5	T45.0X6
Pyridine	T52.8X1	T52.8X2	T52.8X3	T52.8X4	—	—
aldoxime methiodide	T50.6X1	T50.6X2	T50.6X3	T50.6X4	T50.6X5	T50.6X6
aldoxime methyl chloride	T50.6X1	T50.6X2	T50.6X3	T50.6X4	T50.6X5	T50.6X6
vapor	T59.891	T59.892	T59.893	T59.894	—	—
Pyridium	T39.8X1	T39.8X2	T39.8X3	T39.8X4	T39.8X5	T39.8X6
Pyridostigmine bromide	T44.0X1	T44.0X2	T44.0X3	T44.0X4	T44.0X5	T44.0X6
Pyridoxal phosphate	T45.2X1	T45.2X2	T45.2X3	T45.2X4	T45.2X5	T45.2X6
Pyridoxine	T45.2X1	T45.2X2	T45.2X3	T45.2X4	T45.2X5	T45.2X6
Pyrilamine	T45.0X1	T45.0X2	T45.0X3	T45.0X4	T45.0X5	T45.0X6
Pyrimethamine	T37.2X1	T37.2X2	T37.2X3	T37.2X4	T37.2X5	T37.2X6
with sulfadoxine	T37.2X1	T37.2X2	T37.2X3	T37.2X4	T37.2X5	T37.2X6
Pyrimidine antagonist	T45.1X1	T45.1X2	T45.1X3	T45.1X4	T45.1X5	T45.1X6
Pyriminil	T60.4X1	T60.4X2	T60.4X3	T60.4X4	—	—
Pyrithione zinc	T49.4X1	T49.4X2	T49.4X3	T49.4X4	T49.4X5	T49.4X6
Pyrithyldione	T42.6X1	T42.6X2	T42.6X3	T42.6X4	T42.6X5	T42.6X6
Pyrogallic acid	T49.0X1	T49.0X2	T49.0X3	T49.0X4	T49.0X5	T49.0X6
Pyrogallol	T49.0X1	T49.0X2	T49.0X3	T49.0X4	T49.0X5	T49.0X6
Pyroxylin	T49.3X1	T49.3X2	T49.3X3	T49.3X4	T49.3X5	T49.3X6
Pyrrobutamine	T45.0X1	T45.0X2	T45.0X3	T45.0X4	T45.0X5	T45.0X6
Pyrrolizidine alkaloids	T62.8X1	T62.8X2	T62.8X3	T62.8X4	—	—
Pyrvinium chloride	T37.4X1	T37.4X2	T37.4X3	T37.4X4	T37.4X5	T37.4X6
PZI	T38.3X1	T38.3X2	T38.3X3	T38.3X4	T38.3X5	T38.3X6
Quaalude	T42.6X1	T42.6X2	T42.6X3	T42.6X4	T42.6X5	T42.6X6
Quarternary ammonium						
anti-infective	T49.0X1	T49.0X2	T49.0X3	T49.0X4	T49.0X5	T49.0X6
ganglion blocking	T44.2X1	T44.2X2	T44.2X3	T44.2X4	T44.2X5	T44.2X6
parasympatholytic	T44.3X1	T44.3X2	T44.3X3	T44.3X4	T44.3X5	T44.3X6
Quazepam	T42.4X1	T42.4X2	T42.4X3	T42.4X4	T42.4X5	T42.4X6
Quicklime	T54.3X1	T54.3X2	T54.3X3	T54.3X4	—	—
Quillaja extract	T48.4X1	T48.4X2	T48.4X3	T48.4X4	T48.4X5	T48.4X6
Quinacrine	T37.2X1	T37.2X2	T37.2X3	T37.2X4	T37.2X5	T37.2X6
Quinaglute	T46.2X1	T46.2X2	T46.2X3	T46.2X4	T46.2X5	T46.2X6
Quinalbarbital	T42.3X1	T42.3X2	T42.3X3	T42.3X4	T42.3X5	T42.3X6
Quinalbarbitone sodium	T42.3X1	T42.3X2	T42.3X3	T42.3X4	T42.3X5	T42.3X6
Quinalphos	T60.0X1	T60.0X2	T60.0X3	T60.0X4	—	—
Quinapril	T46.4X1	T46.4X2	T46.4X3	T46.4X4	T46.4X5	T46.4X6
Quinestradiol	T38.5X1	T38.5X2	T38.5X3	T38.5X4	T38.5X5	T38.5X6
Quinestradol	T38.5X1	T38.5X2	T38.5X3	T38.5X4	T38.5X5	T38.5X6
Quinestrol	T38.5X1	T38.5X2	T38.5X3	T38.5X4	T38.5X5	T38.5X6
Quinethazone	T50.2X1	T50.2X2	T50.2X3	T50.2X4	T50.2X5	T50.2X6
Quingestanol	T38.4X1	T38.4X2	T38.4X3	T38.4X4	T38.4X5	T38.4X6
Quinidine	T46.2X1	T46.2X2	T46.2X3	T46.2X4	T46.2X5	T46.2X6
Quinine	T37.2X1	T37.2X2	T37.2X3	T37.2X4	T37.2X5	T37.2X6
Quiniobine	T37.8X1	T37.8X2	T37.8X3	T37.8X4	T37.8X5	T37.8X6
Quinisocaine	T49.1X1	T49.1X2	T49.1X3	T49.1X4	T49.1X5	T49.1X6
Quinocide	T37.2X1	T37.2X2	T37.2X3	T37.2X4	T37.2X5	T37.2X6
Quinoline (derivatives) NEC	T37.8X1	T37.8X2	T37.8X3	T37.8X4	T37.8X5	T37.8X6
Quinupramine	T43.011	T43.012	T43.013	T43.014	T43.015	T43.016
Quotane	T41.3X1	T41.3X2	T41.3X3	T41.3X4	T41.3X5	T41.3X6
Rabies						
immune globulin (human)	T50.Z11	T50.Z12	T50.Z13	T50.Z14	T50.Z15	T50.Z16
vaccine	T50.B91	T50.B92	T50.B93	T50.B94	T50.B95	T50.B96
Racemoramide	T40.2X1	T40.2X2	T40.2X3	T40.2X4	—	—
Racemorphan	T40.2X1	T40.2X2	T40.2X3	T40.2X4	T40.2X5	T40.2X6
Racepinefrin	T44.5X1	T44.5X2	T44.5X3	T44.5X4	T44.5X5	T44.5X6
Raclopride	T43.591	T43.592	T43.593	T43.594	T43.595	T43.596
Radiator alcohol	T51.1X1	T51.1X2	T51.1X3	T51.1X4	—	—
Radioactive drug NEC	T50.8X1	T50.8X2	T50.8X3	T50.8X4	T50.8X5	T50.8X6
Radio-opaque (drugs) (materials)	T50.8X1	T50.8X2	T50.8X3	T50.8X4	T50.8X5	T50.8X6
Ramifenazone	T39.2X1	T39.2X2	T39.2X3	T39.2X4	T39.2X5	T39.2X6
Ramipril	T46.4X1	T46.4X2	T46.4X3	T46.4X4	T46.4X5	T46.4X6
Ranitidine	T47.0X1	T47.0X2	T47.0X3	T47.0X4	T47.0X5	T47.0X6
Ranunculus	T62.2X1	T62.2X2	T62.2X3	T62.2X4	—	—
Rat poison NEC	T60.4X1	T60.4X2	T60.4X3	T60.4X4	—	—
Rattlesnake (venom)	T63.011	T63.012	T63.013	T63.014	—	—
Raubasine	T46.7X1	T46.7X2	T46.7X3	T46.7X4	T46.7X5	T46.7X6
Raudixin	T46.5X1	T46.5X2	T46.5X3	T46.5X4	T46.5X5	T46.5X6
Rautensin	T46.5X1	T46.5X2	T46.5X3	T46.5X4	T46.5X5	T46.5X6
Rautina	T46.5X1	T46.5X2	T46.5X3	T46.5X4	T46.5X5	T46.5X6
Rautotal	T46.5X1	T46.5X2	T46.5X3	T46.5X4	T46.5X5	T46.5X6

Substance	Poisoning, Accidental (unintentional)	Poisoning, Intentional Self-harm	Poisoning, Assault	Poisoning, Undetermined	Adverse Effect	Under-dosing
Rauwiloid	T46.5X1	T46.5X2	T46.5X3	T46.5X4	T46.5X5	T46.5X6
Rauwoldin	T46.5X1	T46.5X2	T46.5X3	T46.5X4	T46.5X5	T46.5X6
Rauwolfia (alkaloids)	T46.5X1	T46.5X2	T46.5X3	T46.5X4	T46.5X5	T46.5X6
Razoxane	T45.1X1	T45.1X2	T45.1X3	T45.1X4	T45.1X5	T45.1X6
Realgar	T57.0X1	T57.0X2	T57.0X3	T57.0X4	—	—
Recombinant (R) — see specific protein						
Red blood cells, packed	T45.8X1	T45.8X2	T45.8X3	T45.8X4	T45.8X5	T45.8X6
Red squill (scilliroside)	T60.4X1	T60.4X2	T60.4X3	T60.4X4	—	—
Reducing agent, industrial NEC	T65.891	T65.892	T65.893	T65.894	—	—
Refrigerant gas (chlorofluorocarbon)	T53.5X1	T53.5X2	T53.5X3	T53.5X4	—	—
not chlorofluorocarbon	T59.891	T59.892	T59.893	T59.894	—	—
Regroton	T50.2X1	T50.2X2	T50.2X3	T50.2X4	T50.2X5	T50.2X6
Rehydration salts (oral)	T50.3X1	T50.3X2	T50.3X3	T50.3X4	T50.3X5	T50.3X6
Rela	T42.8X1	T42.8X2	T42.8X3	T42.8X4	T42.8X5	T42.8X6
Relaxant, muscle						
anesthetic	T48.1X1	T48.1X2	T48.1X3	T48.1X4	T48.1X5	T48.1X6
central nervous system	T42.8X1	T42.8X2	T42.8X3	T42.8X4	T42.8X5	T42.8X6
skeletal NEC	T48.1X1	T48.1X2	T48.1X3	T48.1X4	T48.1X5	T48.1X6
smooth NEC	T44.3X1	T44.3X2	T44.3X3	T44.3X4	T44.3X5	T44.3X6
Remoxipride	T43.591	T43.592	T43.593	T43.594	T43.595	T43.596
Renese	T50.2X1	T50.2X2	T50.2X3	T50.2X4	T50.2X5	T50.2X6
Renografin	T50.8X1	T50.8X2	T50.8X3	T50.8X4	T50.8X5	T50.8X6
Replacement solution	T50.3X1	T50.3X2	T50.3X3	T50.3X4	T50.3X5	T50.3X6
Reproterol	T48.6X1	T48.6X2	T48.6X3	T48.6X4	T48.6X5	T48.6X6
Rescinnamine	T46.5X1	T46.5X2	T46.5X3	T46.5X4	T46.5X5	T46.5X6
Reserpin (e)	T46.5X1	T46.5X2	T46.5X3	T46.5X4	T46.5X5	T46.5X6
Resorcin, resorcinol (nonmedicinal)	T65.891	T65.892	T65.893	T65.894	—	—
medicinal	T49.4X1	T49.4X2	T49.4X3	T49.4X4	T49.4X5	T49.4X6
Respaire	T48.4X1	T48.4X2	T48.4X3	T48.4X4	T48.4X5	T48.4X6
Respiratory drug NEC	T48.901	T48.902	T48.903	T48.904	T48.905	T48.906
antiasthmatic NEC	T48.6X1	T48.6X2	T48.6X3	T48.6X4	T48.6X5	T48.6X6
anti-common-cold NEC	T48.5X1	T48.5X2	T48.5X3	T48.5X4	T48.5X5	T48.5X6
expectorant NEC	T48.4X1	T48.4X2	T48.4X3	T48.4X4	T48.4X5	T48.4X6
stimulant	T48.901	T48.902	T48.903	T48.904	T48.905	T48.906
Retinoic acid	T49.0X1	T49.0X2	T49.0X3	T49.0X4	T49.0X5	T49.0X6
Retinol	T45.2X1	T45.2X2	T45.2X3	T45.2X4	T45.2X5	T45.2X6
Rh (D) immune globulin (human)	T50.Z11	T50.Z12	T50.Z13	T50.Z14	T50.Z15	T50.Z16
Rhodine	T39.011	T39.012	T39.013	T39.014	T39.015	T39.016
RhoGAM	T50.Z11	T50.Z12	T50.Z13	T50.Z14	T50.Z15	T50.Z16
Rhubarb						
dry extract	T47.2X1	T47.2X2	T47.2X3	T47.2X4	T47.2X5	T47.2X6
tincture, compound	T47.2X1	T47.2X2	T47.2X3	T47.2X4	T47.2X5	T47.2X6
Ribavirin	T37.5X1	T37.5X2	T37.5X3	T37.5X4	T37.5X5	T37.5X6
Riboflavin	T45.2X1	T45.2X2	T45.2X3	T45.2X4	T45.2X5	T45.2X6
Ribostamycin	T36.5X1	T36.5X2	T36.5X3	T36.5X4	T36.5X5	T36.5X6
Ricin	T62.2X1	T62.2X2	T62.2X3	T62.2X4	—	—
Ricinus communis	T62.2X1	T62.2X2	T62.2X3	T62.2X4	—	—
Rickettsial vaccine NEC	T50.A91	T50.A92	T50.A93	T50.A94	T50.A95	T50.A96
Rifabutin	T36.6X1	T36.6X2	T36.6X3	T36.6X4	T36.6X5	T36.6X6
Rifamide	T36.6X1	T36.6X2	T36.6X3	T36.6X4	T36.6X5	T36.6X6
Rifampicin	T36.6X1	T36.6X2	T36.6X3	T36.6X4	T36.6X5	T36.6X6
with isoniazid	T37.1X1	T37.1X2	T37.1X3	T37.1X4	T37.1X5	T37.1X6
Rifampin	T36.6X1	T36.6X2	T36.6X3	T36.6X4	T36.6X5	T36.6X6
Rifamycin	T36.6X1	T36.6X2	T36.6X3	T36.6X4	T36.6X5	T36.6X6
Rifaximin	T36.6X1	T36.6X2	T36.6X3	T36.6X4	T36.6X5	T36.6X6
Rimantadine	T37.5X1	T37.5X2	T37.5X3	T37.5X4	T37.5X5	T37.5X6
Rimazolium metilsulfate	T39.8X1	T39.8X2	T39.8X3	T39.8X4	T39.8X5	T39.8X6
Rimifon	T37.1X1	T37.1X2	T37.1X3	T37.1X4	T37.1X5	T37.1X6
Rimiterol	T48.6X1	T48.6X2	T48.6X3	T48.6X4	T48.6X5	T48.6X6
Ringer (lactate) solution	T50.3X1	T50.3X2	T50.3X3	T50.3X4	T50.3X5	T50.3X6
Ristocetin	T36.8X1	T36.8X2	T36.8X3	T36.8X4	T36.8X5	T36.8X6
Ritalin	T43.631	T43.632	T43.633	T43.634	T43.635	T43.636
Ritodrine	T44.5X1	T44.5X2	T44.5X3	T44.5X4	T44.5X5	T44.5X6
Roach killer — see Insecticide						
Rociverine	T44.3X1	T44.3X2	T44.3X3	T44.3X4	T44.3X5	T44.3X6
Rocky Mountain spotted fever vaccine	T50.A91	T50.A92	T50.A93	T50.A94	T50.A95	T50.A96
Rodenticide NEC	T60.4X1	T60.4X2	T60.4X3	T60.4X4	—	—
Rohypnol	T42.4X1	T42.4X2	T42.4X3	T42.4X4	T42.4X5	T42.4X6
Rokitamycin	T36.3X1	T36.3X2	T36.3X3	T36.3X4	T36.3X5	T36.3X6
Rolaids	T47.1X1	T47.1X2	T47.1X3	T47.1X4	T47.1X5	T47.1X6
Rolitetracycline	T36.4X1	T36.4X2	T36.4X3	T36.4X4	T36.4X5	T36.4X6
Romilar	T48.3X1	T48.3X2	T48.3X3	T48.3X4	T48.3X5	T48.3X6
Ronifibrate	T46.6X1	T46.6X2	T46.6X3	T46.6X4	T46.6X5	T46.6X6
Rosaprostol	T47.1X1	T47.1X2	T47.1X3	T47.1X4	T47.1X5	T47.1X6
Rose bengal sodium (131I)	T50.8X1	T50.8X2	T50.8X3	T50.8X4	T50.8X5	T50.8X6
Rose water ointment	T49.3X1	T49.3X2	T49.3X3	T49.3X4	T49.3X5	T49.3X6
Rosoxacin	T37.8X1	T37.8X2	T37.8X3	T37.8X4	T37.8X5	T37.8X6

⬇ Subterms under main terms may continue to next column or page   Additional Character May Be Required — Refer to the Tabular List for Character Selection   377

Pyrabital — Rosoxacin

Substance	Poisoning, Accidental (unintentional)	Poisoning, Intentional Self-harm	Poisoning, Assault	Poisoning, Undetermined	Adverse Effect	Under-dosing
Rotenone	T60.2X1	T60.2X2	T60.2X3	T60.2X4	—	—
Rotoxamine	T45.0X1	T45.0X2	T45.0X3	T45.0X4	T45.0X5	T45.0X6
Rough-on-rats	T60.4X1	T60.4X2	T60.4X3	T60.4X4	—	—
Roxatidine	T47.0X1	T47.0X2	T47.0X3	T47.0X4	T47.0X5	T47.0X6
Roxithromycin	T36.3X1	T36.3X2	T36.3X3	T36.3X4	T36.3X5	T36.3X6
Rt-PA	T45.611	T45.612	T45.613	T45.614	T45.615	T45.616
Rubbing alcohol	T51.2X1	T51.2X2	T51.2X3	T51.2X4	—	—
Rubefacient	T49.4X1	T49.4X2	T49.4X3	T49.4X4	T49.4X5	T49.4X6
Rubella vaccine	T50.B91	T50.B92	T50.B93	T50.B94	T50.B95	T50.B96
Rubeola vaccine	T50.B91	T50.B92	T50.B93	T50.B94	T50.B95	T50.B96
Rubidium chloride Rb82	T50.8X1	T50.8X2	T50.8X3	T50.8X4	T50.8X5	T50.8X6
Rubidomycin	T45.1X1	T45.1X2	T45.1X3	T45.1X4	T45.1X5	T45.1X6
Rue	T62.2X1	T62.2X2	T62.2X3	T62.2X4	—	—
Rufocromomycin	T45.1X1	T45.1X2	T45.1X3	T45.1X4	T45.1X5	T45.1X6
Russel's viper venin	T45.7X1	T45.7X2	T45.7X3	T45.7X4	T45.7X5	T45.7X6
Ruta (graveolens)	T62.2X1	T62.2X2	T62.2X3	T62.2X4	—	—
Rutinum	T46.991	T46.992	T46.993	T46.994	T46.995	T46.996
Rutoside	T46.991	T46.992	T46.993	T46.994	T46.995	T46.996
b-sitosterol(s)	T46.6X1	T46.6X2	T46.6X3	T46.6X4	T46.6X5	T46.6X6
Sabadilla (plant)	T62.2X1	T62.2X2	T62.2X3	T62.2X4	—	—
pesticide	T60.2X1	T60.2X2	T60.2X3	T60.2X4	—	—
Saccharated iron oxide	T45.8X1	T45.8X2	T45.8X3	T45.8X4	T45.8X5	T45.8X6
Saccharin	T50.901	T50.902	T50.903	T50.904	T50.905	T50.906
Saccharomyces boulardii	T47.6X1	T47.6X2	T47.6X3	T47.6X4	T47.6X5	T47.6X6
Safflower oil	T46.6X1	T46.6X2	T46.6X3	T46.6X4	T46.6X5	T46.6X6
Safrazine	T43.1X1	T43.1X2	T43.1X3	T43.1X4	T43.1X5	T43.1X6
Salazosulfapyridine	T37.0X1	T37.0X2	T37.0X3	T37.0X4	T37.0X5	T37.0X6
Salbutamol	T48.6X1	T48.6X2	T48.6X3	T48.6X4	T48.6X5	T48.6X6
Salicylamide	T39.091	T39.092	T39.093	T39.094	T39.095	T39.096
Salicylate NEC	T39.091	T39.092	T39.093	T39.094	T39.095	T39.096
methyl	T49.3X1	T49.3X2	T49.3X3	T49.3X4	T49.3X5	T49.3X6
theobromine calcium	T50.2X1	T50.2X2	T50.2X3	T50.2X4	T50.2X5	T50.2X6
Salicylazosulfapyridine	T37.0X1	T37.0X2	T37.0X3	T37.0X4	T37.0X5	T37.0X6
Salicylhydroxamic acid	T49.0X1	T49.0X2	T49.0X3	T49.0X4	T49.0X5	T49.0X6
Salicylic acid	T49.4X1	T49.4X2	T49.4X3	T49.4X4	T49.4X5	T49.4X6
with benzoic acid	T49.4X1	T49.4X2	T49.4X3	T49.4X4	T49.4X5	T49.4X6
congeners	T39.091	T39.092	T39.093	T39.094	T39.095	T39.096
derivative	T39.091	T39.092	T39.093	T39.094	T39.095	T39.096
salts	T39.091	T39.092	T39.093	T39.094	T39.095	T39.096
Salinazid	T37.1X1	T37.1X2	T37.1X3	T37.1X4	T37.1X5	T37.1X6
Salmeterol	T48.6X1	T48.6X2	T48.6X3	T48.6X4	T48.6X5	T48.6X6
Salol	T49.3X1	T49.3X2	T49.3X3	T49.3X4	T49.3X5	T49.3X6
Salsalate	T39.091	T39.092	T39.093	T39.094	T39.095	T39.096
Salt-replacing drug	T50.901	T50.902	T50.903	T50.904	T50.905	T50.906
Salt-retaining mineralocorticoid	T50.0X1	T50.0X2	T50.0X3	T50.0X4	T50.0X5	T50.0X6
Salt substitute	T50.901	T50.902	T50.903	T50.904	T50.905	T50.906
Saluretic NEC	T50.2X1	T50.2X2	T50.2X3	T50.2X4	T50.2X5	T50.2X6
Saluron	T50.2X1	T50.2X2	T50.2X3	T50.2X4	T50.2X5	T50.2X6
Salvarsan 606 (neosilver) (silver)	T37.8X1	T37.8X2	T37.8X3	T37.8X4	T37.8X5	T37.8X6
Sambucus canadensis	T62.2X1	T62.2X2	T62.2X3	T62.2X4	—	—
berry	T62.1X1	T62.1X2	T62.1X3	T62.1X4	—	—
Sandril	T46.5X1	T46.5X2	T46.5X3	T46.5X4	T46.5X5	T46.5X6
Sanguinaria canadensis	T62.2X1	T62.2X2	T62.2X3	T62.2X4	—	—
Saniflush (cleaner)	T54.2X1	T54.2X2	T54.2X3	T54.2X4	—	—
Santonin	T37.4X1	T37.4X2	T37.4X3	T37.4X4	T37.4X5	T37.4X6
Santyl	T49.8X1	T49.8X2	T49.8X3	T49.8X4	T49.8X5	T49.8X6
Saralasin	T46.5X1	T46.5X2	T46.5X3	T46.5X4	T46.5X5	T46.5X6
Sarcolysin	T45.1X1	T45.1X2	T45.1X3	T45.1X4	T45.1X5	T45.1X6
Sarkomycin	T45.1X1	T45.1X2	T45.1X3	T45.1X4	T45.1X5	T45.1X6
Saroten	T43.011	T43.012	T43.013	T43.014	T43.015	T43.016
Saturnine — see Lead						
Savin (oil)	T49.4X1	T49.4X2	T49.4X3	T49.4X4	T49.4X5	T49.4X6
Scammony	T47.2X1	T47.2X2	T47.2X3	T47.2X4	T47.2X5	T47.2X6
Scarlet red	T49.8X1	T49.8X2	T49.8X3	T49.8X4	T49.8X5	T49.8X6
Scheele's green	T57.0X1	T57.0X2	T57.0X3	T57.0X4	—	—
insecticide	T57.0X1	T57.0X2	T57.0X3	T57.0X4	—	—
Schizontozide (blood)	T37.2X1	T37.2X2	T37.2X3	T37.2X4	T37.2X5	T37.2X6
(tissue)	T37.2X1	T37.2X2	T37.2X3	T37.2X4	T37.2X5	T37.2X6
Schradan	T60.0X1	T60.0X2	T60.0X3	T60.0X4	—	—
Schweinfurth green	T57.0X1	T57.0X2	T57.0X3	T57.0X4	—	—
insecticide	T57.0X1	T57.0X2	T57.0X3	T57.0X4	—	—
Scilla, rat poison	T60.4X1	T60.4X2	T60.4X3	T60.4X4	—	—
Scillaren	T60.4X1	T60.4X2	T60.4X3	T60.4X4	—	—
Sclerosing agent	T46.8X1	T46.8X2	T46.8X3	T46.8X4	T46.8X5	T46.8X6
Scombrotoxin	T61.11	T61.12	T61.13	T61.14	—	—
Scopolamine	T44.3X1	T44.3X2	T44.3X3	T44.3X4	T44.3X5	T44.3X6
Scopolia extract	T44.3X1	T44.3X2	T44.3X3	T44.3X4	T44.3X5	T44.3X6
Scouring powder	T65.891	T65.892	T65.893	T65.894	—	—
Sea						
anemone (sting)	T63.631	T63.632	T63.633	T63.634	—	—
cucumber (sting)	T63.691	T63.692	T63.693	T63.694	—	—

Substance	Poisoning, Accidental (unintentional)	Poisoning, Intentional Self-harm	Poisoning, Assault	Poisoning, Undetermined	Adverse Effect	Under-dosing
Sea — continued						
snake (bite) (venom)	T63.091	T63.092	T63.093	T63.094	—	—
urchin spine (puncture)	T63.691	T63.692	T63.693	T63.694	—	—
Seafood	T61.91	T61.92	T61.93	T61.94	—	—
specified NEC	T61.8X1	T61.8X2	T61.8X3	T61.8X4	—	—
Secbutabarbital	T42.3X1	T42.3X2	T42.3X3	T42.3X4	T42.3X5	T42.3X6
Secbutabarbitone	T42.3X1	T42.3X2	T42.3X3	T42.3X4	T42.3X5	T42.3X6
Secnidazole	T37.3X1	T37.3X2	T37.3X3	T37.3X4	T37.3X5	T37.3X6
Secobarbital	T42.3X1	T42.3X2	T42.3X3	T42.3X4	T42.3X5	T42.3X6
Seconal	T42.3X1	T42.3X2	T42.3X3	T42.3X4	T42.3X5	T42.3X6
Secretin	T50.8X1	T50.8X2	T50.8X3	T50.8X4	T50.8X5	T50.8X6
Sedative NEC	T42.71	T42.72	T42.73	T42.74	T42.75	T42.76
mixed NEC	T42.6X1	T42.6X2	T42.6X3	T42.6X4	T42.6X5	T42.6X6
Sedormid	T42.6X1	T42.6X2	T42.6X3	T42.6X4	T42.6X5	T42.6X6
Seed disinfectant or dressing	T60.8X1	T60.8X2	T60.8X3	T60.8X4	—	—
Seeds (poisonous)	T62.2X1	T62.2X2	T62.2X3	T62.2X4	—	—
Selegiline	T42.8X1	T42.8X2	T42.8X3	T42.8X4	T42.8X5	T42.8X6
Selenium NEC	T56.891	T56.892	T56.893	T56.894	—	—
disulfide or sulfide	T49.4X1	T49.4X2	T49.4X3	T49.4X4	T49.4X5	T49.4X6
fumes	T59.891	T59.892	T59.893	T59.894	—	—
sulfide	T49.4X1	T49.4X2	T49.4X3	T49.4X4	T49.4X5	T49.4X6
Selenomethionine (75Se)	T50.8X1	T50.8X2	T50.8X3	T50.8X4	T50.8X5	T50.8X6
Selsun	T49.4X1	T49.4X2	T49.4X3	T49.4X4	T49.4X5	T49.4X6
Semustine	T45.1X1	T45.1X2	T45.1X3	T45.1X4	T45.1X5	T45.1X6
Senega syrup	T48.4X1	T48.4X2	T48.4X3	T48.4X4	T48.4X5	T48.4X6
Senna	T47.2X1	T47.2X2	T47.2X3	T47.2X4	T47.2X5	T47.2X6
Sennoside A+B	T47.2X1	T47.2X2	T47.2X3	T47.2X4	T47.2X5	T47.2X6
Septisol	T49.2X1	T49.2X2	T49.2X3	T49.2X4	T49.2X5	T49.2X6
Seractide	T38.811	T38.812	T38.813	T38.814	T38.815	T38.816
Serax	T42.4X1	T42.4X2	T42.4X3	T42.4X4	T42.4X5	T42.4X6
Serenesil	T42.6X1	T42.6X2	T42.6X3	T42.6X4	T42.6X5	T42.6X6
Serenium (hydrochloride)	T37.91	T37.92	T37.93	T37.94	T37.95	T37.96
Serepax — see Oxazepam						
Sermorelin	T38.891	T38.892	T38.893	T38.894	T38.895	T38.896
Sernyl	T41.1X1	T41.1X2	T41.1X3	T41.1X4	T41.1X5	T41.1X6
Serotonin	T50.991	T50.992	T50.993	T50.994	T50.995	T50.996
Serpasil	T46.5X1	T46.5X2	T46.5X3	T46.5X4	T46.5X5	T46.5X6
Serrapeptase	T45.3X1	T45.3X2	T45.3X3	T45.3X4	T45.3X5	T45.3X6
Serum						
antibotulinus	T50.Z11	T50.Z12	T50.Z13	T50.Z14	T50.Z15	T50.Z16
anticytotoxic	T50.Z11	T50.Z12	T50.Z13	T50.Z14	T50.Z15	T50.Z16
antidiphtheria	T50.Z11	T50.Z12	T50.Z13	T50.Z14	T50.Z15	T50.Z16
antimeningococcus	T50.Z11	T50.Z12	T50.Z13	T50.Z14	T50.Z15	T50.Z16
anti-Rh	T50.Z11	T50.Z12	T50.Z13	T50.Z14	T50.Z15	T50.Z16
anti-snake-bite	T50.Z11	T50.Z12	T50.Z13	T50.Z14	T50.Z15	T50.Z16
antitetanic	T50.Z11	T50.Z12	T50.Z13	T50.Z14	T50.Z15	T50.Z16
antitoxic	T50.Z11	T50.Z12	T50.Z13	T50.Z14	T50.Z15	T50.Z16
complement (inhibitor)	T45.8X1	T45.8X2	T45.8X3	T45.8X4	T45.8X5	T45.8X6
convalescent	T50.Z11	T50.Z12	T50.Z13	T50.Z14	T50.Z15	T50.Z16
hemolytic complement	T45.8X1	T45.8X2	T45.8X3	T45.8X4	T45.8X5	T45.8X6
immune (human)	T50.Z11	T50.Z12	T50.Z13	T50.Z14	T50.Z15	T50.Z16
protective NEC	T50.Z11	T50.Z12	T50.Z13	T50.Z14	T50.Z15	T50.Z16
Setastine	T45.0X1	T45.0X2	T45.0X3	T45.0X4	T45.0X5	T45.0X6
Setoperone	T43.591	T43.592	T43.593	T43.594	T43.595	T43.596
Sewer gas	T59.91	T59.92	T59.93	T59.94	—	—
Shampoo	T55.0X1	T55.0X2	T55.0X3	T55.0X4	—	—
Shellfish, noxious, nonbacterial	T61.781	T61.782	T61.783	T61.784	—	—
Sildenafil	T46.7X1	T46.7X2	T46.7X3	T46.7X4	T46.7X5	T46.7X6
Silibinin	T50.991	T50.992	T50.993	T50.994	T50.995	T50.996
Silicone NEC	T65.891	T65.892	T65.893	T65.894	—	—
medicinal	T49.3X1	T49.3X2	T49.3X3	T49.3X4	T49.3X5	T49.3X6
Silvadene	T49.0X1	T49.0X2	T49.0X3	T49.0X4	T49.0X5	T49.0X6
Silver	T49.0X1	T49.0X2	T49.0X3	T49.0X4	T49.0X5	T49.0X6
anti-infectives	T49.0X1	T49.0X2	T49.0X3	T49.0X4	T49.0X5	T49.0X6
arsphenamine	T37.8X1	T37.8X2	T37.8X3	T37.8X4	T37.8X5	T37.8X6
colloidal	T49.0X1	T49.0X2	T49.0X3	T49.0X4	T49.0X5	T49.0X6
nitrate	T49.0X1	T49.0X2	T49.0X3	T49.0X4	T49.0X5	T49.0X6
ophthalmic preparation	T49.5X1	T49.5X2	T49.5X3	T49.5X4	T49.5X5	T49.5X6
toughened (keratolytic)	T49.4X1	T49.4X2	T49.4X3	T49.4X4	T49.4X5	T49.4X6
nonmedicinal (dust)	T56.891	T56.892	T56.893	T56.894	—	—
protein	T49.5X1	T49.5X2	T49.5X3	T49.5X4	T49.5X5	T49.5X6
salvarsan	T37.8X1	T37.8X2	T37.8X3	T37.8X4	T37.8X5	T37.8X6
sulfadiazine	T49.4X1	T49.4X2	T49.4X3	T49.4X4	T49.4X5	T49.4X6
Silymarin	T50.991	T50.992	T50.993	T50.994	T50.995	T50.996
Simaldrate	T47.1X1	T47.1X2	T47.1X3	T47.1X4	T47.1X5	T47.1X6
Simazine	T60.3X1	T60.3X2	T60.3X3	T60.3X4	—	—
Simethicone	T47.1X1	T47.1X2	T47.1X3	T47.1X4	T47.1X5	T47.1X6
Simfibrate	T46.6X1	T46.6X2	T46.6X3	T46.6X4	T46.6X5	T46.6X6
Simvastatin	T46.6X1	T46.6X2	T46.6X3	T46.6X4	T46.6X5	T46.6X6
Sincalide	T50.8X1	T50.8X2	T50.8X3	T50.8X4	T50.8X5	T50.8X6
Sinequan	T43.011	T43.012	T43.013	T43.014	T43.015	T43.016

Substance	Poisoning, Accidental (unintentional)	Poisoning, Intentional Self-harm	Poisoning, Assault	Poisoning, Undetermined	Adverse Effect	Under-dosing
Singoserp	T46.5X1	T46.5X2	T46.5X3	T46.5X4	T46.5X5	T46.5X6
Sintrom	T45.511	T45.512	T45.513	T45.514	T45.515	T45.516
Sisomicin	T36.5X1	T36.5X2	T36.5X3	T36.5X4	T36.5X5	T36.5X6
Sitosterols	T46.6X1	T46.6X2	T46.6X3	T46.6X4	T46.6X5	T46.6X6
Skeletal muscle relaxants	T48.1X1	T48.1X2	T48.1X3	T48.1X4	T48.1X5	T48.1X6
Skin						
agents (external)	T49.91	T49.92	T49.93	T49.94	T49.95	T49.96
specified NEC	T49.8X1	T49.8X2	T49.8X3	T49.8X4	T49.8X5	T49.8X6
test antigen	T50.8X1	T50.8X2	T50.8X3	T50.8X4	T50.8X5	T50.8X6
Sleep-eze	T45.0X1	T45.0X2	T45.0X3	T45.0X4	T45.0X5	T45.0X6
Sleeping draught, pill	T42.71	T42.72	T42.73	T42.74	T42.75	T42.76
Smallpox vaccine	T50.B11	T50.B12	T50.B13	T50.B14	T50.B15	T50.B16
Smelter fumes NEC	T56.91	T56.92	T56.93	T56.94	—	—
Smog	T59.1X1	T59.1X2	T59.1X3	T59.1X4	—	—
Smoke NEC	T59.811	T59.812	T59.813	T59.814	—	—
Smooth muscle relaxant	T44.3X1	T44.3X2	T44.3X3	T44.3X4	T44.3X5	T44.3X6
Snail killer NEC	T60.8X1	T60.8X2	T60.8X3	T60.8X4	—	—
Snake venom or bite	T63.001	T63.002	T63.003	T63.004		
hemocoagulase	T45.7X1	T45.7X2	T45.7X3	T45.7X4	T45.7X5	T45.7X6
Snuff	T65.211	T65.212	T65.213	T65.214	—	—
Soap (powder) (product)	T55.0X1	T55.0X2	T55.0X3	T55.0X4	—	—
enema	T47.4X1	T47.4X2	T47.4X3	T47.4X4	T47.4X5	T47.4X6
medicinal, soft	T49.2X1	T49.2X2	T49.2X3	T49.2X4	T49.2X5	T49.2X6
superfatted	T49.2X1	T49.2X2	T49.2X3	T49.2X4	T49.2X5	T49.2X6
Sobrerol	T48.4X1	T48.4X2	T48.4X3	T48.4X4	T48.4X5	T48.4X6
Soda (caustic)	T54.3X1	T54.3X2	T54.3X3	T54.3X4	—	—
bicarb	T47.1X1	T47.1X2	T47.1X3	T47.1X4	T47.1X5	T47.1X6
chlorinated — *see* Sodium, hypochlorite						
Sodium						
acetosulfone	T37.1X1	T37.1X2	T37.1X3	T37.1X4	T37.1X5	T37.1X6
acetrizoate	T50.8X1	T50.8X2	T50.8X3	T50.8X4	T50.8X5	T50.8X6
acid phosphate	T50.3X1	T50.3X2	T50.3X3	T50.3X4	T50.3X5	T50.3X6
alginate	T47.8X1	T47.8X2	T47.8X3	T47.8X4	T47.8X5	T47.8X6
amidotrizoate	T50.8X1	T50.8X2	T50.8X3	T50.8X4	T50.8X5	T50.8X6
aminopterin	T45.1X1	T45.1X2	T45.1X3	T45.1X4	T45.1X5	T45.1X6
amylosulfate	T47.8X1	T47.8X2	T47.8X3	T47.8X4	T47.8X5	T47.8X6
amytal	T42.3X1	T42.3X2	T42.3X3	T42.3X4	T42.3X5	T42.3X6
antimony gluconate	T37.3X1	T37.3X2	T37.3X3	T37.3X4	T37.3X5	T37.3X6
arsenate	T57.0X1	T57.0X2	T57.0X3	T57.0X4	—	—
aurothiomalate	T39.4X1	T39.4X2	T39.4X3	T39.4X4	T39.4X5	T39.4X6
aurothiosulfate	T39.4X1	T39.4X2	T39.4X3	T39.4X4	T39.4X5	T39.4X6
barbiturate	T42.3X1	T42.3X2	T42.3X3	T42.3X4	T42.3X5	T42.3X6
basic phosphate	T47.4X1	T47.4X2	T47.4X3	T47.4X4	T47.4X5	T47.4X6
bicarbonate	T47.1X1	T47.1X2	T47.1X3	T47.1X4	T47.1X5	T47.1X6
bichromate	T57.8X1	T57.8X2	T57.8X3	T57.8X4	—	—
biphosphate	T50.3X1	T50.3X2	T50.3X3	T50.3X4	T50.3X5	T50.3X6
bisulfate	T65.891	T65.892	T65.893	T65.894	—	—
borate						
cleanser	T57.8X1	T57.8X2	T57.8X3	T57.8X4	—	—
eye	T49.5X1	T49.5X2	T49.5X3	T49.5X4	T49.5X5	T49.5X6
therapeutic	T49.8X1	T49.8X2	T49.8X3	T49.8X4	T49.8X5	T49.8X6
bromide	T42.6X1	T42.6X2	T42.6X3	T42.6X4	T42.6X5	T42.6X6
cacodylate (nonmedicinal) NEC	T50.8X1	T50.8X2	T50.8X3	T50.8X4	T50.8X5	T50.8X6
anti-infective	T37.8X1	T37.8X2	T37.8X3	T37.8X4	T37.8X5	T37.8X6
herbicide	T60.3X1	T60.3X2	T60.3X3	T60.3X4	—	—
calcium edetate	T45.8X1	T45.8X2	T45.8X3	T45.8X4	T45.8X5	T45.8X6
carbonate NEC	T54.3X1	T54.3X2	T54.3X3	T54.3X4	—	—
chlorate NEC	T65.891	T65.892	T65.893	T65.894	—	—
herbicide	T54.91	T54.92	T54.93	T54.94	—	—
chloride	T50.3X1	T50.3X2	T50.3X3	T50.3X4	T50.3X5	T50.3X6
with glucose	T50.3X1	T50.3X2	T50.3X3	T50.3X4	T50.3X5	T50.3X6
chromate	T65.891	T65.892	T65.893	T65.894	—	—
citrate	T50.991	T50.992	T50.993	T50.994	T50.995	T50.996
cromoglicate	T48.6X1	T48.6X2	T48.6X3	T48.6X4	T48.6X5	T48.6X6
cyanide	T65.0X1	T65.0X2	T65.0X3	T65.0X4	—	—
cyclamate	T50.3X1	T50.3X2	T50.3X3	T50.3X4	T50.3X5	T50.3X6
dehydrocholate	T45.8X1	T45.8X2	T45.8X3	T45.8X4	T45.8X5	T45.8X6
diatrizoate	T50.8X1	T50.8X2	T50.8X3	T50.8X4	T50.8X5	T50.8X6
dibunate	T48.4X1	T48.4X2	T48.4X3	T48.4X4	T48.4X5	T48.4X6
dioctyl sulfosuccinate	T47.4X1	T47.4X2	T47.4X3	T47.4X4	T47.4X5	T47.4X6
dipantoyl ferrate	T45.8X1	T45.8X2	T45.8X3	T45.8X4	T45.8X5	T45.8X6
edetate	T45.8X1	T45.8X2	T45.8X3	T45.8X4	T45.8X5	T45.8X6
ethacrynate	T50.1X1	T50.1X2	T50.1X3	T50.1X4	T50.1X5	T50.1X6
feredetate	T45.8X1	T45.8X2	T45.8X3	T45.8X4	T45.8X5	T45.8X6
Fluoride — *see* Fluoride						
fluoroacetate (dust) (pesticide)	T60.4X1	T60.4X2	T60.4X3	T60.4X4	—	—
free salt	T50.3X1	T50.3X2	T50.3X3	T50.3X4	T50.3X5	T50.3X6
fusidate	T36.8X1	T36.8X2	T36.8X3	T36.8X4	T36.8X5	T36.8X6
glucaldrate	T47.1X1	T47.1X2	T47.1X3	T47.1X4	T47.1X5	T47.1X6
glucosulfone	T37.1X1	T37.1X2	T37.1X3	T37.1X4	T37.1X5	T37.1X6

Substance	Poisoning, Accidental (unintentional)	Poisoning, Intentional Self-harm	Poisoning, Assault	Poisoning, Undetermined	Adverse Effect	Under-dosing
Sodium — *continued*						
glutamate	T45.8X1	T45.8X2	T45.8X3	T45.8X4	T45.8X5	T45.8X6
hydrogen carbonate	T50.3X1	T50.3X2	T50.3X3	T50.3X4	T50.3X5	T50.3X6
hydroxide	T54.3X1	T54.3X2	T54.3X3	T54.3X4	—	—
hypochlorite (bleach) NEC	T54.3X1	T54.3X2	T54.3X3	T54.3X4	—	—
disinfectant	T54.3X1	T54.3X2	T54.3X3	T54.3X4	—	—
medicinal (anti-infective) (external)	T49.0X1	T49.0X2	T49.0X3	T49.0X4	T49.0X5	T49.0X6
vapor	T54.3X1	T54.3X2	T54.3X3	T54.3X4	—	—
hyposulfite	T49.0X1	T49.0X2	T49.0X3	T49.0X4	T49.0X5	T49.0X6
indigotin disulfonate	T50.8X1	T50.8X2	T50.8X3	T50.8X4	T50.8X5	T50.8X6
iodide	T50.991	T50.992	T50.993	T50.994	T50.995	T50.996
I-131	T50.8X1	T50.8X2	T50.8X3	T50.8X4	T50.8X5	T50.8X6
therapeutic	T38.2X1	T38.2X2	T38.2X3	T38.2X4	T38.2X5	T38.2X6
iodohippurate (131I)	T50.8X1	T50.8X2	T50.8X3	T50.8X4	T50.8X5	T50.8X6
iopodate	T50.8X1	T50.8X2	T50.8X3	T50.8X4	T50.8X5	T50.8X6
iothalamate	T50.8X1	T50.8X2	T50.8X3	T50.8X4	T50.8X5	T50.8X6
iron edetate	T45.4X1	T45.4X2	T45.4X3	T45.4X4	T45.4X5	T45.4X6
lactate (compound solution)	T45.8X1	T45.8X2	T45.8X3	T45.8X4	T45.8X5	T45.8X6
lauryl (sulfate)	T49.2X1	T49.2X2	T49.2X3	T49.2X4	T49.2X5	T49.2X6
L-triiodothyronine	T38.1X1	T38.1X2	T38.1X3	T38.1X4	T38.1X5	T38.1X6
magnesium citrate	T50.991	T50.992	T50.993	T50.994	T50.995	T50.996
mersalate	T50.2X1	T50.2X2	T50.2X3	T50.2X4	T50.2X5	T50.2X6
metasilicate	T65.891	T65.892	T65.893	T65.894	—	—
metrizoate	T50.8X1	T50.8X2	T50.8X3	T50.8X4	T50.8X5	T50.8X6
monofluoroacetate (pesticide)	T60.1X1	T60.1X2	T60.1X3	T60.1X4		
morrhuate	T46.8X1	T46.8X2	T46.8X3	T46.8X4	T46.8X5	T46.8X6
nafcillin	T36.0X1	T36.0X2	T36.0X3	T36.0X4	T36.0X5	T36.0X6
nitrate (oxidizing agent)	T65.891	T65.892	T65.893	T65.894	—	—
nitrite	T50.6X1	T50.6X2	T50.6X3	T50.6X4	T50.6X5	T50.6X6
nitroferricyanide	T46.5X1	T46.5X2	T46.5X3	T46.5X4	T46.5X5	T46.5X6
nitroprusside	T46.5X1	T46.5X2	T46.5X3	T46.5X4	T46.5X5	T46.5X6
oxalate	T65.891	T65.892	T65.893	T65.894	—	—
oxide/peroxide	T65.891	T65.892	T65.893	T65.894	—	—
oxybate	T41.291	T41.292	T41.293	T41.294	T41.295	T41.296
para-aminohippurate	T50.8X1	T50.8X2	T50.8X3	T50.8X4	T50.8X5	T50.8X6
perborate (nonmedicinal) NEC	T65.891	T65.892	T65.893	T65.894	—	—
medicinal	T49.0X1	T49.0X2	T49.0X3	T49.0X4	T49.0X5	T49.0X6
soap	T55.0X1	T55.0X2	T55.0X3	T55.0X4	—	—
percarbonate — *see* Sodium, perborate						
pertechnetate Tc99m	T50.8X1	T50.8X2	T50.8X3	T50.8X4	T50.8X5	T50.8X6
phosphate						
cellulose	T45.8X1	T45.8X2	T45.8X3	T45.8X4	T45.8X5	T45.8X6
dibasic	T47.2X1	T47.2X2	T47.2X3	T47.2X4	T47.2X5	T47.2X6
monobasic	T47.2X1	T47.2X2	T47.2X3	T47.2X4	T47.2X5	T47.2X6
phytate	T50.6X1	T50.6X2	T50.6X3	T50.6X4	T50.6X5	T50.6X6
picosulfate	T47.2X1	T47.2X2	T47.2X3	T47.2X4	T47.2X5	T47.2X6
polyhydroxyaluminium monocarbonate	T47.1X1	T47.1X2	T47.1X3	T47.1X4	T47.1X5	T47.1X6
polystyrene sulfonate	T50.3X1	T50.3X2	T50.3X3	T50.3X4	T50.3X5	T50.3X6
propionate	T49.0X1	T49.0X2	T49.0X3	T49.0X4	T49.0X5	T49.0X6
propyl hydroxybenzoate	T50.991	T50.992	T50.993	T50.994	T50.995	T50.996
psylliate	T46.8X1	T46.8X2	T46.8X3	T46.8X4	T46.8X5	T46.8X6
removing resins	T50.3X1	T50.3X2	T50.3X3	T50.3X4	T50.3X5	T50.3X6
salicylate	T39.091	T39.092	T39.093	T39.094	T39.095	T39.096
salt NEC	T50.3X1	T50.3X2	T50.3X3	T50.3X4	T50.3X5	T50.3X6
selenate	T60.2X1	T60.2X2	T60.2X3	T60.2X4	—	—
stibogluconate	T37.3X1	T37.3X2	T37.3X3	T37.3X4	T37.3X5	T37.3X6
sulfate	T47.4X1	T47.4X2	T47.4X3	T47.4X4	T47.4X5	T47.4X6
sulfoxone	T37.1X1	T37.1X2	T37.1X3	T37.1X4	T37.1X5	T37.1X6
tetradecyl sulfate	T46.8X1	T46.8X2	T46.8X3	T46.8X4	T46.8X5	T46.8X6
thiopental	T41.1X1	T41.1X2	T41.1X3	T41.1X4	T41.1X5	T41.1X6
thiosalicylate	T39.091	T39.092	T39.093	T39.094	T39.095	T39.096
thiosulfate	T50.6X1	T50.6X2	T50.6X3	T50.6X4	T50.6X5	T50.6X6
tolbutamide	T38.3X1	T38.3X2	T38.3X3	T38.3X4	T38.3X5	T38.3X6
(L)-triiodothyronine	T38.1X1	T38.1X2	T38.1X3	T38.1X4	T38.1X5	T38.1X6
tyropanoate	T50.8X1	T50.8X2	T50.8X3	T50.8X4	T50.8X5	T50.8X6
valproate	T42.6X1	T42.6X2	T42.6X3	T42.6X4	T42.6X5	T42.6X6
versenate	T50.6X1	T50.6X2	T50.6X3	T50.6X4	T50.6X5	T50.6X6
Sodium-free salt	T50.901	T50.902	T50.903	T50.904	T50.905	T50.906
Sodium-removing resin	T50.3X1	T50.3X2	T50.3X3	T50.3X4	T50.3X5	T50.3X6
Soft soap	T55.0X1	T55.0X2	T55.0X3	T55.0X4	—	—
Solanine	T62.2X1	T62.2X2	T62.2X3	T62.2X4	—	—
berries	T62.1X1	T62.1X2	T62.1X3	T62.1X4	—	—
Solanum dulcamara	T62.2X1	T62.2X2	T62.2X3	T62.2X4	—	—
berries	T62.1X1	T62.1X2	T62.1X3	T62.1X4	—	—
Solapsone	T37.1X1	T37.1X2	T37.1X3	T37.1X4	T37.1X5	T37.1X6
Solar lotion	T49.3X1	T49.3X2	T49.3X3	T49.3X4	T49.3X5	T49.3X6
Solasulfone	T37.1X1	T37.1X2	T37.1X3	T37.1X4	T37.1X5	T37.1X6

Substance	Poisoning, Accidental (unintentional)	Poisoning, Intentional Self-harm	Poisoning, Assault	Poisoning, Undetermined	Adverse Effect	Under-dosing
Soldering fluid	T65.891	T65.892	T65.893	T65.894	—	—
Solid substance	T65.91	T65.92	T65.93	T65.94	—	—
specified NEC	T65.891	T65.892	T65.893	T65.894	—	—
Solvent, industrial NEC	T52.91	T52.92	T52.93	T52.94	—	—
naphtha	T52.0X1	T52.0X2	T52.0X3	T52.0X4	—	—
petroleum	T52.0X1	T52.0X2	T52.0X3	T52.0X4	—	—
specified NEC	T52.8X1	T52.8X2	T52.8X3	T52.8X4	—	—
Soma	T42.8X1	T42.8X2	T42.8X3	T42.8X4	T42.8X5	T42.8X6
Somatorelin	T38.891	T38.892	T38.893	T38.894	T38.895	T38.896
Somatostatin	T38.991	T38.992	T38.993	T38.994	T38.995	T38.996
Somatotropin	T38.811	T38.812	T38.813	T38.814	T38.815	T38.816
Somatrem	T38.811	T38.812	T38.813	T38.814	T38.815	T38.816
Somatropin	T38.811	T38.812	T38.813	T38.814	T38.815	T38.816
Sominex	T45.0X1	T45.0X2	T45.0X3	T45.0X4	T45.0X5	T45.0X6
Somnos	T42.6X1	T42.6X2	T42.6X3	T42.6X4	T42.6X5	T42.6X6
Somonal	T42.3X1	T42.3X2	T42.3X3	T42.3X4	T42.3X5	T42.3X6
Soneryl	T42.3X1	T42.3X2	T42.3X3	T42.3X4	T42.3X5	T42.3X6
Soothing syrup	T50.901	T50.902	T50.903	T50.904	T50.905	T50.906
Sopor	T42.6X1	T42.6X2	T42.6X3	T42.6X4	T42.6X5	T42.6X6
Soporific	T42.71	T42.72	T42.73	T42.74	T42.75	T42.76
Soporific drug	T42.71	T42.72	T42.73	T42.74	T42.75	T42.76
specified type NEC	T42.6X1	T42.6X2	T42.6X3	T42.6X4	T42.6X5	T42.6X6
Sorbide nitrate	T46.3X1	T46.3X2	T46.3X3	T46.3X4	T46.3X5	T46.3X6
Sorbitol	T47.4X1	T47.4X2	T47.4X3	T47.4X4	T47.4X5	T47.4X6
Sotalol	T44.7X1	T44.7X2	T44.7X3	T44.7X4	T44.7X5	T44.7X6
Sotradecol	T46.8X1	T46.8X2	T46.8X3	T46.8X4	T46.8X5	T46.8X6
Soysterol	T46.6X1	T46.6X2	T46.6X3	T46.6X4	T46.6X5	T46.6X6
Spacoline	T44.3X1	T44.3X2	T44.3X3	T44.3X4	T44.3X5	T44.3X6
Spanish fly	T49.8X1	T49.8X2	T49.8X3	T49.8X4	T49.8X5	T49.8X6
Sparine	T43.3X1	T43.3X2	T43.3X3	T43.3X4	T43.3X5	T43.3X6
Sparteine	T48.0X1	T48.0X2	T48.0X3	T48.0X4	T48.0X5	T48.0X6
Spasmolytic						
anticholinergics	T44.3X1	T44.3X2	T44.3X3	T44.3X4	T44.3X5	T44.3X6
autonomic	T44.3X1	T44.3X2	T44.3X3	T44.3X4	T44.3X5	T44.3X6
bronchial NEC	T48.6X1	T48.6X2	T48.6X3	T48.6X4	T48.6X5	T48.6X6
quaternary ammonium	T44.3X1	T44.3X2	T44.3X3	T44.3X4	T44.3X5	T44.3X6
skeletal muscle NEC	T48.1X1	T48.1X2	T48.1X3	T48.1X4	T48.1X5	T48.1X6
Spectinomycin	T36.5X1	T36.5X2	T36.5X3	T36.5X4	T36.5X5	T36.5X6
Speed	T43.621	T43.622	T43.623	T43.624	T43.625	T43.626
Spermicide	T49.8X1	T49.8X2	T49.8X3	T49.8X4	T49.8X5	T49.8X6
Spider (bite) (venom)	T63.391	T63.392	T63.393	T63.394		
antivenin	T50.Z11	T50.Z12	T50.Z13	T50.Z14	T50.Z15	T50.Z16
Spigelia (root)	T37.4X1	T37.4X2	T37.4X3	T37.4X4	T37.4X5	T37.4X6
Spindle inactivator	T50.4X1	T50.4X2	T50.4X3	T50.4X4	T50.4X5	T50.4X6
Spiperone	T43.4X1	T43.4X2	T43.4X3	T43.4X4	T43.4X5	T43.4X6
Spiramycin	T36.3X1	T36.3X2	T36.3X3	T36.3X4	T36.3X5	T36.3X6
Spirapril	T46.4X1	T46.4X2	T46.4X3	T46.4X4	T46.4X5	T46.4X6
Spirilene	T43.591	T43.592	T43.593	T43.594	T43.595	T43.596
Spirit(s) (neutral) NEC	T51.0X1	T51.0X2	T51.0X3	T51.0X4	—	—
beverage	T51.0X1	T51.0X2	T51.0X3	T51.0X4	—	—
industrial	T51.0X1	T51.0X2	T51.0X3	T51.0X4	—	—
mineral	T52.0X1	T52.0X2	T52.0X3	T52.0X4	—	—
of salt — see Hydrochloric acid						
surgical	T51.0X1	T51.0X2	T51.0X3	T51.0X4	—	—
Spironolactone	T50.0X1	T50.0X2	T50.0X3	T50.0X4	T50.0X5	T50.0X6
Spiroperidol	T43.4X1	T43.4X2	T43.4X3	T43.4X4	T43.4X5	T43.4X6
Sponge, absorbable (gelatin)	T45.7X1	T45.7X2	T45.7X3	T45.7X4	T45.7X5	T45.7X6
Sporostacin	T49.0X1	T49.0X2	T49.0X3	T49.0X4	T49.0X5	T49.0X6
Spray (aerosol)	T65.91	T65.92	T65.93	T65.94	—	—
cosmetic	T65.891	T65.892	T65.893	T65.894	—	—
medicinal NEC	T50.901	T50.902	T50.903	T50.904	T50.905	T50.906
pesticides — see Pesticides						
specified content — see specific substance						
Spurge flax	T62.2X1	T62.2X2	T62.2X3	T62.2X4	—	—
Spurges	T62.2X1	T62.2X2	T62.2X3	T62.2X4	—	—
Sputum viscosity-lowering drug	T48.4X1	T48.4X2	T48.4X3	T48.4X4	T48.4X5	T48.4X6
Squill	T46.0X1	T46.0X2	T46.0X3	T46.0X4	T46.0X5	T46.0X6
rat poison	T60.4X1	T60.4X2	T60.4X3	T60.4X4	—	—
Squirting cucumber (cathartic)	T47.2X1	T47.2X2	T47.2X3	T47.2X4	T47.2X5	T47.2X6
Stains	T65.6X1	T65.6X2	T65.6X3	T65.6X4	—	—
Stannous fluoride	T49.7X1	T49.7X2	T49.7X3	T49.7X4	T49.7X5	T49.7X6
Stanolone	T38.7X1	T38.7X2	T38.7X3	T38.7X4	T38.7X5	T38.7X6
Stanozolol	T38.7X1	T38.7X2	T38.7X3	T38.7X4	T38.7X5	T38.7X6
Staphisagria or stavesacre (pediculicide)	T49.0X1	T49.0X2	T49.0X3	T49.0X4	T49.0X5	T49.0X6
Starch	T50.901	T50.902	T50.903	T50.904	T50.905	T50.906
Stelazine	T43.3X1	T43.3X2	T43.3X3	T43.3X4	T43.3X5	T43.3X6
Stemetil	T43.3X1	T43.3X2	T43.3X3	T43.3X4	T43.3X5	T43.3X6
Stepronin	T48.4X1	T48.4X2	T48.4X3	T48.4X4	T48.4X5	T48.4X6
Sterculia	T47.4X1	T47.4X2	T47.4X3	T47.4X4	T47.4X5	T47.4X6
Sternutator gas	T59.891	T59.892	T59.893	T59.894	—	—
Steroid	T38.0X1	T38.0X2	T38.0X3	T38.0X4	T38.0X5	T38.0X6
anabolic	T38.7X1	T38.7X2	T38.7X3	T38.7X4	T38.7X5	T38.7X6
androgenic	T38.7X1	T38.7X2	T38.7X3	T38.7X4	T38.7X5	T38.7X6
antineoplastic, hormone	T38.7X1	T38.7X2	T38.7X3	T38.7X4	T38.7X5	T38.7X6
estrogen	T38.5X1	T38.5X2	T38.5X3	T38.5X4	T38.5X5	T38.5X6
ENT agent	T49.6X1	T49.6X2	T49.6X3	T49.6X4	T49.6X5	T49.6X6
ophthalmic preparation	T49.5X1	T49.5X2	T49.5X3	T49.5X4	T49.5X5	T49.5X6
topical NEC	T49.0X1	T49.0X2	T49.0X3	T49.0X4	T49.0X5	T49.0X6
Stibine	T56.891	T56.892	T56.893	T56.894	—	—
Stibogluconate	T37.3X1	T37.3X2	T37.3X3	T37.3X4	T37.3X5	T37.3X6
Stibophen	T37.4X1	T37.4X2	T37.4X3	T37.4X4	T37.4X5	T37.4X6
Stilbamidine (isetionate)	T37.3X1	T37.3X2	T37.3X3	T37.3X4	T37.3X5	T37.3X6
Stilbestrol	T38.5X1	T38.5X2	T38.5X3	T38.5X4	T38.5X5	T38.5X6
Stilboestrol	T38.5X1	T38.5X2	T38.5X3	T38.5X4	T38.5X5	T38.5X6
Stimulant						
central nervous system — see also Psychostimulant	T43.601	T43.602	T43.603	T43.604	T43.605	T43.606
analeptics	T50.7X1	T50.7X2	T50.7X3	T50.7X4	T50.7X5	T50.7X6
opiate antagonist	T50.7X1	T50.7X2	T50.7X3	T50.7X4	T50.7X5	T50.7X6
psychotherapeutic NEC — see also Psychotherapeutic drug	T43.601	T43.602	T43.603	T43.604	T43.605	T43.606
specified NEC	T43.691	T43.692	T43.693	T43.694	T43.695	T43.696
respiratory	T48.901	T48.902	T48.903	T48.904	T48.905	T48.906
Stone-dissolving drug	T50.901	T50.902	T50.903	T50.904	T50.905	T50.906
Storage battery (cells) (acid)	T54.2X1	T54.2X2	T54.2X3	T54.2X4	—	—
Stovaine	T41.3X1	T41.3X2	T41.3X3	T41.3X4	T41.3X5	T41.3X6
infiltration (subcutaneous)	T41.3X1	T41.3X2	T41.3X3	T41.3X4	T41.3X5	T41.3X6
nerve block (peripheral) (plexus)	T41.3X1	T41.3X2	T41.3X3	T41.3X4	T41.3X5	T41.3X6
spinal	T41.3X1	T41.3X2	T41.3X3	T41.3X4	T41.3X5	T41.3X6
topical (surface)	T41.3X1	T41.3X2	T41.3X3	T41.3X4	T41.3X5	T41.3X6
Stovarsal	T37.8X1	T37.8X2	T37.8X3	T37.8X4	T37.8X5	T37.8X6
Stove gas — see Gas, stove						
Stoxil	T49.5X1	T49.5X2	T49.5X3	T49.5X4	T49.5X5	T49.5X6
Stramonium	T48.6X1	T48.6X2	T48.6X3	T48.6X4	T48.6X5	T48.6X6
natural state	T62.2X1	T62.2X2	T62.2X3	T62.2X4	—	—
Streptodornase	T45.3X1	T45.3X2	T45.3X3	T45.3X4	T45.3X5	T45.3X6
Streptoduocin	T36.5X1	T36.5X2	T36.5X3	T36.5X4	T36.5X5	T36.5X6
Streptokinase	T45.611	T45.612	T45.613	T45.614	T45.615	T45.616
Streptomycin (derivative)	T36.5X1	T36.5X2	T36.5X3	T36.5X4	T36.5X5	T36.5X6
Streptonivicin	T36.5X1	T36.5X2	T36.5X3	T36.5X4	T36.5X5	T36.5X6
Streptovarycin	T36.5X1	T36.5X2	T36.5X3	T36.5X4	T36.5X5	T36.5X6
Streptozocin	T45.1X1	T45.1X2	T45.1X3	T45.1X4	T45.1X5	T45.1X6
Streptozotocin	T45.1X1	T45.1X2	T45.1X3	T45.1X4	T45.1X5	T45.1X6
Stripper (paint) (solvent)	T52.8X1	T52.8X2	T52.8X3	T52.8X4	—	—
Strobane	T60.1X1	T60.1X2	T60.1X3	T60.1X4	—	—
Strofantina	T46.0X1	T46.0X2	T46.0X3	T46.0X4	T46.0X5	T46.0X6
Strophanthin (g) (k)	T46.0X1	T46.0X2	T46.0X3	T46.0X4	T46.0X5	T46.0X6
Strophanthus	T46.0X1	T46.0X2	T46.0X3	T46.0X4	T46.0X5	T46.0X6
Strophantin	T46.0X1	T46.0X2	T46.0X3	T46.0X4	T46.0X5	T46.0X6
Strophantin-g	T46.0X1	T46.0X2	T46.0X3	T46.0X4	T46.0X5	T46.0X6
Strychnine (nonmedicinal) (pesticide) (salts)	T65.1X1	T65.1X2	T65.1X3	T65.1X4	—	—
medicinal	T48.291	T48.292	T48.293	T48.294	T48.295	T48.296
Strychnos (ignatii) — see Strychnine						
Styramate	T42.8X1	T42.8X2	T42.8X3	T42.8X4	T42.8X5	T42.8X6
Styrene	T65.891	T65.892	T65.893	T65.894	—	—
Succinimide, antiepileptic or anticonvulsant	T42.2X1	T42.2X2	T42.2X3	T42.2X4	T42.2X5	T42.2X6
mercuric — see Mercury						
Succinylcholine	T48.1X1	T48.1X2	T48.1X3	T48.1X4	T48.1X5	T48.1X6
Succinylsulfathiazole	T37.0X1	T37.0X2	T37.0X3	T37.0X4	T37.0X5	T37.0X6
Sucralfate	T47.1X1	T47.1X2	T47.1X3	T47.1X4	T47.1X5	T47.1X6
Sucrose	T50.3X1	T50.3X2	T50.3X3	T50.3X4	T50.3X5	T50.3X6
Sufentanil	T40.4X1	T40.4X2	T40.4X3	T40.4X4	T40.4X5	T40.4X6
Sulbactam	T36.0X1	T36.0X2	T36.0X3	T36.0X4	T36.0X5	T36.0X6
Sulbenicillin	T36.0X1	T36.0X2	T36.0X3	T36.0X4	T36.0X5	T36.0X6
Sulbentine	T49.0X1	T49.0X2	T49.0X3	T49.0X4	T49.0X5	T49.0X6
Sulfacetamide	T49.0X1	T49.0X2	T49.0X3	T49.0X4	T49.0X5	T49.0X6
ophthalmic preparation	T49.5X1	T49.5X2	T49.5X3	T49.5X4	T49.5X5	T49.5X6
Sulfachlorpyridazine	T37.0X1	T37.0X2	T37.0X3	T37.0X4	T37.0X5	T37.0X6
Sulfacitine	T37.0X1	T37.0X2	T37.0X3	T37.0X4	T37.0X5	T37.0X6
Sulfadiasulfone sodium	T37.0X1	T37.0X2	T37.0X3	T37.0X4	T37.0X5	T37.0X6
Sulfadiazine	T37.0X1	T37.0X2	T37.0X3	T37.0X4	T37.0X5	T37.0X6
silver (topical)	T49.0X1	T49.0X2	T49.0X3	T49.0X4	T49.0X5	T49.0X6
Sulfadimethoxine	T37.0X1	T37.0X2	T37.0X3	T37.0X4	T37.0X5	T37.0X6
Sulfadimidine	T37.0X1	T37.0X2	T37.0X3	T37.0X4	T37.0X5	T37.0X6
Sulfadoxine	T37.0X1	T37.0X2	T37.0X3	T37.0X4	T37.0X5	T37.0X6
with pyrimethamine	T37.2X1	T37.2X2	T37.2X3	T37.2X4	T37.2X5	T37.2X6

Additional Character May Be Required — Refer to the Tabular List for Character Selection

▽ Subterms under main terms may continue to next column or page

Substance	Poisoning, Accidental (unintentional)	Poisoning, Intentional Self-harm	Poisoning, Assault	Poisoning, Undetermined	Adverse Effect	Under-dosing
Sulfaethidole	T37.0X1	T37.0X2	T37.0X3	T37.0X4	T37.0X5	T37.0X6
Sulfafurazole	T37.0X1	T37.0X2	T37.0X3	T37.0X4	T37.0X5	T37.0X6
Sulfaguanidine	T37.0X1	T37.0X2	T37.0X3	T37.0X4	T37.0X5	T37.0X6
Sulfalene	T37.0X1	T37.0X2	T37.0X3	T37.0X4	T37.0X5	T37.0X6
Sulfaloxate	T37.0X1	T37.0X2	T37.0X3	T37.0X4	T37.0X5	T37.0X6
Sulfaloxic acid	T37.0X1	T37.0X2	T37.0X3	T37.0X4	T37.0X5	T37.0X6
Sulfamazone	T39.2X1	T39.2X2	T39.2X3	T39.2X4	T39.2X5	T39.2X6
Sulfamerazine	T37.0X1	T37.0X2	T37.0X3	T37.0X4	T37.0X5	T37.0X6
Sulfameter	T37.0X1	T37.0X2	T37.0X3	T37.0X4	T37.0X5	T37.0X6
Sulfamethazine	T37.0X1	T37.0X2	T37.0X3	T37.0X4	T37.0X5	T37.0X6
Sulfamethizole	T37.0X1	T37.0X2	T37.0X3	T37.0X4	T37.0X5	T37.0X6
Sulfamethoxazole	T37.0X1	T37.0X2	T37.0X3	T37.0X4	T37.0X5	T37.0X6
with trimethoprim	T36.8X1	T36.8X2	T36.8X3	T36.8X4	T36.8X5	T36.8X6
Sulfamethoxydiazine	T37.0X1	T37.0X2	T37.0X3	T37.0X4	T37.0X5	T37.0X6
Sulfamethoxypyridazine	T37.0X1	T37.0X2	T37.0X3	T37.0X4	T37.0X5	T37.0X6
Sulfamethylthiazole	T37.0X1	T37.0X2	T37.0X3	T37.0X4	T37.0X5	T37.0X6
Sulfametoxydiazine	T37.0X1	T37.0X2	T37.0X3	T37.0X4	T37.0X5	T37.0X6
Sulfamidopyrine	T39.2X1	T39.2X2	T39.2X3	T39.2X4	T39.2X5	T39.2X6
Sulfamonomethoxine	T37.0X1	T37.0X2	T37.0X3	T37.0X4	T37.0X5	T37.0X6
Sulfamoxole	T37.0X1	T37.0X2	T37.0X3	T37.0X4	T37.0X5	T37.0X6
Sulfamylon	T49.0X1	T49.0X2	T49.0X3	T49.0X4	T49.0X5	T49.0X6
Sulfan blue (diagnostic dye)	T50.8X1	T50.8X2	T50.8X3	T50.8X4	T50.8X5	T50.8X6
Sulfanilamide	T37.0X1	T37.0X2	T37.0X3	T37.0X4	T37.0X5	T37.0X6
Sulfanilylguanidine	T37.0X1	T37.0X2	T37.0X3	T37.0X4	T37.0X5	T37.0X6
Sulfaperin	T37.0X1	T37.0X2	T37.0X3	T37.0X4	T37.0X5	T37.0X6
Sulfaphenazole	T37.0X1	T37.0X2	T37.0X3	T37.0X4	T37.0X5	T37.0X6
Sulfaphenylthiazole	T37.0X1	T37.0X2	T37.0X3	T37.0X4	T37.0X5	T37.0X6
Sulfaproxyline	T37.0X1	T37.0X2	T37.0X3	T37.0X4	T37.0X5	T37.0X6
Sulfapyridine	T37.0X1	T37.0X2	T37.0X3	T37.0X4	T37.0X5	T37.0X6
Sulfapyrimidine	T37.0X1	T37.0X2	T37.0X3	T37.0X4	T37.0X5	T37.0X6
Sulfarsphenamine	T37.8X1	T37.8X2	T37.8X3	T37.8X4	T37.8X5	T37.8X6
Sulfasalazine	T37.0X1	T37.0X2	T37.0X3	T37.0X4	T37.0X5	T37.0X6
Sulfasuxidine	T37.0X1	T37.0X2	T37.0X3	T37.0X4	T37.0X5	T37.0X6
Sulfasymazine	T37.0X1	T37.0X2	T37.0X3	T37.0X4	T37.0X5	T37.0X6
Sulfated amylopectin	T47.8X1	T47.8X2	T47.8X3	T47.8X4	T47.8X5	T47.8X6
Sulfathiazole	T37.0X1	T37.0X2	T37.0X3	T37.0X4	T37.0X5	T37.0X6
Sulfatostearate	T49.2X1	T49.2X2	T49.2X3	T49.2X4	T49.2X5	T49.2X6
Sulfinpyrazone	T50.4X1	T50.4X2	T50.4X3	T50.4X4	T50.4X5	T50.4X6
Sulfiram	T49.0X1	T49.0X2	T49.0X3	T49.0X4	T49.0X5	T49.0X6
Sulfisomidine	T37.0X1	T37.0X2	T37.0X3	T37.0X4	T37.0X5	T37.0X6
Sulfisoxazole	T37.0X1	T37.0X2	T37.0X3	T37.0X4	T37.0X5	T37.0X6
ophthalmic preparation	T49.5X1	T49.5X2	T49.5X3	T49.5X4	T49.5X5	T49.5X6
Sulfobromophthalein (sodium)	T50.8X1	T50.8X2	T50.8X3	T50.8X4	T50.8X5	T50.8X6
Sulfobromphthalein	T50.8X1	T50.8X2	T50.8X3	T50.8X4	T50.8X5	T50.8X6
Sulfogaiacol	T48.4X1	T48.4X2	T48.4X3	T48.4X4	T48.4X5	T48.4X6
Sulfomyxin	T36.8X1	T36.8X2	T36.8X3	T36.8X4	T36.8X5	T36.8X6
Sulfonal	T42.6X1	T42.6X2	T42.6X3	T42.6X4	T42.6X5	T42.6X6
Sulfonamide NEC	T37.0X1	T37.0X2	T37.0X3	T37.0X4	T37.0X5	T37.0X6
eye	T49.5X1	T49.5X2	T49.5X3	T49.5X4	T49.5X5	T49.5X6
Sulfonazide	T37.1X1	T37.1X2	T37.1X3	T37.1X4	T37.1X5	T37.1X6
Sulfones	T37.1X1	T37.1X2	T37.1X3	T37.1X4	T37.1X5	T37.1X6
Sulfonethylmethane	T42.6X1	T42.6X2	T42.6X3	T42.6X4	T42.6X5	T42.6X6
Sulfonmethane	T42.6X1	T42.6X2	T42.6X3	T42.6X4	T42.6X5	T42.6X6
Sulfonphthal, sulfonphthol	T50.8X1	T50.8X2	T50.8X3	T50.8X4	T50.8X5	T50.8X6
Sulfonylurea derivatives, oral	T38.3X1	T38.3X2	T38.3X3	T38.3X4	T38.3X5	T38.3X6
Sulforidazine	T43.3X1	T43.3X2	T43.3X3	T43.3X4	T43.3X5	T43.3X6
Sulfoxone	T37.1X1	T37.1X2	T37.1X3	T37.1X4	T37.1X5	T37.1X6
Sulfuric acid	T54.2X1	T54.2X2	T54.2X3	T54.2X4	—	—
Sulfur, sulfurated, sulfuric, sulfurous, sulfuryl (compounds NEC) (medicinal)	T49.4X1	T49.4X2	T49.4X3	T49.4X4	T49.4X5	T49.4X6
acid	T54.2X1	T54.2X2	T54.2X3	T54.2X4	—	—
dioxide (gas)	T59.1X1	T59.1X2	T59.1X3	T59.1X4	—	—
ether — see Ether(s)						
hydrogen	T59.6X1	T59.6X2	T59.6X3	T59.6X4	—	—
medicinal (keratolytic) (ointment) NEC	T49.4X1	T49.4X2	T49.4X3	T49.4X4	T49.4X5	T49.4X6
ointment	T49.0X1	T49.0X2	T49.0X3	T49.0X4	T49.0X5	T49.0X6
pesticide (vapor)	T60.91	T60.92	T60.93	T60.94	—	—
vapor NEC	T59.891	T59.892	T59.893	T59.894	—	—
Sulglicotide	T47.1X1	T47.1X2	T47.1X3	T47.1X4	T47.1X5	T47.1X6
Sulindac	T39.391	T39.392	T39.393	T39.394	T39.395	T39.396
Sulisatin	T47.2X1	T47.2X2	T47.2X3	T47.2X4	T47.2X5	T47.2X6
Sulisobenzone	T49.3X1	T49.3X2	T49.3X3	T49.3X4	T49.3X5	T49.3X6
Sulkowitch's reagent	T50.8X1	T50.8X2	T50.8X3	T50.8X4	T50.8X5	T50.8X6
Sulmetozine	T44.3X1	T44.3X2	T44.3X3	T44.3X4	T44.3X5	T44.3X6
Suloctidil	T46.7X1	T46.7X2	T46.7X3	T46.7X4	T46.7X5	T46.7X6
Sulph- — see also Sulf-						
Sulphadiazine	T37.0X1	T37.0X2	T37.0X3	T37.0X4	T37.0X5	T37.0X6
Sulphadimethoxine	T37.0X1	T37.0X2	T37.0X3	T37.0X4	T37.0X5	T37.0X6

Substance	Poisoning, Accidental (unintentional)	Poisoning, Intentional Self-harm	Poisoning, Assault	Poisoning, Undetermined	Adverse Effect	Under-dosing
Sulphadimidine	T37.0X1	T37.0X2	T37.0X3	T37.0X4	T37.0X5	T37.0X6
Sulphadione	T37.1X1	T37.1X2	T37.1X3	T37.1X4	T37.1X5	T37.1X6
Sulphafurazole	T37.0X1	T37.0X2	T37.0X3	T37.0X4	T37.0X5	T37.0X6
Sulphamethizole	T37.0X1	T37.0X2	T37.0X3	T37.0X4	T37.0X5	T37.0X6
Sulphamethoxazole	T37.0X1	T37.0X2	T37.0X3	T37.0X4	T37.0X5	T37.0X6
Sulphan blue	T50.8X1	T50.8X2	T50.8X3	T50.8X4	T50.8X5	T50.8X6
Sulphaphenazole	T37.0X1	T37.0X2	T37.0X3	T37.0X4	T37.0X5	T37.0X6
Sulphapyridine	T37.0X1	T37.0X2	T37.0X3	T37.0X4	T37.0X5	T37.0X6
Sulphasalazine	T37.0X1	T37.0X2	T37.0X3	T37.0X4	T37.0X5	T37.0X6
Sulphinpyrazone	T50.4X1	T50.4X2	T50.4X3	T50.4X4	T50.4X5	T50.4X6
Sulpiride	T43.591	T43.592	T43.593	T43.594	T43.595	T43.596
Sulprostone	T48.0X1	T48.0X2	T48.0X3	T48.0X4	T48.0X5	T48.0X6
Sulpyrine	T39.2X1	T39.2X2	T39.2X3	T39.2X4	T39.2X5	T39.2X6
Sultamicillin	T36.0X1	T36.0X2	T36.0X3	T36.0X4	T36.0X5	T36.0X6
Sulthiame	T42.6X1	T42.6X2	T42.6X3	T42.6X4	T42.6X5	T42.6X6
Sultiame	T42.6X1	T42.6X2	T42.6X3	T42.6X4	T42.6X5	T42.6X6
Sultopride	T43.591	T43.592	T43.593	T43.594	T43.595	T43.596
Sumatriptan	T39.8X1	T39.8X2	T39.8X3	T39.8X4	T39.8X5	T39.8X6
Sunflower seed oil	T46.6X1	T46.6X2	T46.6X3	T46.6X4	T46.6X5	T46.6X6
Superinone	T48.4X1	T48.4X2	T48.4X3	T48.4X4	T48.4X5	T48.4X6
Suprofen	T39.311	T39.312	T39.313	T39.314	T39.315	T39.316
Suramin (sodium)	T37.4X1	T37.4X2	T37.4X3	T37.4X4	T37.4X5	T37.4X6
Surfacaine	T41.3X1	T41.3X2	T41.3X3	T41.3X4	T41.3X5	T41.3X6
Surital	T41.1X1	T41.1X2	T41.1X3	T41.1X4	T41.1X5	T41.1X6
Sutilains	T45.3X1	T45.3X2	T45.3X3	T45.3X4	T45.3X5	T45.3X6
Suxamethonium (chloride)	T48.1X1	T48.1X2	T48.1X3	T48.1X4	T48.1X5	T48.1X6
Suxethonium (chloride)	T48.1X1	T48.1X2	T48.1X3	T48.1X4	T48.1X5	T48.1X6
Suxibuzone	T39.2X1	T39.2X2	T39.2X3	T39.2X4	T39.2X5	T39.2X6
Sweetener	T50.901	T50.902	T50.903	T50.904	T50.905	T50.906
Sweet niter spirit	T46.3X1	T46.3X2	T46.3X3	T46.3X4	T46.3X5	T46.3X6
Sweet oil (birch)	T49.3X1	T49.3X2	T49.3X3	T49.3X4	T49.3X5	T49.3X6
Sym-dichloroethyl ether	T53.6X1	T53.6X2	T53.6X3	T53.6X4	—	—
Sympatholytic NEC	T44.8X1	T44.8X2	T44.8X3	T44.8X4	T44.8X5	T44.8X6
haloalkylamine	T44.8X1	T44.8X2	T44.8X3	T44.8X4	T44.8X5	T44.8X6
Sympathomimetic NEC	T44.901	T44.902	T44.903	T44.904	T44.905	T44.906
anti-common-cold	T48.5X1	T48.5X2	T48.5X3	T48.5X4	T48.5X5	T48.5X6
bronchodilator	T48.6X1	T48.6X2	T48.6X3	T48.6X4	T48.6X5	T48.6X6
specified NEC	T44.991	T44.992	T44.993	T44.994	T44.995	T44.996
Synagis	T50.B91	T50.B92	T50.B93	T50.B94	T50.B95	T50.B96
Synalar	T49.0X1	T49.0X2	T49.0X3	T49.0X4	T49.0X5	T49.0X6
Synthroid	T38.1X1	T38.1X2	T38.1X3	T38.1X4	T38.1X5	T38.1X6
Syntocinon	T48.0X1	T48.0X2	T48.0X3	T48.0X4	T48.0X5	T48.0X6
Syrosingopine	T46.5X1	T46.5X2	T46.5X3	T46.5X4	T46.5X5	T46.5X6
Systemic drug	T45.91	T45.92	T45.93	T45.94	T45.95	T45.96
specified NEC	T45.8X1	T45.8X2	T45.8X3	T45.8X4	T45.8X5	T45.8X6
Tablets — see also specified substance	T50.901	T50.902	T50.903	T50.904	T50.905	T50.906
Tace	T38.5X1	T38.5X2	T38.5X3	T38.5X4	T38.5X5	T38.5X6
Tacrine	T44.0X1	T44.0X2	T44.0X3	T44.0X4	T44.0X5	T44.0X6
Tadalafil	T46.7X1	T46.7X2	T46.7X3	T46.7X4	T46.7X5	T46.7X6
Talampicillin	T36.0X1	T36.0X2	T36.0X3	T36.0X4	T36.0X5	T36.0X6
Talbutal	T42.3X1	T42.3X2	T42.3X3	T42.3X4	T42.3X5	T42.3X6
Talc powder	T49.3X1	T49.3X2	T49.3X3	T49.3X4	T49.3X5	T49.3X6
Talcum	T49.3X1	T49.3X2	T49.3X3	T49.3X4	T49.3X5	T49.3X6
Taleranol	T38.6X1	T38.6X2	T38.6X3	T38.6X4	T38.6X5	T38.6X6
Tamoxifen	T38.6X1	T38.6X2	T38.6X3	T38.6X4	T38.6X5	T38.6X6
Tamsulosin	T44.6X1	T44.6X2	T44.6X3	T44.6X4	T44.6X5	T44.6X6
Tandearil, tanderil	T39.2X1	T39.2X2	T39.2X3	T39.2X4	T39.2X5	T39.2X6
Tannic acid	T49.2X1	T49.2X2	T49.2X3	T49.2X4	T49.2X5	T49.2X6
medicinal (astringent)	T49.2X1	T49.2X2	T49.2X3	T49.2X4	T49.2X5	T49.2X6
Tannin — see Tannic acid						
Tansy	T62.2X1	T62.2X2	T62.2X3	T62.2X4	—	—
TAO	T36.3X1	T36.3X2	T36.3X3	T36.3X4	T36.3X5	T36.3X6
Tapazole	T38.2X1	T38.2X2	T38.2X3	T38.2X4	T38.2X5	T38.2X6
Taractan	T43.591	T43.592	T43.593	T43.594	T43.595	T43.596
Tarantula (venomous)	T63.321	T63.322	T63.323	T63.324		
Tartar emetic	T37.8X1	T37.8X2	T37.8X3	T37.8X4	T37.8X5	T37.8X6
Tartaric acid	T65.891	T65.892	T65.893	T65.894	—	—
Tartrated antimony (anti-infective)	T37.8X1	T37.8X2	T37.8X3	T37.8X4	T37.8X5	T37.8X6
Tartrate, laxative	T47.4X1	T47.4X2	T47.4X3	T47.4X4	T47.4X5	T47.4X6
Tar NEC	T52.0X1	T52.0X2	T52.0X3	T52.0X4	—	—
camphor	T60.1X1	T60.1X2	T60.1X3	T60.1X4	—	—
distillate	T49.1X1	T49.1X2	T49.1X3	T49.1X4	T49.1X5	T49.1X6
fumes	T59.891	T59.892	T59.893	T59.894	—	—
medicinal	T49.1X1	T49.1X2	T49.1X3	T49.1X4	T49.1X5	T49.1X6
ointment	T49.1X1	T49.1X2	T49.1X3	T49.1X4	T49.1X5	T49.1X6
Tauromustine	T45.1X1	T45.1X2	T45.1X3	T45.1X4	T45.1X5	T45.1X6
TCA — see Trichloroacetic acid						
TCDD	T53.7X1	T53.7X2	T53.7X3	T53.7X4	—	—
TDI (vapor)	T65.0X1	T65.0X2	T65.0X3	T65.0X4	—	—
Tear						
gas	T59.3X1	T59.3X2	T59.3X3	T59.3X4	—	—

Table of Drugs and Chemicals

Substance	Poisoning, Accidental (unintentional)	Poisoning, Intentional Self-harm	Poisoning, Assault	Poisoning, Undetermined	Adverse Effect	Under-dosing
Tear — continued						
solution	T49.5X1	T49.5X2	T49.5X3	T49.5X4	T49.5X5	T49.5X6
Teclothiazide	T50.2X1	T50.2X2	T50.2X3	T50.2X4	T50.2X5	T50.2X6
Teclozan	T37.3X1	T37.3X2	T37.3X3	T37.3X4	T37.3X5	T37.3X6
Tegafur	T45.1X1	T45.1X2	T45.1X3	T45.1X4	T45.1X5	T45.1X6
Tegretol	T42.1X1	T42.1X2	T42.1X3	T42.1X4	T42.1X5	T42.1X6
Teicoplanin	T36.8X1	T36.8X2	T36.8X3	T36.8X4	T36.8X5	T36.8X6
Telepaque	T50.8X1	T50.8X2	T50.8X3	T50.8X4	T50.8X5	T50.8X6
Tellurium	T56.891	T56.892	T56.893	T56.894	—	—
fumes	T56.891	T56.892	T56.893	T56.894	—	—
TEM	T45.1X1	T45.1X2	T45.1X3	T45.1X4	T45.1X5	T45.1X6
Temazepam	T42.4X1	T42.4X2	T42.4X3	T42.4X4	T42.4X5	T42.4X6
Temocillin	T36.0X1	T36.0X2	T36.0X3	T36.0X4	T36.0X5	T36.0X6
Tenamfetamine	T43.621	T43.622	T43.623	T43.624	T43.625	T43.626
Teniposide	T45.1X1	T45.1X2	T45.1X3	T45.1X4	T45.1X5	T45.1X6
Tenitramine	T46.3X1	T46.3X2	T46.3X3	T46.3X4	T46.3X5	T46.3X6
Tenoglicin	T48.4X1	T48.4X2	T48.4X3	T48.4X4	T48.4X5	T48.4X6
Tenonitrozole	T37.3X1	T37.3X2	T37.3X3	T37.3X4	T37.3X5	T37.3X6
Tenoxicam	T39.391	T39.392	T39.393	T39.394	T39.395	T39.396
TEPA	T45.1X1	T45.1X2	T45.1X3	T45.1X4	T45.1X5	T45.1X6
TEPP	T60.0X1	T60.0X2	T60.0X3	T60.0X4	—	—
Teprotide	T46.5X1	T46.5X2	T46.5X3	T46.5X4	T46.5X5	T46.5X6
Terazosin	T44.6X1	T44.6X2	T44.6X3	T44.6X4	T44.6X5	T44.6X6
Terbufos	T60.0X1	T60.0X2	T60.0X3	T60.0X4	—	—
Terbutaline	T48.6X1	T48.6X2	T48.6X3	T48.6X4	T48.6X5	T48.6X6
Terconazole	T49.0X1	T49.0X2	T49.0X3	T49.0X4	T49.0X5	T49.0X6
Terfenadine	T45.0X1	T45.0X2	T45.0X3	T45.0X4	T45.0X5	T45.0X6
Teriparatide (acetate)	T50.991	T50.992	T50.993	T50.994	T50.995	T50.996
Terizidone	T37.1X1	T37.1X2	T37.1X3	T37.1X4	T37.1X5	T37.1X6
Terlipressin	T38.891	T38.892	T38.893	T38.894	T38.895	T38.896
Terodiline	T46.3X1	T46.3X2	T46.3X3	T46.3X4	T46.3X5	T46.3X6
Teroxalene	T37.4X1	T37.4X2	T37.4X3	T37.4X4	T37.4X5	T37.4X6
Terpin (cis) **hydrate**	T48.4X1	T48.4X2	T48.4X3	T48.4X4	T48.4X5	T48.4X6
Terramycin	T36.4X1	T36.4X2	T36.4X3	T36.4X4	T36.4X5	T36.4X6
Tertatolol	T44.7X1	T44.7X2	T44.7X3	T44.7X4	T44.7X5	T44.7X6
Tessalon	T48.3X1	T48.3X2	T48.3X3	T48.3X4	T48.3X5	T48.3X6
Testolactone	T38.7X1	T38.7X2	T38.7X3	T38.7X4	T38.7X5	T38.7X6
Testosterone	T38.7X1	T38.7X2	T38.7X3	T38.7X4	T38.7X5	T38.7X6
Tetanus toxoid or vaccine	T50.A91	T50.A92	T50.A93	T50.A94	T50.A95	T50.A96
antitoxin	T50.Z11	T50.Z12	T50.Z13	T50.Z14	T50.Z15	T50.Z16
immune globulin (human)	T50.Z11	T50.Z12	T50.Z13	T50.Z14	T50.Z15	T50.Z16
toxoid	T50.A91	T50.A92	T50.A93	T50.A94	T50.A95	T50.A96
with diphtheria toxoid	T50.A21	T50.A22	T50.A23	T50.A24	T50.A25	T50.A26
with pertussis	T50.A11	T50.A12	T50.A13	T50.A14	T50.A15	T50.A16
Tetrabenazine	T43.591	T43.592	T43.593	T43.594	T43.595	T43.596
Tetracaine	T41.3X1	T41.3X2	T41.3X3	T41.3X4	T41.3X5	T41.3X6
nerve block (peripheral) (plexus)	T41.3X1	T41.3X2	T41.3X3	T41.3X4	T41.3X5	T41.3X6
regional	T41.3X1	T41.3X2	T41.3X3	T41.3X4	T41.3X5	T41.3X6
spinal	T41.3X1	T41.3X2	T41.3X3	T41.3X4	T41.3X5	T41.3X6
Tetrachlorethylene — see Tetrachloroethylene						
Tetrachlormethiazide	T50.2X1	T50.2X2	T50.2X3	T50.2X4	T50.2X5	T50.2X6
Tetrachloroethane	T53.6X1	T53.6X2	T53.6X3	T53.6X4	—	—
vapor	T53.6X1	T53.6X2	T53.6X3	T53.6X4	—	—
paint or varnish	T53.6X1	T53.6X2	T53.6X3	T53.6X4	—	—
Tetrachloroethylene (liquid)	T53.3X1	T53.3X2	T53.3X3	T53.3X4	—	—
medicinal	T37.4X1	T37.4X2	T37.4X3	T37.4X4	T37.4X5	T37.4X6
vapor	T53.3X1	T53.3X2	T53.3X3	T53.3X4	—	—
Tetrachloromethane — see Carbon tetrachloride						
Tetracosactide	T38.811	T38.812	T38.813	T38.814	T38.815	T38.816
Tetracosactrin	T38.811	T38.812	T38.813	T38.814	T38.815	T38.816
Tetracycline	T36.4X1	T36.4X2	T36.4X3	T36.4X4	T36.4X5	T36.4X6
ophthalmic preparation	T49.5X1	T49.5X2	T49.5X3	T49.5X4	T49.5X5	T49.5X6
topical NEC	T49.0X1	T49.0X2	T49.0X3	T49.0X4	T49.0X5	T49.0X6
Tetradifon	T60.8X1	T60.8X2	T60.8X3	T60.8X4	—	—
Tetradotoxin	T61.771	T61.772	T61.773	T61.774	—	—
Tetraethyl						
lead	T56.0X1	T56.0X2	T56.0X3	T56.0X4	—	—
pyrophosphate	T60.0X1	T60.0X2	T60.0X3	T60.0X4	—	—
Tetraethylammonium **chloride**	T44.2X1	T44.2X2	T44.2X3	T44.2X4	T44.2X5	T44.2X6
Tetraethylthiuram **disulfide**	T50.6X1	T50.6X2	T50.6X3	T50.6X4	T50.6X5	T50.6X6
Tetrahydroaminoacridine	T44.0X1	T44.0X2	T44.0X3	T44.0X4	T44.0X5	T44.0X6
Tetrahydrocannabinol	T40.7X1	T40.7X2	T40.7X3	T40.7X4	T40.7X5	T40.7X6
Tetrahydrofuran	T52.8X1	T52.8X2	T52.8X3	T52.8X4	—	—
Tetrahydronaphthalene	T52.8X1	T52.8X2	T52.8X3	T52.8X4	—	—
Tetrahydrozoline	T49.5X1	T49.5X2	T49.5X3	T49.5X4	T49.5X5	T49.5X6
Tetralin	T52.8X1	T52.8X2	T52.8X3	T52.8X4	—	—
Tetramethrin	T60.2X1	T60.2X2	T60.2X3	T60.2X4	—	—

Substance	Poisoning, Accidental (unintentional)	Poisoning, Intentional Self-harm	Poisoning, Assault	Poisoning, Undetermined	Adverse Effect	Under-dosing
Tetramethylthiuram (disulfide)	T60.3X1	T60.3X2	T60.3X3	T60.3X4	—	—
NEC						
medicinal	T49.0X1	T49.0X2	T49.0X3	T49.0X4	T49.0X5	T49.0X6
Tetramisole	T37.4X1	T37.4X2	T37.4X3	T37.4X4	T37.4X5	T37.4X6
Tetranicotinoyl fructose	T46.7X1	T46.7X2	T46.7X3	T46.7X4	T46.7X5	T46.7X6
Tetrazepam	T42.4X1	T42.4X2	T42.4X3	T42.4X4	T42.4X5	T42.4X6
Tetronal	T42.6X1	T42.6X2	T42.6X3	T42.6X4	T42.6X5	T42.6X6
Tetryl	T65.3X1	T65.3X2	T65.3X3	T65.3X4	—	—
Tetrylammonium chloride	T44.2X1	T44.2X2	T44.2X3	T44.2X4	T44.2X5	T44.2X6
Tetryzoline	T49.5X1	T49.5X2	T49.5X3	T49.5X4	T49.5X5	T49.5X6
Thalidomide	T45.1X1	T45.1X2	T45.1X3	T45.1X4	T45.1X5	T45.1X6
Thallium (compounds) (dust) **NEC**	T56.811	T56.812	T56.813	T56.814		
pesticide	T60.4X1	T60.4X2	T60.4X3	T60.4X4		
THC	T40.7X1	T40.7X2	T40.7X3	T40.7X4	T40.7X5	T40.7X6
Thebacon	T48.3X1	T48.3X2	T48.3X3	T48.3X4	T48.3X5	T48.3X6
Thebaine	T40.2X1	T40.2X2	T40.2X3	T40.2X4	T40.2X5	T40.2X6
Thenoic acid	T49.6X1	T49.6X2	T49.6X3	T49.6X4	T49.6X5	T49.6X6
Thenyldiamine	T45.0X1	T45.0X2	T45.0X3	T45.0X4	T45.0X5	T45.0X6
Theobromine (calcium salicylate)	T48.6X1	T48.6X2	T48.6X3	T48.6X4	T48.6X5	T48.6X6
sodium salicylate	T48.6X1	T48.6X2	T48.6X3	T48.6X4	T48.6X5	T48.6X6
Theophyllamine	T48.6X1	T48.6X2	T48.6X3	T48.6X4	T48.6X5	T48.6X6
Theophylline	T48.6X1	T48.6X2	T48.6X3	T48.6X4	T48.6X5	T48.6X6
aminobenzoic acid	T48.6X1	T48.6X2	T48.6X3	T48.6X4	T48.6X5	T48.6X6
ethylenediamine	T48.6X1	T48.6X2	T48.6X3	T48.6X4	T48.6X5	T48.6X6
piperazine	T48.6X1	T48.6X2	T48.6X3	T48.6X4	T48.6X5	T48.6X6
p-amino-benzoate						
Thiabendazole	T37.4X1	T37.4X2	T37.4X3	T37.4X4	T37.4X5	T37.4X6
Thialbarbital	T41.1X1	T41.1X2	T41.1X3	T41.1X4	T41.1X5	T41.1X6
Thiamazole	T38.2X1	T38.2X2	T38.2X3	T38.2X4	T38.2X5	T38.2X6
Thiambutosine	T37.1X1	T37.1X2	T37.1X3	T37.1X4	T37.1X5	T37.1X6
Thiamine	T45.2X1	T45.2X2	T45.2X3	T45.2X4	T45.2X5	T45.2X6
Thiamphenicol	T36.2X1	T36.2X2	T36.2X3	T36.2X4	T36.2X5	T36.2X6
Thiamylal	T41.1X1	T41.1X2	T41.1X3	T41.1X4	T41.1X5	T41.1X6
sodium	T41.1X1	T41.1X2	T41.1X3	T41.1X4	T41.1X5	T41.1X6
Thiazesim	T43.291	T43.292	T43.293	T43.294	T43.295	T43.296
Thiazides (diuretics)	T50.2X1	T50.2X2	T50.2X3	T50.2X4	T50.2X5	T50.2X6
Thiazinamium metilsulfate	T43.3X1	T43.3X2	T43.3X3	T43.3X4	T43.3X5	T43.3X6
Thiethylperazine	T43.3X1	T43.3X2	T43.3X3	T43.3X4	T43.3X5	T43.3X6
Thimerosal	T49.0X1	T49.0X2	T49.0X3	T49.0X4	T49.0X5	T49.0X6
ophthalmic preparation	T49.5X1	T49.5X2	T49.5X3	T49.5X4	T49.5X5	T49.5X6
Thioacetazone	T37.1X1	T37.1X2	T37.1X3	T37.1X4	T37.1X5	T37.1X6
with isoniazid	T37.1X1	T37.1X2	T37.1X3	T37.1X4	T37.1X5	T37.1X6
Thiobarbital sodium	T41.1X1	T41.1X2	T41.1X3	T41.1X4	T41.1X5	T41.1X6
Thiobarbiturate anesthetic	T41.1X1	T41.1X2	T41.1X3	T41.1X4	T41.1X5	T41.1X6
Thiobismol	T37.8X1	T37.8X2	T37.8X3	T37.8X4	T37.8X5	T37.8X6
Thiobutabarbital sodium	T41.1X1	T41.1X2	T41.1X3	T41.1X4	T41.1X5	T41.1X6
Thiocarbamate (insecticide)	T60.0X1	T60.0X2	T60.0X3	T60.0X4	—	—
Thiocarbamide	T38.2X1	T38.2X2	T38.2X3	T38.2X4	T38.2X5	T38.2X6
Thiocarbarsone	T37.8X1	T37.8X2	T37.8X3	T37.8X4	T37.8X5	T37.8X6
Thiocarlide	T37.1X1	T37.1X2	T37.1X3	T37.1X4	T37.1X5	T37.1X6
Thioctamide	T50.991	T50.992	T50.993	T50.994	T50.995	T50.996
Thioctic acid	T50.991	T50.992	T50.993	T50.994	T50.995	T50.996
Thiofos	T60.0X1	T60.0X2	T60.0X3	T60.0X4	—	—
Thioglycolate	T49.4X1	T49.4X2	T49.4X3	T49.4X4	T49.4X5	T49.4X6
Thioglycolic acid	T65.891	T65.892	T65.893	T65.894	—	—
Thioguanine	T45.1X1	T45.1X2	T45.1X3	T45.1X4	T45.1X5	T45.1X6
Thiomercaptomerin	T50.2X1	T50.2X2	T50.2X3	T50.2X4	T50.2X5	T50.2X6
Thiomerin	T50.2X1	T50.2X2	T50.2X3	T50.2X4	T50.2X5	T50.2X6
Thiomersal	T49.0X1	T49.0X2	T49.0X3	T49.0X4	T49.0X5	T49.0X6
Thionazin	T60.0X1	T60.0X2	T60.0X3	T60.0X4	—	—
Thiopental (sodium)	T41.1X1	T41.1X2	T41.1X3	T41.1X4	T41.1X5	T41.1X6
Thiopentone (sodium)	T41.1X1	T41.1X2	T41.1X3	T41.1X4	T41.1X5	T41.1X6
Thiopropazate	T43.3X1	T43.3X2	T43.3X3	T43.3X4	T43.3X5	T43.3X6
Thioproperazine	T43.3X1	T43.3X2	T43.3X3	T43.3X4	T43.3X5	T43.3X6
Thioridazine	T43.3X1	T43.3X2	T43.3X3	T43.3X4	T43.3X5	T43.3X6
Thiosinamine	T49.3X1	T49.3X2	T49.3X3	T49.3X4	T49.3X5	T49.3X6
Thiotepa	T45.1X1	T45.1X2	T45.1X3	T45.1X4	T45.1X5	T45.1X6
Thiothixene	T43.4X1	T43.4X2	T43.4X3	T43.4X4	T43.4X5	T43.4X6
Thiouracil (benzyl) (methyl) (propyl)	T38.2X1	T38.2X2	T38.2X3	T38.2X4	T38.2X5	T38.2X6
Thiourea	T38.2X1	T38.2X2	T38.2X3	T38.2X4	T38.2X5	T38.2X6
Thiphenamil	T44.3X1	T44.3X2	T44.3X3	T44.3X4	T44.3X5	T44.3X6
Thiram	T60.3X1	T60.3X2	T60.3X3	T60.3X4	—	—
medicinal	T49.2X1	T49.2X2	T49.2X3	T49.2X4	T49.2X5	T49.2X6
Thonzylamine (systemic)	T45.0X1	T45.0X2	T45.0X3	T45.0X4	T45.0X5	T45.0X6
mucosal decongestant	T48.5X1	T48.5X2	T48.5X3	T48.5X4	T48.5X5	T48.5X6
Thorazine	T43.3X1	T43.3X2	T43.3X3	T43.3X4	T43.3X5	T43.3X6
Thorium dioxide **suspension**	T50.8X1	T50.8X2	T50.8X3	T50.8X4	T50.8X5	T50.8X6
Thornapple	T62.2X1	T62.2X2	T62.2X3	T62.2X4		
Throat drug NEC	T49.6X1	T49.6X2	T49.6X3	T49.6X4	T49.6X5	T49.6X6

Additional Character May Be Required — Refer to the Tabular List for Character Selection ▼ Subterms under main terms may continue to next column or page

Tear — Throat drug NEC

Substance	Poisoning, Accidental (unintentional)	Poisoning, Intentional Self-harm	Poisoning, Assault	Poisoning, Undetermined	Adverse Effect	Under-dosing
Thrombin	T45.7X1	T45.7X2	T45.7X3	T45.7X4	T45.7X5	T45.7X6
Thrombolysin	T45.611	T45.612	T45.613	T45.614	T45.615	T45.616
Thromboplastin	T45.7X1	T45.7X2	T45.7X3	T45.7X4	T45.7X5	T45.7X6
Thurfyl nicotinate	T46.7X1	T46.7X2	T46.7X3	T46.7X4	T46.7X5	T46.7X6
Thymol	T49.0X1	T49.0X2	T49.0X3	T49.0X4	T49.0X5	T49.0X6
Thymopentin	T37.5X1	T37.5X2	T37.5X3	T37.5X4	T37.5X5	T37.5X6
Thymoxamine	T46.7X1	T46.7X2	T46.7X3	T46.7X4	T46.7X5	T46.7X6
Thymus extract	T38.891	T38.892	T38.893	T38.894	T38.895	T38.896
Thyreotrophic hormone	T38.811	T38.812	T38.813	T38.814	T38.815	T38.816
Thyroglobulin	T38.1X1	T38.1X2	T38.1X3	T38.1X4	T38.1X5	T38.1X6
Thyroid (hormone)	T38.1X1	T38.1X2	T38.1X3	T38.1X4	T38.1X5	T38.1X6
Thyrolar	T38.1X1	T38.1X2	T38.1X3	T38.1X4	T38.1X5	T38.1X6
Thyrotrophin	T38.811	T38.812	T38.813	T38.814	T38.815	T38.816
Thyrotropic hormone	T38.811	T38.812	T38.813	T38.814	T38.815	T38.816
Thyroxine	T38.1X1	T38.1X2	T38.1X3	T38.1X4	T38.1X5	T38.1X6
Tiabendazole	T37.4X1	T37.4X2	T37.4X3	T37.4X4	T37.4X5	T37.4X6
Tiamizide	T50.2X1	T50.2X2	T50.2X3	T50.2X4	T50.2X5	T50.2X6
Tianeptine	T43.291	T43.292	T43.293	T43.294	T43.295	T43.296
Tiapamil	T46.1X1	T46.1X2	T46.1X3	T46.1X4	T46.1X5	T46.1X6
Tiapride	T43.591	T43.592	T43.593	T43.594	T43.595	T43.596
Tiaprofenic acid	T39.311	T39.312	T39.313	T39.314	T39.315	T39.316
Tiaramide	T39.8X1	T39.8X2	T39.8X3	T39.8X4	T39.8X5	T39.8X6
Ticarcillin	T36.0X1	T36.0X2	T36.0X3	T36.0X4	T36.0X5	T36.0X6
Ticlatone	T49.0X1	T49.0X2	T49.0X3	T49.0X4	T49.0X5	T49.0X6
Ticlopidine	T45.521	T45.522	T45.523	T45.524	T45.525	T45.526
Ticrynafen	T50.1X1	T50.1X2	T50.1X3	T50.1X4	T50.1X5	T50.1X6
Tidiacic	T50.991	T50.992	T50.993	T50.994	T50.995	T50.996
Tiemonium	T44.3X1	T44.3X2	T44.3X3	T44.3X4	T44.3X5	T44.3X6
iodide	T44.3X1	T44.3X2	T44.3X3	T44.3X4	T44.3X5	T44.3X6
Tienilic acid	T50.1X1	T50.1X2	T50.1X3	T50.1X4	T50.1X5	T50.1X6
Tifenamil	T44.3X1	T44.3X2	T44.3X3	T44.3X4	T44.3X5	T44.3X6
Tigan	T45.0X1	T45.0X2	T45.0X3	T45.0X4	T45.0X5	T45.0X6
Tigloidine	T44.3X1	T44.3X2	T44.3X3	T44.3X4	T44.3X5	T44.3X6
Tilactase	T47.5X1	T47.5X2	T47.5X3	T47.5X4	T47.5X5	T47.5X6
Tiletamine	T41.291	T41.292	T41.293	T41.294	T41.295	T41.296
Tilidine	T40.4X1	T40.4X2	T40.4X3	T40.4X4		
Timepidium bromide	T44.3X1	T44.3X2	T44.3X3	T44.3X4	T44.3X5	T44.3X6
Timiperone	T43.4X1	T43.4X2	T43.4X3	T43.4X4	T43.4X5	T43.4X6
Timolol	T44.7X1	T44.7X2	T44.7X3	T44.7X4	T44.7X5	T44.7X6
Tincture, iodine — see Iodine						
Tindal	T43.3X1	T43.3X2	T43.3X3	T43.3X4	T43.3X5	T43.3X6
Tinidazole	T37.3X1	T37.3X2	T37.3X3	T37.3X4	T37.3X5	T37.3X6
Tinoridine	T39.8X1	T39.8X2	T39.8X3	T39.8X4	T39.8X5	T39.8X6
Tin (chloride) (dust) (oxide)	T56.6X1	T56.6X2	T56.6X3	T56.6X4	—	—
NEC						
anti-infectives	T37.8X1	T37.8X2	T37.8X3	T37.8X4	T37.8X5	T37.8X6
Tiocarlide	T37.1X1	T37.1X2	T37.1X3	T37.1X4	T37.1X5	T37.1X6
Tioclomarol	T45.511	T45.512	T45.513	T45.514	T45.515	T45.516
Tioconazole	T49.0X1	T49.0X2	T49.0X3	T49.0X4	T49.0X5	T49.0X6
Tioguanine	T45.1X1	T45.1X2	T45.1X3	T45.1X4	T45.1X5	T45.1X6
Tiopronin	T50.991	T50.992	T50.993	T50.994	T50.995	T50.996
Tiotixene	T43.4X1	T43.4X2	T43.4X3	T43.4X4	T43.4X5	T43.4X6
Tioxolone	T49.4X1	T49.4X2	T49.4X3	T49.4X4	T49.4X5	T49.4X6
Tipepidine	T48.3X1	T48.3X2	T48.3X3	T48.3X4	T48.3X5	T48.3X6
Tiquizium bromide	T44.3X1	T44.3X2	T44.3X3	T44.3X4	T44.3X5	T44.3X6
Tiratricol	T38.1X1	T38.1X2	T38.1X3	T38.1X4	T38.1X5	T38.1X6
Tisopurine	T50.4X1	T50.4X2	T50.4X3	T50.4X4	T50.4X5	T50.4X6
Titanium (compounds)	T56.891	T56.892	T56.893	T56.894	—	—
(vapor)						
dioxide	T49.3X1	T49.3X2	T49.3X3	T49.3X4	T49.3X5	T49.3X6
ointment	T49.3X1	T49.3X2	T49.3X3	T49.3X4	T49.3X5	T49.3X6
oxide	T49.3X1	T49.3X2	T49.3X3	T49.3X4	T49.3X5	T49.3X6
tetrachloride	T56.891	T56.892	T56.893	T56.894	—	—
Titanocene	T56.891	T56.892	T56.893	T56.894	—	—
Titroid	T38.1X1	T38.1X2	T38.1X3	T38.1X4	T38.1X5	T38.1X6
Tizanidine	T42.8X1	T42.8X2	T42.8X3	T42.8X4	T42.8X5	T42.8X6
TMTD	T60.3X1	T60.3X2	T60.3X3	T60.3X4	—	—
TNT (fumes)	T65.3X1	T65.3X2	T65.3X3	T65.3X4	—	—
Toadstool	T62.0X1	T62.0X2	T62.0X3	T62.0X4	—	—
Tobacco NEC	T65.291	T65.292	T65.293	T65.294	—	—
cigarettes	T65.221	T65.222	T65.223	T65.224	—	—
Indian	T62.2X1	T62.2X2	T62.2X3	T62.2X4	—	—
smoke, second-hand	T65.221	T65.222	T65.223	T65.224	—	—
Tobramycin	T36.5X1	T36.5X2	T36.5X3	T36.5X4	T36.5X5	T36.5X6
Tocainide	T46.2X1	T46.2X2	T46.2X3	T46.2X4	T46.2X5	T46.2X6
Tocoferol	T45.2X1	T45.2X2	T45.2X3	T45.2X4	T45.2X5	T45.2X6
Tocopherol	T45.2X1	T45.2X2	T45.2X3	T45.2X4	T45.2X5	T45.2X6
acetate	T45.2X1	T45.2X2	T45.2X3	T45.2X4	T45.2X5	T45.2X6
Tocosamine	T48.0X1	T48.0X2	T48.0X3	T48.0X4	T48.0X5	T48.0X6
Todralazine	T46.5X1	T46.5X2	T46.5X3	T46.5X4	T46.5X5	T46.5X6
Tofisopam	T42.4X1	T42.4X2	T42.4X3	T42.4X4	T42.4X5	T42.4X6
Tofranil	T43.011	T43.012	T43.013	T43.014	T43.015	T43.016
Toilet deodorizer	T65.891	T65.892	T65.893	T65.894	—	—
Tolamolol	T44.7X1	T44.7X2	T44.7X3	T44.7X4	T44.7X5	T44.7X6
Tolazamide	T38.3X1	T38.3X2	T38.3X3	T38.3X4	T38.3X5	T38.3X6
Tolazoline	T46.7X1	T46.7X2	T46.7X3	T46.7X4	T46.7X5	T46.7X6
Tolbutamide (sodium)	T38.3X1	T38.3X2	T38.3X3	T38.3X4	T38.3X5	T38.3X6
Tolciclate	T49.0X1	T49.0X2	T49.0X3	T49.0X4	T49.0X5	T49.0X6
Tolmetin	T39.391	T39.392	T39.393	T39.394	T39.395	T39.396
Tolnaftate	T49.0X1	T49.0X2	T49.0X3	T49.0X4	T49.0X5	T49.0X6
Tolonidine	T46.5X1	T46.5X2	T46.5X3	T46.5X4	T46.5X5	T46.5X6
Toloxatone	T42.6X1	T42.6X2	T42.6X3	T42.6X4	T42.6X5	T42.6X6
Tolperisone	T44.3X1	T44.3X2	T44.3X3	T44.3X4	T44.3X5	T44.3X6
Tolserol	T42.8X1	T42.8X2	T42.8X3	T42.8X4	T42.8X5	T42.8X6
Toluene (liquid)	T52.2X1	T52.2X2	T52.2X3	T52.2X4	—	—
diisocyanate	T65.0X1	T65.0X2	T65.0X3	T65.0X4	—	—
Toluidine	T65.891	T65.892	T65.893	T65.894	—	—
vapor	T59.891	T59.892	T59.893	T59.894	—	—
Toluol (liquid)	T52.2X1	T52.2X2	T52.2X3	T52.2X4	—	—
vapor	T52.2X1	T52.2X2	T52.2X3	T52.2X4	—	—
Toluylenediamine	T65.3X1	T65.3X2	T65.3X3	T65.3X4	—	—
Tolylene-2,4-diisocyanate	T65.0X1	T65.0X2	T65.0X3	T65.0X4	—	—
Tonic NEC	T50.901	T50.902	T50.903	T50.904	T50.905	T50.906
Topical action drug NEC	T49.91	T49.92	T49.93	T49.94	T49.95	T49.96
ear, nose or throat	T49.6X1	T49.6X2	T49.6X3	T49.6X4	T49.6X5	T49.6X6
eye	T49.5X1	T49.5X2	T49.5X3	T49.5X4	T49.5X5	T49.5X6
skin	T49.91	T49.92	T49.93	T49.94	T49.95	T49.96
specified NEC	T49.8X1	T49.8X2	T49.8X3	T49.8X4	T49.8X5	T49.8X6
Toquizine	T44.3X1	T44.3X2	T44.3X3	T44.3X4	T44.3X5	T44.3X6
Toremifene	T38.6X1	T38.6X2	T38.6X3	T38.6X4	T38.6X5	T38.6X6
Tosylchloramide sodium	T49.8X1	T49.8X2	T49.8X3	T49.8X4	T49.8X5	T49.8X6
Toxaphene (dust) (spray)	T60.1X1	T60.1X2	T60.1X3	T60.1X4	—	—
Toxin, diphtheria (Schick Test)	T50.8X1	T50.8X2	T50.8X3	T50.8X4	T50.8X5	T50.8X6
Toxoid						
combined	T50.A21	T50.A22	T50.A23	T50.A24	T50.A25	T50.A26
diphtheria	T50.A91	T50.A92	T50.A93	T50.A94	T50.A95	T50.A96
tetanus	T50.A91	T50.A92	T50.A93	T50.A94	T50.A95	T50.A96
Trace element NEC	T45.8X1	T45.8X2	T45.8X3	T45.8X4	T45.8X5	T45.8X6
Tractor fuel NEC	T52.0X1	T52.0X2	T52.0X3	T52.0X4	—	—
Tragacanth	T50.991	T50.992	T50.993	T50.994	T50.995	T50.996
Tramadol	T40.4X1	T40.4X2	T40.4X3	T40.4X4	T40.4X5	T40.4X6
Tramazoline	T48.5X1	T48.5X2	T48.5X3	T48.5X4	T48.5X5	T48.5X6
Tranexamic acid	T45.621	T45.622	T45.623	T45.624	T45.625	T45.626
Tranilast	T45.0X1	T45.0X2	T45.0X3	T45.0X4	T45.0X5	T45.0X6
Tranquilizer NEC	T43.501	T43.502	T43.503	T43.504	T43.505	T43.506
with hypnotic or sedative	T42.6X1	T42.6X2	T42.6X3	T42.6X4	T42.6X5	T42.6X6
benzodiazepine NEC	T42.4X1	T42.4X2	T42.4X3	T42.4X4	T42.4X5	T42.4X6
butyrophenone NEC	T43.4X1	T43.4X2	T43.4X3	T43.4X4	T43.4X5	T43.4X6
carbamate	T43.591	T43.592	T43.593	T43.594	T43.595	T43.596
dimethylamine	T43.3X1	T43.3X2	T43.3X3	T43.3X4	T43.3X5	T43.3X6
ethylamine	T43.3X1	T43.3X2	T43.3X3	T43.3X4	T43.3X5	T43.3X6
hydroxyzine	T43.591	T43.592	T43.593	T43.594	T43.595	T43.596
major NEC	T43.501	T43.502	T43.503	T43.504	T43.505	T43.506
penothiazine NEC	T43.3X1	T43.3X2	T43.3X3	T43.3X4	T43.3X5	T43.3X6
phenothiazine-based	T43.3X1	T43.3X2	T43.3X3	T43.3X4	T43.3X5	T43.3X6
piperazine NEC	T43.3X1	T43.3X2	T43.3X3	T43.3X4	T43.3X5	T43.3X6
piperidine	T43.3X1	T43.3X2	T43.3X3	T43.3X4	T43.3X5	T43.3X6
propylamine	T43.3X1	T43.3X2	T43.3X3	T43.3X4	T43.3X5	T43.3X6
specified NEC	T43.591	T43.592	T43.593	T43.594	T43.595	T43.596
thioxanthene NEC	T43.591	T43.592	T43.593	T43.594	T43.595	T43.596
Tranxene	T42.4X1	T42.4X2	T42.4X3	T42.4X4	T42.4X5	T42.4X6
Tranylcypromine	T43.1X1	T43.1X2	T43.1X3	T43.1X4	T43.1X5	T43.1X6
Trapidil	T46.3X1	T46.3X2	T46.3X3	T46.3X4	T46.3X5	T46.3X6
Trasentine	T44.3X1	T44.3X2	T44.3X3	T44.3X4	T44.3X5	T44.3X6
Travert	T50.3X1	T50.3X2	T50.3X3	T50.3X4	T50.3X5	T50.3X6
Trazodone	T43.211	T43.212	T43.213	T43.214	T43.215	T43.216
Trecator	T37.1X1	T37.1X2	T37.1X3	T37.1X4	T37.1X5	T37.1X6
Treosulfan	T45.1X1	T45.1X2	T45.1X3	T45.1X4	T45.1X5	T45.1X6
Tretamine	T45.1X1	T45.1X2	T45.1X3	T45.1X4	T45.1X5	T45.1X6
Tretinoin	T49.0X1	T49.0X2	T49.0X3	T49.0X4	T49.0X5	T49.0X6
Tretoquinol	T48.6X1	T48.6X2	T48.6X3	T48.6X4	T48.6X5	T48.6X6
Triacetin	T49.0X1	T49.0X2	T49.0X3	T49.0X4	T49.0X5	T49.0X6
Triacetoxyanthracene	T49.4X1	T49.4X2	T49.4X3	T49.4X4	T49.4X5	T49.4X6
Triacetyloleandomycin	T36.3X1	T36.3X2	T36.3X3	T36.3X4	T36.3X5	T36.3X6
Triamcinolone	T49.0X1	T49.0X2	T49.0X3	T49.0X4	T49.0X5	T49.0X6
ENT agent	T49.6X1	T49.6X2	T49.6X3	T49.6X4	T49.6X5	T49.6X6
hexacetonide	T49.0X1	T49.0X2	T49.0X3	T49.0X4	T49.0X5	T49.0X6
ophthalmic preparation	T49.5X1	T49.5X2	T49.5X3	T49.5X4	T49.5X5	T49.5X6
topical NEC	T49.0X1	T49.0X2	T49.0X3	T49.0X4	T49.0X5	T49.0X6
Triampyzine	T44.3X1	T44.3X2	T44.3X3	T44.3X4	T44.3X5	T44.3X6
Triamterene	T50.2X1	T50.2X2	T50.2X3	T50.2X4	T50.2X5	T50.2X6
Triazine (herbicide)	T60.3X1	T60.3X2	T60.3X3	T60.3X4	—	—
Triaziquone	T45.1X1	T45.1X2	T45.1X3	T45.1X4	T45.1X5	T45.1X6
Triazolam	T42.4X1	T42.4X2	T42.4X3	T42.4X4	T42.4X5	T42.4X6
Triazole (herbicide)	T60.3X1	T60.3X2	T60.3X3	T60.3X4		

⩔ Subterms under main terms may continue to next column or page   Additional Character May Be Required — Refer to the Tabular List for Character Selection   383

Thrombin — Triazole

Substance	Poisoning, Accidental (unintentional)	Poisoning, Intentional Self-harm	Poisoning, Assault	Poisoning, Undetermined	Adverse Effect	Under-dosing
Tribenoside	T46.991	T46.992	T46.993	T46.994	T46.995	T46.996
Tribromacetaldehyde	T42.6X1	T42.6X2	T42.6X3	T42.6X4	T42.6X5	T42.6X6
Tribromoethanol, rectal	T41.291	T41.292	T41.293	T41.294	T41.295	T41.296
Tribromomethane	T42.6X1	T42.6X2	T42.6X3	T42.6X4	T42.6X5	T42.6X6
Trichlorethane	T53.2X1	T53.2X2	T53.2X3	T53.2X4	—	—
Trichlorethylene	T53.2X1	T53.2X2	T53.2X3	T53.2X4	—	—
Trichlorfon	T60.0X1	T60.0X2	T60.0X3	T60.0X4	—	—
Trichlormethiazide	T50.2X1	T50.2X2	T50.2X3	T50.2X4	T50.2X5	T50.2X6
Trichlormethine	T45.1X1	T45.1X2	T45.1X3	T45.1X4	T45.1X5	T45.1X6
Trichloroacetic acid, Trichloracetic acid	T54.2X1	T54.2X2	T54.2X3	T54.2X4	—	—
medicinal	T49.4X1	T49.4X2	T49.4X3	T49.4X4	T49.4X5	T49.4X6
Trichloroethane	T53.2X1	T53.2X2	T53.2X3	T53.2X4	—	—
Trichloroethanol	T42.6X1	T42.6X2	T42.6X3	T42.6X4	T42.6X5	T42.6X6
Trichloroethylene (liquid)	T53.2X1	T53.2X2	T53.2X3	T53.2X4	—	—
(vapor)						
anesthetic (gas)	T41.0X1	T41.0X2	T41.0X3	T41.0X4	T41.0X5	T41.0X6
vapor NEC	T53.2X1	T53.2X2	T53.2X3	T53.2X4	—	—
Trichloroethyl phosphate	T42.6X1	T42.6X2	T42.6X3	T42.6X4	T42.6X5	T42.6X6
Trichlorofluoromethane NEC	T53.5X1	T53.5X2	T53.5X3	T53.5X4	—	—
Trichloronate	T60.0X1	T60.0X2	T60.0X3	T60.0X4	—	—
Trichloropropane	T53.6X1	T53.6X2	T53.6X3	T53.6X4	—	—
Trichlorotriethylamine	T45.1X1	T45.1X2	T45.1X3	T45.1X4	T45.1X5	T45.1X6
Trichomonacides NEC	T37.3X1	T37.3X2	T37.3X3	T37.3X4	T37.3X5	T37.3X6
Trichomycin	T36.7X1	T36.7X2	T36.7X3	T36.7X4	T36.7X5	T36.7X6
Triclobisonium chloride	T49.0X1	T49.0X2	T49.0X3	T49.0X4	T49.0X5	T49.0X6
Triclocarban	T49.0X1	T49.0X2	T49.0X3	T49.0X4	T49.0X5	T49.0X6
Triclofos	T42.6X1	T42.6X2	T42.6X3	T42.6X4	T42.6X5	T42.6X6
Triclosan	T49.0X1	T49.0X2	T49.0X3	T49.0X4	T49.0X5	T49.0X6
Tricresyl phosphate	T65.891	T65.892	T65.893	T65.894	—	—
solvent	T52.91	T52.92	T52.93	T52.94	—	—
Tricyclamol chloride	T44.3X1	T44.3X2	T44.3X3	T44.3X4	T44.3X5	T44.3X6
Tridesilon	T49.0X1	T49.0X2	T49.0X3	T49.0X4	T49.0X5	T49.0X6
Tridihexethyl iodide	T44.3X1	T44.3X2	T44.3X3	T44.3X4	T44.3X5	T44.3X6
Tridione	T42.2X1	T42.2X2	T42.2X3	T42.2X4	T42.2X5	T42.2X6
Trientine	T45.8X1	T45.8X2	T45.8X3	T45.8X4	T45.8X5	T45.8X6
Triethanolamine NEC	T54.3X1	T54.3X2	T54.3X3	T54.3X4	—	—
detergent	T54.3X1	T54.3X2	T54.3X3	T54.3X4	—	—
trinitrate (biphosphate)	T46.3X1	T46.3X2	T46.3X3	T46.3X4	T46.3X5	T46.3X6
Triethanomelamine	T45.1X1	T45.1X2	T45.1X3	T45.1X4	T45.1X5	T45.1X6
Triethylenemelamine	T45.1X1	T45.1X2	T45.1X3	T45.1X4	T45.1X5	T45.1X6
Triethylenephosphoramide	T45.1X1	T45.1X2	T45.1X3	T45.1X4	T45.1X5	T45.1X6
Triethylenethiophosphoramide	T45.1X1	T45.1X2	T45.1X3	T45.1X4	T45.1X5	T45.1X6
Trifluoperazine	T43.3X1	T43.3X2	T43.3X3	T43.3X4	T43.3X5	T43.3X6
Trifluoroethyl vinyl ether	T41.0X1	T41.0X2	T41.0X3	T41.0X4	T41.0X5	T41.0X6
Trifluperidol	T43.4X1	T43.4X2	T43.4X3	T43.4X4	T43.4X5	T43.4X6
Triflupromazine	T43.3X1	T43.3X2	T43.3X3	T43.3X4	T43.3X5	T43.3X6
Trifluridine	T37.5X1	T37.5X2	T37.5X3	T37.5X4	T37.5X5	T37.5X6
Triflusal	T45.521	T45.522	T45.523	T45.524	T45.525	T45.526
Trihexyphenidyl	T44.3X1	T44.3X2	T44.3X3	T44.3X4	T44.3X5	T44.3X6
Triiodothyronine	T38.1X1	T38.1X2	T38.1X3	T38.1X4	T38.1X5	T38.1X6
Trilene	T41.0X1	T41.0X2	T41.0X3	T41.0X4	T41.0X5	T41.0X6
Trilostane	T38.991	T38.992	T38.993	T38.994	T38.995	T38.996
Trimebutine	T44.3X1	T44.3X2	T44.3X3	T44.3X4	T44.3X5	T44.3X6
Trimecaine	T41.3X1	T41.3X2	T41.3X3	T41.3X4	T41.3X5	T41.3X6
Trimeprazine (tartrate)	T44.3X1	T44.3X2	T44.3X3	T44.3X4	T44.3X5	T44.3X6
Trimetaphan camsilate	T44.2X1	T44.2X2	T44.2X3	T44.2X4	T44.2X5	T44.2X6
Trimetazidine	T46.7X1	T46.7X2	T46.7X3	T46.7X4	T46.7X5	T46.7X6
Trimethadione	T42.2X1	T42.2X2	T42.2X3	T42.2X4	T42.2X5	T42.2X6
Trimethaphan	T44.2X1	T44.2X2	T44.2X3	T44.2X4	T44.2X5	T44.2X6
Trimethidinium	T44.2X1	T44.2X2	T44.2X3	T44.2X4	T44.2X5	T44.2X6
Trimethobenzamide	T45.0X1	T45.0X2	T45.0X3	T45.0X4	T45.0X5	T45.0X6
Trimethoprim	T37.8X1	T37.8X2	T37.8X3	T37.8X4	T37.8X5	T37.8X6
with sulfamethoxazole	T36.8X1	T36.8X2	T36.8X3	T36.8X4	T36.8X5	T36.8X6
Trimethylcarbinol	T51.3X1	T51.3X2	T51.3X3	T51.3X4	—	—
Trimethylpsoralen	T49.3X1	T49.3X2	T49.3X3	T49.3X4	T49.3X5	T49.3X6
Trimeton	T45.0X1	T45.0X2	T45.0X3	T45.0X4	T45.0X5	T45.0X6
Trimetrexate	T45.1X1	T45.1X2	T45.1X3	T45.1X4	T45.1X5	T45.1X6
Trimipramine	T43.011	T43.012	T43.013	T43.014	T43.015	T43.016
Trimustine	T45.1X1	T45.1X2	T45.1X3	T45.1X4	T45.1X5	T45.1X6
Trinitrine	T46.3X1	T46.3X2	T46.3X3	T46.3X4	T46.3X5	T46.3X6
Trinitrobenzol	T65.3X1	T65.3X2	T65.3X3	T65.3X4	—	—
Trinitrophenol	T65.3X1	T65.3X2	T65.3X3	T65.3X4	—	—
Trinitrotoluene (fumes)	T65.3X1	T65.3X2	T65.3X3	T65.3X4	—	—
Trional	T42.6X1	T42.6X2	T42.6X3	T42.6X4	T42.6X5	T42.6X6
Triorthocresyl phosphate	T65.891	T65.892	T65.893	T65.894	—	—
Trioxide of arsenic	T57.0X1	T57.0X2	T57.0X3	T57.0X4	—	—
Trioxysalen	T49.4X1	T49.4X2	T49.4X3	T49.4X4	T49.4X5	T49.4X6
Tripamide	T50.2X1	T50.2X2	T50.2X3	T50.2X4	T50.2X5	T50.2X6
Triparanol	T46.6X1	T46.6X2	T46.6X3	T46.6X4	T46.6X5	T46.6X6
Tripelennamine	T45.0X1	T45.0X2	T45.0X3	T45.0X4	T45.0X5	T45.0X6
Triperiden	T44.3X1	T44.3X2	T44.3X3	T44.3X4	T44.3X5	T44.3X6
Triperidol	T43.4X1	T43.4X2	T43.4X3	T43.4X4	T43.4X5	T43.4X6
Triphenylphosphate	T65.891	T65.892	T65.893	T65.894	—	—
Triple						
bromides	T42.6X1	T42.6X2	T42.6X3	T42.6X4	T42.6X5	T42.6X6
carbonate	T47.1X1	T47.1X2	T47.1X3	T47.1X4	T47.1X5	T47.1X6
vaccine						
DPT	T50.A11	T50.A12	T50.A13	T50.A14	T50.A15	T50.A16
including pertussis	T50.A11	T50.A12	T50.A13	T50.A14	T50.A15	T50.A16
MMR	T50.B91	T50.B92	T50.B93	T50.B94	T50.B95	T50.B96
Triprolidine	T45.0X1	T45.0X2	T45.0X3	T45.0X4	T45.0X5	T45.0X6
Trisodium hydrogen edetate	T50.6X1	T50.6X2	T50.6X3	T50.6X4	T50.6X5	T50.6X6
Trisoralen	T49.3X1	T49.3X2	T49.3X3	T49.3X4	T49.3X5	T49.3X6
Trisulfapyrimidines	T37.0X1	T37.0X2	T37.0X3	T37.0X4	T37.0X5	T37.0X6
Trithiozine	T44.3X1	T44.3X2	T44.3X3	T44.3X4	T44.3X5	T44.3X6
Tritiozine	T44.3X1	T44.3X2	T44.3X3	T44.3X4	T44.3X5	T44.3X6
Tritoqualine	T45.0X1	T45.0X2	T45.0X3	T45.0X4	T45.0X5	T45.0X6
Trofosfamide	T45.1X1	T45.1X2	T45.1X3	T45.1X4	T45.1X5	T45.1X6
Troleandomycin	T36.3X1	T36.3X2	T36.3X3	T36.3X4	T36.3X5	T36.3X6
Trolnitrate (phosphate)	T46.3X1	T46.3X2	T46.3X3	T46.3X4	T46.3X5	T46.3X6
Tromantadine	T37.5X1	T37.5X2	T37.5X3	T37.5X4	T37.5X5	T37.5X6
Trometamol	T50.2X1	T50.2X2	T50.2X3	T50.2X4	T50.2X5	T50.2X6
Tromethamine	T50.2X1	T50.2X2	T50.2X3	T50.2X4	T50.2X5	T50.2X6
Tronothane	T41.3X1	T41.3X2	T41.3X3	T41.3X4	T41.3X5	T41.3X6
Tropacine	T44.3X1	T44.3X2	T44.3X3	T44.3X4	T44.3X5	T44.3X6
Tropatepine	T44.3X1	T44.3X2	T44.3X3	T44.3X4	T44.3X5	T44.3X6
Tropicamide	T44.3X1	T44.3X2	T44.3X3	T44.3X4	T44.3X5	T44.3X6
Trospium chloride	T44.3X1	T44.3X2	T44.3X3	T44.3X4	T44.3X5	T44.3X6
Troxerutin	T46.991	T46.992	T46.993	T46.994	T46.995	T46.996
Troxidone	T42.2X1	T42.2X2	T42.2X3	T42.2X4	T42.2X5	T42.2X6
Tryparsamide	T37.3X1	T37.3X2	T37.3X3	T37.3X4	T37.3X5	T37.3X6
Trypsin	T45.3X1	T45.3X2	T45.3X3	T45.3X4	T45.3X5	T45.3X6
Tryptizol	T43.011	T43.012	T43.013	T43.014	T43.015	T43.016
TSH	T38.811	T38.812	T38.813	T38.814	T38.815	T38.816
Tuaminoheptane	T48.5X1	T48.5X2	T48.5X3	T48.5X4	T48.5X5	T48.5X6
Tuberculin, purified protein derivative (PPD)	T50.8X1	T50.8X2	T50.8X3	T50.8X4	T50.8X5	T50.8X6
Tubocurare	T48.1X1	T48.1X2	T48.1X3	T48.1X4	T48.1X5	T48.1X6
Tubocurarine (chloride)	T48.1X1	T48.1X2	T48.1X3	T48.1X4	T48.1X5	T48.1X6
Tulobuterol	T48.6X1	T48.6X2	T48.6X3	T48.6X4	T48.6X5	T48.6X6
Turpentine (spirits of)	T52.8X1	T52.8X2	T52.8X3	T52.8X4	—	—
vapor	T52.8X1	T52.8X2	T52.8X3	T52.8X4	—	—
Tybamate	T43.591	T43.592	T43.593	T43.594	T43.595	T43.596
Tyloxapol	T48.4X1	T48.4X2	T48.4X3	T48.4X4	T48.4X5	T48.4X6
Tymazoline	T48.5X1	T48.5X2	T48.5X3	T48.5X4	T48.5X5	T48.5X6
Typhoid-paratyphoid vaccine	T50.A91	T50.A92	T50.A93	T50.A94	T50.A95	T50.A96
Typhus vaccine	T50.A91	T50.A92	T50.A93	T50.A94	T50.A95	T50.A96
Tyropanoate	T50.8X1	T50.8X2	T50.8X3	T50.8X4	T50.8X5	T50.8X6
Tyrothricin	T49.6X1	T49.6X2	T49.6X3	T49.6X4	T49.6X5	T49.6X6
ENT agent	T49.6X1	T49.6X2	T49.6X3	T49.6X4	T49.6X5	T49.6X6
ophthalmic preparation	T49.5X1	T49.5X2	T49.5X3	T49.5X4	T49.5X5	T49.5X6
Ufenamate	T39.391	T39.392	T39.393	T39.394	T39.395	T39.396
Ultraviolet light protectant	T49.3X1	T49.3X2	T49.3X3	T49.3X4	T49.3X5	T49.3X6
Undecenoic acid	T49.0X1	T49.0X2	T49.0X3	T49.0X4	T49.0X5	T49.0X6
Undecoylium	T49.0X1	T49.0X2	T49.0X3	T49.0X4	T49.0X5	T49.0X6
Undecylenic acid (derivatives)	T49.0X1	T49.0X2	T49.0X3	T49.0X4	T49.0X5	T49.0X6
Unna's boot	T49.3X1	T49.3X2	T49.3X3	T49.3X4	T49.3X5	T49.3X6
Unsaturated fatty acid	T46.6X1	T46.6X2	T46.6X3	T46.6X4	T46.6X5	T46.6X6
Uracil mustard	T45.1X1	T45.1X2	T45.1X3	T45.1X4	T45.1X5	T45.1X6
Uramustine	T45.1X1	T45.1X2	T45.1X3	T45.1X4	T45.1X5	T45.1X6
Urapidil	T46.5X1	T46.5X2	T46.5X3	T46.5X4	T46.5X5	T46.5X6
Urari	T48.1X1	T48.1X2	T48.1X3	T48.1X4	T48.1X5	T48.1X6
Urate oxidase	T50.4X1	T50.4X2	T50.4X3	T50.4X4	T50.4X5	T50.4X6
Urea	T47.3X1	T47.3X2	T47.3X3	T47.3X4	T47.3X5	T47.3X6
peroxide	T49.0X1	T49.0X2	T49.0X3	T49.0X4	T49.0X5	T49.0X6
stibamine	T37.4X1	T37.4X2	T37.4X3	T37.4X4	T37.4X5	T37.4X6
topical	T49.8X1	T49.8X2	T49.8X3	T49.8X4	T49.8X5	T49.8X6
Urethane	T45.1X1	T45.1X2	T45.1X3	T45.1X4	T45.1X5	T45.1X6
Urginea (maritima) (scilla) — see Squill						
Uric acid metabolism drug NEC	T50.4X1	T50.4X2	T50.4X3	T50.4X4	T50.4X5	T50.4X6
Uricosuric agent	T50.4X1	T50.4X2	T50.4X3	T50.4X4	T50.4X5	T50.4X6
Urinary anti-infective	T37.8X1	T37.8X2	T37.8X3	T37.8X4	T37.8X5	T37.8X6
Urofollitropin	T38.811	T38.812	T38.813	T38.814	T38.815	T38.816
Urokinase	T45.611	T45.612	T45.613	T45.614	T45.615	T45.616
Urokon	T50.8X1	T50.8X2	T50.8X3	T50.8X4	T50.8X5	T50.8X6
Ursodeoxycholic acid	T50.991	T50.992	T50.993	T50.994	T50.995	T50.996
Ursodiol	T50.991	T50.992	T50.993	T50.994	T50.995	T50.996
Urtica	T62.2X1	T62.2X2	T62.2X3	T62.2X4	—	—
Utility gas — see Gas, utility						

Additional Character May Be Required — Refer to the Tabular List for Character Selection

▽ Subterms under main terms may continue to next column or page

Substance	Poisoning, Accidental (unintentional)	Poisoning, Intentional Self-harm	Poisoning, Assault	Poisoning, Undetermined	Adverse Effect	Under-dosing
Vaccine NEC	T50.Z91	T50.Z92	T50.Z93	T50.Z94	T50.Z95	T50.Z96
antineoplastic	T50.Z91	T50.Z92	T50.Z93	T50.Z94	T50.Z95	T50.Z96
bacterial NEC	T50.A91	T50.A92	T50.A93	T50.A94	T50.A95	T50.A96
with						
other bacterial component	T50.A21	T50.A22	T50.A23	T50.A24	T50.A25	T50.A26
pertussis component	T50.A11	T50.A12	T50.A13	T50.A14	T50.A15	T50.A16
viral-rickettsial component	T50.A21	T50.A22	T50.A23	T50.A24	T50.A25	T50.A26
mixed NEC	T50.A21	T50.A22	T50.A23	T50.A24	T50.A25	T50.A26
BCG	T50.A91	T50.A92	T50.A93	T50.A94	T50.A95	T50.A96
cholera	T50.A91	T50.A92	T50.A93	T50.A94	T50.A95	T50.A96
diphtheria	T50.A91	T50.A92	T50.A93	T50.A94	T50.A95	T50.A96
with tetanus	T50.A21	T50.A22	T50.A23	T50.A24	T50.A25	T50.A26
and pertussis	T50.A11	T50.A12	T50.A13	T50.A14	T50.A15	T50.A16
influenza	T50.B91	T50.B92	T50.B93	T50.B94	T50.B95	T50.B96
measles	T50.B91	T50.B92	T50.B93	T50.B94	T50.B95	T50.B96
with mumps and rubella	T50.B91	T50.B92	T50.B93	T50.B94	T50.B95	T50.B96
meningococcal	T50.A91	T50.A92	T50.A93	T50.A94	T50.A95	T50.A96
mumps	T50.B91	T50.B92	T50.B93	T50.B94	T50.B95	T50.B96
paratyphoid	T50.A91	T50.A92	T50.A93	T50.A94	T50.A95	T50.A96
pertussis	T50.A11	T50.A12	T50.A13	T50.A14	T50.A15	T50.A16
with diphtheria	T50.A11	T50.A12	T50.A13	T50.A14	T50.A15	T50.A16
and tetanus	T50.A11	T50.A12	T50.A13	T50.A14	T50.A15	T50.A16
with other component	T50.A11	T50.A12	T50.A13	T50.A14	T50.A15	T50.A16
plague	T50.A91	T50.A92	T50.A93	T50.A94	T50.A95	T50.A96
poliomyelitis	T50.B91	T50.B92	T50.B93	T50.B94	T50.B95	T50.B96
poliovirus	T50.B91	T50.B92	T50.B93	T50.B94	T50.B95	T50.B96
rabies	T50.B91	T50.B92	T50.B93	T50.B94	T50.B95	T50.B96
respiratory syncytial virus	T50.B91	T50.B92	T50.B93	T50.B94	T50.B95	T50.B96
rickettsial NEC	T50.A91	T50.A92	T50.A93	T50.A94	T50.A95	T50.A96
with						
bacterial component	T50.A21	T50.A22	T50.A23	T50.A24	T50.A25	T50.A26
Rocky Mountain spotted fever	T50.A91	T50.A92	T50.A93	T50.A94	T50.A95	T50.A96
rubella	T50.B91	T50.B92	T50.B93	T50.B94	T50.B95	T50.B96
sabin oral	T50.B91	T50.B92	T50.B93	T50.B94	T50.B95	T50.B96
smallpox	T50.B11	T50.B12	T50.B13	T50.B14	T50.B15	T50.B16
TAB	T50.A91	T50.A92	T50.A93	T50.A94	T50.A95	T50.A96
tetanus	T50.A91	T50.A92	T50.A93	T50.A94	T50.A95	T50.A96
typhoid	T50.A91	T50.A92	T50.A93	T50.A94	T50.A95	T50.A96
typhus	T50.A91	T50.A92	T50.A93	T50.A94	T50.A95	T50.A96
viral NEC	T50.B91	T50.B92	T50.B93	T50.B94	T50.B95	T50.B96
yellow fever	T50.B91	T50.B92	T50.B93	T50.B94	T50.B95	T50.B96
Vaccinia immune globulin	T50.Z11	T50.Z12	T50.Z13	T50.Z14	T50.Z15	T50.Z16
Vaginal contraceptives	T49.8X1	T49.8X2	T49.8X3	T49.8X4	T49.8X5	T49.8X6
Valerian						
root	T42.6X1	T42.6X2	T42.6X3	T42.6X4	T42.6X5	T42.6X6
tincture	T42.6X1	T42.6X2	T42.6X3	T42.6X4	T42.6X5	T42.6X6
Valethamate bromide	T44.3X1	T44.3X2	T44.3X3	T44.3X4	T44.3X5	T44.3X6
Valisone	T49.0X1	T49.0X2	T49.0X3	T49.0X4	T49.0X5	T49.0X6
Valium	T42.4X1	T42.4X2	T42.4X3	T42.4X4	T42.4X5	T42.4X6
Valmid	T42.6X1	T42.6X2	T42.6X3	T42.6X4	T42.6X5	T42.6X6
Valnoctamide	T42.6X1	T42.6X2	T42.6X3	T42.6X4	T42.6X5	T42.6X6
Valproate (sodium)	T42.6X1	T42.6X2	T42.6X3	T42.6X4	T42.6X5	T42.6X6
Valproic acid	T42.6X1	T42.6X2	T42.6X3	T42.6X4	T42.6X5	T42.6X6
Valpromide	T42.6X1	T42.6X2	T42.6X3	T42.6X4	T42.6X5	T42.6X6
Vanadium	T56.891	T56.892	T56.893	T56.894	—	—
Vancomycin	T36.8X1	T36.8X2	T36.8X3	T36.8X4	T36.8X5	T36.8X6
Vapor — *see also* Gas	T59.91	T59.92	T59.93	T59.94	—	—
kiln (carbon monoxide)	T58.8X1	T58.8X2	T58.8X3	T58.8X4	—	—
lead — *see* lead						
specified source NEC	T59.891	T59.892	T59.893	T59.894	—	—
Vardenafil	T46.7X1	T46.7X2	T46.7X3	T46.7X4	T46.7X5	T46.7X6
Varicose reduction drug	T46.8X1	T46.8X2	T46.8X3	T46.8X4	T46.8X5	T46.8X6
Varnish	T65.4X1	T65.4X2	T65.4X3	T65.4X4	—	—
cleaner	T52.91	T52.92	T52.93	T52.94	—	—
Vaseline	T49.3X1	T49.3X2	T49.3X3	T49.3X4	T49.3X5	T49.3X6
Vasodilan	T46.7X1	T46.7X2	T46.7X3	T46.7X4	T46.7X5	T46.7X6
Vasodilator						
coronary NEC	T46.3X1	T46.3X2	T46.3X3	T46.3X4	T46.3X5	T46.3X6
peripheral NEC	T46.7X1	T46.7X2	T46.7X3	T46.7X4	T46.7X5	T46.7X6
Vasopressin	T38.891	T38.892	T38.893	T38.894	T38.895	T38.896
Vasopressor drugs	T38.891	T38.892	T38.893	T38.894	T38.895	T38.896
Vecuronium bromide	T48.1X1	T48.1X2	T48.1X3	T48.1X4	T48.1X5	T48.1X6
Vegetable extract, astringent	T49.2X1	T49.2X2	T49.2X3	T49.2X4	T49.2X5	T49.2X6
Venlafaxine	T43.211	T43.212	T43.213	T43.214	T43.215	T43.216
Venom, venomous (bite) (sting)	T63.91	T63.92	T63.93	T63.94	—	—
amphibian NEC	T63.831	T63.832	T63.833	T63.834	—	—
animal NEC	T63.891	T63.892	T63.893	T63.894	—	—
ant	T63.421	T63.422	T63.423	T63.424	—	—

Substance	Poisoning, Accidental (unintentional)	Poisoning, Intentional Self-harm	Poisoning, Assault	Poisoning, Undetermined	Adverse Effect	Under-dosing
Venom, venomous — *continued*						
arthropod NEC	T63.481	T63.482	T63.483	T63.484	—	—
bee	T63.441	T63.442	T63.443	T63.444	—	—
centipede	T63.411	T63.412	T63.413	T63.414	—	—
fish	T63.591	T63.592	T63.593	T63.594	—	—
frog	T63.811	T63.812	T63.813	T63.814	—	—
hornet	T63.451	T63.452	T63.453	T63.454	—	—
insect NEC	T63.481	T63.482	T63.483	T63.484	—	—
lizard	T63.121	T63.122	T63.123	T63.124	—	—
marine						
animals	T63.691	T63.692	T63.693	T63.694	—	—
bluebottle	T63.611	T63.612	T63.613	T63.614	—	—
jellyfish NEC	T63.621	T63.622	T63.623	T63.624	—	—
Portugese Man-o-war	T63.611	T63.612	T63.613	T63.614	—	—
sea anemone	T63.631	T63.632	T63.633	T63.634	—	—
specified NEC	T63.691	T63.692	T63.693	T63.694	—	—
fish	T63.591	T63.592	T63.593	T63.594	—	—
plants	T63.711	T63.712	T63.713	T63.714	—	—
sting ray	T63.511	T63.512	T63.513	T63.514	—	—
millipede (tropical)	T63.411	T63.412	T63.413	T63.414	—	—
plant NEC	T63.791	T63.792	T63.793	T63.794	—	—
marine	T63.711	T63.712	T63.713	T63.714	—	—
reptile	T63.191	T63.192	T63.193	T63.194	—	—
gila monster	T63.111	T63.112	T63.113	T63.114	—	—
lizard NEC	T63.121	T63.122	T63.123	T63.124	—	—
scorpion	T63.2X1	T63.2X2	T63.2X3	T63.2X4	—	—
snake	T63.001	T63.002	T63.003	T63.004	—	—
African NEC	T63.081	T63.082	T63.083	T63.084	—	—
American (North) (South) NEC	T63.061	T63.062	T63.063	T63.064	—	—
Asian	T63.081	T63.082	T63.083	T63.084	—	—
Australian	T63.071	T63.072	T63.073	T63.074	—	—
cobra	T63.041	T63.042	T63.043	T63.044	—	—
coral snake	T63.021	T63.022	T63.023	T63.024	—	—
rattlesnake	T63.011	T63.012	T63.013	T63.014	—	—
specified NEC	T63.091	T63.092	T63.093	T63.094	—	—
taipan	T63.031	T63.032	T63.033	T63.034	—	—
specified NEC	T63.891	T63.892	T63.893	T63.894	—	—
spider	T63.301	T63.302	T63.303	T63.304	—	—
black widow	T63.311	T63.312	T63.313	T63.314	—	—
brown recluse	T63.331	T63.332	T63.333	T63.334	—	—
specified NEC	T63.391	T63.392	T63.393	T63.394	—	—
tarantula	T63.321	T63.322	T63.323	T63.324	—	—
sting ray	T63.511	T63.512	T63.513	T63.514	—	—
toad	T63.821	T63.822	T63.823	T63.824	—	—
wasp	T63.461	T63.462	T63.463	T63.464	—	—
Venous sclerosing drug NEC	T46.8X1	T46.8X2	T46.8X3	T46.8X4	T46.8X5	T46.8X6
Ventolin — *see* Albuterol						
Veramon	T42.3X1	T42.3X2	T42.3X3	T42.3X4	T42.3X5	T42.3X6
Verapamil	T46.1X1	T46.1X2	T46.1X3	T46.1X4	T46.1X5	T46.1X6
Veratrine	T46.5X1	T46.5X2	T46.5X3	T46.5X4	T46.5X5	T46.5X6
Veratrum						
album	T62.2X1	T62.2X2	T62.2X3	T62.2X4	—	—
alkaloids	T46.5X1	T46.5X2	T46.5X3	T46.5X4	T46.5X5	T46.5X6
viride	T62.2X1	T62.2X2	T62.2X3	T62.2X4	—	—
Verdigris	T60.3X1	T60.3X2	T60.3X3	T60.3X4	—	—
Veronal	T42.3X1	T42.3X2	T42.3X3	T42.3X4	T42.3X5	T42.3X6
Veroxil	T37.4X1	T37.4X2	T37.4X3	T37.4X4	T37.4X5	T37.4X6
Versenate	T50.6X1	T50.6X2	T50.6X3	T50.6X4	T50.6X5	T50.6X6
Versidyne	T39.8X1	T39.8X2	T39.8X3	T39.8X4	T39.8X5	T39.8X6
Vetrabutine	T48.0X1	T48.0X2	T48.0X3	T48.0X4	T48.0X5	T48.0X6
Vidarabine	T37.5X1	T37.5X2	T37.5X3	T37.5X4	T37.5X5	T37.5X6
Vienna						
green	T57.0X1	T57.0X2	T57.0X3	T57.0X4	—	—
insecticide	T60.2X1	T60.2X2	T60.2X3	T60.2X4	—	—
red	T57.0X1	T57.0X2	T57.0X3	T57.0X4	—	—
pharmaceutical dye	T50.991	T50.992	T50.993	T50.994	T50.995	T50.996
Vigabatrin	T42.6X1	T42.6X2	T42.6X3	T42.6X4	T42.6X5	T42.6X6
Viloxazine	T43.291	T43.292	T43.293	T43.294	T43.295	T43.296
Viminol	T39.8X1	T39.8X2	T39.8X3	T39.8X4	T39.8X5	T39.8X6
Vinbarbital, vinbarbitone	T42.3X1	T42.3X2	T42.3X3	T42.3X4	T42.3X5	T42.3X6
Vinblastine	T45.1X1	T45.1X2	T45.1X3	T45.1X4	T45.1X5	T45.1X6
Vinburnine	T46.7X1	T46.7X2	T46.7X3	T46.7X4	T46.7X5	T46.7X6
Vincamine	T45.1X1	T45.1X2	T45.1X3	T45.1X4	T45.1X5	T45.1X6
Vincristine	T45.1X1	T45.1X2	T45.1X3	T45.1X4	T45.1X5	T45.1X6
Vindesine	T45.1X1	T45.1X2	T45.1X3	T45.1X4	T45.1X5	T45.1X6
Vinesthene, vinethene	T41.0X1	T41.0X2	T41.0X3	T41.0X4	T41.0X5	T41.0X6
Vinorelbine tartrate	T45.1X1	T45.1X2	T45.1X3	T45.1X4	T45.1X5	T45.1X6
Vinpocetine	T46.7X1	T46.7X2	T46.7X3	T46.7X4	T46.7X5	T46.7X6
Vinyl						
acetate	T65.891	T65.892	T65.893	T65.894	—	—
bital	T42.3X1	T42.3X2	T42.3X3	T42.3X4	T42.3X5	T42.3X6

Substance	Poisoning, Accidental (unintentional)	Poisoning, Intentional Self-harm	Poisoning, Assault	Poisoning, Undetermined	Adverse Effect	Under-dosing
Vinyl — *continued*						
bromide	T65.891	T65.892	T65.893	T65.894	—	—
chloride	T59.891	T59.892	T59.893	T59.894	—	—
ether	T41.0X1	T41.0X2	T41.0X3	T41.0X4	T41.0X5	T41.0X6
Vinylbital	T42.3X1	T42.3X2	T42.3X3	T42.3X4	T42.3X5	T42.3X6
Vinylidene chloride	T65.891	T65.892	T65.893	T65.894	—	—
Vioform	T37.8X1	T37.8X2	T37.8X3	T37.8X4	T37.8X5	T37.8X6
topical	T49.0X1	T49.0X2	T49.0X3	T49.0X4	T49.0X5	T49.0X6
Viomycin	T36.8X1	T36.8X2	T36.8X3	T36.8X4	T36.8X5	T36.8X6
Viosterol	T45.2X1	T45.2X2	T45.2X3	T45.2X4	T45.2X5	T45.2X6
Viper (venom)	T63.091	T63.092	T63.093	T63.094	—	—
Viprynium	T37.4X1	T37.4X2	T37.4X3	T37.4X4	T37.4X5	T37.4X6
Viquidil	T46.7X1	T46.7X2	T46.7X3	T46.7X4	T46.7X5	T46.7X6
Viral vaccine NEC	T50.B91	T50.B92	T50.B93	T50.B94	T50.B95	T50.B96
Virginiamycin	T36.8X1	T36.8X2	T36.8X3	T36.8X4	T36.8X5	T36.8X6
Virugon	T37.5X1	T37.5X2	T37.5X3	T37.5X4	T37.5X5	T37.5X6
Viscous agent	T50.901	T50.902	T50.903	T50.904	T50.905	T50.906
Visine	T49.5X1	T49.5X2	T49.5X3	T49.5X4	T49.5X5	T49.5X6
Visnadine	T46.3X1	T46.3X2	T46.3X3	T46.3X4	T46.3X5	T46.3X6
Vitamin NEC	T45.2X1	T45.2X2	T45.2X3	T45.2X4	T45.2X5	T45.2X6
A	T45.2X1	T45.2X2	T45.2X3	T45.2X4	T45.2X5	T45.2X6
B1	T45.2X1	T45.2X2	T45.2X3	T45.2X4	T45.2X5	T45.2X6
B2	T45.2X1	T45.2X2	T45.2X3	T45.2X4	T45.2X5	T45.2X6
B6	T45.2X1	T45.2X2	T45.2X3	T45.2X4	T45.2X5	T45.2X6
B12	T45.2X1	T45.2X2	T45.2X3	T45.2X4	T45.2X5	T45.2X6
B15	T45.2X1	T45.2X2	T45.2X3	T45.2X4	T45.2X5	T45.2X6
B NEC	T45.2X1	T45.2X2	T45.2X3	T45.2X4	T45.2X5	T45.2X6
nicotinic acid	T46.7X1	T46.7X2	T46.7X3	T46.7X4	T46.7X5	T46.7X6
C	T45.2X1	T45.2X2	T45.2X3	T45.2X4	T45.2X5	T45.2X6
D	T45.2X1	T45.2X2	T45.2X3	T45.2X4	T45.2X5	T45.2X6
D2	T45.2X1	T45.2X2	T45.2X3	T45.2X4	T45.2X5	T45.2X6
D3	T45.2X1	T45.2X2	T45.2X3	T45.2X4	T45.2X5	T45.2X6
E	T45.2X1	T45.2X2	T45.2X3	T45.2X4	T45.2X5	T45.2X6
E acetate	T45.2X1	T45.2X2	T45.2X3	T45.2X4	T45.2X5	T45.2X6
hematopoietic	T45.8X1	T45.8X2	T45.8X3	T45.8X4	T45.8X5	T45.8X6
K1	T45.7X1	T45.7X2	T45.7X3	T45.7X4	T45.7X5	T45.7X6
K2	T45.7X1	T45.7X2	T45.7X3	T45.7X4	T45.7X5	T45.7X6
K NEC	T45.7X1	T45.7X2	T45.7X3	T45.7X4	T45.7X5	T45.7X6
PP	T45.2X1	T45.2X2	T45.2X3	T45.2X4	T45.2X5	T45.2X6
ulceroprotectant	T47.1X1	T47.1X2	T47.1X3	T47.1X4	T47.1X5	T47.1X6
Vleminckx's solution	T49.4X1	T49.4X2	T49.4X3	T49.4X4	T49.4X5	T49.4X6
Voltaren — *see* Diclofenac						
sodium						
Warfarin	T45.511	T45.512	T45.513	T45.514	T45.515	T45.516
rodenticide	T60.4X1	T60.4X2	T60.4X3	T60.4X4	—	—
sodium	T60.4X1	T60.4X2	T60.4X3	T60.4X4	—	—
Wasp (sting)	T63.461	T63.462	T63.463	T63.464	—	—
Water						
balance drug	T50.3X1	T50.3X2	T50.3X3	T50.3X4	T50.3X5	T50.3X6
distilled	T50.3X1	T50.3X2	T50.3X3	T50.3X4	T50.3X5	T50.3X6
gas — *see* Gas, water						
incomplete combustion of — *see* Carbon, monoxide, fuel, utility						
hemlock	T62.2X1	T62.2X2	T62.2X3	T62.2X4	—	—
moccasin (venom)	T63.061	T63.062	T63.063	T63.064	—	—
purified	T50.3X1	T50.3X2	T50.3X3	T50.3X4	T50.3X5	T50.3X6
Wax (paraffin) (petroleum)	T52.0X1	T52.0X2	T52.0X3	T52.0X4	—	—
automobile	T65.891	T65.892	T65.893	T65.894	—	—
floor	T52.0X1	T52.0X2	T52.0X3	T52.0X4	—	—
Weed killers NEC	T60.3X1	T60.3X2	T60.3X3	T60.3X4	—	—
Welldorm	T42.6X1	T42.6X2	T42.6X3	T42.6X4	T42.6X5	T42.6X6
White						
arsenic	T57.0X1	T57.0X2	T57.0X3	T57.0X4	—	—
hellebore	T62.2X1	T62.2X2	T62.2X3	T62.2X4	—	—
lotion (keratolytic)	T49.4X1	T49.4X2	T49.4X3	T49.4X4	T49.4X5	T49.4X6
spirit	T52.0X1	T52.0X2	T52.0X3	T52.0X4	—	—
Whitewash	T65.891	T65.892	T65.893	T65.894	—	—
Whole blood (human)	T45.8X1	T45.8X2	T45.8X3	T45.8X4	T45.8X5	T45.8X6
Wild						
black cherry	T62.2X1	T62.2X2	T62.2X3	T62.2X4	—	—
poisonous plants NEC	T62.2X1	T62.2X2	T62.2X3	T62.2X4	—	—
Window cleaning fluid	T65.891	T65.892	T65.893	T65.894	—	—
Wintergreen (oil)	T49.3X1	T49.3X2	T49.3X3	T49.3X4	T49.3X5	T49.3X6
Wisterine	T62.2X1	T62.2X2	T62.2X3	T62.2X4	—	—
Witch hazel	T49.2X1	T49.2X2	T49.2X3	T49.2X4	T49.2X5	T49.2X6
Wood alcohol or spirit	T51.1X1	T51.1X2	T51.1X3	T51.1X4	—	—
Wool fat (hydrous)	T49.3X1	T49.3X2	T49.3X3	T49.3X4	T49.3X5	T49.3X6
Woorali	T48.1X1	T48.1X2	T48.1X3	T48.1X4	T48.1X5	T48.1X6
Wormseed, American	T37.4X1	T37.4X2	T37.4X3	T37.4X4	T37.4X5	T37.4X6
Xamoterol	T44.5X1	T44.5X2	T44.5X3	T44.5X4	T44.5X5	T44.5X6
Xanthine diuretics	T50.2X1	T50.2X2	T50.2X3	T50.2X4	T50.2X5	T50.2X6
Xanthinol nicotinate	T46.7X1	T46.7X2	T46.7X3	T46.7X4	T46.7X5	T46.7X6

Substance	Poisoning, Accidental (unintentional)	Poisoning, Intentional Self-harm	Poisoning, Assault	Poisoning, Undetermined	Adverse Effect	Under-dosing
Xanthotoxin	T49.3X1	T49.3X2	T49.3X3	T49.3X4	T49.3X5	T49.3X6
Xantinol nicotinate	T46.7X1	T46.7X2	T46.7X3	T46.7X4	T46.7X5	T46.7X6
Xantocillin	T36.0X1	T36.0X2	T36.0X3	T36.0X4	T36.0X5	T36.0X6
Xenon (127Xe) (133Xe)	T50.8X1	T50.8X2	T50.8X3	T50.8X4	T50.8X5	T50.8X6
Xenysalate	T49.4X1	T49.4X2	T49.4X3	T49.4X4	T49.4X5	T49.4X6
Xibornol	T37.8X1	T37.8X2	T37.8X3	T37.8X4	T37.8X5	T37.8X6
Xigris	T45.511	T45.512	T45.513	T45.514	T45.515	T45.516
Xipamide	T50.2X1	T50.2X2	T50.2X3	T50.2X4	T50.2X5	T50.2X6
Xylene (vapor)	T52.2X1	T52.2X2	T52.2X3	T52.2X4	—	—
Xylocaine (infiltration)	T41.3X1	T41.3X2	T41.3X3	T41.3X4	T41.3X5	T41.3X6
(topical)						
nerve block (peripheral) (plexus)	T41.3X1	T41.3X2	T41.3X3	T41.3X4	T41.3X5	T41.3X6
spinal	T41.3X1	T41.3X2	T41.3X3	T41.3X4	T41.3X5	T41.3X6
Xylol (vapor)	T52.2X1	T52.2X2	T52.2X3	T52.2X4	—	—
Xylometazoline	T48.5X1	T48.5X2	T48.5X3	T48.5X4	T48.5X5	T48.5X6
Yeast	T45.2X1	T45.2X2	T45.2X3	T45.2X4	T45.2X5	T45.2X6
dried	T45.2X1	T45.2X2	T45.2X3	T45.2X4	T45.2X5	T45.2X6
Yellow						
fever vaccine	T50.B91	T50.B92	T50.B93	T50.B94	T50.B95	T50.B96
jasmine	T62.2X1	T62.2X2	T62.2X3	T62.2X4	—	—
phenolphthalein	T47.2X1	T47.2X2	T47.2X3	T47.2X4	T47.2X5	T47.2X6
Yew	T62.2X1	T62.2X2	T62.2X3	T62.2X4	—	—
Yohimbic acid	T40.991	T40.992	T40.993	T40.994	T40.995	T40.996
Zactane	T39.391	T39.392	T39.393	T39.394	T39.395	T39.396
Zalcitabine	T37.5X1	T37.5X2	T37.5X3	T37.5X4	T37.5X5	T37.5X6
Zaroxolyn	T50.2X1	T50.2X2	T50.2X3	T50.2X4	T50.2X5	T50.2X6
Zephiran (topical)	T49.0X1	T49.0X2	T49.0X3	T49.0X4	T49.0X5	T49.0X6
ophthalmic preparation	T49.5X1	T49.5X2	T49.5X3	T49.5X4	T49.5X5	T49.5X6
Zeranol	T38.7X1	T38.7X2	T38.7X3	T38.7X4	T38.7X5	T38.7X6
Zerone	T51.1X1	T51.1X2	T51.1X3	T51.1X4	—	—
Zidovudine	T37.5X1	T37.5X2	T37.5X3	T37.5X4	T37.5X5	T37.5X6
Zimeldine	T43.221	T43.222	T43.223	T43.224	T43.225	T43.226
Zinc (compounds) (fumes) (vapor)	T56.5X1	T56.5X2	T56.5X3	T56.5X4	—	—
NEC	T49.0X1	T49.0X2	T49.0X3	T49.0X4	T49.0X5	T49.0X6
anti-infectives	T49.0X1	T49.0X2	T49.0X3	T49.0X4	T49.0X5	T49.0X6
antivaricose	T46.8X1	T46.8X2	T46.8X3	T46.8X4	T46.8X5	T46.8X6
bacitracin	T49.0X1	T49.0X2	T49.0X3	T49.0X4	T49.0X5	T49.0X6
chloride (mouthwash)	T49.6X1	T49.6X2	T49.6X3	T49.6X4	T49.6X5	T49.6X6
chromate	T56.5X1	T56.5X2	T56.5X3	T56.5X4	—	—
gelatin	T49.3X1	T49.3X2	T49.3X3	T49.3X4	T49.3X5	T49.3X6
oxide	T49.3X1	T49.3X2	T49.3X3	T49.3X4	T49.3X5	T49.3X6
plaster	T49.3X1	T49.3X2	T49.3X3	T49.3X4	T49.3X5	T49.3X6
peroxide	T49.0X1	T49.0X2	T49.0X3	T49.0X4	T49.0X5	T49.0X6
pesticides	T56.5X1	T56.5X2	T56.5X3	T56.5X4	—	—
phosphide	T60.4X1	T60.4X2	T60.4X3	T60.4X4	—	—
pyrithionate	T49.4X1	T49.4X2	T49.4X3	T49.4X4	T49.4X5	T49.4X6
stearate	T49.3X1	T49.3X2	T49.3X3	T49.3X4	T49.3X5	T49.3X6
sulfate	T49.5X1	T49.5X2	T49.5X3	T49.5X4	T49.5X5	T49.5X6
ENT agent	T49.6X1	T49.6X2	T49.6X3	T49.6X4	T49.6X5	T49.6X6
ophthalmic solution	T49.5X1	T49.5X2	T49.5X3	T49.5X4	T49.5X5	T49.5X6
topical NEC	T49.0X1	T49.0X2	T49.0X3	T49.0X4	T49.0X5	T49.0X6
undecylenate	T49.0X1	T49.0X2	T49.0X3	T49.0X4	T49.0X5	T49.0X6
Zineb	T60.0X1	T60.0X2	T60.0X3	T60.0X4	—	—
Zinostatin	T45.1X1	T45.1X2	T45.1X3	T45.1X4	T45.1X5	T45.1X6
Zipeprol	T48.3X1	T48.3X2	T48.3X3	T48.3X4	T48.3X5	T48.3X6
Zofenopril	T46.4X1	T46.4X2	T46.4X3	T46.4X4	T46.4X5	T46.4X6
Zolpidem	T42.6X1	T42.6X2	T42.6X3	T42.6X4	T42.6X5	T42.6X6
Zomepirac	T39.391	T39.392	T39.393	T39.394	T39.395	T39.396
Zopiclone	T42.6X1	T42.6X2	T42.6X3	T42.6X4	T42.6X5	T42.6X6
Zorubicin	T45.1X1	T45.1X2	T45.1X3	T45.1X4	T45.1X5	T45.1X6
Zotepine	T43.591	T43.592	T43.593	T43.594	T43.595	T43.596
Zovant	T45.511	T45.512	T45.513	T45.514	T45.515	T45.516
Zoxazolamine	T42.8X1	T42.8X2	T42.8X3	T42.8X4	T42.8X5	T42.8X6
Zuclopenthixol	T43.4X1	T43.4X2	T43.4X3	T43.4X4	T43.4X5	T43.4X6
Zygadenus (venenosus)	T62.2X1	T62.2X2	T62.2X3	T62.2X4	—	—
Zyprexa	T43.591	T43.592	T43.593	T43.594	T43.595	T43.596

Additional Character May Be Required — Refer to the Tabular List for Character Selection   ▼ Subterms under main terms may continue to next column or page

A

Abandonment (causing exposure to weather conditions) (with intent to injure or kill) NEC X58 ☑

Abuse (adult) (child) (mental) (physical) (sexual) X58 ☑

Accident (to) X58 ☑

aircraft (in transit) (powered) (see also Accident, transport, aircraft)

  due to, caused by cataclysm — see Forces of nature, by type

animal-drawn vehicle — see Accident, transport, animal-drawn vehicle occupant

animal-rider — see Accident, transport, animal-rider

automobile — see Accident, transport, car occupant

bare foot water skier V94.4 ☑

boat, boating (see also Accident, watercraft)

  striking swimmer

    powered V94.11 ☑

    unpowered V94.12 ☑

bus — see Accident, transport, bus occupant

cable car, not on rails V98.0 ☑

  on rails — see Accident, transport, streetcar occupant

car — see Accident, transport, car occupant

caused by, due to

  animal NEC W64 ☑

  chain hoist W24.0 ☑

  cold (excessive) — see Exposure, cold

  corrosive liquid, substance — see Table of Drugs and Chemicals

  cutting or piercing instrument — see Contact, with, by type of instrument

  drive belt W24.0 ☑

  electric

    current — see Exposure, electric current

    motor (see also Contact, with, by type of machine) W31.3 ☑

      current (of) W86.8 ☑

  environmental factor NEC X58 ☑

  explosive material — see Explosion

  fire, flames — see Exposure, fire

  firearm missile — see Discharge, firearm by type

  heat (excessive) — see Heat

  hot — see Contact, with, hot

  ignition — see Ignition

  lifting device W24.0 ☑

  lightning — see subcategory T75.0 ☑

    causing fire — see Exposure, fire

  machine, machinery — see Contact, with, by type of machine

  natural factor NEC X58 ☑

  pulley (block) W24.0 ☑

  radiation — see Radiation

  steam X13.1 ☑

    inhalation X13.0 ☑

    pipe X16 ☑

  thunderbolt — see subcategory T75.0 ☑

    causing fire — see Exposure, fire

  transmission device W24.1 ☑

coach — see Accident, transport, bus occupant

coal car — see Accident, transport, industrial vehicle occupant

diving (see also Fall, into, water)

  with

    drowning or submersion — see Drowning

forklift — see Accident, transport, industrial vehicle occupant

heavy transport vehicle NOS — see Accident, transport, truck occupant

ice yacht V98.2 ☑

in

  medical, surgical procedure

    as, or due to misadventure — see Misadventure

    causing an abnormal reaction or later complication without mention of misadventure (see also Complication of or following, by type of procedure) Y84.9

land yacht V98.1 ☑

late effect of — see W00-X58 with 7th character S

Accident — continued

logging car — see Accident, transport, industrial vehicle occupant

machine, machinery (see also Contact, with, by type of machine)

  on board watercraft V93.69 ☑

    explosion — see Explosion, in, watercraft

    fire — see Burn, on board watercraft

    powered craft V93.63 ☑

      ferry boat V93.61 ☑

      fishing boat V93.62 ☑

      jetskis V93.63 ☑

      liner V93.61 ☑

      merchant ship V93.60 ☑

      passenger ship V93.61 ☑

      sailboat V93.64 ☑

mine tram — see Accident, transport, industrial vehicle occupant

mobility scooter (motorized) — see Accident, transport, pedestrian, conveyance, specified type NEC

motor scooter — see Accident, transport, motorcyclist

motor vehicle NOS (traffic) (see also Accident, transport) V89.2 ☑

  nontraffic V89.0 ☑

  three-wheeled NOS — see Accident, transport, three-wheeled motor vehicle occupant

motorcycle NOS — see Accident, transport, motorcyclist

nonmotor vehicle NOS (nontraffic) (see also Accident, transport) V89.1 ☑

  traffic NOS V89.3 ☑

nontraffic (victim's mode of transport NOS) V88.9 ☑

  collision (between) V88.7 ☑

    bus and truck V88.5 ☑

    car and:

      bus V88.3 ☑

      pickup V88.2 ☑

      three-wheeled motor vehicle V88.0 ☑

      train V88.6 ☑

      truck V88.4 ☑

      two-wheeled motor vehicle V88.0 ☑

      van V88.2 ☑

    specified vehicle NEC and:

      three-wheeled motor vehicle V88.1 ☑

      two-wheeled motor vehicle V88.1 ☑

  known mode of transport — see Accident, transport, by type of vehicle

  noncollision V88.8 ☑

on board watercraft V93.89 ☑

  powered craft V93.83 ☑

    ferry boat V93.81 ☑

    fishing boat V93.82 ☑

    jetskis V93.83 ☑

    liner V93.81 ☑

    merchant ship V93.80 ☑

    passenger ship V93.81 ☑

  unpowered craft V93.88 ☑

    canoe V93.85 ☑

    inflatable V93.86 ☑

      in tow

        recreational V94.31 ☑

        specified NEC V94.32 ☑

    kayak V93.85 ☑

    sailboat V93.84 ☑

    surf-board V93.88 ☑

    water skis V93.87 ☑

    windsurfer V93.88 ☑

parachutist V97.29 ☑

  entangled in object V97.21 ☑

  injured on landing V97.22 ☑

pedal cycle — see Accident, transport, pedal cyclist

pedestrian (on foot)

  with

    another pedestrian W51 ☑

      with fall W03 ☑

        due to ice or snow W00.0 ☑

    on pedestrian conveyance NEC V00.09 ☑

    roller skater (in-line) V00.01 ☑

    skate boarder V00.02 ☑

    transport vehicle — see Accident, transport

Accident — continued

pedestrian — continued

  on pedestrian conveyance — see Accident, transport, pedestrian, conveyance

pick-up truck or van — see Accident, transport, pickup truck occupant

quarry truck — see Accident, transport, industrial vehicle occupant

railway vehicle (any) (in motion) — see Accident, transport, railway vehicle occupant

  due to cataclysm — see Forces of nature, by type

scooter (non-motorized) — see Accident, transport, pedestrian, conveyance, scooter

sequelae of — see categories W00-X58 with 7th character S

skateboard — see Accident, transport, pedestrian, conveyance, skateboard

ski(ing) — see Accident, transport, pedestrian, conveyance

  lift V98.3 ☑

specified cause NEC X58 ☑

streetcar — see Accident, transport, streetcar occupant

traffic (victim's mode of transport NOS) V87.9 ☑

  collision (between) V87.7 ☑

    bus and truck V87.5 ☑

    car and:

      bus V87.3 ☑

      pickup V87.2 ☑

      three-wheeled motor vehicle V87.0 ☑

      train V87.6 ☑

      truck V87.4 ☑

      two-wheeled motor vehicle V87.0 ☑

      van V87.2 ☑

    specified vehicle NEC and:

      three-wheeled motor vehicle V87.1 ☑

      two-wheeled motor vehicle V87.1 ☑

  known mode of transport — see Accident, transport, by type of vehicle

  noncollision V87.8 ☑

transport (involving injury to) V99 ☑

  18 wheeler — see Accident, transport, truck occupant

  agricultural vehicle occupant (nontraffic) V84.9 ☑

    driver V84.5 ☑

    hanger-on V84.7 ☑

    passenger V84.6 ☑

    traffic V84.3 ☑

      driver V84.0 ☑

      hanger-on V84.2 ☑

      passenger V84.1 ☑

    while boarding or alighting V84.4 ☑

  aircraft NEC V97.89 ☑

    military NEC V97.818 ☑

      with civilian aircraft V97.810 ☑

      civilian injured by V97.811 ☑

    occupant injured (in)

      nonpowered craft accident V96.9 ☑

        balloon V96.00 ☑

          collision V96.03 ☑

          crash V96.01 ☑

          explosion V96.05 ☑

          fire V96.04 ☑

          forced landing V96.02 ☑

          specified type NEC V96.09 ☑

        glider V96.20 ☑

          collision V96.23 ☑

          crash V96.21 ☑

          explosion V96.25 ☑

          fire V96.24 ☑

          forced landing V96.22 ☑

          specified type NEC V96.29 ☑

        hang glider V96.10 ☑

          collision V96.13 ☑

          crash V96.11 ☑

          explosion V96.15 ☑

          fire V96.14 ☑

          forced landing V96.12 ☑

          specified type NEC V96.19 ☑

        specified craft NEC V96.8 ☑

      powered craft accident V95.9 ☑

        fixed wing NEC

Abandonment — Accident

Subterms under main terms may continue to next column or page ☑ Additional Character Required — Refer to the Tabular List for Character Selection 387

Accident — *continued*
　transport — *continued*
　　aircraft — *continued*
　　　occupant injured — *continued*
　　　　powered craft accident — *continued*
　　　　　fixed wing — *continued*
　　　　　　commercial V95.30 ☑
　　　　　　　collision V95.33 ☑
　　　　　　　crash V95.31 ☑
　　　　　　　explosion V95.35 ☑
　　　　　　　fire V95.34 ☑
　　　　　　　forced landing V95.32 ☑
　　　　　　　specified type NEC V95.39 ☑
　　　　　　private V95.20 ☑
　　　　　　　collision V95.23 ☑
　　　　　　　crash V95.21 ☑
　　　　　　　explosion V95.25 ☑
　　　　　　　fire V95.24 ☑
　　　　　　　forced landing V95.22 ☑
　　　　　　　specified type NEC V95.29 ☑
　　　　　glider V95.10 ☑
　　　　　　collision V95.13 ☑
　　　　　　crash V95.11 ☑
　　　　　　explosion V95.15 ☑
　　　　　　fire V95.14 ☑
　　　　　　forced landing V95.12 ☑
　　　　　　specified type NEC V95.19 ☑
　　　　　helicopter V95.00 ☑
　　　　　　collision V95.03 ☑
　　　　　　crash V95.01 ☑
　　　　　　explosion V95.05 ☑
　　　　　　fire V95.04 ☑
　　　　　　forced landing V95.02 ☑
　　　　　　specified type NEC V95.09 ☑
　　　　　spacecraft V95.40 ☑
　　　　　　collision V95.43 ☑
　　　　　　crash V95.41 ☑
　　　　　　explosion V95.45 ☑
　　　　　　fire V95.44 ☑
　　　　　　forced landing V95.42 ☑
　　　　　　specified type NEC V95.49 ☑
　　　　　specified craft NEC V95.8 ☑
　　　　　ultralight V95.10 ☑
　　　　　　collision V95.13 ☑
　　　　　　crash V95.11 ☑
　　　　　　explosion V95.15 ☑
　　　　　　fire V95.14 ☑
　　　　　　forced landing V95.12 ☑
　　　　　　specified type NEC V95.19 ☑
　　　　specified accident NEC V97.0 ☑
　　　　while boarding or alighting V97.1 ☑
　　　person (injured by)
　　　　falling from, in or on aircraft V97.0 ☑
　　　　machinery on aircraft V97.89 ☑
　　　　on ground with aircraft involvement
　　　　　V97.39 ☑
　　　　rotating propeller V97.32 ☑
　　　　struck by object falling from aircraft
　　　　　V97.31 ☑
　　　　sucked into aircraft jet V97.33 ☑
　　　　while boarding or alighting aircraft V97.1 ☑
　　airport (battery-powered) passenger vehicle —
　　　see Accident, transport, industrial vehicle
　　　occupant
　　all-terrain vehicle occupant (nontraffic) V86.99 ☑
　　　driver V86.59 ☑
　　　dune buggy — see Accident, transport, dune
　　　　buggy occupant
　　　hanger-on V86.79 ☑
　　　passenger V86.69 ☑
　　　snowmobile — see Accident, transport, snow-
　　　　mobile occupant
　　　traffic V86.39 ☑
　　　　driver V86.09 ☑
　　　　hanger-on V86.29 ☑
　　　　passenger V86.19 ☑
　　　while boarding or alighting V86.49 ☑
　　ambulance occupant (traffic) V86.31 ☑
　　　driver V86.01 ☑
　　　hanger-on V86.21 ☑
　　　nontraffic V86.91 ☑
　　　　driver V86.51 ☑
　　　　hanger-on V86.71 ☑
　　　　passenger V86.61 ☑
　　　passenger V86.11 ☑
　　　while boarding or alighting V86.41 ☑

Accident — *continued*
　transport — *continued*
　　animal-drawn vehicle occupant (in) V80.929 ☑
　　　collision (with)
　　　　animal V80.12 ☑
　　　　　being ridden V80.711 ☑
　　　　animal-drawn vehicle V80.721 ☑
　　　　bus V80.42 ☑
　　　　car V80.42 ☑
　　　　fixed or stationary object V80.82 ☑
　　　　military vehicle V80.920 ☑
　　　　nonmotor vehicle V80.791 ☑
　　　　pedal cycle V80.22 ☑
　　　　pedestrian V80.12 ☑
　　　　pickup V80.42 ☑
　　　　railway train or vehicle V80.62 ☑
　　　　specified motor vehicle NEC V80.52 ☑
　　　　streetcar V80.731 ☑
　　　　truck V80.42 ☑
　　　　two- or three-wheeled motor vehicle
　　　　　V80.32 ☑
　　　　van V80.42 ☑
　　　noncollision V80.02 ☑
　　　specified circumstance NEC V80.928 ☑
　　animal-rider V80.919 ☑
　　　collision (with)
　　　　animal V80.11 ☑
　　　　　being ridden V80.710 ☑
　　　　animal-drawn vehicle V80.720 ☑
　　　　bus V80.41 ☑
　　　　car V80.41 ☑
　　　　fixed or stationary object V80.81 ☑
　　　　military vehicle V80.910 ☑
　　　　nonmotor vehicle V80.790 ☑
　　　　pedal cycle V80.21 ☑
　　　　pedestrian V80.11 ☑
　　　　pickup V80.41 ☑
　　　　railway train or vehicle V80.61 ☑
　　　　specified motor vehicle NEC V80.51 ☑
　　　　streetcar V80.730 ☑
　　　　truck V80.41 ☑
　　　　two- or three-wheeled motor vehicle
　　　　　V80.31 ☑
　　　　van V80.41 ☑
　　　noncollision V80.018 ☑
　　　　specified as horse rider V80.010 ☑
　　　specified circumstance NEC V80.918 ☑
　　armored car — see Accident, transport, truck occu-
　　　pant
　　battery-powered truck (baggage) (mail) — see
　　　Accident, transport, industrial vehicle occu-
　　　pant
　　bus occupant V79.9 ☑
　　　collision (with)
　　　　animal (traffic) V70.9 ☑
　　　　　being ridden (traffic) V76.9 ☑
　　　　　　nontraffic V76.3 ☑
　　　　　　while boarding or alighting V76.4 ☑
　　　　　nontraffic V70.3 ☑
　　　　　while boarding or alighting V70.4 ☑
　　　　animal-drawn vehicle (traffic) V76.9 ☑
　　　　　nontraffic V76.3 ☑
　　　　　while boarding or alighting V76.4 ☑
　　　　bus (traffic) V74.9 ☑
　　　　　nontraffic V74.3 ☑
　　　　　while boarding or alighting V74.4 ☑
　　　　car (traffic) V73.9 ☑
　　　　　nontraffic V73.3 ☑
　　　　　while boarding or alighting V73.4 ☑
　　　　motor vehicle NOS (traffic) V79.60 ☑
　　　　　nontraffic V79.20 ☑
　　　　　specified type NEC (traffic) V79.69 ☑
　　　　　　nontraffic V79.29 ☑
　　　　pedal cycle (traffic) V71.9 ☑
　　　　　nontraffic V71.3 ☑
　　　　　while boarding or alighting V71.4 ☑
　　　　pickup truck (traffic) V73.9 ☑
　　　　　nontraffic V73.3 ☑
　　　　　while boarding or alighting V73.4 ☑
　　　　railway vehicle (traffic) V75.9 ☑
　　　　　nontraffic V75.3 ☑
　　　　　while boarding or alighting V75.4 ☑
　　　　specified vehicle NEC (traffic) V76.9 ☑
　　　　　nontraffic V76.3 ☑
　　　　　while boarding or alighting V76.4 ☑
　　　　stationary object (traffic) V77.9 ☑

Accident — *continued*
　transport — *continued*
　　bus occupant — *continued*
　　　collision — *continued*
　　　　stationary object — *continued*
　　　　　nontraffic V77.3 ☑
　　　　　while boarding or alighting V77.4 ☑
　　　　streetcar (traffic) V76.9 ☑
　　　　　nontraffic V76.3 ☑
　　　　　while boarding or alighting V76.4 ☑
　　　　three wheeled motor vehicle (traffic)
　　　　　V72.9 ☑
　　　　　nontraffic V72.3 ☑
　　　　　while boarding or alighting V72.4 ☑
　　　　truck (traffic) V74.9 ☑
　　　　　nontraffic V74.3 ☑
　　　　　while boarding or alighting V74.4 ☑
　　　　two wheeled motor vehicle (traffic) V72.9 ☑
　　　　　nontraffic V72.3 ☑
　　　　　while boarding or alighting V72.4 ☑
　　　　van (traffic) V73.9 ☑
　　　　　nontraffic V73.3 ☑
　　　　　while boarding or alighting V73.4 ☑
　　　driver
　　　　collision (with)
　　　　　animal (traffic) V70.5 ☑
　　　　　　being ridden (traffic) V76.5 ☑
　　　　　　　nontraffic V76.0 ☑
　　　　　　nontraffic V70.0 ☑
　　　　　animal-drawn vehicle (traffic) V76.5 ☑
　　　　　　nontraffic V76.0 ☑
　　　　　bus (traffic) V74.5 ☑
　　　　　　nontraffic V74.0 ☑
　　　　　car (traffic) V73.5 ☑
　　　　　　nontraffic V73.0 ☑
　　　　　motor vehicle NOS (traffic) V79.40 ☑
　　　　　　nontraffic V79.00 ☑
　　　　　　specified type NEC (traffic) V79.49 ☑
　　　　　　　nontraffic V79.09 ☑
　　　　　pedal cycle (traffic) V71.5 ☑
　　　　　　nontraffic V71.0 ☑
　　　　　pickup truck (traffic) V73.5 ☑
　　　　　　nontraffic V73.0 ☑
　　　　　railway vehicle (traffic) V75.5 ☑
　　　　　　nontraffic V75.0 ☑
　　　　　specified vehicle NEC (traffic) V76.5 ☑
　　　　　　nontraffic V76.0 ☑
　　　　　stationary object (traffic) V77.5 ☑
　　　　　　nontraffic V77.0 ☑
　　　　　streetcar (traffic) V76.5 ☑
　　　　　　nontraffic V76.0 ☑
　　　　　three wheeled motor vehicle (traffic)
　　　　　　V72.5 ☑
　　　　　　nontraffic V72.0 ☑
　　　　　truck (traffic) V74.5 ☑
　　　　　　nontraffic V74.0 ☑
　　　　　two wheeled motor vehicle (traffic)
　　　　　　V72.5 ☑
　　　　　　nontraffic V72.0 ☑
　　　　　van (traffic) V73.5 ☑
　　　　　　nontraffic V73.0 ☑
　　　　noncollision accident (traffic) V78.5 ☑
　　　　　nontraffic V78.0 ☑
　　　hanger-on
　　　　collision (with)
　　　　　animal (traffic) V70.7 ☑
　　　　　　being ridden (traffic) V76.7 ☑
　　　　　　　nontraffic V76.2 ☑
　　　　　　nontraffic V70.2 ☑
　　　　　animal-drawn vehicle (traffic) V76.7 ☑
　　　　　　nontraffic V76.2 ☑
　　　　　bus (traffic) V74.7 ☑
　　　　　　nontraffic V74.2 ☑
　　　　　car (traffic) V73.7 ☑
　　　　　　nontraffic V73.2 ☑
　　　　　pedal cycle (traffic) V71.7 ☑
　　　　　　nontraffic V71.2 ☑
　　　　　pickup truck (traffic) V73.7 ☑
　　　　　　nontraffic V73.2 ☑
　　　　　railway vehicle (traffic) V75.7 ☑
　　　　　　nontraffic V75.2 ☑
　　　　　specified vehicle NEC (traffic) V76.7 ☑
　　　　　　nontraffic V76.2 ☑
　　　　　stationary object (traffic) V77.7 ☑
　　　　　　nontraffic V77.2 ☑
　　　　　streetcar (traffic) V76.7 ☑

☑ Additional Character Required — Refer to the Tabular List for Character Selection　　　▽ Subterms under main terms may continue to next column or page

Accident — *continued*
  transport — *continued*
    bus occupant — *continued*
      hanger-on — *continued*
        collision — *continued*
          streetcar — *continued*
            nontraffic V76.2 ☑
          three wheeled motor vehicle (traffic)
            V72.7 ☑
            nontraffic V72.2 ☑
          truck (traffic) V74.7 ☑
            nontraffic V74.2 ☑
          two wheeled motor vehicle (traffic)
            V72.7 ☑
            nontraffic V72.2 ☑
          van (traffic) V73.7 ☑
            nontraffic V73.2 ☑
        noncollision accident (traffic) V78.7 ☑
          nontraffic V78.2 ☑
      noncollision accident (traffic) V78.9 ☑
        nontraffic V78.3 ☑
        while boarding or alighting V78.4 ☑
      nontraffic V79.3 ☑
      passenger
        collision (with)
          animal (traffic) V70.6 ☑
            being ridden (traffic) V76.6 ☑
              nontraffic V76.1 ☑
            nontraffic V70.1 ☑
          animal-drawn vehicle (traffic) V76.6 ☑
            nontraffic V76.1 ☑
          bus (traffic) V74.6 ☑
            nontraffic V74.1 ☑
          car (traffic) V73.6 ☑
            nontraffic V73.1 ☑
          motor vehicle NOS (traffic) V79.50 ☑
            nontraffic V79.10 ☑
            specified type NEC (traffic) V79.59 ☑
              nontraffic V79.19 ☑
          pedal cycle (traffic) V71.6 ☑
            nontraffic V71.1 ☑
          pickup truck (traffic) V73.6 ☑
            nontraffic V73.1 ☑
          railway vehicle (traffic) V75.6 ☑
            nontraffic V75.1 ☑
          specified vehicle NEC (traffic) V76.6 ☑
            nontraffic V76.1 ☑
          stationary object (traffic) V77.6 ☑
            nontraffic V77.1 ☑
          streetcar (traffic) V76.6 ☑
            nontraffic V76.1 ☑
          three wheeled motor vehicle (traffic)
            V72.6 ☑
            nontraffic V72.1 ☑
          truck (traffic) V74.6 ☑
            nontraffic V74.1 ☑
          two wheeled motor vehicle (traffic)
            V72.6 ☑
            nontraffic V72.1 ☑
          van (traffic) V73.6 ☑
            nontraffic V73.1 ☑
        noncollision accident (traffic) V78.6 ☑
          nontraffic V78.1 ☑
      specified type NEC V79.88 ☑
      military vehicle V79.81 ☑
    cable car, not on rails V98.0 ☑
      on rails — *see* Accident, transport, streetcar
        occupant
    car occupant V49.9 ☑
      ambulance occupant — *see* Accident, transport,
        ambulance occupant
      collision (with)
        animal (traffic) V40.9 ☑
          being ridden (traffic) V46.9 ☑
            nontraffic V46.3 ☑
            while boarding or alighting V46.4 ☑
          nontraffic V40.3 ☑
          while boarding or alighting V40.4 ☑
        animal-drawn vehicle (traffic) V46.9 ☑
          nontraffic V46.3 ☑
          while boarding or alighting V46.4 ☑
        bus (traffic) V44.9 ☑
          nontraffic V44.3 ☑
          while boarding or alighting V44.4 ☑
        car (traffic) V43.92 ☑
          nontraffic V43.32 ☑

Accident — *continued*
  transport — *continued*
    car occupant — *continued*
      collision — *continued*
        car — *continued*
          while boarding or alighting V43.42 ☑
        motor vehicle NOS (traffic) V49.60 ☑
          nontraffic V49.20 ☑
          specified type NEC (traffic) V49.69 ☑
            nontraffic V49.29 ☑
        pedal cycle (traffic) V41.9 ☑
          nontraffic V41.3 ☑
          while boarding or alighting V41.4 ☑
        pickup truck (traffic) V43.93 ☑
          nontraffic V43.33 ☑
          while boarding or alighting V43.43 ☑
        railway vehicle (traffic) V45.9 ☑
          nontraffic V45.3 ☑
          while boarding or alighting V45.4 ☑
        specified vehicle NEC (traffic) V46.9 ☑
          nontraffic V46.3 ☑
          while boarding or alighting V46.4 ☑
        sport utility vehicle (traffic) V43.91 ☑
          nontraffic V43.31 ☑
          while boarding or alighting V43.41 ☑
        stationary object (traffic) V47.92 ☑
          nontraffic V47.32 ☑
          while boarding or alighting V47.4 ☑
        streetcar (traffic) V46.9 ☑
          nontraffic V46.3 ☑
          while boarding or alighting V46.4 ☑
        three wheeled motor vehicle (traffic)
          V42.9 ☑
          nontraffic V42.3 ☑
          while boarding or alighting V42.4 ☑
        truck (traffic) V44.9 ☑
          nontraffic V44.3 ☑
          while boarding or alighting V44.4 ☑
        two wheeled motor vehicle (traffic) V42.9 ☑
          nontraffic V42.3 ☑
          while boarding or alighting V42.4 ☑
        van (traffic) V43.94 ☑
          nontraffic V43.34 ☑
          while boarding or alighting V43.44 ☑
      driver
        collision (with)
          animal (traffic) V40.5 ☑
            being ridden (traffic) V46.5 ☑
              nontraffic V46.0 ☑
            nontraffic V40.0 ☑
          animal-drawn vehicle (traffic) V46.5 ☑
            nontraffic V46.0 ☑
          bus (traffic) V44.5 ☑
            nontraffic V44.0 ☑
          car (traffic) V43.52 ☑
            nontraffic V43.02 ☑
          motor vehicle NOS (traffic) V49.40 ☑
            nontraffic V49.00 ☑
            specified type NEC (traffic) V49.49 ☑
              nontraffic V49.09 ☑
          pedal cycle (traffic) V41.5 ☑
            nontraffic V41.0 ☑
          pickup truck (traffic) V43.53 ☑
            nontraffic V43.03 ☑
          railway vehicle (traffic) V45.5 ☑
            nontraffic V45.0 ☑
          specified vehicle NEC (traffic) V46.5 ☑
            nontraffic V46.0 ☑
          sport utility vehicle (traffic) V43.51 ☑
            nontraffic V43.01 ☑
          stationary object (traffic) V47.52 ☑
            nontraffic V47.02 ☑
          streetcar (traffic) V46.5 ☑
            nontraffic V46.0 ☑
          three wheeled motor vehicle (traffic)
            V42.5 ☑
            nontraffic V42.0 ☑
          truck (traffic) V44.5 ☑
            nontraffic V44.0 ☑
          two wheeled motor vehicle (traffic)
            V42.5 ☑
            nontraffic V42.0 ☑
          van (traffic) V43.54 ☑
            nontraffic V43.04 ☑
        noncollision accident (traffic) V48.5 ☑
          nontraffic V48.0 ☑

Accident — *continued*
  transport — *continued*
    car occupant — *continued*
      hanger-on
        collision (with)
          animal (traffic) V40.7 ☑
            being ridden (traffic) V46.7 ☑
              nontraffic V46.2 ☑
            nontraffic V40.2 ☑
          animal-drawn vehicle (traffic) V46.7 ☑
            nontraffic V46.2 ☑
          bus (traffic) V44.7 ☑
            nontraffic V44.2 ☑
          car (traffic) V43.72 ☑
            nontraffic V43.22 ☑
          pedal cycle (traffic) V41.7 ☑
            nontraffic V41.2 ☑
          pickup truck (traffic) V43.73 ☑
            nontraffic V43.23 ☑
          railway vehicle (traffic) V45.7 ☑
            nontraffic V45.2 ☑
          specified vehicle NEC (traffic) V46.7 ☑
            nontraffic V46.2 ☑
          sport utility vehicle (traffic) V43.71 ☑
            nontraffic V43.21 ☑
          stationary object (traffic) V47.7 ☑
            nontraffic V47.2 ☑
          streetcar (traffic) V46.7 ☑
            nontraffic V46.2 ☑
          three wheeled motor vehicle (traffic)
            V42.7 ☑
            nontraffic V42.2 ☑
          truck (traffic) V44.7 ☑
            nontraffic V44.2 ☑
          two wheeled motor vehicle (traffic)
            V42.7 ☑
            nontraffic V42.2 ☑
          van (traffic) V43.74 ☑
            nontraffic V43.24 ☑
        noncollision accident (traffic) V48.7 ☑
          nontraffic V48.2 ☑
      noncollision accident (traffic) V48.9 ☑
        nontraffic V48.3 ☑
        while boarding or alighting V48.4 ☑
      nontraffic V49.3 ☑
      passenger
        collision (with)
          animal (traffic) V40.6 ☑
            being ridden (traffic) V46.6 ☑
              nontraffic V46.1 ☑
            nontraffic V40.1 ☑
          animal-drawn vehicle (traffic) V46.6 ☑
            nontraffic V46.1 ☑
          bus (traffic) V44.6 ☑
            nontraffic V44.1 ☑
          car (traffic) V43.62 ☑
            nontraffic V43.12 ☑
          motor vehicle NOS (traffic) V49.50 ☑
            nontraffic V49.10 ☑
            specified type NEC (traffic) V49.59 ☑
              nontraffic V49.19 ☑
          pedal cycle (traffic) V41.6 ☑
            nontraffic V41.1 ☑
          pickup truck (traffic) V43.63 ☑
            nontraffic V43.13 ☑
          railway vehicle (traffic) V45.6 ☑
            nontraffic V45.1 ☑
          specified vehicle NEC (traffic) V46.6 ☑
            nontraffic V46.1 ☑
          sport utility vehicle (traffic) V43.61 ☑
            nontraffic V43.11 ☑
          stationary object (traffic) V47.62 ☑
            nontraffic V47.12 ☑
          streetcar (traffic) V46.6 ☑
            nontraffic V46.1 ☑
          three wheeled motor vehicle (traffic)
            V42.6 ☑
            nontraffic V42.1 ☑
          truck (traffic) V44.6 ☑
            nontraffic V44.1 ☑
          two wheeled motor vehicle (traffic)
            V42.6 ☑
            nontraffic V42.1 ☑
          van (traffic) V43.64 ☑
            nontraffic V43.14 ☑
        noncollision accident (traffic) V48.6 ☑

▽ **Subterms under main terms may continue to next column or page**   ☑ **Additional Character Required — Refer to the Tabular List for Character Selection**

External Causes Index

Accident — Accident

Accident — *continued*
  transport — *continued*
    car occupant — *continued*
      passenger — *continued*
        noncollision accident — *continued*
          nontraffic V48.1 ☑
        specified type NEC V49.88 ☑
        military vehicle V49.81 ☑
    coal car — *see* Accident, transport, industrial vehicle occupant
    construction vehicle occupant (nontraffic) V85.9 ☑
      driver V85.5 ☑
      hanger-on V85.7 ☑
      passenger V85.6 ☑
      traffic V85.3 ☑
        driver V85.0 ☑
        hanger-on V85.2 ☑
        passenger V85.1 ☑
      while boarding or alighting V85.4 ☑
    dirt bike rider — *see* Accident, transport, all-terrain vehicle occupant
    due to cataclysm — *see* Forces of nature, by type
    dune buggy occupant (nontraffic) V86.93 ☑
      driver V86.53 ☑
      hanger-on V86.73 ☑
      passenger V86.63 ☑
      traffic V86.33 ☑
        driver V86.03 ☑
        hanger-on V86.23 ☑
        passenger V86.13 ☑
      while boarding or alighting V86.43 ☑
    forklift — *see* Accident, transport, industrial vehicle occupant
    go cart — *see* Accident, transport, all-terrain vehicle occupant
    golf cart — *see* Accident, transport, all-terrain vehicle occupant
    heavy transport vehicle occupant — *see* Accident, transport, truck occupant
    ice yacht V98.2 ☑
    industrial vehicle occupant (nontraffic) V83.9 ☑
      driver V83.5 ☑
      hanger-on V83.7 ☑
      passenger V83.6 ☑
      traffic V83.3 ☑
        driver V83.0 ☑
        hanger-on V83.2 ☑
        passenger V83.1 ☑
      while boarding or alighting V83.4 ☑
    interurban electric car — *see* Accident, transport, streetcar
    land yacht V98.1 ☑
    logging car — *see* Accident, transport, industrial vehicle occupant
    military vehicle occupant (traffic) V86.34 ☑
      driver V86.04 ☑
      hanger-on V86.24 ☑
      nontraffic V86.94 ☑
        driver V86.54 ☑
        hanger-on V86.74 ☑
        passenger V86.64 ☑
      passenger V86.14 ☑
      while boarding or alighting V86.44 ☑
    mine tram — *see* Accident, transport, industrial vehicle occupant
    motor vehicle NEC occupant (traffic) V86.39 ☑
      driver V86.09 ☑
      hanger-on V86.29 ☑
      nontraffic V86.99 ☑
        driver V86.59 ☑
        hanger-on V86.79 ☑
        passenger V86.69 ☑
      passenger V86.19 ☑
      while boarding or alighting V86.49 ☑
    motorcoach — *see* Accident, transport, bus occupant
    motorcyclist V29.9 ☑
      collision (with)
        animal (traffic) V20.9 ☑
          being ridden (traffic) V26.9 ☑
            nontraffic V26.2 ☑
            while boarding or alighting V26.3 ☑
          nontraffic V20.2 ☑
          while boarding or alighting V20.3 ☑
        animal-drawn vehicle (traffic) V26.9 ☑
          nontraffic V26.2 ☑

Accident — *continued*
  transport — *continued*
    motorcyclist — *continued*
      collision — *continued*
        animal-drawn vehicle — *continued*
          while boarding or alighting V26.3 ☑
        bus (traffic) V24.9 ☑
          nontraffic V24.2 ☑
          while boarding or alighting V24.3 ☑
        car (traffic) V23.9 ☑
          nontraffic V23.2 ☑
          while boarding or alighting V23.3 ☑
        motor vehicle NOS (traffic) V29.60 ☑
          nontraffic V29.20 ☑
          specified type NEC (traffic) V29.69 ☑
            nontraffic V29.29 ☑
        pedal cycle (traffic) V21.9 ☑
          nontraffic V21.2 ☑
          while boarding or alighting V21.3 ☑
        pickup truck (traffic) V23.9 ☑
          nontraffic V23.2 ☑
          while boarding or alighting V23.3 ☑
        railway vehicle (traffic) V25.9 ☑
          nontraffic V25.2 ☑
          while boarding or alighting V25.3 ☑
        specified vehicle NEC (traffic) V26.9 ☑
          nontraffic V26.2 ☑
          while boarding or alighting V26.3 ☑
        stationary object (traffic) V27.9 ☑
          nontraffic V27.2 ☑
          while boarding or alighting V27.3 ☑
        streetcar (traffic) V26.9 ☑
          nontraffic V26.2 ☑
          while boarding or alighting V26.3 ☑
        three wheeled motor vehicle (traffic) V22.9 ☑
          nontraffic V22.2 ☑
          while boarding or alighting V22.3 ☑
        truck (traffic) V24.9 ☑
          nontraffic V24.2 ☑
          while boarding or alighting V24.3 ☑
        two wheeled motor vehicle (traffic) V22.9 ☑
          nontraffic V22.2 ☑
          while boarding or alighting V22.3 ☑
        van (traffic) V23.9 ☑
          nontraffic V23.2 ☑
          while boarding or alighting V23.3 ☑
      driver
        collision (with)
          animal (traffic) V20.4 ☑
            being ridden (traffic) V26.4 ☑
              nontraffic V26.0 ☑
            nontraffic V20.0 ☑
          animal-drawn vehicle (traffic) V26.4 ☑
            nontraffic V26.0 ☑
          bus (traffic) V24.4 ☑
            nontraffic V24.0 ☑
          car (traffic) V23.4 ☑
            nontraffic V23.0 ☑
          motor vehicle NOS (traffic) V29.40 ☑
            nontraffic V29.00 ☑
            specified type NEC (traffic) V29.49 ☑
              nontraffic V29.09 ☑
          pedal cycle (traffic) V21.4 ☑
            nontraffic V21.0 ☑
          pickup truck (traffic) V23.4 ☑
            nontraffic V23.0 ☑
          railway vehicle (traffic) V25.4 ☑
            nontraffic V25.0 ☑
          specified vehicle NEC (traffic) V26.4 ☑
            nontraffic V26.0 ☑
          stationary object (traffic) V27.4 ☑
            nontraffic V27.0 ☑
          streetcar (traffic) V26.4 ☑
            nontraffic V26.0 ☑
          three wheeled motor vehicle (traffic) V22.4 ☑
            nontraffic V22.0 ☑
          truck (traffic) V24.4 ☑
            nontraffic V24.0 ☑
          two wheeled motor vehicle (traffic) V22.4 ☑
            nontraffic V22.0 ☑
          van (traffic) V23.4 ☑
            nontraffic V23.0 ☑
        noncollision accident (traffic) V28.4 ☑

Accident — *continued*
  transport — *continued*
    motorcyclist — *continued*
      driver — *continued*
        noncollision accident — *continued*
          nontraffic V28.0 ☑
      noncollision accident (traffic) V28.9 ☑
        nontraffic V28.2 ☑
        while boarding or alighting V28.3 ☑
      nontraffic V29.3 ☑
      passenger
        collision (with)
          animal (traffic) V20.5 ☑
            being ridden (traffic) V26.5 ☑
              nontraffic V26.1 ☑
            nontraffic V20.1 ☑
          animal-drawn vehicle (traffic) V26.5 ☑
            nontraffic V26.1 ☑
          bus (traffic) V24.5 ☑
            nontraffic V24.1 ☑
          car (traffic) V23.5 ☑
            nontraffic V23.1 ☑
          motor vehicle NOS (traffic) V29.50 ☑
            nontraffic V29.10 ☑
            specified type NEC (traffic) V29.59 ☑
              nontraffic V29.19 ☑
          pedal cycle (traffic) V21.5 ☑
            nontraffic V21.1 ☑
          pickup truck (traffic) V23.5 ☑
            nontraffic V23.1 ☑
          railway vehicle (traffic) V25.5 ☑
            nontraffic V25.1 ☑
          specified vehicle NEC (traffic) V26.5 ☑
            nontraffic V26.1 ☑
          stationary object (traffic) V27.5 ☑
            nontraffic V27.1 ☑
          streetcar (traffic) V26.5 ☑
            nontraffic V26.1 ☑
          three wheeled motor vehicle (traffic) V22.5 ☑
            nontraffic V22.1 ☑
          truck (traffic) V24.5 ☑
            nontraffic V24.1 ☑
          two wheeled motor vehicle (traffic) V22.5 ☑
            nontraffic V22.1 ☑
          van (traffic) V23.5 ☑
            nontraffic V23.1 ☑
        noncollision accident (traffic) V28.5 ☑
          nontraffic V28.1 ☑
      specified type NEC V29.88 ☑
      military vehicle V29.81 ☑
    occupant (of)
      aircraft (powered) V95.9 ☑
        fixed wing
          commercial — *see* Accident, transport, aircraft, occupant, powered, fixed wing, commercial
          private — *see* Accident, transport, aircraft, occupant, powered, fixed wing, private
        nonpowered V96.9 ☑
        specified NEC V95.8 ☑
      airport battery-powered vehicle — *see* Accident, transport, industrial vehicle occupant
      all-terrain vehicle (ATV) — *see* Accident, transport, all-terrain vehicle occupant
      animal-drawn vehicle — *see* Accident, transport, animal-drawn vehicle occupant
      automobile — *see* Accident, transport, car occupant
      balloon V96.00 ☑
      battery-powered vehicle — *see* Accident, transport, industrial vehicle occupant
      bicycle — *see* Accident, transport, pedal cyclist
        motorized — *see* Accident, transport, motorcycle rider
      boat NEC — *see* Accident, watercraft
      bulldozer — *see* Accident, transport, construction vehicle occupant
      bus — *see* Accident, transport, bus occupant
      cable car (on rails) (*see also* Accident, transport, streetcar occupant)
        not on rails V98.0 ☑
      car (*see also* Accident, transport, car occupant)

Accident — *continued*
  transport — *continued*
    occupant — *continued*
      car (*see also* Accident, transport, car occupant) — *continued*
        cable (on rails) (*see also* Accident, transport, streetcar occupant)
          not on rails V98.0 ☑
        coach — *see* Accident, transport, bus occupant
        coal-car — *see* Accident, transport, industrial vehicle occupant
        digger — *see* Accident, transport, construction vehicle occupant
        dump truck — *see* Accident, transport, construction vehicle occupant
        earth-leveler — *see* Accident, transport, construction vehicle occupant
        farm machinery (self-propelled) — *see* Accident, transport, agricultural vehicle occupant
        forklift — *see* Accident, transport, industrial vehicle occupant
        glider (unpowered) V96.20 ☑
          hang V96.10 ☑
          powered (microlight) (ultralight) — *see* Accident, transport, aircraft, occupant, powered, glider
        glider (unpowered) NEC V96.20 ☑
        hang-glider V96.10 ☑
        harvester — *see* Accident, transport, agricultural vehicle occupant
        heavy (transport) vehicle — *see* Accident, transport, truck occupant
        helicopter — *see* Accident, transport, aircraft, occupant, helicopter
        ice-yacht V98.2 ☑
        kite (carrying person) V96.8 ☑
        land-yacht V98.1 ☑
        logging car — *see* Accident, transport, industrial vehicle occupant
        mechanical shovel — *see* Accident, transport, construction vehicle occupant
        microlight — *see* Accident, transport, aircraft, occupant, powered, glider
        minibus — *see* Accident, transport, car occupant
        minivan — *see* Accident, transport, car occupant
        moped — *see* Accident, transport, motorcycle
        motor scooter — *see* Accident, transport, motorcycle
        motorcycle (with sidecar) — *see* Accident, transport, motorcycle
        pedal cycle (*see also* Accident, transport, pedal cyclist)
        pick-up (truck) — *see* Accident, transport, pickup truck occupant
        railway (train) (vehicle) (subterranean) (elevated) — *see* Accident, transport, railway vehicle occupant
        rickshaw — *see* Accident, transport, pedal cycle
          motorized — *see* Accident, transport, three-wheeled motor vehicle
          pedal driven — *see* Accident, transport, pedal cyclist
        road-roller — *see* Accident, transport, construction vehicle occupant
        ship NOS V94.9 ☑
        ski-lift (chair) (gondola) V98.3 ☑
        snowmobile — *see* Accident, transport, snowmobile occupant
        spacecraft, spaceship — *see* Accident, transport, aircraft, occupant, spacecraft
        sport utility vehicle — *see* Accident, transport, car occupant
        streetcar (interurban) (operating on public street or highway) — *see* Accident, transport, streetcar occupant
        SUV — *see* Accident, transport, car occupant
        téléférique V98.0 ☑
        three-wheeled vehicle (motorized) (*see also* Accident, transport, three-wheeled motor vehicle occupant)
          nonmotorized — *see* Accident, transport, pedal cycle
        tractor (farm) (and trailer) — *see* Accident, transport, agricultural vehicle occupant

Accident — *continued*
  transport — *continued*
    occupant — *continued*
      train — *see* Accident, transport, railway vehicle occupant
      tram — *see* Accident, transport, streetcar occupant
        in mine or quarry — *see* Accident, transport, industrial vehicle occupant
      tricycle — *see* Accident, transport, pedal cycle
        motorized — *see* Accident, transport, three-wheeled motor vehicle
      trolley — *see* Accident, transport, streetcar occupant
        in mine or quarry — *see* Accident, transport, industrial vehicle occupant
      tub, in mine or quarry — *see* Accident, transport, industrial vehicle occupant
      ultralight — *see* Accident, transport, aircraft, occupant, powered, glider
      van — *see* Accident, transport, van occupant
      vehicle NEC V89.9 ☑
        heavy transport — *see* Accident, transport, truck occupant
        motor (traffic) NEC V89.2 ☑
          nontraffic NEC V89.0 ☑
      watercraft NOS V94.9 ☑
        causing drowning B — *see* Drowning, resulting from accident to boat
    parachutist V97.29 ☑
      after accident to aircraft — *see* Accident, transport, aircraft
      entangled in object V97.21 ☑
      injured on landing V97.22 ☑
    pedal cyclist V19.9 ☑
      collision (with)
        animal (traffic) V10.9 ☑
          being ridden (traffic) V16.9 ☑
            nontraffic V16.2 ☑
            while boarding or alighting V16.3 ☑
          nontraffic V10.2 ☑
          while boarding or alighting V10.3 ☑
        animal-drawn vehicle (traffic) V16.9 ☑
          nontraffic V16.2 ☑
          while boarding or alighting V16.3 ☑
        bus (traffic) V14.9 ☑
          nontraffic V14.2 ☑
          while boarding or alighting V14.3 ☑
        car (traffic) V13.9 ☑
          nontraffic V13.2 ☑
          while boarding or alighting V13.3 ☑
        motor vehicle NOS (traffic) V19.60 ☑
          nontraffic V19.20 ☑
          specified type NEC (traffic) V19.69 ☑
            nontraffic V19.29 ☑
        pedal cycle (traffic) V11.9 ☑
          nontraffic V11.2 ☑
          while boarding or alighting V11.3 ☑
        pickup truck (traffic) V13.9 ☑
          nontraffic V13.2 ☑
          while boarding or alighting V13.3 ☑
        railway vehicle (traffic) V15.9 ☑
          nontraffic V15.2 ☑
          while boarding or alighting V15.3 ☑
        specified vehicle NEC (traffic) V16.9 ☑
          nontraffic V16.2 ☑
          while boarding or alighting V16.3 ☑
        stationary object (traffic) V17.9 ☑
          nontraffic V17.2 ☑
          while boarding or alighting V17.3 ☑
        streetcar (traffic) V16.9 ☑
          nontraffic V16.2 ☑
          while boarding or alighting V16.3 ☑
        three wheeled motor vehicle (traffic) V12.9 ☑
          nontraffic V12.2 ☑
          while boarding or alighting V12.3 ☑
        truck (traffic) V14.9 ☑
          nontraffic V14.2 ☑
          while boarding or alighting V14.3 ☑
        two wheeled motor vehicle (traffic) V12.9 ☑
          nontraffic V12.2 ☑
          while boarding or alighting V12.3 ☑
        van (traffic) V13.9 ☑
          nontraffic V13.2 ☑
          while boarding or alighting V13.3 ☑

Accident — *continued*
  transport — *continued*
    pedal cyclist — *continued*
      driver
        collision (with)
          animal (traffic) V10.4 ☑
            being ridden (traffic) V16.4 ☑
              nontraffic V16.0 ☑
            nontraffic V10.0 ☑
          animal-drawn vehicle (traffic) V16.4 ☑
            nontraffic V16.0 ☑
          bus (traffic) V14.4 ☑
            nontraffic V14.0 ☑
          car (traffic) V13.4 ☑
            nontraffic V13.0 ☑
          motor vehicle NOS (traffic) V19.40 ☑
            nontraffic V19.00 ☑
            specified type NEC (traffic) V19.49 ☑
              nontraffic V19.09 ☑
          pedal cycle (traffic) V11.4 ☑
            nontraffic V11.0 ☑
          pickup truck (traffic) V13.4 ☑
            nontraffic V13.0 ☑
          railway vehicle (traffic) V15.4 ☑
            nontraffic V15.0 ☑
          specified vehicle NEC (traffic) V16.4 ☑
            nontraffic V16.0 ☑
          stationary object (traffic) V17.4 ☑
            nontraffic V17.0 ☑
          streetcar (traffic) V16.4 ☑
            nontraffic V16.0 ☑
          three wheeled motor vehicle (traffic) V12.4 ☑
            nontraffic V12.0 ☑
          truck (traffic) V14.4 ☑
            nontraffic V14.0 ☑
          two wheeled motor vehicle (traffic) V12.4 ☑
            nontraffic V12.0 ☑
          van (traffic) V13.4 ☑
            nontraffic V13.0 ☑
        noncollision accident (traffic) V18.4 ☑
          nontraffic V18.0 ☑
      noncollision accident (traffic) V18.9 ☑
        nontraffic V18.2 ☑
        while boarding or alighting V18.3 ☑
      nontraffic V19.3 ☑
      passenger
        collision (with)
          animal (traffic) V10.5 ☑
            being ridden (traffic) V16.5 ☑
              nontraffic V16.1 ☑
            nontraffic V10.1 ☑
          animal-drawn vehicle (traffic) V16.5 ☑
            nontraffic V16.1 ☑
          bus (traffic) V14.5 ☑
            nontraffic V14.1 ☑
          car (traffic) V13.5 ☑
            nontraffic V13.1 ☑
          motor vehicle NOS (traffic) V19.50 ☑
            nontraffic V19.10 ☑
            specified type NEC (traffic) V19.59 ☑
              nontraffic V19.19 ☑
          pedal cycle (traffic) V11.5 ☑
            nontraffic V11.1 ☑
          pickup truck (traffic) V13.5 ☑
            nontraffic V13.1 ☑
          railway vehicle (traffic) V15.5 ☑
            nontraffic V15.1 ☑
          specified vehicle NEC (traffic) V16.5 ☑
            nontraffic V16.1 ☑
          stationary object (traffic) V17.5 ☑
            nontraffic V17.1 ☑
          streetcar (traffic) V16.5 ☑
            nontraffic V16.1 ☑
          three wheeled motor vehicle (traffic) V12.5 ☑
            nontraffic V12.1 ☑
          truck (traffic) V14.5 ☑
            nontraffic V14.1 ☑
          two wheeled motor vehicle (traffic) V12.5 ☑
            nontraffic V12.1 ☑
          van (traffic) V13.5 ☑
            nontraffic V13.1 ☑
        noncollision accident (traffic) V18.5 ☑

Accident — *continued*
   transport — *continued*
     pedal cyclist — *continued*
      passenger — *continued*
       noncollision accident — *continued*
        nontraffic V18.1 ☑
       specified type NEC V19.88 ☑
       military vehicle V19.81 ☑
     pedestrian
      conveyance (occupant) V09.9 ☑
       babystroller V00.828 ☑
        collision (with) V09.9 ☑
         animal being ridden or animal drawn vehicle V06.99 ☑
          nontraffic V06.09 ☑
          traffic V06.19 ☑
         bus or heavy transport V04.99 ☑
          nontraffic V04.09 ☑
          traffic V04.19 ☑
         car V03.99 ☑
          nontraffic V03.09 ☑
          traffic V03.19 ☑
         pedal cycle V01.99 ☑
          nontraffic V01.09 ☑
          traffic V01.19 ☑
         pick-up truck or van V03.99 ☑
          nontraffic V03.09 ☑
          traffic V03.19 ☑
         railway (train) (vehicle) V05.99 ☑
          nontraffic V05.09 ☑
          traffic V05.19 ☑
         stationary object V00.822 ☑
         streetcar V06.99 ☑
          nontraffic V06.09 ☑
          traffic V06.19 ☑
         two- or three-wheeled motor vehicle V02.99 ☑
          nontraffic V02.09 ☑
          traffic V02.19 ☑
         vehicle V09.9 ☑
          animal-drawn V06.99 ☑
           nontraffic V06.09 ☑
           traffic V06.19 ☑
          motor
           nontraffic V09.00 ☑
           traffic V09.20 ☑
        fall V00.821 ☑
        nontraffic V09.1 ☑
         involving motor vehicle NEC V09.00 ☑
        traffic V09.3 ☑
         involving motor vehicle NEC V09.20 ☑
       flat-bottomed NEC V00.388 ☑
        collision (with) V09.9 ☑
         animal being ridden or animal drawn vehicle V06.99 ☑
          nontraffic V06.09 ☑
          traffic V06.19 ☑
         bus or heavy transport V04.99 ☑
          nontraffic V04.09 ☑
          traffic V04.19 ☑
         car V03.99 ☑
          nontraffic V03.09 ☑
          traffic V03.19 ☑
         pedal cycle V01.99 ☑
          nontraffic V01.09 ☑
          traffic V01.19 ☑
         pick-up truck or van V03.99 ☑
          nontraffic V03.09 ☑
          traffic V03.19 ☑
         railway (train) (vehicle) V05.99 ☑
          nontraffic V05.09 ☑
          traffic V05.19 ☑
         stationary object V00.382 ☑
         streetcar V06.99 ☑
          nontraffic V06.09 ☑
          traffic V06.19 ☑
         two- or three-wheeled motor vehicle V02.99 ☑
          nontraffic V02.09 ☑
          traffic V02.19 ☑
         vehicle V09.9 ☑
          animal-drawn V06.99 ☑
           nontraffic V06.09 ☑
           traffic V06.19 ☑

Accident — *continued*
   transport — *continued*
     pedestrian — *continued*
      conveyance — *continued*
       flat-bottomed — *continued*
        collision — *continued*
         vehicle — *continued*
          motor
           nontraffic V09.00 ☑
           traffic V09.20 ☑
        fall V00.381 ☑
        nontraffic V09.1 ☑
         involving motor vehicle NEC V09.00 ☑
        snow
         board — *see* Accident, transport, pedestrian, conveyance, snow board
         ski — *see* Accident, transport, pedestrian, conveyance, skis (snow)
        traffic V09.3 ☑
         involving motor vehicle NEC V09.20 ☑
       gliding type NEC V00.288 ☑
        collision (with) V09.9 ☑
         animal being ridden or animal drawn vehicle V06.99 ☑
          nontraffic V06.09 ☑
          traffic V06.19 ☑
         bus or heavy transport V04.99 ☑
          nontraffic V04.09 ☑
          traffic V04.19 ☑
         car V03.99 ☑
          nontraffic V03.09 ☑
          traffic V03.19 ☑
         pedal cycle V01.99 ☑
          nontraffic V01.09 ☑
          traffic V01.19 ☑
         pick-up truck or van V03.99 ☑
          nontraffic V03.09 ☑
          traffic V03.19 ☑
         railway (train) (vehicle) V05.99 ☑
          nontraffic V05.09 ☑
          traffic V05.19 ☑
         stationary object V00.282 ☑
         streetcar V06.99 ☑
          nontraffic V06.09 ☑
          traffic V02.19 ☑
         two- or three-wheeled motor vehicle V02.99 ☑
          nontraffic V02.09 ☑
          traffic V02.19 ☑
         vehicle V09.9 ☑
          animal-drawn V06.99 ☑
           nontraffic V06.09 ☑
           traffic V06.19 ☑
         motor
          nontraffic V09.00 ☑
          traffic V09.20 ☑
       fall V00.281 ☑
       heelies — *see* Accident, transport, pedestrian, conveyance, heelies
       ice skate — *see* Accident, transport, pedestrian, conveyance, ice skate
       nontraffic V09.1 ☑
        involving motor vehicle NEC V09.00 ☑
       sled — *see* Accident, transport, pedestrian, conveyance, sled
       traffic V09.3 ☑
        involving motor vehicle NEC V09.20 ☑
        wheelies — *see* Accident, transport, pedestrian, conveyance, heelies
       heelies V00.158 ☑
        colliding with stationary object V00.152 ☑
        fall V00.151 ☑
       ice skates V00.218 ☑
        collision (with) V09.9 ☑
         animal being ridden or animal drawn vehicle V06.99 ☑
          nontraffic V06.09 ☑
          traffic V06.19 ☑

Accident — *continued*
   transport — *continued*
     pedestrian — *continued*
      conveyance — *continued*
       ice skates — *continued*
        collision — *continued*
         bus or heavy transport V04.99 ☑
          nontraffic V04.09 ☑
          traffic V04.19 ☑
         car V03.99 ☑
          nontraffic V03.09 ☑
          traffic V03.19 ☑
         pedal cycle V01.99 ☑
          nontraffic V01.09 ☑
          traffic V01.19 ☑
         pick-up truck or van V03.99 ☑
          nontraffic V03.09 ☑
          traffic V03.19 ☑
         railway (train) (vehicle) V05.99 ☑
          nontraffic V05.09 ☑
          traffic V05.19 ☑
         stationary object V00.212 ☑
         streetcar V06.99 ☑
          nontraffic V06.09 ☑
          traffic V06.19 ☑
         two- or three-wheeled motor vehicle V02.99 ☑
          nontraffic V02.09 ☑
          traffic V02.19 ☑
         vehicle V09.9 ☑
          animal-drawn V06.99 ☑
           nontraffic V06.09 ☑
           traffic V06.19 ☑
          motor
           nontraffic V09.00 ☑
           traffic V09.20 ☑
       fall V00.211 ☑
       nontraffic V09.1 ☑
        involving motor vehicle NEC V09.00 ☑
       traffic V09.3 ☑
        involving motor vehicle NEC V09.20 ☑
       motorized mobility scooter V00.838 ☑
        collision with stationary object V00.832 ☑
        fall from V00.831 ☑
        nontraffic V09.1 ☑
         involving motor vehicle V09.00 ☑
          military V09.01 ☑
          specified type NEC V09.09 ☑
       roller skates (non in-line) V00.128 ☑
        collision (with) V09.9 ☑
         animal being ridden or animal drawn vehicle V06.91 ☑
          nontraffic V06.01 ☑
          traffic V06.11 ☑
         bus or heavy transport V04.91 ☑
          nontraffic V04.01 ☑
          traffic V04.11 ☑
         car V03.91 ☑
          nontraffic V03.01 ☑
          traffic V03.11 ☑
         pedal cycle V01.91 ☑
          nontraffic V01.01 ☑
          traffic V01.11 ☑
         pick-up truck or van V03.91 ☑
          nontraffic V03.01 ☑
          traffic V03.11 ☑
         railway (train) (vehicle) V05.91 ☑
          nontraffic V05.01 ☑
          traffic V05.11 ☑
         stationary object V00.122 ☑
         streetcar V06.91 ☑
          nontraffic V06.01 ☑
          traffic V06.11 ☑
         two- or three-wheeled motor vehicle V02.91 ☑
          nontraffic V02.01 ☑
          traffic V02.11 ☑
         vehicle V09.9 ☑
          animal-drawn V06.91 ☑
           nontraffic V06.01 ☑
           traffic V06.11 ☑
          motor
           nontraffic V09.00 ☑

☑ **Additional Character Required** — Refer to the Tabular List for Character Selection   ▼ **Subterms under main terms may continue to next column or page**

Accident — *continued*
  transport — *continued*
    pedestrian — *continued*
      conveyance — *continued*
        roller skates — *continued*
          collision — *continued*
            vehicle — *continued*
              motor — *continued*
                traffic V09.20 ☑
            fall V00.121 ☑
            in-line V00.118 ☑
              collision — *see also* Accident, trans-
                port, pedestrian, conveyance
                occupant, roller skates, colli-
                sion
                with stationary object V00.112 ☑
              fall V00.111 ☑
            nontraffic V09.1 ☑
              involving motor vehicle NEC
                V09.00 ☑
            traffic V09.3 ☑
              involving motor vehicle NEC
                V09.20 ☑
        rolling shoes V00.158 ☑
          colliding with stationary object
            V00.152 ☑
          fall V00.151 ☑
        rolling type NEC V00.188 ☑
          collision (with) V09.9 ☑
            animal being ridden or animal drawn
              vehicle V06.99 ☑
              nontraffic V06.09 ☑
              traffic V06.19 ☑
            bus or heavy transport V04.99 ☑
              nontraffic V04.09 ☑
              traffic V04.19 ☑
            car V03.99 ☑
              nontraffic V03.09 ☑
              traffic V03.19 ☑
            pedal cycle V01.99 ☑
              nontraffic V01.09 ☑
              traffic V01.19 ☑
            pick-up truck or van V03.99 ☑
              nontraffic V03.09 ☑
              traffic V03.19 ☑
            railway (train) (vehicle) V05.99 ☑
              nontraffic V05.09 ☑
              traffic V05.19 ☑
            stationary object V00.182 ☑
            streetcar V06.99 ☑
              nontraffic V06.09 ☑
              traffic V06.19 ☑
            two- or three-wheeled motor vehicle
              V02.99 ☑
              nontraffic V02.09 ☑
              traffic V02.19 ☑
            vehicle V09.9 ☑
              animal-drawn V06.99 ☑
                nontraffic V06.09 ☑
                traffic V06.19 ☑
              motor
                nontraffic V09.00 ☑
                traffic V09.20 ☑
          fall V00.181 ☑
          in-line roller skate — *see* Accident,
            transport, pedestrian, conveyance,
            roller skate, in-line
          nontraffic V09.1 ☑
            involving motor vehicle NEC
              V09.00 ☑
          roller skate — *see* Accident, transport,
            pedestrian, conveyance, roller
            skate
          scooter (non-motorized) — *see* Accident,
            transport, pedestrian, conveyance,
            scooter
          skateboard — *see* Accident, transport,
            pedestrian, conveyance, skate-
            board
          traffic V09.3 ☑
            involving motor vehicle NEC
              V09.20 ☑
        scooter (non-motorized) V00.148 ☑
          collision (with) V09.9 ☑
            animal being ridden or animal drawn
              vehicle V06.99 ☑

Accident — *continued*
  transport — *continued*
    pedestrian — *continued*
      conveyance — *continued*
        scooter — *continued*
          collision — *continued*
            animal being ridden or animal drawn
              vehicle — *continued*
                nontraffic V06.09 ☑
                traffic V06.19 ☑
            bus or heavy transport V04.99 ☑
              nontraffic V04.09 ☑
              traffic V04.19 ☑
            car V03.99 ☑
              nontraffic V03.09 ☑
              traffic V03.19 ☑
            pedal cycle V01.99 ☑
              nontraffic V01.09 ☑
              traffic V01.19 ☑
            pick-up truck or van V03.99 ☑
              nontraffic V03.09 ☑
              traffic V03.19 ☑
            railway (train) (vehicle) V05.99 ☑
              nontraffic V05.09 ☑
              traffic V05.19 ☑
            stationary object V00.142 ☑
            streetcar V06.99 ☑
              nontraffic V06.09 ☑
              traffic V06.19 ☑
            two- or three-wheeled motor vehicle
              V02.99 ☑
              nontraffic V02.09 ☑
              traffic V02.19 ☑
            vehicle V09.9 ☑
              animal-drawn V06.99 ☑
                nontraffic V06.09 ☑
                traffic V06.19 ☑
              motor
                nontraffic V09.00 ☑
                traffic V09.20 ☑
          fall V00.141 ☑
          nontraffic V09.1 ☑
            involving motor vehicle NEC
              V09.00 ☑
          traffic V09.3 ☑
            involving motor vehicle NEC
              V09.20 ☑
        skate board V00.138 ☑
          collision (with) V09.9 ☑
            animal being ridden or animal drawn
              vehicle V06.92 ☑
              nontraffic V06.02 ☑
              traffic V06.12 ☑
            bus or heavy transport V04.92 ☑
              nontraffic V04.02 ☑
              traffic V04.12 ☑
            car V03.92 ☑
              nontraffic V03.02 ☑
              traffic V03.12 ☑
            pedal cycle V01.92 ☑
              nontraffic V01.02 ☑
              traffic V01.12 ☑
            pick-up truck or van V03.92 ☑
              nontraffic V03.02 ☑
              traffic V03.12 ☑
            railway (train) (vehicle) V05.92 ☑
              nontraffic V05.02 ☑
              traffic V05.12 ☑
            stationary object V00.132 ☑
            streetcar V06.92 ☑
              nontraffic V06.02 ☑
              traffic V06.12 ☑
            two- or three-wheeled motor vehicle
              V02.92 ☑
              nontraffic V02.02 ☑
              traffic V02.12 ☑
            vehicle V09.9 ☑
              animal-drawn V06.92 ☑
                nontraffic V06.02 ☑
                traffic V06.12 ☑
              motor
                nontraffic V09.00 ☑
                traffic V09.20 ☑
          fall V00.131 ☑
          nontraffic V09.1 ☑

Accident — *continued*
  transport — *continued*
    pedestrian — *continued*
      conveyance — *continued*
        skate board — *continued*
          nontraffic — *continued*
            involving motor vehicle NEC
              V09.00 ☑
          traffic V09.3 ☑
            involving motor vehicle NEC
              V09.20 ☑
        skis (snow) V00.328 ☑
          collision (with) V09.9 ☑
            animal being ridden or animal drawn
              vehicle V06.99 ☑
              nontraffic V06.09 ☑
              traffic V06.19 ☑
            bus or heavy transport V04.99 ☑
              nontraffic V04.09 ☑
              traffic V04.19 ☑
            car V03.99 ☑
              nontraffic V03.09 ☑
              traffic V03.19 ☑
            pedal cycle V01.99 ☑
              nontraffic V01.09 ☑
              traffic V01.19 ☑
            pick-up truck or van V03.99 ☑
              nontraffic V03.09 ☑
              traffic V03.19 ☑
            railway (train) (vehicle) V05.99 ☑
              nontraffic V05.09 ☑
              traffic V05.19 ☑
            stationary object V00.322 ☑
            streetcar V06.99 ☑
              nontraffic V06.09 ☑
              traffic V06.19 ☑
            two- or three-wheeled motor vehicle
              V02.99 ☑
              nontraffic V02.09 ☑
              traffic V02.19 ☑
            vehicle V09.9 ☑
              animal-drawn V06.99 ☑
                nontraffic V06.09 ☑
                traffic V06.19 ☑
              motor
                nontraffic V09.00 ☑
                traffic V09.20 ☑
          fall V00.321 ☑
          nontraffic V09.1 ☑
            involving motor vehicle NEC
              V09.00 ☑
          traffic V09.3 ☑
            involving motor vehicle NEC
              V09.20 ☑
        sled V00.228 ☑
          collision (with) V09.9 ☑
            animal being ridden or animal drawn
              vehicle V06.99 ☑
              nontraffic V06.09 ☑
              traffic V06.19 ☑
            bus or heavy transport V04.99 ☑
              nontraffic V04.09 ☑
              traffic V04.19 ☑
            car V03.99 ☑
              nontraffic V03.09 ☑
              traffic V03.19 ☑
            pedal cycle V01.99 ☑
              nontraffic V01.09 ☑
              traffic V01.19 ☑
            pick-up truck or van V03.99 ☑
              nontraffic V03.09 ☑
              traffic V03.19 ☑
            railway (train) (vehicle) V05.99 ☑
              nontraffic V05.09 ☑
              traffic V05.19 ☑
            stationary object V00.222 ☑
            streetcar V06.99 ☑
              nontraffic V06.09 ☑
              traffic V06.19 ☑
            two- or three-wheeled motor vehicle
              V02.99 ☑
              nontraffic V02.09 ☑
              traffic V02.19 ☑
            vehicle V09.9 ☑
              animal-drawn V06.99 ☑
                nontraffic V06.09 ☑

Accident — *continued*
  transport — *continued*
    pedestrian — *continued*
      conveyance — *continued*
        sled — *continued*
          collision — *continued*
            vehicle — *continued*
              animal-drawn — *continued*
                traffic V06.19 ☑
              motor
                nontraffic V09.00 ☑
                traffic V09.20 ☑
          fall V00.221 ☑
          nontraffic V09.1 ☑
            involving motor vehicle NEC
                V09.00 ☑
          traffic V09.3 ☑
            involving motor vehicle NEC
                V09.20 ☑
        snow board V00.318 ☑
          collision (with) V09.9 ☑
            animal being ridden or animal drawn
                vehicle V06.99 ☑
                nontraffic V06.09 ☑
                traffic V06.19 ☑
            bus or heavy transport V04.99 ☑
                nontraffic V04.09 ☑
                traffic V04.19 ☑
            car V03.99 ☑
                nontraffic V03.09 ☑
                traffic V03.19 ☑
            pedal cycle V01.99 ☑
                nontraffic V01.09 ☑
                traffic V01.19 ☑
            pick-up truck or van V03.99 ☑
                nontraffic V03.09 ☑
                traffic V03.19 ☑
            railway (train) (vehicle) V05.99 ☑
                nontraffic V05.09 ☑
                traffic V05.19 ☑
            stationary object V00.312 ☑
            streetcar V06.99 ☑
                nontraffic V06.09 ☑
                traffic V06.19 ☑
            two- or three-wheeled motor vehicle
                V02.99 ☑
                nontraffic V02.09 ☑
                traffic V02.19 ☑
            vehicle V09.9 ☑
                animal-drawn V06.99 ☑
                  nontraffic V06.09 ☑
                  traffic V06.19 ☑
                motor
                  nontraffic V09.00 ☑
                  traffic V09.20 ☑
          fall V00.311 ☑
          nontraffic V09.1 ☑
            involving motor vehicle NEC
                V09.00 ☑
          traffic V09.3 ☑
            involving motor vehicle NEC
                V09.20 ☑
        specified type NEC V00.898 ☑
          collision (with) V09.9 ☑
            animal being ridden or animal drawn
                vehicle V06.99 ☑
                nontraffic V06.09 ☑
                traffic V06.19 ☑
            bus or heavy transport V04.99 ☑
                nontraffic V04.09 ☑
                traffic V04.19 ☑
            car V03.99 ☑
                nontraffic V03.09 ☑
                traffic V03.19 ☑
            pedal cycle V01.99 ☑
                nontraffic V01.09 ☑
                traffic V01.19 ☑
            pick-up truck or van V03.99 ☑
                nontraffic V03.09 ☑
                traffic V03.19 ☑
            railway (train) (vehicle) V05.99 ☑
                nontraffic V05.09 ☑
                traffic V05.19 ☑
            stationary object V00.892 ☑
            streetcar V06.99 ☑
                nontraffic V06.09 ☑

Accident — *continued*
  transport — *continued*
    pedestrian — *continued*
      conveyance — *continued*
        specified type — *continued*
          collision — *continued*
            streetcar — *continued*
                traffic V06.19 ☑
            two- or three-wheeled motor vehicle
                V02.99 ☑
                nontraffic V02.09 ☑
                traffic V02.19 ☑
            vehicle V09.9 ☑
                animal-drawn V06.99 ☑
                  nontraffic V06.09 ☑
                  traffic V06.19 ☑
                motor
                  nontraffic V09.00 ☑
                  traffic V09.20 ☑
          fall V00.891 ☑
          nontraffic V09.1 ☑
            involving motor vehicle NEC
                V09.00 ☑
          traffic V09.3 ☑
            involving motor vehicle NEC
                V09.20 ☑
        traffic V09.3 ☑
          involving motor vehicle V09.20 ☑
          military V09.21 ☑
          specified type NEC V09.29 ☑
        wheelchair (powered) V00.818 ☑
          collision (with) V09.9 ☑
            animal being ridden or animal drawn
                vehicle V06.99 ☑
                nontraffic V06.09 ☑
                traffic V06.19 ☑
            bus or heavy transport V04.99 ☑
                nontraffic V04.09 ☑
                traffic V04.19 ☑
            car V03.99 ☑
                nontraffic V03.09 ☑
                traffic V03.19 ☑
            pedal cycle V01.99 ☑
                nontraffic V01.09 ☑
                traffic V01.19 ☑
            pick-up truck or van V03.99 ☑
                nontraffic V03.09 ☑
                traffic V03.19 ☑
            railway (train) (vehicle) V05.99 ☑
                nontraffic V05.09 ☑
                traffic V05.19 ☑
            stationary object V00.812 ☑
            streetcar V06.99 ☑
                nontraffic V06.09 ☑
                traffic V06.19 ☑
            two- or three-wheeled motor vehicle
                V02.99 ☑
                nontraffic V02.09 ☑
                traffic V02.19 ☑
            vehicle V09.9 ☑
                animal-drawn V06.99 ☑
                  nontraffic V06.09 ☑
                  traffic V06.19 ☑
                motor
                  nontraffic V09.00 ☑
                  traffic V09.20 ☑
          fall V00.811 ☑
          nontraffic V09.1 ☑
            involving motor vehicle NEC
                V09.00 ☑
          traffic V09.3 ☑
            involving motor vehicle NEC
                V09.20 ☑
        wheeled shoe V00.158 ☑
          colliding with stationary object
                V00.152 ☑
          fall V00.151 ☑
      on foot (*see also* Accident, pedestrian)
        collision (with)
          animal being ridden or animal drawn
                vehicle V06.90 ☑
                nontraffic V06.00 ☑
                traffic V06.10 ☑
          bus or heavy transport V04.90 ☑
                nontraffic V04.00 ☑
                traffic V04.10 ☑

Accident — *continued*
  transport — *continued*
    pedestrian — *continued*
      on foot (*see also* Accident, pedestrian) — *continued*
        collision — *continued*
          car V03.90 ☑
                nontraffic V03.00 ☑
                traffic V03.10 ☑
          pedal cycle V01.90 ☑
                nontraffic V01.00 ☑
                traffic V01.10 ☑
          pick-up truck or van V03.90 ☑
                nontraffic V03.00 ☑
                traffic V03.10 ☑
          railway (train) (vehicle) V05.90 ☑
                nontraffic V05.00 ☑
                traffic V05.10 ☑
          streetcar V06.90 ☑
                nontraffic V06.00 ☑
                traffic V06.10 ☑
          two- or three-wheeled motor vehicle
                V02.90 ☑
                nontraffic V02.00 ☑
                traffic V02.10 ☑
          vehicle V09.9 ☑
                animal-drawn V06.90 ☑
                  nontraffic V06.00 ☑
                  traffic V06.10 ☑
                motor
          nontraffic V09.1 ☑
                involving motor vehicle V09.00 ☑
                military V09.01 ☑
                specified type NEC V09.09 ☑
          traffic V09.3 ☑
                involving motor vehicle V09.20 ☑
                military V09.21 ☑
                specified type NEC V09.29 ☑
    person NEC (unknown way or transportation)
        V99 ☑
      collision (between)
        bus (with)
          heavy transport vehicle (traffic) V87.5 ☑
                nontraffic V88.5 ☑
        car (with)
          bus (traffic) V87.3 ☑
                nontraffic V88.3 ☑
          heavy transport vehicle (traffic) V87.4 ☑
                nontraffic V88.4 ☑
                nontraffic V88.5 ☑
          pick-up truck or van (traffic) V87.2 ☑
                nontraffic V88.2 ☑
          train or railway vehicle (traffic) V87.6 ☑
                nontraffic V88.6 ☑
          two- or three-wheeled motor vehicle
                (traffic) V87.0 ☑
                nontraffic V88.0 ☑
          motor vehicle (traffic) NEC V87.7 ☑
                nontraffic V88.7 ☑
          two- or three-wheeled vehicle (with) (traffic)
                motor vehicle NEC V87.1 ☑
                nontraffic V88.1 ☑
        nonmotor vehicle (collision) (noncollision)
                (traffic) V87.9 ☑
          nontraffic V88.9 ☑
    pickup truck occupant V59.9 ☑
      collision (with)
        animal (traffic) V50.9 ☑
          being ridden (traffic) V56.9 ☑
                nontraffic V56.3 ☑
                while boarding or alighting V56.4 ☑
          nontraffic V50.3 ☑
          while boarding or alighting V50.4 ☑
        animal-drawn vehicle (traffic) V56.9 ☑
                nontraffic V56.3 ☑
                while boarding or alighting V56.4 ☑
        bus (traffic) V54.9 ☑
                nontraffic V54.3 ☑
                while boarding or alighting V54.4 ☑
        car (traffic) V53.9 ☑
                nontraffic V53.3 ☑
                while boarding or alighting V53.4 ☑
        motor vehicle NOS (traffic) V59.60 ☑
                nontraffic V59.20 ☑
                specified type NEC (traffic) V59.69 ☑
                  nontraffic V59.29 ☑

Accident — *continued*
  transport — *continued*
    pickup truck occupant — *continued*
      collision — *continued*
        pedal cycle (traffic) V51.9 ☑
          nontraffic V51.3
          while boarding or alighting V51.4 ☑
        pickup truck (traffic) V53.9 ☑
          nontraffic V53.3
          while boarding or alighting V53.4 ☑
        railway vehicle (traffic) V55.9 ☑
          nontraffic V55.3
          while boarding or alighting V55.4 ☑
        specified vehicle NEC (traffic) V56.9 ☑
          nontraffic V56.3
          while boarding or alighting V56.4 ☑
        stationary object (traffic) V57.9 ☑
          nontraffic V57.3
          while boarding or alighting V57.4 ☑
        streetcar (traffic) V56.9 ☑
          nontraffic V56.3
          while boarding or alighting V56.4 ☑
        three wheeled motor vehicle (traffic) V52.9 ☑
          nontraffic V52.3 ☑
          while boarding or alighting V52.4 ☑
        truck (traffic) V54.9 ☑
          nontraffic V54.3
          while boarding or alighting V54.4 ☑
        two wheeled motor vehicle (traffic) V52.9 ☑
          nontraffic V52.3
          while boarding or alighting V52.4 ☑
        van (traffic) V53.9 ☑
          nontraffic V53.3
          while boarding or alighting V53.4 ☑
     driver
      collision (with)
        animal (traffic) V50.5 ☑
          being ridden (traffic) V56.5 ☑
            nontraffic V56.0 ☑
          nontraffic V50.0 ☑
        animal-drawn vehicle (traffic) V56.5 ☑
          nontraffic V56.0 ☑
        bus (traffic) V54.5 ☑
          nontraffic V54.0 ☑
        car (traffic) V53.5 ☑
          nontraffic V53.0 ☑
        motor vehicle NOS (traffic) V59.40 ☑
          nontraffic V59.00 ☑
          specified type NEC (traffic) V59.49 ☑
            nontraffic V59.09 ☑
        pedal cycle (traffic) V51.5 ☑
          nontraffic V51.0 ☑
        pickup truck (traffic) V53.5 ☑
          nontraffic V53.0 ☑
        railway vehicle (traffic) V55.5 ☑
          nontraffic V55.0 ☑
        specified vehicle NEC (traffic) V56.5 ☑
          nontraffic V56.0 ☑
        stationary object (traffic) V57.5 ☑
          nontraffic V57.0 ☑
        streetcar (traffic) V56.5 ☑
          nontraffic V56.0 ☑
        three wheeled motor vehicle (traffic) V52.5 ☑
          nontraffic V52.0 ☑
        truck (traffic) V54.5 ☑
          nontraffic V54.0 ☑
        two wheeled motor vehicle (traffic) V52.5 ☑
          nontraffic V52.0 ☑
        van (traffic) V53.5 ☑
          nontraffic V53.0 ☑
      noncollision accident (traffic) V58.5 ☑
        nontraffic V58.0 ☑
     hanger-on
      collision (with)
        animal (traffic) V50.7 ☑
          being ridden (traffic) V56.7 ☑
            nontraffic V56.2 ☑
          nontraffic V50.2 ☑
        animal-drawn vehicle (traffic) V56.7 ☑
          nontraffic V56.2 ☑
        bus (traffic) V54.7 ☑
          nontraffic V54.2 ☑
        car (traffic) V53.7 ☑

Accident — *continued*
  transport — *continued*
    pickup truck occupant — *continued*
      hanger-on — *continued*
        collision — *continued*
          car — *continued*
            nontraffic V53.2 ☑
          pedal cycle (traffic) V51.7 ☑
            nontraffic V51.2 ☑
          pickup truck (traffic) V53.7 ☑
            nontraffic V53.2 ☑
          railway vehicle (traffic) V55.7 ☑
            nontraffic V55.2 ☑
          specified vehicle NEC (traffic) V56.7 ☑
            nontraffic V56.2 ☑
          stationary object (traffic) V57.7 ☑
            nontraffic V57.2 ☑
          streetcar (traffic) V56.7 ☑
            nontraffic V56.2 ☑
          three wheeled motor vehicle (traffic) V52.7 ☑
            nontraffic V52.2 ☑
          truck (traffic) V54.7 ☑
            nontraffic V54.2 ☑
          two wheeled motor vehicle (traffic) V52.7 ☑
            nontraffic V52.2 ☑
          van (traffic) V53.7 ☑
            nontraffic V53.2 ☑
        noncollision accident (traffic) V58.7 ☑
          nontraffic V58.2 ☑
      noncollision accident (traffic) V58.9 ☑
        nontraffic V58.3 ☑
        while boarding or alighting V58.4 ☑
      nontraffic V59.3 ☑
      passenger
        collision (with)
          animal (traffic) V50.6 ☑
            being ridden (traffic) V56.6 ☑
              nontraffic V56.1 ☑
            nontraffic V50.1 ☑
          animal-drawn vehicle (traffic) V56.6 ☑
            nontraffic V56.1 ☑
          bus (traffic) V54.6 ☑
            nontraffic V54.1 ☑
          car (traffic) V53.6 ☑
            nontraffic V53.1 ☑
          motor vehicle NOS (traffic) V59.50 ☑
            nontraffic V59.10 ☑
            specified type NEC (traffic) V59.59 ☑
              nontraffic V59.19 ☑
          pedal cycle (traffic) V51.6 ☑
            nontraffic V51.1 ☑
          pickup truck (traffic) V53.6 ☑
            nontraffic V53.1 ☑
          railway vehicle (traffic) V55.6 ☑
            nontraffic V55.1 ☑
          specified vehicle NEC (traffic) V56.6 ☑
            nontraffic V56.1 ☑
          stationary object (traffic) V57.6 ☑
            nontraffic V57.1 ☑
          streetcar (traffic) V56.6 ☑
            nontraffic V56.1 ☑
          three wheeled motor vehicle (traffic) V52.6 ☑
            nontraffic V52.1 ☑
          truck (traffic) V54.6 ☑
            nontraffic V54.1 ☑
          two wheeled motor vehicle (traffic) V52.6 ☑
            nontraffic V52.1 ☑
          van (traffic) V53.6 ☑
            nontraffic V53.1 ☑
      noncollision accident (traffic) V58.6 ☑
        nontraffic V58.1 ☑
      specified type NEC V59.88 ☑
        military vehicle V59.81 ☑
    quarry truck — *see* Accident, transport, industrial vehicle occupant
    race car — *see* Accident, transport, motor vehicle NEC occupant
    railway vehicle occupant V81.9 ☑
      collision (with) V81.3 ☑
        motor vehicle (non-military) (traffic) V81.1 ☑
          military V81.83 ☑

Accident — *continued*
  transport — *continued*
    railway vehicle occupant — *continued*
      collision — *continued*
        motor vehicle — *continued*
          nontraffic V81.0 ☑
        rolling stock V81.2 ☑
        specified object NEC V81.3 ☑
      during derailment V81.7 ☑
        with antecedent collision B — *see* Accident, transport, railway vehicle occupant, collision
      explosion V81.81 ☑
      fall (in railway vehicle) V81.5 ☑
        during derailment V81.7 ☑
          with antecedent collision B — *see* Accident, transport, railway vehicle occupant, collision
        from railway vehicle V81.6 ☑
          during derailment V81.7 ☑
            with antecedent collision B — *see* Accident, transport, railway vehicle occupant, collision
        while boarding or alighting V81.4 ☑
      fire V81.81 ☑
      object falling onto train V81.82 ☑
      specified type NEC V81.89 ☑
      while boarding or alighting V81.4 ☑
    ski lift V98.3 ☑
    snowmobile occupant (nontraffic) V86.92 ☑
      driver V86.52 ☑
      hanger-on V86.72 ☑
      passenger V86.62 ☑
      traffic V86.32 ☑
        driver V86.02 ☑
        hanger-on V86.22 ☑
        passenger V86.12 ☑
      while boarding or alighting V86.42 ☑
    specified NEC V98.8 ☑
    sport utility vehicle occupant (*see also* Accident, transport, car occupant)
      collision (with)
        stationary object (traffic) V47.91 ☑
          nontraffic V47.31 ☑
      driver
        collision (with)
          stationary object (traffic) V47.51 ☑
            nontraffic V47.01 ☑
      passenger
        collision (with)
          stationary object (traffic) V47.61 ☑
            nontraffic V47.11 ☑
    streetcar occupant V82.9 ☑
      collision (with) V82.3 ☑
        motor vehicle (traffic) V82.1 ☑
          nontraffic V82.0 ☑
        rolling stock V82.2 ☑
      during derailment V82.7 ☑
        with antecedent collision B — *see* Accident, transport, streetcar occupant, collision
      fall (in streetcar) V82.5 ☑
        during derailment V82.7 ☑
          with antecedent collision B — *see* Accident, transport, streetcar occupant, collision
        from streetcar V82.6 ☑
          during derailment V82.7 ☑
            with antecedent collision B — *see* Accident, transport, streetcar occupant, collision
        while boarding or alighting V82.4 ☑
      while boarding or alighting V82.4 ☑
    specified type NEC V82.8 ☑
    while boarding or alighting V82.4 ☑
    three-wheeled motor vehicle occupant V39.9 ☑
      collision (with)
        animal (traffic) V30.9 ☑
          being ridden (traffic) V36.9 ☑
            nontraffic V36.3 ☑
            while boarding or alighting V36.4 ☑
          nontraffic V30.3 ☑
          while boarding or alighting V30.4 ☑
        animal-drawn vehicle (traffic) V36.9 ☑
          nontraffic V36.3 ☑
          while boarding or alighting V36.4 ☑
        bus (traffic) V34.9 ☑

Accident — *continued*
 transport — *continued*
  three-wheeled motor vehicle occupant — *continued*
   collision — *continued*
    bus — *continued*
     nontraffic V34.3 ☑
     while boarding or alighting V34.4 ☑
    car (traffic) V33.9 ☑
     nontraffic V33.3 ☑
     while boarding or alighting V33.4 ☑
    motor vehicle NOS (traffic) V39.60 ☑
     nontraffic V39.20 ☑
     specified type NEC (traffic) V39.69 ☑
      nontraffic V39.29 ☑
    pedal cycle (traffic) V31.9 ☑
     nontraffic V31.3 ☑
     while boarding or alighting V31.4 ☑
    pickup truck (traffic) V33.9 ☑
     nontraffic V33.3 ☑
     while boarding or alighting V33.4 ☑
    railway vehicle (traffic) V35.9 ☑
     nontraffic V35.3 ☑
     while boarding or alighting V35.4 ☑
    specified vehicle NEC (traffic) V36.9 ☑
     nontraffic V36.3 ☑
     while boarding or alighting V36.4 ☑
    stationary object (traffic) V37.9 ☑
     nontraffic V37.3 ☑
     while boarding or alighting V37.4 ☑
    streetcar (traffic) V36.9 ☑
     nontraffic V36.3 ☑
     while boarding or alighting V36.4 ☑
    three wheeled motor vehicle (traffic) V32.9 ☑
     nontraffic V32.3 ☑
     while boarding or alighting V32.4 ☑
    truck (traffic) V34.9 ☑
     nontraffic V34.3 ☑
     while boarding or alighting V34.4 ☑
    two wheeled motor vehicle (traffic) V32.9 ☑
     nontraffic V32.3 ☑
     while boarding or alighting V32.4 ☑
    van (traffic) V33.9 ☑
     nontraffic V33.3 ☑
     while boarding or alighting V33.4 ☑
   driver
    collision (with)
     animal (traffic) V30.5 ☑
      being ridden (traffic) V36.5 ☑
       nontraffic V36.0 ☑
      nontraffic V30.0 ☑
     animal-drawn vehicle (traffic) V36.5 ☑
      nontraffic V36.0 ☑
     bus (traffic) V34.5 ☑
      nontraffic V34.0 ☑
     car (traffic) V33.5 ☑
      nontraffic V33.0 ☑
     motor vehicle NOS (traffic) V39.40 ☑
      nontraffic V39.00 ☑
      specified type NEC (traffic) V39.49 ☑
       nontraffic V39.09 ☑
     pedal cycle (traffic) V31.5 ☑
      nontraffic V31.0 ☑
     pickup truck (traffic) V33.5 ☑
      nontraffic V33.0 ☑
     railway vehicle (traffic) V35.5 ☑
      nontraffic V35.0 ☑
     specified vehicle NEC (traffic) V36.5 ☑
      nontraffic V36.0 ☑
     stationary object (traffic) V37.5 ☑
      nontraffic V37.0 ☑
     streetcar (traffic) V36.5 ☑
      nontraffic V36.0 ☑
     three wheeled motor vehicle (traffic) V32.5 ☑
      nontraffic V32.0 ☑
     truck (traffic) V34.5 ☑
      nontraffic V34.0 ☑
     two wheeled motor vehicle (traffic) V32.5 ☑
      nontraffic V32.0 ☑
     van (traffic) V33.5 ☑
      nontraffic V33.0 ☑
    noncollision accident (traffic) V38.5 ☑
     nontraffic V38.0 ☑

Accident — *continued*
 transport — *continued*
  three-wheeled motor vehicle occupant — *continued*
   hanger-on
    collision (with)
     animal (traffic) V30.7 ☑
      being ridden (traffic) V36.7 ☑
       nontraffic V36.2 ☑
      nontraffic V30.2 ☑
     animal-drawn vehicle (traffic) V36.7 ☑
      nontraffic V36.2 ☑
     bus (traffic) V34.7 ☑
      nontraffic V34.2 ☑
     car (traffic) V33.7 ☑
      nontraffic V33.2 ☑
     pedal cycle (traffic) V31.7 ☑
      nontraffic V31.2 ☑
     pickup truck (traffic) V33.7 ☑
      nontraffic V33.2 ☑
     railway vehicle (traffic) V35.7 ☑
      nontraffic V35.2 ☑
     specified vehicle NEC (traffic) V36.7 ☑
      nontraffic V36.2 ☑
     stationary object (traffic) V37.7 ☑
      nontraffic V37.2 ☑
     streetcar (traffic) V36.7 ☑
      nontraffic V36.2 ☑
     three wheeled motor vehicle (traffic) V32.7 ☑
      nontraffic V32.2 ☑
     truck (traffic) V34.7 ☑
      nontraffic V34.2 ☑
     two wheeled motor vehicle (traffic) V32.7 ☑
      nontraffic V32.2 ☑
     van (traffic) V33.7 ☑
      nontraffic V33.2 ☑
    noncollision accident (traffic) V38.7 ☑
     nontraffic V38.2 ☑
   noncollision accident (traffic) V38.9 ☑
    nontraffic V38.3 ☑
    while boarding or alighting V38.4 ☑
   nontraffic V39.3 ☑
   passenger
    collision (with)
     animal (traffic) V30.6 ☑
      being ridden (traffic) V36.6 ☑
       nontraffic V36.1 ☑
      nontraffic V30.1 ☑
     animal-drawn vehicle (traffic) V36.6 ☑
      nontraffic V36.1 ☑
     bus (traffic) V34.6 ☑
      nontraffic V34.1 ☑
     car (traffic) V33.6 ☑
      nontraffic V33.1 ☑
     motor vehicle NOS (traffic) V39.50 ☑
      nontraffic V39.10 ☑
      specified type NEC (traffic) V39.59 ☑
       nontraffic V39.19 ☑
     pedal cycle (traffic) V31.6 ☑
      nontraffic V31.1 ☑
     pickup truck (traffic) V33.6 ☑
      nontraffic V33.1 ☑
     railway vehicle (traffic) V35.6 ☑
      nontraffic V35.1 ☑
     specified vehicle NEC (traffic) V36.6 ☑
      nontraffic V36.1 ☑
     stationary object (traffic) V37.6 ☑
      nontraffic V37.1 ☑
     streetcar (traffic) V36.6 ☑
      nontraffic V36.1 ☑
     three wheeled motor vehicle (traffic) V32.6 ☑
      nontraffic V32.1 ☑
     truck (traffic) V34.6 ☑
      nontraffic V34.1 ☑
     two wheeled motor vehicle (traffic) V32.6 ☑
      nontraffic V32.1 ☑
     van (traffic) V33.6 ☑
      nontraffic V33.1 ☑
    noncollision accident (traffic) V38.6 ☑
     nontraffic V38.1 ☑
   specified type NEC V39.89 ☑
    military vehicle V39.81 ☑

Accident — *continued*
 transport — *continued*
  tractor (farm) (and trailer) — *see* Accident, transport, agricultural vehicle occupant
  tram — *see* Accident, transport, streetcar
   in mine or quarry — *see* Accident, transport, industrial vehicle occupant
  trolley — *see* Accident, transport, streetcar
   in mine or quarry — *see* Accident, transport, industrial vehicle occupant
  truck (heavy) occupant V69.9 ☑
   collision (with)
    animal (traffic) V60.9 ☑
     being ridden (traffic) V66.9 ☑
      nontraffic V66.3 ☑
      while boarding or alighting V66.4 ☑
     nontraffic V60.3 ☑
     while boarding or alighting V60.4 ☑
    animal-drawn vehicle (traffic) V66.9 ☑
     nontraffic V66.3 ☑
     while boarding or alighting V66.4 ☑
    bus (traffic) V64.9 ☑
     nontraffic V64.3 ☑
     while boarding or alighting V64.4 ☑
    car (traffic) V63.9 ☑
     nontraffic V63.3 ☑
     while boarding or alighting V63.4 ☑
    motor vehicle NOS (traffic) V69.60 ☑
     nontraffic V69.20 ☑
     specified type NEC (traffic) V69.69 ☑
      nontraffic V69.29 ☑
    pedal cycle (traffic) V61.9 ☑
     nontraffic V61.3 ☑
     while boarding or alighting V61.4 ☑
    pickup truck (traffic) V63.9 ☑
     nontraffic V63.3 ☑
     while boarding or alighting V63.4 ☑
    railway vehicle (traffic) V65.9 ☑
     nontraffic V65.3 ☑
     while boarding or alighting V65.4 ☑
    specified vehicle NEC (traffic) V66.9 ☑
     nontraffic V66.3 ☑
     while boarding or alighting V66.4 ☑
    stationary object (traffic) V67.9 ☑
     nontraffic V67.3 ☑
     while boarding or alighting V67.4 ☑
    streetcar (traffic) V66.9 ☑
     nontraffic V66.3 ☑
     while boarding or alighting V66.4 ☑
    three wheeled motor vehicle (traffic) V62.9 ☑
     nontraffic V62.3 ☑
     while boarding or alighting V62.4 ☑
    truck (traffic) V64.9 ☑
     nontraffic V64.3 ☑
     while boarding or alighting V64.4 ☑
    two wheeled motor vehicle (traffic) V62.9 ☑
     nontraffic V62.3 ☑
     while boarding or alighting V62.4 ☑
    van (traffic) V63.9 ☑
     nontraffic V63.3 ☑
     while boarding or alighting V63.4 ☑
   driver
    collision (with)
     animal (traffic) V60.5 ☑
      being ridden (traffic) V66.5 ☑
       nontraffic V66.0 ☑
      nontraffic V60.0 ☑
     animal-drawn vehicle (traffic) V66.5 ☑
      nontraffic V66.0 ☑
     bus (traffic) V64.5 ☑
      nontraffic V64.0 ☑
     car (traffic) V63.5 ☑
      nontraffic V63.0 ☑
     motor vehicle NOS (traffic) V69.40 ☑
      nontraffic V69.00 ☑
      specified type NEC (traffic) V69.49 ☑
       nontraffic V69.09 ☑
     pedal cycle (traffic) V61.5 ☑
      nontraffic V61.0 ☑
     pickup truck (traffic) V63.5 ☑
      nontraffic V63.0 ☑
     railway vehicle (traffic) V65.5 ☑
      nontraffic V65.0 ☑
     specified vehicle NEC (traffic) V66.5 ☑
      nontraffic V66.0 ☑

Accident — *continued*
  transport — *continued*
    truck occupant — *continued*
      driver — *continued*
        collision — *continued*
          stationary object (traffic) V67.5 ☑
            nontraffic V67.0 ☑
          streetcar (traffic) V66.5 ☑
            nontraffic V66.0 ☑
          three wheeled motor vehicle (traffic)
            V62.5 ☑
            nontraffic V62.0 ☑
          truck (traffic) V64.5 ☑
            nontraffic V64.0 ☑
          two wheeled motor vehicle (traffic)
            V62.5 ☑
            nontraffic V62.0 ☑
          van (traffic) V63.5 ☑
            nontraffic V63.0 ☑
        noncollision accident (traffic) V68.5 ☑
          nontraffic V68.0 ☑
      dump — *see* Accident, transport, construction
        vehicle occupant
      hanger-on
        collision (with)
          animal (traffic) V60.7 ☑
            being ridden (traffic) V66.7 ☑
              nontraffic V66.2 ☑
            nontraffic V60.2 ☑
          animal-drawn vehicle (traffic) V66.7 ☑
            nontraffic V66.2 ☑
          bus (traffic) V64.7 ☑
            nontraffic V64.2 ☑
          car (traffic) V63.7 ☑
            nontraffic V63.2 ☑
          pedal cycle (traffic) V61.7 ☑
            nontraffic V61.2 ☑
          pickup truck (traffic) V63.7 ☑
            nontraffic V63.2 ☑
          railway vehicle (traffic) V65.7 ☑
            nontraffic V65.2 ☑
          specified vehicle NEC (traffic) V66.7 ☑
            nontraffic V66.2 ☑
          stationary object (traffic) V67.7 ☑
            nontraffic V67.2 ☑
          streetcar (traffic) V66.7 ☑
            nontraffic V66.2 ☑
          three wheeled motor vehicle (traffic)
            V62.7 ☑
            nontraffic V62.2 ☑
          truck (traffic) V64.7 ☑
            nontraffic V64.2 ☑
          two wheeled motor vehicle (traffic)
            V62.7 ☑
            nontraffic V62.2 ☑
          van (traffic) V63.7 ☑
            nontraffic V63.2 ☑
        noncollision accident (traffic) V68.7 ☑
          nontraffic V68.2 ☑
      noncollision accident (traffic) V68.9 ☑
        nontraffic V68.3 ☑
        while boarding or alighting V68.4 ☑
      nontraffic V69.3 ☑
      passenger
        collision (with)
          animal (traffic) V60.6 ☑
            being ridden (traffic) V66.6 ☑
              nontraffic V66.1-
            nontraffic V60.1
          animal-drawn vehicle (traffic) V66.6 ☑
            nontraffic V66.1 ☑
          bus (traffic) V64.6 ☑
            nontraffic V64.1 ☑
          car (traffic) V63.6 ☑
            nontraffic V63.1 ☑
          motor vehicle NOS (traffic) V69.50 ☑
            nontraffic V69.10 ☑
            specified type NEC (traffic) V69.59 ☑
              nontraffic V69.19 ☑
          pedal cycle (traffic) V61.6 ☑
            nontraffic V61.1 ☑
          pickup truck (traffic) V63.6 ☑
            nontraffic V63.1 ☑
          railway vehicle (traffic) V65.6 ☑
            nontraffic V65.1 ☑
          specified vehicle NEC (traffic) V66.6 ☑

Accident — *continued*
  transport — *continued*
    truck occupant — *continued*
      passenger — *continued*
        collision — *continued*
          specified vehicle — *continued*
            nontraffic V66.1 ☑
          stationary object (traffic) V67.6 ☑
            nontraffic V67.1 ☑
          streetcar (traffic) V66.6 ☑
            nontraffic V66.1 ☑
          three wheeled motor vehicle (traffic)
            V62.6 ☑
            nontraffic V62.1 ☑
          truck (traffic) V64.6 ☑
            nontraffic V64.1 ☑
          two wheeled motor vehicle (traffic)
            V62.6 ☑
            nontraffic V62.1 ☑
          van (traffic) V63.6 ☑
            nontraffic V63.1 ☑
        noncollision accident (traffic) V68.6 ☑
          nontraffic V68.1 ☑
      pickup — *see* Accident, transport, pickup truck
        occupant
      specified type NEC V69.88 ☑
        military vehicle V69.81 ☑
    van occupant V59.9 ☑
      collision (with)
        animal (traffic) V50.9 ☑
          being ridden (traffic) V56.9 ☑
            nontraffic V56.3 ☑
            while boarding or alighting V56.4 ☑
          nontraffic V50.3 ☑
          while boarding or alighting V50.4 ☑
        animal-drawn vehicle (traffic) V56.9 ☑
          nontraffic V56.3 ☑
          while boarding or alighting V56.4 ☑
        bus (traffic) V54.9 ☑
          nontraffic V54.3 ☑
          while boarding or alighting V54.4 ☑
        car (traffic) V53.9 ☑
          nontraffic V53.3 ☑
          while boarding or alighting V53.4 ☑
        motor vehicle NOS (traffic) V59.60 ☑
          nontraffic V59.20 ☑
          specified type NEC (traffic) V59.69 ☑
           nontraffic V59.29 ☑
        pedal cycle (traffic) V51.9 ☑
          nontraffic V51.3 ☑
          while boarding or alighting V51.4 ☑
        pickup truck (traffic) V53.9 ☑
          nontraffic V53.3 ☑
          while boarding or alighting V53.4 ☑
        railway vehicle (traffic) V55.9 ☑
          nontraffic V55.3 ☑
          while boarding or alighting V55.4 ☑
        specified vehicle NEC (traffic) V56.9 ☑
          nontraffic V56.3 ☑
          while boarding or alighting V56.4 ☑
        stationary object (traffic) V57.9 ☑
          nontraffic V57.3 ☑
          while boarding or alighting V57.4 ☑
        streetcar (traffic) V56.9 ☑
          nontraffic V56.3 ☑
          while boarding or alighting V56.4 ☑
        three wheeled motor vehicle (traffic)
          V52.9 ☑
          nontraffic V52.3 ☑
          while boarding or alighting V52.4 ☑
        truck (traffic) V54.9 ☑
          nontraffic V54.3 ☑
          while boarding or alighting V54.4 ☑
        two wheeled motor vehicle (traffic) V52.9 ☑
          nontraffic V52.3 ☑
          while boarding or alighting V52.4 ☑
        van (traffic) V53.9 ☑
          nontraffic V53.3 ☑
          while boarding or alighting V53.4 ☑
      driver
        collision (with)
          animal (traffic) V50.5 ☑
            being ridden (traffic) V56.5 ☑
              nontraffic V56.0 ☑
            nontraffic V50.0 ☑
          animal-drawn vehicle (traffic) V56.5 ☑

Accident — *continued*
  transport — *continued*
    van occupant — *continued*
      driver — *continued*
        collision — *continued*
          animal-drawn vehicle — *continued*
            nontraffic V56.0 ☑
          bus (traffic) V54.5 ☑
            nontraffic V54.0 ☑
          car (traffic) V53.5 ☑
            nontraffic V53.0 ☑
          motor vehicle NOS (traffic) V59.40 ☑
            nontraffic V59.00 ☑
            specified type NEC (traffic) V59.49 ☑
              nontraffic V59.09 ☑
          pedal cycle (traffic) V51.5 ☑
            nontraffic V51.0 ☑
          pickup truck (traffic) V53.5 ☑
            nontraffic V53.0 ☑
          railway vehicle (traffic) V55.5 ☑
            nontraffic V55.0 ☑
          specified vehicle NEC (traffic) V56.5 ☑
            nontraffic V56.0 ☑
          stationary object (traffic) V57.5 ☑
            nontraffic V57.0 ☑
          streetcar (traffic) V56.5 ☑
            nontraffic V56.0 ☑
          three wheeled motor vehicle (traffic)
            V52.5 ☑
            nontraffic V52.0 ☑
          truck (traffic) V54.5 ☑
            nontraffic V54.0 ☑
          two wheeled motor vehicle (traffic)
            V52.5 ☑
            nontraffic V52.0 ☑
          van (traffic) V53.5 ☑
            nontraffic V53.0 ☑
        noncollision accident (traffic) V58.5 ☑
          nontraffic V58.0 ☑
      hanger-on
        collision (with)
          animal (traffic) V50.7 ☑
            being ridden (traffic) V56.7 ☑
              nontraffic V56.2 ☑
            nontraffic V50.2 ☑
          animal-drawn vehicle (traffic) V56.7 ☑
            nontraffic V56.2 ☑
          bus (traffic) V54.7 ☑
            nontraffic V54.2 ☑
          car (traffic) V53.7 ☑
            nontraffic V53.2 ☑
          pedal cycle (traffic) V51.7 ☑
            nontraffic V51.2 ☑
          pickup truck (traffic) V53.7 ☑
            nontraffic V53.2 ☑
          railway vehicle (traffic) V55.7 ☑
            nontraffic V55.2 ☑
          specified vehicle NEC (traffic) V56.7 ☑
            nontraffic V56.2 ☑
          stationary object (traffic) V57.7 ☑
            nontraffic V57.2 ☑
          streetcar (traffic) V56.7 ☑
            nontraffic V56.2 ☑
          three wheeled motor vehicle (traffic)
            V52.7 ☑
            nontraffic V52.2 ☑
          truck (traffic) V54.7 ☑
            nontraffic V54.2 ☑
          two wheeled motor vehicle (traffic)
            V52.7 ☑
            nontraffic V52.2 ☑
          van (traffic) V53.7 ☑
            nontraffic V53.2 ☑
        noncollision accident (traffic) V58.7 ☑
          nontraffic V58.2 ☑
      noncollision accident (traffic) V58.9 ☑
        nontraffic V58.3 ☑
        while boarding or alighting V58.4 ☑
      nontraffic V59.3 ☑
      passenger
        collision (with)
          animal (traffic) V50.6 ☑
            being ridden (traffic) V56.6 ☑
              nontraffic V56.1 ☑
            nontraffic V50.1 ☑
          animal-drawn vehicle (traffic) V56.6 ☑

Accident — *continued*
  transport — *continued*
    van occupant — *continued*
      passenger — *continued*
        collision — *continued*
          animal-drawn vehicle — *continued*
            nontraffic V56.1 ☑
          bus (traffic) V54.6 ☑
            nontraffic V54.1 ☑
          car (traffic) V53.6 ☑
            nontraffic V53.1 ☑
          motor vehicle NOS (traffic) V59.50 ☑
            nontraffic V59.10 ☑
            specified type NEC (traffic) V59.59 ☑
              nontraffic V59.19 ☑
          pedal cycle (traffic) V51.6 ☑
            nontraffic V51.1 ☑
          pickup truck (traffic) V53.6 ☑
            nontraffic V53.1 ☑
          railway vehicle (traffic) V55.6 ☑
            nontraffic V55.1 ☑
          specified vehicle NEC (traffic) V56.6 ☑
            nontraffic V56.1 ☑
          stationary object (traffic) V57.6 ☑
            nontraffic V57.1 ☑
          streetcar (traffic) V56.6 ☑
            nontraffic V56.1 ☑
          three wheeled motor vehicle (traffic) V52.6 ☑
            nontraffic V52.1 ☑
          truck (traffic) V54.6 ☑
            nontraffic V54.1 ☑
          two wheeled motor vehicle (traffic) V52.6 ☑
            nontraffic V52.1 ☑
          van (traffic) V53.6 ☑
            nontraffic V53.1 ☑
          noncollision accident (traffic) V58.6 ☑
            nontraffic V58.1 ☑
        specified type NEC V59.88 ☑
          military vehicle V59.81 ☑
    watercraft occupant — *see* Accident, watercraft
    vehicle NEC V89.9 ☑
      animal-drawn NEC — *see* Accident, transport, animal-drawn vehicle occupant
      special
        agricultural — *see* Accident, transport, agricultural vehicle occupant
        construction — *see* Accident, transport, construction vehicle occupant
        industrial — *see* Accident, transport, industrial vehicle occupant
        three-wheeled NEC (motorized) — *see* Accident, transport, three-wheeled motor vehicle occupant
  watercraft V94.9 ☑
    causing
      drowning B — *see* Drowning, due to, accident to, watercraft
      injury NEC V91.89 ☑
        crushed between craft and object V91.19 ☑
          powered craft V91.13 ☑
            ferry boat V91.11 ☑
            fishing boat V91.12 ☑
            jetskis V91.13 ☑
            liner V91.11 ☑
            merchant ship V91.10 ☑
            passenger ship V91.11 ☑
          unpowered craft V91.18 ☑
            canoe V91.15 ☑
            inflatable V91.16 ☑
            kayak V91.15 ☑
            sailboat V91.14 ☑
            surf-board V91.18 ☑
            windsurfer V91.18 ☑
        fall on board V91.29 ☑
          powered craft V91.23 ☑
            ferry boat V91.21 ☑
            fishing boat V91.22 ☑
            jetskis V91.23 ☑
            liner V91.21 ☑
            merchant ship V91.20 ☑
            passenger ship V91.21 ☑
          unpowered craft
            canoe V91.25 ☑
            inflatable V91.26 ☑

Accident — *continued*
  watercraft — *continued*
    causing — *continued*
      injury — *continued*
        fall on board — *continued*
          unpowered craft — *continued*
            kayak V91.25 ☑
            sailboat V91.24 ☑
        fire on board causing burn V91.09 ☑
          powered craft V91.03 ☑
            ferry boat V91.01 ☑
            fishing boat V91.02 ☑
            jetskis V91.03 ☑
            liner V91.01 ☑
            merchant ship V91.00 ☑
            passenger ship V91.01 ☑
          unpowered craft V91.08 ☑
            canoe V91.05 ☑
            inflatable V91.06 ☑
            kayak V91.05 ☑
            sailboat V91.04 ☑
            surf-board V91.08 ☑
            water skis V91.07 ☑
            windsurfer V91.08 ☑
        hit by falling object V91.39 ☑
          powered craft V91.33 ☑
            ferry boat V91.31 ☑
            fishing boat V91.32 ☑
            jetskis V91.33 ☑
            liner V91.31 ☑
            merchant ship V91.30 ☑
            passenger ship V91.31 ☑
          unpowered craft V91.38 ☑
            canoe V91.35 ☑
            inflatable V91.36 ☑
            kayak V91.35 ☑
            sailboat V91.34 ☑
            surf-board V91.38 ☑
            water skis V91.37 ☑
            windsurfer V91.38 ☑
        specified type NEC V91.89 ☑
          powered craft V91.83 ☑
            ferry boat V91.81 ☑
            fishing boat V91.82 ☑
            jetskis V91.83 ☑
            liner V91.81 ☑
            merchant ship V91.80 ☑
            passenger ship V91.81 ☑
          unpowered craft V91.88 ☑
            canoe V91.85 ☑
            inflatable V91.86 ☑
            kayak V91.85 ☑
            sailboat V91.84 ☑
            surf-board V91.88 ☑
            water skis V91.87 ☑
            windsurfer V91.88 ☑
      due to, caused by cataclysm — *see* Forces of nature, by type
      military NEC V94.818 ☑
        with civilian watercraft V94.810 ☑
        civilian in water injured by V94.811 ☑
      nonpowered, struck by
        nonpowered vessel V94.22 ☑
        powered vessel V94.21 ☑
      specified type NEC V94.89 ☑
      striking swimmer
        powered V94.11 ☑
        unpowered V94.12 ☑
Acid throwing (assault) Y08.89 ☑
Activity (involving) (of victim at time of event) Y93.9
  aerobic and step exercise (class) Y93.A3 (*following* Y93.7)
  alpine skiing Y93.23
  animal care NEC Y93.K9 (*following* Y93.7)
  arts and handcrafts NEC Y93.D9 (*following* Y93.7)
  athletics played as a team or group NEC Y93.69
  athletics played individually NEC Y93.59
  athletics NEC Y93.79
  baking Y93.G3 (*following* Y93.7)
  ballet Y93.41
  barbells Y93.B3 (*following* Y93.7)
  BASE (Building, Antenna, Span, Earth) jumping Y93.33
  baseball Y93.64
  basketball Y93.67
  bathing (personal) Y93.E1 (*following* Y93.7)
  beach volleyball Y93.68

Activity — *continued*
  bike riding Y93.55
  boogie boarding Y93.18
  bowling Y93.54
  boxing Y93.71
  brass instrument playing Y93.J4 (*following* Y93.7)
  building construction Y93.H3 (*following* Y93.7)
  bungee jumping Y93.34
  calisthenics Y93.A2 (*following* Y93.7)
  canoeing (in calm and turbulent water) Y93.16
  capture the flag Y93.6A
  cardiorespiratory exercise NEC Y93.A9 (*following* Y93.7)
  caregiving (providing) NEC Y93.F9 (*following* Y93.7)
    bathing Y93.F1 (*following* Y93.7)
    lifting Y93.F2 (*following* Y93.7)
  cellular
    communication device Y93.C2 (*following* Y93.7)
    telephone Y93.C2 (*following* Y93.7)
  challenge course Y93.A5 (*following* Y93.7)
  cheerleading Y93.45
  circuit training Y93.A4 (*following* Y93.7)
  cleaning
    floor Y93.E5 (*following* Y93.7)
  climbing NEC Y93.39
    mountain Y93.31
    rock Y93.31
    wall Y93.31
  clothing care and maintenance NEC Y93.E9 (*following* Y93.7)
  combatives Y93.75
  computer
    keyboarding Y93.C1 (*following* Y93.7)
    technology NEC Y93.C9 (*following* Y93.7)
  confidence course Y93.A5 (*following* Y93.7)
  construction (building) Y93.H3 (*following* Y93.7)
  cooking and baking Y93.G3 (*following* Y93.7)
  cool down exercises Y93.A2 (*following* Y93.7)
  cricket Y93.69
  crocheting Y93.D1 (*following* Y93.7)
  cross country skiing Y93.24
  dancing (all types) Y93.41
  digging
    dirt Y93.H1 (*following* Y93.7)
  dirt digging Y93.H1 (*following* Y93.7)
  dishwashing Y93.G1 (*following* Y93.7)
  diving (platform) (springboard) Y93.12
    underwater Y93.15
  dodge ball Y93.6A
  downhill skiing Y93.23
  drum playing Y93.J2 (*following* Y93.7)
  dumbbells Y93.B3 (*following* Y93.7)
  electronic
    devices NEC Y93.C9 (*following* Y93.7)
      hand held interactive Y93.C2 (*following* Y93.7)
    game playing (using) (with)
      interactive device Y93.C2 (*following* Y93.7)
      keyboard or other stationary device Y93.C1 (*following* Y93.7)
  elliptical machine Y93.A1 (*following* Y93.7)
  exercise(s)
    machines ((primarily) for)
      cardiorespiratory conditioning Y93.A1 (*following* Y93.7)
      muscle strengthening Y93.B1 (*following* Y93.7)
    muscle strengthening (non-machine) NEC Y93.B9 (*following* Y93.7)
  external motion NEC Y93.I9 (*following* Y93.7)
    rollercoaster Y93.I1 (*following* Y93.7)
  field hockey Y93.65
  figure skating (pairs) (singles) Y93.21
  flag football Y93.62
  floor mopping and cleaning Y93.E5 (*following* Y93.7)
  food preparation and clean up Y93.G1 (*following* Y93.7)
  football (American) NOS Y93.61
    flag Y93.62
    tackle Y93.61
    touch Y93.62
  four square Y93.6A
  free weights Y93.B3 (*following* Y93.7)
  frisbee (ultimate) Y93.74
  furniture
    building Y93.D3 (*following* Y93.7)
    finishing Y93.D3 (*following* Y93.7)
    repair Y93.D3 (*following* Y93.7)
  game playing (electronic)
    using interactive device Y93.C2 (*following* Y93.7)
    using keyboard or other stationary device Y93.C1 (*following* Y93.7)

Activity — *continued*
  gardening Y93.H2 (*following* Y93.7)
  golf Y93.53
  grass drills Y93.A6 (*following* Y93.7)
  grilling and smoking food Y93.G2 (*following* Y93.7)
  grooming and shearing an animal Y93.K3 (*following* Y93.7)
  guerilla drills Y93.A6 (*following* Y93.7)
  gymnastics (rhythmic) Y93.43
  hand held interactive electronic device Y93.C2 (*following* Y93.7)
  handball Y93.73
  handcrafts NEC Y93.D9 (*following* Y93.7)
  hang gliding Y93.35
  hiking (on level or elevated terrain) Y93.01
  hockey (ice) Y93.22
    field Y93.65
  horseback riding Y93.52
  household (interior) maintenance NEC Y93.E9 (*following* Y93.7)
  ice NEC Y93.29
    dancing Y93.21
    hockey Y93.22
    skating Y93.21
  inline roller skating Y93.51
  ironing Y93.E4 (*following* Y93.7)
  judo Y93.75
  jumping jacks Y93.A2 (*following* Y93.7)
  jumping rope Y93.56
  jumping (off) NEC Y93.39
    BASE (Building, Antenna, Span, Earth) Y93.33
    bungee Y93.34
    jacks Y93.A2 (*following* Y93.7)
    rope Y93.56
  karate Y93.75
  kayaking (in calm and turbulent water) Y93.16
  keyboarding (computer) Y93.C1 (*following* Y93.7)
  kickball Y93.6A
  knitting Y93.D1 (*following* Y93.7)
  lacrosse Y93.65
  land maintenance NEC Y93.H9 (*following* Y93.7)
  landscaping Y93.H2 (*following* Y93.7)
  laundry Y93.E2 (*following* Y93.7)
  machines (exercise)
    primarily for cardiorespiratory conditioning Y93.A1 (*following* Y93.7)
    primarily for muscle strengthening Y93.B1 (*following* Y93.7)
  maintenance
    exterior building NEC Y93.H9 (*following* Y93.7)
    household (interior) NEC Y93.E9 (*following* Y93.7)
    land Y93.H9 (*following* Y93.7)
    property Y93.H9 (*following* Y93.7)
  marching (on level or elevated terrain) Y93.01
  martial arts Y93.75
  microwave oven Y93.G3 (*following* Y93.7)
  milking an animal Y93.K2 (*following* Y93.7)
  mopping (floor) Y93.E5 (*following* Y93.7)
  mountain climbing Y93.31
  muscle strengthening
    exercises (non-machine) NEC Y93.B9 (*following* Y93.7)
    machines Y93.B1 (*following* Y93.7)
  musical keyboard (electronic) playing Y93.J1 (*following* Y93.7)
  nordic skiing Y93.24
  obstacle course Y93.A5 (*following* Y93.7)
  oven (microwave) Y93.G3 (*following* Y93.7)
  packing up and unpacking in moving to a new residence Y93.E6 (*following* Y93.7)
  parasailing Y93.19
  percussion instrument playing NEC Y93.J2 (*following* Y93.7)
  personal
    bathing and showering Y93.E1 (*following* Y93.7)
    hygiene NEC Y93.E8 (*following* Y93.7)
    showering Y93.E1 (*following* Y93.7)
  physical games generally associated with school recess, summer camp and children Y93.6A
  physical training NEC Y93.A9 (*following* Y93.7)
  piano playing Y93.J1 (*following* Y93.7)
  pilates Y93.B4 (*following* Y93.7)
  platform diving Y93.12
  playing musical instrument
    brass instrument Y93.J4 (*following* Y93.7)
    drum Y93.J2 (*following* Y93.7)
    musical keyboard (electronic) Y93.J1 (*following* Y93.7)

Activity — *continued*
  playing musical instrument — *continued*
    percussion instrument NEC Y93.J2 (*following* Y93.7)
    piano Y93.J1 (*following* Y93.7)
    string instrument Y93.J3 (*following* Y93.7)
    winds instrument Y93.J4 (*following* Y93.7)
  property maintenance
    exterior NEC Y93.H9 (*following* Y93.7)
    interior NEC Y93.E9 (*following* Y93.7)
  pruning (garden and lawn) Y93.H2 (*following* Y93.7)
  pull-ups Y93.B2 (*following* Y93.7)
  push-ups Y93.B2 (*following* Y93.7)
  racquetball Y93.73
  rafting (in calm and turbulent water) Y93.16
  raking (leaves) Y93.H1 (*following* Y93.7)
  rappelling Y93.32
  refereeing a sports activity Y93.81
  residential relocation Y93.E6 (*following* Y93.7)
  rhythmic gymnastics Y93.43
  rhythmic movement NEC Y93.49
  riding
    horseback Y93.52
    rollercoaster Y93.I1 (*following* Y93.7)
  rock climbing Y93.31
  roller skating (inline) Y93.51
  rollercoaster riding Y93.I1 (*following* Y93.7)
  rough housing and horseplay Y93.83
  rowing (in calm and turbulent water) Y93.16
  rugby Y93.63
  running Y93.02
  SCUBA diving Y93.15
  sewing Y93.D2 (*following* Y93.7)
  shoveling Y93.H1 (*following* Y93.7)
    dirt Y93.H1 (*following* Y93.7)
    snow Y93.H1 (*following* Y93.7)
  showering (personal) Y93.E1 (*following* Y93.7)
  sit-ups Y93.B2 (*following* Y93.7)
  skateboarding Y93.51
  skating (ice) Y93.21
    roller Y93.51
  skiing (alpine) (downhill) Y93.23
    cross country Y93.24
    nordic Y93.24
    water Y93.17
  sledding (snow) Y93.23
  sleeping (sleep) Y93.84
  smoking and grilling food Y93.G2 (*following* Y93.7)
  snorkeling Y93.15
  snow NEC Y93.29
    boarding Y93.23
    shoveling Y93.H1 (*following* Y93.7)
    sledding Y93.23
    tubing Y93.23
  soccer Y93.66
  softball Y93.64
  specified NEC Y93.89
  spectator at an event Y93.82
  sports NEC Y93.79
    sports played as a team or group NEC Y93.69
    sports played individually NEC Y93.59
  springboard diving Y93.12
  squash Y93.73
  stationary bike Y93.A1 (*following* Y93.7)
  step (stepping) exercise (class) Y93.A3 (*following* Y93.7)
  stepper machine Y93.A1 (*following* Y93.7)
  stove Y93.G3 (*following* Y93.7)
  string instrument playing Y93.J3 (*following* Y93.7)
  surfing Y93.18
    wind Y93.18
  swimming Y93.11
  tackle football Y93.61
  tap dancing Y93.41
  tennis Y93.73
  tobogganing Y93.23
  touch football Y93.62
  track and field events (non-running) Y93.57
    running Y93.02
  trampoline Y93.44
  treadmill Y93.A1 (*following* Y93.7)
  trimming shrubs Y93.H2 (*following* Y93.7)
  tubing (in calm and turbulent water) Y93.16
    snow Y93.23
  ultimate frisbee Y93.74
  underwater diving Y93.15
  unpacking in moving to a new residence Y93.E6 (*following* Y93.7)
  use of stove, oven and microwave oven Y93.G3 (*following* Y93.7)

Activity — *continued*
  vacuuming Y93.E3 (*following* Y93.7)
  volleyball (beach) (court) Y93.68
  wake boarding Y93.17
  walking (on level or elevated terrain) Y93.01
    an animal Y93.K1 (*following* Y93.7)
  walking an animal Y93.K1 (*following* Y93.7)
  wall climbing Y93.31
  warm up and cool down exercises Y93.A2 (*following* Y93.7)
  water NEC Y93.19
    aerobics Y93.14
    craft NEC Y93.19
    exercise Y93.14
    polo Y93.13
    skiing Y93.17
    sliding Y93.18
    survival training and testing Y93.19
  weeding (garden and lawn) Y93.H2 (*following* Y93.7)
  wind instrument playing Y93.J4 (*following* Y93.7)
  windsurfing Y93.18
  wrestling Y93.72
  yoga Y93.42
Adverse effect of drugs — *see* Table of Drugs and Chemicals
Aerosinusitis — *see* Air, pressure
After-effect, late — *see* Sequelae
Air
  blast in war operations — *see* War operations, air blast
  pressure
    change, rapid
      during
        ascent W94.29 ☑
          while (in) (surfacing from)
            aircraft W94.23 ☑
            deep water diving W94.21 ☑
            underground W94.22 ☑
        descent W94.39 ☑
          in
            aircraft W94.31 ☑
            water W94.32 ☑
    high, prolonged W94.0 ☑
    low, prolonged W94.12 ☑
      due to residence or long visit at high altitude W94.11 ☑
Alpine sickness W94.11 ☑
Altitude sickness W94.11 ☑
Anaphylactic shock, anaphylaxis — *see* Table of Drugs and Chemicals
Andes disease W94.11 ☑
Arachnidism, arachnoidism X58 ☑
Arson (with intent to injure or kill) X97 ☑
Asphyxia, asphyxiation
  by
    food (bone) (seed) — *see* categories T17 and T18 ☑
    gas (*see also* Table of Drugs and Chemicals)
      legal
        execution — *see* Legal, intervention, gas
        intervention — *see* Legal, intervention, gas
  from
    fire (*see also* Exposure, fire)
      in war operations — *see* War operations, fire
    ignition — *see* Ignition
    vomitus T17.81 ☑
  in war operations — *see* War operations, restriction of airway
Aspiration
  food (any type) (into respiratory tract) (with asphyxia, obstruction respiratory tract, suffocation) — *see* categories T17 and T18 ☑
  foreign body — *see* Foreign body, aspiration
  vomitus (with asphyxia, obstruction respiratory tract, suffocation) T17.81 ☑
Assassination (attempt) — *see* Assault
Assault (homicidal) (by) (in) Y09
  arson X97 ☑
  bite (of human being) Y04.1 ☑
  bodily force Y04.8 ☑
    bite Y04.1 ☑
    bumping into Y04.2 ☑
    sexual — *see* subcategories T74.0, T76.0 ☑
    unarmed fight Y04.0 ☑
  bomb X96.9 ☑
    antipersonnel X96.0 ☑
    fertilizer X96.3 ☑
    gasoline X96.1 ☑

Assault — *continued*
- bomb — *continued*
  - letter X96.2 ☑
  - petrol X96.1 ☑
  - pipe X96.3 ☑
  - specified NEC X96.8 ☑
- brawl (hand) (fists) (foot) (unarmed) Y04.0 ☑
- burning, burns (by fire) NEC X97 ☑
  - acid Y08.89 ☑
  - caustic, corrosive substance Y08.89 ☑
  - chemical from swallowing caustic, corrosive substance — *see* Table of Drugs and Chemicals
  - cigarette(s) X97 ☑
  - hot object X98.9 ☑
    - fluid NEC X98.2 ☑
    - household appliance X98.3 ☑
    - specified NEC X98.8 ☑
    - steam X98.0 ☑
    - tap water X98.1 ☑
    - vapors X98.0 ☑
  - scalding — *see* Assault, burning
  - steam X98.0 ☑
  - vitriol Y08.89 ☑
- caustic, corrosive substance (gas) Y08.89 ☑
- crashing of
  - aircraft Y08.81 ☑
  - motor vehicle Y03.8 ☑
    - pushed in front of Y02.0 ☑
    - run over Y03.0 ☑
    - specified NEC Y03.8 ☑
- cutting or piercing instrument X99.9 ☑
  - dagger X99.2 ☑
  - glass X99.0 ☑
  - knife X99.1 ☑
  - specified NEC X99.8 ☑
  - sword X99.2 ☑
- dagger X99.2 ☑
- drowning (in) X92.9 ☑
  - bathtub X92.0 ☑
  - natural water X92.3 ☑
  - specified NEC X92.8 ☑
  - swimming pool X92.1 ☑
    - following fall X92.2 ☑
- dynamite X96.8 ☑
- explosive(s) (material) X96.9 ☑
- fight (hand) (fists) (foot) (unarmed) Y04.0 ☑
  - with weapon — *see* Assault, by type of weapon
- fire X97 ☑
- firearm X95.9 ☑
  - airgun X95.01 ☑
  - handgun X93 ☑
  - hunting rifle X94.1 ☑
  - larger X94.9 ☑
    - specified NEC X94.8 ☑
  - machine gun X94.2 ☑
  - shotgun X94.0 ☑
  - specified NEC X95.8 ☑
- from high place Y01 ☑
- gunshot (wound) NEC — *see* Assault, firearm, by type
- incendiary device X97 ☑
- injury Y09
  - to child due to criminal abortion attempt NEC Y08.89 ☑
- knife X99.1 ☑
- late effect of — *see* categories X92-Y08 with 7th character S
- placing before moving object NEC Y02.8 ☑
  - motor vehicle Y02.0 ☑
- poisoning — *see* categories T36-T65 with 7th character S
- puncture, any part of body — *see* Assault, cutting or piercing instrument
- pushing
  - before moving object NEC Y02.8 ☑
    - motor vehicle Y02.0 ☑
    - subway train Y02.1 ☑
    - train Y02.1 ☑
  - from high place Y01 ☑
- rape T74.2- ☑
- scalding — *see* Assault, burning
- sequelae of — *see* categories X92-Y08 with 7th character S
- sexual (by bodily force) T74.2- ☑
- shooting — *see* Assault, firearm
- specified means NEC Y08.89 ☑

Assault — *continued*
- stab, any part of body — *see* Assault, cutting or piercing instrument
- steam X98.0 ☑
- striking against
  - other person Y04.2 ☑
  - sports equipment Y08.09 ☑
    - baseball bat Y08.02 ☑
    - hockey stick Y08.01 ☑
- struck by
  - sports equipment Y08.09 ☑
    - baseball bat Y08.02 ☑
    - hockey stick Y08.01 ☑
- submersion — *see* Assault, drowning
- violence Y09
- weapon Y09
  - blunt Y00 ☑
  - cutting or piercing — *see* Assault, cutting or piercing instrument
  - firearm — *see* Assault, firearm
- wound Y09
  - cutting — *see* Assault, cutting or piercing instrument
  - gunshot — *see* Assault, firearm
  - knife X99.1 ☑
  - piercing — *see* Assault, cutting or piercing instrument
  - puncture — *see* Assault, cutting or piercing instrument
  - stab — *see* Assault, cutting or piercing instrument

Attack by mammals NEC W55.89 ☑
Avalanche — *see* Landslide
Aviator's disease — *see* Air, pressure

B

Barotitis, barodontalgia, barosinusitis, barotrauma (otitic) (sinus) — *see* Air, pressure
Battered (baby) (child) (person) (syndrome) X58 ☑
Bayonet wound W26.1 ☑
- in
  - legal intervention — *see* Legal, intervention, sharp object, bayonet
  - war operations — *see* War operations, combat
- stated as undetermined whether accidental or intentional Y28.8 ☑
- suicide (attempt) X78.2 ☑

Bean in nose — *see* categories T17 and T18 ☑
Bed set on fire NEC — *see* Exposure, fire, uncontrolled, building, bed
Beheading (by guillotine)
- homicide X99.9 ☑
- legal execution — *see* Legal, intervention

Bending, injury in — *see* Overexertion
Bends — *see* Air, pressure, change
Bite, bitten by
- alligator W58.01 ☑
- arthropod (nonvenomous) NEC W57 ☑
- bull W55.21 ☑
- cat W55.01 ☑
- cow W55.21 ☑
- crocodile W58.11 ☑
- dog W54.0 ☑
- goat W55.31 ☑
- hoof stock NEC W55.31 ☑
- horse W55.11 ☑
- human being (accidentally) W50.3 ☑
  - with intent to injure or kill Y04.1 ☑
    - as, or caused by, a crowd or human stampede (with fall) W52 ☑
    - assault Y04.1 ☑
    - homicide (attempt) Y04.1 ☑
    - in
      - fight Y04.1 ☑
- insect (nonvenomous) W57 ☑
- lizard (nonvenomous) W59.01 ☑
- mammal NEC W55.81 ☑
- mammal NEC W55.81 ☑
  - marine W56.31 ☑
- marine animal (nonvenomous) W56.81 ☑
- millipede W57 ☑
- moray eel W56.51 ☑
- mouse W53.01 ☑
- person(s) (accidentally) W50.3 ☑
  - with intent to injure or kill Y04.1 ☑

Bite, bitten by — *continued*
- person(s) — *continued*
  - as, or caused by, a crowd or human stampede (with fall) W52 ☑
  - assault Y04.1 ☑
  - homicide (attempt) Y04.1 ☑
  - in
    - fight Y04.1 ☑
- pig W55.41 ☑
- raccoon W55.51 ☑
- rat W53.11 ☑
- reptile W59.81 ☑
  - lizard W59.01 ☑
  - snake W59.11 ☑
  - turtle W59.21 ☑
    - terrestrial W59.81 ☑
- rodent W53.81 ☑
  - mouse W53.01 ☑
  - rat W53.11 ☑
  - specified NEC W53.81 ☑
  - squirrel W53.21 ☑
- shark W56.41 ☑
- sheep W55.31 ☑
- snake (nonvenomous) W59.11 ☑
- spider (nonvenomous) W57 ☑
- squirrel W53.21 ☑
Blast (air) in war operations — *see* War operations, blast
Blizzard X37.2 ☑
Blood alcohol level Y90.9
- less than 20mg/100ml Y90.0
- 20-39mg/100ml Y90.1
- 40-59mg/100ml Y90.2
- 60-79mg/100ml Y90.3
- 80-99mg/100ml Y90.4
- 100-119mg/100ml Y90.5
- 120-199mg/100ml Y90.6
- 200-239mg/100ml Y90.7
- presence in blood, level not specified Y90.9
Blow X58 ☑
- by law-enforcing agent, police (on duty) — *see* Legal, intervention, manhandling
  - blunt object — *see* Legal, intervention, blunt object
Blowing up — *see* Explosion
Brawl (hand) (fists) (foot) Y04.0 ☑
Breakage (accidental) (part of)
- ladder (causing fall) W11 ☑
- scaffolding (causing fall) W12 ☑
Broken
- glass, contact with — *see* Contact, with, glass
- power line (causing electric shock) W85 ☑
Bumping against, into (accidentally)
- object NEC W22.8 ☑
  - with fall — *see* Fall, due to, bumping against, object
  - caused by crowd or human stampede (with fall) W52 ☑
  - sports equipment W21.9 ☑
- person(s) W51 ☑
  - with fall W03 ☑
    - due to ice or snow W00.0 ☑
  - assault Y04.2 ☑
  - caused by, a crowd or human stampede (with fall) W52 ☑
  - homicide (attempt) Y04.2 ☑
  - sports equipment W21.9 ☑
Burn, burned, burning (accidental) (by) (from) (on)
- acid NEC — *see* Table of Drugs and Chemicals
- bed linen — *see* Exposure, fire, uncontrolled, in building, bed
- blowtorch X08.8 ☑
  - with ignition of clothing NEC X06.2 ☑
    - nightwear X05 ☑
- bonfire, campfire (controlled) (*see also* Exposure, fire, controlled, not in building)
  - uncontrolled — *see* Exposure, fire, uncontrolled, not in building
- candle X08.8 ☑
  - with ignition of clothing NEC X06.2 ☑
    - nightwear X05 ☑
- caustic liquid, substance (external) (internal) NEC — *see* Table of Drugs and Chemicals
- chemical (external) (internal) (*see also* Table of Drugs and Chemicals)
  - in war operations — *see* War operations. fire
- cigar(s) or cigarette(s) X08.8 ☑

400

☑ Additional Character Required — Refer to the Tabular List for Character Selection   ▽ Subterms under main terms may continue to next column or page

Burn, burned, burning — *continued*
　cigar(s) or cigarette(s) — *continued*
　　with ignition of clothing NEC X06.2 ☑
　　　nightwear X05 ☑
　clothes, clothing NEC (from controlled fire) X06.2 ☑
　　with conflagration — *see* Exposure, fire, uncon-
　　　trolled, building
　　　not in building or structure — *see* Exposure,
　　　　fire, uncontrolled, not in building
　cooker (hot) X15.8 ☑
　　stated as undetermined whether accidental or in-
　　　tentional Y27.3 ☑
　　suicide (attempt) X77.3 ☑
　electric blanket X16 ☑
　engine (hot) X17 ☑
　fire, flames — *see* Exposure, fire
　flare, Very pistol — *see* Discharge, firearm NEC
　heat
　　from appliance (electrical) (household) X15.8 ☑
　　　cooker X15.8 ☑
　　　hotplate X15.2 ☑
　　　kettle X15.8 ☑
　　　light bulb X15.8 ☑
　　　saucepan X15.3 ☑
　　　skillet X15.3 ☑
　　　stated as undetermined whether accidental or
　　　　intentional Y27.3 ☑
　　　stove X15.0 ☑
　　　suicide (attempt) X77.3 ☑
　　　toaster X15.1 ☑
　　in local application or packing during medical or
　　　surgical procedure Y63.5
　heating
　　appliance, radiator or pipe X16 ☑
　homicide (attempt) — *see* Assault, burning
　hot
　　air X14.1 ☑
　　cooker X15.8 ☑
　　drink X10.0 ☑
　　engine X17 ☑
　　fat X10.2 ☑
　　fluid NEC X12 ☑
　　food X10.1 ☑
　　gases X14.1 ☑
　　heating appliance X16 ☑
　　household appliance NEC X15.8 ☑
　　kettle X15.8 ☑
　　liquid NEC X12 ☑
　　machinery X17 ☑
　　metal (molten) (liquid) NEC X18 ☑
　　object (not producing fire or flames) NEC X19 ☑
　　oil (cooking) X10.2 ☑
　　pipe(s) X16 ☑
　　radiator X16 ☑
　　saucepan (glass) (metal) X15.3 ☑
　　stove (kitchen) X15.0 ☑
　　substance NEC X19 ☑
　　　caustic or corrosive NEC — *see* Table of Drugs
　　　　and Chemicals
　　toaster X15.1 ☑
　　tool X17 ☑
　　vapor X13.1 ☑
　　water (tap) — *see* Contact, with, hot, tap water
　hotplate X15.2 ☑
　　suicide (attempt) X77.3 ☑
　ignition — *see* Ignition
　in war operations — *see* War operations, fire
　inflicted by other person X97 ☑
　　by hot objects, hot vapor, and steam — *see* Assault,
　　　burning, hot object
　internal, from swallowed caustic, corrosive liquid,
　　substance — *see* Table of Drugs and Chemicals
　iron (hot) X15.8 ☑
　　stated as undetermined whether accidental or in-
　　　tentional Y27.3 ☑
　　suicide (attempt) X77.3 ☑
　kettle (hot) X15.8 ☑
　　stated as undetermined whether accidental or in-
　　　tentional Y27.3 ☑
　　suicide (attempt) X77.3 ☑
　lamp (flame) X08.8 ☑
　　with ignition of clothing NEC X06.2 ☑
　　　nightwear X05 ☑
　lighter (cigar) (cigarette) X08.8 ☑
　　with ignition of clothing NEC X06.2 ☑
　　　nightwear X05 ☑

Burn, burned, burning — *continued*
　lightning — *see* subcategory T75.0 ☑
　　causing fire — *see* Exposure, fire
　liquid (boiling) (hot) NEC X12 ☑
　　stated as undetermined whether accidental or in-
　　　tentional Y27.2 ☑
　　suicide (attempt) X77.2 ☑
　local application of externally applied substance in
　　medical or surgical care Y63.5
　machinery (hot) X17 ☑
　matches X08.8 ☑
　　with ignition of clothing NEC X06.2 ☑
　　　nightwear X05 ☑
　mattress — *see* Exposure, fire, uncontrolled, building,
　　bed
　medicament, externally applied Y63.5
　metal (hot) (liquid) (molten) NEC X18 ☑
　nightwear (nightclothes, nightdress, gown, pajamas,
　　robe) X05 ☑
　object (hot) NEC X19 ☑
　on board watercraft
　　due to
　　　accident to watercraft V91.09 ☑
　　　　powered craft V91.03 ☑
　　　　　ferry boat V91.01 ☑
　　　　　fishing boat V91.02 ☑
　　　　　jetskis V91.03 ☑
　　　　　liner V91.01 ☑
　　　　　merchant ship V91.00 ☑
　　　　　passenger ship V91.01 ☑
　　　　unpowered craft V91.08 ☑
　　　　　canoe V91.05 ☑
　　　　　inflatable V91.06 ☑
　　　　　kayak V91.05 ☑
　　　　　sailboat V91.04 ☑
　　　　　surf-board V91.08 ☑
　　　　　water skis V91.07 ☑
　　　　　windsurfer V91.08 ☑
　　　fire on board V93.09 ☑
　　　　ferry boat V93.01 ☑
　　　　fishing boat V93.02 ☑
　　　　jetskis V93.03 ☑
　　　　liner V93.01 ☑
　　　　merchant ship V93.00 ☑
　　　　passenger ship V93.01 ☑
　　　　powered craft NEC V93.03 ☑
　　　　sailboat V93.04 ☑
　　　specified heat source NEC on board V93.19 ☑
　　　　ferry boat V93.11 ☑
　　　　fishing boat V93.12 ☑
　　　　jetskis V93.13 ☑
　　　　liner V93.11 ☑
　　　　merchant ship V93.10 ☑
　　　　passenger ship V93.11 ☑
　　　　powered craft NEC V93.13 ☑
　　　　sailboat V93.14 ☑
　pipe (hot) X16 ☑
　　smoking X08.8 ☑
　　　with ignition of clothing NEC X06.2 ☑
　　　　nightwear X05 ☑
　powder — *see* Powder burn
　radiator (hot) X16 ☑
　saucepan (hot) (glass) (metal) X15.3 ☑
　　stated as undetermined whether accidental or in-
　　　tentional Y27.3 ☑
　　suicide (attempt) X77.3 ☑
　self-inflicted X76 ☑
　　stated as undetermined whether accidental or in-
　　　tentional Y26 ☑
　stated as undetermined whether accidental or inten-
　　tional Y27.0 ☑
　steam X13.1 ☑
　　pipe X16 ☑
　　　stated as undetermined whether accidental or
　　　　intentional Y27.8 ☑
　　stated as undetermined whether accidental or in-
　　　tentional Y27.0 ☑
　　suicide (attempt) X77.0 ☑
　stove (hot) (kitchen) X15.0 ☑
　　stated as undetermined whether accidental or in-
　　　tentional Y27.3 ☑
　　suicide (attempt) X77.3 ☑
　substance (hot) NEC X19 ☑
　　boiling X12 ☑
　　　stated as undetermined whether accidental or
　　　　intentional Y27.2 ☑

Burn, burned, burning — *continued*
　substance — *continued*
　　boiling — *continued*
　　　suicide (attempt) X77.2 ☑
　　　molten (metal) X18 ☑
　　suicide (attempt) NEC X76 ☑
　　hot
　　　household appliance X77.3 ☑
　　　object X77.9 ☑
　　therapeutic misadventure
　　　heat in local application or packing during medical
　　　　or surgical procedure Y63.5
　　　overdose of radiation Y63.2
　　toaster (hot) X15.1 ☑
　　　stated as undetermined whether accidental or in-
　　　　tentional Y27.3 ☑
　　　suicide (attempt) X77.3 ☑
　　tool (hot) X17 ☑
　　torch, welding X08.8 ☑
　　　with ignition of clothing NEC X06.2 ☑
　　　　nightwear X05 ☑
　　trash fire (controlled) — *see* Exposure, fire, controlled,
　　　not in building
　　　uncontrolled — *see* Exposure, fire, uncontrolled,
　　　　not in building
　　vapor (hot) X13.1 ☑
　　　stated as undetermined whether accidental or in-
　　　　tentional Y27.0 ☑
　　　suicide (attempt) X77.0 ☑
　　Very pistol — *see* Discharge, firearm NEC
Butted by animal W55.82 ☑
　bull W55.22 ☑
　cow W55.22 ☑
　goat W55.32 ☑
　horse W55.12 ☑
　pig W55.42 ☑
　sheep W55.32 ☑

C

Caisson disease — *see* Air, pressure, change
Campfire (exposure to) (controlled) (*see also* Exposure,
　fire, controlled, not in building)
　uncontrolled — *see* Exposure, fire, uncontrolled, not
　　in building
Capital punishment (any means) — *see* Legal, interven-
　tion
Car sickness T75.3 ☑
Casualty (not due to war) NEC X58 ☑
　war — *see* War operations
Cat
　bite W55.01 ☑
　scratch W55.03 ☑
Cataclysm, cataclysmic (any injury) NEC — *see* Forces
　of nature
Catching fire — *see* Exposure, fire
Caught
　between
　　folding object W23.0 ☑
　　objects (moving) (stationary and moving) W23.0 ☑
　　　and machinery — *see* Contact, with, by type of
　　　　machine
　　　stationary W23.1 ☑
　　sliding door and door frame W23.0 ☑
　by, in
　　machinery (moving parts of) — *see* Contact, with,
　　　by type of machine
　　washing-machine wringer W23.0 ☑
　under packing crate (due to losing grip) W23.1 ☑
Cave-in caused by cataclysmic earth surface move-
　ment or eruption — *see* Landslide
Change(s) in air pressure — *see* Air, pressure, change
Choked, choking (on) (any object except food or vomi-
　tus)
　food (bone) (seed) — *see* categories T17 and T18 ☑
　vomitus T17.81- ☑
Civil insurrection — *see* War operations
Cloudburst (any injury) X37.8 ☑
Cold, exposure to (accidental) (excessive) (extreme)
　(natural) (place) NEC — *see* Exposure, cold
Collapse
　building W20.1 ☑
　　burning (uncontrolled fire) X00.2 ☑
　dam or man-made structure (causing earth movement)
　　X36.0 ☑
　machinery — *see* Contact, with, by type of machine

Collapse — *continued*
structure W20.1 ☑
burning (uncontrolled fire) X00.2 ☑
Collision (accidental) NEC (*see also* Accident, transport)
V89.9 ☑
pedestrian W51 ☑
with fall W03 ☑
due to ice or snow W00.0 ☑
involving pedestrian conveyance — *see* Accident, transport, pedestrian, conveyance
and
crowd or human stampede (with fall) W52 ☑
object W22.8 ☑
with fall — *see* Fall, due to, bumping against, object
person(s) — *see* Collision, pedestrian
transport vehicle NEC V89.9 ☑
and
avalanche, fallen or not moving — *see* Accident, transport
falling or moving — *see* Landslide
landslide, fallen or not moving — *see* Accident, transport
falling or moving — *see* Landslide
due to cataclysm — *see* Forces of nature, by type
intentional, purposeful suicide (attempt) — *see* Suicide, collision
Combustion, spontaneous — *see* Ignition
Complication (delayed) **of or following** (medical or surgical procedure) Y84.9
with misadventure — *see* Misadventure
amputation of limb(s) Y83.5
anastomosis (arteriovenous) (blood vessel) (gastroje-junal) (tendon) (natural or artificial material) Y83.2
aspiration (of fluid) Y84.4
tissue Y84.8
biopsy Y84.8
blood
sampling Y84.7
transfusion
procedure Y84.8
bypass Y83.2
catheterization (urinary) Y84.6
cardiac Y84.0
colostomy Y83.3
cystostomy Y83.3
dialysis (kidney) Y84.1
drug — *see* Table of Drugs and Chemicals
due to misadventure — *see* Misadventure
duodenostomy Y83.3
electroshock therapy Y84.3
external stoma, creation of Y83.3
formation of external stoma Y83.3
gastrostomy Y83.3
graft Y83.2
hypothermia (medically-induced) Y84.8
implant, implantation (of)
artificial
internal device (cardiac pacemaker) (electrodes in brain) (heart valve prosthesis) (ortho-pedic) Y83.1
material or tissue (for anastomosis or bypass) Y83.2
with creation of external stoma Y83.3
natural tissues (for anastomosis or bypass) Y83.2
with creation of external stoma Y83.3
infusion
procedure Y84.8
injection — *see* Table of Drugs and Chemicals
procedure Y84.8
insertion of gastric or duodenal sound Y84.5
insulin-shock therapy Y84.3
paracentesis (abdominal) (thoracic) (aspirative) Y84.4
procedures other than surgical operation — *see* Complication of or following, by type of proce-dure
radiological procedure or therapy Y84.2
removal of organ (partial) (total) NEC Y83.6
sampling
blood Y84.7
fluid NEC Y84.4
tissue Y84.8
shock therapy Y84.3
surgical operation NEC (*see also* Complication of or following, by type of operation) Y83.9
reconstructive NEC Y83.4
with

Complication (delayed) **of or following** — *continued*
surgical operation (*see also* Complication of or follow-ing, by type of operation) — *continued*
reconstructive — *continued*
with — *continued*
anastomosis, bypass or graft Y83.2
formation of external stoma Y83.3
specified NEC Y83.8
transfusion (*see also* Table of Drugs and Chemicals)
procedure Y84.8
transplant, transplantation (heart) (kidney) (liver) (whole organ, any) Y83.0
partial organ Y83.4
ureterostomy Y83.3
vaccination (*see also* Table of Drugs and Chemicals)
procedure Y84.8
Compression
divers' squeeze — *see* Air, pressure, change
trachea by
food (lodged in esophagus) — *see* categories T17 and T18 ☑
vomitus (lodged in esophagus) T17.81- ☑
Conflagration — *see* Exposure, fire, uncontrolled
Constriction (external)
hair W49.01 ☑
jewelry W49.04 ☑
ring W49.04 ☑
rubber band W49.03 ☑
specified item NEC W49.09 ☑
string W49.02 ☑
thread W49.02 ☑
Contact (accidental)
with
abrasive wheel (metalworking) W31.1 ☑
alligator W58.09 ☑
bite W58.01 ☑
crushing W58.03 ☑
strike W58.02 ☑
amphibian W62.9 ☑
frog W62.0 ☑
toad W62.1 ☑
animal (nonvenomous) NEC W64 ☑
marine W56.89 ☑
bite W56.81 ☑
dolphin — *see* Contact, with, dolphin
fish NEC — *see* Contact, with, fish
mammal — *see* Contact, with, mammal, marine
orca — *see* Contact, with, orca
sea lion — *see* Contact, with, sea lion
shark — *see* Contact, with, shark
strike W56.82 ☑
animate mechanical force NEC W64 ☑
arrow W21.89 ☑
not thrown, projected or falling W45.8 ☑
arthropods (nonvenomous) W57 ☑
axe W27.0 ☑
band-saw (industrial) W31.2 ☑
bayonet — *see* Bayonet wound
bee(s) X58 ☑
bench-saw (industrial) W31.2 ☑
bird W61.99 ☑
bite W61.91 ☑
chicken — *see* Contact, with, chicken
duck — *see* Contact, with, duck
goose — *see* Contact, with, goose
macaw — *see* Contact, with, macaw
parrot — *see* Contact, with, parrot
psittacine — *see* Contact, with, psittacine
strike W61.92 ☑
turkey — *see* Contact, with, turkey
blender W29.0 ☑
boiling water X12 ☑
stated as undetermined whether accidental or intentional Y27.2 ☑
suicide (attempt) X77.2 ☑
bore, earth-drilling or mining (land) (seabed) W31.0 ☑
buffalo — *see* Contact, with, hoof stock NEC
bull W55.29 ☑
bite W55.21 ☑
gored W55.22 ☑
strike W55.22 ☑
bumper cars W31.81 ☑
camel — *see* Contact, with, hoof stock NEC

Contact — *continued*
with — *continued*
can
lid W45.2 ☑
opener W27.4 ☑
powered W29.0 ☑
cat W55.09 ☑
bite W55.01 ☑
scratch W55.03 ☑
caterpillar (venomous) X58 ☑
centipede (venomous) X58 ☑
chain
hoist W24.0 ☑
agricultural operations W30.89 ☑
saw W29.3 ☑
chicken W61.39 ☑
peck W61.33 ☑
strike W61.32 ☑
chisel W27.0 ☑
circular saw W31.2 ☑
cobra X58 ☑
combine (harvester) W30.0 ☑
conveyer belt W24.1 ☑
cooker (hot) X15.8 ☑
stated as undetermined whether accidental or intentional Y27.3 ☑
suicide (attempt) X77.3 ☑
coral X58 ☑
cotton gin W31.82 ☑
cow W55.29 ☑
bite W55.21 ☑
strike W55.22 ☑
crane W24.0 ☑
agricultural operations W30.89 ☑
crocodile W58.19 ☑
bite W58.11 ☑
crushing W58.13 ☑
strike W58.12 ☑
dagger W26.1 ☑
stated as undetermined whether accidental or intentional Y28.2 ☑
suicide (attempt) X78.2 ☑
dairy equipment W31.82 ☑
dart W21.89 ☑
not thrown, projected or falling W45.8 ☑
deer — *see* Contact, with, hoof stock NEC
derrick W24.0 ☑
agricultural operations W30.89 ☑
hay W30.2 ☑
dog W54.8 ☑
bite W54.0 ☑
strike W54.1 ☑
dolphin W56.09 ☑
bite W56.01 ☑
strike W56.02 ☑
donkey — *see* Contact, with, hoof stock NEC
drill (powered) W29.8 ☑
earth (land) (seabed) W31.0 ☑
nonpowered W27.8 ☑
drive belt W24.0 ☑
agricultural operations W30.89 ☑
dry ice — *see* Exposure, cold, man-made
dryer (clothes) (powered) (spin) W29.2 ☑
duck W61.69 ☑
bite W61.61 ☑
strike W61.62 ☑
earth (-)
drilling machine (industrial) W31.0 ☑
scraping machine in stationary use W31.83 ☑
edge of stiff paper W45.1 ☑
electric
beater W29.0 ☑
blanket X16 ☑
fan W29.2 ☑
commercial W31.82 ☑
knife W29.1 ☑
mixer W29.0 ☑
elevator (building) W24.0 ☑
agricultural operations W30.89 ☑
grain W30.3 ☑
engine(s), hot NEC X17 ☑
excavating machine W31.0 ☑
farm machine W30.9 ☑
feces — *see* Contact, with, by type of animal
fer de lance X58 ☑

☑ **Additional Character Required** — Refer to the Tabular List for Character Selection
▽ **Subterms under main terms may continue to next column or page**

Contact — *continued*
  with — *continued*
    fish W56.59 ☑
      bite W56.51 ☑
      shark — *see* Contact, with, shark
      strike W56.52 ☑
    flying horses W31.81 ☑
    forging (metalworking) machine W31.1 ☑
    fork W27.4 ☑
    forklift (truck) W24.0 ☑
      agricultural operations W30.89 ☑
    frog W62.0 ☑
    garden
      cultivator (powered) W29.3 ☑
        riding W30.89 ☑
      fork W27.1 ☑
    gas turbine W31.3 ☑
    Gila monster X58 ☑
    giraffe — *see* Contact, with, hoof stock NEC
    glass (sharp) (broken) W25 ☑
      with subsequent fall W18.02 ☑
      assault X99.0 ☑
      due to fall — *see* Fall, by type
      stated as undetermined whether accidental or
        intentional Y28.0 ☑
      suicide (attempt) X78.0 ☑
    goat W55.39 ☑
      bite W55.31 ☑
      strike W55.32 ☑
    goose W61.59 ☑
      bite W61.51 ☑
      strike W61.52 ☑
    hand
      saw W27.0 ☑
      tool (not powered) NEC W27.8 ☑
        powered W29.8 ☑
    harvester W30.0 ☑
    hay-derrick W30.2 ☑
    heating
      appliance (hot) X16 ☑
      pad (electric) X16 ☑
    heat NEC X19 ☑
      from appliance (electrical) (household) — *see*
        Contact, with, hot, household appliance
      heating appliance X16 ☑
    hedge-trimmer (powered) W29.3 ☑
    hoe W27.1 ☑
    hoist (chain) (shaft) NEC W24.0 ☑
      agricultural W30.89 ☑
    hoof stock NEC W55.39 ☑
      bite W55.31 ☑
      strike W55.32 ☑
    hornet(s) X58 ☑
    horse W55.19 ☑
      bite W55.11 ☑
      strike W55.12 ☑
    hot
      air X14.1 ☑
        inhalation X14.0 ☑
      cooker X15.8 ☑
      drinks X10.0 ☑
      engine X17 ☑
      fats X10.2 ☑
      fluids NEC X12 ☑
        assault X98.2 ☑
        suicide (attempt) X77.2 ☑
        undetermined whether accidental or inten-
          tional Y27.2 ☑
      food X10.1 ☑
      gases X14.1 ☑
        inhalation X14.0 ☑
      heating appliance X16 ☑
      household appliance X15.8 ☑
        assault X98.3 ☑
        cooker X15.8 ☑
        hotplate X15.2 ☑
        kettle X15.8 ☑
        light bulb X15.8 ☑
        object NEC X19 ☑
          assault X98.8 ☑
          stated as undetermined whether acciden-
            tal or intentional Y27.9 ☑
          suicide (attempt) X77.8 ☑
        saucepan X15.3 ☑
        skillet X15.3 ☑

Contact — *continued*
  with — *continued*
    hot — *continued*
      household appliance — *continued*
        stated as undetermined whether accidental
          or intentional Y27.3 ☑
        stove X15.0 ☑
        suicide (attempt) X77.3 ☑
        toaster X15.1 ☑
      kettle X15.8 ☑
      light bulb X15.8 ☑
      liquid NEC (*see also* Burn) X12 ☑
        drinks X10.0 ☑
        stated as undetermined whether accidental
          or intentional Y27.2 ☑
        suicide (attempt) X77.2 ☑
        tap water X11.8 ☑
          stated as undetermined whether acciden-
            tal or intentional Y27.1 ☑
          suicide (attempt) X77.1 ☑
      machinery X17 ☑
      metal (molten) (liquid) NEC X18 ☑
      object (not producing fire or flames) NEC X19 ☑
      oil (cooking) X10.2 ☑
      pipe X16 ☑
      plate X15.2 ☑
      radiator X16 ☑
      saucepan (glass) (metal) X15.3 ☑
      skillet X15.3 ☑
      stove (kitchen) X15.0 ☑
      substance NEC X19 ☑
      tap-water X11.8 ☑
        assault X98.1 ☑
        heated on stove X12 ☑
          stated as undetermined whether acciden-
            tal or intentional Y27.2 ☑
          suicide (attempt) X77.2 ☑
        in bathtub X11.0 ☑
        running X11.1 ☑
          stated as undetermined whether accidental
            or intentional Y27.1 ☑
          suicide (attempt) X77.1 ☑
      toaster X15.1 ☑
      tool X17 ☑
      vapors X13.1 ☑
        inhalation X13.0 ☑
      water (tap) X11.8 ☑
        boiling X12 ☑
          stated as undetermined whether acciden-
            tal or intentional Y27.2 ☑
          suicide (attempt) X77.2 ☑
        heated on stove X12 ☑
          stated as undetermined whether acciden-
            tal or intentional Y27.2 ☑
          suicide (attempt) X77.2 ☑
        in bathtub X11.0 ☑
        running X11.1 ☑
          stated as undetermined whether accidental
            or intentional Y27.1 ☑
          suicide (attempt) X77.1 ☑
    hotplate X15.2 ☑
    ice-pick W27.4 ☑
    insect (nonvenomous) NEC W57 ☑
    kettle (hot) X15.8 ☑
    knife W26.0 ☑
      assault X99.1 ☑
      electric W29.1 ☑
      stated as undetermined whether accidental or
        intentional Y28.1 ☑
      suicide (attempt) X78.1 ☑
    lathe (metalworking) W31.1 ☑
      turnings W45.8 ☑
      woodworking W31.2 ☑
    lawnmower (powered) (ridden) W28 ☑
      causing electrocution W86.8 ☑
        suicide (attempt) X83.1 ☑
      unpowered W27.1 ☑
    lift, lifting (devices) W24.0 ☑
      agricultural operations W30.89 ☑
      shaft W24.0 ☑
    liquefied gas — *see* Exposure, cold, man-made
    liquid air, hydrogen, nitrogen — *see* Exposure, cold,
      man-made
    lizard (nonvenomous) W59.09 ☑
      bite W59.01 ☑
      strike W59.02 ☑

Contact — *continued*
  with — *continued*
    llama — *see* Contact, with, hoof stock NEC
    macaw W61.19 ☑
      bite W61.11 ☑
      strike W61.12 ☑
    machine, machinery W31.9 ☑
      abrasive wheel W31.1 ☑
      agricultural including animal-powered
        W30.9 ☑
        combine harvester W30.0 ☑
        grain storage elevator W30.3 ☑
        hay derrick W30.2 ☑
        power take-off device W30.1 ☑
        reaper W30.0 ☑
        specified NEC W30.89 ☑
        thresher W30.0 ☑
        transport vehicle, stationary W30.81 ☑
      band saw W31.2 ☑
      bench saw W31.2 ☑
      circular saw W31.2 ☑
      commercial NEC W31.82 ☑
      drilling, metal (industrial) W31.1 ☑
      earth-drilling W31.0 ☑
      earthmoving or scraping W31.89 ☑
      excavating W31.89 ☑
      forging machine W31.1 ☑
      gas turbine W31.3 ☑
      hot X17 ☑
      internal combustion engine W31.3 ☑
      land drill W31.0 ☑
      lathe W31.1 ☑
      lifting (devices) W24.0 ☑
      metal drill W31.1 ☑
      metalworking (industrial) W31.1 ☑
      milling, metal W31.1 ☑
      mining W31.0 ☑
      molding W31.2 ☑
      overhead plane W31.2 ☑
      power press, metal W31.1 ☑
      prime mover W31.3 ☑
      printing W31.89 ☑
      radial saw W31.2 ☑
      recreational W31.81 ☑
      roller-coaster W31.81 ☑
      rolling mill, metal W31.1 ☑
      sander W31.2 ☑
      seabed drill W31.0 ☑
      shaft
        hoist W31.0 ☑
        lift W31.0 ☑
      specified NEC W31.89 ☑
      spinning W31.89 ☑
      steam engine W31.3 ☑
      transmission W24.1 ☑
      undercutter W31.0 ☑
      water driven turbine W31.3 ☑
      weaving W31.89 ☑
      woodworking or forming (industrial) W31.2 ☑
    mammal (feces) (urine) W55.89 ☑
      bull — *see* Contact, with, bull
      cat — *see* Contact, with, cat
      cow — *see* Contact, with, cow
      goat — *see* Contact, with, goat
      hoof stock — *see* Contact, with, hoof stock
      horse — *see* Contact, with, horse
      marine W56.39 ☑
        dolphin — *see* Contact, with, dolphin
        orca — *see* Contact, with, orca
        sea lion — *see* Contact, with, sea lion
        specified NEC W56.39 ☑
          bite W56.31 ☑
          strike W56.32 ☑
      pig — *see* Contact, with, pig
      raccoon — *see* Contact, with, raccoon
      rodent — *see* Contact, with, rodent
      sheep — *see* Contact, with, sheep
      specified NEC W55.89 ☑
        bite W55.81 ☑
        strike W55.82 ☑
    marine
      animal W56.89 ☑
        bite W56.81 ☑
        dolphin — *see* Contact, with, dolphin
        fish NEC — *see* Contact, with, fish

Contact — *continued*
  with — *continued*
    marine — *continued*
      animal — *continued*
        mammal — *see* Contact, with, mammal, marine
        orca — *see* Contact, with, orca
        sea lion — *see* Contact, with, sea lion
        shark — *see* Contact, with, shark
        strike W56.82 ☑
    meat
      grinder (domestic) W29.0 ☑
        industrial W31.82 ☑
        nonpowered W27.4 ☑
      slicer (domestic) W29.0 ☑
        industrial W31.82 ☑
    merry go round W31.81 ☑
    metal, hot (liquid) (molten) NEC X18 ☑
    millipede W57 ☑
    nail W45.0 ☑
      gun W29.4 ☑
    needle (sewing) W27.3 ☑
      hypodermic W46.0 ☑
        contaminated W46.1 ☑
    object (blunt) NEC
      hot NEC X19 ☑
      legal intervention — *see* Legal, intervention, blunt object
      sharp NEC W45.8 ☑
        inflicted by other person NEC W45.8 ☑
          stated as
            intentional homicide (attempt) — *see* Assault, cutting or piercing instrument
        legal intervention — *see* Legal, intervention, sharp object
        self-inflicted X78.9 ☑
    orca W56.29 ☑
      bite W56.21 ☑
      strike W56.22 ☑
    overhead plane W31.2 ☑
    paper (as sharp object) W45.1 ☑
    paper-cutter W27.5 ☑
    parrot W61.09 ☑
      bite W61.01 ☑
      strike W61.02 ☑
    pig W55.49 ☑
      bite W55.41 ☑
      strike W55.42 ☑
    pipe, hot X16 ☑
    pitchfork W27.1 ☑
    plane (metal) (wood) W27.0 ☑
      overhead W31.2 ☑
    plant thorns, spines, sharp leaves or other mechanisms W60 ☑
    powered
      garden cultivator W29.3 ☑
      household appliance, implement, or machine W29.8 ☑
      saw (industrial) W31.2 ☑
        hand W29.8 ☑
    printing machine W31.89 ☑
    psittacine bird W61.29 ☑
      bite W61.21 ☑
      macaw — *see* Contact, with, macaw
      parrot — *see* Contact, with, parrot
      strike W61.22 ☑
    pulley (block) (transmission) W24.0 ☑
      agricultural operations W30.89 ☑
    raccoon W55.59 ☑
      bite W55.51 ☑
      strike W55.52 ☑
    radial-saw (industrial) W31.2 ☑
    radiator (hot) X16 ☑
    rake W27.1 ☑
    rattlesnake X58 ☑
    reaper W30.0 ☑
    reptile W59.89 ☑
      lizard — *see* Contact, with, lizard
      snake — *see* Contact, with, snake
      specified NEC W59.89 ☑
        bite W59.81 ☑
        crushing W59.83 ☑
        strike W59.82 ☑
      turtle — *see* Contact, with, turtle
    rivet gun (powered) W29.4 ☑

Contact — *continued*
  with — *continued*
    road scraper — *see* Accident, transport, construction vehicle
    rodent (feces) (urine) W53.89 ☑
      bite W53.81 ☑
      mouse W53.09 ☑
        bite W53.01 ☑
      rat W53.19 ☑
        bite W53.11 ☑
      specified NEC W53.89 ☑
        bite W53.81 ☑
      squirrel W53.29 ☑
        bite W53.21 ☑
    roller coaster W31.81 ☑
    rope NEC W24.0 ☑
      agricultural operations W30.89 ☑
    saliva — *see* Contact, with, by type of animal
    sander W29.8 ☑
      industrial W31.2 ☑
    saucepan (hot) (glass) (metal) X15.3 ☑
    saw W27.0 ☑
      band (industrial) W31.2 ☑
      bench (industrial) W31.2 ☑
      chain W29.3 ☑
      hand W27.0 ☑
    sawing machine, metal W31.1 ☑
    scissors W27.2 ☑
    scorpion X58 ☑
    screwdriver W27.0 ☑
      powered W29.8 ☑
    sea
      anemone, cucumber or urchin (spine) X58 ☑
      lion W56.19 ☑
        bite W56.11 ☑
        strike W56.12 ☑
    serpent — *see* Contact, with, snake, by type
    sewing-machine (electric) (powered) W29.2 ☑
      not powered W27.8 ☑
    shaft (hoist) (lift) (transmission) NEC W24.0 ☑
      agricultural W30.89 ☑
    shark W56.49 ☑
      bite W56.41 ☑
      strike W56.42 ☑
    shears (hand) W27.2 ☑
      powered (industrial) W31.1 ☑
        domestic W29.2 ☑
    sheep W55.39 ☑
      bite W55.31 ☑
      strike W55.32 ☑
    shovel W27.8 ☑
      steam — *see* Accident, transport, construction vehicle
    snake (nonvenomous) W59.19 ☑
      bite W59.11 ☑
      crushing W59.13 ☑
      strike W59.12 ☑
    spade W27.1 ☑
    spider (venomous) X58 ☑
    spin-drier W29.2 ☑
    spinning machine W31.89 ☑
    splinter W45.8 ☑
    sports equipment W21.9 ☑
    staple gun (powered) W29.8 ☑
    steam X13.1 ☑
      engine W31.3 ☑
      inhalation X13.0 ☑
      pipe X16 ☑
      shovel W31.89 ☑
    stove (hot) (kitchen) X15.0 ☑
    substance, hot NEC X19 ☑
      molten (metal) X18 ☑
    sword W26.1 ☑
      assault X99.2 ☑
      stated as undetermined whether accidental or intentional Y28.2 ☑
      suicide (attempt) X78.2 ☑
    tarantula X58 ☑
    thresher W30.0 ☑
    tin can lid W45.2 ☑
    toad W62.1 ☑
    toaster (hot) X15.1 ☑
    tool W27.8 ☑
      hand (not powered) W27.8 ☑
        auger W27.0 ☑

Contact — *continued*
  with — *continued*
    tool — *continued*
      hand — *continued*
        axe W27.0 ☑
        can opener W27.4 ☑
        chisel W27.0 ☑
        fork W27.4 ☑
        garden W27.1 ☑
        handsaw W27.0 ☑
        hoe W27.1 ☑
        ice-pick W27.4 ☑
        kitchen utensil W27.4 ☑
        manual
          lawn mower W27.1 ☑
          sewing machine W27.8 ☑
        meat grinder W27.4 ☑
        needle (sewing) W27.3 ☑
          hypodermic W46.0 ☑
            contaminated W46.1 ☑
        paper cutter W27.5 ☑
        pitchfork W27.1 ☑
        rake W27.1 ☑
        scissors W27.2 ☑
        screwdriver W27.0 ☑
        specified NEC W27.8 ☑
        workbench W27.0 ☑
      hot X17 ☑
      powered W29.8 ☑
        blender W29.0 ☑
          commercial W31.82 ☑
        can opener W29.0 ☑
          commercial W31.82 ☑
        chainsaw W29.3 ☑
        clothes dryer W29.2 ☑
          commercial W31.82 ☑
        dishwasher W29.2 ☑
          commercial W31.82 ☑
        edger W29.3 ☑
        electric fan W29.2 ☑
          commercial W31.82 ☑
        electric knife W29.1 ☑
        food processor W29.0 ☑
          commercial W31.82 ☑
        garbage disposal W29.0 ☑
          commercial W31.82 ☑
        garden tool W29.3 ☑
        hedge trimmer W29.3 ☑
        ice maker W29.0 ☑
          commercial W31.82 ☑
        kitchen appliance W29.0 ☑
          commercial W31.82 ☑
        lawn mower W28 ☑
        meat grinder W29.0 ☑
          commercial W31.82 ☑
        mixer W29.0 ☑
          commercial W31.82 ☑
        rototiller W29.3 ☑
        sewing machine W29.2 ☑
          commercial W31.82 ☑
        washing machine W29.2 ☑
          commercial W31.82 ☑
    transmission device (belt, cable, chain, gear, pinion, shaft) W24.1 ☑
      agricultural operations W30.89 ☑
    turbine (gas) (water-driven) W31.3 ☑
    turkey W61.49 ☑
      peck W61.43 ☑
      strike W61.42 ☑
    turtle (nonvenomous) W59.29 ☑
      bite W59.21 ☑
      strike W59.22 ☑
      terrestrial W59.89 ☑
        bite W59.81 ☑
        crushing W59.83 ☑
        strike W59.82 ☑
    under-cutter W31.0 ☑
    urine — *see* Contact, with, by type of animal
    vehicle
      agricultural use (transport) — *see* Accident, transport, agricultural vehicle
        not on public highway W30.81 ☑
      industrial use (transport) — *see* Accident, transport, industrial vehicle
        not on public highway W31.83 ☑

Contact — *continued*
- with — *continued*
  - vehicle — *continued*
    - off-road use (transport) — *see* Accident, transport, all-terrain or off-road vehicle
      - not on public highway W31.83 ☑
    - special construction use (transport) — *see* Accident, transport, construction vehicle
      - not on public highway W31.83 ☑
  - venomous
    - animal X58 ☑
    - arthropods X58 ☑
    - lizard X58 ☑
    - marine animal NEC X58 ☑
    - marine plant NEC X58 ☑
    - millipedes (tropical) X58 ☑
    - plant(s) X58 ☑
    - snake X58 ☑
    - spider X58 ☑
    - viper X58 ☑
  - washing-machine (powered) W29.2 ☑
  - wasp X58 ☑
  - weaving-machine W31.89 ☑
  - winch W24.0 ☑
    - agricultural operations W30.89 ☑
  - wire NEC W24.0 ☑
    - agricultural operations W30.89 ☑
  - wood slivers W45.8 ☑
  - yellow jacket X58 ☑
  - zebra — *see* Contact, with, hoof stock NEC

Coup de soleil X32 ☑

Crash
- aircraft (in transit) (powered) V95.9 ☑
  - balloon V96.01 ☑
  - fixed wing NEC (private) V95.21 ☑
    - commercial V95.31 ☑
  - glider V96.21 ☑
    - hang V96.11 ☑
    - powered V95.11 ☑
  - helicopter V95.01 ☑
  - in war operations — *see* War operations, destruction of aircraft
  - microlight V95.11 ☑
  - nonpowered V96.9 ☑
    - specified NEC V96.8 ☑
  - powered NEC V95.8 ☑
  - stated as
    - homicide (attempt) Y08.81 ☑
    - suicide (attempt) X83.0 ☑
  - ultralight V95.11 ☑
- spacecraft V95.41 ☑
- transport vehicle NEC (*see also* Accident, transport) V89.9 ☑
  - homicide (attempt) Y03.8 ☑
  - motor NEC (traffic) V89.2 ☑
    - homicide (attempt) Y03.8 ☑
  - suicide (attempt) — *see* Suicide, collision

Cruelty (mental) (physical) (sexual) X58 ☑

Crushed (accidentally) X58 ☑
- between objects (moving) (stationary and moving) W23.0 ☑
  - stationary W23.1 ☑
- by
  - alligator W58.03 ☑
  - avalanche NEC — *see* Landslide
  - cave-in W20.0 ☑
    - caused by cataclysmic earth surface movement — *see* Landslide
  - crocodile W58.13 ☑
  - crowd or human stampede W52 ☑
  - falling
    - aircraft V97.39 ☑
      - in war operations — *see* War operations, destruction of aircraft
    - earth, material W20.0 ☑
      - caused by cataclysmic earth surface movement — *see* Landslide
    - object NEC W20.8 ☑
  - landslide NEC — *see* Landslide
  - lizard (nonvenomous) W59.09 ☑
  - machinery — *see* Contact, with, by type of machine
  - reptile NEC W59.89 ☑
  - snake (nonvenomous) W59.13 ☑
- in
  - machinery — *see* Contact, with, by type of machine

Cut, cutting (any part of body) (accidental) (*see also* Contact, with, by object or machine)
- during medical or surgical treatment as misadventure — *see* Index to Diseases and Injuries, Complications
- homicide (attempt) — *see* Assault, cutting or piercing instrument
- inflicted by other person — *see* Assault, cutting or piercing instrument
- legal
  - execution — *see* Legal, intervention
  - intervention — *see* Legal, intervention, sharp object
- machine NEC (*see also* Contact, with, by type of machine) W31.9 ☑
- self-inflicted — *see* Suicide, cutting or piercing instrument
- suicide (attempt) — *see* Suicide, cutting or piercing instrument

Cyclone (any injury) X37.1 ☑

D

Decapitation (accidental circumstances) NEC X58 ☑
- homicide X99.9 ☑
- legal execution — *see* Legal, intervention

Dehydration from lack of water X58 ☑

Deprivation X58 ☑

Derailment (accidental)
- railway (rolling stock) (train) (vehicle) (without antecedent collision) V81.7 ☑
  - with antecedent collision — *see* Accident, transport, railway vehicle occupant
- streetcar (without antecedent collision) V82.7 ☑
  - with antecedent collision — *see* Accident, transport, streetcar occupant

Descent
- parachute (voluntary) (without accident to aircraft) V97.29 ☑
  - due to accident to aircraft — *see* Accident, transport, aircraft

Desertion X58 ☑

Destitution X58 ☑

Disability, late effect or sequela of injury — *see* Sequelae

Discharge (accidental)
- airgun W34.010 ☑
  - assault X95.01 ☑
  - homicide (attempt) X95.01 ☑
  - stated as undetermined whether accidental or intentional Y24.0 ☑
  - suicide (attempt) X74.01 ☑
- BB gun — *see* Discharge, airgun
- firearm (accidental) W34.00 ☑
  - assault X95.9 ☑
  - handgun (pistol) (revolver) W32.0 ☑
    - assault X93 ☑
    - homicide (attempt) X93 ☑
    - legal intervention — *see* Legal, intervention, firearm, handgun
    - stated as undetermined whether accidental or intentional Y22 ☑
    - suicide (attempt) X72 ☑
  - homicide (attempt) X95.9 ☑
  - hunting rifle W33.02 ☑
    - assault X94.1 ☑
    - homicide (attempt) X94.1 ☑
    - legal intervention
      - injuring
        - bystander Y35.032 ☑
        - law enforcement personnel Y35.031 ☑
        - suspect Y35.033 ☑
    - stated as undetermined whether accidental or intentional Y23.1 ☑
    - suicide (attempt) X73.1 ☑
  - larger W33.00 ☑
    - assault X94.9 ☑
    - homicide (attempt) X94.9 ☑
    - hunting rifle — *see* Discharge, firearm, hunting rifle
    - legal intervention — *see* Legal, intervention, firearm by type of firearm
    - machine gun — *see* Discharge, firearm, machine gun
    - shotgun — *see* Discharge, firearm, shotgun
    - specified NEC W33.09 ☑

Discharge — *continued*
- firearm — *continued*
  - larger — *continued*
    - specified — *continued*
      - assault X94.8 ☑
      - homicide (attempt) X94.8 ☑
      - legal intervention
        - injuring
          - bystander Y35.092 ☑
          - law enforcement personnel Y35.091 ☑
          - suspect Y35.093 ☑
      - stated as undetermined whether accidental or intentional Y23.8 ☑
      - suicide (attempt) X73.8 ☑
    - stated as undetermined whether accidental or intentional Y23.9 ☑
    - suicide (attempt) X73.9 ☑
  - legal intervention
    - injuring
      - bystander Y35.002 ☑
      - law enforcement personnel Y35.001 ☑
      - suspect Y35.03 ☑
    - using rubber bullet
      - injuring
        - bystander Y35.042 ☑
        - law enforcement personnel Y35.041 ☑
        - suspect Y35.043 ☑
  - machine gun W33.03 ☑
    - assault X94.2 ☑
    - homicide (attempt) X94.2 ☑
    - legal intervention — *see* Legal, intervention, firearm, machine gun
    - stated as undetermined whether accidental or intentional Y23.3 ☑
    - suicide (attempt) X73.2 ☑
  - pellet gun — *see* Discharge, airgun
  - shotgun W33.01 ☑
    - assault X94.0 ☑
    - homicide (attempt) X94.0 ☑
    - legal intervention — *see* Legal, intervention, firearm, specified NEC
    - stated as undetermined whether accidental or intentional Y23.0 ☑
    - suicide (attempt) X73.0 ☑
  - specified NEC W34.09 ☑
    - assault X95.8 ☑
    - homicide (attempt) X95.8 ☑
    - legal intervention — *see* Legal, intervention, firearm, specified NEC
    - stated as undetermined whether accidental or intentional Y24.8 ☑
    - suicide (attempt) X74.8 ☑
  - stated as undetermined whether accidental or intentional Y24.9 ☑
  - suicide (attempt) X74.9 ☑
  - Very pistol W34.09 ☑
    - assault X95.8 ☑
    - homicide (attempt) X95.8 ☑
    - stated as undetermined whether accidental or intentional Y24.8 ☑
    - suicide (attempt) X74.8 ☑
- firework(s) W39 ☑
  - stated as undetermined whether accidental or intentional Y25 ☑
- gas-operated gun NEC W34.018 ☑
  - airgun — *see* Discharge, airgun
  - assault X95.09 ☑
  - homicide (attempt) X95.09 ☑
  - paintball gun — *see* Discharge, paintball gun
  - stated as undetermined whether accidental or intentional Y24.8 ☑
  - suicide (attempt) X74.09 ☑
- gun NEC (*see also* Discharge, firearm NEC)
  - air — *see* Discharge, airgun
  - BB — *see* Discharge, airgun
  - for single hand use — *see* Discharge, firearm, handgun
  - hand — *see* Discharge, firearm, handgun
  - machine — *see* Discharge, firearm, machine gun
  - other specified — *see* Discharge, firearm NEC
  - paintball — *see* Discharge, paintball gun
  - pellet — *see* Discharge, airgun
- handgun — *see* Discharge, firearm, handgun
- machine gun — *see* Discharge, firearm, machine gun

Discharge — *continued*
paintball gun W34.011 ☑
assault X95.02 ☑
homicide (attempt) X95.02 ☑
stated as undetermined whether accidental or intentional Y24.8 ☑
suicide (attempt) X74.02 ☑
pistol — *see* Discharge, firearm, handgun
flare — *see* Discharge, firearm, Very pistol
pellet — *see* Discharge, airgun
Very — *see* Discharge, firearm, Very pistol
revolver — *see* Discharge, firearm, handgun
rifle (hunting) — *see* Discharge, firearm, hunting rifle
shotgun — *see* Discharge, firearm, shotgun
spring-operated gun NEC W34.018 ☑
assault X95.09 ☑
homicide (attempt) X95.09 ☑
stated as undetermined whether accidental or intentional Y24.8 ☑
suicide (attempt) X74.09 ☑
Disease
Andes W94.11 ☑
aviator's — *see* Air, pressure
range W94.11 ☑
Diver's disease, palsy, paralysis, squeeze — *see* Air, pressure
Diving (into water) — *see* Accident, diving
Dog bite W54.0 ☑
Dragged by transport vehicle NEC (*see also* Accident, transport) V09.9 ☑
Drinking poison (accidental) — *see* Table of Drugs and Chemicals
Dropped (accidentally) **while being carried or supported by other person** W04 ☑
Drowning (accidental) W74 ☑
assault X92.9 ☑
due to
accident (to)
machinery — *see* Contact, with, by type of machine
watercraft V90.89 ☑
burning V90.29 ☑
powered V90.23 ☑
fishing boat V90.22 ☑
jetskis V90.23 ☑
merchant ship V90.20 ☑
passenger ship V90.21 ☑
unpowered V90.28 ☑
canoe V90.25 ☑
inflatable V90.26 ☑
kayak V90.25 ☑
sailboat V90.24 ☑
water skis V90.27 ☑
crushed V90.39 ☑
powered V90.33 ☑
fishing boat V90.32 ☑
jetskis V90.33 ☑
merchant ship V90.30 ☑
passenger ship V90.31 ☑
unpowered V90.38 ☑
canoe V90.35 ☑
inflatable V90.36 ☑
kayak V90.35 ☑
sailboat V90.34 ☑
water skis V90.37 ☑
overturning V90.09 ☑
powered V90.03 ☑
fishing boat V90.02 ☑
jetskis V90.03 ☑
merchant ship V90.00 ☑
passenger ship V90.01 ☑
unpowered V90.08 ☑
canoe V90.05 ☑
inflatable V90.06 ☑
kayak V90.05 ☑
sailboat V90.04 ☑
sinking V90.19 ☑
powered V90.13 ☑
fishing boat V90.12 ☑
jetskis V90.13 ☑
merchant ship V90.10 ☑
passenger ship V90.11 ☑
unpowered V90.18 ☑
canoe V90.15 ☑
inflatable V90.16 ☑
kayak V90.15 ☑

Drowning — *continued*
due to — *continued*
accident — *continued*
watercraft — *continued*
sinking — *continued*
unpowered — *continued*
sailboat V90.14 ☑
specified type NEC V90.89 ☑
powered V90.83 ☑
fishing boat V90.82 ☑
jetskis V90.83 ☑
merchant ship V90.80 ☑
passenger ship V90.81 ☑
unpowered V90.88 ☑
canoe V90.85 ☑
inflatable V90.86 ☑
kayak V90.85 ☑
sailboat V90.84 ☑
water skis V90.87 ☑
avalanche — *see* Landslide
cataclysmic
earth surface movement NEC — *see* Forces of nature, earth movement
storm — *see* Forces of nature, cataclysmic storm
cloudburst X37.8 ☑
cyclone X37.1 ☑
fall overboard (from) V92.09 ☑
powered craft V92.03 ☑
ferry boat V92.01 ☑
fishing boat V92.02 ☑
jetskis V92.03 ☑
liner V92.01 ☑
merchant ship V92.00 ☑
passenger ship V92.01 ☑
resulting from
accident to watercraft — *see* Drowning, due to, accident to, watercraft
being washed overboard (from) V92.29 ☑
powered craft V92.23 ☑
ferry boat V92.21 ☑
fishing boat V92.22 ☑
jetskis V92.23 ☑
liner V92.21 ☑
merchant ship V92.20 ☑
passenger ship V92.21 ☑
unpowered craft V92.28 ☑
canoe V92.25 ☑
inflatable V92.26 ☑
kayak V92.25 ☑
sailboat V92.24 ☑
surf-board V92.28 ☑
water skis V92.27 ☑
windsurfer V92.28 ☑
motion of watercraft V92.19 ☑
powered craft V92.13 ☑
ferry boat V92.11 ☑
fishing boat V92.12 ☑
jetskis V92.13 ☑
liner V92.11 ☑
merchant ship V92.10 ☑
passenger ship V92.11 ☑
unpowered craft
canoe V92.15 ☑
inflatable V92.16 ☑
kayak V92.15 ☑
sailboat V92.14 ☑
unpowered craft V92.08 ☑
canoe V92.05 ☑
inflatable V92.06 ☑
kayak V92.05 ☑
sailboat V92.04 ☑
surf-board V92.08 ☑
water skis V92.07 ☑
windsurfer V92.08 ☑
hurricane X37.0 ☑
jumping into water from watercraft (involved in accident) (*see also* Drowning, due to, accident to, watercraft)
without accident to or on watercraft W16.711 ☑
tidal wave NEC — *see* Forces of nature, tidal wave
torrential rain X37.8 ☑

Drowning — *continued*
following
fall
into
bathtub W16.211 ☑
bucket W16.221 ☑
fountain — *see* Drowning, following, fall, into, water, specified NEC
quarry — *see* Drowning, following, fall, into, water, specified NEC
reservoir — *see* Drowning, following, fall, into, water, specified NEC
swimming-pool W16.011 ☑
stated as undetermined whether accidental or intentional Y21.3 ☑
striking
bottom W16.021 ☑
wall W16.031 ☑
suicide (attempt) X71.2 ☑
water NOS W16.41 ☑
natural (lake) (open sea) (river) (stream) (pond) W16.111 ☑
striking
bottom W16.121 ☑
side W16.131 ☑
specified NEC W16.311 ☑
striking
bottom W16.321 ☑
wall W16.331 ☑
overboard NEC — *see* Drowning, due to, fall overboard
jump or dive
from boat W16.711 ☑
striking bottom W16.721 ☑
into
fountain — *see* Drowning, following, jump or dive, into, water, specified NEC
quarry — *see* Drowning, following, jump or dive, into, water, specified NEC
reservoir — *see* Drowning, following, jump or dive, into, water, specified NEC
swimming-pool W16.511 ☑
striking
bottom W16.521 ☑
wall W16.531 ☑
suicide (attempt) X71.2 ☑
water NOS W16.91 ☑
natural (lake) (open sea) (river) (stream) (pond) W16.611 ☑
specified NEC W16.811 ☑
bottom W16.821 ☑
striking
bottom W16.821 ☑
wall W16.831 ☑
striking
bottom W16.821 ☑
wall W16.831 ☑
striking bottom W16.621 ☑
homicide (attempt) X92.9 ☑
in
bathtub (accidental) W65 ☑
assault X92.0 ☑
following fall W16.211 ☑
stated as undetermined whether accidental or intentional Y21.1 ☑
stated as undetermined whether accidental or intentional Y21.0 ☑
suicide (attempt) X71.0 ☑
lake — *see* Drowning, in, natural water
natural water (lake) (open sea) (river) (stream) (pond) W69 ☑
assault X92.3 ☑
following
dive or jump W16.611 ☑
striking bottom W16.621 ☑
fall W16.111 ☑
striking
bottom W16.121 ☑
side W16.131 ☑
stated as undetermined whether accidental or intentional Y21.4 ☑
suicide (attempt) X71.3 ☑
quarry — *see* Drowning, in, specified place NEC
quenching tank — *see* Drowning, in, specified place NEC
reservoir — *see* Drowning, in, specified place NEC

☑ Additional Character Required — Refer to the Tabular List for Character Selection
🔻 Subterms under main terms may continue to next column or page

Drowning — *continued*
  in — *continued*
      river — *see* Drowning, in, natural water
      sea — *see* Drowning, in, natural water
      specified place NEC W73 ☑
        assault X92.8 ☑
        following
          dive or jump W16.811 ☑
            striking
              bottom W16.821 ☑
              wall W16.831 ☑
          fall W16.311 ☑
            striking
              bottom W16.321 ☑
              wall W16.331 ☑
        stated as undetermined whether accidental or
          intentional Y21.8 ☑
        suicide (attempt) X71.8 ☑
      stream — *see* Drowning, in, natural water
      swimming-pool W67 ☑
        assault X92.1 ☑
          following fall X92.2 ☑
        following
          dive or jump W16.511 ☑
            striking
              bottom W16.521 ☑
              wall W16.531 ☑
          fall W16.011 ☑
            striking
              bottom W16.021 ☑
              wall W16.031 ☑
        stated as undetermined whether accidental or
          intentional Y21.2 ☑
          following fall Y21.3 ☑
        suicide (attempt) X71.1 ☑
          following fall X71.2 ☑
      war operations — *see* War operations, restriction
        of airway
  resulting from accident to watercraft — *see* Drowning,
    due to, accident, watercraft
  self-inflicted X71.9 ☑
  stated as undetermined whether accidental or inten-
    tional Y21.9 ☑
  suicide (attempt) X71.9 ☑

E

Earth falling (on) W20.0 ☑
  caused by cataclysmic earth surface movement or
    eruption — *see* Landslide
Earth (surface) movement NEC — *see* Forces of nature,
  earth movement
Earthquake (any injury) X34 ☑
Effect(s) (adverse) **of**
  air pressure (any) — *see* Air, pressure
  cold, excessive (exposure to) — *see* Exposure, cold
  heat (excessive) — *see* Heat
  hot place (weather) B — *see* Heat
  insolation X30 ☑
  late — *see* Sequelae
  motion — *see* Motion
  nuclear explosion or weapon in war operations — *see*
    War operations, nuclear weapon
  radiation — *see* Radiation
  travel — *see* Travel
Electric shock (accidental) (by) (in) — *see* Exposure,
  electric current
Electrocution (accidental) — *see* Exposure, electric current
Endotracheal tube wrongly placed during anesthetic
  procedure
Entanglement
  in
    bed linen, causing suffocation T71 ☑
    wheel of pedal cycle V19.88 ☑
Entry of foreign body or material — *see* Foreign body
Environmental pollution related condition — *see*
  category Z57
Execution, legal (any method) — *see* Legal, intervention
Exhaustion
  cold — *see* Exposure, cold
  due to excessive exertion — *see* Overexertion
  heat — *see* Heat
Explosion (accidental) (of) (with secondary fire) W40.9 ☑
  acetylene W40.1 ☑
  aerosol can W36.1 ☑

Explosion — *continued*
  air tank (compressed) (in machinery) W36.2 ☑
  aircraft (in transit) (powered) NEC V95.9 ☑
    balloon V96.05 ☑
    fixed wing NEC (private) V95.25 ☑
      commercial V95.35 ☑
    glider V96.25 ☑
      hang V96.15 ☑
      powered V95.15 ☑
    helicopter V95.05 ☑
    in war operations — *see* War operations, destruc-
      tion of aircraft
    microlight V95.15 ☑
    nonpowered V96.9 ☑
      specified NEC V96.8 ☑
    powered NEC V95.8 ☑
    stated as
      homicide (attempt) Y03.8 ☑
      suicide (attempt) X83.0 ☑
    ultralight V95.15 ☑
  anesthetic gas in operating room W40.1 ☑
  antipersonnel bomb W40.8 ☑
    assault X96.0 ☑
    homicide (attempt) X96.0 ☑
    suicide (attempt) X75 ☑
  assault X96.9 ☑
  bicycle tire W37.0 ☑
  blasting (cap) (materials) W40.0 ☑
  boiler (machinery), not on transport vehicle W35 ☑
    on watercraft — *see* Explosion, in, watercraft
  butane W40.1 ☑
  caused by other person X96.9 ☑
  coal gas W40.1 ☑
  detonator W40.0 ☑
  dump (munitions) W40.8 ☑
  dynamite W40.0 ☑
    in
      assault X96.8 ☑
      homicide (attempt) X96.8 ☑
      legal intervention
        injuring
          bystander Y35.112 ☑
          law enforcement personnel Y35.111 ☑
          suspect Y35.113 ☑
      suicide (attempt) X75 ☑
  explosive (material) W40.9 ☑
    gas W40.1 ☑
    in blasting operation W40.0 ☑
    specified NEC W40.8 ☑
      in
        assault X96.8 ☑
        homicide (attempt) X96.8 ☑
        legal intervention
          injuring
            bystander Y35.192 ☑
            law enforcement personnel
              Y35.191 ☑
            suspect Y35.193 ☑
        suicide (attempt) X75 ☑
  factory (munitions) W40.8 ☑
  fertilizer bomb W40.8 ☑
    assault X96.3 ☑
    homicide (attempt) X96.3 ☑
    suicide (attempt) X75 ☑
  firearm (parts) NEC W34.19 ☑
    airgun W34.110 ☑
    BB gun W34.110 ☑
    gas, air or spring-operated gun NEC W34.118 ☑
    hangun W32.1 ☑
    hunting rifle W33.12 ☑
    larger firearm W33.10 ☑
      specified NEC W33.19 ☑
    machine gun W33.13 ☑
    paintball gun W34.111 ☑
    pellet gun W34.110 ☑
    shotgun W33.11 ☑
    Very pistol [flare] W34.19 ☑
  fire-damp W40.1 ☑
  fireworks W39 ☑
  gas (coal) (explosive) W40.1 ☑
    cylinder W36.9 ☑
      aerosol can W36.1 ☑
      air tank W36.2 ☑
      pressurized W36.3 ☑
      specified NEC W36.8 ☑

Explosion — *continued*
  gasoline (fumes) (tank) not in moving motor vehicle
    W40.1 ☑
    bomb W40.8 ☑
      assault X96.1 ☑
      homicide (attempt) X96.1 ☑
      suicide (attempt) X75 ☑
    in motor vehicle — *see* Accident, transport, by type
      of vehicle
  grain store W40.8 ☑
  grenade W40.8 ☑
    in
      assault X96.8 ☑
      homicide (attempt) X96.8 ☑
      legal intervention
        injuring
          bystander Y35.192 ☑
          law enforcement personnel Y35.191 ☑
          suspect Y35.193 ☑
      suicide (attempt) X75 ☑
  handgun (parts) — *see* Explosion, firearm, hangun
    (parts)
  homicide (attempt) X96.9 ☑
    antipersonnel bomb — *see* Explosion, antiperson-
      nel bomb
    fertilizer bomb — *see* Explosion, fertilizer bomb
    gasoline bomb — *see* Explosion, gasoline bomb
    letter bomb — *see* Explosion, letter bomb
    pipe bomb — *see* Explosion, pipe bomb
    specified NEC X96.8 ☑
  hose, pressurized W37.8 ☑
  hot water heater, tank (in machinery) W35 ☑
    on watercraft — *see* Explosion, in, watercraft
  in, on
    dump W40.8 ☑
    factory W40.8 ☑
    mine (of explosive gases) NEC W40.1 ☑
    watercraft V93.59 ☑
      powered craft V93.53 ☑
        ferry boat V93.51 ☑
        fishing boat V93.52 ☑
        jetskis V93.53 ☑
        liner V93.51 ☑
        merchant ship V93.50 ☑
        passenger ship V93.51 ☑
        sailboat V93.54 ☑
  letter bomb W40.8 ☑
    assault X96.2 ☑
    homicide (attempt) X96.2 ☑
    suicide (attempt) X75 ☑
  machinery (*see also* Contact, with, by type of machine)
    on board watercraft — *see* Explosion, in, watercraft
    pressure vessel — *see* Explosion, by type of vessel
  methane W40.1 ☑
  mine W40.1 ☑
  missile NEC W40.8 ☑
  mortar bomb W40.8 ☑
    in
      assault X96.8 ☑
      homicide (attempt) X96.8 ☑
      legal intervention
        injuring
          bystander Y35.192 ☑
          law enforcement personnel Y35.191 ☑
          suspect Y35.193 ☑
      suicide (attempt) X75 ☑
  munitions (dump) (factory) W40.8 ☑
  pipe, pressurized W37.8 ☑
    bomb W40.8 ☑
      assault X96.4 ☑
      homicide (attempt) X96.4 ☑
      suicide (attempt) X75 ☑
  pressure, pressurized
    cooker W38 ☑
    gas tank (in machinery) W36.3 ☑
    hose W37.8 ☑
    pipe W37.8 ☑
    specified device NEC W38 ☑
    tire W37.8 ☑
      bicycle W37.0 ☑
    vessel (in machinery) W38 ☑
  propane W40.1 ☑
  self-inflicted X75 ☑
  shell (artillery) NEC W40.8 ☑
    during war operations — *see* War operations, ex-
      plosion

Explosion — *continued*
  shell — *continued*
    in
      legal intervention
        injuring
          bystander Y35.122 ☑
          law enforcement personnel Y35.121 ☑
          suspect Y35.123 ☑
      war — *see* War operations, explosion
  spacecraft V95.45 ☑
  stated as undetermined whether accidental or intentional Y25 ☑
  steam or water lines (in machinery) W37.8 ☑
  stove W40.9 ☑
  suicide (attempt) X75 ☑
  tire, pressurized W37.8 ☑
    bicycle W37.0 ☑
  undetermined whether accidental or intentional Y25 ☑
  vehicle tire NEC W37.8 ☑
    bicycle W37.0 ☑
  war operations — *see* War operations, explosion
Exposure (to) X58 ☑
  air pressure change — *see* Air, pressure
  cold (accidental) (excessive) (extreme) (natural) (place) X31 ☑
    assault Y08.89 ☑
    due to
      man-made conditions W93.8 ☑
        dry ice (contact) W93.01 ☑
          inhalation W93.02 ☑
        liquid air (contact) (hydrogen) (nitrogen) W93.11 ☑
          inhalation W93.12 ☑
        refrigeration unit (deep freeze) W93.2 ☑
        suicide (attempt) X83.2 ☑
      weather (conditions) X31 ☑
    homicide (attempt) Y08.89 ☑
    self-inflicted X83.2 ☑
  due to abandonment or neglect X58 ☑
  electric current W86.8 ☑
    appliance (faulty) W86.8 ☑
      domestic W86.0 ☑
    caused by other person Y08.89 ☑
    conductor (faulty) W86.1 ☑
    control apparatus (faulty) W86.1 ☑
    electric power generating plant, distribution station W86.1 ☑
    electroshock gun — *see* Exposure, electric current, taser
    high-voltage cable W85 ☑
    homicide (attempt) Y08.89 ☑
    legal execution — *see* Legal, intervention, specified means NEC
    lightning — *see* subcategory T75.0 ☑
    live rail W86.8 ☑
    misadventure in medical or surgical procedure in electroshock therapy Y63.4
    motor (electric) (faulty) W86.8 ☑
      domestic W86.0 ☑
    self-inflicted X83.1 ☑
    specified NEC W86.8 ☑
      domestic W86.0 ☑
    stun gun — *see* Exposure, electric current, taser
    suicide (attempt) X83.1 ☑
    taser W86.8 ☑
      assault Y08.89 ☑
      legal intervention — *see* category Y35 ☑
      self-harm (intentional) X83.8 ☑
      undetermined intent Y33 ☑
    third rail W86.8 ☑
    transformer (faulty) W86.1 ☑
    transmission lines W85 ☑
  environmental tobacco smoke X58 ☑
  excessive
    cold — *see* Exposure, cold
    heat (natural) NEC X30 ☑
      man-made W92 ☑
  factor(s) NOS X58 ☑
    environmental NEC X58 ☑
      man-made NEC W99 ☑
      natural NEC — *see* Forces of nature
    specified NEC X58 ☑
  fire, flames (accidental) X08.8 ☑
    assault X97 ☑

Exposure — *continued*
  fire, flames — *continued*
    campfire — *see* Exposure, fire, controlled, not in building
    controlled (in)
      with ignition (of) clothing (*see also* Ignition, clothes) X06.2 ☑
        nightwear X05 ☑
      bonfire — *see* Exposure, fire, controlled, not in building
      brazier (in building or structure) (*see also* Exposure, fire, controlled, building)
        not in building or structure — *see* Exposure, fire, controlled, not in building
      building or structure X02.0 ☑
        with
          fall from building X02.3 ☑
          from building X02.5 ☑
          injury due to building collapse X02.2 ☑
          smoke inhalation X02.1 ☑
        hit by object from building X02.4 ☑
        specified mode of injury NEC X02.8 ☑
      fireplace, furnace or stove — *see* Exposure, fire, controlled, building
      not in building or structure X03.0 ☑
        with
          fall X03.3 ☑
          smoke inhalation X03.1 ☑
        hit by object X03.4 ☑
        specified mode of injury NEC X03.8 ☑
      trash — *see* Exposure, fire, controlled, not in building
    fireplace — *see* Exposure, fire, controlled, building
    fittings or furniture (in building or structure) (uncontrolled) — *see* Exposure, fire, uncontrolled, building
    forest (uncontrolled) — *see* Exposure, fire, uncontrolled, not in building
    grass (uncontrolled) — *see* Exposure, fire, uncontrolled, not in building
    hay (uncontrolled) — *see* Exposure, fire, uncontrolled, not in building
    homicide (attempt) X97 ☑
    ignition of highly flammable material X04 ☑
    in, of, on, starting in
      machinery — *see* Contact, with, by type of machine
      motor vehicle (in motion) (*see also* Accident, transport, occupant by type of vehicle) V87.8 ☑
        with collision — *see* Collision
      railway rolling stock, train, vehicle V81.81 ☑
        with collision — *see* Accident, transport, railway vehicle occupant
      street car (in motion) V82.8 ☑
        with collision — *see* Accident, transport, streetcar occupant
      transport vehicle NEC (*see also* Accident, transport)
        with collision — *see* Collision
      war operations (*see also* War operations, fire)
        from nuclear explosion — *see* War operations, nuclear weapons
      watercraft (in transit) (not in transit) V91.09 ☑
        localized — *see* Burn, on board watercraft, due to, fire on board
        powered craft V91.03 ☑
          ferry boat V91.01 ☑
          fishing boat V91.02 ☑
          jet skis V91.03 ☑
          liner V91.01 ☑
          merchant ship V91.00 ☑
          passenger ship V91.01 ☑
        unpowered craft V91.08 ☑
          canoe V91.05 ☑
          inflatable V91.06 ☑
          kayak V91.05 ☑
          sailboat V91.04 ☑
          surf-board V91.08 ☑
          waterskis V91.07 ☑
          windsurfer V91.08 ☑
    lumber (uncontrolled) — *see* Exposure, fire, uncontrolled, not in building
    mine (uncontrolled) — *see* Exposure, fire, uncontrolled, not in building

Exposure — *continued*
  fire, flames — *continued*
    prairie (uncontrolled) — *see* Exposure, fire, uncontrolled, not in building
    resulting from
      explosion — *see* Explosion
      lightning X08.8 ☑
    self-inflicted X76 ☑
    specified NEC X08.8 ☑
    started by other person X97 ☑
    stated as undetermined whether accidental or intentional Y26 ☑
    stove — *see* Exposure, fire, controlled, building
    suicide (attempt) X76 ☑
    tunnel (uncontrolled) — *see* Exposure, fire, uncontrolled, not in building
    uncontrolled
      in building or structure X00.0 ☑
        with
          fall from building X00.3 ☑
          injury due to building collapse X00.2 ☑
          jump from building X00.5 ☑
          smoke inhalation X00.1 ☑
        bed X08.00 ☑
          due to
            cigarette X08.01 ☑
            specified material NEC X08.09 ☑
        furniture NEC X08.20 ☑
          due to
            cigarette X08.21 ☑
            specified material NEC X08.29 ☑
        hit by object from building X00.4 ☑
        sofa X08.10 ☑
          due to
            cigarette X08.11 ☑
            specified material NEC X08.19 ☑
        specified mode of injury NEC X00.8 ☑
      not in building or structure (any) X01.0 ☑
        with
          fall X01.3 ☑
          smoke inhalation X01.1 ☑
        hit by object X01.4 ☑
        specified mode of injury NEC X01.8 ☑
    undetermined whether accidental or intentional Y26 ☑
  forces of nature NEC — *see* Forces of nature
  G-forces (abnormal) W49.9 ☑
  gravitational forces (abnormal) W49.9 ☑
  heat (natural) NEC — *see* Heat
  high-pressure jet (hydraulic) (pneumatic) W49.9 ☑
  hydraulic jet W49.9 ☑
  inanimate mechanical force W49.9 ☑
  jet, high-pressure (hydraulic) (pneumatic) W49.9 ☑
  lightning — *see* subcategory T75.0 ☑
    causing fire — *see* Exposure, fire
  mechanical forces NEC W49.9 ☑
    animate NEC W64 ☑
    inanimate NEC W49.9 ☑
  noise W42.9 ☑
    supersonic W42.0 ☑
  noxious substance — *see* Table of Drugs and Chemicals
  pneumatic jet W49.9 ☑
  prolonged in deep-freeze unit or refrigerator W93.2 ☑
  radiation — *see* Radiation
  smoke (*see also* Exposure, fire)
    tobacco, second hand Z77.22
  specified factors NEC X58 ☑
  sunlight X32 ☑
    man-made (sun lamp) W89.8 ☑
      tanning bed W89.1 ☑
  supersonic waves W42.0 ☑
  transmission line(s), electric W85 ☑
  vibration W49.9 ☑
  waves
    infrasound W49.9 ☑
    sound W42.9 ☑
    supersonic W42.0 ☑
  weather NEC — *see* Forces of nature
External cause status Y99.9
  child assisting in compensated work for family Y99.8
  civilian activity done for financial or other compensation Y99.0
  civilian activity done for income or pay Y99.0
  family member assisting in compensated work for other family member Y99.8

External cause status — *continued*
hobby not done for income Y99.8
leisure activity Y99.8
military activity Y99.1
off-duty activity of military personnel Y99.8
recreation or sport not for income or while a student
    Y99.8
specified NEC Y99.8
student activity Y99.8
volunteer activity Y99.2

F

Factors, supplemental
alcohol
  blood level
    less than 20mg/100ml Y90.0
    20-39mg/100ml Y90.1
    40-59mg/100ml Y90.2
    60-79mg/100ml Y90.3
    80-99mg/100ml Y90.4
    100-119mg/100ml Y90.5
    120-199mg/100ml Y90.6
    200-239mg/100ml Y90.7
    240mg/100ml or more Y90.8
    presence in blood, level not specified Y90.9
  presence in blood, but level not specified Y90.9
environmental-pollution-related condition- see Z57 ☑
nosocomial condition Y95
work-related condition Y99.0

Failure
in suture or ligature during surgical procedure Y65.2
mechanical, of instrument or apparatus (any) (during
    any medical or surgical procedure) Y65.8
sterile precautions (during medical and surgical care)
    — *see* Misadventure, failure, sterile precautions,
    by type of procedure
to
  introduce tube or instrument Y65.4
    endotracheal tube during anesthesia Y65.3
  make curve (transport vehicle) NEC — *see* Accident,
    transport
  remove tube or instrument Y65.4

Fall, falling (accidental) W19 ☑
building W20.1 ☑
  burning (uncontrolled fire) X00.3 ☑
down
  embankment W17.81 ☑
  escalator W10.0 ☑
  hill W17.81 ☑
  ladder W11 ☑
  ramp W10.2 ☑
  stairs, steps W10.9 ☑
due to
  bumping against
    object W18.00 ☑
      sharp glass W18.02 ☑
      specified NEC W18.09 ☑
      sports equipment W18.01 ☑
    person W03 ☑
      due to ice or snow W00.0 ☑
      on pedestrian conveyance — *see* Accident,
        transport, pedestrian, conveyance
  collision with another person W03 ☑
    due to ice or snow W00.0 ☑
    involving pedestrian conveyance — *see* Acci-
      dent, transport, pedestrian, conveyance
  grocery cart tipping over W17.82 ☑
  ice or snow W00.9 ☑
    from one level to another W00.2 ☑
    on stairs or steps W00.1 ☑
    involving pedestrian conveyance — *see* Acci-
      dent, transport, pedestrian, conveyance
    on same level W00.0 ☑
  slipping (on moving sidewalk) W01.0 ☑
    with subsequent striking against object
      W01.10 ☑
      furniture W01.190 ☑
      sharp object W01.119 ☑
        glass W01.110 ☑
        power tool or machine W01.111 ☑
        specified NEC W01.118 ☑
      specified NEC W01.198 ☑
  striking against
    object W18.00 ☑
      sharp glass W18.02 ☑
      specified NEC W18.09 ☑

Fall, falling — *continued*
due to — *continued*
  striking against — *continued*
    object — *continued*
      sports equipment W18.01 ☑
    person W03 ☑
      due to ice or snow W00.0 ☑
      on pedestrian conveyance — *see* Accident,
        transport, pedestrian, conveyance
earth (with asphyxia or suffocation (by pressure)) —
    see Earth, falling
from, off, out of
  aircraft NEC (with accident to aircraft NEC) V97.0 ☑
    while boarding or alighting V97.1 ☑
  balcony W13.0 ☑
  bed W06 ☑
  boat, ship, watercraft NEC (with drowning or sub-
    mersion) — *see* Drowning, due to, fall over-
    board
    with hitting bottom or object V94.0 ☑
  bridge W13.1 ☑
  building W13.9 ☑
    burning (uncontrolled fire) X00.3 ☑
  cavity W17.2 ☑
  chair W07 ☑
  cherry picker W17.89 ☑
  cliff W15 ☑
  dock W17.4 ☑
  embankment W17.81 ☑
  escalator W10.0 ☑
  flagpole W13.8 ☑
  furniture NEC W08 ☑
  grocery cart W17.82 ☑
  haystack W17.89 ☑
  high place NEC W17.89 ☑
    stated as undetermined whether accidental or
      intentional Y30 ☑
  hole W17.2 ☑
  incline W10.2 ☑
  ladder W11 ☑
  lifting device W17.89 ☑
  machine, machinery (*see also* Contact, with, by
    type of machine)
    not in operation W17.89 ☑
  manhole W17.1 ☑
  mobile elevated work platform [MEWP] W17.89 ☑
  motorized mobility scooter W05.2 ☑
  one level to another NEC W17.89 ☑
    intentional, purposeful, suicide (attempt)
      X80 ☑
    stated as undetermined whether accidental or
      intentional Y30 ☑
  pit W17.2 ☑
  playground equipment W09.8 ☑
    jungle gym W09.2 ☑
    slide W09.0 ☑
    swing W09.1 ☑
  quarry W17.89 ☑
  railing W13.9 ☑
  ramp W10.2 ☑
  roof W13.2 ☑
  scaffolding W12 ☑
  scooter (nonmotorized) W05.1 ☑
    motorized mobility W05.2 ☑
  sky lift W17.89 ☑
  stairs, steps W10.9 ☑
    curb W10.1 ☑
    due to ice or snow W00.1 ☑
    escalator W10.0 ☑
    incline W10.2 ☑
    ramp W10.2 ☑
    sidewalk curb W10.1 ☑
    specified NEC W10.8 ☑
  stepladder W11 ☑
  storm drain W17.1 ☑
  streetcar NEC V82.6 ☑
    with antecedent collision — *see* Accident,
      transport, streetcar occupant
    while boarding or alighting V82.4 ☑
  structure NEC W13.8 ☑
    burning (uncontrolled fire) X00.3 ☑
  table W08 ☑
  toilet W18.11 ☑
    with subsequent striking against object
      W18.12 ☑

Fall, falling — *continued*
from, off, out of — *continued*
  train NEC V81.6 ☑
    during derailment (without antecedent colli-
      sion) V81.7 ☑
    with antecedent collision — *see* Accident,
      transport, railway vehicle occupant
    while boarding or alighting V81.4 ☑
  transport vehicle after collision — *see* Accident,
    transport, by type of vehicle, collision
  tree W14 ☑
  vehicle (in motion) NEC (*see also* Accident, trans-
    port) V89.9 ☑
    motor NEC (*see also* Accident, transport, occu-
      pant, by type of vehicle) V87.8 ☑
    stationary W17.89 ☑
      while boarding or alighting B — *see* Acci-
        dent, transport, by type of vehicle,
        while boarding or alighting
  viaduct W13.8 ☑
  wall W13.8 ☑
  watercraft (*see also* Drowning, due to, fall over-
    board)
    with hitting bottom or object V94.0 ☑
  well W17.0 ☑
  wheelchair, non-moving W05.0 ☑
    powered — *see* Accident, transport, pedestrian,
      conveyance occupant, specified type NEC
  window W13.4 ☑
in, on
  aircraft NEC V97.0 ☑
    with accident to aircraft V97.0 ☑
    while boarding or alighting V97.1 ☑
  bathtub (empty) W18.2 ☑
    filled W16.212 ☑
      causing drowning W16.211 ☑
  escalator W10.0 ☑
  incline W10.2 ☑
  ladder W11 ☑
  machine, machinery — *see* Contact, with, by type
    of machine
  object, edged, pointed or sharp (with cut) — *see*
    Fall, by type
  playground equipment W09.8 ☑
    jungle gym W09.2 ☑
    slide W09.0 ☑
    swing W09.1 ☑
  ramp W10.2 ☑
  scaffolding W12 ☑
  shower W18.2 ☑
    causing drowning W16.211 ☑
  staircase, stairs, steps W10.9 ☑
    curb W10.1 ☑
    due to ice or snow W00.1 ☑
    escalator W10.0 ☑
    incline W10.2 ☑
    specified NEC W10.8 ☑
  streetcar (without antecedent collision) V82.5 ☑
    with antecedent collision — *see* Accident,
      transport, streetcar occupant
    while boarding or alighting V82.4 ☑
  train (without antecedent collision) V81.5 ☑
    with antecedent collision — *see* Accident,
      transport, railway vehicle occupant
    during derailment (without antecedent colli-
      sion) V81.7 ☑
      with antecedent collision — *see* Accident,
        transport, railway vehicle occupant
    while boarding or alighting V81.4 ☑
  transport vehicle after collision — *see* Accident,
    transport, by type of vehicle, collision
  watercraft V93.39 ☑
    due to
      accident to craft V91.29 ☑
        powered craft V91.23 ☑
          ferry boat V91.21 ☑
          fishing boat V91.22 ☑
          jetskis V91.23 ☑
          liner V91.21 ☑
          merchant ship V91.20 ☑
          passenger ship V91.21 ☑
        unpowered craft
          canoe V91.25 ☑
          inflatable V91.26 ☑
          kayak V91.25 ☑
          sailboat V91.24 ☑

Fall, falling — *continued*
in, on — *continued*
watercraft — *continued*
powered craft V93.33 ☑
ferry boat V93.31 ☑
fishing boat V93.32 ☑
jetskis V93.33 ☑
liner V93.31 ☑
merchant ship V93.30 ☑
passenger ship V93.31 ☑
unpowered craft V93.38 ☑
canoe V93.35 ☑
inflatable V93.36 ☑
kayak V93.35 ☑
sailboat V93.34 ☑
surf-board V93.38 ☑
windsurfer V93.38 ☑
into
cavity W17.2 ☑
dock W17.4 ☑
fire — *see* Exposure, fire, by type
haystack W17.89 ☑
hole W17.2 ☑
lake — *see* Fall, into, water
lake — *see* Fall, into, water
manhole W17.1 ☑
moving part of machinery — *see* Contact, with, by
type of machine
ocean — *see* Fall, into, water
opening in surface NEC W17.89 ☑
pit W17.2 ☑
pond — *see* Fall, into, water
quarry W17.89 ☑
river — *see* Fall, into, water
shaft W17.89 ☑
storm drain W17.1 ☑
stream — *see* Fall, into, water
swimming pool (*see also* Fall, into, water, in,
swimming pool)
empty W17.3 ☑
tank W17.89 ☑
water W16.42 ☑
causing drowning W16.41 ☑
from watercraft — *see* Drowning, due to, fall
overboard
hitting diving board W21.4 ☑
in
bathtub W16.212 ☑
causing drowning W16.211 ☑
bucket W16.222 ☑
causing drowning W16.221 ☑
natural body of water W16.112 ☑
causing drowning W16.111 ☑
striking
bottom W16.122 ☑
causing drowning W16.121 ☑
side W16.132 ☑
causing drowning W16.131 ☑
specified water NEC W16.312 ☑
causing drowning W16.311 ☑
striking
bottom W16.322 ☑
causing drowning W16.321 ☑
wall W16.332 ☑
causing drowning W16.331 ☑
swimming pool W16.012 ☑
causing drowning W16.011 ☑
striking
bottom W16.022 ☑
causing drowning W16.021 ☑
wall W16.032 ☑
causing drowning W16.021 ☑
utility bucket W16.222 ☑
causing drowning W16.221 ☑
well W17.0 ☑
involving
bed W06 ☑
chair W07 ☑
furniture NEC W08 ☑
glass — *see* Fall, by type
playground equipment W09.8 ☑
jungle gym W09.2 ☑
slide W09.0 ☑
swing W09.1 ☑
roller blades — *see* Accident, transport, pedestrian,
conveyance

Fall, falling — *continued*
involving — *continued*
skateboard(s) — *see* Accident, transport, pedestrian, conveyance
skates (ice) (in line) (roller) — *see* Accident, transport, pedestrian, conveyance
skis — *see* Accident, transport, pedestrian, conveyance
table W08 ☑
wheelchair, non-moving W05.0 ☑
powered — *see* Accident, transport, pedestrian,
conveyance, specified type NEC
object — *see* Struck by, object, falling
off
toilet W18.11 ☑
with subsequent striking against object
W18.12 ☑
on same level W18.30 ☑
due to
specified NEC W18.39 ☑
stepping on an object W18.31 ☑
out of
bed W06 ☑
building NEC W13.8 ☑
chair W07 ☑
furniture NEC W08 ☑
wheelchair, non-moving W05.0 ☑
powered — *see* Accident, transport, pedestrian,
conveyance, specified type NEC
window W13.4 ☑
over
animal W01.0 ☑
cliff W15 ☑
embankment W17.81 ☑
small object W01.0 ☑
rock W20.8 ☑
same level W18.30 ☑
from
being crushed, pushed, or stepped on by a
crowd or human stampede W52 ☑
collision, pushing, shoving, by or with other
person W03 ☑
slipping, stumbling, tripping W01.0 ☑
involving ice or snow W00.0 ☑
involving skates (ice) (roller), skateboard, skis
— *see* Accident, transport, pedestrian,
conveyance
snowslide (avalanche) — *see* Landslide
stone W20.8 ☑
structure W20.1 ☑
burning (uncontrolled fire) X00.3 ☑
through
bridge W13.1 ☑
floor W13.3 ☑
roof W13.2 ☑
wall W13.8 ☑
window W13.4 ☑
timber W20.8 ☑
tree (caused by lightning) W20.8 ☑
while being carried or supported by other person(s)
W04 ☑
Fallen on by
animal (not being ridden) NEC W55.89 ☑
Felo-de-se — *see* Suicide
Fight (hand) (fists) (foot) — *see* Assault, fight
Fire (accidental) — *see* Exposure, fire
Firearm discharge — *see* Discharge, firearm
**Fireball effects from nuclear explosion in war oper-
ations** — *see* War operations, nuclear weapons
Fireworks (explosion) W39 ☑
Flash burns from explosion — *see* Explosion
Flood (any injury) (caused by) X38 ☑
collapse of man-made structure causing earth movement X36.0 ☑
tidal wave — *see* Forces of nature, tidal wave
Food (any type) **in**
air passages (with asphyxia, obstruction, or suffocation) — *see* categories T17 and T18 ☑
alimentary tract causing asphyxia (due to compression
of trachea) — *see* categories T17 and T18 ☑
Forces of nature X39.8 ☑
avalanche X36.1 ☑
causing transport accident — *see* Accident, transport, by type of vehicle
blizzard X37.2 ☑

Forces of nature — *continued*
cataclysmic storm X37.9 ☑
with flood X38 ☑
blizzard X37.2 ☑
cloudburst X37.8 ☑
cyclone X37.1 ☑
dust storm X37.3 ☑
hurricane X37.0 ☑
specified storm NEC X37.8 ☑
storm surge X37.0 ☑
tornado X37.1 ☑
twister X37.1 ☑
typhoon X37.0 ☑
cloudburst X37.8 ☑
cold (natural) X31 ☑
cyclone X37.1 ☑
dam collapse causing earth movement X36.0 ☑
dust storm X37.3 ☑
earth movement X36.1 ☑
caused by dam or structure collapse X36.0 ☑
earthquake X34 ☑
earthquake X34 ☑
flood (caused by) X38 ☑
dam collapse X36.0 ☑
tidal wave B — *see* Forces of nature, tidal wave
heat (natural) X30 ☑
hurricane X37.0 ☑
landslide X36.1 ☑
causing transport accident — *see* Accident, transport, by type of vehicle
lightning — *see* subcategory T75.0 ☑
causing fire — *see* Exposure, fire
mudslide X36.1 ☑
causing transport accident — *see* Accident, transport, by type of vehicle
radiation (natural) X39.08 ☑
radon X39.01 ☑
radon X39.01 ☑
specified force NEC X39.8 ☑
storm surge X37.0 ☑
structure collapse causing earth movement X36.0 ☑
sunlight X32 ☑
tidal wave X37.41 ☑
due to
earthquake X37.41 ☑
landslide X37.43 ☑
storm X37.42 ☑
volcanic eruption X37.41 ☑
tornado X37.1 ☑
tsunami X37.41 ☑
twister X37.1 ☑
typhoon X37.0 ☑
volcanic eruption X35 ☑
Foreign body
aspiration — *see* Index to Diseases and Injuries, Foreign body, respiratory tract
entering through skin W45.8 ☑
can lid W45.2 ☑
nail W45.0 ☑
paper W45.1 ☑
specified NEC W45.8 ☑
splinter W45.8 ☑
Forest fire (exposure to) — *see* Exposure, fire, uncontrolled, not in building
Found injured X58 ☑
from exposure (to) — *see* Exposure
on
highway, road(way), street V89.9 ☑
railway right of way V81.9 ☑
Fracture (circumstances unknown or unspecified) X58 ☑
due to specified cause NEC X58 ☑
Freezing — *see* Exposure, cold
Frostbite X31 ☑
due to man-made conditions — *see* Exposure, cold,
man-made
Frozen — *see* Exposure, cold

G

Gored by bull W55.22 ☑
Gunshot wound W34.00 ☑

H

Hailstones, injured by X39.8 ☑

Hanged herself or himself — *see* Hanging, self-inflicted
Hanging (accidental) (*see also* category) T71 ☑
    legal execution — *see* Legal, intervention, specified
        means NEC
Heat (effects of) (excessive) X30 ☑
    due to
        man-made conditions W92 ☑
            on board watercraft V93.29 ☑
                fishing boat V93.22 ☑
                merchant ship V93.20 ☑
                passenger ship V93.21 ☑
                sailboat V93.24 ☑
                specified powered craft NEC V93.23 ☑
        weather (conditions) X30 ☑
    from
        electric heating apparatus causing burning X16 ☑
        nuclear explosion in war operations — *see* War
            operations, nuclear weapons
    inappropriate in local application or packing in medical
        or surgical procedure Y63.5
Hemorrhage
    delayed following medical or surgical treatment
        without mention of misadventure — *see* Index
        to Diseases and Injuries, Complication(s)
    during medical or surgical treatment as misadventure
        — *see* Index to Diseases and Injuries, Complica-
        tion(s)
High
    altitude (effects) — *see* Air, pressure, low
    level of radioactivity, effects — *see* Radiation
    pressure (effects) — *see* Air, pressure, high
    temperature, effects — *see* Heat
Hit, hitting (accidental) by — *see* Struck by
Hitting against — *see* Striking against
Homicide (attempt) (justifiable) — *see* Assault
Hot
    place, effects (*see also* Heat)
    weather, effects X30 ☑
House fire (uncontrolled) — *see* Exposure, fire, uncon-
      trolled, building
Humidity, causing problem X39.8 ☑
Hunger X58 ☑
Hurricane (any injury) X37.0 ☑
Hypobarism, hypobaropathy — *see* Air, pressure, low

I

Ictus
    caloris (*see also* Heat)
    solaris X30 ☑
Ignition (accidental) (*see also* Exposure, fire) X08.8 ☑
    anesthetic gas in operating room W40.1 ☑
    apparel X06.2 ☑
        from highly flammable material X04 ☑
        nightwear X05 ☑
    bed linen (sheets) (spreads) (pillows) (mattress) — *see*
        Exposure, fire, uncontrolled, building, bed
    benzine X04 ☑
    clothes, clothing NEC (from controlled fire) X06.2 ☑
        from
            highly flammable material X04 ☑
    ether X04 ☑
        in operating room W40.1 ☑
    explosive material — *see* Explosion
    gasoline X04 ☑
    jewelry (plastic) (any) X06.0 ☑
    kerosene X04 ☑
    material
        explosive — *see* Explosion
        highly flammable with secondary explosion X04 ☑
    nightwear X05 ☑
    paraffin X04 ☑
    petrol X04 ☑
Immersion (accidental) (*see also* Drowning)
    hand or foot due to cold (excessive) X31 ☑
Implantation of quills of porcupine W55.89 ☑
Inanition (from) (hunger) X58 ☑
    thirst X58 ☑
Inappropriate operation performed
    correct operation on wrong side or body part (wrong
        side) (wrong site) Y65.53
    operation intended for another patient done on wrong
        patient Y65.52
    wrong operation performed on correct patient Y65.51
Inattention after, at birth (homicidal intent) (infantici-
      dal intent) X58 ☑

Incident, adverse
    device
        anesthesiology Y70.8
            accessory Y70.2
            diagnostic Y70.0
            miscellaneous Y70.8
            monitoring Y70.0
            prosthetic Y70.2
            rehabilitative Y70.1
            surgical Y70.3
            therapeutic Y70.1
        cardiovascular Y71.8
            accessory Y71.2
            diagnostic Y71.0
            miscellaneous Y71.8
            monitoring Y71.0
            prosthetic Y71.2
            rehabilitative Y71.1
            surgical Y71.3
            therapeutic Y71.1
        gastroenterology Y73.8
            accessory Y73.2
            diagnostic Y73.0
            miscellaneous Y73.8
            monitoring Y73.0
            prosthetic Y73.2
            rehabilitative Y73.1
            surgical Y73.3
            therapeutic Y73.1
        general
            hospital Y74.8
                accessory Y74.2
                diagnostic Y74.0
                miscellaneous Y74.8
                monitoring Y74.0
                prosthetic Y74.2
                rehabilitative Y74.1
                surgical Y74.3
                therapeutic Y74.1
            surgical Y81.8
                accessory Y81.2
                diagnostic Y81.0
                miscellaneous Y81.8
                monitoring Y81.0
                prosthetic Y81.2
                rehabilitative Y81.1
                surgical Y81.3
                therapeutic Y81.1
        gynecological Y76.8
            accessory Y76.2
            diagnostic Y76.0
            miscellaneous Y76.8
            monitoring Y76.0
            prosthetic Y76.2
            rehabilitative Y76.1
            surgical Y76.3
            therapeutic Y76.1
        medical Y82.9
            specified type NEC Y82.8
        neurological Y75.8
            accessory Y75.2
            diagnostic Y75.0
            miscellaneous Y75.8
            monitoring Y75.0
            prosthetic Y75.2
            rehabilitative Y75.1
            surgical Y75.3
            therapeutic Y75.1
        obstetrical Y76.8
            accessory Y76.2
            diagnostic Y76.0
            miscellaneous Y76.8
            monitoring Y76.0
            prosthetic Y76.2
            rehabilitative Y76.1
            surgical Y76.3
            therapeutic Y76.1
        ophthalmic Y77.8
            accessory Y77.2
            diagnostic Y77.0
            miscellaneous Y77.8
            monitoring Y77.0
            prosthetic Y77.2
            rehabilitative Y77.1
            surgical Y77.3
            therapeutic Y77.1
        orthopedic Y79.8
            accessory Y79.2

Incident, adverse — *continued*
    device — *continued*
        orthopedic — *continued*
            diagnostic Y79.0
            miscellaneous Y79.8
            monitoring Y79.0
            prosthetic Y79.2
            rehabilitative Y79.1
            surgical Y79.3
            therapeutic Y79.1
        otorhinolaryngological Y72.8
            accessory Y72.2
            diagnostic Y72.0
            miscellaneous Y72.8
            monitoring Y72.0
            prosthetic Y72.2
            rehabilitative Y72.1
            surgical Y72.3
            therapeutic Y72.1
        personal use Y74.8
            accessory Y74.2
            diagnostic Y74.0
            miscellaneous Y74.8
            monitoring Y74.0
            prosthetic Y74.2
            rehabilitative Y74.1
            surgical Y74.3
            therapeutic Y74.1
        physical medicine Y80.8
            accessory Y80.2
            diagnostic Y80.0
            miscellaneous Y80.8
            monitoring Y80.0
            prosthetic Y80.2
            rehabilitative Y80.1
            surgical Y80.3
            therapeutic Y80.1
        plastic surgical Y81.8
            accessory Y81.2
            diagnostic Y81.0
            miscellaneous Y81.8
            monitoring Y81.0
            prosthetic Y81.2
            rehabilitative Y81.1
            surgical Y81.3
            therapeutic Y81.1
        radiological Y78.8
            accessory Y78.2
            diagnostic Y78.0
            miscellaneous Y78.8
            monitoring Y78.0
            prosthetic Y78.2
            rehabilitative Y78.1
            surgical Y78.3
            therapeutic Y78.1
        urology Y73.8
            accessory Y73.2
            diagnostic Y73.0
            miscellaneous Y73.8
            monitoring Y73.0
            prosthetic Y73.2
            rehabilitative Y73.1
            surgical Y73.3
            therapeutic Y73.1
Incineration (accidental) — *see* Exposure, fire
Infanticide — *see* Assault
Infrasound waves (causing injury) W49.9 ☑
Ingestion
    foreign body (causing injury) (with obstruction) — *see*
        Foreign body, alimentary canal
    poisonous
        plant(s) X58 ☑
        substance NEC — *see* Table of Drugs and Chemicals
Inhalation
    excessively cold substance, man-made — *see* Expo-
        sure, cold, man-made
    food (any type) (into respiratory tract) (with asphyxia,
        obstruction respiratory tract, suffocation) — *see*
        categories T17 and T18 ☑
    foreign body — *see* Foreign body, aspiration
    gastric contents (with asphyxia, obstruction respiratory
        passage, suffocation) T17.81- ☑
    hot air or gases X14.0 ☑
    liquid air, hydrogen, nitrogen W93.12 ☑
        suicide (attempt) X83.2 ☑
    steam X13.0 ☑
        assault X98.0 ☑

Inhalation — *continued*
  steam — *continued*
    stated as undetermined whether accidental or intentional Y27.0 ☑
    suicide (attempt) X77.0 ☑
  toxic gas — *see* Table of Drugs and Chemicals
  vomitus (with asphyxia, obstruction respiratory passage, suffocation) T17.81- ☑
Injury, injured (accidental(ly)) NOS X58 ☑
  by, caused by, from
    assault — *see* Assault
    law-enforcing agent, police, in course of legal intervention — *see* Legal intervention
    suicide (attempt) X83.8 ☑
  due to, in
    civil insurrection — *see* War operations
    fight (*see also* Assault, fight) Y04.0 ☑
    war operations — *see* War operations
  homicide (*see also* Assault) Y09
  inflicted (by)
    in course of arrest (attempted), suppression of disturbance, maintenance of order, by law-enforcing agents — *see* Legal intervention
    other person
      stated as
        accidental X58 ☑
        intentional, homicide (attempt) — *see* Assault
        undetermined whether accidental or intentional Y33 ☑
    purposely (inflicted) by other person(s) — *see* Assault
  self-inflicted X83.8 ☑
    stated as accidental X58 ☑
  specified cause NEC X58 ☑
  undetermined whether accidental or intentional Y33 ☑
Insolation, effects X30 ☑
Insufficient nourishment X58 ☑
Interruption of respiration (by)
  food (lodged in esophagus) — *see* categories T17 and T18 ☑
  vomitus (lodged in esophagus) T17.81- ☑
Intervention, legal — *see* Legal intervention
Intoxication
  drug — *see* Table of Drugs and Chemicals
  poison — *see* Table of Drugs and Chemicals

J

Jammed (accidentally)
  between objects (moving) (stationary and moving) W23.0 ☑
    stationary W23.1 ☑
Jumped, jumping
  before moving object NEC X81.8 ☑
    motor vehicle X81.0 ☑
    subway train X81.1 ☑
    train X81.1 ☑
    undetermined whether accidental or intentional Y31 ☑
  from
    boat (into water) voluntarily, without accident (to or on boat) W16.712 ☑
      with
        accident to or on boat — *see* Accident, watercraft
        drowning or submersion W16.711 ☑
          suicide (attempt) X71.3 ☑
      striking bottom W16.722 ☑
        causing drowning W16.721 ☑
    building (*see also* Jumped, from, high place) W13.9 ☑
      burning (uncontrolled fire) X00.5 ☑
    high place NEC W17.89 ☑
      suicide (attempt) X80 ☑
      undetermined whether accidental or intentional Y30 ☑
    structure (*see also* Jumped, from, high place) W13.9 ☑
      burning (uncontrolled fire) X00.5 ☑
  into water W16.92 ☑
    causing drowning W16.91 ☑
    from, off watercraft — *see* Jumped, from, boat
    in
      natural body W16.612 ☑
        causing drowning W16.611 ☑

Jumped, jumping — *continued*
  into water — *continued*
    in — *continued*
      natural body — *continued*
        striking bottom W16.622 ☑
          causing drowning W16.621 ☑
      specified place NEC W16.812 ☑
        causing drowning W16.811 ☑
        striking
          bottom W16.822 ☑
            causing drowning W16.821 ☑
          wall W16.832 ☑
            causing drowning W16.831 ☑
      swimming pool W16.512 ☑
        causing drowning W16.511 ☑
        striking
          bottom W16.522 ☑
            causing drowning W16.521 ☑
          wall W16.532 ☑
            causing drowning W16.531 ☑
  suicide (attempt) X71.3 ☑

K

Kicked by
  animal NEC W55.82 ☑
  person(s) (accidentally) W50.1 ☑
    with intent to injure or kill Y04.0 ☑
    as, or caused by, a crowd or human stampede (with fall) W52 ☑
    assault Y04.0 ☑
    homicide (attempt) Y04.0 ☑
    in
      fight Y04.0 ☑
      legal intervention
        injuring
          bystander Y35.812 ☑
          law enforcement personnel Y35.811 ☑
          suspect Y35.813 ☑
Kicking against
  object W22.8 ☑
    sports equipment W21.9 ☑
    stationary wW22.09
      sports equipment W21.89 ☑
  person — *see* Striking against, person
  sports equipment W21.9 ☑
Killed, killing (accidentally) NOS (*see also* Injury) X58 ☑
  in
    action — *see* War operations
    brawl, fight (hand) (fists) (foot) Y04.0 ☑
      by weapon (*see also* Assault)
        cutting, piercing — *see* Assault, cutting or piercing instrument
        firearm — *see* Discharge, firearm, by type, homicide
  self
    stated as
      accident NOS X58 ☑
      suicide — *see* Suicide
      undetermined whether accidental or intentional Y33 ☑
Knocked down (accidentally) (by) NOS X58 ☑
  animal (not being ridden) NEC (*see also* Struck by, by type of animal)
  crowd or human stampede W52 ☑
  person W51 ☑
    in brawl, fight Y04.0 ☑
  transport vehicle NEC (*see also* Accident, transport) V09.9 ☑

L

Laceration NEC — *see* Injury
Lack of
  care (helpless person) (infant) (newborn) X58 ☑
  food except as result of abandonment or neglect X58 ☑
    due to abandonment or neglect X58 ☑
  water except as result of transport accident X58 ☑
    due to transport accident B — *see* Accident, transport, by type
    helpless person, infant, newborn X58 ☑
Landslide (falling on transport vehicle) X36.1 ☑
  caused by collapse of man-made structure X36.0 ☑
Late effect — *see* Sequelae

Legal
  execution (any method) — *see* Legal, intervention
  intervention (by)
    baton — *see* Legal, intervention, blunt object, baton
    bayonet — *see* Legal, intervention, sharp object, bayonet
    blow — *see* Legal, intervention, manhandling
    blunt object
      baton
        injuring
          bystander Y35.312 ☑
          law enforcement personnel Y35.311 ☑
          suspect Y35.313 ☑
      injuring
        bystander Y35.302 ☑
        law enforcement personnel Y35.301 ☑
        suspect Y35.303 ☑
      specified NEC
        injuring
          bystander Y35.392 ☑
          law enforcement personnel Y35.391 ☑
          suspect Y35.393 ☑
      stave
        injuring
          bystander Y35.392 ☑
          law enforcement personnel Y35.391 ☑
          suspect Y35.393 ☑
    bomb — *see* Legal, intervention, explosive
    cutting or piercing instrument — *see* Legal, intervention, sharp object
    dynamite — *see* Legal, intervention, explosive, dynamite
    explosive(s)
      dynamite
        injuring
          bystander Y35.112 ☑
          law enforcement personnel Y35.111 ☑
          suspect Y35.113 ☑
      grenade
        injuring
          bystander Y35.192 ☑
          law enforcement personnel Y35.191 ☑
          suspect Y35.193 ☑
      injuring
        bystander Y35.102 ☑
        law enforcement personnel Y35.101 ☑
        suspect Y35.103 ☑
      mortar bomb
        injuring
          bystander Y35.192 ☑
          law enforcement personnel Y35.191 ☑
          suspect Y35.193 ☑
      shell
        injuring
          bystander Y35.122 ☑
          law enforcement personnel Y35.121 ☑
          suspect Y35.123 ☑
      specified NEC
        injuring
          bystander Y35.192 ☑
          law enforcement personnel Y35.191 ☑
          suspect Y35.193 ☑
    firearm(s) (discharge)
      handgun
        injuring
          bystander Y35.022 ☑
          law enforcement personnel Y35.021 ☑
          suspect Y35.023 ☑
      injuring
        bystander Y35.002 ☑
        law enforcement personnel Y35.001 ☑
        suspect Y35.003 ☑
      machine gun
        injuring
          bystander Y35.012 ☑
          law enforcement personnel Y35.011 ☑
          suspect Y35.013 ☑
      rifle pellet
        injuring
          bystander Y35.032 ☑
          law enforcement personnel Y35.031 ☑
          suspect Y35.033 ☑
      rubber bullet
        injuring
          bystander Y35.042 ☑
          law enforcement personnel Y35.041 ☑

External Causes Index

Legal — *continued*
  intervention — *continued*
    firearm(s) — *continued*
      rubber bullet — *continued*
        injuring — *continued*
          suspect Y35.043 ☑
      shotgun — *see* Legal, intervention, firearm,
        specified NEC
      specified NEC
        injuring
          bystander Y35.092 ☑
          law enforcement personnel Y35.091 ☑
          suspect Y35.093 ☑
    gas (asphyxiation) (poisoning)
      injuring
        bystander Y35.202 ☑
        law enforcement personnel Y35.201 ☑
        suspect Y35.203 ☑
      specified NEC
        injuring
          bystander Y35.292 ☑
          law enforcement personnel Y35.291 ☑
          suspect Y35.293 ☑
      tear gas
        injuring
          bystander Y35.212 ☑
          law enforcement personnel Y35.211 ☑
          suspect Y35.213 ☑
    grenade — *see* Legal, intervention, explosive,
      grenade
    injuring
      bystander Y35.92 ☑
      law enforcement personnel Y35.91 ☑
      suspect Y35.93 ☑
    late effect (of) — *see with 7th character S* Y35 ☑
    manhandling
      injuring
        bystander Y35.812 ☑
        law enforcement personnel Y35.811 ☑
        suspect Y35.813 ☑
    sequelae (of) — *see with 7th character S* Y35 ☑
    sharp objects
      bayonet
        injuring
          bystander Y35.412 ☑
          law enforcement personnel Y35.411 ☑
          suspect Y35.413 ☑
      injuring
        bystander Y35.402 ☑
        law enforcement personnel Y35.401 ☑
        suspect Y35.403 ☑
      specified NEC
        injuring
          bystander Y35.492 ☑
          law enforcement personnel Y35.491 ☑
          suspect Y35.493 ☑
    specified means NEC
      injuring
        bystander Y35.892 ☑
        law enforcement personnel Y35.891 ☑
        suspect Y35.893 ☑
    stabbing — *see* Legal, intervention, sharp object
    stave — *see* Legal, intervention, blunt object, stave
    tear gas — *see* Legal, intervention, gas, tear gas
    truncheon — *see* Legal, intervention, blunt object,
      stave
Lightning (shock) (stroke) (struck by) — *see subcategory*
  T75.0 ☑
  causing fire — *see* Exposure, fire
Loss of control (transport vehicle) NEC — *see* Accident,
  transport
Lost at sea NOS — *see* Drowning, due to, fall overboard
Low
  pressure (effects) — *see* Air, pressure, low
  temperature (effects) — *see* Exposure, cold
Lying before train, vehicle or other moving object
  X81.8 ☑
  subway train X81.1 ☑
  train X81.1 ☑
  undetermined whether accidental or intentional
    Y31 ☑
Lynching — *see* Assault

M

Malfunction (mechanism or component) (of)
  firearm W34.10 ☑
    airgun W34.110 ☑
    BB gun W34.110 ☑
    gas, air or spring-operated gun NEC W34.118 ☑
    handgun W32.1 ☑
    hunting rifle W33.12 ☑
    larger firearm W33.10 ☑
      specified NEC W33.19 ☑
    machine gun W33.13 ☑
    paintball gun W34.111 ☑
    pellet gun W34.110 ☑
    shotgun W33.11 ☑
    specified NEC W34.19 ☑
    Very pistol (flare) W34.19 ☑
  handgun — *see* Malfunction, firearm, handgun
Maltreatment — *see* Perpetrator
Mangled (accidentally) NOS X58 ☑
Manhandling (in brawl, fight) Y04.0 ☑
  legal intervention — *see* Legal, intervention, manhan-
    dling
Manslaughter (nonaccidental) — *see* Assault
Mauled by animal NEC W55.89 ☑
Medical procedure, complication of (delayed or as an
  abnormal reaction without mention of misadventure) — *see* Complication of or following, by specified type of procedure
  due to or as a result of misadventure — *see* Misadven-
    ture
Melting (due to fire) (*see also* Exposure, fire)
  apparel NEC X06.3 ☑
  clothes, clothing NEC X06.3 ☑
    nightwear X05 ☑
  fittings or furniture (burning building) (uncontrolled
    fire) X00.8 ☑
  nightwear X05 ☑
  plastic jewelry X06.1 ☑
Mental cruelty X58 ☑
Military operations (injuries to military and civilians
  occuring during peacetime on military property
  and during routine military exercises and operations) (by) (from) (involving) Y37.90- ☑
  air blast Y37.20- ☑
  aircraft
    destruction — *see* Military operations, destruction
      of aircraft
    airway restriction — *see* Military operations, restriction
      of airways
  asphyxiation — *see* Military operations, restriction of
    airways
  biological weapons Y37.6X- ☑
  blast Y37.20- ☑
  blast fragments Y37.20- ☑
  blast wave Y37.20- ☑
  blast wind Y37.20- ☑
  bomb Y37.20- ☑
    dirty Y37.50- ☑
    gasoline Y37.31- ☑
    incendiary Y37.31- ☑
    petrol Y37.31- ☑
  bullet Y37.43- ☑
    incendiary Y37.32- ☑
    rubber Y37.41- ☑
  chemical weapons Y37.7X- ☑
  combat
    hand to hand (unarmed) combat Y37.44- ☑
    using blunt or piercing object Y37.45- ☑
  conflagration — *see* Military operations, fire
  conventional warfare NEC Y37.49- ☑
  depth-charge Y37.01- ☑
  destruction of aircraft Y37.10- ☑
    due to
      air to air missile Y37.11- ☑
      collision with other aircraft Y37.12- ☑
      detonation (accidental) of onboard munitions
        and explosives Y37.14- ☑
      enemy fire or explosives Y37.11- ☑
      explosive placed on aircraft Y37.11- ☑
      onboard fire Y37.13- ☑
      rocket propelled grenade [RPG] Y37.11- ☑
      small arms fire Y37.11- ☑
      surface to air missile Y37.11- ☑
    specified NEC Y37.19- ☑

Military operations — *continued*
  detonation (accidental) of
    onboard marine weapons Y37.05- ☑
    own munitions or munitions launch device Y37.24- ☑
  dirty bomb Y37.50- ☑
  explosion (of) Y37.20- ☑
    aerial bomb Y37.21- ☑
    bomb NOS (*see also* Military operations, bomb(s))
      Y37.20- ☑
    fragments Y37.20- ☑
    grenade Y37.29- ☑
    guided missile Y37.22- ☑
    improvised explosive device [IED] (person-borne)
      (roadside) (vehicle-borne) Y37.23- ☑
    land mine Y37.29- ☑
    marine mine (at sea) (in harbor) Y37.02- ☑
    marine weapon Y37.00- ☑
      specified NEC Y37.09- ☑
    own munitions or munitions launch device (acci-
      dental) Y37.24- ☑
    sea-based artillery shell Y37.03- ☑
    specified NEC Y37.29- ☑
    torpedo Y37.04- ☑
  fire Y37.30- ☑
    specified NEC Y37.39- ☑
  firearms
    discharge Y37.43- ☑
    pellets Y37.42- ☑
  flamethrower Y37.33- ☑
  fragments (from) (of)
    improvised explosive device [IED] (person-borne)
      (roadside) (vehicle-borne) Y37.26- ☑
    munitions Y37.25- ☑
    specified NEC Y37.29- ☑
    weapons Y37.27- ☑
  friendly fire Y37.92- ☑
  hand to hand (unarmed) combat Y37.44- ☑
  hot substances — *see* Military operations, fire
  incendiary bullet Y37.32- ☑
  nuclear weapon (effects of) Y37.50- ☑
    acute radiation exposure Y37.54- ☑
    blast pressure Y37.51- ☑
    direct blast Y37.51- ☑
    direct heat Y37.53- ☑
    fallout exposure Y37.54- ☑
    fireball Y37.53- ☑
    indirect blast (struck or crushed by blast debris)
      (being thrown by blast) Y37.52- ☑
    ionizing radiation (immediate exposure) Y37.54- ☑
    nuclear radiation Y37.54- ☑
    radiation
      ionizing (immediate exposure) Y37.54- ☑
      nuclear Y37.54- ☑
      thermal Y37.53- ☑
    secondary effects Y37.54- ☑
    specified NEC Y37.59- ☑
    thermal radiation Y37.53- ☑
  restriction of air (airway)
    intentional Y37.46- ☑
    unintentional Y37.47- ☑
  rubber bullets Y37.41- ☑
  shrapnel NOS Y37.29- ☑
  suffocation — *see* Military operations, restriction of
    airways
  unconventional warfare NEC Y37.7X- ☑
  underwater blast NOS Y37.00- ☑
  warfare
    conventional NEC Y37.49- ☑
    unconventional NEC Y37.7X- ☑
  weapon of mass destruction [WMD] Y37.91- ☑
  weapons
    biological weapons Y37.6X- ☑
    chemical Y37.7X- ☑
    nuclear (effects of) Y37.50- ☑
      acute radiation exposure Y37.54- ☑
      blast pressure Y37.51- ☑
      direct blast Y37.51- ☑
      direct heat Y37.53- ☑
      fallout exposure Y37.54- ☑
      fireball Y37.53- ☑
      indirect blast (struck or crushed by blast debris)
        (being thrown by blast) Y37.52- ☑
      radiation
        ionizing (immediate exposure) Y37.54- ☑
        nuclear Y37.54- ☑
        thermal Y37.53- ☑

Legal — Military operations

Military operations — *continued*
  weapons — *continued*
    nuclear — *continued*
      secondary effects Y37.54- ☑
      specified NEC Y37.59- ☑
    of mass destruction [WMD] Y37.91- ☑
Misadventure(s) **to patient**(s) **during surgical or medical care** Y69
  contaminated medical or biological substance (blood, drug, fluid) Y64.9
    administered (by) NEC Y64.9
      immunization Y64.1
      infusion Y64.0
      injection Y64.1
      specified means NEC Y64.8
      transfusion Y64.0
      vaccination Y64.1
  excessive amount of blood or other fluid during transfusion or infusion Y63.0
  failure
    in dosage Y63.9
      electroshock therapy Y63.4
      inappropriate temperature (too hot or too cold) in local application and packing Y63.5
      infusion
        excessive amount of fluid Y63.0
        incorrect dilution of fluid Y63.1
      insulin-shock therapy Y63.4
      nonadministration of necessary drug or biological substance Y63.6
      overdose — *see* Table of Drugs and Chemicals
        radiation, in therapy Y63.2
      radiation
        overdose Y63.2
      specified procedure NEC Y63.8
      transfusion
        excessive amount of blood Y63.0
    mechanical, of instrument or apparatus (any) (during any procedure) Y65.8
    sterile precautions (during procedure) Y62.9
      aspiration of fluid or tissue (by puncture or catheterization, except heart) Y62.6
      biopsy (except needle aspiration) Y62.8
        needle (aspirating) Y62.6
      blood sampling Y62.6
      catheterization Y62.6
        heart Y62.5
      dialysis (kidney) Y62.2
      endoscopic examination Y62.4
      enema Y62.8
      immunization Y62.3
      infusion Y62.1
      injection Y62.3
      needle biopsy Y62.6
      paracentesis (abdominal) (thoracic) Y62.6
      perfusion Y62.2
      puncture (lumbar) Y62.6
      removal of catheter or packing Y62.8
      specified procedure NEC Y62.8
      surgical operation Y62.0
      transfusion Y62.1
      vaccination Y62.3
    suture or ligature during surgical procedure Y65.2
    to introduce or to remove tube or instrument B — *see* Failure, to
  hemorrhage — *see* Index to Diseases and Injuries, Complication(s)
  inadvertent exposure of patient to radiation Y63.3
  inappropriate
    operation performed — *see* Inappropriate operation performed
    temperature (too hot or too cold) in local application or packing Y63.5
  infusion (*see also* Misadventure, by type, infusion) Y69
    excessive amount of fluid Y63.0
    incorrect dilution of fluid Y63.1
    wrong fluid Y65.1
  mismatched blood in transfusion Y65.0
  nonadministration of necessary drug or biological substance
    overdose — *see* Table of Drugs and Chemicals
      radiation (in therapy) Y63.2
  perforation — *see* Index to Diseases and Injuries, Complication(s)
  performance of inappropriate operation — *see* Inappropriate operation performed
  puncture — *see* Index to Diseases and Injuries, Complication(s)

Misadventure(s) **to patient**(s) **during surgical or medical care** — *continued*
  specified type NEC Y65.8
    failure
      suture or ligature during surgical operation Y65.2
      to introduce or to remove tube or instrument B — *see* Failure, to
    infusion of wrong fluid Y65.1
    performance of inappropriate operation — *see* Inappropriate operation performed
    transfusion of mismatched blood Y65.0
    wrong
      fluid in infusion Y65.1
      placement of endotracheal tube during anesthetic procedure Y65.3
  transfusion — *see* Misadventure, by type, transfusion
    excessive amount of blood Y63.0
    mismatched blood Y65.0
  wrong
    drug given in error — *see* Table of Drugs and Chemicals
    fluid in infusion Y65.1
    placement of endotracheal tube during anesthetic procedure Y65.3
Mismatched blood in transfusion Y65.0
Motion sickness T75.3 ☑
Mountain sickness W94.11 ☑
Mudslide (of cataclysmic nature) — *see* Landslide
Murder (attempt) — *see* Assault

N

Nail, contact with W45.0 ☑
  gun W29.4 ☑
Neglect (criminal) (homicidal intent) X58 ☑
Noise (causing injury) (pollution) W42.9 ☑
  supersonic W42.0 ☑
Nonadministration (of)
  drug or biological substance (necessary) Y63.6
  surgical and medical care Y66
Nosocomial condition Y95

O

Object
  falling
    from, in, on, hitting
      machinery — *see* Contact, with, by type of machine
  set in motion by
    accidental explosion or rupture of pressure vessel W38 ☑
    firearm — *see* Discharge, firearm, by type
    machine(ry) — *see* Contact, with, by type of machine
Overdose (drug) — *see* Table of Drugs and Chemicals
  radiation Y63.2
Overexertion — *see* category Y93 ☑
Overexposure (accidental) (to)
  cold (*see also* Exposure, cold) X31 ☑
    due to man-made conditions — *see* Exposure, cold, man-made
  heat (*see also* Heat) X30 ☑
  radiation — *see* Radiation
  radioactivity W88.0 ☑
  sun (sunburn) X32 ☑
  weather NEC — *see* Forces of nature
  wind NEC — *see* Forces of nature
Overheated — *see* Heat
Overturning (accidental)
  machinery — *see* Contact, with, by type of machine
  transport vehicle NEC (*see also* Accident, transport) V89.9 ☑
  watercraft (causing drowning, submersion) (*see also* Drowning, due to, accident to, watercraft, overturning)
    causing injury except drowning or submersion B — *see* Accident, watercraft, causing, injury NEC

P

Parachute descent (voluntary) (without accident to aircraft) V97.29 ☑
Pecked by bird W61.99 ☑

Perforation during medical or surgical treatment as misadventure — *see* Index to Diseases and Injuries, Complication(s)

Perpetrator, perpetration, of assault, maltreatment and neglect (by) Y07.9
  boyfriend Y07.03
  brother Y07.410
    stepbrother Y07.435
  coach Y07.53
  cousin
    female Y07.491
    male Y07.490
  daycare provider Y07.519
    at-home
      adult care Y07.512
      childcare Y07.510
    care center
      adult care Y07.513
      childcare Y07.511
  family member NEC Y07.499
  father Y07.11
    adoptive Y07.13
    foster Y07.420
    stepfather Y07.430
  foster father Y07.420
  foster mother Y07.421
  girl friend Y07.04
  healthcare provider Y07.529
    mental health Y07.521
    specified NEC Y07.528
  husband Y07.01
  instructor Y07.53
  mother Y07.12
    adoptive Y07.14
    foster Y07.421
    stepmother Y07.433
  nonfamily member Y07.50
    specified NEC Y07.59
  nurse Y07.528
  occupational therapist Y07.528
  partner of parent
    female Y07.434
    male Y07.432
  physical therapist Y07.528
  sister Y07.411
  speech therapist Y07.528
  stepbrother Y07.435
  stepfather Y07.430
  stepmother Y07.433
  stepsister Y07.436
  teacher Y07.53
  wife Y07.02

Piercing — *see* Contact, with, by type of object or machine

Pinched
  between objects (moving) (stationary and moving) W23.0 ☑
  stationary W23.1 ☑

Pinned under machine(ry) — *see* Contact, with, by type of machine

Place of occurrence Y92.9
  abandoned house Y92.89
  airplane Y92.813
  airport Y92.520
  ambulatory health services establishment NEC Y92.538
  ambulatory surgery center Y92.530
  amusement park Y92.831
  apartment (co-op) — *see* Place of occurrence, residence, apartment
  assembly hall Y92.29
  bank Y92.510
  barn Y92.71
  baseball field Y92.320
  basketball court Y92.310
  beach Y92.832
  boarding house — *see* Place of occurrence, residence, boarding house
  boat Y92.814
  bowling alley Y92.39
  bridge Y92.89
  building under construction Y92.61
  bus Y92.811
    station Y92.521
  cafe Y92.511

Place of occurrence — *continued*
  campsite Y92.833
  campus — *see* Place of occurrence, school
  canal Y92.89
  car Y92.810
  casino Y92.59
  children's home — *see* Place of occurrence, residence, institutional, orphanage
  church Y92.22
  cinema Y92.26
  clubhouse Y92.29
  coal pit Y92.64
  college (community) Y92.214
  condominium — *see* Place of occurrence, residence, apartment
  construction area — *see* Place of occurrence, industrial and construction area
  convalescent home — *see* Place of occurrence, residence, institutional, nursing home
  court-house Y92.240
  cricket ground Y92.328
  cultural building Y92.258
    art gallery Y92.250
    museum Y92.251
    music hall Y92.252
    opera house Y92.253
    specified NEC Y92.258
    theater Y92.254
  dancehall Y92.252
  day nursery Y92.210
  dentist office Y92.531
  derelict house Y92.89
  desert Y92.820
  dockyard Y92.62
  dock NOS Y92.89
  doctor's office Y92.531
  dormitory — *see* Place of occurrence, residence, institutional, school dormitory
  dry dock Y92.62
  factory (building) (premises) Y92.63
  farm (land under cultivation) (outbuildings) Y92.79
    barn Y92.71
    chicken coop Y92.72
    field Y92.73
    hen house Y92.72
    house — *see* Place of occurrence, residence, house
    orchard Y92.74
    specified NEC Y92.79
  football field Y92.321
  forest Y92.821
  freeway Y92.411
  gallery Y92.250
  garage (commercial) Y92.59
    boarding house Y92.044
    military base Y92.135
    mobile home Y92.025
    nursing home Y92.124
    orphanage Y92.114
    private house Y92.015
    reform school Y92.155
  gas station Y92.524
  gasworks Y92.69
  golf course Y92.39
  gravel pit Y92.64
  grocery Y92.512
  gymnasium Y92.39
  handball court Y92.318
  harbor Y92.89
  harness racing course Y92.39
  healthcare provider office Y92.531
  highway (interstate) Y92.411
  hill Y92.828
  hockey rink Y92.330
  home — *see* Place of occurrence, residence
  hospice — *see* Place of occurrence, residence, institutional, nursing home
  hospital Y92.239
    cafeteria Y92.233
    corridor Y92.232
    operating room Y92.234
    patient
      bathroom Y92.231
      room Y92.230
    specified NEC Y92.238
  hotel Y92.59
  house (*see also* Place of occurrence, residence)
    abandoned Y92.89
    under construction Y92.61

Place of occurrence — *continued*
  industrial and construction area (yard) Y92.69
    building under construction Y92.61
    dock Y92.62
    dry dock Y92.62
    factory Y92.63
    gasworks Y92.69
    mine Y92.64
    oil rig Y92.65
    pit Y92.64
    power station Y92.69
    shipyard Y92.62
    specified NEC Y92.69
    tunnel under construction Y92.69
    workshop Y92.69
  kindergarten Y92.211
  lacrosse field Y92.328
  lake Y92.828
  library Y92.241
  mall Y92.59
  market Y92.512
  marsh Y92.828
  military
    base — *see* Place of occurrence, residence, institutional, military base
    training ground Y92.84
  mine Y92.64
  mosque Y92.22
  motel Y92.59
  motorway (interstate) Y92.411
  mountain Y92.828
  movie-house Y92.26
  museum Y92.251
  music-hall Y92.252
  not applicable Y92.9
  nuclear power station Y92.69
  nursing home — *see* Place of occurrence, residence, institutional, nursing home
  office building Y92.59
  offshore installation Y92.65
  oil rig Y92.65
  old people's home — *see* Place of occurrence, residence, institutional, specified NEC
  opera-house Y92.253
  orphanage — *see* Place of occurrence, residence, institutional, orphanage
  outpatient surgery center Y92.530
  park (public) Y92.830
    amusement Y92.831
  parking garage Y92.89
    lot Y92.481
  pavement Y92.480
  physician office Y92.531
  polo field Y92.328
  pond Y92.828
  post office Y92.242
  power station Y92.69
  prairie Y92.828
  prison — *see* Place of occurrence, residence, institutional, prison
  public
    administration building Y92.248
      city hall Y92.243
      courthouse Y92.240
      library Y92.241
      post office Y92.242
      specified NEC Y92.248
    building NEC Y92.29
    hall Y92.29
    place NOS Y92.89
  race course Y92.39
  radio station Y92.59
  railway line (bridge) Y92.85
  ranch (outbuildings) — *see* Place of occurrence, farm
  recreation area Y92.838
    amusement park Y92.831
    beach Y92.832
    campsite Y92.833
    park (public) Y92.830
    seashore Y92.832
    specified NEC Y92.838
  reform school - — *see* Place of occurrence, residence, institutional, reform school
  religious institution Y92.22
  residence (non-institutional) (private) Y92.009
    apartment Y92.039
      bathroom Y92.031
      bedroom Y92.032

Place of occurrence — *continued*
  residence — *continued*
    apartment — *continued*
      kitchen Y92.030
      specified NEC Y92.038
    bathroom Y92.002
    bedroom Y92.003
    boarding house Y92.049
      bathroom Y92.041
      bedroom Y92.042
      driveway Y92.043
      garage Y92.044
      garden Y92.046
      kitchen Y92.040
      specified NEC Y92.048
      swimming pool Y92.045
      yard Y92.046
    dining room Y92.001
    garden Y92.007
    home Y92.009
    house, single family Y92.019
      bathroom Y92.012
      bedroom Y92.013
      dining room Y92.011
      driveway Y92.014
      garage Y92.015
      garden Y92.017
      kitchen Y92.010
      specified NEC Y92.018
      swimming pool Y92.016
      yard Y92.017
    institutional Y92.10
      children's home — *see* Place of occurrence, residence, institutional, orphanage
      hospice — *see* Place of occurrence, residence, institutional, nursing home
      military base Y92.139
        barracks Y92.133
        garage Y92.135
        garden Y92.137
        kitchen Y92.130
        mess hall Y92.131
        specified NEC Y92.138
        swimming pool Y92.136
        yard Y92.137
      nursing home Y92.129
        bathroom Y92.121
        bedroom Y92.122
        driveway Y92.123
        garage Y92.124
        garden Y92.126
        kitchen Y92.120
        specified NEC Y92.128
        swimming pool Y92.125
        yard Y92.126
      orphanage Y92.119
        bathroom Y92.111
        bedroom Y92.112
        driveway Y92.113
        garage Y92.114
        garden Y92.116
        kitchen Y92.110
        specified NEC Y92.118
        swimming pool Y92.115
        yard Y92.116
      prison Y92.149
        bathroom Y92.142
        cell Y92.143
        courtyard Y92.147
        dining room Y92.141
        kitchen Y92.140
        specified NEC Y92.148
        swimming pool Y92.146
      reform school Y92.159
        bathroom Y92.152
        bedroom Y92.153
        dining room Y92.151
        driveway Y92.154
        garage Y92.155
        garden Y92.157
        kitchen Y92.150
        specified NEC Y92.158
        swimming pool Y92.156
        yard Y92.157
      school dormitory Y92.169
        bathroom Y92.162
        bedroom Y92.163
        dining room Y92.161

External Causes Index

Place of occurrence — Prolonged

Place of occurrence — *continued*
  residence — *continued*
    institutional — *continued*
      school dormitory — *continued*
        kitchen Y92.160
        specified NEC Y92.168
      specified NEC Y92.199
        bathroom Y92.192
        bedroom Y92.193
        dining room Y92.191
        driveway Y92.194
        garage Y92.195
        garden Y92.197
        kitchen Y92.190
        specified NEC Y92.198
        swimming pool Y92.196
        yard Y92.197
    kitchen Y92.000
    mobile home Y92.029
      bathroom Y92.022
      bedroom Y92.023
      dining room Y92.021
      driveway Y92.024
      garage Y92.025
      garden Y92.027
      kitchen Y92.020
      specified NEC Y92.028
      swimming pool Y92.026
      yard Y92.027
    specified place in residence NEC Y92.009
    specified residence type NEC Y92.099
      bathroom Y92.091
      bedroom Y92.092
      driveway Y92.093
      garage Y92.094
      garden Y92.096
      kitchen Y92.090
      specified NEC Y92.098
      swimming pool Y92.095
      yard Y92.096
  restaurant Y92.511
  riding school Y92.39
  river Y92.828
  road Y92.488
  rodeo ring Y92.39
  rugby field Y92.328
  same day surgery center Y92.530
  sand pit Y92.64
  school (private) (public) (state) Y92.219
    college Y92.214
    daycare center Y92.210
    elementary school Y92.211
    high school Y92.213
    kindergarten Y92.211
    middle school Y92.212
    specified NEC Y92.218
    trace school Y92.215
    university Y92.214
    vocational school Y92.215
  sea (shore) Y92.832
  senior citizen center Y92.29
  service area
    airport Y92.520
    bus station Y92.521
    gas station Y92.524
    highway rest stop Y92.523
    railway station Y92.522
  shipyard Y92.62
  shop (commercial) Y92.513
  sidewalk Y92.480
  silo Y92.79
  skating rink (roller) Y92.331
    ice Y92.330
  slaughter house Y92.86
  soccer field Y92.322
  specified place NEC Y92.89
  sports area Y92.39
    athletic
      court Y92.318
        basketball Y92.310
        specified NEC Y92.318
        squash Y92.311
        tennis Y92.312
      field Y92.328
        baseball Y92.320
        cricket ground Y92.328
        football Y92.321
        hockey Y92.328

Place of occurrence — *continued*
  sports area — *continued*
    athletic — *continued*
      field — *continued*
        soccer Y92.322
        specified NEC Y92.328
    golf course Y92.39
    gymnasium Y92.39
    riding school Y92.39
    skating rink (roller) Y92.331
      ice Y92.330
    stadium Y92.39
    swimming pool Y92.34
  squash court Y92.311
  stadium Y92.39
  steeplechasing course Y92.39
  store Y92.512
  stream Y92.828
  street and highway Y92.410
    bike path Y92.482
    freeway Y92.411
    highway ramp Y92.415
    interstate highway Y92.411
    local residential or business street Y92.414
    motorway Y92.411
    parking lot Y92.481
    parkway Y92.412
    sidewalk Y92.480
    specified NEC Y92.488
    state road Y92.413
  subway car Y92.816
  supermarket Y92.512
  swamp Y92.828
  swimming pool (public) Y92.34
    private (at) Y92.095
      boarding house Y92.045
      military base Y92.136
      mobile home Y92.026
      nursing home Y92.125
      orphanage Y92.115
      prison Y92.146
      reform school Y92.156
      single family residence Y92.016
  synagogue Y92.22
  television station Y92.59
  tennis court Y92.312
  theater Y92.254
  trade area Y92.59
    bank Y92.510
    cafe Y92.511
    casino Y92.59
    garage Y92.59
    hotel Y92.59
    market Y92.512
    office building Y92.59
    radio station Y92.59
    restaurant Y92.511
    shop Y92.513
    shopping mall Y92.59
    store Y92.512
    supermarket Y92.512
    television station Y92.59
    warehouse Y92.59
  trailer park, residential — *see* Place of occurrence, residence, mobile home
  trailer site NOS Y92.89
  train Y92.815
    station Y92.522
  truck Y92.812
  tunnel under construction Y92.69
  university Y92.214
  urgent (health) care center Y92.532
  vehicle (transport) Y92.818
    airplane Y92.813
    boat Y92.814
    bus Y92.811
    car Y92.810
    specified NEC Y92.818
    subway car Y92.816
    train Y92.815
    truck Y92.812
  warehouse Y92.59
  water reservoir Y92.89
  wilderness area Y92.828
    desert Y92.820
    forest Y92.821
    marsh Y92.828
    mountain Y92.828

Place of occurrence — *continued*
  wilderness area — *continued*
    prairie Y92.828
    specified NEC Y92.828
    swamp Y92.828
  workshop Y92.69
  yard, private Y92.096
    boarding house Y92.046
    mobile home Y92.027
    single family house Y92.017
  youth center Y92.29
  zoo (zoological garden) Y92.834
Plumbism — *see* Table of Drugs and Chemicals, lead
Poisoning (accidental) (by) (*see also* Table of Drugs and Chemicals)
  by plant, thorns, spines, sharp leaves or other mechanisms NEC X58 ☑
  carbon monoxide
    generated by
      motor vehicle — *see* Accident, transport
      watercraft (in transit) (not in transit) V93.89 ☑
        ferry boat V93.81 ☑
        fishing boat V93.82 ☑
        jet skis V93.83 ☑
        liner V93.81 ☑
        merchant ship V93.80 ☑
        passenger ship V93.81 ☑
        powered craft NEC V93.83 ☑
  caused by injection of poisons into skin by plant thorns, spines, sharp leaves X58 ☑
    marine or sea plants (venomous) X58 ☑
  execution — *see* Legal, intervention, gas
  intervention
    by gas — *see* Legal, intervention, gas
    other specified means — *see* Legal, intervention, specified means NEC
  exhaust gas
    generated by
      motor vehicle — *see* Accident, transport
      watercraft (in transit) (not in transit) V93.89 ☑
        ferry boat V93.81 ☑
        fishing boat V93.82 ☑
        jet skis V93.83 ☑
        liner V93.81 ☑
        merchant ship V93.80 ☑
        passenger ship V93.81 ☑
        powered craft NEC V93.83 ☑
  fumes or smoke due to
    explosion (*see also* Explosion) W40.9 ☑
    fire — *see* Exposure, fire
    ignition — *see* Ignition
  gas
    in legal intervention — *see* Legal, intervention, gas
    legal execution — *see* Legal, intervention, gas
  in war operations — *see* War operations
  legal
Powder burn (by) (from)
  airgun W34.110 ☑
  BB gun W34.110 ☑
  firearm NEC W34.19 ☑
  gas, air or spring-operated gun NEC W34.118 ☑
  handgun W32.1 ☑
  hunting rifle W33.12 ☑
  larger firearm W33.10 ☑
    specified NEC W33.19 ☑
  machine gun W33.13 ☑
  paintball gun W34.111 ☑
  pellet gun W34.110 ☑
  shotgun W33.11 ☑
  Very pistol [flare] W34.19 ☑
Premature cessation (of) **surgical and medical care** Y66
Privation (food) (water) X58 ☑
Procedure (operation)
  correct, on wrong side or body part (wrong side) (wrong site) Y65.53
  intended for another patient done on wrong patient Y65.52
  performed on patient not scheduled for surgery Y65.52
  performed on wrong patient Y65.52
  wrong, performed on correct patient Y65.51
Prolonged
  sitting in transport vehicle — *see* Travel, by type of vehicle
  stay in
    high altitude as cause of anoxia, barodontalgia, barotitis or hypoxia W94.11 ☑

☑ Additional Character Required — Refer to the Tabular List for Character Selection   ▽ Subterms under main terms may continue to next column or page

Prolonged — *continued*
  stay in — *continued*
    weightless environment X52 ☑
Pulling, excessive — *see* Overexertion
Puncture, puncturing (*see also* Contact, with, by type
    of object or machine)
  by
    plant thorns, spines, sharp leaves or other mecha-
      nisms NEC W60 ☑
  during medical or surgical treatment as misadventure
    — *see* Index to Diseases and Injuries, Complica-
    tion(s)
Pushed, pushing (accidental) (injury in) (overexertion)
  (*see also* Overexertion)
  by other person(s) (accidental) W51 ☑
    with fall W03 ☑
      due to ice or snow W00.0 ☑
    as, or caused by, a crowd or human stampede (with
      fall) W52 ☑
    before moving object NEC Y02.8 ☑
      motor vehicle Y02.0 ☑
      subway train Y02.1 ☑
      train Y02.1 ☑
    from
      high place NEC
        in accidental circumstances W17.89 ☑
        stated as
          intentional, homicide (attempt) Y01 ☑
          undetermined whether accidental or
            intentional Y30 ☑
      transport vehicle NEC (*see also* Accident, trans-
        port) V89.9 ☑
        stated as
          intentional, homicide (attempt)
            Y08.89 ☑

R

Radiation (exposure to)
  arc lamps W89.0 ☑
  atomic power plant (malfunction) NEC W88.1 ☑
  complication of or abnormal reaction to medical radio-
    therapy Y84.2
  electromagnetic, ionizing W88.0 ☑
  gamma rays W88.1 ☑
  in
    war operations (from or following nuclear explo-
      sion) — *see* War operations
  inadvertent exposure of patient (receiving test or
    therapy) Y63.3
  infrared (heaters and lamps) W90.1 ☑
    excessive heat from W92 ☑
  ionized, ionizing (particles, artificially accelerated)
    radioisotopes W88.1 ☑
    specified NEC W88.8 ☑
    x-rays W88.0 ☑
  isotopes, radioactive — *see* Radiation, radioactive
    isotopes
  laser(s) W90.2 ☑
    in war operations — *see* War operations
    misadventure in medical care Y63.2
  light sources (man-made visible and ultraviolet)
    W89.9 ☑
    natural X32 ☑
    specified NEC W89.8 ☑
    tanning bed W89.1 ☑
    welding light W89.0 ☑
  man-made visible light W89.9 ☑
    specified NEC W89.8 ☑
    tanning bed W89.1 ☑
    welding light W89.0 ☑
  microwave W90.8 ☑
  misadventure in medical or surgical procedure Y63.2
  natural NEC X39.08 ☑
    radon X39.01 ☑
  overdose (in medical or surgical procedure) Y63.2
  radar W90.0 ☑
  radioactive isotopes (any) W88.1 ☑
    atomic power plant malfunction W88.1 ☑
    misadventure in medical or surgical treatment
      Y63.2
  radiofrequency W90.0 ☑
  radium NEC W88.1 ☑
  sun X32 ☑
  ultraviolet (light) (man-made) W89.9 ☑
    natural X32 ☑

Radiation — *continued*
  ultraviolet — *continued*
    specified NEC W89.8 ☑
    tanning bed W89.1 ☑
    welding light W89.0 ☑
  welding arc, torch, or light W89.0 ☑
    excessive heat from W92 ☑
  x-rays (hard) (soft) W88.0 ☑
Range disease W94.11 ☑
Rape (attempted) T74.2- ☑
Rat bite W53.11 ☑
Reaction, abnormal to medical procedure (*see also*
    Complication of or following, by type of procedure)
    Y84.9
  with misadventure — *see* Misadventure
  biologicals — *see* Table of Drugs and Chemicals
  drugs — *see* Table of Drugs and Chemicals
  vaccine — *see* Table of Drugs and Chemicals
Recoil
  airgun W34.110 ☑
  BB gun W34.110 ☑
  firearm NEC W34.19 ☑
  gas, air or spring-operated gun NEC W34.118 ☑
  handgun W32.1 ☑
  hunting rifle W33.12 ☑
  larger firearm W33.10 ☑
    specified NEC W33.19 ☑
  machine gun W33.13 ☑
  paintball gun W34.111 ☑
  pellet W34.110 ☑
  shotgun W33.11 ☑
  Very pistol [flare] W34.19 ☑
Reduction in
  atmospheric pressure — *see* Air, pressure, change
Rock falling on or hitting (accidentally) (person)
    W20.8 ☑
  in cave-in W20.0 ☑
Run over (accidentally) (by)
  animal (not being ridden) NEC W55.89 ☑
  machinery — *see* Contact, with, by specified type of
    machine
  transport vehicle NEC (*see also* Accident, transport)
    V09.9 ☑
    intentional homicide (attempt) Y03.0 ☑
    motor NEC V09.20 ☑
      intentional homicide (attempt) Y03.0 ☑
Running
  before moving object X81.8 ☑
    motor vehicle X81.0 ☑
Running off, away
  animal (being ridden) (*see also* Accident, transport)
    V80.918 ☑
    not being ridden W55.89 ☑
  animal-drawn vehicle NEC (*see also* Accident, trans-
    port) V80.928 ☑
  highway, road(way), street
    transport vehicle NEC (*see also* Accident, transport)
      V89.9 ☑
Rupture pressurized devices — *see* Explosion, by type
    of device

S

Saturnism — *see* Table of Drugs and Chemicals, lead
Scald, scalding (accidental) (by) (from) (in) X19 ☑
  air (hot) X14.1 ☑
  gases (hot) X14.1 ☑
  homicide (attempt) — *see* Assault, burning, hot object
  inflicted by other person
    stated as intentional, homicide (attempt) — *see*
      Assault, burning, hot object
  liquid (boiling) (hot) NEC X12 ☑
    stated as undetermined whether accidental or in-
      tentional Y27.2 ☑
    suicide (attempt) X77.2 ☑
  local application of externally applied substance in
    medical or surgical care Y63.5
  metal (molten) (liquid) (hot) NEC X18 ☑
  self-inflicted X77.9 ☑
  stated as undetermined whether accidental or inten-
    tional Y27.8 ☑
  steam X13.1 ☑
    assault X98.0 ☑
    stated as undetermined whether accidental or in-
      tentional Y27.0 ☑
    suicide (attempt) X77.0 ☑

Scald, scalding — *continued*
  suicide (attempt) X77.9 ☑
  vapor (hot) X13.1 ☑
    assault X98.0 ☑
    stated as undetermined whether accidental or in-
      tentional Y27.0 ☑
    suicide (attempt) X77.0 ☑
Scratched by
  cat W55.03 ☑
  person(s) (accidentally) W50.4 ☑
    with intent to injure or kill Y04.0 ☑
    as, or caused by, a crowd or human stampede (with
      fall) W52 ☑
    assault Y04.0 ☑
    homicide (attempt) Y04.0 ☑
    in
      fight Y04.0 ☑
      legal intervention
        injuring
          bystander Y35.892 ☑
          law enforcement personnel Y35.891 ☑
          suspect Y35.893 ☑
Seasickness T75.3 ☑
Self-harm NEC (*see also* External cause by type, undeter-
    mined whether accidental or intentional)
  intentional — *see* Suicide
  poisoning NEC — *see* Table of Drugs and Chemicals,
    poisoning, accidental
Self-inflicted (injury) **NEC** (*see also* External cause by
    type, undetermined whether accidental or inten-
    tional)
  intentional — *see* Suicide
  poisoning NEC — *see* Table of Drugs and Chemicals,
    poisoning, accidental
Sequelae (of)
  accident NEC — *see* W00-X58 with 7th character S
  assault (homicidal) (any means) — *see* X92-Y08 with
    7th character S
  homicide, attempt (any means) — *see* X92-Y08 with
    7th character S
  injury undetermined whether accidentally or purposely
    inflicted — *see* Y21-Y33 with 7th character S
  intentional self-harm (classifiable to X71-X83) — *see*
    X71-X83 with 7th character S
  legal intervention — *see* with 7th character S Y35 ☑
  motor vehicle accident — *see* V00-V99 with 7th char-
    acter S
  suicide, attempt (any means) — *see* X71-X83 with 7th
    character S
  transport accident — *see* V00-V99 with 7th character
    S
  war operations — *see* War operations
Shock
  electric — *see* Exposure, electric current
  from electric appliance (any) (faulty) W86.8 ☑
    domestic W86.0 ☑
    suicide (attempt) X83.1 ☑
Shooting, shot (accidental(ly)) (*see also* Discharge,
    firearm, by type)
  herself or himself — *see* Discharge, firearm by type,
    self-inflicted
  homicide (attempt) — *see* Discharge, firearm by type,
    homicide
  in war operations — *see* War operations
  inflicted by other person — *see* Discharge, firearm by
    type, homicide
    accidental — *see* Discharge, firearm, by type of
      firearm
  legal
    execution — *see* Legal, intervention, firearm
    intervention — *see* Legal, intervention, firearm
  self-inflicted — *see* Discharge, firearm by type, suicide
    accidental — *see* Discharge, firearm, by type of
      firearm
  suicide (attempt) — *see* Discharge, firearm by type,
    suicide
Shoving (accidentally) **by other person** — *see* Pushed,
    by other person
Sickness
  alpine W94.11 ☑
  motion — *see* Motion
  mountain W94.11 ☑

Sinking (accidental)
watercraft (causing drowning, submersion) (*see also* Drowning, due to, accident to, watercraft, sinking)
causing injury except drowning or submersion B — *see* Accident, watercraft, causing, injury NEC
Siriasis X32 ☑
Slashed wrists — *see* Cut, self-inflicted
Slipping (accidental) (on same level) (with fall) W01.0 ☑
without fall W18.40 ☑
due to
specified NEC W18.49 ☑
stepping from one level to another W18.43 ☑
stepping into hole or opening W18.42 ☑
stepping on object W18.41 ☑
on
ice W00.0 ☑
with skates — *see* Accident, transport, pedestrian, conveyance
mud W01.0 ☑
oil W01.0 ☑
snow W00.0 ☑
with skis — *see* Accident, transport, pedestrian, conveyance
surface (slippery) (wet) NEC W01.0 ☑
Sliver, wood, contact with W45.8 ☑
Smoldering (due to fire) — *see* Exposure, fire
Sodomy (attempted) **by force** T74.2 ☑
Sound waves (causing injury) W42.9 ☑
supersonic W42.0 ☑
Splinter, contact with W45.8 ☑
Stab, stabbing B — *see* Cut
Starvation X58 ☑
Status of external cause Y99.9
child assisting in compensated work for family Y99.8
civilian activity done for financial or other compensation Y99.0
civilian activity done for income or pay Y99.0
family member assisting in compensated work for other family member Y99.8
hobby not done for income Y99.8
leisure activity Y99.8
military activity Y99.1
off-duty activity of military personnel Y99.8
recreation or sport not for income or while a student Y99.8
specified NEC Y99.8
student activity Y99.8
volunteer activity Y99.2
Stepped on
by
animal (not being ridden) NEC W55.89 ☑
crowd or human stampede W52 ☑
person W50.0 ☑
Stepping on
object W22.8 ☑
with fall W18.31 ☑
sports equipment W21.9 ☑
stationary W22.09 ☑
sports equipment W21.89 ☑
person W51 ☑
by crowd or human stampede W52 ☑
sports equipment W21.9 ☑
Sting
arthropod, nonvenomous W57 ☑
insect, nonvenomous W57 ☑
Storm (cataclysmic) B — *see* Forces of nature, cataclysmic storm
Straining, excessive — *see* Overexertion
Strangling — *see* Strangulation
Strangulation (accidental) T71 ☑
Strenuous movements — *see* category Y93
Striking against
airbag (automobile) W22.10 ☑
driver side W22.11 ☑
front passenger side W22.12 ☑
specified NEC W22.19 ☑
bottom when
diving or jumping into water (in) W16.822 ☑
causing drowning W16.821 ☑
from boat W16.722 ☑
causing drowning W16.721 ☑
natural body W16.622 ☑
causing drowning W16.821 ☑
swimming pool W16.522 ☑
causing drowning W16.521 ☑

Striking against — *continued*
bottom when — *continued*
falling into water (in) W16.322 ☑
causing drowning W16.321 ☑
fountain — *see* Striking against, bottom when, falling into water, specified NEC
natural body W16.122 ☑
causing drowning W16.121 ☑
reservoir — *see* Striking against, bottom when, falling into water, specified NEC
specified NEC W16.322 ☑
causing drowning W16.321 ☑
swimming pool W16.022 ☑
causing drowning W16.021 ☑
diving board (swimming-pool) W21.4 ☑
object W22.8 ☑
with
drowning or submersion — *see* Drowning
fall — *see* Fall, due to, bumping against, object
caused by crowd or human stampede (with fall) W52 ☑
furniture W22.03 ☑
lamppost W22.02 ☑
sports equipment W21.9 ☑
stationary W22.09 ☑
sports equipment W21.89 ☑
wall W22.01 ☑
person(s) W51 ☑
with fall W03 ☑
due to ice or snow W00.0 ☑
as, or caused by, a crowd or human stampede (with fall) W52 ☑
assault Y04.2 ☑
homicide (attempt) Y04.2 ☑
sports equipment W21.9 ☑
wall (when) W22.01 ☑
diving or jumping into water (in) W16.832 ☑
causing drowning W16.831 ☑
swimming pool W16.532 ☑
causing drowning W16.531 ☑
falling into water (in) W16.332 ☑
causing drowning W16.331 ☑
fountain — *see* Striking against, wall when, falling into water, specified NEC
natural body W16.132 ☑
causing drowning W16.131 ☑
reservoir — *see* Striking against, wall when, falling into water, specified NEC
specified NEC W16.332 ☑
causing drowning W16.331 ☑
swimming pool W16.032 ☑
causing drowning W16.031 ☑
swimming pool (when) W22.042 ☑
causing drowning W22.041 ☑
diving or jumping into water W16.532 ☑
causing drowning W16.531 ☑
falling into water W16.032 ☑
causing drowning W16.031 ☑
Struck (accidentally) **by**
airbag (automobile) W22.10 ☑
driver side W22.11 ☑
front passenger side W22.12 ☑
specified NEC W22.19 ☑
alligator W58.02 ☑
animal (not being ridden) NEC W55.89 ☑
avalanche — *see* Landslide
ball (hit) (thrown) W21.00 ☑
assault Y08.09 ☑
baseball W21.03 ☑
basketball W21.05 ☑
football W21.01 ☑
golf ball W21.04 ☑
soccer W21.02 ☑
softball W21.07 ☑
specified NEC W21.09 ☑
volleyball W21.06 ☑
bat or racquet
baseball bat W21.11 ☑
assault Y08.02 ☑
golf club W21.13 ☑
assault Y08.09 ☑
specified NEC W21.19 ☑
assault Y08.09 ☑
tennis racquet W21.12 ☑
assault Y08.09 ☑

Struck (accidentally) **by** — *continued*
bullet (*see also* Discharge, firearm by type)
in war operations — *see* War operations
crocodile W58.12 ☑
dog W54.1 ☑
flare, Very pistol — *see* Discharge, firearm NEC
hailstones X39.8 ☑
hockey (ice)
field
puck W21.221 ☑
stick W21.211 ☑
puck W21.220 ☑
stick W21.210 ☑
assault Y08.01 ☑
landslide — *see* Landslide
law-enforcement agent (on duty) — *see* Legal, intervention, manhandling
with blunt object — *see* Legal, intervention, blunt object
lightning T75.0 ☑
causing fire — *see* Exposure, fire
machine — *see* Contact, with, by type of machine
mammal NEC W55.89 ☑
marine W56.32 ☑
marine animal W56.82 ☑
missile
firearm — *see* Discharge, firearm by type
in war operations — *see* War operations, missile
object W22.8 ☑
blunt W22.8 ☑
assault Y00 ☑
suicide (attempt) X79 ☑
undetermined whether accidental or intentional Y29 ☑
falling W20.8 ☑
from, in, on
building W20.1 ☑
burning (uncontrolled fire) X00.4 ☑
cataclysmic
earth surface movement NEC — *see* Landslide
storm — *see* Forces of nature, cataclysmic storm
cave-in W20.0 ☑
earthquake X34 ☑
machine (in operation) — *see* Contact, with, by type of machine
structure W20.1 ☑
burning X00.4 ☑
transport vehicle (in motion) — *see* Accident, transport, by type of vehicle
watercraft V93.49 ☑
due to
accident to craft V91.39 ☑
powered craft V91.33 ☑
ferry boat V91.31 ☑
fishing boat V91.32 ☑
jetskis V91.33 ☑
liner V91.31 ☑
merchant ship V91.30 ☑
passenger ship V91.31 ☑
unpowered craft V91.38 ☑
canoe V91.35 ☑
inflatable V91.36 ☑
kayak V91.35 ☑
sailboat V91.34 ☑
surf-board V91.38 ☑
windsurfer V91.38 ☑
powered craft V93.43 ☑
ferry boat V93.41 ☑
fishing boat V93.42 ☑
jetskis V93.43 ☑
liner V93.41 ☑
merchant ship V93.40 ☑
passenger ship V93.41 ☑
unpowered craft V93.48 ☑
sailboat V93.44 ☑
surf-board V93.48 ☑
windsurfer V93.48 ☑
moving NEC W20.8 ☑
projected W20.8 ☑
assault Y00 ☑
in sports W21.9 ☑
assault Y08.09 ☑
ball W21.00 ☑

☑ **Additional Character Required** — Refer to the Tabular List for Character Selection   ◥ **Subterms under main terms may continue to next column or page**

Struck (accidentally) **by** — *continued*
  object — *continued*
    projected — *continued*
      in sports — *continued*
        ball — *continued*
          baseball W21.03 ☑
          basketball W21.05 ☑
          football W21.01 ☑
          golf ball W21.04 ☑
          soccer W21.02 ☑
          softball W21.07 ☑
          specified NEC W21.09 ☑
          volleyball W21.06 ☑
        bat or racquet
          baseball bat W21.11 ☑
            assault Y08.02 ☑
          golf club W21.13 ☑
            assault Y08.09 ☑
          specified NEC W21.19 ☑
            assault Y08.09 ☑
          tennis racquet W21.12 ☑
            assault Y08.09 ☑
        hockey (ice)
          field
            puck W21.221 ☑
            stick W21.211 ☑
          puck W21.220 ☑
          stick W21.210 ☑
            assault Y08.01 ☑
        specified NEC W21.89 ☑
    set in motion by explosion — *see* Explosion
    thrown W20.8 ☑
      assault Y00 ☑
      in sports W21.9 ☑
        assault Y08.09 ☑
        ball W21.00 ☑
          baseball W21.03 ☑
          basketball W21.05 ☑
          football W21.01 ☑
          golf ball W21.04 ☑
          soccer W21.02 ☑
          soft ball W21.07 ☑
          specified NEC W21.09 ☑
          volleyball W21.06 ☑
        bat or racquet
          baseball bat W21.11 ☑
            assault Y08.02 ☑
          golf club W21.13 ☑
            assault Y08.09 ☑
          specified NEC W21.19 ☑
            assault Y08.09 ☑
          tennis racquet W21.12 ☑
            assault Y08.09 ☑
        hockey (ice)
          field
            puck W21.221 ☑
            stick W21.211 ☑
          puck W21.220 ☑
          stick W21.210 ☑
            assault Y08.01 ☑
        specified NEC W21.89 ☑
  other person(s) W50.0 ☑
    with
      blunt object W22.8 ☑
        intentional, homicide (attempt) Y00 ☑
      sports equipment W21.9 ☑
      undetermined whether accidental or intentional Y29 ☑
    fall W03 ☑
      due to ice or snow W00.0 ☑
    as, or caused by, a crowd or human stampede (with fall) W52 ☑
    assault Y04.2 ☑
    homicide (attempt) Y04.2 ☑
    in legal intervention
      injuring
        bystander Y35.812 ☑
        law enforcement personnel Y35.811 ☑
        suspect Y35.813 ☑
    sports equipment W21.9 ☑
    police (on duty) — *see* Legal, intervention, manhandling
      with blunt object — *see* Legal, intervention, blunt object
    sports equipment W21.9 ☑
      assault Y08.09 ☑

Struck (accidentally) **by** — *continued*
  sports equipment — *continued*
    ball W21.00 ☑
      baseball W21.03 ☑
      basketball W21.05 ☑
      football W21.01 ☑
      golf ball W21.04 ☑
      soccer W21.02 ☑
      soft ball W21.07 ☑
      specified NEC W21.09 ☑
      volleyball W21.06 ☑
    bat or racquet
      baseball bat W21.11 ☑
        assault Y08.02 ☑
      golf club W21.13 ☑
        assault Y08.09 ☑
      specified NEC W21.19 ☑
      tennis racquet W21.12 ☑
        assault Y08.09 ☑
    cleats (shoe) W21.31 ☑
    foot wear NEC W21.39 ☑
    football helmet W21.81 ☑
    hockey (ice)
      field
        puck W21.221 ☑
        stick W21.211 ☑
      puck W21.220 ☑
      stick W21.210 ☑
        assault Y08.01 ☑
    skate blades W21.32 ☑
    specified NEC W21.89 ☑
      assault Y08.09 ☑
  thunderbolt — *see* subcategory T75.0 ☑
    causing fire — *see* Exposure, fire
  transport vehicle NEC (*see also* Accident, transport) V09.9 ☑
    intentional, homicide (attempt) Y03.0 ☑
    motor NEC (*see also* Accident, transport) V09.20 ☑
      homicide Y03.0 ☑
  vehicle (transport) NEC — *see* Accident, transport, by type of vehicle
    stationary (falling from jack, hydraulic lift, ramp) W20.8 ☑
Stumbling
  without fall W18.40 ☑
    due to
      specified NEC W18.49 ☑
      stepping from one level to another W18.43 ☑
      stepping into hole or opening W18.42 ☑
      stepping on object W18.41 ☑
    over
      animal NEC W01.0 ☑
        with fall W18.09 ☑
      carpet, rug or (small) object W22.8 ☑
        with fall W18.09 ☑
      person W51 ☑
        with fall W03 ☑
          due to ice or snow W00.0 ☑
Submersion (accidental) — *see* Drowning
Suffocation (accidental) (by external means) (by pressure) (mechanical) (*see also* category) T71 ☑
  due to, by
    avalanche — *see* Landslide
    explosion — *see* Explosion
    fire — *see* Exposure, fire
    food, any type (aspiration) (ingestion) (inhalation) — *see* categories T17 and T18 ☑
    ignition — *see* Ignition
    landslide — *see* Landslide
    machine(ry) — *see* Contact, with, by type of machine
    vomitus (aspiration) (inhalation) T17.81- ☑
  in
    burning building X00.8 ☑
Suicide, suicidal (attempted) (by) X83.8 ☑
  blunt object X79 ☑
  burning, burns X76 ☑
    hot object X77.9 ☑
      fluid NEC X77.2 ☑
      household appliance X77.3 ☑
      specified NEC X77.8 ☑
      steam X77.0 ☑
      tap water X77.1 ☑
      vapors X77.0 ☑
  caustic substance — *see* Table of Drugs and Chemicals
  cold, extreme X83.2 ☑

Suicide, suicidal — *continued*
  collision of motor vehicle with
    motor vehicle X82.0 ☑
    specified NEC X82.8 ☑
    train X82.1 ☑
    tree X82.2 ☑
  crashing of aircraft X83.0 ☑
  cut (any part of body) X78.9 ☑
  cutting or piercing instrument X78.9 ☑
    dagger X78.2 ☑
    glass X78.0 ☑
    knife X78.1 ☑
    specified NEC X78.8 ☑
    sword X78.2 ☑
  drowning (in) X71.9 ☑
    bathtub X71.0 ☑
    natural water X71.3 ☑
    specified NEC X71.8 ☑
    swimming pool X71.1 ☑
      following fall X71.2 ☑
  electrocution X83.1 ☑
  explosive(s) (material) X75 ☑
  fire, flames X76 ☑
  firearm X74.9 ☑
    airgun X74.01 ☑
    handgun X72 ☑
    hunting rifle X73.1 ☑
    larger X73.9 ☑
      specified NEC X73.8 ☑
    machine gun X73.2 ☑
    shotgun X73.0 ☑
    specified NEC X74.8 ☑
  hanging X83.8 ☑
  hot object — *see* Suicide, burning, hot object
  jumping
    before moving object X81.8 ☑
      motor vehicle X81.0 ☑
      subway train X81.1 ☑
      train X81.1 ☑
    from high place X80 ☑
  late effect of attempt — *see* X71-X83 with 7th character S
  lying before moving object, train, vehicle X81.8 ☑
  poisoning — *see* Table of Drugs and Chemicals
  puncture (any part of body) — *see* Suicide, cutting or piercing instrument
  scald — *see* Suicide, burning, hot object
  sequelae of attempt — *see* X71-X83 with 7th character S
  sharp object (any) — *see* Suicide, cutting or piercing instrument
  shooting — *see* Suicide, firearm
  specified means NEC X83.8 ☑
  stab (any part of body) — *see* Suicide, cutting or piercing instrument
  steam, hot vapors X77.0 ☑
  strangulation X83.8 ☑
  submersion — *see* Suicide, drowning
  suffocation X83.8 ☑
  wound NEC X83.8 ☑
Sunstroke X32 ☑
Supersonic waves (causing injury) W42.0 ☑
Surgical procedure, complication of (delayed or as an abnormal reaction without mention of misadventure) (*see also* Complication of or following, by type of procedure)
  due to or as a result of misadventure — *see* Misadventure
Swallowed, swallowing
  foreign body — *see* Foreign body, alimentary canal
  poison — *see* Table of Drugs and Chemicals
  substance
    caustic or corrosive — *see* Table of Drugs and Chemicals
    poisonous — *see* Table of Drugs and Chemicals

T

Tackle in sport W03 ☑
Terrorism (involving) Y38.80 ☑
  biological weapons Y38.6X- ☑
  chemical weapons Y38.7X- ☑
  conflagration Y38.3X- ☑
  explosion Y38.2X- ☑
    destruction of aircraft Y38.1X- ☑
    marine weapons Y38.0X- ☑

Terrorism — *continued*
  fire Y38.3X- ☑
  firearms Y38.4X- ☑
  hot substances Y38.5X- ☑
  nuclear weapons Y38.5X- ☑
  specified method NEC Y38.89- ☑
Thirst X58 ☑
Threat to breathing
  aspiration — *see* Aspiration
  due to cave-in, falling earth or substance NEC T71 ☑
Thrown (accidentally)
  against part (any) of or object in transport vehicle (in
        motion) NEC (*see also* Accident, transport)
  from
    high place, homicide (attempt) Y01 ☑
    machinery — *see* Contact, with, by type of machine
    transport vehicle NEC (*see also* Accident, transport)
        V89.9 ☑
  off — *see* Thrown, from
Thunderbolt — *see* subcategory T75.0 ☑
  causing fire — *see* Exposure, fire
Tidal wave (any injury) NEC — *see* Forces of nature, tidal
        wave
Took
  overdose (drug) — *see* Table of Drugs and Chemicals
  poison — *see* Table of Drugs and Chemicals
Tornado (any injury) X37.1 ☑
Torrential rain (any injury) X37.8 ☑
Torture X58 ☑
Trampled by animal NEC W55.89 ☑
Trapped (accidentally)
  between objects (moving) (stationary and moving) —
        see Caught
  by part (any) of
    motorcycle V29.88 ☑
    pedal cycle V19.88 ☑
    transport vehicle NEC (*see also* Accident, transport)
        V89.9 ☑
Travel (effects) (sickness) T75.3 ☑
Tree falling on or hitting (accidentally) (person)
        W20.8 ☑
Tripping
  without fall W18.40 ☑
    due to
      specified NEC W18.49 ☑
      stepping from one level to another W18.43 ☑
      stepping into hole or opening W18.42 ☑
      stepping on object W18.41 ☑
    over
      animal W01.0 ☑
        with fall W01.0 ☑
      carpet, rug or (small) object W22.8 ☑
        with fall W18.09 ☑
      person W51 ☑
        with fall W03 ☑
    due to ice or snow W00.0 ☑
Twisted by person(s) (accidentally) W50.2 ☑
  with intent to injure or kill Y04.0 ☑
  as, or caused by, a crowd or human stampede (with
        fall) W52 ☑
  assault Y04.0 ☑
  homicide (attempt) Y04.0 ☑
  in
    fight Y04.0 ☑
    legal intervention — *see* Legal, intervention,
        manhandling
Twisting, excessive — *see* Overexertion

U

**Underdosing of necessary drugs, medicaments or
        biological substances** Y63.6
Undetermined intent (contact) (exposure)
  automobile collision Y32 ☑
  blunt object Y29 ☑
  drowning (submersion) (in) Y21.9 ☑
    bathtub Y21.0 ☑
      after fall Y21.1 ☑
    natural water (lake) (ocean) (pond) (river) (stream)
        Y21.4 ☑
    specified place NEC Y21.8 ☑
    swimming pool Y21.2 ☑
      after fall Y21.3 ☑
  explosive material Y25 ☑
  fall, jump or push from high place Y30 ☑
  falling, lying or running before moving object Y31 ☑

Undetermined intent — *continued*
  fire Y26 ☑
  firearm discharge Y24.9 ☑
    airgun (BB) (pellet) Y24.0 ☑
    handgun (pistol) (revolver) Y22 ☑
    hunting rifle Y23.1 ☑
    larger Y23.9 ☑
      hunting rifle Y23.1 ☑
      machine gun Y23.3 ☑
      military Y23.2 ☑
      shotgun Y23.0 ☑
      specified type NEC Y23.8 ☑
    machine gun Y23.3 ☑
    military Y23.2 ☑
    shotgun Y23.0 ☑
    specified type NEC Y24.8 ☑
    Very pistol Y24.8 ☑
  hot object Y27.9 ☑
    fluid NEC Y27.2 ☑
    household appliance Y27.3 ☑
    specified object NEC Y27.8 ☑
    steam Y27.0 ☑
    tap water Y27.1 ☑
    vapor Y27.0 ☑
  jump, fall or push from high place Y30 ☑
  lying, falling or running before moving object Y31 ☑
  motor vehicle crash Y32 ☑
  push, fall or jump from high place Y30 ☑
  running, falling or lying before moving object Y31 ☑
  sharp object Y28.9 ☑
    dagger Y28.2 ☑
    glass Y28.0 ☑
    knife Y28.1 ☑
    specified object NEC Y28.8 ☑
    sword Y28.2 ☑
  smoke Y26 ☑
  specified event NEC Y33 ☑

V

Vibration (causing injury) W49.9 ☑
Victim (of)
  avalanche — *see* Landslide
  earth movements NEC — *see* Forces of nature, earth
        movement
  earthquake X34 ☑
  flood — *see* Flood
  landslide — *see* Landslide
  lightning — *see* subcategory T75.0 ☑
    causing fire — *see* Exposure, fire
  storm (cataclysmic) NEC — *see* Forces of nature, cata-
        clysmic storm
  volcanic eruption X35 ☑
Volcanic eruption (any injury) X35 ☑
Vomitus, gastric contents in air passages (with as-
        phyxia, obstruction or suffocation) T17.81- ☑

W

Walked into stationary object (any) W22.09 ☑
  furniture W22.03 ☑
  lamppost W22.02 ☑
  wall W22.01 ☑
War operations (injuries to military personnel and civil-
        ians during war, civil insurrection and peacekeeping
        missions) (by) (from) (involving) Y36.90 ☑
  after cessation of hostilities Y36.89- ☑
    explosion (of)
      bomb placed during war operations Y36.82- ☑
      mine placed during war operations Y36.81- ☑
      specified NEC Y36.88- ☑
  air blast Y36.20- ☑
  aircraft
    destruction — *see* War operations, destruction of
        aircraft
    airway restriction — *see* War operations, restriction
        of airways
    asphyxiation — *see* War operations, restriction of air-
        ways
  biological weapons Y36.6X- ☑
  blast Y36.20- ☑
  blast fragments Y36.20- ☑
  blast wave Y36.20- ☑
  blast wind Y36.20- ☑

War operations — *continued*
  bomb Y36.20- ☑
    dirty Y36.50- ☑
    gasoline Y36.31- ☑
    incendiary Y36.31- ☑
    petrol Y36.31- ☑
  bullet Y36.43- ☑
    incendiary Y36.32- ☑
    rubber Y36.41- ☑
  chemical weapons Y36.7X- ☑
  combat
    hand to hand (unarmed) combat Y36.44- ☑
    using blunt or piercing object Y36.45- ☑
  conflagration — *see* War operations, fire
  conventional warfare NEC Y36.49- ☑
  depth-charge Y36.01- ☑
  destruction of aircraft Y36.10- ☑
    due to
      air to air missile Y36.11- ☑
      collision with other aircraft Y36.12- ☑
      detonation (accidental) of onboard munitions
        and explosives Y36.14- ☑
      enemy fire or explosives Y36.11- ☑
      explosive placed on aircraft Y36.11- ☑
      onboard fire Y36.13- ☑
      rocket propelled grenade [RPG] Y36.11- ☑
      small arms fire Y36.11- ☑
      surface to air missile Y36.11- ☑
      specified NEC Y36.19- ☑
  detonation (accidental) of
    onboard marine weapons Y36.05- ☑
    own munitions or munitions launch device
        Y36.24- ☑
  dirty bomb Y36.50- ☑
  explosion (of) Y36.20- ☑
    aerial bomb Y36.21- ☑
    after cessation of hostilities
      bomb placed during war operations Y36.82- ☑
      mine placed during war operations Y36.81- ☑
    bomb NOS (*see also* War operations, bomb(s))
        Y36.20- ☑
    fragments Y36.20- ☑
    grenade Y36.29- ☑
    guided missile Y36.22- ☑
    improvised explosive device [IED] (person-borne)
        (roadside) (vehicle-borne) Y36.23- ☑
    land mine Y36.29- ☑
    marine mine (at sea) (in harbor) Y36.02- ☑
    marine weapon Y36.00- ☑
      specified NEC Y36.09- ☑
    own munitions or munitions launch device (acci-
        dental) Y36.24- ☑
    sea-based artillery shell Y36.03- ☑
    specified NEC Y36.29- ☑
    torpedo Y36.04- ☑
  fire Y36.30- ☑
    specified NEC Y36.39- ☑
  firearms
    discharge Y36.43- ☑
    pellets Y36.42- ☑
  flamethrower Y36.33- ☑
  fragments (from) (of)
    improvised explosive device [IED] (person-borne)
        (roadside) (vehicle-borne) Y36.26- ☑
    munitions Y36.25- ☑
    specified NEC Y36.29- ☑
    weapons Y36.27- ☑
  friendly fire Y36.92 ☑
  hand to hand (unarmed) combat Y36.44- ☑
  hot substances — *see* War operations, fire
  incendiary bullet Y36.32- ☑
  nuclear weapon (effects of) Y36.50- ☑
    acute radiation exposure Y36.54- ☑
    blast pressure Y36.51- ☑
    direct blast Y36.51- ☑
    direct heat Y36.53- ☑
    fallout exposure Y36.54- ☑
    fireball Y36.53- ☑
    indirect blast (struck or crushed by blast debris)
        (being thrown by blast) Y36.52- ☑
    ionizing radiation (immediate exposure) Y36.54- ☑
    nuclear radiation Y36.54- ☑
    radiation
      ionizing (immediate exposure) Y36.54- ☑
      nuclear Y36.54- ☑
      thermal Y36.53- ☑

War operations — *continued*
  nuclear weapon — *continued*
    secondary effects Y36.54- ☑
    specified NEC Y36.59- ☑
    thermal radiation Y36.53- ☑
  restriction of air (airway)
    intentional Y36.46- ☑
    unintentional Y36.47- ☑
  rubber bullets Y36.41- ☑
  shrapnel NOS Y36.29- ☑
  suffocation — *see* War operations, restriction of airways
  unconventional warfare NEC Y36.7X- ☑
  underwater blast NOS Y36.00- ☑
  warfare
    conventional NEC Y36.49- ☑
    unconventional NEC Y36.7X- ☑
  weapon of mass destruction [WMD] Y36.91 ☑
  weapons
    biological weapons Y36.6X- ☑

War operations — *continued*
  weapons — *continued*
    chemical Y36.7X- ☑
    nuclear (effects of) Y36.50- ☑
      acute radiation exposure Y36.54- ☑
      blast pressure Y36.51- ☑
      direct blast Y36.51- ☑
      direct heat Y36.53- ☑
      fallout exposure Y36.54- ☑
      fireball Y36.53- ☑
      indirect blast (struck or crushed by blast debris) (being thrown by blast) Y36.52- ☑
      radiation
        ionizing (!immediate exposure) Y36.54- ☑
        nuclear Y36.54- ☑
        thermal Y36.53- ☑
      secondary effects Y36.54- ☑
      specified NEC Y36.59- ☑
    of mass destruction [WMD] Y36.91 ☑

Washed
  away by flood — *see* Flood
  off road by storm (transport vehicle) — *see* Forces of nature, cataclysmic storm
Weather exposure NEC — *see* Forces of nature
Weightlessness (causing injury) (effects of) (in spacecraft, real or simulated) X52 ☑
Work related condition Y99.0
Wound (accidental) NEC (*see also* Injury) X58 ☑
  battle (*see also* War operations) Y36.90 ☑
  gunshot — *see* Discharge, firearm by type
Wreck transport vehicle NEC (*see also* Accident, transport) V89.9 ☑
Wrong
  device implanted into correct surgical site Y65.51
  fluid in infusion Y65.1
  patient, procedure performed on Y65.52
  procedure (operation) on correct patient Y65.51

Chapter Specific Guidelines with Coding Examples

The chapter specific guidelines from the ICD-10-CM Official Guidelines for Coding and Reporting have been provided below. Along with these guidelines are coding examples, contained in the shaded boxes, that have been developed to help illustrate the coding and/or sequencing guidance found in these guidelines.

a. Human immunodeficiency virus (HIV) infections

1) Code only confirmed cases

Code only confirmed cases of HIV infection/illness. This is an exception to the hospital inpatient guideline Section II, H.

In this context, "confirmation" does not require documentation of positive serology or culture for HIV; the provider's diagnostic statement that the patient is HIV positive, or has an HIV-related illness is sufficient.

> Patient admitted with anemia with possible HIV infection
>
> **D64.9   Anemia, unspecified**
>
> *Explanation:* Only the anemia is coded in this scenario because it has not been confirmed that an HIV infection is present. This is an exception to the guideline Section II, H for hospital inpatient coding.

2) Selection and sequencing of HIV codes

(a) Patient admitted for HIV-related condition

If a patient is admitted for an HIV-related condition, the principal diagnosis should be B20, Human immunodeficiency virus [HIV] disease followed by additional diagnosis codes for all reported HIV-related conditions.

> HIV with PCP
>
> **B20   Human immunodeficiency virus [HIV] disease**
>
> **B59   Pneumocystosis**
>
> *Explanation:* Pneumonia due to *Pneumocystis carinii* is an HIV related condition, so the HIV diagnosis code is reported first, followed by the code for the pneumonia.

(b) Patient with HIV disease admitted for unrelated condition

If a patient with HIV disease is admitted for an unrelated condition (such as a traumatic injury), the code for the unrelated condition (e.g., the nature of injury code) should be the principal diagnosis. Other diagnoses would be B20 followed by additional diagnosis codes for all reported HIV-related conditions.

> Unstable angina, native coronary artery atherosclerosis, HIV
>
> **I25.110   Atherosclerotic heart disease of native coronary artery with unstable angina pectoris**
>
> **B20   Human immunodeficiency virus [HIV] disease**
>
> *Explanation:* The arteriosclerotic coronary artery disease and the unstable angina are not related to HIV, so those conditions are reported first using a combination code, and HIV is reported secondarily.

(c) Whether the patient is newly diagnosed

Whether the patient is newly diagnosed or has had previous admissions/encounters for HIV conditions is irrelevant to the sequencing decision.

> Newly diagnosed multiple cutaneous Kaposi's sarcoma lesions in previously diagnosed HIV disease
>
> **B20   Human immunodeficiency virus [HIV] disease**
>
> **C46.0   Kaposi's sarcoma of skin**
>
> *Explanation:* Even though the HIV was diagnosed on a previous encounter, it is still sequenced first when coded with an HIV related condition. Kaposi's sarcoma is an HIV-related condition.

(d) Asymptomatic human immunodeficiency virus

Z21, Asymptomatic human immunodeficiency virus [HIV] infection status, is to be applied when the patient without any documentation of symptoms is listed as being "HIV positive," "known HIV," "HIV test positive," or similar terminology. Do not use this code if the term "AIDS" is used or if the patient is treated for any HIV-related illness or is described as having any condition(s) resulting from his/her HIV positive status; use B20 in these cases.

> Patient admitted with acute appendicitis. Status positive HIV test on Atripla, with no prior symptoms
>
> **K35.80   Unspecified acute appendicitis**
>
> **Z21   Asymptomatic human immunodeficiency virus [HIV] infection status**
>
> *Explanation:* Code Z21 is sequenced second since documentation indicates that the patient has had a positive HIV test but has been asymptomatic. Being on medication for HIV is not an indication that code B20 is used instead of Z21. Unless there has been documentation that the patient has had current or prior symptoms or HIV-related complications, code B20 is not used. The appendicitis is not an AIDS-related complication and is sequenced first.

(e) Patients with inconclusive HIV serology

Patients with inconclusive HIV serology, but no definitive diagnosis or manifestations of the illness, may be assigned code R75, Inconclusive laboratory evidence of human immunodeficiency virus [HIV].

(f) Previously diagnosed HIV-related illness

Patients with any known prior diagnosis of an HIV-related illness should be coded to B20. Once a patient has developed an HIV-related illness, the patient should always be assigned code B20 on every subsequent admission/encounter. Patients previously diagnosed with any HIV illness (B20) should never be assigned to R75 or Z21, Asymptomatic human immunodeficiency virus [HIV] infection status

(g) HIV infection in pregnancy, childbirth and the puerperium

During pregnancy, childbirth or the puerperium, a patient admitted (or presenting for a health care encounter) because of an HIV-related illness should receive a principal diagnosis code of O98.7-, Human immunodeficiency [HIV] disease complicating pregnancy, childbirth and the puerperium, followed by B20 and the code(s) for the HIV-related illness(es). Codes from Chapter 15 always take sequencing priority.

Patients with asymptomatic HIV infection status admitted (or presenting for a health care encounter) during pregnancy, childbirth, or the puerperium should receive codes of O98.7- and Z21.

(h) Encounters for testing for HIV

If a patient is being seen to determine his/her HIV status, use code Z11.4, Encounter for screening for human immunodeficiency virus [HIV]. Use additional codes for any associated high risk behavior.

If a patient with signs or symptoms is being seen for HIV testing, code the signs and symptoms. An additional counseling code Z71.7, Human immunodeficiency virus [HIV] counseling, may be used if counseling is provided during the encounter for the test.

When a patient returns to be informed of his/her HIV test results and the test result is negative, use code Z71.7, Human immunodeficiency virus [HIV] counseling.

If the results are positive, see previous guidelines and assign codes as appropriate.

b. Infectious agents as the cause of diseases classified to other chapters

Certain infections are classified in chapters other than Chapter 1 and no organism is identified as part of the infection code. In these instances, it is necessary to use an additional code from Chapter 1 to identify the organism. A code from category B95, Streptococcus, Staphylococcus, and Enterococcus as the cause of diseases classified to other chapters, B96, Other bacterial agents as the cause of diseases classified to other chapters, or B97, Viral agents as the cause of diseases classified to other chapters, is to be used as an additional code to identify the organism. An instructional note will be found at the infection code advising that an additional organism code is required.

E. coli UTI

N39.Ø	Urinary tract infection, site not specified
B96.2Ø	Unspecified Escherichia coli [E.coli] as the cause of diseases classified elsewhere

Explanation: An instructional note under the code for the urinary tract infection indicates to code also the specific organism.

c. Infections resistant to antibiotics

Many bacterial infections are resistant to current antibiotics. It is necessary to identify all infections documented as antibiotic resistant. Assign a code from category Z16, Resistance to antimicrobial drugs, following the infection code only if the infection code does not identify drug resistance.

Antimycobacterial-resistant primary pulmonary tuberculosis

A15.Ø	Tuberculosis of lung
Z16.341	Resistance to single antimycobacterial drug

Explanation: Code Z16.341 is assigned as a secondary code to represent the antimycobacterial resistance. This code includes resistance to antimycobacterial drug "NOS"; if multiple drug resistance is not specified, classification defaults to the single drug resistance code.

d. Sepsis, severe sepsis, and septic shock

1) Coding of Sepsis and Severe Sepsis

(a) Sepsis

For a diagnosis of sepsis, assign the appropriate code for the underlying systemic infection. If the type of infection or causal organism is not further specified, assign code A41.9, Sepsis, unspecified organism.

A code from subcategory R65.2, Severe sepsis, should not be assigned unless severe sepsis or an associated acute organ dysfunction is documented.

Gram-negative sepsis

A41.5Ø	Gram-negative sepsis, unspecified

Staphylococcal sepsis

A41.2	Sepsis due to unspecified staphylococcus

Explanation: In both examples above the organism causing the sepsis is identified, therefore A41.9 Sepsis, unspecified organism, would not be appropriate as this code would not capture the highest degree of specificity found in the documentation. Do not use the additional code for severe sepsis unless documented as severe sepsis with acute organ dysfunction.

(i) Negative or inconclusive blood cultures and sepsis

Negative or inconclusive blood cultures do not preclude a diagnosis of sepsis in patients with clinical evidence of the condition; however, the provider should be queried.

(ii) Urosepsis

The term urosepsis is a nonspecific term. It is not to be considered synonymous with sepsis. It has no default code in the Alphabetic Index. Should a provider use this term, he/she must be queried for clarification.

(iii) Sepsis with organ dysfunction

If a patient has sepsis and associated acute organ dysfunction or multiple organ dysfunction (MOD), follow the instructions for coding severe sepsis.

(iv) Acute organ dysfunction that is not clearly associated with the sepsis

If a patient has sepsis and an acute organ dysfunction, but the medical record documentation indicates that the acute organ dysfunction is related to a medical condition other than the sepsis, do not assign a code from subcategory R65.2, Severe sepsis. An acute organ dysfunction must be associated with the sepsis in order to assign the severe sepsis code. If the documentation is not clear as to whether an acute organ dysfunction is related to the sepsis or another medical condition, query the provider.

Sepsis and acute respiratory failure due to COPD exacerbation

A41.9	Sepsis, unspecified organism
J44.1	Chronic obstructive pulmonary disease with (acute) exacerbation
J96.ØØ	Acute respiratory failure, unspecified whether with hypoxia or hypercapnia

Explanation: Although acute organ dysfunction is present in the form of acute respiratory failure, severe sepsis (R65.2) is not coded in this example, as the acute respiratory failure is attributed to the COPD exacerbation rather than the sepsis. Sequencing of these codes would be determined by the circumstances of the admission.

(b) Severe sepsis

The coding of severe sepsis requires a minimum of 2 codes: first a code for the underlying systemic infection, followed by a code from subcategory R65.2, Severe sepsis. If the causal organism is not documented, assign code A41.9, Sepsis, unspecified organism, for the infection. Additional code(s) for the associated acute organ dysfunction are also required.

Due to the complex nature of severe sepsis, some cases may require querying the provider prior to assignment of the codes.

2) Septic shock

(a) Septic shock generally refers to circulatory failure associated with severe sepsis, and therefore, it represents a type of acute organ dysfunction.

For cases of septic shock, the code for the systemic infection should be sequenced first, followed by code R65.21, Severe sepsis with septic shock or code T81.12, Postprocedural septic shock. Any additional codes for the other acute organ dysfunctions should also be assigned. As noted in the sequencing instructions in the Tabular List, the code for septic shock cannot be assigned as a principal diagnosis.

Sepsis with septic shock

A41.9	Sepsis, unspecified organism
R65.21	Severe sepsis with septic shock

Explanation: Documentation of septic shock automatically implies severe sepsis as it is a form of acute organ dysfunction. Septic shock is not coded as the principal diagnosis; it is always preceded by the code for the systemic infection.

3) Sequencing of severe sepsis

If severe sepsis is present on admission, and meets the definition of principal diagnosis, the underlying systemic infection should be assigned as principal diagnosis followed by the appropriate code from subcategory R65.2 as required by the sequencing rules in the Tabular List. A code from subcategory R65.2 can never be assigned as a principal diagnosis.

When severe sepsis develops during an encounter (it was not present on admission), the underlying systemic infection and the appropriate code from subcategory R65.2 should be assigned as secondary diagnoses.

Severe sepsis may be present on admission, but the diagnosis may not be confirmed until sometime after admission. If the documentation is not clear whether severe sepsis was present on admission, the provider should be queried.

4) Sepsis and severe sepsis with a localized infection

If the reason for admission is both sepsis or severe sepsis and a localized infection, such as pneumonia or cellulitis, a code(s) for the underlying systemic infection should be assigned first and the code for the localized infection should be assigned as a secondary diagnosis. If the patient has severe sepsis, a code from subcategory R65.2 should also be assigned as a secondary diagnosis. If the patient is admitted with a localized infection, such as pneumonia, and sepsis/severe sepsis doesn't develop until after admission, the localized infection should be assigned first, followed by the appropriate sepsis/severe sepsis codes.

Patient presents with acute renal failure due to severe sepsis from *Pseudomonas pneumonia*

A41.9	**Sepsis, unspecified organism**
J15.1	**Pneumonia due to Pseudomonas**
R65.20	**Severe sepsis without septic shock**
N17.9	**Acute kidney failure, unspecified**

Explanation: If all conditions are present on admission, the systemic infection (sepsis) is sequenced first followed by the codes for the localized infection (pneumonia), severe sepsis and any organ dysfunction. If only the pneumonia was present on admission with the sepsis and resulting renal failure developing later in the admission, then the pneumonia would be sequenced first.

5) Sepsis due to a postprocedural infection

(a) Documentation of causal relationship

As with all postprocedural complications, code assignment is based on the provider's documentation of the relationship between the infection and the procedure.

(b) Sepsis due to a postprocedural infection

For such cases, the postprocedural infection code, such as T80.2, Infections following infusion, transfusion, and therapeutic injection, T81.4, Infection following a procedure, T88.0, Infection following immunization, or O86.0, Infection of obstetric surgical wound, should be coded first, followed by the code for the specific infection. If the patient has severe sepsis, the appropriate code from subcategory R65.2 should also be assigned with the additional code(s) for any acute organ dysfunction.

(c) Postprocedural infection and postprocedural septic shock

In cases where a postprocedural infection has occurred and has resulted in severe sepsis the code for the precipitating complication such as code T81.4, Infection following a procedure, or O86.0, Infection of obstetrical surgical wound should be coded first followed by code R65.20, Severe sepsis without septic shock. A code for the systemic infection should also be assigned.

If a postprocedural infection has resulted in postprocedural septic shock, the code for the precipitating complication such as code T81.4, Infection following a procedure, or O86.0, Infection of obstetrical surgical wound should be coded first followed by code T81.12-, Postprocedural septic shock. A code for the systemic infection should also be assigned.

6) Sepsis and severe sepsis associated with a noninfectious process (condition)

In some cases a noninfectious process (condition), such as trauma, may lead to an infection which can result in sepsis or severe sepsis. If sepsis or severe sepsis is documented as associated with a noninfectious condition, such as a burn or serious injury, and this condition meets the definition for principal diagnosis, the code for the noninfectious condition should be sequenced first, followed by the code for the resulting infection. If severe sepsis is present, a code from subcategory R65.2 should also be assigned with any associated organ dysfunction(s) codes. It is not necessary to assign a code from subcategory R65.1, Systemic inflammatory response syndrome (SIRS) of non-infectious origin, for these cases.

If the infection meets the definition of principal diagnosis, it should be sequenced before the non-infectious condition. When both the associated non-infectious condition and the infection meet the definition of principal diagnosis, either may be assigned as principal diagnosis.

Only one code from category R65, Symptoms and signs specifically associated with systemic inflammation and infection, should be assigned. Therefore, when a non-infectious condition leads to an infection resulting in severe sepsis, assign the appropriate code from subcategory R65.2, Severe sepsis. Do not additionally assign a code from subcategory R65.1, Systemic inflammatory response syndrome (SIRS) of non-infectious origin.

See Section I.C.18. SIRS due to non-infectious process

Patient admitted with multiple third-degree burns of upper arm develops severe MSSA sepsis with septic shock, three days into admission

T22.391A	**Burn of third degree of multiple sites of right shoulder and upper arm limb, except wrist and hand, initial encounter**
A41.01	**Sepsis due to methicillin susceptible Staphylococcus aureus**
R65.21	**Severe sepsis with septic shock**

Explanation: Severe sepsis is coded rather than SIRS from R65 because it is documented as a severe systemic infectious response with septic shock to a noninfectious condition. The code for the systemic infection is not used as the principal diagnosis because it was not present on admission. The patient was admitted for the burn injury.

7) Sepsis and septic shock complicating abortion, pregnancy, childbirth, and the puerperium

See Section I.C.15. Sepsis and septic shock complicating abortion, pregnancy, childbirth and the puerperium

8) Newborn sepsis

See Section I.C.16. f. Bacterial sepsis of Newborn

e. Methicillin resistant *Staphylococcus aureus* (MRSA) conditions

1) Selection and sequencing of MRSA codes

(a) Combination codes for MRSA infection

When a patient is diagnosed with an infection that is due to methicillin resistant *Staphylococcus aureus* (MRSA), and that infection has a combination code that includes the causal organism (e.g., sepsis, pneumonia) assign the appropriate combination code for the condition (e.g., code A41.02, Sepsis due to Methicillin resistant Staphylococcus aureus or code J15.212, Pneumonia due to Methicillin resistant Staphylococcus aureus). Do not assign code B95.62, Methicillin resistant Staphylococcus aureus infection as the cause of diseases classified elsewhere, as an additional code, because the combination code includes the type of infection and the MRSA organism. Do not assign a code from subcategory Z16.11, Resistance to penicillins, as an additional diagnosis.

See Section C.1. for instructions on coding and sequencing of sepsis and severe sepsis.

(b) Other codes for MRSA infection

When there is documentation of a current infection (e.g., wound infection, stitch abscess, urinary tract infection) due to MRSA, and that infection does not have a combination code that includes the causal organism, assign the appropriate code to identify the condition along with code B95.62, Methicillin resistant Staphylococcus aureus infection as the cause of diseases classified elsewhere for the MRSA infection. Do not assign a code from subcategory Z16.11, Resistance to penicillins.

(c) Methicillin susceptible Staphylococcus aureus (MSSA) and MRSA colonization

The condition or state of being colonized or carrying MSSA or MRSA is called colonization or carriage, while an individual person is described as being colonized or being a carrier. Colonization means that MSSA or MSRA is present on or in the body without necessarily causing illness. A positive MRSA colonization test might be documented by the provider as "MRSA screen positive" or "MRSA nasal swab positive".

Assign code Z22.322, Carrier or suspected carrier of Methicillin resistant Staphylococcus aureus, for patients documented as having MRSA colonization. Assign code Z22.321, Carrier or suspected carrier of Methicillin susceptible Staphylococcus aureus, for patient documented as having MSSA colonization. Colonization is not necessarily indicative of a disease process or as the cause of a specific condition the patient may have unless documented as such by the provider.

(d) MRSA colonization and infection

If a patient is documented as having both MRSA colonization and infection during a hospital admission, code Z22.322, Carrier or suspected carrier of Methicillin resistant Staphylococcus aureus, and a code for the MRSA infection may both be assigned.

Chapter 1. Certain Infectious and Parasitic Diseases (A00-B99)

INCLUDES diseases generally recognized as communicable or transmissible
Use additional code to identify resistance to antimicrobial drugs (Z16.-)
EXCLUDES 1 certain localized infections—see body system-related chapters
EXCLUDES 2 carrier or suspected carrier of infectious disease (Z22.-)
infectious and parasitic diseases specific to the perinatal period (P35-P39)
infectious and parasitic diseases complicating pregnancy, childbirth and the puerperium (O98.-)
influenza and other acute respiratory infections (J00-J22)

This chapter contains the following blocks:

A00-A09   Intestinal infectious diseases
A15-A19   Tuberculosis
A20-A28   Certain zoonotic bacterial diseases
A30-A49   Other bacterial diseases
A50-A64   Infections with a predominantly sexual mode of transmission
A65-A69   Other spirochetal diseases
A70-A74   Other diseases caused by chlamydiae
A75-A79   Rickettsioses
A80-A89   Viral infections of the central nervous system
A90-A99   Arthropod-borne viral fevers and viral hemorrhagic fevers
B00-B09   Viral infections characterized by skin and mucous membrane lesions
B10   Other human herpesviruses
B15-B19   Viral hepatitis
B20   Human immunodeficiency virus [HIV] disease
B25-B34   Other viral diseases
B35-B49   Mycoses
B50-B64   Protozoal diseases
B65-B83   Helminthiases
B85-B89   Pediculosis, acariasis and other infestations
B90-B94   Sequelae of infectious and parasitic diseases
B95-B97   Bacterial and viral infectious agents
B99   Other infectious diseases

Intestinal Infectious Diseases (A00-A09)

✓4ᵗʰ **A00 Cholera**

A00.0 Cholera due to Vibrio cholerae 01, biovar cholerae
Classical cholera

A00.1 Cholera due to Vibrio cholerae 01, biovar eltor
Cholera eltor

A00.9 Cholera, unspecified ▽

✓4ᵗʰ **A01 Typhoid and paratyphoid fevers**

✓5ᵗʰ **A01.0 Typhoid fever**
Infection due to Salmonella typhi

    A01.00 Typhoid fever, unspecified ▽

    A01.01 Typhoid meningitis

    A01.02 Typhoid fever with heart involvement
Typhoid endocarditis
Typhoid myocarditis

   ²,⁸ **A01.03 Typhoid pneumonia**

    A01.04 Typhoid arthritis

    A01.05 Typhoid osteomyelitis

    A01.09 Typhoid fever with other complications

A01.1 Paratyphoid fever A

A01.2 Paratyphoid fever B

A01.3 Paratyphoid fever C

A01.4 Paratyphoid fever, unspecified ▽
Infection due to Salmonella paratyphi NOS

✓4ᵗʰ **A02 Other salmonella infections**
INCLUDES infection or foodborne intoxication due to any Salmonella species other than S. typhi and S. paratyphi

A02.0 Salmonella enteritis
Salmonellosis

A02.1 Salmonella sepsis CC

✓5ᵗʰ **A02.2 Localized salmonella infections**

    A02.20 Localized salmonella infection, unspecified ▽

    A02.21 Salmonella meningitis

   ²,⁸ **A02.22 Salmonella pneumonia**

    A02.23 Salmonella arthritis

    A02.24 Salmonella osteomyelitis

    A02.25 Salmonella pyelonephritis
Salmonella tubulo-interstitial nephropathy

    A02.29 Salmonella with other localized infection

A02.8 Other specified salmonella infections

A02.9 Salmonella infection, unspecified ▽

✓4ᵗʰ **A03 Shigellosis**

A03.0 Shigellosis due to Shigella dysenteriae
Group A shigellosis [Shiga-Kruse dysentery]

A03.1 Shigellosis due to Shigella flexneri
Group B shigellosis

A03.2 Shigellosis due to Shigella boydii
Group C shigellosis

A03.3 Shigellosis due to Shigella sonnei
Group D shigellosis

A03.8 Other shigellosis

A03.9 Shigellosis, unspecified ▽
Bacillary dysentery NOS

✓4ᵗʰ **A04 Other bacterial intestinal infections**
EXCLUDES 1 bacterial foodborne intoxications, NEC (A05.-)
tuberculous enteritis (A18.32)

A04.0 Enteropathogenic Escherichia coli infection

A04.1 Enterotoxigenic Escherichia coli infection

A04.2 Enteroinvasive Escherichia coli infection

A04.3 Enterohemorrhagic Escherichia coli infection

A04.4 Other intestinal Escherichia coli infections
Escherichia coli enteritis NOS

A04.5 Campylobacter enteritis

A04.6 Enteritis due to Yersinia enterocolitica
EXCLUDES 1 extraintestinal yersiniosis (A28.2)

A04.7 Enterocolitis due to Clostridium difficile CC
Foodborne intoxication by Clostridium difficile
Pseudomembraneous colitis

A04.8 Other specified bacterial intestinal infections CC

A04.9 Bacterial intestinal infection, unspecified ▽
Bacterial enteritis NOS

✓4ᵗʰ **A05 Other bacterial foodborne intoxications, not elsewhere classified**
EXCLUDES 1 Clostridium difficile foodborne intoxication and infection (A04.7)
Escherichia coli infection (A04.0-A04.4)
listeriosis (A32.-)
salmonella foodborne intoxication and infection (A02.-)
toxic effect of noxious foodstuffs (T61-T62)

A05.0 Foodborne staphylococcal intoxication

A05.1 Botulism food poisoning
Botulism NOS
Classical foodborne intoxication due to Clostridium botulinum
EXCLUDES 1 infant botulism (A48.51)
wound botulism (A48.52)

A05.2 Foodborne Clostridium perfringens [Clostridium welchii] intoxication
Enteritis necroticans
Pig-bel

A05.3 Foodborne Vibrio parahaemolyticus intoxication

A05.4 Foodborne Bacillus cereus intoxication

A05.5 Foodborne Vibrio vulnificus intoxication

A05.8 Other specified bacterial foodborne intoxications

A05.9 Bacterial foodborne intoxication, unspecified ▽

✓4ᵗʰ **A06 Amebiasis**
INCLUDES infection due to Entamoeba histolytica
EXCLUDES 1 other protozoal intestinal diseases (A07.-)
EXCLUDES 2 acanthamebiasis (B60.1-)
Naegleriasis (B60.2)

A06.0 Acute amebic dysentery
Acute amebiasis
Intestinal amebiasis NOS

A06.1 Chronic intestinal amebiasis

A06.2 Amebic nondysenteric colitis

A06.3 Ameboma of intestine
Ameboma NOS

A06.4 Amebic liver abscess
Hepatic amebiasis

A06.5 Amebic lung abscess
Amebic abscess of lung (and liver)

---

² Special Care High = With fever

⁸ Clinically Complex = Without fever

N Newborn   P Pediatric   M Maternity   A Adult   RIC RIC Dx   NC Dx Noncancer Dx   PDx Primary Dx   CC RIC CC Condition   ►◄ Revised Text   ● New Code   ▲ Revised Code Title

426   ICD-10-CM 2016

A06.6 Amebic brain abscess
Amebic abscess of brain (and liver) (and lung)

A06.7 Cutaneous amebiasis

✓5ᵗʰ **A06.8 Amebic infection of other sites**

    A06.81 Amebic cystitis

    A06.82 Other amebic genitourinary infections
        Amebic balanitis
        Amebic vesiculitis
        Amebic vulvovaginitis

    A06.89 Other amebic infections
        Amebic appendicitis
        Amebic splenic abscess

A06.9 Amebiasis, unspecified ▽

✓4ᵗʰ **A07 Other protozoal intestinal diseases**

A07.0 Balantidiasis
    Balantidial dysentery

A07.1 Giardiasis [lambliasis]

A07.2 Cryptosporidiosis

A07.3 Isosporiasis
    Infection due to Isospora belli and Isospora hominis
    Intestinal coccidiosis
    Isosporosis

A07.4 Cyclosporiasis

A07.8 Other specified protozoal intestinal diseases
    Intestinal microsporidiosis   Sarcocystosis
    Intestinal trichomoniasis   Sarcosporidiosis

A07.9 Protozoal intestinal disease, unspecified ▽
    Flagellate diarrhea   Protozoal diarrhea
    Protozoal colitis   Protozoal dysentery

✓4ᵗʰ **A08 Viral and other specified intestinal infections**
    EXCLUDES 1 *influenza with involvement of gastrointestinal tract (J09.X3, J10.2, J11.2)*

A08.0 Rotaviral enteritis

✓5ᵗʰ **A08.1 Acute gastroenteropathy due to Norwalk agent and other small round viruses**

    A08.11 Acute gastroenteropathy due to Norwalk agent
        Acute gastroenteropathy due to Norovirus
        Acute gastroenteropathy due to Norwalk-like agent

    A08.19 Acute gastroenteropathy due to other small round viruses
        Acute gastroenteropathy due to small round virus [SRV] NOS

A08.2 Adenoviral enteritis

✓5ᵗʰ **A08.3 Other viral enteritis**

    A08.31 Calicivirus enteritis

    A08.32 Astrovirus enteritis

    A08.39 Other viral enteritis
        Coxsackie virus enteritis
        Echovirus enteritis
        Enterovirus enteritis NEC
        Torovirus enteritis

A08.4 Viral intestinal infection, unspecified ▽
    Viral enteritis NOS
    Viral gastroenteritis NOS
    Viral gastroenteropathy NOS

A08.8 Other specified intestinal infections

A09 Infectious gastroenteritis and colitis, unspecified ▽
    Infectious colitis NOS
    Infectious enteritis NOS
    Infectious gastroenteritis NOS
    EXCLUDES 1 *colitis NOS (K52.9)*
        diarrhea NOS (R19.7)
        enteritis NOS (K52.9)
        gastroenteritis NOS (K52.9)
        noninfective gastroenteritis and colitis, unspecified (K52.9)

Tuberculosis (A15-A19)

INCLUDES   infections due to Mycobacterium tuberculosis and Mycobacterium bovis

EXCLUDES 1   *congenital tuberculosis (P37.0)*
nonspecific reaction to test for tuberculosis without active tuberculosis (R76.1-)
pneumoconiosis associated with tuberculosis, any type in A15 (J65)
positive PPD (R76.11)
positive tuberculin skin test without active tuberculosis (R76.11)
sequelae of tuberculosis (B90.-)
silicotuberculosis (J65)

✓4ᵗʰ **A15 Respiratory tuberculosis**

²,⁸ **A15.0 Tuberculosis of lung**   cc
    Tuberculous bronchiectasis
    Tuberculous fibrosis of lung
    Tuberculous pneumonia
    Tuberculous pneumothorax
    RIC Excl: 15 Pulmonary

A15.4 Tuberculosis of intrathoracic lymph nodes   cc
    Tuberculosis of hilar lymph nodes
    Tuberculosis of mediastinal lymph nodes
    Tuberculosis of tracheobronchial lymph nodes
    EXCLUDES 1 *tuberculosis specified as primary (A15.7)*
    RIC Excl: 15 Pulmonary

A15.5 Tuberculosis of larynx, trachea and bronchus   cc
    Tuberculosis of bronchus
    Tuberculosis of glottis
    Tuberculosis of larynx
    Tuberculosis of trachea
    RIC Excl: 15 Pulmonary

A15.6 Tuberculous pleurisy   cc
    Tuberculosis of pleura Tuberculous empyema
    EXCLUDES 1 *primary respiratory tuberculosis (A15.7)*
    RIC Excl: 15 Pulmonary

A15.7 Primary respiratory tuberculosis

A15.8 Other respiratory tuberculosis   cc
    Mediastinal tuberculosis
    Nasopharyngeal tuberculosis
    Tuberculosis of nose
    Tuberculosis of sinus [any nasal]
    RIC Excl: 15 Pulmonary

A15.9 Respiratory tuberculosis unspecified   cc ▽
    RIC Excl: 15 Pulmonary

✓4ᵗʰ **A17 Tuberculosis of nervous system**

A17.0 Tuberculous meningitis   cc
    Tuberculosis of meninges (cerebral)(spinal)
    Tuberculous leptomeningitis
    EXCLUDES 1 *tuberculous meningoencephalitis (A17.82)*
    RIC Excl: 03 Non-traumatic brain injury; 05 Non-traumatic spinal cord injury

A17.1 Meningeal tuberculoma   cc
    Tuberculoma of meninges (cerebral) (spinal)
    EXCLUDES 2 *tuberculoma of brain and spinal cord (A17.81)*
    RIC Excl: 03 Non-traumatic brain injury; 05 Non-traumatic spinal cord injury

✓5ᵗʰ **A17.8 Other tuberculosis of nervous system**

    A17.81 Tuberculoma of brain and spinal cord   cc
        Tuberculous abscess of brain and spinal cord
        RIC Excl: 03 Non-traumatic brain injury; 05 Non-traumatic spinal cord injury

    A17.82 Tuberculous meningoencephalitis   cc
        Tuberculous myelitis
        RIC Excl: 03 Non-traumatic brain injury

    A17.83 Tuberculous neuritis   cc
        Tuberculous mononeuropathy
        RIC Excl: 03 Non-traumatic brain injury

    A17.89 Other tuberculosis of nervous system   cc
        Tuberculous polyneuropathy
        RIC Excl: 03 Non-traumatic brain injury; 05 Non-traumatic spinal cord injury

A17.9 Tuberculosis of nervous system, unspecified   cc ▽
    RIC Excl: 03 Non-traumatic brain injury; 05 Non-traumatic spinal cord injury

---

² Special Care High = With fever

⁸ Clinically Complex = Without fever

☑ Add'l Character Required   ✓x7ᵗʰ Placeholder Alert   RUG IV Special Care High Dx   RUG IV Clinically Complex Dx   RUG IV Special Care Low Dx   Manifestation Code   Other Specified Code   ▽ Unspecified Code

Chapter 1. Certain Infectious and Parasitic Diseases

√4ᵗʰ **A18 Tuberculosis of** other organs

  √5ᵗʰ **A18.0 Tuberculosis of** bones and joints

    A18.01 Tuberculosis of spine   CC
Pott's disease or curvature of spine
Tuberculous arthritis
Tuberculous osteomyelitis of spine
Tuberculous spondylitis
RIC Excl: 03 Non-traumatic brain injury; 09 Other orthopedic

    A18.02 Tuberculous arthritis of other joints   CC
Tuberculosis of hip (joint)
Tuberculosis of knee (joint)
RIC Excl: 09 Other orthopedic

    A18.03 Tuberculosis of other bones   CC
Tuberculous mastoiditis
Tuberculous osteomyelitis
RIC Excl: 09 Other orthopedic; 10 Amputation, lower extremity; 11 Amputation, non-lower extremity

    A18.09 Other musculoskeletal tuberculosis   CC
Tuberculous myositis
Tuberculous synovitis
Tuberculous tenosynovitis
RIC Excl: 09 Other orthopedic

  √5ᵗʰ **A18.1 Tuberculosis of** genitourinary system

    A18.10 Tuberculosis of genitourinary system, unspecified   CC ▽

    A18.11 Tuberculosis of kidney and ureter   CC

    A18.12 Tuberculosis of bladder   CC

    A18.13 Tuberculosis of other urinary organs   CC
Tuberculous urethritis

    A18.14 Tuberculosis of prostate   CC A♂

    A18.15 Tuberculosis of other male genital organs   CC ♂

    A18.16 Tuberculosis of cervix   CC ♀

    A18.17 Tuberculous female pelvic inflammatory disease   CC ♀
Tuberculous endometritis
Tuberculous oophoritis and salpingitis

    A18.18 Tuberculosis of other female genital organs   CC ♀
Tuberculous ulceration of vulva

  A18.2 Tuberculous peripheral lymphadenopathy   CC
Tuberculous adenitis
EXCLUDES 2 tuberculosis of bronchial and mediastinal lymph nodes (A15.4)
tuberculosis of mesenteric and retroperitoneal lymph nodes (A18.39)
tuberculous tracheobronchial adenopathy (A15.4)

  √5ᵗʰ **A18.3 Tuberculosis of** intestines, peritoneum and mesenteric glands

    A18.31 Tuberculous peritonitis   CC
Tuberculous ascites

    A18.32 Tuberculous enteritis   CC
Tuberculosis of anus and rectum
Tuberculosis of intestine (large) (small)

    A18.39 Retroperitoneal tuberculosis   CC
Tuberculosis of mesenteric glands
Tuberculosis of retroperitoneal (lymph glands)

  A18.4 Tuberculosis of skin and subcutaneous tissue'   CC
Erythema induratum, tuberculous
Lupus excedens
Lupus vulgaris NOS
Lupus vulgaris of eyelid
Scrofuloderma
Tuberculosis of external ear
EXCLUDES 2 lupus erythematosus (L93.-)
lupus NOS (M32.9)
systemic (M32.-)

  √5ᵗʰ **A18.5 Tuberculosis of** eye
EXCLUDES 2 lupus vulgaris of eyelid (A18.4)

    A18.50 Tuberculosis of eye, unspecified   CC ▽

    A18.51 Tuberculous episcleritis   CC

    A18.52 Tuberculous keratitis   CC
Tuberculous interstitial keratitis
Tuberculous keratoconjunctivitis (interstitial) (phlyctenular)

    A18.53 Tuberculous chorioretinitis   CC

    A18.54 Tuberculous iridocyclitis   CC

    A18.59 Other tuberculosis of eye   CC
Tuberculous conjunctivitis

    A18.6 Tuberculosis of (inner) (middle) ear   CC
Tuberculous otitis media
EXCLUDES 2 tuberculosis of external ear (A18.4)
tuberculous mastoiditis (A18.03)

    A18.7 Tuberculosis of adrenal glands   CC
Tuberculous Addison's disease

  √5ᵗʰ **A18.8 Tuberculosis of** other specified organs

    A18.81 Tuberculosis of thyroid gland   CC

    A18.82 Tuberculosis of other endocrine glands   CC
Tuberculosis of pituitary gland
Tuberculosis of thymus gland

    A18.83 Tuberculosis of digestive tract organs, **not elsewhere classified**   CC
EXCLUDES 1 tuberculosis of intestine (A18.32)

    A18.84 Tuberculosis of heart   CC
Tuberculous cardiomyopathy
Tuberculous endocarditis
Tuberculous myocarditis
Tuberculous pericarditis

    A18.85 Tuberculosis of spleen   CC

    A18.89 Tuberculosis of other sites   CC
Tuberculosis of muscle
Tuberculous cerebral arteritis

√4ᵗʰ **A19 Miliary tuberculosis**
INCLUDES disseminated tuberculosis
generalized tuberculosis
tuberculous polyserositis

  A19.0 Acute miliary tuberculosis of a single specified site   CC

  A19.1 Acute miliary tuberculosis of multiple sites   CC

  A19.2 Acute miliary tuberculosis, unspecified   CC ▽

  A19.8 Other miliary tuberculosis   CC

  A19.9 Miliary tuberculosis, unspecified   CC ▽

Certain zoonotic bacterial diseases (A20-A28)

√4ᵗʰ **A20 Plague**
INCLUDES infection due to Yersinia pestis

  A20.0 Bubonic plague

  A20.1 Cellulocutaneous plague

  A20.2 Pneumonic plague

  A20.3 Plague meningitis

  A20.7 Septicemic plague

  A20.8 Other forms of plague
Abortive plague
Asymptomatic plague
Pestis minor

  A20.9 Plague, unspecified   ▽

√4ᵗʰ **A21 Tularemia**
INCLUDES deer-fly fever
infection due to Francisella tularensis
rabbit fever

  A21.0 Ulceroglandular tularemia

  A21.1 Oculoglandular tularemia
Ophthalmic tularemia

  A21.2 Pulmonary tularemia

  A21.3 Gastrointestinal tularemia
Abdominal tularemia

  A21.7 Generalized tularemia

  A21.8 Other forms of tularemia

  A21.9 Tularemia, unspecified   ▽

√4ᵗʰ **A22 Anthrax**
INCLUDES infection due to Bacillus anthracis

  A22.0 Cutaneous anthrax
Malignant carbuncle
Malignant pustule

  A22.1 Pulmonary anthrax   CC
Inhalation anthrax
Ragpicker's disease
Woolsorter's disease
RIC Excl: 15 Pulmonary

  A22.2 Gastrointestinal anthrax

  A22.7 Anthrax sepsis   CC

  A22.8 Other forms of anthrax
Anthrax meningitis

  A22.9 Anthrax, unspecified   ▽

N Newborn   P Pediatric   M Maternity   A Adult   RIC RIC Dx   NCDx Noncancer Dx   PDx Primary Dx   CC RIC CC Condition   ►◄ Revised Text   ● New Code   ▲ Revised Code Title

428   ICD-10-CM 2016

✓4th **A23 Brucellosis**
Malta fever
Mediterranean fever
Undulant fever
- **A23.0 Brucellosis due to** Brucella melitensis
- **A23.1 Brucellosis due to** Brucella abortus
- **A23.2 Brucellosis due to** Brucella suis
- **A23.3 Brucellosis due to** Brucella canis
- **A23.8 Other brucellosis**
- **A23.9 Brucellosis, unspecified** ▽

✓4th **A24 Glanders and melioidosis**
- **A24.0 Glanders**
Infection due to Pseudomonas mallei
Malleus
- 2,8 **A24.1 Acute and fulminating melioidosis**
Melioidosis pneumonia
Melioidosis sepsis
- **A24.2 Subacute and chronic melioidosis**
- **A24.3 Other melioidosis**
- **A24.9 Melioidosis, unspecified** ▽
Infection due to Pseudomonas pseudomallei NOS
Whitmore's disease

✓4th **A25 Rat-bite fevers**
- **A25.0 Spirillosis**
Sodoku
- **A25.1 Streptobacillosis**
Epidemic arthritic erythema
Haverhill fever
Streptobacillary rat-bite fever
- **A25.9 Rat-bite fever, unspecified** ▽

✓4th **A26 Erysipeloid**
- **A26.0 Cutaneous erysipeloid** CC
Erythema migrans
- **A26.7 Erysipelothrix sepsis** CC
- **A26.8 Other forms of erysipeloid** CC
- **A26.9 Erysipeloid, unspecified** CC ▽

✓4th **A27 Leptospirosis**
- **A27.0 Leptospirosis icterohemorrhagica**
Leptospiral or spirochetal jaundice (hemorrhagic)
Weil's disease
- ✓5th **A27.8 Other forms of leptospirosis**
  - **A27.81 Aseptic meningitis in leptospirosis**
  - **A27.89 Other forms of leptospirosis**
- **A27.9 Leptospirosis, unspecified** ▽

✓4th **A28 Other zoonotic bacterial diseases, not elsewhere classified**
- **A28.0 Pasteurellosis** CC
- **A28.1 Cat-scratch disease**
Cat-scratch fever
- **A28.2 Extraintestinal yersiniosis** CC
EXCLUDES 1 enteritis due to Yersinia enterocolitica (A04.6)
plague (A20.-)
- **A28.8 Other specified zoonotic bacterial diseases, not elsewhere classified** CC
- **A28.9 Zoonotic bacterial disease, unspecified** CC ▽

Other bacterial diseases (A30-A49)

✓4th **A30 Leprosy [Hansen's disease]**
INCLUDES infection due to Mycobacterium leprae
EXCLUDES 1 sequelae of leprosy (B92)
- **A30.0 Indeterminate leprosy**
I leprosy
- **A30.1 Tuberculoid leprosy**
TT leprosy
- **A30.2 Borderline tuberculoid leprosy**
BT leprosy
- **A30.3 Borderline leprosy**
BB leprosy
- **A30.4 Borderline lepromatous leprosy**
BL leprosy

- **A30.5 Lepromatous leprosy**
LL leprosy
- **A30.8 Other forms of leprosy**
- **A30.9 Leprosy, unspecified** ▽

✓4th **A31 Infection due to other mycobacteria**
EXCLUDES 2 leprosy (A30.-)
tuberculosis (A15-A19)
- **A31.0 Pulmonary mycobacterial infection**
Infection due to Mycobacterium avium
Infection due to Mycobacterium intracellulare [Battey bacillus]
Infection due to Mycobacterium kansasii
- **A31.1 Cutaneous mycobacterial infection**
Buruli ulcer
Infection due to Mycobacterium marinum
Infection due to Mycobacterium ulcerans
- **A31.2 Disseminated mycobacterium avium-intracellulare complex (DMAC)**
MAC sepsis
- **A31.8 Other mycobacterial infections**
- **A31.9 Mycobacterial infection, unspecified** ▽
Atypical mycobacterial infection NOS
Mycobacteriosis NOS

✓4th **A32 Listeriosis**
INCLUDES listerial foodborne infection
EXCLUDES 1 neonatal (disseminated) listeriosis (P37.2)
- **A32.0 Cutaneous listeriosis** CC
- ✓5th **A32.1 Listerial meningitis and meningoencephalitis**
  - **A32.11 Listerial meningitis** CC
  - **A32.12 Listerial meningoencephalitis** CC
- **A32.7 Listerial sepsis** CC
- ✓5th **A32.8 Other forms of listeriosis**
  - **A32.81 Oculoglandular listeriosis** CC
  - **A32.82 Listerial endocarditis** CC
  - **A32.89 Other forms of listeriosis** CC
Listerial cerebral arteritis
- **A32.9 Listeriosis, unspecified** CC ▽

A33 Tetanus neonatorum N

A34 Obstetrical tetanus M ♀

A35 Other tetanus CC
Tetanus NOS
EXCLUDES 1 obstetrical tetanus (A34)
tetanus neonatorum (A33)
RIC Excl: 06 Neurological

✓4th **A36 Diphtheria**
- **A36.0 Pharyngeal diphtheria**
Diphtheritic membranous angina
Tonsillar diphtheria
- **A36.1 Nasopharyngeal diphtheria**
- **A36.2 Laryngeal diphtheria**
Diphtheritic laryngotracheitis
- **A36.3 Cutaneous diphtheria**
EXCLUDES 2 erythrasma (L08.1)
- ✓5th **A36.8 Other diphtheria**
  - **A36.81 Diphtheritic cardiomyopathy**
Diphtheritic myocarditis
  - **A36.82 Diphtheritic radiculomyelitis**
  - **A36.83 Diphtheritic polyneuritis**
  - **A36.84 Diphtheritic tubulo-interstitial nephropathy**
  - **A36.85 Diphtheritic cystitis**
  - **A36.86 Diphtheritic conjunctivitis**
  - **A36.89 Other diphtheritic complications**
Diphtheritic peritonitis
- **A36.9 Diphtheria, unspecified** ▽

✓4th **A37 Whooping cough**
- ✓5th **A37.0 Whooping cough due to** Bordetella pertussis
  - **A37.00 Whooping cough due to Bordetella pertussis without pneumonia**
  - 2,8 **A37.01 Whooping cough due to Bordetella pertussis with pneumonia** CC

---

2 Special Care High = With fever

8 Clinically Complex = Without fever

☑ Add'l Character Required   ✓x7th Placeholder Alert   RUG IV Special Care High Dx   RUG IV Clinically Complex Dx   RUG IV Special Care Low Dx   Manifestation Code   Other Specified Code   ▽ Unspecified Code

Chapter 1. Certain Infectious and Parasitic Diseases

A37.1–A43.8

✓5ᵗʰ **A37.1 Whooping cough due to** Bordetella parapertussis

    A37.10 Whooping cough due to Bordetella parapertussis without pneumonia

2,8 **A37.11 Whooping cough due to Bordetella parapertussis** with pneumonia   cc

✓5ᵗʰ **A37.8 Whooping cough due to** other **Bordetella species**

    A37.80 Whooping cough due to other Bordetella species without pneumonia

2,8 **A37.81 Whooping cough due to other Bordetella species** with pneumonia   cc
        RIC Excl: 15 Pulmonary

✓5ᵗʰ **A37.9 Whooping cough,** unspecified **species**

    A37.90 Whooping cough, unspecified species without pneumonia   ▽

2,8 **A37.91 Whooping cough, unspecified species with** pneumonia   cc ▽
        RIC Excl: 15 Pulmonary

✓4ᵗʰ **A38 Scarlet fever**
    INCLUDES scarlatina
    EXCLUDES 2 streptococcal sore throat (J02.0)

A38.0 Scarlet fever with otitis media

A38.1 Scarlet fever with myocarditis

A38.8 Scarlet fever with other complications

A38.9 Scarlet fever, uncomplicated
    Scarlet fever, NOS

✓4ᵗʰ **A39 Meningococcal infection**

A39.0 Meningococcal meningitis   cc
    RIC Excl: 03 Non-traumatic brain injury;
    05 Non-traumatic spinal cord injury

A39.1 Waterhouse-Friderichsen **syndrome**   cc
    Meningococcal hemorrhagic adrenalitis
    Meningococcic adrenal syndrome
    RIC Excl: 05 Non-traumatic spinal cord injury

A39.2 Acute **meningococcemia**   cc
    RIC Excl: 03 Non-traumatic brain injury;
    05 Non-traumatic spinal cord injury

A39.3 Chronic **meningococcemia**   cc
    RIC Excl: 03 Non-traumatic brain injury;
    05 Non-traumatic spinal cord injury

A39.4 Meningococcemia, unspecified   cc ▽
    RIC Excl: 03 Non-traumatic brain injury;
    05 Non-traumatic spinal cord injury

✓5ᵗʰ **A39.5 Meningococcal** heart disease

    A39.50 Meningococcal carditis, unspecified   cc ▽
        RIC Excl: 14 Cardiac

    A39.51 Meningococcal endocarditis   cc
        RIC Excl: 14 Cardiac

    A39.52 Meningococcal myocarditis   cc
        RIC Excl: 14 Cardiac

    A39.53 Meningococcal pericarditis

✓5ᵗʰ **A39.8** Other **meningococcal infections**

    A39.81 Meningococcal encephalitis

    A39.82 Meningococcal retrobulbar neuritis

    A39.83 Meningococcal arthritis

    A39.84 Postmeningococcal arthritis

    A39.89 Other meningococcal infections
        Meningococcal conjunctivitis

A39.9 Meningococcal infection, unspecified   ▽
    Meningococcal disease NOS

✓4ᵗʰ **A40 Streptococcal sepsis**
    Code first: postprocedural streptococcal sepsis (T81.4)
        streptococcal sepsis during labor (O75.3)
        streptococcal sepsis following abortion or ectopic or molar pregnancy (O03-O07, O08.0)
        streptococcal sepsis following immunization (T88.0)
        streptococcal sepsis following infusion, transfusion or therapeutic injection (T80.2-)
    EXCLUDES 1 neonatal (P36.0-P36.1)
        puerperal sepsis (O85)
        sepsis due to Streptococcus, group D (A41.81)

A40.0 Sepsis due to streptococcus, group A   cc

A40.1 Sepsis due to streptococcus, group B   cc

A40.3 Sepsis due to Streptococcus pneumoniae   cc
    Pneumococcal sepsis

A40.8 Other streptococcal sepsis   cc

A40.9 Streptococcal sepsis, unspecified   cc ▽

✓4ᵗʰ **A41 Other sepsis**
    Code first: postprocedural sepsis (T81.4)
        sepsis during labor (O75.3)
        sepsis following abortion, ectopic or molar pregnancy (O03-O07, O08.0)
        sepsis following immunization (T88.0)
        sepsis following infusion, transfusion or therapeutic injection (T80.2-)
    EXCLUDES 1 bacteremia NOS (R78.81)
        neonatal (P36.-)
        puerperal sepsis (O85)
        sepsis NOS (A41.9)
        streptococcal sepsis (A40.-)
    EXCLUDES 2 sepsis (due to) (in) actinomycotic (A42.7)
        sepsis (due to) (in) anthrax (A22.7)
        sepsis (due to) (in) candidal (B37.7)
        sepsis (due to) (in) Erysipelothrix (A26.7)
        sepsis (due to) (in) extraintestinal yersiniosis (A28.2)
        sepsis (due to) (in) gonococcal (A54.86)
        sepsis (due to) (in) herpesviral (B00.7)
        sepsis (due to) (in) listerial (A32.7)
        sepsis (due to) (in) melioidosis (A24.1)
        sepsis (due to) (in) meningococcal (A39.2-A39.4)
        sepsis (due to) (in) plague (A20.7)
        sepsis (due to) (in) tularemia (A21.7)
        toxic shock syndrome (A48.3)
    AHA: 2014, 2Q, 13

✓5ᵗʰ **A41.0 Sepsis due to** Staphylococcus aureus

    A41.01 Sepsis due to methicillin susceptible **Staphylococcus aureus**   cc
        MSSA sepsis
        Staphylococcus aureus sepsis NOS

    A41.02 Sepsis due to methicillin resistant **Staphylococcus aureus**   cc

A41.1 Sepsis due to other specified staphylococcus   cc
    Coagulase negative staphylococcus sepsis

A41.2 Sepsis due to unspecified staphylococcus   cc ▽

A41.3 Sepsis due to Hemophilus influenzae   cc

A41.4 Sepsis due to anaerobes   cc
    EXCLUDES 1 gas gangrene (A48.0)

✓5ᵗʰ **A41.5 Sepsis due to other** Gram-negative organisms

    A41.50 Gram-negative sepsis, unspecified   cc ▽
        Gram-negative sepsis NOS

    A41.51 Sepsis due to Escherichia coli [E. coli]   cc

    A41.52 Sepsis due to Pseudomonas   cc
        Pseudomonas aeroginosa

    A41.53 Sepsis due to Serratia   cc

    A41.59 Other Gram-negative sepsis   cc

✓5ᵗʰ **A41.8** Other **specified sepsis**

    A41.81 Sepsis due to Enterococcus   cc

    A41.89 Other specified sepsis   cc

A41.9 Sepsis, unspecified organism   cc ▽
    Septicemia NOS

✓4ᵗʰ **A42 Actinomycosis**
    EXCLUDES 1 actinomycetoma (B47.1)

A42.0 Pulmonary **actinomycosis**

A42.1 Abdominal **actinomycosis**

A42.2 Cervicofacial **actinomycosis**

A42.7 Actinomycotic sepsis   cc

✓5ᵗʰ **A42.8 Other forms of actinomycosis**

    A42.81 Actinomycotic meningitis

    A42.82 Actinomycotic encephalitis

    A42.89 Other forms of actinomycosis

A42.9 Actinomycosis, unspecified   ▽

✓4ᵗʰ **A43 Nocardiosis**

A43.0 Pulmonary **nocardiosis**

A43.1 Cutaneous **nocardiosis**

A43.8 Other forms of nocardiosis

---

2 Special Care High = With fever

8 Clinically Complex = Without fever

Ⓝ Newborn   Ⓟ Pediatric   Ⓜ Maternity   Ⓐ Adult   **RIC** RIC Dx   **NC Dx** Noncancer Dx   **PDx** Primary Dx   **CC** RIC CC Condition   ▶◀ Revised Text   ● New Code   ▲ Revised Code Title

A43.9   **Nocardiosis, unspecified**   ▽

✓4ᵗʰ **A44 Bartonellosis**

   A44.0   Systemic **bartonellosis**
     Oroya fever

   A44.1   Cutaneous and mucocutaneous **bartonellosis**
     Verruga peruana

   A44.8   Other forms of bartonellosis

   A44.9   **Bartonellosis, unspecified**   ▽

A46 Erysipelas
   EXCLUDES 1   *postpartum or puerperal erysipelas (O86.89)*

✓4ᵗʰ **A48 Other bacterial diseases, not elsewhere classified**
   EXCLUDES 1   *actinomycetoma (B47.1)*

   A48.0   **Gas gangrene**
     Clostridial cellulitis
     Clostridial myonecrosis

   A48.1   **Legionnaires' disease**   cc
     RIC Excl: 15 Pulmonary

   A48.2   **Nonpneumonic Legionnaires' disease [Pontiac fever]**

   A48.3   **Toxic shock syndrome**
     Use additional code to identify the organism (B95, B96)
     EXCLUDES 1   *endotoxic shock NOS (R57.8)*
         sepsis NOS (A41.9)

   A48.4   **Brazilian purpuric fever**
     Systemic Hemophilus aegyptius infection

   ✓5ᵗʰ A48.5   **Other specified botulism**
     Non-foodborne intoxication due to toxins of Clostridium
     botulinum [C. botulinum]
     EXCLUDES 1   *food poisoning due to toxins of Clostridium botulinum*
         (A05.1)

     A48.51   Infant **botulism**   P

     A48.52   Wound **botulism**
       Non-foodborne botulism NOS
       Use additional code for associated wound

   A48.8   Other specified bacterial diseases

✓4ᵗʰ **A49 Bacterial infection of unspecified site**
   EXCLUDES 1   *bacterial agents as the cause of diseases classified elsewhere*
       (B95-B96)
       chlamydial infection NOS (A74.9)
       meningococcal infection NOS (A39.9)
       rickettsial infection NOS (A79.9)
       spirochetal infection NOS (A69.9)

   ✓5ᵗʰ A49.0   Staphylococcal **infection, unspecified site**

     A49.01   Methicillin susceptible **Staphylococcus aureus**
       infection, unspecified site
       Methicillin susceptible Staphylococcus aureus (MSSA)
       infection
       Staphylococcus aureus infection NOS

     A49.02   Methicillin resistant **Staphylococcus aureus**
       infection, unspecified site
       Methicillin resistant Staphylococcus aureus (MRSA)
       infection

   A49.1   Streptococcal **infection, unspecified site**

   A49.2   Hemophilus influenzae **infection, unspecified site**

   A49.3   Mycoplasma **infection, unspecified site**

   A49.8   Other bacterial infections of unspecified site

   A49.9   **Bacterial infection, unspecified**   ▽
     EXCLUDES 1   *bacteremia NOS (R78.81)*

Infections with a predominantly sexual mode of transmission (A50-A64)

   EXCLUDES 1   *human immunodeficiency virus [HIV] disease (B20)*
     nonspecific and nongonococcal urethritis (N34.1)
     Reiter's disease (M02.3-)

✓4ᵗʰ **A50 Congenital syphilis**

   ✓5ᵗʰ A50.0   Early **congenital syphilis,** symptomatic
     Any congenital syphilitic condition specified as early or manifest
     less than two years after birth.

     A50.01   Early congenital syphilitic oculopathy

     A50.02   Early congenital syphilitic osteochondropathy

     A50.03   Early congenital syphilitic pharyngitis
       Early congenital syphilitic laryngitis

     2,8 A50.04   **Early congenital syphilitic** pneumonia

---

2 Special Care High = With fever

8 Clinically Complex = Without fever

A50.05   **Early congenital syphilitic** rhinitis

A50.06   **Early** cutaneous **congenital syphilis**

A50.07   **Early** mucocutaneous **congenital syphilis**

A50.08   **Early** visceral **congenital syphilis**

A50.09   **Other early congenital syphilis, symptomatic**

A50.1   Early **congenital syphilis,** latent
   Congenital syphilis without clinical manifestations, with positive
   serological reaction and negative spinal fluid test, less than
   two years after birth.

A50.2   **Early congenital syphilis, unspecified**   ▽
   Congenital syphilis NOS less than two years after birth.

✓5ᵗʰ A50.3   Late **congenital syphilitic** oculopathy
   EXCLUDES 1   *Hutchinson's triad (A50.53)*

   A50.30   **Late congenital syphilitic oculopathy,**   ▽
     unspecified

   A50.31   **Late congenital syphilitic** interstitial keratitis

   A50.32   **Late congenital syphilitic** chorioretinitis

   A50.39   **Other late congenital syphilitic oculopathy**

✓5ᵗʰ A50.4   Late **congenital neurosyphilis [juvenile neurosyphilis]**
   Use additional code to identify any associated mental disorder
   EXCLUDES 1   *Hutchinson's triad (A50.53)*

   A50.40   **Late congenital neurosyphilis, unspecified**   ▽
     Juvenile neurosyphilis NOS

   A50.41   **Late congenital syphilitic** meningitis   cc
     RIC Excl: 03 Non-traumatic brain injury;
     05 Non-traumatic spinal cord injury

   A50.42   **Late congenital syphilitic** encephalitis

   A50.43   **Late congenital syphilitic** polyneuropathy

   A50.44   **Late congenital syphilitic** optic nerve atrophy

   A50.45   Juvenile general paresis
     Dementia paralytica juvenilis
     Juvenile tabetoparetic neurosyphilis

   A50.49   **Other late congenital neurosyphilis**
     Juvenile tabes dorsalis

✓5ᵗʰ A50.5   Other late **congenital syphilis,** symptomatic
   Any congenital syphilitic condition specified as late or manifest
   two years or more after birth.

   A50.51   **Clutton's joints**

   A50.52   **Hutchinson's teeth**

   A50.53   **Hutchinson's triad**

   A50.54   **Late congenital cardiovascular syphilis**

   A50.55   **Late congenital syphilitic arthropathy**

   A50.56   **Late congenital syphilitic osteochondropathy**

   A50.57   **Syphilitic saddle nose**

   A50.59   **Other late congenital syphilis, symptomatic**

A50.6   Late **congenital syphilis,** latent
   Congenital syphilis without clinical manifestations, with positive
   serological reaction and negative spinal fluid test, two
   years or more after birth.

A50.7   Late **congenital syphilis, unspecified**   ▽
   Congenital syphilis NOS two years or more after birth.

A50.9   Congenital **syphilis, unspecified**   ▽

✓4ᵗʰ **A51 Early syphilis**

   A51.0   Primary genital **syphilis**
     Syphilitic chancre NOS

   A51.1   Primary anal **syphilis**

   A51.2   Primary **syphilis of other sites**

   ✓5ᵗʰ A51.3   Secondary **syphilis of** skin and mucous membranes

     A51.31   **Condyloma latum**

     A51.32   **Syphilitic alopecia**

     A51.39   **Other secondary syphilis of skin**
       Syphilitic leukoderma
       Syphilitic mucous patch
       EXCLUDES 1   *late syphilitic leukoderma (A52.79)*

   ✓5ᵗʰ A51.4   Other secondary **syphilis**

     A51.41   **Secondary syphilitic** meningitis

     A51.42   **Secondary syphilitic** female pelvic disease   ♀

     A51.43   **Secondary syphilitic** oculopathy
       Secondary syphilitic chorioretinitis
       Secondary syphilitic iridocyclitis, iritis
       Secondary syphilitic uveitis

☑ Add'l Character Required   ✓ₓ7ᵗʰ Placeholder Alert   RUG IV Special Care High Dx   RUG IV Clinically Complex Dx   RUG IV Special Care Low Dx   Manifestation Code   Other Specified Code   ▽ Unspecified Code

ICD-10-CM 2016   431

Chapter 1. Certain Infectious and Parasitic Diseases

A51.44 Secondary syphilitic **nephritis**

A51.45 Secondary syphilitic **hepatitis**

A51.46 Secondary syphilitic **osteopathy**

A51.49 **Other secondary syphilitic conditions**
Secondary syphilitic lymphadenopathy
Secondary syphilitic myositis

A51.5 Early **syphilis, latent**
Syphilis (acquired) without clinical manifestations, with positive serological reaction and negative spinal fluid test, less than two years after infection.

A51.9 Early **syphilis, unspecified** ▽

✓4th **A52** **Late syphilis**

✓5th **A52.0** Cardiovascular and cerebrovascular **syphilis**

A52.00 **Cardiovascular syphilis, unspecified** ▽

A52.01 **Syphilitic aneurysm of aorta**

A52.02 **Syphilitic aortitis**

A52.03 **Syphilitic endocarditis** CC
Syphilitic aortic valve incompetence or stenosis
Syphilitic mitral valve stenosis
Syphilitic pulmonary valve regurgitation
RIC Excl: 14 Cardiac

A52.04 **Syphilitic cerebral arteritis**

A52.05 Other cerebrovascular **syphilis**
Syphilitic cerebral aneurysm (ruptured) (non-ruptured)
Syphilitic cerebral thrombosis

A52.06 Other **syphilitic heart involvement** CC
Syphilitic coronary artery disease
Syphilitic myocarditis
Syphilitic pericarditis
RIC Excl: 14 Cardiac

A52.09 Other **cardiovascular syphilis**

✓5th **A52.1** Symptomatic **neurosyphilis**

A52.10 **Symptomatic neurosyphilis, unspecified** ▽

A52.11 **Tabes dorsalis**
Locomotor ataxia (progressive)
Tabetic neurosyphilis

A52.12 Other **cerebrospinal syphilis**

A52.13 **Late syphilitic meningitis** CC
RIC Excl: 03 Non-traumatic brain injury; 05 Non-traumatic spinal cord injury

A52.14 **Late syphilitic encephalitis**

A52.15 **Late syphilitic neuropathy**
Late syphilitic acoustic neuritis
Late syphilitic optic (nerve) atrophy
Late syphilitic polyneuropathy
Late syphilitic retrobulbar neuritis

A52.16 **Charcôt's arthropathy (tabetic)**

A52.17 **General paresis**
Dementia paralytica

A52.19 **Other symptomatic neurosyphilis** CC
Syphilitic parkinsonism
RIC Excl: 01 Stroke; 03 Nontraumatic brain injury

A52.2 Asymptomatic **neurosyphilis**

A52.3 **Neurosyphilis, unspecified** ▽
Gumma (syphilitic)
Syphilis (late)
Syphiloma

✓5th **A52.7** Other **symptomatic late syphilis**

A52.71 **Late syphilitic oculopathy**
Late syphilitic chorioretinitis
Late syphilitic episcleritis

A52.72 **Syphilis of lung and bronchus**

A52.73 **Symptomatic late syphilis of other respiratory organs**

A52.74 **Syphilis of liver and other viscera**
Late syphilitic peritonitis

A52.75 **Syphilis of kidney and ureter**
Syphilitic glomerular disease

A52.76 Other genitourinary **symptomatic late syphilis**
Late syphilitic female pelvic inflammatory disease

A52.77 **Syphilis of bone and joint**

A52.78 **Syphilis of other musculoskeletal tissue**
Late syphilitic bursitis
Syphilis [stage unspecified] of bursa
Syphilis [stage unspecified] of muscle
Syphilis [stage unspecified] of synovium
Syphilis [stage unspecified] of tendon

A52.79 **Other symptomatic late syphilis**
Late syphilitic leukoderma
Syphilis of adrenal gland
Syphilis of pituitary gland
Syphilis of thyroid gland
Syphilitic splenomegaly
EXCLUDES 1 syphilitic leukoderma (secondary) (A51.39)

A52.8 Late **syphilis, latent**
Syphilis (acquired) without clinical manifestations, with positive serological reaction and negative spinal fluid test, two years or more after infection

A52.9 Late **syphilis, unspecified** ▽

✓4th **A53** Other and unspecified **syphilis**

A53.0 Latent **syphilis, unspecified as early or late**
Latent syphilis NOS
Positive serological reaction for syphilis

A53.9 **Syphilis, unspecified** ▽
Infection due to Treponema pallidum NOS
Syphilis (acquired) NOS
EXCLUDES 1 syphilis NOS under two years of age (A50.2)

✓4th **A54** **Gonococcal infection**

✓5th **A54.0** **Gonococcal infection of lower genitourinary tract without periurethral or accessory gland abscess**
EXCLUDES 1 gonococcal infection with genitourinary gland abscess (A54.1)
gonococcal infection with periurethral abscess (A54.1)

A54.00 **Gonococcal infection of lower genitourinary tract, unspecified** ▽

A54.01 **Gonococcal cystitis and urethritis, unspecified**

A54.02 **Gonococcal vulvovaginitis, unspecified** ♀

A54.03 **Gonococcal cervicitis, unspecified** ♀

A54.09 **Other gonococcal infection of lower genitourinary tract**

A54.1 **Gonococcal infection of lower genitourinary tract with periurethral and accessory gland abscess**
Gonococcal Bartholin's gland abscess

✓5th **A54.2** **Gonococcal pelviperitonitis and other gonococcal genitourinary infection**

A54.21 **Gonococcal infection of kidney and ureter**

A54.22 **Gonococcal prostatitis** ♂

A54.23 **Gonococcal infection of other male genital organs** ♂
Gonococcal epididymitis
Gonococcal orchitis

A54.24 **Gonococcal female pelvic inflammatory disease** ♀
Gonococcal pelviperitonitis
EXCLUDES 1 gonococcal peritonitis (A54.85)

A54.29 **Other gonococcal genitourinary infections**

✓5th **A54.3** **Gonococcal infection of eye**

A54.30 **Gonococcal infection of eye, unspecified** ▽

A54.31 **Gonococcal conjunctivitis**
Ophthalmia neonatorum due to gonococcus

A54.32 **Gonococcal iridocyclitis**

A54.33 **Gonococcal keratitis**

A54.39 **Other gonococcal eye infection**
Gonococcal endophthalmia

✓5th **A54.4** **Gonococcal infection of musculoskeletal system**

A54.40 **Gonococcal infection of musculoskeletal system, unspecified** ▽

A54.41 **Gonococcal spondylopathy**

A54.42 **Gonococcal arthritis**
EXCLUDES 2 gonococcal infection of spine (A54.41)

A54.43 **Gonococcal osteomyelitis**
EXCLUDES 2 gonococcal infection of spine (A54.41)

A54.49 **Gonococcal infection of other musculoskeletal tissue**
Gonococcal bursitis
Gonococcal myositis
Gonococcal synovitis
Gonococcal tenosynovitis

A54.5 **Gonococcal pharyngitis**

A54.6 **Gonococcal infection of anus and rectum**

N Newborn   P Pediatric   M Maternity   A Adult   RIC RIC Dx   NCDx Noncancer Dx   PDx Primary Dx   CC RIC CC Condition   ►◄ Revised Text   ● New Code   ▲ Revised Code Title

432   ICD-10-CM 2016

✓5ᵗʰ **A54.8 Other gonococcal infections**

    A54.81 Gonococcal meningitis

    A54.82 Gonococcal brain abscess   CC

    A54.83 Gonococcal heart infection
        Gonococcal endocarditis
        Gonococcal myocarditis
        Gonococcal pericarditis

2,8   **A54.84 Gonococcal pneumonia**   CC

    A54.85 Gonococcal peritonitis
        EXCLUDES1   gonococcal pelviperitonitis (A54.24)

    A54.86 Gonococcal sepsis   CC

    A54.89 Other gonococcal infections   CC
        Gonococcal keratoderma
        Gonococcal lymphadenitis

  A54.9 Gonococcal infection, unspecified   CC ▽

A55 Chlamydial lymphogranuloma (venereum)
    Climatic or tropical bubo
    Durand-Nicolas-Favre disease
    Esthiomene
    Lymphogranuloma inguinale

✓4ᵗʰ **A56 Other sexually transmitted chlamydial diseases**
    INCLUDES   sexually transmitted diseases due to Chlamydia trachomatis
    EXCLUDES1   neonatal chlamydial conjunctivitis (P39.1)
        neonatal chlamydial pneumonia (P23.1)
    EXCLUDES2   chlamydial lymphogranuloma (A55)
        conditions classified to A74-

✓5ᵗʰ **A56.0 Chlamydial infection of lower genitourinary tract**

    A56.00 Chlamydial infection of lower genitourinary tract, unspecified   ▽

    A56.01 Chlamydial cystitis and urethritis

    A56.02 Chlamydial vulvovaginitis   ♀

    A56.09 Other chlamydial infection of lower genitourinary tract
        Chlamydial cervicitis

✓5ᵗʰ **A56.1 Chlamydial infection of pelviperitoneum and other genitourinary organs**

    A56.11 Chlamydial female pelvic inflammatory disease   ♀

    A56.19 Other chlamydial genitourinary infection
        Chlamydial epididymitis
        Chlamydial orchitis

  A56.2 Chlamydial infection of genitourinary tract, unspecified   ▽

  A56.3 Chlamydial infection of anus and rectum

  A56.4 Chlamydial infection of pharynx

  A56.8 Sexually transmitted chlamydial infection of other sites

A57 Chancroid
    Ulcus molle

A58 Granuloma inguinale
    Donovanosis

✓4ᵗʰ **A59 Trichomoniasis**
    EXCLUDES2   intestinal trichomoniasis (A07.8)

✓5ᵗʰ **A59.0 Urogenital trichomoniasis**

    A59.00 Urogenital trichomoniasis, unspecified   ▽
        Fluor (vaginalis) due to Trichomonas
        Leukorrhea (vaginalis) due to Trichomonas

    A59.01 Trichomonal vulvovaginitis   ♀

    A59.02 Trichomonal prostatitis   ♂

    A59.03 Trichomonal cystitis and urethritis

    A59.09 Other urogenital trichomoniasis
        Trichomonas cervicitis

  A59.8 Trichomoniasis of other sites

  A59.9 Trichomoniasis, unspecified   ▽

✓4ᵗʰ **A60 Anogenital herpesviral [herpes simplex] infections**

✓5ᵗʰ **A60.0 Herpesviral infection of genitalia and urogenital tract**

    A60.00 Herpesviral infection of urogenital system, unspecified   ▽

    A60.01 Herpesviral infection of penis   ♂

    A60.02 Herpesviral infection of other male genital organs   ♂

    A60.03 Herpesviral cervicitis   ♀

    A60.04 Herpesviral vulvovaginitis   ♀
        Herpesviral [herpes simplex] ulceration
        Herpesviral [herpes simplex] vaginitis
        Herpesviral [herpes simplex] vulvitis

    A60.09 Herpesviral infection of other urogenital tract

  A60.1 Herpesviral infection of perianal skin and rectum

  A60.9 Anogenital herpesviral infection, unspecified   ▽

✓4ᵗʰ **A63 Other predominantly sexually transmitted diseases, not elsewhere classified**
    EXCLUDES2   molluscum contagiosum (B08.1)
        papilloma of cervix (D26.0)

  A63.0 Anogenital (venereal) warts
    Anogenital warts due to (human) papillomavirus [HPV]
    Condyloma acuminatum

  A63.8 Other specified predominantly sexually transmitted diseases

A64 Unspecified sexually transmitted disease   ▽

Other spirochetal diseases (A65-A69)

    EXCLUDES2   leptospirosis (A27.-)
        syphilis (A50-A53)

A65 Nonvenereal syphilis
    Bejel   Njovera
    Endemic syphilis

✓4ᵗʰ **A66 Yaws**
    INCLUDES   bouba
        frambesia (tropica)
        pian

  A66.0 Initial lesions of yaws
    Chancre of yaws
    Frambesia, initial or primary
    Initial frambesial ulcer
    Mother yaw

  A66.1 Multiple papillomata and wet crab yaws
    Frambesioma
    Pianoma
    Plantar or palmar papilloma of yaws

  A66.2 Other early skin lesions of yaws
    Cutaneous yaws, less than five years after infection
    Early yaws (cutaneous) (macular) (maculopapular)
        (micropapular) (papular)
    Frambeside of early yaws

  A66.3 Hyperkeratosis of yaws
    Ghoul hand
    Hyperkeratosis, palmar or plantar (early) (late) due to yaws
    Worm-eaten soles

  A66.4 Gummata and ulcers of yaws
    Gummatous frambeside
    Nodular late yaws (ulcerated)

  A66.5 Gangosa
    Rhinopharyngitis mutilans

  A66.6 Bone and joint lesions of yaws
    Yaws ganglion   Yaws hydrarthrosis
    Yaws goundou   Yaws osteitis
    Yaws gumma, bone   Yaws periostitis (hypertrophic)
    Yaws gummatous osteitis
        or periostitis

  A66.7 Other manifestations of yaws
    Juxta-articular nodules of yaws
    Mucosal yaws

  A66.8 Latent yaws
    Yaws without clinical manifestations, with positive serology

  A66.9 Yaws, unspecified   ▽

✓4ᵗʰ **A67 Pinta [carate]**

  A67.0 Primary lesions of pinta
    Chancre (primary) of pinta
    Papule (primary) of pinta

  A67.1 Intermediate lesions of pinta
    Erythematous plaques of pinta
    Hyperchromic lesions of pinta
    Hyperkeratosis of pinta
    Pintids

  A67.2 Late lesions of pinta
    Achromic skin lesions of pinta
    Cicatricial skin lesions of pinta
    Dyschromic skin lesions of pinta

---

2 Special Care High = With fever

8 Clinically Complex = Without fever

☑ Add'l Character Required   ✓7ᵗʰ Placeholder Alert   RUG IV Special Care High Dx   RUG IV Clinically Complex Dx   RUG IV Special Care Low Dx   Manifestation Code   Other Specified Code   ▽ Unspecified Code

A67.3 Mixed lesions of pinta
Achromic with hyperchromic skin lesions of pinta [carate]

A67.9 Pinta, unspecified ▽

✓4th **A68 Relapsing fevers**
INCLUDES recurrent fever
EXCLUDES 2 *Lyme disease (A69.2-)*

A68.0 Louse-borne relapsing fever
Relapsing fever due to Borrelia recurrentis

A68.1 Tick-borne relapsing fever
Relapsing fever due to any Borrelia species other than Borrelia recurrentis

A68.9 Relapsing fever, unspecified ▽

✓4th **A69 Other spirochetal infections**

A69.0 Necrotizing ulcerative stomatitis
Cancrum oris
Fusospirochetal gangrene
Noma
Stomatitis gangrenosa

A69.1 Other Vincent's infections
Fusospirochetal pharyngitis
Necrotizing ulcerative (acute) gingivitis
Necrotizing ulcerative (acute) gingivostomatitis
Spirochetal stomatitis
Trench mouth
Vincent's angina
Vincent's gingivitis

✓5th **A69.2 Lyme disease**
Erythema chronicum migrans due to Borrelia burgdorferi

A69.20 Lyme disease, unspecified ▽

A69.21 Meningitis due to Lyme disease

A69.22 Other neurologic disorders in Lyme disease
Cranial neuritis
Meningoencephalitis
Polyneuropathy

A69.23 Arthritis due to Lyme disease

A69.29 Other conditions associated with Lyme disease
Myopericarditis due to Lyme disease

A69.8 Other specified spirochetal infections

A69.9 Spirochetal infection, unspecified ▽

Other diseases caused by chlamydiae (A70-A74)
EXCLUDES 1 *sexually transmitted chlamydial diseases (A55-A56)*

A70 Chlamydia psittaci infections
Ornithosis
Parrot fever
Psittacosis

✓4th **A71 Trachoma**
EXCLUDES 1 *sequelae of trachoma (B94.0)*

A71.0 Initial stage of trachoma
Trachoma dubium

A71.1 Active stage of trachoma
Granular conjunctivitis (trachomatous)
Trachomatous follicular conjunctivitis
Trachomatous pannus

A71.9 Trachoma, unspecified ▽

✓4th **A74 Other diseases caused by chlamydiae**
EXCLUDES 1 *neonatal chlamydial conjunctivitis (P39.1)*
neonatal chlamydial pneumonia (P23.1)
Reiter's disease (M02.3-)
sexually transmitted chlamydial diseases (A55-A56)
EXCLUDES 2 *chlamydial pneumonia (J16.0)*

A74.0 Chlamydial conjunctivitis
Paratrachoma

✓5th **A74.8 Other chlamydial diseases**

A74.81 Chlamydial peritonitis

A74.89 Other chlamydial diseases

A74.9 Chlamydial infection, unspecified ▽
Chlamydiosis NOS

Rickettsioses (A75-A79)

✓4th **A75 Typhus fever**
EXCLUDES 1 *rickettsiosis due to Ehrlichia sennetsu (A79.81)*

A75.0 Epidemic louse-borne typhus fever due to Rickettsia prowazekii
Classical typhus (fever)
Epidemic (louse-borne) typhus

A75.1 Recrudescent typhus [Brill's disease]
Brill-Zinsser disease

A75.2 Typhus fever due to Rickettsia typhi
Murine (flea-borne) typhus

A75.3 Typhus fever due to Rickettsia tsutsugamushi
Scrub (mite-borne) typhus
Tsutsugamushi fever

A75.9 Typhus fever, unspecified ▽
Typhus (fever) NOS

✓4th **A77 Spotted fever [tick-borne rickettsioses]**

A77.0 Spotted fever due to Rickettsia rickettsii
Rocky Mountain spotted fever
Sao Paulo fever

A77.1 Spotted fever due to Rickettsia conorii
African tick typhus
Boutonneuse fever
India tick typhus
Kenya tick typhus
Marseilles fever
Mediterranean tick fever

A77.2 Spotted fever due to Rickettsia siberica
North Asian tick fever
Siberian tick typhus

A77.3 Spotted fever due to Rickettsia australis
Queensland tick typhus

✓5th **A77.4 Ehrlichiosis**
EXCLUDES 1 *Rickettsiosis due to Ehrlichia sennetsu (A79.81)*

A77.40 Ehrlichiosis, unspecified ▽

A77.41 Ehrlichiosis chafeensis [E. chafeensis]

A77.49 Other ehrlichiosis

A77.8 Other spotted fevers

A77.9 Spotted fever, unspecified ▽
Tick-borne typhus NOS

A78 Q fever
Infection due to Coxiella burnetii
Nine Mile fever
Quadrilateral fever

✓4th **A79 Other rickettsioses**

A79.0 Trench fever
Quintan fever
Wolhynian fever

A79.1 Rickettsialpox due to Rickettsia akari
Kew Garden fever
Vesicular rickettsiosis

✓5th **A79.8 Other specified rickettsioses**

A79.81 Rickettsiosis due to Ehrlichia sennetsu

A79.89 Other specified rickettsioses

A79.9 Rickettsiosis, unspecified ▽
Rickettsial infection NOS

Viral and prion infections of the central nervous system (A80-A89)
EXCLUDES 1 *postpolio syndrome (G14)*
sequelae of poliomyelitis (B91)
sequelae of viral encephalitis (B94.1)

✓4th **A80 Acute poliomyelitis**

A80.0 Acute paralytic poliomyelitis, vaccine-associated

A80.1 Acute paralytic poliomyelitis, wild virus, imported

A80.2 Acute paralytic poliomyelitis, wild virus, indigenous

✓5th **A80.3 Acute paralytic poliomyelitis, other and unspecified**

A80.30 Acute paralytic poliomyelitis, unspecified ▽

A80.39 Other acute paralytic poliomyelitis

A80.4 Acute nonparalytic poliomyelitis

A80.9 Acute poliomyelitis, unspecified ▽

✓4th **A81 Atypical virus infections of central nervous system**
INCLUDES diseases of the central nervous system caused by prions
Use additional code to identify:
dementia with behavioral disturbance (F02.81)
dementia without behavioral disturbance (F02.80)

✓5th **A81.0 Creutzfeldt-Jakob disease**

A81.00 Creutzfeldt-Jakob disease, unspecified ▽
Jakob-Creutzfeldt disease, unspecified

A81.01 Variant Creutzfeldt-Jakob disease
vCJD

A81.09 **Other Creutzfeldt-Jakob disease**
CJD
Familial Creutzfeldt-Jakob disease
Iatrogenic Creutzfeldt-Jakob disease
Sporadic Creutzfeldt-Jakob disease
Subacute spongiform encephalopathy (with dementia)

A81.1 **Subacute sclerosing panencephalitis**
Dawson's inclusion body encephalitis
Van Bogaert's sclerosing leukoencephalopathy

A81.2 **Progressive multifocal leukoencephalopathy**
Multifocal leukoencephalopathy NOS

✓5ᵗʰ A81.8 **Other atypical virus infections of central nervous system**

A81.81 **Kuru**

A81.82 **Gerstmann-Sträussler-Scheinker syndrome**
GSS syndrome

A81.83 **Fatal familial insomnia**
FFI

A81.89 **Other atypical virus infections of central nervous system**

A81.9 **Atypical virus infection of central nervous system, unspecified** ▽
Prion diseases of the central nervous system NOS

✓4ᵗʰ A82 **Rabies**

A82.0 **Sylvatic rabies**

A82.1 **Urban rabies**

A82.9 **Rabies, unspecified** ▽

✓4ᵗʰ A83 **Mosquito-borne viral encephalitis**
INCLUDES mosquito-borne viral meningoencephalitis
EXCLUDES2 *Venezuelan equine encephalitis (A92.2)*
West Nile fever (A92.3-)
West Nile virus (A92.3-)

A83.0 **Japanese encephalitis**

A83.1 **Western equine encephalitis**

A83.2 **Eastern equine encephalitis**

A83.3 **St Louis encephalitis**

A83.4 **Australian encephalitis**
Kunjin virus disease

A83.5 **California encephalitis**
California meningoencephalitis
La Crosse encephalitis

A83.6 **Rocio virus disease**

A83.8 **Other mosquito-borne viral encephalitis**

A83.9 **Mosquito-borne viral encephalitis, unspecified** ▽

✓4ᵗʰ A84 **Tick-borne viral encephalitis**
INCLUDES tick-borne viral meningoencephalitis

A84.0 **Far Eastern tick-borne encephalitis [Russian spring-summer encephalitis]**

A84.1 **Central European tick-borne encephalitis**

A84.8 **Other tick-borne viral encephalitis**
Louping ill
Powassan virus disease

A84.9 **Tick-borne viral encephalitis, unspecified** ▽

✓4ᵗʰ A85 **Other viral encephalitis, not elsewhere classified**
INCLUDES specified viral encephalomyelitis NEC
specified viral meningoencephalitis NEC
EXCLUDES1 *benign myalgic encephalomyelitis (G93.3)*
encephalitis due to cytomegalovirus (B25.8)
encephalitis due to herpesvirus NEC (B10.0-)
encephalitis due to herpesvirus [herpes simplex] (B00.4)
encephalitis due to measles virus (B05.0)
encephalitis due to mumps virus (B26.2)
encephalitis due to poliomyelitis virus (A80.-)
encephalitis due to zoster (B02.0
lymphocytic choriomeningitis (A87.2)

A85.0 **Enteroviral encephalitis**
Enteroviral encephalomyelitis

A85.1 **Adenoviral encephalitis**
Adenoviral meningoencephalitis

A85.2 **Arthropod-borne viral encephalitis, unspecified** ▽
EXCLUDES1 *West nile virus with encephalitis (A92.31)*

A85.8 **Other specified viral encephalitis**
Encephalitis lethargica
Von Economo-Cruchet disease

A86 **Unspecified viral encephalitis** CC ▽
Viral encephalomyelitis NOS
Viral meningoencephalitis NOS
RIC Excl: 03 Non-traumatic brain injury

✓4ᵗʰ A87 **Viral meningitis**
EXCLUDES1 *meningitis due to herpesvirus [herpes simplex] (B00.3)*
meningitis due to measles virus (B05.1)
meningitis due to mumps virus (B26.1)
meningitis due to poliomyelitis virus (A80.-)
meningitis due to zoster (B02.1)

A87.0 **Enteroviral meningitis** CC
Coxsackievirus meningitis
Echovirus meningitis
RIC Excl: 03 Non-traumatic brain injury;
05 Non-traumatic spinal cord injury

A87.1 **Adenoviral meningitis**

A87.2 **Lymphocytic choriomeningitis** CC
Lymphocytic meningoencephalitis
RIC Excl: 03 Non-traumatic brain injury;
05 Non-traumatic spinal cord injury

A87.8 **Other viral meningitis** CC
RIC Excl: 03 Non-traumatic brain injury;
05 Non-traumatic spinal cord injury

A87.9 **Viral meningitis, unspecified** CC ▽
RIC Excl: 03 Non-traumatic brain injury;
05 Non-traumatic spinal cord injury

✓4ᵗʰ A88 **Other viral infections of central nervous system, not elsewhere classified**
EXCLUDES1 *viral encephalitis NOS (A86)*
viral meningitis NOS (A87.9)

A88.0 **Enteroviral exanthematous fever [Boston exanthem]** CC
RIC Excl: 03 Non-traumatic brain injury;
05 Non-traumatic spinal cord injury

A88.1 **Epidemic vertigo**

A88.8 **Other specified viral infections of central nervous system**

A89 **Unspecified viral infection of central nervous system** CC ▽
RIC Excl: 03 Non-traumatic brain injury

Arthropod-borne viral fevers and viral hemorrhagic fevers (A90-A99)

A90 **Dengue fever [classical dengue]**
EXCLUDES1 *dengue hemorrhagic fever (A91)*

A91 **Dengue hemorrhagic fever**

✓4ᵗʰ A92 **Other mosquito-borne viral fevers**
EXCLUDES1 *Ross River disease (B33.1)*

A92.0 **Chikungunya virus disease**
Chikungunya (hemorrhagic) fever

A92.1 **O'nyong-nyong fever**

A92.2 **Venezuelan equine fever**
Venezuelan equine encephalitis
Venezuelan equine encephalomyelitis virus disease

✓5ᵗʰ A92.3 **West Nile virus infection**
West Nile fever

A92.30 **West Nile virus infection, unspecified** ▽
West Nile fever NOS
West Nile fever without complications
West Nile virus NOS

A92.31 **West Nile virus infection with encephalitis**
West Nile encephalitis
West Nile encephalomyelitis

A92.32 **West Nile virus infection with other neurologic manifestation**
Use additional code to specify the neurologic manifestation

A92.39 **West Nile virus infection with other complications**
Use additional code to specify the other conditions

A92.4 **Rift Valley fever**

A92.8 **Other specified mosquito-borne viral fevers**

A92.9 **Mosquito-borne viral fever, unspecified** ▽

✓4ᵗʰ A93 **Other arthropod-borne viral fevers, not elsewhere classified**

A93.0 **Oropouche virus disease**
Oropouche fever

A93.1 **Sandfly fever**
Pappataci fever
Phlebotomus fever

A93.2 **Colorado tick fever**

A93.8 Other specified arthropod-borne viral fevers
    Piry virus disease
    Vesicular stomatitis virus disease [Indiana fever]

A94 Unspecified arthropod-borne viral fever ▽
    Arboviral fever NOS
    Arbovirus infection NOS

✓4ᵗʰ **A95 Yellow fever**
  A95.0 Sylvatic yellow fever
    Jungle yellow fever
  A95.1 Urban yellow fever
  A95.9 Yellow fever, unspecified ▽

✓4ᵗʰ **A96 Arenaviral hemorrhagic fever**
  A96.0 Junin hemorrhagic fever
    Argentinian hemorrhagic fever
  A96.1 Machupo hemorrhagic fever
    Bolivian hemorrhagic fever
  A96.2 Lassa fever
  A96.8 Other arenaviral hemorrhagic fevers
  A96.9 Arenaviral hemorrhagic fever, unspecified ▽

✓4ᵗʰ **A98 Other viral hemorrhagic fevers, not elsewhere classified**
  EXCLUDES 1 chikungunya hemorrhagic fever (A92.0)
    dengue hemorrhagic fever (A91)
  A98.0 Crimean-Congo hemorrhagic fever
    Central Asian hemorrhagic fever
  A98.1 Omsk hemorrhagic fever
  A98.2 Kyasanur Forest disease
  A98.3 Marburg virus disease
  A98.4 Ebola virus disease
  A98.5 Hemorrhagic fever with renal syndrome
    Epidemic hemorrhagic fever
    Korean hemorrhagic fever
    Russian hemorrhagic fever
    Hantaan virus disease
    Hantavirus disease with renal manifestations
    Nephropathia epidemica
    Songo fever
    EXCLUDES 1 hantavirus (cardio)-pulmonary syndrome (B33.4)
  A98.8 Other specified viral hemorrhagic fevers

A99 Unspecified viral hemorrhagic fever ▽

Viral infections characterized by skin and mucous membrane lesions (B00-B09)

✓4ᵗʰ **B00 Herpesviral [herpes simplex] infections**
  EXCLUDES 1 congenital herpesviral infections (P35.2)
  EXCLUDES 2 anogenital herpesviral infection (A60.-)
    gammaherpesviral mononucleosis (B27.0-)
    herpangina (B08.5)
  B00.0 Eczema herpeticum
    Kaposi's varicelliform eruption
  B00.1 Herpesviral vesicular dermatitis
    Herpes simplex facialis   Vesicular dermatitis of ear
    Herpes simplex labialis   Vesicular dermatitis of lip
    Herpes simplex otitis externa
  B00.2 Herpesviral gingivostomatitis and pharyngotonsillitis
    Herpesviral pharyngitis
  B00.3 Herpesviral meningitis CC
    RIC Excl: 03 Non-traumatic brain injury;
    05 Non-traumatic spinal cord injury
  B00.4 Herpesviral encephalitis CC
    Herpesviral meningoencephalitis
    Simian B disease
    EXCLUDES 1 herpesviral encephalitis due to herpesvirus 6 and 7 (B10.01, B10.09)
    non-simplex herpesviral encephalitis (B10.0-)
    RIC Excl: 03 Non-traumatic brain injury
✓5ᵗʰ **B00.5 Herpesviral ocular disease**
    B00.50 Herpesviral ocular disease, unspecified ▽
    B00.51 Herpesviral iridocyclitis
      Herpesviral iritis
      Herpesviral uveitis, anterior
    B00.52 Herpesviral keratitis
      Herpesviral keratoconjunctivitis
    B00.53 Herpesviral conjunctivitis

    B00.59 Other herpesviral disease of eye
      Herpesviral dermatitis of eyelid
  B00.7 Disseminated herpesviral disease CC
    Herpesviral sepsis
    RIC Excl: 03 Non-traumatic brain injury
✓5ᵗʰ **B00.8 Other forms of herpesviral infections**
    B00.81 Herpesviral hepatitis
    B00.82 Herpes simplex myelitis CC
    B00.89 Other herpesviral infection CC
      Herpesviral whitlow
  B00.9 Herpesviral infection, unspecified ▽
    Herpes simplex infection NOS

✓4ᵗʰ **B01 Varicella [chickenpox]**
  B01.0 Varicella meningitis
✓5ᵗʰ **B01.1 Varicella encephalitis, myelitis and encephalomyelitis**
    Postchickenpox encephalitis, myelitis and encephalomyelitis
    B01.11 Varicella encephalitis and encephalomyelitis CC
      Postchickenpox encephalitis and encephalomyelitis
      RIC Excl: 03 Non-traumatic brain injury
    B01.12 Varicella myelitis
      Postchickenpox myelitis
2,8 **B01.2 Varicella pneumonia** CC
    RIC Excl: 15 Pulmonary
✓5ᵗʰ **B01.8 Varicella with other complications**
    B01.81 Varicella keratitis
    B01.89 Other varicella complications
  B01.9 Varicella without complication ▽
    Varicella NOS

✓4ᵗʰ **B02 Zoster [herpes zoster]**
  INCLUDES shingles
    zona
  B02.0 Zoster encephalitis
    Zoster meningoencephalitis
  B02.1 Zoster meningitis CC
    RIC Excl: 03 Non-traumatic brain injury;
    05 Non-traumatic spinal cord injury
✓5ᵗʰ **B02.2 Zoster with other nervous system involvement**
    B02.21 Postherpetic geniculate ganglionitis
    B02.22 Postherpetic trigeminal neuralgia
    B02.23 Postherpetic polyneuropathy CC
      RIC Excl: 06 Neurological
    B02.24 Postherpetic myelitis
      Herpes zoster myelitis
    B02.29 Other postherpetic nervous system involvement
      Postherpetic radiculopathy
✓5ᵗʰ **B02.3 Zoster ocular disease**
    B02.30 Zoster ocular disease, unspecified ▽
    B02.31 Zoster conjunctivitis
    B02.32 Zoster iridocyclitis
    B02.33 Zoster keratitis
      Herpes zoster keratoconjunctivitis
    B02.34 Zoster scleritis
    B02.39 Other herpes zoster eye disease
      Zoster blepharitis
  B02.7 Disseminated zoster
  B02.8 Zoster with other complications
    Herpes zoster otitis externa
  B02.9 Zoster without complications ▽
    Zoster NOS

B03 Smallpox
  NOTE In 1980 the 33rd World Health Assembly declared that smallpox had been eradicated. The classification is maintained for surveillance purposes.

B04 Monkeypox

✓4ᵗʰ **B05 Measles**
  INCLUDES morbilli
  EXCLUDES 1 subacute sclerosing panencephalitis (A81.1)
  B05.0 Measles complicated by encephalitis CC
    Postmeasles encephalitis
    RIC Excl: 03 Non-traumatic brain injury
  B05.1 Measles complicated by meningitis
    Postmeasles meningitis

---

² Special Care High = With fever

⁸ Clinically Complex = Without fever

Ⓝ Newborn   Ⓟ Pediatric   Ⓜ Maternity   Ⓐ Adult   **RIC** RIC Dx   **NCDx** Noncancer Dx   **PDx** Primary Dx   **CC** RIC CC Condition   ▶◀ Revised Text   ● New Code   ▲ Revised Code Title

2,8 B05.2 Measles complicated by pneumonia
     Postmeasles pneumonia
     RIC Excl: 15 Pulmonary   `CC`

B05.3 Measles complicated by otitis media
     Postmeasles otitis media

B05.4 Measles with intestinal **complications**

B05.8 Measles with other **complications**
     B05.81 Measles keratitis and keratoconjunctivitis
     B05.89 Other measles complications

B05.9 Measles without complication   ▽
     Measles NOS

B06 Rubella [German measles]
     EXCLUDES 1   congenital rubella (P35.0)

B06.0 Rubella with neurological complications
     B06.00 Rubella with neurological complication, unspecified   ▽
     B06.01 Rubella encephalitis
         Rubella meningoencephalitis
     B06.02 Rubella meningitis
     B06.09 Other neurological complications of rubella

B06.8 Rubella with other **complications**
     2,8 B06.81 Rubella pneumonia
     B06.82 Rubella arthritis
     B06.89 Other rubella complications

B06.9 Rubella without complication   ▽
     Rubella NOS

B07 Viral warts
     INCLUDES   verruca simplex
         verruca vulgaris
         viral warts due to human papillomavirus
     EXCLUDES 2   anogenital (venereal) warts (A63.0)
         papilloma of bladder (D41.4)
         papilloma of cervix (D26.0)
         papilloma larynx (D14.1)

B07.0 Plantar wart
     Verruca plantaris

B07.8 Other viral warts
     Common wart
     Flat wart
     Verruca plana

B07.9 Viral wart, unspecified   ▽

B08 Other viral infections characterized by skin and mucous membrane lesions, not elsewhere classified
     EXCLUDES 1   vesicular stomatitis virus disease (A93.8)

B08.0 Other orthopoxvirus infections
     EXCLUDES 2   monkeypox (B04)
     B08.01 Cowpox and vaccinia not from vaccine
         B08.010 Cowpox
         B08.011 Vaccinia not from vaccine
             EXCLUDES 1   vaccinia (from vaccination) (generalized) (T88.1)
     B08.02 Orf virus disease
         Contagious pustular dermatitis
         Ecthyma contagiosum
     B08.03 Pseudocowpox [milker's node]
     B08.04 Paravaccinia, unspecified   ▽
     B08.09 Other orthopoxvirus infections
         Orthopoxvirus infection NOS

B08.1 Molluscum contagiosum

B08.2 Exanthema subitum [sixth disease]
     Roseola infantum
     B08.20 Exanthema subitum [sixth disease], unspecified   `P` ▽
         Roseola infantum, unspecified
     B08.21 Exanthema subitum [sixth disease] due to human herpesvirus 6   `P`
         Roseola infantum due to human herpesvirus 6
     B08.22 Exanthema subitum [sixth disease] due to human herpesvirus 7   `P`
         Roseola infantum due to human herpesvirus 7

B08.3 Erythema infectiosum [fifth disease]

B08.4 Enteroviral vesicular stomatitis with exanthem
     Hand, foot and mouth disease

B08.5 Enteroviral vesicular pharyngitis
     Herpangina

B08.6 Parapoxvirus infections
     B08.60 Parapoxvirus infection, unspecified   ▽
     B08.61 Bovine stomatitis
     B08.62 Sealpox
     B08.69 Other parapoxvirus infections

B08.7 Yatapoxvirus infections
     B08.70 Yatapoxvirus infection, unspecified   ▽
     B08.71 Tanapox virus disease
     B08.72 Yaba pox virus disease
         Yaba monkey tumor disease
     B08.79 Other yatapoxvirus infections

B08.8 Other specified viral infections characterized by skin and mucous membrane lesions
     Enteroviral lymphonodular pharyngitis
     Foot-and-mouth disease
     Poxvirus NEC

B09 Unspecified viral infection characterized by skin and mucous membrane lesions   ▽
     Viral enanthema NOS   Viral exanthema NOS

Other human herpesviruses (B10)

B10 Other human herpesviruses
     EXCLUDES 2   cytomegalovirus (B25.9)
         Epstein-Barr virus (B27.0-)
         herpes NOS (B00.9)
         herpes simplex (B00.-)
         herpes zoster (B02.-)
         human herpesvirus NOS (B00.-)
         human herpesvirus 1 and 2 (B00.-)
         human herpesvirus 3 (B01.-, B02.-)
         human herpesvirus 4 (B27.0-)
         human herpesvirus 5 (B25.-)
         varicella (B01.-)
         zoster (B02.-)

B10.0 Other human herpesvirus encephalitis
     EXCLUDES 2   herpes encephalitis NOS (B00.4)
         herpes simplex encephalitis (B00.4)
         human herpesvirus encephalitis (B00.4)
         simian B herpes virus encephalitis (B00.4)
     B10.01 Human herpesvirus 6 **encephalitis**   `CC`
         RIC Excl: 03 Non-traumatic brain injury
     B10.09 Other human herpesvirus encephalitis   `CC`
         Human herpesvirus 7 encephalitis
         RIC Excl: 03 Non-traumatic brain injury

B10.8 Other human herpesvirus infection
     B10.81 Human herpesvirus 6 **infection**
     B10.82 Human herpesvirus 7 **infection**
     B10.89 Other human herpesvirus infection
         Human herpesvirus 8 infection
         Kaposi's sarcoma-associated herpesvirus infection

Viral hepatitis (B15-B19)

     EXCLUDES 1   sequelae of viral hepatitis (B94.2)
     EXCLUDES 2   cytomegaloviral hepatitis (B25.1)
         herpesviral [herpes simplex] hepatitis (B00.81)

B15 Acute hepatitis A
     B15.0 Hepatitis A with hepatic coma
     B15.9 Hepatitis A without hepatic coma
         Hepatitis A (acute)(viral) NOS

B16 Acute hepatitis B
     B16.0 Acute hepatitis B with delta-agent with hepatic coma   `CC`
         RIC Excl: 03 Non-traumatic brain injury
     B16.1 Acute hepatitis B with delta-agent without hepatic coma
     B16.2 Acute hepatitis B without delta-agent with hepatic coma   `CC`
         RIC Excl: 03 Non-traumatic brain injury
     B16.9 Acute hepatitis B without delta-agent and without hepatic coma
         Hepatitis B (acute) (viral) NOS

---

2 Special Care High = With fever

8 Clinically Complex = Without fever

✔ Add'l Character Required   ✔7th Placeholder Alert   RUG IV Special Care High Dx   RUG IV Clinically Complex Dx   RUG IV Special Care Low Dx   Manifestation Code   Other Specified Code   ▽ Unspecified Code

Chapter 1. Certain Infectious and Parasitic Diseases

✓4ᵗʰ **B17** Other acute **viral hepatitis**

B17.0 Acute delta-(super) infection of hepatitis B carrier   CC
RIC Excl: 03 Non-traumatic brain injury

✓5ᵗʰ **B17.1** Acute hepatitis C

  B17.10 Acute hepatitis C without hepatic coma
Acute hepatitis C NOS

  B17.11 Acute hepatitis C with hepatic coma   CC
RIC Excl: 03 Non-traumatic brain injury

B17.2 Acute hepatitis E   CC
RIC Excl: 03 Non-traumatic brain injury

B17.8 Other specified acute viral hepatitis   CC
Hepatitis non-A non-B (acute) (viral) NEC
RIC Excl: 03 Non-traumatic brain injury

B17.9 Acute viral hepatitis, unspecified   ▽
Acute hepatitis NOS

✓4ᵗʰ **B18** Chronic **viral hepatitis**

B18.0 Chronic viral hepatitis B with delta-agent   CC
RIC Excl: 03 Non-traumatic brain injury

B18.1 Chronic viral hepatitis B without delta-agent   CC
Chronic (viral) hepatitis B
RIC Excl: 03 Non-traumatic brain injury

B18.2 Chronic viral hepatitis C   CC
RIC Excl: 03 Non-traumatic brain injury

B18.8 Other chronic viral hepatitis

B18.9 Chronic viral hepatitis, unspecified   ▽

✓4ᵗʰ **B19** Unspecified **viral hepatitis**

B19.0 Unspecified viral hepatitis with hepatic coma   CC ▽
RIC Excl: 03 Non-traumatic brain injury

✓5ᵗʰ **B19.1** Unspecified viral hepatitis B

  B19.10 Unspecified viral hepatitis B without hepatic coma   ▽
Unspecified viral hepatitis B NOS

  B19.11 Unspecified viral hepatitis B with hepatic coma   CC ▽
RIC Excl: 03 Non-traumatic brain injury

✓5ᵗʰ **B19.2** Unspecified viral hepatitis C

  B19.20 Unspecified viral hepatitis C without hepatic coma   ▽
Viral hepatitis C NOS

  B19.21 Unspecified viral hepatitis C with hepatic coma   CC ▽
RIC Excl: 03 Non-traumatic brain injury

B19.9 Unspecified viral hepatitis without hepatic coma   ▽
Viral hepatitis NOS

Human immunodeficiency virus [HIV] disease (B20)

B20 Human immunodeficiency virus [HIV] disease   CC NC Dx
INCLUDES   acquired immune deficiency syndrome [AIDS]
AIDS-related complex [ARC]
HIV infection, symptomatic
Code first human immunodeficiency virus [HIV] disease complicating pregnancy, childbirth and the puerperium, if applicable (O98.7-)
Use additional code(s) to identify all manifestations of HIV infection
EXCLUDES 1   asymptomatic human immunodeficiency virus [HIV] infection status (Z21)
exposure to HIV virus (Z20.6)
inconclusive serologic evidence of HIV (R75)

Other viral diseases (B25-B34)

✓4ᵗʰ **B25** Cytomegaloviral disease
EXCLUDES 1   congenital cytomegalovirus infection (P35.1)
cytomegaloviral mononucleosis (B27.1-)

B25.0 Cytomegaloviral pneumonitis   CC
RIC Excl: 15 Pulmonary

B25.1 Cytomegaloviral hepatitis

B25.2 Cytomegaloviral pancreatitis

B25.8 Other cytomegaloviral diseases
Cytomegaloviral encephalitis

B25.9 Cytomegaloviral disease, unspecified   ▽

✓4ᵗʰ **B26** Mumps
INCLUDES   epidemic parotitis
infectious parotitis

B26.0 Mumps orchitis   ♂

B26.1 Mumps meningitis   CC
RIC Excl: 03 Non-traumatic brain injury; 05 Non-traumatic spinal cord injury

B26.2 Mumps encephalitis   CC
RIC Excl: 03 Non-traumatic brain injury

B26.3 Mumps pancreatitis   CC

✓5ᵗʰ **B26.8** Mumps with other complications

  B26.81 Mumps hepatitis

  B26.82 Mumps myocarditis

  B26.83 Mumps nephritis

  B26.84 Mumps polyneuropathy

  B26.85 Mumps arthritis

  B26.89 Other mumps complications

B26.9 Mumps without complication   ▽
Mumps NOS
Mumps parotitis NOS

✓4ᵗʰ **B27** Infectious mononucleosis
INCLUDES   glandular fever
monocytic angina
Pfeiffer's disease

✓5ᵗʰ **B27.0** Gammaherpesviral mononucleosis
Mononucleosis due to Epstein-Barr virus

  B27.00 Gammaherpesviral mononucleosis without complication

  B27.01 Gammaherpesviral mononucleosis with polyneuropathy

  B27.02 Gammaherpesviral mononucleosis with meningitis

  B27.09 Gammaherpesviral mononucleosis with other complications
Hepatomegaly in gammaherpesviral mononucleosis

✓5ᵗʰ **B27.1** Cytomegaloviral mononucleosis

  B27.10 Cytomegaloviral mononucleosis without complications

  B27.11 Cytomegaloviral mononucleosis with polyneuropathy

  B27.12 Cytomegaloviral mononucleosis with meningitis

  B27.19 Cytomegaloviral mononucleosis with other complication
Hepatomegaly in cytomegaloviral mononucleosis

✓5ᵗʰ **B27.8** Other infectious mononucleosis

  B27.80 Other infectious mononucleosis without complication

  B27.81 Other infectious mononucleosis with polyneuropathy

  B27.82 Other infectious mononucleosis with meningitis

  B27.89 Other infectious mononucleosis with other complication
Hepatomegaly in other infectious mononucleosis

✓5ᵗʰ **B27.9** Infectious mononucleosis, unspecified

  B27.90 Infectious mononucleosis, unspecified without complication   ▽

  B27.91 Infectious mononucleosis, unspecified with polyneuropathy   ▽

  B27.92 Infectious mononucleosis, unspecified with meningitis   ▽

  B27.99 Infectious mononucleosis, unspecified with other complication   ▽
Hepatomegaly in unspecified infectious mononucleosis

✓4ᵗʰ **B30** Viral conjunctivitis
EXCLUDES 1   herpesviral [herpes simplex] ocular disease (B00.5)
ocular zoster (B02.3)

B30.0 Keratoconjunctivitis due to adenovirus
Epidemic keratoconjunctivitis
Shipyard eye

B30.1 Conjunctivitis due to adenovirus
Acute adenoviral follicular conjunctivitis
Swimming-pool conjunctivitis

B30.2 Viral pharyngoconjunctivitis

B30.3 Acute epidemic hemorrhagic conjunctivitis (enteroviral)
Conjunctivitis due to coxsackievirus 24
Conjunctivitis due to enterovirus 70
Hemorrhagic conjunctivitis (acute)(epidemic)

B30.8 Other viral conjunctivitis
Newcastle conjunctivitis

B30.9 Viral conjunctivitis, unspecified   ▽

Ⓝ Newborn   Ⓟ Pediatric   Ⓜ Maternity   Ⓐ Adult   RIC RIC Dx   NC Dx Noncancer Dx   PDx Primary Dx   CC RIC CC Condition   ►◄ Revised Text   ● New Code   ▲ Revised Code Title

438   ICD-10-CM 2016

✓4ᵗʰ B33 Other viral diseases, not elsewhere classified

    B33.0 Epidemic myalgia
        Bornholm disease

    B33.1 Ross River disease
        Epidemic polyarthritis and exanthema
        Ross River fever

    ✓5ᵗʰ B33.2 Viral carditis
        Coxsackie (virus) carditis

        B33.20 Viral carditis, unspecified   ▽
        B33.21 Viral endocarditis
        B33.22 Viral myocarditis
        B33.23 Viral pericarditis
        B33.24 Viral cardiomyopathy

    B33.3 Retrovirus infections, not elsewhere classified   CC
        Retrovirus infection NOS

    B33.4 Hantavirus (cardio)-pulmonary syndrome [HPS] [HCPS]
        Hantavirus disease with pulmonary manifestations
        Sin nombre virus disease
        Use additional code to identify any associated acute kidney
           failure (N17.9)
        EXCLUDES 1 *hantavirus disease with renal manifestations (A98.5)*
           hemorrhagic fever with renal manifestations (A98.5)

    B33.8 Other specified viral diseases
        EXCLUDES 1 *anogenital human papillomavirus infection (A63.0)*
           viral warts due to human papillomavirus infection
             (B07)

✓4ᵗʰ B34 Viral infection of unspecified site
    EXCLUDES 1 *anogenital human papillomavirus infection (A63.0)*
        cytomegaloviral disease NOS (B25.9)
        herpesvirus [herpes simplex] infection NOS (B00.9)
        retrovirus infection NOS (B33.3)
        viral agents as the cause of diseases classified elsewhere (B97.-)
        viral warts due to human papillomavirus infection (B07)

    B34.0 Adenovirus infection, unspecified

    B34.1 Enterovirus infection, unspecified
        Coxsackievirus infection NOS
        Echovirus infection NOS

    B34.2 Coronavirus infection, unspecified
        EXCLUDES 1 *pneumonia due to SARS-associated coronavirus*
             (J12.81)

    B34.3 Parvovirus infection, unspecified

    B34.4 Papovavirus infection, unspecified

    B34.8 Other viral infections of unspecified site

    B34.9 Viral infection, unspecified   ▽
        Viremia NOS

Mycoses (B35-B49)

EXCLUDES 2 *hypersensitivity pneumonitis due to organic dust (J67.-)*
       mycosis fungoides (C84.0-)

✓4ᵗʰ B35 Dermatophytosis
    INCLUDES favus
        infections due to species of Epidermophyton, Micro-sporum
          and Trichophyton
        tinea, any type except those in B36-

    B35.0 Tinea barbae and tinea capitis
        Beard ringworm   Scalp ringworm
        Kerion   Sycosis, mycotic

    B35.1 Tinea unguium
        Dermatophytic onychia   Onychomycosis
        Dermatophytosis of nail   Ringworm of nails

    B35.2 Tinea manuum
        Dermatophytosis of hand   Hand ringworm

    B35.3 Tinea pedis
        Athlete's foot
        Dermatophytosis of foot
        Foot ringworm

    B35.4 Tinea corporis
        Ringworm of the body

    B35.5 Tinea imbricata
        Tokelau

    B35.6 Tinea cruris
        Dhobi itch   Jock itch
        Groin ringworm

    B35.8 Other dermatophytoses
        Disseminated dermatophytosis
        Granulomatous dermatophytosis

    B35.9 Dermatophytosis, unspecified   ▽
        Ringworm NOS

✓4ᵗʰ B36 Other superficial mycoses

    B36.0 Pityriasis versicolor
        Tinea flava   Tinea versicolor

    B36.1 Tinea nigra
        Keratomycosis nigricans palmaris
        Microsporosis nigra
        Pityriasis nigra

    B36.2 White piedra
        Tinea blanca

    B36.3 Black piedra

    B36.8 Other specified superficial mycoses

    B36.9 Superficial mycosis, unspecified   ▽

✓4ᵗʰ B37 Candidiasis
    INCLUDES candidosis
        moniliasis
    EXCLUDES 1 *neonatal candidiasis (P37.5)*

    B37.0 Candidal stomatitis
        Oral thrush

    2,8 B37.1 Pulmonary candidiasis   CC
        Candidal bronchitis   Candidal pneumonia
        RIC Excl: 15 Pulmonary

    B37.2 Candidiasis of skin and nail
        Candidal onychia   Candidal paronychia
        EXCLUDES 2 *diaper dermatitis (L22)*

    B37.3 Candidiasis of vulva and vagina   ♀
        Candidal vulvovaginitis   Vaginal thrush
        Monilial vulvovaginitis

    ✓5ᵗʰ B37.4 Candidiasis of other urogenital sites
        B37.41 Candidal cystitis and urethritis
        B37.42 Candidal balanitis
        B37.49 Other urogenital candidiasis
           Candidal pyelonephritis

    B37.5 Candidal meningitis   CC
        RIC Excl: 03 Non-traumatic brain injury; 05 Non-traumatic spinal
          cord injury

    B37.6 Candidal endocarditis   CC
        RIC Excl: 14 Cardiac

    B37.7 Candidal sepsis   CC
        Disseminated candidiasis   Systemic candidiasis
        AHA: 2014, 4Q, 46

    ✓5ᵗʰ B37.8 Candidiasis of other sites
        B37.81 Candidal esophagitis   CC
        B37.82 Candidal enteritis
           Candidal proctitis
        B37.83 Candidal cheilitis
        B37.84 Candidal otitis externa
        B37.89 Other sites of candidiasis
           Candidal osteomyelitis

    B37.9 Candidiasis, unspecified   ▽
        Thrush NOS

✓4ᵗʰ B38 Coccidioidomycosis

    B38.0 Acute pulmonary coccidioidomycosis

    B38.1 Chronic pulmonary coccidioidomycosis

    B38.2 Pulmonary coccidioidomycosis, unspecified

    B38.3 Cutaneous coccidioidomycosis

    B38.4 Coccidioidomycosis meningitis   CC
        RIC Excl: 03 Non-traumatic brain injury; 05 Non-traumatic spinal
          cord injury

    B38.7 Disseminated coccidioidomycosis
        Generalized coccidioidomycosis

    ✓5ᵗʰ B38.8 Other forms of coccidioidomycosis
        B38.81 Prostatic coccidioidomycosis   ♂
        B38.89 Other forms of coccidioidomycosis

    B38.9 Coccidioidomycosis, unspecified   ▽

---

[2] Special Care High = With fever

[0] Clinically Complex = Without fever

✔ Add'l Character Required   ✔x7ᵗʰ Placeholder Alert   RUG IV Special Care High Dx   RUG IV Clinically Complex Dx   RUG IV Special Care Low Dx   Manifestation Code   Other Specified Code   ▽ Unspecified Code

✓4ᵗʰ **B39** **Histoplasmosis**
Code first associated AIDS (B20)
Use additional code for any associated manifestations, such as:
endocarditis (I39)
meningitis (G02)
pericarditis (I32)
retinitits (H32)

B39.0 **Acute pulmonary histoplasmosis capsulati** `CC`
RIC Excl: 15 Pulmonary

B39.1 **Chronic pulmonary histoplasmosis capsulati** `CC`
RIC Excl: 15 Pulmonary

B39.2 **Pulmonary histoplasmosis capsulati, unspecified** `CC`
RIC Excl: 15 Pulmonary

B39.3 **Disseminated histoplasmosis capsulati** `CC`
Generalized histoplasmosis capsulati
RIC Excl: 15 Pulmonary

B39.4 **Histoplasmosis capsulati, unspecified** `CC`
American histoplasmosis
RIC Excl: 15 Pulmonary

B39.5 **Histoplasmosis duboisii** `CC`
African histoplasmosis

B39.9 **Histoplasmosis, unspecified** `CC` ▽
RIC Excl: 15 Pulmonary

✓4ᵗʰ **B40** **Blastomycosis**
EXCLUDES 1 Brazilian blastomycosis (B41.-)
keloidal blastomycosis (B48.0)

B40.0 **Acute pulmonary blastomycosis**

B40.1 **Chronic pulmonary blastomycosis**

B40.2 **Pulmonary blastomycosis, unspecified**

B40.3 **Cutaneous blastomycosis**

B40.7 **Disseminated blastomycosis**
Generalized blastomycosis

✓5ᵗʰ **B40.8** **Other forms of blastomycosis**

B40.81 **Blastomycotic meningoencephalitis**
Meningomyelitis due to blastomycosis

B40.89 **Other forms of blastomycosis**

B40.9 **Blastomycosis, unspecified** ▽

✓4ᵗʰ **B41** **Paracoccidioidomycosis**
INCLUDES Brazilian blastomycosis
Lutz' disease

B41.0 **Pulmonary paracoccidioidomycosis**

B41.7 **Disseminated paracoccidioidomycosis**
Generalized paracoccidioidomycosis

B41.8 **Other forms of paracoccidioidomycosis**

B41.9 **Paracoccidioidomycosis, unspecified** ▽

✓4ᵗʰ **B42** **Sporotrichosis**

B42.0 **Pulmonary sporotrichosis**

B42.1 **Lymphocutaneous sporotrichosis**

B42.7 **Disseminated sporotrichosis**
Generalized sporotrichosis

✓5ᵗʰ **B42.8** **Other forms of sporotrichosis**

B42.81 **Cerebral sporotrichosis**
Meningitis due to sporotrichosis

B42.82 **Sporotrichosis arthritis**

B42.89 **Other forms of sporotrichosis**

B42.9 **Sporotrichosis, unspecified** ▽

✓4ᵗʰ **B43** **Chromomycosis and pheomycotic abscess**

B43.0 **Cutaneous chromomycosis**
Dermatitis verrucosa

B43.1 **Pheomycotic brain abscess**
Cerebral chromomycosis

B43.2 **Subcutaneous pheomycotic abscess and cyst**

B43.8 **Other forms of chromomycosis**

B43.9 **Chromomycosis, unspecified** ▽

✓4ᵗʰ **B44** **Aspergillosis**
INCLUDES aspergilloma

B44.0 **Invasive pulmonary aspergillosis** `CC`
RIC Excl: 15 Pulmonary

B44.1 **Other pulmonary aspergillosis**

B44.2 **Tonsillar aspergillosis**

B44.7 **Disseminated aspergillosis**
Generalized aspergillosis

✓5ᵗʰ **B44.8** **Other forms of aspergillosis**

B44.81 **Allergic bronchopulmonary aspergillosis**

B44.89 **Other forms of aspergillosis**

B44.9 **Aspergillosis, unspecified** ▽

✓4ᵗʰ **B45** **Cryptococcosis**

B45.0 **Pulmonary cryptococcosis**

B45.1 **Cerebral cryptococcosis** `CC`
Cryptococcal meningitis
Cryptococcosis meningocerebralis
RIC Excl: 03 Non-traumatic brain injury; 05 Non-traumatic spinal cord injury

B45.2 **Cutaneous cryptococcosis**

B45.3 **Osseous cryptococcosis**

B45.7 **Disseminated cryptococcosis**
Generalized cryptococcosis

B45.8 **Other forms of cryptococcosis**

B45.9 **Cryptococcosis, unspecified** ▽

✓4ᵗʰ **B46** **Zygomycosis**

B46.0 **Pulmonary mucormycosis**

B46.1 **Rhinocerebral mucormycosis**

B46.2 **Gastrointestinal mucormycosis**

B46.3 **Cutaneous mucormycosis**
Subcutaneous mucormycosis

B46.4 **Disseminated mucormycosis**
Generalized mucormycosis

B46.5 **Mucormycosis, unspecified**

B46.8 **Other zygomycoses**
Entomophthoromycosis

B46.9 **Zygomycosis, unspecified** ▽
Phycomycosis NOS

✓4ᵗʰ **B47** **Mycetoma**

B47.0 **Eumycetoma**
Madura foot, mycotic   Maduromycosis

B47.1 **Actinomycetoma**

B47.9 **Mycetoma, unspecified** ▽
Madura foot NOS

✓4ᵗʰ **B48** **Other mycoses, not elsewhere classified**

B48.0 **Lobomycosis**
Keloidal blastomycosis   Lobo's disease

B48.1 **Rhinosporidiosis**

B48.2 **Allescheriasis**
Infection due to Pseudallescheria boydii
EXCLUDES 1 eumycetoma (B47.0)

B48.3 **Geotrichosis**
Geotrichum stomatitis

B48.4 **Penicillosis**

B48.8 **Other specified mycoses**
Adiaspiromycosis
Infection of tissue and organs by Alternaria
Infection of tissue and organs by Drechslera
Infection of tissue and organs by Fusarium
Infection of tissue and organs by saprophytic fungi NEC
AHA: 2014, 4Q, 46; 2014, 2Q, 13

B49 **Unspecified mycosis** ▽
Fungemia NOS

Protozoal diseases (B50-B64)

EXCLUDES 1 amebiasis (A06.-)
other protozoal intestinal diseases (A07.-)

✓4ᵗʰ **B50** **Plasmodium falciparum malaria**
INCLUDES mixed infections of Plasmodium falciparum with any other Plasmodium species

B50.0 **Plasmodium falciparum malaria with cerebral complications**
Cerebral malaria NOS

B50.8 **Other severe and complicated Plasmodium falciparum malaria**
Severe or complicated Plasmodium falciparum malaria NOS

B50.9 **Plasmodium falciparum malaria, unspecified** ▽

✓4ᵗʰ **B51** **Plasmodium vivax malaria**
INCLUDES mixed infections of Plasmodium vivax with other Plasmodium species, except Plasmodium falciparum
EXCLUDES 1 plasmodium vivax with Plasmodium falciparum (B50.-)

B51.0 **Plasmodium vivax malaria with rupture of spleen**

B51.8 **Plasmodium vivax malaria with other complications**

B51.9 **Plasmodium vivax malaria without complication**
Plasmodium vivax malaria NOS

Ⓝ Newborn | Ⓟ Pediatric | Ⓜ Maternity | Ⓐ Adult | **RIC** RIC Dx | **NCDx** Noncancer Dx | **PDx** Primary Dx | **CC** RIC CC Condition | ▶◀ Revised Text | ● New Code | ▲ Revised Code Title

440

ICD-10-CM 2016

Chapter 1. Certain Infectious and Parasitic Diseases

☑4ᵗʰ **B52 Plasmodium** malariae **malaria**
     INCLUDES   mixed infections of Plasmodium malariae with other Plasmodium species, except Plasmodium falciparum and Plasmodium vivax
     EXCLUDES 1   Plasmodium falciparum (B50.-)
                  Plasmodium vivax (B51.-)

     B52.0 Plasmodium malariae **malaria with** nephropathy

     B52.8 Plasmodium malariae **malaria with** other complications

     B52.9 Plasmodium malariae **malaria** without complication
         Plasmodium malariae malaria NOS

☑4ᵗʰ **B53** Other specified **malaria**

     B53.0 Plasmodium ovale **malaria**
         EXCLUDES 1   Plasmodium ovale with Plasmodium falciparum (B50.-)
                  Plasmodium ovale with Plasmodium malariae (B52.-)
                  Plasmodium ovale with Plasmodium vivax (B51.-)

     B53.1 Malaria due to simian plasmodia
         EXCLUDES 1   Malaria due to simian plasmodia with Plasmodium falciparum (B50.-)
                  Malaria due to simian plasmodia with Plasmodium malariae (B52.-)
                  Malaria due to simian plasmodia with Plasmodium ovale (B53.0)
                  Malaria due to simian plasmodia with Plasmodium vivax (B51.-)

     B53.8 Other malaria, not elsewhere classified

     B54 Unspecified malaria   ▽

☑4ᵗʰ **B55 Leishmaniasis**

     B55.0 Visceral **leishmaniasis**
         Kala-azar
         Post-kala-azar dermal leishmaniasis

     B55.1 Cutaneous **leishmaniasis**

     B55.2 Mucocutaneous **leishmaniasis**

     B55.9 Leishmaniasis, unspecified   ▽

☑4ᵗʰ **B56 African trypanosomiasis**

     B56.0 Gambiense **trypanosomiasis**
         Infection due to Trypanosoma brucei gambiense
         West African sleeping sickness

     B56.1 Rhodesiense **trypanosomiasis**
         East African sleeping sickness
         Infection due to Trypanosoma brucei rhodesiense

     B56.9 African **trypanosomiasis, unspecified**   ▽
         Sleeping sickness NOS

☑4ᵗʰ **B57 Chagas' disease**
     INCLUDES   American trypanosomiasis
                infection due to Trypanosoma cruzi

     B57.0 Acute **Chagas' disease with heart** involvement
         Acute Chagas' disease with myocarditis

     B57.1 Acute **Chagas' disease without heart** involvement
         Acute Chagas' disease NOS

     B57.2 Chagas' disease (chronic) **with heart** involvement
         American trypanosomiasis NOS
         Chagas' disease (chronic) NOS
         Chagas' disease (chronic) with myocarditis
         Trypanosomiasis NOS

☑5ᵗʰ **B57.3 Chagas' disease** (chronic) **with** digestive system **involvement**
         B57.30 Chagas' disease with digestive system involvement, unspecified   ▽
         B57.31 Megaesophagus **in Chagas' disease**
         B57.32 Megacolon **in Chagas' disease**
         B57.39 Other digestive system involvement in Chagas' disease

☑5ᵗʰ **B57.4 Chagas' disease** (chronic) **with** nervous system **involvement**
         B57.40 Chagas' disease with nervous system involvement, unspecified   ▽
         B57.41 Meningitis **in Chagas' disease**
         B57.42 Meningoencephalitis **in Chagas' disease**
         B57.49 Other nervous system involvement in Chagas' disease

     B57.5 Chagas' disease (chronic) **with other organ involvement**

☑4ᵗʰ **B58 Toxoplasmosis**
     INCLUDES   infection due to Toxoplasma gondii
     EXCLUDES 1   congenital toxoplasmosis (P37.1)

☑5ᵗʰ **B58.0 Toxoplasma** oculopathy
         B58.00 Toxoplasma oculopathy, unspecified   ▽
         B58.01 Toxoplasma chorioretinitis
         B58.09 Other toxoplasma oculopathy
                Toxoplasma uveitis

     B58.1 Toxoplasma hepatitis

     B58.2 Toxoplasma meningoencephalitis   cc
         RIC Excl: 03 Non-traumatic brain injury; 05 Non-traumatic spinal cord injury

     B58.3 Pulmonary **toxoplasmosis**   cc
         RIC Excl: 15 Pulmonary

☑5ᵗʰ **B58.8 Toxoplasmosis with** other organ involvement
         B58.81 Toxoplasma myocarditis   cc
                RIC Excl: 14 Cardiac
         B58.82 Toxoplasma myositis
         B58.83 Toxoplasma tubulo-interstitial nephropathy
                Toxoplasma pyelonephritis
         B58.89 Toxoplasmosis with other organ involvement

     B58.9 Toxoplasmosis, unspecified   ▽

2,8 **B59 Pneumocystosis**   cc
         Pneumonia due to Pneumocystis carinii
         Pneumonia due to Pneumocystis jiroveci
         RIC Excl: 15 Pulmonary

☑4ᵗʰ **B60** Other protozoal diseases, not elsewhere classified
     EXCLUDES 1   cryptosporidiosis (A07.2)
                intestinal microsporidiosis (A07.8)
                isosporiasis (A07.3)

     B60.0 Babesiosis
         Piroplasmosis

☑5ᵗʰ **B60.1** Acanthamebiasis
         B60.10 Acanthamebiasis, unspecified   ▽
         B60.11 Meningoencephalitis **due to Acanthamoeba (culbertsoni)**
         B60.12 Conjunctivitis **due to Acanthamoeba**
         B60.13 Keratoconjunctivitis **due to Acanthamoeba**
         B60.19 Other acanthamebic disease

     B60.2 Naegleriasis
         Primary amebic meningoencephalitis

     B60.8 Other specified protozoal diseases
         Microsporidiosis

     B64 Unspecified protozoal disease   ▽

Helminthiases (B65-B83)

☑4ᵗʰ **B65 Schistosomiasis [bilharziasis]**
     INCLUDES   snail fever

     B65.0 Schistosomiasis due to Schistosoma haematobium [urinary schistosomiasis]

     B65.1 Schistosomiasis due to Schistosoma mansoni [intestinal schistosomiasis]

     B65.2 Schistosomiasis due to Schistosoma japonicum
         Asiatic schistosomiasis

     B65.3 Cercarial dermatitis
         Swimmer's itch

     B65.8 Other schistosomiasis
         Infection due to Schistosoma intercalatum
         Infection due to Schistosoma mattheei
         Infection due to Schistosoma mekongi

     B65.9 Schistosomiasis, unspecified   ▽

☑4ᵗʰ **B66 Other fluke infections**
     B66.0 Opisthorchiasis
         Infection due to cat liver fluke
         Infection due to Opisthorchis (felineus)(viverrini)

     B66.1 Clonorchiasis
         Chinese liver fluke disease
         Infection due to Clonorchis sinensis
         Oriental liver fluke disease

     B66.2 Dicroceliasis
         Infection due to Dicrocoelium dendriticum
         Lancet fluke infection

---

2 Special Care High = With fever
8 Clinically Complex = Without fever

☑ Add'l Character Required   ☑✔7ᵗʰ Placeholder Alert   **RUG IV Special Care High Dx**   RUG IV Clinically Complex Dx   RUG IV Special Care Low Dx   Manifestation Code   Other Specified Code   ▽ Unspecified Code

B66.3 Fascioliasis
Infection due to Fasciola gigantica
Infection due to Fasciola hepatica
Infection due to Fasciola indica
Sheep liver fluke disease

B66.4 Paragonimiasis
Infection due to Paragonimus species
Lung fluke disease
Pulmonary distomiasis

B66.5 Fasciolopsiasis
Infection due to Fasciolopsis buski
Intestinal distomiasis

B66.8 Other specified fluke infections
Echinostomiasis
Heterophyiasis
Metagonimiasis
Nanophyetiasis
Watsoniasis

B66.9 Fluke infection, unspecified ▽

✓4ᵗʰ **B67 Echinococcosis**
INCLUDES hydatidosis

B67.0 Echinococcus granulosus infection of liver

B67.1 Echinococcus granulosus infection of lung

B67.2 Echinococcus granulosus infection of bone

✓5ᵗʰ **B67.3 Echinococcus granulosus infection, other and multiple sites**

B67.31 Echinococcus granulosus infection, thyroid gland

B67.32 Echinococcus granulosus infection, multiple sites

B67.39 Echinococcus granulosus infection, other sites

B67.4 Echinococcus granulosus infection, unspecified ▽
Dog tapeworm (infection)

B67.5 Echinococcus multilocularis **infection of** liver

✓5ᵗʰ **B67.6 Echinococcus** multilocularis **infection, other and multiple sites**

B67.61 Echinococcus multilocularis infection, multiple sites

B67.69 Echinococcus multilocularis infection, other sites

B67.7 Echinococcus multilocularis **infection,** unspecified

B67.8 Echinococcosis, unspecified, **of** liver

✓5ᵗʰ **B67.9 Echinococcosis, other and unspecified**

B67.90 Echinococcosis, unspecified ▽
Echinococcosis NOS

B67.99 Other echinococcosis

✓4ᵗʰ **B68 Taeniasis**
EXCLUDES 1 cysticercosis (B69.-)

B68.0 Taenia solium **taeniasis**
Pork tapeworm (infection)

B68.1 Taenia saginata **taeniasis**
Beef tapeworm (infection)
Infection due to adult tapeworm Taenia saginata

B68.9 Taeniasis, unspecified ▽

✓4ᵗʰ **B69 Cysticercosis**
INCLUDES cysticerciasis infection due to larval form of Taenia solium

B69.0 Cysticercosis of central nervous system

B69.1 Cysticercosis of eye

✓5ᵗʰ **B69.8 Cysticercosis of** other sites

B69.81 Myositis in cysticercosis

B69.89 Cysticercosis of other sites

B69.9 Cysticercosis, unspecified ▽

✓4ᵗʰ **B70 Diphyllobothriasis and sparganosis**

B70.0 Diphyllobothriasis
Diphyllobothrium (adult) (latum) (pacificum) infection
Fish tapeworm (infection)
EXCLUDES 2 larval diphyllobothriasis (B70.1)

B70.1 Sparganosis
Infection due to Sparganum (mansoni) (proliferum)
Infection due to Spirometra larva
Larval diphyllobothriasis
Spirometrosis

✓4ᵗʰ **B71 Other cestode infections**

B71.0 Hymenolepiasis
Dwarf tapeworm infection   Rat tapeworm (infection)

B71.1 Dipylidiasis

B71.8 Other specified cestode infections
Coenurosis

B71.9 Cestode infection, unspecified ▽
Tapeworm (infection) NOS

B72 Dracunculiasis
INCLUDES guinea worm infection
infection due to Dracunculus medinensis

✓4ᵗʰ **B73 Onchocerciasis**
INCLUDES onchocerca volvulus infection
onchocercosis
river blindness

✓5ᵗʰ **B73.0 Onchocerciasis** with eye disease

B73.00 Onchocerciasis with eye involvement, unspecified ▽

B73.01 Onchocerciasis with endophthalmitis

B73.02 Onchocerciasis with glaucoma

B73.09 Onchocerciasis with other eye involvement
Infestation of eyelid due to onchocerciasis

B73.1 Onchocerciasis without eye disease

✓4ᵗʰ **B74 Filariasis**
EXCLUDES 2 onchocerciasis (B73)
tropical (pulmonary) eosinophilia NOS (J82)

B74.0 Filariasis due to Wuchereria bancrofti
Bancroftian elephantiasis   Bancroftian filariasis

B74.1 Filariasis due to Brugia malayi

B74.2 Filariasis due to Brugia timori

B74.3 Loiasis
Calabar swelling
Eyeworm disease of Africa
Loa loa infection

B74.4 Mansonelliasis
Infection due to Mansonella ozzardi
Infection due to Mansonella perstans
Infection due to Mansonella streptocerca

B74.8 Other filariases
Dirofilariasis

B74.9 Filariasis, unspecified ▽

B75 Trichinellosis
INCLUDES infection due to Trichinella species
trichiniasis

✓4ᵗʰ **B76 Hookworm diseases**
INCLUDES uncinariasis

B76.0 Ancylostomiasis
Infection due to Ancylostoma species

B76.1 Necatoriasis
Infection due to Necator americanus

B76.8 Other hookworm diseases

B76.9 Hookworm disease, unspecified ▽
Cutaneous larva migrans NOS

✓4ᵗʰ **B77 Ascariasis**
INCLUDES ascaridiasis
roundworm infection

B77.0 Ascariasis with intestinal complications

✓5ᵗʰ **B77.8 Ascariasis with** other complications

2,8 **B77.81 Ascariasis** pneumonia   CC
RIC Excl: 15 Pulmonary

B77.89 Ascariasis with other complications

B77.9 Ascariasis, unspecified ▽

✓4ᵗʰ **B78 Strongyloidiasis**
EXCLUDES 1 trichostrongyliasis (B81.2)

B78.0 Intestinal strongyloidiasis

B78.1 Cutaneous strongyloidiasis

B78.7 Disseminated strongyloidiasis

B78.9 Strongyloidiasis, unspecified ▽

B79 Trichuriasis
INCLUDES trichocephaliasis
whipworm (disease)(infection)

B80 Enterobiasis
INCLUDES oxyuriasis
pinworm infection
threadworm infection

---

2 Special Care High = With fever

8 Clinically Complex = Without fever

N Newborn   P Pediatric   M Maternity   A Adult   RIC RIC Dx   NC Dx Noncancer Dx   PDx Primary Dx   CC RIC CC Condition   ►◄ Revised Text   ● New Code   ▲ Revised Code Title

442

ICD-10-CM 2016

✓4th **B81** **Other intestinal helminthiases, not elsewhere classified**
    EXCLUDES 1   *angiostrongyliasis due to Parastrongylus cantonensis (B83.2)*

   B81.0 **Anisakiasis**
     Infection due to Anisakis larva

   B81.1 **Intestinal capillariasis**
     Capillariasis NOS
     Infection due to Capillaria philippinensis
     EXCLUDES 2   *hepatic capillariasis (B83.8)*

   B81.2 **Trichostrongyliasis**

   B81.3 **Intestinal angiostrongyliasis**
     Angiostrongyliasis due to Parastrongylus costaricensis

   B81.4 **Mixed intestinal helminthiases**
     Infection due to intestinal helminths classified to more than one
       of the categories B65.0-B81.3 and B81.8
     Mixed helminthiasis NOS

   B81.8 **Other specified intestinal helminthiases**
     Infection due to Oesophagostomum species
       [esophagostomiasis]
     Infection due to Ternidens diminutus [ternidensiasis]

✓4th **B82** **Unspecified intestinal parasitism**

   B82.0 **Intestinal** helminthiasis, **unspecified** ▽

   B82.9 **Intestinal** parasitism, **unspecified** ▽

✓4th **B83** **Other helminthiases**
    EXCLUDES 1   *capillariasis NOS (B81.1)*
    EXCLUDES 2   *intestinal capillariasis (B81.1)*

   B83.0 **Visceral larva migrans**
     Toxocariasis

   B83.1 **Gnathostomiasis**
     Wandering swelling

   B83.2 **Angiostrongyliasis due to Parastrongylus cantonensis**
     Eosinophilic meningoencephalitis due to Parastrongylus
       cantonensis
     EXCLUDES 2   *intestinal angiostrongyliasis (B81.3)*

   B83.3 **Syngamiasis**
     Syngamosis

   B83.4 **Internal hirudiniasis**
     EXCLUDES 2   *external hirudiniasis (B88.3)*

   B83.8 **Other specified helminthiases**
     Acanthocephaliasis   Metastrongyliasis
     Gongylonemiasis   Thelaziasis
     Hepatic capillariasis

   B83.9 **Helminthiasis, unspecified** ▽
     Worms NOS
     EXCLUDES 1   *intestinal helminthiasis NOS (B82.0)*

Pediculosis, acariasis and other infestations (B85-B89)

✓4th **B85** **Pediculosis and phthiriasis**

   B85.0 **Pediculosis due to** Pediculus humanus capitis
     Head-louse infestation

   B85.1 **Pediculosis due to** Pediculus humanus corporis
     Body-louse infestation

   B85.2 **Pediculosis, unspecified** ▽

   B85.3 **Phthiriasis**
     Infestation by crab-louse
     Infestation by Phthirus pubis

   B85.4 **Mixed pediculosis and phthiriasis**
     Infestation classifiable to more than one of the categories B85.0-
       B85.3

   B86 **Scabies**
     Sarcoptic itch

✓4th **B87** **Myiasis**
    INCLUDES   infestation by larva of flies

   B87.0 **Cutaneous myiasis**
     Creeping myiasis

   B87.1 **Wound myiasis**
     Traumatic myiasis

   B87.2 **Ocular myiasis**

   B87.3 **Nasopharyngeal myiasis**
     Laryngeal myiasis

   B87.4 **Aural myiasis**

   ✓5th **B87.8** **Myiasis of** other sites

     B87.81 **Genitourinary myiasis**

     B87.82 **Intestinal myiasis**

     B87.89 **Myiasis of other sites**

   B87.9 **Myiasis, unspecified** ▽

✓4th **B88** **Other infestations**

   B88.0 **Other acariasis**
     Acarine dermatitis
     Dermatitis due to Demodex species
     Dermatitis due to Dermanyssus gallinae
     Dermatitis due to Liponyssoides sanguineus
     Trombiculosis
     EXCLUDES 2   *scabies (B86)*

   B88.1 **Tungiasis [sandflea infestation]**

   B88.2 **Other arthropod infestations**
     Scarabiasis

   B88.3 **External hirudiniasis**
     Leech infestation NOS
     EXCLUDES 2   *internal hirudiniasis (B83.4)*

   B88.8 **Other specified infestations**
     Ichthyoparasitism due to Vandellia cirrhosa
     Linguatulosis
     Porocephaliasis

   B88.9 **Infestation, unspecified** ▽
     Infestation (skin) NOS
     Infestation by mites NOS
     Skin parasites NOS

   B89 **Unspecified parasitic disease** ▽

Sequelae of infectious and parasitic diseases (B90-B94)

    NOTE   Categories B90-B94 are to be used to indicate conditions in
     categories A00-B89 as the cause of sequelae, which are themselves
     classified elsewhere. The "sequelae" include conditions specified as
     such; they also include residuals of diseases classifiable to the above
     categories if there is evidence that the disease itself is no longer
     present. Codes from these categories are not to be used for chronic
     infections. Code chronic current infections to active infectious
     disease as appropriate.

    Code first condition resulting from (sequela) the infectious or parasitic disease

✓4th **B90** **Sequelae of** tuberculosis

   B90.0 **Sequelae of** central nervous system **tuberculosis**

   B90.1 **Sequelae of** genitourinary **tuberculosis**

   B90.2 **Sequelae of tuberculosis of** bones and joints

   B90.8 **Sequelae of tuberculosis of other organs**
     EXCLUDES 2   *sequelae of respiratory tuberculosis (B90.9)*

   B90.9 **Sequelae of** respiratory **and unspecified tuberculosis** ▽
     Sequelae of tuberculosis NOS

   B91 **Sequelae of** poliomyelitis
     EXCLUDES 1   *postpolio syndrome (G14)*

   B92 **Sequelae of** leprosy

✓4th **B94** **Sequelae of** other and unspecified **infectious and parasitic diseases**

   B94.0 **Sequelae of** trachoma

   B94.1 **Sequelae of** viral encephalitis   CC
     RIC Excl: 03 Non-traumatic brain injury

   B94.2 **Sequelae of** viral hepatitis

   B94.8 **Sequelae of other specified infectious and parasitic diseases**

   B94.9 **Sequelae of unspecified infectious and parasitic disease** ▽

Bacterial and viral infectious agents (B95-B97)

    NOTE   These categories are provided for use as supplementary or
     additional codes to identify the infectious agent(s) in diseases
     classified elsewhere.

✓4th **B95** **Streptococcus, Staphylococcus, and Enterococcus as the cause of diseases classified elsewhere**

   B95.0 **Streptococcus, group A, as the cause of diseases classified elsewhere**

   B95.1 **Streptococcus, group B, as the cause of diseases classified elsewhere**

   B95.2 **Enterococcus as the cause of diseases classified elsewhere**

   B95.3 **Streptococcus pneumoniae as the cause of diseases classified elsewhere**

   B95.4 **Other streptococcus as the cause of diseases classified elsewhere**

   B95.5 **Unspecified streptococcus as the cause of diseases classified elsewhere** ▽

✔ Add'l Character Required   ✔x7th Placeholder Alert   RUG IV Special Care High Dx   RUG IV Clinically Complex Dx   RUG IV Special Care Low Dx   Manifestation Code   Other Specified Code   ▽ Unspecified Code

ICD-10-CM 2016   443

Chapter 1. Certain Infectious and Parasitic Diseases

✓5ᵗʰ **B95.6** Staphylococcus aureus **as the cause of diseases classified elsewhere**

     B95.61 Methicillin susceptible **Staphylococcus aureus infection as the cause of diseases classified elsewhere**

        Methicillin susceptible Staphylococcus aureus (MSSA) infection as the cause of diseases classified elsewhere

        Staphylococcus aureus infection NOS as the cause of diseases classified elsewhere

     B95.62 Methicillin resistant **Staphylococcus aureus infection as the cause of diseases classified elsewhere**

        Methicillin resistant Staphylococcus aureus (MRSA) infection as the cause of diseases classified elsewhere

B95.7 **Other staphylococcus as the cause of diseases classified elsewhere**

B95.8 **Unspecified staphylococcus as the cause of diseases classified elsewhere** ▽

✓4ᵗʰ **B96** **Other bacterial agents as the cause of diseases classified elsewhere**

B96.0 Mycoplasma pneumoniae [M. pneumoniae] **as the cause of diseases classified elsewhere**

     Pleuro-pneumonia-like-organism [PPLO]

B96.1 Klebsiella pneumoniae [K. pneumoniae] **as the cause of diseases classified elsewhere**

✓5ᵗʰ **B96.2** Escherichia coli [E. coli] **as the cause of diseases classified elsewhere**

     B96.20 **Unspecified Escherichia coli [E. coli] as the cause of diseases classified elsewhere** ▽

        Escherichia coli [E. coli] NOS

     B96.21 Shiga toxin-producing **Escherichia coli [E. coli] (STEC) O157 as the cause of diseases classified elsewhere**

        E. coli O157:H- (nonmotile) with confirmation of Shiga toxin

        E. coli O157 with confirmation of Shiga toxin when H antigen is unknown, or is not H7

        O157:H7 Escherichia coli [E.coli] with or without confirmation of Shiga toxin-production

        Shiga toxin-producing Escherichia coli [E.coli] O157:H7 with or without confirmation of Shiga toxin-production

        STEC O157:H7 with or without confirmation of Shiga toxin-production

     B96.22 Other specified Shiga toxin-producing **Escherichia coli [E. coli] (STEC) as the cause of diseases classified elsewhere**

        Non-O157 Shiga toxin-producing Escherichia coli [E.coli]

        Non-O157 Shiga toxin-producing Escherichia coli [E.coli] with known O group

     B96.23 Unspecified Shiga toxin-producing **Escherichia coli [E. coli] (STEC) as the cause of diseases classified elsewhere** ▽

        Shiga toxin-producing Escherichia coli [E. coli] with unspecified O group

        STEC NOS

     B96.29 **Other Escherichia coli [E. coli] as the cause of diseases classified elsewhere**

        Non-Shiga toxin-producing E. coli

B96.3 Hemophilus influenzae [H. influenzae] **as the cause of diseases classified elsewhere**

B96.4 Proteus (mirabilis) (morganii) **as the cause of diseases classified elsewhere**

B96.5 Pseudomonas (aeruginosa) (mallei) (pseudomallei) **as the cause of diseases classified elsewhere** CC

     AHA: 2015, 1Q, 18

B96.6 Bacteroides fragilis [B. fragilis] **as the cause of diseases classified elsewhere**

B96.7 Clostridium perfringens [C. perfringens] **as the cause of diseases classified elsewhere**

✓5ᵗʰ **B96.8** **Other specified bacterial agents as the cause of diseases classified elsewhere**

     B96.81 Helicobacter pylori [H. pylori] **as the cause of diseases classified elsewhere**

     B96.82 Vibrio vulnificus **as the cause of diseases classified elsewhere**

     B96.89 **Other specified bacterial agents as the cause of diseases classified elsewhere**

✓4ᵗʰ **B97** **Viral agents as the cause of diseases classified elsewhere**

B97.0 Adenovirus **as the cause of diseases classified elsewhere**

✓5ᵗʰ **B97.1** Enterovirus **as the cause of diseases classified elsewhere**

     B97.10 **Unspecified enterovirus as the cause of diseases classified elsewhere** ▽

     B97.11 Coxsackievirus **as the cause of diseases classified elsewhere**

     B97.12 Echovirus **as the cause of diseases classified elsewhere**

     B97.19 **Other enterovirus as the cause of diseases classified elsewhere**

✓5ᵗʰ **B97.2** Coronavirus **as the cause of diseases classified elsewhere**

     B97.21 SARS-associated **coronavirus as the cause of diseases classified elsewhere**

        EXCLUDES 1 pneumonia due to SARS-associated coronavirus (J12.81)

     B97.29 **Other coronavirus as the cause of diseases classified elsewhere**

✓5ᵗʰ **B97.3** Retrovirus **as the cause of diseases classified elsewhere**

     EXCLUDES 1 human immunodeficiency virus [HIV} disease (B20)

     B97.30 **Unspecified retrovirus as the cause of diseases classified elsewhere** CC ▽

     B97.31 Lentivirus **as the cause of diseases classified elsewhere** CC

     B97.32 Oncovirus **as the cause of diseases classified elsewhere** CC

     B97.33 Human T-cell lymphotrophic virus, type I [HTLV-I] **as the cause of diseases classified elsewhere** CC

        RIC Excl: 06 Neurological

     B97.34 Human T-cell lymphotrophic virus, type II [HTLV-II] **as the cause of diseases classified elsewhere** CC

        RIC Excl: 06 Neurological

     B97.35 Human immunodeficiency virus, type 2 [HIV 2] **as the cause of diseases classified elsewhere** CC

     B97.39 **Other retrovirus as the cause of diseases classified elsewhere** CC

B97.4 Respiratory syncytial **virus as the cause of diseases classified elsewhere**

B97.5 Reovirus **as the cause of diseases classified elsewhere**

B97.6 Parvovirus **as the cause of diseases classified elsewhere**

B97.7 Papillomavirus **as the cause of diseases classified elsewhere**

✓5ᵗʰ **B97.8** Other **viral agents as the cause of diseases classified elsewhere**

     B97.81 Human metapneumovirus **as the cause of diseases classified elsewhere**

     B97.89 **Other viral agents as the cause of diseases classified elsewhere**

Other infectious diseases (B99)

✓4ᵗʰ **B99** **Other and unspecified infectious diseases**

B99.8 **Other infectious disease**

B99.9 **Unspecified infectious disease** ▽

Ⓝ Newborn   Ⓟ Pediatric   Ⓜ Maternity   Ⓐ Adult   **RIC** RIC Dx   **NCDx** Noncancer Dx   **PDx** Primary Dx   **CC** RIC CC Condition   ▶◀ Revised Text   ● New Code   ▲ Revised Code Title

Chapter 2. Neoplasms (C00–D49)

Chapter Specific Guidelines with Coding Examples

The chapter specific guidelines from the ICD-10-CM Official Guidelines for Coding and Reporting have been provided below. Along with these guidelines are coding examples, contained in the shaded boxes, that have been developed to help illustrate the coding and/or sequencing guidance found in these guidelines.

General guidelines

Chapter 2 of the ICD-10-CM contains the codes for most benign and all malignant neoplasms. Certain benign neoplasms, such as prostatic adenomas, may be found in the specific body system chapters. To properly code a neoplasm it is necessary to determine from the record if the neoplasm is benign, in-situ, malignant, or of uncertain histologic behavior. If malignant, any secondary (metastatic) sites should also be determined.

Primary malignant neoplasms overlapping site boundaries

A primary malignant neoplasm that overlaps two or more contiguous (next to each other) sites should be classified to the subcategory/code .8 ('overlapping lesion'), unless the combination is specifically indexed elsewhere. For multiple neoplasms of the same site that are not contiguous such as tumors in different quadrants of the same breast, codes for each site should be assigned.

> A 73-year-old white female with a large rapidly growing malignant tumor in the left breast extending from the upper outer quadrant into the axillary tail
>
> **C50.812** **Malignant neoplasm of overlapping sites of left female breast**
>
> *Explanation*: Because this is a single large tumor that overlaps two contiguous sites, a single code for overlapping sites is assigned.

> A 52-year old white female with two distinct lesions of the right breast, one (0.5 cm) in the upper outer quadrant and a second (1.5 cm) in the lower outer quadrant; path report indicates both lesions are malignant
>
> **C50.411** **Malignant neoplasm of upper-outer quadrant of breast, female**
>
> **C50.511** **Malignant neoplasm of lower-outer quadrant of breast, female**
>
> *Explanation*: This patient has two distinct malignant lesions of right breast in adjacent quadrants. Because the lesions are not contiguous, two codes are reported.

Malignant neoplasm of ectopic tissue

Malignant neoplasms of ectopic tissue are to be coded to the site of origin mentioned, e.g., ectopic pancreatic malignant neoplasms involving the stomach are coded to pancreas, unspecified (C25.9).

The neoplasm table in the Alphabetic Index should be referenced first. However, if the histological term is documented, that term should be referenced first, rather than going immediately to the Neoplasm Table, in order to determine which column in the Neoplasm Table is appropriate. For example, if the documentation indicates "adenoma," refer to the term in the Alphabetic Index to review the entries under this term and the instructional note to "see also neoplasm, by site, benign." The table provides the proper code based on the type of neoplasm and the site. It is important to select the proper column in the table that corresponds to the type of neoplasm. The Tabular List should then be referenced to verify that the correct code has been selected from the table and that a more specific site code does not exist.

See Section I.C.21. Factors influencing health status and contact with health services, Status, for information regarding Z15.0, codes for genetic susceptibility to cancer.

a. Treatment directed at the malignancy

If the treatment is directed at the malignancy, designate the malignancy as the principal diagnosis.

The only exception to this guideline is if a patient admission/encounter is solely for the administration of chemotherapy, immunotherapy or radiation therapy, assign the appropriate Z51.-- code as the first-listed or principal diagnosis, and the diagnosis or problem for which the service is being performed as a secondary diagnosis.

b. Treatment of secondary site

When a patient is admitted because of a primary neoplasm with metastasis and treatment is directed toward the secondary site only, the secondary neoplasm is designated as the principal diagnosis even though the primary malignancy is still present.

> Patient with primary prostate cancer with metastasis to lungs admitted for wedge resection of mass in right lung
>
> **C78.01** **Secondary malignant neoplasm of right lung**
>
> **C61** **Malignant neoplasm of prostate**
>
> *Explanation*: Since the admission is for treatment of the lung metastasis, the secondary lung metastasis is sequenced before the primary prostate cancer.

c. Coding and sequencing of complications

Coding and sequencing of complications associated with the malignancies or with the therapy thereof are subject to the following guidelines:

1) Anemia associated with malignancy

When admission/encounter is for management of an anemia associated with the malignancy, and the treatment is only for anemia, the appropriate code for the malignancy is sequenced as the principal or first-listed diagnosis followed by the appropriate code for the anemia (such as code D63.0, Anemia in neoplastic disease).

> Patient is admitted for treatment of anemia in advanced colon cancer
>
> **C18.9** **Malignant neoplasm of colon, unspecified**
>
> **D63.0** **Anemia in neoplastic disease**
>
> *Explanation*: Even though the admission was solely to treat the anemia, this guideline indicates that the code for the malignancy is sequenced first.

2) Anemia associated with chemotherapy, immunotherapy and radiation therapy

When the admission/encounter is for management of an anemia associated with an adverse effect of the administration of chemotherapy or immunotherapy and the only treatment is for the anemia, the anemia code is sequenced first followed by the appropriate codes for the neoplasm and the adverse effect (T45.1X5, Adverse effect of antineoplastic and immunosuppressive drugs).

> A 56-year-old Hispanic male with grade II follicular lymphoma involving multiple lymph node sites referred for blood transfusion to treat anemia due to chemotherapy
>
> **D64.81** **Anemia due to antineoplastic chemotherapy**
>
> **C82.18** **Follicular lymphoma grade II, lymph nodes of multiple sites**
>
> **T45.1X5A** **Adverse effect of antineoplastic and immunosuppressive drugs, initial encounter**
>
> *Explanation*: The code for the anemia is sequenced first followed by the code for the malignant neoplasm and lastly the code for the adverse effect.

When the admission/encounter is for management of an anemia associated with an adverse effect of radiotherapy, the anemia code should be sequenced first, followed by the appropriate neoplasm code and code Y84.2, Radiological procedure and radiotherapy as the cause of abnormal reaction of the patient, or of later complication, without mention of misadventure at the time of the procedure.

A 55-year-old male with a large malignant rectal tumor has been receiving external radiation therapy to shrink the tumor prior to planned surgery. He is admitted today for a blood transfusion to treat anemia related to radiation therapy.

D64.89   Other specified anemia

C20   Malignant neoplasm of rectum

Y84.2   Radiological procedure and radiotherapy as the cause of abnormal reaction of the patient, or of later complication, without mention of misadventure at the time of the procedure

Explanation: The code for the anemia is sequenced first, followed by the code for the malignancy, and lastly the code for the abnormal reaction due to radiotherapy.

3) Management of dehydration due to the malignancy

When the admission/encounter is for management of dehydration due to the malignancy and only the dehydration is being treated (intravenous rehydration), the dehydration is sequenced first, followed by the code(s) for the malignancy.

4) Treatment of a complication resulting from a surgical procedure

When the admission/encounter is for treatment of a complication resulting from a surgical procedure, designate the complication as the principal or first-listed diagnosis if treatment is directed at resolving the complication.

d. Primary malignancy previously excised

When a primary malignancy has been previously excised or eradicated from its site and there is no further treatment directed to that site and there is no evidence of any existing primary malignancy, a code from category Z85, Personal history of malignant neoplasm, should be used to indicate the former site of the malignancy. Any mention of extension, invasion, or metastasis to another site is coded as a secondary malignant neoplasm to that site. The secondary site may be the principal or first-listed with the Z85 code used as a secondary code.

History of breast cancer, left radical mastectomy 18 months ago with no current treatment; bronchoscopy with lung biopsy shows metastatic disease in the right lung

C78.01   Secondary malignant neoplasm of right lung

Z85.3   Personal history of malignant neoplasm of breast

Explanation: The patient has undergone a diagnostic procedure that revealed metastatic breast cancer in the right lung. The code for the secondary (metastatic) site is sequenced first followed by a personal history code to identify the former site of the primary malignancy.

e. Admissions/Encounters involving chemotherapy, immunotherapy and radiation therapy

1) Episode of care involves surgical removal of neoplasm

When an episode of care involves the surgical removal of a neoplasm, primary or secondary site, followed by adjunct chemotherapy or radiation treatment during the same episode of care, the code for the neoplasm should be assigned as principal or first-listed diagnosis.

2) Patient admission/encounter solely for administration of chemotherapy, immunotherapy and radiation therapy

If a patient admission/encounter is solely for the administration of chemotherapy, immunotherapy or radiation therapy assign code Z51.0, Encounter for antineoplastic radiation therapy, or Z51.11, Encounter for antineoplastic chemotherapy, or Z51.12, Encounter for antineoplastic immunotherapy as the first-listed or principal diagnosis. If a patient receives more than one of these therapies during the same admission more than one of these codes may be assigned, in any sequence.

The malignancy for which the therapy is being administered should be assigned as a secondary diagnosis.

Patient is admitted for second round of rituximab and fludarabine for his chronic B cell lymphocytic leukemia

Z51.11   Encounter for antineoplastic chemotherapy

Z51.12   Encounter for antineoplastic immunotherapy

C91.10   Chronic lymphocytic leukemia of B-cell type not having achieved remission

Explanation: Rituximab is an antineoplastic immunotherapy while fludarabine is an antineoplastic chemotherapy. The two treatments are often used together. The admission was solely for the purpose of administering this treatment and either can be sequenced first, before the neoplastic condition.

3) Patient admitted for radiation therapy, chemotherapy or immunotherapy and develops complications

When a patient is admitted for the purpose of radiotherapy, immunotherapy or chemotherapy and develops complications such as uncontrolled nausea and vomiting or dehydration, the principal or first-listed diagnosis is Z51.0, Encounter for antineoplastic radiation therapy, or Z51.11, Encounter for antineoplastic chemotherapy, or Z51.12, Encounter for antineoplastic immunotherapy followed by any codes for the complications.

f. Admission/encounter to determine extent of malignancy

When the reason for admission/encounter is to determine the extent of the malignancy, or for a procedure such as paracentesis or thoracentesis, the primary malignancy or appropriate metastatic site is designated as the principal or first-listed diagnosis, even though chemotherapy or radiotherapy is administered.

Patient with left lung cancer with malignant pleural effusion admitted for paracentesis and initiation/administration of chemotherapy

C34.92   Malignant neoplasm of unspecified part of left bronchus or lung

J91.0   Malignant pleural effusion

Z51.11   Encounter for antineoplastic chemotherapy

Explanation: The lung cancer is sequenced before the chemotherapy in this instance because the paracentesis for the malignant effusion is also being performed. An instructional note under the malignant effusion instructs that the lung cancer be sequenced first.

g. Symptoms, signs, and abnormal findings listed in Chapter 18 associated with neoplasms

Symptoms, signs, and ill-defined conditions listed in Chapter 18 characteristic of, or associated with, an existing primary or secondary site malignancy cannot be used to replace the malignancy as principal or first-listed diagnosis, regardless of the number of admissions or encounters for treatment and care of the neoplasm.

See Section I.C.21. Factors influencing health status and contact with health services, Encounter for prophylactic organ removal.

h. Admission/encounter for pain control/management

See Section I.C.6. for information on coding admission/encounter for pain control/management.

i. Malignancy in two or more noncontiguous sites

A patient may have more than one malignant tumor in the same organ. These tumors may represent different primaries or metastatic disease, depending on the site. Should the documentation be unclear, the provider should be queried as to the status of each tumor so that the correct codes can be assigned.

j. Disseminated malignant neoplasm, unspecified

Code C80.0, Disseminated malignant neoplasm, unspecified, is for use only in those cases where the patient has advanced metastatic disease and no known primary or secondary sites are specified. It should not be used in place of assigning codes for the primary site and all known secondary sites.

Patient who has had no medical care for many years is seen today and diagnosed with carcinomatosis

C80.0   Disseminated malignant neoplasm, unspecified

Explanation: Carcinomatosis NOS is an "includes" note under this code. Should seldom be used but is available for use in cases such as this.

k. Malignant neoplasm without specification of site

Code C80.1, Malignant (primary) neoplasm, unspecified, equates to Cancer, unspecified. This code should only be used when no determination can be made as to the primary site of a malignancy. This code should rarely be used in the inpatient setting.

> Evaluation of painful hip leads to diagnosis of a metastatic bone lesion from an unknown primary neoplasm source
>
> **C79.51**   **Secondary malignant neoplasm of bone**
>
> **C80.1**   **Malignant (primary) neoplasm, unspecified**
>
> *Explanation*: If only the secondary site is known, use code C80.1 for the unknown primary site.

l. Sequencing of neoplasm codes

1) Encounter for treatment of primary malignancy

If the reason for the encounter is for treatment of a primary malignancy, assign the malignancy as the principal/first-listed diagnosis. The primary site is to be sequenced first, followed by any metastatic sites.

2) Encounter for treatment of secondary malignancy

When an encounter is for a primary malignancy with metastasis and treatment is directed toward the metastatic (secondary) site(s) only, the metastatic site(s) is designated as the principal/first-listed diagnosis. The primary malignancy is coded as an additional code.

> Patient has primary colon cancer with metastasis to rib and is evaluated for possible excision of portion of rib bone
>
> **C79.51**   **Secondary malignant neoplasm of bone**
>
> **C18.9**   **Malignant neoplasm of colon, unspecified**
>
> *Explanation*: The treatment for this encounter is focused on the metastasis to the rib bone rather than the primary colon cancer, thus indicating that the bone metastasis is sequenced as the first-listed code.

3) Malignant neoplasm in a pregnant patient

When a pregnant woman has a malignant neoplasm, a code from subcategory O9A.1-, Malignant neoplasm complicating pregnancy, childbirth, and the puerperium, should be sequenced first, followed by the appropriate code from Chapter 2 to indicate the type of neoplasm.

> A 30-year-old pregnant female in second trimester evaluated for thyroid malignancy
>
> **O9A.112**   **Malignant neoplasm complicating pregnancy, second trimester**
>
> **C73**   **Malignant neoplasm of thyroid gland**
>
> *Explanation*: Codes from chapter 15 describing complications of pregnancy are sequenced as first-listed codes, further specified by codes from other chapters such as neoplastic, unless the pregnancy is documented as incidental to the condition. See also guideline 1.C.15.a.1.

4) Encounter for complication associated with a neoplasm

When an encounter is for management of a complication associated with a neoplasm, such as dehydration, and the treatment is only for the complication, the complication is coded first, followed by the appropriate code(s) for the neoplasm.

The exception to this guideline is anemia. When the admission/encounter is for management of an anemia associated with the malignancy, and the treatment is only for anemia, the appropriate code for the malignancy is sequenced as the principal or first-listed diagnosis followed by code D63.0, Anemia in neoplastic disease.

> Patient with pancreatic cancer is seen for initiation of TPN for cancer-related moderate protein-calorie malnutrition
>
> **E44.0**   **Moderate protein-calorie malnutrition**
>
> **C25.9**   **Malignant neoplasm of pancreas, unspecified**
>
> *Explanation*: The encounter is to initiate treatment for malnutrition, a common complication of many types of neoplasms, and is sequenced first.

5) Complication from surgical procedure for treatment of a neoplasm

When an encounter is for treatment of a complication resulting from a surgical procedure performed for the treatment of the neoplasm, designate the complication as the principal/first-listed diagnosis. See guideline regarding the coding of a current malignancy versus personal history to determine if the code for the neoplasm should also be assigned.

6) Pathologic fracture due to a neoplasm

When an encounter is for a pathological fracture due to a neoplasm, and the focus of treatment is the fracture, a code from subcategory M84.5, Pathological fracture in neoplastic disease, should be sequenced first, followed by the code for the neoplasm.

If the focus of treatment is the neoplasm with an associated pathological fracture, the neoplasm code should be sequenced first, followed by a code from M84.5 for the pathological fracture.

m. Current malignancy versus personal history of malignancy

When a primary malignancy has been excised but further treatment, such as an additional surgery for the malignancy, radiation therapy or chemotherapy is directed to that site, the primary malignancy code should be used until treatment is completed.

When a primary malignancy has been previously excised or eradicated from its site, there is no further treatment (of the malignancy) directed to that site, and there is no evidence of any existing primary malignancy, a code from category Z85, Personal history of malignant neoplasm, should be used to indicate the former site of the malignancy.

See Section I.C.21. Factors influencing health status and contact with health services, History (of)

> Female patient with ongoing chemotherapy after right mastectomy for breast cancer
>
> **C50.911**   **Malignant neoplasm of unspecified site of right female breast**
>
> *Explanation*: Even though the breast has been removed, the breast cancer is still being treated with chemotherapy and therefore is still coded as a current condition rather than personal history.

n. Leukemia, multiple myeloma, and malignant plasma cell neoplasms in remission versus personal history

The categories for leukemia, and category C90, Multiple myeloma and malignant plasma cell neoplasms, have codes indicating whether or not the leukemia has achieved remission. There are also codes Z85.6, Personal history of leukemia, and Z85.79, Personal history of other malignant neoplasms of lymphoid, hematopoietic and related tissues. If the documentation is unclear as to whether the leukemia has achieved remission, the provider should be queried.

See Section I.C.21. Factors influencing health status and contact with health services, History (of)

o. Aftercare following surgery for neoplasm

See Section I.C.21. Factors influencing health status and contact with health services, Aftercare

p. Follow-up care for completed treatment of a malignancy

See Section I.C.21. Factors influencing health status and contact with health services, Follow-up

q. Prophylactic organ removal for prevention of malignancy

See Section I.C. 21, Factors influencing health status and contact with health services, Prophylactic organ removal

r. Malignant neoplasm associated with transplanted organ

A malignant neoplasm of a transplanted organ should be coded as a transplant complication. Assign first the appropriate code from category T86.-, Complications of transplanted organs and tissue, followed by code C80.2, Malignant neoplasm associated with transplanted organ. Use an additional code for the specific malignancy.

Chapter 2. Neoplasms (C00-D49)

NOTE

Functional activity

All neoplasms are classified in this chapter, whether they are functionally active or not. An additional code from Chapter 4 may be used, to identify functional activity associated with any neoplasm.

Morphology [Histology]

Chapter 2 classifies neoplasms primarily by site (topography), with broad groupings for behavior, malignant, in situ, benign, etc. The Table of Neoplasms should be used to identify the correct topography code. In a few cases, such as for malignant melanoma and certain neuroendocrine tumors, the morphology (histologic type) is included in the category and codes.

Primary malignant neoplasms overlapping site boundaries

A primary malignant neoplasm that overlaps two or more contiguous (next to each other) sites should be classified to the subcategory/code .8 ("overlapping lesion"), unless the combination is specifically indexed elsewhere. For multiple neoplasms of the same site that are not contiguous, such as tumors in different quadrants of the same breast, codes for each site should be assigned.

Malignant neoplasm of ectopic tissue

Malignant neoplasms of ectopic tissue are to be coded to the site mentioned, e.g., ectopic pancreatic malignant neoplasms are coded to pancreas, unspecified (C25.9).

This chapter contains the following blocks:

C00-C14	Malignant neoplasms of lip, oral cavity and pharynx
C15-C26	Malignant neoplasms of digestive organs
C30-C39	Malignant neoplasms of respiratory and intrathoracic organs
C40-C41	Malignant neoplasms of bone and articular cartilage
C43-C44	Melanoma and other malignant neoplasms of skin
C45-C49	Malignant neoplasms of mesothelial and soft tissue
C50	Malignant neoplasms of breast
C51-C58	Malignant neoplasms of female genital organs
C60-C63	Malignant neoplasms of male genital organs
C64-C68	Malignant neoplasms of urinary tract
C69-C72	Malignant neoplasms of eye, brain and other parts of central nervous system
C73-C75	Malignant neoplasms of thyroid and other endocrine glands
C7A	Malignant neuroendocrine tumors
C7B	Secondary neuroendocrine tumors
C76-C80	Malignant neoplasms of ill-defined, other secondary and unspecified sites
C81-C96	Malignant neoplasms of lymphoid, hematopoietic and related tissue
D00-D09	In situ neoplasms
D10-D36	Benign neoplasms, except benign neuroendocrine tumors
D3A	Benign neuroendocrine tumors
D37-D48	Neoplasms of uncertain behavior, polycythemia vera and myelodysplastic syndromes
D49	Neoplasms of unspecified behavior

MALIGNANT NEOPLASMS (C00-C96)

Malignant neoplasms, stated or presumed to be primary (of specified sites), and certain specified histologies, except neuroendocrine, and of lymphoid, hematopoietic and related tissue (C00-C75)

Malignant neoplasms of lip, oral cavity and pharynx (C00-C14)

✓4ᵗʰ C00 **Malignant neoplasm of** lip
    Use additional code to identify:
       alcohol abuse and dependence (F10.-)
       history of tobacco use (Z87.891)
       tobacco dependence (F17.-)
       tobacco use (Z72.0)
    EXCLUDES 1   malignant melanoma of lip (C43.0)
             Merkel cell carcinoma of lip (C4A.0)
             other and unspecified malignant neoplasm of skin of lip (C44.0-)

    C00.0 **Malignant neoplasm of** external upper lip
       Malignant neoplasm of lipstick area of upper lip
       Malignant neoplasm of upper lip NOS
       Malignant neoplasm of vermilion border of upper lip

    C00.1 **Malignant neoplasm of** external lower lip
       Malignant neoplasm of lower lip NOS
       Malignant neoplasm of lipstick area of lower lip
       Malignant neoplasm of vermilion border of lower lip

    C00.2 **Malignant neoplasm of** external lip, unspecified   ▽
       Malignant neoplasm of vermilion border of lip NOS

    C00.3 **Malignant neoplasm of** upper lip, inner aspect
       Malignant neoplasm of buccal aspect of upper lip
       Malignant neoplasm of frenulum of upper lip
       Malignant neoplasm of mucosa of upper lip
       Malignant neoplasm of oral aspect of upper lip

    C00.4 **Malignant neoplasm of** lower lip, inner aspect
       Malignant neoplasm of buccal aspect of lower lip
       Malignant neoplasm of frenulum of lower lip
       Malignant neoplasm of mucosa of lower lip
       Malignant neoplasm of oral aspect of lower lip

    C00.5 **Malignant neoplasm of** lip, unspecified, inner aspect   ▽
       Malignant neoplasm of buccal aspect of lip, unspecified
       Malignant neoplasm of frenulum of lip, unspecified
       Malignant neoplasm of mucosa of lip, unspecified
       Malignant neoplasm of oral aspect of lip, unspecified

    C00.6 **Malignant neoplasm of** commissure of lip, unspecified

    C00.8 **Malignant neoplasm of** overlapping sites of lip

    C00.9 **Malignant neoplasm of** lip, unspecified   ▽

C01 **Malignant neoplasm of** base of tongue
    Malignant neoplasm of dorsal surface of base of tongue
    Malignant neoplasm of fixed part of tongue NOS
    Malignant neoplasm of posterior third of tongue
    Use additional code to identify:
       alcohol abuse and dependence (F10.-)
       history of tobacco use (Z87.891)
       tobacco dependence (F17.-)
       tobacco use (Z72.0)

✓4ᵗʰ C02 **Malignant neoplasm of** other and unspecified parts of tongue
    Use additional code to identify:
       alcohol abuse and dependence (F10.-)
       history of tobacco use (Z87.891)
       tobacco dependence (F17.-)
       tobacco use (Z72.0)

    C02.0 **Malignant neoplasm of** dorsal surface of tongue
       Malignant neoplasm of anterior two-thirds of tongue, dorsal surface
       EXCLUDES 2   malignant neoplasm of dorsal surface of base of tongue (C01)

    C02.1 **Malignant neoplasm of** border of tongue
       Malignant neoplasm of tip of tongue

    C02.2 **Malignant neoplasm of** ventral surface of tongue
       Malignant neoplasm of anterior two-thirds of tongue, ventral surface
       Malignant neoplasm of frenulum linguae

    C02.3 **Malignant neoplasm of** anterior two-thirds of tongue, part unspecified
       Malignant neoplasm of middle third of tongue NOS
       Malignant neoplasm of mobile part of tongue NOS

    C02.4 **Malignant neoplasm of** lingual tonsil
       EXCLUDES 2   malignant neoplasm of tonsil NOS (C09.9)

    C02.8 **Malignant neoplasm of** overlapping sites of tongue
       Malignant neoplasm of two or more contiguous sites of tongue

    C02.9 **Malignant neoplasm of** tongue, unspecified   ▽

✓4ᵗʰ C03 **Malignant neoplasm of** gum
    INCLUDES   malignant neoplasm of alveolar (ridge) mucosa
              malignant neoplasm of gingiva
    Use additional code to identify:
       alcohol abuse and dependence (F10.-)
       history of tobacco use (Z87.891)
       tobacco dependence (F17.-)
       tobacco use (Z72.0)
    EXCLUDES 2   malignant odontogenic neoplasms (C41.0-C41.1)

    C03.0 **Malignant neoplasm of** upper gum

    C03.1 **Malignant neoplasm of** lower gum

    C03.9 **Malignant neoplasm of** gum, unspecified   ▽

✓4ᵗʰ C04 **Malignant neoplasm of** floor of mouth
    Use additional code to identify:
       alcohol abuse and dependence (F10.-)
       history of tobacco use (Z87.891)
       tobacco dependence (F17.-)
       tobacco use (Z72.0)

    C04.0 **Malignant neoplasm of** anterior floor of mouth
       Malignant neoplasm of anterior to the premolar-canine junction

    C04.1 **Malignant neoplasm of** lateral floor of mouth

    C04.8 **Malignant neoplasm of** overlapping sites of floor of mouth

    C04.9 **Malignant neoplasm of** floor of mouth, unspecified   ▽

☑4ᵗʰ C05 Malignant neoplasm of palate
Use additional code to identify:
alcohol abuse and dependence (F10.-)
history of tobacco use (Z87.891)
tobacco dependence (F17.-)
tobacco use (Z72.0)
EXCLUDES 1 *Kaposi's sarcoma of palate (C46.2)*

C05.0 Malignant neoplasm of hard palate
C05.1 Malignant neoplasm of soft palate
EXCLUDES 2 *malignant neoplasm of nasopharyngeal surface of soft palate (C11.3)*
C05.2 Malignant neoplasm of uvula
C05.8 Malignant neoplasm of overlapping sites **of palate**
C05.9 Malignant neoplasm of palate, unspecified ▽
Malignant neoplasm of roof of mouth

☑4ᵗʰ C06 Malignant neoplasm of other and unspecified parts of mouth
Use additional code to identify:
alcohol abuse and dependence (F10.-)
history of tobacco use (Z87.891)
tobacco dependence (F17.-)
tobacco use (Z72.0)

C06.0 Malignant neoplasm of cheek mucosa
Malignant neoplasm of buccal mucosa NOS
Malignant neoplasm of internal cheek
C06.1 Malignant neoplasm of vestibule **of mouth**
Malignant neoplasm of buccal sulcus (upper) (lower)
Malignant neoplasm of labial sulcus (upper) (lower)
C06.2 Malignant neoplasm of retromolar area
☑5ᵗʰ C06.8 Malignant neoplasm of overlapping sites of other and unspecified **parts of mouth**
C06.80 Malignant neoplasm of overlapping sites of ▽ **unspecified parts of mouth**
C06.89 Malignant neoplasm of overlapping sites of other parts of mouth
"book leaf" neoplasm [ventral surface of tongue and floor of mouth]
C06.9 Malignant neoplasm of mouth, unspecified ▽
Malignant neoplasm of minor salivary gland, unspecified site
Malignant neoplasm of oral cavity NOS

C07 Malignant neoplasm of parotid gland
Use additional code to identify:
alcohol abuse and dependence (F10.-)
exposure to environmental tobacco smoke (Z77.22)
exposure to tobacco smoke in the perinatal period (P96.81)
history of tobacco use (Z87.891)
occupational exposure to environmental tobacco smoke (Z57.31)
tobacco dependence (F17.-)
tobacco use (Z72.0)

☑4ᵗʰ C08 Malignant neoplasm of other and unspecified major salivary glands
INCLUDES malignant neoplasm of salivary ducts
Use additional code to identify:
alcohol abuse and dependence (F10.-)
exposure to environmental tobacco smoke (Z77.22)
exposure to tobacco smoke in the perinatal period (P96.81)
history of tobacco use (Z87.891)
occupational exposure to environmental tobacco smoke (Z57.31)
tobacco dependence (F17.-)
tobacco use (Z72.0)
EXCLUDES 1 *malignant neoplasms of specified minor salivary glands which are classified according to their anatomical location*
EXCLUDES 2 *malignant neoplasms of minor salivary glands NOS (C06.9) malignant neoplasm of parotid gland (C07)*

C08.0 Malignant neoplasm of submandibular **gland**
Malignant neoplasm of submaxillary gland
C08.1 Malignant neoplasm of sublingual **gland**
C08.9 Malignant neoplasm of major salivary gland, **unspecified** ▽
Malignant neoplasm of salivary gland (major) NOS

☑4ᵗʰ C09 Malignant neoplasm of tonsil
Use additional code to identify:
alcohol abuse and dependence (F10.-)
exposure to environmental tobacco smoke (Z77.22)
exposure to tobacco smoke in the perinatal period (P96.81)
history of tobacco use (Z87.891)
occupational exposure to environmental tobacco smoke (Z57.31)
tobacco dependence (F17.-)
tobacco use (Z72.0)
EXCLUDES 2 *malignant neoplasm of linguai tonsil (C02.4) malignant neoplasm of pharyngeal tonsil (C11.1)*

C09.0 Malignant neoplasm of tonsillar fossa
C09.1 Malignant neoplasm of tonsillar pillar **(anterior) (posterior)**
C09.8 Malignant neoplasm of overlapping sites **of tonsil**
C09.9 Malignant neoplasm of tonsil, unspecified ▽
Malignant neoplasm of tonsil NOS
Malignant neoplasm of faucial tonsils
Malignant neoplasm of palatine tonsils

☑4ᵗʰ C10 Malignant neoplasm of oropharynx
Use additional code to identify:
alcohol abuse and dependence (F10.-)
exposure to environmental tobacco smoke (Z77.22)
exposure to tobacco smoke in the perinatal period (P96.81)
history of tobacco use (Z87.891)
occupational exposure to environmental tobacco smoke (Z57.31)
tobacco dependence (F17.-)
tobacco use (Z72.0)
EXCLUDES 2 *malignant neoplasm of tonsil (C09.-)*

C10.0 Malignant neoplasm of vallecula
C10.1 Malignant neoplasm of anterior surface of epiglottis
Malignant neoplasm of epiglottis, free border [margin]
Malignant neoplasm of glossoepiglottic fold(s)
EXCLUDES 2 *malignant neoplasm of epiglottis (suprahyoid portion) NOS (C32.1)*
C10.2 Malignant neoplasm of lateral wall **of oropharynx**
C10.3 Malignant neoplasm of posterior wall **of oropharynx**
C10.4 Malignant neoplasm of branchial cleft
Malignant neoplasm of branchial cyst [site of neoplasm]
C10.8 Malignant neoplasm of overlapping sites **of oropharynx**
Malignant neoplasm of junctional region of oropharynx
C10.9 Malignant neoplasm of oropharynx, unspecified ▽

☑4ᵗʰ C11 Malignant neoplasm of nasopharynx
Use additional code to identify:
exposure to environmental tobacco smoke (Z77.22)
exposure to tobacco smoke in the perinatal period (P96.81)
history of tobacco use (Z87.891)
occupational exposure to environmental tobacco smoke (Z57.31)
tobacco dependence (F17.-)
tobacco use (Z72.0)

C11.0 Malignant neoplasm of superior wall **of nasopharynx**
Malignant neoplasm of roof of nasopharynx
C11.1 Malignant neoplasm of posterior wall **of nasopharynx**
Malignant neoplasm of adenoid
Malignant neoplasm of pharyngeal tonsil
C11.2 Malignant neoplasm of lateral wall **of nasopharynx**
Malignant neoplasm of fossa of Rosenmüller
Malignant neoplasm of opening of auditory tube
Malignant neoplasm of pharyngeal recess
C11.3 Malignant neoplasm of anterior wall **of nasopharynx**
Malignant neoplasm of floor of nasopharynx
Malignant neoplasm of nasopharyngeal (anterior) (posterior) surface of soft palate
Malignant neoplasm of posterior margin of nasal choana
Malignant neoplasm of posterior margin of nasal septum
C11.8 Malignant neoplasm of overlapping sites **of nasopharynx**
C11.9 Malignant neoplasm of nasopharynx, unspecified ▽
Malignant neoplasm of nasopharyngeal wall NOS

C12 Malignant neoplasm of pyriform sinus
Malignant neoplasm of pyriform fossa
Use additional code to identify:
exposure to environmental tobacco smoke (Z77.22)
exposure to tobacco smoke in the perinatal period (P96.81)
history of tobacco use (Z87.891)
occupational exposure to environmental tobacco smoke (Z57.31)
tobacco dependence (F17.-)
tobacco use (Z72.0)

☑ Add'l Character Required ☑x7ᵗʰ Placeholder Alert RUG IV Special Care High Dx RUG IV Clinically Complex Dx RUG IV Special Care Low Dx Manifestation Code Other Specified Code ▽ Unspecified Code

ICD-10-CM 2016   449

C05–C12

Chapter 2. Neoplasms

☑4ᵗʰ **C13** **Malignant neoplasm of** hypopharynx

Use additional code to identify:
exposure to environmental tobacco smoke (Z77.22)
exposure to tobacco smoke in the perinatal period (P96.81)
history of tobacco use (Z87.891)
occupational exposure to environmental tobacco smoke (Z57.31)
tobacco dependence (F17.-)
tobacco use (Z72.0)

EXCLUDES 2   *malignant neoplasm of pyriform sinus (C12)*

C13.0 **Malignant neoplasm of** postcricoid region

C13.1 **Malignant neoplasm of** aryepiglottic fold, hypopharyngeal aspect

Malignant neoplasm of aryepiglottic fold, marginal zone
Malignant neoplasm of aryepiglottic fold NOS
Malignant neoplasm of interarytenoid fold, marginal zone
Malignant neoplasm of interarytenoid fold NOS

EXCLUDES 2   *malignant neoplasm of aryepiglottic fold or interarytenoid fold, laryngeal aspect (C32.1)*

C13.2 **Malignant neoplasm of** posterior wall of hypopharynx

C13.8 **Malignant neoplasm of** overlapping sites of hypopharynx

C13.9 **Malignant neoplasm of hypopharynx, unspecified** ▽
Malignant neoplasm of hypopharyngeal wall NOS

☑4ᵗʰ **C14** **Malignant neoplasm of** other and ill-defined sites in the lip, oral cavity and pharynx

Use additional code to identify:
alcohol abuse and dependence (F10.-)
exposure to environmental tobacco smoke (Z77.22)
exposure to tobacco smoke in the perinatal period (P96.81)
history of tobacco use (Z87.891)
occupational exposure to environmental tobacco smoke (Z57.31)
tobacco dependence (F17.-)
tobacco use (Z72.0)

EXCLUDES 1   *malignant neoplasm of oral cavity NOS (C06.9)*

C14.0 **Malignant neoplasm of pharynx, unspecified** ▽

C14.2 **Malignant neoplasm of** Waldeyer's ring

C14.8 **Malignant neoplasm of** overlapping sites of lip, oral cavity and pharynx

Primary malignant neoplasm of two or more contiguous sites of lip, oral cavity and pharynx

EXCLUDES 1   *"book leaf" neoplasm [ventral surface of tongue and floor of mouth] (C06.89)*

Malignant neoplasms of digestive organs (C15-C26)

EXCLUDES 1   *Kaposi's sarcoma of gastrointestinal sites (C46.4)*

☑4ᵗʰ **C15** **Malignant neoplasm of** esophagus

Use additional code to identify:
alcohol abuse and dependence (F10.-)

C15.3 **Malignant neoplasm of** upper third of esophagus

C15.4 **Malignant neoplasm of** middle third of esophagus

C15.5 **Malignant neoplasm of** lower third of esophagus

EXCLUDES 1   *malignant neoplasm of cardio-esophageal junction (C16.0)*

C15.8 **Malignant neoplasm of** overlapping sites of esophagus

C15.9 **Malignant neoplasm of esophagus, unspecified** ▽

☑4ᵗʰ **C16** **Malignant neoplasm of** stomach

Use additional code to identify:
alcohol abuse and dependence (F10.-)

EXCLUDES 2   *malignant carcinoid tumor of the stomach (C7A.092)*

C16.0 **Malignant neoplasm of** cardia
Malignant neoplasm of cardiac orifice
Malignant neoplasm of cardio-esophageal junction
Malignant neoplasm of esophagus and stomach
Malignant neoplasm of gastro-esophageal junction

C16.1 **Malignant neoplasm of** fundus of stomach

C16.2 **Malignant neoplasm of** body of stomach

C16.3 **Malignant neoplasm of** pyloric antrum
Malignant neoplasm of gastric antrum

C16.4 **Malignant neoplasm of** pylorus
Malignant neoplasm of prepylorus
Malignant neoplasm of pyloric canal

C16.5 **Malignant neoplasm of** lesser curvature of stomach, unspecified
Malignant neoplasm of lesser curvature of stomach, not classifiable to C16.1-C16.4

C16.6 **Malignant neoplasm of** greater curvature of stomach, unspecified
Malignant neoplasm of greater curvature of stomach, not classifiable to C16.0-C16.4

C16.8 **Malignant neoplasm of** overlapping sites of stomach

C16.9 **Malignant neoplasm of stomach, unspecified** ▽
Gastric cancer NOS

☑4ᵗʰ **C17** **Malignant neoplasm of** small intestine

EXCLUDES 1   *malignant carcinoid tumors of the small intestine (C7A.01)*

C17.0 **Malignant neoplasm of** duodenum

C17.1 **Malignant neoplasm of** jejunum

C17.2 **Malignant neoplasm of** ileum

EXCLUDES 1   *malignant neoplasm of ileocecal valve (C18.0)*

C17.3 **Meckel's diverticulum, malignant**

EXCLUDES 1   *Meckel's diverticulum, congenital (Q43.0)*

C17.8 **Malignant neoplasm of** overlapping sites of small intestine

C17.9 **Malignant neoplasm of small intestine, unspecified** ▽

☑4ᵗʰ **C18** **Malignant neoplasm of** colon

EXCLUDES 1   *malignant carcinoid tumors of the colon (C7A.02-)*

C18.0 **Malignant neoplasm of** cecum
Malignant neoplasm of ileocecal valve

C18.1 **Malignant neoplasm of** appendix

C18.2 **Malignant neoplasm of** ascending colon

C18.3 **Malignant neoplasm of** hepatic flexure

C18.4 **Malignant neoplasm of** transverse colon

C18.5 **Malignant neoplasm of** splenic flexure

C18.6 **Malignant neoplasm of** descending colon

C18.7 **Malignant neoplasm of** sigmoid colon
Malignant neoplasm of sigmoid (flexure)

EXCLUDES 1   *malignant neoplasm of rectosigmoid junction (C19)*

C18.8 **Malignant neoplasm of** overlapping sites of colon

C18.9 **Malignant neoplasm of colon, unspecified** ▽
Malignant neoplasm of large intestine NOS

C19 **Malignant neoplasm of** rectosigmoid junction
Malignant neoplasm of colon with rectum
Malignant neoplasm of rectosigmoid (colon)

EXCLUDES 1   *malignant carcinoid tumors of the colon (C7A.02-)*

C20 **Malignant neoplasm of** rectum
Malignant neoplasm of rectal ampulla

EXCLUDES 1   *malignant carcinoid tumor of the rectum (C7A.026)*

☑4ᵗʰ **C21** **Malignant neoplasm of** anus and anal canal

EXCLUDES 2   *malignant carcinoid tumors of the colon (C7A.02-)*
malignant melanoma of anal margin (C43.51)
malignant melanoma of anal skin (C43.51)
malignant melanoma of perianal skin (C43.51)
other and unspecified malignant neoplasm of anal margin (C44.500, C44.510, C44.520, C44.590)
other and unspecified malignant neoplasm of anal skin (C44.500, C44.510, C44.520, C44.590)
other and unspecified malignant neoplasm of perianal skin (C44.500, C44.510, C44.520, C44.590)

C21.0 **Malignant neoplasm of anus, unspecified** ▽

C21.1 **Malignant neoplasm of** anal canal
Malignant neoplasm of anal sphincter

C21.2 **Malignant neoplasm of** cloacogenic zone

C21.8 **Malignant neoplasm of** overlapping sites of rectum, anus and anal canal
Malignant neoplasm of anorectal junction
Malignant neoplasm of anorectum
Primary malignant neoplasm of two or more contiguous sites of rectum, anus and anal canal

☑4ᵗʰ **C22** **Malignant neoplasm of** liver and intrahepatic bile ducts

Use additional code to identify:
alcohol abuse and dependence (F10.-)
hepatitis B (B16.-, B18.0-B18.1)
hepatitis C (B17.1-, B18.2)

EXCLUDES 1   *malignant neoplasm of biliary tract NOS (C24.9)*
secondary malignant neoplasm of liver and intrahepatic bile duct (C78.7)

C22.0 Liver cell **carcinoma**
Hepatocellular carcinoma
Hepatoma

C22.1 Intrahepatic bile duct **carcinoma**
Cholangiocarcinoma

EXCLUDES 1   *malignant neoplasm of hepatic duct (C24.0)*

C22.2 Hepatoblastoma

C22.3 Angiosarcoma **of liver**
Kupffer cell sarcoma

C22.4 Other sarcomas **of liver**

Ⓝ Newborn   Ⓟ Pediatric   Ⓜ Maternity   Ⓐ Adult   **RIC** RIC Dx   **NCDx** Noncancer Dx   **PDx** Primary Dx   **CC** RIC CC Condition   ►◄ Revised Text   ● New Code   ▲ Revised Code Title

450   ICD-10-CM 2016

C22.7   Other specified carcinomas of liver

C22.8   Malignant neoplasm of liver, **primary, unspecified** as to type   ▽

C22.9   Malignant neoplasm of liver, **not specified as** primary or secondary   ▽

C23   **Malignant neoplasm of** gallbladder

☑4ᵗʰ **C24**   **Malignant neoplasm of** other and unspecified parts of biliary tract
> **EXCLUDES 1**   *malignant neoplasm of intrahepatic bile duct (C22.1)*

C24.0   **Malignant neoplasm of** extrahepatic bile duct
> Malignant neoplasm of biliary duct or passage NOS
> Malignant neoplasm of common bile duct
> Malignant neoplasm of cystic duct
> Malignant neoplasm of hepatic duct

C24.1   **Malignant neoplasm of** ampulla of Vater

C24.8   **Malignant neoplasm of** overlapping sites of biliary tract
> Malignant neoplasm involving both intrahepatic and extrahepatic bile duct
> Primary malignant neoplasm of two or more contiguous sites of biliary tract

C24.9   **Malignant neoplasm of** biliary tract, unspecified   ▽

☑4ᵗʰ **C25**   **Malignant neoplasm of** pancreas
> Use additional code to identify:
>   alcohol abuse and dependence (F10.-)

C25.0   **Malignant neoplasm of** head of pancreas

C25.1   **Malignant neoplasm of** body of pancreas

C25.2   **Malignant neoplasm of** tail of pancreas

C25.3   **Malignant neoplasm of** pancreatic duct

C25.4   **Malignant neoplasm of** endocrine pancreas
> Malignant neoplasm of islets of Langerhans
> Use additional code to identify any functional activity

C25.7   **Malignant neoplasm of other parts of pancreas**
> Malignant neoplasm of neck of pancreas

C25.8   **Malignant neoplasm of** overlapping sites of pancreas

C25.9   **Malignant neoplasm of** pancreas, unspecified   ▽

☑4ᵗʰ **C26**   **Malignant neoplasm of** other and ill-defined digestive organs
> **EXCLUDES 1**   *malignant neoplasm of peritoneum and retroperitoneum (C48.-)*

C26.0   **Malignant neoplasm of** intestinal tract, part unspecified
> Malignant neoplasm of intestine NOS

C26.1   **Malignant neoplasm of** spleen
> **EXCLUDES 1**   *Hodgkin lymphoma (C81.-)*
>   *non-Hodgkin lymphoma (C82-C85)*

C26.9   **Malignant neoplasm of** ill-defined sites within the digestive system
> Malignant neoplasm of alimentary canal or tract NOS
> Malignant neoplasm of gastrointestinal tract NOS
> **EXCLUDES 1**   *malignant neoplasm of abdominal NOS (C76.2)*
>   *malignant neoplasm of intra-abdominal NOS (C76.2)*

Malignant neoplasms of respiratory and intrathoracic organs (C30-C39)

> **INCLUDES**   malignant neoplasm of middle ear
> **EXCLUDES 1**   *mesothelioma (C45.-)*

☑4ᵗʰ **C30**   **Malignant neoplasm of** nasal cavity and middle ear

C30.0   **Malignant neoplasm of** nasal cavity
> Malignant neoplasm of cartilage of nose
> Malignant neoplasm of nasal concha
> Malignant neoplasm of internal nose
> Malignant neoplasm of septum of nose
> Malignant neoplasm of vestibule of nose
> **EXCLUDES 1**   *malignant melanoma of skin of nose (C43.31)*
>   *malignant neoplasm of nasal bone (C41.0)*
>   *malignant neoplasm of nose NOS (C76.0)*
>   *malignant neoplasm of olfactory bulb (C72.2-)*
>   *malignant neoplasm of posterior margin of nasal septum and choana (C11.3)*
>   *malignant neoplasm of turbinates (C41.0)*
>   *other and unspecified malignant neoplasm of skin of nose (C44.301, C44.311, C44.321, C44.391)*

C30.1   **Malignant neoplasm of** middle ear
> Malignant neoplasm of antrum tympanicum
> Malignant neoplasm of auditory tube
> Malignant neoplasm of eustachian tube
> Malignant neoplasm of inner ear
> Malignant neoplasm of mastoid air cells
> Malignant neoplasm of tympanic cavity
> **EXCLUDES 1**   *malignant melanoma of skin of (external) ear (C43.2-)*
>   *malignant neoplasm of auricular canal (external) (C43.2-,C44.2-)*
>   *malignant neoplasm of bone of ear (meatus) (C41.0)*
>   *malignant neoplasm of cartilage of ear (C49.0)*
>   *other and unspecified malignant neoplasm of skin of (external) ear (C44.2-)*

☑4ᵗʰ **C31**   **Malignant neoplasm of accessory sinuses**

C31.0   **Malignant neoplasm of** maxillary sinus
> Malignant neoplasm of antrum (Highmore) (maxillary)

C31.1   **Malignant neoplasm of** ethmoidal sinus

C31.2   **Malignant neoplasm of** frontal sinus

C31.3   **Malignant neoplasm of** sphenoid sinus

C31.8   **Malignant neoplasm of** overlapping sites of accessory sinuses

C31.9   **Malignant neoplasm of** accessory sinus, unspecified   ▽

☑4ᵗʰ **C32**   **Malignant neoplasm of larynx**
> Use additional code to identify:
>   alcohol abuse and dependence (F10.-)
>   exposure to environmental tobacco smoke (Z77.22)
>   exposure to tobacco smoke in the perinatal period (P96.81)
>   history of tobacco use (Z87.891)
>   occupational exposure to environmental tobacco smoke (Z57.31)
>   tobacco dependence (F17.-)
>   tobacco use (Z72.0)

C32.0   **Malignant neoplasm of** glottis
> Malignant neoplasm of intrinsic larynx
> Malignant neoplasm of laryngeal commissure (anterior) (posterior)
> Malignant neoplasm of vocal cord (true) NOS

C32.1   **Malignant neoplasm of** supraglottis
> Malignant neoplasm of aryepiglottic fold or interarytenoid fold, laryngeal aspect
> Malignant neoplasm of epiglottis (suprahyoid portion) NOS
> Malignant neoplasm of extrinsic larynx
> Malignant neoplasm of false vocal cord
> Malignant neoplasm of posterior (laryngeal) surface of epiglottis
> Malignant neoplasm of ventricular bands
> **EXCLUDES 2**   *malignant neoplasm of anterior surface of epiglottis (C10.1)*
>   *malignant neoplasm of aryepiglottic fold or interarytenoid fold, hypopharyngeal aspect (C13.1)*
>   *malignant neoplasm of aryepiglottic fold or interarytenoid fold, marginal zone (C13.1)*
>   *malignant neoplasm of aryepiglottic fold or interarytenoid fold NOS (C13.1)*

C32.2   **Malignant neoplasm of** subglottis

C32.3   **Malignant neoplasm of** laryngeal cartilage

C32.8   **Malignant neoplasm of** overlapping sites of larynx

C32.9   **Malignant neoplasm of** larynx, unspecified   ▽

C33   **Malignant neoplasm of** trachea
> Use additional code to identify:
>   exposure to environmental tobacco smoke (Z77.22)
>   exposure to tobacco smoke in the perinatal period (P96.81)
>   history of tobacco use (Z87.891)
>   occupational exposure to environmental tobacco smoke (Z57.31)
>   tobacco dependence (F17.-)
>   tobacco use (Z72.0)

☑4ᵗʰ **C34**   **Malignant neoplasm of** bronchus and lung
> Use additional code to identify:
>   exposure to environmental tobacco smoke (Z77.22)
>   exposure to tobacco smoke in the perinatal period (P96.81)
>   history of tobacco use (Z87.891)
>   occupational exposure to environmental tobacco smoke (Z57.31)
>   tobacco dependence (F17.-)
>   tobacco use (Z72.0)
> **EXCLUDES 1**   *Kaposi's sarcoma of lung (C46.5-)*
>   *malignant carcinoid tumor of the bronchus and lung (C7A.090)*

☑5ᵗʰ **C34.0**   **Malignant neoplasm of** main bronchus
> Malignant neoplasm of carina
> Malignant neoplasm of hilus (of lung)

C34.00   **Malignant neoplasm of unspecified main bronchus**   ▽

C34.01   Malignant neoplasm of right main bronchus

C34.02   Malignant neoplasm of left main bronchus

√5ᵗʰ **C34.1**   Malignant neoplasm of upper lobe, bronchus or lung

C34.10   Malignant neoplasm of upper lobe, unspecified bronchus or lung ▽

C34.11   Malignant neoplasm of upper lobe, right bronchus or lung

C34.12   Malignant neoplasm of upper lobe, left bronchus or lung

C34.2   Malignant neoplasm of middle lobe, bronchus or lung

√5ᵗʰ **C34.3**   Malignant neoplasm of lower lobe, bronchus or lung

C34.30   Malignant neoplasm of lower lobe, unspecified bronchus or lung ▽

C34.31   Malignant neoplasm of lower lobe, right bronchus or lung

C34.32   Malignant neoplasm of lower lobe, left bronchus or lung

√5ᵗʰ **C34.8**   Malignant neoplasm of overlapping sites of bronchus and lung

C34.80   Malignant neoplasm of overlapping sites of unspecified bronchus and lung ▽

C34.81   Malignant neoplasm of overlapping sites of right bronchus and lung

C34.82   Malignant neoplasm of overlapping sites of left bronchus and lung

√5ᵗʰ **C34.9**   Malignant neoplasm of unspecified part of bronchus or lung

C34.90   Malignant neoplasm of unspecified part of unspecified bronchus or lung ▽
  Lung cancer NOS

C34.91   Malignant neoplasm of unspecified part of right bronchus or lung ▽

C34.92   Malignant neoplasm of unspecified part of left bronchus or lung ▽

C37   **Malignant neoplasm of thymus**
  EXCLUDES 1   malignant carcinoid tumor of the thymus (C7A.091)

√4ᵗʰ **C38**   **Malignant neoplasm of heart, mediastinum and pleura**
  EXCLUDES 1   mesothelioma (C45.-)

C38.0   Malignant neoplasm of heart
  Malignant neoplasm of pericardium
  EXCLUDES 1   malignant neoplasm of great vessels (C49.3)

C38.1   Malignant neoplasm of anterior mediastinum

C38.2   Malignant neoplasm of posterior mediastinum

C38.3   Malignant neoplasm of mediastinum, part unspecified ▽

C38.4   Malignant neoplasm of pleura

C38.8   Malignant neoplasm of overlapping sites of heart, mediastinum and pleura

√4ᵗʰ **C39**   **Malignant neoplasm of other and ill-defined sites in the respiratory system and intrathoracic organs**
  Use additional code to identify:
    exposure to environmental tobacco smoke (Z77.22)
    exposure to tobacco smoke in the perinatal period (P96.81)
    history of tobacco use (Z87.891)
    occupational exposure to environmental tobacco smoke (Z57.31)
    tobacco dependence (F17.-)
    tobacco use (Z72.0)
  EXCLUDES 1   intrathoracic malignant neoplasm NOS (C76.1)
    thoracic malignant neoplasm NOS (C76.1)

C39.0   Malignant neoplasm of upper respiratory tract, part unspecified ▽

C39.9   Malignant neoplasm of lower respiratory tract, part unspecified ▽
  Malignant neoplasm of respiratory tract NOS

Malignant neoplasms of bone and articular cartilage (C40-C41)

INCLUDES   malignant neoplasm of cartilage (articular) (joint)
  malignant neoplasm of periosteum
EXCLUDES 1   malignant neoplasm of bone marrow NOS (C96.9)
  malignant neoplasm of synovia (C49.-)

√4ᵗʰ **C40**   **Malignant neoplasm of bone and articular cartilage of limbs**
  Use additional code to identify major osseous defect, if applicable (M89.7-)

√5ᵗʰ **C40.0**   Malignant neoplasm of scapula and long bones of upper limb

C40.00   Malignant neoplasm of scapula and long bones of unspecified upper limb ▽

C40.01   Malignant neoplasm of scapula and long bones of right upper limb

C40.02   Malignant neoplasm of scapula and long bones of left upper limb

√5ᵗʰ **C40.1**   Malignant neoplasm of short bones of upper limb

C40.10   Malignant neoplasm of short bones of unspecified upper limb ▽

C40.11   Malignant neoplasm of short bones of right upper limb

C40.12   Malignant neoplasm of short bones of left upper limb

√5ᵗʰ **C40.2**   Malignant neoplasm of long bones of lower limb

C40.20   Malignant neoplasm of long bones of unspecified lower limb ▽

C40.21   Malignant neoplasm of long bones of right lower limb

C40.22   Malignant neoplasm of long bones of left lower limb

√5ᵗʰ **C40.3**   Malignant neoplasm of short bones of lower limb

C40.30   Malignant neoplasm of short bones of unspecified lower limb ▽

C40.31   Malignant neoplasm of short bones of right lower limb

C40.32   Malignant neoplasm of short bones of left lower limb

√5ᵗʰ **C40.8**   Malignant neoplasm of overlapping sites of bone and articular cartilage of limb

C40.80   Malignant neoplasm of overlapping sites of bone and articular cartilage of unspecified limb ▽

C40.81   Malignant neoplasm of overlapping sites of bone and articular cartilage of right limb

C40.82   Malignant neoplasm of overlapping sites of bone and articular cartilage of left limb

√5ᵗʰ **C40.9**   Malignant neoplasm of unspecified bones and articular cartilage of limb

C40.90   Malignant neoplasm of unspecified bones and articular cartilage of unspecified limb ▽

C40.91   Malignant neoplasm of unspecified bones and articular cartilage of right limb ▽

C40.92   Malignant neoplasm of unspecified bones and articular cartilage of left limb ▽

√4ᵗʰ **C41**   **Malignant neoplasm of bone and articular cartilage of other and unspecified sites**
  EXCLUDES 1   malignant neoplasm of bones of limbs (C40.-)
    malignant neoplasm of cartilage of ear (C49.0)
    malignant neoplasm of cartilage of eyelid (C49.0)
    malignant neoplasm of cartilage of larynx (C32.3)
    malignant neoplasm of cartilage of limbs (C40.-)
    malignant neoplasm of cartilage of nose (C30.0)

C41.0   Malignant neoplasm of bones of skull and face
  Malignant neoplasm of maxilla (superior)
  Malignant neoplasm of orbital bone
  EXCLUDES 2   carcinoma, any type except intraosseous or odontogenic of:
    maxillary sinus (C31.0)
    upper jaw (C03.0)
    malignant neoplasm of jaw bone (lower) (C41.1)

C41.1   Malignant neoplasm of mandible
  Malignant neoplasm of inferior maxilla
  Malignant neoplasm of lower jaw bone
  EXCLUDES 2   carcinoma, any type except intraosseous or odontogenic of:
    jaw NOS (C03.9)
    lower (C03.1)
    malignant neoplasm of upper jaw bone (C41.0)

C41.2   Malignant neoplasm of vertebral column
  EXCLUDES 1   malignant neoplasm of sacrum and coccyx (C41.4)

C41.3   Malignant neoplasm of ribs, sternum and clavicle

C41.4   Malignant neoplasm of pelvic bones, sacrum and coccyx

C41.9   Malignant neoplasm of bone and articular cartilage, unspecified ▽

Melanoma and other malignant neoplasms of skin (C43-C44)

☑️4ᵗʰ C43   **Malignant melanoma of** skin
> EXCLUDES 1   melanoma in situ (D03.-)
> EXCLUDES 2   malignant melanoma of skin of genital organs (C51-C52, C60.-, C63.-)
> Merkel cell carcinoma (C4A.-)
> sites other than skin—code to malignant neoplasm of the site

C43.0   **Malignant melanoma of** lip
> EXCLUDES 1   malignant neoplasm of vermilion border of lip (C00.0-C00.2)

☑️5ᵗʰ C43.1   **Malignant melanoma of** eyelid, including canthus ▽
- **C43.10**   **Malignant melanoma of unspecified eyelid, including canthus**
- **C43.11**   **Malignant melanoma of** right **eyelid, including canthus**
- **C43.12**   **Malignant melanoma of** left **eyelid, including canthus**

☑️5ᵗʰ C43.2   **Malignant melanoma of** ear and external auricular canal ▽
- **C43.20**   **Malignant melanoma of unspecified ear and external auricular canal**
- **C43.21**   **Malignant melanoma of** right **ear and external auricular canal**
- **C43.22**   **Malignant melanoma of** left **ear and external auricular canal**

☑️5ᵗʰ C43.3   **Malignant melanoma of other and unspecified** parts of face
- **C43.30**   **Malignant melanoma of unspecified part of face** ▽
- **C43.31**   **Malignant melanoma of** nose
- **C43.39**   Malignant melanoma of other parts of face

C43.4   **Malignant melanoma of** scalp and neck

☑️5ᵗʰ C43.5   **Malignant melanoma of** trunk
> EXCLUDES 2   malignant neoplasm of anus NOS (C21.0)
> malignant neoplasm of scrotum (C63.2)
- **C43.51**   **Malignant melanoma of** anal skin
> Malignant melanoma of anal margin
> Malignant melanoma of perianal skin
- **C43.52**   **Malignant melanoma of** skin of breast
- **C43.59**   Malignant melanoma of other part of trunk

☑️5ᵗʰ C43.6   **Malignant melanoma of** upper limb, including shoulder
- **C43.60**   **Malignant melanoma of unspecified upper limb, including shoulder** ▽
- **C43.61**   **Malignant melanoma of** right **upper limb, including shoulder**
- **C43.62**   **Malignant melanoma of** left **upper limb, including shoulder**

☑️5ᵗʰ C43.7   **Malignant melanoma of** lower limb, including hip
- **C43.70**   **Malignant melanoma of unspecified lower limb, including hip** ▽
- **C43.71**   **Malignant melanoma of** right **lower limb, including hip**
- **C43.72**   **Malignant melanoma of** left **lower limb, including hip**

C43.8   **Malignant melanoma of** overlapping sites **of skin** ▽

C43.9   **Malignant melanoma of skin, unspecified** ▽
> Malignant melanoma of unspecified site of skin

☑️4ᵗʰ C4A   **Merkel cell carcinoma**

C4A.0   **Merkel cell carcinoma of** lip
> EXCLUDES 1   malignant neoplasm of vermilion border of lip (C00.0-C00.2)

☑️5ᵗʰ C4A.1   **Merkel cell carcinoma of** eyelid, including canthus
- **C4A.10**   **Merkel cell carcinoma of unspecified eyelid, including canthus** ▽
- **C4A.11**   **Merkel cell carcinoma of** right **eyelid, including canthus**
- **C4A.12**   **Merkel cell carcinoma of** left **eyelid, including canthus**

☑️5ᵗʰ C4A.2   **Merkel cell carcinoma of** ear and external auricular canal
- **C4A.20**   **Merkel cell carcinoma of unspecified ear and external auricular canal** ▽
- **C4A.21**   **Merkel cell carcinoma of** right **ear and external auricular canal**
- **C4A.22**   **Merkel cell carcinoma of** left **ear and external auricular canal**

☑️5ᵗʰ C4A.3   **Merkel cell carcinoma of** other and unspecified **parts of face**
- **C4A.30**   Merkel cell carcinoma of unspecified part of face ▽

- **C4A.31**   **Merkel cell carcinoma of** nose
- **C4A.39**   Merkel cell carcinoma of other parts of face

C4A.4   **Merkel cell carcinoma of** scalp and neck

☑️5ᵗʰ C4A.5   **Merkel cell carcinoma of** trunk
> EXCLUDES 2   malignant neoplasm of anus NOS (C21.0)
> malignant neoplasm of scrotum (C63.2)
- **C4A.51**   **Merkel cell carcinoma of** anal skin
> Merkel cell carcinoma of anal margin
> Merkel cell carcinoma of perianal skin
- **C4A.52**   **Merkel cell carcinoma of** skin of breast
- **C4A.59**   Merkel cell carcinoma of other part of trunk

☑️5ᵗʰ C4A.6   **Merkel cell carcinoma of** upper limb, including shoulder
- **C4A.60**   **Merkel cell carcinoma of unspecified upper limb, including shoulder** ▽
- **C4A.61**   **Merkel cell carcinoma of** right **upper limb, including shoulder**
- **C4A.62**   **Merkel cell carcinoma of** left **upper limb, including shoulder**

☑️5ᵗʰ C4A.7   **Merkel cell carcinoma of** lower limb, including hip
- **C4A.70**   **Merkel cell carcinoma of unspecified lower limb, including hip** ▽
- **C4A.71**   **Merkel cell carcinoma of** right **lower limb, including hip**
- **C4A.72**   **Merkel cell carcinoma of** left **lower limb, including hip**

C4A.8   **Merkel cell carcinoma of** overlapping sites

C4A.9   **Merkel cell carcinoma, unspecified** ▽
> Merkel cell carcinoma of unspecified site

☑️4ᵗʰ C44   **Other and unspecified** malignant neoplasm **of skin**
> INCLUDES   malignant neoplasm of sebaceous glands
> malignant neoplasm of sweat glands
> EXCLUDES 1   Kaposi's sarcoma of skin (C46.0)
> malignant melanoma of skin (C43.-)
> malignant neoplasm of skin of genital organs (C51-C52, C60-, C63.2)
> Merkel cell carcinoma (C4A.-)

☑️5ᵗʰ C44.0   **Other and unspecified malignant neoplasm of skin of** lip
> EXCLUDES 1   malignant neoplasm of lip (C00.-)
- **C44.00**   **Unspecified malignant neoplasm of skin of lip** ▽
- **C44.01**   Basal cell carcinoma **of skin of lip**
- **C44.02**   Squamous cell carcinoma **of skin of lip**
- **C44.09**   Other specified malignant neoplasm of skin of lip

☑️5ᵗʰ C44.1   **Other and unspecified malignant neoplasm of skin of** eyelid, including canthus
> EXCLUDES 1   connective tissue of eyelid (C49.0)
- **☑️6ᵗʰ C44.10**   Unspecified **malignant neoplasm of skin of eyelid, including canthus**
  - **C44.101**   **Unspecified malignant neoplasm of skin of unspecified eyelid, including canthus** ▽
  - **C44.102**   **Unspecified malignant neoplasm of skin of** right **eyelid, including canthus** ▽
  - **C44.109**   **Unspecified malignant neoplasm of skin of** left **eyelid, including canthus** ▽
- **☑️6ᵗʰ C44.11**   Basal cell carcinoma **of skin of eyelid, including canthus**
  - **C44.111**   **Basal cell carcinoma of skin of unspecified eyelid, including canthus** ▽
  - **C44.112**   **Basal cell carcinoma of skin of** right **eyelid, including canthus**
  - **C44.119**   **Basal cell carcinoma of skin of** left **eyelid, including canthus**
- **☑️6ᵗʰ C44.12**   Squamous cell carcinoma **of skin of eyelid, including canthus**
  - **C44.121**   **Squamous cell carcinoma of skin of unspecified eyelid, including canthus** ▽
  - **C44.122**   **Squamous cell carcinoma of skin of** right **eyelid, including canthus**
  - **C44.129**   **Squamous cell carcinoma of skin of** left **eyelid, including canthus**
- **☑️6ᵗʰ C44.19**   Other specified malignant neoplasm of skin of **eyelid, including canthus**
  - **C44.191**   Other specified malignant neoplasm of skin of unspecified eyelid, including canthus ▽

☑️ Add'l Character Required   ☑️x7ᵗʰ Placeholder Alert   RUG IV Special Care High Dx   RUG IV Clinically Complex Dx   RUG IV Special Care Low Dx   Manifestation Code   Other Specified Code   ▽ Unspecified Code

Chapter 2. Neoplasms

C44.192　**Other specified malignant neoplasm of skin of** right **eyelid, including canthus**

C44.199　**Other specified malignant neoplasm of skin of** left **eyelid, including canthus**

☑5ᵗʰ **C44.2　Other and unspecified malignant neoplasm of** skin of ear and external auricular canal

　EXCLUDES 1　*connective tissue of ear (C49.0)*

　☑6ᵗʰ **C44.20**　Unspecified **malignant neoplasm of skin of ear and external auricular canal**

　　C44.201　**Unspecified malignant neoplasm of skin of unspecified ear and external auricular canal**　▽

　　C44.202　**Unspecified malignant neoplasm of skin of** right **ear and external auricular canal**　▽

　　C44.209　**Unspecified malignant neoplasm of skin of** left **ear and external auricular canal**　▽

　☑6ᵗʰ **C44.21**　Basal cell carcinoma **of skin of ear and external auricular canal**

　　C44.211　**Basal cell carcinoma of skin of unspecified ear and external auricular canal**　▽

　　C44.212　**Basal cell carcinoma of skin of** right **ear and external auricular canal**

　　C44.219　**Basal cell carcinoma of skin of** left **ear and external auricular canal**

　☑6ᵗʰ **C44.22**　Squamous cell carcinoma **of skin of ear and external auricular canal**

　　C44.221　**Squamous cell carcinoma of skin of unspecified ear and external auricular canal**　▽

　　C44.222　**Squamous cell carcinoma of skin of** right **ear and external auricular canal**

　　C44.229　**Squamous cell carcinoma of skin of** left **ear and external auricular canal**

　☑6ᵗʰ **C44.29**　Other **specified malignant neoplasm of skin of ear and external auricular canal**

　　C44.291　**Other specified malignant neoplasm of skin of unspecified ear and external auricular canal**　▽

　　C44.292　**Other specified malignant neoplasm of skin of** right **ear and external auricular canal**

　　C44.299　**Other specified malignant neoplasm of skin of** left **ear and external auricular canal**

☑5ᵗʰ **C44.3　Other and unspecified malignant neoplasm of skin of** other and unspecified parts of face

　☑6ᵗʰ **C44.30**　Unspecified **malignant neoplasm of skin of other and unspecified parts of face**

　　C44.300　**Unspecified malignant neoplasm of skin of unspecified part of face**　▽

　　C44.301　**Unspecified malignant neoplasm of skin of** nose　▽

　　C44.309　**Unspecified malignant neoplasm of skin of other parts of face**　▽

　☑6ᵗʰ **C44.31**　Basal cell carcinoma **of skin of other and unspecified parts of face**

　　C44.310　**Basal cell carcinoma of skin of unspecified parts of face**　▽

　　C44.311　**Basal cell carcinoma of skin of** nose

　　C44.319　**Basal cell carcinoma of skin of other parts of face**

　☑6ᵗʰ **C44.32**　Squamous cell carcinoma **of skin of other and unspecified parts of face**

　　C44.320　**Squamous cell carcinoma of skin of unspecified parts of face**　▽

　　C44.321　**Squamous cell carcinoma of skin of** nose

　　C44.329　**Squamous cell carcinoma of skin of other parts of face**

　☑6ᵗʰ **C44.39**　Other **specified malignant neoplasm of skin of other and unspecified parts of face**

　　C44.390　**Other specified malignant neoplasm of skin of unspecified parts of face**　▽

　　C44.391　**Other specified malignant neoplasm of skin of** nose

　　C44.399　**Other specified malignant neoplasm of skin of other parts of face**

☑5ᵗʰ **C44.4　Other and unspecified malignant neoplasm of skin of** scalp and neck

　C44.40　**Unspecified malignant neoplasm of skin of scalp and neck**　▽

　C44.41　Basal cell carcinoma **of skin of scalp and neck**

　C44.42　Squamous cell carcinoma **of skin of scalp and neck**

　C44.49　**Other specified malignant neoplasm of skin of scalp and neck**

☑5ᵗʰ **C44.5　Other and unspecified malignant neoplasm of** skin of trunk

　EXCLUDES 1　*anus NOS (C21.0)*
　　　　　　scrotum (C63.2)

　☑6ᵗʰ **C44.50**　Unspecified **malignant neoplasm of skin of trunk**

　　C44.500　**Unspecified malignant neoplasm of** anal skin　▽
　　　　　　Unspecified malignant neoplasm of anal margin
　　　　　　Unspecified malignant neoplasm of perianal skin

　　C44.501　**Unspecified malignant neoplasm of** skin of breast　▽

　　C44.509　**Unspecified malignant neoplasm of skin of other part of trunk**　▽

　☑6ᵗʰ **C44.51**　Basal cell carcinoma **of skin of trunk**

　　C44.510　**Basal cell carcinoma of** anal skin
　　　　　　Basal cell carcinoma of anal margin
　　　　　　Basal cell carcinoma of perianal skin

　　C44.511　**Basal cell carcinoma of** skin of breast

　　C44.519　**Basal cell carcinoma of skin of other part of trunk**

　☑6ᵗʰ **C44.52**　Squamous cell carcinoma **of skin of trunk**

　　C44.520　**Squamous cell carcinoma of** anal skin
　　　　　　Squamous cell carcinoma of anal margin
　　　　　　Squamous cell carcinoma of perianal skin

　　C44.521　**Squamous cell carcinoma of** skin of breast

　　C44.529　**Squamous cell carcinoma of skin of other part of trunk**

　☑6ᵗʰ **C44.59**　Other **specified malignant neoplasm of skin of trunk**

　　C44.590　**Other specified malignant neoplasm of** anal skin
　　　　　　Other specified malignant neoplasm of anal margin
　　　　　　Other specified malignant neoplasm of perianal skin

　　C44.591　**Other specified malignant neoplasm of** skin of breast

　　C44.599　**Other specified malignant neoplasm of skin of other part of trunk**

☑5ᵗʰ **C44.6　Other and unspecified malignant neoplasm of skin of** upper limb, including shoulder

　☑6ᵗʰ **C44.60**　Unspecified **malignant neoplasm of skin of upper limb, including shoulder**

　　C44.601　**Unspecified malignant neoplasm of skin of unspecified upper limb, including shoulder**　▽

　　C44.602　**Unspecified malignant neoplasm of skin of** right **upper limb, including shoulder**　▽

　　C44.609　**Unspecified malignant neoplasm of skin of** left **upper limb, including shoulder**　▽

　☑6ᵗʰ **C44.61**　Basal cell carcinoma **of skin of upper limb, including shoulder**

　　C44.611　**Basal cell carcinoma of skin of unspecified upper limb, including shoulder**　▽

　　C44.612　**Basal cell carcinoma of skin of** right **upper limb, including shoulder**

　　C44.619　**Basal cell carcinoma of skin of** left **upper limb, including shoulder**

　☑6ᵗʰ **C44.62**　Squamous cell carcinoma **of skin of upper limb, including shoulder**

　　C44.621　**Squamous cell carcinoma of skin of unspecified upper limb, including shoulder**　▽

　　C44.622　**Squamous cell carcinoma of skin of** right **upper limb, including shoulder**

　　C44.629　**Squamous cell carcinoma of skin of** left **upper limb, including shoulder**

Ⓝ Newborn　Ⓟ Pediatric　Ⓜ Maternity　Ⓐ Adult　RIC RIC Dx　NC Dx Noncancer Dx　PDx Primary Dx　CC RIC CC Condition　►◄ Revised Text　● New Code　▲ Revised Code Title

454　　　　　　　　　　　　　　　　　　　　　　　　　　　　　　　　　　　ICD-10-CM 2016

☑6ᵗʰ **C44.69** Other specified malignant neoplasm of skin of upper limb, including shoulder

    C44.691 Other specified malignant neoplasm of skin of unspecified upper limb, including shoulder ▽

    C44.692 Other specified malignant neoplasm of skin of right upper limb, including shoulder ▽

    C44.699 Other specified malignant neoplasm of skin of left upper limb, including shoulder ▽

☑5ᵗʰ **C44.7** Other and unspecified malignant neoplasm of skin of lower limb, including hip

  ☑6ᵗʰ **C44.70** Unspecified malignant neoplasm of skin of lower limb, including hip

    C44.701 Unspecified malignant neoplasm of skin of unspecified lower limb, including hip ▽

    C44.702 Unspecified malignant neoplasm of skin of right lower limb, including hip ▽

    C44.709 Unspecified malignant neoplasm of skin of left lower limb, including hip ▽

  ☑6ᵗʰ **C44.71** Basal cell carcinoma of skin of lower limb, including hip

    C44.711 Basal cell carcinoma of skin of unspecified lower limb, including hip ▽

    C44.712 Basal cell carcinoma of skin of right lower limb, including hip

    C44.719 Basal cell carcinoma of skin of left lower limb, including hip

  ☑6ᵗʰ **C44.72** Squamous cell carcinoma of skin of lower limb, including hip

    C44.721 Squamous cell carcinoma of skin of unspecified lower limb, including hip ▽

    C44.722 Squamous cell carcinoma of skin of right lower limb, including hip

    C44.729 Squamous cell carcinoma of skin of left lower limb, including hip

  ☑6ᵗʰ **C44.79** Other specified malignant neoplasm of skin of lower limb, including hip

    C44.791 Other specified malignant neoplasm of skin of unspecified lower limb, including hip ▽

    C44.792 Other specified malignant neoplasm of skin of right lower limb, including hip

    C44.799 Other specified malignant neoplasm of skin of left lower limb, including hip

☑5ᵗʰ **C44.8** Other and unspecified malignant neoplasm of overlapping sites of skin

  C44.80 Unspecified malignant neoplasm of overlapping sites of skin ▽

  C44.81 Basal cell carcinoma of overlapping sites of skin

  C44.82 Squamous cell carcinoma of overlapping sites of skin

  C44.89 Other specified malignant neoplasm of overlapping sites of skin

☑5ᵗʰ **C44.9** Other and unspecified malignant neoplasm of skin, unspecified

  C44.90 Unspecified malignant neoplasm of skin, unspecified ▽
    Malignant neoplasm of unspecified site of skin

  C44.91 Basal cell carcinoma of skin, unspecified

  C44.92 Squamous cell carcinoma of skin, unspecified

  C44.99 Other specified malignant neoplasm of skin, unspecified

Malignant neoplasms of mesothelial and soft tissue (C45-C49)

☑4ᵗʰ **C45 Mesothelioma**

  C45.0 Mesothelioma of pleura
    EXCLUDES 1   *other malignant neoplasm of pleura (C38.4)*

  C45.1 Mesothelioma of peritoneum
    Mesothelioma of cul-de-sac
    Mesothelioma of mesentery
    Mesothelioma of mesocolon
    Mesothelioma of omentum
    Mesothelioma of peritoneum (parietal) (pelvic)
    EXCLUDES 1   *other malignant neoplasm of soft tissue of peritoneum (C48.-)*

  C45.2 Mesothelioma of pericardium
    EXCLUDES 1   *other malignant neoplasm of pericardium (C38.0)*

  C45.7 Mesothelioma of other sites

  C45.9 Mesothelioma, unspecified ▽

☑4ᵗʰ **C46 Kaposi's sarcoma**
  Code first any human immunodeficiency virus [HIV] disease (B20)

  C46.0 Kaposi's sarcoma of skin

  C46.1 Kaposi's sarcoma of soft tissue
    Kaposi's sarcoma of blood vessel
    Kaposi's sarcoma of connective tissue
    Kaposi's sarcoma of fascia
    Kaposi's sarcoma of ligament
    Kaposi's sarcoma of lymphatic(s) NEC
    Kaposi's sarcoma of muscle
    EXCLUDES 2   *Kaposi's sarcoma of lymph glands and nodes (C46.3)*

  C46.2 Kaposi's sarcoma of palate

  C46.3 Kaposi's sarcoma of lymph nodes

  C46.4 Kaposi's sarcoma of gastrointestinal sites

☑5ᵗʰ **C46.5 Kaposi's sarcoma of** lung

    C46.50 Kaposi's sarcoma of unspecified lung ▽

    C46.51 Kaposi's sarcoma of right lung

    C46.52 Kaposi's sarcoma of left lung

  C46.7 Kaposi's sarcoma of other sites

  C46.9 Kaposi's sarcoma, unspecified ▽
    Kaposi's sarcoma of unspecified site

☑4ᵗʰ **C47 Malignant neoplasm of peripheral nerves and autonomic nervous system**
  INCLUDES   malignant neoplasm of sympathetic and parasympathetic nerves and ganglia
  EXCLUDES 1   *Kaposi's sarcoma of soft tissue (C46.1)*

  C47.0 Malignant neoplasm of peripheral nerves of head, face and neck
    EXCLUDES 1   *malignant neoplasm of peripheral nerves of orbit (C69.6-)*

☑5ᵗʰ **C47.1 Malignant neoplasm of peripheral nerves of** upper limb, including shoulder

    C47.10 Malignant neoplasm of peripheral nerves of unspecified upper limb, including shoulder ▽

    C47.11 Malignant neoplasm of peripheral nerves of right upper limb, including shoulder

    C47.12 Malignant neoplasm of peripheral nerves of left upper limb, including shoulder

☑5ᵗʰ **C47.2 Malignant neoplasm of peripheral nerves of** lower limb, including hip

    C47.20 Malignant neoplasm of peripheral nerves of unspecified lower limb, including hip ▽

    C47.21 Malignant neoplasm of peripheral nerves of right lower limb, including hip

    C47.22 Malignant neoplasm of peripheral nerves of left lower limb, including hip

  C47.3 Malignant neoplasm of peripheral nerves of thorax

  C47.4 Malignant neoplasm of peripheral nerves of abdomen

  C47.5 Malignant neoplasm of peripheral nerves of pelvis

  C47.6 Malignant neoplasm of peripheral nerves of trunk, unspecified ▽
    Malignant neoplasm of peripheral nerves of unspecified part of trunk

  C47.8 Malignant neoplasm of overlapping sites **of peripheral nerves and autonomic nervous system**

  C47.9 Malignant neoplasm of peripheral nerves and autonomic nervous system, unspecified ▽
    Malignant neoplasm of unspecified site of peripheral nerves and autonomic nervous system

☑4ᵗʰ **C48 Malignant neoplasm of** retroperitoneum and peritoneum
  EXCLUDES 1   *Kaposi's sarcoma of connective tissue (C46.1)*
              mesothelioma (C45.-)

  C48.0 Malignant neoplasm of retroperitoneum

  C48.1 Malignant neoplasm of specified parts of peritoneum
    Malignant neoplasm of cul-de-sac
    Malignant neoplasm of mesentery
    Malignant neoplasm of mesocolon
    Malignant neoplasm of omentum
    Malignant neoplasm of parietal peritoneum
    Malignant neoplasm of pelvic peritoneum

  C48.2 Malignant neoplasm of peritoneum, **unspecified** ▽

☑ Add'l Character Required   ☑ᵗʰ Placeholder Alert   RUG IV Special Care High Dx   RUG IV Clinically Complex Dx   RUG IV Special Care Low Dx   Manifestation Code   Other Specified Code   ▽ Unspecified Code

Chapter 2. Neoplasms (side tab)

C48.8 **Malignant neoplasm of** overlapping sites **of retroperitoneum and peritoneum**

✓4ᵗʰ **C49** **Malignant neoplasm of** other connective and soft tissue

INCLUDES   malignant neoplasm of blood vessel
malignant neoplasm of bursa
malignant neoplasm of cartilage
malignant neoplasm of fascia
malignant neoplasm of fat
malignant neoplasm of ligament, except uterine
malignant neoplasm of lymphatic vessel
malignant neoplasm of muscle
malignant neoplasm of synovia
malignant neoplasm of tendon (sheath)

EXCLUDES 1   malignant neoplasm of cartilage (of):
articular (C40-C41)
larynx (C32.3)
nose (C30.0)
malignant neoplasm of connective tissue of breast (C50.-)

EXCLUDES 2   Kaposi's sarcoma of soft tissue (C46.1)
malignant neoplasm of heart (C38.0)
malignant neoplasm of peripheral nerves and autonomic
nervous system (C47.-)
malignant neoplasm of peritoneum (C48.2)
malignant neoplasm of retroperitoneum (C48.0)
malignant neoplasm of uterine ligament (C57.3)
mesothelioma (C45.-)

C49.0 **Malignant neoplasm of connective and soft tissue of** head, face and neck
Malignant neoplasm of connective tissue of ear
Malignant neoplasm of connective tissue of eyelid
EXCLUDES 1   connective tissue of orbit (C69.6-)

✓5ᵗʰ **C49.1** **Malignant neoplasm of connective and soft tissue of** upper limb, including shoulder

C49.10 **Malignant neoplasm of connective and soft tissue** ▽ **of unspecified upper limb, including shoulder**

C49.11 **Malignant neoplasm of connective and soft tissue of** right **upper limb, including shoulder**

C49.12 **Malignant neoplasm of connective and soft tissue of** left **upper limb, including shoulder**

✓5ᵗʰ **C49.2** **Malignant neoplasm of connective and soft tissue of** lower limb, including hip

C49.20 **Malignant neoplasm of connective and soft tissue** ▽ **of unspecified lower limb, including hip**

C49.21 **Malignant neoplasm of connective and soft tissue of** right **lower limb, including hip**

C49.22 **Malignant neoplasm of connective and soft tissue of** left **lower limb, including hip**

C49.3 **Malignant neoplasm of connective and soft tissue of** thorax
Malignant neoplasm of axilla
Malignant neoplasm of diaphragm
Malignant neoplasm of great vessels
EXCLUDES 1   malignant neoplasm of breast (C50.-)
malignant neoplasm of heart (C38.0)
malignant neoplasm of mediastinum (C38.1-C38.3)
malignant neoplasm of thymus (C37)

C49.4 **Malignant neoplasm of connective and soft tissue of** abdomen
Malignant neoplasm of abdominal wall
Malignant neoplasm of hypochondrium

C49.5 **Malignant neoplasm of connective and soft tissue of** pelvis
Malignant neoplasm of buttock
Malignant neoplasm of groin
Malignant neoplasm of perineum

C49.6 **Malignant neoplasm of connective and soft tissue of** ▽ trunk, unspecified
Malignant neoplasm of back NOS

C49.8 **Malignant neoplasm of** overlapping sites **of connective and soft tissue**
Primary malignant neoplasm of two or more contiguous sites of connective and soft tissue

C49.9 **Malignant neoplasm of connective and soft tissue,** ▽ unspecified

Malignant neoplasms of breast (C50)

✓4ᵗʰ **C50** **Malignant neoplasm of** breast
INCLUDES   connective tissue of breast
Paget's disease of breast
Paget's disease of nipple
Use additional code to identify estrogen receptor status (Z17.0, Z17.1)
EXCLUDES 1   skin of breast (C44.501, C44.511, C44.521, C44.591)

✓5ᵗʰ **C50.0** **Malignant neoplasm of** nipple and areola

✓6ᵗʰ **C50.01** **Malignant neoplasm of nipple and areola,** female

C50.011 **Malignant neoplasm of nipple and**   ♀
areola, right **female breast**

C50.012 **Malignant neoplasm of nipple and**   ♀
areola, left **female breast**

C50.019 **Malignant neoplasm of nipple and**   ♀▽
areola, unspecified female breast

✓6ᵗʰ **C50.02** **Malignant neoplasm of nipple and areola,** male

C50.021 **Malignant neoplasm of nipple and**   ♂
areola, right **male breast**

C50.022 **Malignant neoplasm of nipple and**   ♂
areola, left **male breast**

C50.029 **Malignant neoplasm of nipple and**   ♂▽
areola, unspecified male breast

✓5ᵗʰ **C50.1** **Malignant neoplasm of** central portion **of breast**

✓6ᵗʰ **C50.11** **Malignant neoplasm of central portion of breast,** female

C50.111 **Malignant neoplasm of central portion**   ♀
of right **female breast**

C50.112 **Malignant neoplasm of central portion**   ♀
of left **female breast**

C50.119 **Malignant neoplasm of central**   ♀▽
portion of unspecified female breast

✓6ᵗʰ **C50.12** **Malignant neoplasm of central portion of breast,** male

C50.121 **Malignant neoplasm of central portion**   ♂
of right **male breast**

C50.122 **Malignant neoplasm of central portion**   ♂
of left **male breast**

C50.129 **Malignant neoplasm of central**   ♂▽
portion of unspecified male breast

✓5ᵗʰ **C50.2** **Malignant neoplasm of** upper-inner quadrant **of breast**

✓6ᵗʰ **C50.21** **Malignant neoplasm of upper-inner quadrant of breast,** female

C50.211 **Malignant neoplasm of upper-inner**   ♀
quadrant of right **female breast**

C50.212 **Malignant neoplasm of upper-inner**   ♀
quadrant of left **female breast**

C50.219 **Malignant neoplasm of upper-inner**   ♀▽
quadrant of unspecified female breast

✓6ᵗʰ **C50.22** **Malignant neoplasm of upper-inner quadrant of breast,** male

C50.221 **Malignant neoplasm of upper-inner**   ♂
quadrant of right **male breast**

C50.222 **Malignant neoplasm of upper-inner**   ♂
quadrant of left **male breast**

C50.229 **Malignant neoplasm of upper-inner**   ♂▽
quadrant of unspecified male breast

✓5ᵗʰ **C50.3** **Malignant neoplasm of** lower-inner quadrant **of breast**

✓6ᵗʰ **C50.31** **Malignant neoplasm of lower-inner quadrant of breast,** female

C50.311 **Malignant neoplasm of lower-inner**   ♀
quadrant of right **female breast**

C50.312 **Malignant neoplasm of lower-inner**   ♀
quadrant of left **female breast**

C50.319 **Malignant neoplasm of lower-inner**   ♀▽
quadrant of unspecified female breast

✓6ᵗʰ **C50.32** **Malignant neoplasm of lower-inner quadrant of breast,** male

C50.321 **Malignant neoplasm of lower-inner**   ♂
quadrant of right **male breast**

C50.322 **Malignant neoplasm of lower-inner**   ♂
quadrant of left **male breast**

C50.329 **Malignant neoplasm of lower-inner**   ♂▽
quadrant of unspecified male breast

Ⓝ Newborn   Ⓟ Pediatric   Ⓜ Maternity   Ⓐ Adult   RIC RIC Dx   NC Dx Noncancer Dx   PDx Primary Dx   CC RIC CC Condition   ►◄ Revised Text   ● New Code   ▲ Revised Code Title

456   ICD-10-CM 2016

✓5ᵗʰ **C50.4 Malignant neoplasm of upper-outer quadrant of breast**

    ✓6ᵗʰ **C50.41 Malignant neoplasm of upper-outer quadrant of breast, female**

        C50.411 Malignant neoplasm of upper-outer quadrant of right female breast ♀

        C50.412 Malignant neoplasm of upper-outer quadrant of left female breast ♀

        C50.419 Malignant neoplasm of upper-outer quadrant of unspecified female breast ♀▽

    ✓6ᵗʰ **C50.42 Malignant neoplasm of upper-outer quadrant of breast, male**

        C50.421 Malignant neoplasm of upper-outer quadrant of right male breast ♂

        C50.422 Malignant neoplasm of upper-outer quadrant of left male breast ♂

        C50.429 Malignant neoplasm of upper-outer quadrant of unspecified male breast ♂▽

✓5ᵗʰ **C50.5 Malignant neoplasm of lower-outer quadrant of breast**

    ✓6ᵗʰ **C50.51 Malignant neoplasm of lower-outer quadrant of breast, female**

        C50.511 Malignant neoplasm of lower-outer quadrant of right female breast ♀

        C50.512 Malignant neoplasm of lower-outer quadrant of left female breast ♀

        C50.519 Malignant neoplasm of lower-outer quadrant of unspecified female breast ♀▽

    ✓6ᵗʰ **C50.52 Malignant neoplasm of lower-outer quadrant of breast, male**

        C50.521 Malignant neoplasm of lower-outer quadrant of right male breast ♂

        C50.522 Malignant neoplasm of lower-outer quadrant of left male breast ♂

        C50.529 Malignant neoplasm of lower-outer quadrant of unspecified male breast ♂▽

✓5ᵗʰ **C50.6 Malignant neoplasm of axillary tail of breast**

    ✓6ᵗʰ **C50.61 Malignant neoplasm of axillary tail of breast, female**

        C50.611 Malignant neoplasm of axillary tail of right female breast ♀

        C50.612 Malignant neoplasm of axillary tail of left female breast ♀

        C50.619 Malignant neoplasm of axillary tail of unspecified female breast ♀▽

    ✓6ᵗʰ **C50.62 Malignant neoplasm of axillary tail of breast, male**

        C50.621 Malignant neoplasm of axillary tail of right male breast ♂

        C50.622 Malignant neoplasm of axillary tail of left male breast ♂

        C50.629 Malignant neoplasm of axillary tail of unspecified male breast ♂▽

✓5ᵗʰ **C50.8 Malignant neoplasm of overlapping sites of breast**

    ✓6ᵗʰ **C50.81 Malignant neoplasm of overlapping sites of breast, female**

        C50.811 Malignant neoplasm of overlapping sites of right female breast ♀

        C50.812 Malignant neoplasm of overlapping sites of left female breast ♀

        C50.819 Malignant neoplasm of overlapping sites of unspecified female breast ♀▽

    ✓6ᵗʰ **C50.82 Malignant neoplasm of overlapping sites of breast, male**

        C50.821 Malignant neoplasm of overlapping sites of right male breast ♂

        C50.822 Malignant neoplasm of overlapping sites of left male breast ♂

        C50.829 Malignant neoplasm of overlapping sites of unspecified male breast ♂▽

✓5ᵗʰ **C50.9 Malignant neoplasm of breast of unspecified site**

    ✓6ᵗʰ **C50.91 Malignant neoplasm of breast of unspecified site, female**

        C50.911 Malignant neoplasm of unspecified site of right female breast ♀

        C50.912 Malignant neoplasm of unspecified site of left female breast ♀

        C50.919 Malignant neoplasm of unspecified site of unspecified female breast ♀▽

    ✓6ᵗʰ **C50.92 Malignant neoplasm of breast of unspecified site, male**

        C50.921 Malignant neoplasm of unspecified site of right male breast ♂

        C50.922 Malignant neoplasm of unspecified site of left male breast ♂

        C50.929 Malignant neoplasm of unspecified site of unspecified male breast ♂▽

Malignant neoplasms of female genital organs (C51-C58)

INCLUDES   malignant neoplasm of skin of female genital organs

✓4ᵗʰ **C51 Malignant neoplasm of vulva**

EXCLUDES 1   carcinoma in situ of vulva (D07.1)

    C51.0 Malignant neoplasm of labium majus ♀
        Malignant neoplasm of Bartholin's [greater vestibular] gland

    C51.1 Malignant neoplasm of labium minus ♀

    C51.2 Malignant neoplasm of clitoris ♀

    C51.8 Malignant neoplasm of overlapping sites of vulva ♀

    C51.9 Malignant neoplasm of vulva, unspecified ♀▽
        Malignant neoplasm of external female genitalia NOS
        Malignant neoplasm of pudendum

    C52 Malignant neoplasm of vagina ♀
    EXCLUDES 1   carcinoma in situ of vagina (D07.2)

✓4ᵗʰ **C53 Malignant neoplasm of cervix uteri**
    EXCLUDES 1   carcinoma in situ of cervix uteri (D06.-)

    C53.0 Malignant neoplasm of endocervix ♀

    C53.1 Malignant neoplasm of exocervix ♀

    C53.8 Malignant neoplasm of overlapping sites of cervix uteri ♀

    C53.9 Malignant neoplasm of cervix uteri, unspecified ♀▽

✓4ᵗʰ **C54 Malignant neoplasm of corpus uteri**

    C54.0 Malignant neoplasm of isthmus uteri ♀
        Malignant neoplasm of lower uterine segment

    C54.1 Malignant neoplasm of endometrium ♀

    C54.2 Malignant neoplasm of myometrium ♀

    C54.3 Malignant neoplasm of fundus uteri ♀

    C54.8 Malignant neoplasm of overlapping sites of corpus uteri ♀

    C54.9 Malignant neoplasm of corpus uteri, unspecified ♀▽

    C55 Malignant neoplasm of uterus, part unspecified ♀▽

✓4ᵗʰ **C56 Malignant neoplasm of ovary**
    Use additional code to identify any functional activity

    C56.1 Malignant neoplasm of right ovary ♀

    C56.2 Malignant neoplasm of left ovary ♀

    C56.9 Malignant neoplasm of unspecified ovary ♀▽

✓4ᵗʰ **C57 Malignant neoplasm of other and unspecified female genital organs**

    ✓5ᵗʰ **C57.0 Malignant neoplasm of fallopian tube**
        Malignant neoplasm of oviduct
        Malignant neoplasm of uterine tube

        C57.00 Malignant neoplasm of unspecified fallopian tube ♀▽

        C57.01 Malignant neoplasm of right fallopian tube ♀

        C57.02 Malignant neoplasm of left fallopian tube ♀

    ✓5ᵗʰ **C57.1 Malignant neoplasm of broad ligament**

        C57.10 Malignant neoplasm of unspecified broad ligament ♀▽

        C57.11 Malignant neoplasm of right broad ligament ♀

        C57.12 Malignant neoplasm of left broad ligament ♀

    ✓5ᵗʰ **C57.2 Malignant neoplasm of round ligament**

        C57.20 Malignant neoplasm of unspecified round ligament ♀▽

        C57.21 Malignant neoplasm of right round ligament ♀

        C57.22 Malignant neoplasm of left round ligament ♀

    C57.3 Malignant neoplasm of parametrium ♀
        Malignant neoplasm of uterine ligament NOS

    C57.4 Malignant neoplasm of uterine adnexa, unspecified ♀▽

    C57.7 Malignant neoplasm of other specified female genital organs ♀
        Malignant neoplasm of wolffian body or duct

✓ Add'l Character Required   ✗x7ᵗʰ Placeholder Alert   RUG IV Special Care High Dx   RUG IV Clinically Complex Dx   RUG IV Special Care Low Dx   Manifestation Code   Other Specified Code   ▽ Unspecified Code

C57.8 Malignant neoplasm of overlapping sites **of female genital organs** ♀

Primary malignant neoplasm of two or more contiguous sites of the female genital organs whose point of origin cannot be determined

Primary tubo-ovarian malignant neoplasm whose point of origin cannot be determined

Primary utero-ovarian malignant neoplasm whose point of origin cannot be determined

C57.9 Malignant neoplasm of female genital organ, unspecified ♀▽

Malignant neoplasm of female genitourinary tract NOS

C58 Malignant neoplasm of placenta ♀

INCLUDES choriocarcinoma NOS
chorionepithelioma NOS

EXCLUDES 1 chorioadenoma (destruens) (D39.2)
hydatidiform mole NOS (O01.9)
invasive hydatidiform mole (D39.2)
male choriocarcinoma NOS (C62.9-)
malignant hydatidiform mole (D39.2)

Malignant neoplasms of male genital organs (C60-C63)

INCLUDES malignant neoplasm of skin of male genital organs

✓4ᵗʰ **C60 Malignant neoplasm of** penis

C60.0 Malignant neoplasm of prepuce ♂
Malignant neoplasm of foreskin

C60.1 Malignant neoplasm of glans **penis** ♂

C60.2 Malignant neoplasm of body **of penis** ♂
Malignant neoplasm of corpus cavernosum

C60.8 Malignant neoplasm of overlapping sites **of penis** ♂

C60.9 Malignant neoplasm of penis, unspecified ♂▽
Malignant neoplasm of skin of penis NOS

C61 Malignant neoplasm of prostate ♂
EXCLUDES 1 malignant neoplasm of seminal vesicle (C63.7)

✓4ᵗʰ **C62 Malignant neoplasm of** testis
Use additional code to identify any functional activity

  ✓5ᵗʰ **C62.0 Malignant neoplasm of** undescended **testis**
Malignant neoplasm of ectopic testis
Malignant neoplasm of retained testis

    C62.00 Malignant neoplasm of unspecified undescended testis ♂▽

    C62.01 Malignant neoplasm of undescended right **testis** ♂

    C62.02 Malignant neoplasm of undescended left **testis** ♂

  ✓5ᵗʰ **C62.1 Malignant neoplasm of** descended **testis**
Malignant neoplasm of scrotal testis

    C62.10 Malignant neoplasm of unspecified descended testis ♂▽

    C62.11 Malignant neoplasm of descended right **testis** ♂

    C62.12 Malignant neoplasm of descended left **testis** ♂

  ✓5ᵗʰ **C62.9 Malignant neoplasm of testis, unspecified whether** descended or undescended

    C62.90 Malignant neoplasm of unspecified testis, unspecified whether descended or undescended ♂▽
Malignant neoplasm of testis NOS

    C62.91 Malignant neoplasm of right **testis, unspecified whether descended or undescended** ♂

    C62.92 Malignant neoplasm of left **testis, unspecified whether descended or undescended** ♂

✓4ᵗʰ **C63 Malignant neoplasm of** other and unspecified male genital organs

  ✓5ᵗʰ **C63.0 Malignant neoplasm of** epididymis

    C63.00 Malignant neoplasm of unspecified epididymis ♂▽

    C63.01 Malignant neoplasm of right **epididymis** ♂

    C63.02 Malignant neoplasm of left **epididymis** ♂

  ✓5ᵗʰ **C63.1 Malignant neoplasm of** spermatic cord

    C63.10 Malignant neoplasm of unspecified spermatic cord ♂▽

    C63.11 Malignant neoplasm of right **spermatic cord** ♂

    C63.12 Malignant neoplasm of left **spermatic cord** ♂

  C63.2 Malignant neoplasm of scrotum ♂
Malignant neoplasm of skin of scrotum

  C63.7 Malignant neoplasm of other specified **male genital organs** ♂
Malignant neoplasm of seminal vesicle
Malignant neoplasm of tunica vaginalis

C63.8 Malignant neoplasm of overlapping sites **of male genital organs** ♂

Primary malignant neoplasm of two or more contiguous sites of male genital organs whose point of origin cannot be determined

C63.9 Malignant neoplasm of male genital organ, unspecified ♂▽
Malignant neoplasm of male genitourinary tract NOS

Malignant neoplasms of urinary tract (C64-C68)

✓4ᵗʰ **C64 Malignant neoplasm of** kidney, except renal pelvis
EXCLUDES 1 malignant carcinoid tumor of the kidney (C7A.093)
malignant neoplasm of renal calyces (C65.-)
malignant neoplasm of renal pelvis (C65.-)

C64.1 Malignant neoplasm of right **kidney, except renal pelvis**

C64.2 Malignant neoplasm of left **kidney, except renal pelvis**

C64.9 Malignant neoplasm of unspecified kidney, except renal pelvis ▽

✓4ᵗʰ **C65 Malignant neoplasm of** renal pelvis
INCLUDES malignant neoplasm of pelviureteric junction
malignant neoplasm of renal calyces

C65.1 Malignant neoplasm of right **renal pelvis**

C65.2 Malignant neoplasm of left **renal pelvis**

C65.9 Malignant neoplasm of unspecified renal pelvis ▽

✓4ᵗʰ **C66 Malignant neoplasm of** ureter
EXCLUDES 1 malignant neoplasm of ureteric orifice of bladder (C67.6)

C66.1 Malignant neoplasm of right **ureter**

C66.2 Malignant neoplasm of left **ureter**

C66.9 Malignant neoplasm of unspecified ureter ▽

✓4ᵗʰ **C67 Malignant neoplasm of** bladder

C67.0 Malignant neoplasm of trigone **of bladder**

C67.1 Malignant neoplasm of dome **of bladder**

C67.2 Malignant neoplasm of lateral wall **of bladder**

C67.3 Malignant neoplasm of anterior wall **of bladder**

C67.4 Malignant neoplasm of posterior wall **of bladder**

C67.5 Malignant neoplasm of bladder neck
Malignant neoplasm of internal urethral orifice

C67.6 Malignant neoplasm of ureteric orifice

C67.7 Malignant neoplasm of urachus

C67.8 Malignant neoplasm of overlapping sites **of bladder**

C67.9 Malignant neoplasm of bladder, unspecified ▽

✓4ᵗʰ **C68 Malignant neoplasm of** other and unspecified urinary organs
EXCLUDES 1 malignant neoplasm of female genitourinary tract NOS (C57.9)
malignant neoplasm of male genitourinary tract NOS (C63.9)

C68.0 Malignant neoplasm of urethra
EXCLUDES 1 malignant neoplasm of urethral orifice of bladder (C67.5)

C68.1 Malignant neoplasm of paraurethral glands

C68.8 Malignant neoplasm of overlapping sites **of urinary organs**
Primary malignant neoplasm of two or more contiguous sites of urinary organs whose point of origin cannot be determined

C68.9 Malignant neoplasm of urinary organ, unspecified ▽
Malignant neoplasm of urinary system NOS

Malignant neoplasms of eye, brain and other parts of central nervous system (C69-C72)

✓4ᵗʰ **C69 Malignant neoplasm of** eye and adnexa
EXCLUDES 1 malignant neoplasm of connective tissue of eyelid (C49.0)
malignant neoplasm of eyelid (skin) (C43.1-, C44.1-)
malignant neoplasm of optic nerve (C72.3-)

  ✓5ᵗʰ **C69.0 Malignant neoplasm of** conjunctiva

    C69.00 Malignant neoplasm of unspecified conjunctiva ▽

    C69.01 Malignant neoplasm of right **conjunctiva**

    C69.02 Malignant neoplasm of left **conjunctiva**

  ✓5ᵗʰ **C69.1 Malignant neoplasm of** cornea

    C69.10 Malignant neoplasm of unspecified cornea ▽

    C69.11 Malignant neoplasm of right **cornea**

    C69.12 Malignant neoplasm of left **cornea**

Ⓝ Newborn   Ⓟ Pediatric   Ⓜ Maternity   Ⓐ Adult   RIC RIC Dx   NCDx Noncancer Dx   PDx Primary Dx   CC RIC CC Condition   ▶◀ Revised Text   ● New Code   ▲ Revised Code Title

458   ICD-10-CM 2016

✓5ᵗʰ C69.2 Malignant neoplasm of retina

    EXCLUDES 1   dark area on retina (D49.81)
                     neoplasm of unspecified behavior of retina and choroid
                         (D49.81)
                     retinal freckle (D49.81)

    C69.20 Malignant neoplasm of unspecified retina ▽
    C69.21 Malignant neoplasm of right **retina**
    C69.22 Malignant neoplasm of left **retina**

✓5ᵗʰ C69.3 Malignant neoplasm of choroid

    C69.30 Malignant neoplasm of unspecified choroid ▽
    C69.31 Malignant neoplasm of right **choroid**
    C69.32 Malignant neoplasm of left **choroid**

✓5ᵗʰ C69.4 Malignant neoplasm of ciliary body

    C69.40 Malignant neoplasm of unspecified ciliary body ▽
    C69.41 Malignant neoplasm of right **ciliary body**
    C69.42 Malignant neoplasm of left **ciliary body**

✓5ᵗʰ C69.5 Malignant neoplasm of lacrimal gland and duct

    Malignant neoplasm of lacrimal sac
    Malignant neoplasm of nasolacrimal duct

    C69.50 Malignant neoplasm of unspecified lacrimal ▽
         gland and duct
    C69.51 Malignant neoplasm of right **lacrimal gland and duct**
    C69.52 Malignant neoplasm of left **lacrimal gland and duct**

✓5ᵗʰ C69.6 Malignant neoplasm of orbit

    Malignant neoplasm of connective tissue of orbit
    Malignant neoplasm of extraocular muscle
    Malignant neoplasm of peripheral nerves of orbit
    Malignant neoplasm of retrobulbar tissue
    Malignant neoplasm of retro-ocular tissue
    EXCLUDES 1   malignant neoplasm of orbital bone (C41.0)

    C69.60 Malignant neoplasm of unspecified orbit ▽
    C69.61 Malignant neoplasm of right **orbit**
    C69.62 Malignant neoplasm of left **orbit**

✓5ᵗʰ C69.8 Malignant neoplasm of overlapping sites **of eye and adnexa**

    C69.80 Malignant neoplasm of overlapping sites of ▽
         unspecified eye and adnexa
    C69.81 Malignant neoplasm of overlapping sites of right
         eye and adnexa
    C69.82 Malignant neoplasm of overlapping sites of left **eye and adnexa**

✓5ᵗʰ C69.9 Malignant neoplasm of unspecified **site of eye**

    Malignant neoplasm of eyeball

    C69.90 Malignant neoplasm of unspecified site of ▽
         unspecified eye
    C69.91 Malignant neoplasm of unspecified site of right **eye**
    C69.92 Malignant neoplasm of unspecified site of left **eye**

✓4ᵗʰ C70 Malignant neoplasm of meninges

    C70.0 Malignant neoplasm of cerebral **meninges**
    C70.1 Malignant neoplasm of spinal **meninges**
    C70.9 Malignant neoplasm of meninges, unspecified ▽

✓4ᵗʰ C71 Malignant neoplasm of brain

    EXCLUDES 1   malignant neoplasm of cranial nerves (C72.2-C72.5)
                retrobulbar malignant neoplasm (C69.6-)

    C71.0 Malignant neoplasm of cerebrum, except lobes and ventricles
         Malignant neoplasm of supratentorial NOS
    C71.1 Malignant neoplasm of frontal **lobe**
    C71.2 Malignant neoplasm of temporal **lobe**
    C71.3 Malignant neoplasm of parietal **lobe**
    C71.4 Malignant neoplasm of occipital **lobe**
    C71.5 Malignant neoplasm of cerebral **ventricle**
         EXCLUDES 1   malignant neoplasm of fourth cerebral ventricle (C71.7)
    C71.6 Malignant neoplasm of cerebellum
    C71.7 Malignant neoplasm of brain stem
         Malignant neoplasm of fourth cerebral ventricle
         Infratentorial malignant neoplasm NOS
    C71.8 Malignant neoplasm of overlapping sites **of brain**
    C71.9 Malignant neoplasm of brain, unspecified ▽
         AHA: 2014, 3Q, 3

✓4ᵗʰ C72 Malignant neoplasm of spinal cord, cranial nerves and other **parts of central nervous system**

    EXCLUDES 1   malignant neoplasm of meninges (C70.-)
                malignant neoplasm of peripheral nerves and autonomic
                    nervous system (C47.-)

    C72.0 Malignant neoplasm of spinal cord
    C72.1 Malignant neoplasm of cauda equina

✓5ᵗʰ C72.2 Malignant neoplasm of olfactory nerve

    Malignant neoplasm of olfactory bulb

    C72.20 Malignant neoplasm of unspecified olfactory ▽
         nerve
    C72.21 Malignant neoplasm of right **olfactory nerve**
    C72.22 Malignant neoplasm of left **olfactory nerve**

✓5ᵗʰ C72.3 Malignant neoplasm of optic nerve

    C72.30 Malignant neoplasm of unspecified optic nerve ▽
    C72.31 Malignant neoplasm of right **optic nerve**
    C72.32 Malignant neoplasm of left **optic nerve**

✓5ᵗʰ C72.4 Malignant neoplasm of acoustic nerve

    C72.40 Malignant neoplasm of unspecified acoustic ▽
         nerve
    C72.41 Malignant neoplasm of right **acoustic nerve**
    C72.42 Malignant neoplasm of left **acoustic nerve**

✓5ᵗʰ C72.5 Malignant neoplasm of other and unspecified cranial nerves

    C72.50 Malignant neoplasm of unspecified cranial nerve ▽
         Malignant neoplasm of cranial nerve NOS
    C72.59 Malignant neoplasm of other cranial nerves

    C72.9 Malignant neoplasm of central nervous system, ▽
    unspecified
         Malignant neoplasm of unspecified site of central nervous
           system
         Malignant neoplasm of nervous system NOS

Malignant neoplasms of thyroid and other endocrine glands (C73-C75)

C73 Malignant neoplasm of thyroid gland

    Use additional code to identify any functional activity

✓4ᵗʰ C74 Malignant neoplasm of adrenal gland

✓5ᵗʰ C74.0 Malignant neoplasm of cortex **of adrenal gland**

    C74.00 Malignant neoplasm of cortex of unspecified ▽
         adrenal gland
    C74.01 Malignant neoplasm of cortex of right **adrenal gland**
    C74.02 Malignant neoplasm of cortex of left **adrenal gland**

✓5ᵗʰ C74.1 Malignant neoplasm of medulla **of adrenal gland**

    C74.10 Malignant neoplasm of medulla of unspecified ▽
         adrenal gland
    C74.11 Malignant neoplasm of medulla of right **adrenal gland**
    C74.12 Malignant neoplasm of medulla of left **adrenal gland**

✓5ᵗʰ C74.9 Malignant neoplasm of unspecified part **of adrenal gland**

    C74.90 Malignant neoplasm of unspecified part of ▽
         unspecified adrenal gland
    C74.91 Malignant neoplasm of unspecified part of right **adrenal gland**
    C74.92 Malignant neoplasm of unspecified part of left **adrenal gland**

✓4ᵗʰ C75 Malignant neoplasm of other endocrine glands and related **structures**

    EXCLUDES 1   malignant carcinoid tumors (C7A.0-)
                malignant neoplasm of adrenal gland (C74.-)
                malignant neoplasm of endocrine pancreas (C25.4)
                malignant neoplasm of islets of Langerhans (C25.4)
                malignant neoplasm of ovary (C56.-)
                malignant neoplasm of testis (C62.-)
                malignant neoplasm of thymus (C37)
                malignant neoplasm of thyroid gland (C73)
                malignant neuroendocrine tumors (C7A.-)

    C75.0 Malignant neoplasm of parathyroid **gland**
    C75.1 Malignant neoplasm of pituitary **gland**
    C75.2 Malignant neoplasm of craniopharyngeal duct
    C75.3 Malignant neoplasm of pineal **gland**
    C75.4 Malignant neoplasm of carotid body
    C75.5 Malignant neoplasm of aortic body and other paraganglia
    C75.8 Malignant neoplasm with pluriglandular involvement, unspecified

---

☑ Add'l Character Required   ✓x7ᵗʰ Placeholder Alert   RUG IV Special Care High Dx   RUG IV Clinically Complex Dx   RUG IV Special Care Low Dx   Manifestation Code   Other Specified Code   ▽ Unspecified Code

ICD-10-CM 2016   459

C75.9 Malignant neoplasm of endocrine gland, unspecified ▽

Malignant neuroendocrine tumors (C7A)

✓4th C7A Malignant neuroendocrine tumors
Code also any associated multiple endocrine neoplasia [MEN] syndromes (E31.2-)
Use additional code to identify any associated endocrine syndrome, such as:
carcinoid syndrome (E34.0)
EXCLUDES 2   *malignant pancreatic islet cell tumors (C25.4)*
Merkel cell carcinoma (C4A.-)

✓5th C7A.0 Malignant carcinoid tumors

    C7A.00 Malignant carcinoid tumor of unspecified site ▽

    ✓6th C7A.01 Malignant carcinoid tumors of the small intestine

        C7A.010 Malignant carcinoid tumor of the duodenum

        C7A.011 Malignant carcinoid tumor of the jejunum

        C7A.012 Malignant carcinoid tumor of the ileum

        C7A.019 Malignant carcinoid tumor of the small ▽ intestine, unspecified portion

    ✓6th C7A.02 Malignant carcinoid tumors of the appendix, large intestine, and rectum

        C7A.020 Malignant carcinoid tumor of the appendix

        C7A.021 Malignant carcinoid tumor of the cecum

        C7A.022 Malignant carcinoid tumor of the ascending colon

        C7A.023 Malignant carcinoid tumor of the transverse colon

        C7A.024 Malignant carcinoid tumor of the descending colon

        C7A.025 Malignant carcinoid tumor of the sigmoid colon

        C7A.026 Malignant carcinoid tumor of the rectum

        C7A.029 Malignant carcinoid tumor of the ▽ large intestine, unspecified portion
             Malignant carcinoid tumor of the colon NOS

    ✓6th C7A.09 Malignant carcinoid tumors of other sites

        C7A.090 Malignant carcinoid tumor of the bronchus and lung

        C7A.091 Malignant carcinoid tumor of the thymus

        C7A.092 Malignant carcinoid tumor of the stomach

        C7A.093 Malignant carcinoid tumor of the kidney

        C7A.094 Malignant carcinoid tumor of the foregut NOS

        C7A.095 Malignant carcinoid tumor of the midgut NOS

        C7A.096 Malignant carcinoid tumor of the hindgut NOS

        C7A.098 Malignant carcinoid tumors of other sites

    C7A.1 Malignant poorly differentiated neuroendocrine tumors
         High grade neuroendocrine carcinoma, any site
         Malignant poorly differentiated neuroendocrine tumor NOS
         Malignant poorly differentiated neuroendocrine carcinoma, any site

    C7A.8 Other malignant neuroendocrine tumors

Secondary neuroendocrine tumors (C7B)

✓4th C7B Secondary neuroendocrine tumors
Use additional code to identify any functional activity

✓5th C7B.0 Secondary carcinoid tumors

    C7B.00 Secondary carcinoid tumors, unspecified site ▽

    C7B.01 Secondary carcinoid tumors of distant lymph nodes

    C7B.02 Secondary carcinoid tumors of liver

    C7B.03 Secondary carcinoid tumors of bone

    C7B.04 Secondary carcinoid tumors of peritoneum
         Mesentery metastasis of carcinoid tumor

    C7B.09 Secondary carcinoid tumors of other sites

    C7B.1 Secondary Merkel cell carcinoma
         Merkel cell carcinoma nodal presentation
         Merkel cell carcinoma visceral metastatic presentation

    C7B.8 Other secondary neuroendocrine tumors

Malignant neoplasms of ill-defined, other secondary and unspecified sites (C76-C80)

✓4th C76 Malignant neoplasm of other and ill-defined sites
EXCLUDES 1   *malignant neoplasm of female genitourinary tract NOS (C57.9)*
malignant neoplasm of male genitourinary tract NOS (C63.9)
malignant neoplasm of lymphoid, hematopoietic and related tissue (C81-C96)
malignant neoplasm of skin (C44.-)
malignant neoplasm of unspecified site NOS (C80.1)

  C76.0 Malignant neoplasm of head, face and neck
      Malignant neoplasm of cheek NOS
      Malignant neoplasm of nose NOS

  C76.1 Malignant neoplasm of thorax
      Intrathoracic malignant neoplasm NOS
      Malignant neoplasm of axilla NOS
      Thoracic malignant neoplasm NOS

  C76.2 Malignant neoplasm of abdomen

  C76.3 Malignant neoplasm of pelvis
      Malignant neoplasm of groin NOS
      Malignant neoplasm of sites overlapping systems within the pelvis
      Rectovaginal (septum) malignant neoplasm
      Rectovesical (septum) malignant neoplasm

  ✓5th C76.4 Malignant neoplasm of upper limb

    C76.40 Malignant neoplasm of unspecified upper limb ▽

    C76.41 Malignant neoplasm of right upper limb

    C76.42 Malignant neoplasm of left upper limb

  ✓5th C76.5 Malignant neoplasm of lower limb

    C76.50 Malignant neoplasm of unspecified lower limb ▽

    C76.51 Malignant neoplasm of right lower limb

    C76.52 Malignant neoplasm of left lower limb

  C76.8 Malignant neoplasm of other specified ill-defined sites
      Malignant neoplasm of overlapping ill-defined sites

✓4th C77 Secondary and unspecified malignant neoplasm of lymph nodes
EXCLUDES 1   *malignant neoplasm of lymph nodes, specified as primary (C81-C86, C88, C96.-)*
mesentery metastasis of carcinoid tumor (C7B.04)
secondary carcinoid tumors of distant lymph nodes (C7B.01)

  C77.0 Secondary and unspecified malignant neoplasm of lymph nodes of head, face and neck
      Secondary and unspecified malignant neoplasm of supraclavicular lymph nodes

  C77.1 Secondary and unspecified malignant neoplasm of intrathoracic lymph nodes

  C77.2 Secondary and unspecified malignant neoplasm of intra-abdominal lymph nodes

  C77.3 Secondary and unspecified malignant neoplasm of axilla and upper limb lymph nodes
      Secondary and unspecified malignant neoplasm of pectoral lymph nodes

  C77.4 Secondary and unspecified malignant neoplasm of inguinal and lower limb lymph nodes

  C77.5 Secondary and unspecified malignant neoplasm of intrapelvic lymph nodes

  C77.8 Secondary and unspecified malignant neoplasm of lymph nodes of multiple regions

  C77.9 Secondary and unspecified malignant neoplasm of ▽ lymph node, unspecified

✓4th C78 Secondary malignant neoplasm of respiratory and digestive organs
EXCLUDES 1   *lymph node metastases (C77.0)*
secondary carcinoid tumors of liver (C7B.02)
secondary carcinoid tumors of peritoneum (C7B.04)

  ✓5th C78.0 Secondary malignant neoplasm of lung

    C78.00 Secondary malignant neoplasm of unspecified ▽ lung

    C78.01 Secondary malignant neoplasm of right lung

    C78.02 Secondary malignant neoplasm of left lung

  C78.1 Secondary malignant neoplasm of mediastinum

  C78.2 Secondary malignant neoplasm of pleura

  ✓5th C78.3 Secondary malignant neoplasm of other and unspecified respiratory organs

    C78.30 Secondary malignant neoplasm of unspecified ▽ respiratory organ

    C78.39 Secondary malignant neoplasm of other respiratory organs

---

N Newborn   **P** Pediatric   **M** Maternity   **A** Adult   **RIC** RIC Dx   **NCDx** Noncancer Dx   **PDx** Primary Dx   **CC** RIC CC Condition   ►◄ Revised Text   ● New Code   ▲ Revised Code Title

C78.4 Secondary malignant neoplasm of small intestine

C78.5 Secondary malignant neoplasm of large intestine and rectum

C78.6 Secondary malignant neoplasm of retroperitoneum and peritoneum

C78.7 Secondary malignant neoplasm of liver and intrahepatic bile duct

✓5ᵗʰ **C78.8** Secondary malignant neoplasm of other and unspecified digestive organs

     C78.80 Secondary malignant neoplasm of unspecified ▽ digestive organ

     C78.89 Secondary malignant neoplasm of other digestive organs

✓4ᵗʰ **C79** Secondary malignant neoplasm of other and unspecified sites

     EXCLUDES 1   *lymph node metastases (C77.0)*
       secondary carcinoid tumors (C7B.-)
       secondary neuroendocrine tumors (C7B.-)

✓5ᵗʰ **C79.0** Secondary malignant neoplasm of kidney and renal pelvis

     C79.00 Secondary malignant neoplasm of unspecified ▽ kidney and renal pelvis

     C79.01 Secondary malignant neoplasm of right kidney and renal pelvis

     C79.02 Secondary malignant neoplasm of left kidney and renal pelvis

✓5ᵗʰ **C79.1** Secondary malignant neoplasm of bladder and other and unspecified urinary organs

     C79.10 Secondary malignant neoplasm of unspecified ▽ urinary organs

     C79.11 Secondary malignant neoplasm of bladder

     C79.19 Secondary malignant neoplasm of other urinary organs

C79.2 Secondary malignant neoplasm of skin

     EXCLUDES 1   *secondary Merkel cell carcinoma (C7B.1)*

✓5ᵗʰ **C79.3** Secondary malignant neoplasm of brain and cerebral meninges

     C79.31 Secondary malignant neoplasm of brain

     C79.32 Secondary malignant neoplasm of cerebral meninges

✓5ᵗʰ **C79.4** Secondary malignant neoplasm of other and unspecified parts of nervous system

     C79.40 Secondary malignant neoplasm of unspecified ▽ part of nervous system

     C79.49 Secondary malignant neoplasm of other parts of nervous system

✓5ᵗʰ **C79.5** Secondary malignant neoplasm of bone and bone marrow

     EXCLUDES 1   *secondary carcinoid tumors of bone (C7B.03)*

     C79.51 Secondary malignant neoplasm of bone

     C79.52 Secondary malignant neoplasm of bone marrow

✓5ᵗʰ **C79.6** Secondary malignant neoplasm of ovary

     C79.60 Secondary malignant neoplasm of unspecified ♀▽ ovary

     C79.61 Secondary malignant neoplasm of right ovary ♀

     C79.62 Secondary malignant neoplasm of left ovary ♀

✓5ᵗʰ **C79.7** Secondary malignant neoplasm of adrenal gland

     C79.70 Secondary malignant neoplasm of unspecified ▽ adrenal gland

     C79.71 Secondary malignant neoplasm of right adrenal gland

     C79.72 Secondary malignant neoplasm of left adrenal gland

✓5ᵗʰ **C79.8** Secondary malignant neoplasm of other specified sites

     C79.81 Secondary malignant neoplasm of breast

     C79.82 Secondary malignant neoplasm of genital organs

     C79.89 Secondary malignant neoplasm of other specified sites

C79.9 Secondary malignant neoplasm of unspecified site ▽
     Metastatic cancer NOS
     Metastatic disease NOS
     EXCLUDES 1   *carcinomatosis NOS (C80.0)*
       generalized cancer NOS (C80.0)
       malignant (primary) neoplasm of unspecified site
       (C80.1)

✓4ᵗʰ **C80** Malignant neoplasm without specification of site

     EXCLUDES 1   *malignant carcinoid tumor of unspecified site (C7A.00)*
       malignant neoplasm of specified multiple sites—code to each
       site

C80.0 Disseminated malignant neoplasm, unspecified ▽
     Carcinomatosis NOS
     Generalized cancer, unspecified site (primary) (secondary)
     Generalized malignancy, unspecified site (primary) (secondary)

C80.1 Malignant (primary) neoplasm, unspecified ▽
     Cancer NOS
     Cancer unspecified site (primary)
     Carcinoma unspecified site (primary)
     Malignancy unspecified site (primary)
     EXCLUDES 1   *secondary malignant neoplasm of unspecified site*
       (C79.9)

C80.2 Malignant neoplasm associated with transplanted organ
     Code first complication of transplanted organ (T86.-)
     Use additional code to identify the specific malignancy

Malignant neoplasms of lymphoid, hematopoietic and related tissue (C81-C96)

     EXCLUDES 2   *Kaposi's sarcoma of lymph nodes (C46.3)*
       secondary and unspecified neoplasm of lymph nodes (C77.-)
       secondary neoplasm of bone marrow (C79.52)
       secondary neoplasm of spleen (C78.89)

✓4ᵗʰ **C81** Hodgkin lymphoma

     EXCLUDES 1   *personal history of Hodgkin lymphoma (Z85.71)*

✓5ᵗʰ **C81.0** Nodular lymphocyte predominant Hodgkin lymphoma

     C81.00 Nodular lymphocyte predominant Hodgkin ▽ lymphoma, unspecified site

     C81.01 Nodular lymphocyte predominant Hodgkin lymphoma, lymph nodes of head, face, and neck

     C81.02 Nodular lymphocyte predominant Hodgkin lymphoma, intrathoracic lymph nodes

     C81.03 Nodular lymphocyte predominant Hodgkin lymphoma, intra-abdominal lymph nodes

     C81.04 Nodular lymphocyte predominant Hodgkin lymphoma, lymph nodes of axilla and upper limb

     C81.05 Nodular lymphocyte predominant Hodgkin lymphoma, lymph nodes of inguinal region and lower limb

     C81.06 Nodular lymphocyte predominant Hodgkin lymphoma, intrapelvic lymph nodes

     C81.07 Nodular lymphocyte predominant Hodgkin lymphoma, spleen

     C81.08 Nodular lymphocyte predominant Hodgkin lymphoma, lymph nodes of multiple sites

     C81.09 Nodular lymphocyte predominant Hodgkin lymphoma, extranodal and solid organ sites

✓5ᵗʰ **C81.1** Nodular sclerosis classical Hodgkin lymphoma

     C81.10 Nodular sclerosis classical Hodgkin lymphoma, ▽ unspecified site

     C81.11 Nodular sclerosis classical Hodgkin lymphoma, lymph nodes of head, face, and neck

     C81.12 Nodular sclerosis classical Hodgkin lymphoma, intrathoracic lymph nodes

     C81.13 Nodular sclerosis classical Hodgkin lymphoma, intra-abdominal lymph nodes

     C81.14 Nodular sclerosis classical Hodgkin lymphoma, lymph nodes of axilla and upper limb

     C81.15 Nodular sclerosis classical Hodgkin lymphoma, lymph nodes of inguinal region and lower limb

     C81.16 Nodular sclerosis classical Hodgkin lymphoma, intrapelvic lymph nodes

     C81.17 Nodular sclerosis classical Hodgkin lymphoma, spleen

     C81.18 Nodular sclerosis classical Hodgkin lymphoma, lymph nodes of multiple sites

     C81.19 Nodular sclerosis classical Hodgkin lymphoma, extranodal and solid organ sites

✓5ᵗʰ **C81.2** Mixed cellularity classical Hodgkin lymphoma

     C81.20 Mixed cellularity classical Hodgkin lymphoma, ▽ unspecified site

     C81.21 Mixed cellularity classical Hodgkin lymphoma, lymph nodes of head, face, and neck

     C81.22 Mixed cellularity classical Hodgkin lymphoma, intrathoracic lymph nodes

☑ Add'l Character Required   ✔x 7ᵗʰ Placeholder Alert   RUG IV Special Care High Dx   RUG IV Clinically Complex Dx   RUG IV Special Care Low Dx   Manifestation Code   Other Specified Code   ▽ Unspecified Code

ICD-10-CM 2016   **461**

Chapter 2. Neoplasms

C81.23 Mixed cellularity classical Hodgkin lymphoma, intra-abdominal lymph nodes

C81.24 Mixed cellularity classical Hodgkin lymphoma, lymph nodes of axilla and upper limb

C81.25 Mixed cellularity classical Hodgkin lymphoma, lymph nodes of inguinal region and lower limb

C81.26 Mixed cellularity classical Hodgkin lymphoma, intrapelvic lymph nodes

C81.27 Mixed cellularity classical Hodgkin lymphoma, spleen

C81.28 Mixed cellularity classical Hodgkin lymphoma, lymph nodes of multiple sites

C81.29 Mixed cellularity classical Hodgkin lymphoma, extranodal and solid organ sites

✓5ᵗʰ **C81.3 Lymphocyte-depleted classical Hodgkin lymphoma**

C81.30 Lymphocyte-depleted classical Hodgkin lymphoma, unspecified site ▽

C81.31 Lymphocyte-depleted classical Hodgkin lymphoma, lymph nodes of head, face, and neck

C81.32 Lymphocyte-depleted classical Hodgkin lymphoma, intrathoracic lymph nodes

C81.33 Lymphocyte-depleted classical Hodgkin lymphoma, intra-abdominal lymph nodes

C81.34 Lymphocyte-depleted classical Hodgkin lymphoma, lymph nodes of axilla and upper limb

C81.35 Lymphocyte-depleted classical Hodgkin lymphoma, lymph nodes of inguinal region and lower limb

C81.36 Lymphocyte-depleted classical Hodgkin lymphoma, intrapelvic lymph nodes

C81.37 Lymphocyte-depleted classical Hodgkin lymphoma, spleen

C81.38 Lymphocyte-depleted classical Hodgkin lymphoma, lymph nodes of multiple sites

C81.39 Lymphocyte-depleted classical Hodgkin lymphoma, extranodal and solid organ sites

✓5ᵗʰ **C81.4 Lymphocyte-rich classical Hodgkin lymphoma**

EXCLUDES 1 *nodular lymphocyte predominant Hodgkin lymphoma (C81.0-)*

C81.40 Lymphocyte-rich classical Hodgkin lymphoma, unspecified site ▽

C81.41 Lymphocyte-rich classical Hodgkin lymphoma, lymph nodes of head, face, and neck

C81.42 Lymphocyte-rich classical Hodgkin lymphoma, intrathoracic lymph nodes

C81.43 Lymphocyte-rich classical Hodgkin lymphoma, intra-abdominal lymph nodes

C81.44 Lymphocyte-rich classical Hodgkin lymphoma, lymph nodes of axilla and upper limb

C81.45 Lymphocyte-rich classical Hodgkin lymphoma, lymph nodes of inguinal region and lower limb

C81.46 Lymphocyte-rich classical Hodgkin lymphoma, intrapelvic lymph nodes

C81.47 Lymphocyte-rich classical Hodgkin lymphoma, spleen

C81.48 Lymphocyte-rich classical Hodgkin lymphoma, lymph nodes of multiple sites

C81.49 Lymphocyte-rich classical Hodgkin lymphoma, extranodal and solid organ sites

✓5ᵗʰ **C81.7 Other classical Hodgkin lymphoma**

Classical Hodgkin lymphoma NOS

C81.70 Other classical Hodgkin lymphoma, unspecified site ▽

C81.71 Other classical Hodgkin lymphoma, lymph nodes of head, face, and neck

C81.72 Other classical Hodgkin lymphoma, intrathoracic lymph nodes

C81.73 Other classical Hodgkin lymphoma, intra-abdominal lymph nodes

C81.74 Other classical Hodgkin lymphoma, lymph nodes of axilla and upper limb

C81.75 Other classical Hodgkin lymphoma, lymph nodes of inguinal region and lower limb

C81.76 Other classical Hodgkin lymphoma, intrapelvic lymph nodes

C81.77 Other classical Hodgkin lymphoma, spleen

C81.78 Other classical Hodgkin lymphoma, lymph nodes of multiple sites

C81.79 Other classical Hodgkin lymphoma, extranodal and solid organ sites

✓5ᵗʰ **C81.9 Hodgkin lymphoma, unspecified**

C81.90 Hodgkin lymphoma, unspecified, unspecified site ▽

C81.91 Hodgkin lymphoma, unspecified, lymph nodes of head, face, and neck ▽

C81.92 Hodgkin lymphoma, unspecified, intrathoracic lymph nodes ▽

C81.93 Hodgkin lymphoma, unspecified, intra-abdominal lymph nodes ▽

C81.94 Hodgkin lymphoma, unspecified, lymph nodes of axilla and upper limb ▽

C81.95 Hodgkin lymphoma, unspecified, lymph nodes of inguinal region and lower limb ▽

C81.96 Hodgkin lymphoma, unspecified, intrapelvic lymph nodes ▽

C81.97 Hodgkin lymphoma, unspecified, spleen ▽

C81.98 Hodgkin lymphoma, unspecified, lymph nodes of multiple sites ▽

C81.99 Hodgkin lymphoma, unspecified, extranodal and solid organ sites ▽

✓4ᵗʰ **C82 Follicular lymphoma**

INCLUDES follicular lymphoma with or without diffuse areas

EXCLUDES 1 *mature T/NK-cell lymphomas (C84.-)*
personal history of non-Hodgkin lymphoma (Z85.72)

✓5ᵗʰ **C82.0 Follicular lymphoma grade I**

C82.00 Follicular lymphoma grade I, unspecified site ▽

C82.01 Follicular lymphoma grade I, lymph nodes of head, face, and neck

C82.02 Follicular lymphoma grade I, intrathoracic lymph nodes

C82.03 Follicular lymphoma grade I, intra-abdominal lymph nodes

C82.04 Follicular lymphoma grade I, lymph nodes of axilla and upper limb

C82.05 Follicular lymphoma grade I, lymph nodes of inguinal region and lower limb

C82.06 Follicular lymphoma grade I, intrapelvic lymph nodes

C82.07 Follicular lymphoma grade I, spleen

C82.08 Follicular lymphoma grade I, lymph nodes of multiple sites

C82.09 Follicular lymphoma grade I, extranodal and solid organ sites

✓5ᵗʰ **C82.1 Follicular lymphoma grade II**

C82.10 Follicular lymphoma grade II, unspecified site ▽

C82.11 Follicular lymphoma grade II, lymph nodes of head, face, and neck

C82.12 Follicular lymphoma grade II, intrathoracic lymph nodes

C82.13 Follicular lymphoma grade II, intra-abdominal lymph nodes

C82.14 Follicular lymphoma grade II, lymph nodes of axilla and upper limb

C82.15 Follicular lymphoma grade II, lymph nodes of inguinal region and lower limb

C82.16 Follicular lymphoma grade II, intrapelvic lymph nodes

C82.17 Follicular lymphoma grade II, spleen

C82.18 Follicular lymphoma grade II, lymph nodes of multiple sites

C82.19 Follicular lymphoma grade II, extranodal and solid organ sites

✓5ᵗʰ **C82.2 Follicular lymphoma grade III, unspecified**

C82.20 Follicular lymphoma grade III, unspecified, unspecified site ▽

C82.21 Follicular lymphoma grade III, unspecified, lymph nodes of head, face, and neck ▽

C82.22 Follicular lymphoma grade III, unspecified, intrathoracic lymph nodes ▽

C82.23 Follicular lymphoma grade III, unspecified, intra-abdominal lymph nodes ▽

C82.24 Follicular lymphoma grade III, unspecified, lymph nodes of axilla and upper limb ▽

N Newborn   P Pediatric   M Maternity   A Adult   RIC RIC Dx   NC Dx Noncancer Dx   PDx Primary Dx   CC RIC CC Condition   ►◄ Revised Text   ● New Code   ▲ Revised Code Title

462

ICD-10-CM 2016

C82.25   Follicular lymphoma grade III, unspecified, lymph nodes of inguinal region and lower limb ▽

C82.26   Follicular lymphoma grade III, unspecified, intrapelvic lymph nodes ▽

C82.27   Follicular lymphoma grade III, unspecified, spleen ▽

C82.28   Follicular lymphoma grade III, unspecified, lymph nodes of multiple sites ▽

C82.29   Follicular lymphoma grade III, unspecified, extranodal and solid organ sites ▽

✓5ᵗʰ C82.3   Follicular lymphoma grade IIIa

C82.3Ø   Follicular lymphoma grade IIIa, unspecified site ▽

C82.31   Follicular lymphoma grade IIIa, lymph nodes of head, face, and neck

C82.32   Follicular lymphoma grade IIIa, intrathoracic lymph nodes

C82.33   Follicular lymphoma grade IIIa, intra-abdominal lymph nodes

C82.34   Follicular lymphoma grade IIIa, lymph nodes of axilla and upper limb

C82.35   Follicular lymphoma grade IIIa, lymph nodes of inguinal region and lower limb

C82.36   Follicular lymphoma grade IIIa, intrapelvic lymph nodes

C82.37   Follicular lymphoma grade IIIa, spleen

C82.38   Follicular lymphoma grade IIIa, lymph nodes of multiple sites

C82.39   Follicular lymphoma grade IIIa, extranodal and solid organ sites

✓5ᵗʰ C82.4   Follicular lymphoma grade IIIb

C82.4Ø   Follicular lymphoma grade IIIb, unspecified site ▽

C82.41   Follicular lymphoma grade IIIb, lymph nodes of head, face, and neck

C82.42   Follicular lymphoma grade IIIb, intrathoracic lymph nodes

C82.43   Follicular lymphoma grade IIIb, intra-abdominal lymph nodes

C82.44   Follicular lymphoma grade IIIb, lymph nodes of axilla and upper limb

C82.45   Follicular lymphoma grade IIIb, lymph nodes of inguinal region and lower limb

C82.46   Follicular lymphoma grade IIIb, intrapelvic lymph nodes

C82.47   Follicular lymphoma grade IIIb, spleen

C82.48   Follicular lymphoma grade IIIb, lymph nodes of multiple sites

C82.49   Follicular lymphoma grade IIIb, extranodal and solid organ sites

✓5ᵗʰ C82.5   Diffuse follicle center lymphoma

C82.5Ø   Diffuse follicle center lymphoma, unspecified site ▽

C82.51   Diffuse follicle center lymphoma, lymph nodes of head, face, and neck

C82.52   Diffuse follicle center lymphoma, intrathoracic lymph nodes

C82.53   Diffuse follicle center lymphoma, intra-abdominal lymph nodes

C82.54   Diffuse follicle center lymphoma, lymph nodes of axilla and upper limb

C82.55   Diffuse follicle center lymphoma, lymph nodes of inguinal region and lower limb

C82.56   Diffuse follicle center lymphoma, intrapelvic lymph nodes

C82.57   Diffuse follicle center lymphoma, spleen

C82.58   Diffuse follicle center lymphoma, lymph nodes of multiple sites

C82.59   Diffuse follicle center lymphoma, extranodal and solid organ sites

✓5ᵗʰ C82.6   Cutaneous follicle center lymphoma

C82.6Ø   Cutaneous follicle center lymphoma, unspecified site ▽

C82.61   Cutaneous follicle center lymphoma, lymph nodes of head, face, and neck

C82.62   Cutaneous follicle center lymphoma, intrathoracic lymph nodes

C82.63   Cutaneous follicle center lymphoma, intra-abdominal lymph nodes

C82.64   Cutaneous follicle center lymphoma, lymph nodes of axilla and upper limb

C82.65   Cutaneous follicle center lymphoma, lymph nodes of inguinal region and lower limb

C82.66   Cutaneous follicle center lymphoma, intrapelvic lymph nodes

C82.67   Cutaneous follicle center lymphoma, spleen

C82.68   Cutaneous follicle center lymphoma, lymph nodes of multiple sites

C82.69   Cutaneous follicle center lymphoma, extranodal and solid organ sites

✓5ᵗʰ C82.8   Other types of follicular lymphoma

C82.8Ø   Other types of follicular lymphoma, unspecified site ▽

C82.81   Other types of follicular lymphoma, lymph nodes of head, face, and neck

C82.82   Other types of follicular lymphoma, intrathoracic lymph nodes

C82.83   Other types of follicular lymphoma, intra-abdominal lymph nodes

C82.84   Other types of follicular lymphoma, lymph nodes of axilla and upper limb

C82.85   Other types of follicular lymphoma, lymph nodes of inguinal region and lower limb

C82.86   Other types of follicular lymphoma, intrapelvic lymph nodes

C82.87   Other types of follicular lymphoma, spleen

C82.88   Other types of follicular lymphoma, lymph nodes of multiple sites

C82.89   Other types of follicular lymphoma, extranodal and solid organ sites

✓5ᵗʰ C82.9   Follicular lymphoma, unspecified

C82.9Ø   Follicular lymphoma, unspecified, unspecified site ▽

C82.91   Follicular lymphoma, unspecified, lymph nodes of head, face, and neck ▽

C82.92   Follicular lymphoma, unspecified, intrathoracic lymph nodes ▽

C82.93   Follicular lymphoma, unspecified, intra-abdominal lymph nodes ▽

C82.94   Follicular lymphoma, unspecified, lymph nodes of axilla and upper limb ▽

C82.95   Follicular lymphoma, unspecified, lymph nodes of inguinal region and lower limb ▽

C82.96   Follicular lymphoma, unspecified, intrapelvic lymph nodes ▽

C82.97   Follicular lymphoma, unspecified, spleen ▽

C82.98   Follicular lymphoma, unspecified, lymph nodes of multiple sites ▽

C82.99   Follicular lymphoma, unspecified, extranodal and solid organ sites ▽

✓4ᵗʰ C83   Non-follicular lymphoma

     EXCLUDES 1   personal history of non-Hodgkin lymphoma (Z85.72)

✓5ᵗʰ C83.Ø   Small cell B-cell lymphoma

     Lymphoplasmacytic lymphoma
     Nodal marginal zone lymphoma
     Non-leukemic variant of B-CLL
     Splenic marginal zone lymphoma

     EXCLUDES 1   chronic lymphocytic leukemia (C91.1)
             mature T/NK-cell lymphomas (C84.-)
             Waldenström macroglobulinemia (C88.Ø)

C83.ØØ   Small cell B-cell lymphoma, unspecified site ▽

C83.Ø1   Small cell B-cell lymphoma, lymph nodes of head, face, and neck

C83.Ø2   Small cell B-cell lymphoma, intrathoracic lymph nodes

C83.Ø3   Small cell B-cell lymphoma, intra-abdominal lymph nodes

C83.Ø4   Small cell B-cell lymphoma, lymph nodes of axilla and upper limb

C83.Ø5   Small cell B-cell lymphoma, lymph nodes of inguinal region and lower limb

C83.Ø6   Small cell B-cell lymphoma, intrapelvic lymph nodes

C83.Ø7   Small cell B-cell lymphoma, spleen

C83.Ø8   Small cell B-cell lymphoma, lymph nodes of multiple sites

Chapter 2. Neoplasms

C83.09   **Small cell B-cell lymphoma,** extranodal and solid organ sites

✓5ᵗʰ **C83.1**   Mantle cell **lymphoma**
Centrocytic lymphoma
Malignant lymphomatous polyposis

C83.10   **Mantle cell lymphoma, unspecified site** ▽

C83.11   **Mantle cell lymphoma, lymph nodes of** head, face, and neck

C83.12   **Mantle cell lymphoma,** intrathoracic **lymph nodes**

C83.13   **Mantle cell lymphoma,** intra-abdominal **lymph nodes**

C83.14   **Mantle cell lymphoma, lymph nodes of** axilla and upper limb

C83.15   **Mantle cell lymphoma, lymph nodes of** inguinal region and lower limb

C83.16   **Mantle cell lymphoma,** intrapelvic **lymph nodes**

C83.17   **Mantle cell lymphoma,** spleen

C83.18   **Mantle cell lymphoma, lymph nodes of** multiple sites

C83.19   **Mantle cell lymphoma,** extranodal and solid organ sites

✓5ᵗʰ **C83.3**   Diffuse large B-cell **lymphoma**
Anaplastic diffuse large B-cell lymphoma
CD30-positive diffuse large B-cell lymphoma
Centroblastic diffuse large B-cell lymphoma
Diffuse large B-cell lymphoma, subtype not specified
Immunoblastic diffuse large B-cell lymphoma
Plasmablastic diffuse large B-cell lymphoma
T-cell rich diffuse large B-cell lymphoma
EXCLUDES 1   *mature T/NK-cell lymphomas (C84.-)*
      mediastinal (thymic) large B-cell lymphoma (C85.2-)

C83.30   **Diffuse large B-cell lymphoma, unspecified site** ▽

C83.31   **Diffuse large B-cell lymphoma, lymph nodes of** head, face, and neck

C83.32   **Diffuse large B-cell lymphoma,** intrathoracic **lymph nodes**

C83.33   **Diffuse large B-cell lymphoma,** intra-abdominal **lymph nodes**

C83.34   **Diffuse large B-cell lymphoma, lymph nodes of** axilla and upper limb

C83.35   **Diffuse large B-cell lymphoma, lymph nodes of** inguinal region and lower limb

C83.36   **Diffuse large B-cell lymphoma,** intrapelvic **lymph nodes**

C83.37   **Diffuse large B-cell lymphoma,** spleen

C83.38   **Diffuse large B-cell lymphoma, lymph nodes of** multiple sites

C83.39   **Diffuse large B-cell lymphoma,** extranodal and solid organ sites

✓5ᵗʰ **C83.5**   Lymphoblastic (diffuse) **lymphoma**
B-precursor lymphoma
Lymphoblastic B-cell lymphoma
Lymphoblastic lymphoma NOS
Lymphoblastic T-cell lymphoma
T-precursor lymphoma

C83.50   **Lymphoblastic (diffuse) lymphoma, unspecified site** ▽

C83.51   **Lymphoblastic (diffuse) lymphoma, lymph nodes of** head, face, and neck

C83.52   **Lymphoblastic (diffuse) lymphoma,** intrathoracic **lymph nodes**

C83.53   **Lymphoblastic (diffuse) lymphoma,** intra-abdominal **lymph nodes**

C83.54   **Lymphoblastic (diffuse) lymphoma, lymph nodes of** axilla and upper limb

C83.55   **Lymphoblastic (diffuse) lymphoma, lymph nodes of** inguinal region and lower limb

C83.56   **Lymphoblastic (diffuse) lymphoma,** intrapelvic **lymph nodes**

C83.57   **Lymphoblastic (diffuse) lymphoma,** spleen

C83.58   **Lymphoblastic (diffuse) lymphoma, lymph nodes of** multiple sites

C83.59   **Lymphoblastic (diffuse) lymphoma,** extranodal and solid organ sites

✓5ᵗʰ **C83.7**   Burkitt **lymphoma**
Atypical Burkitt lymphoma
Burkitt-like lymphoma
EXCLUDES 1   *mature B-cell leukemia Burkitt type (C91.A-)*

C83.70   **Burkitt lymphoma, unspecified site** ▽

C83.71   **Burkitt lymphoma, lymph nodes of** head, face, and neck

C83.72   **Burkitt lymphoma,** intrathoracic **lymph nodes**

C83.73   **Burkitt lymphoma,** intra-abdominal **lymph nodes**

C83.74   **Burkitt lymphoma, lymph nodes of** axilla and upper limb

C83.75   **Burkitt lymphoma, lymph nodes of** inguinal region and lower limb

C83.76   **Burkitt lymphoma,** intrapelvic **lymph nodes**

C83.77   **Burkitt lymphoma,** spleen

C83.78   **Burkitt lymphoma, lymph nodes of** multiple sites

C83.79   **Burkitt lymphoma,** extranodal and solid organ sites

✓5ᵗʰ **C83.8**   Other non-follicular **lymphoma**
Intravascular large B-cell lymphoma
Lymphoid granulomatosis
Primary effusion B-cell lymphoma
EXCLUDES 1   *mediastinal (thymic) large B-cell lymphoma (C85.2-)*
      T-cell rich B-cell lymphoma (C83.3-)

C83.80   **Other non-follicular lymphoma, unspecified site** ▽

C83.81   **Other non-follicular lymphoma, lymph nodes of** head, face, and neck

C83.82   **Other non-follicular lymphoma,** intrathoracic **lymph nodes**

C83.83   **Other non-follicular lymphoma,** intra-abdominal **lymph nodes**

C83.84   **Other non-follicular lymphoma, lymph nodes of** axilla and upper limb

C83.85   **Other non-follicular lymphoma, lymph nodes of** inguinal region and lower limb

C83.86   **Other non-follicular lymphoma,** intrapelvic **lymph nodes**

C83.87   **Other non-follicular lymphoma,** spleen

C83.88   **Other non-follicular lymphoma, lymph nodes of** multiple sites

C83.89   **Other non-follicular lymphoma,** extranodal and solid organ sites

✓5ᵗʰ **C83.9**   Non-follicular (diffuse) **lymphoma,** unspecified

C83.90   **Non-follicular (diffuse) lymphoma, unspecified, unspecified site** ▽

C83.91   **Non-follicular (diffuse) lymphoma, unspecified, lymph nodes of** head, face, and neck ▽

C83.92   **Non-follicular (diffuse) lymphoma, unspecified,** intrathoracic **lymph nodes** ▽

C83.93   **Non-follicular (diffuse) lymphoma, unspecified,** intra-abdominal **lymph nodes** ▽

C83.94   **Non-follicular (diffuse) lymphoma, unspecified, lymph nodes of** axilla and upper limb ▽

C83.95   **Non-follicular (diffuse) lymphoma, unspecified, lymph nodes of** inguinal region and lower limb ▽

C83.96   **Non-follicular (diffuse) lymphoma, unspecified,** intrapelvic **lymph nodes** ▽

C83.97   **Non-follicular (diffuse) lymphoma, unspecified,** spleen ▽

C83.98   **Non-follicular (diffuse) lymphoma, unspecified, lymph nodes of** multiple sites ▽

C83.99   **Non-follicular (diffuse) lymphoma, unspecified,** extranodal and solid organ sites ▽

✓4ᵗʰ **C84**   **Mature T/NK-cell lymphomas**
EXCLUDES 1   *personal history of non-Hodgkin lymphoma (Z85.72)*

✓5ᵗʰ **C84.0**   **Mycosis fungoides**
EXCLUDES 1   *peripheral T-cell lymphoma, not classified (C84.4-)*

C84.00   **Mycosis fungoides, unspecified site** ▽

C84.01   **Mycosis fungoides, lymph nodes of** head, face, and neck

C84.02   **Mycosis fungoides,** intrathoracic **lymph nodes**

C84.03   **Mycosis fungoides,** intra-abdominal **lymph nodes**

C84.04   **Mycosis fungoides, lymph nodes of** axilla and upper limb

C84.05   **Mycosis fungoides, lymph nodes of** inguinal region and lower limb

N Newborn   P Pediatric   M Maternity   A Adult   RIC RIC Dx   NC Dx Noncancer Dx   PDx Primary Dx   CC RIC CC Condition   ►◄ Revised Text   ● New Code   ▲ Revised Code Title

464   ICD-10-CM 2016

C84.06   Mycosis fungoides, intrapelvic lymph nodes
C84.07   Mycosis fungoides, spleen
C84.08   Mycosis fungoides, lymph nodes of multiple sites
C84.09   Mycosis fungoides, extranodal and solid organ sites

✓5ᵗʰ **C84.1**   Sézary disease
C84.10   Sézary disease, unspecified site ▽
C84.11   Sézary disease, lymph nodes of head, face, and neck
C84.12   Sézary disease, intrathoracic lymph nodes
C84.13   Sézary disease, intra-abdominal lymph nodes
C84.14   Sézary disease, lymph nodes of axilla and upper limb
C84.15   Sézary disease, lymph nodes of inguinal region and lower limb
C84.16   Sézary disease, intrapelvic lymph nodes
C84.17   Sézary disease, spleen
C84.18   Sézary disease, lymph nodes of multiple sites
C84.19   Sézary disease, extranodal and solid organ sites

✓5ᵗʰ **C84.4**   Peripheral T-cell lymphoma, not classified
Lennert's lymphoma
Lymphoepithelioid lymphoma
Mature T-cell lymphoma, not elsewhere classified
C84.40   Peripheral T-cell lymphoma, not classified, unspecified site ▽
C84.41   Peripheral T-cell lymphoma, not classified, lymph nodes of head, face, and neck
C84.42   Peripheral T-cell lymphoma, not classified, intrathoracic lymph nodes
C84.43   Peripheral T-cell lymphoma, not classified, intra-abdominal lymph nodes
C84.44   Peripheral T-cell lymphoma, not classified, lymph nodes of axilla and upper limb
C84.45   Peripheral T-cell lymphoma, not classified, lymph nodes of inguinal region and lower limb
C84.46   Peripheral T-cell lymphoma, not classified, intrapelvic lymph nodes
C84.47   Peripheral T-cell lymphoma, not classified, spleen
C84.48   Peripheral T-cell lymphoma, not classified, lymph nodes of multiple sites
C84.49   Peripheral T-cell lymphoma, not classified, extranodal and solid organ sites

✓5ᵗʰ **C84.6**   Anaplastic large cell lymphoma, ALK-positive
Anaplastic large cell lymphoma, CD30-positive
C84.60   Anaplastic large cell lymphoma, ALK-positive, unspecified site ▽
C84.61   Anaplastic large cell lymphoma, ALK-positive, lymph nodes of head, face, and neck
C84.62   Anaplastic large cell lymphoma, ALK-positive, intrathoracic lymph nodes
C84.63   Anaplastic large cell lymphoma, ALK-positive, intra-abdominal lymph nodes
C84.64   Anaplastic large cell lymphoma, ALK-positive, lymph nodes of axilla and upper limb
C84.65   Anaplastic large cell lymphoma, ALK-positive, lymph nodes of inguinal region and lower limb
C84.66   Anaplastic large cell lymphoma, ALK-positive, intrapelvic lymph nodes
C84.67   Anaplastic large cell lymphoma, ALK-positive, spleen
C84.68   Anaplastic large cell lymphoma, ALK-positive, lymph nodes of multiple sites
C84.69   Anaplastic large cell lymphoma, ALK-positive, extranodal and solid organ sites

✓5ᵗʰ **C84.7**   Anaplastic large cell lymphoma, ALK-negative
EXCLUDES 1   primary cutaneous CD30-positive T-cell proliferations (C86.6-)
C84.70   Anaplastic large cell lymphoma, ALK-negative, unspecified site ▽
C84.71   Anaplastic large cell lymphoma, ALK-negative, lymph nodes of head, face, and neck
C84.72   Anaplastic large cell lymphoma, ALK-negative, intrathoracic lymph nodes
C84.73   Anaplastic large cell lymphoma, ALK-negative, intra-abdominal lymph nodes
C84.74   Anaplastic large cell lymphoma, ALK-negative, lymph nodes of axilla and upper limb
C84.75   Anaplastic large cell lymphoma, ALK-negative, lymph nodes of inguinal region and lower limb

C84.76   Anaplastic large cell lymphoma, ALK-negative, intrapelvic lymph nodes
C84.77   Anaplastic large cell lymphoma, ALK-negative, spleen
C84.78   Anaplastic large cell lymphoma, ALK-negative, lymph nodes of multiple sites
C84.79   Anaplastic large cell lymphoma, ALK-negative, extranodal and solid organ sites

✓5ᵗʰ **C84.A**   Cutaneous T-cell lymphoma, unspecified
C84.A0   Cutaneous T-cell lymphoma, unspecified, unspecified site ▽
C84.A1   Cutaneous T-cell lymphoma, unspecified lymph nodes of head, face, and neck ▽
C84.A2   Cutaneous T-cell lymphoma, unspecified, intrathoracic lymph nodes ▽
C84.A3   Cutaneous T-cell lymphoma, unspecified, intra-abdominal lymph nodes ▽
C84.A4   Cutaneous T-cell lymphoma, unspecified, lymph nodes of axilla and upper limb ▽
C84.A5   Cutaneous T-cell lymphoma, unspecified, lymph nodes of inguinal region and lower limb ▽
C84.A6   Cutaneous T-cell lymphoma, unspecified, intrapelvic lymph nodes ▽
C84.A7   Cutaneous T-cell lymphoma, unspecified, spleen ▽
C84.A8   Cutaneous T-cell lymphoma, unspecified, lymph nodes of multiple sites ▽
C84.A9   Cutaneous T-cell lymphoma, unspecified, extranodal and solid organ sites ▽

✓5ᵗʰ **C84.Z**   Other mature T/NK-cell lymphomas
NOTE   If T-cell lineage or involvement is mentioned in conjunction with a specific lymphoma, code to the more specific description.
EXCLUDES 1   angioimmunoblastic T-cell lymphoma (C86.5)
blastic NK-cell lymphoma (C86.4)
enteropathy-type T-cell lymphoma (C86.2)
extranodal NK-cell lymphoma, nasal type (C86.0)
hepatosplenic T-cell lymphoma (C86.1)
primary cutaneous CD30-positive T-cell proliferations (C86.6)
subcutaneous panniculitis-like T-cell lymphoma (C86.3)
T-cell leukemia (C91.1-)
C84.Z0   Other mature T/NK-cell lymphomas, unspecified site ▽
C84.Z1   Other mature T/NK-cell lymphomas, lymph nodes of head, face, and neck
C84.Z2   Other mature T/NK-cell lymphomas, intrathoracic lymph nodes
C84.Z3   Other mature T/NK-cell lymphomas, intra-abdominal lymph nodes
C84.Z4   Other mature T/NK-cell lymphomas, lymph nodes of axilla and upper limb
C84.Z5   Other mature T/NK-cell lymphomas, lymph nodes of inguinal region and lower limb
C84.Z6   Other mature T/NK-cell lymphomas, intrapelvic lymph nodes
C84.Z7   Other mature T/NK-cell lymphomas, spleen
C84.Z8   Other mature T/NK-cell lymphomas, lymph nodes of multiple sites
C84.Z9   Other mature T/NK-cell lymphomas, extranodal and solid organ sites

✓5ᵗʰ **C84.9**   Mature T/NK-cell lymphomas, unspecified
NK/T cell lymphoma NOS
EXCLUDES 1   mature T-cell lymphoma, not elsewhere classified (C84.4-)
C84.90   Mature T/NK-cell lymphomas, unspecified, unspecified site ▽
C84.91   Mature T/NK-cell lymphomas, unspecified, lymph nodes of head, face, and neck ▽
C84.92   Mature T/NK-cell lymphomas, unspecified, intrathoracic lymph nodes ▽
C84.93   Mature T/NK-cell lymphomas, unspecified, intra-abdominal lymph nodes ▽
C84.94   Mature T/NK-cell lymphomas, unspecified, lymph nodes of axilla and upper limb ▽
C84.95   Mature T/NK-cell lymphomas, unspecified, lymph nodes of inguinal region and lower limb ▽
C84.96   Mature T/NK-cell lymphomas, unspecified, intrapelvic lymph nodes ▽

☑ Add'l Character Required   ✓7ᵗʰ Placeholder Alert   RUG IV Special Care High Dx   RUG IV Clinically Complex Dx   RUG IV Special Care Low Dx   Manifestation Code   Other Specified Code   ▽ Unspecified Code

C84.97   Mature T/NK-cell lymphomas, unspecified, spleen ▽

C84.98   Mature T/NK-cell lymphomas, unspecified, lymph nodes of multiple sites ▽

C84.99   Mature T/NK-cell lymphomas, unspecified, extranodal and solid organ sites ▽

✓4ᵗʰ C85   Other specified and unspecified types of non-Hodgkin lymphoma

> **EXCLUDES 1**   other specified types of T/NK-cell lymphoma (C86.-)
> personal history of non-Hodgkin lymphoma (Z85.72)

✓5ᵗʰ C85.1   Unspecified B-cell lymphoma

> **NOTE**   If B-cell lineage or involvement is mentioned in conjunction with a specific lymphoma, code to the more specific description.

C85.10   Unspecified B-cell lymphoma, unspecified site ▽

C85.11   Unspecified B-cell lymphoma, lymph nodes of head, face, and neck ▽

C85.12   Unspecified B-cell lymphoma, intrathoracic lymph nodes ▽

C85.13   Unspecified B-cell lymphoma, intra-abdominal lymph nodes ▽

C85.14   Unspecified B-cell lymphoma, lymph nodes of axilla and upper limb ▽

C85.15   Unspecified B-cell lymphoma, lymph nodes of inguinal region and lower limb ▽

C85.16   Unspecified B-cell lymphoma, intrapelvic lymph nodes ▽

C85.17   Unspecified B-cell lymphoma, spleen ▽

C85.18   Unspecified B-cell lymphoma, lymph nodes of multiple sites ▽

C85.19   Unspecified B-cell lymphoma, extranodal and solid organ sites ▽

✓5ᵗʰ C85.2   Mediastinal (thymic) large B-cell lymphoma

C85.20   Mediastinal (thymic) large B-cell lymphoma, unspecified site ▽

C85.21   Mediastinal (thymic) large B-cell lymphoma, lymph nodes of head, face, and neck

C85.22   Mediastinal (thymic) large B-cell lymphoma, intrathoracic lymph nodes

C85.23   Mediastinal (thymic) large B-cell lymphoma, intra-abdominal lymph nodes

C85.24   Mediastinal (thymic) large B-cell lymphoma, lymph nodes of axilla and upper limb

C85.25   Mediastinal (thymic) large B-cell lymphoma, lymph nodes of inguinal region and lower limb

C85.26   Mediastinal (thymic) large B-cell lymphoma, intrapelvic lymph nodes

C85.27   Mediastinal (thymic) large B-cell lymphoma, spleen

C85.28   Mediastinal (thymic) large B-cell lymphoma, lymph nodes of multiple sites

C85.29   Mediastinal (thymic) large B-cell lymphoma, extranodal and solid organ sites

✓5ᵗʰ C85.8   Other specified types of non-Hodgkin lymphoma

C85.80   Other specified types of non-Hodgkin lymphoma, unspecified site ▽

C85.81   Other specified types of non-Hodgkin lymphoma, lymph nodes of head, face, and neck

C85.82   Other specified types of non-Hodgkin lymphoma, intrathoracic lymph nodes

C85.83   Other specified types of non-Hodgkin lymphoma, intra-abdominal lymph nodes

C85.84   Other specified types of non-Hodgkin lymphoma, lymph nodes of axilla and upper limb

C85.85   Other specified types of non-Hodgkin lymphoma, lymph nodes of inguinal region and lower limb

C85.86   Other specified types of non-Hodgkin lymphoma, intrapelvic lymph nodes

C85.87   Other specified types of non-Hodgkin lymphoma, spleen

C85.88   Other specified types of non-Hodgkin lymphoma, lymph nodes of multiple sites

C85.89   Other specified types of non-Hodgkin lymphoma, extranodal and solid organ sites

✓5ᵗʰ C85.9   Non-Hodgkin lymphoma, unspecified

Lymphoma NOS
Malignant lymphoma NOS
Non-Hodgkin lymphoma NOS

C85.90   Non-Hodgkin lymphoma, unspecified, unspecified site ▽

C85.91   Non-Hodgkin lymphoma, unspecified, lymph nodes of head, face, and neck ▽

C85.92   Non-Hodgkin lymphoma, unspecified, intrathoracic lymph nodes ▽

C85.93   Non-Hodgkin lymphoma, unspecified, intra-abdominal lymph nodes ▽

C85.94   Non-Hodgkin lymphoma, unspecified, lymph nodes of axilla and upper limb ▽

C85.95   Non-Hodgkin lymphoma, unspecified, lymph nodes of inguinal region and lower limb ▽

C85.96   Non-Hodgkin lymphoma, unspecified, intrapelvic lymph nodes ▽

C85.97   Non-Hodgkin lymphoma, unspecified, spleen ▽

C85.98   Non-Hodgkin lymphoma, unspecified, lymph nodes of multiple sites ▽

C85.99   Non-Hodgkin lymphoma, unspecified, extranodal and solid organ sites ▽

✓4ᵗʰ C86   Other specified types of T/NK-cell lymphoma

> **EXCLUDES 1**   anaplastic large cell lymphoma, ALK negative (C84.7-)
> anaplastic large cell lymphoma, ALK positive (C84.6-)
> mature T/NK-cell lymphomas (C84.-)
> other specified types of non-Hodgkin lymphoma (C85.8-)

C86.0   Extranodal NK/T-cell lymphoma, nasal type

C86.1   Hepatosplenic T-cell lymphoma
Alpha-beta and gamma delta types

C86.2   Enteropathy-type (intestinal) T-cell lymphoma
Enteropathy associated T-cell lymphoma

C86.3   Subcutaneous panniculitis-like T-cell lymphoma

C86.4   Blastic NK-cell lymphoma

C86.5   Angioimmunoblastic T-cell lymphoma
Angioimmunoblastic lymphadenopathy with dysproteinemia [AILD]

C86.6   Primary cutaneous CD30-positive T-cell proliferations
Lymphomatoid papulosis
Primary cutaneous anaplastic large cell lymphoma
Primary cutaneous CD30-positive large T-cell lymphoma

✓4ᵗʰ C88   Malignant immunoproliferative diseases and certain other B-cell lymphomas

> **EXCLUDES 1**   B-cell lymphoma, unspecified (C85.1-)
> personal history of other malignant neoplasms of lymphoid, hematopoietic and related tissues (Z85.79)

C88.0   Waldenström macroglobulinemia
Lymphoplasmacytic lymphoma with IgM-production
Macroglobulinemia (idiopathic) (primary)
> **EXCLUDES 1**   small cell B-cell lymphoma (C83.0)

C88.2   Heavy chain disease
Franklin disease
Gamma heavy chain disease
Mu heavy chain disease

C88.3   Immunoproliferative small intestinal disease
Alpha heavy chain disease
Mediterranean lymphoma

C88.4   Extranodal marginal zone B-cell lymphoma of mucosa-associated lymphoid tissue [MALT-lymphoma]
Lymphoma of skin-associated lymphoid tissue [SALT-lymphoma]
Lymphoma of bronchial-associated lymphoid tissue [BALT-lymphoma]
> **EXCLUDES 1**   high malignant (diffuse large B-cell) lymphoma (C83.3-)

C88.8   Other malignant immunoproliferative diseases

C88.9   Malignant immunoproliferative disease, unspecified ▽
Immunoproliferative disease NOS

Ⓝ Newborn   Ⓟ Pediatric   Ⓜ Maternity   Ⓐ Adult   RIC RIC Dx   NC Dx Noncancer Dx   PDx Primary Dx   CC RIC CC Condition   ►◄ Revised Text   ● New Code   ▲ Revised Code Title

466   ICD-10-CM 2016

☑4ᵗʰ **C90 Multiple myeloma and malignant plasma cell neoplasms**
> **EXCLUDES 1** *personal history of other malignant neoplasms of lymphoid, hematopoietic and related tissues (Z85.79)*

☑5ᵗʰ **C90.0 Multiple myeloma**
Kahler's disease   Myelomatosis
Medullary plasmacytoma   Plasma cell myeloma
> **EXCLUDES 1** *solitary myeloma (C90.3-)*
> *solitary plasmacytoma (C90.3-)*

    C90.00 Multiple myeloma not having achieved remission
        Multiple myeloma with failed remission
        Multiple myeloma NOS

    C90.01 Multiple myeloma in remission

    C90.02 Multiple myeloma in relapse

☑5ᵗʰ **C90.1 Plasma cell leukemia**
Plasmacytic leukemia

    C90.10 Plasma cell leukemia not having achieved remission
        Plasma cell leukemia with failed remission
        Plasma cell leukemia NOS

    C90.11 Plasma cell leukemia in remission

    C90.12 Plasma cell leukemia in relapse

☑5ᵗʰ **C90.2 Extramedullary plasmacytoma**

    C90.20 Extramedullary plasmacytoma not having achieved remission
        Extramedullary plasmacytoma with failed remission
        Extramedullary plasmacytoma NOS

    C90.21 Extramedullary plasmacytoma in remission

    C90.22 Extramedullary plasmacytoma in relapse

☑5ᵗʰ **C90.3 Solitary plasmacytoma**
Localized malignant plasma cell tumor NOS
Plasmacytoma NOS
Solitary myeloma

    C90.30 Solitary plasmacytoma not having achieved remission
        Solitary plasmacytoma with failed remission
        Solitary plasmacytoma NOS

    C90.31 Solitary plasmacytoma in remission

    C90.32 Solitary plasmacytoma in relapse

☑4ᵗʰ **C91 Lymphoid leukemia**
> **EXCLUDES 1** *personal history of leukemia (Z85.6)*

☑5ᵗʰ **C91.0 Acute lymphoblastic leukemia [ALL]**
> **NOTE** Code C91.0 should only be used for T-cell and B-cell precursor leukemia.

    C91.00 Acute lymphoblastic leukemia not having achieved remission `CC`
        Acute lymphoblastic leukemia with failed remission
        Acute lymphoblastic leukemia NOS

    C91.01 Acute lymphoblastic leukemia, in remission

    C91.02 Acute lymphoblastic leukemia, in relapse `CC`

☑5ᵗʰ **C91.1 Chronic lymphocytic leukemia of B-cell type**
Lymphoplasmacytic leukemia
Richter syndrome
> **EXCLUDES 1** *lymphoplasmacytic lymphoma (C83.0-)*

    C91.10 Chronic lymphocytic leukemia of B-cell type not having achieved remission
        Chronic lymphocytic leukemia of B-cell type with failed remission
        Chronic lymphocytic leukemia of B-cell type NOS

    C91.11 Chronic lymphocytic leukemia of B-cell type in remission

    C91.12 Chronic lymphocytic leukemia of B-cell type in relapse

☑5ᵗʰ **C91.3 Prolymphocytic leukemia of B-cell type**

    C91.30 Prolymphocytic leukemia of B-cell type not having achieved remission
        Prolymphocytic leukemia of B-cell type with failed remission
        Prolymphocytic leukemia of B-cell type NOS

    C91.31 Prolymphocytic leukemia of B-cell type, in remission

    C91.32 Prolymphocytic leukemia of B-cell type, in relapse

☑5ᵗʰ **C91.4 Hairy cell leukemia**
Leukemic reticuloendotheliosis

    C91.40 Hairy cell leukemia not having achieved remission
        Hairy cell leukemia with failed remission
        Hairy cell leukemia NOS

    C91.41 Hairy cell leukemia, in remission

    C91.42 Hairy cell leukemia, in relapse

☑5ᵗʰ **C91.5 Adult T-cell lymphoma/leukemia (HTLV-1-associated)**
Acute variant of adult T-cell lymphoma/leukemia (HTLV-1-associated)
Chronic variant of adult T-cell lymphoma/leukemia (HTLV-1-associated)
Lymphomatoid variant of adult T-cell lymphoma/leukemia (HTLV-1-associated)
Smouldering variant of adult T-cell lymphoma/leukemia (HTLV-1-associated)

    C91.50 Adult T-cell lymphoma/leukemia (HTLV-1-associated) not having achieved remission `A`
        Adult T-cell lymphoma/leukemia (HTLV-1-associated) with failed remission
        Adult T-cell lymphoma/leukemia (HTLV-1-associated) NOS

    C91.51 Adult T-cell lymphoma/leukemia (HTLV-1-associated), in remission `A`

    C91.52 Adult T-cell lymphoma/leukemia (HTLV-1-associated), in relapse `A`

☑5ᵗʰ **C91.6 Prolymphocytic leukemia of T-cell type**

    C91.60 Prolymphocytic leukemia of T-cell type not having achieved remission
        Prolymphocytic leukemia of T-cell type with failed remission
        Prolymphocytic leukemia of T-cell type NOS

    C91.61 Prolymphocytic leukemia of T-cell type, in remission

    C91.62 Prolymphocytic leukemia of T-cell type, in relapse

☑5ᵗʰ **C91.A Mature B-cell leukemia Burkitt-type**
> **EXCLUDES 1** *Burkitt lymphoma (C83.7-)*

    C91.A0 Mature B-cell leukemia Burkitt-type not having achieved remission
        Mature B-cell leukemia Burkitt-type with failed remission
        Mature B-cell leukemia Burkitt-type NOS

    C91.A1 Mature B-cell leukemia Burkitt-type, in remission

    C91.A2 Mature B-cell leukemia Burkitt-type, in relapse

☑5ᵗʰ **C91.Z Other lymphoid leukemia**
T-cell large granular lymphocytic leukemia (associated with rheumatoid arthritis)

    C91.Z0 Other lymphoid leukemia not having achieved remission
        Other lymphoid leukemia with failed remission
        Other lymphoid leukemia NOS

    C91.Z1 Other lymphoid leukemia, in remission

    C91.Z2 Other lymphoid leukemia, in relapse

☑5ᵗʰ **C91.9 Lymphoid leukemia, unspecified**

    C91.90 Lymphoid leukemia, unspecified not having achieved remission ▽
        Lymphoid leukemia with failed remission
        Lymphoid leukemia NOS

    C91.91 Lymphoid leukemia, unspecified, in remission ▽

    C91.92 Lymphoid leukemia, unspecified, in relapse ▽

☑4ᵗʰ **C92 Myeloid leukemia**
> **INCLUDES** granulocytic leukemia
> myelogenous leukemia
> **EXCLUDES 1** *personal history of leukemia (Z85.6)*

☑5ᵗʰ **C92.0 Acute myeloblastic leukemia**
Acute myeloblastic leukemia, minimal differentiation
Acute myeloblastic leukemia (with maturation)
Acute myeloblastic leukemia 1/ETO
Acute myeloblastic leukemia M0
Acute myeloblastic leukemia M1
Acute myeloblastic leukemia M2
Acute myeloblastic leukemia with t(8;21)
Acute myeloblastic leukemia (without a FAB classification) NOS
Refractory anemia with excess blasts in transformation [RAEB T]
> **EXCLUDES 1** *acute exacerbation of chronic myeloid leukemia (C92.10)*
> *refractory anemia with excess of blasts not in transformation (D46.2-)*

    C92.00 Acute myeloblastic leukemia, not having achieved remission `CC`
        Acute myeloblastic leukemia with failed remission
        Acute myeloblastic leukemia NOS

    C92.01 Acute myeloblastic leukemia, in remission

    C92.02 Acute myeloblastic leukemia, in relapse `CC`

☑ Add'l Character Required   ☑x7ᵗʰ Placeholder Alert   RUG IV Special Care High Dx   RUG IV Clinically Complex Dx   RUG IV Special Care Low Dx   Manifestation Code   Other Specified Code   ▽ Unspecified Code

Chapter 2. Neoplasms

C92.1–C94.Ø1

✓5ᵗʰ **C92.1** Chronic **myeloid leukemia**, BCR/ABL-positive
Chronic myelogenous leukemia, Philadelphia chromosome (Ph1) positive
Chronic myelogenous leukemia, t(9;22) (q34;q11)
Chronic myelogenous leukemia with crisis of blast cells

> EXCLUDES 1   *atypical chronic myeloid leukemia BCR/ABL-negative (C92.2-)*
> *chronic myelomonocytic leukemia (C93.1-)*
> *chronic myeloproliferative disease (D47.1)*

     C92.1Ø Chronic myeloid leukemia, BCR/ABL-positive, not having achieved remission
        Chronic myeloid leukemia, BCR/ABL-positive with failed remission
        Chronic myeloid leukemia, BCR/ABL-positive NOS

     C92.11 Chronic myeloid leukemia, BCR/ABL-positive, in remission

     C92.12 Chronic myeloid leukemia, BCR/ABL-positive, in relapse

✓5ᵗʰ **C92.2** Atypical chronic **myeloid** leukemia, BCR/ABL-negative

     C92.2Ø Atypical chronic myeloid leukemia, BCR/ABL-negative, not having achieved remission
        Atypical chronic myeloid leukemia, BCR/ABL-negative with failed remission
        Atypical chronic myeloid leukemia, BCR/ABL-negative NOS

     C92.21 Atypical chronic myeloid leukemia, BCR/ABL-negative, in remission

     C92.22 Atypical chronic myeloid leukemia, BCR/ABL-negative, in relapse

✓5ᵗʰ **C92.3** Myeloid sarcoma
A malignant tumor of immature myeloid cells
Chloroma
Granulocytic sarcoma

     C92.3Ø Myeloid sarcoma, not having achieved remission
        Myeloid sarcoma with failed remission
        Myeloid sarcoma NOS

     C92.31 Myeloid sarcoma, in remission

     C92.32 Myeloid sarcoma, in relapse

✓5ᵗʰ **C92.4** Acute promyelocytic **leukemia**
AML M3
AML Me with t(15;17) and variants

     C92.4Ø Acute promyelocytic leukemia, not having achieved remission   [CC]
        Acute promyelocytic leukemia with failed remission
        Acute promyelocytic leukemia NOS

     C92.41 Acute promyelocytic leukemia, in remission

     C92.42 Acute promyelocytic leukemia, in relapse   [CC]

✓5ᵗʰ **C92.5** Acute myelomonocytic **leukemia**
AML M4
AML M4 Eo with inv(16) or t(16;16)

     C92.5Ø Acute myelomonocytic leukemia, not having achieved remission   [CC]
        Acute myelomonocytic leukemia with failed remission
        Acute myelomonocytic leukemia NOS

     C92.51 Acute myelomonocytic leukemia, in remission

     C92.52 Acute myelomonocytic leukemia, in relapse   [CC]

✓5ᵗʰ **C92.6** Acute myeloid **leukemia with** 11q23-abnormality
Acute myeloid leukemia with variation of MLL-gene

     C92.6Ø Acute myeloid leukemia with 11q23-abnormality not having achieved remission   [CC]
        Acute myeloid leukemia with 11q23-abnormality with failed remission
        Acute myeloid leukemia with 11q23-abnormality NOS

     C92.61 Acute myeloid leukemia with 11q23-abnormality in remission

     C92.62 Acute myeloid leukemia with 11q23-abnormality in relapse   [CC]

✓5ᵗʰ **C92.A** Acute myeloid **leukemia with** multilineage dysplasia
Acute myeloid leukemia with dysplasia of remaining hematopoesis and/or myelodysplastic disease in its history

     C92.AØ Acute myeloid leukemia with multilineage dysplasia, not having achieved remission   [CC]
        Acute myeloid leukemia with multilineage dysplasia with failed remission
        Acute myeloid leukemia with multilineage dysplasia NOS

     C92.A1 Acute myeloid leukemia with multilineage dysplasia, in remission

     C92.A2 Acute myeloid leukemia with multilineage dysplasia, in relapse   [CC]

✓5ᵗʰ **C92.Z** Other **myeloid leukemia**

     C92.ZØ Other myeloid leukemia not having achieved remission
        Myeloid leukemia NEC with failed remission
        Myeloid leukemia NEC

     C92.Z1 Other myeloid leukemia, in remission

     C92.Z2 Other myeloid leukemia, in relapse

✓5ᵗʰ **C92.9** Myeloid leukemia, unspecified

     C92.9Ø Myeloid leukemia, unspecified, not having achieved remission   ▽
        Myeloid leukemia, unspecified with failed remission
        Myeloid leukemia, unspecified NOS

     C92.91 Myeloid leukemia, unspecified in remission   ▽

     C92.92 Myeloid leukemia, unspecified in relapse   ▽

✓4ᵗʰ **C93** Monocytic leukemia

> INCLUDES   monocytoid leukemia
> EXCLUDES 1   *personal history of leukemia (Z85.6)*

✓5ᵗʰ **C93.Ø** Acute **monoblastic/monocytic leukemia**
AML M5   AML M5b
AML M5a

     C93.ØØ Acute monoblastic/monocytic leukemia, not having achieved remission   [CC]
        Acute monoblastic/monocytic leukemia with failed remission
        Acute monoblastic/monocytic leukemia NOS

     C93.Ø1 Acute monoblastic/monocytic leukemia, in remission

     C93.Ø2 Acute monoblastic/monocytic leukemia, in relapse   [CC]

✓5ᵗʰ **C93.1** Chronic **myelomonocytic leukemia**
Chronic monocytic leukemia
CMML-1
CMML-2
CMML with eosinophilia

     C93.1Ø Chronic myelomonocytic leukemia not having achieved remission
        Chronic myelomonocytic leukemia with failed remission
        Chronic myelomonocytic leukemia NOS

     C93.11 Chronic myelomonocytic leukemia, in remission

     C93.12 Chronic myelomonocytic leukemia, in relapse

✓5ᵗʰ **C93.3** Juvenile **myelomonocytic leukemia**

     C93.3Ø Juvenile myelomonocytic leukemia, not having achieved remission   [P]
        Juvenile myelomonocytic leukemia with failed remission
        Juvenile myelomonocytic leukemia NOS

     C93.31 Juvenile myelomonocytic leukemia, in remission   [P]

     C93.32 Juvenile myelomonocytic leukemia, in relapse   [P]

✓5ᵗʰ **C93.Z** Other **monocytic leukemia**

     C93.ZØ Other monocytic leukemia, not having achieved remission
        Other monocytic leukemia NOS

     C93.Z1 Other monocytic leukemia, in remission

     C93.Z2 Other monocytic leukemia, in relapse

✓5ᵗʰ **C93.9** Monocytic leukemia, unspecified

     C93.9Ø Monocytic leukemia, unspecified, not having achieved remission   ▽
        Monocytic leukemia, unspecified with failed remission
        Monocytic leukemia, unspecified NOS

     C93.91 Monocytic leukemia, unspecified in remission   ▽

     C93.92 Monocytic leukemia, unspecified in relapse   ▽

✓4ᵗʰ **C94** Other **leukemias of** specified cell type

> EXCLUDES 1   *leukemic reticuloendotheliosis (C91.4-)*
> *myelodysplastic syndromes (D46.-)*
> *personal history of leukemia (Z85.6)*
> *plasma cell leukemia (C9Ø.1-)*

✓5ᵗʰ **C94.Ø** Acute **erythroid leukemia**
Acute myeloid leukemia M6(a)(b)
Erythroleukemia

     C94.ØØ Acute erythroid leukemia, not having achieved remission   [CC]
        Acute erythroid leukemia with failed remission
        Acute erythroid leukemia NOS

     C94.Ø1 Acute erythroid leukemia, in remission

[N] Newborn   [P] Pediatric   [M] Maternity   [A] Adult   [RIC] RIC Dx   [NC Dx] Noncancer Dx   [PDx] Primary Dx   [CC] RIC CC Condition   ►◄ Revised Text   ● New Code   ▲ Revised Code Title

468   ICD-10-CM 2016

C94.02   **Acute erythroid leukemia,** in relapse   `CC`

✓5ᵗʰ **C94.2**   **Acute megakaryoblastic leukemia**
Acute myeloid leukemia M7
Acute megakaryocytic leukemia

     C94.20   **Acute megakaryoblastic leukemia** not having achieved remission
Acute megakaryoblastic leukemia with failied remission
Acute megakaryoblastic leukemia NOS

     C94.21   **Acute megakaryoblastic leukemia,** in remission

     C94.22   **Acute megakaryoblastic leukemia,** in relapse

✓5ᵗʰ **C94.3**   **Mast cell leukemia**

     C94.30   **Mast cell leukemia** not having achieved remission
Mast cell leukemia with failed remission
Mast cell leukemia NOS

     C94.31   **Mast cell leukemia,** in remission

     C94.32   **Mast cell leukemia,** in relapse

✓5ᵗʰ **C94.4**   **Acute panmyelosis with myelofibrosis**
Acute myelofibrosis
   EXCLUDES 1   myelofibrosis NOS (D75.81)
              secondary myelofibrosis NOS (D75.81)

     C94.40   **Acute panmyelosis with myelofibrosis** not having achieved remission
Acute myelofibrosis NOS
Acute panmyelosis with myelofibrosis with failed remission
Acute panmyelosis NOS

     C94.41   **Acute panmyelosis with myelofibrosis,** in remission

     C94.42   **Acute panmyelosis with myelofibrosis,** in relapse

C94.6   **Myelodysplastic disease, not classified**
Myeloproliferative disease, not classified

✓5ᵗʰ **C94.8**   **Other specified leukemias**
Aggressive NK-cell leukemia
Acute basophilic leukemia

     C94.80   **Other specified leukemias** not having achieved remission
Other specified leukemia with failed remission
Other specified leukemias NOS

     C94.81   **Other specified leukemias,** in remission

     C94.82   **Other specified leukemias,** in relapse

✓4ᵗʰ **C95**   **Leukemia of** unspecified cell type
   EXCLUDES 1   personal history of leukemia (Z85.6)

✓5ᵗʰ **C95.0**   Acute **leukemia of unspecified cell type**
Acute bilineal leukemia
Acute mixed lineage leukemia
Biphenotypic acute leukemia
Stem cell leukemia of unclear lineage
   EXCLUDES 1   acute exacerbation of unspecified chronic leukemia (C95.10)

     C95.00   **Acute leukemia of unspecified cell type** not having achieved remission   `CC`
Acute leukemia of unspecified cell type with failed remission
Acute leukemia NOS

     C95.01   **Acute leukemia of unspecified cell type,** in remission

     C95.02   **Acute leukemia of unspecified cell type,** in relapse   `CC`

✓5ᵗʰ **C95.1**   Chronic **leukemia of unspecified cell type**

     C95.10   **Chronic leukemia of unspecified cell type** not having achieved remission
Chronic leukemia of unspecified cell type with failed remission
Chronic leukemia NOS

     C95.11   **Chronic leukemia of unspecified cell type,** in remission

     C95.12   **Chronic leukemia of unspecified cell type,** in relapse

✓5ᵗʰ **C95.9**   **Leukemia,** unspecified

     C95.90   **Leukemia, unspecified** not having achieved remission   ▽
Leukemia, unspecified with failed remission
Leukemia NOS

     C95.91   **Leukemia, unspecified,** in remission   ▽

     C95.92   **Leukemia, unspecified,** in relapse   ▽

✓4ᵗʰ **C96**   **Other and unspecified malignant neoplasms of lymphoid, hematopoietic and related tissue**
   EXCLUDES 1   personal history of other malignant neoplasms of lymphoid, hematopoietic and related tissues (Z85.79)

C96.0   **Multifocal and multisystemic (disseminated) Langerhans-cell histiocytosis**
Histiocytosis X, multisystemic
Letterer-Siwe disease
   EXCLUDES 1   adult pulmonary Langerhans cell histiocytosis (J84.82)
            multifocal and unisystemic Langerhans-cell histiocytosis (C96.5)
            unifocal Langerhans-cell histiocytosis (C96.6)

C96.2   **Malignant mast cell tumor**
Aggressive systemic mastocytosis
Mast cell sarcoma
   EXCLUDES 1   indolent mastocytosis (D47.0)
            mast cell leukemia (C94.30)
            mastocytosis (congenital) (cutaneous) (Q82.2)

C96.4   **Sarcoma of dendritic cells (accessory cells)**
Follicular dendritic cell sarcoma
Interdigitating dendritic cell sarcoma
Langerhans cell sarcoma

C96.5   **Multifocal and unisystemic Langerhans-cell histiocytosis**
Hand-Schüller-Christian disease
Histiocytosis X, multifocal
   EXCLUDES 1   multifocal and multisystemic (disseminated) Langerhans-cell histiocytosis (C96.0)
            unifocal Langerhans-cell histiocytosis (C96.6)

C96.6   **Unifocal Langerhans-cell histiocytosis**
Eosinophilic granuloma
Histiocytosis X, unifocal
Histiocytosis X NOS
Langerhans-cell histiocytosis NOS
   EXCLUDES 1   multifocal and multisysemic (disseminated) Langerhans-cell histiocytosis (C96.0)
            multifocal and unisystemic Langerhans-cell histiocytosis (C96.5)

C96.A   **Histiocytic sarcoma**
Malignant histiocytosis

C96.Z   **Other specified malignant neoplasms of lymphoid, hematopoietic and related tissue**

C96.9   **Malignant neoplasm of lymphoid, hematopoietic and related tissue, unspecified**   ▽

In situ neoplasms (D00-D09)

   INCLUDES   Bowen's disease
            erythroplasia
            grade III intraepithelial neoplasia
            Queyrat's erythroplasia

✓4ᵗʰ **D00**   **Carcinoma in situ of** oral cavity, esophagus and stomach
   EXCLUDES 1   melanoma in situ (D03.-)

✓5ᵗʰ **D00.0**   **Carcinoma in situ of** lip, oral cavity and pharynx
Use additional code to identify:
   exposure to environmental tobacco smoke (Z77.22)
   exposure to tobacco smoke in the perinatal period (P96.81)
   history of tobacco use (Z87.891)
   occupational exposure to environmental tobacco smoke (Z57.31)
   tobacco dependence (F17.-)
   tobacco use (Z72.0)
   EXCLUDES 1   carcinoma in situ of aryepiglottic fold or interarytenoid fold, laryngeal aspect (D02.0)
            carcinoma in situ of epiglottis NOS (D02.0)
            carcinoma in situ of epiglottis suprahyoid portion (D02.0)
            carcinoma in situ of skin of lip (D03.0, D04.0)

     D00.00   **Carcinoma in situ of oral cavity, unspecified site**   ▽

     D00.01   **Carcinoma in situ of** labial mucosa and vermilion border

     D00.02   **Carcinoma in situ of** buccal mucosa

     D00.03   **Carcinoma in situ of** gingiva and edentulous alveolar ridge

     D00.04   **Carcinoma in situ of** soft palate

     D00.05   **Carcinoma in situ of** hard palate

     D00.06   **Carcinoma in situ of** floor of mouth

     D00.07   **Carcinoma in situ of** tongue

     D00.08   **Carcinoma in situ of** pharynx
Carcinoma in situ of aryepiglottic fold NOS
Carcinoma in situ of hypopharyngeal aspect of aryepiglottic fold
Carcinoma in situ of marginal zone of aryepiglottic fold

D00.1   **Carcinoma in situ of** esophagus

D00.2   **Carcinoma in situ of** stomach

☑4ᵗʰ **D01** **Carcinoma in situ of** other and unspecified digestive organs
     EXCLUDES 1   *melanoma in situ (D03.-)*

   D01.0 **Carcinoma in situ of** colon
     EXCLUDES 1   *carcinoma in situ of rectosigmoid junction (D01.1)*

   D01.1 **Carcinoma in situ of** rectosigmoid junction

   D01.2 **Carcinoma in situ of** rectum

   D01.3 **Carcinoma in situ of** anus and anal canal
     EXCLUDES 1   *carcinoma in situ of anal margin (D04.5)*
           carcinoma in situ of anal skin (D04.5)
           carcinoma in situ of perianal skin (D04.5)

   ☑5ᵗʰ **D01.4** **Carcinoma in situ of other and unspecified parts of** intestine
     EXCLUDES 1   *carcinoma in situ of ampulla of Vater (D01.5)*

     D01.40 **Carcinoma in situ of unspecified part of intestine** ▽
     D01.49 **Carcinoma in situ of other parts of intestine**

   D01.5 **Carcinoma in situ of** liver, gallbladder and bile ducts
     Carcinoma in situ of ampulla of Vater

   D01.7 **Carcinoma in situ of other specified digestive organs**
     Carcinoma in situ of pancreas

   D01.9 **Carcinoma in situ of digestive organ, unspecified** ▽

☑4ᵗʰ **D02** **Carcinoma in situ of** middle ear and respiratory system
     Use additional code to identify:
     exposure to environmental tobacco smoke (Z77.22)
     exposure to tobacco smoke in the perinatal period (P96.81)
     history of tobacco use (Z87.891)
     occupational exposure to environmental tobacco smoke (Z57.31)
     tobacco dependence (F17.-)
     tobacco use (Z72.0)
     EXCLUDES 1   *melanoma in situ (D03.-)*

   D02.0 **Carcinoma in situ of** larynx
     Carcinoma in situ of aryepiglottic fold or interarytenoid fold,
       laryngeal aspect
     Carcinoma in situ of epiglottis (suprahyoid portion)
     EXCLUDES 1   *carcinoma in situ of aryepiglottic fold or interarytenoid*
           fold NOS (D00.08)
           carcinoma in situ of hypopharyngeal aspect (D00.08)
           carcinoma in situ of marginal zone (D00.08)

   D02.1 **Carcinoma in situ of** trachea

   ☑5ᵗʰ **D02.2** **Carcinoma in situ of** bronchus and lung
     D02.20 **Carcinoma in situ of unspecified bronchus** ▽
       and lung
     D02.21 **Carcinoma in situ of** right **bronchus and lung**
     D02.22 **Carcinoma in situ of** left **bronchus and lung**

   D02.3 **Carcinoma in situ of other parts of respiratory system**
     Carcinoma in situ of accessory sinuses
     Carcinoma in situ of middle ear
     Carcinoma in situ of nasal cavities
     EXCLUDES 1   *carcinoma in situ of ear (external) (skin) (D04.2-)*
           carcinoma in situ of nose NOS (D09.8)
           carcinoma in situ of skin of nose (D04.3)

   D02.4 **Carcinoma in situ of respiratory system, unspecified** ▽

☑4ᵗʰ **D03** Melanoma **in situ**

   D03.0 **Melanoma in situ of** lip

   ☑5ᵗʰ **D03.1** **Melanoma in situ of** eyelid, including canthus
     D03.10 **Melanoma in situ of unspecified eyelid, including** ▽
       canthus
     D03.11 **Melanoma in situ of** right **eyelid, including canthus**
     D03.12 **Melanoma in situ of** left **eyelid, including canthus**

   ☑5ᵗʰ **D03.2** **Melanoma in situ of** ear and external auricular canal
     D03.20 **Melanoma in situ of unspecified ear and external** ▽
       auricular canal
     D03.21 **Melanoma in situ of** right **ear and external auricular**
       canal
     D03.22 **Melanoma in situ of** left **ear and external auricular**
       canal

   ☑5ᵗʰ **D03.3** **Melanoma in situ of** other and unspecified parts of face
     D03.30 **Melanoma in situ of unspecified part of face** ▽
     D03.39 **Melanoma in situ of other parts of face**

   D03.4 **Melanoma in situ of** scalp and neck

   ☑5ᵗʰ **D03.5** **Melanoma in situ of** trunk
     D03.51 **Melanoma in situ of** anal skin
       Melanoma in situ of anal margin
       Melanoma in situ of perianal skin
     D03.52 **Melanoma in situ of** breast (skin) (soft tissue)
     D03.59 **Melanoma in situ of other part of trunk**

   ☑5ᵗʰ **D03.6** **Melanoma in situ of** upper limb, including shoulder
     D03.60 **Melanoma in situ of unspecified upper limb,** ▽
       including shoulder
     D03.61 **Melanoma in situ of** right **upper limb, including**
       shoulder
     D03.62 **Melanoma in situ of** left **upper limb, including**
       shoulder

   ☑5ᵗʰ **D03.7** **Melanoma in situ of** lower limb, including hip
     D03.70 **Melanoma in situ of unspecified lower limb,** ▽
       including hip
     D03.71 **Melanoma in situ of** right **lower limb, including hip**
     D03.72 **Melanoma in situ of** left **lower limb, including hip**

   D03.8 **Melanoma in situ of other sites**
     Melanoma in situ of scrotum
     EXCLUDES 1   *carcinoma in situ of scrotum (D07.61)*

   D03.9 **Melanoma in situ, unspecified** ▽

☑4ᵗʰ **D04** **Carcinoma in situ of** skin
     EXCLUDES 1   *erythroplasia of Queyrat (penis) NOS (D07.4)*
           melanoma in situ (D03.-)

   D04.0 **Carcinoma in situ of skin of** lip
     EXCLUDES 1   *carcinoma in situ of vermilion border of lip (D00.01)*

   ☑5ᵗʰ **D04.1** **Carcinoma in situ of skin of** eyelid, including canthus
     D04.10 **Carcinoma in situ of skin of unspecified eyelid,** ▽
       including canthus
     D04.11 **Carcinoma in situ of skin of** right **eyelid, including**
       canthus
     D04.12 **Carcinoma in situ of skin of** left **eyelid, including**
       canthus

   ☑5ᵗʰ **D04.2** **Carcinoma in situ of skin of** ear and external auricular canal
     D04.20 **Carcinoma in situ of skin of unspecified ear and** ▽
       external auricular canal
     D04.21 **Carcinoma in situ of skin of** right **ear and external**
       auricular canal
     D04.22 **Carcinoma in situ of skin of** left **ear and external**
       auricular canal

   ☑5ᵗʰ **D04.3** **Carcinoma in situ of skin of** other and unspecified parts of
     face
     D04.30 **Carcinoma in situ of skin of unspecified** ▽
       part of face
     D04.39 **Carcinoma in situ of skin of other parts of face**

   D04.4 **Carcinoma in situ of skin of** scalp and neck

   D04.5 **Carcinoma in situ of skin of** trunk
     Carcinoma in situ of anal margin
     Carcinoma in situ of anal skin
     Carcinoma in situ of perianal skin
     Carcinoma in situ of skin of breast
     EXCLUDES 1   *carcinoma in situ of anus NOS (D01.3)*
           carcinoma in situ of scrotum (D07.61)
           carcinoma in situ of skin of genital organs (D07.-)

   ☑5ᵗʰ **D04.6** **Carcinoma in situ of skin of** upper limb, including shoulder
     D04.60 **Carcinoma in situ of skin of unspecified upper** ▽
       limb, including shoulder
     D04.61 **Carcinoma in situ of skin of** right **upper limb,**
       including shoulder
     D04.62 **Carcinoma in situ of skin of** left **upper limb, including**
       shoulder

   ☑5ᵗʰ **D04.7** **Carcinoma in situ of skin of** lower limb, including hip
     D04.70 **Carcinoma in situ of skin of unspecified lower** ▽
       limb, including hip
     D04.71 **Carcinoma in situ of skin of** right **lower limb,**
       including hip
     D04.72 **Carcinoma in situ of skin of** left **lower limb, including**
       hip

   D04.8 **Carcinoma in situ of skin of other sites**

   D04.9 **Carcinoma in situ of skin, unspecified** ▽

☑4ᵗʰ **D05** **Carcinoma in situ of** breast
     EXCLUDES 1   *carcinoma in situ of skin of breast (D04.5)*
           melanoma in situ of breast (skin) (D03.5)
           Paget's disease of breast or nipple (C50.-)

   ☑5ᵗʰ **D05.0** Lobular **carcinoma in situ of breast**
     D05.00 **Lobular carcinoma in situ of unspecified breast** ▽
     D05.01 **Lobular carcinoma in situ of** right **breast**
     D05.02 **Lobular carcinoma in situ of** left **breast**

Ⓝ Newborn   Ⓟ Pediatric   Ⓜ Maternity   Ⓐ Adult   RIC RIC Dx   NCDx Noncancer Dx   PDx Primary Dx   CC RIC CC Condition   ►◄ Revised Text   ● New Code   ▲ Revised Code Title

470   ICD-10-CM 2016

☑5ᵗʰ **D05.1** Intraductal carcinoma in situ of breast
    D05.10 Intraductal carcinoma in situ of unspecified breast ▽
    D05.11 Intraductal carcinoma in situ of right breast
    D05.12 Intraductal carcinoma in situ of left breast

☑5ᵗʰ **D05.8** Other specified type of carcinoma in situ of breast
    D05.80 Other specified type of carcinoma in situ of unspecified breast ▽
    D05.81 Other specified type of carcinoma in situ of right breast
    D05.82 Other specified type of carcinoma in situ of left breast

☑5ᵗʰ **D05.9** Unspecified type of carcinoma in situ of breast
    D05.90 Unspecified type of carcinoma in situ of unspecified breast ▽
    D05.91 Unspecified type of carcinoma in situ of right breast ▽
    D05.92 Unspecified type of carcinoma in situ of left breast ▽

☑4ᵗʰ **D06** Carcinoma in situ of cervix uteri
    INCLUDES cervical adenocarcinoma in situ
        cervical intraepithelial glandular neoplasia
        cervical intraepithelial neoplasia III [CIN III]
        severe dysplasia of cervix uteri
    EXCLUDES 1 *cervical intraepithelial neoplasia II [CIN II] (N87.1)*
        cytologic evidence of malignancy of cervix without histologic confirmation (R87.614)
        high grade squamous intraepithelial lesion (HGSIL) of cervix (R87.613)
        melanoma in situ of cervix (D03.5)
        moderate cervical dysplasia (N87.1)

  D06.0 Carcinoma in situ of endocervix ♀
  D06.1 Carcinoma in situ of exocervix ♀
  D06.7 Carcinoma in situ of other parts of cervix ♀
  D06.9 Carcinoma in situ of cervix, unspecified ♀▽

☑4ᵗʰ **D07** Carcinoma in situ of other and unspecified genital organs
    EXCLUDES 1 *melanoma in situ of trunk (D03.5)*

  D07.0 Carcinoma in situ of endometrium ♀

  D07.1 Carcinoma in situ of vulva ♀
    Severe dysplasia of vulva
    Vulvar intraepithelial neoplasia III [VIN III]
    EXCLUDES 1 *moderate dysplasia of vulva (N90.1)*
        vulvar intraepithelial neoplasia II [VIN II] (N90.1)

  D07.2 Carcinoma in situ of vagina ♀
    Severe dysplasia of vagina
    Vaginal intraepithelial neoplasia III [VAIN III]
    EXCLUDES 1 *moderate dysplasia of vagina (N89.1)*
        vaginal intraepithelial neoplasia II [VIN II] (N89.1)

☑5ᵗʰ **D07.3** Carcinoma in situ of other and unspecified female genital organs
    D07.30 Carcinoma in situ of unspecified female genital organs ♀▽
    D07.39 Carcinoma in situ of other female genital organs ♀

  D07.4 Carcinoma in situ of penis ♂
    Erythroplasia of Queyrat NOS

  D07.5 Carcinoma in situ of prostate ♂
    Prostatic intraepithelial neoplasia III (PIN III)
    Severe dysplasia of prostate
    EXCLUDES 1 *dysplasia (mild) (moderate) of prostate (N42.3)*

☑5ᵗʰ **D07.6** Carcinoma in situ of other and unspecified male genital organs
    D07.60 Carcinoma in situ of unspecified male genital organs ♂▽
    D07.61 Carcinoma in situ of scrotum ♂
    D07.69 Carcinoma in situ of other male genital organs ♂

☑4ᵗʰ **D09** Carcinoma in situ of other and unspecified sites
    EXCLUDES 1 *melanoma in situ (D03.-)*

  D09.0 Carcinoma in situ of bladder

☑5ᵗʰ **D09.1** Carcinoma in situ of other and unspecified urinary organs
    D09.10 Carcinoma in situ of unspecified urinary organ ▽
    D09.19 Carcinoma in situ of other urinary organs

☑5ᵗʰ **D09.2** Carcinoma in situ of eye
    EXCLUDES 1 *carcinoma in situ of skin of eyelid (D04.1-)*
    D09.20 Carcinoma in situ of unspecified eye ▽

    D09.21 Carcinoma in situ of right eye
    D09.22 Carcinoma in situ of left eye

  D09.3 Carcinoma in situ of thyroid and other endocrine glands
    EXCLUDES 1 *carcinoma in situ of endocrine pancreas (D01.7)*
        carcinoma in situ of ovary (D07.39)
        carcinoma in situ of testis (D07.69)

  D09.8 Carcinoma in situ of other specified sites
  D09.9 Carcinoma in situ, unspecified ▽

Benign neoplasms, except benign neuroendocrine tumors (D10-D36)

☑4ᵗʰ **D10** Benign neoplasm of mouth and pharynx
  D10.0 Benign neoplasm of lip
    Benign neoplasm of lip (frenulum) (inner aspect) (mucosa) (vermilion border)
    EXCLUDES 1 *benign neoplasm of skin of lip (D22.0, D23.0)*

  D10.1 Benign neoplasm of tongue
    Benign neoplasm of lingual tonsil

  D10.2 Benign neoplasm of floor of mouth

☑5ᵗʰ **D10.3** Other and unspecified parts of mouth
    D10.30 Benign neoplasm of unspecified part of mouth ▽
    D10.39 Benign neoplasm of other parts of mouth
        Benign neoplasm of minor salivary gland NOS
        EXCLUDES 1 *benign odontogenic neoplasms (D16.4-D16.5)*
            benign neoplasm of mucosa of lip (D10.0)
            benign neoplasm of nasopharyngeal surface of soft palate (D10.6)

  D10.4 Benign neoplasm of tonsil
    Benign neoplasm of tonsil (faucial) (palatine)
    EXCLUDES 1 *benign neoplasm of lingual tonsil (D10.1)*
        benign neoplasm of pharyngeal tonsil (D10.6)
        benign neoplasm of tonsillar fossa (D10.5)
        benign neoplasm of tonsillar pillars (D10.5)

  D10.5 Benign neoplasm of other parts of oropharynx
    Benign neoplasm of epiglottis, anterior aspect
    Benign neoplasm of tonsillar fossa
    Benign neoplasm of tonsillar pillars
    Benign neoplasm of vallecula
    EXCLUDES 1 *benign neoplasm of epiglottis NOS (D14.1)*
        benign neoplasm of epiglottis, suprahyoid portion (D14.1)

  D10.6 Benign neoplasm of nasopharynx
    Benign neoplasm of pharyngeal tonsil
    Benign neoplasm of posterior margin of septum and choanae

  D10.7 Benign neoplasm of hypopharynx
  D10.9 Benign neoplasm of pharynx, unspecified ▽

☑4ᵗʰ **D11** Benign neoplasm of major salivary glands
    EXCLUDES 1 *benign neoplasms of specified minor salivary glands which are classified according to their anatomical location*
        benign neoplasms of minor salivary glands NOS (D10.39)

  D11.0 Benign neoplasm of parotid gland

  D11.7 Benign neoplasm of other major salivary glands
    Benign neoplasm of sublingual salivary gland
    Benign neoplasm of submandibular salivary gland

  D11.9 Benign neoplasm of major salivary gland, unspecified ▽

☑4ᵗʰ **D12** Benign neoplasm of colon, rectum, anus and anal canal
    EXCLUDES 1 *benign carcinoid tumors of the large intestine, and rectum (D3A.02-)*

  D12.0 Benign neoplasm of cecum
    Benign neoplasm of ileocecal valve

  D12.1 Benign neoplasm of appendix
    EXCLUDES 1 *benign carcinoid tumor of the appendix (D3A.020)*

  D12.2 Benign neoplasm of ascending colon

  D12.3 Benign neoplasm of transverse colon
    Benign neoplasm of hepatic flexure
    Benign neoplasm of splenic flexure

  D12.4 Benign neoplasm of descending colon

  D12.5 Benign neoplasm of sigmoid colon

  D12.6 Benign neoplasm of colon, unspecified ▽
    Adenomatosis of colon
    Benign neoplasm of large intestine NOS
    Polyposis (hereditary) of colon
    EXCLUDES 1 *inflammatory polyp of colon (K51.4-)*
        polyp of colon NOS (K63.5)

  D12.7 Benign neoplasm of rectosigmoid junction

☑ Add'l Character Required   ᴠₓ7ᵗʰ Placeholder Alert   RUG IV Special Care High Dx   RUG IV Clinically Complex Dx   RUG IV Special Care Low Dx   Manifestation Code   Other Specified Code   ▽ Unspecified Code

ICD-10-CM 2016   471

Chapter 2. Neoplasms

D12.8   Benign neoplasm of rectum
- *EXCLUDES 1*   *benign carcinoid tumor of the rectum (D3A.026)*

D12.9   Benign neoplasm of anus and anal canal
- Benign neoplasm of anus NOS
- *EXCLUDES 1*   *benign neoplasm of anal margin (D22.5, D23.5)*
  - *benign neoplasm of anal skin (D22.5, D23.5)*
  - *benign neoplasm of perianal skin (D22.5, D23.5)*

✓4ᵗʰ **D13**   **Benign neoplasm of** other and ill-defined parts of digestive system
- *EXCLUDES 1*   *benign stromal tumors of digestive system (D21.4)*

D13.0   Benign neoplasm of esophagus

D13.1   Benign neoplasm of stomach
- *EXCLUDES 1*   *benign carcinoid tumor of the stomach (D3A.092)*

D13.2   Benign neoplasm of duodenum
- *EXCLUDES 1*   *benign carcinoid tumor of the duodenum (D3A.010)*

✓5ᵗʰ **D13.3**   Benign neoplasm of other and unspecified parts of small intestine
- *EXCLUDES 1*   *benign carcinoid tumors of the small intestine (D3A.01-)*
  - *benign neoplasm of ileocecal valve (D12.0)*

     D13.30   Benign neoplasm of unspecified part of small intestine   ▽

     D13.39   Benign neoplasm of other parts of small intestine

D13.4   Benign neoplasm of liver
- Benign neoplasm of intrahepatic bile ducts

D13.5   Benign neoplasm of extrahepatic bile ducts

D13.6   Benign neoplasm of pancreas
- *EXCLUDES 1*   *benign neoplasm of endocrine pancreas (D13.7)*

D13.7   Benign neoplasm of endocrine pancreas
- Islet cell tumor
- Benign neoplasm of islets of Langerhans
- Use additional code to identify any functional activity

D13.9   Benign neoplasm of ill-defined sites within the digestive system
- Benign neoplasm of digestive system NOS
- Benign neoplasm of intestine NOS
- Benign neoplasm of spleen

✓4ᵗʰ **D14**   **Benign neoplasm of** middle ear and respiratory system

D14.0   **Benign neoplasm of** middle ear, nasal cavity and accessory sinuses
- Benign neoplasm of cartilage of nose
- *EXCLUDES 1*   *benign neoplasm of auricular canal (external) (D22.2-, D23.2-)*
  - *benign neoplasm of bone of ear (D16.4)*
  - *benign neoplasm of bone of nose (D16.4)*
  - *benign neoplasm of cartilage of ear (D21.0)*
  - *benign neoplasm of ear (external)(skin) (D22.2-, D23.2-)*
  - *benign neoplasm of nose NOS (D36.7)*
  - *benign neoplasm of skin of nose (D22.39, D23.39)*
  - *benign neoplasm of olfactory bulb (D33.3)*
  - *benign neoplasm of posterior margin of septum and choanae (D10.6)*
  - *polyp of accessory sinus (J33.8)*
  - *polyp of ear (middle) (H74.4)*
  - *polyp of nasal (cavity) (J33.-)*

D14.1   Benign neoplasm of larynx
- Adenomatous polyp of larynx
- Benign neoplasm of epiglottis (suprahyoid portion)
- *EXCLUDES 1*   *benign neoplasm of epiglottis, anterior aspect (D10.5)*
  - *polyp (nonadenomatous) of vocal cord or larynx (J38.1)*

D14.2   Benign neoplasm of trachea

✓5ᵗʰ **D14.3**   Benign neoplasm of bronchus and lung
- *EXCLUDES 1*   *benign carcinoid tumor of the bronchus and lung (D3A.090)*

     D14.30   Benign neoplasm of unspecified bronchus and lung   ▽

     D14.31   Benign neoplasm of right bronchus and lung

     D14.32   Benign neoplasm of left bronchus and lung

D14.4   Benign neoplasm of respiratory system, unspecified   ▽

✓4ᵗʰ **D15**   **Benign neoplasm of** other and unspecified intrathoracic organs
- *EXCLUDES 1*   *benign neoplasm of mesothelial tissue (D19.-)*

D15.0   Benign neoplasm of thymus
- *EXCLUDES 1*   *benign carcinoid tumor of the thymus (D3A.091)*

D15.1   Benign neoplasm of heart
- *EXCLUDES 1*   *benign neoplasm of great vessels (D21.3)*

D15.2   Benign neoplasm of mediastinum

D15.7   Benign neoplasm of other specified intrathoracic organs

D15.9   Benign neoplasm of intrathoracic organ, unspecified   ▽

✓4ᵗʰ **D16**   **Benign neoplasm of** bone and articular cartilage
- *EXCLUDES 1*   *benign neoplasm of connective tissue of ear (D21.0)*
  - *benign neoplasm of connective tissue of eyelid (D21.0)*
  - *benign neoplasm of connective tissue of larynx (D14.1)*
  - *benign neoplasm of connective tissue of nose (D14.0)*
  - *benign neoplasm of synovia (D21.-)*

✓5ᵗʰ **D16.0**   Benign neoplasm of scapula and long bones of upper limb

     D16.00   Benign neoplasm of scapula and long bones of unspecified upper limb   ▽

     D16.01   Benign neoplasm of scapula and long bones of right upper limb

     D16.02   Benign neoplasm of scapula and long bones of left upper limb

✓5ᵗʰ **D16.1**   Benign neoplasm of short bones of upper limb

     D16.10   Benign neoplasm of short bones of unspecified upper limb   ▽

     D16.11   Benign neoplasm of short bones of right upper limb

     D16.12   Benign neoplasm of short bones of left upper limb

✓5ᵗʰ **D16.2**   Benign neoplasm of long bones of lower limb

     D16.20   Benign neoplasm of long bones of unspecified lower limb   ▽

     D16.21   Benign neoplasm of long bones of right lower limb

     D16.22   Benign neoplasm of long bones of left lower limb

✓5ᵗʰ **D16.3**   Benign neoplasm of short bones of lower limb

     D16.30   Benign neoplasm of short bones of unspecified lower limb   ▽

     D16.31   Benign neoplasm of short bones of right lower limb

     D16.32   Benign neoplasm of short bones of left lower limb

D16.4   Benign neoplasm of bones of skull and face
- Benign neoplasm of maxilla (superior)
- Benign neoplasm of orbital bone
- Keratocyst of maxilla
- Keratocystic odontogenic tumor of maxilla
- *EXCLUDES 1*   *benign neoplasm of lower jaw bone (D16.5)*

D16.5   Benign neoplasm of lower jaw bone
- Keratocyst of mandible
- Keratocystic odontogenic tumor of mandible

D16.6   Benign neoplasm of vertebral column
- *EXCLUDES 1*   *benign neoplasm of sacrum and coccyx (D16.8)*

D16.7   Benign neoplasm of ribs, sternum and clavicle

D16.8   Benign neoplasm of pelvic bones, sacrum and coccyx

D16.9   Benign neoplasm of bone and articular cartilage, unspecified   ▽

✓4ᵗʰ **D17**   **Benign** lipomatous **neoplasm**

D17.0   Benign lipomatous neoplasm of skin and subcutaneous tissue of head, face and neck

D17.1   Benign lipomatous neoplasm of skin and subcutaneous tissue of trunk

✓5ᵗʰ **D17.2**   Benign lipomatous neoplasm of skin and subcutaneous tissue of limb

     D17.20   Benign lipomatous neoplasm of skin and subcutaneous tissue of unspecified limb   ▽

     D17.21   Benign lipomatous neoplasm of skin and subcutaneous tissue of right arm

     D17.22   Benign lipomatous neoplasm of skin and subcutaneous tissue of left arm

     D17.23   Benign lipomatous neoplasm of skin and subcutaneous tissue of right leg

     D17.24   Benign lipomatous neoplasm of skin and subcutaneous tissue of left leg

✓5ᵗʰ **D17.3**   Benign lipomatous neoplasm of skin and subcutaneous tissue of other and unspecified sites

     D17.30   Benign lipomatous neoplasm of skin and subcutaneous tissue of unspecified sites   ▽

     D17.39   Benign lipomatous neoplasm of skin and subcutaneous tissue of other sites

D17.4   Benign lipomatous neoplasm of intrathoracic organs

D17.5   Benign lipomatous neoplasm of intra-abdominal organs
- *EXCLUDES 1*   *benign lipomatous neoplasm of peritoneum and retroperitoneum (D17.79)*

D17.6   Benign lipomatous neoplasm of spermatic cord   ♂

✓5ᵗʰ **D17.7**   Benign lipomatous neoplasm of other sites

     D17.71   Benign lipomatous neoplasm of kidney

Ⓝ Newborn   Ⓟ Pediatric   Ⓜ Maternity   Ⓐ Adult   **RIC** RIC Dx   **NCDx** Noncancer Dx   **PDx** Primary Dx   **CC** RIC CC Condition   ▶◀ Revised Text   ● New Code   ▲ Revised Code Title

D17.72   **Benign lipomatous neoplasm of other genitourinary organ**

D17.79   **Benign lipomatous neoplasm of other sites**
Benign lipomatous neoplasm of peritoneum
Benign lipomatous neoplasm of retroperitoneum

D17.9   **Benign lipomatous neoplasm, unspecified** ▽
Lipoma NOS

✓4ᵗʰ **D18**   **Hemangioma and lymphangioma, any site**
EXCLUDES 1   *benign neoplasm of glomus jugulare (D35.6)*
blue or pigmented nevus (D22.-)
nevus NOS (D22.-)
vascular nevus (Q82.5)

✓5ᵗʰ **D18.0**   **Hemangioma**
Angioma NOS
Cavernous nevus

D18.00   **Hemangioma unspecified site** ▽

D18.01   **Hemangioma of skin and subcutaneous tissue**

D18.02   **Hemangioma of intracranial structures**

D18.03   **Hemangioma of intra-abdominal structures**

D18.09   **Hemangioma of other sites**

D18.1   **Lymphangioma, any site**

✓4ᵗʰ **D19**   **Benign neoplasm of mesothelial tissue**

D19.0   **Benign neoplasm of mesothelial tissue of pleura**

D19.1   **Benign neoplasm of mesothelial tissue of peritoneum**

D19.7   **Benign neoplasm of mesothelial tissue of other sites**

D19.9   **Benign neoplasm of mesothelial tissue, unspecified** ▽
Benign mesothelioma NOS

✓4ᵗʰ **D20**   **Benign neoplasm of soft tissue of retroperitoneum and peritoneum**
EXCLUDES 1   *benign lipomatous neoplasm of peritoneum and retroperitoneum (D17.79)*
benign neoplasm of mesothelial tissue (D19.-)

D20.0   **Benign neoplasm of soft tissue of retroperitoneum**

D20.1   **Benign neoplasm of soft tissue of peritoneum**

✓4ᵗʰ **D21**   **Other benign neoplasms of connective and other soft tissue**
INCLUDES   benign neoplasm of blood vessel
benign neoplasm of bursa
benign neoplasm of cartilage
benign neoplasm of fascia
benign neoplasm of fat
benign neoplasm of ligament, except uterine
benign neoplasm of lymphatic channel
benign neoplasm of muscle
benign neoplasm of synovia
benign neoplasm of tendon (sheath)
benign stromal tumors
EXCLUDES 1   *benign neoplasm of articular cartilage (D16.-)*
benign neoplasm of cartilage of larynx (D14.1)
benign neoplasm of cartilage of nose (D14.0)
benign neoplasm of connective tissue of breast (D24.-)
benign neoplasm of peripheral nerves and autonomic nervous system (D36.1-)
benign neoplasm of peritoneum (D20.1)
benign neoplasm of retroperitoneum (D20.0)
benign neoplasm of uterine ligament, any (D28.2)
benign neoplasm of vascular tissue (D18.-)
hemangioma (D18.0-)
lipomatous neoplasm (D17.-)
lymphangioma (D18.1)
uterine leiomyoma (D25.-)

D21.0   **Benign neoplasm of connective and other soft tissue of head, face and neck**
Benign neoplasm of connective tissue of ear
Benign neoplasm of connective tissue of eyelid
EXCLUDES 1   *benign neoplasm of connective tissue of orbit (D31.6-)*

✓5ᵗʰ **D21.1**   **Benign neoplasm of connective and other soft tissue of upper limb, including shoulder**

D21.10   **Benign neoplasm of connective and other soft tissue of unspecified upper limb, including shoulder** ▽

D21.11   **Benign neoplasm of connective and other soft tissue of right upper limb, including shoulder**

D21.12   **Benign neoplasm of connective and other soft tissue of left upper limb, including shoulder**

✓5ᵗʰ **D21.2**   **Benign neoplasm of connective and other soft tissue of lower limb, including hip**

D21.20   **Benign neoplasm of connective and other soft tissue of unspecified lower limb, including hip** ▽

D21.21   **Benign neoplasm of connective and other soft tissue of right lower limb, including hip**

D21.22   **Benign neoplasm of connective and other soft tissue of left lower limb, including hip**

D21.3   **Benign neoplasm of connective and other soft tissue of thorax**
Benign neoplasm of axilla
Benign neoplasm of diaphragm
Benign neoplasm of great vessels
EXCLUDES 1   *benign neoplasm of heart (D15.1)*
benign neoplasm of mediastinum (D15.2)
benign neoplasm of thymus (D15.0)

D21.4   **Benign neoplasm of connective and other soft tissue of abdomen**
Benign stromal tumors of abdomen

D21.5   **Benign neoplasm of connective and other soft tissue of pelvis**
EXCLUDES 1   *benign neoplasm of any uterine ligament (D28.2)*
uterine leiomyoma (D25.-)

D21.6   **Benign neoplasm of connective and other soft tissue of trunk, unspecified** ▽
Benign neoplasm of back NOS

D21.9   **Benign neoplasm of connective and other soft tissue, unspecified** ▽

✓4ᵗʰ **D22**   **Melanocytic nevi**
INCLUDES   atypical nevus
blue hairy pigmented nevus
nevus NOS

D22.0   **Melanocytic nevi of lip**

✓5ᵗʰ **D22.1**   **Melanocytic nevi of eyelid, including canthus**

D22.10   **Melanocytic nevi of unspecified eyelid, including canthus** ▽

D22.11   **Melanocytic nevi of right eyelid, including canthus**

D22.12   **Melanocytic nevi of left eyelid, including canthus**

✓5ᵗʰ **D22.2**   **Melanocytic nevi of ear and external auricular canal**

D22.20   **Melanocytic nevi of unspecified ear and external auricular canal** ▽

D22.21   **Melanocytic nevi of right ear and external auricular canal**

D22.22   **Melanocytic nevi of left ear and external auricular canal**

✓5ᵗʰ **D22.3**   **Melanocytic nevi of other and unspecified parts of face**

D22.30   **Melanocytic nevi of unspecified part of face** ▽

D22.39   **Melanocytic nevi of other parts of face**

D22.4   **Melanocytic nevi of scalp and neck**

D22.5   **Melanocytic nevi of trunk**
Melanocytic nevi of anal margin
Melanocytic nevi of anal skin
Melanocytic nevi of perianal skin
Melanocytic nevi of skin of breast

✓5ᵗʰ **D22.6**   **Melanocytic nevi of upper limb, including shoulder**

D22.60   **Melanocytic nevi of unspecified upper limb, including shoulder** ▽

D22.61   **Melanocytic nevi of right upper limb, including shoulder**

D22.62   **Melanocytic nevi of left upper limb, including shoulder**

✓5ᵗʰ **D22.7**   **Melanocytic nevi of lower limb, including hip**

D22.70   **Melanocytic nevi of unspecified lower limb, including hip** ▽

D22.71   **Melanocytic nevi of right lower limb, including hip**

D22.72   **Melanocytic nevi of left lower limb, including hip**

D22.9   **Melanocytic nevi, unspecified** ▽

✓4ᵗʰ **D23**   **Other benign neoplasms of skin**
INCLUDES   benign neoplasm of hair follicles
benign neoplasm of sebaceous glands
benign neoplasm of sweat glands
EXCLUDES 1   *benign lipomatous neoplasms of skin (D17.0-D17.3)*
melanocytic nevi (D22.-)

D23.0   **Other benign neoplasm of skin of lip**
EXCLUDES 1   *benign neoplasm of vermilion border of lip (D10.0)*

✓5ᵗʰ **D23.1**   **Other benign neoplasm of skin of eyelid, including canthus**

D23.10   **Other benign neoplasm of skin of unspecified eyelid, including canthus** ▽

D23.11   **Other benign neoplasm of skin of right eyelid, including canthus**

✓ Add'l Character Required   ✓x7ᵗʰ Placeholder Alert   RUG IV Special Care High Dx   RUG IV Clinically Complex Dx   RUG IV Special Care Low Dx   Manifestation Code   Other Specified Code   ▽ Unspecified Code

D23.12 Other benign neoplasm of skin of left eyelid, including canthus

√5ᵗʰ D23.2 Other benign neoplasm of skin of ear and external auricular canal

D23.20 Other benign neoplasm of skin of unspecified ear and external auricular canal ▽

D23.21 Other benign neoplasm of skin of right ear and external auricular canal

D23.22 Other benign neoplasm of skin of left ear and external auricular canal

√5ᵗʰ D23.3 Other benign neoplasm of skin of other and unspecified parts of face

D23.30 Other benign neoplasm of skin of unspecified part of face ▽

D23.39 Other benign neoplasm of skin of other parts of face

D23.4 Other benign neoplasm of skin of scalp and neck

D23.5 Other benign neoplasm of skin of trunk
Other benign neoplasm of anal margin
Other benign neoplasm of anal skin
Other benign neoplasm of perianal skin
Other benign neoplasm of skin of breast
EXCLUDES 1 *benign neoplasm of anus NOS (D12.9)*

√5ᵗʰ D23.6 Other benign neoplasm of skin of upper limb, including shoulder

D23.60 Other benign neoplasm of skin of unspecified upper limb, including shoulder ▽

D23.61 Other benign neoplasm of skin of right upper limb, including shoulder

D23.62 Other benign neoplasm of skin of left upper limb, including shoulder

√5ᵗʰ D23.7 Other benign neoplasm of skin of lower limb, including hip

D23.70 Other benign neoplasm of skin of unspecified lower limb, including hip ▽

D23.71 Other benign neoplasm of skin of right lower limb, including hip

D23.72 Other benign neoplasm of skin of left lower limb, including hip

D23.9 Other benign neoplasm of skin, unspecified ▽

√4ᵗʰ D24 Benign neoplasm of breast
INCLUDES benign neoplasm of connective tissue of breast
benign neoplasm of soft parts of breast
fibroadenoma of breast
EXCLUDES 2 *adenofibrosis of breast (N60.2)*
benign cyst of breast (N60.-)
benign mammary dysplasia (N60.-)
benign neoplasm of skin of breast (D22.5, D23.5)
fibrocystic disease of breast (N60.-)

D24.1 Benign neoplasm of right breast

D24.2 Benign neoplasm of left breast

D24.9 Benign neoplasm of unspecified breast ▽

√4ᵗʰ D25 Leiomyoma of uterus
INCLUDES uterine fibroid
uterine fibromyoma
uterine myoma

D25.0 Submucous leiomyoma of uterus ♀

D25.1 Intramural leiomyoma of uterus ♀
Interstitial leiomyoma of uterus

D25.2 Subserosal leiomyoma of uterus ♀
Subperitoneal leiomyoma of uterus

D25.9 Leiomyoma of uterus, unspecified ♀▽

√4ᵗʰ D26 Other benign neoplasms of uterus

D26.0 Other benign neoplasm of cervix uteri ♀

D26.1 Other benign neoplasm of corpus uteri ♀

D26.7 Other benign neoplasm of other parts of uterus ♀

D26.9 Other benign neoplasm of uterus, unspecified ♀▽

√4ᵗʰ D27 Benign neoplasm of ovary
Use additional code to identify any functional activity
EXCLUDES 2 *corpus albicans cyst (N83.2)*
corpus luteum cyst (N83.1)
endometrial cyst (N80.1)
follicular (atretic) cyst (N83.0)
graafian follicle cyst (N83.0)
ovarian cyst NEC (N83.2)
ovarian retention cyst (N83.2)

D27.0 Benign neoplasm of right ovary ♀

D27.1 Benign neoplasm of left ovary ♀

D27.9 Benign neoplasm of unspecified ovary ♀▽

√4ᵗʰ D28 Benign neoplasm of other and unspecified female genital organs
INCLUDES adenomatous polyp
benign neoplasm of skin of female genital organs
benign teratoma
EXCLUDES 1 *epoophoron cyst (Q50.5)*
fimbrial cyst (Q50.4)
Gartner's duct cyst (Q52.4)
parovarian cyst (Q50.5)

D28.0 Benign neoplasm of vulva ♀

D28.1 Benign neoplasm of vagina ♀

D28.2 Benign neoplasm of uterine tubes and ligaments ♀
Benign neoplasm of fallopian tube
Benign neoplasm of uterine ligament (broad) (round)

D28.7 Benign neoplasm of other specified female genital organs ♀

D28.9 Benign neoplasm of female genital organ, unspecified ♀▽

√4ᵗʰ D29 Benign neoplasm of male genital organs
INCLUDES benign neoplasm of skin of male genital organs

D29.0 Benign neoplasm of penis ♂

D29.1 Benign neoplasm of prostate ♂
EXCLUDES 1 *enlarged prostate (N40.-)*

√5ᵗʰ D29.2 Benign neoplasm of testis
Use additional code to identify any functional activity

D29.20 Benign neoplasm of unspecified testis ♂▽

D29.21 Benign neoplasm of right testis ♂

D29.22 Benign neoplasm of left testis ♂

√5ᵗʰ D29.3 Benign neoplasm of epididymis

D29.30 Benign neoplasm of unspecified epididymis ♂▽

D29.31 Benign neoplasm of right epididymis ♂

D29.32 Benign neoplasm of left epididymis ♂

D29.4 Benign neoplasm of scrotum ♂
Benign neoplasm of skin of scrotum

D29.8 Benign neoplasm of other specified male genital organs ♂
Benign neoplasm of seminal vesicle
Benign neoplasm of spermatic cord
Benign neoplasm of tunica vaginalis

D29.9 Benign neoplasm of male genital organ, unspecified ♂▽

√4ᵗʰ D30 Benign neoplasm of urinary organs

√5ᵗʰ D30.0 Benign neoplasm of kidney
EXCLUDES 1 *benign carcinoid tumor of the kidney (D3A.093)*
benign neoplasm of renal calyces (D30.1-)
benign neoplasm of renal pelvis (D30.1-)

D30.00 Benign neoplasm of unspecified kidney ▽

D30.01 Benign neoplasm of right kidney

D30.02 Benign neoplasm of left kidney

√5ᵗʰ D30.1 Benign neoplasm of renal pelvis

D30.10 Benign neoplasm of unspecified renal pelvis ▽

D30.11 Benign neoplasm of right renal pelvis

D30.12 Benign neoplasm of left renal pelvis

√5ᵗʰ D30.2 Benign neoplasm of ureter
EXCLUDES 1 *benign neoplasm of ureteric orifice of bladder (D30.3)*

D30.20 Benign neoplasm of unspecified ureter ▽

D30.21 Benign neoplasm of right ureter

D30.22 Benign neoplasm of left ureter

D30.3 Benign neoplasm of bladder
Benign neoplasm of ureteric orifice of bladder
Benign neoplasm of urethral orifice of bladder

D30.4 Benign neoplasm of urethra
EXCLUDES 1 *benign neoplasm of urethral orifice of bladder (D30.3)*

D30.8 Benign neoplasm of other specified urinary organs
Benign neoplasm of paraurethral glands

D30.9 Benign neoplasm of urinary organ, unspecified ▽
Benign neoplasm of urinary system NOS

√4ᵗʰ D31 Benign neoplasm of eye and adnexa
EXCLUDES 1 *benign neoplasm of connective tissue of eyelid (D21.0)*
benign neoplasm of optic nerve (D33.3)
benign neoplasm of skin of eyelid (D22.1-, D23.1-)

√5ᵗʰ D31.0 Benign neoplasm of conjunctiva

D31.00 Benign neoplasm of unspecified conjunctiva ▽

D31.01 Benign neoplasm of right conjunctiva

D31.02 Benign neoplasm of left conjunctiva

✓5ᵗʰ **D31.1** **Benign neoplasm of** cornea

    D31.1Ø **Benign neoplasm of unspecified cornea** ▽

    D31.11 **Benign neoplasm of** right **cornea**

    D31.12 **Benign neoplasm of** left **cornea**

✓5ᵗʰ **D31.2** **Benign neoplasm of** retina

    EXCLUDES 1   dark area on retina (D49.81)
                hemangioma of retina (D49.81)
                neoplasm of unspecified behavior of retina and choroid
                   (D49.81)
                retinal freckle (D49.81)

    D31.2Ø **Benign neoplasm of unspecified retina** ▽

    D31.21 **Benign neoplasm of** right **retina**

    D31.22 **Benign neoplasm of** left **retina**

✓5ᵗʰ **D31.3** **Benign neoplasm of** choroid

    D31.3Ø **Benign neoplasm of unspecified choroid** ▽

    D31.31 **Benign neoplasm of** right **choroid**

    D31.32 **Benign neoplasm of** left **choroid**

✓5ᵗʰ **D31.4** **Benign neoplasm of** ciliary body

    D31.4Ø **Benign neoplasm of unspecified ciliary body** ▽

    D31.41 **Benign neoplasm of** right **ciliary body**

    D31.42 **Benign neoplasm of** left **ciliary body**

✓5ᵗʰ **D31.5** **Benign neoplasm of** lacrimal gland and duct
    Benign neoplasm of lacrimal sac
    Benign neoplasm of nasolacrimal duct

    D31.5Ø **Benign neoplasm of unspecified lacrimal gland** ▽
            and duct

    D31.51 **Benign neoplasm of** right **lacrimal gland and duct**

    D31.52 **Benign neoplasm of** left **lacrimal gland and duct**

✓5ᵗʰ **D31.6** **Benign neoplasm of unspecified site of** orbit
    Benign neoplasm of connective tissue of orbit
    Benign neoplasm of extraocular muscle
    Benign neoplasm of peripheral nerves of orbit
    Benign neoplasm of retrobulbar tissue
    Benign neoplasm of retro-ocular tissue
    EXCLUDES 1   benign neoplasm of orbital bone (D16.4)

    D31.6Ø **Benign neoplasm of unspecified site of** ▽
            unspecified orbit

    D31.61 **Benign neoplasm of unspecified site of** right **orbit**

    D31.62 **Benign neoplasm of unspecified site of** left **orbit**

✓5ᵗʰ **D31.9** **Benign neoplasm of** unspecified part of eye
    Benign neoplasm of eyeball

    D31.9Ø **Benign neoplasm of unspecified part of** ▽
            unspecified eye

    D31.91 **Benign neoplasm of unspecified part of** right **eye**

    D31.92 **Benign neoplasm of unspecified part of** left **eye**

✓4ᵗʰ **D32** **Benign neoplasm of** meninges

    D32.Ø **Benign neoplasm of** cerebral **meninges**

    D32.1 **Benign neoplasm of** spinal **meninges**

    D32.9 **Benign neoplasm of meninges, unspecified** ▽
        Meningioma NOS

✓4ᵗʰ **D33** **Benign neoplasm of** brain and other parts of central nervous system

    EXCLUDES 1   angioma (D18.Ø-)
                benign neoplasm of meninges (D32.-)
                benign neoplasm of peripheral nerves and autonomic nervous
                   system (D36.1-)
                hemangioma (D18.Ø-)
                neurofibromatosis (Q85.Ø-)
                retro-ocular benign neoplasm (D31.6-)

    D33.Ø **Benign neoplasm of** brain, supratentorial
        Benign neoplasm of cerebral ventricle
        Benign neoplasm of cerebrum
        Benign neoplasm of frontal lobe
        Benign neoplasm of occipital lobe
        Benign neoplasm of parietal lobe
        Benign neoplasm of temporal lobe
        EXCLUDES 1   benign neoplasm of fourth ventricle (D33.1)

    D33.1 **Benign neoplasm of** brain, infratentorial
        Benign neoplasm of brain stem
        Benign neoplasm of cerebellum
        Benign neoplasm of fourth ventricle

    D33.2 **Benign neoplasm of brain, unspecified** ▽

    D33.3 **Benign neoplasm of** cranial nerves
        Benign neoplasm of olfactory bulb

    D33.4 **Benign neoplasm of** spinal cord

    D33.7 **Benign neoplasm of other specified parts of central nervous system**

    D33.9 **Benign neoplasm of central nervous system, unspecified** ▽
        Benign neoplasm of nervous system (central) NOS

D34 **Benign neoplasm of** thyroid gland
    Use additional code to identify any functional activity

✓4ᵗʰ **D35** **Benign neoplasm of** other and unspecified endocrine glands
    Use additional code to identify any functional activity
    EXCLUDES 1   benign neoplasm of endocrine pancreas (D13.7)
                benign neoplasm of ovary (D27.-)
                benign neoplasm of testis (D29.2-)
                benign neoplasm of thymus (D15.Ø)

    ✓5ᵗʰ **D35.Ø** **Benign neoplasm of** adrenal gland

        D35.ØØ **Benign neoplasm of unspecified adrenal gland** ▽

        D35.Ø1 **Benign neoplasm of** right **adrenal gland**

        D35.Ø2 **Benign neoplasm of** left **adrenal gland**

    D35.1 **Benign neoplasm of** parathyroid gland

    D35.2 **Benign neoplasm of** pituitary gland
        AHA: 2014, 3Q, 22

    D35.3 **Benign neoplasm of** craniopharyngeal duct

    D35.4 **Benign neoplasm of** pineal gland

    D35.5 **Benign neoplasm of** carotid body

    D35.6 **Benign neoplasm of** aortic body and other paraganglia
        Benign tumor of glomus jugulare

    D35.7 **Benign neoplasm of other specified endocrine glands**

    D35.9 **Benign neoplasm of endocrine gland, unspecified** ▽
        Benign neoplasm of unspecified endocrine gland

✓4ᵗʰ **D36** **Benign neoplasm of** other and unspecified sites

    D36.Ø **Benign neoplasm of** lymph nodes
        EXCLUDES 1   lymphangioma (D18.1)

    ✓5ᵗʰ **D36.1** **Benign neoplasm of** peripheral nerves and autonomic nervous system
        EXCLUDES 1   benign neoplasm of peripheral nerves of orbit (D31.6-)
                    neurofibromatosis (Q85.Ø-)

        D36.1Ø **Benign neoplasm of peripheral nerves and** ▽
            autonomic nervous system, unspecified

        D36.11 **Benign neoplasm of peripheral nerves and autonomic nervous system of** face, head, and neck

        D36.12 **Benign neoplasm of peripheral nerves and autonomic nervous system,** upper limb, including shoulder

        D36.13 **Benign neoplasm of peripheral nerves and autonomic nervous system of** lower limb, including hip

        D36.14 **Benign neoplasm of peripheral nerves and autonomic nervous system of** thorax

        D36.15 **Benign neoplasm of peripheral nerves and autonomic nervous system of** abdomen

        D36.16 **Benign neoplasm of peripheral nerves and autonomic nervous system of** pelvis

        D36.17 **Benign neoplasm of peripheral nerves and** ▽
            autonomic nervous system of trunk, unspecified

    D36.7 **Benign neoplasm of other specified sites**
        Benign neoplasm of nose NOS

    D36.9 **Benign neoplasm, unspecified site** ▽

Benign neuroendocrine tumors (D3A)

✓4ᵗʰ **D3A** **Benign neuroendocrine tumors**
    Code also any associated multiple endocrine neoplasia [MEN]
        syndromes (E31.2-)
    Use additional code to identify any associated endocrine syndrome,
        such as:
        carcinoid syndrome (E34.Ø)
    EXCLUDES 2   benign pancreatic islet cell tumors (D13.7)

    ✓5ᵗʰ **D3A.Ø** **Benign** carcinoid tumors

        D3A.ØØ **Benign carcinoid tumor of unspecified site** ▽
            Carcinoid tumor NOS

        ✓6ᵗʰ **D3A.Ø1** **Benign carcinoid tumors of the** small intestine

            D3A.Ø1Ø **Benign carcinoid tumor of the** duodenum

            D3A.Ø11 **Benign carcinoid tumor of the** jejunum

            D3A.Ø12 **Benign carcinoid tumor of the** ileum

            D3A.Ø19 **Benign carcinoid tumor of the small** ▽
                    intestine, unspecified portion

☑ Add'l Character Required   ✗ˣ⁷ᵗʰ Placeholder Alert   RUG IV Special Care High Dx   RUG IV Clinically Complex Dx   RUG IV Special Care Low Dx   Manifestation Code   Other Specified Code   ▽ Unspecified Code

ICD-10-CM 2016   475

D31.1–D3A.Ø19

✓6ᵗʰ **D3A.Ø2**   **Benign carcinoid tumors of the** appendix, large intestine, and rectum

    D3A.Ø2Ø   **Benign carcinoid tumor of the** appendix

    D3A.Ø21   **Benign carcinoid tumor of the** cecum

    D3A.Ø22   **Benign carcinoid tumor of the** ascending colon

    D3A.Ø23   **Benign carcinoid tumor of the** transverse colon

    D3A.Ø24   **Benign carcinoid tumor of the** descending colon

    D3A.Ø25   **Benign carcinoid tumor of the** sigmoid colon

    D3A.Ø26   **Benign carcinoid tumor of the** rectum

    D3A.Ø29   **Benign carcinoid tumor of the large** ▽ **intestine, unspecified portion**
       Benign carcinoid tumor of the colon NOS

✓6ᵗʰ **D3A.Ø9**   **Benign carcinoid tumors of** other sites

    D3A.Ø9Ø   **Benign carcinoid tumor of the** bronchus and lung

    D3A.Ø91   **Benign carcinoid tumor of the** thymus

    D3A.Ø92   **Benign carcinoid tumor of the** stomach

    D3A.Ø93   **Benign carcinoid tumor of the** kidney

    D3A.Ø94   **Benign carcinoid tumor of the** foregut NOS

    D3A.Ø95   **Benign carcinoid tumor of the** midgut NOS

    D3A.Ø96   **Benign carcinoid tumor of the** hindgut NOS

    D3A.Ø98   **Benign carcinoid tumors of other sites**

D3A.8   **Other benign neuroendocrine tumors** ▽
    Neuroendocrine tumor NOS

Neoplasms of uncertain behavior, polycythemia vera and myelodysplastic syndromes (D37-D48)

NOTE   Categories D37-D44, and D48 classify by site neoplasms of uncertain behavior, i.e., histologic confirmation whether the neoplasm is malignant or benign cannot be made.

EXCLUDES 1   *neoplasms of unspecified behavior (D49.-)*

✓4ᵗʰ **D37**   **Neoplasm of uncertain behavior of** oral cavity and digestive organs

   EXCLUDES 1   *stromal tumors of uncertain behavior of digestive system (D48.1)*

✓5ᵗʰ **D37.Ø**   **Neoplasm of uncertain behavior of** lip, oral cavity and pharynx

   EXCLUDES 1   *neoplasm of uncertain behavior of aryepiglottic fold or interarytenoid fold, laryngeal aspect (D38.Ø)*
     neoplasm of uncertain behavior of epiglottis NOS (D38.Ø)
     neoplasm of uncertain behavior of skin of lip (D48.5)
     neoplasm of uncertain behavior of suprahyoid portion of epiglottis (D38.Ø)

    D37.Ø1   **Neoplasm of uncertain behavior of** lip
       Neoplasm of uncertain behavior of vermilion border of lip

    D37.Ø2   **Neoplasm of uncertain behavior of** tongue

    ✓6ᵗʰ **D37.Ø3**   **Neoplasm of uncertain behavior of the** major salivary glands

      D37.Ø3Ø   **Neoplasm of uncertain behavior of the** parotid salivary glands

      D37.Ø31   **Neoplasm of uncertain behavior of the** sublingual salivary glands

      D37.Ø32   **Neoplasm of uncertain behavior of the** submandibular salivary glands

      D37.Ø39   **Neoplasm of uncertain behavior of the** ▽ **major salivary glands, unspecified**

    D37.Ø4   **Neoplasm of uncertain behavior of the** minor salivary glands
       Neoplasm of uncertain behavior of submucosal salivary glands of lip
       Neoplasm of uncertain behavior of submucosal salivary glands of cheek
       Neoplasm of uncertain behavior of submucosal salivary glands of hard palate
       Neoplasm of uncertain behavior of submucosal salivary glands of soft palate

    D37.Ø5   **Neoplasm of uncertain behavior of** pharynx
       Neoplasm of uncertain behavior of aryepiglottic fold of pharynx NOS
       Neoplasm of uncertain behavior of hypopharyngeal aspect of aryepiglottic fold of pharynx
       Neoplasm of uncertain behavior of marginal zone of aryepiglottic fold of pharynx

    D37.Ø9   **Neoplasm of uncertain behavior of other specified sites of the oral cavity**

D37.1   **Neoplasm of uncertain behavior of** stomach

D37.2   **Neoplasm of uncertain behavior of** small intestine

D37.3   **Neoplasm of uncertain behavior of** appendix

D37.4   **Neoplasm of uncertain behavior of** colon

D37.5   **Neoplasm of uncertain behavior of** rectum
    Neoplasm of uncertain behavior of rectosigmoid junction

D37.6   **Neoplasm of uncertain behavior of** liver, gallbladder and bile ducts
    Neoplasm of uncertain behavior of ampulla of Vater

D37.8   **Neoplasm of uncertain behavior of other specified digestive organs**
    Neoplasm of uncertain behavior of anal canal
    Neoplasm of uncertain behavior of anal sphincter
    Neoplasm of uncertain behavior of anus NOS
    Neoplasm of uncertain behavior of esophagus
    Neoplasm of uncertain behavior of intestine NOS
    Neoplasm of uncertain behavior of pancreas

   EXCLUDES 1   *neoplasm of uncertain behavior of anal margin (D48.5)*
     neoplasm of uncertain behavior of anal skin (D48.5)
     neoplasm of uncertain behavior of perianal skin (D48.5)

D37.9   **Neoplasm of uncertain behavior of** digestive organ, ▽ unspecified

✓4ᵗʰ **D38**   **Neoplasm of uncertain behavior of** middle ear and respiratory and intrathoracic organs

   EXCLUDES 1   *neoplasm of uncertain behavior of heart (D48.7)*

D38.Ø   **Neoplasm of uncertain behavior of** larynx
    Neoplasm of uncertain behavior of aryepiglottic fold or interarytenoid fold, laryngeal aspect
    Neoplasm of uncertain behavior of epiglottis (suprahyoid portion)

   EXCLUDES 1   *neoplasm of uncertain behavior of aryepiglottic fold or interarytenoid fold NOS (D37.Ø5)*
     neoplasm of uncertain behavior of hypopharyngeal aspect of aryepiglottic fold (D37.Ø5)
     neoplasm of uncertain behavior of marginal zone of aryepiglottic fold (D37.Ø5)

D38.1   **Neoplasm of uncertain behavior of** trachea, bronchus and lung

D38.2   **Neoplasm of uncertain behavior of** pleura

D38.3   **Neoplasm of uncertain behavior of** mediastinum

D38.4   **Neoplasm of uncertain behavior of** thymus

D38.5   **Neoplasm of uncertain behavior of other respiratory organs**
    Neoplasm of uncertain behavior of accessory sinuses
    Neoplasm of uncertain behavior of cartilage of nose
    Neoplasm of uncertain behavior of middle ear
    Neoplasm of uncertain behavior of nasal cavities

   EXCLUDES 1   *neoplasm of uncertain behavior of ear (external) (skin) (D48.5)*
     neoplasm of uncertain behavior of nose NOS (D48.7)
     neoplasm of uncertain behavior of skin of nose (D48.5)

D38.6   **Neoplasm of uncertain behavior of** respiratory organ, ▽ unspecified

✓4ᵗʰ **D39**   **Neoplasm of uncertain behavior of** female genital organs

D39.Ø   **Neoplasm of uncertain behavior of** uterus   ♀

✓5ᵗʰ **D39.1**   **Neoplasm of uncertain behavior of** ovary
    Use additional code to identify any functional activity

    D39.1Ø   **Neoplasm of uncertain behavior of unspecified** ♀▽ **ovary**

    D39.11   **Neoplasm of uncertain behavior of** right **ovary**   ♀

    D39.12   **Neoplasm of uncertain behavior of** left **ovary**   ♀

D39.2   **Neoplasm of uncertain behavior of** placenta   ♀
    Chorioadenoma destruens
    Invasive hydatidiform mole
    Malignant hydatidiform mole

   EXCLUDES 1   *hydatidiform mole NOS (OØ1.9)*

D39.8   **Neoplasm of uncertain behavior of other specified**   ♀ **female genital organs**
    Neoplasm of uncertain behavior of skin of female genital organs

D39.9   **Neoplasm of uncertain behavior of** female genital organ, ♀▽ unspecified

Ⓝ Newborn   Ⓟ Pediatric   Ⓜ Maternity   Ⓐ Adult   **RIC** RIC Dx   **NCDx** Noncancer Dx   **PDx** Primary Dx   **CC** RIC CC Condition   ►◄ Revised Text   ● New Code   ▲ Revised Code Title

476   ICD-10-CM 2016

✓4ᵗʰ D40 Neoplasm of uncertain behavior of male genital organs

  D40.0 Neoplasm of uncertain behavior of prostate ♂

  ✓5ᵗʰ D40.1 Neoplasm of uncertain behavior of testis

    D40.10 Neoplasm of uncertain behavior of unspecified testis ♂▽

    D40.11 Neoplasm of uncertain behavior of right testis ♂

    D40.12 Neoplasm of uncertain behavior of left testis ♂

  D40.8 Neoplasm of uncertain behavior of other specified male genital organs ♂

    Neoplasm of uncertain behavior of skin of male genital organs

  D40.9 Neoplasm of uncertain behavior of male genital organ, unspecified ♂▽

✓4ᵗʰ D41 Neoplasm of uncertain behavior of urinary organs

  ✓5ᵗʰ D41.0 Neoplasm of uncertain behavior of kidney

    EXCLUDES 1   neoplasm of uncertain behavior of renal pelvis (D41.1-)

    D41.00 Neoplasm of uncertain behavior of unspecified kidney ▽

    D41.01 Neoplasm of uncertain behavior of right kidney

    D41.02 Neoplasm of uncertain behavior of left kidney

  ✓5ᵗʰ D41.1 Neoplasm of uncertain behavior of renal pelvis

    D41.10 Neoplasm of uncertain behavior of unspecified renal pelvis ▽

    D41.11 Neoplasm of uncertain behavior of right renal pelvis

    D41.12 Neoplasm of uncertain behavior of left renal pelvis

  ✓5ᵗʰ D41.2 Neoplasm of uncertain behavior of ureter

    D41.20 Neoplasm of uncertain behavior of unspecified ureter ▽

    D41.21 Neoplasm of uncertain behavior of right ureter

    D41.22 Neoplasm of uncertain behavior of left ureter

  D41.3 Neoplasm of uncertain behavior of urethra

  D41.4 Neoplasm of uncertain behavior of bladder

  D41.8 Neoplasm of uncertain behavior of other specified urinary organs

  D41.9 Neoplasm of uncertain behavior of unspecified urinary organ ▽

✓4ᵗʰ D42 Neoplasm of uncertain behavior of meninges

  D42.0 Neoplasm of uncertain behavior of cerebral meninges

  D42.1 Neoplasm of uncertain behavior of spinal meninges

  D42.9 Neoplasm of uncertain behavior of meninges, unspecified ▽

✓4ᵗʰ D43 Neoplasm of uncertain behavior of brain and central nervous system

  EXCLUDES 1   neoplasm of uncertain behavior of peripheral nerves and autonomic nervous system (D48.2)

  D43.0 Neoplasm of uncertain behavior of brain, supratentorial

    Neoplasm of uncertain behavior of cerebral ventricle

    Neoplasm of uncertain behavior of cerebrum

    Neoplasm of uncertain behavior of frontal lobe

    Neoplasm of uncertain behavior of occipital lobe

    Neoplasm of uncertain behavior of parietal lobe

    Neoplasm of uncertain behavior of temporal lobe

    EXCLUDES 1   neoplasm of uncertain behavior of fourth ventricle (D43.1)

  D43.1 Neoplasm of uncertain behavior of brain, infratentorial

    Neoplasm of uncertain behavior of brain stem

    Neoplasm of uncertain behavior of cerebellum

    Neoplasm of uncertain behavior of fourth ventricle

  D43.2 Neoplasm of uncertain behavior of brain, unspecified ▽

  D43.3 Neoplasm of uncertain behavior of cranial nerves

  D43.4 Neoplasm of uncertain behavior of spinal cord

  D43.8 Neoplasm of uncertain behavior of other specified parts of central nervous system

  D43.9 Neoplasm of uncertain behavior of central nervous system, unspecified ▽

    Neoplasm of uncertain behavior of nervous system (central) NOS

✓4ᵗʰ D44 Neoplasm of uncertain behavior of endocrine glands

  EXCLUDES 1   multiple endocrine adenomatosis (E31.2-)

     multiple endocrine neoplasia (E31.2-)

     neoplasm of uncertain behavior of endocrine pancreas (D37.8)

     neoplasm of uncertain behavior of ovary (D39.1-)

     neoplasm of uncertain behavior of testis (D40.1-)

     neoplasm of uncertain behavior of thymus (D38.4)

  D44.0 Neoplasm of uncertain behavior of thyroid gland

✓5ᵗʰ D44.1 Neoplasm of uncertain behavior of adrenal gland

  Use additional code to identify any functional activity

  D44.10 Neoplasm of uncertain behavior of unspecified adrenal gland ▽

  D44.11 Neoplasm of uncertain behavior of right adrenal gland

  D44.12 Neoplasm of uncertain behavior of left adrenal gland

D44.2 Neoplasm of uncertain behavior of parathyroid gland

D44.3 Neoplasm of uncertain behavior of pituitary gland

  Use additional code to identify any functional activity

D44.4 Neoplasm of uncertain behavior of craniopharyngeal duct

D44.5 Neoplasm of uncertain behavior of pineal gland

D44.6 Neoplasm of uncertain behavior of carotid body

D44.7 Neoplasm of uncertain behavior of aortic body and other paraganglia

D44.9 Neoplasm of uncertain behavior of unspecified endocrine gland ▽

D45 Polycythemia vera

  EXCLUDES 1   familial polycythemia (D75.0)

     secondary polycythemia (D75.1)

✓4ᵗʰ D46 Myelodysplastic syndromes

  Use additional code for adverse effect, if applicable, to identify drug (T36-T50 with fifth or sixth character 5)

  EXCLUDES 2   drug-induced aplastic anemia (D61.1)

  D46.0 Refractory anemia without ring sideroblasts, so stated

    Refractory anemia without sideroblasts, without excess of blasts

  D46.1 Refractory anemia with ring sideroblasts

    RARS

  ✓5ᵗʰ D46.2 Refractory anemia with excess of blasts

    D46.20 Refractory anemia with excess of blasts, unspecified ▽

     RAEB NOS

    D46.21 Refractory anemia with excess of blasts 1

     RAEB 1

    D46.22 Refractory anemia with excess of blasts 2

     RAEB 2

  D46.A Refractory cytopenia with multilineage dysplasia

  D46.B Refractory cytopenia with multilineage dysplasia and ring sideroblasts

    RCMD RS

  D46.C Myelodysplastic syndrome with isolated del(5q) chromosomal abnormality

    Myelodysplastic syndrome with 5q deletion

    5q minus syndrome NOS

  D46.4 Refractory anemia, unspecified ▽

  D46.Z Other myelodysplastic syndromes

    EXCLUDES 1   chronic myelomonocytic leukemia (C93.1-)

  D46.9 Myelodysplastic syndrome, unspecified ▽

    Myelodysplasia NOS

✓4ᵗʰ D47 Other neoplasms of uncertain behavior of lymphoid, hematopoietic and related tissue

  D47.0 Histiocytic and mast cell tumors of uncertain behavior ▽

    Indolent systemic mastocytosis

    Mast cell tumor NOS

    Mastocytoma NOS

    EXCLUDES 1   malignant mast cell tumor (C96.2)

     mastocytosis (congenital) (cutaneous) (Q82.2)

  D47.1 Chronic myeloproliferative disease

    Chronic neutrophilic leukemia

    Myeloproliferative disease, unspecified

    EXCLUDES 1   atypical chronic myeloid leukemia BCR/ABL-negative (C92.2-)

     chronic myeloid leukemia BCR/ABL-positive (C92.1-)

     myelofibrosis NOS (D75.81)

     myelophthisic anemia (D61.82)

     myelophthisis (D61.82)

     secondary myelofibrosis NOS (D75.81)

  D47.2 Monoclonal gammopathy

    Monoclonal gammopathy of undetermined significance [MGUS]

  D47.3 Essential (hemorrhagic) thrombocythemia

    Essential thrombocytosis

    Idiopathic hemorrhagic thrombocythemia

Chapter 2. Neoplasms

D47.4 Osteomyelofibrosis
Chronic idiopathic myelofibrosis
Myelofibrosis (idiopathic) (with myeloid metaplasia)
Myelosclerosis (megakaryocytic) with myeloid metaplasia
Secondary myelofibrosis in myeloproliferative disease
EXCLUDES 1   *acute myelofibrosis (C94.4-)*

☑5ᵗʰ **D47.Z Other specified neoplasms of uncertain behavior of lymphoid, hematopoietic and related tissue**

    D47.Z1 Post-transplant lymphoproliferative disorder (PTLD)
Code first complications of transplanted organs and tissue (T86.-)

    D47.Z9 Other specified neoplasms of uncertain behavior of lymphoid, hematopoietic and related tissue
Histiocytic tumors of uncertain behavior

D47.9 Neoplasm of uncertain behavior of lymphoid, hematopoietic and related tissue, unspecified ▽
Lymphoproliferative disease NOS

☑4ᵗʰ **D48 Neoplasm of uncertain behavior of other and unspecified sites**
EXCLUDES 1   *neurofibromatosis (nonmalignant) (Q85.0-)*

D48.0 Neoplasm of uncertain behavior of bone and articular cartilage
EXCLUDES 1   *neoplasm of uncertain behavior of cartilage of ear (D48.1)*
neoplasm of uncertain behavior of cartilage of larynx (D38.0)
neoplasm of uncertain behavior of cartilage of nose (D38.5)
neoplasm of uncertain behavior of connective tissue of eyelid (D48.1)
neoplasm of uncertain behavior of synovia (D48.1)

D48.1 Neoplasm of uncertain behavior of connective and other soft tissue
Neoplasm of uncertain behavior of connective tissue of ear
Neoplasm of uncertain behavior of connective tissue of eyelid
Stromal tumors of uncertain behavior of digestive system
EXCLUDES 1   *neoplasm of uncertain behavior of articular cartilage (D48.0)*
neoplasm of uncertain behavior of cartilage of larynx (D38.0)
neoplasm of uncertain behavior of cartilage of nose (D38.5)
neoplasm of uncertain behavior of connective tissue of breast (D48.6-)

D48.2 Neoplasm of uncertain behavior of peripheral nerves and autonomic nervous system
EXCLUDES 1   *neoplasm of uncertain behavior of peripheral nerves of orbit (D48.7)*

D48.3 Neoplasm of uncertain behavior of retroperitoneum

D48.4 Neoplasm of uncertain behavior of peritoneum

D48.5 Neoplasm of uncertain behavior of skin
Neoplasm of uncertain behavior of anal margin
Neoplasm of uncertain behavior of anal skin
Neoplasm of uncertain behavior of perianal skin
Neoplasm of uncertain behavior of skin of breast
EXCLUDES 1   *neoplasm of uncertain behavior of anus NOS (D37.8)*
neoplasm of uncertain behavior of skin of genital organs (D39.8, D40.8)
neoplasm of uncertain behavior of vermilion border of lip (D37.0)

☑5ᵗʰ **D48.6 Neoplasm of uncertain behavior of breast**
Neoplasm of uncertain behavior of connective tissue of breast
Cystosarcoma phyllodes
EXCLUDES 1   *neoplasm of uncertain behavior of skin of breast (D48.5)*

    D48.60 Neoplasm of uncertain behavior of unspecified breast ▽

    D48.61 Neoplasm of uncertain behavior of right breast

    D48.62 Neoplasm of uncertain behavior of left breast

D48.7 Neoplasm of uncertain behavior of other specified sites
Neoplasm of uncertain behavior of eye
Neoplasm of uncertain behavior of heart
Neoplasm of uncertain behavior of peripheral nerves of orbit
EXCLUDES 1   *neoplasm of uncertain behavior of connective tissue (D48.1)*
neoplasm of uncertain behavior of skin of eyelid (D48.5)

D48.9 Neoplasm of uncertain behavior, unspecified ▽

Neoplasms of uncertain behavior (D49)

☑4ᵗʰ **D49 Neoplasms of unspecified behavior**
NOTE   Category D49 classifies by site neoplasms of unspecified morphology and behavior. The term "mass", unless otherwise stated, is not to be regarded as a neoplastic growth.
INCLUDES   "growth" NOS
neoplasm NOS
new growth NOS
tumor NOS
EXCLUDES 1   *neoplasms of uncertain behavior (D37-D44, D48)*

D49.0 Neoplasm of unspecified behavior of digestive system
EXCLUDES 1   *neoplasm of unspecified behavior of margin of anus (D49.2)*
neoplasm of unspecified behavior of perianal skin (D49.2)
neoplasm of unspecified behavior of skin of anus (D49.2)

D49.1 Neoplasm of unspecified behavior of respiratory system

D49.2 Neoplasm of unspecified behavior of bone, soft tissue, and skin
EXCLUDES 1   *neoplasm of unspecified behavior of anal canal (D49.0)*
neoplasm of unspecified behavior of anus NOS (D49.0)
neoplasm of unspecified behavior of bone marrow (D49.89)
neoplasm of unspecified behavior of cartilage of larynx (D49.1)
neoplasm of unspecified behavior of cartilage of nose (D49.1)
neoplasm of unspecified behavior of connective tissue of breast (D49.3)
neoplasm of unspecified behavior of skin of genital organs (D49.5)
neoplasm of unspecified behavior of vermilion border of lip (D49.0)

D49.3 Neoplasm of unspecified behavior of breast
EXCLUDES 1   *neoplasm of unspecified behavior of skin of breast (D49.2)*

D49.4 Neoplasm of unspecified behavior of bladder

D49.5 Neoplasm of unspecified behavior of other genitourinary organs

D49.6 Neoplasm of unspecified behavior of brain
EXCLUDES 1   *neoplasm of unspecified behavior of cerebral meninges (D49.7)*
neoplasm of unspecified behavior of cranial nerves (D49.7)

D49.7 Neoplasm of unspecified behavior of endocrine glands and other parts of nervous system
EXCLUDES 1   *neoplasm of unspecified behavior of peripheral, sympathetic, and parasympathetic nerves and ganglia (D49.2)*

☑5ᵗʰ **D49.8 Neoplasm of unspecified behavior of other specified sites**
EXCLUDES 1   *neoplasm of unspecified behavior of eyelid (skin) (D49.2)*
neoplasm of unspecified behavior of eyelid cartilage (D49.2)
neoplasm of unspecified behavior of great vessels (D49.2)
neoplasm of unspecified behavior of optic nerve (D49.7)

    D49.81 Neoplasm of unspecified behavior of retina and choroid
Dark area on retina
Retinal freckle

    D49.89 Neoplasm of unspecified behavior of other specified sites ▽

D49.9 Neoplasm of unspecified behavior of unspecified site ▽

Ⓝ Newborn   Ⓟ Pediatric   Ⓜ Maternity   Ⓐ Adult   **RIC** RIC Dx   **NCDx** Noncancer Dx   **PDx** Primary Dx   **CC** RIC CC Condition   ▶◀ Revised Text   ● New Code   ▲ Revised Code Title

478   ICD-10-CM 2016

Chapter 3. Disease of the Blood and Blood-Forming Organs and Certain Disorders Involving the Immune Mechanism (D50–D89)

Chapter Specific Coding Guidelines and Examples
Reserved for future guideline expansion

Chapter 3. Disease of the Blood and Blood-Forming Organs *(left margin, vertical)*

D50–D56.3 *(left margin, vertical)*

Chapter 3. Diseases of the Blood and Blood-forming Organs and Certain Disorders Involving the Immune Mechanism (D50-D89)

EXCLUDES 2   *autoimmune disease (systemic) NOS (M35.9)*
certain conditions originating in the perinatal period (P00-P96)
complications of pregnancy, childbirth and the puerperium (O00-O9A)
congenital malformations, deformations and chromosomal abnormalities (Q00-Q99)
endocrine, nutritional and metabolic diseases (E00-E88)
human immunodeficiency virus [HIV] disease (B20)
injury, poisoning and certain other consequences of external causes (S00-T88)
neoplasms (C00-D49)
symptoms, signs and abnormal clinical and laboratory findings, not elsewhere classified (R00-R94)

This chapter contains the following blocks:

D50-D53	Nutritional anemias
D55-D59	Hemolytic anemias
D60-D64	Aplastic and other anemias and other bone marrow failure syndromes
D65-D69	Coagulation defects, purpura and other hemorrhagic conditions
D70-D77	Other disorders of blood and blood-forming organs
D78	Intraoperative and postprocedural complications of the spleen
D80-D89	Certain disorders involving the immune mechanism

Nutritional anemias (D50-D53)

✓4th **D50**   **Iron deficiency anemia**
INCLUDES   asiderotic anemia
hypochromic anemia

D50.0   **Iron deficiency anemia secondary to blood loss (chronic)**
Posthemorrhagic anemia (chronic)
EXCLUDES 1   *acute posthemorrhagic anemia (D62)*
congenital anemia from fetal blood loss (P61.3)

D50.1   **Sideropenic dysphagia**
Kelly-Paterson syndrome
Plummer-Vinson syndrome

D50.8   **Other iron deficiency anemias**
Iron deficiency anemia due to inadequate dietary iron intake

D50.9   **Iron deficiency anemia, unspecified**   ▽

✓4th **D51**   **Vitamin B12 deficiency anemia**
EXCLUDES 1   *vitamin B12 deficiency (E53.8)*

D51.0   **Vitamin B12 deficiency anemia due to intrinsic factor deficiency**
Addison anemia
Biermer anemia
Pernicious (congenital) anemia
Congenital intrinsic factor deficiency

D51.1   **Vitamin B12 deficiency anemia due to selective vitamin B12 malabsorption with proteinuria**
Imerslund (Gräsbeck) syndrome
Megaloblastic hereditary anemia

D51.2   **Transcobalamin II deficiency**

D51.3   **Other dietary vitamin B12 deficiency anemia**
Vegan anemia

D51.8   **Other vitamin B12 deficiency anemias**

D51.9   **Vitamin B12 deficiency anemia, unspecified**   ▽

✓4th **D52**   **Folate deficiency anemia**
EXCLUDES 1   *folate deficiency without anemia (E53.8)*

D52.0   **Dietary folate deficiency anemia**
Nutritional megaloblastic anemia

D52.1   **Drug-induced folate deficiency anemia**
Use additional code for adverse effect, if applicable, to identify drug (T36-T50 with fifth or sixth character 5)

D52.8   **Other folate deficiency anemias**

D52.9   **Folate deficiency anemia, unspecified**   ▽
Folic acid deficiency anemia NOS

✓4th **D53**   **Other nutritional anemias**
INCLUDES   megaloblastic anemia unresponsive to vitamin B12 or folate therapy

D53.0   **Protein deficiency anemia**
Amino-acid deficiency anemia
Orotaciduric anemia
EXCLUDES 1   *Lesch-Nyhan syndrome (E79.1)*

D53.1   **Other megaloblastic anemias, not elsewhere classified**
Megaloblastic anemia NOS
EXCLUDES 1   *Di Guglielmo's disease (C94.0)*

D53.2   **Scorbutic anemia**
EXCLUDES 1   *scurvy (E54)*

D53.8   **Other specified nutritional anemias**
Anemia associated with deficiency of copper
Anemia associated with deficiency of molybdenum
Anemia associated with deficiency of zinc
EXCLUDES 1   *nutritional deficiencies without anemia, such as:*
copper deficiency NOS (E61.0)
molybdenum deficiency NOS (E61.5)
zinc deficiency NOS (E60)

D53.9   **Nutritional anemia, unspecified**   ▽
Simple chronic anemia
EXCLUDES 1   *anemia NOS (D64.9)*

Hemolytic anemias (D55-D59)

✓4th **D55**   **Anemia due to enzyme disorders**
EXCLUDES 1   *drug-induced enzyme deficiency anemia (D59.2)*

D55.0   **Anemia due to glucose-6-phosphate dehydrogenase [G6PD] deficiency**
Favism
G6PD deficiency anemia

D55.1   **Anemia due to other disorders of glutathione metabolism**
Anemia (due to) enzyme deficiencies, except G6PD, related to the hexose monophosphate [HMP] shunt pathway
Anemia (due to) hemolytic nonspherocytic (hereditary), type I

D55.2   **Anemia due to disorders of glycolytic enzymes**
Hemolytic nonspherocytic (hereditary) anemia, type II
Hexokinase deficiency anemia
Pyruvate kinase [PK] deficiency anemia
Triose-phosphate isomerase deficiency anemia
EXCLUDES 1   *disorders of glycolysis not associated with anemia (E74.8)*

D55.3   **Anemia due to disorders of nucleotide metabolism**

D55.8   **Other anemias due to enzyme disorders**

D55.9   **Anemia due to enzyme disorder, unspecified**   ▽

✓4th **D56**   **Thalassemia**
EXCLUDES 1   *sickle-cell thalassemia (D57.4-)*

D56.0   **Alpha thalassemia**
Alpha thalassemia major
Hemoglobin H Constant Spring
Hemoglobin H disease
Hydrops fetalis due to alpha thalassemia
Severe alpha thalassemia
Triple gene defect alpha thalassemia
Use additional code, if applicable, for hydrops fetalis due to alpha thalassemia (P56.99)
EXCLUDES 1   *alpha thalassemia trait or minor (D56.3)*
asymptomatic alpha thalassemia (D56.3)
hydrops fetalis due to isoimmunization (P56.0)
hydrops fetalis not due to immune hemolysis (P83.2)

D56.1   **Beta thalassemia**
Beta thalassemia major
Cooley's anemia
Homozygous beta thalassemia
Severe beta thalassemia
Thalassemia intermedia
Thalassemia major
EXCLUDES 1   *beta thalassemia minor (D56.3)*
beta thalassemia trait (D56.3)
delta-beta thalassemia (D56.2)
hemoglobin E-beta thalassemia (D56.5)
sickle-cell beta thalassemia (D57.4-)

D56.2   **Delta-beta thalassemia**
Homozygous delta-beta thalassemia
EXCLUDES 1   *delta-beta thalassemia minor (D56.3)*
delta-beta thalassemia trait (D56.3)

D56.3   **Thalassemia minor**
Alpha thalassemia minor
Alpha thalassemia silent carrier
Alpha thalassemia trait
Beta thalassemia minor
Beta thalassemia trait
Delta-beta thalassemia minor
Delta-beta thalassemia trait
Thalassemia trait NOS
EXCLUDES 1   *alpha thalassemia (D56.0)*
beta thalassemia (D56.1)
delta-beta thalassemia (D56.2)
hemoglobin E-beta thalassemia (D56.5)
sickle-cell trait (D57.3)

N Newborn   P Pediatric   M Maternity   A Adult   RIC RIC Dx   NCDx Noncancer Dx   PDx Primary Dx   CC RIC CC Condition   ►◄ Revised Text   ● New Code   ▲ Revised Code Title

D56.4   Hereditary persistence of fetal hemoglobin [HPFH]

D56.5   Hemoglobin E-beta thalassemia
     EXCLUDES 1   *beta thalassemia (D56.1)*
                   beta thalassemia minor (D56.3)
                   beta thalassemia trait (D56.3)
                   delta-beta thalassemia (D56.2)
                   delta-beta thalassemia trait (D56.3)
                   hemoglobin E disease (D58.2)
                   other hemoglobinopathies (D58.2)
                   sickle-cell beta thalassemia (D57.4-)

D56.8   **Other thalassemias**
     Dominant thalassemia
     Hemoglobin C thalassemia
     Mixed thalassemia
     Thalassemia with other hemoglobinopathy
     EXCLUDES 1   *hemoglobin C disease (D58.2)*
                   hemoglobin E disease (D58.2)
                   other hemoglobinopathies (D58.2)
                   sickle-cell anemia (D57.-)
                   sickle-cell thalassemia (D57.4)

D56.9   **Thalassemia, unspecified**   ▽
     Mediterranean anemia (with other hemoglobinopathy)

✓4ᵗʰ D57   **Sickle-cell disorders**
     Use additional code for any associated fever (R50.81)
     EXCLUDES 1   *other hemoglobinopathies (D58.-)*

    ✓5ᵗʰ D57.0   **Hb-SS disease with crisis**
        Sickle-cell disease NOS with crisis
        Hb-SS disease with vasoocclusive pain

        D57.00   **Hb-SS disease with crisis, unspecified**   `CC` ▽
        D57.01   **Hb-SS disease with** acute chest syndrome   `CC`
        D57.02   **Hb-SS disease with** splenic sequestration   `CC`

    D57.1   **Sickle-cell disease** without crisis   `CC`
        Hb-SS disease without crisis
        Sickle-cell anemia NOS
        Sickle-cell disease NOS
        Sickle-cell disorder NOS

    ✓5ᵗʰ D57.2   **Sickle-cell/Hb-C disease**
        Hb-SC disease
        Hb-S/Hb-C disease

        D57.20   **Sickle-cell/Hb-C disease** without crisis   `CC`

      ✓6ᵗʰ D57.21   **Sickle-cell/Hb-C disease** with crisis
           D57.211   **Sickle-cell/Hb-C disease with** acute   `CC`
                  chest syndrome
           D57.212   **Sickle-cell/Hb-C disease with** splenic   `CC`
                  sequestration
           D57.219   **Sickle-cell/Hb-C disease with crisis,**   `CC` ▽
                  unspecified
                     Sickle-cell/Hb-C disease with crisis NOS

    D57.3   **Sickle-cell** trait
        Hb-S trait
        Heterozygous hemoglobin S

    ✓5ᵗʰ D57.4   **Sickle-cell** thalassemia
        Sickle-cell beta thalassemia
        Thalassemia Hb-S disease

        D57.40   **Sickle-cell thalassemia** without crisis
              Microdrepanocytosis
              Sickle-cell thalassemia NOS

      ✓6ᵗʰ D57.41   **Sickle-cell thalassemia** with crisis
              Sickle-cell thalassemia with vasoocclusive pain
           D57.411   **Sickle-cell thalassemia with** acute   `CC`
                  chest syndrome
           D57.412   **Sickle-cell thalassemia with** splenic   `CC`
                  sequestration
           D57.419   **Sickle-cell thalassemia with crisis,**   ▽
                  unspecified
                     Sickle-cell thalassemia with crisis NOS

    ✓5ᵗʰ D57.8   **Other sickle-cell disorders**
        Hb-SD disease
        Hb-SE disease

        D57.80   **Other sickle-cell disorders** without crisis   `CC`

      ✓6ᵗʰ D57.81   **Other sickle-cell disorders** with crisis
           D57.811   **Other sickle-cell disorders with** acute   `CC`
                  chest syndrome
           D57.812   **Other sickle-cell disorders with**   `CC`
                  splenic sequestration
           D57.819   **Other sickle-cell disorders with**   `CC` ▽
                  crisis, unspecified
                     Other sickle-cell disorders with crisis NOS

✓4ᵗʰ D58   **Other hereditary hemolytic anemias**
     EXCLUDES 1   *hemolytic anemia of the newborn (P55.-)*

    D58.0   **Hereditary spherocytosis**
        Acholuric (familial) jaundice
        Congenital (spherocytic) hemolytic icterus
        Minkowski-Chauffard syndrome

    D58.1   **Hereditary elliptocytosis**
        Elliptocytosis (congenital)
        Ovalocytosis (congenital) (hereditary)

    D58.2   **Other hemoglobinopathies**
        Abnormal hemoglobin NOS
        Congenital Heinz body anemia
        Hb-C disease
        Hb-D disease
        Hb-E disease
        Hemoglobinopathy NOS
        Unstable hemoglobin hemolytic disease
        EXCLUDES 1   *familial polycythemia (D75.0)*
                   Hb-M disease (D74.0)
                   hemoglobin E-beta thalassemia (D56.5)
                   hereditary persistence of fetal hemoglobin [HPFH]
                     (D56.4)
                   high-altitude polycythemia (D75.1)
                   methemoglobinemia (D74.-)
                   other hemoglobinopathies with thalassemia (D56.8)

    D58.8   **Other specified hereditary hemolytic anemias**
        Stomatocytosis

    D58.9   **Hereditary hemolytic anemia, unspecified**   ▽

✓4ᵗʰ D59   **Acquired hemolytic anemia**

    D59.0   **Drug-induced autoimmune hemolytic anemia**
        Use additional code for adverse effect, if applicable, to identify
           drug (T36-T50 with fifth or sixth character 5)

    D59.1   **Other autoimmune hemolytic anemias**
        Autoimmune hemolytic disease (cold type) (warm type)
        Chronic cold hemagglutinin disease
        Cold agglutinin disease
        Cold agglutinin hemoglobinuria
        Cold type (secondary) (symptomatic) hemolytic anemia
        Warm type (secondary) (symptomatic) hemolytic anemia
        EXCLUDES 1   *Evans syndrome (D69.41)*
                   hemolytic disease of newborn (P55.-)
                   paroxysmal cold hemoglobinuria (D59.6)

    D59.2   **Drug-induced nonautoimmune hemolytic anemia**
        Drug-induced enzyme deficiency anemia
        Use additional code for adverse effect, if applicable, to identify
           drug (T36-T50 with fifth or sixth character 5)

    D59.3   **Hemolytic-uremic syndrome**
        Use additional code to identify associated:
           E. coli infection (B96.2-)
           Pneumococcal pneumonia (J13)
           Shigella dysenteriae (A03.9)

    D59.4   **Other nonautoimmune hemolytic anemias**
        Mechanical hemolytic anemia
        Microangiopathic hemolytic anemia
        Toxic hemolytic anemia

    D59.5   **Paroxysmal nocturnal hemoglobinuria [Marchiafava-Micheli]**
        EXCLUDES 1   *hemoglobinuria NOS (R82.3)*

    D59.6   **Hemoglobinuria due to hemolysis from other external causes**
        Hemoglobinuria from exertion
        March hemoglobinuria
        Paroxysmal cold hemoglobinuria
        Use additional code (Chapter 20) to identify external cause
        EXCLUDES 1   *hemoglobinuria NOS (R82.3)*

    D59.8   **Other acquired hemolytic anemias**

    D59.9   **Acquired hemolytic anemia, unspecified**   ▽
        Idiopathic hemolytic anemia, chronic

Aplastic and other anemias and other bone marrow failure syndromes (D60-D64)

✓4ᵗʰ D60   **Acquired pure red cell aplasia [erythroblastopenia]**
     INCLUDES   red cell aplasia (acquired) (adult) (with thymoma)
     EXCLUDES 1   *congenital red cell aplasia (D61.01)*

    D60.0   **Chronic acquired pure red cell aplasia**   `CC`
    D60.1   **Transient acquired pure red cell aplasia**   `CC`
    D60.8   **Other acquired pure red cell aplasias**   `CC`
    D60.9   **Acquired pure red cell aplasia, unspecified**   `CC` ▽

Chapter 3. Disease of the Blood and Blood-Forming Organs

D61–D68.0

✓4ᵗʰ **D61** **Other aplastic anemias and other bone marrow failure syndromes**
- EXCLUDES 1   neutropenia (D70.-)
- AHA: 2014, 4Q, 22

  ✓5ᵗʰ **D61.0** **Constitutional aplastic anemia**

    D61.01 **Constitutional (pure) red blood cell aplasia**   CC
- Blackfan-Diamond syndrome
- Congenital (pure) red cell aplasia
- Familial hypoplastic anemia
- Primary (pure) red cell aplasia
- Red cell (pure) aplasia of infants
- EXCLUDES 1   acquired red cell aplasia (D60.9)

    D61.09 **Other constitutional aplastic anemia**   CC
- Fanconi's anemia
- Pancytopenia with malformations

  D61.1 **Drug-induced aplastic anemia**   CC
- Use additional code for adverse effect, if applicable, to identify drug (T36-T50 with fifth or sixth character 5)

  D61.2 **Aplastic anemia due to other external agents**   CC
- Code first, if applicable, toxic effects of substances chiefly nonmedicinal as to source (T51-T65)

  D61.3 **Idiopathic aplastic anemia**   CC

  ✓5ᵗʰ **D61.8** **Other specified aplastic anemias and other bone marrow failure syndromes**

    ✓6ᵗʰ **D61.81** **Pancytopenia**
- EXCLUDES 1   pancytopenia (due to) (with) aplastic anemia (D61.9)
- pancytopenia (due to) (with) bone marrow infiltration (D61.82)
- pancytopenia (due to) (with) congenital (pure) red cell aplasia (D61.01)
- pancytopenia (due to) (with) hairy cell leukemia (C91.4-)
- pancytopenia (due to) (with) human immunodeficiency virus disease (B20)
- pancytopenia (due to) (with) leukoerythroblastic anemia (D61.82)
- pancytopenia (due to) (with) myelodysplastic syndromes (D46.-)
- pancytopenia (due to) (with) myeloproliferative disease (D47.1)

      D61.810 **Antineoplastic chemotherapy induced pancytopenia**   CC
- EXCLUDES 2   aplastic anemia due to antineoplastic chemotherapy (D61.1)

      D61.811 **Other drug-induced pancytopenia**   CC
- EXCLUDES 2   aplastic anemia due to drugs (D61.1)

      D61.818 **Other pancytopenia**   CC

    D61.82 **Myelophthisis**   CC
- Leukoerythroblastic anemia
- Myelophthisic anemia
- Panmyelophthisis
- Code also the underlying disorder, such as:
  - malignant neoplasm of breast (C50.-)
  - tuberculosis (A15.-)
- EXCLUDES 1   idiopathic myelofibrosis (D47.1)
- myelofibrosis NOS (D75.81)
- myelofibrosis with myeloid metaplasia (D47.4)
- primary myelofibrosis (D47.1)
- secondary myelofibrosis (D75.81)

    D61.89 **Other specified aplastic anemias and other bone marrow failure syndromes**   CC

  D61.9 **Aplastic anemia, unspecified**   CC ▽
- Hypoplastic anemia NOS   Medullary hypoplasia

D62 **Acute posthemorrhagic anemia**
- EXCLUDES 1   anemia due to chronic blood loss (D50.0)
- blood loss anemia NOS (D50.0)
- congenital anemia from fetal blood loss (P61.3)

✓4ᵗʰ **D63** **Anemia in chronic diseases classified elsewhere**

  D63.0 **Anemia in neoplastic disease**
- Code first neoplasm (C00-D49)
- EXCLUDES 1   anemia due to antineoplastic chemotherapy (D64.81)
- aplastic anemia due to antineoplastic chemotherapy (D61.1)

  D63.1 **Anemia in chronic kidney disease**
- Erythropoietin resistant anemia (EPO resistant anemia)
- Code first underlying chronic kidney disease (CKD) (N18.-)

  D63.8 **Anemia in other chronic diseases classified elsewhere**
- Code first underlying disease, such as:
  - diphyllobothriasis (B70.0)
  - hookworm disease (B76.0-B76.9)
  - hypothyroidism (E00.0-E03.9)
  - malaria (B50.0-B54)
  - symptomatic late syphilis (A52.79)
  - tuberculosis (A18.89)

✓4ᵗʰ **D64** **Other anemias**
- EXCLUDES 1   refractory anemia (D46.-)
- refractory anemia with excess blasts in transformation [RAEB T] (C92.0-)

  D64.0 **Hereditary sideroblastic anemia**
- Sex-linked hypochromic sideroblastic anemia

  D64.1 **Secondary sideroblastic anemia due to disease**
- Code first underlying disease

  D64.2 **Secondary sideroblastic anemia due to drugs and toxins**
- Code first poisoning due to drug or toxin, if applicable (T36-T65 with fifth or sixth character 1-4 or 6)
- Use additional code for adverse effect, if applicable, to identify drug (T36-T50 with fifth or sixth character 5)

  D64.3 **Other sideroblastic anemias**
- Sideroblastic anemia NOS
- Pyridoxine-responsive sideroblastic anemia NEC

  D64.4 **Congenital dyserythropoietic anemia**
- Dyshematopoietic anemia (congenital)
- EXCLUDES 1   Blackfan-Diamond syndrome (D61.01)
- Di Guglielmo's disease (C94.0)

  ✓5ᵗʰ **D64.8** **Other specified anemias**

    D64.81 **Anemia due to antineoplastic chemotherapy**   CC
- Antineoplastic chemotherapy induced anemia
- EXCLUDES 1   anemia in neoplastic disease (D63.0)
- aplastic anemia due to antineoplastic chemotherapy (D61.1)
- AHA: 2014, 4Q, 22

    D64.89 **Other specified anemias**
- Infantile pseudoleukemia

  D64.9 **Anemia, unspecified**   ▽

Coagulation defects, purpura and other hemorrhagic conditions (D65-D69)

D65 **Disseminated intravascular coagulation [defibrination syndrome]**   CC
- Afibrinogenemia, acquired
- Consumption coagulopathy
- Diffuse or disseminated intravascular coagulation [DIC]
- Fibrinolytic hemorrhage, acquired
- Fibrinolytic purpura
- Purpura fulminans
- EXCLUDES 1   disseminated intravascular coagulation (complicating):
  - abortion or ectopic or molar pregnancy (O00-O07, O08.1)
  - in newborn (P60)
  - pregnancy, childbirth and the puerperium (O45.0, O46.0, O67.0, O72.3)

D66 **Hereditary factor VIII deficiency**   CC
- Classical hemophilia
- Deficiency factor VIII (with functional defect)
- Hemophilia A
- Hemophilia NOS
- EXCLUDES 1   factor VIII deficiency with vascular defect (D68.0)

D67 **Hereditary factor IX deficiency**   CC
- Christmas disease
- Factor IX deficiency (with functional defect)
- Hemophilia B
- Plasma thromboplastin component [PTC] deficiency

✓4ᵗʰ **D68** **Other coagulation defects**
- EXCLUDES 1   abnormal coagulation profile (R79.1)
- coagulation defects complicating abortion or ectopic or molar pregnancy (O00-O07, O08.1)
- coagulation defects complicating pregnancy, childbirth and the puerperium (O45.0, O46.0, O67.0, O72.3)

  D68.0 **Von Willebrand's disease**
- Angiohemophilia
- Factor VIII deficiency with vascular defect
- Vascular hemophilia
- EXCLUDES 1   capillary fragility (hereditary) (D69.8)
- factor VIII deficiency NOS (D66)
- factor VIII deficiency with functional defect (D66)

Ⓝ Newborn   Ⓟ Pediatric   Ⓜ Maternity   Ⓐ Adult   RIC RIC Dx   NCDx Noncancer Dx   PDx Primary Dx   CC RIC CC Condition   ▶◀ Revised Text   ● New Code   ▲ Revised Code Title

482   ICD-10-CM 2016

D68.1   Hereditary factor XI deficiency
  Hemophilia C
  Plasma thromboplastin antecedent [PTA] deficiency
  Rosenthal's disease

D68.2   Hereditary deficiency of other clotting factors
  AC globulin deficiency
  Congenital afibrinogenemia
  Deficiency of factor I [fibrinogen]
  Deficiency of factor II [prothrombin]
  Deficiency of factor V [labile]
  Deficiency of factor VII [stable]
  Deficiency of factor X [Stuart-Prower]
  Deficiency of factor XII [Hageman]
  Deficiency of factor XIII [fibrin stabilizing]
  Dysfibrinogenemia (congenital)
  Hypoproconvertinemia
  Owren's disease
  Proaccelerin deficiency

☑5ᵗʰ **D68.3**   Hemorrhagic disorder due to circulating anticoagulants

  ☑6ᵗʰ **D68.31**   Hemorrhagic disorder due to intrinsic circulating anticoagulants, antibodies, or inhibitors

    D68.311   Acquired hemophilia
  Autoimmune hemophilia
  Autoimmune inhibitors to clotting factors
  Secondary hemophilia

    D68.312   Antiphospholipid antibody with hemorrhagic disorder
  Lupus anticoagulant (LAC) with hemorrhagic disorder
  Systemic lupus erythematosus [SLE] inhibitor with hemorrhagic disorder
  EXCLUDES 1   *antiphospholipid antibody, finding without diagnosis (R76.0)*
  antiphospholipid antibody syndrome (D68.61)
  antiphospholipid antibody with hypercoagulable state (D68.61)
  lupus anticoagulant (LAC) finding without diagnosis (R76.0)
  lupus anticoagulant (LAC) with hypercoagulable state (D68.62)
  systemic lupus erythematosus [SLE] inhibitor finding without diagnosis (R76.0)
  systemic lupus erythematosus [SLE] inhibitor with hypercoagulable state (D68.62)

    D68.318   Other hemorrhagic disorder due to intrinsic circulating anticoagulants, antibodies, or inhibitors
  Antithromboplastinemia
  Antithromboplastinogenemia
  Hemorrhagic disorder due to intrinsic increase in antithrombin
  Hemorrhagic disorder due to intrinsic increase in anti-VIIIa
  Hemorrhagic disorder due to intrinsic increase in anti-IXa
  Hemorrhagic disorder due to intrinsic increase in anti-XIa

  D68.32   Hemorrhagic disorder due to extrinsic circulating anticoagulants
  Drug-induced hemorrhagic disorder
  Hemorrhagic disorder due to increase in anti-IIa
  Hemorrhagic disorder due to increase in anti-Xa
  Hyperheparinemia
  Use additional code for adverse effect, if applicable, to identify drug (T45.515, T45.525)

D68.4   Acquired coagulation factor deficiency
  Deficiency of coagulation factor due to liver disease
  Deficiency of coagulation factor due to vitamin K deficiency
  EXCLUDES 1   *vitamin K deficiency of newborn (P53)*

☑5ᵗʰ **D68.5**   Primary thrombophilia
  Primary hypercoagulable states
  EXCLUDES 1   *antiphospholipid syndrome (D68.61)*
  lupus anticoagulant (D68.62)
  secondary activated protein C resistance (D68.69)
  secondary antiphospholipid antibody syndrome (D68.69)
  secondary lupus anticoagulant with hypercoagulable state (D68.69)
  secondary systemic lupus erythematosus [SLE] inhibitor with hypercoagulable state (D68.69)
  systemic lupus erythematosus [SLE] inhibitor finding without diagnosis (R76.0)
  systemic lupus erythematosus [SLE] inhibitor with hemorrhagic disorder (D68.312)
  thrombotic thrombocytopenic purpura (M31.1)

  D68.51   Activated protein C resistance
  Factor V Leiden mutation

  D68.52   Prothrombin gene mutation

  D68.59   Other primary thrombophilia
  Antithrombin III deficiencyProtein C deficiency
  Hypercoagulable state NOSProtein S deficiency
  Primary hypercoagulable Thrombophilia NOS state NEC
  Primary thrombophilia NEC

☑5ᵗʰ **D68.6**   Other thrombophilia
  Other hypercoagulable states
  EXCLUDES 1   *diffuse or disseminated intravascular coagulation [DIC] (D65)*
  heparin induced thrombocytopenia (HIT) (D75.82)
  hyperhomocysteinemia (E72.11)

  D68.61   Antiphospholipid syndrome
  Anticardiolipin syndrome
  Antiphospholipid antibody syndrome
  EXCLUDES 1   *antiphospholipid antibody, finding without diagnosis (R76.0)*
  antiphospholipid antibody with hemorrhagic disorder (D68.312)
  lupus anticoagulant syndrome (D68.62)

  D68.62   Lupus anticoagulant syndrome
  Lupus anticoagulant
  Presence of systemic lupus erythematosus [SLE] inhibitor
  EXCLUDES 1   *anticardiolipin syndrome (D68.61)*
  antiphospholipid syndrome (D68.61)
  lupus anticoagulant (LAC) finding without diagnosis (R79.0)
  lupus anticoagulant (LAC) with hemorrhagic disorder (D68.312)

  D68.69   Other thrombophilia
  Hypercoagulable states NEC
  Secondary hypercoagulable state NOS

D68.8   Other specified coagulation defects
  EXCLUDES 1   *hemorrhagic disease of newborn (P53)*

D68.9   Coagulation defect, unspecified   ▽

☑4ᵗʰ **D69**   Purpura and other hemorrhagic conditions
  EXCLUDES 1   *benign hypergammaglobulinemic purpura (D89.0)*
  cryoglobulinemic purpura (D89.1)
  essential (hemorrhagic) thrombocythemia (D47.3)
  hemorrhagic thrombocythemia (D47.3)
  purpura fulminans (D65)
  thrombotic thrombocytopenic purpura (M31.1)
  Waldenström hypergammaglobulinemic purpura (D89.0)

D69.0   Allergic purpura
  Allergic vasculitis
  Nonthrombocytopenic hemorrhagic purpura
  Nonthrombocytopenic idiopathic purpura
  Purpura anaphylactoid
  Purpura Henoch(-Schönlein)
  Purpura rheumatica
  Vascular purpura
  EXCLUDES 1   *thrombocytopenic hemorrhagic purpura (D69.3)*

D69.1   Qualitative platelet defects
  Bernard-Soulier [giant platelet] syndrome
  Glanzmann's disease
  Grey platelet syndrome
  Thromboasthenia (hemorrhagic) (hereditary)
  Thrombocytopathy
  EXCLUDES 1   *von Willebrand's disease (D68.0)*

D69.2   Other nonthrombocytopenic purpura   ▽
  Purpura NOS   Senile purpura
  Purpura simplex

☑ Add'l Character Required   ☑x7ᵗʰ Placeholder Alert   RUG IV Special Care High Dx   RUG IV Clinically Complex Dx   RUG IV Special Care Low Dx   Manifestation Code   Other Specified Code   ▽ Unspecified Code

D69.3   Immune thrombocytopenic purpura
Hemorrhagic (thrombocytopenic) purpura
Idiopathic thrombocytopenic purpura
Tidal platelet dysgenesis

✓5ᵗʰ **D69.4   Other primary thrombocytopenia**
EXCLUDES 1   *transient neonatal thrombocytopenia (P61.0)*
Wiskott-Aldrich syndrome (D82.0)

D69.41   Evans syndrome

D69.42   Congenital and hereditary thrombocytopenia purpura
Congenital thrombocytopenia
Hereditary thrombocytopenia
Code first congenital or hereditary disorder, such as:
thrombocytopenia with absent radius (TAR syndrome) (Q87.2)

D69.49   Other primary thrombocytopenia
Megakaryocytic hypoplasia
Primary thrombocytopenia NOS

✓5ᵗʰ **D69.5   Secondary thrombocytopenia**
EXCLUDES 1   *heparin induced thrombocytopenia (HIT) (D75.82)*
transient thrombocytopenia of newborn (P61.0)

D69.51   Posttransfusion purpura
Posttransfusion purpura from whole blood (fresh) or blood products
PTP

D69.59   Other secondary thrombocytopenia
AHA: 2014, 4Q, 22

D69.6   Thrombocytopenia, unspecified ▽

D69.8   Other specified hemorrhagic conditions
Capillary fragility (hereditary)   Vascular pseudohemophilia

D69.9   Hemorrhagic condition, unspecified ▽

Other disorders of blood and blood-forming organs (D70-D77)

✓4ᵗʰ **D70   Neutropenia**
[INCLUDES]   agranulocytosis
decreased absolute neurophile count (ANC)
Use additional code for any associated:
fever (R50.81)
mucositis (J34.81, K12.3-, K92.81, N76.81)
EXCLUDES 1   *neutropenic splenomegaly (D73.81)*
transient neonatal neutropenia (P61.5)

D70.0   Congenital agranulocytosis
Congenital neutropenia
Infantile genetic agranulocytosis
Kostmann's disease

D70.1   Agranulocytosis secondary to cancer chemotherapy
Code also underlying neoplasm
Use additional code for adverse effect, if applicable, to identify drug (T45.1X5)
AHA: 2014, 4Q, 22

D70.2   Other drug-induced agranulocytosis
Use additional code for adverse effect, if applicable, to identify drug (T36-T50 with fifth or sixth character 5)

D70.3   Neutropenia due to infection

D70.4   Cyclic neutropenia
Cyclic hematopoiesis   Periodic neutropenia

D70.8   Other neutropenia

D70.9   Neutropenia, unspecified ▽

D71   Functional disorders of polymorphonuclear neutrophils
Cell membrane receptor complex [CR3] defect
Chronic (childhood) granulomatous disease
Congenital dysphagocytosis
Progressive septic granulomatosis

✓4ᵗʰ **D72   Other disorders of white blood cells**
EXCLUDES 1   *basophilia (D72.824)*
immunity disorders (D80-D89)
neutropenia (D70)
preleukemia (syndrome) (D46.9)

D72.0   Genetic anomalies of leukocytes
Alder (granulation) (granulocyte) anomaly
Alder syndrome
Hereditary leukocytic hypersegmentation
Hereditary leukocytic hyposegmentation
Hereditary leukomelanopathy
May-Hegglin (granulation) (granulocyte) anomaly
May-Hegglin syndrome
Pelger-Huët (granulation) (granulocyte) anomaly
Pelger-Huët syndrome
EXCLUDES 1   *Chédiak (-Steinbrinck)-Higashi syndrome (E70.330)*

D72.1   Eosinophilia
Allergic eosinophilia
Hereditary eosinophilia
EXCLUDES 1   *Löffler's syndrome (J82)*
pulmonary eosinophilia (J82)

✓5ᵗʰ **D72.8   Other specified disorders of white blood cells**
EXCLUDES 1   *leukemia (C91-C95)*

✓6ᵗʰ **D72.81   Decreased white blood cell count**
EXCLUDES 1   *neutropenia (D70.-)*

D72.810   Lymphocytopenia
Decreased lymphocytes

D72.818   Other decreased white blood cell count
Basophilic leukopenia
Eosinophilic leukopenia
Monocytopenia
Other decreased leukocytes
Plasmacytopenia

D72.819   Decreased white blood cell count, unspecified ▽
Decreased leukocytes, unspecified
Leukocytopenia, unspecified
Leukopenia
EXCLUDES 1   *malignant leukopenia (D70.9)*

✓6ᵗʰ **D72.82   Elevated white blood cell count**
EXCLUDES 1   *eosinophilia (D72.1)*

D72.820   Lymphocytosis (symptomatic)
Elevated lymphocytes

D72.821   Monocytosis (symptomatic)
EXCLUDES 1   *infectious mononucleosis (B27.-)*

D72.822   Plasmacytosis

D72.823   Leukemoid reaction
Basophilic leukemoid reaction
Leukemoid reaction NOS
Lymphocytic leukemoid reaction
Monocytic leukemoid reaction
Myelocytic leukemoid reaction
Neutrophilic leukemoid reaction

D72.824   Basophilia

D72.825   Bandemia
Bandemia without diagnosis of specific infection
EXCLUDES 1   *confirmed infection—code to infection*
leukemia (C91.-, C92.-, C93.-, C94.-, C95.-)

D72.828   Other elevated white blood cell count

D72.829   Elevated white blood cell count, unspecified ▽
Elevated leukocytes, unspecified
Leukocytosis, unspecified

D72.89   Other specified disorders of white blood cells
Abnormality of white blood cells NEC

D72.9   Disorder of white blood cells, unspecified ▽
Abnormal leukocyte differential NOS

✓4ᵗʰ **D73   Diseases of spleen**

D73.0   Hyposplenism
Atrophy of spleen
EXCLUDES 1   *asplenia (congenital) (Q89.01)*
postsurgical absence of spleen (Z90.81)

D73.1   Hypersplenism
EXCLUDES 1   *neutropenic splenomegaly (D73.81)*
primary splenic neutropenia (D73.81)
splenitis, splenomegaly in late syphilis (A52.79)
splenitis, splenomegaly in tuberculosis (A18.85)
splenomegaly NOS (R16.1)
splenomegaly congenital (Q89.0)

D73.2   Chronic congestive splenomegaly

D73.3   Abscess of spleen

D73.4   Cyst of spleen

D73.5   Infarction of spleen
Splenic rupture, nontraumatic
Torsion of spleen
EXCLUDES 1   *rupture of spleen due to Plasmodium vivax malaria (B51.0)*
traumatic rupture of spleen (S36.03-)

✓5ᵗʰ **D73.8   Other diseases of spleen**

D73.81   Neutropenic splenomegaly
Werner-Schultz disease

[N] Newborn   [P] Pediatric   [M] Maternity   [A] Adult   [RIC] RIC Dx   [NCDx] Noncancer Dx   [PDx] Primary Dx   [CC] RIC CC Condition   ▶◀ Revised Text   ● New Code   ▲ Revised Code Title

D73.89 Other diseases of spleen
Fibrosis of spleen NOS
Perisplenitis
Splenitis NOS

D73.9 Disease of spleen, unspecified ▽

✓4ᵗʰ D74 Methemoglobinemia

D74.0 Congenital methemoglobinemia
Congenital NADH-methemoglobin reductase deficiency
Hemoglobin-M [Hb-M] disease
Methemoglobinemia, hereditary

D74.8 Other methemoglobinemias
Acquired methemoglobinemia (with sulfhemoglobinemia)
Toxic methemoglobinemia

D74.9 Methemoglobinemia, unspecified ▽

✓4ᵗʰ D75 Other and unspecified diseases of blood and blood-forming organs
EXCLUDES 2   acute lymphadenitis (L04.-)
chronic lymphadenitis (I88.1)
enlarged lymph nodes (R59.-)
hypergammaglobulinemia NOS (D89.2)
lymphadenitis NOS (I88.9)
mesenteric lymphadenitis (acute) (chronic) (I88.0)

D75.0 Familial erythrocytosis
Benign polycythemia
Familial polycythemia
EXCLUDES 1   hereditary ovalocytosis (D58.1)

D75.1 Secondary polycythemia
Acquired polycythemia
Emotional polycythemia
Erythrocytosis NOS
Hypoxemic polycythemia
Nephrogenous polycythemia
Polycythemia due to erythropoietin
Polycythemia due to fall in plasma volume
Polycythemia due to high altitude
Polycythemia due to stress
Polycythemia NOS
Relative polycythemia
EXCLUDES 1   polycythemia neonatorum (P61.1)
polycythemia vera (D45)

✓5ᵗʰ D75.8 Other specified diseases of blood and blood-forming organs

D75.81 Myelofibrosis
Myelofibrosis NOS
Secondary myelofibrosis NOS
Code first the underlying disorder, such as:
malignant neoplasm of breast (C50.-)
Use additional code, if applicable, for associated therapy-related myelodysplastic syndrome (D46.-)
Use additional code for adverse effect, if applicable, to identify drug (T45.1X5)
EXCLUDES 1   acute myelofibrosis (C94.4-)
idiopathic myelofibrosis (D47.1)
leukoerythroblastic anemia (D61.82)
myelofibrosis with myeloid metaplasia (D47.4)
myelophthisic anemia (D61.82)
myelophthisis (D61.82)
primary myelofibrosis (D47.1)

D75.82 Heparin induced thrombocytopenia (HIT)

D75.89 Other specified diseases of blood and blood-forming organs

D75.9 Disease of blood and blood-forming organs, unspecified ▽

✓4ᵗʰ D76 Other specified diseases with participation of lymphoreticular and reticulohistiocytic tissue
EXCLUDES 1   (Abt-) Letterer-Siwe disease (C96.0)
eosinophilic granuloma (C96.6)
Hand-Schüller-Christian disease (C96.5)
histiocytic sarcoma (C96.A)
histiocytosis X, multifocal (C96.5)
histiocytosis X, unifocal (C96.6)
Langerhans-cell histiocytosis, multifocal (C96.5)
Langerhans-cell histiocytosis NOS (C96.6)
Langerhans-cell histiocytosis, unifocal (C96.6)
leukemic reticuloendotheliosis or reticulosis (C91.4-)
lipomelanotic reticuloendotheliosis or reticulosis (I89.8)
malignant histiocytosis (C96.A)

D76.1 Hemophagocytic lymphohistiocytosis
Familial hemophagocytic reticulosis
Histiocytoses of mononuclear phagocytes

D76.2 Hemophagocytic syndrome, infection-associated
Use additional code to identify infectious agent or disease

D76.3 Other histiocytosis syndromes
Reticulohistiocytoma (giant-cell)
Sinus histiocytosis with massive lymphadenopathy
Xanthogranuloma

D77 Other disorders of blood and blood-forming organs in diseases classified elsewhere
Code first underlying disease, such as:
amyloidosis (E85.-)
congenital early syphilis (A50.0)
echinococcosis (B67.0-B67.9)
malaria (B50.0-B54)
schistosomiasis [bilharziasis] (B65.0-B65.9)
vitamin C deficiency (E54)
EXCLUDES 1   rupture of spleen due to Plasmodium vivax malaria (B51.0)
splenitis, splenomegaly in late syphilis (A52.79)
splenitis, splenomegaly in tuberculosis (A18.85)

Intraoperative and postprocedural complications of the spleen (D78)

✓4ᵗʰ D78 Intraoperative and postprocedural complications of the spleen

✓5ᵗʰ D78.0 Intraoperative hemorrhage and hematoma of the spleen complicating a procedure
EXCLUDES 1   intraoperative hemorrhage and hematoma of the spleen due to accidental puncture or laceration during a procedure (D78.1-)

D78.01 Intraoperative hemorrhage and hematoma of the spleen complicating a procedure on the spleen

D78.02 Intraoperative hemorrhage and hematoma of the spleen complicating other procedure

✓5ᵗʰ D78.1 Accidental puncture and laceration of the spleen during a procedure

D78.11 Accidental puncture and laceration of the spleen during a procedure on the spleen

D78.12 Accidental puncture and laceration of the spleen during other procedure

✓5ᵗʰ D78.2 Postprocedural hemorrhage and hematoma of the spleen following a procedure

D78.21 Postprocedural hemorrhage and hematoma of the spleen following a procedure on the spleen

D78.22 Postprocedural hemorrhage and hematoma of the spleen following other procedure

✓5ᵗʰ D78.8 Other intraoperative and postprocedural complications of the spleen
Use additional code, if applicable, to further specify disorder

D78.81 Other intraoperative complications of the spleen

D78.89 Other postprocedural complications of the spleen

Certain disorders involving the immune mechanism (D80-D89)
INCLUDES   defects in the complement system
immunodeficiency disorders, except human immunodeficiency virus [HIV] disease
sarcoidosis
EXCLUDES 1   autoimmune disease (systemic) NOS (M35.9)
functional disorders of polymorphonuclear neutrophils (D71)
human immunodeficiency virus [HIV] disease (B20)

✓4ᵗʰ D80 Immunodeficiency with predominantly antibody defects

D80.0 Hereditary hypogammaglobulinemia
Autosomal recessive agammaglobulinemia (Swiss type)
X-linked agammaglobulinemia [Bruton] (with growth hormone deficiency)

D80.1 Nonfamilial hypogammaglobulinemia
Agammaglobulinemia with immunoglobulin-bearing B-lymphocytes
Common variable agammaglobulinemia [CVAgamma]
Hypogammaglobulinemia NOS

D80.2 Selective deficiency of immunoglobulin A [IgA]

D80.3 Selective deficiency of immunoglobulin G [IgG] subclasses

D80.4 Selective deficiency of immunoglobulin M [IgM]

D80.5 Immunodeficiency with increased immunoglobulin M [IgM]

D80.6 Antibody deficiency with near-normal immunoglobulins or with hyperimmunoglobulinemia

D80.7 Transient hypogammaglobulinemia of infancy Ⓝ

D80.8 Other immunodeficiencies with predominantly antibody defects
Kappa light chain deficiency

☑ Add'l Character Required   ✓×7ᵗʰ Placeholder Alert   RUG IV Special Care High Dx   RUG IV Clinically Complex Dx   RUG IV Special Care Low Dx   Manifestation Code   Other Specified Code   ▽ Unspecified Code

ICD-10-CM 2016   485

Chapter 3. Disease of the Blood and Blood-Forming Organs

D80.9   **Immunodeficiency with predominantly antibody defects, unspecified** ▽

✓4ᵗʰ **D81 Combined immunodeficiencies**
   EXCLUDES 1   *autosomal recessive agammaglobulinemia (Swiss type) (D80.0)*

D81.0   Severe **combined immunodeficiency [SCID] with reticular dysgenesis**

D81.1   Severe **combined immunodeficiency [SCID] with low T- and B-cell numbers**

D81.2   Severe **combined immunodeficiency [SCID] with low or normal B-cell numbers**

D81.3   **Adenosine deaminase [ADA] deficiency**

D81.4   **Nezelof's syndrome**

D81.5   **Purine nucleoside phosphorylase [PNP] deficiency**

D81.6   **Major histocompatibility complex class I deficiency**
    Bare lymphocyte syndrome

D81.7   **Major histocompatibility complex class II deficiency**

✓5ᵗʰ D81.8   Other **combined immunodeficiencies**

    ✓6ᵗʰ **D81.81 Biotin-dependent carboxylase deficiency**
      Multiple carboxylase deficiency
      EXCLUDES 1   *biotin-dependent carboxylase deficiency due to dietary deficiency of biotin (E53.8)*

     D81.810   **Biotinidase deficiency**

     D81.818   **Other biotin-dependent carboxylase deficiency**
       Holocarboxylase synthetase deficiency
       Other multiple carboxylase deficiency

     D81.819   **Biotin-dependent carboxylase deficiency, unspecified** ▽
       Multiple carboxylase deficiency, unspecified

    D81.89   **Other combined immunodeficiencies**

D81.9   **Combined immunodeficiency, unspecified** ▽
    Severe combined immunodeficiency disorder [SCID] NOS

✓4ᵗʰ **D82 Immunodeficiency associated with other major defects**
   EXCLUDES 1   *ataxia telangiectasia [Louis-Bar] (G11.3)*

D82.0   **Wiskott-Aldrich syndrome**
    Immunodeficiency with thrombocytopenia and eczema

D82.1   **Di George's syndrome**
    Pharyngeal pouch syndrome   Thymic aplasia or hypoplasia
    Thymic alymphoplasia   with immunodeficiency

D82.2   **Immunodeficiency with short-limbed stature**

D82.3   **Immunodeficiency following hereditary defective response to Epstein-Barr virus**
    X-linked lymphoproliferative disease

D82.4   **Hyperimmunoglobulin E [IgE] syndrome**

D82.8   **Immunodeficiency associated with other specified major defects**

D82.9   **Immunodeficiency associated with major defect, unspecified** ▽

✓4ᵗʰ **D83 Common variable immunodeficiency**

D83.0   **Common variable immunodeficiency with predominant abnormalities of B-cell numbers and function**

D83.1   **Common variable immunodeficiency with predominant immunoregulatory T-cell disorders**

D83.2   **Common variable immunodeficiency with autoantibodies to B- or T-cells**

D83.8   **Other common variable immunodeficiencies**

D83.9   **Common variable immunodeficiency, unspecified** ▽

✓4ᵗʰ **D84 Other immunodeficiencies**

D84.0   **Lymphocyte function antigen-1 [LFA-1] defect**

D84.1   **Defects in the complement system**
    C1 esterase inhibitor [C1-INH] deficiency

D84.8   **Other specified immunodeficiencies**

D84.9   **Immunodeficiency, unspecified** ▽

✓4ᵗʰ **D86 Sarcoidosis**

D86.0   **Sarcoidosis of lung**

D86.1   **Sarcoidosis of lymph nodes**

D86.2   **Sarcoidosis of lung with sarcoidosis of lymph nodes**

D86.3   **Sarcoidosis of skin**

✓5ᵗʰ D86.8   **Sarcoidosis of other sites**

    D86.81   **Sarcoid meningitis**

    D86.82   **Multiple cranial nerve palsies in sarcoidosis**

    D86.83   **Sarcoid iridocyclitis**

    D86.84   **Sarcoid pyelonephritis**
      Tubulo-interstitial nephropathy in sarcoidosis

    D86.85   **Sarcoid myocarditis**

    D86.86   **Sarcoid arthropathy**
      Polyarthritis in sarcoidosis

    D86.87   **Sarcoid myositis**

    D86.89   **Sarcoidosis of other sites**
      Hepatic granulomaUveoparotid fever [Heerfordt]

D86.9   **Sarcoidosis, unspecified** ▽

✓4ᵗʰ **D89 Other disorders involving the immune mechanism, not elsewhere classified**
   EXCLUDES 1   *hyperglobulinemia NOS (R77.1)*
        monoclonal gammopathy (of undetermined significance) (D47.2)
   EXCLUDES 2   *transplant failure and rejection (T86.-)*

D89.0   **Polyclonal hypergammaglobulinemia**
    Benign hypergammaglobulinemic purpura
    Polyclonal gammopathy NOS

D89.1   **Cryoglobulinemia**
    Cryoglobulinemic purpura   Mixed cryoglobulinemia
    Cryoglobulinemic vasculitis   Primary cryoglobulinemia
    Essential cryoglobulinemia   Secondary cryoglobulinemia
    Idiopathic cryoglobulinemia

D89.2   **Hypergammaglobulinemia, unspecified**

D89.3   **Immune reconstitution syndrome**
    Immune reconstitution inflammatory syndrome [IRIS]
    Use additional code for adverse effect, if applicable, to identify drug (T36-T50 with fifth or sixth character 5)

✓5ᵗʰ D89.8   **Other specified disorders involving the immune mechanism, not elsewhere classified**

    ✓6ᵗʰ **D89.81 Graft-versus-host disease**
      Code first underlying cause, such as:
       complications of transplanted organs and tissue (T86.-)
       complications of blood transfusion (T80.89)
      Use additional code to identify associated manifestations, such as:
       desquamative dermatitis (L30.8)
       diarrhea (R19.7)
       elevated bilirubin (R17)
       hair loss (L65.9)

     D89.810   **Acute graft-versus-host disease**

     D89.811   **Chronic graft-versus-host disease**

     D89.812   **Acute on chronic graft-versus-host disease**

     D89.813   **Graft-versus-host disease, unspecified** ▽

    D89.82   **Autoimmune lymphoproliferative syndrome [ALPS]**

    D89.89   **Other specified disorders involving the immune mechanism, not elsewhere classified**
      EXCLUDES 1   *human immunodeficiency virus disease (B20)*

D89.9   **Disorder involving the immune mechanism, unspecified** ▽
    Immune disease NOS

N Newborn   P Pediatric   M Maternity   A Adult   RIC RIC Dx   NCDx Noncancer Dx   PDx Primary Dx   CC RIC CC Condition   ▶◀ Revised Text   ● New Code   ▲ Revised Code Title

486   ICD-10-CM 2016

Chapter 4. Endocrine, Nutritional, and Metabolic Diseases (E00–E89)

Chapter Specific Guidelines with Coding Examples

The chapter specific guidelines from the ICD-10-CM Official Guidelines for Coding and Reporting have been provided below. Along with these guidelines are coding examples, contained in the shaded boxes, that have been developed to help illustrate the coding and/or sequencing guidance found in these guidelines.

a. Diabetes mellitus

The diabetes mellitus codes are combination codes that include the type of diabetes mellitus, the body system affected, and the complications affecting that body system. As many codes within a particular category as are necessary to describe all of the complications of the disease may be used. They should be sequenced based on the reason for a particular encounter. Assign as many codes from categories E08–E13 as needed to identify all of the associated conditions that the patient has.

> Patient is seen for uncontrolled diabetes, type 2, with diabetic polyneuropathy and diabetic retinopathy with macular edema
>
> **E11.65**   **Type 2 diabetes mellitus with hyperglycemia**
>
> **E11.311**   **Type 2 diabetes mellitus with unspecified diabetic retinopathy with macular edema**
>
> **E11.42**   **Type 2 diabetes mellitus with diabetic polyneuropathy**
>
> *Explanation*: Use as many codes to describe the diabetic complications as needed. Many are combination codes that describe more than one condition. Code first the reason for the encounter. "Uncontrolled" is described as "with hyperglycemia."

1) Type of diabetes

The age of a patient is not the sole determining factor, though most type 1 diabetics develop the condition before reaching puberty. For this reason type 1 diabetes mellitus is also referred to as juvenile diabetes.

> A 45-year-old patient is diagnosed with Type 1 diabetes
>
> **E10.9**   **Type 1 diabetes mellitus without complications**
>
> *Explanation*: Although most type 1 diabetics are diagnosed in childhood or adolescence, it can also begin in adults.

2) Type of diabetes mellitus not documented

If the type of diabetes mellitus is not documented in the medical record the default is E11.-, Type 2 diabetes mellitus.

> Office visit lists diabetes and hypertension on patient problem list
>
> **E11.9**   **Type 2 diabetes mellitus without complications**
>
> **I10**   **Essential (primary) hypertension**
>
> *Explanation*: Since the type of diabetes was not documented and no complications were noted, the default code is E11.9.

3) Diabetes mellitus and the use of insulin

If the documentation in a medical record does not indicate the type of diabetes but does indicate that the patient uses insulin, code E11, Type 2 diabetes mellitus, should be assigned. Code Z79.4, Long-term (current) use of insulin, should also be assigned to indicate that the patient uses insulin. Code Z79.4 should not be assigned if insulin is given temporarily to bring a type 2 patient's blood sugar under control during an encounter.

> Office visit lists chronic diabetes with daily insulin use on patient problem list
>
> **E11.9**   **Type 2 diabetes mellitus without complications**
>
> **Z79.4**   **Long-term (current) use of insulin**
>
> *Explanation*: Do not assume that a patient on insulin must have type 1 diabetes. The default for diabetes without further specification defaults to type 2. Add the code for long-term use of insulin.

4) Diabetes mellitus in pregnancy and gestational diabetes

See Section I.C.15. Diabetes mellitus in pregnancy.

See Section I.C.15. Gestational (pregnancy induced) diabetes

5) Complications due to insulin pump malfunction

(a) Underdose of insulin due to insulin pump failure

An underdose of insulin due to an insulin pump failure should be assigned to a code from subcategory T85.6, Mechanical complication of other specified internal and external prosthetic devices, implants and grafts, that specifies the type of pump malfunction, as the principal or first-listed code, followed by code T38.3X6-, Underdosing of insulin and oral hypoglycemic [antidiabetic] drugs. Additional codes for the type of diabetes mellitus and any associated complications due to the underdosing should also be assigned.

> A 24-year-old type 1 diabetic male treated in ED for hyperglycemia; insulin pump found to be malfunctioning and underdosing
>
> **T85.614A**   **Breakdown (mechanical) of insulin pump, initial encounter**
>
> **T38.3X6A**   **Underdosing of insulin and oral hypoglycemic [antidiabetic] drugs, initial encounter**
>
> **E10.65**   **Type 1 diabetes mellitus with hyperglycemia**
>
> *Explanation*: The complication code for the mechanical breakdown of the pump is sequenced first, followed by the underdosing code and type of diabetes with complication. Code all other diabetic complication codes necessary to describe the patient's condition.

(b) Overdose of insulin due to insulin pump failure

The principal or first-listed code for an encounter due to an insulin pump malfunction resulting in an overdose of insulin, should also be T85.6-, Mechanical complication of other specified internal and external prosthetic devices, implants and grafts, followed by code T38.3X1-, Poisoning by insulin and oral hypoglycemic [antidiabetic] drugs, accidental (unintentional).

> A 24-year-old type 1 diabetic male found down with diabetic coma, brought into ED and treated for hypoglycemia; insulin pump found to be malfunctioning and overdosing
>
> **T85.614A**   **Breakdown (mechanical) of insulin pump, initial encounter**
>
> **T38.3X1A**   **Poisoning by insulin and oral hypoglycemic [antidiabetic] drugs, accidental (unintentional), initial encounter**
>
> **E10.641**   **Type 1 diabetes mellitus with hypoglycemia with coma**
>
> *Explanation*: The complication code for the mechanical breakdown of the pump is sequenced first, followed by the poisoning code and type of diabetes with complication. All the characters in the combination code must be used to form a valid code and to fully describe the type of diabetes, the hypoglycemia, and the coma.

6) Secondary diabetes mellitus

Codes under categories E08, Diabetes mellitus due to underlying condition, E09, Drug or chemical induced diabetes mellitus, and E13, Other specified diabetes mellitus, identify complications/manifestations associated with secondary diabetes mellitus. Secondary diabetes is always caused by another condition or event (e.g., cystic fibrosis, malignant neoplasm of pancreas, pancreatectomy, adverse effect of drug, or poisoning).

(a) Secondary diabetes mellitus and the use of insulin

For patients who routinely use insulin, code Z79.4, Long-term (current) use of insulin, should also be assigned. Code Z79.4 should not be assigned if insulin is given temporarily to bring a patient's blood sugar under control during an encounter.

Chapter 4. Endocrine, Nutritional, and Metabolic Diseases

Type 2 diabetic with no complications, normally only on oral metformin, is given insulin for three days to maintain glucose control while in the hospital recovering from surgery

E11.9   Type 2 diabetes mellitus without complications

No code is used for insulin use

Explanation: Do not code the long term (current) use of insulin when only provided temporarily.

Type 2 diabetic with diabetic polyneuropathy on insulin

E11.42   Type 2 diabetes mellitus with diabetic polyneuropathy

Z79.4   Long-term (current) use of insulin

Explanation: Add the Z code for the long-term use of insulin because the insulin is taken chronically.

(b) Assigning and sequencing secondary diabetes codes and its causes

The sequencing of the secondary diabetes codes in relationship to codes for the cause of the diabetes is based on the Tabular List instructions for categories E08, E09 and E13.

(i) Secondary diabetes mellitus due to pancreatectomy

For postpancreatectomy diabetes mellitus (lack of insulin due to the surgical removal of all or part of the pancreas), assign code E89.1, Postprocedural hypoinsulinemia. Assign a code from category E13 and a code from subcategory Z90.41-, Acquired absence of pancreas, as additional codes.

Patient with newly diagnosed diabetes after surgical removal of part of pancreas

E89.1   Postprocedural hypoinsulinemia

E13.9   Other specified diabetes mellitus without complications

Z90.411   Acquired partial absence of pancreas

Explanation: Sequence the postprocedural complication of the hypoinsulinemia due to the partial removal of the pancreas as the first-listed code, followed by the other specified diabetes (NEC) with or without complications and the partial or total acquired absence of the pancreas.

(ii) Secondary diabetes due to drugs

Secondary diabetes may be caused by an adverse effect of correctly administered medications, poisoning or sequela of poisoning.

See section I.C.19.e for coding of adverse effects and poisoning, and section I.C.20 for external cause code reporting.

Initial encounter for corticosteroid-induced diabetes mellitus

E09.9   Drug or chemical induced diabetes mellitus without complications

T38.0X5A   Adverse effect of glucocorticoids and synthetic analogues, initial encounter

Explanation: If the diabetes is caused by an adverse effect of a drug, the diabetic condition is coded first. If it occurs from a poisoning or overdose, the poisoning code causing the diabetes is sequenced first.

Chapter 4. Endocrine, Nutritional and Metabolic Diseases (E00-E89)

NOTE All neoplasms, whether functionally active or not, are classified in Chapter 2. Appropriate codes in this chapter (i.e. E05.8, E07.0, E16-E31, E34-) may be used as additional codes to indicate either functional activity by neoplasms and ectopic endocrine tissue or hyperfunction and hypofunction of endocrine glands associated with neoplasms and other conditions classified elsewhere.

EXCLUDES 1 *transitory endocrine and metabolic disorders specific to newborn (P70-P74)*

This chapter contains the following blocks:

E00-E07   Disorders of thyroid gland
E08-E13   Diabetes mellitus
E15-E16   Other disorders of glucose regulation and pancreatic internal secretion
E20-E35   Disorders of other endocrine glands
E36   Intraoperative complications of endocrine system
E40-E46   Malnutrition
E50-E64   Other nutritional deficiencies
E65-E68   Overweight, obesity and other hyperalimentation
E70-E88   Metabolic disorders
E89   Postprocedural endocrine and metabolic complications and disorders, not elsewhere classified

Disorders of thyroid gland (E00-E07)

☑4ᵗʰ E00 Congenital iodine-deficiency syndrome
Use additional code (F70-F79) to identify associated intellectual disabilities
EXCLUDES 1 *subclinical iodine-deficiency hypothyroidism (E02)*

E00.0 Congenital iodine-deficiency syndrome, neurological type
Endemic cretinism, neurological type

E00.1 Congenital iodine-deficiency syndrome, myxedematous type
Endemic hypothyroid cretinism
Endemic cretinism, myxedematous type

E00.2 Congenital iodine-deficiency syndrome, mixed type
Endemic cretinism, mixed type

E00.9 Congenital iodine-deficiency syndrome, unspecified ▽
Congenital iodine-deficiency hypothyroidism NOS
Endemic cretinism NOS

☑4ᵗʰ E01 Iodine-deficiency related thyroid disorders and allied conditions
EXCLUDES 1 *congenital iodine-deficiency syndrome (E00.-)*
subclinical iodine-deficiency hypothyroidism (E02)

E01.0 Iodine-deficiency related diffuse (endemic) goiter

E01.1 Iodine-deficiency related multinodular (endemic) goiter
Iodine-deficiency related nodular goiter

E01.2 Iodine-deficiency related (endemic) goiter, unspecified ▽
Endemic goiter NOS

E01.8 Other iodine-deficiency related thyroid disorders and allied conditions
Acquired iodine-deficiency hypothyroidism NOS

E02 Subclinical iodine-deficiency hypothyroidism

☑4ᵗʰ E03 Other hypothyroidism
EXCLUDES 1 *iodine-deficiency related hypothyroidism (E00-E02)*
postprocedural hypothyroidism (E89.0)

E03.0 Congenital hypothyroidism with diffuse goiter
Congenital parenchymatous goiter (nontoxic)
Congenital goiter (nontoxic) NOS
EXCLUDES 1 *transitory congenital goiter with normal function (P72.0)*

E03.1 Congenital hypothyroidism without goiter
Aplasia of thyroid (with myxedema)
Congenital atrophy of thyroid
Congenital hypothyroidism NOS

E03.2 Hypothyroidism due to medicaments and other exogenous substances
Code first poisoning due to drug or toxin, if applicable (T36-T65 with fifth or sixth character 1-4 or 6)
Use additional code for adverse effect, if applicable, to identify drug (T36-T50 with fifth or sixth character 5)

E03.3 Postinfectious hypothyroidism

E03.4 Atrophy of thyroid (acquired)
EXCLUDES 1 *congenital atrophy of thyroid (E03.1)*

E03.5 Myxedema coma   **NC Dx**

E03.8 Other specified hypothyroidism

E03.9 Hypothyroidism, unspecified ▽
Myxedema NOS

☑4ᵗʰ E04 Other nontoxic goiter
EXCLUDES 1 *congenital goiter (NOS) (diffuse) (parenchymatous) (E03.0)*
iodine-deficiency related goiter (E00-E02)

E04.0 Nontoxic diffuse goiter
Diffuse (colloid) nontoxic goiter
Simple nontoxic goiter

E04.1 Nontoxic single thyroid nodule
Colloid nodule (cystic) (thyroid)
Nontoxic uninodular goiter
Thyroid (cystic) nodule NOS

E04.2 Nontoxic multinodular goiter
Cystic goiter NOS
Multinodular (cystic) goiter NOS

E04.8 Other specified nontoxic goiter

E04.9 Nontoxic goiter, unspecified ▽
Goiter NOS
Nodular goiter (nontoxic) NOS

☑4ᵗʰ E05 Thyrotoxicosis [hyperthyroidism]
EXCLUDES 1 *chronic thyroiditis with transient thyrotoxicosis (E06.2)*
neonatal thyrotoxicosis (P72.1)

✓5ᵗʰ E05.0 Thyrotoxicosis with diffuse goiter
Exophthalmic or toxic goiter NOS   Graves' disease
                      Toxic diffuse goiter

E05.00 Thyrotoxicosis with diffuse goiter without thyrotoxic crisis or storm

E05.01 Thyrotoxicosis with diffuse goiter with thyrotoxic crisis or storm

✓5ᵗʰ E05.1 Thyrotoxicosis with toxic single thyroid nodule
Thyrotoxicosis with toxic uninodular goiter

E05.10 Thyrotoxicosis with toxic single thyroid nodule without thyrotoxic crisis or storm

E05.11 Thyrotoxicosis with toxic single thyroid nodule with thyrotoxic crisis or storm

✓5ᵗʰ E05.2 Thyrotoxicosis with toxic multinodular goiter
Toxic nodular goiter NOS

E05.20 Thyrotoxicosis with toxic multinodular goiter without thyrotoxic crisis or storm

E05.21 Thyrotoxicosis with toxic multinodular goiter with thyrotoxic crisis or storm

✓5ᵗʰ E05.3 Thyrotoxicosis from ectopic thyroid tissue

E05.30 Thyrotoxicosis from ectopic thyroid tissue without thyrotoxic crisis or storm

E05.31 Thyrotoxicosis from ectopic thyroid tissue with thyrotoxic crisis or storm

✓5ᵗʰ E05.4 Thyrotoxicosis factitia

E05.40 Thyrotoxicosis factitia without thyrotoxic crisis or storm

E05.41 Thyrotoxicosis factitia with thyrotoxic crisis or storm

✓5ᵗʰ E05.8 Other thyrotoxicosis
Overproduction of thyroid-stimulating hormone

E05.80 Other thyrotoxicosis without thyrotoxic crisis or storm

E05.81 Other thyrotoxicosis with thyrotoxic crisis or storm

✓5ᵗʰ E05.9 Thyrotoxicosis, unspecified
Hyperthyroidism NOS

E05.90 Thyrotoxicosis, unspecified without thyrotoxic crisis or storm ▽

E05.91 Thyrotoxicosis, unspecified with thyrotoxic crisis or storm ▽

☑4ᵗʰ E06 Thyroiditis
EXCLUDES 1 *postpartum thyroiditis (O90.5)*

E06.0 Acute thyroiditis
Abscess of thyroid   Suppurative thyroiditis
Pyogenic thyroiditis
Use additional code (B95-B97) to identify infectious agent

E06.1 Subacute thyroiditis
de Quervain thyroiditis   Nonsuppurative thyroiditis
Giant-cell thyroiditis   Viral thyroiditis
Granulomatous thyroiditis
EXCLUDES 1 *autoimmune thyroiditis (E06.3)*

E06.2 Chronic thyroiditis with transient thyrotoxicosis
EXCLUDES 1 *autoimmune thyroiditis (E06.3)*

E06.3 Autoimmune thyroiditis
Hashimoto's thyroiditis   Lymphocytic thyroiditis
Hashitoxicosis (transient)   Struma lymphomatosa
Lymphadenoid goiter

☑ Add'l Character Required   ☑x7ᵗʰ Placeholder Alert   **RUG IV Special Care High Dx**   RUG IV Clinically Complex Dx   RUG IV Special Care Low Dx   Manifestation Code   Other Specified Code   ▽ Unspecified Code

E06.4 Drug-induced thyroiditis
Use additional code for adverse effect, if applicable, to identify drug (T36-T50 with fifth or sixth character 5)

E06.5 Other chronic thyroiditis
Chronic fibrous thyroiditis   Ligneous thyroiditis
Chronic thyroiditis NOS   Riedel thyroiditis

E06.9 Thyroiditis, unspecified ▽

✓4th **E07 Other disorders of thyroid**

E07.0 Hypersecretion of calcitonin
C-cell hyperplasia of thyroid
Hypersecretion of thyrocalcitonin

E07.1 Dyshormogenetic goiter
Familial dyshormogenetic goiter
Pendred's syndrome
EXCLUDES 1 *transitory congenital goiter with normal function (P72.0)*

✓5th **E07.8 Other specified disorders of thyroid**

E07.81 Sick-euthyroid syndrome
Euthyroid sick-syndrome

E07.89 Other specified disorders of thyroid
Abnormality of thyroid-binding globulin
Hemorrhage of thyroid
Infarction of thyroid

E07.9 Disorder of thyroid, unspecified ▽

Diabetes mellitus (E08-E13)

✓4th **E08 Diabetes mellitus due to underlying condition**
Code first the underlying condition, such as:
congenital rubella (P35.0)
cushing's syndrome (E24.-)
cystic fibrosis (E84.-)
malignant neoplasm (C00-C96)
malnutrition (E40-E46)
pancreatitis and other diseases of the pancreas (K85.-, K86.-)
Use additional code to identify any insulin use (Z79.4)
EXCLUDES 1 *drug or chemical induced diabetes mellitus (E09.-)*
gestational diabetes (O24.4-)
neonatal diabetes mellitus (P70.2)
postpancreatectomy diabetes mellitus (E13.-)
postprocedural diabetes mellitus (E13.-)
secondary diabetes mellitus NEC (E13.-)
type 1 diabetes mellitus (E10.-)
type 2 diabetes mellitus (E11.-)
AHA: 2013, 4Q, 114; 2013, 3Q, 20

✓5th **E08.0 Diabetes mellitus due to underlying condition with hyperosmolarity**

[1] **E08.00 Diabetes mellitus due to underlying condition with hyperosmolarity without nonketotic hyperglycemic-hyperosmolar coma (NKHHC)**

E08.01 Diabetes mellitus due to underlying condition with hyperosmolarity with coma

✓5th **E08.1 Diabetes mellitus due to underlying condition with ketoacidosis**

[1] **E08.10 Diabetes mellitus due to underlying condition with ketoacidosis without coma**

E08.11 Diabetes mellitus due to underlying condition with ketoacidosis with coma

✓5th **E08.2 Diabetes mellitus due to underlying condition with kidney complications**

[1] **E08.21 Diabetes mellitus due to underlying condition with diabetic nephropathy** CC
Diabetes mellitus due to underlying condition with intercapillary glomerulosclerosis
Diabetes mellitus due to underlying condition with intracapillary glomerulonephrosis
Diabetes mellitus due to underlying condition with Kimmelstiel-Wilson disease

[1] **E08.22 Diabetes mellitus due to underlying condition with diabetic chronic kidney disease** CC
Use additional code to identify stage of chronic kidney disease (N18.1-N18.6)

[1] **E08.29 Diabetes mellitus due to underlying condition with other diabetic kidney complication** CC
Renal tubular degeneration in diabetes mellitus due to underlying condition

✓5th **E08.3 Diabetes mellitus due to underlying condition with ophthalmic complications**

✓6th **E08.31 Diabetes mellitus due to underlying condition with unspecified diabetic retinopathy**

[1] **E08.311 Diabetes mellitus due to underlying condition with unspecified diabetic retinopathy with macular edema** CC ▽

[1] **E08.319 Diabetes mellitus due to underlying condition with unspecified diabetic retinopathy without macular edema** CC ▽

✓6th **E08.32 Diabetes mellitus due to underlying condition with mild nonproliferative diabetic retinopathy**
Diabetes mellitus due to underlying condition with nonproliferative diabetic retinopathy NOS

[1] **E08.321 Diabetes mellitus due to underlying condition with mild nonproliferative diabetic retinopathy with macular edema** CC

[1] **E08.329 Diabetes mellitus due to underlying condition with mild nonproliferative diabetic retinopathy without macular edema** CC

✓6th **E08.33 Diabetes mellitus due to underlying condition with moderate nonproliferative diabetic retinopathy**

[1] **E08.331 Diabetes mellitus due to underlying condition with moderate nonproliferative diabetic retinopathy with macular edema** CC

[1] **E08.339 Diabetes mellitus due to underlying condition with moderate nonproliferative diabetic retinopathy without macular edema** CC

✓6th **E08.34 Diabetes mellitus due to underlying condition with severe nonproliferative diabetic retinopathy**

[1] **E08.341 Diabetes mellitus due to underlying condition with severe nonproliferative diabetic retinopathy with macular edema** CC

[1] **E08.349 Diabetes mellitus due to underlying condition with severe nonproliferative diabetic retinopathy without macular edema** CC

✓6th **E08.35 Diabetes mellitus due to underlying condition with proliferative diabetic retinopathy**

[1] **E08.351 Diabetes mellitus due to underlying condition with proliferative diabetic retinopathy with macular edema** CC

[1] **E08.359 Diabetes mellitus due to underlying condition with proliferative diabetic retinopathy without macular edema** CC

[1] **E08.36 Diabetes mellitus due to underlying condition with diabetic cataract** CC

[1] **E08.39 Diabetes mellitus due to underlying condition with other diabetic ophthalmic complication** CC
Use additional code to identify manifestation, such as: diabetic glaucoma (H40-H42)

✓5th **E08.4 Diabetes mellitus due to underlying condition with neurological complications**

[1] **E08.40 Diabetes mellitus due to underlying condition with diabetic neuropathy, unspecified** CC ▽
RIC Excl: 06 Neurological

[1] **E08.41 Diabetes mellitus due to underlying condition with diabetic mononeuropathy** CC

[1] **E08.42 Diabetes mellitus due to underlying condition with diabetic polyneuropathy** CC
Diabetes mellitus due to underlying condition with diabetic neuralgia
RIC Excl: 06 Neurological

[1] **E08.43 Diabetes mellitus due to underlying condition with diabetic autonomic (poly)neuropathy** CC
Diabetes mellitus due to underlying condition with diabetic gastroparesis
AHA: 2013, 4Q, 114

[1] **E08.44 Diabetes mellitus due to underlying condition with diabetic amyotrophy** CC

[1] **E08.49 Diabetes mellitus due to underlying condition with other diabetic neurological complication** CC

---

[1] Special Care High = With insulin injection and order changes

Ⓝ Newborn   Ⓟ Pediatric   Ⓜ Maternity   Ⓐ Adult   RIC RIC Dx   NCDx Noncancer Dx   PDx Primary Dx   CC RIC CC Condition   ▶◀ Revised Text   ● New Code   ▲ Revised Code Title

490   ICD-10-CM 2016

√5th **E08.5** **Diabetes mellitus due to underlying condition with** circulatory complications

> [1] **E08.51** **Diabetes mellitus due to underlying condition** CC **with diabetic** peripheral angiopathy without gangrene

> [1] **E08.52** **Diabetes mellitus due to underlying condition** CC **with diabetic** peripheral angiopathy with gangrene
>> Diabetes mellitus due to underlying condition with diabetic gangrene

> [1] **E08.59** **Diabetes mellitus due to underlying condition** CC **with other circulatory complications**

√5th **E08.6** **Diabetes mellitus due to underlying condition with** other specified complications

> √6th **E08.61** **Diabetes mellitus due to underlying condition with** diabetic arthropathy

>> [1] **E08.610** **Diabetes mellitus due to underlying** CC **condition with diabetic** neuropathic arthropathy
>>> Diabetes mellitus due to underlying condition with Charcôt's joints

>> [1] **E08.618** **Diabetes mellitus due to underlying** CC **condition with other diabetic arthropathy**

> √6th **E08.62** **Diabetes mellitus due to underlying condition with** skin complications

>> [1] **E08.620** **Diabetes mellitus due to underlying** CC **condition with** diabetic dermatitis
>>> Diabetes mellitus due to underlying condition with diabetic necrobiosis lipoidica

>> [1,6] **E08.621** **Diabetes mellitus due to underlying** CC **condition with** foot ulcer
>>> Use additional code to identify site of ulcer (L97.4-, L97.5-)

>> [1,6] **E08.622** **Diabetes mellitus due to underlying** CC **condition with** other skin ulcer
>>> Use additional code to identify site of ulcer (L97.1-L97.9, L98.41-L98.49)

>> [1] **E08.628** **Diabetes mellitus due to underlying** CC **condition with other skin complications**

> √6th **E08.63** **Diabetes mellitus due to underlying condition with** oral complications

>> [1] **E08.630** **Diabetes mellitus due to underlying** CC **condition with** periodontal disease

>> [1] **E08.638** **Diabetes mellitus due to underlying** CC **condition with other oral complications**

> √6th **E08.64** **Diabetes mellitus due to underlying condition with** hypoglycemia

>> **E08.641** **Diabetes mellitus due to underlying condition with hypoglycemia** with coma

>> [1] **E08.649** **Diabetes mellitus due to underlying** CC **condition with hypoglycemia** without coma

> [1] **E08.65** **Diabetes mellitus due to underlying condition** CC **with** hyperglycemia

> [1] **E08.69** **Diabetes mellitus due to underlying condition** CC **with other specified complication**
>> Use additional code to identify complication

[1] **E08.8** **Diabetes mellitus due to underlying condition** with ▽ unspecified complications

[1] **E08.9** **Diabetes mellitus due to underlying condition** without complications

√4th **E09** **Drug or chemical induced diabetes mellitus**
> Code first poisoning due to drug or toxin, if applicable (T36-T65 with fifth or sixth character 1-4 or 6)
> Use additional code for adverse effect, if applicable, to identify drug (T36-T50 with fifth or sixth character 5)
> Use additional code to identify any insulin use (Z79.4)
> **EXCLUDES 1** diabetes mellitus due to underlying condition (E08.-)
>> gestational diabetes (O24.4-)
>> neonatal diabetes mellitus (P70.2)
>> postpancreatectomy diabetes mellitus (E13.-)
>> postprocedural diabetes mellitus (E13.-)
>> secondary diabetes mellitus NEC (E13.-)
>> type 1 diabetes mellitus (E10.-)
>> type 2 diabetes mellitus (E11.-)
> **AHA:** 2013, 4Q, 114; 2013, 3Q, 20

√5th **E09.0** **Drug or chemical induced diabetes mellitus with** hyperosmolarity

> [1] **E09.00** **Drug or chemical induced diabetes mellitus with** hyperosmolarity without nonketotic hyperglycemic-hyperosmolar coma (NKHHC)

> **E09.01** **Drug or chemical induced diabetes mellitus with** hyperosmolarity with coma

√5th **E09.1** **Drug or chemical induced diabetes mellitus with** ketoacidosis

> [1] **E09.10** **Drug or chemical induced diabetes mellitus with** ketoacidosis without coma

> **E09.11** **Drug or chemical induced diabetes mellitus with** ketoacidosis with coma

√5th **E09.2** **Drug or chemical induced diabetes mellitus with** kidney complications

> [1] **E09.21** **Drug or chemical induced diabetes mellitus** CC **with** diabetic nephropathy
>> Drug or chemical induced diabetes mellitus with intercapillary glomerulosclerosis
>> Drug or chemical induced diabetes mellitus with intracapillary glomerulonephrosis
>> Drug or chemical induced diabetes mellitus with Kimmelstiel-Wilson disease

> [1] **E09.22** **Drug or chemical induced diabetes mellitus** CC **with** diabetic chronic kidney disease
>> Use additional code to identify stage of chronic kidney disease (N18.1-N18.6)

> [1] **E09.29** **Drug or chemical induced diabetes mellitus** CC **with other diabetic kidney complication**
>> Drug or chemical induced diabetes mellitus with renal tubular degeneration

√5th **E09.3** **Drug or chemical induced diabetes mellitus with** ophthalmic complications

> √6th **E09.31** **Drug or chemical induced diabetes mellitus with** unspecified diabetic retinopathy

>> [1] **E09.311** **Drug or chemical induced diabetes** CC ▽ **mellitus with unspecified diabetic retinopathy** with macular edema

>> [1] **E09.319** **Drug or chemical induced diabetes** CC ▽ **mellitus with unspecified diabetic retinopathy** without macular edema

> √6th **E09.32** **Drug or chemical induced diabetes mellitus with** mild nonproliferative diabetic retinopathy
>> Drug or chemical induced diabetes mellitus with nonproliferative diabetic retinopathy NOS

>> [1] **E09.321** **Drug or chemical induced diabetes** CC **mellitus with mild nonproliferative diabetic retinopathy** with macular edema

>> [1] **E09.329** **Drug or chemical induced diabetes** CC **mellitus with mild nonproliferative diabetic retinopathy** without macular edema

> √6th **E09.33** **Drug or chemical induced diabetes mellitus with** moderate nonproliferative diabetic retinopathy

>> [1] **E09.331** **Drug or chemical induced diabetes** CC **mellitus with moderate nonproliferative diabetic retinopathy** with macular edema

>> [1] **E09.339** **Drug or chemical induced diabetes** CC **mellitus with moderate nonproliferative diabetic retinopathy** without macular edema

> √6th **E09.34** **Drug or chemical induced diabetes mellitus with** severe nonproliferative diabetic retinopathy

>> [1] **E09.341** **Drug or chemical induced diabetes** CC **mellitus with severe nonproliferative diabetic retinopathy** with macular edema

>> [1] **E09.349** **Drug or chemical induced diabetes** CC **mellitus with severe nonproliferative diabetic retinopathy** without macular edema

> √6th **E09.35** **Drug or chemical induced diabetes mellitus with** proliferative diabetic retinopathy

>> [1] **E09.351** **Drug or chemical induced diabetes** CC **mellitus with proliferative diabetic retinopathy** with macular edema

>> [1] **E09.359** **Drug or chemical induced diabetes** CC **mellitus with proliferative diabetic retinopathy** without macular edema

---

[1] Special Care High = With insulin injection and order changes

[6] Special Care Low = Without insulin injection and order changes

---

☑ Add'l Character Required √7th Placeholder Alert RUG IV Special Care High Dx RUG IV Clinically Complex Dx RUG IV Special Care Low Dx Manifestation Code Other Specified Code ▽ Unspecified Code

ICD-10-CM 2016

491

E08.5–E09.359

[1] E09.36 Drug or chemical induced diabetes mellitus with diabetic cataract CC

[1] E09.39 Drug or chemical induced diabetes mellitus with other diabetic ophthalmic complication CC
Use additional code to identify manifestation, such as: diabetic glaucoma (H40-H42)

✓5th E09.4 Drug or chemical induced diabetes mellitus with neurological complications

[1] E09.40 Drug or chemical induced diabetes mellitus with neurological complications with diabetic neuropathy, unspecified CC ▽
RIC Excl: 06 Neurological

[1] E09.41 Drug or chemical induced diabetes mellitus with neurological complications with diabetic mononeuropathy CC

[1] E09.42 Drug or chemical induced diabetes mellitus with neurological complications with diabetic polyneuropathy CC
Drug or chemical induced diabetes mellitus with diabetic neuralgia
RIC Excl: 06 Neurological

[1] E09.43 Drug or chemical induced diabetes mellitus with neurological complications with diabetic autonomic (poly)neuropathy CC
Drug or chemical induced diabetes mellitus with diabetic gastroparesis
AHA: 2013, 4Q, 114

[1] E09.44 Drug or chemical induced diabetes mellitus with neurological complications with diabetic amyotrophy CC

[1] E09.49 Drug or chemical induced diabetes mellitus with neurological complications with other diabetic neurological complication CC

✓5th E09.5 Drug or chemical induced diabetes mellitus with circulatory complications

[1] E09.51 Drug or chemical induced diabetes mellitus with diabetic peripheral angiopathy without gangrene CC

[1] E09.52 Drug or chemical induced diabetes mellitus with diabetic peripheral angiopathy with gangrene CC
Drug or chemical induced diabetes mellitus with diabetic gangrene

[1] E09.59 Drug or chemical induced diabetes mellitus with other circulatory complications CC

✓5th E09.6 Drug or chemical induced diabetes mellitus with other specified complications

✓6th E09.61 Drug or chemical induced diabetes mellitus with diabetic arthropathy

[1] E09.610 Drug or chemical induced diabetes mellitus with diabetic neuropathic arthropathy CC
Drug or chemical induced diabetes mellitus with Charcôt's joints

[1] E09.618 Drug or chemical induced diabetes mellitus with other diabetic arthropathy CC

✓6th E09.62 Drug or chemical induced diabetes mellitus with skin complications

[1] E09.620 Drug or chemical induced diabetes mellitus with diabetic dermatitis CC
Drug or chemical induced diabetes mellitus with diabetic necrobiosis lipoidica

[1,6] E09.621 Drug or chemical induced diabetes mellitus with foot ulcer CC
Use additional code to identify site of ulcer (L97.4-, L97.5-)

[1,6] E09.622 Drug or chemical induced diabetes mellitus with other skin ulcer CC
Use additional code to identify site of ulcer (L97.1-L97.9, L98.41-L98.49)

[1] E09.628 Drug or chemical induced diabetes mellitus with other skin complications CC

✓6th E09.63 Drug or chemical induced diabetes mellitus with oral complications

[1] E09.630 Drug or chemical induced diabetes mellitus with periodontal disease CC

[1] E09.638 Drug or chemical induced diabetes mellitus with other oral complications CC

✓6th E09.64 Drug or chemical induced diabetes mellitus with hypoglycemia

E09.641 Drug or chemical induced diabetes mellitus with hypoglycemia with coma

[1] E09.649 Drug or chemical induced diabetes mellitus with hypoglycemia without coma

[1] E09.65 Drug or chemical induced diabetes mellitus with hyperglycemia CC

[1] E09.69 Drug or chemical induced diabetes mellitus with other specified complication CC
Use additional code to identify complication

[1] E09.8 Drug or chemical induced diabetes mellitus with unspecified complications ▽

[1] E09.9 Drug or chemical induced diabetes mellitus without complications

✓4th E10 Type 1 diabetes mellitus
INCLUDES
brittle diabetes (mellitus)
diabetes (mellitus) due to autoimmune process
diabetes (mellitus) due to immune mediated pancreatic islet beta-cell destruction
idiopathic diabetes (mellitus)
juvenile onset diabetes (mellitus)
ketosis-prone diabetes (mellitus)
EXCLUDES 1
diabetes mellitus due to underlying condition (E08.-)
drug or chemical induced diabetes mellitus (E09.-)
gestational diabetes (O24.4-)
hyperglycemia NOS (R73.9)
neonatal diabetes mellitus (P70.2)
postpancreatectomy diabetes mellitus (E13.-)
postprocedural diabetes mellitus (E13.-)
secondary diabetes mellitus NEC (E13.-)
type 2 diabetes mellitus (E11.-)
AHA: 2013, 4Q, 114; 2013, 3Q, 20

✓5th E10.1 Type 1 diabetes mellitus with ketoacidosis
AHA: 2013, 3Q, 20

[1] E10.10 Type 1 diabetes mellitus with ketoacidosis without coma

E10.11 Type 1 diabetes mellitus with ketoacidosis with coma

✓5th E10.2 Type 1 diabetes mellitus with kidney complications

[1] E10.21 Type 1 diabetes mellitus with diabetic nephropathy CC
Type 1 diabetes mellitus with intercapillary glomerulosclerosis
Type 1 diabetes mellitus with intracapillary glomerulonephrosis
Type 1 diabetes mellitus with Kimmelstiel-Wilson disease

[1] E10.22 Type 1 diabetes mellitus with diabetic chronic kidney disease CC
Use additional code to identify stage of chronic kidney disease (N18.1-N18.6)

[1] E10.29 Type 1 diabetes mellitus with other diabetic kidney complication CC
Type 1 diabetes mellitus with renal tubular degeneration

✓5th E10.3 Type 1 diabetes mellitus with ophthalmic complications

✓6th E10.31 Type 1 diabetes mellitus with unspecified diabetic retinopathy

[1] E10.311 Type 1 diabetes mellitus with unspecified diabetic retinopathy with macular edema CC

[1] E10.319 Type 1 diabetes mellitus with unspecified diabetic retinopathy without macular edema CC

✓6th E10.32 Type 1 diabetes mellitus with mild nonproliferative diabetic retinopathy
Type 1 diabetes mellitus with nonproliferative diabetic retinopathy NOS

[1] E10.321 Type 1 diabetes mellitus with mild nonproliferative diabetic retinopathy with macular edema CC

[1] E10.329 Type 1 diabetes mellitus with mild nonproliferative diabetic retinopathy without macular edema CC

---

[1] Special Care High = With insulin injection and order changes
[6] Special Care Low = Without insulin injection and order changes

✓6th **E10.33**   **Type 1 diabetes mellitus with moderate nonproliferative diabetic retinopathy**

[1] **E10.331**   **Type 1 diabetes mellitus with moderate nonproliferative diabetic retinopathy with macular edema**   CC

[1] **E10.339**   **Type 1 diabetes mellitus with moderate nonproliferative diabetic retinopathy without macular edema**   CC

✓6th **E10.34**   **Type 1 diabetes mellitus with severe nonproliferative diabetic retinopathy**

[1] **E10.341**   **Type 1 diabetes mellitus with severe nonproliferative diabetic retinopathy with macular edema**   CC

[1] **E10.349**   **Type 1 diabetes mellitus with severe nonproliferative diabetic retinopathy without macular edema**   CC

✓6th **E10.35**   **Type 1 diabetes mellitus with proliferative diabetic retinopathy**

[1] **E10.351**   **Type 1 diabetes mellitus with proliferative diabetic retinopathy with macular edema**   CC

[1] **E10.359**   **Type 1 diabetes mellitus with proliferative diabetic retinopathy without macular edema**   CC

[1] **E10.36**   **Type 1 diabetes mellitus with diabetic cataract**   CC

[1] **E10.39**   **Type 1 diabetes mellitus with other diabetic ophthalmic complication**   CC

Use additional code to identify manifestation, such as: diabetic glaucoma (H40-H42)

✓5th **E10.4**   **Type 1 diabetes mellitus with neurological complications**

[1] **E10.40**   **Type 1 diabetes mellitus with diabetic neuropathy, unspecified**   CC ▽

RIC Excl: 06 Neurological

[1] **E10.41**   **Type 1 diabetes mellitus with diabetic mononeuropathy**   CC

RIC Excl: 06 Neurological

[1] **E10.42**   **Type 1 diabetes mellitus with diabetic polyneuropathy**   CC

Type 1 diabetes mellitus with diabetic neuralgia

RIC Excl: 06 Neurological

[1] **E10.43**   **Type 1 diabetes mellitus with diabetic autonomic (poly)neuropathy**   CC

Type 1 diabetes mellitus with diabetic gastroparesis

AHA: 2013, 4Q, 114

RIC Excl: 06 Neurological

[1] **E10.44**   **Type 1 diabetes mellitus with diabetic amyotrophy**   CC

RIC Excl: 06 Neurological

[1] **E10.49**   **Type 1 diabetes mellitus with other diabetic neurological complication**   CC

RIC Excl: 06 Neurological

✓5th **E10.5**   **Type 1 diabetes mellitus with circulatory complications**

[1] **E10.51**   **Type 1 diabetes mellitus with diabetic peripheral angiopathy without gangrene**   CC

[1] **E10.52**   **Type 1 diabetes mellitus with diabetic peripheral angiopathy with gangrene**   CC

Type 1 diabetes melli tus with diabetic gangrene

[1] **E10.59**   **Type 1 diabetes mellitus with other circulatory complications**   CC

✓5th **E10.6**   **Type 1 diabetes mellitus with other specified complications**

✓6th **E10.61**   **Type 1 diabetes mellitus with diabetic arthropathy**

[1] **E10.610**   **Type 1 diabetes mellitus with diabetic neuropathic arthropathy**   CC

Type 1 diabetes mellitus with Charcôt's joints

RIC Excl: 06 Neurological

[1] **E10.618**   **Type 1 diabetes mellitus with other diabetic arthropathy**   CC

✓6th **E10.62**   **Type 1 diabetes mellitus with skin complications**

[1] **E10.620**   **Type 1 diabetes mellitus with diabetic dermatitis**   CC

Type 1 diabetes mellitus with diabetic necrobiosis lipoidica

[1,6] **E10.621**   **Type 1 diabetes mellitus with foot ulcer**   CC

Use additional code to identify site of ulcer (L97.4-, L97.5-)

[1,6] **E10.622**   **Type 1 diabetes mellitus with other skin ulcer**   CC

Use additional code to identify site of ulcer (L97.1-L97.9, L98.41-L98.49)

[1] **E10.628**   **Type 1 diabetes mellitus with other skin complications**   CC

✓6th **E10.63**   **Type 1 diabetes mellitus with oral complications**

[1] **E10.630**   **Type 1 diabetes mellitus with periodontal disease**   CC

[1] **E10.638**   **Type 1 diabetes mellitus with other oral complications**   CC

✓6th **E10.64**   **Type 1 diabetes mellitus with hypoglycemia**

E10.641   **Type 1 diabetes mellitus with hypoglycemia with coma**   CC

[1] **E10.649**   **Type 1 diabetes mellitus with hypoglycemia without coma**   CC

[1] **E10.65**   **Type 1 diabetes mellitus with hyperglycemia**   CC

AHA: 2013, 3Q, 20

[1] **E10.69**   **Type 1 diabetes mellitus with other specified complication**   CC

Use additional code to identify complication

[1] **E10.8**   **Type 1 diabetes mellitus with unspecified complications**   CC ▽

[1] **E10.9**   **Type 1 diabetes mellitus without complications**   CC

✓4th **E11**   **Type 2 diabetes mellitus**

INCLUDES   diabetes (mellitus) due to insulin secretory defect

diabetes NOS

insulin resistant diabetes (mellitus)

Use additional code to identify any insulin use (Z79.4)

EXCLUDES 1   *diabetes mellitus due to underlying condition (E08.-)*

drug or chemical induced diabetes mellitus (E09.-)

gestational diabetes (O24.4-)

neonatal diabetes mellitus (P70.2)

postpancreatectomy diabetes mellitus (E13.-)

postprocedural diabetes mellitus (E13.-)

secondary diabetes mellitus NEC (E13.-)

type 1 diabetes mellitus (E10.-)

AHA: 2013, 4Q, 114; 2013, 3Q, 20; 2013, 1Q, 26

✓5th **E11.0**   **Type 2 diabetes mellitus with hyperosmolarity**

[1] **E11.00**   **Type 2 diabetes mellitus with hyperosmolarity without nonketotic hyperglycemic-hyperosmolar coma (NKHHC)**

E11.01   **Type 2 diabetes mellitus with hyperosmolarity with coma**

✓5th **E11.2**   **Type 2 diabetes mellitus with kidney complications**

[1] **E11.21**   **Type 2 diabetes mellitus with diabetic nephropathy**   CC

Type 2 diabetes mellitus with intercapillary glomerulosclerosis

Type 2 diabetes mellitus with intracapillary glomerulonephrosis

Type 2 diabetes mellitus with Kimmelstiel-Wilson disease

[1] **E11.22**   **Type 2 diabetes mellitus with diabetic chronic kidney disease**   CC

Use additional code to identify stage of chronic kidney disease (N18.1-N18.6)

[1] **E11.29**   **Type 2 diabetes mellitus with other diabetic kidney complication**   CC

Type 2 diabetes mellitus with renal tubular degeneration

✓5th **E11.3**   **Type 2 diabetes mellitus with ophthalmic complications**

✓6th **E11.31**   **Type 2 diabetes mellitus with unspecified diabetic retinopathy**

[1] **E11.311**   **Type 2 diabetes mellitus with unspecified diabetic retinopathy with macular edema**   CC ▽

[1] **E11.319**   **Type 2 diabetes mellitus with unspecified diabetic retinopathy without macular edema**   CC ▽

---

[1] Special Care High = With insulin injection and order changes

[6] Special Care Low = Without insulin injection and order changes

---

☑ Add'l Character Required   ✓x7th Placeholder Alert   RUG IV Special Care High Dx   RUG IV Clinically Complex Dx   RUG IV Special Care Low Dx   Manifestation Code   Other Specified Code   ▽ Unspecified Code

√6ᵗʰ **E11.32 Type 2 diabetes mellitus with mild nonproliferative diabetic retinopathy**
Type 2 diabetes mellitus with nonproliferative diabetic retinopathy NOS

[1] **E11.321 Type 2 diabetes mellitus with mild nonproliferative diabetic retinopathy with macular edema** CC

[1] **E11.329 Type 2 diabetes mellitus with mild nonproliferative diabetic retinopathy without macular edema**

√6ᵗʰ **E11.33 Type 2 diabetes mellitus with moderate nonproliferative diabetic retinopathy**

[1] **E11.331 Type 2 diabetes mellitus with moderate nonproliferative diabetic retinopathy with macular edema** CC

[1] **E11.339 Type 2 diabetes mellitus with moderate nonproliferative diabetic retinopathy without macular edema** CC

√6ᵗʰ **E11.34 Type 2 diabetes mellitus with severe nonproliferative diabetic retinopathy**

[1] **E11.341 Type 2 diabetes mellitus with severe nonproliferative diabetic retinopathy with macular edema** CC

[1] **E11.349 Type 2 diabetes mellitus with severe nonproliferative diabetic retinopathy without macular edema** CC

√6ᵗʰ **E11.35 Type 2 diabetes mellitus with proliferative diabetic retinopathy**

[1] **E11.351 Type 2 diabetes mellitus with proliferative diabetic retinopathy with macular edema** CC

[1] **E11.359 Type 2 diabetes mellitus with proliferative diabetic retinopathy without macular edema**

[1] **E11.36 Type 2 diabetes mellitus with diabetic cataract** CC

[1] **E11.39 Type 2 diabetes mellitus with other diabetic ophthalmic complication** CC
Use additional code to identify manifestation, such as: diabetic glaucoma (H40-H42)

√5ᵗʰ **E11.4 Type 2 diabetes mellitus with neurological complications**

[1] **E11.40 Type 2 diabetes mellitus with diabetic neuropathy, unspecified** CC ▽
AHA: 2013, 4Q, 129
RIC Excl: 06 Neurological

[1] **E11.41 Type 2 diabetes mellitus with diabetic mononeuropathy** CC
RIC Excl: 06 Neurological

[1] **E11.42 Type 2 diabetes mellitus with diabetic polyneuropathy** CC
Type 2 diabetes mellitus with diabetic neuralgia
RIC Excl: 06 Neurological

[1] **E11.43 Type 2 diabetes mellitus with diabetic autonomic (poly)neuropathy** CC
Type 2 diabetes mellitus with diabetic gastroparesis
AHA: 2013, 4Q, 114
RIC Excl: 06 Neurological

[1] **E11.44 Type 2 diabetes mellitus with diabetic amyotrophy** CC
RIC Excl: 06 Neurological

[1] **E11.49 Type 2 diabetes mellitus with other diabetic neurological complication** CC
RIC Excl: 06 Neurological

√5ᵗʰ **E11.5 Type 2 diabetes mellitus with circulatory complications**

[1] **E11.51 Type 2 diabetes mellitus with diabetic peripheral angiopathy without gangrene** CC

[1] **E11.52 Type 2 diabetes mellitus with diabetic peripheral angiopathy with gangrene** CC
Type 2 diabetes mellitus with diabetic gangrene

[1] **E11.59 Type 2 diabetes mellitus with other circulatory complications** CC

√5ᵗʰ **E11.6 Type 2 diabetes mellitus with other specified complications**

√6ᵗʰ **E11.61 Type 2 diabetes mellitus with diabetic arthropathy**

[1] **E11.610 Type 2 diabetes mellitus with diabetic neuropathic arthropathy** CC
Type 2 diabetes mellitus with Charcôt's joints
RIC Excl: 06 Neurological

[1] **E11.618 Type 2 diabetes mellitus with other diabetic arthropathy** CC

√6ᵗʰ **E11.62 Type 2 diabetes mellitus with skin complications**

[1] **E11.620 Type 2 diabetes mellitus with diabetic dermatitis** CC
Type 2 diabetes mellitus with diabetic necrobiosis lipoidica

[1,6] **E11.621 Type 2 diabetes mellitus with foot ulcer** CC
Use additional code to identify site of ulcer (L97.4-, L97.5-)

[1,6] **E11.622 Type 2 diabetes mellitus with other skin ulcer** CC
Use additional code to identify site of ulcer (L97.1-L97.9, L98.41-L98.49)

[1] **E11.628 Type 2 diabetes mellitus with other skin complications** CC

√6ᵗʰ **E11.63 Type 2 diabetes mellitus with oral complications**

[1] **E11.630 Type 2 diabetes mellitus with periodontal disease** CC

[1] **E11.638 Type 2 diabetes mellitus with other oral complications** CC

√6ᵗʰ **E11.64 Type 2 diabetes mellitus with hypoglycemia**

E11.641 Type 2 diabetes mellitus with hypoglycemia with coma

[1] **E11.649 Type 2 diabetes mellitus with hypoglycemia without coma** CC

[1] **E11.65 Type 2 diabetes mellitus with hyperglycemia** CC
AHA: 2013, 3Q, 20

[1] **E11.69 Type 2 diabetes mellitus with other specified complication** CC
Use additional code to identify complication

[1] **E11.8 Type 2 diabetes mellitus with unspecified complications** ▽

[1] **E11.9 Type 2 diabetes mellitus without complications**

√4ᵗʰ **E13 Other specified diabetes mellitus**
Diabetes mellitus due to genetic defects of beta-cell function
Diabetes mellitus due to genetic defects in insulin action
Postpancreatectomy diabetes mellitus
Postprocedural diabetes mellitus
Secondary diabetes mellitus NEC
Use additional code to identify any insulin use (Z79.4)
EXCLUDES 1 *diabetes (mellitus) due to autoimmune process (E10.-)*
diabetes (mellitus) due to immune mediated pancreatic islet beta-cell destruction (E10.-)
diabetes mellitus due to underlying condition (E08.-)
drug or chemical induced diabetes mellitus (E09.-)
gestational diabetes (O24.4-)
neonatal diabetes mellitus (P70.2)
type 2 diabetes mellitus (E11.-)
AHA: 2013, 4Q, 114; 2013, 3Q, 20

√5ᵗʰ **E13.0 Other specified diabetes mellitus with hyperosmolarity**

[1] **E13.00 Other specified diabetes mellitus with hyperosmolarity without nonketotic hyperglycemic-hyperosmolar coma (NKHHC)**

E13.01 Other specified diabetes mellitus with hyperosmolarity with coma

√5ᵗʰ **E13.1 Other specified diabetes mellitus with ketoacidosis**
AHA: 2013, 1Q, 26

[1] **E13.10 Other specified diabetes mellitus with ketoacidosis without coma**

E13.11 Other specified diabetes mellitus with ketoacidosis with coma

√5ᵗʰ **E13.2 Other specified diabetes mellitus with kidney complications**

[1] **E13.21 Other specified diabetes mellitus with diabetic nephropathy** CC
Other specified diabetes mellitus with intercapillary glomerulosclerosis
Other specified diabetes mellitus with intracapillary glomerulonephrosis
Other specified diabetes mellitus with Kimmelstiel-Wilson disease

[1] **E13.22 Other specified diabetes mellitus with diabetic chronic kidney disease** CC
Use additional code to identify stage of chronic kidney disease (N18.1-N18.6)

---

[1] Special Care High = With insulin injection and order changes

[6] Special Care Low = Without insulin injection and order changes

Ⓝ Newborn   Ⓟ Pediatric   Ⓜ Maternity   Ⓐ Adult   RIC RIC Dx   NCDx Noncancer Dx   PDx Primary Dx   CC RIC CC Condition   ▶◀ Revised Text   ● New Code   ▲ Revised Code Title

494   ICD-10-CM 2016

[1] **E13.29** **Other specified diabetes mellitus with other diabetic** kidney complication   cc
Other specified diabetes mellitus with renal tubular degeneration

✓5th **E13.3** **Other specified diabetes mellitus with** ophthalmic complications

✓6th **E13.31** **Other specified diabetes mellitus with** unspecified diabetic retinopathy

[1] **E13.311** **Other specified diabetes mellitus with unspecified diabetic retinopathy** with macular edema   cc ▽

[1] **E13.319** **Other specified diabetes mellitus with unspecified diabetic retinopathy** without macular edema   cc ▽

✓6th **E13.32** **Other specified diabetes mellitus with** mild nonproliferative diabetic retinopathy
Other specified diabetes mellitus with nonproliferative diabetic retinopathy NOS

[1] **E13.321** **Other specified diabetes mellitus with mild nonproliferative diabetic retinopathy** with macular edema   cc

[1] **E13.329** **Other specified diabetes mellitus with mild nonproliferative diabetic retinopathy** without macular edema   cc

✓6th **E13.33** **Other specified diabetes mellitus with** moderate nonproliferative **diabetic retinopathy**

[1] **E13.331** **Other specified diabetes mellitus with moderate nonproliferative diabetic retinopathy** with macular edema   cc

[1] **E13.339** **Other specified diabetes mellitus with moderate nonproliferative diabetic retinopathy** without macular edema   cc

✓6th **E13.34** **Other specified diabetes mellitus with** severe nonproliferative **diabetic retinopathy**

[1] **E13.341** **Other specified diabetes mellitus with severe nonproliferative diabetic retinopathy** with macular edema   cc

[1] **E13.349** **Other specified diabetes mellitus with severe nonproliferative diabetic retinopathy** without macular edema   cc

✓6th **E13.35** **Other specified diabetes mellitus with proliferative diabetic** retinopathy

[1] **E13.351** **Other specified diabetes mellitus with proliferative diabetic retinopathy** with macular edema   cc

[1] **E13.359** **Other specified diabetes mellitus with proliferative diabetic retinopathy** without macular edema   cc

[1] **E13.36** **Other specified diabetes mellitus with** diabetic cataract   cc

[1] **E13.39** **Other specified diabetes mellitus with** other diabetic ophthalmic complication   cc
Use additional code to identify manifestation, such as: diabetic glaucoma (H40-H42)

✓5th **E13.4** **Other specified diabetes mellitus with** neurological complications

[1] **E13.40** **Other specified diabetes mellitus with** diabetic neuropathy, unspecified   cc ▽
RIC Excl: 06 Neurological

[1] **E13.41** **Other specified diabetes mellitus with diabetic** mononeuropathy   cc
RIC Excl: 06 Neurological

[1] **E13.42** **Other specified diabetes mellitus with diabetic** polyneuropathy   cc
Other specified diabetes mellitus with diabetic neuralgia
RIC Excl: 06 Neurological

[1] **E13.43** **Other specified diabetes mellitus with diabetic** autonomic (poly)neuropathy   cc
Other specified diabetes mellitus with diabetic gastroparesis
AHA: 2013, 4Q, 114
RIC Excl: 06 Neurological

[1] **E13.44** **Other specified diabetes mellitus with diabetic** amyotrophy   cc
RIC Excl: 06 Neurological

[1] **E13.49** **Other specified diabetes mellitus with other diabetic neurological complication**   cc
RIC Excl: 06 Neurological

✓5th **E13.5** **Other specified diabetes mellitus with** circulatory complications

[1] **E13.51** **Other specified diabetes mellitus with diabetic** peripheral angiopathy without gangrene   cc

[1] **E13.52** **Other specified diabetes mellitus with diabetic** peripheral angiopathy with gangrene   cc
Other specified diabetes mellitus with diabetic gangrene

[1] **E13.59** **Other specified diabetes mellitus with other circulatory complications**   cc

✓5th **E13.6** **Other specified diabetes mellitus with** other specified complications

✓6th **E13.61** **Other specified diabetes mellitus with diabetic** arthropathy

[1] **E13.610** **Other specified diabetes mellitus with diabetic** neuropathic **arthropathy**   cc
Other specified diabetes mellitus with Charcôt's joints
RIC Excl: 06 Neurological

[1] **E13.618** **Other specified diabetes mellitus with other diabetic arthropathy**   cc

✓6th **E13.62** **Other specified diabetes mellitus with** skin complications

[1] **E13.620** **Other specified diabetes mellitus with** dermatitis   cc
Other specified diabetes mellitus with diabetic necrobiosis lipoidica

[1,6] **E13.621** **Other specified diabetes mellitus with** foot ulcer   cc
Use additional code to identify site of ulcer (L97.4-, L97.5-)

[1,6] **E13.622** **Other specified diabetes mellitus with** other skin ulcer   cc
Use additional code to identify site of ulcer (L97.1-L97.9, L98.41-L98.49)

[1] **E13.628** **Other specified diabetes mellitus with other skin complications**   cc

✓6th **E13.63** **Other specified diabetes mellitus with** oral complications

[1] **E13.630** **Other specified diabetes mellitus with** periodontal disease   cc

[1] **E13.638** **Other specified diabetes mellitus with** other oral complications   cc

✓6th **E13.64** **Other specified diabetes mellitus with** hypoglycemia

E13.641 **Other specified diabetes mellitus with hypoglycemia** with coma

[1] **E13.649** **Other specified diabetes mellitus with hypoglycemia** without coma   cc

[1] **E13.65** **Other specified diabetes mellitus with** hyperglycemia

[1] **E13.69** **Other specified diabetes mellitus with other** specified complication   cc
Use additional code to identify complication

[1] **E13.8** **Other specified diabetes mellitus with unspecified** complications   ▽

[1] **E13.9** **Other specified diabetes mellitus** without complications

Other disorders of glucose regulation and pancreatic internal secretion (E15-E16)

E15 **Nondiabetic hypoglycemic coma**
INCLUDES drug-induced insulin coma in nondiabetic hyperinsulinism with hypoglycemic coma hypoglycemic coma NOS

✓4th **E16** **Other disorders of pancreatic internal secretion**

E16.0 **Drug-induced hypoglycemia without coma**
Use additional code for adverse effect, if applicable, to identify drug (T36-T50 with fifth or sixth character 5)

---

[1] Special Care High = With insulin injection and order changes
[6] Special Care Low = Without insulin injection and order changes

---

✓ Add'l Character Required   ✓7th Placeholder Alert   RUG IV Special Care High Dx   RUG IV Clinically Complex Dx   RUG IV Special Care Low Dx   Manifestation Code   Other Specified Code   ▽ Unspecified Code

E16.1 **Other hypoglycemia**
Functional hyperinsulinism
Functional nonhyperinsulinemic hypoglycemia
Hyperinsulinism NOS
Hyperplasia of pancreatic islet beta cells NOS
   EXCLUDES 1   *hypoglycemia in infant of diabetic mother (P70.1)*
                neonatal hypoglycemia (P70.4)

E16.2 **Hypoglycemia, unspecified** ▽

E16.3 **Increased secretion of glucagon**
Hyperplasia of pancreatic endocrine cells with glucagon excess

E16.4 **Increased secretion of gastrin**
Hypergastrinemia
Hyperplasia of pancreatic endocrine cells with gastrin excess
Zollinger-Ellison syndrome

E16.8 **Other specified disorders of pancreatic internal secretion**
Increased secretion from endocrine pancreas of growth
   hormone-releasing hormone
Increased secretion from endocrine pancreas of pancreatic
   polypeptide
Increased secretion from endocrine pancreas of somatostatin
Increased secretion from endocrine pancreas of
   vasoactive-intestinal polypeptide

E16.9 **Disorder of pancreatic internal secretion, unspecified** ▽
Islet-cell hyperplasia NOS
Pancreatic endocrine cell hyperplasia NOS

Disorders of other endocrine glands (E20-E35)

   EXCLUDES 1   *galactorrhea (N64.3)*
                gynecomastia (N62)

✓4th **E20** **Hypoparathyroidism**
   EXCLUDES 1   *Di George's syndrome (D82.1)*
                postprocedural hypoparathyroidism (E89.2)
                tetany NOS (R29.0)
                transitory neonatal hypoparathyroidism (P71.4)

E20.0 **Idiopathic hypoparathyroidism**

E20.1 **Pseudohypoparathyroidism**

E20.8 **Other hypoparathyroidism**

E20.9 **Hypoparathyroidism, unspecified** ▽
Parathyroid tetany

✓4th **E21** **Hyperparathyroidism and other disorders of parathyroid gland**
   EXCLUDES 1   *adult osteomalacia (M83.-)*
                ectopic hyperparathyroidism (E34.2)
                familial hypocalciuric hypercalcemia (E83.52)
                hungry bone syndrome (E83.81)
                infantile and juvenile osteomalacia (E55.0)

E21.0 **Primary hyperparathyroidism**
Hyperplasia of parathyroid
Osteitis fibrosa cystica generalisata [von Recklinghausen's
   disease of bone]

E21.1 **Secondary hyperparathyroidism, not elsewhere classified**
   EXCLUDES 1   *secondary hyperparathyroidism of renal origin (N25.81)*

E21.2 **Other hyperparathyroidism**
Tertiary hyperparathyroidism
   EXCLUDES 1   *familial hypocalciuric hypercalcemia (E83.52)*

E21.3 **Hyperparathyroidism, unspecified** ▽

E21.4 **Other specified disorders of parathyroid gland**

E21.5 **Disorder of parathyroid gland, unspecified** ▽

✓4th **E22** **Hyperfunction of pituitary gland**
   EXCLUDES 1   *Cushing's syndrome (E24.-)*
                Nelson's syndrome (E24.1)
                overproduction of ACTH not associated with Cushing's disease
                (E27.0)
                overproduction of pituitary ACTH (E24.0)
                overproduction of thyroid-stimulating hormone (E05.8-)

E22.0 **Acromegaly and pituitary gigantism**
Overproduction of growth hormone
   EXCLUDES 1   *constitutional gigantism (E34.4)*
                constitutional tall stature (E34.4)
                increased secretion from endocrine pancreas of growth
                hormone-releasing hormone (E16.8)

E22.1 **Hyperprolactinemia**
Use additional code for adverse effect, if applicable, to identify
   drug (T36-T50 with fifth or sixth character 5)

E22.2 **Syndrome of inappropriate secretion of antidiuretic hormone**

E22.8 **Other hyperfunction of pituitary gland**
Central precocious puberty

E22.9 **Hyperfunction of pituitary gland, unspecified** ▽

✓4th **E23** **Hypofunction and other disorders of the pituitary gland**
   INCLUDES   the listed conditions whether the disorder is in the pituitary
                or the hypothalamus
   EXCLUDES 1   *postprocedural hypopituitarism (E89.3)*

E23.0 **Hypopituitarism**
Fertile eunuch syndrome
Hypogonadotropic hypogonadism
Idiopathic growth hormone deficiency
Isolated deficiency of gonadotropin
Isolated deficiency of growth hormone
Isolated deficiency of pituitary hormone
Kallmann's syndrome
Lorain-Levi short stature
Necrosis of pituitary gland (postpartum)
Panhypopituitarism
Pituitary cachexia
Pituitary insufficiency NOS
Pituitary short stature
Sheehan's syndrome
Simmonds' disease

E23.1 **Drug-induced hypopituitarism**
Use additional code for adverse effect, if applicable, to identify
   drug (T36-T50 with fifth or sixth character 5)

E23.2 **Diabetes insipidus**
   EXCLUDES 1   *nephrogenic diabetes insipidus (N25.1)*

E23.3 **Hypothalamic dysfunction, not elsewhere classified**
   EXCLUDES 1   *Prader-Willi syndrome (Q87.1)*
                Russell-Silver syndrome (Q87.1)

E23.6 **Other disorders of pituitary gland**
Abscess of pituitary   Adiposogenital dystrophy

E23.7 **Disorder of pituitary gland, unspecified** ▽

✓4th **E24** **Cushing's syndrome**
   EXCLUDES 1   *congenital adrenal hyperplasia (E25.0)*

E24.0 **Pituitary-dependent Cushing's disease**
Overproduction of pituitary ACTH
Pituitary-dependent hypercorticalism

E24.1 **Nelson's syndrome**

E24.2 **Drug-induced Cushing's syndrome**
Use additional code for adverse effect, if applicable, to identify
   drug (T36-T50 with fifth or sixth character 5)

E24.3 **Ectopic ACTH syndrome**

E24.4 **Alcohol-induced pseudo-Cushing's syndrome**

E24.8 **Other Cushing's syndrome**

E24.9 **Cushing's syndrome, unspecified** ▽

✓4th **E25** **Adrenogenital disorders**
   INCLUDES   adrenogenital syndromes, virilizing or feminizing, whether
                acquired or due to adrenal hyperplasia
                consequent on inborn enzyme defects in hormone synthesis
                female adrenal pseudohermaphroditism
                female heterosexual precocious pseudopuberty
                male isosexual precocious pseudopuberty
                male macrogenitosomia praecox
                male sexual precocity with adrenal hyperplasia
                male virilization (female)
   EXCLUDES 1   *indeterminate sex and pseudohermaphroditism (Q56)*
                chromosomal abnormalities (Q90-Q99)

E25.0 **Congenital adrenogenital disorders associated with enzyme
deficiency**
Congenital adrenal hyperplasia
21-Hydroxylase deficiency
Salt-losing congenital adrenal hyperplasia

E25.8 **Other adrenogenital disorders**
Idiopathic adrenogenital disorder
Use additional code for adverse effect, if applicable, to identify
   drug (T36-T50 with fifth or sixth character 5)

E25.9 **Adrenogenital disorder, unspecified** ▽
Adrenogenital syndrome NOS

✓4th **E26** **Hyperaldosteronism**

✓5th **E26.0** **Primary hyperaldosteronism**

   E26.01 **Conn's syndrome**
        Code also adrenal adenoma (D35.0-)

   E26.02 **Glucocorticoid-remediable aldosteronism**
        Familial aldosteronism type I

   E26.09 **Other primary hyperaldosteronism**
        Primary aldosteronism due to adrenal hyperplasia
        (bilateral)

E26.1 **Secondary hyperaldosteronism**

Ⓝ Newborn   Ⓟ Pediatric   Ⓜ Maternity   Ⓐ Adult   RIC RIC Dx   NCDx Noncancer Dx   PDx Primary Dx   CC RIC CC Condition   ▶◀ Revised Text   ● New Code   ▲ Revised Code Title

496   ICD-10-CM 2016

✓5th **E26.8** **Other hyperaldosteronism**

    E26.81 **Bartter's syndrome**

    E26.89 **Other hyperaldosteronism**

E26.9 **Hyperaldosteronism, unspecified** ▽

    Aldosteronism NOS   Hyperaldosteronism NOS

✓4th **E27** **Other disorders of adrenal gland**

E27.0 **Other adrenocortical overactivity**

    Overproduction of ACTH, not associated with Cushing's disease

    Premature adrenarche

    EXCLUDES 1   Cushing's syndrome (E24.-)

E27.1 **Primary adrenocortical insufficiency**

    Addison's disease

    Autoimmune adrenalitis

    EXCLUDES 1   Addison only phenotype adrenoleukodystrophy

             (E71.528)

           amyloidosis (E85.-)

           tuberculous Addison's disease (A18.7)

           Waterhouse-Friderichsen syndrome (A39.1)

E27.2 **Addisonian crisis**

    Adrenal crisis

    Adrenocortical crisis

E27.3 **Drug-induced adrenocortical insufficiency**

    Use additional code for adverse effect, if applicable, to identify drug (T36-T50 with fifth or sixth character 5)

✓5th **E27.4** **Other and unspecified adrenocortical insufficiency**

    EXCLUDES 1   adrenoleukodystrophy [Addison-Schilder] (E71.528)

           Waterhouse-Friderichsen syndrome (A39.1)

    E27.40 **Unspecified adrenocortical insufficiency** ▽

        Adrenocortical insufficiency NOS

        Hypoaldosteronism

    E27.49 **Other adrenocortical insufficiency**

        Adrenal hemorrhage

        Adrenal infarction

E27.5 **Adrenomedullary hyperfunction**

    Adrenomedullary hyperplasia

    Catecholamine hypersecretion

E27.8 **Other specified disorders of adrenal gland**

    Abnormality of cortisol-binding globulin

E27.9 **Disorder of adrenal gland, unspecified** ▽

✓4th **E28** **Ovarian dysfunction**

    EXCLUDES 1   isolated gonadotropin deficiency (E23.0)

         postprocedural ovarian failure (E89.4-)

E28.0 **Estrogen excess** ♀

    Use additional code for adverse effect, if applicable, to identify drug (T36-T50 with fifth or sixth character 5)

E28.1 **Androgen excess** ♀

    Hypersecretion of ovarian androgens

    Use additional code for adverse effect, if applicable, to identify drug (T36-T50 with fifth or sixth character 5)

E28.2 **Polycystic ovarian syndrome** ♀

    Sclerocystic ovary syndrome

    Stein-Leventhal syndrome

✓5th **E28.3** **Primary ovarian failure**

    EXCLUDES 1   pure gonadal dysgenesis (Q99.1)

         Turner's syndrome (Q96.-)

    ✓6th **E28.31** **Premature menopause**

        E28.310 **Symptomatic premature menopause** ♀

            Symptoms such as flushing, sleeplessness, headache, lack of concentration, associated with premature menopause

        E28.319 **Asymptomatic premature menopause** ♀

            Premature menopause NOS

    E28.39 **Other primary ovarian failure** ♀

        Decreased estrogen

        Resistant ovary syndrome

E28.8 **Other ovarian dysfunction** ♀

    Ovarian hyperfunction NOS

    EXCLUDES 1   postprocedural ovarian failure (E89.4-)

E28.9 **Ovarian dysfunction, unspecified** ♀▽

✓4th **E29** **Testicular dysfunction**

    EXCLUDES 1   androgen insensitivity syndrome (E34.5-)

         azoospermia or oligospermia NOS (N46.0-N46.1)

         isolated gonadotropin deficiency (E23.0)

         Klinefelter's syndrome (Q98.0-Q98.2, Q98.4)

E29.0 **Testicular hyperfunction** ♂

    Hypersecretion of testicular hormones

E29.1 **Testicular hypofunction** ♂

    Defective biosynthesis of testicular androgen NOS

    5-delta-Reductase deficiency (with male pseudohermaphroditism)

    Testicular hypogonadism NOS

    Use additional code for adverse effect, if applicable, to identify drug (T36-T50 with fifth or sixth character 5)

    EXCLUDES 1   postprocedural testicular hypofunction (E89.5)

E29.8 **Other testicular dysfunction** ♂

E29.9 **Testicular dysfunction, unspecified** ♂▽

✓4th **E30** **Disorders of puberty, not elsewhere classified**

E30.0 **Delayed puberty**

    Constitutional delay of puberty

    Delayed sexual development

E30.1 **Precocious puberty** P

    Precocious menstruation

    EXCLUDES 1   Albright (-McCune) (-Sternberg) syndrome (Q78.1)

         central precocious puberty (E22.8)

         congenital adrenal hyperplasia (E25.0)

         female heterosexual precocious pseudopuberty (E25.-)

         male isosexual precocious pseudopuberty (E25.-)

E30.8 **Other disorders of puberty** P

    Premature thelarche

E30.9 **Disorder of puberty, unspecified** ▽

✓4th **E31** **Polyglandular dysfunction**

    EXCLUDES 1   ataxia telangiectasia [Louis-Bar] (G11.3)

         dystrophia myotonica [Steinert] (G71.11)

         pseudohypoparathyroidism (E20.1)

E31.0 **Autoimmune polyglandular failure**

    Schmidt's syndrome

E31.1 **Polyglandular hyperfunction**

    EXCLUDES 1   multiple endocrine adenomatosis (E31.2-)

         multiple endocrine neoplasia (E31.2-)

✓5th **E31.2** **Multiple endocrine neoplasia [MEN] syndromes**

    Multiple endocrine adenomatosis

    Code also any associated malignancies and other conditions associated with the syndromes

    E31.20 **Multiple endocrine neoplasia [MEN] syndrome, unspecified** ▽

        Multiple endocrine adenomatosis NOS

        Multiple endocrine neoplasia [MEN] syndrome NOS

    E31.21 **Multiple endocrine neoplasia [MEN] type I**

        Wermer's syndrome

    E31.22 **Multiple endocrine neoplasia [MEN] type IIA**

        Sipple's syndrome

    E31.23 **Multiple endocrine neoplasia [MEN] type IIB**

E31.8 **Other polyglandular dysfunction**

E31.9 **Polyglandular dysfunction, unspecified** ▽

✓4th **E32** **Diseases of thymus**

    EXCLUDES 1   aplasia or hypoplasia of thymus with immunodeficiency (D82.1)

         myasthenia gravis (G70.0)

E32.0 **Persistent hyperplasia of thymus**

    Hypertrophy of thymus

E32.1 **Abscess of thymus**

E32.8 **Other diseases of thymus**

    EXCLUDES 1   aplasia or hypoplasia with immunodeficiency (D82.1)

         thymoma (D15.0)

E32.9 **Disease of thymus, unspecified** ▽

✓4th **E34** **Other endocrine disorders**

    EXCLUDES 1   pseudohypoparathyroidism (E20.1)

E34.0 **Carcinoid syndrome**

    NOTE   May be used as an additional code to identify functional activity associated with a carcinoid tumor.

E34.1 **Other hypersecretion of intestinal hormones**

E34.2 **Ectopic hormone secretion, not elsewhere classified**

    EXCLUDES 1   ectopic ACTH syndrome (E24.3)

✓ Add'l Character Required   ✓x7th Placeholder Alert   RUG IV Special Care High Dx   RUG IV Clinically Complex Dx   RUG IV Special Care Low Dx   Manifestation Code   Other Specified Code   ▽ Unspecified Code

E34.3 Short stature due to endocrine disorder
Constitutional short stature
Laron-type short stature
EXCLUDES 1 *achondroplastic short stature (Q77.4)*
hypochondroplastic short stature (Q77.4)
nutritional short stature (E45)
pituitary short stature (E23.0)
progeria (E34.8)
renal short stature (N25.0)
Russell-Silver syndrome (Q87.1)
short-limbed stature with immunodeficiency (D82.2)
short stature in specific dysmorphic syndromes— code to syndrome—see Alphabetical Index
short stature NOS (R62.52)

E34.4 Constitutional tall stature
Constitutional gigantism

✓5ᵗʰ E34.5 Androgen insensitivity syndrome

E34.50 Androgen insensitivity syndrome, unspecified ▽
Androgen insensitivity NOS

E34.51 Complete androgen insensitivity syndrome
Complete androgen insensitivity
de Quervain syndrome
Goldberg-Maxwell syndrome

E34.52 Partial androgen insensitivity syndrome
Partial androgen insensitivity
Reifenstein syndrome

E34.8 Other specified endocrine disorders
Pineal gland dysfunction
Progeria
EXCLUDES 2 *pseudohypoparathyroidism (E20.1)*

E34.9 Endocrine disorder, unspecified ▽
Endocrine disturbance NOS
Hormone disturbance NOS

E35 *Disorders of endocrine glands in diseases classified elsewhere*
Code first underlying disease, such as:
late congenital syphilis of thymus gland [Dubois disease] (A50.5)
Use additional code, if applicable, to identify:
sequelae of tuberculosis of other organs (B90.8)
EXCLUDES 1 *Echinococcus granulosus infection of thyroid gland (B67.3)*
meningococcal hemorrhagic adrenalitis (A39.1)
syphilis of endocrine gland (A52.79)
tuberculosis of adrenal gland, except calcification (A18.7)
tuberculosis of endocrine gland NEC (A18.82)
tuberculosis of thyroid gland (A18.81)
Waterhouse-Friderichsen syndrome (A39.1)

✓4ᵗʰ E36 Intraoperative complications of endocrine system
EXCLUDES 2 *postprocedural endocrine and metabolic complications and disorders, not elsewhere classified (E89.-)*

✓5ᵗʰ E36.0 Intraoperative hemorrhage and hematoma of an endocrine system organ or structure complicating a procedure
EXCLUDES 1 *intraoperative hemorrhage and hematoma of an endocrine system organ or structure due to accidental puncture or laceration during a procedure (E36.1-)*

E36.01 Intraoperative hemorrhage and hematoma of an endocrine system organ or structure complicating an endocrine system procedure

E36.02 Intraoperative hemorrhage and hematoma of an endocrine system organ or structure complicating other procedure

✓5ᵗʰ E36.1 Accidental puncture and laceration of an endocrine system organ or structure during a procedure

E36.11 Accidental puncture and laceration of an endocrine system organ or structure during an endocrine system procedure

E36.12 Accidental puncture and laceration of an endocrine system organ or structure during other procedure

E36.8 Other intraoperative complications of endocrine system
Use additional code, if applicable, to further specify disorder

Malnutrition (E40-E46)

EXCLUDES 1 *intestinal malabsorption (K90.-)*
sequelae of protein-calorie malnutrition (E64.0)
EXCLUDES 2 *nutritional anemias (D50-D53)*
starvation (T73.0)

E40 Kwashiorkor
Severe malnutrition with nutritional edema with dyspigmentation of skin and hair
EXCLUDES 1 *marasmic kwashiorkor (E42)*

E41 Nutritional marasmus
Severe malnutrition with marasmus
EXCLUDES 1 *marasmic kwashiorkor (E42)*

E42 Marasmic kwashiorkor
Intermediate form severe protein-calorie malnutrition
Severe protein-calorie malnutrition with signs of both kwashiorkor and marasmus

E43 Unspecified severe protein-calorie malnutrition ▽
Starvation edema

✓4ᵗʰ E44 Protein-calorie malnutrition of moderate and mild degree

E44.0 Moderate protein-calorie malnutrition

E44.1 Mild protein-calorie malnutrition

E45 Retarded development following protein-calorie malnutrition
Nutritional short stature
Nutritional stunting
Physical retardation due to malnutrition

E46 Unspecified protein-calorie malnutrition ▽
Malnutrition NOS
Protein-calorie imbalance NOS
EXCLUDES 1 *nutritional deficiency NOS (E63.9)*

Other nutritional deficiencies (E50-E64)

EXCLUDES 2 *nutritional anemias (D50-D53)*

✓4ᵗʰ E50 Vitamin A deficiency
EXCLUDES 1 *sequelae of vitamin A deficiency (E64.1)*

E50.0 Vitamin A deficiency with conjunctival xerosis

E50.1 Vitamin A deficiency with Bitot's spot and conjunctival xerosis
Bitot's spot in the young child

E50.2 Vitamin A deficiency with corneal xerosis

E50.3 Vitamin A deficiency with corneal ulceration and xerosis

E50.4 Vitamin A deficiency with keratomalacia

E50.5 Vitamin A deficiency with night blindness

E50.6 Vitamin A deficiency with xerophthalmic scars of cornea

E50.7 Other ocular manifestations of vitamin A deficiency
Xerophthalmia NOS

E50.8 Other manifestations of vitamin A deficiency
Follicular keratosis
Xeroderma

E50.9 Vitamin A deficiency, unspecified ▽
Hypovitaminosis A NOS

✓4ᵗʰ E51 Thiamine deficiency
EXCLUDES 1 *sequelae of thiamine deficiency (E64.8)*

✓5ᵗʰ E51.1 Beriberi

E51.11 Dry beriberi
Beriberi NOS
Beriberi with polyneuropathy

E51.12 Wet beriberi
Beriberi with cardiovascular manifestations
Cardiovascular beriberi
Shoshin disease

E51.2 Wernicke's encephalopathy

E51.8 Other manifestations of thiamine deficiency

E51.9 Thiamine deficiency, unspecified ▽

E52 Niacin deficiency [pellagra]
Niacin (-tryptophan) deficiency
Nicotinamide deficiency
Pellagra (alcoholic)
EXCLUDES 1 *sequelae of niacin deficiency (E64.8)*

✓4ᵗʰ E53 Deficiency of other B group vitamins
EXCLUDES 1 *sequelae of vitamin B deficiency (E64.8)*

E53.0 Riboflavin deficiency
Ariboflavinosis
Vitamin B2 deficiency

E53.1 Pyridoxine deficiency
Vitamin B6 deficiency
EXCLUDES 1 *pyridoxine-responsive sideroblastic anemia (D64.3)*

E53.8 Deficiency of other specified B group vitamins
Biotin deficiency   Folic acid deficiency
Cyanocobalamin deficiency   Pantothenic acid deficiency
Folate deficiency   Vitamin B12 deficiency
EXCLUDES 1 *folate deficiency anemia (D52.-)*
vitamin B12 deficiency anemia (D51.-)

E53.9 Vitamin B deficiency, unspecified ▽

Ⓝ Newborn   Ⓟ Pediatric   Ⓜ Maternity   Ⓐ Adult   **RIC** RIC Dx   **NC Dx** Noncancer Dx   **PDx** Primary Dx   **CC** RIC CC Condition   ►◄ Revised Text   ● New Code   ▲ Revised Code Title

498

ICD-10-CM 2016

E54   **Ascorbic acid** deficiency
     Deficiency of vitamin C
     Scurvy
     EXCLUDES 1   scorbutic anemia (D53.2)
          sequelae of vitamin C deficiency (E64.2)

✓4ᵗʰ **E55**   **Vitamin D** deficiency
     EXCLUDES 1   adult osteomalacia (M83.-)
          osteoporosis (M80.-)
          sequelae of rickets (E64.3)

     E55.0   **Rickets,** active
          Infantile osteomalacia
          Juvenile osteomalacia
          EXCLUDES 1   celiac rickets (K90.0)
                 Crohn's rickets (K50.-)
                 hereditary vitamin D-dependent rickets (E83.32)
                 inactive rickets (E64.3)
                 renal rickets (N25.0)
                 sequelae of rickets (E64.3)
                 vitamin D-resistant rickets (E83.31)

     E55.9   **Vitamin D deficiency,** unspecified   ▽
          Avitaminosis D

✓4ᵗʰ **E56**   **Other vitamin** deficiencies
     EXCLUDES 1   sequelae of other vitamin deficiencies (E64.8)

     E56.0   **Deficiency of vitamin E**
     E56.1   **Deficiency of vitamin K**
          EXCLUDES 1   deficiency of coagulation factor due to vitamin K
                 deficiency (D68.4)
                 vitamin K deficiency of newborn (P53)

     E56.8   **Deficiency of other vitamins**
     E56.9   **Vitamin deficiency,** unspecified   ▽

E58   **Dietary calcium** deficiency
     EXCLUDES 1   disorders of calcium metabolism (E83.5-)
          sequelae of calcium deficiency (E64.8)

E59   **Dietary selenium** deficiency
     Keshan disease
     EXCLUDES 1   sequelae of selenium deficiency (E64.8)

E60   **Dietary zinc** deficiency

✓4ᵗʰ **E61**   **Deficiency of other nutrient elements**
     Use additional code for adverse effect, if applicable, to identify drug
          (T36-T50 with fifth or sixth character 5)
     EXCLUDES 1   disorders of mineral metabolism (E83.-)
          iodine deficiency related thyroid disorders (E00-E02)
          sequelae of malnutrition and other nutritional deficiencies
              (E64.-)

     E61.0   **Copper deficiency**
     E61.1   **Iron deficiency**
          EXCLUDES 1   iron deficiency anemia (D50.-)

     E61.2   **Magnesium deficiency**
     E61.3   **Manganese deficiency**
     E61.4   **Chromium deficiency**
     E61.5   **Molybdenum deficiency**
     E61.6   **Vanadium deficiency**
     E61.7   **Deficiency of multiple nutrient elements**
     E61.8   **Deficiency of other specified nutrient elements**
     E61.9   **Deficiency of nutrient element, unspecified**   ▽

✓4ᵗʰ **E63**   **Other nutritional deficiencies**
     EXCLUDES 1   dehydration (E86.0)
          failure to thrive, adult (R62.7)
          failure to thrive, child (R62.51)
          feeding problems in newborn (P92.-)
          sequelae of malnutrition and other nutritional deficiencies
              (E64.-)

     E63.0   **Essential fatty acid [EFA] deficiency**
     E63.1   **Imbalance of constituents of food intake**
     E63.8   **Other specified nutritional deficiencies**
     E63.9   **Nutritional deficiency, unspecified**   ▽

✓4ᵗʰ **E64**   **Sequelae of malnutrition and other nutritional deficiencies**
     NOTE   This category is to be used to indicate conditions in
          categories E43, E44, E46, E50-E63 as the cause of sequelae,
          which are themselves classified elsewhere. The 'sequelae'
          include conditions specified as such; they also include the
          late effects of diseases classifiable to the above categories if
          the disease itself is no longer present.
     Code first condition resulting from (sequela) of malnutrition and other
          nutritional deficiencies

     E64.0   **Sequelae of protein-calorie malnutrition**
          EXCLUDES 2   retarded development following protein-calorie
                 malnutrition (E45)

     E64.1   **Sequelae of vitamin A deficiency**
     E64.2   **Sequelae of vitamin C deficiency**
     E64.3   **Sequelae of rickets**
     E64.8   **Sequelae of other nutritional deficiencies**
     E64.9   **Sequelae of unspecified nutritional deficiency**   ▽

Overweight, obesity and other hyperalimentation (E65-E68)

E65   **Localized adiposity**
     Fat pad

✓4ᵗʰ **E66**   **Overweight and obesity**
     Code first obesity complicating pregnancy, childbirth and the
          puerperium, if applicable (O99.21-)
     Use additional code to identify body mass index (BMI), if known (Z68.-)
     EXCLUDES 1   adiposogenital dystrophy (E23.6)
          lipomatosis NOS (E88.2)
          lipomatosis dolorosa [Dercum] (E88.2)
          Prader-Willi syndrome (Q87.1)

     ✓5ᵗʰ **E66.0**   **Obesity due to excess calories**
          E66.01   **Morbid (severe) obesity due to excess calories**   CC
              EXCLUDES 1   morbid (severe) obesity with alveolar
                    hypoventilation (E66.2)

          E66.09   **Other obesity due to excess calories**

     E66.1   **Drug-induced obesity**
          Use additional code for adverse effect, if applicable, to identify
          drug (T36-T50 with fifth or sixth character 5)

     E66.2   **Morbid (severe) obesity with alveolar hypoventilation**
          Pickwickian syndrome

     E66.3   **Overweight**
     E66.8   **Other obesity**
     E66.9   **Obesity, unspecified**   ▽
          Obesity NOS

✓4ᵗʰ **E67**   **Other hyperalimentation**
     EXCLUDES 1   hyperalimentation NOS (R63.2)
          sequelae of hyperalimentation (E68)

     E67.0   **Hypervitaminosis A**
     E67.1   **Hypercarotinemia**
     E67.2   **Megavitamin-B6 syndrome**
     E67.3   **Hypervitaminosis D**
     E67.8   **Other specified hyperalimentation**

E68   **Sequelae of hyperalimentation**
     Code first condition resulting from (sequela) of hyperalimentation

Metabolic disorders (E70-E88)

     EXCLUDES 1   androgen insensitivity syndrome (E34.5-)
          congenital adrenal hyperplasia (E25.0)
          Ehlers-Danlos syndrome (Q79.6)
          hemolytic anemias attributable to enzyme disorders (D55.-)
          Marfan's syndrome (Q87.4)
          5-alpha-reductase deficiency (E29.1)

✓4ᵗʰ **E70**   **Disorders of aromatic amino-acid metabolism**
     E70.0   **Classical phenylketonuria**
     E70.1   **Other hyperphenylalaninemias**
     ✓5ᵗʰ **E70.2**   **Disorders of tyrosine metabolism**
          EXCLUDES 1   transitory tyrosinemia of newborn (P74.5)
          E70.20   **Disorder of tyrosine metabolism, unspecified**   ▽
          E70.21   **Tyrosinemia**
              Hypertyrosinemia
          E70.29   **Other disorders of tyrosine metabolism**
              Alkaptonuria   Ochronosis

     ✓5ᵗʰ **E70.3**   **Albinism**
          E70.30   **Albinism, unspecified**   ▽
          ✓6ᵗʰ **E70.31**   **Ocular albinism**
              E70.310   **X-linked ocular albinism**
              E70.311   **Autosomal recessive ocular albinism**
              E70.318   **Other ocular albinism**
              E70.319   **Ocular albinism, unspecified**   ▽

☑ Add'l Character Required   ✓ˣ⁷ᵗʰ Placeholder Alert   RUG IV Special Care High Dx   RUG IV Clinically Complex Dx   RUG IV Special Care Low Dx   Manifestation Code   Other Specified Code   ▽ Unspecified Code

✓6th **E70.32** Oculocutaneous albinism
> EXCLUDES 1   Chediak-Higashi syndrome (E70.330)
> Hermansky-Pudlak syndrome (E70.331)

E70.320 Tyrosinase negative oculocutaneous albinism
Albinism I
Oculocutaneous albinism ty-neg

E70.321 Tyrosinase positive oculocutaneous albinism
Albinism II
Oculocutaneous albinism ty-pos

E70.328 Other oculocutaneous albinism
Cross syndrome

E70.329 Oculocutaneous albinism, unspecified ▽

✓6th **E70.33** Albinism with hematologic abnormality

E70.330 Chediak-Higashi syndrome

E70.331 Hermansky-Pudlak syndrome

E70.338 Other albinism with hematologic abnormality

E70.339 Albinism with hematologic abnormality, unspecified ▽

E70.39 Other specified albinism
Piebaldism

✓5th **E70.4** Disorders of histidine metabolism

E70.40 Disorders of histidine metabolism, unspecified ▽

E70.41 Histidinemia

E70.49 Other disorders of histidine metabolism

E70.5 Disorders of tryptophan metabolism

E70.8 Other disorders of aromatic amino-acid metabolism

E70.9 Disorder of aromatic amino-acid metabolism, unspecified ▽

✓4th **E71** Disorders of branched-chain amino-acid metabolism and fatty-acid metabolism

E71.0 Maple-syrup-urine disease

✓5th **E71.1** Other disorders of branched-chain amino-acid metabolism

✓6th **E71.11** Branched-chain organic acidurias

E71.110 Isovaleric acidemia

E71.111 3-methylglutaconic aciduria

E71.118 Other branched-chain organic acidurias

✓6th **E71.12** Disorders of propionate metabolism

E71.120 Methylmalonic acidemia

E71.121 Propionic acidemia

E71.128 Other disorders of propionate metabolism

E71.19 Other disorders of branched-chain amino-acid metabolism
Hyperleucine-isoleucinemia
Hypervalinemia

E71.2 Disorder of branched-chain amino-acid metabolism, unspecified ▽

✓5th **E71.3** Disorders of fatty-acid metabolism
> EXCLUDES 1   peroxisomal disorders (E71.5)
> Refsum's disease (G60.1)
> Schilder's disease (G37.0)
> EXCLUDES 2   carnitine deficiency due to inborn error of metabolism (E71.42)

E71.30 Disorder of fatty-acid metabolism, unspecified ▽

✓6th **E71.31** Disorders of fatty-acid oxidation

E71.310 Long chain/very long chain acyl CoA dehydrogenase deficiency
LCAD   VLCAD

E71.311 Medium chain acyl CoA dehydrogenase deficiency
MCAD

E71.312 Short chain acyl CoA dehydrogenase deficiency
SCAD

E71.313 Glutaric aciduria type II
Glutaric aciduria type II A
Glutaric aciduria type II B
Glutaric aciduria type II C
> EXCLUDES 1   glutaric aciduria (type 1) NOS (E72.3)

E71.314 Muscle carnitine palmitoyltransferase deficiency

E71.318 Other disorders of fatty-acid oxidation

E71.32 Disorders of ketone metabolism

E71.39 Other disorders of fatty-acid metabolism

✓5th **E71.4** Disorders of carnitine metabolism
> EXCLUDES 1   muscle carnitine palmitoyltransferase deficiency (E71.314)

E71.40 Disorder of carnitine metabolism, unspecified ▽

E71.41 Primary carnitine deficiency

E71.42 Carnitine deficiency due to inborn errors of metabolism
Code also associated inborn error or metabolism

E71.43 Iatrogenic carnitine deficiency
Carnitine deficiency due to hemodialysis
Carnitine deficiency due to Valproic acid therapy

✓6th **E71.44** Other secondary carnitine deficiency

E71.440 Ruvalcaba-Myhre-Smith syndrome

E71.448 Other secondary carnitine deficiency

✓5th **E71.5** Peroxisomal disorders
> EXCLUDES 1   Schilder's disease (G37.0)

E71.50 Peroxisomal disorder, unspecified ▽

✓6th **E71.51** Disorders of peroxisome biogenesis
Group 1 peroxisomal disorders
> EXCLUDES 1   Refsum's disease (G60.1)

E71.510 Zellweger syndrome

E71.511 Neonatal adrenoleukodystrophy   N
> EXCLUDES 1   X-linked adrenoleuko- dystrophy (E71.52-)

E71.518 Other disorders of peroxisome biogenesis

✓6th **E71.52** X-linked adrenoleukodystrophy

E71.520 Childhood cerebral X-linked adrenoleukodystrophy

E71.521 Adolescent X-linked adrenoleukodystrophy

E71.522 Adrenomyeloneuropathy

E71.528 Other X-linked adrenoleukodystrophy
Addison only phenotype adrenoleukodystrophy
Addison-Schilder adrenoleukodystrophy

E71.529 X-linked adrenoleukodystrophy, unspecified type ▽

E71.53 Other group 2 peroxisomal disorders

✓6th **E71.54** Other peroxisomal disorders

E71.540 Rhizomelic chondrodysplasia punctata
> EXCLUDES 1   chondrodysplasia punctata NOS (Q77.3)

E71.541 Zellweger-like syndrome

E71.542 Other group 3 peroxisomal disorders

E71.548 Other peroxisomal disorders

✓4th **E72** Other disorders of amino-acid metabolism
> EXCLUDES 1   disorders of:
> aromatic amino-acid metabolism (E70.-)
> branched-chain amino-acid metabolism (E71.0-E71.2)
> fatty-acid metabolism (E71.3)
> purine and pyrimidine metabolism (E79.-)
> gout (M1A.-, M10.-)

✓5th **E72.0** Disorders of amino-acid transport
> EXCLUDES 1   disorders of tryptophan metabolism (E70.5)

E72.00 Disorders of amino-acid transport, unspecified ▽

E72.01 Cystinuria

E72.02 Hartnup's disease

E72.03 Lowe's syndrome
Use additional code for associated glaucoma (H42)

E72.04 Cystinosis
Fanconi (-de Toni) (-Debré) syndrome with cystinosis
> EXCLUDES 1   Fanconi (-de Toni) (-Debré) syndrome without cystinosis (E72.09)

E72.09 Other disorders of amino-acid transport
Fanconi (-de Toni) (-Debré) syndrome, unspecified

✓5th **E72.1** Disorders of sulfur-bearing amino-acid metabolism
> EXCLUDES 1   cystinosis (E72.04)
> cystinuria (E72.01)
> transcobalamin II deficiency (D51.2)

E72.10 Disorders of sulfur-bearing amino-acid metabolism, unspecified ▽

E72.11 Homocystinuria
Cystathionine synthase deficiency

E72.12 Methylenetetrahydrofolate reductase deficiency

N Newborn   P Pediatric   M Maternity   A Adult   RIC RIC Dx   NC Dx Noncancer Dx   PDx Primary Dx   CC RIC CC Condition   ►◄ Revised Text   ● New Code   ▲ Revised Code Title

500   ICD-10-CM 2016

E72.19　Other disorders of sulfur-bearing amino-acid metabolism
　　　Cystathioninuria
　　　Methioninemia
　　　Sulfite oxidase deficiency

✓5ᵗʰ **E72.2　Disorders of urea cycle metabolism**
　　EXCLUDES 1　*disorders of ornithine metabolism (E72.4)*

E72.20　Disorder of urea cycle metabolism, unspecified ▽
　　　Hyperammonemia
　　　EXCLUDES 1　*hyperammonemia- hyperornithinemia-homocitrullinemia syndrome (E72.4)*
　　　　　　transient hyperammonemia of newborn (P74.6)

E72.21　Argininemia

E72.22　Arginosuccinic aciduria

E72.23　Citrullinemia

E72.29　Other disorders of urea cycle metabolism

E72.3　Disorders of lysine and hydroxylysine metabolism
　　　Glutaric aciduria NOS　　　Hydroxylysinemia
　　　Glutaric aciduria (type I)　Hyperlysinemia
　　EXCLUDES 1　*glutaric aciduria type II (E71.313)*
　　　　　　Refsum's disease (G60.1)
　　　　　　Zellweger syndrome (E71.510)

E72.4　Disorders of ornithine metabolism
　　　Hyperammonemia-hyperornithinemia-homocitrullinemia syndrome
　　　Ornithinemia (types I, II)
　　　Ornithine transcarbamylase deficiency
　　EXCLUDES 1　*hereditary choroidal dystrophy (H31.2-)*

✓5ᵗʰ **E72.5　Disorders of glycine metabolism**

E72.50　Disorder of glycine metabolism, unspecified ▽

E72.51　Non-ketotic hyperglycinemia

E72.52　Trimethylaminuria

E72.53　Hyperoxaluria
　　　Oxalosis
　　　Oxaluria

E72.59　Other disorders of glycine metabolism
　　　D-glycericacidemia
　　　Hyperhydroxyprolinemia
　　　Hyperprolinemia (types I, II)
　　　Sarcosinemia

E72.8　Other specified disorders of amino-acid metabolism
　　　Disorders of beta-amino-acid metabolism
　　　Disorders of gamma-glutamyl cycle

E72.9　Disorder of amino-acid metabolism, unspecified ▽

✓4ᵗʰ **E73　Lactose intolerance**

E73.0　Congenital lactase deficiency

E73.1　Secondary lactase deficiency

E73.8　Other lactose intolerance

E73.9　Lactose intolerance, unspecified ▽

✓4ᵗʰ **E74　Other disorders of carbohydrate metabolism**
　　EXCLUDES 1　*diabetes mellitus (E08-E13)*
　　　　　　hypoglycemia NOS (E16.2)
　　　　　　increased secretion of glucagon (E16.3)
　　　　　　mucopolysaccharidosis (E76.0-E76.3)

✓5ᵗʰ **E74.0　Glycogen storage disease**

E74.00　Glycogen storage disease, unspecified ▽

E74.01　von Gierke disease
　　　Type I glycogen storage disease

E74.02　Pompe disease
　　　Cardiac glycogenosis
　　　Type II glycogen storage disease

E74.03　Cori disease
　　　Forbes disease
　　　Type III glycogen storage disease

E74.04　McArdle disease
　　　Type V glycogen storage disease

E74.09　Other glycogen storage disease
　　　Andersen disease
　　　Hers disease
　　　Tauri disease
　　　Glycogen storage disease, types 0, IV, VI-XI
　　　Liver phosphorylase deficiency
　　　Muscle phosphofructokinase deficiency

✓5ᵗʰ **E74.1　Disorders of fructose metabolism**
　　EXCLUDES 1　*muscle phosphofructokinase deficiency (E74.09)*

E74.10　Disorder of fructose metabolism, unspecified ▽

E74.11　Essential fructosuria
　　　Fructokinase deficiency

E74.12　Hereditary fructose intolerance
　　　Fructosemia

E74.19　Other disorders of fructose metabolism
　　　Fructose-1, 6-diphosphatase deficiency

✓5ᵗʰ **E74.2　Disorders of galactose metabolism**

E74.20　Disorders of galactose metabolism, unspecified ▽

E74.21　Galactosemia

E74.29　Other disorders of galactose metabolism
　　　Galactokinase deficiency

✓5ᵗʰ **E74.3　Other disorders of intestinal carbohydrate absorption**
　　EXCLUDES 2　*lactose intolerance (E73.-)*

E74.31　Sucrase-isomaltase deficiency

E74.39　Other disorders of intestinal carbohydrate absorption
　　　Disorder of intestinal carbohydrate absorption NOS
　　　Glucose-galactose malabsorption
　　　Sucrase deficiency

E74.4　Disorders of pyruvate metabolism and gluconeogenesis
　　　Deficiency of phosphoenolpyruvate carboxykinase
　　　Deficiency of pyruvate carboxylase
　　　Deficiency of pyruvate dehydrogenase
　　EXCLUDES 1　*disorders of pyruvate metabolism and gluconeogenesis with anemia (D55.-)*
　　　　　　Leigh's syndrome (G31.82)

E74.8　Other specified disorders of carbohydrate metabolism
　　　Essential pentosuria
　　　Renal glycosuria

E74.9　Disorder of carbohydrate metabolism, unspecified ▽

✓4ᵗʰ **E75　Disorders of sphingolipid metabolism and other lipid storage disorders**
　　EXCLUDES 1　*mucolipidosis, types I-III (E77.0-E77.1)*
　　　　　　Refsum's disease (G60.1)

✓5ᵗʰ **E75.0　GM2 gangliosidosis**

E75.00　GM2 gangliosidosis, unspecified ▽

E75.01　Sandhoff disease

E75.02　Tay-Sachs disease

E75.09　Other GM2 gangliosidosis
　　　Adult GM2 gangliosidosis
　　　Juvenile GM2 gangliosidosis

✓5ᵗʰ **E75.1　Other and unspecified gangliosidosis**

E75.10　Unspecified gangliosidosis ▽
　　　Gangliosidosis NOS

E75.11　Mucolipidosis IV

E75.19　Other gangliosidosis
　　　GM1 gangliosidosis　　　GM3 gangliosidosis

✓5ᵗʰ **E75.2　Other sphingolipidosis**
　　EXCLUDES 1　*adrenoleukodystrophy [Addison-Schilder] (E71.528)*

E75.21　Fabry (-Anderson) disease

E75.22　Gaucher disease

E75.23　Krabbe disease

✓6ᵗʰ **E75.24　Niemann-Pick disease**

E75.240　Niemann-Pick disease type A

E75.241　Niemann-Pick disease type B

E75.242　Niemann-Pick disease type C

E75.243　Niemann-Pick disease type D

E75.248　Other Niemann-Pick disease

E75.249　Niemann-Pick disease, unspecified ▽

E75.25　Metachromatic leukodystrophy

E75.29　Other sphingolipidosis
　　　Farber's syndrome
　　　Sulfatase deficiency
　　　Sulfatide lipidosis

E75.3　Sphingolipidosis, unspecified ▽

E75.4　Neuronal ceroid lipofuscinosis
　　　Batten disease　　　　　　Kufs disease
　　　Bielschowsky-Jansky disease　Spielmeyer-Vogt disease

E75.5　Other lipid storage disorders
　　　Cerebrotendinous cholesterosis [van Bogaert-Scherer-Epstein]
　　　Wolman's disease

E75.6　Lipid storage disorder, unspecified ▽

✓4ᵗʰ **E76　Disorders of glycosaminoglycan metabolism**

✓5ᵗʰ **E76.0　Mucopolysaccharidosis, type I**

E76.01　Hurler's syndrome

E76.02   Hurler-Scheie **syndrome**

E76.03   Scheie's **syndrome**

E76.1   **Mucopolysaccharidosis, type II**
Hunter's syndrome

✓5th **E76.2**   Other **mucopolysaccharidoses**

   ✓6th **E76.21**   Morquio **mucopolysaccharidoses**

     E76.210   **Morquio A mucopolysaccharidoses**
Classic Morquio syndrome
Morquio syndrome A
Mucopolysaccharidosis, type IVA

     E76.211   **Morquio B mucopolysaccharidoses**
Morquio-like mucopolysaccharidoses
Morquio-like syndrome
Morquio syndrome B
Mucopolysaccharidosis, type IVB

     E76.219   **Morquio mucopolysaccharidoses, unspecified** ▽
Morquio syndrome
Mucopolysaccharidosis, type IV

   E76.22   Sanfilippo **mucopolysaccharidoses**
Mucopolysaccharidosis, type III (A) (B) (C) (D)
Sanfilippo A syndrome
Sanfilippo B syndrome
Sanfilippo C syndrome
Sanfilippo D syndrome

   E76.29   **Other mucopolysaccharidoses**
beta-Glucuronidase deficiency
Maroteaux-Lamy (mild) (severe) syndrome
Mucopolysaccharidosis, types VI, VII

E76.3   **Mucopolysaccharidosis, unspecified** ▽

E76.8   **Other disorders of glucosaminoglycan metabolism**

E76.9   **Glucosaminoglycan metabolism disorder, unspecified** ▽

✓4th **E77**   **Disorders of** glycoprotein **metabolism**

E77.0   Defects in post-translational modification of lysosomal enzymes
Mucolipidosis II [I-cell disease]
Mucolipidosis III [pseudo-Hurler polydystrophy]

E77.1   Defects in glycoprotein degradation
Aspartylglucosaminuria
Fucosidosis
Mannosidosis
Sialidosis [mucolipidosis I]

E77.8   **Other disorders of glycoprotein metabolism**

E77.9   **Disorder of glycoprotein metabolism, unspecified** ▽

✓4th **E78**   **Disorders of** lipoprotein **metabolism and other lipidemias**
EXCLUDES 1   *sphingolipidosis (E75.0-E75.3)*

E78.0   **Pure hypercholesterolemia**
Familial hypercholesterolemia
Fredrickson's hyperlipoproteinemia, type IIa
Hyperbetalipoproteinemia
Hyperlipidemia, Group A
Low-density-lipoprotein-type [LDL] hyperlipoproteinemia

E78.1   **Pure hyperglyceridemia**
Elevated fasting triglycerides
Endogenous hyperglyceridemia
Fredrickson's hyperlipoproteinemia, type IV
Hyperlipidemia, group B
Hyperprebetalipoproteinemia
Very-low-density-lipoprotein-type [VLDL] hyperlipoproteinemia

E78.2   **Mixed hyperlipidemia**
Broad- or floating-betalipoproteinemia
Combined hyperlipidemia NOS
Elevated cholesterol with elevated triglycerides NEC
Fredrickson's hyperlipoproteinemia, type IIb or III
Hyperbetalipoproteinemia with prebetalipoproteinemia
Hypercholesteremia with endogenous hyperglyceridemia
Hyperlipidemia, group C
Tubo-eruptive xanthoma
Xanthoma tuberosum
   EXCLUDES 1   *cerebrotendinous cholesterosis [van Bogaert-Scherer-Epstein] (E75.5)*
     familial combined hyperlipidemia (E78.4)

E78.3   **Hyperchylomicronemia**
Chylomicron retention disease
Fredrickson's hyperlipoproteinemia, type I or V
Hyperlipidemia, group D
Mixed hyperglyceridemia

E78.4   **Other hyperlipidemia**
Familial combined hyperlipidemia

E78.5   **Hyperlipidemia, unspecified** ▽

E78.6   **Lipoprotein deficiency**
Abetalipoproteinemia
Depressed HDL cholesterol
High-density lipoprotein deficiency
Hypoalphalipoproteinemia
Hypobetalipoproteinemia (familial)
Lecithin cholesterol acyltransferase deficiency
Tangier disease

✓5th **E78.7**   **Disorders of** bile acid and cholesterol **metabolism**
EXCLUDES 1   *Niemann-Pick disease type C (E75.242)*

   E78.70   **Disorder of bile acid and cholesterol metabolism, unspecified** ▽

   E78.71   **Barth syndrome**

   E78.72   **Smith-Lemli-Opitz syndrome**

   E78.79   **Other disorders of bile acid and cholesterol metabolism**

✓5th **E78.8**   **Other disorders of lipoprotein metabolism**

   E78.81   **Lipoid dermatoarthritis**

   E78.89   **Other lipoprotein metabolism disorders**

E78.9   **Disorder of lipoprotein metabolism, unspecified** ▽

✓4th **E79**   **Disorders of** purine and pyrimidine **metabolism**
EXCLUDES 1   *Ataxia-telangiectasia (Q87.1)*
   Bloom's syndrome (Q82.8)
   Cockayne's syndrome (Q87.1)
   calculus of kidney (N20.0)
   combined immunodeficiency disorders (D81.-)
   Fanconi's anemia (D61.09)
   gout (M1A.-, M10.-)
   orotaciduric anemia (D53.0)
   progeria (E34.8)
   Werner's syndrome (E34.8)
   xeroderma pigmentosum (Q82.1)

E79.0   **Hyperuricemia without signs of inflammatory arthritis and tophaceous disease**
Asymptomatic hyperuricemia

E79.1   **Lesch-Nyhan syndrome**
HGPRT deficiency

E79.2   **Myoadenylate deaminase deficiency**

E79.8   **Other disorders of purine and pyrimidine metabolism**
Hereditary xanthinuria

E79.9   **Disorder of purine and pyrimidine metabolism, unspecified** ▽

✓4th **E80**   **Disorders of** porphyrin and bilirubin **metabolism**
INCLUDES   defects of catalase and peroxidase

E80.0   **Hereditary erythropoietic porphyria**
Congenital erythropoietic porphyria
Erythropoietic protoporphyria

E80.1   **Porphyria cutanea tarda**

✓5th **E80.2**   **Other and unspecified porphyria**

   E80.20   **Unspecified porphyria** ▽
Porphyria NOS

   E80.21   Acute intermittent **(hepatic) porphyria**

   E80.29   **Other porphyria**
Hereditary coproporphyria

E80.3   **Defects of catalase and peroxidase**
Acatalasia [Takahara]

E80.4   **Gilbert syndrome**

E80.5   **Crigler-Najjar syndrome**

E80.6   **Other disorders of bilirubin metabolism**
Dubin-Johnson syndrome
Rotor's syndrome

E80.7   **Disorder of bilirubin metabolism, unspecified** ▽

✓4th **E83**   **Disorders of** mineral **metabolism**
EXCLUDES 1   *dietary mineral deficiency (E58-E61)*
   parathyroid disorders (E20-E21)
   vitamin D deficiency (E55.-)

✓5th **E83.0**   **Disorders of** copper **metabolism**

   E83.00   **Disorder of copper metabolism, unspecified** ▽

   E83.01   **Wilson's disease**
Code also associated Kayser Fleischer ring (H18.04-)

   E83.09   **Other disorders of copper metabolism**
Menkes' (kinky hair) (steely hair) disease

✓5th **E83.1**   **Disorders of** iron **metabolism**
EXCLUDES 1   *iron deficiency anemia (D50.-)*
   sideroblastic anemia (D64.0-D64.3)

   E83.10   **Disorder of iron metabolism, unspecified** ▽

N Newborn   P Pediatric   M Maternity   A Adult   RIC RIC Dx   NC-Dx Noncancer Dx   PDx Primary Dx   CC RIC CC Condition   ▶◀ Revised Text   ● New Code   ▲ Revised Code Title

502   ICD-10-CM 2016

√6th **E83.11 Hemochromatosis**

     E83.110 Hereditary hemochromatosis
         Bronzed diabetes
         Pigmentary cirrhosis (of liver)
         Primary (hereditary) hemochromatosis

     E83.111 Hemochromatosis due to repeated red blood cell transfusions
         Iron overload due to repeated red blood cell transfusions
         Transfusion (red blood cell) associated hemochromatosis

     E83.118 Other hemochromatosis

     E83.119 Hemochromatosis, unspecified ▽

E83.19 Other disorders of iron metabolism
     Use additional code, if applicable, for idiopathic pulmonary hemosiderosis (J84.03)

E83.2 Disorders of zinc metabolism
     Acrodermatitis enteropathica

√5th **E83.3 Disorders of phosphorus metabolism and phosphatases**
     EXCLUDES 1 *adult osteomalacia (M83.-)*
                 osteoporosis (M80.-)

     E83.30 Disorder of phosphorus metabolism, unspecified ▽

     E83.31 Familial hypophosphatemia
         Vitamin D-resistant osteomalacia
         Vitamin D-resistant rickets
         EXCLUDES 1 *vitamin D-deficiency rickets (E55.0)*

     E83.32 Hereditary vitamin D-dependent rickets (type 1) (type 2)
         25-hydroxyvitamin D 1-alpha-hydroxylase deficiency
         Pseudovitamin D deficiency
         Vitamin D receptor defect

     E83.39 Other disorders of phosphorus metabolism
         Acid phosphatase deficiency
         Hypophosphatasia

√5th **E83.4 Disorders of magnesium metabolism**

     E83.40 Disorders of magnesium metabolism, unspecified ▽

     E83.41 Hypermagnesemia

     E83.42 Hypomagnesemia

     E83.49 Other disorders of magnesium metabolism

√5th **E83.5 Disorders of calcium metabolism**
     EXCLUDES 1 *chondrocalcinosis (M11.1-M11.2)*
                 hungry bone syndrome (E83.81)
                 hyperparathyroidism (E21.0-E21.3)

     E83.50 Unspecified disorder of calcium metabolism ▽

     E83.51 Hypocalcemia

     E83.52 Hypercalcemia
         Familial hypocalciuric hypercalcemia

     E83.59 Other disorders of calcium metabolism
         Idiopathic hypercalciuria

√5th **E83.8 Other disorders of mineral metabolism**

     E83.81 Hungry bone syndrome

     E83.89 Other disorders of mineral metabolism

E83.9 Disorder of mineral metabolism, unspecified ▽

√4th **E84 Cystic fibrosis**
     INCLUDES mucoviscidosis

E84.0 Cystic fibrosis with pulmonary manifestations CC
     Use additional code to identify any infectious organism present, such as:
     Pseudomonas (B96.5)
     RIC Excl: 15 Pulmonary

√5th **E84.1 Cystic fibrosis with intestinal manifestations**

     E84.11 Meconium ileus in cystic fibrosis CC N
         EXCLUDES 1 *meconium ileus not due to cystic fibrosis (P76.0)*
         RIC Excl: 15 Pulmonary

     E84.19 Cystic fibrosis with other intestinal manifestations CC
         Distal intestinal obstruction syndrome
         RIC Excl: 15 Pulmonary

E84.8 Cystic fibrosis with other manifestations CC
     RIC Excl: 15 Pulmonary

E84.9 Cystic fibrosis, unspecified CC ▽
     RIC Excl: 15 Pulmonary

√4th **E85 Amyloidosis**
     EXCLUDES 1 *Alzheimer's disease (G30.0-)*

E85.0 Non-neuropathic heredofamilial amyloidosis
     Familial Mediterranean fever
     Hereditary amyloid nephropathy

E85.1 Neuropathic heredofamilial amyloidosis
     Amyloid polyneuropathy (Portuguese)
     AHA: 2012, 4Q, 99

E85.2 Heredofamilial amyloidosis, unspecified ▽

E85.3 Secondary systemic amyloidosis
     Hemodialysis-associated amyloidosis

E85.4 Organ-limited amyloidosis
     Localized amyloidosis

E85.8 Other amyloidosis

E85.9 Amyloidosis, unspecified ▽

√4th **E86 Volume depletion**
     EXCLUDES 1 *dehydration of newborn (P74.1)*
                 hypovolemic shock NOS (R57.1)
                 postprocedural hypovolemic shock (T81.19)
                 traumatic hypovolemic shock (T79.4)

E86.0 Dehydration
     AHA: 2014, 1Q, 7

E86.1 Hypovolemia
     Depletion of volume of plasma

E86.9 Volume depletion, unspecified ▽

√4th **E87 Other disorders of fluid, electrolyte and acid-base balance**
     EXCLUDES 1 *diabetes insipidus (E23.2)*
                 electrolyte imbalance associated with hyperemesis gravidarum (O21.1)
                 electrolyte imbalance following ectopic or molar pregnancy (O08.5)
                 familial periodic paralysis (G72.3)

E87.0 Hyperosmolality and hypernatremia
     Sodium [Na] excess
     Sodium [Na] overload
     AHA: 2014, 1Q, 7

E87.1 Hypo-osmolality and hyponatremia
     Sodium [Na] deficiency
     EXCLUDES 1 *syndrome of inappropriate secretion of antidiuretic hormone (E22.2)*
     AHA: 2014, 1Q, 7

E87.2 Acidosis
     Acidosis NOS   Metabolic acidosis
     Lactic acidosis   Respiratory acidosis
     EXCLUDES 1 *diabetic acidosis—see categories E08-E10, E13 with ketoacidosis*

E87.3 Alkalosis
     Alkalosis NOS   Respiratory alkalosis
     Metabolic alkalosis

E87.4 Mixed disorder of acid-base balance

E87.5 Hyperkalemia
     Potassium [K] excess   Potassium [K] overload

E87.6 Hypokalemia
     Potassium [K] deficiency

√5th **E87.7 Fluid overload**
     EXCLUDES 1 *edema NOS (R60.9)*
                 fluid retention (R60.9)

     E87.70 Fluid overload, unspecified ▽

     E87.71 Transfusion associated circulatory overload
         Fluid overload due to transfusion (blood) (blood components)
         TACO

     E87.79 Other fluid overload

E87.8 Other disorders of electrolyte and fluid balance, not elsewhere classified
     Electrolyte imbalance NOS
     Hyperchloremia
     Hypochloremia

☑ Add'l Character Required   √7th Placeholder Alert   RUG IV Special Care High Dx   RUG IV Clinically Complex Dx   RUG IV Special Care Low Dx   Manifestation Code   Other Specified Code   ▽ Unspecified Code

Chapter 4. Endocrine, Nutritional, and Metabolic Diseases

☑4ᵗʰ **E88 Other and unspecified metabolic disorders**
Use additional codes for associated conditions
EXCLUDES 1 histiocytosis X (chronic) (C96.6)

☑5ᵗʰ **E88.0 Disorders of plasma-protein metabolism, not elsewhere classified**
EXCLUDES 1 disorder of lipoprotein metabolism (E78.-)
monoclonal gammopathy (of undetermined significance) (D47.2)
polyclonal hypergammaglobulinemia (D89.0)
Waldenström's macroglobulinemia (C88.0)

E88.01 Alpha-1-antitrypsin deficiency
AAT deficiency

E88.09 Other disorders of plasma-protein metabolism, not elsewhere classified
Bisalbuminemia

E88.1 Lipodystrophy, not elsewhere classified
Lipodystrophy NOS
EXCLUDES 1 Whipple's disease (K90.81)

E88.2 Lipomatosis, not elsewhere classified
Lipomatosis NOS
Lipomatosis (Check) dolorosa [Dercum]

E88.3 Tumor lysis syndrome
Tumor lysis syndrome (spontaneous)
Tumor lysis syndrome following antineoplastic drug chemotherapy
Use additional code for adverse effect, if applicable, to identify drug (T45.1X5)

☑5ᵗʰ **E88.4 Mitochondrial metabolism disorders**
EXCLUDES 1 disorders of pyruvate metabolism (E74.4)
Kearns-Sayre syndrome (H49.81)
Leber's disease (H47.22)
Leigh's encephalopathy (G31.82)
Mitochondrial myopathy, NEC (G71.3)
Reye's syndrome (G93.7)

E88.40 Mitochondrial metabolism disorder, unspecified ▽

E88.41 MELAS syndrome
Mitochondrial myopathy, encephalopathy, lactic acidosis and stroke-like episodes

E88.42 MERRF syndrome
Myoclonic epilepsy associated with ragged-red fibers
Code also myoclonic epilepsy (G40.3-)

E88.49 Other mitochondrial metabolism disorders

☑5ᵗʰ **E88.8 Other specified metabolic disorders**
E88.81 Metabolic syndrome
Dysmetabolic syndrome X
Use additional codes for associated manifestations, such as:
obesity (E66.-)

E88.89 Other specified metabolic disorders
Launois-Bensaude adenolipomatosis
EXCLUDES 1 adult pulmonary Langerhans cell histiocytosis (J84.82)

E88.9 Metabolic disorder, unspecified ▽

☑4ᵗʰ **E89 Postprocedural endocrine and metabolic complications and disorders, not elsewhere classified**
EXCLUDES 2 intraoperative complications of endocrine system organ or structure (E36.0-, E36.1-, E36.8)

E89.0 Postprocedural hypothyroidism
Postirradiation hypothyroidism
Postsurgical hypothyroidism

E89.1 Postprocedural hypoinsulinemia
Postpancreatectomy hyperglycemia
Postsurgical hypoinsulinemia
Use additional code, if applicable, to identify:
acquired absence of pancreas (Z90.41-)
diabetes mellitus (postpancreatectomy) (postprocedural) (E13.-)
insulin use (Z79.4)
EXCLUDES 1 transient postprocedural hyperglycemia (R73.9)
transient postprocedural hypoglycemia (E16.2)

E89.2 Postprocedural hypoparathyroidism
Parathyroprival tetany

E89.3 Postprocedural hypopituitarism
Postirradiation hypopituitarism

☑5ᵗʰ **E89.4 Postprocedural ovarian failure**
E89.40 Asymptomatic postprocedural ovarian failure ♀
Postprocedural ovarian failure NOS

E89.41 Symptomatic postprocedural ovarian failure ♀
Symptoms such as flushing, sleeplessness, headache, lack of concentration, associated with postprocedural menopause

E89.5 Postprocedural testicular hypofunction ♂

E89.6 Postprocedural adrenocortical (-medullary) hypofunction

☑5ᵗʰ **E89.8 Other postprocedural endocrine and metabolic complications and disorders**
☑6ᵗʰ **E89.81 Postprocedural hemorrhage and hematoma of an endocrine system organ or structure following a procedure**
E89.810 Postprocedural hemorrhage and hematoma of an endocrine system organ or structure following an endocrine system procedure
E89.811 Postprocedural hemorrhage and hematoma of an endocrine system organ or structure following other procedure

E89.89 Other postprocedural endocrine and metabolic complications and disorders
Use additional code, if applicable, to further specify disorder

Ⓝ Newborn   Ⓟ Pediatric   Ⓜ Maternity   Ⓐ Adult   RIC RIC Dx   NCDx Noncancer Dx   PDx Primary Dx   CC RIC CC Condition   ►◄ Revised Text   ● New Code   ▲ Revised Code Title

504
ICD-10-CM 2016

Chapter 5. Mental, Behavioral and Neurodevelopmental Disorders (F01–F99)

Chapter Specific Guidelines with Coding Examples

The chapter specific guidelines from the ICD-10-CM Official Guidelines for Coding and Reporting have been provided below. Along with these guidelines are coding examples, contained in the shaded boxes, that have been developed to help illustrate the coding and/or sequencing guidance found in these guidelines.

a. Pain disorders related to psychological factors

Assign code F45.41, for pain that is exclusively related to psychological disorders. As indicated by the Excludes 1 note under category G89, a code from category G89 should not be assigned with code F45.41.

Perceived abdominal pain determined to be persistent somatoform pain disorder

F45.41   Pain disorder exclusively related to psychological factors

Explanation: This pain was diagnosed as being exclusively psychological; therefore, no code from category G89 is added.

Code F45.42, Pain disorders with related psychological factors, should be used with a code from category G89, Pain, not elsewhere classified, if there is documentation of a psychological component for a patient with acute or chronic pain.

See Section I.C.6. Pain

b. Mental and behavioral disorders due to psychoactive substance use

1) In remission

Selection of codes for "in remission" for categories F10-F19, Mental and behavioral disorders due to psychoactive substance use (categories F10-F19 with -.21) requires the provider's clinical judgment. The appropriate codes for "in remission" are assigned only on the basis of provider documentation (as defined in the Official Guidelines for Coding and Reporting).

Medical history: Opioid dependence in remission

F11.21   Opioid dependence, in remission

Explanation: The "in remission" codes are assigned when the provider documents the remission.

2) Psychoactive substance use, abuse and dependence

When the provider documentation refers to use, abuse and dependence of the same substance (e.g. alcohol, opioid, cannabis, etc.), only one code should be assigned to identify the pattern of use based on the following hierarchy:

- If both use and abuse are documented, assign only the code for abuse
- If both abuse and dependence are documented, assign only the code for dependence
- If use, abuse and dependence are all documented, assign only the code for dependence
- If both use and dependence are documented, assign only the code for dependence.

History and physical notes cannabis dependence; progress note says cannabis abuse

F12.20   Cannabis dependence, uncomplicated

Explanation: In the hierarchy, the dependence code is used if both abuse and dependence are documented.

Discharge summary says cocaine abuse; progress notes list cocaine use

F14.10   Cocaine abuse, uncomplicated

Explanation: In the hierarchy, the abuse code is used if both abuse and use are documented.

3) Psychoactive Substance Use

As with all other diagnoses, the codes for psychoactive substance use (F10.9-, F11.9-, F12.9-, F13.9-, F14.9-, F15.9-, F16.9-) should only be assigned based on provider documentation and when they meet the definition of a reportable diagnosis (see Section III, Reporting Additional Diagnoses). The codes are to be used only when the psychoactive substance use is associated with a mental or behavioral disorder, and such a relationship is documented by the provider.

ED reports that a 27-year-old female tripped and broke her right ankle. Her friends reported that they were drinking and dancing at a nightclub.

S82.891A   Other fracture of right lower leg, initial encounter for closed fracture

W01.0XXA   Fall on same level from slipping, tripping and stumbling, initial encounter

Y92.252   Music hall as the place of occurrence of the external cause

Y93.41   Activity, dancing

Explanation: Note that no code was added for alcohol use or abuse. Unless it is specifically associated with a diagnosis by provider documentation and meets the definition of a reportable diagnosis, it is not assigned. However, if the documentation from the provider stated: "The patient tripped, fell and fractured her right ankle while dancing due to her elevated blood alcohol, consistent with her ongoing alcohol abuse," the following code would be added:

F10.10   Alcohol abuse, uncomplicated

Chapter 5. Mental, Behavioral, and Neurodevelopmental Disorders (F01-F99)

INCLUDES disorders of psychological development
EXCLUDES 2 *symptoms, signs and abnormal clinical laboratory findings, not elsewhere classified (RØØ-R99)*

This chapter contains the following blocks:

F01-F09 Mental disorders due to known physiological conditions
F10-F19 Mental and behavioral disorders due to psychoactive substance use
F20-F29 Schizophrenia, schizotypal, delusional, and other non-mood psychotic disorders
F30-F39 Mood [affective] disorders
F40-F48 Anxiety, dissociative, stress-related, somatoform and other nonpsychotic mental disorders
F50-F59 Behavioral syndromes associated with physiological disturbances and physical factors
F60-F69 Disorders of adult personality and behavior
F70-F79 Intellectual disabilities
F80-F89 Pervasive and specific developmental disorders
F90-F98 Behavioral and emotional disorders with onset usually occurring in childhood and adolescence
F99 Unspecified mental disorder

Mental disorders due to known physiological conditions (F01-F09)

NOTE This block comprises a range of mental disorders grouped together on the basis of their having in common a demonstrable etiology in cerebral disease, brain injury, or other insult leading to cerebral dysfunction. The dysfunction may be primary, as in diseases, injuries, and insults that affect the brain directly and selectively; or secondary, as in systemic diseases and disorders that attack the brain only as one of the multiple organs or systems of the body that are involved.

✓4ᵗʰ F01 Vascular dementia

Vascular dementia as a result of infarction of the brain due to vascular disease, including hypertensive cerebrovascular disease.
INCLUDES arteriosclerotic dementia
Code first the underlying physiological condition or sequelae of cerebrovascular disease.

✓5ᵗʰ F01.5 Vascular dementia

F01.5Ø Vascular dementia without behavioral disturbance [A]

F01.51 Vascular dementia with behavioral disturbance [A]
Vascular dementia with aggressive behavior
Vascular dementia with combative behavior
Vascular dementia with violent behavior
Use additional code, if applicable, to identify wandering in vascular dementia (Z91.83)

✓4ᵗʰ F02 Dementia in other diseases classified elsewhere

➡ Code first the underlying physiological condition, such as:
Alzheimer's (G3Ø.-)
cerebral lipidosis (E75.4)
Creutzfeldt-Jakob disease (A81.Ø-)
dementia with Lewy bodies (G31.83)
epilepsy and recurrent seizures (G4Ø.-)
frontotemporal dementia (G31.Ø9)
hepatolenticular degeneration (E83.Ø)
human immunodeficiency virus [HIV] disease (B2Ø)
hypercalcemia (E83.52)
hypothyroidism, acquired (EØØ-EØ3.-)
intoxications (T36-T65)
Jakob-Creutzfeldt disease (A81.Ø-)
multiple sclerosis (G35)
neurosyphilis (A52.17)
niacin deficiency [pellagra] (E52)
Parkinson's disease (G2Ø)
Pick's disease (G31.Ø1)
polyarteritis nodosa (M3Ø.Ø)
systemic lupus erythematosus (M32.-)
trypanosomiasis (B56.-, B57.-)
vitamin B deficiency (E53.8)
EXCLUDES 1 dementia with Parkinsonism (G31.83)
EXCLUDES 2 dementia in alcohol and psychoactive substance disorders (F1Ø-F19, with .17, .27, .97)
vascular dementia (F01.5-)

✓5ᵗʰ F02.8 Dementia in other diseases classified elsewhere

F02.8Ø Dementia in other diseases classified elsewhere without behavioral disturbance
Dementia in other diseases classified elsewhere NOS

F02.81 Dementia in other diseases classified elsewhere with behavioral disturbance
Dementia in other diseases classified elsewhere with aggressive behavior
Dementia in other diseases classified elsewhere with combative behavior
Dementia in other diseases classified elsewhere with violent behavior
Use additional code, if applicable, to identify wandering in dementia in conditions classified elsewhere (Z91.83)

✓4ᵗʰ F03 Unspecified dementia

Presenile dementia NOS
Presenile psychosis NOS
Primary degenerative dementia NOS
Senile dementia NOS
Senile dementia depressed or paranoid type
Senile psychosis NOS
EXCLUDES 1 senility NOS (R41.81)
EXCLUDES 2 mild memory disturbance due to known physiological condition (FØ6.8)
senile dementia with delirium or acute confusional state (FØ5)

✓5ᵗʰ F03.9 Unspecified dementia

F03.9Ø Unspecified dementia without behavioral disturbance [A][▽]
Dementia NOS
AHA: 2012, 4Q, 92

F03.91 Unspecified dementia with behavioral disturbance [A][▽]
Unspecified dementia with aggressive behavior
Unspecified dementia with combative behavior
Unspecified dementia with violent behavior
Use additional code, if applicable, to identify wandering in unspecified dementia (Z91.83)

F04 Amnestic disorder due to known physiological condition

Korsakov's psychosis or syndrome, nonalcoholic
Code first the underlying physiological condition
EXCLUDES 1 amnesia NOS (R41.3)
anterograde amnesia (R41.1)
dissociative amnesia (F44.Ø)
retrograde amnesia (R41.2)
EXCLUDES 2 alcohol-induced or unspecified Korsakov's syndrome (F1Ø.26, F1Ø.96)
Korsakov's syndrome induced by other psychoactive substances (F13.26, F13.96, F19.16, F19.26, F19.96)

F05 Delirium due to known physiological condition

Acute or subacute brain syndrome
Acute or subacute confusional state (nonalcoholic)
Acute or subacute infective psychosis
Acute or subacute organic reaction
Acute or subacute psycho-organic syndrome
Delirium of mixed etiology
Delirium superimposed on dementia
Sundowning
Code first the underlying physiological condition
EXCLUDES 1 delirium NOS (R41.Ø)
EXCLUDES 2 delirium tremens alcohol-induced or unspecified (F1Ø.231, F1Ø.921)

✓4ᵗʰ F06 Other mental disorders due to known physiological condition

INCLUDES mental disorders due to endocrine disorder
mental disorders due to exogenous hormone
mental disorders due to exogenous toxic substance
mental disorders due to primary cerebral disease
mental disorders due to somatic illness
mental disorders due to systemic disease affecting the brain
Code first the underlying physiological condition
EXCLUDES 1 unspecified dementia (FØ3)
EXCLUDES 2 delirium due to known physiological condition (FØ5)
dementia as classified in F01-F02
other mental disorders associated with alcohol and other psychoactive substances (F1Ø-F19)

F06.Ø Psychotic disorder with hallucinations due to known physiological condition
Organic hallucinatory state (nonalcoholic)
EXCLUDES 2 hallucinations and perceptual disturbance induced by alcohol and other psychoactive substances (F1Ø-F19 with .151, .251, .951)
schizophrenia (F2Ø.-)

[N] Newborn   [P] Pediatric   [M] Maternity   [A] Adult   [RIC] RIC Dx   [NCDx] Noncancer Dx   [PDx] Primary Dx   [CC] RIC CC Condition   ▶◀ Revised Text   ● New Code   ▲ Revised Code Title

506   ICD-10-CM 2016

F06.1 Catatonic **disorder due to known physiological condition**
    EXCLUDES 1   catatonic stupor (R40.1)
       stupor NOS (R40.1)
    EXCLUDES 2   catatonic schizophrenia (F20.2)
       dissociative stupor (F44.2)

F06.2 Psychotic disorder with delusions **due to known physiological condition**
    Paranoid and paranoid-hallucinatory organic states
    Schizophrenia-like psychosis in epilepsy
    EXCLUDES 2   alcohol and drug-induced psychotic disorder (F10-F19
       with .150, .250, .950)
       brief psychotic disorder (F23)
       delusional disorder (F22)
       schizophrenia (F20.-)

✓5ᵗʰ F06.3 Mood **disorder due to known physiological condition**
    EXCLUDES 2   mood disorders due to alcohol and other psychoactive
       substances (F10-F19 with .14, .24, .94)
       mood disorders, not due to known physiological
       condition or unspecified (F30-F39)

    F06.30 Mood disorder due to known physiological ▽
       condition, unspecified

    F06.31 Mood disorder due to known physiological
       condition with depressive features

    F06.32 Mood disorder due to known physiological
       condition with major depressive-like episode

    F06.33 Mood disorder due to known physiological
       condition with manic features

    F06.34 Mood disorder due to known physiological
       condition with mixed features

F06.4 Anxiety **disorder due to known physiological condition**
    EXCLUDES 2   anxiety disorders due to alcohol and other psychoactive
       substances (F10-F19 with .180, .280, .980)
       anxiety disorders, not due to known physiological
       condition or unspecified (F40.-, F41.-)

F06.8 Other specified mental disorders due to known physiological condition
    Epileptic psychosis NOS
    Organic dissociative disorder
    Organic emotionally labile [asthenic] disorder

✓4ᵗʰ F07 Personality and behavioral disorders due to known physiological condition
    Code first the underlying physiological condition

F07.0 Personality **change due to known physiological condition**
    Frontal lobe syndrome
    Limbic epilepsy personality syndrome
    Lobotomy syndrome
    Organic personality disorder
    Organic pseudopsychopathic personality
    Organic pseudoretarded personality
    Postleucotomy syndrome
    Code first underlying physiological condition
    EXCLUDES 1   mild cognitive impairment (G31.84)
       postconcussional syndrome (F07.81)
       postencephalitic syndrome (F07.89)
       signs and symptoms involving emotional state (R45.-)
    EXCLUDES 2   specific personality disorder (F60.-)

✓5ᵗʰ F07.8 Other **personality and behavioral disorders due to known physiological condition**

    F07.81 Postconcussional syndrome
       Postcontusional syndrome (encephalopathy)
       Post-traumatic brain syndrome, nonpsychotic
       Use additional code to identify associated
       post-traumatic headache, if applicable (G44.3-)
       EXCLUDES 1   current concussion (brain) (S06.0-)
         postencephalitic syndrome (F07.89)

    F07.89 Other personality and behavioral disorders due to known physiological condition
       Postencephalitic syndrome
       Right hemispheric organic affective disorder

F07.9 Unspecified personality and behavioral disorder due to ▽
known physiological condition
    Organic psychosyndrome

F09 Unspecified mental disorder due to known physiological ▽
condition
    Mental disorder NOS due to known physiological condition
    Organic brain syndrome NOS
    Organic mental disorder NOS
    Organic psychosis NOS
    Symptomatic psychosis NOS
    Code first the underlying physiological condition
    EXCLUDES 1   psychosis NOS (F29)

Mental and behavioral disorders due to psychoactive substance use (F10-F19)

✓4ᵗʰ F10 Alcohol **related disorders**
    Use additional code for blood alcohol level, if applicable (Y90.-)

✓5ᵗʰ F10.1 Alcohol abuse
    EXCLUDES 1   alcohol dependence (F10.2-)
       alcohol use, unspecified (F10.9-)

    F10.10 Alcohol abuse, uncomplicated

    ✓6ᵗʰ F10.12 Alcohol abuse with intoxication
       F10.120 Alcohol abuse with intoxication,
         uncomplicated
       F10.121 Alcohol abuse with intoxication delirium
       F10.129 Alcohol abuse with intoxication, ▽
         unspecified

    F10.14 Alcohol abuse with alcohol-induced mood disorder

    ✓6ᵗʰ F10.15 Alcohol abuse with alcohol-induced psychotic
       disorder
       F10.150 Alcohol abuse with alcohol-induced
         psychotic disorder with delusions
       F10.151 Alcohol abuse with alcohol-induced
         psychotic disorder with hallucinations
       F10.159 Alcohol abuse with alcohol-induced ▽
         psychotic disorder, unspecified

    ✓6ᵗʰ F10.18 Alcohol abuse with other alcohol-induced **disorders**
       F10.180 Alcohol abuse with alcohol-induced
         anxiety disorder
       F10.181 Alcohol abuse with alcohol-induced sexual
         dysfunction
       F10.182 Alcohol abuse with alcohol-induced sleep
         disorder
       F10.188 Alcohol abuse with other alcohol-induced disorder

    F10.19 Alcohol abuse with unspecified alcohol-induced ▽
       disorder

✓5ᵗʰ F10.2 Alcohol dependence
    EXCLUDES 1   alcohol abuse (F10.1-)
       alcohol use, unspecified (F10.9-)
    EXCLUDES 2   toxic effect of alcohol (T51.0-)

    F10.20 Alcohol dependence, uncomplicated

    F10.21 Alcohol dependence, in remission

    ✓6ᵗʰ F10.22 Alcohol dependence with intoxication
       Acute drunkenness (in alcoholism)
       EXCLUDES 1   alcohol dependence with withdrawal
         (F10.23-)
       F10.220 Alcohol dependence with intoxication,
         uncomplicated
       F10.221 Alcohol dependence with intoxication
         delirium
       F10.229 Alcohol dependence with intoxication, ▽
         unspecified

    ✓6ᵗʰ F10.23 Alcohol dependence with withdrawal
       EXCLUDES 1   Alcohol dependence with intoxication
         (F10.22-)
       F10.230 Alcohol dependence with withdrawal,
         uncomplicated
       F10.231 Alcohol dependence with withdrawal
         delirium
       F10.232 Alcohol dependence with withdrawal with
         perceptual disturbance
       F10.239 Alcohol dependence with withdrawal, ▽
         unspecified

    F10.24 Alcohol dependence with alcohol-induced mood
       disorder

☑ Add'l Character Required   ✓x7ᵗʰ Placeholder Alert   RUG IV Special Care High Dx   RUG IV Clinically Complex Dx   RUG IV Special Care Low Dx   Manifestation Code   Other Specified Code   ▽ Unspecified Code

Chapter 5. Mental, Behavioral and Neurodevelopmental Disorders

✓6ᵗʰ **F10.25**   Alcohol dependence with alcohol-induced psychotic disorder
    F10.250   Alcohol dependence with alcohol-induced psychotic disorder with delusions
    F10.251   Alcohol dependence with alcohol-induced psychotic disorder with hallucinations
    F10.259   Alcohol dependence with alcohol-induced psychotic disorder, unspecified ▽

F10.26   Alcohol dependence with alcohol-induced persisting amnestic disorder

F10.27   Alcohol dependence with alcohol-induced persisting dementia

✓6ᵗʰ **F10.28**   Alcohol dependence with other alcohol-induced disorders
    F10.280   Alcohol dependence with alcohol-induced anxiety disorder
    F10.281   Alcohol dependence with alcohol-induced sexual dysfunction
    F10.282   Alcohol dependence with alcohol-induced sleep disorder
    F10.288   Alcohol dependence with other alcohol-induced disorder

F10.29   Alcohol dependence with unspecified alcohol-induced disorder ▽

✓5ᵗʰ **F10.9**   Alcohol use, unspecified
    EXCLUDES 1   alcohol abuse (F10.1-)
              alcohol dependence (F10.2-)

✓6ᵗʰ **F10.92**   Alcohol use, unspecified with intoxication
    F10.920   Alcohol use, unspecified with intoxication, uncomplicated
    F10.921   Alcohol use, unspecified with intoxication delirium
    F10.929   Alcohol use, unspecified with intoxication, unspecified ▽

F10.94   Alcohol use, unspecified with alcohol-induced mood disorder

✓6ᵗʰ **F10.95**   Alcohol use, unspecified with alcohol-induced psychotic disorder
    F10.950   Alcohol use, unspecified with alcohol-induced psychotic disorder with delusions
    F10.951   Alcohol use, unspecified with alcohol-induced psychotic disorder with hallucinations
    F10.959   Alcohol use, unspecified with alcohol-induced psychotic disorder, unspecified ▽

F10.96   Alcohol use, unspecified with alcohol-induced persisting amnestic disorder

F10.97   Alcohol use, unspecified with alcohol-induced persisting dementia

✓6ᵗʰ **F10.98**   Alcohol use, unspecified with other alcohol-induced disorders
    F10.980   Alcohol use, unspecified with alcohol-induced anxiety disorder
    F10.981   Alcohol use, unspecified with alcohol-induced sexual dysfunction
    F10.982   Alcohol use, unspecified with alcohol-induced sleep disorder
    F10.988   Alcohol use, unspecified with other alcohol-induced disorder

F10.99   Alcohol use, unspecified with unspecified alcohol-induced disorder ▽

✓4ᵗʰ **F11**   **Opioid related disorders**

✓5ᵗʰ **F11.1**   Opioid abuse
    EXCLUDES 1   opioid dependence (F11.2-)
              opioid use, unspecified (F11.9-)

F11.10   Opioid abuse, uncomplicated

✓6ᵗʰ **F11.12**   Opioid abuse with intoxication
    F11.120   Opioid abuse with intoxication, uncomplicated
    F11.121   Opioid abuse with intoxication delirium
    F11.122   Opioid abuse with intoxication with perceptual disturbance
    F11.129   Opioid abuse with intoxication, unspecified ▽

F11.14   Opioid abuse with opioid-induced mood disorder

✓6ᵗʰ **F11.15**   Opioid abuse with opioid-induced psychotic disorder
    F11.150   Opioid abuse with opioid-induced psychotic disorder with delusions
    F11.151   Opioid abuse with opioid-induced psychotic disorder with hallucinations
    F11.159   Opioid abuse with opioid-induced psychotic disorder, unspecified ▽

✓6ᵗʰ **F11.18**   Opioid abuse with other opioid-induced disorder
    F11.181   Opioid abuse with opioid-induced sexual dysfunction
    F11.182   Opioid abuse with opioid-induced sleep disorder
    F11.188   Opioid abuse with other opioid-induced disorder

F11.19   Opioid abuse with unspecified opioid-induced disorder ▽

✓5ᵗʰ **F11.2**   Opioid dependence
    EXCLUDES 1   opioid abuse (F11.1-)
              opioid use, unspecified (F11.9-)
    EXCLUDES 2   opioid poisoning (T40.0-T40.2-)

F11.20   Opioid dependence, uncomplicated

F11.21   Opioid dependence, in remission

✓6ᵗʰ **F11.22**   Opioid dependence with intoxication
    EXCLUDES 1   opioid dependence with withdrawal (F11.23)
    F11.220   Opioid dependence with intoxication, uncomplicated
    F11.221   Opioid dependence with intoxication delirium
    F11.222   Opioid dependence with intoxication with perceptual disturbance
    F11.229   Opioid dependence with intoxication, unspecified ▽

F11.23   Opioid dependence with withdrawal
    EXCLUDES 1   opioid dependence with intoxication (F11.22-)

F11.24   Opioid dependence with opioid-induced mood disorder

✓6ᵗʰ **F11.25**   Opioid dependence with opioid-induced psychotic disorder
    F11.250   Opioid dependence with opioid-induced psychotic disorder with delusions
    F11.251   Opioid dependence with opioid-induced psychotic disorder with hallucinations
    F11.259   Opioid dependence with opioid-induced psychotic disorder, unspecified ▽

✓6ᵗʰ **F11.28**   Opioid dependence with other opioid-induced disorder
    F11.281   Opioid dependence with opioid-induced sexual dysfunction
    F11.282   Opioid dependence with opioid-induced sleep disorder
    F11.288   Opioid dependence with other opioid-induced disorder

F11.29   Opioid dependence with unspecified opioid-induced disorder ▽

✓5ᵗʰ **F11.9**   Opioid use, unspecified
    EXCLUDES 1   opioid abuse (F11.1-)
              opioid dependence (F11.2-)

F11.90   Opioid use, unspecified, uncomplicated ▽

✓6ᵗʰ **F11.92**   Opioid use, unspecified with intoxication
    EXCLUDES 1   opioid use, unspecified with withdrawal (F11.93)
    F11.920   Opioid use, unspecified with intoxication, uncomplicated
    F11.921   Opioid use, unspecified with intoxication delirium
    F11.922   Opioid use, unspecified with intoxication with perceptual disturbance
    F11.929   Opioid use, unspecified with intoxication, unspecified ▽

F11.93   Opioid use, unspecified with withdrawal
    EXCLUDES 1   opioid use, unspecified with intoxication (F11.92-)

Ⓝ Newborn   Ⓟ Pediatric   Ⓜ Maternity   Ⓐ Adult   **RIC** RIC Dx   **NC Dx** Noncancer Dx   **PDx** Primary Dx   **CC** RIC CC Condition   ▶◀ Revised Text   ● New Code   ▲ Revised Code Title

508   ICD-10-CM 2016

F11.94   Opioid use, unspecified with opioid-induced mood disorder ▽

✓6ᵗʰ F11.95   Opioid use, unspecified with opioid-induced psychotic disorder
    F11.950   Opioid use, unspecified with opioid-induced psychotic disorder with delusions
    F11.951   Opioid use, unspecified with opioid-induced psychotic disorder with hallucinations
    F11.959   Opioid use, unspecified with opioid-induced psychotic disorder, unspecified ▽

✓6ᵗʰ F11.98   Opioid use, unspecified with other specified opioid-induced disorder
    F11.981   Opioid use, unspecified with opioid-induced sexual dysfunction
    F11.982   Opioid use, unspecified with opioid-induced sleep disorder
    F11.988   Opioid use, unspecified with other opioid-induced disorder

F11.99   Opioid use, unspecified with unspecified opioid-induced disorder ▽

✓4ᵗʰ **F12**   Cannabis **related disorders**
   INCLUDES   marijuana

✓5ᵗʰ F12.1   **Cannabis** abuse
   EXCLUDES 1   cannabis dependence (F12.2-)
             cannabis use, unspecified (F12.9-)

    F12.10   Cannabis abuse, uncomplicated

✓6ᵗʰ F12.12   Cannabis abuse with intoxication
    F12.120   Cannabis abuse with intoxication, uncomplicated
    F12.121   Cannabis abuse with intoxication delirium
    F12.122   Cannabis abuse with intoxication with perceptual disturbance
    F12.129   Cannabis abuse with intoxication, unspecified ▽

✓6ᵗʰ F12.15   Cannabis abuse with psychotic disorder
    F12.150   Cannabis abuse with psychotic disorder with delusions
    F12.151   Cannabis abuse with psychotic disorder with hallucinations
    F12.159   Cannabis abuse with psychotic disorder, unspecified ▽

✓6ᵗʰ F12.18   Cannabis abuse with other cannabis-induced disorder
    F12.180   Cannabis abuse with cannabis-induced anxiety disorder
    F12.188   Cannabis abuse with other cannabis-induced disorder

F12.19   Cannabis abuse with unspecified cannabis-induced disorder ▽

✓5ᵗʰ F12.2   **Cannabis** dependence
   EXCLUDES 1   cannabis abuse (F12.1-)
             cannabis use, unspecified (F12.9-)
   EXCLUDES 2   cannabis poisoning (T40.7-)

    F12.20   Cannabis dependence, uncomplicated
    F12.21   Cannabis dependence, in remission

✓6ᵗʰ F12.22   Cannabis dependence with intoxication
    F12.220   Cannabis dependence with intoxication, uncomplicated
    F12.221   Cannabis dependence with intoxication delirium
    F12.222   Cannabis dependence with intoxication with perceptual disturbance
    F12.229   Cannabis dependence with intoxication, unspecified ▽

✓6ᵗʰ F12.25   Cannabis dependence with psychotic disorder
    F12.250   Cannabis dependence with psychotic disorder with delusions
    F12.251   Cannabis dependence with psychotic disorder with hallucinations
    F12.259   Cannabis dependence with psychotic disorder, unspecified ▽

✓6ᵗʰ F12.28   Cannabis dependence with other cannabis-induced disorder
    F12.280   Cannabis dependence with cannabis-induced anxiety disorder
    F12.288   Cannabis dependence with other cannabis-induced disorder

F12.29   Cannabis dependence with unspecified cannabis-induced disorder ▽

✓5ᵗʰ F12.9   Cannabis use, unspecified
   EXCLUDES 1   cannabis abuse (F12.1-)
             cannabis dependence (F12.2-)

    F12.90   Cannabis use, unspecified, uncomplicated

✓6ᵗʰ F12.92   Cannabis use, unspecified with intoxication
    F12.920   Cannabis use, unspecified with intoxication, uncomplicated
    F12.921   Cannabis use, unspecified with intoxication delirium
    F12.922   Cannabis use, unspecified with intoxication with perceptual disturbance
    F12.929   Cannabis use, unspecified with intoxication, unspecified

✓6ᵗʰ F12.95   Cannabis use, unspecified with psychotic disorder
    F12.950   Cannabis use, unspecified with psychotic disorder with delusions
    F12.951   Cannabis use, unspecified with psychotic disorder with hallucinations
    F12.959   Cannabis use, unspecified with psychotic disorder, unspecified ▽

✓6ᵗʰ F12.98   Cannabis use, unspecified with other cannabis-induced disorder
    F12.980   Cannabis use, unspecified with anxiety disorder
    F12.988   Cannabis use, unspecified with other cannabis-induced disorder

F12.99   Cannabis use, unspecified with unspecified cannabis-induced disorder ▽

✓4ᵗʰ **F13**   Sedative, hypnotic, or anxiolytic **related disorders**

✓5ᵗʰ F13.1   **Sedative, hypnotic or anxiolytic-related** abuse
   EXCLUDES 1   sedative, hypnotic or anxiolytic-related dependence (F13.2-)
             sedative, hypnotic, or anxiolytic use, unspecified (F13.9-)

    F13.10   Sedative, hypnotic or anxiolytic abuse, uncomplicated

✓6ᵗʰ F13.12   Sedative, hypnotic or anxiolytic abuse with intoxication
    F13.120   Sedative, hypnotic or anxiolytic abuse with intoxication, uncomplicated
    F13.121   Sedative, hypnotic or anxiolytic abuse with intoxication delirium
    F13.129   Sedative, hypnotic or anxiolytic abuse with intoxication, unspecified ▽

    F13.14   Sedative, hypnotic or anxiolytic abuse with sedative, hypnotic or anxiolytic-induced mood disorder

✓6ᵗʰ F13.15   Sedative, hypnotic or anxiolytic abuse with sedative, hypnotic or anxiolytic-induced psychotic disorder
    F13.150   Sedative, hypnotic or anxiolytic abuse with sedative, hypnotic or anxiolytic-induced psychotic disorder with delusions
    F13.151   Sedative, hypnotic or anxiolytic abuse with sedative, hypnotic or anxiolytic-induced psychotic disorder with hallucinations
    F13.159   Sedative, hypnotic or anxiolytic abuse with sedative, hypnotic or anxiolytic-induced psychotic disorder, unspecified ▽

✓6ᵗʰ F13.18   Sedative, hypnotic or anxiolytic abuse with other sedative, hypnotic or anxiolytic-induced disorders
    F13.180   Sedative, hypnotic or anxiolytic abuse with sedative, hypnotic or anxiolytic-induced anxiety disorder
    F13.181   Sedative, hypnotic or anxiolytic abuse with sedative, hypnotic or anxiolytic-induced sexual dysfunction

☑ Add'l Character Required   ✓x7ᵗʰ Placeholder Alert   RUG IV Special Care High Dx   RUG IV Clinically Complex Dx   RUG IV Special Care Low Dx   Manifestation Code   Other Specified Code   ▽ Unspecified Code

ICD-10-CM 2016   **509**

Chapter 5. Mental, Behavioral and Neurodevelopmental Disorders

F13.182 Sedative, hypnotic or anxiolytic abuse with sedative, hypnotic or anxiolytic-induced sleep disorder

F13.188 Sedative, hypnotic or anxiolytic abuse with other sedative, hypnotic or anxiolytic-induced disorder

F13.19 Sedative, hypnotic or anxiolytic abuse with unspecified sedative, hypnotic or anxiolytic-induced disorder △

✓5ᵗʰ **F13.2** Sedative, hypnotic or anxiolytic-related dependence

> **EXCLUDES 1** *sedative, hypnotic or anxiolytic-related abuse (F13.1-)*
> *sedative, hypnotic, or anxiolytic use, unspecified (F13.9-)*
>
> **EXCLUDES 2** *sedative, hypnotic, or anxiolytic poisoning (T42.-)*

F13.20 Sedative, hypnotic or anxiolytic dependence, uncomplicated

F13.21 Sedative, hypnotic or anxiolytic dependence, in remission

✓6ᵗʰ **F13.22** Sedative, hypnotic or anxiolytic dependence with intoxication

> **EXCLUDES 1** *sedative, hypnotic or anxiolytic dependence with withdrawal (F13.23-)*

F13.220 Sedative, hypnotic or anxiolytic dependence with intoxication, uncomplicated

F13.221 Sedative, hypnotic or anxiolytic dependence with intoxication delirium

F13.229 Sedative, hypnotic or anxiolytic dependence with intoxication, unspecified △

✓6ᵗʰ **F13.23** Sedative, hypnotic or anxiolytic dependence with withdrawal

> **EXCLUDES 1** *sedative, hypnotic or anxiolytic dependence with intoxication (F13.22-)*

F13.230 Sedative, hypnotic or anxiolytic dependence with withdrawal, uncomplicated

F13.231 Sedative, hypnotic or anxiolytic dependence with withdrawal delirium

F13.232 Sedative, hypnotic or anxiolytic dependence with withdrawal with perceptual disturbance

F13.239 Sedative, hypnotic or anxiolytic dependence with withdrawal, unspecified △

F13.24 Sedative, hypnotic or anxiolytic dependence with sedative, hypnotic or anxiolytic-induced mood disorder

✓6ᵗʰ **F13.25** Sedative, hypnotic or anxiolytic dependence with sedative, hypnotic or anxiolytic-induced psychotic disorder

F13.250 Sedative, hypnotic or anxiolytic dependence with sedative, hypnotic or anxiolytic-induced psychotic disorder with delusions

F13.251 Sedative, hypnotic or anxiolytic dependence with sedative, hypnotic or anxiolytic-induced psychotic disorder with hallucinations

F13.259 Sedative, hypnotic or anxiolytic dependence with sedative, hypnotic or anxiolytic-induced psychotic disorder, unspecified △

F13.26 Sedative, hypnotic or anxiolytic dependence with sedative, hypnotic or anxiolytic-induced persisting amnestic disorder

F13.27 Sedative, hypnotic or anxiolytic dependence with sedative, hypnotic or anxiolytic-induced persisting dementia

✓6ᵗʰ **F13.28** Sedative, hypnotic or anxiolytic dependence with other sedative, hypnotic or anxiolytic-induced disorders

F13.280 Sedative, hypnotic or anxiolytic dependence with sedative, hypnotic or anxiolytic-induced anxiety disorder

F13.281 Sedative, hypnotic or anxiolytic dependence with sedative, hypnotic or anxiolytic-induced sexual dysfunction

F13.282 Sedative, hypnotic or anxiolytic dependence with sedative, hypnotic or anxiolytic-induced sleep disorder

F13.288 Sedative, hypnotic or anxiolytic dependence with other sedative, hypnotic or anxiolytic-induced disorder

F13.29 Sedative, hypnotic or anxiolytic dependence with unspecified sedative, hypnotic or anxiolytic-induced disorder △

✓5ᵗʰ **F13.9** Sedative, hypnotic or anxiolytic-related use, unspecified

> **EXCLUDES 1** *sedative, hypnotic or anxiolytic-related abuse (F13.1-)*
> *sedative, hypnotic or anxiolytic-related dependence (F13.2-)*

F13.90 Sedative, hypnotic, or anxiolytic use, unspecified, uncomplicated

✓6ᵗʰ **F13.92** Sedative, hypnotic or anxiolytic use, unspecified with intoxication

> **EXCLUDES 1** *sedative, hypnotic or anxiolytic use, unspecified with withdrawal (F13.93-)*

F13.920 Sedative, hypnotic or anxiolytic use, unspecified with intoxication, uncomplicated

F13.921 Sedative, hypnotic or anxiolytic use, unspecified with intoxication delirium

F13.929 Sedative, hypnotic or anxiolytic use, unspecified with intoxication, unspecified △

✓6ᵗʰ **F13.93** Sedative, hypnotic or anxiolytic use, unspecified with withdrawal

> **EXCLUDES 1** *sedative, hypnotic or anxiolytic use, unspecified with intoxication (F13.92-)*

F13.930 Sedative, hypnotic or anxiolytic use, unspecified with withdrawal, uncomplicated

F13.931 Sedative, hypnotic or anxiolytic use, unspecified with withdrawal delirium

F13.932 Sedative, hypnotic or anxiolytic use, unspecified with withdrawal with perceptual disturbances

F13.939 Sedative, hypnotic or anxiolytic use, unspecified with withdrawal, unspecified △

F13.94 Sedative, hypnotic or anxiolytic use, unspecified with sedative, hypnotic or anxiolytic-induced mood disorder

✓6ᵗʰ **F13.95** Sedative, hypnotic or anxiolytic use, unspecified with sedative, hypnotic or anxiolytic-induced psychotic disorder

F13.950 Sedative, hypnotic or anxiolytic use, unspecified with sedative, hypnotic or anxiolytic-induced psychotic disorder with delusions

F13.951 Sedative, hypnotic or anxiolytic use, unspecified with sedative, hypnotic or anxiolytic-induced psychotic disorder with hallucinations

F13.959 Sedative, hypnotic or anxiolytic use, unspecified with sedative, hypnotic or anxiolytic-induced psychotic disorder, unspecified △

F13.96 Sedative, hypnotic or anxiolytic use, unspecified with sedative, hypnotic or anxiolytic-induced persisting amnestic disorder

F13.97 Sedative, hypnotic or anxiolytic use, unspecified with sedative, hypnotic or anxiolytic-induced persisting dementia

✓6ᵗʰ **F13.98** Sedative, hypnotic or anxiolytic use, unspecified with other sedative, hypnotic or anxiolytic-induced disorders

F13.980 Sedative, hypnotic or anxiolytic use, unspecified with sedative, hypnotic or anxiolytic-induced anxiety disorder

F13.981 Sedative, hypnotic or anxiolytic use, unspecified with sedative, hypnotic or anxiolytic-induced sexual dysfunction

F13.982 Sedative, hypnotic or anxiolytic use, unspecified with sedative, hypnotic or anxiolytic-induced sleep disorder

F13.988 Sedative, hypnotic or anxiolytic use, unspecified with other sedative, hypnotic or anxiolytic-induced disorder

Ⓝ Newborn   Ⓟ Pediatric   Ⓜ Maternity   Ⓐ Adult   **RIC** RIC Dx   **NC Dx** Noncancer Dx   **PDx** Primary Dx   **CC** RIC CC Condition   ▶◀ Revised Text   ● New Code   ▲ Revised Code Title

510   ICD-10-CM 2016

F13.99   Sedative, hypnotic or anxiolytic use, unspecified ▽
with unspecified sedative, hypnotic or
anxiolytic-induced disorder

✓4ᵗʰ **F14**   Cocaine **related disorders**
     EXCLUDES 2   *other stimulant-related disorders (F15.-)*

✓5ᵗʰ   **F14.1**   Cocaine abuse
      EXCLUDES 1   *cocaine dependence (F14.2-)*
              cocaine use, unspecified (F14.9-)

     F14.10   Cocaine abuse, uncomplicated

✓6ᵗʰ   F14.12   Cocaine abuse with intoxication
         F14.120   Cocaine abuse with intoxication,
uncomplicated
         F14.121   Cocaine abuse with intoxication with
delirium
         F14.122   Cocaine abuse with intoxication with
perceptual disturbance
         F14.129   Cocaine abuse with intoxication, ▽
unspecified

     F14.14   Cocaine abuse with cocaine-induced mood disorder

✓6ᵗʰ   F14.15   Cocaine abuse with cocaine-induced psychotic
disorder
         F14.150   Cocaine abuse with cocaine-induced
psychotic disorder with delusions
         F14.151   Cocaine abuse with cocaine-induced
psychotic disorder with hallucinations
         F14.159   Cocaine abuse with cocaine-induced ▽
psychotic disorder, unspecified

✓6ᵗʰ   F14.18   Cocaine abuse with other cocaine-induced disorder
         F14.180   Cocaine abuse with cocaine-induced
anxiety disorder
         F14.181   Cocaine abuse with cocaine-induced
sexual dysfunction
         F14.182   Cocaine abuse with cocaine-induced sleep
disorder
         F14.188   Cocaine abuse with other cocaine-induced
disorder

     F14.19   Cocaine abuse with unspecified cocaine-induced ▽
disorder

✓5ᵗʰ   **F14.2**   Cocaine dependence
      EXCLUDES 1   *cocaine abuse (F14.1-)*
              cocaine use, unspecified (F14.9-)
      EXCLUDES 2   *cocaine poisoning (T40.5-)*

     F14.20   Cocaine dependence, uncomplicated
     F14.21   Cocaine dependence, in remission

✓6ᵗʰ   F14.22   Cocaine dependence with intoxication
         EXCLUDES 1   *cocaine dependence with withdrawal
(F14.23)*
         F14.220   Cocaine dependence with intoxication,
uncomplicated
         F14.221   Cocaine dependence with intoxication
delirium
         F14.222   Cocaine dependence with intoxication
with perceptual disturbance
         F14.229   Cocaine dependence with intoxication, ▽
unspecified

     F14.23   Cocaine dependence with withdrawal
         EXCLUDES 1   *cocaine dependence with intoxication
(F14.22-)*

     F14.24   Cocaine dependence with cocaine-induced mood
disorder

✓6ᵗʰ   F14.25   Cocaine dependence with cocaine-induced psychotic
disorder
         F14.250   Cocaine dependence with
cocaine-induced psychotic disorder with
delusions
         F14.251   Cocaine dependence with
cocaine-induced psychotic disorder with
hallucinations
         F14.259   Cocaine dependence with ▽
cocaine-induced psychotic disorder,
unspecified

✓6ᵗʰ   F14.28   Cocaine dependence with other cocaine-induced
disorder
         F14.280   Cocaine dependence with
cocaine-induced anxiety disorder
         F14.281   Cocaine dependence with
cocaine-induced sexual dysfunction

         F14.282   Cocaine dependence with
cocaine-induced sleep disorder
         F14.288   Cocaine dependence with other
cocaine-induced disorder

     F14.29   Cocaine dependence with unspecified ▽
cocaine-induced disorder

✓5ᵗʰ   **F14.9**   Cocaine use, unspecified
      EXCLUDES 1   *cocaine abuse (F14.1-)*
              cocaine dependence (F14.2-)

     F14.90   Cocaine use, unspecified, uncomplicated

✓6ᵗʰ   F14.92   Cocaine use, unspecified with intoxication
         F14.920   Cocaine use, unspecified with
intoxication, uncomplicated
         F14.921   Cocaine use, unspecified with
intoxication delirium
         F14.922   Cocaine use, unspecified with
intoxication with perceptual disturbance
         F14.929   Cocaine use, unspecified with ▽
intoxication, unspecified

     F14.94   Cocaine use, unspecified with cocaine-induced
mood disorder

✓6ᵗʰ   F14.95   Cocaine use, unspecified with cocaine-induced
psychotic disorder
         F14.950   Cocaine use, unspecified with
cocaine-induced psychotic disorder with
delusions
         F14.951   Cocaine use, unspecified with
cocaine-induced psychotic disorder with
hallucinations
         F14.959   Cocaine use, unspecified with ▽
cocaine-induced psychotic disorder,
unspecified

✓6ᵗʰ   F14.98   Cocaine use, unspecified with other specified
cocaine-induced disorder
         F14.980   Cocaine use, unspecified with
cocaine-induced anxiety disorder
         F14.981   Cocaine use, unspecified with
cocaine-induced sexual dysfunction
         F14.982   Cocaine use, unspecified with
cocaine-induced sleep disorder
         F14.988   Cocaine use, unspecified with other
cocaine-induced disorder

     F14.99   Cocaine use, unspecified with unspecified ▽
cocaine-induced disorder

✓4ᵗʰ **F15**   Other stimulant **related disorders**
     INCLUDES   amphetamine-related disorders
              caffeine
     EXCLUDES 2   *cocaine-related disorders (F14.-)*

✓5ᵗʰ   **F15.1**   Other stimulant abuse
      EXCLUDES 1   *other stimulant dependence (F15.2-)*
              other stimulant use, unspecified (F15.9-)

     F15.10   Other stimulant abuse, uncomplicated

✓6ᵗʰ   F15.12   Other stimulant abuse with intoxication
         F15.120   Other stimulant abuse with intoxication,
uncomplicated
         F15.121   Other stimulant abuse with intoxication
delirium
         F15.122   Other stimulant abuse with intoxication
with perceptual disturbance
         F15.129   Other stimulant abuse with ▽
intoxication, unspecified

     F15.14   Other stimulant abuse with stimulant-induced mood
disorder

✓6ᵗʰ   F15.15   Other stimulant abuse with stimulant-induced
psychotic disorder
         F15.150   Other stimulant abuse with
stimulant-induced psychotic disorder
with delusions
         F15.151   Other stimulant abuse with
stimulant-induced psychotic disorder
with hallucinations
         F15.159   Other stimulant abuse with ▽
stimulant-induced psychotic disorder,
unspecified

☑ Add'l Character Required   ✓x7ᵗʰ Placeholder Alert   RUG IV Special Care High Dx   RUG IV Clinically Complex Dx   RUG IV Special Care Low Dx   Manifestation Code   Other Specified Code   ▽ Unspecified Code

F15.18–F16.229 | Chapter 5. Mental, Behavioral and Neurodevelopmental Disorders

✓6th **F15.18** **Other stimulant abuse with other stimulant-induced disorder**
- **F15.180** **Other stimulant abuse with stimulant-induced anxiety disorder**
- **F15.181** **Other stimulant abuse with stimulant-induced sexual dysfunction**
- **F15.182** **Other stimulant abuse with stimulant-induced sleep disorder**
- **F15.188** **Other stimulant abuse with other stimulant-induced disorder**

F15.19 **Other stimulant abuse with unspecified stimulant-induced disorder** ▽

✓5th **F15.2** **Other stimulant dependence**
> EXCLUDES 1   *other stimulant abuse (F15.1-)*
> *other stimulant use, unspecified (F15.9-)*

F15.20 **Other stimulant dependence, uncomplicated**

F15.21 **Other stimulant dependence, in remission**

✓6th **F15.22** **Other stimulant dependence with intoxication**
> EXCLUDES 1   *other stimulant dependence with withdrawal (F15.23)*
- **F15.220** **Other stimulant dependence with intoxication, uncomplicated**
- **F15.221** **Other stimulant dependence with intoxication delirium**
- **F15.222** **Other stimulant dependence with intoxication with perceptual disturbance**
- **F15.229** **Other stimulant dependence with intoxication, unspecified** ▽

F15.23 **Other stimulant dependence with withdrawal**
> EXCLUDES 1   *other stimulant dependence with intoxication (F15.22-)*

F15.24 **Other stimulant dependence with stimulant-induced mood disorder**

✓6th **F15.25** **Other stimulant dependence with stimulant-induced psychotic disorder**
- **F15.250** **Other stimulant dependence with stimulant-induced psychotic disorder with delusions**
- **F15.251** **Other stimulant dependence with stimulant-induced psychotic disorder with hallucinations**
- **F15.259** **Other stimulant dependence with stimulant-induced psychotic disorder, unspecified** ▽

✓6th **F15.28** **Other stimulant dependence with other stimulant-induced disorder**
- **F15.280** **Other stimulant dependence with stimulant-induced anxiety disorder**
- **F15.281** **Other stimulant dependence with stimulant-induced sexual dysfunction**
- **F15.282** **Other stimulant dependence with stimulant-induced sleep disorder**
- **F15.288** **Other stimulant dependence with other stimulant-induced disorder**

F15.29 **Other stimulant dependence with unspecified stimulant-induced disorder** ▽

✓5th **F15.9** **Other stimulant use, unspecified**
> EXCLUDES 1   *other stimulant abuse (F15.1-)*
> *other stimulant dependence (F15.2-)*

F15.90 **Other stimulant use, unspecified, uncomplicated**

✓6th **F15.92** **Other stimulant use, unspecified with intoxication**
> EXCLUDES 1   *other stimulant use, unspecified with withdrawal (F15.93)*
- **F15.920** **Other stimulant use, unspecified with intoxication, uncompl icated**
- **F15.921** **Other stimulant use, unspecified with intoxication delirium**
- **F15.922** **Other stimulant use, unspecified with intoxication with perceptual disturbance**
- **F15.929** **Other stimulant use, unspecified with intoxication, unspecified** ▽

F15.93 **Other stimulant use, unspecified with withdrawal**
> EXCLUDES 1   *other stimulant use, unspecified with intoxication (F15.92-)*

F15.94 **Other stimulant use, unspecified with stimulant-induced mood disorder**

✓6th **F15.95** **Other stimulant use, unspecified with stimulant-induced psychotic disorder**
- **F15.950** **Other stimulant use, unspecified with stimulant-induced psychotic disorder with delusions**
- **F15.951** **Other stimulant use, unspecified with stimulant-induced psychotic disorder with hallucinations**
- **F15.959** **Other stimulant use, unspecified with stimulant-induced psychotic disorder, unspecified** ▽

✓6th **F15.98** **Other stimulant use, unspecified with other stimulant-induced disorder**
- **F15.980** **Other stimulant use, unspecified with stimulant-induced anxiety disorder**
- **F15.981** **Other stimulant use, unspecified with stimulant-induced sexual dysfunction**
- **F15.982** **Other stimulant use, unspecified with stimulant-induced sleep disorder**
- **F15.988** **Other stimulant use, unspecified with other stimulant-induced disorder**

F15.99 **Other stimulant use, unspecified with unspecified stimulant-induced disorder** ▽

✓4th **F16** **Hallucinogen related disorders**
> INCLUDES   ecstasy
> PCP
> phencyclidine

✓5th **F16.1** **Hallucinogen abuse**
> EXCLUDES 1   *hallucinogen dependence (F16.2-)*
> *hallucinogen use, unspecified (F16.9-)*

F16.10 **Hallucinogen abuse, uncomplicated**

✓6th **F16.12** **Hallucinogen abuse with intoxication**
- **F16.120** **Hallucinogen abuse with intoxication, uncomplicated**
- **F16.121** **Hallucinogen abuse with intoxication with delirium**
- **F16.122** **Hallucinogen abuse with intoxication with perceptual disturbance**
- **F16.129** **Hallucinogen abuse with intoxication, unspecified** ▽

F16.14 **Hallucinogen abuse with hallucinogen-induced mood disorder**

✓6th **F16.15** **Hallucinogen abuse with hallucinogen-induced psychotic disorder**
- **F16.150** **Hallucinogen abuse with hallucinogen-induced psychotic disorder with delusions**
- **F16.151** **Hallucinogen abuse with hallucinogen-induced psychotic disorder with hallucinations**
- **F16.159** **Hallucinogen abuse with hallucinogen-induced psychotic disorder, unspecified** ▽

✓6th **F16.18** **Hallucinogen abuse with other hallucinogen-induced disorder**
- **F16.180** **Hallucinogen abuse with hallucinogen-induced anxiety disorder**
- **F16.183** **Hallucinogen abuse with hallucinogen persisting perception disorder (flashbacks)**
- **F16.188** **Hallucinogen abuse with other hallucinogen-induced disorder**

F16.19 **Hallucinogen abuse with unspecified hallucinogen-induced disorder** ▽

✓5th **F16.2** **Hallucinogen dependence**
> EXCLUDES 1   *hallucinogen abuse (F16.1-)*
> *hallucinogen use, unspecified (F16.9-)*

F16.20 **Hallucinogen dependence, uncomplicated**

F16.21 **Hallucinogen dependence, in remission**

✓6th **F16.22** **Hallucinogen dependence with intoxication**
- **F16.220** **Hallucinogen dependence with intoxication, uncomplicated**
- **F16.221** **Hallucinogen dependence with intoxication with delirium**
- **F16.229** **Hallucinogen dependence with intoxication, unspecified** ▽

N Newborn   P Pediatric   M Maternity   A Adult   RIC RIC Dx   NC Dx Noncancer Dx   PDx Primary Dx   CC RIC CC Condition   ▶◀ Revised Text   ● New Code   ▲ Revised Code Title

512   ICD-10-CM 2016

F16.24   Hallucinogen dependence with hallucinogen-induced mood disorder

√6ᵗʰ   F16.25   Hallucinogen dependence with hallucinogen-induced psychotic disorder

     F16.250   Hallucinogen dependence with hallucinogen-induced psychotic disorder with delusions

     F16.251   Hallucinogen dependence with hallucinogen-induced psychotic disorder with hallucinations

     F16.259   Hallucinogen dependence with hallucinogen-induced psychotic disorder, unspecified   ▽

√6ᵗʰ   F16.28   Hallucinogen dependence with other hallucinogen-induced disorder

     F16.280   Hallucinogen dependence with hallucinogen-induced anxiety disorder

     F16.283   Hallucinogen dependence with hallucinogen persisting perception disorder (flashbacks)

     F16.288   Hallucinogen dependence with other hallucinogen-induced disorder

F16.29   Hallucinogen dependence with unspecified hallucinogen-induced disorder   ▽

√5ᵗʰ   F16.9   Hallucinogen use, unspecified
     EXCLUDES 1   hallucinogen abuse (F16.1-)
                hallucinogen dependence (F16.2-)

F16.90   Hallucinogen use, unspecified, uncomplicated

√6ᵗʰ   F16.92   Hallucinogen use, unspecified with intoxication

     F16.920   Hallucinogen use, unspecified with intoxication, uncomplicated

     F16.921   Hallucinogen use, unspecified with intoxication with delirium

     F16.929   Hallucinogen use, unspecified with intoxication, unspecified   ▽

F16.94   Hallucinogen use, unspecified with hallucinogen-induced mood disorder

√6ᵗʰ   F16.95   Hallucinogen use, unspecified with hallucinogen-induced psychotic disorder

     F16.950   Hallucinogen use, unspecified with hallucinogen-induced psychotic disorder with delusions

     F16.951   Hallucinogen use, unspecified with hallucinogen-induced psychotic disorder with hallucinations

     F16.959   Hallucinogen use, unspecified with hallucinogen-induced psychotic disorder, unspecified   ▽

√6ᵗʰ   F16.98   Hallucinogen use, unspecified with other specified hallucinogen-induced disorder

     F16.980   Hallucinogen use, unspecified with hallucinogen-induced anxiety disorder

     F16.983   Hallucinogen use, unspecified with hallucinogen persisting perception disorder (flashbacks)

     F16.988   Hallucinogen use, unspecified with other hallucinogen-induced disorder

F16.99   Hallucinogen use, unspecified with unspecified hallucinogen-induced disorder   ▽

√4ᵗʰ   **F17**   Nicotine dependence
     EXCLUDES 1   history of tobacco dependence (Z87.891)
                tobacco use NOS (Z72.0)
     EXCLUDES 2   tobacco use (smoking) during pregnancy, childbirth and the puerperium (O99.33-)
                toxic effect of nicotine (T65.2-)
     AHA: 2013, 4Q, 108-109

√5ᵗʰ   F17.2   Nicotine dependence

√6ᵗʰ   F17.20   Nicotine dependence, unspecified

     F17.200   Nicotine dependence, unspecified, uncomplicated

     F17.201   Nicotine dependence, unspecified, in remission

     F17.203   Nicotine dependence unspecified, with withdrawal

     F17.208   Nicotine dependence, unspecified, with other nicotine-induced disorders

     F17.209   Nicotine dependence, unspecified, with unspecified nicotine-induced disorders   ▽

√6ᵗʰ   F17.21   Nicotine dependence, cigarettes

     F17.210   Nicotine dependence, cigarettes, uncomplicated

     F17.211   Nicotine dependence, cigarettes, in remission

     F17.213   Nicotine dependence, cigarettes, with withdrawal

     F17.218   Nicotine dependence, cigarettes, with other nicotine-induced disorders

     F17.219   Nicotine dependence, cigarettes, with unspecified nicotine-induced disorders   ▽

√6ᵗʰ   F17.22   Nicotine dependence, chewing tobacco

     F17.220   Nicotine dependence, chewing tobacco, uncomplicated

     F17.221   Nicotine dependence, chewing tobacco, in remission

     F17.223   Nicotine dependence, chewing tobacco, with withdrawal

     F17.228   Nicotine dependence, chewing tobacco, with other nicotine-induced disorders

     F17.229   Nicotine dependence, chewing tobacco, with unspecified nicotine-induced disorders   ▽

√6ᵗʰ   F17.29   Nicotine dependence, other tobacco product

     F17.290   Nicotine dependence, other tobacco product, uncomplicated

     F17.291   Nicotine dependence, other tobacco product, in remission

     F17.293   Nicotine dependence, other tobacco product, with withdrawal

     F17.298   Nicotine dependence, other tobacco product, with other nicotine-induced disorders

     F17.299   Nicotine dependence, other tobacco product, with unspecified nicotine-induced disorders   ▽

√4ᵗʰ   **F18**   Inhalant related disorders
     INCLUDES   volatile solvents

√5ᵗʰ   F18.1   Inhalant abuse
     EXCLUDES 1   inhalant dependence (F18.2-)
                inhalant use, unspecified (F18.9-)

     F18.10   Inhalant abuse, uncomplicated

√6ᵗʰ   F18.12   Inhalant abuse with intoxication

     F18.120   Inhalant abuse with intoxication, uncomplicated

     F18.121   Inhalant abuse with intoxication delirium

     F18.129   Inhalant abuse with intoxication, unspecified   ▽

     F18.14   Inhalant abuse with inhalant-induced mood disorder

√6ᵗʰ   F18.15   Inhalant abuse with inhalant-induced psychotic disorder

     F18.150   Inhalant abuse with inhalant-induced psychotic disorder with delusions

     F18.151   Inhalant abuse with inhalant-induced psychotic disorder with hallucinations

     F18.159   Inhalant abuse with inhalant-induced psychotic disorder, unspecified   ▽

     F18.17   Inhalant abuse with inhalant-induced dementia

√6ᵗʰ   F18.18   Inhalant abuse with other inhalant-induced disorders

     F18.180   Inhalant abuse with inhalant-induced anxiety disorder

     F18.188   Inhalant abuse with other inhalant-induced disorder

     F18.19   Inhalant abuse with unspecified inhalant-induced disorder   ▽

√5ᵗʰ   F18.2   Inhalant dependence
     EXCLUDES 1   inhalant abuse (F18.1-)
                inhalant use, unspecified (F18.9-)

     F18.20   Inhalant dependence, uncomplicated

     F18.21   Inhalant dependence, in remission

☑ Add'l Character Required   √x7ᵗʰ Placeholder Alert   RUG IV Special Care High Dx   RUG IV Clinically Complex Dx   RUG IV Special Care Low Dx   Manifestation Code   Other Specified Code   ▽ Unspecified Code

ICD-10-CM 2016   513

✓6ᵗʰ **F18.22**   **Inhalant dependence with** intoxication
- **F18.220**   **Inhalant dependence with intoxication, uncomplicated**
- **F18.221**   **Inhalant dependence with intoxication delirium**
- **F18.229**   **Inhalant dependence with intoxication,** ▽ **unspecified**

F18.24   **Inhalant dependence with inhalant-induced** mood disorder

✓6ᵗʰ **F18.25**   **Inhalant dependence with inhalant-induced** psychotic disorder
- **F18.250**   **Inhalant dependence with inhalant-induced psychotic disorder with delusions**
- **F18.251**   **Inhalant dependence with inhalant-induced psychotic disorder with** hallucinations
- **F18.259**   **Inhalant dependence with** ▽ **inhalant-induced psychotic disorder, unspecified**

F18.27   **Inhalant dependence with inhalant-induced** dementia

✓6ᵗʰ **F18.28**   **Inhalant dependence with** other **inhalant-induced disorders**
- **F18.280**   **Inhalant dependence with inhalant-induced** anxiety disorder
- **F18.288**   **Inhalant dependence with other inhalant-induced disorder**

F18.29   **Inhalant dependence with unspecified** ▽ **inhalant-induced disorder**

✓5ᵗʰ **F18.9**   **Inhalant use,** unspecified
> EXCLUDES1   *inhalant abuse (F18.1-)*
>   *inhalant dependence (F18.2-)*

F18.90   **Inhalant use, unspecified,** uncomplicated

✓6ᵗʰ **F18.92**   **Inhalant use, unspecified with** intoxication
- **F18.920**   **Inhalant use, unspecified with intoxication, uncomplicated**
- **F18.921**   **Inhalant use, unspecified with intoxication with** delirium
- **F18.929**   **Inhalant use, unspecified with** ▽ **intoxication, unspecified**

F18.94   **Inhalant use, unspecified with inhalant-induced** mood disorder

✓6ᵗʰ **F18.95**   **Inhalant use, unspecified with inhalant-induced** psychotic disorder
- **F18.950**   **Inhalant use, unspecified with inhalant-induced psychotic disorder with delusions**
- **F18.951**   **Inhalant use, unspecified with inhalant-induced psychotic disorder with hallucinations**
- **F18.959**   **Inhalant use, unspecified with** ▽ **inhalant-induced psychotic disorder, unspecified**

F18.97   **Inhalant use, unspecified with inhalant-induced** persisting dementia

✓6ᵗʰ **F18.98**   **Inhalant use, unspecified with** other **inhalant-induced disorders**
- **F18.980**   **Inhalant use, unspecified with inhalant-induced** anxiety disorder
- **F18.988**   **Inhalant use, unspecified with other inhalant-induced disorder**

F18.99   **Inhalant use, unspecified with unspecified** ▽ **inhalant-induced disorder**

✓4ᵗʰ **F19**   **Other psychoactive substance related disorders**
> INCLUDES   polysubstance drug use (indiscriminate drug use)

✓5ᵗʰ **F19.1**   **Other psychoactive substance** abuse
> EXCLUDES1   *other psychoactive substance dependence (F19.2-)*
>   *other psychoactive substance use, unspecified (F19.9-)*

F19.10   **Other psychoactive substance abuse,** uncomplicated

✓6ᵗʰ **F19.12**   **Other psychoactive substance abuse with** intoxication
- **F19.120**   **Other psychoactive substance abuse with intoxication,** uncomplicated
- **F19.121**   **Other psychoactive substance abuse with intoxication** delirium

F19.122   **Other psychoactive substance abuse with intoxication with** perceptual disturbances

F19.129   **Other psychoactive substance abuse** ▽ **with intoxication, unspecified**

F19.14   **Other psychoactive substance abuse with psychoactive substance-induced** mood disorder

✓6ᵗʰ **F19.15**   **Other psychoactive substance abuse with psychoactive substance-induced** psychotic disorder
- **F19.150**   **Other psychoactive substance abuse with psychoactive substance-induced psychotic disorder with** delusions
- **F19.151**   **Other psychoactive substance abuse with psychoactive substance-induced psychotic disorder with** hallucinations
- **F19.159**   **Other psychoactive substance abuse** ▽ **with psychoactive substance-induced psychotic disorder, unspecified**

F19.16   **Other psychoactive substance abuse with psychoactive substance-induced** persisting amnestic disorder

F19.17   **Other psychoactive substance abuse with psychoactive substance-induced** persisting dementia

✓6ᵗʰ **F19.18**   **Other psychoactive substance abuse with** other **psychoactive substance-induced disorders**
- **F19.180**   **Other psychoactive substance abuse with psychoactive substance-induced** anxiety disorder
- **F19.181**   **Other psychoactive substance abuse with psychoactive substance-induced** sexual dysfunction
- **F19.182**   **Other psychoactive substance abuse with psychoactive substance-induced** sleep disorder
- **F19.188**   **Other psychoactive substance abuse with other psychoactive substance-induced disorder**

F19.19   **Other psychoactive substance abuse with** ▽ **unspecified psychoactive substance-induced disorder**

✓5ᵗʰ **F19.2**   **Other psychoactive substance** dependence
> EXCLUDES1   *other psychoactive substance abuse (F19.1-)*
>   *other psychoactive substance use, unspecified (F19.9-)*

F19.20   **Other psychoactive substance dependence,** uncomplicated

F19.21   **Other psychoactive substance dependence,** in remission

✓6ᵗʰ **F19.22**   **Other psychoactive substance dependence with** intoxication
> EXCLUDES1   *other psychoactive substance dependence with withdrawal (F19.23-)*
- **F19.220**   **Other psychoactive substance dependence with intoxication,** uncomplicated
- **F19.221**   **Other psychoactive substance dependence with intoxication** delirium
- **F19.222**   **Other psychoactive substance dependence with intoxication with** perceptual disturbance
- **F19.229**   **Other psychoactive substance** ▽ **dependence with intoxication, unspecified**

✓6ᵗʰ **F19.23**   **Other psychoactive substance dependence with** withdrawal
> EXCLUDES1   *other psychoactive substance dependence with intoxication (F19.22-)*
- **F19.230**   **Other psychoactive substance dependence with withdrawal, uncomplicated**
- **F19.231**   **Other psychoactive substance dependence with withdrawal** delirium
- **F19.232**   **Other psychoactive substance dependence with withdrawal with** perceptual disturbance
- **F19.239**   **Other psychoactive substance** ▽ **dependence with withdrawal, unspecified**

F19.24 Other psychoactive substance dependence with psychoactive substance-induced mood disorder

☑6ᵗʰ **F19.25** Other psychoactive substance dependence with psychoactive substance-induced psychotic disorder

    F19.250 Other psychoactive substance dependence with psychoactive substance-induced psychotic disorder with delusions

    F19.251 Other psychoactive substance dependence with psychoactive substance-induced psychotic disorder with hallucinations

    F19.259 Other psychoactive substance dependence with psychoactive substance-induced psychotic disorder, unspecified ▽

F19.26 Other psychoactive substance dependence with psychoactive substance-induced persisting amnestic disorder

F19.27 Other psychoactive substance dependence with psychoactive substance-induced persisting dementia

☑6ᵗʰ **F19.28** Other psychoactive substance dependence with other psychoactive substance-induced disorders

    F19.280 Other psychoactive substance dependence with psychoactive substance-induced anxiety disorder

    F19.281 Other psychoactive substance dependence with psychoactive substance-induced sexual dysfunction

    F19.282 Other psychoactive substance dependence with psychoactive substance-induced sleep disorder

    F19.288 Other psychoactive substance dependence with other psychoactive substance-induced disorder

F19.29 Other psychoactive substance dependence with unspecified psychoactive substance-induced disorder ▽

☑5ᵗʰ **F19.9** Other psychoactive substance use, unspecified
    EXCLUDES 1 other psychoactive substance abuse (F19.1-)
          other psychoactive substance dependence (F19.2-)

F19.90 Other psychoactive substance use, unspecified, uncomplicated

☑6ᵗʰ **F19.92** Other psychoactive substance use, unspecified with intoxication
    EXCLUDES 1 other psychoactive substance use, unspecified with withdrawal (F19.93)

    F19.920 Other psychoactive substance use, unspecified with intoxication, uncomplicated

    F19.921 Other psychoactive substance use, unspecified with intoxication with delirium

    F19.922 Other psychoactive substance use, unspecified with intoxication with perceptual disturbance

    F19.929 Other psychoactive substance use, unspecified with intoxication, unspecified ▽

☑6ᵗʰ **F19.93** Other psychoactive substance use, unspecified with withdrawal
    EXCLUDES 1 other psychoactive substance use, unspecified with intoxication (F19.92-)

    F19.930 Other psychoactive substance use, unspecified with withdrawal, uncomplicated

    F19.931 Other psychoactive substance use, unspecified with withdrawal delirium

    F19.932 Other psychoactive substance use, unspecified with withdrawal with perceptual disturbance

    F19.939 Other psychoactive substance use, unspecified with withdrawal, unspecified ▽

F19.94 Other psychoactive substance use, unspecified with psychoactive substance-induced mood disorder

☑6ᵗʰ **F19.95** Other psychoactive substance use, unspecified with psychoactive substance-induced psychotic disorder

    F19.950 Other psychoactive substance use, unspecified with psychoactive substance-induced psychotic disorder with delusions

    F19.951 Other psychoactive substance use, unspecified with psychoactive substance-induced psychotic disorder with hallucinations

    F19.959 Other psychoactive substance use, unspecified with psychoactive substance-induced psychotic disorder, unspecified ▽

F19.96 Other psychoactive substance use, unspecified with psychoactive substance-induced persisting amnestic disorder

F19.97 Other psychoactive substance use, unspecified with psychoactive substance-induced persisting dementia

☑6ᵗʰ **F19.98** Other psychoactive substance use, unspecified with other psychoactive substance-induced disorders

    F19.980 Other psychoactive substance use, unspecified with psychoactive substance-induced anxiety disorder

    F19.981 Other psychoactive substance use, unspecified with psychoactive substance-induced sexual dysfunction

    F19.982 Other psychoactive substance use, unspecified with psychoactive substance-induced sleep disorder

    F19.988 Other psychoactive substance use, unspecified with other psychoactive substance-induced disorder

F19.99 Other psychoactive substance use, unspecified with unspecified psychoactive substance-induced disorder ▽

Schizophrenia, schizotypal, delusional, and other non-mood psychotic disorders (F20-F29)

☑4ᵗʰ **F20** Schizophrenia
    EXCLUDES 1 brief psychotic disorder (F23)
          cyclic schizophrenia (F25.0)
          mood [affective] disorders with psychotic symptoms (F30.2, F31.2, F31.5, F31.64, F32.3, F33.3)
          schizoaffective disorder (F25.-)
          schizophrenic reaction NOS (F23)
    EXCLUDES 2 schizophrenic reaction in:
          alcoholism (F10.15-, F10.25-, F10.95-)
          brain disease (F06.2)
          epilepsy (F06.2)
          psychoactive drug use (F11-F19 with .15, .25, .95)
          schizotypal disorder (F21)

F20.0 Paranoid schizophrenia
    Paraphrenic schizophrenia
    EXCLUDES 1 involutional paranoid state (F22)
          paranoia (F22)

F20.1 Disorganized schizophrenia
    Hebephrenic schizophrenia
    Hebephrenia

F20.2 Catatonic schizophrenia
    Schizophrenic catalepsy
    Schizophrenic catatonia
    Schizophrenic flexibilitas cerea
    EXCLUDES 1 catatonic stupor (R40.1)

F20.3 Undifferentiated schizophrenia
    Atypical schizophrenia
    EXCLUDES 1 acute schizophrenia-like psychotic disorder (F23)
    EXCLUDES 2 post-schizophrenic depression (F32.8)

F20.5 Residual schizophrenia
    Restzustand (schizophrenic)
    Schizophrenic residual state

☑5ᵗʰ **F20.8** Other schizophrenia

    F20.81 Schizophreniform disorder
       Schizophreniform psychosis NOS

    F20.89 Other schizophrenia
       Cenesthopathic schizophrenia
       Simple schizophrenia

F20.9 Schizophrenia, unspecified ▽

F21 **Schizotypal disorder**
Borderline schizophrenia
Latent schizophrenia
Latent schizophrenic reaction
Prepsychotic schizophrenia
Prodromal schizophrenia
Pseudoneurotic schizophrenia
Pseudopsychopathic schizophrenia
Schizotypal personality disorder
> EXCLUDES 2 *Asperger's syndrome (F84.5)*
> *schizoid personality disorder (F60.1)*

F22 **Delusional disorders**
Delusional dysmorphophobia
Involutional paranoid state
Paranoia
Paranoia querulans
Paranoid psychosis
Paranoid state
Paraphrenia (late)
Sensitiver Beziehungswahn
> EXCLUDES 1 *mood [affective] disorders with psychotic symptoms (F30.2, F31.2, F31.5, F31.64, F32.3, F33.3)*
> *paranoid schizophrenia (F20.0)*
> EXCLUDES 2 *paranoid personality disorder (F60.0)*
> *paranoid psychosis, psychogenic (F23)*
> *paranoid reaction (F23)*

F23 **Brief psychotic disorder**
Paranoid reaction
Psychogenic paranoid psychosis
> EXCLUDES 2 *mood [affective] disorders with psychotic symptoms (F30.2, F31.2, F31.5, F31.64, F32.3, F33.3)*

F24 **Shared psychotic disorder**
Folie à deux
Induced paranoid disorder
Induced psychotic disorder

✓4th F25 **Schizoaffective disorders**
> EXCLUDES 1 *mood [affective] disorders with psychotic symptoms (F30.2, F31.2, F31.5, F31.64, F32.3, F33.3)*
> *schizophrenia (F20.-)*

F25.0 **Schizoaffective disorder,** bipolar type
Cyclic schizophrenia
Schizoaffective disorder, manic type
Schizoaffective disorder, mixed type
Schizoaffective psychosis, bipolar type
Schizophreniform psychosis, manic type

F25.1 **Schizoaffective disorder,** depressive type
Schizoaffective psychosis, depressive type
Schizophreniform psychosis, depressive type

F25.8 **Other schizoaffective disorders**

F25.9 **Schizoaffective disorder, unspecified** ▽
Schizoaffective psychosis NOS

F28 **Other psychotic disorder not due to a substance or known physiological condition**
Chronic hallucinatory psychosis

F29 **Unspecified psychosis not due to a substance or known** ▽ **physiological condition**
Psychosis NOS
> EXCLUDES 1 *mental disorder NOS (F99)*
> *unspecified mental disorder due to known physiological condition (F09)*

Mood [affective] disorders (F30-F39)

✓4th F30 **Manic episode**
> INCLUDES bipolar disorder, single manic episode
> mixed affective episode
> EXCLUDES 1 *bipolar disorder (F31.-)*
> *major depressive disorder, recurrent (F33.-)*
> *major depressive disorder, single episode (F32.-)*

✓5th F30.1 **Manic episode** without psychotic symptoms
F30.10 **Manic episode without psychotic symptoms,** ▽ **unspecified**
F30.11 **Manic episode without psychotic symptoms,** mild
F30.12 **Manic episode without psychotic symptoms,** moderate
F30.13 **Manic episode,** severe, **without psychotic symptoms**

F30.2 **Manic episode,** severe with psychotic symptoms
Manic stupor
Mania with mood-congruent psychotic symptoms
Mania with mood-incongruent psychotic symptoms

F30.3 **Manic episode** in partial remission

F30.4 **Manic episode** in full remission

F30.8 **Other manic episodes**
Hypomania

F30.9 **Manic episode, unspecified** ▽
Mania NOS

✓4th F31 **Bipolar disorder**
> INCLUDES manic-depressive illness
> manic-depressive psychosis
> manic-depressive reaction
> EXCLUDES 1 *bipolar disorder, single manic episode (F30.-)*
> *major depressive disorder, single episode (F32.-)*
> *major depressive disorder, recurrent (F33.-)*
> EXCLUDES 2 *cyclothymia (F34.0)*

F31.0 **Bipolar disorder, current episode** hypomanic

✓5th F31.1 **Bipolar disorder, current episode** manic without psychotic features
F31.10 **Bipolar disorder, current episode manic without** ▽ **psychotic features, unspecified**
F31.11 **Bipolar disorder, current episode manic without psychotic features,** mild
F31.12 **Bipolar disorder, current episode manic without psychotic features,** moderate
F31.13 **Bipolar disorder, current episode manic without psychotic features,** severe

F31.2 **Bipolar disorder, current episode** manic severe with psychotic features
Bipolar disorder, current episode manic with mood-congruent psychotic symptoms
Bipolar disorder, current episode manic with mood-incongruent psychotic symptoms

✓5th F31.3 **Bipolar disorder, current episode** depressed, mild or moderate severity
F31.30 **Bipolar disorder, current episode depressed,** ▽ **mild or moderate severity, unspecified**
F31.31 **Bipolar disorder, current episode depressed,** mild
⟩ F31.32 **Bipolar disorder, current episode depressed,** moderate

F31.4 **Bipolar disorder, current episode** depressed, severe, without psychotic features

F31.5 **Bipolar disorder, current episode** depressed, severe, with psychotic features
Bipolar disorder, current episode depressed with mood-incongruent psychotic symptoms
Bipolar disorder, current episode depressed with mood-congruent psychotic symptoms

✓5th F31.6 **Bipolar disorder, current episode** mixed
F31.60 **Bipolar disorder, current episode mixed,** ▽ **unspecified**
F31.61 **Bipolar disorder, current episode mixed,** mild
F31.62 **Bipolar disorder, current episode mixed,** moderate
F31.63 **Bipolar disorder, current episode mixed,** severe, without psychotic features
F31.64 **Bipolar disorder, current episode mixed,** severe, with psychotic features
Bipolar disorder, current episode mixed with mood-congruent psychotic symptoms
Bipolar disorder, current episode mixed with mood-incongruent psychotic symptoms

✓5th F31.7 **Bipolar disorder, currently** in remission
F31.70 **Bipolar disorder, currently in remission,** ▽ **most recent episode unspecified**
F31.71 **Bipolar disorder,** in partial remission, **most recent episode** hypomanic
F31.72 **Bipolar disorder,** in full remission, **most recent episode** hypomanic
F31.73 **Bipolar disorder,** in partial remission, **most recent episode** manic
F31.74 **Bipolar disorder,** in full remission, **most recent episode** manic
F31.75 **Bipolar disorder,** in partial remission, **most recent episode** depressed
F31.76 **Bipolar disorder,** in full remission, **most recent episode** depressed
F31.77 **Bipolar disorder,** in partial remission, **most recent episode** mixed
F31.78 **Bipolar disorder,** in full remission, **most recent episode** mixed

✓5th F31.8 **Other bipolar disorders**
F31.81 **Bipolar II disorder**
F31.89 **Other bipolar disorder**
Recurrent manic episodes NOS

F31.9 **Bipolar disorder, unspecified** ▽

N Newborn   P Pediatric   M Maternity   A Adult   RIC RIC Dx   NCDx Noncancer Dx   PDx Primary Dx   CC RIC CC Condition   ►◄ Revised Text   ● New Code   ▲ Revised Code Title

516   ICD-10-CM 2016

✅4ᵗʰ **F32 Major depressive disorder, single episode**
    INCLUDES single episode of agitated depression
              single episode of depressive reaction
              single episode of major depression
              single episode of psychogenic depression
              single episode of reactive depression
              single episode of vital depression
    EXCLUDES 1 *bipolar disorder (F31.-)*
              manic episode (F30.-)
              recurrent depressive disorder (F33.-)
    EXCLUDES 2 *adjustment disorder (F43.2)*

    F32.0 Major depressive disorder, single episode, mild

    F32.1 Major depressive disorder, single episode, moderate

    F32.2 Major depressive disorder, single episode, severe without psychotic features

    F32.3 Major depressive disorder, single episode, severe with psychotic features
         Single episode of major depression with mood-congruent psychotic symptoms
         Single episode of major depression with mood-incongruent psychotic symptoms
         Single episode of major depression with psychotic symptoms
         Single episode of psychogenic depressive psychosis
         Single episode of psychotic depression
         Single episode of reactive depressive psychosis

    F32.4 Major depressive disorder, single episode, in partial remission

    F32.5 Major depressive disorder, single episode, in full remission

    F32.8 Other depressive episodes
         Atypical depression
         Post-schizophrenic depression
         Single episode of 'masked' depression NOS

    F32.9 Major depressive disorder, single episode, unspecified ▽
         Depression NOS
         Depressive disorder NOS
         Major depression NOS
         AHA: 2013, 4Q, 107

✅4ᵗʰ **F33 Major depressive disorder, recurrent**
     Recurrent episodes of depressive reaction
     Recurrent episodes of endogenous depression
     Recurrent episodes of major depression
     Recurrent episodes of psychogenic depression
     Recurrent episodes of reactive depression
     Recurrent episodes of seasonal depressive disorder
     Recurrent episodes of vital depression
    EXCLUDES 1 *bipolar disorder (F31.-)*
              manic episode (F30.-)

    F33.0 Major depressive disorder, recurrent, mild

    F33.1 Major depressive disorder, recurrent, moderate

    F33.2 Major depressive disorder, recurrent, severe without psychotic features

    F33.3 Major depressive disorder, recurrent, severe with psychotic symptoms
         Endogenous depression with psychotic symptoms
         Recurrent severe episodes of major depression with mood-congruent psychotic symptoms
         Recurrent severe episodes of major depression with mood-incongruent psychotic symptoms
         Recurrent severe episodes of major depression with psychotic symptoms
         Recurrent severe episodes of psychogenic depressive psychosis
         Recurrent severe episodes of psychotic depression
         Recurrent severe episodes of reactive depressive psychosis

✅5ᵗʰ **F33.4 Major depressive disorder, recurrent, in remission**
        F33.40 Major depressive disorder, recurrent, in remission, unspecified
        F33.41 Major depressive disorder, recurrent, in partial remission
        F33.42 Major depressive disorder, recurrent, in full remission

    F33.8 Other recurrent depressive disorders
         Recurrent brief depressive episodes

    F33.9 Major depressive disorder, recurrent, unspecified ▽
         Monopolar depression NOS

✅4ᵗʰ **F34 Persistent mood [affective] disorders**
    F34.0 Cyclothymic disorder
         Affective personality disorder
         Cycloid personality
         Cyclothymia
         Cyclothymic personality

    F34.1 Dysthymic disorder
         Depressive neurosis
         Depressive personality disorder
         Dysthymia
         Neurotic depression
         Persistent anxiety depression
         EXCLUDES 2 *anxiety depression (mild or not persistent) (F41.8)*

    F34.8 Other persistent mood [affective] disorders

    F34.9 Persistent mood [affective] disorder, unspecified ▽

  F39 Unspecified mood [affective] disorder ▽
     Affective psychosis NOS

Anxiety, dissociative, stress-related, somatoform and other nonpsychotic mental disorders (F40-F48)

✅4ᵗʰ **F40 Phobic anxiety disorders**
  ✅5ᵗʰ **F40.0 Agoraphobia**
        F40.00 Agoraphobia, unspecified ▽
        F40.01 Agoraphobia with panic disorder
             Panic disorder with agoraphobia
             EXCLUDES 1 *panic disorder without agoraphobia (F41.0)*
        F40.02 Agoraphobia without panic disorder

  ✅5ᵗʰ **F40.1 Social phobias**
         Anthropophobia
         Social anxiety disorder of childhood
         Social neurosis
        F40.10 Social phobia, unspecified ▽
        F40.11 Social phobia, generalized

  ✅5ᵗʰ **F40.2 Specific (isolated) phobias**
         EXCLUDES 2 *dysmorphophobia (nondelusional) (F45.22)*
               nosophobia (F45.22)
    ✅6ᵗʰ **F40.21 Animal type phobia**
        F40.210 Arachnophobia
             Fear of spiders
        F40.218 Other animal type phobia
    ✅6ᵗʰ **F40.22 Natural environment type phobia**
        F40.220 Fear of thunderstorms
        F40.228 Other natural environment type phobia
    ✅6ᵗʰ **F40.23 Blood, injection, injury type phobia**
        F40.230 Fear of blood
        F40.231 Fear of injections and transfusions
        F40.232 Fear of other medical care
        F40.233 Fear of injury
    ✅6ᵗʰ **F40.24 Situational type phobia**
        F40.240 Claustrophobia
        F40.241 Acrophobia
        F40.242 Fear of bridges
        F40.243 Fear of flying
        F40.248 Other situational type phobia
    ✅6ᵗʰ **F40.29 Other specified phobia**
        F40.290 Androphobia
             Fear of men
        F40.291 Gynephobia
             Fear of women
        F40.298 Other specified phobia

    F40.8 Other phobic anxiety disorders
         Phobic anxiety disorder of childhood

    F40.9 Phobic anxiety disorder, unspecified ▽
         Phobia NOS
         Phobic state NOS

✅4ᵗʰ **F41 Other anxiety disorders**
    EXCLUDES 2 *anxiety in:*
           acute stress reaction (F43.0)
           transient adjustment reaction (F43.2)
           neurasthenia (F48.8)
           psychophysiologic disorders (F45.-)
           separation anxiety (F93.0)

    F41.0 Panic disorder [episodic paroxysmal anxiety] without agoraphobia
         Panic attack   Panic state
         EXCLUDES 1 *panic disorder with agoraphobia (F40.01)*

    F41.1 Generalized anxiety disorder
         Anxiety neurosis   Anxiety state
         Anxiety reaction   Overanxious disorder
         EXCLUDES 2 *neurasthenia (F48.8)*

☑ Add'l Character Required   **✓x7ᵗʰ** Placeholder Alert   RUG IV Special Care High Dx   RUG IV Clinically Complex Dx   RUG IV Special Care Low Dx   Manifestation Code   Other Specified Code   ▽ Unspecified Code

Chapter 5. Mental, Behavioral and Neurodevelopmental Disorders

F41.3 **Other** mixed **anxiety disorders**

F41.8 **Other specified anxiety disorders**
Anxiety depression (mild or not persistent)
Anxiety hysteria
Mixed anxiety and depressive disorder

F41.9 **Anxiety disorder, unspecified** ▽
Anxiety NOS

F42 **Obsessive-compulsive disorder**
Anancastic neurosis
Obsessive-compulsive neurosis
EXCLUDES 2 *obsessive-compulsive personality (disorder) (F60.5)*
obsessive-compulsive symptoms occurring in depression (F32-F33)
obsessive-compulsive symptoms occurring in schizophrenia (F20.-)

✓4ᵗʰ **F43** **Reaction to severe stress, and adjustment disorders**

F43.0 **Acute stress reaction**
Acute crisis reaction
Acute reaction to stress
Combat and operational stress reaction
Combat fatigue
Crisis state
Psychic shock

✓5ᵗʰ **F43.1** **Post-traumatic stress disorder (PTSD)**
Traumatic neurosis

F43.10 **Post-traumatic stress disorder, unspecified** ▽

F43.11 **Post-traumatic stress disorder, acute**

F43.12 **Post-traumatic stress disorder, chronic**

✓5ᵗʰ **F43.2** **Adjustment disorders**
Culture shock
Grief reaction
Hospitalism in children
EXCLUDES 2 *separation anxiety disorder of childhood (F93.0)*

F43.20 **Adjustment disorder, unspecified** ▽

F43.21 **Adjustment disorder with** depressed mood
AHA: 2014, 1Q, 25

F43.22 **Adjustment disorder with** anxiety

F43.23 **Adjustment disorder with** mixed anxiety and depressed mood

F43.24 **Adjustment disorder with** disturbance of conduct

F43.25 **Adjustment disorder with** mixed disturbance of emotions and conduct

F43.29 **Adjustment disorder with other symptoms**

F43.8 **Other reactions to severe stress**

F43.9 **Reaction to severe stress, unspecified** ▽

✓4ᵗʰ **F44** **Dissociative and conversion disorders**
INCLUDES conversion hysteria
conversion reaction
hysteria
hysterical psychosis
EXCLUDES 2 *malingering [conscious simulation] (Z76.5)*

F44.0 **Dissociative** amnesia
EXCLUDES 1 *amnesia NOS (R41.3)*
anterograde amnesia (R41.1)
retrograde amnesia (R41.2)
EXCLUDES 2 *alcohol-or other psychoactive substance-induced amnestic disorder (F10, F13, F19 with .26, .96)*
amnestic disorder due to known physiological condition (F04)
postictal amnesia in epilepsy (G40.-)

F44.1 **Dissociative** fugue
EXCLUDES 2 *postictal fugue in epilepsy (G40.-)*

F44.2 **Dissociative** stupor
EXCLUDES 1 *catatonic stupor (R40.1)*
stupor NOS (R40.1)
EXCLUDES 2 *catatonic disorder due to known physiological condition (F06.1)*
depressive stupor (F32, F33)
manic stupor (F30, F31)

F44.4 **Conversion disorder with** motor symptom or deficit
Dissociative motor disorders
Psychogenic aphonia
Psychogenic dysphonia

F44.5 **Conversion disorder with** seizures or convulsions
Dissociative convulsions

F44.6 **Conversion disorder with** sensory symptom or deficit
Dissociative anesthesia and sensory loss
Psychogenic deafness

F44.7 **Conversion disorder with** mixed symptom presentation

✓5ᵗʰ **F44.8** Other **dissociative and conversion disorders**

F44.81 **Dissociative** identity **disorder**
Multiple personality disorder

F44.89 **Other dissociative and conversion disorders**
Ganser's syndrome
Psychogenic confusion
Psychogenic twilight state
Trance and possession disorders

F44.9 **Dissociative and conversion disorder, unspecified** ▽
Dissociative disorder NOS

✓4ᵗʰ **F45** **Somatoform disorders**
EXCLUDES 2 *dissociative and conversion disorders (F44.-)*
factitious disorders (F68.1-)
hair-plucking (F63.3)
lalling (F80.0)
lisping (F80.0)
malingering [conscious simulation] (Z76.5)
nail-biting (F98.8)
psychological or behavioral factors associated with disorders or diseases classified elsewhere (F54)
sexual dysfunction, not due to a substance or known physiological condition (F52.-)
thumb-sucking (F98.8)
tic disorders (in childhood and adolescence) (F95.-)
Tourette's syndrome (F95.2)
trichotillomania (F63.3)

F45.0 **Somatization disorder**
Briquet's disorder
Multiple psychosomatic disorder

F45.1 **Undifferentiated somatoform disorder**
Undifferentiated psychosomatic disorder

✓5ᵗʰ **F45.2** **Hypochondriacal disorders**
EXCLUDES 2 *delusional dysmorphophobia (F22)*
fixed delusions about bodily functions or shape (F22)

F45.20 **Hypochondriacal disorder, unspecified** ▽

F45.21 **Hypochondriasis**
Hypochondriacal neurosis

F45.22 **Body dysmorphic disorder**
Dysmorphophobia (nondelusional)
Nosophobia

F45.29 **Other hypochondriacal disorders**

✓5ᵗʰ **F45.4** **Pain disorders related to psychological factors**
EXCLUDES 1 *pain NOS (R52)*

F45.41 **Pain disorder exclusively related to psychological factors**
Somatoform pain disorder (persistent)

F45.42 **Pain disorder with related psychological factors**
Code also associated acute or chronic pain (G89.-)

F45.8 **Other somatoform disorders**
Psychogenic dysmenorrhea
Psychogenic dysphagia, including "globus hystericus"
Psychogenic pruritus
Psychogenic torticollis
Somatoform autonomic dysfunction
Teeth grinding
EXCLUDES 1 *sleep related teeth grinding (G47.63)*

F45.9 **Somatoform disorder, unspecified** ▽
Psychosomatic disorder NOS

✓4ᵗʰ **F48** **Other nonpsychotic mental disorders**

F48.1 **Depersonalization-derealization syndrome**

F48.2 **Pseudobulbar affect**
Involuntary emotional expression disorder
Code first underlying cause, if known, such as:
amyotrophic lateral sclerosis (G12.21)
multiple sclerosis (G35)
sequelae of cerebrovascular disease (I69.-)
sequelae of traumatic intracranial injury (S06.-)

Ⓝ Newborn   Ⓟ Pediatric   Ⓜ Maternity   Ⓐ Adult   RIC RIC Dx   NCDx Noncancer Dx   PDx Primary Dx   CC RIC CC Condition   ►◄ Revised Text   ● New Code   ▲ Revised Code Title

518
ICD-10-CM 2016

F48.8   **Other specified nonpsychotic mental disorders**
Dhat syndrome
Neurasthenia
Occupational neurosis, including writer's cramp
Psychasthenia
Psychasthenic neurosis
Psychogenic syncope

F48.9   **Nonpsychotic mental disorder, unspecified**   ▽
Neurosis NOS

Behavioral syndromes associated with physiological disturbances and physical factors (F50-F59)

✓4ᵗʰ **F50**   **Eating disorders**
    EXCLUDES 1   *anorexia NOS (R63.0)*
                feeding difficulties (R63.3)
                polyphagia (R63.2)
    EXCLUDES 2   *feeding disorder in infancy or childhood (F98.2-)*

✓5ᵗʰ **F50.0**   **Anorexia nervosa**
       EXCLUDES 1   *loss of appetite (R63.0)*
                   psychogenic loss of appetite (F50.8)

   F50.00   **Anorexia nervosa, unspecified**   ▽
   F50.01   **Anorexia nervosa, restricting type**
   F50.02   **Anorexia nervosa, binge eating/purging type**
         EXCLUDES 1   *bulimia nervosa (F50.2)*

F50.2   **Bulimia nervosa**
Bulimia NOS
Hyperorexia nervosa
     EXCLUDES 1   *anorexia nervosa, binge eating/purging type (F50.02)*

F50.8   **Other eating disorders**
Pica in adults
Psychogenic loss of appetite
     EXCLUDES 2   *pica of infancy and childhood (F98.3)*

F50.9   **Eating disorder, unspecified**   ▽
Atypical anorexia nervosa
Atypical bulimia nervosa

✓4ᵗʰ **F51**   **Sleep disorders not due to a substance or known physiological condition**
    EXCLUDES 2   *organic sleep disorders (G47.-)*

✓5ᵗʰ **F51.0**   **Insomnia not due to a substance or known physiological condition**
       EXCLUDES 2   *alcohol related insomnia (F10.182, F10.282, F10.982)*
                   drug-related insomnia (F11.182, F11.282, F11.982,
                        F13.182, F13.282, F13.982, F14.182, F14.282,
                        F14.982, F15.182, F15.282, F15.982, F19.182,
                        F19.282, F19.982)
                   insomnia NOS (G47.0-)
                   insomnia due to known physiological condition
                        (G47.0-)
                   organic insomnia (G47.0-)
                   sleep deprivation (Z72.820)

   F51.01   **Primary insomnia**
         Idiopathic insomnia
   F51.02   **Adjustment insomnia**
   F51.03   **Paradoxical insomnia**
   F51.04   **Psychophysiologic insomnia**
   F51.05   **Insomnia due to other mental disorder**
         Code also associated mental disorder
   F51.09   **Other insomnia not due to a substance or known physiological condition**

✓5ᵗʰ **F51.1**   **Hypersomnia not due to a substance or known physiological condition**
       EXCLUDES 2   *alcohol related hypersomnia (F10.182, F10.282,*
                   F10.982)
                   drug-related hypersomnia (F11.182, F11.282, F11.982,
                        F13.182, F13.282, F13.982, F14.182, F14.282,
                        F14.982, F15.182, F15.282, F15.982, F19.182,
                        F19.282, F19.982)
                   hypersomnia NOS (G47.10)
                   hypersomnia due to known physiological condition
                        (G47.10)
                   idiopathic hypersomnia (G47.11, G47.12)
                   narcolepsy (G47.4-)

   F51.11   **Primary hypersomnia**
   F51.12   **Insufficient sleep syndrome**
         EXCLUDES 1   *sleep deprivation (Z72.820)*

   F51.13   **Hypersomnia due to other mental disorder**
         Code also associated mental disorder
   F51.19   **Other hypersomnia not due to a substance or known physiological condition**

F51.3   **Sleepwalking [somnambulism]**
F51.4   **Sleep terrors [night terrors]**
F51.5   **Nightmare disorder**
Dream anxiety disorder

F51.8   **Other sleep disorders not due to a substance or known physiological condition**

F51.9   **Sleep disorder not due to a substance or known physiological condition, unspecified**   ▽
Emotional sleep disorder NOS

✓4ᵗʰ **F52**   **Sexual dysfunction not due to a substance or known physiological condition**
    EXCLUDES 2   *Dhat syndrome (F48.8)*

F52.0   **Hypoactive sexual desire disorder**
Anhedonia (sexual)
Lack or loss of sexual desire
     EXCLUDES 1   *decreased libido (R68.82)*

F52.1   **Sexual aversion disorder**
Sexual aversion and lack of sexual enjoyment

✓5ᵗʰ **F52.2**   **Sexual arousal disorders**
Failure of genital response

   F52.21   **Male erectile disorder**   ♂
         Psychogenic impotence
         EXCLUDES 1   *impotence of organic origin (N52.-)*
                   impotence NOS (N52.-)

   F52.22   **Female sexual arousal disorder**   ♀
         Frigidity

✓5ᵗʰ **F52.3**   **Orgasmic disorder**
Inhibited orgasm
Psychogenic anorgasmy

   F52.31   **Female orgasmic disorder**   ♀
   F52.32   **Male orgasmic disorder**   ♂

F52.4   **Premature ejaculation**   ♂
F52.5   **Vaginismus not due to a substance or known physiological condition**   ♀
Psychogenic vaginismus
     EXCLUDES 2   *vaginismus (due to a known physiological condition)*
                   (N94.2)

F52.6   **Dyspareunia not due to a substance or known physiological condition**   ♀
Psychogenic dyspareunia
     EXCLUDES 2   *dyspareunia (due to a known physiological condition)*
                   (N94.1)

F52.8   **Other sexual dysfunction not due to a substance or known physiological condition**
Excessive sexual drive
Nymphomania
Satyriasis

F52.9   **Unspecified sexual dysfunction not due to a substance or known physiological condition**   ▽
Sexual dysfunction NOS

F53   **Puerperal psychosis**   ♀
Postpartum depression
    EXCLUDES 1   *mood disorders with psychotic features (F30.2, F31.2, F31.5,*
                   F31.64, F32.3, F33.3)
                   postpartum dysphoria (O90.6)
                   psychosis in schizophrenia, schizotypal, delusional, and other
                      psychotic disorders (F20-F29)

F54   *Psychological and behavioral factors associated with disorders or diseases classified elsewhere*
Psychological factors affecting physical conditions
Code first the associated physical disorder, such as:
    asthma (J45.-)
    dermatitis (L23-L25)
    gastric ulcer (K25.-)
    mucous colitis (K58.-)
    ulcerative colitis (K51.-)
    urticaria (L50.-)
    EXCLUDES 2   *tension-type headache (G44.2)*

✓4ᵗʰ **F55**   **Abuse of non-psychoactive substances**
    EXCLUDES 2   *abuse of psychoactive substances (F10-F19)*

F55.0   **Abuse of antacids**
F55.1   **Abuse of herbal or folk remedies**

F55.2   **Abuse of** laxatives

F55.3   **Abuse of** steroids or hormones

F55.4   **Abuse of** vitamins

F55.8   **Abuse of other non-psychoactive substances**

F59   Unspecified behavioral syndromes associated with physiological disturbances and physical factors ▽
Psychogenic physiological dysfunction NOS

Disorders of adult personality and behavior (F60-F69)

✓4ᵗʰ **F60   Specific personality disorders**

F60.0   **Paranoid personality disorder**
Expansive paranoid personality (disorder)
Fanatic personality (disorder)
Paranoid personality (disorder)
Querulant personality (disorder)
Sensitive paranoid personality (disorder)
EXCLUDES 2   paranoia (F22)
paranoia querulans (F22)
paranoid psychosis (F22)
paranoid schizophrenia (F20.0)
paranoid state (F22)

F60.1   **Schizoid personality disorder**
EXCLUDES 2   Asperger's syndrome (F84.5)
delusional disorder (F22)
schizoid disorder of childhood (F84.5)
schizophrenia (F20.-)
schizotypal disorder (F21)

F60.2   **Antisocial personality disorder**
Amoral personality (disorder)
Asocial personality (disorder)
Dissocial personality disorder
Psychopathic personality (disorder)
Sociopathic personality (disorder)
EXCLUDES 1   conduct disorders (F91.-)
EXCLUDES 2   borderline personality disorder (F60.3)

F60.3   **Borderline personality disorder**
Aggressive personality (disorder)
Emotionally unstable personality disorder
Explosive personality (disorder)
EXCLUDES 2   antisocial personality disorder (F60.2)

F60.4   **Histrionic personality disorder**
Hysterical personality (disorder)
Psychoinfantile personality (disorder)

F60.5   **Obsessive-compulsive personality disorder**
Anankastic personality (disorder)
Compulsive personality (disorder)
Obsessional personality (disorder)
EXCLUDES 2   obsessive-compulsive disorder (F42)

F60.6   **Avoidant personality disorder**
Anxious personality disorder

F60.7   **Dependent personality disorder**
Asthenic personality (disorder)
Inadequate personality (disorder)
Passive personality (disorder)

✓5ᵗʰ **F60.8   Other specific personality disorders**

F60.81   **Narcissistic personality disorder**

F60.89   **Other specific personality disorders**
Eccentric personality disorder
"Haltlose" type personality disorder
Immature personality disorder
Passive-aggressive personality disorder
Psychoneurotic personality disorder
Self-defeating personality disorder

F60.9   **Personality disorder, unspecified** ▽
Character disorder NOS
Character neurosis NOS
Pathological personality NOS

✓4ᵗʰ **F63   Impulse disorders**
EXCLUDES 2   habitual excessive use of alcohol or psychoactive substances (F10-F19)
impulse disorders involving sexual behavior (F65.-)

F63.0   **Pathological gambling**
Compulsive gambling
EXCLUDES 1   gambling and betting NOS (Z72.6)
EXCLUDES 2   excessive gambling by manic patients (F30, F31)
gambling in antisocial personality disorder (F60.2)

F63.1   **Pyromania**
Pathological fire-setting
EXCLUDES 2   fire-setting (by) (in):
adult with antisocial personality disorder (F60.2)
alcohol or psychoactive substance intoxication (F10-F19)
conduct disorders (F91.-)
mental disorders due to known physiological condition (F01-F09)
schizophrenia (F20.-)

F63.2   **Kleptomania**
Pathological stealing
EXCLUDES 1   shoplifting as the reason for observation for suspected mental disorder (Z03.8)
EXCLUDES 2   depressive disorder with stealing (F31-F33)
stealing due to underlying mental condition—code to mental condition
stealing in mental disorders due to known physiological condition (F01-F09)

F63.3   **Trichotillomania**
Hair plucking
EXCLUDES 2   other stereotyped movement disorder (F98.4)

✓5ᵗʰ **F63.8   Other impulse disorders**

F63.81   **Intermittent explosive disorder**

F63.89   **Other impulse disorders**

F63.9   **Impulse disorder, unspecified** ▽
Impulse control disorder NOS

✓4ᵗʰ **F64   Gender identity disorders**

F64.1   **Gender identity disorder in adolescence and adulthood**
Dual role transvestism
Transsexualism
Use additional code to identify sex reassignment status (Z87.890)
EXCLUDES 1   gender identity disorder in childhood (F64.2)
EXCLUDES 2   fetishistic transvestism (F65.1)

F64.2   **Gender identity disorder of childhood** P
EXCLUDES 1   gender identity disorder in adolescence and adulthood (F64.1)
EXCLUDES 2   sexual maturation disorder (F66)

F64.8   **Other gender identity disorders**

F64.9   **Gender identity disorder, unspecified** ▽
Gender-role disorder NOS

✓4ᵗʰ **F65   Paraphilias**

F65.0   **Fetishism**

F65.1   **Transvestic fetishism**
Fetishistic transvestism

F65.2   **Exhibitionism**

F65.3   **Voyeurism**

F65.4   **Pedophilia**

✓5ᵗʰ **F65.5   Sadomasochism**

F65.50   **Sadomasochism, unspecified** ▽

F65.51   **Sexual masochism**

F65.52   **Sexual sadism**

✓5ᵗʰ **F65.8   Other paraphilias**

F65.81   **Frotteurism**

F65.89   **Other paraphilias**
Necrophilia

F65.9   **Paraphilia, unspecified** ▽
Sexual deviation NOS

F66   Other sexual disorders
Sexual maturation disorder
Sexual relationship disorder

✓4ᵗʰ **F68   Other disorders of adult personality and behavior**

✓5ᵗʰ **F68.1   Factitious disorder**
Compensation neurosis
Elaboration of physical symptoms for psychological reasons
Hospital hopper syndrome
Münchhausen's syndrome
Peregrinating patient
EXCLUDES 2   factitial dermatitis (L98.1)
person feigning illness (with obvious motivation) (Z76.5)

F68.10   **Factitious disorder, unspecified** ▽

N Newborn   P Pediatric   M Maternity   A Adult   RIC RIC Dx   NC Dx Noncancer Dx   PDx Primary Dx   CC RIC CC Condition   ►◄ Revised Text   ● New Code   ▲ Revised Code Title

520   ICD-10-CM 2016

F68.11   **Factitious disorder** with predominantly psychological signs and symptoms

F68.12   **Factitious disorder** with predominantly physical signs and symptoms

F68.13   **Factitious disorder** with combined psychological and physical signs and symptoms

F68.8   **Other specified disorders of adult personality and behavior**

F69   **Unspecified disorder of adult personality and behavior**   Ⓐ▽

Intellectual Disabilities (F70-F79)

Code first any associated physical or developmental disorders

EXCLUDES 1   *borderline intellectual functioning, IQ above 70 to 84 (R41.83)*

F70   **Mild intellectual disabilities**
IQ level 50-55 to approximately 70
Mild mental subnormality

F71   **Moderate intellectual disabilities**
IQ level 35-40 to 50-55
Moderate mental subnormality

F72   **Severe intellectual disabilities**
IQ 20-25 to 35-40
Severe mental subnormality

F73   **Profound intellectual disabilities**
IQ level below 20-25
Profound mental subnormality

F78   **Other intellectual disabilities**

F79   **Unspecified intellectual disabilities**   ▽
Mental deficiency NOS
Mental subnormality NOS

Pervasive and specific developmental disorders (F80-F89)

✔4ᵗʰ **F80**   **Specific developmental disorders of speech and language**

F80.0   **Phonological disorder**
Dyslalia
Functional speech articulation disorder
Lalling
Lisping
Phonological developmental disorder
Speech articulation developmental disorder
EXCLUDES 1   *speech articulation impairment due to aphasia NOS (R47.01)*
speech articulation impairment due to apraxia (R48.2)
EXCLUDES 2   *speech articulation impairment due to hearing loss (F80.4)*
speech articulation impairment due to intellectual disabilities (F70-F79)
speech articulation impairment with expressive language developmental disorder (F80.1)
speech articulation impairment with mixed receptive expressive language developmental disorder (F80.2)

F80.1   **Expressive language disorder**
Developmental dysphasia or aphasia, expressive type
EXCLUDES 1   *dysphasia and aphasia NOS (R47.-)*
mixed receptive-expressive language disorder (F80.2)
EXCLUDES 2   *acquired aphasia with epilepsy [Landau-Kleffner] (G40.80-)*
intellectual disabilities (F70-F79)
pervasive developmental disorders (F84.-)
selective mutism (F94.0)

F80.2   **Mixed receptive-expressive language disorder**
Developmental dysphasia or aphasia, receptive type
Developmental Wernicke's aphasia
EXCLUDES 1   *central auditory processing disorder (H93.25)*
dysphasia or aphasia NOS (R47.-)
expressive language disorder (F80.1)
expressive type dysphasia or aphasia (F80.1)
word deafness (H93.25)
EXCLUDES 2   *acquired aphasia with epilepsy [Landau-Kleffner] (G40.80-)*
intellectual disabilities (F70-F79)
pervasive developmental disorders (F84.-)
selective mutism (F94.0)

F80.4   **Speech and language development delay** due to hearing loss
Code also type of hearing loss (H90.-, H91.-)

✔5ᵗʰ   F80.8   **Other** developmental disorders of speech and language

F80.81   **Childhood onset fluency disorder**
Cluttering NOS
Stuttering NOS
EXCLUDES 1   *adult onset fluency disorder (F98.5)*
fluency disorder in conditions classified elsewhere (R47.82)
fluency disorder (stuttering) following cerebrovascular disease (I69. with final characters-23)

F80.89   **Other developmental disorders of speech and language**

F80.9   **Developmental disorder of speech and language, unspecified**   ▽
Communication disorder NOS
Language disorder NOS

✔4ᵗʰ **F81**   **Specific developmental disorders of scholastic skills**

F81.0   **Specific reading disorder**
"Backward reading"
Developmental dyslexia
Specific reading retardation
EXCLUDES 1   *alexia NOS (R48.0)*
dyslexia NOS (R48.0)

F81.2   **Mathematics disorder**
Developmental acalculia
Developmental arithmetical disorder
Developmental Gerstmann's syndrome
EXCLUDES 1   *acalculia NOS (R48.8)*
EXCLUDES 2   *arithmetical difficulties associated with a reading disorder (F81.0)*
arithmetical difficulties associated with a spelling disorder (F81.81)
arithmetical difficulties due to inadequate teaching (Z55.8)

✔5ᵗʰ   F81.8   **Other developmental disorders of scholastic skills**

F81.81   **Disorder of written expression**
Specific spelling disorder

F81.89   **Other developmental disorders of scholastic skills**

F81.9   **Developmental disorder of scholastic skills, unspecified**   ▽
Knowledge acquisition disability NOS
Learning disability NOS
Learning disorder NOS

F82   **Specific developmental disorder of motor function**
Clumsy child syndrome
Developmental coordination disorder
Developmental dyspraxia
EXCLUDES 1   *abnormalities of gait and mobility (R26.-)*
lack of coordination (R27.-)
EXCLUDES 2   *lack of coordination secondary to intellectual disabilities (F70-F79)*

✔4ᵗʰ **F84**   **Pervasive developmental disorders**
Use additional code to identify any associated medical condition and intellectual disabilities

F84.0   **Autistic disorder**
Infantile autism
Infantile psychosis
Kanner's syndrome
EXCLUDES 1   *Asperger's syndrome (F84.5)*

F84.2   **Rett's syndrome**
EXCLUDES 1   *Asperger's syndrome (F84.5)*
Autistic disorder (F84.0)
Other childhood disintegrative disorder (F84.3)

F84.3   **Other childhood disintegrative disorder**   Ⓟ
Dementia infantilis
Disintegrative psychosis
Heller's syndrome
Symbiotic psychosis
Use additional code to identify any associated neurological condition
EXCLUDES 1   *Asperger's syndrome (F84.5)*
Autistic disorder (F84.0)
Rett's syndrome (F84.2)

F84.5   **Asperger's syndrome**
Asperger's disorder
Autistic psychopathy
Schizoid disorder of childhood

✔ Add'l Character Required   ✔×7ᵗʰ Placeholder Alert   RUG IV Special Care High Dx   RUG IV Clinically Complex Dx   RUG IV Special Care Low Dx   Manifestation Code   Other Specified Code   ▽Unspecified Code

ICD-10-CM 2016   521

Chapter 5. Mental, Behavioral and Neurodevelopmental Disorders

F84.8   **Other pervasive developmental disorders**
Overactive disorder associated with intellectual disabilities and stereotyped movements

F84.9   **Pervasive developmental disorder, unspecified** ▽
Atypical autism

F88   **Other disorders of psychological development**
Developmental agnosia

F89   **Unspecified disorder of psychological development** ▽
Developmental disorder NOS

Behavioral and emotional disorders with onset usually occurring in childhood and adolescence (F90-F98)

NOTE   Codes within categories F90-F98 may be used regardless of the age of a patient. These disorders generally have onset within the childhood or adolescent years, but may continue throughout life or not be diagnosed until adulthood.

✓4ᵗʰ **F90**   **Attention-deficit hyperactivity disorders**
    INCLUDES attention deficit disorder with hyperactivity
                attention deficit syndrome with hyperactivity
    EXCLUDES 2 *anxiety disorders (F40.-, F41.-)*
                mood [affective] disorders (F30-F39)
                pervasive developmental disorders (F84.-)
                schizophrenia (F20.-)

F90.0   **Attention-deficit hyperactivity disorder, predominantly inattentive type**

F90.1   **Attention-deficit hyperactivity disorder, predominantly hyperactive type**

F90.2   **Attention-deficit hyperactivity disorder, combined type**

F90.8   **Attention-deficit hyperactivity disorder, other type**

F90.9   **Attention-deficit hyperactivity disorder, unspecified type** ▽
Attention-deficit hyperactivity disorder of childhood or adolescence NOS
Attention-deficit hyperactivity disorder NOS

✓4ᵗʰ **F91**   **Conduct disorders**
    EXCLUDES 1 *antisocial behavior (Z72.81-)*
                antisocial personality disorder (F60.2)
    EXCLUDES 2 *conduct problems associated with attention-deficit hyperactivity disorder (F90.-)*
                mood [affective] disorders (F30-F39)
                pervasive developmental disorders (F84.-)
                schizophrenia (F20.-)

F91.0   **Conduct disorder confined to family context**

F91.1   **Conduct disorder, childhood-onset type**
Unsocialized conduct disorder
Conduct disorder, solitary aggressive type
Unsocialized aggressive disorder

F91.2   **Conduct disorder, adolescent-onset type**
Socialized conduct disorder
Conduct disorder, group type

F91.3   **Oppositional defiant disorder**

F91.8   **Other conduct disorders**

F91.9   **Conduct disorder, unspecified** ▽
Behavioral disorder NOS
Conduct disorder NOS
Disruptive behavior disorder NOS

✓4ᵗʰ **F93**   **Emotional disorders with onset specific to childhood**

F93.0   **Separation anxiety disorder of childhood** P
    EXCLUDES 2 *mood [affective] disorders (F30-F39)*
                nonpsychotic mental disorders (F40-F48)
                phobic anxiety disorder of childhood (F40.8)
                social phobia (F40.1)

F93.8   **Other childhood emotional disorders** P
Identity disorder
    EXCLUDES 2 *gender identity disorder of childhood (F64.2)*

F93.9   **Childhood emotional disorder, unspecified** P ▽

✓4ᵗʰ **F94**   **Disorders of social functioning with onset specific to childhood and adolescence**

F94.0   **Selective mutism**
Elective mutism
    EXCLUDES 2 *pervasive developmental disorders (F84.-)*
                schizophrenia (F20.-)
                specific developmental disorders of speech and language (F80.-)
                transient mutism as part of separation anxiety in young children (F93.0)

F94.1   **Reactive attachment disorder of childhood** P
Use additional code to identify any associated failure to thrive or growth retardation
    EXCLUDES 1 *disinhibited attachment disorder of childhood (F94.1)*
                normal variation in pattern of selective attachment
    EXCLUDES 2 *Asperger's syndrome (F84.5)*
                maltreatment syndromes (T74.-)
                sexual or physical abuse in childhood, resulting in psychosocial problems (Z62.81-)

F94.2   **Disinhibited attachment disorder of childhood** P
Affectionless psychopathy
Institutional syndrome
    EXCLUDES 1 *reactive attachment disorder of childhood (F94.1)*
    EXCLUDES 2 *Asperger's syndrome (F84.5)*
                attention-deficit hyperactivity disorders (F90.-)
                hospitalism in children (F43.2-)

F94.8   **Other childhood disorders of social functioning** P

F94.9   **Childhood disorder of social functioning, unspecified** P ▽

✓4ᵗʰ **F95**   **Tic disorder**

F95.0   **Transient tic disorder**

F95.1   **Chronic motor or vocal tic disorder**

F95.2   **Tourette's disorder**
Combined vocal and multiple motor tic disorder [de la Tourette]
Tourette's syndrome

F95.8   **Other tic disorders**

F95.9   **Tic disorder, unspecified** ▽
Tic NOS

✓4ᵗʰ **F98**   **Other behavioral and emotional disorders with onset usually occurring in childhood and adolescence**
    EXCLUDES 2 *breath-holding spells (R06.89)*
                gender identity disorder of childhood (F64.2)
                Kleine-Levin syndrome (G47.13)
                obsessive-compulsive disorder (F42)
                sleep disorders not due to a substance or known physiological condition (F51.-)

F98.0   **Enuresis not due to a substance or known physiological condition**
Enuresis (primary) (secondary) of nonorganic origin
Functional enuresis
Psychogenic enuresis
Urinary incontinence of nonorganic origin
    EXCLUDES 1 *enuresis NOS (R32)*

F98.1   **Encopresis not due to a substance or known physiological condition**
Functional encopresis
Incontinence of feces of nonorganic origin
Psychogenic encopresis
Use additional code to identify the cause of any coexisting constipation
    EXCLUDES 1 *encopresis NOS (R15.-)*

✓5ᵗʰ **F98.2**   **Other feeding disorders of infancy and childhood**
    EXCLUDES 1 *feeding difficulties (R63.3)*
    EXCLUDES 2 *anorexia nervosa and other eating disorders (F50.-)*
                feeding problems of newborn (P92.-)
                pica of infancy or childhood (F98.3)

F98.21   **Rumination disorder of infancy** P

F98.29   **Other feeding disorders of infancy and early childhood** P

F98.3   **Pica of infancy and childhood** P

F98.4   **Stereotyped movement disorders**
Stereotype/habit disorder
    EXCLUDES 1 *abnormal involuntary movements (R25.-)*
    EXCLUDES 2 *compulsions in obsessive-compulsive disorder (F42)*
                hair plucking (F63.3)
                movement disorders of organic origin (G20-G25)
                nail-biting (F98.8)
                nose-picking (F98.8)
                stereotypies that are part of a broader psychiatric condition (F01-F95)
                thumb-sucking (F98.8)
                tic disorders (F95.-)
                trichotillomania (F63.3)

N Newborn   P Pediatric   M Maternity   A Adult   RIC RIC Dx   NCDx Noncancer Dx   PDx Primary Dx   CC RIC CC Condition   ►◄ Revised Text   ● New Code   ▲ Revised Code Title

522   ICD-10-CM 2016

Chapter 5. Mental, Behavioral and Neurodevelopmental Disorders   F84.8–F98.4

F98.5 **Adult onset fluency disorder**
  EXCLUDES 1 childhood onset fluency disorder (F80.81)
       dysphasia (R47.02)
       fluency disorder in conditions classified elsewhere
           (R47.82)
       fluency disorder (stuttering) following cerebrovascular
           disease (I69. with final characters -23)
       tic disorders (F95.-)

F98.8 **Other specified behavioral and emotional disorders with** P
       onset usually occurring in childhood and adolescence
       Excessive masturbation
       Nail-biting
       Nose-picking
       Thumb-sucking

F98.9 **Unspecified behavioral and emotional disorders with** P ▽
       onset usually occurring in childhood and adolescence

Unspecified mental disorder (F99)

F99 **Mental disorder, not otherwise specified** ▽
       Mental illness NOS
       EXCLUDES 1 unspecified mental disorder due to known physiological
            condition (F09)

☑ Add'l Character Required **EXCLUDES 1** **x7th** Placeholder Alert RUG IV Special Care High Dx RUG IV Clinically Complex Dx RUG IV Special Care Low Dx Manifestation Code Other Specified Code ▽Unspecified Code

ICD-10-CM 2016   523

Chapter 6. Diseases of the Nervous System (G00-G99)

Chapter Specific Guidelines with Coding Examples

The chapter specific guidelines from the ICD-10-CM Official Guidelines for Coding and Reporting have been provided below. Along with these guidelines are coding examples, contained in the shaded boxes, that have been developed to help illustrate the coding and/or sequencing guidance found in these guidelines.

a. Dominant/nondominant side

Codes from category G81, Hemiplegia and hemiparesis, and subcategories G83.1, Monoplegia of lower limb, G83.2, Monoplegia of upper limb, and G83.3, Monoplegia, unspecified, identify whether the dominant or nondominant side is affected. Should the affected side be documented, but not specified as dominant or nondominant, and the classification system does not indicate a default, code selection is as follows:

- For ambidextrous patients, the default should be dominant.
- If the left side is affected, the default is non-dominant.
- If the right side is affected, the default is dominant.

> Hemiplegia affecting left side of ambidextrous patient
>
> **G81.92 Hemiplegia, unspecified affecting left dominant side**
>
> *Explanation*: Documentation states that the left side is affected and dominant is used for ambidextrous persons.

> Right spastic hemiplegia, unknown whether patient is right- or left-handed
>
> **G81.11 Spastic hemiplegia affecting right dominant side**
>
> *Explanation*: Since it is unknown whether the patient is right- or left-handed, if the right side is affected, the default is dominant.

b. Pain—Category G89

1) General coding information

Codes in category G89, Pain, not elsewhere classified, may be used in conjunction with codes from other categories and chapters to provide more detail about acute or chronic pain and neoplasm-related pain, unless otherwise indicated below.

If the pain is not specified as acute or chronic, post-thoracotomy, postprocedural, or neoplasm-related, do not assign codes from category G89.

A code from category G89 should not be assigned if the underlying (definitive) diagnosis is known, unless the reason for the encounter is pain control/ management and not management of the underlying condition.

When an admission or encounter is for a procedure aimed at treating the underlying condition (e.g., spinal fusion, kyphoplasty), a code for the underlying condition (e.g., vertebral fracture, spinal stenosis) should be assigned as the principal diagnosis. No code from category G89 should be assigned.

> Elderly patient with back pain is admitted for outpatient kyphoplasty for age-related osteopathic compression fracture at vertebra T3
>
> **M80.08XA Age-related osteoporosis with current pathological fracture, vertebra(e), initial encounter**
>
> *Explanation*: No code is assigned for the pain as it is inherent in the underlying condition being treated.

(a) Category G89 codes as principal or first-listed diagnosis

Category G89 codes are acceptable as principal diagnosis or the first-listed code:

- When pain control or pain management is the reason for the admission/encounter (e.g., a patient with displaced intervertebral disc, nerve impingement and severe back pain presents for injection of steroid into the spinal canal). The underlying cause of the pain should be reported as an additional diagnosis, if known.

> Patient presents for a steroid injection for control of pain of chronic right knee due to primary degenerative joint disease
>
> **G89.29 Other chronic pain**
>
> **M17.11 Unilateral primary osteoarthritis, right knee**
>
> *Explanation*: Since the encounter is for control of pain, not treating the underlying condition, the pain code is sequenced first followed by the underlying condition. The M25 pain code is not necessary as the underlying condition code represents the specific site.

- When a patient is admitted for the insertion of a neurostimulator for pain control, assign the appropriate pain code as the principal or first-listed diagnosis. When an admission or encounter is for a procedure aimed at treating the underlying condition and a neurostimulator is inserted for pain control during the same admission/encounter, a code for the underlying condition should be assigned as the principal diagnosis and the appropriate pain code should be assigned as a secondary diagnosis.

(b) Use of category G89 codes in conjunction with site specific pain codes

(i) Assigning category G89 and site-specific pain codes

Codes from category G89 may be used in conjunction with codes that identify the site of pain (including codes from chapter 18) if the category G89 code provides additional information. For example, if the code describes the site of the pain, but does not fully describe whether the pain is acute or chronic, then both codes should be assigned.

> Patient is seen to evaluate chronic left shoulder pain
>
> **M25.512 Pain in left shoulder**
>
> **G89.29 Other chronic pain**
>
> *Explanation*: No underlying condition has been determined yet so the pain would be the reason for the visit. The M25 pain code in this instance does not fully describe the condition as it does not represent that the pain is chronic. The G89 chronic pain code is assigned to provide specificity.

(ii) Sequencing of category G89 codes with site-specific pain codes

The sequencing of category G89 codes with site-specific pain codes (including chapter 18 codes), is dependent on the circumstances of the encounter/admission as follows:

- If the encounter is for pain control or pain management, assign the code from category G89 followed by the code identifying the specific site of pain (e.g., encounter for pain management for acute neck pain from trauma is assigned code G89.11, Acute pain due to trauma, followed by code M54.2, Cervicalgia, to identify the site of pain).

> Management of acute, traumatic right knee pain
>
> **G89.11 Acute pain due to trauma**
>
> **M25.561 Pain in right knee**
>
> *Explanation*: The reason for the encounter is to manage or control the pain, not to treat or evaluate an underlying condition. The G89 pain code is assigned as the principal diagnosis but in this instance does not fully describe the condition as it does not include the site and laterality. The M25 pain code is added to provide this information.

- If the encounter is for any other reason except pain control or pain management, and a related definitive diagnosis has not been established (confirmed) by the provider, assign the code for the specific site of pain first, followed by the appropriate code from category G89.

> Tests are performed to investigate the source of the patient's chronic epigastric abdominal pain
>
> **R10.13   Epigastric pain**
>
> **G89.29   Other chronic pain**
>
> *Explanation*: In this instance the patient's epigastric pain is not being treated; rather the source of the pain is being investigated. A code from chapter 18 for epigastric pain is sequenced before the additional specificity of the G89 code for the chronic pain.

2) Pain due to devices, implants and grafts

See Section I.C.19. Pain due to medical devices

3) Postoperative Pain

The provider's documentation should be used to guide the coding of postoperative pain, as well as *Section III. Reporting Additional Diagnoses* and *Section IV. Diagnostic Coding and Reporting in the Outpatient Setting.*

The default for post-thoracotomy and other postoperative pain not specified as acute or chronic is the code for the acute form.

Routine or expected postoperative pain immediately after surgery should not be coded.

> Pain pump dose is increased for the patient's unexpected, extreme pain post-thoracotomy
>
> **G89.12   Acute post-thoracotomy pain**
>
> *Explanation*: When acute or chronic is not documented, default to acute. The use of "unexpected, extreme" and the increase of medication dosage indicate that the pain was more than routine or expected.

(a) Postoperative pain not associated with specific postoperative complication

Postoperative pain not associated with a specific postoperative complication is assigned to the appropriate postoperative pain code in category G89.

(b) Postoperative pain associated with specific postoperative complication

Postoperative pain associated with a specific postoperative complication (such as painful wire sutures) is assigned to the appropriate code(s) found in Chapter 19, Injury, poisoning, and certain other consequences of external causes. If appropriate, use additional code(s) from category G89 to identify acute or chronic pain (G89.18 or G89.28).

4) Chronic pain

Chronic pain is classified to subcategory G89.2. There is no time frame defining when pain becomes chronic pain. The provider's documentation should be used to guide use of these codes.

5) Neoplasm related pain

Code G89.3 is assigned to pain documented as being related, associated or due to cancer, primary or secondary malignancy, or tumor. This code is assigned regardless of whether the pain is acute or chronic.

This code may be assigned as the principal or first-listed code when the stated reason for the admission/encounter is documented as pain control/pain management. The underlying neoplasm should be reported as an additional diagnosis.

> Pain medication adjustment for chronic pain from bone metastasis
>
> **G89.3   Neoplasm related pain (acute)(chronic)**
>
> **C79.51   Secondary malignant neoplasm of bone**
>
> *Explanation*: Since the encounter was for pain medication management, the pain, rather than the neoplasm, was the reason for the encounter and is sequenced first. This "neoplasm-related pain" code includes both acute and chronic pain.

When the reason for the admission/encounter is management of the neoplasm and the pain associated with the neoplasm is also documented, code G89.3 may be assigned as an additional diagnosis. It is not necessary to assign an additional code for the site of the pain.

See Section I.C.2 for instructions on the sequencing of neoplasms for all other stated reasons for the admission/encounter (except for pain control/pain management).

> Patient with lung cancer presents with acute hip pain and is evaluated and found to have iliac bone metastasis
>
> **C79.51   Secondary malignant neoplasm of bone**
>
> **C34.90   Malignant neoplasm of unspecified part of unspecified bronchus or lung**
>
> **G89.3   Neoplasm related pain (acute)(chronic)**
>
> *Explanation*: The reason for the encounter was the evaluation and diagnosis of the bone metastasis, whose code would be assigned as first-listed, followed by codes for the primary neoplasm and the pain due to the iliac bone metastasis.

6) Chronic pain syndrome

Central pain syndrome (G89.0) and chronic pain syndrome (G89.4) are different than the term "chronic pain," and therefore codes should only be used when the provider has specifically documented this condition.

See Section I.C.5. Pain disorders related to psychological factors

Chapter 6. Diseases of the Nervous System (G00-G99)

EXCLUDES 2   certain conditions originating in the perinatal period (P04-P96)
certain infectious and parasitic diseases (A00-B99)
complications of pregnancy, childbirth and the puerperium (O00-O9A)
congenital malformations, deformations, and chromosomal
abnormalities (Q00-Q99)
endocrine, nutritional and metabolic diseases (E00-E88)
injury, poisoning and certain other consequences of external causes
(S00-T88)
neoplasms (C00-D49)
symptoms, signs and abnormal clinical and laboratory findings, not
elsewhere classified (R00-R94)

This chapter contains the following blocks:

G00-G09	Inflammatory diseases of the central nervous system
G10-G14	Systemic atrophies primarily affecting the central nervous system
G20-G26	Extrapyramidal and movement disorders
G30-G32	Other degenerative diseases of the nervous system
G35-G37	Demyelinating diseases of the central nervous system
G40-G47	Episodic and paroxysmal disorders
G50-G59	Nerve, nerve root and plexus disorders
G60-G65	Polyneuropathies and other disorders of the peripheral nervous system
G70-G73	Diseases of myoneural junction and muscle
G80-G83	Cerebral palsy and other paralytic syndromes
G89-G99	Other disorders of the nervous system

Inflammatory diseases of the central nervous system (G00-G09)

✓4th G00 Bacterial meningitis, not elsewhere classified

INCLUDES   bacterial arachnoiditis
bacterial leptomeningitis
bacterial meningitis
bacterial pachymeningitis

EXCLUDES 1   bacterial:
meningoencephalitis (G04.2)
meningomyelitis (G04.2)

G00.0 Hemophilus meningitis   cc
Meningitis due to Hemophilus influenzae
RIC Excl: 03 Non-traumatic brain injury; 05 Non-traumatic spinal cord injury

G00.1 Pneumococcal meningitis   cc
RIC Excl: 03 Non-traumatic brain injury; 05 Non-traumatic spinal cord injury

G00.2 Streptococcal meningitis   cc
Use additional code to further identify organism (B95.0-B95.5)
RIC Excl: 03 Non-traumatic brain injury; 05 Non-traumatic spinal cord injury

G00.3 Staphylococcal meningitis   cc
Use additional code to further identify organism (B95.61-B95.8)
RIC Excl: 03 Non-traumatic brain injury; 05 Non-traumatic spinal cord injury

G00.8 Other bacterial meningitis   cc
Meningitis due to Escherichia coli
Meningitis due to Friedländer's bacillus
Meningitis due to Klebsiella
Use additional code to further identify organism (B96.-)
RIC Excl: 03 Non-traumatic brain injury; 05 Non-traumatic spinal cord injury

G00.9 Bacterial meningitis, unspecified   cc ▽
Meningitis due to gram-negative bacteria, unspecified
Purulent meningitis NOS
Pyogenic meningitis NOS
Suppurative meningitis NOS
RIC Excl: 03 Non-traumatic brain injury; 05 Non-traumatic spinal cord injury

G01 Meningitis in bacterial diseases classified elsewhere   cc
Code first underlying disease
EXCLUDES 1   meningitis (in):
gonococcal (A54.81)
leptospirosis (A27.81)
listeriosis (A32.11)
Lyme disease (A69.21)
meningococcal (A39.0)
neurosyphilis (A52.13)
tuberculosis (A17.0)
meningoencephalitis and meningomyelitis in bacterial diseases
classified elsewhere (G05)
RIC Excl: 03 Non-traumatic brain injury; 05 Non-traumatic spinal cord injury

G02 Meningitis in other infectious and parasitic diseases classified elsewhere   cc
Code first underlying disease, such as:
African trypanosomiasis (B56.-)
poliovirus infection (A80.-)
EXCLUDES 1   candidal meningitis (B37.5)
coccidioidomycosis meningitis (B38.4)
cryptococcal meningitis (B45.1)
herpesviral [herpes simplex] meningitis (B00.3)
infectious mononucleosis complicated by meningitis (B27.- with
fourth character 2)
measles complicated by meningitis (B05.1)
meningoencephalitis and meningomyelitis in other infectious
and parasitic diseases classified elsewhere (G05)
mumps meningitis (B26.1)
rubella meningitis (B06.02)
varicella [chickenpox] meningitis (B01.0)
zoster meningitis (B02.1)
RIC Excl: 03 Non-traumatic brain injury; 05 Non-traumatic spinal cord injury

✓4th G03 Meningitis due to other and unspecified causes
INCLUDES   arachnoiditis NOS
leptomeningitis NOS
meningitis NOS
pachymeningitis NOS
EXCLUDES 1   meningoencephalitis (G04.-)
meningomyelitis (G04.-)

G03.0 Nonpyogenic meningitis   cc
Aseptic meningitis
Nonbacterial meningitis
RIC Excl: 03 Non-traumatic brain injury; 05 Non-traumatic spinal cord injury

G03.1 Chronic meningitis   cc
RIC Excl: 03 Non-traumatic brain injury; 05 Non-traumatic spinal cord injury

G03.2 Benign recurrent meningitis [Mollaret]   cc
RIC Excl: 03 Non-traumatic brain injury; 05 Non-traumatic spinal cord injury

G03.8 Meningitis due to other specified causes

G03.9 Meningitis, unspecified   cc ▽
Arachnoiditis (spinal) NOS
RIC Excl: 03 Non-traumatic brain injury; 05 Non-traumatic spinal cord injury

✓4th G04 Encephalitis, myelitis and encephalomyelitis
INCLUDES   acute ascending myelitis
meningoencephalitis
meningomyelitis
EXCLUDES 1   encephalopathy NOS (G93.40)
EXCLUDES 2   acute transverse myelitis (G37.3-)
alcoholic encephalopathy (G31.2)
benign myalgic encephalomyelitis (G93.3)
multiple sclerosis (G35)
subacute necrotizing myelitis (G37.4)
toxic encephalitis (G92)
toxic encephalopathy (G92)

✓5th G04.0 Acute disseminated encephalitis and encephalomyelitis (ADEM)
EXCLUDES 1   acute necrotizing hemorrhagic encephalopathy
(G04.3-)
other noninfectious acute disseminated
encephalomyelitis (noninfectious ADEM)
(G04.81)

G04.00 Acute disseminated encephalitis and   cc ▽
encephalomyelitis, unspecified
RIC Excl: 03 Non-traumatic brain injury

G04.01 Postinfectious acute disseminated encephalitis   cc
and encephalomyelitis (postinfectious ADEM)
EXCLUDES 1   post chickenpox encephalitis (B01.1)
post measles encephalitis (B05.0)
post measles myelitis (B05.1)
RIC Excl: 03 Non-traumatic brain injury

G04.02 Postimmunization acute disseminated encephalitis,   cc
myelitis and encephalomyelitis
Encephalitis, postimmunization
Encephalomyelitis, postimmunization
Use additional code to identify the vaccine (T50.A-,
T50.B-, T50.Z-)

G04.1 Tropical spastic paraplegia

G04.2 Bacterial meningoencephalitis and meningomyelitis,   cc
not elsewhere classified
RIC Excl: 03 Non-traumatic brain injury; 05 Non-traumatic spinal cord injury

N Newborn   P Pediatric   M Maternity   A Adult   RIC RIC Dx   NCDx Noncancer Dx   PDx Primary Dx   cc RIC CC Condition   ▶◀ Revised Text   ● New Code   ▲ Revised Code Title

526   ICD-10-CM 2016

✔5th **G04.3 Acute necrotizing hemorrhagic encephalopathy**
> *EXCLUDES 1* *acute disseminated encephalitis and encephalomyelitis (G04.0-)*

G04.30 Acute necrotizing hemorrhagic CC ▽
encephalopathy, unspecified
RIC Excl: 03 Non-traumatic brain injury

G04.31 Postinfectious acute necrotizing hemorrhagic CC
encephalopathy
RIC Excl: 03 Non-traumatic brain injury

G04.32 Postimmunization acute necrotizing
hemorrhagic encephalopathy
Use additional code to identify the vaccine (T50.A-, T50.B-, T50.Z-)

G04.39 Other acute necrotizing hemorrhagic CC
encephalopathy
Code also underlying etiology, if applicable
RIC Excl: 03 Non-traumatic brain injury

✔5th **G04.8 Other encephalitis, myelitis and encephalomyelitis**
Code also any associated seizure (G40.-, R56.9)

G04.81 Other encephalitis and encephalomyelitis CC NC Dx
Noninfectious acute disseminated encephalomyelitis (noninfectious ADEM)
RIC Excl: 03 Non-traumatic brain injury

G04.89 Other myelitis CC NC Dx
RIC Excl: 03 Non-traumatic brain injury

✔5th **G04.9 Encephalitis, myelitis and encephalomyelitis, unspecified**

G04.90 Encephalitis and encephalomyelitis, CC ▽
unspecified
Ventriculitis (cerebral) NOS
RIC Excl: 03 Non-traumatic brain injury

G04.91 Myelitis, unspecified CC ▽
RIC Excl: 03 Non-traumatic brain injury

✔4th **G05 Encephalitis, myelitis and encephalomyelitis in diseases classified elsewhere**
Code first underlying disease, such as:
human immunodeficiency virus [HIV] disease (B20)
poliovirus (A80.-)
suppurative otitis media (H66.01-H66.4)
trichinellosis (B75)
> *EXCLUDES 1* *adenoviral encephalitis, myelitis and encephalomyelitis (A85.1)*
> *congenital toxoplasmosis encephalitis, myelitis and encephalomyelitis (P37.1)*
> *cytomegaloviral encephalitis, myelitis and encephalomyelitis (B25.8)*
> *encephalitis, myelitis and encephalomyelitis (in) measles (B05.0)*
> *encephalitis, myelitis and encephalomyelitis (in) systemic lupus erythematosus (M32.19)*
> *enteroviral encephalitis, myelitis and encephalomyelitis (A85.0)*
> *eosinophilic meningoencephalitis (B83.2)*
> *herpesviral [herpes simplex] encephalitis, myelitis and encephalomyelitis (B00.4)*
> *listerial encephalitis, myelitis and encephalomyelitis (A32.12)*
> *meningococcal encephalitis, myelitis and encephalomyelitis (A39.81)*
> *mumps encephalitis, myelitis and encephalomyelitis (B26.2)*
> *postchickenpox encephalitis, myelitis and encephalomyelitis (B01.1-)*
> *rubella encephalitis, myelitis and encephalomyelitis (B06.01)*
> *toxoplasmosis encephalitis, myelitis and encephalomyelitis (B58.2)*
> *zoster encephalitis, myelitis and encephalomyelitis (B02.0)*

G05.3 Encephalitis and encephalomyelitis in diseases classified elsewhere
Meningoencephalitis in diseases classified elsewhere

G05.4 Myelitis in diseases classified elsewhere CC
Meningomyelitis in diseases classified elsewhere
RIC Excl: 03 Non-traumatic brain injury

✔4th **G06 Intracranial and intraspinal abscess and granuloma**
Use additional code (B95-B97) to identify infectious agent

G06.0 Intracranial abscess and granuloma CC
Brain [any part] abscess (embolic)
Cerebellar abscess (embolic)
Cerebral abscess (embolic)
Intracranial epidural abscess or granuloma
Intracranial extradural abscess or granuloma
Intracranial subdural abscess or granuloma
Otogenic abscess (embolic)
> *EXCLUDES 1* *tuberculous intracranial abscess and granuloma (A17.81)*

RIC Excl: 03 Non-traumatic brain injury

G06.1 Intraspinal abscess and granuloma CC
Abscess (embolic) of spinal cord [any part]
Intraspinal epidural abscess or granuloma
Intraspinal extradural abscess or granuloma
Intraspinal subdural abscess or granuloma
> *EXCLUDES 1* *tuberculous intraspinal abscess and granuloma (A17.81)*

RIC Excl: 03 Non-traumatic brain injury

G06.2 Extradural and subdural abscess, unspecified CC ▽
RIC Excl: 03 Non-traumatic brain injury

G07 Intracranial and intraspinal abscess and granuloma CC
in diseases classified elsewhere
Code first underlying disease, such as:
schistosomiasis granuloma of brain (B65.-)
> *EXCLUDES 1* *abscess of brain:*
> *amebic (A06.6)*
> *chromomycotic (B43.1)*
> *gonococcal (A54.82)*
> *tuberculous (A17.81)*
> *tuberculoma of meninges (A17.1)*

RIC Excl: 03 Non-traumatic brain injury

G08 Intracranial and intraspinal phlebitis and thrombophlebitis
Septic embolism of intracranial or intraspinal venous sinuses and veins
Septic endophlebitis of intracranial or intraspinal venous sinuses and veins
Septic phlebitis of intracranial or intraspinal venous sinuses and veins
Septic thrombophlebitis of intracranial or intraspinal venous sinuses and veins
Septic thrombosis of intracranial or intraspinal venous sinuses and veins
> *EXCLUDES 1* *intracranial phlebitis and thrombophlebitis complicating:*
> *abortion, ectopic or molar pregnancy (O00-O07, O08.7)*
> *pregnancy, childbirth and the puerperium (O22.5, O87.3)*
> *nonpyogenic intracranial phlebitis and thrombophlebitis (I67.6)*
> *EXCLUDES 2* *intracranial phlebitis and thrombophlebitis complicating nonpyogenic intraspinal phlebitis and thrombophlebitis (G95.1)*

G09 Sequelae of inflammatory diseases of central nervous system
> **NOTE** Category G09 is to be used to indicate conditions whose primary classification is to G00-G08 as the cause of sequelae, themselves classifiable elsewhere. The "sequelae" include conditions specified as residuals.

Code first condition resulting from (sequela) of inflammatory diseases of central nervous system

Systemic atrophies primarily affecting the central nervous system (G10-G14)

G10 Huntington's disease
Huntington's chorea
Huntington's dementia

✔4th **G11 Hereditary ataxia**
> *EXCLUDES 2* *cerebral palsy (G80.-)*
> *hereditary and idiopathic neuropathy (G60.-)*
> *metabolic disorders (E70-E88)*

G11.0 Congenital nonprogressive ataxia

G11.1 Early-onset cerebellar ataxia
Early-onset cerebellar ataxia with essential tremor
Early-onset cerebellar ataxia with myoclonus [Hunt's ataxia]
Early-onset cerebellar ataxia with retained tendon reflexes
Friedreich's ataxia (autosomal recessive)
X-linked recessive spinocerebellar ataxia

G11.2 Late-onset cerebellar ataxia A

G11.3 Cerebellar ataxia with defective DNA repair
Ataxia telangiectasia [Louis-Bar]
> *EXCLUDES 2* *Cockayne's syndrome (Q87.1)*
> *other disorders of purine and pyrimidine metabolism (E79.-)*
> *xeroderma pigmentosum (Q82.1)*

G11.4 Hereditary spastic paraplegia

G11.8 Other hereditary ataxias

G11.9 Hereditary ataxia, unspecified ▽
Hereditary cerebellar ataxia NOS
Hereditary cerebellar degeneration
Hereditary cerebellar disease
Hereditary cerebellar syndrome

✔4th **G12 Spinal muscular atrophy and related syndromes**

G12.0 Infantile spinal muscular atrophy, type I [Werdnig-Hoffman]

Chapter 6. Diseases of the Nervous System

G12.1 **Other** inherited **spinal muscular atrophy**
Adult form spinal muscular atrophy
Childhood form, type II spinal muscular atrophy
Distal spinal muscular atrophy
Juvenile form, type III spinal muscular atrophy
[Kugelberg-Welander]
Progressive bulbar palsy of childhood [Fazio-Londe]
Scapuloperoneal form spinal muscular atrophy

✓5ᵗʰ **G12.2** Motor neuron disease

    G12.20 **Motor neuron disease, unspecified** ▽

    G12.21 Amyotrophic lateral sclerosis   NC Dx A
Progressive spinal muscle atrophy

    G12.22 Progressive bulbar palsy

    G12.29 **Other motor neuron disease**
Familial motor neuron disease
Primary lateral sclerosis

G12.8 **Other spinal muscular atrophies and related syndromes**

G12.9 **Spinal muscular atrophy, unspecified** ▽

✓4ᵗʰ **G13** **Systemic atrophies primarily affecting central nervous system in diseases classified elsewhere**

G13.0 *Paraneoplastic neuromyopathy and neuropathy*
Carcinomatous neuromyopathy
Sensorial paraneoplastic neuropathy [Denny Brown]
Code first underlying neoplasm (C00-D49)

G13.1 *Other systemic atrophy primarily affecting central nervous system in neoplastic disease*
Paraneoplastic limbic encephalopathy
Code first underlying neoplasm (C00-D49)

G13.2 *Systemic atrophy primarily affecting the central nervous system in myxedema*
Code first underlying disease, such as:
hypothyroidism (E03.-)
myxedematous congenital iodine deficiency (E00.1)

G13.8 *Systemic atrophy primarily affecting central nervous system in other diseases classified elsewhere*
Code first underlying disease

G14 **Postpolio syndrome**
Postpolio myelitic syndrome
EXCLUDES 1   *sequelae of poliomyelitis (B91)*

Extrapyramidal and movement disorders (G20-G26)

G20 **Parkinson's disease**   NC Dx
Hemiparkinsonism
Idiopathic Parkinsonism or Parkinson's disease
Paralysis agitans
Parkinsonism or Parkinson's disease NOS
Primary Parkinsonism or Parkinson's disease
EXCLUDES 1   *dementia with Parkinsonism (G31.83)*

✓4ᵗʰ **G21** **Secondary parkinsonism**
EXCLUDES 1   *dementia with Parkinsonism (G31.83)*
Huntington's disease (G10)
Shy-Drager syndrome (G90.3)
syphilitic Parkinsonism (A52.19)

G21.0 Malignant neuroleptic **syndrome**
Use additional code for adverse effect, if applicable, to identify drug (T43.3X5, T43.4X5, T43.505, T43.595)
EXCLUDES 1   *neuroleptic induced parkinsonism (G21.11)*

✓5ᵗʰ **G21.1** Other drug-induced **secondary parkinsonism**

    G21.11 **Neuroleptic** induced **parkinsonism**
Use additional code for adverse effect, if applicable, to identify drug (T43.3X5, T43.4X5, T43.505, T43.595)
EXCLUDES 1   *malignant neuroleptic syndrome (G21.0)*

    G21.19 **Other drug induced secondary parkinsonism**
Use additional code for adverse effect, if applicable, to identify drug (T36-T50 with fifth or sixth character 5)

G21.2 **Secondary parkinsonism due to** other external agents
Code first (T51-T65) to identify external agent

G21.3 Postencephalitic **parkinsonism**

G21.4 Vascular **parkinsonism**

G21.8 **Other secondary parkinsonism**

G21.9 **Secondary parkinsonism, unspecified** ▽

✓4ᵗʰ **G23** **Other degenerative diseases of basal ganglia**
EXCLUDES 2   *multi-system degeneration of the autonomic nervous system (G90.3)*

G23.0 **Hallervorden-Spatz disease**
Pigmentary pallidal degeneration

G23.1 **Progressive supranuclear ophthalmoplegia [Steele-Richardson-Olszewski]**
Progressive supranuclear palsy

G23.2 **Striatonigral degeneration**

G23.8 **Other specified degenerative diseases of basal ganglia**
Calcification of basal ganglia

G23.9 **Degenerative disease of basal ganglia, unspecified** ▽

✓4ᵗʰ **G24** **Dystonia**
INCLUDES   dyskinesia
EXCLUDES 2   *athetoid cerebral palsy (G80.3)*

✓5ᵗʰ **G24.0** Drug induced **dystonia**
Use additional code for adverse effect, if applicable, to identify drug (T36-T50 with fifth or sixth character5)

    G24.01 **Drug induced** subacute **dyskinesia**
Drug induced blepharospasm
Drug induced orofacial dyskinesia
Neuroleptic induced tardive dyskinesia
Tardive dyskinesia

    G24.02 **Drug induced** acute **dystonia**
Acute dystonic reaction to drugs
Neuroleptic induced acute dystonia

    G24.09 **Other drug induced dystonia**

G24.1 Genetic torsion **dystonia**
Dystonia deformans progressiva
Dystonia musculorum deformans
Familial torsion dystonia
Idiopathic familial dystonia
Idiopathic (torsion) dystonia NOS
(Schwalbe-) Ziehen-Oppenheim disease

G24.2 Idiopathic nonfamilial **dystonia**

G24.3 Spasmodic **torticollis**
EXCLUDES 1   *congenital torticollis (Q68.0)*
hysterical torticollis (F44.4)
ocular torticollis (R29.891)
psychogenic torticollis (F45.8)
torticollis NOS (M43.6)
traumatic recurrent torticollis (S13.4)

G24.4 Idiopathic orofacial **dystonia**
Orofacial dyskinesia
EXCLUDES 1   *drug induced orofacial dyskinesia (G24.01)*

G24.5 Blepharospasm
EXCLUDES 1   *drug induced blepharospasm (G24.01)*

G24.8 **Other dystonia**
Acquired torsion dystonia NOS

G24.9 **Dystonia, unspecified** ▽
Dyskinesia NOS

✓4ᵗʰ **G25** **Other extrapyramidal and movement disorders**
EXCLUDES 2   *sleep related movement disorders (G47.6-)*

G25.0 **Essential** tremor
Familial tremor
EXCLUDES 1   *tremor NOS (R25.1)*

G25.1 **Drug-induced** tremor
Use additional code for adverse effect, if applicable, to identify drug (T36-T50 with fifth or sixth character 5)

G25.2 **Other specified forms of tremor**
Intention tremor

G25.3 **Myoclonus**
Drug-induced myoclonus
Palatal myoclonus
Use additional code for adverse effect, if applicable, to identify drug (T36-T50 with fifth or sixth character 5)
EXCLUDES 1   *facial myokymia (G51.4)*
myoclonic epilepsy (G40.-)

G25.4 **Drug-induced chorea**
Use additional code for adverse effect, if applicable, to identify drug (T36-T50 with fifth or sixth character 5)

G25.5 **Other chorea**
Chorea NOS
EXCLUDES 1   *chorea NOS with heart involvement (I02.0)*
Huntington's chorea (G10)
rheumatic chorea (I02.-)
Sydenham's chorea (I02.-)

N Newborn   P Pediatric   M Maternity   A Adult   RIC RIC Dx   NC Dx Noncancer Dx   PDx Primary Dx   CC RIC CC Condition   ►◄ Revised Text   ● New Code   ▲ Revised Code Title

528   ICD-10-CM 2016

✓5ᵗʰ **G25.6 Drug induced tics and other tics of organic origin**

    G25.61 Drug induced tics

        Use additional code for adverse effect, if applicable, to identify drug (T36-T50 with fifth or sixth character 5)

    G25.69 Other tics of organic origin

        EXCLUDES 1 habit spasm (F95.9)
                tic NOS (F95.9)
                Tourette's syndrome (F95.2)

✓5ᵗʰ **G25.7 Other and unspecified drug induced movement disorders**

    Use additional code for adverse effect, if applicable, to identify drug (T36-T50 with fifth or sixth character 5)

    G25.70 Drug induced movement disorder, unspecified ▽

    G25.71 Drug induced akathisia

        Drug induced acathisia
        Neuroleptic induced acute akathisia

    G25.79 Other drug induced movement disorders

✓5ᵗʰ **G25.8 Other specified extrapyramidal and movement disorders**

    G25.81 Restless legs syndrome

    G25.82 Stiff-man syndrome

    G25.83 Benign shuddering attacks

    G25.89 Other specified extrapyramidal and movement disorders

G25.9 Extrapyramidal and movement disorder, unspecified ▽

G26 Extrapyramidal and movement disorders in diseases classified elsewhere

    Code first underlying disease

Other degenerative diseases of the nervous system (G30-G32)

✓4ᵗʰ **G30 Alzheimer's disease**

    INCLUDES Alzheimer's dementia senile and presenile forms

    Use additional code to identify:
        delirium, if applicable (F05)
        dementia with behavioral disturbance (F02.81)
        dementia without behavioral disturbance (F02.80)

    EXCLUDES 1 senile degeneration of brain NEC (G31.1)
                senile dementia NOS (F03)
                senility NOS (R41.81)

    G30.0 Alzheimer's disease with early onset NC Dx

    G30.1 Alzheimer's disease with late onset NC Dx A

    G30.8 Other Alzheimer's disease NC Dx

    G30.9 Alzheimer's disease, unspecified NC Dx ▽
        AHA: 2012, 4Q, 95

✓4ᵗʰ **G31 Other degenerative diseases of nervous system, not elsewhere classified**

    Use additional code to identify:
        dementia with behavioral disturbance (F02.81)
        dementia without behavioral disturbance (F02.80)

    EXCLUDES 2 Reye's syndrome (G93.7)

  ✓5ᵗʰ **G31.0 Frontotemporal dementia**

    G31.01 Pick's disease NC Dx
        Primary progressive aphasia
        Progressive isolated aphasia

    G31.09 Other frontotemporal dementia NC Dx
        Frontal dementia

    G31.1 Senile degeneration of brain, not elsewhere classified NC Dx
        EXCLUDES 1 Alzheimer's disease (G30.-)
                senility NOS (R41.81)

    G31.2 Degeneration of nervous system due to alcohol
        Alcoholic cerebellar ataxia
        Alcoholic cerebellar degeneration
        Alcoholic cerebral degeneration
        Alcoholic encephalopathy
        Dysfunction of the autonomic nervous system due to alcohol
        Code also associated alcoholism (F10.-)

  ✓5ᵗʰ **G31.8 Other specified degenerative diseases of nervous system**

    G31.81 Alpers disease
        Grey-matter degeneration

    G31.82 Leigh's disease
        Subacute necrotizing encephalopathy

    G31.83 Dementia with Lewy bodies NC Dx
        Dementia with Parkinsonism
        Lewy body dementia
        Lewy body disease

    G31.84 Mild cognitive impairment, so stated
        EXCLUDES 1 age related cognitive decline (R41.81)
                 altered mental status (R41.82)
                 cerebral degeneration (G31.9)
                 change in mental status (R41.82)
                 cognitive deficits following (sequelae of) cerebral hemorrhage or infarction (I69.01, I69.11, I69.21, I69.31, I69.81, I69.91)
                 cognitive impairment due to intracranial or head injury (S06.-)
                 dementia (F01.-, F02.-, F03)
                 mild memory disturbance (F06.8)
                 neurologic neglect syndrome (R41.4)
                 personality change, nonpsychotic (F68.8)

    G31.85 Corticobasal degeneration NC Dx

    G31.89 Other specified degenerative diseases of nervous system

  G31.9 Degenerative disease of nervous system, unspecified ▽

✓4ᵗʰ **G32 Other degenerative disorders of nervous system in diseases classified elsewhere**

  G32.0 Subacute combined degeneration of spinal cord in diseases classified elsewhere
    Dana-Putnam syndrome
    Sclerosis of spinal cord (combined) (dorsolateral) (posterolateral)

    Code first underlying disease, such as:
        vitamin B12 deficiency (E53.8)
        vitamin B12 deficiency:
            anemia (D51.9)
                dietary (D51.3)
                pernicious (D51.0)

    EXCLUDES 1 syphilitic combined degeneration of spinal cord (A52.11)

  ✓5ᵗʰ **G32.8 Other specified degenerative disorders of nervous system in diseases classified elsewhere**

    Code first underlying disease, such as:
        amyloidosis cerebral degeneration (E85.-)
        cerebral degeneration (due to) hypothyroidism (E00.0-E03.9)
        cerebral degeneration (due to) neoplasm (C00-D49)
        cerebral degeneration (due to) vitamin B deficiency, except thiamine (E52-E53.-)

    EXCLUDES 1 superior hemorrhagic polioencephalitis [Wernicke's encephalopathy] (E51.2)

    G32.81 Cerebellar ataxia in diseases classified elsewhere
        Code first underlying disease, such as:
            celiac disease (with gluten ataxia) (K90.0)
            cerebellar ataxia (in) neoplastic disease (paraneoplastic cerebellar degeneration) (C00-D49)
            non-celiac gluten ataxia (M35.9)
        EXCLUDES 1 systemic atrophy primarily affecting the central nervous system in alcoholic cerebellar ataxia (G31.2)
                systemic atrophy primarily affecting the central nervous system in myxedema (G13.2)

    G32.89 Other specified degenerative disorders of nervous system in diseases classified elsewhere
        Degenerative encephalopathy in diseases classified elsewhere

Demyelinating diseases of the central nervous system (G35-G37)

G35 Multiple sclerosis
    Disseminated multiple sclerosis
    Generalized multiple sclerosis
    Multiple sclerosis NOS
    Multiple sclerosis of brain stem
    Multiple sclerosis of cord

✓4ᵗʰ **G36 Other acute disseminated demyelination**
    EXCLUDES 1 postinfectious encephalitis and encephalomyelitis NOS (G04.01)

  G36.0 Neuromyelitis optica [Devic]
    Demyelination in optic neuritis
    EXCLUDES 1 optic neuritis NOS (H46)

  G36.1 Acute and subacute hemorrhagic leukoencephalitis [Hurst]

  G36.8 Other specified acute disseminated demyelination

  G36.9 Acute disseminated demyelination, unspecified ▽

✔ Add'l Character Required   ✓x7ᵗʰ Placeholder Alert   RUG IV Special Care High Dx   RUG IV Clinically Complex Dx   RUG IV Special Care Low Dx   Manifestation Code   Other Specified Code   ▽ Unspecified Code

Chapter 6. Diseases of the Nervous System

✓4ᵗʰ **G37** **Other demyelinating diseases of central nervous system**

  G37.0 **Diffuse sclerosis of central nervous system**
Periaxial encephalitis
Schilder's disease
EXCLUDES 1 *X linked adrenoleukodystrophy (E71.52-)*

  G37.1 **Central demyelination of corpus callosum**

  G37.2 **Central pontine myelinolysis**

  G37.3 **Acute transverse myelitis in demyelinating disease**   CC
of central nervous system
Acute transverse myelitis NOS
Acute transverse myelopathy
EXCLUDES 1 *multiple sclerosis (G35)*
neuromyelitis optica [Devic] (G36.0)
RIC Excl: 03 Non-traumatic brain injury

  G37.4 **Subacute necrotizing myelitis of central nervous system**   CC
RIC Excl: 03 Non-traumatic brain injury

  G37.5 **Concentric sclerosis [Balo] of central nervous system**

  G37.8 **Other specified demyelinating diseases of central nervous system**

  G37.9 **Demyelinating disease of central nervous system,**   ▽
unspecified

Episodic and paroxysmal disorders (G40-G47)

✓4ᵗʰ **G40** **Epilepsy and recurrent seizures**
NOTE The following terms are to be considered equivalent to
intractable: pharmacoresistant (pharmacologically resistant),
treatment resistant, refractory (medically) and poorly
controlled
EXCLUDES 1 *conversion disorder with seizures (F44.5)*
convulsions NOS (R56.9)
hippocampal sclerosis (G93.81)
mesial temporal sclerosis (G93.81)
post traumatic seizures (R56.1)
seizure (convulsive) NOS (R56.9)
seizure of newborn (P90)
temporal sclerosis (G93.81)
Todd's paralysis (G83.8)

  ✓5ᵗʰ **G40.0** **Localization-related (focal) (partial) idiopathic epilepsy and**
epileptic syndromes with seizures of localized onset
Benign childhood epilepsy with centrotemporal EEG spikes
Childhood epilepsy with occipital EEG paroxysms
EXCLUDES 1 *adult onset localization-related epilepsy (G40.1-,*
G40.2-)

    ✓6ᵗʰ **G40.00** **Localization-related (focal) (partial) idiopathic**
epilepsy and epileptic syndromes with seizures of
localized onset, not intractable
Localization-related (focal) (partial) idiopathic epilepsy
and epileptic syndromes with seizures of
localized onset without intractability

      G40.001 **Localization-related (focal) (partial)**
idiopathic epilepsy and epileptic
syndromes with seizures of localized
onset, not intractable, with status
epilepticus

      G40.009 **Localization-related (focal) (partial)**
idiopathic epilepsy and epileptic
syndromes with seizures of localized
onset, not intractable, without status
epilepticus
Localization-related (focal) (partial)
idiopathic epilepsy and epileptic
syndromes with seizures of localized
onset NOS

    ✓6ᵗʰ **G40.01** **Localization-related (focal) (partial) idiopathic**
epilepsy and epileptic syndromes with seizures of
localized onset, intractable

      G40.011 **Localization-related (focal) (partial)**
idiopathic epilepsy and epileptic
syndromes with seizures of localized
onset, intractable, with status epilepticus

      G40.019 **Localization-related (focal) (partial)**
idiopathic epilepsy and epileptic
syndromes with seizures of localized
onset, intractable, without status
epilepticus

  ✓5ᵗʰ **G40.1** **Localization-related (focal) (partial) symptomatic epilepsy**
and epileptic syndromes with simple partial seizures
Attacks without alteration of consciousness
Epilepsia partialis continua [Kozhevnikof]
Simple partial seizures developing into secondarily generalized
seizures

    ✓6ᵗʰ **G40.10** **Localization-related (focal) (partial) symptomatic**
epilepsy and epileptic syndromes with simple partial
seizures, not intractable
Localization-related (focal) (partial) symptomatic
epilepsy and epileptic syndromes with simple
partial seizures without intractability

      G40.101 **Localization-related (focal) (partial)**
symptomatic epilepsy and epileptic
syndromes with simple partial seizures,
not intractable, with status epilepticus

      G40.109 **Localization-related (focal) (partial)**
symptomatic epilepsy and epileptic
syndromes with simple partial seizures,
not intractable, without status epilepticus
Localization-related (focal) (partial)
symptomatic epilepsy and epileptic
syndromes with simple partial seizures
NOS

    ✓6ᵗʰ **G40.11** **Localization-related (focal) (partial) symptomatic**
epilepsy and epileptic syndromes with simple partial
seizures, intractable

      G40.111 **Localization-related (focal) (partial)**
symptomatic epilepsy and epileptic
syndromes with simple partial seizures,
intractable, with status epilepticus

      G40.119 **Localization-related (focal) (partial)**
symptomatic epilepsy and epileptic
syndromes with simple partial seizures,
intractable, without status epilepticus

  ✓5ᵗʰ **G40.2** **Localization-related (focal) (partial) symptomatic epilepsy**
and epileptic syndromes with complex partial seizures
Attacks with alteration of consciousness, often with
automatisms
Complex partial seizures developing into secondarily
generalized seizures

    ✓6ᵗʰ **G40.20** **Localization-related (focal) (partial) symptomatic**
epilepsy and epileptic syndromes with complex
partial seizures, not intractable
Localization-related (focal) (partial) symptomatic
epilepsy and epileptic syndromes with complex
partial seizures without intractability

      G40.201 **Localization-related (focal) (partial)**
symptomatic epilepsy and epileptic
syndromes with complex partial seizures,
not intractable, with status epilepticus

      G40.209 **Localization-related (focal) (partial)**
symptomatic epilepsy and epileptic
syndromes with complex partial seizures,
not intractable, without status epilepticus
Localization-related (focal) (partial)
symptomatic epilepsy and epileptic
syndromes with complex partial
seizures NOS

    ✓6ᵗʰ **G40.21** **Localization-related (focal) (partial) symptomatic**
epilepsy and epileptic syndromes with complex
partial seizures, intractable

      G40.211 **Localization-related (focal) (partial)**
symptomatic epilepsy and epileptic
syndromes with complex partial seizures,
intractable, with status epilepticus

      G40.219 **Localization-related (focal) (partial)**
symptomatic epilepsy and epileptic
syndromes with complex partial seizures,
intractable, without status epilepticus

  ✓5ᵗʰ **G40.3** **Generalized idiopathic epilepsy and epileptic syndromes**
Code also MERRF syndrome, if applicable (E88.42)

    ✓6ᵗʰ **G40.30** **Generalized idiopathic epilepsy and epileptic**
syndromes, not intractable
Generalized idiopathic epilepsy and epileptic
syndromes without intractability

      G40.301 **Generalized idiopathic epilepsy and**   CC
epileptic syndromes, not intractable,
with status epilepticus
RIC Excl: 02 Traumatic brain injury; 03
Non-traumatic brain injury

      G40.309 **Generalized idiopathic epilepsy and**
epileptic syndromes, not intractable,
without status epilepticus
Generalized idiopathic epilepsy and
epileptic syndromes NOS

N Newborn   P Pediatric   M Maternity   A Adult   RIC RIC Dx   NC Dx Noncancer Dx   PDx Primary Dx   CC RIC CC Condition   ►◄ Revised Text   ● New Code   ▲ Revised Code Title

530   ICD-10-CM 2016

G40.31 **Generalized idiopathic epilepsy and epileptic syndromes,** intractable

    G40.311 **Generalized idiopathic epilepsy and epileptic syndromes, intractable, with status epilepticus** `CC`
       RIC Excl: 02 Traumatic brain injury; 03 Non-traumatic brain injury

    G40.319 **Generalized idiopathic epilepsy and epileptic syndromes, intractable, without status epilepticus** `CC`
       RIC Excl: 02 Traumatic brain injury; 03 Non-traumatic brain injury

G40.A Absence **epileptic syndrome**
   Childhood absence epilepsy [pyknolepsy]
   Juvenile absence epilepsy
   Absence epileptic syndrome, NOS

   G40.A0 **Absence epileptic syndrome,** not intractable
     G40.A01 **Absence epileptic syndrome, not intractable, with status epilepticus**
     G40.A09 **Absence epileptic syndrome, not intractable, without status epilepticus**

   G40.A1 **Absence epileptic syndrome,** intractable
     G40.A11 **Absence epileptic syndrome, intractable, with status epilepticus**
     G40.A19 **Absence epileptic syndrome, intractable, without status epilepticus**

G40.B Juvenile myoclonic epilepsy [impulsive petit mal]

   G40.B0 **Juvenile myoclonic epilepsy,** not intractable
     G40.B01 **Juvenile myoclonic epilepsy, not intractable, with status epilepticus**
     G40.B09 **Juvenile myoclonic epilepsy, not intractable, without status epilepticus**

   G40.B1 **Juvenile myoclonic epilepsy,** intractable
     G40.B11 **Juvenile myoclonic epilepsy, intractable, with status epilepticus**
     G40.B19 **Juvenile myoclonic epilepsy, intractable, without status epilepticus**

G40.4 Other generalized **epilepsy and epileptic syndromes**
   Epilepsy with grand mal seizures on awakening
   Epilepsy with myoclonic absences
   Epilepsy with myoclonic-astatic seizures
   Grand mal seizure NOS
   Nonspecific atonic epileptic seizures
   Nonspecific clonic epileptic seizures
   Nonspecific myoclonic epileptic seizures
   Nonspecific tonic epileptic seizures
   Nonspecific tonic-clonic epileptic seizures
   Symptomatic early myoclonic encephalopathy

   G40.40 **Other generalized epilepsy and epileptic syndromes,** not intractable
     Other generalized epilepsy and epileptic syndromes without intractability
     Other generalized epilepsy and epileptic syndromes NOS
     G40.401 **Other generalized epilepsy and epileptic syndromes, not intractable, with status epilepticus**
     G40.409 **Other generalized epilepsy and epileptic syndromes, not intractable, without status epilepticus**

   G40.41 **Other generalized epilepsy and epileptic syndromes,** intractable
     G40.411 **Other generalized epilepsy and epileptic syndromes, intractable, with status epilepticus** `CC`
       RIC Excl: 02 Traumatic brain injury; 03 Non-traumatic brain injury
     G40.419 **Other generalized epilepsy and epileptic syndromes, intractable, without status epilepticus** `CC`
       RIC Excl: 02 Traumatic brain injury; 03 Non-traumatic brain injury

G40.5 **Epileptic seizures related to** external causes
   Epileptic seizures related to alcohol
   Epileptic seizures related to drugs
   Epileptic seizures related to hormonal changes
   Epileptic seizures related to sleep deprivation
   Epileptic seizures related to stress
   Code also, if applicable, associated epilepsy and recurrent seizures (G40.-)
   Use additional code for adverse effect, if applicable, to identify drug (T36-T50 with fifth or sixth character 5)

   G40.50 **Epileptic seizures related to external causes,** not intractable
     G40.501 **Epileptic seizures related to external causes, not intractable, with status epilepticus**
     G40.509 **Epileptic seizures related to external causes, not intractable, without status epilepticus**
       Epileptic seizures related to external causes, NOS

G40.8 **Other epilepsy and recurrent seizures**
   Epilepsies and epileptic syndromes undetermined as to whether they are focal or generalized
   Landau-Kleffner syndrome

   G40.80 **Other epilepsy**
     G40.801 **Other epilepsy, not intractable, with status epilepticus**
       Other epilepsy without intractability with status epilepticus
     G40.802 **Other epilepsy, not intractable, without status epilepticus**
       Other epilepsy without intractability without status epilepticus
     G40.803 **Other epilepsy, intractable, with status epilepticus**
     G40.804 **Other epilepsy, intractable, without status epilepticus**

   G40.81 **Lennox-Gastaut syndrome**
     G40.811 **Lennox-Gastaut syndrome,** not intractable, with status epilepticus
     G40.812 **Lennox-Gastaut syndrome,** not intractable, without status epilepticus
     G40.813 **Lennox-Gastaut syndrome,** intractable, with status epilepticus
     G40.814 **Lennox-Gastaut syndrome,** intractable, without status epilepticus

   G40.82 **Epileptic spasms**
     Infantile spasms
     Salaam attacks
     West's syndrome
     G40.821 **Epileptic spasms,** not intractable, with status epilepticus
     G40.822 **Epileptic spasms,** not intractable, without status epilepticus
     G40.823 **Epileptic spasms,** intractable, with status epilepticus
     G40.824 **Epileptic spasms,** intractable, without status epilepticus

   G40.89 **Other seizures**
     `EXCLUDES 1` post traumatic seizures (R56.1)
       recurrent seizures NOS (G40.909)
       seizure NOS (R56.9)

G40.9 **Epilepsy,** unspecified

   G40.90 **Epilepsy, unspecified,** not intractable
     Epilepsy, unspecified, without intractability
     G40.901 **Epilepsy, unspecified, not intractable, with status epilepticus** ▽
     G40.909 **Epilepsy, unspecified, not intractable, without status epilepticus** ▽
       Epilepsy NOS
       Epileptic convulsions NOS
       Epileptic fits NOS
       Epileptic seizures NOS
       Recurrent seizures NOS
       Seizure disorder NOS

   G40.91 **Epilepsy, unspecified,** intractable
     Intractable seizure disorder NOS
     G40.911 **Epilepsy, unspecified, intractable, with status epilepticus** ▽

☑ Add'l Character Required   `✓x7th` Placeholder Alert   RUG IV Special Care High Dx   RUG IV Clinically Complex Dx   RUG IV Special Care Low Dx   Manifestation Code   Other Specified Code   ▽ Unspecified Code

G40.919   **Epilepsy, unspecified, intractable,** ▽
           without status epilepticus

✓4ᵗʰ **G43 Migraine**
       NOTE   The following terms are to be considered equivalent to
                  intractable: pharmacoresistant (pharmacologically resistant),
                  treatment resistant, refractory (medically) and poorly
                  controlled.
       Use additional code for adverse effect, if applicable, to identify drug
       (T36-T50 with fifth or sixth character 5)
       EXCLUDES 1   headache NOS (R51)
                        lower half migraine (G44.00)
       EXCLUDES 2   headache syndromes (G44.-)

✓5ᵗʰ **G43.0 Migraine** without aura
            Common migraine
            EXCLUDES 1   chronic migraine without aura (G43.7-)

   ✓6ᵗʰ **G43.00   Migraine without aura,** not intractable
                   Migraine without aura without mention of refractory
                   migraine
         G43.001   Migraine without aura, not intractable,
                     with status migrainosus
         G43.009   Migraine without aura, not intractable,
                     without status migrainosus
                     Migraine without aura NOS

   ✓6ᵗʰ **G43.01   Migraine without aura,** intractable
                   Migraine without aura with refractory migraine
         G43.011   Migraine without aura, intractable, with
                     status migrainosus
         G43.019   Migraine without aura, intractable,
                     without status migrainosus

✓5ᵗʰ **G43.1 Migraine** with aura
            Basilar migraine
            Classical migraine
            Migraine equivalents
            Migraine preceded or accompanied by transient focal
                neurological phenomena
            Migraine triggered seizures
            Migraine with acute-onset aura
            Migraine with aura without headache (migraine equivalents)
            Migraine with prolonged aura
            Migraine with typical aura
            Retinal migraine
            Code also any associated seizure (G40.-, R56.9)
            EXCLUDES 1   persistent migraine aura (G43.5-, G43.6-)

   ✓6ᵗʰ **G43.10   Migraine with aura,** not intractable
                   Migraine with aura without mention of refractory
                   migraine
         G43.101   Migraine with aura, not intractable, with
                     status migrainosus
         G43.109   Migraine with aura, not intractable,
                     without status migrainosus
                     Migraine with aura NOS

   ✓6ᵗʰ **G43.11   Migraine with aura,** intractable
                   Migraine with aura with refractory migraine
         G43.111   Migraine with aura, intractable, with
                     status migrainosus
         G43.119   Migraine with aura, intractable, without
                     status migrainosus

✓5ᵗʰ **G43.4 Hemiplegic migraine**
            Familial migraine
            Sporadic migraine

   ✓6ᵗʰ **G43.40   Hemiplegic migraine,** not intractable
                   Hemiplegic migraine without refractory migraine
         G43.401   Hemiplegic migraine, not intractable, with
                     status migrainosus
         G43.409   Hemiplegic migraine, not intractable,
                     without status migrainosus
                     Hemiplegic migraine NOS

   ✓6ᵗʰ **G43.41   Hemiplegic migraine,** intractable
                   Hemiplegic migraine with refractory migraine
         G43.411   Hemiplegic migraine, intractable, with
                     status migrainosus
         G43.419   Hemiplegic migraine, intractable, without
                     status migrainosus

✓5ᵗʰ **G43.5 Persistent migraine** aura without cerebral infarction

   ✓6ᵗʰ **G43.50   Persistent migraine aura without cerebral infarction,**
                   not intractable
                   Persistent migraine aura without cerebral infarction,
                   without refractory migraine

         G43.501   Persistent migraine aura without cerebral
                     infarction, not intractable, with status
                     migrainosus
         G43.509   Persistent migraine aura without cerebral
                     infarction, not intractable, without status
                     migrainosus
                     Persistent migraine aura NOS

   ✓6ᵗʰ **G43.51   Persistent migraine aura without cerebral infarction,**
                   intractable
                   Persistent migraine aura without cerebral infarction,
                   with refractory migraine
         G43.511   Persistent migraine aura without cerebral
                     infarction, intractable, with status
                     migrainosus
         G43.519   Persistent migraine aura without cerebral
                     infarction, intractable, without status
                     migrainosus

✓5ᵗʰ **G43.6 Persistent migraine** aura with cerebral infarction
            Code also the type of cerebral infarction (I63.-)

   ✓6ᵗʰ **G43.60   Persistent migraine aura with cerebral infarction,**
                   not intractable
                   Persistent migraine aura with cerebral infarction,
                   without refractory migraine
         G43.601   Persistent migraine aura with cerebral
                     infarction, not intractable, with status
                     migrainosus
         G43.609   Persistent migraine aura with cerebral
                     infarction, not intractable, without status
                     migrainosus

   ✓6ᵗʰ **G43.61   Persistent migraine aura with cerebral infarction,**
                   intractable
                   Persistent migraine aura with cerebral infarction, with
                   refractory migraine
         G43.611   Persistent migraine aura with cerebral
                     infarction, intractable, with status
                     migrainosus
         G43.619   Persistent migraine aura with cerebral
                     infarction, intractable, without status
                     migrainosus

✓5ᵗʰ **G43.7 Chronic migraine** without aura
            Transformed migraine
            EXCLUDES 1   migraine without aura (G43.0-)

   ✓6ᵗʰ **G43.70   Chronic migraine without aura,** not intractable
                   Chronic migraine without aura, without refractory
                   migraine
         G43.701   Chronic migraine without aura, not
                     intractable, with status migrainosus
         G43.709   Chronic migraine without aura, not
                     intractable, without status migrainosus
                     Chronic migraine without aura NOS

   ✓6ᵗʰ **G43.71   Chronic migraine without aura,** intractable
                   Chronic migraine without aura, with refractory
                   migraine
         G43.711   Chronic migraine without aura,
                     intractable, with status migrainosus
         G43.719   Chronic migraine without aura,
                     intractable, without status migrainosus

✓5ᵗʰ **G43.A Cyclical vomiting**
         G43.A0   Cyclical vomiting, not intractable
                   Cyclical vomiting, without refractory migraine
         G43.A1   Cyclical vomiting, intractable
                   Cyclical vomiting, with refractory migraine

✓5ᵗʰ **G43.B Ophthalmoplegic migraine**
         G43.B0   Ophthalmoplegic migraine, not intractable
                   Ophthalmoplegic migraine, without refractory
                   migraine
         G43.B1   Ophthalmoplegic migraine, intractable
                   Ophthalmoplegic migraine, with refractory migraine

✓5ᵗʰ **G43.C Periodic headache syndromes** in child or adult
         G43.C0   Periodic headache syndromes in child or adult, not
                   intractable
                   Periodic headache syndromes in child or adult,
                   without refractory migraine
         G43.C1   Periodic headache syndromes in child or adult,
                   intractable
                   Periodic headache syndromes in child or adult, with
                   refractory migraine

✓5ᵗʰ **G43.D** Abdominal **migraine**

    G43.D0 Abdominal **migraine,** not intractable
        Abdominal migraine, without refractory migraine

    G43.D1 Abdominal **migraine,** intractable
        Abdominal migraine, with refractory migraine

✓5ᵗʰ **G43.8** Other **migraine**

  ✓6ᵗʰ **G43.80** Other **migraine,** not intractable
      Other migraine, without refractory migraine

      G43.801 **Other migraine, not intractable, with status migrainosus**

      G43.809 **Other migraine, not intractable,** without **status migrainosus**

  ✓6ᵗʰ **G43.81** Other **migraine,** intractable
      Other migraine, with refractory migraine

      G43.811 **Other migraine, intractable, with status migrainosus**

      G43.819 **Other migraine, intractable,** without **status migrainosus**

  ✓6ᵗʰ **G43.82** Menstrual **migraine,** not intractable
      Menstrual headache, not intractable
      Menstrual migraine, without refractory migraine
      Menstrually related migraine, not intractable
      Pre-menstrual headache, not intractable
      Pre-menstrual migraine, not intractable
      Pure menstrual migraine, not intractable
      Code also associated premenstrual tension syndrome (N94.3)

      G43.821 **Menstrual migraine, not intractable, with status migrainosus** ♀

      G43.829 **Menstrual migraine, not intractable, without status migrainosus** ♀
        Menstrual migraine NOS

  ✓6ᵗʰ **G43.83** Menstrual **migraine,** intractable
      Menstrual headache, intractable
      Menstrual migraine, with refractory migraine
      Menstrually related migraine, intractable
      Pre-menstrual headache, intractable
      Pre-menstrual migraine, intractable
      Pure menstrual migraine, intractable
      Code also associated premenstrual tension syndrome (N94.3)

      G43.831 **Menstrual migraine, intractable, with status migrainosus** ♀

      G43.839 **Menstrual migraine, intractable, without status migrainosus** ♀

✓5ᵗʰ **G43.9** **Migraine, unspecified**

  ✓6ᵗʰ **G43.90** **Migraine, unspecified,** not intractable
      Migraine, unspecified, without refractory migraine

      G43.901 **Migraine, unspecified, not intractable, with status migrainosus** ▽
        Status migrainosus NOS

      G43.909 **Migraine, unspecified, not intractable, without status migrainosus** ▽
        Migraine NOS

  ✓6ᵗʰ **G43.91** **Migraine, unspecified,** intractable
      Migraine, unspecified, with refractory migraine

      G43.911 **Migraine, unspecified, intractable, with status migrainosus** ▽

      G43.919 **Migraine, unspecified, intractable, without status migrainosus** ▽

✓4ᵗʰ **G44** Other headache **syndromes**
    EXCLUDES 1 headache NOS (R51)
    EXCLUDES 2 atypical facial pain (G50.1)
        headache due to lumbar puncture (G97.1)
        migraines (G43.-)
        trigeminal neuralgia (G50.0)

  ✓5ᵗʰ **G44.0** Cluster headaches **and other trigeminal autonomic cephalgias (TAC)**

    ✓6ᵗʰ **G44.00** **Cluster headache syndrome,** unspecified
        Ciliary neuralgia
        Cluster headache NOS
        Histamine cephalgia
        Lower half migraine
        Migrainous neuralgia

        G44.001 **Cluster headache syndrome, unspecified,** intractable ▽

        G44.009 **Cluster headache syndrome, unspecified,** not intractable ▽
            Cluster headache syndrome NOS

  ✓6ᵗʰ **G44.01** Episodic **cluster headache**

      G44.011 **Episodic cluster headache,** intractable

      G44.019 **Episodic cluster headache,** not intractable
        Episodic cluster headache NOS

  ✓6ᵗʰ **G44.02** Chronic **cluster headache**

      G44.021 **Chronic cluster headache,** intractable

      G44.029 **Chronic cluster headache,** not intractable
        Chronic cluster headache NOS

  ✓6ᵗʰ **G44.03** Episodic paroxysmal **hemicrania**
      Paroxysmal hemicrania NOS

      G44.031 **Episodic paroxysmal hemicrania,** intractable

      G44.039 **Episodic paroxysmal hemicrania,** not intractable
        Episodic paroxysmal hemicrania NOS

  ✓6ᵗʰ **G44.04** Chronic paroxysmal **hemicrania**

      G44.041 **Chronic paroxysmal hemicrania,** intractable

      G44.049 **Chronic paroxysmal hemicrania,** not intractable
        Chronic paroxysmal hemicrania NOS

  ✓6ᵗʰ **G44.05** Short lasting unilateral **neuralgiform headache with conjunctival injection and tearing (SUNCT)**

      G44.051 **Short lasting unilateral neuralgiform headache with conjunctival injection and tearing (SUNCT),** intractable

      G44.059 **Short lasting unilateral neuralgiform headache with conjunctival injection and tearing (SUNCT),** not intractable
        Short lasting unilateral neuralgiform headache with conjunctival injection and tearing (SUNCT) NOS

  ✓6ᵗʰ **G44.09** Other trigeminal autonomic cephalgias **(TAC)**

      G44.091 **Other trigeminal autonomic cephalgias (TAC),** intractable

      G44.099 **Other trigeminal autonomic cephalgias syndrome (TAC),** not intractable

  G44.1 Vascular **headache, not elsewhere classified**
    EXCLUDES 2 cluster headache (G44.0)
        complicated headache syndromes (G44.5-)
        drug-induced headache (G44.4-)
        migraine (G43.-)
        other specified headache syndromes (G44.8-)
        post-traumatic headache (G44.3-)
        tension-type headache (G44.2-)

  ✓5ᵗʰ **G44.2** Tension-type **headache**

    ✓6ᵗʰ **G44.20** **Tension-type headache,** unspecified

      G44.201 **Tension-type headache, unspecified,** intractable ▽

      G44.209 **Tension-type headache, unspecified,** not intractable ▽
        Tension headache NOS

    ✓6ᵗʰ **G44.21** Episodic **tension-type headache**

      G44.211 **Episodic tension-type headache,** intractable

      G44.219 **Episodic tension-type headache,** not intractable
        Episodic tension-type headache NOS

    ✓6ᵗʰ **G44.22** Chronic **tension-type headache**

      G44.221 **Chronic tension-type headache,** intractable

      G44.229 **Chronic tension-type headache,** not intractable
        Chronic tension-type headache NOS

  ✓5ᵗʰ **G44.3** Post-traumatic **headache**

    ✓6ᵗʰ **G44.30** **Post-traumatic headache,** unspecified

      G44.301 **Post-traumatic headache, unspecified,** intractable ▽

      G44.309 **Post-traumatic headache, unspecified,** not intractable ▽
        Post-traumatic headache NOS

    ✓6ᵗʰ **G44.31** Acute **post-traumatic headache**

      G44.311 **Acute post-traumatic headache,** intractable

      G44.319 **Acute post-traumatic headache,** not intractable
        Acute post-traumatic headache NOS

Chapter 6. Diseases of the Nervous System

☑6ᵗʰ **G44.32**   Chronic post-traumatic headache

> **G44.321**   **Chronic post-traumatic headache, intractable**
>
> **G44.329**   **Chronic post-traumatic headache, not intractable**
> > Chronic post-traumatic headache NOS

☑5ᵗʰ **G44.4**   **Drug-induced headache, not elsewhere classified**
> Medication overuse headache
>
> Use additional code for adverse effect, if applicable, to identify drug (T36-T50 with fifth or sixth character 5)

> **G44.40**   **Drug-induced headache, not elsewhere classified, not intractable**
>
> **G44.41**   **Drug-induced headache, not elsewhere classified, intractable**

☑5ᵗʰ **G44.5**   Complicated headache syndromes

> **G44.51**   Hemicrania continua
>
> **G44.52**   New daily persistent headache (NDPH)
>
> **G44.53**   Primary thunderclap headache
>
> **G44.59**   Other complicated headache syndrome

☑5ᵗʰ **G44.8**   Other specified headache syndromes

> **G44.81**   Hypnic headache
>
> **G44.82**   Headache associated with sexual activity
> > Orgasmic headache
> > Preorgasmic headache
>
> **G44.83**   Primary cough headache
>
> **G44.84**   Primary exertional headache
>
> **G44.85**   Primary stabbing headache
>
> **G44.89**   Other headache syndrome

☑4ᵗʰ **G45**   **Transient cerebral ischemic attacks and related syndromes**
> EXCLUDES 1   neonatal cerebral ischemia (P91.0)
> > transient retinal artery occlusion (H34.0-)

> **G45.0**   **Vertebro-basilar artery syndrome**
>
> **G45.1**   **Carotid artery syndrome (hemispheric)**   🅰
>
> **G45.2**   **Multiple and bilateral precerebral artery syndromes**   🅰
>
> **G45.3**   **Amaurosis fugax**
>
> **G45.4**   **Transient global amnesia**   NC Dx
> > EXCLUDES 1   amnesia NOS (R41.3)
>
> **G45.8**   **Other transient cerebral ischemic attacks and related syndromes**   🅰
>
> **G45.9**   **Transient cerebral ischemic attack, unspecified**   🅰▽
> > Spasm of cerebral artery
> > TIA
> > Transient cerebral ischemia NOS

☑4ᵗʰ **G46**   **Vascular syndromes of brain in cerebrovascular diseases**
> Code first underlying cerebrovascular disease (I60-I69)

> **G46.0**   Middle cerebral artery syndrome   🅰
>
> **G46.1**   Anterior cerebral artery syndrome   🅰
>
> **G46.2**   Posterior cerebral artery syndrome   🅰
>
> **G46.3**   Brain stem stroke syndrome   NC Dx
> > Benedikt syndrome
> > Claude syndrome
> > Foville syndrome
> > Millard-Gubler syndrome
> > Wallenberg syndrome
> > Weber syndrome
>
> **G46.4**   Cerebellar stroke syndrome   NC Dx
>
> **G46.5**   Pure motor lacunar syndrome   NC Dx
>
> **G46.6**   Pure sensory lacunar syndrome   NC Dx
>
> **G46.7**   Other lacunar syndromes   NC Dx
>
> **G46.8**   Other vascular syndromes of brain in cerebrovascular diseases   NC Dx

☑4ᵗʰ **G47**   **Sleep disorders**
> EXCLUDES 2   nightmares (F51.5)
> > nonorganic sleep disorders (F51.-)
> > sleep terrors (F51.4)
> > sleepwalking (F51.3)

☑5ᵗʰ **G47.0**   **Insomnia**
> EXCLUDES 2   alcohol related insomnia (F10.182, F10.282, F10.982)
> > drug-related insomnia (F11.182, F11.282, F11.982, F13.182, F13.282, F13.982, F14.182, F14.282,F14.982, F15.182, F15.282, F15.982, F19.182, F19.282, F19.982)
> > idiopathic insomnia (F51.01)
> > insomnia due to a mental disorder (F51.05)
> > insomnia not due to a substance or known physiological condition (F51.0-)
> > nonorganic insomnia (F51.0-)
> > primary insomnia (F51.01)
> > sleep apnea (G47.3-)

> **G47.00**   **Insomnia, unspecified**   ▽
> > Insomnia NOS
>
> **G47.01**   **Insomnia** due to medical condition
> > Code also associated medical condition
>
> **G47.09**   **Other insomnia**

☑5ᵗʰ **G47.1**   **Hypersomnia**
> EXCLUDES 2   alcohol-related hypersomnia (F10.182, F10.282, F10.982)
> > drug-related hypersomnia (F11.182, F11.282, F11.982, F13.182, F13.282, F13.982, F14.182,F14.282, F14.982, F15.182, F15.282, F15.982, F19.182, F19.282, F19.982)
> > hypersomnia due to a mental disorder (F51.13)
> > hypersomnia not due to a substance or known physiological condition (F51.1-)
> > primary hypersomnia (F51.11)
> > sleep apnea (G47.3-)

> **G47.10**   **Hypersomnia, unspecified**   ▽
> > Hypersomnia NOS
>
> **G47.11**   Idiopathic hypersomnia with long sleep time
> > Idiopathic hypersomnia NOS
>
> **G47.12**   Idiopathic hypersomnia without long sleep time
>
> **G47.13**   Recurrent hypersomnia
> > Kleine-Levin syndrome
> > Menstrual related hypersomnia
>
> **G47.14**   Hypersomnia due to medical condition
> > Code also associated medical condition
>
> **G47.19**   Other hypersomnia

☑5ᵗʰ **G47.2**   **Circadian rhythm sleep disorders**
> Disorders of the sleep wake schedule
> Inversion of nyctohemeral rhythm
> Inversion of sleep rhythm

> **G47.20**   **Circadian rhythm sleep disorder, unspecified type** ▽
> > Sleep wake schedule disorder NOS
>
> **G47.21**   **Circadian rhythm sleep disorder, delayed sleep phase type**
> > Delayed sleep phase syndrome
>
> **G47.22**   **Circadian rhythm sleep disorder, advanced sleep phase type**
>
> **G47.23**   **Circadian rhythm sleep disorder, irregular sleep wake type**
> > Irregular sleep-wake pattern
>
> **G47.24**   **Circadian rhythm sleep disorder, free running type**
>
> **G47.25**   **Circadian rhythm sleep disorder, jet lag type**
>
> **G47.26**   **Circadian rhythm sleep disorder, shift work type**
>
> **G47.27**   *Circadian rhythm sleep disorder in conditions classified elsewhere*
> > *Code first underlying condition*
>
> **G47.29**   **Other circadian rhythm sleep disorder**

☑5ᵗʰ **G47.3**   **Sleep apnea**
> Code also any associated underlying condition
> EXCLUDES 1   apnea NOS (R06.81)
> > Cheyne-Stokes breathing (R06.3)
> > pickwickian syndrome (E66.2)
> > sleep apnea of newborn (P28.3)

> **G47.30**   **Sleep apnea, unspecified**   ▽
> > Sleep apnea NOS
>
> **G47.31**   Primary central sleep apnea
>
> **G47.32**   High altitude periodic breathing
>
> **G47.33**   Obstructive sleep apnea (adult) (pediatric)
> > EXCLUDES 1   obstructive sleep apnea of newborn (P28.3)
>
> **G47.34**   Idiopathic sleep related nonobstructive alveolar hypoventilation
> > Sleep related hypoxia
>
> **G47.35**   Congenital central alveolar hypoventilation syndrome

Ⓝ Newborn   Ⓟ Pediatric   Ⓜ Maternity   🅰 Adult   RIC RIC Dx   NC Dx Noncancer Dx   PDx Primary Dx   CC RIC CC Condition   ▶◀ Revised Text   ● New Code   ▲ Revised Code Title

534   ICD-10-CM 2016

G47.36 *Sleep related hypoventilation in conditions classified elsewhere*
  Sleep related hypoxemia in conditions classified elsewhere
  Code first underlying condition

G47.37 *Central sleep apnea in conditions classified elsewhere*
  Code first underlying condition

G47.39 **Other sleep apnea**

✓5ᵗʰ **G47.4 Narcolepsy and cataplexy**

✓6ᵗʰ **G47.41** **Narcolepsy**

G47.411 **Narcolepsy with cataplexy**

G47.419 **Narcolepsy without cataplexy**
  Narcolepsy NOS

✓6ᵗʰ **G47.42** **Narcolepsy in conditions classified elsewhere**
  Code first underlying condition

G47.421 *Narcolepsy in conditions classified elsewhere with cataplexy*

G47.429 *Narcolepsy in conditions classified elsewhere without cataplexy*

✓5ᵗʰ **G47.5 Parasomnia**
  EXCLUDES 1 alcohol induced parasomnia (F10.182, F10.282, F10.982)
    drug induced parasomnia (F11.182, F11.282, F11.982, F13.182, F13.282, F13.982, F14.182, F14.282, F14.982, F15.182, F15.282, F15.982, F19.182, F19.282, F19.982)
    parasomnia not due to a substance or known physiological condition (F51.8)

G47.50 **Parasomnia, unspecified** ▽
  Parasomnia NOS

G47.51 **Confusional arousals**

G47.52 **REM sleep behavior disorder**

G47.53 **Recurrent isolated sleep paralysis**

G47.54 *Parasomnia in conditions classified elsewhere*
  Code first underlying condition

G47.59 **Other parasomnia**

✓5ᵗʰ **G47.6 Sleep related movement disorders**
  EXCLUDES 2 restless legs syndrome (G25.81)

G47.61 **Periodic limb movement disorder**

G47.62 **Sleep related leg cramps**

G47.63 **Sleep related bruxism**
  EXCLUDES 1 psychogenic bruxism (F45.8)

G47.69 **Other sleep related movement disorders**

G47.8 Other sleep disorders

G47.9 Sleep disorder, unspecified ▽
  Sleep disorder NOS

Nerve, nerve root and plexus disorders (G50-G59)

EXCLUDES 1 current traumatic nerve, nerve root and plexus disorders—see Injury, nerve by body region
  neuralgia NOS (M79.2)
  neuritis NOS (M79.2)
  peripheral neuritis in pregnancy (O26.82-)
  radiculitis NOS (M54.1-)

✓4ᵗʰ **G50 Disorders of trigeminal nerve**
  INCLUDES disorders of 5th cranial nerve

G50.0 **Trigeminal neuralgia**
  Syndrome of paroxysmal facial pain
  Tic douloureux

G50.1 **Atypical facial pain**

G50.8 **Other disorders of trigeminal nerve**

G50.9 **Disorder of trigeminal nerve, unspecified** ▽

✓4ᵗʰ **G51 Facial nerve disorders**
  INCLUDES disorders of 7th cranial nerve

G51.0 **Bell's palsy**
  Facial palsy

G51.1 **Geniculate ganglionitis**
  EXCLUDES 1 postherpetic geniculate ganglionitis (B02.21)

G51.2 **Melkersson's syndrome**
  Melkersson-Rosenthal syndrome

G51.3 **Clonic hemifacial spasm**

G51.4 **Facial myokymia**

G51.8 **Other disorders of facial nerve**

G51.9 **Disorder of facial nerve, unspecified** ▽

✓4ᵗʰ **G52 Disorders of other cranial nerves**
  EXCLUDES 2 disorders of acoustic [8th] nerve (H93.3)
    disorders of optic [2nd] nerve (H46, H47.0)
    paralytic strabismus due to nerve palsy (H49.0-H49.2)

G52.0 **Disorders of olfactory nerve**
  Disorders of 1st cranial nerve

G52.1 **Disorders of glossopharyngeal nerve**
  Disorder of 9th cranial nerve
  Glossopharyngeal neuralgia

G52.2 **Disorders of vagus nerve**
  Disorders of pneumogastric [10th] nerve

G52.3 **Disorders of hypoglossal nerve**
  Disorders of 12th cranial nerve

G52.7 **Disorders of multiple cranial nerves**
  Polyneuritis cranialis

G52.8 **Disorders of other specified cranial nerves**

G52.9 **Cranial nerve disorder, unspecified** ▽

G53 *Cranial nerve disorders in diseases classified elsewhere*
  Code first underlying disease, such as:
    neoplasm (C00-D49)
  EXCLUDES 1 multiple cranial nerve palsy in sarcoidosis (D86.82)
    multiple cranial nerve palsy in syphilis (A52.15)
    postherpetic geniculate ganglionitis (B02.21)
    postherpetic trigeminal neuralgia (B02.22)

✓4ᵗʰ **G54 Nerve root and plexus disorders**
  EXCLUDES 1 current traumatic nerve root and plexus disorders—see nerve injury by body region
    intervertebral disc disorders (M50-M51)
    neuralgia or neuritis NOS (M79.2)
    neuritis or radiculitis brachial NOS (M54.13)
    neuritis or radiculitis lumbar NOS (M54.16)
    neuritis or radiculitis lumbosacral NOS (M54.17)
    neuritis or radiculitis thoracic NOS (M54.14)
    radiculitis NOS (M54.10)
    radiculopathy NOS (M54.10)
    spondylosis (M47.-)

G54.0 **Brachial plexus disorders**
  Thoracic outlet syndrome

G54.1 **Lumbosacral plexus disorders**

G54.2 **Cervical root disorders, not elsewhere classified**

G54.3 **Thoracic root disorders, not elsewhere classified**

G54.4 **Lumbosacral root disorders, not elsewhere classified**

G54.5 **Neuralgic amyotrophy**
  Parsonage-Aldren-Turner syndrome
  Shoulder-girdle neuritis
  EXCLUDES 1 neuralgic amyotrophy in diabetes mellitus (E08-E13 with .44)

G54.6 **Phantom limb syndrome with pain**

G54.7 **Phantom limb syndrome without pain**
  Phantom limb syndrome NOS

G54.8 **Other nerve root and plexus disorders**

G54.9 **Nerve root and plexus disorder, unspecified** ▽

G55 *Nerve root and plexus compressions in diseases classified elsewhere*
  Code first underlying disease, such as:
    neoplasm (C00-D49)
  EXCLUDES 1 nerve root compression (due to) (in) ankylosing spondylitis (M45.-)
    nerve root compression (due to) (in) dorsopathies (M53.-, M54.-)
    nerve root compression (due to) (in) intervertebral disc disorders (M50.1-, M51.1-)
    nerve root compression (due to) (in) spondylopathies (M46.-, M48.-)

✓4ᵗʰ **G56 Mononeuropathies of upper limb**
  EXCLUDES 1 current traumatic nerve disorder—see nerve injury by body region

✓5ᵗʰ **G56.0 Carpal tunnel syndrome**

G56.00 **Carpal tunnel syndrome, unspecified upper limb** ▽

G56.01 **Carpal tunnel syndrome, right upper limb**

G56.02 **Carpal tunnel syndrome, left upper limb**

✓5ᵗʰ **G56.1 Other lesions of median nerve**

G56.10 **Other lesions of median nerve, unspecified upper limb** ▽

G56.11 **Other lesions of median nerve, right upper limb**

G56.12 **Other lesions of median nerve, left upper limb**

Chapter 6. Diseases of the Nervous System

G56.2–G61.1

√5ᵗʰ G56.2 Lesion of ulnar nerve
Tardy ulnar nerve palsy

    G56.20 Lesion of ulnar nerve, unspecified upper limb ▽

    G56.21 Lesion of ulnar nerve, right upper limb

    G56.22 Lesion of ulnar nerve, left upper limb

√5ᵗʰ G56.3 Lesion of radial nerve

    G56.30 Lesion of radial nerve, unspecified upper limb ▽

    G56.31 Lesion of radial nerve, right upper limb

    G56.32 Lesion of radial nerve, left upper limb

√5ᵗʰ G56.4 Causalgia of upper limb
Complex regional pain syndrome II of upper limb

    EXCLUDES 1 *complex regional pain syndrome I of lower limb (G90.52-)*
      complex regional pain syndrome I of upper limb (G90.51-)
      complex regional pain syndrome II of lower limb (G57.7-)
      reflex sympathetic dystrophy of lower limb (G90.52-)
      reflex sympathetic dystrophy of upper limb (G90.51-)

    G56.40 Causalgia of unspecified upper limb ▽

    G56.41 Causalgia of right upper limb

    G56.42 Causalgia of left upper limb

√5ᵗʰ G56.8 Other specified mononeuropathies of upper limb
Interdigital neuroma of upper limb

    G56.80 Other specified mononeuropathies of unspecified ▽
    upper limb

    G56.81 Other specified mononeuropathies of right upper limb

    G56.82 Other specified mononeuropathies of left upper limb

√5ᵗʰ G56.9 Unspecified mononeuropathy of upper limb

    G56.90 Unspecified mononeuropathy of unspecified upper limb ▽

    G56.91 Unspecified mononeuropathy of right upper limb ▽

    G56.92 Unspecified mononeuropathy of left upper limb ▽

√4ᵗʰ G57 Mononeuropathies of lower limb

    EXCLUDES 1 *current traumatic nerve disorder—see nerve injury by body region*

√5ᵗʰ G57.0 Lesion of sciatic nerve

    EXCLUDES 1 *sciatica NOS (M54.3-)*
    EXCLUDES 2 *sciatica attributed to intervertebral disc disorder (M51.1-)*

    G57.00 Lesion of sciatic nerve, unspecified lower limb ▽

    G57.01 Lesion of sciatic nerve, right lower limb

    G57.02 Lesion of sciatic nerve, left lower limb

√5ᵗʰ G57.1 Meralgia paresthetica
Lateral cutaneous nerve of thigh syndrome

    G57.10 Meralgia paresthetica, unspecified lower limb ▽

    G57.11 Meralgia paresthetica, right lower limb

    G57.12 Meralgia paresthetica, left lower limb

√5ᵗʰ G57.2 Lesion of femoral nerve

    G57.20 Lesion of femoral nerve, unspecified lower limb ▽

    G57.21 Lesion of femoral nerve, right lower limb

    G57.22 Lesion of femoral nerve, left lower limb

√5ᵗʰ G57.3 Lesion of lateral popliteal nerve
Peroneal nerve palsy

    G57.30 Lesion of lateral popliteal nerve, unspecified lower limb ▽

    G57.31 Lesion of lateral popliteal nerve, right lower limb

    G57.32 Lesion of lateral popliteal nerve, left lower limb

√5ᵗʰ G57.4 Lesion of medial popliteal nerve

    G57.40 Lesion of medial popliteal nerve, unspecified lower limb ▽

    G57.41 Lesion of medial popliteal nerve, right lower limb

    G57.42 Lesion of medial popliteal nerve, left lower limb

√5ᵗʰ G57.5 Tarsal tunnel syndrome

    G57.50 Tarsal tunnel syndrome, unspecified lower limb ▽

    G57.51 Tarsal tunnel syndrome, right lower limb

    G57.52 Tarsal tunnel syndrome, left lower limb

√5ᵗʰ G57.6 Lesion of plantar nerve
Morton's metatarsalgia

    G57.60 Lesion of plantar nerve, unspecified lower limb ▽

    G57.61 Lesion of plantar nerve, right lower limb

    G57.62 Lesion of plantar nerve, left lower limb

√5ᵗʰ G57.7 Causalgia of lower limb
Complex regional pain syndrome II of lower limb

    EXCLUDES 1 *complex regional pain syndrome I of lower limb (G90.52-)*
      complex regional pain syndrome I of upper limb (G90.51-)
      complex regional pain syndrome II of upper limb (G56.4-)
      reflex sympathetic dystrophy of lower limb (G90.52-)
      reflex sympathetic dystrophy of upper limb (G90.51-)

    G57.70 Causalgia of unspecified lower limb ▽

    G57.71 Causalgia of right lower limb

    G57.72 Causalgia of left lower limb

√5ᵗʰ G57.8 Other specified mononeuropathies of lower limb
Interdigital neuroma of lower limb

    G57.80 Other specified mononeuropathies of unspecified lower limb ▽

    G57.81 Other specified mononeuropathies of right lower limb

    G57.82 Other specified mononeuropathies of left lower limb

√5ᵗʰ G57.9 Unspecified mononeuropathy of lower limb

    G57.90 Unspecified mononeuropathy of unspecified lower limb ▽

    G57.91 Unspecified mononeuropathy of right lower limb ▽

    G57.92 Unspecified mononeuropathy of left lower limb ▽

√4ᵗʰ G58 Other mononeuropathies

    G58.0 Intercostal neuropathy

    G58.7 Mononeuritis multiplex

    G58.8 Other specified mononeuropathies

    G58.9 Mononeuropathy, unspecified ▽

G59 *Mononeuropathy in diseases classified elsewhere*
Code first underlying disease

    EXCLUDES 1 *diabetic mononeuropathy (E08-E13 with .41)*
      syphilitic nerve paralysis (A52.19)
      syphilitic neuritis (A52.15)
      tuberculous mononeuropathy (A17.83)

Polyneuropathies and other disorders of the peripheral nervous system (G60-G65)

    EXCLUDES 1 *neuralgia NOS (M79.2)*
      neuritis NOS (M79.2)
      peripheral neuritis in pregnancy (O26.82-)
      radiculitis NOS (M54.10)

√4ᵗʰ G60 Hereditary and idiopathic neuropathy

    G60.0 Hereditary motor and sensory neuropathy
      Charcôt-Marie-Tooth disease
      Déjérine-Sottas disease
      Hereditary motor and sensory neuropathy, types I-IV
      Hypertrophic neuropathy of infancy
      Peroneal muscular atrophy (axonal type) (hypertrophic type)
      Roussy-Levy syndrome

    G60.1 Refsum's disease
      Infantile Refsum disease

    G60.2 Neuropathy in association with hereditary ataxia

    G60.3 Idiopathic progressive neuropathy

    G60.8 Other hereditary and idiopathic neuropathies
      Dominantly inherited sensory neuropathy
      Morvan's disease
      Nelaton's syndrome
      Recessively inherited sensory neuropathy

    G60.9 Hereditary and idiopathic neuropathy, unspecified ▽

√4ᵗʰ G61 Inflammatory polyneuropathy

    G61.0 Guillain-Barre syndrome
      Acute (post-)infective polyneuritis
      Miller Fisher syndrome
      AHA: 2014, 2Q, 4

    G61.1 Serum neuropathy
      Use additional code for adverse effect, if applicable, to identify serum (T50.-)

N Newborn   P Pediatric   M Maternity   A Adult   **RIC** RIC Dx   **NC Dx** Noncancer Dx   **PDx** Primary Dx   **CC** RIC CC Condition   ►◄ Revised Text   ● New Code   ▲ Revised Code Title

536   ICD-10-CM 2016

☑5ᵗʰ   **G61.8**   Other **inflammatory polyneuropathies**

     G61.81   Chronic inflammatory **demyelinating polyneuritis**

     G61.89   Other inflammatory polyneuropathies

     G61.9   **Inflammatory polyneuropathy, unspecified**   ▽

☑4ᵗʰ   **G62**   Other **and unspecified polyneuropathies**

     G62.0   **Drug-induced** polyneuropathy

        Use additional code for adverse effect, if applicable, to identify drug (T36-T50 with fifth or sixth character 5)

     G62.1   Alcoholic **polyneuropathy**

     G62.2   **Polyneuropathy** due to other toxic agents

        Code first (T51-T65) to identify toxic agent

☑5ᵗʰ   **G62.8**   Other **specified polyneuropathies**

     G62.81   Critical illness **polyneuropathy**

        Acute motor neuropathy

     G62.82   Radiation-induced **polyneuropathy**

        Use additional external cause code (W88-W90, X39.0-) to identify cause

     G62.89   Other specified polyneuropathies

     G62.9   **Polyneuropathy, unspecified**   ▽

        Neuropathy NOS

G63   *Polyneuropathy in diseases classified elsewhere*

     Code first underlying disease, such as:

        amyloidosis (E85.-)

        endocrine disease, except diabetes (E00-E07, E15-E16, E20-E34)

        metabolic diseases (E70-E88)

        neoplasm (C00-D49)

        nutritional deficiency (E40-E64)

        EXCLUDES 1   *polyneuropathy (in):*

           diabetes mellitus (E08-E13 with .42)

           diphtheria (A36.83)

           infectious mononucleosis (B27.0-B27.9 with 1)

           Lyme disease (A69.22)

           mumps (B26.84)

           postherpetic (B02.23)

           rheumatoid arthritis (M05.33)

           scleroderma (M34.83)

           systemic lupus erythematosus (M32.19)

     AHA: 2012, 4Q, 99

G64   Other disorders of peripheral nervous system

     Disorder of peripheral nervous system NOS

☑4ᵗʰ   **G65**   Sequelae of inflammatory and toxic polyneuropathies

     Code first condition resulting from (sequela) of inflammatory and toxic polyneuropathies

     G65.0   Sequelae of Guillain-Barré syndrome

     G65.1   **Sequelae of other inflammatory polyneuropathy**

     G65.2   Sequelae of toxic polyneuropathy

Diseases of myoneural junction and muscle (G70-G73)

☑4ᵗʰ   **G70**   Myasthenia gravis and other myoneural disorders

     EXCLUDES 1   *botulism (A05.1, A48.51-A48.52)*

           transient neonatal myasthenia gravis (P94.0)

☑5ᵗʰ   **G70.0**   Myasthenia gravis

     G70.00   **Myasthenia gravis** without (acute) exacerbation

        Myasthenia gravis NOS

     G70.01   **Myasthenia gravis** with (acute) exacerbation

        Myasthenia gravis in crisis

     G70.1   **Toxic myoneural disorders**

        Code first (T51-T65) to identify toxic agent

     G70.2   **Congenital and developmental myasthenia**

☑5ᵗʰ   **G70.8**   **Other specified myoneural disorders**

     G70.80   **Lambert-Eaton syndrome, unspecified**   ▽

        Lambert-Eaton syndrome NOS

     G70.81   *Lambert-Eaton syndrome in disease classified elsewhere*

        Code first underlying disease

        EXCLUDES 1   *Lambert-Eaton syndrome in neoplastic disease (G73.1)*

     G70.89   Other specified myoneural disorders

     G70.9   **Myoneural disorder, unspecified**   ▽

☑4ᵗʰ   **G71**   **Primary disorders of muscles**

     EXCLUDES 2   *arthrogryposis multiplex congenita (Q74.3)*

           metabolic disorders (E70-E88)

           myositis (M60.-)

     G71.0   Muscular dystrophy

        Autosomal recessive, childhood type, muscular dystrophy resembling Duchenne or Becker muscular dystrophy

        Benign [Becker] muscular dystrophy

        Benign scapuloperoneal muscular dystrophy with early contractures [Emery-Dreifuss]

        Congenital muscular dystrophy NOS

        Congenital muscular dystrophy with specific morphological abnormalities of the muscle fiber

        Distal muscular dystrophy

        Facioscapulohumeral muscular dystrophy

        Limb-girdle muscular dystrophy

        Ocular muscular dystrophy

        Oculopharyngeal muscular dystrophy

        Scapuloperoneal muscular dystrophy

        Severe [Duchenne] muscular dystrophy

☑5ᵗʰ   **G71.1**   Myotonic **disorders**

     G71.11   **Myotonic muscular dystrophy**

        Dystrophia myotonica [Steinert]

        Myotonia atrophica

        Myotonic dystrophy

        Proximal myotonic myopathy (PROMM)

        Steinert disease

     G71.12   **Myotonia** congenita

        Acetazolamide responsive myotonia congenita

        Dominant myotonia congenita [Thomsen disease]

        Myotonia levior

        Recessive myotonia congenita [Becker disease]

     G71.13   **Myotonic** chondrodystrophy

        Chondrodystrophic myotonia

        Congenital myotonic chondrodystrophy

        Schwartz-Jampel disease

     G71.14   Drug induced **myotonia**

        Use additional code for adverse effect, if applicable, to identify drug (T36-T50 with fifth or sixth character 5)

     G71.19   Other specified myotonic disorders

        Myotonia fluctuans

        Myotonia permanens

        Neuromyotonia [Isaacs]

        Paramyotonia congenita (of von Eulenburg)

        Pseudomyotonia

        Symptomatic myotonia

     G71.2   Congenital myopathies

        Central core disease

        Fiber-type disproportion

        Minicore disease

        Multicore disease

        Myotubular (centronuclear) myopathy

        Nemaline myopathy

        EXCLUDES 1   *arthrogryposis multiplex congenita (Q74.3)*

     G71.3   Mitochondrial myopathy, **not elsewhere classified**

        EXCLUDES 1   *Kearns-Sayre syndrome (H49.81)*

           Leber's disease (H47.21)

           Leigh's encephalopathy (G31.82)

           mitochondrial metabolism disorders (E88.4-)

           Reye's syndrome (G93.7)

     G71.8   Other primary disorders of muscles

     G71.9   **Primary disorder of muscle, unspecified**   ▽

        Hereditary myopathy NOS

☑4ᵗʰ   **G72**   Other **and unspecified myopathies**

     EXCLUDES 1   *arthrogryposis multiplex congenita (Q74.3)*

           dermatopolymyositis (M33.-)

           ischemic infarction of muscle (M62.2-)

           myositis (M60.-)

           polymyositis (M33.2-)

     G72.0   Drug-induced **myopathy**

        Use additional code for adverse effect, if applicable, to identify drug (T36-T50 with fifth or sixth character 5)

     G72.1   Alcoholic **myopathy**

        Use additional code to identify alcoholism (F10.-)

     G72.2   **Myopathy** due to other toxic agents

        Code first (T51-T65) to identify toxic agent

     G72.3   Periodic paralysis

        Familial periodic paralysis

        Hyperkalemic periodic paralysis (familial)

        Hypokalemic periodic paralysis (familial)

        Myotonic periodic paralysis (familial)

        Normokalemic paralysis (familial)

        Potassium sensitive periodic paralysis

        EXCLUDES 1   *paramyotonia congenita (of von Eulenburg) (G71.19)*

☑ Add'l Character Required   ☑ˣ⁷ᵗ Placeholder Alert   RUG IV Special Care High Dx   RUG IV Clinically Complex Dx   RUG IV Special Care Low Dx   Manifestation Code   Other Specified Code   ▽ Unspecified Code

✓5ᵗʰ **G72.4** Inflammatory and immune **myopathies, not elsewhere classified**

    G72.41 Inclusion body myositis [IBM]

    G72.49 **Other inflammatory and immune myopathies, not elsewhere classified**
        Inflammatory myopathy NOS

✓5ᵗʰ **G72.8** Other specified **myopathies**

    G72.81 Critical illness **myopathy**
        Acute necrotizing myopathy
        Acute quadriplegic myopathy
        Intensive care (ICU) myopathy
        Myopathy of critical illness

    G72.89 **Other specified myopathies**

G72.9 Myopathy, unspecified ▽

✓4ᵗʰ **G73** Disorders of myoneural junction and muscle in diseases classified elsewhere

    G73.1 *Lambert-Eaton syndrome in neoplastic disease*
        Code first underlying neoplasm (C00-D49)
        EXCLUDES 1   *Lambert-Eaton syndrome not associated with neoplasm (G70.80-G70.81)*

    G73.3 *Myasthenic syndromes in other diseases classified elsewhere*
        Code first underlying disease, such as:
          neoplasm (C00-D49)
          thyrotoxicosis (E05.-)

    G73.7 *Myopathy in diseases classified elsewhere*
        Code first underlying disease, such as:
          hyperparathyroidism (E21.0, E21.3)
          hypoparathyroidism (E20.-)
          glycogen storage disease (E74.0)
          lipid storage disorders (E75.-)
        EXCLUDES 1   *myopathy in:*
          rheumatoid arthritis (M05.4-)
          sarcoidosis (D86.87)
          scleroderma (M34.82)
          sicca syndrome [Sjögren] (M35.03)
          systemic lupus erythematosus (M32.19)

Cerebral palsy and other paralytic syndromes (G80-G83)

✓4ᵗʰ **G80** Cerebral palsy
    EXCLUDES 1   *hereditary spastic paraplegia (G11.4)*

    G80.0 Spastic quadriplegic **cerebral palsy**
        Congenital spastic paralysis (cerebral)

    G80.1 Spastic diplegic **cerebral palsy**
        Spastic cerebral palsy NOS

    G80.2 Spastic hemiplegic **cerebral palsy**

    G80.3 Athetoid **cerebral palsy**
        Double athetosis (syndrome)
        Dyskinetic cerebral palsy
        Dystonic cerebral palsy
        Vogt disease

    G80.4 Ataxic **cerebral palsy**

    G80.8 **Other cerebral palsy**
        Mixed cerebral palsy syndromes

    G80.9 **Cerebral palsy, unspecified** ▽
        Cerebral palsy NOS

✓4ᵗʰ **G81** Hemiplegia and hemiparesis
    NOTE   This category is to be used only when hemiplegia (complete)(incomplete) is reported without further specification, or is stated to be old or longstanding but of unspecified cause. The category is also for use in multiple coding to identify these types of hemiplegia resulting from any cause.
    EXCLUDES 1   *congenital cerebral palsy (G80.-)*
        hemiplegia and hemiparesis due to sequela of cerebrovascular disease (I69.05-, I69.15-, I69.25-, I69.35-, I69.85-, I69.95-)
    AHA: 2015, 1Q, 25

    ✓5ᵗʰ **G81.0** Flaccid **hemiplegia**

        G81.00 **Flaccid hemiplegia affecting unspecified side** CC ▽
            RIC Excl: 01 Stroke

        G81.01 **Flaccid hemiplegia affecting** right **dominant side** CC
            RIC Excl: 01 Stroke

        G81.02 **Flaccid hemiplegia affecting** left **dominant side** CC
            RIC Excl: 01 Stroke

        G81.03 **Flaccid hemiplegia affecting** right **nondominant side** CC
            RIC Excl: 01 Stroke

        G81.04 **Flaccid hemiplegia affecting** left **nondominant side** CC
            RIC Excl: 01 Stroke

    ✓5ᵗʰ **G81.1** Spastic **hemiplegia**

        G81.10 **Spastic hemiplegia affecting unspecified side** CC ▽
            RIC Excl: 01 Stroke

        G81.11 **Spastic hemiplegia affecting** right **dominant side** CC
            RIC Excl: 01 Stroke

        G81.12 **Spastic hemiplegia affecting** left **dominant side** CC
            RIC Excl: 01 Stroke

        G81.13 **Spastic hemiplegia affecting** right **nondominant side** CC
            RIC Excl: 01 Stroke

        G81.14 **Spastic hemiplegia affecting** left **nondominant side** CC
            RIC Excl: 01 Stroke

    ✓5ᵗʰ **G81.9** Hemiplegia, **unspecified**
        AHA: 2014, 1Q, 23

        G81.90 **Hemiplegia, unspecified affecting unspecified side** CC ▽
            RIC Excl: 01 Stroke

        G81.91 **Hemiplegia, unspecified affecting** right **dominant side** CC ▽
            RIC Excl: 01 Stroke

        G81.92 **Hemiplegia, unspecified affecting** left **dominant side** CC ▽
            RIC Excl: 01 Stroke

        G81.93 **Hemiplegia, unspecified affecting** right **nondominant side** CC ▽
            RIC Excl: 01 Stroke

        G81.94 **Hemiplegia, unspecified affecting** left **nondominant side** CC ▽
            RIC Excl: 01 Stroke

✓4ᵗʰ **G82** Paraplegia (paraparesis) and quadriplegia (quadriparesis)
    NOTE   This category is to be used only when the listed conditions are reported without further specification, or are stated to be old or longstanding but of unspecified cause. The category is also for use in multiple coding to identify these conditions resulting from any cause.
    EXCLUDES 1   *congenital cerebral palsy (G80.-)*
        functional quadriplegia (R53.2)
        hysterical paralysis (F44.4)

    ✓5ᵗʰ **G82.2** Paraplegia
        Paralysis of both lower limbs NOS
        Paraparesis (lower) NOS
        Paraplegia (lower) NOS

        G82.20 **Paraplegia, unspecified** ▽

        G82.21 **Paraplegia,** complete

        G82.22 **Paraplegia,** incomplete

    ✓5ᵗʰ **G82.5** Quadriplegia

        G82.50 **Quadriplegia, unspecified** ▽

        G82.51 **Quadriplegia,** C1-C4 complete

        G82.52 **Quadriplegia,** C1-C4 incomplete

        G82.53 **Quadriplegia,** C5-C7 complete

        G82.54 **Quadriplegia,** C5-C7 incomplete

✓4ᵗʰ **G83** Other **paralytic syndromes**
    NOTE   This category is to be used only when the listed conditions are reported without further specification, or are stated to be old or longstanding but of unspecified cause. The category is also for use in multiple coding to identify these conditions resulting from any cause.
    INCLUDES   *paralysis (complete) (incomplete), except as in G80-G82*

    G83.0 Diplegia **of upper limbs**
        Diplegia (upper)
        Paralysis of both upper limbs

    ✓5ᵗʰ **G83.1** Monoplegia **of lower limb**
        Paralysis of lower limb
        EXCLUDES 1   *monoplegia of lower limbs due to sequela of cerebrovascular disease (I69.04-, I69.14-, I69.24-, I69.34-, I69.84-, I69.94-)*

        G83.10 **Monoplegia of lower limb affecting unspecified side** ▽

        G83.11 **Monoplegia of lower limb affecting** right **dominant side**

        G83.12 **Monoplegia of lower limb affecting** left **dominant side**

N Newborn   P Pediatric   M Maternity   A Adult   RIC RIC Dx   NC Dx Noncancer Dx   PD Primary Dx   CC RIC CC Condition   ►◄ Revised Text   ● New Code   ▲ Revised Code Title

538   ICD-10-CM 2016

G83.13   **Monoplegia of lower limb affecting right nondominant side**

G83.14   **Monoplegia of lower limb affecting left nondominant side**

✓5ᵗʰ   **G83.2**   Monoplegia **of upper limb**
Paralysis of upper limb
EXCLUDES 1   *monoplegia of upper limbs due to sequela of cerebrovascular disease (I69.03-, I69.13-, I69.23-, I69.33-, I69.83-, I69.93-)*

G83.20   **Monoplegia of upper limb affecting unspecified side** ▽

G83.21   **Monoplegia of upper limb affecting right dominant side**

G83.22   **Monoplegia of upper limb affecting left dominant side**

G83.23   **Monoplegia of upper limb affecting right nondominant side**

G83.24   **Monoplegia of upper limb affecting left nondominant side**

✓5ᵗʰ   **G83.3**   Monoplegia, unspecified

G83.30   **Monoplegia, unspecified affecting unspecified side** ▽

G83.31   **Monoplegia, unspecified affecting right dominant side** ▽

G83.32   **Monoplegia, unspecified affecting left dominant side** ▽

G83.33   **Monoplegia, unspecified affecting right nondominant side** ▽

G83.34   **Monoplegia, unspecified affecting left nondominant side** ▽

G83.4   **Cauda equina syndrome**
Neurogenic bladder due to cauda equina syndrome
EXCLUDES 1   *cord bladder NOS (G95.89)*
neurogenic bladder NOS (N31.9)

G83.5   **Locked-in state**

✓5ᵗʰ   **G83.8**   **Other specified paralytic syndromes**
EXCLUDES 1   *paralytic syndromes due to current spinal cord injury—code to spinal cord injury (S14, S24, S34)*

G83.81   **Brown-Séquard syndrome**
G83.82   **Anterior cord syndrome**
G83.83   **Posterior cord syndrome**
G83.84   **Todd's paralysis (postepileptic)**
G83.89   **Other specified paralytic syndromes**

G83.9   **Paralytic syndrome, unspecified** ▽

Other disorders of the nervous system (G89-G99)

✓4ᵗʰ   **G89**   **Pain, not elsewhere classified**
Code also related psychological factors associated with pain (F45.42)
EXCLUDES 1   *generalized pain NOS (R52)*
pain disorders exclusively related to psychological factors (F45.41)
pain NOS (R52)
EXCLUDES 2   *atypical face pain (G50.1)*
headache syndromes (G44.-)
localized pain, unspecified type—code to pain by site, such as:
abdomen pain (R10.-)
back pain (M54.9)
breast pain (N64.4)
chest pain (R07.1-R07.9)
ear pain (H92.0-)
eye pain (H57.1)
headache (R51)
joint pain (M25.5-)
limb pain (M79.6-)
lumbar region pain (M54.5)
painful urination (R30.9)
pelvic and perineal pain (R10.2)
renal colic (N23)
shoulder pain (M25.51-)
spine pain (M54.-)
throat pain (R07.0)
tongue pain (K14.6)
tooth pain (K08.8)
migraines (G43.-)
myalgia (M79.1)
pain from prosthetic devices, implants, and grafts (T82.84, T83.84, T84.84, T85.84)
phantom limb syndrome with pain (G54.6)
vulvar vestibulitis (N94.810)
vulvodynia (N94.81-)

G89.0   **Central pain syndrome**
Déjérine-Roussy syndrome
Myelopathic pain syndrome
Thalamic pain syndrome (hyperesthetic)

✓5ᵗʰ   **G89.1**   Acute pain, **not elsewhere classified**
G89.11   **Acute pain due to trauma**
G89.12   **Acute post-thoracotomy pain**
Post-thoracotomy pain NOS
G89.18   **Other acute postprocedural pain**
Postoperative pain NOS
Postprocedural pain NOS

✓5ᵗʰ   **G89.2**   Chronic pain, **not elsewhere classified**
EXCLUDES 1   *causalgia, lower limb (G57.7-)*
causalgia, upper limb (G56.4-)
central pain syndrome (G89.0)
chronic pain syndrome (G89.4)
complex regional pain syndrome II, lower limb (G57.7-)
complex regional pain syndrome II, upper limb (G56.4-)
neoplasm related chronic pain (G89.3)
reflex sympathetic dystrophy (G90.5-)

G89.21   **Chronic pain due to trauma**
G89.22   **Chronic post-thoracotomy pain**
G89.28   **Other chronic postprocedural pain**
Other chronic postoperative pain
G89.29   **Other chronic pain**

G89.3   **Neoplasm related pain (acute) (chronic)**
Cancer associated pain
Pain due to malignancy (primary) (secondary)
Tumor associated pain

G89.4   **Chronic pain syndrome**
Chronic pain associated with significant psychosocial dysfunction

✓4ᵗʰ   **G90**   **Disorders of autonomic nervous system**
EXCLUDES 1   *dysfunction of the autonomic nervous system due to alcohol (G31.2)*

✓5ᵗʰ   **G90.0**   **Idiopathic peripheral autonomic neuropathy**
G90.01   **Carotid sinus syncope**
Carotid sinus syndrome
G90.09   **Other idiopathic peripheral autonomic neuropathy**
Idiopathic peripheral autonomic neuropathy NOS

G90.1   **Familial dysautonomia [Riley-Day]**
G90.2   **Horner's syndrome**
Bernard(-Horner) syndrome
Cervical sympathetic dystrophy or paralysis

G90.3 Multi-system degeneration of the autonomic nervous system
Neurogenic orthostatic hypotension [Shy-Drager]
EXCLUDES 1   orthostatic hypotension NOS (I95.1)

G90.4 Autonomic dysreflexia
Use additional code to identify the cause, such as:
    fecal impaction (K56.41)
    pressure ulcer (pressure area) (L89.-)
    urinary tract infection (N39.0)

✓5ᵗʰ **G90.5 Complex regional pain syndrome I (CRPS I)**
Reflex sympathetic dystrophy
EXCLUDES 1   causalgia of lower limb (G57.7-)
    causalgia of upper limb (G56.4-)
    complex regional pain syndrome II of lower limb (G57.7-)
    complex regional pain syndrome II of upper limb (G56.4-)

G90.50 Complex regional pain syndrome I, unspecified ▽

✓6ᵗʰ **G90.51 Complex regional pain syndrome I of upper limb**

G90.511 Complex regional pain syndrome I of right upper limb

G90.512 Complex regional pain syndrome I of left upper limb

G90.513 Complex regional pain syndrome I of upper limb, bilateral

G90.519 Complex regional pain syndrome I of unspecified upper limb ▽

✓6ᵗʰ **G90.52 Complex regional pain syndrome I of lower limb**

G90.521 Complex regional pain syndrome I of right lower limb

G90.522 Complex regional pain syndrome I of left lower limb

G90.523 Complex regional pain syndrome I of lower limb, bilateral

G90.529 Complex regional pain syndrome I of unspecified lower limb ▽

G90.59 Complex regional pain syndrome I of other specified site

G90.8 Other disorders of autonomic nervous system

G90.9 Disorder of the autonomic nervous system, unspecified ▽

✓4ᵗʰ **G91 Hydrocephalus**
INCLUDES   acquired hydrocephalus
EXCLUDES 1   Arnold-Chiari syndrome with hydrocephalus (Q07.-)
    congenital hydrocephalus (Q03.-)
    spina bifida with hydrocephalus (Q05.-)

G91.0 Communicating hydrocephalus
Secondary normal pressure hydrocephalus

G91.1 Obstructive hydrocephalus

G91.2 (Idiopathic) normal pressure hydrocephalus
Normal pressure hydrocephalus NOS

G91.3 Post-traumatic hydrocephalus, unspecified

G91.4 Hydrocephalus in diseases classified elsewhere
Code first underlying condition, such as:
    congenital syphilis (A50.4-)
    neoplasm (C00-D49)
EXCLUDES 1   hydrocephalus due to congenital toxoplasmosis (P37.1)
AHA: 2014, 3Q, 3

G91.8 Other hydrocephalus

G91.9 Hydrocephalus, unspecified ▽

G92 Toxic encephalopathy
Toxic encephalitis
Toxic metabolic encephalopathy
Code first (T51-T65) to identify toxic agent

✓4ᵗʰ **G93 Other disorders of brain**

G93.0 Cerebral cysts
Arachnoid cyst
Porencephalic cyst, acquired
EXCLUDES 1   acquired periventricular cysts of newborn (P91.1)
    congenital cerebral cysts (Q04.6)

G93.1 Anoxic brain damage, not elsewhere classified CC
EXCLUDES 1   cerebral anoxia due to anesthesia during labor and delivery (O74.3)
    cerebral anoxia due to anesthesia during the puerperium (O89.2)
    neonatal anoxia (P84)
RIC Excl: 02 Traumatic brain injury; 03 Non-traumatic brain injury

G93.2 Benign intracranial hypertension
EXCLUDES 1   hypertensive encephalopathy (I67.4)

G93.3 Postviral fatigue syndrome
Benign myalgic encephalomyelitis
EXCLUDES 1   chronic fatigue syndrome NOS (R53.82)

✓5ᵗʰ **G93.4 Other and unspecified encephalopathy**
EXCLUDES 1   alcoholic encephalopathy (G31.2)
    encephalopathy in diseases classified elsewhere (G94)
    hypertensive encephalopathy (I67.4)
    toxic (metabolic) encephalopathy (G92)

G93.40 Encephalopathy, unspecified ▽

G93.41 Metabolic encephalopathy
Septic encephalopathy

G93.49 Other encephalopathy
Encephalopathy NEC

G93.5 Compression of brain
Arnold-Chiari type 1 compression of brain
Compression of brain (stem)
Herniation of brain (stem)
EXCLUDES 1   diffuse traumatic compression of brain (S06.2-)
    focal traumatic compression of brain (S06.3-)

G93.6 Cerebral edema
EXCLUDES 1   cerebral edema due to birth injury (P11.0)
    traumatic cerebral edema (S06.1-)

G93.7 Reye's syndrome P
Code first (T39.0-), if salicylates-induced

✓5ᵗʰ **G93.8 Other specified disorders of brain**

G93.81 Temporal sclerosis
Hippocampal sclerosis
Mesial temporal sclerosis

G93.82 Brain death

G93.89 Other specified disorders of brain
Postradiation encephalopathy

G93.9 Disorder of brain, unspecified ▽

G94 Other disorders of brain in diseases classified elsewhere
Code first underlying disease
EXCLUDES 1   encephalopathy in congenital syphilis (A50.49)
    encephalopathy in influenza (J09.X9, J10.81, J11.81)
    encephalopathy in syphilis (A52.19)
    hydrocephalus in diseases classified elsewhere (G91.4)

✓4ᵗʰ **G95 Other and unspecified diseases of spinal cord**
EXCLUDES 2   myelitis (G04.-)

G95.0 Syringomyelia and syringobulbia

✓5ᵗʰ **G95.1 Vascular myelopathies**
EXCLUDES 2   intraspinal phlebitis and thrombophlebitis, except non-pyogenic (G08)

G95.11 Acute infarction of spinal cord (embolic) (nonembolic)
Anoxia of spinal cord
Arterial thrombosis of spinal cord

G95.19 Other vascular myelopathies
Edema of spinal cord
Hematomyelia
Nonpyogenic intraspinal phlebitis and thrombophlebitis
Subacute necrotic myelopathy

✓5ᵗʰ **G95.2 Other and unspecified cord compression**

G95.20 Unspecified cord compression ▽

G95.29 Other cord compression

✓5ᵗʰ **G95.8 Other specified diseases of spinal cord**
EXCLUDES 1   neurogenic bladder NOS (N31.9)
    neurogenic bladder due to cauda equina syndrome (G83.4)
    neuromuscular dysfunction of bladder without spinal cord lesion (N31.-)

G95.81 Conus medullaris syndrome

G95.89 Other specified diseases of spinal cord
Cord bladder NOS
Drug-induced myelopathy
Radiation-induced myelopathy
EXCLUDES 1   myelopathy NOS (G95.9)

G95.9 Disease of spinal cord, unspecified ▽
Myelopathy NOS

N Newborn   P Pediatric   M Maternity   A Adult   RIC RIC Dx   NC Dx Noncancer Dx   PDx Primary Dx   CC RIC CC Condition   ▶◀ Revised Text   ● New Code   ▲ Revised Code Title

540

ICD-10-CM 2016

✓4ᵗʰ **G96 Other disorders of central nervous system**

    G96.0 Cerebrospinal fluid leak
        EXCLUDES 1   *cerebrospinal fluid leak from spinal puncture (G97.0)*

    ✓5ᵗʰ **G96.1 Disorders of meninges, not elsewhere classified**
        G96.11 Dural tear
            EXCLUDES 1   *accidental puncture or laceration of dura during a procedure (G97.41)*
            AHA: 2014, 4Q, 24
        G96.12 Meningeal adhesions (cerebral) (spinal)
        G96.19 Other disorders of meninges, not elsewhere classified

    G96.8 Other specified disorders of central nervous system

    G96.9 Disorder of central nervous system, unspecified   ▽

✓4ᵗʰ **G97 Intraoperative and postprocedural complications and disorders of nervous system, not elsewhere classified**
    EXCLUDES 2   *intraoperative and postprocedural cerebrovascular infarction (I97.81-, I97.82-)*

    G97.0 Cerebrospinal fluid leak from spinal puncture

    G97.1 Other reaction to spinal and lumbar puncture
        Headache due to lumbar puncture

    G97.2 Intracranial hypotension following ventricular shunting

    ✓5ᵗʰ **G97.3 Intraoperative hemorrhage and hematoma of a nervous system organ or structure complicating a procedure**
        EXCLUDES 1   *intraoperative hemorrhage and hematoma of a nervous system organ or structure due to accidental puncture and laceration during a procedure (G97.4-)*
        G97.31 Intraoperative hemorrhage and hematoma of a nervous system organ or structure complicating a nervous system procedure
        G97.32 Intraoperative hemorrhage and hematoma of a nervous system organ or structure complicating other procedure

    ✓5ᵗʰ **G97.4 Accidental puncture and laceration of a nervous system organ or structure during a procedure**
        G97.41 Accidental puncture or laceration of dura during a procedure
            Incidental (inadvertent) durotomy
            AHA: 2014, 4Q, 24
        G97.48 Accidental puncture and laceration of other nervous system organ or structure during a nervous system procedure
        G97.49 Accidental puncture and laceration of other nervous system organ or structure during other procedure

    ✓5ᵗʰ **G97.5 Postprocedural hemorrhage and hematoma of a nervous system organ or structure following a procedure**
        G97.51 Postprocedural hemorrhage and hematoma of a nervous system organ or structure following a nervous system procedure
        G97.52 Postprocedural hemorrhage and hematoma of a nervous system organ or structure following other procedure

    ✓5ᵗʰ **G97.8 Other intraoperative and postprocedural complications and disorders of nervous system**
        Use additional code to further specify disorder
        G97.81 Other intraoperative complications of nervous system
        G97.82 Other postprocedural complications and disorders of nervous system

✓4ᵗʰ **G98 Other disorders of nervous system not elsewhere classified**
    INCLUDES   nervous system disorder NOS

    G98.0 Neurogenic arthritis, not elsewhere classified
        Nonsyphilitic neurogenic arthropathy NEC
        Nonsyphilitic neurogenic spondylopathy NEC
        EXCLUDES 1   *spondylopathy (in):*
            syringomyelia and syringobulbia (G95.0)
            tabes dorsalis (A52.11)

    G98.8 Other disorders of nervous system
        Nervous system disorder NOS

✓4ᵗʰ **G99 Other disorders of nervous system in diseases classified elsewhere**

    G99.0 Autonomic neuropathy in diseases classified elsewhere
        Code first underlying disease, such as:
            amyloidosis (E85.-)
            gout (M1A.-, M10.-)
            hyperthyroidism (E05.-)
        EXCLUDES 1   *diabetic autonomic neuropathy (E08-E13 with .43)*

    G99.2 Myelopathy in diseases classified elsewhere
        Code first underlying disease, such as:
            neoplasm (C00-D49)
        EXCLUDES 1   *myelopathy in:*
            intervertebral disease (M50.0-, M51.0-)
            spondylosis (M47.0-, M47.1-)

    G99.8 Other specified disorders of nervous system in diseases classified elsewhere
        Code first underlying disorder, such as:
            amyloidosis (E85.-)
            avitaminosis (E56.9)
        EXCLUDES 1   *nervous system involvement in:*
            cysticercosis (B69.0)
            rubella (B06.0-)
            syphilis (A52.1-)

Chapter 7. Diseases of the Eye and Adnexa (H00–H59)

Chapter Specific Guidelines with Coding Examples

The chapter specific guidelines from the ICD-10-CM Official Guidelines for Coding and Reporting have been provided below. Along with these guidelines are coding examples, contained in the shaded boxes, that have been developed to help illustrate the coding and/or sequencing guidance found in these guidelines.

a. Glaucoma

1) Assigning glaucoma codes

Assign as many codes from category H40, Glaucoma, as needed to identify the type of glaucoma, the affected eye, and the glaucoma stage.

2) Bilateral glaucoma with same type and stage

When a patient has bilateral glaucoma and both eyes are documented as being the same type and stage, and there is a code for bilateral glaucoma, report only the code for the type of glaucoma, bilateral, with the seventh character for the stage.

> Bilateral severe stage pigmentary glaucoma
>
> **H40.1333   Pigmentary glaucoma, bilateral, severe stage**
>
> *Explanation*: In this scenario, the patient has the same type and stage of glaucoma in both eyes. As this type of glaucoma has a code for bilateral, assign only the code for the bilateral glaucoma with the seventh character for the stage.

When a patient has bilateral glaucoma and both eyes are documented as being the same type and stage, and the classification does not provide a code for bilateral glaucoma (i.e. subcategories H40.10, H40.11 and H40.20) report only one code for the type of glaucoma with the appropriate seventh character for the stage.

> Bilateral, mild stage, primary open-angle glaucoma
>
> **H40.11X1   Primary open-angle glaucoma, mild stage**
>
> *Explanation*: In this scenario, the patient has glaucoma of the same type and stage of both eyes, but there is no code specifically for bilateral glaucoma. Only one code is assigned with the appropriate seventh character for the stage.

3) Bilateral glaucoma stage with different types or stages

When a patient has bilateral glaucoma and each eye is documented as having a different type or stage, and the classification distinguishes laterality, assign the appropriate code for each eye rather than the code for bilateral glaucoma.

> Bilateral chronic angle-closure glaucoma; right eye is documented as mild stage and left eye as moderate stage
>
> **H40.2211   Chronic angle-closure glaucoma, right eye, mild stage**
>
> **H40.2222   Chronic angle-closure glaucoma, left eye, moderate stage**
>
> *Explanation*: In this scenario the patient has the same type of glaucoma in both eyes, but each eye is at a different stage. Because the subcategory for this condition identifies laterality, one code is assigned for the right eye and one code is assigned for the left eye, each with the appropriate seventh character for the stage appended.

When a patient has bilateral glaucoma and each eye is documented as having a different type, and the classification does not distinguish laterality (i.e. subcategories H40.10, H40.11 and H40.20), assign one code for each type of glaucoma with the appropriate seventh character for the stage.

> Documentation relates mild, unspecified primary angle-closure glaucoma of the left eye with mild primary open-angle glaucoma of the right eye
>
> **H40.20X1   Unspecified primary angle-closure glaucoma, mild stage**
>
> **H40.11X1   Primary open-angle glaucoma, mild stage**
>
> *Explanation*: In this scenario the patient has a different type of glaucoma in each eye and the classification does not distinguish laterality. A code for each type of glaucoma is assigned, each with the appropriate seventh character for the stage.

When a patient has bilateral glaucoma and each eye is documented as having the same type, but different stage, and the classification does not distinguish laterality (i.e. subcategories H40.10, H40.11 and H40.20), assign a code for the type of glaucoma for each eye with the seventh character for the specific glaucoma stage documented for each eye.

> Bilateral primary open-angle glaucoma; the right eye is documented to be in mild stage and the left eye as being in moderate stage
>
> **H40.11X2   Primary open-angle glaucoma, moderate stage**
>
> **H40.11X1   Primary open-angle glaucoma, mild stage**
>
> *Explanation*: In this scenario the patient has the same type of glaucoma in each eye but each eye is at a different stage, and the classification does not distinguish laterality at this subcategory level. Two codes are assigned; both codes represent the same type of glaucoma but each has a different seventh character identifying the appropriate stage for each eye.

4) Patient admitted with glaucoma and stage evolves during the admission

If a patient is admitted with glaucoma and the stage progresses during the admission, assign the code for highest stage documented.

> Patient admitted with mild low-tension glaucoma of the right eye, which progresses to moderate stage during the patient's stay
>
> **H40.1212   Low-tension glaucoma, right eye, moderate stage**
>
> *Explanation*: When the glaucoma stage progresses during an admission, assign only the code for the highest stage documented.

5) Indeterminate stage glaucoma

Assignment of the seventh character "4" for "indeterminate stage" should be based on the clinical documentation. The seventh character "4" is used for glaucomas whose stage cannot be clinically determined. This seventh character should not be confused with the seventh character "0", unspecified, which should be assigned when there is no documentation regarding the stage of the glaucoma.

Chapter 7. Diseases of the Eye and Adnexa (H00-H59)

NOTE   Use an external cause code following the code for the eye condition, if applicable, to identify the cause of the eye condition.

EXCLUDES 2   *certain conditions originating in the perinatal period (P04-P96)*
certain infectious and parasitic diseases (A00-B99)
complications of pregnancy, childbirth and the puerperium (O00-O9A)
congenital malformations, deformations, and chromosomal
*   abnormalities (Q00-Q99)*
diabetes mellitus related eye conditions (E09.3-, E10.3-, E11.3-, E13.3-)
endocrine, nutritional and metabolic diseases (E00-E88)
injury (trauma) of eye and orbit (S05.-)
injury, poisoning and certain other consequences of external causes
*   (S00-T88)*
neoplasms (C00-D49)
symptoms, signs and abnormal clinical and laboratory findings, not
*   elsewhere classified (R00-R94)*
syphilis related eye disorders (A50.01, A50.3-, A51.43, A52.71)

This chapter contains the following blocks:

H00-H05	Disorders of eyelid, lacrimal system and orbit
H10-H11	Disorders of conjunctiva
H15-H22	Disorders of sclera, cornea, iris and ciliary body
H25-H28	Disorders of lens
H30-H36	Disorders of choroid and retina
H40-H42	Glaucoma
H43-H44	Disorders of vitreous body and globe
H46-H47	Disorders of optic nerve and visual pathways
H49-H52	Disorders of ocular muscles, binocular movement, accommodation and refraction
H53-H54	Visual disturbances and blindness
H55-H57	Other disorders of eye and adnexa
H59	Intraoperative and postprocedural complications and disorders of eye and adnexa, not elsewhere classified

Disorders of eyelid, lacrimal system and orbit (H00-H05)

EXCLUDES 2   *open wound of eyelid (S01.1-)*
superficial injury of eyelid (S00.1-, S00.2-)

✓4ᵗʰ **H00 Hordeolum and chalazion**

  ✓5ᵗʰ **H00.0** Hordeolum (externum) (internum) of eyelid

    ✓6ᵗʰ **H00.01** **Hordeolum** externum
         Hordeolum NOS
         Stye

        H00.011 **Hordeolum externum** right upper **eyelid**
        H00.012 **Hordeolum externum** right lower **eyelid**
        H00.013 **Hordeolum externum** right eye, **unspecified eyelid** ▽
        H00.014 **Hordeolum externum** left upper **eyelid**
        H00.015 **Hordeolum externum** left lower **eyelid**
        H00.016 **Hordeolum externum** left eye, **unspecified eyelid** ▽
        H00.019 **Hordeolum externum unspecified eye, unspecified eyelid** ▽

    ✓6ᵗʰ **H00.02** **Hordeolum** internum
         Infection of meibomian gland

        H00.021 **Hordeolum internum** right upper **eyelid**
        H00.022 **Hordeolum internum** right lower **eyelid**
        H00.023 **Hordeolum internum** right eye, **unspecified eyelid** ▽
        H00.024 **Hordeolum internum** left upper **eyelid**
        H00.025 **Hordeolum internum** left lower **eyelid**
        H00.026 **Hordeolum internum** left eye, **unspecified eyelid** ▽
        H00.029 **Hordeolum internum unspecified eye, unspecified eyelid** ▽

    ✓6ᵗʰ **H00.03** **Abscess** of eyelid
         Furuncle of eyelid

        H00.031 **Abscess of** right upper **eyelid**
        H00.032 **Abscess of** right lower **eyelid**
        H00.033 **Abscess of eyelid** right eye, **unspecified eyelid** ▽
        H00.034 **Abscess of** left upper **eyelid**
        H00.035 **Abscess of** left lower **eyelid**
        H00.036 **Abscess of eyelid** left eye, **unspecified eyelid** ▽
        H00.039 **Abscess of eyelid unspecified eye, unspecified eyelid** ▽

        H01.126 **Discoid lupus erythematosus of** left ▽

✓5ᵗʰ **H00.1 Chalazion**
    Meibomian (gland) cyst
    EXCLUDES 2   *infected meibomian gland (H00.02-)*

  H00.11 **Chalazion** right upper **eyelid**
  H00.12 **Chalazion** right lower **eyelid**
  H00.13 **Chalazion** right eye, **unspecified eyelid** ▽
  H00.14 **Chalazion** left upper **eyelid**
  H00.15 **Chalazion** left lower **eyelid**
  H00.16 **Chalazion** left eye, **unspecified eyelid** ▽
  H00.19 **Chalazion unspecified eye, unspecified eyelid** ▽

✓4ᵗʰ **H01 Other inflammation of eyelid**

  ✓5ᵗʰ **H01.0 Blepharitis**
    EXCLUDES 1   *blepharoconjunctivitis (H10.5-)*

    ✓6ᵗʰ **H01.00** **Unspecified blepharitis**
        H01.001 **Unspecified blepharitis** right upper **eyelid** ▽
        H01.002 **Unspecified blepharitis** right lower **eyelid** ▽
        H01.003 **Unspecified blepharitis** right eye, **unspecified eyelid** ▽
        H01.004 **Unspecified blepharitis** left upper **eyelid** ▽
        H01.005 **Unspecified blepharitis** left lower **eyelid** ▽
        H01.006 **Unspecified blepharitis** left eye, **unspecified eyelid** ▽
        H01.009 **Unspecified blepharitis unspecified eye, unspecified eyelid** ▽

    ✓6ᵗʰ **H01.01** **Ulcerative blepharitis**
        H01.011 **Ulcerative blepharitis** right upper **eyelid**
        H01.012 **Ulcerative blepharitis** right lower **eyelid**
        H01.013 **Ulcerative blepharitis** right eye, **unspecified eyelid** ▽
        H01.014 **Ulcerative blepharitis** left upper **eyelid**
        H01.015 **Ulcerative blepharitis** left lower **eyelid**
        H01.016 **Ulcerative blepharitis** left eye, **unspecified eyelid** ▽
        H01.019 **Ulcerative blepharitis unspecified eye, unspecified eyelid** ▽

    ✓6ᵗʰ **H01.02** **Squamous blepharitis**
        H01.021 **Squamous blepharitis** right upper **eyelid**
        H01.022 **Squamous blepharitis** right lower **eyelid**
        H01.023 **Squamous blepharitis** right eye, **unspecified eyelid** ▽
        H01.024 **Squamous blepharitis** left upper **eyelid**
        H01.025 **Squamous blepharitis** left lower **eyelid**
        H01.026 **Squamous blepharitis** left eye, **unspecified eyelid** ▽
        H01.029 **Squamous blepharitis unspecified eye, unspecified eyelid** ▽

  ✓5ᵗʰ **H01.1 Noninfectious dermatoses of eyelid**

    ✓6ᵗʰ **H01.11** **Allergic dermatitis of eyelid**
         Contact dermatitis of eyelid

        H01.111 **Allergic dermatitis of** right upper **eyelid**
        H01.112 **Allergic dermatitis of** right lower **eyelid**
        H01.113 **Allergic dermatitis of** right eye, **unspecified eyelid** ▽
        H01.114 **Allergic dermatitis of** left upper **eyelid**
        H01.115 **Allergic dermatitis of** left lower **eyelid**
        H01.116 **Allergic dermatitis of** left eye, **unspecified eyelid** ▽
        H01.119 **Allergic dermatitis of unspecified eye, unspecified eyelid** ▽

    ✓6ᵗʰ **H01.12** **Discoid lupus erythematosus of eyelid**
        H01.121 **Discoid lupus erythematosus of** right upper **eyelid**
        H01.122 **Discoid lupus erythematosus of** right lower **eyelid**
        H01.123 **Discoid lupus erythematosus of** right eye, **unspecified eyelid** ▽
        H01.124 **Discoid lupus erythematosus of** left upper **eyelid**
        H01.125 **Discoid lupus erythematosus of** left lower **eyelid**
            eye, unspecified eyelid

☑ **Add'l Character Required** ☑ᵥₓ⁷ᵗʰ **Placeholder Alert** **RUG IV Special Care High Dx** **RUG IV Clinically Complex Dx** **RUG IV Special Care Low Dx** **Manifestation Code** **Other Specified Code** ▽**Unspecified Code**

ICD-10-CM 2016   **543**

Chapter 7. Diseases of the Eye and Adnexa

H01.129 Discoid lupus erythematosus of ▽
unspecified eye, unspecified eyelid

✓6ᵗʰ **H01.13 Eczematous dermatitis of eyelid**

H01.131 Eczematous dermatitis of right upper eyelid

H01.132 Eczematous dermatitis of right lower eyelid

H01.133 Eczematous dermatitis of right eye, ▽
unspecified eyelid

H01.134 Eczematous dermatitis of left upper eyelid

H01.135 Eczematous dermatitis of left lower eyelid

H01.136 Eczematous dermatitis of left eye, ▽
unspecified eyelid

H01.139 Eczematous dermatitis of unspecified ▽
eye, unspecified eyelid

✓6ᵗʰ **H01.14 Xeroderma of eyelid**

H01.141 Xeroderma of right upper eyelid

H01.142 Xeroderma of right lower eyelid

H01.143 Xeroderma of right eye, unspecified ▽
eyelid

H01.144 Xeroderma of left upper eyelid

H01.145 Xeroderma of left lower eyelid

H01.146 Xeroderma of left eye, unspecified ▽
eyelid

H01.149 Xeroderma of unspecified eye, ▽
unspecified eyelid

H01.8 Other specified inflammations of eyelid

H01.9 Unspecified inflammation of eyelid ▽
Inflammation of eyelid NOS

✓4ᵗʰ **H02 Other disorders of eyelid**

EXCLUDES 1   congenital malformations of eyelid (Q10.0-Q10.3)

✓5ᵗʰ **H02.0 Entropion and trichiasis of eyelid**

✓6ᵗʰ **H02.00 Unspecified entropion of eyelid**

H02.001 Unspecified entropion of right upper ▽
eyelid

H02.002 Unspecified entropion of right lower ▽
eyelid

H02.003 Unspecified entropion of right eye, ▽
unspecified eyelid

H02.004 Unspecified entropion of left upper ▽
eyelid

H02.005 Unspecified entropion of left lower ▽
eyelid

H02.006 Unspecified entropion of left eye, ▽
unspecified eyelid

H02.009 Unspecified entropion of unspecified ▽
eye, unspecified eyelid

✓6ᵗʰ **H02.01 Cicatricial entropion of eyelid**

H02.011 Cicatricial entropion of right upper eyelid

H02.012 Cicatricial entropion of right lower eyelid

H02.013 Cicatricial entropion of right eye, ▽
unspecified eyelid

H02.014 Cicatricial entropion of left upper eyelid

H02.015 Cicatricial entropion of left lower eyelid

H02.016 Cicatricial entropion of left eye, ▽
unspecified eyelid

H02.019 Cicatricial entropion of unspecified ▽
eye, unspecified eyelid

✓6ᵗʰ **H02.02 Mechanical entropion of eyelid**

H02.021 Mechanical entropion of right upper eyelid

H02.022 Mechanical entropion of right lower eyelid

H02.023 Mechanical entropion of right eye, ▽
unspecified eyelid

H02.024 Mechanical entropion of left upper eyelid

H02.025 Mechanical entropion of left lower eyelid

H02.026 Mechanical entropion of left eye, ▽
unspecified eyelid

H02.029 Mechanical entropion of unspecified ▽
eye, unspecified eyelid

✓6ᵗʰ **H02.03 Senile entropion of eyelid**

H02.031 Senile entropion of right upper eyelid Ⓐ

H02.032 Senile entropion of right lower eyelid Ⓐ

H02.033 Senile entropion of right eye, Ⓐ▽
unspecified eyelid

H02.034 Senile entropion of left upper eyelid Ⓐ

H02.035 Senile entropion of left lower eyelid Ⓐ

H02.036 Senile entropion of left eye, Ⓐ▽
unspecified eyelid

H02.039 Senile entropion of unspecified eye, Ⓐ▽
unspecified eyelid

✓6ᵗʰ **H02.04 Spastic entropion of eyelid**

H02.041 Spastic entropion of right upper eyelid

H02.042 Spastic entropion of right lower eyelid

H02.043 Spastic entropion of right eye, ▽
unspecified eyelid

H02.044 Spastic entropion of left upper eyelid

H02.045 Spastic entropion of left lower eyelid

H02.046 Spastic entropion of left eye, ▽
unspecified eyelid

H02.049 Spastic entropion of unspecified eye, ▽
unspecified eyelid

✓6ᵗʰ **H02.05 Trichiasis without entropian**

H02.051 Trichiasis without entropian right upper eyelid

H02.052 Trichiasis without entropian right lower eyelid

H02.053 Trichiasis without entropian right eye, ▽
unspecified eyelid

H02.054 Trichiasis without entropian left upper eyelid

H02.055 Trichiasis without entropian left lower eyelid

H02.056 Trichiasis without entropian left eye, ▽
unspecified eyelid

H02.059 Trichiasis without entropian ▽
unspecified eye, unspecified eyelid

✓5ᵗʰ **H02.1 Ectropion of eyelid**

✓6ᵗʰ **H02.10 Unspecified ectropion of eyelid**

H02.101 Unspecified ectropion of right upper ▽
eyelid

H02.102 Unspecified ectropion of right lower ▽
eyelid

H02.103 Unspecified ectropion of right eye, ▽
unspecified eyelid

H02.104 Unspecified ectropion of left upper ▽
eyelid

H02.105 Unspecified ectropion of left lower ▽
eyelid

H02.106 Unspecified ectropion of left eye, ▽
unspecified eyelid

H02.109 Unspecified ectropion of unspecified ▽
eye, unspecified eyelid

✓6ᵗʰ **H02.11 Cicatricial ectropion of eyelid**

H02.111 Cicatricial ectropion of right upper eyelid

H02.112 Cicatricial ectropion of right lower eyelid

H02.113 Cicatricial ectropion of right eye, ▽
unspecified eyelid

H02.114 Cicatricial ectropion of left upper eyelid

H02.115 Cicatricial ectropion of left lower eyelid

H02.116 Cicatricial ectropion of left eye, ▽
unspecified eyelid

H02.119 Cicatricial ectropion of unspecified ▽
eye, unspecified eyelid

✓6ᵗʰ **H02.12 Mechanical ectropion of eyelid**

H02.121 Mechanical ectropion of right upper eyelid

H02.122 Mechanical ectropion of right lower eyelid

H02.123 Mechanical ectropion of right eye, ▽
unspecified eyelid

H02.124 Mechanical ectropion of left upper eyelid

H02.125 Mechanical ectropion of left lower eyelid

H02.126 Mechanical ectropion of left eye, ▽
unspecified eyelid

H02.129 Mechanical ectropion of unspecified ▽
eye, unspecified eyelid

✓6ᵗʰ **H02.13 Senile ectropion of eyelid**

H02.131 Senile ectropion of right upper eyelid Ⓐ

H02.132 Senile ectropion of right lower eyelid Ⓐ

H02.133 Senile ectropion of right eye, Ⓐ▽
unspecified eyelid

H02.134 Senile ectropion of left upper eyelid Ⓐ

H02.135 Senile ectropion of left lower eyelid Ⓐ

Ⓝ Newborn   Ⓟ Pediatric   Ⓜ Maternity   Ⓐ Adult   **RIC** RIC Dx   **NC Dx** Noncancer Dx   **PDx** Primary Dx   **CC** RIC CC Condition   ▶◀ Revised Text   ● New Code   ▲ Revised Code Title

544

ICD-10-CM 2016

H02.136   Senile ectropion of left eye, 🅰▽
           unspecified eyelid
H02.139   Senile ectropion of unspecified eye, 🅰▽
           unspecified eyelid

✓6ᵗʰ H02.14   Spastic ectropion of eyelid
H02.141   Spastic ectropion of right upper eyelid
H02.142   Spastic ectropion of right lower eyelid
H02.143   Spastic ectropion of right eye, ▽
           unspecified eyelid
H02.144   Spastic ectropion of left upper eyelid
H02.145   Spastic ectropion of left lower eyelid
H02.146   Spastic ectropion of left eye, ▽
           unspecified eyelid
H02.149   Spastic ectropion of unspecified eye, ▽
           unspecified eyelid

✓5ᵗʰ H02.2   Lagophthalmos
✓6ᵗʰ H02.20   Unspecified lagophthalmos
H02.201   Unspecified lagophthalmos ▽
           right upper eyelid
H02.202   Unspecified lagophthalmos ▽
           right lower eyelid
H02.203   Unspecified lagophthalmos ▽
           right eye, unspecified eyelid
H02.204   Unspecified lagophthalmos ▽
           left upper eyelid
H02.205   Unspecified lagophthalmos ▽
           left lower eyelid
H02.206   Unspecified lagophthalmos left eye, ▽
           unspecified eyelid
H02.209   Unspecified lagophthalmos ▽
           unspecified eye, unspecified eyelid

✓6ᵗʰ H02.21   Cicatricial lagophthalmos
H02.211   Cicatricial lagophthalmos right upper
           eyelid
H02.212   Cicatricial lagophthalmos right lower
           eyelid
H02.213   Cicatricial lagophthalmos right eye, ▽
           unspecified eyelid
H02.214   Cicatricial lagophthalmos left upper eyelid
H02.215   Cicatricial lagophthalmos left lower eyelid
H02.216   Cicatricial lagophthalmos left eye, ▽
           unspecified eyelid
H02.219   Cicatricial lagophthalmos unspecified ▽
           eye, unspecified eyelid

✓6ᵗʰ H02.22   Mechanical lagophthalmos
H02.221   Mechanical lagophthalmos right
           upper eyelid
H02.222   Mechanical lagophthalmos right
           lower eyelid
H02.223   Mechanical lagophthalmos right eye, ▽
           unspecified eyelid
H02.224   Mechanical lagophthalmos left
           upper eyelid
H02.225   Mechanical lagophthalmos left
           lower eyelid
H02.226   Mechanical lagophthalmos left eye, ▽
           unspecified eyelid
H02.229   Mechanical lagophthalmos unspecified ▽
           eye, unspecified eyelid

✓6ᵗʰ H02.23   Paralytic lagophthalmos
H02.231   Paralytic lagophthalmos right upper
           eyelid
H02.232   Paralytic lagophthalmos right lower
           eyelid
H02.233   Paralytic lagophthalmos right eye, ▽
           unspecified eyelid
H02.234   Paralytic lagophthalmos left upper eyelid
H02.235   Paralytic lagophthalmos left lower eyelid
H02.236   Paralytic lagophthalmos left eye, ▽
           unspecified eyelid
H02.239   Paralytic lagophthalmos unspecified ▽
           eye, unspecified eyelid

✓5ᵗʰ H02.3   Blepharochalasis
        Pseudoptosis
H02.30   Blepharochalasis unspecified eye, unspecified ▽
           eyelid
H02.31   Blepharochalasis right upper eyelid

H02.32   Blepharochalasis right lower eyelid
H02.33   Blepharochalasis right eye, unspecified eyelid ▽
H02.34   Blepharochalasis left upper eyelid
H02.35   Blepharochalasis left lower eyelid
H02.36   Blepharochalasis left eye, unspecified eyelid ▽

✓5ᵗʰ H02.4   Ptosis of eyelid
✓6ᵗʰ H02.40   Unspecified ptosis of eyelid
H02.401   Unspecified ptosis of right eyelid ▽
H02.402   Unspecified ptosis of left eyelid ▽
H02.403   Unspecified ptosis of bilateral eyelids ▽
H02.409   Unspecified ptosis of unspecified eyelid ▽

✓6ᵗʰ H02.41   Mechanical ptosis of eyelid
H02.411   Mechanical ptosis of right eyelid
H02.412   Mechanical ptosis of left eyelid
H02.413   Mechanical ptosis of bilateral eyelids
H02.419   Mechanical ptosis of unspecified eyelid ▽

✓6ᵗʰ H02.42   Myogenic ptosis of eyelid
H02.421   Myogenic ptosis of right eyelid
H02.422   Myogenic ptosis of left eyelid
H02.423   Myogenic ptosis of bilateral eyelids
H02.429   Myogenic ptosis of unspecified eyelid ▽

✓6ᵗʰ H02.43   Paralytic ptosis of eyelid
        Neurogenic ptosis of eyelid
H02.431   Paralytic ptosis of right eyelid
H02.432   Paralytic ptosis of left eyelid
H02.433   Paralytic ptosis of bilateral eyelids
H02.439   Paralytic ptosis unspecified eyelid ▽

✓5ᵗʰ H02.5   Other disorders affecting eyelid function
        EXCLUDES 2   blepharospasm (G24.5)
                     organic tic (G25.69)
                     psychogenic tic (F95.-)

✓6ᵗʰ H02.51   Abnormal innervation syndrome
H02.511   Abnormal innervation syndrome right
           upper eyelid
H02.512   Abnormal innervation syndrome right
           lower eyelid
H02.513   Abnormal innervation syndrome right ▽
           eye, unspecified eyelid
H02.514   Abnormal innervation syndrome left
           upper eyelid
H02.515   Abnormal innervation syndrome left
           lower eyelid
H02.516   Abnormal innervation syndrome left ▽
           eye, unspecified eyelid
H02.519   Abnormal innervation syndrome ▽
           unspecified eye, unspecified eyelid

✓6ᵗʰ H02.52   Blepharophimosis
        Ankyloblepharon
H02.521   Blepharophimosis right upper eyelid
H02.522   Blepharophimosis right lower eyelid
H02.523   Blepharophimosis right eye, ▽
           unspecified eyelid
H02.524   Blepharophimosis left upper eyelid
H02.525   Blepharophimosis left lower eyelid
H02.526   Blepharophimosis left eye, ▽
           unspecified eyelid
H02.529   Blepharophimosis unspecified eye, ▽
           unspecified lid

✓6ᵗʰ H02.53   Eyelid retraction
        Eyelid lag
H02.531   Eyelid retraction right upper eyelid
H02.532   Eyelid retraction right lower eyelid
H02.533   Eyelid retraction right eye, unspecified ▽
           eyelid
H02.534   Eyelid retraction left upper eyelid
H02.535   Eyelid retraction left lower eyelid
H02.536   Eyelid retraction left eye, unspecified ▽
           eyelid
H02.539   Eyelid retraction unspecified eye, ▽
           unspecified lid

H02.59   Other disorders affecting eyelid function
           Deficient blink reflex   Sensory disorders

✓5ᵗʰ H02.6   Xanthelasma of eyelid
H02.60   Xanthelasma of unspecified eye, unspecified ▽
           eyelid

Chapter 7. Diseases of the Eye and Adnexa

H02.61 Xanthelasma of right upper eyelid
H02.62 Xanthelasma of right lower eyelid
H02.63 Xanthelasma of right eye, unspecified eyelid ▽
H02.64 Xanthelasma of left upper eyelid
H02.65 Xanthelasma of left lower eyelid
H02.66 Xanthelasma of left eye, unspecified eyelid ▽

✓5th H02.7 **Other and unspecified degenerative disorders of eyelid and periocular area**

H02.70 Unspecified degenerative disorders of eyelid and periocular area ▽

✓6th H02.71 Chloasma of eyelid and periocular area
Dyspigmentation of eyelid
Hyperpigmentation of eyelid
H02.711 Chloasma of right upper eyelid and periocular area
H02.712 Chloasma of right lower eyelid and periocular area
H02.713 Chloasma of right eye, unspecified eyelid and periocular area ▽
H02.714 Chloasma of left upper eyelid and periocular area
H02.715 Chloasma of left lower eyelid and periocular area
H02.716 Chloasma of left eye, unspecified eyelid and periocular area ▽
H02.719 Chloasma of unspecified eye, unspecified eyelid and periocular area ▽

✓6th H02.72 Madarosis of eyelid and periocular area
Hypotrichosis of eyelid
H02.721 Madarosis of right upper eyelid and periocular area
H02.722 Madarosis of right lower eyelid and periocular area
H02.723 Madarosis of right eye, unspecified eyelid and periocular area
H02.724 Madarosis of left upper eyelid and periocular area
H02.725 Madarosis of left lower eyelid and periocular area
H02.726 Madarosis of left eye, unspecified eyelid and periocular area ▽
H02.729 Madarosis of unspecified eye, unspecified eyelid and periocular area ▽

✓6th H02.73 Vitiligo of eyelid and periocular area
Hypopigmentation of eyelid
H02.731 Vitiligo of right upper eyelid and periocular area
H02.732 Vitiligo of right lower eyelid and periocular area
H02.733 Vitiligo of right eye, unspecified eyelid ▽ and periocular area
H02.734 Vitiligo of left upper eyelid and periocular area
H02.735 Vitiligo of left lower eyelid and periocular area
H02.736 Vitiligo of left eye, unspecified eyelid ▽ and periocular area
H02.739 Vitiligo of unspecified eye, unspecified ▽ eyelid and periocular area

H02.79 **Other degenerative disorders of eyelid and periocular area**

✓5th H02.8 **Other specified disorders of eyelid**

✓6th H02.81 Retained foreign body in eyelid
Use additional code to identify the type of retained foreign body (Z18.-)
EXCLUDES 1 laceration of eyelid with foreign body (S01.12-)
retained intraocular foreign body (H44.6-, H44.7-)
superficial foreign body of eyelid and periocular area (S00.25-)
H02.811 Retained foreign body in right upper eyelid
H02.812 Retained foreign body in right lower eyelid
H02.813 Retained foreign body in right eye, unspecified eyelid ▽
H02.814 Retained foreign body in left upper eyelid
H02.815 Retained foreign body in left lower eyelid

H02.816 Retained foreign body in left eye, ▽ unspecified eyelid
H02.819 Retained foreign body in unspecified ▽ eye, unspecified eyelid

✓6th H02.82 Cysts of eyelid
Sebaceous cyst of eyelid
H02.821 Cysts of right upper eyelid
H02.822 Cysts of right lower eyelid
H02.823 Cysts of right eye, unspecified eyelid ▽
H02.824 Cysts of left upper eyelid
H02.825 Cysts of left lower eyelid
H02.826 Cysts of left eye, unspecified eyelid ▽
H02.829 Cysts of unspecified eye, unspecified ▽ eyelid

✓6th H02.83 Dermatochalasis of eyelid
H02.831 Dermatochalasis of right upper eyelid
H02.832 Dermatochalasis of right lower eyelid
H02.833 Dermatochalasis of right eye, ▽ unspecified eyelid
H02.834 Dermatochalasis of left upper eyelid
H02.835 Dermatochalasis of left lower eyelid
H02.836 Dermatochalasis of left eye, ▽ unspecified eyelid
H02.839 Dermatochalasis of unspecified eye, ▽ unspecified eyelid

✓6th H02.84 Edema of eyelid
Hyperemia of eyelid
H02.841 Edema of right upper eyelid
H02.842 Edema of right lower eyelid
H02.843 Edema of right eye, unspecified eyelid ▽
H02.844 Edema of left upper eyelid
H02.845 Edema of left lower eyelid
H02.846 Edema of left eye, unspecified eyelid ▽
H02.849 Edema of unspecified eye, unspecified ▽ eyelid

✓6th H02.85 Elephantiasis of eyelid
H02.851 Elephantiasis of right upper eyelid
H02.852 Elephantiasis of right lower eyelid
H02.853 Elephantiasis of right eye, unspecified ▽ eyelid
H02.854 Elephantiasis of left upper eyelid
H02.855 Elephantiasis of left lower eyelid
H02.856 Elephantiasis of left eye, unspecified ▽ eyelid
H02.859 Elephantiasis of unspecified eye, ▽ unspecified eyelid

✓6th H02.86 Hypertrichosis of eyelid
H02.861 Hypertrichosis of right upper eyelid
H02.862 Hypertrichosis of right lower eyelid
H02.863 Hypertrichosis of right eye, ▽ unspecified eyelid
H02.864 Hypertrichosis of left upper eyelid
H02.865 Hypertrichosis of left lower eyelid
H02.866 Hypertrichosis of left eye, ▽ unspecified eyelid
H02.869 Hypertrichosis of unspecified eye, ▽ unspecified eyelid

✓6th H02.87 Vascular anomalies of eyelid
H02.871 Vascular anomalies of right upper eyelid
H02.872 Vascular anomalies of right lower eyelid
H02.873 Vascular anomalies of right eye, ▽ unspecified eyelid
H02.874 Vascular anomalies of left upper eyelid
H02.875 Vascular anomalies of left lower eyelid
H02.876 Vascular anomalies of left eye, ▽ unspecified eyelid
H02.879 Vascular anomalies of unspecified eye, ▽ unspecified eyelid

H02.89 **Other specified disorders of eyelid**
Hemorrhage of eyelid

H02.9 **Unspecified disorder of eyelid** ▽
Disorder of eyelid NOS

N Newborn   P Pediatric   M Maternity   A Adult   RIC RIC Dx   NCDx Noncancer Dx   PDx Primary Dx   CC RIC CC Condition   ►◄ Revised Text   ● New Code   ▲ Revised Code Title

546
ICD-10-CM 2016

H02.61–H02.9

✔4th **H04 Disorders of lacrimal system**
     EXCLUDES 1   *congenital malformations of lacrimal system (Q10.4-Q10.6)*

   ✔5th **H04.0 Dacryoadenitis**

     ✔6th **H04.00 Unspecified dacryoadenitis**
       H04.001 Unspecified dacryoadenitis, right lacrimal gland ▽
       H04.002 Unspecified dacryoadenitis, left lacrimal gland ▽
       H04.003 Unspecified dacryoadenitis, bilateral lacrimal glands ▽
       H04.009 Unspecified dacryoadenitis, unspecified lacrimal gland ▽

     ✔6th **H04.01 Acute dacryoadenitis**
       H04.011 Acute dacryoadenitis, right lacrimal gland
       H04.012 Acute dacryoadenitis, left lacrimal gland
       H04.013 Acute dacryoadenitis, bilateral lacrimal glands
       H04.019 Acute dacryoadenitis, unspecified lacrimal gland ▽

     ✔6th **H04.02 Chronic dacryoadenitis**
       H04.021 Chronic dacryoadenitis, right lacrimal gland
       H04.022 Chronic dacryoadenitis, left lacrimal gland
       H04.023 Chronic dacryoadenitis, bilateral lacrimal glands
       H04.029 Chronic dacryoadenitis, unspecified lacrimal gland ▽

     ✔6th **H04.03 Chronic enlargement of lacrimal gland**
       H04.031 Chronic enlargement of right lacrimal gland
       H04.032 Chronic enlargement of left lacrimal gland
       H04.033 Chronic enlargement of bilateral lacrimal glands
       H04.039 Chronic enlargement of unspecified lacrimal gland ▽

   ✔5th **H04.1 Other disorders of lacrimal gland**

     ✔6th **H04.11 Dacryops**
       H04.111 Dacryops of right lacrimal gland
       H04.112 Dacryops of left lacrimal gland
       H04.113 Dacryops of bilateral lacrimal glands
       H04.119 Dacryops of unspecified lacrimal gland ▽

     ✔6th **H04.12 Dry eye syndrome**
       Tear film insufficiency, NOS
       H04.121 Dry eye syndrome of right lacrimal gland
       H04.122 Dry eye syndrome of left lacrimal gland
       H04.123 Dry eye syndrome of bilateral lacrimal glands
       H04.129 Dry eye syndrome of unspecified lacrimal gland ▽

     ✔6th **H04.13 Lacrimal cyst**
       Lacrimal cystic degeneration
       H04.131 Lacrimal cyst, right lacrimal gland
       H04.132 Lacrimal cyst, left lacrimal gland
       H04.133 Lacrimal cyst, bilateral lacrimal glands
       H04.139 Lacrimal cyst, unspecified lacrimal gland ▽

     ✔6th **H04.14 Primary lacrimal gland atrophy**
       H04.141 Primary lacrimal gland atrophy, right lacrimal gland
       H04.142 Primary lacrimal gland atrophy, left lacrimal gland
       H04.143 Primary lacrimal gland atrophy, bilateral lacrimal glands
       H04.149 Primary lacrimal gland atrophy, unspecified lacrimal gland ▽

     ✔6th **H04.15 Secondary lacrimal gland atrophy**
       H04.151 Secondary lacrimal gland atrophy, right lacrimal gland
       H04.152 Secondary lacrimal gland atrophy, left lacrimal gland
       H04.153 Secondary lacrimal gland atrophy, bilateral lacrimal glands
       H04.159 Secondary lacrimal gland atrophy, unspecified lacrimal gland ▽

     ✔6th **H04.16 Lacrimal gland dislocation**
       H04.161 Lacrimal gland dislocation, right lacrimal gland
       H04.162 Lacrimal gland dislocation, left lacrimal gland
       H04.163 Lacrimal gland dislocation, bilateral lacrimal glands
       H04.169 Lacrimal gland dislocation, unspecified lacrimal gland ▽

     H04.19 Other specified disorders of lacrimal gland

   ✔5th **H04.2 Epiphora**

     ✔6th **H04.20 Unspecified epiphora**
       H04.201 Unspecified epiphora, right lacrimal gland ▽
       H04.202 Unspecified epiphora, left lacrimal gland ▽
       H04.203 Unspecified epiphora, bilateral lacrimal glands ▽
       H04.209 Unspecified epiphora, unspecified lacrimal gland ▽

     ✔6th **H04.21 Epiphora due to excess lacrimation**
       H04.211 Epiphora due to excess lacrimation, right lacrimal gland
       H04.212 Epiphora due to excess lacrimation, left lacrimal gland
       H04.213 Epiphora due to excess lacrimation, bilateral lacrimal glands
       H04.219 Epiphora due to excess lacrimation, unspecified lacrimal gland ▽

     ✔6th **H04.22 Epiphora due to insufficient drainage**
       H04.221 Epiphora due to insufficient drainage, right lacrimal gland
       H04.222 Epiphora due to insufficient drainage, left lacrimal gland
       H04.223 Epiphora due to insufficient drainage, bilateral lacrimal glands
       H04.229 Epiphora due to insufficient drainage, unspecified lacrimal gland ▽

   ✔5th **H04.3 Acute and unspecified inflammation of lacrimal passages**
     EXCLUDES 1   *neonatal dacryocystitis (P39.1)*

     ✔6th **H04.30 Unspecified dacryocystitis**
       H04.301 Unspecified dacryocystitis of right lacrimal passage ▽
       H04.302 Unspecified dacryocystitis of left lacrimal passage ▽
       H04.303 Unspecified dacryocystitis of bilateral lacrimal passages ▽
       H04.309 Unspecified dacryocystitis of unspecified lacrimal passage ▽

     ✔6th **H04.31 Phlegmonous dacryocystitis**
       H04.311 Phlegmonous dacryocystitis of right lacrimal passage
       H04.312 Phlegmonous dacryocystitis of left lacrimal passage
       H04.313 Phlegmonous dacryocystitis of bilateral lacrimal passages
       H04.319 Phlegmonous dacryocystitis of unspecified lacrimal passage ▽

     ✔6th **H04.32 Acute dacryocystitis**
       Acute dacryopericystitis
       H04.321 Acute dacryocystitis of right lacrimal passage
       H04.322 Acute dacryocystitis of left lacrimal passage
       H04.323 Acute dacryocystitis of bilateral lacrimal passages
       H04.329 Acute dacryocystitis of unspecified lacrimal passage ▽

     ✔6th **H04.33 Acute lacrimal canaliculitis**
       H04.331 Acute lacrimal canaliculitis of right lacrimal passage
       H04.332 Acute lacrimal canaliculitis of left lacrimal passage
       H04.333 Acute lacrimal canaliculitis of bilateral lacrimal passages
       H04.339 Acute lacrimal canaliculitis of unspecified lacrimal passage ▽

✔ Add'l Character Required   ✔x7th Placeholder Alert   RUG IV Special Care High Dx   RUG IV Clinically Complex Dx   RUG IV Special Care Low Dx   Manifestation Code   Other Specified Code   ▽ Unspecified Code

✓5ᵗʰ **H04.4 Chronic inflammation of lacrimal passages**

✓6ᵗʰ **H04.41** Chronic dacryocystitis
- **H04.411** Chronic dacryocystitis of right lacrimal passage
- **H04.412** Chronic dacryocystitis of left lacrimal passage
- **H04.413** Chronic dacryocystitis of bilateral lacrimal passages
- **H04.419** Chronic dacryocystitis of unspecified lacrimal passage ▽

✓6ᵗʰ **H04.42** Chronic lacrimal canaliculitis
- **H04.421** Chronic lacrimal canaliculitis of right lacrimal passage
- **H04.422** Chronic lacrimal canaliculitis of left lacrimal passage
- **H04.423** Chronic lacrimal canaliculitis of bilateral lacrimal passages
- **H04.429** Chronic lacrimal canaliculitis of unspecified lacrimal passage ▽

✓6ᵗʰ **H04.43** Chronic lacrimal mucocele
- **H04.431** Chronic lacrimal mucocele of right lacrimal passage
- **H04.432** Chronic lacrimal mucocele of left lacrimal passage
- **H04.433** Chronic lacrimal mucocele of bilateral lacrimal passages
- **H04.439** Chronic lacrimal mucocele of unspecified lacrimal passage ▽

✓5ᵗʰ **H04.5 Stenosis and insufficiency of lacrimal passages**

✓6ᵗʰ **H04.51** Dacryolith
- **H04.511** Dacryolith of right lacrimal passage
- **H04.512** Dacryolith of left lacrimal passage
- **H04.513** Dacryolith of bilateral lacrimal passages
- **H04.519** Dacryolith of unspecified lacrimal passage ▽

✓6ᵗʰ **H04.52** Eversion of lacrimal punctum
- **H04.521** Eversion of right lacrimal punctum
- **H04.522** Eversion of left lacrimal punctum
- **H04.523** Eversion of bilateral lacrimal punctum
- **H04.529** Eversion of unspecified lacrimal punctum ▽

✓6ᵗʰ **H04.53** Neonatal obstruction of nasolacrimal duct
> **EXCLUDES 1** *congenital stenosis and stricture of lacrimal duct (Q10.5)*
- **H04.531** Neonatal obstruction of right nasolacrimal duct Ⓝ
- **H04.532** Neonatal obstruction of left nasolacrimal duct Ⓝ
- **H04.533** Neonatal obstruction of bilateral nasolacrimal duct Ⓝ
- **H04.539** Neonatal obstruction of unspecified nasolacrimal duct Ⓝ▽

✓6ᵗʰ **H04.54** Stenosis of lacrimal canaliculi
- **H04.541** Stenosis of right lacrimal canaliculi
- **H04.542** Stenosis of left lacrimal canaliculi
- **H04.543** Stenosis of bilateral lacrimal canaliculi
- **H04.549** Stenosis of unspecified lacrimal canaliculi ▽

✓6ᵗʰ **H04.55** Acquired stenosis of nasolacrimal duct
- **H04.551** Acquired stenosis of right nasolacrimal duct
- **H04.552** Acquired stenosis of left nasolacrimal duct
- **H04.553** Acquired stenosis of bilateral nasolacrimal duct
- **H04.559** Acquired stenosis of unspecified nasolacrimal duct ▽

✓6ᵗʰ **H04.56** Stenosis of lacrimal punctum
- **H04.561** Stenosis of right lacrimal punctum
- **H04.562** Stenosis of left lacrimal punctum
- **H04.563** Stenosis of bilateral lacrimal punctum
- **H04.569** Stenosis of unspecified lacrimal punctum ▽

✓6ᵗʰ **H04.57** Stenosis of lacrimal sac
- **H04.571** Stenosis of right lacrimal sac
- **H04.572** Stenosis of left lacrimal sac
- **H04.573** Stenosis of bilateral lacrimal sac
- **H04.579** Stenosis of unspecified lacrimal sac ▽

✓5ᵗʰ **H04.6 Other changes of lacrimal passages**

✓6ᵗʰ **H04.61** Lacrimal fistula
- **H04.611** Lacrimal fistula right lacrimal passage
- **H04.612** Lacrimal fistula left lacrimal passage
- **H04.613** Lacrimal fistula bilateral lacrimal passages
- **H04.619** Lacrimal fistula unspecified lacrimal passage ▽

- **H04.69** Other changes of lacrimal passages

✓5ᵗʰ **H04.8 Other disorders of lacrimal system**

✓6ᵗʰ **H04.81** Granuloma of lacrimal passages
- **H04.811** Granuloma of right lacrimal passage
- **H04.812** Granuloma of left lacrimal passage
- **H04.813** Granuloma of bilateral lacrimal passages
- **H04.819** Granuloma of unspecified lacrimal passage ▽

- **H04.89** Other disorders of lacrimal system

H04.9 Disorder of lacrimal system, unspecified ▽

✓4ᵗʰ **H05 Disorders of orbit**
> **EXCLUDES 1** *congenital malformation of orbit (Q10.7)*

✓5ᵗʰ **H05.0 Acute inflammation of orbit**
- **H05.00** Unspecified acute inflammation of orbit ▽

✓6ᵗʰ **H05.01** Cellulitis of orbit
     Abscess of orbit
- **H05.011** Cellulitis of right orbit 🅲🅲
- **H05.012** Cellulitis of left orbit 🅲🅲
- **H05.013** Cellulitis of bilateral orbits 🅲🅲
- **H05.019** Cellulitis of unspecified orbit 🅲🅲▽

✓6ᵗʰ **H05.02** Osteomyelitis of orbit
- **H05.021** Osteomyelitis of right orbit 🅲🅲
- **H05.022** Osteomyelitis of left orbit 🅲🅲
- **H05.023** Osteomyelitis of bilateral orbits 🅲🅲
- **H05.029** Osteomyelitis of unspecified orbit 🅲🅲▽

✓6ᵗʰ **H05.03** Periostitis of orbit
- **H05.031** Periostitis of right orbit 🅲🅲
- **H05.032** Periostitis of left orbit 🅲🅲
- **H05.033** Periostitis of bilateral orbits 🅲🅲
- **H05.039** Periostitis of unspecified orbit 🅲🅲▽

✓6ᵗʰ **H05.04** Tenonitis of orbit
- **H05.041** Tenonitis of right orbit
- **H05.042** Tenonitis of left orbit
- **H05.043** Tenonitis of bilateral orbits
- **H05.049** Tenonitis of unspecified orbit ▽

✓5ᵗʰ **H05.1 Chronic inflammatory disorders of orbit**
- **H05.10** Unspecified chronic inflammatory disorders of orbit ▽

✓6ᵗʰ **H05.11** Granuloma of orbit
     Pseudotumor (inflammatory) of orbit
- **H05.111** Granuloma of right orbit
- **H05.112** Granuloma of left orbit
- **H05.113** Granuloma of bilateral orbits
- **H05.119** Granuloma of unspecified orbit ▽

✓6ᵗʰ **H05.12** Orbital myositis
- **H05.121** Orbital myositis, right orbit
- **H05.122** Orbital myositis, left orbit
- **H05.123** Orbital myositis, bilateral
- **H05.129** Orbital myositis, unspecified orbit ▽

✓5ᵗʰ **H05.2 Exophthalmic conditions**
- **H05.20** Unspecified exophthalmos ▽

✓6ᵗʰ **H05.21** Displacement (lateral) of globe
- **H05.211** Displacement (lateral) of globe, right eye
- **H05.212** Displacement (lateral) of globe, left eye
- **H05.213** Displacement (lateral) of globe, bilateral
- **H05.219** Displacement (lateral) of globe, unspecified eye ▽

✓6ᵗʰ **H05.22** Edema of orbit
     Orbital congestion
- **H05.221** Edema of right orbit
- **H05.222** Edema of left orbit
- **H05.223** Edema of bilateral orbit
- **H05.229** Edema of unspecified orbit ▽

Ⓝ Newborn   Ⓟ Pediatric   Ⓜ Maternity   Ⓐ Adult   **RIC** RIC Dx   **NC Dx** Noncancer Dx   **PD Dx** Primary Dx   🅲🅲 RIC CC Condition   ▶◀ Revised Text   ● New Code   ▲ Revised Code Title

548

ICD-10-CM 2016

✓6ᵗʰ **H05.23 Hemorrhage of orbit**
    H05.231 Hemorrhage of right orbit
    H05.232 Hemorrhage of left orbit
    H05.233 Hemorrhage of bilateral orbit
    H05.239 Hemorrhage of unspecified orbit ▽

✓6ᵗʰ **H05.24 Constant exophthalmos**
    H05.241 Constant exophthalmos, right eye
    H05.242 Constant exophthalmos, left eye
    H05.243 Constant exophthalmos, bilateral
    H05.249 Constant exophthalmos, unspecified eye ▽

✓6ᵗʰ **H05.25 Intermittent exophthalmos**
    H05.251 Intermittent exophthalmos, right eye
    H05.252 Intermittent exophthalmos, left eye
    H05.253 Intermittent exophthalmos, bilateral
    H05.259 Intermittent exophthalmos, unspecified eye ▽

✓6ᵗʰ **H05.26 Pulsating exophthalmos**
    H05.261 Pulsating exophthalmos, right eye
    H05.262 Pulsating exophthalmos, left eye
    H05.263 Pulsating exophthalmos, bilateral
    H05.269 Pulsating exophthalmos, unspecified eye ▽

✓5ᵗʰ **H05.3 Deformity of orbit**
    EXCLUDES 1   *congenital deformity of orbit (Q10.7)*
        hypertelorism (Q75.2)
    H05.30 Unspecified deformity of orbit ▽

✓6ᵗʰ **H05.31 Atrophy of orbit**
    H05.311 Atrophy of right orbit
    H05.312 Atrophy of left orbit
    H05.313 Atrophy of bilateral orbit
    H05.319 Atrophy of unspecified orbit ▽

✓6ᵗʰ **H05.32 Deformity of orbit due to bone disease**
    Code also associated bone disease
    H05.321 Deformity of right orbit due to bone disease
    H05.322 Deformity of left orbit due to bone disease
    H05.323 Deformity of bilateral orbits due to bone disease
    H05.329 Deformity of unspecified orbit due to bone disease ▽

✓6ᵗʰ **H05.33 Deformity of orbit due to trauma or surgery**
    H05.331 Deformity of right orbit due to trauma or surgery
    H05.332 Deformity of left orbit due to trauma or surgery
    H05.333 Deformity of bilateral orbits due to trauma or surgery
    H05.339 Deformity of unspecified orbit due to trauma or surgery ▽

✓6ᵗʰ **H05.34 Enlargement of orbit**
    H05.341 Enlargement of right orbit
    H05.342 Enlargement of left orbit
    H05.343 Enlargement of bilateral orbits
    H05.349 Enlargement of unspecified orbit ▽

✓6ᵗʰ **H05.35 Exostosis of orbit**
    H05.351 Exostosis of right orbit
    H05.352 Exostosis of left orbit
    H05.353 Exostosis of bilateral orbits
    H05.359 Exostosis of unspecified orbit ▽

✓5ᵗʰ **H05.4 Enophthalmos**
  ✓6ᵗʰ **H05.40 Unspecified enophthalmos**
    H05.401 Unspecified enophthalmos, right eye ▽
    H05.402 Unspecified enophthalmos, left eye ▽
    H05.403 Unspecified enophthalmos, bilateral ▽
    H05.409 Unspecified enophthalmos, unspecified eye ▽

  ✓6ᵗʰ **H05.41 Enophthalmos due to atrophy of orbital tissue**
    H05.411 Enophthalmos due to atrophy of orbital tissue, right eye
    H05.412 Enophthalmos due to atrophy of orbital tissue, left eye
    H05.413 Enophthalmos due to atrophy of orbital tissue, bilateral

    H05.419 Enophthalmos due to atrophy of orbital tissue, unspecified eye ▽

  ✓6ᵗʰ **H05.42 Enophthalmos due to trauma or surgery**
    H05.421 Enophthalmos due to trauma or surgery, right eye
    H05.422 Enophthalmos due to trauma or surgery, left eye
    H05.423 Enophthalmos due to trauma or surgery, bilateral
    H05.429 Enophthalmos due to trauma or surgery, unspecified eye ▽

✓5ᵗʰ **H05.5 Retained (old) foreign body following penetrating wound of orbit**
    Retrobulbar foreign body
    Use additional code to identify the type of retained foreign body (Z18.-)
    EXCLUDES 1   *current penetrating wound of orbit (S05.4-)*
    EXCLUDES 2   *retained foreign body of eyelid (H02.81-)*
        retained intraocular foreign body (H44.6-, H44.7-)
    H05.50 Retained (old) foreign body following penetrating wound of unspecified orbit ▽
    H05.51 Retained (old) foreign body following penetrating wound of right orbit
    H05.52 Retained (old) foreign body following penetrating wound of left orbit
    H05.53 Retained (old) foreign body following penetrating wound of bilateral orbits

✓5ᵗʰ **H05.8 Other disorders of orbit**
  ✓6ᵗʰ **H05.81 Cyst of orbit**
    Encephalocele of orbit
    H05.811 Cyst of right orbit
    H05.812 Cyst of left orbit
    H05.813 Cyst of bilateral orbits
    H05.819 Cyst of unspecified orbit ▽

  ✓6ᵗʰ **H05.82 Myopathy of extraocular muscles**
    H05.821 Myopathy of extraocular muscles, right orbit
    H05.822 Myopathy of extraocular muscles, left orbit
    H05.823 Myopathy of extraocular muscles, bilateral
    H05.829 Myopathy of extraocular muscles, unspecified orbit ▽

    H05.89 Other disorders of orbit
  H05.9 Unspecified disorder of orbit ▽

Disorders of conjunctiva (H10-H11)

✓4ᵗʰ **H10 Conjunctivitis**
    EXCLUDES 1   *keratoconjunctivitis (H16.2-)*
  ✓5ᵗʰ **H10.0 Mucopurulent conjunctivitis**
    ✓6ᵗʰ **H10.01 Acute follicular conjunctivitis**
      H10.011 Acute follicular conjunctivitis, right eye
      H10.012 Acute follicular conjunctivitis, left eye
      H10.013 Acute follicular conjunctivitis, bilateral
      H10.019 Acute follicular conjunctivitis, unspecified eye ▽

    ✓6ᵗʰ **H10.02 Other mucopurulent conjunctivitis**
      H10.021 Other mucopurulent conjunctivitis, right eye
      H10.022 Other mucopurulent conjunctivitis, left eye
      H10.023 Other mucopurulent conjunctivitis, bilateral
      H10.029 Other mucopurulent conjunctivitis, unspecified eye ▽

  ✓5ᵗʰ **H10.1 Acute atopic conjunctivitis**
    Acute papillary conjunctivitis
    H10.10 Acute atopic conjunctivitis, unspecified eye ▽
    H10.11 Acute atopic conjunctivitis, right eye
    H10.12 Acute atopic conjunctivitis, left eye
    H10.13 Acute atopic conjunctivitis, bilateral
  ✓5ᵗʰ **H10.2 Other acute conjunctivitis**

Chapter 7. Diseases of the Eye and Adnexa

H10.21–H11.059

✓6ᵗʰ **H10.21 Acute toxic conjunctivitis**
Acute chemical conjunctivitis
Code first (T51-T65) to identify chemical and intent
EXCLUDES 1   *burn and corrosion of eye and adnexa (T26.-)*

H10.211 Acute toxic conjunctivitis, right eye
H10.212 Acute toxic conjunctivitis, left eye
H10.213 Acute toxic conjunctivitis, bilateral
H10.219 Acute toxic conjunctivitis, unspecified eye ▽

✓6ᵗʰ **H10.22 Pseudomembranous conjunctivitis**
H10.221 Pseudomembranous conjunctivitis, right eye
H10.222 Pseudomembranous conjunctivitis, left eye
H10.223 Pseudomembranous conjunctivitis, bilateral
H10.229 Pseudomembranous conjunctivitis, unspecified eye ▽

✓6ᵗʰ **H10.23 Serous conjunctivitis, except viral**
EXCLUDES 1   *viral conjunctivitis (B30.-)*
H10.231 Serous conjunctivitis, except viral, right eye
H10.232 Serous conjunctivitis, except viral, left eye
H10.233 Serous conjunctivitis, except viral, bilateral
H10.239 Serous conjunctivitis, except viral, unspecified eye ▽

✓5ᵗʰ **H10.3 Unspecified acute conjunctivitis**
EXCLUDES 1   *ophthalmia neonatorum NOS (P39.1)*
H10.30 Unspecified acute conjunctivitis, unspecified eye ▽
H10.31 Unspecified acute conjunctivitis, right eye ▽
H10.32 Unspecified acute conjunctivitis, left eye ▽
H10.33 Unspecified acute conjunctivitis, bilateral ▽

✓5ᵗʰ **H10.4 Chronic conjunctivitis**
✓6ᵗʰ **H10.40 Unspecified chronic conjunctivitis**
H10.401 Unspecified chronic conjunctivitis, right eye ▽
H10.402 Unspecified chronic conjunctivitis, left eye ▽
H10.403 Unspecified chronic conjunctivitis, bilateral ▽
H10.409 Unspecified chronic conjunctivitis, unspecified eye ▽

✓6ᵗʰ **H10.41 Chronic giant papillary conjunctivitis**
H10.411 Chronic giant papillary conjunctivitis, right eye
H10.412 Chronic giant papillary conjunctivitis, left eye
H10.413 Chronic giant papillary conjunctivitis, bilateral
H10.419 Chronic giant papillary conjunctivitis, unspecified eye ▽

✓6ᵗʰ **H10.42 Simple chronic conjunctivitis**
H10.421 Simple chronic conjunctivitis, right eye
H10.422 Simple chronic conjunctivitis, left eye
H10.423 Simple chronic conjunctivitis, bilateral
H10.429 Simple chronic conjunctivitis, unspecified eye ▽

✓6ᵗʰ **H10.43 Chronic follicular conjunctivitis**
H10.431 Chronic follicular conjunctivitis, right eye
H10.432 Chronic follicular conjunctivitis, left eye
H10.433 Chronic follicular conjunctivitis, bilateral
H10.439 Chronic follicular conjunctivitis, unspecified eye ▽

H10.44 Vernal conjunctivitis
EXCLUDES 1   *vernal keratoconjunctivitis with limbar and corneal involvement (H16.26-)*

H10.45 Other chronic allergic conjunctivitis

✓5ᵗʰ **H10.5 Blepharoconjunctivitis**
✓6ᵗʰ **H10.50 Unspecified blepharoconjunctivitis**
H10.501 Unspecified blepharoconjunctivitis, right eye ▽
H10.502 Unspecified blepharoconjunctivitis, left eye ▽

H10.503 Unspecified blepharoconjunctivitis, bilateral ▽
H10.509 Unspecified blepharoconjunctivitis, unspecified eye ▽

✓6ᵗʰ **H10.51 Ligneous conjunctivitis**
H10.511 Ligneous conjunctivitis, right eye
H10.512 Ligneous conjunctivitis, left eye
H10.513 Ligneous conjunctivitis, bilateral
H10.519 Ligneous conjunctivitis, unspecified eye ▽

✓6ᵗʰ **H10.52 Angular blepharoconjunctivitis**
H10.521 Angular blepharoconjunctivitis, right eye
H10.522 Angular blepharoconjunctivitis, left eye
H10.523 Angular blepharoconjunctivitis, bilateral
H10.529 Angular blepharoconjunctivitis, unspecified eye ▽

✓6ᵗʰ **H10.53 Contact blepharoconjunctivitis**
H10.531 Contact blepharoconjunctivitis, right eye
H10.532 Contact blepharoconjunctivitis, left eye
H10.533 Contact blepharoconjunctivitis, bilateral
H10.539 Contact blepharoconjunctivitis, unspecified eye ▽

✓5ᵗʰ **H10.8 Other conjunctivitis**
✓6ᵗʰ **H10.81 Pingueculitis**
EXCLUDES 1   *pinguecula (H11.15-)*
H10.811 Pingueculitis, right eye
H10.812 Pingueculitis, left eye
H10.813 Pingueculitis, bilateral
H10.819 Pingueculitis, unspecified eye ▽

H10.89 Other conjunctivitis

H10.9 Unspecified conjunctivitis ▽

✓4ᵗʰ **H11 Other disorders of conjunctiva**
EXCLUDES 1   *keratoconjunctivitis (H16.2-)*

✓5ᵗʰ **H11.0 Pterygium of eye**
EXCLUDES 1   *pseudopterygium (H11.81-)*

✓6ᵗʰ **H11.00 Unspecified pterygium of eye**
H11.001 Unspecified pterygium of right eye ▽
H11.002 Unspecified pterygium of left eye ▽
H11.003 Unspecified pterygium of eye, bilateral ▽
H11.009 Unspecified pterygium of unspecified eye ▽

✓6ᵗʰ **H11.01 Amyloid pterygium**
H11.011 Amyloid pterygium of right eye
H11.012 Amyloid pterygium of left eye
H11.013 Amyloid pterygium of eye, bilateral
H11.019 Amyloid pterygium of unspecified eye ▽

✓6ᵗʰ **H11.02 Central pterygium of eye**
H11.021 Central pterygium of right eye
H11.022 Central pterygium of left eye
H11.023 Central pterygium of eye, bilateral
H11.029 Central pterygium of unspecified eye ▽

✓6ᵗʰ **H11.03 Double pterygium of eye**
H11.031 Double pterygium of right eye
H11.032 Double pterygium of left eye
H11.033 Double pterygium of eye, bilateral
H11.039 Double pterygium of unspecified eye ▽

✓6ᵗʰ **H11.04 Peripheral pterygium of eye, stationary**
H11.041 Peripheral pterygium, stationary, right eye
H11.042 Peripheral pterygium, stationary, left eye
H11.043 Peripheral pterygium, stationary, bilateral
H11.049 Peripheral pterygium, stationary, unspecified eye ▽

✓6ᵗʰ **H11.05 Peripheral pterygium of eye, progressive**
H11.051 Peripheral pterygium, progressive, right eye
H11.052 Peripheral pterygium, progressive, left eye
H11.053 Peripheral pterygium, progressive, bilateral
H11.059 Peripheral pterygium, progressive, unspecified eye ▽

Ⓝ Newborn   Ⓟ Pediatric   Ⓜ Maternity   Ⓐ Adult   RIC RIC Dx   NC Dx Noncancer Dx   PDx Primary Dx   CC RIC CC Condition   ►◄ Revised Text   ● New Code   ▲ Revised Code Title

550   ICD-10-CM 2016

✓6th **H11.06　Recurrent pterygium of eye**
　　　　H11.061　Recurrent pterygium of right eye
　　　　H11.062　Recurrent pterygium of left eye
　　　　H11.063　Recurrent pterygium of eye, bilateral
　　　　H11.069　Recurrent pterygium of unspecified eye ▽

✓5th **H11.1　Conjunctival degenerations and deposits**
　　　EXCLUDES 2　*pseudopterygium (H11.81)*
　　　　H11.10　Unspecified conjunctival degenerations ▽

✓6th **H11.11　Conjunctival deposits**
　　　　H11.111　Conjunctival deposits, right eye
　　　　H11.112　Conjunctival deposits, left eye
　　　　H11.113　Conjunctival deposits, bilateral
　　　　H11.119　Conjunctival deposits, unspecified eye ▽

✓6th **H11.12　Conjunctival concretions**
　　　　H11.121　Conjunctival concretions, right eye
　　　　H11.122　Conjunctival concretions, left eye
　　　　H11.123　Conjunctival concretions, bilateral
　　　　H11.129　Conjunctival concretions, unspecified ▽
　　　　　　　　　eye

✓6th **H11.13　Conjunctival pigmentations**
　　　　Conjunctival argyrosis [argyria]
　　　　H11.131　Conjunctival pigmentations, right eye
　　　　H11.132　Conjunctival pigmentations, left eye
　　　　H11.133　Conjunctival pigmentations, bilateral
　　　　H11.139　Conjunctival pigmentations, ▽
　　　　　　　　　unspecified eye

✓6th **H11.14　Conjunctival xerosis, unspecified**
　　　EXCLUDES 1　*xerosis of conjunctiva due to vitamin A
　　　　　　　　　deficiency (E50.0, E50.1)*
　　　　H11.141　Conjunctival xerosis, unspecified, right ▽
　　　　　　　　　eye
　　　　H11.142　Conjunctival xerosis , unspecified, left ▽
　　　　　　　　　eye
　　　　H11.143　Conjunctival xerosis, unspecified, ▽
　　　　　　　　　bilateral
　　　　H11.149　Conjunctival xerosis, unspecified, ▽
　　　　　　　　　unspecified eye

✓6th **H11.15　Pinguecula**
　　　EXCLUDES 1　*pingueculitis (H10.81-)*
　　　　H11.151　Pinguecula, right eye
　　　　H11.152　Pinguecula, left eye
　　　　H11.153　Pinguecula, bilateral
　　　　H11.159　Pinguecula, unspecified eye ▽

✓5th **H11.2　Conjunctival scars**
　✓6th **H11.21　Conjunctival adhesions and strands (localized)**
　　　　H11.211　Conjunctival adhesions and strands
　　　　　　　　　(localized), right eye
　　　　H11.212　Conjunctival adhesions and strands
　　　　　　　　　(localized), left eye
　　　　H11.213　Conjunctival adhesions and strands
　　　　　　　　　(localized), bilateral
　　　　H11.219　Conjunctival adhesions and strands ▽
　　　　　　　　　(localized), unspecified eye

　✓6th **H11.22　Conjunctival granuloma**
　　　　H11.221　Conjunctival granuloma, right eye
　　　　H11.222　Conjunctival granuloma, left eye
　　　　H11.223　Conjunctival granuloma, bilateral
　　　　H11.229　Conjunctival granuloma, unspecified ▽

　✓6th **H11.23　Symblepharon**
　　　　H11.231　Symblepharon, right eye
　　　　H11.232　Symblepharon, left eye
　　　　H11.233　Symblepharon, bilateral
　　　　H11.239　Symblepharon, unspecified eye ▽

　✓6th **H11.24　Scarring of conjunctiva**
　　　　H11.241　Scarring of conjunctiva, right eye
　　　　H11.242　Scarring of conjunctiva, left eye
　　　　H11.243　Scarring of conjunctiva, bilateral
　　　　H11.249　Scarring of conjunctiva, unspecified ▽
　　　　　　　　　eye

✓5th **H11.3　Conjunctival hemorrhage**
　　　　Subconjunctival hemorrhage
　　　　H11.30　Conjunctival hemorrhage, unspecified eye ▽
　　　　H11.31　Conjunctival hemorrhage, right eye

　　　　H11.32　Conjunctival hemorrhage, left eye
　　　　H11.33　Conjunctival hemorrhage, bilateral

✓5th **H11.4　Other conjunctival vascular disorders and cysts**
　✓6th **H11.41　Vascular abnormalities of conjunctiva**
　　　　Conjunctival aneurysm
　　　　H11.411　Vascular abnormalities of conjunctiva,
　　　　　　　　　right eye
　　　　H11.412　Vascular abnormalities of conjunctiva, left
　　　　　　　　　eye
　　　　H11.413　Vascular abnormalities of conjunctiva,
　　　　　　　　　bilateral
　　　　H11.419　Vascular abnormalities of conjunctiva, ▽
　　　　　　　　　unspecified eye

　✓6th **H11.42　Conjunctival edema**
　　　　H11.421　Conjunctival edema, right eye
　　　　H11.422　Conjunctival edema, left eye
　　　　H11.423　Conjunctival edema, bilateral
　　　　H11.429　Conjunctival edema, unspecified eye ▽

　✓6th **H11.43　Conjunctival hyperemia**
　　　　H11.431　Conjunctival hyperemia, right eye
　　　　H11.432　Conjunctival hyperemia, left eye
　　　　H11.433　Conjunctival hyperemia, bilateral
　　　　H11.439　Conjunctival hyperemia, unspecified ▽
　　　　　　　　　eye

　✓6th **H11.44　Conjunctival cysts**
　　　　H11.441　Conjunctival cysts, right eye
　　　　H11.442　Conjunctival cysts, left eye
　　　　H11.443　Conjunctival cysts, bilateral
　　　　H11.449　Conjunctival cysts, unspecified eye ▽

✓5th **H11.8　Other specified disorders of conjunctiva**
　✓6th **H11.81　Pseudopterygium of conjunctiva**
　　　　H11.811　Pseudopterygium of conjunctiva, right
　　　　　　　　　eye
　　　　H11.812　Pseudopterygium of conjunctiva, left eye
　　　　H11.813　Pseudopterygium of conjunctiva, bilateral
　　　　H11.819　Pseudopterygium of conjunctiva, ▽
　　　　　　　　　unspecified eye

　✓6th **H11.82　Conjunctivochalasis**
　　　　H11.821　Conjunctivochalasis, right eye
　　　　H11.822　Conjunctivochalasis, left eye
　　　　H11.823　Conjunctivochalasis, bilateral
　　　　H11.829　Conjunctivochalasis, unspecified eye ▽
　　　　H11.89　Other specified disorders of conjunctiva
　　　　H11.9　Unspecified disorder of conjunctiva ▽

Disorders of sclera, cornea, iris and ciliary body (H15-H22)

✓4th **H15　Disorders of sclera**
　✓5th **H15.0　Scleritis**
　　✓6th **H15.00　Unspecified scleritis**
　　　　H15.001　Unspecified scleritis, right eye ▽
　　　　H15.002　Unspecified scleritis, left eye ▽
　　　　H15.003　Unspecified scleritis, bilateral ▽
　　　　H15.009　Unspecified scleritis, unspecified eye ▽

　　✓6th **H15.01　Anterior scleritis**
　　　　H15.011　Anterior scleritis, right eye
　　　　H15.012　Anterior scleritis, left eye
　　　　H15.013　Anterior scleritis, bilateral
　　　　H15.019　Anterior scleritis, unspecified eye ▽

　　✓6th **H15.02　Brawny scleritis**
　　　　H15.021　Brawny scleritis, right eye
　　　　H15.022　Brawny scleritis, left eye
　　　　H15.023　Brawny scleritis, bilateral
　　　　H15.029　Brawny scleritis, unspecified eye ▽

　　✓6th **H15.03　Posterior scleritis**
　　　　Sclerotenonitis
　　　　H15.031　Posterior scleritis, right eye
　　　　H15.032　Posterior scleritis, left eye
　　　　H15.033　Posterior scleritis, bilateral
　　　　H15.039　Posterior scleritis, unspecified eye ▽

　　✓6th **H15.04　Scleritis with corneal involvement**
　　　　H15.041　Scleritis with corneal involvement, right
　　　　　　　　　eye

H15.042 Scleritis with corneal involvement, left eye

H15.043 Scleritis with corneal involvement, bilateral

H15.049 Scleritis with corneal involvement, unspecified eye ▽

√6th **H15.05** Scleromalacia perforans

H15.051 Scleromalacia perforans, right eye

H15.052 Scleromalacia perforans, left eye

H15.053 Scleromalacia perforans, bilateral

H15.059 Scleromalacia perforans, unspecified eye ▽

√6th **H15.09** Other scleritis
Scleral abscess

H15.091 Other scleritis, right eye

H15.092 Other scleritis, left eye

H15.093 Other scleritis, bilateral

H15.099 Other scleritis, unspecified eye ▽

√5th **H15.1** Episcleritis

√6th **H15.10** Unspecified episcleritis

H15.101 Unspecified episcleritis, right eye ▽

H15.102 Unspecified episcleritis, left eye ▽

H15.103 Unspecified episcleritis, bilateral ▽

H15.109 Unspecified episcleritis, unspecified eye ▽

√6th **H15.11** Episcleritis periodica fugax

H15.111 Episcleritis periodica fugax, right eye

H15.112 Episcleritis periodica fugax, left eye

H15.113 Episcleritis periodica fugax, bilateral

H15.119 Episcleritis periodica fugax, unspecified eye ▽

√6th **H15.12** Nodular episcleritis

H15.121 Nodular episcleritis, right eye

H15.122 Nodular episcleritis, left eye

H15.123 Nodular episcleritis, bilateral

H15.129 Nodular episcleritis, unspecified eye ▽

√5th **H15.8** Other disorders of sclera
EXCLUDES 2 blue sclera (Q13.5)
degenerative myopia (H44.2-)

√6th **H15.81** Equatorial staphyloma

H15.811 Equatorial staphyloma, right eye

H15.812 Equatorial staphyloma, left eye

H15.813 Equatorial staphyloma, bilateral

H15.819 Equatorial staphyloma, unspecified eye ▽

√6th **H15.82** Localized anterior staphyloma

H15.821 Localized anterior staphyloma, right eye

H15.822 Localized anterior staphyloma, left eye

H15.823 Localized anterior staphyloma, bilateral

H15.829 Localized anterior staphyloma, unspecified eye ▽

√6th **H15.83** Staphyloma posticum

H15.831 Staphyloma posticum, right eye

H15.832 Staphyloma posticum, left eye

H15.833 Staphyloma posticum, bilateral

H15.839 Staphyloma posticum, unspecified eye ▽

√6th **H15.84** Scleral ectasia

H15.841 Scleral ectasia, right eye

H15.842 Scleral ectasia, left eye

H15.843 Scleral ectasia, bilateral

H15.849 Scleral ectasia, unspecified eye ▽

√6th **H15.85** Ring staphyloma

H15.851 Ring staphyloma, right eye

H15.852 Ring staphyloma, left eye

H15.853 Ring staphyloma, bilateral

H15.859 Ring staphyloma, unspecified eye ▽

H15.89 Other disorders of sclera

H15.9 Unspecified disorder of sclera ▽

√4th **H16** Keratitis

√5th **H16.0** Corneal ulcer

√6th **H16.00** Unspecified corneal ulcer

H16.001 Unspecified corneal ulcer, right eye ▽

H16.002 Unspecified corneal ulcer, left eye ▽

H16.003 Unspecified corneal ulcer, bilateral ▽

H16.009 Unspecified corneal ulcer, unspecified eye ▽

√6th **H16.01** Central corneal ulcer

H16.011 Central corneal ulcer, right eye

H16.012 Central corneal ulcer, left eye

H16.013 Central corneal ulcer, bilateral

H16.019 Central corneal ulcer, unspecified eye ▽

√6th **H16.02** Ring corneal ulcer

H16.021 Ring corneal ulcer, right eye

H16.022 Ring corneal ulcer, left eye

H16.023 Ring corneal ulcer, bilateral

H16.029 Ring corneal ulcer, unspecified eye ▽

√6th **H16.03** Corneal ulcer with hypopyon

H16.031 Corneal ulcer with hypopyon, right eye

H16.032 Corneal ulcer with hypopyon, left eye

H16.033 Corneal ulcer with hypopyon, bilateral

H16.039 Corneal ulcer with hypopyon, unspecified eye ▽

√6th **H16.04** Marginal corneal ulcer

H16.041 Marginal corneal ulcer, right eye

H16.042 Marginal corneal ulcer, left eye

H16.043 Marginal corneal ulcer, bilateral

H16.049 Marginal corneal ulcer, unspecified eye ▽

√6th **H16.05** Mooren's corneal ulcer

H16.051 Mooren's corneal ulcer, right eye

H16.052 Mooren's corneal ulcer, left eye

H16.053 Mooren's corneal ulcer, bilateral

H16.059 Mooren's corneal ulcer, unspecified eye ▽

√6th **H16.06** Mycotic corneal ulcer

H16.061 Mycotic corneal ulcer, right eye

H16.062 Mycotic corneal ulcer, left eye

H16.063 Mycotic corneal ulcer, bilateral

H16.069 Mycotic corneal ulcer, unspecified eye ▽

√6th **H16.07** Perforated corneal ulcer

H16.071 Perforated corneal ulcer, right eye

H16.072 Perforated corneal ulcer, left eye

H16.073 Perforated corneal ulcer, bilateral

H16.079 Perforated corneal ulcer, unspecified eye ▽

√5th **H16.1** Other and unspecified superficial keratitis without conjunctivitis

√6th **H16.10** Unspecified superficial keratitis

H16.101 Unspecified superficial keratitis, right eye ▽

H16.102 Unspecified superficial keratitis, left eye ▽

H16.103 Unspecified superficial keratitis, bilateral ▽

H16.109 Unspecified superficial keratitis, unspecified eye ▽

√6th **H16.11** Macular keratitis
Areolar keratitis
Nummular keratitis
Stellate keratitis
Striate keratitis

H16.111 Macular keratitis, right eye

H16.112 Macular keratitis, left eye

H16.113 Macular keratitis, bilateral

H16.119 Macular keratitis, unspecified eye ▽

√6th **H16.12** Filamentary keratitis

H16.121 Filamentary keratitis, right eye

H16.122 Filamentary keratitis, left eye

H16.123 Filamentary keratitis, bilateral

H16.129 Filamentary keratitis, unspecified eye ▽

√6th **H16.13** Photokeratitis
Snow blindness
Welders keratitis

H16.131 Photokeratitis, right eye

H16.132 Photokeratitis, left eye

H16.133 Photokeratitis, bilateral

H16.139 Photokeratitis, unspecified eye ▽

Ⓝ Newborn   Ⓟ Pediatric   Ⓜ Maternity   Ⓐ Adult   RIC RIC Dx   NC Dx Noncancer Dx   PDx Primary Dx   CC RIC CC Condition   ►◄ Revised Text   ● New Code   ▲ Revised Code Title

552   ICD-10-CM 2016

✓6ᵗʰ **H16.14** Punctate keratitis
     H16.141 Punctate keratitis, right eye
     H16.142 Punctate keratitis, left eye
     H16.143 Punctate keratitis, bilateral
     H16.149 Punctate keratitis, unspecified eye ▽

✓5ᵗʰ **H16.2** Keratoconjunctivitis
   ✓6ᵗʰ **H16.20** Unspecified keratoconjunctivitis
       Superficial keratitis with conjunctivitis NOS
     H16.201 Unspecified keratoconjunctivitis, right eye ▽
     H16.202 Unspecified keratoconjunctivitis, left eye ▽
     H16.203 Unspecified keratoconjunctivitis, bilateral ▽
     H16.209 Unspecified keratoconjunctivitis, unspecified eye ▽

   ✓6ᵗʰ **H16.21** Exposure keratoconjunctivitis
     H16.211 Exposure keratoconjunctivitis, right eye
     H16.212 Exposure keratoconjunctivitis, left eye
     H16.213 Exposure keratoconjunctivitis, bilateral
     H16.219 Exposure keratoconjunctivitis, unspecified eye

   ✓6ᵗʰ **H16.22** Keratoconjunctivitis sicca, not specified as Sjögren's
       EXCLUDES 1   Sjögren's syndrome (M35.Ø1)
     H16.221 Keratoconjunctivitis sicca, not specified as Sjögren's, right eye
     H16.222 Keratoconjunctivitis sicca, not specified as Sjögren's, left eye
     H16.223 Keratoconjunctivitis sicca, not specified as Sjögren's, bilateral
     H16.229 Keratoconjunctivitis sicca, not specified as Sjögren's, unspecified eye ▽

   ✓6ᵗʰ **H16.23** Neurotrophic keratoconjunctivitis
     H16.231 Neurotrophic keratoconjunctivitis, right eye
     H16.232 Neurotrophic keratoconjunctivitis, left eye
     H16.233 Neurotrophic keratoconjunctivitis, bilateral
     H16.239 Neurotrophic keratoconjunctivitis, unspecified eye ▽

   ✓6ᵗʰ **H16.24** Ophthalmia nodosa
     H16.241 Ophthalmia nodosa, right eye
     H16.242 Ophthalmia nodosa, left eye
     H16.243 Ophthalmia nodosa, bilateral
     H16.249 Ophthalmia nodosa, unspecified eye ▽

   ✓6ᵗʰ **H16.25** Phlyctenular keratoconjunctivitis
     H16.251 Phlyctenular keratoconjunctivitis, right eye
     H16.252 Phlyctenular keratoconjunctivitis, left eye
     H16.253 Phlyctenular keratoconjunctivitis, bilateral
     H16.259 Phlyctenular keratoconjunctivitis, unspecified eye ▽

   ✓6ᵗʰ **H16.26** Vernal keratoconjunctivitis, with limbar and corneal involvement
       EXCLUDES 1   vernal conjunctivitis without limbar and corneal involvement (H1Ø.44)
     H16.261 Vernal keratoconjunctivitis, with limbar and corneal involvement, right eye
     H16.262 Vernal keratoconjunctivitis, with limbar and corneal involvement, left eye
     H16.263 Vernal keratoconjunctivitis, with limbar and corneal involvement, bilateral
     H16.269 Vernal keratoconjunctivitis, with limbar and corneal involvement, unspecified eye ▽

   ✓6ᵗʰ **H16.29** Other keratoconjunctivitis
     H16.291 Other keratoconjunctivitis, right eye
     H16.292 Other keratoconjunctivitis, left eye
     H16.293 Other keratoconjunctivitis, bilateral
     H16.299 Other keratoconjunctivitis, unspecified eye ▽

✓5ᵗʰ **H16.3** Interstitial and deep keratitis
   ✓6ᵗʰ **H16.30** Unspecified interstitial keratitis
     H16.301 Unspecified interstitial keratitis, right eye ▽
     H16.302 Unspecified interstitial keratitis, left eye ▽
     H16.303 Unspecified interstitial keratitis, bilateral ▽
     H16.309 Unspecified interstitial keratitis, unspecified eye ▽

   ✓6ᵗʰ **H16.31** Corneal abscess
     H16.311 Corneal abscess, right eye
     H16.312 Corneal abscess, left eye
     H16.313 Corneal abscess, bilateral
     H16.319 Corneal abscess, unspecified eye ▽

   ✓6ᵗʰ **H16.32** Diffuse interstitial keratitis
       Cogan's syndrome
     H16.321 Diffuse interstitial keratitis, right eye
     H16.322 Diffuse interstitial keratitis, left eye
     H16.323 Diffuse interstitial keratitis, bilateral
     H16.329 Diffuse interstitial keratitis, unspecified eye ▽

   ✓6ᵗʰ **H16.33** Sclerosing keratitis
     H16.331 Sclerosing keratitis, right eye
     H16.332 Sclerosing keratitis, left eye
     H16.333 Sclerosing keratitis, bilateral
     H16.339 Sclerosing keratitis, unspecified eye ▽

   ✓6ᵗʰ **H16.39** Other interstitial and deep keratitis
     H16.391 Other interstitial and deep keratitis, right eye
     H16.392 Other interstitial and deep keratitis, left eye
     H16.393 Other interstitial and deep keratitis, bilateral
     H16.399 Other interstitial and deep keratitis, unspecified eye ▽

✓5ᵗʰ **H16.4** Corneal neovascularization
   ✓6ᵗʰ **H16.40** Unspecified corneal neovascularization
     H16.401 Unspecified corneal neovascularization, right eye ▽
     H16.402 Unspecified corneal neovascularization, left eye ▽
     H16.403 Unspecified corneal neovascularization, bilateral ▽
     H16.409 Unspecified corneal neovascularization, unspecified eye ▽

   ✓6ᵗʰ **H16.41** Ghost vessels (corneal)
     H16.411 Ghost vessels (corneal), right eye
     H16.412 Ghost vessels (corneal), left eye
     H16.413 Ghost vessels (corneal), bilateral
     H16.419 Ghost vessels (corneal), unspecified eye ▽

   ✓6ᵗʰ **H16.42** Pannus (corneal)
     H16.421 Pannus (corneal), right eye
     H16.422 Pannus (corneal), left eye
     H16.423 Pannus (corneal), bilateral
     H16.429 Pannus (corneal), unspecified eye ▽

   ✓6ᵗʰ **H16.43** Localized vascularization of cornea
     H16.431 Localized vascularization of cornea, right eye
     H16.432 Localized vascularization of cornea, left eye
     H16.433 Localized vascularization of cornea, bilateral
     H16.439 Localized vascularization of cornea, unspecified eye ▽

   ✓6ᵗʰ **H16.44** Deep vascularization of cornea
     H16.441 Deep vascularization of cornea, right eye
     H16.442 Deep vascularization of cornea, left eye
     H16.443 Deep vascularization of cornea, bilateral
     H16.449 Deep vascularization of cornea, unspecified eye ▽

H16.8 **Other keratitis**
H16.9 Unspecified keratitis ▽

☑ Add'l Character Required   ✓7ᵗʰ Placeholder Alert   **RUG IV Special Care High Dx**   **RUG IV Clinically Complex Dx**   **RUG IV Special Care Low Dx**   Manifestation Code   Other Specified Code   ▽ Unspecified Code

Chapter 7. Diseases of the Eye and Adnexa

☑4ᵗʰ **H17** **Corneal scars and opacities**

  ☑5ᵗʰ **H17.0** **Adherent leukoma**
- **H17.00** Adherent leukoma, unspecified eye ▽
- **H17.01** Adherent leukoma, right eye
- **H17.02** Adherent leukoma, left eye
- **H17.03** Adherent leukoma, bilateral

  ☑5ᵗʰ **H17.1** **Central corneal opacity**
- **H17.10** Central corneal opacity, unspecified eye ▽
- **H17.11** Central corneal opacity, right eye
- **H17.12** Central corneal opacity, left eye
- **H17.13** Central corneal opacity, bilateral

  ☑5ᵗʰ **H17.8** **Other corneal scars and opacities**
-   ☑6ᵗʰ **H17.81** Minor opacity of cornea
  - Corneal nebula
  - **H17.811** Minor opacity of cornea, right eye
  - **H17.812** Minor opacity of cornea, left eye
  - **H17.813** Minor opacity of cornea, bilateral
  - **H17.819** Minor opacity of cornea, unspecified eye ▽
-   ☑6ᵗʰ **H17.82** Peripheral opacity of cornea
  - **H17.821** Peripheral opacity of cornea, right eye
  - **H17.822** Peripheral opacity of cornea, left eye
  - **H17.823** Peripheral opacity of cornea, bilateral
  - **H17.829** Peripheral opacity of cornea, unspecified eye ▽
- **H17.89** Other corneal scars and opacities

  H17.9 Unspecified corneal scar and opacity ▽

☑4ᵗʰ **H18** **Other disorders of cornea**

  ☑5ᵗʰ **H18.0** **Corneal pigmentations and deposits**
-   ☑6ᵗʰ **H18.00** Unspecified corneal deposit
  - **H18.001** Unspecified corneal deposit, right eye ▽
  - **H18.002** Unspecified corneal deposit, left eye ▽
  - **H18.003** Unspecified corneal deposit, bilateral ▽
  - **H18.009** Unspecified corneal deposit, unspecified eye ▽
-   ☑6ᵗʰ **H18.01** Anterior corneal pigmentations
  - Staehli's line
  - **H18.011** Anterior corneal pigmentations, right eye
  - **H18.012** Anterior corneal pigmentations, left eye
  - **H18.013** Anterior corneal pigmentations, bilateral
  - **H18.019** Anterior corneal pigmentations, unspecified eye ▽
-   ☑6ᵗʰ **H18.02** Argentous corneal deposits
  - **H18.021** Argentous corneal deposits, right eye
  - **H18.022** Argentous corneal deposits, left eye
  - **H18.023** Argentous corneal deposits, bilateral
  - **H18.029** Argentous corneal deposits, unspecified eye ▽
-   ☑6ᵗʰ **H18.03** Corneal deposits in metabolic disorders
  - Code also associated metabolic disorder
  - **H18.031** Corneal deposits in metabolic disorders, right eye
  - **H18.032** Corneal deposits in metabolic disorders, left eye
  - **H18.033** Corneal deposits in metabolic disorders, bilateral
  - **H18.039** Corneal deposits in metabolic disorders, unspecified eye ▽
-   ☑6ᵗʰ **H18.04** Kayser-Fleischer ring
  - Code also associated Wilson's disease (E83.01)
  - **H18.041** Kayser-Fleischer ring, right eye
  - **H18.042** Kayser-Fleischer ring, left eye
  - **H18.043** Kayser-Fleischer ring, bilateral
  - **H18.049** Kayser-Fleischer ring, unspecified eye ▽
-   ☑6ᵗʰ **H18.05** Posterior corneal pigmentations
  - Krukenberg's spindle
  - **H18.051** Posterior corneal pigmentations, right eye
  - **H18.052** Posterior corneal pigmentations, left eye
  - **H18.053** Posterior corneal pigmentations, bilateral
  - **H18.059** Posterior corneal pigmentations, unspecified eye ▽

  ☑6ᵗʰ **H18.06** Stromal corneal pigmentations
- Hematocornea
- **H18.061** Stromal corneal pigmentations, right eye
- **H18.062** Stromal corneal pigmentations, left eye
- **H18.063** Stromal corneal pigmentations, bilateral
- **H18.069** Stromal corneal pigmentations, unspecified eye ▽

  ☑5ᵗʰ **H18.1** **Bullous keratopathy**
- **H18.10** Bullous keratopathy, unspecified eye ▽
- **H18.11** Bullous keratopathy, right eye
- **H18.12** Bullous keratopathy, left eye
- **H18.13** Bullous keratopathy, bilateral

  ☑5ᵗʰ **H18.2** **Other and unspecified corneal edema**
- **H18.20** Unspecified corneal edema ▽
-   ☑6ᵗʰ **H18.21** Corneal edema secondary to contact lens
  - **EXCLUDES 2** other corneal disorders due to contact lens (H18.82-)
  - **H18.211** Corneal edema secondary to contact lens, right eye
  - **H18.212** Corneal edema secondary to contact lens, left eye
  - **H18.213** Corneal edema secondary to contact lens, bilateral
  - **H18.219** Corneal edema secondary to contact lens, unspecified eye ▽
-   ☑6ᵗʰ **H18.22** Idiopathic corneal edema
  - **H18.221** Idiopathic corneal edema, right eye
  - **H18.222** Idiopathic corneal edema, left eye
  - **H18.223** Idiopathic corneal edema, bilateral
  - **H18.229** Idiopathic corneal edema, unspecified eye ▽
-   ☑6ᵗʰ **H18.23** Secondary corneal edema
  - **H18.231** Secondary corneal edema, right eye
  - **H18.232** Secondary corneal edema, left eye
  - **H18.233** Secondary corneal edema, bilateral
  - **H18.239** Secondary corneal edema, unspecified eye ▽

  ☑5ᵗʰ **H18.3** **Changes of corneal membranes**
- **H18.30** Unspecified corneal membrane change ▽
-   ☑6ᵗʰ **H18.31** Folds and rupture in Bowman's membrane
  - **H18.311** Folds and rupture in Bowman's membrane, right eye
  - **H18.312** Folds and rupture in Bowman's membrane, left eye
  - **H18.313** Folds and rupture in Bowman's membrane, bilateral
  - **H18.319** Folds and rupture in Bowman's membrane, unspecified eye ▽
-   ☑6ᵗʰ **H18.32** Folds in Descemet's membrane
  - **H18.321** Folds in Descemet's membrane, right eye
  - **H18.322** Folds in Descemet's membrane, left eye
  - **H18.323** Folds in Descemet's membrane, bilateral
  - **H18.329** Folds in Descemet's membrane, unspecified eye ▽
-   ☑6ᵗʰ **H18.33** Rupture in Descemet's membrane
  - **H18.331** Rupture in Descemet's membrane, right eye
  - **H18.332** Rupture in Descemet's membrane, left eye
  - **H18.333** Rupture in Descemet's membrane, bilateral
  - **H18.339** Rupture in Descemet's membrane, unspecified eye ▽

  ☑5ᵗʰ **H18.4** **Corneal degeneration**
- **EXCLUDES 1** Mooren's ulcer (H16.0-)
  - recurrent erosion of cornea (H18.83-)
- **H18.40** Unspecified corneal degeneration ▽
-   ☑6ᵗʰ **H18.41** Arcus senilis
  - Senile corneal changes
  - **H18.411** Arcus senilis, right eye
  - **H18.412** Arcus senilis, left eye
  - **H18.413** Arcus senilis, bilateral
  - **H18.419** Arcus senilis, unspecified eye ▽
-   ☑6ᵗʰ **H18.42** Band keratopathy
  - **H18.421** Band keratopathy, right eye

Ⓝ Newborn Ⓟ Pediatric Ⓜ Maternity Ⓐ Adult **RIC** RIC Dx **NC Dx** Noncancer Dx **PDx** Primary Dx **CC** RIC CC Condition ►◄ Revised Text ● New Code ▲ Revised Code Title

554   ICD-10-CM 2016

H18.422   **Band keratopathy, left eye**
H18.423   **Band keratopathy, bilateral**
H18.429   **Band keratopathy, unspecified eye** ▽

H18.43   **Other calcerous corneal degeneration**

☑6ᵗʰ H18.44   **Keratomalacia**
     EXCLUDES 1   *keratomalacia due to vitamin A deficiency (E50.4)*
H18.441   **Keratomalacia, right eye**
H18.442   **Keratomalacia, left eye**
H18.443   **Keratomalacia, bilateral**
H18.449   **Keratomalacia, unspecified eye** ▽

☑6ᵗʰ H18.45   **Nodular corneal degeneration**
H18.451   **Nodular corneal degeneration, right eye**
H18.452   **Nodular corneal degeneration, left eye**
H18.453   **Nodular corneal degeneration, bilateral**
H18.459   **Nodular corneal degeneration, unspecified eye** ▽

☑6ᵗʰ H18.46   **Peripheral corneal degeneration**
H18.461   **Peripheral corneal degeneration, right eye**
H18.462   **Peripheral corneal degeneration, left eye**
H18.463   **Peripheral corneal degeneration, bilateral**
H18.469   **Peripheral corneal degeneration, unspecified eye** ▽

H18.49   **Other corneal degeneration**

☑5ᵗʰ H18.5   **Hereditary corneal dystrophies**
H18.50   **Unspecified hereditary corneal dystrophies** ▽
H18.51   **Endothelial corneal dystrophy**
     Fuchs' dystrophy
H18.52   **Epithelial (juvenile) corneal dystrophy**
H18.53   **Granular corneal dystrophy**
H18.54   **Lattice corneal dystrophy**
H18.55   **Macular corneal dystrophy**
H18.59   **Other hereditary corneal dystrophies**

☑5ᵗʰ H18.6   **Keratoconus**
☑6ᵗʰ H18.60   **Keratoconus, unspecified**
H18.601   **Keratoconus, unspecified, right eye** ▽
H18.602   **Keratoconus, unspecified, left eye** ▽
H18.603   **Keratoconus, unspecified, bilateral** ▽
H18.609   **Keratoconus, unspecified, unspecified eye** ▽

☑6ᵗʰ H18.61   **Keratoconus, stable**
H18.611   **Keratoconus, stable, right eye**
H18.612   **Keratoconus, stable, left eye**
H18.613   **Keratoconus, stable, bilateral**
H18.619   **Keratoconus, stable, unspecified eye** ▽

☑6ᵗʰ H18.62   **Keratoconus, unstable**
     Acute hydrops
H18.621   **Keratoconus, unstable, right eye**
H18.622   **Keratoconus, unstable, left eye**
H18.623   **Keratoconus, unstable, bilateral**
H18.629   **Keratoconus, unstable, unspecified eye** ▽

☑5ᵗʰ H18.7   **Other and unspecified corneal deformities**
     EXCLUDES 1   *congenital malformations of cornea (Q13.3-Q13.4)*
H18.70   **Unspecified corneal deformity** ▽
☑6ᵗʰ H18.71   **Corneal ectasia**
H18.711   **Corneal ectasia, right eye**
H18.712   **Corneal ectasia, left eye**
H18.713   **Corneal ectasia, bilateral**
H18.719   **Corneal ectasia, unspecified eye** ▽

☑6ᵗʰ H18.72   **Corneal staphyloma**
H18.721   **Corneal staphyloma, right eye**
H18.722   **Corneal staphyloma, left eye**
H18.723   **Corneal staphyloma, bilateral**
H18.729   **Corneal staphyloma, unspecified eye** ▽

☑6ᵗʰ H18.73   **Descemetocele**
H18.731   **Descemetocele, right eye**
H18.732   **Descemetocele, left eye**
H18.733   **Descemetocele, bilateral**
H18.739   **Descemetocele, unspecified eye** ▽

☑6ᵗʰ H18.79   **Other corneal deformities**
H18.791   **Other corneal deformities, right eye**

H18.792   **Other corneal deformities, left eye**
H18.793   **Other corneal deformities, bilateral** ▽
H18.799   **Other corneal deformities, unspecified eye**

☑5ᵗʰ H18.8   **Other specified disorders of cornea**
☑6ᵗʰ H18.81   **Anesthesia and hypoesthesia of cornea**
H18.811   **Anesthesia and hypoesthesia of cornea, right eye**
H18.812   **Anesthesia and hypoesthesia of cornea, left eye**
H18.813   **Anesthesia and hypoesthesia of cornea, bilateral**
H18.819   **Anesthesia and hypoesthesia of cornea, unspecified eye** ▽

☑6ᵗʰ H18.82   **Corneal disorder due to contact lens**
     EXCLUDES 2   *corneal edema due to contact lens (H18.21-)*
H18.821   **Corneal disorder due to contact lens, right eye**
H18.822   **Corneal disorder due to contact lens, left eye**
H18.823   **Corneal disorder due to contact lens, bilateral**
H18.829   **Corneal disorder due to contact lens, unspecified eye** ▽

☑6ᵗʰ H18.83   **Recurrent erosion of cornea**
H18.831   **Recurrent erosion of cornea, right eye**
H18.832   **Recurrent erosion of cornea, left eye**
H18.833   **Recurrent erosion of cornea, bilateral**
H18.839   **Recurrent erosion of cornea, unspecified eye** ▽

☑6ᵗʰ H18.89   **Other specified disorders of cornea**
H18.891   **Other specified disorders of cornea, right eye**
H18.892   **Other specified disorders of cornea, left eye**
H18.893   **Other specified disorders of cornea, bilateral**
H18.899   **Other specified disorders of cornea, unspecified eye** ▽

H18.9   **Unspecified disorder of cornea** ▽

☑4ᵗʰ **H20 Iridocyclitis**
☑5ᵗʰ H20.0   **Acute and subacute iridocyclitis**
     Acute anterior uveitis
     Acute cyclitis
     Acute iritis
     Subacute anterior uveitis
     Subacute cyclitis
     Subacute iritis
     EXCLUDES 1   *iridocyclitis, iritis, uveitis (due to) (in) diabetes mellitus (E08-E13 with .39)*
         iridocyclitis, iritis, uveitis (due to) (in) diphtheria (A36.89)
         iridocyclitis, iritis, uveitis (due to) (in) gonococcal (A54.32)
         iridocyclitis, iritis, uveitis (due to) (in) herpes (simplex) (B00.51)
         iridocyclitis, iritis, uveitis (due to) (in) herpes zoster (B02.32)
         iridocyclitis, iritis, uveitis (due to) (in) late congenital syphilis (A50.39)
         iridocyclitis, iritis, uveitis (due to) (in) late syphilis (A52.71)
         iridocyclitis, iritis, uveitis (due to) (in) sarcoidosis (D86.83)
         iridocyclitis, iritis, uveitis (due to) (in) syphilis (A51.43)
         iridocyclitis, iritis, uveitis (due to) (in) toxoplasmosis (B58.09)
         iridocyclitis, iritis, uveitis (due to) (in) tuberculosis (A18.54)

H20.00   **Unspecified acute and subacute iridocyclitis** ▽
☑6ᵗʰ H20.01   **Primary iridocyclitis**
H20.011   **Primary iridocyclitis, right eye**
H20.012   **Primary iridocyclitis, left eye**
H20.013   **Primary iridocyclitis, bilateral**
H20.019   **Primary iridocyclitis, unspecified eye** ▽
☑6ᵗʰ H20.02   **Recurrent acute iridocyclitis**
H20.021   **Recurrent acute iridocyclitis, right eye**
H20.022   **Recurrent acute iridocyclitis, left eye**

☑ Add'l Character Required   ☑x7ᵗʰ Placeholder Alert   ▨ RUG IV Special Care High Dx   RUG IV Clinically Complex Dx   RUG IV Special Care Low Dx   Manifestation Code   Other Specified Code   ▽ Unspecified Code

ICD-10-CM 2016   555

H20.023   Recurrent acute iridocyclitis, bilateral

H20.029   Recurrent acute iridocyclitis, unspecified eye ▽

✓6ᵗʰ H20.03   Secondary infectious iridocyclitis

H20.031   Secondary infectious iridocyclitis, right eye

H20.032   Secondary infectious iridocyclitis, left eye

H20.033   Secondary infectious iridocyclitis, bilateral

H20.039   Secondary infectious iridocyclitis, unspecified eye ▽

✓6ᵗʰ H20.04   Secondary noninfectious iridocyclitis

H20.041   Secondary noninfectious iridocyclitis, right eye

H20.042   Secondary noninfectious iridocyclitis, left eye

H20.043   Secondary noninfectious iridocyclitis, bilateral

H20.049   Secondary noninfectious iridocyclitis, unspecified eye ▽

✓6ᵗʰ H20.05   Hypopyon

H20.051   Hypopyon, right eye

H20.052   Hypopyon, left eye

H20.053   Hypopyon, bilateral

H20.059   Hypopyon, unspecified eye ▽

✓5ᵗʰ H20.1   Chronic iridocyclitis

Use additional code for any associated cataract (H26.21-)

EXCLUDES 2   posterior cyclitis (H30.2-)

H20.10   Chronic iridocyclitis, unspecified eye ▽

H20.11   Chronic iridocyclitis, right eye

H20.12   Chronic iridocyclitis, left eye

H20.13   Chronic iridocyclitis, bilateral

✓5ᵗʰ H20.2   Lens-induced iridocyclitis

H20.20   Lens-induced iridocyclitis, unspecified eye ▽

H20.21   Lens-induced iridocyclitis, right eye

H20.22   Lens-induced iridocyclitis, left eye

H20.23   Lens-induced iridocyclitis, bilateral

✓5ᵗʰ H20.8   Other iridocyclitis

EXCLUDES 2   glaucomatocyclitis crises (H40.4-)

posterior cyclitis (H30.2-)

sympathetic uveitis (H44.13-)

✓6ᵗʰ H20.81   Fuchs' heterochromic cyclitis

H20.811   Fuchs' heterochromic cyclitis, right eye

H20.812   Fuchs' heterochromic cyclitis, left eye

H20.813   Fuchs' heterochromic cyclitis, bilateral

H20.819   Fuchs' heterochromic cyclitis, unspecified eye ▽

✓6ᵗʰ H20.82   Vogt-Koyanagi syndrome

H20.821   Vogt-Koyanagi syndrome, right eye

H20.822   Vogt-Koyanagi syndrome, left eye

H20.823   Vogt-Koyanagi syndrome, bilateral

H20.829   Vogt-Koyanagi syndrome, unspecified eye ▽

H20.9   Unspecified iridocyclitis ▽

Uveitis NOS

✓4ᵗʰ H21   Other disorders of iris and ciliary body

EXCLUDES 2   sympathetic uveitis (H44.1-)

✓5ᵗʰ H21.0   Hyphema

EXCLUDES 1   traumatic hyphema (S05.1-)

H21.00   Hyphema, unspecified eye ▽

H21.01   Hyphema, right eye

H21.02   Hyphema, left eye

H21.03   Hyphema, bilateral

✓5ᵗʰ H21.1   Other vascular disorders of iris and ciliary body

Neovascularization of iris or ciliary body

Rubeosis iridis

Rubeosis of iris

✓6ᵗʰ H21.1X   Other vascular disorders of iris and ciliary body

H21.1X1   Other vascular disorders of iris and ciliary body, right eye

H21.1X2   Other vascular disorders of iris and ciliary body, left eye

H21.1X3   Other vascular disorders of iris and ciliary body, bilateral

H21.1X9   Other vascular disorders of iris and ciliary body, unspecified eye ▽

✓5ᵗʰ H21.2   Degeneration of iris and ciliary body

✓6ᵗʰ H21.21   Degeneration of chamber angle

H21.211   Degeneration of chamber angle, right eye

H21.212   Degeneration of chamber angle, left eye

H21.213   Degeneration of chamber angle, bilateral

H21.219   Degeneration of chamber angle, unspecified eye ▽

✓6ᵗʰ H21.22   Degeneration of ciliary body

H21.221   Degeneration of ciliary body, right eye

H21.222   Degeneration of ciliary body, left eye

H21.223   Degeneration of ciliary body, bilateral

H21.229   Degeneration of ciliary body, unspecified eye ▽

✓6ᵗʰ H21.23   Degeneration of iris (pigmentary)

Translucency of iris

H21.231   Degeneration of iris (pigmentary), right eye

H21.232   Degeneration of iris (pigmentary), left eye

H21.233   Degeneration of iris (pigmentary), bilateral

H21.239   Degeneration of iris (pigmentary), unspecified eye ▽

✓6ᵗʰ H21.24   Degeneration of pupillary margin

H21.241   Degeneration of pupillary margin, right eye

H21.242   Degeneration of pupillary margin, left eye

H21.243   Degeneration of pupillary margin, bilateral

H21.249   Degeneration of pupillary margin, unspecified eye ▽

✓6ᵗʰ H21.25   Iridoschisis

H21.251   Iridoschisis, right eye

H21.252   Iridoschisis, left eye

H21.253   Iridoschisis, bilateral

H21.259   Iridoschisis, unspecified eye ▽

✓6ᵗʰ H21.26   Iris atrophy (essential) (progressive)

H21.261   Iris atrophy (essential) (progressive), right eye

H21.262   Iris atrophy (essential) (progressive), left eye

H21.263   Iris atrophy (essential) (progressive), bilateral

H21.269   Iris atrophy (essential) (progressive), unspecified eye ▽

✓6ᵗʰ H21.27   Miotic pupillary cyst

H21.271   Miotic pupillary cyst, right eye

H21.272   Miotic pupillary cyst, left eye

H21.273   Miotic pupillary cyst, bilateral

H21.279   Miotic pupillary cyst, unspecified eye ▽

H21.29   Other iris atrophy

✓5ᵗʰ H21.3   Cyst of iris, ciliary body and anterior chamber

EXCLUDES 2   miotic pupillary cyst (H21.27-)

✓6ᵗʰ H21.30   Idiopathic cysts of iris, ciliary body or anterior chamber

Cyst of iris, ciliary body or anterior chamber NOS

H21.301   Idiopathic cysts of iris, ciliary body or anterior chamber, right eye

H21.302   Idiopathic cysts of iris, ciliary body or anterior chamber, left eye

H21.303   Idiopathic cysts of iris, ciliary body or anterior chamber, bilateral

H21.309   Idiopathic cysts of iris, ciliary body or anterior chamber, unspecified eye ▽

✓6ᵗʰ H21.31   Exudative cysts of iris or anterior chamber

H21.311   Exudative cysts of iris or anterior chamber, right eye

H21.312   Exudative cysts of iris or anterior chamber, left eye

H21.313   Exudative cysts of iris or anterior chamber, bilateral

H21.319   Exudative cysts of iris or anterior chamber, unspecified eye ▽

Ⓝ Newborn   Ⓟ Pediatric   Ⓜ Maternity   Ⓐ Adult   RIC Dx RIC Dx   NC Dx Noncancer Dx   PDx Primary Dx   CC RIC CC Condition   ►◄ Revised Text   ● New Code   ▲ Revised Code Title

556   ICD-10-CM 2016

✓6ᵗʰ H21.32 Implantation cysts of iris, ciliary body or anterior chamber
- H21.321 Implantation cysts of iris, ciliary body or anterior chamber, **right** eye
- H21.322 Implantation cysts of iris, ciliary body or anterior chamber, **left** eye
- H21.323 Implantation cysts of iris, ciliary body or anterior chamber, **bilateral**
- H21.329 Implantation cysts of iris, ciliary body or anterior chamber, unspecified eye ▽

✓6ᵗʰ H21.33 Parasitic cyst of iris, ciliary body or anterior chamber
- H21.331 Parasitic cyst of iris, ciliary body or anterior chamber, **right** eye
- H21.332 Parasitic cyst of iris, ciliary body or anterior chamber, **left** eye
- H21.333 Parasitic cyst of iris, ciliary body or anterior chamber, **bilateral**
- H21.339 Parasitic cyst of iris, ciliary body or anterior chamber, unspecified eye ▽

✓6ᵗʰ H21.34 Primary cyst of **pars plana**
- H21.341 Primary cyst of pars plana, **right** eye
- H21.342 Primary cyst of pars plana, **left** eye
- H21.343 Primary cyst of pars plana, **bilateral**
- H21.349 Primary cyst of pars plana, unspecified eye ▽

✓6ᵗʰ H21.35 Exudative cyst of **pars plana**
- H21.351 Exudative cyst of pars plana, **right** eye
- H21.352 Exudative cyst of pars plana, **left** eye
- H21.353 Exudative cyst of pars plana, **bilateral**
- H21.359 Exudative cyst of pars plana, unspecified eye ▽

✓5ᵗʰ H21.4 Pupillary membranes
Iris bombé   Pupillary seclusion
Pupillary occlusion
EXCLUDES 1 congenital pupillary membranes (Q13.8)
- H21.40 Pupillary membranes, unspecified eye ▽
- H21.41 Pupillary membranes, **right** eye
- H21.42 Pupillary membranes, **left** eye
- H21.43 Pupillary membranes, **bilateral**

✓5ᵗʰ H21.5 Other and unspecified adhesions and disruptions of iris and ciliary body
EXCLUDES 1 corectopia (Q13.2)

✓6ᵗʰ H21.50 Unspecified adhesions of iris
Synechia (iris) NOS
- H21.501 Unspecified adhesions of iris, **right** eye ▽
- H21.502 Unspecified adhesions of iris, **left** eye ▽
- H21.503 Unspecified adhesions of iris, **bilateral** ▽
- H21.509 Unspecified adhesions of iris and ciliary body, unspecified eye ▽

✓6ᵗʰ H21.51 Anterior synechiae (iris)
- H21.511 Anterior synechiae (iris), **right** eye
- H21.512 Anterior synechiae (iris), **left** eye
- H21.513 Anterior synechiae (iris), **bilateral**
- H21.519 Anterior synechiae (iris), unspecified eye ▽

✓6ᵗʰ H21.52 Goniosynechiae
- H21.521 Goniosynechiae, **right** eye
- H21.522 Goniosynechiae, **left** eye
- H21.523 Goniosynechiae, **bilateral**
- H21.529 Goniosynechiae, unspecified eye ▽

✓6ᵗʰ H21.53 Iridodialysis
- H21.531 Iridodialysis, **right** eye
- H21.532 Iridodialysis, **left** eye
- H21.533 Iridodialysis, **bilateral**
- H21.539 Iridodialysis, unspecified eye ▽

✓6ᵗʰ H21.54 Posterior synechiae (iris)
- H21.541 Posterior synechiae (iris), **right** eye
- H21.542 Posterior synechiae (iris), **left** eye
- H21.543 Posterior synechiae (iris), **bilateral**
- H21.549 Posterior synechiae (iris), unspecified eye ▽

✓6ᵗʰ H21.55 Recession of chamber angle
- H21.551 Recession of chamber angle, **right** eye
- H21.552 Recession of chamber angle, **left** eye
- H21.553 Recession of chamber angle, **bilateral**
- H21.559 Recession of chamber angle, unspecified eye ▽

✓6ᵗʰ H21.56 Pupillary abnormalities
Deformed pupil
Ectopic pupil
Rupture of sphincter, pupil
EXCLUDES 1 congenital deformity of pupil (Q13.2-)
- H21.561 Pupillary abnormality, **right** eye
- H21.562 Pupillary abnormality, **left** eye
- H21.563 Pupillary abnormality, **bilateral**
- H21.569 Pupillary abnormality, unspecified eye ▽

✓5ᵗʰ H21.8 Other specified disorders of iris and ciliary body
- H21.81 **Floppy iris syndrome**
Intraoperative floppy iris syndrome (IFIS)
Use additional code for adverse effect, if applicable, to identify drug (T36-T50 with fifth or sixth character 5)
- H21.82 **Plateau iris syndrome (post-iridectomy) (postprocedural)**
- H21.89 **Other specified disorders of iris and ciliary body**

H21.9 Unspecified disorder of iris and ciliary body ▽

H22 Disorders of iris and ciliary body in diseases classified elsewhere
Code first underlying disease, such as:
gout (M1A.-, M10.-)
leprosy (A30.-)
parasitic disease (B89)

Disorders of lens (H25-H28)

✓4ᵗʰ H25 Age-related cataract
Senile cataract
EXCLUDES 2 capsular glaucoma with pseudoexfoliation of lens (H40.1-)

✓5ᵗʰ H25.0 Age-related incipient cataract

✓6ᵗʰ H25.01 Cortical age-related cataract
- H25.011 Cortical age-related cataract, **right** eye ▣
- H25.012 Cortical age-related cataract, **left** eye ▣
- H25.013 Cortical age-related cataract, **bilateral** ▣
- H25.019 Cortical age-related cataract, unspecified eye ▣▽

✓6ᵗʰ H25.03 Anterior subcapsular polar age-related cataract
- H25.031 Anterior subcapsular polar age-related cataract, **right** eye ▣
- H25.032 Anterior subcapsular polar age-related cataract, **left** eye ▣
- H25.033 Anterior subcapsular polar age-related cataract, **bilateral** ▣
- H25.039 Anterior subcapsular polar age-related cataract, unspecified eye ▣▽

✓6ᵗʰ H25.04 Posterior subcapsular polar age-related cataract
- H25.041 Posterior subcapsular polar age-related cataract, **right** eye ▣
- H25.042 Posterior subcapsular polar age-related cataract, **left** eye ▣
- H25.043 Posterior subcapsular polar age-related cataract, **bilateral** ▣
- H25.049 Posterior subcapsular polar age-related cataract, unspecified eye ▣▽

✓6ᵗʰ H25.09 Other age-related incipient cataract
Coronary age-related cataract
Punctate age-related cataract
Water clefts
- H25.091 Other age-related incipient cataract, **right eye** ▣
- H25.092 Other age-related incipient cataract, **left eye** ▣
- H25.093 Other age-related incipient cataract, **bilateral** ▣
- H25.099 Other age-related incipient cataract, unspecified eye ▣▽

☑ Add'l Character Required   ✓7ᵗʰ Placeholder Alert   **RUG IV Special Care High Dx**   **RUG IV Clinically Complex Dx**   **RUG IV Special Care Low Dx**   Manifestation Code   Other Specified Code   ▽ Unspecified Code

ICD-10-CM 2016   557

Chapter 7. Diseases of the Eye and Adnexa

H21.32–H25.099

Chapter 7. Diseases of the Eye and Adnexa

√5ᵗʰ **H25.1 Age-related nuclear cataract**
Cataracta brunescens
Nuclear sclerosis cataract

     H25.10 Age-related nuclear cataract, unspecified eye   A ▽

     H25.11 Age-related nuclear cataract, right eye   A

     H25.12 Age-related nuclear cataract, left eye   A

     H25.13 Age-related nuclear cataract, bilateral   A

√5ᵗʰ **H25.2 Age-related cataract, morgagnian type**
Age-related hypermature cataract

     H25.20 Age-related cataract, morgagnian type, unspecified eye   A ▽

     H25.21 Age-related cataract, morgagnian type, right eye   A

     H25.22 Age-related cataract, morgagnian type, left eye   A

     H25.23 Age-related cataract, morgagnian type, bilateral   A

√5ᵗʰ **H25.8 Other age-related cataract**

     √6ᵗʰ **H25.81 Combined forms of age-related cataract**

         H25.811 Combined forms of age-related cataract, right eye   A

         H25.812 Combined forms of age-related cataract, left eye   A

         H25.813 Combined forms of age-related cataract, bilateral   A

         H25.819 Combined forms of age-related cataract, unspecified eye   A ▽

     H25.89 Other age-related cataract   A

     H25.9 Unspecified age-related cataract   A ▽

√4ᵗʰ **H26 Other cataract**
     EXCLUDES 1   congenital cataract (Q12.0)

     √5ᵗʰ **H26.0 Infantile and juvenile cataract**

         √6ᵗʰ **H26.00 Unspecified infantile and juvenile cataract**

            H26.001 Unspecified infantile and juvenile cataract, right eye   P ▽

            H26.002 Unspecified infantile and juvenile cataract, left eye   P ▽

            H26.003 Unspecified infantile and juvenile cataract, bilateral   P ▽

            H26.009 Unspecified infantile and juvenile cataract, unspecified eye   P ▽

         √6ᵗʰ **H26.01 Infantile and juvenile cortical, lamellar, or zonular cataract**

            H26.011 Infantile and juvenile cortical, lamellar, or zonular cataract, right eye   P

            H26.012 Infantile and juvenile cortical, lamellar, or zonular cataract, left eye   P

            H26.013 Infantile and juvenile cortical, lamellar, or zonular cataract, bilateral   P

            H26.019 Infantile and juvenile cortical, lamellar, or zonular cataract, unspecified eye   P ▽

         √6ᵗʰ **H26.03 Infantile and juvenile nuclear cataract**

            H26.031 Infantile and juvenile nuclear cataract, right eye   P

            H26.032 Infantile and juvenile nuclear cataract, left eye   P

            H26.033 Infantile and juvenile nuclear cataract, bilateral   P

            H26.039 Infantile and juvenile nuclear cataract, unspecified eye   P ▽

         √6ᵗʰ **H26.04 Anterior subcapsular polar infantile and juvenile cataract**

            H26.041 Anterior subcapsular polar infantile and juvenile cataract, right eye   P

            H26.042 Anterior subcapsular polar infantile and juvenile cataract, left eye   P

            H26.043 Anterior subcapsular polar infantile and juvenile cataract, bilateral   P

            H26.049 Anterior subcapsular polar infantile and juvenile cataract, unspecified eye   P ▽

         √6ᵗʰ **H26.05 Posterior subcapsular polar infantile and juvenile cataract**

            H26.051 Posterior subcapsular polar infantile and juvenile cataract, right eye   P

            H26.052 Posterior subcapsular polar infantile and juvenile cataract, left eye   P

            H26.053 Posterior subcapsular polar infantile and juvenile cataract, bilateral   P

            H26.059 Posterior subcapsular polar infantile and juvenile cataract, unspecified eye   P ▽

         √6ᵗʰ **H26.06 Combined forms of infantile and juvenile cataract**

            H26.061 Combined forms of infantile and juvenile cataract, right eye   P

            H26.062 Combined forms of infantile and juvenile cataract, left eye   P

            H26.063 Combined forms of infantile and juvenile cataract, bilateral   P

            H26.069 Combined forms of infantile and juvenile cataract, unspecified eye   P ▽

         H26.09 Other infantile and juvenile cataract   P

     √5ᵗʰ **H26.1 Traumatic cataract**
         Use additional code (Chapter 20) to identify external cause

         √6ᵗʰ **H26.10 Unspecified traumatic cataract**

            H26.101 Unspecified traumatic cataract, right eye   ▽

            H26.102 Unspecified traumatic cataract, left eye   ▽

            H26.103 Unspecified traumatic cataract, bilateral   ▽

            H26.109 Unspecified traumatic cataract, unspecified eye   ▽

         √6ᵗʰ **H26.11 Localized traumatic opacities**

            H26.111 Localized traumatic opacities, right eye

            H26.112 Localized traumatic opacities, left eye

            H26.113 Localized traumatic opacities, bilateral

            H26.119 Localized traumatic opacities, unspecified eye   ▽

         √6ᵗʰ **H26.12 Partially resolved traumatic cataract**

            H26.121 Partially resolved traumatic cataract, right eye

            H26.122 Partially resolved traumatic cataract, left eye

            H26.123 Partially resolved traumatic cataract, bilateral

            H26.129 Partially resolved traumatic cataract, unspecified eye   ▽

         √6ᵗʰ **H26.13 Total traumatic cataract**

            H26.131 Total traumatic cataract, right eye

            H26.132 Total traumatic cataract, left eye

            H26.133 Total traumatic cataract, bilateral

            H26.139 Total traumatic cataract, unspecified eye   ▽

     √5ᵗʰ **H26.2 Complicated cataract**

         H26.20 Unspecified complicated cataract   ▽
            Cataracta complicata NOS

         √6ᵗʰ **H26.21 Cataract with neovascularization**
            Code also associated condition, such as:
            chronic iridocyclitis (H20.1-)

            H26.211 Cataract with neovascularization, right eye

            H26.212 Cataract with neovascularization, left eye

            H26.213 Cataract with neovascularization, bilateral

            H26.219 Cataract with neovascularization, unspecified eye   ▽

         √6ᵗʰ **H26.22 Cataract secondary to ocular disorders (degenerative) (inflammatory)**
            Code also associated ocular disorder

            H26.221 Cataract secondary to ocular disorders (degenerative) (inflammatory), right eye

            H26.222 Cataract secondary to ocular disorders (degenerative) (inflammatory), left eye

            H26.223 Cataract secondary to ocular disorders (degenerative) (inflammatory), bilateral

            H26.229 Cataract secondary to ocular disorders (degenerative) (inflammatory), unspecified eye   ▽

         √6ᵗʰ **H26.23 Glaucomatous flecks (subcapsular)**
            Code first underlying glaucoma (H40-H42)

            H26.231 Glaucomatous flecks (subcapsular), right eye

            H26.232 Glaucomatous flecks (subcapsular), left eye

            H26.233 Glaucomatous flecks (subcapsular), bilateral

N Newborn   P Pediatric   M Maternity   A Adult   RIC RIC Dx   NC Dx Noncancer Dx   PDx Primary Dx   CC RIC CC Condition   ▶◀ Revised Text   ● New Code   ▲ Revised Code Title

558   ICD-10-CM 2016

    H26.239   **Glaucomatous flecks (subcapsular),** ▽
            unspecified eye

✓5ᵗʰ **H26.3 Drug-induced cataract**
    Toxic cataract
    Use additional code for adverse effect, if applicable, to identify
        drug (T36-T50 with fifth or sixth character 5)
    H26.30   **Drug-induced cataract, unspecified eye** ▽
    H26.31   **Drug-induced cataract, right eye**
    H26.32   **Drug-induced cataract, left eye**
    H26.33   **Drug-induced cataract, bilateral**

✓5ᵗʰ **H26.4 Secondary cataract**
    H26.40   **Unspecified secondary cataract** ▽
    ✓6ᵗʰ H26.41   **Soemmering's ring**
        H26.411   **Soemmering's ring, right eye**
        H26.412   **Soemmering's ring, left eye**
        H26.413   **Soemmering's ring, bilateral**
        H26.419   **Soemmering's ring, unspecified eye** ▽
    ✓6ᵗʰ H26.49   **Other secondary cataract**
        H26.491   **Other secondary cataract, right eye**
        H26.492   **Other secondary cataract, left eye**
        H26.493   **Other secondary cataract, bilateral**
        H26.499   **Other secondary cataract,** ▽
             unspecified eye

H26.8 Other specified cataract
H26.9 Unspecified cataract ▽

✓4ᵗʰ **H27 Other disorders of lens**
    EXCLUDES 1 *congenital lens malformations (Q12.-)*
        mechanical complications of intraocular lens implant (T85.2)
        pseudophakia (Z96.1)

    ✓5ᵗʰ **H27.0 Aphakia**
        Acquired absence of lens
        Acquired aphakia
        Aphakia due to trauma
        EXCLUDES 1 *cataract extraction status (Z98.4-)*
            congenital absence of lens (Q12.3)
            congenital aphakia (Q12.3)
        H27.00   **Aphakia, unspecified eye** ▽
        H27.01   **Aphakia, right eye**
        H27.02   **Aphakia, left eye**
        H27.03   **Aphakia, bilateral**

    ✓5ᵗʰ **H27.1 Dislocation of lens**
        H27.10   **Unspecified dislocation of lens** ▽
        ✓6ᵗʰ H27.11   **Subluxation of lens**
            H27.111   **Subluxation of lens, right eye**
            H27.112   **Subluxation of lens, left eye**
            H27.113   **Subluxation of lens, bilateral**
            H27.119   **Subluxation of lens, unspecified eye** ▽
        ✓6ᵗʰ H27.12   **Anterior dislocation of lens**
            H27.121   **Anterior dislocation of lens, right eye**
            H27.122   **Anterior dislocation of lens, left eye**
            H27.123   **Anterior dislocation of lens, bilateral**
            H27.129   **Anterior dislocation of lens, unspecified** ▽
                 eye
        ✓6ᵗʰ H27.13   **Posterior dislocation of lens**
            H27.131   **Posterior dislocation of lens, right eye**
            H27.132   **Posterior dislocation of lens, left eye**
            H27.133   **Posterior dislocation of lens, bilateral**
            H27.139   **Posterior dislocation of lens,** ▽
                 unspecified eye

    H27.8 Other specified disorders of lens
    H27.9 Unspecified disorder of lens ▽

H28 *Cataract in diseases classified elsewhere*
    Code first underlying disease, such as:
        hypoparathyroidism (E20.-)
        myotonia (G71.1-)
        myxedema (E03.-)
        protein-calorie malnutrition (E40-E46)
    EXCLUDES 1 *cataract in diabetes mellitus (E08.36, E09.36, E10.36, E11.36,*
        E13.36)

Disorders of choroid and retina (H30-H36)

✓4ᵗʰ **H30 Chorioretinal inflammation**
    ✓5ᵗʰ **H30.0 Focal chorioretinal inflammation**
        Focal chorioretinitis
        Focal choroiditis
        Focal retinitis
        Focal retinochoroiditis
        ✓6ᵗʰ **H30.00 Unspecified focal chorioretinal inflammation**
            Focal chorioretinitis NOS
            Focal choroiditis NOS
            Focal retinitis NOS
            Focal retinochoroiditis NOS
            H30.001   **Unspecified focal chorioretinal** ▽
                 inflammation, right eye
            H30.002   **Unspecified focal chorioretinal** ▽
                 inflammation, left eye
            H30.003   **Unspecified focal chorioretinal** ▽
                 inflammation, bilateral
            H30.009   **Unspecified focal chorioretinal** ▽
                 inflammation, unspecified eye
        ✓6ᵗʰ **H30.01 Focal chorioretinal inflammation, juxtapapillary**
            H30.011   **Focal chorioretinal inflammation,**
                 juxtapapillary, right eye
            H30.012   **Focal chorioretinal inflammation,**
                 juxtapapillary, left eye
            H30.013   **Focal chorioretinal inflammation,**
                 juxtapapillary, bilateral
            H30.019   **Focal chorioretinal inflammation,** ▽
                 juxtapapillary, unspecified eye
        ✓6ᵗʰ **H30.02 Focal chorioretinal inflammation of posterior pole**
            H30.021   **Focal chorioretinal inflammation of**
                 posterior pole, right eye
            H30.022   **Focal chorioretinal inflammation of**
                 posterior pole, left eye
            H30.023   **Focal chorioretinal inflammation of**
                 posterior pole, bilateral
            H30.029   **Focal chorioretinal inflammation of** ▽
                 posterior pole, unspecified eye
        ✓6ᵗʰ **H30.03 Focal chorioretinal inflammation, peripheral**
            H30.031   **Focal chorioretinal inflammation,**
                 peripheral, right eye
            H30.032   **Focal chorioretinal inflammation,**
                 peripheral, left eye
            H30.033   **Focal chorioretinal inflammation,**
                 peripheral, bilateral
            H30.039   **Focal chorioretinal inflammation,** ▽
                 peripheral, unspecified eye
        ✓6ᵗʰ **H30.04 Focal chorioretinal inflammation, macular or**
        paramacular
            H30.041   **Focal chorioretinal inflammation, macular**
                 or paramacular, right eye
            H30.042   **Focal chorioretinal inflammation, macular**
                 or paramacular, left eye
            H30.043   **Focal chorioretinal inflammation, macular**
                 or paramacular, bilateral
            H30.049   **Focal chorioretinal inflammation,** ▽
                 macular or paramacular, unspecified
                 eye

    ✓5ᵗʰ **H30.1 Disseminated chorioretinal inflammation**
        Disseminated chorioretinitis
        Disseminated choroiditis
        Disseminated retinitis
        Disseminated retinochoroiditis
        EXCLUDES 2 *exudative retinopathy (H35.02-)*
        ✓6ᵗʰ **H30.10 Unspecified disseminated chorioretinal**
        inflammation
            Disseminated chorioretinitis NOS
            Disseminated choroiditis NOS
            Disseminated retinitis NOS
            Disseminated retinochoroiditis NOS
            H30.101   **Unspecified disseminated** ▽
                 chorioretinal inflammation, right eye
            H30.102   **Unspecified disseminated** ▽
                 chorioretinal inflammation, left eye
            H30.103   **Unspecified disseminated** ▽
                 chorioretinal inflammation, bilateral

Chapter 7. Diseases of the Eye and Adnexa

H30.109–H31.29

H30.109   **Unspecified disseminated chorioretinal inflammation, unspecified eye** ▽

✓6ᵗʰ **H30.11**   **Disseminated chorioretinal inflammation of** posterior pole
- H30.111   **Disseminated chorioretinal inflammation of posterior pole,** right **eye**
- H30.112   **Disseminated chorioretinal inflammation of posterior pole,** left **eye**
- H30.113   **Disseminated chorioretinal inflammation of posterior pole,** bilateral
- H30.119   **Disseminated chorioretinal inflammation of posterior pole, unspecified eye** ▽

✓6ᵗʰ **H30.12**   **Disseminated chorioretinal inflammation,** peripheral
- H30.121   **Disseminated chorioretinal inflammation, peripheral** right **eye**
- H30.122   **Disseminated chorioretinal inflammation, peripheral,** left **eye**
- H30.123   **Disseminated chorioretinal inflammation, peripheral,** bilateral
- H30.129   **Disseminated chorioretinal inflammation, peripheral, unspecified eye** ▽

✓6ᵗʰ **H30.13**   **Disseminated chorioretinal inflammation,** generalized
- H30.131   **Disseminated chorioretinal inflammation, generalized,** right **eye**
- H30.132   **Disseminated chorioretinal inflammation, generalized,** left **eye**
- H30.133   **Disseminated chorioretinal inflammation, generalized,** bilateral
- H30.139   **Disseminated chorioretinal inflammation, generalized, unspecified eye** ▽

✓6ᵗʰ **H30.14**   Acute posterior multifocal placoid pigment epitheliopathy
- H30.141   **Acute posterior multifocal placoid pigment epitheliopathy,** right **eye**
- H30.142   **Acute posterior multifocal placoid pigment epitheliopathy,** left **eye**
- H30.143   **Acute posterior multifocal placoid pigment epitheliopathy,** bilateral
- H30.149   **Acute posterior multifocal placoid pigment epitheliopathy, unspecified eye** ▽

✓5ᵗʰ **H30.2**   Posterior cyclitis
   Pars planitis
- H30.20   **Posterior cyclitis, unspecified eye** ▽
- H30.21   **Posterior cyclitis,** right **eye**
- H30.22   **Posterior cyclitis,** left **eye**
- H30.23   **Posterior cyclitis,** bilateral

✓5ᵗʰ **H30.8**   Other chorioretinal inflammations

✓6ᵗʰ **H30.81**   Harada's disease
- H30.811   **Harada's disease,** right **eye**
- H30.812   **Harada's disease,** left **eye**
- H30.813   **Harada's disease,** bilateral
- H30.819   **Harada's disease, unspecified eye** ▽

✓6ᵗʰ **H30.89**   Other chorioretinal inflammations
- H30.891   **Other chorioretinal inflammations,** right **eye**
- H30.892   **Other chorioretinal inflammations,** left **eye**
- H30.893   **Other chorioretinal inflammations,** bilateral
- H30.899   **Other chorioretinal inflammations, unspecified eye** ▽

✓5ᵗʰ **H30.9**   Unspecified chorioretinal inflammation
Chorioretinitis NOS	Retinitis NOS
Choroiditis NOS	Retinochoroiditis NOS
Neuroretinitis NOS	
- H30.90   **Unspecified chorioretinal inflammation, unspecified eye** ▽
- H30.91   **Unspecified chorioretinal inflammation,** right **eye** ▽
- H30.92   **Unspecified chorioretinal inflammation,** left **eye** ▽
- H30.93   **Unspecified chorioretinal inflammation,** bilateral ▽

✓4ᵗʰ **H31**   **Other disorders of choroid**

✓5ᵗʰ **H31.0**   **Chorioretinal** scars
   EXCLUDES 2   postsurgical chorioretinal scars (H59.81-)

✓6ᵗʰ **H31.00**   **Unspecified** chorioretinal scars
- H31.001   **Unspecified chorioretinal scars,** right **eye** ▽
- H31.002   **Unspecified chorioretinal scars,** left **eye** ▽
- H31.003   **Unspecified chorioretinal scars,** bilateral ▽
- H31.009   **Unspecified chorioretinal scars, unspecified eye** ▽

✓6ᵗʰ **H31.01**   **Macula scars of posterior pole (postinflammatory) (post-traumatic)**
   EXCLUDES 1   postprocedural chorioretinal scar (H59.81-)
- H31.011   **Macula scars of posterior pole (postinflammatory) (post-traumatic),** right **eye**
- H31.012   **Macula scars of posterior pole (postinflammatory) (post-traumatic),** left **eye**
- H31.013   **Macula scars of posterior pole (postinflammatory) (post-traumatic),** bilateral
- H31.019   **Macula scars of posterior pole (postinflammatory) (post-traumatic), unspecified eye** ▽

✓6ᵗʰ **H31.02**   **Solar retinopathy**
- H31.021   **Solar retinopathy,** right **eye**
- H31.022   **Solar retinopathy,** left **eye**
- H31.023   **Solar retinopathy,** bilateral
- H31.029   **Solar retinopathy, unspecified eye** ▽

✓6ᵗʰ **H31.09**   **Other chorioretinal scars**
- H31.091   **Other chorioretinal scars,** right **eye**
- H31.092   **Other chorioretinal scars,** left **eye**
- H31.093   **Other chorioretinal scars,** bilateral
- H31.099   **Other chorioretinal scars, unspecified eye** ▽

✓5ᵗʰ **H31.1**   **Choroidal** degeneration
   EXCLUDES 2   angioid streaks of macula (H35.33)

✓6ᵗʰ **H31.10**   Unspecified **choroidal degeneration**
   Choroidal sclerosis NOS
- H31.101   **Choroidal degeneration, unspecified,** right **eye** ▽
- H31.102   **Choroidal degeneration, unspecified,** left **eye** ▽
- H31.103   **Choroidal degeneration, unspecified,** bilateral ▽
- H31.109   **Choroidal degeneration, unspecified, unspecified eye** ▽

✓6ᵗʰ **H31.11**   Age-related **choroidal atrophy**
- H31.111   **Age-related choroidal atrophy,** right **eye** Ⓐ
- H31.112   **Age-related choroidal atrophy,** left **eye** Ⓐ
- H31.113   **Age-related choroidal atrophy,** bilateral Ⓐ
- H31.119   **Age-related choroidal atrophy, unspecified eye** Ⓐ▽

✓6ᵗʰ **H31.12**   Diffuse secondary **atrophy of choroid**
- H31.121   **Diffuse secondary atrophy of choroid,** right **eye**
- H31.122   **Diffuse secondary atrophy of choroid,** left **eye**
- H31.123   **Diffuse secondary atrophy of choroid,** bilateral
- H31.129   **Diffuse secondary atrophy of choroid, unspecified eye** ▽

✓5ᵗʰ **H31.2**   **Hereditary choroidal dystrophy**
   EXCLUDES 2   hyperornithinemia (E72.4)
                 ornithinemia (E72.4)
- H31.20   **Hereditary choroidal dystrophy, unspecified** ▽
- H31.21   **Choroideremia**
- H31.22   **Choroidal dystrophy (central areolar) (generalized) (peripapillary)**
- H31.23   **Gyrate atrophy, choroid**
- H31.29   **Other hereditary choroidal dystrophy**

Ⓝ Newborn   Ⓟ Pediatric   Ⓜ Maternity   Ⓐ Adult   **RIC** RIC Dx   **NCDx** Noncancer Dx   **PDx** Primary Dx   **CC** RIC CC Condition   ▶◀ Revised Text   ● New Code   ▲ Revised Code Title

560   ICD-10-CM 2016

☑5ᵗʰ H31.3 Choroidal hemorrhage and rupture

  ☑6ᵗʰ H31.30 Unspecified choroidal hemorrhage

    H31.301 **Unspecified choroidal hemorrhage, right eye** ▽

    H31.302 **Unspecified choroidal hemorrhage, left eye** ▽

    H31.303 **Unspecified choroidal hemorrhage, bilateral** ▽

    H31.309 **Unspecified choroidal hemorrhage, unspecified eye** ▽

  ☑6ᵗʰ H31.31 Expulsive choroidal hemorrhage

    H31.311 **Expulsive choroidal hemorrhage, right eye**

    H31.312 **Expulsive choroidal hemorrhage, left eye**

    H31.313 **Expulsive choroidal hemorrhage, bilateral**

    H31.319 **Expulsive choroidal hemorrhage, unspecified eye** ▽

  ☑6ᵗʰ H31.32 Choroidal rupture

    H31.321 **Choroidal rupture, right eye**

    H31.322 **Choroidal rupture, left eye**

    H31.323 **Choroidal rupture, bilateral**

    H31.329 **Choroidal rupture, unspecified eye** ▽

☑5ᵗʰ H31.4 Choroidal detachment

  ☑6ᵗʰ H31.40 Unspecified choroidal detachment

    H31.401 **Unspecified choroidal detachment, right eye** ▽

    H31.402 **Unspecified choroidal detachment, left eye** ▽

    H31.403 **Unspecified choroidal detachment, bilateral** ▽

    H31.409 **Unspecified choroidal detachment, unspecified eye** ▽

  ☑6ᵗʰ H31.41 Hemorrhagic choroidal detachment

    H31.411 **Hemorrhagic choroidal detachment, right eye**

    H31.412 **Hemorrhagic choroidal detachment, left eye**

    H31.413 **Hemorrhagic choroidal detachment, bilateral**

    H31.419 **Hemorrhagic choroidal detachment, unspecified eye** ▽

  ☑6ᵗʰ H31.42 Serous choroidal detachment

    H31.421 **Serous choroidal detachment, right eye**

    H31.422 **Serous choroidal detachment, left eye**

    H31.423 **Serous choroidal detachment, bilateral**

    H31.429 **Serous choroidal detachment, unspecified eye** ▽

H31.8 Other specified disorders of choroid

H31.9 Unspecified disorder of choroid ▽

H32 *Chorioretinal disorders in diseases classified elsewhere*

Code first underlying disease, such as:
* congenital toxoplasmosis (P37.1)*
* histoplasmosis (B39.-)*
* leprosy (A30.-)*

  EXCLUDES 1 *chorioretinitis (in):*
*   toxoplasmosis (acquired) (B58.01)*
*   tuberculosis (A18.53)*

☑4ᵗʰ H33 Retinal detachments and breaks

  EXCLUDES 1 *detachment of retinal pigment epithelium (H35.72-, H35.73-)*

☑5ᵗʰ H33.0 Retinal detachment with retinal break

  Rhegmatogenous retinal detachment

    EXCLUDES 1 *serous retinal detachment (without retinal break) (H33.2-)*

  ☑6ᵗʰ H33.00 Unspecified retinal detachment with retinal break

    H33.001 **Unspecified retinal detachment with retinal break, right eye** ▽

    H33.002 **Unspecified retinal detachment with retinal break, left eye** ▽

    H33.003 **Unspecified retinal detachment with retinal break, bilateral** ▽

    H33.009 **Unspecified retinal detachment with retinal break, unspecified eye** ▽

  ☑6ᵗʰ H33.01 Retinal detachment with single break

    H33.011 **Retinal detachment with single break, right eye**

    H33.012 **Retinal detachment with single break, left eye**

    H33.013 **Retinal detachment with single break, bilateral**

    H33.019 **Retinal detachment with single break, unspecified eye** ▽

  ☑6ᵗʰ H33.02 Retinal detachment with multiple breaks

    H33.021 **Retinal detachment with multiple breaks, right eye**

    H33.022 **Retinal detachment with multiple breaks, left eye**

    H33.023 **Retinal detachment with multiple breaks, bilateral**

    H33.029 **Retinal detachment with multiple breaks, unspecified eye** ▽

  ☑6ᵗʰ H33.03 Retinal detachment with giant retinal tear

    H33.031 **Retinal detachment with giant retinal tear, right eye**

    H33.032 **Retinal detachment with giant retinal tear, left eye**

    H33.033 **Retinal detachment with giant retinal tear, bilateral**

    H33.039 **Retinal detachment with giant retinal tear, unspecified eye** ▽

  ☑6ᵗʰ H33.04 Retinal detachment with retinal dialysis

    H33.041 **Retinal detachment with retinal dialysis, right eye**

    H33.042 **Retinal detachment with retinal dialysis, left eye**

    H33.043 **Retinal detachment with retinal dialysis, bilateral**

    H33.049 **Retinal detachment with retinal dialysis, unspecified eye** ▽

  ☑6ᵗʰ H33.05 Total retinal detachment

    H33.051 **Total retinal detachment, right eye**

    H33.052 **Total retinal detachment, left eye**

    H33.053 **Total retinal detachment, bilateral**

    H33.059 **Total retinal detachment, unspecified eye** ▽

☑5ᵗʰ H33.1 Retinoschisis and retinal cysts

  EXCLUDES 1 *congenital retinoschisis (Q14.1)*
*   microcystoid degeneration of retina (H35.42-)*

  ☑6ᵗʰ H33.10 Unspecified retinoschisis

    H33.101 **Unspecified retinoschisis, right eye** ▽

    H33.102 **Unspecified retinoschisis, left eye** ▽

    H33.103 **Unspecified retinoschisis, bilateral** ▽

    H33.109 **Unspecified retinoschisis, unspecified eye** ▽

  ☑6ᵗʰ H33.11 Cyst of ora serrata

    H33.111 **Cyst of ora serrata, right eye**

    H33.112 **Cyst of ora serrata, left eye**

    H33.113 **Cyst of ora serrata, bilateral**

    H33.119 **Cyst of ora serrata, unspecified eye** ▽

  ☑6ᵗʰ H33.12 Parasitic cyst of retina

    H33.121 **Parasitic cyst of retina, right eye**

    H33.122 **Parasitic cyst of retina, left eye**

    H33.123 **Parasitic cyst of retina, bilateral**

    H33.129 **Parasitic cyst of retina, unspecified eye** ▽

  ☑6ᵗʰ H33.19 Other retinoschisis and retinal cysts

  Pseudocyst of retina

    H33.191 **Other retinoschisis and retinal cysts, right eye**

    H33.192 **Other retinoschisis and retinal cysts, left eye**

    H33.193 **Other retinoschisis and retinal cysts, bilateral**

    H33.199 **Other retinoschisis and retinal cysts, unspecified eye** ▽

☑5ᵗʰ H33.2 Serous retinal detachment

  Retinal detachment NOS
  Retinal detachment without retinal break

    EXCLUDES 1 *central serous chorioretinopathy (H35.71-)*

  H33.20 **Serous retinal detachment, unspecified eye** ▽

  H33.21 **Serous retinal detachment, right eye**

  H33.22 **Serous retinal detachment, left eye**

  H33.23 **Serous retinal detachment, bilateral**

☑ Add'l Character Required   ☑6ᵗʰ7ᵗʰ Placeholder Alert   RUG IV Special Care High Dx   RUG IV Clinically Complex Dx   RUG IV Special Care Low Dx   Manifestation Code   Other Specified Code   ▽ Unspecified Code

ICD-10-CM 2016   561

✓5ᵗʰ H33.3 Retinal breaks without detachment
     EXCLUDES 1 chorioretinal scars after surgery for detachment (H59.81-)
            peripheral retinal degeneration without break (H35.4-)

   ✓6ᵗʰ H33.30 Unspecified retinal break
     H33.301 Unspecified retinal break, right eye ▽
     H33.302 Unspecified retinal break, left eye ▽
     H33.303 Unspecified retinal break, bilateral ▽
     H33.309 Unspecified retinal break, unspecified eye ▽

   ✓6ᵗʰ H33.31 Horseshoe tear of retina without detachment
     Operculum of retina without detachment
     H33.311 Horseshoe tear of retina without detachment, right eye
     H33.312 Horseshoe tear of retina without detachment, left eye
     H33.313 Horseshoe tear of retina without detachment, bilateral
     H33.319 Horseshoe tear of retina without detachment, unspecified eye ▽

   ✓6ᵗʰ H33.32 Round hole of retina without detachment
     H33.321 Round hole, right eye
     H33.322 Round hole, left eye
     H33.323 Round hole, bilateral
     H33.329 Round hole, unspecified eye ▽

   ✓6ᵗʰ H33.33 Multiple defects of retina without detachment
     H33.331 Multiple defects of retina without detachment, right eye
     H33.332 Multiple defects of retina without detachment, left eye
     H33.333 Multiple defects of retina without detachment, bilateral
     H33.339 Multiple defects of retina without detachment, unspecified eye ▽

✓5ᵗʰ H33.4 Traction detachment of retina
     Proliferative vitreo-retinopathy with retinal detachment
     H33.40 Traction detachment of retina, unspecified eye ▽
     H33.41 Traction detachment of retina, right eye
     H33.42 Traction detachment of retina, left eye
     H33.43 Traction detachment of retina, bilateral

H33.8 Other retinal detachments

✓4ᵗʰ H34 Retinal vascular occlusions
     EXCLUDES 1 amaurosis fugax (G45.3)

   ✓5ᵗʰ H34.0 Transient retinal artery occlusion
     H34.00 Transient retinal artery occlusion, unspecified eye ▽
     H34.01 Transient retinal artery occlusion, right eye
     H34.02 Transient retinal artery occlusion, left eye
     H34.03 Transient retinal artery occlusion, bilateral

   ✓5ᵗʰ H34.1 Central retinal artery occlusion
     H34.10 Central retinal artery occlusion, unspecified eye ▽
     H34.11 Central retinal artery occlusion, right eye
     H34.12 Central retinal artery occlusion, left eye
     H34.13 Central retinal artery occlusion, bilateral

   ✓5ᵗʰ H34.2 Other retinal artery occlusions
   ✓6ᵗʰ H34.21 Partial retinal artery occlusion
     Hollenhorst's plaque
     Retinal microembolism
     H34.211 Partial retinal artery occlusion, right eye
     H34.212 Partial retinal artery occlusion, left eye
     H34.213 Partial retinal artery occlusion, bilateral
     H34.219 Partial retinal artery occlusion, unspecified eye ▽

   ✓6ᵗʰ H34.23 Retinal artery branch occlusion
     H34.231 Retinal artery branch occlusion, right eye
     H34.232 Retinal artery branch occlusion, left eye
     H34.233 Retinal artery branch occlusion, bilateral
     H34.239 Retinal artery branch occlusion, unspecified eye ▽

   ✓5ᵗʰ H34.8 Other retinal vascular occlusions
   ✓6ᵗʰ H34.81 Central retinal vein occlusion
     H34.811 Central retinal vein occlusion, right eye
     H34.812 Central retinal vein occlusion, left eye
     H34.813 Central retinal vein occlusion, bilateral

     H34.819 Central retinal vein occlusion, unspecified eye ▽

   ✓6ᵗʰ H34.82 Venous engorgement
     Incipient retinal vein occlusion
     Partial retinal vein occlusion
     H34.821 Venous engorgement, right eye
     H34.822 Venous engorgement, left eye
     H34.823 Venous engorgement, bilateral
     H34.829 Venous engorgement, unspecified eye ▽

   ✓6ᵗʰ H34.83 Tributary (branch) retinal vein occlusion
     H34.831 Tributary (branch) retinal vein occlusion, right eye
     H34.832 Tributary (branch) retinal vein occlusion, left eye
     H34.833 Tributary (branch) retinal vein occlusion, bilateral
     H34.839 Tributary (branch) retinal vein occlusion, unspecified eye ▽

H34.9 Unspecified retinal vascular occlusion ▽

✓4ᵗʰ H35 Other retinal disorders
     EXCLUDES 2 diabetic retinal disorders (E08.311- E08.359, E09.311- E09.359, E10.311- E10.359, E11.311- E11.359, E13.311- E13.359)

   ✓5ᵗʰ H35.0 Background retinopathy and retinal vascular changes
     Code also any associated hypertension (I10.-)
     H35.00 Unspecified background retinopathy ▽

   ✓6ᵗʰ H35.01 Changes in retinal vascular appearance
     Retinal vascular sheathing
     H35.011 Changes in retinal vascular appearance, right eye
     H35.012 Changes in retinal vascular appearance, left eye
     H35.013 Changes in retinal vascular appearance, bilateral
     H35.019 Changes in retinal vascular appearance, unspecified eye ▽

   ✓6ᵗʰ H35.02 Exudative retinopathy
     Coats retinopathy
     H35.021 Exudative retinopathy, right eye
     H35.022 Exudative retinopathy, left eye
     H35.023 Exudative retinopathy, bilateral
     H35.029 Exudative retinopathy, unspecified eye ▽

   ✓6ᵗʰ H35.03 Hypertensive retinopathy
     H35.031 Hypertensive retinopathy, right eye
     H35.032 Hypertensive retinopathy, left eye
     H35.033 Hypertensive retinopathy, bilateral
     H35.039 Hypertensive retinopathy, unspecified eye ▽

   ✓6ᵗʰ H35.04 Retinal micro-aneurysms, unspecified
     H35.041 Retinal micro-aneurysms, unspecified, right eye ▽
     H35.042 Retinal micro-aneurysms, unspecified, left eye ▽
     H35.043 Retinal micro-aneurysms, unspecified, bilateral ▽
     H35.049 Retinal micro-aneurysms, unspecified, unspecified eye ▽

   ✓6ᵗʰ H35.05 Retinal neovascularization, unspecified
     H35.051 Retinal neovascularization, unspecified, right eye ▽
     H35.052 Retinal neovascularization, unspecified, left eye ▽
     H35.053 Retinal neovascularization, unspecified, bilateral ▽
     H35.059 Retinal neovascularization, unspecified, unspecified eye ▽

   ✓6ᵗʰ H35.06 Retinal vasculitis
     Eales disease   Retinal perivasculitis
     H35.061 Retinal vasculitis, right eye
     H35.062 Retinal vasculitis, left eye
     H35.063 Retinal vasculitis, bilateral
     H35.069 Retinal vasculitis, unspecified eye ▽

   ✓6ᵗʰ H35.07 Retinal telangiectasis
     H35.071 Retinal telangiectasis, right eye
     H35.072 Retinal telangiectasis, left eye
     H35.073 Retinal telangiectasis, bilateral

        H35.079   Retinal telangiectasis, unspecified eye ▽
    H35.09   **Other intraretinal microvascular abnormalities**
           Retinal varices

✓5th **H35.1**   **Retinopathy of prematurity**
  ✓6th **H35.10**   **Retinopathy of prematurity,** unspecified
           Retinopathy of prematurity NOS
       H35.101   Retinopathy of prematurity, unspecified, right eye ▽
       H35.102   Retinopathy of prematurity, unspecified, left eye ▽
       H35.103   Retinopathy of prematurity, unspecified, bilateral ▽
       H35.109   Retinopathy of prematurity, unspecified, unspecified eye ▽
  ✓6th **H35.11**   **Retinopathy of prematurity,** stage 0
       H35.111   Retinopathy of prematurity, stage 0, right eye
       H35.112   Retinopathy of prematurity, stage 0, left eye
       H35.113   Retinopathy of prematurity, stage 0, bilateral
       H35.119   Retinopathy of prematurity, stage 0, unspecified eye ▽
  ✓6th **H35.12**   **Retinopathy of prematurity,** stage 1
       H35.121   Retinopathy of prematurity, stage 1, right eye
       H35.122   Retinopathy of prematurity, stage 1, left eye
       H35.123   Retinopathy of prematurity, stage 1, bilateral
       H35.129   Retinopathy of prematurity, stage 1, unspecified eye ▽
  ✓6th **H35.13**   **Retinopathy of prematurity,** stage 2
       H35.131   Retinopathy of prematurity, stage 2, right eye
       H35.132   Retinopathy of prematurity, stage 2, left eye
       H35.133   Retinopathy of prematurity, stage 2, bilateral
       H35.139   Retinopathy of prematurity, stage 2, unspecified eye ▽
  ✓6th **H35.14**   **Retinopathy of prematurity,** stage 3
       H35.141   Retinopathy of prematurity, stage 3, right eye
       H35.142   Retinopathy of prematurity, stage 3, left eye
       H35.143   Retinopathy of prematurity, stage 3, bilateral
       H35.149   Retinopathy of prematurity, stage 3, unspecified eye ▽
  ✓6th **H35.15**   **Retinopathy of prematurity,** stage 4
       H35.151   Retinopathy of prematurity, stage 4, right eye
       H35.152   Retinopathy of prematurity, stage 4, left eye
       H35.153   Retinopathy of prematurity, stage 4, bilateral
       H35.159   Retinopathy of prematurity, stage 4, unspecified eye ▽
  ✓6th **H35.16**   **Retinopathy of prematurity,** stage 5
       H35.161   Retinopathy of prematurity, stage 5, right eye
       H35.162   Retinopathy of prematurity, stage 5, left eye
       H35.163   Retinopathy of prematurity, stage 5, bilateral
       H35.169   Retinopathy of prematurity, stage 5, unspecified eye ▽
  ✓6th **H35.17**   **Retrolental fibroplasia**
       H35.171   Retrolental fibroplasia, right eye
       H35.172   Retrolental fibroplasia, left eye
       H35.173   Retrolental fibroplasia, bilateral
       H35.179   Retrolental fibroplasia, unspecified eye ▽

✓5th **H35.2**   **Other non-diabetic proliferative retinopathy**
    Proliferative vitreo-retinopathy
    EXCLUDES 1   *proliferative vitreo-retinopathy with retinal detachment (H33.4-)*
    H35.20   **Other non-diabetic proliferative retinopathy, unspecified eye** ▽
    H35.21   **Other non-diabetic proliferative retinopathy, right eye**
    H35.22   **Other non-diabetic proliferative retinopathy, left eye**
    H35.23   **Other non-diabetic proliferative retinopathy, bilateral**

✓5th **H35.3**   **Degeneration of macula and posterior pole**
    H35.30   **Unspecified macular degeneration** A ▽
        Age-related macular degeneration
    H35.31   **Nonexudative age-related** macular degeneration A
        Atrophic age-related macular degeneration
    H35.32   **Exudative age-related** macular degeneration A
    H35.33   **Angioid streaks** of macula
  ✓6th **H35.34**   **Macular cyst, hole, or pseudohole**
       H35.341   Macular cyst, hole, or pseudohole, right eye
       H35.342   Macular cyst, hole, or pseudohole, left eye
       H35.343   Macular cyst, hole, or pseudohole, bilateral
       H35.349   Macular cyst, hole, or pseudohole, unspecified eye ▽
  ✓6th **H35.35**   **Cystoid macular degeneration**
       EXCLUDES 1   *cystoid macular edema following cataract surgery (H59.03-)*
       H35.351   Cystoid macular degeneration, right eye
       H35.352   Cystoid macular degeneration, left eye
       H35.353   Cystoid macular degeneration, bilateral
       H35.359   Cystoid macular degeneration, unspecified eye ▽
  ✓6th **H35.36**   **Drusen (degenerative) of macula**
       H35.361   Drusen (degenerative) of macula, right eye
       H35.362   Drusen (degenerative) of macula, left eye
       H35.363   Drusen (degenerative) of macula, bilateral
       H35.369   Drusen (degenerative) of macula, unspecified eye ▽
  ✓6th **H35.37**   **Puckering of macula**
       H35.371   Puckering of macula, right eye
       H35.372   Puckering of macula, left eye
       H35.373   Puckering of macula, bilateral
       H35.379   Puckering of macula, unspecified eye ▽
  ✓6th **H35.38**   **Toxic maculopathy**
       Code first poisoning due to drug or toxin, if applicable (T36-T65 with fifth or sixth character 1-4 or 6)
       Use additional code for adverse effect, if applicable, to identify drug (T36-T50 with fifth or sixth character 5)
       H35.381   Toxic maculopathy, right eye
       H35.382   Toxic maculopathy, left eye
       H35.383   Toxic maculopathy, bilateral
       H35.389   Toxic maculopathy, unspecified eye ▽

✓5th **H35.4**   **Peripheral retinal degeneration**
    EXCLUDES 1   *hereditary retinal degeneration (dystrophy) (H35.5-)*
           peripheral retinal degeneration with retinal break (H33.3-)
    H35.40   **Unspecified peripheral retinal degeneration** ▽
  ✓6th **H35.41**   **Lattice** degeneration of retina
        Palisade degeneration of retina
       H35.411   Lattice degeneration of retina, right eye
       H35.412   Lattice degeneration of retina, left eye
       H35.413   Lattice degeneration of retina, bilateral
       H35.419   Lattice degeneration of retina, unspecified eye ▽
  ✓6th **H35.42**   **Microcystoid** degeneration of retina
       H35.421   Microcystoid degeneration of retina, right eye
       H35.422   Microcystoid degeneration of retina, left eye

---

☑ Add'l Character Required   ✓x7th Placeholder Alert   RUG IV Special Care High Dx   RUG IV Clinically Complex Dx   RUG IV Special Care Low Dx   Manifestation Code   Other Specified Code   ▽ Unspecified Code

ICD-10-CM 2016   563

Chapter 7. Diseases of the Eye and Adnexa

H35.423 **Microcystoid degeneration of retina, bilateral**

H35.429 **Microcystoid degeneration of retina, unspecified eye** ▽

✓6ᵗʰ H35.43 Paving stone **degeneration of retina**

H35.431 **Paving stone degeneration of retina, right eye**

H35.432 **Paving stone degeneration of retina, left eye**

H35.433 **Paving stone degeneration of retina, bilateral**

H35.439 **Paving stone degeneration of retina, unspecified eye** ▽

✓6ᵗʰ H35.44 Age-related reticular **degeneration of retina**

H35.441 **Age-related reticular degeneration of retina, right eye** 🄰

H35.442 **Age-related reticular degeneration of retina, left eye** 🄰

H35.443 **Age-related reticular degeneration of retina, bilateral** 🄰

H35.449 **Age-related reticular degeneration of retina, unspecified eye** 🄰▽

✓6ᵗʰ H35.45 Secondary pigmentary **degeneration**

H35.451 **Secondary pigmentary degeneration, right eye**

H35.452 **Secondary pigmentary degeneration, left eye**

H35.453 **Secondary pigmentary degeneration, bilateral**

H35.459 **Secondary pigmentary degeneration, unspecified eye** ▽

✓6ᵗʰ H35.46 Secondary vitreoretinal **degeneration**

H35.461 **Secondary vitreoretinal degeneration, right eye**

H35.462 **Secondary vitreoretinal degeneration, left eye**

H35.463 **Secondary vitreoretinal degeneration, bilateral**

H35.469 **Secondary vitreoretinal degeneration, unspecified eye** ▽

✓5ᵗʰ H35.5 **Hereditary retinal dystrophy**

EXCLUDES 1   dystrophies primarily involving Bruch's membrane (H31.1-)

H35.50 **Unspecified hereditary retinal dystrophy** ▽

H35.51 Vitreoretinal **dystrophy**

H35.52 Pigmentary **retinal dystrophy**
Albipunctate retinal dystrophy
Retinitis pigmentosa
Tapetoretinal dystrophy

H35.53 **Other dystrophies primarily involving the sensory retina**
Stargardt's disease

H35.54 **Dystrophies primarily involving the** retinal pigment epithelium
Vitelliform retinal dystrophy

✓5ᵗʰ H35.6 **Retinal hemorrhage**

H35.60 **Retinal hemorrhage, unspecified eye** ▽

H35.61 **Retinal hemorrhage, right eye**

H35.62 **Retinal hemorrhage, left eye**

H35.63 **Retinal hemorrhage, bilateral**

✓5ᵗʰ H35.7 **Separation of retinal layers**

EXCLUDES 1   retinal detachment (serous) (H33.2-)
rhegmatogenous retinal detachment (H33.0-)

H35.70 **Unspecified separation of retinal layers** ▽

✓6ᵗʰ H35.71 Central serous **chorioretinopathy**

H35.711 **Central serous chorioretinopathy, right eye**

H35.712 **Central serous chorioretinopathy, left eye**

H35.713 **Central serous chorioretinopathy, bilateral**

H35.719 **Central serous chorioretinopathy, unspecified eye** ▽

✓6ᵗʰ H35.72 Serous **detachment of retinal pigment epithelium**

H35.721 **Serous detachment of retinal pigment epithelium, right eye**

H35.722 **Serous detachment of retinal pigment epithelium, left eye**

H35.723 **Serous detachment of retinal pigment epithelium, bilateral**

H35.729 **Serous detachment of retinal pigment epithelium, unspecified eye** ▽

✓6ᵗʰ H35.73 Hemorrhagic **detachment of retinal pigment epithelium**

H35.731 **Hemorrhagic detachment of retinal pigment epithelium, right eye**

H35.732 **Hemorrhagic detachment of retinal pigment epithelium, left eye**

H35.733 **Hemorrhagic detachment of retinal pigment epithelium, bilateral**

H35.739 **Hemorrhagic detachment of retinal pigment epithelium, unspecified eye** ▽

✓5ᵗʰ H35.8 **Other specified retinal disorders**

EXCLUDES 2   retinal hemorrhage (H35.6-)

H35.81 **Retinal edema**
Retinal cotton wool spots

H35.82 **Retinal ischemia**

H35.89 **Other specified retinal disorders**

H35.9 **Unspecified retinal disorder** ▽

H36 Retinal disorders in diseases classified elsewhere

Code first underlying disease, such as:
lipid storage disorders (E75.-)
sickle-cell disorders (D57.-)

EXCLUDES 1   arteriosclerotic retinopathy (H35.0-)
diabetic retinopathy (E08.3-, E09.3-, E10.3-, E11.3-, E13.3-)

Glaucoma (H40-H42)

✓4ᵗʰ **H40 Glaucoma**

EXCLUDES 1   absolute glaucoma (H44.51-)
congenital glaucoma (Q15.0)
traumatic glaucoma due to birth injury (P15.3)

✓5ᵗʰ H40.0 **Glaucoma** suspect

✓6ᵗʰ H40.00 **Preglaucoma,** unspecified

H40.001 **Preglaucoma, unspecified, right eye** ▽

H40.002 **Preglaucoma, unspecified, left eye** ▽

H40.003 **Preglaucoma, unspecified, bilateral** ▽

H40.009 **Preglaucoma, unspecified, unspecified eye** ▽

✓6ᵗʰ H40.01 Open angle **with borderline findings, low risk**
Open angle, low risk

H40.011 **Open angle with borderline findings, low risk, right eye**

H40.012 **Open angle with borderline findings, low risk, left eye**

H40.013 **Open angle with borderline findings, low risk, bilateral**

H40.019 **Open angle with borderline findings, low risk, unspecified eye** ▽

✓6ᵗʰ H40.02 Open angle **with borderline findings, high risk**
Open angle, high risk

H40.021 **Open angle with borderline findings, high risk, right eye**

H40.022 **Open angle with borderline findings, high risk, left eye**

H40.023 **Open angle with borderline findings, high risk, bilateral**

H40.029 **Open angle with borderline findings, high risk, unspecified eye** ▽

✓6ᵗʰ H40.03 Anatomical narrow **angle**
Primary angle closure suspect

H40.031 **Anatomical narrow angle, right eye**

H40.032 **Anatomical narrow angle, left eye**

H40.033 **Anatomical narrow angle, bilateral**

H40.039 **Anatomical narrow angle, unspecified eye** ▽

✓6ᵗʰ H40.04 Steroid **responder**

H40.041 **Steroid responder, right eye**

H40.042 **Steroid responder, left eye**

H40.043 **Steroid responder, bilateral**

H40.049 **Steroid responder, unspecified eye** ▽

✓6ᵗʰ H40.05 Ocular **hypertension**

H40.051 **Ocular hypertension, right eye**

H40.052 **Ocular hypertension, left eye**

🄽 Newborn   🄿 Pediatric   🄼 Maternity   🄰 Adult   **RIC** RIC Dx   **NC Dx** Noncancer Dx   **PDx** Primary Dx   **CC** RIC CC Condition   ►◄ Revised Text   ● New Code   ▲ Revised Code Title

564   ICD-10-CM 2016

H35.423–H40.052

H40.053   Ocular hypertension, bilateral

H40.059   Ocular hypertension, unspecified eye ▽

√6ᵗʰ   **H40.06**   Primary angle closure without glaucoma damage

H40.061   Primary angle closure without glaucoma damage, right eye

H40.062   Primary angle closure without glaucoma damage, left eye

H40.063   Primary angle closure without glaucoma damage, bilateral

H40.069   Primary angle closure without glaucoma damage, unspecified eye ▽

√5ᵗʰ   **H40.1**   Open-angle glaucoma

> One of the following 7th characters is to be assigned to each code in subcategories H40.10, H40.11, H40.12-, H40.13-, and H40.14- to designate the stage of glaucoma.
> 0   stage unspecified
> 1   mild stage
> 2   moderate stage
> 3   severe stage
> 4   indeterminate stage

√x7ᵗʰ   **H40.10**   Unspecified open-angle glaucoma   ▽

√x7ᵗʰ   **H40.11**   Primary open-angle glaucoma
Chronic simple glaucoma

√6ᵗʰ   **H40.12**   Low-tension glaucoma

√7ᵗʰ   H40.121   Low-tension glaucoma, right eye

√7ᵗʰ   H40.122   Low-tension glaucoma, left eye

√7ᵗʰ   H40.123   Low-tension glaucoma, bilateral

√7ᵗʰ   H40.129   Low-tension glaucoma, unspecified eye ▽

√6ᵗʰ   **H40.13**   Pigmentary glaucoma

√7ᵗʰ   H40.131   Pigmentary glaucoma, right eye

√7ᵗʰ   H40.132   Pigmentary glaucoma, left eye

√7ᵗʰ   H40.133   Pigmentary glaucoma, bilateral

√7ᵗʰ   H40.139   Pigmentary glaucoma, unspecified eye ▽

√6ᵗʰ   **H40.14**   Capsular glaucoma with pseudoexfoliation of lens

√7ᵗʰ   H40.141   Capsular glaucoma with pseudoexfoliation of lens, right eye

√7ᵗʰ   H40.142   Capsular glaucoma with pseudoexfoliation of lens, left eye

√7ᵗʰ   H40.143   Capsular glaucoma with pseudoexfoliation of lens, bilateral

√7ᵗʰ   H40.149   Capsular glaucoma with pseudoexfoliation of lens, unspecified eye ▽

√6ᵗʰ   **H40.15**   Residual stage of open-angle glaucoma

H40.151   Residual stage of open-angle glaucoma, right eye

H40.152   Residual stage of open-angle glaucoma, left eye

H40.153   Residual stage of open-angle glaucoma, bilateral

H40.159   Residual stage of open-angle glaucoma, unspecified eye ▽

√5ᵗʰ   **H40.2**   Primary angle-closure glaucoma

> **EXCLUDES 1**   aqueous misdirection (H40.83-)
> malignant glaucoma (H40.83-)

> One of the following 7th characters is to be assigned to each code in subcategories H40.20 and H40.22- to designate the stage of glaucoma.
> 0   stage unspecified
> 1   mild stage
> 2   moderate stage
> 3   severe stage
> 4   indeterminate stage

√x7ᵗʰ   **H40.20**   Unspecified primary angle-closure glaucoma ▽

√6ᵗʰ   **H40.21**   Acute angle-closure glaucoma
Acute angle-closure glaucoma attack
Acute angle-closure glaucoma crisis

H40.211   Acute angle-closure glaucoma, right eye

H40.212   Acute angle-closure glaucoma, left eye

H40.213   Acute angle-closure glaucoma, bilateral

H40.219   Acute angle-closure glaucoma, unspecified eye ▽

√6ᵗʰ   **H40.22**   Chronic angle-closure glaucoma
Chronic primary angle-closure glaucoma

√7ᵗʰ   H40.221   Chronic angle-closure glaucoma, right eye

√7ᵗʰ   H40.222   Chronic angle-closure glaucoma, left eye

√7ᵗʰ   H40.223   Chronic angle-closure glaucoma, bilateral

√7ᵗʰ   H40.229   Chronic angle-closure glaucoma, unspecified eye ▽

√6ᵗʰ   **H40.23**   Intermittent angle-closure glaucoma

H40.231   Intermittent angle-closure glaucoma, right eye

H40.232   Intermittent angle-closure glaucoma, left eye

H40.233   Intermittent angle-closure glaucoma, bilateral

H40.239   Intermittent angle-closure glaucoma, unspecified eye ▽

√6ᵗʰ   **H40.24**   Residual stage of angle-closure glaucoma

H40.241   Residual stage of angle-closure glaucoma, right eye

H40.242   Residual stage of angle-closure glaucoma, left eye

H40.243   Residual stage of angle-closure glaucoma, bilateral

H40.249   Residual stage of angle-closure glaucoma, unspecified eye ▽

√5ᵗʰ   **H40.3**   Glaucoma secondary to eye trauma
Code also underlying condition

> One of the following 7th characters is to be assigned to each code in subcategory H40.3- to designate the stage of glaucoma.
> 0   stage unspecified
> 1   mild stage
> 2   moderate stage
> 3   severe stage
> 4   indeterminate stage

√x7ᵗʰ   **H40.30**   Glaucoma secondary to eye trauma, unspecified eye ▽

√x7ᵗʰ   **H40.31**   Glaucoma secondary to eye trauma, right eye

√x7ᵗʰ   **H40.32**   Glaucoma secondary to eye trauma, left eye

√x7ᵗʰ   **H40.33**   Glaucoma secondary to eye trauma, bilateral

√5ᵗʰ   **H40.4**   Glaucoma secondary to eye inflammation
Code also underlying condition

> One of the following 7th characters is to be assigned to each code in subcategory H40.4- to designate the stage of glaucoma.
> 0   stage unspecified
> 1   mild stage
> 2   moderate stage
> 3   severe stage
> 4   indeterminate stage

√x7ᵗʰ   **H40.40**   Glaucoma secondary to eye inflammation, unspecified eye ▽

√x7ᵗʰ   **H40.41**   Glaucoma secondary to eye inflammation, right eye

√x7ᵗʰ   **H40.42**   Glaucoma secondary to eye inflammation, left eye

√x7ᵗʰ   **H40.43**   Glaucoma secondary to eye inflammation, bilateral

√5ᵗʰ   **H40.5**   Glaucoma secondary to other eye disorders
Code also underlying eye disorder

> One of the following 7th characters is to be assigned to each code in subcategory H40.5- to designate the stage of glaucoma.
> 0   stage unspecified
> 1   mild stage
> 2   moderate stage
> 3   severe stage
> 4   indeterminate stage

√x7ᵗʰ   **H40.50**   Glaucoma secondary to other eye disorders, unspecified eye ▽

√x7ᵗʰ   **H40.51**   Glaucoma secondary to other eye disorders, right eye

√x7ᵗʰ   **H40.52**   Glaucoma secondary to other eye disorders, left eye

√x7ᵗʰ   **H40.53**   Glaucoma secondary to other eye disorders, bilateral

☑ Add'l Character Required   √x7ᵗʰ Placeholder Alert   RUG IV Special Care High Dx   RUG IV Clinically Complex Dx   RUG IV Special Care Low Dx   Manifestation Code   Other Specified Code   ▽ Unspecified Code

ICD-10-CM 2016   565

Chapter 7. Diseases of the Eye and Adnexa

H40.6–H44.122

✓5ᵗʰ **H40.6** **Glaucoma** secondary to drugs
Use additional code for adverse effect, if applicable, to identify drug (T36-T50 with fifth or sixth character 5)

> One of the following 7th characters is to be assigned to each code in subcategory H40.6- to designate the stage of glaucoma.
> 0   stage unspecified
> 1   mild stage
> 2   moderate stage
> 3   severe stage
> 4   indeterminate stage

✓x7ᵗʰ **H40.60** **Glaucoma secondary to drugs, unspecified eye** ▽
✓x7ᵗʰ **H40.61** **Glaucoma secondary to drugs, right eye**
✓x7ᵗʰ **H40.62** **Glaucoma secondary to drugs, left eye**
✓x7ᵗʰ **H40.63** **Glaucoma secondary to drugs, bilateral**

✓5ᵗʰ **H40.8** **Other** glaucoma
✓6ᵗʰ **H40.81** **Glaucoma with** increased episcleral venous pressure
H40.811 **Glaucoma with increased episcleral venous pressure, right eye**
H40.812 **Glaucoma with increased episcleral venous pressure, left eye**
H40.813 **Glaucoma with increased episcleral venous pressure, bilateral**
H40.819 **Glaucoma with increased episcleral venous pressure, unspecified eye** ▽

✓6ᵗʰ **H40.82** **Hypersecretion glaucoma**
H40.821 **Hypersecretion glaucoma, right eye**
H40.822 **Hypersecretion glaucoma, left eye**
H40.823 **Hypersecretion glaucoma, bilateral**
H40.829 **Hypersecretion glaucoma, unspecified eye** ▽

✓6ᵗʰ **H40.83** **Aqueous misdirection**
Malignant glaucoma
H40.831 **Aqueous misdirection, right eye**
H40.832 **Aqueous misdirection, left eye**
H40.833 **Aqueous misdirection, bilateral**
H40.839 **Aqueous misdirection, unspecified eye** ▽

H40.89 **Other specified glaucoma**
H40.9 **Unspecified glaucoma** ▽

H42 *Glaucoma in diseases classified elsewhere*
Code first underlying condition, such as:
amyloidosis (E85.-)
aniridia (Q13.1)
Lowe's syndrome (E72.03)
Reiger's anomaly (Q13.81)
specified metabolic disorder (E70-E88)
EXCLUDES1 *glaucoma (in):*
diabetes mellitus (E08.39, E09.39, E10.39, E11.39, E13.39)
onchocerciasis (B73.02)
syphilis (A52.71)
tuberculous (A18.59)

Disorders of vitreous body and globe (H43-H44)

✓4ᵗʰ **H43** **Disorders of vitreous body**
✓5ᵗʰ **H43.0** **Vitreous** prolapse
EXCLUDES1 *traumatic vitreous prolapse (S05.2-)*
vitreous syndrome following cataract surgery (H59.0-)
H43.00 **Vitreous prolapse, unspecified eye** ▽
H43.01 **Vitreous prolapse, right eye**
H43.02 **Vitreous prolapse, left eye**
H43.03 **Vitreous prolapse, bilateral**

✓5ᵗʰ **H43.1** **Vitreous** hemorrhage
H43.10 **Vitreous hemorrhage, unspecified eye** ▽
H43.11 **Vitreous hemorrhage, right eye**
H43.12 **Vitreous hemorrhage, left eye**
H43.13 **Vitreous hemorrhage, bilateral**

✓5ᵗʰ **H43.2** **Crystalline deposits** in vitreous body
H43.20 **Crystalline deposits in vitreous body, unspecified eye** ▽
H43.21 **Crystalline deposits in vitreous body, right eye**
H43.22 **Crystalline deposits in vitreous body, left eye**
H43.23 **Crystalline deposits in vitreous body, bilateral**

✓5ᵗʰ **H43.3** **Other** vitreous opacities
✓6ᵗʰ **H43.31** **Vitreous** membranes and strands
H43.311 **Vitreous membranes and strands, right eye**
H43.312 **Vitreous membranes and strands, left eye**
H43.313 **Vitreous membranes and strands, bilateral**
H43.319 **Vitreous membranes and strands, unspecified eye** ▽

✓6ᵗʰ **H43.39** **Other** vitreous opacities
Vitreous floaters
H43.391 **Other vitreous opacities, right eye**
H43.392 **Other vitreous opacities, left eye**
H43.393 **Other vitreous opacities, bilateral**
H43.399 **Other vitreous opacities, unspecified eye** ▽

✓5ᵗʰ **H43.8** **Other** disorders of vitreous body
EXCLUDES1 *proliferative vitreo-retinopathy with retinal detachment (H33.4-)*
EXCLUDES2 *vitreous abscess (H44.02-)*
✓6ᵗʰ **H43.81** **Vitreous** degeneration
Vitreous detachment
H43.811 **Vitreous degeneration, right eye**
H43.812 **Vitreous degeneration, left eye**
H43.813 **Vitreous degeneration, bilateral**
H43.819 **Vitreous degeneration, unspecified eye** ▽

✓6ᵗʰ **H43.82** **Vitreomacular** adhesion
Vitreomacular traction
H43.821 **Vitreomacular adhesion, right eye** 🅰
H43.822 **Vitreomacular adhesion, left eye** 🅰
H43.823 **Vitreomacular adhesion, bilateral** 🅰
H43.829 **Vitreomacular adhesion, unspecified eye** 🅰▽

H43.89 **Other disorders of vitreous body**
H43.9 **Unspecified disorder of vitreous body** ▽

✓4ᵗʰ **H44** **Disorders of globe**
INCLUDES disorders affecting multiple structures of eye
✓5ᵗʰ **H44.0** **Purulent endophthalmitis**
Use additional code to identify organism
EXCLUDES1 *bleb associated endophthalmitis (H59.4-)*
✓6ᵗʰ **H44.00** **Unspecified purulent endophthalmitis**
H44.001 **Unspecified purulent endophthalmitis, right eye** ▽
H44.002 **Unspecified purulent endophthalmitis, left eye** ▽
H44.003 **Unspecified purulent endophthalmitis, bilateral** ▽
H44.009 **Unspecified purulent endophthalmitis, unspecified eye** ▽

✓6ᵗʰ **H44.01** **Panophthalmitis (acute)**
H44.011 **Panophthalmitis (acute), right eye**
H44.012 **Panophthalmitis (acute), left eye**
H44.013 **Panophthalmitis (acute), bilateral**
H44.019 **Panophthalmitis (acute), unspecified eye** ▽

✓6ᵗʰ **H44.02** **Vitreous abscess (chronic)**
H44.021 **Vitreous abscess (chronic), right eye**
H44.022 **Vitreous abscess (chronic), left eye**
H44.023 **Vitreous abscess (chronic), bilateral**
H44.029 **Vitreous abscess (chronic), unspecified eye** ▽

✓5ᵗʰ **H44.1** **Other endophthalmitis**
EXCLUDES1 *bleb associated endophthalmitis (H59.4-)*
EXCLUDES2 *ophthalmia nodosa (H16.2-)*
✓6ᵗʰ **H44.11** **Panuveitis**
H44.111 **Panuveitis, right eye**
H44.112 **Panuveitis, left eye**
H44.113 **Panuveitis, bilateral**
H44.119 **Panuveitis, unspecified eye** ▽

✓6ᵗʰ **H44.12** **Parasitic endophthalmitis, unspecified**
H44.121 **Parasitic endophthalmitis, unspecified, right eye** ▽
H44.122 **Parasitic endophthalmitis, unspecified, left eye** ▽

Ⓝ Newborn   Ⓟ Pediatric   Ⓜ Maternity   🅰 Adult   RIC RIC Dx   NCDx Noncancer Dx   PDx Primary Dx   CC RIC CC Condition   ►◄ Revised Text   ● New Code   ▲ Revised Code Title

566   ICD-10-CM 2016

H44.123   Parasitic endophthalmitis, unspecified, ▽
bilateral

H44.129   Parasitic endophthalmitis, unspecified, ▽
unspecified eye

✓6ᵗʰ   **H44.13**   **Sympathetic uveitis**

H44.131   Sympathetic uveitis, right eye

H44.132   Sympathetic uveitis, left eye

H44.133   Sympathetic uveitis, bilateral

H44.139   Sympathetic uveitis, unspecified eye ▽

H44.19   Other endophthalmitis

✓5ᵗʰ   **H44.2**   **Degenerative myopia**
Malignant myopia

H44.20   Degenerative myopia, unspecified eye ▽

H44.21   Degenerative myopia, right eye

H44.22   Degenerative myopia, left eye

H44.23   Degenerative myopia, bilateral

✓5ᵗʰ   **H44.3**   **Other and unspecified degenerative disorders of globe**

H44.30   Unspecified degenerative disorder of globe ▽

✓6ᵗʰ   **H44.31**   **Chalcosis**

H44.311   Chalcosis, right eye

H44.312   Chalcosis, left eye

H44.313   Chalcosis, bilateral

H44.319   Chalcosis, unspecified eye ▽

✓6ᵗʰ   **H44.32**   **Siderosis of eye**

H44.321   Siderosis of eye, right eye

H44.322   Siderosis of eye, left eye

H44.323   Siderosis of eye, bilateral

H44.329   Siderosis of eye, unspecified eye ▽

✓6ᵗʰ   **H44.39**   **Other degenerative disorders of globe**

H44.391   Other degenerative disorders of globe,
right eye

H44.392   Other degenerative disorders of globe,
left eye

H44.393   Other degenerative disorders of globe,
bilateral

H44.399   Other degenerative disorders of globe, ▽
unspecified eye

✓5ᵗʰ   **H44.4**   **Hypotony of eye**

H44.40   Unspecified hypotony of eye ▽

✓6ᵗʰ   **H44.41**   **Flat anterior chamber hypotony of eye**

H44.411   Flat anterior chamber hypotony of right
eye

H44.412   Flat anterior chamber hypotony of left eye

H44.413   Flat anterior chamber hypotony of eye,
bilateral

H44.419   Flat anterior chamber hypotony of ▽
unspecified eye

✓6ᵗʰ   **H44.42**   **Hypotony of eye due to ocular fistula**

H44.421   Hypotony of right eye due to ocular fistula

H44.422   Hypotony of left eye due to ocular fistula

H44.423   Hypotony of eye due to ocular fistula,
bilateral

H44.429   Hypotony of unspecified eye due to ▽
ocular fistula

✓6ᵗʰ   **H44.43**   **Hypotony of eye due to other ocular disorders**

H44.431   Hypotony of eye due to other ocular
disorders, right eye

H44.432   Hypotony of eye due to other ocular
disorders, left eye

H44.433   Hypotony of eye due to other ocular
disorders, bilateral

H44.439   Hypotony of eye due to other ocular ▽
disorders, unspecified eye

✓6ᵗʰ   **H44.44**   **Primary hypotony of eye**

H44.441   Primary hypotony of right eye

H44.442   Primary hypotony of left eye

H44.443   Primary hypotony of eye, bilateral

H44.449   Primary hypotony of unspecified eye ▽

✓5ᵗʰ   **H44.5**   **Degenerated conditions of globe**

H44.50   Unspecified degenerated conditions of globe ▽

✓6ᵗʰ   **H44.51**   **Absolute glaucoma**

H44.511   Absolute glaucoma, right eye

H44.512   Absolute glaucoma, left eye

H44.513   Absolute glaucoma, bilateral

H44.519   Absolute glaucoma, unspecified eye ▽

✓6ᵗʰ   **H44.52**   **Atrophy of globe**
Phthisis bulbi

H44.521   Atrophy of globe, right eye

H44.522   Atrophy of globe, left eye

H44.523   Atrophy of globe, bilateral

H44.529   Atrophy of globe, unspecified eye ▽

✓6ᵗʰ   **H44.53**   **Leucocoria**

H44.531   Leucocoria, right eye

H44.532   Leucocoria, left eye

H44.533   Leucocoria, bilateral

H44.539   Leucocoria, unspecified eye ▽

✓5ᵗʰ   **H44.6**   **Retained (old) intraocular foreign body, magnetic**
Use additional code to identify magnetic foreign body (Z18.11)

EXCLUDES 1   current intraocular foreign body (S05.-)

EXCLUDES 2   retained foreign body in eyelid (H02.81-)
retained (old) foreign body following penetrating
wound of orbit (H05.5-)
retained (old) intraocular foreign body, nonmagnetic
(H44.7-)

✓6ᵗʰ   **H44.60**   **Unspecified retained (old) intraocular foreign body,
magnetic**

H44.601   Unspecified retained (old) intraocular ▽
foreign body, magnetic, right eye

H44.602   Unspecified retained (old) intraocular ▽
foreign body, magnetic, left eye

H44.603   Unspecified retained (old) intraocular ▽
foreign body, magnetic, bilateral

H44.609   Unspecified retained (old) intraocular ▽
foreign body, magnetic, unspecified eye

✓6ᵗʰ   **H44.61**   **Retained (old) magnetic foreign body in anterior
chamber**

H44.611   Retained (old) magnetic foreign body in
anterior chamber, right eye

H44.612   Retained (old) magnetic foreign body in
anterior chamber, left eye

H44.613   Retained (old) magnetic foreign body in
anterior chamber, bilateral

H44.619   Retained (old) magnetic foreign body ▽
in anterior chamber, unspecified eye

✓6ᵗʰ   **H44.62**   **Retained (old) magnetic foreign body in iris or ciliary
body**

H44.621   Retained (old) magnetic foreign body in
iris or ciliary body, right eye

H44.622   Retained (old) magnetic foreign body in
iris or ciliary body, left eye

H44.623   Retained (old) magnetic foreign body in
iris or ciliary body, bilateral

H44.629   Retained (old) magnetic foreign body ▽
in iris or ciliary body, unspecified eye

✓6ᵗʰ   **H44.63**   **Retained (old) magnetic foreign body in lens**

H44.631   Retained (old) magnetic foreign body in
lens, right eye

H44.632   Retained (old) magnetic foreign body in
lens, left eye

H44.633   Retained (old) magnetic foreign body in
lens, bilateral

H44.639   Retained (old) magnetic foreign body ▽
in lens, unspecified eye

✓6ᵗʰ   **H44.64**   **Retained (old) magnetic foreign body in posterior
wall of globe**

H44.641   Retained (old) magnetic foreign body in
posterior wall of globe, right eye

H44.642   Retained (old) magnetic foreign body in
posterior wall of globe, left eye

H44.643   Retained (old) magnetic foreign body in
posterior wall of globe, bilateral

H44.649   Retained (old) magnetic foreign body ▽
in posterior wall of globe, unspecified
eye

✓6ᵗʰ   **H44.65**   **Retained (old) magnetic foreign body in vitreous
body**

H44.651   Retained (old) magnetic foreign body in
vitreous body, right eye

H44.652   Retained (old) magnetic foreign body in
vitreous body, left eye

H44.653   Retained (old) magnetic foreign body in vitreous body, bilateral

H44.659   Retained (old) magnetic foreign body in vitreous body, unspecified eye ▽

✓6th **H44.69**   Retained (old) intraocular foreign body, magnetic, in other or multiple sites

H44.691   Retained (old) intraocular foreign body, magnetic, in other or multiple sites, right eye

H44.692   Retained (old) intraocular foreign body, magnetic, in other or multiple sites, left eye

H44.693   Retained (old) intraocular foreign body, magnetic, in other or multiple sites, bilateral

H44.699   Retained (old) intraocular foreign body, magnetic, in other or multiple sites, unspecified eye ▽

✓5th **H44.7**   Retained (old) intraocular foreign body, nonmagnetic
Use additional code to identify nonmagnetic foreign body (Z18.01-Z18.10, Z18.12, Z18.2-Z18.9)
> EXCLUDES1   current intraocular foreign body (S05.-)
> EXCLUDES2   retained foreign body in eyelid (H02.81-)
> retained (old) foreign body following penetrating wound of orbit (H05.5-)
> retained (old) intraocular foreign body, magnetic (H44.6-)

✓6th **H44.70**   Unspecified retained (old) intraocular foreign body, nonmagnetic

H44.701   Unspecified retained (old) intraocular foreign body, nonmagnetic, right eye ▽

H44.702   Unspecified retained (old) intraocular foreign body, nonmagnetic, left eye ▽

H44.703   Unspecified retained (old) intraocular foreign body, nonmagnetic, bilateral ▽

H44.709   Unspecified retained (old) intraocular foreign body, nonmagnetic, unspecified eye ▽
> Retained (old) intraocular foreign body NOS

✓6th **H44.71**   Retained (nonmagnetic) (old) foreign body in anterior chamber

H44.711   Retained (nonmagnetic) (old) foreign body in anterior chamber, right eye

H44.712   Retained (nonmagnetic) (old) foreign body in anterior chamber, left eye

H44.713   Retained (nonmagnetic) (old) foreign body in anterior chamber, bilateral

H44.719   Retained (nonmagnetic) (old) foreign body in anterior chamber, unspecified eye ▽

✓6th **H44.72**   Retained (nonmagnetic) (old) foreign body in iris or ciliary body

H44.721   Retained (nonmagnetic) (old) foreign body in iris or ciliary body, right eye

H44.722   Retained (nonmagnetic) (old) foreign body in iris or ciliary body, left eye

H44.723   Retained (nonmagnetic) (old) foreign body in iris or ciliary body, bilateral

H44.729   Retained (nonmagnetic) (old) foreign body in iris or ciliary body, unspecified eye ▽

✓6th **H44.73**   Retained (nonmagnetic) (old) foreign body in lens

H44.731   Retained (nonmagnetic) (old) foreign body in lens, right eye

H44.732   Retained (nonmagnetic) (old) foreign body in lens, left eye

H44.733   Retained (nonmagnetic) (old) foreign body in lens, bilateral

H44.739   Retained (nonmagnetic) (old) foreign body in lens, unspecified eye ▽

✓6th **H44.74**   Retained (nonmagnetic) (old) foreign body in posterior wall of globe

H44.741   Retained (nonmagnetic) (old) foreign body in posterior wall of globe, right eye

H44.742   Retained (nonmagnetic) (old) foreign body in posterior wall of globe, left eye

H44.743   Retained (nonmagnetic) (old) foreign body in posterior wall of globe, bilateral

H44.749   Retained (nonmagnetic) (old) foreign body in posterior wall of globe, unspecified eye ▽

✓6th **H44.75**   Retained (nonmagnetic) (old) foreign body in vitreous body

H44.751   Retained (nonmagnetic) (old) foreign body in vitreous body, right eye

H44.752   Retained (nonmagnetic) (old) foreign body in vitreous body, left eye

H44.753   Retained (nonmagnetic) (old) foreign body in vitreous body, bilateral

H44.759   Retained (nonmagnetic) (old) foreign body in vitreous body, unspecified eye ▽

✓6th **H44.79**   Retained (old) intraocular foreign body, nonmagnetic, in other or multiple sites

H44.791   Retained (old) intraocular foreign body, nonmagnetic, in other or multiple sites, right eye

H44.792   Retained (old) intraocular foreign body, nonmagnetic, in other or multiple sites, left eye

H44.793   Retained (old) intraocular foreign body, nonmagnetic, in other or multiple sites, bilateral

H44.799   Retained (old) intraocular foreign body, nonmagnetic, in other or multiple sites, unspecified eye ▽

✓5th **H44.8**   Other disorders of globe

✓6th **H44.81**   Hemophthalmos

H44.811   Hemophthalmos, right eye

H44.812   Hemophthalmos, left eye

H44.813   Hemophthalmos, bilateral

H44.819   Hemophthalmos, unspecified eye ▽

✓6th **H44.82**   Luxation of globe

H44.821   Luxation of globe, right eye

H44.822   Luxation of globe, left eye

H44.823   Luxation of globe, bilateral

H44.829   Luxation of globe, unspecified eye ▽

H44.89   Other disorders of globe

H44.9   Unspecified disorder of globe ▽

Disorders of optic nerve and visual pathways (H46-H47)

✓4th **H46**   Optic neuritis
> EXCLUDES2   ischemic optic neuropathy (H47.01-)
> neuromyelitis optica [Devic] (G36.0)

✓5th **H46.0**   Optic papillitis

H46.00   Optic papillitis, unspecified eye ▽

H46.01   Optic papillitis, right eye

H46.02   Optic papillitis, left eye

H46.03   Optic papillitis, bilateral

✓5th **H46.1**   Retrobulbar neuritis
> Retrobulbar neuritis NOS
> EXCLUDES1   syphilitic retrobulbar neuritis (A52.15)

H46.10   Retrobulbar neuritis, unspecified eye ▽

H46.11   Retrobulbar neuritis, right eye

H46.12   Retrobulbar neuritis, left eye

H46.13   Retrobulbar neuritis, bilateral

H46.2   Nutritional optic neuropathy

H46.3   Toxic optic neuropathy
> Code first (T51-T65) to identify cause

H46.8   Other optic neuritis

H46.9   Unspecified optic neuritis ▽

✓4th **H47**   Other disorders of optic [2nd] nerve and visual pathways

✓5th **H47.0**   Disorders of optic nerve, not elsewhere classified

✓6th **H47.01**   Ischemic optic neuropathy

H47.011   Ischemic optic neuropathy, right eye

H47.012   Ischemic optic neuropathy, left eye

H47.013   Ischemic optic neuropathy, bilateral

H47.019   Ischemic optic neuropathy, unspecified eye ▽

✓6th **H47.02**   Hemorrhage in optic nerve sheath

H47.021   Hemorrhage in optic nerve sheath, right eye

H47.022   Hemorrhage in optic nerve sheath, left eye

N Newborn   P Pediatric   M Maternity   A Adult   RIC RIC Dx   NCDx Noncancer Dx   PDx Primary Dx   CC RIC CC Condition   ►◄ Revised Text   ● New Code   ▲ Revised Code Title

568   ICD-10-CM 2016

H47.023　Hemorrhage in optic nerve sheath, bilateral
H47.029　Hemorrhage in optic nerve sheath, unspecified eye ▽

✓6ᵗʰ H47.03　Optic nerve hypoplasia
H47.031　Optic nerve hypoplasia, right eye
H47.032　Optic nerve hypoplasia, left eye
H47.033　Optic nerve hypoplasia, bilateral
H47.039　Optic nerve hypoplasia, unspecified eye ▽

✓6ᵗʰ H47.09　Other disorders of optic nerve, not elsewhere classified
　　Compression of optic nerve
H47.091　Other disorders of optic nerve, not elsewhere classified, right eye
H47.092　Other disorders of optic nerve, not elsewhere classified, left eye
H47.093　Other disorders of optic nerve, not elsewhere classified, bilateral
H47.099　Other disorders of optic nerve, not elsewhere classified, unspecified eye ▽

✓5ᵗʰ H47.1　Papilledema
H47.10　Unspecified papilledema ▽
H47.11　Papilledema associated with increased intracranial pressure
H47.12　Papilledema associated with decreased ocular pressure
H47.13　Papilledema associated with retinal disorder

✓6ᵗʰ H47.14　Foster-Kennedy syndrome
H47.141　Foster-Kennedy syndrome, right eye
H47.142　Foster-Kennedy syndrome, left eye
H47.143　Foster-Kennedy syndrome, bilateral
H47.149　Foster-Kennedy syndrome, unspecified eye ▽

✓5ᵗʰ H47.2　Optic atrophy
H47.20　Unspecified optic atrophy ▽

✓6ᵗʰ H47.21　Primary optic atrophy
H47.211　Primary optic atrophy, right eye
H47.212　Primary optic atrophy, left eye
H47.213　Primary optic atrophy, bilateral
H47.219　Primary optic atrophy, unspecified eye ▽

H47.22　Hereditary optic atrophy
　　Leber's optic atrophy

✓6ᵗʰ H47.23　Glaucomatous optic atrophy
H47.231　Glaucomatous optic atrophy, right eye
H47.232　Glaucomatous optic atrophy, left eye
H47.233　Glaucomatous optic atrophy, bilateral
H47.239　Glaucomatous optic atrophy, unspecified eye ▽

✓6ᵗʰ H47.29　Other optic atrophy
　　Temporal pallor of optic disc
H47.291　Other optic atrophy, right eye
H47.292　Other optic atrophy, left eye
H47.293　Other optic atrophy, bilateral
H47.299　Other optic atrophy, unspecified eye ▽

✓5ᵗʰ H47.3　Other disorders of optic disc

✓6ᵗʰ H47.31　Coloboma of optic disc
H47.311　Coloboma of optic disc, right eye
H47.312　Coloboma of optic disc, left eye
H47.313　Coloboma of optic disc, bilateral
H47.319　Coloboma of optic disc, unspecified eye ▽

✓6ᵗʰ H47.32　Drusen of optic disc
H47.321　Drusen of optic disc, right eye
H47.322　Drusen of optic disc, left eye
H47.323　Drusen of optic disc, bilateral
H47.329　Drusen of optic disc, unspecified eye ▽

✓6ᵗʰ H47.33　Pseudopapilledema of optic disc
H47.331　Pseudopapilledema of optic disc, right eye
H47.332　Pseudopapilledema of optic disc, left eye
H47.333　Pseudopapilledema of optic disc, bilateral
H47.339　Pseudopapilledema of optic disc, unspecified eye ▽

✓6ᵗʰ H47.39　Other disorders of optic disc
H47.391　Other disorders of optic disc, right eye
H47.392　Other disorders of optic disc, left eye
H47.393　Other disorders of optic disc, bilateral
H47.399　Other disorders of optic disc, unspecified eye ▽

✓5ᵗʰ H47.4　Disorders of optic chiasm
　　Code also underlying condition
H47.41　Disorders of optic chiasm in (due to) inflammatory disorders
H47.42　Disorders of optic chiasm in (due to) neoplasm
H47.43　Disorders of optic chiasm in (due to) vascular disorders
H47.49　Disorders of optic chiasm in (due to) other disorders

✓5ᵗʰ H47.5　Disorders of other visual pathways
　　Disorders of optic tracts, geniculate nuclei and optic radiations
　　Code also underlying condition

✓6ᵗʰ H47.51　Disorders of visual pathways in (due to) inflammatory disorders
H47.511　Disorders of visual pathways in (due to) inflammatory disorders, right side
H47.512　Disorders of visual pathways in (due to) inflammatory disorders, left side
H47.519　Disorders of visual pathways in (due to) inflammatory disorders, unspecified side ▽

✓6ᵗʰ H47.52　Disorders of visual pathways in (due to) neoplasm
H47.521　Disorders of visual pathways in (due to) neoplasm, right side
H47.522　Disorders of visual pathways in (due to) neoplasm, left side
H47.529　Disorders of visual pathways in (due to) neoplasm, unspecified side ▽

✓6ᵗʰ H47.53　Disorders of visual pathways in (due to) vascular disorders
H47.531　Disorders of visual pathways in (due to) vascular disorders, right side
H47.532　Disorders of visual pathways in (due to) vascular disorders, left side
H47.539　Disorders of visual pathways in (due to) vascular disorders, unspecified side ▽

✓5ᵗʰ H47.6　Disorders of visual cortex
　　Code also underlying condition
　　EXCLUDES 1　injury to visual cortex S04.04

✓6ᵗʰ H47.61　Cortical blindness
H47.611　Cortical blindness, right side of brain
H47.612　Cortical blindness, left side of brain
H47.619　Cortical blindness, unspecified side of brain ▽

✓6ᵗʰ H47.62　Disorders of visual cortex in (due to) inflammatory disorders
H47.621　Disorders of visual cortex in (due to) inflammatory disorders, right side of brain
H47.622　Disorders of visual cortex in (due to) inflammatory disorders, left side of brain
H47.629　Disorders of visual cortex in (due to) inflammatory disorders, unspecified side of brain ▽

✓6ᵗʰ H47.63　Disorders of visual cortex in (due to) neoplasm
H47.631　Disorders of visual cortex in (due to) neoplasm, right side of brain
H47.632　Disorders of visual cortex in (due to) neoplasm, left side of brain
H47.639　Disorders of visual cortex in (due to) neoplasm, unspecified side of brain ▽

✓6ᵗʰ H47.64　Disorders of visual cortex in (due to) vascular disorders
H47.641　Disorders of visual cortex in (due to) vascular disorders, right side of brain
H47.642　Disorders of visual cortex in (due to) vascular disorders, left side of brain
H47.649　Disorders of visual cortex in (due to) vascular disorders, unspecified side of brain ▽

H47.9　Unspecified disorder of visual pathways ▽

Chapter 7. Diseases of the Eye and Adnexa

H47.023–H47.9

Disorders of ocular muscles, binocular movement, accommodation and refraction (H49-H52)

EXCLUDES 2   nystagmus and other irregular eye movements (H55)

✓4ᵗʰ H49 Paralytic strabismus
> **EXCLUDES 2**   internal ophthalmoplegia (H52.51-)
> internuclear ophthalmoplegia (H51.2-)
> progressive supranuclear ophthalmoplegia (G23.1)

✓5ᵗʰ H49.0 Third [oculomotor] nerve palsy
- H49.00   Third [oculomotor] nerve palsy, unspecified eye ▽
- H49.01   Third [oculomotor] nerve palsy, right eye
- H49.02   Third [oculomotor] nerve palsy, left eye
- H49.03   Third [oculomotor] nerve palsy, bilateral

✓5ᵗʰ H49.1 Fourth [trochlear] nerve palsy
- H49.10   Fourth [trochlear] nerve palsy, unspecified eye ▽
- H49.11   Fourth [trochlear] nerve palsy, right eye
- H49.12   Fourth [trochlear] nerve palsy, left eye
- H49.13   Fourth [trochlear] nerve palsy, bilateral

✓5ᵗʰ H49.2 Sixth [abducent] nerve palsy
- H49.20   Sixth [abducent] nerve palsy, unspecified eye ▽
- H49.21   Sixth [abducent] nerve palsy, right eye
- H49.22   Sixth [abducent] nerve palsy, left eye
- H49.23   Sixth [abducent] nerve palsy, bilateral

✓5ᵗʰ H49.3 Total (external) ophthalmoplegia
- H49.30   Total (external) ophthalmoplegia, unspecified eye ▽
- H49.31   Total (external) ophthalmoplegia, right eye
- H49.32   Total (external) ophthalmoplegia, left eye
- H49.33   Total (external) ophthalmoplegia, bilateral

✓5ᵗʰ H49.4 Progressive external ophthalmoplegia
> **EXCLUDES 1**   Kearns-Sayre syndrome (H49.81-)
- H49.40   Progressive external ophthalmoplegia, unspecified eye ▽
- H49.41   Progressive external ophthalmoplegia, right eye
- H49.42   Progressive external ophthalmoplegia, left eye
- H49.43   Progressive external ophthalmoplegia, bilateral

✓5ᵗʰ H49.8 Other paralytic strabismus
- **✓6ᵗʰ H49.81 Kearns-Sayre syndrome**
  > Progressive external ophthalmoplegia with pigmentary retinopathy
  > Use additional code for other manifestation, such as: heart block (I45.9)
  - H49.811   Kearns-Sayre syndrome, right eye
  - H49.812   Kearns-Sayre syndrome, left eye
  - H49.813   Kearns-Sayre syndrome, bilateral
  - H49.819   Kearns-Sayre syndrome, unspecified eye ▽
- **✓6ᵗʰ H49.88 Other paralytic strabismus**
  > External ophthalmoplegia NOS
  - H49.881   Other paralytic strabismus, right eye
  - H49.882   Other paralytic strabismus, left eye
  - H49.883   Other paralytic strabismus, bilateral
  - H49.889   Other paralytic strabismus, unspecified eye ▽

H49.9 Unspecified paralytic strabismus ▽

✓4ᵗʰ H50 Other strabismus
✓5ᵗʰ H50.0 Esotropia
> Convergent concomitant strabismus
> **EXCLUDES 1**   intermittent esotropia (H50.31-, H50.32)
- H50.00   Unspecified esotropia ▽
- **✓6ᵗʰ H50.01 Monocular esotropia**
  - H50.011   Monocular esotropia, right eye
  - H50.012   Monocular esotropia, left eye
- **✓6ᵗʰ H50.02 Monocular esotropia with A pattern**
  - H50.021   Monocular esotropia with A pattern, right eye
  - H50.022   Monocular esotropia with A pattern, left eye
- **✓6ᵗʰ H50.03 Monocular esotropia with V pattern**
  - H50.031   Monocular esotropia with V pattern, right eye
  - H50.032   Monocular esotropia with V pattern, left eye

✓6ᵗʰ H50.04 Monocular esotropia with other noncomitancies
- H50.041   Monocular esotropia with other noncomitancies, right eye
- H50.042   Monocular esotropia with other noncomitancies, left eye
- H50.05   Alternating esotropia
- H50.06   Alternating esotropia with A pattern
- H50.07   Alternating esotropia with V pattern
- H50.08   Alternating esotropia with other noncomitancies

✓5ᵗʰ H50.1 Exotropia
> Divergent concomitant strabismus
> **EXCLUDES 1**   intermittent exotropia (H50.33-, H50.34)
- H50.10   Unspecified exotropia ▽
- **✓6ᵗʰ H50.11 Monocular exotropia**
  - H50.111   Monocular exotropia, right eye
  - H50.112   Monocular exotropia, left eye
- **✓6ᵗʰ H50.12 Monocular exotropia with A pattern**
  - H50.121   Monocular exotropia with A pattern, right eye
  - H50.122   Monocular exotropia with A pattern, left eye
- **✓6ᵗʰ H50.13 Monocular exotropia with V pattern**
  - H50.131   Monocular exotropia with V pattern, right eye
  - H50.132   Monocular exotropia with V pattern, left eye
- **✓6ᵗʰ H50.14 Monocular exotropia with other noncomitancies**
  - H50.141   Monocular exotropia with other noncomitancies, right eye
  - H50.142   Monocular exotropia with other noncomitancies, left eye
- H50.15   Alternating exotropia
- H50.16   Alternating exotropia with A pattern
- H50.17   Alternating exotropia with V pattern
- H50.18   Alternating exotropia with other noncomitancies

✓5ᵗʰ H50.2 Vertical strabismus
> Hypertropia
- H50.21   Vertical strabismus, right eye
- H50.22   Vertical strabismus, left eye

✓5ᵗʰ H50.3 Intermittent heterotropia
- H50.30   Unspecified intermittent heterotropia ▽
- **✓6ᵗʰ H50.31 Intermittent monocular esotropia**
  - H50.311   Intermittent monocular esotropia, right eye
  - H50.312   Intermittent monocular esotropia, left eye
- H50.32   Intermittent alternating esotropia
- **✓6ᵗʰ H50.33 Intermittent monocular exotropia**
  - H50.331   Intermittent monocular exotropia, right eye
  - H50.332   Intermittent monocular exotropia, left eye
- H50.34   Intermittent alternating exotropia

✓5ᵗʰ H50.4 Other and unspecified heterotropia
- H50.40   Unspecified heterotropia ▽
- **✓6ᵗʰ H50.41 Cyclotropia**
  - H50.411   Cyclotropia, right eye
  - H50.412   Cyclotropia, left eye
- H50.42   Monofixation syndrome
- H50.43   Accommodative component in esotropia

✓5ᵗʰ H50.5 Heterophoria
- H50.50   Unspecified heterophoria ▽
- H50.51   Esophoria
- H50.52   Exophoria
- H50.53   Vertical heterophoria
- H50.54   Cyclophoria
- H50.55   Alternating heterophoria

✓5ᵗʰ H50.6 Mechanical strabismus
- H50.60   Mechanical strabismus, unspecified ▽
- **✓6ᵗʰ H50.61 Brown's sheath syndrome**
  - H50.611   Brown's sheath syndrome, right eye
  - H50.612   Brown's sheath syndrome, left eye

Ⓝ Newborn   Ⓟ Pediatric   Ⓜ Maternity   Ⓐ Adult   **RIC** RIC Dx   **NC Dx** Noncancer Dx   **PDx** Primary Dx   **CC** RIC CC Condition   ▶◀ Revised Text   ● New Code   ▲ Revised Code Title

570   ICD-10-CM 2016

H50.69   **Other mechanical strabismus**
Strabismus due to adhesions
Traumatic limitation of duction of eye muscle

✓5th **H50.8**   **Other specified strabismus**

   ✓6th **H50.81**   **Duane's syndrome**
     H50.811   Duane's syndrome, right eye
     H50.812   Duane's syndrome, left eye
   H50.89   **Other specified strabismus**

H50.9   **Unspecified strabismus**   ▽

✓4th **H51**   **Other disorders of binocular movement**

H51.0   **Palsy (spasm) of conjugate gaze**

✓5th **H51.1**   **Convergence insufficiency and excess**
   H51.11   Convergence insufficiency
   H51.12   Convergence excess

✓5th **H51.2**   **Internuclear ophthalmoplegia**
   H51.20   Internuclear ophthalmoplegia, unspecified eye   ▽
   H51.21   Internuclear ophthalmoplegia, right eye
   H51.22   Internuclear ophthalmoplegia, left eye
   H51.23   Internuclear ophthalmoplegia, bilateral

H51.8   **Other specified disorders of binocular movement**

H51.9   **Unspecified disorder of binocular movement**   ▽

✓4th **H52**   **Disorders of refraction and accommodation**

✓5th **H52.0**   **Hypermetropia**
   H52.00   Hypermetropia, unspecified eye   ▽
   H52.01   Hypermetropia, right eye
   H52.02   Hypermetropia, left eye
   H52.03   Hypermetropia, bilateral

✓5th **H52.1**   **Myopia**
   EXCLUDES 1   *degenerative myopia (H44.2-)*
   H52.10   Myopia, unspecified eye   ▽
   H52.11   Myopia, right eye
   H52.12   Myopia, left eye
   H52.13   Myopia, bilateral

✓5th **H52.2**   **Astigmatism**

   ✓6th **H52.20**   **Unspecified astigmatism**
     H52.201   Unspecified astigmatism, right eye   ▽
     H52.202   Unspecified astigmatism, left eye   ▽
     H52.203   Unspecified astigmatism, bilateral   ▽
     H52.209   Unspecified astigmatism, unspecified eye   ▽

   ✓6th **H52.21**   **Irregular astigmatism**
     H52.211   Irregular astigmatism, right eye
     H52.212   Irregular astigmatism, left eye
     H52.213   Irregular astigmatism, bilateral
     H52.219   Irregular astigmatism, unspecified eye   ▽

   ✓6th **H52.22**   **Regular astigmatism**
     H52.221   Regular astigmatism, right eye
     H52.222   Regular astigmatism, left eye
     H52.223   Regular astigmatism, bilateral
     H52.229   Regular astigmatism, unspecified eye   ▽

✓5th **H52.3**   **Anisometropia and aniseikonia**
   H52.31   Anisometropia
   H52.32   Aniseikonia

H52.4   **Presbyopia**

✓5th **H52.5**   **Disorders of accommodation**

   ✓6th **H52.51**   **Internal ophthalmoplegia (complete) (total)**
     H52.511   Internal ophthalmoplegia (complete) (total), right eye
     H52.512   Internal ophthalmoplegia (complete) (total), left eye
     H52.513   Internal ophthalmoplegia (complete) (total), bilateral
     H52.519   Internal ophthalmoplegia (complete) (total), unspecified eye   ▽

   ✓6th **H52.52**   **Paresis of accommodation**
     H52.521   Paresis of accommodation, right eye
     H52.522   Paresis of accommodation, left eye
     H52.523   Paresis of accommodation, bilateral
     H52.529   Paresis of accommodation, unspecified eye   ▽

   ✓6th **H52.53**   **Spasm of accommodation**
     H52.531   Spasm of accommodation, right eye
     H52.532   Spasm of accommodation, left eye
     H52.533   Spasm of accommodation, bilateral
     H52.539   Spasm of accommodation, unspecified eye   ▽

H52.6   **Other disorders of refraction**

H52.7   **Unspecified disorder of refraction**   ▽

Visual disturbances and blindness (H53-H54)

✓4th **H53**   **Visual disturbances**

✓5th **H53.0**   **Amblyopia ex anopsia**
   EXCLUDES 1   *amblyopia due to vitamin A deficiency (E50.5)*

   ✓6th **H53.00**   **Unspecified amblyopia**
     H53.001   Unspecified amblyopia, right eye   ▽
     H53.002   Unspecified amblyopia, left eye   ▽
     H53.003   Unspecified amblyopia, bilateral   ▽
     H53.009   Unspecified amblyopia, unspecified eye   ▽

   ✓6th **H53.01**   **Deprivation amblyopia**
     H53.011   Deprivation amblyopia, right eye
     H53.012   Deprivation amblyopia, left eye
     H53.013   Deprivation amblyopia, bilateral
     H53.019   Deprivation amblyopia, unspecified eye   ▽

   ✓6th **H53.02**   **Refractive amblyopia**
     H53.021   Refractive amblyopia, right eye
     H53.022   Refractive amblyopia, left eye
     H53.023   Refractive amblyopia, bilateral
     H53.029   Refractive amblyopia, unspecified eye   ▽

   ✓6th **H53.03**   **Strabismic amblyopia**
     EXCLUDES 1   *strabismus (H50.-)*
     H53.031   Strabismic amblyopia, right eye
     H53.032   Strabismic amblyopia, left eye
     H53.033   Strabismic amblyopia, bilateral
     H53.039   Strabismic amblyopia, unspecified eye   ▽

✓5th **H53.1**   **Subjective visual disturbances**
   EXCLUDES 1   *subjective visual disturbances due to vitamin A deficiency (E50.5)*
           visual hallucinations (R44.1)

   H53.10   Unspecified subjective visual disturbances   ▽

   H53.11   **Day blindness**
     Hemeralopia

   ✓6th **H53.12**   **Transient visual loss**
     Scintillating scotoma
     EXCLUDES 1   *amaurosis fugax (G45.3-)*
           transient retinal artery occlusion (H34.0-)
     H53.121   Transient visual loss, right eye
     H53.122   Transient visual loss, left eye
     H53.123   Transient visual loss, bilateral
     H53.129   Transient visual loss, unspecified eye   ▽

   ✓6th **H53.13**   **Sudden visual loss**
     H53.131   Sudden visual loss, right eye
     H53.132   Sudden visual loss, left eye
     H53.133   Sudden visual loss, bilateral
     H53.139   Sudden visual loss, unspecified eye   ▽

   ✓6th **H53.14**   **Visual discomfort**
     Asthenopia
     Photophobia
     H53.141   Visual discomfort, right eye
     H53.142   Visual discomfort, left eye
     H53.143   Visual discomfort, bilateral
     H53.149   Visual discomfort, unspecified   ▽

   H53.15   **Visual distortions of shape and size**
     Metamorphopsia

   H53.16   **Psychophysical visual disturbances**

   H53.19   **Other subjective visual disturbances**
     Visual halos

H53.2   **Diplopia**
   Double vision

✓ Add'l Character Required   ✗x7th Placeholder Alert   RUG IV Special Care High Dx   RUG IV Clinically Complex Dx   RUG IV Special Care Low Dx   Manifestation Code   Other Specified Code   ▽ Unspecified Code

Chapter 7. Diseases of the Eye and Adnexa

✓5ᵗʰ **H53.3 Other and unspecified disorders of binocular vision**
    H53.30 Unspecified disorder of binocular vision ▽
    H53.31 Abnormal retinal correspondence
    H53.32 Fusion with defective stereopsis
    H53.33 Simultaneous visual perception without fusion
    H53.34 Suppression of binocular vision

✓5ᵗʰ **H53.4 Visual field defects**
    H53.40 Unspecified visual field defects ▽
    ✓6ᵗʰ **H53.41 Scotoma involving** central area
         Central scotoma
        H53.411 Scotoma involving central area, right eye
        H53.412 Scotoma involving central area, left eye
        H53.413 Scotoma involving central area, bilateral
        H53.419 Scotoma involving central area, ▽
        unspecified eye
    ✓6ᵗʰ **H53.42 Scotoma of** blind spot **area**
         Enlarged blind spot
        H53.421 Scotoma of blind spot area, right **eye**
        H53.422 Scotoma of blind spot area, left **eye**
        H53.423 Scotoma of blind spot area, bilateral
        H53.429 Scotoma of blind spot area, unspecified ▽
        eye
    ✓6ᵗʰ **H53.43 Sector or arcuate defects**
         Arcuate scotoma
         Bjerrum scotoma
        H53.431 Sector or arcuate defects, right **eye**
        H53.432 Sector or arcuate defects, left **eye**
        H53.433 Sector or arcuate defects, bilateral
        H53.439 Sector or arcuate defects, unspecified ▽
        eye
    ✓6ᵗʰ **H53.45 Other localized visual field defect**
         Peripheral visual field defect
         Ring scotoma NOS
         Scotoma NOS
        H53.451 Other localized visual field defect, right
        eye
        H53.452 Other localized visual field defect, left **eye**
        H53.453 Other localized visual field defect,
        bilateral
        H53.459 Other localized visual field defect, ▽
        unspecified eye
    ✓6ᵗʰ **H53.46 Homonymous bilateral field defects**
         Homonymous hemianopia
         Homonymous hemianopsia
         Quadrant anopia
         Quadrant anopsia
        H53.461 Homonymous bilateral field defects, right
        side
        H53.462 Homonymous bilateral field defects, left
        side
        H53.469 Homonymous bilateral field defects, ▽
        unspecified side
             Homonymous bilateral field defects NOS
    H53.47 Heteronymous bilateral field defects
         Heteronymous hemianop(s)ia
    ✓6ᵗʰ **H53.48 Generalized contraction of visual field**
        H53.481 Generalized contraction of visual field,
        right eye
        H53.482 Generalized contraction of visual field, left
        eye
        H53.483 Generalized contraction of visual field,
        bilateral
        H53.489 Generalized contraction of visual field, ▽
        unspecified eye

✓5ᵗʰ **H53.5 Color vision deficiencies**
     Color blindness
    EXCLUDES 2 day blindness (H53.11)
    H53.50 Unspecified color vision deficiencies ▽
         Color blindness NOS
    H53.51 Achromatopsia
    H53.52 Acquired color vision deficiency
    H53.53 Deuteranomaly
         Deuteranopia
    H53.54 Protanomaly
         Protanopia

    H53.55 Tritanomaly
         Tritanopia
    H53.59 Other color vision deficiencies

✓5ᵗʰ **H53.6 Night blindness**
    EXCLUDES 1 night blindness due to vitamin A deficiency (E50.5)
    H53.60 Unspecified night blindness ▽
    H53.61 Abnormal dark adaptation curve
    H53.62 Acquired night blindness
    H53.63 Congenital night blindness
    H53.69 Other night blindness

✓5ᵗʰ **H53.7 Vision** sensitivity **deficiencies**
    H53.71 Glare sensitivity
    H53.72 Impaired contrast sensitivity

H53.8 Other visual disturbances
H53.9 Unspecified visual disturbance ▽

✓4ᵗʰ **H54 Blindness and low vision**
    NOTE For definition of visual impairment categories see table below
     Code first any associated underlying cause of the blindness
    EXCLUDES 1 amaurosis fugax (G45.3)
    H54.0 Blindness, both eyes
         Visual impairment categories 3, 4, 5 in both eyes.
    ✓5ᵗʰ **H54.1 Blindness,** one eye, low vision other eye
         Visual impairment categories 3, 4, 5 in one eye, with categories 1 or 2 in the other eye.
        H54.10 Blindness, one eye, low vision other eye, ▽
        unspecified eyes
        H54.11 Blindness, right **eye, low vision** left **eye**
        H54.12 Blindness, left **eye, low vision** right **eye**
    H54.2 Low vision, both eyes
         Visual impairment categories 1 or 2 in both eyes.
    H54.3 Unqualified visual loss, both eyes
         Visual impairment category 9 in both eyes.
    ✓5ᵗʰ **H54.4 Blindness,** one eye
         Visual impairment categories 3, 4, 5 in one eye [normal vision in other eye]
        H54.40 Blindness, one eye, unspecified eye ▽
        H54.41 Blindness, right **eye, normal vision** left **eye**
        H54.42 Blindness, left **eye, normal vision** right **eye**
    ✓5ᵗʰ **H54.5 Low vision,** one eye
         Visual impairment categories 1 or 2 in one eye [normal vision in other eye].
        H54.50 Low vision, one eye, unspecified eye ▽
        H54.51 Low vision, right **eye, normal vision** left **eye**
        H54.52 Low vision, left **eye, normal vision** right **eye**
    ✓5ᵗʰ **H54.6 Unqualified visual loss,** one eye
         Visual impairment category 9 in one eye [normal vision in other eye].
        H54.60 Unqualified visual loss, one eye, unspecified ▽
        H54.61 Unqualified visual loss, right **eye, normal vision**
        left **eye**
        H54.62 Unqualified visual loss, left **eye, normal vision**
        right **eye**
    H54.7 Unspecified visual loss ▽
         Visual impairment category 9 NOS
    H54.8 Legal blindness, as defined in USA
         Blindness NOS according to USA definition
        EXCLUDES 1 legal blindness with specification of impairment level (H54.0-H54.7)
    NOTE The following table gives a classification of severity of visual impairment recommended by a WHO Study Group on the Prevention of Blindness, Geneva, 6-10 November l972.
         The term "low vision" in category H54 comprises categories 1 and 2 of the table, the term "blindness" categories 3, 4 and 5, and the term "unqualified visual loss" category 9.
         If the extent of the visual field is taken into account, patients with a field no greater than 10 but greater than 5 around central fixation should be placed in category 3 and patients with a field no category greater than 5 around central fixation should be placed in 4, even if the central acuity is not impaired.

N Newborn   P Pediatric   M Maternity   A Adult   RIC RIC Dx   NCDx Noncancer Dx   PDx Primary Dx   CC RIC CC Condition   ►◄ Revised Text   ● New Code   ▲ Revised Code Title

572   ICD-10-CM 2016

H53.3–H54.8

Category of visual impairment	Visual acuity with best possible correction	
	Maximum less than:	Minimum equal to or better than:
1	6/18 3/10 (0.3) 20/70	6/60 1/10 (0.1) 20/200
2	6/60 1/10 (0.1) 20/200	3/60 1/20 (0.5) 20/400
3	3/60 1/20 (0.05) 20/400	1/60 (finger counting at one meter) 1/50 (0.02) 5/300 (20/1200)
4	1/60 (finger counting at one meter) 1/50 (0.02) 5/300	Light perception
5	No light perception	
9	Undetermined or unspecified	

Other disorders of eye and adnexa (H55-H59)

✓4ᵗʰ H55 Nystagmus and other irregular eye movements

  ✓5ᵗʰ H55.0 Nystagmus

    H55.00 Unspecified nystagmus ▽

    H55.01 Congenital **nystagmus**

    H55.02 Latent nystagmus

    H55.03 Visual deprivation **nystagmus**

    H55.04 Dissociated **nystagmus**

    H55.09 Other forms of nystagmus

  ✓5ᵗʰ H55.8 Other irregular eye movements

    H55.81 Saccadic **eye movements**

    H55.89 Other irregular eye movements

✓4ᵗʰ H57 Other disorders of eye and adnexa

  ✓5ᵗʰ H57.0 Anomalies of pupillary function

    H57.00 Unspecified anomaly of pupillary function ▽

    H57.01 Argyll Robertson pupil, atypical

        EXCLUDES 1   syphilitic Argyll Robertson pupil (A52.19)

    H57.02 Anisocoria

    H57.03 Miosis

    H57.04 Mydriasis

    ✓6ᵗʰ H57.05 Tonic pupil

      H57.051 Tonic pupil, right eye

      H57.052 Tonic pupil, left eye

      H57.053 Tonic pupil, bilateral

      H57.059 Tonic pupil, unspecified eye ▽

    H57.09 Other anomalies of pupillary function

  ✓5ᵗʰ H57.1 Ocular pain

    H57.10 Ocular pain, unspecified eye ▽

    H57.11 Ocular pain, right eye

    H57.12 Ocular pain, left eye

    H57.13 Ocular pain, bilateral

  H57.8 Other specified disorders of eye and adnexa

  H57.9 Unspecified disorder of eye and adnexa ▽

✓4ᵗʰ H59 Intraoperative and postprocedural complications and disorders of eye and adnexa, not elsewhere classified

    EXCLUDES 1   mechanical complication of intraocular lens (T85.2)
            mechanical complication of other ocular prosthetic devices, implants and grafts (T85.3)
            pseudophakia (Z96.1)
            secondary cataracts (H26.4-)

  ✓5ᵗʰ H59.0 Disorders of the eye following cataract surgery

    ✓6ᵗʰ H59.01 Keratopathy (bullous aphakic) following cataract surgery

         Vitreal corneal syndrome

         Vitreous (touch) syndrome

      H59.011 Keratopathy (bullous aphakic) following cataract surgery, right eye

      H59.012 Keratopathy (bullous aphakic) following cataract surgery, left eye

      H59.013 Keratopathy (bullous aphakic) following cataract surgery, bilateral

      H59.019 Keratopathy (bullous aphakic) following cataract surgery, unspecified eye ▽

    ✓6ᵗʰ H59.02 Cataract (lens) fragments in eye following cataract surgery

      H59.021 Cataract (lens) fragments in eye following cataract surgery, right eye

      H59.022 Cataract (lens) fragments in eye following cataract surgery, left eye

      H59.023 Cataract (lens) fragments in eye following cataract surgery, bilateral

      H59.029 Cataract (lens) fragments in eye following cataract surgery, unspecified eye ▽

    ✓6ᵗʰ H59.03 Cystoid macular edema following cataract surgery

      H59.031 Cystoid macular edema following cataract surgery, right eye

      H59.032 Cystoid macular edema following cataract surgery, left eye

      H59.033 Cystoid macular edema following cataract surgery, bilateral

      H59.039 Cystoid macular edema following cataract surgery, unspecified eye ▽

    ✓6ᵗʰ H59.09 Other disorders of the eye following cataract surgery

      H59.091 Other disorders of the right eye following cataract surgery

      H59.092 Other disorders of the left eye following cataract surgery

      H59.093 Other disorders of the eye following cataract surgery, bilateral

      H59.099 Other disorders of unspecified eye following cataract surgery ▽

  ✓5ᵗʰ H59.1 Intraoperative hemorrhage and hematoma of eye and adnexa complicating a procedure

      EXCLUDES 1   intraoperative hemorrhage and hematoma of eye and adnexa due to accidental puncture or laceration during a procedure (H59.2-)

    ✓6ᵗʰ H59.11 Intraoperative hemorrhage and hematoma of eye and adnexa complicating an ophthalmic procedure

      H59.111 Intraoperative hemorrhage and hematoma of right eye and adnexa complicating an ophthalmic procedure

      H59.112 Intraoperative hemorrhage and hematoma of left eye and adnexa complicating an ophthalmic procedure

      H59.113 Intraoperative hemorrhage and hematoma of eye and adnexa complicating an ophthalmic procedure, bilateral

      H59.119 Intraoperative hemorrhage and hematoma of unspecified eye and adnexa complicating an ophthalmic procedure ▽

    ✓6ᵗʰ H59.12 Intraoperative hemorrhage and hematoma of eye and adnexa complicating other procedure

      H59.121 Intraoperative hemorrhage and hematoma of right eye and adnexa complicating other procedure

      H59.122 Intraoperative hemorrhage and hematoma of left eye and adnexa complicating other procedure

      H59.123 Intraoperative hemorrhage and hematoma of eye and adnexa complicating other procedure, bilateral

      H59.129 Intraoperative hemorrhage and hematoma of unspecified eye and adnexa complicating other procedure ▽

  ✓5ᵗʰ H59.2 Accidental puncture and laceration of eye and adnexa during a procedure

    ✓6ᵗʰ H59.21 Accidental puncture and laceration of eye and adnexa during an ophthalmic procedure

      H59.211 Accidental puncture and laceration of right eye and adnexa during an ophthalmic procedure

      H59.212 Accidental puncture and laceration of left eye and adnexa during an ophthalmic procedure

✓ Add'l Character Required ✓×7ᵗʰ Placeholder Alert RUG IV Special Care High Dx RUG IV Clinically Complex Dx RUG IV Special Care Low Dx Manifestation Code Other Specified Code ▽ Unspecified Code

CD-10-CM 2016   573

Chapter 7. Diseases of the Eye and Adnexa

H59.213 Accidental puncture and laceration of eye and adnexa during an ophthalmic procedure, bilateral

H59.219 Accidental puncture and laceration of unspecified eye and adnexa during an ophthalmic procedure ▽

✓6th H59.22 Accidental puncture and laceration of eye and adnexa during other procedure

H59.221 Accidental puncture and laceration of right eye and adnexa during other procedure

H59.222 Accidental puncture and laceration of left eye and adnexa during other procedure

H59.223 Accidental puncture and laceration of eye and adnexa during other procedure, bilateral

H59.229 Accidental puncture and laceration of unspecified eye and adnexa during other procedure ▽

✓5th H59.3 Postprocedural hemorrhage and hematoma of eye and adnexa following a procedure

✓6th H59.31 Postprocedural hemorrhage and hematoma of eye and adnexa following an ophthalmic procedure

H59.311 Postprocedural hemorrhage and hematoma of right eye and adnexa following an ophthalmic procedure

H59.312 Postprocedural hemorrhage and hematoma of left eye and adnexa following an ophthalmic procedure

H59.313 Postprocedural hemorrhage and hematoma of eye and adnexa following an ophthalmic procedure, bilateral

H59.319 Postprocedural hemorrhage and hematoma of unspecified eye and adnexa following an ophthalmic procedure ▽

✓6th H59.32 Postprocedural hemorrhage and hematoma of eye and adnexa following other procedure

H59.321 Postprocedural hemorrhage and hematoma of right eye and adnexa following other procedure

H59.322 Postprocedural hemorrhage and hematoma of left eye and adnexa following other procedure

H59.323 Postprocedural hemorrhage and hematoma of eye and adnexa following other procedure, bilateral

H59.329 Postprocedural hemorrhage and hematoma of unspecified eye and adnexa following other procedure ▽

✓5th H59.4 Inflammation (infection) of postprocedural bleb
Postprocedural blebitis
EXCLUDES 1 filtering (vitreous) bleb after glaucoma surgery status (Z98.83)

H59.40 Inflammation (infection) of postprocedural bleb, unspecified ▽

H59.41 Inflammation (infection) of postprocedural bleb, stage 1

H59.42 Inflammation (infection) of postprocedural bleb, stage 2

H59.43 Inflammation (infection) of postprocedural bleb, stage 3
Bleb endophthalmitis

✓5th H59.8 Other intraoperative and postprocedural complications and disorders of eye and adnexa, not elsewhere classified

✓6th H59.81 Chorioretinal scars after surgery for detachment

H59.811 Chorioretinal scars after surgery for detachment, right eye

H59.812 Chorioretinal scars after surgery for detachment, left eye

H59.813 Chorioretinal scars after surgery for detachment, bilateral

H59.819 Chorioretinal scars after surgery for detachment, unspecified eye ▽

H59.88 Other intraoperative complications of eye and adnexa, not elsewhere classified

H59.89 Other postprocedural complications and disorders of eye and adnexa, not elsewhere classified

Chapter 8. Diseases of the Ear and Mastoid Process (H60–H95)

Chapter Specific Coding Guidelines and Examples
Reserved for future guideline expansion.

Chapter 8. Diseases of the Ear and Mastoid Process (H60–H95)

NOTE   Use an external cause code following the code for the ear condition, if applicable, to identify the cause of the ear condition.

EXCLUDES 2   *certain conditions originating in the perinatal period (P04-P96)*
certain infectious and parasitic diseases (A00-B99)
complications of pregnancy, childbirth and the puerperium (O00-O9A)
congenital malformations, deformations and chromosomal abnormalities (Q00-Q99)
endocrine, nutritional and metabolic diseases (E00-E88)
injury, poisoning and certain other consequences of external causes (S00-T88)
neoplasms (C00-D49)
symptoms, signs and abnormal clinical and laboratory findings, not elsewhere classified (R00-R94)

This chapter contains the following blocks:

H60-H62   Diseases of external ear
H65-H75   Diseases of middle ear and mastoid
H80-H83   Diseases of inner ear
H90-H94   Other disorders of ear
H95   Intraoperative and postprocedural complications and disorders of ear and mastoid process, not elsewhere classified

Diseases of external ear (H60-H62)

√4ᵗ **H60**   **Otitis externa**

√5ᵗ **H60.0**   Abscess of external ear
Boil of external ear
Carbuncle of auricle or external auditory canal
Furuncle of external ear
- **H60.00**   Abscess of external ear, unspecified ear   ▽
- **H60.01**   Abscess of right external ear
- **H60.02**   Abscess of left external ear
- **H60.03**   Abscess of external ear, bilateral

√5ᵗ **H60.1**   Cellulitis of external ear
Cellulitis of auricle
Cellulitis of external auditory canal
- **H60.10**   Cellulitis of external ear, unspecified ear   ▽
- **H60.11**   Cellulitis of right external ear
- **H60.12**   Cellulitis of left external ear
- **H60.13**   Cellulitis of external ear, bilateral

√5ᵗ **H60.2**   Malignant otitis externa
- **H60.20**   Malignant otitis externa, unspecified ear   ▽
- **H60.21**   Malignant otitis externa, right ear
- **H60.22**   Malignant otitis externa, left ear
- **H60.23**   Malignant otitis externa, bilateral

√5ᵗ **H60.3**   Other infective otitis externa
√6ᵗ **H60.31**   Diffuse otitis externa
- **H60.311**   Diffuse otitis externa, right ear
- **H60.312**   Diffuse otitis externa, left ear
- **H60.313**   Diffuse otitis externa, bilateral
- **H60.319**   Diffuse otitis externa, unspecified ear   ▽

√6ᵗ **H60.32**   Hemorrhagic otitis externa
- **H60.321**   Hemorrhagic otitis externa, right ear
- **H60.322**   Hemorrhagic otitis externa, left ear
- **H60.323**   Hemorrhagic otitis externa, bilateral
- **H60.329**   Hemorrhagic otitis externa, unspecified ear   ▽

√6ᵗ **H60.33**   Swimmer's ear
- **H60.331**   Swimmer's ear, right ear
- **H60.332**   Swimmer's ear, left ear
- **H60.333**   Swimmer's ear, bilateral
- **H60.339**   Swimmer's ear, unspecified ear   ▽

√6ᵗ **H60.39**   Other infective otitis externa
- **H60.391**   Other infective otitis externa, right ear
- **H60.392**   Other infective otitis externa, left ear
- **H60.393**   Other infective otitis externa, bilateral
- **H60.399**   Other infective otitis externa, unspecified ear   ▽

√5ᵗ **H60.4**   Cholesteatoma of external ear
Keratosis obturans of external ear (canal)
EXCLUDES 2   *cholesteatoma of middle ear (H71.-)*
recurrent cholesteatoma of postmastoidectomy cavity (H95.0-)
- **H60.40**   Cholesteatoma of external ear, unspecified ear   ▽
- **H60.41**   Cholesteatoma of right external ear
- **H60.42**   Cholesteatoma of left external ear
- **H60.43**   Cholesteatoma of external ear, bilateral

√5ᵗ **H60.5**   Acute noninfective otitis externa
√6ᵗ **H60.50**   Unspecified acute noninfective otitis externa
Acute otitis externa NOS
- **H60.501**   Unspecified acute noninfective otitis externa, right ear   ▽
- **H60.502**   Unspecified acute noninfective otitis externa, left ear   ▽
- **H60.503**   Unspecified acute noninfective otitis externa, bilateral   ▽
- **H60.509**   Unspecified acute noninfective otitis externa, unspecified ear   ▽

√6ᵗ **H60.51**   Acute actinic otitis externa
- **H60.511**   Acute actinic otitis externa, right ear
- **H60.512**   Acute actinic otitis externa, left ear
- **H60.513**   Acute actinic otitis externa, bilateral
- **H60.519**   Acute actinic otitis externa, unspecified ear   ▽

√6ᵗ **H60.52**   Acute chemical otitis externa
- **H60.521**   Acute chemical otitis externa, right ear
- **H60.522**   Acute chemical otitis externa, left ear
- **H60.523**   Acute chemical otitis externa, bilateral
- **H60.529**   Acute chemical otitis externa, unspecified ear   ▽

√6ᵗ **H60.53**   Acute contact otitis externa
- **H60.531**   Acute contact otitis externa, right ear
- **H60.532**   Acute contact otitis externa, left ear
- **H60.533**   Acute contact otitis externa, bilateral
- **H60.539**   Acute contact otitis externa, unspecified ear   ▽

√6ᵗ **H60.54**   Acute eczematoid otitis externa
- **H60.541**   Acute eczematoid otitis externa, right ear
- **H60.542**   Acute eczematoid otitis externa, left ear
- **H60.543**   Acute eczematoid otitis externa, bilateral
- **H60.549**   Acute eczematoid otitis externa, unspecified ear   ▽

√6ᵗ **H60.55**   Acute reactive otitis externa
- **H60.551**   Acute reactive otitis externa, right ear
- **H60.552**   Acute reactive otitis externa, left ear
- **H60.553**   Acute reactive otitis externa, bilateral
- **H60.559**   Acute reactive otitis externa, unspecified ear   ▽

√6ᵗ **H60.59**   Other noninfective acute otitis externa
- **H60.591**   Other noninfective acute otitis externa, right ear
- **H60.592**   Other noninfective acute otitis externa, left ear
- **H60.593**   Other noninfective acute otitis externa, bilateral
- **H60.599**   Other noninfective acute otitis externa, unspecified ear   ▽

√5ᵗ **H60.6**   Unspecified chronic otitis externa
- **H60.60**   Unspecified chronic otitis externa, unspecified ear   ▽
- **H60.61**   Unspecified chronic otitis externa, right ear   ▽
- **H60.62**   Unspecified chronic otitis externa, left ear   ▽
- **H60.63**   Unspecified chronic otitis externa, bilateral   ▽

√5ᵗ **H60.8**   Other otitis externa
√6ᵗ **H60.8X**   Other otitis externa
- **H60.8X1**   Other otitis externa, right ear
- **H60.8X2**   Other otitis externa, left ear
- **H60.8X3**   Other otitis externa, bilateral
- **H60.8X9**   Other otitis externa, unspecified ear   ▽

√5ᵗ **H60.9**   Unspecified otitis externa
- **H60.90**   Unspecified otitis externa, unspecified ear   ▽
- **H60.91**   Unspecified otitis externa, right ear   ▽

Ⓝ Newborn   Ⓟ Pediatric   Ⓜ Maternity   Ⓐ Adult   **RIC** RIC Dx   **NCDx** Noncancer Dx   **PDx** Primary Dx   **CC** RIC CC Condition   ►◄ Revised Text   ● New Code   ▲ Revised Code Title

576   ICD-10-CM 2016

H60.92   **Unspecified otitis externa,** left **ear** ▽

H60.93   **Unspecified otitis externa,** bilateral ▽

✓4ᵗʰ **H61   Other disorders of external ear**

   ✓5ᵗʰ **H61.0   Chondritis and perichondritis of external ear**
      Chondrodermatitis nodularis chronica helicis
      Perichondritis of auricle
      Perichondritis of pinna

     ✓6ᵗʰ **H61.00   Unspecified perichondritis of external ear**
       H61.001   Unspecified perichondritis of right **external ear** ▽
       H61.002   Unspecified perichondritis of left **external ear** ▽
       H61.003   Unspecified perichondritis of external ear, bilateral ▽
       H61.009   Unspecified perichondritis of external ear, unspecified ear ▽

     ✓6ᵗʰ **H61.01   Acute perichondritis of external ear**
       H61.011   Acute perichondritis of right **external ear**
       H61.012   Acute perichondritis of left **external ear**
       H61.013   Acute perichondritis of external ear, bilateral
       H61.019   Acute perichondritis of external ear, unspecified ear ▽

     ✓6ᵗʰ **H61.02   Chronic perichondritis of external ear**
       H61.021   Chronic perichondritis of right **external ear**
       H61.022   Chronic perichondritis of left **external ear**
       H61.023   Chronic perichondritis of external ear, bilateral
       H61.029   Chronic perichondritis of external ear, unspecified ear ▽

     ✓6ᵗʰ **H61.03   Chondritis of external ear**
       Chondritis of auricle
       Chondritis of pinna
       AHA: 2015, 1Q, 18
       H61.031   Chondritis of right **external ear**
       H61.032   Chondritis of left **external ear**
       H61.033   Chondritis of external ear, bilateral
       H61.039   Chondritis of external ear, unspecified ear ▽

   ✓5ᵗʰ **H61.1   Noninfective disorders of pinna**
      EXCLUDES 2   cauliflower ear (M95.1-)
              gouty tophi of ear (M1A.-)

     ✓6ᵗʰ **H61.10   Unspecified noninfective disorders of pinna**
       Disorder of pinna NOS
       H61.101   Unspecified noninfective disorders of pinna, right **ear** ▽
       H61.102   Unspecified noninfective disorders of pinna, left **ear** ▽
       H61.103   Unspecified noninfective disorders of pinna, bilateral ▽
       H61.109   Unspecified noninfective disorders of pinna, unspecified ear ▽

     ✓6ᵗʰ **H61.11   Acquired deformity of pinna**
       Acquired deformity of auricle
       EXCLUDES 2   cauliflower ear (M95.1-)
       H61.111   Acquired deformity of pinna, right **ear**
       H61.112   Acquired deformity of pinna, left **ear**
       H61.113   Acquired deformity of pinna, bilateral
       H61.119   Acquired deformity of pinna, unspecified ear ▽

     ✓6ᵗʰ **H61.12   Hematoma of pinna**
       Hematoma of auricle
       H61.121   Hematoma of pinna, right **ear**
       H61.122   Hematoma of pinna, left **ear**
       H61.123   Hematoma of pinna, bilateral
       H61.129   Hematoma of pinna, unspecified ear ▽

     ✓6ᵗʰ **H61.19   Other noninfective disorders of pinna**
       H61.191   Noninfective disorders of pinna, right **ear**
       H61.192   Noninfective disorders of pinna, left **ear**
       H61.193   Noninfective disorders of pinna, bilateral
       H61.199   Noninfective disorders of pinna, unspecified ear ▽

   ✓5ᵗʰ **H61.2   Impacted cerumen**
      Wax in ear
      H61.20   Impacted cerumen, unspecified ear ▽
      H61.21   Impacted cerumen, right **ear**
      H61.22   Impacted cerumen, left **ear**
      H61.23   Impacted cerumen, bilateral

   ✓5ᵗʰ **H61.3   Acquired stenosis of external ear canal**
      Collapse of external ear canal
      EXCLUDES 1   postprocedural stenosis of external ear canal (H95.81-)

     ✓6ᵗʰ **H61.30   Acquired stenosis of external ear canal,** unspecified
       H61.301   Acquired stenosis of right **external ear canal, unspecified** ▽
       H61.302   Acquired stenosis of left **external ear canal, unspecified** ▽
       H61.303   Acquired stenosis of external ear canal, unspecified, bilateral ▽
       H61.309   Acquired stenosis of external ear canal, unspecified, unspecified ear ▽

     ✓6ᵗʰ **H61.31   Acquired stenosis of external ear canal** secondary to trauma
       H61.311   Acquired stenosis of right **external ear canal secondary to trauma**
       H61.312   Acquired stenosis of left **external ear canal secondary to trauma**
       H61.313   Acquired stenosis of external ear canal secondary to trauma, bilateral
       H61.319   Acquired stenosis of external ear canal secondary to trauma, unspecified ear ▽

     ✓6ᵗʰ **H61.32   Acquired stenosis of external ear canal** secondary to inflammation and infection
       H61.321   Acquired stenosis of right **external ear canal secondary to inflammation and infection**
       H61.322   Acquired stenosis of left **external ear canal secondary to inflammation and infection**
       H61.323   Acquired stenosis of external ear canal secondary to inflammation and infection, bilateral
       H61.329   Acquired stenosis of external ear canal secondary to inflammation and infection, unspecified ear ▽

     ✓6ᵗʰ **H61.39   Other acquired stenosis of external ear canal**
       H61.391   Other acquired stenosis of right **external ear canal**
       H61.392   Other acquired stenosis of left **external ear canal**
       H61.393   Other acquired stenosis of external ear canal, bilateral
       H61.399   Other acquired stenosis of external ear canal, unspecified ear ▽

   ✓5ᵗʰ **H61.8   Other specified disorders of external ear**
     ✓6ᵗʰ **H61.81   Exostosis of external canal**
       H61.811   Exostosis of right **external canal**
       H61.812   Exostosis of left **external canal**
       H61.813   Exostosis of external canal, bilateral
       H61.819   Exostosis of external canal, unspecified ear ▽

     ✓6ᵗʰ **H61.89   Other specified disorders of external ear**
       H61.891   Other specified disorders of right **external ear**
       H61.892   Other specified disorders of left **external ear**
       H61.893   Other specified disorders of external ear, bilateral
       H61.899   Other specified disorders of external ear, unspecified ear ▽

   ✓5ᵗʰ **H61.9   Disorder of external ear, unspecified**
      H61.90   Disorder of external ear, unspecified, unspecified ear ▽
      H61.91   Disorder of right **external ear, unspecified** ▽
      H61.92   Disorder of left **external ear, unspecified** ▽
      H61.93   Disorder of external ear, unspecified, bilateral ▽

✓ Add'l Character Required   ✓x7ᵗʰ Placeholder Alert   RUG IV Special Care High Dx   RUG IV Clinically Complex Dx   RUG IV Special Care Low Dx   Manifestation Code   Other Specified Code   ▽ Unspecified Code

ICD-10-CM 2016   577

Chapter 8. Diseases of the Ear and Mastoid Process

✓4ᵗʰ **H62 Disorders of external ear in diseases classified elsewhere**

  ✓5ᵗʰ **H62.4 Otitis externa in other diseases classified elsewhere**

    Code first underlying disease, such as:
      erysipelas (A46)
      impetigo (LØ1.Ø)
    EXCLUDES 1 *otitis externa (in):*
      candidiasis (B37.84)
      herpes viral [herpes simplex] (BØØ.1)
      herpes zoster (BØ2.8)

    H62.4Ø *Otitis externa in other diseases classified elsewhere, unspecified ear*

    H62.41 *Otitis externa in other diseases classified elsewhere, right ear*

    H62.42 *Otitis externa in other diseases classified elsewhere, left ear*

    H62.43 *Otitis externa in other diseases classified elsewhere, bilateral*

  ✓5ᵗʰ **H62.8 Other disorders of external ear in diseases classified elsewhere**

    Code first underlying disease, such as:
      gout (M1A.-, M1Ø.-)

    ✓6ᵗʰ **H62.8X Other disorders of external ear in diseases classified elsewhere**

      H62.8X1 *Other disorders of right external ear in diseases classified elsewhere*

      H62.8X2 *Other disorders of left external ear in diseases classified elsewhere*

      H62.8X3 *Other disorders of external ear in diseases classified elsewhere, bilateral*

      H62.8X9 *Other disorders of external ear in diseases classified elsewhere, unspecified ear* ▽

Diseases of middle ear and mastoid (H65-H75)

✓4ᵗʰ **H65 Nonsuppurative otitis media**

  INCLUDES nonsuppurative otitis media with myringitis
  Use additional code for any associated perforated tympanic membrane (H72.-)
  Use additional code to identify:
    exposure to environmental tobacco smoke (Z77.22)
    exposure to tobacco smoke in the perinatal period (P96.81)
    history of tobacco use (Z87.891)
    occupational exposure to environmental tobacco smoke (Z57.31)
    tobacco dependence (F17.-)
    tobacco use (Z72.Ø)

  ✓5ᵗʰ **H65.Ø Acute serous otitis media**

    Acute and subacute secretory otitis

    H65.ØØ Acute serous otitis media, unspecified ear ▽
    H65.Ø1 Acute serous otitis media, right ear
    H65.Ø2 Acute serous otitis media, left ear
    H65.Ø3 Acute serous otitis media, bilateral
    H65.Ø4 Acute serous otitis media, recurrent, right ear
    H65.Ø5 Acute serous otitis media, recurrent, left ear
    H65.Ø6 Acute serous otitis media, recurrent, bilateral
    H65.Ø7 Acute serous otitis media, recurrent, unspecified ear ▽

  ✓5ᵗʰ **H65.1 Other acute nonsuppurative otitis media**

    EXCLUDES 1 *otitic barotrauma (T7Ø.Ø)*
      otitis media (acute) NOS (H66.9)

    ✓6ᵗʰ **H65.11 Acute and subacute allergic otitis media (mucoid) (sanguinous) (serous)**

      H65.111 Acute and subacute allergic otitis media (mucoid) (sanguinous) (serous), right ear
      H65.112 Acute and subacute allergic otitis media (mucoid) (sanguinous) (serous), left ear
      H65.113 Acute and subacute allergic otitis media (mucoid) (sanguinous) (serous), bilateral
      H65.114 Acute and subacute allergic otitis media (mucoid) (sanguinous) (serous), recurrent, right ear
      H65.115 Acute and subacute allergic otitis media (mucoid) (sanguinous) (serous), recurrent, left ear
      H65.116 Acute and subacute allergic otitis media (mucoid) (sanguinous) (serous), recurrent, bilateral

      H65.117 Acute and subacute allergic otitis media (mucoid) (sanguinous) (serous), recurrent, unspecified ear ▽
      H65.119 Acute and subacute allergic otitis media (mucoid) (sanguinous) (serous), unspecified ear ▽

    ✓6ᵗʰ **H65.19 Other acute nonsuppurative otitis media**
      Acute and subacute mucoid otitis media
      Acute and subacute nonsuppurative otitis media NOS
      Acute and subacute sanguinous otitis media
      Acute and subacute seromucinous otitis media

      H65.191 Other acute nonsuppurative otitis media, right ear
      H65.192 Other acute nonsuppurative otitis media, left ear
      H65.193 Other acute nonsuppurative otitis media, bilateral
      H65.194 Other acute nonsuppurative otitis media, recurrent, right ear
      H65.195 Other acute nonsuppurative otitis media, recurrent, left ear
      H65.196 Other acute nonsuppurative otitis media, recurrent, bilateral
      H65.197 Other acute nonsuppurative otitis media recurrent, unspecified ear ▽
      H65.199 Other acute nonsuppurative otitis media, unspecified ear ▽

  ✓5ᵗʰ **H65.2 Chronic serous otitis media**
    Chronic tubotympanal catarrh

    H65.2Ø Chronic serous otitis media, unspecified ear ▽
    H65.21 Chronic serous otitis media, right ear
    H65.22 Chronic serous otitis media, left ear
    H65.23 Chronic serous otitis media, bilateral

  ✓5ᵗʰ **H65.3 Chronic mucoid otitis media**
    Chronic mucinous otitis media
    Chronic secretory otitis media
    Glue ear
    Chronic transudative otitis media
    EXCLUDES 1 *adhesive middle ear disease (H74.1)*

    H65.3Ø Chronic mucoid otitis media, unspecified ear ▽
    H65.31 Chronic mucoid otitis media, right ear
    H65.32 Chronic mucoid otitis media, left ear
    H65.33 Chronic mucoid otitis media, bilateral

  ✓5ᵗʰ **H65.4 Other chronic nonsuppurative otitis media**

    ✓6ᵗʰ **H65.41 Chronic allergic otitis media**

      H65.411 Chronic allergic otitis media, right ear
      H65.412 Chronic allergic otitis media, left ear
      H65.413 Chronic allergic otitis media, bilateral
      H65.419 Chronic allergic otitis media, unspecified ear ▽

    ✓6ᵗʰ **H65.49 Other chronic nonsuppurative otitis media**
      Chronic exudative otitis media
      Chronic nonsuppurative otitis media NOS
      Chronic otitis media with effusion (nonpurulent)
      Chronic seromucinous otitis media

      H65.491 Other chronic nonsuppurative otitis media, right ear
      H65.492 Other chronic nonsuppurative otitis media, left ear
      H65.493 Other chronic nonsuppurative otitis media, bilateral
      H65.499 Other chronic nonsuppurative otitis media, unspecified ear ▽

  ✓5ᵗʰ **H65.9 Unspecified nonsuppurative otitis media**
    Allergic otitis media NOS   Secretory otitis media NOS
    Catarrhal otitis media NOS   Seromucinous otitis media NOS
    Exudative otitis media NOS   Serous otitis media NOS
    Mucoid otitis media NOS   Transudative otitis media NOS
    Otitis media with effusion (nonpurulent) NOS

    H65.9Ø Unspecified nonsuppurative otitis media, unspecified ear ▽
    H65.91 Unspecified nonsuppurative otitis media, right ear ▽
    H65.92 Unspecified nonsuppurative otitis media, left ear ▽
    H65.93 Unspecified nonsuppurative otitis media, bilateral ▽

Ⓝ Newborn   Ⓟ Pediatric   Ⓜ Maternity   Ⓐ Adult   **RIC** RIC Dx   **NC Dx** Noncancer Dx   **PDx** Primary Dx   **CC** RIC CC Condition   ▶◀ Revised Text   ● New Code   ▲ Revised Code Title

578   ICD-10-CM 2016

✓4ᵗʰ **H66　Suppurative and unspecified otitis media**
　　INCLUDES　suppurative and unspecified otitis media with myringitis
　　Use additional code to identify:
　　　exposure to environmental tobacco smoke (Z77.22)
　　　exposure to tobacco smoke in the perinatal period (P96.81)
　　　history of tobacco use (Z87.891)
　　　occupational exposure to environmental tobacco smoke (Z57.31)
　　　tobacco dependence (F17.-)
　　　tobacco use (Z72.0)

✓5ᵗʰ **H66.0　Acute suppurative otitis media**
　　✓6ᵗʰ **H66.00　Acute suppurative otitis media without spontaneous rupture of ear drum**
　　　　H66.001　Acute suppurative otitis media without spontaneous rupture of ear drum, right ear
　　　　H66.002　Acute suppurative otitis media without spontaneous rupture of ear drum, left ear
　　　　H66.003　Acute suppurative otitis media without spontaneous rupture of ear drum, bilateral
　　　　H66.004　Acute suppurative otitis media without spontaneous rupture of ear drum, recurrent, right ear
　　　　H66.005　Acute suppurative otitis media without spontaneous rupture of ear drum, recurrent, left ear
　　　　H66.006　Acute suppurative otitis media without spontaneous rupture of ear drum, recurrent, bilateral
　　　　H66.007　Acute suppurative otitis media without ▽ spontaneous rupture of ear drum, recurrent, unspecified ear
　　　　H66.009　Acute suppurative otitis media without ▽ spontaneous rupture of ear drum, unspecified ear
　　✓6ᵗʰ **H66.01　Acute suppurative otitis media with spontaneous rupture of ear drum**
　　　　H66.011　Acute suppurative otitis media with spontaneous rupture of ear drum, right ear
　　　　H66.012　Acute suppurative otitis media with spontaneous rupture of ear drum, left ear
　　　　H66.013　Acute suppurative otitis media with spontaneous rupture of ear drum, bilateral
　　　　H66.014　Acute suppurative otitis media with spontaneous rupture of ear drum, recurrent, right ear
　　　　H66.015　Acute suppurative otitis media with spontaneous rupture of ear drum, recurrent, left ear
　　　　H66.016　Acute suppurative otitis media with spontaneous rupture of ear drum, recurrent, bilateral
　　　　H66.017　Acute suppurative otitis media with ▽ spontaneous rupture of ear drum, recurrent, unspecified ear
　　　　H66.019　Acute suppurative otitis media with ▽ spontaneous rupture of ear drum, unspecified ear

✓5ᵗʰ **H66.1　Chronic tubotympanic suppurative otitis media**
　　　Benign chronic suppurative otitis media
　　　Chronic tubotympanic disease
　　　Use additional code for any associated perforated tympanic membrane (H72.-)
　　　H66.10　Chronic tubotympanic suppurative otitis media, ▽ unspecified
　　　H66.11　Chronic tubotympanic suppurative otitis media, right ear
　　　H66.12　Chronic tubotympanic suppurative otitis media, left ear
　　　H66.13　Chronic tubotympanic suppurative otitis media, bilateral

✓5ᵗʰ **H66.2　Chronic atticoantral suppurative otitis media**
　　　Chronic atticoantral disease
　　　Use additional code for any associated perforated tympanic membrane (H72.-)
　　　H66.20　Chronic atticoantral suppurative otitis media, ▽ unspecified ear

H66.21　Chronic atticoantral suppurative otitis media, right ear
H66.22　Chronic atticoantral suppurative otitis media, left ear
H66.23　Chronic atticoantral suppurative otitis media, bilateral

✓5ᵗʰ **H66.3　Other chronic suppurative otitis media**
　　　Chronic suppurative otitis media NOS
　　　Use additional code for any associated perforated tympanic membrane (H72.-)
　　　EXCLUDES 1　tuberculous otitis media (A18.6)
　　✓6ᵗʰ **H66.3X　Other chronic suppurative otitis media**
　　　　H66.3X1　Other chronic suppurative otitis media, right ear
　　　　H66.3X2　Other chronic suppurative otitis media, left ear
　　　　H66.3X3　Other chronic suppurative otitis media, bilateral
　　　　H66.3X9　Other chronic suppurative otitis media, ▽ unspecified ear

✓5ᵗʰ **H66.4　Suppurative otitis media, unspecified**
　　　Purulent otitis media NOS
　　　Use additional code for any associated perforated tympanic membrane (H72.-)
　　　H66.40　Suppurative otitis media, unspecified, ▽ unspecified ear
　　　H66.41　Suppurative otitis media, unspecified, right ear
　　　H66.42　Suppurative otitis media, unspecified, left ear
　　　H66.43　Suppurative otitis media, unspecified, bilateral

✓5ᵗʰ **H66.9　Otitis media, unspecified**
　　　Otitis media NOS
　　　Acute otitis media NOS
　　　Chronic otitis media NOS
　　　Use additional code for any associated perforated tympanic membrane (H72.-)
　　　H66.90　Otitis media, unspecified, unspecified ear ▽
　　　H66.91　Otitis media, unspecified, right ear ▽
　　　H66.92　Otitis media, unspecified, left ear ▽
　　　H66.93　Otitis media, unspecified, bilateral ▽

✓4ᵗʰ **H67　Otitis media in diseases classified elsewhere**
　　　Code first underlying disease, such as:
　　　　viral disease NEC (B00-B34)
　　　Use additional code for any associated perforated tympanic membrane (H72.-)
　　　EXCLUDES 1　otitis media in:
　　　　　influenza (J09.X9, J10.83, J11.83)
　　　　　measles (B05.3)
　　　　　scarlet fever (A38.0)
　　　　　tuberculosis (A18.6)
　　　H67.1　Otitis media in diseases classified elsewhere, right ear
　　　H67.2　Otitis media in diseases classified elsewhere, left ear
　　　H67.3　Otitis media in diseases classified elsewhere, bilateral
　　　H67.9　Otitis media in diseases classified elsewhere, unspecified ear ▽

✓4ᵗʰ **H68　Eustachian salpingitis and obstruction**
　　✓5ᵗʰ **H68.0　Eustachian salpingitis**
　　　✓6ᵗʰ **H68.00　Unspecified Eustachian salpingitis**
　　　　H68.001　Unspecified Eustachian salpingitis, ▽ right ear
　　　　H68.002　Unspecified Eustachian salpingitis, ▽ left ear
　　　　H68.003　Unspecified Eustachian salpingitis, ▽ bilateral
　　　　H68.009　Unspecified Eustachian salpingitis, ▽ unspecified ear
　　　✓6ᵗʰ **H68.01　Acute Eustachian salpingitis**
　　　　H68.011　Acute Eustachian salpingitis, right ear
　　　　H68.012　Acute Eustachian salpingitis, left ear
　　　　H68.013　Acute Eustachian salpingitis, bilateral
　　　　H68.019　Acute Eustachian salpingitis, ▽ unspecified ear
　　　✓6ᵗʰ **H68.02　Chronic Eustachian salpingitis**
　　　　H68.021　Chronic Eustachian salpingitis, right ear
　　　　H68.022　Chronic Eustachian salpingitis, left ear
　　　　H68.023　Chronic Eustachian salpingitis, bilateral

H68.029　Chronic Eustachian salpingitis, unspecified ear　▽

✓5th **H68.1**　Obstruction **of Eustachian tube**
　　Stenosis of Eustachian tube　　Stricture of Eustachian tube

✓6th **H68.10**　Unspecified **obstruction of Eustachian tube**

H68.101　Unspecified obstruction of Eustachian tube, right ear　▽

H68.102　Unspecified obstruction of Eustachian tube, left ear　▽

H68.103　Unspecified obstruction of Eustachian tube, bilateral　▽

H68.109　Unspecified obstruction of Eustachian tube, unspecified ear　▽

✓6th **H68.11**　Osseous **obstruction of Eustachian tube**

H68.111　Osseous obstruction of Eustachian tube, right ear

H68.112　Osseous obstruction of Eustachian tube, left ear

H68.113　Osseous obstruction of Eustachian tube, bilateral

H68.119　Osseous obstruction of Eustachian tube, unspecified ear　▽

✓6th **H68.12**　Intrinsic cartilagenous **obstruction of Eustachian tube**

H68.121　Intrinsic cartilagenous obstruction of Eustachian tube, right ear

H68.122　Intrinsic cartilagenous obstruction of Eustachian tube, left ear

H68.123　Intrinsic cartilagenous obstruction of Eustachian tube, bilateral

H68.129　Intrinsic cartilagenous obstruction of Eustachian tube, unspecified ear　▽

✓6th **H68.13**　Extrinsic cartilagenous **obstruction of Eustachian tube**
　　Compression of Eustachian tube

H68.131　Extrinsic cartilagenous obstruction of Eustachian tube, right ear

H68.132　Extrinsic cartilagenous obstruction of Eustachian tube, left ear

H68.133　Extrinsic cartilagenous obstruction of Eustachian tube, bilateral

H68.139　Extrinsic cartilagenous obstruction of Eustachian tube, unspecified ear　▽

✓4th **H69**　**Other and unspecified disorders of Eustachian tube**

✓5th **H69.0**　Patulous **Eustachian tube**

H69.00　Patulous Eustachian tube, unspecified ear　▽

H69.01　Patulous Eustachian tube, right ear

H69.02　Patulous Eustachian tube, left ear

H69.03　Patulous Eustachian tube, bilateral

✓5th **H69.8**　Other specified **disorders of Eustachian tube**

H69.80　Other specified disorders of Eustachian tube, unspecified ear　▽

H69.81　Other specified disorders of Eustachian tube, right ear

H69.82　Other specified disorders of Eustachian tube, left ear

H69.83　Other specified disorders of Eustachian tube, bilateral

✓5th **H69.9**　Unspecified **Eustachian tube disorder**

H69.90　Unspecified Eustachian tube disorder, unspecified ear　▽

H69.91　Unspecified Eustachian tube disorder, right ear　▽

H69.92　Unspecified Eustachian tube disorder, left ear　▽

H69.93　Unspecified Eustachian tube disorder, bilateral　▽

✓4th **H70**　**Mastoiditis and related conditions**

✓5th **H70.0**　Acute **mastoiditis**
　　Abscess of mastoid
　　Empyema of mastoid

✓6th **H70.00**　Acute mastoiditis **without complications**

H70.001　Acute mastoiditis without complications, right ear

H70.002　Acute mastoiditis without complications, left ear

H70.003　Acute mastoiditis without complications, bilateral

H70.009　Acute mastoiditis without complications, unspecified ear　▽

✓6th **H70.01**　Subperiosteal abscess **of mastoid**

H70.011　Subperiosteal abscess of mastoid, right ear

H70.012　Subperiosteal abscess of mastoid, left ear

H70.013　Subperiosteal abscess of mastoid, bilateral

H70.019　Subperiosteal abscess of mastoid, unspecified ear　▽

✓6th **H70.09**　Acute mastoiditis with other complications

H70.091　Acute mastoiditis with other complications, right ear

H70.092　Acute mastoiditis with other complications, left ear

H70.093　Acute mastoiditis with other complications, bilateral

H70.099　Acute mastoiditis with other complications, unspecified ear　▽

✓5th **H70.1**　Chronic **mastoiditis**
　　Caries of mastoid
　　Fistula of mastoid
　　EXCLUDES 1　tuberculous mastoiditis (A18.03)

H70.10　Chronic mastoiditis, unspecified ear　▽

H70.11　Chronic mastoiditis, right ear

H70.12　Chronic mastoiditis, left ear

H70.13　Chronic mastoiditis, bilateral

✓5th **H70.2**　Petrositis
　　Inflammation of petrous bone

✓6th **H70.20**　Unspecified petrositisH70.201

H70.201　Unspecified petrositis, right ear　▽

H70.202　Unspecified petrositis, left ear　▽

H70.203　Unspecified petrositis, bilateral　▽

H70.209　Unspecified petrositis, unspecified ear　▽

✓6th **H70.21**　Acute petrositis

H70.211　Acute petrositis, right ear

H70.212　Acute petrositis, left ear

H70.213　Acute petrositis, bilateral

H70.219　Acute petrositis, unspecified ear　▽

✓6th **H70.22**　Chronic petrositis

H70.221　Chronic petrositis, right ear

H70.222　Chronic petrositis, left ear

H70.223　Chronic petrositis, bilateral

H70.229　Chronic petrositis, unspecified ear　▽

✓5th **H70.8**　**Other mastoiditis and related conditions**
　　EXCLUDES 1　preauricular sinus and cyst (Q18.1)
　　　　sinus, fistula, and cyst of branchial cleft (Q18.0)

✓6th **H70.81**　Postauricular fistula

H70.811　Postauricular fistula, right ear

H70.812　Postauricular fistula, left ear

H70.813　Postauricular fistula, bilateral

H70.819　Postauricular fistula, unspecified ear　▽

✓6th **H70.89**　Other **mastoiditis and related conditions**

H70.891　Other mastoiditis and related conditions, right ear

H70.892　Other mastoiditis and related conditions, left ear

H70.893　Other mastoiditis and related conditions, bilateral

H70.899　Other mastoiditis and related conditions, unspecified ear　▽

✓5th **H70.9**　Unspecified **mastoiditis**

H70.90　Unspecified mastoiditis, unspecified ear　▽

H70.91　Unspecified mastoiditis, right ear　▽

H70.92　Unspecified mastoiditis, left ear　▽

H70.93　Unspecified mastoiditis, bilateral　▽

✓4th **H71**　**Cholesteatoma of middle ear**
　　EXCLUDES 2　cholesteatoma of external ear (H60.4-)
　　　　recurrent cholesteatoma of postmastoidectomy cavity (H95.0-)

✓5th **H71.0**　Cholesteatoma of attic

H71.00　Cholesteatoma of attic, unspecified ear　▽

H71.01　Cholesteatoma of attic, right ear

H71.02　Cholesteatoma of attic, left ear

Ⓝ Newborn　Ⓟ Pediatric　Ⓜ Maternity　Ⓐ Adult　**RIC** RIC Dx　**NCDx** Noncancer Dx　**PDx** Primary Dx　**CC** RIC CC Condition　►◄ Revised Text　● New Code　▲ Revised Code Title

580　　　　ICD-10-CM 2016

H71.03   **Cholesteatoma of attic,** bilateral

☑5ᵗʰ H71.1 **Cholesteatoma of** tympanum
H71.10   **Cholesteatoma of tympanum, unspecified ear**
H71.11   **Cholesteatoma of tympanum,** right **ear**
H71.12   **Cholesteatoma of tympanum,** left **ear**
H71.13   **Cholesteatoma of tympanum,** bilateral

☑5ᵗʰ H71.2 **Cholesteatoma of** mastoid
H71.20   **Cholesteatoma of mastoid, unspecified ear** ▽
H71.21   **Cholesteatoma of mastoid,** right **ear**
H71.22   **Cholesteatoma of mastoid,** left **ear**
H71.23   **Cholesteatoma of mastoid,** bilateral

☑5ᵗʰ H71.3 **Diffuse cholesteatosis**
H71.30   **Diffuse cholesteatosis, unspecified ear** ▽
H71.31   **Diffuse cholesteatosis,** right **ear**
H71.32   **Diffuse cholesteatosis,** left **ear**
H71.33   **Diffuse cholesteatosis,** bilateral

☑5ᵗʰ H71.9 **Unspecified cholesteatoma**
H71.90   **Unspecified cholesteatoma, unspecified ear** ▽
H71.91   **Unspecified cholesteatoma,** right **ear** ▽
H71.92   **Unspecified cholesteatoma,** left **ear** ▽
H71.93   **Unspecified cholesteatoma,** bilateral ▽

☑4ᵗʰ **H72 Perforation of tympanic membrane**
INCLUDES   persistent post-traumatic perforation of ear drum
postinflammatory perforation of ear drum
Code first any associated otitis media (H65.-, H66.1-, H66.2-, H66.3-, H66.4-, H66.9-, H67.-)
EXCLUDES 1   *acute suppurative otitis media with rupture of the tympanic membrane (H66.01-)*
traumatic rupture of ear drum (S09.2-)

☑5ᵗʰ H72.0 **Central perforation of tympanic membrane**
H72.00   **Central perforation of tympanic membrane, unspecified ear** ▽
H72.01   **Central perforation of tympanic membrane,** right **ear**
H72.02   **Central perforation of tympanic membrane,** left **ear**
H72.03   **Central perforation of tympanic membrane,** bilateral

☑5ᵗʰ H72.1 **Attic perforation of tympanic membrane**
Perforation of pars flaccida
H72.10   **Attic perforation of tympanic membrane, unspecified ear** ▽
H72.11   **Attic perforation of tympanic membrane,** right **ear**
H72.12   **Attic perforation of tympanic membrane,** left **ear**
H72.13   **Attic perforation of tympanic membrane,** bilateral

☑5ᵗʰ H72.2 **Other marginal perforations of tympanic membrane**
☑6ᵗʰ H72.2X   **Other marginal perforations of tympanic membrane**
H72.2X1   **Other marginal perforations of tympanic membrane,** right **ear**
H72.2X2   **Other marginal perforations of tympanic membrane,** left **ear**
H72.2X3   **Other marginal perforations of tympanic membrane,** bilateral
H72.2X9   **Other marginal perforations of tympanic membrane, unspecified ear** ▽

☑5ᵗʰ H72.8 **Other perforations of tympanic membrane**
☑6ᵗʰ H72.81   **Multiple perforations of tympanic membrane**
H72.811   **Multiple perforations of tympanic membrane,** right **ear**
H72.812   **Multiple perforations of tympanic membrane,** left **ear**
H72.813   **Multiple perforations of tympanic membrane,** bilateral
H72.819   **Multiple perforations of tympanic membrane, unspecified ear** ▽
☑6ᵗʰ H72.82   **Total perforations of tympanic membrane**
H72.821   **Total perforations of tympanic membrane,** right **ear**
H72.822   **Total perforations of tympanic membrane,** left **ear**
H72.823   **Total perforations of tympanic membrane,** bilateral
H72.829   **Total perforations of tympanic membrane, unspecified ear** ▽

☑5ᵗʰ H72.9 **Unspecified perforation of tympanic membrane**
H72.90   **Unspecified perforation of tympanic membrane, unspecified ear** ▽
H72.91   **Unspecified perforation of tympanic membrane,** right **ear** ▽
H72.92   **Unspecified perforation of tympanic membrane,** left **ear** ▽
H72.93   **Unspecified perforation of tympanic membrane,** bilateral ▽

☑4ᵗʰ **H73 Other disorders of tympanic membrane**
☑5ᵗʰ H73.0 **Acute myringitis**
EXCLUDES 1   *acute myringitis with otitis media (H65, H66)*
☑6ᵗʰ H73.00   **Unspecified acute myringitis**
Acute tympanitis NOS
H73.001   **Acute myringitis,** right **ear**
H73.002   **Acute myringitis,** left **ear**
H73.003   **Acute myringitis,** bilateral
H73.009   **Acute myringitis, unspecified ear** ▽
☑6ᵗʰ H73.01   **Bullous myringitis**
H73.011   **Bullous myringitis,** right **ear**
H73.012   **Bullous myringitis,** left **ear**
H73.013   **Bullous myringitis,** bilateral
H73.019   **Bullous myringitis, unspecified ear** ▽
☑6ᵗʰ H73.09   **Other acute myringitis**
H73.091   **Other acute myringitis,** right **ear**
H73.092   **Other acute myringitis,** left **ear**
H73.093   **Other acute myringitis,** bilateral
H73.099   **Other acute myringitis, unspecified ear** ▽

☑5ᵗʰ H73.1 **Chronic myringitis**
Chronic tympanitis
EXCLUDES 1   *chronic myringitis with otitis media (H65, H66)*
H73.10   **Chronic myringitis, unspecified ear** ▽
H73.11   **Chronic myringitis,** right **ear**
H73.12   **Chronic myringitis,** left **ear**
H73.13   **Chronic myringitis,** bilateral

☑5ᵗʰ H73.2 **Unspecified myringitis**
H73.20   **Unspecified myringitis, unspecified ear** ▽
H73.21   **Unspecified myringitis,** right **ear** ▽
H73.22   **Unspecified myringitis,** left **ear** ▽
H73.23   **Unspecified myringitis,** bilateral ▽

☑5ᵗʰ H73.8 **Other specified disorders of tympanic membrane**
☑6ᵗʰ H73.81   **Atrophic flaccid tympanic membrane**
H73.811   **Atrophic flaccid tympanic membrane,** right **ear**
H73.812   **Atrophic flaccid tympanic membrane,** left **ear**
H73.813   **Atrophic flaccid tympanic membrane,** bilateral
H73.819   **Atrophic flaccid tympanic membrane, unspecified ear** ▽
☑6ᵗʰ H73.82   **Atrophic nonflaccid tympanic membrane**
H73.821   **Atrophic nonflaccid tympanic membrane,** right **ear**
H73.822   **Atrophic nonflaccid tympanic membrane,** left **ear**
H73.823   **Atrophic nonflaccid tympanic membrane,** bilateral
H73.829   **Atrophic nonflaccid tympanic membrane, unspecified ear** ▽
☑6ᵗʰ H73.89   **Other specified disorders of tympanic membrane**
H73.891   **Other specified disorders of tympanic membrane,** right **ear**
H73.892   **Other specified disorders of tympanic membrane,** left **ear**
H73.893   **Other specified disorders of tympanic membrane,** bilateral
H73.899   **Other specified disorders of tympanic membrane, unspecified ear** ▽

☑5ᵗʰ H73.9 **Unspecified disorder of tympanic membrane**
H73.90   **Unspecified disorder of tympanic membrane, unspecified ear** ▽
H73.91   **Unspecified disorder of tympanic membrane,** right **ear** ▽

☑ Add'l Character Required ☑x7ᵗʰ Placeholder Alert RUG IV Special Care High Dx RUG IV Clinically Complex Dx RUG IV Special Care Low Dx Manifestation Code Other Specified Code ▽Unspecified Code

Chapter 8. Diseases of the Ear and Mastoid Process

H73.92   Unspecified disorder of tympanic membrane, left ear   ▽

H73.93   Unspecified disorder of tympanic membrane, bilateral   ▽

✓4ᵗʰ **H74**   **Other disorders of middle ear mastoid**
    EXCLUDES 2   mastoiditis (H70.-)

✓5ᵗʰ **H74.0**   **Tympanosclerosis**

    H74.01   **Tympanosclerosis, right ear**

    H74.02   **Tympanosclerosis, left ear**

    H74.03   **Tympanosclerosis, bilateral**

    H74.09   **Tympanosclerosis, unspecified ear**   ▽

✓5ᵗʰ **H74.1**   **Adhesive middle ear disease**
    Adhesive otitis
      EXCLUDES 1   glue ear (H65.3-)

    H74.11   **Adhesive right middle ear disease**

    H74.12   **Adhesive left middle ear disease**

    H74.13   **Adhesive middle ear disease, bilateral**

    H74.19   **Adhesive middle ear disease, unspecified ear**   ▽

✓5ᵗʰ **H74.2**   **Discontinuity and dislocation of ear ossicles**

    H74.20   **Discontinuity and dislocation of ear ossicles, unspecified ear**   ▽

    H74.21   **Discontinuity and dislocation of right ear ossicles**

    H74.22   **Discontinuity and dislocation of left ear ossicles**

    H74.23   **Discontinuity and dislocation of ear ossicles, bilateral**

✓5ᵗʰ **H74.3**   **Other acquired abnormalities of ear ossicles**

    ✓6ᵗʰ **H74.31**   **Ankylosis of ear ossicles**

      H74.311   **Ankylosis of ear ossicles, right ear**

      H74.312   **Ankylosis of ear ossicles, left ear**

      H74.313   **Ankylosis of ear ossicles, bilateral**

      H74.319   **Ankylosis of ear ossicles, unspecified ear**   ▽

    ✓6ᵗʰ **H74.32**   **Partial loss of ear ossicles**

      H74.321   **Partial loss of ear ossicles, right ear**

      H74.322   **Partial loss of ear ossicles, left ear**

      H74.323   **Partial loss of ear ossicles, bilateral**

      H74.329   **Partial loss of ear ossicles, unspecified ear**   ▽

    ✓6ᵗʰ **H74.39**   **Other acquired abnormalities of ear ossicles**

      H74.391   **Other acquired abnormalities of right ear ossicles**

      H74.392   **Other acquired abnormalities of left ear ossicles**

      H74.393   **Other acquired abnormalities of ear ossicles, bilateral**

      H74.399   **Other acquired abnormalities of ear ossicles, unspecified ear**   ▽

✓5ᵗʰ **H74.4**   **Polyp of middle ear**

    H74.40   **Polyp of middle ear, unspecified ear**   ▽

    H74.41   **Polyp of right middle ear**

    H74.42   **Polyp of left middle ear**

    H74.43   **Polyp of middle ear, bilateral**

✓5ᵗʰ **H74.8**   **Other specified disorders of middle ear and mastoid**

    ✓6ᵗʰ **H74.8X**   **Other specified disorders of middle ear and mastoid**

      H74.8X1   **Other specified disorders of right middle ear and mastoid**

      H74.8X2   **Other specified disorders of left middle ear and mastoid**

      H74.8X3   **Other specified disorders of middle ear and mastoid, bilateral**

      H74.8X9   **Other specified disorders of middle ear and mastoid, unspecified ear**   ▽

✓5ᵗʰ **H74.9**   **Unspecified disorder of middle ear and mastoid**

    H74.90   **Unspecified disorder of middle ear and mastoid, unspecified ear**   ▽

    H74.91   **Unspecified disorder of right middle ear and mastoid**   ▽

    H74.92   **Unspecified disorder of left middle ear and mastoid**   ▽

    H74.93   **Unspecified disorder of middle ear and mastoid, bilateral**   ▽

✓4ᵗʰ **H75**   **Other disorders of middle ear and mastoid in diseases classified elsewhere**
    Code first underlying disease

✓5ᵗʰ **H75.0**   **Mastoiditis in infectious and parasitic diseases classified elsewhere**
      EXCLUDES 1   mastoiditis (in):
        syphilis (A52.77)
        tuberculosis (A18.03)

    H75.00   *Mastoiditis in infectious and parasitic diseases classified elsewhere, unspecified ear*   ▽

    H75.01   *Mastoiditis in infectious and parasitic diseases classified elsewhere, right ear*

    H75.02   *Mastoiditis in infectious and parasitic diseases classified elsewhere, left ear*

    H75.03   *Mastoiditis in infectious and parasitic diseases classified elsewhere, bilateral*

✓5ᵗʰ **H75.8**   **Other specified disorders of middle ear and mastoid in diseases classified elsewhere**

    H75.80   *Other specified disorders of middle ear and mastoid in diseases classified elsewhere, unspecified ear*   ▽

    H75.81   *Other specified disorders of right middle ear and mastoid in diseases classified elsewhere*

    H75.82   *Other specified disorders of left middle ear and mastoid in diseases classified elsewhere*

    H75.83   *Other specified disorders of middle ear and mastoid in diseases classified elsewhere, bilateral*

Diseases of inner ear (H80-H83)

✓4ᵗʰ **H80**   **Otosclerosis**
    INCLUDES   Otospongiosis

✓5ᵗʰ **H80.0**   **Otosclerosis involving oval window, nonobliterative**

    H80.00   **Otosclerosis involving oval window, nonobliterative, unspecified ear**   ▽

    H80.01   **Otosclerosis involving oval window, nonobliterative, right ear**

    H80.02   **Otosclerosis involving oval window, nonobliterative, left ear**

    H80.03   **Otosclerosis involving oval window, nonobliterative, bilateral**

✓5ᵗʰ **H80.1**   **Otosclerosis involving oval window, obliterative**

    H80.10   **Otosclerosis involving oval window, obliterative, unspecified ear**   ▽

    H80.11   **Otosclerosis involving oval window, obliterative, right ear**

    H80.12   **Otosclerosis involving oval window, obliterative, left ear**

    H80.13   **Otosclerosis involving oval window, obliterative, bilateral**

✓5ᵗʰ **H80.2**   **Cochlear otosclerosis**
    Otosclerosis involving otic capsule
    Otosclerosis involving round window

    H80.20   **Cochlear otosclerosis, unspecified ear**   ▽

    H80.21   **Cochlear otosclerosis, right ear**

    H80.22   **Cochlear otosclerosis, left ear**

    H80.23   **Cochlear otosclerosis, bilateral**

✓5ᵗʰ **H80.8**   **Other otosclerosis**

    H80.80   **Other otosclerosis, unspecified ear**   ▽

    H80.81   **Other otosclerosis, right ear**

    H80.82   **Other otosclerosis, left ear**

    H80.83   **Other otosclerosis, bilateral**

✓5ᵗʰ **H80.9**   **Unspecified otosclerosis**

    H80.90   **Unspecified otosclerosis, unspecified ear**   ▽

    H80.91   **Unspecified otosclerosis, right ear**   ▽

    H80.92   **Unspecified otosclerosis, left ear**   ▽

    H80.93   **Unspecified otosclerosis, bilateral**   ▽

✓4ᵗʰ **H81**   **Disorders of vestibular function**
    EXCLUDES 1   epidemic vertigo (A88.1)
       vertigo NOS (R42)

✓5ᵗʰ **H81.0**   **Ménière's disease**
    Labyrinthine hydrops
    Ménière's syndrome or vertigo

    H81.01   **Ménière's disease, right ear**

    H81.02   **Ménière's disease, left ear**

N Newborn   P Pediatric   M Maternity   A Adult   RIC RIC Dx   NC Dx Noncancer Dx   PDx Primary Dx   CC RIC CC Condition   ▶◀ Revised Text   ● New Code   ▲ Revised Code Title

582

ICD-10-CM 2016

         H81.03   Ménière's disease, bilateral
         H81.09   Ménière's disease, unspecified ear ▽

✓5th H81.1   Benign paroxysmal vertigo
         H81.10   Benign paroxysmal vertigo, unspecified ear ▽
         H81.11   Benign paroxysmal vertigo, right ear
         H81.12   Benign paroxysmal vertigo, left ear
         H81.13   Benign paroxysmal vertigo, bilateral

✓5th H81.2   Vestibular neuronitis
         H81.20   Vestibular neuronitis, unspecified ear ▽
         H81.21   Vestibular neuronitis, right ear
         H81.22   Vestibular neuronitis, left ear
         H81.23   Vestibular neuronitis, bilateral

✓5th H81.3   Other peripheral vertigo
    ✓6th H81.31   Aural vertigo
             H81.311   Aural vertigo, right ear
             H81.312   Aural vertigo, left ear
             H81.313   Aural vertigo, bilateral
             H81.319   Aural vertigo, unspecified ear ▽
    ✓6th H81.39   Other peripheral vertigo
             Lermoyez' syndrome
             Otogenic vertigo
             Peripheral vertigo NOS
             H81.391   Other peripheral vertigo, right ear
             H81.392   Other peripheral vertigo, left ear
             H81.393   Other peripheral vertigo, bilateral
             H81.399   Other peripheral vertigo, unspecified ear ▽

✓5th H81.4   Vertigo of central origin
         Central positional nystagmus
         H81.41   Vertigo of central origin, right ear
         H81.42   Vertigo of central origin, left ear
         H81.43   Vertigo of central origin, bilateral
         H81.49   Vertigo of central origin, unspecified ear ▽

✓5th H81.8   Other disorders of vestibular function
    ✓6th H81.8X   Other disorders of vestibular function
             H81.8X1   Other disorders of vestibular function, right ear
             H81.8X2   Other disorders of vestibular function, left ear
             H81.8X3   Other disorders of vestibular function, bilateral
             H81.8X9   Other disorders of vestibular function, unspecified ear ▽

✓5th H81.9   Unspecified disorder of vestibular function
         Vertiginous syndrome NOS
         H81.90   Unspecified disorder of vestibular function, unspecified ear ▽
         H81.91   Unspecified disorder of vestibular function, right ear ▽
         H81.92   Unspecified disorder of vestibular function, left ear ▽
         H81.93   Unspecified disorder of vestibular function, bilateral ▽

✓4th H82   Vertiginous syndromes in diseases classified elsewhere
         Code first underlying disease
         EXCLUDES 1   epidemic vertigo (A88.1)
         H82.1   *Vertiginous syndromes in diseases classified elsewhere, right ear*
         H82.2   *Vertiginous syndromes in diseases classified elsewhere, left ear*
         H82.3   *Vertiginous syndromes in diseases classified elsewhere, bilateral*
         H82.9   *Vertiginous syndromes in diseases classified elsewhere, unspecified ear* ▽

✓4th H83   Other diseases of inner ear
    ✓5th H83.0   Labyrinthitis
         H83.01   Labyrinthitis, right ear
         H83.02   Labyrinthitis, left ear
         H83.03   Labyrinthitis, bilateral
         H83.09   Labyrinthitis, unspecified ear ▽
    ✓5th H83.1   Labyrinthine fistula
         H83.11   Labyrinthine fistula, right ear

         H83.12   Labyrinthine fistula, left ear
         H83.13   Labyrinthine fistula, bilateral
         H83.19   Labyrinthine fistula, unspecified ear ▽

✓5th H83.2   Labyrinthine dysfunction
         Labyrinthine hypersensitivity
         Labyrinthine hypofunction
         Labyrinthine loss of function
    ✓6th H83.2X   Labyrinthine dysfunction
             H83.2X1   Labyrinthine dysfunction, right ear
             H83.2X2   Labyrinthine dysfunction, left ear
             H83.2X3   Labyrinthine dysfunction, bilateral
             H83.2X9   Labyrinthine dysfunction, unspecified ear ▽

✓5th H83.3   Noise effects on inner ear
         Acoustic trauma of inner ear
         Noise-induced hearing loss of inner ear
    ✓6th H83.3X   Noise effects on inner ear
             H83.3X1   Noise effects on right inner ear
             H83.3X2   Noise effects on left inner ear
             H83.3X3   Noise effects on inner ear, bilateral
             H83.3X9   Noise effects on inner ear, unspecified ear ▽

✓5th H83.8   Other specified diseases of inner ear
    ✓6th H83.8X   Other specified diseases of inner ear
             H83.8X1   Other specified diseases of right inner ear
             H83.8X2   Other specified diseases of left inner ear
             H83.8X3   Other specified diseases of inner ear, bilateral
             H83.8X9   Other specified diseases of inner ear, unspecified ear ▽

✓5th H83.9   Unspecified disease of inner ear
         H83.90   Unspecified disease of inner ear, unspecified ear ▽
         H83.91   Unspecified disease of right inner ear ▽
         H83.92   Unspecified disease of left inner ear ▽
         H83.93   Unspecified disease of inner ear, bilateral ▽

Other disorders of ear (H90-H94)

✓4th H90   Conductive and sensorineural hearing loss
         EXCLUDES 1   *deaf nonspeaking NEC (H91.3)*
                 deafness NOS (H91.9-)
                 hearing loss NOS (H91.9-)
                 noise-induced hearing loss (H83.3-)
                 ototoxic hearing loss (H91.0-)
                 sudden (idiopathic) hearing loss (H91.2-)

         H90.0   Conductive hearing loss, bilateral

    ✓5th H90.1   Conductive hearing loss, unilateral with unrestricted hearing on the contralateral side
         H90.11   Conductive hearing loss, unilateral, right ear, with unrestricted hearing on the contralateral side
         H90.12   Conductive hearing loss, unilateral, left ear, with unrestricted hearing on the contralateral side

         H90.2   Conductive hearing loss, unspecified ▽
         Conductive deafness NOS

         H90.3   Sensorineural hearing loss, bilateral

    ✓5th H90.4   Sensorineural hearing loss, unilateral with unrestricted hearing on the contralateral side
         H90.41   Sensorineural hearing loss, unilateral, right ear, with unrestricted hearing on the contralateral side
         H90.42   Sensorineural hearing loss, unilateral, left ear, with unrestricted hearing on the contralateral side

         H90.5   Unspecified sensorineural hearing loss ▽
         Central hearing loss NOS
         Congenital deafness NOS
         Neural hearing loss NOS
         Perceptive hearing loss NOS
         Sensorineural deafness NOS
         Sensory hearing loss NOS
         EXCLUDES 1   *abnormal auditory perception (H93.2-)*
                 psychogenic deafness (F44.6)

         H90.6   Mixed conductive and sensorineural hearing loss, bilateral

    ✓5th H90.7   Mixed conductive and sensorineural hearing loss, unilateral with unrestricted hearing on the contralateral side
         H90.71   Mixed conductive and sensorineural hearing loss, unilateral, right ear, with unrestricted hearing on the contralateral side

Chapter 8. Diseases of the Ear and Mastoid Process

H90.72–H93.8X9

H90.72   Mixed conductive and sensorineural hearing loss, unilateral, left ear, with unrestricted hearing on the contralateral side

H90.8   Mixed conductive and sensorineural hearing loss, unspecified   ▽

☑4ᵗʰ **H91**   **Other and unspecified hearing loss**
> EXCLUDES 1   *abnormal auditory perception (H93.2-)*
> *hearing loss as classified in H90-*
> *impacted cerumen (H61.2-)*
> *noise-induced hearing loss (H83.3-)*
> *psychogenic deafness (F44.6)*
> *transient ischemic deafness (H93.01-)*

☑5ᵗʰ **H91.0**   **Ototoxic hearing loss**
> Code first poisoning due to drug or toxin, if applicable (T36-T65 with fifth or sixth character 1-4 or 6)
> Use additional code for adverse effect, if applicable, to identify drug (T36-T50 with fifth or sixth character 5)

    H91.01   Ototoxic hearing loss, right ear
    H91.02   Ototoxic hearing loss, left ear
    H91.03   Ototoxic hearing loss, bilateral
    H91.09   Ototoxic hearing loss, unspecified ear   ▽

☑5ᵗʰ **H91.1**   **Presbycusis**
> Presbyacusia

    H91.10   Presbycusis, unspecified ear   ▽
    H91.11   Presbycusis, right ear
    H91.12   Presbycusis, left ear
    H91.13   Presbycusis, bilateral

☑5ᵗʰ **H91.2**   **Sudden idiopathic hearing loss**
> Sudden hearing loss NOS

    H91.20   Sudden idiopathic hearing loss, unspecified ear   ▽
    H91.21   Sudden idiopathic hearing loss, right ear
    H91.22   Sudden idiopathic hearing loss, left ear
    H91.23   Sudden idiopathic hearing loss, bilateral

H91.3   Deaf nonspeaking, not elsewhere classified

☑5ᵗʰ **H91.8**   **Other specified hearing loss**
    ☑6ᵗʰ **H91.8X**   Other specified hearing loss
       H91.8X1   Other specified hearing loss, right ear
       H91.8X2   Other specified hearing loss, left ear
       H91.8X3   Other specified hearing loss, bilateral
       H91.8X9   Other specified hearing loss, unspecified ear   ▽

☑5ᵗʰ **H91.9**   **Unspecified hearing loss**
> Deafness NOS
> High frequency deafness
> Low frequency deafness

    H91.90   Unspecified hearing loss, unspecified ear   ▽
    H91.91   Unspecified hearing loss, right ear   ▽
    H91.92   Unspecified hearing loss, left ear   ▽
    H91.93   Unspecified hearing loss, bilateral   ▽

☑4ᵗʰ **H92**   **Otalgia and effusion of ear**
☑5ᵗʰ **H92.0**   **Otalgia**
    H92.01   Otalgia, right ear
    H92.02   Otalgia, left ear
    H92.03   Otalgia, bilateral
    H92.09   Otalgia, unspecified ear   ▽

☑5ᵗʰ **H92.1**   **Otorrhea**
> EXCLUDES 1   *leakage of cerebrospinal fluid through ear (G96.0)*

    H92.10   Otorrhea, unspecified ear   ▽
    H92.11   Otorrhea, right ear
    H92.12   Otorrhea, left ear
    H92.13   Otorrhea, bilateral

☑5ᵗʰ **H92.2**   **Otorrhagia**
> EXCLUDES 1   *traumatic otorrhagia—code to injury*

    H92.20   Otorrhagia, unspecified ear   ▽
    H92.21   Otorrhagia, right ear
    H92.22   Otorrhagia, left ear
    H92.23   Otorrhagia, bilateral

☑4ᵗʰ **H93**   **Other disorders of ear, not elsewhere classified**
☑5ᵗʰ **H93.0**   **Degenerative and vascular disorders of ear**
> EXCLUDES 1   *presbycusis (H91.1)*

    ☑6ᵗʰ **H93.01**   Transient ischemic deafness
       H93.011   Transient ischemic deafness, right ear

H93.012   Transient ischemic deafness, left ear
H93.013   Transient ischemic deafness, bilateral
H93.019   Transient ischemic deafness, unspecified ear   ▽

☑6ᵗʰ **H93.09**   Unspecified degenerative and vascular disorders of ear
    H93.091   Unspecified degenerative and vascular disorders of right ear   ▽
    H93.092   Unspecified degenerative and vascular disorders of left ear   ▽
    H93.093   Unspecified degenerative and vascular disorders of ear, bilateral   ▽
    H93.099   Unspecified degenerative and vascular disorders of unspecified ear   ▽

☑5ᵗʰ **H93.1**   **Tinnitus**
    H93.11   Tinnitus, right ear
    H93.12   Tinnitus, left ear
    H93.13   Tinnitus, bilateral
    H93.19   Tinnitus, unspecified ear   ▽

☑5ᵗʰ **H93.2**   **Other abnormal auditory perceptions**
> EXCLUDES 2   *auditory hallucinations (R44.0)*

    ☑6ᵗʰ **H93.21**   Auditory recruitment
       H93.211   Auditory recruitment, right ear
       H93.212   Auditory recruitment, left ear
       H93.213   Auditory recruitment, bilateral
       H93.219   Auditory recruitment, unspecified ear   ▽

    ☑6ᵗʰ **H93.22**   Diplacusis
       H93.221   Diplacusis, right ear
       H93.222   Diplacusis, left ear
       H93.223   Diplacusis, bilateral
       H93.229   Diplacusis, unspecified ear   ▽

    ☑6ᵗʰ **H93.23**   Hyperacusis
       H93.231   Hyperacusis, right ear
       H93.232   Hyperacusis, left ear
       H93.233   Hyperacusis, bilateral
       H93.239   Hyperacusis, unspecified ear   ▽

    ☑6ᵗʰ **H93.24**   Temporary auditory threshold shift
       H93.241   Temporary auditory threshold shift, right ear
       H93.242   Temporary auditory threshold shift, left ear
       H93.243   Temporary auditory threshold shift, bilateral
       H93.249   Temporary auditory threshold shift, unspecified ear   ▽

       H93.25   Central auditory processing disorder
> Congenital auditory imperception
> Word deafness
> EXCLUDES 1   *mixed receptive-expressive language disorder (F80.2)*

    ☑6ᵗʰ **H93.29**   Other abnormal auditory perceptions
       H93.291   Other abnormal auditory perceptions, right ear
       H93.292   Other abnormal auditory perceptions, left ear
       H93.293   Other abnormal auditory perceptions, bilateral
       H93.299   Other abnormal auditory perceptions, unspecified ear   ▽

☑5ᵗʰ **H93.3**   **Disorders of acoustic nerve**
> Disorder of 8th cranial nerve
> EXCLUDES 1   *acoustic neuroma (D33.3)*
> *syphilitic acoustic neuritis (A52.15)*

    ☑6ᵗʰ **H93.3X**   Disorders of acoustic nerve
       H93.3X1   Disorders of right acoustic nerve
       H93.3X2   Disorders of left acoustic nerve
       H93.3X3   Disorders of bilateral acoustic nerves
       H93.3X9   Disorders of unspecified acoustic nerve   ▽

☑5ᵗʰ **H93.8**   **Other specified disorders of ear**
    ☑6ᵗʰ **H93.8X**   Other specified disorders of ear
       H93.8X1   Other specified disorders of right ear
       H93.8X2   Other specified disorders of left ear
       H93.8X3   Other specified disorders of ear, bilateral
       H93.8X9   Other specified disorders of ear, unspecified ear   ▽

Ⓝ Newborn   Ⓟ Pediatric   Ⓜ Maternity   Ⓐ Adult   **RIC** RIC Dx   **NC Dx** Noncancer Dx   **PDx** Primary Dx   **CC** RIC CC Condition   ▶◀ Revised Text   ● New Code   ▲ Revised Code Title

584   ICD-10-CM 2016

✓5ᵗʰ **H93.9** **Unspecified disorder of ear**

     H93.90 Unspecified disorder of ear, unspecified ear ▽

     H93.91 Unspecified disorder of right ear ▽

     H93.92 Unspecified disorder of left ear ▽

     H93.93 Unspecified disorder of ear, bilateral ▽

✓4ᵗʰ **H94** **Other disorders of ear in diseases classified elsewhere**

   ✓5ᵗʰ **H94.0** **Acoustic neuritis in infectious and parasitic diseases classified elsewhere**

     Code first underlying disease, such as:
     parasitic disease (B65-B89)

     EXCLUDES 1   *acoustic neuritis (in):*
        herpes zoster (B02.29)
        syphilis (A52.15)

     H94.00 Acoustic neuritis in infectious and parasitic diseases classified elsewhere, unspecified ear ▽

     H94.01 Acoustic neuritis in infectious and parasitic diseases classified elsewhere, right ear

     H94.02 Acoustic neuritis in infectious and parasitic diseases classified elsewhere, left ear

     H94.03 Acoustic neuritis in infectious and parasitic diseases classified elsewhere, bilateral

   ✓5ᵗʰ **H94.8** **Other specified disorders of ear in diseases classified elsewhere**

     Code first underlying disease, such as:
     congenital syphilis (A50.0)

     EXCLUDES 1   *aural myiasis (B87.4)*
        syphilitic labyrinthitis (A52.79)

     H94.80 Other specified disorders of ear in diseases classified elsewhere, unspecified ear ▽

     H94.81 Other specified disorders of right ear in diseases classified elsewhere

     H94.82 Other specified disorders of left ear in diseases classified elsewhere

     H94.83 Other specified disorders of ear in diseases classified elsewhere, bilateral

Intraoperative and postprocedural complications and disorders of ear and mastoid process, not elsewhere classified (H95)

✓4ᵗʰ **H95** **Intraoperative and postprocedural complications and disorders of ear and mastoid process, not elsewhere classified**

   ✓5ᵗʰ **H95.0** **Recurrent cholesteatoma of postmastoidectomy cavity**

     H95.00 Recurrent cholesteatoma of postmastoidectomy cavity, unspecified ear ▽

     H95.01 Recurrent cholesteatoma of postmastoidectomy cavity, right ear

     H95.02 Recurrent cholesteatoma of postmastoidectomy cavity, left ear

     H95.03 Recurrent cholesteatoma of postmastoidectomy cavity, bilateral ears

   ✓5ᵗʰ **H95.1** **Other disorders of ear and mastoid process following mastoidectomy**

    ✓6ᵗʰ **H95.11** Chronic inflammation of postmastoidectomy cavity

     H95.111 Chronic inflammation of postmastoidectomy cavity, right ear

     H95.112 Chronic inflammation of postmastoidectomy cavity, left ear

     H95.113 Chronic inflammation of postmastoidectomy cavity, bilateral ears

     H95.119 Chronic inflammation of postmastoidectomy cavity, unspecified ear ▽

    ✓6ᵗʰ **H95.12** Granulation of postmastoidectomy cavity

     H95.121 Granulation of postmastoidectomy cavity, right ear

     H95.122 Granulation of postmastoidectomy cavity, left ear

     H95.123 Granulation of postmastoidectomy cavity, bilateral ears

     H95.129 Granulation of postmastoidectomy cavity, unspecified ear ▽

    ✓6ᵗʰ **H95.13** Mucosal cyst of postmastoidectomy cavity

     H95.131 Mucosal cyst of postmastoidectomy cavity, right ear

     H95.132 Mucosal cyst of postmastoidectomy cavity, left ear

     H95.133 Mucosal cyst of postmastoidectomy cavity, bilateral ears

     H95.139 Mucosal cyst of postmastoidectomy cavity, unspecified ear ▽

    ✓6ᵗʰ **H95.19** Other disorders following mastoidectomy

     H95.191 Other disorders following mastoidectomy, right ear

     H95.192 Other disorders following mastoidectomy, left ear

     H95.193 Other disorders following mastoidectomy, bilateral ears

     H95.199 Other disorders following mastoidectomy, unspecified ear ▽

   ✓5ᵗʰ **H95.2** Intraoperative hemorrhage and hematoma of ear and mastoid process complicating a procedure

     EXCLUDES 1   *intraoperative hemorrhage and hematoma of ear and mastoid process due to accidental puncture or laceration during a procedure (H95.3-)*

     H95.21 Intraoperative hemorrhage and hematoma of ear and mastoid process complicating a procedure on the ear and mastoid process

     H95.22 Intraoperative hemorrhage and hematoma of ear and mastoid process complicating other procedure

   ✓5ᵗʰ **H95.3** Accidental puncture and laceration of ear and mastoid process during a procedure

     H95.31 Accidental puncture and laceration of the ear and mastoid process during a procedure on the ear and mastoid process

     H95.32 Accidental puncture and laceration of the ear and mastoid process during other procedure

   ✓5ᵗʰ **H95.4** Postprocedural hemorrhage and hematoma of ear and mastoid process following a procedure

     H95.41 Postprocedural hemorrhage and hematoma of ear and mastoid process following a procedure on the ear and mastoid process

     H95.42 Postprocedural hemorrhage and hematoma of ear and mastoid process following other procedure

   ✓5ᵗʰ **H95.8** Other intraoperative and postprocedural complications and disorders of the ear and mastoid process, not elsewhere classified

     EXCLUDES 2   *postprocedural complications and disorders following mastoidectomy (H95.0-, H95.1-)*

    ✓6ᵗʰ **H95.81** Postprocedural stenosis of external ear canal

     H95.811 Postprocedural stenosis of right external ear canal

     H95.812 Postprocedural stenosis of left external ear canal

     H95.813 Postprocedural stenosis of external ear canal, bilateral

     H95.819 Postprocedural stenosis of unspecified external ear canal ▽

     H95.88 Other intraoperative complications and disorders of the ear and mastoid process, not elsewhere classified

       Use additional code, if applicable, to further specify disorder

     H95.89 Other postprocedural complications and disorders of the ear and mastoid process, not elsewhere classified

       Use additional code, if applicable, to further specify disorder

---

✓ Add'l Character Required   ✓x7ᵗʰ Placeholder Alert   RUG IV Special Care High Dx   RUG IV Clinically Complex Dx   RUG IV Special Care Low Dx   Manifestation Code   Other Specified Code   ▽ Unspecified Code

Chapter 9. Diseases of the Circulatory System (I00–I99)

Chapter 9. Diseases of the Circulatory System

Chapter Specific Guidelines with Coding Examples

The chapter specific guidelines from the ICD-10-CM Official Guidelines for Coding and Reporting have been provided below. Along with these guidelines are coding examples, contained in the shaded boxes, that have been developed to help illustrate the coding and/or sequencing guidance found in these guidelines.

a. Hypertension

1) Hypertension with heart disease

Heart conditions classified to I50.- or I51.4-I51.9, are assigned to a code from category I11, Hypertensive heart disease, when a causal relationship is stated (due to hypertension) or implied (hypertensive). Use an additional code from category I50, Heart failure, to identify the type of heart failure in those patients with heart failure.

The same heart conditions (I50.-, I51.4-I51.9) with hypertension, but without a stated causal relationship, are coded separately. Sequence according to the circumstances of the admission/encounter.

> Hypertensive heart disease with left heart failure
>
> **I11.0**   **Hypertensive heart disease with heart failure**
>
> **I50.1**   **Left ventricular failure**
>
> *Explanation*: A causal relationship between hypertension and heart disease must be stated or implied to report codes from category I11 Hypertensive heart disease. Use an additional code to identify type of heart failure (I50.-).

2) Hypertensive chronic kidney disease

Assign codes from category I12, Hypertensive chronic kidney disease, when both hypertension and a condition classifiable to category N18, Chronic kidney disease (CKD), are present. Unlike hypertension with heart disease, ICD-10-CM presumes a cause-and-effect relationship and classifies chronic kidney disease with hypertension as hypertensive chronic kidney disease.

The appropriate code from category N18 should be used as a secondary code with a code from category I12 to identify the stage of chronic kidney disease.

See Section I.C.14. Chronic kidney disease.

If a patient has hypertensive chronic kidney disease and acute renal failure, an additional code for the acute renal failure is required.

> Patient is admitted with stage IV chronic kidney disease (CKD). The physician has also documented hypertension for this patient.
>
> **I12.9**   **Hypertensive chronic kidney disease with stage 1 through stage 4 chronic kidney disease, or unspecified chronic kidney disease**
>
> **N18.4**   **Chronic kidney disease, stage 4 (severe)**
>
> *Explanation*: A causal relationship between hypertension and chronic kidney disease (CKD) is **assumed** unless otherwise documented. Use an additional code to identify the stage of chronic kidney disease.

3) Hypertensive heart and chronic kidney disease

Assign codes from combination category I13, Hypertensive heart and chronic kidney disease, when both hypertensive kidney disease and hypertensive heart disease are stated in the diagnosis. Assume a relationship between the hypertension and the chronic kidney disease, whether or not the condition is so designated. If heart failure is present, assign an additional code from category I50 to identify the type of heart failure.

The appropriate code from category N18, Chronic kidney disease, should be used as a secondary code with a code from category I13 to identify the stage of chronic kidney disease.

See Section I.C.14. Chronic kidney disease.

The codes in category I13, Hypertensive heart and chronic kidney disease, are combination codes that include hypertension, heart disease and chronic kidney disease. The Includes note at I13 specifies that the conditions included at I11 and I12 are included together in I13. If a patient has hypertension, heart disease and chronic kidney disease then a code from I13 should be used, not individual codes for hypertension, heart disease and chronic kidney disease, or codes from I11 or I12.

For patients with both acute renal failure and chronic kidney disease an additional code for acute renal failure is required.

> Hypertensive heart and kidney disease with congestive heart failure and stage 2 chronic kidney disease
>
> **I13.0**   **Hypertensive heart and chronic kidney disease with heart failure and stage 1 through stage 4 chronic kidney disease, or unspecified chronic kidney disease**
>
> **I50.9**   **Heart failure, unspecified**
>
> **N18.2**   **Chronic kidney disease, stage 2 (mild)**
>
> *Explanation*: Combination codes in category I13 are used to report conditions classifiable to *both* categories I11 and I12. Do not report conditions classifiable to I11 and I12 separately. Use additional codes to report type of heart failure and stage of CKD.

4) Hypertensive cerebrovascular disease

For hypertensive cerebrovascular disease, first assign the appropriate code from categories I60-I69, followed by the appropriate hypertension code.

> Rupture of cerebral aneurysm caused by malignant hypertension
>
> **I60.8**   **Other nontraumatic subarachnoid hemorrhage**
>
> **I10**   **Essential (primary) hypertension**
>
> *Explanation*: Hypertensive cerebrovascular disease requires two codes: the appropriate I60–I69 code followed by the appropriate hypertension code.

5) Hypertensive retinopathy

Subcategory H35.0, Background retinopathy and retinal vascular changes, should be used with a code from category I10 – I15, Hypertensive disease to include the systemic hypertension. The sequencing is based on the reason for the encounter.

> Hypertensive retinopathy of the right eye
>
> **H35.031**   **Hypertensive retinopathy, right eye**
>
> **I10**   **Essential (primary) hypertension**
>
> *Explanation*: Hypertensive retinopathy requires two codes: the appropriate subcategory H35.0 code and a code for the hypertension.

6) Hypertension, secondary

Secondary hypertension is due to an underlying condition. Two codes are required: one to identify the underlying etiology and one from category I15 to identify the hypertension. Sequencing of codes is determined by the reason for admission/encounter.

> Renovascular hypertension due to renal artery atherosclerosis
>
> **I15.0**   **Renovascular hypertension**
>
> **I70.1**   **Atherosclerosis of renal artery**
>
> *Explanation*: Secondary hypertension requires two codes: a code to identify the etiology and the appropriate I15 code.

7) Hypertension, transient

Assign code R03.0, Elevated blood pressure reading without diagnosis of hypertension, unless patient has an established diagnosis of hypertension. Assign code O13.-, Gestational [pregnancy-induced] hypertension without significant proteinuria, or O14.-, Pre-eclampsia, for transient hypertension of pregnancy.

8) Hypertension, controlled

This diagnostic statement usually refers to an existing state of hypertension under control by therapy. Assign the appropriate code from categories I10-I15, Hypertensive diseases.

9) Hypertension, uncontrolled

Uncontrolled hypertension may refer to untreated hypertension or hypertension not responding to current therapeutic regimen. In either case, assign the appropriate code from categories I10-I15, Hypertensive diseases.

b. Atherosclerotic coronary artery disease and angina

ICD-10-CM has combination codes for atherosclerotic heart disease with angina pectoris. The subcategories for these codes are I25.11, Atherosclerotic heart disease of native coronary artery with angina pectoris and I25.7,

Atherosclerosis of coronary artery bypass graft(s) and coronary artery of transplanted heart with angina pectoris.

When using one of these combination codes it is not necessary to use an additional code for angina pectoris. A causal relationship can be assumed in a patient with both atherosclerosis and angina pectoris, unless the documentation indicates the angina is due to something other than the atherosclerosis.

If a patient with coronary artery disease is admitted due to an acute myocardial infarction (AMI), the AMI should be sequenced before the coronary artery disease.

See Section I.C.9. Acute myocardial infarction (AMI)

Patient is being seen for spastic angina pectoris. She also has a documented history of progressive coronary artery disease of the native vessels.

I25.111   **Atherosclerotic heart disease of native coronary artery with angina pectoris with documented spasm**

Explanation: Report the combination code for atherosclerotic heart disease (coronary artery disease) with angina pectoris. A causal relationship is assumed in a patient with both atherosclerosis and angina pectoris, unless the documentation indicates the angina is due to something other than the atherosclerosis. When using one of these combination codes, it is not necessary to use an additional code for angina pectoris.

---

c. Intraoperative and postprocedural cerebrovascular accident

Medical record documentation should clearly specify the cause- and- effect relationship between the medical intervention and the cerebrovascular accident in order to assign a code for intraoperative or postprocedural cerebrovascular accident.

Proper code assignment depends on whether it was an infarction or hemorrhage and whether it occurred intraoperatively or postoperatively. If it was a cerebral hemorrhage, code assignment depends on the type of procedure performed.

Embolic cerebral infarction of the right middle cerebral artery that occurred during hip replacement surgery. The surgeon documented as due to the surgery.

I97.811   **Intraoperative cerebrovascular infarction during other surgery**

I63.411   **Cerebral infarction due to embolism of right middle cerebral artery**

Explanation: Code assignment for intraoperative or postprocedural cerebrovascular accident is based on the provider's documentation of a cause-and-effect relationship between the condition and the procedure. Proper code assignment also depends on whether the cerebrovascular accident was an infarction or hemorrhage, occurred intraoperatively or postoperatively, and the type of procedure performed.

---

d. Sequelae of cerebrovascular disease

1) Category I69, Sequelae of cerebrovascular disease

Category I69 is used to indicate conditions classifiable to categories I60-I67 as the causes of sequela (neurologic deficits), themselves classified elsewhere. These "late effects" include neurologic deficits that persist after initial onset of conditions classifiable to categories I60-I67. The neurologic deficits caused by cerebrovascular disease may be present from the onset or may arise at any time after the onset of the condition classifiable to categories I60-I67.

Codes from category I69, Sequelae of cerebrovascular disease, that specify hemiplegia, hemiparesis and monoplegia identify whether the dominant or nondominant side is affected. Should the affected side be documented, but not specified as dominant or nondominant, and the classification system does not indicate a default, code selection is as follows:

- For ambidextrous patients, the default should be dominant.
- If the left side is affected, the default is non-dominant.
- If the right side is affected, the default is dominant.

2) Codes from category I69 with codes from I60–I67

Codes from category I69 may be assigned on a health care record with codes from I60-I67, if the patient has a current cerebrovascular disease and deficits from an old cerebrovascular disease.

3) Codes from category I69 and Personal history of transient ischemic attack (TIA) and cerebral infarction (Z86.73)

Codes from category I69 should not be assigned if the patient does not have neurologic deficits.

See Section I.C.21. 4. History (of) for use of personal history codes

---

Flaccid hemiparesis of the right side due to old cerebral infarction

I69.351   **Hemiplegia and hemiparesis following cerebral infarction affecting right dominant side**

Explanation: Sequela codes specify the residual effect that remains after the acute phase of a previous illness or injury (I60–I67). The "sequelae" include conditions specified as such or as residuals, which may occur at any time, even months or years, after the onset of the causal condition. There is no time limit restricting the reporting of sequela (late effect) codes. For this scenario, the documentation indicates that the right side is affected but does not note which side is the patient's dominant side, e.g., right or left. The default is to assume the right side is the dominant side.

---

e. Acute myocardial infarction (AMI)

1) ST elevation myocardial infarction (STEMI) and non ST elevation myocardial infarction (NSTEMI)

The ICD-10-CM codes for acute myocardial infarction (AMI) identify the site, such as anterolateral wall or true posterior wall. Subcategories I21.0-I21.2 and code I21.3 are used for ST elevation myocardial infarction (STEMI). Code I21.4, Non-ST elevation (NSTEMI) myocardial infarction, is used for non ST elevation myocardial infarction (NSTEMI) and nontransmural MIs.

If NSTEMI evolves to STEMI, assign the STEMI code. If STEMI converts to NSTEMI due to thrombolytic therapy, it is still coded as STEMI.

For encounters occurring while the myocardial infarction is equal to, or less than, four weeks old, including transfers to another acute setting or a postacute setting, and the patient requires continued care for the myocardial infarction, codes from category I21 may continue to be reported. For encounters after the 4 week time frame and the patient is still receiving care related to the myocardial infarction, the appropriate aftercare code should be assigned, rather than a code from category I21. For old or healed myocardial infarctions not requiring further care, code I25.2, Old myocardial infarction, may be assigned.

Acute inferior NSTEMI evolved into STEMI

I21.19   **ST elevation (STEMI) myocardial infarction involving other coronary artery of inferior wall**

Explanation: If an NSTEMI converts to a STEMI, report only the STEMI code.

---

2) Acute myocardial infarction, unspecified

Code I21.3, ST elevation (STEMI) myocardial infarction of unspecified site, is the default for unspecified acute myocardial infarction. If only STEMI or transmural MI without the site is documented, assign code I21.3.

3) AMI documented as nontransmural or subendocardial but site provided

If an AMI is documented as nontransmural or subendocardial, but the site is provided, it is still coded as a subendocardial AMI.

See Section I.C.21.3 for information on coding status post administration of tPA in a different facility within the last 24 hours.

Acute inferior subendocardial myocardial infarction (NSTEMI)

I21.4   **Non-ST elevation (NSTEMI) myocardial infarction**

Explanation: An AMI documented as subendocardial or nontransmural is coded as such (I21.4, I22.2), even if the site of infarction is specified.

---

4) Subsequent acute myocardial infarction

A code from category I22, Subsequent ST elevation (STEMI) and non ST elevation (NSTEMI) myocardial infarction, is to be used when a patient who has suffered an AMI has a new AMI within the 4 week time frame of the initial AMI. A code from category I22 must be used in conjunction with a code from category I21. The sequencing of the I22 and I21 codes depends on the circumstances of the encounter.

Acute inferior STEMI status post acute NSTEMI two weeks ago.

I22.1   **Subsequent ST elevation (STEMI) myocardial infarction of inferior wall**

I21.4   **Non-ST elevation (NSTEMI) myocardial infarction**

Explanation: A code from I22 must be used in conjunction with a code from I21 when a patient who has suffered an AMI has a new AMI within four weeks of the initial one. Category I22 is never reported alone. The guidelines for assigning the correct I22 code are the same as those for reporting the initial MI (I21). Sequencing is determined by the circumstances of the encounter.

Chapter 9. Diseases of the Circulatory System(I00–I99)

EXCLUDES 2   certain conditions originating in the perinatal period (P04-P96)
certain infectious and parasitic diseases (A00-B99)
complications of pregnancy, childbirth and the puerperium (O00-O9A)
congenital malformations, deformations, and chromosomal abnormalities (Q00-Q99)
endocrine, nutritional and metabolic diseases (E00-E88)
injury, poisoning and certain other consequences of external causes (S00-T88)
neoplasms (C00-D49)
symptoms, signs and abnormal clinical and laboratory findings, not elsewhere classified (R00-R94)
systemic connective tissue disorders (M30-M36)
transient cerebral ischemic attacks and related syndromes (G45.-)

This chapter contains the following blocks:

I00-I02	Acute rheumatic fever
I05-I09	Chronic rheumatic heart diseases
I10-I15	Hypertensive diseases
I20-I25	Ischemic heart diseases
I26-I28	Pulmonary heart disease and diseases of pulmonary circulation
I30-I52	Other forms of heart disease
I60-I69	Cerebrovascular diseases
I70-I79	Diseases of arteries, arterioles and capillaries
I80-I89	Diseases of veins, lymphatic vessels and lymph nodes, not elsewhere classified
I95-I99	Other and unspecified disorders of the circulatory system

Acute rheumatic fever (I00–I02)

I00   **Rheumatic fever without heart involvement**
    INCLUDES   arthritis, rheumatic, acute or subacute
    EXCLUDES 1   rheumatic fever with heart involvement (I01.0-I01.9)

✓4ᵗʰ **I01**   **Rheumatic fever with heart involvement**
    EXCLUDES 1   chronic diseases of rheumatic origin (I05-I09) unless rheumatic fever is also present or there is evidence of reactivation or activity of the rheumatic process.

   I01.0   **Acute rheumatic pericarditis**
      Any condition in I00 with pericarditis
      Rheumatic pericarditis (acute)
      EXCLUDES 1   acute pericarditis not specified as rheumatic (I30.-)

   I01.1   **Acute rheumatic endocarditis**
      Any condition in I00 with endocarditis or valvulitis
      Acute rheumatic valvulitis

   I01.2   **Acute rheumatic myocarditis**
      Any condition in I00 with myocarditis

   I01.8   **Other acute rheumatic heart disease**
      Any condition in I00 with other or multiple types of heart involvement
      Acute rheumatic pancarditis

   I01.9   **Acute rheumatic heart disease, unspecified**   ▽
      Any condition in I00 with unspecified type of heart involvement
      Rheumatic carditis, acute
      Rheumatic heart disease, active or acute

✓4ᵗʰ **I02**   **Rheumatic chorea**
    INCLUDES   Sydenham's chorea
    EXCLUDES 1   chorea NOS (G25.5)
               Huntington's chorea (G10)

   I02.0   **Rheumatic chorea with heart involvement**
      Chorea NOS with heart involvement
      Rheumatic chorea with heart involvement of any type classifiable under I01-

   I02.9   **Rheumatic chorea without heart involvement**
      Rheumatic chorea NOS

Chronic rheumatic heart diseases (I05–I09)

✓4ᵗʰ **I05**   **Rheumatic mitral valve diseases**
    INCLUDES   conditions classifiable to both I05.0 and I05.2-I05.9, whether specified as rheumatic or not
    EXCLUDES 1   mitral valve disease specified as nonrheumatic (I34.-)
               mitral valve disease with aortic and/or tricuspid valve involvement (I08.-)

   I05.0   **Rheumatic mitral stenosis**
      Mitral (valve) obstruction (rheumatic)

   I05.1   **Rheumatic mitral insufficiency**
      Rheumatic mitral incompetence
      Rheumatic mitral regurgitation
      EXCLUDES 1   mitral insufficiency not specified as rheumatic (I34.0)

   I05.2   **Rheumatic mitral stenosis with insufficiency**
      Rheumatic mitral stenosis with incompetence or regurgitation

   I05.8   **Other rheumatic mitral valve diseases**
      Rheumatic mitral (valve) failure

   I05.9   **Rheumatic mitral valve disease, unspecified**   ▽
      Rheumatic mitral (valve) disorder (chronic) NOS

✓4ᵗʰ **I06**   **Rheumatic aortic valve diseases**
    EXCLUDES 1   aortic valve disease not specified as rheumatic (I35.-)
               aortic valve disease with mitral and/or tricuspid valve involvement (I08.-)

   I06.0   **Rheumatic aortic stenosis**
      Rheumatic aortic (valve) obstruction

   I06.1   **Rheumatic aortic insufficiency**
      Rheumatic aortic incompetence
      Rheumatic aortic regurgitation

   I06.2   **Rheumatic aortic stenosis with insufficiency**
      Rheumatic aortic stenosis with incompetence or regurgitation

   I06.8   **Other rheumatic aortic valve diseases**

   I06.9   **Rheumatic aortic valve disease, unspecified**   ▽
      Rheumatic aortic (valve) disease NOS

✓4ᵗʰ **I07**   **Rheumatic tricuspid valve diseases**
    INCLUDES   rheumatic tricuspid valve diseases specified as rheumatic or unspecified
    EXCLUDES 1   tricuspid valve disease specified as nonrheumatic (I36.-)
               tricuspid valve disease with aortic and/or mitral valve involvement (I08.-)

   I07.0   **Rheumatic tricuspid stenosis**
      Tricuspid (valve) stenosis (rheumatic)

   I07.1   **Rheumatic tricuspid insufficiency**
      Tricuspid (valve) insufficiency (rheumatic)

   I07.2   **Rheumatic tricuspid stenosis and insufficiency**

   I07.8   **Other rheumatic tricuspid valve diseases**

   I07.9   **Rheumatic tricuspid valve disease, unspecified**   ▽
      Rheumatic tricuspid valve disorder NOS

✓4ᵗʰ **I08**   **Multiple valve diseases**
    INCLUDES   multiple valve diseases specified as rheumatic or unspecified
    EXCLUDES 1   endocarditis, valve unspecified (I38)
               multiple valve disease specified a nonrheumatic (I34.-, I35.-, I36.-, I37.-, I38.-, Q22.-, Q23.-, Q24.8-)
               rheumatic valve disease NOS (I09.1)

   I08.0   **Rheumatic disorders of both mitral and aortic valves**
      Involvement of both mitral and aortic valves specified as rheumatic or unspecified

   I08.1   **Rheumatic disorders of both mitral and tricuspid valves**

   I08.2   **Rheumatic disorders of both aortic and tricuspid valves**

   I08.3   **Combined rheumatic disorders of mitral, aortic and tricuspid valves**

   I08.8   **Other rheumatic multiple valve diseases**

   I08.9   **Rheumatic multiple valve disease, unspecified**   ▽

✓4ᵗʰ **I09**   **Other rheumatic heart diseases**

   I09.0   **Rheumatic myocarditis**   [CC]
      EXCLUDES 1   myocarditis not specified as rheumatic (I51.4)
      RIC Excl: 14 Cardiac

   I09.1   **Rheumatic diseases of endocardium, valve unspecified**   ▽
      Rheumatic endocarditis (chronic)
      Rheumatic valvulitis (chronic)
      EXCLUDES 1   endocarditis, valve unspecified (I38)

   I09.2   **Chronic rheumatic pericarditis**
      Adherent pericardium, rheumatic
      Chronic rheumatic mediastinopericarditis
      Chronic rheumatic myopericarditis
      EXCLUDES 1   chronic pericarditis not specified as rheumatic (I31.-)

✓5ᵗʰ **I09.8**   **Other specified rheumatic heart diseases**

     I09.81   **Rheumatic heart failure**
        Use additional code to identify type of heart failure (I50.-)

     I09.89   **Other specified rheumatic heart diseases**
        Rheumatic disease of pulmonary valve

   I09.9   **Rheumatic heart disease, unspecified**   ▽
      Rheumatic carditis
      EXCLUDES 1   rheumatoid carditis (M05.31)

Ⓝ Newborn   Ⓟ Pediatric   Ⓜ Maternity   Ⓐ Adult   **RIC** RIC Dx   **NC Dx** Noncancer Dx   **PDx** Primary Dx   **CC** RIC CC Condition   ▶◀ Revised Text   ● New Code   ▲ Revised Code Title

588   ICD-10-CM 2016

Hypertensive diseases (I10-I15)

Use additional code to identify:
   exposure to environmental tobacco smoke (Z77.22)
   history of tobacco use (Z87.891)
   occupational exposure to environmental tobacco smoke (Z57.31)
   tobacco dependence (F17.-)
   tobacco use (Z72.Ø)
   EXCLUDES 1   hypertensive disease complicating pregnancy, childbirth and the
            puerperium (O1Ø-O11, O13-O16)
            neonatal hypertension (P29.2)
            primary pulmonary hypertension (I27.Ø)

I1Ø   Essential (primary) hypertension
   INCLUDES   high blood pressure
             hypertension (arterial) (benign) (essential) (malignant)
               (primary) (systemic)
   EXCLUDES 1   hypertensive disease complicating pregnancy, childbirth and
            the puerperium (O1Ø-O11, O13-O16)
   EXCLUDES 2   essential (primary) hypertension involving vessels of brain
            (I6Ø-I69)
            essential (primary) hypertension involving vessels of eye
            (H35.Ø-)

✓4ᵗʰ I11   Hypertensive heart disease
   INCLUDES   any condition in I51.4-I51.9 due to hypertension

   I11.Ø   **Hypertensive heart disease with heart failure**   `NC Dx`
       Hypertensive heart failure
       Use additional code to identify type of heart failure (I5Ø.-)

   I11.9   **Hypertensive heart disease without heart failure**
       Hypertensive heart disease NOS

✓4ᵗʰ I12   Hypertensive chronic kidney disease
   INCLUDES   any condition in N18- and N26- due to hypertension
            arteriosclerosis of kidney
            arteriosclerotic nephritis (chronic) (interstitial)
            hypertensive nephropathy
            nephrosclerosis
   EXCLUDES 1   hypertension due to kidney disease (I15.Ø, I15.1)
            renovascular hypertension (I15.Ø)
            secondary hypertension (I15.-)
   EXCLUDES 2   acute kidney failure (N17.-)

   I12.Ø   **Hypertensive chronic kidney disease with stage 5**   `CC` `NC Dx`
       chronic kidney disease or end stage renal disease
         Use additional code to identify the stage of chronic kidney
           disease (N18.5, N18.6)

   I12.9   **Hypertensive chronic kidney disease with stage 1 through**
       stage 4 chronic kidney disease, or unspecified chronic kidney
       disease
       Hypertensive chronic kidney disease NOS
       Hypertensive renal disease NOS
       Use additional code to identify the stage of chronic kidney
         disease (N18.1-N18.4, N18.9)

✓4ᵗʰ I13   Hypertensive heart and chronic kidney disease
   INCLUDES   any condition in I11- with any condition in I12-
            cardiorenal disease
            cardiovascular renal disease

   I13.Ø   **Hypertensive heart and chronic kidney disease**   `CC` `NC Dx`
       with heart failure and stage 1 through stage 4 chronic
       kidney disease, or unspecified chronic kidney disease
       Use additional code to identify type of heart failure (I5Ø.-)
       Use additional code to identify stage of chronic kidney disease
         (N18.1-N18.4, N18.9)
       RIC Excl: 14 Cardiac

   ✓5ᵗʰ I13.1   **Hypertensive heart and chronic kidney disease**
       without heart failure

      I13.1Ø   **Hypertensive heart and chronic kidney disease**
          without heart failure, with stage 1 through stage 4
          chronic kidney disease, or unspecified chronic
          kidney disease
          Hypertensive heart disease and hypertensive chronic
            kidney disease NOS
          Use additional code to identify the stage of chronic
            kidney disease (N18.1-N18.4, N18.9)

      I13.11   **Hypertensive heart and chronic kidney disease**   `NC Dx`
          without heart failure, with stage 5 chronic kidney
          disease, or end stage renal disease
          Use additional code to identify the stage of chronic
            kidney disease (N18.5, N18.6)

   I13.2   **Hypertensive heart and chronic kidney disease**   `CC` `NC Dx`
       with heart failure and with stage 5 chronic kidney
       disease, or end stage renal disease
       Use additional code to identify type of heart failure (I5Ø.-)
       Use additional code to identify the stage of chronic kidney
         disease (N18.5, N18.6)
       RIC Excl: 14 Cardiac

✓4ᵗʰ I15   Secondary hypertension
   Code also underlying condition
   EXCLUDES 1   postprocedural hypertension (I97.3)
   EXCLUDES 2   secondary hypertension involving vessels of brain (I6Ø-I69)
            secondary hypertension involving vessels of eye (H35.Ø-)

   I15.Ø   **Renovascular hypertension**

   I15.1   **Hypertension secondary to other renal disorders**

   I15.2   **Hypertension secondary to endocrine disorders**

   I15.8   **Other secondary hypertension**

   I15.9   **Secondary hypertension, unspecified**   ▽

Ischemic heart diseases (I2Ø-I25)

Use additional code to identify presence of hypertension (I1Ø-I15)

✓4ᵗʰ I2Ø   Angina pectoris
   Use additional code to identify:
      exposure to environmental tobacco smoke (Z77.22)
      history of tobacco use (Z87.891)
      occupational exposure to environmental tobacco smoke (Z57.31)
      tobacco dependence (F17.-)
      tobacco use (Z72.Ø)
   EXCLUDES 1   angina pectoris with atherosclerotic heart disease of native
            coronary arteries (I25.1-)
            atherosclerosis of coronary artery bypass graft(s) and coronary
              artery of transplanted heart with angina pectoris (I25.7-)
            postinfarction angina (I23.7)

   I2Ø.Ø   **Unstable angina**   `A`
       Accelerated angina
       Crescendo angina
       De novo effort angina
       Intermediate coronary syndrome
       Preinfarction syndrome
       Worsening effort angina

   I2Ø.1   **Angina pectoris with documented spasm**   `A`
       Angiospastic angina
       Prinzmetal angina
       Spasm-induced angina
       Variant angina

   I2Ø.8   **Other forms of angina pectoris**   `A`
       Angina equivalent
       Angina of effort
       Coronary slow flow syndrome
       Stenocardia
       Use additional code(s) for symptoms associated with angina
         equivalent

   I2Ø.9   **Angina pectoris, unspecified**   `A` ▽
       Angina NOS
       Anginal syndrome
       Cardiac angina
       Ischemic chest pain

✓4ᵗʰ I21   ST elevation (STEMI) and non-ST elevation (NSTEMI) myocardial infarction
   INCLUDES   cardiac infarction
            coronary (artery) embolism
            coronary (artery) occlusion
            coronary (artery) rupture
            coronary (artery) thrombosis
            infarction of heart, myocardium, or ventricle
            myocardial infarction specified as acute or with a stated
               duration of 4 weeks (28 days) or less from onset
   Use additional code, if applicable, to identify:
      exposure to environmental tobacco smoke (Z77.22)
      history of tobacco use (Z87.891)
      occupational exposure to environmental tobacco smoke (Z57.31)
      status post administration of tPA (rtPA) in a different facility within
         the last 24 hours prior to admission to current facility (Z92.82)
      tobacco dependence (F17.-)
      tobacco use (Z72.Ø)
   EXCLUDES 2   old myocardial infarction (I25.2)
            postmyocardial infarction syndrome (I24.1)
            subsequent myocardial infarction (I22.-)
   AHA: 2013, 1Q, 25; 2012, 4Q, 96, 102-103

☑ Add'l Character Required   **✓x7ᵗʰ** Placeholder Alert   `RUG IV Special Care High Dx`   RUG IV Clinically Complex Dx   `RUG IV Special Care Low Dx`   Manifestation Code   Other Specified Code   ▽ Unspecified Code

ICD-10-CM 2016   589

Chapter 9. Diseases of the Circulatory System

✓5ᵗʰ I21.0 ST elevation (STEMI) myocardial infarction of anterior wall

I21.01 ST elevation (STEMI) myocardial infarction involving left main coronary artery Ⓐ

I21.02 ST elevation (STEMI) myocardial infarction involving left anterior descending coronary artery Ⓐ
ST elevation (STEMI) myocardial infarction involving diagonal coronary artery
AHA: 2013, 1Q, 25

I21.09 ST elevation (STEMI) myocardial infarction involving other coronary artery of anterior wall Ⓐ
Acute transmural myocardial infarction of anterior wall
Anteroapical transmural (Q wave) infarction (acute)
Anterolateral transmural (Q wave) infarction (acute)
Anteroseptal transmural (Q wave) infarction (acute)
Transmural (Q wave) infarction (acute) (of) anterior (wall) NOS
AHA: 2012, 4Q, 102-103

✓5ᵗʰ I21.1 ST elevation (STEMI) myocardial infarction of inferior wall

I21.11 ST elevation (STEMI) myocardial infarction involving right coronary artery Ⓐ
Inferoposterior transmural (Q wave) infarction (acute)

I21.19 ST elevation (STEMI) myocardial infarction involving other coronary artery of inferior wall Ⓐ
Acute transmural myocardial infarction of inferior wall
Inferolateral transmural (Q wave) infarction (acute)
Transmural (Q wave) infarction (acute) (of) diaphragmatic wall
Transmural (Q wave) infarction (acute) (of) inferior (wall) NOS
EXCLUDES 2   ST elevation (STEMI) myocardial infarction involving left circumflex coronary artery (I21.21)
AHA: 2012, 4Q, 96

✓5ᵗʰ I21.2 ST elevation (STEMI) myocardial infarction of other sites

I21.21 ST elevation (STEMI) myocardial infarction involving left circumflex coronary artery Ⓐ
ST elevation (STEMI) myocardial infarction involving oblique marginal coronary artery

I21.29 ST elevation (STEMI) myocardial infarction involving other sites Ⓐ
Acute transmural myocardial infarction of other sites
Apical-lateral transmural (Q wave) infarction (acute)
Basal-lateral transmural (Q wave) infarction (acute)
High lateral transmural (Q wave) infarction (acute)
Lateral (wall) NOS transmural (Q wave) infarction (acute)
Posterior (true) transmural (Q wave) infarction (acute)
Posterobasal transmural (Q wave) infarction (acute)
Posterolateral transmural (Q wave) infarction (acute)
Posteroseptal transmural (Q wave) infarction (acute)
Septal transmural (Q wave) infarction (acute) NOS

I21.3 ST elevation (STEMI) myocardial infarction of unspecified site Ⓐ▽
Acute transmural myocardial infarction of unspecified site
Myocardial infarction (acute) NOS
Transmural (Q wave) myocardial infarction NOS

I21.4 Non-ST elevation (NSTEMI) myocardial infarction Ⓐ
Acute subendocardial myocardial infarction
Non-Q wave myocardial infarction NOS
Nontransmural myocardial infarction NOS

✓4ᵗʰ I22 Subsequent ST elevation (STEMI) and non-ST elevation (NSTEMI) myocardial infarction
INCLUDES   acute myocardial infarction occurring within four weeks (28 days) of a previous acute myocardial infarction, regardless of site
cardiac infarction
coronary (artery) embolism
coronary (artery) occlusion
coronary (artery) rupture
coronary (artery) thrombosis
infarction of heart, myocardium, or ventricle
recurrent myocardial infarction
reinfarction of myocardium
rupture of heart, myocardium, or ventricle
Use additional code, if applicable, to identify:
exposure to environmental tobacco smoke (Z77.22)
history of tobacco use (Z87.891)
occupational exposure to environmental tobacco smoke (Z57.31)
status post administration of tPA (rtPA) in a different facility within the last 24 hours prior to admission to current facility (Z92.82)
tobacco dependence (F17.-)
tobacco use (Z72.0)
AHA: 2013, 1Q, 25; 2012, 4Q, 97, 102-103

I22.0 Subsequent ST elevation (STEMI) myocardial infarction of anterior wall Ⓐ
Subsequent acute transmural myocardial infarction of anterior wall
Subsequent transmural (Q wave) infarction (acute)(of) anterior (wall) NOS
Subsequent anteroapical transmural (Q wave) infarction (acute)
Subsequent anterolateral transmural (Q wave) infarction (acute)
Subsequent anteroseptal transmural (Q wave) infarction (acute)

I22.1 Subsequent ST elevation (STEMI) myocardial infarction of inferior wall Ⓐ
Subsequent acute transmural myocardial infarction of inferior wall
Subsequent transmural (Q wave) infarction (acute)(of) diaphragmatic wall
Subsequent transmural (Q wave) infarction (acute)(of) inferior (wall) NOS
Subsequent inferolateral transmural (Q wave) infarction (acute)
Subsequent inferoposterior transmural (Q wave) infarction (acute)
AHA: 2012, 4Q, 102

I22.2 Subsequent non-ST elevation (NSTEMI) myocardial infarction Ⓐ
Subsequent acute subendocardial myocardial infarction
Subsequent non-Q wave myocardial infarction NOS
Subsequent nontransmural myocardial infarction NOS

I22.8 Subsequent ST elevation (STEMI) myocardial infarction of other sites Ⓐ
Subsequent acute transmural myocardial infarction of other sites
Subsequent apical-lateral transmural (Q wave) myocardial infarction (acute)
Subsequent basal-lateral transmural (Q wave) myocardial infarction (acute)
Subsequent high lateral transmural (Q wave) myocardial infarction (acute)
Subsequent transmural (Q wave) myocardial infarction (acute)(of) lateral (wall) NOS
Subsequent posterior (true)transmural (Q wave) myocardial infarction (acute)
Subsequent posterobasal transmural (Q wave) myocardial infarction (acute)
Subsequent posterolateral transmural (Q wave) myocardial infarction (acute)
Subsequent posteroseptal transmural (Q wave) myocardial infarction (acute)
Subsequent septal NOS transmural (Q wave) myocardial infarction (acute)

I22.9 Subsequent ST elevation (STEMI) myocardial infarction of unspecified site Ⓐ▽
Subsequent acute myocardial infarction of unspecified site
Subsequent myocardial infarction (acute) NOS

✓4ᵗʰ I23 Certain current complications following ST elevation (STEMI) and non-ST elevation (NSTEMI) myocardial infarction (within the 28 day period)

I23.0 Hemopericardium as current complication following acute myocardial infarction NC Dx Ⓐ
EXCLUDES 1   hemopericardium not specified as current complication following acute myocardial infarction (I31.2)

I23.1 Atrial septal defect as current complication following acute myocardial infarction NC Dx Ⓐ
EXCLUDES 1   acquired atrial septal defect not specified as current complication following acute myocardial infarction (I51.0)

I23.2 Ventricular septal defect as current complication following acute myocardial infarction NC Dx Ⓐ
EXCLUDES 1   acquired ventricular septal defect not specified as current complication following acute myocardial infarction (I51.0)

I23.3 Rupture of cardiac wall without hemopericardium as current complication following acute myocardial infarction NC Dx Ⓐ

I23.4 Rupture of chordae tendineae as current complication following acute myocardial infarction NC Dx
EXCLUDES 1   rupture of chordae tendineae not specified as current complication following acute myocardial infarction (I51.1)

I23.5 Rupture of papillary muscle as current complication following acute myocardial infarction NC Dx
EXCLUDES 1   rupture of papillary muscle not specified as current complication following acute myocardial infarction (I51.2)▪

I23.6   Thrombosis of atrium, auricular appendage, and ventricle as current complications following acute myocardial infarction   NC Dx   A
> EXCLUDES 1   *thrombosis of atrium, auricular appendage, and ventricle not specified as current complication following acute myocardial infarction (I51.3)*

I23.7   Postinfarction angina   NC Dx   A

I23.8   Other current complications following acute myocardial infarction   A

✓4ᵗʰ I24   **Other acute ischemic heart diseases**
> EXCLUDES 1   *angina pectoris (I20.-)*
> *transient myocardial ischemia in newborn (P29.4)*

I24.0   Acute coronary thrombosis not resulting in myocardial infarction   A
> Acute coronary (artery) (vein) embolism not resulting in myocardial infarction
> Acute coronary (artery) (vein) occlusion not resulting in myocardial infarction
> Acute coronary (artery) (vein) thromboembolism not resulting in myocardial infarction
> EXCLUDES 1   *atherosclerotic heart disease (I25.1-)*
> **AHA:** 2013, 1Q, 24

I24.1   Dressler's syndrome   A
> Postmyocardial infarction syndrome
> EXCLUDES 1   *postinfarction angina (I23.7)*

I24.8   Other forms of acute ischemic heart disease   A

I24.9   Acute ischemic heart disease, unspecified   A ▽
> EXCLUDES 1   *ischemic heart disease (chronic) NOS (I25.9)*

✓4ᵗʰ I25   **Chronic ischemic heart disease**
> Use additional code to identify:
> chronic total occlusion of coronary artery (I25.82)
> exposure to environmental tobacco smoke (Z77.22)
> history of tobacco use (Z87.891)
> occupational exposure to environmental tobacco smoke (Z57.31)
> tobacco dependence (F17.-)
> tobacco use (Z72.0)

I25.1   Atherosclerotic heart disease of native coronary artery
> Atherosclerotic cardiovascular disease
> Coronary (artery) atheroma
> Coronary (artery) atherosclerosis
> Coronary (artery) disease
> Coronary (artery) sclerosis
> Use additional code, if applicable, to identify:
> coronary atherosclerosis due to calcified coronary lesion (I25.84)
> coronary atherosclerosis due to lipid rich plaque (I25.83)
> EXCLUDES 2   *atheroembolism (I75.-)*
> *atherosclerosis of coronary artery bypass graft(s) and transplanted heart (I25.7-)*

  I25.10   Atherosclerotic heart disease of native coronary artery without angina pectoris   A
> Atherosclerotic heart disease NOS
> **AHA:** 2012, 4Q, 92

  ✓6ᵗʰ I25.11   Atherosclerotic heart disease of native coronary artery with angina pectoris

    I25.110   Atherosclerotic heart disease of native coronary artery with unstable angina pectoris   A
> EXCLUDES 1   *unstable angina without atherosclerotic heart disease (I20.0)*

    I25.111   Atherosclerotic heart disease of native coronary artery with angina pectoris with documented spasm   A
> EXCLUDES 1   *angina pectoris with documented spasm without atherosclerotic heart disease (I20.1)*

    I25.118   Atherosclerotic heart disease of native coronary artery with other forms of angina pectoris   A
> EXCLUDES 1   *other forms of angina pectoris without atherosclerotic heart disease (I20.8)*

    I25.119   Atherosclerotic heart disease of native coronary artery with unspecified angina pectoris   A ▽
> Atherosclerotic heart disease with angina NOS
> Atherosclerotic heart disease with ischemic chest pain
> EXCLUDES 1   *unspecified angina pectoris without atherosclerotic heart disease (I20.9)*

I25.2   Old myocardial infarction   A
> Healed myocardial infarction
> Past myocardial infarction diagnosed by ECG or other investigation, but currently presenting no symptoms

I25.3   Aneurysm of heart   NC Dx
> Mural aneurysm
> Ventricular aneurysm

✓5ᵗʰ I25.4   Coronary artery aneurysm and dissection

  I25.41   Coronary artery aneurysm   NC Dx
> Coronary arteriovenous fistula, acquired
> EXCLUDES 1   *congenital coronary (artery) aneurysm (Q24.5)*

  I25.42   Coronary artery dissection

I25.5   Ischemic cardiomyopathy   NC Dx
> EXCLUDES 2   *coronary atherosclerosis (I25.1-, I25.7-)*

I25.6   Silent myocardial ischemia   NC Dx

✓5ᵗʰ I25.7   Atherosclerosis of coronary artery bypass graft(s) and coronary artery of transplanted heart with angina pectoris
> Use additional code, if applicable, to identify:
> coronary atherosclerosis due to calcified coronary lesion (I25.84)
> coronary atherosclerosis due to lipid rich plaque (I25.83)
> EXCLUDES 1   *atherosclerosis of bypass graft(s) of transplanted heart without angina pectoris (I25.812)*
> *atherosclerosis of coronary artery bypass graft(s) without angina pectoris (I25.810)*
> *atherosclerosis of native coronary artery of transplanted heart without angina pectoris (I25.811)*
> *embolism or thrombus of coronary artery bypass graft(s) (T82.8-)*

  ✓6ᵗʰ I25.70   Atherosclerosis of coronary artery bypass graft(s), unspecified, with angina pectoris

    I25.700   Atherosclerosis of coronary artery bypass graft(s), unspecified, with unstable angina pectoris   A ▽
> EXCLUDES 1   *unstable angina pectoris without atherosclerosis of coronary artery bypass graft (I20.0)*

    I25.701   Atherosclerosis of coronary artery bypass graft(s), unspecified, with angina pectoris with documented spasm   A ▽
> EXCLUDES 1   *angina pectoris with documented spasm without atherosclerosis of coronary artery bypass graft (I20.1)*

    I25.708   Atherosclerosis of coronary artery bypass graft(s), unspecified, with other forms of angina pectoris   A ▽
> EXCLUDES 1   *other forms of angina pectoris without atherosclerosis of coronary artery bypass graft (I20.8)*

    I25.709   Atherosclerosis of coronary artery bypass graft(s), unspecified, with unspecified angina pectoris   A ▽
> EXCLUDES 1   *unspecified angina pectoris without atherosclerosis of coronary artery bypass graft (I20.9)*

  ✓6ᵗʰ I25.71   Atherosclerosis of autologous vein coronary artery bypass graft(s) with angina pectoris

    I25.710   Atherosclerosis of autologous vein coronary artery bypass graft(s) with unstable angina pectoris   A
> EXCLUDES 1   *unstable angina without atherosclerosis of autologous vein coronary artery bypass graft(s) (I20.0)*

☑ Add'l Character Required   ☑×7ᵗʰ Placeholder Alert   RUG IV Special Care High Dx   RUG IV Clinically Complex Dx   RUG IV Special Care Low Dx   Manifestation Code   Other Specified Code   ▽ Unspecified Code

Chapter 9. Diseases of the Circulatory System

I25.711–I25.799

I25.711   **Atherosclerosis of autologous vein coronary artery bypass graft(s) with angina pectoris with** documented spasm 🅰
> **EXCLUDES 1**   angina pectoris with documented spasm without atherosclerosis of autologous vein coronary artery bypass graft(s) (I20.1)

I25.718   **Atherosclerosis of autologous vein coronary artery bypass graft(s) with other forms of angina pectoris** 🅰
> **EXCLUDES 1**   other forms of angina pectoris without atherosclerosis of autologous vein coronary artery bypass graft(s) (I20.8)

I25.719   **Atherosclerosis of autologous vein coronary artery bypass graft(s) with unspecified angina pectoris** 🅰▽
> **EXCLUDES 1**   unspecified angina pectoris without atherosclerosis of autologous vein coronary artery bypass graft(s) (I20.9)

✓6ᵗʰ **I25.72**   **Atherosclerosis of** autologous artery **coronary artery bypass graft(s) with angina pectoris**
> Atherosclerosis of internal mammary artery graft with angina pectoris

I25.720   **Atherosclerosis of autologous artery coronary artery bypass graft(s) with** unstable **angina pectoris** 🅰
> **EXCLUDES 1**   unstable angina without atherosclerosis of autologous artery coronary artery bypass graft(s) (I20.0)

I25.721   **Atherosclerosis of autologous artery coronary artery bypass graft(s) with angina pectoris with** documented spasm 🅰
> **EXCLUDES 1**   angina pectoris with documented spasm without atherosclerosis of autologous artery coronary artery bypass graft(s) (I20.1)

I25.728   **Atherosclerosis of autologous artery coronary artery bypass graft(s) with other forms of angina pectoris** 🅰
> **EXCLUDES 1**   other forms of angina pectoris without atherosclerosis of autologous artery coronary artery bypass graft(s) (I20.8)

I25.729   **Atherosclerosis of autologous artery coronary artery bypass graft(s) with unspecified angina pectoris** 🅰▽
> **EXCLUDES 1**   unspecified angina pectoris without atherosclerosis of autologous artery coronary artery bypass graft(s) (I20.9)

✓6ᵗʰ **I25.73**   **Atherosclerosis of** nonautologous biological **coronary artery bypass graft(s) with angina pectoris**

I25.730   **Atherosclerosis of nonautologous biological coronary artery bypass graft(s) with** unstable **angina pectoris** 🅰
> **EXCLUDES 1**   unstable angina without atherosclerosis of nonautologous biological coronary artery bypass graft(s) (I20.0)

I25.731   **Atherosclerosis of nonautologous biological coronary artery bypass graft(s) with angina pectoris with** documented spasm 🅰
> **EXCLUDES 1**   angina pectoris with documented spasm without atherosclerosis of nonautologous biological coronary artery bypass graft(s) (I20.1)

I25.738   **Atherosclerosis of nonautologous biological coronary artery bypass graft(s) with other forms of angina pectoris** 🅰
> **EXCLUDES 1**   other forms of angina pectoris without atherosclerosis of nonautologous biological coronary artery bypass graft(s) (I20.8)

I25.739   **Atherosclerosis of nonautologous biological coronary artery bypass graft(s) with unspecified angina pectoris** 🅰▽
> **EXCLUDES 1**   unspecified angina pectoris without atherosclerosis of nonautologous biological coronary artery bypass graft(s) (I20.9)

✓6ᵗʰ **I25.75**   **Atherosclerosis of** native **coronary artery of** transplanted heart **with angina pectoris**
> **EXCLUDES 1**   atherosclerosis of native coronary artery of transplanted heart without angina pectoris (I25.811)

I25.750   **Atherosclerosis of native coronary artery of transplanted heart with** unstable **angina** 🅰

I25.751   **Atherosclerosis of native coronary artery of transplanted heart with angina pectoris with** documented spasm 🅰

I25.758   **Atherosclerosis of native coronary artery of transplanted heart with other forms of angina pectoris** 🅰

I25.759   **Atherosclerosis of native coronary artery of transplanted heart with unspecified angina pectoris** 🅰▽

✓6ᵗʰ **I25.76**   **Atherosclerosis of** bypass graft **of coronary artery of** transplanted heart **with angina pectoris**
> **EXCLUDES 1**   atherosclerosis of bypass graft of coronary artery of transplanted heart without angina pectoris (I25.812)

I25.760   **Atherosclerosis of bypass graft of coronary artery of transplanted heart with** unstable **angina** 🅰

I25.761   **Atherosclerosis of bypass graft of coronary artery of transplanted heart with angina pectoris with** documented spasm 🅰

I25.768   **Atherosclerosis of bypass graft of coronary artery of transplanted heart with other forms of angina pectoris** 🅰

I25.769   **Atherosclerosis of bypass graft of coronary artery of transplanted heart with unspecified angina pectoris** 🅰▽

✓6ᵗʰ **I25.79**   **Atherosclerosis of** other **coronary artery bypass graft(s) with angina pectoris**

I25.790   **Atherosclerosis of other coronary artery bypass graft(s) with** unstable **angina pectoris** 🅰
> **EXCLUDES 1**   unstable angina without atherosclerosis of other coronary artery bypass graft(s) (I20.0)

I25.791   **Atherosclerosis of other coronary artery bypass graft(s) with angina pectoris with** documented spasm 🅰
> **EXCLUDES 1**   angina pectoris with documented spasm without atherosclerosis of other coronary artery bypass graft(s) (I20.1)

I25.798   **Atherosclerosis of other coronary artery bypass graft(s) with other forms of angina pectoris** 🅰
> **EXCLUDES 1**   other forms of angina pectoris without atherosclerosis of other coronary artery bypass graft(s) (I20.8)

I25.799   **Atherosclerosis of other coronary artery bypass graft(s) with unspecified angina pectoris** 🅰▽
> **EXCLUDES 1**   unspecified angina pectoris without atherosclerosis of other coronary artery bypass graft(s) (I20.9)

Ⓝ Newborn   Ⓟ Pediatric   Ⓜ Maternity   🅰 Adult   **RIC** RIC Dx   **NCDx** Noncancer Dx   **PDx** Primary Dx   **CC** RIC CC Condition   ▶◀ Revised Text   ● New Code   ▲ Revised Code Title

592   ICD-10-CM 2016

Chapter 9. Diseases of the Circulatory System

✓5th **I25.8** **Other forms of chronic ischemic heart disease**

    ✓6th **I25.81** **Atherosclerosis of** other **coronary vessels** without angina pectoris
        Use additional code, if applicable, to identify:
           coronary atherosclerosis due to calcified coronary lesion (I25.84)
           coronary atherosclerosis due to lipid rich plaque (I25.83)
        EXCLUDES 1   atherosclerotic heart disease of native coronary artery without angina pectoris (I25.10)

        I25.810 **Atherosclerosis of coronary artery bypass graft(s) without angina pectoris** `A`
             Atherosclerosis of coronary artery bypass graft NOS
             EXCLUDES 1   atherosclerosis of coronary bypass graft(s) with angina pectoris (I25.70–I25.73-, I25.79-)

        I25.811 **Atherosclerosis of** native **coronary artery of** transplanted heart **without angina pectoris** `A`
             Atherosclerosis of native coronary artery of transplanted heart NOS
             EXCLUDES 1   atherosclerosis of native coronary artery of transplanted heart with angina pectoris (I25.75-)

        I25.812 **Atherosclerosis of** bypass graft **of coronary artery of** transplanted heart **without angina pectoris** `A`
             Atherosclerosis of bypass graft of transplanted heart NOS
             EXCLUDES 1   atherosclerosis of bypass graft of transplanted heart with angina pectoris (I25.76)

    I25.82 **Chronic total occlusion of coronary artery** `NC Dx`
        Complete occlusion of coronary artery
        Total occlusion of coronary artery
        Code first coronary atherosclerosis (I25.1-, I25.7-, I25.81-)
        EXCLUDES 1   acute coronary occlusion with myocardial infarction (I21.-, I22.-)
                 acute coronary occlusion without myocardial infarction (I24.0)

    I25.83 **Coronary atherosclerosis due to** lipid rich plaque `NC Dx` `A`
        Code first coronary atherosclerosis (I25.1-, I25.7-, I25.81-)

    I25.84 **Coronary atherosclerosis due to** calcified coronary lesion `NC Dx`
        Coronary atherosclerosis due to severely calcified coronary lesion
        Code first coronary atherosclerosis (I25.1-, I25.7-, I25.81-)

    I25.89 **Other forms of chronic ischemic heart disease** `NC Dx`

  I25.9 **Chronic ischemic heart disease, unspecified** `NC Dx` ▽
      Ischemic heart disease (chronic) NOS

Pulmonary heart disease and diseases of pulmonary circulation (I26-I28)

✓4th **I26** **Pulmonary embolism**
    Pulmonary (acute) (artery)(vein) infarction
    Pulmonary (acute) (artery)(vein) thromboembolism
    Pulmonary (acute) (artery)(vein) thrombosis
    EXCLUDES 2   chronic pulmonary embolism (I27.82)
           personal history of pulmonary embolism (Z86.711)
           pulmonary embolism due to trauma (T79.0, T79.1)
           pulmonary embolism due to complications of surgical and medical care (T80.0, T81.7-, T82.8-)
           pulmonary embolism complicating abortion, ectopic or molar pregnancy (O00-O07, O08.2)
           pulmonary embolism complicating pregnancy, childbirth and the puerperium (O88.-)
           septic (non-pulmonary) arterial embolism (I76)

  ✓5th **I26.0** **Pulmonary embolism** with acute cor pulmonale

    I26.01 Septic **pulmonary embolism with acute cor pulmonale** `CC`
        Code first underlying infection
        RIC Excl: 15 Pulmonary

    I26.02 Saddle **embolus of pulmonary artery with acute cor pulmonale** `CC` `NC Dx`
        RIC Excl: 15 Pulmonary

    I26.09 **Other pulmonary embolism with acute cor pulmonale** `CC` `NC Dx`
        Acute cor pulmonale NOS
        AHA: 2014, 4Q, 21
        RIC Excl: 15 Pulmonary

  ✓5th **I26.9** **Pulmonary embolism** without acute cor pulmonale

    I26.90 Septic **pulmonary embolism without acute cor pulmonale** `CC`
        Code first underlying infection
        RIC Excl: 15 Pulmonary

    I26.92 Saddle **embolus of pulmonary artery without acute cor pulmonale** `CC` `NC Dx`
        RIC Excl: 15 Pulmonary

    I26.99 **Other pulmonary embolism without acute cor pulmonale** `CC` `NC Dx`
        Acute pulmonary embolism NOS
        Pulmonary embolism NOS
        RIC Excl: 15 Pulmonary

✓4th **I27** **Other pulmonary heart diseases**

  I27.0 **Primary pulmonary hypertension** `NC Dx`
    EXCLUDES 1   pulmonary hypertension NOS (I27.2)
           secondary pulmonary hypertension (I27.2)

  I27.1 **Kyphoscoliotic heart disease** `NC Dx`

  I27.2 **Other secondary pulmonary hypertension** `NC Dx`
    Pulmonary hypertension NOS
    Code also associated underlying condition
    AHA: 2014, 4Q, 21

  ✓5th **I27.8** **Other specified pulmonary heart diseases**

    I27.81 **Cor pulmonale (chronic)** `NC Dx`
        Cor pulmonale NOS
        EXCLUDES 1   acute cor pulmonale (I26.0-)
        AHA: 2014, 4Q, 21

    I27.82 **Chronic pulmonary embolism** `CC` `NC Dx`
        Use additional code, if applicable, for associated long-term (current) use of anticoagulants (Z79.01)
        EXCLUDES 1   personal history of pulmonary embolism (Z86.711)
        RIC Excl: 15 Pulmonary

    I27.89 **Other specified pulmonary heart diseases** `NC Dx`
        Eisenmenger's complex
        Eisenmenger's syndrome
        EXCLUDES 1   Eisenmenger's defect (Q21.8)

  I27.9 **Pulmonary heart disease, unspecified** `NC Dx` ▽
    Chronic cardiopulmonary disease

✓4th **I28** **Other diseases of pulmonary vessels**

  I28.0 **Arteriovenous fistula of pulmonary vessels** `NC Dx`
    EXCLUDES 1   congenital arteriovenous fistula (Q25.72)

  I28.1 **Aneurysm of pulmonary artery** `NC Dx`
    EXCLUDES 1   congenital aneurysm (Q25.79)
           congenital arteriovenous aneurysm (Q25.72)

  I28.8 **Other diseases of pulmonary vessels**
    Pulmonary arteritis
    Pulmonary endarteritis
    Rupture of pulmonary vessels
    Stenosis of pulmonary vessels
    Stricture of pulmonary vessels

  I28.9 **Disease of pulmonary vessels, unspecified** ▽

Other forms of heart disease (I30-I52)

✓4th **I30** **Acute pericarditis**
    INCLUDES   acute mediastinopericarditis
           acute myopericarditis
           acute pericardial effusion
           acute pleuropericarditis
           acute pneumopericarditis
    EXCLUDES 1   Dressler's syndrome (I24.1)
           rheumatic pericarditis (acute) (I01.0)

  I30.0 **Acute** nonspecific idiopathic **pericarditis**

Chapter 9. Diseases of the Circulatory System

I25.8–I30.0

Chapter 9. Diseases of the Circulatory System

I30.1   **Infective pericarditis**
Pneumococcal pericarditis
Pneumopyopericardium
Purulent pericarditis
Pyopericarditis
Pyopericardium
Pyopneumopericardium
Staphylococcal pericarditis
Streptococcal pericarditis
Suppurative pericarditis
Viral pericarditis
Use additional code (B95-B97) to identify infectious agent

I30.8   **Other forms of acute pericarditis**

I30.9   **Acute pericarditis, unspecified** ▽

✓4ᵗʰ **I31**   **Other diseases of pericardium**
EXCLUDES 1   *diseases of pericardium specified as rheumatic (I09.2)*
postcardiotomy syndrome (I97.0)
traumatic injury to pericardium (S26.-)

I31.0   **Chronic adhesive pericarditis**
Accretio cordis
Adherent pericardium
Adhesive mediastinopericarditis

I31.1   **Chronic constrictive pericarditis**
Concretio cordis
Pericardial calcification

I31.2   **Hemopericardium, not elsewhere classified**
EXCLUDES 1   *hemopericardium as current complication following*
acute myocardial infarction (I23.0)

I31.3   **Pericardial effusion (noninflammatory)**
Chylopericardium
EXCLUDES 1   *acute pericardial effusion (I30.9)*

I31.4   **Cardiac tamponade**
Code first underlying cause

I31.8   **Other specified diseases of pericardium**
Epicardial plaques
Focal pericardial adhesions

I31.9   **Disease of pericardium, unspecified** ▽
Pericarditis (chronic) NOS

I32   **Pericarditis in diseases classified elsewhere**
Code first underlying disease
EXCLUDES 1   *pericarditis (in):*
coxsackie (virus) (B33.23)
gonococcal (A54.83)
meningococcal (A39.53)
rheumatoid (arthritis) (M05.31)
syphilitic (A52.06)
systemic lupus erythematosus (M32.12)
tuberculosis (A18.84)

✓4ᵗʰ **I33**   **Acute and subacute endocarditis**
EXCLUDES 1   *acute rheumatic endocarditis (I01.1)*
endocarditis NOS (I38)

I33.0   **Acute and subacute infective endocarditis**   CC
Bacterial endocarditis (acute) (subacute)
Infective endocarditis (acute) (subacute) NOS
Endocarditis lenta (acute) (subacute)
Malignant endocarditis (acute) (subacute)
Purulent endocarditis (acute) (subacute)
Septic endocarditis (acute) (subacute)
Ulcerative endocarditis (acute) (subacute)
Vegetative endocarditis (acute) (subacute)
Use additional code (B95-B97) to identify infectious agent
RIC Excl: 14 Cardiac

I33.9   **Acute and subacute endocarditis, unspecified**   CC ▽
Acute endocarditis NOS
Acute myoendocarditis NOS
Acute periendocarditis NOS
Subacute endocarditis NOS
Subacute myoendocarditis NOS
Subacute periendocarditis NOS
RIC Excl: 14 Cardiac

✓4ᵗʰ **I34**   **Nonrheumatic mitral valve disorders**
EXCLUDES 1   *mitral valve disease (I05.9)*
mitral valve failure (I05.8)
mitral valve stenosis (I05.0)
mitral valve disorder of unspecified cause with diseases of aortic
and/or tricuspid valve(s) (I08.-)
mitral valve disorder of unspecified cause with mitral stenosis or
obstruction (I05.0)
mitral valve disorder specified as congenital (Q23.2, Q23.3)
mitral valve disorder specified as rheumatic (I05.-)

I34.0   **Nonrheumatic mitral (valve) insufficiency**
Nonrheumatic mitral (valve) incompetence NOS
Nonrheumatic mitral (valve) regurgitation NOS

I34.1   **Nonrheumatic mitral (valve) prolapse**
Floppy nonrheumatic mitral valve syndrome
EXCLUDES 1   *Marfan's syndrome (Q87.4-)*

I34.2   **Nonrheumatic mitral (valve) stenosis**

I34.8   **Other nonrheumatic mitral valve disorders**

I34.9   **Nonrheumatic mitral valve disorder, unspecified** ▽

✓4ᵗʰ **I35**   **Nonrheumatic aortic valve disorders**
EXCLUDES 1   *aortic valve disorder of unspecified cause but with diseases of*
mitral and/or tricuspid valve(s) (I08.-)
aortic valve disorder specified as congenital (Q23.0, Q23.1)
aortic valve disorder specified as rheumatic (I06.-)
hypertrophic subaortic stenosis (I42.1)

I35.0   **Nonrheumatic aortic (valve) stenosis**

I35.1   **Nonrheumatic aortic (valve) insufficiency**
Nonrheumatic aortic (valve) incompetence NOS
Nonrheumatic aortic (valve) regurgitation NOS

I35.2   **Nonrheumatic aortic (valve) stenosis with insufficiency**

I35.8   **Other nonrheumatic aortic valve disorders**

I35.9   **Nonrheumatic aortic valve disorder, unspecified** ▽

✓4ᵗʰ **I36**   **Nonrheumatic tricuspid valve disorders**
EXCLUDES 1   *tricuspid valve disorders of unspecified cause (I07.-)*
tricuspid valve disorders specified as congenital (Q22.4, Q22.8,
Q22.9)
tricuspid valve disorders specified as rheumatic (I07.-)
tricuspid valve disorders with aortic and/or mitral valve
involvement (I08.-)

I36.0   **Nonrheumatic tricuspid (valve) stenosis**

I36.1   **Nonrheumatic tricuspid (valve) insufficiency**
Nonrheumatic tricuspid (valve) incompetence
Nonrheumatic tricuspid (valve) regurgitation

I36.2   **Nonrheumatic tricuspid (valve) stenosis with insufficiency**

I36.8   **Other nonrheumatic tricuspid valve disorders**

I36.9   **Nonrheumatic tricuspid valve disorder, unspecified** ▽

✓4ᵗʰ **I37**   **Nonrheumatic pulmonary valve disorders**
EXCLUDES 1   *pulmonary valve disorder specified as congenital (Q22.1, Q22.2,*
Q22.3)
pulmonary valve disorder specified as rheumatic (I09.89)

I37.0   **Nonrheumatic pulmonary valve stenosis**

I37.1   **Nonrheumatic pulmonary valve insufficiency**
Nonrheumatic pulmonary valve incompetence
Nonrheumatic pulmonary valve regurgitation

I37.2   **Nonrheumatic pulmonary valve stenosis with insufficiency**

I37.8   **Other nonrheumatic pulmonary valve disorders**

I37.9   **Nonrheumatic pulmonary valve disorder, unspecified** ▽

I38   **Endocarditis, valve unspecified** ▽
INCLUDES   endocarditis (chronic) NOS
valvular incompetence NOS
valvular insufficiency NOS
valvular regurgitation NOS
valvular stenosis NOS
valvulitis (chronic) NOS
EXCLUDES 1   *congenital insufficiency of cardiac valve NOS (Q24.8)*
congenital stenosis of cardiac valve NOS (Q24.8)
endocardial fibroelastosis (I42.4)
endocarditis specified as rheumatic (I09.1)

Chapter 9. Diseases of the Circulatory System

I30.1–I38

Ⓝ Newborn   Ⓟ Pediatric   Ⓜ Maternity   Ⓐ Adult   **RIC** RIC Dx   **NC Dx** Noncancer Dx   **PDx** Primary Dx   **CC** RIC CC Condition   ▶◀ Revised Text   ● New Code   ▲ Revised Code Title

594   ICD-10-CM 2016

I39   *Endocarditis and heart valve disorders in diseases classified*   CC
elsewhere
> *Code first underlying disease, such as:*
> Q fever (A78)
> > **EXCLUDES 1**   endocardial involvement in:
> > > candidiasis (B37.6)
> > > gonococcal infection (A54.83)
> > > Libman-Sacks disease (M32.11)
> > > listerosis (A32.82)
> > > meningococcal infection (A39.51)
> > > rheumatoid arthritis (M05.31)
> > > syphilis (A52.03)
> > > tuberculosis (A18.84)
> > > typhoid fever (A01.02)
> > **RIC Excl:** 14 Cardiac

✓4ᵗʰ I40   **Acute myocarditis**
> **INCLUDES**   subacute myocarditis
> > **EXCLUDES 1**   acute rheumatic myocarditis (I01.2)

I40.0   **Infective** myocarditis   CC
> Septic myocarditis
> Use additional code (B95-B97) to identify infectious agent
> **RIC Excl:** 14 Cardiac

I40.1   **Isolated** myocarditis   CC
> Fiedler's myocarditis
> Giant cell myocarditis
> Idiopathic myocarditis
> **RIC Excl:** 14 Cardiac

I40.8   **Other acute myocarditis**   CC
> **RIC Excl:** 14 Cardiac

I40.9   **Acute myocarditis, unspecified**   CC ▽
> **RIC Excl:** 14 Cardiac

I41   *Myocarditis in diseases classified elsewhere*   CC
> *Code first underlying disease, such as:*
> typhus (A75.0-A75.9)
> > **EXCLUDES 1**   myocarditis (in):
> > > Chagas' disease (chronic) (B57.2)
> > > > acute (B57.0)
> > > coxsackie (virus) infection (B33.22)
> > > diphtheritic (A36.81)
> > > gonococcal (A54.83)
> > > influenzal (J09.X9, J10.82, J11.82)
> > > meningococcal (A39.52)
> > > mumps (B26.82)
> > > rheumatoid arthritis (M05.31)
> > > sarcoid (D86.85)
> > > syphilis (A52.06)
> > > toxoplasmosis (B58.81)
> > > tuberculous (A18.84)
> > **RIC Excl:** 14 Cardiac

✓4ᵗʰ I42   **Cardiomyopathy**
> **INCLUDES**   myocardiopathy
> Code first pre-existing cardiomyopathy complicating pregnancy and
> puerperium (O99.4)
> > **EXCLUDES 1**   ischemic cardiomyopathy (I25.5)
> > > peripartum cardiomyopathy (O90.3)
> > **EXCLUDES 2**   ventricular hypertrophy (I51.7)

I42.0   **Dilated** cardiomyopathy
> Congestive cardiomyopathy

I42.1   **Obstructive hypertrophic** cardiomyopathy
> Hypertrophic subaortic stenosis (idiopathic)

I42.2   **Other hypertrophic** cardiomyopathy
> Nonobstructive hypertrophic cardiomyopathy

I42.3   **Endomyocardial (eosinophilic) disease**
> Endomyocardial (tropical) fibrosis
> Löffler's endocarditis

I42.4   **Endocardial fibroelastosis**
> Congenital cardiomyopathy
> Elastomyofibrosis

I42.5   **Other restrictive** cardiomyopathy
> Constrictive cardiomyopathy NOS

I42.6   **Alcoholic** cardiomyopathy
> Code also presence of alcoholism (F10.-)

I42.7   **Cardiomyopathy** due to drug and external agent
> Code first poisoning due to drug or toxin, if applicable (T36-T65
> with fifth or sixth character 1-4 or 6)
> Use additional code for adverse effect, if applicable, to identify
> drug (T36-T50 with fifth or sixth character 5)

I42.8   **Other cardiomyopathies**

I42.9   **Cardiomyopathy, unspecified**   ▽
> Cardiomyopathy (primary) (secondary) NOS

I43   *Cardiomyopathy in diseases classified elsewhere*
> *Code first underlying disease, such as:*
> amyloidosis (E85.-)
> glycogen storage disease (E74.0)
> gout (M10.0-)
> thyrotoxicosis (E05.0-E05.9-)
> > **EXCLUDES 1**   cardiomyopathy (in):
> > > coxsackie (virus) (B33.24)
> > > diphtheria (A36.81)
> > > sarcoidosis (D86.85)
> > > tuberculosis (A18.84)

✓4ᵗʰ I44   **Atrioventricular and left bundle-branch block**

I44.0   **Atrioventricular block, first degree**

I44.1   **Atrioventricular block, second degree**
> Atrioventricular block, type I and II
> Möbitz block, type I and II
> Second degree block, type I and II
> Wenckebach's block

I44.2   **Atrioventricular block, complete**
> Complete heart block NOS
> Third degree block

✓5ᵗʰ I44.3   **Other and unspecified atrioventricular block**
> Atrioventricular block NOS

I44.30   Unspecified atrioventricular block   ▽

I44.39   Other atrioventricular block

I44.4   Left anterior fascicular block

I44.5   Left posterior fascicular block

✓5ᵗʰ I44.6   **Other and unspecified fascicular block**

I44.60   Unspecified fascicular block   ▽
> Left bundle-branch hemiblock NOS

I44.69   Other fascicular block

I44.7   Left bundle-branch block, unspecified   ▽

✓4ᵗʰ I45   **Other conduction disorders**

I45.0   **Right fascicular block**

✓5ᵗʰ I45.1   **Other and unspecified right bundle-branch block**

I45.10   Unspecified right bundle-branch block   ▽
> Right bundle-branch block NOS

I45.19   Other right bundle-branch block

I45.2   **Bifascicular block**

I45.3   **Trifascicular block**

I45.4   **Nonspecific intraventricular block**
> Bundle-branch block NOS

I45.5   **Other specified heart block**
> Sinoatrial block   Sinoauricular block
> > **EXCLUDES 1**   heart block NOS (I45.9)

I45.6   **Pre-excitation syndrome**
> Accelerated atrioventricular conduction
> Accessory atrioventricular conduction
> Anomalous atrioventricular excitation
> Lown-Ganong-Levine syndrome
> Pre-excitation atrioventricular conduction
> Wolff-Parkinson-White syndrome

✓5ᵗʰ I45.8   **Other specified conduction disorders**

I45.81   **Long QT syndrome**

I45.89   **Other specified conduction disorders**
> Atrioventricular [AV] dissociation
> Interference dissociation
> Isorhythmic dissociation
> Nonparoxysmal AV nodal tachycardia
> **AHA:** 2013, 2Q, 31

I45.9   **Conduction disorder, unspecified**   ▽
> Heart block NOS
> Stokes-Adams syndrome

✓4ᵗʰ I46   **Cardiac arrest**
> **EXCLUDES 1**   cardiogenic shock (R57.0)

I46.2   **Cardiac arrest** due to underlying cardiac condition   CC
> Code first underlying cardiac condition
> **RIC Excl:** 14 Cardiac

I46.8   **Cardiac arrest due to other underlying condition**   CC
> Code first underlying condition
> **RIC Excl:** 14 Cardiac

I46.9   **Cardiac arrest, cause unspecified**   CC ▽
> **RIC Excl:** 14 Cardiac

✓ Add'l Character Required   ✓x7ᵗʰ Placeholder Alert   RUG IV Special Care High Dx   RUG IV Clinically Complex Dx   RUG IV Special Care Low Dx   Manifestation Code   Other Specified Code   ▽ Unspecified Code

Chapter 9. Diseases of the Circulatory System

☑4ᵗʰ I47   Paroxysmal tachycardia
Code first tachycardia complicating:
   abortion or ectopic or molar pregnancy (O00-O07, O08.8)
   obstetric surgery and procedures (O75.4)
   EXCLUDES 1   *tachycardia NOS (R00.0)*
            sinoauricular tachycardia NOS (R00.0)
            sinus [sinusal] tachycardia NOS (R00.0)

I47.0   Re-entry ventricular arrhythmia

I47.1   Supraventricular tachycardia
   Atrial (paroxysmal) tachycardia
   Atrioventricular [AV] (paroxysmal) tachycardia
   Atrioventricular re-entrant (nodal) tachycardia [AVNRT] [AVRT]
   Junctional (paroxysmal) tachycardia
   Nodal (paroxysmal) tachycardia

I47.2   Ventricular tachycardia
   AHA: 2013, 3Q, 23

I47.9   Paroxysmal tachycardia, unspecified   ▽
   Bouveret (-Hoffman) syndrome

☑4ᵗʰ I48   Atrial fibrillation and flutter

I48.0   Paroxysmal atrial fibrillation

I48.1   Persistent atrial fibrillation

I48.2   Chronic atrial fibrillation
   Permanent atrial fibrillation

I48.3   Typical atrial flutter
   Type I atrial flutter

I48.4   Atypical atrial flutter
   Type II atrial flutter

☑5ᵗʰ I48.9   Unspecified atrial fibrillation and atrial flutter
   I48.91   Unspecified atrial fibrillation   ▽
   I48.92   Unspecified atrial flutter   ▽

☑4ᵗʰ I49   Other cardiac arrhythmias
Code first cardiac arrhythmia complicating:
   abortion or ectopic or molar pregnancy (O00-O07, O08.8)
   obstetric surgery and procedures (O75.4)
   EXCLUDES 1   *bradycardia NOS (R00.1)*
            neonatal dysrhythmia (P29.1-)
            sinoatrial bradycardia (R00.1)
            sinus bradycardia (R00.1)
            vagal bradycardia (R00.1)

☑5ᵗʰ I49.0   Ventricular fibrillation and flutter
   I49.01   Ventricular fibrillation   CC
      RIC Excl: 14 Cardiac
   I49.02   Ventricular flutter

I49.1   Atrial premature depolarization
   Atrial premature beats

I49.2   Junctional premature depolarization

I49.3   Ventricular premature depolarization

☑5ᵗʰ I49.4   Other and unspecified premature depolarization
   I49.40   Unspecified premature depolarization   ▽
      Premature beats NOS
   I49.49   Other premature depolarization
      Ectopic beats
      Extrasystoles
      Extrasystolic arrhythmias
      Premature contractions

I49.5   Sick sinus syndrome
   Tachycardia-bradycardia syndrome

I49.8   Other specified cardiac arrhythmias
   Coronary sinus rhythm disorder
   Ectopic rhythm disorder
   Nodal rhythm disorder

I49.9   Cardiac arrhythmia, unspecified   ▽
   Arrhythmia (cardiac) NOS

☑4ᵗʰ I50   Heart failure
Code first:
   heart failure complicating abortion or ectopic or molar pregnancy
      (O00-O07, O08.8)
   heart failure following surgery (I97.13-)
   heart failure due to hypertension (I11.0)
   heart failure due to hypertension with chronic kidney disease (I13.-)
   obstetric surgery and procedures (O75.4)
   rheumatic heart failure (I09.81)
   EXCLUDES 1   *cardiac arrest (I46.-)*
            neonatal cardiac failure (P29.0)
   AHA: 2014, 1Q, 25; 2013, 2Q, 33

I50.1   Left ventricular failure   CC NC Dx
   Cardiac asthma
   Edema of lung with heart disease NOS
   Edema of lung with heart failure
   Left heart failure
   Pulmonary edema with heart disease NOS
   Pulmonary edema with heart failure
   EXCLUDES 1   *edema of lung without heart disease or heart failure*
            (J81.-)
            pulmonary edema without heart disease or failure
            (J81.-)
   RIC Excl: 14 Cardiac

☑5ᵗʰ I50.2   Systolic (congestive) heart failure
   EXCLUDES 1   *combined systolic (congestive) and diastolic*
            (congestive) heart failure (I50.4-)
   ¹⁰ **I50.20   Unspecified systolic (congestive) heart failure**   CC ▽
      RIC Excl: 14 Cardiac
   I50.21   Acute systolic (congestive) heart failure   CC NC Dx
      RIC Excl: 14 Cardiac
   I50.22   Chronic systolic (congestive) heart failure   CC NC Dx
      RIC Excl: 14 Cardiac
   I50.23   Acute on chronic systolic (congestive)   CC NC Dx
      heart failure
      RIC Excl: 14 Cardiac

☑5ᵗʰ I50.3   Diastolic (congestive) heart failure
   EXCLUDES 1   *combined systolic (congestive) and diastolic*
            (congestive) heart failure (I50.4-)
   ¹⁰ **I50.30   Unspecified diastolic (congestive) heart**   CC ▽
      failure
      RIC Excl: 14 Cardiac
   I50.31   Acute diastolic (congestive) heart failure   CC NC Dx
      RIC Excl: 14 Cardiac
   I50.32   Chronic diastolic (congestive) heart failure   CC NC Dx
      RIC Excl: 14 Cardiac
   I50.33   Acute on chronic diastolic (congestive)   CC NC Dx
      heart failure
      RIC Excl: 14 Cardiac

☑5ᵗʰ I50.4   Combined systolic (congestive) and diastolic (congestive)
   heart failure
   ¹⁰ **I50.40   Unspecified combined systolic (congestive)**   CC ▽
      and diastolic (congestive) heart failure
      RIC Excl: 14 Cardiac
   I50.41   Acute combined systolic (congestive) and   CC NC Dx
      diastolic (congestive) heart failure
      RIC Excl: 14 Cardiac
   I50.42   Chronic combined systolic (congestive) and   CC NC Dx
      diastolic (congestive) heart failure
      RIC Excl: 14 Cardiac
   I50.43   Acute on chronic combined systolic   CC NC Dx
      (congestive) and diastolic (congestive) heart failure
      RIC Excl: 14 Cardiac

¹⁰ **I50.9   Heart failure, unspecified**   ▽
   Biventricular (heart) failure NOS
   Cardiac, heart or myocardial failure NOS
   Congestive heart disease
   Congestive heart failure NOS
   Right ventricular failure (secondary to left heart failure)
   EXCLUDES 1   *fluid overload (E87.70)*
   AHA: 2014, 4Q, 21; 2012, 4Q, 92

☑4ᵗʰ I51   Complications and ill-defined descriptions of heart disease
   EXCLUDES 1   *any condition in I51.4-I51.9 due to hypertension (I11.-)*
            any condition in I51.4-I51.9 due to hypertension and chronic
            kidney disease (I13.-)
            heart disease specified as rheumatic (I00-I09)

I51.0   Cardiac septal defect, acquired   A
   Acquired septal atrial defect (old)
   Acquired septal auricular defect (old)
   Acquired septal ventricular defect (old)
   EXCLUDES 1   *cardiac septal defect as current complication following*
            acute myocardial infarction (I23.1, I23.2)

I51.1   Rupture of chordae tendineae, not elsewhere classified   NC Dx
   EXCLUDES 1   *rupture of chordae tendineae as current complication*
            following acute myocardial infarction (I23.4)

I51.2   Rupture of papillary muscle, not elsewhere classified   NC Dx
   EXCLUDES 1   *rupture of papillary muscle as current complication*
            following acute myocardial infarction (I23.5)

----

¹⁰ Hospice questionable admission diagnosis

I51.3 Intracardiac thrombosis, not elsewhere classified   NC Dx A
   Apical thrombosis (old)
   Atrial thrombosis (old)
   Auricular thrombosis (old)
   Mural thrombosis (old)
   Ventricular thrombosis (old)
   EXCLUDES 1 intracardiac thrombosis as current complication
        following acute myocardial infarction (I23.6)
   AHA: 2013, 1Q, 24

I51.4 Myocarditis, unspecified   NC Dx ▽
   Chronic (interstitial) myocarditis   Myocarditis NOS
   Myocardial fibrosis
   EXCLUDES 1 acute or subacute myocarditis (I40.-)

I51.5 Myocardial degeneration   NC Dx
   Fatty degeneration of heart or myocardium
   Myocardial disease
   Senile degeneration of heart or myocardium

I51.7 Cardiomegaly
   Cardiac dilatation
   Cardiac hypertrophy
   Ventricular dilatation

✓5ᵗʰ **I51.8 Other ill-defined heart diseases**

   I51.81 Takotsubo syndrome
      Reversible left ventricular dysfunction following
         sudden emotional stress
      Stress induced cardiomyopathy
      Takotsubo cardiomyopathy
      Transient left ventricular apical ballooning syndrome

   I51.89 Other ill-defined heart diseases
      Carditis (acute)(chronic)
      Pancarditis (acute)(chronic)

I51.9 Heart disease, unspecified   ▽

I52 Other heart disorders in diseases classified elsewhere
   Code first underlying disease, such as:
      congenital syphilis (A50.5)
      mucopolysaccharidosis (E76.3)
      schistosomiasis (B65.0-B65.9)
   EXCLUDES 1 heart disease (in):
         gonococcal infection (A54.83)
         meningococcal infection (A39.50)
         rheumatoid arthritis (M05.31)
         syphilis (A52.06)

Cerebrovascular diseases (I60-I69)

Use additional code to identify presence of:
   alcohol abuse and dependence (F10.-)
   exposure to environmental tobacco smoke (Z77.22)
   history of tobacco use (Z87.891)
   hypertension (I10-I15)
   occupational exposure to environmental tobacco smoke (Z57.31)
   tobacco dependence (F17.-)
   tobacco use (Z72.0)
   EXCLUDES 1 transient cerebral ischemic attacks and related syndromes (G45.-)
      traumatic intracranial hemorrhage (S06.-)
   AHA: 2014, 3Q, 5; 2012, 4Q, 91-92

✓4ᵗʰ **I60 Nontraumatic subarachnoid hemorrhage**
   INCLUDES ruptured cerebral aneurysm
   EXCLUDES 1 sequelae of subarachnoid hemorrhage (I69.0-)
      syphilitic ruptured cerebral aneurysm (A52.05)

   ✓5ᵗʰ **I60.0 Nontraumatic subarachnoid hemorrhage from carotid siphon and bifurcation**

      I60.00 Nontraumatic subarachnoid hemorrhage   CC NC Dx ▽
         from unspecified carotid siphon and bifurcation
         RIC Excl: 01 Stroke; 02 Traumatic brain injury; 03
         Non-traumatic brain injury

      I60.01 Nontraumatic subarachnoid hemorrhage   CC NC Dx
         from right carotid siphon and bifurcation
         RIC Excl: 01 Stroke; 02 Traumatic brain injury; 03
         Non-traumatic brain injury

      I60.02 Nontraumatic subarachnoid hemorrhage   CC NC Dx
         from left carotid siphon and bifurcation
         RIC Excl: 01 Stroke; 02 Traumatic brain injury; 03
         Non-traumatic brain injury

   ✓5ᵗʰ **I60.1 Nontraumatic subarachnoid hemorrhage from middle cerebral artery**

      I60.10 Nontraumatic subarachnoid hemorrhage   CC NC Dx ▽
         from unspecified middle cerebral artery
         RIC Excl: 01 Stroke; 02 Traumatic brain injury; 03
         Non-traumatic brain injury

      I60.11 Nontraumatic subarachnoid hemorrhage   CC NC Dx
         from right middle cerebral artery
         RIC Excl: 01 Stroke; 02 Traumatic brain injury; 03
         Non-traumatic brain injury

      I60.12 Nontraumatic subarachnoid hemorrhage   CC NC Dx
         from left middle cerebral artery
         RIC Excl: 01 Stroke; 02 Traumatic brain injury; 03
         Non-traumatic brain injury

   ✓5ᵗʰ **I60.2 Nontraumatic subarachnoid hemorrhage from anterior communicating artery**

      I60.20 Nontraumatic subarachnoid hemorrhage   CC NC Dx ▽
         from unspecified anterior communicating artery
         RIC Excl: 01 Stroke; 02 Traumatic brain injury; 03
         Non-traumatic brain injury

      I60.21 Nontraumatic subarachnoid hemorrhage   CC NC Dx
         from right anterior communicating artery
         RIC Excl: 01 Stroke; 02 Traumatic brain injury; 03
         Non-traumatic brain injury

      I60.22 Nontraumatic subarachnoid hemorrhage   CC NC Dx
         from left anterior communicating artery
         RIC Excl: 01 Stroke; 02 Traumatic brain injury; 03
         Non-traumatic brain injury

   ✓5ᵗʰ **I60.3 Nontraumatic subarachnoid hemorrhage from posterior communicating artery**

      I60.30 Nontraumatic subarachnoid hemorrhage   CC NC Dx ▽
         from unspecified posterior communicating artery
         RIC Excl: 01 Stroke; 02 Traumatic brain injury; 03
         Non-traumatic brain injury

      I60.31 Nontraumatic subarachnoid hemorrhage   CC NC Dx
         from right posterior communicating artery
         RIC Excl: 01 Stroke; 02 Traumatic brain injury; 03
         Non-traumatic brain injury

      I60.32 Nontraumatic subarachnoid hemorrhage   CC NC Dx
         from left posterior communicating artery
         RIC Excl: 01 Stroke; 02 Traumatic brain injury; 03
         Non-traumatic brain injury

   I60.4 Nontraumatic subarachnoid hemorrhage from basilar artery   CC NC Dx
      RIC Excl: 01 Stroke; 02 Traumatic brain injury; 03 Non-traumatic
      brain injury

   ✓5ᵗʰ **I60.5 Nontraumatic subarachnoid hemorrhage from vertebral artery**

      I60.50 Nontraumatic subarachnoid hemorrhage   CC NC Dx ▽
         from unspecified vertebral artery
         RIC Excl: 01 Stroke; 02 Traumatic brain injury; 03
         Non-traumatic brain injury

      I60.51 Nontraumatic subarachnoid hemorrhage   CC NC Dx
         from right vertebral artery
         RIC Excl: 01 Stroke; 02 Traumatic brain injury; 03
         Non-traumatic brain injury

      I60.52 Nontraumatic subarachnoid hemorrhage   CC NC Dx
         from left vertebral artery
         RIC Excl: 01 Stroke; 02 Traumatic brain injury; 03
         Non-traumatic brain injury

   I60.6 Nontraumatic subarachnoid hemorrhage from other intracranial arteries   CC NC Dx
      RIC Excl: 01 Stroke; 02 Traumatic brain injury; 03 Non-traumatic
      brain injury

   I60.7 Nontraumatic subarachnoid hemorrhage from unspecified intracranial artery   CC NC Dx ▽
      Ruptured (congenital) berry aneurysm
      Ruptured (congenital) cerebral aneurysm
      Subarachnoid hemorrhage (nontraumatic) from cerebral artery
         NOS
      Subarachnoid hemorrhage (nontraumatic) from communicating
         artery NOS
      EXCLUDES 1 berry aneurysm, nonruptured (I67.1)
      RIC Excl: 01 Stroke; 02 Traumatic brain injury; 03 Non-traumatic
      brain injury

   I60.8 Other nontraumatic subarachnoid hemorrhage   CC NC Dx
      Meningeal hemorrhage
      Rupture of cerebral arteriovenous malformation
      RIC Excl: 01 Stroke; 02 Traumatic brain injury; 03 Non-traumatic
      brain injury

   I60.9 Nontraumatic subarachnoid hemorrhage, unspecified   CC NC Dx ▽
      RIC Excl: 01 Stroke; 02 Traumatic brain injury; 03 Non-traumatic
      brain injury

✓4th I61 **Nontraumatic intracerebral hemorrhage**
    EXCLUDES 1 *sequelae of intracerebral hemorrhage (I69.1-)*

  I61.0 **Nontraumatic intracerebral hemorrhage in** `CC` `NC Dx`
    hemisphere, subcortical
    Deep intracerebral hemorrhage (nontraumatic)
    RIC Excl: 01 Stroke; 02 Traumatic brain injury; 03 Non-traumatic brain injury

  I61.1 **Nontraumatic intracerebral hemorrhage in** `CC` `NC Dx`
    hemisphere, cortical
    Cerebral lobe hemorrhage (nontraumatic)
    Superficial intracerebral hemorrhage (nontraumatic)
    RIC Excl: 01 Stroke; 02 Traumatic brain injury; 03 Non-traumatic brain injury

  I61.2 **Nontraumatic intracerebral hemorrhage in** `CC` `NC Dx` ▽
    hemisphere, unspecified
    RIC Excl: 01 Stroke; 02 Traumatic brain injury; 03 Non-traumatic brain injury

  I61.3 **Nontraumatic intracerebral hemorrhage in** `CC` `NC Dx`
    brain stem
    RIC Excl: 01 Stroke; 02 Traumatic brain injury; 03 Non-traumatic brain injury

  I61.4 **Nontraumatic intracerebral hemorrhage in** `CC` `NC Dx`
    cerebellum
    RIC Excl: 01 Stroke; 02 Traumatic brain injury; 03 Non-traumatic brain injury

  I61.5 **Nontraumatic intracerebral hemorrhage,** `CC` `NC Dx`
    intraventricular
    RIC Excl: 01 Stroke; 02 Traumatic brain injury; 03 Non-traumatic brain injury

  I61.6 **Nontraumatic intracerebral hemorrhage,** `CC` `NC Dx`
    multiple localized
    RIC Excl: 01 Stroke; 02 Traumatic brain injury; 03 Non-traumatic brain injury

  I61.8 **Other nontraumatic intracerebral hemorrhage** `CC` `NC Dx`
    RIC Excl: 01 Stroke; 02 Traumatic brain injury; 03 Non-traumatic brain injury

  I61.9 **Nontraumatic intracerebral hemorrhage,** `CC` `NC Dx` ▽
    unspecified
    RIC Excl: 01 Stroke; 02 Traumatic brain injury; 03 Non-traumatic brain injury

✓4th I62 **Other and unspecified nontraumatic intracranial hemorrhage**
    EXCLUDES 1 *sequelae of intracranial hemorrhage (I69.2)*

  ✓5th I62.0 **Nontraumatic subdural hemorrhage**

    I62.00 **Nontraumatic subdural hemorrhage,** `CC` `NC Dx` ▽
      unspecified
      RIC Excl: 01 Stroke; 02 Traumatic brain injury; 03 Non-traumatic brain injury

    I62.01 **Nontraumatic acute subdural hemorrhage** `CC` `NC Dx`
      RIC Excl: 01 Stroke; 02 Traumatic brain injury; 03 Non-traumatic brain injury

    I62.02 **Nontraumatic subacute subdural** `CC` `NC Dx`
      hemorrhage
      RIC Excl: 01 Stroke; 02 Traumatic brain injury; 03 Non-traumatic brain injury

    I62.03 **Nontraumatic chronic subdural** `CC` `NC Dx`
      hemorrhage
      RIC Excl: 01 Stroke; 02 Traumatic brain injury; 03 Non-traumatic brain injury

  I62.1 **Nontraumatic extradural hemorrhage** `CC` `NC Dx`
    Nontraumatic epidural hemorrhage
    RIC Excl: 01 Stroke; 02 Traumatic brain injury; 03 Non-traumatic brain injury

  ¹⁰ **I62.9** **Nontraumatic intracranial hemorrhage, unspecified** ▽

✓4th I63 **Cerebral infarction**
    INCLUDES occlusion and stenosis of cerebral and precerebral arteries, resulting in cerebral infarction
    Use additional code, if applicable, to identify status post administration of tPA (rtPA) in a different facility within the last 24 hours prior to admission to current facility (Z92.82)
    EXCLUDES 1 *sequelae of cerebral infarction (I69.3-)*
    AHA: 2014, 1Q, 23

  ✓5th I63.0 **Cerebral infarction due to thrombosis of precerebral arteries**

    I63.00 **Cerebral infarction due to thrombosis of** `CC` `NC Dx` ▽
      unspecified precerebral artery
      RIC Excl: 01 Stroke

    ✓6th I63.01 **Cerebral infarction due to thrombosis of vertebral artery**

      I63.011 **Cerebral infarction due to** `CC` `NC Dx` `A`
        thrombosis of right vertebral artery
        RIC Excl: 01 Stroke

      I63.012 **Cerebral infarction due to** `CC` `NC Dx` `A`
        thrombosis of left vertebral artery
        RIC Excl: 01 Stroke

      I63.019 **Cerebral infarction due to** `CC` `NC Dx` `A` ▽
        thrombosis of unspecified vertebral artery
        RIC Excl: 01 Stroke

    I63.02 **Cerebral infarction due to thrombosis of** `CC` `NC Dx` `A`
      basilar artery
      RIC Excl: 01 Stroke

    ✓6th I63.03 **Cerebral infarction due to thrombosis of carotid artery**

      I63.031 **Cerebral infarction due to** `CC` `NC Dx`
        thrombosis of right carotid artery
        RIC Excl: 01 Stroke

      I63.032 **Cerebral infarction due to** `CC` `NC Dx`
        thrombosis of left carotid artery
        RIC Excl: 01 Stroke

      I63.039 **Cerebral infarction due to** `CC` `NC Dx` ▽
        thrombosis of unspecified carotid artery
        RIC Excl: 01 Stroke

    I63.09 **Cerebral infarction due to thrombosis of** `CC` `NC Dx`
      other precerebral artery
      RIC Excl: 01 Stroke

  ✓5th I63.1 **Cerebral infarction due to embolism of precerebral arteries**

    I63.10 **Cerebral infarction due to embolism of** `CC` `NC Dx` ▽
      unspecified precerebral artery
      RIC Excl: 01 Stroke

    ✓6th I63.11 **Cerebral infarction due to embolism of vertebral artery**

      I63.111 **Cerebral infarction due to** `CC` `NC Dx` `A`
        embolism of right vertebral artery
        RIC Excl: 01 Stroke

      I63.112 **Cerebral infarction due to** `CC` `NC Dx` `A`
        embolism of left vertebral artery
        RIC Excl: 01 Stroke

      I63.119 **Cerebral infarction due to** `CC` `NC Dx` `A` ▽
        embolism of unspecified vertebral artery
        RIC Excl: 01 Stroke

    I63.12 **Cerebral infarction due to embolism of** `CC` `NC Dx` `A`
      basilar artery
      RIC Excl: 01 Stroke

    ✓6th I63.13 **Cerebral infarction due to embolism of carotid artery**

      I63.131 **Cerebral infarction due to** `CC` `NC Dx`
        embolism of right carotid artery
        RIC Excl: 01 Stroke

      I63.132 **Cerebral infarction due to** `CC` `NC Dx`
        embolism of left carotid artery
        RIC Excl: 01 Stroke

      I63.139 **Cerebral infarction due to** `CC` `NC Dx` ▽
        embolism of unspecified carotid artery
        RIC Excl: 01 Stroke

    I63.19 **Cerebral infarction due to embolism of** `CC` `NC Dx`
      other precerebral artery
      RIC Excl: 01 Stroke

  ✓5th I63.2 **Cerebral infarction due to unspecified occlusion or stenosis of precerebral arteries**

    I63.20 **Cerebral infarction due to unspecified** `CC` `NC Dx` ▽
      occlusion or stenosis of unspecified precerebral arteries
      RIC Excl: 01 Stroke

    ✓6th I63.21 **Cerebral infarction due to unspecified occlusion or stenosis of vertebral arteries**

      I63.211 **Cerebral infarction due to** `CC` `NC Dx` `A`
        unspecified occlusion or stenosis of right vertebral arteries
        RIC Excl: 01 Stroke

---

¹⁰ Hospice questionable admission diagnosis

I63.212	Cerebral infarction due to unspecified occlusion or stenosis of left vertebral arteries	CC NC Dx A

RIC Excl: 01 Stroke

I63.219	Cerebral infarction due to unspecified occlusion or stenosis of unspecified vertebral arteries	CC NC Dx A ▽

RIC Excl: 01 Stroke

I63.22 Cerebral infarction due to unspecified occlusion or stenosis of basilar arteries   CC NC Dx A
RIC Excl: 01 Stroke

✓6ᵗʰ **I63.23** Cerebral infarction due to unspecified occlusion or stenosis of carotid arteries

I63.231	Cerebral infarction due to unspecified occlusion or stenosis of right carotid arteries	CC NC Dx

RIC Excl: 01 Stroke

I63.232	Cerebral infarction due to unspecified occlusion or stenosis of left carotid arteries	CC NC Dx

RIC Excl: 01 Stroke

I63.239	Cerebral infarction due to unspecified occlusion or stenosis of unspecified carotid arteries	CC NC Dx ▽

RIC Excl: 01 Stroke

I63.29 Cerebral infarction due to unspecified occlusion or stenosis of other precerebral arteries   CC NC Dx
RIC Excl: 01 Stroke

✓5ᵗʰ **I63.3** Cerebral infarction due to thrombosis of cerebral arteries

I63.30	Cerebral infarction due to thrombosis of unspecified cerebral artery	CC NC Dx A ▽

RIC Excl: 01 Stroke

✓6ᵗʰ **I63.31** Cerebral infarction due to thrombosis of middle cerebral artery

I63.311	Cerebral infarction due to thrombosis of right middle cerebral artery	CC NC Dx A

RIC Excl: 01 Stroke

I63.312	Cerebral infarction due to thrombosis of left middle cerebral artery	CC NC Dx A

RIC Excl: 01 Stroke

I63.319	Cerebral infarction due to thrombosis of unspecified middle cerebral artery	CC NC Dx A ▽

RIC Excl: 01 Stroke

✓6ᵗʰ **I63.32** Cerebral infarction due to thrombosis of anterior cerebral artery

I63.321	Cerebral infarction due to thrombosis of right anterior cerebral artery	CC NC Dx A

RIC Excl: 01 Stroke

I63.322	Cerebral infarction due to thrombosis of left anterior cerebral artery	CC NC Dx A

RIC Excl: 01 Stroke

I63.329	Cerebral infarction due to thrombosis of unspecified anterior cerebral artery	CC NC Dx A ▽

RIC Excl: 01 Stroke

✓6ᵗʰ **I63.33** Cerebral infarction due to thrombosis of posterior cerebral artery

I63.331	Cerebral infarction due to thrombosis of right posterior cerebral artery	CC NC Dx A

RIC Excl: 01 Stroke

I63.332	Cerebral infarction due to thrombosis of left posterior cerebral artery	CC NC Dx A

RIC Excl: 01 Stroke

I63.339	Cerebral infarction due to thrombosis of unspecified posterior cerebral artery	CC NC Dx A ▽

RIC Excl: 01 Stroke

✓6ᵗʰ **I63.34** Cerebral infarction due to thrombosis of cerebellar artery

I63.341	Cerebral infarction due to thrombosis of right cerebellar artery	CC NC Dx A

RIC Excl: 01 Stroke

I63.342	Cerebral infarction due to thrombosis of left cerebellar artery	CC NC Dx A

RIC Excl: 01 Stroke

I63.349	Cerebral infarction due to thrombosis of unspecified cerebellar artery	CC NC Dx A ▽

RIC Excl: 01 Stroke

I63.39 Cerebral infarction due to thrombosis of other cerebral artery   CC NC Dx A
RIC Excl: 01 Stroke

✓5ᵗʰ **I63.4** Cerebral infarction due to embolism of cerebral arteries

I63.40	Cerebral infarction due to embolism of unspecified cerebral artery	CC NC Dx A ▽

RIC Excl: 01 Stroke

✓6ᵗʰ **I63.41** Cerebral infarction due to embolism of middle cerebral artery

I63.411	Cerebral infarction due to embolism of right middle cerebral artery	CC NC Dx A

RIC Excl: 01 Stroke

I63.412	Cerebral infarction due to embolism of left middle cerebral artery	CC NC Dx A

RIC Excl: 01 Stroke

I63.419	Cerebral infarction due to embolism of unspecified middle cerebral artery	CC NC Dx A ▽

RIC Excl: 01 Stroke

✓6ᵗʰ **I63.42** Cerebral infarction due to embolism of anterior cerebral artery

I63.421	Cerebral infarction due to embolism of right anterior cerebral artery	CC NC Dx A

RIC Excl: 01 Stroke

I63.422	Cerebral infarction due to embolism of left anterior cerebral artery	CC NC Dx A

RIC Excl: 01 Stroke

I63.429	Cerebral infarction due to embolism of unspecified anterior cerebral artery	CC NC Dx A ▽

RIC Excl: 01 Stroke

✓6ᵗʰ **I63.43** Cerebral infarction due to embolism of posterior cerebral artery

I63.431	Cerebral infarction due to embolism of right posterior cerebral artery	CC NC Dx A

RIC Excl: 01 Stroke

I63.432	Cerebral infarction due to embolism of left posterior cerebral artery	CC NC Dx A

RIC Excl: 01 Stroke

I63.439	Cerebral infarction due to unspecified embolism of posterior cerebral artery	CC NC Dx A ▽

RIC Excl: 01 Stroke

✓6ᵗʰ **I63.44** Cerebral infarction due to embolism of cerebellar artery

I63.441	Cerebral infarction due to embolism of right cerebellar artery	CC NC Dx A

RIC Excl: 01 Stroke

I63.442	Cerebral infarction due to embolism of left cerebellar artery	CC NC Dx A

RIC Excl: 01 Stroke

I63.449	Cerebral infarction due to unspecified embolism of cerebellar artery	CC NC Dx A ▽

RIC Excl: 01 Stroke

I63.49 Cerebral infarction due to embolism of other cerebral artery   CC NC Dx A
RIC Excl: 01 Stroke

☑ Add'l Character Required   ✓x7ᵗʰ Placeholder Alert   RUG IV Special Care High Dx   RUG IV Clinically Complex Dx   RUG IV Special Care Low Dx   Manifestation Code   Other Specified Code   ▽ Unspecified Code

Chapter 9. Diseases of the Circulatory System

I63.5–I66.9

✓5ᵗʰ **I63.5 Cerebral infarction due to** unspecified occlusion or stenosis of cerebral **arteries**

    I63.50 Cerebral infarction due to unspecified occlusion or stenosis of unspecified cerebral artery CC NC Dx ▽
      RIC Excl: 01 Stroke

    ✓6ᵗʰ **I63.51 Cerebral infarction due to unspecified occlusion or stenosis of** middle **cerebral artery**

      I63.511 Cerebral infarction due to unspecified occlusion or stenosis of right **middle cerebral artery** CC NC Dx
       RIC Excl: 01 Stroke

      I63.512 Cerebral infarction due to unspecified occlusion or stenosis of left **middle cerebral artery** CC NC Dx
       RIC Excl: 01 Stroke

      I63.519 Cerebral infarction due to unspecified occlusion or stenosis of unspecified middle cerebral artery CC NC Dx ▽
       RIC Excl: 01 Stroke

    ✓6ᵗʰ **I63.52 Cerebral infarction due to unspecified occlusion or stenosis of** anterior **cerebral artery**

      I63.521 Cerebral infarction due to unspecified occlusion or stenosis of right **anterior cerebral artery** CC NC Dx
       RIC Excl: 01 Stroke

      I63.522 Cerebral infarction due to unspecified occlusion or stenosis of left **anterior cerebral artery** CC NC Dx
       RIC Excl: 01 Stroke

      I63.529 Cerebral infarction due to unspecified occlusion or stenosis of unspecified anterior cerebral artery CC NC Dx ▽
       RIC Excl: 01 Stroke

    ✓6ᵗʰ **I63.53 Cerebral infarction due to unspecified occlusion or stenosis of** posterior **cerebral artery**

      I63.531 Cerebral infarction due to unspecified occlusion or stenosis of right **posterior cerebral artery** CC NC Dx
       RIC Excl: 01 Stroke

      I63.532 Cerebral infarction due to unspecified occlusion or stenosis of left **posterior cerebral artery** CC NC Dx
       RIC Excl: 01 Stroke

      I63.539 Cerebral infarction due to unspecified occlusion or stenosis of unspecified posterior cerebral artery CC NC Dx ▽
       RIC Excl: 01 Stroke

    ✓6ᵗʰ **I63.54 Cerebral infarction due to unspecified occlusion or stenosis of** cerebellar **artery**

      I63.541 Cerebral infarction due to unspecified occlusion or stenosis of right **cerebellar artery** CC NC Dx
       RIC Excl: 01 Stroke

      I63.542 Cerebral infarction due to unspecified occlusion or stenosis of left **cerebellar artery** CC NC Dx
       RIC Excl: 01 Stroke

      I63.549 Cerebral infarction due to unspecified occlusion or stenosis of unspecified cerebellar artery CC NC Dx ▽
       RIC Excl: 01 Stroke

    I63.59 Cerebral infarction due to unspecified occlusion or stenosis of other cerebral artery CC NC Dx
      RIC Excl: 01 Stroke

I63.6 Cerebral infarction due to cerebral venous thrombosis, nonpyogenic CC NC Dx A
    RIC Excl: 01 Stroke

I63.8 Other cerebral infarction CC NC Dx
    RIC Excl: 01 Stroke

I63.9 Cerebral infarction, unspecified CC NC Dx ▽
    Stroke NOS
    AHA: 2015, 1Q, 25
    RIC Excl: 01 Stroke

✓4ᵗʰ **I65 Occlusion and stenosis of** precerebral **arteries, not resulting in** cerebral **infarction**
    INCLUDES   embolism of precerebral artery
      narrowing of precerebral artery
      obstruction (complete) (partial) of precerebral artery
      thrombosis of precerebral artery
    EXCLUDES 1   insufficiency, NOS, of precerebral artery (G45.-)
      insufficiency of precerebral arteries causing cerebral infarction (I63.0-I63.2)

    ✓5ᵗʰ **I65.0 Occlusion and stenosis of** vertebral **artery**

      I65.01 Occlusion and stenosis of right **vertebral artery** A
      I65.02 Occlusion and stenosis of left **vertebral artery** A
      I65.03 Occlusion and stenosis of bilateral **vertebral arteries** A
      I65.09 Occlusion and stenosis of unspecified vertebral artery A ▽

    I65.1 Occlusion and stenosis of basilar **artery** NC Dx A

    ✓5ᵗʰ **I65.2 Occlusion and stenosis of** carotid **artery**

      I65.21 Occlusion and stenosis of right **carotid artery** A
      I65.22 Occlusion and stenosis of left **carotid artery** A
      I65.23 Occlusion and stenosis of bilateral **carotid arteries** A
      I65.29 Occlusion and stenosis of unspecified carotid artery A ▽

    I65.8 Occlusion and stenosis of other precerebral arteries NC Dx A

    I65.9 Occlusion and stenosis of unspecified precerebral artery A ▽
      Occlusion and stenosis of precerebral artery NOS

✓4ᵗʰ **I66 Occlusion and stenosis of** cerebral **arteries, not resulting in** cerebral **infarction**
    INCLUDES   embolism of cerebral artery
      narrowing of cerebral artery
      obstruction (complete) (partial) of cerebral artery
      thrombosis of cerebral artery
    EXCLUDES 1   occlusion and stenosis of cerebral artery causing cerebral infarction (I63.3-I63.5)

    ✓5ᵗʰ **I66.0 Occlusion and stenosis of** middle **cerebral artery**

      I66.01 Occlusion and stenosis of right **middle cerebral artery** A
      I66.02 Occlusion and stenosis of left **middle cerebral artery** A
      I66.03 Occlusion and stenosis of bilateral **middle cerebral arteries** A
      I66.09 Occlusion and stenosis of unspecified middle cerebral artery A ▽

    ✓5ᵗʰ **I66.1 Occlusion and stenosis of** anterior **cerebral artery**

      I66.11 Occlusion and stenosis of right **anterior cerebral artery** A
      I66.12 Occlusion and stenosis of left **anterior cerebral artery** A
      I66.13 Occlusion and stenosis of bilateral **anterior cerebral arteries** A
      I66.19 Occlusion and stenosis of unspecified anterior cerebral artery A ▽

    ✓5ᵗʰ **I66.2 Occlusion and stenosis of** posterior **cerebral artery**

      I66.21 Occlusion and stenosis of right **posterior cerebral artery** A
      I66.22 Occlusion and stenosis of left **posterior cerebral artery** A
      I66.23 Occlusion and stenosis of bilateral **posterior cerebral arteries** A
      I66.29 Occlusion and stenosis of unspecified posterior cerebral artery A ▽

    I66.3 Occlusion and stenosis of cerebellar **arteries** A

    I66.8 Occlusion and stenosis of other cerebral arteries A
      Occlusion and stenosis of perforating arteries

    I66.9 Occlusion and stenosis of unspecified cerebral artery A ▽

N Newborn   P Pediatric   M Maternity   A Adult   RIC RIC Dx   NC Dx Noncancer Dx   PDx Primary Dx   CC RIC CC Condition   ►◄ Revised Text   ● New Code   ▲ Revised Code Title

600   ICD-10-CM 2016

☑4ᵗʰ I67 Other cerebrovascular diseases

    EXCLUDES 1   *sequelae of the listed conditions (I69.8)*

  I67.0 Dissection of cerebral arteries, nonruptured

    EXCLUDES 1   *ruptured cerebral arteries (I60.7)*

  I67.1 Cerebral aneurysm, nonruptured

    Cerebral aneurysm NOS
    Cerebral arteriovenous fistula, acquired
    Internal carotid artery aneurysm, intracranial portion
    Internal carotid artery aneurysm, NOS

    EXCLUDES 1   *congenital cerebral aneurysm, nonruptured (Q28.-)*
        ruptured cerebral aneurysm (I60.7)

  I67.2 Cerebral atherosclerosis   `NC Dx` `A`

    Atheroma of cerebral and precerebral arteries

  I67.3 Progressive vascular leukoencephalopathy

    Binswanger's disease

  I67.4 Hypertensive encephalopathy   `NC Dx`

  I67.5 Moyamoya disease   `NC Dx`

  I67.6 Nonpyogenic thrombosis of intracranial venous system   `NC Dx`

    Nonpyogenic thrombosis of cerebral vein
    Nonpyogenic thrombosis of intracranial venous sinus

    EXCLUDES 1   *nonpyogenic thrombosis of intracranial venous system*
        causing infarction (I63.6)

  I67.7 Cerebral arteritis, not elsewhere classified   `NC Dx`

    Granulomatous angiitis of the nervous system

    EXCLUDES 1   *allergic granulomatous angiitis (M30.1)*

  ☑5ᵗʰ I67.8 Other specified cerebrovascular diseases

    I67.81 Acute cerebrovascular insufficiency   `NC Dx`

      Acute cerebrovascular insufficiency unspecified
      as to location or reversibility

    I67.82 Cerebral ischemia   `NC Dx`

      Chronic cerebral ischemia

    I67.83 Posterior reversible encephalopathy syndrome

      PRES

    ☑6ᵗʰ I67.84 Cerebral vasospasm and vasoconstriction

      I67.841 Reversible cerebrovascular   `A`
        vasoconstriction syndrome

        Call-Fleming syndrome
        Code first underlying condition, if
          applicable, such as eclampsia
          (O15.00-O15.9)

      I67.848 Other cerebrovascular vasospasm   `A`
        and vasoconstriction

    I67.89 Other cerebrovascular disease   `CC` `NC Dx`

      RIC Excl: 01 Stroke

  ¹⁰ I67.9 Cerebrovascular disease, unspecified   ▽

☑4ᵗʰ I68 Cerebrovascular disorders in diseases classified elsewhere

  I68.0 Cerebral amyloid angiopathy

    Code first underlying amyloidosis (E85.-)

  I68.2 Cerebral arteritis in other diseases classified elsewhere

    Code first underlying disease

    EXCLUDES 1   *cerebral arteritis (in):*
        listerosis (A32.89)
        systemic lupus erythematosus (M32.19)
        syphilis (A52.04)
        tuberculosis (A18.89)

  I68.8 Other cerebrovascular disorders in diseases classified elsewhere

    Code first underlying disease

    EXCLUDES 1   *syphilitic cerebral aneurysm (A52.05)*

☑4ᵗʰ I69 Sequelae of cerebrovascular disease

  NOTE   Category I69 is to be used to indicate conditions in I60-I67 as
    the cause of sequelae. The "sequelae" include conditions
    specified as such or as residuals which may occur at any time
    after the onset of the causal condition

  EXCLUDES 1   *personal history of cerebral infarction without residual deficit*
    (Z86.73)
    personal history of prolonged reversible ischemic neurologic
      deficit (PRIND) (Z86.73)
    personal history of reversible ischemic neurologcial deficit
      (RIND) (Z86.73)
    sequelae of traumatic intracranial injury (S06.-)
    transient ischemic attack (TIA) (G45.9)

  AHA: 2012, 4Q, 106

☑5ᵗʰ I69.0 Sequelae of nontraumatic subarachnoid hemorrhage

  I69.00 Unspecified sequelae of nontraumatic   ▽
    subarachnoid hemorrhage

  I69.01 Cognitive deficits following nontraumatic
    subarachnoid hemorrhage

  ☑6ᵗʰ I69.02 Speech and language deficits following
    nontraumatic subarachnoid hemorrhage

    I69.020 Aphasia following nontraumatic
      subarachnoid hemorrhage

    I69.021 Dysphasia following nontraumatic
      subarachnoid hemorrhage

    I69.022 Dysarthria following nontraumatic
      subarachnoid hemorrhage

    I69.023 Fluency disorder following nontraumatic
      subarachnoid hemorrhage

      Stuttering following nontraumatic
      subarachnoid hemorrhage

    I69.028 Other speech and language deficits
      following nontraumatic subarachnoid
      hemorrhage

  ☑6ᵗʰ I69.03 Monoplegia of upper limb following nontraumatic
    subarachnoid hemorrhage

    I69.031 Monoplegia of upper limb following
      nontraumatic subarachnoid hemorrhage
      affecting right dominant side

    I69.032 Monoplegia of upper limb following
      nontraumatic subarachnoid hemorrhage
      affecting left dominant side

    I69.033 Monoplegia of upper limb following
      nontraumatic subarachnoid hemorrhage
      affecting right non-dominant side

    I69.034 Monoplegia of upper limb following
      nontraumatic subarachnoid hemorrhage
      affecting left non-dominant side

    I69.039 Monoplegia of upper limb following   ▽
      nontraumatic subarachnoid hemorrhage
      affecting unspecified side

  ☑6ᵗʰ I69.04 Monoplegia of lower limb following nontraumatic
    subarachnoid hemorrhage

    I69.041 Monoplegia of lower limb following
      nontraumatic subarachnoid hemorrhage
      affecting right dominant side

    I69.042 Monoplegia of lower limb following
      nontraumatic subarachnoid hemorrhage
      affecting left dominant side

    I69.043 Monoplegia of lower limb following
      nontraumatic subarachnoid hemorrhage
      affecting right non-dominant side

    I69.044 Monoplegia of lower limb following
      nontraumatic subarachnoid hemorrhage
      affecting left non-dominant side

    I69.049 Monoplegia of lower limb following   ▽
      nontraumatic subarachnoid
      hemorrhage affecting unspecified side

  ☑6ᵗʰ I69.05 Hemiplegia and hemiparesis following
    nontraumatic subarachnoid hemorrhage

    AHA: 2015, 1Q, 25

    I69.051 Hemiplegia and hemiparesis following
      nontraumatic subarachnoid hemorrhage
      affecting right dominant side

    I69.052 Hemiplegia and hemiparesis following
      nontraumatic subarachnoid hemorrhage
      affecting left dominant side

    I69.053 Hemiplegia and hemiparesis following
      nontraumatic subarachnoid hemorrhage
      affecting right non-dominant side

    I69.054 Hemiplegia and hemiparesis following
      nontraumatic subarachnoid hemorrhage
      affecting left non-dominant side

    I69.059 Hemiplegia and hemiparesis following   ▽
      nontraumatic subarachnoid
      hemorrhage affecting unspecified side

---

¹⁰ Hospice questionable admission diagnosis

☑ Add'l Character Required   ✗ʑᵗʰ Placeholder Alert   `RUG IV Special Care High Dx`   `RUG IV Clinically Complex Dx`   `RUG IV Special Care Low Dx`   Manifestation Code   Other Specified Code   ▽ Unspecified Code

✓6ᵗʰ **I69.06** **Other paralytic syndrome** following nontraumatic subarachnoid hemorrhage
  Use additional code to identify type of paralytic syndrome, such as:
    locked-in state (G83.5)
    quadriplegia (G82.5-)
    EXCLUDES 1 *hemiplegia/hemiparesis following nontraumatic subarachnoid hemorrhage (I69.05-)*
    monoplegia of lower limb following nontraumatic subarachnoid hemorrhage (I69.04-)
    monoplegia of upper limb following nontraumatic subarachnoid hemorrhage (I69.03-)

  I69.061 **Other paralytic syndrome following nontraumatic subarachnoid hemorrhage affecting right dominant side**

  I69.062 **Other paralytic syndrome following nontraumatic subarachnoid hemorrhage affecting left dominant side**

  I69.063 **Other paralytic syndrome following nontraumatic subarachnoid hemorrhage affecting right non-dominant side**

  I69.064 **Other paralytic syndrome following nontraumatic subarachnoid hemorrhage affecting left non-dominant side**

  I69.065 **Other paralytic syndrome following nontraumatic subarachnoid hemorrhage, bilateral**

  I69.069 **Other paralytic syndrome following nontraumatic subarachnoid hemorrhage affecting unspecified side** ▽

✓6ᵗʰ **I69.09** **Other** sequelae of nontraumatic subarachnoid hemorrhage

  I69.090 **Apraxia following nontraumatic subarachnoid hemorrhage**

  I69.091 **Dysphagia following nontraumatic subarachnoid hemorrhage** CC
    Use additional code to identify the type of dysphagia, if known (R13.1-)
    RIC Excl: 01 Stroke

  I69.092 **Facial weakness following nontraumatic subarachnoid hemorrhage**
    Facial droop following nontraumatic subarachnoid hemorrhage

  I69.093 **Ataxia following nontraumatic subarachnoid hemorrhage**

  I69.098 **Other sequelae following nontraumatic subarachnoid hemorrhage**
    Alterations of sensation following nontraumatic subarachnoid hemorrhage
    Disturbance of vision following nontraumatic subarachnoid hemorrhage
    Use additional code to identify the sequelae

✓5ᵗʰ **I69.1** **Sequelae of nontraumatic intracerebral hemorrhage**

  I69.10 **Unspecified sequelae of nontraumatic intracerebral hemorrhage** ▽

  I69.11 **Cognitive deficits following nontraumatic intracerebral hemorrhage**

✓6ᵗʰ **I69.12** **Speech and language deficits following nontraumatic intracerebral hemorrhage**

  I69.120 **Aphasia following nontraumatic intracerebral hemorrhage**

  I69.121 **Dysphasia following nontraumatic intracerebral hemorrhage**

  I69.122 **Dysarthria following nontraumatic intracerebral hemorrhage**

  I69.123 **Fluency disorder following nontraumatic intracerebral hemorrhage**
    Stuttering following nontraumatic subarachnoid hemorrhage

  I69.128 **Other speech and language deficits following nontraumatic intracerebral hemorrhage**

✓6ᵗʰ **I69.13** **Monoplegia of upper limb following nontraumatic intracerebral hemorrhage**

  I69.131 **Monoplegia of upper limb following nontraumatic intracerebral hemorrhage affecting right dominant side**

  I69.132 **Monoplegia of upper limb following nontraumatic intracerebral hemorrhage affecting left dominant side**

  I69.133 **Monoplegia of upper limb following nontraumatic intracerebral hemorrhage affecting right non-dominant side**

  I69.134 **Monoplegia of upper limb following nontraumatic intracerebral hemorrhage affecting left non-dominant side**

  I69.139 **Monoplegia of upper limb following nontraumatic intracerebral hemorrhage affecting unspecified side** ▽

✓6ᵗʰ **I69.14** **Monoplegia of lower limb following nontraumatic intracerebral hemorrhage**

  I69.141 **Monoplegia of lower limb following nontraumatic intracerebral hemorrhage affecting right dominant side**

  I69.142 **Monoplegia of lower limb following nontraumatic intracerebral hemorrhage affecting left dominant side**

  I69.143 **Monoplegia of lower limb following nontraumatic intracerebral hemorrhage affecting right non-dominant side**

  I69.144 **Monoplegia of lower limb following nontraumatic intracerebral hemorrhage affecting left non-dominant side**

  I69.149 **Monoplegia of lower limb following nontraumatic intracerebral hemorrhage affecting unspecified side** ▽

✓6ᵗʰ **I69.15** **Hemiplegia and hemiparesis following nontraumatic intracerebral hemorrhage**
    AHA: 2015, 1Q, 25

  I69.151 **Hemiplegia and hemiparesis following nontraumatic intracerebral hemorrhage affecting right dominant side**

  I69.152 **Hemiplegia and hemiparesis following nontraumatic intracerebral hemorrhage affecting left dominant side**

  I69.153 **Hemiplegia and hemiparesis following nontraumatic intracerebral hemorrhage affecting right non-dominant side**

  I69.154 **Hemiplegia and hemiparesis following nontraumatic intracerebral hemorrhage affecting left non-dominant side**

  I69.159 **Hemiplegia and hemiparesis following nontraumatic intracerebral hemorrhage affecting unspecified side** ▽

✓6ᵗʰ **I69.16** **Other paralytic syndrome** following nontraumatic intracerebral hemorrhage
  Use additional code to identify type of paralytic syndrome, such as:
    locked-in state (G83.5)
    quadriplegia (G82.5-)
    EXCLUDES 1 *hemiplegia/hemiparesis following nontraumatic intracerebral hemorrhage (I69.15-)*
    monoplegia of lower limb following nontraumatic intracerebral hemorrhage (I69.14-)
    monoplegia of upper limb following nontraumatic intracerebral hemorrhage (I69.13-)

  I69.161 **Other paralytic syndrome following nontraumatic intracerebral hemorrhage affecting right dominant side**

  I69.162 **Other paralytic syndrome following nontraumatic intracerebral hemorrhage affecting left dominant side**

  I69.163 **Other paralytic syndrome following nontraumatic intracerebral hemorrhage affecting right non-dominant side**

  I69.164 **Other paralytic syndrome following nontraumatic intracerebral hemorrhage affecting left non-dominant side**

  I69.165 **Other paralytic syndrome following nontraumatic intracerebral hemorrhage, bilateral**

  I69.169 **Other paralytic syndrome following nontraumatic intracerebral hemorrhage affecting unspecified side** ▽

☑ 6ᵗʰ I69.19 Other sequelae of nontraumatic intracerebral hemorrhage

  I69.19Ø Apraxia following nontraumatic intracerebral hemorrhage

  I69.191 Dysphagia following nontraumatic   `CC` intracerebral hemorrhage
    Use additional code to identify the type of dysphagia, if known (R13.1-)
    RIC Excl: 01 Stroke

  I69.192 Facial weakness following nontraumatic intracerebral hemorrhage
    Facial droop following nontraumatic intracerebral hemorrhage

  I69.193 Ataxia following nontraumatic intracerebral hemorrhage

  I69.198 Other sequelae of nontraumatic intracerebral hemorrhage
    Alteration of sensations following nontraumatic intracerebral hemorrhage
    Disturbance of vision following nontraumatic intracerebral hemorrhage
    Use additional code to identify the sequelae

☑ 5ᵗʰ I69.2 Sequelae of other nontraumatic intracranial hemorrhage

  I69.2Ø Unspecified sequelae of other nontraumatic   ▽ **intracranial hemorrhage**

  I69.21 Cognitive deficits following other nontraumatic intracranial hemorrhage

  ☑ 6ᵗʰ I69.22 Speech and language deficits following other nontraumatic intracranial hemorrhage

    I69.22Ø Aphasia following other nontraumatic intracranial hemorrhage

    I69.221 Dysphasia following other nontraumatic intracranial hemorrhage

    I69.222 Dysarthria following other nontraumatic intracranial hemorrhage

    I69.223 Fluency disorder following other nontraumatic intracranial hemorrhage
      Stuttering following nontraumatic subarachnoid hemorrhage

    I69.228 Other speech and language deficits following other nontraumatic intracranial hemorrhage

  ☑ 6ᵗʰ I69.23 Monoplegia of upper limb following other nontraumatic intracranial hemorrhage

    I69.231 Monoplegia of upper limb following other nontraumatic intracranial hemorrhage affecting right dominant side

    I69.232 Monoplegia of upper limb following other nontraumatic intracranial hemorrhage affecting left dominant side

    I69.233 Monoplegia of upper limb following other nontraumatic intracranial hemorrhage affecting right non-dominant side

    I69.234 Monoplegia of upper limb following other nontraumatic intracranial hemorrhage affecting left non-dominant side

    I69.239 Monoplegia of upper limb following   ▽ **other nontraumatic intracranial hemorrhage affecting unspecified side**

  ☑ 6ᵗʰ I69.24 Monoplegia of lower limb following other nontraumatic intracranial hemorrhage

    I69.241 Monoplegia of lower limb following other nontraumatic intracranial hemorrhage affecting right dominant side

    I69.242 Monoplegia of lower limb following other nontraumatic intracranial hemorrhage affecting left dominant side

    I69.243 Monoplegia of lower limb following other nontraumatic intracranial hemorrhage affecting right non-dominant side

    I69.244 Monoplegia of lower limb following other nontraumatic intracranial hemorrhage affecting left non-dominant side

    I69.249 Monoplegia of lower limb following   ▽ **other nontraumatic intracranial hemorrhage affecting unspecified side**

☑ 6ᵗʰ I69.25 Hemiplegia and hemiparesis following other nontraumatic intracranial hemorrhage
  AHA: 2015, 1Q, 25

  I69.251 Hemiplegia and hemiparesis following other nontraumatic intracranial hemorrhage affecting right dominant side

  I69.252 Hemiplegia and hemiparesis following other nontraumatic intracranial hemorrhage affecting left dominant side

  I69.253 Hemiplegia and hemiparesis following other nontraumatic intracranial hemorrhage affecting right non-dominant side

  I69.254 Hemiplegia and hemiparesis following other nontraumatic intracranial hemorrhage affecting left non-dominant side

  I69.259 Hemiplegia and hemiparesis following   ▽ **other nontraumatic intracranial hemorrhage affecting unspecified side**

☑ 6ᵗʰ I69.26 Other paralytic syndrome following other nontraumatic intracranial hemorrhage
  Use additional code to identify type of paralytic syndrome, such as:
  locked-in state (G83.5)
  quadriplegia (G82.5-)
  EXCLUDES 1 hemiplegia/hemiparesis following other nontraumatic intracranial hemorrhage (I69.25-)
    monoplegia of lower limb following other nontraumatic intracranial hemorrhage (I69.24-)
    monoplegia of upper limb following other nontraumatic intracranial hemorrhage (I69.23-)

  I69.261 Other paralytic syndrome following other nontraumatic intracranial hemorrhage affecting right dominant side

  I69.262 Other paralytic syndrome following other nontraumatic intracranial hemorrhage affecting left dominant side

  I69.263 Other paralytic syndrome following other nontraumatic intracranial hemorrhage affecting right non-dominant side

  I69.264 Other paralytic syndrome following other nontraumatic intracranial hemorrhage affecting left non-dominant side

  I69.265 Other paralytic syndrome following other nontraumatic intracranial hemorrhage, bilateral

  I69.269 Other paralytic syndrome following   ▽ **other nontraumatic intracranial hemorrhage affecting unspecified side**

☑ 6ᵗʰ I69.29 Other sequelae of other nontraumatic intracranial hemorrhage

  I69.29Ø Apraxia following other nontraumatic intracranial hemorrhage

  I69.291 Dysphagia following other   `CC` **nontraumatic intracranial hemorrhage**
    Use additional code to identify the type of dysphagia, if known (R13.1-)
    RIC Excl: 01 Stroke

  I69.292 Facial weakness following other nontraumatic intracranial hemorrhage
    Facial droop following other nontraumatic intracranial hemorrhage

  I69.293 Ataxia following other nontraumatic intracranial hemorrhage

  I69.298 Other sequelae of other nontraumatic intracranial hemorrhage
    Alteration of sensation following other nontraumatic intracranial hemorrhage
    Disturbance of vision following other nontraumatic intracranial hemorrhage
    Use additional code to identify the sequelae

☑ 5ᵗʰ I69.3 Sequelae of cerebral infarction
  Sequelae of stroke NOS
  AHA: 2013, 4Q, 127-128; 2012, 4Q, 92, 94

  I69.3Ø Unspecified sequelae of cerebral infarction   ▽

  I69.31 Cognitive deficits following cerebral infarction

☑ Add'l Character Required   ✓ᴬᵀᴴ Placeholder Alert   RUG IV Special Care High Dx   RUG IV Clinically Complex Dx   RUG IV Special Care Low Dx   Manifestation Code   Other Specified Code   ▽ Unspecified Code

ICD-10-CM 2016   603

Chapter 9. Diseases of the Circulatory System

✓6ᵗʰ **I69.32** Speech and language deficits following cerebral infarction

I69.320 Aphasia following cerebral infarction

I69.321 Dysphasia following cerebral infarction
AHA: 2012, 4Q, 91

I69.322 Dysarthria following cerebral infarction

I69.323 Fluency disorder following cerebral infarction
Stuttering following nontraumatic subarachnoid hemorrhage

I69.328 Other speech and language deficits following cerebral infarction

✓6ᵗʰ **I69.33** Monoplegia of upper limb following cerebral infarction

I69.331 Monoplegia of upper limb following cerebral infarction affecting right dominant side

I69.332 Monoplegia of upper limb following cerebral infarction affecting left dominant side

I69.333 Monoplegia of upper limb following cerebral infarction affecting right non-dominant side

I69.334 Monoplegia of upper limb following cerebral infarction affecting left non-dominant side

I69.339 Monoplegia of upper limb following ▽ cerebral infarction affecting unspecified side

✓6ᵗʰ **I69.34** Monoplegia of lower limb following cerebral infarction

I69.341 Monoplegia of lower limb following cerebral infarction affecting right dominant side

I69.342 Monoplegia of lower limb following cerebral infarction affecting left dominant side

I69.343 Monoplegia of lower limb following cerebral infarction affecting right non-dominant side

I69.344 Monoplegia of lower limb following cerebral infarction affecting left non-dominant side

I69.349 Monoplegia of lower limb following ▽ cerebral infarction affecting unspecified side

✓6ᵗʰ **I69.35** Hemiplegia and hemiparesis following cerebral infarction
AHA: 2015, 1Q, 25

I69.351 Hemiplegia and hemiparesis following cerebral infarction affecting right dominant side

I69.352 Hemiplegia and hemiparesis following cerebral infarction affecting left dominant side

I69.353 Hemiplegia and hemiparesis following cerebral infarction affecting right non-dominant side

I69.354 Hemiplegia and hemiparesis following cerebral infarction affecting left non-dominant side
AHA: 2012, 4Q, 91

I69.359 Hemiplegia and hemiparesis following ▽ cerebral infarction affecting unspecified side

✓6ᵗʰ **I69.36** Other paralytic syndrome following cerebral infarction
Use additional code to identify type of paralytic syndrome, such as:
locked-in state (G83.5)
quadriplegia (G82.5-)
EXCLUDES 1 *hemiplegia/hemiparesis following cerebral infarction (I69.35-)*
monoplegia of lower limb following cerebral infarction (I69.34-)
monoplegia of upper limb following cerebral infarction (I69.33-)

I69.361 Other paralytic syndrome following cerebral infarction affecting right dominant side

I69.362 Other paralytic syndrome following cerebral infarction affecting left dominant side

I69.363 Other paralytic syndrome following cerebral infarction affecting right non-dominant side

I69.364 Other paralytic syndrome following cerebral infarction affecting left non-dominant side

I69.365 Other paralytic syndrome following cerebral infarction, bilateral

I69.369 Other paralytic syndrome following ▽ cerebral infarction affecting unspecified side

✓6ᵗʰ **I69.39** Other sequelae of cerebral infarction

I69.390 Apraxia following cerebral infarction

I69.391 Dysphagia following cerebral CC infarction
Use additional code to identify the type of dysphagia, if known (R13.1-)
RIC Excl: 01 Stroke

I69.392 Facial weakness following cerebral infarction
Facial droop following cerebral infarction

I69.393 Ataxia following cerebral infarction

I69.398 Other sequelae of cerebral infarction
Alteration of sensation following cerebral infarction
Disturbance of vision following cerebral infarction
Use additional code to identify the sequelae

✓5ᵗʰ **I69.8** Sequelae of other cerebrovascular diseases
EXCLUDES 1 *sequelae of traumatic intracranial injury (S06.-)*

I69.80 Unspecified sequelae of other cerebrovascular ▽ disease

I69.81 Cognitive deficits following other cerebrovascular disease

✓6ᵗʰ **I69.82** Speech and language deficits following other cerebrovascular disease

I69.820 Aphasia following other cerebrovascular disease

I69.821 Dysphasia following other cerebrovascular disease

I69.822 Dysarthria following other cerebrovascular disease

I69.823 Fluency disorder following other cerebrovascular disease
Stuttering following nontraumatic subarachnoid hemorrhage

I69.828 Other speech and language deficits following other cerebrovascular disease

✓6ᵗʰ **I69.83** Monoplegia of upper limb following other cerebrovascular disease

I69.831 Monoplegia of upper limb following other cerebrovascular disease affecting right dominant side

I69.832 Monoplegia of upper limb following other cerebrovascular disease affecting left dominant side

I69.833 Monoplegia of upper limb following other cerebrovascular disease affecting right non-dominant side

I69.834 Monoplegia of upper limb following other cerebrovascular disease affecting left non-dominant side

I69.839 Monoplegia of upper limb following ▽ other cerebrovascular disease affecting unspecified side

✓6ᵗʰ **I69.84** Monoplegia of lower limb following other cerebrovascular disease

I69.841 Monoplegia of lower limb following other cerebrovascular disease affecting right dominant side

I69.842 Monoplegia of lower limb following other cerebrovascular disease affecting left dominant side

I69.843 Monoplegia of lower limb following other cerebrovascular disease affecting right non-dominant side

Ⓝ Newborn   Ⓟ Pediatric   Ⓜ Maternity   Ⓐ Adult   **RIC** RIC Dx   **NC Dx** Noncancer Dx   **PDx** Primary Dx   **CC** RIC CC Condition   ►◄ Revised Text   ● New Code   ▲ Revised Code Title

604   ICD-10-CM 2016

I69.844   **Monoplegia of lower limb following other cerebrovascular disease affecting left non-dominant side**

I69.849   **Monoplegia of lower limb following other cerebrovascular disease affecting unspecified side** ▽

✓6ᵗʰ **I69.85**   Hemiplegia and hemiparesis following other cerebrovascular disease
     AHA: 2015, 1Q, 25

I69.851   **Hemiplegia and hemiparesis following other cerebrovascular disease affecting right dominant side**

I69.852   **Hemiplegia and hemiparesis following other cerebrovascular disease affecting left dominant side**

I69.853   **Hemiplegia and hemiparesis following other cerebrovascular disease affecting right non-dominant side**

I69.854   **Hemiplegia and hemiparesis following other cerebrovascular disease affecting left non-dominant side**

I69.859   **Hemiplegia and hemiparesis following other cerebrovascular disease affecting unspecified side** ▽

✓6ᵗʰ **I69.86**   Other paralytic syndrome following other cerebrovascular disease
     Use additional code to identify type of paralytic syndrome, such as:
       locked-in state (G83.5)
       quadriplegia (G82.5-)
     EXCLUDES 1   hemiplegia/hemiparesis following other cerebrovascular disease (I69.85-)
         monoplegia of lower limb following other cerebrovascular disease (I69.84-)
         monoplegia of upper limb following other cerebrovascular disease (I69.83-)

I69.861   **Other paralytic syndrome following other cerebrovascular disease affecting right dominant side**

I69.862   **Other paralytic syndrome following other cerebrovascular disease affecting left dominant side**

I69.863   **Other paralytic syndrome following other cerebrovascular disease affecting right non-dominant side**

I69.864   **Other paralytic syndrome following other cerebrovascular disease affecting left non-dominant side**

I69.865   **Other paralytic syndrome following other cerebrovascular disease, bilateral**

I69.869   **Other paralytic syndrome following other cerebrovascular disease affecting unspecified side** ▽

✓6ᵗʰ **I69.89**   Other sequelae of other cerebrovascular disease

I69.890   Apraxia following other cerebrovascular disease

I69.891   Dysphagia following other cerebrovascular disease   **CC**
     Use additional code to identify the type of dysphagia, if known (R13.1-)
     RIC Excl: 01 Stroke

I69.892   Facial weakness following other cerebrovascular disease
     Facial droop following other cerebrovascular disease

I69.893   Ataxia following other cerebrovascular disease

I69.898   Other sequelae of other cerebrovascular disease
     Alteration of sensation following other cerebrovascular disease
     Disturbance of vision following other cerebrovascular disease
     Use additional code to identify the sequelae

✓5ᵗʰ **I69.9**   Sequelae of unspecified cerebrovascular diseases
     EXCLUDES 1   sequelae of stroke (I69.3)
         sequelae of traumatic intracranial injury (S06.-)

I69.90   Unspecified sequelae of unspecified cerebrovascular disease ▽

I69.91   Cognitive deficits following unspecified cerebrovascular disease

✓6ᵗʰ **I69.92**   Speech and language deficits following unspecified cerebrovascular disease

I69.920   Aphasia following unspecified cerebrovascular disease

I69.921   Dysphasia following unspecified cerebrovascular disease

I69.922   Dysarthria following unspecified cerebrovascular disease

I69.923   Fluency disorder following unspecified cerebrovascular disease
     Stuttering following nontraumatic subarachnoid hemorrhage

I69.928   **Other speech and language deficits following unspecified cerebrovascular disease** ▽

✓6ᵗʰ **I69.93**   Monoplegia of upper limb following unspecified cerebrovascular disease

I69.931   **Monoplegia of upper limb following unspecified cerebrovascular disease affecting right dominant side**

I69.932   **Monoplegia of upper limb following unspecified cerebrovascular disease affecting left dominant side**

I69.933   **Monoplegia of upper limb following unspecified cerebrovascular disease affecting right non-dominant side**

I69.934   **Monoplegia of upper limb following unspecified cerebrovascular disease affecting left non-dominant side**

I69.939   **Monoplegia of upper limb following unspecified cerebrovascular disease affecting unspecified side** ▽

✓6ᵗʰ **I69.94**   Monoplegia of lower limb following unspecified cerebrovascular disease

I69.941   **Monoplegia of lower limb following unspecified cerebrovascular disease affecting right dominant side**

I69.942   **Monoplegia of lower limb following unspecified cerebrovascular disease affecting left dominant side**

I69.943   **Monoplegia of lower limb following unspecified cerebrovascular disease affecting right non-dominant side**

I69.944   **Monoplegia of lower limb following unspecified cerebrovascular disease affecting left non-dominant side**

I69.949   **Monoplegia of lower limb following unspecified cerebrovascular disease affecting unspecified side** ▽

✓6ᵗʰ **I69.95**   Hemiplegia and hemiparesis following unspecified cerebrovascular disease
     AHA: 2015, 1Q, 25

I69.951   **Hemiplegia and hemiparesis following unspecified cerebrovascular disease affecting right dominant side**

I69.952   **Hemiplegia and hemiparesis following unspecified cerebrovascular disease affecting left dominant side**

I69.953   **Hemiplegia and hemiparesis following unspecified cerebrovascular disease affecting right non-dominant side**

I69.954   **Hemiplegia and hemiparesis following unspecified cerebrovascular disease affecting left non-dominant side**

I69.959   **Hemiplegia and hemiparesis following unspecified cerebrovascular disease affecting unspecified side** ▽

☑ Add'l Character Required   ✓×7ᵗʰ Placeholder Alert   RUG IV Special Care High Dx   RUG IV Clinically Complex Dx   RUG IV Special Care Low Dx   Manifestation Code   Other Specified Code   ▽ Unspecified Code

ICD-10-CM 2016   **605**

✓6ᵗʰ **I69.96** Other paralytic syndrome **following unspecified cerebrovascular disease**
  Use additional code to identify type of paralytic syndrome, such as:
    locked-in state (G83.5)
    quadriplegia (G82.5-)
  EXCLUDES 1 *hemiplegia/hemiparesis following unspecified cerebrovascular disease (I69.95-)*
    monoplegia of lower limb following unspecified cerebrovascular disease (I69.94-)
    monoplegia of upper limb following unspecified cerebrovascular disease (I69.93-)

  I69.961 **Other paralytic syndrome following unspecified cerebrovascular disease affecting right dominant side**

  I69.962 **Other paralytic syndrome following unspecified cerebrovascular disease affecting left dominant side**

  I69.963 **Other paralytic syndrome following unspecified cerebrovascular disease affecting right non-dominant side**

  I69.964 **Other paralytic syndrome following unspecified cerebrovascular disease affecting left non-dominant side**

  I69.965 **Other paralytic syndrome following unspecified cerebrovascular disease, bilateral**

  I69.969 **Other paralytic syndrome following unspecified cerebrovascular disease affecting unspecified side** ▽

✓6ᵗʰ **I69.99** Other **sequelae of unspecified cerebrovascular disease**

  I69.990 **Apraxia following unspecified cerebrovascular disease**

  I69.991 **Dysphagia following unspecified cerebrovascular disease** CC
    Use additional code to identify the type of dysphagia, if known (R13.1-)
    RIC Excl: 01 Stroke

  I69.992 **Facial weakness following unspecified cerebrovascular disease**
    Facial droop following unspecified cerebrovascular disease

  I69.993 **Ataxia following unspecified cerebrovascular disease**

  I69.998 **Other sequelae following unspecified cerebrovascular disease**
    Alteration in sensation following unspecified cerebrovascular disease
    Disturbance of vision following unspecified cerebrovascular disease
    Use additional code to identify the sequelae

Diseases of arteries, arterioles and capillaries (I70-I79)

✓4ᵗʰ **I70** **Atherosclerosis**
  INCLUDES arteriolosclerosis
    arterial degeneration
    arteriosclerosis
    arteriosclerotic vascular disease
    arteriovascular degeneration
    atheroma
    endarteritis deformans or obliterans
    senile arteritis
    senile endarteritis
    vascular degeneration
  Use additional code to identify:
    exposure to environmental tobacco smoke (Z77.22)
    history of tobacco use (Z87.891)
    occupational exposure to environmental tobacco smoke (Z57.31)
    tobacco dependence (F17.-)
    tobacco use (Z72.0)
  EXCLUDES 2 *arteriosclerotic cardiovascular disease (I25.1-)*
    arteriosclerotic heart disease (I25.1-)
    atheroembolism (I75.-)
    cerebral atherosclerosis (I67.2)
    coronary atherosclerosis (I25.1-)
    mesenteric atherosclerosis (K55.1)
    precerebral atherosclerosis (I67.2)
    primary pulmonary atherosclerosis (I27.0)

  I70.0 **Atherosclerosis of aorta** Ⓐ

  I70.1 **Atherosclerosis of renal artery** Ⓐ
    Goldblatt's kidney
    EXCLUDES 2 *atherosclerosis of renal arterioles (I12.-)*

✓5ᵗʰ **I70.2** **Atherosclerosis of native arteries of the extremities**
    Mönckeberg's (medial) sclerosis
    Use additional code, if applicable, to identify chronic total occlusion of artery of extremity (I70.92)
    EXCLUDES 2 *atherosclerosis of bypass graft of extremities (I70.30-I70.79)*

  ✓6ᵗʰ **I70.20** Unspecified **atherosclerosis of native arteries of extremities**

    I70.201 **Unspecified atherosclerosis of native arteries of extremities, right leg** Ⓐ▽

    I70.202 **Unspecified atherosclerosis of native arteries of extremities, left leg** Ⓐ▽

    I70.203 **Unspecified atherosclerosis of native arteries of extremities, bilateral legs** Ⓐ▽

    I70.208 **Unspecified atherosclerosis of native arteries of extremities, other extremity** Ⓐ▽

    I70.209 **Unspecified atherosclerosis of native arteries of extremities, unspecified extremity** Ⓐ▽

  ✓6ᵗʰ **I70.21** **Atherosclerosis of native arteries of extremities with intermittent claudication**

    I70.211 **Atherosclerosis of native arteries of extremities with intermittent claudication, right leg** Ⓐ

    I70.212 **Atherosclerosis of native arteries of extremities with intermittent claudication, left leg** Ⓐ

    I70.213 **Atherosclerosis of native arteries of extremities with intermittent claudication, bilateral legs** Ⓐ

    I70.218 **Atherosclerosis of native arteries of extremities with intermittent claudication, other extremity** Ⓐ

    I70.219 **Atherosclerosis of native arteries of extremities with intermittent claudication, unspecified extremity** Ⓐ▽

  ✓6ᵗʰ **I70.22** **Atherosclerosis of native arteries of extremities with rest pain**
      INCLUDES any condition classifiable to I70.21-

    I70.221 **Atherosclerosis of native arteries of extremities with rest pain, right leg** Ⓐ

    I70.222 **Atherosclerosis of native arteries of extremities with rest pain, left leg** Ⓐ

    I70.223 **Atherosclerosis of native arteries of extremities with rest pain, bilateral legs** Ⓐ

Ⓝ Newborn   Ⓟ Pediatric   Ⓜ Maternity   Ⓐ Adult   RIC RIC Dx   NC Dx Noncancer Dx   PDx Primary Dx   CC RIC CC Condition   ▶◀ Revised Text   ● New Code   ▲ Revised Code Title

606   ICD-10-CM 2016

I70.228   **Atherosclerosis of native arteries of extremities with rest pain, other extremity**   A

I70.229   **Atherosclerosis of native arteries of extremities with rest pain, unspecified extremity**   A ▽

✓6th **I70.23**   **Atherosclerosis of native arteries of right leg with ulceration**
> INCLUDES   any condition classifiable to I70.211 and I70.221
> Use additional code to identify severity of ulcer (L97.-)

I70.231   **Atherosclerosis of native arteries of right leg with ulceration of thigh**   cc A
> RIC Excl: 10 Amputation, lower extremity; 11 Amputation, non-lower extremity

I70.232   **Atherosclerosis of native arteries of right leg with ulceration of calf**   cc A
> RIC Excl: 10 Amputation, lower extremity; 11 Amputation, non-lower extremity

I70.233   **Atherosclerosis of native arteries of right leg with ulceration of ankle**   cc A
> RIC Excl: 10 Amputation, lower extremity; 11 Amputation, non-lower extremity

I70.234   **Atherosclerosis of native arteries of right leg with ulceration of heel and midfoot**   cc A
> Atherosclerosis of native arteries of right leg with ulceration of plantar surface of midfoot
> RIC Excl: 10 Amputation, lower extremity; 11 Amputation, non-lower extremity

I70.235   **Atherosclerosis of native arteries of right leg with ulceration of other part of foot**   cc A
> Atherosclerosis of native arteries of right leg extremities with ulceration of toe
> RIC Excl: 10 Amputation, lower extremity; 11 Amputation, non-lower extremity

I70.238   **Atherosclerosis of native arteries of right leg with ulceration of other part of lower right leg**   cc A
> RIC Excl: 10 Amputation, lower extremity; 11 Amputation, non-lower extremity

I70.239   **Atherosclerosis of native arteries of right leg with ulceration of unspecified site**   cc A ▽
> RIC Excl: 10 Amputation, lower extremity; 11 Amputation, non-lower extremity

✓6th **I70.24**   **Atherosclerosis of native arteries of left leg with ulceration**
> INCLUDES   any condition classifiable to I70.212 and I70.222
> Use additional code to identify severity of ulcer (L97.-)

I70.241   **Atherosclerosis of native arteries of left leg with ulceration of thigh**   cc A
> RIC Excl: 10 Amputation, lower extremity; 11 Amputation, non-lower extremity

I70.242   **Atherosclerosis of native arteries of left leg with ulceration of calf**   cc A
> RIC Excl: 10 Amputation, lower extremity; 11 Amputation, non-lower extremity

I70.243   **Atherosclerosis of native arteries of left leg with ulceration of ankle**   cc A
> RIC Excl: 10 Amputation, lower extremity; 11 Amputation, non-lower extremity

I70.244   **Atherosclerosis of native arteries of left leg with ulceration of heel and midfoot**   cc A
> Atherosclerosis of native arteries of left leg with ulceration of plantar surface of midfoot
> RIC Excl: 10 Amputation, lower extremity; 11 Amputation, non-lower extremity

I70.245   **Atherosclerosis of native arteries of left leg with ulceration of other part of foot**   cc A
> Atherosclerosis of native arteries of left leg extremities with ulceration of toe
> RIC Excl: 10 Amputation, lower extremity; 11 Amputation, non-lower extremity

I70.248   **Atherosclerosis of native arteries of left leg with ulceration of other part of lower left leg**   cc A
> RIC Excl: 10 Amputation, lower extremity; 11 Amputation, non-lower extremity

I70.249   **Atherosclerosis of native arteries of left leg with ulceration of unspecified site**   cc A ▽
> RIC Excl: 10 Amputation, lower extremity; 11 Amputation, non-lower extremity

I70.25   **Atherosclerosis of native arteries of other extremities with ulceration**   cc A
> INCLUDES   any condition classifiable to I70.218 and I70.228
> Use additional code to identify the severity of the ulcer (L98.49-)
> RIC Excl: 10 Amputation, lower extremity; 11 Amputation, non-lower extremity

✓6th **I70.26**   **Atherosclerosis of native arteries of extremities with gangrene**
> INCLUDES   any condition classifiable to I70.21-, I70.22-, I70.23-, I70.24-, and I70.25-
> Use additional code to identify the severity of any ulcer (L97.-, L98.49-), if applicable

I70.261   **Atherosclerosis of native arteries of extremities with gangrene, right leg**   cc A
> RIC Excl: 10 Amputation, lower extremity; 11 Amputation, non-lower extremity

I70.262   **Atherosclerosis of native arteries of extremities with gangrene, left leg**   cc A
> RIC Excl: 10 Amputation, lower extremity; 11 Amputation, non-lower extremity

I70.263   **Atherosclerosis of native arteries of extremities with gangrene, bilateral legs**   cc A
> RIC Excl: 10 Amputation, lower extremity; 11 Amputation, non-lower extremity

I70.268   **Atherosclerosis of native arteries of extremities with gangrene, other extremity**   cc A
> RIC Excl: 10 Amputation, lower extremity; 11 Amputation, non-lower extremity

I70.269   **Atherosclerosis of native arteries of extremities with gangrene, unspecified extremity**   cc A ▽
> RIC Excl: 10 Amputation, lower extremity; 11 Amputation, non-lower extremity

✓6th **I70.29**   **Other atherosclerosis of native arteries of extremities**

I70.291   **Other atherosclerosis of native arteries of extremities, right leg**   A

I70.292   **Other atherosclerosis of native arteries of extremities, left leg**   A

I70.293   **Other atherosclerosis of native arteries of extremities, bilateral legs**   A

I70.298   **Other atherosclerosis of native arteries of extremities, other extremity**   A

I70.299   **Other atherosclerosis of native arteries of extremities, unspecified extremity**   A ▽

✓5th **I70.3**   **Atherosclerosis of unspecified type of bypass graft(s) of the extremities**
> Use additional code, if applicable, to identify chronic total occlusion of artery of extremity (I70.92)
> EXCLUDES 1   embolism or thrombus of bypass graft(s) of extremities (T82.8-)

✓6th **I70.30**   **Unspecified atherosclerosis of unspecified type of bypass graft(s) of the extremities**

I70.301   **Unspecified atherosclerosis of unspecified type of bypass graft(s) of the extremities, right leg**   A

I70.302   **Unspecified atherosclerosis of unspecified type of bypass graft(s) of the extremities, left leg**   A

I70.303   **Unspecified atherosclerosis of unspecified type of bypass graft(s) of the extremities, bilateral legs**   A

I70.308   **Unspecified atherosclerosis of unspecified type of bypass graft(s) of the extremities, other extremity**   A

I70.309   **Unspecified atherosclerosis of unspecified type of bypass graft(s) of the extremities, unspecified extremity**   A ▽

☑ Add'l Character Required   ✓x7th Placeholder Alert   RUG IV Special Care High Dx   RUG IV Clinically Complex Dx   RUG IV Special Care Low Dx   Manifestation Code   Other Specified Code   ▽ Unspecified Code

Chapter 9. Diseases of the Circulatory System

I70.31 Atherosclerosis of unspecified type of bypass graft(s) of the extremities with intermittent claudication

- **I70.311 Atherosclerosis of unspecified type of bypass graft(s) of the extremities with intermittent claudication, right leg** Ⓐ
- **I70.312 Atherosclerosis of unspecified type of bypass graft(s) of the extremities with intermittent claudication, left leg** Ⓐ
- **I70.313 Atherosclerosis of unspecified type of bypass graft(s) of the extremities with intermittent claudication, bilateral legs** Ⓐ
- **I70.318 Atherosclerosis of unspecified type of bypass graft(s) of the extremities with intermittent claudication, other extremity** Ⓐ
- **I70.319 Atherosclerosis of unspecified type of bypass graft(s) of the extremities with intermittent claudication, unspecified extremity** Ⓐ▽

I70.32 Atherosclerosis of unspecified type of bypass graft(s) of the extremities with rest pain
INCLUDES any condition classifiable to I70.31-

- **I70.321 Atherosclerosis of unspecified type of bypass graft(s) of the extremities with rest pain, right leg** Ⓐ
- **I70.322 Atherosclerosis of unspecified type of bypass graft(s) of the extremities with rest pain, left leg** Ⓐ
- **I70.323 Atherosclerosis of unspecified type of bypass graft(s) of the extremities with rest pain, bilateral legs** Ⓐ
- **I70.328 Atherosclerosis of unspecified type of bypass graft(s) of the extremities with rest pain, other extremity** Ⓐ
- **I70.329 Atherosclerosis of unspecified type of bypass graft(s) of the extremities with rest pain, unspecified extremity** Ⓐ▽

I70.33 Atherosclerosis of unspecified type of bypass graft(s) of the right leg with ulceration
INCLUDES any condition classifiable to I70.311 and I70.321
Use additional code to identify severity of ulcer (L97.-)

- **I70.331 Atherosclerosis of unspecified type of bypass graft(s) of the right leg with ulceration of thigh** Ⓐ
- **I70.332 Atherosclerosis of unspecified type of bypass graft(s) of the right leg with ulceration of calf** Ⓐ
- **I70.333 Atherosclerosis of unspecified type of bypass graft(s) of the right leg with ulceration of ankle** Ⓐ
- **I70.334 Atherosclerosis of unspecified type of bypass graft(s) of the right leg with ulceration of heel and midfoot** Ⓐ
  Atherosclerosis of unspecified type of bypass graft(s) of right leg with ulceration of plantar surface of midfoot
- **I70.335 Atherosclerosis of unspecified type of bypass graft(s) of the right leg with ulceration of other part of foot** Ⓐ
  Atherosclerosis of unspecified type of bypass graft(s) of the right leg with ulceration of toe
- **I70.338 Atherosclerosis of unspecified type of bypass graft(s) of the right leg with ulceration of other part of lower leg** Ⓐ
- **I70.339 Atherosclerosis of unspecified type of bypass graft(s) of the right leg with ulceration of unspecified site** Ⓐ▽

I70.34 Atherosclerosis of unspecified type of bypass graft(s) of the left leg with ulceration
INCLUDES any condition classifiable to I70.312 and I70.322
Use additional code to identify severity of ulcer (L97.-)

- **I70.341 Atherosclerosis of unspecified type of bypass graft(s) of the left leg with ulceration of thigh** Ⓐ
- **I70.342 Atherosclerosis of unspecified type of bypass graft(s) of the left leg with ulceration of calf** Ⓐ
- **I70.343 Atherosclerosis of unspecified type of bypass graft(s) of the left leg with ulceration of ankle** Ⓐ
- **I70.344 Atherosclerosis of unspecified type of bypass graft(s) of the left leg with ulceration of heel and midfoot** Ⓐ
  Atherosclerosis of unspecified type of bypass graft(s) of left leg with ulceration of plantar surface of midfoot
- **I70.345 Atherosclerosis of unspecified type of bypass graft(s) of the left leg with ulceration of other part of foot** Ⓐ
  Atherosclerosis of unspecified type of bypass graft(s) of the left leg with ulceration of toe
- **I70.348 Atherosclerosis of unspecified type of bypass graft(s) of the left leg with ulceration of other part of lower leg** Ⓐ
- **I70.349 Atherosclerosis of unspecified type of bypass graft(s) of the left leg with ulceration of unspecified site** Ⓐ▽

I70.35 Atherosclerosis of unspecified type of bypass graft(s) of other extremity with ulceration Ⓐ
INCLUDES any condition classifiable to I70.318 and I70.328
Use additional code to identify severity of ulcer (L98.49-)

I70.36 Atherosclerosis of unspecified type of bypass graft(s) of the extremities with gangrene
INCLUDES any condition classifiable to I70.31-, I70.32-, I70.33-, I70.34-, I70.35
Use additional code to identify the severity of any ulcer (L97.-, L98.49-), if applicable

- **I70.361 Atherosclerosis of unspecified type of bypass graft(s) of the extremities with gangrene, right leg** Ⓐ
- **I70.362 Atherosclerosis of unspecified type of bypass graft(s) of the extremities with gangrene, left leg** Ⓐ
- **I70.363 Atherosclerosis of unspecified type of bypass graft(s) of the extremities with gangrene, bilateral legs** Ⓐ
- **I70.368 Atherosclerosis of unspecified type of bypass graft(s) of the extremities with gangrene, other extremity** Ⓐ
- **I70.369 Atherosclerosis of unspecified type of bypass graft(s) of the extremities with gangrene, unspecified extremity** Ⓐ▽

I70.39 Other atherosclerosis of unspecified type of bypass graft(s) of the extremities

- **I70.391 Other atherosclerosis of unspecified type of bypass graft(s) of the extremities, right leg** Ⓐ
- **I70.392 Other atherosclerosis of unspecified type of bypass graft(s) of the extremities, left leg** Ⓐ
- **I70.393 Other atherosclerosis of unspecified type of bypass graft(s) of the extremities, bilateral legs** Ⓐ
- **I70.398 Other atherosclerosis of unspecified type of bypass graft(s) of the extremities, other extremity** Ⓐ
- **I70.399 Other atherosclerosis of unspecified type of bypass graft(s) of the extremities, unspecified extremity** Ⓐ▽

I70.4 Atherosclerosis of autologous vein bypass graft(s) of the extremities
Use additional code, if applicable, to identify chronic total occlusion of artery of extremity (I70.92)

I70.40 Unspecified atherosclerosis of autologous vein bypass graft(s) of the extremities

- **I70.401 Unspecified atherosclerosis of autologous vein bypass graft(s) of the extremities, right leg** Ⓐ▽
- **I70.402 Unspecified atherosclerosis of autologous vein bypass graft(s) of the extremities, left leg** Ⓐ▽
- **I70.403 Unspecified atherosclerosis of autologous vein bypass graft(s) of the extremities, bilateral legs** Ⓐ▽

Ⓝ Newborn   Ⓟ Pediatric   Ⓜ Maternity   Ⓐ Adult   **RIC** RIC Dx   **NCDx** Noncancer Dx   **PDx** Primary Dx   **CC** RIC CC Condition   ►◄ Revised Text   ● New Code   ▲ Revised Code Title

608

ICD-10-CM 2016

I70.408   **Unspecified atherosclerosis of autologous vein bypass graft(s) of the extremities, other extremity**   A ▽

I70.409   **Unspecified atherosclerosis of autologous vein bypass graft(s) of the extremities, unspecified extremity**   A ▽

✓6ᵗʰ   **I70.41**   **Atherosclerosis of autologous vein bypass graft(s) of the extremities with intermittent claudication**

I70.411   **Atherosclerosis of autologous vein bypass graft(s) of the extremities with intermittent claudication, right leg**   A

I70.412   **Atherosclerosis of autologous vein bypass graft(s) of the extremities with intermittent claudication, left leg**   A

I70.413   **Atherosclerosis of autologous vein bypass graft(s) of the extremities with intermittent claudication, bilateral legs**   A

I70.418   **Atherosclerosis of autologous vein bypass graft(s) of the extremities with intermittent claudication, other extremity**   A

I70.419   **Atherosclerosis of autologous vein bypass graft(s) of the extremities with intermittent claudication, unspecified extremity**   A ▽

✓6ᵗʰ   **I70.42**   **Atherosclerosis of autologous vein bypass graft(s) of the extremities with rest pain**
    INCLUDES   any condition classifiable to I70.41-

I70.421   **Atherosclerosis of autologous vein bypass graft(s) of the extremities with rest pain, right leg**   A

I70.422   **Atherosclerosis of autologous vein bypass graft(s) of the extremities with rest pain, left leg**   A

I70.423   **Atherosclerosis of autologous vein bypass graft(s) of the extremities with rest pain, bilateral legs**   A

I70.428   **Atherosclerosis of autologous vein bypass graft(s) of the extremities with rest pain, other extremity**   A

I70.429   **Atherosclerosis of autologous vein bypass graft(s) of the extremities with rest pain, unspecified extremity**   A ▽

✓6ᵗʰ   **I70.43**   **Atherosclerosis of autologous vein bypass graft(s) of the right leg with ulceration**
    INCLUDES   any condition classifiable to I70.411 and I70.421
    Use additional code to identify severity of ulcer (L97.-)

I70.431   **Atherosclerosis of autologous vein bypass graft(s) of the right leg with ulceration of thigh**

I70.432   **Atherosclerosis of autologous vein bypass graft(s) of the right leg with ulceration of calf**   A

I70.433   **Atherosclerosis of autologous vein bypass graft(s) of the right leg with ulceration of ankle**   A

I70.434   **Atherosclerosis of autologous vein bypass graft(s) of the right leg with ulceration of heel and midfoot**   A
    Atherosclerosis of autologous vein bypass graft(s) of right leg with ulceration of plantar surface of midfoot

I70.435   **Atherosclerosis of autologous vein bypass graft(s) of the right leg with ulceration of other part of foot**   A
    Atherosclerosis of autologous vein bypass graft(s) of right leg with ulceration of toe

I70.438   **Atherosclerosis of autologous vein bypass graft(s) of the right leg with ulceration of other part of lower leg**   A

I70.439   **Atherosclerosis of autologous vein bypass graft(s) of the right leg with ulceration of unspecified site**   A ▽

✓6ᵗʰ   **I70.44**   **Atherosclerosis of autologous vein bypass graft(s) of the left leg with ulceration**
    INCLUDES   any condition classifiable to I70.412 and I70.422
    Use additional code to identify severity of ulcer (L97.-)

I70.441   **Atherosclerosis of autologous vein bypass graft(s) of the left leg with ulceration of thigh**   A

I70.442   **Atherosclerosis of autologous vein bypass graft(s) of the left leg with ulceration of calf**   A

I70.443   **Atherosclerosis of autologous vein bypass graft(s) of the left leg with ulceration of ankle**   A

I70.444   **Atherosclerosis of autologous vein bypass graft(s) of the left leg with ulceration of heel and midfoot**   A
    Atherosclerosis of autologous vein bypass graft(s) of left leg with ulceration of plantar surface of midfoot

I70.445   **Atherosclerosis of autologous vein bypass graft(s) of the left leg with ulceration of other part of foot**   A
    Atherosclerosis of autologous vein bypass graft(s) of left leg with ulceration of toe

I70.448   **Atherosclerosis of autologous vein bypass graft(s) of the left leg with ulceration of other part of lower leg**   A

I70.449   **Atherosclerosis of autologous vein bypass graft(s) of the left leg with ulceration of unspecified site**   A ▽

I70.45   **Atherosclerosis of autologous vein bypass graft(s) of other extremity with ulceration**   A
    INCLUDES   any condition classifiable to I70.418, I70.428, and I70.438
    Use additional code to identify severity of ulcer (L98.49)

✓6ᵗʰ   **I70.46**   **Atherosclerosis of autologous vein bypass graft(s) of the extremities with gangrene**
    INCLUDES   any condition classifiable to I70.41-, I70.42-, and I70.43-, I70.44-, I70.45
    Use additional code to identify the severity of any ulcer (L97.-, L98.49-), if applicable

I70.461   **Atherosclerosis of autologous vein bypass graft(s) of the extremities with gangrene, right leg**   A

I70.462   **Atherosclerosis of autologous vein bypass graft(s) of the extremities with gangrene, left leg**   A

I70.463   **Atherosclerosis of autologous vein bypass graft(s) of the extremities with gangrene, bilateral legs**   A

I70.468   **Atherosclerosis of autologous vein bypass graft(s) of the extremities with gangrene, other extremity**   A

I70.469   **Atherosclerosis of autologous vein bypass graft(s) of the extremities with gangrene, unspecified extremity**   A ▽

✓6ᵗʰ   **I70.49**   **Other atherosclerosis of autologous vein bypass graft(s) of the extremities**

I70.491   **Other atherosclerosis of autologous vein bypass graft(s) of the extremities, right leg**   A

I70.492   **Other atherosclerosis of autologous vein bypass graft(s) of the extremities, left leg**   A

I70.493   **Other atherosclerosis of autologous vein bypass graft(s) of the extremities, bilateral legs**   A

I70.498   **Other atherosclerosis of autologous vein bypass graft(s) of the extremities, other extremity**   A

I70.499   **Other atherosclerosis of autologous vein bypass graft(s) of the extremities, unspecified extremity**   A ▽

Chapter 9. Diseases of the Circulatory System

√5ᵗʰ **I70.5 Atherosclerosis of nonautologous biological bypass graft(s) of the extremities**

Use additional code, if applicable, to identify chronic total occlusion of artery of extremity (I70.92)

√6ᵗʰ **I70.50 Unspecified atherosclerosis of nonautologous biological bypass graft(s) of the extremities**

I70.501 Unspecified atherosclerosis of nonautologous biological bypass graft(s) of the extremities, right leg 🅰▽

I70.502 Unspecified atherosclerosis of nonautologous biological bypass graft(s) of the extremities, left leg 🅰▽

I70.503 Unspecified atherosclerosis of nonautologous biological bypass graft(s) of the extremities, bilateral legs 🅰▽

I70.508 Unspecified atherosclerosis of nonautologous biological bypass graft(s) of the extremities, other extremity 🅰▽

I70.509 Unspecified atherosclerosis of nonautologous biological bypass graft(s) of the extremities, unspecified extremity 🅰▽

√6ᵗʰ **I70.51 Atherosclerosis of nonautologous biological bypass graft(s) of the extremities with intermittent claudication**

I70.511 Atherosclerosis of nonautologous biological bypass graft(s) of the extremities with intermittent claudication, right leg 🅰

I70.512 Atherosclerosis of nonautologous biological bypass graft(s) of the extremities with intermittent claudication, left leg 🅰

I70.513 Atherosclerosis of nonautologous biological bypass graft(s) of the extremities with intermittent claudication, bilateral legs 🅰

I70.518 Atherosclerosis of nonautologous biological bypass graft(s) of the extremities with intermittent claudication, other extremity 🅰

I70.519 Atherosclerosis of nonautologous biological bypass graft(s) of the extremities with intermittent claudication, unspecified extremity 🅰▽

√6ᵗʰ **I70.52 Atherosclerosis of nonautologous biological bypass graft(s) of the extremities with rest pain**

INCLUDES any condition classifiable to I70.51-

I70.521 Atherosclerosis of nonautologous biological bypass graft(s) of the extremities with rest pain, right leg 🅰

I70.522 Atherosclerosis of nonautologous biological bypass graft(s) of the extremities with rest pain, left leg 🅰

I70.523 Atherosclerosis of nonautologous biological bypass graft(s) of the extremities with rest pain, bilateral legs 🅰

I70.528 Atherosclerosis of nonautologous biological bypass graft(s) of the extremities with rest pain, other extremity 🅰

I70.529 Atherosclerosis of nonautologous biological bypass graft(s) of the extremities with rest pain, unspecified extremity 🅰▽

√6ᵗʰ **I70.53 Atherosclerosis of nonautologous biological bypass graft(s) of the right leg with ulceration**

INCLUDES any condition classifiable to I70.511 and I70.521

Use additional code to identify severity of ulcer (L97.-)

I70.531 Atherosclerosis of nonautologous biological bypass graft(s) of the right leg with ulceration of thigh 🅰

I70.532 Atherosclerosis of nonautologous biological bypass graft(s) of the right leg with ulceration of calf 🅰

I70.533 Atherosclerosis of nonautologous biological bypass graft(s) of the right leg with ulceration of ankle 🅰

I70.534 Atherosclerosis of nonautologous biological bypass graft(s) of the right leg with ulceration of heel and midfoot 🅰

Atherosclerosis of nonautologous biological bypass graft(s) of right leg with ulceration of plantar surface of midfoot

I70.535 Atherosclerosis of nonautologous biological bypass graft(s) of the right leg with ulceration of other part of foot 🅰

Atherosclerosis of nonautologous biological bypass graft(s) of the right leg with ulceration of toe

I70.538 Atherosclerosis of nonautologous biological bypass graft(s) of the right leg with ulceration of other part of lower leg 🅰

I70.539 Atherosclerosis of nonautologous biological bypass graft(s) of the right leg with ulceration of unspecified site 🅰▽

√6ᵗʰ **I70.54 Atherosclerosis of nonautologous biological bypass graft(s) of the left leg with ulceration**

INCLUDES any condition classifiable to I70.512 and I70.522

Use additional code to identify severity of ulcer (L97.-)

I70.541 Atherosclerosis of nonautologous biological bypass graft(s) of the left leg with ulceration of thigh 🅰

I70.542 Atherosclerosis of nonautologous biological bypass graft(s) of the left leg with ulceration of calf 🅰

I70.543 Atherosclerosis of nonautologous biological bypass graft(s) of the left leg with ulceration of ankle 🅰

I70.544 Atherosclerosis of nonautologous biological bypass graft(s) of the left leg with ulceration of heel and midfoot 🅰

Atherosclerosis of nonautologous biological bypass graft(s) of left leg with ulceration of plantar surface of midfoot

I70.545 Atherosclerosis of nonautologous biological bypass graft(s) of the left leg with ulceration of other part of foot 🅰

Atherosclerosis of nonautologous biological bypass graft(s) of the left leg with ulceration of toe

I70.548 Atherosclerosis of nonautologous biological bypass graft(s) of the left leg with ulceration of other part of lower leg 🅰

I70.549 Atherosclerosis of nonautologous biological bypass graft(s) of the left leg with ulceration of unspecified site 🅰▽

I70.55 Atherosclerosis of nonautologous biological bypass graft(s) of other extremity with ulceration 🅰

INCLUDES any condition classifiable to I70.518, I70.528, and I70.538

Use additional code to identify severity of ulcer (L98.49)

√6ᵗʰ **I70.56 Atherosclerosis of nonautologous biological bypass graft(s) of the extremities with gangrene**

INCLUDES any condition classifiable to I70.51-, I70.52-, and I70.53-, I70.54-, I70.55

Use additional code to identify the severity of any ulcer (L97.-, L98.49-), if applicable

I70.561 Atherosclerosis of nonautologous biological bypass graft(s) of the extremities with gangrene, right leg 🅰

I70.562 Atherosclerosis of nonautologous biological bypass graft(s) of the extremities with gangrene, left leg 🅰

I70.563 Atherosclerosis of nonautologous biological bypass graft(s) of the extremities with gangrene, bilateral legs 🅰

I70.568 Atherosclerosis of nonautologous biological bypass graft(s) of the extremities with gangrene, other extremity 🅰

Ⓝ Newborn Ⓟ Pediatric Ⓜ Maternity 🅰 Adult RIC RIC Dx NCDx Noncancer Dx PDx Primary Dx CC RIC CC Condition ▶◀ Revised Text ● New Code ▲ Revised Code Title

610 ICD-10-CM 2016

I70.569   Atherosclerosis of nonautologous biological bypass graft(s) of the extremities with gangrene, unspecified extremity △▽

✓6ᵗʰ **I70.59**   Other atherosclerosis of nonautologous biological bypass graft(s) of the extremities

     I70.591   Other atherosclerosis of nonautologous biological bypass graft(s) of the extremities, right leg △

     I70.592   Other atherosclerosis of nonautologous biological bypass graft(s) of the extremities, left leg △

     I70.593   Other atherosclerosis of nonautologous biological bypass graft(s) of the extremities, bilateral legs △

     I70.598   Other atherosclerosis of nonautologousbiological bypass graft(s) of the extremities, other extremity △

     I70.599   Other atherosclerosis of nonautologous biological bypass graft(s) of the extremities, unspecified extremity △▽

✓5ᵗʰ **I70.6**   Atherosclerosis of nonbiological bypass graft(s) of the extremities

     Use additional code, if applicable, to identify chronic total occlusion of artery of extremity (I70.92)

✓6ᵗʰ **I70.60**   Unspecified atherosclerosis of nonbiological bypass graft(s) of the extremities

     I70.601   Unspecified atherosclerosis of nonbiological bypass graft(s) of the extremities, right leg △▽

     I70.602   Unspecified atherosclerosis of nonbiological bypass graft(s) of the extremities, left leg △▽

     I70.603   Unspecified atherosclerosis of nonbiological bypass graft(s) of the extremities, bilateral legs △▽

     I70.608   Unspecified atherosclerosis of nonbiological bypass graft(s) of the extremities, other extremity △▽

     I70.609   Unspecified atherosclerosis of nonbiological bypass graft(s) of the extremities, unspecified extremity △▽

✓6ᵗʰ **I70.61**   Atherosclerosis of nonbiological bypass graft(s) of the extremities with intermittent claudication

     I70.611   Atherosclerosis of nonbiological bypass graft(s) of the extremities with intermittent claudication, right leg △

     I70.612   Atherosclerosis of nonbiological bypass graft(s) of the extremities with intermittent claudication, left leg △

     I70.613   Atherosclerosis of nonbiological bypass graft(s) of the extremities with intermittent claudication, bilateral legs △

     I70.618   Atherosclerosis of nonbiological bypass graft(s) of the extremities with intermittent claudication, other extremity △

     I70.619   Atherosclerosis of nonbiological bypassgraft(s) of the extremities with intermittent claudication, unspecified extremity △▽

✓6ᵗʰ **I70.62**   Atherosclerosis of nonbiological bypass graft(s) of the extremities with rest pain

     INCLUDES   any condition classifiable to I70.61-

     I70.621   Atherosclerosis of nonbiological bypass graft(s) of the extremities with rest pain, right leg △

     I70.622   Atherosclerosis of nonbiological bypass graft(s) of the extremities with rest pain, left leg △

     I70.623   Atherosclerosis of nonbiological bypass graft(s) of the extremities with rest pain, bilateral legs △

     I70.628   Atherosclerosis of nonbiological bypass graft(s) of the extremities with rest pain, other extremity △

     I70.629   Atherosclerosis of nonbiological bypass graft(s) of the extremities with rest pain, unspecified extremity △▽

✓6ᵗʰ **I70.63**   Atherosclerosis of nonbiological bypass graft(s) of the right leg with ulceration

     INCLUDES   any condition classifiable to I70.611 and I70.621

     Use additional code to identify severity of ulcer (L97.-)

     I70.631   Atherosclerosis of nonbiological bypass graft(s) of the right leg with ulceration of thigh △

     I70.632   Atherosclerosis of nonbiological bypass graft(s) of the right leg with ulceration of calf △

     I70.633   Atherosclerosis of nonbiological bypass graft(s) of the right leg with ulceration of ankle △

     I70.634   Atherosclerosis of nonbiological bypass graft(s) of the right leg with ulceration of heel and midfoot △
       Atherosclerosis of nonbiological bypass graft(s) of right leg with ulceration of plantar surface of midfoot

     I70.635   Atherosclerosis of nonbiological bypass graft(s) of the right leg with ulceration of other part of foot △
       Atherosclerosis of nonbiological bypass graft(s) of the right leg with ulceration of toe

     I70.638   Atherosclerosis of nonbiological bypass graft(s) of the right leg with ulceration of other part of lower leg △

     I70.639   Atherosclerosis of nonbiological bypass graft(s) of the right leg with ulceration of unspecified site △▽

✓6ᵗʰ **I70.64**   Atherosclerosis of nonbiological bypass graft(s) of the left leg with ulceration

     INCLUDES   any condition classifiable to I70.612 and I70.622

     Use additional code to identify severity of ulcer (L97.-)

     I70.641   Atherosclerosis of nonbiological bypass graft(s) of the left leg with ulceration of thigh △

     I70.642   Atherosclerosis of nonbiological bypass graft(s) of the left leg with ulceration of calf △

     I70.643   Atherosclerosis of nonbiological bypass graft(s) of the left leg with ulceration of ankle △

     I70.644   Atherosclerosis of nonbiological bypass graft(s) of the left leg with ulceration of heel and midfoot △
       Atherosclerosis of nonbiological bypass graft(s) of left leg with ulceration of plantar surface of midfoot

     I70.645   Atherosclerosis of nonbiological bypassgraft(s) of the left leg with ulceration of other part of foot △
       Atherosclerosis of nonbiological bypass graft(s) of the left leg with ulceration of toe

     I70.648   Atherosclerosis of nonbiological bypass graft(s) of the left leg with ulceration of other part of lower leg △

     I70.649   Atherosclerosis of nonbiological bypass graft(s) of the left leg with ulceration of unspecified site △▽

I70.65   Atherosclerosis of nonbiological bypass graft(s) of other extremity with ulceration △

     INCLUDES   any condition classifiable to I70.618 and I70.628

     Use additional code to identify severity of ulcer (L98.49)

✓6ᵗʰ **I70.66**   Atherosclerosis of nonbiological bypass graft(s) of the extremities with gangrene

     INCLUDES   any condition classifiable to I70.61-, I70.62-, I70.63-, I70.64-, I70.65

     Use additional code to identify the severity of any ulcer (L97.-, L98.49-), if applicable

     I70.661   Atherosclerosis of nonbiological bypass graft(s) of the extremities with gangrene, right leg △

     I70.662   Atherosclerosis of nonbiological bypass graft(s) of the extremities with gangrene, left leg △

✔ Add'l Character Required   ✗x7ᵗʰ Placeholder Alert   RUG IV Special Care High Dx   RUG IV Clinically Complex Dx   RUG IV Special Care Low Dx   Manifestation Code   Other Specified Code   ▽ Unspecified Code

ICD-10-CM 2016   611

Chapter 9. Diseases of the Circulatory System

I70.663 Atherosclerosis of nonbiological bypass graft(s) of the extremities with gangrene, bilateral legs ⒶＡ

I70.668 Atherosclerosis of nonbiological bypass graft(s) of the extremities with gangrene, other extremity Ⓐ

I70.669 Atherosclerosis of nonbiological bypass graft(s) of the extremities with gangrene, unspecified extremity Ⓐ▽

✓6ᵗʰ **I70.69** Other atherosclerosis of nonbiological bypass graft(s) of the extremities

I70.691 Other atherosclerosis of nonbiological bypass graft(s) of the extremities, right leg Ⓐ

I70.692 Other atherosclerosis of nonbiological bypass graft(s) of the extremities, left leg Ⓐ

I70.693 Other atherosclerosis of nonbiological bypass graft(s) of the extremities, bilateral legs Ⓐ

I70.698 Other atherosclerosis of nonbiological bypass graft(s) of the extremities, other extremity Ⓐ

I70.699 Other atherosclerosis of nonbiological bypass graft(s) of the extremities, unspecified extremity Ⓐ▽

✓5ᵗʰ **I70.7** Atherosclerosis of other type of bypass graft(s) of the extremities
Use additional code, if applicable, to identify chronic total occlusion of artery of extremity (I70.92)

✓6ᵗʰ **I70.70** Unspecified atherosclerosis of other type of bypass graft(s) of the extremities

I70.701 Unspecified atherosclerosis of other type of bypass graft(s) of the extremities, right leg Ⓐ▽

I70.702 Unspecified atherosclerosis of other type of bypass graft(s) of the extremities, left leg Ⓐ▽

I70.703 Unspecified atherosclerosis of other type of bypass graft(s) of the extremities, bilateral legs Ⓐ▽

I70.708 Unspecified atherosclerosis of other type of bypass graft(s) of the extremities, other extremity Ⓐ▽

I70.709 Unspecified atherosclerosis of other type of bypass graft(s) of the extremities, unspecified extremity Ⓐ▽

✓6ᵗʰ **I70.71** Atherosclerosis of other type of bypass graft(s) of the extremities with intermittent claudication

I70.711 Atherosclerosis of other type of bypass graft(s) of the extremities with intermittent claudication, right leg Ⓐ

I70.712 Atherosclerosis of other type of bypass graft(s) of the extremities with intermittent claudication, left leg Ⓐ

I70.713 Atherosclerosis of other type of bypass graft(s) of the extremities with intermittent claudication, bilateral legs Ⓐ

I70.718 Atherosclerosis of other type of bypass graft(s) of the extremities with intermittent claudication, other extremity Ⓐ

I70.719 Atherosclerosis of other type of graft(s) bypass of the extremities with intermittent claudication, unspecified extremity Ⓐ▽

✓6ᵗʰ **I70.72** Atherosclerosis of other type of bypass graft(s) of the extremities with rest pain
INCLUDES any condition classifiable to I70.71-

I70.721 Atherosclerosis of other type of bypass graft(s) of the extremities with rest pain, right leg Ⓐ

I70.722 Atherosclerosis of other type of bypass graft(s) of the extremities with rest pain, left leg Ⓐ

I70.723 Atherosclerosis of other type of bypass graft(s) of the extremities with rest pain, bilateral legs Ⓐ

I70.728 Atherosclerosis of other type of bypass graft(s) of the extremities with rest pain, other extremity Ⓐ

I70.729 Atherosclerosis of other type of bypass graft(s) of the extremities with rest pain, unspecified extremity Ⓐ▽

✓6ᵗʰ **I70.73** Atherosclerosis of other type of bypass graft(s) of the right leg with ulceration
INCLUDES any condition classifiable to I70.711 and I70.721
Use additional code to identify severity of ulcer (L97.-)

I70.731 Atherosclerosis of other type of bypass graft(s) of the right leg with ulceration of thigh Ⓐ

I70.732 Atherosclerosis of other type of bypass graft(s) of the right leg with ulceration of calf Ⓐ

I70.733 Atherosclerosis of other type of bypass graft(s) of the right leg with ulceration of ankle Ⓐ

I70.734 Atherosclerosis of other type of bypass graft(s) of the right leg with ulceration of heel and midfoot Ⓐ
Atherosclerosis of other type of bypass graft(s) of right leg with ulceration of plantar surface of midfoot

I70.735 Atherosclerosis of other type of bypass graft(s) of the right leg with ulceration of other part of foot Ⓐ
Atherosclerosis of other type of bypass graft(s) of right leg with ulceration of toe

I70.738 Atherosclerosis of other type of bypass graft(s) of the right leg with ulceration of other part of lower leg Ⓐ

I70.739 Atherosclerosis of other type of bypass graft(s) of the right leg with ulceration of unspecified site Ⓐ▽

✓6ᵗʰ **I70.74** Atherosclerosis of other type of bypass graft(s) of the left leg with ulceration
INCLUDES any condition classifiable to I70.712 and I70.722
Use additional code to identify severity of ulcer (L97.-)

I70.741 Atherosclerosis of other type of bypass graft(s) of the left leg with ulceration of thigh Ⓐ

I70.742 Atherosclerosis of other type of bypass graft(s) of the left leg with ulceration of calf Ⓐ

I70.743 Atherosclerosis of other type of bypass graft(s) of the left leg with ulceration of ankle Ⓐ

I70.744 Atherosclerosis of other type of bypass graft(s) of the left leg with ulceration of heel and midfoot Ⓐ
Atherosclerosis of other type of bypass graft(s) of left leg with ulceration of plantar surface of midfoot

I70.745 Atherosclerosis of other type of bypass graft(s) of the left leg with ulceration of other part of foot Ⓐ
Atherosclerosis of other type of bypass graft(s) of left leg with ulceration of toe

I70.748 Atherosclerosis of other type of bypass graft(s) of the left leg with ulceration of other part of lower leg Ⓐ

I70.749 Atherosclerosis of other type of bypass graft(s) of the left leg with ulceration of unspecified site Ⓐ▽

I70.75 Atherosclerosis of other type of bypass graft(s) of other extremity with ulceration Ⓐ
INCLUDES any condition classifiable to I70.718 and I70.728
Use additional code to identify severity of ulcer (L98.49)

✓6ᵗʰ **I70.76** Atherosclerosis of other type of bypass graft(s) of the extremities with gangrene
INCLUDES any condition classifiable to I70.71-, I70.72-, I70.73-, I70.74-, I70.75
Use additional code to identify the severity of any ulcer (L97.-, L98.49-), if applicable

I70.761 Atherosclerosis of other type of bypass graft(s) of the extremities with gangrene, right leg Ⓐ

Ⓝ Newborn   Ⓟ Pediatric   Ⓜ Maternity   Ⓐ Adult   **RIC** RIC Dx   **NCDx** Noncancer Dx   **PDx** Primary Dx   **CC** RIC CC Condition   ▶◀ Revised Text   ● New Code   ▲ Revised Code Title

612   ICD-10-CM 2016

I70.762 Atherosclerosis of other type of bypass graft(s) of the extremities with gangrene, left leg 🅰

I70.763 Atherosclerosis of other type of bypass graft(s) of the extremities with gangrene, bilateral legs 🅰

I70.768 Atherosclerosis of other type of bypass graft(s) of the extremities with gangrene, other extremity 🅰

I70.769 Atherosclerosis of other type of bypass graft(s) of the extremities with gangrene, unspecified extremity 🅰 ▽

✓6th I70.79 Other atherosclerosis of other type of bypass graft(s) of the extremities

I70.791 Other atherosclerosis of other type of bypass graft(s) of the extremities, right leg 🅰

I70.792 Other atherosclerosis of other type of bypass graft(s) of the extremities, left leg 🅰

I70.793 Other atherosclerosis of other type of bypass graft(s) of the extremities, bilateral legs 🅰

I70.798 Other atherosclerosis of other type of bypass graft(s) of the extremities, other extremity 🅰

I70.799 Other atherosclerosis of other type of bypass graft(s) of the extremities, unspecified extremity 🅰 ▽

I70.8 **Atherosclerosis of other arteries** 🅰

✓5th I70.9 **Other and unspecified atherosclerosis**

I70.90 Unspecified atherosclerosis 🅰 ▽

I70.91 Generalized atherosclerosis 🅰

I70.92 Chronic total occlusion of artery of the extremities cc 🅰
Complete occlusion of artery of the extremities
Total occlusion of artery of the extremities
Code first atherosclerosis of arteries of the extremities (I70.2-, I70.3-, I70.4-, I70.5-, I70.6-, I70.7-)
RIC Excl: 10 Amputation, lower extremity; 11 Amputation, non-lower extremity

✓4th **I71 Aortic aneurysm and dissection**
EXCLUDES 1 aortic ectasia (I77.81-)
syphilitic aortic aneurysm (A52.01)
traumatic aortic aneurysm (S25.09, S35.09)

✓5th I71.0 Dissection of aorta

I71.00 **Dissection of unspecified site of aorta** cc 🅰 ▽
RIC Excl: 05 Non-traumatic spinal cord injury

I71.01 **Dissection of thoracic aorta** cc 🅰
RIC Excl: 05 Non-traumatic spinal cord injury

I71.02 **Dissection of abdominal aorta** cc 🅰
RIC Excl: 05 Non-traumatic spinal cord injury

I71.03 **Dissection of thoracoabdominal aorta** cc 🅰
RIC Excl: 05 Non-traumatic spinal cord injury

I71.1 Thoracic **aortic aneurysm, ruptured** cc 🅰
RIC Excl: 05 Non-traumatic spinal cord injury

I71.2 Thoracic **aortic aneurysm, without rupture** 🅰

I71.3 Abdominal **aortic aneurysm, ruptured** cc 🅰
RIC Excl: 05 Non-traumatic spinal cord injury

I71.4 Abdominal **aortic aneurysm, without rupture** 🅰

I71.5 Thoracoabdominal **aortic aneurysm, ruptured** cc 🅰
RIC Excl: 05 Non-traumatic spinal cord injury

I71.6 Thoracoabdominal **aortic aneurysm, without rupture** 🅰

I71.8 **Aortic aneurysm of unspecified site, ruptured** cc 🅰 ▽
Rupture of aorta NOS

I71.9 **Aortic aneurysm of unspecified site, without rupture** 🅰 ▽
Aneurysm of aorta
Dilatation of aorta
Hyaline necrosis of aorta

✓4th **I72 Other aneurysm**
INCLUDES aneurysm (cirsoid) (false) (ruptured)
EXCLUDES 2 acquired aneurysm (I77.0)
aneurysm (of) aorta (I71.-)
aneurysm (of) arteriovenous NOS (Q27.3-)
carotid artery dissection (I77.71)
cerebral (nonruptured) aneurysm (I67.1)
coronary aneurysm (I25.4)
coronary artery dissection (I25.42)
dissection of artery NEC (I77.79)
heart aneurysm (I25.3)
iliac artery dissection (I77.72)
pulmonary artery aneurysm (I28.1)
renal artery dissection (I77.73)
retinal aneurysm (H35.0)
ruptured cerebral aneurysm (I60.7)
varicose aneurysm (I77.0)
vertebral artery dissection (I77.74)

I72.0 **Aneurysm of carotid artery** 🅰
Aneurysm of common carotid artery
Aneurysm of external carotid artery
Aneurysm of internal carotid artery, extracranial portion
EXCLUDES 1 aneurysm of internal carotid artery, intracranial portion (I67.1)
aneurysm of internal carotid artery NOS (I67.1)

I72.1 **Aneurysm of artery of upper extremity** 🅰

I72.2 **Aneurysm of renal artery** 🅰

I72.3 **Aneurysm of iliac artery** 🅰

I72.4 **Aneurysm of artery of lower extremity** 🅰

I72.8 **Aneurysm of other specified arteries** 🅰

I72.9 **Aneurysm of unspecified site** 🅰 ▽

✓4th **I73 Other peripheral vascular diseases**
EXCLUDES 2 chilblains (T69.1)
frostbite (T33- T34)
immersion hand or foot (T69.0-)
spasm of cerebral artery (G45.9)

✓5th I73.0 **Raynaud's syndrome**
Raynaud's disease
Raynaud's phenomenon (secondary)

I73.00 **Raynaud's syndrome without gangrene**

I73.01 **Raynaud's syndrome with gangrene**

I73.1 **Thromboangiitis obliterans [Buerger's disease]**

✓5th I73.8 **Other specified peripheral vascular diseases**
EXCLUDES 1 diabetic (peripheral) angiopathy (E08-E13 with .51-.52)

I73.81 **Erythromelalgia**

I73.89 **Other specified peripheral vascular diseases**
Acrocyanosis
Erythrocyanosis
Simple acroparesthesia [Schultze's type]
Vasomotor acroparesthesia [Nothnagel's type]

I73.9 **Peripheral vascular disease, unspecified** ▽
Intermittent claudication
Peripheral angiopathy NOS
Spasm of artery
EXCLUDES 1 atherosclerosis of the extremities (I70.2--I70.7-)

✓4th **I74 Arterial embolism and thrombosis**
Embolic infarction
Embolic occlusion
Thrombotic infarction
Thrombotic occlusion
Code first:
embolism and thrombosis complicating abortion or ectopic or molar pregnancy (O00-O07, O08.2)
embolism and thrombosis complicating pregnancy, childbirth and the puerperium (O88.-)
EXCLUDES 2 atheroembolism (I75.-)
basilar embolism and thrombosis (I63.0-I63.2, I65.1)
carotid embolism and thrombosis (I63.0-I63.2, I65.2)
cerebral embolism and thrombosis (I63.3-I63.5, I66-)
coronary embolism and thrombosis (I21-I25)
mesenteric embolism and thrombosis (K55.0)
ophthalmic embolism and thrombosis (H34.-)
precerebral embolism and thrombosis NOS (I63.0-I63.2, I65.9)
pulmonary embolism and thrombosis (I26.-)
renal embolism and thrombosis (N28.0)
retinal embolism and thrombosis (H34.-)
septic embolism and thrombosis (I76)
vertebral embolism and thrombosis (I63.0-I63.2, I65.0)

✅ Add'l Character Required ✓x7th Placeholder Alert RUG IV Special Care High Dx RUG IV Clinically Complex Dx RUG IV Special Care Low Dx Manifestation Code Other Specified Code ▽ Unspecified Code

Chapter 9. Diseases of the Circulatory System *(side tab)*

✓5th I74.0 Embolism and thrombosis of abdominal aorta

   I74.01 Saddle **embolus of abdominal aorta**

   I74.09 Other arterial **embolism and thrombosis of abdominal aorta**
      Aortic bifurcation syndrome
      Aortoiliac obstruction
      Leriche's syndrome

✓5th I74.1 Embolism and thrombosis of other and unspecified parts **of aorta**

   I74.10 Embolism and thrombosis of unspecified parts of aorta ▽

   I74.11 Embolism and thrombosis of thoracic **aorta**

   I74.19 Embolism and thrombosis of other parts of aorta

I74.2 Embolism and thrombosis of arteries of the upper extremities

I74.3 Embolism and thrombosis of arteries of the lower extremities

I74.4 Embolism and thrombosis of arteries of extremities, unspecified ▽
   Peripheral arterial embolism NOS

I74.5 Embolism and thrombosis of iliac **artery**

I74.8 Embolism and thrombosis of other arteries

I74.9 Embolism and thrombosis of unspecified artery ▽

✓4th I75 Atheroembolism
   Atherothrombotic microembolism
   Cholesterol embolism

✓5th I75.0 Atheroembolism of extremities

   ✓6th I75.01 Atheroembolism of upper **extremity**

      I75.011 Atheroembolism of right **upper extremity**

      I75.012 Atheroembolism of left **upper extremity**

      I75.013 Atheroembolism of bilateral **upper extremities**

      I75.019 Atheroembolism of unspecified upper extremity ▽

   ✓6th I75.02 Atheroembolism of lower **extremity**

      I75.021 Atheroembolism of right **lower extremity**

      I75.022 Atheroembolism of left **lower extremity**

      I75.023 Atheroembolism of bilateral **lower extremities**

      I75.029 Atheroembolism of unspecified lower extremity ▽

✓5th I75.8 Atheroembolism of other sites

   I75.81 Atheroembolism of kidney
      Use additional code for any associated acute kidney failure and chronic kidney disease (N17.-, N18.-)

   I75.89 Atheroembolism of other site

I76 Septic arterial embolism   CC
   Code first underlying infection, such as:
     infective endocarditis (I33.0)
     lung abscess (J85.-)
   Use additional code to identify the site of the embolism (I74.-)
   EXCLUDES 2 septic pulmonary embolism (I26.01, I26.90)

✓4th I77 Other disorders of arteries and arterioles
   EXCLUDES 2 collagen (vascular) diseases (M30-M36)
     hypersensitivity angiitis (M31.0)
     pulmonary artery (I28.-)

I77.0 Arteriovenous fistula, acquired
   Aneurysmal varix   Arteriovenous aneurysm, acquired
   EXCLUDES 1 arteriovenous aneurysm NOS (Q27.3-)
     presence of arteriovenous shunt (fistula) for dialysis (Z99.2)
     traumatic—see injury of blood vessel by body region
   EXCLUDES 2 cerebral (I67.1)
     coronary (I25.4)

I77.1 Stricture of artery
   Narrowing of artery

I77.2 Rupture of artery
   Erosion of artery
   Fistula of artery
   Ulcer of artery
   EXCLUDES 1 traumatic rupture of artery—see injury of blood vessel by body region

I77.3 Arterial fibromuscular dysplasia
   Fibromuscular hyperplasia (of) carotid artery
   Fibromuscular hyperplasia (of) renal artery

I77.4 Celiac artery compression syndrome

I77.5 Necrosis of artery

I77.6 Arteritis, unspecified ▽
   Aortitis NOS
   Endarteritis NOS
   EXCLUDES 1 arteritis or endarteritis:
     aortic arch (M31.4)
     cerebral NEC (I67.7)
     coronary (I25.89)
     deformans (I70.-)
     giant cell (M31.5., M31.6)
     obliterans (I70.-)
     senile (I70.-)

✓5th I77.7 Other arterial dissection
   EXCLUDES 2 dissection of aorta (I71.0-)
     dissection of coronary artery (I25.42)

   I77.71 Dissection of carotid **artery**

   I77.72 Dissection of iliac **artery**

   I77.73 Dissection of renal **artery**

   I77.74 Dissection of vertebral **artery**

   I77.79 Dissection of other artery

✓5th I77.8 Other specified disorders of arteries and arterioles

   ✓6th I77.81 Aortic ectasia
      Ectasis aorta
      EXCLUDES 1 aortic aneurysm and dissection (I71.0-)

      I77.810 Thoracic aortic ectasia

      I77.811 Abdominal aortic ectasia

      I77.812 Thoracoabdominal aortic ectasia

      I77.819 Aortic ectasia, unspecified site ▽

   I77.89 Other specified disorders of arteries and arterioles

I77.9 Disorder of arteries and arterioles, unspecified ▽

✓4th I78 Diseases of capillaries

I78.0 Hereditary hemorrhagic telangiectasia
   Rendu-Osler-Weber disease

I78.1 Nevus, non-neoplastic
   Araneus nevus
   Senile nevus
   Spider nevus
   Stellar nevus
   EXCLUDES 1 nevus NOS (D22.-)
     vascular NOS (Q82.5)
   EXCLUDES 2 blue nevus (D22.-)
     flammeus nevus (Q82.5)
     hairy nevus (D22.-)
     melanocytic nevus (D22.-)
     pigmented nevus (D22.-)
     portwine nevus (Q82.5)
     sanguineous nevus (Q82.5)
     strawberry nevus (Q82.5)
     verrucous nevus (Q82.5)

I78.8 Other diseases of capillaries

I78.9 Disease of capillaries, unspecified ▽

✓4th I79 Disorders of arteries, arterioles and capillaries in diseases classified elsewhere

I79.0 Aneurysm of aorta in diseases classified elsewhere   A
   Code first underlying disease
   EXCLUDES 1 syphilitic aneurysm (A52.01)

I79.1 Aortitis in diseases classified elsewhere
   Code first underlying disease
   EXCLUDES 1 syphilitic aortitis (A52.02)

I79.8 Other disorders of arteries, arterioles and capillaries in diseases classified elsewhere
   Code first underlying disease, such as:
     amyloidosis (E85.-)
   EXCLUDES 1 diabetic (peripheral) angiopathy (E08-E13 with .51-.52)
     syphilitic endarteritis (A52.09)
     tuberculous endarteritis (A18.89)

N Newborn   P Pediatric   M Maternity   A Adult   RIC RIC Dx   NC Dx Noncancer Dx   PDx Primary Dx   CC RIC CC Condition   ►◄ Revised Text   ● New Code   ▲ Revised Code Title

I74.0–I79.8

614   ICD-10-CM 2016

☑️4ᵗʰ **I80 Phlebitis and thrombophlebitis**
    INCLUDES endophlebitis
            inflammation, vein
            periphlebitis
            suppurative phlebitis
    Code first:
        phlebitis and thrombophlebitis complicating abortion, ectopic or
            molar pregnancy (O00–O07, O08.7)
        phlebitis and thrombophlebitis complicating pregnancy, childbirth
            and the puerperium (O22.-, O87.-)
      EXCLUDES 1 *venous embolism and thrombosis of lower extremities ((I82.4-,*
            I82.5-, I82.81-)

☑️5ᵗʰ **I80.0 Phlebitis and thrombophlebitis of** superficial vessels of lower
      extremities
    Phlebitis and thrombophlebitis of femoropopliteal vein
    I80.00 Phlebitis and thrombophlebitis of superficial ▽
        vessels of unspecified lower extremity
    I80.01 Phlebitis and thrombophlebitis of superficial
        vessels of right **lower extremity**
    I80.02 Phlebitis and thrombophlebitis of superficial
        vessels of left **lower extremity**
    I80.03 Phlebitis and thrombophlebitis of superficial
        vessels of lower extremities, bilateral

☑️5ᵗʰ **I80.1 Phlebitis and thrombophlebitis of** femoral vein
    I80.10 Phlebitis and thrombophlebitis of unspecified ▽
        femoral vein
    I80.11 Phlebitis and thrombophlebitis of right **femoral vein**
    I80.12 Phlebitis and thrombophlebitis of left **femoral vein**
    I80.13 Phlebitis and thrombophlebitis of femoral vein,
        bilateral

☑️5ᵗʰ **I80.2 Phlebitis and thrombophlebitis of** other and unspecified deep
    vessels of lower extremities
    ☑️6ᵗʰ **I80.20 Phlebitis and thrombophlebitis of** unspecified **deep**
        vessels of lower extremities
        I80.201 Phlebitis and thrombophlebitis of
            unspecified deep vessels of right **lower**
            extremity
        I80.202 Phlebitis and thrombophlebitis of
            unspecified deep vessels of left **lower**
            extremity
        I80.203 Phlebitis and thrombophlebitis of
            unspecified deep vessels of lower
            extremities, bilateral
        I80.209 Phlebitis and thrombophlebitis of ▽
            unspecified deep vessels of unspecified
            lower extremity
    ☑️6ᵗʰ **I80.21 Phlebitis and thrombophlebitis of** iliac vein
        I80.211 Phlebitis and thrombophlebitis of right
            iliac vein
         I80.212 Phlebitis and thrombophlebitis of left **iliac**
            vein
        I80.213 Phlebitis and thrombophlebitis of iliac
            vein, bilateral
        I80.219 Phlebitis and thrombophlebitis of ▽
            unspecified iliac vein
    ☑️6ᵗʰ **I80.22 Phlebitis and thrombophlebitis of** popliteal vein
        I80.221 Phlebitis and thrombophlebitis of right
            popliteal vein
        I80.222 Phlebitis and thrombophlebitis of left
            popliteal vein
        I80.223 Phlebitis and thrombophlebitis of
            popliteal vein, bilateral
        I80.229 Phlebitis and thrombophlebitis of ▽
            unspecified popliteal vein
    ☑️6ᵗʰ **I80.23 Phlebitis and thrombophlebitis of** tibial vein
        I80.231 Phlebitis and thrombophlebitis of right
            tibial vein
        I80.232 Phlebitis and thrombophlebitis of left
            tibial vein
        I80.233 Phlebitis and thrombophlebitis of tibial
            vein, bilateral
        I80.239 Phlebitis and thrombophlebitis of ▽
            unspecified tibial vein
    ☑️6ᵗʰ **I80.29 Phlebitis and thrombophlebitis of** other **deep**
        vessels of lower extremities
        I80.291 Phlebitis and thrombophlebitis of other
            deep vessels of right **lower extremity**

        I80.292 Phlebitis and thrombophlebitis of other
            deep vessels of left **lower extremity**
        I80.293 Phlebitis and thrombophlebitis of other
            deep vessels of lower extremity, bilateral
        I80.299 Phlebitis and thrombophlebitis of ▽
            other deep vessels of unspecified
            lower extremity
    I80.3 Phlebitis and thrombophlebitis of lower extremities, ▽
      unspecified
    I80.8 Phlebitis and thrombophlebitis of other sites
    I80.9 Phlebitis and thrombophlebitis of unspecified site ▽

I81 Portal vein thrombosis   CC
    Portal (vein) obstruction
      EXCLUDES 2 *hepatic vein thrombosis (I82.0)*
              phlebitis of portal vein (K75.1)

☑️4ᵗʰ **I82 Other venous embolism and thrombosis**
    Code first venous embolism and thrombosis complicating:
      abortion, ectopic or molar pregnancy (O00–O07, O08.7)
      pregnancy, childbirth and the puerperium (O22.-, O87.-)
      EXCLUDES 2 *venous embolism and thrombosis (of):*
            cerebral (I63.6, I67.6)
            coronary (I21–I25)
            intracranial and intraspinal, septic or NOS (G08)
            intracranial, nonpyogenic (I67.6)
            intraspinal, nonpyogenic (G95.1)
            mesenteric (K55.0)
            portal (I81)
            pulmonary (I26.-)

    I82.0 Budd-Chiari syndrome   CC
      Hepatic vein thrombosis
    I82.1 Thrombophlebitis migrans   CC
    ☑️5ᵗʰ **I82.2 Embolism and thrombosis of** vena cava **and** other thoracic
      veins
      ☑️6ᵗʰ **I82.21 Embolism and thrombosis of** superior vena cava
        I82.210 Acute embolism and thrombosis of
            superior vena cava
            Embolism and thrombosis of superior vena
            cava NOS
        I82.211 Chronic embolism and thrombosis of
            superior vena cava
      ☑️6ᵗʰ **I82.22 Embolism and thrombosis of** inferior vena cava
        I82.220 Acute embolism and thrombosis of   CC
            inferior vena cava
             Embolism and thrombosis of inferior vena
            cava NOS
        I82.221 Chronic embolism and thrombosis of   CC
            inferior vena cava
      ☑️6ᵗʰ **I82.29 Embolism and thrombosis of** other thoracic veins
        Embolism and thrombosis of brachiocephalic
        (innominate) vein
        I82.290 Acute embolism and thrombosis of
            other thoracic veins
        I82.291 Chronic embolism and thrombosis
            of other thoracic veins
    I82.3 Embolism and thrombosis of renal vein   CC
    ☑️5ᵗʰ **I82.4 Acute embolism and thrombosis of** deep veins of lower
      extremity
      ☑️6ᵗʰ **I82.40 Acute embolism and thrombosis of** unspecified **deep**
        veins of lower extremity
        Deep vein thrombosis NOS
        DVT NOS
          EXCLUDES 1 *acute embolism and thrombosis of*
              unspecified deep veins of distal lower
              extremity (I82.4Z-)
            acute embolism and thrombosis of
              unspecified deep veins of proximal lower
              extremity (I82.4Y-)
        I82.401 Acute embolism and thrombosis of
            unspecified deep veins of right **lower**
            extremity
        I82.402 Acute embolism and thrombosis of
            unspecified deep veins of left **lower**
            extremity
        I82.403 Acute embolism and thrombosis of
            unspecified deep veins of lower extremity,
            bilateral
        I82.409 Acute embolism and thrombosis of ▽
            unspecified deep veins of unspecified
            lower extremity

☑️ Add'l Character Required   ☑️x7ᵗʰ Placeholder Alert   RUG IV Special Care High Dx   RUG IV Clinically Complex Dx   RUG IV Special Care Low Dx   Manifestation Code   Other Specified Code   ▽ Unspecified Code

ICD-10-CM 2016   **615**

Chapter 9. Diseases of the Circulatory System

✓6ᵗʰ **I82.41** Acute embolism and thrombosis of femoral vein

    I82.411 Acute embolism and thrombosis of right femoral vein

    I82.412 Acute embolism and thrombosis of left femoral vein

    I82.413 Acute embolism and thrombosis of femoral vein, bilateral

    I82.419 Acute embolism and thrombosis of unspecified femoral vein ▽

✓6ᵗʰ **I82.42** Acute embolism and thrombosis of iliac vein

    I82.421 Acute embolism and thrombosis of right iliac vein

    I82.422 Acute embolism and thrombosis of left iliac vein

    I82.423 Acute embolism and thrombosis of iliac vein, bilateral

    I82.429 Acute embolism and thrombosis of unspecified iliac vein ▽

✓6ᵗʰ **I82.43** Acute embolism and thrombosis of popliteal vein

    I82.431 Acute embolism and thrombosis of right popliteal vein

    I82.432 Acute embolism and thrombosis of left popliteal vein

    I82.433 Acute embolism and thrombosis of popliteal vein, bilateral

    I82.439 Acute embolism and thrombosis of unspecified popliteal vein ▽

✓6ᵗʰ **I82.44** Acute embolism and thrombosis of tibial vein

    I82.441 Acute embolism and thrombosis of right tibial vein

    I82.442 Acute embolism and thrombosis of left tibial vein

    I82.443 Acute embolism and thrombosis of tibial vein, bilateral

    I82.449 Acute embolism and thrombosis of unspecified tibial vein ▽

✓6ᵗʰ **I82.49** Acute embolism and thrombosis of other specified deep vein of lower extremity

    I82.491 Acute embolism and thrombosis of other specified deep vein of right lower extremity

    I82.492 Acute embolism and thrombosis of other specified deep vein of left lower extremity

    I82.493 Acute embolism and thrombosis of other specified deep vein of lower extremity, bilateral

    I82.499 Acute embolism and thrombosis of other specified deep vein of unspecified lower extremity ▽

✓6ᵗʰ **I82.4Y** Acute embolism and thrombosis of unspecified deep veins of proximal lower extremity

    Acute embolism and thrombosis of deep vein of thigh NOS

    Acute embolism and thrombosis of deep vein of upper leg NOS

    I82.4Y1 Acute embolism and thrombosis of unspecified deep veins of right proximal lower extremity

    I82.4Y2 Acute embolism and thrombosis of unspecified deep veins of left proximal lower extremity

    I82.4Y3 Acute embolism and thrombosis of unspecified deep veins of proximal lower extremity, bilateral

    I82.4Y9 Acute embolism and thrombosis of unspecified deep veins of unspecified proximal lower extremity ▽

✓6ᵗʰ **I82.4Z** Acute embolism and thrombosis of unspecified deep veins of distal lower extremity

    Acute embolism and thrombosis of deep vein of calf NOS

    Acute embolism and thrombosis of deep vein of lower leg NOS

    I82.4Z1 Acute embolism and thrombosis of unspecified deep veins of right distal lower extremity

    I82.4Z2 Acute embolism and thrombosis of unspecified deep veins of left distal lower extremity

    I82.4Z3 Acute embolism and thrombosis of unspecified deep veins of distal lower extremity, bilateral

    I82.4Z9 Acute embolism and thrombosis of unspecified deep veins of unspecified distal lower extremity ▽

✓5ᵗʰ **I82.5** Chronic embolism and thrombosis of deep veins of lower extremity

    Use additional code, if applicable, for associated long-term (current) use of anticoagulants (Z79.01)

    EXCLUDES 1 personal history of venous embolism and thrombosis (Z86.718)

✓6ᵗʰ **I82.50** Chronic embolism and thrombosis of unspecified deep veins of lower extremity

    EXCLUDES 1 chronic embolism and thrombosis of unspecified deep veins of distal lower extremity (I82.5Z-)

        chronic embolism and thrombosis of unspecified deep veins of proximal lower extremity (I82.5Y-)

    I82.501 Chronic embolism and thrombosis of unspecified deep veins of right lower extremity

    I82.502 Chronic embolism and thrombosis of unspecified deep veins of left lower extremity

    I82.503 Chronic embolism and thrombosis of unspecified deep veins of lower extremity, bilateral

    I82.509 Chronic embolism and thrombosis of unspecified deep veins of unspecified lower extremity ▽

✓6ᵗʰ **I82.51** Chronic embolism and thrombosis of femoral vein

    I82.511 Chronic embolism and thrombosis of right femoral vein

    I82.512 Chronic embolism and thrombosis of left femoral vein

    I82.513 Chronic embolism and thrombosis of femoral vein, bilateral

    I82.519 Chronic embolism and thrombosis of unspecified femoral vein ▽

✓6ᵗʰ **I82.52** Chronic embolism and thrombosis of iliac vein

    I82.521 Chronic embolism and thrombosis of right iliac vein

    I82.522 Chronic embolism and thrombosis of left iliac vein

    I82.523 Chronic embolism and thrombosis of iliac vein, bilateral

    I82.529 Chronic embolism and thrombosis of unspecified iliac vein ▽

✓6ᵗʰ **I82.53** Chronic embolism and thrombosis of popliteal vein

    I82.531 Chronic embolism and thrombosis of right popliteal vein

    I82.532 Chronic embolism and thrombosis of left popliteal vein

    I82.533 Chronic embolism and thrombosis of popliteal vein, bilateral

    I82.539 Chronic embolism and thrombosis of unspecified popliteal vein ▽

✓6ᵗʰ **I82.54** Chronic embolism and thrombosis of tibial vein

    I82.541 Chronic embolism and thrombosis of right tibial vein

    I82.542 Chronic embolism and thrombosis of left tibial vein

    I82.543 Chronic embolism and thrombosis of tibial vein, bilateral

    I82.549 Chronic embolism and thrombosis of unspecified tibial vein ▽

✓6ᵗʰ **I82.59** Chronic embolism and thrombosis of other specified deep vein of lower extremity

    I82.591 Chronic embolism and thrombosis of other specified deep vein of right lower extremity

    I82.592 Chronic embolism and thrombosis of other specified deep vein of left lower extremity

    I82.593 Chronic embolism and thrombosis of other specified deep vein of lower extremity, bilateral

Ⓝ Newborn   Ⓟ Pediatric   Ⓜ Maternity   Ⓐ Adult   **RIC** RIC Dx   **NC Dx** Noncancer Dx   **PDx** Primary Dx   **CC** RIC CC Condition   ►◄ Revised Text   ● New Code   ▲ Revised Code Title

616   ICD-10-CM 2016

I82.599   Chronic embolism and thrombosis of ▽
other specified deep vein of
unspecified lower extremity

✓6ᵗʰ **I82.5Y**   **Chronic embolism and thrombosis of** unspecified
deep veins of proximal lower extremity
Chronic embolism and thrombosis of deep veins of
thigh NOS
Chronic embolism and thrombosis of deep veins of
upper leg NOS

I82.5Y1   **Chronic embolism and thrombosis of
unspecified deep veins of** right **proximal
lower extremity**

I82.5Y2   **Chronic embolism and thrombosis of
unspecified deep veins of** left **proximal
lower extremity**

I82.5Y3   **Chronic embolism and thrombosis of
unspecified deep veins of proximal lower
extremity,** bilateral

I82.5Y9   **Chronic embolism and thrombosis of** ▽
**unspecified deep veins of unspecified
proximal lower extremity**

✓6ᵗʰ **I82.5Z**   **Chronic embolism and thrombosis of** unspecified
deep veins of distal lower extremity
Chronic embolism and thrombosis of deep veins of
calf NOS
Chronic embolism and thrombosis of deep veins of
lower leg NOS

I82.5Z1   **Chronic embolism and thrombosis of
unspecified deep veins of** right **distal
lower extremity**

I82.5Z2   **Chronic embolism and thrombosis of
unspecified deep veins of** left **distal lower
extremity**

I82.5Z3   **Chronic embolism and thrombosis of
unspecified deep veins of distal lower
extremity,** bilateral

I82.5Z9   **Chronic embolism and thrombosis of** ▽
**unspecified deep veins of unspecified
distal lower extremity**

✓5ᵗʰ **I82.6**   Acute **embolism and thrombosis of veins of** upper extremity

✓6ᵗʰ **I82.60**   **Acute embolism and thrombosis of** unspecified **veins
of upper extremity**

I82.601   **Acute embolism and thrombosis of
unspecified veins of** right **upper extremity**

I82.602   **Acute embolism and thrombosis of
unspecified veins of** left **upper extremity**

I82.603   **Acute embolism and thrombosis of
unspecified veins of upper extremity,**
bilateral

I82.609   **Acute embolism and thrombosis of** ▽
**unspecified veins of unspecified upper
extremity**

✓6ᵗʰ **I82.61**   **Acute embolism and thrombosis of** superficial veins
of upper extremity
Acute embolism and thrombosis of antecubital vein
Acute embolism and thrombosis of basilic vein
Acute embolism and thrombosis of cephalic vein

I82.611   **Acute embolism and thrombosis of
superficial veins of** right **upper extremity**

I82.612   **Acute embolism and thrombosis of
superficial veins of** left **upper extremity**

I82.613   **Acute embolism and thrombosis of
superficial veins of upper extremity,**
bilateral

I82.619   **Acute embolism and thrombosis of** ▽
**superficial veins of unspecified upper
extremity**

✓6ᵗʰ **I82.62**   **Acute embolism and thrombosis of** deep veins **of
upper extremity**
Acute embolism and thrombosis of brachial vein
Acute embolism and thrombosis of radial vein
Acute embolism and thrombosis of ulnar vein

I82.621   **Acute embolism and thrombosis of deep
veins of** right **upper extremity**

I82.622   **Acute embolism and thrombosis of deep
veins of** left **upper extremity**

I82.623   **Acute embolism and thrombosis of deep
veins of upper extremity,** bilateral

I82.629   **Acute embolism and thrombosis of** ▽
**deep veins of unspecified upper
extremity**

✓5ᵗʰ **I82.7**   Chronic **embolism and thrombosis of veins of** upper extremity
Use additional code, if applicable, for associated long-term
(current) use of anticoagulants (Z79.Ø1)
EXCLUDES 1   *personal history of venous embolism and thrombosis
(Z86.718)*

✓6ᵗʰ **I82.7Ø**   **Chronic embolism and thrombosis of** unspecified
veins of upper extremity

I82.7Ø1   **Chronic embolism and thrombosis of
unspecified veins of** right **upper extremity**

I82.7Ø2   **Chronic embolism and thrombosis of
unspecified veins of** left **upper extremity**

I82.7Ø3   **Chronic embolism and thrombosis of
unspecified veins of upper extremity,**
bilateral

I82.7Ø9   **Chronic embolism and thrombosis of** ▽
**unspecified veins of unspecified upper
extremity**

✓6ᵗʰ **I82.71**   **Chronic embolism and thrombosis of** superficial
veins **of upper extremity**
Chronic embolism and thrombosis of antecubital vein
Chronic embolism and thrombosis of basilic vein
Chronic embolism and thrombosis of cephalic vein

I82.711   **Chronic embolism and thrombosis of
superficial veins of** right **upper extremity**

I82.712   **Chronic embolism and thrombosis of
superficial veins of** left **upper extremity**

I82.713   **Chronic embolism and thrombosis of
superficial veins of upper extremity,**
bilateral

I82.719   **Chronic embolism and thrombosis of** ▽
**superficial veins of unspecified upper
extremity**

✓6ᵗʰ **I82.72**   **Chronic embolism and thrombosis of** deep veins **of
upper extremity**
Chronic embolism and thrombosis of brachial vein
Chronic embolism and thrombosis of radial vein
Chronic embolism and thrombosis of ulnar vein

I82.721   **Chronic embolism and thrombosis of deep
veins of** right **upper extremity**

I82.722   **Chronic embolism and thrombosis of deep
veins of** left **upper extremity**

I82.723   **Chronic embolism and thrombosis of deep
veins of** upper **extremity, bilateral**

I82.729   **Chronic embolism and thrombosis of** ▽
**deep veins of unspecified upper
extremity**

✓5ᵗʰ **I82.A**   **Embolism and thrombosis of** axillary vein

✓6ᵗʰ **I82.A1**   Acute **embolism and thrombosis of axillary vein**

I82.A11   **Acute embolism and thrombosis of** right
axillary vein

I82.A12   **Acute embolism and thrombosis of** left
axillary vein

I82.A13   **Acute embolism and thrombosis of
axillary vein,** bilateral

I82.A19   **Acute embolism and thrombosis of** ▽
unspecified axillary vein

✓6ᵗʰ **I82.A2**   Chronic **embolism and thrombosis of axillary vein**

I82.A21   **Chronic embolism and thrombosis of** right
axillary vein

I82.A22   **Chronic embolism and thrombosis of** left
axillary vein

I82.A23   **Chronic embolism and thrombosis of
axillary vein,** bilateral

I82.A29   **Chronic embolism and thrombosis of** ▽
unspecified axillary vein

✓5ᵗʰ **I82.B**   **Embolism and thrombosis of** subclavian vein

✓6ᵗʰ **I82.B1**   Acute **embolism and thrombosis of subclavian vein**

I82.B11   **Acute embolism and thrombosis of** right
subclavian vein

I82.B12   **Acute embolism and thrombosis of** left
subclavian vein

I82.B13   **Acute embolism and thrombosis of
subclavian vein,** bilateral

I82.B19   **Acute embolism and thrombosis of** ▽
unspecified subclavian vein

☑ Add'l Character Required   ✓x7ᵗʰ Placeholder Alert   RUG IV Special Care High Dx   RUG IV Clinically Complex Dx   RUG IV Special Care Low Dx   Manifestation Code   Other Specified Code   ▽Unspecified Code

✓6th **I82.B2** Chronic embolism and thrombosis of subclavian vein

I82.B21 Chronic embolism and thrombosis of right subclavian vein

I82.B22 Chronic embolism and thrombosis of left subclavian vein

I82.B23 Chronic embolism and thrombosis of subclavian vein, bilateral

I82.B29 Chronic embolism and thrombosis of ▽ unspecified subclavian vein

✓5th **I82.C** Embolism and thrombosis of internal jugular vein

✓6th **I82.C1** Acute embolism and thrombosis of internal jugular vein

I82.C11 Acute embolism and thrombosis of right internal jugular vein

I82.C12 Acute embolism and thrombosis of left internal jugular vein

I82.C13 Acute embolism and thrombosis of internal jugular vein, bilateral

I82.C19 Acute embolism and thrombosis of ▽ unspecified internal jugular vein

✓6th **I82.C2** Chronic embolism and thrombosis of internal jugular vein

I82.C21 Chronic embolism and thrombosis of right internal jugular vein

I82.C22 Chronic embolism and thrombosis of left internal jugular vein

I82.C23 Chronic embolism and thrombosis of internal jugular vein, bilateral

I82.C29 Chronic embolism and thrombosis of ▽ unspecified internal jugular vein

✓5th **I82.8** Embolism and thrombosis of other specified veins
Use additional code, if applicable, for associated long-term (current) use of anticoagulants (Z79.01)

✓6th **I82.81** Embolism and thrombosis of superficial veins of lower extremities
Embolism and thrombosis of saphenous vein (greater) (lesser)

I82.811 Embolism and thrombosis of superficial veins of right lower extremities

I82.812 Embolism and thrombosis of superficial veins of left lower extremities

I82.813 Embolism and thrombosis of superficial veins of lower extremities, bilateral

I82.819 Embolism and thrombosis of ▽ superficial veins of unspecified lower extremities

✓6th **I82.89** Embolism and thrombosis of other specified veins

I82.890 Acute embolism and thrombosis of other specified veins

I82.891 Chronic embolism and thrombosis of other specified veins

✓5th **I82.9** Embolism and thrombosis of unspecified vein

I82.90 Acute embolism and thrombosis of unspecified ▽ vein
Embolism of vein NOS
Thrombosis (vein) NOS

I82.91 Chronic embolism and thrombosis of unspecified ▽ vein

✓4th **I83** Varicose veins of lower extremities
EXCLUDES 1 varicose veins complicating pregnancy (O22.0-)
varicose veins complicating the puerperium (O87.4)

✓5th **I83.0** Varicose veins of lower extremities with ulcer
Use additional code to identify severity of ulcer (L97.-)

✓6th **I83.00** Varicose veins of unspecified lower extremity with ulcer

I83.001 Varicose veins of unspecified lower 🅐 extremity with ulcer of thigh

I83.002 Varicose veins of unspecified lower 🅐 extremity with ulcer of calf

I83.003 Varicose veins of unspecified lower 🅐 extremity with ulcer of ankle

I83.004 Varicose veins of unspecified lower 🅐 extremity with ulcer of heel and midfoot
Varicose veins of unspecified lower extremity with ulcer of plantar surface of midfoot

I83.005 Varicose veins of unspecified lower 🅐 extremity with ulcer other part of foot
Varicose veins of unspecified lower extremity with ulcer of toe

I83.008 Varicose veins of unspecified lower 🅐 extremity with ulcer other part of lower leg

I83.009 Varicose veins of unspecified lower 🅐▽ extremity with ulcer of unspecified site

✓6th **I83.01** Varicose veins of right lower extremity with ulcer

I83.011 Varicose veins of right lower extremity 🅐 with ulcer of thigh

I83.012 Varicose veins of right lower extremity 🅐 with ulcer of calf

I83.013 Varicose veins of right lower extremity 🅐 with ulcer of ankle

I83.014 Varicose veins of right lower extremity 🅐 with ulcer of heel and midfoot
Varicose veins of right lower extremity with ulcer of plantar surface of midfoot

I83.015 Varicose veins of right lower extremity 🅐 with ulcer other part of foot
Varicose veins of right lower extremity with ulcer of toe

I83.018 Varicose veins of right lower extremity 🅐 with ulcer other part of lower leg

I83.019 Varicose veins of right lower 🅐▽ extremity with ulcer of unspecified site

✓6th **I83.02** Varicose veins of left lower extremity with ulcer

I83.021 Varicose veins of left lower extremity 🅐 with ulcer of thigh

I83.022 Varicose veins of left lower extremity 🅐 with ulcer of calf

I83.023 Varicose veins of left lower extremity 🅐 with ulcer of ankle

I83.024 Varicose veins of left lower extremity 🅐 with ulcer of heel and midfoot
Varicose veins of left lower extremity with ulcer of plantar surface of midfoot

I83.025 Varicose veins of left lower extremity 🅐 with ulcer other part of foot
Varicose veins of left lower extremity with ulcer of toe

I83.028 Varicose veins of left lower extremity 🅐 with ulcer other part of lower leg

I83.029 Varicose veins of left lower extremity 🅐▽ with ulcer of unspecified site

✓5th **I83.1** Varicose veins of lower extremities with inflammation
Stasis dermatitis

I83.10 Varicose veins of unspecified lower extremity 🅐▽ with inflammation

I83.11 Varicose veins of right lower extremity with 🅐 inflammation

I83.12 Varicose veins of left lower extremity with 🅐 inflammation

✓5th **I83.2** Varicose veins of lower extremities with both ulcer and inflammation
Use additional code to identify severity of ulcer (L97.-)

✓6th **I83.20** Varicose veins of unspecified lower extremity with both ulcer and inflammation

I83.201 Varicose veins of unspecified lower 🅐 extremity with both ulcer of thigh and inflammation

I83.202 Varicose veins of unspecified lower 🅐 extremity with both ulcer of calf and inflammation

I83.203 Varicose veins of unspecified lower 🅐 extremity with both ulcer of ankle and inflammation

I83.204 Varicose veins of unspecified lower 🅐 extremity with both ulcer of heel and midfoot and inflammation
Varicose veins of unspecified lower extremity with both ulcer of plantar surface of midfoot and inflammation

Ⓝ Newborn   Ⓟ Pediatric   Ⓜ Maternity   🅐 Adult   RIC RIC Dx   HC Dx Noncancer Dx   PDx Primary Dx   CC RIC CC Condition   ►◄ Revised Text   ● New Code   ▲ Revised Code Title

618   ICD-10-CM 2016

I83.205   **Varicose veins of unspecified lower extremity with both ulcer of other part of foot and inflammation**   A
     Varicose veins of unspecified lower extremity with both ulcer of toe and inflammation

I83.208   **Varicose veins of unspecified lower extremity with both ulcer of other part of lower extremity and inflammation**   A

I83.209   **Varicose veins of unspecified lower extremity with both ulcer of unspecified site and inflammation**   A ▽

✓6th **I83.21**   **Varicose veins of right lower extremity with both ulcer and inflammation**

   I83.211   **Varicose veins of right lower extremity with both ulcer of thigh and inflammation**   A

   I83.212   **Varicose veins of right lower extremity with both ulcer of calf and inflammation**   A

   I83.213   **Varicose veins of right lower extremity with both ulcer of ankle and inflammation**   A

   I83.214   **Varicose veins of right lower extremity with both ulcer of heel and midfoot and inflammation**   A
     Varicose veins of right lower extremity with both ulcer of plantar surface of midfoot and inflammation

   I83.215   **Varicose veins of right lower extremity with both ulcer other part of foot and inflammation**   A
     Varicose veins of right lower extremity with both ulcer of toe and inflammation

   I83.218   **Varicose veins of right lower extremity with both ulcer of other part of lower extremity and inflammation**   A

   I83.219   **Varicose veins of right lower extremity with both ulcer of unspecified site and inflammation**   A ▽

✓6th **I83.22**   **Varicose veins of left lower extremity with both ulcer and inflammation**

   I83.221   **Varicose veins of left lower extremity with both ulcer of thigh and inflammation**   A

   I83.222   **Varicose veins of left lower extremity with both ulcer of calf and inflammation**   A

   I83.223   **Varicose veins of left lower extremity with both ulcer of ankle and inflammation**   A

   I83.224   **Varicose veins of left lower extremity with both ulcer of heel and midfoot and inflammation**   A
     Varicose veins of left lower extremity with both ulcer of plantar surface of midfoot and inflammation

   I83.225   **Varicose veins of left lower extremity with both ulcer other part of foot and inflammation**   A
     Varicose veins of left lower extremity with both ulcer of toe and inflammation

   I83.228   **Varicose veins of left lower extremity with both ulcer of other part of lower extremity and inflammation**   A

   I83.229   **Varicose veins of left lower extremity with both ulcer of unspecified site and inflammation**   A ▽

✓5th **I83.8**   **Varicose veins of lower extremities with other complications**

 ✓6th **I83.81**   **Varicose veins of lower extremities with pain**

   I83.811   **Varicose veins of right lower extremities with pain**   A

   I83.812   **Varicose veins of left lower extremities with pain**   A

   I83.813   **Varicose veins of bilateral lower extremities with pain**   A

   I83.819   **Varicose veins of unspecified lower extremities with pain**   A ▽

 ✓6th **I83.89**   **Varicose veins of lower extremities with other complications**
     Varicose veins of lower extremities with edema
     Varicose veins of lower extremities with swelling

   I83.891   **Varicose veins of right lower extremities with other complications**   A

   I83.892   **Varicose veins of left lower extremities with other complications**   A

   I83.893   **Varicose veins of bilateral lower extremities with other complications**   A

   I83.899   **Varicose veins of unspecified lower extremities with other complications**   A ▽

✓5th **I83.9**   **Asymptomatic varicose veins of lower extremities**
     Phlebectasia of lower extremities
     Varicose veins of lower extremities
     Varix of lower extremities

   I83.90   **Asymptomatic varicose veins of unspecified lower extremity**   A ▽
     Varicose veins NOS

   I83.91   **Asymptomatic varicose veins of right lower extremity**   A

   I83.92   **Asymptomatic varicose veins of left lower extremity**   A

   I83.93   **Asymptomatic varicose veins of bilateral lower extremities**   A

✓4th **I85**   **Esophageal varices**
     Use additional code to identify:
     alcohol abuse and dependence (F10.-)

 ✓5th **I85.0**   **Esophageal varices**
     Idiopathic esophageal varices   Primary esophageal varices

   I85.00   **Esophageal varices without bleeding**
     Esophageal varices NOS

   I85.01   **Esophageal varices with bleeding**

 ✓5th **I85.1**   **Secondary esophageal varices**
     Esophageal varices secondary to alcoholic liver disease
     Esophageal varices secondary to cirrhosis of liver
     Esophageal varices secondary to schistosomiasis
     Esophageal varices secondary to toxic liver disease
     Code first underlying disease

   I85.10   **Secondary esophageal varices without bleeding**

   I85.11   **Secondary esophageal varices with bleeding**

✓4th **I86**   **Varicose veins of other sites**
   EXCLUDES 1   varicose veins of unspecified site (I83.9-)
   EXCLUDES 2   retinal varices (H35.0-)

  I86.0   **Sublingual varices**

  I86.1   **Scrotal varices**   ♂
     Varicocele

  I86.2   **Pelvic varices**

  I86.3   **Vulval varices**   A ♀
   EXCLUDES 1   vulval varices complicating childbirth and the puerperium (O87.8)
             vulval varices complicating pregnancy (O22.1-)

  I86.4   **Gastric varices**

  I86.8   **Varicose veins of other specified sites**   A
     Varicose ulcer of nasal septum

✓4th **I87**   **Other disorders of veins**

 ✓5th **I87.0**   **Postthrombotic syndrome**
     Chronic venous hypertension due to deep vein thrombosis
     Postphlebitic syndrome
   EXCLUDES 1   chronic venous hypertension without deep vein thrombosis (I87.3-)

  ✓6th **I87.00**   **Postthrombotic syndrome without complications**
     Asymptomatic postthrombotic syndrome

    I87.001   **Postthrombotic syndrome without complications of right lower extremity**

    I87.002   **Postthrombotic syndrome without complications of left lower extremity**

    I87.003   **Postthrombotic syndrome without complications of bilateral lower extremity**

    I87.009   **Postthrombotic syndrome without complications of unspecified extremity**   ▽
     Postthrombotic syndrome NOS

  ✓6th **I87.01**   **Postthrombotic syndrome with ulcer**
     Use additional code to specify site and severity of ulcer (L97.-)

    I87.011   **Postthrombotic syndrome with ulcer of right lower extremity**

    I87.012   **Postthrombotic syndrome with ulcer of left lower extremity**

    I87.013   **Postthrombotic syndrome with ulcer of bilateral lower extremity**

    I87.019   **Postthrombotic syndrome with ulcer of unspecified lower extremity**   ▽

☑ Add'l Character Required   ✓x7th Placeholder Alert   RUG IV Special Care High Dx   RUG IV Clinically Complex Dx   RUG IV Special Care Low Dx   Manifestation Code   Other Specified Code   ▽ Unspecified Code

ICD-10-CM 2016   619

Chapter 9. Diseases of the Circulatory System

I87.02–I89.8

✓6ᵗʰ **I87.02 Postthrombotic syndrome with** inflammation

I87.021 **Postthrombotic syndrome with inflammation of** right lower **extremity**

I87.022 **Postthrombotic syndrome with inflammation of** left lower **extremity**

I87.023 **Postthrombotic syndrome with inflammation of** bilateral lower **extremity**

I87.029 **Postthrombotic syndrome with inflammation of unspecified lower extremity** ▽

✓6ᵗʰ **I87.03 Postthrombotic syndrome with** ulcer and inflammation
Use additional code to specify site and severity of ulcer (L97.-)

I87.031 **Postthrombotic syndrome with ulcer and inflammation of** right lower **extremity**

I87.032 **Postthrombotic syndrome with ulcer and inflammation of** left lower **extremity**

I87.033 **Postthrombotic syndrome with ulcer and inflammation of** bilateral lower **extremity**

I87.039 **Postthrombotic syndrome with ulcer and inflammation of unspecified lower extremity** ▽

✓6ᵗʰ **I87.09 Postthrombotic syndrome with** other complications

I87.091 **Postthrombotic syndrome with other complications of** right lower **extremity**

I87.092 **Postthrombotic syndrome with other complications of** left lower **extremity**

I87.093 **Postthrombotic syndrome with other complications of** bilateral lower **extremity**

I87.099 **Postthrombotic syndrome with other complications of unspecified lower extremity** ▽

I87.1 Compression of vein
Stricture of vein
Vena cava syndrome (inferior) (superior)
EXCLUDES 2 compression of pulmonary vein (I28.8)

I87.2 Venous insufficiency (chronic) (peripheral)

✓5ᵗʰ **I87.3 Chronic venous hypertension (idiopathic)**
Stasis edema
EXCLUDES 1 chronic venous hypertension due to deep vein thrombosis (I87.0-)
varicose veins of lower extremities (I83.-)

✓6ᵗʰ **I87.30 Chronic venous hypertension (idiopathic)** without complications
Asymptomatic chronic venous hypertension (idiopathic)

I87.301 **Chronic venous hypertension (idiopathic) without complications of** right lower **extremity**

I87.302 **Chronic venous hypertension (idiopathic) without complications of** left lower **extremity**

I87.303 **Chronic venous hypertension (idiopathic) without complications of** bilateral lower **extremity**

I87.309 **Chronic venous hypertension (idiopathic) without complications of unspecified lower extremity** ▽
Chronic venous hypertension NOS

✓6ᵗʰ **I87.31 Chronic venous hypertension (idiopathic)** with ulcer
Use additional code to specify site and severity of ulcer (L97.-)

I87.311 **Chronic venous hypertension (idiopathic) with ulcer of** right lower **extremity**

I87.312 **Chronic venous hypertension (idiopathic) with ulcer of** left lower **extremity**

I87.313 **Chronic venous hypertension (idiopathic) with ulcer of** bilateral lower **extremity**

I87.319 **Chronic venous hypertension (idiopathic) with ulcer of unspecified lower extremity** ▽

✓6ᵗʰ **I87.32 Chronic venous hypertension (idiopathic) with** inflammation

I87.321 **Chronic venous hypertension (idiopathic) with inflammation of** right lower **extremity**

I87.322 **Chronic venous hypertension (idiopathic) with inflammation of** left lower **extremity**

I87.323 **Chronic venous hypertension (idiopathic) with inflammation of** bilateral lower **extremity**

I87.329 **Chronic venous hypertension (idiopathic) with inflammation of unspecified lower extremity** ▽

✓6ᵗʰ **I87.33 Chronic venous hypertension (idiopathic) with** ulcer and inflammation
Use additional code to specify site and severity of ulcer (L97.-)

I87.331 **Chronic venous hypertension (idiopathic) with ulcer and inflammation of** right lower **extremity**

I87.332 **Chronic venous hypertension (idiopathic) with ulcer and inflammation of** left lower **extremity**

I87.333 **Chronic venous hypertension (idiopathic) with ulcer and inflammation of** bilateral lower **extremity**

I87.339 **Chronic venous hypertension (idiopathic) with ulcer and inflammation of unspecified lower extremity** ▽

✓6ᵗʰ **I87.39 Chronic venous hypertension (idiopathic) with** other complications

I87.391 **Chronic venous hypertension (idiopathic) with other complications of** right lower **extremity**

I87.392 **Chronic venous hypertension (idiopathic) with other complications of** left lower **extremity**

I87.393 **Chronic venous hypertension (idiopathic) with other complications of** bilateral lower **extremity**

I87.399 **Chronic venous hypertension (idiopathic) with other complications of unspecified lower extremity** ▽

I87.8 Other specified disorders of veins
Phlebosclerosis
Venofibrosis

I87.9 Disorder of vein, unspecified ▽

✓4ᵗʰ **I88 Nonspecific lymphadenitis**
EXCLUDES 1 acute lymphadenitis, except mesenteric (L04.-)
enlarged lymph nodes NOS (R59.-)
human immunodeficiency virus [HIV] disease resulting in generalized lymphadenopathy (B20)

I88.0 Nonspecific mesenteric lymphadenitis
Mesenteric lymphadenitis (acute)(chronic)

I88.1 Chronic lymphadenitis, except mesenteric
Adenitis
Lymphadenitis

I88.8 Other nonspecific lymphadenitis

I88.9 Nonspecific lymphadenitis, unspecified ▽
Lymphadenitis NOS

✓4ᵗʰ **I89 Other noninfective disorders of lymphatic vessels and lymph nodes**
EXCLUDES 1 chylocele, tunica vaginalis (nonfilarial) NOS (N50.8)
enlarged lymph nodes NOS (R59.-)
filarial chylocele (B74.-)
hereditary lymphedema (Q82.0)

I89.0 Lymphedema, not elsewhere classified
Elephantiasis (nonfilarial) NOS
Lymphangiectasis
Obliteration, lymphatic vessel
Praecox lymphedema
Secondary lymphedema
EXCLUDES 1 postmastectomy lymphedema (I97.2)

I89.1 Lymphangitis
Chronic lymphangitis
Lymphangitis NOS
Subacute lymphangitis
EXCLUDES 1 acute lymphangitis (L03.-)

I89.8 Other specified noninfective disorders of lymphatic vessels and lymph nodes
Chylocele (nonfilarial)
Chylous ascites
Chylous cyst
Lipomelanotic reticulosis
Lymph node or vessel fistula
Lymph node or vessel infarction
Lymph node or vessel rupture

Ⓝ Newborn   Ⓟ Pediatric   Ⓜ Maternity   Ⓐ Adult   **RIC** RIC Dx   **NCDx** Noncancer Dx   **PDx** Primary Dx   **CC** RIC CC Condition   ►◄ Revised Text   ● New Code   ▲ Revised Code Title

620   ICD-10-CM 2016

I89.9 **Noninfective disorder of lymphatic vessels and lymph nodes, unspecified** ▽
Disease of lymphatic vessels NOS

Other and unspecified disorders of the circulatory system (I95-I99)

☑4ᵗʰ I95 **Hypotension**
> EXCLUDES 1 *cardiovascular collapse (R57.9)*
> *maternal hypotension syndrome (O26.5-)*
> *nonspecific low blood pressure reading NOS (R03.1)*

I95.0 **Idiopathic hypotension**

I95.1 **Orthostatic hypotension**
Hypotension, postural
> EXCLUDES 1 *neurogenic orthostatic hypotension [Shy-Drager] (G90.3)*
> *orthostatic hypotension due to drugs (I95.2)*

I95.2 **Hypotension due to drugs**
Orthostatic hypotension due to drugs
Use additional code for adverse effect, if applicable, to identify drug (T36-T50 with fifth or sixth character 5)

I95.3 **Hypotension of hemodialysis**
Intra-dialytic hypotension

☑5ᵗʰ I95.8 **Other hypotension**

I95.81 **Postprocedural hypotension**

I95.89 **Other hypotension**
Chronic hypotension

I95.9 **Hypotension, unspecified** ▽

☑4ᵗʰ I96 **Gangrene, not elsewhere classified** CC ▽
Gangrenous cellulitis
> EXCLUDES 1 *gangrene in atherosclerosis of native arteries of the extremities (I70.26)*
> *gangrene in diabetes mellitus (E08-E13)*
> *gangrene in hernia (K40.1, K40.4, K41.1, K41.4, K42.1, K43.1-, K44.1, K45.1, K46.1)*
> *gangrene in other peripheral vascular diseases (I73.-)*
> *gangrene of certain specified sites—see Alphabetical Index*
> *gas gangrene (A48.0)*
> *pyoderma gangrenosum (L88)*

AHA: 2013, 2Q, 34
RIC Excl: 10 Amputation, lower extremity; 11 Amputation, non-lower extremity

☑4ᵗʰ I97 **Intraoperative and postprocedural complications and disorders of circulatory system, not elsewhere classified**
> EXCLUDES 2 *postprocedural shock (T81.1-)*

I97.0 **Postcardiotomy syndrome**

☑5ᵗʰ I97.1 **Other postprocedural cardiac functional disturbances**
> EXCLUDES 2 *acute pulmonary insufficiency following thoracic surgery (J95.1)*
> *intraoperative cardiac functional disturbances (I97.7-)*

☑6ᵗʰ I97.11 **Postprocedural cardiac insufficiency**

I97.110 **Postprocedural cardiac insufficiency following cardiac surgery** NC Dx

I97.111 **Postprocedural cardiac insufficiency following other surgery** NC Dx

☑6ᵗʰ I97.12 **Postprocedural cardiac arrest**

I97.120 **Postprocedural cardiac arrest following cardiac surgery** NC Dx

I97.121 **Postprocedural cardiac arrest following other surgery** NC Dx

☑6ᵗʰ I97.13 **Postprocedural heart failure**
Use additional code to identify the heart failure (I50.-)

I97.130 **Postprocedural heart failure following cardiac surgery** NC Dx

I97.131 **Postprocedural heart failure following other surgery** NC Dx

☑6ᵗʰ I97.19 **Other postprocedural cardiac functional disturbances**
Use additional code, if applicable, to further specify disorder

I97.190 **Other postprocedural cardiac functional disturbances following cardiac surgery** NC Dx

I97.191 **Other postprocedural cardiac functional disturbances following other surgery** NC Dx

I97.2 **Postmastectomy lymphedema syndrome** A
Elephantiasis due to mastectomy
Obliteration of lymphatic vessels

I97.3 **Postprocedural hypertension**

☑5ᵗʰ I97.4 **Intraoperative hemorrhage and hematoma of a circulatory system organ or structure complicating a procedure**
> EXCLUDES 1 *intraoperative hemorrhage and hematoma of a circulatory system organ or structure due to accidental puncture and laceration during a procedure (I97.5-)*
> EXCLUDES 2 *intraoperative cerebrovascular hemorrhage complicating a procedure (G97.3-)*

☑6ᵗʰ I97.41 **Intraoperative hemorrhage and hematoma of a circulatory system organ or structure complicating a circulatory system procedure**

I97.410 **Intraoperative hemorrhage and hematoma of a circulatory system organ or structure complicating a cardiac catheterization**

I97.411 **Intraoperative hemorrhage and hematoma of a circulatory system organ or structure complicating a cardiac bypass**

I97.418 **Intraoperative hemorrhage and hematoma of a circulatory system organ or structure complicating other circulatory system procedure**

I97.42 **Intraoperative hemorrhage and hematoma of a circulatory system organ or structure complicating other procedure**

☑5ᵗʰ I97.5 **Accidental puncture and laceration of a circulatory system organ or structure during a procedure**
> EXCLUDES 2 *accidental puncture and laceration of brain during a procedure (G97.4-)*

I97.51 **Accidental puncture and laceration of a circulatory system organ or structure during a circulatory system procedure**

I97.52 **Accidental puncture and laceration of a circulatory system organ or structure during other procedure**

☑5ᵗʰ I97.6 **Postprocedural hemorrhage and hematoma of a circulatory system organ or structure following a procedure**
> EXCLUDES 2 *postprocedural cerebrovascular hemorrhage complicating a procedure (G97.5-)*

☑6ᵗʰ I97.61 **Postprocedural hemorrhage and hematoma of a circulatory system organ or structure following a circulatory system procedure**

I97.610 **Postprocedural hemorrhage and hematoma of a circulatory system organ or structure following a cardiac catheterization**

I97.611 **Postprocedural hemorrhage and hematoma of a circulatory system organ or structure following cardiac bypass**

I97.618 **Postprocedural hemorrhage and hematoma of a circulatory system organ or structure following other circulatory system procedure**

I97.62 **Postprocedural hemorrhage and hematoma of a circulatory system organ or structure following other procedure**

☑5ᵗʰ I97.7 **Intraoperative cardiac functional disturbances**
> EXCLUDES 2 *acute pulmonary insufficiency following thoracic surgery (J95.1)*
> *postprocedural cardiac functional disturbances (I97.1-)*

☑6ᵗʰ I97.71 **Intraoperative cardiac arrest**

I97.710 **Intraoperative cardiac arrest during cardiac surgery**

I97.711 **Intraoperative cardiac arrest during other surgery**

☑6ᵗʰ I97.79 **Other intraoperative cardiac functional disturbances**
Use additional code, if applicable, to further specify disorder

I97.790 **Other intraoperative cardiac functional disturbances during cardiac surgery**

I97.791 **Other intraoperative cardiac functional disturbances during other surgery**

✓5ᵗʰ **I97.8** Other intraoperative and postprocedural complications and disorders of the circulatory system, not elsewhere classified
Use additional code, if applicable, to further specify disorder

     ✓6ᵗʰ **I97.81** Intraoperative cerebrovascular infarction

         I97.810 Intraoperative cerebrovascular infarction during cardiac surgery

         I97.811 Intraoperative cerebrovascular infarction during other surgery

     ✓6ᵗʰ **I97.82** Postprocedural cerebrovascular infarction

         I97.820 Postprocedural cerebrovascular infarction during cardiac surgery

         I97.821 Postprocedural cerebrovascular infarction during other surgery

     I97.88 Other intraoperative complications of the circulatory system, not elsewhere classified

     I97.89 Other postprocedural complications and disorders of the circulatory system, not elsewhere classified

✓4ᵗʰ **I99** Other and unspecified disorders of circulatory system

     I99.8 Other disorder of circulatory system

     I99.9 Unspecified disorder of circulatory system   ▽

Ⓝ Newborn   Ⓟ Pediatric   Ⓜ Maternity   Ⓐ Adult   **RIC** RIC Dx   **NC Dx** Noncancer Dx   **PDx** Primary Dx   **CC** RIC CC Condition   ►◄ Revised Text   ● New Code   ▲ Revised Code Title

622   ICD-10-CM 2016

Chapter 10. Diseases of the Respiratory System (J00–J99)

Chapter Specific Guidelines with Coding Examples

The chapter specific guidelines from the ICD-10-CM Official Guidelines for Coding and Reporting have been provided below. Along with these guidelines are coding examples, contained in the shaded boxes, that have been developed to help illustrate the coding and/or sequencing guidance found in these guidelines.

a. Chronic obstructive pulmonary disease [COPD] and asthma

1) Acute exacerbation of chronic obstructive bronchitis and asthma

The codes in categories J44 and J45 distinguish between uncomplicated cases and those in acute exacerbation. An acute exacerbation is a worsening or a decompensation of a chronic condition. An acute exacerbation is not equivalent to an infection superimposed on a chronic condition, though an exacerbation may be triggered by an infection.

> Acute streptococcal bronchitis with acute exacerbation of COPD
>
> **J20.2**   **Acute bronchitis due to streptococcus**
>
> **J44.0**   **Chronic obstructive pulmonary disease with acute lower respiratory infection**
>
> **J44.1**   **Chronic obstructive pulmonary disease with (acute) exacerbation**
>
> *Explanation*: ICD-10-CM uses combination codes to create organism-specific classifications for acute bronchitis. Category J44 codes include combination codes with severity components, which differentiate between COPD with acute lower respiratory infection (acute bronchitis), COPD with acute exacerbation, and COPD without mention of a complication (unspecified).
>
> An acute exacerbation is a worsening or a decompensation of a chronic condition. An acute exacerbation is not equivalent to an infection superimposed on a chronic condition, though an exacerbation may be triggered by an infection, as in this example.

> Exacerbation of moderate persistent asthma with status asthmaticus
>
> **J45.42**   **Moderate persistent asthma with status asthmaticus**
>
> *Explanation*: Category J45 Asthma includes severity-specific subcategories and fifth-character codes to distinguish between uncomplicated cases, those in acute exacerbation, and those with status asthmaticus.

b. Acute respiratory failure

1) Acute respiratory failure as principal diagnosis

A code from subcategory J96.0, Acute respiratory failure, or subcategory J96.2, Acute and chronic respiratory failure, may be assigned as a principal diagnosis when it is the condition established after study to be chiefly responsible for occasioning the admission to the hospital, and the selection is supported by the Alphabetic Index and Tabular List. However, chapter-specific coding guidelines (such as obstetrics, poisoning, HIV, newborn) that provide sequencing direction take precedence.

> Acute hypoxic respiratory failure due to COPD exacerbation
>
> **J96.01**   **Acute respiratory failure with hypoxia**
>
> **J44.1**   **Chronic obstructive pulmonary disease with (acute) exacerbation**
>
> *Explanation*: Category J96 classifies respiratory failure with combination codes that designate the severity and the presence of hypoxia and hypercapnia. Code J96.01 is sequenced as the first-listed diagnosis, as the reason for the admission. Respiratory failure may be assigned as a principal diagnosis when it is the condition established after study to be chiefly responsible for occasioning the admission to the hospital and the selection is supported by the Alphabetic Index and Tabular List.

2) Acute respiratory failure as secondary diagnosis

Respiratory failure may be listed as a secondary diagnosis if it occurs after admission, or if it is present on admission, but does not meet the definition of principal diagnosis.

> Acute respiratory failure due to accidental oxycodone overdose
>
> **T40.2X1A**   **Poisoning by other opioids, accidental (unintentional), initial encounter**
>
> **J96.00**   **Acute respiratory failure, unspecified whether with hypoxia or hypercapnia**
>
> *Explanation*: Respiratory failure may be assigned as a principal diagnosis when it is the condition established after study to be chiefly responsible for occasioning the admission to the hospital, and the selection is supported by the Alphabetic Index and Tabular List. However, chapter-specific coding guidelines, such as poisoning, that provide sequencing direction take precedence. When coding a poisoning or reaction to the improper use of a medication (e.g. overdose, wrong substance given or taken in error, wrong route of administration), first assign the appropriate code from categories T36–T50. Use additional code(s) for all manifestations of the poisoning. In this instance, the respiratory failure is a manifestation of the poisoning and is sequenced as a secondary diagnosis.

> Acute pneumococcal pneumonia with subsequent development of acute respiratory failure
>
> **J13**   **Pneumonia due to Streptococcus pneumoniae**
>
> **J96.00**   **Acute respiratory failure, unspecified whether with hypoxia or hypercapnia**
>
> *Explanation*: Acute respiratory failure may be listed as a secondary diagnosis if it occurs after admission, or if it is present on admission but does not meet the definition of principal diagnosis.

3) Sequencing of acute respiratory failure and another acute condition

When a patient is admitted with respiratory failure and another acute condition, (e.g., myocardial infarction, cerebrovascular accident, aspiration pneumonia), the principal diagnosis will not be the same in every situation. This applies whether the other acute condition is a respiratory or nonrespiratory condition. Selection of the principal diagnosis will be dependent on the circumstances of admission. If both the respiratory failure and the other acute condition are equally responsible for occasioning the admission to the hospital, and there are no chapter-specific sequencing rules, the guideline regarding two or more diagnoses that equally meet the definition for principal diagnosis (Section II, C.) may be applied in these situations.

If the documentation is not clear as to whether acute respiratory failure and another condition are equally responsible for occasioning the admission, query the provider for clarification.

> Acute pneumococcal pneumonia and acute respiratory failure, both present on admission
>
> **J96.00**   **Acute respiratory failure, unspecified whether with hypoxia or hypercapnia**
>
> **J13**   **Pneumonia due to Streptococcus pneumoniae**
>
> *Explanation*: When a patient is admitted with respiratory failure and another acute condition, such as a bacterial pneumonia, the principal diagnosis is not the same in every situation. This applies whether the other acute condition is a respiratory or nonrespiratory condition. The principal diagnosis depends on the circumstances of admission.

c. Influenza due to certain identified influenza viruses

Code only confirmed cases of influenza due to certain identified influenza viruses (category J09), and due to other identified influenza virus (category J10). This is an exception to the hospital inpatient guideline Section II, H. (Uncertain Diagnosis).

In this context, "confirmation" does not require documentation of positive laboratory testing specific for avian or other novel influenza A or other identified influenza virus. However, coding should be based on the provider's diagnostic statement that the patient has avian influenza, or other novel influenza A, for category J09, or has another particular identified strain of influenza, such as H1N1 or H3N2, but not identified as novel or variant, for category J10.

If the provider records "suspected" or "possible" or "probable" avian influenza, or novel influenza, or other identified influenza, then the appropriate influenza code from category J11, Influenza due to unidentified influenza virus, should be assigned. A code from category J09, Influenza due to certain identified influenza viruses, should not be assigned nor should a code from category J10, Influenza due to other identified influenza virus.

Influenza due to avian influenza virus with pneumonia

J09.X1   **Influenza due to identified novel influenza A virus with pneumonia**

Explanation: Codes in category J09 Influenza due to certain identified influenza viruses should be assigned only for confirmed cases. "Confirmation" does not require positive laboratory testing of a specific influenza virus but does need to be based on the provider's diagnostic statement, which should not include terms such as "possible," "probable," or "suspected."

d. Ventilator associated pneumonia

1) Documentation of ventilator associated pneumonia

As with all procedural or postprocedural complications, code assignment is based on the provider's documentation of the relationship between the condition and the procedure.

Code J95.851, Ventilator associated pneumonia, should be assigned only when the provider has documented ventilator associated pneumonia (VAP). An additional code to identify the organism (e.g., Pseudomonas aeruginosa, code B96.5) should also be assigned. Do not assign an additional code from categories J12-J18 to identify the type of pneumonia.

Code J95.851 should not be assigned for cases where the patient has pneumonia and is on a mechanical ventilator and the provider has not specifically stated that the pneumonia is ventilator-associated pneumonia. If the documentation is unclear as to whether the patient has a pneumonia that is a complication attributable to the mechanical ventilator, query the provider.

2) Ventilator associated pneumonia develops after admission

A patient may be admitted with one type of pneumonia (e.g., code J13, Pneumonia due to Streptococcus pneumonia) and subsequently develop VAP. In this instance, the principal diagnosis would be the appropriate code from categories J12-J18 for the pneumonia diagnosed at the time of admission. Code J95.851, Ventilator associated pneumonia, would be assigned as an additional diagnosis when the provider has also documented the presence of ventilator associated pneumonia.

Patient with pneumonia due to *Klebsiella pneumoniae* develops superimposed MRSA ventilator-associated pneumonia

J15.0   **Pneumonia due to Klebsiella pneumoniae**

J95.851   **Ventilator associated pneumonia**

B95.62   **Methicillin resistant Staphylococcus aureus infection as the cause of diseases classified elsewhere**

Explanation: Code assignment for ventilator-associated pneumonia is based on the provider's documentation of the relationship between the condition and the procedure and is reported only when the provider has documented ventilator-associated pneumonia (VAP).

A patient may be admitted with one type of pneumonia and subsequently develop VAP. In this example, the principal diagnosis code describes the pneumonia diagnosed at the time of admission, with code J95.851 Ventilator associated pneumonia, assigned as secondary.

Chapter 10. Diseases of the Respiratory System (J00-J99)

> **NOTE** When a respiratory condition is described as occurring in more than one site and is not specifically indexed, it should be classified to the lower anatomic site (e.g. tracheobronchitis to bronchitis in J40).

Use additional code, where applicable, to identify:
exposure to environmental tobacco smoke (Z77.22)
exposure to tobacco smoke in the perinatal period (P96.81)
history of tobacco use (Z87.891)
occupational exposure to environmental tobacco smoke (Z57.31)
tobacco dependence (F17.-)
tobacco use (Z72.0)

EXCLUDES 2 certain conditions originating in the perinatal period (P04-P96)
certain infectious and parasitic diseases (A00-B99)
complications of pregnancy, childbirth and the puerperium (O00-O9A)
congenital malformations, deformations and chromosomal abnormalities (Q00-Q99)
endocrine, nutritional and metabolic diseases (E00-E88)
injury, poisoning and certain other consequences of external causes (S00-T88)
neoplasms (C00-D49)
smoke inhalation (T59.81-)
symptoms, signs and abnormal clinical and laboratory findings, not elsewhere classified (R00-R94)

This chapter contains the following blocks:

J00-J06   Acute upper respiratory infections
J09-J18   Influenza and pneumonia
J20-J22   Other acute lower respiratory infections
J30-J39   Other diseases of upper respiratory tract
J40-J47   Chronic lower respiratory diseases
J60-J70   Lung diseases due to external agents
J80-J84   Other respiratory diseases principally affecting the interstitium
J85-J86   Suppurative and necrotic conditions of the lower respiratory tract
J90-J94   Other diseases of the pleura
J95   Intraoperative and postprocedural complications and disorders of respiratory system, not elsewhere classified
J96-J99   Other diseases of the respiratory system

Acute upper respiratory infections (J00-J06)

EXCLUDES 1 influenza virus with other respiratory manifestations (J09.X2, J10.1, J11.1)
EXCLUDES 2 chronic obstructive pulmonary disease with acute lower respiratory infection (J44.0)

J00   Acute nasopharyngitis (common cold)
Acute rhinitis
Coryza (acute)
Infective nasopharyngitis NOS
Infective rhinitis
Nasal catarrh, acute
Nasopharyngitis NOS
EXCLUDES 1 acute pharyngitis (J02.-)
acute sore throat NOS (J02.9)
pharyngitis NOS (J02.9)
rhinitis NOS (J31.0)
sore throat NOS (J02.9)
EXCLUDES 2 allergic rhinitis (J30.1-J30.9)
chronic pharyngitis (J31.2)
chronic rhinitis (J31.0)
chronic sore throat (J31.2)
nasopharyngitis, chronic (J31.1)
vasomotor rhinitis (J30.0)

✓4th J01   Acute sinusitis
INCLUDES acute abscess of sinus
acute empyema of sinus
acute infection of sinus
acute inflammation of sinus
acute suppuration of sinus
Use additional code (B95-B97) to identify infectious agent
EXCLUDES 1 sinusitis NOS (J32.9)
EXCLUDES 2 chronic sinusitis (J32.0-J32.8)

✓5th J01.0   Acute maxillary sinusitis
Acute antritis
J01.00   Acute maxillary sinusitis, unspecified ▽
J01.01   Acute recurrent maxillary sinusitis

✓5th J01.1   Acute frontal sinusitis
J01.10   Acute frontal sinusitis, unspecified ▽
J01.11   Acute recurrent frontal sinusitis

✓5th J01.2   Acute ethmoidal sinusitis
J01.20   Acute ethmoidal sinusitis, unspecified ▽
J01.21   Acute recurrent ethmoidal sinusitis

✓5th J01.3   Acute sphenoidal sinusitis
J01.30   Acute sphenoidal sinusitis, unspecified ▽
J01.31   Acute recurrent sphenoidal sinusitis

✓5th J01.4   Acute pansinusitis
J01.40   Acute pansinusitis, unspecified ▽
J01.41   Acute recurrent pansinusitis

✓5th J01.8   Other acute sinusitis
J01.80   Other acute sinusitis
Acute sinusitis involving more than one sinus but not pansinusitis
J01.81   Other acute recurrent sinusitis
Acute recurrent sinusitis involving more than one sinus but not pansinusitis

✓5th J01.9   Acute sinusitis, unspecified
J01.90   Acute sinusitis, unspecified ▽
J01.91   Acute recurrent sinusitis, unspecified ▽

✓4th J02   Acute pharyngitis
INCLUDES acute sore throat
EXCLUDES 1 acute laryngopharyngitis (J06.0)
peritonsillar abscess (J36)
pharyngeal abscess (J39.1)
retropharyngeal abscess (J39.0)
EXCLUDES 2 chronic pharyngitis (J31.2)

J02.0   Streptococcal pharyngitis
Septic pharyngitis
Streptococcal sore throat
EXCLUDES 2 scarlet fever (A38.-)

J02.8   Acute pharyngitis due to other specified organisms
Use additional code (B95-B97) to identify infectious agent
EXCLUDES 1 acute pharyngitis due to coxsackie virus (B08.5)
acute pharyngitis due to gonococcus (A54.5)
acute pharyngitis due to herpes [simplex] virus (B00.2)
acute pharyngitis due to infectious mononucleosis (B27.-)
enteroviral vesicular pharyngitis (B08.5)

J02.9   Acute pharyngitis, unspecified ▽
Gangrenous pharyngitis (acute)
Infective pharyngitis (acute) NOS
Pharyngitis (acute) NOS
Sore throat (acute) NOS
Suppurative pharyngitis (acute)
Ulcerative pharyngitis (acute)

✓4th J03   Acute tonsillitis
EXCLUDES 1 acute sore throat (J02.-)
hypertrophy of tonsils (J35.1)
peritonsillar abscess (J36)
sore throat NOS (J02.9)
streptococcal sore throat (J02.0)
EXCLUDES 2 chronic tonsillitis (J35.0)

✓5th J03.0   Streptococcal tonsillitis
J03.00   Acute streptococcal tonsillitis, unspecified ▽
J03.01   Acute recurrent streptococcal tonsillitis

✓5th J03.8   Acute tonsillitis due to other specified organisms
Use additional code (B95-B97) to identify infectious agent
EXCLUDES 1 diphtheritic tonsillitis (A36.0)
herpesviral pharyngotonsillitis (B00.2)
streptococcal tonsillitis (J03.0)
tuberculous tonsillitis (A15.8)
Vincent's tonsillitis (A69.1)
J03.80   Acute tonsillitis due to other specified organisms
J03.81   Acute recurrent tonsillitis due to other specified organisms

✓5th J03.9   Acute tonsillitis, unspecified
Follicular tonsillitis (acute)
Gangrenous tonsillitis (acute)
Infective tonsillitis (acute)
Tonsillitis (acute) NOS
Ulcerative tonsillitis (acute)
J03.90   Acute tonsillitis, unspecified ▽
J03.91   Acute recurrent tonsillitis, unspecified ▽

✓4ᵗʰ **J04**   **Acute laryngitis and tracheitis**
      Use additional code (B95-B97) to identify infectious agent
        EXCLUDES 1   *acute obstructive laryngitis [croup] and epiglottitis (J05.-)*
        EXCLUDES 2   *laryngismus (stridulus) (J38.5)*

    J04.0   **Acute laryngitis**
        Edematous laryngitis (acute)
        Laryngitis (acute) NOS
        Subglottic laryngitis (acute)
        Suppurative laryngitis (acute)
        Ulcerative laryngitis (acute)
          EXCLUDES 1   *acute obstructive laryngitis (J05.0)*
          EXCLUDES 2   *chronic laryngitis (J37.0)*

    ✓5ᵗʰ **J04.1**   **Acute tracheitis**
        Acute viral tracheitis
        Catarrhal tracheitis (acute)
        Tracheitis (acute) NOS
          EXCLUDES 2   *chronic tracheitis (J42)*

        J04.10   **Acute tracheitis without obstruction**

        J04.11   **Acute tracheitis with obstruction**   CC
          RIC Excl: 15 Pulmonary

    J04.2   **Acute laryngotracheitis**
        Laryngotracheitis NOS
        Tracheitis (acute) with laryngitis (acute)
          EXCLUDES 1   *acute obstructive laryngotracheitis (J05.0)*
          EXCLUDES 2   *chronic laryngotracheitis (J37.1)*

    ✓5ᵗʰ **J04.3**   **Supraglottitis, unspecified**
        J04.30   **Supraglottitis, unspecified, without obstruction** ▽
        J04.31   **Supraglottitis, unspecified, with obstruction** ▽

✓4ᵗʰ **J05**   **Acute obstructive laryngitis [croup] and epiglottitis**
      Use additional code (B95-B97) to identify infectious agent

    J05.0   **Acute obstructive laryngitis [croup]**   CC
        Obstructive laryngitis (acute) NOS
        Obstructive laryngotracheitis NOS
        RIC Excl: 15 Pulmonary

    ✓5ᵗʰ **J05.1**   **Acute epiglottitis**
          EXCLUDES 2   *epiglottitis, chronic (J37.0)*

        J05.10   **Acute epiglottitis without obstruction**
          Epiglottitis NOS

        J05.11   **Acute epiglottitis with obstruction**   CC
          RIC Excl: 15 Pulmonary

✓4ᵗʰ **J06**   **Acute upper respiratory infections of multiple and unspecified sites**
        EXCLUDES 1   *acute respiratory infection NOS (J22)*
            streptococcal pharyngitis (J02.0)3

    J06.0   **Acute laryngopharyngitis**

    J06.9   **Acute upper respiratory infection, unspecified**   ▽
        Upper respiratory disease, acute
        Upper respiratory infection NOS

Influenza and pneumonia (J09-J18)

    EXCLUDES 2   *allergic or eosinophilic pneumonia (J82)*
        aspiration pneumonia NOS (J69.0)
        congenital pneumonia (P23.9)
        lipid pneumonia (J69.1)
        meconium pneumonia (P24.01)
        neonatal aspiration pneumonia (P24.-)
        pneumonia due to solids and liquids (J69.-)
        rheumatic pneumonia (I00)
        ventilator associated pneumonia (J95.851)

✓4ᵗʰ **J09**   **Influenza due to certain identified influenza viruses**
        EXCLUDES 1   *seasonal influenza due to other identified influenza virus (J10.-)*
            seasonal influenza due to unidentified influenza virus (J11.-)

    ✓5ᵗʰ **J09.X**   **Influenza due to identified novel influenza A virus**
        Avian influenza
        Bird influenza
        Influenza A/H5N1
        Influenza of other animal origin, not bird or swine
        Swine influenza virus (viruses that normally cause infections in pigs)

        2,8 **J09.X1**   **Influenza due to identified novel influenza A virus with pneumonia**   CC
          Code also, if applicable, associated:
            lung abscess (J85.1)
            other specified type of pneumonia
          RIC Excl: 15 Pulmonary

        J09.X2   **Influenza due to identified novel influenza A virus with other respiratory manifestations**   CC
          Influenza due to identified novel influenza A virus NOS
          Influenza due to identified novel influenza A virus with laryngitis
          Influenza due to identified novel influenza A virus with pharyngitis
          Influenza due to identified novel influenza A virus with upper respiratory symptoms
          Use additional code, if applicable, for associated:
            pleural effusion (J91.8)
            sinusitis (J01.-)
          RIC Excl: 15 Pulmonary

        J09.X3   **Influenza due to identified novel influenza A virus with gastrointestinal manifestations**   CC
          Influenza due to identified novel influenza A virus gastroenteritis
           EXCLUDES 1   *'intestinal flu' [viral gastroenteritis] (A08.-)*
          RIC Excl: 15 Pulmonary

        J09.X9   **Influenza due to identified novel influenza A virus with other manifestations**   CC
          Influenza due to identified novel influenza A virus with encephalopathy
          Influenza due to identified novel influenza A virus with myocarditis
          Influenza due to identified novel influenza A virus with otitis media
          Use additional code to identify manifestation
          RIC Excl: 15 Pulmonary

✓4ᵗʰ **J10**   **Influenza due to other identified influenza virus**
        EXCLUDES 1   *influenza due to avian influenza virus (J09.X-)*
            influenza due to swine flu (J09.X-)
            influenza due to unidentifed influenza virus (J11.-)

    ✓5ᵗʰ **J10.0**   **Influenza due to other identified influenza virus with pneumonia**
        Code also associated lung abscess, if applicable (J85.1)

        2,8 **J10.00**   **Influenza due to other identified influenza virus with unspecified type of pneumonia**   CC ▽
          RIC Excl: 15 Pulmonary

        2,8 **J10.01**   **Influenza due to other identified influenza virus with the same other identified influenza virus pneumonia**

        2,8 **J10.08**   **Influenza due to other identified influenza virus with other specified pneumonia**   CC
          Code also other specified type of pneumonia
          RIC Excl: 15 Pulmonary

    J10.1   **Influenza due to other identified influenza virus with other respiratory manifestations**   CC
        Influenza due to other identified influenza virus NOS
        Influenza due to other identified influenza virus with laryngitis
        Influenza due to other identified influenza virus with pharyngitis
        Influenza due to other identified influenza virus with upper respiratory symptoms
        Use additional code for associated pleural effusion, if applicable (J91.8)
        Use additional code for associated sinusitis, if applicable (J01.-)
        RIC Excl: 15 Pulmonary

    J10.2   **Influenza due to other identified influenza virus with gastrointestinal manifestations**
        Influenza due to other identified influenza virus gastroenteritis
          EXCLUDES 1   *'intestinal flu' [viral gastroenteritis] (A08.-)*

    ✓5ᵗʰ **J10.8**   **Influenza due to other identified influenza virus with other manifestations**

        J10.81   **Influenza due to other identified influenza virus with encephalopathy**

        J10.82   **Influenza due to other identified influenza virus with myocarditis**

        J10.83   **Influenza due to other identified influenza virus with otitis media**
          Use additional code for any associated perforated tympanic membrane (H72.-)

        J10.89   **Influenza due to other identified influenza virus with other manifestations**
          Use additional codes to identify the manifestations

---

² Special Care High = With fever

⁸ Clinically Complex = Without fever

✓4th **J11** **Influenza due to** unidentified **influenza virus**

✓5th **J11.Ø** **Influenza due to unidentified influenza virus with** pneumonia
Code also associated lung abscess, if applicable (J85.1)

2,8 **J11.ØØ** **Influenza due to unidentified influenza virus with unspecified type of pneumonia** cc ▽
Influenza with pneumonia NOS
RIC Excl: 15 Pulmonary

2,8 **J11.Ø8** **Influenza due to unidentified influenza virus with** specified **pneumonia** cc
Code also other specified type of pneumonia
RIC Excl: 15 Pulmonary

J11.1 **Influenza due to unidentified influenza virus with other** respiratory manifestations
Influenza NOS
Influenzal laryngitis NOS
Influenzal pharyngitis NOS
Influenza with upper respiratory symptoms NOS
Use additional code for associated pleural effusion, if applicable (J91.8)
Use additional code for associated sinusitis, if applicable (JØ1.-)

J11.2 **Influenza due to unidentified influenza virus with** gastrointestinal manifestations
Influenza gastroenteritis NOS
EXCLUDES 1 'intestinal flu' [viral gastroenteritis] (AØ8.-)

✓5th **J11.8** **Influenza due to unidentified influenza virus with** other manifestations

J11.81 **Influenza due to unidentified influenza virus with** encephalopathy
Influenzal encephalopathy NOS

J11.82 **Influenza due to unidentified influenza virus with** myocarditis
Influenzal myocarditis NOS

J11.83 **Influenza due to unidentified influenza virus with** otitis media
Influenzal otitis media NOS
Use additional code for any associated perforated tympanic membrane (H72.-)

J11.89 **Influenza due to unidentified influenza virus with other manifestations**
Use additional codes to identify the manifestations

✓4th **J12** **Viral pneumonia, not elsewhere classified**
INCLUDES bronchopneumonia due to viruses other than influenza viruses
Code first associated influenza, if applicable (JØ9.X1, J1Ø.Ø-, J11.Ø-)
Code also associated abscess, if applicable (J85.1)
EXCLUDES 1 aspiration pneumonia due to anesthesia during labor and delivery (O74.Ø)
aspiration pneumonia due to anesthesia during pregnancy (O29)
aspiration pneumonia due to anesthesia during puerperium (O89.Ø)
aspiration pneumonia due to solids and liquids (J69.-)
aspiration pneumonia NOS (J69.Ø)
congenital pneumonia (P23.Ø)
congenital rubella pneumonitis (P35.Ø)
interstitial pneumonia NOS (J84.9)
lipid pneumonia (J69.1)
neonatal aspiration pneumonia (P24.-)
AHA: 2013, 4Q, 118

2,8 **J12.Ø** Adenoviral **pneumonia** cc
RIC Excl: 15 Pulmonary

2,8 **J12.1** Respiratory syncytial **virus pneumonia** cc
RIC Excl: 15 Pulmonary

2,8 **J12.2** Parainfluenza **virus pneumonia** cc
RIC Excl: 15 Pulmonary

2,8 **J12.3** Human metapneumovirus **pneumonia** cc
RIC Excl: 15 Pulmonary

✓5th **J12.8** Other **viral pneumonia**

2,8 **J12.81** **Pneumonia due to SARS-associated coronavirus**
Severe acute respiratory syndrome NOS

2,8 **J12.89** **Other viral pneumonia** cc
RIC Excl: 15 Pulmonary

2,8 **J12.9** **Viral pneumonia, unspecified** cc ▽
RIC Excl: 15 Pulmonary

2,8 **J13** **Pneumonia due to** Streptococcus pneumoniae cc
Bronchopneumonia due to S. pneumoniae
Code first associated influenza, if applicable (JØ9.X1, J1Ø.Ø-, J11.Ø-)
Code also associated lung abscess, if applicable (J85.1)
EXCLUDES 1 congenital pneumonia due to S. pneumoniae (P23.6)
lobar pneumonia, unspecified organism (J18.1)
pneumonia due to other streptococci (J15.3-J15.4)
AHA: 2013, 4Q, 118
RIC Excl: 15 Pulmonary

2,8 **J14** **Pneumonia due to** Hemophilus influenzae cc
Bronchopneumonia due to H. influenzae
Code first associated influenza, if applicable (JØ9.X1, J1Ø.Ø-, J11.Ø-)
Code also associated lung abscess, if applicable (J85.1)
EXCLUDES 1 congenital pneumonia due to H. influenzae (P23.6)
AHA: 2013, 4Q, 118
RIC Excl: 15 Pulmonary

✓4th **J15** Bacterial **pneumonia, not elsewhere classified**
Bronchopneumonia due to bacteria other than S. pneumoniae and H. influenzae
Code first associated influenza, if applicable (JØ9.X1, J1Ø.Ø-, J11.Ø-)
Code also associated lung abscess, if applicable (J85.1)
EXCLUDES 1 chlamydial pneumonia (J16.Ø)
congenital pneumonia (P23.-)
Legionnaires' disease (A48.1)
spirochetal pneumonia (A69.8)
AHA: 2013, 4Q, 118

2,8 **J15.Ø** **Pneumonia due to** Klebsiella pneumoniae cc
RIC Excl: 15 Pulmonary

2,8 **J15.1** **Pneumonia due to** Pseudomonas cc
RIC Excl: 15 Pulmonary

✓5th **J15.2** **Pneumonia due to** staphylococcus

2,8 **J15.2Ø** **Pneumonia due to staphylococcus, unspecified** cc ▽
RIC Excl: 15 Pulmonary

✓6th **J15.21** **Pneumonia due to Staphylococcus** aureus

2,8 **J15.211** **Pneumonia due to** methicillin susceptible **Staphylococcus aureus** cc
MSSA pneumonia
Pneumonia due to Staphylococcus aureus NOS
RIC Excl: 15 Pulmonary

2,8 **J15.212** **Pneumonia due to** methicillin resistant **Staphylococcus aureus** cc
RIC Excl: 15 Pulmonary

2,8 **J15.29** **Pneumonia due to** other **staphylococcus** cc
RIC Excl: 15 Pulmonary

2,8 **J15.3** **Pneumonia due to streptococcus,** group B cc
RIC Excl: 15 Pulmonary

2,8 **J15.4** **Pneumonia due to** other **streptococci** cc
EXCLUDES 1 pneumonia due to streptococcus, group B (J15.3)
pneumonia due to Streptococcus pneumoniae (J13)
RIC Excl: 15 Pulmonary

2,8 **J15.5** **Pneumonia due to** Escherichia coli cc
RIC Excl: 15 Pulmonary

2,8 **J15.6** **Pneumonia due to** other aerobic Gram-negative bacteria cc
Pneumonia due to Serratia marcescens
RIC Excl: 15 Pulmonary

2,8 **J15.7** **Pneumonia due to** Mycoplasma pneumoniae cc
RIC Excl: 15 Pulmonary

2,8 **J15.8** **Pneumonia due to other specified bacteria** cc
RIC Excl: 15 Pulmonary

2,8 **J15.9** **Unspecified bacterial pneumonia** cc ▽
Pneumonia due to gram-positive bacteria
RIC Excl: 15 Pulmonary

✓4th **J16** **Pneumonia due to other infectious organisms, not elsewhere classified**
Code first associated influenza, if applicable (JØ9.X1, J1Ø.Ø-, J11.Ø-)
Code also associated lung abscess, if applicable (J85.1)
EXCLUDES 1 congenital pneumonia (P23.-)
ornithosis (A7Ø)
pneumocystosis (B59)
pneumonia NOS (J18.9)
AHA: 2013, 4Q, 118

2,8 **J16.Ø** Chlamydial **pneumonia** cc
RIC Excl: 15 Pulmonary

2,8 **J16.8** **Pneumonia due to other** specified infectious organisms cc
RIC Excl: 15 Pulmonary

---

2 Special Care High = With fever

8 Clinically Complex = Without fever

✓ Add'l Character Required ✓x7th Placeholder Alert RUG IV Special Care High Dx　RUG IV Clinically Complex Dx　RUG IV Special Care Low Dx　Manifestation Code　Other Specified Code　▽Unspecified Code

Chapter 10. Diseases of the Respiratory System

J17   Pneumonia in diseases classified elsewhere   cc

Code first underlying disease, such as:
Q fever (A78)
rheumatic fever (I00)
schistosomiasis (B65.0-B65.9)

EXCLUDES 1   candidial pneumonia (B37.1)
chlamydial pneumonia (J16.0)
gonorrheal pneumonia (A54.84)
histoplasmosis pneumonia (B39.0-B39.2)
measles pneumonia (B05.2)
nocardiosis pneumonia (A43.0)
pneumocystosis (B59)
pneumonia due to Pneumocystis carinii (B59)
pneumonia due to Pneumocystis jiroveci (B59)
pneumonia in actinomycosis (A42.0)
pneumonia in anthrax (A22.1)
pneumonia in ascariasis (B77.81)
pneumonia in aspergillosis (B44.0-B44.1)
pneumonia in coccidioidomycosis (B38.0-B38.2)
pneumonia in cytomegalovirus disease (B25.0)
pneumonia in toxoplasmosis (B58.3)
rubella pneumonia (B06.81)
salmonella pneumonia (A02.22)
spirochetal infection NEC with pneumonia (A69.8)
tularemia pneumonia (A21.2)
typhoid fever with pneumonia (A01.03)
varicella pneumonia (B01.2)
whooping cough with pneumonia (A37 with fifth-character 1)

AHA: 2013, 4Q, 118
RIC Excl: 15 Pulmonary

✓4ᵗʰ J18   Pneumonia, unspecified organism

Code first associated influenza, if applicable (J09.X1, J10.0-, J11.0-)

EXCLUDES 1   abscess of lung with pneumonia (J85.1)
aspiration pneumonia due to anesthesia during labor and delivery (O74.0)
aspiration pneumonia due to anesthesia during pregnancy (O29)
aspiration pneumonia due to anesthesia during puerperium (O89.0)
aspiration pneumonia due to solids and liquids (J69.-)
aspiration pneumonia NOS (J69.0)
congenital pneumonia (P23.0)
drug-induced interstitial lung disorder (J70.2-J70.4)
interstitial pneumonia NOS (J84.9)
lipid pneumonia (J69.1)
neonatal aspiration pneumonia (P24.-)
pneumonitis due to external agents (J67-J70)
pneumonitis due to fumes and vapors (J68.0)
usual interstitial pneumonia (J84.17)

AHA: 2013, 4Q, 118

2,8 J18.0   Bronchopneumonia, unspecified organism   cc ▽

EXCLUDES 1   hypostatic bronchopneumonia (J18.2)
lipid pneumonia (J69.1)
EXCLUDES 2   acute bronchiolitis (J21.-)
chronic bronchiolitis (J44.9)

RIC Excl: 15 Pulmonary

2,8 J18.1   Lobar pneumonia, unspecified organism   cc ▽
RIC Excl: 15 Pulmonary

2,8 J18.2   Hypostatic pneumonia, unspecified organism   cc ▽
Hypostatic bronchopneumonia
Passive pneumonia
RIC Excl: 15 Pulmonary

2,8 J18.8   Other pneumonia, unspecified organism   cc ▽
RIC Excl: 15 Pulmonary

2,8 J18.9   Pneumonia, unspecified organism   cc ▽
AHA: 2014, 3Q, 4; 2013, 4Q, 119; 2012, 4Q, 94
RIC Excl: 15 Pulmonary

Other acute lower respiratory infections (J20-J22)

EXCLUDES 2   chronic obstructive pulmonary disease with acute lower respiratory infection (J44.0)

✓4ᵗʰ J20   Acute bronchitis

INCLUDES   acute and subacute bronchitis (with) bronchospasm
acute and subacute bronchitis (with) tracheitis
acute and subacute bronchitis (with) tracheobronchitis, acute
acute and subacute fibrinous bronchitis
acute and subacute membranous bronchitis
acute and subacute purulent bronchitis
acute and subacute septic bronchitis

EXCLUDES 1   bronchitis NOS (J40)
tracheobronchitis NOS (J40)
EXCLUDES 2   acute bronchitis with bronchiectasis (J47.0)
acute bronchitis with chronic obstructive asthma (J44.0)
acute bronchitis with chronic obstructive pulmonary disease (J44.0)
allergic bronchitis NOS (J45.909)
bronchitis due to chemicals, fumes and vapors (J68.0)
chronic bronchitis NOS (J42)
chronic mucopurulent bronchitis (J41.1)
chronic obstructive bronchitis (J44.-)
chronic obstructive tracheobronchitis (J44.-)
chronic simple bronchitis (J41.0)
chronic tracheobronchitis (J42)

J20.0   Acute bronchitis due to Mycoplasma pneumoniae

J20.1   Acute bronchitis due to Hemophilus influenzae

J20.2   Acute bronchitis due to streptococcus

J20.3   Acute bronchitis due to coxsackievirus

J20.4   Acute bronchitis due to parainfluenza virus

J20.5   Acute bronchitis due to respiratory syncytial virus

J20.6   Acute bronchitis due to rhinovirus

J20.7   Acute bronchitis due to echovirus

J20.8   Acute bronchitis due to other specified organisms

J20.9   Acute bronchitis, unspecified   ▽

✓4ᵗʰ J21   Acute bronchiolitis

Acute bronchiolitis with bronchospasm
EXCLUDES 2   respiratory bronchiolitis interstitial lung disease (J84.115)

J21.0   Acute bronchiolitis due to respiratory syncytial virus   cc
RIC Excl: 15 Pulmonary

J21.1   Acute bronchiolitis due to human metapneumovirus   cc
RIC Excl: 15 Pulmonary

J21.8   Acute bronchiolitis due to other specified organisms   cc
RIC Excl: 15 Pulmonary

J21.9   Acute bronchiolitis, unspecified   cc ▽
Bronchiolitis (acute)
EXCLUDES 1   chronic bronchiolitis (J44.-)
RIC Excl: 15 Pulmonary

J22   Unspecified acute lower respiratory infection   ▽
Acute (lower) respiratory (tract) infection NOS
EXCLUDES 1   upper respiratory infection (acute) (J06.9)

Other diseases of upper respiratory tract (J30-J39)

✓4ᵗʰ J30   Vasomotor and allergic rhinitis

INCLUDES   spasmodic rhinorrhea
EXCLUDES 1   allergic rhinitis with asthma (bronchial) (J45.909)
rhinitis NOS (J31.0)

J30.0   Vasomotor rhinitis

J30.1   Allergic rhinitis due to pollen
Allergy NOS due to pollen
Hay fever
Pollinosis

J30.2   Other seasonal allergic rhinitis

J30.5   Allergic rhinitis due to food

✓5ᵗʰ J30.8   Other allergic rhinitis

J30.81   Allergic rhinitis due to animal (cat) (dog) hair and dander

J30.89   Other allergic rhinitis
Perennial allergic rhinitis

J30.9   Allergic rhinitis, unspecified   ▽

---

² Special Care High = With fever

⁸ Clinically Complex = Without fever

Ⓝ Newborn   Ⓟ Pediatric   Ⓜ Maternity   Ⓐ Adult   RIC RIC Dx   NCDx Noncancer Dx   PDx Primary Dx   cc RIC CC Condition   ▶◀ Revised Text   ● New Code   ▲ Revised Code Title

628   ICD-10-CM 2016

J17–J30.9

✓4ᵗʰ **J31   Chronic rhinitis, nasopharyngitis and pharyngitis**
     Use additional code to identify:
       exposure to environmental tobacco smoke (Z77.22)
       exposure to tobacco smoke in the perinatal period (P96.81)
       history of tobacco use (Z87.891)
       occupational exposure to environmental tobacco smoke (Z57.31)
       tobacco dependence (F17.-)
       tobacco use (Z72.0)

     J31.0   Chronic rhinitis
       Atrophic rhinitis (chronic)
       Granulomatous rhinitis (chronic)
       Hypertrophic rhinitis (chronic)
       Obstructive rhinitis (chronic)
       Ozena
       Purulent rhinitis (chronic)
       Rhinitis (chronic) NOS
       Ulcerative rhinitis (chronic)
       EXCLUDES 1   *allergic rhinitis (J30.1-J30.9)*
          vasomotor rhinitis (J30.0)

     J31.1   Chronic nasopharyngitis
       EXCLUDES 2   *acute nasopharyngitis (J00)*

     J31.2   Chronic pharyngitis
       Atrophic pharyngitis (chronic)
       Chronic sore throat
       Granular pharyngitis (chronic)
       Hypertrophic pharyngitis (chronic)
       EXCLUDES 2   *acute pharyngitis (J02.9)*

✓4ᵗʰ **J32   Chronic sinusitis**
     INCLUDES   sinus abscess
          sinus empyema
          sinus infection
          sinus suppuration
     Use additional code to identify:
       exposure to environmental tobacco smoke (Z77.22)
       exposure to tobacco smoke in the perinatal period (P96.81)
       history of tobacco use (Z87.891)
       infectious agent (B95-B97)
       occupational exposure to environmental tobacco smoke (Z57.31)
       tobacco dependence (F17.-)
       tobacco use (Z72.0)
     EXCLUDES 2   *acute sinusitis (J01.-)*

     J32.0   Chronic maxillary sinusitis
       Antritis (chronic)
       Maxillary sinusitis NOS

     J32.1   Chronic frontal sinusitis
       Frontal sinusitis NOS

     J32.2   Chronic ethmoidal sinusitis
       Ethmoidal sinusitis NOS
       EXCLUDES 1   *Woakes' ethmoiditis (J33.1)*

     J32.3   Chronic sphenoidal sinusitis
       Sphenoidal sinusitis NOS

     J32.4   Chronic pansinusitis
       Pansinusitis NOS

     J32.8   Other chronic sinusitis
       Sinusitis (chronic) involving more than one sinus but not
         pansinusitis

     J32.9   Chronic sinusitis, unspecified   ▽
       Sinusitis (chronic) NOS

✓4ᵗʰ **J33   Nasal polyp**
     Use additional code to identify:
       exposure to environmental tobacco smoke (Z77.22)
       exposure to tobacco smoke in the perinatal period (P96.81)
       history of tobacco use (Z87.891)
       occupational exposure to environmental tobacco smoke (Z57.31)
       tobacco dependence (F17.-)
       tobacco use (Z72.0)
     EXCLUDES 1   *adenomatous polyps (D14.0)*

     J33.0   Polyp of nasal cavity
       Choanal polyp
       Nasopharyngeal polyp

     J33.1   Polypoid sinus degeneration
       Woakes' syndrome or ethmoiditis

     J33.8   Other polyp of sinus
       Accessory polyp of sinus
       Ethmoidal polyp of sinus
       Maxillary polyp of sinus
       Sphenoidal polyp of sinus

     J33.9   Nasal polyp, unspecified   ▽

✓4ᵗʰ **J34   Other and unspecified disorders of nose and nasal sinuses**
     EXCLUDES 2   *varicose ulcer of nasal septum (I86.8)*

     J34.0   Abscess, furuncle and carbuncle of nose
       Cellulitis of nose
       Necrosis of nose
       Ulceration of nose

     J34.1   Cyst and mucocele of nose and nasal sinus

     J34.2   Deviated nasal septum
       Deflection or deviation of septum (nasal) (acquired)
       EXCLUDES 1   *congenital deviated nasal septum (Q67.4)*

     J34.3   Hypertrophy of nasal turbinates

✓5ᵗʰ   **J34.8   Other specified disorders of nose and nasal sinuses**
       J34.81   Nasal mucositis (ulcerative)
          Code also type of associated therapy, such as:
            antineoplastic and immunosuppressive drugs
              (T45.1X-)
            radiological procedure and radiotherapy (Y84.2)
          EXCLUDES 2   *gastrointestinal mucositis (ulcerative)*
            (K92.81)
            mucositis (ulcerative) of vagina and vulva
            (N76.81)
            oral mucositis (ulcerative) (K12.3-)

       J34.89   Other specified disorders of nose and nasal sinuses
          Perforation of nasal septum NOS
          Rhinolith

     J34.9   Unspecified disorder of nose and nasal sinuses   ▽

✓4ᵗʰ **J35   Chronic diseases of tonsils and adenoids**
     Use additional code to identify:
       exposure to environmental tobacco smoke (Z77.22)
       exposure to tobacco smoke in the perinatal period (P96.81)
       history of tobacco use (Z87.891)
       occupational exposure to environmental tobacco smoke (Z57.31)
       tobacco dependence (F17.-)
       tobacco use (Z72.0)

✓5ᵗʰ   **J35.0   Chronic tonsillitis and adenoiditis**
       EXCLUDES 2   *acute tonsillitis (J03.-)*

       J35.01   Chronic tonsillitis

       J35.02   Chronic adenoiditis

       J35.03   Chronic tonsillitis and adenoiditis

     J35.1   Hypertrophy of tonsils
       Enlargement of tonsils
       EXCLUDES 1   *hypertrophy of tonsils with tonsillitis (J35.0-)*

     J35.2   Hypertrophy of adenoids
       Enlargement of adenoids
       EXCLUDES 1   *hypertrophy of adenoids with adenoiditis (J35.0-)*

     J35.3   Hypertrophy of tonsils with hypertrophy of adenoids
       EXCLUDES 1   *hypertrophy of tonsils and adenoids with tonsillitis and*
          adenoiditis (J35.03)

     J35.8   Other chronic diseases of tonsils and adenoids
       Adenoid vegetations
       Amygdalolith
       Calculus, tonsil
       Cicatrix of tonsil (and adenoid)
       Tonsillar tag
       Ulcer of tonsil

     J35.9   Chronic disease of tonsils and adenoids, unspecified   ▽
       Disease (chronic) of tonsils and adenoids NOS

J36   Peritonsillar abscess
     INCLUDES   abscess of tonsil
          peritonsillar cellulitis
          quinsy
     Use additional code (B95-B97) to identify infectious agent
     EXCLUDES 1   *acute tonsillitis (J03.-)*
       chronic tonsillitis (J35.0)
       retropharyngeal abscess (J39.0)
       tonsillitis NOS (J03.9-)

☑ Add'l Character Required   ☑x7ᵗʰ Placeholder Alert   RUG IV Special Care High Dx   RUG IV Clinically Complex Dx   RUG IV Special Care Low Dx   Manifestation Code   Other Specified Code   ▽ Unspecified Code

ICD-10-CM 2016   629

Chapter 10. Diseases of the Respiratory System

J37–J42

☑4th J37   Chronic laryngitis and laryngotracheitis

Use additional code to identify:
exposure to environmental tobacco smoke (Z77.22)
exposure to tobacco smoke in the perinatal period (P96.81)
history of tobacco use (Z87.891)
infectious agent (B95-B97)
occupational exposure to environmental tobacco smoke (Z57.31)
tobacco dependence (F17.-)
tobacco use (Z72.0)

J37.0   Chronic laryngitis
Catarrhal laryngitis
Hypertrophic laryngitis
Sicca laryngitis
EXCLUDES 2   *acute laryngitis (J04.0)*
obstructive (acute) laryngitis (J05.0)

J37.1   Chronic laryngotracheitis
Laryngitis, chronic, with tracheitis (chronic)
Tracheitis, chronic, with laryngitis
EXCLUDES 1   *chronic tracheitis (J42)*
EXCLUDES 2   *acute laryngotracheitis (J04.2)*
acute tracheitis (J04.1)

☑4th J38   Diseases of vocal cords and larynx, not elsewhere classified

Use additional code to identify:
exposure to environmental tobacco smoke (Z77.22)
exposure to tobacco smoke in the perinatal period (P96.81)
history of tobacco use (Z87.891)
occupational exposure to environmental tobacco smoke (Z57.31)
tobacco dependence (F17.-)
tobacco use (Z72.0)
EXCLUDES 1   *congenital laryngeal stridor (P28.89)*
obstructive laryngitis (acute) (J05.0)
postprocedural subglottic stenosis (J95.5)
stridor (R06.1)
ulcerative laryngitis (J04.0)

☑5th J38.0   Paralysis of vocal cords and larynx
Laryngoplegia
Paralysis of glottis

    J38.00   Paralysis of vocal cords and larynx, unspecified   CC ▽
       RIC Excl: 15 Pulmonary

    J38.01   Paralysis of vocal cords and larynx, unilateral   CC
       RIC Excl: 15 Pulmonary

    J38.02   Paralysis of vocal cords and larynx, bilateral   CC
       RIC Excl: 15 Pulmonary

J38.1   Polyp of vocal cord and larynx
EXCLUDES 1   *adenomatous polyps (D14.1)*

J38.2   Nodules of vocal cords
Chorditis (fibrinous)(nodosa)(tuberosa)
Singer's nodes
Teacher's nodes

J38.3   Other diseases of vocal cords
Abscess of vocal cords
Cellulitis of vocal cords
Granuloma of vocal cords
Leukokeratosis of vocal cords
Leukoplakia of vocal cords

J38.4   Edema of larynx   CC
Edema (of) glottis
Subglottic edema
Supraglottic edema
EXCLUDES 1   *acute obstructive laryngitis [croup] (J05.0)*
edematous laryngitis (J04.0)
RIC Excl: 15 Pulmonary

J38.5   Laryngeal spasm
Laryngismus (stridulus)

J38.6   Stenosis of larynx

J38.7   Other diseases of larynx
Abscess of larynx
Cellulitis of larynx
Disease of larynx NOS
Necrosis of larynx
Pachyderma of larynx
Perichondritis of larynx
Ulcer of larynx

☑4th J39   Other diseases of upper respiratory tract

EXCLUDES 1   *acute respiratory infection NOS (J22)*
acute upper respiratory infection (J06.9)
upper respiratory inflammation due to chemicals, gases, fumes or vapors (J68.2)

J39.0   Retropharyngeal and parapharyngeal abscess
Peripharyngeal abscess
EXCLUDES 1   *peritonsillar abscess (J36)*

J39.1   Other abscess of pharynx
Cellulitis of pharynx
Nasopharyngeal abscess

J39.2   Other diseases of pharynx
Cyst of pharynx
Edema of pharynx
EXCLUDES 2   *chronic pharyngitis (J31.2)*
ulcerative pharyngitis (J02.9)

J39.3   Upper respiratory tract hypersensitivity reaction, site unspecified   ▽
EXCLUDES 1   *hypersensitivity reaction of upper respiratory tract, such as:*
extrinsic allergic alveolitis (J67.9)
pneumoconiosis (J60-J67.9)

J39.8   Other specified diseases of upper respiratory tract

J39.9   Disease of upper respiratory tract, unspecified   ▽

Chronic lower respiratory diseases (J40-J47)

EXCLUDES 1   *bronchitis due to chemicals, gases, fumes and vapors (J68.0)*
EXCLUDES 2   *cystic fibrosis (E84.-)*

J40   Bronchitis, not specified as acute or chronic

Bronchitis NOS
Bronchitis with tracheitis NOS
Catarrhal bronchitis
Tracheobronchitis NOS
Use additional code to identify:
exposure to environmental tobacco smoke (Z77.22)
exposure to tobacco smoke in the perinatal period (P96.81)
history of tobacco use (Z87.891)
occupational exposure to environmental tobacco smoke (Z57.31)
tobacco dependence (F17.-)
tobacco use (Z72.0)
EXCLUDES 1   *acute bronchitis (J20.-)*
allergic bronchitis NOS (J45.909)
asthmatic bronchitis NOS (J45.9-)
bronchitis due to chemicals, gases, fumes and vapors (J68.0)

☑4th J41   Simple and mucopurulent chronic bronchitis

Use additional code to identify:
exposure to environmental tobacco smoke (Z77.22)
exposure to tobacco smoke in the perinatal period (P96.81)
history of tobacco use (Z87.891)
occupational exposure to environmental tobacco smoke (Z57.31)
tobacco dependence (F17.-)
tobacco use (Z72.0)
EXCLUDES 1   *chronic bronchitis NOS (J42)*
chronic obstructive bronchitis (J44.-)

J41.0   Simple chronic bronchitis

J41.1   Mucopurulent chronic bronchitis

J41.8   Mixed simple and mucopurulent chronic bronchitis

J42   Unspecified chronic bronchitis   ▽

Chronic bronchitis NOS
Chronic tracheitis
Chronic tracheobronchitis
Use additional code to identify:
exposure to environmental tobacco smoke (Z77.22)
exposure to tobacco smoke in the perinatal period (P96.81)
history of tobacco use (Z87.891)
occupational exposure to environmental tobacco smoke (Z57.31)
tobacco dependence (F17.-)
tobacco use (Z72.0)
EXCLUDES 1   *chronic asthmatic bronchitis (J44.-)*
chronic bronchitis with airways obstruction (J44.-)
chronic emphysematous bronchitis (J44.-)
chronic obstructive pulmonary disease NOS (J44.9)
simple and mucopurulent chronic bronchitis (J41.-)

Ⓝ Newborn   Ⓟ Pediatric   Ⓜ Maternity   Ⓐ Adult   RIC RIC Dx   NCDx Noncancer Dx   PDx Primary Dx   CC RIC CC Condition   ►◄ Revised Text   ● New Code   ▲ Revised Code Title

630   ICD-10-CM 2016

✓4th **J43 Emphysema**

Use additional code to identify:
exposure to environmental tobacco smoke (Z77.22)
history of tobacco use (Z87.891)
occupational exposure to environmental tobacco smoke (Z57.31)
tobacco dependence (F17.-)
tobacco use (Z72.0)

EXCLUDES1   *compensatory emphysema (J98.3)*
emphysema due to inhalation of chemicals, gases, fumes or
vapors (J68.4)
emphysema with chronic (obstructive) bronchitis (J44.-)
emphysematous (obstructive) bronchitis (J44.-)
interstitial emphysema (J98.2)
mediastinal emphysema (J98.2)
neonatal interstitial emphysema (P25.0)
surgical (subcutaneous) emphysema (T81.82)
traumatic subcutaneous emphysema (T79.7)

J43.0 Unilateral pulmonary emphysema [MacLeod's syndrome]
Swyer-James syndrome
Unilateral emphysema
Unilateral hyperlucent lung
Unilateral pulmonary artery functional hypoplasia
Unilateral transparency of lung

J43.1 Panlobular emphysema
Panacinar emphysema

J43.2 Centrilobular emphysema

J43.8 Other emphysema

J43.9 Emphysema, unspecified ▽
Bullous emphysema (lung)(pulmonary)
Emphysema (lung)(pulmonary) NOS
Emphysematous bleb
Vesicular emphysema (lung)(pulmonary)

✓4th **J44 Other chronic obstructive pulmonary disease**
INCLUDES   asthma with chronic obstructive pulmonary disease
chronic asthmatic (obstructive) bronchitis
chronic bronchitis with airways obstruction
chronic bronchitis with emphysema
chronic emphysematous bronchitis
chronic obstructive asthma
chronic obstructive bronchitis
chronic obstructive tracheobronchitis

Code also type of asthma, if applicable (J45.-)
Use additional code to identify:
exposure to environmental tobacco smoke (Z77.22)
history of tobacco use (Z87.891)
occupational exposure to environmental tobacco smoke (Z57.31)
tobacco dependence (F17.-)
tobacco use (Z72.0)

EXCLUDES1   *bronchiectasis (J47.-)*
chronic bronchitis NOS (J42)
chronic simple and mucopurulent bronchitis (J41.-)
chronic tracheitis (J42)
chronic tracheobronchitis (J42)
emphysema without chronic bronchitis (J43.-)
lung diseases due to external agents (J60-J70)

AHA: 2013, 4Q, 109

J44.0 Chronic obstructive pulmonary disease with acute lower respiratory infection   NC Dx
Use additional code to identify the infection

J44.1 Chronic obstructive pulmonary disease with (acute) exacerbation   NC Dx
Decompensated COPD
Decompensated COPD with (acute) exacerbation
EXCLUDES2   *chronic obstructive pulmonary disease [COPD] with*
acute bronchitis (J44.0)

J44.9 Chronic obstructive pulmonary disease, unspecified   NC Dx ▽
Chronic obstructive airway disease NOS
Chronic obstructive lung disease NOS
AHA: 2014, 4Q, 21; 2013, 4Q, 129

✓4th **J45 Asthma**
INCLUDES   allergic (predominantly) asthma
allergic bronchitis nos
allergic rhinitis with asthma
atopic asthma
extrinsic allergic asthma
hay fever with asthma
idiosyncratic asthma
intrinsic nonallergic asthma
nonallergic asthma

Use additional code to identify:
exposure to environmental tobacco smoke (Z77.22)
exposure to tobacco smoke in the perinatal period (P96.81)
history of tobacco use (Z87.891)
occupational exposure to environmental tobacco smoke (Z57.31)
tobacco dependence (F17.-)
tobacco use (Z72.0)

EXCLUDES1   *detergent asthma (J69.8)*
eosinophilic asthma (J82)
lung diseases due to external agents (J60-J70)
miner's asthma (J60)
wheezing NOS (R06.2)
wood asthma (J67.8)

EXCLUDES2   *asthma with chronic obstructive pulmonary disease (J44.9)*
chronic asthmatic (obstructive) bronchitis (J44.9)
chronic obstructive asthma (J44.9)

✓5th **J45.2 Mild intermittent asthma**

J45.20 Mild intermittent asthma, uncomplicated
Mild intermittent asthma NOS

J45.21 Mild intermittent asthma with (acute) exacerbation

J45.22 Mild intermittent asthma with status asthmaticus

✓5th **J45.3 Mild persistent asthma**

J45.30 Mild persistent asthma, uncomplicated
Mild persistent asthma NOS

J45.31 Mild persistent asthma with (acute) exacerbation

J45.32 Mild persistent asthma with status asthmaticus

✓5th **J45.4 Moderate persistent asthma**

J45.40 Moderate persistent asthma, uncomplicated
Moderate persistent asthma NOS

J45.41 Moderate persistent asthma with (acute) exacerbation

J45.42 Moderate persistent asthma with status asthmaticus

✓5th **J45.5 Severe persistent asthma**

J45.50 Severe persistent asthma, uncomplicated
Severe persistent asthma NOS

J45.51 Severe persistent asthma with (acute) exacerbation

J45.52 Severe persistent asthma with status asthmaticus

✓5th **J45.9 Other and unspecified asthma**

✓6th **J45.90 Unspecified asthma**
Asthmatic bronchitis NOS   Late onset asthma
Childhood asthma NOS

J45.901 Unspecified asthma with (acute) exacerbation ▽

J45.902 Unspecified asthma with status asthmaticus ▽

J45.909 Unspecified asthma, uncomplicated ▽
Asthma NOS

✓6th **J45.99 Other asthma**

J45.990 Exercise induced bronchospasm

J45.991 Cough variant asthma

J45.998 Other asthma

✓4th **J47 Bronchiectasis**
INCLUDES   bronchiolectasis
Use additional code to identify:
exposure to environmental tobacco smoke (Z77.22)
exposure to tobacco smoke in the perinatal period (P96.81)
history of tobacco use (Z87.891)
occupational exposure to environmental tobacco smoke (Z57.31)
tobacco dependence (F17.-)
tobacco use (Z72.0)

EXCLUDES1   *congenital bronchiectasis (Q33.4)*
tuberculous bronchiectasis (current disease) (A15.0)

J47.0 Bronchiectasis with acute lower respiratory infection
Bronchiectasis with acute bronchitis

J47.1 Bronchiectasis with (acute) exacerbation

J47.9 Bronchiectasis, uncomplicated
Bronchiectasis NOS

✓ Add'l Character Required   ✓x7th Placeholder Alert   RUG IV Special Care High Dx   RUG IV Clinically Complex Dx   RUG IV Special Care Low Dx   Manifestation Code   Other Specified Code   ▽ Unspecified Code

Chapter 10. Diseases of the Respiratory System

Lung diseases due to external agents (J60-J70)

EXCLUDES 2 asthma (J45.-)
malignant neoplasm of bronchus and lung (C34.-)

J60 Coalworker's pneumoconiosis 🅰
Anthracosilicosis
Anthracosis
Black lung disease
Coalworker's lung
EXCLUDES 1 coalworker pneumoconiosis with tuberculosis, any type in A15 (J65)

J61 Pneumoconiosis due to asbestos and other mineral fibers 🅰
Asbestosis
EXCLUDES 1 pleural plaque with asbestosis (J92.0)
pneumoconiosis with tuberculosis, any type in A15 (J65)

✓4ᵗʰ **J62 Pneumoconiosis due to dust containing silica**
INCLUDES silicotic fibrosis (massive) of lung
EXCLUDES 1 pneumoconiosis with tuberculosis, any type in A15 (J65)

J62.0 Pneumoconiosis due to talc dust

J62.8 Pneumoconiosis due to other dust containing silica
Silicosis NOS

✓4ᵗʰ **J63 Pneumoconiosis due to other inorganic dusts**
EXCLUDES 1 pneumoconiosis with tuberculosis, any type in A15 (J65)

J63.0 Aluminosis (of lung)

J63.1 Bauxite fibrosis (of lung)

J63.2 Berylliosis

J63.3 Graphite fibrosis (of lung)

J63.4 Siderosis

J63.5 Stannosis

J63.6 Pneumoconiosis due to other specified inorganic dusts

J64 Unspecified pneumoconiosis ▽
EXCLUDES 1 pneumonoconiosis with tuberculosis, any type in A15 (J65)

J65 Pneumoconiosis associated with tuberculosis
Any condition in J60-J64 with tuberculosis, any type in A15
Silicotuberculosis

✓4ᵗʰ **J66 Airway disease due to specific organic dust**
EXCLUDES 2 allergic alveolitis (J67.-)
asbestosis (J61)
bagassosis (J67.1)
farmer's lung (J67.0)
hypersensitivity pneumonitis due to organic dust (J67.-)
reactive airways dysfunction syndrome (J68.3)

J66.0 Byssinosis
Airway disease due to cotton dust

J66.1 Flax-dressers' disease

J66.2 Cannabinosis

J66.8 Airway disease due to other specific organic dusts

✓4ᵗʰ **J67 Hypersensitivity pneumonitis due to organic dust**
INCLUDES allergic alveolitis and pneumonitis due to inhaled organic dust and particles of fungal, actinomycetic or other origin
EXCLUDES 1 pneumonitis due to inhalation of chemicals, gases, fumes or vapors (J68.0)

J67.0 Farmer's lung
Harvester's lung
Haymaker's lung
Moldy hay disease

J67.1 Bagassosis
Bagasse disease
Bagasse pneumonitis

J67.2 Bird fancier's lung
Budgerigar fancier's disease or lung
Pigeon fancier's disease or lung

J67.3 Suberosis
Corkhandler's disease or lung
Corkworker's disease or lung

J67.4 Maltworker's lung
Alveolitis due to Aspergillus clavatus

J67.5 Mushroom-worker's lung

J67.6 Maple-bark-stripper's lung
Alveolitis due to Cryptostroma corticale
Cryptostromosis

J67.7 Air conditioner and humidifier lung
Allergic alveolitis due to fungal, thermophilic actinomycetes and other organisms growing in ventilation [air conditioning] systems

J67.8 Hypersensitivity pneumonitis due to other organic dusts
Cheese-washer's lung
Coffee-worker's lung
Fish-meal worker's lung
Furrier's lung
Sequoiosis

J67.9 Hypersensitivity pneumonitis due to unspecified organic dust ▽
Allergic alveolitis (extrinsic) NOS
Hypersensitivity pneumonitis NOS

✓4ᵗʰ **J68 Respiratory conditions due to inhalation of chemicals, gases, fumes and vapors**
Code first (T51-T65) to identify cause
Use additional code to identify associated respiratory conditions, such as:
acute respiratory failure (J96.0-)

J68.0 Bronchitis and pneumonitis due to chemicals, gases, fumes and vapors CC
Chemical bronchitis (acute)
RIC Excl: 15 Pulmonary

J68.1 Pulmonary edema due to chemicals, gases, fumes and vapors CC
Chemical pulmonary edema (acute) (chronic)
EXCLUDES 1 pulmonary edema (acute) (chronic) NOS (J81.-)
RIC Excl: 15 Pulmonary

J68.2 Upper respiratory inflammation due to chemicals, gases, fumes and vapors, not elsewhere classified

J68.3 Other acute and subacute respiratory conditions due to chemicals, gases, fumes and vapors
Reactive airways dysfunction syndrome

J68.4 Chronic respiratory conditions due to chemicals, gases, fumes and vapors
Emphysema (diffuse) (chronic) due to inhalation of chemicals, gases, fumes and vapors
Obliterative bronchiolitis (chronic) (subacute) due to inhalation of chemicals, gases, fumes and vapors
Pulmonary fibrosis (chronic) due to inhalation of chemicals, gases, fumes and vapors
EXCLUDES 1 chronic pulmonary edema due to chemicals, gases, fumes and vapors (J68.1)

J68.8 Other respiratory conditions due to chemicals, gases, fumes and vapors

J68.9 Unspecified respiratory condition due to chemicals, gases, fumes and vapors ▽

✓4ᵗʰ **J69 Pneumonitis due to solids and liquids**
EXCLUDES 1 neonatal aspiration syndromes (P24.-)
postprocedural pneumonitis (J95.4)

2,8 **J69.0 Pneumonitis due to inhalation of food and vomit** CC
Aspiration pneumonia NOS
Aspiration pneumonia (due to) food (regurgitated)
Aspiration pneumonia (due to) gastric secretions
Aspiration pneumonia (due to) milk
Aspiration pneumonia (due to) vomit
Code also any associated foreign body in respiratory tract (T17.-)
EXCLUDES 1 chemical pneumonitis due to anesthesia (J95.4)
obstetric aspiration pneumonia (O74.0)
RIC Excl: 15 Pulmonary

2,8 **J69.1 Pneumonitis due to inhalation of oils and essences** CC
Exogenous lipoid pneumonia
Lipid pneumonia NOS
Code first (T51-T65) to identify substance
EXCLUDES 1 endogenous lipoid pneumonia (J84.89)
RIC Excl: 15 Pulmonary

2,8 **J69.8 Pneumonitis due to inhalation of other solids and liquids** CC
Pneumonitis due to aspiration of blood
Pneumonitis due to aspiration of detergent
Code first (T51-T65) to identify substance
RIC Excl: 15 Pulmonary

---

² Special Care High = With fever

⁸ Clinically Complex = Without fever

Ⓝ Newborn   Ⓟ Pediatric   Ⓜ Maternity   🅰 Adult   RIC RIC Dx   NC Dx Noncancer Dx   PDx Primary Dx   CC RIC CC Condition   ►◄ Revised Text   ● New Code   ▲ Revised Code Title

632

ICD-10-CM 2016

J60–J69.8

✓4ᵗʰ **J70 Respiratory conditions due to other external agents**

J70.0 Acute **pulmonary manifestations due to** radiation
Radiation pneumonitis
Use additional code (W88-W90, X39.0-) to identify the external cause

J70.1 Chronic **and other pulmonary manifestations due to** radiation
Fibrosis of lung following radiation
Use additional code (W88-W90, X39.0-) to identify the external cause

J70.2 Acute drug-induced interstitial lung **disorders**
Use additional code for adverse effect, if applicable, to identify drug (T36-T50 with fifth or sixth character 5)
EXCLUDES 1   *interstitial pneumonia NOS (J84.9)*
lymphoid interstitial pneumonia (J84.2)

J70.3 Chronic drug-induced interstitial **lung disorders**
Use additional code for adverse effect, if applicable, to identify drug (T36-T50 with fifth or sixth character 5)
EXCLUDES 1   *interstitial pneumonia NOS (J84.9)*
lymphoid interstitial pneumonia (J84.2)

J70.4 Drug-induced interstitial lung disorders, unspecified ▽
Use additional code for adverse effect, if applicable, to identify drug (T36-T50 with fifth or sixth character 5)
EXCLUDES 1   *interstitial pneumonia NOS (J84.9)*
lymphoid interstitial pneumonia (J84.2)

J70.5 Respiratory conditions due to smoke inhalation
Smoke inhalation NOS
EXCLUDES 1   *smoke inhalation due to chemicals, gases, fumes and vapors (J68.9)*
AHA: 2013, 4Q, 121

J70.8 Respiratory conditions due to other specified external agents
Code first (T51-T65) to identify the external agent

J70.9 Respiratory conditions due to unspecified external agent ▽
Code first (T51-T65) to identify the external agent

Other respiratory diseases principally affecting the interstitium (J80-J84)

J80 Acute respiratory distress syndrome
Acute respiratory distress syndrome in adult or child
Adult hyaline membrane disease
EXCLUDES 1   *respiratory distress syndrome in newborn (perinatal) (P22.0)*

✓4ᵗʰ **J81 Pulmonary edema**
Use additional code to identify:
exposure to environmental tobacco smoke (Z77.22)
history of tobacco use (Z87.891)
occupational exposure to environmental tobacco smoke (Z57.31)
tobacco dependence (F17.-)
tobacco use (Z72.0)
EXCLUDES 1   *chemical (acute) pulmonary edema (J68.1)*
hypostatic pneumonia (J18.2)
passive pneumonia (J18.2)
pulmonary edema due to external agents (J60-J70)
pulmonary edema with heart disease NOS (I50.1)
pulmonary edema with heart failure (I50.1)

J81.0 Acute pulmonary edema
Acute edema of lung

J81.1 Chronic pulmonary edema   cc
Pulmonary congestion (chronic) (passive)
Pulmonary edema NOS
RIC Excl: 15 Pulmonary

2,8 **J82 Pulmonary eosinophilia, not elsewhere classified**   cc
Allergic pneumonia
Eosinophilic asthma
Eosinophilic pneumonia
Löffler's pneumonia
Tropical (pulmonary) eosinophilia NOS
EXCLUDES 1   *pulmonary eosinophilia due to aspergillosis (B44.-)*
pulmonary eosinophilia due to drugs (J70.2-J70.4)
pulmonary eosinophilia due to specified parasitic infection (B50-B83)
pulmonary eosinophilia due to systemic connective tissue disorders (M30-M36)
pulmonary infiltrate NOS (R91.8)
RIC Excl: 15 Pulmonary

✓4ᵗʰ **J84 Other interstitial pulmonary diseases**
EXCLUDES 1   *drug-induced interstitial lung disorders (J70.2-J70.4)*
interstitial emphysema (J98.2)
lung diseases due to external agents (J60-J70)

✓5ᵗʰ **J84.0 Alveolar and parieto-alveolar conditions**

J84.01 Alveolar proteinosis

J84.02 Pulmonary alveolar microlithiasis

J84.03 Idiopathic pulmonary hemosiderosis
Essential brown induration of lung
Code first underlying disease, such as:
disorders of iron metabolism (E83.1-)
EXCLUDES 1   *acute idiopathic pulmonary hemorrhage in infants [AIPHI] (R04.81)*

J84.09 Other alveolar and parieto-alveolar conditions

✓5ᵗʰ **J84.1 Other interstitial pulmonary diseases with fibrosis**
EXCLUDES 1   *pulmonary fibrosis (chronic) due to inhalation of chemicals, gases, fumes or vapors (J68.4)*
pulmonary fibrosis (chronic) following radiation (J70.1)

J84.10 Pulmonary fibrosis, unspecified   cc ▽
Capillary fibrosis of lung
Cirrhosis of lung (chronic) NOS
Fibrosis of lung (atrophic) (chronic) (confluent) (massive) (perialveolar) (peribronchial) NOS
Induration of lung (chronic) NOS
Postinflammatory pulmonary fibrosis
RIC Excl: 15 Pulmonary

✓6ᵗʰ **J84.11 Idiopathic interstitial pneumonia**
EXCLUDES 1   *lymphoid interstitial pneumonia (J84.2)*
pneumocystis pneumonia (B59)

2,8 **J84.111 Idiopathic interstitial pneumonia, not otherwise specified**

J84.112 Idiopathic pulmonary fibrosis   cc
Cryptogenic fibrosing alveolitis
Idiopathic fibrosing alveolitis
RIC Excl: 15 Pulmonary

J84.113 Idiopathic non-specific interstitial pneumonitis   cc
EXCLUDES 1   *non-specific interstitial pneumonia NOS, or due to known underlying cause (J84.89)*
RIC Excl: 15 Pulmonary

2,8 **J84.114 Acute interstitial pneumonitis**   cc
Hamman-Rich syndrome
EXCLUDES 1   *pneumocystis pneumonia (B59)*
RIC Excl: 15 Pulmonary

J84.115 Respiratory bronchiolitis interstitial lung disease   cc
RIC Excl: 15 Pulmonary

2,8 **J84.116 Cryptogenic organizing pneumonia**
EXCLUDES 1   *organizing pneumonia NOS, or due to known cause (J84.89)*

2,8 **J84.117 Desquamative interstitial pneumonia**

J84.17 Other interstitial pulmonary diseases with fibrosis in diseases classified elsewhere   cc
Interstitial pneumonia (nonspecific) (usual) due to collagen vascular disease
Interstitial pneumonia (nonspecific) (usual) in diseases classified elsewhere
Organizing pneumonia due to collagen vascular disease
Organizing pneumonia in diseases classified elsewhere
Code first underlying disease, such as:
progressive systemic sclerosis (M34.0)
rheumatoid arthritis (M05.00-M06.9)
systemic lupus erythematosis (M32.0-M32.9)
RIC Excl: 15 Pulmonary

2,8 **J84.2 Lymphoid interstitial pneumonia**
Lymphoid interstitial pneumonitis

✓5ᵗʰ **J84.8 Other specified interstitial pulmonary diseases**
EXCLUDES 1   *exogenous lipoid pneumonia (J69.1)*
unspecified lipoid pneumonia (J69.1)

J84.81 Lymphangioleiomyomatosis   ♀
Lymphangiomyomatosis

J84.82 Adult pulmonary Langerhans cell histiocytosis   A
Adult PLCH

---
2 Special Care High = With fever

8 Clinically Complex = Without fever

Chapter 10. Diseases of the Respiratory System

J84.83   **Surfactant mutations of the lung**

✓6ᵗʰ J84.84   **Other interstitial lung diseases of childhood**

J84.841   **Neuroendocrine cell hyperplasia of infancy**

J84.842   **Pulmonary interstitial glycogenesis**

J84.843   **Alveolar capillary dysplasia with vein misalignment**

J84.848   **Other interstitial lung diseases of childhood**   P

2,8 J84.89   **Other specified interstitial pulmonary diseases**   CC

Endogenous lipoid pneumonia
Interstitial pneumonitis
Non-specific interstitial pneumonitis NOS
Organizing pneumonia due to known underlying cause
Organizing pneumonia NOS
Code first, if applicable:
   poisoning due to drug or toxin (T51-T65 with fifth or sixth character to indicate intent), for toxic pneumonopathy
   underlying cause of pneumonopathy, if known
Use additional code, for adverse effect, to identify drug (T36-T50 with fifth or sixth character 5), if drug-induced

EXCLUDES 1   *cryptogenic organizing pneumonia (J84.116)*
     idiopathic non-specific interstitial pneumonitis (J84.113)
     lipoid pneumonia, exogenous or unspecified (J69.1)
     lymphoid interstitial pneumonia (J84.2)

RIC Excl: 15 Pulmonary

2,8 J84.9   **Interstitial pulmonary disease, unspecified**   ▽

Interstitial pneumonia NOS

Suppurative and necrotic conditions of the lower respiratory tract (J85-J86)

✓4ᵗʰ J85   **Abscess of lung and mediastinum**

Use additional code (B95-B97) to identify infectious agent.

J85.0   **Gangrene and necrosis of lung**   CC

RIC Excl: 15 Pulmonary

2,8 J85.1   **Abscess of lung with pneumonia**   CC

Code also the type of pneumonia
RIC Excl: 15 Pulmonary

J85.2   **Abscess of lung without pneumonia**   CC

Abscess of lung NOS
RIC Excl: 15 Pulmonary

J85.3   **Abscess of mediastinum**   CC

RIC Excl: 15 Pulmonary

✓4ᵗʰ J86   **Pyothorax**

Use additional code (B95-B97) to identify infectious agent.

EXCLUDES 1   *abscess of lung (J85.-)*
     pyothorax due to tuberculosis (A15.6)

J86.0   **Pyothorax with fistula**   CC

Bronchocutaneous fistula
Bronchopleural fistula
Hepatopleural fistula
Mediastinal fistula
Pleural fistula
Thoracic fistula
Any condition classifiable to J86.9 with fistula
RIC Excl: 15 Pulmonary

J86.9   **Pyothorax without fistula**   CC

Abscess of pleura
Abscess of thorax
Empyema (chest) (lung) (pleura)
Fibrinopurulent pleurisy
Purulent pleurisy
Pyopneumothorax
Septic pleurisy
Seropurulent pleurisy
Suppurative pleurisy
RIC Excl: 15 Pulmonary

Other diseases of the pleura (J90-J94)

J90   **Pleural effusion, not elsewhere classified**   CC

Encysted pleurisy
Pleural effusion NOS
Pleurisy with effusion (exudative) (serous)

EXCLUDES 1   *chylous (pleural) effusion (J94.0)*
     malignant pleural effusion (J91.0))
     pleurisy NOS (R09.1)
     tuberculous pleural effusion (A15.6)

RIC Excl: 15 Pulmonary

✓4ᵗʰ J91   **Pleural effusion in conditions classified elsewhere**

EXCLUDES 2   *pleural effusion in heart failure (I50.-)*
     pleural effusion in systemic lupus erythematosus (M32.13)

J91.0   *Malignant pleural effusion*

Code first underlying neoplasm

J91.8   *Pleural effusion in other conditions classified elsewhere*

Code first underlying disease, such as:
filariasis (B74.0-B74.9)
influenza (J09.X2, J10.1, J11.1)

✓4ᵗʰ J92   **Pleural plaque**

INCLUDES   pleural thickening

J92.0   **Pleural plaque** with presence of asbestos

J92.9   **Pleural plaque** without asbestos

Pleural plaque NOS

✓4ᵗʰ J93   **Pneumothorax and air leak**

EXCLUDES 1   *congenital or perinatal pneumothorax (P25.1)*
     postprocedural air leak (J95.812)
     postprocedural pneumothorax (J95.811)
     traumatic pneumothorax (S27.0)
     tuberculous (current disease) pneumothorax (A15.-)
     pyopneumothorax (J86.-)

J93.0   **Spontaneous tension** pneumothorax

✓5ᵗʰ J93.1   **Other spontaneous** pneumothorax

J93.11   **Primary** spontaneous pneumothorax

J93.12   **Secondary** spontaneous pneumothorax

Code first underlying condition, such as:
   catamenial pneumothorax due to endometriosis (N80.8)
   cystic fibrosis (E84.-)
   eosinophilic pneumonia (J82)
   lymphangioleiomyomatosis (J84.81)
   malignant neoplasm of bronchus and lung (C34.-)
   Marfan's syndrome (Q87.4)
   pneumonia due to Pneumocystis carinii (B59)
   secondary malignant neoplasm of lung (C78.0-)
   spontaneous rupture of the esophagus (K22.3)

✓5ᵗʰ J93.8   **Other pneumothorax and** air leak

J93.81   **Chronic** pneumothorax

J93.82   **Other** air leak

Persistent air leak

J93.83   **Other** pneumothorax

Acute pneumothorax
Spontaneous pneumothorax NOS

J93.9   **Pneumothorax, unspecified**   ▽

Pneumothorax NOS

✓4ᵗʰ J94   **Other pleural conditions**

EXCLUDES 1   *pleurisy NOS (R09.1)*
     traumatic hemopneumothorax (S27.2)
     traumatic hemothorax (S27.1)
     tuberculous pleural conditions (current disease) (A15.-)

J94.0   **Chylous effusion**

Chyliform effusion

J94.1   **Fibrothorax**

J94.2   **Hemothorax**   CC

Hemopneumothorax
RIC Excl: 15 Pulmonary

J94.8   **Other specified pleural conditions**

Hydropneumothorax
Hydrothorax

J94.9   **Pleural condition, unspecified**   ▽

---

² Special Care High = With fever

⁸ Clinically Complex = Without fever

Ⓝ Newborn   Ⓟ Pediatric   Ⓜ Maternity   Ⓐ Adult   **RIC** RIC Dx   **NC Dx** Noncancer Dx   **PDx** Primary Dx   **CC** RIC CC Condition   ►◄ Revised Text   ● New Code   ▲ Revised Code Title

634   ICD-10-CM 2016

Intraoperative and postprocedural complications and disorders of respiratory system, not elsewhere classified (J95)

✓4ᵗʰ J95   Intraoperative and postprocedural complications and disorders of respiratory system, not elsewhere classified

> EXCLUDES 2   aspiration pneumonia (J69.-)
> emphysema (subcutaneous) resulting from a procedure (T81.82)
> hypostatic pneumonia (J18.2)
> pulmonary manifestations due to radiation (J70.0- J70.1)

✓5ᵗʰ J95.0   Tracheostomy complications

     J95.00   Unspecified tracheostomy complication   ▽

     J95.01   Hemorrhage from tracheostomy stoma

     J95.02   Infection of tracheostomy stoma
> Use additional code to identify type of infection, such as:
> cellulitis of neck (L03.8)
> sepsis (A40, A41-)

     J95.03   Malfunction of tracheostomy stoma
> Mechanical complication of tracheostomy stoma
> Obstruction of tracheostomy airway
> Tracheal stenosis due to tracheostomy

     J95.04   Tracheo-esophageal fistula following tracheostomy

     J95.09   Other tracheostomy complication

J95.1   Acute pulmonary insufficiency following thoracic surgery   cc
> EXCLUDES 2   functional disturbances following cardiac surgery (I97.0, I97.1-)
> **RIC Excl:** 15 Pulmonary

J95.2   Acute pulmonary insufficiency following nonthoracic surgery   cc
> EXCLUDES 2   functional disturbances following cardiac surgery (I97.0, I97.1-)
> **RIC Excl:** 15 Pulmonary

J95.3   Chronic pulmonary insufficiency following surgery   cc
> EXCLUDES 2   functional disturbances following cardiac surgery (I97.0, I97.1-)
> **RIC Excl:** 15 Pulmonary

J95.4   Chemical pneumonitis due to anesthesia
> Mendelson's syndrome
> Postprocedural aspiration pneumonia
> Use additional code for adverse effect, if applicable, to identify drug (T41.- with fifth or sixth character 5)
> EXCLUDES 1   aspiration pneumonitis due to anesthesia complicating labor and delivery (O74.0)
> aspiration pneumonitis due to anesthesia complicating pregnancy (O29)
> aspiration pneumonitis due to anesthesia complicating the puerperium (O89.01)

J95.5   Postprocedural subglottic stenosis

✓5ᵗʰ J95.6   Intraoperative hemorrhage and hematoma of a respiratory system organ or structure complicating a procedure
> EXCLUDES 1   intraoperative hemorrhage and hematoma of a respiratory system organ or structure due to accidental puncture and laceration during procedure (J95.7-)

     J95.61   Intraoperative hemorrhage and hematoma of a respiratory system organ or structure complicating a respiratory system procedure

     J95.62   Intraoperative hemorrhage and hematoma of a respiratory system organ or structure complicating other procedure

✓5ᵗʰ J95.7   Accidental puncture and laceration of a respiratory system organ or structure during a procedure
> EXCLUDES 2   postprocedural pneumothorax (J95.811)

     J95.71   Accidental puncture and laceration of a respiratory system organ or structure during a respiratory system procedure

     J95.72   Accidental puncture and laceration of a respiratory system organ or structure during other procedure

✓5ᵗʰ J95.8   Other intraoperative and postprocedural complications and disorders of respiratory system, not elsewhere classified

     ✓6ᵗʰ J95.81   Postprocedural pneumothorax and air leak

         J95.811   Postprocedural pneumothorax

         J95.812   Postprocedural air leak

✓6ᵗʰ J95.82   Postprocedural respiratory failure
> EXCLUDES 1   respiratory failure in other conditions (J96.-)

     J95.821   Acute postprocedural respiratory failure   cc
> Postprocedural respiratory failure NOS
> **RIC Excl:** 15 Pulmonary

     J95.822   Acute and chronic postprocedural respiratory failure   cc
> **RIC Excl:** 15 Pulmonary

✓6ᵗʰ J95.83   Postprocedural hemorrhage and hematoma of a respiratory system organ or structure following a procedure

     J95.830   Postprocedural hemorrhage and hematoma of a respiratory system organ or structure following a respiratory system procedure

     J95.831   Postprocedural hemorrhage and hematoma of a respiratory system organ or structure following other procedure

J95.84   Transfusion-related acute lung injury (TRALI)

✓6ᵗʰ J95.85   Complication of respirator [ventilator]

     J95.850   Mechanical complication of respirator
> EXCLUDES 1   encounter for respirator [ventilator] dependence during power failure (Z99.12)

     [2,8] **J95.851   Ventilator associated pneumonia**
> Ventilator associated pneumonitis
> Use additional code to identify the organism, if known (B95.-, B96.-, B97.-)
> EXCLUDES 1   ventilator lung in newborn (P27.8)

     J95.859   Other complication of respirator [ventilator]

J95.88   Other intraoperative complications of respiratory system, not elsewhere classified

J95.89   Other postprocedural complications and disorders of respiratory system, not elsewhere classified
> Use additional code to identify disorder, such as:
> aspiration pneumonia (J69.-)
> bacterial or viral pneumonia (J12-J18)
> EXCLUDES 2   acute pulmonary insufficiency following thoracic surgery (J95.1)
> postprocedural subglottic stenosis (J95.5)

Other diseases of the respiratory system (J96-J99)

✓4ᵗʰ J96   Respiratory failure, not elsewhere classified
> EXCLUDES 1   acute respiratory distress syndrome (J80)
> cardiorespiratory failure (R09.2)
> newborn respiratory distress syndrome (P22.0)
> postprocedural respiratory failure (J95.82-)
> respiratory arrest (R09.2)
> respiratory arrest of newborn (P28.81)
> respiratory failure of newborn (P28.5)

✓5ᵗʰ J96.0   Acute respiratory failure

     [5] **J96.00   Acute respiratory failure, unspecified whether with hypoxia or hypercapnia**   cc
> **AHA:** 2013, 4Q, 121
> **RIC Excl:** 15 Pulmonary

     [5] **J96.01   Acute respiratory failure with hypoxia**   cc
> **RIC Excl:** 15 Pulmonary

     [5] **J96.02   Acute respiratory failure with hypercapnia**   cc
> **RIC Excl:** 15 Pulmonary

✓5ᵗʰ J96.1   Chronic respiratory failure

     [5] **J96.10   Chronic respiratory failure, unspecified whether with hypoxia or hypercapnia**
> **AHA:** 2015, 1Q, 21

     [5] **J96.11   Chronic respiratory failure with hypoxia**
> **AHA:** 2013, 4Q, 129

     [5] **J96.12   Chronic respiratory failure with hypercapnia**

---

[2] Special Care High = With fever

[5] Special Care Low = With oxygen therapy

[8] Clinically Complex = Without fever

Chapter 10. Diseases of the Respiratory System

✓5ᵗʰ **J96.2** Acute and chronic **respiratory failure**
 Acute on chronic respiratory failure

 5 **J96.20** **Acute and chronic respiratory failure, unspecified whether with hypoxia or hypercapnia** CC
  RIC Excl: 15 Pulmonary

 5 **J96.21** **Acute and chronic respiratory failure with hypoxia** CC
  RIC Excl: 15 Pulmonary

 5 **J96.22** **Acute and chronic respiratory failure with hypercapnia** CC
  RIC Excl: 15 Pulmonary

✓5ᵗʰ **J96.9** **Respiratory failure, unspecified**

 5 **J96.90** **Respiratory failure, unspecified, unspecified whether with hypoxia or hypercapnia** CC ▽
  RIC Excl: 15 Pulmonary

 5 **J96.91** **Respiratory failure, unspecified with hypoxia** CC ▽
  RIC Excl: 15 Pulmonary

 5 **J96.92** **Respiratory failure, unspecified with hypercapnia** CC ▽
  RIC Excl: 15 Pulmonary

✓4ᵗʰ **J98** **Other respiratory disorders**
 Use additional code to identify:
  exposure to environmental tobacco smoke (Z77.22)
  exposure to tobacco smoke in the perinatal period (P96.81)
  history of tobacco use (Z87.891)
  occupational exposure to environmental tobacco smoke (Z57.31)
  tobacco dependence (F17.-)
  tobacco use (Z72.0)
  EXCLUDES 1 newborn apnea (P28.4)
   newborn sleep apnea (P28.3)
  EXCLUDES 2 apnea NOS (R06.81)
   sleep apnea (G47.3-)

✓5ᵗʰ **J98.0** **Diseases of bronchus, not elsewhere classified**

 J98.01 **Acute bronchospasm**
  EXCLUDES 1 acute bronchiolitis with bronchospasm (J21.-)
   acute bronchitis with bronchospasm (J20.-)
   asthma (J45.-)
   exercise induced bronchospasm (J45.990)

 J98.09 **Other diseases of bronchus, not elsewhere classified**
  Broncholithiasis
  Calcification of bronchus
  Stenosis of bronchus
  Tracheobronchial collapse
  Tracheobronchial dyskinesia
  Ulcer of bronchus

✓5ᵗʰ **J98.1** **Pulmonary collapse**
 EXCLUDES 1 therapeutic collapse of lung status (Z98.3)

 J98.11 **Atelectasis**
  EXCLUDES 1 newborn atelectasis
   tuberculous atelectasis (current disease) (A15)

 J98.19 **Other pulmonary collapse**

J98.2 **Interstitial emphysema**
 Mediastinal emphysema
 EXCLUDES 1 emphysema NOS (J43.9)
  emphysema in newborn (P25.0)
  surgical emphysema (subcutaneous) (T81.82)
  traumatic subcutaneous emphysema (T79.7)

J98.3 **Compensatory emphysema**

J98.4 **Other disorders of lung**
 Calcification of lung
 Cystic lung disease (acquired)
 Lung disease NOS
 Pulmolithiasis
 EXCLUDES 1 acute interstitial pneumonitis (J84.114)
  pulmonary insufficiency following surgery (J95.1-J95.2)

J98.5 **Diseases of mediastinum, not elsewhere classified** CC
 Fibrosis of mediastinum
 Hernia of mediastinum
 Retraction of mediastinum
 Mediastinitis
 EXCLUDES 2 abscess of mediastinum (J85.3)
 RIC Excl: 15 Pulmonary

J98.6 **Disorders of diaphragm**
 Diaphragmatitis
 Paralysis of diaphragm
 Relaxation of diaphragm
 EXCLUDES 1 congenital malformation of diaphragm NEC (Q79.1)
  congenital diaphragmatic hernia (Q79.0)
 EXCLUDES 2 diaphragmatic hernia (K44.-)

J98.8 **Other specified respiratory disorders**

J98.9 **Respiratory disorder, unspecified** ▽
 Respiratory disease (chronic) NOS

J99 ***Respiratory disorders in diseases classified elsewhere***
 Code first underlying disease, such as:
  amyloidosis (E85.-)
  ankylosing spondylitis (M45)
  congenital syphilis (A50.5)
  cryoglobulinemia (D89.1)
  early congenital syphilis (A50.0)
  schistosomiasis (B65.0-B65.9)
  EXCLUDES 1 *respiratory disorders in:*
   amebiasis (A06.5)
   blastomycosis (B40.0-B40.2)
   candidiasis (B37.1)
   coccidioidomycosis (B38.0-B38.2)
   cystic fibrosis with pulmonary manifestations (E84.0)
   dermatomyositis (M33.01, M33.11)
   histoplasmosis (B39.0-B39.2)
   late syphilis (A52.72, A52.73)
   polymyositis (M33.21)
   sicca syndrome (M35.02)
   systemic lupus erythematosus (M32.13)
   systemic sclerosis (M34.81)
   Wegener's granulomatosis (M31.30-M31.31)

---

⁵ Special Care Low = With oxygen therapy

Chapter 11. Diseases of the Digestive System (K00–K95)

Chapter Specific Coding Guidelines and Examples
Reserved for future guideline expansion.

Chapter 11. Diseases of the Digestive System (K00-K95)

EXCLUDES 2   certain conditions originating in the perinatal period (P04-P96)
certain infectious and parasitic diseases (A00-B99)
complications of pregnancy, childbirth and the puerperium (O00-O9A)
congenital malformations, deformations and chromosomal abnormalities (Q00-Q99)
endocrine, nutritional and metabolic diseases (E00-E88)
injury, poisoning and certain other consequences of external causes (S00-T88)
neoplasms (C00-D49)
symptoms, signs and abnormal clinical and laboratory findings, not elsewhere classified (R00-R94)

This chapter contains the following blocks:

K00-K14   Diseases of oral cavity and salivary glands
K20-K31   Diseases of esophagus, stomach and duodenum
K35-K38   Diseases of appendix
K40-K46   Hernia
K50-K52   Noninfective enteritis and colitis
K55-K64   Other diseases of intestines
K65-K68   Diseases of peritoneum and retroperitoneum
K70-K77   Diseases of liver
K80-K87   Disorders of gallbladder, biliary tract and pancreas
K90-K95   Other diseases of the digestive system

Diseases of oral cavity and salivary glands (K00-K14)

✓4ᵗʰ **K00 Disorders of tooth development and eruption**
EXCLUDES 2   embedded and impacted teeth (K01.-)

K00.0 Anodontia
Hypodontia
Oligodontia
EXCLUDES 1   acquired absence of teeth (K08.1-)

K00.1 Supernumerary teeth
Distomolar
Fourth molar
Mesiodens
Paramolar
Supplementary teeth
EXCLUDES 2   supernumerary roots (K00.2)

K00.2 Abnormalities of size and form of teeth
Concrescence of teeth
Dens evaginatus
Dens in dente
Dens invaginatus
Enamel pearls
Fusion of teeth
Gemination of teeth
Macrodontia
Microdontia
Peg-shaped [conical] teeth
Supernumerary roots
Taurodontism
Tuberculum paramolare
EXCLUDES 1   abnormalities of teeth due to congenital syphilis (A50.5)
tuberculum Carabelli, which is regarded as a normal variation and should not be coded

K00.3 Mottled teeth
Dental fluorosis
Mottling of enamel
Nonfluoride enamel opacities
EXCLUDES 2   deposits [accretions] on teeth (K03.6)

K00.4 Disturbances in tooth formation
Aplasia and hypoplasia of cementum
Dilaceration of tooth
Enamel hypoplasia (neonatal) (postnatal) (prenatal)
Regional odontodysplasia
Turner's tooth
EXCLUDES 1   Hutchinson's teeth and mulberry molars in congenital syphilis (A50.5)
EXCLUDES 2   mottled teeth (K00.3)

K00.5 Hereditary disturbances in tooth structure, not elsewhere classified
Amelogenesis imperfecta
Dentinogenesis imperfecta
Odontogenesis imperfecta
Dentinal dysplasia
Shell teeth

K00.6 Disturbances in tooth eruption
Dentia praecox
Natal tooth
Neonatal tooth
Premature eruption of tooth
Premature shedding of primary [deciduous] tooth
Prenatal teeth
Retained [persistent] primary tooth
EXCLUDES 2   embedded and impacted teeth (K01.-)

K00.7 Teething syndrome

K00.8 Other disorders of tooth development
Color changes during tooth formation
Intrinsic staining of teeth NOS
EXCLUDES 2   posteruptive color changes (K03.7)

K00.9 Disorder of tooth development, unspecified   ▽
Disorder of odontogenesis NOS

✓4ᵗʰ **K01 Embedded and impacted teeth**
EXCLUDES 1   abnormal position of fully erupted teeth (M26.3-)

K01.0 Embedded teeth

K01.1 Impacted teeth

✓4ᵗʰ **K02 Dental caries**
Dental cavities
Tooth decay

K02.3 Arrested dental caries
Arrested coronal and root caries

✓5ᵗʰ **K02.5 Dental caries on pit and fissure surface**
Dental caries on chewing surface of tooth

K02.51 Dental caries on pit and fissure surface limited to enamel
White spot lesions [initial caries] on pit and fissure surface of tooth

K02.52 Dental caries on pit and fissure surface penetrating into dentin

K02.53 Dental caries on pit and fissure surface penetrating into pulp

✓5ᵗʰ **K02.6 Dental caries on smooth surface**

K02.61 Dental caries on smooth surface limited to enamel
White spot lesions [initial caries] on smooth surface of tooth

K02.62 Dental caries on smooth surface penetrating into dentin

K02.63 Dental caries on smooth surface penetrating into pulp

K02.7 Dental root caries

K02.9 Dental caries, unspecified   ▽

✓4ᵗʰ **K03 Other diseases of hard tissues of teeth**
EXCLUDES 2   bruxism (F45.8)
dental caries (K02.-)
teeth-grinding NOS (F45.8)

K03.0 Excessive attrition of teeth
Approximal wear of teeth
Occlusal wear of teeth

K03.1 Abrasion of teeth
Dentifrice abrasion of teeth
Habitual abrasion of teeth
Occupational abrasion of teeth
Ritual abrasion of teeth
Traditional abrasion of teeth
Wedge defect NOS

K03.2 Erosion of teeth
Erosion of teeth due to diet
Erosion of teeth due to drugs and medicaments
Erosion of teeth due to persistent vomiting
Erosion of teeth NOS
Idiopathic erosion of teeth
Occupational erosion of teeth

K03.3 Pathological resorption of teeth
Internal granuloma of pulp
Resorption of teeth (external)

K03.4 Hypercementosis
Cementation hyperplasia

K03.5 Ankylosis of teeth

Ⓝ Newborn   Ⓟ Pediatric   Ⓜ Maternity   Ⓐ Adult   RIC RIC Dx   NCDx Noncancer Dx   PDx Primary Dx   CC RIC CC Condition   ►◄ Revised Text   ● New Code   ▲ Revised Code Title

638   ICD-10-CM 2016

K03.6 Deposits [accretions] on teeth
Betel deposits [accretions] on teeth
Black deposits [accretions] on teeth
Extrinsic staining of teeth NOS
Green deposits [accretions] on teeth
Materia alba deposits [accretions] on teeth
Orange deposits [accretions] on teeth
Staining of teeth NOS
Subgingival dental calculus
Supragingival dental calculus
Tobacco deposits [accretions] on teeth

K03.7 Posteruptive color changes of dental hard tissues
EXCLUDES 2   deposits [accretions] on teeth (K03.6)

✓5th **K03.8 Other specified diseases of hard tissues of teeth**
  K03.81 Cracked tooth
    EXCLUDES 1   asymptomatic craze lines in enamel—omit code
           broken or fractured tooth due to trauma (S02.5)
  K03.89 Other specified diseases of hard tissues of teeth

K03.9 Disease of hard tissues of teeth, unspecified ▽

✓4th **K04 Diseases of pulp and periapical tissues**
K04.0 Pulpitis
Acute pulpitis
Chronic (hyperplastic) (ulcerative) pulpitis
Irreversible pulpitis
Reversible pulpitis

K04.1 Necrosis of pulp
Pulpal gangrene

K04.2 Pulp degeneration
Denticles
Pulpal calcifications
Pulpal stones

K04.3 Abnormal hard tissue formation in pulp
Secondary or irregular dentine

K04.4 Acute apical periodontitis of pulpal origin
Acute apical periodontitis NOS
EXCLUDES 1   acute periodontitis (K05.2-)

K04.5 Chronic apical periodontitis
Apical or periapical granuloma
Apical periodontitis NOS
EXCLUDES 1   chronic periodontitis (K05.3-)

K04.6 Periapical abscess with sinus
Dental abscess with sinus
Dentoalveolar abscess with sinus

K04.7 Periapical abscess without sinus
Dental abscess without sinus
Dentoalveolar abscess without sinus
Periapical abscess without sinus

K04.8 Radicular cyst
Apical (periodontal) cyst
Periapical cyst
Residual radicular cyst
EXCLUDES 2   lateral periodontal cyst (K09.0)

✓5th **K04.9 Other and unspecified diseases of pulp and periapical tissues**
  K04.90 Unspecified diseases of pulp and periapical tissues ▽
  K04.99 Other diseases of pulp and periapical tissues

✓4th **K05 Gingivitis and periodontal diseases**
Use additional code to identify:
alcohol abuse and dependence (F10.-)
exposure to environmental tobacco smoke (Z77.22)
exposure to tobacco smoke in the perinatal period (P96.81)
history of tobacco use (Z87.891)
occupational exposure to environmental tobacco smoke (Z57.31)
tobacco dependence (F17.-)
tobacco use (Z72.0)

✓5th **K05.0 Acute gingivitis**
EXCLUDES 1   acute necrotizing ulcerative gingivitis (A69.1)
           herpesviral [herpes simplex] gingivostomatitis (B00.2)
  K05.00 Acute gingivitis, plaque induced
Acute gingivitis NOS
  K05.01 Acute gingivitis, non-plaque induced

✓5th **K05.1 Chronic gingivitis**
Desquamative gingivitis (chronic)
Gingivitis (chronic) NOS
Hyperplastic gingivitis (chronic)
Simple marginal gingivitis (chronic)
Ulcerative gingivitis (chronic)
  K05.10 Chronic gingivitis, plaque induced
Chronic gingivitis NOS
Gingivitis NOS
  K05.11 Chronic gingivitis, non-plaque induced

✓5th **K05.2 Aggressive periodontitis**
Acute pericoronitis
EXCLUDES 1   acute apical periodontitis (K04.4)
           periapical abscess (K04.7)
           periapical abscess with sinus (K04.6)
  K05.20 Aggressive periodontitis, unspecified ▽
  K05.21 Aggressive periodontitis, localized
Periodontal abscess
  K05.22 Aggressive periodontitis, generalized

✓5th **K05.3 Chronic periodontitis**
Chronic pericoronitis
Complex periodontitis
Periodontitis NOS
Simplex periodontitis
EXCLUDES 1   chronic apical periodontitis (K04.5)
  K05.30 Chronic periodontitis, unspecified ▽
  K05.31 Chronic periodontitis, localized
  K05.32 Chronic periodontitis, generalized

K05.4 Periodontosis
Juvenile periodontosis

K05.5 Other periodontal diseases
EXCLUDES 2   leukoplakia of gingiva (K13.21)

K05.6 Periodontal disease, unspecified ▽

✓4th **K06 Other disorders of gingiva and edentulous alveolar ridge**
EXCLUDES 2   acute gingivitis (K05.0)
           atrophy of edentulous alveolar ridge (K08.2)
           chronic gingivitis (K05.1)
           gingivitis NOS (K05.1)

K06.0 Gingival recession
Gingival recession (generalized) (localized) (postinfective) (postprocedural)

K06.1 Gingival enlargement
Gingival fibromatosis

K06.2 Gingival and edentulous alveolar ridge lesions associated with trauma
Irritative hyperplasia of edentulous ridge [denture hyperplasia]
Use additional code (Chapter 20) to identify external cause or denture status (Z97.2)

K06.8 Other specified disorders of gingiva and edentulous alveolar ridge
Fibrous epulis
Flabby alveolar ridge
Giant cell epulis
Peripheral giant cell granuloma of gingiva
Pyogenic granuloma of gingiva
EXCLUDES 2   gingival cyst (K09.0)

K06.9 Disorder of gingiva and edentulous alveolar ridge, unspecified ▽

✓4th **K08 Other disorders of teeth and supporting structures**
EXCLUDES 2   dentofacial anomalies [including malocclusion] (M26.-)
           disorders of jaw (M27.-)

K08.0 Exfoliation of teeth due to systemic causes
Code also underlying systemic condition

✓5th **K08.1 Complete loss of teeth**
Acquired loss of teeth, complete
EXCLUDES 1   congenital absence of teeth (K00.0)
           exfoliation of teeth due to systemic causes (K08.0)
           partial loss of teeth (K08.4-)
  ✓6th **K08.10 Complete loss of teeth, unspecified cause**
    K08.101 Complete loss of teeth, unspecified cause, class I
    K08.102 Complete loss of teeth, unspecified cause, class II
    K08.103 Complete loss of teeth, unspecified cause, class III
    K08.104 Complete loss of teeth, unspecified cause, class IV

Chapter 11. Diseases of the Digestive System

K08.109   **Complete loss of teeth, unspecified cause, unspecified class** ▽
Edentulism NOS

✓6ᵗʰ **K08.11   Complete loss of teeth** due to trauma
K08.111   **Complete loss of teeth due to trauma, class I**
K08.112   **Complete loss of teeth due to trauma, class II**
K08.113   **Complete loss of teeth due to trauma, class III**
K08.114   **Complete loss of teeth due to trauma, class IV**
K08.119   **Complete loss of teeth due to trauma, unspecified class** ▽

✓6ᵗʰ **K08.12   Complete loss of teeth due to** periodontal diseases
K08.121   **Complete loss of teeth due to periodontal diseases, class I**
K08.122   **Complete loss of teeth due to periodontal diseases, class II**
K08.123   **Complete loss of teeth due to periodontal diseases, class III**
K08.124   **Complete loss of teeth due to periodontal diseases, class IV**
K08.129   **Complete loss of teeth due to periodontal diseases, unspecified class** ▽

✓6ᵗʰ **K08.13   Complete loss of teeth due to** caries
K08.131   **Complete loss of teeth due to caries, class I**
K08.132   **Complete loss of teeth due to caries, class II**
K08.133   **Complete loss of teeth due to caries, class III**
K08.134   **Complete loss of teeth due to caries, class IV**
K08.139   **Complete loss of teeth due to caries, unspecified class** ▽

✓6ᵗʰ **K08.19   Complete loss of teeth due to** other specified **cause**
K08.191   **Complete loss of teeth due to other specified cause, class I**
K08.192   **Complete loss of teeth due to other specified cause, class II**
K08.193   **Complete loss of teeth due to other specified cause, class III**
K08.194   **Complete loss of teeth due to other specified cause, class IV**
K08.199   **Complete loss of teeth due to other specified cause, unspecified class** ▽

✓5ᵗʰ **K08.2   Atrophy of edentulous alveolar ridge**
K08.20   **Unspecified atrophy of edentulous alveolar ridge** ▽
Atrophy of the mandible NOS
Atrophy of the maxilla NOS
K08.21   **Minimal atrophy of the** mandible
Minimal atrophy of the edentulous mandible
K08.22   **Moderate atrophy of the** mandible
Moderate atrophy of the edentulous mandible
K08.23   **Severe atrophy of the** mandible
Severe atrophy of the edentulous mandible
K08.24   **Minimal atrophy of** maxilla
Minimal atrophy of the edentulous maxilla
K08.25   **Moderate atrophy of the** maxilla
Moderate atrophy of the edentulous maxilla
K08.26   **Severe atrophy of the** maxilla
Severe atrophy of the edentulous maxilla

K08.3   **Retained dental root**

✓5ᵗʰ **K08.4   Partial loss of teeth**
Acquired loss of teeth, partial
EXCLUDES 1   complete loss of teeth (K08.1-)
congenital absence of teeth (K00.0)
EXCLUDES 2   exfoliation of teeth due to systemic causes (K08.0)

✓6ᵗʰ **K08.40   Partial loss of teeth,** unspecified cause
K08.401   **Partial loss of teeth, unspecified cause, class I**
K08.402   **Partial loss of teeth, unspecified cause, class II**
K08.403   **Partial loss of teeth, unspecified cause, class III**
K08.404   **Partial loss of teeth, unspecified cause, class IV**

K08.409   **Partial loss of teeth, unspecified cause, unspecified class** ▽
Tooth extraction status NOS

✓6ᵗʰ **K08.41   Partial loss of teeth due to** trauma
K08.411   **Partial loss of teeth due to trauma,** class I
K08.412   **Partial loss of teeth due to trauma,** class II
K08.413   **Partial loss of teeth due to trauma,** class III
K08.414   **Partial loss of teeth due to trauma,** class IV
K08.419   **Partial loss of teeth due to trauma, unspecified class** ▽

✓6ᵗʰ **K08.42   Partial loss of teeth due to** periodontal diseases
K08.421   **Partial loss of teeth due to periodontal diseases,** class I
K08.422   **Partial loss of teeth due to periodontal diseases,** class II
K08.423   **Partial loss of teeth due to periodontal diseases,** class III
K08.424   **Partial loss of teeth due to periodontal diseases,** class IV
K08.429   **Partial loss of teeth due to periodontal diseases, unspecified class** ▽

✓6ᵗʰ **K08.43   Partial loss of teeth due to** caries
K08.431   **Partial loss of teeth due to caries,** class I
K08.432   **Partial loss of teeth due to caries,** class II
K08.433   **Partial loss of teeth due to caries,** class III
K08.434   **Partial loss of teeth due to caries,** class IV
K08.439   **Partial loss of teeth due to caries, unspecified class** ▽

✓6ᵗʰ **K08.49   Partial loss of teeth due to** other specified cause
K08.491   **Partial loss of teeth due to other specified cause,** class I
K08.492   **Partial loss of teeth due to other specified cause,** class II
K08.493   **Partial loss of teeth due to other specified cause,** class III
K08.494   **Partial loss of teeth due to other specified cause,** class IV
K08.499   **Partial loss of teeth due to other specified cause, unspecified class** ▽

✓5ᵗʰ **K08.5   Unsatisfactory restoration of tooth**
Defective bridge, crown, filling
Defective dental restoration
EXCLUDES 1   dental restoration status (Z98.811)
EXCLUDES 2   endosseous dental implant failure (M27.6-)
unsatisfactory endodontic treatment (M27.5-)

K08.50   **Unsatisfactory restoration of tooth, unspecified** ▽
Defective dental restoration NOS

K08.51   **Open restoration margins of tooth**
Dental restoration failure of marginal integrity
Open margin on tooth restoration
Poor gingival margin to tooth restoration

K08.52   **Unrepairable overhanging of dental restorative materials**
Overhanging of tooth restoration

✓6ᵗʰ **K08.53   Fractured dental restorative material**
EXCLUDES 1   cracked tooth (K03.81)
traumatic fracture of tooth (S02.5)
K08.530   **Fractured dental restorative material** without loss of material
K08.531   **Fractured dental restorative material** with loss of material
K08.539   **Fractured dental restorative material, unspecified** ▽

K08.54   **Contour of existing restoration of tooth biologically incompatible with oral health**
Dental restoration failure of periodontal anatomical integrity
Unacceptable contours of existing restoration of tooth
Unacceptable morphology of existing restoration of tooth

K08.55   **Allergy to existing dental restorative material**
Use additional code to identify the specific type of allergy

K08.56   **Poor aesthetic of existing restoration of tooth**
Dental restoration aesthetically inadequate or displeasing

K08.59   **Other unsatisfactory restoration of tooth**
Other defective dental restoration

K08.8 Other specified disorders of teeth and supporting structures
Enlargement of alveolar ridge NOS
Irregular alveolar process
Toothache NOS

K08.9 Disorder of teeth and supporting structures, unspecified ▽

✓4ᵗʰ **K09 Cysts of oral region, not elsewhere classified**
INCLUDES lesions showing histological features both of aneurysmal cyst and of another fibro-osseous lesion
EXCLUDES 2 *cysts of jaw (M27.0-, M27.4-)*
radicular cyst (K04.8)

K09.0 Developmental odontogenic cysts
Dentigerous cyst
Eruption cyst
Follicular cyst
Gingival cyst
Lateral periodontal cyst
Primordial cyst
EXCLUDES 2 *keratocysts (D16.4, D16.5)*
odontogenic keratocystic tumors (D16.4, D16.5)

K09.1 Developmental (nonodontogenic) cysts of oral region
Cyst (of) incisive canal
Cyst (of) palatine of papilla
Globulomaxillary cyst
Median palatal cyst
Nasoalveolar cyst
Nasolabial cyst
Nasopalatine duct cyst

K09.8 Other cysts of oral region, not elsewhere classified
Dermoid cyst
Epidermoid cyst
Lymphoepithelial cyst
Epstein's pearl

K09.9 Cyst of oral region, unspecified ▽

✓4ᵗʰ **K11 Diseases of salivary glands**
Use additional code to identify:
alcohol abuse and dependence (F10.-)
exposure to environmental tobacco smoke (Z77.22)
exposure to tobacco smoke in the perinatal period (P96.81)
history of tobacco use (Z87.891)
occupational exposure to environmental tobacco smoke (Z57.31)
tobacco dependence (F17.-)
tobacco use (Z72.0)

K11.0 Atrophy of salivary gland

K11.1 Hypertrophy of salivary gland

✓5ᵗʰ **K11.2 Sialoadenitis**
Parotitis
EXCLUDES 1 *epidemic parotitis (B26.-)*
mumps (B26.-)
uveoparotid fever [Heerfordt] (D86.89)

K11.20 Sialoadenitis, unspecified ▽

K11.21 Acute sialoadenitis
EXCLUDES 1 *acute recurrent sialoadenitis (K11.22)*

K11.22 Acute recurrent sialoadenitis

K11.23 Chronic sialoadenitis

K11.3 Abscess of salivary gland

K11.4 Fistula of salivary gland
EXCLUDES 1 *congenital fistula of salivary gland (Q38.4)*

K11.5 Sialolithiasis
Calculus of salivary gland or duct
Stone of salivary gland or duct

K11.6 Mucocele of salivary gland
Mucous extravasation cyst of salivary gland
Mucous retention cyst of salivary gland
Ranula

K11.7 Disturbances of salivary secretion
Hypoptyalism
Ptyalism
Xerostomia
EXCLUDES 2 *dry mouth NOS (R68.2)*

K11.8 Other diseases of salivary glands
Benign lymphoepithelial lesion of salivary gland
Mikulicz' disease
Necrotizing sialometaplasia
Sialectasia
Stenosis of salivary duct
Stricture of salivary duct
EXCLUDES 1 *sicca syndrome [Sjögren] (M35.0-)*

K11.9 Disease of salivary gland, unspecified ▽
Sialoadenopathy NOS

✓4ᵗʰ **K12 Stomatitis and related lesions**
Use additional code to identify:
alcohol abuse and dependence (F10.-)
exposure to environmental tobacco smoke (Z77.22)
exposure to tobacco smoke in the perinatal period (P96.81)
history of tobacco use (Z87.891)
occupational exposure to environmental tobacco smoke (Z57.31)
tobacco dependence (F17.-)
tobacco use (Z72.0)
EXCLUDES 1 *cancrum oris (A69.0)*
cheilitis (K13.0)
gangrenous stomatitis (A69.0)
herpesviral [herpes simplex] gingivostomatitis (B00.2)
noma (A69.0)

K12.0 Recurrent oral aphthae
Aphthous stomatitis (major) (minor)
Bednar's aphthae
Periadenitis mucosa necrotica recurrens
Recurrent aphthous ulcer
Stomatitis herpetiformis

K12.1 Other forms of stomatitis
Stomatitis NOS   Ulcerative stomatitis
Denture stomatitis   Vesicular stomatitis
EXCLUDES 1 *acute necrotizing ulcerative stomatitis (A69.1)*
Vincent's stomatitis (A69.1)

K12.2 Cellulitis and abscess of mouth   CC
Cellulitis of mouth (floor)
Submandibular abscess
EXCLUDES 2 *abscess of salivary gland (K11.3)*
abscess of tongue (K14.0)
periapical abscess (K04.6-K04.7)
periodontal abscess (K05.21)
peritonsillar abscess (J36)

✓5ᵗʰ **K12.3 Oral mucositis (ulcerative)**
Mucositis (oral) (oropharyneal)
EXCLUDES 2 *gastrointestinal mucositis (ulcerative) (K92.81)*
mucositis (ulcerative) of vagina and vulva (N76.81)
nasal mucositis (ulcerative) (J34.81)

K12.30 Oral mucositis (ulcerative), unspecified ▽

K12.31 Oral mucositis (ulcerative) due to antineoplastic therapy
Use additional code for adverse effect, if applicable, to identify antineoplastic and immunosuppressive drugs (T45.1X5)
Use additional code for other antineoplastic therapy, such as:
radiological procedure and radiotherapy (Y84.2)

K12.32 Oral mucositis (ulcerative) due to other drugs
Use additional code for adverse effect, if applicable, to identify drug (T36-T50 with fifth or sixth character 5)

K12.33 Oral mucositis (ulcerative) due to radiation
Use additional external cause code (W88-W90, X39.0-) to identify cause

K12.39 Other oral mucositis (ulcerative)
Viral oral mucositis (ulcerative)

☑4ᵗʰ K13 Other diseases of lip and oral mucosa

INCLUDES epithelial disturbances of tongue

Use additional code to identify:
alcohol abuse and dependence (F10.-)
exposure to environmental tobacco smoke (Z77.22)
exposure to tobacco smoke in the perinatal period (P96.81)
history of tobacco use (Z87.891)
occupational exposure to environmental tobacco smoke (Z57.31)
tobacco dependence (F17.-)
tobacco use (Z72.0)

EXCLUDES 2 certain disorders of gingiva and edentulous alveolar ridge
(K05-K06)
cysts of oral region (K09.-)
diseases of tongue (K14.-)
stomatitis and related lesions (K12.-)

K13.0 Diseases of lips
Abscess of lips
Angular cheilitis
Cellulitis of lips
Cheilitis NOS
Cheilodynia
Cheilosis
Exfoliative cheilitis
Fistula of lips
Glandular cheilitis
Hypertrophy of lips
Perlèche NEC

EXCLUDES 1 ariboflavinosis (E53.0)
cheilitis due to radiation-related disorders (L55-L59)
congenital fistula of lips (Q38.0)
congenital hypertrophy of lips (Q18.6)
Perlèche due to candidiasis (B37.83)
Perlèche due to riboflavin deficiency (E53.0)

K13.1 Cheek and lip biting

☑5ᵗʰ K13.2 Leukoplakia and other disturbances of oral epithelium, including tongue

EXCLUDES 1 carcinoma in situ of oral epithelium (D00.0-)
hairy leukoplakia (K13.3)

K13.21 Leukoplakia of oral mucosa, including tongue
Leukokeratosis of oral mucosa
Leukoplakia of gingiva, lips, tongue

EXCLUDES 1 hairy leukoplakia (K13.3)
leukokeratosis nicotina palati (K13.24)

K13.22 Minimal keratinized residual ridge mucosa
Minimal keratinization of alveolar ridge mucosa

K13.23 Excessive keratinized residual ridge mucosa
Excessive keratinization of alveolar ridge mucosa

K13.24 Leukokeratosis nicotina palati
Smoker's palate

K13.29 Other disturbances of oral epithelium, including tongue
Erythroplakia of mouth or tongue
Focal epithelial hyperplasia of mouth or tongue
Leukoedema of mouth or tongue
Other oral epithelium disturbances

K13.3 Hairy leukoplakia

K13.4 Granuloma and granuloma-like lesions of oral mucosa
Eosinophilic granuloma   Verrucous xanthoma
Granuloma pyogenicum

K13.5 Oral submucous fibrosis
Submucous fibrosis of tongue

K13.6 Irritative hyperplasia of oral mucosa

EXCLUDES 2 irritative hyperplasia of edentulous ridge [denture
hyperplasia] (K06.2)

☑5ᵗʰ K13.7 Other and unspecified lesions of oral mucosa

K13.70 Unspecified lesions of oral mucosa ▽

K13.79 Other lesions of oral mucosa
Focal oral mucinosis

☑4ᵗʰ K14 Diseases of tongue

Use additional code to identify:
alcohol abuse and dependence (F10.-)
exposure to environmental tobacco smoke (Z77.22)
history of tobacco use (Z87.891)
occupational exposure to environmental tobacco smoke (Z57.31)
tobacco dependence (F17.-)
tobacco use (Z72.0)

EXCLUDES 2 erythroplakia (K13.29)
focal epithelial hyperplasia (K13.29)
leukedema of tongue (K13.29)
leukoplakia of tongue (K13.21)
hairy leukoplakia (K13.3)
macroglossia (congenital) (Q38.2)
submucous fibrosis of tongue (K13.5)

K14.0 Glossitis
Abscess of tongue   Ulceration (traumatic) of tongue

EXCLUDES 1 atrophic glossitis (K14.4)

K14.1 Geographic tongue
Benign migratory glossitis
Glossitis areata exfoliativa

K14.2 Median rhomboid glossitis

K14.3 Hypertrophy of tongue papillae
Black hairy tongue
Coated tongue
Hypertrophy of foliate papillae
Lingua villosa nigra

K14.4 Atrophy of tongue papillae
Atrophic glossitis

K14.5 Plicated tongue
Fissured tongue
Furrowed tongue
Scrotal tongue

EXCLUDES 1 fissured tongue, congenital (Q38.3)

K14.6 Glossodynia
Glossopyrosis
Painful tongue

K14.8 Other diseases of tongue
Atrophy of tongue
Crenated tongue
Enlargement of tongue
Glossocele
Glossoptosis
Hypertrophy of tongue

K14.9 Disease of tongue, unspecified ▽
Glossopathy NOS

Diseases of esophagus, stomach and duodenum (K20-K31)

EXCLUDES 2 hiatus hernia (K44.-)

☑4ᵗʰ K20 Esophagitis

Use additional code to identify:
alcohol abuse and dependence (F10.-)

EXCLUDES 1 erosion of esophagus (K22.1-)
esophagitis with gastro-esophageal reflux disease (K21.0)
reflux esophagitis (K21.0)
ulcerative esophagitis (K22.1-)

EXCLUDES 2 eosinophilic gastritis or gastroenteritis (K52.81)

K20.0 Eosinophilic esophagitis

K20.8 Other esophagitis
Abscess of esophagus

K20.9 Esophagitis, unspecified ▽
Esophagitis NOS

☑4ᵗʰ K21 Gastro-esophageal reflux disease

EXCLUDES 1 newborn esophageal reflux (P78.83)

K21.0 Gastro-esophageal reflux disease with esophagitis
Reflux esophagitis

K21.9 Gastro-esophageal reflux disease without esophagitis
Esophageal reflux NOS

☑4ᵗʰ K22 Other diseases of esophagus

EXCLUDES 2 esophageal varices (I85.-)

K22.0 Achalasia of cardia
Achalasia NOS
Cardiospasm

EXCLUDES 1 congenital cardiospasm (Q39.5)

N Newborn   P Pediatric   M Maternity   A Adult   RIC RIC Dx   NCDx Noncancer Dx   PDx Primary Dx   CC RIC CC Condition   ►◄ Revised Text   ● New Code   ▲ Revised Code Title

642   ICD-10-CM 2016

Chapter 11. Diseases of the Digestive System

√5th K22.1 Ulcer of esophagus
Barrett's ulcer
Erosion of esophagus
Fungal ulcer of esophagus
Peptic ulcer of esophagus
Ulcer of esophagus due to ingestion of chemicals
Ulcer of esophagus due to ingestion of drugs and medicaments
Ulcerative esophagitis
Code first poisoning due to drug or toxin, if applicable (T36-T65 with fifth or sixth character 1-4 or 6)
Use additional code for adverse effect, if applicable, to identify drug (T36-T50 with fifth or sixth character 5)
EXCLUDES1 Barrett's esophagus (K22.7-)

    K22.10 Ulcer of esophagus without bleeding
Ulcer of esophagus NOS

    K22.11 Ulcer of esophagus with bleeding
EXCLUDES2 bleeding esophageal varices (I85.01, I85.11)

K22.2 Esophageal obstruction
Compression of esophagus
Constriction of esophagus
Stenosis of esophagus
Stricture of esophagus
EXCLUDES1 congenital stenosis or stricture of esophagus (Q39.3)

K22.3 Perforation of esophagus   cc
Rupture of esophagus
EXCLUDES1 traumatic perforation of (thoracic) esophagus (S27.8-)

K22.4 Dyskinesia of esophagus
Corkscrew esophagus
Diffuse esophageal spasm
Spasm of esophagus
EXCLUDES1 cardiospasm (K22.0)

K22.5 Diverticulum of esophagus, acquired
Esophageal pouch, acquired
EXCLUDES1 diverticulum of esophagus (congenital) (Q39.6)

K22.6 Gastro-esophageal laceration-hemorrhage syndrome
Mallory-Weiss syndrome

√5th K22.7 Barrett's esophagus
Barrett's disease
Barrett's syndrome
EXCLUDES1 Barrett's ulcer (K22.1)
malignant neoplasm of esophagus (C15.-)

    K22.70 Barrett's esophagus without dysplasia
Barrett's esophagus NOS

    √6th K22.71 Barrett's esophagus with dysplasia
        K22.710 Barrett's esophagus with low grade dysplasia
        K22.711 Barrett's esophagus with high grade dysplasia
        K22.719 Barrett's esophagus with dysplasia, unspecified   ▽

K22.8 Other specified diseases of esophagus   cc
Hemorrhage of esophagus NOS
EXCLUDES2 esophageal varices (I85.-)
Paterson-Kelly syndrome (D50.1)
RIC Excl: 15 Pulmonary

K22.9 Disease of esophagus, unspecified   ▽

K23 Disorders of esophagus in diseases classified elsewhere
Code first underlying disease, such as:
congenital syphilis (A50.5)
EXCLUDES1 late syphilis (A52.79)
megaesophagus due to Chagas' disease (B57.31)
tuberculosis (A18.83)

√4th K25 Gastric ulcer
INCLUDES   erosion (acute) of stomach
pylorus ulcer (peptic)
stomach ulcer (peptic)
Use additional code to identify:
alcohol abuse and dependence (F10.-)
EXCLUDES1 acute gastritis (K29.0-)
peptic ulcer NOS (K27.-)

K25.0 Acute gastric ulcer with hemorrhage   cc
K25.1 Acute gastric ulcer with perforation   cc
K25.2 Acute gastric ulcer with both hemorrhage and perforation   cc
K25.3 Acute gastric ulcer without hemorrhage or perforation
K25.4 Chronic or unspecified gastric ulcer with hemorrhage   cc
K25.5 Chronic or unspecified gastric ulcer with perforation   cc

K25.6 Chronic or unspecified gastric ulcer with both hemorrhage and perforation   cc
K25.7 Chronic gastric ulcer without hemorrhage or perforation
K25.9 Gastric ulcer, unspecified as acute or chronic, without hemorrhage or perforation   ▽

√4th K26 Duodenal ulcer
INCLUDES   erosion (acute) of duodenum
duodenum ulcer (peptic)
postpyloric ulcer (peptic)
Use additional code to identify:
alcohol abuse and dependence (F10.-)
EXCLUDES1 peptic ulcer NOS (K27.-)

K26.0 Acute duodenal ulcer with hemorrhage   cc
K26.1 Acute duodenal ulcer with perforation   cc
K26.2 Acute duodenal ulcer with both hemorrhage and perforation   cc
K26.3 Acute duodenal ulcer without hemorrhage or perforation
K26.4 Chronic or unspecified duodenal ulcer with hemorrhage   cc
K26.5 Chronic or unspecified duodenal ulcer with perforation   cc
K26.6 Chronic or unspecified duodenal ulcer with both hemorrhage and perforation   cc
K26.7 Chronic duodenal ulcer without hemorrhage or perforation
K26.9 Duodenal ulcer, unspecified as acute or chronic, without hemorrhage or perforation   ▽

√4th K27 Peptic ulcer, site unspecified
INCLUDES   gastroduodenal ulcer NOS
peptic ulcer NOS
Use additional code to identify:
alcohol abuse and dependence (F10.-)
EXCLUDES1 peptic ulcer of newborn (P78.82)

K27.0 Acute peptic ulcer, site unspecified, with hemorrhage   cc
K27.1 Acute peptic ulcer, site unspecified, with perforation   cc
K27.2 Acute peptic ulcer, site unspecified, with both hemorrhage and perforation   cc
K27.3 Acute peptic ulcer, site unspecified, without hemorrhage or perforation
K27.4 Chronic or unspecified peptic ulcer, site unspecified, with hemorrhage   cc
K27.5 Chronic or unspecified peptic ulcer, site unspecified, with perforation   cc
K27.6 Chronic or unspecified peptic ulcer, site unspecified, with both hemorrhage and perforation   cc
K27.7 Chronic peptic ulcer, site unspecified, without hemorrhage or perforation
K27.9 Peptic ulcer, site unspecified, unspecified as acute or chronic, without hemorrhage or perforation   ▽

√4th K28 Gastrojejunal ulcer
INCLUDES   anastomotic ulcer (peptic) or erosion
gastrocolic ulcer (peptic) or erosion
gastrointestinal ulcer (peptic) or erosion
gastrojejunal ulcer (peptic) or erosion
jejunal ulcer (peptic) or erosion
marginal ulcer (peptic) or erosion
stomal ulcer (peptic) or erosion
Use additional code to identify:
alcohol abuse and dependence (F10.-)
EXCLUDES1 primary ulcer of small intestine (K63.3)

K28.0 Acute gastrojejunal ulcer with hemorrhage   cc
K28.1 Acute gastrojejunal ulcer with perforation   cc
K28.2 Acute gastrojejunal ulcer with both hemorrhage and perforation   cc
K28.3 Acute gastrojejunal ulcer without hemorrhage or perforation
K28.4 Chronic or unspecified gastrojejunal ulcer with hemorrhage   cc
K28.5 Chronic or unspecified gastrojejunal ulcer with perforation   cc
K28.6 Chronic or unspecified gastrojejunal ulcer with both hemorrhage and perforation   cc
K28.7 Chronic gastrojejunal ulcer without hemorrhage or perforation
K28.9 Gastrojejunal ulcer, unspecified as acute or chronic, without hemorrhage or perforation   ▽

☑ Add'l Character Required   √x7th Placeholder Alert   RUG IV Special Care High Dx   RUG IV Clinically Complex Dx   RUG IV Special Care Low Dx   Manifestation Code   Other Specified Code   ▽ Unspecified Code

Chapter 11. Diseases of the Digestive System

K29–K38.9

✓4th K29 Gastritis and duodenitis
EXCLUDES 1   *eosinophilic gastritis or gastroenteritis (K52.81)*
      Zollinger-Ellison syndrome (E16.4)

✓5th **K29.0 Acute gastritis**
    Use additional code to identify:
      alcohol abuse and dependence (F10.-)
    EXCLUDES 1   *erosion (acute) of stomach (K25.-)*

    K29.00 Acute gastritis without bleeding
    K29.01 Acute gastritis with bleeding   CC

✓5th **K29.2 Alcoholic gastritis**
    Use additional code to identify:
      alcohol abuse and dependence (F10.-)

    K29.20 Alcoholic gastritis without bleeding
    K29.21 Alcoholic gastritis with bleeding   CC

✓5th **K29.3 Chronic superficial gastritis**
    K29.30 Chronic superficial gastritis without bleeding
    K29.31 Chronic superficial gastritis with bleeding   CC

✓5th **K29.4 Chronic atrophic gastritis**
    Gastric atrophy
    K29.40 Chronic atrophic gastritis without bleeding
    K29.41 Chronic atrophic gastritis with bleeding   CC

✓5th **K29.5 Unspecified chronic gastritis**
    Chronic antral gastritis
    Chronic fundal gastritis
    K29.50 Unspecified chronic gastritis without bleeding   ▽
    K29.51 Unspecified chronic gastritis with bleeding   CC ▽

✓5th **K29.6 Other gastritis**
    Giant hypertrophic gastritis
    Granulomatous gastritis
    Ménétrier's disease
    K29.60 Other gastritis without bleeding
    K29.61 Other gastritis with bleeding   CC

✓5th **K29.7 Gastritis, unspecified**
    K29.70 Gastritis, unspecified, without bleeding   ▽
    K29.71 Gastritis, unspecified, with bleeding   CC ▽

✓5th **K29.8 Duodenitis**
    K29.80 Duodenitis without bleeding
    K29.81 Duodenitis with bleeding   CC

✓5th **K29.9 Gastroduodenitis, unspecified**
    K29.90 Gastroduodenitis, unspecified, without bleeding   ▽
    K29.91 Gastroduodenitis, unspecified, with bleeding   CC ▽

K30 Functional dyspepsia
Indigestion
EXCLUDES 1   *dyspepsia NOS (R10.13)*
      heartburn (R12)
      nervous dyspepsia (F45.8)
      neurotic dyspepsia (F45.8)
      psychogenic dyspepsia (F45.8)

✓4th K31 Other diseases of stomach and duodenum
INCLUDES   functional disorders of stomach
EXCLUDES 2   *diabetic gastroparesis (E08.43, E09.43, E10.43, E11.43, E13.43)*
      diverticulum of duodenum (K57.00-K57.13)

K31.0 Acute dilatation of stomach
    Acute distention of stomach

K31.1 Adult hypertrophic pyloric stenosis   A
    Pyloric stenosis NOS
    EXCLUDES 1   *congenital or infantile pyloric stenosis (Q40.0)*

K31.2 Hourglass stricture and stenosis of stomach
    EXCLUDES 1   *congenital hourglass stomach (Q40.2)*
      hourglass contraction of stomach (K31.89)

K31.3 Pylorospasm, not elsewhere classified
    EXCLUDES 1   *congenital or infantile pylorospasm (Q40.0)*
      neurotic pylorospasm (F45.8)
      psychogenic pylorospasm (F45.8)

K31.4 Gastric diverticulum
    EXCLUDES 1   *congenital diverticulum of stomach (Q40.2)*

K31.5 Obstruction of duodenum
    Constriction of duodenum
    Duodenal ileus (chronic)
    Stenosis of duodenum
    Stricture of duodenum
    Volvulus of duodenum
    EXCLUDES 1   *congenital stenosis of duodenum (Q41.0)*

K31.6 Fistula of stomach and duodenum   CC
    Gastrocolic fistula
    Gastrojejunocolic fistula

K31.7 Polyp of stomach and duodenum
    EXCLUDES 1   *adenomatous polyp of stomach (D13.1)*

✓5th **K31.8 Other specified diseases of stomach and duodenum**
    ✓6th **K31.81 Angiodysplasia of stomach and duodenum**
      K31.811 Angiodysplasia of stomach and duodenum with bleeding   CC
      K31.819 Angiodysplasia of stomach and duodenum without bleeding
        Angiodysplasia of stomach and duodenum NOS

    K31.82 Dieulafoy lesion (hemorrhagic) of stomach and duodenum   CC
      EXCLUDES 2   *Dieulafoy lesion of intestine (K63.81)*

    K31.83 Achlorhydria

    K31.84 Gastroparesis
      Gastroparalysis
      Code first underlying disease, if known, such as:
        anorexia nervosa (F50.0-)
        diabetes mellitus (E08.43, E09.43, E10.43, E11.43, E13.43)
        scleroderma (M34.-)
      AHA: 2013, 4Q, 114

    K31.89 Other diseases of stomach and duodenum

K31.9 Disease of stomach and duodenum, unspecified   ▽

Diseases of appendix (K35-K38)

✓4th K35 Acute appendicitis
K35.2 Acute appendicitis with generalized peritonitis   CC
    Appendicitis (acute) with generalized (diffuse) peritonitis following rupture or perforation of appendix
    Perforated appendix NOS
    Ruptured appendix NOS

K35.3 Acute appendicitis with localized peritonitis
    Acute appendicitis with or without perforation or rupture NOS
    Acute appendicitis with or without perforation or rupture with localized peritonitis
    Acute appendicitis with peritoneal abscess

✓5th **K35.8 Other and unspecified acute appendicitis**
    K35.80 Unspecified acute appendicitis   ▽
      Acute appendicitis NOS
      Acute appendicitis without (localized) (generalized) peritonitis

    K35.89 Other acute appendicitis

K36 Other appendicitis
Chronic appendicitis
Recurrent appendicitis

K37 Unspecified appendicitis   ▽
EXCLUDES 1   *unspecified appendicitis with peritonitis (K35.2-K35.3)*

✓4th K38 Other diseases of appendix
K38.0 Hyperplasia of appendix

K38.1 Appendicular concretions
    Fecalith of appendix
    Stercolith of appendix

K38.2 Diverticulum of appendix

K38.3 Fistula of appendix

K38.8 Other specified diseases of appendix
    Intussusception of appendix

K38.9 Disease of appendix, unspecified   ▽

N Newborn   P Pediatric   M Maternity   A Adult   RIC RIC Dx   NC Dx Noncancer Dx   PDx Primary Dx   CC RIC CC Condition   ►◄ Revised Text   ● New Code   ▲ Revised Code Title

644   ICD-10-CM 2016

Hernia (K40-K46)

NOTE   Hernia with both gangrene and obstruction is classified to hernia with gangrene.

INCLUDES   acquired hernia
congenital [except diaphragmatic or hiatus] hernia
recurrent hernia

✓4ᵗʰ **K40**   **Inguinal hernia**
    INCLUDES   bubonocele
            direct inguinal hernia
            double inguinal hernia
            indirect inguinal hernia
            inguinal hernia NOS
            oblique inguinal hernia
            scrotal hernia

✓5ᵗʰ **K40.0**   **Bilateral inguinal hernia, with obstruction, without gangrene**
    Inguinal hernia (bilateral) causing obstruction without gangrene
    Incarcerated inguinal hernia (bilateral) without gangrene
    Irreducible inguinal hernia (bilateral) without gangrene
    Strangulated inguinal hernia (bilateral) without gangrene

    K40.00   **Bilateral inguinal hernia, with obstruction, without gangrene, not specified as recurrent**
       Bilateral inguinal hernia, with obstruction, without gangrene NOS

    K40.01   **Bilateral inguinal hernia, with obstruction, without gangrene, recurrent**

✓5ᵗʰ **K40.1**   **Bilateral inguinal hernia, with gangrene**
    K40.10   **Bilateral inguinal hernia, with gangrene, not specified as recurrent**
       Bilateral inguinal hernia, with gangrene NOS

    K40.11   **Bilateral inguinal hernia, with gangrene, recurrent**

✓5ᵗʰ **K40.2**   **Bilateral inguinal hernia, without obstruction or gangrene**
    K40.20   **Bilateral inguinal hernia, without obstruction or gangrene, not specified as recurrent**
       Bilateral inguinal hernia NOS

    K40.21   **Bilateral inguinal hernia, without obstruction or gangrene, recurrent**

✓5ᵗʰ **K40.3**   **Unilateral inguinal hernia, with obstruction, without gangrene**
    Inguinal hernia (unilateral) causing obstruction without gangrene
    Incarcerated inguinal hernia (unilateral) without gangrene
    Irreducible inguinal hernia (unilateral) without gangrene
    Strangulated inguinal hernia (unilateral) without gangrene

    K40.30   **Unilateral inguinal hernia, with obstruction, without gangrene, not specified as recurrent**
       Inguinal hernia, with obstruction NOS
       Unilateral inguinal hernia, with obstruction, without gangrene NOS

    K40.31   **Unilateral inguinal hernia, with obstruction, without gangrene, recurrent**

✓5ᵗʰ **K40.4**   **Unilateral inguinal hernia, with gangrene**
    K40.40   **Unilateral inguinal hernia, with gangrene, not specified as recurrent**
       Inguinal hernia with gangrene NOS
       Unilateral inguinal hernia with gangrene NOS

    K40.41   **Unilateral inguinal hernia, with gangrene, recurrent**

✓5ᵗʰ **K40.9**   **Unilateral inguinal hernia, without obstruction or gangrene**
    K40.90   **Unilateral inguinal hernia, without obstruction or gangrene, not specified as recurrent**
       Inguinal hernia NOS
       Unilateral inguinal hernia NOS

    K40.91   **Unilateral inguinal hernia, without obstruction or gangrene, recurrent**

✓4ᵗʰ **K41**   **Femoral hernia**

✓5ᵗʰ **K41.0**   **Bilateral femoral hernia, with obstruction, without gangrene**
    Femoral hernia (bilateral) causing obstruction, without gangrene
    Incarcerated femoral hernia (bilateral), without gangrene
    Irreducible femoral hernia (bilateral), without gangrene
    Strangulated femoral hernia (bilateral), without gangrene

    K41.00   **Bilateral femoral hernia, with obstruction, without gangrene, not specified as recurrent**
       Bilateral femoral hernia, with obstruction, without gangrene NOS

    K41.01   **Bilateral femoral hernia, with obstruction, without gangrene, recurrent**

✓5ᵗʰ **K41.1**   **Bilateral femoral hernia, with gangrene**
    K41.10   **Bilateral femoral hernia, with gangrene, not specified as recurrent**
       Bilateral femoral hernia, with gangrene NOS

    K41.11   **Bilateral femoral hernia, with gangrene, recurrent**

✓5ᵗʰ **K41.2**   **Bilateral femoral hernia, without obstruction or gangrene**
    K41.20   **Bilateral femoral hernia, without obstruction or gangrene, not specified as recurrent**
       Bilateral femoral hernia NOS

    K41.21   **Bilateral femoral hernia, without obstruction or gangrene, recurrent**

✓5ᵗʰ **K41.3**   **Unilateral femoral hernia, with obstruction, without gangrene**
    Femoral hernia (unilateral) causing obstruction, without gangrene
    Incarcerated femoral hernia (unilateral), without gangrene
    Irreducible femoral hernia (unilateral), without gangrene
    Strangulated femoral hernia (unilateral), without gangrene

    K41.30   **Unilateral femoral hernia, with obstruction, without gangrene, not specified as recurrent**
       Femoral hernia, with obstruction NOS
       Unilateral femoral hernia, with obstruction NOS

    K41.31   **Unilateral femoral hernia, with obstruction, without gangrene, recurrent**

✓5ᵗʰ **K41.4**   **Unilateral femoral hernia, with gangrene**
    K41.40   **Unilateral femoral hernia, with gangrene, not specified as recurrent**
       Femoral hernia, with gangrene NOS
       Unilateral femoral hernia, with gangrene NOS

    K41.41   **Unilateral femoral hernia, with gangrene, recurrent**

✓5ᵗʰ **K41.9**   **Unilateral femoral hernia, without obstruction or gangrene**
    K41.90   **Unilateral femoral hernia, without obstruction or gangrene, not specified as recurrent**
       Femoral hernia NOS
       Unilateral femoral hernia NOS

    K41.91   **Unilateral femoral hernia, without obstruction or gangrene, recurrent**

✓4ᵗʰ **K42**   **Umbilical hernia**
    INCLUDES   paraumbilical hernia
    EXCLUDES 1   omphalocele (Q79.2)

    K42.0   **Umbilical hernia with obstruction, without gangrene**
       Umbilical hernia causing obstruction, without gangrene
       Incarcerated umbilical hernia, without gangrene
       Irreducible umbilical hernia, without gangrene
       Strangulated umbilical hernia, without gangrene

    K42.1   **Umbilical hernia with gangrene**
       Gangrenous umbilical hernia

    K42.9   **Umbilical hernia without obstruction or gangrene**
       Umbilical hernia NOS

✓4ᵗʰ **K43**   **Ventral hernia**

    K43.0   **Incisional hernia with obstruction, without gangrene**
       Incisional hernia causing obstruction, without gangrene
       Incarcerated incisional hernia, without gangrene
       Irreducible incisional hernia, without gangrene
       Strangulated incisional hernia, without gangrene

    K43.1   **Incisional hernia with gangrene**
       Gangrenous incisional hernia

    K43.2   **Incisional hernia without obstruction or gangrene**
       Incisional hernia NOS

    K43.3   **Parastomal hernia with obstruction, without gangrene**
       Incarcerated parastomal hernia, without gangrene
       Irreducible parastomal hernia, without gangrene
       Parastomal hernia causing obstruction, without gangrene
       Strangulated parastomal hernia, without gangrene

    K43.4   **Parastomal hernia with gangrene**
       Gangrenous parastomal hernia

    K43.5   **Parastomal hernia without obstruction or gangrene**
       Parastomal hernia NOS

Chapter 11. Diseases of the Digestive System (side margin)

K43.6 **Other and unspecified ventral hernia with obstruction, without gangrene** ▽
  Epigastric hernia causing obstruction, without gangrene
  Hypogastric hernia causing obstruction, without gangrene
  Incarcerated epigastric hernia without gangrene
  Incarcerated hypogastric hernia without gangrene
  Incarcerated midline hernia without gangrene
  Incarcerated spigelian hernia without gangrene
  Incarcerated subxiphoid hernia without gangrene
  irreducible epigastric hernia without gangrene
  Irreducible hypogastric hernia without gangrene
  Irreducible midline hernia without gangrene
  Irreducible spigelian hernia without gangrene
  Irreducible subxiphoid hernia without gangrene
  Midline hernia causing obstruction, without gangrene
  Spigelian hernia causing obstruction, without gangrene
  Strangulated epigastric hernia without gangrene ·
  Strangulated hypogastric hernia without gangrene
  Strangulated midline hernia without gangrene
  Strangulated spigelian hernia without gangrene
  Strangulated subxiphoid hernia without gangrene
  Subxiphoid hernia causing obstruction, without gangrene

K43.7 **Other and unspecified ventral hernia with gangrene** ▽
  Any condition listed under K43.6 specified as gangrenous

K43.9 **Ventral hernia without obstruction or gangrene** ▽
  Epigastric hernia
  Ventral hernia NOS

✓4ᵗʰ **K44** **Diaphragmatic hernia**
  INCLUDES hiatus hernia (esophageal) (sliding)
    paraesophageal hernia
  EXCLUDES 1 congenital diaphragmatic hernia (Q79.0)
    congenital hiatus hernia (Q40.1)

K44.0 **Diaphragmatic hernia with obstruction, without gangrene**
  Diaphragmatic hernia causing obstruction
  Incarcerated diaphragmatic hernia
  Irreducible diaphragmatic hernia
  Strangulated diaphragmatic hernia

K44.1 **Diaphragmatic hernia with gangrene**
  Gangrenous diaphragmatic hernia

K44.9 **Diaphragmatic hernia without obstruction or gangrene**
  Diaphragmatic hernia NOS

✓4ᵗʰ **K45** **Other abdominal hernia**
  INCLUDES abdominal hernia, specified site NEC
    lumbar hernia
    obturator hernia
    pudendal hernia
    retroperitoneal hernia
    sciatic hernia

K45.0 **Other specified abdominal hernia with obstruction, without gangrene**
  Other specified abdominal hernia causing obstruction
  Other specified incarcerated abdominal hernia
  Other specified irreducible abdominal hernia
  Other specified strangulated abdominal hernia

K45.1 **Other specified abdominal hernia with gangrene**
  Any condition listed under K45 specified as gangrenous

K45.8 **Other specified abdominal hernia without obstruction or gangrene**

✓4ᵗʰ **K46** **Unspecified abdominal hernia**
  INCLUDES enterocele
    epiplocele
    hernia NOS
    interstitial hernia
    intestinal hernia
    intra-abdominal hernia
  EXCLUDES 1 vaginal enterocele (N81.5)

K46.0 **Unspecified abdominal hernia with obstruction, without gangrene** ▽
  Unspecified abdominal hernia causing obstruction
  Unspecified incarcerated abdominal hernia
  Unspecified irreducible abdominal hernia
  Unspecified strangulated abdominal hernia

K46.1 **Unspecified abdominal hernia with gangrene** ▽
  Any condition listed under K46 specified as gangrenous

K46.9 **Unspecified abdominal hernia without obstruction or gangrene** ▽
  Abdominal hernia NOS

Noninfective enteritis and colitis (K50-K52)

INCLUDES noninfective inflammatory bowel disease
EXCLUDES 1 irritable bowel syndrome (K58.-)
  megacolon (K59.3)

✓4ᵗʰ **K50** **Crohn's disease [regional enteritis]**
  INCLUDES granulomatous enteritis
  Use additional code to identify manifestations, such as:
    pyoderma gangrenosum (L88)
  EXCLUDES 1 ulcerative colitis (K51.-)
  AHA: 2012, 4Q, 104

✓5ᵗʰ **K50.0** **Crohn's disease of small intestine**
  Crohn's disease [regional enteritis] of duodenum
  Crohn's disease [regional enteritis] of ileum
  Crohn's disease [regional enteritis] of jejunum
  Regional ileitis
  Terminal ileitis
  EXCLUDES 1 Crohn's disease of both small and large intestine (K50.8-)

  K50.00 **Crohn's disease of small intestine without complications**

  ✓6ᵗʰ **K50.01** **Crohn's disease of small intestine with complications**
    K50.011 **Crohn's disease of small intestine with rectal bleeding**
    K50.012 **Crohn's disease of small intestine with intestinal obstruction**
    K50.013 **Crohn's disease of small intestine with fistula**
    K50.014 **Crohn's disease of small intestine with abscess**
      AHA: 2012, 4Q, 104
    K50.018 **Crohn's disease of small intestine with other complication**
    K50.019 **Crohn's disease of small intestine with unspecified complications** ▽

✓5ᵗʰ **K50.1** **Crohn's disease of large intestine**
  Crohn's disease [regional enteritis] of colon
  Crohn's disease [regional enteritis] of large bowel
  Crohn's disease [regional enteritis] of rectum
  Granulomatous colitis
  Regional colitis
  EXCLUDES 1 Crohn's disease of both small and large intestine (K50.8)

  K50.10 **Crohn's disease of large intestine without complications**

  ✓6ᵗʰ **K50.11** **Crohn's disease of large intestine with complications**
    K50.111 **Crohn's disease of large intestine with rectal bleeding**
    K50.112 **Crohn's disease of large intestine with intestinal obstruction**
    K50.113 **Crohn's disease of large intestine with fistula**
    K50.114 **Crohn's disease of large intestine with abscess**
    K50.118 **Crohn's disease of large intestine with other complication**
    K50.119 **Crohn's disease of large intestine with unspecified complications** ▽

✓5ᵗʰ **K50.8** **Crohn's disease of both small and large intestine**
  K50.80 **Crohn's disease of both small and large intestine without complications**

  ✓6ᵗʰ **K50.81** **Crohn's disease of both small and large intestine with complications**
    K50.811 **Crohn's disease of both small and large intestine with rectal bleeding**
    K50.812 **Crohn's disease of both small and large intestine with intestinal obstruction**
    K50.813 **Crohn's disease of both small and large intestine with fistula**
    K50.814 **Crohn's disease of both small and large intestine with abscess**
    K50.818 **Crohn's disease of both small and large intestine with other complication**
    K50.819 **Crohn's disease of both small and large intestine with unspecified complications** ▽

N Newborn P Pediatric M Maternity A Adult RIC RIC Dx NCDx Noncancer Dx PDx Primary Dx CC RIC CC Condition ►◄ Revised Text ● New Code ▲ Revised Code Title

646   ICD-10-CM 2016

K43.6–K50.819 (side margin)

✓5th **K50.9** **Crohn's disease,** unspecified

     K50.90 **Crohn's disease, unspecified,** without complications
         Crohn's disease NOS
         Regional enteritis NOS

     ✓6th **K50.91** **Crohn's disease, unspecified,** with complications

         K50.911 **Crohn's disease, unspecified, with** rectal bleeding

         K50.912 **Crohn's disease, unspecified, with** intestinal obstruction

         K50.913 **Crohn's disease, unspecified, with** fistula

         K50.914 **Crohn's disease, unspecified, with** abscess

         K50.918 **Crohn's disease, unspecified, with other complication**

         K50.919 **Crohn's disease, unspecified, with unspecified complications** ▽

✓4th **K51** **Ulcerative colitis**

     Use additional code to identify manifestations, such as: pyoderma gangrenosum (L88)
     EXCLUDES 1 *Crohn's disease [regional enteritis] (K50.-)*

     ✓5th **K51.0** **Ulcerative (chronic)** pancolitis
         Backwash ileitis

         K51.00 **Ulcerative (chronic) pancolitis** without complications
             Ulcerative (chronic) pancolitis NOS

         ✓6th **K51.01** **Ulcerative (chronic) pancolitis** with complications

             K51.011 **Ulcerative (chronic) pancolitis with** rectal bleeding

             K51.012 **Ulcerative (chronic) pancolitis with** intestinal obstruction

             K51.013 **Ulcerative (chronic) pancolitis with** fistula

             K51.014 **Ulcerative (chronic) pancolitis with abscess**

             K51.018 **Ulcerative (chronic) pancolitis with other complication**

             K51.019 **Ulcerative (chronic) pancolitis with unspecified complications** ▽

     ✓5th **K51.2** **Ulcerative (chronic)** proctitis

         K51.20 **Ulcerative (chronic) proctitis** without complications
             Ulcerative (chronic) proctitis NOS

         ✓6th **K51.21** **Ulcerative (chronic) proctitis** with complications

             K51.211 **Ulcerative (chronic) proctitis with** rectal bleeding

             K51.212 **Ulcerative (chronic) proctitis with** intestinal obstruction

             K51.213 **Ulcerative (chronic) proctitis with** fistula

             K51.214 **Ulcerative (chronic) proctitis with** abscess

             K51.218 **Ulcerative (chronic) proctitis with other complication**

             K51.219 **Ulcerative (chronic) proctitis with unspecified complications** ▽

     ✓5th **K51.3** **Ulcerative (chronic)** rectosigmoiditis

         K51.30 **Ulcerative (chronic) rectosigmoiditis** without complications
             Ulcerative (chronic) rectosigmoiditis NOS

         ✓6th **K51.31** **Ulcerative (chronic) rectosigmoiditis** with complications

             K51.311 **Ulcerative (chronic) rectosigmoiditis with** rectal bleeding

             K51.312 **Ulcerative (chronic) rectosigmoiditis with** intestinal obstruction

             K51.313 **Ulcerative (chronic) rectosigmoiditis with** fistula

             K51.314 **Ulcerative (chronic) rectosigmoiditis with** abscess

             K51.318 **Ulcerative (chronic) rectosigmoiditis with other complication**

             K51.319 **Ulcerative (chronic) rectosigmoiditis with unspecified complications** ▽

     ✓5th **K51.4** **Inflammatory polyps of colon**
         EXCLUDES 1 *adenomatous polyp of colon (D12.6)*
                   polyposis of colon (D12.6)
                   polyps of colon NOS (K63.5)

         K51.40 **Inflammatory polyps of colon** without complications
             Inflammatory polyps of colon NOS

     ✓6th **K51.41** **Inflammatory polyps of colon** with complications

         K51.411 **Inflammatory polyps of colon with** rectal bleeding

         K51.412 **Inflammatory polyps of colon with** intestinal obstruction

         K51.413 **Inflammatory polyps of colon with** fistula

         K51.414 **Inflammatory polyps of colon with** abscess

         K51.418 **Inflammatory polyps of colon with other complication**

         K51.419 **Inflammatory polyps of colon with unspecified complications** ▽

     ✓5th **K51.5** **Left sided colitis**
         Left hemicolitis

         K51.50 **Left sided colitis** without complications
             Left sided colitis NOS

     ✓6th **K51.51** **Left sided colitis** with complications

         K51.511 **Left sided colitis with** rectal bleeding

         K51.512 **Left sided colitis with** intestinal obstruction

         K51.513 **Left sided colitis with** fistula

         K51.514 **Left sided colitis with** abscess

         K51.518 **Left sided colitis with other complication**

         K51.519 **Left sided colitis with unspecified complications** ▽

     ✓5th **K51.8** **Other ulcerative colitis**

         K51.80 **Other ulcerative colitis** without complications

     ✓6th **K51.81** **Other ulcerative colitis** with complications

         K51.811 **Other ulcerative colitis with** rectal bleeding

         K51.812 **Other ulcerative colitis with** intestinal obstruction

         K51.813 **Other ulcerative colitis with** fistula

         K51.814 **Other ulcerative colitis with** abscess

         K51.818 **Other ulcerative colitis with other complication**

         K51.819 **Other ulcerative colitis with unspecified complications** ▽

     ✓5th **K51.9** **Ulcerative colitis, unspecified**

         K51.90 **Ulcerative colitis, unspecified,** without complications

     ✓6th **K51.91** **Ulcerative colitis, unspecified,** with complications

         K51.911 **Ulcerative colitis, unspecified with** rectal bleeding

         K51.912 **Ulcerative colitis, unspecified with** intestinal obstruction

         K51.913 **Ulcerative colitis, unspecified with** fistula

         K51.914 **Ulcerative colitis, unspecified with** abscess

         K51.918 **Ulcerative colitis, unspecified with other complication**

         K51.919 **Ulcerative colitis, unspecified with unspecified complications** ▽

✓4th **K52** **Other and unspecified noninfective gastroenteritis and colitis**

     K52.0 **Gastroenteritis and colitis due to** radiation

     K52.1 **Toxic** **gastroenteritis and colitis**
         Drug-induced gastroenteritis and colitis
         Code first (T51-T65) to identify toxic agent
         Use additional code for adverse effect, if applicable, to identify drug (T36-T50 with fifth or sixth character 5)

     K52.2 **Allergic and dietetic** **gastroenteritis and colitis**
         Food hypersensitivity gastroenteritis or colitis
         Use additional code to identify type of food allergy (Z91.01-, Z91.02-)

     ✓5th **K52.8** **Other specified noninfective gastroenteritis and colitis**

         K52.81 **Eosinophilic gastritis or gastroenteritis**   CC
             Eosinophilic enteritis
             EXCLUDES 1 *eosinophilic esophagitis (K20.0)*

         K52.82 **Eosinophilic colitis**

         K52.89 **Other specified noninfective gastroenteritis and colitis**
             Collagenous colitis
             Lymphocytic colitis
             Microscopic colitis (collagenous or lymphocytic)

☑ Add'l Character Required   ✓x7th Placeholder Alert   RUG IV Special Care High Dx   RUG IV Clinically Complex Dx   RUG IV Special Care Low Dx   Manifestation Code   Other Specified Code   ▽ Unspecified Code

ICD-10-CM 2016   647

K52.9 Noninfective gastroenteritis and colitis, unspecified ▽

    Colitis NOS   Ileitis NOS

    Enteritis NOS   Jejunitis NOS

    Gastroenteritis NOS   Sigmoiditis NOS

    EXCLUDES 1   *diarrhea NOS (R19.7)*

                 functional diarrhea (K59.1)

                 infectious gastroenteritis and colitis NOS (A09)

                 neonatal diarrhea (noninfective) (P78.3)

                 psychogenic diarrhea (F45.8)

Other diseases of intestines (K55-K64)

✓4ᵗʰ K55 Vascular disorders of intestine

    EXCLUDES 1   *necrotizing enterocolitis of newborn (P77.-)*

K55.0 Acute vascular disorders of intestine   CC

    Acute fulminant ischemic colitis

    Acute intestinal infarction

    Acute small intestine ischemia

    Infarction of appendices epiploicae

    Mesenteric (artery) (vein) embolism

    Mesenteric (artery) (vein) infarction

    Mesenteric (artery) (vein) thrombosis

    Necrosis of intestine

    Subacute ischemic colitis

K55.1 Chronic vascular disorders of intestine

    Chronic ischemic colitis   Mesenteric atherosclerosis

    Chronic ischemic enteritis   Mesenteric vascular

    Chronic ischemic enterocolitis   insufficiency

    Ischemic stricture of intestine

✓5ᵗʰ K55.2 Angiodysplasia of colon

    K55.20 Angiodysplasia of colon without hemorrhage

    K55.21 Angiodysplasia of colon with hemorrhage   CC

K55.8 Other vascular disorders of intestine

K55.9 Vascular disorder of intestine, unspecified ▽

    Ischemic colitis

    Ischemic enteritis

    Ischemic enterocolitis

✓4ᵗʰ K56 Paralytic ileus and intestinal obstruction without hernia

    EXCLUDES 1   *congenital stricture or stenosis of intestine (Q41-Q42)*

                 cystic fibrosis with meconium ileus (E84.11)

                 intestinal obstruction with hernia (K40-K46)

                 ischemic stricture of intestine (K55.1)

                 meconium ileus NOS (P76.0)

                 neonatal intestinal obstructions classifiable to P76-

                 obstruction of duodenum (K31.5)

                 postprocedural intestinal obstruction (K91.3)

                 stenosis of anus or rectum (K62.4)

K56.0 Paralytic ileus

    Paralysis of bowel

    Paralysis of colon

    Paralysis of intestine

    EXCLUDES 1   *gallstone ileus (K56.3)*

                 ileus NOS (K56.7)

                 obstructive ileus NOS (K56.69)

K56.1 Intussusception

    Intussusception or invagination of bowel

    Intussusception or invagination of colon

    Intussusception or invagination of intestine

    Intussusception or invagination of rectum

    EXCLUDES 2   *intussusception of appendix (K38.8)*

K56.2 Volvulus

    Strangulation of colon or intestine

    Torsion of colon or intestine

    Twist of colon or intestine

    EXCLUDES 2   *volvulus of duodenum (K31.5)*

K56.3 Gallstone ileus

    Obstruction of intestine by gallstone

✓5ᵗʰ K56.4 Other impaction of intestine

    K56.41 Fecal impaction

        EXCLUDES 1   *constipation (K59.0-)*

                  incomplete defecation (R15.0)

    K56.49 Other impaction of intestine

K56.5 Intestinal adhesions [bands] with obstruction (postprocedural) (postinfection)

    Abdominal hernia due to adhesions with obstruction

    Peritoneal adhesions [bands] with intestinal obstruction

       (postprocedural) (postinfection)

✓5ᵗʰ K56.6 Other and unspecified intestinal obstruction

    K56.60 Unspecified intestinal obstruction ▽

        Intestinal obstruction NOS

        EXCLUDES 1   *intestinal obstruction due to specified*

                  condition—code to condition

    K56.69 Other intestinal obstruction

        Enterostenosis NOS

        Obstructive ileus NOS

        Occlusion of colon or intestine NOS

        Stenosis of colon or intestine NOS

        Stricture of colon or intestine NOS

        EXCLUDES 1   *intestinal obstruction due to specified*

                  condition—code to condition

K56.7 Ileus, unspecified ▽

    EXCLUDES 1   *obstructive ileus (K56.69)*

✓4ᵗʰ K57 Diverticular disease of intestine

    EXCLUDES 1   *congenital diverticulum of intestine (Q43.8)*

                 Meckel's diverticulum (Q43.0)

    EXCLUDES 2   *diverticulum of appendix (K38.2)*

✓5ᵗʰ K57.0 Diverticulitis of small intestine with perforation and abscess

    Diverticulitis of small intestine with peritonitis

    EXCLUDES 1   *diverticulitis of both small and large intestine with*

                 perforation and abscess (K57.4-)

    K57.00 Diverticulitis of small intestine with perforation and abscess without bleeding

    K57.01 Diverticulitis of small intestine with perforation and abscess with bleeding   CC

✓5ᵗʰ K57.1 Diverticular disease of small intestine without perforation or abscess

    EXCLUDES 1   *diverticular disease of both small and large intestine*

                 without perforation or abscess (K57.5-)

    K57.10 Diverticulosis of small intestine without perforation or abscess without bleeding

        Diverticular disease of small intestine NOS

    K57.11 Diverticulosis of small intestine without perforation or abscess with bleeding   CC

    K57.12 Diverticulitis of small intestine without perforation or abscess without bleeding

    K57.13 Diverticulitis of small intestine without perforation or abscess with bleeding   CC

✓5ᵗʰ K57.2 Diverticulitis of large intestine with perforation and abscess

    Diverticulitis of colon with peritonitis

    EXCLUDES 1   *diverticulitis of both small and large intestine with*

                 perforation and abscess (K57.4-)

    K57.20 Diverticulitis of large intestine with perforation and abscess without bleeding

    K57.21 Diverticulitis of large intestine with perforation and abscess with bleeding   CC

✓5ᵗʰ K57.3 Diverticular disease of large intestine without perforation or abscess

    EXCLUDES 1   *diverticular disease of both small and large intestine*

                 without perforation or abscess (K57.5-)

    K57.30 Diverticulosis of large intestine without perforation or abscess without bleeding

        Diverticular disease of colon NOS

    K57.31 Diverticulosis of large intestine without perforation or abscess with bleeding   CC

    K57.32 Diverticulitis of large intestine without perforation or abscess without bleeding

    K57.33 Diverticulitis of large intestine without perforation or abscess with bleeding   CC

✓5ᵗʰ K57.4 Diverticulitis of both small and large intestine with perforation and abscess

    Diverticulitis of both small and large intestine with peritonitis

    K57.40 Diverticulitis of both small and large intestine with perforation and abscess without bleeding

    K57.41 Diverticulitis of both small and large intestine with perforation and abscess with bleeding   CC

✓5ᵗʰ K57.5 Diverticular disease of both small and large intestine without perforation or abscess

    K57.50 Diverticulosis of both small and large intestine without perforation or abscess without bleeding

        Diverticular disease of both small and large intestine NOS

    K57.51 Diverticulosis of both small and large intestine without perforation or abscess with bleeding   CC

    K57.52 Diverticulitis of both small and large intestine without perforation or abscess without bleeding

N Newborn   P Pediatric   M Maternity   A Adult   RIC RIC Dx   NC Dx Noncancer Dx   PDx Primary Dx   CC RIC CC Condition   ►◄ Revised Text   ● New Code   ▲ Revised Code Title

648   ICD-10-CM 2016

K57.53   Diverticulitis **of both small and large intestine** **without perforation or abscess** with bleeding   `CC`

✓5ᵗʰ **K57.8**   **Diverticulitis of intestine,** part unspecified, with perforation and abscess
    Diverticulitis of intestine NOS with peritonitis

K57.80   **Diverticulitis of intestine, part unspecified, with perforation and abscess** without bleeding   ▽

K57.81   **Diverticulitis of intestine, part unspecified, with perforation and abscess** with bleeding   `CC` ▽

✓5ᵗʰ **K57.9**   **Diverticular disease of intestine,** part unspecified, without perforation or abscess

K57.90   **Diverticulosis of intestine, part unspecified, without perforation or abscess** without bleeding   ▽
    Diverticular disease of intestine NOS

K57.91   **Diverticulosis of intestine, part unspecified, without perforation or abscess** with bleeding   `CC` ▽

K57.92   **Diverticulitis of intestine, part unspecified, without perforation or abscess** without bleeding   ▽

K57.93   **Diverticulitis of intestine, part unspecified, without perforation or abscess** with bleeding   `CC` ▽

✓4ᵗʰ **K58**   **Irritable bowel syndrome**
   `INCLUDES`   irritable colon
          spastic colon

K58.0   **Irritable bowel syndrome** with diarrhea

K58.9   **Irritable bowel syndrome** without diarrhea
    Irritable bowel syndrome NOS

✓4ᵗʰ **K59**   **Other functional intestinal disorders**
   `EXCLUDES 1`   change in bowel habit NOS (R19.4)
          intestinal malabsorption (K90.-)
          psychogenic intestinal disorders (F45.8)
   `EXCLUDES 2`   functional disorders of stomach (K31.-)

✓5ᵗʰ **K59.0**   **Constipation**
   `EXCLUDES 1`   fecal impaction (K56.41)
          incomplete defecation (R15.0)

K59.00   **Constipation, unspecified**   ▽

K59.01   **Slow transit constipation**

K59.02   **Outlet dysfunction constipation**

K59.09   **Other constipation**

K59.1   **Functional diarrhea**
   `EXCLUDES 1`   diarrhea NOS (R19.7)
          irritable bowel syndrome with diarrhea (K58.0)

K59.2   **Neurogenic bowel, not elsewhere classified**

K59.3   **Megacolon, not elsewhere classified**
    Dilatation of colon
    Toxic megacolon
    Code first (T51-T65) to identify toxic agent
   `EXCLUDES 1`   congenital megacolon (aganglionic) (Q43.1)
          megacolon (due to) (in) Chagas' disease (B57.32)
          megacolon (due to) (in) Clostridium difficile (A04.7)
          megacolon (due to) (in) Hirschsprung's disease (Q43.1)

K59.4   **Anal spasm**
    Proctalgia fugax

K59.8   **Other specified functional intestinal disorders**
    Atony of colon
    Pseudo-obstruction (acute) (chronic) of intestine

K59.9   **Functional intestinal disorder, unspecified**   ▽

✓4ᵗʰ **K60**   **Fissure and fistula of anal and rectal regions**
   `EXCLUDES 1`   fissure and fistula of anal and rectal regions with abscess or cellulitis (K61.-)
   `EXCLUDES 2`   anal sphincter tear (healed) (nontraumatic) (old) (K62.81)

K60.0   **Acute anal fissure**

K60.1   **Chronic anal fissure**

K60.2   **Anal fissure, unspecified**   ▽

K60.3   **Anal fistula**

K60.4   **Rectal fistula**
    Fistula of rectum to skin
   `EXCLUDES 1`   rectovaginal fistula (N82.3)
          vesicorectal fistual (N32.1)

K60.5   **Anorectal fistula**

✓4ᵗʰ **K61**   **Abscess of anal and rectal regions**
   `INCLUDES`   abscess of anal and rectal regions
          cellulitis of anal and rectal regions

K61.0   **Anal abscess**
    Perianal abscess
   `EXCLUDES 1`   intrasphincteric abscess (K61.4)

K61.1   **Rectal abscess**
    Perirectal abscess
   `EXCLUDES 1`   ischiorectal abscess (K61.3)
    AHA: 2012, 4Q, 104

K61.2   **Anorectal abscess**

K61.3   **Ischiorectal abscess**
    Abscess of ischiorectal fossa

K61.4   **Intrasphincteric abscess**

✓4ᵗʰ **K62**   **Other diseases of anus and rectum**
   `INCLUDES`   anal canal
   `EXCLUDES 2`   colostomy and enterostomy malfunction (K94.0-, K94.1-)
          fecal incontinence (R15.-)
          hemorrhoids (K64.-)

K62.0   **Anal polyp**

K62.1   **Rectal polyp**
   `EXCLUDES 1`   adenomatous polyp (D12.8)

K62.2   **Anal prolapse**
    Prolapse of anal canal

K62.3   **Rectal prolapse**
    Prolapse of rectal mucosa

K62.4   **Stenosis of anus and rectum**
    Stricture of anus (sphincter)

K62.5   **Hemorrhage of anus and rectum**
   `EXCLUDES 1`   gastrointestinal bleeding NOS (K92.2)
          melena (K92.1)
          neonatal rectal hemorrhage (P54.2)

K62.6   **Ulcer of anus and rectum**
    Solitary ulcer of anus and rectum
    Stercoral ulcer of anus and rectum
   `EXCLUDES 1`   fissure and fistula of anus and rectum (K60.-)
          ulcerative colitis (K51.-)

K62.7   **Radiation proctitis**
    Use additional code to identify the type of radiation (W90.-)

✓5ᵗʰ **K62.8**   **Other specified diseases of anus and rectum**
   `EXCLUDES 2`   ulcerative proctitis (K51.2)

K62.81   **Anal sphincter tear (healed) (nontraumatic) (old)**
    Tear of anus, nontraumatic
    Use additional code for any associated fecal incontinence (R15.-)
   `EXCLUDES 2`   anal fissure (K60.-)
          anal sphincter tear (healed) (old) complicating delivery (O34.7-)
          traumatic tear of anal sphincter (S31.831)

K62.82   **Dysplasia of anus**
    Anal intraepithelial neoplasia I and II (AIN I and II) (histologically confirmed)
    Dysplasia of anus NOS
    Mild and moderate dysplasia of anus (histologically confirmed)
   `EXCLUDES 1`   abnormal results from anal cytologic examination without histologic confirmation (R85.61-)
          anal intraepithelial neoplasia III (D01.3)
          carcinoma in situ of anus (D01.3)
          HGSIL of anus (R85.613)
          severe dysplasia of anus (D01.3)

K62.89   **Other specified diseases of anus and rectum**
    Proctitis NOS
    Use additional code for any associated fecal incontinence (R15.-)

K62.9   **Disease of anus and rectum, unspecified**   ▽

✓4ᵗʰ **K63**   **Other diseases of intestine**

K63.0   **Abscess of intestine**
   `EXCLUDES 1`   abscess of intestine with Crohn's disease (K50.014, K50.114, K50.814, K50.914)
          abscess of intestine with diverticular disease (K57.0, K57.2, K57.4, K57.8)
          abscess of intestine with ulcerative colitis (K51.014, K51.214, K51.314, K51.414, K51.514, K51.814, K51.914)
   `EXCLUDES 2`   abscess of anal and rectal regions (K61.-)
          abscess of appendix (K35.3)

K63.1   **Perforation of intestine (nontraumatic)**   `CC`
    Perforation (nontraumatic) of rectum
   `EXCLUDES 1`   perforation (nontraumatic) of duodenum (K26.-)
          perforation (nontraumatic) of intestine with diverticular disease (K57.0, K57.2, K57.4, K57.8)
   `EXCLUDES 2`   perforation (nontraumatic) of appendix (K35.2, K35.3)

Chapter 11. Diseases of the Digestive System

K63.2 Fistula of intestine
> EXCLUDES 1 fistula of duodenum (K31.6)
> fistula of intestine with Crohn's disease (K50.013, K50.113, K50.813, K50.913)
> fistula of intestine with ulcerative colitis (K51.013, K51.213, K51.313, K51.413, K51.513, K51.813, K51.913)

> EXCLUDES 2 fistula of anal and rectal regions (K60.-)
> fistula of appendix (K38.3)
> intestinal-genital fistula, female (N82.2-N82.4)
> vesicointestinal fistula (N32.1)

K63.3 Ulcer of intestine
Primary ulcer of small intestine
> EXCLUDES 1 duodenal ulcer (K26.-)
> gastrointestinal ulcer (K28.-)
> gastrojejunal ulcer (K28.-)
> jejunal ulcer (K28.-)
> peptic ulcer, site unspecified (K27.-)
> ulcer of intestine with perforation (K63.1)
> ulcer of anus or rectum (K62.6)
> ulcerative colitis (K51.-)

K63.4 Enteroptosis

K63.5 Polyp of colon
> EXCLUDES 1 adenomatous polyp of colon (D12.6)
> inflammatory polyp of colon (K51.4-)
> polyposis of colon (D12.6)

✓5ᵗʰ K63.8 Other specified diseases of intestine

K63.81 Dieulafoy lesion of intestine
> EXCLUDES 2 Dieulafoy lesion of stomach and duodenum (K31.82)

K63.89 Other specified diseases of intestine
AHA: 2013, 2Q, 31

K63.9 Disease of intestine, unspecified ▽

✓4ᵗʰ K64 Hemorrhoids and perianal venous thrombosis
> INCLUDES piles
> EXCLUDES 1 hemorrhoids complicating childbirth and the puerperium (O87.2)
> hemorrhoids complicating pregnancy (O22.4)

K64.0 First degree hemorrhoids
Grade/stage I hemorrhoids
Hemorrhoids (bleeding) without prolapse outside of anal canal

K64.1 Second degree hemorrhoids
Grade/stage II hemorrhoids
Hemorrhoids (bleeding) that prolapse with straining, but retract spontaneously

K64.2 Third degree hemorrhoids
Grade/stage III hemorrhoids
Hemorrhoids (bleeding) that prolapse with straining and require manual replacement back inside anal canal

K64.3 Fourth degree hemorrhoids
Grade/stage IV hemorrhoids
Hemorrhoids (bleeding) with prolapsed tissue that cannot be manually replaced

K64.4 Residual hemorrhoidal skin tags
External hemorrhoids, NOS
Skin tags of anus

K64.5 Perianal venous thrombosis
External hemorrhoids with thrombosis
Perianal hematoma
Thrombosed hemorrhoids NOS

K64.8 Other hemorrhoids
Internal hemorrhoids, without mention of degree
Prolapsed hemorrhoids, degree not specified

K64.9 Unspecified hemorrhoids ▽
Hemorrhoids (bleeding) NOS
Hemorrhoids (bleeding) without mention of degree

Diseases of peritoneum and retroperitoneum (K65-K68)

✓4ᵗʰ K65 Peritonitis
Use additional code (B95-B97), to identify infectious agent
> EXCLUDES 1 acute appendicitis with generalized peritonitis (K35.2)
> aseptic peritonitis (T81.6)
> benign paroxysmal peritonitis (E85.0)
> chemical peritonitis (T81.6)
> diverticulitis of both small and large intestine with peritonitis (K57.4-)
> diverticulitis of colon with peritonitis (K57.2-)
> diverticulitis of intestine, NOS, with peritonitis (K57.8-)
> diverticulitis of small intestine with peritonitis (K57.0-)
> gonococcal peritonitis (A54.85)
> neonatal peritonitis (P78.0-P78.1)
> pelvic peritonitis, female (N73.3-N73.5)
> periodic familial peritonitis (E85.0)
> peritonitis due to talc or other foreign substance (T81.6)
> peritonitis in chlamydia (A74.81)
> peritonitis in diphtheria (A36.89)
> peritonitis in syphilis (late) (A52.74)
> peritonitis in tuberculosis (A18.31)
> peritonitis with or following abortion or ectopic or molar pregnancy (O00-O07, O08.0)
> peritonitis with or following appendicitis (K35.-)
> peritonitis with or following diverticular disease of intestine (K57.-)
> puerperal peritonitis (O85)
> retroperitoneal infections (K68.-)

K65.0 Generalized (acute) peritonitis CC
Pelvic peritonitis (acute), male
Subphrenic peritonitis (acute)
Suppurative peritonitis (acute)

K65.1 Peritoneal abscess CC
Abdominopelvic abscess   Subdiaphragmatic abscess
Abscess (of) omentum   Subhepatic abscess
Abscess (of) peritoneum   Subphrenic abscess
Mesenteric abscess
Retrocecal abscess

K65.2 Spontaneous bacterial peritonitis CC
> EXCLUDES 1 bacterial peritonitis NOS (K65.9)

K65.3 Choleperitonitis CC
Peritonitis due to bile

K65.4 Sclerosing mesenteritis CC
Fat necrosis of peritoneum
(Idiopathic) sclerosing mesenteric fibrosis
Mesenteric lipodystrophy
Mesenteric panniculitis
Retractile mesenteritis

K65.8 Other peritonitis CC
Chronic proliferative peritonitis
Peritonitis due to urine

K65.9 Peritonitis, unspecified CC ▽
Bacterial peritonitis NOS
AHA: 2013, 2Q, 31

✓4ᵗʰ K66 Other disorders of peritoneum
> EXCLUDES 2 ascites (R18.-)
> peritoneal effusion (chronic) (R18.8)

K66.0 Peritoneal adhesions (postprocedural) (postinfection)
Adhesions (of) abdominal (wall) Adhesions (of) omentum
Adhesions (of) diaphragm   Adhesions (of) stomach
Adhesions (of) intestine   Adhesive bands
Adhesions (of) male pelvis   Mesenteric adhesions
> EXCLUDES 1 female pelvic adhesions [bands] (N73.6)
> peritoneal adhesions with intestinal obstruction (K56.5)

K66.1 Hemoperitoneum
> EXCLUDES 1 traumatic hemoperitoneum (S36.8-)

K66.8 Other specified disorders of peritoneum

K66.9 Disorder of peritoneum, unspecified ▽

K67 *Disorders of peritoneum in infectious diseases classified elsewhere* CC
Code first underlying disease, such as :
congenital syphilis (A50.0)
helminthiasis (B65.0-B83.9)
> EXCLUDES 1 peritonitis in chlamydia (A74.81)
> peritonitis in diphtheria (A36.89)
> peritonitis in gonococcal (A54.85)
> peritonitis in syphilis (late) (A52.74)
> peritonitis in tuberculosis (A18.31)

Ⓝ Newborn   Ⓟ Pediatric   Ⓜ Maternity   Ⓐ Adult   RIC RIC Dx   NCDx Noncancer Dx   PDx Primary Dx   CC RIC CC Condition   ►◄ Revised Text   ● New Code   ▲ Revised Code Title

650

ICD-10-CM 2016

✓4ᵗʰ **K68 Disorders of retroperitoneum**

  ✓5ᵗʰ **K68.1 Retroperitoneal abscess**

    K68.11 Postprocedural retroperitoneal abscess   `CC`

    K68.12 Psoas muscle abscess

    K68.19 Other retroperitoneal abscess   `CC`

  K68.9 Other disorders of retroperitoneum   `CC`

Diseases of liver (K70-K77)

EXCLUDES 1   jaundice NOS (R17)
EXCLUDES 2   hemochromatosis (E83.11-)
     Reye's syndrome (G93.7)
     viral hepatitis (B15-B19)
     Wilson's disease (E83.Ø)

✓4ᵗʰ **K70 Alcoholic liver disease**

  Use additional code to identify:
  alcohol abuse and dependence (F10.-)

  K70.Ø Alcoholic fatty liver   `A`

  ✓5ᵗʰ **K70.1 Alcoholic hepatitis**

    K70.10 Alcoholic hepatitis without ascites   `A`

    K70.11 Alcoholic hepatitis with ascites   `A`

  K70.2 Alcoholic fibrosis and sclerosis of liver   `NC Dx` `A`

  ✓5ᵗʰ **K70.3 Alcoholic cirrhosis of liver**
    Alcoholic cirrhosis NOS

    K70.30 Alcoholic cirrhosis of liver without ascites   `NC Dx` `A`

    K70.31 Alcoholic cirrhosis of liver with ascites   `NC Dx` `A`

  ✓5ᵗʰ **K70.4 Alcoholic hepatic failure**
    Acute alcoholic hepatic failure
    Alcoholic hepatic failure NOS
    Chronic alcoholic hepatic failure
    Subacute alcoholic hepatic failure

    K70.40 Alcoholic hepatic failure without coma   `NC Dx` `A`

    K70.41 Alcoholic hepatic failure with coma   `NC Dx` `A`

  K70.9 Alcoholic liver disease, unspecified   `A` ▽

✓4ᵗʰ **K71 Toxic liver disease**

  INCLUDES   drug-induced idiosyncratic (unpredictable) liver disease
           drug-induced toxic (predictable) liver disease

  Code first poisoning due to drug or toxin, if applicable (T36-T65 with
  fifth or sixth character 1-4 or 6)

  Use additional code for adverse effect, if applicable, to identify drug
  (T36-T50 with fifth or sixth character 5)

  EXCLUDES 2   alcoholic liver disease (K70.-)
           Budd-Chiari syndrome (I82.Ø)

  K71.Ø Toxic liver disease with cholestasis   `NC Dx`
    Cholestasis with hepatocyte injury
    "Pure" cholestasis

  ✓5ᵗʰ **K71.1 Toxic liver disease with hepatic necrosis**
    Hepatic failure (acute) (chronic) due to drugs

    K71.10 Toxic liver disease with hepatic necrosis, without coma   `NC Dx`

    K71.11 Toxic liver disease with hepatic necrosis, with coma   `NC Dx`

  K71.2 Toxic liver disease with acute hepatitis   `NC Dx`

  K71.3 Toxic liver disease with chronic persistent hepatitis   `NC Dx`

  K71.4 Toxic liver disease with chronic lobular hepatitis   `NC Dx`

  ✓5ᵗʰ **K71.5 Toxic liver disease with chronic active hepatitis**
    Toxic liver disease with lupoid hepatitis

    K71.50 Toxic liver disease with chronic active hepatitis without ascites   `NC Dx`

    K71.51 Toxic liver disease with chronic active hepatitis with ascites   `NC Dx`

  K71.6 Toxic liver disease with hepatitis, not elsewhere classified   `NC Dx`

  K71.7 Toxic liver disease with fibrosis and cirrhosis of liver   `NC Dx`

  K71.8 Toxic liver disease with other disorders of liver   `NC Dx`
    Toxic liver disease with focal nodular hyperplasia
    Toxic liver disease with hepatic granulomas
    Toxic liver disease with peliosis hepatis
    Toxic liver disease with veno-occlusive disease of liver

  K71.9 Toxic liver disease, unspecified   `NC Dx` ▽

✓4ᵗʰ **K72 Hepatic failure, not elsewhere classified**

  INCLUDES   acute hepatitis NEC, with hepatic failure
           fulminant hepatitis NEC, with hepatic failure
           hepatic encephalopathy NOS
           liver (cell) necrosis with hepatic failure
           malignant hepatitis NEC, with hepatic failure
           yellow liver atrophy or dystrophy

  EXCLUDES 1   alcoholic hepatic failure (K70.4)
           hepatic failure with toxic liver disease (K71.1-)
           icterus of newborn (P55-P59)
           postprocedural hepatic failure (K91.82)
           viral hepatitis with hepatic coma (B15-B19)

  EXCLUDES 2   hepatic failure complicating abortion or ectopic or molar
           pregnancy (O00-O07, O08.8)
           hepatic failure complicating pregnancy, childbirth and the
           puerperium (O26.6-)

  ✓5ᵗʰ **K72.Ø Acute and subacute hepatic failure**
    AHA: 2014, 2Q, 13

    K72.00 Acute and subacute hepatic failure without coma   `CC`

    K72.01 Acute and subacute hepatic failure with coma   `CC` `NC Dx`

  ✓5ᵗʰ **K72.1 Chronic hepatic failure**

    K72.10 Chronic hepatic failure without coma

    K72.11 Chronic hepatic failure with coma   `NC Dx`

  ✓5ᵗʰ **K72.9 Hepatic failure, unspecified**

    K72.90 Hepatic failure, unspecified without coma   `NC Dx` ▽

    K72.91 Hepatic failure, unspecified with coma   `NC Dx` ▽
      Hepatic coma NOS

✓4ᵗʰ **K73 Chronic hepatitis, not elsewhere classified**

  EXCLUDES 1   alcoholic hepatitis (chronic) (K70.1-)
           drug-induced hepatitis (chronic) (K71.-)
           granulomatous hepatitis (chronic) NEC (K75.3)
           reactive, nonspecific hepatitis (chronic) (K75.2)
           viral hepatitis (chronic) (B15-B19)

  K73.Ø Chronic persistent hepatitis, not elsewhere classified   `NC Dx`

  K73.1 Chronic lobular hepatitis, not elsewhere classified   `NC Dx`

  K73.2 Chronic active hepatitis, not elsewhere classified   `NC Dx`

  K73.8 Other chronic hepatitis, not elsewhere classified   `NC Dx`

  K73.9 Chronic hepatitis, unspecified   `NC Dx` ▽

✓4ᵗʰ **K74 Fibrosis and cirrhosis of liver**

  Code also, if applicable, viral hepatitis (acute) (chronic) (B15-B19)

  EXCLUDES 1   alcoholic cirrhosis (of liver) (K70.3)
           alcoholic fibrosis of liver (K70.2)
           cardiac sclerosis of liver (K76.1)
           cirrhosis (of liver) with toxic liver disease (K71.7)
           congenital cirrhosis (of liver) (P78.81)
           pigmentary cirrhosis (of liver) (E83.110)

  K74.Ø Hepatic fibrosis   `NC Dx`

  K74.1 Hepatic sclerosis

  K74.2 Hepatic fibrosis with hepatic sclerosis

  K74.3 Primary biliary cirrhosis   `NC Dx`
    Chronic nonsuppurative destructive cholangitis

  K74.4 Secondary biliary cirrhosis   `NC Dx`

  K74.5 Biliary cirrhosis, unspecified   `NC Dx` ▽

  ✓5ᵗʰ **K74.6 Other and unspecified cirrhosis of liver**

    K74.60 Unspecified cirrhosis of liver   `NC Dx` ▽
      Cirrhosis (of liver) NOS

    K74.69 Other cirrhosis of liver   `NC Dx`
      Cryptogenic cirrhosis (of liver)
      Macronodular cirrhosis (of liver)
      Micronodular cirrhosis (of liver)
      Mixed type cirrhosis (of liver)
      Portal cirrhosis (of liver)
      Postnecrotic cirrhosis (of liver)

✓4ᵗʰ **K75 Other inflammatory liver diseases**

  EXCLUDES 2   toxic liver disease (K71.-)

  K75.Ø Abscess of liver   `CC`
    Cholangitic hepatic abscess
    Hematogenic hepatic abscess
    Hepatic abscess NOS
    Lymphogenic hepatic abscess
    Pylephlebitic hepatic abscess

    EXCLUDES 1   amebic liver abscess (A06.4)
           cholangitis without liver abscess (K83.Ø)
           pylephlebitis without liver abscess (K75.1)

✔ Add'l Character Required   ✔x7ᵗʰ Placeholder Alert   RUG IV Special Care High Dx   RUG IV Clinically Complex Dx   RUG IV Special Care Low Dx   Manifestation Code   Other Specified Code   ▽ Unspecified Code

ICD-10-CM 2016   651

K75.1 Phlebitis of portal vein
Pylephlebitis
EXCLUDES 1 pylephlebitic liver abscess (K75.0)

K75.2 Nonspecific reactive hepatitis `NC Dx`
EXCLUDES 1 acute or subacute hepatitis (K72.0-)
chronic hepatitis NEC (K73.-)
viral hepatitis (B15-B19)

K75.3 Granulomatous hepatitis, not elsewhere classified `NC Dx`
EXCLUDES 1 acute or subacute hepatitis (K72.0-)
chronic hepatitis NEC (K73.-)
viral hepatitis (B15-B19)

K75.4 Autoimmune hepatitis `NC Dx`
Lupoid hepatitis NEC

✓5ᵗʰ **K75.8 Other specified inflammatory liver diseases**
K75.81 Nonalcoholic steatohepatitis (NASH) `NC Dx`
K75.89 Other specified inflammatory liver diseases `NC Dx`

K75.9 Inflammatory liver disease, unspecified `NC Dx` ▽
Hepatitis NOS
EXCLUDES 1 acute or subacute hepatitis (K72.0-)
chronic hepatitis NEC (K73.-)
viral hepatitis (B15-B19)

✓4ᵗʰ **K76 Other diseases of liver**
EXCLUDES 2 alcoholic liver disease (K70.-)
amyloid degeneration of liver (E85.-)
cystic disease of liver (congenital) (Q44.6)
hepatic vein thrombosis (I82.0)
hepatomegaly NOS (R16.0)
pigmentary cirrhosis (of liver) (E83.110)
portal vein thrombosis (I81)
toxic liver disease (K71.-)

K76.0 Fatty (change of) liver, not elsewhere classified
Nonalcoholic fatty liver disease (NAFLD)
EXCLUDES 1 nonalcoholic steatohepatitis (NASH) (K75.81)

K76.1 Chronic passive congestion of liver
Cardiac cirrhosis
Cardiac sclerosis

K76.2 Central hemorrhagic necrosis of liver `CC`
EXCLUDES 1 liver necrosis with hepatic failure (K72.-)

K76.3 Infarction of liver

K76.4 Peliosis hepatis `NC Dx`
Hepatic angiomatosis

K76.5 Hepatic veno-occlusive disease
EXCLUDES 1 Budd-Chiari syndrome (I82.0)

K76.6 Portal hypertension
Use additional code for any associated complications, such as:
portal hypertensive gastropathy (K31.89)

K76.7 Hepatorenal syndrome `CC` `NC Dx`
EXCLUDES 1 hepatorenal syndrome following labor and delivery
(O90.4)
postprocedural hepatorenal syndrome (K91.82)

✓5ᵗʰ **K76.8 Other specified diseases of liver**
K76.81 Hepatopulmonary syndrome
Code first underlying liver disease, such as:
alcoholic cirrhosis of liver (K70.3-)
cirrhosis of liver without mention of alcohol (K74.6-)

K76.89 Other specified diseases of liver
Cyst (simple) of liver
Focal nodular hyperplasia of liver
Hepatoptosis

K76.9 Liver disease, unspecified ▽

K77 Liver disorders in diseases classified elsewhere
Code first underlying disease, such as:
amyloidosis (E85.-)
congenital syphilis (A50.0, A50.5)
congenital toxoplasmosis (P37.1)
schistosomiasis (B65.0-B65.9)
EXCLUDES 1 alcoholic hepatitis (K70.1-)
alcoholic liver disease (K70.-)
cytomegaloviral hepatitis (B25.1)
herpesviral [herpes simplex] hepatitis (B00.81)
infectious mononucleosis with liver disease
(B27.0-B27.9 with .9)
mumps hepatitis (B26.81)
sarcoidosis with liver disease (D86.89)
secondary syphilis with liver disease (A51.45)
syphilis (late) with liver disease (A52.74)
toxoplasmosis (acquired) hepatitis (B58.1)
tuberculosis with liver disease (A18.83)

Disorders of gallbladder, biliary tract and pancreas (K80-K87)

✓4ᵗʰ **K80 Cholelithiasis**
EXCLUDES 1 retained cholelithiasis following cholecystectomy (K91.86)

✓5ᵗʰ **K80.0 Calculus of gallbladder with acute cholecystitis**
Any condition listed in K80.2 with acute cholecystitis
**K80.00 Calculus of gallbladder with acute cholecystitis
without obstruction**
**K80.01 Calculus of gallbladder with acute cholecystitis with
obstruction**

✓5ᵗʰ **K80.1 Calculus of gallbladder with other cholecystitis**
**K80.10 Calculus of gallbladder with chronic cholecystitis
without obstruction**
Cholelithiasis with cholecystitis NOS
**K80.11 Calculus of gallbladder with chronic cholecystitis
with obstruction**
**K80.12 Calculus of gallbladder with acute and chronic
cholecystitis without obstruction**
**K80.13 Calculus of gallbladder with acute and chronic
cholecystitis with obstruction**
**K80.18 Calculus of gallbladder with other cholecystitis
without obstruction**
**K80.19 Calculus of gallbladder with other cholecystitis
with obstruction**

✓5ᵗʰ **K80.2 Calculus of gallbladder without cholecystitis**
Cholecystolithiasis without cholecystitis
Cholelithiasis (without cholecystitis)
Colic (recurrent) of gallbladder (without cholecystitis)
Gallstone (impacted) of cystic duct (without cholecystitis)
Gallstone (impacted) of gallbladder (without cholecystitis)
**K80.20 Calculus of gallbladder without cholecystitis
without obstruction**
**K80.21 Calculus of gallbladder without cholecystitis
with obstruction**

✓5ᵗʰ **K80.3 Calculus of bile duct with cholangitis**
Any condition listed in K80.5 with cholangitis
**K80.30 Calculus of bile duct with cholangitis,
unspecified, without obstruction** ▽
**K80.31 Calculus of bile duct with cholangitis,
unspecified, with obstruction** ▽
**K80.32 Calculus of bile duct with acute cholangitis without
obstruction**
**K80.33 Calculus of bile duct with acute cholangitis with
obstruction**
**K80.34 Calculus of bile duct with chronic cholangitis
without obstruction**
**K80.35 Calculus of bile duct with chronic cholangitis with
obstruction**
**K80.36 Calculus of bile duct with acute and chronic
cholangitis without obstruction**
**K80.37 Calculus of bile duct with acute and chronic
cholangitis with obstruction**

✓5ᵗʰ **K80.4 Calculus of bile duct with cholecystitis**
Any condition listed in K80.5 with cholecystitis (with cholangitis)
**K80.40 Calculus of bile duct with cholecystitis,
unspecified, without obstruction** ▽
**K80.41 Calculus of bile duct with cholecystitis,
unspecified, with obstruction** ▽
**K80.42 Calculus of bile duct with acute cholecystitis
without obstruction**
**K80.43 Calculus of bile duct with acute cholecystitis
with obstruction**
**K80.44 Calculus of bile duct with chronic cholecystitis
without obstruction**
**K80.45 Calculus of bile duct with chronic cholecystitis
with obstruction**
**K80.46 Calculus of bile duct with acute and chronic
cholecystitis without obstruction**
**K80.47 Calculus of bile duct with acute and chronic
cholecystitis with obstruction**

N Newborn   P Pediatric   M Maternity   A Adult   RIC RIC Dx   NC Dx Noncancer Dx   PDx Primary Dx   CC RIC CC Condition   ►◄ Revised Text   ● New Code   ▲ Revised Code Title

652   ICD-10-CM 2016

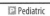

✓5th **K80.5** **Calculus of** bile duct without cholangitis or cholecystitis
     Choledocholithiasis (without cholangitis or cholecystitis)
     Gallstone (impacted) of bile duct NOS (without cholangitis or cholecystitis)
     Gallstone (impacted) of common duct (without cholangitis or cholecystitis)
     Gallstone (impacted) of hepatic duct (without cholangitis or cholecystitis)
     Hepatic cholelithiasis (without cholangitis or cholecystitis)
     Hepatic colic (recurrent) (without cholangitis or cholecystitis)

     K80.50 **Calculus of bile duct without cholangitis or cholecystitis** without obstruction

     K80.51 **Calculus of bile duct without cholangitis or cholecystitis** with obstruction

✓5th **K80.6** **Calculus of** gallbladder and bile duct with cholecystitis

     K80.60 **Calculus of gallbladder and bile duct with cholecystitis, unspecified,** without obstruction ▽

     K80.61 **Calculus of gallbladder and bile duct with cholecystitis, unspecified,** with obstruction ▽

     K80.62 **Calculus of gallbladder and bile duct with** acute **cholecystitis** without obstruction

     K80.63 **Calculus of gallbladder and bile duct with** acute **cholecystitis** with obstruction

     K80.64 **Calculus of gallbladder and bile duct with** chronic **cholecystitis** without obstruction

     K80.65 **Calculus of gallbladder and bile duct with** chronic **cholecystitis** with obstruction

     K80.66 **Calculus of gallbladder and bile duct with** acute and chronic **cholecystitis** without obstruction

     K80.67 **Calculus of gallbladder and bile duct with** acute and chronic **cholecystitis** with obstruction

✓5th **K80.7** **Calculus of** gallbladder and bile duct without cholecystitis

     K80.70 **Calculus of gallbladder and bile duct without cholecystitis** without obstruction

     K80.71 **Calculus of gallbladder and bile duct without cholecystitis** with obstruction

✓5th **K80.8** Other cholelithiasis

     K80.80 **Other cholelithiasis** without obstruction

     K80.81 **Other cholelithiasis** with obstruction

✓4th **K81** **Cholecystitis**
     EXCLUDES 1   *cholecystitis with cholelithiasis (K80.-)*

     K81.0 Acute **cholecystitis**
         Abscess of gallbladder
         Angiocholecystitis
         Emphysematous (acute) cholecystitis
         Empyema of gallbladder
         Gangrene of gallbladder
         Gangrenous cholecystitis
         Suppurative cholecystitis

     K81.1 Chronic **cholecystitis**

     K81.2 Acute **cholecystitis** with chronic **cholecystitis**

     K81.9 **Cholecystitis, unspecified** ▽

✓4th **K82** **Other diseases of gallbladder**
     EXCLUDES 1   *nonvisualization of gallbladder (R93.2)*
         postcholecystectomy syndrome (K91.5)

     K82.0 **Obstruction of gallbladder**
         Occlusion of cystic duct or gallbladder without cholelithiasis
         Stenosis of cystic duct or gallbladder without cholelithiasis
         Stricture of cystic duct or gallbladder without cholelithiasis
         EXCLUDES 1   *obstruction of gallbladder with cholelithiasis (K80.-)*

     K82.1 **Hydrops of gallbladder**
         Mucocele of gallbladder

     K82.2 **Perforation of gallbladder**   CC
         Rupture of cystic duct or gallbladder

     K82.3 **Fistula of gallbladder**
         Cholecystocolic fistula
         Cholecystoduodenal fistula

     K82.4 **Cholesterolosis of gallbladder**
         Strawberry gallbladder
         EXCLUDES 1   *cholesterolosis of gallbladder with cholecystitis (K81.-)*
         cholesterolosis of gallbladder with cholelithiasis (K80.-)

K82.8 **Other specified diseases of gallbladder**
     Adhesions of cystic duct or gallbladder
     Atrophy of cystic duct or gallbladder
     Cyst of cystic duct or gallbladder
     Dyskinesia of cystic duct or gallbladder
     Hypertrophy of cystic duct or gallbladder
     Nonfunctioning of cystic duct or gallbladder
     Ulcer of cystic duct or gallbladder

K82.9 **Disease of gallbladder, unspecified** ▽

✓4th **K83** **Other diseases of biliary tract**
     EXCLUDES 1   *postcholecystectomy syndrome (K91.5)*
     EXCLUDES 2   *conditions involving the gallbladder (K81-K82)*
         conditions involving the cystic duct (K81-K82)

     K83.0 **Cholangitis**
         Ascending cholangitis
         Cholangitis NOS
         Primary cholangitis
         Recurrent cholangitis
         Sclerosing cholangitis
         Secondary cholangitis
         Stenosing cholangitis
         Suppurative cholangitis
         EXCLUDES 1   *cholangitic liver abscess (K75.0)*
         cholangitis with choledocholithiasis (K80.3-, K80.4-)
         chronic nonsuppurative destructive cholangitis (K74.3)

     K83.1 **Obstruction of bile duct**
         Occlusion of bile duct without cholelithiasis
         Stenosis of bile duct without cholelithiasis
         Stricture of bile duct without cholelithiasis
         EXCLUDES 1   *congenital obstruction of bile duct (Q44.3)*
         obstruction of bile duct with cholelithiasis (K80.-)

     K83.2 **Perforation of bile duct**   CC
         Rupture of bile duct

     K83.3 **Fistula of bile duct**
         Choledochoduodenal fistula

     K83.4 **Spasm of sphincter of Oddi**

     K83.5 **Biliary cyst**

     K83.8 **Other specified diseases of biliary tract**
         Adhesions of biliary tract
         Atrophy of biliary tract
         Hypertrophy of biliary tract
         Ulcer of biliary tract

     K83.9 **Disease of biliary tract, unspecified** ▽

✓4th **K85** **Acute pancreatitis**
     Abscess of pancreas
     Acute necrosis of pancreas
     Acute (recurrent) pancreatitis
     Gangrene of (gangrenous) pancreas
     Hemorrhagic pancreatitis
     Infective necrosis of pancreas
     Subacute pancreatitis
     Suppurative pancreatitis

     K85.0 **Idiopathic** acute pancreatitis

     K85.1 **Biliary** acute pancreatitis
         Gallstone pancreatitis

     K85.2 **Alcohol induced** acute pancreatitis
         EXCLUDES 2   *alcohol induced chronic pancreatitis (K86.0)*

     K85.3 **Drug induced** acute pancreatitis
         Use additional code for adverse effect, if applicable, to identify drug (T36-T50 with fifth or sixth character 5)
         Use additional code to identify drug abuse and dependence (F11.- F17.-)

     K85.8 **Other acute pancreatitis**

     K85.9 **Acute pancreatitis, unspecified** ▽
         Pancreatitis NOS

✓4th **K86** **Other diseases of pancreas**
     EXCLUDES 2   *fibrocystic disease of pancreas (E84.-)*
         islet cell tumor (of pancreas) (D13.7)
         pancreatic steatorrhea (K90.3)

     K86.0 **Alcohol-induced chronic pancreatitis**
         Use additional code to identify:
         alcohol abuse and dependence (F10.-)
         EXCLUDES 2   *alcohol induced acute pancreatitis (K85.2)*

     K86.1 **Other chronic pancreatitis**
         Chronic pancreatitis NOS
         Infectious chronic pancreatitis
         Recurrent chronic pancreatitis
         Relapsing chronic pancreatitis

     K86.2 **Cyst of pancreas**   CC

✓ Add'l Character Required   ✓x7th Placeholder Alert   RUG IV Special Care High Dx   RUG IV Clinically Complex Dx   RUG IV Special Care Low Dx   Manifestation Code   Other Specified Code   ▽ Unspecified Code

Chapter 11. Diseases of the Digestive System

K86.3   **Pseudocyst of pancreas**   cc

K86.8   **Other specified diseases of pancreas**
Aseptic pancreatic necrosis
Atrophy of pancreas
Calculus of pancreas
Cirrhosis of pancreas
Fibrosis of pancreas
Pancreatic fat necrosis
Pancreatic infantilism
Pancreatic necrosis NOS

K86.9   **Disease of pancreas, unspecified**   ▽

K87   *Disorders of gallbladder, biliary tract and pancreas in diseases classified elsewhere*
Code first underlying disease
EXCLUDES 1   *cytomegaloviral pancreatitis (B25.2)*
mumps pancreatitis (B26.3)
syphilitic gallbladder (A52.74)
syphilitic pancreas (A52.74)
tuberculosis of gallbladder (A18.83)
tuberculosis of pancreas (A18.83)

Other diseases of the digestive system (K90-K95)

☑4ᵗʰ **K90**   **Intestinal malabsorption**
EXCLUDES 1   *intestinal malabsorption following gastrointestinal surgery (K91.2)*

K90.0   **Celiac disease**
Gluten-sensitive enteropathy
Idiopathic steatorrhea
Nontropical sprue
Use additional code for associated disorders including:
dermatitis herpetiformis (L13.0)
gluten ataxia (G32.81)

K90.1   **Tropical sprue**
Sprue NOS
Tropical steatorrhea

K90.2   **Blind loop syndrome, not elsewhere classified**
Blind loop syndrome NOS
EXCLUDES 1   *congenital blind loop syndrome (Q43.8)*
postsurgical blind loop syndrome (K91.2)

K90.3   **Pancreatic steatorrhea**

K90.4   **Malabsorption due to intolerance, not elsewhere classified**
Malabsorption due to intolerance to carbohydrate
Malabsorption due to intolerance to fat
Malabsorption due to intolerance to protein
Malabsorption due to intolerance to starch
EXCLUDES 2   *gluten-sensitive enteropathy (K90.0)*
lactose intolerance (E73.-)

☑5ᵗʰ **K90.8**   **Other intestinal malabsorption**
K90.81   **Whipple's disease**
K90.89   **Other intestinal malabsorption**

K90.9   **Intestinal malabsorption, unspecified**   ▽

☑4ᵗʰ **K91**   **Intraoperative and postprocedural complications and disorders of digestive system, not elsewhere classified**
EXCLUDES 2   *complications of artificial opening of digestive system (K94.-)*
complications of bariatric procedures (K95.-)
gastrojejunal ulcer (K28.-)
postprocedural (radiation) retroperitoneal abscess (K68.11)
radiation colitis (K52.0)
radiation gastroenteritis (K52.0)
radiation proctitis (K62.7)

K91.0   **Vomiting following gastrointestinal surgery**

K91.1   **Postgastric surgery syndromes**
Dumping syndrome
Postgastrectomy syndrome
Postvagotomy syndrome

K91.2   **Postsurgical malabsorption, not elsewhere classified**   cc
Postsurgical blind loop syndrome
EXCLUDES 1   *malabsorption osteomalacia in adults (M83.2)*
malabsorption osteoporosis, postsurgical (M80.8-, M81.8)

K91.3   **Postprocedural intestinal obstruction**

K91.5   **Postcholecystectomy syndrome**

☑5ᵗʰ **K91.6**   **Intraoperative hemorrhage and hematoma of a digestive system organ or structure complicating a procedure**
EXCLUDES 1   *intraoperative hemorrhage and hematoma of a digestive system organ or structure due to accidental puncture and laceration during a procedure (K91.7-)*

K91.61   **Intraoperative hemorrhage and hematoma of a digestive system organ or structure complicating a digestive system procedure**

K91.62   **Intraoperative hemorrhage and hematoma of a digestive system organ or structure complicating other procedure**

☑5ᵗʰ **K91.7**   **Accidental puncture and laceration of a digestive system organ or structure during a procedure**

K91.71   **Accidental puncture and laceration of a digestive system organ or structure during a digestive system procedure**

K91.72   **Accidental puncture and laceration of a digestive system organ or structure during other procedure**

☑5ᵗʰ **K91.8**   **Other intraoperative and postprocedural complications and disorders of digestive system**

K91.81   **Other intraoperative complications of digestive system**

K91.82   **Postprocedural hepatic failure**

K91.83   **Postprocedural hepatorenal syndrome**

☑6ᵗʰ **K91.84**   **Postprocedural hemorrhage and hematoma of a digestive system organ or structure following a procedure**

K91.840   **Postprocedural hemorrhage and hematoma of a digestive system organ or structure following a digestive system procedure**

K91.841   **Postprocedural hemorrhage and hematoma of a digestive system organ or structure following other procedure**

☑6ᵗʰ **K91.85**   **Complications of intestinal pouch**

K91.850   **Pouchitis**
Inflammation of internal ileoanal pouch

K91.858   **Other complications of intestinal pouch**

K91.86   **Retained cholelithiasis following cholecystectomy**

K91.89   **Other postprocedural complications and disorders of digestive system**
Use additional code, if applicable, to further specify disorder
EXCLUDES 2   *postprocedural retroperitoneal abscess (K68.11)*

☑4ᵗʰ **K92**   **Other diseases of digestive system**
EXCLUDES 1   *neonatal gastrointestinal hemorrhage (P54.0-P54.3)*

K92.0   **Hematemesis**

K92.1   **Melena**
EXCLUDES 1   *occult blood in feces (R19.5)*

K92.2   **Gastrointestinal hemorrhage, unspecified**   ▽
Gastric hemorrhage NOS
Intestinal hemorrhage NOS
EXCLUDES 1   *acute hemorrhagic gastritis (K29.01)*
hemorrhage of anus and rectum (K62.5)
angiodysplasia of stomach with hemorrhage (K31.811)
diverticular disease with hemorrhage (K57.-)
gastritis and duodenitis with hemorrhage (K29.-)
peptic ulcer with hemorrhage (K25-K28)

☑5ᵗʰ **K92.8**   **Other specified diseases of the digestive system**

K92.81   **Gastrointestinal mucositis (ulcerative)**
Code also type of associated therapy, such as:
antineoplastic and immunosuppressive drugs (T45.1X-)
radiological procedure and radiotherapy (Y84.2)
EXCLUDES 2   *mucositis (ulcerative) of vagina and vulva (N76.81)*
nasal mucositis (ulcerative) (J34.81)
oral mucositis (ulcerative) (K12.3-)

K92.89   **Other specified diseases of the digestive system**

K92.9   **Disease of digestive system, unspecified**   ▽

☑4ᵗʰ **K94**   **Complications of artificial openings of the digestive system**

☑5ᵗʰ **K94.0**   **Colostomy complications**

K94.00   **Colostomy complication, unspecified**   cc ▽

K94.01   **Colostomy hemorrhage**   cc

🆕 Newborn   🅿 Pediatric   Ⓜ Maternity   🅰 Adult   **RIC** RIC Dx   **NC Dx** Noncancer Dx   **PDx** Primary Dx   **CC** RIC CC Condition   ▶◀ Revised Text   ● New Code   ▲ Revised Code Title

654   ICD-10-CM 2016

K94.02   **Colostomy** infection   `CC`
Use additional code to specify type of infection, such
as:
cellulitis of abdominal wall (L03.311)
sepsis (A40-, A41-)

K94.03   **Colostomy** malfunction   `CC`
Mechanical complication of colostomy

K94.09   **Other complications of colostomy**   `CC`

`✓5ᵗʰ` **K94.1**   Enterostomy **complications**

K94.10   **Enterostomy complication, unspecified**   `CC` ▽

K94.11   **Enterostomy** hemorrhage   `CC`

K94.12   **Enterostomy** infection   `CC`
Use additional code to specify type of infection, such
as:
cellulitis of abdominal wall (L03.311)
sepsis (A40-, A41-)

K94.13   **Enterostomy** malfunction   `CC`
Mechanical complication of enterostomy

K94.19   **Other complications of enterostomy**   `CC`

`✓5ᵗʰ` **K94.2**   Gastrostomy **complications**

K94.20   **Gastrostomy complication, unspecified**   ▽

K94.21   **Gastrostomy** hemorrhage

K94.22   **Gastrostomy** infection
Use additional code to specify type of infection, such
as:
cellulitis of abdominal wall (L03.311)
sepsis (A40-, A41-)

K94.23   **Gastrostomy** malfunction
Mechanical complication of gastrostomy

K94.29   **Other complications of gastrostomy**

`✓5ᵗʰ` **K94.3**   Esophagostomy **complications**

K94.30   **Esophagostomy complications, unspecified**   ▽

K94.31   **Esophagostomy** hemorrhage

K94.32   **Esophagostomy** infection
Use additional code to identify the infection

K94.33   **Esophagostomy** malfunction
Mechanical complication of esophagostomy

K94.39   **Other complications of esophagostomy**

`✓4ᵗʰ` **K95**   **Complications of bariatric procedures**

`✓5ᵗʰ` **K95.0**   **Complications of** gastric band procedure

K95.01   Infection **due to gastric band procedure**
Use additional code to specify type of infection or
organism, such as:
bacterial and viral infectious agents (B95.-, B96.-)
cellulitis of abdominal wall (L03.311)
sepsis (A40.-, A41.-)

K95.09   **Other complications of gastric band procedure**
Use additional code, if applicable, to further specify
complication

`✓5ᵗʰ` **K95.8**   **Complications of** other bariatric procedure

> *EXCLUDES 1*   complications of gastric band surgery (K95.0-)

K95.81   Infection **due to other bariatric procedure**
Use additional code to specify type of infection or
organism, such as:
bacterial and viral infectious agents (B95.-, B96.-)
cellulitis of abdominal wall (L03.311)
sepsis (A40.-, A41.-)

K95.89   **Other complications of other bariatric procedure**
Use additional code, if applicable, to further specify
complication

☑ Add'l Character Required `✓x7ᵗʰ` Placeholder Alert RUG IV Special Care High Dx   RUG IV Clinically Complex Dx   RUG IV Special Care Low Dx   Manifestation Code   Other Specified Code   ▽ Unspecified Code

Chapter 12. Diseases of the Skin and Subcutaneous Tissue (L00–L99)

Chapter Specific Guidelines with Coding Examples

The chapter specific guidelines from the ICD-10-CM Official Guidelines for Coding and Reporting have been provided below. Along with these guidelines are coding examples, contained in the shaded boxes, that have been developed to help illustrate the coding and/or sequencing guidance found in these guidelines.

a. Pressure ulcer stage codes

1) Pressure ulcer stages

Codes from category L89, Pressure ulcer, are combination codes that identify the site of the pressure ulcer as well as the stage of the ulcer.

The ICD-10-CM classifies pressure ulcer stages based on severity, which is designated by stages 1-4, unspecified stage and unstageable.

Assign as many codes from category L89 as needed to identify all the pressure ulcers the patient has, if applicable.

> Stage 4 pressure ulcer right heel, 9 x 10 cm that invades the muscle and fascia; stage 2 pressure ulcer of left elbow
>
> **L89.614   Pressure ulcer of right heel, stage 4**
>
> **L89.022   Pressure ulcer of left elbow, stage 2**
>
> *Explanation:* Patient has a right heel pressure ulcer documented as stage 4 and a left elbow pressure ulcer documented as stage 2. Combination codes from category L89 Pressure ulcer, identify the site of the pressure ulcer as well as the stage. Assign as many codes from category L89 as needed to identify all the pressure ulcers the patient has.

2) Unstageable pressure ulcers

Assignment of the code for unstageable pressure ulcer (L89.--0) should be based on the clinical documentation. These codes are used for pressure ulcers whose stage cannot be clinically determined (e.g., the ulcer is covered by eschar or has been treated with a skin or muscle graft) and pressure ulcers that are documented as deep tissue injury but not documented as due to trauma. This code should not be confused with the codes for unspecified stage (L89.--9). When there is no documentation regarding the stage of the pressure ulcer, assign the appropriate code for unspecified stage (L89.--9).

> Pressure ulcer of the right lower back documented as unstageable due to the presence of thick eschar covering the ulcer
>
> **L89.130   Pressure ulcer of right lower back, unstageable**
>
> *Explanation:* Codes for unstageable pressure ulcers are assigned when the stage cannot be clinically determined (e.g., the ulcer is covered by eschar or has been treated with a skin or muscle graft).

3) Documented pressure ulcer stage

Assignment of the pressure ulcer stage code should be guided by clinical documentation of the stage or documentation of the terms found in the Alphabetic Index. For clinical terms describing the stage that are not found in the Alphabetic Index, and there is no documentation of the stage, the provider should be queried.

> Left heel pressure ulcer with partial thickness skin loss involving the dermis
>
> **L89.622   Pressure ulcer of left heel, stage 2**
>
> *Explanation:* Code assignment for the pressure ulcer stage should be guided by either the clinical documentation of the stage or the documentation of terms found in the Alphabetic Index. The clinical documentation describing the left heel pressure ulcer "partial thickness skin loss involving the dermis" matches the ICD-10-CM index parenthetical description for stage 2 "(abrasion, blister, partial thickness skin loss involving epidermis and/or dermis)."

4) Patients admitted with pressure ulcers documented as healed

No code is assigned if the documentation states that the pressure ulcer is completely healed.

> Patient receiving follow-up examination of a completely healed pressure ulcer of the foot
>
> **Z09   Encounter for follow-up examination after completed treatment for conditions other than malignant neoplasm**
>
> **Z87.2   Personal history of diseases of the skin and subcutaneous tissue**
>
> *Explanation:* Assign only codes for the reason for the encounter and the personal history of the pressure ulcer. Personal history code Z87.2 includes conditions classifiable to L00–L99 such as pressure ulcer. No code is assigned for a pressure ulcer documented as completely healed.

5) Patients admitted with pressure ulcers documented as healing

Pressure ulcers described as healing should be assigned the appropriate pressure ulcer stage code based on the documentation in the medical record. If the documentation does not provide information about the stage of the healing pressure ulcer, assign the appropriate code for unspecified stage.

If the documentation is unclear as to whether the patient has a current (new) pressure ulcer or if the patient is being treated for a healing pressure ulcer, query the provider.

> Healing stage 2 sacral pressure ulcer
>
> **L89.152   Pressure ulcer of sacral region, stage 2**
>
> *Explanation:* Pressure ulcers described as healing should be assigned the appropriate code for the pressure ulcer stage as documented.

6) Patient admitted with pressure ulcer evolving into another stage during the admission

If a patient is admitted with a pressure ulcer at one stage and it progresses to a higher stage, assign the code for the highest stage reported for that site.

> Stage 3 right hip pressure ulcer worsened during admission to a stage 4 pressure ulcer
>
> **L89.214   Pressure ulcer of right hip, stage 4**
>
> *Explanation:* A pressure ulcer that progresses from a lower stage to a higher stage is assigned only the code for the highest stage reported for that site.

Chapter 12. Diseases of the Skin and Subcutaneous Tissue (L00-L99)

EXCLUDES 2   *certain conditions originating in the perinatal period (P04-P96)*
certain infectious and parasitic diseases (A00-B99)
complications of pregnancy, childbirth and the puerperium (O00-O9A)
congenital malformations, deformations, and chromosomal abnormalities (Q00-Q99)
endocrine, nutritional and metabolic diseases (E00-E88)
lipomelanotic reticulosis (I89.8)
neoplasms (C00-D49)
symptoms, signs and abnormal clinical and laboratory findings, not elsewhere classified (R00-R94)
systemic connective tissue disorders (M30-M36)
viral warts (B07.-)

This chapter contains the following blocks:

L00-L08   Infections of the skin and subcutaneous tissue
L10-L14   Bullous disorders
L20-L30   Dermatitis and eczema
L40-L45   Papulosquamous disorders
L49-L54   Urticaria and erythema
L55-L59   Radiation-related disorders of the skin and subcutaneous tissue
L60-L75   Disorders of skin appendages
L76   Intraoperative and postprocedural complications of skin and subcutaneous tissue
L80-L99   Other disorders of the skin and subcutaneous tissue

Infections of the skin and subcutaneous tissue (L00-L08)

Use additional code (B95-B97) to identify infectious agent

EXCLUDES 2   *hordeolum (H00.0)*
infective dermatitis (L30.3)
local infections of skin classified in Chapter 1
lupus panniculitis (L93.2)
panniculitis NOS (M79.3)
panniculitis of neck and back (M54.0-)
Perlèche NOS (K13.0)
Perlèche due to candidiasis (B37.0)
Perlèche due to riboflavin deficiency (E53.0)
pyogenic granuloma (L98.0)
relapsing panniculitis [Weber-Christian] (M35.6)
viral warts (B07.-)
zoster (B02.-)

L00   Staphylococcal scalded skin syndrome
Ritter's disease
Use additional code to identify percentage of skin exfoliation (L49.-)

EXCLUDES 1   *bullous impetigo (L01.03)*
pemphigus neonatorum (L01.03)
toxic epidermal necrolysis [Lyell] (L51.2)

✓4ᵗʰ L01   Impetigo
EXCLUDES 1   *impetigo herpetiformis (L40.1)*

✓5ᵗʰ L01.0   Impetigo
Impetigo contagiosa
Impetigo vulgaris

    L01.00   Impetigo, unspecified   ▽
       Impetigo NOS

    L01.01   Non-bullous impetigo

    L01.02   Bockhart's impetigo
       Impetigo follicularis
       Perifolliculitis NOS
       Superficial pustular perifolliculitis

    L01.03   Bullous impetigo
       Impetigo neonatorum
       Pemphigus neonatorum

    L01.09   Other impetigo
       Ulcerative impetigo

L01.1   Impetiginization of other dermatoses

✓4ᵗʰ L02   Cutaneous abscess, furuncle and carbuncle
Use additional code to identify organism (B95-B96)

EXCLUDES 2   *abscess of anus and rectal regions (K61.-)*
abscess of female genital organs (external) (N76.4)
abscess of male genital organs (external) (N48.2, N49-)

✓5ᵗʰ L02.0   Cutaneous abscess, furuncle and carbuncle of face

EXCLUDES 2   *abscess of ear, external (H60.0)*
abscess of eyelid (H00.0)
abscess of head [any part, except face] (L02.8)
abscess of lacrimal gland (H04.0)
abscess of lacrimal passages (H04.3)
abscess of mouth (K12.2)
abscess of nose (J34.0)
abscess of orbit (H05.0)
submandibular abscess (K12.2)

    L02.01   Cutaneous abscess of face   cc

    L02.02   Furuncle of face
       Boil of face
       Folliculitis of face

    L02.03   Carbuncle of face

✓5ᵗʰ L02.1   Cutaneous abscess, furuncle and carbuncle of neck

    L02.11   Cutaneous abscess of neck   cc

    L02.12   Furuncle of neck
       Boil of neck
       Folliculitis of neck

    L02.13   Carbuncle of neck

✓5ᵗʰ L02.2   Cutaneous abscess, furuncle and carbuncle of trunk

EXCLUDES 1   *non-newborn omphalitis (L08.82)*
omphalitis of newborn (P38.-)

EXCLUDES 2   *abscess of breast (N61)*
abscess of buttocks (L02.3)
abscess of female external genital organs (N76.4)
abscess of hip (L02.4)
abscess of male external genital organs (N48.2, N49-)

   ✓6ᵗʰ L02.21   Cutaneous abscess of trunk

      L02.211   Cutaneous abscess of abdominal wall   cc
      L02.212   Cutaneous abscess of back [any part, except buttock]   cc
      L02.213   Cutaneous abscess of chest wall   cc
      L02.214   Cutaneous abscess of groin   cc
      L02.215   Cutaneous abscess of perineum   cc
      L02.216   Cutaneous abscess of umbilicus   cc
      L02.219   Cutaneous abscess of trunk, unspecified   cc ▽

   ✓6ᵗʰ L02.22   Furuncle of trunk
      Boil of trunk
      Folliculitis of trunk

      L02.221   Furuncle of abdominal wall
      L02.222   Furuncle of back [any part, except buttock]
      L02.223   Furuncle of chest wall
      L02.224   Furuncle of groin
      L02.225   Furuncle of perineum
      L02.226   Furuncle of umbilicus
      L02.229   Furuncle of trunk, unspecified   ▽

   ✓6ᵗʰ L02.23   Carbuncle of trunk

      L02.231   Carbuncle of abdominal wall
      L02.232   Carbuncle of back [any part, except buttock]
      L02.233   Carbuncle of chest wall
      L02.234   Carbuncle of groin
      L02.235   Carbuncle of perineum
      L02.236   Carbuncle of umbilicus
      L02.239   Carbuncle of trunk, unspecified   ▽

✓5ᵗʰ L02.3   Cutaneous abscess, furuncle and carbuncle of buttock

EXCLUDES 1   *pilonidal cyst with abscess (L05.01)*

    L02.31   Cutaneous abscess of buttock   cc
       Cutaneous abscess of gluteal region

    L02.32   Furuncle of buttock
       Boil of buttock
       Folliculitis of buttock
       Furuncle of gluteal region

    L02.33   Carbuncle of buttock
       Carbuncle of gluteal region

☑ Add'l Character Required   ✓ 7ᵗʰ Placeholder Alert   **RUG IV Special Care High Dx**   RUG IV Clinically Complex Dx   RUG IV Special Care Low Dx   Manifestation Code   Other Specified Code   ▽ Unspecified Code

√5ᵗʰ L02.4 Cutaneous abscess, furuncle and carbuncle of limb

    EXCLUDES 2   cutaneous abscess, furuncle and carbuncle of groin (L02.214, L02.224, L02.234)
       cutaneous abscess, furuncle and carbuncle of hand (L02.5-)
       cutaneous abscess, furuncle and carbuncle of foot (L02.6-)

  √6ᵗʰ L02.41 Cutaneous abscess of limb

    L02.411 Cutaneous abscess of right axilla   cc
    L02.412 Cutaneous abscess of left axilla   cc
    L02.413 Cutaneous abscess of right upper limb   cc
    L02.414 Cutaneous abscess of left upper limb   cc
    L02.415 Cutaneous abscess of right lower limb   cc
         RIC Excl: 10 Amputation, lower extremity
    L02.416 Cutaneous abscess of left lower limb   cc
         RIC Excl: 10 Amputation, lower extremity
    L02.419 Cutaneous abscess of limb, unspecified   cc ▽
         RIC Excl: 10 Amputation, lower extremity

  √6ᵗʰ L02.42 Furuncle of limb
    Boil of limb
    Folliculitis of limb

    L02.421 Furuncle of right axilla
    L02.422 Furuncle of left axilla
    L02.423 Furuncle of right upper limb
    L02.424 Furuncle of left upper limb
    L02.425 Furuncle of right lower limb
    L02.426 Furuncle of left lower limb
    L02.429 Furuncle of limb, unspecified   ▽

  √6ᵗʰ L02.43 Carbuncle of limb

    L02.431 Carbuncle of right axilla
    L02.432 Carbuncle of left axilla
    L02.433 Carbuncle of right upper limb
    L02.434 Carbuncle of left upper limb
    L02.435 Carbuncle of right lower limb
    L02.436 Carbuncle of left lower limb
    L02.439 Carbuncle of limb, unspecified   ▽

√5ᵗʰ L02.5 Cutaneous abscess, furuncle and carbuncle of hand

  √6ᵗʰ L02.51 Cutaneous abscess of hand

    L02.511 Cutaneous abscess of right hand   cc
    L02.512 Cutaneous abscess of left hand   cc
    L02.519 Cutaneous abscess of unspecified hand   cc ▽

  √6ᵗʰ L02.52 Furuncle hand
    Boil of hand
    Folliculitis of hand

    L02.521 Furuncle right hand
    L02.522 Furuncle left hand
    L02.529 Furuncle unspecified hand   ▽

  √6ᵗʰ L02.53 Carbuncle of hand

    L02.531 Carbuncle of right hand
    L02.532 Carbuncle of left hand
    L02.539 Carbuncle of unspecified hand   ▽

√5ᵗʰ L02.6 Cutaneous abscess, furuncle and carbuncle of foot

  √6ᵗʰ L02.61 Cutaneous abscess of foot

    L02.611 Cutaneous abscess of right foot   cc
         RIC Excl: 10 Amputation, lower extremity
    L02.612 Cutaneous abscess of left foot   cc
         RIC Excl: 10 Amputation, lower extremity
    L02.619 Cutaneous abscess of unspecified foot   cc ▽
         RIC Excl: 10 Amputation, lower extremity

  √6ᵗʰ L02.62 Furuncle of foot
    Boil of foot
    Folliculitis of foot

    L02.621 Furuncle of right foot
    L02.622 Furuncle of left foot
    L02.629 Furuncle of unspecified foot   ▽

  √6ᵗʰ L02.63 Carbuncle of foot

    L02.631 Carbuncle of right foot
    L02.632 Carbuncle of left foot
    L02.639 Carbuncle of unspecified foot   ▽

√5ᵗʰ L02.8 Cutaneous abscess, furuncle and carbuncle of other sites

  √6ᵗʰ L02.81 Cutaneous abscess of other sites

    L02.811 Cutaneous abscess of head [any part, except face]   cc
    L02.818 Cutaneous abscess of other sites   cc

  √6ᵗʰ L02.82 Furuncle of other sites
    Boil of other sites
    Folliculitis of other sites

    L02.821 Furuncle of head [any part, except face]
    L02.828 Furuncle of other sites

  √6ᵗʰ L02.83 Carbuncle of other sites

    L02.831 Carbuncle of head [any part, except face]
    L02.838 Carbuncle of other sites

√5ᵗʰ L02.9 Cutaneous abscess, furuncle and carbuncle, unspecified

  L02.91 Cutaneous abscess, unspecified   ▽
  L02.92 Furuncle, unspecified   ▽
    Boil NOS
    Furunculosis NOS
  L02.93 Carbuncle, unspecified   ▽

√4ᵗʰ L03 Cellulitis and acute lymphangitis

  EXCLUDES 2   cellulitis of anal and rectal region (K61.-)
     cellulitis of external auditory canal (H60.1)
     cellulitis of eyelid (H00.03-)
     cellulitis of female external genital organs (N76.4)
     cellulitis of lacrimal apparatus (H04.3)
     cellulitis of male external genital organs (N48.2, N49-)
     cellulitis of mouth (K12.2)
     cellulitis of nose (J34.0)
     eosinophilic cellulitis [Wells] (L98.3)
     febrile neutrophilic dermatosis [Sweet] (L98.2)
     lymphangitis (chronic) (subacute) (I89.1)

  √5ᵗʰ L03.0 Cellulitis and acute lymphangitis of finger and toe
    Infection of nail
    Onychia
    Paronychia
    Perionychia

    √6ᵗʰ L03.01 Cellulitis of finger
      Felon
      Whitlow
      EXCLUDES 1   herpetic whitlow (B00.89)

      L03.011 Cellulitis of right finger
      L03.012 Cellulitis of left finger
      L03.019 Cellulitis of unspecified finger   ▽

    √6ᵗʰ L03.02 Acute lymphangitis of finger
      Hangnail with lymphangitis of finger

      L03.021 Acute lymphangitis of right finger
      L03.022 Acute lymphangitis of left finger
      L03.029 Acute lymphangitis of unspecified finger   ▽

    √6ᵗʰ L03.03 Cellulitis of toe

      L03.031 Cellulitis of right toe
      L03.032 Cellulitis of left toe
      L03.039 Cellulitis of unspecified toe   ▽

    √6ᵗʰ L03.04 Acute lymphangitis of toe
      Hangnail with lymphangitis of toe

      L03.041 Acute lymphangitis of right toe
      L03.042 Acute lymphangitis of left toe
      L03.049 Acute lymphangitis of unspecified toe   ▽

  √5ᵗʰ L03.1 Cellulitis and acute lymphangitis of other parts of limb

    √6ᵗʰ L03.11 Cellulitis of other parts of limb
      EXCLUDES 2   cellulitis of fingers (L03.01-)
         cellulitis of toes (L03.03-)
         groin (L03.314)

      L03.111 Cellulitis of right axilla   cc
      L03.112 Cellulitis of left axilla   cc
      L03.113 Cellulitis of right upper limb   cc
      L03.114 Cellulitis of left upper limb   cc
      L03.115 Cellulitis of right lower limb   cc
         RIC Excl: 10 Amputation, lower extremity
      L03.116 Cellulitis of left lower limb   cc
         RIC Excl: 10 Amputation, lower extremity
      L03.119 Cellulitis of unspecified part of limb   cc ▽
         RIC Excl: 10 Amputation, lower extremity

Ⓝ Newborn   Ⓟ Pediatric   Ⓜ Maternity   Ⓐ Adult   **RIC** RIC Dx   **NC Dx** Noncancer Dx   **PDx** Primary Dx   **CC** RIC CC Condition   ▶◀ Revised Text   ● New Code   ▲ Revised Code Title

658   ICD-10-CM 2016

√6th **L03.12**   Acute lymphangitis of other parts of limb
    EXCLUDES 2   *acute lymphangitis of fingers (L03.02-)*
       acute lymphangitis of groin (L03.324)
       acute lymphangitis of toes (L03.04-)

   L03.121   Acute lymphangitis of right axilla   CC
   L03.122   Acute lymphangitis of left axilla   CC
   L03.123   Acute lymphangitis of right upper limb   CC
   L03.124   Acute lymphangitis of left upper limb   CC
   L03.125   Acute lymphangitis of right lower limb   CC
      RIC Excl: 10 Amputation, lower extremity
   L03.126   Acute lymphangitis of left lower limb   CC
      RIC Excl: 10 Amputation, lower extremity
   L03.129   Acute lymphangitis of unspecified part of limb   CC ▽
      RIC Excl: 10 Amputation, lower extremity

√5th **L03.2**   Cellulitis and acute lymphangitis of face and neck

√6th **L03.21**   Cellulitis and acute lymphangitis of face

   L03.211   Cellulitis of face   CC
     EXCLUDES 2   *cellulitis of ear (H60.1-)*
       cellulitis of eyelid (H00.03-)
       cellulitis of head (L03.811)
       cellulitis of lacrimal apparatus (H04.3)
       cellulitis of lip (K13.0)
       cellulitis of mouth (K12.2)
       cellulitis of nose (internal) (J34.0)
       cellulitis of orbit (H05.0)
       cellulitis of scalp (L03.811)
     AHA: 2013, 4Q, 123

   L03.212   Acute lymphangitis of face   CC

√6th **L03.22**   Cellulitis and acute lymphangitis of neck

   L03.221   Cellulitis of neck   CC
   L03.222   Acute lymphangitis of neck   CC

√5th **L03.3**   Cellulitis and acute lymphangitis of trunk

√6th **L03.31**   Cellulitis of trunk
     EXCLUDES 2   *cellulitis of anal and rectal regions (K61.-)*
       cellulitis of breast NOS (N61)
       cellulitis of female external genital organs (N76.4)
       cellulitis of male external genital organs (N48.2, N49-)
       omphalitis of newborn (P38.-)
       puerperal cellulitis of breast (O91.2)

   L03.311   Cellulitis of abdominal wall   CC
     EXCLUDES 2   *cellulitis of umbilicus (L03.316)*
       cellulitis of groin (L03.314)
   L03.312   Cellulitis of back [any part except buttock]   CC
   L03.313   Cellulitis of chest wall   CC
   L03.314   Cellulitis of groin   CC
   L03.315   Cellulitis of perineum   CC
   L03.316   Cellulitis of umbilicus   CC
   L03.317   Cellulitis of buttock   CC
   L03.319   Cellulitis of trunk, unspecified   CC ▽

√6th **L03.32**   Acute lymphangitis of trunk

   L03.321   Acute lymphangitis of abdominal wall   CC
   L03.322   Acute lymphangitis of back [any part except buttock]   CC
   L03.323   Acute lymphangitis of chest wall   CC
   L03.324   Acute lymphangitis of groin   CC
   L03.325   Acute lymphangitis of perineum   CC
   L03.326   Acute lymphangitis of umbilicus   CC
   L03.327   Acute lymphangitis of buttock   CC
   L03.329   Acute lymphangitis of trunk, unspecified   CC ▽

√5th **L03.8**   Cellulitis and acute lymphangitis of other sites

√6th **L03.81**   Cellulitis of other sites

   L03.811   Cellulitis of head [any part, except face]   CC
     Cellulitis of scalp
     EXCLUDES 2   *cellulitis of face (L03.211)*
   L03.818   Cellulitis of other sites   CC

√6th **L03.89**   Acute lymphangitis of other sites

   L03.891   Acute lymphangitis of head [any part, except face]   CC
   L03.898   Acute lymphangitis of other sites   CC

√5th **L03.9**   Cellulitis and acute lymphangitis, unspecified

   L03.90   Cellulitis, unspecified   ▽
   L03.91   Acute lymphangitis, unspecified   ▽
     EXCLUDES 1   *lymphangitis NOS (I89.1)*

√4th **L04**   **Acute lymphadenitis**
   INCLUDES   abscess (acute) of lymph nodes, except mesenteric
       acute lymphadenitis, except mesenteric
   EXCLUDES 1   *chronic or subacute lymphadenitis, except mesenteric (I88.1)*
       enlarged lymph nodes (R59.-)
       human immunodeficiency virus [HIV] disease resulting in generalized lymphadenopathy (B20)
       lymphadenitis NOS (I88.9)
       nonspecific mesenteric lymphadenitis (I88.0)

   L04.0   Acute lymphadenitis of face, head and neck
   L04.1   Acute lymphadenitis of trunk
   L04.2   Acute lymphadenitis of upper limb
     Acute lymphadenitis of axilla
     Acute lymphadenitis of shoulder
   L04.3   Acute lymphadenitis of lower limb
     Acute lymphadenitis of hip
     EXCLUDES 2   *acute lymphadenitis of groin (L04.1)*
   L04.8   Acute lymphadenitis of other sites
   L04.9   Acute lymphadenitis, unspecified   ▽

√4th **L05**   **Pilonidal cyst and sinus**

√5th **L05.0**   Pilonidal cyst and sinus with abscess

   L05.01   Pilonidal cyst with abscess
     Parasacral dimple with abscess
     Pilonidal abscess
     Pilonidal dimple with abscess
     Postanal dimple with abscess

   L05.02   Pilonidal sinus with abscess
     Coccygeal fistula with abscess
     Coccygeal sinus with abscess
     Pilonidal fistula with abscess

√5th **L05.9**   Pilonidal cyst and sinus without abscess

   L05.91   Pilonidal cyst without abscess
     Parasacral dimple
     Pilonidal dimple
     Postanal dimple
     Pilonidal cyst NOS

   L05.92   Pilonidal sinus without abscess
     Coccygeal fistula
     Coccygeal sinus without abscess
     Pilonidal fistula

√4th **L08**   **Other local infections of skin and subcutaneous tissue**

   L08.0   Pyoderma
     Dermatitis gangrenosa
     Purulent dermatitis
     Septic dermatitis
     Suppurative dermatitis
     EXCLUDES 1   *pyoderma gangrenosum (L88)*
       pyoderma vegetans (L08.81)

   L08.1   Erythrasma

√5th **L08.8**   Other specified local infections of the skin and subcutaneous tissue

   L08.81   Pyoderma vegetans
     EXCLUDES 1   *pyoderma gangrenosum (L88)*
       pyoderma NOS (L08.0)
   L08.82   Omphalitis not of newborn
     EXCLUDES 1   *omphalitis of newborn (P38.-)*
   L08.89   Other specified local infections of the skin and subcutaneous tissue

   L08.9   Local infection of the skin and subcutaneous tissue, unspecified   ▽

☑ Add'l Character Required   √x7th Placeholder Alert   RUG IV Special Care High Dx   RUG IV Clinically Complex Dx   RUG IV Special Care Low Dx   Manifestation Code   Other Specified Code   ▽ Unspecified Code

Bullous disorders (L10-L14)

EXCLUDES 1   benign familial pemphigus [Hailey-Hailey] (Q82.8)
staphylococcal scalded skin syndrome (L00)
toxic epidermal necrolysis [Lyell] (L51.2)

✓4ᵗʰ **L10　Pemphigus**
     EXCLUDES 1   pemphigus neonatorum (L01.03)

     L10.0　Pemphigus vulgaris
     L10.1　Pemphigus vegetans
     L10.2　Pemphigus foliaceous
     L10.3　Brazilian pemphigus [fogo selvagem]
     L10.4　Pemphigus erythematosus
         Senear-Usher syndrome
     L10.5　Drug-induced pemphigus
         Use additional code for adverse effect, if applicable, to identify drug (T36-T50 with fifth or sixth character 5)
     ✓5ᵗʰ **L10.8　Other pemphigus**
         L10.81　Paraneoplastic pemphigus
         L10.89　Other pemphigus
     L10.9　Pemphigus, unspecified ▽

✓4ᵗʰ **L11　Other acantholytic disorders**
     L11.0　Acquired keratosis follicularis
         EXCLUDES 1   keratosis follicularis (congenital) [Darier-White] (Q82.8)
     L11.1　Transient acantholytic dermatosis [Grover]
     L11.8　Other specified acantholytic disorders
     L11.9　Acantholytic disorder, unspecified ▽

✓4ᵗʰ **L12　Pemphigoid**
     EXCLUDES 1   herpes gestationis (O26.4-)
            impetigo herpetiformis (L40.1)

     L12.0　Bullous pemphigoid
     L12.1　Cicatricial pemphigoid
         Benign mucous membrane pemphigoid
     L12.2　Chronic bullous disease of childhood 🄿
         Juvenile dermatitis herpetiformis
     ✓5ᵗʰ **L12.3　Acquired epidermolysis bullosa**
         EXCLUDES 1   epidermolysis bullosa (congenital) (Q81.-) ▽
         L12.30　Acquired epidermolysis bullosa, unspecified
         L12.31　Epidermolysis bullosa due to drug
            Use additional code for adverse effect, if applicable, to identify drug (T36-T50 with fifth or sixth character 5)
         L12.35　Other acquired epidermolysis bullosa
     L12.8　Other pemphigoid
     L12.9　Pemphigoid, unspecified ▽

✓4ᵗʰ **L13　Other bullous disorders**
     L13.0　Dermatitis herpetiformis
         Duhring's disease
         Hydroa herpetiformis
         EXCLUDES 1   juvenile dermatitis herpetiformis (L12.2)
            senile dermatitis herpetiformis (L12.0)
     L13.1　Subcorneal pustular dermatitis
         Sneddon-Wilkinson disease
     L13.8　Other specified bullous disorders
     L13.9　Bullous disorder, unspecified ▽

L14　Bullous disorders in diseases classified elsewhere
     Code first underlying disease

Dermatitis and eczema (L20-L30)

NOTE   In this block the terms dermatitis and eczema are used synonymously and interchangeably.

EXCLUDES 2   chronic (childhood) granulomatous disease (D71)
dermatitis gangrenosa (L08.0)
dermatitis herpetiformis (L13.0)
dry skin dermatitis (L85.3)
factitial dermatitis (L98.1)
perioral dermatitis (L71.0)
radiation-related disorders of the skin and subcutaneous tissue (L55-L59)
stasis dermatitis (I83.1-I83.2)

✓4ᵗʰ **L20　Atopic dermatitis**
     L20.0　Besnier's prurigo
     ✓5ᵗʰ **L20.8　Other atopic dermatitis**
         EXCLUDES 2   circumscribed neurodermatitis (L28.0)
         L20.81　Atopic neurodermatitis
            Diffuse neurodermatitis
         L20.82　Flexural eczema
         L20.83　Infantile (acute) (chronic) eczema 🄿
         L20.84　Intrinsic (allergic) eczema
         L20.89　Other atopic dermatitis
     L20.9　Atopic dermatitis, unspecified ▽

✓4ᵗʰ **L21　Seborrheic dermatitis**
     EXCLUDES 2   infective dermatitis (L30.3)
            seborrheic keratosis (L82.-)
     L21.0　Seborrhea capitis 🄿
         Cradle cap
     L21.1　Seborrheic infantile dermatitis 🄿
     L21.8　Other seborrheic dermatitis
     L21.9　Seborrheic dermatitis, unspecified ▽
         Seborrhea NOS

L22　Diaper dermatitis
     Diaper erythema
     Diaper rash
     Psoriasiform diaper rash

✓4ᵗʰ **L23　Allergic contact dermatitis**
     EXCLUDES 1   allergy NOS (T78.40)
            contact dermatitis NOS (L25.9)
            dermatitis NOS (L30.9)
     EXCLUDES 2   dermatitis due to substances taken internally (L27.-)
            dermatitis of eyelid (H01.1-)
            diaper dermatitis (L22)
            eczema of external ear (H60.5-)
            irritant contact dermatitis (L24.-)
            perioral dermatitis (L71.0)
            radiation-related disorders of the skin and subcutaneous tissue (L55-L59)
     L23.0　Allergic contact dermatitis due to metals
         Allergic contact dermatitis due to chromium
         Allergic contact dermatitis due to nickel
     L23.1　Allergic contact dermatitis due to adhesives
     L23.2　Allergic contact dermatitis due to cosmetics
     L23.3　Allergic contact dermatitis due to drugs in contact with skin
         Use additional code for adverse effect, if applicable, to identify drug (T36-T50 with fifth or sixth character 5)
         EXCLUDES 2   dermatitis due to ingested drugs and medicaments (L27.0-L27.1)
     L23.4　Allergic contact dermatitis due to dyes
     L23.5　Allergic contact dermatitis due to other chemical products
         Allergic contact dermatitis due to cement
         Allergic contact dermatitis due to insecticide
         Allergic contact dermatitis due to plastic
         Allergic contact dermatitis due to rubber
     L23.6　Allergic contact dermatitis due to food in contact with the skin
         EXCLUDES 2   dermatitis due to ingested food (L27.2)
     L23.7　Allergic contact dermatitis due to plants, except food
         EXCLUDES 2   allergy NOS due to pollen (J30.1)
     ✓5ᵗʰ **L23.8　Allergic contact dermatitis due to other agents**
         L23.81　Allergic contact dermatitis due to animal (cat) (dog) dander
            Allergic contact dermatitis due to animal (cat) (dog) hair
         L23.89　Allergic contact dermatitis due to other agents

🅝 Newborn　🄿 Pediatric　🄼 Maternity　🄰 Adult　**RIC** RIC Dx　**NC Dx** Noncancer Dx　**PDx** Primary Dx　**CC** RIC CC Condition　►◄ Revised Text　● New Code　▲ Revised Code Title

660　　　　ICD-10-CM 2016

L23.9   Allergic contact dermatitis, unspecified cause ▽
     Allergic contact eczema NOS

☑4ᵗʰ **L24   Irritant contact dermatitis**
     EXCLUDES 1   *allergy NOS (T78.40)*
                contact dermatitis NOS (L25.9)
                dermatitis NOS (L30.9)
     EXCLUDES 2   *allergic contact dermatitis (L23.-)*
                dermatitis due to substances taken internally (L27.-)
                dermatitis of eyelid (H01.1-)
                diaper dermatitis (L22)
                eczema of external ear (H60.5-)
                perioral dermatitis (L71.0)
                radiation-related disorders of the skin and subcutaneous tissue
                  (L55-L59)

L24.0   Irritant contact dermatitis due to detergents

L24.1   Irritant contact dermatitis due to oils and greases

L24.2   Irritant contact dermatitis due to solvents
     Irritant contact dermatitis due to chlorocompound
     Irritant contact dermatitis due to cyclohexane
     Irritant contact dermatitis due to ester
     Irritant contact dermatitis due to glycol
     Irritant contact dermatitis due to hydrocarbon
     Irritant contact dermatitis due to ketone

L24.3   Irritant contact dermatitis due to cosmetics

L24.4   Irritant contact dermatitis due to drugs in contact with skin
     Use additional code for adverse effect, if applicable, to identify
         drug (T36-T50 with fifth or sixth character 5)

L24.5   Irritant contact dermatitis due to other chemical products
     Irritant contact dermatitis due to cement
     Irritant contact dermatitis due to insecticide
     Irritant contact dermatitis due to plastic
     Irritant contact dermatitis due to rubber

L24.6   Irritant contact dermatitis due to food in contact with skin
     EXCLUDES 2   *dermatitis due to ingested food (L27.2)*

L24.7   Irritant contact dermatitis due to plants, except food
     EXCLUDES 2   *allergy NOS to pollen (J30.1)*

☑5ᵗʰ **L24.8   Irritant contact dermatitis due to** other agents

     L24.81   Irritant contact dermatitis due to metals
          Irritant contact dermatitis due to chromium
          Irritant contact dermatitis due to nickel

     L24.89   Irritant contact dermatitis due to other agents
          Irritant contact dermatitis due to dyes

L24.9   Irritant contact dermatitis, unspecified cause ▽
     Irritant contact eczema NOS

☑4ᵗʰ **L25   Unspecified contact dermatitis**
     EXCLUDES 1   *allergic contact dermatitis (L23.-)*
                allergy NOS (T78.40)
                dermatitis NOS (L30.9)
                irritant contact dermatitis (L24.-)
     EXCLUDES 2   *dermatitis due to ingested substances (L27.-)*
                dermatitis of eyelid (H01.1-)
                eczema of external ear (H60.5-)
                perioral dermatitis (L71.0)
                radiation-related disorders of the skin and subcutaneous tissue
                  (L55-L59)

L25.0   Unspecified contact dermatitis due to cosmetics   ▽

L25.1   Unspecified contact dermatitis due to drugs in contact   ▽
     with skin
     Use additional code for adverse effect, if applicable, to identify
         drug (T36-T50 with fifth or sixth character 5)
     EXCLUDES 2   *dermatitis due to ingested drugs and medicaments*
                  (L27.0-L27.1)

L25.2   Unspecified contact dermatitis due to dyes   ▽

L25.3   Unspecified contact dermatitis due to other chemical   ▽
     products
     Unspecified contact dermatitis due to cement
     Unspecified contact dermatitis due to insecticide

L25.4   Unspecified contact dermatitis due to food in contact with   ▽
     skin
     EXCLUDES 2   *dermatitis due to ingested food (L27.2)*

L25.5   Unspecified contact dermatitis due to plants, except food   ▽
     EXCLUDES 1   *nettle rash (L50.9)*
     EXCLUDES 2   *allergy NOS due to pollen (J30.1)*

L25.8   Unspecified contact dermatitis due to other agents   ▽

L25.9   Unspecified contact dermatitis, unspecified cause   ▽
     Contact dermatitis (occupational) NOS
     Contact eczema (occupational) NOS

☑4ᵗʰ **L26   Exfoliative dermatitis**
     Hebra's pityriasis
     EXCLUDES 1   *Ritter's disease (L00)*

☑4ᵗʰ **L27   Dermatitis due to substances taken internally**
     EXCLUDES 1   *allergy NOS (T78.40)*
     EXCLUDES 2   *adverse food reaction, except dermatitis (T78.0-T78.1)*
                contact dermatitis (L23-L25)
                drug photoallergic response (L56.1)
                drug phototoxic response (L56.0)
                urticaria (L50.-)

**L27.0   Generalized skin eruption due to drugs and medicaments
     taken internally**
     Use additional code for adverse effect, if applicable, to identify
         drug (T36-T50 with fifth or sixth character 5)

**L27.1   Localized skin eruption due to drugs and medicaments
     taken internally**
     Use additional code for adverse effect, if applicable, to identify
         drug (T36-T50 with fifth or sixth character 5)

L27.2   Dermatitis due to ingested food
     EXCLUDES 2   *dermatitis due to food in contact with skin (L23.6, L24.6,*
                L25.4)

L27.8   Dermatitis due to other substances taken internally

L27.9   Dermatitis due to unspecified substance taken internally   ▽

☑4ᵗʰ **L28   Lichen simplex chronicus and prurigo**

L28.0   Lichen simplex chronicus
     Circumscribed neurodermatitis
     Lichen NOS

L28.1   Prurigo nodularis

L28.2   Other prurigo
     Prurigo NOS
     Prurigo Hebra
     Prurigo mitis
     Urticaria papulosa

☑4ᵗʰ **L29   Pruritus**
     EXCLUDES 1   *neurotic excoriation (L98.1)*
                psychogenic pruritus (F45.8)

L29.0   Pruritus ani

L29.1   Pruritus scroti   ♂

L29.2   Pruritus vulvae   ♀

L29.3   Anogenital pruritus, unspecified   ▽

L29.8   Other pruritus

L29.9   Pruritus, unspecified   ▽
     Itch NOS

☑4ᵗʰ **L30   Other and unspecified dermatitis**
     EXCLUDES 2   *contact dermatitis (L23-L25)*
                dry skin dermatitis (L85.3)
                small plaque parapsoriasis (L41.3)
                stasis dermatitis (I83.1-.2)

L30.0   Nummular dermatitis

L30.1   Dyshidrosis [pompholyx]

L30.2   Cutaneous autosensitization
     Candidid [levurid]
     Dermatophytid
     Eczematid

L30.3   Infective dermatitis
     Infectious eczematoid dermatitis

L30.4   Erythema intertrigo

L30.5   Pityriasis alba

L30.8   Other specified dermatitis

L30.9   Dermatitis, unspecified   ▽
     Eczema NOS

Papulosquamous disorders (L40-L45)

☑4ᵗʰ **L40   Psoriasis**

L40.0   Psoriasis vulgaris
     Nummular psoriasis
     Plaque psoriasis

L40.1   Generalized pustular psoriasis
     Impetigo herpetiformis
     Von Zumbusch's disease

L40.2   Acrodermatitis continua

L40.3   Pustulosis palmaris et plantaris

L40.4   Guttate psoriasis

Chapter 12. Diseases of the Skin and Subcutaneous Tissue

L23.9–L40.4

☑ Add'l Character Required   ☑x7ᵗʰ Placeholder Alert   RUG IV Special Care High Dx   RUG IV Clinically Complex Dx   RUG IV Special Care Low Dx   Manifestation Code   Other Specified Code   ▽Unspecified Code

ICD-10-CM 2016   661

✓5ᵗʰ **L40.5** Arthropathic psoriasis
L40.50 Arthropathic psoriasis, unspecified ▽
L40.51 Distal interphalangeal psoriatic arthropathy
L40.52 Psoriatic arthritis mutilans
L40.53 Psoriatic spondylitis
L40.54 Psoriatic juvenile arthropathy
L40.59 Other psoriatic arthropathy
L40.8 Other psoriasis
Flexural psoriasis
L40.9 Psoriasis, unspecified ▽

✓4ᵗʰ **L41** Parapsoriasis
EXCLUDES 1 poikiloderma vasculare atrophicans (L94.5)
L41.0 Pityriasis lichenoides et varioliformis acuta
Mucha-Habermann disease
L41.1 Pityriasis lichenoides chronica
L41.3 Small plaque parapsoriasis
L41.4 Large plaque parapsoriasis
L41.5 Retiform parapsoriasis
L41.8 Other parapsoriasis
L41.9 Parapsoriasis, unspecified ▽

L42 Pityriasis rosea

✓4ᵗʰ **L43** Lichen planus
EXCLUDES 1 lichen planopilaris (L66.1)
L43.0 Hypertrophic lichen planus
L43.1 Bullous lichen planus
L43.2 Lichenoid drug reaction
Use additional code for adverse effect, if applicable, to identify drug (T36-T50 with fifth or sixth character 5)
L43.3 Subacute (active) lichen planus
Lichen planus tropicus
L43.8 Other lichen planus
L43.9 Lichen planus, unspecified ▽

✓4ᵗʰ **L44** Other papulosquamous disorders
L44.0 Pityriasis rubra pilaris
L44.1 Lichen nitidus
L44.2 Lichen striatus
L44.3 Lichen ruber moniliformis
L44.4 Infantile papular acrodermatitis [Gianotti-Crosti] ℗
L44.8 Other specified papulosquamous disorders
L44.9 Papulosquamous disorder, unspecified ▽

L45 *Papulosquamous disorders in diseases classified elsewhere*
Code first underlying disease

Urticaria and erythema (L49-L54)
EXCLUDES 1 Lyme disease (A69.2-)
rosacea (L71.-)

✓4ᵗʰ **L49** Exfoliation due to erythematous conditions according to extent of body surface involved
Code first erythematous condition causing exfoliation, such as:
Ritter's disease (L00)
(Staphylococcal) scalded skin syndrom (L00)
Stevens-Johnson syndrome (L51.1)
Stevens-Johnson syndrome-toxic epidermal necrolysis overlap syndrome (L51.3)
toxic epidermal necrolysis (L51.2)
L49.0 Exfoliation due to erythematous condition involving less than 10 percent of body surface
Exfoliation due to erythematous condition NOS
L49.1 Exfoliation due to erythematous condition involving 10-19 percent of body surface
L49.2 Exfoliation due to erythematous condition involving 20-29 percent of body surface
L49.3 Exfoliation due to erythematous condition involving 30-39 percent of body surface
L49.4 Exfoliation due to erythematous condition involving 40-49 percent of body surface
L49.5 Exfoliation due to erythematous condition involving 50-59 percent of body surface
L49.6 Exfoliation due to erythematous condition involving 60-69 percent of body surface
L49.7 Exfoliation due to erythematous condition involving 70-79 percent of body surface

L49.8 Exfoliation due to erythematous condition involving 80-89 percent of body surface
L49.9 Exfoliation due to erythematous condition involving 90 or more percent of body surface

✓4ᵗʰ **L50** Urticaria
EXCLUDES 1 allergic contact dermatitis (L23.-)
angioneurotic edema (T78.3)
giant urticaria (T78.3)
hereditary angio-edema (D84.1)
Quincke's edema (T78.3)
serum urticaria (T80.6-)
solar urticaria (L56.3)
urticaria neonatorum (P83.8)
urticaria papulosa (L28.2)
urticaria pigmentosa (Q82.2)
L50.0 Allergic urticaria
L50.1 Idiopathic urticaria
L50.2 Urticaria due to cold and heat
L50.3 Dermatographic urticaria
L50.4 Vibratory urticaria
L50.5 Cholinergic urticaria
L50.6 Contact urticaria
L50.8 Other urticaria
Chronic urticaria
Recurrent periodic urticaria
L50.9 Urticaria, unspecified ▽

✓4ᵗʰ **L51** Erythema multiforme
Use additional code for adverse effect, if applicable, to identify drug (T36-T50 with fifth or sixth character 5)
Use additional code to identify associated manifestations, such as:
arthropathy associated with dermatological disorders (M14.8-)
conjunctival edema (H11.42)
conjunctivitis (H10.22-)
corneal scars and opacities (H17.-)
corneal ulcer (H16.0-)
edema of eyelid (H02.84)
inflammation of eyelid (H01.8)
keratoconjunctivitis sicca (H16.22-)
mechanical lagophthalmos (H02.22-)
stomatitis (K12.-)
symblepharon (H11.23-)
Use additional code to identify percentage of skin exfoliation (L49.-)
EXCLUDES 1 staphylococcal scalded skin syndrome (L00)
Ritter's disease (L00)
L51.0 Nonbullous erythema multiforme
L51.1 Stevens-Johnson syndrome
L51.2 Toxic epidermal necrolysis [Lyell]
L51.3 Stevens-Johnson syndrome-toxic epidermal necrolysis overlap syndrome
SJS-TEN overlap syndrome
L51.8 Other erythema multiforme
L51.9 Erythema multiforme, unspecified ▽
Erythema iris
Erythema multiforme major NOS
Erythema multiforme minor NOS
Herpes iris

L52 Erythema nodosum
EXCLUDES 1 tuberculous erythema nodosum (A18.4)

✓4ᵗʰ **L53** Other erythematous conditions
EXCLUDES 1 erythema ab igne (L59.0)
erythema due to external agents in contact with skin (L23-L25)
erythema intertrigo (L30.4)
L53.0 Toxic erythema
Code first poisoning due to drug or toxin, if applicable (T36-T65 with fifth or sixth character 1-4 or 6)
Use additional code for adverse effect, if applicable, to identify drug (T36-T50 with fifth or sixth character 5)
EXCLUDES 1 neonatal erythema toxicum (P83.1)
L53.1 Erythema annulare centrifugum
L53.2 Erythema marginatum
L53.3 Other chronic figurate erythema
L53.8 Other specified erythematous conditions
L53.9 Erythematous condition, unspecified ▽
Erythema NOS
Erythroderma NOS

L54 *Erythema in diseases classified elsewhere*
Code first underlying disease

Ⓝ Newborn   ℗ Pediatric   Ⓜ Maternity   Ⓐ Adult   **RIC** RIC Dx   **NCDx** Noncancer Dx   **PDx** Primary Dx   **CC** RIC CC Condition   ▶◀ Revised Text   ● New Code   ▲ Revised Code Title

662   ICD-10-CM 2016

Chapter 12. Diseases of the Skin and Subcutaneous Tissue

Radiation-related disorders of the skin and subcutaneous tissue (L55-L59)

✓4ᵗʰ L55   Sunburn
- **L55.0   Sunburn of** first degree
- **L55.1   Sunburn of** second degree
- **L55.2   Sunburn of** third degree
- **L55.9   Sunburn, unspecified**   ▽

✓4ᵗʰ L56   Other acute skin changes due to ultraviolet radiation
Use additional code to identify the source of the ultraviolet radiation (W89, X32)
- **L56.0   Drug phototoxic response**
 Use additional code for adverse effect, if applicable, to identify drug (T36-T50 with fifth or sixth character 5)
- **L56.1   Drug photoallergic response**
 Use additional code for adverse effect, if applicable, to identify drug (T36-T50 with fifth or sixth character 5)
- **L56.2   Photocontact dermatitis [berloque dermatitis]**
- **L56.3   Solar urticaria**
- **L56.4   Polymorphous light eruption**
- **L56.5   Disseminated superficial actinic porokeratosis (DSAP)**
- **L56.8   Other specified acute skin changes due to ultraviolet radiation**
- **L56.9   Acute skin change due to ultraviolet radiation, unspecified** ▽

✓4ᵗʰ L57   Skin changes due to chronic exposure to nonionizing radiation
Use additional code to identify the source of the ultraviolet radiation (W89, X32)
- **L57.0   Actinic keratosis**
 Keratosis NOS
 Senile keratosis
 Solar keratosis
- **L57.1   Actinic reticuloid**
- **L57.2   Cutis rhomboidalis nuchae**
- **L57.3   Poikiloderma of Civatte**
- **L57.4   Cutis laxa senilis**
 Elastosis senilis
- **L57.5   Actinic granuloma**
- **L57.8   Other skin changes due to chronic exposure to nonionizing radiation**
 Farmer's skin
 Sailor's skin
 Solar dermatitis
- **L57.9   Skin changes due to chronic exposure to nonionizing radiation, unspecified** ▽

✓4ᵗʰ L58   Radiodermatitis
Use additional code to identify the source of the radiation (W88, W90)
- **L58.0   Acute radiodermatitis**
- **L58.1   Chronic radiodermatitis**
- **L58.9   Radiodermatitis, unspecified**   ▽

✓4ᵗʰ L59   Other disorders of skin and subcutaneous tissue related to radiation
- **L59.0   Erythema ab igne [dermatitis ab igne]**
- **L59.8   Other specified disorders of the skin and subcutaneous tissue related to radiation**
- **L59.9   Disorder of the skin and subcutaneous tissue related to radiation, unspecified** ▽

Disorders of skin appendages (L60-L75)
EXCLUDES 1   congenital malformations of integument (Q84.-)

✓4ᵗʰ L60   Nail disorders
EXCLUDES 2   clubbing of nails (R68.3)
 onychia and paronychia (L03.0-)
- **L60.0   Ingrowing nail**
- **L60.1   Onycholysis**
- **L60.2   Onychogryphosis**
- **L60.3   Nail dystrophy**
- **L60.4   Beau's lines**
- **L60.5   Yellow nail syndrome**
- **L60.8   Other nail disorders**
- **L60.9   Nail disorder, unspecified**   ▽

L62   Nail disorders in diseases classified elsewhere
Code first underlying disease, such as:
 pachydermoperiostosis (M89.4-)

✓4ᵗʰ L63   Alopecia areata
- **L63.0   Alopecia (capitis)** totalis
- **L63.1   Alopecia** universalis
- **L63.2   Ophiasis**
- **L63.8   Other alopecia areata**
- **L63.9   Alopecia areata, unspecified**   ▽

✓4ᵗʰ L64   Androgenic alopecia
INCLUDES   male-pattern baldness
- **L64.0   Drug-induced androgenic alopecia**
 Use additional code for adverse effect, if applicable, to identify drug (T36-T50 with fifth or sixth character 5)
- **L64.8   Other androgenic alopecia**
- **L64.9   Androgenic alopecia, unspecified**   ▽

✓4ᵗʰ L65   Other nonscarring hair loss
Use additional code for adverse effect, if applicable, to identify drug (T36-T50 with fifth or sixth character 5)
EXCLUDES 1   trichotillomania (F63.3)
- **L65.0   Telogen effluvium**
- **L65.1   Anagen effluvium**
- **L65.2   Alopecia mucinosa**
- **L65.8   Other specified nonscarring hair loss**
- **L65.9   Nonscarring hair loss, unspecified**   ▽
 Alopecia NOS

✓4ᵗʰ L66   Cicatricial alopecia [scarring hair loss]
- **L66.0   Pseudopelade**
- **L66.1   Lichen planopilaris**
 Follicular lichen planus
- **L66.2   Folliculitis decalvans**
- **L66.3   Perifolliculitis capitis abscedens**
- **L66.4   Folliculitis ulerythematosa reticulata**
- **L66.8   Other cicatricial alopecia**
 AHA: 2015, 1Q, 19
- **L66.9   Cicatricial alopecia, unspecified**   ▽

✓4ᵗʰ L67   Hair color and hair shaft abnormalities
EXCLUDES 1   monilethrix (Q84.1)
 pili annulati (Q84.1)
 telogen effluvium (L65.0)
- **L67.0   Trichorrhexis nodosa**
- **L67.1   Variations in hair color**
 Canities
 Greyness, hair (premature)
 Heterochromia of hair
 Poliosis circumscripta, acquired
 Poliosis NOS
- **L67.8   Other hair color and hair shaft abnormalities**
 Fragilitas crinium
- **L67.9   Hair color and hair shaft abnormality, unspecified**   ▽

✓4ᵗʰ L68   Hypertrichosis
INCLUDES   excess hair
EXCLUDES 1   congenital hypertrichosis (Q84.2)
 persistent lanugo (Q84.2)
- **L68.0   Hirsutism**
- **L68.1   Acquired hypertrichosis lanuginosa**
- **L68.2   Localized hypertrichosis**
- **L68.3   Polytrichia**
- **L68.8   Other hypertrichosis**
- **L68.9   Hypertrichosis, unspecified**   ▽

✓4ᵗʰ L70   Acne
EXCLUDES 2   acne keloid (L73.0)
- **L70.0   Acne vulgaris**
- **L70.1   Acne conglobata**
- **L70.2   Acne varioliformis**
 Acne necrotica miliaris
- **L70.3   Acne tropica**
- **L70.4   Infantile acne**   Ⓟ
- **L70.5   Acné excoriée des jeunes filles**
 Picker's acne
- **L70.8   Other acne**
- **L70.9   Acne, unspecified**   ▽

Chapter 12. Diseases of the Skin and Subcutaneous Tissue

L55–L70.9

Chapter 12. Diseases of the Skin and Subcutaneous Tissue

✓4th **L71 Rosacea**
Use additional code for adverse effect, if applicable, to identify drug (T36-T50 with fifth or sixth character 5)

     L71.0 Perioral dermatitis
     L71.1 Rhinophyma
     L71.8 Other rosacea
     L71.9 Rosacea, unspecified ▽

✓4th **L72 Follicular cysts of skin and subcutaneous tissue**
     L72.0 Epidermal cyst
     ✓5th **L72.1 Pilar and trichodermal cyst**
         L72.11 Pilar cyst
         L72.12 Trichodermal cyst
             Trichilemmal (proliferating) cyst
     L72.2 Steatocystoma multiplex
     L72.3 Sebaceous cyst
         EXCLUDES 2   pilar cyst (L72.11)
                 trichilemmal (proliferating) cyst (L72.12)
     L72.8 Other follicular cysts of the skin and subcutaneous tissue
     L72.9 Follicular cyst of the skin and subcutaneous tissue, unspecified ▽

✓4th **L73 Other follicular disorders**
     L73.0 Acne keloid
     L73.1 Pseudofolliculitis barbae
     L73.2 Hidradenitis suppurativa
     L73.8 Other specified follicular disorders
         Sycosis barbae
     L73.9 Follicular disorder, unspecified ▽

✓4th **L74 Eccrine sweat disorders**
     EXCLUDES 2   generalized hyperhidrosis (R61)
     L74.0 Miliaria rubra
     L74.1 Miliaria crystallina
     L74.2 Miliaria profunda
         Miliaria tropicalis
     L74.3 Miliaria, unspecified ▽
     L74.4 Anhidrosis
         Hypohidrosis
     ✓5th **L74.5 Focal hyperhidrosis**
         ✓6th **L74.51 Primary focal hyperhidrosis**
             L74.510 Primary focal hyperhidrosis, axilla
             L74.511 Primary focal hyperhidrosis, face
             L74.512 Primary focal hyperhidrosis, palms
             L74.513 Primary focal hyperhidrosis, soles
             L74.519 Primary focal hyperhidrosis, unspecified ▽
         L74.52 Secondary focal hyperhidrosis
             Frey's syndrome
     L74.8 Other eccrine sweat disorders
     L74.9 Eccrine sweat disorder, unspecified ▽
         Sweat gland disorder NOS

✓4th **L75 Apocrine sweat disorders**
     EXCLUDES 1   dyshidrosis (L30.1)
                 hidradenitis suppurativa (L73.2)
     L75.0 Bromhidrosis
     L75.1 Chromhidrosis
     L75.2 Apocrine miliaria
         Fox-Fordyce disease
     L75.8 Other apocrine sweat disorders
     L75.9 Apocrine sweat disorder, unspecified ▽

Intraoperative and postprocedural complications of skin and subcutaneous tissue (L76)

✓4th **L76 Intraoperative and postprocedural complications of skin and subcutaneous tissue**
     ✓5th **L76.0 Intraoperative hemorrhage and hematoma of skin and subcutaneous tissue complicating a procedure**
         EXCLUDES 1   intraoperative hemorrhage and hematoma of skin and subcutaneous tissue due to accidental puncture and laceration during a procedure (L76.1-)
         L76.01 Intraoperative hemorrhage and hematoma of skin and subcutaneous tissue complicating a dermatologic procedure

L76.02 Intraoperative hemorrhage and hematoma of skin and subcutaneous tissue complicating other procedure

✓5th **L76.1 Accidental puncture and laceration of skin and subcutaneous tissue during a procedure**
     L76.11 Accidental puncture and laceration of skin and subcutaneous tissue during a dermatologic procedure
     L76.12 Accidental puncture and laceration of skin and subcutaneous tissue during other procedure

✓5th **L76.2 Postprocedural hemorrhage and hematoma of skin and subcutaneous tissue following a procedure**
     L76.21 Postprocedural hemorrhage and hematoma of skin and subcutaneous tissue following a dermatologic procedure
     L76.22 Postprocedural hemorrhage and hematoma of skin and subcutaneous tissue following other procedure

✓5th **L76.8 Other intraoperative and postprocedural complications of skin and subcutaneous tissue**
     Use additional code, if applicable, to further specify disorder
     L76.81 Other intraoperative complications of skin and subcutaneous tissue
     L76.82 Other postprocedural complications of skin and subcutaneous tissue

Other disorders of the skin and subcutaneous tissue (L80-L99)

L80 Vitiligo
     EXCLUDES 2   vitiligo of eyelids (H02.73-)
                 vitiligo of vulva (N90.89)

✓4th **L81 Other disorders of pigmentation**
     EXCLUDES 1   birthmark NOS (Q82.5)
                 Peutz-Jeghers syndrome (Q85.8)
     EXCLUDES 2   nevus—see Alphabetical Index
     L81.0 Postinflammatory hyperpigmentation
     L81.1 Chloasma
     L81.2 Freckles
     L81.3 Café au lait spots
     L81.4 Other melanin hyperpigmentation
         Lentigo
     L81.5 Leukoderma, not elsewhere classified
     L81.6 Other disorders of diminished melanin formation
     L81.7 Pigmented purpuric dermatosis
         Angioma serpiginosum
     L81.8 Other specified disorders of pigmentation
         Iron pigmentation
         Tattoo pigmentation
     L81.9 Disorder of pigmentation, unspecified ▽

✓4th **L82 Seborrheic keratosis**
     INCLUDES   dermatosis papulosa nigra
                 Leser-Trélat disease
     EXCLUDES 2   seborrheic dermatitis (L21.-)
     L82.0 Inflamed seborrheic keratosis
     L82.1 Other seborrheic keratosis
         Seborrheic keratosis NOS

L83 Acanthosis nigricans
     Confluent and reticulated papillomatosis

L84 Corns and callosities
     Callus
     Clavus

✓4th **L85 Other epidermal thickening**
     EXCLUDES 2   hypertrophic disorders of the skin (L91.-)
     L85.0 Acquired ichthyosis
         EXCLUDES 1   congenital ichthyosis (Q80.-)
     L85.1 Acquired keratosis [keratoderma] palmaris et plantaris
         EXCLUDES 1   inherited keratosis palmaris et plantaris (Q82.8)
     L85.2 Keratosis punctata (palmaris et plantaris)
     L85.3 Xerosis cutis
         Dry skin dermatitis
     L85.8 Other specified epidermal thickening
         Cutaneous horn
     L85.9 Epidermal thickening, unspecified ▽

N Newborn   P Pediatric   M Maternity   A Adult   RIC RIC Dx   NCDx Noncancer Dx   PDx Primary Dx   CC RIC CC Condition   ▶◀ Revised Text   ● New Code   ▲ Revised Code Title

ICD-10-CM 2016

664

L71–L85.9

L86   *Keratoderma in diseases classified elsewhere*
> *Code first underlying disease, such as:*
> *Reiter's disease (M02.3-)*
> **EXCLUDES 1**   *gonococcal keratoderma (A54.89)*
> *gonococcal keratosis (A54.89)*
> *keratoderma due to vitamin A deficiency (E50.8)*
> *keratosis due to vitamin A deficiency (E50.8)*
> *xeroderma due to vitamin A deficiency (E50.8)*

✓4ᵗʰ L87   **Transepidermal elimination disorders**
> **EXCLUDES 1**   *granuloma annulare (perforating) (L92.0)*

L87.0   **Keratosis follicularis et parafollicularis in cutem penetrans**
> Hyperkeratosis follicularis penetrans
> Kyrle disease

L87.1   **Reactive perforating collagenosis**

L87.2   **Elastosis perforans serpiginosa**

L87.8   **Other transepidermal elimination disorders**

L87.9   **Transepidermal elimination disorder, unspecified**   ▽

L88   **Pyoderma gangrenosum**
> Phagedenic pyoderma
> **EXCLUDES 1**   *dermatitis gangrenosa (L08.0)*

✓4ᵗʰ L89   **Pressure ulcer**
> Bed sore
> Decubitus ulcer
> Plaster ulcer
> Pressure area
> Pressure sore
> Code first any associated gangrene (I96)
> **EXCLUDES 2**   *decubitus (trophic) ulcer of cervix (uteri) (N86)*
> *diabetic ulcers (E08.621, E08.622, E09.621, E09.622, E10.621,*
> *E10.622, E11.621, E11.622, E13.621, E13.622)*
> *non-pressure chronic ulcer of skin (L97.-)*
> *skin infections (L00-L08)*
> *varicose ulcer (I83.0, I83.2)*

✓5ᵗʰ L89.0   **Pressure ulcer of elbow**

   ✓6ᵗʰ L89.00   **Pressure ulcer of unspecified elbow**

      L89.000   **Pressure ulcer of unspecified elbow,**   ▽
         unstageable

      L89.001   **Pressure ulcer of unspecified elbow,**   ▽
         stage 1
> Healing pressure ulcer of unspecified
>   elbow, stage 1
> Pressure pre-ulcer skin changes limited to
>   persistent focal edema, unspecified
>   elbow

      L89.002   **Pressure ulcer of unspecified elbow,**   ▽
         stage 2
> Healing pressure ulcer of unspecified
>   elbow, stage 2
> Pressure ulcer with abrasion, blister, partial
>   thickness skin loss involving epidermis
>   and/or dermis, unspecified elbow

      L89.003   **Pressure ulcer of unspecified elbow,**   ▽
         stage 3
> Healing pressure ulcer of unspecified
>   elbow, stage 3
> Pressure ulcer with full thickness skin loss
>   involving damage or necrosis of
>   subcutaneous tissue, unspecified
>   elbow

      L89.004   **Pressure ulcer of unspecified elbow,**   ▽
         stage 4
> Healing pressure ulcer of unspecified
>   elbow, stage 4
> Pressure ulcer with necrosis of soft tissues
>   through to underlying muscle,
>   tendon, or bone, unspecified elbow

      L89.009   **Pressure ulcer of unspecified elbow,**   ▽
         unspecified stage
> Healing pressure ulcer of elbow NOS
> Healing pressure ulcer of unspecified,
>   elbow, unspecified stage

   ✓6ᵗʰ L89.01   **Pressure ulcer of right elbow**

      L89.010   **Pressure ulcer of right elbow, unstageable**

      L89.011   **Pressure ulcer of right elbow, stage 1**
> Healing pressure ulcer of right elbow,
>   stage 1
> Pressure pre-ulcer skin changes limited to
>   persistent focal edema, right elbow

      L89.012   **Pressure ulcer of right elbow, stage 2**
> Healing pressure ulcer of right elbow,
>   stage 2
> Pressure ulcer with abrasion, blister, partial
>   thickness skin loss involving epidermis
>   and/or dermis, right elbow

      L89.013   **Pressure ulcer of right elbow, stage 3**
> Healing pressure ulcer of right elbow,
>   stage 3
> Pressure ulcer with full thickness skin loss
>   involving damage or necrosis of
>   subcutaneous tissue, right elbow

      L89.014   **Pressure ulcer of right elbow, stage 4**
> Healing pressure ulcer of right elbow,
>   stage 4
> Pressure ulcer with necrosis of soft tissues
>   through to underlying muscle,
>   tendon, or bone, right elbow

      L89.019   **Pressure ulcer of right elbow,**   ▽
         unspecified stage
> Healing pressure right of elbow NOS
> Healing pressure ulcer of unspecified
>   elbow, unspecified stage

   ✓6ᵗʰ L89.02   **Pressure ulcer of left elbow**

      L89.020   **Pressure ulcer of left elbow, unstageable**

      L89.021   **Pressure ulcer of left elbow, stage 1**
> Healing pressure ulcer of left elbow, stage 1
> Pressure pre-ulcer skin changes limited to
>   persistent focal edema, left elbow

      L89.022   **Pressure ulcer of left elbow, stage 2**
> Healing pressure ulcer of left elbow, stage 2
> Pressure ulcer with abrasion, blister, partial
>   thickness skin loss involving epidermis
>   and/or dermis, left elbow

      L89.023   **Pressure ulcer of left elbow, stage 3**
> Healing pressure ulcer of left elbow, stage 3
> Pressure ulcer with full thickness skin loss
>   involving damage or necrosis of
>   subcutaneous tissue, left elbow

      L89.024   **Pressure ulcer of left elbow, stage 4**
> Healing pressure ulcer of left elbow, stage 4
> Pressure ulcer with necrosis of soft tissues
>   through to underlying muscle,
>   tendon, or bone, left elbow

      L89.029   **Pressure ulcer of left elbow,**   ▽
         unspecified stage
> Healing pressure ulcer of left of elbow NOS
> Healing pressure ulcer of unspecified
>   elbow, unspecified stage

✓5ᵗʰ L89.1   **Pressure ulcer of back**

   ✓6ᵗʰ L89.10   **Pressure ulcer of unspecified part of back**

      L89.100   **Pressure ulcer of unspecified part of**   ▽
         back, unstageable

      L89.101   **Pressure ulcer of unspecified part of**   ▽
         back, stage 1
> Healing pressure ulcer of unspecified part
>   of back, stage 1
> Pressure pre-ulcer skin changes limited to
>   persistent focal edema, unspecified
>   part of back

      L89.102   **Pressure ulcer of unspecified part of**   ▽
         back, stage 2
> Healing pressure ulcer of unspecified part
>   of back, stage 2
> Pressure ulcer with abrasion, blister, partial
>   thickness skin loss involving epidermis
>   and/or dermis, unspecified part of
>   back

      L89.103   **Pressure ulcer of unspecified part of**   ▽
         back, stage 3
> Healing pressure ulcer of unspecified part
>   of back, stage 3
> Pressure ulcer with full thickness skin loss
>   involving damage or necrosis of
>   subcutaneous tissue, unspecified part
>   of back

      L89.104   **Pressure ulcer of unspecified part of**   ▽
         back, stage 4
> Healing pressure ulcer of unspecified part
>   of back, stage 4
> Pressure ulcer with necrosis of soft tissues
>   through to underlying muscle, tendon,
>   or bone, unspecified part of back

✓ Add'l Character Required   ✓7ᵗʰ Placeholder Alert   RUG IV Special Care High Dx   RUG IV Clinically Complex Dx   RUG IV Special Care Low Dx   Manifestation Code   Other Specified Code   ▽ Unspecified Code

L89.109 **Pressure ulcer of unspecified part of back, unspecified stage** ▽
   Healing pressure ulcer of unspecified part of back NOS
   Healing pressure ulcer of unspecified part of back, unspecified stage

✓6ᵗʰ **L89.11** **Pressure ulcer of** right upper back
   Pressure ulcer of right shoulder blade

L89.110 **Pressure ulcer of right upper back,** unstageable

L89.111 **Pressure ulcer of right upper back,** stage 1
   Healing pressure ulcer of right upper back, stage 1
   Pressure pre-ulcer skin changes limited to persistent focal edema, right upper back

L89.112 **Pressure ulcer of right upper back,** stage 2
   Healing pressure ulcer of right upper back, stage 2
   Pressure ulcer with abrasion, blister, partial thickness skin loss involving epidermis and/or dermis, right upper back

L89.113 **Pressure ulcer of right upper back,** stage 3
   Healing pressure ulcer of right upper back, stage 3
   Pressure ulcer with full thickness skin loss involving damage or necrosis of subcutaneous tissue, right upper back

L89.114 **Pressure ulcer of right upper back,** stage 4
   Healing pressure ulcer of right upper back, stage 4
   Pressure ulcer with necrosis of soft tissues through to underlying muscle, tendon, or bone, right upper back

L89.119 **Pressure ulcer of right upper back, unspecified stage** ▽
   Healing pressure ulcer of right upper back NOS
   Healing pressure ulcer of right upper back, unspecified stage

✓6ᵗʰ **L89.12** **Pressure ulcer of** left upper back
   Pressure ulcer of left shoulder blade

L89.120 **Pressure ulcer of left upper back,** unstageable

L89.121 **Pressure ulcer of left upper back,** stage 1
   Healing pressure ulcer of left upper back, stage 1
   Pressure pre-ulcer skin changes limited to persistent focal edema, left upper back

L89.122 **Pressure ulcer of left upper back,** stage 2
   Healing pressure ulcer of left upper back, stage 2
   Pressure ulcer with abrasion, blister, partial thickness skin loss involving epidermis and/or dermis, left upper back

L89.123 **Pressure ulcer of left upper back,** stage 3
   Healing pressure ulcer of left upper back, stage 3
   Pressure ulcer with full thickness skin loss involving damage or necrosis of subcutaneous tissue, left upper back

L89.124 **Pressure ulcer of left upper back,** stage 4
   Healing pressure ulcer of left upper back, stage 4
   Pressure ulcer with necrosis of soft tissues through to underlying muscle, tendon, or bone, left upper back

L89.129 **Pressure ulcer of left upper back, unspecified stage** ▽
   Healing pressure ulcer of left upper back NOS
   Healing pressure ulcer of left upper back, unspecified stage

✓6ᵗʰ **L89.13** **Pressure ulcer of** right lower back

L89.130 **Pressure ulcer of right lower back,** unstageable

L89.131 **Pressure ulcer of right lower back,** stage 1
   Healing pressure ulcer of right lower back, stage 1
   Pressure pre-ulcer skin changes limited to persistent focal edema, right lower back

L89.132 **Pressure ulcer of right lower back,** stage 2
   Healing pressure ulcer of right lower back, stage 2
   Pressure ulcer with abrasion, blister, partial thickness skin loss involving epidermis and/or dermis, right lower back

L89.133 **Pressure ulcer of right lower back,** stage 3
   Healing pressure ulcer of right lower back, stage 3
   Pressure ulcer with full thickness skin loss involving damage or necrosis of subcutaneous tissue, right lower back

L89.134 **Pressure ulcer of right lower back,** stage 4
   Healing pressure ulcer of right lower back, stage 4
   Pressure ulcer with necrosis of soft tissues through to underlying muscle, tendon, or bone, right lower back

L89.139 **Pressure ulcer of right lower back, unspecified stage** ▽
   Healing pressure ulcer of right lower back NOS
   Healing pressure ulcer of right lower back, unspecified stage

✓6ᵗʰ **L89.14** **Pressure ulcer of** left lower back

L89.140 **Pressure ulcer of left lower back,** unstageable

L89.141 **Pressure ulcer of left lower back,** stage 1
   Healing pressure ulcer of left lower back, stage 1
   Pressure pre-ulcer skin changes limited to persistent focal edema, left lower back

L89.142 **Pressure ulcer of left lower back,** stage 2
   Healing pressure ulcer of left lower back, stage 2
   Pressure ulcer with abrasion, blister, partial thickness skin loss involving epidermis and/or dermis, left lower back

L89.143 **Pressure ulcer of left lower back,** stage 3
   Healing pressure ulcer of left lower back, stage 3
   Pressure ulcer with full thickness skin loss involving damage or necrosis of subcutaneous tissue, left lower back

L89.144 **Pressure ulcer of left lower back,** stage 4
   Healing pressure ulcer of left lower back, stage 4
   Pressure ulcer with necrosis of soft tissues through to underlying muscle, tendon, or bone, left lower back

L89.149 **Pressure ulcer of left lower back, unspecified stage** ▽
   Healing pressure ulcer of left lower back NOS
   Healing pressure ulcer of left lower back, unspecified stage

✓6ᵗʰ **L89.15** **Pressure ulcer of** sacral region
   Pressure ulcer of coccyx
   Pressure ulcer of tailbone

L89.150 **Pressure ulcer of sacral region,** unstageable

L89.151 **Pressure ulcer of sacral region,** stage 1
   Healing pressure ulcer of sacral region, stage 1
   Pressure pre-ulcer skin changes limited to persistent focal edema, sacral region

L89.152 **Pressure ulcer of sacral region,** stage 2
   Healing pressure ulcer of sacral region, stage 2
   Pressure ulcer with abrasion, blister, partial thickness skin loss involving epidermis and/or dermis, sacral region

L89.153 **Pressure ulcer of sacral region,** stage 3
   Healing pressure ulcer of sacral region, stage 3
   Pressure ulcer with full thickness skin loss involving damage or necrosis of subcutaneous tissue, sacral region

L89.154 **Pressure ulcer of sacral region,** stage 4
     Healing pressure ulcer of sacral region, stage 4
     Pressure ulcer with necrosis of soft tissues through to underlying muscle, tendon, or bone, sacral region

L89.159 **Pressure ulcer of sacral region, unspecified stage** ▽
     Healing pressure ulcer of sacral region NOS
     Healing pressure ulcer of sacral region, unspecified stage

✓5ᵗʰ **L89.2** **Pressure ulcer of** hip

✓6ᵗʰ **L89.20** **Pressure ulcer of** unspecified hip

L89.200 **Pressure ulcer of unspecified hip,** unstageable ▽

L89.201 **Pressure ulcer of unspecified hip,** stage 1 ▽
     Healing pressure ulcer of unspecified hip, stage 1
     Pressure pre-ulcer skin changes limited to persistent focal edema, unspecified hip

L89.202 **Pressure ulcer of unspecified hip,** stage 2 ▽
     Healing pressure ulcer of unspecified hip, stage 2
     Pressure ulcer with abrasion, blister, partial thickness skin loss involving epidermis and/or dermis, unspecified hip

L89.203 **Pressure ulcer of unspecified hip,** stage 3 ▽
     Healing pressure ulcer of unspecified hip, stage 3
     Pressure ulcer with full thickness skin loss involving damage or necrosis of subcutaneous tissue, unspecified hip

L89.204 **Pressure ulcer of unspecified hip,** stage 4 ▽
     Healing pressure ulcer of unspecified hip, stage 4
     Pressure ulcer with necrosis of soft tissues through to underlying muscle, tendon, or bone, unspecified hip

L89.209 **Pressure ulcer of unspecified hip, unspecified stage** ▽
     Healing pressure ulcer of unspecified hip NOS
     Healing pressure ulcer of unspecified hip, unspecified stage

✓6ᵗʰ **L89.21** **Pressure ulcer of** right hip

L89.210 **Pressure ulcer of right hip,** unstageable

L89.211 **Pressure ulcer of right hip,** stage 1
     Healing pressure ulcer of right hip, stage 1
     Pressure pre-ulcer skin changes limited to persistent focal edema, right hip

L89.212 **Pressure ulcer of right hip,** stage 2
     Healing pressure ulcer of right hip, stage 2
     Pressure ulcer with abrasion, blister, partial thickness skin loss involving epidermis and/or dermis, right hip

L89.213 **Pressure ulcer of right hip,** stage 3
     Healing pressure ulcer of right hip, stage 3
     Pressure ulcer with full thickness skin loss involving damage or necrosis of subcutaneous tissue, right hip

L89.214 **Pressure ulcer of right hip,** stage 4
     Healing pressure ulcer of right hip, stage 4
     Pressure ulcer with necrosis of soft tissues through to underlying muscle, tendon, or bone, right hip

L89.219 **Pressure ulcer of right hip, unspecified stage** ▽
     Healing pressure ulcer of right hip NOS
     Healing pressure ulcer of right hip, unspecified stage

✓6ᵗʰ **L89.22** **Pressure ulcer of** left hip

L89.220 **Pressure ulcer of left hip,** unstageable

L89.221 **Pressure ulcer of left hip,** stage 1
     Healing pressure ulcer of left hip, stage 1
     Pressure pre-ulcer skin changes limited to persistent focal edema, left hip

L89.222 **Pressure ulcer of left hip,** stage 2
     Healing pressure ulcer of left hip, stage 2
     Pressure ulcer with abrasion, blister, partial thickness skin loss involving epidermis and/or dermis, left hip

L89.223 **Pressure ulcer of left hip,** stage 3
     Healing pressure ulcer of left hip, stage 3
     Pressure ulcer with full thickness skin loss involving damage or necrosis of subcutaneous tissue, left hip

L89.224 **Pressure ulcer of left hip,** stage 4
     Healing pressure ulcer of left hip, stage 4
     Pressure ulcer with necrosis of soft tissues through to underlying muscle, tendon, or bone, left hip

L89.229 **Pressure ulcer of left hip, unspecified stage** ▽
     Healing pressure ulcer of left hip NOS
     Healing pressure ulcer of left hip, unspecified stage

✓5ᵗʰ **L89.3** **Pressure ulcer of** buttock

✓6ᵗʰ **L89.30** **Pressure ulcer of** unspecified buttock

L89.300 **Pressure ulcer of unspecified buttock, unstageable** ▽

L89.301 **Pressure ulcer of unspecified buttock,** stage 1 ▽
     Healing pressure ulcer of unspecified buttock, stage 1
     Pressure pre-ulcer skin changes limited to persistent focal edema, unspecified buttock

L89.302 **Pressure ulcer of unspecified buttock,** stage 2 ▽
     Healing pressure ulcer of unspecified buttock, stage 2
     Pressure ulcer with abrasion, blister, partial thickness skin loss involving epidermis and/or dermis, unspecified buttock

L89.303 **Pressure ulcer of unspecified buttock,** stage 3 ▽
     Healing pressure ulcer of unspecified buttock, stage 3
     Pressure ulcer with full thickness skin loss involving damage or necrosis of subcutaneous tissue, unspecified buttock

L89.304 **Pressure ulcer of unspecified buttock,** stage 4 ▽
     Healing pressure ulcer of unspecified buttock, stage 4
     Pressure ulcer with necrosis of soft tissues through to underlying muscle, tendon, or bone, unspecified buttock

L89.309 **Pressure ulcer of unspecified buttock, unspecified stage** ▽
     Healing pressure ulcer of unspecified buttock NOS
     Healing pressure ulcer of unspecified buttock, unspecified stage

✓6ᵗʰ **L89.31** **Pressure ulcer of** right buttock

L89.310 **Pressure ulcer of right buttock,** unstageable

L89.311 **Pressure ulcer of right buttock,** stage 1
     Healing pressure ulcer of right buttock, stage 1
     Pressure pre-ulcer skin changes limited to persistent focal edema, right buttock

L89.312 **Pressure ulcer of right buttock,** stage 2
     Healing pressure ulcer of right buttock, stage 2
     Pressure ulcer with abrasion, blister, partial thickness skin loss involving epidermis and/or dermis, right buttock

L89.313 **Pressure ulcer of right buttock,** stage 3
     Healing pressure ulcer of right buttock, stage 3
     Pressure ulcer with full thickness skin loss involving damage or necrosis of subcutaneous tissue, right buttock

---

✓ Add'l Character Required   ✓x7ᵗʰ Placeholder Alert   RUG IV Special Care High Dx   RUG IV Clinically Complex Dx   RUG IV Special Care Low Dx   Manifestation Code   Other Specified Code   ▽ Unspecified Code

L89.314 Pressure ulcer of right buttock, stage 4
Healing pressure ulcer of right buttock, stage 4
Pressure ulcer with necrosis of soft tissues through to underlying muscle, tendon, or bone, right buttock

L89.319 Pressure ulcer of right buttock, unspecified stage ▽
Healing pressure ulcer of right buttock NOS
Healing pressure ulcer of right buttock, unspecified stage

✓6th **L89.32 Pressure ulcer of left buttock**

L89.320 Pressure ulcer of left buttock, unstageable

L89.321 Pressure ulcer of left buttock, stage 1
Healing pressure ulcer of left buttock, stage 1
Pressure pre-ulcer skin changes limited to persistent focal edema, left buttock

L89.322 Pressure ulcer of left buttock, stage 2
Healing pressure ulcer of left buttock, stage 2
Pressure ulcer with abrasion, blister, partial thickness skin loss involving epidermis and/or dermis, left buttock

L89.323 Pressure ulcer of left buttock, stage 3
Healing pressure ulcer of left buttock, stage 3
Pressure ulcer with full thickness skin loss involving damage or necrosis of subcutaneous tissue, left buttock

L89.324 Pressure ulcer of left buttock, stage 4
Healing pressure ulcer of left buttock, stage 4
Pressure ulcer with necrosis of soft tissues through to underlying muscle, tendon, or bone, left buttock

L89.329 Pressure ulcer of left buttock, unspecified stage ▽
Healing pressure ulcer of left buttock NOS
Healing pressure ulcer of left buttock, unspecified stage

✓5th **L89.4 Pressure ulcer of contiguous site of back, buttock and hip** ▽

L89.40 Pressure ulcer of contiguous site of back, buttock and hip, unspecified stage ▽
Healing pressure ulcer of contiguous site of back, buttock and hip NOS
Healing pressure ulcer of contiguous site of back, buttock and hip, unspecified stage

L89.41 Pressure ulcer of contiguous site of back, buttock and hip, stage 1
Healing pressure ulcer of contiguous site of back, buttock and hip, stage 1
Pressure pre-ulcer skin changes limited to persistent focal edema, contiguous site of back, buttock and hip

L89.42 Pressure ulcer of contiguous site of back, buttock and hip, stage 2
Healing pressure ulcer of contiguous site of back, buttock and hip, stage 2
Pressure ulcer with abrasion, blister, partial thickness skin loss involving epidermis and/or dermis, contiguous site of back, buttock and hip

L89.43 Pressure ulcer of contiguous site of back, buttock and hip, stage 3
Healing pressure ulcer of contiguous site of back, buttock and hip, stage 3
Pressure ulcer with full thickness skin loss involving damage or necrosis of subcutaneous tissue, contiguous site of back, buttock and hip

L89.44 Pressure ulcer of contiguous site of back, buttock and hip, stage 4
Healing pressure ulcer of contiguous site of back, buttock and hip, stage 4
Pressure ulcer with necrosis of soft tissues through to underlying muscle, tendon, or bone, contiguous site of back, buttock and hip

L89.45 Pressure ulcer of contiguous site of back, buttock and hip, unstageable

✓5th **L89.5 Pressure ulcer of ankle**

✓6th **L89.50 Pressure ulcer of unspecified ankle**

L89.500 Pressure ulcer of unspecified ankle, unstageable ▽

L89.501 Pressure ulcer of unspecified ankle, stage 1 ▽
Healing pressure ulcer of unspecified ankle, stage 1
Pressure pre-ulcer skin changes limited to persistent focal edema, unspecified ankle

L89.502 Pressure ulcer of unspecified ankle, stage 2 ▽
Healing pressure ulcer of unspecified ankle, stage 2
Pressure ulcer with abrasion, blister, partial thickness skin loss involving epidermis and/or dermis, unspecified ankle

L89.503 Pressure ulcer of unspecified ankle, stage 3 ▽
Healing pressure ulcer of unspecified ankle, stage 3
Pressure ulcer with full thickness skin loss involving damage or necrosis of subcutaneous tissue, unspecified ankle

L89.504 Pressure ulcer of unspecified ankle, stage 4 ▽
Healing pressure ulcer of unspecified ankle, stage 4
Pressure ulcer with necrosis of soft tissues through to underlying muscle, tendon, or bone, unspecified ankle

L89.509 Pressure ulcer of unspecified ankle, unspecified stage ▽
Healing pressure ulcer of unspecified ankle NOS
Healing pressure ulcer of unspecified ankle, unspecified stage

✓6th **L89.51 Pressure ulcer of right ankle**

L89.510 Pressure ulcer of right ankle, unstageable

L89.511 Pressure ulcer of right ankle, stage 1
Healing pressure ulcer of right ankle, stage 1
Pressure pre-ulcer skin changes limited to persistent focal edema, right ankle

L89.512 Pressure ulcer of right ankle, stage 2
Healing pressure ulcer of right ankle, stage 2
Pressure ulcer with abrasion, blister, partial thickness skin loss involving epidermis and/or dermis, right ankle

L89.513 Pressure ulcer of right ankle, stage 3
Healing pressure ulcer of right ankle, stage 3
Pressure ulcer with full thickness skin loss involving damage or necrosis of subcutaneous tissue, right ankle

L89.514 Pressure ulcer of right ankle, stage 4
Healing pressure ulcer of right ankle, stage 4
Pressure ulcer with necrosis of soft tissues through to underlying muscle, tendon, or bone, right ankle

L89.519 Pressure ulcer of right ankle, unspecified stage ▽
Healing pressure ulcer of right ankle NOS
Healing pressure ulcer of right ankle, unspecified stage

✓6th **L89.52 Pressure ulcer of left ankle**

L89.520 Pressure ulcer of left ankle, unstageable

L89.521 Pressure ulcer of left ankle, stage 1
Healing pressure ulcer of left ankle, stage 1
Pressure pre-ulcer skin changes limited to persistnt focal edema, left ankle

L89.522 Pressure ulcer of left ankle, stage 2
Healing pressure ulcer of left ankle, stage 2
Pressure ulcer with abrasion, blister, partial thickness skin loss involving epidermis and/or dermis, left ankle

L89.523 Pressure ulcer of left ankle, stage 3
Healing pressure ulcer of left ankle, stage 3
Pressure ulcer with full thickness skin loss involving damage or necrosis of subcutaneous tissue, left ankle

N Newborn   P Pediatric   M Maternity   A Adult   RIC RIC Dx   NCDx Noncancer Dx   PDx Primary Dx   CC RIC CC Condition   ▶◀ Revised Text   ● New Code   ▲ Revised Code Title

668   ICD-10-CM 2016

L89.524   **Pressure ulcer of left ankle,** stage 4
Healing pressure ulcer of left ankle, stage 4
Pressure ulcer with necrosis of soft tissues
through to underlying muscle,
tendon, or bone, left ankle

L89.529   **Pressure ulcer of left ankle, unspecified** ▽
stage
Healing pressure ulcer of left ankle NOS
Healing pressure ulcer of left ankle,
unspecified stage

✓5ᵗʰ **L89.6**   **Pressure ulcer of** heel

   ✓6ᵗʰ **L89.60**   **Pressure ulcer of** unspecified heel

L89.600   **Pressure ulcer of unspecified heel,** ▽
unstageable

L89.601   **Pressure ulcer of unspecified heel,** ▽
stage 1
Healing pressure ulcer of unspecified heel,
stage 1
Pressure pre-ulcer skin changes limited to
persistent focal edema, unspecified
heel

L89.602   **Pressure ulcer of unspecified heel,** ▽
stage 2
Healing pressure ulcer of unspecified heel,
stage 2
Pressure ulcer with abrasion, blister, partial
thickness skin loss involving epidermis
and/or dermis, unspecified heel

L89.603   **Pressure ulcer of unspecified heel,** ▽
stage 3
Healing pressure ulcer of unspecified heel,
stage 3
Pressure ulcer with full thickness skin loss
involving damage or necrosis of
subcutaneous tissue, unspecified heel

L89.604   **Pressure ulcer of unspecified heel,** ▽
stage 4
Healing pressure ulcer of unspecified heel,
stage 4
Pressure ulcer with necrosis of soft tissues
through to underlying muscle,
tendon, or bone, unspecified heel

L89.609   **Pressure ulcer of unspecified heel,** ▽
unspecified stage
Healing pressure ulcer of unspecified heel
NOS
Healing pressure ulcer of unspecified heel,
unspecified stage

   ✓6ᵗʰ **L89.61**   **Pressure ulcer of** right heel

L89.610   **Pressure ulcer of right heel,** unstageable

L89.611   **Pressure ulcer of right heel,** stage 1
Healing pressure ulcer of right heel, stage 1
Pressure pre-ulcer skin changes limited to
persistent focal edema, right heel

L89.612   **Pressure ulcer of right heel,** stage 2
Healing pressure ulcer of right heel, stage 2
Pressure ulcer with abrasion, blister, partial
thickness skin loss involving epidermis
and/or dermis, right heel

L89.613   **Pressure ulcer of right heel,** stage 3
Healing pressure ulcer of right heel, stage 3
Pressure ulcer with full thickness skin loss
involving damage or necrosis of
subcutaneous tissue, right heel

L89.614   **Pressure ulcer of right heel,** stage 4
Healing pressure ulcer of right heel, stage 4
Pressure ulcer with necrosis of soft tissues
through to underlying muscle,
tendon, or bone, right heel

L89.619   **Pressure ulcer of right heel,** ▽
unspecified stage
Healing pressure ulcer of right heel NOS
Healing pressure ulcer of unspecified heel,
right stage

   ✓6ᵗʰ **L89.62**   **Pressure ulcer of** left heel

L89.620   **Pressure ulcer of left heel,** unstageable

L89.621   **Pressure ulcer of left heel,** stage 1
Healing pressure ulcer of left heel, stage 1
Pressure pre-ulcer skin changes limited to
persistent focal edema, left heel

L89.622   **Pressure ulcer of left heel,** stage 2
Healing pressure ulcer of left heel, stage 2
Pressure ulcer with abrasion, blister, partial
thickness skin loss involving epidermis
and/or dermis, left heel

L89.623   **Pressure ulcer of left heel,** stage 3
Healing pressure ulcer of left heel, stage 3
Pressure ulcer with full thickness skin loss
involving damage or necrosis of
subcutaneous tissue, left heel

L89.624   **Pressure ulcer of left heel,** stage 4
Healing pressure ulcer of left heel, stage 4
Pressure ulcer with necrosis of soft tissues
through to underlying muscle,
tendon, or bone, left heel

L89.629   **Pressure ulcer of left heel, unspecified** ▽
stage
Healing pressure ulcer of left heel NOS
Healing pressure ulcer of left heel,
unspecified stage

✓5ᵗʰ **L89.8**   **Pressure ulcer of** other site

   ✓6ᵗʰ **L89.81**   **Pressure ulcer of** head
Pressure ulcer of face

L89.810   **Pressure ulcer of head,** unstageable

L89.811   **Pressure ulcer of head,** stage 1
Healing pressure ulcer of head, stage 1
Pressure pre-ulcer skin changes limited to
persistent focal edema, head

L89.812   **Pressure ulcer of head,** stage 2
Healing pressure ulcer of head, stage 2
Pressure ulcer with abrasion, blister, partial
thickness skin loss involving epidermis
and/or dermis, head

L89.813   **Pressure ulcer of head,** stage 3
Healing pressure ulcer of head, stage 3
Pressure ulcer with full thickness skin loss
involving damage or necrosis of
subcutaneous tissue, head

L89.814   **Pressure ulcer of head,** stage 4
Healing pressure ulcer of head, stage 4
Pressure ulcer with necrosis of soft tissues
through to underlying muscle,
tendon, or bone, head

L89.819   **Pressure ulcer of head, unspecified** ▽
stage
Healing pressure ulcer of head NOS
Healing pressure ulcer of head, unspecified
stage

   ✓6ᵗʰ **L89.89**   **Pressure ulcer of** other site

L89.890   **Pressure ulcer of other site,** unstageable

L89.891   **Pressure ulcer of other site,** stage 1
Healing pressure ulcer of other site, stage 1
Pressure pre-ulcer skin changes limited to
persistent focal edema, other site

L89.892   **Pressure ulcer of other site,** stage 2
Healing pressure ulcer of other site, stage 2
Pressure ulcer with abrasion, blister, partial
thickness skin loss involving epidermis
and/or dermis, other site

L89.893   **Pressure ulcer of other site,** stage 3
Healing pressure ulcer of other site, stage 3
Pressure ulcer with full thickness skin loss
involving damage or necrosis of
subcutaneous tissue, other site

L89.894   **Pressure ulcer of other site,** stage 4
Healing pressure ulcer of other site, stage 4
Pressure ulcer with necrosis of soft tissues
through to underlying muscle,
tendon, or bone, other site

L89.899   **Pressure ulcer of other site,** ▽
unspecified stage
Healing pressure ulcer of other site NOS
Healing pressure ulcer of other site,
unspecified stage

✓5ᵗʰ **L89.9 Pressure ulcer of** unspecified site

L89.90 Pressure ulcer of unspecified site, unspecified stage ▽
Healing pressure ulcer of unspecified site NOS
Healing pressure ulcer of unspecified site, unspecified stage

L89.91 Pressure ulcer of unspecified site, stage 1 ▽
Healing pressure ulcer of unspecified site, stage 1
Pressure pre-ulcer skin changes limited to persistent focal edema, unspecified site

L89.92 Pressure ulcer of unspecified site, stage 2 ▽
Healing pressure ulcer of unspecified site, stage 2
Pressure ulcer with abrasion, blister, partial thickness skin loss involving epidermis and/or dermis, unspecified site

L89.93 Pressure ulcer of unspecified site, stage 3 ▽
Healing pressure ulcer of unspecified site, stage 3
Pressure ulcer with full thickness skin loss involving damage or necrosis of subcutaneous tissue, unspecified site

L89.94 Pressure ulcer of unspecified site, stage 4 ▽
Healing pressure ulcer of unspecified site, stage 4
Pressure ulcer with necrosis of soft tissues through to underlying muscle, tendon, or bone, unspecified site

L89.95 Pressure ulcer of unspecified site, unstageable ▽

✓4ᵗʰ **L90 Atrophic disorders of skin**

L90.0 Lichen sclerosus et atrophicus
EXCLUDES 2   *lichen sclerosus of external female genital organs (N90.4)*
lichen sclerosus of external male genital organs (N48.0)

L90.1 Anetoderma of Schweninger-Buzzi

L90.2 Anetoderma of Jadassohn-Pellizzari

L90.3 Atrophoderma of Pasini and Pierini

L90.4 Acrodermatitis chronica atrophicans

L90.5 Scar conditions and fibrosis of skin
Adherent scar (skin)
Cicatrix
Disfigurement of skin due to scar
Fibrosis of skin NOS
Scar NOS
EXCLUDES 2   *hypertrophic scar (L91.0)*
keloid scar (L91.0)
AHA: 2015, 1Q, 19

L90.6 Striae atrophicae

L90.8 Other atrophic disorders of skin

L90.9 Atrophic disorder of skin, unspecified ▽

✓4ᵗʰ **L91 Hypertrophic disorders of skin**

L91.0 Hypertrophic scar
Keloid
Keloid scar
EXCLUDES 2   *acne keloid (L73.0)*
scar NOS (L90.5)

L91.8 Other hypertrophic disorders of the skin

L91.9 Hypertrophic disorder of the skin, unspecified ▽

✓4ᵗʰ **L92 Granulomatous disorders of skin and subcutaneous tissue**
EXCLUDES 2   *actinic granuloma (L57.5)*

L92.0 Granuloma annulare
Perforating granuloma annulare

L92.1 Necrobiosis lipoidica, not elsewhere classified
EXCLUDES 1   *necrobiosis lipoidica associated with diabetes mellitus (E08-E13 with .620)*

L92.2 Granuloma faciale [eosinophilic granuloma of skin]

L92.3 Foreign body granuloma of the skin and subcutaneous tissue
Use additional code to identify the type of retained foreign body (Z18.-)

L92.8 Other granulomatous disorders of the skin and subcutaneous tissue

L92.9 Granulomatous disorder of the skin and subcutaneous tissue, unspecified ▽

✓4ᵗʰ **L93 Lupus erythematosus**
Use additional code for adverse effect, if applicable, to identify drug (T36-T50 with fifth or sixth character 5)
EXCLUDES 1   *lupus exedens (A18.4)*
lupus vulgaris (A18.4)
scleroderma (M34.-)
systemic lupus erythematosus (M32.-)

L93.0 Discoid lupus erythematosus
Lupus erythematosus NOS

L93.1 Subacute cutaneous lupus erythematosus

L93.2 Other local lupus erythematosus
Lupus erythematosus profundus
Lupus panniculitis

✓4ᵗʰ **L94 Other localized connective tissue disorders**
EXCLUDES 1   *systemic connective tissue disorders (M30-M36)*

L94.0 Localized scleroderma [morphea]
Circumscribed scleroderma

L94.1 Linear scleroderma
En coup de sabre lesion

L94.2 Calcinosis cutis

L94.3 Sclerodactyly

L94.4 Gottron's papules

L94.5 Poikiloderma vasculare atrophicans

L94.6 Ainhum

L94.8 Other specified localized connective tissue disorders

L94.9 Localized connective tissue disorder, unspecified ▽

✓4ᵗʰ **L95 Vasculitis limited to skin, not elsewhere classified**
EXCLUDES 1   *angioma serpiginosum (L81.7)*
Henoch(-Schönlein) purpura (D69.0)
hypersensitivity angiitis (M31.0)
lupus panniculitis (L93.2)
panniculitis NOS (M79.3)
panniculitis of neck and back (M54.0-)
polyarteritis nodosa (M30.0)
relapsing panniculitis (M35.6)
rheumatoid vasculitis (M05.2)
serum sickness (T80.6-)
urticaria (L50.-)
Wegener's granulomatosis (M31.3-)

L95.0 Livedoid vasculitis
Atrophie blanche (en plaque)

L95.1 Erythema elevatum diutinum

L95.8 Other vasculitis limited to the skin

L95.9 Vasculitis limited to the skin, unspecified ▽

✓4ᵗʰ **L97 Non-pressure chronic ulcer of lower limb, not elsewhere classified**
INCLUDES   chronic ulcer of skin of lower limb NOS
non-healing ulcer of skin
non-infected sinus of skin
trophic ulcer NOS
tropical ulcer NOS
ulcer of skin of lower limb NOS
Code first any associated underlying condition, such as:
atherosclerosis of the lower extremities (I70.23-, I70.24-, I70.33-, I70.34-, I70.43-, I70.44-, I70.53-, I70.54-, I70.63-, I70.64-, I70.73-, I70.74-)
chronic venous hypertension (I87.31-, I87.33-)
diabetic ulcers (E08.621, E08.622, E09.621, E09.622, E10.621, E10.622, E11.621, E11.622, E13.621, E13.622)
postphlebitic syndrome (I87.01-, I87.03-)
postthrombotic syndrome (I87.01-, I87.03-)
varicose ulcer (I83.0-, I83.2-)
Code first any associated gangrene (I96)
EXCLUDES 2   *pressure ulcer (pressure area) (L89.-)*
skin infections (L00-L08)
specific infections classified to A00-B99

✓5ᵗʰ **L97.1 Non-pressure chronic ulcer of** thigh

✓6ᵗʰ **L97.10 Non-pressure chronic ulcer of** unspecified thigh

L97.101 Non-pressure chronic ulcer of unspecified thigh limited to breakdown of skin ▽

L97.102 Non-pressure chronic ulcer of unspecified thigh with fat layer exposed ▽

L97.103 Non-pressure chronic ulcer of unspecified thigh with necrosis of muscle ▽

L97.104 Non-pressure chronic ulcer of unspecified thigh with necrosis of bone ▽

L97.109   **Non-pressure chronic ulcer of** unspecified thigh with unspecified severity ▽

√6ᵗʰ   L97.11   **Non-pressure chronic ulcer of** right thigh

L97.111   **Non-pressure chronic ulcer of right thigh** limited to breakdown of skin

L97.112   **Non-pressure chronic ulcer of right thigh** with fat layer exposed

L97.113   **Non-pressure chronic ulcer of right thigh** with necrosis of muscle

L97.114   **Non-pressure chronic ulcer of right thigh** with necrosis of bone

L97.119   **Non-pressure chronic ulcer of right** thigh with unspecified severity ▽

√6ᵗʰ   L97.12   **Non-pressure chronic ulcer of** left thigh

L97.121   **Non-pressure chronic ulcer of left thigh** limited to breakdown of skin

L97.122   **Non-pressure chronic ulcer of left thigh** with fat layer exposed

L97.123   **Non-pressure chronic ulcer of left thigh** with necrosis of muscle

L97.124   **Non-pressure chronic ulcer of left thigh** with necrosis of bone

L97.129   **Non-pressure chronic ulcer of left** thigh with unspecified severity ▽

√5ᵗʰ   **L97.2 Non-pressure chronic ulcer of** calf

√6ᵗʰ   L97.20   **Non-pressure chronic ulcer of** unspecified calf

L97.201   **Non-pressure chronic ulcer of** unspecified calf limited to breakdown of skin ▽

L97.202   **Non-pressure chronic ulcer of** unspecified calf with fat layer exposed ▽

L97.203   **Non-pressure chronic ulcer of** unspecified calf with necrosis of muscle ▽

L97.204   **Non-pressure chronic ulcer of** unspecified calf with necrosis of bone

L97.209   **Non-pressure chronic ulcer of** unspecified calf with unspecified severity ▽

√6ᵗʰ   L97.21   **Non-pressure chronic ulcer of** right calf

L97.211   **Non-pressure chronic ulcer of right calf** limited to breakdown of skin

L97.212   **Non-pressure chronic ulcer of right calf** with fat layer exposed

L97.213   **Non-pressure chronic ulcer of right calf** with necrosis of muscle

L97.214   **Non-pressure chronic ulcer of right calf** with necrosis of bone

L97.219   **Non-pressure chronic ulcer of right calf** with unspecified severity ▽

√6ᵗʰ   L97.22   **Non-pressure chronic ulcer of** left calf

L97.221   **Non-pressure chronic ulcer of left calf** limited to breakdown of skin

L97.222   **Non-pressure chronic ulcer of left calf** with fat layer exposed

L97.223   **Non-pressure chronic ulcer of left calf** with necrosis of muscle

L97.224   **Non-pressure chronic ulcer of left calf** with necrosis of bone

L97.229   **Non-pressure chronic ulcer of left calf** with unspecified severity ▽

√5ᵗʰ   **L97.3 Non-pressure chronic ulcer of** ankle

√6ᵗʰ   L97.30   **Non-pressure chronic ulcer of** unspecified ankle

L97.301   **Non-pressure chronic ulcer of** unspecified ankle limited to breakdown of skin ▽

L97.302   **Non-pressure chronic ulcer of** unspecified ankle with fat layer exposed ▽

L97.303   **Non-pressure chronic ulcer of** unspecified ankle with necrosis of muscle ▽

L97.304   **Non-pressure chronic ulcer of** unspecified ankle with necrosis of bone ▽

L97.309   **Non-pressure chronic ulcer of** unspecified ankle with unspecified severity ▽

√6ᵗʰ   L97.31   **Non-pressure chronic ulcer of** right ankle

L97.311   **Non-pressure chronic ulcer of right ankle** limited to breakdown of skin

L97.312   **Non-pressure chronic ulcer of right ankle** with fat layer exposed

L97.313   **Non-pressure chronic ulcer of right ankle** with necrosis of muscle

L97.314   **Non-pressure chronic ulcer of right ankle** with necrosis of bone

L97.319   **Non-pressure chronic ulcer of right** ankle with unspecified severity ▽

√6ᵗʰ   L97.32   **Non-pressure chronic ulcer of** left ankle

L97.321   **Non-pressure chronic ulcer of left ankle** limited to breakdown of skin

L97.322   **Non-pressure chronic ulcer of left ankle** with fat layer exposed

L97.323   **Non-pressure chronic ulcer of left ankle** with necrosis of muscle

L97.324   **Non-pressure chronic ulcer of left ankle** with necrosis of bone

L97.329   **Non-pressure chronic ulcer of left** ankle with unspecified severity ▽

√5ᵗʰ   **L97.4 Non-pressure chronic ulcer of** heel and midfoot
Non-pressure chronic ulcer of plantar surface of midfoot

√6ᵗʰ   L97.40   **Non-pressure chronic ulcer of** unspecified heel and midfoot

L97.401   **Non-pressure chronic ulcer of** unspecified heel and midfoot limited to breakdown of skin ▽

L97.402   **Non-pressure chronic ulcer of** unspecified heel and midfoot with fat layer exposed ▽

L97.403   **Non-pressure chronic ulcer of** unspecified heel and midfoot with necrosis of muscle ▽

L97.404   **Non-pressure chronic ulcer of** unspecified heel and midfoot with necrosis of bone ▽

L97.409   **Non-pressure chronic ulcer of** unspecified heel and midfoot with unspecified severity ▽

√6ᵗʰ   L97.41   **Non-pressure chronic ulcer of** right heel and midfoot

L97.411   **Non-pressure chronic ulcer of right heel and midfoot** limited to breakdown of skin

L97.412   **Non-pressure chronic ulcer of right heel and midfoot** with fat layer exposed

L97.413   **Non-pressure chronic ulcer of right heel and midfoot** with necrosis of muscle

L97.414   **Non-pressure chronic ulcer of right heel and midfoot** with necrosis of bone

L97.419   **Non-pressure chronic ulcer of right** heel and midfoot with unspecified severity ▽

√6ᵗʰ   L97.42   **Non-pressure chronic ulcer of** left heel and midfoot

L97.421   **Non-pressure chronic ulcer of left heel and midfoot** limited to breakdown of skin

L97.422   **Non-pressure chronic ulcer of left heel and midfoot** with fat layer exposed

L97.423   **Non-pressure chronic ulcer of left heel and midfoot** with necrosis of muscle

L97.424   **Non-pressure chronic ulcer of left heel and midfoot** with necrosis of bone

L97.429   **Non-pressure chronic ulcer of left heel and midfoot** with unspecified severity ▽

√5ᵗʰ   **L97.5 Non-pressure chronic ulcer of** other part of foot
Non-pressure chronic ulcer of toe

√6ᵗʰ   L97.50   **Non-pressure chronic ulcer of** other part of unspecified foot

L97.501   **Non-pressure chronic ulcer of other** part of unspecified foot limited to breakdown of skin ▽

L97.502   **Non-pressure chronic ulcer of other** part of unspecified foot with fat layer exposed ▽

L97.503   **Non-pressure chronic ulcer of other** part of unspecified foot with necrosis of muscle ▽

✔ Add'l Character Required   √x7ᵗʰ Placeholder Alert   RUG IV Special Care High Dx   RUG IV Clinically Complex Dx   RUG IV Special Care Low Dx   Manifestation Code   Other Specified Code   ▽ Unspecified Code

Chapter 12. Diseases of the Skin and Subcutaneous Tissue

L97.504 Non-pressure chronic ulcer of other part of unspecified foot with necrosis of bone ▽

L97.509 Non-pressure chronic ulcer of other part of unspecified foot with unspecified severity ▽

✓6ᵗʰ L97.51 Non-pressure chronic ulcer of other part of right foot

L97.511 Non-pressure chronic ulcer of other part of right foot limited to breakdown of skin

L97.512 Non-pressure chronic ulcer of other part of right foot with fat layer exposed

L97.513 Non-pressure chronic ulcer of other part of right foot with necrosis of muscle

L97.514 Non-pressure chronic ulcer of other part of right foot with necrosis of bone

L97.519 Non-pressure chronic ulcer of other part of right foot with unspecified severity ▽

✓6ᵗʰ L97.52 Non-pressure chronic ulcer of other part of left foot

L97.521 Non-pressure chronic ulcer of other part of left foot limited to breakdown of skin

L97.522 Non-pressure chronic ulcer of other part of left foot with fat layer exposed

L97.523 Non-pressure chronic ulcer of other part of left foot with necrosis of muscle

L97.524 Non-pressure chronic ulcer of other part of left foot with necrosis of bone

L97.529 Non-pressure chronic ulcer of other part of left foot with unspecified severity ▽

✓5ᵗʰ L97.8 Non-pressure chronic ulcer of other part of lower leg

✓6ᵗʰ L97.80 Non-pressure chronic ulcer of other part of unspecified lower leg

L97.801 Non-pressure chronic ulcer of other part of unspecified lower leg limited to breakdown of skin ▽

L97.802 Non-pressure chronic ulcer of other part of unspecified lower leg with fat layer exposed ▽

L97.803 Non-pressure chronic ulcer of other part of unspecified lower leg with necrosis of muscle ▽

L97.804 Non-pressure chronic ulcer of other part of unspecified lower leg with necrosis of bone ▽

L97.809 Non-pressure chronic ulcer of other part of unspecified lower leg with unspecified severity ▽

✓6ᵗʰ L97.81 Non-pressure chronic ulcer of other part of right lower leg

L97.811 Non-pressure chronic ulcer of other part of right lower leg limited to breakdown of skin

L97.812 Non-pressure chronic ulcer of other part of right lower leg with fat layer exposed

L97.813 Non-pressure chronic ulcer of other part of right lower leg with necrosis of muscle

L97.814 Non-pressure chronic ulcer of other part of right lower leg with necrosis of bone

L97.819 Non-pressure chronic ulcer of other part of right lower leg with unspecified severity ▽

✓6ᵗʰ L97.82 Non-pressure chronic ulcer of other part of left lower leg

L97.821 Non-pressure chronic ulcer of other part of left lower leg limited to breakdown of skin

L97.822 Non-pressure chronic ulcer of other part of left lower leg with fat layer exposed

L97.823 Non-pressure chronic ulcer of other part of left lower leg with necrosis of muscle

L97.824 Non-pressure chronic ulcer of other part of left lower leg with necrosis of bone

L97.829 Non-pressure chronic ulcer of other part of left lower leg with unspecified severity ▽

✓5ᵗʰ L97.9 Non-pressure chronic ulcer of unspecified part of lower leg

✓6ᵗʰ L97.90 Non-pressure chronic ulcer of unspecified part of unspecified lower leg

L97.901 Non-pressure chronic ulcer of unspecified part of unspecified lower leg limited to breakdown of skin ▽

L97.902 Non-pressure chronic ulcer of unspecified part of unspecified lower leg with fat layer exposed ▽

L97.903 Non-pressure chronic ulcer of unspecified part of unspecified lower leg with necrosis of muscle ▽

L97.904 Non-pressure chronic ulcer of unspecified part of unspecified lower leg with necrosis of bone ▽

L97.909 Non-pressure chronic ulcer of unspecified part of unspecified lower leg with unspecified severity ▽

✓6ᵗʰ L97.91 Non-pressure chronic ulcer of unspecified part of right lower leg

L97.911 Non-pressure chronic ulcer of unspecified part of right lower leg limited to breakdown of skin ▽

L97.912 Non-pressure chronic ulcer of unspecified part of right lower leg with fat layer exposed ▽

L97.913 Non-pressure chronic ulcer of unspecified part of right lower leg with necrosis of muscle ▽

L97.914 Non-pressure chronic ulcer of unspecified part of right lower leg with necrosis of bone ▽

L97.919 Non-pressure chronic ulcer of unspecified part of right lower leg with unspecified severity ▽

✓6ᵗʰ L97.92 Non-pressure chronic ulcer of unspecified part of left lower leg

L97.921 Non-pressure chronic ulcer of unspecified part of left lower leg limited to breakdown of skin ▽

L97.922 Non-pressure chronic ulcer of unspecified part of left lower leg with fat layer exposed ▽

L97.923 Non-pressure chronic ulcer of unspecified part of left lower leg with necrosis of muscle ▽

L97.924 Non-pressure chronic ulcer of unspecified part of left lower leg with necrosis of bone ▽

L97.929 Non-pressure chronic ulcer of unspecified part of left lower leg with unspecified severity ▽

✓4ᵗʰ L98 Other disorders of skin and subcutaneous tissue, not elsewhere classified

L98.0 Pyogenic granuloma

EXCLUDES 2 pyogenic granuloma of gingiva (K06.8)
pyogenic granuloma of maxillary alveolar ridge (K04.5)
pyogenic granuloma of oral mucosa (K13.4)

L98.1 Factitial dermatitis
Neurotic excoriation

L98.2 Febrile neutrophilic dermatosis [Sweet]

L98.3 Eosinophilic cellulitis [Wells]

✓5ᵗʰ L98.4 Non-pressure chronic ulcer of skin, not elsewhere classified
Chronic ulcer of skin NOS
Tropical ulcer NOS
Ulcer of skin NOS

EXCLUDES 2 pressure ulcer (pressure area) (L89.-)
gangrene (I96)
skin infections (L00-L08)
specific infections classified to A00-B99
ulcer of lower limb NEC (L97.-)
varicose ulcer (I83.0-I82.2)

✓6ᵗʰ L98.41 Non-pressure chronic ulcer of buttock

L98.411 Non-pressure chronic ulcer of buttock limited to breakdown of skin

L98.412 Non-pressure chronic ulcer of buttock with fat layer exposed

L98.413 Non-pressure chronic ulcer of buttock with necrosis of muscle

Ⓝ Newborn Ⓟ Pediatric Ⓜ Maternity Ⓐ Adult RIC RIC Dx NC Dx Noncancer Dx PDx Primary Dx CC RIC CC Condition ►◄ Revised Text ● New Code ▲ Revised Code Title

672 | ICD-10-CM 2016

	L98.414	**Non-pressure chronic ulcer of buttock with necrosis of bone**
	L98.419	**Non-pressure chronic ulcer of buttock with unspecified severity** ▽

✓6ᵗʰ **L98.42**   **Non-pressure chronic ulcer of back**

	L98.421	**Non-pressure chronic ulcer of back limited to breakdown of skin**
	L98.422	**Non-pressure chronic ulcer of back with fat layer exposed**
	L98.423	**Non-pressure chronic ulcer of back with necrosis of muscle**
	L98.424	**Non-pressure chronic ulcer of back with necrosis of bone**
	L98.429	**Non-pressure chronic ulcer of back with unspecified severity** ▽

✓6ᵗʰ **L98.49**   **Non-pressure chronic ulcer of skin of other sites**
Non-pressure chronic ulcer of skin NOS

	L98.491	**Non-pressure chronic ulcer of skin of other sites limited to breakdown of skin**
	L98.492	**Non-pressure chronic ulcer of skin of other sites with fat layer exposed**
	L98.493	**Non-pressure chronic ulcer of skin of other sites with necrosis of muscle**
	L98.494	**Non-pressure chronic ulcer of skin of other sites with necrosis of bone**

	L98.499	**Non-pressure chronic ulcer of skin of other sites with unspecified severity** ▽

L98.5   **Mucinosis of the skin**
Focal mucinosis
Lichen myxedematosus
Reticular erythematous mucinosis
EXCLUDES 1   *focal oral mucinosis (K13.79)*
myxedema (E03.9)

L98.6   **Other infiltrative disorders of the skin and subcutaneous tissue**
EXCLUDES 1   *hyalinosis cutis et mucosae (E78.89)*

L98.8   **Other specified disorders of the skin and subcutaneous tissue**
AHA: 2013, 2Q, 32

L98.9   **Disorder of the skin and subcutaneous tissue, unspecified** ▽

L99   *Other disorders of skin and subcutaneous tissue in diseases classified elsewhere*
Code first underlying disease, such as:
amyloidosis (E85.-)
EXCLUDES 1   *skin disorders in diabetes (E08-E13 with .62)*
skin disorders in gonorrhea (A54.89)
skin disorders in syphilis (A51.31, A52.79)

☑ Add'l Character Required ✓x7ᵗʰ Placeholder Alert RUG IV Special Care High Dx   RUG IV Clinically Complex Dx   RUG IV Special Care Low Dx   Manifestation Code   Other Specified Code   ▽ Unspecified Code

Chapter 13. Diseases of the Musculoskeletal System and Connective Tissue (M00–M99)

Chapter Specific Guidelines with Coding Examples

The chapter specific guidelines from the ICD-10-CM Official Guidelines for Coding and Reporting have been provided below. Along with these guidelines are coding examples, contained in the shaded boxes, that have been developed to help illustrate the coding and/or sequencing guidance found in these guidelines.

a. Site and laterality

Most of the codes within Chapter 13 have site and laterality designations. The site represents the bone, joint or the muscle involved. For some conditions where more than one bone, joint or muscle is usually involved, such as osteoarthritis, there is a "multiple sites" code available. For categories where no multiple site code is provided and more than one bone, joint or muscle is involved, multiple codes should be used to indicate the different sites involved.

Right elbow infective bursitis

M71.121   Other infective bursitis, right elbow

Explanation: Most of the codes within chapter 13 have site and laterality designations. The site represents the bone, joint, or the muscle involved.

Rheumatoid arthritis of multiple sites without rheumatoid factor

M06.09   Rheumatoid arthritis without rheumatoid factor, multiple sites

Explanation: For some conditions where more than one bone, joint or muscle is usually involved, such as osteoarthritis, there is a "multiple sites" code available.

Osteomyelitis of the fourth thoracic and second lumbar vertebrae

M46.24   Osteomyelitis of vertebra, thoracic region

M46.26   Osteomyelitis of vertebra, lumbar region

Explanation: For categories without a multiple site code and more than one bone, joint, or muscle is involved, multiple codes should be used to indicate the different sites involved.

1) Bone versus joint

For certain conditions, the bone may be affected at the upper or lower end, (e.g., avascular necrosis of bone, M87, Osteoporosis, M80, M81). Though the portion of the bone affected may be at the joint, the site designation will be the bone, not the joint.

Idiopathic avascular necrosis of the femoral head of the left hip joint

M87.052   Idiopathic aseptic necrosis of left femur

Explanation: For certain conditions such as avascular necrosis, the bone may be affected at the joint, but the site designation is the bone, not the joint.

b. Acute traumatic versus chronic or recurrent musculoskeletal conditions

Many musculoskeletal conditions are a result of previous injury or trauma to a site, or are recurrent conditions. Bone, joint or muscle conditions that are the result of a healed injury are usually found in chapter 13. Recurrent bone, joint or muscle conditions are also usually found in chapter 13. Any current, acute injury should be coded to the appropriate injury code from chapter 19. Chronic or recurrent conditions should generally be coded with a code from chapter 13. If it is difficult to determine from the documentation in the record which code is best to describe a condition, query the provider.

Acute traumatic bucket handle tear of right medial meniscus

S83.211A   Bucket-handle tear of medial meniscus, current injury, right knee, initial encounter

Explanation: Any current, acute injury is not coded in chapter 13. It should instead be coded to the appropriate injury code from chapter 19.

Old bucket handle tear of right medial meniscus

M23.203   Derangement of unspecified medial meniscus due to old tear or injury, right knee

Explanation: Chronic or recurrent conditions should generally be coded with a code from chapter 13.

c. Coding of Pathologic Fractures

7th character A is for use as long as the patient is receiving active treatment for the fracture. Examples of active treatment are: surgical treatment, emergency department encounter, evaluation and

continuing treatment by the same or a different physician. While the patient may be seen by a new or different provider over the course of treatment for a pathological fracture, assignment of the 7th character is based on whether the patient is undergoing active treatment and not whether the provider is seeing the patient for the first time.

7th character, D is to be used for encounters after the patient has completed active treatment. The other 7th characters, listed under each subcategory in the Tabular List, are to be used for subsequent encounters for treatment of problems associated with the healing, such as malunions, nonunions, and sequelae.

Care for complications of surgical treatment for fracture repairs during the healing or recovery phase should be coded with the appropriate complication codes.

See Section I.C.19. Coding of traumatic fractures.

Pathologic fracture of left foot, unknown cause, currently under active treatment by a follow-up provider

M84.475A   Pathological fracture, left foot, initial encounter for fracture

Explanation: Seventh character A is for use as long as the patient is receiving active treatment for a pathologic fracture. Examples of active treatment are surgical treatment, emergency department encounter, evaluation, and continuing treatment by the same or a different physician.

The seventh character is based on whether the patient is undergoing active treatment and not whether the provider is seeing the patient for the first time.

d. Osteoporosis

Osteoporosis is a systemic condition, meaning that all bones of the musculoskeletal system are affected. Therefore, site is not a component of the codes under category M81, Osteoporosis without current pathological fracture. The site codes under category M80, Osteoporosis with current pathological fracture, identify the site of the fracture, not the osteoporosis.

1) Osteoporosis without pathological fracture

Category M81, Osteoporosis without current pathological fracture, is for use for patients with osteoporosis who do not currently have a pathologic fracture due to the osteoporosis, even if they have had a fracture in the past. For patients with a history of osteoporosis fractures, status code Z87.310, Personal history of (healed) osteoporosis fracture, should follow the code from M81.

Age-related osteoporosis with healed osteoporotic fracture of the lumbar vertebra

M81.0   Age-related osteoporosis without current pathological fracture

Z87.310   Personal history of (healed) osteoporosis fracture

Explanation: Category M81 is used for patients with osteoporosis who do not currently have a pathologic fracture due to the osteoporosis. To report a previous (healed) fracture, status code Z87.310 Personal history of (healed) osteoporosis fracture, should follow the code from M81.

2) Osteoporosis with current pathological fracture

Category M80, Osteoporosis with current pathological fracture, is for patients who have a current pathologic fracture at the time of an encounter. The codes under M80 identify the site of the fracture. A code from category M80, not a traumatic fracture code, should be used for any patient with known osteoporosis who suffers a fracture, even if the patient had a minor fall or trauma, if that fall or trauma would not usually break a normal, healthy bone.

Disuse osteoporosis with current fracture of right shoulder sustained lifting a grocery bag, initial encounter

M80.811A   Other osteoporosis with current pathological fracture, right shoulder, initial encounter for fracture

Explanation: A code from category M80, not a traumatic fracture code, should be used for any patient with known osteoporosis who suffers a fracture, even if the patient had a minor fall or trauma, if that fall or trauma would not usually break a normal, healthy bone.

Muscle/Tendon Table

ICD-10-CM categorizes certain muscles and tendons in the upper and lower extremities by their action (e.g., extension, flexion), their anatomical location (e.g., posterior, anterior), and/or whether they are intrinsic or extrinsic to a certain anatomical area. The Muscle/Tendon Table is provided at the beginning of chapters 13 and 19 as a resource to help users when code selection depends on one or more of these characteristics. The categories and/or subcategories that relate to this table are identified by the icon ✦. Please note that this table is not all-inclusive, and proper code assignment should be based on the provider's documentation.

Body Region	Muscle	Extensor Tendon	Flexor Tendon	Other Tendon
Shoulder				
	Deltoid	Posterior deltoid	Anterior deltoid	
	Rotator cuff			
	Infraspinatus			Infraspinatus
	Subscapularis			Subscapularis
	Supraspinatus			Supraspinatus
	Teres minor			Teres minor
	Teres major	Teres major		
Upper arm				
	Anterior muscles			
	Biceps brachii — long head		Biceps brachii — long head	
	Biceps brachii — short head		Biceps brachii — short head	
	Brachialis		Brachialis	
	Coracobrachialis		Coracobrachialis	
	Posterior muscles			
	Triceps brachii	Triceps brachii		
Forearm				
	Anterior muscles			
	Flexors			
	Deep			
	Flexor digitorum profundus		Flexor digitorum profundus	
	Flexor pollicis longus		Flexor pollicis longus	
	Intermediate			
	Flexor digitorum superficialis		Flexor digitorum superficialis	
	Superficial			
	Flexor carpi radialis		Flexor carpi radialis	
	Flexor carpi ulnaris		Flexor carpi ulnaris	
	Palmaris longus		Palmaris longus	
	Pronators			
	Pronator quadratus			Pronator quadratus
	Pronator teres			Pronator teres
	Posterior muscles			
	Extensors			
	Deep			
	Abductor pollicis longus			Abductor pollicis longus
	Extensor indicis	Extensor indicis		
	Extensor pollicis brevis	Extensor pollicis brevis		
	Extensor pollicis longus	Extensor pollicis longus		
	Superficial			
	Brachioradialis			Brachioradialis
	Extensor carpi radialis brevis	Extensor carpi radialis brevis		
	Extensor carpi radialis longus	Extensor carpi radialis longus		
	Extensor carpi ulnaris	Extensor carpi ulnaris		
	Extensor digiti minimi	Extensor digiti minimi		
	Extensor digitorum	Extensor digitorum		
	Anconeus	Anconeus		
	Supinator			Supinator

Chapter 13. Diseases of the Musculoskeletal System and Connective Tissue

Body Region	Muscle	Extensor Tendon	Flexor Tendon	Other Tendon
Hand				
Extrinsic — attach to a site in the forearm as well as a site in the hand with action related to hand movement at the wrist				
	Extensor carpi radialis brevis	Extensor carpi radialis brevis		
	Extensor carpi radialis longus	Extensor carpie radialis longus		
	Extensor carpi ulnaris	Extensor carpi ulnaris		
	Flexor carpi radialis		Flexor carpi radialis	
	Flexor carpi ulnaris		Flexor carpi ulnaris	
	Flexor digitorum superficialis		Flexor digitorum superficialis	
	Palmaris longus		Palmaris longus	
Extrinsic — attach to a site in the forearm as well as a site in the hand with action in the hand related to finger movement				
	Adductor pollicis longus			Adductor pollicis longus
	Extensor digiti minimi	Extensor digiti minimi		
	Extensor digitorum	Extensor digitorum		
	Extensor indicis	Extensor indicis		
	Flexor digitorum profundus		Flexor digitorum profundus	
	Flexor digitorum superficialis		Flexor digitorum superficialis	
Extrinsic — attach to a site in the forearm as well as a site in the hand with action in the hand related to thumb movement				
	Extensor pollicis brevis	Extensor pollicis brevis		
	Extensor pollicis longus	Extensor pollicis longus		
	Flexor pollicis longus		Flexor pollicis longus	
Intrinsic — found within the hand only				
	Adductor pollicis			Adductor pollicis
	Dorsal interossei	Dorsal interossei	Dorsal interossei	
	Lumbricals	Lumbricals	Lumbricals	
	Palmaris brevis			Palmaris brevis
	Palmar interossei	Palmar interossei	Palmar interossei	
	Hypothenar muscles			
	Abductor digiti minimi			Abductor digiti minimi
	Flexor digiti minimi brevis		Flexor digiti minimi brevis	
	Oppenens digiti minimi		Oppenens digiti minimi	
	Thenar muscles			
	Abductor pollicis brevis			Abductor pollicis brevis
	Flexor pollicis brevis		Flexor pollicis brevis	
	Oppenens pollicis		Oppenens pollicis	
Thigh				
	Anterior muscles			
	Iliopsoas		Iliopsoas	
	Pectineus		Pectineus	
	Quadriceps	Quadriceps		
	Rectus femoris	Rectus femoris — Extends knee	Rectus femoris — Flexes hip	
	Vastus intermedius	Vastus intermedius		
	Vastus lateralis	Vastus lateralis		
	Vastus medialis	Vastus medialis		
	Sartorius		Sartorius	
	Medial muscles			
	Adductor brevis			Adductor brevis
	Adductor longus			Adductor longus
	Adductor magnus			Adductor magnus
	Gracilis			Gracilis
	Obturator externus			Obturator externus
	Posterior muscles			
	Hamstring	Hamstring — Extends hip	Hamstring — Flexes knee	
	Biceps femoris	Biceps femoris	Biceps femoris	
	Semimembranosus	Semimembranosus	Semimembranosus	
	Semitendinosus	Semitendinosus	Semitendinosus	

Body Region	Muscle	Extensor Tendon	Flexor Tendon	Other Tendon
Lower leg				
	Anterior muscles			
	Extensor digitorum longus	Extensor digitorum longus		
	Extensor hallucis longus	Extensor hallucis longus		
	Fibularis (peroneus) tertius	Fibularis (peroneus) tertius		
	Tibialis anterior	Tibialis anterior		Tibialis anterior
	Lateral muscles			
	Fibularis (peroneus) brevis		Fibularis (peroneus) brevis	
	Fibularis (peroneus) longus		Fibularis (peroneus) longus	
	Posterior muscles			
	Deep			
	Flexor digitorum longus		Flexor digitorum longus	
	Flexor hallucis longus		Flexor hallucis longus	
	Popliteus		Popliteus	
	Tibialis posterior		Tibialis posterior	
	Superficial			
	Gastrocnemius		Gastrocnemius	
	Plantaris		Plantaris	
	Soleus		Soleus	
				Calcaneal (Achilles)
Ankle/Foot				
Extrinsic — attach to a site in the lower leg as well as a site in the foot with action related to foot movement at the ankle				
	Plantaris		Plantaris	
	Soleus		Soleus	
	Tibialis anterior	Tibialis anterior		
	Tibialis posterior		Tibialis posterior	
Extrinsic — attach to a site in the lower leg as well as a site in the foot with action in the foot related to toe movement				
	Extensor digitorum longus	Extensor digitorum longus		
	Extensor hallicus longus	Extensor hallicus longus		
	Flexor digitorum longus		Flexor digitorum longus	
	Flexor hallucis longus		Flexor hallucis longus	
Intrinsic — found within the ankle/foot only				
	Dorsal muscles			
	Extensor digitorum brevis	Extensor digitorum brevis		
	Extensor hallucis brevis	Extensor hallucis brevis		
	Plantar muscles			
	Abductor digiti minimi		Abductor digiti minimi	
	Abductor hallucis		Abductor hallucis	
	Dorsal interossei	Dorsal interossei	Dorsal interossei	
	Flexor digiti minimi brevis		Flexor digiti minimi brevis	
	Flexor digitorum brevis		Flexor digitorum brevis	
	Flexor hallucis brevis		Flexor hallucis brevis	
	Lumbricals	Lumbricals	Lumbricals	
	Quadratus plantae		Quadratus plantae	
	Plantar interossei	Plantar interossei	Plantar interossei	

Chapter 13. Diseases of the Musculoskeletal System and Connective Tissue (M00-M99)

NOTE Use an external cause code following the code for the musculoskeletal condition, if applicable, to identify the cause of the musculoskeletal condition.

EXCLUDES 2 *arthropathic psoriasis (L40.5-)*
certain conditions originating in the perinatal period (P04-P96)
certain infectious and parasitic diseases (A00-B99)
compartment syndrome (traumatic) (T79.A-)
complications of pregnancy, childbirth and the puerperium (O00-O9A)
congenital malformations, deformations, and chromosomal abnormalities (Q00-Q99)
endocrine, nutritional and metabolic diseases (E00-E88)
injury, poisoning and certain other consequences of external causes (S00-T88)
neoplasms (C00-D49)
symptoms, signs and abnormal clinical and laboratory findings, not elsewhere classified (R00-R94)

This chapter contains the following blocks:

M00-M02	Infectious arthropathies
M05-M14	Inflammatory polyarthropathies
M15-M19	Osteoarthritis
M20-M25	Other joint disorders
M26-M27	Dentofacial anomalies [including malocclusion] and other disorders of jaw
M30-M36	Systemic connective tissue disorders
M40-M43	Deforming dorsopathies
M45-M49	Spondylopathies
M50-M54	Other dorsopathies
M60-M63	Disorders of muscles
M65-M67	Disorders of synovium and tendon
M70-M79	Other soft tissue disorders
M80-M85	Disorders of bone density and structure
M86-M90	Other osteopathies
M91-M94	Chondropathies
M95	Other disorders of the musculoskeletal system and connective tissue
M96	Intraoperative and postprocedural complications and disorders of musculoskeletal system, not elsewhere classified
M99	Biomechanical lesions, not elsewhere classified

ARTHROPATHIES (M00-M25)

INCLUDES disorders affecting predominantly peripheral (limb) joints

Infectious arthropathies (M00-M02)

NOTE This block comprises arthropathies due to microbiological agents. Distinction is made between the following types of etiological relationship:

a) direct infection of joint, where organisms invade synovial tissue and microbial antigen is present in the joint;

b) indirect infection, which may be of two types: a reactive arthropathy, where microbial infection of the body is established but neither organisms nor antigens can be identified in the joint, and a postinfective arthropathy, where microbial antigen is present but recovery of an organism is inconstant and evidence of local multiplication is lacking.

✓4ᵗʰ **M00 Pyogenic arthritis**

✓5ᵗʰ **M00.0 Staphylococcal arthritis and polyarthritis**
Use additional code (B95.61-B95.8) to identify bacterial agent
EXCLUDES 2 *infection and inflammatory reaction due to internal joint prosthesis (T84.5-)*

     M00.00 Staphylococcal arthritis, unspecified joint ▽

✓6ᵗʰ **M00.01 Staphylococcal arthritis,** shoulder
     M00.011 Staphylococcal arthritis, right shoulder
     M00.012 Staphylococcal arthritis, left shoulder
     M00.019 Staphylococcal arthritis, unspecified ▽ **shoulder**

✓6ᵗʰ **M00.02 Staphylococcal arthritis,** elbow
     M00.021 Staphylococcal arthritis, right elbow
     M00.022 Staphylococcal arthritis, left elbow
     M00.029 Staphylococcal arthritis, unspecified ▽ **elbow**

✓6ᵗʰ **M00.03 Staphylococcal arthritis,** wrist
Staphylococcal arthritis of carpal bones
     M00.031 Staphylococcal arthritis, right wrist
     M00.032 Staphylococcal arthritis, left wrist
     M00.039 Staphylococcal arthritis, unspecified ▽ **wrist**

✓6ᵗʰ **M00.04 Staphylococcal arthritis,** hand
Staphylococcal arthritis of metacarpus and phalanges
     M00.041 Staphylococcal arthritis, right hand
     M00.042 Staphylococcal arthritis, left hand
     M00.049 Staphylococcal arthritis, unspecified ▽ **hand**

✓6ᵗʰ **M00.05 Staphylococcal arthritis,** hip
     M00.051 Staphylococcal arthritis, right hip
     M00.052 Staphylococcal arthritis, left hip
     M00.059 Staphylococcal arthritis, unspecified ▽ **hip**

✓6ᵗʰ **M00.06 Staphylococcal arthritis,** knee
     M00.061 Staphylococcal arthritis, right knee
     M00.062 Staphylococcal arthritis, left knee
     M00.069 Staphylococcal arthritis, unspecified ▽ **knee**

✓6ᵗʰ **M00.07 Staphylococcal arthritis,** ankle and foot
Staphylococcal arthritis, tarsus, metatarsus and phalanges
     M00.071 Staphylococcal arthritis, right ankle and foot
     M00.072 Staphylococcal arthritis, left ankle and foot
     M00.079 Staphylococcal arthritis, unspecified ▽ **ankle and foot**

     M00.08 Staphylococcal arthritis, vertebrae

     M00.09 Staphylococcal polyarthritis

✓5ᵗʰ **M00.1 Pneumococcal arthritis and polyarthritis**
     M00.10 Pneumococcal arthritis, unspecified joint ▽

✓6ᵗʰ **M00.11 Pneumococcal arthritis,** shoulder
     M00.111 Pneumococcal arthritis, right shoulder
     M00.112 Pneumococcal arthritis, left shoulder
     M00.119 Pneumococcal arthritis, unspecified ▽ **shoulder**

✓6ᵗʰ **M00.12 Pneumococcal arthritis,** elbow
     M00.121 Pneumococcal arthritis, right elbow
     M00.122 Pneumococcal arthritis, left elbow
     M00.129 Pneumococcal arthritis, unspecified ▽ **elbow**

✓6ᵗʰ **M00.13 Pneumococcal arthritis,** wrist
Pneumococcal arthritis of carpal bones
     M00.131 Pneumococcal arthritis, right wrist
     M00.132 Pneumococcal arthritis, left wrist
     M00.139 Pneumococcal arthritis, unspecified ▽ **wrist**

✓6ᵗʰ **M00.14 Pneumococcal arthritis,** hand
Pneumococcal arthritis of metacarpus and phalanges
     M00.141 Pneumococcal arthritis, right hand
     M00.142 Pneumococcal arthritis, left hand
     M00.149 Pneumococcal arthritis, unspecified ▽ **hand**

✓6ᵗʰ **M00.15 Pneumococcal arthritis,** hip
     M00.151 Pneumococcal arthritis, right hip
     M00.152 Pneumococcal arthritis, left hip
     M00.159 Pneumococcal arthritis, unspecified ▽ **hip**

✓6ᵗʰ **M00.16 Pneumococcal arthritis,** knee
     M00.161 Pneumococcal arthritis, right knee
     M00.162 Pneumococcal arthritis, left knee
     M00.169 Pneumococcal arthritis, unspecified ▽ **knee**

✓6ᵗʰ **M00.17 Pneumococcal arthritis,** ankle and foot
Pneumococcal arthritis, tarsus, metatarsus and phalanges
     M00.171 Pneumococcal arthritis, right ankle and foot
     M00.172 Pneumococcal arthritis, left ankle and foot
     M00.179 Pneumococcal arthritis, unspecified ▽ **ankle and foot**

     M00.18 Pneumococcal arthritis, vertebrae

     M00.19 Pneumococcal polyarthritis

N Newborn   P Pediatric   M Maternity   A Adult   RIC RIC Dx   NCDx Noncancer Dx   PDx Primary Dx   CC RIC CC Condition   ►◄ Revised Text   ● New Code   ▲ Revised Code Title

678   ICD-10-CM 2016

✓5ᵗʰ **M00.2** **Other streptococcal arthritis and polyarthritis**
Use additional code (B95.0-B95.2, B95.4-B95.5) to identify bacterial agent

    M00.20 **Other streptococcal arthritis, unspecified** joint ▽

✓6ᵗʰ   **M00.21** **Other streptococcal arthritis, shoulder**
      M00.211 **Other streptococcal arthritis, right shoulder**
      M00.212 **Other streptococcal arthritis, left shoulder**
      M00.219 **Other streptococcal arthritis, unspecified shoulder** ▽

✓6ᵗʰ   **M00.22** **Other streptococcal arthritis, elbow**
      M00.221 **Other streptococcal arthritis, right elbow**
      M00.222 **Other streptococcal arthritis, left elbow**
      M00.229 **Other streptococcal arthritis, unspecified elbow** ▽

✓6ᵗʰ   **M00.23** **Other streptococcal arthritis, wrist**
     Other streptococcal arthritis of carpal bones
      M00.231 **Other streptococcal arthritis, right wrist**
      M00.232 **Other streptococcal arthritis, left wrist**
      M00.239 **Other streptococcal arthritis, unspecified wrist** ▽

✓6ᵗʰ   **M00.24** **Other streptococcal arthritis, hand**
     Other streptococcal arthritis metacarpus and phalanges
      M00.241 **Other streptococcal arthritis, right hand**
      M00.242 **Other streptococcal arthritis, left hand**
      M00.249 **Other streptococcal arthritis, unspecified hand** ▽

✓6ᵗʰ   **M00.25** **Other streptococcal arthritis, hip**
      M00.251 **Other streptococcal arthritis, right hip**
      M00.252 **Other streptococcal arthritis, left hip**
      M00.259 **Other streptococcal arthritis, unspecified hip** ▽

✓6ᵗʰ   **M00.26** **Other streptococcal arthritis, knee**
      M00.261 **Other streptococcal arthritis, right knee**
      M00.262 **Other streptococcal arthritis, left knee**
      M00.269 **Other streptococcal arthritis, unspecified knee** ▽

✓6ᵗʰ   **M00.27** **Other streptococcal arthritis, ankle and foot**
     Other streptococcal arthritis, tarsus, metatarsus and phalanges
      M00.271 **Other streptococcal arthritis, right ankle and foot**
      M00.272 **Other streptococcal arthritis, left ankle and foot**
      M00.279 **Other streptococcal arthritis, unspecified ankle and foot** ▽

    M00.28 **Other streptococcal arthritis, vertebrae**
    M00.29 **Other streptococcal polyarthritis**

✓5ᵗʰ **M00.8** **Arthritis and polyarthritis due to other bacteria**
Use additional code (B96) to identify bacteria

    M00.80 **Arthritis due to other bacteria, unspecified joint** ▽

✓6ᵗʰ   **M00.81** **Arthritis due to other bacteria, shoulder**
      M00.811 **Arthritis due to other bacteria, right shoulder**
      M00.812 **Arthritis due to other bacteria, left shoulder**
      M00.819 **Arthritis due to other bacteria, unspecified shoulder** ▽

✓6ᵗʰ   **M00.82** **Arthritis due to other bacteria, elbow**
      M00.821 **Arthritis due to other bacteria, right elbow**
      M00.822 **Arthritis due to other bacteria, left elbow**
      M00.829 **Arthritis due to other bacteria, unspecified elbow** ▽

✓6ᵗʰ   **M00.83** **Arthritis due to other bacteria, wrist**
     Arthritis due to other bacteria, carpal bones
      M00.831 **Arthritis due to other bacteria, right wrist**
      M00.832 **Arthritis due to other bacteria, left wrist**
      M00.839 **Arthritis due to other bacteria, unspecified wrist** ▽

✓6ᵗʰ   **M00.84** **Arthritis due to other bacteria, hand**
     Arthritis due to other bacteria, metacarpus and phalanges
      M00.841 **Arthritis due to other bacteria, right hand**

      M00.842 **Arthritis due to other bacteria, left hand**
      M00.849 **Arthritis due to other bacteria, unspecified hand** ▽

✓6ᵗʰ   **M00.85** **Arthritis due to other bacteria, hip**
      M00.851 **Arthritis due to other bacteria, right hip**
      M00.852 **Arthritis due to other bacteria, left hip**
      M00.859 **Arthritis due to other bacteria, unspecified hip** ▽

✓6ᵗʰ   **M00.86** **Arthritis due to other bacteria, knee**
      M00.861 **Arthritis due to other bacteria, right knee**
      M00.862 **Arthritis due to other bacteria, left knee**
      M00.869 **Arthritis due to other bacteria, unspecified knee** ▽

✓6ᵗʰ   **M00.87** **Arthritis due to other bacteria, ankle and foot**
     Arthritis due to other bacteria, tarsus, metatarsus, and phalanges
      M00.871 **Arthritis due to other bacteria, right ankle and foot**
      M00.872 **Arthritis due to other bacteria, left ankle and foot**
      M00.879 **Arthritis due to other bacteria, unspecified ankle and foot** ▽

    M00.88 **Arthritis due to other bacteria, vertebrae**
    M00.89 **Polyarthritis due to other bacteria**

M00.9 **Pyogenic arthritis, unspecified** ▽
    Infective arthritis NOS

✓4ᵗʰ **M01** **Direct infections of joint in infectious and parasitic diseases classified elsewhere**
Code first underlying disease, such as:
* leprosy [Hansen's disease] (A30.-)*
* mycoses (B35-B49)*
* O'nyong-nyong fever (A92.1)*
* paratyphoid fever (A01.1-A01.4)*
  EXCLUDES 1 *arthropathy in Lyme disease (A69.23)*
        gonococcal arthritis (A54.42)
        meningococcal arthritis (A39.83)
        mumps arthritis (B26.85)
        postinfective arthropathy (M02.-)
        postmeningococcal arthritis (A39.84)
        reactive arthritis (M02.3)
        rubella arthritis (B06.82)
        sarcoidosis arthritis (D86.86)
        typhoid fever arthritis (A01.04)
        tuberculosis arthritis (A18.01-A18.02)

✓5ᵗʰ **M01.X** **Direct infection of joint in infectious and parasitic diseases classified elsewhere**

    M01.X0 *Direct infection of unspecified joint in infectious and parasitic diseases classified elsewhere* ▽

✓6ᵗʰ   *M01.X1* *Direct infection of shoulder joint in infectious and parasitic diseases classified elsewhere*
      M01.X11 *Direct infection of right shoulder in infectious and parasitic diseases classified elsewhere*
      M01.X12 *Direct infection of left shoulder in infectious and parasitic diseases classified elsewhere*
      M01.X19 *Direct infection of unspecified shoulder in infectious and parasitic diseases classified elsewhere* ▽

✓6ᵗʰ   *M01.X2* *Direct infection of elbow in infectious and parasitic diseases classified elsewhere*
      M01.X21 *Direct infection of right elbow in infectious and parasitic diseases classified elsewhere*
      M01.X22 *Direct infection of left elbow in infectious and parasitic diseases classified elsewhere*
      M01.X29 *Direct infection of unspecified elbow in infectious and parasitic diseases classified elsewhere* ▽

✓6ᵗʰ   *M01.X3* *Direct infection of wrist in infectious and parasitic diseases classified elsewhere*
     Direct infection of carpal bones in infectious and parasitic diseases classified elsewhere
      M01.X31 *Direct infection of right wrist in infectious and parasitic diseases classified elsewhere*
      M01.X32 *Direct infection of left wrist in infectious and parasitic diseases classified elsewhere*
      M01.X39 *Direct infection of unspecified wrist in infectious and parasitic diseases classified elsewhere* ▽

☑ Add'l Character Required ✓7ᵗʰ Placeholder Alert   RUG IV Special Care High Dx   RUG IV Clinically Complex Dx   RUG IV Special Care Low Dx   Manifestation Code   Other Specified Code ▽ Unspecified Code

✓6ᵗʰ **M01.X4** **Direct infection of hand in infectious and parasitic diseases classified elsewhere**
Direct infection of metacarpus and phalanges in infectious and parasitic diseases classified elsewhere

M01.X41   *Direct infection of right hand in infectious and parasitic diseases classified elsewhere*

M01.X42   *Direct infection of left hand in infectious and parasitic diseases classified elsewhere*

M01.X49   *Direct infection of unspecified hand in infectious and parasitic diseases classified elsewhere* ▽

✓6ᵗʰ **M01.X5** **Direct infection of hip in infectious and parasitic diseases classified elsewhere**

M01.X51   *Direct infection of right hip in infectious and parasitic diseases classified elsewhere*

M01.X52   *Direct infection of left hip in infectious and parasitic diseases classified elsewhere*

M01.X59   *Direct infection of unspecified hip in infectious and parasitic diseases classified elsewhere* ▽

✓6ᵗʰ **M01.X6** **Direct infection of knee in infectious and parasitic diseases classified elsewhere**

M01.X61   *Direct infection of right knee in infectious and parasitic diseases classified elsewhere*

M01.X62   *Direct infection of left knee in infectious and parasitic diseases classified elsewhere*

M01.X69   *Direct infection of unspecified knee in infectious and parasitic diseases classified elsewhere* ▽

✓6ᵗʰ **M01.X7** **Direct infection of ankle and foot in infectious and parasitic diseases classified elsewhere**
Direct infection of tarsus, metatarsus and phalanges in infectious and parasitic diseases classified elsewhere

M01.X71   *Direct infection of right ankle and foot in infectious and parasitic diseases classified elsewhere*

M01.X72   *Direct infection of left ankle and foot in infectious and parasitic diseases classified elsewhere*

M01.X79   *Direct infection of unspecified ankle and foot in infectious and parasitic diseases classified elsewhere* ▽

M01.X8   *Direct infection of vertebrae in infectious and parasitic diseases classified elsewhere*

M01.X9   *Direct infection of multiple joints in infectious and parasitic diseases classified elsewhere*

✓4ᵗʰ **M02** **Postinfective and reactive arthropathies**
Code first underlying disease, such as:
    congenital syphilis [Clutton's joints] (A50.5)
    enteritis due to Yersinia enterocolitica (A04.6)
    infective endocarditis (I33.0)
    viral hepatitis (B15-B19)

  EXCLUDES 1   *Behçet's disease (M35.2)*
    direct infections of joint in infectious and parasitic diseases classified elsewhere (M01.-)
    postmeningococcal arthritis (A39.84)
    mumps arthritis (B26.85)
    rheumatic fever (I00)
    rubella arthritis (B06.82)
    syphilis arthritis (late) (A52.77)
    tabetic arthropathy [Charcôt's] (A52.16)

✓5ᵗʰ **M02.0** **Arthropathy following intestinal bypass**

M02.00   **Arthropathy following intestinal bypass, unspecified site** ▽

✓6ᵗʰ **M02.01**   **Arthropathy following intestinal bypass, shoulder**

M02.011   **Arthropathy following intestinal bypass, right shoulder**

M02.012   **Arthropathy following intestinal bypass, left shoulder**

M02.019   **Arthropathy following intestinal bypass, unspecified shoulder** ▽

✓6ᵗʰ **M02.02**   **Arthropathy following intestinal bypass, elbow**

M02.021   **Arthropathy following intestinal bypass, right elbow**

M02.022   **Arthropathy following intestinal bypass, left elbow**

M02.029   **Arthropathy following intestinal bypass, unspecified elbow** ▽

✓6ᵗʰ **M02.03**   **Arthropathy following intestinal bypass, wrist**
Arthropathy following intestinal bypass, carpal bones

M02.031   **Arthropathy following intestinal bypass, right wrist**

M02.032   **Arthropathy following intestinal bypass, left wrist**

M02.039   **Arthropathy following intestinal bypass, unspecified wrist** ▽

✓6ᵗʰ **M02.04**   **Arthropathy following intestinal bypass, hand**
Arthropathy following intestinal bypass, metacarpals and phalanges

M02.041   **Arthropathy following intestinal bypass, right hand**

M02.042   **Arthropathy following intestinal bypass, left hand**

M02.049   **Arthropathy following intestinal bypass, unspecified hand** ▽

✓6ᵗʰ **M02.05**   **Arthropathy following intestinal bypass, hip**

M02.051   **Arthropathy following intestinal bypass, right hip**

M02.052   **Arthropathy following intestinal bypass, left hip**

M02.059   **Arthropathy following intestinal bypass, unspecified hip** ▽

✓6ᵗʰ **M02.06**   **Arthropathy following intestinal bypass, knee**

M02.061   **Arthropathy following intestinal bypass, right knee**

M02.062   **Arthropathy following intestinal bypass, left knee**

M02.069   **Arthropathy following intestinal bypass, unspecified knee** ▽

✓6ᵗʰ **M02.07**   **Arthropathy following intestinal bypass, ankle and foot**
Arthropathy following intestinal bypass, tarsus, metatarsus and phalanges

M02.071   **Arthropathy following intestinal bypass, right ankle and foot**

M02.072   **Arthropathy following intestinal bypass, left ankle and foot**

M02.079   **Arthropathy following intestinal bypass, unspecified ankle and foot** ▽

M02.08   **Arthropathy following intestinal bypass, vertebrae**

M02.09   **Arthropathy following intestinal bypass, multiple sites**

✓5ᵗʰ **M02.1** **Postdysenteric arthropathy**

M02.10   **Postdysenteric arthropathy, unspecified site** ▽

✓6ᵗʰ **M02.11**   **Postdysenteric arthropathy, shoulder**

M02.111   **Postdysenteric arthropathy, right shoulder**

M02.112   **Postdysenteric arthropathy, left shoulder**

M02.119   **Postdysenteric arthropathy, unspecified shoulder** ▽

✓6ᵗʰ **M02.12**   **Postdysenteric arthropathy, elbow**

M02.121   **Postdysenteric arthropathy, right elbow**

M02.122   **Postdysenteric arthropathy, left elbow**

M02.129   **Postdysenteric arthropathy, unspecified elbow** ▽

✓6ᵗʰ **M02.13**   **Postdysenteric arthropathy, wrist**
Postdysenteric arthropathy, carpal bones

M02.131   **Postdysenteric arthropathy, right wrist**

M02.132   **Postdysenteric arthropathy, left wrist**

M02.139   **Postdysenteric arthropathy, unspecified wrist** ▽

✓6ᵗʰ **M02.14**   **Postdysenteric arthropathy, hand**
Postdysenteric arthropathy, metacarpus and phalanges

M02.141   **Postdysenteric arthropathy, right hand**

M02.142   **Postdysenteric arthropathy, left hand**

M02.149   **Postdysenteric arthropathy, unspecified hand** ▽

✓6ᵗʰ **M02.15**   **Postdysenteric arthropathy, hip**

M02.151   **Postdysenteric arthropathy, right hip**

M02.152   **Postdysenteric arthropathy, left hip**

M02.159   **Postdysenteric arthropathy, unspecified hip** ▽

✓6ᵗʰ **M02.16** **Postdysenteric arthropathy,** knee
    M02.161 **Postdysenteric arthropathy,** right **knee**
    M02.162 **Postdysenteric arthropathy,** left **knee**
    M02.169 **Postdysenteric arthropathy,** ▽
       unspecified knee

✓6ᵗʰ **M02.17** **Postdysenteric arthropathy,** ankle and foot
    Postdysenteric arthropathy, tarsus, metatarsus and
    phalanges
    M02.171 **Postdysenteric arthropathy,** right **ankle**
       and foot
    M02.172 **Postdysenteric arthropathy,** left **ankle and**
       foot
    M02.179 **Postdysenteric arthropathy,** ▽
       unspecified ankle and foot

   M02.18 **Postdysenteric arthropathy,** vertebrae

   M02.19 **Postdysenteric arthropathy,** multiple sites

✓5ᵗʰ **M02.2** Postimmunization arthropathy
   M02.20 **Postimmunization arthropathy, unspecified site** ▽

✓6ᵗʰ **M02.21** **Postimmunization arthropathy,** shoulder
    M02.211 **Postimmunization arthropathy,** right
       shoulder
    M02.212 **Postimmunization arthropathy,** left
       shoulder
    M02.219 **Postimmunization arthropathy,** ▽
       unspecified shoulder

✓6ᵗʰ **M02.22** **Postimmunization arthropathy,** elbow
    M02.221 **Postimmunization arthropathy,** right
       elbow
    M02.222 **Postimmunization arthropathy,** left **elbow**
    M02.229 **Postimmunization arthropathy,** ▽
       unspecified elbow

✓6ᵗʰ **M02.23** **Postimmunization arthropathy,** wrist
    Postimmunization arthropathy, carpal bones
    M02.231 **Postimmunization arthropathy,** right
       wrist
    M02.232 **Postimmunization arthropathy,** left **wrist**
    M02.239 **Postimmunization arthropathy,** ▽
       unspecified wrist

✓6ᵗʰ **M02.24** **Postimmunization arthropathy,** hand
    Postimmunization arthropathy, metacarpus and
    phalanges
    M02.241 **Postimmunization arthropathy,** right
       hand
    M02.242 **Postimmunization arthropathy,** left **hand**
    M02.249 **Postimmunization arthropathy,** ▽
       unspecified hand

✓6ᵗʰ **M02.25** **Postimmunization arthropathy,** hip
    M02.251 **Postimmunization arthropathy,** right **hip**
    M02.252 **Postimmunization arthropathy,** left **hip**
    M02.259 **Postimmunization arthropathy,** ▽
       unspecified hip

✓6ᵗʰ **M02.26** **Postimmunization arthropathy,** knee
    M02.261 **Postimmunization arthropathy,** right
       knee
    M02.262 **Postimmunization arthropathy,** left **knee**
    M02.269 **Postimmunization arthropathy,** ▽
       unspecified knee

✓6ᵗʰ **M02.27** **Postimmunization arthropathy,** ankle and foot
    Postimmunization arthropathy, tarsus, metatarsus and
    phalanges
    M02.271 **Postimmunization arthropathy,** right
       ankle and foot
    M02.272 **Postimmunization arthropathy,** left **ankle**
       and foot
    M02.279 **Postimmunization arthropathy,** ▽
       unspecified ankle and foot

   M02.28 **Postimmunization arthropathy,** vertebrae

   M02.29 **Postimmunization arthropathy,** multiple sites

✓5ᵗʰ **M02.3** Reiter's disease
    Reactive arthritis
   M02.30 **Reiter's disease, unspecified site** ▽

✓6ᵗʰ **M02.31** **Reiter's disease,** shoulder
    M02.311 **Reiter's disease, right shoulder**
    M02.312 **Reiter's disease,** left **shoulder**
    M02.319 **Reiter's disease, unspecified shoulder** ▽

✓6ᵗʰ **M02.32** **Reiter's disease,** elbow
    M02.321 **Reiter's disease,** right **elbow**
    M02.322 **Reiter's disease,** left **elbow**
    M02.329 **Reiter's disease, unspecified elbow** ▽

✓6ᵗʰ **M02.33** **Reiter's disease,** wrist
    Reiter's disease, carpal bones
    M02.331 **Reiter's disease, right wrist**
    M02.332 **Reiter's disease,** left **wrist**
    M02.339 **Reiter's disease, unspecified wrist** ▽

✓6ᵗʰ **M02.34** **Reiter's disease,** hand
    Reiter's disease, metacarpus and phalanges
    M02.341 **Reiter's disease, right hand**
    M02.342 **Reiter's disease,** left **hand**
    M02.349 **Reiter's disease, unspecified hand** ▽

✓6ᵗʰ **M02.35** **Reiter's disease,** hip
    M02.351 **Reiter's disease, right hip**
    M02.352 **Reiter's disease,** left **hip**
    M02.359 **Reiter's disease, unspecified hip** ▽

✓6ᵗʰ **M02.36** **Reiter's disease,** knee
    M02.361 **Reiter's disease, right knee**
    M02.362 **Reiter's disease,** left **knee**
    M02.369 **Reiter's disease, unspecified knee** ▽

✓6ᵗʰ **M02.37** **Reiter's disease,** ankle and foot
    Reiter's disease, tarsus, metatarsus and phalanges
    M02.371 **Reiter's disease,** right **ankle and foot**
    M02.372 **Reiter's disease,** left **ankle and foot**
    M02.379 **Reiter's disease, unspecified ankle** ▽
       and foot

   M02.38 **Reiter's disease,** vertebrae

   M02.39 **Reiter's disease,** multiple sites

✓5ᵗʰ **M02.8** Other reactive arthropathies
   M02.80 **Other reactive arthropathies, unspecified site** ▽

✓6ᵗʰ **M02.81** **Other reactive arthropathies,** shoulder
    M02.811 **Other reactive arthropathies,** right
       shoulder
    M02.812 **Other reactive arthropathies,** left
       shoulder
    M02.819 **Other reactive arthropathies,** ▽
       unspecified shoulder

✓6ᵗʰ **M02.82** **Other reactive arthropathies,** elbow
    M02.821 **Other reactive arthropathies,** right **elbow**
    M02.822 **Other reactive arthropathies,** left **elbow**
    M02.829 **Other reactive arthropathies,** ▽
       unspecified elbow

✓6ᵗʰ **M02.83** **Other reactive arthropathies,** wrist
    Other reactive arthropathies, carpal bones
    M02.831 **Other reactive arthropathies,** right **wrist**
    M02.832 **Other reactive arthropathies,** left **wrist**
    M02.839 **Other reactive arthropathies,** ▽
       unspecified wrist

✓6ᵗʰ **M02.84** **Other reactive arthropathies,** hand
    Other reactive arthropathies, metacarpus and
    phalanges
    M02.841 **Other reactive arthropathies,** right **hand**
    M02.842 **Other reactive arthropathies,** left **hand**
    M02.849 **Other reactive arthropathies,** ▽
       unspecified hand

✓6ᵗʰ **M02.85** **Other reactive arthropathies,** hip
    M02.851 **Other reactive arthropathies,** right **hip**
    M02.852 **Other reactive arthropathies,** left **hip**
    M02.859 **Other reactive arthropathies,** ▽
       unspecified hip

✓6ᵗʰ **M02.86** **Other reactive arthropathies,** knee
    M02.861 **Other reactive arthropathies,** right **knee**
    M02.862 **Other reactive arthropathies,** left **knee**
    M02.869 **Other reactive arthropathies,** ▽
       unspecified knee

✓6ᵗʰ **M02.87** **Other reactive arthropathies,** ankle and foot
    Other reactive arthropathies, tarsus, metatarsus and
    phalanges
    M02.871 **Other reactive arthropathies,** right **ankle**
       and foot
    M02.872 **Other reactive arthropathies,** left **ankle**
       and foot

☑ Add'l Character Required   ✓7ᵗʰ Placeholder Alert   RUG IV Special Care High Dx   RUG IV Clinically Complex Dx   RUG IV Special Care Low Dx   Manifestation Code   Other Specified Code   ▽ Unspecified Code

M02.879   **Other reactive arthropathies, unspecified ankle and foot** ▽

M02.88   *Other reactive arthropathies, vertebrae*

M02.89   *Other reactive arthropathies, multiple sites*

M02.9   *Reactive arthropathy, unspecified* ▽

Inflammatory polyarthropathies (M05-M14)

✓4ᵗʰ **M05   Rheumatoid arthritis with rheumatoid factor**

    EXCLUDES 1   rheumatic fever (I00)
          juvenile rheumatoid arthritis (M08.-)
          rheumatoid arthritis of spine (M45.-)

✓5ᵗʰ **M05.0   Felty's syndrome**
       Rheumatoid arthritis with splenoadenomegaly and leukopenia

   M05.00   Felty's syndrome, unspecified site ▽

   ✓6ᵗʰ **M05.01   Felty's syndrome, shoulder**

     M05.011   Felty's syndrome, right shoulder

     M05.012   Felty's syndrome, left shoulder

     M05.019   Felty's syndrome, unspecified shoulder ▽

   ✓6ᵗʰ **M05.02   Felty's syndrome, elbow**

     M05.021   Felty's syndrome, right elbow

     M05.022   Felty's syndrome, left elbow

     M05.029   Felty's syndrome, unspecified elbow ▽

   ✓6ᵗʰ **M05.03   Felty's syndrome, wrist**
       Felty's syndrome, carpal bones

     M05.031   Felty's syndrome, right wrist

     M05.032   Felty's syndrome, left wrist

     M05.039   Felty's syndrome, unspecified wrist ▽

   ✓6ᵗʰ **M05.04   Felty's syndrome, hand**
       Felty's syndrome, metacarpus and phalanges

     M05.041   Felty's syndrome, right hand

     M05.042   Felty's syndrome, left hand

     M05.049   Felty's syndrome, unspecified hand ▽

   ✓6ᵗʰ **M05.05   Felty's syndrome, hip**

     M05.051   Felty's syndrome, right hip

     M05.052   Felty's syndrome, left hip

     M05.059   Felty's syndrome, unspecified hip ▽

   ✓6ᵗʰ **M05.06   Felty's syndrome, knee**

     M05.061   Felty's syndrome, right knee

     M05.062   Felty's syndrome, left knee

     M05.069   Felty's syndrome, unspecified knee ▽

   ✓6ᵗʰ **M05.07   Felty's syndrome, ankle and foot**
       Felty's syndrome, tarsus, metatarsus and phalanges

     M05.071   Felty's syndrome, right ankle and foot

     M05.072   Felty's syndrome, left ankle and foot

     M05.079   Felty's syndrome, unspecified ankle and foot ▽

   M05.09   Felty's syndrome, multiple sites

✓5ᵗʰ **M05.1   Rheumatoid lung disease with rheumatoid arthritis**

   M05.10   Rheumatoid lung disease with rheumatoid arthritis of unspecified site ▽

   ✓6ᵗʰ **M05.11   Rheumatoid lung disease with rheumatoid arthritis of shoulder**

     M05.111   Rheumatoid lung disease with rheumatoid arthritis of right shoulder

     M05.112   Rheumatoid lung disease with rheumatoid arthritis of left shoulder

     M05.119   Rheumatoid lung disease with rheumatoid arthritis of unspecified shoulder ▽

   ✓6ᵗʰ **M05.12   Rheumatoid lung disease with rheumatoid arthritis of elbow**

     M05.121   Rheumatoid lung disease with rheumatoid arthritis of right elbow

     M05.122   Rheumatoid lung disease with rheumatoid arthritis of left elbow

     M05.129   Rheumatoid lung disease with rheumatoid arthritis of unspecified elbow ▽

   ✓6ᵗʰ **M05.13   Rheumatoid lung disease with rheumatoid arthritis of wrist**
       Rheumatoid lung disease with rheumatoid arthritis, carpal bones

     M05.131   Rheumatoid lung disease with rheumatoid arthritis of right wrist

     M05.132   Rheumatoid lung disease with rheumatoid arthritis of left wrist

     M05.139   Rheumatoid lung disease with rheumatoid arthritis of unspecified wrist ▽

   ✓6ᵗʰ **M05.14   Rheumatoid lung disease with rheumatoid arthritis of hand**
       Rheumatoid lung disease with rheumatoid arthritis, metacarpus and phalanges

     M05.141   Rheumatoid lung disease with rheumatoid arthritis of right hand

     M05.142   Rheumatoid lung disease with rheumatoid arthritis of left hand

     M05.149   Rheumatoid lung disease with rheumatoid arthritis of unspecified hand ▽

   ✓6ᵗʰ **M05.15   Rheumatoid lung disease with rheumatoid arthritis of hip**

     M05.151   Rheumatoid lung disease with rheumatoid arthritis of right hip

     M05.152   Rheumatoid lung disease with rheumatoid arthritis of left hip

     M05.159   Rheumatoid lung disease with rheumatoid arthritis of unspecified hip ▽

   ✓6ᵗʰ **M05.16   Rheumatoid lung disease with rheumatoid arthritis of knee**

     M05.161   Rheumatoid lung disease with rheumatoid arthritis of right knee

     M05.162   Rheumatoid lung disease with rheumatoid arthritis of left knee

     M05.169   Rheumatoid lung disease with rheumatoid arthritis of unspecified knee ▽

   ✓6ᵗʰ **M05.17   Rheumatoid lung disease with rheumatoid arthritis of ankle and foot**
       Rheumatoid lung disease with rheumatoid arthritis, tarsus, metatarsus and phalanges

     M05.171   Rheumatoid lung disease with rheumatoid arthritis of right ankle and foot

     M05.172   Rheumatoid lung disease with rheumatoid arthritis of left ankle and foot

     M05.179   Rheumatoid lung disease with rheumatoid arthritis of unspecified ankle and foot ▽

   M05.19   Rheumatoid lung disease with rheumatoid arthritis of multiple sites

✓5ᵗʰ **M05.2   Rheumatoid vasculitis with rheumatoid arthritis**

   M05.20   Rheumatoid vasculitis with rheumatoid arthritis of unspecified site ▽

   ✓6ᵗʰ **M05.21   Rheumatoid vasculitis with rheumatoid arthritis of shoulder**

     M05.211   Rheumatoid vasculitis with rheumatoid arthritis of right shoulder

     M05.212   Rheumatoid vasculitis with rheumatoid arthritis of left shoulder

     M05.219   Rheumatoid vasculitis with rheumatoid arthritis of unspecified shoulder ▽

   ✓6ᵗʰ **M05.22   Rheumatoid vasculitis with rheumatoid arthritis of elbow**

     M05.221   Rheumatoid vasculitis with rheumatoid arthritis of right elbow

     M05.222   Rheumatoid vasculitis with rheumatoid arthritis of left elbow

     M05.229   Rheumatoid vasculitis with rheumatoid arthritis of unspecified elbow ▽

   ✓6ᵗʰ **M05.23   Rheumatoid vasculitis with rheumatoid arthritis of wrist**
       Rheumatoid vasculitis with rheumatoid arthritis, carpal bones

     M05.231   Rheumatoid vasculitis with rheumatoid arthritis of right wrist

     M05.232   Rheumatoid vasculitis with rheumatoid arthritis of left wrist

     M05.239   Rheumatoid vasculitis with rheumatoid arthritis of unspecified wrist ▽

Ⓝ Newborn   Ⓟ Pediatric   Ⓜ Maternity   Ⓐ Adult   **RIC** RIC Dx   **NCDx** Noncancer Dx   **PDx** Primary Dx   **CC** RIC CC Condition   ▶◀ Revised Text   ● New Code   ▲ Revised Code Title

682   ICD-10-CM 2016

✓6ᵗʰ **M05.24 Rheumatoid vasculitis with rheumatoid arthritis of hand**
Rheumatoid vasculitis with rheumatoid arthritis, metacarpus and phalanges

     M05.241 Rheumatoid vasculitis with rheumatoid arthritis of right hand

     M05.242 Rheumatoid vasculitis with rheumatoid arthritis of left hand

     M05.249 Rheumatoid vasculitis with rheumatoid arthritis of unspecified hand ▽

✓6ᵗʰ **M05.25 Rheumatoid vasculitis with rheumatoid arthritis of hip**

     M05.251 Rheumatoid vasculitis with rheumatoid arthritis of right hip

     M05.252 Rheumatoid vasculitis with rheumatoid arthritis of left hip

     M05.259 Rheumatoid vasculitis with rheumatoid arthritis of unspecified hip ▽

✓6ᵗʰ **M05.26 Rheumatoid vasculitis with rheumatoid arthritis of knee**

     M05.261 Rheumatoid vasculitis with rheumatoid arthritis of right knee

     M05.262 Rheumatoid vasculitis with rheumatoid arthritis of left knee

     M05.269 Rheumatoid vasculitis with rheumatoid arthritis of unspecified knee ▽

✓6ᵗʰ **M05.27 Rheumatoid vasculitis with rheumatoid arthritis of ankle and foot**
Rheumatoid vasculitis with rheumatoid arthritis, tarsus, metatarsus and phalanges

     M05.271 Rheumatoid vasculitis with rheumatoid arthritis of right ankle and foot

     M05.272 Rheumatoid vasculitis with rheumatoid arthritis of left ankle and foot

     M05.279 Rheumatoid vasculitis with rheumatoid arthritis of unspecified ankle and foot ▽

M05.29 Rheumatoid vasculitis with rheumatoid arthritis of multiple sites

✓5ᵗʰ **M05.3 Rheumatoid heart disease with rheumatoid arthritis**
Rheumatoid carditis   Rheumatoid myocarditis
Rheumatoid endocarditis   Rheumatoid pericarditis

     M05.30 Rheumatoid heart disease with rheumatoid arthritis of unspecified site ▽

✓6ᵗʰ **M05.31 Rheumatoid heart disease with rheumatoid arthritis of shoulder**

     M05.311 Rheumatoid heart disease with rheumatoid arthritis of right shoulder

     M05.312 Rheumatoid heart disease with rheumatoid arthritis of left shoulder

     M05.319 Rheumatoid heart disease with rheumatoid arthritis of unspecified shoulder ▽

✓6ᵗʰ **M05.32 Rheumatoid heart disease with rheumatoid arthritis of elbow**

     M05.321 Rheumatoid heart disease with rheumatoid arthritis of right elbow

     M05.322 Rheumatoid heart disease with rheumatoid arthritis of left elbow

     M05.329 Rheumatoid heart disease with rheumatoid arthritis of unspecified elbow ▽

✓6ᵗʰ **M05.33 Rheumatoid heart disease with rheumatoid arthritis of wrist**
Rheumatoid heart disease with rheumatoid arthritis, carpal bones

     M05.331 Rheumatoid heart disease with rheumatoid arthritis of right wrist

     M05.332 Rheumatoid heart disease with rheumatoid arthritis of left wrist

     M05.339 Rheumatoid heart disease with rheumatoid arthritis of unspecified wrist ▽

✓6ᵗʰ **M05.34 Rheumatoid heart disease with rheumatoid arthritis of hand**
Rheumatoid heart disease with rheumatoid arthritis, metacarpus and phalanges

     M05.341 Rheumatoid heart disease with rheumatoid arthritis of right hand

     M05.342 Rheumatoid heart disease with rheumatoid arthritis of left hand

     M05.349 Rheumatoid heart disease with rheumatoid arthritis of unspecified hand ▽

✓6ᵗʰ **M05.35 Rheumatoid heart disease with rheumatoid arthritis of hip**

     M05.351 Rheumatoid heart disease with rheumatoid arthritis of right hip

     M05.352 Rheumatoid heart disease with rheumatoid arthritis of left hip

     M05.359 Rheumatoid heart disease with rheumatoid arthritis of unspecified hip ▽

✓6ᵗʰ **M05.36 Rheumatoid heart disease with rheumatoid arthritis of knee**

     M05.361 Rheumatoid heart disease with rheumatoid arthritis of right knee

     M05.362 Rheumatoid heart disease with rheumatoid arthritis of left knee

     M05.369 Rheumatoid heart disease with rheumatoid arthritis of unspecified knee ▽

✓6ᵗʰ **M05.37 Rheumatoid heart disease with rheumatoid arthritis of ankle and foot**
Rheumatoid heart disease with rheumatoid arthritis, tarsus, metatarsus and phalanges

     M05.371 Rheumatoid heart disease with rheumatoid arthritis of right ankle and foot

     M05.372 Rheumatoid heart disease with rheumatoid arthritis of left ankle and foot

     M05.379 Rheumatoid heart disease with rheumatoid arthritis of unspecified ankle and foot ▽

M05.39 Rheumatoid heart disease with rheumatoid arthritis of multiple sites

✓5ᵗʰ **M05.4 Rheumatoid myopathy with rheumatoid arthritis**

     M05.40 Rheumatoid myopathy with rheumatoid arthritis of unspecified site ▽

✓6ᵗʰ **M05.41 Rheumatoid myopathy with rheumatoid arthritis of shoulder**

     M05.411 Rheumatoid myopathy with rheumatoid arthritis of right shoulder

     M05.412 Rheumatoid myopathy with rheumatoid arthritis of left shoulder

     M05.419 Rheumatoid myopathy with rheumatoid arthritis of unspecified shoulder ▽

✓6ᵗʰ **M05.42 Rheumatoid myopathy with rheumatoid arthritis of elbow**

     M05.421 Rheumatoid myopathy with rheumatoid arthritis of right elbow

     M05.422 Rheumatoid myopathy with rheumatoid arthritis of left elbow

     M05.429 Rheumatoid myopathy with rheumatoid arthritis of unspecified elbow ▽

✓6ᵗʰ **M05.43 Rheumatoid myopathy with rheumatoid arthritis of wrist**
Rheumatoid myopathy with rheumatoid arthritis, carpal bones

     M05.431 Rheumatoid myopathy with rheumatoid arthritis of right wrist

     M05.432 Rheumatoid myopathy with rheumatoid arthritis of left wrist

     M05.439 Rheumatoid myopathy with rheumatoid arthritis of unspecified wrist ▽

✓6ᵗʰ **M05.44 Rheumatoid myopathy with rheumatoid arthritis of hand**
Rheumatoid myopathy with rheumatoid arthritis, metacarpus and phalanges

     M05.441 Rheumatoid myopathy with rheumatoid arthritis of right hand

Chapter 13. Diseases of the Musculoskeletal System and Connective Tissue

M05.442–M05.649

M05.442   **Rheumatoid myopathy with rheumatoid arthritis of** left **hand**

M05.449   **Rheumatoid myopathy with rheumatoid arthritis of unspecified hand** ▽

✓6ᵗʰ   **M05.45   Rheumatoid myopathy with rheumatoid arthritis of** hip

    M05.451   **Rheumatoid myopathy with rheumatoid arthritis of** right **hip**

    M05.452   **Rheumatoid myopathy with rheumatoid arthritis of** left **hip**

    M05.459   **Rheumatoid myopathy with rheumatoid arthritis of unspecified hip** ▽

✓6ᵗʰ   **M05.46   Rheumatoid myopathy with rheumatoid arthritis of** knee

    M05.461   **Rheumatoid myopathy with rheumatoid arthritis of** right **knee**

    M05.462   **Rheumatoid myopathy with rheumatoid arthritis of** left **knee**

    M05.469   **Rheumatoid myopathy with rheumatoid arthritis of unspecified knee** ▽

✓6ᵗʰ   **M05.47   Rheumatoid myopathy with rheumatoid arthritis of** ankle and foot

    Rheumatoid myopathy with rheumatoid arthritis, tarsus, metatarsus and phalanges

    M05.471   **Rheumatoid myopathy with rheumatoid arthritis of** right **ankle and foot**

    M05.472   **Rheumatoid myopathy with rheumatoid arthritis of** left **ankle and foot**

    M05.479   **Rheumatoid myopathy with rheumatoid arthritis of unspecified ankle and foot** ▽

   M05.49   **Rheumatoid myopathy with rheumatoid arthritis of** multiple sites

✓5ᵗʰ   **M05.5   Rheumatoid** polyneuropathy with rheumatoid arthritis

   M05.50   **Rheumatoid polyneuropathy with rheumatoid arthritis of unspecified site** ▽

✓6ᵗʰ   **M05.51   Rheumatoid polyneuropathy with rheumatoid arthritis of** shoulder

    M05.511   **Rheumatoid polyneuropathy with rheumatoid arthritis of** right **shoulder**

    M05.512   **Rheumatoid polyneuropathy with rheumatoid arthritis of** left **shoulder**

    M05.519   **Rheumatoid polyneuropathy with rheumatoid arthritis of unspecified shoulder** ▽

✓6ᵗʰ   **M05.52   Rheumatoid polyneuropathy with rheumatoid arthritis of** elbow

    M05.521   **Rheumatoid polyneuropathy with rheumatoid arthritis of** right **elbow**

    M05.522   **Rheumatoid polyneuropathy with rheumatoid arthritis of** left **elbow**

    M05.529   **Rheumatoid polyneuropathy with rheumatoid arthritis of unspecified elbow** ▽

✓6ᵗʰ   **M05.53   Rheumatoid polyneuropathy with rheumatoid arthritis of** wrist

    Rheumatoid polyneuropathy with rheumatoid arthritis, carpal bones

    M05.531   **Rheumatoid polyneuropathy with rheumatoid arthritis of** right **wrist**

    M05.532   **Rheumatoid polyneuropathy with rheumatoid arthritis of** left **wrist**

    M05.539   **Rheumatoid polyneuropathy with rheumatoid arthritis of unspecified wrist** ▽

✓6ᵗʰ   **M05.54   Rheumatoid polyneuropathy with rheumatoid arthritis of** hand

    Rheumatoid polyneuropathy with rheumatoid arthritis, metacarpus and phalanges

    M05.541   **Rheumatoid polyneuropathy with rheumatoid arthritis of** right **hand**

    M05.542   **Rheumatoid polyneuropathy with rheumatoid arthritis of** left **hand**

    M05.549   **Rheumatoid polyneuropathy with rheumatoid arthritis of unspecified hand** ▽

✓6ᵗʰ   **M05.55   Rheumatoid polyneuropathy with rheumatoid arthritis of** hip

    M05.551   **Rheumatoid polyneuropathy with rheumatoid arthritis of** right **hip**

    M05.552   **Rheumatoid polyneuropathy with rheumatoid arthritis of** left **hip**

    M05.559   **Rheumatoid polyneuropathy with rheumatoid arthritis of unspecified hip** ▽

✓6ᵗʰ   **M05.56   Rheumatoid polyneuropathy with rheumatoid arthritis of** knee

    M05.561   **Rheumatoid polyneuropathy with rheumatoid arthritis of** right **knee**

    M05.562   **Rheumatoid polyneuropathy with rheumatoid arthritis of** left **knee**

    M05.569   **Rheumatoid polyneuropathy with rheumatoid arthritis of unspecified knee** ▽

✓6ᵗʰ   **M05.57   Rheumatoid polyneuropathy with rheumatoid arthritis of** ankle and foot

    Rheumatoid polyneuropathy with rheumatoid arthritis, tarsus, metatarsus and phalanges

    M05.571   **Rheumatoid polyneuropathy with rheumatoid arthritis of** right **ankle and foot**

    M05.572   **Rheumatoid polyneuropathy with rheumatoid arthritis of** left **ankle and foot**

    M05.579   **Rheumatoid polyneuropathy with rheumatoid arthritis of unspecified ankle and foot** ▽

   M05.59   **Rheumatoid polyneuropathy with rheumatoid arthritis of** multiple sites

✓5ᵗʰ   **M05.6   Rheumatoid arthritis** with involvement of other organs and systems

   M05.60   **Rheumatoid arthritis of unspecified site with involvement of other organs and systems** ▽

✓6ᵗʰ   **M05.61   Rheumatoid arthritis of** shoulder **with involvement of other organs and systems**

    M05.611   **Rheumatoid arthritis of** right **shoulder with involvement of other organs and systems**

    M05.612   **Rheumatoid arthritis of** left **shoulder with involvement of other organs and systems**

    M05.619   **Rheumatoid arthritis of unspecified shoulder with involvement of other organs and systems** ▽

✓6ᵗʰ   **M05.62   Rheumatoid arthritis of** elbow **with involvement of other organs and systems**

    M05.621   **Rheumatoid arthritis of** right **elbow with involvement of other organs and systems**

    M05.622   **Rheumatoid arthritis of** left **elbow with involvement of other organs and systems**

    M05.629   **Rheumatoid arthritis of unspecified elbow with involvement of other organs and systems** ▽

✓6ᵗʰ   **M05.63   Rheumatoid arthritis of** wrist **with involvement of other organs and systems**

    Rheumatoid arthritis of carpal bones with involvement of other organs and systems

    M05.631   **Rheumatoid arthritis of** right **wrist with involvement of other organs and systems**

    M05.632   **Rheumatoid arthritis of** left **wrist with involvement of other organs and systems**

    M05.639   **Rheumatoid arthritis of unspecified wrist with involvement of other organs and systems** ▽

✓6ᵗʰ   **M05.64   Rheumatoid arthritis of** hand **with involvement of other organs and systems**

    Rheumatoid arthritis of metacarpus and phalanges with involvement of other organs and systems

    M05.641   **Rheumatoid arthritis of** right **hand with involvement of other organs and systems**

    M05.642   **Rheumatoid arthritis of** left **hand with involvement of other organs and systems**

    M05.649   **Rheumatoid arthritis of unspecified hand with involvement of other organs and systems** ▽

Ⓝ Newborn   Ⓟ Pediatric   Ⓜ Maternity   Ⓐ Adult   **RIC** RIC Dx   **NC Dx** Noncancer Dx   **PDx** Primary Dx   **CC** RIC CC Condition   ▶◀ Revised Text   ● New Code   ▲ Revised Code Title

684   ICD-10-CM 2016

✓6ᵗʰ **M05.65** **Rheumatoid arthritis of hip with involvement of other organs and systems**

     M05.651 Rheumatoid arthritis of right hip with involvement of other organs and systems

     M05.652 Rheumatoid arthritis of left hip with involvement of other organs and systems

     M05.659 Rheumatoid arthritis of unspecified hip with involvement of other organs and systems ▽

✓6ᵗʰ **M05.66** **Rheumatoid arthritis of knee with involvement of other organs and systems**

     M05.661 Rheumatoid arthritis of right knee with involvement of other organs and systems

     M05.662 Rheumatoid arthritis of left knee with involvement of other organs and systems

     M05.669 Rheumatoid arthritis of unspecified knee with involvement of other organs and systems ▽

✓6ᵗʰ **M05.67** **Rheumatoid arthritis of ankle and foot with involvement of other organs and systems**

     Rheumatoid arthritis of tarsus, metatarsus and phalanges with involvement of other organs and systems

     M05.671 Rheumatoid arthritis of right ankle and foot with involvement of other organs and systems

     M05.672 Rheumatoid arthritis of left ankle and foot with involvement of other organs and systems

     M05.679 Rheumatoid arthritis of unspecified ankle and foot with involvement of other organs and systems ▽

     M05.69 Rheumatoid arthritis of multiple sites with involvement of other organs and systems

✓5ᵗʰ **M05.7** **Rheumatoid arthritis with rheumatoid factor without organ or systems involvement**

     M05.70 Rheumatoid arthritis with rheumatoid factor of unspecified site without organ or systems involvement ▽

✓6ᵗʰ **M05.71** **Rheumatoid arthritis with rheumatoid factor of shoulder without organ or systems involvement**

     M05.711 Rheumatoid arthritis with rheumatoid factor of right shoulder without organ or systems involvement

     M05.712 Rheumatoid arthritis with rheumatoid factor of left shoulder without organ or systems involvement

     M05.719 Rheumatoid arthritis with rheumatoid factor of unspecified shoulder without organ or systems involvement ▽

✓6ᵗʰ **M05.72** **Rheumatoid arthritis with rheumatoid factor of elbow without organ or systems involvement**

     M05.721 Rheumatoid arthritis with rheumatoid factor of right elbow without organ or systems involvement

     M05.722 Rheumatoid arthritis with rheumatoid factor of left elbow without organ or systems involvement

     M05.729 Rheumatoid arthritis with rheumatoid factor of unspecified elbow without organ or systems involvement ▽

✓6ᵗʰ **M05.73** **Rheumatoid arthritis with rheumatoid factor of wrist without organ or systems involvement**

     M05.731 Rheumatoid arthritis with rheumatoid factor of right wrist without organ or systems involvement

     M05.732 Rheumatoid arthritis with rheumatoid factor of left wrist without organ or systems involvement

     M05.739 Rheumatoid arthritis with rheumatoid factor of unspecified wrist without organ or systems involvement ▽

✓6ᵗʰ **M05.74** **Rheumatoid arthritis with rheumatoid factor of hand without organ or systems involvement**

     M05.741 Rheumatoid arthritis with rheumatoid factor of right hand without organ or systems involvement

     M05.742 Rheumatoid arthritis with rheumatoid factor of left hand without organ or systems involvement

     M05.749 Rheumatoid arthritis with rheumatoid factor of unspecified hand without organ or systems involvement ▽

✓6ᵗʰ **M05.75** **Rheumatoid arthritis with rheumatoid factor of hip without organ or systems involvement**

     M05.751 Rheumatoid arthritis with rheumatoid factor of right hip without organ or systems involvement

     M05.752 Rheumatoid arthritis with rheumatoid factor of left hip without organ or systems involvement

     M05.759 Rheumatoid arthritis with rheumatoid factor of unspecified hip without organ or systems involvement ▽

✓6ᵗʰ **M05.76** **Rheumatoid arthritis with rheumatoid factor of knee without organ or systems involvement**

     M05.761 Rheumatoid arthritis with rheumatoid factor of right knee without organ or systems involvement

     M05.762 Rheumatoid arthritis with rheumatoid factor of left knee without organ or systems involvement

     M05.769 Rheumatoid arthritis with rheumatoid factor of unspecified knee without organ or systems involvement ▽

✓6ᵗʰ **M05.77** **Rheumatoid arthritis with rheumatoid factor of ankle and foot without organ or systems involvement**

     M05.771 Rheumatoid arthritis with rheumatoid factor of right ankle and foot without organ or systems involvement

     M05.772 Rheumatoid arthritis with rheumatoid factor of left ankle and foot without organ or systems involvement

     M05.779 Rheumatoid arthritis with rheumatoid factor of unspecified ankle and foot without organ or systems involvement ▽

     M05.79 Rheumatoid arthritis with rheumatoid factor of multiple sites without organ or systems involvement

✓5ᵗʰ **M05.8** **Other rheumatoid arthritis with rheumatoid factor**

     M05.80 Other rheumatoid arthritis with rheumatoid factor of unspecified site ▽

✓6ᵗʰ **M05.81** **Other rheumatoid arthritis with rheumatoid factor of shoulder**

     M05.811 Other rheumatoid arthritis with rheumatoid factor of right shoulder

     M05.812 Other rheumatoid arthritis with rheumatoid factor of left shoulder

     M05.819 Other rheumatoid arthritis with rheumatoid factor of unspecified shoulder ▽

✓6ᵗʰ **M05.82** **Other rheumatoid arthritis with rheumatoid factor of elbow**

     M05.821 Other rheumatoid arthritis with rheumatoid factor of right elbow

     M05.822 Other rheumatoid arthritis with rheumatoid factor of left elbow

     M05.829 Other rheumatoid arthritis with rheumatoid factor of unspecified elbow ▽

✓6ᵗʰ **M05.83** **Other rheumatoid arthritis with rheumatoid factor of wrist**

     M05.831 Other rheumatoid arthritis with rheumatoid factor of right wrist

     M05.832 Other rheumatoid arthritis with rheumatoid factor of left wrist

     M05.839 Other rheumatoid arthritis with rheumatoid factor of unspecified wrist ▽

✓6ᵗʰ **M05.84** **Other rheumatoid arthritis with rheumatoid factor of hand**

     M05.841 Other rheumatoid arthritis with rheumatoid factor of right hand

     M05.842 Other rheumatoid arthritis with rheumatoid factor of left hand

     M05.849 Other rheumatoid arthritis with rheumatoid factor of unspecified hand ▽

☑ Add'l Character Required ✓x7ᵗʰ Placeholder Alert   RUG IV Special Care High Dx   RUG IV Clinically Complex Dx   RUG IV Special Care Low Dx   Manifestation Code   Other Specified Code   ▽ Unspecified Code

ICD-10-CM 2016   685

✓6ᵗʰ **M05.85** Other rheumatoid arthritis with rheumatoid factor of hip

     M05.851 Other rheumatoid arthritis with rheumatoid factor of right hip

     M05.852 Other rheumatoid arthritis with rheumatoid factor of left hip

     M05.859 Other rheumatoid arthritis with rheumatoid factor of unspecified hip ▽

✓6ᵗʰ **M05.86** Other rheumatoid arthritis with rheumatoid factor of knee

     M05.861 Other rheumatoid arthritis with rheumatoid factor of right knee

     M05.862 Other rheumatoid arthritis with rheumatoid factor of left knee

     M05.869 Other rheumatoid arthritis with rheumatoid factor of unspecified knee ▽

✓6ᵗʰ **M05.87** Other rheumatoid arthritis with rheumatoid factor of ankle and foot

     M05.871 Other rheumatoid arthritis with rheumatoid factor of right ankle and foot

     M05.872 Other rheumatoid arthritis with rheumatoid factor of left ankle and foot

     M05.879 Other rheumatoid arthritis with rheumatoid factor of unspecified ankle and foot ▽

     M05.89 Other rheumatoid arthritis with rheumatoid factor of multiple sites

M05.9 Rheumatoid arthritis with rheumatoid factor, unspecified ▽

✓4ᵗʰ **M06** Other rheumatoid arthritis

✓5ᵗʰ **M06.0** Rheumatoid arthritis without rheumatoid factor

     M06.00 Rheumatoid arthritis without rheumatoid factor, unspecified site ▽

  ✓6ᵗʰ **M06.01** Rheumatoid arthritis without rheumatoid factor, shoulder

     M06.011 Rheumatoid arthritis without rheumatoid factor, right shoulder

     M06.012 Rheumatoid arthritis without rheumatoid factor, left shoulder

     M06.019 Rheumatoid arthritis without rheumatoid factor, unspecified shoulder ▽

  ✓6ᵗʰ **M06.02** Rheumatoid arthritis without rheumatoid factor, elbow

     M06.021 Rheumatoid arthritis without rheumatoid factor, right elbow

     M06.022 Rheumatoid arthritis without rheumatoid factor, left elbow

     M06.029 Rheumatoid arthritis without rheumatoid factor, unspecified elbow ▽

  ✓6ᵗʰ **M06.03** Rheumatoid arthritis without rheumatoid factor, wrist

     M06.031 Rheumatoid arthritis without rheumatoid factor, right wrist

     M06.032 Rheumatoid arthritis without rheumatoid factor, left wrist

     M06.039 Rheumatoid arthritis without rheumatoid factor, unspecified wrist ▽

  ✓6ᵗʰ **M06.04** Rheumatoid arthritis without rheumatoid factor, hand

     M06.041 Rheumatoid arthritis without rheumatoid factor, right hand

     M06.042 Rheumatoid arthritis without rheumatoid factor, left hand

     M06.049 Rheumatoid arthritis without rheumatoid factor, unspecified hand ▽

  ✓6ᵗʰ **M06.05** Rheumatoid arthritis without rheumatoid factor, hip

     M06.051 Rheumatoid arthritis without rheumatoid factor, right hip

     M06.052 Rheumatoid arthritis without rheumatoid factor, left hip

     M06.059 Rheumatoid arthritis without rheumatoid factor, unspecified hip ▽

  ✓6ᵗʰ **M06.06** Rheumatoid arthritis without rheumatoid factor, knee

     M06.061 Rheumatoid arthritis without rheumatoid factor, right knee

     M06.062 Rheumatoid arthritis without rheumatoid factor, left knee

     M06.069 Rheumatoid arthritis without rheumatoid factor, unspecified knee ▽

  ✓6ᵗʰ **M06.07** Rheumatoid arthritis without rheumatoid factor, ankle and foot

     M06.071 Rheumatoid arthritis without rheumatoid factor, right ankle and foot

     M06.072 Rheumatoid arthritis without rheumatoid factor, left ankle and foot

     M06.079 Rheumatoid arthritis without rheumatoid factor, unspecified ankle and foot ▽

     M06.08 Rheumatoid arthritis without rheumatoid factor, vertebrae

     M06.09 Rheumatoid arthritis without rheumatoid factor, multiple sites

M06.1 Adult-onset Still's disease   Ⓐ

   EXCLUDES 1   Still's disease NOS (M08.2-)

✓5ᵗʰ **M06.2** Rheumatoid bursitis

     M06.20 Rheumatoid bursitis, unspecified site ▽

  ✓6ᵗʰ **M06.21** Rheumatoid bursitis, shoulder

     M06.211 Rheumatoid bursitis, right shoulder

     M06.212 Rheumatoid bursitis, left shoulder

     M06.219 Rheumatoid bursitis, unspecified shoulder ▽

  ✓6ᵗʰ **M06.22** Rheumatoid bursitis, elbow

     M06.221 Rheumatoid bursitis, right elbow

     M06.222 Rheumatoid bursitis, left elbow

     M06.229 Rheumatoid bursitis, unspecified elbow ▽

  ✓6ᵗʰ **M06.23** Rheumatoid bursitis, wrist

     M06.231 Rheumatoid bursitis, right wrist

     M06.232 Rheumatoid bursitis, left wrist

     M06.239 Rheumatoid bursitis, unspecified wrist ▽

  ✓6ᵗʰ **M06.24** Rheumatoid bursitis, hand

     M06.241 Rheumatoid bursitis, right hand

     M06.242 Rheumatoid bursitis, left hand

     M06.249 Rheumatoid bursitis, unspecified hand ▽

  ✓6ᵗʰ **M06.25** Rheumatoid bursitis, hip

     M06.251 Rheumatoid bursitis, right hip

     M06.252 Rheumatoid bursitis, left hip

     M06.259 Rheumatoid bursitis, unspecified hip ▽

  ✓6ᵗʰ **M06.26** Rheumatoid bursitis, knee

     M06.261 Rheumatoid bursitis, right knee

     M06.262 Rheumatoid bursitis, left knee

     M06.269 Rheumatoid bursitis, unspecified knee ▽

  ✓6ᵗʰ **M06.27** Rheumatoid bursitis, ankle and foot

     M06.271 Rheumatoid bursitis, right ankle and foot

     M06.272 Rheumatoid bursitis, left ankle and foot

     M06.279 Rheumatoid bursitis, unspecified ankle and foot ▽

     M06.28 Rheumatoid bursitis, vertebrae

     M06.29 Rheumatoid bursitis, multiple sites

✓5ᵗʰ **M06.3** Rheumatoid nodule

     M06.30 Rheumatoid nodule, unspecified site ▽

  ✓6ᵗʰ **M06.31** Rheumatoid nodule, shoulder

     M06.311 Rheumatoid nodule, right shoulder

     M06.312 Rheumatoid nodule, left shoulder

     M06.319 Rheumatoid nodule, unspecified shoulder ▽

  ✓6ᵗʰ **M06.32** Rheumatoid nodule, elbow

     M06.321 Rheumatoid nodule, right elbow

     M06.322 Rheumatoid nodule, left elbow

     M06.329 Rheumatoid nodule, unspecified elbow ▽

  ✓6ᵗʰ **M06.33** Rheumatoid nodule, wrist

     M06.331 Rheumatoid nodule, right wrist

     M06.332 Rheumatoid nodule, left wrist

     M06.339 Rheumatoid nodule, unspecified wrist ▽

  ✓6ᵗʰ **M06.34** Rheumatoid nodule, hand

     M06.341 Rheumatoid nodule, right hand

     M06.342 Rheumatoid nodule, left hand

     M06.349 Rheumatoid nodule, unspecified hand ▽

Ⓝ Newborn   Ⓟ Pediatric   Ⓜ Maternity   Ⓐ Adult   **RIC** RIC Dx   **NC Dx** Noncancer Dx   **PD Dx** Primary Dx   **CC** RIC CC Condition   ►◄ Revised Text   ● New Code   ▲ Revised Code Title

686   ICD-10-CM 2016

✓6ᵗʰ **M06.35** **Rheumatoid nodule,** hip
　　　　M06.351 **Rheumatoid nodule,** right **hip**
　　　　M06.352 **Rheumatoid nodule,** left **hip**
　　　　M06.359 **Rheumatoid nodule,** unspecified hip ▽

✓6ᵗʰ **M06.36** **Rheumatoid nodule,** knee
　　　　M06.361 **Rheumatoid nodule,** right **knee**
　　　　M06.362 **Rheumatoid nodule,** left **knee**
　　　　M06.369 **Rheumatoid nodule,** unspecified knee ▽

✓6ᵗʰ **M06.37** **Rheumatoid nodule,** ankle and foot
　　　　M06.371 **Rheumatoid nodule,** right **ankle and foot**
　　　　M06.372 **Rheumatoid nodule,** left **ankle and foot**
　　　　M06.379 **Rheumatoid nodule,** unspecified ▽
　　　　　　　　ankle and foot

　　　　M06.38 **Rheumatoid nodule,** vertebrae
　　　　M06.39 **Rheumatoid nodule,** multiple sites

M06.4 **Inflammatory polyarthropathy**
　　EXCLUDES 1 *polyarthritis NOS (M13.0)*

✓5ᵗʰ **M06.8** **Other** specified rheumatoid arthritis
　　　M06.80 **Other specified rheumatoid arthritis,** ▽
　　　　　unspecified site

✓6ᵗʰ **M06.81** **Other specified rheumatoid arthritis,** shoulder
　　　　M06.811 **Other specified rheumatoid arthritis,** right
　　　　　　　shoulder
　　　　M06.812 **Other specified rheumatoid arthritis,** left
　　　　　　　shoulder
　　　　M06.819 **Other specified rheumatoid arthritis,** ▽
　　　　　　　unspecified shoulder

✓6ᵗʰ **M06.82** **Other specified rheumatoid arthritis,** elbow
　　　　M06.821 **Other specified rheumatoid arthritis,** right
　　　　　　　elbow
　　　　M06.822 **Other specified rheumatoid arthritis,** left
　　　　　　　elbow
　　　　M06.829 **Other specified rheumatoid arthritis,** ▽
　　　　　　　unspecified elbow

✓6ᵗʰ **M06.83** **Other specified rheumatoid arthritis,** wrist
　　　　M06.831 **Other specified rheumatoid arthritis,** right
　　　　　　　wrist
　　　　M06.832 **Other specified rheumatoid arthritis,** left
　　　　　　　wrist
　　　　M06.839 **Other specified rheumatoid arthritis,** ▽
　　　　　　　unspecified wrist

✓6ᵗʰ **M06.84** **Other specified rheumatoid arthritis,** hand
　　　　M06.841 **Other specified rheumatoid arthritis,** right
　　　　　　　hand
　　　　M06.842 **Other specified rheumatoid arthritis,** left
　　　　　　　hand
　　　　M06.849 **Other specified rheumatoid arthritis,** ▽
　　　　　　　unspecified hand

✓6ᵗʰ **M06.85** **Other specified rheumatoid arthritis,** hip
　　　　M06.851 **Other specified rheumatoid arthritis,** right
　　　　　　　hip
　　　　M06.852 **Other specified rheumatoid arthritis,** left
　　　　　　　hip
　　　　M06.859 **Other specified rheumatoid arthritis,** ▽
　　　　　　　unspecified hip

✓6ᵗʰ **M06.86** **Other specified rheumatoid arthritis,** knee
　　　　M06.861 **Other specified rheumatoid arthritis,** right
　　　　　　　knee
　　　　M06.862 **Other specified rheumatoid arthritis,** left
　　　　　　　knee
　　　　M06.869 **Other specified rheumatoid arthritis,** ▽
　　　　　　　unspecified knee

✓6ᵗʰ **M06.87** **Other specified rheumatoid arthritis,** ankle and foot
　　　　M06.871 **Other specified rheumatoid arthritis,** right
　　　　　　　ankle and foot
　　　　M06.872 **Other specified rheumatoid arthritis,** left
　　　　　　　ankle and foot
　　　　M06.879 **Other specified rheumatoid arthritis,** ▽
　　　　　　　unspecified ankle and foot

　　　　M06.88 **Other specified rheumatoid arthritis,** vertebrae
　　　　M06.89 **Other specified rheumatoid arthritis,** multiple sites

M06.9 **Rheumatoid arthritis, unspecified** ▽

✓4ᵗʰ **M07** **Enteropathic arthropathies**
　　Code also associated enteropathy, such as:
　　　regional enteritis [Crohn's disease] (K50.-)
　　　ulcerative colitis (K51.-)
　　　EXCLUDES 1 *psoriatic arthropathies (L40.5-)*

✓5ᵗʰ **M07.6** **Enteropathic arthropathies**
　　　M07.60 **Enteropathic arthropathies,** unspecified site ▽

✓6ᵗʰ **M07.61** **Enteropathic arthropathies,** shoulder
　　　　M07.611 **Enteropathic arthropathies,** right shoulder
　　　　M07.612 **Enteropathic arthropathies,** left **shoulder**
　　　　M07.619 **Enteropathic arthropathies,** ▽
　　　　　　　unspecified shoulder

✓6ᵗʰ **M07.62** **Enteropathic arthropathies,** elbow
　　　　M07.621 **Enteropathic arthropathies,** right **elbow**
　　　　M07.622 **Enteropathic arthropathies,** left **elbow**
　　　　M07.629 **Enteropathic arthropathies,** ▽
　　　　　　　unspecified elbow

✓6ᵗʰ **M07.63** **Enteropathic arthropathies,** wrist
　　　　M07.631 **Enteropathic arthropathies,** right **wrist**
　　　　M07.632 **Enteropathic arthropathies,** left **wrist**
　　　　M07.639 **Enteropathic arthropathies,** ▽
　　　　　　　unspecified wrist

✓6ᵗʰ **M07.64** **Enteropathic arthropathies,** hand
　　　　M07.641 **Enteropathic arthropathies,** right **hand**
　　　　M07.642 **Enteropathic arthropathies,** left **hand**
　　　　M07.649 **Enteropathic arthropathies,** ▽
　　　　　　　unspecified hand

✓6ᵗʰ **M07.65** **Enteropathic arthropathies,** hip
　　　　M07.651 **Enteropathic arthropathies,** right **hip**
　　　　M07.652 **Enteropathic arthropathies,** left **hip**
　　　　M07.659 **Enteropathic arthropathies,** ▽
　　　　　　　unspecified hip

✓6ᵗʰ **M07.66** **Enteropathic arthropathies,** knee
　　　　M07.661 **Enteropathic arthropathies,** right **knee**
　　　　M07.662 **Enteropathic arthropathies,** left **knee**
　　　　M07.669 **Enteropathic arthropathies,** ▽
　　　　　　　unspecified knee

✓6ᵗʰ **M07.67** **Enteropathic arthropathies,** ankle and foot
　　　　M07.671 **Enteropathic arthropathies,** right **ankle**
　　　　　　　and foot
　　　　M07.672 **Enteropathic arthropathies,** left **ankle and**
　　　　　　　foot
　　　　M07.679 **Enteropathic arthropathies,** ▽
　　　　　　　unspecified ankle and foot

　　　　M07.68 **Enteropathic arthropathies,** vertebrae
　　　　M07.69 **Enteropathic arthropathies,** multiple sites

✓4ᵗʰ **M08** **Juvenile arthritis**
　　Code also any associated underlying condition, such as:
　　　regional enteritis [Crohn's disease] (K50.-)
　　　ulcerative colitis (K51.-)
　　　EXCLUDES 1 *arthropathy in Whipple's disease (M14.8)*
　　　　Felty's syndrome (M05.0)
　　　　juvenile dermatomyositis (M33.0-)
　　　　psoriatic juvenile arthropathy (L40.54)

✓5ᵗʰ **M08.0** **Unspecified juvenile** rheumatoid arthritis
　　　Juvenile rheumatoid arthritis with or without rheumatoid factor
　　　M08.00 **Unspecified juvenile rheumatoid arthritis of** ▽
　　　　　unspecified site

✓6ᵗʰ **M08.01** **Unspecified juvenile rheumatoid arthritis,** shoulder
　　　　M08.011 **Unspecified juvenile rheumatoid** ▽
　　　　　　　arthritis, right **shoulder**
　　　　M08.012 **Unspecified juvenile rheumatoid** ▽
　　　　　　　arthritis, left **shoulder**
　　　　M08.019 **Unspecified juvenile rheumatoid** ▽
　　　　　　　arthritis, unspecified shoulder

✓6ᵗʰ **M08.02** **Unspecified juvenile rheumatoid arthritis of** elbow
　　　　M08.021 **Unspecified juvenile rheumatoid** ▽
　　　　　　　arthritis, right **elbow**
　　　　M08.022 **Unspecified juvenile rheumatoid** ▽
　　　　　　　arthritis, left **elbow**
　　　　M08.029 **Unspecified juvenile rheumatoid** ▽
　　　　　　　arthritis, unspecified elbow

✔ Add'l Character Required　✓✗7ᵗʰ Placeholder Alert　RUG IV Special Care High Dx　RUG IV Clinically Complex Dx　RUG IV Special Care Low Dx　Manifestation Code　Other Specified Code　▽ Unspecified Code

ICD-10-CM 2016　　　　　　　　　　687

Chapter 13. Diseases of the Musculoskeletal System and Connective Tissue

M08.03–M08.462

✓6ᵗʰ **M08.03 Unspecified juvenile rheumatoid arthritis, wrist**
  M08.031 Unspecified juvenile rheumatoid arthritis, right wrist ▽
  M08.032 Unspecified juvenile rheumatoid arthritis, left wrist ▽
  M08.039 Unspecified juvenile rheumatoid arthritis, unspecified wrist ▽

✓6ᵗʰ **M08.04 Unspecified juvenile rheumatoid arthritis, hand**
  M08.041 Unspecified juvenile rheumatoid arthritis, right hand ▽
  M08.042 Unspecified juvenile rheumatoid arthritis, left hand ▽
  M08.049 Unspecified juvenile rheumatoid arthritis, unspecified hand ▽

✓6ᵗʰ **M08.05 Unspecified juvenile rheumatoid arthritis, hip**
  M08.051 Unspecified juvenile rheumatoid arthritis, right hip ▽
  M08.052 Unspecified juvenile rheumatoid arthritis, left hip ▽
  M08.059 Unspecified juvenile rheumatoid arthritis, unspecified hip ▽

✓6ᵗʰ **M08.06 Unspecified juvenile rheumatoid arthritis, knee**
  M08.061 Unspecified juvenile rheumatoid arthritis, right knee ▽
  M08.062 Unspecified juvenile rheumatoid arthritis, left knee ▽
  M08.069 Unspecified juvenile rheumatoid arthritis, unspecified knee ▽

✓6ᵗʰ **M08.07 Unspecified juvenile rheumatoid arthritis, ankle and foot**
  M08.071 Unspecified juvenile rheumatoid arthritis, right ankle and foot ▽
  M08.072 Unspecified juvenile rheumatoid arthritis, left ankle and foot ▽
  M08.079 Unspecified juvenile rheumatoid arthritis, unspecified ankle and foot ▽

  M08.08 Unspecified juvenile rheumatoid arthritis, vertebrae ▽
  M08.09 Unspecified juvenile rheumatoid arthritis, multiple sites ▽

M08.1 Juvenile ankylosing spondylitis
  EXCLUDES 1 ankylosing spondylitis in adults (M45.0-)

✓5ᵗʰ **M08.2 Juvenile rheumatoid arthritis with systemic onset**
  Still's disease NOS
  EXCLUDES 1 adult-onset Still's disease (M06.1-)
  M08.20 Juvenile rheumatoid arthritis with systemic onset, unspecified site ▽

✓6ᵗʰ **M08.21 Juvenile rheumatoid arthritis with systemic onset, shoulder**
  M08.211 Juvenile rheumatoid arthritis with systemic onset, right shoulder
  M08.212 Juvenile rheumatoid arthritis with systemic onset, left shoulder
  M08.219 Juvenile rheumatoid arthritis with systemic onset, unspecified shoulder ▽

✓6ᵗʰ **M08.22 Juvenile rheumatoid arthritis with systemic onset, elbow**
  M08.221 Juvenile rheumatoid arthritis with systemic onset, right elbow
  M08.222 Juvenile rheumatoid arthritis with systemic onset, left elbow
  M08.229 Juvenile rheumatoid arthritis with systemic onset, unspecified elbow ▽

✓6ᵗʰ **M08.23 Juvenile rheumatoid arthritis with systemic onset, wrist**
  M08.231 Juvenile rheumatoid arthritis with systemic onset, right wrist
  M08.232 Juvenile rheumatoid arthritis with systemic onset, left wrist
  M08.239 Juvenile rheumatoid arthritis with systemic onset, unspecified wrist ▽

✓6ᵗʰ **M08.24 Juvenile rheumatoid arthritis with systemic onset, hand**
  M08.241 Juvenile rheumatoid arthritis with systemic onset, right hand
  M08.242 Juvenile rheumatoid arthritis with systemic onset, left hand

  M08.249 Juvenile rheumatoid arthritis with systemic onset, unspecified hand ▽

✓6ᵗʰ **M08.25 Juvenile rheumatoid arthritis with systemic onset, hip**
  M08.251 Juvenile rheumatoid arthritis with systemic onset, right hip
  M08.252 Juvenile rheumatoid arthritis with systemic onset, left hip
  M08.259 Juvenile rheumatoid arthritis with systemic onset, unspecified hip ▽

✓6ᵗʰ **M08.26 Juvenile rheumatoid arthritis with systemic onset, knee**
  M08.261 Juvenile rheumatoid arthritis with systemic onset, right knee
  M08.262 Juvenile rheumatoid arthritis with systemic onset, left knee
  M08.269 Juvenile rheumatoid arthritis with systemic onset, unspecified knee ▽

✓6ᵗʰ **M08.27 Juvenile rheumatoid arthritis with systemic onset, ankle and foot**
  M08.271 Juvenile rheumatoid arthritis with systemic onset, right ankle and foot
  M08.272 Juvenile rheumatoid arthritis with systemic onset, left ankle and foot
  M08.279 Juvenile rheumatoid arthritis with systemic onset, unspecified ankle and foot ▽

  M08.28 Juvenile rheumatoid arthritis with systemic onset, vertebrae
  M08.29 Juvenile rheumatoid arthritis with systemic onset, multiple sites

M08.3 Juvenile rheumatoid polyarthritis (seronegative)

✓5ᵗʰ **M08.4 Pauciarticular juvenile rheumatoid arthritis**
  M08.40 Pauciarticular juvenile rheumatoid arthritis, unspecified site ▽

✓6ᵗʰ **M08.41 Pauciarticular juvenile rheumatoid arthritis, shoulder**
  M08.411 Pauciarticular juvenile rheumatoid arthritis, right shoulder
  M08.412 Pauciarticular juvenile rheumatoid arthritis, left shoulder
  M08.419 Pauciarticular juvenile rheumatoid arthritis, unspecified shoulder ▽

✓6ᵗʰ **M08.42 Pauciarticular juvenile rheumatoid arthritis, elbow**
  M08.421 Pauciarticular juvenile rheumatoid arthritis, right elbow
  M08.422 Pauciarticular juvenile rheumatoid arthritis, left elbow
  M08.429 Pauciarticular juvenile rheumatoid arthritis, unspecified elbow ▽

✓6ᵗʰ **M08.43 Pauciarticular juvenile rheumatoid arthritis, wrist**
  M08.431 Pauciarticular juvenile rheumatoid arthritis, right wrist
  M08.432 Pauciarticular juvenile rheumatoid arthritis, left wrist
  M08.439 Pauciarticular juvenile rheumatoid arthritis, unspecified wrist ▽

✓6ᵗʰ **M08.44 Pauciarticular juvenile rheumatoid arthritis, hand**
  M08.441 Pauciarticular juvenile rheumatoid arthritis, right hand
  M08.442 Pauciarticular juvenile rheumatoid arthritis, left hand
  M08.449 Pauciarticular juvenile rheumatoid arthritis, unspecified hand ▽

✓6ᵗʰ **M08.45 Pauciarticular juvenile rheumatoid arthritis, hip**
  M08.451 Pauciarticular juvenile rheumatoid arthritis, right hip
  M08.452 Pauciarticular juvenile rheumatoid arthritis, left hip
  M08.459 Pauciarticular juvenile rheumatoid arthritis, unspecified hip ▽

✓6ᵗʰ **M08.46 Pauciarticular juvenile rheumatoid arthritis, knee**
  M08.461 Pauciarticular juvenile rheumatoid arthritis, right knee
  M08.462 Pauciarticular juvenile rheumatoid arthritis, left knee

Ⓝ Newborn   Ⓟ Pediatric   Ⓜ Maternity   Ⓐ Adult   **RIC** RIC Dx   **NC Dx** Noncancer Dx   **PDx** Primary Dx   **CC** RIC CC Condition   ►◄ Revised Text   ● New Code   ▲ Revised Code Title

688

ICD-10-CM 2016

M08.469 Pauciarticular juvenile rheumatoid arthritis, unspecified knee ▽

✓6ᵗʰ M08.47 Pauciarticular juvenile rheumatoid arthritis, ankle and foot

M08.471 Pauciarticular juvenile rheumatoid arthritis, right ankle and foot

M08.472 Pauciarticular juvenile rheumatoid arthritis, left ankle and foot

M08.479 Pauciarticular juvenile rheumatoid arthritis, unspecified ankle and foot ▽

M08.48 Pauciarticular juvenile rheumatoid arthritis, vertebrae

✓5ᵗʰ M08.8 Other juvenile arthritis

M08.80 Other juvenile arthritis, unspecified site ▽

✓6ᵗʰ M08.81 Other juvenile arthritis, shoulder

M08.811 Other juvenile arthritis, right shoulder

M08.812 Other juvenile arthritis, left shoulder

M08.819 Other juvenile arthritis, unspecified shoulder ▽

✓6ᵗʰ M08.82 Other juvenile arthritis, elbow

M08.821 Other juvenile arthritis, right elbow

M08.822 Other juvenile arthritis, left elbow

M08.829 Other juvenile arthritis, unspecified elbow ▽

✓6ᵗʰ M08.83 Other juvenile arthritis, wrist

M08.831 Other juvenile arthritis, right wrist

M08.832 Other juvenile arthritis, left wrist

M08.839 Other juvenile arthritis, unspecified wrist ▽

✓6ᵗʰ M08.84 Other juvenile arthritis, hand

M08.841 Other juvenile arthritis, right hand

M08.842 Other juvenile arthritis, left hand

M08.849 Other juvenile arthritis, unspecified hand ▽

✓6ᵗʰ M08.85 Other juvenile arthritis, hip

M08.851 Other juvenile arthritis, right hip

M08.852 Other juvenile arthritis, left hip

M08.859 Other juvenile arthritis, unspecified hip ▽

✓6ᵗʰ M08.86 Other juvenile arthritis, knee

M08.861 Other juvenile arthritis, right knee

M08.862 Other juvenile arthritis, left knee

M08.869 Other juvenile arthritis, unspecified knee ▽

✓6ᵗʰ M08.87 Other juvenile arthritis, ankle and foot

M08.871 Other juvenile arthritis, right ankle and foot

M08.872 Other juvenile arthritis, left ankle and foot

M08.879 Other juvenile arthritis, unspecified ankle and foot ▽

M08.88 Other juvenile arthritis, other specified site
Other juvenile arthritis, vertebrae

M08.89 Other juvenile arthritis, multiple sites

✓5ᵗʰ M08.9 Juvenile arthritis, unspecified

EXCLUDES 1 juvenile rheumatoid arthritis, unspecified (M08.0-)

M08.90 Juvenile arthritis, unspecified, unspecified site ▽

✓6ᵗʰ M08.91 Juvenile arthritis, unspecified, shoulder

M08.911 Juvenile arthritis, unspecified, right shoulder

M08.912 Juvenile arthritis, unspecified, left shoulder

M08.919 Juvenile arthritis, unspecified, unspecified shoulder ▽

✓6ᵗʰ M08.92 Juvenile arthritis, unspecified, elbow

M08.921 Juvenile arthritis, unspecified, right elbow

M08.922 Juvenile arthritis, unspecified, left elbow

M08.929 Juvenile arthritis, unspecified, unspecified elbow ▽

✓6ᵗʰ M08.93 Juvenile arthritis, unspecified, wrist

M08.931 Juvenile arthritis, unspecified, right wrist

M08.932 Juvenile arthritis, unspecified, left wrist

M08.939 Juvenile arthritis, unspecified, unspecified wrist ▽

✓6ᵗʰ M08.94 Juvenile arthritis, unspecified, hand

M08.941 Juvenile arthritis, unspecified, right hand

M08.942 Juvenile arthritis, unspecified, left hand

M08.949 Juvenile arthritis, unspecified, unspecified hand ▽

✓6ᵗʰ M08.95 Juvenile arthritis, unspecified, hip

M08.951 Juvenile arthritis, unspecified, right hip

M08.952 Juvenile arthritis, unspecified, left hip

M08.959 Juvenile arthritis, unspecified, unspecified hip ▽

✓6ᵗʰ M08.96 Juvenile arthritis, unspecified, knee

M08.961 Juvenile arthritis, unspecified, right knee

M08.962 Juvenile arthritis, unspecified, left knee

M08.969 Juvenile arthritis, unspecified, unspecified knee ▽

✓6ᵗʰ M08.97 Juvenile arthritis, unspecified, ankle and foot

M08.971 Juvenile arthritis, unspecified, right ankle and foot

M08.972 Juvenile arthritis, unspecified, left ankle and foot

M08.979 Juvenile arthritis, unspecified, unspecified ankle and foot ▽

M08.98 Juvenile arthritis, unspecified, vertebrae

M08.99 Juvenile arthritis, unspecified, multiple sites

✓4ᵗʰ M1A Chronic gout

Use additional code to identify:
autonomic neuropathy in diseases classified elsewhere (G99.0)
calculus of urinary tract in diseases classified elsewhere (N22)
cardiomyopathy in diseases classified elsewhere (I43)
disorders of external ear in diseases classified elsewhere (H61.1-, H62.8-)
disorders of iris and ciliary body in diseases classified elsewhere (H22)
glomerular disorders in diseases classified elsewhere (N08)

EXCLUDES 1 acute gout (M10.-)
gout NOS (M10.-)

The appropriate 7th character is to be added to each code from category M1A.
0   without tophus (tophi)
1   with tophus (tophi)

✓5ᵗʰ M1A.0 Idiopathic chronic gout
Chronic gouty bursitis   Primary chronic gout

✓x7ᵗʰ M1A.00 Idiopathic chronic gout, unspecified site ▽

✓6ᵗʰ M1A.01 Idiopathic chronic gout, shoulder

✓7ᵗʰ M1A.011 Idiopathic chronic gout, right shoulder

✓7ᵗʰ M1A.012 Idiopathic chronic gout, left shoulder

✓7ᵗʰ M1A.019 Idiopathic chronic gout, unspecified shoulder ▽

✓6ᵗʰ M1A.02 Idiopathic chronic gout, elbow

✓7ᵗʰ M1A.021 Idiopathic chronic gout, right elbow

✓7ᵗʰ M1A.022 Idiopathic chronic gout, left elbow

✓7ᵗʰ M1A.029 Idiopathic chronic gout, unspecified elbow ▽

✓6ᵗʰ M1A.03 Idiopathic chronic gout, wrist

✓7ᵗʰ M1A.031 Idiopathic chronic gout, right wrist

✓7ᵗʰ M1A.032 Idiopathic chronic gout, left wrist

✓7ᵗʰ M1A.039 Idiopathic chronic gout, unspecified wrist ▽

✓6ᵗʰ M1A.04 Idiopathic chronic gout, hand

✓7ᵗʰ M1A.041 Idiopathic chronic gout, right hand

✓7ᵗʰ M1A.042 Idiopathic chronic gout, left hand

✓7ᵗʰ M1A.049 Idiopathic chronic gout, unspecified hand ▽

✓6ᵗʰ M1A.05 Idiopathic chronic gout, hip

✓7ᵗʰ M1A.051 Idiopathic chronic gout, right hip

✓7ᵗʰ M1A.052 Idiopathic chronic gout, left hip

✓7ᵗʰ M1A.059 Idiopathic chronic gout, unspecified hip ▽

✓6ᵗʰ M1A.06 Idiopathic chronic gout, knee

✓7ᵗʰ M1A.061 Idiopathic chronic gout, right knee

✓7ᵗʰ M1A.062 Idiopathic chronic gout, left knee

✓7ᵗʰ M1A.069 Idiopathic chronic gout, unspecified knee ▽

√6ᵗʰ **M1A.Ø7 Idiopathic chronic gout,** ankle and foot

    √7ᵗʰ **M1A.Ø71 Idiopathic chronic gout,** right **ankle and foot**

    √7ᵗʰ **M1A.Ø72 Idiopathic chronic gout,** left **ankle and foot**

    √7ᵗʰ **M1A.Ø79 Idiopathic chronic gout, unspecified ankle and foot** ▽

√x7ᵗʰ **M1A.Ø8 Idiopathic chronic gout,** vertebrae

√x7ᵗʰ **M1A.Ø9 Idiopathic chronic gout,** multiple sites

√5ᵗʰ **M1A.1 Lead-induced chronic gout**

    Code first toxic effects of lead and its compounds (T56.Ø-)

√x7ᵗʰ **M1A.1Ø Lead-induced chronic gout, unspecified site** ▽

√6ᵗʰ **M1A.11 Lead-induced chronic gout,** shoulder

    √7ᵗʰ **M1A.111 Lead-induced chronic gout,** right **shoulder**

    √7ᵗʰ **M1A.112 Lead-induced chronic gout,** left **shoulder**

    √7ᵗʰ **M1A.119 Lead-induced chronic gout, unspecified shoulder** ▽

√6ᵗʰ **M1A.12 Lead-induced chronic gout,** elbow

    √7ᵗʰ **M1A.121 Lead-induced chronic gout,** right **elbow**

    √7ᵗʰ **M1A.122 Lead-induced chronic gout,** left **elbow**

    √7ᵗʰ **M1A.129 Lead-induced chronic gout, unspecified elbow** ▽

√6ᵗʰ **M1A.13 Lead-induced chronic gout,** wrist

    √7ᵗʰ **M1A.131 Lead-induced chronic gout,** right **wrist**

    √7ᵗʰ **M1A.132 Lead-induced chronic gout,** left **wrist**

    √7ᵗʰ **M1A.139 Lead-induced chronic gout, unspecified wrist** ▽

√6ᵗʰ **M1A.14 Lead-induced chronic gout,** hand

    √7ᵗʰ **M1A.141 Lead-induced chronic gout,** right **hand**

    √7ᵗʰ **M1A.142 Lead-induced chronic gout,** left **hand**

    √7ᵗʰ **M1A.149 Lead-induced chronic gout, unspecified hand** ▽

√6ᵗʰ **M1A.15 Lead-induced chronic gout,** hip

    √7ᵗʰ **M1A.151 Lead-induced chronic gout,** right **hip**

    √7ᵗʰ **M1A.152 Lead-induced chronic gout,** left **hip**

    √7ᵗʰ **M1A.159 Lead-induced chronic gout, unspecified hip** ▽

√6ᵗʰ **M1A.16 Lead-induced chronic gout,** knee

    √7ᵗʰ **M1A.161 Lead-induced chronic gout,** right **knee**

    √7ᵗʰ **M1A.162 Lead-induced chronic gout,** left **knee**

    √7ᵗʰ **M1A.169 Lead-induced chronic gout, unspecified knee** ▽

√6ᵗʰ **M1A.17 Lead-induced chronic gout,** ankle and foot

    √7ᵗʰ **M1A.171 Lead-induced chronic gout,** right **ankle and foot**

    √7ᵗʰ **M1A.172 Lead-induced chronic gout,** left **ankle and foot**

    √7ᵗʰ **M1A.179 Lead-induced chronic gout, unspecified ankle and foot** ▽

√x7ᵗʰ **M1A.18 Lead-induced chronic gout,** vertebrae

√x7ᵗʰ **M1A.19 Lead-induced chronic gout,** multiple sites

√5ᵗʰ **M1A.2 Drug-induced chronic gout**

    Use additional code for adverse effect, if applicable, to identify drug (T36-T5Ø with fifth or sixth character 5)

√x7ᵗʰ **M1A.2Ø Drug-induced chronic gout, unspecified site** ▽

√6ᵗʰ **M1A.21 Drug-induced chronic gout,** shoulder

    √7ᵗʰ **M1A.211 Drug-induced chronic gout,** right **shoulder**

    √7ᵗʰ **M1A.212 Drug-induced chronic gout,** left **shoulder**

    √7ᵗʰ **M1A.219 Drug-induced chronic gout, unspecified shoulder** ▽

√6ᵗʰ **M1A.22 Drug-induced chronic gout,** elbow

    √7ᵗʰ **M1A.221 Drug-induced chronic gout,** right **elbow**

    √7ᵗʰ **M1A.222 Drug-induced chronic gout,** left **elbow**

    √7ᵗʰ **M1A.229 Drug-induced chronic gout, unspecified elbow** ▽

√6ᵗʰ **M1A.23 Drug-induced chronic gout,** wrist

    √7ᵗʰ **M1A.231 Drug-induced chronic gout,** right **wrist**

    √7ᵗʰ **M1A.232 Drug-induced chronic gout,** left **wrist**

    √7ᵗʰ **M1A.239 Drug-induced chronic gout, unspecified wrist** ▽

√6ᵗʰ **M1A.24 Drug-induced chronic gout,** hand

    √7ᵗʰ **M1A.241 Drug-induced chronic gout,** right **hand**

    √7ᵗʰ **M1A.242 Drug-induced chronic gout,** left **hand**

    √7ᵗʰ **M1A.249 Drug-induced chronic gout, unspecified hand** ▽

√6ᵗʰ **M1A.25 Drug-induced chronic gout,** hip

    √7ᵗʰ **M1A.251 Drug-induced chronic gout,** right **hip**

    √7ᵗʰ **M1A.252 Drug-induced chronic gout,** left **hip**

    √7ᵗʰ **M1A.259 Drug-induced chronic gout, unspecified hip** ▽

√6ᵗʰ **M1A.26 Drug-induced chronic gout,** knee

    √7ᵗʰ **M1A.261 Drug-induced chronic gout,** right **knee**

    √7ᵗʰ **M1A.262 Drug-induced chronic gout,** left **knee**

    √7ᵗʰ **M1A.269 Drug-induced chronic gout, unspecified knee** ▽

√6ᵗʰ **M1A.27 Drug-induced chronic gout,** ankle and foot

    √7ᵗʰ **M1A.271 Drug-induced chronic gout,** right **ankle and foot**

    √7ᵗʰ **M1A.272 Drug-induced chronic gout,** left **ankle and foot**

    √7ᵗʰ **M1A.279 Drug-induced chronic gout, unspecified ankle and foot** ▽

√x7ᵗʰ **M1A.28 Drug-induced chronic gout,** vertebrae

√x7ᵗʰ **M1A.29 Drug-induced chronic gout,** multiple sites

√5ᵗʰ **M1A.3 Chronic gout** due to renal impairment

    Code first associated renal disease

√x7ᵗʰ **M1A.3Ø Chronic gout due to renal impairment, unspecified site** ▽

√6ᵗʰ **M1A.31 Chronic gout due to renal impairment,** shoulder

    √7ᵗʰ **M1A.311 Chronic gout due to renal impairment,** right **shoulder**

    √7ᵗʰ **M1A.312 Chronic gout due to renal impairment,** left **shoulder**

    √7ᵗʰ **M1A.319 Chronic gout due to renal impairment, unspecified shoulder** ▽

√6ᵗʰ **M1A.32 Chronic gout due to renal impairment,** elbow

    √7ᵗʰ **M1A.321 Chronic gout due to renal impairment,** right **elbow**

    √7ᵗʰ **M1A.322 Chronic gout due to renal impairment,** left **elbow**

    √7ᵗʰ **M1A.329 Chronic gout due to renal impairment, unspecified elbow** ▽

√6ᵗʰ **M1A.33 Chronic gout due to renal impairment,** wrist

    √7ᵗʰ **M1A.331 Chronic gout due to renal impairment,** right **wrist**

    √7ᵗʰ **M1A.332 Chronic gout due to renal impairment,** left **wrist**

    √7ᵗʰ **M1A.339 Chronic gout due to renal impairment,** ▽ **unspecified wrist**

√6ᵗʰ **M1A.34 Chronic gout due to renal impairment,** hand

    √7ᵗʰ **M1A.341 Chronic gout due to renal impairment,** right **hand**

    √7ᵗʰ **M1A.342 Chronic gout due to renal impairment,** left **hand**

    √7ᵗʰ **M1A.349 Chronic gout due to renal impairment, unspecified hand** ▽

√6ᵗʰ **M1A.35 Chronic gout due to renal impairment,** hip

    √7ᵗʰ **M1A.351 Chronic gout due to renal impairment,** right **hip**

    √7ᵗʰ **M1A.352 Chronic gout due to renal impairment,** left **hip**

    √7ᵗʰ **M1A.359 Chronic gout due to renal impairment, unspecified hip** ▽

Ⓝ Newborn   🄟 Pediatric   🄜 Maternity   🄐 Adult   **RIC** RIC Dx   **NCDx** Noncancer Dx   **PDx** Primary Dx   **CC** RIC CC Condition   ▶◀ Revised Text   ● New Code   ▲ Revised Code Title

690   ICD-10-CM 2016

✓6ᵗʰ **M1A.36** Chronic gout due to renal impairment, knee

     ✓7ᵗʰ **M1A.361** Chronic gout due to renal impairment, right knee

     ✓7ᵗʰ **M1A.362** Chronic gout due to renal impairment, left knee

     ✓7ᵗʰ **M1A.369** Chronic gout due to renal impairment, unspecified knee ▽

✓6ᵗʰ **M1A.37** Chronic gout due to renal impairment, ankle and foot

     ✓7ᵗʰ **M1A.371** Chronic gout due to renal impairment, right ankle and foot

     ✓7ᵗʰ **M1A.372** Chronic gout due to renal impairment, left ankle and foot

     ✓7ᵗʰ **M1A.379** Chronic gout due to renal impairment, unspecified ankle and foot ▽

✓x7ᵗʰ **M1A.38** Chronic gout due to renal impairment, vertebrae

✓x7ᵗʰ **M1A.39** Chronic gout due to renal impairment, multiple sites

✓5ᵗʰ **M1A.4** Other secondary chronic gout

     Code first associated condition

✓x7ᵗʰ **M1A.40** Other secondary chronic gout, unspecified site ▽

✓6ᵗʰ **M1A.41** Other secondary chronic gout, shoulder

     ✓7ᵗʰ **M1A.411** Other secondary chronic gout, right shoulder

     ✓7ᵗʰ **M1A.412** Other secondary chronic gout, left shoulder

     ✓7ᵗʰ **M1A.419** Other secondary chronic gout, unspecified shoulder ▽

✓6ᵗʰ **M1A.42** Other secondary chronic gout, elbow

     ✓7ᵗʰ **M1A.421** Other secondary chronic gout, right elbow

     ✓7ᵗʰ **M1A.422** Other secondary chronic gout, left elbow

     ✓7ᵗʰ **M1A.429** Other secondary chronic gout, unspecified elbow ▽

✓6ᵗʰ **M1A.43** Other secondary chronic gout, wrist

     ✓7ᵗʰ **M1A.431** Other secondary chronic gout, right wrist

     ✓7ᵗʰ **M1A.432** Other secondary chronic gout, left wrist

     ✓7ᵗʰ **M1A.439** Other secondary chronic gout, unspecified wrist ▽

✓6ᵗʰ **M1A.44** Other secondary chronic gout, hand

     ✓7ᵗʰ **M1A.441** Other secondary chronic gout, right hand

     ✓7ᵗʰ **M1A.442** Other secondary chronic gout, left hand

     ✓7ᵗʰ **M1A.449** Other secondary chronic gout, unspecified hand ▽

✓6ᵗʰ **M1A.45** Other secondary chronic gout, hip

     ✓7ᵗʰ **M1A.451** Other secondary chronic gout, right hip

     ✓7ᵗʰ **M1A.452** Other secondary chronic gout, left hip

     ✓7ᵗʰ **M1A.459** Other secondary chronic gout, unspecified hip ▽

✓6ᵗʰ **M1A.46** Other secondary chronic gout, knee

     ✓7ᵗʰ **M1A.461** Other secondary chronic gout, right knee

     ✓7ᵗʰ **M1A.462** Other secondary chronic gout, left knee

     ✓7ᵗʰ **M1A.469** Other secondary chronic gout, unspecified knee ▽

✓6ᵗʰ **M1A.47** Other secondary chronic gout, ankle and foot

     ✓7ᵗʰ **M1A.471** Other secondary chronic gout, right ankle and foot

     ✓7ᵗʰ **M1A.472** Other secondary chronic gout, left ankle and foot

     ✓7ᵗʰ **M1A.479** Other secondary chronic gout, unspecified ankle and foot ▽

✓x7ᵗʰ **M1A.48** Other secondary chronic gout, vertebrae

✓x7ᵗʰ **M1A.49** Other secondary chronic gout, multiple sites

✓x7ᵗʰ **M1A.9** Chronic gout, unspecified ▽

✓4ᵗʰ **M10 Gout**

     Acute gout   Gout NOS

     Gout attack   Podagra

     Gout flare

     Use additional code to identify:

       autonomic neuropathy in diseases classified elsewhere (G99.0)

       calculus of urinary tract in diseases classified elsewhere (N22)

       cardiomyopathy in diseases classified elsewhere (I43)

       disorders of external ear in diseases classified elsewhere (H61.1-, H62.8-)

       disorders of iris and ciliary body in diseases classified elsewhere (H22)

       glomerular disorders in diseases classified elsewhere (N08)

     EXCLUDES 1   chronic gout (M1A.-)

✓5ᵗʰ **M10.0** Idiopathic gout

     Gouty bursitis

     Primary gout

     M10.00 Idiopathic gout, unspecified site

✓6ᵗʰ **M10.01** Idiopathic gout, shoulder

     M10.011 Idiopathic gout, right shoulder

     M10.012 Idiopathic gout, left shoulder

     M10.019 Idiopathic gout, unspecified shoulder ▽

✓6ᵗʰ **M10.02** Idiopathic gout, elbow

     M10.021 Idiopathic gout, right elbow

     M10.022 Idiopathic gout, left elbow

     M10.029 Idiopathic gout, unspecified elbow ▽

✓6ᵗʰ **M10.03** Idiopathic gout, wrist

     M10.031 Idiopathic gout, right wrist

     M10.032 Idiopathic gout, left wrist

     M10.039 Idiopathic gout, unspecified wrist ▽

✓6ᵗʰ **M10.04** Idiopathic gout, hand

     M10.041 Idiopathic gout, right hand

     M10.042 Idiopathic gout, left hand

     M10.049 Idiopathic gout, unspecified hand ▽

✓6ᵗʰ **M10.05** Idiopathic gout, hip

     M10.051 Idiopathic gout, right hip

     M10.052 Idiopathic gout, left hip

     M10.059 Idiopathic gout, unspecified hip ▽

✓6ᵗʰ **M10.06** Idiopathic gout, knee

     M10.061 Idiopathic gout, right knee

     M10.062 Idiopathic gout, left knee

     M10.069 Idiopathic gout, unspecified knee ▽

✓6ᵗʰ **M10.07** Idiopathic gout, ankle and foot

     M10.071 Idiopathic gout, right ankle and foot

     M10.072 Idiopathic gout, left ankle and foot

     M10.079 Idiopathic gout, unspecified ankle and foot ▽

     M10.08 Idiopathic gout, vertebrae

     M10.09 Idiopathic gout, multiple sites

✓5ᵗʰ **M10.1** Lead-induced gout

     Code first toxic effects of lead and its compounds (T56.0-)

     M10.10 Lead-induced gout, unspecified site ▽

✓6ᵗʰ **M10.11** Lead-induced gout, shoulder

     M10.111 Lead-induced gout, right shoulder

     M10.112 Lead-induced gout, left shoulder

     M10.119 Lead-induced gout, unspecified shoulder ▽

✓6ᵗʰ **M10.12** Lead-induced gout, elbow

     M10.121 Lead-induced gout, right elbow

     M10.122 Lead-induced gout, left elbow

     M10.129 Lead-induced gout, unspecified elbow ▽

✓6ᵗʰ **M10.13** Lead-induced gout, wrist

     M10.131 Lead-induced gout, right wrist

     M10.132 Lead-induced gout, left wrist

     M10.139 Lead-induced gout, unspecified wrist ▽

✓6ᵗʰ **M10.14** Lead-induced gout, hand

     M10.141 Lead-induced gout, right hand

     M10.142 Lead-induced gout, left hand

     M10.149 Lead-induced gout, unspecified hand ▽

✓6ᵗʰ **M10.15** Lead-induced gout, hip

     M10.151 Lead-induced gout, right hip

     M10.152 Lead-induced gout, left hip

     M10.159 Lead-induced gout, unspecified hip ▽

✅ Add'l Character Required   ✓x7ᵗʰ Placeholder Alert   RUG IV Special Care High Dx   RUG IV Clinically Complex Dx   RUG IV Special Care Low Dx   Manifestation Code   Other Specified Code   ▽Unspecified Code

Chapter 13. Diseases of the Musculoskeletal System and Connective Tissue

M10.16–M11.019

✓6ᵗʰ **M10.16 Lead-induced gout,** knee
     M10.161 **Lead-induced gout,** right **knee**
     M10.162 **Lead-induced gout,** left **knee**
     M10.169 **Lead-induced gout, unspecified knee** ▽

✓6ᵗʰ **M10.17 Lead-induced gout,** ankle and foot
     M10.171 **Lead-induced gout,** right **ankle and foot**
     M10.172 **Lead-induced gout,** left **ankle and foot**
     M10.179 **Lead-induced gout, unspecified ankle** ▽
                and foot

     M10.18 Lead-induced gout, vertebrae
     M10.19 Lead-induced gout, multiple sites

✓5ᵗʰ **M10.2 Drug-induced gout**
     Use additional code for adverse effect, if applicable, to identify drug (T36-T50 with fifth or sixth character 5)
     M10.20 Drug-induced gout, unspecified site ▽

✓6ᵗʰ **M10.21 Drug-induced gout,** shoulder
     M10.211 **Drug-induced gout,** right **shoulder**
     M10.212 **Drug-induced gout,** left **shoulder**
     M10.219 **Drug-induced gout, unspecified** ▽
                shoulder

✓6ᵗʰ **M10.22 Drug-induced gout,** elbow
     M10.221 **Drug-induced gout,** right **elbow**
     M10.222 **Drug-induced gout,** left **elbow**
     M10.229 **Drug-induced gout, unspecified elbow** ▽

✓6ᵗʰ **M10.23 Drug-induced gout,** wrist
     M10.231 **Drug-induced gout,** right **wrist**
     M10.232 **Drug-induced gout,** left **wrist**
     M10.239 **Drug-induced gout, unspecified wrist** ▽

✓6ᵗʰ **M10.24 Drug-induced gout,** hand
     M10.241 **Drug-induced gout,** right **hand**
     M10.242 **Drug-induced gout,** left **hand**
     M10.249 **Drug-induced gout, unspecified hand** ▽

✓6ᵗʰ **M10.25 Drug-induced gout,** hip
     M10.251 **Drug-induced gout,** right **hip**
     M10.252 **Drug-induced gout,** left **hip**
     M10.259 **Drug-induced gout, unspecified hip** ▽

✓6ᵗʰ **M10.26 Drug-induced gout,** knee
     M10.261 **Drug-induced gout,** right **knee**
     M10.262 **Drug-induced gout,** left **knee**
     M10.269 **Drug-induced gout, unspecified knee** ▽

✓6ᵗʰ **M10.27 Drug-induced gout,** ankle and foot
     M10.271 **Drug-induced gout,** right **ankle and foot**
     M10.272 **Drug-induced gout,** left **ankle and foot**
     M10.279 **Drug-induced gout, unspecified ankle** ▽
                and foot

     M10.28 Drug-induced gout, vertebrae
     M10.29 Drug-induced gout, multiple sites

✓5ᵗʰ **M10.3 Gout due to** renal impairment
     Code first associated renal disease
     M10.30 Gout due to renal impairment, unspecified site ▽

✓6ᵗʰ **M10.31 Gout due to renal impairment,** shoulder
     M10.311 **Gout due to renal impairment,** right **shoulder**
     M10.312 **Gout due to renal impairment,** left **shoulder**
     M10.319 **Gout due to renal impairment,** ▽
                unspecified shoulder

✓6ᵗʰ **M10.32 Gout due to renal impairment,** elbow
     M10.321 **Gout due to renal impairment,** right **elbow**
     M10.322 **Gout due to renal impairment,** left **elbow**
     M10.329 **Gout due to renal impairment,** ▽
                unspecified elbow

✓6ᵗʰ **M10.33 Gout due to renal impairment,** wrist
     M10.331 **Gout due to renal impairment,** right **wrist**
     M10.332 **Gout due to renal impairment,** left **wrist**
     M10.339 **Gout due to renal impairment,** ▽
                unspecified wrist

✓6ᵗʰ **M10.34 Gout due to renal impairment,** hand
     M10.341 **Gout due to renal impairment,** right **hand**
     M10.342 **Gout due to renal impairment,** left **hand**
     M10.349 **Gout due to renal impairment,** ▽
                unspecified hand

✓6ᵗʰ **M10.35 Gout due to renal impairment,** hip
     M10.351 **Gout due to renal impairment,** right **hip**
     M10.352 **Gout due to renal impairment,** left **hip**
     M10.359 **Gout due to renal impairment,** ▽
                unspecified hip

✓6ᵗʰ **M10.36 Gout due to renal impairment,** knee
     M10.361 **Gout due to renal impairment,** right **knee**
     M10.362 **Gout due to renal impairment,** left **knee**
     M10.369 **Gout due to renal impairment,** ▽
                unspecified knee

✓6ᵗʰ **M10.37 Gout due to renal impairment,** ankle and foot
     M10.371 **Gout due to renal impairment,** right **ankle and foot**
     M10.372 **Gout due to renal impairment,** left **ankle and foot**
     M10.379 **Gout due to renal impairment,** ▽
                unspecified ankle and foot

     M10.38 Gout due to renal impairment, vertebrae
     M10.39 Gout due to renal impairment, multiple sites

✓5ᵗʰ **M10.4 Other secondary** gout
     Code first associated condition
     M10.40 Other secondary gout, unspecified site ▽

✓6ᵗʰ **M10.41 Other secondary gout,** shoulder
     M10.411 **Other secondary gout,** right **shoulder**
     M10.412 **Other secondary gout,** left **shoulder**
     M10.419 **Other secondary gout, unspecified** ▽
                shoulder

✓6ᵗʰ **M10.42 Other secondary gout,** elbow
     M10.421 **Other secondary gout,** right **elbow**
     M10.422 **Other secondary gout,** left **elbow**
     M10.429 **Other secondary gout, unspecified** ▽
                elbow

✓6ᵗʰ **M10.43 Other secondary gout,** wrist
     M10.431 **Other secondary gout,** right **wrist**
     M10.432 **Other secondary gout,** left **wrist**
     M10.439 **Other secondary gout, unspecified** ▽
                wrist

✓6ᵗʰ **M10.44 Other secondary gout,** hand
     M10.441 **Other secondary gout,** right **hand**
     M10.442 **Other secondary gout,** left **hand**
     M10.449 **Other secondary gout, unspecified** ▽
                hand

✓6ᵗʰ **M10.45 Other secondary gout,** hip
     M10.451 **Other secondary gout,** right **hip**
     M10.452 **Other secondary gout,** left **hip**
     M10.459 **Other secondary gout, unspecified hip** ▽

✓6ᵗʰ **M10.46 Other secondary gout,** knee
     M10.461 **Other secondary gout,** right **knee**
     M10.462 **Other secondary gout,** left **knee**
     M10.469 **Other secondary gout, unspecified** ▽
                knee

✓6ᵗʰ **M10.47 Other secondary gout,** ankle and foot
     M10.471 **Other secondary gout,** right **ankle and foot**
     M10.472 **Other secondary gout,** left **ankle and foot**
     M10.479 **Other secondary gout, unspecified** ▽
                ankle and foot

     M10.48 Other secondary gout, vertebrae
     M10.49 Other secondary gout, multiple sites

     M10.9 Gout, unspecified ▽
         Gout NOS

✓4ᵗʰ **M11 Other crystal arthropathies**

✓5ᵗʰ **M11.0 Hydroxyapatite deposition disease**
     M11.00 Hydroxyapatite deposition disease, ▽
                unspecified site

✓6ᵗʰ **M11.01 Hydroxyapatite deposition disease,** shoulder
     M11.011 **Hydroxyapatite deposition disease,** right **shoulder**
     M11.012 **Hydroxyapatite deposition disease,** left **shoulder**
     M11.019 **Hydroxyapatite deposition disease,** ▽
                unspecified shoulder

Ⓝ Newborn   Ⓟ Pediatric   Ⓜ Maternity   Ⓐ Adult   **RIC** RIC Dx   **NCDx** Noncancer Dx   **PDx** Primary Dx   **CC** RIC CC Condition   ▶◀ Revised Text   ● New Code   ▲ Revised Code Title

692   ICD-10-CM 2016

☑6ᵗʰ **M11.02 Hydroxyapatite deposition disease,** elbow
- **M11.021 Hydroxyapatite deposition disease,** right **elbow**
- **M11.022 Hydroxyapatite deposition disease,** left **elbow**
- **M11.029 Hydroxyapatite deposition disease,** unspecified **elbow** ▽

☑6ᵗʰ **M11.03 Hydroxyapatite deposition disease,** wrist
- **M11.031 Hydroxyapatite deposition disease,** right **wrist**
- **M11.032 Hydroxyapatite deposition disease,** left **wrist**
- **M11.039 Hydroxyapatite deposition disease,** unspecified **wrist** ▽

☑6ᵗʰ **M11.04 Hydroxyapatite deposition disease,** hand
- **M11.041 Hydroxyapatite deposition disease,** right **hand**
- **M11.042 Hydroxyapatite deposition disease,** left **hand**
- **M11.049 Hydroxyapatite deposition disease,** unspecified **hand** ▽

☑6ᵗʰ **M11.05 Hydroxyapatite deposition disease,** hip
- **M11.051 Hydroxyapatite deposition disease,** right **hip**
- **M11.052 Hydroxyapatite deposition disease,** left **hip**
- **M11.059 Hydroxyapatite deposition disease,** unspecified **hip** ▽

☑6ᵗʰ **M11.06 Hydroxyapatite deposition disease,** knee
- **M11.061 Hydroxyapatite deposition disease,** right **knee**
- **M11.062 Hydroxyapatite deposition disease,** left **knee**
- **M11.069 Hydroxyapatite deposition disease,** unspecified **knee** ▽

☑6ᵗʰ **M11.07 Hydroxyapatite deposition disease,** ankle and foot
- **M11.071 Hydroxyapatite deposition disease,** right **ankle and foot**
- **M11.072 Hydroxyapatite deposition disease,** left **ankle and foot**
- **M11.079 Hydroxyapatite deposition disease,** unspecified **ankle and foot** ▽

M11.08 Hydroxyapatite deposition disease, vertebrae
M11.09 Hydroxyapatite deposition disease, multiple sites

☑5ᵗʰ **M11.1 Familial chondrocalcinosis**
- **M11.10 Familial chondrocalcinosis, unspecified site** ▽

☑6ᵗʰ **M11.11 Familial chondrocalcinosis,** shoulder
- **M11.111 Familial chondrocalcinosis,** right **shoulder**
- **M11.112 Familial chondrocalcinosis,** left **shoulder**
- **M11.119 Familial chondrocalcinosis,** unspecified **shoulder** ▽

☑6ᵗʰ **M11.12 Familial chondrocalcinosis,** elbow
- **M11.121 Familial chondrocalcinosis,** right **elbow**
- **M11.122 Familial chondrocalcinosis,** left **elbow**
- **M11.129 Familial chondrocalcinosis,** unspecified **elbow** ▽

☑6ᵗʰ **M11.13 Familial chondrocalcinosis,** wrist
- **M11.131 Familial chondrocalcinosis,** right **wrist**
- **M11.132 Familial chondrocalcinosis,** left **wrist**
- **M11.139 Familial chondrocalcinosis,** unspecified **wrist** ▽

☑6ᵗʰ **M11.14 Familial chondrocalcinosis,** hand
- **M11.141 Familial chondrocalcinosis,** right **hand**
- **M11.142 Familial chondrocalcinosis,** left **hand**
- **M11.149 Familial chondrocalcinosis,** unspecified **hand** ▽

☑6ᵗʰ **M11.15 Familial chondrocalcinosis,** hip
- **M11.151 Familial chondrocalcinosis,** right **hip**
- **M11.152 Familial chondrocalcinosis,** left **hip**
- **M11.159 Familial chondrocalcinosis,** unspecified **hip** ▽

☑6ᵗʰ **M11.16 Familial chondrocalcinosis,** knee
- **M11.161 Familial chondrocalcinosis,** right **knee**
- **M11.162 Familial chondrocalcinosis,** left **knee**
- **M11.169 Familial chondrocalcinosis,** unspecified **knee** ▽

☑6ᵗʰ **M11.17 Familial chondrocalcinosis,** ankle and foot
- **M11.171 Familial chondrocalcinosis,** right **ankle and foot**
- **M11.172 Familial chondrocalcinosis,** left **ankle and foot**
- **M11.179 Familial chondrocalcinosis,** unspecified **ankle and foot** ▽

M11.18 Familial chondrocalcinosis, vertebrae
M11.19 Familial chondrocalcinosis, multiple sites

☑5ᵗʰ **M11.2 Other chondrocalcinosis**
    Chondrocalcinosis NOS
- **M11.20 Other chondrocalcinosis, unspecified site** ▽
- **M11.21 Other chondrocalcinosis,** shoulder
  - **M11.211 Other chondrocalcinosis,** right **shoulder**
  - **M11.212 Other chondrocalcinosis,** left **shoulder**
  - **M11.219 Other chondrocalcinosis,** unspecified **shoulder** ▽

☑6ᵗʰ **M11.22 Other chondrocalcinosis,** elbow
- **M11.221 Other chondrocalcinosis,** right **elbow**
- **M11.222 Other chondrocalcinosis,** left **elbow**
- **M11.229 Other chondrocalcinosis,** unspecified **elbow** ▽

☑6ᵗʰ **M11.23 Other chondrocalcinosis,** wrist
- **M11.231 Other chondrocalcinosis,** right **wrist**
- **M11.232 Other chondrocalcinosis,** left **wrist**
- **M11.239 Other chondrocalcinosis,** unspecified **wrist** ▽

☑6ᵗʰ **M11.24 Other chondrocalcinosis,** hand
- **M11.241 Other chondrocalcinosis,** right **hand**
- **M11.242 Other chondrocalcinosis,** left **hand**
- **M11.249 Other chondrocalcinosis,** unspecified **hand** ▽

☑6ᵗʰ **M11.25 Other chondrocalcinosis,** hip
- **M11.251 Other chondrocalcinosis,** right **hip**
- **M11.252 Other chondrocalcinosis,** left **hip**
- **M11.259 Other chondrocalcinosis,** unspecified **hip** ▽

☑6ᵗʰ **M11.26 Other chondrocalcinosis,** knee
- **M11.261 Other chondrocalcinosis,** right **knee**
- **M11.262 Other chondrocalcinosis,** left **knee**
- **M11.269 Other chondrocalcinosis,** unspecified **knee** ▽

☑6ᵗʰ **M11.27 Other chondrocalcinosis,** ankle and foot
- **M11.271 Other chondrocalcinosis,** right **ankle and foot**
- **M11.272 Other chondrocalcinosis,** left **ankle and foot**
- **M11.279 Other chondrocalcinosis,** unspecified **ankle and foot** ▽

M11.28 Other chondrocalcinosis, vertebrae
M11.29 Other chondrocalcinosis, multiple sites

☑5ᵗʰ **M11.8 Other specified crystal arthropathies**
- **M11.80 Other specified crystal arthropathies, unspecified site** ▽

☑6ᵗʰ **M11.81 Other specified crystal arthropathies,** shoulder
- **M11.811 Other specified crystal arthropathies,** right **shoulder**
- **M11.812 Other specified crystal arthropathies,** left **shoulder**
- **M11.819 Other specified crystal arthropathies,** unspecified **shoulder** ▽

☑6ᵗʰ **M11.82 Other specified crystal arthropathies,** elbow
- **M11.821 Other specified crystal arthropathies,** right **elbow**
- **M11.822 Other specified crystal arthropathies,** left **elbow**
- **M11.829 Other specified crystal arthropathies,** unspecified **elbow** ▽

☑6ᵗʰ **M11.83 Other specified crystal arthropathies,** wrist
- **M11.831 Other specified crystal arthropathies,** right **wrist**
- **M11.832 Other specified crystal arthropathies,** left **wrist**

☑ Add'l Character Required   ☑x7ᵗʰ Placeholder Alert   RUG IV Special Care High Dx   RUG IV Clinically Complex Dx   RUG IV Special Care Low Dx   Manifestation Code   Other Specified Code   ▽ Unspecified Code

M11.839 **Other specified crystal arthropathies, unspecified wrist** ▽

✓6ᵗʰ M11.84 **Other specified crystal arthropathies,** hand

    M11.841 **Other specified crystal arthropathies,** right **hand**

    M11.842 **Other specified crystal arthropathies,** left **hand**

    M11.849 **Other specified crystal arthropathies, unspecified hand** ▽

✓6ᵗʰ M11.85 **Other specified crystal arthropathies,** hip

    M11.851 **Other specified crystal arthropathies,** right **hip**

    M11.852 **Other specified crystal arthropathies,** left **hip**

    M11.859 **Other specified crystal arthropathies, unspecified hip** ▽

✓6ᵗʰ M11.86 **Other specified crystal arthropathies,** knee

    M11.861 **Other specified crystal arthropathies,** right **knee**

    M11.862 **Other specified crystal arthropathies,** left **knee**

    M11.869 **Other specified crystal arthropathies, unspecified knee** ▽

✓6ᵗʰ M11.87 **Other specified crystal arthropathies,** ankle and foot

    M11.871 **Other specified crystal arthropathies,** right **ankle and foot**

    M11.872 **Other specified crystal arthropathies,** left **ankle and foot**

    M11.879 **Other specified crystal arthropathies, unspecified ankle and foot** ▽

M11.88 **Other specified crystal arthropathies,** vertebrae

M11.89 **Other specified crystal arthropathies,** multiple sites

M11.9 **Crystal arthropathy, unspecified** ▽

✓4ᵗʰ **M12 Other and unspecified arthropathy**

    EXCLUDES 1   arthrosis (M15-M19)

                 cricoarytenoid arthropathy (J38.7)

✓5ᵗʰ M12.0 **Chronic postrheumatic arthropathy [Jaccoud]**

    M12.00 **Chronic postrheumatic arthropathy [Jaccoud], unspecified site** ▽

    ✓6ᵗʰ M12.01 **Chronic postrheumatic arthropathy [Jaccoud],** shoulder

        M12.011 **Chronic postrheumatic arthropathy [Jaccoud],** right **shoulder**

        M12.012 **Chronic postrheumatic arthropathy [Jaccoud],** left **shoulder**

        M12.019 **Chronic postrheumatic arthropathy [Jaccoud], unspecified shoulder** ▽

    ✓6ᵗʰ M12.02 **Chronic postrheumatic arthropathy [Jaccoud],** elbow

        M12.021 **Chronic postrheumatic arthropathy [Jaccoud],** right **elbow**

        M12.022 **Chronic postrheumatic arthropathy [Jaccoud],** left **elbow**

        M12.029 **Chronic postrheumatic arthropathy [Jaccoud], unspecified elbow** ▽

    ✓6ᵗʰ M12.03 **Chronic postrheumatic arthropathy [Jaccoud],** wrist

        M12.031 **Chronic postrheumatic arthropathy [Jaccoud],** right **wrist**

        M12.032 **Chronic postrheumatic arthropathy [Jaccoud],** left **wrist**

        M12.039 **Chronic postrheumatic arthropathy [Jaccoud], unspecified wrist** ▽

    ✓6ᵗʰ M12.04 **Chronic postrheumatic arthropathy [Jaccoud],** hand

        M12.041 **Chronic postrheumatic arthropathy [Jaccoud],** right **hand**

        M12.042 **Chronic postrheumatic arthropathy [Jaccoud],** left **hand**

        M12.049 **Chronic postrheumatic arthropathy [Jaccoud], unspecified hand** ▽

    ✓6ᵗʰ M12.05 **Chronic postrheumatic arthropathy [Jaccoud],** hip

        M12.051 **Chronic postrheumatic arthropathy [Jaccoud],** right **hip**

        M12.052 **Chronic postrheumatic arthropathy [Jaccoud],** left **hip**

        M12.059 **Chronic postrheumatic arthropathy [Jaccoud], unspecified hip** ▽

✓6ᵗʰ M12.06 **Chronic postrheumatic arthropathy [Jaccoud],** knee

    M12.061 **Chronic postrheumatic arthropathy [Jaccoud],** right **knee**

    M12.062 **Chronic postrheumatic arthropathy [Jaccoud],** left **knee**

    M12.069 **Chronic postrheumatic arthropathy [Jaccoud], unspecified knee** ▽

✓6ᵗʰ M12.07 **Chronic postrheumatic arthropathy [Jaccoud],** ankle and foot

    M12.071 **Chronic postrheumatic arthropathy [Jaccoud],** right **ankle and foot**

    M12.072 **Chronic postrheumatic arthropathy [Jaccoud],** left **ankle and foot**

    M12.079 **Chronic postrheumatic arthropathy [Jaccoud], unspecified ankle and foot** ▽

M12.08 **Chronic postrheumatic arthropathy [Jaccoud], other specified site**

    Chronic postrheumatic arthropathy [Jaccoud], vertebrae

M12.09 **Chronic postrheumatic arthropathy [Jaccoud],** multiple sites

✓5ᵗʰ M12.1 **Kaschin-Beck disease**

    Osteochondroarthrosis deformans endemica

    M12.10 **Kaschin-Beck disease, unspecified site** ▽

    ✓6ᵗʰ M12.11 **Kaschin-Beck disease,** shoulder

        M12.111 **Kaschin-Beck disease,** right **shoulder**

        M12.112 **Kaschin-Beck disease,** left **shoulder**

        M12.119 **Kaschin-Beck disease, unspecified shoulder** ▽

    ✓6ᵗʰ M12.12 **Kaschin-Beck disease,** elbow

        M12.121 **Kaschin-Beck disease,** right **elbow**

        M12.122 **Kaschin-Beck disease,** left **elbow**

        M12.129 **Kaschin-Beck disease, unspecified elbow** ▽

    ✓6ᵗʰ M12.13 **Kaschin-Beck disease,** wrist

        M12.131 **Kaschin-Beck disease,** right **wrist**

        M12.132 **Kaschin-Beck disease,** left **wrist**

        M12.139 **Kaschin-Beck disease, unspecified wrist** ▽

    ✓6ᵗʰ M12.14 **Kaschin-Beck disease,** hand

        M12.141 **Kaschin-Beck disease,** right **hand**

        M12.142 **Kaschin-Beck disease,** left **hand**

        M12.149 **Kaschin-Beck disease, unspecified hand** ▽

    ✓6ᵗʰ M12.15 **Kaschin-Beck disease,** hip

        M12.151 **Kaschin-Beck disease,** right **hip**

        M12.152 **Kaschin-Beck disease,** left **hip**

        M12.159 **Kaschin-Beck disease, unspecified hip** ▽

    ✓6ᵗʰ M12.16 **Kaschin-Beck disease,** knee

        M12.161 **Kaschin-Beck disease,** right **knee**

        M12.162 **Kaschin-Beck disease,** left **knee**

        M12.169 **Kaschin-Beck disease, unspecified knee** ▽

    ✓6ᵗʰ M12.17 **Kaschin-Beck disease,** ankle and foot

        M12.171 **Kaschin-Beck disease,** right **ankle and foot**

        M12.172 **Kaschin-Beck disease,** left **ankle and foot**

        M12.179 **Kaschin-Beck disease, unspecified ankle and foot** ▽

    M12.18 **Kaschin-Beck disease,** vertebrae

    M12.19 **Kaschin-Beck disease,** multiple sites

✓5ᵗʰ M12.2 **Villonodular synovitis (pigmented)**

    M12.20 **Villonodular synovitis (pigmented), unspecified site** ▽

    ✓6ᵗʰ M12.21 **Villonodular synovitis (pigmented),** shoulder

        M12.211 **Villonodular synovitis (pigmented),** right **shoulder**

        M12.212 **Villonodular synovitis (pigmented),** left **shoulder**

        M12.219 **Villonodular synovitis (pigmented), unspecified shoulder** ▽

    ✓6ᵗʰ M12.22 **Villonodular synovitis (pigmented),** elbow

        M12.221 **Villonodular synovitis (pigmented),** right **elbow**

        M12.222 **Villonodular synovitis (pigmented),** left **elbow**

Ⓝ Newborn   Ⓟ Pediatric   Ⓜ Maternity   Ⓐ Adult   **RIC** RIC Dx   **NCDx** Noncancer Dx   **PDx** Primary Dx   **CC** RIC CC Condition   ▶◀ Revised Text   ● New Code   ▲ Revised Code Title

694

ICD-10-CM 2016

M12.229   Villonodular synovitis (pigmented), unspecified elbow   ▽

✓6ᵗʰ M12.23   Villonodular synovitis (pigmented), wrist

     M12.231   Villonodular synovitis (pigmented), right wrist

     M12.232   Villonodular synovitis (pigmented), left wrist

     M12.239   Villonodular synovitis (pigmented), unspecified wrist   ▽

✓6ᵗʰ M12.24   Villonodular synovitis (pigmented), hand

     M12.241   Villonodular synovitis (pigmented), right hand

     M12.242   Villonodular synovitis (pigmented), left hand

     M12.249   Villonodular synovitis (pigmented), unspecified hand   ▽

✓6ᵗʰ M12.25   Villonodular synovitis (pigmented), hip

     M12.251   Villonodular synovitis (pigmented), right hip

     M12.252   Villonodular synovitis (pigmented), left hip

     M12.259   Villonodular synovitis (pigmented), unspecified hip   ▽

✓6ᵗʰ M12.26   Villonodular synovitis (pigmented), knee

     M12.261   Villonodular synovitis (pigmented), right knee

     M12.262   Villonodular synovitis (pigmented), left knee

     M12.269   Villonodular synovitis (pigmented), unspecified knee   ▽

✓6ᵗʰ M12.27   Villonodular synovitis (pigmented), ankle and foot

     M12.271   Villonodular synovitis (pigmented), right ankle and foot

     M12.272   Villonodular synovitis (pigmented), left ankle and foot

     M12.279   Villonodular synovitis (pigmented), unspecified ankle and foot   ▽

M12.28   Villonodular synovitis (pigmented), other specified site

     Villonodular synovitis (pigmented), vertebrae

M12.29   Villonodular synovitis (pigmented), multiple sites

✓5ᵗʰ M12.3   Palindromic rheumatism

     M12.30   Palindromic rheumatism, unspecified site   ▽

✓6ᵗʰ M12.31   Palindromic rheumatism, shoulder

     M12.311   Palindromic rheumatism, right shoulder

     M12.312   Palindromic rheumatism, left shoulder

     M12.319   Palindromic rheumatism, unspecified shoulder   ▽

✓6ᵗʰ M12.32   Palindromic rheumatism, elbow

     M12.321   Palindromic rheumatism, right elbow

     M12.322   Palindromic rheumatism, left elbow

     M12.329   Palindromic rheumatism, unspecified elbow   ▽

✓6ᵗʰ M12.33   Palindromic rheumatism, wrist

     M12.331   Palindromic rheumatism, right wrist

     M12.332   Palindromic rheumatism, left wrist

     M12.339   Palindromic rheumatism, unspecified wrist   ▽

✓6ᵗʰ M12.34   Palindromic rheumatism, hand

     M12.341   Palindromic rheumatism, right hand

     M12.342   Palindromic rheumatism, left hand

     M12.349   Palindromic rheumatism, unspecified hand   ▽

✓6ᵗʰ M12.35   Palindromic rheumatism, hip

     M12.351   Palindromic rheumatism, right hip

     M12.352   Palindromic rheumatism, left hip

     M12.359   Palindromic rheumatism, unspecified hip   ▽

✓6ᵗʰ M12.36   Palindromic rheumatism, knee

     M12.361   Palindromic rheumatism, right knee

     M12.362   Palindromic rheumatism, left knee

     M12.369   Palindromic rheumatism, unspecified knee   ▽

✓6ᵗʰ M12.37   Palindromic rheumatism, ankle and foot

     M12.371   Palindromic rheumatism, right ankle and foot

     M12.372   Palindromic rheumatism, left ankle and foot

     M12.379   Palindromic rheumatism, unspecified ankle and foot   ▽

M12.38   Palindromic rheumatism, other specified site

     Palindromic rheumatism, vertebrae

M12.39   Palindromic rheumatism, multiple sites

✓5ᵗʰ M12.4   Intermittent hydrarthrosis

     M12.40   Intermittent hydrarthrosis, unspecified site   ▽

✓6ᵗʰ M12.41   Intermittent hydrarthrosis, shoulder

     M12.411   Intermittent hydrarthrosis, right shoulder

     M12.412   Intermittent hydrarthrosis, left shoulder

     M12.419   Intermittent hydrarthrosis, unspecified shoulder   ▽

✓6ᵗʰ M12.42   Intermittent hydrarthrosis, elbow

     M12.421   Intermittent hydrarthrosis, right elbow

     M12.422   Intermittent hydrarthrosis, left elbow

     M12.429   Intermittent hydrarthrosis, unspecified elbow   ▽

✓6ᵗʰ M12.43   Intermittent hydrarthrosis, wrist

     M12.431   Intermittent hydrarthrosis, right wrist

     M12.432   Intermittent hydrarthrosis, left wrist

     M12.439   Intermittent hydrarthrosis, unspecified wrist   ▽

✓6ᵗʰ M12.44   Intermittent hydrarthrosis, hand

     M12.441   Intermittent hydrarthrosis, right hand

     M12.442   Intermittent hydrarthrosis, left hand

     M12.449   Intermittent hydrarthrosis, unspecified hand   ▽

✓6ᵗʰ M12.45   Intermittent hydrarthrosis, hip

     M12.451   Intermittent hydrarthrosis, right hip

     M12.452   Intermittent hydrarthrosis, left hip

     M12.459   Intermittent hydrarthrosis, unspecified hip   ▽

✓6ᵗʰ M12.46   Intermittent hydrarthrosis, knee

     M12.461   Intermittent hydrarthrosis, right knee

     M12.462   Intermittent hydrarthrosis, left knee

     M12.469   Intermittent hydrarthrosis, unspecified knee   ▽

✓6ᵗʰ M12.47   Intermittent hydrarthrosis, ankle and foot

     M12.471   Intermittent hydrarthrosis, right ankle and foot

     M12.472   Intermittent hydrarthrosis, left ankle and foot

     M12.479   Intermittent hydrarthrosis, unspecified ankle and foot   ▽

M12.48   Intermittent hydrarthrosis, other site

M12.49   Intermittent hydrarthrosis, multiple sites

✓5ᵗʰ M12.5   Traumatic arthropathy

     EXCLUDES 1   *current injury–see Alphabetic Index*
     post-traumatic osteoarthritis NOS (M19.1-)
     post-traumatic osteoarthritis of first carpometacarpal joint (M18.2-M18.3)
     post-traumatic osteoarthritis of hip (M16.4-M16.5)
     post-traumatic osteoarthritis of knee (M17.2-M17.3)
     post-traumatic osteoarthritis of other single joints (M19.1-)

     AHA: 2015, 1Q, 17

     M12.50   Traumatic arthropathy, unspecified site   ▽

✓6ᵗʰ M12.51   Traumatic arthropathy, shoulder

     M12.511   Traumatic arthropathy, right shoulder

     M12.512   Traumatic arthropathy, left shoulder

     M12.519   Traumatic arthropathy, unspecified shoulder   ▽

✓6ᵗʰ M12.52   Traumatic arthropathy, elbow

     M12.521   Traumatic arthropathy, right elbow

     M12.522   Traumatic arthropathy, left elbow

     M12.529   Traumatic arthropathy, unspecified elbow   ▽

✓6ᵗʰ M12.53   Traumatic arthropathy, wrist

     M12.531   Traumatic arthropathy, right wrist

     M12.532   Traumatic arthropathy, left wrist

☑ Add'l Character Required   ✓ₓ7ᵗʰ Placeholder Alert   RUG IV Special Care High Dx   RUG IV Clinically Complex Dx   RUG IV Special Care Low Dx   Manifestation Code   Other Specified Code   ▽ Unspecified Code

ICD-10-CM 2016   695

M12.539 Traumatic arthropathy, unspecified wrist ▽

✓6ᵗʰ M12.54 Traumatic arthropathy, hand
     M12.541 Traumatic arthropathy, right hand
     M12.542 Traumatic arthropathy, left hand
     M12.549 Traumatic arthropathy, unspecified hand ▽

✓6ᵗʰ M12.55 Traumatic arthropathy, hip
     M12.551 Traumatic arthropathy, right hip
     M12.552 Traumatic arthropathy, left hip
     M12.559 Traumatic arthropathy, unspecified hip ▽

✓6ᵗʰ M12.56 Traumatic arthropathy, knee
     M12.561 Traumatic arthropathy, right knee
     M12.562 Traumatic arthropathy, left knee
     M12.569 Traumatic arthropathy, unspecified knee ▽

✓6ᵗʰ M12.57 Traumatic arthropathy, ankle and foot
     M12.571 Traumatic arthropathy, right ankle and foot
     M12.572 Traumatic arthropathy, left ankle and foot
     M12.579 Traumatic arthropathy, unspecified ankle and foot ▽

M12.58 Traumatic arthropathy, other specified site
     Traumatic arthropathy, vertebrae

M12.59 Traumatic arthropathy, multiple sites

✓5ᵗʰ M12.8 Other specific arthropathies, not elsewhere classified
     Transient arthropathy

M12.80 Other specific arthropathies, not elsewhere classified, unspecified site ▽

✓6ᵗʰ M12.81 Other specific arthropathies, not elsewhere classified, shoulder
     M12.811 Other specific arthropathies, not elsewhere classified, right shoulder
     M12.812 Other specific arthropathies, not elsewhere classified, left shoulder
     M12.819 Other specific arthropathies, not elsewhere classified, unspecified shoulder ▽

✓6ᵗʰ M12.82 Other specific arthropathies, not elsewhere classified, elbow
     M12.821 Other specific arthropathies, not elsewhere classified, right elbow
     M12.822 Other specific arthropathies, not elsewhere classified, left elbow
     M12.829 Other specific arthropathies, not elsewhere classified, unspecified elbow ▽

✓6ᵗʰ M12.83 Other specific arthropathies, not elsewhere classified, wrist
     M12.831 Other specific arthropathies, not elsewhere classified, right wrist
     M12.832 Other specific arthropathies, not elsewhere classified, left wrist
     M12.839 Other specific arthropathies, not elsewhere classified, unspecified wrist ▽

✓6ᵗʰ M12.84 Other specific arthropathies, not elsewhere classified, hand
     M12.841 Other specific arthropathies, not elsewhere classified, right hand
     M12.842 Other specific arthropathies, not elsewhere classified, left hand
     M12.849 Other specific arthropathies, not elsewhere classified, unspecified hand ▽

✓6ᵗʰ M12.85 Other specific arthropathies, not elsewhere classified, hip
     M12.851 Other specific arthropathies, not elsewhere classified, right hip
     M12.852 Other specific arthropathies, not elsewhere classified, left hip
     M12.859 Other specific arthropathies, not elsewhere classified, unspecified hip ▽

✓6ᵗʰ M12.86 Other specific arthropathies, not elsewhere classified, knee
     M12.861 Other specific arthropathies, not elsewhere classified, right knee
     M12.862 Other specific arthropathies, not elsewhere classified, left knee
     M12.869 Other specific arthropathies, not elsewhere classified, unspecified knee ▽

✓6ᵗʰ M12.87 Other specific arthropathies, not elsewhere classified, ankle and foot
     M12.871 Other specific arthropathies, not elsewhere classified, right ankle and foot
     M12.872 Other specific arthropathies, not elsewhere classified, left ankle and foot
     M12.879 Other specific arthropathies, not elsewhere classified, unspecified ankle and foot ▽

M12.88 Other specific arthropathies, not elsewhere classified, other specified site
     Other specific arthropathies, not elsewhere classified, vertebrae

M12.89 Other specific arthropathies, not elsewhere classified, multiple sites

M12.9 Arthropathy, unspecified ▽

✓4ᵗʰ **M13 Other arthritis**
     EXCLUDES 1   arthrosis (M15-M19)
                  osteoarthritis (M15-M19)

M13.0 Polyarthritis, unspecified ▽

✓5ᵗʰ M13.1 Monoarthritis, not elsewhere classified
     M13.10 Monoarthritis, not elsewhere classified, unspecified site ▽

✓6ᵗʰ M13.11 Monoarthritis, not elsewhere classified, shoulder
     M13.111 Monoarthritis, not elsewhere classified, right shoulder
     M13.112 Monoarthritis, not elsewhere classified, left shoulder
     M13.119 Monoarthritis, not elsewhere classified, unspecified shoulder ▽

✓6ᵗʰ M13.12 Monoarthritis, not elsewhere classified, elbow
     M13.121 Monoarthritis, not elsewhere classified, right elbow
     M13.122 Monoarthritis, not elsewhere classified, left elbow
     M13.129 Monoarthritis, not elsewhere classified, unspecified elbow ▽

✓6ᵗʰ M13.13 Monoarthritis, not elsewhere classified, wrist
     M13.131 Monoarthritis, not elsewhere classified, right wrist
     M13.132 Monoarthritis, not elsewhere classified, left wrist
     M13.139 Monoarthritis, not elsewhere classified, unspecified wrist ▽

✓6ᵗʰ M13.14 Monoarthritis, not elsewhere classified, hand
     M13.141 Monoarthritis, not elsewhere classified, right hand
     M13.142 Monoarthritis, not elsewhere classified, left hand
     M13.149 Monoarthritis, not elsewhere classified, unspecified hand ▽

✓6ᵗʰ M13.15 Monoarthritis, not elsewhere classified, hip
     M13.151 Monoarthritis, not elsewhere classified, right hip
     M13.152 Monoarthritis, not elsewhere classified, left hip
     M13.159 Monoarthritis, not elsewhere classified, unspecified hip ▽

✓6ᵗʰ M13.16 Monoarthritis, not elsewhere classified, knee
     M13.161 Monoarthritis, not elsewhere classified, right knee
     M13.162 Monoarthritis, not elsewhere classified, left knee
     M13.169 Monoarthritis, not elsewhere classified, unspecified knee ▽

Ⓝ Newborn   Ⓟ Pediatric   Ⓜ Maternity   Ⓐ Adult   **RIC** RIC Dx   **NC Dx** Noncancer Dx   **PDx** Primary Dx   **CC** RIC CC Condition   ▶◀ Revised Text   ● New Code   ▲ Revised Code Title

696   ICD-10-CM 2016

√6ᵗʰ **M13.17** Monoarthritis, not elsewhere classified, ankle and foot

  M13.171 Monoarthritis, not elsewhere classified, right ankle and foot

  M13.172 Monoarthritis, not elsewhere classified, left ankle and foot

  M13.179 Monoarthritis, not elsewhere classified, unspecified ankle and foot ▽

√5ᵗʰ **M13.8** **Other specified arthritis**
  Allergic arthritis
  EXCLUDES 1 osteoarthritis (M15-M19)

 M13.80 Other specified arthritis, unspecified site ▽

√6ᵗʰ **M13.81** Other specified arthritis, shoulder
  M13.811 Other specified arthritis, right shoulder
  M13.812 Other specified arthritis, left shoulder
  M13.819 Other specified arthritis, unspecified shoulder ▽

√6ᵗʰ **M13.82** Other specified arthritis, elbow
  M13.821 Other specified arthritis, right elbow
  M13.822 Other specified arthritis, left elbow
  M13.829 Other specified arthritis, unspecified elbow ▽

√6ᵗʰ **M13.83** Other specified arthritis, wrist
  M13.831 Other specified arthritis, right wrist
  M13.832 Other specified arthritis, left wrist
  M13.839 Other specified arthritis, unspecified wrist ▽

√6ᵗʰ **M13.84** Other specified arthritis, hand
  M13.841 Other specified arthritis, right hand
  M13.842 Other specified arthritis, left hand
  M13.849 Other specified arthritis, unspecified hand ▽

√6ᵗʰ **M13.85** Other specified arthritis, hip
  M13.851 Other specified arthritis, right hip
  M13.852 Other specified arthritis, left hip
  M13.859 Other specified arthritis, unspecified hip ▽

√6ᵗʰ **M13.86** Other specified arthritis, knee
  M13.861 Other specified arthritis, right knee
  M13.862 Other specified arthritis, left knee
  M13.869 Other specified arthritis, unspecified knee ▽

√6ᵗʰ **M13.87** Other specified arthritis, ankle and foot
  M13.871 Other specified arthritis, right ankle and foot
  M13.872 Other specified arthritis, left ankle and foot
  M13.879 Other specified arthritis, unspecified ankle and foot ▽

 M13.88 Other specified arthritis, other site

 M13.89 Other specified arthritis, multiple sites

√4ᵗʰ **M14** **Arthropathies in other diseases classified elsewhere**
  EXCLUDES 1 arthropathy in:
   diabetes mellitus (E08-E13 with .61-)
   hematological disorders (M36.2-M36.3)
   hypersensitivity reactions (M36.4)
   neoplastic disease (M36.1)
   neurosyphillis (A52.16)
   sarcoidosis (D86.86)
  enteropathic arthropathies (M07.-)
  juvenile psoriatic arthropathy (L40.54)
  lipoid dermatoarthritis (E78.81)

√5ᵗʰ **M14.6** **Charcôt's joint**
  Neuropathic arthropathy
  EXCLUDES 1 Charcôt's joint in diabetes mellitus (E08-E13 with .610)
   Charcôt's joint in tabes dorsalis (A52.16)

 M14.60 Charcôt's joint, unspecified site ▽

√6ᵗʰ **M14.61** Charcôt's joint, shoulder
  M14.611 Charcôt's joint, right shoulder
  M14.612 Charcôt's joint, left shoulder
  M14.619 Charcôt's joint, unspecified shoulder ▽

√6ᵗʰ **M14.62** Charcôt's joint, elbow
  M14.621 Charcôt's joint, right elbow
  M14.622 Charcôt's joint, left elbow
  M14.629 Charcôt's joint, unspecified elbow ▽

√6ᵗʰ **M14.63** Charcôt's joint, wrist
  M14.631 Charcôt's joint, right wrist
  M14.632 Charcôt's joint, left wrist
  M14.639 Charcôt's joint, unspecified wrist ▽

√6ᵗʰ **M14.64** Charcôt's joint, hand
  M14.641 Charcôt's joint, right hand
  M14.642 Charcôt's joint, left hand
  M14.649 Charcôt's joint, unspecified hand ▽

√6ᵗʰ **M14.65** Charcôt's joint, hip
  M14.651 Charcôt's joint, right hip
  M14.652 Charcôt's joint, left hip
  M14.659 Charcôt's joint, unspecified hip ▽

√6ᵗʰ **M14.66** Charcôt's joint, knee
  M14.661 Charcôt's joint, right knee
  M14.662 Charcôt's joint, left knee
  M14.669 Charcôt's joint, unspecified knee ▽

√6ᵗʰ **M14.67** Charcôt's joint, ankle and foot
  M14.671 Charcôt's joint, right ankle and foot
  M14.672 Charcôt's joint, left ankle and foot
  M14.679 Charcôt's joint, unspecified ankle and foot ▽

 M14.68 Charcôt's joint, vertebrae

 M14.69 Charcôt's joint, multiple sites

√5ᵗʰ **M14.8** **Arthropathies in other specified diseases classified elsewhere**
  Code first underlying disease, such as:
   amyloidosis (E85.-)
   erythema multiforme (L51.-)
   erythema nodosum (L52)
   hemochromatosis (E83.11-)
   hyperparathyroidism (E21.-)
   hypothyroidism (E00-E03)
   sickle-cell disorders (D57.-)
   thyrotoxicosis [hyperthyroidism] (E05.-)
   Whipple's disease (K90.81)

 M14.80 *Arthropathies in other specified diseases classified elsewhere, unspecified site* ▽

√6ᵗʰ **M14.81** *Arthropathies in other specified diseases classified elsewhere, shoulder*
  M14.811 *Arthropathies in other specified diseases classified elsewhere, right shoulder*
  M14.812 *Arthropathies in other specified diseases classified elsewhere, left shoulder*
  M14.819 *Arthropathies in other specified diseases classified elsewhere, unspecified shoulder* ▽

√6ᵗʰ **M14.82** *Arthropathies in other specified diseases classified elsewhere, elbow*
  M14.821 *Arthropathies in other specified diseases classified elsewhere, right elbow*
  M14.822 *Arthropathies in other specified diseases classified elsewhere, left elbow*
  M14.829 *Arthropathies in other specified diseases classified elsewhere, unspecified elbow* ▽

√6ᵗʰ **M14.83** *Arthropathies in other specified diseases classified elsewhere, wrist*
  M14.831 *Arthropathies in other specified diseases classified elsewhere, right wrist*
  M14.832 *Arthropathies in other specified diseases classified elsewhere, left wrist*
  M14.839 *Arthropathies in other specified diseases classified elsewhere, unspecified wrist* ▽

√6ᵗʰ **M14.84** *Arthropathies in other specified diseases classified elsewhere, hand*
  M14.841 *Arthropathies in other specified diseases classified elsewhere, right hand*
  M14.842 *Arthropathies in other specified diseases classified elsewhere, left hand*
  M14.849 *Arthropathies in other specified diseases classified elsewhere, unspecified hand* ▽

☑ Add'l Character Required √x7ᵗʰ Placeholder Alert RUG IV Special Care High Dx RUG IV Clinically Complex Dx RUG IV Special Care Low Dx Manifestation Code Other Specified Code ▽ Unspecified Code

ICD-10-CM 2016   **697**

M13.17–M14.849

✓6ᵗʰ **M14.85** Arthropathies in other specified diseases classified elsewhere, hip

　　M14.851 **Arthropathies in other specified diseases classified elsewhere, right hip**

　　M14.852 **Arthropathies in other specified diseases classified elsewhere, left hip**

　　M14.859 **Arthropathies in other specified diseases classified elsewhere, unspecified hip** ▽

✓6ᵗʰ **M14.86** Arthropathies in other specified diseases classified elsewhere, knee

　　M14.861 **Arthropathies in other specified diseases classified elsewhere, right knee**

　　M14.862 **Arthropathies in other specified diseases classified elsewhere, left knee**

　　M14.869 **Arthropathies in other specified diseases classified elsewhere, unspecified knee** ▽

✓6ᵗʰ **M14.87** Arthropathies in other specified diseases classified elsewhere, ankle and foot

　　M14.871 **Arthropathies in other specified diseases classified elsewhere, right ankle and foot**

　　M14.872 **Arthropathies in other specified diseases classified elsewhere, left ankle and foot**

　　M14.879 **Arthropathies in other specified diseases classified elsewhere, unspecified ankle and foot** ▽

　　M14.88 *Arthropathies in other specified diseases classified elsewhere, vertebrae*

　　M14.89 *Arthropathies in other specified diseases classified elsewhere, multiple sites*

Osteoarthritis (M15-M19)

EXCLUDES 2　osteoarthritis of spine (M47.-)

✓4ᵗʰ **M15** **Polyosteoarthritis**

　INCLUDES　arthritis of multiple sites

　EXCLUDES 1　bilateral involvement of single joint (M16-M19)

　M15.0 **Primary generalized (osteo)arthritis**

　M15.1 **Heberden's nodes (with arthropathy)**
　　Interphalangeal distal osteoarthritis

　M15.2 **Bouchard's nodes (with arthropathy)**
　　Juxtaphalangeal distal osteoarthritis

　M15.3 **Secondary multiple arthritis**
　　Post-traumatic polyosteoarthritis

　M15.4 **Erosive (osteo)arthritis**

　M15.8 **Other polyosteoarthritis**

　M15.9 **Polyosteoarthritis, unspecified** ▽
　　Generalized osteoarthritis NOS

✓4ᵗʰ **M16** **Osteoarthritis of hip**

　M16.0 **Bilateral primary osteoarthritis of hip**

✓5ᵗʰ **M16.1** **Unilateral primary osteoarthritis of hip**
　　Primary osteoarthritis of hip NOS

　　M16.10 **Unilateral primary osteoarthritis, unspecified hip** ▽

　　M16.11 **Unilateral primary osteoarthritis, right hip**

　　M16.12 **Unilateral primary osteoarthritis, left hip**

　M16.2 **Bilateral osteoarthritis resulting from hip dysplasia**

✓5ᵗʰ **M16.3** **Unilateral osteoarthritis resulting from hip dysplasia**
　　Dysplastic osteoarthritis of hip NOS

　　M16.30 **Unilateral osteoarthritis resulting from hip dysplasia, unspecified hip** ▽

　　M16.31 **Unilateral osteoarthritis resulting from hip dysplasia, right hip**

　　M16.32 **Unilateral osteoarthritis resulting from hip dysplasia, left hip**

　M16.4 **Bilateral post-traumatic osteoarthritis of hip**

✓5ᵗʰ **M16.5** **Unilateral post-traumatic osteoarthritis of hip**
　　Post-traumatic osteoarthritis of hip NOS

　　M16.50 **Unilateral post-traumatic osteoarthritis, unspecified hip** ▽

　　M16.51 **Unilateral post-traumatic osteoarthritis, right hip**

　　M16.52 **Unilateral post-traumatic osteoarthritis, left hip**

　M16.6 **Other bilateral secondary osteoarthritis of hip**

　M16.7 **Other unilateral secondary osteoarthritis of hip**
　　Secondary osteoarthritis of hip NOS

　M16.9 **Osteoarthritis of hip, unspecified** ▽

✓4ᵗʰ **M17** **Osteoarthritis of knee**

　M17.0 **Bilateral primary osteoarthritis of knee**

✓5ᵗʰ **M17.1** **Unilateral primary osteoarthritis of knee**
　　Primary osteoarthritis of knee NOS

　　M17.10 **Unilateral primary osteoarthritis, unspecified knee** ▽

　　M17.11 **Unilateral primary osteoarthritis, right knee**

　　M17.12 **Unilateral primary osteoarthritis, left knee**

　M17.2 **Bilateral post-traumatic osteoarthritis of knee**

✓5ᵗʰ **M17.3** **Unilateral post-traumatic osteoarthritis of knee**
　　Post-traumatic osteoarthritis of knee NOS

　　M17.30 **Unilateral post-traumatic osteoarthritis, unspecified knee** ▽

　　M17.31 **Unilateral post-traumatic osteoarthritis, right knee**

　　M17.32 **Unilateral post-traumatic osteoarthritis, left knee**

　M17.4 **Other bilateral secondary osteoarthritis of knee**

　M17.5 **Other unilateral secondary osteoarthritis of knee**
　　Secondary osteoarthritis of knee NOS

　M17.9 **Osteoarthritis of knee, unspecified** ▽

✓4ᵗʰ **M18** **Osteoarthritis of first carpometacarpal joint**

　M18.0 **Bilateral primary osteoarthritis of first carpometacarpal joints**

✓5ᵗʰ **M18.1** **Unilateral primary osteoarthritis of first carpometacarpal joint**
　　Primary osteoarthritis of first carpometacarpal joint NOS

　　M18.10 **Unilateral primary osteoarthritis of first carpometacarpal joint, unspecified hand** ▽

　　M18.11 **Unilateral primary osteoarthritis of first carpometacarpal joint, right hand**

　　M18.12 **Unilateral primary osteoarthritis of first carpometacarpal joint, left hand**

　M18.2 **Bilateral post-traumatic osteoarthritis of first carpometacarpal joints**

✓5ᵗʰ **M18.3** **Unilateral post-traumatic osteoarthritis of first carpometacarpal joint**
　　Post-traumatic osteoarthritis of first carpometacarpal joint NOS

　　M18.30 **Unilateral post-traumatic osteoarthritis of first carpometacarpal joint, unspecified hand** ▽

　　M18.31 **Unilateral post-traumatic osteoarthritis of first carpometacarpal joint, right hand**

　　M18.32 **Unilateral post-traumatic osteoarthritis of first carpometacarpal joint, left hand**

　M18.4 **Other bilateral secondary osteoarthritis of first carpometacarpal joints**

✓5ᵗʰ **M18.5** **Other unilateral secondary osteoarthritis of first carpometacarpal joint**
　　Secondary osteoarthritis of first carpometacarpal joint NOS

　　M18.50 **Other unilateral secondary osteoarthritis of first carpometacarpal joint, unspecified hand** ▽

　　M18.51 **Other unilateral secondary osteoarthritis of first carpometacarpal joint, right hand**

　　M18.52 **Other unilateral secondary osteoarthritis of first carpometacarpal joint, left hand**

　M18.9 **Osteoarthritis of first carpometacarpal joint, unspecified** ▽

✓4ᵗʰ **M19** **Other and unspecified osteoarthritis**

　EXCLUDES 1　polyarthritis (M15.-)

　EXCLUDES 2　arthrosis of spine (M47.-)
　　　hallux rigidus (M20.2)
　　　osteoarthritis of spine (M47.-)

✓5ᵗʰ **M19.0** **Primary osteoarthritis of other joints**

　　✓6ᵗʰ **M19.01** **Primary osteoarthritis, shoulder**

　　　　M19.011 **Primary osteoarthritis, right shoulder**

　　　　M19.012 **Primary osteoarthritis, left shoulder**

　　　　M19.019 **Primary osteoarthritis, unspecified shoulder** ▽

　　✓6ᵗʰ **M19.02** **Primary osteoarthritis, elbow**

　　　　M19.021 **Primary osteoarthritis, right elbow**

　　　　M19.022 **Primary osteoarthritis, left elbow**

　　　　M19.029 **Primary osteoarthritis, unspecified elbow** ▽

Ⓝ Newborn　Ⓟ Pediatric　Ⓜ Maternity　Ⓐ Adult　RIC RIC Dx　NC Dx Noncancer Dx　PDx Primary Dx　CC RIC CC Condition　▶◀ Revised Text　● New Code　▲ Revised Code Title

698　　ICD-10-CM 2016

✓6th **M19.03 Primary osteoarthritis, wrist**
     M19.031 **Primary osteoarthritis, right wrist**
     M19.032 **Primary osteoarthritis, left wrist**
     M19.039 **Primary osteoarthritis, unspecified wrist** ▽

✓6th **M19.04 Primary osteoarthritis, hand**
     EXCLUDES 2 *primary osteoarthritis of first carpometacarpal joint (M18.0-, M18.1-)*
     M19.041 **Primary osteoarthritis, right hand**
     M19.042 **Primary osteoarthritis, left hand**
     M19.049 **Primary osteoarthritis, unspecified hand** ▽

✓6th **M19.07 Primary osteoarthritis ankle and foot**
     M19.071 **Primary osteoarthritis, right ankle and foot**
     M19.072 **Primary osteoarthritis, left ankle and foot**
     M19.079 **Primary osteoarthritis, unspecified ankle and foot** ▽

✓5th **M19.1 Post-traumatic osteoarthritis of other joints**

✓6th **M19.11 Post-traumatic osteoarthritis, shoulder**
     M19.111 **Post-traumatic osteoarthritis, right shoulder**
     M19.112 **Post-traumatic osteoarthritis, left shoulder**
     M19.119 **Post-traumatic osteoarthritis, unspecified shoulder** ▽

✓6th **M19.12 Post-traumatic osteoarthritis, elbow**
     M19.121 **Post-traumatic osteoarthritis, right elbow**
     M19.122 **Post-traumatic osteoarthritis, left elbow**
     M19.129 **Post-traumatic osteoarthritis, unspecified elbow** ▽

✓6th **M19.13 Post-traumatic osteoarthritis, wrist**
     M19.131 **Post-traumatic osteoarthritis, right wrist**
     M19.132 **Post-traumatic osteoarthritis, left wrist**
     M19.139 **Post-traumatic osteoarthritis, unspecified wrist** ▽

✓6th **M19.14 Post-traumatic osteoarthritis, hand**
     EXCLUDES 2 *post-traumatic osteoarthritis of first carpometacarpal joint (M18.2-, M18.3-)*
     M19.141 **Post-traumatic osteoarthritis, right hand**
     M19.142 **Post-traumatic osteoarthritis, left hand**
     M19.149 **Post-traumatic osteoarthritis, unspecified hand** ▽

✓6th **M19.17 Post-traumatic osteoarthritis ankle and foot**
     M19.171 **Post-traumatic osteoarthritis, right ankle and foot**
     M19.172 **Post-traumatic osteoarthritis, left ankle and foot**
     M19.179 **Post-traumatic osteoarthritis, unspecified ankle and foot** ▽

✓5th **M19.2 Secondary osteoarthritis of other joints**

✓6th **M19.21 Secondary osteoarthritis, shoulder**
     M19.211 **Secondary osteoarthritis, right shoulder**
     M19.212 **Secondary osteoarthritis, left shoulder**
     M19.219 **Secondary osteoarthritis, unspecified shoulder** ▽

✓6th **M19.22 Secondary osteoarthritis, elbow**
     M19.221 **Secondary osteoarthritis, right elbow**
     M19.222 **Secondary osteoarthritis, left elbow**
     M19.229 **Secondary osteoarthritis, unspecified elbow** ▽

✓6th **M19.23 Secondary osteoarthritis, wrist**
     M19.231 **Secondary osteoarthritis, right wrist**
     M19.232 **Secondary osteoarthritis, left wrist**
     M19.239 **Secondary osteoarthritis, unspecified wrist** ▽

✓6th **M19.24 Secondary osteoarthritis, hand**
     M19.241 **Secondary osteoarthritis, right hand**
     M19.242 **Secondary osteoarthritis, left hand**
     M19.249 **Secondary osteoarthritis, unspecified hand** ▽

✓6th **M19.27 Secondary osteoarthritis, ankle and foot**
     M19.271 **Secondary osteoarthritis, right ankle and foot**
     M19.272 **Secondary osteoarthritis, left ankle and foot**
     M19.279 **Secondary osteoarthritis, unspecified ankle and foot** ▽

✓5th **M19.9 Osteoarthritis, unspecified site**
     M19.90 **Unspecified osteoarthritis, unspecified site** ▽
     Arthrosis NOS
     Arthritis NOS
     Osteoarthritis NOS
     M19.91 **Primary osteoarthritis, unspecified site** ▽
     Primary osteoarthritis NOS
     M19.92 **Post-traumatic osteoarthritis, unspecified site** ▽
     Post-traumatic osteoarthritis NOS
     M19.93 **Secondary osteoarthritis, unspecified site** ▽
     Secondary osteoarthritis NOS

Other joint disorders (M20-M25)

EXCLUDES 2 *joints of the spine (M40-M54)*

✓4th **M20 Acquired deformities of fingers and toes**
     EXCLUDES 1 *acquired absence of fingers and toes (Z89.-)*
     congenital absence of fingers and toes (Q71.3-, Q72.3-)
     congenital deformities and malformations of fingers and toes (Q66-, Q68-Q70, Q74-)

✓5th **M20.0 Deformity of finger(s)**
     EXCLUDES 1 *clubbing of fingers (R68.3)*
     palmar fascial fibromatosis [Dupuytren] (M72.0)
     trigger finger (M65.3)

✓6th **M20.00 Unspecified deformity of finger(s)**
     M20.001 **Unspecified deformity of right finger(s)**
     M20.002 **Unspecified deformity of left finger(s)**
     M20.009 **Unspecified deformity of unspecified finger(s)** ▽

✓6th **M20.01 Mallet finger**
     M20.011 **Mallet finger of right finger(s)**
     M20.012 **Mallet finger of left finger(s)**
     M20.019 **Mallet finger of unspecified finger(s)** ▽

✓6th **M20.02 Boutonnière deformity**
     M20.021 **Boutonnière deformity of right finger(s)**
     M20.022 **Boutonnière deformity of left finger(s)**
     M20.029 **Boutonnière deformity of unspecified finger(s)** ▽

✓6th **M20.03 Swan-neck deformity**
     M20.031 **Swan-neck deformity of right finger(s)**
     M20.032 **Swan-neck deformity of left finger(s)**
     M20.039 **Swan-neck deformity of unspecified finger(s)** ▽

✓6th **M20.09 Other deformity of finger(s)**
     M20.091 **Other deformity of right finger(s)**
     M20.092 **Other deformity of left finger(s)**
     M20.099 **Other deformity of finger(s), unspecified finger(s)** ▽

✓5th **M20.1 Hallux valgus (acquired)**
     Bunion
     M20.10 **Hallux valgus (acquired), unspecified foot** ▽
     M20.11 **Hallux valgus (acquired), right foot**
     M20.12 **Hallux valgus (acquired), left foot**

✓5th **M20.2 Hallux rigidus**
     M20.20 **Hallux rigidus, unspecified foot** ▽
     M20.21 **Hallux rigidus, right foot**
     M20.22 **Hallux rigidus, left foot**

✓5th **M20.3 Hallux varus (acquired)**
     M20.30 **Hallux varus (acquired), unspecified foot** ▽
     M20.31 **Hallux varus (acquired), right foot**
     M20.32 **Hallux varus (acquired), left foot**

✓5th **M20.4 Other hammer toe(s) (acquired)**
     M20.40 **Other hammer toe(s) (acquired), unspecified foot** ▽
     M20.41 **Other hammer toe(s) (acquired), right foot**
     M20.42 **Other hammer toe(s) (acquired), left foot**

☑ Add'l Character Required   ✓x7th Placeholder Alert   RUG IV Special Care High Dx   RUG IV Clinically Complex Dx   RUG IV Special Care Low Dx   Manifestation Code   Other Specified Code   ▽ Unspecified Code

ICD-10-CM 2016   **699**

✓5ᵗʰ **M20.5** Other deformities of toe(s) (acquired)
　✓6ᵗʰ **M20.5X** Other deformities of toe(s) (acquired)
　　　M20.5X1 Other deformities of toe(s) (acquired), right foot
　　　M20.5X2 Other deformities of toe(s) (acquired), left foot
　　　M20.5X9 Other deformities of toe(s) (acquired), unspecified foot ▽

✓5ᵗʰ **M20.6** Acquired deformities of toe(s), unspecified
　　　M20.60 Acquired deformities of toe(s), unspecified, unspecified foot ▽
　　　M20.61 Acquired deformities of toe(s), unspecified, right foot ▽
　　　M20.62 Acquired deformities of toe(s), unspecified, left foot ▽

✓4ᵗʰ **M21** **Other acquired deformities of limbs**
　　EXCLUDES 1 acquired absence of limb (Z89.-)
　　　congenital absence of limbs (Q71-Q73)
　　　congenital deformities and malformations of limbs (Q65-Q66, Q68-Q74)
　　EXCLUDES 2 acquired deformities of fingers or toes (M20.-)
　　　coxa plana (M91.2)

✓5ᵗʰ **M21.0** Valgus deformity, not elsewhere classified
　　EXCLUDES 1 metatarsus valgus (Q66.6)
　　　talipes calcaneovalgus (Q66.4)
　　　M21.00 Valgus deformity, not elsewhere classified, unspecified site ▽
　✓6ᵗʰ **M21.02** Valgus deformity, not elsewhere classified, elbow
　　　　Cubitus valgus
　　　M21.021 Valgus deformity, not elsewhere classified, right elbow
　　　M21.022 Valgus deformity, not elsewhere classified, left elbow
　　　M21.029 Valgus deformity, not elsewhere classified, unspecified elbow ▽
　✓6ᵗʰ **M21.05** Valgus deformity, not elsewhere classified, hip
　　　M21.051 Valgus deformity, not elsewhere classified, right hip
　　　M21.052 Valgus deformity, not elsewhere classified, left hip
　　　M21.059 Valgus deformity, not elsewhere classified, unspecified hip ▽
　✓6ᵗʰ **M21.06** Valgus deformity, not elsewhere classified, knee
　　　　Genu valgumKnock knee
　　　M21.061 Valgus deformity, not elsewhere classified, right knee
　　　M21.062 Valgus deformity, not elsewhere classified, left knee
　　　M21.069 Valgus deformity, not elsewhere classified, unspecified knee ▽
　✓6ᵗʰ **M21.07** Valgus deformity, not elsewhere classified, ankle
　　　M21.071 Valgus deformity, not elsewhere classified, right ankle
　　　M21.072 Valgus deformity, not elsewhere classified, left ankle
　　　M21.079 Valgus deformity, not elsewhere classified, unspecified ankle ▽

✓5ᵗʰ **M21.1** Varus deformity, not elsewhere classified
　　EXCLUDES 1 metatarsus varus (Q66.2)
　　　tibia vara (M92.5)
　　　M21.10 Varus deformity, not elsewhere classified, unspecified site ▽
　✓6ᵗʰ **M21.12** Varus deformity, not elsewhere classified, elbow
　　　　Cubitus varus, elbow
　　　M21.121 Varus deformity, not elsewhere classified, right elbow
　　　M21.122 Varus deformity, not elsewhere classified, left elbow
　　　M21.129 Varus deformity, not elsewhere classified, unspecified elbow ▽
　✓6ᵗʰ **M21.15** Varus deformity, not elsewhere classified, hip
　　　M21.151 Varus deformity, not elsewhere classified, right hip
　　　M21.152 Varus deformity, not elsewhere classified, left hip
　　　M21.159 Varus deformity, not elsewhere classified, unspecified ▽

✓6ᵗʰ **M21.16** Varus deformity, not elsewhere classified, knee
　　　Bow leg
　　　Genu varum
　　　M21.161 Varus deformity, not elsewhere classified, right knee
　　　M21.162 Varus deformity, not elsewhere classified, left knee
　　　M21.169 Varus deformity, not elsewhere classified, unspecified knee ▽
✓6ᵗʰ **M21.17** Varus deformity, not elsewhere classified, ankle
　　　M21.171 Varus deformity, not elsewhere classified, right ankle
　　　M21.172 Varus deformity, not elsewhere classified, left ankle
　　　M21.179 Varus deformity, not elsewhere classified, unspecified ankle ▽

✓5ᵗʰ **M21.2** Flexion deformity
　　　M21.20 Flexion deformity, unspecified site ▽
　✓6ᵗʰ **M21.21** Flexion deformity, shoulder
　　　M21.211 Flexion deformity, right shoulder
　　　M21.212 Flexion deformity, left shoulder
　　　M21.219 Flexion deformity, unspecified shoulder ▽
　✓6ᵗʰ **M21.22** Flexion deformity, elbow
　　　M21.221 Flexion deformity, right elbow
　　　M21.222 Flexion deformity, left elbow
　　　M21.229 Flexion deformity, unspecified elbow ▽
　✓6ᵗʰ **M21.23** Flexion deformity, wrist
　　　M21.231 Flexion deformity, right wrist
　　　M21.232 Flexion deformity, left wrist
　　　M21.239 Flexion deformity, unspecified wrist ▽
　✓6ᵗʰ **M21.24** Flexion deformity, finger joints
　　　M21.241 Flexion deformity, right finger joints
　　　M21.242 Flexion deformity, left finger joints
　　　M21.249 Flexion deformity, unspecified finger joints ▽
　✓6ᵗʰ **M21.25** Flexion deformity, hip
　　　M21.251 Flexion deformity, right hip
　　　M21.252 Flexion deformity, left hip
　　　M21.259 Flexion deformity, unspecified hip ▽
　✓6ᵗʰ **M21.26** Flexion deformity, knee
　　　M21.261 Flexion deformity, right knee
　　　M21.262 Flexion deformity, left knee
　　　M21.269 Flexion deformity, unspecified knee ▽
　✓6ᵗʰ **M21.27** Flexion deformity, ankle and toes
　　　M21.271 Flexion deformity, right ankle and toes
　　　M21.272 Flexion deformity, left ankle and toes
　　　M21.279 Flexion deformity, unspecified ankle and toes ▽

✓5ᵗʰ **M21.3** Wrist or foot drop (acquired)
　✓6ᵗʰ **M21.33** Wrist drop (acquired)
　　　M21.331 Wrist drop, right wrist
　　　M21.332 Wrist drop, left wrist
　　　M21.339 Wrist drop, unspecified wrist ▽
　✓6ᵗʰ **M21.37** Foot drop (acquired)
　　　M21.371 Foot drop, right foot
　　　M21.372 Foot drop, left foot
　　　M21.379 Foot drop, unspecified foot ▽

✓5ᵗʰ **M21.4** Flat foot [pes planus] (acquired)
　　EXCLUDES 1 congenital pes planus (Q66.5-)
　　　M21.40 Flat foot [pes planus] (acquired), unspecified foot ▽
　　　M21.41 Flat foot [pes planus] (acquired), right foot
　　　M21.42 Flat foot [pes planus] (acquired), left foot

✓5ᵗʰ **M21.5** Acquired clawhand, clubhand, clawfoot and clubfoot
　　EXCLUDES 1 clubfoot, not specified as acquired (Q66.89)
　✓6ᵗʰ **M21.51** Acquired clawhand
　　　M21.511 Acquired clawhand, right hand
　　　M21.512 Acquired clawhand, left hand
　　　M21.519 Acquired clawhand, unspecified hand ▽

| N Newborn | P Pediatric | M Maternity | A Adult | RIC RIC Dx | NC Dx Noncancer Dx | PDx Primary Dx | CC RIC CC Condition | ►◄ Revised Text | ● New Code | ▲ Revised Code Title |

700　　ICD-10-CM 2016

✓6ᵗʰ **M21.52** **Acquired** clubhand
    M21.521 **Acquired clubhand,** right **hand**
    M21.522 **Acquired clubhand,** left **hand**
    M21.529 **Acquired clubhand, unspecified hand** ▽

✓6ᵗʰ **M21.53** **Acquired** clawfoot
    M21.531 **Acquired clawfoot,** right **foot**
    M21.532 **Acquired clawfoot,** left **foot**
    M21.539 **Acquired clawfoot, unspecified foot** ▽

✓6ᵗʰ **M21.54** **Acquired** clubfoot
    M21.541 **Acquired clubfoot,** right **foot**
    M21.542 **Acquired clubfoot,** left **foot**
    M21.549 **Acquired clubfoot, unspecified foot** ▽

✓5ᵗʰ **M21.6** Other **acquired deformities of foot**
    EXCLUDES 2 deformities of toe (acquired) (M20.1-M20.6)

✓6ᵗʰ **M21.6X** **Other acquired deformities of** foot
    M21.6X1 **Other acquired deformities of** right **foot**
    M21.6X2 **Other acquired deformities of** left **foot**
    M21.6X9 **Other acquired deformities of unspecified foot** ▽

✓5ᵗʰ **M21.7** Unequal limb length **(acquired)**
    NOTE The site used should correspond to the shorter limb.
    M21.70 **Unequal limb length (acquired), unspecified site** ▽

✓6ᵗʰ **M21.72** **Unequal limb length (acquired),** humerus
    M21.721 **Unequal limb length (acquired),** right **humerus**
    M21.722 **Unequal limb length (acquired),** left **humerus**
    M21.729 **Unequal limb length (acquired), unspecified humerus** ▽

✓6ᵗʰ **M21.73** **Unequal limb length (acquired),** ulna and radius
    M21.731 **Unequal limb length (acquired),** right ulna
    M21.732 **Unequal limb length (acquired),** left ulna
    M21.733 **Unequal limb length (acquired),** right radius
    M21.734 **Unequal limb length (acquired),** left radius
    M21.739 **Unequal limb length (acquired), unspecified ulna and radius** ▽

✓6ᵗʰ **M21.75** **Unequal limb length (acquired),** femur
    M21.751 **Unequal limb length (acquired),** right **femur**
    M21.752 **Unequal limb length (acquired),** left **femur**
    M21.759 **Unequal limb length (acquired), unspecified femur** ▽

✓6ᵗʰ **M21.76** **Unequal limb length (acquired),** tibia and fibula
    M21.761 **Unequal limb length (acquired),** right tibia
    M21.762 **Unequal limb length (acquired),** left tibia
    M21.763 **Unequal limb length (acquired),** right fibula
    M21.764 **Unequal limb length (acquired),** left fibula
    M21.769 **Unequal limb length (acquired), unspecified tibia and fibula** ▽

✓5ᵗʰ **M21.8** Other **specified acquired deformities of** limbs
    EXCLUDES 2 coxa plana (M91.2)

    M21.80 **Other specified acquired deformities of unspecified limb** ▽

✓6ᵗʰ **M21.82** **Other specified acquired deformities of** upper arm
    M21.821 **Other specified acquired deformities of** right **upper arm**
    M21.822 **Other specified acquired deformities of** left **upper arm**
    M21.829 **Other specified acquired deformities of unspecified upper arm** ▽

✓6ᵗʰ **M21.83** **Other specified acquired deformities of** forearm
    M21.831 **Other specified acquired deformities of** right **forearm**
    M21.832 **Other specified acquired deformities of** left **forearm**
    M21.839 **Other specified acquired deformities of unspecified forearm** ▽

✓6ᵗʰ **M21.85** **Other specified acquired deformities of** thigh
    M21.851 **Other specified acquired deformities of** right **thigh**
    M21.852 **Other specified acquired deformities of** left **thigh**

    M21.859 **Other specified acquired deformities of unspecified thigh** ▽

✓6ᵗʰ **M21.86** **Other specified acquired deformities of** lower leg
    M21.861 **Other specified acquired deformities of** right **lower leg**
    M21.862 **Other specified acquired deformities of** left **lower leg**
    M21.869 **Other specified acquired deformities of unspecified lower leg** ▽

✓5ᵗʰ **M21.9** **Unspecified acquired deformity of** limb and hand
    M21.90 **Unspecified acquired deformity of unspecified limb** ▽

✓6ᵗʰ **M21.92** **Unspecified acquired deformity of** upper arm
    M21.921 **Unspecified acquired deformity of** right **upper arm** ▽
    M21.922 **Unspecified acquired deformity of** left **upper arm** ▽
    M21.929 **Unspecified acquired deformity of unspecified upper arm** ▽

✓6ᵗʰ **M21.93** **Unspecified acquired deformity of** forearm
    M21.931 **Unspecified acquired deformity of** right **forearm** ▽
    M21.932 **Unspecified acquired deformity of** left **forearm** ▽
    M21.939 **Unspecified acquired deformity of unspecified forearm** ▽

✓6ᵗʰ **M21.94** **Unspecified acquired deformity of** hand
    M21.941 **Unspecified acquired deformity of hand,** right **hand** ▽
    M21.942 **Unspecified acquired deformity of hand,** left **hand** ▽
    M21.949 **Unspecified acquired deformity of hand, unspecified hand** ▽

✓6ᵗʰ **M21.95** **Unspecified acquired deformity of** thigh
    M21.951 **Unspecified acquired deformity of** right **thigh** ▽
    M21.952 **Unspecified acquired deformity of** left **thigh** ▽
    M21.959 **Unspecified acquired deformity of unspecified thigh** ▽

✓6ᵗʰ **M21.96** **Unspecified acquired deformity of** lower leg
    M21.961 **Unspecified acquired deformity of** right **lower leg** ▽
    M21.962 **Unspecified acquired deformity of** left **lower leg** ▽
    M21.969 **Unspecified acquired deformity of unspecified lower leg** ▽

✓4ᵗʰ **M22** **Disorder of patella**
    EXCLUDES 1 traumatic dislocation of patella (S83.0-)

✓5ᵗʰ **M22.0** Recurrent dislocation **of patella**
    M22.00 **Recurrent dislocation of patella, unspecified knee** ▽
    M22.01 **Recurrent dislocation of patella,** right **knee**
    M22.02 **Recurrent dislocation of patella,** left **knee**

✓5ᵗʰ **M22.1** Recurrent subluxation **of patella**
    Incomplete dislocation of patella
    M22.10 **Recurrent subluxation of patella, unspecified knee** ▽
    M22.11 **Recurrent subluxation of patella,** right **knee**
    M22.12 **Recurrent subluxation of patella,** left **knee**

✓5ᵗʰ **M22.2** Patellofemoral **disorders**

✓6ᵗʰ **M22.2X** **Patellofemoral disorders**
    M22.2X1 **Patellofemoral disorders,** right **knee**
    M22.2X2 **Patellofemoral disorders,** left **knee**
    M22.2X9 **Patellofemoral disorders, unspecified knee** ▽

✓5ᵗʰ **M22.3** Other derangements **of patella**

✓6ᵗʰ **M22.3X** **Other derangements of patella**
    M22.3X1 **Other derangements of patella,** right **knee**
    M22.3X2 **Other derangements of patella,** left **knee**
    M22.3X9 **Other derangements of patella, unspecified knee** ▽

Chapter 13. Diseases of the Musculoskeletal System and Connective Tissue

M21.52–M22.3X9

✓5ᵗʰ **M22.4** Chondromalacia **patellae**

    M22.40 Chondromalacia patellae, unspecified knee ▽

    M22.41 Chondromalacia patellae, right knee

    M22.42 Chondromalacia patellae, left knee

✓5ᵗʰ **M22.8** Other **disorders of patella**

    ✓6ᵗʰ **M22.8X** Other disorders of patella

      M22.8X1 Other disorders of patella, right knee

      M22.8X2 Other disorders of patella, left knee

      M22.8X9 Other disorders of patella, unspecified knee ▽

✓5ᵗʰ **M22.9** Unspecified **disorder of patella**

    M22.90 Unspecified disorder of patella, unspecified knee ▽

    M22.91 Unspecified disorder of patella, right knee ▽

    M22.92 Unspecified disorder of patella, left knee ▽

✓4ᵗʰ **M23** Internal **derangement of knee**

    EXCLUDES 1   ankylosis (M24.66)
                  current injury—see injury of knee and lower leg (S80-S89)
                  deformity of knee (M21.-)
                  osteochondritis dissecans (M93.2)
                  recurrent dislocation or subluxation of joints (M24.4)
                  recurrent dislocation or subluxation of patella (M22.0-M22.1)

  ✓5ᵗʰ **M23.0** Cystic **meniscus**

    ✓6ᵗʰ **M23.00** Cystic meniscus, unspecified meniscus

      Cystic meniscus, unspecified lateral meniscus
      Cystic meniscus, unspecified medial meniscus

      M23.000 Cystic meniscus, unspecified lateral meniscus, right knee

      M23.001 Cystic meniscus, unspecified lateral meniscus, left knee

      M23.002 Cystic meniscus, unspecified lateral meniscus, unspecified knee ▽

      M23.003 Cystic meniscus, unspecified medial meniscus, right knee

      M23.004 Cystic meniscus, unspecified medial meniscus, left knee

      M23.005 Cystic meniscus, unspecified medial meniscus, unspecified knee ▽

      M23.006 Cystic meniscus, unspecified meniscus, right knee

      M23.007 Cystic meniscus, unspecified meniscus, left knee

      M23.009 Cystic meniscus, unspecified meniscus, unspecified knee ▽

    ✓6ᵗʰ **M23.01** Cystic meniscus, anterior horn of medial meniscus

      M23.011 Cystic meniscus, anterior horn of medial meniscus, right knee

      M23.012 Cystic meniscus, anterior horn of medial meniscus, left knee

      M23.019 Cystic meniscus, anterior horn of medial meniscus, unspecified knee ▽

    ✓6ᵗʰ **M23.02** Cystic meniscus, posterior horn of medial meniscus

      M23.021 Cystic meniscus, posterior horn of medial meniscus, right knee

      M23.022 Cystic meniscus, posterior horn of medial meniscus, left knee

      M23.029 Cystic meniscus, posterior horn of medial meniscus, unspecified knee ▽

    ✓6ᵗʰ **M23.03** Cystic meniscus, other medial meniscus

      M23.031 Cystic meniscus, other medial meniscus, right knee

      M23.032 Cystic meniscus, other medial meniscus, left knee

      M23.039 Cystic meniscus, other medial meniscus, unspecified knee ▽

    ✓6ᵗʰ **M23.04** Cystic meniscus, anterior horn of lateral meniscus

      M23.041 Cystic meniscus, anterior horn of lateral meniscus, right knee

      M23.042 Cystic meniscus, anterior horn of lateral meniscus, left knee

      M23.049 Cystic meniscus, anterior horn of lateral meniscus, unspecified knee ▽

    ✓6ᵗʰ **M23.05** Cystic meniscus, posterior horn of lateral meniscus

      M23.051 Cystic meniscus, posterior horn of lateral meniscus, right knee

      M23.052 Cystic meniscus, posterior horn of lateral meniscus, left knee

      M23.059 Cystic meniscus, posterior horn of lateral meniscus, unspecified knee ▽

    ✓6ᵗʰ **M23.06** Cystic meniscus, other lateral meniscus

      M23.061 Cystic meniscus, other lateral meniscus, right knee

      M23.062 Cystic meniscus, other lateral meniscus, left knee

      M23.069 Cystic meniscus, other lateral meniscus, unspecified knee ▽

  ✓5ᵗʰ **M23.2** Derangement **of meniscus due to old tear or injury**

    Old bucket-handle tear

    ✓6ᵗʰ **M23.20** Derangement of unspecified meniscus due to old tear or injury

      Derangement of unspecified lateral meniscus due to old tear or injury
      Derangement of unspecified medial meniscus due to old tear or injury

      M23.200 Derangement of unspecified lateral meniscus due to old tear or injury, right knee

      M23.201 Derangement of unspecified lateral meniscus due to old tear or injury, left knee

      M23.202 Derangement of unspecified lateral meniscus due to old tear or injury, unspecified knee ▽

      M23.203 Derangement of unspecified medial meniscus due to old tear or injury, right knee

      M23.204 Derangement of unspecified medial meniscus due to old tear or injury, left knee

      M23.205 Derangement of unspecified medial meniscus due to old tear or injury, unspecified knee ▽

      M23.206 Derangement of unspecified meniscus due to old tear or injury, right knee

      M23.207 Derangement of unspecified meniscus due to old tear or injury, left knee

      M23.209 Derangement of unspecified meniscus due to old tear or injury, unspecified knee ▽

    ✓6ᵗʰ **M23.21** Derangement of anterior horn of medial meniscus due to old tear or injury

      M23.211 Derangement of anterior horn of medial meniscus due to old tear or injury, right knee

      M23.212 Derangement of anterior horn of medial meniscus due to old tear or injury, left knee

      M23.219 Derangement of anterior horn of medial meniscus due to old tear or injury, unspecified knee ▽

    ✓6ᵗʰ **M23.22** Derangement of posterior horn of medial meniscus due to old tear or injury

      M23.221 Derangement of posterior horn of medial meniscus due to old tear or injury, right knee

      M23.222 Derangement of posterior horn of medial meniscus due to old tear or injury, left knee

      M23.229 Derangement of posterior horn of medial meniscus due to old tear or injury, unspecified knee ▽

    ✓6ᵗʰ **M23.23** Derangement of other medial meniscus due to old tear or injury

      M23.231 Derangement of other medial meniscus due to old tear or injury, right knee

      M23.232 Derangement of other medial meniscus due to old tear or injury, left knee

      M23.239 Derangement of other medial meniscus due to old tear or injury, unspecified knee ▽

N Newborn   P Pediatric   M Maternity   A Adult   **RIC** RIC Dx   **NC Dx** Noncancer Dx   **PDx** Primary Dx   **CC** RIC CC Condition   ▶◀ Revised Text   ● New Code   ▲ Revised Code Title

702   ICD-10-CM 2016

✓6ᵗʰ **M23.24** **Derangement of** anterior horn of lateral **meniscus due to old tear or injury**

     M23.241 Derangement of anterior horn of lateral meniscus due to old tear or injury, right knee

     M23.242 Derangement of anterior horn of lateral meniscus due to old tear or injury, left knee

     M23.249 Derangement of anterior horn of lateral meniscus due to old tear or injury, unspecified knee ▽

✓6ᵗʰ **M23.25** **Derangement of** posterior horn of lateral **meniscus due to old tear or injury**

     M23.251 Derangement of posterior horn of lateral meniscus due to old tear or injury, right knee

     M23.252 Derangement of posterior horn of lateral meniscus due to old tear or injury, left knee

     M23.259 Derangement of posterior horn of lateral meniscus due to old tear or injury, unspecified knee ▽

✓6ᵗʰ **M23.26** **Derangement of** other lateral **meniscus due to old tear or injury**

     M23.261 Derangement of other lateral meniscus due to old tear or injury, right knee

     M23.262 Derangement of other lateral meniscus due to old tear or injury, left knee

     M23.269 Derangement of other lateral meniscus due to old tear or injury, unspecified knee ▽

✓5ᵗʰ **M23.3** **Other meniscus derangements**
     Degenerate meniscus
     Detached meniscus
     Retained meniscus

✓6ᵗʰ **M23.30** **Other meniscus derangements,** unspecified meniscus
     Other meniscus derangements, unspecified lateral meniscus
     Other meniscus derangements, unspecified medial meniscus

     M23.300 Other meniscus derangements, unspecified lateral meniscus, right knee ▽

     M23.301 Other meniscus derangements, unspecified lateral meniscus, left knee ▽

     M23.302 Other meniscus derangements, unspecified lateral meniscus, unspecified knee ▽

     M23.303 Other meniscus derangements, unspecified medial meniscus, right knee ▽

     M23.304 Other meniscus derangements, unspecified medial meniscus, left knee ▽

     M23.305 Other meniscus derangements, unspecified medial meniscus, unspecified knee ▽

     M23.306 Other meniscus derangements, unspecified meniscus, right knee ▽

     M23.307 Other meniscus derangements, unspecified meniscus, left knee ▽

     M23.309 Other meniscus derangements, unspecified meniscus, unspecified knee ▽

✓6ᵗʰ **M23.31** **Other meniscus derangements,** anterior horn of medial **meniscus**

     M23.311 Other meniscus derangements, anterior horn of medial meniscus, right knee

     M23.312 Other meniscus derangements, anterior horn of medial meniscus, left knee

     M23.319 Other meniscus derangements, anterior horn of medial meniscus, unspecified knee ▽

✓6ᵗʰ **M23.32** **Other meniscus derangements,** posterior horn of medial **meniscus**

     M23.321 Other meniscus derangements, posterior horn of medial meniscus, right knee

     M23.322 Other meniscus derangements, posterior horn of medial meniscus, left knee

     M23.329 Other meniscus derangements, posterior horn of medial meniscus, unspecified knee ▽

✓6ᵗʰ **M23.33** **Other meniscus derangements,** other medial **meniscus**

     M23.331 Other meniscus derangements, other medial meniscus, right knee

     M23.332 Other meniscus derangements, other medial meniscus, left knee

     M23.339 Other meniscus derangements, other medial meniscus, unspecified knee ▽

✓6ᵗʰ **M23.34** **Other meniscus derangements,** anterior horn of lateral **meniscus**

     M23.341 Other meniscus derangements, anterior horn of lateral meniscus, right knee

     M23.342 Other meniscus derangements, anterior horn of lateral meniscus, left knee

     M23.349 Other meniscus derangements, anterior horn of lateral meniscus, unspecified knee ▽

✓6ᵗʰ **M23.35** **Other meniscus derangements,** posterior horn of lateral **meniscus**

     M23.351 Other meniscus derangements, posterior horn of lateral meniscus, right knee

     M23.352 Other meniscus derangements, posterior horn of lateral meniscus, left knee

     M23.359 Other meniscus derangements, posterior horn of lateral meniscus, unspecified knee ▽

✓6ᵗʰ **M23.36** **Other meniscus derangements,** other lateral **meniscus**

     M23.361 Other meniscus derangements, other lateral meniscus, right knee

     M23.362 Other meniscus derangements, other lateral meniscus, left knee

     M23.369 Other meniscus derangements, other lateral meniscus, unspecified knee ▽

✓5ᵗʰ **M23.4** **Loose body in knee**

     M23.40 Loose body in knee, unspecified knee ▽

     M23.41 Loose body in knee, right knee

     M23.42 Loose body in knee, left knee

✓5ᵗʰ **M23.5** **Chronic instability of knee**

     M23.50 Chronic instability of knee, unspecified knee ▽

     M23.51 Chronic instability of knee, right knee

     M23.52 Chronic instability of knee, left knee

✓5ᵗʰ **M23.6** **Other spontaneous disruption of ligament(s) of knee**

✓6ᵗʰ **M23.60** **Other spontaneous disruption of** unspecified ligament **of knee**

     M23.601 Other spontaneous disruption of unspecified ligament of right knee ▽

     M23.602 Other spontaneous disruption of unspecified ligament of left knee ▽

     M23.609 Other spontaneous disruption of unspecified ligament of unspecified knee ▽

✓6ᵗʰ **M23.61** **Other spontaneous disruption of** anterior cruciate **ligament of knee**

     M23.611 Other spontaneous disruption of anterior cruciate ligament of right knee

     M23.612 Other spontaneous disruption of anterior cruciate ligament of left knee

     M23.619 Other spontaneous disruption of anterior cruciate ligament of unspecified knee ▽

✓6ᵗʰ **M23.62** **Other spontaneous disruption of** posterior cruciate **ligament of knee**

     M23.621 Other spontaneous disruption of posterior cruciate ligament of right knee

     M23.622 Other spontaneous disruption of posterior cruciate ligament of left knee

     M23.629 Other spontaneous disruption of posterior cruciate ligament of unspecified knee ▽

✓6ᵗʰ **M23.63** **Other spontaneous disruption of** medial collateral **ligament of knee**

     M23.631 Other spontaneous disruption of medial collateral ligament of right knee

     M23.632 Other spontaneous disruption of medial collateral ligament of left knee

☑ Add'l Character Required   ✓x7ᵗʰ Placeholder Alert   RUG IV Special Care High Dx   RUG IV Clinically Complex Dx   RUG IV Special Care Low Dx   Manifestation Code   Other Specified Code   ▽ Unspecified Code

ICD-10-CM 2016   **703**

M23.639 Other spontaneous disruption of medial collateral ligament of unspecified knee ▽

✓6th **M23.64** Other spontaneous disruption of lateral collateral ligament of knee

    M23.641 Other spontaneous disruption of lateral collateral ligament of right knee

    M23.642 Other spontaneous disruption of lateral collateral ligament of left knee

    M23.649 Other spontaneous disruption of lateral collateral ligament of unspecified knee ▽

✓6th **M23.67** Other spontaneous disruption of capsular ligament of knee

    M23.671 Other spontaneous disruption of capsular ligament of right knee

    M23.672 Other spontaneous disruption of capsular ligament of left knee

    M23.679 Other spontaneous disruption of capsular ligament of unspecified knee ▽

✓5th **M23.8** Other internal derangements of knee
    Laxity of ligament of knee
    Snapping knee

  ✓6th **M23.8X** Other internal derangements of knee

    M23.8X1 Other internal derangements of right knee

    M23.8X2 Other internal derangements of left knee

    M23.8X9 Other internal derangements of unspecified knee ▽

✓5th **M23.9** Unspecified internal derangement of knee

    M23.90 Unspecified internal derangement of unspecified knee ▽

    M23.91 Unspecified internal derangement of right knee ▽

    M23.92 Unspecified internal derangement of left knee ▽

✓4th **M24** Other specific joint derangements
    EXCLUDES 1 current injury—see injury of joint by body region
    EXCLUDES 2 ganglion (M67.4)
            snapping knee (M23.8-)
            temporomandibular joint disorders (M26.6-)

✓5th **M24.0** Loose body in joint
    EXCLUDES 2 loose body in knee (M23.4)

    M24.00 Loose body in unspecified joint ▽

  ✓6th **M24.01** Loose body in shoulder
    M24.011 Loose body in right shoulder
    M24.012 Loose body in left shoulder
    M24.019 Loose body in unspecified shoulder ▽

  ✓6th **M24.02** Loose body in elbow
    M24.021 Loose body in right elbow
    M24.022 Loose body in left elbow
    M24.029 Loose body in unspecified elbow ▽

  ✓6th **M24.03** Loose body in wrist
    M24.031 Loose body in right wrist
    M24.032 Loose body in left wrist
    M24.039 Loose body in unspecified wrist ▽

  ✓6th **M24.04** Loose body in finger joints
    M24.041 Loose body in right finger joint(s)
    M24.042 Loose body in left finger joint(s)
    M24.049 Loose body in unspecified finger joint(s) ▽

  ✓6th **M24.05** Loose body in hip
    M24.051 Loose body in right hip
    M24.052 Loose body in left hip
    M24.059 Loose body in unspecified hip ▽

  ✓6th **M24.07** Loose body in ankle and toe joints
    M24.071 Loose body in right ankle
    M24.072 Loose body in left ankle
    M24.073 Loose body in unspecified ankle ▽
    M24.074 Loose body in right toe joint(s)
    M24.075 Loose body in left toe joint(s)
    M24.076 Loose body in unspecified toe joints ▽

    M24.08 Loose body, other site

✓5th **M24.1** Other articular cartilage disorders
    EXCLUDES 2 chondrocalcinosis (M11.1, M11.2-)
            internal derangement of knee (M23.-)
            metastatic calcification (E83.5)
            ochronosis (E70.2)

    M24.10 Other articular cartilage disorders, unspecified site ▽

  ✓6th **M24.11** Other articular cartilage disorders, shoulder
    M24.111 Other articular cartilage disorders, right shoulder
    M24.112 Other articular cartilage disorders, left shoulder
    M24.119 Other articular cartilage disorders, unspecified shoulder ▽

  ✓6th **M24.12** Other articular cartilage disorders, elbow
    M24.121 Other articular cartilage disorders, right elbow
    M24.122 Other articular cartilage disorders, left elbow
    M24.129 Other articular cartilage disorders, unspecified elbow ▽

  ✓6th **M24.13** Other articular cartilage disorders, wrist
    M24.131 Other articular cartilage disorders, right wrist
    M24.132 Other articular cartilage disorders, left wrist
    M24.139 Other articular cartilage disorders, unspecified wrist ▽

  ✓6th **M24.14** Other articular cartilage disorders, hand
    M24.141 Other articular cartilage disorders, right hand
    M24.142 Other articular cartilage disorders, left hand
    M24.149 Other articular cartilage disorders, unspecified hand ▽

  ✓6th **M24.15** Other articular cartilage disorders, hip
    M24.151 Other articular cartilage disorders, right hip
    M24.152 Other articular cartilage disorders, left hip
    M24.159 Other articular cartilage disorders, unspecified hip ▽

  ✓6th **M24.17** Other articular cartilage disorders, ankle and foot
    M24.171 Other articular cartilage disorders, right ankle
    M24.172 Other articular cartilage disorders, left ankle
    M24.173 Other articular cartilage disorders, unspecified ankle ▽
    M24.174 Other articular cartilage disorders, right foot
    M24.175 Other articular cartilage disorders, left foot
    M24.176 Other articular cartilage disorders, unspecified foot ▽

✓5th **M24.2** Disorder of ligament
    Instability secondary to old ligament injury
    Ligamentous laxity NOS
    EXCLUDES 1 familial ligamentous laxity (M35.7)
    EXCLUDES 2 internal derangement of knee (M23.5-M23.89)

    M24.20 Disorder of ligament, unspecified site ▽

  ✓6th **M24.21** Disorder of ligament, shoulder
    M24.211 Disorder of ligament, right shoulder
    M24.212 Disorder of ligament, left shoulder
    M24.219 Disorder of ligament, unspecified shoulder ▽

  ✓6th **M24.22** Disorder of ligament, elbow
    M24.221 Disorder of ligament, right elbow
    M24.222 Disorder of ligament, left elbow
    M24.229 Disorder of ligament, unspecified elbow ▽

  ✓6th **M24.23** Disorder of ligament, wrist
    M24.231 Disorder of ligament, right wrist
    M24.232 Disorder of ligament, left wrist
    M24.239 Disorder of ligament, unspecified wrist ▽

Ⓝ Newborn   Ⓟ Pediatric   Ⓜ Maternity   Ⓐ Adult   **RIC** RIC Dx   **NCDx** Noncancer Dx   **PDx** Primary Dx   **CC** RIC CC Condition   ►◄ Revised Text   ● New Code   ▲ Revised Code Title

704   ICD-10-CM 2016

✓6ᵗʰ **M24.24 Disorder of ligament, hand**
     M24.241 Disorder of ligament, right hand
     M24.242 Disorder of ligament, left hand
     M24.249 Disorder of ligament, unspecified ▽
           hand

✓6ᵗʰ **M24.25 Disorder of ligament, hip**
     M24.251 Disorder of ligament, right hip
     M24.252 Disorder of ligament, left hip
     M24.259 Disorder of ligament, unspecified hip ▽

✓6ᵗʰ **M24.27 Disorder of ligament, ankle and foot**
     M24.271 Disorder of ligament, right ankle
     M24.272 Disorder of ligament, left ankle
     M24.273 Disorder of ligament, unspecified ▽
           ankle
     M24.274 Disorder of ligament, right foot
     M24.275 Disorder of ligament, left foot
     M24.276 Disorder of ligament, unspecified ▽
           foot

     M24.28 Disorder of ligament, vertebrae

✓5ᵗʰ **M24.3 Pathological dislocation of joint, not elsewhere classified**
     EXCLUDES 1 congenital dislocation or displacement of joint—see
           congenital malformations and deformations of
           the musculoskeletal system (Q65-Q79)
           current injury—see injury of joints and ligaments by
           body region
           recurrent dislocation of joint (M24.4-)
     M24.30 Pathological dislocation of unspecified joint, ▽
           not elsewhere classified

✓6ᵗʰ **M24.31 Pathological dislocation of shoulder, not
elsewhere classified**
     M24.311 Pathological dislocation of right
           shoulder, not elsewhere classified
     M24.312 Pathological dislocation of left
           shoulder, not elsewhere classified
     M24.319 Pathological dislocation of unspecified ▽
           shoulder, not elsewhere classified

✓6ᵗʰ **M24.32 Pathological dislocation of elbow, not elsewhere
classified**
     M24.321 Pathological dislocation of right elbow,
           not elsewhere classified
     M24.322 Pathological dislocation of left elbow,
           not elsewhere classified
     M24.329 Pathological dislocation of unspecified ▽
           elbow, not elsewhere classified

✓6ᵗʰ **M24.33 Pathological dislocation of wrist, not elsewhere
classified**
     M24.331 Pathological dislocation of right wrist,
           not elsewhere classified
     M24.332 Pathological dislocation of left wrist,
           not elsewhere classified
     M24.339 Pathological dislocation of unspecified ▽
           wrist, not elsewhere classified

✓6ᵗʰ **M24.34 Pathological dislocation of hand, not elsewhere
classified**
     M24.341 Pathological dislocation of right hand,
           not elsewhere classified
     M24.342 Pathological dislocation of left hand,
           not elsewhere classified
     M24.349 Pathological dislocation of unspecified ▽
           hand, not elsewhere classified

✓6ᵗʰ **M24.35 Pathological dislocation of hip, not elsewhere
classified**
     M24.351 Pathological dislocation of right hip,
           not elsewhere classified
     M24.352 Pathological dislocation of left hip,
           not elsewhere classified
     M24.359 Pathological dislocation of unspecified ▽
           hip, not elsewhere classified

✓6ᵗʰ **M24.36 Pathological dislocation of knee, not elsewhere
classified**
     M24.361 Pathological dislocation of right knee,
           not elsewhere classified
     M24.362 Pathological dislocation of left knee,
           not elsewhere classified
     M24.369 Pathological dislocation of unspecified ▽
           knee, not elsewhere classified

✓6ᵗʰ **M24.37 Pathological dislocation of ankle and foot, not
elsewhere classified**
     M24.371 Pathological dislocation of right ankle,
           not elsewhere classified
     M24.372 Pathological dislocation of left ankle,
           not elsewhere classified
     M24.373 Pathological dislocation of unspecified ▽
           ankle, not elsewhere classified
     M24.374 Pathological dislocation of right foot,
           not elsewhere classified
     M24.375 Pathological dislocation of left foot,
           not elsewhere classified
     M24.376 Pathological dislocation of unspecified ▽
           foot, not elsewhere classified

✓5ᵗʰ **M24.4 Recurrent dislocation of joint**
     Recurrent subluxation of joint
     EXCLUDES 2 recurrent dislocation of patella (M22.0-M22.1)
           recurrent vertebral dislocation (M43.3-, M43.4, M43.5-)
     M24.40 Recurrent dislocation, unspecified joint ▽

✓6ᵗʰ **M24.41 Recurrent dislocation, shoulder**
     M24.411 Recurrent dislocation, right shoulder
     M24.412 Recurrent dislocation, left shoulder
     M24.419 Recurrent dislocation, unspecified ▽
           shoulder

✓6ᵗʰ **M24.42 Recurrent dislocation, elbow**
     M24.421 Recurrent dislocation, right elbow
     M24.422 Recurrent dislocation, left elbow
     M24.429 Recurrent dislocation, unspecified ▽
           elbow

✓6ᵗʰ **M24.43 Recurrent dislocation, wrist**
     M24.431 Recurrent dislocation, right wrist
     M24.432 Recurrent dislocation, left wrist
     M24.439 Recurrent dislocation, unspecified ▽
           wrist

✓6ᵗʰ **M24.44 Recurrent dislocation, hand and finger(s)**
     M24.441 Recurrent dislocation, right hand
     M24.442 Recurrent dislocation, left hand
     M24.443 Recurrent dislocation, unspecified ▽
           hand
     M24.444 Recurrent dislocation, right finger
     M24.445 Recurrent dislocation, left finger
     M24.446 Recurrent dislocation, unspecified ▽
           finger

✓6ᵗʰ **M24.45 Recurrent dislocation, hip**
     M24.451 Recurrent dislocation, right hip
     M24.452 Recurrent dislocation, left hip
     M24.459 Recurrent dislocation, unspecified hip ▽

✓6ᵗʰ **M24.46 Recurrent dislocation, knee**
     M24.461 Recurrent dislocation, right knee
     M24.462 Recurrent dislocation, left knee
     M24.469 Recurrent dislocation, unspecified ▽
           knee

✓6ᵗʰ **M24.47 Recurrent dislocation, ankle, foot and toes**
     M24.471 Recurrent dislocation, right ankle
     M24.472 Recurrent dislocation, left ankle
     M24.473 Recurrent dislocation, unspecified ▽
           ankle
     M24.474 Recurrent dislocation, right foot
     M24.475 Recurrent dislocation, left foot
     M24.476 Recurrent dislocation, unspecified ▽
           foot
     M24.477 Recurrent dislocation, right toe(s)
     M24.478 Recurrent dislocation, left toe(s)
     M24.479 Recurrent dislocation, unspecified ▽
           toe(s)

☑ Add'l Character Required   ✓7ᵗʰ Placeholder Alert   RUG IV Special Care High Dx   RUG IV Clinically Complex Dx   RUG IV Special Care Low Dx   Manifestation Code   Other Specified Code   ▽ Unspecified Code

✓5ᵗʰ M24.5 Contracture of joint
    EXCLUDES 1   *contracture of muscle without contracture of joint (M62.4-)*
            contracture of tendon (sheath) without contracture of joint (M62.4-)
            Dupuytren's contracture (M72.0)
    EXCLUDES 2   *acquired deformities of limbs (M20-M21)*

     M24.50   Contracture, unspecified joint ▽

    ✓6ᵗʰ M24.51   Contracture, shoulder
        M24.511   Contracture, right shoulder
        M24.512   Contracture, left shoulder
        M24.519   Contracture, unspecified shoulder

    ✓6ᵗʰ M24.52   Contracture, elbow
        M24.521   Contracture, right elbow
        M24.522   Contracture, left elbow
        M24.529   Contracture, unspecified elbow ▽

    ✓6ᵗʰ M24.53   Contracture, wrist
        M24.531   Contracture, right wrist
        M24.532   Contracture, left wrist
        M24.539   Contracture, unspecified wrist ▽

    ✓6ᵗʰ M24.54   Contracture, hand
        M24.541   Contracture, right hand
        M24.542   Contracture, left hand
        M24.549   Contracture, unspecified hand ▽

    ✓6ᵗʰ M24.55   Contracture, hip
        M24.551   Contracture, right hip
        M24.552   Contracture, left hip
        M24.559   Contracture, unspecified hip ▽

    ✓6ᵗʰ M24.56   Contracture, knee
        M24.561   Contracture, right knee
        M24.562   Contracture, left knee
        M24.569   Contracture, unspecified knee ▽

    ✓6ᵗʰ M24.57   Contracture, ankle and foot
        M24.571   Contracture, right ankle
        M24.572   Contracture, left ankle
        M24.573   Contracture, unspecified ankle ▽
        M24.574   Contracture, right foot
        M24.575   Contracture, left foot
        M24.576   Contracture, unspecified foot ▽

✓5ᵗʰ M24.6 Ankylosis of joint
    EXCLUDES 1   *stiffness of joint without ankylosis (M25.6-)*
    EXCLUDES 2   *spine (M43.2-)*

     M24.60   Ankylosis, unspecified joint ▽

    ✓6ᵗʰ M24.61   Ankylosis, shoulder
        M24.611   Ankylosis, right shoulder
        M24.612   Ankylosis, left shoulder
        M24.619   Ankylosis, unspecified shoulder ▽

    ✓6ᵗʰ M24.62   Ankylosis, elbow
        M24.621   Ankylosis, right elbow
        M24.622   Ankylosis, left elbow
        M24.629   Ankylosis, unspecified elbow ▽

    ✓6ᵗʰ M24.63   Ankylosis, wrist
        M24.631   Ankylosis, right wrist
        M24.632   Ankylosis, left wrist
        M24.639   Ankylosis, unspecified wrist ▽

    ✓6ᵗʰ M24.64   Ankylosis, hand
        M24.641   Ankylosis, right hand
        M24.642   Ankylosis, left hand
        M24.649   Ankylosis, unspecified hand ▽

    ✓6ᵗʰ M24.65   Ankylosis, hip
        M24.651   Ankylosis, right hip
        M24.652   Ankylosis, left hip
        M24.659   Ankylosis, unspecified hip ▽

    ✓6ᵗʰ M24.66   Ankylosis, knee
        M24.661   Ankylosis, right knee
        M24.662   Ankylosis, left knee
        M24.669   Ankylosis, unspecified knee ▽

    ✓6ᵗʰ M24.67   Ankylosis, ankle and foot
        M24.671   Ankylosis, right ankle
        M24.672   Ankylosis, left ankle
        M24.673   Ankylosis, unspecified ankle ▽
        M24.674   Ankylosis, right foot

        M24.675   Ankylosis, left foot
        M24.676   Ankylosis, unspecified foot ▽

M24.7 Protrusio acetabuli

✓5ᵗʰ M24.8 Other specific joint derangements, not elsewhere classified
    EXCLUDES 2   *iliotibial band syndrome (M76.3)*

     M24.80   Other specific joint derangements of unspecified joint, not elsewhere classified

    ✓6ᵗʰ M24.81   Other specific joint derangements of shoulder, not elsewhere classified
        M24.811   Other specific joint derangements of right shoulder, not elsewhere classified
        M24.812   Other specific joint derangements of left shoulder, not elsewhere classified
        M24.819   Other specific joint derangements of unspecified shoulder, not elsewhere classified ▽

    ✓6ᵗʰ M24.82   Other specific joint derangements of elbow, not elsewhere classified
        M24.821   Other specific joint derangements of right elbow, not elsewhere classified
        M24.822   Other specific joint derangements of left elbow, not elsewhere classified
        M24.829   Other specific joint derangements of unspecified elbow, not elsewhere classified ▽

    ✓6ᵗʰ M24.83   Other specific joint derangements of wrist, not elsewhere classified
        M24.831   Other specific joint derangements of right wrist, not elsewhere classified
        M24.832   Other specific joint derangements of left wrist, not elsewhere classified
        M24.839   Other specific joint derangements of unspecified wrist, not elsewhere classified ▽

    ✓6ᵗʰ M24.84   Other specific joint derangements of hand, not elsewhere classified
        M24.841   Other specific joint derangements of right hand, not elsewhere classified
        M24.842   Other specific joint derangements of left hand, not elsewhere classified
        M24.849   Other specific joint derangements of unspecified hand, not elsewhere classified ▽

    ✓6ᵗʰ M24.85   Other specific joint derangements of hip, not elsewhere classified
        Irritable hip
        M24.851   Other specific joint derangements of right hip, not elsewhere classified
        M24.852   Other specific joint derangements of left hip, not elsewhere classified
        M24.859   Other specific joint derangements of unspecified hip, not elsewhere classified ▽

    ✓6ᵗʰ M24.87   Other specific joint derangements of ankle and foot, not elsewhere classified
        M24.871   Other specific joint derangements of right ankle, not elsewhere classified
        M24.872   Other specific joint derangements of left ankle, not elsewhere classified
        M24.873   Other specific joint derangements of unspecified ankle, not elsewhere classified ▽
        M24.874   Other specific joint derangements of right foot, not elsewhere classified
        M24.875   Other specific joint derangements left foot, not elsewhere classified
        M24.876   Other specific joint derangements of unspecified foot, not elsewhere classified ▽

M24.9 Joint derangement, unspecified ▽

Ⓝ Newborn   Ⓟ Pediatric   Ⓜ Maternity   Ⓐ Adult   RIC RIC Dx   NC Dx Noncancer Dx   PDx Primary Dx   CC RIC CC Condition   ▶◀ Revised Text   ● New Code   ▲ Revised Code Title

706   ICD-10-CM 2016

☑️4ᵗʰ **M25 Other joint disorder, not elsewhere classified**

     EXCLUDES 2   *abnormality of gait and mobility (R26.-)*
                acquired deformities of limb (M20-M21)
                calcification of bursa (M71.4-)
                calcification of shoulder (joint) (M75.3)
                calcification of tendon (M65.2-)
                difficulty in walking (R26.2)
                temporomandibular joint disorder (M26.6-)

☑️5ᵗʰ   **M25.0 Hemarthrosis**

     EXCLUDES 1   *current injury—see injury of joint by body region*
                hemophilic arthropathy (M36.2)

     M25.00 Hemarthrosis, unspecified joint ▽

     ☑️6ᵗʰ   **M25.01 Hemarthrosis,** shoulder
         M25.011 Hemarthrosis, right shoulder
         M25.012 Hemarthrosis, left shoulder
         M25.019 Hemarthrosis, unspecified shoulder ▽

     ☑️6ᵗʰ   **M25.02 Hemarthrosis,** elbow
         M25.021 Hemarthrosis, right elbow
         M25.022 Hemarthrosis, left elbow
         M25.029 Hemarthrosis, unspecified elbow ▽

     ☑️6ᵗʰ   **M25.03 Hemarthrosis,** wrist
         M25.031 Hemarthrosis, right wrist
         M25.032 Hemarthrosis, left wrist
         M25.039 Hemarthrosis, unspecified wrist ▽

     ☑️6ᵗʰ   **M25.04 Hemarthrosis,** hand
         M25.041 Hemarthrosis, right hand
         M25.042 Hemarthrosis, left hand
         M25.049 Hemarthrosis, unspecified hand ▽

     ☑️6ᵗʰ   **M25.05 Hemarthrosis,** hip
         M25.051 Hemarthrosis, right hip
         M25.052 Hemarthrosis, left hip
         M25.059 Hemarthrosis, unspecified hip ▽

     ☑️6ᵗʰ   **M25.06 Hemarthrosis,** knee
         M25.061 Hemarthrosis, right knee
         M25.062 Hemarthrosis, left knee
         M25.069 Hemarthrosis, unspecified knee ▽

     ☑️6ᵗʰ   **M25.07 Hemarthrosis,** ankle and foot
         M25.071 Hemarthrosis, right ankle
         M25.072 Hemarthrosis, left ankle
         M25.073 Hemarthrosis, unspecified ankle ▽
         M25.074 Hemarthrosis, right foot
         M25.075 Hemarthrosis, left foot
         M25.076 Hemarthrosis, unspecified foot ▽

     M25.08 Hemarthrosis, other specified site
         Hemarthrosis, vertebrae

☑️5ᵗʰ   **M25.1 Fistula of joint**

     M25.10 Fistula, unspecified joint ▽

     ☑️6ᵗʰ   **M25.11 Fistula,** shoulder
         M25.111 Fistula, right shoulder
         M25.112 Fistula, left shoulder
         M25.119 Fistula, unspecified shoulder ▽

     ☑️6ᵗʰ   **M25.12 Fistula,** elbow
         M25.121 Fistula, right elbow
         M25.122 Fistula, left elbow
         M25.129 Fistula, unspecified elbow ▽

     ☑️6ᵗʰ   **M25.13 Fistula,** wrist
         M25.131 Fistula, right wrist
         M25.132 Fistula, left wrist
         M25.139 Fistula, unspecified wrist ▽

     ☑️6ᵗʰ   **M25.14 Fistula,** hand
         M25.141 Fistula, right hand
         M25.142 Fistula, left hand
         M25.149 Fistula, unspecified hand ▽

     ☑️6ᵗʰ   **M25.15 Fistula,** hip
         M25.151 Fistula, right hip
         M25.152 Fistula, left hip
         M25.159 Fistula, unspecified hip ▽

     ☑️6ᵗʰ   **M25.16 Fistula,** knee
         M25.161 Fistula, right knee
         M25.162 Fistula, left knee
         M25.169 Fistula, unspecified knee ▽

     ☑️6ᵗʰ   **M25.17 Fistula,** ankle and foot
         M25.171 Fistula, right ankle
         M25.172 Fistula, left ankle
         M25.173 Fistula, unspecified ankle ▽
         M25.174 Fistula, right foot
         M25.175 Fistula, left foot
         M25.176 Fistula, unspecified foot ▽

     M25.18 Fistula, other specified site
         Fistula, vertebrae

☑️5ᵗʰ   **M25.2 Flail joint**

     M25.20 Flail joint, unspecified joint ▽

     ☑️6ᵗʰ   **M25.21 Flail joint,** shoulder
         M25.211 Flail joint, right shoulder
         M25.212 Flail joint, left shoulder
         M25.219 Flail joint, unspecified shoulder ▽

     ☑️6ᵗʰ   **M25.22 Flail joint,** elbow
         M25.221 Flail joint, right elbow
         M25.222 Flail joint, left elbow
         M25.229 Flail joint, unspecified elbow ▽

     ☑️6ᵗʰ   **M25.23 Flail joint,** wrist
         M25.231 Flail joint, right wrist
         M25.232 Flail joint, left wrist
         M25.239 Flail joint, unspecified wrist ▽

     ☑️6ᵗʰ   **M25.24 Flail joint,** hand
         M25.241 Flail joint, right hand
         M25.242 Flail joint, left hand
         M25.249 Flail joint, unspecified hand ▽

     ☑️6ᵗʰ   **M25.25 Flail joint,** hip
         M25.251 Flail joint, right hip
         M25.252 Flail joint, left hip
         M25.259 Flail joint, unspecified hip ▽

     ☑️6ᵗʰ   **M25.26 Flail joint,** knee
         M25.261 Flail joint, right knee
         M25.262 Flail joint, left knee
         M25.269 Flail joint, unspecified knee ▽

     ☑️6ᵗʰ   **M25.27 Flail joint,** ankle and foot
         M25.271 Flail joint, right ankle and foot
         M25.272 Flail joint, left ankle and foot
         M25.279 Flail joint, unspecified ankle and foot ▽

     M25.28 Flail joint, other site

☑️5ᵗʰ   **M25.3 Other instability of joint**

     EXCLUDES 1   *instability of joint secondary to old ligament injury*
                (M24.2-)
                instability of joint secondary to removal of joint
                prosthesis (M96.8-)
     EXCLUDES 2   *spinal instabilities (M53.2-)*

     M25.30 Other instability, unspecified joint ▽

     ☑️6ᵗʰ   **M25.31 Other instability,** shoulder
         M25.311 Other instability, right shoulder
         M25.312 Other instability, left shoulder
         M25.319 Other instability, unspecified shoulder ▽

     ☑️6ᵗʰ   **M25.32 Other instability,** elbow
         M25.321 Other instability, right elbow
         M25.322 Other instability, left elbow
         M25.329 Other instability, unspecified elbow ▽

     ☑️6ᵗʰ   **M25.33 Other instability,** wrist
         M25.331 Other instability, right wrist
         M25.332 Other instability, left wrist
         M25.339 Other instability, unspecified wrist ▽

     ☑️6ᵗʰ   **M25.34 Other instability,** hand
         M25.341 Other instability, right hand
         M25.342 Other instability, left hand
         M25.349 Other instability, unspecified hand ▽

     ☑️6ᵗʰ   **M25.35 Other instability,** hip
         M25.351 Other instability, right hip
         M25.352 Other instability, left hip
         M25.359 Other instability, unspecified hip ▽

     ☑️6ᵗʰ   **M25.36 Other instability,** knee
         M25.361 Other instability, right knee
         M25.362 Other instability, left knee
         M25.369 Other instability, unspecified knee ▽

☑️ Add'l Character Required   ✗x7ᵗʰ Placeholder Alert   RUG IV Special Care High Dx   RUG IV Clinically Complex Dx   RUG IV Special Care Low Dx   Manifestation Code   Other Specified Code   ▽Unspecified Code

ICD-10-CM 2016   707

✓6ᵗʰ **M25.37** **Other instability,** ankle and foot
- **M25.371** **Other instability,** right ankle
- **M25.372** **Other instability,** left ankle
- **M25.373** **Other instability, unspecified ankle**
- **M25.374** **Other instability,** right foot
- **M25.375** **Other instability,** left foot
- **M25.376** **Other instability, unspecified foot** ▽

✓5ᵗʰ **M25.4** **Effusion of joint**
> EXCLUDES 1   hydrarthrosis in yaws (A66.6)
> intermittent hydrarthrosis (M12.4-)
> other infective (teno)synovitis (M65.1-)

- **M25.40** **Effusion, unspecified joint** ▽
- ✓6ᵗʰ **M25.41** **Effusion,** shoulder
  - **M25.411** **Effusion,** right shoulder
  - **M25.412** **Effusion,** left shoulder
  - **M25.419** **Effusion, unspecified shoulder** ▽
- ✓6ᵗʰ **M25.42** **Effusion,** elbow
  - **M25.421** **Effusion,** right elbow
  - **M25.422** **Effusion,** left elbow
  - **M25.429** **Effusion, unspecified elbow** ▽
- ✓6ᵗʰ **M25.43** **Effusion,** wrist
  - **M25.431** **Effusion,** right wrist
  - **M25.432** **Effusion,** left wrist
  - **M25.439** **Effusion, unspecified wrist** ▽
- ✓6ᵗʰ **M25.44** **Effusion,** hand
  - **M25.441** **Effusion,** right hand
  - **M25.442** **Effusion,** left hand
  - **M25.449** **Effusion, unspecified hand** ▽
- ✓6ᵗʰ **M25.45** **Effusion,** hip
  - **M25.451** **Effusion,** right hip
  - **M25.452** **Effusion,** left hip
  - **M25.459** **Effusion, unspecified hip** ▽
- ✓6ᵗʰ **M25.46** **Effusion,** knee
  - **M25.461** **Effusion,** right knee
  - **M25.462** **Effusion,** left knee
  - **M25.469** **Effusion, unspecified knee** ▽
- ✓6ᵗʰ **M25.47** **Effusion,** ankle and foot
  - **M25.471** **Effusion,** right ankle
  - **M25.472** **Effusion,** left ankle
  - **M25.473** **Effusion, unspecified ankle** ▽
  - **M25.474** **Effusion,** right foot
  - **M25.475** **Effusion,** left foot
  - **M25.476** **Effusion, unspecified foot** ▽
- **M25.48** **Effusion, other site**

✓5ᵗʰ **M25.5** **Pain in joint**
> EXCLUDES 2   pain in hand (M79.64-)
> pain in fingers (M79.64-)
> pain in foot (M79.67-)
> pain in limb (M79.6-)
> pain in toes (M79.67-)

- **M25.50** **Pain in unspecified joint** ▽
- ✓6ᵗʰ **M25.51** **Pain in** shoulder
  - **M25.511** **Pain in** right shoulder
  - **M25.512** **Pain in** left shoulder
  - **M25.519** **Pain in unspecified shoulder** ▽
- ✓6ᵗʰ **M25.52** **Pain in** elbow
  - **M25.521** **Pain in** right elbow
  - **M25.522** **Pain in** left elbow
  - **M25.529** **Pain in unspecified elbow** ▽
- ✓6ᵗʰ **M25.53** **Pain in** wrist
  - **M25.531** **Pain in** right wrist
  - **M25.532** **Pain in** left wrist
  - **M25.539** **Pain in unspecified wrist** ▽
- ✓6ᵗʰ **M25.55** **Pain in** hip
  - **M25.551** **Pain in** right hip
  - **M25.552** **Pain in** left hip
  - **M25.559** **Pain in unspecified hip** ▽
- ✓6ᵗʰ **M25.56** **Pain in** knee
  - **M25.561** **Pain in** right knee
  - **M25.562** **Pain in** left knee
  - **M25.569** **Pain in unspecified knee** ▽

✓6ᵗʰ **M25.57** **Pain in** ankle and joints of foot
- **M25.571** **Pain in** right ankle and joints of right foot
- **M25.572** **Pain in** left ankle and joints of left foot
- **M25.579** **Pain in unspecified ankle and joints of unspecified foot** ▽

✓5ᵗʰ **M25.6** **Stiffness of joint, not elsewhere classified**
> EXCLUDES 1   ankylosis of joint (M24.6-)
> contracture of joint (M24.5-)

- **M25.60** **Stiffness of unspecified joint, not elsewhere classified** ▽
- ✓6ᵗʰ **M25.61** **Stiffness of** shoulder, **not elsewhere classified**
  - **M25.611** **Stiffness of** right shoulder, **not elsewhere classified**
  - **M25.612** **Stiffness of** left shoulder, **not elsewhere classified**
  - **M25.619** **Stiffness of unspecified shoulder, not elsewhere classified** ▽
- ✓6ᵗʰ **M25.62** **Stiffness of** elbow, **not elsewhere classified**
  - **M25.621** **Stiffness of** right elbow, **not elsewhere classified**
  - **M25.622** **Stiffness of** left elbow, **not elsewhere classified**
  - **M25.629** **Stiffness of unspecified elbow, not elsewhere classified** ▽
- ✓6ᵗʰ **M25.63** **Stiffness of** wrist, **not elsewhere classified**
  - **M25.631** **Stiffness of** right wrist, **not elsewhere classified**
  - **M25.632** **Stiffness of** left wrist, **not elsewhere classified**
  - **M25.639** **Stiffness of unspecified wrist, not elsewhere classified** ▽
- ✓6ᵗʰ **M25.64** **Stiffness of** hand, **not elsewhere classified**
  - **M25.641** **Stiffness of** right hand, **not elsewhere classified**
  - **M25.642** **Stiffness of** left hand, **not elsewhere classified**
  - **M25.649** **Stiffness of unspecified hand, not elsewhere classified** ▽
- ✓6ᵗʰ **M25.65** **Stiffness of** hip, **not elsewhere classified**
  - **M25.651** **Stiffness of** right hip, **not elsewhere classified**
  - **M25.652** **Stiffness of** left hip, **not elsewhere classified**
  - **M25.659** **Stiffness of unspecified hip, not elsewhere classified** ▽
- ✓6ᵗʰ **M25.66** **Stiffness of** knee, **not elsewhere classified**
  - **M25.661** **Stiffness of** right knee, **not elsewhere classified**
  - **M25.662** **Stiffness of** left knee, **not elsewhere classified**
  - **M25.669** **Stiffness of unspecified knee, not elsewhere classified** ▽
- ✓6ᵗʰ **M25.67** **Stiffness of** ankle and foot, **not elsewhere classified**
  - **M25.671** **Stiffness of** right ankle, **not elsewhere classified**
  - **M25.672** **Stiffness of** left ankle, **not elsewhere classified**
  - **M25.673** **Stiffness of unspecified ankle, not elsewhere classified** ▽
  - **M25.674** **Stiffness of** right foot, **not elsewhere classified**
  - **M25.675** **Stiffness of** left foot, **not elsewhere classified**
  - **M25.676** **Stiffness of unspecified foot, not elsewhere classified** ▽

✓5ᵗʰ **M25.7** **Osteophyte**
- **M25.70** **Osteophyte, unspecified joint** ▽
- ✓6ᵗʰ **M25.71** **Osteophyte,** shoulder
  - **M25.711** **Osteophyte,** right shoulder
  - **M25.712** **Osteophyte,** left shoulder
  - **M25.719** **Osteophyte, unspecified shoulder** ▽
- ✓6ᵗʰ **M25.72** **Osteophyte,** elbow
  - **M25.721** **Osteophyte,** right elbow
  - **M25.722** **Osteophyte,** left elbow
  - **M25.729** **Osteophyte, unspecified elbow** ▽

Ⓝ Newborn   Ⓟ Pediatric   Ⓜ Maternity   Ⓐ Adult   **RIC** RIC Dx   **NC Dx** Noncancer Dx   **PDx** Primary Dx   **CC** RIC CC Condition   ►◄ Revised Text   ● New Code   ▲ Revised Code Title

708   ICD-10-CM 2016

√6th **M25.73 Osteophyte,** wrist
    M25.731 Osteophyte, right wrist
    M25.732 Osteophyte, left wrist
    M25.739 Osteophyte, unspecified wrist ▽

√6th **M25.74 Osteophyte,** hand
    M25.741 Osteophyte, right hand
    M25.742 Osteophyte, left hand
    M25.749 Osteophyte, unspecified hand ▽

√6th **M25.75 Osteophyte,** hip
    M25.751 Osteophyte, right hip
    M25.752 Osteophyte, left hip
    M25.759 Osteophyte, unspecified hip ▽

√6th **M25.76 Osteophyte,** knee
    M25.761 Osteophyte, right knee
    M25.762 Osteophyte, left knee
    M25.769 Osteophyte, unspecified knee ▽

√6th **M25.77 Osteophyte,** ankle and foot
    M25.771 Osteophyte, right ankle
    M25.772 Osteophyte, left ankle
    M25.773 Osteophyte, unspecified ankle ▽
    M25.774 Osteophyte, right foot
    M25.775 Osteophyte, left foot
    M25.776 Osteophyte, unspecified foot ▽
    M25.78 Osteophyte, vertebrae

√5th **M25.8 Other specified joint disorders**
    M25.80 **Other specified joint disorders, unspecified joint** ▽

√6th **M25.81 Other specified joint disorders,** shoulder
    M25.811 **Other specified joint disorders, right shoulder**
    M25.812 **Other specified joint disorders, left shoulder**
    M25.819 **Other specified joint disorders, unspecified shoulder** ▽

√6th **M25.82 Other specified joint disorders,** elbow
    M25.821 **Other specified joint disorders, right elbow**
    M25.822 **Other specified joint disorders, left elbow**
    M25.829 **Other specified joint disorders, unspecified elbow** ▽

√6th **M25.83 Other specified joint disorders,** wrist
    M25.831 **Other specified joint disorders,** right wrist
    M25.832 **Other specified joint disorders,** left wrist
    M25.839 **Other specified joint disorders, unspecified wrist** ▽

√6th **M25.84 Other specified joint disorders,** hand
    M25.841 **Other specified joint disorders, right hand**
    M25.842 **Other specified joint disorders, left hand**
    M25.849 **Other specified joint disorders, unspecified hand** ▽

√6th **M25.85 Other specified joint disorders,** hip
    AHA: 2014, 4Q, 25
    M25.851 **Other specified joint disorders,** right hip
    M25.852 **Other specified joint disorders,** left hip
    M25.859 **Other specified joint disorders, unspecified hip** ▽

√6th **M25.86 Other specified joint disorders,** knee
    M25.861 **Other specified joint disorders,** right knee
    M25.862 **Other specified joint disorders,** left knee
    M25.869 **Other specified joint disorders, unspecified knee** ▽

√6th **M25.87 Other specified joint disorders,** ankle and foot
    M25.871 **Other specified joint disorders, right ankle and foot**
    M25.872 **Other specified joint disorders, left ankle and foot**
    M25.879 **Other specified joint disorders, unspecified ankle and foot** ▽

M25.9 Joint disorder, unspecified ▽

Dentofacial anomalies [including malocclusion] and other disorders of jaw (M26-M27)

EXCLUDES 1   hemifacial atrophy or hypertrophy (Q67.4)
         unilateral condylar hyperplasia or hypoplasia (M27.8)

√4th **M26 Dentofacial anomalies [including malocclusion]**

√5th **M26.0 Major anomalies of jaw size**
    EXCLUDES 1   acromegaly (E22.0)
                Robin's syndrome (Q87.0)
    M26.00 **Unspecified anomaly of jaw size** ▽
    M26.01 **Maxillary hyperplasia**
    M26.02 **Maxillary hypoplasia**
        AHA: 2014, 3Q, 23
    M26.03 **Mandibular hyperplasia**
    M26.04 **Mandibular hypoplasia**
    M26.05 **Macrogenia**
    M26.06 **Microgenia**
    M26.07 **Excessive tuberosity of jaw**
        Entire maxillary tuberosity
    M26.09 **Other specified anomalies of jaw size**

√5th **M26.1 Anomalies of jaw-cranial base relationship**
    M26.10 **Unspecified anomaly of jaw-cranial base relationship** ▽
    M26.11 **Maxillary asymmetry**
    M26.12 **Other jaw asymmetry**
    M26.19 **Other specified anomalies of jaw-cranial base relationship**

√5th **M26.2 Anomalies of dental arch relationship**
    M26.20 **Unspecified anomaly of dental arch relationship** ▽

√6th **M26.21 Malocclusion, Angle's class**
    M26.211 **Malocclusion, Angle's** class I
        Neutro-occlusion
    M26.212 **Malocclusion, Angle's** class II
        Disto-occlusion Division I
        Disto-occlusion Division II
    M26.213 **Malocclusion, Angle's** class III
        Mesio-occlusion
    M26.219 **Malocclusion, Angle's class, unspecified** ▽

√6th **M26.22 Open occlusal relationship**
    M26.220 **Open** anterior **occlusal relationship**
        Anterior openbite
    M26.221 **Open** posterior **occlusal relationship**
        Posterior openbite
    M26.23 **Excessive horizontal overlap**
        Excessive horizontal overjet
    M26.24 **Reverse articulation**
        Crossbite (anterior) (posterior)
    M26.25 **Anomalies of interarch distance**
    M26.29 **Other anomalies of dental arch relationship**
        Midline deviation of dental arch
        Overbite (excessive) deep
        Overbite (excessive) horizontal
        Overbite (excessive) vertical
        Posterior lingual occlusion of mandibular teeth

√5th **M26.3 Anomalies of tooth position of fully erupted tooth or teeth**
    EXCLUDES 2   embedded and impacted teeth (K01.-)
    M26.30 **Unspecified anomaly of tooth position of fully erupted tooth or teeth** ▽
        Abnormal spacing of fully erupted tooth or teeth NOS
        Displacement of fully erupted tooth or teeth NOS
        Transposition of fully erupted tooth or teeth NOS
    M26.31 **Crowding of fully erupted teeth**
    M26.32 **Excessive spacing of fully erupted teeth**
        Diastema of fully erupted tooth or teeth NOS
    M26.33 **Horizontal displacement of fully erupted tooth or teeth**
        Tipped tooth or teeth
        Tipping of fully erupted tooth
    M26.34 **Vertical displacement of fully erupted tooth or teeth**
        Extruded tooth
        Infraeruption of tooth or teeth
        Supraeruption of tooth or teeth
    M26.35 **Rotation of fully erupted tooth or teeth**

Chapter 13. Diseases of the Musculoskeletal System and Connective Tissue

M26.36 Insufficient **interocclusal distance of fully erupted teeth (ridge)**
Lack of adequate intermaxillary vertical dimension of fully erupted teeth

M26.37 Excessive **interocclusal distance of fully erupted teeth**
Excessive intermaxillary vertical dimension of fully erupted teeth
Loss of occlusal vertical dimension of fully erupted teeth

M26.39 **Other anomalies of tooth position of fully erupted tooth or teeth**

M26.4 **Malocclusion, unspecified** ▽

✓5ᵗʰ **M26.5** **Dentofacial functional abnormalities**
EXCLUDES 1   *bruxism (F45.8)*
teeth-grinding NOS (F45.8)

     M26.50 **Dentofacial functional abnormalities, unspecified** ▽

     M26.51 **Abnormal jaw closure**

     M26.52 **Limited mandibular range of motion**

     M26.53 **Deviation in opening and closing of the mandible**

     M26.54 **Insufficient anterior guidance**
Insufficient anterior occlusal guidance

     M26.55 **Centric occlusion maximum intercuspation discrepancy**
EXCLUDES 1   *centric occlusion NOS (M26.59)*

     M26.56 **Non-working side interference**
Balancing side interference

     M26.57 **Lack of posterior occlusal support**

     M26.59 **Other dentofacial functional abnormalities**
Centric occlusion (of teeth) NOS
Malocclusion due to abnormal swallowing
Malocclusion due to mouth breathing
Malocclusion due to tongue, lip or finger habits

✓5ᵗʰ **M26.6** **Temporomandibular joint disorders**
EXCLUDES 2   *current temporomandibular joint dislocation (S03.0)*
current temporomandibular joint sprain (S03.4)

     M26.60 **Temporomandibular joint disorder, unspecified** ▽

     M26.61 **Adhesions and ankylosis of temporomandibular joint**

     M26.62 **Arthralgia of temporomandibular joint**

     M26.63 **Articular disc disorder of temporomandibular joint**

     M26.69 **Other specified disorders of temporomandibular joint**

✓5ᵗʰ **M26.7** **Dental alveolar anomalies**

     M26.70 **Unspecified alveolar anomaly** ▽

     M26.71 **Alveolar** maxillary hyperplasia

     M26.72 **Alveolar** mandibular hyperplasia

     M26.73 **Alveolar** maxillary hypoplasia

     M26.74 **Alveolar** mandibular hypoplasia

     M26.79 **Other specified alveolar anomalies**

✓5ᵗʰ **M26.8** **Other dentofacial anomalies**

     M26.81 **Anterior soft tissue impingement**
Anterior soft tissue impingement on teeth

     M26.82 **Posterior soft tissue impingement**
Posterior soft tissue impingement on teeth

     M26.89 **Other dentofacial anomalies**

M26.9 **Dentofacial anomaly, unspecified** ▽

✓4ᵗʰ **M27** **Other diseases of jaws**

M27.0 **Developmental disorders of jaws**
Latent bone cyst of jaw   Torus mandibularis
Stafne's cyst   Torus palatinus

M27.1 **Giant cell granuloma, central**
Giant cell granuloma NOS
EXCLUDES 1   *peripheral giant cell granuloma (K06.8)*

M27.2 **Inflammatory conditions of jaws**
Osteitis of jaw(s)   Periostitis jaw(s)
Osteomyelitis (neonatal) jaw(s)   Sequestrum of jaw bone
Osteoradionecrosis jaw(s)
Use additional code (W88-W90, X39.0) to identify radiation, if radiation-induced
EXCLUDES 2   *osteonecrosis of jaw due to drug (M87.180)*

M27.3 **Alveolitis of jaws**
Alveolar osteitis
Dry socket

✓5ᵗʰ **M27.4** **Other and unspecified cysts of jaw**
EXCLUDES 1   *cysts of oral region (K09.-)*
latent bone cyst of jaw (M27.0)
Stafne's cyst (M27.0)

     M27.40 **Unspecified cyst of jaw** ▽
Cyst of jaw NOS

     M27.49 **Other cysts of jaw**
Aneurysmal cyst of jaw
Hemorrhagic cyst of jaw
Traumatic cyst of jaw

✓5ᵗʰ **M27.5** **Periradicular pathology associated with previous endodontic treatment**

     M27.51 **Perforation of root canal space due to endodontic treatment**

     M27.52 **Endodontic overfill**

     M27.53 **Endodontic underfill**

     M27.59 **Other periradicular pathology associated with previous endodontic treatment**

✓5ᵗʰ **M27.6** **Endosseous dental implant failure**

     M27.61 Osseointegration **failure of dental implant**
Hemorrhagic complications of dental implant placement
Iatrogenic osseointegration failure of dental implant
Osseointegration failure of dental implant due to complications of systemic disease
Osseointegration failure of dental implant due to poor bone quality
Pre-integration failure of dental implant NOS
Pre-osseointegration failure of dental implant

     M27.62 Post-osseointegration biological **failure of dental implant**
Failure of dental implant due to lack of attached gingiva
Failure of dental implant due to occlusal trauma (caused by poor prosthetic design)
Failure of dental implant due to parafunctional habits
Failure of dental implant due to periodontal infection (peri-implantitis)
Failure of dental implant due to poor oral hygiene
Iatrogenic post-osseointegration failure of dental implant
Post-osseointegration failure of dental implant due to complications of systemic disease

     M27.63 Post-osseointegration mechanical **failure of dental implant**
Failure of dental prosthesis causing loss of dental implant
Fracture of dental implant
EXCLUDES 2   *cracked tooth (K03.81)*
fractured dental restorative material with loss of material (K08.531)
fractured dental restorative material without loss of material (K08.530)
fractured tooth (S02.5)

     M27.69 **Other endosseous dental implant failure**
Dental implant failure NOS

M27.8 **Other specified diseases of jaws**
Cherubism   Unilateral condylar hyperplasia
Exostosis   Unilateral condylar hypoplasia
Fibrous dysplasia
EXCLUDES 1   *jaw pain (R68.84)*

M27.9 **Disease of jaws, unspecified** ▽

Systemic connective tissue disorders (M30-M36)

INCLUDES   autoimmune disease NOS
collagen (vascular) disease NOS
systemic autoimmune disease
systemic collagen (vascular) disease

EXCLUDES 1   *autoimmune disease, single organ or single cell-type—code to relevant condition category*

✓4ᵗʰ **M30** **Polyarteritis nodosa and related conditions**
EXCLUDES 1   *microscopic polyarteritis (M31.7)*

M30.0 **Polyarteritis nodosa**

M30.1 **Polyarteritis with lung involvement [Churg-Strauss]**
Allergic granulomatous angiitis

M30.2 **Juvenile polyarteritis**

M30.3 **Mucocutaneous lymph node syndrome [Kawasaki]**

M30.8 **Other conditions related to polyarteritis nodosa**
Polyangiitis overlap syndrome

Ⓝ Newborn   Ⓟ Pediatric   Ⓜ Maternity   Ⓐ Adult   **RIC** RIC Dx   **NCDx** Noncancer Dx   **PDx** Primary Dx   **CC** RIC CC Condition   ►◄ Revised Text   ● New Code   ▲ Revised Code Title

710   ICD-10-CM 2016

✓4ᵗʰ M31 Other necrotizing vasculopathies

M31.0 Hypersensitivity angiitis
Goodpasture's syndrome

M31.1 Thrombotic microangiopathy
Thrombotic thrombocytopenic purpura

M31.2 Lethal midline granuloma   cc

✓5ᵗʰ **M31.3 Wegener's granulomatosis**
Necrotizing respiratory granulomatosis

    M31.30 Wegener's granulomatosis without renal involvement
Wegener's granulomatosis NOS

    M31.31 Wegener's granulomatosis with renal involvement

M31.4 Aortic arch syndrome [Takayasu]

M31.5 Giant cell arteritis with polymyalgia rheumatica

M31.6 Other giant cell arteritis

M31.7 Microscopic polyangiitis
Microscopic polyarteritis
EXCLUDES 1   polyarteritis nodosa (M30.0)

M31.8 Other specified necrotizing vasculopathies
Hypocomplementemic vasculitis
Septic vasculitis

M31.9 Necrotizing vasculopathy, unspecified ▽

✓4ᵗʰ M32 Systemic lupus erythematosus (SLE)

EXCLUDES 1   lupus erythematosus (discoid) (NOS) (L93.0)

M32.0 Drug-induced systemic lupus erythematosus
Use additional code for adverse effect, if applicable, to identify drug (T36-T50 with fifth or sixth character 5)

✓5ᵗʰ **M32.1 Systemic lupus erythematosus with organ or system involvement**

    M32.10 Systemic lupus erythematosus, organ or system involvement unspecified ▽

    M32.11 Endocarditis in systemic lupus erythematosus
Libman-Sacks disease

    M32.12 Pericarditis in systemic lupus erythematosus
Lupus pericarditis

    M32.13 Lung involvement in systemic lupus erythematosus
Pleural effusion due to systemic lupus erythematosus

    M32.14 Glomerular disease in systemic lupus erythematosus
Lupus renal disease NOS
AHA: 2013, 4Q, 125

    M32.15 Tubulo-interstitial nephropathy in systemic lupus erythematosus

    M32.19 Other organ or system involvement in systemic lupus erythematosus

M32.8 Other forms of systemic lupus erythematosus

M32.9 Systemic lupus erythematosus, unspecified ▽
SLE NOS
Systemic lupus erythematosus NOS
Systemic lupus erythematosus without organ involvement

✓4ᵗʰ M33 Dermatopolymyositis

✓5ᵗʰ **M33.0 Juvenile dermatopolymyositis**

    M33.00 Juvenile dermatopolymyositis, organ involvement unspecified ▽

    M33.01 Juvenile dermatopolymyositis with respiratory involvement

    M33.02 Juvenile dermatopolymyositis with myopathy

    M33.09 Juvenile dermatopolymyositis with other organ involvement

✓5ᵗʰ **M33.1 Other dermatopolymyositis**

    M33.10 Other dermatopolymyositis, organ involvement unspecified ▽

    M33.11 Other dermatopolymyositis with respiratory involvement

    M33.12 Other dermatopolymyositis with myopathy

    M33.19 Other dermatopolymyositis with other organ involvement

✓5ᵗʰ **M33.2 Polymyositis**

    M33.20 Polymyositis, organ involvement unspecified ▽

    M33.21 Polymyositis with respiratory involvement

    M33.22 Polymyositis with myopathy

    M33.29 Polymyositis with other organ involvement

✓5ᵗʰ **M33.9 Dermatopolymyositis, unspecified**

    M33.90 Dermatopolymyositis, unspecified, organ involvement unspecified ▽

    M33.91 Dermatopolymyositis, unspecified with respiratory involvement ▽

    M33.92 Dermatopolymyositis, unspecified with myopathy ▽

    M33.99 Dermatopolymyositis, unspecified with other organ involvement ▽

✓4ᵗʰ M34 Systemic sclerosis [scleroderma]

EXCLUDES 1   circumscribed scleroderma (L94.0)
        neonatal scleroderma (P83.8)

M34.0 Progressive systemic sclerosis

M34.1 CR(E)ST syndrome
Combination of calcinosis, Raynaud's phenomenon, esophageal dysfunction, sclerodactyly, telangiectasia

M34.2 Systemic sclerosis induced by drug and chemical
Code first poisoning due to drug or toxin, if applicable (T36-T65 with fifth or sixth character 1-4 or 6)
Use additional code for adverse effect, if applicable, to identify drug (T36-T50 with fifth or sixth character 5)

✓5ᵗʰ **M34.8 Other forms of systemic sclerosis**

    M34.81 Systemic sclerosis with lung involvement

    M34.82 Systemic sclerosis with myopathy

    M34.83 Systemic sclerosis with polyneuropathy

    M34.89 Other systemic sclerosis

M34.9 Systemic sclerosis, unspecified ▽

✓4ᵗʰ M35 Other systemic involvement of connective tissue

EXCLUDES 1   reactive perforating collagenosis (L87.1)

✓5ᵗʰ **M35.0 Sicca syndrome [Sjögren]**

    M35.00 Sicca syndrome, unspecified ▽

    M35.01 Sicca syndrome with keratoconjunctivitis

    M35.02 Sicca syndrome with lung involvement

    M35.03 Sicca syndrome with myopathy

    M35.04 Sicca syndrome with tubulo-interstitial nephropathy
Renal tubular acidosis in sicca syndrome

    M35.09 Sicca syndrome with other organ involvement

M35.1 Other overlap syndromes
Mixed connective tissue disease
EXCLUDES 1   polyangiitis overlap syndrome (M30.8)

M35.2 Behçet's disease

M35.3 Polymyalgia rheumatica
EXCLUDES 1   polymyalgia rheumatica with giant cell arteritis (M31.5)

M35.4 Diffuse (eosinophilic) fasciitis

M35.5 Multifocal fibrosclerosis

M35.6 Relapsing panniculitis [Weber-Christian]
EXCLUDES 1   lupus panniculitis (L93.2)
        panniculitis NOS (M79.3-)

M35.7 Hypermobility syndrome
Familial ligamentous laxity
EXCLUDES 1   Ehlers-Danlos syndrome (Q79.6)
        ligamentous laxity, NOS (M24.2-)

M35.8 Other specified systemic involvement of connective tissue

M35.9 Systemic involvement of connective tissue, unspecified ▽
Autoimmune disease (systemic) NOS
Collagen (vascular) disease NOS

✓4ᵗʰ M36 Systemic disorders of connective tissue in diseases classified elsewhere

EXCLUDES 2   arthropathies in diseases classified elsewhere (M14.-)

M36.0 Dermato(poly)myositis in neoplastic disease
Code first underlying neoplasm (C00-D49)

M36.1 Arthropathy in neoplastic disease
Code first underlying neoplasm, such as:
leukemia (C91-C95)
malignant histiocytosis (C96.A)
multiple myeloma (C90.0)

Chapter 13. Diseases of the Musculoskeletal System and Connective Tissue

M36.2 Hemophilic arthropathy
Hemarthrosis in hemophilic arthropathy
Code first underlying disease, such as:
factor VIII deficiency (D66)
with vascular defect (D68.0)
factor IX deficiency (D67)
hemophilia (classical) (D66)
hemophilia B (D67)
hemophilia C (D68.1)

M36.3 Arthropathy in other blood disorders

M36.4 Arthropathy in hypersensitivity reactions classified elsewhere
Code first underlying disease, such as:
Henoch (-Schönlein) purpura (D69.0)
serum sickness (T80.6-)

M36.8 Systemic disorders of connective tissue in other diseases classified elsewhere
Code first underlying disease, such as:
alkaptonuria (E70.2)
hypogammaglobulinemia (D80.-)
ochronosis (E70.2)

DORSOPATHIES (M40-M54)

Deforming dorsopathies (M40-M43)

✓4ᵗʰ **M40 Kyphosis and lordosis**
EXCLUDES 1 congenital kyphosis and lordosis (Q76.4)
kyphoscoliosis (M41.-)
postprocedural kyphosis and lordosis (M96.-)

✓5ᵗʰ **M40.0 Postural kyphosis**
EXCLUDES 1 osteochondrosis of spine (M42.-)
M40.00 Postural kyphosis, site unspecified ▽
M40.03 Postural kyphosis, cervicothoracic region
M40.04 Postural kyphosis, thoracic region
M40.05 Postural kyphosis, thoracolumbar region

✓5ᵗʰ **M40.1 Other secondary kyphosis**
M40.10 Other secondary kyphosis, site unspecified ▽
M40.12 Other secondary kyphosis, cervical region
M40.13 Other secondary kyphosis, cervicothoracic region
M40.14 Other secondary kyphosis, thoracic region
M40.15 Other secondary kyphosis, thoracolumbar region

✓5ᵗʰ **M40.2 Other and unspecified kyphosis**
✓6ᵗʰ **M40.20 Unspecified kyphosis**
M40.202 Unspecified kyphosis, cervical region ▽
M40.203 Unspecified kyphosis, cervicothoracic region ▽
M40.204 Unspecified kyphosis, thoracic region ▽
M40.205 Unspecified kyphosis, thoracolumbar region ▽
M40.209 Unspecified kyphosis, site unspecified ▽
✓6ᵗʰ **M40.29 Other kyphosis**
M40.292 Other kyphosis, cervical region
M40.293 Other kyphosis, cervicothoracic region
M40.294 Other kyphosis, thoracic region
M40.295 Other kyphosis, thoracolumbar region
M40.299 Other kyphosis, site unspecified ▽

✓5ᵗʰ **M40.3 Flatback syndrome**
M40.30 Flatback syndrome, site unspecified ▽
M40.35 Flatback syndrome, thoracolumbar region
M40.36 Flatback syndrome, lumbar region
M40.37 Flatback syndrome, lumbosacral region

✓5ᵗʰ **M40.4 Postural lordosis**
Acquired lordosis
M40.40 Postural lordosis, site unspecified ▽
M40.45 Postural lordosis, thoracolumbar region
M40.46 Postural lordosis, lumbar region
M40.47 Postural lordosis, lumbosacral region

✓5ᵗʰ **M40.5 Lordosis, unspecified**
M40.50 Lordosis, unspecified, site unspecified ▽
M40.55 Lordosis, unspecified, thoracolumbar region
M40.56 Lordosis, unspecified, lumbar region
M40.57 Lordosis, unspecified, lumbosacral region

✓4ᵗʰ **M41 Scoliosis**
INCLUDES kyphoscoliosis
EXCLUDES 1 congenital scoliosis due to bony malformation (Q76.3)
congenital scoliosis NOS (Q67.5)
kyphoscoliotic heart disease (I27.1)
postprocedural scoliosis (M96.-)
postural congenital scoliosis (Q67.5)

✓5ᵗʰ **M41.0 Infantile idiopathic scoliosis**
AHA: 2014, 4Q, 26
M41.00 Infantile idiopathic scoliosis, site unspecified ▽
M41.02 Infantile idiopathic scoliosis, cervical region
M41.03 Infantile idiopathic scoliosis, cervicothoracic region
M41.04 Infantile idiopathic scoliosis, thoracic region
M41.05 Infantile idiopathic scoliosis, thoracolumbar region
M41.06 Infantile idiopathic scoliosis, lumbar region
M41.07 Infantile idiopathic scoliosis, lumbosacral region
M41.08 Infantile idiopathic scoliosis, sacral and sacrococcygeal region

✓5ᵗʰ **M41.1 Juvenile and adolescent idiopathic scoliosis**
✓6ᵗʰ **M41.11 Juvenile idiopathic scoliosis**
AHA: 2014, 4Q, 28
M41.112 Juvenile idiopathic scoliosis, cervical region
M41.113 Juvenile idiopathic scoliosis, cervicothoracic region
M41.114 Juvenile idiopathic scoliosis, thoracic region
M41.115 Juvenile idiopathic scoliosis, thoracolumbar region
M41.116 Juvenile idiopathic scoliosis, lumbar region
M41.117 Juvenile idiopathic scoliosis, lumbosacral region
M41.119 Juvenile idiopathic scoliosis, site unspecified ▽
✓6ᵗʰ **M41.12 Adolescent scoliosis**
M41.122 Adolescent idiopathic scoliosis, cervical region
M41.123 Adolescent idiopathic scoliosis, cervicothoracic region
M41.124 Adolescent idiopathic scoliosis, thoracic region
M41.125 Adolescent idiopathic scoliosis, thoracolumbar region
M41.126 Adolescent idiopathic scoliosis, lumbar region
M41.127 Adolescent idiopathic scoliosis, lumbosacral region
M41.129 Adolescent idiopathic scoliosis, site unspecified ▽

✓5ᵗʰ **M41.2 Other idiopathic scoliosis**
M41.20 Other idiopathic scoliosis, site unspecified ▽
M41.22 Other idiopathic scoliosis, cervical region
M41.23 Other idiopathic scoliosis, cervicothoracic region
M41.24 Other idiopathic scoliosis, thoracic region
M41.25 Other idiopathic scoliosis, thoracolumbar region
M41.26 Other idiopathic scoliosis, lumbar region
M41.27 Other idiopathic scoliosis, lumbosacral region

✓5ᵗʰ **M41.3 Thoracogenic scoliosis**
M41.30 Thoracogenic scoliosis, site unspecified ▽
M41.34 Thoracogenic scoliosis, thoracic region
M41.35 Thoracogenic scoliosis, thoracolumbar region

✓5ᵗʰ **M41.4 Neuromuscular scoliosis**
Scoliosis secondary to cerebral palsy, Friedreich's ataxia, poliomyelitis and other neuromuscular disorders
Code also underlying condition
AHA: 2014, 4Q, 27
M41.40 Neuromuscular scoliosis, site unspecified ▽
M41.41 Neuromuscular scoliosis, occipito-atlanto-axial region
M41.42 Neuromuscular scoliosis, cervical region
M41.43 Neuromuscular scoliosis, cervicothoracic region
M41.44 Neuromuscular scoliosis, thoracic region
M41.45 Neuromuscular scoliosis, thoracolumbar region
M41.46 Neuromuscular scoliosis, lumbar region

N Newborn   P Pediatric   M Maternity   A Adult   RIC RIC Dx   NCDx Noncancer Dx   PDx Primary Dx   CC RIC CC Condition   ▶◀ Revised Text   ● New Code   ▲ Revised Code Title

712   ICD-10-CM 2016

     M41.47   Neuromuscular scoliosis, lumbosacral region

✓5ᵗʰ   **M41.5**   Other secondary scoliosis

     M41.50   **Other secondary scoliosis, site unspecified** ▽

     M41.52   **Other secondary scoliosis, cervical region**

     M41.53   **Other secondary scoliosis, cervicothoracic region**

     M41.54   **Other secondary scoliosis, thoracic region**

     M41.55   **Other secondary scoliosis, thoracolumbar region**

     M41.56   **Other secondary scoliosis, lumbar region**

     M41.57   **Other secondary scoliosis, lumbosacral region**

✓5ᵗʰ   **M41.8**   Other forms of scoliosis

     M41.80   **Other forms of scoliosis, site unspecified** ▽

     M41.82   **Other forms of scoliosis, cervical region**

     M41.83   **Other forms of scoliosis, cervicothoracic region**

     M41.84   **Other forms of scoliosis, thoracic region**

     M41.85   **Other forms of scoliosis, thoracolumbar region**

     M41.86   **Other forms of scoliosis, lumbar region**

     M41.87   **Other forms of scoliosis, lumbosacral region**

   M41.9   Scoliosis, unspecified ▽

✓4ᵗʰ **M42**   Spinal osteochondrosis

✓5ᵗʰ   **M42.0**   Juvenile osteochondrosis of spine
     Calvé's disease
     Scheuermann's disease
     EXCLUDES 1   postural kyphosis (M40.0)

     M42.00   **Juvenile osteochondrosis of spine, site unspecified** ▽

     M42.01   **Juvenile osteochondrosis of spine, occipito-atlanto-axial region**

     M42.02   **Juvenile osteochondrosis of spine, cervical region**

     M42.03   **Juvenile osteochondrosis of spine, cervicothoracic region**

     M42.04   **Juvenile osteochondrosis of spine, thoracic region**

     M42.05   **Juvenile osteochondrosis of spine, thoracolumbar region**

     M42.06   **Juvenile osteochondrosis of spine, lumbar region**

     M42.07   **Juvenile osteochondrosis of spine, lumbosacral region**

     M42.08   **Juvenile osteochondrosis of spine, sacral and sacrococcygeal region**

     M42.09   **Juvenile osteochondrosis of spine, multiple sites in spine**

✓5ᵗʰ   **M42.1**   Adult osteochondrosis of spine

     M42.10   **Adult osteochondrosis of spine, site unspecified** Ⓐ▽

     M42.11   **Adult osteochondrosis of spine, occipito-atlanto-axial region** Ⓐ

     M42.12   **Adult osteochondrosis of spine, cervical region** Ⓐ

     M42.13   **Adult osteochondrosis of spine, cervicothoracic region** Ⓐ

     M42.14   **Adult osteochondrosis of spine, thoracic region** Ⓐ

     M42.15   **Adult osteochondrosis of spine, thoracolumbar region** Ⓐ

     M42.16   **Adult osteochondrosis of spine, lumbar region** Ⓐ

     M42.17   **Adult osteochondrosis of spine, lumbosacral region** Ⓐ

     M42.18   **Adult osteochondrosis of spine, sacral and sacrococcygeal region** Ⓐ

     M42.19   **Adult osteochondrosis of spine, multiple sites in spine** Ⓐ

   M42.9   Spinal osteochondrosis, unspecified ▽

✓4ᵗʰ **M43**   Other deforming dorsopathies
     EXCLUDES 1   congenital spondylolysis and spondylolisthesis (Q76.2)
       hemivertebra (Q76.3-Q76.4)
       Klippel-Feil syndrome (Q76.1)
       lumbarization and sacralization (Q76.4)
       platyspondylisis (Q76.4)
       spina bifida occulta (Q76.0)
       spinal curvature in osteoporosis (M80.-)
       spinal curvature in Paget's disease of bone [osteitis deformans] (M88.-)

✓5ᵗʰ   **M43.0**   Spondylolysis
     EXCLUDES 1   congenital spondylolysis (Q76.2)
       spondylolisthesis (M43.1)

     M43.00   **Spondylolysis, site unspecified** ▽

     M43.01   Spondylolysis, occipito-atlanto-axial region

     M43.02   Spondylolysis, cervical region

     M43.03   Spondylolysis, cervicothoracic region

     M43.04   Spondylolysis, thoracic region

     M43.05   Spondylolysis, thoracolumbar region

     M43.06   Spondylolysis, lumbar region

     M43.07   Spondylolysis, lumbosacral region

     M43.08   Spondylolysis, sacral and sacrococcygeal region

     M43.09   Spondylolysis, multiple sites in spine

✓5ᵗʰ   **M43.1**   Spondylolisthesis
     EXCLUDES 1   acute traumatic of lumbosacral region (S33.1)
       acute traumatic of sites other than lumbosacral— code to Fracture, vertebra, by region
       congenital spondylolisthesis (Q76.2)

     M43.10   **Spondylolisthesis, site unspecified** ▽

     M43.11   **Spondylolisthesis, occipito-atlanto-axial region**

     M43.12   **Spondylolisthesis, cervical region**

     M43.13   **Spondylolisthesis, cervicothoracic region**

     M43.14   **Spondylolisthesis, thoracic region**

     M43.15   **Spondylolisthesis, thoracolumbar region**

     M43.16   **Spondylolisthesis, lumbar region**

     M43.17   **Spondylolisthesis, lumbosacral region**

     M43.18   **Spondylolisthesis, sacral and sacrococcygeal region**

     M43.19   **Spondylolisthesis, multiple sites in spine**

✓5ᵗʰ   **M43.2**   Fusion of spine
     Ankylosis of spinal joint
     EXCLUDES 1   ankylosing spondylitis (M45.0-)
       congenital fusion of spine (Q76.4)
     EXCLUDES 2   arthrodesis status (Z98.1)
       pseudoarthrosis after fusion or arthrodesis (M96.0)

     M43.20   **Fusion of spine, site unspecified** ▽

     M43.21   **Fusion of spine, occipito-atlanto-axial region**

     M43.22   **Fusion of spine, cervical region**

     M43.23   **Fusion of spine, cervicothoracic region**

     M43.24   **Fusion of spine, thoracic region**

     M43.25   **Fusion of spine, thoracolumbar region**

     M43.26   **Fusion of spine, lumbar region**

     M43.27   **Fusion of spine, lumbosacral region**

     M43.28   **Fusion of spine, sacral and sacrococcygeal region**

   M43.3   Recurrent atlantoaxial dislocation with myelopathy

   M43.4   Other recurrent atlantoaxial dislocation

✓5ᵗʰ   **M43.5**   Other recurrent vertebral dislocation
     EXCLUDES 1   biomechanical lesions NEC (M99.-)

     ✓6ᵗʰ   **M43.5X**   Other recurrent vertebral dislocation

       M43.5X2   **Other recurrent vertebral dislocation, cervical region**

       M43.5X3   **Other recurrent vertebral dislocation, cervicothoracic region**

       M43.5X4   **Other recurrent vertebral dislocation, thoracic region**

       M43.5X5   **Other recurrent vertebral dislocation, thoracolumbar region**

       M43.5X6   **Other recurrent vertebral dislocation, lumbar region**

       M43.5X7   **Other recurrent vertebral dislocation, lumbosacral region**

       M43.5X8   **Other recurrent vertebral dislocation, sacral and sacrococcygeal region**

       M43.5X9   **Other recurrent vertebral dislocation, site unspecified** ▽

   M43.6   Torticollis
     EXCLUDES 1   congenital (sternomastoid) torticollis (Q68.0)
       current injury—see Injury, of spine, by body region
       ocular torticollis (R29.891)
       psychogenic torticollis (F45.8)
       spasmodic torticollis (G24.3)
       torticollis due to birth injury (P15.2)

☑ Add'l Character Required   ☑x7ᵗʰ Placeholder Alert   RUG IV Special Care High Dx   RUG IV Clinically Complex Dx   RUG IV Special Care Low Dx   Manifestation Code   Other Specified Code   ▽Unspecified Code

ICD-10-CM 2016   713

Chapter 13. Diseases of the Musculoskeletal System and Connective Tissue

M43.8–M46.89

✓5ᵗʰ **M43.8 Other specified deforming dorsopathies**
> EXCLUDES 2 *kyphosis and lordosis (M40.-)*
> *scoliosis (M41.-)*

    ✓6ᵗʰ **M43.8X Other specified deforming dorsopathies**

      M43.8X1 Other specified deforming dorsopathies, occipito-atlanto-axial region

      M43.8X2 Other specified deforming dorsopathies, cervical region

      M43.8X3 Other specified deforming dorsopathies, cervicothoracic region

      M43.8X4 Other specified deforming dorsopathies, thoracic region

      M43.8X5 Other specified deforming dorsopathies, thoracolumbar region

      M43.8X6 Other specified deforming dorsopathies, lumbar region

      M43.8X7 Other specified deforming dorsopathies, lumbosacral region

      M43.8X8 Other specified deforming dorsopathies, sacral and sacrococcygeal region

      M43.8X9 Other specified deforming dorsopathies, site unspecified ▽

M43.9 Deforming dorsopathy, unspecified ▽
> Curvature of spine NOS

Spondylopathies (M45-M49)

✓4ᵗʰ **M45 Ankylosing spondylitis**
> Rheumatoid arthritis of spine
> EXCLUDES 1 *arthropathy in Reiter's disease (M02.3-)*
> *juvenile (ankylosing) spondylitis (M08.1)*
> EXCLUDES 2 *Behçet's disease (M35.2)*

M45.0 Ankylosing spondylitis of multiple sites in spine

M45.1 Ankylosing spondylitis of occipito-atlanto-axial region

M45.2 Ankylosing spondylitis of cervical region

M45.3 Ankylosing spondylitis of cervicothoracic region

M45.4 Ankylosing spondylitis of thoracic region

M45.5 Ankylosing spondylitis of thoracolumbar region

M45.6 Ankylosing spondylitis lumbar region

M45.7 Ankylosing spondylitis of lumbosacral region

M45.8 Ankylosing spondylitis sacral and sacrococcygeal region

M45.9 Ankylosing spondylitis of unspecified sites in spine ▽

✓4ᵗʰ **M46 Other inflammatory spondylopathies**

    ✓5ᵗʰ **M46.0 Spinal enthesopathy**
> Disorder of ligamentous or muscular attachments of spine

      M46.00 Spinal enthesopathy, site unspecified ▽

      M46.01 Spinal enthesopathy, occipito-atlanto-axial region

      M46.02 Spinal enthesopathy, cervical region

      M46.03 Spinal enthesopathy, cervicothoracic region

      M46.04 Spinal enthesopathy, thoracic region

      M46.05 Spinal enthesopathy, thoracolumbar region

      M46.06 Spinal enthesopathy, lumbar region

      M46.07 Spinal enthesopathy, lumbosacral region

      M46.08 Spinal enthesopathy, sacral and sacrococcygeal region

      M46.09 Spinal enthesopathy, multiple sites in spine

M46.1 Sacroiliitis, not elsewhere classified

    ✓5ᵗʰ **M46.2 Osteomyelitis of vertebra**

      M46.20 Osteomyelitis of vertebra, site unspecified ▽

      M46.21 Osteomyelitis of vertebra, occipito-atlanto-axial region

      M46.22 Osteomyelitis of vertebra, cervical region

      M46.23 Osteomyelitis of vertebra, cervicothoracic region

      M46.24 Osteomyelitis of vertebra, thoracic region

      M46.25 Osteomyelitis of vertebra, thoracolumbar region

      M46.26 Osteomyelitis of vertebra, lumbar region

      M46.27 Osteomyelitis of vertebra, lumbosacral region

      M46.28 Osteomyelitis of vertebra, sacral and sacrococcygeal region

✓5ᵗʰ **M46.3 Infection of intervertebral disc (pyogenic)**
> Use additional code (B95-B97) to identify infectious agent

    M46.30 Infection of intervertebral disc (pyogenic), site unspecified ▽

    M46.31 Infection of intervertebral disc (pyogenic), occipito-atlanto-axial region

    M46.32 Infection of intervertebral disc (pyogenic), cervical region

    M46.33 Infection of intervertebral disc (pyogenic), cervicothoracic region

    M46.34 Infection of intervertebral disc (pyogenic), thoracic region

    M46.35 Infection of intervertebral disc (pyogenic), thoracolumbar region

    M46.36 Infection of intervertebral disc (pyogenic), lumbar region

    M46.37 Infection of intervertebral disc (pyogenic), lumbosacral region

    M46.38 Infection of intervertebral disc (pyogenic), sacral and sacrococcygeal region

    M46.39 Infection of intervertebral disc (pyogenic), multiple sites in spine

✓5ᵗʰ **M46.4 Discitis, unspecified**

    M46.40 Discitis, unspecified, site unspecified Ⓐ▽

    M46.41 Discitis, unspecified, occipito-atlanto-axial region Ⓐ▽

    M46.42 Discitis, unspecified, cervical region Ⓐ▽

    M46.43 Discitis, unspecified, cervicothoracic region Ⓐ▽

    M46.44 Discitis, unspecified, thoracic region Ⓐ▽

    M46.45 Discitis, unspecified, thoracolumbar region Ⓐ▽

    M46.46 Discitis, unspecified, lumbar region Ⓐ▽

    M46.47 Discitis, unspecified, lumbosacral region Ⓐ▽

    M46.48 Discitis, unspecified, sacral and sacrococcygeal region Ⓐ▽

    M46.49 Discitis, unspecified, multiple sites in spine Ⓐ▽

✓5ᵗʰ **M46.5 Other infective spondylopathies**

    M46.50 Other infective spondylopathies, site unspecified ▽

    M46.51 Other infective spondylopathies, occipito-atlanto-axial region

    M46.52 Other infective spondylopathies, cervical region

    M46.53 Other infective spondylopathies, cervicothoracic region

    M46.54 Other infective spondylopathies, thoracic region

    M46.55 Other infective spondylopathies, thoracolumbar region

    M46.56 Other infective spondylopathies, lumbar region

    M46.57 Other infective spondylopathies, lumbosacral region

    M46.58 Other infective spondylopathies, sacral and sacrococcygeal region

    M46.59 Other infective spondylopathies, multiple sites in spine

✓5ᵗʰ **M46.8 Other specified inflammatory spondylopathies**

    M46.80 Other specified inflammatory spondylopathies, site unspecified ▽

    M46.81 Other specified inflammatory spondylopathies, occipito-atlanto-axial region

    M46.82 Other specified inflammatory spondylopathies, cervical region

    M46.83 Other specified inflammatory spondylopathies, cervicothoracic region

    M46.84 Other specified inflammatory spondylopathies, thoracic region

    M46.85 Other specified inflammatory spondylopathies, thoracolumbar region

    M46.86 Other specified inflammatory spondylopathies, lumbar region

    M46.87 Other specified inflammatory spondylopathies, lumbosacral region

    M46.88 Other specified inflammatory spondylopathies, sacral and sacrococcygeal region

    M46.89 Other specified inflammatory spondylopathies, multiple sites in spine

Ⓝ Newborn   Ⓟ Pediatric   Ⓜ Maternity   Ⓐ Adult   **RIC** RIC Dx   **NC Dx** Noncancer Dx   **PDx** Primary Dx   **CC** RIC CC Condition   ►◄ Revised Text   ● New Code   ▲ Revised Code Title

714   ICD-10-CM 2016

✓5th **M46.9 Unspecified inflammatory spondylopathy**

M46.90 Unspecified inflammatory spondylopathy, site unspecified ▽

M46.91 Unspecified inflammatory spondylopathy, occipito-atlanto-axial region ▽

M46.92 Unspecified inflammatory spondylopathy, cervical region ▽

M46.93 Unspecified inflammatory spondylopathy, cervicothoracic region ▽

M46.94 Unspecified inflammatory spondylopathy, thoracic region ▽

M46.95 Unspecified inflammatory spondylopathy, thoracolumbar region ▽

M46.96 Unspecified inflammatory spondylopathy, lumbar region ▽

M46.97 Unspecified inflammatory spondylopathy, lumbosacral region ▽

M46.98 Unspecified inflammatory spondylopathy, sacral and sacrococcygeal region ▽

M46.99 Unspecified inflammatory spondylopathy, multiple sites in spine ▽

✓4th **M47 Spondylosis**

INCLUDES   arthrosis or osteoarthritis of spine
degeneration of facet joints

✓5th **M47.0 Anterior spinal and vertebral artery compression syndromes**

✓6th **M47.01 Anterior spinal artery compression syndromes**

M47.011 Anterior spinal artery compression syndromes, occipito-atlanto-axial region

M47.012 Anterior spinal artery compression syndromes, cervical region

M47.013 Anterior spinal artery compression syndromes, cervicothoracic region

M47.014 Anterior spinal artery compression syndromes, thoracic region

M47.015 Anterior spinal artery compression syndromes, thoracolumbar region

M47.016 Anterior spinal artery compression syndromes, lumbar region

M47.019 Anterior spinal artery compression syndromes, site unspecified ▽

✓6th **M47.02 Vertebral artery compression syndromes**

M47.021 Vertebral artery compression syndromes, occipito-atlanto-axial region

M47.022 Vertebral artery compression syndromes, cervical region

M47.029 Vertebral artery compression syndromes, site unspecified ▽

✓5th **M47.1 Other spondylosis with myelopathy**

Spondylogenic compression of spinal cord

EXCLUDES 1   vertebral subluxation (M43.3-M43.5X9)

M47.10 Other spondylosis with myelopathy, site unspecified ▽

M47.11 Other spondylosis with myelopathy, occipito-atlanto-axial region

M47.12 Other spondylosis with myelopathy, cervical region

M47.13 Other spondylosis with myelopathy, cervicothoracic region

M47.14 Other spondylosis with myelopathy, thoracic region

M47.15 Other spondylosis with myelopathy, thoracolumbar region

M47.16 Other spondylosis with myelopathy, lumbar region

✓5th **M47.2 Other spondylosis with radiculopathy**

M47.20 Other spondylosis with radiculopathy, site unspecified ▽

M47.21 Other spondylosis with radiculopathy, occipito-atlanto-axial region

M47.22 Other spondylosis with radiculopathy, cervical region

M47.23 Other spondylosis with radiculopathy, cervicothoracic region

M47.24 Other spondylosis with radiculopathy, thoracic region

M47.25 Other spondylosis with radiculopathy, thoracolumbar region

M47.26 Other spondylosis with radiculopathy, lumbar region

M47.27 Other spondylosis with radiculopathy, lumbosacral region

M47.28 Other spondylosis with radiculopathy, sacral and sacrococcygeal region

✓5th **M47.8 Other spondylosis**

✓6th **M47.81 Spondylosis without myelopathy or radiculopathy**

M47.811 Spondylosis without myelopathy or radiculopathy, occipito-atlanto-axial region

M47.812 Spondylosis without myelopathy or radiculopathy, cervical region

M47.813 Spondylosis without myelopathy or radiculopathy, cervicothoracic region

M47.814 Spondylosis without myelopathy or radiculopathy, thoracic region

M47.815 Spondylosis without myelopathy or radiculopathy, thoracolumbar region

M47.816 Spondylosis without myelopathy or radiculopathy, lumbar region

M47.817 Spondylosis without myelopathy or radiculopathy, lumbosacral region

M47.818 Spondylosis without myelopathy or radiculopathy, sacral and sacrococcygeal region

M47.819 Spondylosis without myelopathy or radiculopathy, site unspecified ▽

✓6th **M47.89 Other spondylosis**

M47.891 Other spondylosis, occipito-atlanto-axial region

M47.892 Other spondylosis, cervical region

M47.893 Other spondylosis, cervicothoracic region

M47.894 Other spondylosis, thoracic region

M47.895 Other spondylosis, thoracolumbar region

M47.896 Other spondylosis, lumbar region

M47.897 Other spondylosis, lumbosacral region

M47.898 Other spondylosis, sacral and sacrococcygeal region

M47.899 Other spondylosis, site unspecified ▽

M47.9 Spondylosis, unspecified ▽

✓4th **M48 Other spondylopathies**

✓5th **M48.0 Spinal stenosis**

Caudal stenosis

M48.00 Spinal stenosis, site unspecified A ▽

M48.01 Spinal stenosis, occipito-atlanto-axial region

M48.02 Spinal stenosis, cervical region

M48.03 Spinal stenosis, cervicothoracic region

M48.04 Spinal stenosis, thoracic region A

M48.05 Spinal stenosis, thoracolumbar region A

M48.06 Spinal stenosis, lumbar region A

M48.07 Spinal stenosis, lumbosacral region A

M48.08 Spinal stenosis, sacral and sacrococcygeal region A

✓5th **M48.1 Ankylosing hyperostosis [Forestier]**

Diffuse idiopathic skeletal hyperostosis [DISH]

M48.10 Ankylosing hyperostosis [Forestier], site unspecified ▽

M48.11 Ankylosing hyperostosis [Forestier], occipito-atlanto-axial region

M48.12 Ankylosing hyperostosis [Forestier], cervical region

M48.13 Ankylosing hyperostosis [Forestier], cervicothoracic region

M48.14 Ankylosing hyperostosis [Forestier], thoracic region

M48.15 Ankylosing hyperostosis [Forestier], thoracolumbar region

M48.16 Ankylosing hyperostosis [Forestier], lumbar region

M48.17 Ankylosing hyperostosis [Forestier], lumbosacral region

M48.18 Ankylosing hyperostosis [Forestier], sacral and sacrococcygeal region

M48.19 Ankylosing hyperostosis [Forestier], multiple sites in spine

✓ Add'l Character Required   ✓x7th Placeholder Alert   RUG IV Special Care High Dx   RUG IV Clinically Complex Dx   RUG IV Special Care Low Dx   Manifestation Code   Other Specified Code   ▽ Unspecified Code

√5ᵗʰ **M48.2 Kissing spine**
 M48.20 Kissing spine, site unspecified ▽
 M48.21 Kissing spine, occipito-atlanto-axial region
 M48.22 Kissing spine, cervical region
 M48.23 Kissing spine, cervicothoracic region
 M48.24 Kissing spine, thoracic region
 M48.25 Kissing spine, thoracolumbar region
 M48.26 Kissing spine, lumbar region
 M48.27 Kissing spine, lumbosacral region

√5ᵗʰ **M48.3 Traumatic spondylopathy**
 M48.30 Traumatic spondylopathy, site unspecified ▽
 M48.31 Traumatic spondylopathy, occipito-atlanto-axial region
 M48.32 Traumatic spondylopathy, cervical region
 M48.33 Traumatic spondylopathy, cervicothoracic region
 M48.34 Traumatic spondylopathy, thoracic region
 M48.35 Traumatic spondylopathy, thoracolumbar region
 M48.36 Traumatic spondylopathy, lumbar region
 M48.37 Traumatic spondylopathy, lumbosacral region
 M48.38 Traumatic spondylopathy, sacral and sacrococcygeal region

√5ᵗʰ **M48.4 Fatigue fracture of vertebra**
 Stress fracture of vertebra
 EXCLUDES 1 *pathological fracture NOS (M84.4-)*
 pathological fracture of vertebra due to neoplasm (M84.58)
 pathological fracture of vertebra due to other diagnosis (M84.68)
 pathological fracture of vertebra due to osteoporosis (M80.-)
 traumatic fracture of vertebrae (S12.0-S12.3-, S22.0-, S32.0-)

 The appropriate 7th character is to be added to each code from subcategory M48.4.
 A initial encounter for fracture
 D subsequent encounter for fracture with routine healing
 G subsequent encounter for fracture with delayed healing
 S sequela of fracture

 √x7ᵗʰ **M48.40 Fatigue fracture of vertebra, site unspecified** ▽
 √x7ᵗʰ **M48.41 Fatigue fracture of vertebra, occipito-atlanto-axial region**
 √x7ᵗʰ **M48.42 Fatigue fracture of vertebra, cervical region**
 √x7ᵗʰ **M48.43 Fatigue fracture of vertebra, cervicothoracic region**
 √x7ᵗʰ **M48.44 Fatigue fracture of vertebra, thoracic region**
 √x7ᵗʰ **M48.45 Fatigue fracture of vertebra, thoracolumbar region**
 √x7ᵗʰ **M48.46 Fatigue fracture of vertebra, lumbar region**
 √x7ᵗʰ **M48.47 Fatigue fracture of vertebra, lumbosacral region**
 √x7ᵗʰ **M48.48 Fatigue fracture of vertebra, sacral and sacrococcygeal region**

√5ᵗʰ **M48.5 Collapsed vertebra, not elsewhere classified**
 Collapsed vertebra NOS
 Wedging of vertebra NOS
 EXCLUDES 1 *current injury—see Injury of spine, by body region*
 fatigue fracture of vertebra (M48.4)
 pathological fracture of vertebra due to neoplasm (M84.58)
 pathological fracture of vertebra due to other diagnosis (M84.68)
 pathological fracture of vertebra due to osteoporosis (M80.-)
 pathological fracture NOS (M84.4-)
 stress fracture of vertebra (M48.4-)
 traumatic fracture of vertebra (S12-, S22-, S32-)

 The appropriate 7th character is to be added to each code from subcategory M48.5.
 A initial encounter for fracture
 D subsequent encounter for fracture with routine healing
 G subsequent encounter for fracture with delayed healing
 S sequela of fracture

 √x7ᵗʰ **M48.50 Collapsed vertebra, not elsewhere classified, site unspecified** ▽
 √x7ᵗʰ **M48.51 Collapsed vertebra, not elsewhere classified, occipito-atlanto-axial region**
 √x7ᵗʰ **M48.52 Collapsed vertebra, not elsewhere classified, cervical region**
 √x7ᵗʰ **M48.53 Collapsed vertebra, not elsewhere classified, cervicothoracic region**
 √x7ᵗʰ **M48.54 Collapsed vertebra, not elsewhere classified, thoracic region**
 √x7ᵗʰ **M48.55 Collapsed vertebra, not elsewhere classified, thoracolumbar region**
 √x7ᵗʰ **M48.56 Collapsed vertebra, not elsewhere classified, lumbar region**
 √x7ᵗʰ **M48.57 Collapsed vertebra, not elsewhere classified, lumbosacral region**
 √x7ᵗʰ **M48.58 Collapsed vertebra, not elsewhere classified, sacral and sacrococcygeal region**

√5ᵗʰ **M48.8 Other specified spondylopathies**
 Ossification of posterior longitudinal ligament
 √6ᵗʰ **M48.8X Other specified spondylopathies**
 M48.8X1 Other specified spondylopathies, occipito-atlanto-axial region
 M48.8X2 Other specified spondylopathies, cervical region
 M48.8X3 Other specified spondylopathies, cervicothoracic region
 M48.8X4 Other specified spondylopathies, thoracic region
 M48.8X5 Other specified spondylopathies, thoracolumbar region
 M48.8X6 Other specified spondylopathies, lumbar region
 M48.8X7 Other specified spondylopathies, lumbosacral region
 M48.8X8 Other specified spondylopathies, sacral and sacrococcygeal region
 M48.8X9 Other specified spondylopathies, site unspecified ▽

 M48.9 Spondylopathy, unspecified ▽

√4ᵗʰ **M49 Spondylopathies in diseases classified elsewhere**
 INCLUDES curvature of spine in diseases classified elsewhere
 deformity of spine in diseases classified elsewhere
 kyphosis in diseases classified elsewhere
 scoliosis in diseases classified elsewhere
 spondylopathy in diseases classified elsewhere
 Code first underlying disease, such as:
 brucellosis (A23.-)
 Charcôt-Marie-Tooth disease (G60.0)
 enterobacterial infections (A01-A04)
 osteitis fibrosa cystica (E21.0)
 EXCLUDES 1 *curvature of spine in tuberculosis [Pott's] (A18.01)*
 enteropathic arthropathies (M07.-)
 gonococcal spondylitis (A54.41)
 neuropathic [tabes dorsalis] spondylitis (A52.11)
 neuropathic spondylopathy in syringomyelia (G95.0)
 neuropathic spondylopathy in tabes dorsalis (A52.11)
 nonsyphilitic neuropathic spondylopathy NEC (G98.0)
 spondylitis in syphilis (acquired) (A52.77)
 tuberculous spondylitis (A18.01)
 typhoid fever spondylitis (A01.05)

√5ᵗʰ **M49.8 Spondylopathy in diseases classified elsewhere**
 M49.80 Spondylopathy in diseases classified elsewhere, site unspecified ▽
 M49.81 Spondylopathy in diseases classified elsewhere, occipito-atlanto-axial region
 M49.82 Spondylopathy in diseases classified elsewhere, cervical region
 M49.83 Spondylopathy in diseases classified elsewhere, cervicothoracic region
 M49.84 Spondylopathy in diseases classified elsewhere, thoracic region
 M49.85 Spondylopathy in diseases classified elsewhere, thoracolumbar region
 M49.86 Spondylopathy in diseases classified elsewhere, lumbar region
 M49.87 Spondylopathy in diseases classified elsewhere, lumbosacral region

N Newborn **P** Pediatric **M** Maternity **A** Adult **RIC** RIC Dx **NC Dx** Noncancer Dx **PDx** Primary Dx **CC** RIC CC Condition ▶◀ Revised Text ● New Code ▲ Revised Code Title

ICD-10-CM 2016
716

M49.88 *Spondylopathy in diseases classified elsewhere, sacral and sacrococcygeal region*

M49.89 *Spondylopathy in diseases classified elsewhere, multiple sites in spine*

Other dorsopathies (M50-M54)

EXCLUDES 1   current injury—see injury of spine by body region
discitis NOS (M46.4-)

✓4ᵗʰ M50   Cervical disc disorders

    NOTE   Code to the most superior level of disorder.

    INCLUDES   cervicothoracic disc disorders with cervicalgia
cervicothoracic disc disorders

    ✓5ᵗʰ M50.0   Cervical disc disorder with myelopathy

      M50.00   Cervical disc disorder with myelopathy, unspecified cervical region   A ▽

      M50.01   Cervical disc disorder with myelopathy, high cervical region   A
         C2-C3 disc disorder with myelopathy
         C3-C4 disc disorder with myelopathy

      M50.02   Cervical disc disorder with myelopathy, mid-cervical region   A
         C4-C5 disc disorder with myelopathy
         C5-C6 disc disorder with myelopathy
         C6-C7 disc disorder with myelopathy

      M50.03   Cervical disc disorder with myelopathy, cervicothoracic region   A
         C7-T1 disc disorder with myelopathy

    ✓5ᵗʰ M50.1   Cervical disc disorder with radiculopathy

        EXCLUDES 2   brachial radiculitis NOS (M54.13)

      M50.10   Cervical disc disorder with radiculopathy, unspecified cervical region   ▽

      M50.11   Cervical disc disorder with radiculopathy, high cervical region
         C2-C3 disc disorder with radiculopathy
         C3 radiculopathy due to disc disorder
         C3-C4 disc disorder with radiculopathy
         C4 radiculopathy due to disc disorder

      M50.12   Cervical disc disorder with radiculopathy, mid-cervical region
         C4-C5 disc disorder with radiculopathy
         C5 radiculopathy due to disc disorder
         C5-C6 disc disorder with radiculopathy
         C6 radiculopathy due to disc disorder
         C6-C7 disc disorder with radiculopathy
         C7 radiculopathy due to disc disorder

      M50.13   Cervical disc disorder with radiculopathy, cervicothoracic region
         C7-T1 disc disorder with radiculopathy
         C8 radiculopathy due to disc disorder

    ✓5ᵗʰ M50.2   Other cervical disc displacement

      M50.20   Other cervical disc displacement, unspecified cervical region   A ▽

      M50.21   Other cervical disc displacement, high cervical region   A
         Other C2-C3 cervical disc displacement
         Other C3-C4 cervical disc displacement

      M50.22   Other cervical disc displacement, mid-cervical region   A
         Other C4-C5 cervical disc displacement
         Other C5-C6 cervical disc displacement
         Other C6-C7 cervical disc displacement

      M50.23   Other cervical disc displacement, cervicothoracic region   A
         Other C7-T1 cervical disc displacement

    ✓5ᵗʰ M50.3   Other cervical disc degeneration

      M50.30   Other cervical disc degeneration, unspecified cervical region   A ▽

      M50.31   Other cervical disc degeneration, high cervical region   A
         Other C2-C3 cervical disc degeneration
         Other C3-C4 cervical disc degeneration

      M50.32   Other cervical disc degeneration, mid-cervical region   A
         Other C4-C5 cervical disc degeneration
         Other C5-C6 cervical disc degeneration
         Other C6-C7 cervical disc degeneration

      M50.33   Other cervical disc degeneration, cervicothoracic region   A
         Other C7-T1 cervical disc degeneration

    ✓5ᵗʰ M50.8   Other cervical disc disorders

      M50.80   Other cervical disc disorders, unspecified cervical region   A ▽

      M50.81   Other cervical disc disorders, high cervical region   A
         Other C2-C3 cervical disc disorders
         Other C3-C4 cervical disc disorders

      M50.82   Other cervical disc disorders, mid-cervical region   A
         Other C4-C5 cervical disc disorders
         Other C5-C6 cervical disc disorders
         Other C6-C7 cervical disc disorders

      M50.83   Other cervical disc disorders, cervicothoracic region   A
         Other C7-T1 cervical disc disorders

    ✓5ᵗʰ M50.9   Cervical disc disorder, unspecified

      M50.90   Cervical disc disorder, unspecified, unspecified cervical region   A ▽

      M50.91   Cervical disc disorder, unspecified, high cervical region   A ▽
         C2-C3 cervical disc disorder, unspecified
         C3-C4 cervical disc disorder, unspecified

      M50.92   Cervical disc disorder, unspecified, mid-cervical region   A ▽
         C4-C5 cervical disc disorder, unspecified
         C5-C6 cervical disc disorder, unspecified
         C6-C7 cervical disc disorder, unspecified

      M50.93   Cervical disc disorder, unspecified, cervicothoracic region   A ▽
         C7-T1 cervical disc disorder, unspecified

✓4ᵗʰ M51   Thoracic, thoracolumbar, and lumbosacral intervertebral disc disorders

        EXCLUDES 2   cervical and cervicothoracic disc disorders (M50.-)
              sacral and sacrococcygeal disorders (M53.3)

    ✓5ᵗʰ M51.0   Thoracic, thoracolumbar and lumbosacral intervertebral disc disorders with myelopathy

      M51.04   Intervertebral disc disorders with myelopathy, thoracic region   A

      M51.05   Intervertebral disc disorders with myelopathy, thoracolumbar region   A

      M51.06   Intervertebral disc disorders with myelopathy, lumbar region   A

    ✓5ᵗʰ M51.1   Thoracic, thoracolumbar and lumbosacral intervertebral disc disorders with radiculopathy
        Sciatica due to intervertebral disc disorder

        EXCLUDES 1   lumbar radiculitis NOS (M54.16)
              sciatica NOS (M54.3)

      M51.14   Intervertebral disc disorders with radiculopathy, thoracic region

      M51.15   Intervertebral disc disorders with radiculopathy, thoracolumbar region

      M51.16   Intervertebral disc disorders with radiculopathy, lumbar region

      M51.17   Intervertebral disc disorders with radiculopathy, lumbosacral region

    ✓5ᵗʰ M51.2   Other thoracic, thoracolumbar and lumbosacral intervertebral disc displacement
        Lumbago due to displacement of intervertebral disc

      M51.24   Other intervertebral disc displacement, thoracic region   A

      M51.25   Other intervertebral disc displacement, thoracolumbar region   A

      M51.26   Other intervertebral disc displacement, lumbar region   A

      M51.27   Other intervertebral disc displacement, lumbosacral region   A

    ✓5ᵗʰ M51.3   Other thoracic, thoracolumbar and lumbosacral intervertebral disc degeneration
        AHA: 2013, 3Q, 22

      M51.34   Other intervertebral disc degeneration, thoracic region   A

      M51.35   Other intervertebral disc degeneration, thoracolumbar region   A

      M51.36   Other intervertebral disc degeneration, lumbar region

      M51.37   Other intervertebral disc degeneration, lumbosacral region

✓ Add'l Character Required   ✓x7ᵗʰ Placeholder Alert   RUG IV Special Care High Dx   RUG IV Clinically Complex Dx   RUG IV Special Care Low Dx   Manifestation Code   Other Specified Code   ▽ Unspecified Code

ICD-10-CM 2016   717

✓5ᵗʰ **M51.4 Schmorl's nodes**

    M51.44 Schmorl's nodes, thoracic region 🅐

    M51.45 Schmorl's nodes, thoracolumbar region 🅐

    M51.46 Schmorl's nodes, lumbar region 🅐

    M51.47 Schmorl's nodes, lumbosacral region 🅐

✓5ᵗʰ **M51.8 Other thoracic, thoracolumbar and lumbosacral intervertebral disc disorders**

    M51.84 Other intervertebral disc disorders, thoracic region 🅐

    M51.85 Other intervertebral disc disorders, thoracolumbar region 🅐

    M51.86 Other intervertebral disc disorders, lumbar region 🅐

    M51.87 Other intervertebral disc disorders, lumbosacral region 🅐

  M51.9 Unspecified thoracic, thoracolumbar and lumbosacral intervertebral disc disorder ▽

✓4ᵗʰ **M53 Other and unspecified dorsopathies, not elsewhere classified**

  M53.0 Cervicocranial syndrome
    Posterior cervical sympathetic syndrome

  M53.1 Cervicobrachial syndrome
    EXCLUDES 2   *cervical disc disorder (M50.-)*
              thoracic outlet syndrome (G54.0)

✓5ᵗʰ **M53.2 Spinal instabilities**

  ✓6ᵗʰ **M53.2X Spinal instabilities**

    M53.2X1 Spinal instabilities, occipito-atlanto-axial region

    M53.2X2 Spinal instabilities, cervical region

    M53.2X3 Spinal instabilities, cervicothoracic region

    M53.2X4 Spinal instabilities, thoracic region

    M53.2X5 Spinal instabilities, thoracolumbar region

    M53.2X6 Spinal instabilities, lumbar region

    M53.2X7 Spinal instabilities, lumbosacral region

    M53.2X8 Spinal instabilities, sacral and sacrococcygeal region

    M53.2X9 Spinal instabilities, site unspecified ▽

  M53.3 Sacrococcygeal disorders, not elsewhere classified
    Coccygodynia

✓5ᵗʰ **M53.8 Other specified dorsopathies**

    M53.80 Other specified dorsopathies, site unspecified ▽

    M53.81 Other specified dorsopathies, occipito-atlanto-axial region

    M53.82 Other specified dorsopathies, cervical region

    M53.83 Other specified dorsopathies, cervicothoracic region

    M53.84 Other specified dorsopathies, thoracic region

    M53.85 Other specified dorsopathies, thoracolumbar region

    M53.86 Other specified dorsopathies, lumbar region

    M53.87 Other specified dorsopathies, lumbosacral region

    M53.88 Other specified dorsopathies, sacral and sacrococcygeal region

  M53.9 Dorsopathy, unspecified ▽

✓4ᵗʰ **M54 Dorsalgia**
    EXCLUDES 1   *psychogenic dorsalgia (F45.41)*

  ✓5ᵗʰ **M54.0 Panniculitis affecting regions of neck and back**
    EXCLUDES 1   *lupus panniculitis (L93.2)*
              panniculitis NOS (M79.3)
              relapsing [Weber-Christian] panniculitis (M35.6)

    M54.00 Panniculitis affecting regions of neck and back, site unspecified ▽

    M54.01 Panniculitis affecting regions of neck and back, occipito-atlanto-axial region

    M54.02 Panniculitis affecting regions of neck and back, cervical region

    M54.03 Panniculitis affecting regions of neck and back, cervicothoracic region

    M54.04 Panniculitis affecting regions of neck and back, thoracic region

    M54.05 Panniculitis affecting regions of neck and back, thoracolumbar region

    M54.06 Panniculitis affecting regions of neck and back, lumbar region

    M54.07 Panniculitis affecting regions of neck and back, lumbosacral region

    M54.08 Panniculitis affecting regions of neck and back, sacral and sacrococcygeal region

    M54.09 Panniculitis affecting regions, neck and back, multiple sites in spine

  ✓5ᵗʰ **M54.1 Radiculopathy**
    Brachial neuritis or radiculitis NOS
    Lumbar neuritis or radiculitis NOS
    Lumbosacral neuritis or radiculitis NOS
    Thoracic neuritis or radiculitis NOS
    Radiculitis NOS
    EXCLUDES 1   *neuralgia and neuritis NOS (M79.2)*
              radiculopathy with cervical disc disorder (M50.1)
              radiculopathy with lumbar and other intervertebral disc disorder (M51.1-)
              radiculopathy with spondylosis (M47.2-)

    M54.10 Radiculopathy, site unspecified ▽

    M54.11 Radiculopathy, occipito-atlanto-axial region

    M54.12 Radiculopathy, cervical region

    M54.13 Radiculopathy, cervicothoracic region

    M54.14 Radiculopathy, thoracic region

    M54.15 Radiculopathy, thoracolumbar region

    M54.16 Radiculopathy, lumbar region

    M54.17 Radiculopathy, lumbosacral region

    M54.18 Radiculopathy, sacral and sacrococcygeal region

  M54.2 Cervicalgia
    EXCLUDES 1   *cervicalgia due to intervertebral cervical disc disorder (M50.-)*

  ✓5ᵗʰ **M54.3 Sciatica**
    EXCLUDES 1   *lesion of sciatic nerve (G57.0)*
              sciatica due to intervertebral disc disorder (M51.1-)
              sciatica with lumbago (M54.4-)

    M54.30 Sciatica, unspecified side ▽

    M54.31 Sciatica, right side

    M54.32 Sciatica, left side

  ✓5ᵗʰ **M54.4 Lumbago with sciatica**
    EXCLUDES 1   *lumbago with sciatica due to intervertebral disc disorder (M51.1-)*

    M54.40 Lumbago with sciatica, unspecified side ▽

    M54.41 Lumbago with sciatica, right side

    M54.42 Lumbago with sciatica, left side

  M54.5 Low back pain
    Loin pain
    Lumbago NOS
    EXCLUDES 1   *low back strain (S39.012)*
              lumbago due to intervertebral disc displacement (M51.2-)
              lumbago with sciatica (M54.4-)

  M54.6 Pain in thoracic spine
    EXCLUDES 1   *pain in thoracic spine due to intervertebral disc disorder (M51.-)*

  ✓5ᵗʰ **M54.8 Other dorsalgia**
    EXCLUDES 1   *dorsalgia in thoracic region (M54.6)*
              low back pain (M54.5)

    M54.81 Occipital neuralgia

    M54.89 Other dorsalgia

  M54.9 Dorsalgia, unspecified ▽
    Backache NOS   Back pain NOS

ℕ Newborn   ℙ Pediatric   Ⓜ Maternity   🅐 Adult   **RIC** RIC Dx   **NC Dx** Noncancer Dx   **PDx** Primary Dx   **CC** RIC CC Condition   ►◄ Revised Text   ● New Code   ▲ Revised Code Title

718   ICD-10-CM 2016

SOFT TISSUE DISORDERS (M60-M79)

Disorders of muscles (M60-M63)

EXCLUDES 1   dermatopolymyositis (M33.-)
muscular dystrophies and myopathies (G71-G72)
myopathy in amyloidosis (E85.-)
myopathy in polyarteritis nodosa (M30.0)
myopathy in rheumatoid arthritis (M05.32)
myopathy in scleroderma (M34.-)
myopathy in Sjögren's syndrome (M35.03)
myopathy in systemic lupus erythematosus (M32.-)

✓4ᵗʰ **M60 Myositis**
    EXCLUDES 2   inclusion body myositis [IBM] (G72.41)

✓5ᵗʰ **M60.0 Infective myositis**
    Tropical pyomyositis
    Use additional code (B95-B97) to identify infectious agent

   ✓6ᵗʰ **M60.00 Infective myositis,** unspecified site
       M60.000 Infective myositis, unspecified right arm
         Infective myositis, right upper limb NOS
       M60.001 Infective myositis, unspecified left arm
         Infective myositis, left upper limb NOS
       M60.002 Infective myositis, unspecified arm   ▽
         Infective myositis, upper limb NOS
       M60.003 Infective myositis, unspecified right leg
         Infective myositis, right lower limb NOS
       M60.004 Infective myositis, unspecified left leg
         Infective myositis, left lower limb NOS
       M60.005 Infective myositis, unspecified leg   ▽
         Infective myositis, lower limb NOS
       M60.009 Infective myositis, unspecified site   ▽

   ✓6ᵗʰ **M60.01 Infective myositis,** shoulder
       M60.011 Infective myositis, right shoulder
       M60.012 Infective myositis, left shoulder
       M60.019 Infective myositis, unspecified   ▽
         shoulder

   ✓6ᵗʰ **M60.02 Infective myositis,** upper arm
       M60.021 Infective myositis, right upper arm
       M60.022 Infective myositis, left upper arm
       M60.029 Infective myositis, unspecified   ▽
         upper arm

   ✓6ᵗʰ **M60.03 Infective myositis,** forearm
       M60.031 Infective myositis, right forearm
       M60.032 Infective myositis, left forearm
       M60.039 Infective myositis, unspecified   ▽
         forearm

   ✓6ᵗʰ **M60.04 Infective myositis,** hand and fingers
       M60.041 Infective myositis, right hand
       M60.042 Infective myositis, left hand
       M60.043 Infective myositis, unspecified hand   ▽
       M60.044 Infective myositis, right finger(s)
       M60.045 Infective myositis, left finger(s)
       M60.046 Infective myositis, unspecified   ▽
         finger(s)

   ✓6ᵗʰ **M60.05 Infective myositis,** thigh
       M60.051 Infective myositis, right thigh
       M60.052 Infective myositis, left thigh
       M60.059 Infective myositis, unspecified thigh   ▽

   ✓6ᵗʰ **M60.06 Infective myositis,** lower leg
       M60.061 Infective myositis, right lower leg
       M60.062 Infective myositis, left lower leg
       M60.069 Infective myositis, unspecified   ▽
         lower leg

   ✓6ᵗʰ **M60.07 Infective myositis,** ankle, foot and toes
       M60.070 Infective myositis, right ankle
       M60.071 Infective myositis, left ankle
       M60.072 Infective myositis, unspecified ankle   ▽
       M60.073 Infective myositis, right foot
       M60.074 Infective myositis, left foot
       M60.075 Infective myositis, unspecified foot   ▽
       M60.076 Infective myositis, right toe(s)
       M60.077 Infective myositis, left toe(s)
       M60.078 Infective myositis, unspecified toe(s)   ▽
    M60.08 Infective myositis, other site
    M60.09 Infective myositis, multiple sites

✓5ᵗʰ **M60.1 Interstitial myositis**
    M60.10 Interstitial myositis of unspecified site   ▽
   ✓6ᵗʰ **M60.11 Interstitial myositis,** shoulder
       M60.111 Interstitial myositis, right shoulder
       M60.112 Interstitial myositis, left shoulder
       M60.119 Interstitial myositis, unspecified   ▽
         shoulder

   ✓6ᵗʰ **M60.12 Interstitial myositis,** upper arm
       M60.121 Interstitial myositis, right upper arm
       M60.122 Interstitial myositis, left upper arm
       M60.129 Interstitial myositis, unspecified   ▽
         upper arm

   ✓6ᵗʰ **M60.13 Interstitial myositis,** forearm
       M60.131 Interstitial myositis, right forearm
       M60.132 Interstitial myositis, left forearm
       M60.139 Interstitial myositis, unspecified   ▽
         forearm

   ✓6ᵗʰ **M60.14 Interstitial myositis,** hand
       M60.141 Interstitial myositis, right hand
       M60.142 Interstitial myositis, left hand
       M60.149 Interstitial myositis, unspecified   ▽
         hand

   ✓6ᵗʰ **M60.15 Interstitial myositis,** thigh
       M60.151 Interstitial myositis, right thigh
       M60.152 Interstitial myositis, left thigh
       M60.159 Interstitial myositis, unspecified   ▽
         thigh

   ✓6ᵗʰ **M60.16 Interstitial myositis,** lower leg
       M60.161 Interstitial myositis, right lower leg
       M60.162 Interstitial myositis, left lower leg
       M60.169 Interstitial myositis, unspecified   ▽
         lower leg

   ✓6ᵗʰ **M60.17 Interstitial myositis,** ankle and foot
       M60.171 Interstitial myositis, right ankle and foot
       M60.172 Interstitial myositis, left ankle and foot
       M60.179 Interstitial myositis, unspecified   ▽
         ankle and foot
    M60.18 Interstitial myositis, other site
    M60.19 Interstitial myositis, multiple sites

✓5ᵗʰ **M60.2 Foreign body granuloma of soft tissue, not elsewhere classified**
    Use additional code to identify the type of retained foreign body (Z18.-)
    EXCLUDES 1   foreign body granuloma of skin and subcutaneous tissue (L92.3)

    M60.20 Foreign body granuloma of soft tissue, not   ▽
       elsewhere classified, unspecified site

   ✓6ᵗʰ **M60.21 Foreign body granuloma of soft tissue, not**
       elsewhere classified, shoulder
       M60.211 Foreign body granuloma of soft tissue,
         not elsewhere classified, right shoulder
       M60.212 Foreign body granuloma of soft tissue,
         not elsewhere classified, left shoulder
       M60.219 Foreign body granuloma of soft   ▽
         tissue, not elsewhere classified, unspecified shoulder

   ✓6ᵗʰ **M60.22 Foreign body granuloma of soft tissue, not**
       elsewhere classified, upper arm
       M60.221 Foreign body granuloma of soft tissue,
         not elsewhere classified, right upper arm
       M60.222 Foreign body granuloma of soft tissue,
         not elsewhere classified, left upper arm
       M60.229 Foreign body granuloma of soft   ▽
         tissue, not elsewhere classified, unspecified upper arm

   ✓6ᵗʰ **M60.23 Foreign body granuloma of soft tissue, not**
       elsewhere classified, forearm
       M60.231 Foreign body granuloma of soft tissue,
         not elsewhere classified, right forearm
       M60.232 Foreign body granuloma of soft tissue,
         not elsewhere classified, left forearm
       M60.239 Foreign body granuloma of soft   ▽
         tissue, not elsewhere classified, unspecified forearm

✓6ᵗʰ **M60.24** Foreign body granuloma of soft tissue, not elsewhere classified, **hand**

M60.241 Foreign body granuloma of soft tissue, not elsewhere classified, **right hand**

M60.242 Foreign body granuloma of soft tissue, not elsewhere classified, **left hand**

M60.249 Foreign body granuloma of soft tissue, not elsewhere classified, unspecified hand ▽

✓6ᵗʰ **M60.25** Foreign body granuloma of soft tissue, not elsewhere classified, **thigh**

M60.251 Foreign body granuloma of soft tissue, not elsewhere classified, **right thigh**

M60.252 Foreign body granuloma of soft tissue, not elsewhere classified, **left thigh**

M60.259 Foreign body granuloma of soft tissue, not elsewhere classified, unspecified thigh ▽

✓6ᵗʰ **M60.26** Foreign body granuloma of soft tissue, not elsewhere classified, **lower leg**

M60.261 Foreign body granuloma of soft tissue, not elsewhere classified, **right lower leg**

M60.262 Foreign body granuloma of soft tissue, not elsewhere classified, **left lower leg**

M60.269 Foreign body granuloma of soft tissue, not elsewhere classified, unspecified lower leg ▽

✓6ᵗʰ **M60.27** Foreign body granuloma of soft tissue, not elsewhere classified, **ankle and foot**

M60.271 Foreign body granuloma of soft tissue, not elsewhere classified, **right ankle and foot**

M60.272 Foreign body granuloma of soft tissue, not elsewhere classified, **left ankle and foot**

M60.279 Foreign body granuloma of soft tissue, not elsewhere classified, unspecified ankle and foot ▽

M60.28 Foreign body granuloma of soft tissue, not elsewhere classified, other site

✓5ᵗʰ **M60.8** Other myositis

M60.80 Other myositis, unspecified site ▽

✓6ᵗʰ **M60.81** Other myositis, **shoulder**

M60.811 Other myositis, **right shoulder**

M60.812 Other myositis, **left shoulder**

M60.819 Other myositis, unspecified shoulder ▽

✓6ᵗʰ **M60.82** Other myositis, **upper arm**

M60.821 Other myositis, **right upper arm**

M60.822 Other myositis, **left upper arm**

M60.829 Other myositis, unspecified upper arm ▽

✓6ᵗʰ **M60.83** Other myositis, **forearm**

M60.831 Other myositis, **right forearm**

M60.832 Other myositis, **left forearm**

M60.839 Other myositis, unspecified forearm ▽

✓6ᵗʰ **M60.84** Other myositis, **hand**

M60.841 Other myositis, **right hand**

M60.842 Other myositis, **left hand**

M60.849 Other myositis, unspecified hand ▽

✓6ᵗʰ **M60.85** Other myositis, **thigh**

M60.851 Other myositis, **right thigh**

M60.852 Other myositis, **left thigh**

M60.859 Other myositis, unspecified thigh ▽

✓6ᵗʰ **M60.86** Other myositis, **lower leg**

M60.861 Other myositis, **right lower leg**

M60.862 Other myositis, **left lower leg**

M60.869 Other myositis, unspecified lower leg ▽

✓6ᵗʰ **M60.87** Other myositis, **ankle and foot**

M60.871 Other myositis, **right ankle and foot**

M60.872 Other myositis, **left ankle and foot**

M60.879 Other myositis, unspecified ankle and foot ▽

M60.88 Other myositis, other site

M60.89 Other myositis, **multiple sites**

M60.9 Myositis, unspecified ▽

✓4ᵗʰ **M61 Calcification and ossification of muscle**

✓5ᵗʰ **M61.0** Myositis ossificans traumatica

M61.00 Myositis ossificans traumatica, unspecified site ▽

✓6ᵗʰ **M61.01** Myositis ossificans traumatica, **shoulder**

M61.011 Myositis ossificans traumatica, **right shoulder**

M61.012 Myositis ossificans traumatica, **left shoulder**

M61.019 Myositis ossificans traumatica, unspecified shoulder ▽

✓6ᵗʰ **M61.02** Myositis ossificans traumatica, **upper arm**

M61.021 Myositis ossificans traumatica, **right upper arm**

M61.022 Myositis ossificans traumatica, **left upper arm**

M61.029 Myositis ossificans traumatica, unspecified upper arm ▽

✓6ᵗʰ **M61.03** Myositis ossificans traumatica, **forearm**

M61.031 Myositis ossificans traumatica, **right forearm**

M61.032 Myositis ossificans traumatica, **left forearm**

M61.039 Myositis ossificans traumatica, unspecified forearm ▽

✓6ᵗʰ **M61.04** Myositis ossificans traumatica, **hand**

M61.041 Myositis ossificans traumatica, **right hand**

M61.042 Myositis ossificans traumatica, **left hand**

M61.049 Myositis ossificans traumatica, unspecified hand ▽

✓6ᵗʰ **M61.05** Myositis ossificans traumatica, **thigh**

M61.051 Myositis ossificans traumatica, **right thigh**

M61.052 Myositis ossificans traumatica, **left thigh**

M61.059 Myositis ossificans traumatica, unspecified thigh ▽

✓6ᵗʰ **M61.06** Myositis ossificans traumatica, **lower leg**

M61.061 Myositis ossificans traumatica, **right lower leg**

M61.062 Myositis ossificans traumatica, **left lower leg**

M61.069 Myositis ossificans traumatica, unspecified lower leg ▽

✓6ᵗʰ **M61.07** Myositis ossificans traumatica, **ankle and foot**

M61.071 Myositis ossificans traumatica, **right ankle and foot**

M61.072 Myositis ossificans traumatica, **left ankle and foot**

M61.079 Myositis ossificans traumatica, unspecified ankle and foot ▽

M61.08 Myositis ossificans traumatica, other site

M61.09 Myositis ossificans traumatica, **multiple sites**

✓5ᵗʰ **M61.1** Myositis ossificans progressiva
Fibrodysplasia ossificans progressiva

M61.10 Myositis ossificans progressiva, unspecified site ▽

✓6ᵗʰ **M61.11** Myositis ossificans progressiva, **shoulder**

M61.111 Myositis ossificans progressiva, **right shoulder**

M61.112 Myositis ossificans progressiva, **left shoulder**

M61.119 Myositis ossificans progressiva, unspecified shoulder ▽

✓6ᵗʰ **M61.12** Myositis ossificans progressiva, **upper arm**

M61.121 Myositis ossificans progressiva, **right upper arm**

M61.122 Myositis ossificans progressiva, **left upper arm**

M61.129 Myositis ossificans progressiva, unspecified arm ▽

✓6ᵗʰ **M61.13** Myositis ossificans progressiva, **forearm**

M61.131 Myositis ossificans progressiva, **right forearm**

M61.132 Myositis ossificans progressiva, **left forearm**

M61.139 Myositis ossificans progressiva, unspecified forearm ▽

Ⓝ Newborn   Ⓟ Pediatric   Ⓜ Maternity   Ⓐ Adult   **RIC** RIC Dx   **NC Dx** Noncancer Dx   **PDx** Primary Dx   **CC** RIC CC Condition   ▶◀ Revised Text   ● New Code   ▲ Revised Code Title

720   ICD-10-CM 2016

✓6ᵗʰ **M61.14 Myositis ossificans progressiva, hand and finger(s)**
     M61.141 Myositis ossificans progressiva, right hand
     M61.142 Myositis ossificans progressiva, left hand
     M61.143 Myositis ossificans progressiva, unspecified hand ▽
     M61.144 Myositis ossificans progressiva, right finger(s)
     M61.145 Myositis ossificans progressiva, left finger(s)
     M61.146 Myositis ossificans progressiva, unspecified finger(s) ▽

✓6ᵗʰ **M61.15 Myositis ossificans progressiva, thigh**
     M61.151 Myositis ossificans progressiva, right thigh
     M61.152 Myositis ossificans progressiva, left thigh
     M61.159 Myositis ossificans progressiva, unspecified thigh ▽

✓6ᵗʰ **M61.16 Myositis ossificans progressiva, lower leg**
     M61.161 Myositis ossificans progressiva, right lower leg
     M61.162 Myositis ossificans progressiva, left lower leg
     M61.169 Myositis ossificans progressiva, unspecified lower leg ▽

✓6ᵗʰ **M61.17 Myositis ossificans progressiva, ankle, foot and toe(s)**
     M61.171 Myositis ossificans progressiva, right ankle
     M61.172 Myositis ossificans progressiva, left ankle
     M61.173 Myositis ossificans progressiva, unspecified ankle ▽
     M61.174 Myositis ossificans progressiva, right foot
     M61.175 Myositis ossificans progressiva, left foot
     M61.176 Myositis ossificans progressiva, unspecified foot ▽
     M61.177 Myositis ossificans progressiva, right toe(s)
     M61.178 Myositis ossificans progressiva, left toe(s)
     M61.179 Myositis ossificans progressiva, unspecified toe(s) ▽

M61.18 Myositis ossificans progressiva, other site
M61.19 Myositis ossificans progressiva, multiple sites

✓5ᵗʰ **M61.2 Paralytic calcification and ossification of muscle**
     Myositis ossificans associated with quadriplegia or paraplegia
     M61.20 Paralytic calcification and ossification of muscle, unspecified site ▽
✓6ᵗʰ **M61.21 Paralytic calcification and ossification of muscle, shoulder**
     M61.211 Paralytic calcification and ossification of muscle, right shoulder
     M61.212 Paralytic calcification and ossification of muscle, left shoulder
     M61.219 Paralytic calcification and ossification of muscle, unspecified shoulder ▽
✓6ᵗʰ **M61.22 Paralytic calcification and ossification of muscle, upper arm**
     M61.221 Paralytic calcification and ossification of muscle, right upper arm
     M61.222 Paralytic calcification and ossification of muscle, left upper arm
     M61.229 Paralytic calcification and ossification of muscle, unspecified upper arm ▽
✓6ᵗʰ **M61.23 Paralytic calcification and ossification of muscle, forearm**
     M61.231 Paralytic calcification and ossification of muscle, right forearm
     M61.232 Paralytic calcification and ossification of muscle, left forearm
     M61.239 Paralytic calcification and ossification of muscle, unspecified forearm ▽
✓6ᵗʰ **M61.24 Paralytic calcification and ossification of muscle, hand**
     M61.241 Paralytic calcification and ossification of muscle, right hand
     M61.242 Paralytic calcification and ossification of muscle, left hand

     M61.249 Paralytic calcification and ossification of muscle, unspecified hand ▽
✓6ᵗʰ **M61.25 Paralytic calcification and ossification of muscle, thigh**
     M61.251 Paralytic calcification and ossification of muscle, right thigh
     M61.252 Paralytic calcification and ossification of muscle, left thigh
     M61.259 Paralytic calcification and ossification of muscle, unspecified thigh ▽
✓6ᵗʰ **M61.26 Paralytic calcification and ossification of muscle, lower leg**
     M61.261 Paralytic calcification and ossification of muscle, right lower leg
     M61.262 Paralytic calcification and ossification of muscle, left lower leg
     M61.269 Paralytic calcification and ossification of muscle, unspecified lower leg ▽
✓6ᵗʰ **M61.27 Paralytic calcification and ossification of muscle, ankle and foot**
     M61.271 Paralytic calcification and ossification of muscle, right ankle and foot
     M61.272 Paralytic calcification and ossification of muscle, left ankle and foot
     M61.279 Paralytic calcification and ossification of muscle, unspecified ankle and foot ▽
     M61.28 Paralytic calcification and ossification of muscle, other site
     M61.29 Paralytic calcification and ossification of muscle, multiple sites

✓5ᵗʰ **M61.3 Calcification and ossification of muscles associated with burns**
     Myositis ossificans associated with burns
     M61.30 Calcification and ossification of muscles associated with burns, unspecified site ▽
✓6ᵗʰ **M61.31 Calcification and ossification of muscles associated with burns, shoulder**
     M61.311 Calcification and ossification of muscles associated with burns, right shoulder
     M61.312 Calcification and ossification of muscles associated with burns, left shoulder
     M61.319 Calcification and ossification of muscles associated with burns, unspecified shoulder ▽
✓6ᵗʰ **M61.32 Calcification and ossification of muscles associated with burns, upper arm**
     M61.321 Calcification and ossification of muscles associated with burns, right upper arm
     M61.322 Calcification and ossification of muscles associated with burns, left upper arm
     M61.329 Calcification and ossification of muscles associated with burns, unspecified upper arm ▽
✓6ᵗʰ **M61.33 Calcification and ossification of muscles associated with burns, forearm**
     M61.331 Calcification and ossification of muscles associated with burns, right forearm
     M61.332 Calcification and ossification of muscles associated with burns, left forearm
     M61.339 Calcification and ossification of muscles associated with burns, unspecified forearm ▽
✓6ᵗʰ **M61.34 Calcification and ossification of muscles associated with burns, hand**
     M61.341 Calcification and ossification of muscles associated with burns, right hand
     M61.342 Calcification and ossification of muscles associated with burns, left hand
     M61.349 Calcification and ossification of muscles associated with burns, unspecified hand ▽
✓6ᵗʰ **M61.35 Calcification and ossification of muscles associated with burns, thigh**
     M61.351 Calcification and ossification of muscles associated with burns, right thigh
     M61.352 Calcification and ossification of muscles associated with burns, left thigh

---

☑ Add'l Character Required   ✓ᵡ7ᵗʰ Placeholder Alert   RUG IV Special Care High Dx   RUG IV Clinically Complex Dx   RUG IV Special Care Low Dx   Manifestation Code   Other Specified Code   ▽ Unspecified Code

M61.359   Calcification and ossification of muscles associated with burns, unspecified thigh ▽

✓6ᵗʰ **M61.36**   Calcification and ossification of muscles associated with burns, lower leg

     M61.361   Calcification and ossification of muscles associated with burns, right lower leg

     M61.362   Calcification and ossification of muscles associated with burns, left lower leg

     M61.369   Calcification and ossification of muscles associated with burns, unspecified lower leg ▽

✓6ᵗʰ **M61.37**   Calcification and ossification of muscles associated with burns, ankle and foot

     M61.371   Calcification and ossification of muscles associated with burns, right ankle and foot

     M61.372   Calcification and ossification of muscles associated with burns, left ankle and foot

     M61.379   Calcification and ossification of muscles associated with burns, unspecified ankle and foot ▽

M61.38   Calcification and ossification of muscles associated with burns, other site

M61.39   Calcification and ossification of muscles associated with burns, multiple sites

✓5ᵗʰ **M61.4**   Other calcification of muscle

     EXCLUDES 1   calcific tendinitis NOS (M65.2-)
                 calcific tendinitis of shoulder (M75.3)

M61.40   Other calcification of muscle, unspecified site ▽

✓6ᵗʰ **M61.41**   Other calcification of muscle, shoulder

     M61.411   Other calcification of muscle, right shoulder

     M61.412   Other calcification of muscle, left shoulder

     M61.419   Other calcification of muscle, unspecified shoulder ▽

✓6ᵗʰ **M61.42**   Other calcification of muscle, upper arm

     M61.421   Other calcification of muscle, right upper arm

     M61.422   Other calcification of muscle, left upper arm

     M61.429   Other calcification of muscle, unspecified upper arm ▽

✓6ᵗʰ **M61.43**   Other calcification of muscle, forearm

     M61.431   Other calcification of muscle, right forearm

     M61.432   Other calcification of muscle, left forearm

     M61.439   Other calcification of muscle, unspecified forearm ▽

✓6ᵗʰ **M61.44**   Other calcification of muscle, hand

     M61.441   Other calcification of muscle, right hand

     M61.442   Other calcification of muscle, left hand

     M61.449   Other calcification of muscle, unspecified hand ▽

✓6ᵗʰ **M61.45**   Other calcification of muscle, thigh

     M61.451   Other calcification of muscle, right thigh

     M61.452   Other calcification of muscle, left thigh

     M61.459   Other calcification of muscle, unspecified thigh ▽

✓6ᵗʰ **M61.46**   Other calcification of muscle, lower leg

     M61.461   Other calcification of muscle, right lower leg

     M61.462   Other calcification of muscle, left lower leg

     M61.469   Other calcification of muscle, unspecified lower leg ▽

✓6ᵗʰ **M61.47**   Other calcification of muscle, ankle and foot

     M61.471   Other calcification of muscle, right ankle and foot

     M61.472   Other calcification of muscle, left ankle and foot

     M61.479   Other calcification of muscle, unspecified ankle and foot ▽

M61.48   Other calcification of muscle, other site

M61.49   Other calcification of muscle, multiple sites

✓5ᵗʰ **M61.5**   Other ossification of muscle

M61.50   Other ossification of muscle, unspecified site ▽

✓6ᵗʰ **M61.51**   Other ossification of muscle, shoulder

     M61.511   Other ossification of muscle, right shoulder

     M61.512   Other ossification of muscle, left shoulder

     M61.519   Other ossification of muscle, unspecified shoulder ▽

✓6ᵗʰ **M61.52**   Other ossification of muscle, upper arm

     M61.521   Other ossification of muscle, right upper arm

     M61.522   Other ossification of muscle, left upper arm

     M61.529   Other ossification of muscle, unspecified upper arm ▽

✓6ᵗʰ **M61.53**   Other ossification of muscle, forearm

     M61.531   Other ossification of muscle, right forearm

     M61.532   Other ossification of muscle, left forearm

     M61.539   Other ossification of muscle, unspecified forearm ▽

✓6ᵗʰ **M61.54**   Other ossification of muscle, hand

     M61.541   Other ossification of muscle, right hand

     M61.542   Other ossification of muscle, left hand

     M61.549   Other ossification of muscle, unspecified hand ▽

✓6ᵗʰ **M61.55**   Other ossification of muscle, thigh

     M61.551   Other ossification of muscle, right thigh

     M61.552   Other ossification of muscle, left thigh

     M61.559   Other ossification of muscle, unspecified thigh ▽

✓6ᵗʰ **M61.56**   Other ossification of muscle, lower leg

     M61.561   Other ossification of muscle, right lower leg

     M61.562   Other ossification of muscle, left lower leg

     M61.569   Other ossification of muscle, unspecified lower leg ▽

✓6ᵗʰ **M61.57**   Other ossification of muscle, ankle and foot

     M61.571   Other ossification of muscle, right ankle and foot

     M61.572   Other ossification of muscle, left ankle and foot

     M61.579   Other ossification of muscle, unspecified ankle and foot ▽

M61.58   Other ossification of muscle, other site

M61.59   Other ossification of muscle, multiple sites

M61.9   Calcification and ossification of muscle, unspecified ▽

✓4ᵗʰ **M62**   Other disorders of muscle

     EXCLUDES 1   alcoholic myopathy (G72.1)
                 cramp and spasm (R25.2)
                 drug-induced myopathy (G72.0)
                 myalgia (M79.1)
                 stiff-man syndrome (G25.82)
     EXCLUDES 2   nontraumatic hematoma of muscle (M79.81)

✓5ᵗʰ **M62.0**   Separation of muscle (nontraumatic)

     Diastasis of muscle

     EXCLUDES 1   diastasis recti complicating pregnancy, labor and delivery (O71.8)
                 traumatic separation of muscle—see strain of muscle by body region

M62.00   Separation of muscle (nontraumatic), unspecified site ▽

✓6ᵗʰ **M62.01**   Separation of muscle (nontraumatic), shoulder

     M62.011   Separation of muscle (nontraumatic), right shoulder

     M62.012   Separation of muscle (nontraumatic), left shoulder

     M62.019   Separation of muscle (nontraumatic), unspecified shoulder ▽

✓6ᵗʰ **M62.02**   Separation of muscle (nontraumatic), upper arm

     M62.021   Separation of muscle (nontraumatic), right upper arm

| Ⓝ Newborn | Ⓟ Pediatric | Ⓜ Maternity | Ⓐ Adult | **RIC** RIC Dx | **NC Dx** Noncancer Dx | **PDx** Primary Dx | **CC** RIC CC Condition | ►◄ Revised Text | ● New Code | ▲ Revised Code Title |

722   ICD-10-CM 2016

M62.022 Separation of muscle (nontraumatic), left upper arm

M62.029 Separation of muscle (nontraumatic), unspecified upper arm ▽

✓6ᵗʰ M62.03 Separation of muscle (nontraumatic), forearm

M62.031 Separation of muscle (nontraumatic), right forearm

M62.032 Separation of muscle (nontraumatic), left forearm

M62.039 Separation of muscle (nontraumatic), unspecified forearm ▽

✓6ᵗʰ M62.04 Separation of muscle (nontraumatic), hand

M62.041 Separation of muscle (nontraumatic), right hand

M62.042 Separation of muscle (nontraumatic), left hand

M62.049 Separation of muscle (nontraumatic), unspecified hand ▽

✓6ᵗʰ M62.05 Separation of muscle (nontraumatic), thigh

M62.051 Separation of muscle (nontraumatic), right thigh

M62.052 Separation of muscle (nontraumatic), left thigh

M62.059 Separation of muscle (nontraumatic), unspecified thigh ▽

✓6ᵗʰ M62.06 Separation of muscle (nontraumatic), lower leg

M62.061 Separation of muscle (nontraumatic), right lower leg

M62.062 Separation of muscle (nontraumatic), left lower leg

M62.069 Separation of muscle (nontraumatic), unspecified lower leg ▽

✓6ᵗʰ M62.07 Separation of muscle (nontraumatic), ankle and foot

M62.071 Separation of muscle (nontraumatic), right ankle and foot

M62.072 Separation of muscle (nontraumatic), left ankle and foot

M62.079 Separation of muscle (nontraumatic), unspecified ankle and foot ▽

M62.08 Separation of muscle (nontraumatic), other site

✓5ᵗʰ M62.1 Other rupture of muscle (nontraumatic)

EXCLUDES 1 traumatic rupture of muscle—see strain of muscle by body region

EXCLUDES 2 rupture of tendon (M66.-)

M62.10 Other rupture of muscle (nontraumatic), unspecified site ▽

✓6ᵗʰ M62.11 Other rupture of muscle (nontraumatic), shoulder

M62.111 Other rupture of muscle (nontraumatic), right shoulder

M62.112 Other rupture of muscle (nontraumatic), left shoulder

M62.119 Other rupture of muscle (nontraumatic), unspecified shoulder ▽

✓6ᵗʰ M62.12 Other rupture of muscle (nontraumatic), upper arm

M62.121 Other rupture of muscle (nontraumatic), right upper arm

M62.122 Other rupture of muscle (nontraumatic), left upper arm

M62.129 Other rupture of muscle (nontraumatic), unspecified upper arm ▽

✓6ᵗʰ M62.13 Other rupture of muscle (nontraumatic), forearm

M62.131 Other rupture of muscle (nontraumatic), right forearm

M62.132 Other rupture of muscle (nontraumatic), left forearm

M62.139 Other rupture of muscle (nontraumatic), unspecified forearm ▽

✓6ᵗʰ M62.14 Other rupture of muscle (nontraumatic), hand

M62.141 Other rupture of muscle (nontraumatic), right hand

M62.142 Other rupture of muscle (nontraumatic), left hand

M62.149 Other rupture of muscle (nontraumatic), unspecified hand ▽

✓6ᵗʰ M62.15 Other rupture of muscle (nontraumatic), thigh

M62.151 Other rupture of muscle (nontraumatic), right thigh

M62.152 Other rupture of muscle (nontraumatic), left thigh

M62.159 Other rupture of muscle (nontraumatic), unspecified thigh ▽

✓6ᵗʰ M62.16 Other rupture of muscle (nontraumatic), lower leg

M62.161 Other rupture of muscle (nontraumatic), right lower leg

M62.162 Other rupture of muscle (nontraumatic), left lower leg

M62.169 Other rupture of muscle (nontraumatic), unspecified lower leg ▽

✓6ᵗʰ M62.17 Other rupture of muscle (nontraumatic), ankle and foot

M62.171 Other rupture of muscle (nontraumatic), right ankle and foot

M62.172 Other rupture of muscle (nontraumatic), left ankle and foot

M62.179 Other rupture of muscle (nontraumatic), unspecified ankle and foot ▽

M62.18 Other rupture of muscle (nontraumatic), other site

✓5ᵗʰ M62.2 Nontraumatic ischemic infarction of muscle

EXCLUDES 1 compartment syndrome (traumatic) (T79.A-)
nontraumatic compartment syndrome (M79.A-)
rhabdomyolysis (M62.82)
traumatic ischemia of muscle (T79.6)
Volkmann's ischemic contracture (T79.6)

M62.20 Nontraumatic ischemic infarction of muscle, unspecified site ▽

✓6ᵗʰ M62.21 Nontraumatic ischemic infarction of muscle, shoulder

M62.211 Nontraumatic ischemic infarction of muscle, right shoulder

M62.212 Nontraumatic ischemic infarction of muscle, left shoulder

M62.219 Nontraumatic ischemic infarction of muscle, unspecified shoulder ▽

✓6ᵗʰ M62.22 Nontraumatic ischemic infarction of muscle, upper arm

M62.221 Nontraumatic ischemic infarction of muscle, right upper arm

M62.222 Nontraumatic ischemic infarction of muscle, left upper arm

M62.229 Nontraumatic ischemic infarction of muscle, unspecified upper arm ▽

✓6ᵗʰ M62.23 Nontraumatic ischemic infarction of muscle, forearm

M62.231 Nontraumatic ischemic infarction of muscle, right forearm

M62.232 Nontraumatic ischemic infarction of muscle, left forearm

M62.239 Nontraumatic ischemic infarction of muscle, unspecified forearm ▽

✓6ᵗʰ M62.24 Nontraumatic ischemic infarction of muscle, hand

M62.241 Nontraumatic ischemic infarction of muscle, right hand

M62.242 Nontraumatic ischemic infarction of muscle, left hand

M62.249 Nontraumatic ischemic infarction of muscle, unspecified hand ▽

✓6ᵗʰ M62.25 Nontraumatic ischemic infarction of muscle, thigh

M62.251 Nontraumatic ischemic infarction of muscle, right thigh

M62.252 Nontraumatic ischemic infarction of muscle, left thigh

M62.259 Nontraumatic ischemic infarction of muscle, unspecified thigh ▽

✓6ᵗʰ M62.26 Nontraumatic ischemic infarction of muscle, lower leg

M62.261 Nontraumatic ischemic infarction of muscle, right lower leg

M62.262 Nontraumatic ischemic infarction of muscle, left lower leg

M62.269 Nontraumatic ischemic infarction of muscle, unspecified lower leg ▽

✓6ᵗʰ M62.27 Nontraumatic ischemic infarction of muscle, ankle and foot

M62.271 Nontraumatic ischemic infarction of muscle, right ankle and foot

☑ Add'l Character Required   x7ᵗʰ Placeholder Alert   RUG IV Special Care High Dx   RUG IV Clinically Complex Dx   RUG IV Special Care Low Dx   Manifestation Code   Other Specified Code   ▽ Unspecified Code

ICD-10-CM 2016   723

M62.022–M62.271

      M62.272   **Nontraumatic ischemic infarction of muscle, left ankle and foot**

      M62.279   **Nontraumatic ischemic infarction of muscle, unspecified ankle and foot** ▽

   M62.28   **Nontraumatic ischemic infarction of muscle, other site**

  M62.3   **Immobility syndrome (paraplegic)**

✓5ᵗʰ   M62.4   **Contracture of muscle**
Contracture of tendon (sheath)
EXCLUDES 1   contracture of joint (M24.5-)

   M62.40   **Contracture of muscle, unspecified site** ▽

   ✓6ᵗʰ   M62.41   **Contracture of muscle, shoulder**
      M62.411   **Contracture of muscle, right shoulder**
      M62.412   **Contracture of muscle, left shoulder**
      M62.419   **Contracture of muscle, unspecified shoulder** ▽

   ✓6ᵗʰ   M62.42   **Contracture of muscle, upper arm**
      M62.421   **Contracture of muscle, right upper arm**
      M62.422   **Contracture of muscle, left upper arm**
      M62.429   **Contracture of muscle, unspecified upper arm** ▽

   ✓6ᵗʰ   M62.43   **Contracture of muscle, forearm**
      M62.431   **Contracture of muscle, right forearm**
      M62.432   **Contracture of muscle, left forearm**
      M62.439   **Contracture of muscle, unspecified forearm** ▽

   ✓6ᵗʰ   M62.44   **Contracture of muscle, hand**
      M62.441   **Contracture of muscle, right hand**
      M62.442   **Contracture of muscle, left hand**
      M62.449   **Contracture of muscle, unspecified hand** ▽

   ✓6ᵗʰ   M62.45   **Contracture of muscle, thigh**
      M62.451   **Contracture of muscle, right thigh**
      M62.452   **Contracture of muscle, left thigh**
      M62.459   **Contracture of muscle, unspecified thigh** ▽

   ✓6ᵗʰ   M62.46   **Contracture of muscle, lower leg**
      M62.461   **Contracture of muscle, right lower leg**
      M62.462   **Contracture of muscle, left lower leg**
      M62.469   **Contracture of muscle, unspecified lower leg** ▽

   ✓6ᵗʰ   M62.47   **Contracture of muscle, ankle and foot**
      M62.471   **Contracture of muscle, right ankle and foot**
      M62.472   **Contracture of muscle, left ankle and foot**
      M62.479   **Contracture of muscle, unspecified ankle and foot** ▽

   M62.48   **Contracture of muscle, other site**
   M62.49   **Contracture of muscle, multiple sites**

✓5ᵗʰ   M62.5   **Muscle wasting and atrophy, not elsewhere classified**
Disuse atrophy NEC
EXCLUDES 1   neuralgic amyotrophy (G54.5)
        progressive muscular atrophy (G12.29)
EXCLUDES 2   pelvic muscle wasting (N81.84)

   M62.50   **Muscle wasting and atrophy, not elsewhere classified, unspecified site** ▽

   ✓6ᵗʰ   M62.51   **Muscle wasting and atrophy, not elsewhere classified, shoulder**
      M62.511   **Muscle wasting and atrophy, not elsewhere classified, right shoulder**
      M62.512   **Muscle wasting and atrophy, not elsewhere classified, left shoulder**
      M62.519   **Muscle wasting and atrophy, not elsewhere classified, unspecified shoulder** ▽

   ✓6ᵗʰ   M62.52   **Muscle wasting and atrophy, not elsewhere classified, upper arm**
      M62.521   **Muscle wasting and atrophy, not elsewhere classified, right upper arm**
      M62.522   **Muscle wasting and atrophy, not elsewhere classified, left upper arm**
      M62.529   **Muscle wasting and atrophy, not elsewhere classified, unspecified upper arm** ▽

   ✓6ᵗʰ   M62.53   **Muscle wasting and atrophy, not elsewhere classified, forearm**
      M62.531   **Muscle wasting and atrophy, not elsewhere classified, right forearm**
      M62.532   **Muscle wasting and atrophy, not elsewhere classified, left forearm**
      M62.539   **Muscle wasting and atrophy, not elsewhere classified, unspecified forearm** ▽

   ✓6ᵗʰ   M62.54   **Muscle wasting and atrophy, not elsewhere classified, hand**
      M62.541   **Muscle wasting and atrophy, not elsewhere classified, right hand**
      M62.542   **Muscle wasting and atrophy, not elsewhere classified, left hand**
      M62.549   **Muscle wasting and atrophy, not elsewhere classified, unspecified hand** ▽

   ✓6ᵗʰ   M62.55   **Muscle wasting and atrophy, not elsewhere classified, thigh**
      M62.551   **Muscle wasting and atrophy, not elsewhere classified, right thigh**
      M62.552   **Muscle wasting and atrophy, not elsewhere classified, left thigh**
      M62.559   **Muscle wasting and atrophy, not elsewhere classified, unspecified thigh** ▽

   ✓6ᵗʰ   M62.56   **Muscle wasting and atrophy, not elsewhere classified, lower leg**
      M62.561   **Muscle wasting and atrophy, not elsewhere classified, right lower leg**
      M62.562   **Muscle wasting and atrophy, not elsewhere classified, left lower leg**
      M62.569   **Muscle wasting and atrophy, not elsewhere classified, unspecified lower leg** ▽

   ✓6ᵗʰ   M62.57   **Muscle wasting and atrophy, not elsewhere classified, ankle and foot**
      M62.571   **Muscle wasting and atrophy, not elsewhere classified, right ankle and foot**
      M62.572   **Muscle wasting and atrophy, not elsewhere classified, left ankle and foot**
      M62.579   **Muscle wasting and atrophy, not elsewhere classified, unspecified ankle and foot** ▽

   M62.58   **Muscle wasting and atrophy, not elsewhere classified, other site**

   M62.59   **Muscle wasting and atrophy, not elsewhere classified, multiple sites**

✓5ᵗʰ   M62.8   **Other specified disorders of muscle**
EXCLUDES 2   nontraumatic hematoma of muscle (M79.81)

   M62.81   **Muscle weakness (generalized)**

   M62.82   **Rhabdomyolysis**
EXCLUDES 1   traumatic rhabdomyolysis (T79.6)

   ✓6ᵗʰ   M62.83   **Muscle spasm**
      M62.830   **Muscle spasm of back**
      M62.831   **Muscle spasm of calf**
          Charley-horse
      M62.838   **Other muscle spasm**

   M62.89   **Other specified disorders of muscle**
Muscle (sheath) hernia

  M62.9   **Disorder of muscle, unspecified** ▽

✓4ᵗʰ   **M63   Disorders of muscle in diseases classified elsewhere**
Code first underlying disease, such as:
   leprosy (A30.-)
   neoplasm (C49-, C79.89, D21-, D48.1)
   schistosomiasis (B65.-)
   trichinellosis (B75)
EXCLUDES 1   myopathy in cysticercosis (B69.81)
        myopathy in endocrine diseases (G73.7)
        myopathy in metabolic diseases (G73.7)
        myopathy in sarcoidosis (D86.87)
        myopathy in secondary syphilis (A51.49)
        myopathy in syphilis (late) (A52.78)
        myopathy in toxoplasmosis (B58.82)
        myopathy in tuberculosis (A18.09)

Ⓝ Newborn   Ⓟ Pediatric   Ⓜ Maternity   Ⓐ Adult   **RIC** RIC Dx   **NC-Dx** Noncancer Dx   **PDx** Primary Dx   **CC** RIC CC Condition   ►◄ Revised Text   ● New Code   ▲ Revised Code Title

724   ICD-10-CM 2016

✓5ᵗʰ **M63.8 Disorders of muscle in diseases classified elsewhere**

M63.80 Disorders of muscle in diseases classified elsewhere, unspecified site ▽

✓6ᵗʰ **M63.81 Disorders of muscle in diseases classified elsewhere, shoulder**

M63.811 Disorders of muscle in diseases classified elsewhere, right shoulder

M63.812 Disorders of muscle in diseases classified elsewhere, left shoulder

M63.819 Disorders of muscle in diseases classified elsewhere, unspecified shoulder ▽

✓6ᵗʰ **M63.82 Disorders of muscle in diseases classified elsewhere, upper arm**

M63.821 Disorders of muscle in diseases classified elsewhere, right upper arm

M63.822 Disorders of muscle in diseases classified elsewhere, left upper arm

M63.829 Disorders of muscle in diseases classified elsewhere, unspecified upper arm ▽

✓6ᵗʰ **M63.83 Disorders of muscle in diseases classified elsewhere, forearm**

M63.831 Disorders of muscle in diseases classified elsewhere, right forearm

M63.832 Disorders of muscle in diseases classified elsewhere, left forearm

M63.839 Disorders of muscle in diseases classified elsewhere, unspecified forearm ▽

✓6ᵗʰ **M63.84 Disorders of muscle in diseases classified elsewhere, hand**

M63.841 Disorders of muscle in diseases classified elsewhere, right hand

M63.842 Disorders of muscle in diseases classified elsewhere, left hand

M63.849 Disorders of muscle in diseases classified elsewhere, unspecified hand ▽

✓6ᵗʰ **M63.85 Disorders of muscle in diseases classified elsewhere, thigh**

M63.851 Disorders of muscle in diseases classified elsewhere, right thigh

M63.852 Disorders of muscle in diseases classified elsewhere, left thigh

M63.859 Disorders of muscle in diseases classified elsewhere, unspecified thigh ▽

✓6ᵗʰ **M63.86 Disorders of muscle in diseases classified elsewhere, lower leg**

M63.861 Disorders of muscle in diseases classified elsewhere, right lower leg

M63.862 Disorders of muscle in diseases classified elsewhere, left lower leg

M63.869 Disorders of muscle in diseases classified elsewhere, unspecified lower leg ▽

✓6ᵗʰ **M63.87 Disorders of muscle in diseases classified elsewhere, ankle and foot**

M63.871 Disorders of muscle in diseases classified elsewhere, right ankle and foot

M63.872 Disorders of muscle in diseases classified elsewhere, left ankle and foot

M63.879 Disorders of muscle in diseases classified elsewhere, unspecified ankle and foot ▽

M63.88 Disorders of muscle in diseases classified elsewhere, other site

M63.89 Disorders of muscle in diseases classified elsewhere, multiple sites

Disorders of synovium and tendon (M65-M67)

✓4ᵗʰ **M65 Synovitis and tenosynovitis**

EXCLUDES 1 chronic crepitant synovitis of hand and wrist (M70.0-)
current injury—see injury of ligament or tendon by body region
soft tissue disorders related to use, overuse and pressure (M70.-)

✓5ᵗʰ **M65.0 Abscess of tendon sheath**

Use additional code (B95-B96) to identify bacterial agent.

M65.00 Abscess of tendon sheath, unspecified site ▽

✓6ᵗʰ **M65.01 Abscess of tendon sheath, shoulder**

M65.011 Abscess of tendon sheath, right shoulder

M65.012 Abscess of tendon sheath, left shoulder

M65.019 Abscess of tendon sheath, unspecified shoulder ▽

✓6ᵗʰ **M65.02 Abscess of tendon sheath, upper arm**

M65.021 Abscess of tendon sheath, right upper arm

M65.022 Abscess of tendon sheath, left upper arm

M65.029 Abscess of tendon sheath, unspecified upper arm ▽

✓6ᵗʰ **M65.03 Abscess of tendon sheath, forearm**

M65.031 Abscess of tendon sheath, right forearm

M65.032 Abscess of tendon sheath, left forearm

M65.039 Abscess of tendon sheath, unspecified forearm ▽

✓6ᵗʰ **M65.04 Abscess of tendon sheath, hand**

M65.041 Abscess of tendon sheath, right hand

M65.042 Abscess of tendon sheath, left hand

M65.049 Abscess of tendon sheath, unspecified hand ▽

✓6ᵗʰ **M65.05 Abscess of tendon sheath, thigh**

M65.051 Abscess of tendon sheath, right thigh

M65.052 Abscess of tendon sheath, left thigh

M65.059 Abscess of tendon sheath, unspecified thigh ▽

✓6ᵗʰ **M65.06 Abscess of tendon sheath, lower leg**

M65.061 Abscess of tendon sheath, right lower leg

M65.062 Abscess of tendon sheath, left lower leg

M65.069 Abscess of tendon sheath, unspecified lower leg ▽

✓6ᵗʰ **M65.07 Abscess of tendon sheath, ankle and foot**

M65.071 Abscess of tendon sheath, right ankle and foot

M65.072 Abscess of tendon sheath, left ankle and foot

M65.079 Abscess of tendon sheath, unspecified ankle and foot ▽

M65.08 Abscess of tendon sheath, other site

✓5ᵗʰ **M65.1 Other infective (teno)synovitis**

M65.10 Other infective (teno)synovitis, unspecified site ▽

✓6ᵗʰ **M65.11 Other infective (teno)synovitis, shoulder**

M65.111 Other infective (teno)synovitis, right shoulder

M65.112 Other infective (teno)synovitis, left shoulder

M65.119 Other infective (teno)synovitis, unspecified shoulder ▽

✓6ᵗʰ **M65.12 Other infective (teno)synovitis, elbow**

M65.121 Other infective (teno)synovitis, right elbow

M65.122 Other infective (teno)synovitis, left elbow

M65.129 Other infective (teno)synovitis, unspecified elbow ▽

✓6ᵗʰ **M65.13 Other infective (teno)synovitis, wrist**

M65.131 Other infective (teno)synovitis, right wrist

M65.132 Other infective (teno)synovitis, left wrist

M65.139 Other infective (teno)synovitis, unspecified wrist ▽

✓6ᵗʰ **M65.14 Other infective (teno)synovitis, hand**

M65.141 Other infective (teno)synovitis, right hand

M65.142 Other infective (teno)synovitis, left hand

M65.149 Other infective (teno)synovitis, unspecified hand ▽

✓6ᵗʰ **M65.15 Other infective (teno)synovitis, hip**

M65.151 Other infective (teno)synovitis, right hip

M65.152 Other infective (teno)synovitis, left hip

M65.159 Other infective (teno)synovitis, unspecified hip ▽

✓6ᵗʰ **M65.16 Other infective (teno)synovitis, knee**

M65.161 Other infective (teno)synovitis, right knee

M65.162 Other infective (teno)synovitis, left knee

M65.169 Other infective (teno)synovitis, unspecified knee ▽

✓6ᵗʰ **M65.17 Other infective (teno)synovitis, ankle and foot**

M65.171 Other infective (teno)synovitis, right ankle and foot

✓ Add'l Character Required ✓7ᵗʰ Placeholder Alert RUG IV Special Care High Dx RUG IV Clinically Complex Dx RUG IV Special Care Low Dx Manifestation Code Other Specified Code ▽ Unspecified Code

ICD-10-CM 2016 725

Chapter 13. Diseases of the Musculoskeletal System and Connective Tissue

M65.172–M66.132

       M65.172 Other infective (teno)synovitis, left ankle and foot

       M65.179 Other infective (teno)synovitis, unspecified ankle and foot ▽

    M65.18 Other infective (teno)synovitis, other site

    M65.19 Other infective (teno)synovitis, multiple sites

✓5ᵗʰ **M65.2 Calcific tendinitis**
> EXCLUDES 1   tendinitis as classified in M75-M77
> calcified tendinitis of shoulder (M75.3)

    M65.20 Calcific tendinitis, unspecified site ▽

✓6ᵗʰ **M65.22** Calcific tendinitis, upper arm
       M65.221 Calcific tendinitis, right upper arm
       M65.222 Calcific tendinitis, left upper arm
       M65.229 Calcific tendinitis, unspecified upper arm ▽

✓6ᵗʰ **M65.23** Calcific tendinitis, forearm
       M65.231 Calcific tendinitis, right forearm
       M65.232 Calcific tendinitis, left forearm
       M65.239 Calcific tendinitis, unspecified forearm ▽

✓6ᵗʰ **M65.24** Calcific tendinitis, hand
       M65.241 Calcific tendinitis, right hand
       M65.242 Calcific tendinitis, left hand
       M65.249 Calcific tendinitis, unspecified hand ▽

✓6ᵗʰ **M65.25** Calcific tendinitis, thigh
       M65.251 Calcific tendinitis, right thigh
       M65.252 Calcific tendinitis, left thigh
       M65.259 Calcific tendinitis, unspecified thigh ▽

✓6ᵗʰ **M65.26** Calcific tendinitis, lower leg
       M65.261 Calcific tendinitis, right lower leg
       M65.262 Calcific tendinitis, left lower leg
       M65.269 Calcific tendinitis, unspecified lower leg ▽

✓6ᵗʰ **M65.27** Calcific tendinitis, ankle and foot
       M65.271 Calcific tendinitis, right ankle and foot
       M65.272 Calcific tendinitis, left ankle and foot
       M65.279 Calcific tendinitis, unspecified ankle and foot ▽

    M65.28 Calcific tendinitis, other site

    M65.29 Calcific tendinitis, multiple sites

M65.3 Trigger finger
    Nodular tendinous disease

    M65.30 Trigger finger, unspecified finger ▽

✓6ᵗʰ **M65.31** Trigger thumb
       M65.311 Trigger thumb, right thumb
       M65.312 Trigger thumb, left thumb
       M65.319 Trigger thumb, unspecified thumb ▽

✓6ᵗʰ **M65.32** Trigger finger, index finger
       M65.321 Trigger finger, right index finger
       M65.322 Trigger finger, left index finger
       M65.329 Trigger finger, unspecified index finger ▽

✓6ᵗʰ **M65.33** Trigger finger, middle finger
       M65.331 Trigger finger, right middle finger
       M65.332 Trigger finger, left middle finger
       M65.339 Trigger finger, unspecified middle finger ▽

✓6ᵗʰ **M65.34** Trigger finger, ring finger
       M65.341 Trigger finger, right ring finger
       M65.342 Trigger finger, left ring finger
       M65.349 Trigger finger, unspecified ring finger ▽

✓6ᵗʰ **M65.35** Trigger finger, little finger
       M65.351 Trigger finger, right little finger
       M65.352 Trigger finger, left little finger
       M65.359 Trigger finger, unspecified little finger ▽

M65.4 Radial styloid tenosynovitis [de Quervain]

✓5ᵗʰ **M65.8 Other synovitis and tenosynovitis**
    M65.80 Other synovitis and tenosynovitis, unspecified site ▽

✓6ᵗʰ **M65.81** Other synovitis and tenosynovitis, shoulder
       M65.811 Other synovitis and tenosynovitis, right shoulder
       M65.812 Other synovitis and tenosynovitis, left shoulder
       M65.819 Other synovitis and tenosynovitis, unspecified shoulder ▽

✓6ᵗʰ **M65.82** Other synovitis and tenosynovitis, upper arm
       M65.821 Other synovitis and tenosynovitis, right upper arm
       M65.822 Other synovitis and tenosynovitis, left upper arm
       M65.829 Other synovitis and tenosynovitis, unspecified upper arm ▽

✓6ᵗʰ **M65.83** Other synovitis and tenosynovitis, forearm
       M65.831 Other synovitis and tenosynovitis, right forearm
       M65.832 Other synovitis and tenosynovitis, left forearm
       M65.839 Other synovitis and tenosynovitis, unspecified forearm ▽

✓6ᵗʰ **M65.84** Other synovitis and tenosynovitis, hand
       M65.841 Other synovitis and tenosynovitis, right hand
       M65.842 Other synovitis and tenosynovitis, left hand
       M65.849 Other synovitis and tenosynovitis, unspecified hand ▽

✓6ᵗʰ **M65.85** Other synovitis and tenosynovitis, thigh
       M65.851 Other synovitis and tenosynovitis, right thigh
       M65.852 Other synovitis and tenosynovitis, left thigh
       M65.859 Other synovitis and tenosynovitis, unspecified thigh ▽

✓6ᵗʰ **M65.86** Other synovitis and tenosynovitis, lower leg
       M65.861 Other synovitis and tenosynovitis, right lower leg
       M65.862 Other synovitis and tenosynovitis, left lower leg
       M65.869 Other synovitis and tenosynovitis, unspecified lower leg ▽

✓6ᵗʰ **M65.87** Other synovitis and tenosynovitis, ankle and foot
       M65.871 Other synovitis and tenosynovitis, right ankle and foot
       M65.872 Other synovitis and tenosynovitis, left ankle and foot
       M65.879 Other synovitis and tenosynovitis, unspecified ankle and foot ▽

    M65.88 Other synovitis and tenosynovitis, other site

    M65.89 Other synovitis and tenosynovitis, multiple sites

M65.9 Synovitis and tenosynovitis, unspecified ▽

✓4ᵗʰ **M66 Spontaneous rupture of synovium and tendon**
> INCLUDES   rupture that occurs when a normal force is applied to tissues that are inferred to have less than normal strength
> EXCLUDES 2   rotator cuff syndrome (M75.1-)
> rupture where an abnormal force is applied to normal tissue—see injury of tendon by body region

M66.0 Rupture of popliteal cyst

✓5ᵗʰ **M66.1 Rupture of synovium**
    Rupture of synovial cyst
> EXCLUDES 2   rupture of popliteal cyst (M66.0)

    M66.10 Rupture of synovium, unspecified joint ▽

✓6ᵗʰ **M66.11** Rupture of synovium, shoulder
       M66.111 Rupture of synovium, right shoulder
       M66.112 Rupture of synovium, left shoulder
       M66.119 Rupture of synovium, unspecified shoulder ▽

✓6ᵗʰ **M66.12** Rupture of synovium, elbow
       M66.121 Rupture of synovium, right elbow
       M66.122 Rupture of synovium, left elbow
       M66.129 Rupture of synovium, unspecified elbow ▽

✓6ᵗʰ **M66.13** Rupture of synovium, wrist
       M66.131 Rupture of synovium, right wrist
       M66.132 Rupture of synovium, left wrist

Ⓝ Newborn   Ⓟ Pediatric   Ⓜ Maternity   Ⓐ Adult   **RIC** RIC Dx   **NCDx** Noncancer Dx   **PDx** Primary Dx   **CC** RIC CC Condition   ▶◀ Revised Text   ● New Code   ▲ Revised Code Title

726   ICD-10-CM 2016

M66.139   Rupture of synovium, unspecified wrist ▽

✓6ᵗʰ **M66.14**   **Rupture of synovium, hand and fingers**
    M66.141   Rupture of synovium, right hand
    M66.142   Rupture of synovium, left hand
    M66.143   Rupture of synovium, unspecified hand ▽
    M66.144   Rupture of synovium, right finger(s)
    M66.145   Rupture of synovium, left finger(s)
    M66.146   Rupture of synovium, unspecified finger(s) ▽

✓6ᵗʰ **M66.15**   **Rupture of synovium, hip**
    M66.151   Rupture of synovium, right hip
    M66.152   Rupture of synovium, left hip
    M66.159   Rupture of synovium, unspecified hip ▽

✓6ᵗʰ **M66.17**   **Rupture of synovium, ankle, foot and toes**
    M66.171   Rupture of synovium, right ankle
    M66.172   Rupture of synovium, left ankle
    M66.173   Rupture of synovium, unspecified ankle ▽
    M66.174   Rupture of synovium, right foot
    M66.175   Rupture of synovium, left foot
    M66.176   Rupture of synovium, unspecified foot ▽
    M66.177   Rupture of synovium, right toe(s)
    M66.178   Rupture of synovium, left toe(s)
    M66.179   Rupture of synovium, unspecified toe(s) ▽

    M66.18   **Rupture of synovium, other site**

✦ ✓5ᵗʰ **M66.2**   **Spontaneous rupture of extensor tendons**
    M66.20   Spontaneous rupture of extensor tendons, unspecified site ▽

✓6ᵗʰ **M66.21**   **Spontaneous rupture of extensor tendons, shoulder**
    M66.211   Spontaneous rupture of extensor tendons, right shoulder
    M66.212   Spontaneous rupture of extensor tendons, left shoulder
    M66.219   Spontaneous rupture of extensor tendons, unspecified shoulder ▽

✓6ᵗʰ **M66.22**   **Spontaneous rupture of extensor tendons, upper arm**
    M66.221   Spontaneous rupture of extensor tendons, right upper arm
    M66.222   Spontaneous rupture of extensor tendons, left upper arm
    M66.229   Spontaneous rupture of extensor tendons, unspecified upper arm ▽

✓6ᵗʰ **M66.23**   **Spontaneous rupture of extensor tendons, forearm**
    M66.231   Spontaneous rupture of extensor tendons, right forearm
    M66.232   Spontaneous rupture of extensor tendons, left forearm
    M66.239   Spontaneous rupture of extensor tendons, unspecified forearm ▽

✓6ᵗʰ **M66.24**   **Spontaneous rupture of extensor tendons, hand**
    M66.241   Spontaneous rupture of extensor tendons, right hand
    M66.242   Spontaneous rupture of extensor tendons, left hand
    M66.249   Spontaneous rupture of extensor tendons, unspecified hand ▽

✓6ᵗʰ **M66.25**   **Spontaneous rupture of extensor tendons, thigh**
    M66.251   Spontaneous rupture of extensor tendons, right thigh
    M66.252   Spontaneous rupture of extensor tendons, left thigh
    M66.259   Spontaneous rupture of extensor tendons, unspecified thigh ▽

✓6ᵗʰ **M66.26**   **Spontaneous rupture of extensor tendons, lower leg**
    M66.261   Spontaneous rupture of extensor tendons, right lower leg
    M66.262   Spontaneous rupture of extensor tendons, left lower leg

M66.269   Spontaneous rupture of extensor tendons, unspecified lower leg ▽

✓6ᵗʰ **M66.27**   **Spontaneous rupture of extensor tendons, ankle and foot**
    M66.271   Spontaneous rupture of extensor tendons, right ankle and foot
    M66.272   Spontaneous rupture of extensor tendons, left ankle and foot
    M66.279   Spontaneous rupture of extensor tendons, unspecified ankle and foot ▽

    M66.28   **Spontaneous rupture of extensor tendons, other site**
    M66.29   Spontaneous rupture of extensor tendons, multiple sites

✦ ✓5ᵗʰ **M66.3**   **Spontaneous rupture of flexor tendons**
    M66.30   Spontaneous rupture of flexor tendons, unspecified site ▽

✓6ᵗʰ **M66.31**   **Spontaneous rupture of flexor tendons, shoulder**
    M66.311   Spontaneous rupture of flexor tendons, right shoulder
    M66.312   Spontaneous rupture of flexor tendons, left shoulder
    M66.319   Spontaneous rupture of flexor tendons, unspecified shoulder ▽

✓6ᵗʰ **M66.32**   **Spontaneous rupture of flexor tendons, upper arm**
    M66.321   Spontaneous rupture of flexor tendons, right upper arm
    M66.322   Spontaneous rupture of flexor tendons, left upper arm
    M66.329   Spontaneous rupture of flexor tendons, unspecified upper arm ▽

✓6ᵗʰ **M66.33**   **Spontaneous rupture of flexor tendons, forearm**
    M66.331   Spontaneous rupture of flexor tendons, right forearm
    M66.332   Spontaneous rupture of flexor tendons, left forearm
    M66.339   Spontaneous rupture of flexor tendons, unspecified forearm ▽

✓6ᵗʰ **M66.34**   **Spontaneous rupture of flexor tendons, hand**
    M66.341   Spontaneous rupture of flexor tendons, right hand
    M66.342   Spontaneous rupture of flexor tendons, left hand
    M66.349   Spontaneous rupture of flexor tendons, unspecified hand ▽

✓6ᵗʰ **M66.35**   **Spontaneous rupture of flexor tendons, thigh**
    M66.351   Spontaneous rupture of flexor tendons, right thigh
    M66.352   Spontaneous rupture of flexor tendons, left thigh
    M66.359   Spontaneous rupture of flexor tendons, unspecified thigh ▽

✓6ᵗʰ **M66.36**   **Spontaneous rupture of flexor tendons, lower leg**
    M66.361   Spontaneous rupture of flexor tendons, right lower leg
    M66.362   Spontaneous rupture of flexor tendons, left lower leg
    M66.369   Spontaneous rupture of flexor tendons, unspecified lower leg ▽

✓6ᵗʰ **M66.37**   **Spontaneous rupture of flexor tendons, ankle and foot**
    M66.371   Spontaneous rupture of flexor tendons, right ankle and foot
    M66.372   Spontaneous rupture of flexor tendons, left ankle and foot
    M66.379   Spontaneous rupture of flexor tendons, unspecified ankle and foot ▽

    M66.38   **Spontaneous rupture of flexor tendons, other site**
    M66.39   Spontaneous rupture of flexor tendons, multiple sites

✦ ✓5ᵗʰ **M66.8**   **Spontaneous rupture of other tendons**
    M66.80   Spontaneous rupture of other tendons, unspecified site ▽

✓6ᵗʰ **M66.81**   **Spontaneous rupture of other tendons, shoulder**
    M66.811   Spontaneous rupture of other tendons, right shoulder

---

✦ Refer to the Muscle/Tendon Table at beginning of this chapter.

      M66.812   **Spontaneous rupture of other tendons, left shoulder**

      M66.819   **Spontaneous rupture of other tendons, unspecified shoulder** ▽

✓6ᵗʰ   **M66.82**   **Spontaneous rupture of other tendons, upper arm**

      M66.821   **Spontaneous rupture of other tendons, right upper arm**

      M66.822   **Spontaneous rupture of other tendons, left upper arm**

      M66.829   **Spontaneous rupture of other tendons, unspecified upper arm** ▽

✓6ᵗʰ   **M66.83**   **Spontaneous rupture of other tendons, forearm**

      M66.831   **Spontaneous rupture of other tendons, right forearm**

      M66.832   **Spontaneous rupture of other tendons, left forearm**

      M66.839   **Spontaneous rupture of other tendons, unspecified forearm** ▽

✓6ᵗʰ   **M66.84**   **Spontaneous rupture of other tendons, hand**

      M66.841   **Spontaneous rupture of other tendons, right hand**

      M66.842   **Spontaneous rupture of other tendons, left hand**

      M66.849   **Spontaneous rupture of other tendons, unspecified hand** ▽

✓6ᵗʰ   **M66.85**   **Spontaneous rupture of other tendons, thigh**

      M66.851   **Spontaneous rupture of other tendons, right thigh**

      M66.852   **Spontaneous rupture of other tendons, left thigh**

      M66.859   **Spontaneous rupture of other tendons, unspecified thigh** ▽

✓6ᵗʰ   **M66.86**   **Spontaneous rupture of other tendons, lower leg**

      M66.861   **Spontaneous rupture of other tendons, right lower leg**

      M66.862   **Spontaneous rupture of other tendons, left lower leg**

      M66.869   **Spontaneous rupture of other tendons, unspecified lower leg** ▽

✓6ᵗʰ   **M66.87**   **Spontaneous rupture of other tendons, ankle and foot**

      M66.871   **Spontaneous rupture of other tendons, right ankle and foot**

      M66.872   **Spontaneous rupture of other tendons, left ankle and foot**

      M66.879   **Spontaneous rupture of other tendons, unspecified ankle and foot** ▽

    M66.88   **Spontaneous rupture of other tendons, other**

    M66.89   **Spontaneous rupture of other tendons, multiple sites**

M66.9   **Spontaneous rupture of unspecified tendon** ▽
        Rupture at musculotendinous junction, nontraumatic

✓4ᵗʰ   **M67**   **Other disorders of synovium and tendon**
    EXCLUDES 1   palmar fascial fibromatosis [Dupuytren] (M72.0)
                tendinitis NOS (M77.9-)
                xanthomatosis localized to tendons (E78.2)

✓5ᵗʰ   **M67.0**   **Short Achilles tendon (acquired)**

    M67.00   **Short Achilles tendon (acquired), unspecified ankle** ▽

    M67.01   **Short Achilles tendon (acquired), right ankle**

    M67.02   **Short Achilles tendon (acquired), left ankle**

✓5ᵗʰ   **M67.2**   **Synovial hypertrophy, not elsewhere classified**
      EXCLUDES 1   villonodular synovitis (pigmented) (M12.2-)

    M67.20   **Synovial hypertrophy, not elsewhere classified, unspecified site** ▽

✓6ᵗʰ   **M67.21**   **Synovial hypertrophy, not elsewhere classified, shoulder**

      M67.211   **Synovial hypertrophy, not elsewhere classified, right shoulder**

      M67.212   **Synovial hypertrophy, not elsewhere classified, left shoulder**

      M67.219   **Synovial hypertrophy, not elsewhere classified, unspecified shoulder** ▽

✓6ᵗʰ   **M67.22**   **Synovial hypertrophy, not elsewhere classified, upper arm**

      M67.221   **Synovial hypertrophy, not elsewhere classified, right upper arm**

      M67.222   **Synovial hypertrophy, not elsewhere classified, left upper arm**

      M67.229   **Synovial hypertrophy, not elsewhere classified, unspecified upper arm** ▽

✓6ᵗʰ   **M67.23**   **Synovial hypertrophy, not elsewhere classified, forearm**

      M67.231   **Synovial hypertrophy, not elsewhere classified, right forearm**

      M67.232   **Synovial hypertrophy, not elsewhere classified, left forearm**

      M67.239   **Synovial hypertrophy, not elsewhere classified, unspecified forearm** ▽

✓6ᵗʰ   **M67.24**   **Synovial hypertrophy, not elsewhere classified, hand**

      M67.241   **Synovial hypertrophy, not elsewhere classified, right hand**

      M67.242   **Synovial hypertrophy, not elsewhere classified, left hand**

      M67.249   **Synovial hypertrophy, not elsewhere classified, unspecified hand** ▽

✓6ᵗʰ   **M67.25**   **Synovial hypertrophy, not elsewhere classified, thigh**

      M67.251   **Synovial hypertrophy, not elsewhere classified, right thigh**

      M67.252   **Synovial hypertrophy, not elsewhere classified, left thigh**

      M67.259   **Synovial hypertrophy, not elsewhere classified, unspecified thigh** ▽

✓6ᵗʰ   **M67.26**   **Synovial hypertrophy, not elsewhere classified, lower leg**

      M67.261   **Synovial hypertrophy, not elsewhere classified, right lower leg**

      M67.262   **Synovial hypertrophy, not elsewhere classified, left lower leg**

      M67.269   **Synovial hypertrophy, not elsewhere classified, unspecified lower leg** ▽

✓6ᵗʰ   **M67.27**   **Synovial hypertrophy, not elsewhere classified, ankle and foot**

      M67.271   **Synovial hypertrophy, not elsewhere classified, right ankle and foot**

      M67.272   **Synovial hypertrophy, not elsewhere classified, left ankle and foot**

      M67.279   **Synovial hypertrophy, not elsewhere classified, unspecified ankle and foot** ▽

    M67.28   **Synovial hypertrophy, not elsewhere classified, other site**

    M67.29   **Synovial hypertrophy, not elsewhere classified, multiple sites**

✓5ᵗʰ   **M67.3**   **Transient synovitis**
        Toxic synovitis
      EXCLUDES 1   palindromic rheumatism (M12.3-)

    M67.30   **Transient synovitis, unspecified site** ▽

✓6ᵗʰ   **M67.31**   **Transient synovitis, shoulder**

      M67.311   **Transient synovitis, right shoulder**

      M67.312   **Transient synovitis, left shoulder**

      M67.319   **Transient synovitis, unspecified shoulder** ▽

✓6ᵗʰ   **M67.32**   **Transient synovitis, elbow**

      M67.321   **Transient synovitis, right elbow**

      M67.322   **Transient synovitis, left elbow**

      M67.329   **Transient synovitis, unspecified elbow** ▽

✓6ᵗʰ   **M67.33**   **Transient synovitis, wrist**

      M67.331   **Transient synovitis, right wrist**

      M67.332   **Transient synovitis, left wrist**

      M67.339   **Transient synovitis, unspecified wrist** ▽

✓6ᵗʰ   **M67.34**   **Transient synovitis, hand**

      M67.341   **Transient synovitis, right hand**

      M67.342   **Transient synovitis, left hand**

      M67.349   **Transient synovitis, unspecified hand** ▽

✓6ᵗʰ   **M67.35**   **Transient synovitis, hip**

      M67.351   **Transient synovitis, right hip**

N Newborn   P Pediatric   M Maternity   A Adult   **RIC** RIC Dx   **NC Dx** Noncancer Dx   **PDx** Primary Dx   **CC** RIC CC Condition   ►◄ Revised Text   ● New Code   ▲ Revised Code Title

728   ICD-10-CM 2016

M67.352   Transient synovitis, left hip

M67.359   Transient synovitis, unspecified hip ▽

✓6ᵗʰ **M67.36**   **Transient synovitis, knee**

M67.361   Transient synovitis, right knee

M67.362   Transient synovitis, left knee

M67.369   Transient synovitis, unspecified knee ▽

✓6ᵗʰ **M67.37**   **Transient synovitis, ankle and foot**

M67.371   Transient synovitis, right ankle and foot

M67.372   Transient synovitis, left ankle and foot

M67.379   Transient synovitis, unspecified ▽
ankle and foot

M67.38   **Transient synovitis, other site**

M67.39   **Transient synovitis, multiple sites**

✓5ᵗʰ **M67.4**   **Ganglion**

Ganglion of joint or tendon (sheath)

EXCLUDES 1   *ganglion in yaws (A66.6)*

EXCLUDES 2   *cyst of bursa (M71.2-M71.3)*
cyst of synovium (M71.2-M71.3)

M67.4Ø   **Ganglion, unspecified site** ▽

✓6ᵗʰ **M67.41**   **Ganglion, shoulder**

M67.411   Ganglion, right shoulder

M67.412   Ganglion, left shoulder

M67.419   Ganglion, unspecified shoulder ▽

✓6ᵗʰ **M67.42**   **Ganglion, elbow**

M67.421   Ganglion, right elbow

M67.422   Ganglion, left elbow

M67.429   Ganglion, unspecified elbow ▽

✓6ᵗʰ **M67.43**   **Ganglion, wrist**

M67.431   Ganglion, right wrist

M67.432   Ganglion, left wrist

M67.439   Ganglion, unspecified wrist ▽

✓6ᵗʰ **M67.44**   **Ganglion, hand**

M67.441   Ganglion, right hand

M67.442   Ganglion, left hand

M67.449   Ganglion, unspecified hand ▽

✓6ᵗʰ **M67.45**   **Ganglion, hip**

M67.451   Ganglion, right hip

M67.452   Ganglion, left hip

M67.459   Ganglion, unspecified hip ▽

✓6ᵗʰ **M67.46**   **Ganglion, knee**

M67.461   Ganglion, right knee

M67.462   Ganglion, left knee

M67.469   Ganglion, unspecified knee ▽

✓6ᵗʰ **M67.47**   **Ganglion, ankle and foot**

M67.471   Ganglion, right ankle and foot

M67.472   Ganglion, left ankle and foot

M67.479   Ganglion, unspecified ankle and foot ▽

M67.48   **Ganglion, other site**

M67.49   **Ganglion, multiple sites**

✓5ᵗʰ **M67.5**   **Plica syndrome**

Plica knee

M67.5Ø   **Plica syndrome, unspecified knee** ▽

M67.51   **Plica syndrome, right knee**

M67.52   **Plica syndrome, left knee**

✓5ᵗʰ **M67.8**   **Other specified disorders of synovium and tendon**

M67.8Ø   **Other specified disorders of synovium and** ▽
tendon, unspecified site

✓6ᵗʰ **M67.81**   **Other specified disorders of synovium and tendon, shoulder**

M67.811   **Other specified disorders of synovium, right shoulder**

M67.812   **Other specified disorders of synovium, left shoulder**

M67.813   **Other specified disorders of tendon, right shoulder**

M67.814   **Other specified disorders of tendon, left shoulder**

M67.819   **Other specified disorders of synovium** ▽
and tendon, unspecified shoulder

✓6ᵗʰ **M67.82**   **Other specified disorders of synovium and tendon, elbow**

M67.821   **Other specified disorders of synovium, right elbow**

M67.822   **Other specified disorders of synovium, left elbow**

M67.823   **Other specified disorders of tendon, right elbow**

M67.824   **Other specified disorders of tendon, left elbow**

M67.829   **Other specified disorders of synovium** ▽
and tendon, unspecified elbow

✓6ᵗʰ **M67.83**   **Other specified disorders of synovium and tendon, wrist**

M67.831   **Other specified disorders of synovium, right wrist**

M67.832   **Other specified disorders of synovium, left wrist**

M67.833   **Other specified disorders of tendon, right wrist**

M67.834   **Other specified disorders of tendon, left wrist**

M67.839   **Other specified disorders of synovium** ▽
and tendon, unspecified forearm

✓6ᵗʰ **M67.84**   **Other specified disorders of synovium and tendon, hand**

M67.841   **Other specified disorders of synovium, right hand**

M67.842   **Other specified disorders of synovium, left hand**

M67.843   **Other specified disorders of tendon, right hand**

M67.844   **Other specified disorders of tendon, left hand**

M67.849   **Other specified disorders of synovium** ▽
and tendon, unspecified hand

✓6ᵗʰ **M67.85**   **Other specified disorders of synovium and tendon, hip**

M67.851   **Other specified disorders of synovium, right hip**

M67.852   **Other specified disorders of synovium, left hip**

M67.853   **Other specified disorders of tendon, right hip**

M67.854   **Other specified disorders of tendon, left hip**

M67.859   **Other specified disorders of synovium** ▽
and tendon, unspecified hip

✓6ᵗʰ **M67.86**   **Other specified disorders of synovium and tendon, knee**

M67.861   **Other specified disorders of synovium, right knee**

M67.862   **Other specified disorders of synovium, left knee**

M67.863   **Other specified disorders of tendon, right knee**

M67.864   **Other specified disorders of tendon, left knee**

M67.869   **Other specified disorders of synovium** ▽
and tendon, unspecified knee

✓6ᵗʰ **M67.87**   **Other specified disorders of synovium and tendon, ankle and foot**

M67.871   **Other specified disorders of synovium, right ankle and foot**

M67.872   **Other specified disorders of synovium, left ankle and foot**

M67.873   **Other specified disorders of tendon, right ankle and foot**

M67.874   **Other specified disorders of tendon, left ankle and foot**

M67.879   **Other specified disorders of synovium** ▽
and tendon, unspecified ankle and foot

M67.88   **Other specified disorders of synovium and tendon, other site**

M67.89   **Other specified disorders of synovium and tendon, multiple sites**

✓5ᵗʰ **M67.9**   **Unspecified disorder of synovium and tendon**

M67.9Ø   **Unspecified disorder of synovium and tendon,** ▽
unspecified site

☑ Add'l Character Required   ☑✗7ᵗʰ Placeholder Alert   RUG IV Special Care High Dx   RUG IV Clinically Complex Dx   RUG IV Special Care Low Dx   Manifestation Code   Other Specified Code   ▽ Unspecified Code

√6ᵗʰ **M67.91** Unspecified disorder of synovium and tendon, shoulder
- **M67.911** Unspecified disorder of synovium and tendon, right shoulder ▽
- **M67.912** Unspecified disorder of synovium and tendon, left shoulder ▽
- **M67.919** Unspecified disorder of synovium and tendon, unspecified shoulder ▽

√6ᵗʰ **M67.92** Unspecified disorder of synovium and tendon, upper arm
- **M67.921** Unspecified disorder of synovium and tendon, right upper arm ▽
- **M67.922** Unspecified disorder of synovium and tendon, left upper arm ▽
- **M67.929** Unspecified disorder of synovium and tendon, unspecified upper arm ▽

√6ᵗʰ **M67.93** Unspecified disorder of synovium and tendon, forearm
- **M67.931** Unspecified disorder of synovium and tendon, right forearm ▽
- **M67.932** Unspecified disorder of synovium and tendon, left forearm ▽
- **M67.939** Unspecified disorder of synovium and tendon, unspecified forearm ▽

√6ᵗʰ **M67.94** Unspecified disorder of synovium and tendon, hand
- **M67.941** Unspecified disorder of synovium and tendon, right hand ▽
- **M67.942** Unspecified disorder of synovium and tendon, left hand ▽
- **M67.949** Unspecified disorder of synovium and tendon, unspecified hand ▽

√6ᵗʰ **M67.95** Unspecified disorder of synovium and tendon, thigh
- **M67.951** Unspecified disorder of synovium and tendon, right thigh ▽
- **M67.952** Unspecified disorder of synovium and tendon, left thigh ▽
- **M67.959** Unspecified disorder of synovium and tendon, unspecified thigh ▽

√6ᵗʰ **M67.96** Unspecified disorder of synovium and tendon, lower leg
- **M67.961** Unspecified disorder of synovium and tendon, right lower leg ▽
- **M67.962** Unspecified disorder of synovium and tendon, left lower leg ▽
- **M67.969** Unspecified disorder of synovium and tendon, unspecified lower leg ▽

√6ᵗʰ **M67.97** Unspecified disorder of synovium and tendon, ankle and foot
- **M67.971** Unspecified disorder of synovium and tendon, right ankle and foot ▽
- **M67.972** Unspecified disorder of synovium and tendon, left ankle and foot ▽
- **M67.979** Unspecified disorder of synovium and tendon, unspecified ankle and foot ▽

M67.98 Unspecified disorder of synovium and tendon, other site ▽

M67.99 Unspecified disorder of synovium and tendon, multiple sites ▽

Other soft tissue disorders (M70-M79)

√4ᵗʰ **M70** Soft tissue disorders related to use, overuse and pressure

    INCLUDES soft tissue disorders of occupational origin

    Use additional external cause code to identify activity causing disorder (Y93.-)

    EXCLUDES 1 bursitis NOS (M71.9-)

    EXCLUDES 2 bursitis of shoulder (M75.5)
    enthesopathies (M76-M77)
    pressure ulcer (pressure area) (L89.-)

√5ᵗʰ **M70.0** Crepitant synovitis (acute) (chronic) of hand and wrist
- √6ᵗʰ **M70.03** Crepitant synovitis (acute) (chronic), wrist
  - **M70.031** Crepitant synovitis (acute) (chronic), right wrist
  - **M70.032** Crepitant synovitis (acute) (chronic), left wrist

    M70.039 Crepitant synovitis (acute) (chronic), unspecified wrist ▽

- √6ᵗʰ **M70.04** Crepitant synovitis (acute) (chronic), hand
  - **M70.041** Crepitant synovitis (acute) (chronic), right hand
  - **M70.042** Crepitant synovitis (acute) (chronic), left hand
  - **M70.049** Crepitant synovitis (acute) (chronic), unspecified hand ▽

√5ᵗʰ **M70.1** Bursitis of hand
- **M70.10** Bursitis, unspecified hand ▽
- **M70.11** Bursitis, right hand
- **M70.12** Bursitis, left hand

√5ᵗʰ **M70.2** Olecranon bursitis
- **M70.20** Olecranon bursitis, unspecified elbow ▽
- **M70.21** Olecranon bursitis, right elbow
- **M70.22** Olecranon bursitis, left elbow

√5ᵗʰ **M70.3** Other bursitis of elbow
- **M70.30** Other bursitis of elbow, unspecified elbow ▽
- **M70.31** Other bursitis of elbow, right elbow
- **M70.32** Other bursitis of elbow, left elbow

√5ᵗʰ **M70.4** Prepatellar bursitis
- **M70.40** Prepatellar bursitis, unspecified knee ▽
- **M70.41** Prepatellar bursitis, right knee
- **M70.42** Prepatellar bursitis, left knee

√5ᵗʰ **M70.5** Other bursitis of knee
- **M70.50** Other bursitis of knee, unspecified knee ▽
- **M70.51** Other bursitis of knee, right knee
- **M70.52** Other bursitis of knee, left knee

√5ᵗʰ **M70.6** Trochanteric bursitis
    Trochanteric tendinitis
- **M70.60** Trochanteric bursitis, unspecified hip ▽
- **M70.61** Trochanteric bursitis, right hip
- **M70.62** Trochanteric bursitis, left hip

√5ᵗʰ **M70.7** Other bursitis of hip
    Ischial bursitis
- **M70.70** Other bursitis of hip, unspecified hip ▽
- **M70.71** Other bursitis of hip, right hip
- **M70.72** Other bursitis of hip, left hip

√5ᵗʰ **M70.8** Other soft tissue disorders related to use, overuse and pressure
- **M70.80** Other soft tissue disorders related to use, overuse and pressure of unspecified site ▽
- √6ᵗʰ **M70.81** Other soft tissue disorders related to use, overuse and pressure of shoulder
  - **M70.811** Other soft tissue disorders related to use, overuse and pressure, right shoulder
  - **M70.812** Other soft tissue disorders related to use, overuse and pressure, left shoulder
  - **M70.819** Other soft tissue disorders related to use, overuse and pressure, unspecified shoulder ▽
- √6ᵗʰ **M70.82** Other soft tissue disorders related to use, overuse and pressure of upper arm
  - **M70.821** Other soft tissue disorders related to use, overuse and pressure, right upper arm
  - **M70.822** Other soft tissue disorders related to use, overuse and pressure, left upper arm
  - **M70.829** Other soft tissue disorders related to use, overuse and pressure, unspecified upper arms ▽
- √6ᵗʰ **M70.83** Other soft tissue disorders related to use, overuse and pressure of forearm
  - **M70.831** Other soft tissue disorders related to use, overuse and pressure, right forearm
  - **M70.832** Other soft tissue disorders related to use, overuse and pressure, left forearm
  - **M70.839** Other soft tissue disorders related to use, overuse and pressure, unspecified forearm ▽
- √6ᵗʰ **M70.84** Other soft tissue disorders related to use, overuse and pressure of hand
  - **M70.841** Other soft tissue disorders related to use, overuse and pressure, right hand

N Newborn   P Pediatric   M Maternity   A Adult   **RIC** RIC Dx   **NCDx** Noncancer Dx   **PDx** Primary Dx   **CC** RIC CC Condition   ▶◀ Revised Text   ● New Code   ▲ Revised Code Title

730   ICD-10-CM 2016

M70.842   Other soft tissue disorders related to use, overuse and pressure, left hand

M70.849   Other soft tissue disorders related to use, overuse and pressure, unspecified hand ▽

✓6ᵗʰ   M70.85   Other soft tissue disorders related to use, overuse and pressure of thigh

M70.851   Other soft tissue disorders related to use, overuse and pressure, right thigh

M70.852   Other soft tissue disorders related to use, overuse and pressure, left thigh

M70.859   Other soft tissue disorders related to use, overuse and pressure, unspecified thigh ▽

✓6ᵗʰ   M70.86   Other soft tissue disorders related to use, overuse and pressure lower leg

M70.861   Other soft tissue disorders related to use, overuse and pressure, right lower leg

M70.862   Other soft tissue disorders related to use, overuse and pressure, left lower leg

M70.869   Other soft tissue disorders related to use, overuse and pressure, unspecified leg ▽

✓6ᵗʰ   M70.87   Other soft tissue disorders related to use, overuse and pressure of ankle and foot

M70.871   Other soft tissue disorders related to use, overuse and pressure, right ankle and foot

M70.872   Other soft tissue disorders related to use, overuse and pressure, left ankle and foot

M70.879   Other soft tissue disorders related to use, overuse and pressure, unspecified ankle and foot ▽

M70.88   Other soft tissue disorders related to use, overuse and pressure other site

M70.89   Other soft tissue disorders related to use, overuse and pressure multiple sites

✓5ᵗʰ   M70.9   Unspecified soft tissue disorder related to use, overuse and pressure

M70.90   Unspecified soft tissue disorder related to use, overuse and pressure of unspecified site ▽

✓6ᵗʰ   M70.91   Unspecified soft tissue disorder related to use, overuse and pressure of shoulder

M70.911   Unspecified soft tissue disorder related to use, overuse and pressure, right shoulder ▽

M70.912   Unspecified soft tissue disorder related to use, overuse and pressure, left shoulder ▽

M70.919   Unspecified soft tissue disorder related to use, overuse and pressure, unspecified shoulder ▽

✓6ᵗʰ   M70.92   Unspecified soft tissue disorder related to use, overuse and pressure of upper arm

M70.921   Unspecified soft tissue disorder related to use, overuse and pressure, right upper arm ▽

M70.922   Unspecified soft tissue disorder related to use, overuse and pressure, left upper arm ▽

M70.929   Unspecified soft tissue disorder related to use, overuse and pressure, unspecified upper arm ▽

✓6ᵗʰ   M70.93   Unspecified soft tissue disorder related to use, overuse and pressure of forearm

M70.931   Unspecified soft tissue disorder related to use, overuse and pressure, right forearm ▽

M70.932   Unspecified soft tissue disorder related to use, overuse and pressure, left forearm ▽

M70.939   Unspecified soft tissue disorder related to use, overuse and pressure, unspecified forearm ▽

✓6ᵗʰ   M70.94   Unspecified soft tissue disorder related to use, overuse and pressure of hand

M70.941   Unspecified soft tissue disorder related to use, overuse and pressure, right hand ▽

M70.942   Unspecified soft tissue disorder related to use, overuse and pressure, left hand ▽

M70.949   Unspecified soft tissue disorder related to use, overuse and pressure, unspecified hand ▽

✓6ᵗʰ   M70.95   Unspecified soft tissue disorder related to use, overuse and pressure of thigh

M70.951   Unspecified soft tissue disorder related to use, overuse and pressure, right thigh ▽

M70.952   Unspecified soft tissue disorder related to use, overuse and pressure, left thigh ▽

M70.959   Unspecified soft tissue disorder related to use, overuse and pressure, unspecified thigh ▽

✓6ᵗʰ   M70.96   Unspecified soft tissue disorder related to use, overuse and pressure lower leg

M70.961   Unspecified soft tissue disorder related to use, overuse and pressure, right lower leg ▽

M70.962   Unspecified soft tissue disorder related to use, overuse and pressure, left lower leg ▽

M70.969   Unspecified soft tissue disorder related to use, overuse and pressure, unspecified lower leg ▽

✓6ᵗʰ   M70.97   Unspecified soft tissue disorder related to use, overuse and pressure of ankle and foot

M70.971   Unspecified soft tissue disorder related to use, overuse and pressure, right ankle and foot ▽

M70.972   Unspecified soft tissue disorder related to use, overuse and pressure, left ankle and foot ▽

M70.979   Unspecified soft tissue disorder related to use, overuse and pressure, unspecified ankle and foot ▽

M70.98   Unspecified soft tissue disorder related to use, overuse and pressure other ▽

M70.99   Unspecified soft tissue disorder related to use, overuse and pressure multiple sites ▽

✓4ᵗʰ   M71   Other bursopathies

EXCLUDES 1   bunion (M20.1)
bursitis related to use, overuse or pressure (M70.-)
enthesopathies (M76-M77)

✓5ᵗʰ   M71.0   Abscess of bursa

Use additional code (B95.-, B96.-) to identify causative organism

M71.00   Abscess of bursa, unspecified site ▽

✓6ᵗʰ   M71.01   Abscess of bursa, shoulder

M71.011   Abscess of bursa, right shoulder

M71.012   Abscess of bursa, left shoulder

M71.019   Abscess of bursa, unspecified shoulder ▽

✓6ᵗʰ   M71.02   Abscess of bursa, elbow

M71.021   Abscess of bursa, right elbow

M71.022   Abscess of bursa, left elbow

M71.029   Abscess of bursa, unspecified elbow ▽

✓6ᵗʰ   M71.03   Abscess of bursa, wrist

M71.031   Abscess of bursa, right wrist

M71.032   Abscess of bursa, left wrist

M71.039   Abscess of bursa, unspecified wrist ▽

✓6ᵗʰ   M71.04   Abscess of bursa, hand

M71.041   Abscess of bursa, right hand

M71.042   Abscess of bursa, left hand

M71.049   Abscess of bursa, unspecified hand ▽

✓6ᵗʰ   M71.05   Abscess of bursa, hip

M71.051   Abscess of bursa, right hip

M71.052   Abscess of bursa, left hip

M71.059   Abscess of bursa, unspecified hip ▽

✓6ᵗʰ   M71.06   Abscess of bursa, knee

M71.061   Abscess of bursa, right knee

M71.062   Abscess of bursa, left knee

M71.069   Abscess of bursa, unspecified knee ▽

☑ Add'l Character Required   ✓×7ᵗʰ Placeholder Alert   RUG IV Special Care High Dx   RUG IV Clinically Complex Dx   RUG IV Special Care Low Dx   Manifestation Code   Other Specified Code   ▽ Unspecified Code

ICD-10-CM 2016   731

✓6ᵗʰ **M71.Ø7** **Abscess of bursa,** ankle and foot
    M71.Ø71 **Abscess of bursa,** right **ankle and foot**
    M71.Ø72 **Abscess of bursa,** left **ankle and foot**
    M71.Ø79 **Abscess of bursa, unspecified ankle and foot** ▽
M71.Ø8 **Abscess of bursa, other site**
M71.Ø9 **Abscess of bursa,** multiple sites

✓5ᵗʰ **M71.1** **Other infective bursitis**
    Use additional code (B95.-, B96.-) to identify causative organism
M71.1Ø **Other infective bursitis, unspecified site** ▽
✓6ᵗʰ **M71.11** **Other infective bursitis,** shoulder
    M71.111 **Other infective bursitis,** right **shoulder**
    M71.112 **Other infective bursitis,** left **shoulder**
    M71.119 **Other infective bursitis, unspecified shoulder** ▽
✓6ᵗʰ **M71.12** **Other infective bursitis,** elbow
    M71.121 **Other infective bursitis,** right **elbow**
    M71.122 **Other infective bursitis,** left **elbow**
    M71.129 **Other infective bursitis, unspecified elbow** ▽
✓6ᵗʰ **M71.13** **Other infective bursitis,** wrist
    M71.131 **Other infective bursitis,** right **wrist**
    M71.132 **Other infective bursitis,** left **wrist**
    M71.139 **Other infective bursitis, unspecified wrist** ▽
✓6ᵗʰ **M71.14** **Other infective bursitis,** hand
    M71.141 **Other infective bursitis,** right **hand**
    M71.142 **Other infective bursitis,** left **hand**
    M71.149 **Other infective bursitis, unspecified hand** ▽
✓6ᵗʰ **M71.15** **Other infective bursitis,** hip
    M71.151 **Other infective bursitis,** right **hip**
    M71.152 **Other infective bursitis,** left **hip**
    M71.159 **Other infective bursitis, unspecified hip** ▽
✓6ᵗʰ **M71.16** **Other infective bursitis,** knee
    M71.161 **Other infective bursitis,** right **knee**
    M71.162 **Other infective bursitis,** left **knee**
    M71.169 **Other infective bursitis, unspecified knee** ▽
✓6ᵗʰ **M71.17** **Other infective bursitis,** ankle and foot
    M71.171 **Other infective bursitis,** right **ankle and foot**
    M71.172 **Other infective bursitis,** left **ankle and foot**
    M71.179 **Other infective bursitis, unspecified ankle and foot** ▽
M71.18 **Other infective bursitis, other site**
M71.19 **Other infective bursitis,** multiple sites

✓5ᵗʰ **M71.2** **Synovial cyst of popliteal space [Baker]**
    EXCLUDES 1   synovial cyst of popliteal space with rupture (M66.Ø)
M71.2Ø **Synovial cyst of popliteal space [Baker], unspecified knee** ▽
M71.21 **Synovial cyst of popliteal space [Baker],** right **knee**
M71.22 **Synovial cyst of popliteal space [Baker],** left **knee**

✓5ᵗʰ **M71.3** **Other bursal cyst**
    Synovial cyst NOS
    EXCLUDES 1   synovial cyst with rupture (M66.1-)
M71.3Ø **Other bursal cyst, unspecified site** ▽
✓6ᵗʰ **M71.31** **Other bursal cyst,** shoulder
    M71.311 **Other bursal cyst,** right **shoulder**
    M71.312 **Other bursal cyst,** left **shoulder**
    M71.319 **Other bursal cyst, unspecified shoulder** ▽
✓6ᵗʰ **M71.32** **Other bursal cyst,** elbow
    M71.321 **Other bursal cyst,** right **elbow**
    M71.322 **Other bursal cyst,** left **elbow**
    M71.329 **Other bursal cyst, unspecified elbow** ▽
✓6ᵗʰ **M71.33** **Other bursal cyst,** wrist
    M71.331 **Other bursal cyst,** right **wrist**
    M71.332 **Other bursal cyst,** left **wrist**
    M71.339 **Other bursal cyst, unspecified wrist** ▽
✓6ᵗʰ **M71.34** **Other bursal cyst,** hand
    M71.341 **Other bursal cyst,** right **hand**

M71.342 **Other bursal cyst,** left **hand**
M71.349 **Other bursal cyst, unspecified hand** ▽
✓6ᵗʰ **M71.35** **Other bursal cyst,** hip
    M71.351 **Other bursal cyst,** right **hip**
    M71.352 **Other bursal cyst,** left **hip**
    M71.359 **Other bursal cyst, unspecified hip** ▽
✓6ᵗʰ **M71.37** **Other bursal cyst,** ankle and foot
    M71.371 **Other bursal cyst,** right **ankle and foot**
    M71.372 **Other bursal cyst,** left **ankle and foot**
    M71.379 **Other bursal cyst, unspecified ankle and foot** ▽
M71.38 **Other bursal cyst, other site**
M71.39 **Other bursal cyst,** multiple sites

✓5ᵗʰ **M71.4** **Calcium deposit in bursa**
    EXCLUDES 2   calcium deposit in bursa of shoulder (M75.3)
M71.4Ø **Calcium deposit in bursa, unspecified site** ▽
✓6ᵗʰ **M71.42** **Calcium deposit in bursa,** elbow
    M71.421 **Calcium deposit in bursa,** right **elbow**
    M71.422 **Calcium deposit in bursa,** left **elbow**
    M71.429 **Calcium deposit in bursa, unspecified elbow** ▽
✓6ᵗʰ **M71.43** **Calcium deposit in bursa,** wrist
    M71.431 **Calcium deposit in bursa,** right **wrist**
    M71.432 **Calcium deposit in bursa,** left **wrist**
    M71.439 **Calcium deposit in bursa, unspecified wrist** ▽
✓6ᵗʰ **M71.44** **Calcium deposit in bursa,** hand
    M71.441 **Calcium deposit in bursa,** right **hand**
    M71.442 **Calcium deposit in bursa,** left **hand**
    M71.449 **Calcium deposit in bursa, unspecified hand** ▽
✓6ᵗʰ **M71.45** **Calcium deposit in bursa,** hip
    M71.451 **Calcium deposit in bursa,** right **hip**
    M71.452 **Calcium deposit in bursa,** left **hip**
    M71.459 **Calcium deposit in bursa, unspecified hip** ▽
✓6ᵗʰ **M71.46** **Calcium deposit in bursa,** knee
    M71.461 **Calcium deposit in bursa,** right **knee**
    M71.462 **Calcium deposit in bursa,** left **knee**
    M71.469 **Calcium deposit in bursa, unspecified knee** ▽
✓6ᵗʰ **M71.47** **Calcium deposit in bursa,** ankle and foot
    M71.471 **Calcium deposit in bursa,** right **ankle and foot**
    M71.472 **Calcium deposit in bursa,** left **ankle and foot**
    M71.479 **Calcium deposit in bursa, unspecified ankle and foot** ▽
M71.48 **Calcium deposit in bursa, other site**
M71.49 **Calcium deposit in bursa,** multiple sites

✓5ᵗʰ **M71.5** **Other bursitis, not elsewhere classified**
    EXCLUDES 1   bursitis NOS (M71.9-)
    EXCLUDES 2   bursitis of shoulder (M75.5)
             bursitis of tibial collateral [Pellegrini-Stieda] (M76.4)
M71.5Ø **Other bursitis, not elsewhere classified, unspecified site** ▽
✓6ᵗʰ **M71.52** **Other bursitis, not elsewhere classified,** elbow
    M71.521 **Other bursitis, not elsewhere classified,** right **elbow**
    M71.522 **Other bursitis, not elsewhere classified,** left **elbow**
    M71.529 **Other bursitis, not elsewhere classified, unspecified elbow** ▽
✓6ᵗʰ **M71.53** **Other bursitis, not elsewhere classified,** wrist
    M71.531 **Other bursitis, not elsewhere classified,** right **wrist**
    M71.532 **Other bursitis, not elsewhere classified,** left **wrist**
    M71.539 **Other bursitis, not elsewhere classified, unspecified wrist** ▽
✓6ᵗʰ **M71.54** **Other bursitis, not elsewhere classified,** hand
    M71.541 **Other bursitis, not elsewhere classified,** right **hand**

M71.542   **Other bursitis, not elsewhere classified, left hand**

M71.549   **Other bursitis, not elsewhere classified, unspecified hand** ▽

✓6th **M71.55   Other bursitis, not elsewhere classified, hip**

M71.551   **Other bursitis, not elsewhere classified, right hip**

M71.552   **Other bursitis, not elsewhere classified, left hip**

M71.559   **Other bursitis, not elsewhere classified, unspecified hip** ▽

✓6th **M71.56   Other bursitis, not elsewhere classified, knee**

M71.561   **Other bursitis, not elsewhere classified, right knee**

M71.562   **Other bursitis, not elsewhere classified, left knee**

M71.569   **Other bursitis, not elsewhere classified, unspecified knee** ▽

✓6th **M71.57   Other bursitis, not elsewhere classified, ankle and foot**

M71.571   **Other bursitis, not elsewhere classified, right ankle and foot**

M71.572   **Other bursitis, not elsewhere classified, left ankle and foot**

M71.579   **Other bursitis, not elsewhere classified, unspecified ankle and foot** ▽

M71.58   **Other bursitis, not elsewhere classified, other site**

✓5th **M71.8 Other specified bursopathies**

M71.80   **Other specified bursopathies, unspecified site** ▽

✓6th **M71.81   Other specified bursopathies, shoulder**

M71.811   **Other specified bursopathies, right shoulder**

M71.812   **Other specified bursopathies, left shoulder**

M71.819   **Other specified bursopathies, unspecified shoulder** ▽

✓6th **M71.82   Other specified bursopathies, elbow**

M71.821   **Other specified bursopathies, right elbow**

M71.822   **Other specified bursopathies, left elbow**

M71.829   **Other specified bursopathies, unspecified elbow** ▽

✓6th **M71.83   Other specified bursopathies, wrist**

M71.831   **Other specified bursopathies, right wrist**

M71.832   **Other specified bursopathies, left wrist**

M71.839   **Other specified bursopathies, unspecified wrist** ▽

✓6th **M71.84   Other specified bursopathies, hand**

M71.841   **Other specified bursopathies, right hand**

M71.842   **Other specified bursopathies, left hand**

M71.849   **Other specified bursopathies, unspecified hand** ▽

✓6th **M71.85   Other specified bursopathies, hip**

M71.851   **Other specified bursopathies, right hip**

M71.852   **Other specified bursopathies, left hip**

M71.859   **Other specified bursopathies, unspecified hip** ▽

✓6th **M71.86   Other specified bursopathies, knee**

M71.861   **Other specified bursopathies, right knee**

M71.862   **Other specified bursopathies, left knee**

M71.869   **Other specified bursopathies, unspecified knee** ▽

✓6th **M71.87   Other specified bursopathies, ankle and foot**

M71.871   **Other specified bursopathies, right ankle and foot**

M71.872   **Other specified bursopathies, left ankle and foot**

M71.879   **Other specified bursopathies, unspecified ankle and foot** ▽

M71.88   **Other specified bursopathies, other site**

M71.89   **Other specified bursopathies, multiple sites**

M71.9 Bursopathy, unspecified ▽
Bursitis NOS

✓4th **M72 Fibroblastic disorders**
EXCLUDES 2   retroperitoneal fibromatosis (D48.3)

M72.0 Palmar fascial fibromatosis [Dupuytren] Ⓐ

M72.1 Knuckle pads

M72.2 Plantar fascial fibromatosis
Plantar fasciitis

M72.4 Pseudosarcomatous fibromatosis
Nodular fasciitis

M72.6 Necrotizing fasciitis
Use additional code (B95.-, B96.-) to identify causative organism

M72.8 Other fibroblastic disorders
Abscess of fascia
Fasciitis NEC
Other infective fasciitis
Use additional code to (B95.-, B96.-) identify causative organism
EXCLUDES 1   diffuse (eosinophilic) fasciitis (M35.4)
necrotizing fasciitis (M72.6)
nodular fasciitis (M72.4)
perirenal fasciitis NOS (N13.5)
perirenal fasciitis with infection (N13.6)
plantar fasciitis (M72.2)

M72.9 Fibroblastic disorder, unspecified ▽
Fasciitis NOS
Fibromatosis NOS

✓4th **M75 Shoulder lesions**
EXCLUDES 2   shoulder-hand syndrome (M89.0-)

✓5th **M75.0 Adhesive capsulitis of shoulder**
Frozen shoulder
Periarthritis of shoulder

M75.00   **Adhesive capsulitis of unspecified shoulder** ▽

M75.01   **Adhesive capsulitis of right shoulder**

M75.02   **Adhesive capsulitis of left shoulder**

✓5th **M75.1 Rotator cuff tear or rupture, not specified as traumatic**
Rotator cuff syndrome
Supraspinatus syndrome
Supraspinatus tear or rupture, not specified as traumatic
EXCLUDES 1   tear of rotator cuff, traumatic (S46.01-)

✓6th **M75.10   Unspecified rotator cuff tear or rupture, not specified as traumatic**

M75.100   **Unspecified rotator cuff tear or rupture of unspecified shoulder, not specified as traumatic** ▽

M75.101   **Unspecified rotator cuff tear or rupture of right shoulder, not specified as traumatic** ▽

M75.102   **Unspecified rotator cuff tear or rupture of left shoulder, not specified as traumatic** ▽

✓6th **M75.11   Incomplete rotator cuff tear or rupture not specified as traumatic**

M75.110   **Incomplete rotator cuff tear or rupture of unspecified shoulder, not specified as traumatic** ▽

M75.111   **Incomplete rotator cuff tear or rupture of right shoulder, not specified as traumatic**

M75.112   **Incomplete rotator cuff tear or rupture of left shoulder, not specified as traumatic**

✓6th **M75.12   Complete rotator cuff tear or rupture not specified as traumatic**

M75.120   **Complete rotator cuff tear or rupture of unspecified shoulder, not specified as traumatic** ▽

M75.121   **Complete rotator cuff tear or rupture of right shoulder, not specified as traumatic**

M75.122   **Complete rotator cuff tear or rupture of left shoulder, not specified as traumatic**

✓5th **M75.2 Bicipital tendinitis**

M75.20   **Bicipital tendinitis, unspecified shoulder** ▽

M75.21   **Bicipital tendinitis, right shoulder**

M75.22   **Bicipital tendinitis, left shoulder**

✓5th **M75.3 Calcific tendinitis of shoulder**
Calcified bursa of shoulder

M75.30   **Calcific tendinitis of unspecified shoulder** ▽

M75.31   **Calcific tendinitis of right shoulder**

M75.32   **Calcific tendinitis of left shoulder**

✓5th **M75.4 Impingement syndrome of shoulder**

M75.40   **Impingement syndrome of unspecified shoulder** ▽

M75.41   Impingement syndrome of right shoulder
M75.42   Impingement syndrome of left shoulder

✓5ᵗʰ M75.5   Bursitis of shoulder
    M75.50   Bursitis of unspecified shoulder ▽
    M75.51   Bursitis of right shoulder
    M75.52   Bursitis of left shoulder

✓5ᵗʰ M75.8   Other shoulder lesions
    M75.80   Other shoulder lesions, unspecified shoulder ▽
    M75.81   Other shoulder lesions, right shoulder
    M75.82   Other shoulder lesions, left shoulder

✓5ᵗʰ M75.9   Shoulder lesion, unspecified
    M75.90   Shoulder lesion, unspecified, unspecified shoulder ▽
    M75.91   Shoulder lesion, unspecified, right shoulder ▽
    M75.92   Shoulder lesion, unspecified, left shoulder ▽

✓4ᵗʰ **M76   Enthesopathies, lower limb, excluding foot**
    EXCLUDES 2   *bursitis due to use, overuse and pressure (M70.-)*
          enthesopathies of ankle and foot (M77.5-)

✓5ᵗʰ M76.0   Gluteal tendinitis
    M76.00   Gluteal tendinitis, unspecified hip ▽
    M76.01   Gluteal tendinitis, right hip
    M76.02   Gluteal tendinitis, left hip

✓5ᵗʰ M76.1   Psoas tendinitis
    M76.10   Psoas tendinitis, unspecified hip ▽
    M76.11   Psoas tendinitis, right hip
    M76.12   Psoas tendinitis, left hip

✓5ᵗʰ M76.2   Iliac crest spur
    M76.20   Iliac crest spur, unspecified hip ▽
    M76.21   Iliac crest spur, right hip
    M76.22   Iliac crest spur, left hip

✓5ᵗʰ M76.3   Iliotibial band syndrome
    M76.30   Iliotibial band syndrome, unspecified leg ▽
    M76.31   Iliotibial band syndrome, right leg
    M76.32   Iliotibial band syndrome, left leg

✓5ᵗʰ M76.4   Tibial collateral bursitis [Pellegrini-Stieda]
    M76.40   Tibial collateral bursitis [Pellegrini-Stieda], unspecified leg ▽
    M76.41   Tibial collateral bursitis [Pellegrini-Stieda], right leg
    M76.42   Tibial collateral bursitis [Pellegrini-Stieda], left leg

✓5ᵗʰ M76.5   Patellar tendinitis
    M76.50   Patellar tendinitis, unspecified knee ▽
    M76.51   Patellar tendinitis, right knee
    M76.52   Patellar tendinitis, left knee

✓5ᵗʰ M76.6   Achilles tendinitis
    Achilles bursitis
    M76.60   Achilles tendinitis, unspecified leg ▽
    M76.61   Achilles tendinitis, right leg
    M76.62   Achilles tendinitis, left leg

✓5ᵗʰ M76.7   Peroneal tendinitis
    M76.70   Peroneal tendinitis, unspecified leg ▽
    M76.71   Peroneal tendinitis, right leg
    M76.72   Peroneal tendinitis, left leg

✓5ᵗʰ M76.8   Other specified enthesopathies of lower limb, excluding foot
    ✓6ᵗʰ M76.81   Anterior tibial syndrome
        M76.811   Anterior tibial syndrome, right leg
        M76.812   Anterior tibial syndrome, left leg
        M76.819   Anterior tibial syndrome, unspecified leg ▽
    ✓6ᵗʰ M76.82   Posterior tibial tendinitis
        M76.821   Posterior tibial tendinitis, right leg
        M76.822   Posterior tibial tendinitis, left leg
        M76.829   Posterior tibial tendinitis, unspecified leg ▽
    ✓6ᵗʰ M76.89   Other specified enthesopathies of lower limb, excluding foot
        M76.891   Other specified enthesopathies of right lower limb, excluding foot
        M76.892   Other specified enthesopathies of left lower limb, excluding foot
        M76.899   Other specified enthesopathies of unspecified lower limb, excluding foot ▽

M76.9   Unspecified enthesopathy, lower limb, excluding foot ▽

✓4ᵗʰ **M77   Other enthesopathies**
    EXCLUDES 1   *bursitis NOS (M71.9-)*
    EXCLUDES 2   *bursitis due to use, overuse and pressure (M70.-)*
          osteophyte (M25.7)
          spinal enthesopathy (M46.0-)

✓5ᵗʰ M77.0   Medial epicondylitis
    M77.00   Medial epicondylitis, unspecified elbow ▽
    M77.01   Medial epicondylitis, right elbow
    M77.02   Medial epicondylitis, left elbow

✓5ᵗʰ M77.1   Lateral epicondylitis
    Tennis elbow
    M77.10   Lateral epicondylitis, unspecified elbow ▽
    M77.11   Lateral epicondylitis, right elbow
    M77.12   Lateral epicondylitis, left elbow

✓5ᵗʰ M77.2   Periarthritis of wrist
    M77.20   Periarthritis, unspecified wrist ▽
    M77.21   Periarthritis, right wrist
    M77.22   Periarthritis, left wrist

✓5ᵗʰ M77.3   Calcaneal spur
    M77.30   Calcaneal spur, unspecified foot ▽
    M77.31   Calcaneal spur, right foot
    M77.32   Calcaneal spur, left foot

✓5ᵗʰ M77.4   Metatarsalgia
    EXCLUDES 1   *Morton's metatarsalgia (G57.6)*
    M77.40   Metatarsalgia, unspecified foot ▽
    M77.41   Metatarsalgia, right foot
    M77.42   Metatarsalgia, left foot

✓5ᵗʰ M77.5   Other enthesopathy of foot
    M77.50   Other enthesopathy of unspecified foot ▽
    M77.51   Other enthesopathy of right foot
    M77.52   Other enthesopathy of left foot

M77.8   Other enthesopathies, not elsewhere classified
M77.9   Enthesopathy, unspecified ▽
    Bone spur NOS   Periarthritis NOS
    Capsulitis NOS   Tendinitis NOS

✓4ᵗʰ **M79   Other and unspecified soft tissue disorders, not elsewhere classified**
    EXCLUDES 1   *psychogenic rheumatism (F45.8)*
          soft tissue pain, psychogenic (F45.41)

M79.0   Rheumatism, unspecified ▽
    EXCLUDES 1   *fibromyalgia (M79.7)*
          palindromic rheumatism (M12.3-)

M79.1   Myalgia
    Myofascial pain syndrome
    EXCLUDES 1   *fibromyalgia (M79.7)*
          myositis (M60.-)

M79.2   Neuralgia and neuritis, unspecified ▽
    EXCLUDES 1   *brachial radiculitis NOS (M54.1)*
          lumbosacral radiculitis NOS (M54.1)
          mononeuropathies (G56-G58)
          radiculitis NOS (M54.1)
          sciatica (M54.3-M54.4)

M79.3   Panniculitis, unspecified ▽
    EXCLUDES 1   *lupus panniculitis (L93.2)*
          neck and back panniculitis (M54.0-)
          relapsing [Weber-Christian] panniculitis (M35.6)

M79.4   Hypertrophy of (infrapatellar) fat pad
M79.5   Residual foreign body in soft tissue
    EXCLUDES 1   *foreign body granuloma of skin and subcutaneous tissue (L92.3)*
          foreign body granuloma of soft tissue (M60.2-)

✓5ᵗʰ M79.6   Pain in limb, hand, foot, fingers and toes
    EXCLUDES 2   *pain in joint (M25.5-)*
    ✓6ᵗʰ M79.60   Pain in limb, unspecified
        M79.601   Pain in right arm
          Pain in right upper limb NOS
        M79.602   Pain in left arm
          Pain in left upper limb NOS
        M79.603   Pain in arm, unspecified ▽
          Pain in upper limb NOS
        M79.604   Pain in right leg
          Pain in right lower limb NOS

Ⓝ Newborn   Ⓟ Pediatric   Ⓜ Maternity   Ⓐ Adult   RIC RIC Dx   NCDx Noncancer Dx   P Dx Primary Dx   CC RIC CC Condition   ►◄ Revised Text   ● New Code   ▲ Revised Code Title

734   ICD-10-CM 2016

M79.605   **Pain in** left leg
  Pain in left lower limb NOS

M79.606   **Pain in leg, unspecified**   ▽
  Pain in lower limb NOS

M79.609   **Pain in unspecified limb**   ▽
  Pain in limb NOS

✓6ᵗʰ **M79.62**   **Pain in** upper arm
  Pain in axillary region

M79.621   **Pain in** right **upper arm**

M79.622   **Pain in** left **upper arm**

M79.629   **Pain in unspecified upper arm**   ▽

✓6ᵗʰ **M79.63**   **Pain in** forearm

M79.631   **Pain in** right **forearm**

M79.632   **Pain in** left **forearm**

M79.639   **Pain in unspecified forearm**   ▽

✓6ᵗʰ **M79.64**   **Pain in** hand and fingers

M79.641   **Pain in** right **hand**

M79.642   **Pain in** left **hand**

M79.643   **Pain in unspecified hand**   ▽

M79.644   **Pain in** right **finger(s)**

M79.645   **Pain in** left **finger(s)**

M79.646   **Pain in unspecified finger(s)**   ▽

✓6ᵗʰ **M79.65**   **Pain in** thigh

M79.651   **Pain in** right **thigh**

M79.652   **Pain in** left **thigh**

M79.659   **Pain in unspecified thigh**   ▽

✓6ᵗʰ **M79.66**   **Pain in** lower leg

M79.661   **Pain in** right **lower leg**

M79.662   **Pain in** left **lower leg**

M79.669   **Pain in unspecified lower leg**   ▽

✓6ᵗʰ **M79.67**   **Pain in** foot and toes

M79.671   **Pain in** right **foot**

M79.672   **Pain in** left **foot**

M79.673   **Pain in unspecified foot**   ▽

M79.674   **Pain in** right **toe(s)**

M79.675   **Pain in** left **toe(s)**

M79.676   **Pain in unspecified toe(s)**   ▽

M79.7 Fibromyalgia
  Fibromyositis   Myofibrositis
  Fibrositis

✓5ᵗʰ **M79.A Nontraumatic compartment syndrome**
  Code first, if applicable, associated postprocedural complication
  EXCLUDES 1   *compartment syndrome NOS (T79.A-)*
    fibromyalgia (M79.7)
    nontraumatic ischemic infarction of muscle (M62.2-)
    traumatic compartment syndrome (T79.A-)

✓6ᵗʰ **M79.A1**   **Nontraumatic compartment syndrome of** upper **extremity**
  Nontraumatic compartment syndrome of shoulder, arm, forearm, wrist, hand, and fingers

M79.A11   **Nontraumatic compartment syndrome of** right **upper extremity**

M79.A12   **Nontraumatic compartment syndrome of** left **upper extremity**

M79.A19   **Nontraumatic compartment syndrome of unspecified upper extremity**   ▽

✓6ᵗʰ **M79.A2**   **Nontraumatic compartment syndrome of** lower **extremity**
  Nontraumatic compartment syndrome of hip, buttock, thigh, leg, foot, and toes

M79.A21   **Nontraumatic compartment syndrome of** right **lower extremity**

M79.A22   **Nontraumatic compartment syndrome of** left **lower extremity**

M79.A29   **Nontraumatic compartment syndrome of unspecified lower extremity**   ▽

M79.A3   **Nontraumatic compartment syndrome of** abdomen

M79.A9   **Nontraumatic compartment syndrome of other sites**

✓5ᵗʰ **M79.8 Other specified soft tissue disorders**

M79.81   **Nontraumatic hematoma of soft tissue**
  Nontraumatic hematoma of muscle
  Nontraumatic seroma of muscle and soft tissue

M79.89   **Other specified soft tissue disorders**
  Polyalgia

M79.9   **Soft tissue disorder, unspecified**   ▽

OSTEOPATHIES AND CHONDROPATHIES (M80-M94)

Disorders of bone density and structure (M80-M85)

✓4ᵗʰ **M80 Osteoporosis** with current pathological fracture
  INCLUDES osteoporosis with current fragility fracture
  Use additional code to identify major osseous defect, if applicable (M89.7-)
  EXCLUDES 1   *collapsed vertebra NOS (M48.5)*
    pathological fracture NOS (M84.4)
    wedging of vertebra NOS (M48.5)
  EXCLUDES 2   *personal history of (healed) osteoporosis fracture (Z87.310)*

The appropriate 7th character is to be added to each code from category M80.
A   initial encounter for fracture
D   subsequent encounter for fracture with routine healing
G   subsequent encounter for fracture with delayed healing
K   subsequent encounter for fracture with nonunion
P   subsequent encounter for fracture with malunion
S   sequela

✓5ᵗʰ **M80.0**   Age-related **osteoporosis with current pathological fracture**
  Involutional osteoporosis with current pathological fracture
  Osteoporosis NOS with current pathological fracture
  Postmenopausal osteoporosis with current pathological fracture
  Senile osteoporosis with current pathological fracture

✓✗7ᵗʰ **M80.00**   **Age-related osteoporosis with current pathological fracture, unspecified site**   A ▽

✓6ᵗʰ **M80.01**   **Age-related osteoporosis with current pathological fracture,** shoulder

✓7ᵗʰ **M80.011**   **Age-related osteoporosis with current pathological fracture,** right **shoulder**   A

✓7ᵗʰ **M80.012**   **Age-related osteoporosis with current pathological fracture,** left **shoulder**   A

✓7ᵗʰ **M80.019**   **Age-related osteoporosis with current pathological fracture, unspecified shoulder**   A ▽

✓6ᵗʰ **M80.02**   **Age-related osteoporosis with current pathological fracture,** humerus

✓7ᵗʰ **M80.021**   **Age-related osteoporosis with current pathological fracture,** right **humerus**   A

✓7ᵗʰ **M80.022**   **Age-related osteoporosis with current pathological fracture,** left **humerus**   A

✓7ᵗʰ **M80.029**   **Age-related osteoporosis with current pathological fracture, unspecified humerus**   A ▽

✓6ᵗʰ **M80.03**   **Age-related osteoporosis with current pathological fracture,** forearm
  Age-related osteoporosis with current pathological fracture of wrist

✓7ᵗʰ **M80.031**   **Age-related osteoporosis with current pathological fracture,** right **forearm**   A

✓7ᵗʰ **M80.032**   **Age-related osteoporosis with current pathological fracture,** left **forearm**   A

✓7ᵗʰ **M80.039**   **Age-related osteoporosis with current pathological fracture, unspecified forearm**   A ▽

✓6ᵗʰ **M80.04**   **Age-related osteoporosis with current pathological fracture,** hand

✓7ᵗʰ **M80.041**   **Age-related osteoporosis with current pathological fracture,** right **hand**   A

✓7ᵗʰ **M80.042**   **Age-related osteoporosis with current pathological fracture,** left **hand**   A

✓7ᵗʰ **M80.049**   **Age-related osteoporosis with current pathological fracture, unspecified hand**   A ▽

✓6ᵗʰ **M80.05**   **Age-related osteoporosis with current pathological fracture,** femur
  Age-related osteoporosis with current pathological fracture of hip

✓7ᵗʰ **M80.051**   **Age-related osteoporosis with current pathological fracture,** right **femur**   A

✓7ᵗʰ **M80.052**   **Age-related osteoporosis with current pathological fracture,** left **femur**   A

☑ Add'l Character Required   ✓✗7ᵗʰ Placeholder Alert   RUG IV Special Care High Dx   RUG IV Clinically Complex Dx   RUG IV Special Care Low Dx   Manifestation Code   Other Specified Code   ▽ Unspecified Code

ICD-10-CM 2016   **735**

Chapter 13. Diseases of the Musculoskeletal System and Connective Tissue

M80.059–M83.9

✓7th **M80.059** Age-related osteoporosis with current pathological fracture, unspecified femur Ⓐ ▽

✓6th **M80.06** Age-related osteoporosis with current pathological fracture, lower leg

    ✓7th **M80.061** Age-related osteoporosis with current pathological fracture, right lower leg Ⓐ

    ✓7th **M80.062** Age-related osteoporosis with current pathological fracture, left lower leg Ⓐ

    ✓7th **M80.069** Age-related osteoporosis with current pathological fracture, unspecified lower leg Ⓐ ▽

✓6th **M80.07** Age-related osteoporosis with current pathological fracture, ankle and foot

    ✓7th **M80.071** Age-related osteoporosis with current pathological fracture, right ankle and foot Ⓐ

    ✓7th **M80.072** Age-related osteoporosis with current pathological fracture, left ankle and foot Ⓐ

    ✓7th **M80.079** Age-related osteoporosis with current pathological fracture, unspecified ankle and foot Ⓐ ▽

✓x7th **M80.08** Age-related osteoporosis with current pathological fracture, vertebra(e) Ⓐ

✓5th **M80.8** Other osteoporosis with current pathological fracture
Drug-induced osteoporosis with current pathological fracture
Idiopathic osteoporosis with current pathological fracture
Osteoporosis of disuse with current pathological fracture
Postoophorectomy osteoporosis with current pathological fracture
Postsurgical malabsorption osteoporosis with current pathological fracture
Post-traumatic osteoporosis with current pathological fracture
Use additional code for adverse effect, if applicable, to identify drug (T36-T50 with fifth or sixth character 5)

✓x7th **M80.80** Other osteoporosis with current pathological fracture, unspecified site ▽

✓6th **M80.81** Other osteoporosis with pathological fracture, shoulder

    ✓7th **M80.811** Other osteoporosis with current pathological fracture, right shoulder

    ✓7th **M80.812** Other osteoporosis with current pathological fracture, left shoulder

    ✓7th **M80.819** Other osteoporosis with current pathological fracture, unspecified shoulder ▽

✓6th **M80.82** Other osteoporosis with current pathological fracture, humerus

    ✓7th **M80.821** Other osteoporosis with current pathological fracture, right humerus

    ✓7th **M80.822** Other osteoporosis with current pathological fracture, left humerus

    ✓7th **M80.829** Other osteoporosis with current pathological fracture, unspecified humerus ▽

✓6th **M80.83** Other osteoporosis with current pathological fracture, forearm
Other osteoporosis with current pathological fracture of wrist

    ✓7th **M80.831** Other osteoporosis with current pathological fracture, right forearm

    ✓7th **M80.832** Other osteoporosis with current pathological fracture, left forearm

    ✓7th **M80.839** Other osteoporosis with current pathological fracture, unspecified forearm ▽

✓6th **M80.84** Other osteoporosis with current pathological fracture, hand

    ✓7th **M80.841** Other osteoporosis with current pathological fracture, right hand

    ✓7th **M80.842** Other osteoporosis with current pathological fracture, left hand

    ✓7th **M80.849** Other osteoporosis with current pathological fracture, unspecified hand ▽

✓6th **M80.85** Other osteoporosis with current pathological fracture, femur
Other osteoporosis with current pathological fracture of hip

    ✓7th **M80.851** Other osteoporosis with current pathological fracture, right femur

    ✓7th **M80.852** Other osteoporosis with current pathological fracture, left femur

    ✓7th **M80.859** Other osteoporosis with current pathological fracture, unspecified femur ▽

✓6th **M80.86** Other osteoporosis with current pathological fracture, lower leg

    ✓7th **M80.861** Other osteoporosis with current pathological fracture, right lower leg

    ✓7th **M80.862** Other osteoporosis with current pathological fracture, left lower leg

    ✓7th **M80.869** Other osteoporosis with current pathological fracture, unspecified lower leg ▽

✓6th **M80.87** Other osteoporosis with current pathological fracture, ankle and foot

    ✓7th **M80.871** Other osteoporosis with current pathological fracture, right ankle and foot

    ✓7th **M80.872** Other osteoporosis with current pathological fracture, left ankle and foot

    ✓7th **M80.879** Other osteoporosis with current pathological fracture, unspecified ankle and foot ▽

✓x7th **M80.88** Other osteoporosis with current pathological fracture, vertebra(e)

✓4th **M81** Osteoporosis without current pathological fracture
Use additional code to identify:
major osseous defect, if applicable (M89.7-)
personal history of (healed) osteoporosis fracture, if applicable (Z87.310)
   EXCLUDES 1   osteoporosis with current pathological fracture (M80.-)
         Sudeck's atrophy (M89.0)

M81.0 Age-related osteoporosis without current pathological fracture Ⓐ
Involutional osteoporosis without current pathological fracture
Osteoporosis NOS
Postmenopausal osteoporosis without current pathological fracture
Senile osteoporosis without current pathological fracture

M81.6 Localized osteoporosis [Lequesne]
   EXCLUDES 1   Sudeck's atrophy (M89.0)

M81.8 Other osteoporosis without current pathological fracture
Drug-induced osteoporosis without current pathological fracture
Idiopathic osteoporosis without current pathological fracture
Osteoporosis of disuse without current pathological fracture
Postoophorectomy osteoporosis without current pathological fracture
Postsurgical malabsorption osteoporosis without current pathological fracture
Post-traumatic osteoporosis without current pathological fracture
Use additional code for adverse effect, if applicable, to identify drug (T36-T50 with fifth or sixth character 5)

✓4th **M83** Adult osteomalacia
   EXCLUDES 1   infantile and juvenile osteomalacia (E55.0)
         renal osteodystrophy (N25.0)
         rickets (active) (E55.0)
         rickets (active) sequelae (E64.3)
         vitamin D-resistant osteomalacia (E83.3)
         vitamin D-resistant rickets (active) (E83.3)

M83.0 Puerperal osteomalacia Ⓜ♀

M83.1 Senile osteomalacia Ⓐ

M83.2 Adult osteomalacia due to malabsorption Ⓐ
Postsurgical malabsorption osteomalacia in adults

M83.3 Adult osteomalacia due to malnutrition Ⓐ

M83.4 Aluminum bone disease

M83.5 Other drug-induced osteomalacia in adults Ⓐ
Use additional code for adverse effect, if applicable, to identify drug (T36-T50 with fifth or sixth character 5)

M83.8 Other adult osteomalacia Ⓐ

M83.9 Adult osteomalacia, unspecified Ⓐ ▽

Ⓝ Newborn   Ⓟ Pediatric   Ⓜ Maternity   Ⓐ Adult   **RIC** RIC Dx   **NCDx** Noncancer Dx   **PDx** Primary Dx   **CC** RIC CC Condition   ▶◀ Revised Text   ● New Code   ▲ Revised Code Title

736   ICD-10-CM 2016

✓4ᵗʰ M84 Disorder of continuity of bone

EXCLUDES 2   *traumatic fracture of bone-see fracture, by site*

✓5ᵗʰ M84.3 Stress fracture

Fatigue fracture   Stress fracture NOS
March fracture   Stress reaction

Use additional external cause code(s) to identify the cause of the stress fracture

EXCLUDES 1   *pathological fracture NOS (M84.4-)*
            pathological fracture due to osteoporosis (M80.-)
            traumatic fracture (S12-, S22-, S32-, S42-, S52-, S62-,
            S72-, S82-, S92-)

EXCLUDES 2   *personal history of (healed) stress (fatigue) fracture*
            (Z87.312)
            stress fracture of vertebra (M48.4-)

The appropriate 7th character is to be added to each code from subcategory M84.3.
A   initial encounter for fracture
D   subsequent encounter for fracture with routine healing
G   subsequent encounter for fracture with delayed healing
K   subsequent encounter for fracture with nonunion
P   subsequent encounter for fracture with malunion
S   sequela

✓x7ᵗʰ **M84.30**   Stress fracture, unspecified site ▽

✓6ᵗʰ **M84.31**   Stress fracture, shoulder
    ✓7ᵗʰ **M84.311**   Stress fracture, right shoulder
    ✓7ᵗʰ **M84.312**   Stress fracture, left shoulder
    ✓7ᵗʰ **M84.319**   Stress fracture, unspecified shoulder ▽

✓6ᵗʰ **M84.32**   Stress fracture, humerus
    ✓7ᵗʰ **M84.321**   Stress fracture, right humerus
    ✓7ᵗʰ **M84.322**   Stress fracture, left humerus
    ✓7ᵗʰ **M84.329**   Stress fracture, unspecified humerus ▽

✓6ᵗʰ **M84.33**   Stress fracture, ulna and radius
    ✓7ᵗʰ **M84.331**   Stress fracture, right ulna
    ✓7ᵗʰ **M84.332**   Stress fracture, left ulna
    ✓7ᵗʰ **M84.333**   Stress fracture, right radius
    ✓7ᵗʰ **M84.334**   Stress fracture, left radius
    ✓7ᵗʰ **M84.339**   Stress fracture, unspecified ulna and radius ▽

✓6ᵗʰ **M84.34**   Stress fracture, hand and fingers
    ✓7ᵗʰ **M84.341**   Stress fracture, right hand
    ✓7ᵗʰ **M84.342**   Stress fracture, left hand
    ✓7ᵗʰ **M84.343**   Stress fracture, unspecified hand ▽
    ✓7ᵗʰ **M84.344**   Stress fracture, right finger(s)
    ✓7ᵗʰ **M84.345**   Stress fracture, left finger(s)
    ✓7ᵗʰ **M84.346**   Stress fracture, unspecified finger(s) ▽

✓6ᵗʰ **M84.35**   Stress fracture, pelvis and femur
              Stress fracture, hip
    ✓7ᵗʰ **M84.350**   Stress fracture, pelvis
    ✓7ᵗʰ **M84.351**   Stress fracture, right femur
    ✓7ᵗʰ **M84.352**   Stress fracture, left femur
    ✓7ᵗʰ **M84.353**   Stress fracture, unspecified femur ▽
    ✓7ᵗʰ **M84.359**   Stress fracture, hip, unspecified ▽

✓6ᵗʰ **M84.36**   Stress fracture, tibia and fibula
    ✓7ᵗʰ **M84.361**   Stress fracture, right tibia
    ✓7ᵗʰ **M84.362**   Stress fracture, left tibia
    ✓7ᵗʰ **M84.363**   Stress fracture, right fibula
    ✓7ᵗʰ **M84.364**   Stress fracture, left fibula
    ✓7ᵗʰ **M84.369**   Stress fracture, unspecified tibia and fibula ▽

✓6ᵗʰ **M84.37**   Stress fracture, ankle, foot and toes
    ✓7ᵗʰ **M84.371**   Stress fracture, right ankle
    ✓7ᵗʰ **M84.372**   Stress fracture, left ankle
    ✓7ᵗʰ **M84.373**   Stress fracture, unspecified ankle ▽
    ✓7ᵗʰ **M84.374**   Stress fracture, right foot
    ✓7ᵗʰ **M84.375**   Stress fracture, left foot
    ✓7ᵗʰ **M84.376**   Stress fracture, unspecified foot ▽
    ✓7ᵗʰ **M84.377**   Stress fracture, right toe(s)
    ✓7ᵗʰ **M84.378**   Stress fracture, left toe(s)
    ✓7ᵗʰ **M84.379**   Stress fracture, unspecified toe(s) ▽

✓x7ᵗʰ M84.38 Stress fracture, other site

EXCLUDES 2   *stress fracture of vertebra (M48.4-)*

✓5ᵗʰ M84.4 Pathological fracture, not elsewhere classified

Chronic fracture
Pathological fracture NOS

EXCLUDES 1   *collapsed vertebra NEC (M48.5)*
            pathological fracture in neoplastic disease (M84.5-)
            pathological fracture in osteoporosis (M80.-)
            pathological fracture in other disease (M84.6-)
            stress fracture (M84.3-)
            traumatic fracture (S12.-, S22.-, S32.-, S42.-, S52.-, S62.-,
            S72.-, S82.-, S92.-)

EXCLUDES 2   *personal history of (healed) pathological fracture*
            (Z87.311)

The appropriate 7th character is to be added to each code from subcategory M84.4.
A   initial encounter for fracture
D   subsequent encounter for fracture with routine healing
G   subsequent encounter for fracture with delayed healing
K   subsequent encounter for fracture with nonunion
P   subsequent encounter for fracture with malunion
S   sequela

✓x7ᵗʰ **M84.40**   Pathological fracture, unspecified site ▽

✓6ᵗʰ **M84.41**   Pathological fracture, shoulder
    ✓7ᵗʰ **M84.411**   Pathological fracture, right shoulder
    ✓7ᵗʰ **M84.412**   Pathological fracture, left shoulder
    ✓7ᵗʰ **M84.419**   Pathological fracture, unspecified shoulder ▽

✓6ᵗʰ **M84.42**   Pathological fracture, humerus
    ✓7ᵗʰ **M84.421**   Pathological fracture, right humerus
    ✓7ᵗʰ **M84.422**   Pathological fracture, left humerus
    ✓7ᵗʰ **M84.429**   Pathological fracture, unspecified humerus ▽

✓6ᵗʰ **M84.43**   Pathological fracture, ulna and radius
    ✓7ᵗʰ **M84.431**   Pathological fracture, right ulna
    ✓7ᵗʰ **M84.432**   Pathological fracture, left ulna
    ✓7ᵗʰ **M84.433**   Pathological fracture, right radius
    ✓7ᵗʰ **M84.434**   Pathological fracture, left radius
    ✓7ᵗʰ **M84.439**   Pathological fracture, unspecified ulna and radius ▽

✓6ᵗʰ **M84.44**   Pathological fracture, hand and fingers
    ✓7ᵗʰ **M84.441**   Pathological fracture, right hand
    ✓7ᵗʰ **M84.442**   Pathological fracture, left hand
    ✓7ᵗʰ **M84.443**   Pathological fracture, unspecified hand ▽
    ✓7ᵗʰ **M84.444**   Pathological fracture, right finger(s)
    ✓7ᵗʰ **M84.445**   Pathological fracture, left finger(s)
    ✓7ᵗʰ **M84.446**   Pathological fracture, unspecified finger(s) ▽

✓6ᵗʰ **M84.45**   Pathological fracture, femur and pelvis
    ✓7ᵗʰ **M84.451**   Pathological fracture, right femur
    ✓7ᵗʰ **M84.452**   Pathological fracture, left femur
    ✓7ᵗʰ **M84.453**   Pathological fracture, unspecified femur ▽
    ✓7ᵗʰ **M84.454**   Pathological fracture, pelvis
    ✓7ᵗʰ **M84.459**   Pathological fracture, hip, unspecified ▽

✓6ᵗʰ **M84.46**   Pathological fracture, tibia and fibula
    ✓7ᵗʰ **M84.461**   Pathological fracture, right tibia
    ✓7ᵗʰ **M84.462**   Pathological fracture, left tibia
    ✓7ᵗʰ **M84.463**   Pathological fracture, right fibula
    ✓7ᵗʰ **M84.464**   Pathological fracture, left fibula
    ✓7ᵗʰ **M84.469**   Pathological fracture, unspecified tibia and fibula ▽

✓6ᵗʰ **M84.47**   Pathological fracture, ankle, foot and toes
    ✓7ᵗʰ **M84.471**   Pathological fracture, right ankle
    ✓7ᵗʰ **M84.472**   Pathological fracture, left ankle
    ✓7ᵗʰ **M84.473**   Pathological fracture, unspecified ankle ▽
    ✓7ᵗʰ **M84.474**   Pathological fracture, right foot
    ✓7ᵗʰ **M84.475**   Pathological fracture, left foot

☑ Add'l Character Required   ✓x7ᵗʰ Placeholder Alert   RUG IV Special Care High Dx   RUG IV Clinically Complex Dx   RUG IV Special Care Low Dx   Manifestation Code   Other Specified Code   ▽ Unspecified Code

☑7ᵗʰ **M84.476** Pathological fracture, unspecified foot ▽

☑7ᵗʰ **M84.477** Pathological fracture, right toe(s)

☑7ᵗʰ **M84.478** Pathological fracture, left toe(s)

☑7ᵗʰ **M84.479** Pathological fracture, unspecified toe(s) ▽

☑x7ᵗʰ **M84.48** Pathological fracture, other site

☑5ᵗʰ **M84.5** Pathological fracture in neoplastic disease
Code also underlying neoplasm

> The appropriate 7th character is to be added to each code from subcategory M84.5.
> A   initial encounter for fracture
> D   subsequent encounter for fracture with routine healing
> G   subsequent encounter for fracture with delayed healing
> K   subsequent encounter for fracture with nonunion
> P   subsequent encounter for fracture with malunion
> S   sequela

☑x7ᵗʰ **M84.50** Pathological fracture in neoplastic disease, unspecified site ▽

☑6ᵗʰ **M84.51** Pathological fracture in neoplastic disease, shoulder

☑7ᵗʰ **M84.511** Pathological fracture in neoplastic disease, right shoulder

☑7ᵗʰ **M84.512** Pathological fracture in neoplastic disease, left shoulder

☑7ᵗʰ **M84.519** Pathological fracture in neoplastic disease, unspecified shoulder ▽

☑6ᵗʰ **M84.52** Pathological fracture in neoplastic disease, humerus

☑7ᵗʰ **M84.521** Pathological fracture in neoplastic disease, right humerus

☑7ᵗʰ **M84.522** Pathological fracture in neoplastic disease, left humerus

☑7ᵗʰ **M84.529** Pathological fracture in neoplastic disease, unspecified humerus ▽

☑6ᵗʰ **M84.53** Pathological fracture in neoplastic disease, ulna and radius

☑7ᵗʰ **M84.531** Pathological fracture in neoplastic disease, right ulna

☑7ᵗʰ **M84.532** Pathological fracture in neoplastic disease, left ulna

☑7ᵗʰ **M84.533** Pathological fracture in neoplastic disease, right radius

☑7ᵗʰ **M84.534** Pathological fracture in neoplastic disease, left radius

☑7ᵗʰ **M84.539** Pathological fracture in neoplastic disease, unspecified ulna and radius ▽

☑6ᵗʰ **M84.54** Pathological fracture in neoplastic disease, hand

☑7ᵗʰ **M84.541** Pathological fracture in neoplastic disease, right hand

☑7ᵗʰ **M84.542** Pathological fracture in neoplastic disease, left hand

☑7ᵗʰ **M84.549** Pathological fracture in neoplastic disease, unspecified hand ▽

☑6ᵗʰ **M84.55** Pathological fracture in neoplastic disease, pelvis and femur

☑7ᵗʰ **M84.550** Pathological fracture in neoplastic disease, pelvis

☑7ᵗʰ **M84.551** Pathological fracture in neoplastic disease, right femur

☑7ᵗʰ **M84.552** Pathological fracture in neoplastic disease, left femur

☑7ᵗʰ **M84.553** Pathological fracture in neoplastic disease, unspecified femur ▽

☑7ᵗʰ **M84.559** Pathological fracture in neoplastic disease, hip, unspecified ▽

☑6ᵗʰ **M84.56** Pathological fracture in neoplastic disease, tibia and fibula

☑7ᵗʰ **M84.561** Pathological fracture in neoplastic disease, right tibia

☑7ᵗʰ **M84.562** Pathological fracture in neoplastic disease, left tibia

☑7ᵗʰ **M84.563** Pathological fracture in neoplastic disease, right fibula

☑7ᵗʰ **M84.564** Pathological fracture in neoplastic disease, left fibula

☑7ᵗʰ **M84.569** Pathological fracture in neoplastic disease, unspecified tibia and fibula ▽

☑6ᵗʰ **M84.57** Pathological fracture in neoplastic disease, ankle and foot

☑7ᵗʰ **M84.571** Pathological fracture in neoplastic disease, right ankle

☑7ᵗʰ **M84.572** Pathological fracture in neoplastic disease, left ankle

☑7ᵗʰ **M84.573** Pathological fracture in neoplastic disease, unspecified ankle ▽

☑7ᵗʰ **M84.574** Pathological fracture in neoplastic disease, right foot

☑7ᵗʰ **M84.575** Pathological fracture in neoplastic disease, left foot

☑7ᵗʰ **M84.576** Pathological fracture in neoplastic disease, unspecified foot ▽

☑x7ᵗʰ **M84.58** Pathological fracture in neoplastic disease, other specified site
Pathological fracture in neoplastic disease, vertebrae

☑5ᵗʰ **M84.6** Pathological fracture in other disease
Code also underlying condition
EXCLUDES 1 pathological fracture in osteoporosis (M80.-)

> The appropriate 7th character is to be added to each code from subcategory M84.6.
> A   initial encounter for fracture
> D   subsequent encounter for fracture with routine healing
> G   subsequent encounter for fracture with delayed healing
> K   subsequent encounter for fracture with nonunion
> P   subsequent encounter for fracture with malunion
> S   sequela

☑x7ᵗʰ **M84.60** Pathological fracture in other disease, unspecified site ▽

☑6ᵗʰ **M84.61** Pathological fracture in other disease, shoulder

☑7ᵗʰ **M84.611** Pathological fracture in other disease, right shoulder

☑7ᵗʰ **M84.612** Pathological fracture in other disease, left shoulder

☑7ᵗʰ **M84.619** Pathological fracture in other disease, unspecified shoulder ▽

☑6ᵗʰ **M84.62** Pathological fracture in other disease, humerus

☑7ᵗʰ **M84.621** Pathological fracture in other disease, right humerus

☑7ᵗʰ **M84.622** Pathological fracture in other disease, left humerus

☑7ᵗʰ **M84.629** Pathological fracture in other disease, unspecified humerus ▽

☑6ᵗʰ **M84.63** Pathological fracture in other disease, ulna and radius

☑7ᵗʰ **M84.631** Pathological fracture in other disease, right ulna

☑7ᵗʰ **M84.632** Pathological fracture in other disease, left ulna

☑7ᵗʰ **M84.633** Pathological fracture in other disease, right radius

☑7ᵗʰ **M84.634** Pathological fracture in other disease, left radius

☑7ᵗʰ **M84.639** Pathological fracture in other disease, unspecified ulna and radius ▽

☑6ᵗʰ **M84.64** Pathological fracture in other disease, hand

☑7ᵗʰ **M84.641** Pathological fracture in other disease, right hand

☑7ᵗʰ **M84.642** Pathological fracture in other disease, left hand

☑7ᵗʰ **M84.649** Pathological fracture in other disease, unspecified hand ▽

☑6ᵗʰ **M84.65** Pathological fracture in other disease, pelvis and femur

☑7ᵗʰ **M84.650** Pathological fracture in other disease, pelvis

☑7ᵗʰ **M84.651** Pathological fracture in other disease, right femur

---

Ⓝ Newborn   Ⓟ Pediatric   Ⓜ Maternity   Ⓐ Adult   **RIC** RIC Dx   **NCDx** Noncancer Dx   **PDx** Primary Dx   **CC** RIC CC Condition   ►◄ Revised Text   ● New Code   ▲ Revised Code Title

✓7ᵗʰ **M84.652** Pathological fracture in other disease, left femur

✓7ᵗʰ **M84.653** Pathological fracture in other disease, unspecified femur △

✓7ᵗʰ **M84.659** Pathological fracture in other disease, hip, unspecified △

✓6ᵗʰ **M84.66** Pathological fracture in other disease, tibia and fibula

    ✓7ᵗʰ **M84.661** Pathological fracture in other disease, right tibia

    ✓7ᵗʰ **M84.662** Pathological fracture in other disease, left tibia

    ✓7ᵗʰ **M84.663** Pathological fracture in other disease, right fibula

    ✓7ᵗʰ **M84.664** Pathological fracture in other disease, left fibula

    ✓7ᵗʰ **M84.669** Pathological fracture in other disease, unspecified tibia and fibula △

✓6ᵗʰ **M84.67** Pathological fracture in other disease, ankle and foot

    ✓7ᵗʰ **M84.671** Pathological fracture in other disease, right ankle

    ✓7ᵗʰ **M84.672** Pathological fracture in other disease, left ankle

    ✓7ᵗʰ **M84.673** Pathological fracture in other disease, unspecified ankle △

    ✓7ᵗʰ **M84.674** Pathological fracture in other disease, right foot

    ✓7ᵗʰ **M84.675** Pathological fracture in other disease, left foot

    ✓7ᵗʰ **M84.676** Pathological fracture in other disease, unspecified foot △

✓x7ᵗʰ **M84.68** Pathological fracture in other disease, other site

✓5ᵗʰ **M84.8** Other disorders of continuity of bone

    M84.80 Other disorders of continuity of bone, unspecified site △

✓6ᵗʰ **M84.81** Other disorders of continuity of bone, shoulder

    M84.811 Other disorders of continuity of bone, right shoulder

    M84.812 Other disorders of continuity of bone, left shoulder

    M84.819 Other disorders of continuity of bone, unspecified shoulder △

✓6ᵗʰ **M84.82** Other disorders of continuity of bone, humerus

    M84.821 Other disorders of continuity of bone, right humerus

    M84.822 Other disorders of continuity of bone, left humerus

    M84.829 Other disorders of continuity of bone, unspecified humerus △

✓6ᵗʰ **M84.83** Other disorders of continuity of bone, ulna and radius

    M84.831 Other disorders of continuity of bone, right ulna

    M84.832 Other disorders of continuity of bone, left ulna

    M84.833 Other disorders of continuity of bone, right radius

    M84.834 Other disorders of continuity of bone, left radius

    M84.839 Other disorders of continuity of bone, unspecified ulna and radius △

✓6ᵗʰ **M84.84** Other disorders of continuity of bone, hand

    M84.841 Other disorders of continuity of bone, right hand

    M84.842 Other disorders of continuity of bone, left hand

    M84.849 Other disorders of continuity of bone, unspecified hand △

✓6ᵗʰ **M84.85** Other disorders of continuity of bone, pelvic region and thigh

    M84.851 Other disorders of continuity of bone, right pelvic region and thigh

    M84.852 Other disorders of continuity of bone, left pelvic region and thigh

M84.859 Other disorders of continuity of bone, unspecified pelvic region and thigh △

✓6ᵗʰ **M84.86** Other disorders of continuity of bone, tibia and fibula

    M84.861 Other disorders of continuity of bone, right tibia

    M84.862 Other disorders of continuity of bone, left tibia

    M84.863 Other disorders of continuity of bone, right fibula

    M84.864 Other disorders of continuity of bone, left fibula

    M84.869 Other disorders of continuity of bone, unspecified tibia and fibula △

✓6ᵗʰ **M84.87** Other disorders of continuity of bone, ankle and foot

    M84.871 Other disorders of continuity of bone, right ankle and foot

    M84.872 Other disorders of continuity of bone, left ankle and foot

    M84.879 Other disorders of continuity of bone, unspecified ankle and foot △

M84.88 Other disorders of continuity of bone, other site

M84.9 Disorder of continuity of bone, unspecified △

✓4ᵗʰ **M85** **Other disorders of bone density and structure**

    EXCLUDES 1   osteogenesis imperfecta (Q78.0)
         osteopetrosis (Q78.2)
         osteopoikilosis (Q78.8)
         polyostotic fibrous dysplasia (Q78.1)

✓5ᵗʰ **M85.0** Fibrous dysplasia (monostotic)

    EXCLUDES 2   fibrous dysplasia of jaw (M27.8)

    M85.00 Fibrous dysplasia (monostotic), unspecified site △

✓6ᵗʰ **M85.01** Fibrous dysplasia (monostotic), shoulder

    M85.011 Fibrous dysplasia (monostotic), right shoulder

    M85.012 Fibrous dysplasia (monostotic), left shoulder

    M85.019 Fibrous dysplasia (monostotic), unspecified shoulder △

✓6ᵗʰ **M85.02** Fibrous dysplasia (monostotic), upper arm

    M85.021 Fibrous dysplasia (monostotic), right upper arm

    M85.022 Fibrous dysplasia (monostotic), left upper arm

    M85.029 Fibrous dysplasia (monostotic), unspecified upper arm △

✓6ᵗʰ **M85.03** Fibrous dysplasia (monostotic), forearm

    M85.031 Fibrous dysplasia (monostotic), right forearm

    M85.032 Fibrous dysplasia (monostotic), left forearm

    M85.039 Fibrous dysplasia (monostotic), unspecified forearm △

✓6ᵗʰ **M85.04** Fibrous dysplasia (monostotic), hand

    M85.041 Fibrous dysplasia (monostotic), right hand

    M85.042 Fibrous dysplasia (monostotic), left hand

    M85.049 Fibrous dysplasia (monostotic), unspecified hand △

✓6ᵗʰ **M85.05** Fibrous dysplasia (monostotic), thigh

    M85.051 Fibrous dysplasia (monostotic), right thigh

    M85.052 Fibrous dysplasia (monostotic), left thigh

    M85.059 Fibrous dysplasia (monostotic), unspecified thigh △

✓6ᵗʰ **M85.06** Fibrous dysplasia (monostotic), lower leg

    M85.061 Fibrous dysplasia (monostotic), right lower leg

    M85.062 Fibrous dysplasia (monostotic), left lower leg

    M85.069 Fibrous dysplasia (monostotic), unspecified lower leg △

✓6ᵗʰ **M85.07** Fibrous dysplasia (monostotic), ankle and foot

    M85.071 Fibrous dysplasia (monostotic), right ankle and foot

    M85.072 Fibrous dysplasia (monostotic), left ankle and foot

M85.079   Fibrous dysplasia (monostotic), unspecified ankle and foot ▽

M85.08   **Fibrous dysplasia (monostotic), other site**

M85.09   Fibrous dysplasia (monostotic), multiple sites

√5ᵗʰ   **M85.1   Skeletal fluorosis**

M85.10   Skeletal fluorosis, unspecified site ▽

√6ᵗʰ   M85.11   Skeletal fluorosis, shoulder

M85.111   Skeletal fluorosis, right shoulder

M85.112   Skeletal fluorosis, left shoulder

M85.119   Skeletal fluorosis, unspecified shoulder ▽

√6ᵗʰ   M85.12   Skeletal fluorosis, upper arm

M85.121   Skeletal fluorosis, right upper arm

M85.122   Skeletal fluorosis, left upper arm

M85.129   Skeletal fluorosis, unspecified upper arm ▽

√6ᵗʰ   M85.13   Skeletal fluorosis, forearm

M85.131   Skeletal fluorosis, right forearm

M85.132   Skeletal fluorosis, left forearm

M85.139   Skeletal fluorosis, unspecified forearm ▽

√6ᵗʰ   M85.14   Skeletal fluorosis, hand

M85.141   Skeletal fluorosis, right hand

M85.142   Skeletal fluorosis, left hand

M85.149   Skeletal fluorosis, unspecified hand ▽

√6ᵗʰ   M85.15   Skeletal fluorosis, thigh

M85.151   Skeletal fluorosis, right thigh

M85.152   Skeletal fluorosis, left thigh

M85.159   Skeletal fluorosis, unspecified thigh ▽

√6ᵗʰ   M85.16   Skeletal fluorosis, lower leg

M85.161   Skeletal fluorosis, right lower leg

M85.162   Skeletal fluorosis, left lower leg

M85.169   Skeletal fluorosis, unspecified lower leg ▽

√6ᵗʰ   M85.17   Skeletal fluorosis, ankle and foot

M85.171   Skeletal fluorosis, right ankle and foot

M85.172   Skeletal fluorosis, left ankle and foot

M85.179   Skeletal fluorosis, unspecified ankle and foot ▽

M85.18   **Skeletal fluorosis, other site**

M85.19   Skeletal fluorosis, multiple sites

M85.2   Hyperostosis of skull

√5ᵗʰ   **M85.3   Osteitis condensans**

M85.30   Osteitis condensans, unspecified site ▽

√6ᵗʰ   M85.31   Osteitis condensans, shoulder

M85.311   Osteitis condensans, right shoulder

M85.312   Osteitis condensans, left shoulder

M85.319   Osteitis condensans, unspecified shoulder ▽

√6ᵗʰ   M85.32   Osteitis condensans, upper arm

M85.321   Osteitis condensans, right upper arm

M85.322   Osteitis condensans, left upper arm

M85.329   Osteitis condensans, unspecified upper arm ▽

√6ᵗʰ   M85.33   Osteitis condensans, forearm

M85.331   Osteitis condensans, right forearm

M85.332   Osteitis condensans, left forearm

M85.339   Osteitis condensans, unspecified forearm ▽

√6ᵗʰ   M85.34   Osteitis condensans, hand

M85.341   Osteitis condensans, right hand

M85.342   Osteitis condensans, left hand

M85.349   Osteitis condensans, unspecified hand ▽

√6ᵗʰ   M85.35   Osteitis condensans, thigh

M85.351   Osteitis condensans, right thigh

M85.352   Osteitis condensans, left thigh

M85.359   Osteitis condensans, unspecified thigh ▽

√6ᵗʰ   M85.36   Osteitis condensans, lower leg

M85.361   Osteitis condensans, right lower leg

M85.362   Osteitis condensans, left lower leg

M85.369   Osteitis condensans, unspecified lower leg ▽

√6ᵗʰ   M85.37   Osteitis condensans, ankle and foot

M85.371   Osteitis condensans, right ankle and foot

M85.372   Osteitis condensans, left ankle and foot

M85.379   Osteitis condensans, unspecified ankle and foot ▽

M85.38   **Osteitis condensans, other site**

M85.39   Osteitis condensans, multiple sites

√5ᵗʰ   **M85.4   Solitary bone cyst**

EXCLUDES 2   solitary cyst of jaw (M27.4)

M85.40   Solitary bone cyst, unspecified site ▽

√6ᵗʰ   M85.41   Solitary bone cyst, shoulder

M85.411   Solitary bone cyst, right shoulder

M85.412   Solitary bone cyst, left shoulder

M85.419   Solitary bone cyst, unspecified shoulder ▽

√6ᵗʰ   M85.42   Solitary bone cyst, humerus

M85.421   Solitary bone cyst, right humerus

M85.422   Solitary bone cyst, left humerus

M85.429   Solitary bone cyst, unspecified humerus ▽

√6ᵗʰ   M85.43   Solitary bone cyst, ulna and radius

M85.431   Solitary bone cyst, right ulna and radius

M85.432   Solitary bone cyst, left ulna and radius

M85.439   Solitary bone cyst, unspecified ulna and radius ▽

√6ᵗʰ   M85.44   Solitary bone cyst, hand

M85.441   Solitary bone cyst, right hand

M85.442   Solitary bone cyst, left hand

M85.449   Solitary bone cyst, unspecified hand ▽

√6ᵗʰ   M85.45   Solitary bone cyst, pelvis

M85.451   Solitary bone cyst, right pelvis

M85.452   Solitary bone cyst, left pelvis

M85.459   Solitary bone cyst, unspecified pelvis ▽

√6ᵗʰ   M85.46   Solitary bone cyst, tibia and fibula

M85.461   Solitary bone cyst, right tibia and fibula

M85.462   Solitary bone cyst, left tibia and fibula

M85.469   Solitary bone cyst, unspecified tibia and fibula ▽

√6ᵗʰ   M85.47   Solitary bone cyst, ankle and foot

M85.471   Solitary bone cyst, right ankle and foot

M85.472   Solitary bone cyst, left ankle and foot

M85.479   Solitary bone cyst, unspecified ankle and foot ▽

M85.48   **Solitary bone cyst, other site**

√5ᵗʰ   **M85.5   Aneurysmal bone cyst**

EXCLUDES 2   aneurysmal cyst of jaw (M27.4)

M85.50   Aneurysmal bone cyst, unspecified site ▽

√6ᵗʰ   M85.51   Aneurysmal bone cyst, shoulder

M85.511   Aneurysmal bone cyst, right shoulder

M85.512   Aneurysmal bone cyst, left shoulder

M85.519   Aneurysmal bone cyst, unspecified shoulder ▽

√6ᵗʰ   M85.52   Aneurysmal bone cyst, upper arm

M85.521   Aneurysmal bone cyst, right upper arm

M85.522   Aneurysmal bone cyst, left upper arm

M85.529   Aneurysmal bone cyst, unspecified upper arm ▽

√6ᵗʰ   M85.53   Aneurysmal bone cyst, forearm

M85.531   Aneurysmal bone cyst, right forearm

M85.532   Aneurysmal bone cyst, left forearm

M85.539   Aneurysmal bone cyst, unspecified forearm ▽

√6ᵗʰ   M85.54   Aneurysmal bone cyst, hand

M85.541   Aneurysmal bone cyst, right hand

M85.542   Aneurysmal bone cyst, left hand

M85.549   Aneurysmal bone cyst, unspecified hand ▽

√6ᵗʰ   M85.55   Aneurysmal bone cyst, thigh

M85.551   Aneurysmal bone cyst, right thigh

M85.552   Aneurysmal bone cyst, left thigh

Ⓝ Newborn   Ⓟ Pediatric   Ⓜ Maternity   Ⓐ Adult   RIC RIC Dx   NC Dx Noncancer Dx   PDx Primary Dx   CC RIC CC Condition   ▶◀ Revised Text   ● New Code   ▲ Revised Code Title

740   ICD-10-CM 2016

M85.559   Aneurysmal bone cyst, unspecified thigh   ▽

✓6ᵗʰ M85.56   Aneurysmal bone cyst, lower leg
    M85.561   Aneurysmal bone cyst, right lower leg
    M85.562   Aneurysmal bone cyst, left lower leg
    M85.569   Aneurysmal bone cyst, unspecified lower leg   ▽

✓6ᵗʰ M85.57   Aneurysmal bone cyst, ankle and foot
    M85.571   Aneurysmal bone cyst, right ankle and foot
    M85.572   Aneurysmal bone cyst, left ankle and foot
    M85.579   Aneurysmal bone cyst, unspecified ankle and foot   ▽

M85.58   Aneurysmal bone cyst, other site
M85.59   Aneurysmal bone cyst, multiple sites

✓5ᵗʰ M85.6   Other cyst of bone
    EXCLUDES 1   cyst of jaw NEC (M27.4)
       osteitis fibrosa cystica generalisata [von Recklinghausen's disease of bone] (E21.0)

M85.60   Other cyst of bone, unspecified site   ▽

✓6ᵗʰ M85.61   Other cyst of bone, shoulder
    M85.611   Other cyst of bone, right shoulder
    M85.612   Other cyst of bone, left shoulder
    M85.619   Other cyst of bone, unspecified shoulder   ▽

✓6ᵗʰ M85.62   Other cyst of bone, upper arm
    M85.621   Other cyst of bone, right upper arm
    M85.622   Other cyst of bone, left upper arm
    M85.629   Other cyst of bone, unspecified upper arm   ▽

✓6ᵗʰ M85.63   Other cyst of bone, forearm
    M85.631   Other cyst of bone, right forearm
    M85.632   Other cyst of bone, left forearm
    M85.639   Other cyst of bone, unspecified forearm   ▽

✓6ᵗʰ M85.64   Other cyst of bone, hand
    M85.641   Other cyst of bone, right hand
    M85.642   Other cyst of bone, left hand
    M85.649   Other cyst of bone, unspecified hand   ▽

✓6ᵗʰ M85.65   Other cyst of bone, thigh
    M85.651   Other cyst of bone, right thigh
    M85.652   Other cyst of bone, left thigh
    M85.659   Other cyst of bone, unspecified thigh   ▽

✓6ᵗʰ M85.66   Other cyst of bone, lower leg
    M85.661   Other cyst of bone, right lower leg
    M85.662   Other cyst of bone, left lower leg
    M85.669   Other cyst of bone, unspecified lower leg   ▽

✓6ᵗʰ M85.67   Other cyst of bone, ankle and foot
    M85.671   Other cyst of bone, right ankle and foot
    M85.672   Other cyst of bone, left ankle and foot
    M85.679   Other cyst of bone, unspecified ankle and foot   ▽

M85.68   Other cyst of bone, other site
M85.69   Other cyst of bone, multiple sites

✓5ᵗʰ M85.8   Other specified disorders of bone density and structure
    Hyperostosis of bones, except skull
    Osteosclerosis, acquired
    EXCLUDES 1   diffuse idiopathic skeletal hyperostosis [DISH] (M48.1)
       osteosclerosis congenita (Q77.4)
       osteosclerosis fragilitas (generalisata) (Q78.2)
       osteosclerosis myelofibrosis (D75.81)

M85.80   Other specified disorders of bone density and structure, unspecified site   ▽

✓6ᵗʰ M85.81   Other specified disorders of bone density and structure, shoulder
    M85.811   Other specified disorders of bone density and structure, right shoulder
    M85.812   Other specified disorders of bone density and structure, left shoulder
    M85.819   Other specified disorders of bone density and structure, unspecified shoulder   ▽

✓6ᵗʰ M85.82   Other specified disorders of bone density and structure, upper arm
    M85.821   Other specified disorders of bone density and structure, right upper arm
    M85.822   Other specified disorders of bone density and structure, left upper arm
    M85.829   Other specified disorders of bone density and structure, unspecified upper arm   ▽

✓6ᵗʰ M85.83   Other specified disorders of bone density and structure, forearm
    M85.831   Other specified disorders of bone density and structure, right forearm
    M85.832   Other specified disorders of bone density and structure, left forearm
    M85.839   Other specified disorders of bone density and structure, unspecified forearm   ▽

✓6ᵗʰ M85.84   Other specified disorders of bone density and structure, hand
    M85.841   Other specified disorders of bone density and structure, right hand
    M85.842   Other specified disorders of bone density and structure, left hand
    M85.849   Other specified disorders of bone density and structure, unspecified hand   ▽

✓6ᵗʰ M85.85   Other specified disorders of bone density and structure, thigh
    M85.851   Other specified disorders of bone density and structure, right thigh
    M85.852   Other specified disorders of bone density and structure, left thigh
    M85.859   Other specified disorders of bone density and structure, unspecified thigh   ▽

✓6ᵗʰ M85.86   Other specified disorders of bone density and structure, lower leg
    M85.861   Other specified disorders of bone density and structure, right lower leg
    M85.862   Other specified disorders of bone density and structure, left lower leg
    M85.869   Other specified disorders of bone density and structure, unspecified lower leg   ▽

✓6ᵗʰ M85.87   Other specified disorders of bone density and structure, ankle and foot
    M85.871   Other specified disorders of bone density and structure, right ankle and foot
    M85.872   Other specified disorders of bone density and structure, left ankle and foot
    M85.879   Other specified disorders of bone density and structure, unspecified ankle and foot   ▽

M85.88   Other specified disorders of bone density and structure, other site
M85.89   Other specified disorders of bone density and structure, multiple sites

M85.9   Disorder of bone density and structure, unspecified   ▽

Other osteopathies (M86-M90)

EXCLUDES 1   postprocedural osteopathies (M96.-)

✓4ᵗʰ **M86 Osteomyelitis**
    Use additional code (B95-B97) to identify infectious agent
    Use additional code to identify major osseous defect, if applicable (M89.7-)
    EXCLUDES 1   osteomyelitis due to:
       echinococcus (B67.2)
       gonococcus (A54.43)
       salmonella (A02.24)
    EXCLUDES 2   ostemyelitis of:
       orbit (H05.0-)
       petrous bone (H70.2-)
       vertebra (M46.2-)

✓5ᵗʰ M86.0   Acute hematogenous osteomyelitis
    M86.00   Acute hematogenous osteomyelitis, unspecified site   ▽

    ✓6ᵗʰ M86.01   Acute hematogenous osteomyelitis, shoulder
       M86.011   Acute hematogenous osteomyelitis, right shoulder

---

✓ Add'l Character Required   ✓×7ᵗʰ Placeholder Alert   RUG IV Special Care High Dx   RUG IV Clinically Complex Dx   RUG IV Special Care Low Dx   Manifestation Code   Other Specified Code   ▽ Unspecified Code

M86.012   Acute hematogenous osteomyelitis, left shoulder

M86.019   Acute hematogenous osteomyelitis, unspecified shoulder ▽

✓6ᵗʰ   M86.02   Acute hematogenous osteomyelitis, humerus

M86.021   Acute hematogenous osteomyelitis, right humerus

M86.022   Acute hematogenous osteomyelitis, left humerus

M86.029   Acute hematogenous osteomyelitis, unspecified humerus ▽

✓6ᵗʰ   M86.03   Acute hematogenous osteomyelitis, radius and ulna

M86.031   Acute hematogenous osteomyelitis, right radius and ulna

M86.032   Acute hematogenous osteomyelitis, left radius and ulna

M86.039   Acute hematogenous osteomyelitis, unspecified radius and ulna ▽

✓6ᵗʰ   M86.04   Acute hematogenous osteomyelitis, hand

M86.041   Acute hematogenous osteomyelitis, right hand

M86.042   Acute hematogenous osteomyelitis, left hand

M86.049   Acute hematogenous osteomyelitis, unspecified hand ▽

✓6ᵗʰ   M86.05   Acute hematogenous osteomyelitis, femur

M86.051   Acute hematogenous osteomyelitis, right femur

M86.052   Acute hematogenous osteomyelitis, left femur

M86.059   Acute hematogenous osteomyelitis, unspecified femur ▽

✓6ᵗʰ   M86.06   Acute hematogenous osteomyelitis, tibia and fibula

M86.061   Acute hematogenous osteomyelitis, right tibia and fibula

M86.062   Acute hematogenous osteomyelitis, left tibia and fibula

M86.069   Acute hematogenous osteomyelitis, unspecified tibia and fibula ▽

✓6ᵗʰ   M86.07   Acute hematogenous osteomyelitis, ankle and foot

M86.071   Acute hematogenous osteomyelitis, right ankle and foot

M86.072   Acute hematogenous osteomyelitis, left ankle and foot

M86.079   Acute hematogenous osteomyelitis, unspecified ankle and foot ▽

M86.08   Acute hematogenous osteomyelitis, other sites

M86.09   Acute hematogenous osteomyelitis, multiple sites

✓5ᵗʰ   M86.1   Other acute osteomyelitis

M86.10   Other acute osteomyelitis, unspecified site ▽

✓6ᵗʰ   M86.11   Other acute osteomyelitis, shoulder

M86.111   Other acute osteomyelitis, right shoulder

M86.112   Other acute osteomyelitis, left shoulder

M86.119   Other acute osteomyelitis, unspecified shoulder ▽

✓6ᵗʰ   M86.12   Other acute osteomyelitis, humerus

M86.121   Other acute osteomyelitis, right humerus

M86.122   Other acute osteomyelitis, left humerus

M86.129   Other acute osteomyelitis, unspecified humerus ▽

✓6ᵗʰ   M86.13   Other acute osteomyelitis, radius and ulna

M86.131   Other acute osteomyelitis, right radius and ulna

M86.132   Other acute osteomyelitis, left radius and ulna

M86.139   Other acute osteomyelitis, unspecified radius and ulna ▽

✓6ᵗʰ   M86.14   Other acute osteomyelitis, hand

M86.141   Other acute osteomyelitis, right hand

M86.142   Other acute osteomyelitis, left hand

M86.149   Other acute osteomyelitis, unspecified hand ▽

✓6ᵗʰ   M86.15   Other acute osteomyelitis, femur

M86.151   Other acute osteomyelitis, right femur

M86.152   Other acute osteomyelitis, left femur

M86.159   Other acute osteomyelitis, unspecified femur ▽

✓6ᵗʰ   M86.16   Other acute osteomyelitis, tibia and fibula

M86.161   Other acute osteomyelitis, right tibia and fibula

M86.162   Other acute osteomyelitis, left tibia and fibula

M86.169   Other acute osteomyelitis, unspecified tibia and fibula ▽

✓6ᵗʰ   M86.17   Other acute osteomyelitis, ankle and foot

M86.171   Other acute osteomyelitis, right ankle and foot

M86.172   Other acute osteomyelitis, left ankle and foot

M86.179   Other acute osteomyelitis, unspecified ankle and foot ▽

M86.18   Other acute osteomyelitis, other site

M86.19   Other acute osteomyelitis, multiple sites

✓5ᵗʰ   M86.2   Subacute osteomyelitis

M86.20   Subacute osteomyelitis, unspecified site ▽

✓6ᵗʰ   M86.21   Subacute osteomyelitis, shoulder

M86.211   Subacute osteomyelitis, right shoulder

M86.212   Subacute osteomyelitis, left shoulder

M86.219   Subacute osteomyelitis, unspecified shoulder ▽

✓6ᵗʰ   M86.22   Subacute osteomyelitis, humerus

M86.221   Subacute osteomyelitis, right humerus

M86.222   Subacute osteomyelitis, left humerus

M86.229   Subacute osteomyelitis, unspecified humerus ▽

✓6ᵗʰ   M86.23   Subacute osteomyelitis, radius and ulna

M86.231   Subacute osteomyelitis, right radius and ulna

M86.232   Subacute osteomyelitis, left radius and ulna

M86.239   Subacute osteomyelitis, unspecified radius and ulna ▽

✓6ᵗʰ   M86.24   Subacute osteomyelitis, hand

M86.241   Subacute osteomyelitis, right hand

M86.242   Subacute osteomyelitis, left hand

M86.249   Subacute osteomyelitis, unspecified hand ▽

✓6ᵗʰ   M86.25   Subacute osteomyelitis, femur

M86.251   Subacute osteomyelitis, right femur

M86.252   Subacute osteomyelitis, left femur

M86.259   Subacute osteomyelitis, unspecified femur ▽

✓6ᵗʰ   M86.26   Subacute osteomyelitis, tibia and fibula

M86.261   Subacute osteomyelitis, right tibia and fibula

M86.262   Subacute osteomyelitis, left tibia and fibula

M86.269   Subacute osteomyelitis, unspecified tibia and fibula ▽

✓6ᵗʰ   M86.27   Subacute osteomyelitis, ankle and foot

M86.271   Subacute osteomyelitis, right ankle and foot

M86.272   Subacute osteomyelitis, left ankle and foot

M86.279   Subacute osteomyelitis, unspecified ankle and foot ▽

M86.28   Subacute osteomyelitis, other site

M86.29   Subacute osteomyelitis, multiple sites

✓5ᵗʰ   M86.3   Chronic multifocal osteomyelitis

M86.30   Chronic multifocal osteomyelitis, unspecified site ▽

✓6ᵗʰ   M86.31   Chronic multifocal osteomyelitis, shoulder

M86.311   Chronic multifocal osteomyelitis, right shoulder

M86.312   Chronic multifocal osteomyelitis, left shoulder

M86.319   Chronic multifocal osteomyelitis, unspecified shoulder ▽

Ⓝ Newborn   Ⓟ Pediatric   Ⓜ Maternity   Ⓐ Adult   RIC RIC Dx   NCDx Noncancer Dx   PDx Primary Dx   CC RIC CC Condition   ▶◀ Revised Text   ● New Code   ▲ Revised Code Title

742   ICD-10-CM 2016

✓6ᵗʰ **M86.32 Chronic multifocal osteomyelitis, humerus**
    M86.321 Chronic multifocal osteomyelitis, right humerus
    M86.322 Chronic multifocal osteomyelitis, left humerus
    M86.329 Chronic multifocal osteomyelitis, unspecified humerus ▽

✓6ᵗʰ **M86.33 Chronic multifocal osteomyelitis, radius and ulna**
    M86.331 Chronic multifocal osteomyelitis, right radius and ulna
    M86.332 Chronic multifocal osteomyelitis, left radius and ulna
    M86.339 Chronic multifocal osteomyelitis, unspecified radius and ulna ▽

✓6ᵗʰ **M86.34 Chronic multifocal osteomyelitis, hand**
    M86.341 Chronic multifocal osteomyelitis, right hand
    M86.342 Chronic multifocal osteomyelitis, left hand
    M86.349 Chronic multifocal osteomyelitis, unspecified hand ▽

✓6ᵗʰ **M86.35 Chronic multifocal osteomyelitis, femur**
    M86.351 Chronic multifocal osteomyelitis, right femur
    M86.352 Chronic multifocal osteomyelitis, left femur
    M86.359 Chronic multifocal osteomyelitis, unspecified femur ▽

✓6ᵗʰ **M86.36 Chronic multifocal osteomyelitis, tibia and fibula**
    M86.361 Chronic multifocal osteomyelitis, right tibia and fibula
    M86.362 Chronic multifocal osteomyelitis, left tibia and fibula
    M86.369 Chronic multifocal osteomyelitis, unspecified tibia and fibula ▽

✓6ᵗʰ **M86.37 Chronic multifocal osteomyelitis, ankle and foot**
    M86.371 Chronic multifocal osteomyelitis, right ankle and foot
    M86.372 Chronic multifocal osteomyelitis, left ankle and foot
    M86.379 Chronic multifocal osteomyelitis, unspecified ankle and foot ▽

    M86.38 Chronic multifocal osteomyelitis, other site
    M86.39 Chronic multifocal osteomyelitis, multiple sites

✓5ᵗʰ **M86.4 Chronic osteomyelitis with draining sinus**
    M86.40 Chronic osteomyelitis with draining sinus, unspecified site ▽

✓6ᵗʰ **M86.41 Chronic osteomyelitis with draining sinus, shoulder**
    M86.411 Chronic osteomyelitis with draining sinus, right shoulder
    M86.412 Chronic osteomyelitis with draining sinus, left shoulder
    M86.419 Chronic osteomyelitis with draining sinus, unspecified shoulder ▽

✓6ᵗʰ **M86.42 Chronic osteomyelitis with draining sinus, humerus**
    M86.421 Chronic osteomyelitis with draining sinus, right humerus
    M86.422 Chronic osteomyelitis with draining sinus, left humerus
    M86.429 Chronic osteomyelitis with draining sinus, unspecified humerus ▽

✓6ᵗʰ **M86.43 Chronic osteomyelitis with draining sinus, radius and ulna**
    M86.431 Chronic osteomyelitis with draining sinus, right radius and ulna
    M86.432 Chronic osteomyelitis with draining sinus, left radius and ulna
    M86.439 Chronic osteomyelitis with draining sinus, unspecified radius and ulna ▽

✓6ᵗʰ **M86.44 Chronic osteomyelitis with draining sinus, hand**
    M86.441 Chronic osteomyelitis with draining sinus, right hand
    M86.442 Chronic osteomyelitis with draining sinus, left hand
    M86.449 Chronic osteomyelitis with draining sinus, unspecified hand ▽

✓6ᵗʰ **M86.45 Chronic osteomyelitis with draining sinus, femur**
    M86.451 Chronic osteomyelitis with draining sinus, right femur
    M86.452 Chronic osteomyelitis with draining sinus, left femur
    M86.459 Chronic osteomyelitis with draining sinus, unspecified femur ▽

✓6ᵗʰ **M86.46 Chronic osteomyelitis with draining sinus, tibia and fibula**
    M86.461 Chronic osteomyelitis with draining sinus, right tibia and fibula
    M86.462 Chronic osteomyelitis with draining sinus, left tibia and fibula
    M86.469 Chronic osteomyelitis with draining sinus, unspecified tibia and fibula ▽

✓6ᵗʰ **M86.47 Chronic osteomyelitis with draining sinus, ankle and foot**
    M86.471 Chronic osteomyelitis with draining sinus, right ankle and foot
    M86.472 Chronic osteomyelitis with draining sinus, left ankle and foot
    M86.479 Chronic osteomyelitis with draining sinus, unspecified ankle and foot ▽

    M86.48 Chronic osteomyelitis with draining sinus, other site
    M86.49 Chronic osteomyelitis with draining sinus, multiple sites

✓5ᵗʰ **M86.5 Other chronic hematogenous osteomyelitis**
    M86.50 Other chronic hematogenous osteomyelitis, unspecified site ▽

✓6ᵗʰ **M86.51 Other chronic hematogenous osteomyelitis, shoulder**
    M86.511 Other chronic hematogenous osteomyelitis, right shoulder
    M86.512 Other chronic hematogenous osteomyelitis, left shoulder
    M86.519 Other chronic hematogenous osteomyelitis, unspecified shoulder ▽

✓6ᵗʰ **M86.52 Other chronic hematogenous osteomyelitis, humerus**
    M86.521 Other chronic hematogenous osteomyelitis, right humerus
    M86.522 Other chronic hematogenous osteomyelitis, left humerus
    M86.529 Other chronic hematogenous osteomyelitis, unspecified humerus ▽

✓6ᵗʰ **M86.53 Other chronic hematogenous osteomyelitis, radius and ulna**
    M86.531 Other chronic hematogenous osteomyelitis, right radius and ulna
    M86.532 Other chronic hematogenous osteomyelitis, left radius and ulna
    M86.539 Other chronic hematogenous osteomyelitis, unspecified radius and ulna ▽

✓6ᵗʰ **M86.54 Other chronic hematogenous osteomyelitis, hand**
    M86.541 Other chronic hematogenous osteomyelitis, right hand
    M86.542 Other chronic hematogenous osteomyelitis, left hand
    M86.549 Other chronic hematogenous osteomyelitis, unspecified hand ▽

✓6ᵗʰ **M86.55 Other chronic hematogenous osteomyelitis, femur**
    M86.551 Other chronic hematogenous osteomyelitis, right femur
    M86.552 Other chronic hematogenous osteomyelitis, left femur
    M86.559 Other chronic hematogenous osteomyelitis, unspecified femur ▽

✓6ᵗʰ **M86.56 Other chronic hematogenous osteomyelitis, tibia and fibula**
    M86.561 Other chronic hematogenous osteomyelitis, right tibia and fibula
    M86.562 Other chronic hematogenous osteomyelitis, left tibia and fibula
    M86.569 Other chronic hematogenous osteomyelitis, unspecified tibia and fibula ▽

☑ Add'l Character Required   ☑x7ᵗʰ Placeholder Alert   RUG IV Special Care High Dx   RUG IV Clinically Complex Dx   RUG IV Special Care Low Dx   Manifestation Code   Other Specified Code   ▽ Unspecified Code

√6ᵗʰ **M86.57** **Other chronic hematogenous osteomyelitis,** ankle and foot

    M86.571 **Other chronic hematogenous osteomyelitis,** right **ankle and foot**

    M86.572 **Other chronic hematogenous osteomyelitis,** left **ankle and foot**

    M86.579 **Other chronic hematogenous osteomyelitis, unspecified ankle and foot** ▽

  M86.58 **Other chronic hematogenous osteomyelitis, other site**

  M86.59 **Other chronic hematogenous osteomyelitis,** multiple sites

√5ᵗʰ **M86.6** Other chronic **osteomyelitis**

  M86.60 **Other chronic osteomyelitis, unspecified site** ▽

  √6ᵗʰ **M86.61** **Other chronic osteomyelitis,** shoulder

    M86.611 **Other chronic osteomyelitis,** right **shoulder**

    M86.612 **Other chronic osteomyelitis,** left **shoulder**

    M86.619 **Other chronic osteomyelitis, unspecified shoulder** ▽

  √6ᵗʰ **M86.62** **Other chronic osteomyelitis,** humerus

    M86.621 **Other chronic osteomyelitis,** right **humerus**

    M86.622 **Other chronic osteomyelitis,** left **humerus**

    M86.629 **Other chronic osteomyelitis, unspecified humerus** ▽

  √6ᵗʰ **M86.63** **Other chronic osteomyelitis,** radius and ulna

    M86.631 **Other chronic osteomyelitis,** right **radius and ulna**

    M86.632 **Other chronic osteomyelitis,** left **radius and ulna**

    M86.639 **Other chronic osteomyelitis, unspecified radius and ulna** ▽

  √6ᵗʰ **M86.64** **Other chronic osteomyelitis,** hand

    M86.641 **Other chronic osteomyelitis,** right **hand**

    M86.642 **Other chronic osteomyelitis,** left **hand**

    M86.649 **Other chronic osteomyelitis, unspecified hand** ▽

  √6ᵗʰ **M86.65** **Other chronic osteomyelitis,** thigh

    M86.651 **Other chronic osteomyelitis,** right **thigh**

    M86.652 **Other chronic osteomyelitis,** left **thigh**

    M86.659 **Other chronic osteomyelitis, unspecified thigh** ▽

  √6ᵗʰ **M86.66** **Other chronic osteomyelitis,** tibia and fibula

    M86.661 **Other chronic osteomyelitis,** right **tibia and fibula**

    M86.662 **Other chronic osteomyelitis,** left **tibia and fibula**

    M86.669 **Other chronic osteomyelitis, unspecified tibia and fibula** ▽

  √6ᵗʰ **M86.67** **Other chronic osteomyelitis,** ankle and foot

    M86.671 **Other chronic osteomyelitis,** right **ankle and foot**

    M86.672 **Other chronic osteomyelitis,** left **ankle and foot**

    M86.679 **Other chronic osteomyelitis, unspecified ankle and foot** ▽

  M86.68 **Other chronic osteomyelitis, other site**

  M86.69 **Other chronic osteomyelitis,** multiple sites

√5ᵗʰ **M86.8** Other **osteomyelitis**

  Brodie's abscess

  √6ᵗʰ **M86.8X** **Other osteomyelitis**

    M86.8X0 **Other osteomyelitis,** multiple sites

    M86.8X1 **Other osteomyelitis,** shoulder

    M86.8X2 **Other osteomyelitis,** upper arm

    M86.8X3 **Other osteomyelitis,** forearm

    M86.8X4 **Other osteomyelitis,** hand

    M86.8X5 **Other osteomyelitis,** thigh

    M86.8X6 **Other osteomyelitis,** lower leg

    M86.8X7 **Other osteomyelitis,** ankle and foot

    M86.8X8 **Other osteomyelitis, other site**

    M86.8X9 **Other osteomyelitis, unspecified sites** ▽

M86.9 **Osteomyelitis, unspecified** ▽

  Infection of bone NOS   Periostitis without osteomyelitis

√4ᵗʰ **M87** **Osteonecrosis**

  INCLUDES   avascular necrosis of bone

  Use additional code to identify major osseous defect, if applicable (M89.7-)

  EXCLUDES 1   *juvenile osteonecrosis (M91-M92)*

    osteochondropathies (M90-M93)

√5ᵗʰ **M87.0** Idiopathic aseptic **necrosis of bone**

  M87.00 **Idiopathic aseptic necrosis of unspecified bone** ▽

  √6ᵗʰ **M87.01** **Idiopathic aseptic necrosis of** shoulder

    Idiopathic aseptic necrosis of clavicle and scapula

    M87.011 **Idiopathic aseptic necrosis of** right **shoulder**

    M87.012 **Idiopathic aseptic necrosis of** left **shoulder**

    M87.019 **Idiopathic aseptic necrosis of unspecified shoulder** ▽

  √6ᵗʰ **M87.02** **Idiopathic aseptic necrosis of** humerus

    M87.021 **Idiopathic aseptic necrosis of** right **humerus**

    M87.022 **Idiopathic aseptic necrosis of** left **humerus**

    M87.029 **Idiopathic aseptic necrosis of unspecified humerus** ▽

  √6ᵗʰ **M87.03** **Idiopathic aseptic necrosis of** radius, ulna and carpus

    M87.031 **Idiopathic aseptic necrosis of** right radius

    M87.032 **Idiopathic aseptic necrosis of** left radius

    M87.033 **Idiopathic aseptic necrosis of unspecified radius** ▽

    M87.034 **Idiopathic aseptic necrosis of** right ulna

    M87.035 **Idiopathic aseptic necrosis of** left ulna

    M87.036 **Idiopathic aseptic necrosis of unspecified ulna** ▽

    M87.037 **Idiopathic aseptic necrosis of** right carpus

    M87.038 **Idiopathic aseptic necrosis of** left carpus

    M87.039 **Idiopathic aseptic necrosis of unspecified carpus** ▽

  √6ᵗʰ **M87.04** **Idiopathic aseptic necrosis of** hand and fingers

    Idiopathic aseptic necrosis of metacarpals and phalanges of hands

    M87.041 **Idiopathic aseptic necrosis of** right hand

    M87.042 **Idiopathic aseptic necrosis of** left hand

    M87.043 **Idiopathic aseptic necrosis of unspecified hand** ▽

    M87.044 **Idiopathic aseptic necrosis of** right finger(s)

    M87.045 **Idiopathic aseptic necrosis of** left finger(s)

    M87.046 **Idiopathic aseptic necrosis of unspecified finger(s)**

  √6ᵗʰ **M87.05** **Idiopathic aseptic necrosis of** pelvis and femur

    M87.050 **Idiopathic aseptic necrosis of** pelvis

    M87.051 **Idiopathic aseptic necrosis of** right femur

    M87.052 **Idiopathic aseptic necrosis of** left femur

    M87.059 **Idiopathic aseptic necrosis of unspecified femur** ▽

    Idiopathic aseptic necrosis of hip NOS

  √6ᵗʰ **M87.06** **Idiopathic aseptic necrosis of** tibia and fibula

    M87.061 **Idiopathic aseptic necrosis of** right tibia

    M87.062 **Idiopathic aseptic necrosis of** left tibia

    M87.063 **Idiopathic aseptic necrosis of unspecified tibia** ▽

    M87.064 **Idiopathic aseptic necrosis of** right fibula

    M87.065 **Idiopathic aseptic necrosis of** left fibula

    M87.066 **Idiopathic aseptic necrosis of unspecified fibula** ▽

  √6ᵗʰ **M87.07** **Idiopathic aseptic necrosis of** ankle, foot and toes

    Idiopathic aseptic necrosis of metatarsus, tarsus, and phalanges of toes

    M87.071 **Idiopathic aseptic necrosis of** right ankle

    M87.072 **Idiopathic aseptic necrosis of** left ankle

    M87.073 **Idiopathic aseptic necrosis of unspecified ankle** ▽

    M87.074 **Idiopathic aseptic necrosis of** right foot

    M87.075 **Idiopathic aseptic necrosis of** left foot

    M87.076 **Idiopathic aseptic necrosis of unspecified foot** ▽

    M87.077 **Idiopathic aseptic necrosis of** right toe(s)

Ⓝ Newborn   Ⓟ Pediatric   Ⓜ Maternity   Ⓐ Adult   **RIC** RIC Dx   **NC Dx** Noncancer Dx   **PDx** Primary Dx   **CC** RIC CC Condition   ►◄ Revised Text   ● New Code   ▲ Revised Code Title

744   ICD-10-CM 2016

M87.078 **Idiopathic aseptic necrosis of** left toe(s)

M87.079 **Idiopathic aseptic necrosis of unspecified toe(s)** ▽

M87.08 Idiopathic aseptic necrosis of bone, other site

M87.09 **Idiopathic aseptic necrosis of bone,** multiple sites

✓5ᵗʰ **M87.1 Osteonecrosis** due to drugs

> Use additional code for adverse effect, if applicable, to identify drug (T36-T50 with fifth or sixth character 5)

M87.10 **Osteonecrosis due to drugs, unspecified bone** ▽

✓6ᵗʰ **M87.11 Osteonecrosis due to drugs,** shoulder

M87.111 **Osteonecrosis due to drugs,** right **shoulder**

M87.112 **Osteonecrosis due to drugs,** left **shoulder**

M87.119 **Osteonecrosis due to drugs, unspecified shoulder** ▽

✓6ᵗʰ **M87.12 Osteonecrosis due to drugs,** humerus

M87.121 **Osteonecrosis due to drugs,** right **humerus**

M87.122 **Osteonecrosis due to drugs,** left **humerus**

M87.129 **Osteonecrosis due to drugs, unspecified humerus** ▽

✓6ᵗʰ **M87.13 Osteonecrosis due to drugs of** radius, ulna and carpus

M87.131 **Osteonecrosis due to drugs of** right radius

M87.132 **Osteonecrosis due to drugs of** left radius

M87.133 **Osteonecrosis due to drugs of unspecified radius** ▽

M87.134 **Osteonecrosis due to drugs of** right ulna

M87.135 **Osteonecrosis due to drugs of** left ulna

M87.136 **Osteonecrosis due to drugs of unspecified ulna** ▽

M87.137 **Osteonecrosis due to drugs of** right carpus

M87.138 **Osteonecrosis due to drugs of** left carpus

M87.139 **Osteonecrosis due to drugs of unspecified carpus** ▽

✓6ᵗʰ **M87.14 Osteonecrosis due to drugs,** hand and fingers

M87.141 **Osteonecrosis due to drugs,** right hand

M87.142 **Osteonecrosis due to drugs,** left hand

M87.143 **Osteonecrosis due to drugs, unspecified hand** ▽

M87.144 **Osteonecrosis due to drugs,** right finger(s)

M87.145 **Osteonecrosis due to drugs,** left finger(s)

M87.146 **Osteonecrosis due to drugs, unspecified finger(s)** ▽

✓6ᵗʰ **M87.15 Osteonecrosis due to drugs,** pelvis and femur

M87.150 **Osteonecrosis due to drugs,** pelvis

M87.151 **Osteonecrosis due to drugs,** right femur

M87.152 **Osteonecrosis due to drugs,** left femur

M87.159 **Osteonecrosis due to drugs, unspecified femur**

✓6ᵗʰ **M87.16 Osteonecrosis due to drugs,** tibia and fibula

M87.161 **Osteonecrosis due to drugs,** right tibia

M87.162 **Osteonecrosis due to drugs,** left tibia

M87.163 **Osteonecrosis due to drugs, unspecified tibia** ▽

M87.164 **Osteonecrosis due to drugs,** right fibula

M87.165 **Osteonecrosis due to drugs,** left fibula

M87.166 **Osteonecrosis due to drugs, unspecified fibula** ▽

✓6ᵗʰ **M87.17 Osteonecrosis due to drugs,** ankle, foot and toes

M87.171 **Osteonecrosis due to drugs,** right ankle

M87.172 **Osteonecrosis due to drugs,** left ankle

M87.173 **Osteonecrosis due to drugs, unspecified ankle** ▽

M87.174 **Osteonecrosis due to drugs,** right foot

M87.175 **Osteonecrosis due to drugs,** left foot

M87.176 **Osteonecrosis due to drugs, unspecified foot** ▽

M87.177 **Osteonecrosis due to drugs,** right toe(s)

M87.178 **Osteonecrosis due to drugs,** left toe(s)

M87.179 **Osteonecrosis due to drugs, unspecified toe(s)** ▽

✓6ᵗʰ **M87.18 Osteonecrosis due to drugs,** other site

M87.180 **Osteonecrosis due to drugs,** jaw

M87.188 **Osteonecrosis due to drugs, other site**

M87.19 **Osteonecrosis due to drugs,** multiple sites

✓5ᵗʰ **M87.2 Osteonecrosis** due to previous trauma

M87.20 **Osteonecrosis due to previous trauma, unspecified bone** ▽

✓6ᵗʰ **M87.21 Osteonecrosis due to previous trauma,** shoulder

M87.211 **Osteonecrosis due to previous trauma, right shoulder**

M87.212 **Osteonecrosis due to previous trauma, left shoulder**

M87.219 **Osteonecrosis due to previous trauma, unspecified shoulder** ▽

✓6ᵗʰ **M87.22 Osteonecrosis due to previous trauma,** humerus

M87.221 **Osteonecrosis due to previous trauma, right humerus**

M87.222 **Osteonecrosis due to previous trauma, left humerus**

M87.229 **Osteonecrosis due to previous trauma, unspecified humerus** ▽

✓6ᵗʰ **M87.23 Osteonecrosis due to previous trauma of** radius, ulna and carpus

M87.231 **Osteonecrosis due to previous trauma of right radius**

M87.232 **Osteonecrosis due to previous trauma of left radius**

M87.233 **Osteonecrosis due to previous trauma of unspecified radius** ▽

M87.234 **Osteonecrosis due to previous trauma of right ulna**

M87.235 **Osteonecrosis due to previous trauma of left ulna**

M87.236 **Osteonecrosis due to previous trauma of unspecified ulna** ▽

M87.237 **Osteonecrosis due to previous trauma of right carpus**

M87.238 **Osteonecrosis due to previous trauma of left carpus**

M87.239 **Osteonecrosis due to previous trauma of unspecified carpus** ▽

✓6ᵗʰ **M87.24 Osteonecrosis due to previous trauma,** hand and fingers

M87.241 **Osteonecrosis due to previous trauma, right hand**

M87.242 **Osteonecrosis due to previous trauma, left hand**

M87.243 **Osteonecrosis due to previous trauma, unspecified hand** ▽

M87.244 **Osteonecrosis due to previous trauma, right finger(s)**

M87.245 **Osteonecrosis due to previous trauma, left finger(s)**

M87.246 **Osteonecrosis due to previous trauma, unspecified finger(s)** ▽

✓6ᵗʰ **M87.25 Osteonecrosis due to previous trauma,** pelvis and femur

M87.250 **Osteonecrosis due to previous trauma, pelvis**

M87.251 **Osteonecrosis due to previous trauma, right femur**

M87.252 **Osteonecrosis due to previous trauma, left femur**

M87.256 **Osteonecrosis due to previous trauma, unspecified femur** ▽

✓6ᵗʰ **M87.26 Osteonecrosis due to previous trauma,** tibia and fibula

M87.261 **Osteonecrosis due to previous trauma, right tibia**

M87.262 **Osteonecrosis due to previous trauma, left tibia**

M87.263 **Osteonecrosis due to previous trauma, unspecified tibia** ▽

M87.264 **Osteonecrosis due to previous trauma, right fibula**

M87.265 **Osteonecrosis due to previous trauma, left fibula**

M87.266 **Osteonecrosis due to previous trauma, unspecified fibula** ▽

☑ Add'l Character Required ☑ₓ₇ᵗʰ Placeholder Alert RUG IV Special Care High Dx RUG IV Clinically Complex Dx RUG IV Special Care Low Dx Manifestation Code Other Specified Code ▽ Unspecified Code

Chapter 13. Diseases of the Musculoskeletal System and Connective Tissue

√6ᵗʰ **M87.27** **Osteonecrosis due to previous trauma,** ankle, foot and toes

    M87.271 **Osteonecrosis due to previous trauma,** right ankle

    M87.272 **Osteonecrosis due to previous trauma,** left ankle

    M87.273 **Osteonecrosis due to previous trauma, unspecified ankle** ▽

    M87.274 **Osteonecrosis due to previous trauma,** right foot

    M87.275 **Osteonecrosis due to previous trauma,** left foot

    M87.276 **Osteonecrosis due to previous trauma, unspecified foot** ▽

    M87.277 **Osteonecrosis due to previous trauma,** right toe(s)

    M87.278 **Osteonecrosis due to previous trauma,** left toe(s)

    M87.279 **Osteonecrosis due to previous trauma, unspecified toe(s)** ▽

M87.28 **Osteonecrosis due to previous trauma, other site**

M87.29 **Osteonecrosis due to previous trauma,** multiple sites

√5ᵗʰ **M87.3** Other secondary osteonecrosis

    M87.30 **Other secondary osteonecrosis, unspecified bone** ▽

√6ᵗʰ **M87.31** **Other secondary osteonecrosis,** shoulder

    M87.311 **Other secondary osteonecrosis,** right shoulder

    M87.312 **Other secondary osteonecrosis,** left shoulder

    M87.319 **Other secondary osteonecrosis, unspecified shoulder** ▽

√6ᵗʰ **M87.32** **Other secondary osteonecrosis,** humerus

    M87.321 **Other secondary osteonecrosis,** right humerus

    M87.322 **Other secondary osteonecrosis,** left humerus

    M87.329 **Other secondary osteonecrosis, unspecified humerus** ▽

√6ᵗʰ **M87.33** **Other secondary osteonecrosis of** radius, ulna and carpus

    M87.331 **Other secondary osteonecrosis of** right radius

    M87.332 **Other secondary osteonecrosis of** left radius

    M87.333 **Other secondary osteonecrosis of unspecified radius** ▽

    M87.334 **Other secondary osteonecrosis of** right ulna

    M87.335 **Other secondary osteonecrosis of** left ulna

    M87.336 **Other secondary osteonecrosis of unspecified ulna** ▽

    M87.337 **Other secondary osteonecrosis of** right carpus

    M87.338 **Other secondary osteonecrosis of** left carpus

    M87.339 **Other secondary osteonecrosis of unspecified carpus** ▽

√6ᵗʰ **M87.34** **Other secondary osteonecrosis,** hand and fingers

    M87.341 **Other secondary osteonecrosis,** right hand

    M87.342 **Other secondary osteonecrosis,** left hand

    M87.343 **Other secondary osteonecrosis, unspecified hand** ▽

    M87.344 **Other secondary osteonecrosis,** right finger(s)

    M87.345 **Other secondary osteonecrosis,** left finger(s)

    M87.346 **Other secondary osteonecrosis, unspecified finger(s)** ▽

√6ᵗʰ **M87.35** **Other secondary osteonecrosis,** pelvis and femur

    M87.350 **Other secondary osteonecrosis,** pelvis

    M87.351 **Other secondary osteonecrosis,** right femur

    M87.352 **Other secondary osteonecrosis,** left femur

    M87.353 **Other secondary osteonecrosis, unspecified femur** ▽

√6ᵗʰ **M87.36** **Other secondary osteonecrosis,** tibia and fibula

    M87.361 **Other secondary osteonecrosis,** right tibia

    M87.362 **Other secondary osteonecrosis,** left tibia

    M87.363 **Other secondary osteonecrosis, unspecified tibia** ▽

    M87.364 **Other secondary osteonecrosis,** right fibula

    M87.365 **Other secondary osteonecrosis,** left fibula

    M87.366 **Other secondary osteonecrosis, unspecified fibula** ▽

√6ᵗʰ **M87.37** **Other secondary osteonecrosis,** ankle and foot

    M87.371 **Other secondary osteonecrosis,** right ankle

    M87.372 **Other secondary osteonecrosis,** left ankle

    M87.373 **Other secondary osteonecrosis, unspecified ankle** ▽

    M87.374 **Other secondary osteonecrosis,** right foot

    M87.375 **Other secondary osteonecrosis,** left foot

    M87.376 **Other secondary osteonecrosis, unspecified foot** ▽

    M87.377 **Other secondary osteonecrosis,** right toe(s)

    M87.378 **Other secondary osteonecrosis,** left toe(s)

    M87.379 **Other secondary osteonecrosis, unspecified toe(s)** ▽

M87.38 **Other secondary osteonecrosis, other site**

M87.39 **Other secondary osteonecrosis,** multiple sites

√5ᵗʰ **M87.8** Other osteonecrosis

    M87.80 **Other osteonecrosis, unspecified bone** ▽

√6ᵗʰ **M87.81** **Other osteonecrosis,** shoulder

    M87.811 **Other osteonecrosis,** right **shoulder**

    M87.812 **Other osteonecrosis,** left **shoulder**

    M87.819 **Other osteonecrosis, unspecified shoulder** ▽

√6ᵗʰ **M87.82** **Other osteonecrosis,** humerus

    M87.821 **Other osteonecrosis,** right **humerus**

    M87.822 **Other osteonecrosis,** left **humerus**

    M87.829 **Other osteonecrosis, unspecified humerus** ▽

√6ᵗʰ **M87.83** **Other osteonecrosis of** radius, ulna and carpus

    M87.831 **Other osteonecrosis of** right radius

    M87.832 **Other osteonecrosis of** left radius

    M87.833 **Other osteonecrosis of unspecified radius** ▽

    M87.834 **Other osteonecrosis of** right ulna

    M87.835 **Other osteonecrosis of** left ulna

    M87.836 **Other osteonecrosis of unspecified ulna** ▽

    M87.837 **Other osteonecrosis of** right carpus

    M87.838 **Other osteonecrosis of** left carpus

    M87.839 **Other osteonecrosis of unspecified carpus** ▽

√6ᵗʰ **M87.84** **Other osteonecrosis,** hand and fingers

    M87.841 **Other osteonecrosis,** right hand

    M87.842 **Other osteonecrosis,** left hand

    M87.843 **Other osteonecrosis, unspecified hand** ▽

    M87.844 **Other osteonecrosis,** right finger(s)

    M87.845 **Other osteonecrosis,** left finger(s)

    M87.849 **Other osteonecrosis, unspecified finger(s)** ▽

√6ᵗʰ **M87.85** **Other osteonecrosis,** pelvis and femur

    M87.850 **Other osteonecrosis,** pelvis

    M87.851 **Other osteonecrosis,** right femur

    M87.852 **Other osteonecrosis,** left femur

    M87.859 **Other osteonecrosis, unspecified femur** ▽

√6ᵗʰ **M87.86** **Other osteonecrosis,** tibia and fibula

    M87.861 **Other osteonecrosis,** right tibia

Ⓝ Newborn   Ⓟ Pediatric   Ⓜ Maternity   Ⓐ Adult   **RIC** RIC Dx   **NCDx** Noncancer Dx   **PDx** Primary Dx   **CC** RIC CC Condition   ▶◀ Revised Text   ● New Code   ▲ Revised Code Title

746   ICD-10-CM 2016

     M87.862   **Other osteonecrosis,** left tibia
     M87.863   **Other osteonecrosis, unspecified tibia** ▽
     M87.864   **Other osteonecrosis,** right fibula
     M87.865   **Other osteonecrosis,** left fibula
     M87.869   **Other osteonecrosis, unspecified fibula** ▽

✓6ᵗʰ **M87.87**   **Other osteonecrosis, ankle, foot and toes**
     M87.871   **Other osteonecrosis,** right ankle
     M87.872   **Other osteonecrosis,** left ankle
     M87.873   **Other osteonecrosis, unspecified ankle** ▽
     M87.874   **Other osteonecrosis,** right foot
     M87.875   **Other osteonecrosis,** left foot
     M87.876   **Other osteonecrosis, unspecified foot** ▽
     M87.877   **Other osteonecrosis,** right toe(s)
     M87.878   **Other osteonecrosis,** left toe(s)
     M87.879   **Other osteonecrosis, unspecified toe(s)** ▽

   M87.88   **Other osteonecrosis, other site**
   M87.89   **Other osteonecrosis,** multiple sites

M87.9 Osteonecrosis, unspecified ▽
     Necrosis of bone NOS

✓4ᵗʰ **M88 Osteitis deformans [Paget's disease of bone]**
   EXCLUDES 1   osteitis deformans in neoplastic disease (M90.6)

M88.0 Osteitis deformans of skull
M88.1 Osteitis deformans of vertebrae

✓5ᵗʰ **M88.8 Osteitis deformans of other bones**

✓6ᵗʰ **M88.81**   **Osteitis deformans of** shoulder
     M88.811   **Osteitis deformans of** right shoulder
     M88.812   **Osteitis deformans of** left shoulder
     M88.819   **Osteitis deformans of unspecified shoulder** ▽

✓6ᵗʰ **M88.82**   **Osteitis deformans of** upper arm
     M88.821   **Osteitis deformans of** right upper arm
     M88.822   **Osteitis deformans of** left upper arm
     M88.829   **Osteitis deformans of unspecified upper arm** ▽

✓6ᵗʰ **M88.83**   **Osteitis deformans of** forearm
     M88.831   **Osteitis deformans of** right forearm
     M88.832   **Osteitis deformans of** left forearm
     M88.839   **Osteitis deformans of unspecified forearm** ▽

✓6ᵗʰ **M88.84**   **Osteitis deformans of** hand
     M88.841   **Osteitis deformans of** right hand
     M88.842   **Osteitis deformans of** left hand
     M88.849   **Osteitis deformans of unspecified hand** ▽

✓6ᵗʰ **M88.85**   **Osteitis deformans of** thigh
     M88.851   **Osteitis deformans of** right thigh
     M88.852   **Osteitis deformans of** left thigh
     M88.859   **Osteitis deformans of unspecified thigh** ▽

✓6ᵗʰ **M88.86**   **Osteitis deformans of** lower leg
     M88.861   **Osteitis deformans of** right lower leg
     M88.862   **Osteitis deformans of** left lower leg
     M88.869   **Osteitis deformans of unspecified lower leg** ▽

✓6ᵗʰ **M88.87**   **Osteitis deformans of** ankle and foot
     M88.871   **Osteitis deformans of** right ankle and foot
     M88.872   **Osteitis deformans of** left ankle and foot
     M88.879   **Osteitis deformans of unspecified ankle and foot** ▽

   M88.88   **Osteitis deformans of other bones**
     EXCLUDES 2   osteitis deformans of skull (M88.0)
       osteitis deformans of vertebrae (M88.1)

   M88.89   **Osteitis deformans of** multiple sites
M88.9 Osteitis deformans of unspecified bone ▽

✓4ᵗʰ **M89 Other disorders of bone**

✓5ᵗʰ **M89.0 Algoneurodystrophy**
     Shoulder-hand syndrome
     Sudeck's atrophy
     EXCLUDES 1   causalgia, lower limb (G57.7-)
       causalgia, upper limb (G56.4-)
       complex regional pain syndrome II, lower limb (G57.7-)
       complex regional pain syndrome II, upper limb (G56.4-)
       reflex sympathetic dystrophy (G90.5-)

   M89.00   **Algoneurodystrophy, unspecified site** ▽

✓6ᵗʰ **M89.01**   **Algoneurodystrophy,** shoulder
     M89.011   **Algoneurodystrophy,** right shoulder
     M89.012   **Algoneurodystrophy,** left shoulder
     M89.019   **Algoneurodystrophy, unspecified shoulder** ▽

✓6ᵗʰ **M89.02**   **Algoneurodystrophy,** upper arm
     M89.021   **Algoneurodystrophy,** right upper arm
     M89.022   **Algoneurodystrophy,** left upper arm
     M89.029   **Algoneurodystrophy, unspecified upper arm** ▽

✓6ᵗʰ **M89.03**   **Algoneurodystrophy,** forearm
     M89.031   **Algoneurodystrophy,** right forearm
     M89.032   **Algoneurodystrophy,** left forearm
     M89.039   **Algoneurodystrophy, unspecified forearm** ▽

✓6ᵗʰ **M89.04**   **Algoneurodystrophy,** hand
     M89.041   **Algoneurodystrophy,** right hand
     M89.042   **Algoneurodystrophy,** left hand
     M89.049   **Algoneurodystrophy, unspecified hand** ▽

✓6ᵗʰ **M89.05**   **Algoneurodystrophy,** thigh
     M89.051   **Algoneurodystrophy,** right thigh
     M89.052   **Algoneurodystrophy,** left thigh
     M89.059   **Algoneurodystrophy, unspecified thigh** ▽

✓6ᵗʰ **M89.06**   **Algoneurodystrophy,** lower leg
     M89.061   **Algoneurodystrophy,** right lower leg
     M89.062   **Algoneurodystrophy,** left lower leg
     M89.069   **Algoneurodystrophy, unspecified lower leg** ▽

✓6ᵗʰ **M89.07**   **Algoneurodystrophy,** ankle and foot
     M89.071   **Algoneurodystrophy,** right ankle and foot
     M89.072   **Algoneurodystrophy,** left ankle and foot
     M89.079   **Algoneurodystrophy, unspecified ankle and foot** ▽

   M89.08   **Algoneurodystrophy, other site**
   M89.09   **Algoneurodystrophy,** multiple sites

✓5ᵗʰ **M89.1 Physeal arrest**
     Arrest of growth plate
     Epiphyseal arrest
     Growth plate arrest

✓6ᵗʰ **M89.12**   **Physeal arrest,** humerus
     M89.121   **Complete physeal arrest,** right proximal humerus
     M89.122   **Complete physeal arrest,** left proximal humerus
     M89.123   **Partial physeal arrest,** right proximal humerus
     M89.124   **Partial physeal arrest,** left proximal humerus
     M89.125   **Complete physeal arrest,** right distal humerus
     M89.126   **Complete physeal arrest,** left distal humerus
     M89.127   **Partial physeal arrest,** right distal humerus
     M89.128   **Partial physeal arrest,** left distal humerus
     M89.129   **Physeal arrest, humerus, unspecified** ▽

✓6ᵗʰ **M89.13**   **Physeal arrest,** forearm
     M89.131   **Complete physeal arrest,** right distal radius
     M89.132   **Complete physeal arrest,** left distal radius
     M89.133   **Partial physeal arrest,** right distal radius
     M89.134   **Partial physeal arrest,** left distal radius
     M89.138   **Other physeal arrest of forearm**

☑ Add'l Character Required   ✓x7ᵗʰ Placeholder Alert   RUG IV Special Care High Dx   RUG IV Clinically Complex Dx   RUG IV Special Care Low Dx   Manifestation Code   Other Specified Code   ▽ Unspecified Code

ICD-10-CM 2016   **747**

M89.139 Physeal arrest, forearm, unspecified ▽

✓6ᵗʰ M89.15 Physeal arrest, femur
- M89.151 Complete physeal arrest, right proximal femur
- M89.152 Complete physeal arrest, left proximal femur
- M89.153 Partial physeal arrest, right proximal femur
- M89.154 Partial physeal arrest, left proximal femur
- M89.155 Complete physeal arrest, right distal femur
- M89.156 Complete physeal arrest, left distal femur
- M89.157 Partial physeal arrest, right distal femur
- M89.158 Partial physeal arrest, left distal femur
- M89.159 Physeal arrest, femur, unspecified ▽

✓6ᵗʰ M89.16 Physeal arrest, lower leg
- M89.160 Complete physeal arrest, right proximal tibia
- M89.161 Complete physeal arrest, left proximal tibia
- M89.162 Partial physeal arrest, right proximal tibia
- M89.163 Partial physeal arrest, left proximal tibia
- M89.164 Complete physeal arrest, right distal tibia
- M89.165 Complete physeal arrest, left distal tibia
- M89.166 Partial physeal arrest, right distal tibia
- M89.167 Partial physeal arrest, left distal tibia
- M89.168 Other physeal arrest of lower leg
- M89.169 Physeal arrest, lower leg, unspecified ▽

M89.18 Physeal arrest, other site

✓5ᵗʰ M89.2 Other disorders of bone development and growth
- M89.20 Other disorders of bone development and growth, unspecified site ▽

✓6ᵗʰ M89.21 Other disorders of bone development and growth, shoulder
- M89.211 Other disorders of bone development and growth, right shoulder
- M89.212 Other disorders of bone development and growth, left shoulder
- M89.219 Other disorders of bone development and growth, unspecified shoulder ▽

✓6ᵗʰ M89.22 Other disorders of bone development and growth, humerus
- M89.221 Other disorders of bone development and growth, right humerus
- M89.222 Other disorders of bone development and growth, left humerus
- M89.229 Other disorders of bone development and growth, unspecified humerus ▽

✓6ᵗʰ M89.23 Other disorders of bone development and growth, ulna and radius
- M89.231 Other disorders of bone development and growth, right ulna
- M89.232 Other disorders of bone development and growth, left ulna
- M89.233 Other disorders of bone development and growth, right radius
- M89.234 Other disorders of bone development and growth, left radius
- M89.239 Other disorders of bone development and growth, unspecified ulna and radius ▽

✓6ᵗʰ M89.24 Other disorders of bone development and growth, hand
- M89.241 Other disorders of bone development and growth, right hand
- M89.242 Other disorders of bone development and growth, left hand
- M89.249 Other disorders of bone development and growth, unspecified hand ▽

✓6ᵗʰ M89.25 Other disorders of bone development and growth, femur
- M89.251 Other disorders of bone development and growth, right femur

M89.252 Other disorders of bone development and growth, left femur
- M89.259 Other disorders of bone development and growth, unspecified femur ▽

✓6ᵗʰ M89.26 Other disorders of bone development and growth, tibia and fibula
- M89.261 Other disorders of bone development and growth, right tibia
- M89.262 Other disorders of bone development and growth, left tibia
- M89.263 Other disorders of bone development and growth, right fibula
- M89.264 Other disorders of bone development and growth, left fibula
- M89.269 Other disorders of bone development and growth, unspecified lower leg ▽

✓6ᵗʰ M89.27 Other disorders of bone development and growth, ankle and foot
- M89.271 Other disorders of bone development and growth, right ankle and foot
- M89.272 Other disorders of bone development and growth, left ankle and foot
- M89.279 Other disorders of bone development and growth, unspecified ankle and foot ▽

M89.28 Other disorders of bone development and growth, other site

M89.29 Other disorders of bone development and growth, multiple sites

✓5ᵗʰ M89.3 Hypertrophy of bone
- M89.30 Hypertrophy of bone, unspecified site ▽

✓6ᵗʰ M89.31 Hypertrophy of bone, shoulder
- M89.311 Hypertrophy of bone, right shoulder
- M89.312 Hypertrophy of bone, left shoulder
- M89.319 Hypertrophy of bone, unspecified shoulder ▽

✓6ᵗʰ M89.32 Hypertrophy of bone, humerus
- M89.321 Hypertrophy of bone, right humerus
- M89.322 Hypertrophy of bone, left humerus
- M89.329 Hypertrophy of bone, unspecified humerus ▽

✓6ᵗʰ M89.33 Hypertrophy of bone, ulna and radius
- M89.331 Hypertrophy of bone, right ulna
- M89.332 Hypertrophy of bone, left ulna
- M89.333 Hypertrophy of bone, right radius
- M89.334 Hypertrophy of bone, left radius
- M89.339 Hypertrophy of bone, unspecified ulna and radius ▽

✓6ᵗʰ M89.34 Hypertrophy of bone, hand
- M89.341 Hypertrophy of bone, right hand
- M89.342 Hypertrophy of bone, left hand
- M89.349 Hypertrophy of bone, unspecified hand ▽

✓6ᵗʰ M89.35 Hypertrophy of bone, femur
- M89.351 Hypertrophy of bone, right femur
- M89.352 Hypertrophy of bone, left femur
- M89.359 Hypertrophy of bone, unspecified femur ▽

✓6ᵗʰ M89.36 Hypertrophy of bone, tibia and fibula
- M89.361 Hypertrophy of bone, right tibia
- M89.362 Hypertrophy of bone, left tibia
- M89.363 Hypertrophy of bone, right fibula
- M89.364 Hypertrophy of bone, left fibula
- M89.369 Hypertrophy of bone, unspecified tibia and fibula ▽

✓6ᵗʰ M89.37 Hypertrophy of bone, ankle and foot
- M89.371 Hypertrophy of bone, right ankle and foot
- M89.372 Hypertrophy of bone, left ankle and foot
- M89.379 Hypertrophy of bone, unspecified ankle and foot ▽

M89.38 Hypertrophy of bone, other site

M89.39 Hypertrophy of bone, multiple sites

✓5ᵗʰ **M89.4 Other hypertrophic osteoarthropathy**
    Marie-Bamberger disease   Pachydermoperiostosis

M89.40 Other hypertrophic osteoarthropathy, unspecified site ▽

✓6ᵗʰ **M89.41 Other hypertrophic osteoarthropathy, shoulder**
  M89.411 Other hypertrophic osteoarthropathy, right shoulder
  M89.412 Other hypertrophic osteoarthropathy, left shoulder
  M89.419 Other hypertrophic osteoarthropathy, unspecified shoulder ▽

✓6ᵗʰ **M89.42 Other hypertrophic osteoarthropathy, upper arm**
  M89.421 Other hypertrophic osteoarthropathy, right upper arm
  M89.422 Other hypertrophic osteoarthropathy, left upper arm
  M89.429 Other hypertrophic osteoarthropathy, unspecified upper arm ▽

✓6ᵗʰ **M89.43 Other hypertrophic osteoarthropathy, forearm**
  M89.431 Other hypertrophic osteoarthropathy, right forearm
  M89.432 Other hypertrophic osteoarthropathy, left forearm
  M89.439 Other hypertrophic osteoarthropathy, unspecified forearm ▽

✓6ᵗʰ **M89.44 Other hypertrophic osteoarthropathy, hand**
  M89.441 Other hypertrophic osteoarthropathy, right hand
  M89.442 Other hypertrophic osteoarthropathy, left hand
  M89.449 Other hypertrophic osteoarthropathy, unspecified hand ▽

✓6ᵗʰ **M89.45 Other hypertrophic osteoarthropathy, thigh**
  M89.451 Other hypertrophic osteoarthropathy, right thigh
  M89.452 Other hypertrophic osteoarthropathy, left thigh
  M89.459 Other hypertrophic osteoarthropathy, unspecified thigh ▽

✓6ᵗʰ **M89.46 Other hypertrophic osteoarthropathy, lower leg**
  M89.461 Other hypertrophic osteoarthropathy, right lower leg
  M89.462 Other hypertrophic osteoarthropathy, left lower leg
  M89.469 Other hypertrophic osteoarthropathy, unspecified lower leg ▽

✓6ᵗʰ **M89.47 Other hypertrophic osteoarthropathy, ankle and foot**
  M89.471 Other hypertrophic osteoarthropathy, right ankle and foot
  M89.472 Other hypertrophic osteoarthropathy, left ankle and foot
  M89.479 Other hypertrophic osteoarthropathy, unspecified ankle and foot ▽

M89.48 Other hypertrophic osteoarthropathy, other site

M89.49 Other hypertrophic osteoarthropathy, multiple sites

✓5ᵗʰ **M89.5 Osteolysis**
  Use additional code to identify major osseous defect, if applicable (M89.7-)
  EXCLUDES 2 *periprosthetic osteolysis of internal prosthetic joint (T84.05-)*

M89.50 Osteolysis, unspecified site ▽

✓6ᵗʰ **M89.51 Osteolysis, shoulder**
  M89.511 Osteolysis, right shoulder
  M89.512 Osteolysis, left shoulder
  M89.519 Osteolysis, unspecified shoulder ▽

✓6ᵗʰ **M89.52 Osteolysis, upper arm**
  M89.521 Osteolysis, right upper arm
  M89.522 Osteolysis, left upper arm
  M89.529 Osteolysis, unspecified upper arm ▽

✓6ᵗʰ **M89.53 Osteolysis, forearm**
  M89.531 Osteolysis, right forearm
  M89.532 Osteolysis, left forearm
  M89.539 Osteolysis, unspecified forearm ▽

✓6ᵗʰ **M89.54 Osteolysis, hand**
  M89.541 Osteolysis, right hand
  M89.542 Osteolysis, left hand
  M89.549 Osteolysis, unspecified hand ▽

✓6ᵗʰ **M89.55 Osteolysis, thigh**
  M89.551 Osteolysis, right thigh
  M89.552 Osteolysis, left thigh
  M89.559 Osteolysis, unspecified thigh ▽

✓6ᵗʰ **M89.56 Osteolysis, lower leg**
  M89.561 Osteolysis, right lower leg
  M89.562 Osteolysis, left lower leg
  M89.569 Osteolysis, unspecified lower leg ▽

✓6ᵗʰ **M89.57 Osteolysis, ankle and foot**
  M89.571 Osteolysis, right ankle and foot
  M89.572 Osteolysis, left ankle and foot
  M89.579 Osteolysis, unspecified ankle and foot ▽

M89.58 Osteolysis, other site

M89.59 Osteolysis, multiple sites

✓5ᵗʰ **M89.6 Osteopathy after poliomyelitis**
  Use additional code (B91) to identify previous poliomyelitis
  EXCLUDES 1 *postpolio syndrome (G14)*

M89.60 Osteopathy after poliomyelitis, unspecified site ▽

✓6ᵗʰ **M89.61 Osteopathy after poliomyelitis, shoulder**
  M89.611 Osteopathy after poliomyelitis, right shoulder
  M89.612 Osteopathy after poliomyelitis, left shoulder
  M89.619 Osteopathy after poliomyelitis, unspecified shoulder ▽

✓6ᵗʰ **M89.62 Osteopathy after poliomyelitis, upper arm**
  M89.621 Osteopathy after poliomyelitis, right upper arm
  M89.622 Osteopathy after poliomyelitis, left upper arm
  M89.629 Osteopathy after poliomyelitis, unspecified upper arm ▽

✓6ᵗʰ **M89.63 Osteopathy after poliomyelitis, forearm**
  M89.631 Osteopathy after poliomyelitis, right forearm
  M89.632 Osteopathy after poliomyelitis, left forearm
  M89.639 Osteopathy after poliomyelitis, unspecified forearm ▽

✓6ᵗʰ **M89.64 Osteopathy after poliomyelitis, hand**
  M89.641 Osteopathy after poliomyelitis, right hand
  M89.642 Osteopathy after poliomyelitis, left hand
  M89.649 Osteopathy after poliomyelitis, unspecified hand ▽

✓6ᵗʰ **M89.65 Osteopathy after poliomyelitis, thigh**
  M89.651 Osteopathy after poliomyelitis, right thigh
  M89.652 Osteopathy after poliomyelitis, left thigh
  M89.659 Osteopathy after poliomyelitis, unspecified thigh ▽

✓6ᵗʰ **M89.66 Osteopathy after poliomyelitis, lower leg**
  M89.661 Osteopathy after poliomyelitis, right lower leg
  M89.662 Osteopathy after poliomyelitis, left lower leg
  M89.669 Osteopathy after poliomyelitis, unspecified lower leg ▽

✓6ᵗʰ **M89.67 Osteopathy after poliomyelitis, ankle and foot**
  M89.671 Osteopathy after poliomyelitis, right ankle and foot
  M89.672 Osteopathy after poliomyelitis, left ankle and foot
  M89.679 Osteopathy after poliomyelitis, unspecified ankle and foot ▽

M89.68 Osteopathy after poliomyelitis, other site

M89.69 Osteopathy after poliomyelitis, multiple sites

☑ Add'l Character Required   ✓x7ᵗʰ Placeholder Alert   RUG IV Special Care High Dx   RUG IV Clinically Complex Dx   RUG IV Special Care Low Dx   Manifestation Code   Other Specified Code   ▽ Unspecified Code

☑5ᵗʰ M89.7 Major osseous defect
Code first underlying disease, if known, such as:
aseptic necrosis of bone (M87.-)
malignant neoplasm of bone (C40.-)
osteolysis (M89.5)
osteomyelitis (M86.-)
osteonecrosis (M87.-)
osteoporosis (M80.-, M81.-)
periprosthetic osteolysis (T84.05-)

M89.70 Major osseous defect, unspecified site ▽

☑6ᵗʰ M89.71 Major osseous defect, shoulder region
Major osseous defect clavicle or scapula

M89.711 Major osseous defect, right shoulder region

M89.712 Major osseous defect, left shoulder region

M89.719 Major osseous defect, unspecified shoulder region ▽

☑6ᵗʰ M89.72 Major osseous defect, humerus

M89.721 Major osseous defect, right humerus

M89.722 Major osseous defect, left humerus

M89.729 Major osseous defect, unspecified humerus ▽

☑6ᵗʰ M89.73 Major osseous defect, forearm
Major osseous defect of radius and ulna

M89.731 Major osseous defect, right forearm

M89.732 Major osseous defect, left forearm

M89.739 Major osseous defect, unspecified forearm ▽

☑6ᵗʰ M89.74 Major osseous defect, hand
Major osseous defect of carpus, fingers, metacarpus

M89.741 Major osseous defect, right hand

M89.742 Major osseous defect, left hand

M89.749 Major osseous defect, unspecified hand ▽

☑6ᵗʰ M89.75 Major osseous defect, pelvic region and thigh
Major osseous defect of femur and pelvis

M89.751 Major osseous defect, right pelvic region and thigh

M89.752 Major osseous defect, left pelvic region and thigh

M89.759 Major osseous defect, unspecified pelvic region and thigh ▽

☑6ᵗʰ M89.76 Major osseous defect, lower leg
Major osseous defect of fibula and tibia

M89.761 Major osseous defect, right lower leg

M89.762 Major osseous defect, left lower leg

M89.769 Major osseous defect, unspecified lower leg ▽

☑6ᵗʰ M89.77 Major osseous defect, ankle and foot
Major osseous defect of metatarsus, tarsus, toes

M89.771 Major osseous defect, right ankle and foot

M89.772 Major osseous defect, left ankle and foot

M89.779 Major osseous defect, unspecified ankle and foot ▽

M89.78 Major osseous defect, other site

M89.79 Major osseous defect, multiple sites

☑5ᵗʰ M89.8 Other specified disorders of bone
Infantile cortical hyperostoses
Post-traumatic subperiosteal ossification

☑6ᵗʰ M89.8X Other specified disorders of bone

M89.8X0 Other specified disorders of bone, multiple sites

M89.8X1 Other specified disorders of bone, shoulder

M89.8X2 Other specified disorders of bone, upper arm

M89.8X3 Other specified disorders of bone, forearm

M89.8X4 Other specified disorders of bone, hand

M89.8X5 Other specified disorders of bone, thigh

M89.8X6 Other specified disorders of bone, lower leg

M89.8X7 Other specified disorders of bone, ankle and foot

M89.8X8 Other specified disorders of bone, other site

M89.8X9 Other specified disorders of bone, unspecified site ▽

M89.9 Disorder of bone, unspecified ▽

☑4ᵗʰ M90 Osteopathies in diseases classified elsewhere
EXCLUDES 1 osteochondritis, osteomyelitis, and osteopathy (in):
cryptococcosis (B45.3)
diabetes mellitus (E08-E13 with .61-)
gonococcal (A54.43)
neurogenic syphilis (A52.11)
renal osteodystrophy (N25.0)
salmonellosis (A02.24)
secondary syphilis (A51.46)
syphilis (late) (A52.77)

☑5ᵗʰ M90.5 Osteonecrosis in diseases classified elsewhere
Code first underlying disease, such as:
caisson disease (T70.3)
hemoglobinopathy (D50-D64)

M90.50 *Osteonecrosis in diseases classified elsewhere, unspecified site* ▽

☑6ᵗʰ M90.51 *Osteonecrosis in diseases classified elsewhere, shoulder*

M90.511 *Osteonecrosis in diseases classified elsewhere, right shoulder*

M90.512 *Osteonecrosis in diseases classified elsewhere, left shoulder*

M90.519 *Osteonecrosis in diseases classified elsewhere, unspecified shoulder* ▽

☑6ᵗʰ M90.52 *Osteonecrosis in diseases classified elsewhere, upper arm*

M90.521 *Osteonecrosis in diseases classified elsewhere, right upper arm*

M90.522 *Osteonecrosis in diseases classified elsewhere, left upper arm*

M90.529 *Osteonecrosis in diseases classified elsewhere, unspecified upper arm* ▽

☑6ᵗʰ M90.53 *Osteonecrosis in diseases classified elsewhere, forearm*

M90.531 *Osteonecrosis in diseases classified elsewhere, right forearm*

M90.532 *Osteonecrosis in diseases classified elsewhere, left forearm*

M90.539 *Osteonecrosis in diseases classified elsewhere, unspecified forearm* ▽

☑6ᵗʰ M90.54 *Osteonecrosis in diseases classified elsewhere, hand*

M90.541 *Osteonecrosis in diseases classified elsewhere, right hand*

M90.542 *Osteonecrosis in diseases classified elsewhere, left hand*

M90.549 *Osteonecrosis in diseases classified elsewhere, unspecified hand* ▽

☑6ᵗʰ M90.55 *Osteonecrosis in diseases classified elsewhere, thigh*

M90.551 *Osteonecrosis in diseases classified elsewhere, right thigh*

M90.552 *Osteonecrosis in diseases classified elsewhere, left thigh*

M90.559 *Osteonecrosis in diseases classified elsewhere, unspecified thigh* ▽

☑6ᵗʰ M90.56 *Osteonecrosis in diseases classified elsewhere, lower leg*

M90.561 *Osteonecrosis in diseases classified elsewhere, right lower leg*

M90.562 *Osteonecrosis in diseases classified elsewhere, left lower leg*

M90.569 *Osteonecrosis in diseases classified elsewhere, unspecified lower leg* ▽

☑6ᵗʰ M90.57 *Osteonecrosis in diseases classified elsewhere, ankle and foot*

M90.571 *Osteonecrosis in diseases classified elsewhere, right ankle and foot*

M90.572 *Osteonecrosis in diseases classified elsewhere, left ankle and foot*

M90.579 *Osteonecrosis in diseases classified elsewhere, unspecified ankle and foot* ▽

M90.58 *Osteonecrosis in diseases classified elsewhere, other site*

M90.59 *Osteonecrosis in diseases classified elsewhere, multiple sites*

Ⓝ Newborn   Ⓟ Pediatric   Ⓜ Maternity   Ⓐ Adult   **RIC** RIC Dx   **NC Dx** Noncancer Dx   **PDx** Primary Dx   **CC** RIC CC Condition   ►◄ Revised Text   ● New Code   ▲ Revised Code Title

750   ICD-10-CM 2016

✓5ᵗʰ **M90.6 Osteitis deformans in neoplastic diseases**
Osteitis deformans in malignant neoplasm of bone
Code first the neoplasm (C40-, C41-)
EXCLUDES 1   osteitis deformans [Paget's disease of bone] (M88.-)

  M90.60 Osteitis deformans in neoplastic diseases, unspecified site ▽

  ✓6ᵗʰ **M90.61 Osteitis deformans in neoplastic diseases, shoulder**
    M90.611 Osteitis deformans in neoplastic diseases, right shoulder
    M90.612 Osteitis deformans in neoplastic diseases, left shoulder
    M90.619 Osteitis deformans in neoplastic diseases, unspecified shoulder ▽

  ✓6ᵗʰ **M90.62 Osteitis deformans in neoplastic diseases, upper arm**
    M90.621 Osteitis deformans in neoplastic diseases, right upper arm
    M90.622 Osteitis deformans in neoplastic diseases, left upper arm
    M90.629 Osteitis deformans in neoplastic diseases, unspecified upper arm ▽

  ✓6ᵗʰ **M90.63 Osteitis deformans in neoplastic diseases, forearm**
    M90.631 Osteitis deformans in neoplastic diseases, right forearm
    M90.632 Osteitis deformans in neoplastic diseases, left forearm
    M90.639 Osteitis deformans in neoplastic diseases, unspecified forearm ▽

  ✓6ᵗʰ **M90.64 Osteitis deformans in neoplastic diseases, hand**
    M90.641 Osteitis deformans in neoplastic diseases, right hand
    M90.642 Osteitis deformans in neoplastic diseases, left hand
    M90.649 Osteitis deformans in neoplastic diseases, unspecified hand ▽

  ✓6ᵗʰ **M90.65 Osteitis deformans in neoplastic diseases, thigh**
    M90.651 Osteitis deformans in neoplastic diseases, right thigh
    M90.652 Osteitis deformans in neoplastic diseases, left thigh
    M90.659 Osteitis deformans in neoplastic diseases, unspecified thigh ▽

  ✓6ᵗʰ **M90.66 Osteitis deformans in neoplastic diseases, lower leg**
    M90.661 Osteitis deformans in neoplastic diseases, right lower leg
    M90.662 Osteitis deformans in neoplastic diseases, left lower leg
    M90.669 Osteitis deformans in neoplastic diseases, unspecified lower leg ▽

  ✓6ᵗʰ **M90.67 Osteitis deformans in neoplastic diseases, ankle and foot**
    M90.671 Osteitis deformans in neoplastic diseases, right ankle and foot
    M90.672 Osteitis deformans in neoplastic diseases, left ankle and foot
    M90.679 Osteitis deformans in neoplastic diseases, unspecified ankle and foot ▽

  M90.68 Osteitis deformans in neoplastic diseases, other site
  M90.69 Osteitis deformans in neoplastic diseases, multiple sites

✓5ᵗʰ **M90.8 Osteopathy in diseases classified elsewhere**
Code first underlying disease, such as:
rickets (E55.0)
vitamin-D-resistant rickets (E83.3)

  M90.80 Osteopathy in diseases classified elsewhere, unspecified site ▽

  ✓6ᵗʰ **M90.81 Osteopathy in diseases classified elsewhere, shoulder**
    M90.811 Osteopathy in diseases classified elsewhere, right shoulder
    M90.812 Osteopathy in diseases classified elsewhere, left shoulder
    M90.819 Osteopathy in diseases classified elsewhere, unspecified shoulder ▽

  ✓6ᵗʰ **M90.82 Osteopathy in diseases classified elsewhere, upper arm**
    M90.821 Osteopathy in diseases classified elsewhere, right upper arm
    M90.822 Osteopathy in diseases classified elsewhere, left upper arm
    M90.829 Osteopathy in diseases classified elsewhere, unspecified upper arm ▽

  ✓6ᵗʰ **M90.83 Osteopathy in diseases classified elsewhere, forearm**
    M90.831 Osteopathy in diseases classified elsewhere, right forearm
    M90.832 Osteopathy in diseases classified elsewhere, left forearm
    M90.839 Osteopathy in diseases classified elsewhere, unspecified forearm ▽

  ✓6ᵗʰ **M90.84 Osteopathy in diseases classified elsewhere, hand**
    M90.841 Osteopathy in diseases classified elsewhere, right hand
    M90.842 Osteopathy in diseases classified elsewhere, left hand
    M90.849 Osteopathy in diseases classified elsewhere, unspecified hand ▽

  ✓6ᵗʰ **M90.85 Osteopathy in diseases classified elsewhere, thigh**
    M90.851 Osteopathy in diseases classified elsewhere, right thigh
    M90.852 Osteopathy in diseases classified elsewhere, left thigh
    M90.859 Osteopathy in diseases classified elsewhere, unspecified thigh ▽

  ✓6ᵗʰ **M90.86 Osteopathy in diseases classified elsewhere, lower leg**
    M90.861 Osteopathy in diseases classified elsewhere, right lower leg
    M90.862 Osteopathy in diseases classified elsewhere, left lower leg
    M90.869 Osteopathy in diseases classified elsewhere, unspecified lower leg ▽

  ✓6ᵗʰ **M90.87 Osteopathy in diseases classified elsewhere, ankle and foot**
    M90.871 Osteopathy in diseases classified elsewhere, right ankle and foot
    M90.872 Osteopathy in diseases classified elsewhere, left ankle and foot
    M90.879 Osteopathy in diseases classified elsewhere, unspecified ankle and foot ▽

  M90.88 Osteopathy in diseases classified elsewhere, other site
  M90.89 Osteopathy in diseases classified elsewhere, multiple sites

Chondropathies (M91-M94)

EXCLUDES 1   postprocedural chondropathies (M96.-)

✓4ᵗʰ **M91 Juvenile osteochondrosis of hip and pelvis**
  EXCLUDES 1   slipped upper femoral epiphysis (nontraumatic) (M93.0)

  M91.0 Juvenile osteochondrosis of pelvis
    Osteochondrosis (juvenile) of acetabulum
    Osteochondrosis (juvenile) of iliac crest [Buchanan]
    Osteochondrosis (juvenile) of ischiopubic synchondrosis [van Neck]
    Osteochondrosis (juvenile) of symphysis pubis [Pierson]

  ✓5ᵗʰ **M91.1 Juvenile osteochondrosis of head of femur [Legg-Calvé-Perthes]**
    M91.10 Juvenile osteochondrosis of head of femur [Legg-Calvé-Perthes], unspecified leg ▽
    M91.11 Juvenile osteochondrosis of head of femur [Legg-Calvé-Perthes], right leg
    M91.12 Juvenile osteochondrosis of head of femur [Legg-Calvé-Perthes], left leg

  ✓5ᵗʰ **M91.2 Coxa plana**
    Hip deformity due to previous juvenile osteochondrosis
    M91.20 Coxa plana, unspecified hip ▽
    M91.21 Coxa plana, right hip
    M91.22 Coxa plana, left hip

  ✓5ᵗʰ **M91.3 Pseudocoxalgia**
    M91.30 Pseudocoxalgia, unspecified hip ▽
    M91.31 Pseudocoxalgia, right hip
    M91.32 Pseudocoxalgia, left hip

  ✓5ᵗʰ **M91.4 Coxa magna**
    M91.40 Coxa magna, unspecified hip ▽
    M91.41 Coxa magna, right hip
    M91.42 Coxa magna, left hip

☑ Add'l Character Required   ✓x7ᵗʰ Placeholder Alert   RUG IV Special Care High Dx   RUG IV Clinically Complex Dx   RUG IV Special Care Low Dx   Manifestation Code   Other Specified Code   ▽ Unspecified Code

Chapter 13. Diseases of the Musculoskeletal System and Connective Tissue

✓5th **M91.8 Other** juvenile osteochondrosis of hip and pelvis
     Juvenile osteochondrosis after reduction of congenital dislocation of hip

     M91.80 Other juvenile osteochondrosis of hip and pelvis, unspecified leg ▽

     M91.81 Other juvenile osteochondrosis of hip and pelvis, right leg

     M91.82 Other juvenile osteochondrosis of hip and pelvis, left leg

✓5th **M91.9 Juvenile osteochondrosis of hip and pelvis, unspecified**

     M91.90 Juvenile osteochondrosis of hip and pelvis, unspecified, unspecified leg ▽

     M91.91 Juvenile osteochondrosis of hip and pelvis, unspecified, right leg ▽

     M91.92 Juvenile osteochondrosis of hip and pelvis, unspecified, left leg ▽

✓4th **M92 Other juvenile osteochondrosis**

✓5th **M92.0 Juvenile osteochondrosis of humerus**
     Osteochondrosis (juvenile) of capitulum of humerus [Panner]
     Osteochondrosis (juvenile) of head of humerus [Haas]

     M92.00 Juvenile osteochondrosis of humerus, unspecified arm ▽

     M92.01 Juvenile osteochondrosis of humerus, right arm

     M92.02 Juvenile osteochondrosis of humerus, left arm

✓5th **M92.1 Juvenile osteochondrosis of radius and ulna**
     Osteochondrosis (juvenile) of lower ulna [Burns]
     Osteochondrosis (juvenile) of radial head [Brailsford]

     M92.10 Juvenile osteochondrosis of radius and ulna, unspecified arm ▽

     M92.11 Juvenile osteochondrosis of radius and ulna, right arm

     M92.12 Juvenile osteochondrosis of radius and ulna, left arm

✓5th **M92.2 Juvenile osteochondrosis, hand**

     ✓6th **M92.20 Unspecified juvenile osteochondrosis, hand**

         M92.201 Unspecified juvenile osteochondrosis, right hand ▽

         M92.202 Unspecified juvenile osteochondrosis, left hand ▽

         M92.209 Unspecified juvenile osteochondrosis, unspecified hand ▽

     ✓6th **M92.21 Osteochondrosis (juvenile) of carpal lunate [Kienböck]**

         M92.211 Osteochondrosis (juvenile) of carpal lunate [Kienböck], right hand

         M92.212 Osteochondrosis (juvenile) of carpal lunate [Kienböck], left hand

         M92.219 Osteochondrosis (juvenile) of carpal lunate [Kienböck], unspecified hand ▽

     ✓6th **M92.22 Osteochondrosis (juvenile) of metacarpal heads [Mauclaire]**

         M92.221 Osteochondrosis (juvenile) of metacarpal heads [Mauclaire], right hand

         M92.222 Osteochondrosis (juvenile) of metacarpal heads [Mauclaire], left hand

         M92.229 Osteochondrosis (juvenile) of metacarpal heads [Mauclaire], unspecified hand ▽

     ✓6th **M92.29 Other juvenile osteochondrosis, hand**

         M92.291 Other juvenile osteochondrosis, right hand

         M92.292 Other juvenile osteochondrosis, left hand

         M92.299 Other juvenile osteochondrosis, unspecified hand ▽

✓5th **M92.3 Other juvenile osteochondrosis, upper limb**

     M92.30 Other juvenile osteochondrosis, unspecified upper limb ▽

     M92.31 Other juvenile osteochondrosis, right upper limb

     M92.32 Other juvenile osteochondrosis, left upper limb

✓5th **M92.4 Juvenile osteochondrosis of patella**
     Osteochondrosis (juvenile) of primary patellar center [Köhler]
     Osteochondrosis (juvenile) of secondary patellar centre [Sinding Larsen]

     M92.40 Juvenile osteochondrosis of patella, unspecified knee ▽

     M92.41 Juvenile osteochondrosis of patella, right knee

M92.42 Juvenile osteochondrosis of patella, left knee

✓5th **M92.5 Juvenile osteochondrosis of tibia and fibula**
     Osteochondrosis (juvenile) of proximal tibia [Blount]
     Osteochondrosis (juvenile) of tibial tubercle [Osgood-Schlatter]
     Tibia vara

     M92.50 Juvenile osteochondrosis of tibia and fibula, unspecified leg ▽

     M92.51 Juvenile osteochondrosis of tibia and fibula, right leg

     M92.52 Juvenile osteochondrosis of tibia and fibula, left leg

✓5th **M92.6 Juvenile osteochondrosis of tarsus**
     Osteochondrosis (juvenile) of calcaneum [Sever]
     Osteochondrosis (juvenile) of os tibiale externum [Haglund]
     Osteochondrosis (juvenile) of talus [Diaz]
     Osteochondrosis (juvenile) of tarsal navicular [Köhler]

     M92.60 Juvenile osteochondrosis of tarsus, unspecified ankle ▽

     M92.61 Juvenile osteochondrosis of tarsus, right ankle

     M92.62 Juvenile osteochondrosis of tarsus, left ankle

✓5th **M92.7 Juvenile osteochondrosis of metatarsus**
     Osteochondrosis (juvenile) of fifth metatarsus [Iselin]
     Osteochondrosis (juvenile) of second metatarsus [Freiberg]

     M92.70 Juvenile osteochondrosis of metatarsus, unspecified foot ▽

     M92.71 Juvenile osteochondrosis of metatarsus, right foot

     M92.72 Juvenile osteochondrosis of metatarsus, left foot

M92.8 Other specified juvenile osteochondrosis
     Calcaneal apophysitis

M92.9 Juvenile osteochondrosis, unspecified ▽
     Juvenile apophysitis NOS
     Juvenile epiphysitis NOS
     Juvenile osteochondritis NOS
     Juvenile osteochondrosis NOS

✓4th **M93 Other osteochondropathies**
     EXCLUDES 2   osteochondrosis of spine (M42.-)

✓5th **M93.0 Slipped upper femoral epiphysis (nontraumatic)**
     Use additional code for associated chondrolysis (M94.3)

     ✓6th **M93.00 Unspecified slipped upper femoral epiphysis (nontraumatic)**

         M93.001 Unspecified slipped upper femoral epiphysis (nontraumatic), right hip ▽

         M93.002 Unspecified slipped upper femoral epiphysis (nontraumatic), left hip ▽

         M93.003 Unspecified slipped upper femoral epiphysis (nontraumatic), unspecified hip ▽

     ✓6th **M93.01 Acute slipped upper femoral epiphysis (nontraumatic)**

         M93.011 Acute slipped upper femoral epiphysis (nontraumatic), right hip

         M93.012 Acute slipped upper femoral epiphysis (nontraumatic), left hip

         M93.013 Acute slipped upper femoral epiphysis (nontraumatic), unspecified hip ▽

     ✓6th **M93.02 Chronic slipped upper femoral epiphysis (nontraumatic)**

         M93.021 Chronic slipped upper femoral epiphysis (nontraumatic), right hip

         M93.022 Chronic slipped upper femoral epiphysis (nontraumatic), left hip

         M93.023 Chronic slipped upper femoral epiphysis (nontraumatic), unspecified hip ▽

     ✓6th **M93.03 Acute on chronic slipped upper femoral epiphysis (nontraumatic)**

         M93.031 Acute on chronic slipped upper femoral epiphysis (nontraumatic), right hip

         M93.032 Acute on chronic slipped upper femoral epiphysis (nontraumatic), left hip

         M93.033 Acute on chronic slipped upper femoral epiphysis (nontraumatic), unspecified hip ▽

M93.1 Kienböck's disease of adults Ⓐ
     Adult osteochondrosis of carpal lunates

✓5th **M93.2 Osteochondritis dissecans**

     M93.20 Osteochondritis dissecans of unspecified site ▽

     ✓6th **M93.21 Osteochondritis dissecans of shoulder**

Ⓝ Newborn   Ⓟ Pediatric   Ⓜ Maternity   Ⓐ Adult   RIC RIC Dx   NC Dx Noncancer Dx   PDx Primary Dx   CC RIC CC Condition   ►◄ Revised Text   ● New Code   ▲ Revised Code Title

752   ICD-10-CM 2016

M93.211   Osteochondritis dissecans, right shoulder
M93.212   Osteochondritis dissecans, left shoulder
M93.219   Osteochondritis dissecans, unspecified shoulder ▽

✓6ᵗʰ   M93.22   Osteochondritis dissecans of elbow
M93.221   Osteochondritis dissecans, right elbow
M93.222   Osteochondritis dissecans, left elbow
M93.229   Osteochondritis dissecans, unspecified elbow ▽

✓6ᵗʰ   M93.23   Osteochondritis dissecans of wrist
M93.231   Osteochondritis dissecans, right wrist
M93.232   Osteochondritis dissecans, left wrist
M93.239   Osteochondritis dissecans, unspecified wrist ▽

✓6ᵗʰ   M93.24   Osteochondritis dissecans of joints of hand
M93.241   Osteochondritis dissecans, joints of right hand
M93.242   Osteochondritis dissecans, joints of left hand
M93.249   Osteochondritis dissecans, joints of unspecified hand ▽

✓6ᵗʰ   M93.25   Osteochondritis dissecans of hip
M93.251   Osteochondritis dissecans, right hip
M93.252   Osteochondritis dissecans, left hip
M93.259   Osteochondritis dissecans, unspecified hip ▽

✓6ᵗʰ   M93.26   Osteochondritis dissecans knee
M93.261   Osteochondritis dissecans, right knee
M93.262   Osteochondritis dissecans, left knee
M93.269   Osteochondritis dissecans, unspecified knee ▽

✓6ᵗʰ   M93.27   Osteochondritis dissecans of ankle and joints of foot
M93.271   Osteochondritis dissecans, right ankle and joints of right foot
M93.272   Osteochondritis dissecans, left ankle and joints of left foot
M93.279   Osteochondritis dissecans, unspecified ankle and joints of foot ▽

M93.28   Osteochondritis dissecans other site
M93.29   Osteochondritis dissecans multiple sites

✓5ᵗʰ   M93.8   Other specified osteochondropathies
M93.80   Other specified osteochondropathies of unspecified site ▽

✓6ᵗʰ   M93.81   Other specified osteochondropathies of shoulder
M93.811   Other specified osteochondropathies, right shoulder
M93.812   Other specified osteochondropathies, left shoulder
M93.819   Other specified osteochondropathies, unspecified shoulder ▽

✓6ᵗʰ   M93.82   Other specified osteochondropathies of upper arm
M93.821   Other specified osteochondropathies, right upper arm
M93.822   Other specified osteochondropathies, left upper arm
M93.829   Other specified osteochondropathies, unspecified upper arm ▽

✓6ᵗʰ   M93.83   Other specified osteochondropathies of forearm
M93.831   Other specified osteochondropathies, right forearm
M93.832   Other specified osteochondropathies, left forearm
M93.839   Other specified osteochondropathies, unspecified forearm ▽

✓6ᵗʰ   M93.84   Other specified osteochondropathies of hand
M93.841   Other specified osteochondropathies, right hand
M93.842   Other specified osteochondropathies, left hand
M93.849   Other specified osteochondropathies, unspecified hand ▽

✓6ᵗʰ   M93.85   Other specified osteochondropathies of thigh
M93.851   Other specified osteochondropathies, right thigh

M93.852   Other specified osteochondropathies, left thigh
M93.859   Other specified osteochondropathies, unspecified thigh ▽

✓6ᵗʰ   M93.86   Other specified osteochondropathies lower leg
M93.861   Other specified osteochondropathies, right lower leg
M93.862   Other specified osteochondropathies, left lower leg
M93.869   Other specified osteochondropathies, unspecified lower leg ▽

✓6ᵗʰ   M93.87   Other specified osteochondropathies of ankle and foot
M93.871   Other specified osteochondropathies, right ankle and foot
M93.872   Other specified osteochondropathies, left ankle and foot
M93.879   Other specified osteochondropathies, unspecified ankle and foot ▽

M93.88   Other specified osteochondropathies other site
M93.89   Other specified osteochondropathies multiple sites

✓5ᵗʰ   M93.9   Osteochondropathy, unspecified
Apophysitis NOS   Osteochondritis NOS
Epiphysitis NOS   Osteochondrosis NOS
M93.90   Osteochondropathy, unspecified of unspecified site ▽

✓6ᵗʰ   M93.91   Osteochondropathy, unspecified of shoulder
M93.911   Osteochondropathy, unspecified, right shoulder ▽
M93.912   Osteochondropathy, unspecified, left shoulder ▽
M93.919   Osteochondropathy, unspecified, unspecified shoulder ▽

✓6ᵗʰ   M93.92   Osteochondropathy, unspecified of upper arm
M93.921   Osteochondropathy, unspecified, right upper arm ▽
M93.922   Osteochondropathy, unspecified, left upper arm ▽
M93.929   Osteochondropathy, unspecified, unspecified upper arm ▽

✓6ᵗʰ   M93.93   Osteochondropathy, unspecified of forearm
M93.931   Osteochondropathy, unspecified, right forearm ▽
M93.932   Osteochondropathy, unspecified, left forearm ▽
M93.939   Osteochondropathy, unspecified, unspecified forearm ▽

✓6ᵗʰ   M93.94   Osteochondropathy, unspecified of hand
M93.941   Osteochondropathy, unspecified, right hand ▽
M93.942   Osteochondropathy, unspecified, left hand ▽
M93.949   Osteochondropathy, unspecified, unspecified hand ▽

✓6ᵗʰ   M93.95   Osteochondropathy, unspecified of thigh
M93.951   Osteochondropathy, unspecified, right thigh ▽
M93.952   Osteochondropathy, unspecified, left thigh ▽
M93.959   Osteochondropathy, unspecified, unspecified thigh ▽

✓6ᵗʰ   M93.96   Osteochondropathy, unspecified lower leg
M93.961   Osteochondropathy, unspecified, right lower leg ▽
M93.962   Osteochondropathy, unspecified, left lower leg ▽
M93.969   Osteochondropathy, unspecified, unspecified lower leg ▽

✓6ᵗʰ   M93.97   Osteochondropathy, unspecified of ankle and foot
M93.971   Osteochondropathy, unspecified, right ankle and foot ▽
M93.972   Osteochondropathy, unspecified, left ankle and foot ▽
M93.979   Osteochondropathy, unspecified, unspecified ankle and foot ▽

M93.98   Osteochondropathy, unspecified other site ▽
M93.99   Osteochondropathy, unspecified multiple sites ▽

☑4ᵗʰ M94 Other disorders of cartilage

M94.0 Chondrocostal junction syndrome [Tietze]
Costochondritis

M94.1 Relapsing polychondritis

☑5ᵗʰ M94.2 Chondromalacia
EXCLUDES 1 chondromalacia patellae (M22.4)

    M94.20 Chondromalacia, unspecified site ▽

    ☑6ᵗʰ M94.21 Chondromalacia, shoulder
        M94.211 Chondromalacia, right shoulder
        M94.212 Chondromalacia, left shoulder
        M94.219 Chondromalacia, unspecified shoulder ▽

    ☑6ᵗʰ M94.22 Chondromalacia, elbow
        M94.221 Chondromalacia, right elbow
        M94.222 Chondromalacia, left elbow
        M94.229 Chondromalacia, unspecified elbow ▽

    ☑6ᵗʰ M94.23 Chondromalacia, wrist
        M94.231 Chondromalacia, right wrist
        M94.232 Chondromalacia, left wrist
        M94.239 Chondromalacia, unspecified wrist ▽

    ☑6ᵗʰ M94.24 Chondromalacia, joints of hand
        M94.241 Chondromalacia, joints of right hand
        M94.242 Chondromalacia, joints of left hand
        M94.249 Chondromalacia, joints of unspecified hand ▽

    ☑6ᵗʰ M94.25 Chondromalacia, hip
        M94.251 Chondromalacia, right hip
        M94.252 Chondromalacia, left hip
        M94.259 Chondromalacia, unspecified hip ▽

    ☑6ᵗʰ M94.26 Chondromalacia, knee
        M94.261 Chondromalacia, right knee
        M94.262 Chondromalacia, left knee
        M94.269 Chondromalacia, unspecified knee ▽

    ☑6ᵗʰ M94.27 Chondromalacia, ankle and joints of foot
        M94.271 Chondromalacia, right ankle and joints of right foot
        M94.272 Chondromalacia, left ankle and joints of left foot
        M94.279 Chondromalacia, unspecified ankle and joints of foot ▽

    M94.28 Chondromalacia, other site

    M94.29 Chondromalacia, multiple sites

☑5ᵗʰ M94.3 Chondrolysis
Code first any associated slipped upper femoral epiphysis (nontraumatic) (M93.0-)

    ☑6ᵗʰ M94.35 Chondrolysis, hip
        M94.351 Chondrolysis, right hip
        M94.352 Chondrolysis, left hip
        M94.359 Chondrolysis, unspecified hip ▽

☑5ᵗʰ M94.8 Other specified disorders of cartilage

    ☑6ᵗʰ M94.8X Other specified disorders of cartilage
        M94.8X0 Other specified disorders of cartilage, multiple sites
        M94.8X1 Other specified disorders of cartilage, shoulder
        M94.8X2 Other specified disorders of cartilage, upper arm
        M94.8X3 Other specified disorders of cartilage, forearm
        M94.8X4 Other specified disorders of cartilage, hand
        M94.8X5 Other specified disorders of cartilage, thigh
        M94.8X6 Other specified disorders of cartilage, lower leg
        M94.8X7 Other specified disorders of cartilage, ankle and foot
        M94.8X8 Other specified disorders of cartilage, other site
        M94.8X9 Other specified disorders of cartilage, unspecified sites ▽

M94.9 Disorder of cartilage, unspecified ▽

Other disorders of the musculoskeletal system and connective tissue (M95)

☑4ᵗʰ M95 Other acquired deformities of musculoskeletal system and connective tissue
EXCLUDES 2 acquired absence of limbs and organs (Z89-Z90)
acquired deformities of limbs (M20-M21)
congenital malformations and deformations of the musculoskeletal system (Q65-Q79)
deforming dorsopathies (M40-M43)
dentofacial anomalies [including malocclusion] (M26.-)
postprocedural musculoskeletal disorders (M96.-)

M95.0 Acquired deformity of nose
EXCLUDES 2 deviated nasal septum (J34.2)

☑5ᵗʰ M95.1 Cauliflower ear
EXCLUDES 2 other acquired deformities of ear (H61.1)

    M95.10 Cauliflower ear, unspecified ear ▽
    M95.11 Cauliflower ear, right ear
    M95.12 Cauliflower ear, left ear

M95.2 Other acquired deformity of head

M95.3 Acquired deformity of neck

M95.4 Acquired deformity of chest and rib
AHA: 2014, 4Q, 26-27

M95.5 Acquired deformity of pelvis
EXCLUDES 1 maternal care for known or suspected disproportion (O33.-)

M95.8 Other specified acquired deformities of musculoskeletal system

M95.9 Acquired deformity of musculoskeletal system, unspecified ▽

Intraoperative and postprocedural complications and disorders of musculoskeletal system, not elsewhere classified (M96)

☑4ᵗʰ M96 Intraoperative and postprocedural complications and disorders of musculoskeletal system, not elsewhere classified
EXCLUDES 2 arthropathy following intestinal bypass (M02.0-)
complications of internal orthopedic prosthetic devices, implants and grafts (T84.-)
disorders associated with osteoporosis (M80)
presence of functional implants and other devices (Z96-Z97)

M96.0 Pseudarthrosis after fusion or arthrodesis

M96.1 Postlaminectomy syndrome, not elsewhere classified ▲

M96.2 Postradiation kyphosis

M96.3 Postlaminectomy kyphosis

M96.4 Postsurgical lordosis

M96.5 Postradiation scoliosis

☑5ᵗʰ M96.6 Fracture of bone following insertion of orthopedic implant, joint prosthesis, or bone plate
Intraoperative fracture of bone during insertion of orthopedic implant, joint prosthesis, or bone plate
EXCLUDES 2 complication of internal orthopedic devices, implants or grafts (T84.-)

    ☑6ᵗʰ M96.62 Fracture of humerus following insertion of orthopedic implant, joint prosthesis, or bone plate
        M96.621 Fracture of humerus following insertion of orthopedic implant, joint prosthesis, or bone plate, right arm
        M96.622 Fracture of humerus following insertion of orthopedic implant, joint prosthesis, or bone plate, left arm
        M96.629 Fracture of humerus following insertion of orthopedic implant, joint prosthesis, or bone plate, unspecified arm ▽

    ☑6ᵗʰ M96.63 Fracture of radius or ulna following insertion of orthopedic implant, joint prosthesis, or bone plate
        M96.631 Fracture of radius or ulna following insertion of orthopedic implant, joint prosthesis, or bone plate, right arm
        M96.632 Fracture of radius or ulna following insertion of orthopedic implant, joint prosthesis, or bone plate, left arm
        M96.639 Fracture of radius or ulna following insertion of orthopedic implant, joint prosthesis, or bone plate, unspecified arm ▽

    M96.65 Fracture of pelvis following insertion of orthopedic implant, joint prosthesis, or bone plate

---

✓6ᵗʰ **M96.66** Fracture of femur following insertion of orthopedic implant, joint prosthesis, or bone plate

    M96.661 Fracture of femur following insertion of orthopedic implant, joint prosthesis, or bone plate, right leg

    M96.662 Fracture of femur following insertion of orthopedic implant, joint prosthesis, or bone plate, left leg

    M96.669 Fracture of femur following insertion of orthopedic implant, joint prosthesis, or bone plate, unspecified leg ▽

✓6ᵗʰ **M96.67** Fracture of tibia or fibula following insertion of orthopedic implant, joint prosthesis, or bone plate

    M96.671 Fracture of tibia or fibula following insertion of orthopedic implant, joint prosthesis, or bone plate, right leg

    M96.672 Fracture of tibia or fibula following insertion of orthopedic implant, joint prosthesis, or bone plate, left leg

    M96.679 Fracture of tibia or fibula following insertion of orthopedic implant, joint prosthesis, or bone plate, unspecified leg ▽

M96.69 Fracture of other bone following insertion of orthopedic implant, joint prosthesis, or bone plate

✓5ᵗʰ **M96.8** Other intraoperative and postprocedural complications and disorders of musculoskeletal system, not elsewhere classified

  ✓6ᵗʰ **M96.81** Intraoperative hemorrhage and hematoma of a musculoskeletal structure complicating a procedure

      EXCLUDES 1   intraoperative hemorrhage and hematoma of a musculoskeletal structure due to accidental puncture and laceration during a procedure (M96.82-)

    M96.810 Intraoperative hemorrhage and hematoma of a musculoskeletal structure complicating a musculoskeletal system procedure

    M96.811 Intraoperative hemorrhage and hematoma of a musculoskeletal structure complicating other procedure

  ✓6ᵗʰ **M96.82** Accidental puncture and laceration of a musculoskeletal structure during a procedure

    M96.820 Accidental puncture and laceration of a musculoskeletal structure during a musculoskeletal system procedure

    M96.821 Accidental puncture and laceration of a musculoskeletal structure during other procedure

  ✓6ᵗʰ **M96.83** Postprocedural hemorrhage and hematoma of a musculoskeletal structure following a procedure

    M96.830 Postprocedural hemorrhage and hematoma of a musculoskeletal structure following a musculoskeletal system procedure

    M96.831 Postprocedural hemorrhage and hematoma of a musculoskeletal structure following other procedure

M96.89 Other intraoperative and postprocedural complications and disorders of the musculoskeletal system

    Instability of joint secondary to removal of joint prosthesis

    Use additional code, if applicable, to further specify disorder

Biomechanical lesions, not elsewhere classified (M99)

✓4ᵗʰ **M99 Biomechanical lesions, not elsewhere classified**

    NOTE   This category should not be used if the condition can be classified elsewhere.

  ✓5ᵗʰ **M99.0** Segmental and somatic dysfunction

    M99.00 Segmental and somatic dysfunction of head region

    M99.01 Segmental and somatic dysfunction of cervical region

    M99.02 Segmental and somatic dysfunction of thoracic region

    M99.03 Segmental and somatic dysfunction of lumbar region

    M99.04 Segmental and somatic dysfunction of sacral region

    M99.05 Segmental and somatic dysfunction of pelvic region

    M99.06 Segmental and somatic dysfunction of lower extremity

    M99.07 Segmental and somatic dysfunction of upper extremity

    M99.08 Segmental and somatic dysfunction of rib cage

    M99.09 Segmental and somatic dysfunction of abdomen and other regions

✓5ᵗʰ **M99.1** Subluxation complex (vertebral)

    M99.10 Subluxation complex (vertebral) of head region

    M99.11 Subluxation complex (vertebral) of cervical region

    M99.12 Subluxation complex (vertebral) of thoracic region

    M99.13 Subluxation complex (vertebral) of lumbar region

    M99.14 Subluxation complex (vertebral) of sacral region

    M99.15 Subluxation complex (vertebral) of pelvic region

    M99.16 Subluxation complex (vertebral) of lower extremity

    M99.17 Subluxation complex (vertebral) of upper extremity

    M99.18 Subluxation complex (vertebral) of rib cage

    M99.19 Subluxation complex (vertebral) of abdomen and other regions

✓5ᵗʰ **M99.2** Subluxation stenosis of neural canal

    M99.20 Subluxation stenosis of neural canal of head region

    M99.21 Subluxation stenosis of neural canal of cervical region

    M99.22 Subluxation stenosis of neural canal of thoracic region 🅰

    M99.23 Subluxation stenosis of neural canal of lumbar region 🅰

    M99.24 Subluxation stenosis of neural canal of sacral region 🅰

    M99.25 Subluxation stenosis of neural canal of pelvic region 🅰

    M99.26 Subluxation stenosis of neural canal of lower extremity 🅰

    M99.27 Subluxation stenosis of neural canal of upper extremity 🅰

    M99.28 Subluxation stenosis of neural canal of rib cage 🅰

    M99.29 Subluxation stenosis of neural canal of abdomen and other regions 🅰

✓5ᵗʰ **M99.3** Osseous stenosis of neural canal

    M99.30 Osseous stenosis of neural canal of head region

    M99.31 Osseous stenosis of neural canal of cervical region

    M99.32 Osseous stenosis of neural canal of thoracic region 🅰

    M99.33 Osseous stenosis of neural canal of lumbar region 🅰

    M99.34 Osseous stenosis of neural canal of sacral region 🅰

    M99.35 Osseous stenosis of neural canal of pelvic region 🅰

    M99.36 Osseous stenosis of neural canal of lower extremity 🅰

    M99.37 Osseous stenosis of neural canal of upper extremity 🅰

    M99.38 Osseous stenosis of neural canal of rib cage 🅰

    M99.39 Osseous stenosis of neural canal of abdomen and other regions 🅰

✓5ᵗʰ **M99.4** Connective tissue stenosis of neural canal

    M99.40 Connective tissue stenosis of neural canal of head region

    M99.41 Connective tissue stenosis of neural canal of cervical region

    M99.42 Connective tissue stenosis of neural canal of thoracic region 🅰

    M99.43 Connective tissue stenosis of neural canal of lumbar region 🅰

    M99.44 Connective tissue stenosis of neural canal of sacral region 🅰

    M99.45 Connective tissue stenosis of neural canal of pelvic region 🅰

    M99.46 Connective tissue stenosis of neural canal of lower extremity 🅰

    M99.47 Connective tissue stenosis of neural canal of upper extremity 🅰

    M99.48 Connective tissue stenosis of neural canal of rib cage 🅰

    M99.49 Connective tissue stenosis of neural canal of abdomen and other regions 🅰

☑ Add'l Character Required   ✓x7ᵗʰ Placeholder Alert   RUG IV Special Care High Dx   RUG IV Clinically Complex Dx   RUG IV Special Care Low Dx   Manifestation Code   Other Specified Code   ▽ Unspecified Code

ICD-10-CM 2016   755

✓5ᵗʰ **M99.5 Intervertebral disc stenosis of neural canal**

    M99.50 Intervertebral disc stenosis of neural canal of head region

    M99.51 Intervertebral disc stenosis of neural canal of cervical region

    M99.52 Intervertebral disc stenosis of neural canal of thoracic region   🅐

    M99.53 Intervertebral disc stenosis of neural canal of lumbar region   🅐

    M99.54 Intervertebral disc stenosis of neural canal of sacral region   🅐

    M99.55 Intervertebral disc stenosis of neural canal of pelvic region   🅐

    M99.56 Intervertebral disc stenosis of neural canal of lower extremity   🅐

    M99.57 Intervertebral disc stenosis of neural canal of upper extremity   🅐

    M99.58 Intervertebral disc stenosis of neural canal of rib cage   🅐

    M99.59 Intervertebral disc stenosis of neural canal of abdomen and other regions   🅐

✓5ᵗʰ **M99.6 Osseous and subluxation stenosis of intervertebral foramina**

    M99.60 Osseous and subluxation stenosis of intervertebral foramina of head region

    M99.61 Osseous and subluxation stenosis of intervertebral foramina of cervical region

    M99.62 Osseous and subluxation stenosis of intervertebral foramina of thoracic region   🅐

    M99.63 Osseous and subluxation stenosis of intervertebral foramina of lumbar region   🅐

    M99.64 Osseous and subluxation stenosis of intervertebral foramina of sacral region   🅐

    M99.65 Osseous and subluxation stenosis of intervertebral foramina of pelvic region   🅐

    M99.66 Osseous and subluxation stenosis of intervertebral foramina of lower extremity   🅐

    M99.67 Osseous and subluxation stenosis of intervertebral foramina of upper extremity   🅐

    M99.68 Osseous and subluxation stenosis of intervertebral foramina of rib cage   🅐

    M99.69 Osseous and subluxation stenosis of intervertebral foramina of abdomen and other regions   🅐

✓5ᵗʰ **M99.7 Connective tissue and disc stenosis of intervertebral foramina**

    M99.70 Connective tissue and disc stenosis of intervertebral foramina of head region

    M99.71 Connective tissue and disc stenosis of intervertebral foramina of cervical region

    M99.72 Connective tissue and disc stenosis of intervertebral foramina of thoracic region   🅐

    M99.73 Connective tissue and disc stenosis of intervertebral foramina of lumbar region   🅐

    M99.74 Connective tissue and disc stenosis of intervertebral foramina of sacral region   🅐

    M99.75 Connective tissue and disc stenosis of intervertebral foramina of pelvic region   🅐

    M99.76 Connective tissue and disc stenosis of intervertebral foramina of lower extremity   🅐

    M99.77 Connective tissue and disc stenosis of intervertebral foramina of upper extremity   🅐

    M99.78 Connective tissue and disc stenosis of intervertebral foramina of rib cage   🅐

    M99.79 Connective tissue and disc stenosis of intervertebral foramina of abdomen and other regions   🅐

✓5ᵗʰ **M99.8 Other biomechanical lesions**

    M99.80 Other biomechanical lesions of head region

    M99.81 Other biomechanical lesions of cervical region

    M99.82 Other biomechanical lesions of thoracic region

    M99.83 Other biomechanical lesions of lumbar region

    M99.84 Other biomechanical lesions of sacral region

    M99.85 Other biomechanical lesions of pelvic region

    M99.86 Other biomechanical lesions of lower extremity

    M99.87 Other biomechanical lesions of upper extremity

    M99.88 Other biomechanical lesions of rib cage

    M99.89 Other biomechanical lesions of abdomen and other regions

  M99.9 Biomechanical lesion, unspecified   ▽

Ⓝ Newborn   Ⓟ Pediatric   Ⓜ Maternity   🅐 Adult   **RIC** RIC Dx   **NC Dx** Noncancer Dx   **PDx** Primary Dx   **CC** RIC CC Condition   ▶◀ Revised Text   ● New Code   ▲ Revised Code Title

756   ICD-10-CM 2016

Chapter 14. Diseases of Genitourinary System (NØØ–N99)

Chapter Specific Guidelines with Coding Examples

The chapter specific guidelines from the ICD-10-CM Official Guidelines for Coding and Reporting have been provided below. Along with these guidelines are coding examples, contained in the shaded boxes, that have been developed to help illustrate the coding and/or sequencing guidance found in these guidelines.

a. Chronic kidney disease

1) Stages of chronic kidney disease (CKD)

The ICD-10-CM classifies CKD based on severity. The severity of CKD is designated by stages 1-5. Stage 2, code N18.2, equates to mild CKD; stage 3, code N18.3, equates to moderate CKD; and stage 4, code N18.4, equates to severe CKD. Code N18.6, End stage renal disease (ESRD), is assigned when the provider has documented end-stage-renal disease (ESRD).

If both a stage of CKD and ESRD are documented, assign code N18.6 only.

> Stage 5 chronic kidney disease with ESRD requiring chronic dialysis
>
> **N18.6**   **End stage renal disease**
>
> **Z99.2**   **Dependence on renal dialysis**
>
> *Explanation:* The diagnostic statement indicates the patient has chronic kidney disease, documented both as stage 5 and as ESRD requiring chronic dialysis. Code N18.6 End stage renal disease (ESRD), is assigned when the provider has documented end-stage-renal disease (ESRD). If both a stage of CKD and ESRD are documented, assign code N18.6 only.

2) Chronic kidney disease and kidney transplant status

Patients who have undergone kidney transplant may still have some form of chronic kidney disease (CKD) because the kidney transplant may not fully restore kidney function. Therefore, the presence of CKD alone does not constitute a transplant complication. Assign the appropriate N18 code for the patient's stage of CKD and code Z94.Ø, Kidney transplant status. If a transplant complication such as failure or rejection or other transplant complication is documented, see section I.C.19.g for information on coding complications of a kidney transplant. If the documentation is unclear as to whether the patient has a complication of the transplant, query the provider.

> Patient with residual chronic kidney disease stage 1 after kidney transplant
>
> **N18.1**   **Chronic kidney disease, stage 1**
>
> **Z94.Ø**   **Kidney transplant status**
>
> *Explanation:* Patients who have undergone kidney transplant may still have some form of chronic kidney disease (CKD) because the kidney transplant may not fully restore kidney function. The presence of CKD alone does not constitute a transplant complication. Assign the appropriate N18 code for the patient's stage of CKD and code Z94.Ø Kidney transplant status.

3) Chronic kidney disease with other conditions

Patients with CKD may also suffer from other serious conditions, most commonly diabetes mellitus and hypertension. The sequencing of the CKD code in relationship to codes for other contributing conditions is based on the conventions in the Tabular List.

See I.C.9. Hypertensive chronic kidney disease.

See I.C.19. Chronic kidney disease and kidney transplant complications.

> Type 1 diabetic chronic kidney disease, stage 2
>
> **E10.22**   **Type 1 diabetes mellitus with diabetic chronic kidney disease**
>
> **N18.2**   **Chronic kidney disease, stage 2 (mild)**
>
> *Explanation:* Patients with CKD may also suffer from other serious conditions such as diabetes mellitus. The sequencing of the CKD code in relationship to codes for other contributing conditions is based on the conventions in the Tabular List. Diabetic CKD code E10.22 includes an instructional note to "Use additional code to identify stage of chronic kidney disease (N18.1–N18.6)," thus providing sequencing direction.

Chapter 14. Diseases of the Genitourinary System (N00-N99)

EXCLUDES 2
certain conditions originating in the perinatal period (P04-P96)
certain infectious and parasitic diseases (A00-B99)
complications of pregnancy, childbirth and the puerperium (O00-O9A)
congenital malformations, deformations and chromosomal abnormalities (Q00-Q99)
endocrine, nutritional and metabolic diseases (E00-E88)
injury, poisoning and certain other consequences of external causes (S00-T88)
neoplasms (C00-D49)
symptoms, signs and abnormal clinical and laboratory findings, not elsewhere classified (R00-R94)

This chapter contains the following blocks:

N00-N08	Glomerular diseases
N10-N16	Renal tubulo-interstitial diseases
N17-N19	Acute kidney failure and chronic kidney disease
N20-N23	Urolithiasis
N25-N29	Other disorders of kidney and ureter
N30-N39	Other diseases of the urinary system
N40-N53	Diseases of male genital organs
N60-N65	Disorders of breast
N70-N77	Inflammatory diseases of female pelvic organs
N80-N98	Noninflammatory disorders of female genital tract
N99	Intraoperative and postprocedural complications and disorders of genitourinary system, not elsewhere classified

Glomerular diseases (N00-N08)

Code also any associated kidney failure (N17-N19).
EXCLUDES 1   hypertensive chronic kidney disease (I12.-)

✓4th **N00**   Acute nephritic syndrome
   INCLUDES   acute glomerular disease
     acute glomerulonephritis
     acute nephritis
   EXCLUDES 1   acute tubulo-interstitial nephritis (N10)
     nephritic syndrome NOS (N05.-)

   N00.0   **Acute nephritic syndrome with** minor glomerular abnormality   CC
     Acute nephritic syndrome with minimal change lesion

   N00.1   **Acute nephritic syndrome with** focal and segmental glomerular lesions   CC
     Acute nephritic syndrome with focal and segmental hyalinosis
     Acute nephritic syndrome with focal and segmental sclerosis
     Acute nephritic syndrome with focal glomerulonephritis

   N00.2   **Acute nephritic syndrome with** diffuse membranous glomerulonephritis   CC

   N00.3   **Acute nephritic syndrome with** diffuse mesangial proliferative glomerulonephritis   CC

   N00.4   **Acute nephritic syndrome with** diffuse endocapillary proliferative glomerulonephritis   CC

   N00.5   **Acute nephritic syndrome with** diffuse mesangiocapillary glomerulonephritis   CC
     Acute nephritic syndrome with membranoproliferative glomerulonephritis, types 1 and 3, or NOS

   N00.6   **Acute nephritic syndrome with** dense deposit disease   CC
     Acute nephritic syndrome with membranoproliferative glomerulonephritis, type 2

   N00.7   **Acute nephritic syndrome with** diffuse crescentic glomerulonephritis   CC
     Acute nephritic syndrome with extracapillary glomerulonephritis

   N00.8   **Acute nephritic syndrome with other morphologic changes**   CC
     Acute nephritic syndrome with proliferative glomerulonephritis NOS

   N00.9   **Acute nephritic syndrome with unspecified morphologic changes**   CC ▽

✓4th **N01**   Rapidly progressive nephritic syndrome
   INCLUDES   rapidly progressive glomerular disease
     rapidly progressive glomerulonephritis
     rapidly progressive nephritis
   EXCLUDES 1   nephritic syndrome NOS (N05.-)

   N01.0   **Rapidly progressive nephritic syndrome with** minor glomerular abnormality   CC
     Rapidly progressive nephritic syndrome with minimal change lesion

   N01.1   **Rapidly progressive nephritic syndrome with** focal and segmental glomerular lesions   CC
     Rapidly progressive nephritic syndrome with focal and segmental hyalinosis
     Rapidly progressive nephritic syndrome with focal and segmental sclerosis
     Rapidly progressive nephritic syndrome with focal glomerulonephritis

   N01.2   **Rapidly progressive nephritic syndrome with** diffuse membranous glomerulonephritis   CC

   N01.3   **Rapidly progressive nephritic syndrome with** diffuse mesangial proliferative glomerulonephritis   CC

   N01.4   **Rapidly progressive nephritic syndrome with** diffuse endocapillary proliferative glomerulonephritis   CC

   N01.5   **Rapidly progressive nephritic syndrome with** diffuse mesangiocapillary glomerulonephritis   CC
     Rapidly progressive nephritic syndrome with membranoproliferative glomerulonephritis, types 1 and 3, or NOS

   N01.6   **Rapidly progressive nephritic syndrome with** dense deposit disease   CC
     Rapidly progressive nephritic syndrome with membranoproliferative glomerulonephritis, type 2

   N01.7   **Rapidly progressive nephritic syndrome with** diffuse crescentic glomerulonephritis   CC
     Rapidly progressive nephritic syndrome with extracapillary glomerulonephritis

   N01.8   **Rapidly progressive nephritic syndrome with other morphologic changes**   CC
     Rapidly progressive nephritic syndrome with proliferative glomerulonephritis NOS

   N01.9   **Rapidly progressive nephritic syndrome with unspecified morphologic changes**   CC ▽

✓4th **N02**   Recurrent and persistent hematuria
   EXCLUDES 1   acute cystitis with hematuria (N30.01)
     hematuria NOS (R31.9)
     hematuria not associated with specified morphologic lesions (R31.-)

   N02.0   **Recurrent and persistent hematuria with** minor glomerular abnormality
     Recurrent and persistent hematuria with minimal change lesion

   N02.1   **Recurrent and persistent hematuria with** focal and segmental glomerular lesions
     Recurrent and persistent hematuria with focal and segmental hyalinosis
     Recurrent and persistent hematuria with focal and segmental sclerosis
     Recurrent and persistent hematuria with focal glomerulonephritis

   N02.2   **Recurrent and persistent hematuria with** diffuse membranous glomerulonephritis

   N02.3   **Recurrent and persistent hematuria with** diffuse mesangial proliferative glomerulonephritis

   N02.4   **Recurrent and persistent hematuria with** diffuse endocapillary proliferative glomerulonephritis

   N02.5   **Recurrent and persistent hematuria with** diffuse mesangiocapillary glomerulonephritis
     Recurrent and persistent hematuria with membranoproliferative glomerulonephritis, types 1 and 3, or NOS

   N02.6   **Recurrent and persistent hematuria with** dense deposit disease
     Recurrent and persistent hematuria with membranoproliferative glomerulonephritis, type 2

   N02.7   **Recurrent and persistent hematuria with** diffuse crescentic glomerulonephritis
     Recurrent and persistent hematuria with extracapillary glomerulonephritis

   N02.8   **Recurrent and persistent hematuria with other morphologic changes**
     Recurrent and persistent hematuria with proliferative glomerulonephritis NOS

   N02.9   **Recurrent and persistent hematuria with unspecified morphologic changes**   ▽

Ⓝ Newborn   Ⓟ Pediatric   Ⓜ Maternity   Ⓐ Adult   RIC RIC Dx   NCDx Noncancer Dx   PDx Primary Dx   CC RIC CC Condition   ▶◀ Revised Text   ● New Code   ▲ Revised Code Title

758   ICD-10-CM 2016

✓4ᵗʰ **N03** **Chronic** nephritic syndrome
> INCLUDES   chronic glomerular disease
> chronic glomerulonephritis
> chronic nephritis
>
> EXCLUDES 1   *chronic tubulo-interstitial nephritis (N11.-)*
> *diffuse sclerosing glomerulonephritis (N05.8-)*
> *nephritic syndrome NOS (N05.-)*

N03.0 **Chronic** nephritic syndrome with minor glomerular abnormality
> Chronic nephritic syndrome with minimal change lesion

N03.1 **Chronic** nephritic syndrome with focal and segmental glomerular lesions
> Chronic nephritic syndrome with focal and segmental hyalinosis
> Chronic nephritic syndrome with focal and segmental sclerosis
> Chronic nephritic syndrome with focal glomerulonephritis

N03.2 **Chronic** nephritic syndrome with diffuse membranous glomerulonephritis

N03.3 **Chronic** nephritic syndrome with diffuse mesangial proliferative glomerulonephritis

N03.4 **Chronic** nephritic syndrome with diffuse endocapillary proliferative glomerulonephritis

N03.5 **Chronic** nephritic syndrome with diffuse mesangiocapillary glomerulonephritis
> Chronic nephritic syndrome with membranoproliferative glomerulonephritis, types 1 and 3, or NOS

N03.6 **Chronic** nephritic syndrome with dense deposit disease
> Chronic nephritic syndrome with membranoproliferative glomerulonephritis, type 2

N03.7 **Chronic** nephritic syndrome with diffuse crescentic glomerulonephritis
> Chronic nephritic syndrome with extracapillary glomerulonephritis

N03.8 **Chronic nephritic syndrome with other morphologic changes**
> Chronic nephritic syndrome with proliferative glomerulonephritis NOS

N03.9 **Chronic** nephritic syndrome with unspecified morphologic changes   ▽

✓4ᵗʰ **N04** **Nephrotic syndrome**
> INCLUDES   congenital nephrotic syndrome
> lipoid nephrosis

N04.0 **Nephrotic syndrome with** minor glomerular abnormality
> Nephrotic syndrome with minimal change lesion

N04.1 **Nephrotic syndrome with** focal and segmental glomerular lesions
> Nephrotic syndrome with focal and segmental hyalinosis
> Nephrotic syndrome with focal and segmental sclerosis
> Nephrotic syndrome with focal glomerulonephritis

N04.2 **Nephrotic syndrome with** diffuse membranous glomerulonephritis

N04.3 **Nephrotic syndrome with** diffuse mesangial proliferative glomerulonephritis

N04.4 **Nephrotic syndrome with** diffuse endocapillary proliferative glomerulonephritis

N04.5 **Nephrotic syndrome with** diffuse mesangiocapillary glomerulonephritis
> Nephrotic syndrome with membranoproliferative glomerulonephritis, types 1 and 3, or NOS

N04.6 **Nephrotic syndrome with** dense deposit disease
> Nephrotic syndrome with membranoproliferative glomerulonephritis, type 2

N04.7 **Nephrotic syndrome with** diffuse crescentic glomerulonephritis
> Nephrotic syndrome with extracapillary glomerulonephritis

N04.8 **Nephrotic syndrome with other morphologic changes**
> Nephrotic syndrome with proliferative glomerulonephritis NOS

N04.9 **Nephrotic syndrome with** unspecified morphologic changes   ▽

✓4ᵗʰ **N05** **Unspecified** nephritic syndrome
> INCLUDES   glomerular disease NOS
> glomerulonephritis NOS
> nephritis NOS
> nephropathy NOS and renal disease NOS with morphological lesion specified in .0-.8
>
> EXCLUDES 1   *nephropathy NOS with no stated morphological lesion (N28.9)*
> *renal disease NOS with no stated morphological lesion (N28.9)*
> *tubulo-interstitial nephritis NOS (N12)*

N05.0 **Unspecified** nephritic syndrome with minor glomerular   ▽
abnormality
> Unspecified nephritic syndrome with minimal change lesion

N05.1 **Unspecified** nephritic syndrome with focal and   ▽
segmental glomerular lesions
> Unspecified nephritic syndrome with focal and segmental hyalinosis
> Unspecified nephritic syndrome with focal and segmental sclerosis
> Unspecified nephritic syndrome with focal glomerulonephritis

N05.2 **Unspecified** nephritic syndrome with diffuse   ▽
membranous glomerulonephritis

N05.3 **Unspecified** nephritic syndrome with diffuse   ▽
mesangial proliferative glomerulonephritis

N05.4 **Unspecified** nephritic syndrome with diffuse   ▽
endocapillary proliferative glomerulonephritis

N05.5 **Unspecified** nephritic syndrome with diffuse   ▽
mesangiocapillary glomerulonephritis
> Unspecified nephritic syndrome with membranoproliferative glomerulonephritis, types 1 and 3, or NOS

N05.6 **Unspecified** nephritic syndrome with dense deposit   ▽
disease
> Unspecified nephritic syndrome with membranoproliferative glomerulonephritis, type 2

N05.7 **Unspecified** nephritic syndrome with diffuse   ▽
crescentic glomerulonephritis
> Unspecified nephritic syndrome with extracapillary glomerulonephritis

N05.8 **Unspecified nephritic syndrome with other morphologic**   ▽
changes
> Unspecified nephritic syndrome with proliferative glomerulonephritis NOS

N05.9 **Unspecified** nephritic syndrome with unspecified   CC ▽
morphologic changes

✓4ᵗʰ **N06** **Isolated proteinuria with specified morphological lesion**
> EXCLUDES 1   *proteinuria not associated with specific morphologic lesions (R80.0)*

N06.0 **Isolated proteinuria with** minor glomerular abnormality
> Isolated proteinuria with minimal change lesion

N06.1 **Isolated proteinuria with** focal and segmental glomerular lesions
> Isolated proteinuria with focal and segmental hyalinosis
> Isolated proteinuria with focal and segmental sclerosis
> Isolated proteinuria with focal glomerulonephritis

N06.2 **Isolated proteinuria with** diffuse membranous glomerulonephritis

N06.3 **Isolated proteinuria with** diffuse mesangial proliferative glomerulonephritis

N06.4 **Isolated proteinuria with** diffuse endocapillary proliferative glomerulonephritis

N06.5 **Isolated proteinuria with** diffuse mesangiocapillary glomerulonephritis
> Isolated proteinuria with membranoproliferative glomerulonephritis, types 1 and 3, or NOS

N06.6 **Isolated proteinuria with** dense deposit disease
> Isolated proteinuria with membranoproliferative glomerulonephritis, type 2

N06.7 **Isolated proteinuria with** diffuse crescentic glomerulonephritis
> Isolated proteinuria with extracapillary glomerulonephritis

N06.8 **Isolated proteinuria with other morphologic lesion**
> Isolated proteinuria with proliferative glomerulonephritis NOS

N06.9 **Isolated proteinuria with** unspecified morphologic   ▽
lesion

✓4ᵗʰ **N07** **Hereditary nephropathy, not elsewhere classified**
> EXCLUDES 2   *Alport's syndrome (Q87.81-)*
> *hereditary amyloid nephropathy (E85.-)*
> *nail patella syndrome (Q87.2)*
> *non-neuropathic heredofamilial amyloidosis (E85.-)*

N07.0 **Hereditary nephropathy, not elsewhere classified with** minor glomerular abnormality
> Hereditary nephropathy, not elsewhere classified with minimal change lesion

N07.1 **Hereditary nephropathy, not elsewhere classified with** focal and segmental glomerular lesions
> Hereditary nephropathy, not elsewhere classified with focal and segmental hyalinosis
> Hereditary nephropathy, not elsewhere classified with focal and segmental sclerosis
> Hereditary nephropathy, not elsewhere classified with focal glomerulonephritis

N07.2 **Hereditary nephropathy, not elsewhere classified with** diffuse membranous glomerulonephritis

☑ Add'l Character Required   ✓7ᵗʰ Placeholder Alert   RUG IV Special Care High Dx   RUG IV Clinically Complex Dx   RUG IV Special Care Low Dx   Manifestation Code   Other Specified Code   ▽ Unspecified Code

ICD-10-CM 2016   759

NØ7.3 Hereditary nephropathy, not elsewhere classified with diffuse mesangial proliferative glomerulonephritis

NØ7.4 Hereditary nephropathy, not elsewhere classified with diffuse endocapillary proliferative glomerulonephritis

NØ7.5 Hereditary nephropathy, not elsewhere classified with diffuse mesangiocapillary glomerulonephritis
Hereditary nephropathy, not elsewhere classified with membranoproliferative glomerulonephritis, types 1 and 3, or NOS

NØ7.6 Hereditary nephropathy, not elsewhere classified with dense deposit disease
Hereditary nephropathy, not elsewhere classified with membranoproliferative glomerulonephritis, type 2

NØ7.7 Hereditary nephropathy, not elsewhere classified with diffuse crescentic glomerulonephritis
Hereditary nephropathy, not elsewhere classified with extracapillary glomerulonephritis

NØ7.8 Hereditary nephropathy, not elsewhere classified with other morphologic lesions
Hereditary nephropathy, not elsewhere classified with proliferative glomerulonephritis NOS

NØ7.9 Hereditary nephropathy, not elsewhere classified with unspecified morphologic lesions ▽

NØ8 Glomerular disorders in diseases classified elsewhere cc
Glomerulonephritis
Nephritis
Nephropathy
Code first underlying disease, such as:
amyloidosis (E85.-)
congenital syphilis (A50.5)
cryoglobulinemia (D89.1)
disseminated intravascular coagulation (D65)
gout (M1A.-, M10.-)
microscopic polyangiitis (M31.7)
multiple myeloma (C90.0-)
sepsis (A40.0-A41.9)
sickle-cell disease (D57.0-D57.8)
EXCLUDES 1 *glomerulonephritis, nephritis and nephropathy (in):*
antiglomerular basement membrane disease (M31.0)
diabetes (E08-E13 with .21)
gonococcal (A54.21)
Goodpasture's syndrome (M31.0)
hemolytic-uremic syndrome (D59.3)
lupus (M32.14)
mumps (B26.83)
syphilis (A52.75)
systemic lupus erythematosus (M32.14)
Wegener's granulomatosis (M31.31)
pyelonephritis in diseases classified elsewhere (N16)
renal tubulo-interstitial disorders classified elsewhere (N16)

Renal tubulo-interstitial diseases (N10-N16)

INCLUDES *pyelonephritis*
EXCLUDES 1 *pyeloureteritis cystica (N28.85)*

N10 Acute tubulo-interstitial nephritis
Acute infectious interstitial nephritis
Acute pyelitis
Acute pyelonephritis
Hemoglobin nephrosis
Myoglobin nephrosis
Use additional code (B95-B97), to identify infectious agent

☑4th N11 Chronic tubulo-interstitial nephritis
INCLUDES chronic infectious interstitial nephritis
chronic pyelitis
chronic pyelonephritis
Use additional code (B95-B97), to identify infectious agent

N11.0 Nonobstructive reflux-associated chronic pyelonephritis
Pyelonephritis (chronic) associated with (vesicoureteral) reflux
EXCLUDES 1 *vesicoureteral reflux NOS (N13.70)*

N11.1 Chronic obstructive pyelonephritis
Pyelonephritis (chronic) associated with anomaly of pelviureteric junction
Pyelonephritis (chronic) associated with anomaly of pyeloureteric junction
Pyelonephritis (chronic) associated with crossing of vessel
Pyelonephritis (chronic) associated with kinking of ureter
Pyelonephritis (chronic) associated with obstruction of ureter
Pyelonephritis (chronic) associated with stricture of pelviureteric junction
Pyelonephritis (chronic) associated with stricture of ureter
EXCLUDES 1 *calculus pyelonephritis (N20.9)*
obstructive uropathy (N13.-)

N11.8 Other chronic tubulo-interstitial nephritis
Nonobstructive chronic pyelonephritis NOS

N11.9 Chronic tubulo-interstitial nephritis, unspecified ▽
Chronic interstitial nephritis NOS
Chronic pyelitis NOS
Chronic pyelonephritis NOS

N12 Tubulo-interstitial nephritis, not specified as acute or chronic
Interstitial nephritis NOS
Pyelitis NOS
Pyelonephritis NOS
EXCLUDES 1 *calculous pyelonephritis (N20.9)*

☑4th N13 Obstructive and reflux uropathy
EXCLUDES 2 *calculus of kidney and ureter without hydronephrosis (N20.-)*
congenital obstructive defects of renal pelvis and ureter (Q62.0-Q62.3)
hydronephrosis with ureteropelvic junction obstruction (Q62.1)
obstructive pyelonephritis (N11.1)

N13.1 Hydronephrosis with ureteral stricture, not elsewhere classified
EXCLUDES 1 *hydronephrosis with ureteral stricture with infection (N13.6)*

N13.2 Hydronephrosis with renal and ureteral calculous obstruction
EXCLUDES 1 *hydronephrosis with renal and ureteral calculous obstruction with infection (N13.6)*

☑5th N13.3 Other and unspecified hydronephrosis
EXCLUDES 1 *hydronephrosis with infection (N13.6)*

N13.30 Unspecified hydronephrosis ▽

N13.39 Other hydronephrosis

N13.4 Hydroureter
EXCLUDES 1 *congenital hydroureter (Q62.3-)*
hydroureter with infection (N13.6)
vesicoureteral-reflux with hydroureter (N13.73-)

N13.5 Crossing vessel and stricture of ureter without hydronephrosis
Kinking and stricture of ureter without hydronephrosis
EXCLUDES 1 *crossing vessel and stricture of ureter without hydronephrosis with infection (N13.6)*

N13.6 Pyonephrosis
Conditions in N13.1-N13.5 with infection
Obstructive uropathy with infection
Use additional code (B95-B97), to identify infectious agent

☑5th N13.7 Vesicoureteral-reflux
EXCLUDES 1 *reflux-associated pyelonephritis (N11.0)*

N13.70 Vesicoureteral-reflux, unspecified ▽
Vesicoureteral-reflux NOS

N13.71 Vesicoureteral-reflux without reflux nephropathy

☑6th N13.72 Vesicoureteral-reflux with reflux nephropathy without hydroureter

N13.721 Vesicoureteral-reflux with reflux nephropathy without hydroureter, unilateral

N13.722 Vesicoureteral-reflux with reflux nephropathy without hydroureter, bilateral

N13.729 Vesicoureteral-reflux with reflux nephropathy without hydroureter, unspecified ▽

☑6th N13.73 Vesicoureteral-reflux with reflux nephropathy with hydroureter

N13.731 Vesicoureteral-reflux with reflux nephropathy with hydroureter, unilateral

N13.732 Vesicoureteral-reflux with reflux nephropathy with hydroureter, bilateral

N13.739 Vesicoureteral-reflux with reflux nephropathy with hydroureter, unspecified ▽

N13.8 Other obstructive and reflux uropathy
Urinary tract obstruction due to specified cause
Code first, if applicable, any causal condition, such as:
enlarged prostate (N40.1)

N13.9 Obstructive and reflux uropathy, unspecified ▽
Urinary tract obstruction NOS

N Newborn P Pediatric M Maternity A Adult RIC RIC Dx NCDx Noncancer Dx PDx Primary Dx CC RIC CC Condition ►◄ Revised Text ● New Code ▲ Revised Code Title

760 ICD-10-CM 2016

✓4ᵗʰ **N14 Drug- and heavy-metal-induced tubulo-interstitial and tubular conditions**

Code first poisoning due to drug or toxin, if applicable (T36-T65 with fifth or sixth character 1-4 or 6)

Use additional code for adverse effect, if applicable, to identify drug (T36-T5Ø with fifth or sixth character 5)

N14.Ø Analgesic nephropathy

N14.1 Nephropathy induced by other drugs, medicaments and biological substances

N14.2 Nephropathy induced by unspecified drug, medicament or biological substance ▽

N14.3 Nephropathy induced by heavy metals

N14.4 Toxic nephropathy, not elsewhere classified

✓4ᵗʰ **N15 Other renal tubulo-interstitial diseases**

N15.Ø Balkan nephropathy
Balkan endemic nephropathy

N15.1 Renal and perinephric abscess CC

N15.8 Other specified renal tubulo-interstitial diseases

N15.9 Renal tubulo-interstitial disease, unspecified ▽
Infection of kidney NOS
EXCLUDES 1 *urinary tract infection NOS (N39.Ø)*

N16 Renal tubulo-interstitial disorders in diseases classified elsewhere
Pyelonephritis
Tubulo-interstitial nephritis
Code first underlying disease, such as:
brucellosis (A23.Ø-A23.9)
cryoglobulinemia (D89.1)
glycogen storage disease (E74.Ø)
leukemia (C91-C95)
lymphoma (C81.Ø-C85.9, C96.Ø-C96.9)
multiple myeloma (C9Ø.Ø-)
sepsis (A4Ø.Ø-A41.9)
Wilson's disease (E83.Ø)
EXCLUDES 1 *diphtheritic pyelonephritis and tubulo-interstitial nephritis (A36.84)*
pyelonephritis and tubulo-interstitial nephritis in candidiasis (B37.49)
pyelonephritis and tubulo-interstitial nephritis in cystinosis (E72.Ø4)
pyelonephritis and tubulo-interstitial nephritis in salmonella infection (AØ2.25)
pyelonephritis and tubulo-interstitial nephritis in sarcoidosis (D86.84)
pyelonephritis and tubulo-interstitial nephritis in sicca syndrome [Sjogren's] (M35.Ø4)
pyelonephritis and tubulo-interstitial nephritis in systemic lupus erythematosus (M32.15)
pyelonephritis and tubulo-interstitial nephritis in toxoplasmosis (B58.83)
renal tubular degeneration in diabetes (EØ8-E13 with .29)
syphilitic pyelonephritis and tubulo-interstitial nephritis (A52.75)

Acute kidney failure and chronic kidney disease (N17-N19)

EXCLUDES 2 *congenital renal failure (P96.Ø)*
drug- and heavy-metal-induced tubulo-interstitial and tubular conditions (N14.-)
extrarenal uremia (R39.2)
hemolytic-uremic syndrome (D59.3)
hepatorenal syndrome (K76.7)
postpartum hepatorenal syndrome (O9Ø.4)
posttraumatic renal failure (T79.5)
prerenal uremia (R39.2)
renal failure complicating abortion or ectopic or molar pregnancy (OØØ-OØ7, OØ8.4)
renal failure following labor and delivery (O9Ø.4)
renal failure postprocedural (N99.Ø)

✓4ᵗʰ **N17 Acute kidney failure**
Code also associated underlying condition
EXCLUDES 1 *posttraumatic renal failure (T79.5)*
AHA: 2013, 4Q, 124

N17.Ø Acute kidney failure with tubular necrosis CC NC Dx
Acute tubular necrosis
Renal tubular necrosis
Tubular necrosis NOS

N17.1 Acute kidney failure with acute cortical necrosis CC NC Dx
Acute cortical necrosis
Cortical necrosis NOS
Renal cortical necrosis

N17.2 Acute kidney failure with medullary necrosis CC NC Dx
Medullary [papillary] necrosis NOS
Acute medullary [papillary] necrosis
Renal medullary [papillary] necrosis

N17.8 Other acute kidney failure CC NC Dx

N17.9 Acute kidney failure, unspecified CC NC Dx ▽
Acute kidney injury (nontraumatic)
EXCLUDES 2 *traumatic kidney injury (S37.Ø-)*

✓4ᵗʰ **N18 Chronic kidney disease (CKD)**
Code first any associated:
diabetic chronic kidney disease (EØ8.22, EØ9.22, E1Ø.22, E11.22, E13.22)
hypertensive chronic kidney disease (I12-, I13-)
Use additional code to identify kidney transplant status, if applicable, (Z94.Ø)
AHA: 2013, 1Q, 24

N18.1 Chronic kidney disease, stage 1

N18.2 Chronic kidney disease, stage 2 (mild)

N18.3 Chronic kidney disease, stage 3 (moderate)

N18.4 Chronic kidney disease, stage 4 (severe)

N18.5 Chronic kidney disease, stage 5 NC Dx
EXCLUDES 1 *chronic kidney disease, stage 5 requiring chronic dialysis (N18.6)*

N18.6 End stage renal disease NC Dx
Chronic kidney disease requiring chronic dialysis
Use additional code to identify dialysis status (Z99.2)
AHA: 2013, 4Q, 124-125

N18.9 Chronic kidney disease, unspecified NC Dx ▽
Chronic renal disease
Chronic renal failure NOS
Chronic renal insufficiency
Chronic uremia

[10] **N19 Unspecified kidney failure** ▽
Uremia NOS
EXCLUDES 1 *acute kidney failure (N17.-)*
chronic kidney disease (N18.-)
chronic uremia (N18.9)
extrarenal uremia (R39.2)
prerenal uremia (R39.2)
renal insufficiency (acute) (N28.9)
uremia of newborn (P96.Ø)

Urolithiasis (N2Ø-N23)

✓4ᵗʰ **N2Ø Calculus of kidney and ureter**
Calculous pyelonephritis
EXCLUDES 1 *nephrocalcinosis (E83.5)*
that with hydronephrosis (N13.2)

N2Ø.Ø Calculus of kidney
Nephrolithiasis NOS
Renal calculus
Renal stone
Staghorn calculus
Stone in kidney

N2Ø.1 Calculus of ureter
Ureteric stone

N2Ø.2 Calculus of kidney with calculus of ureter

N2Ø.9 Urinary calculus, unspecified ▽

✓4ᵗʰ **N21 Calculus of lower urinary tract**
Calculus of lower urinary tract with cystitis and urethritis

N21.Ø Calculus in bladder
Calculus in diverticulum of bladder
Urinary bladder stone
EXCLUDES 2 *staghorn calculus (N2Ø.Ø)*

N21.1 Calculus in urethra
EXCLUDES 2 *calculus of prostate (N42.Ø)*

N21.8 Other lower urinary tract calculus

N21.9 Calculus of lower urinary tract, unspecified ▽
EXCLUDES 1 *calculus of urinary tract NOS (N2Ø.9)*

N22 Calculus of urinary tract in diseases classified elsewhere
Code first underlying disease, such as:
gout (M1A.-, M1Ø.-)
schistosomiasis (B65.Ø-B65.9)

N23 Unspecified renal colic ▽

───────────
[10] Hospice questionable admission diagnosis

✓ Add'l Character Required ✓x7ᵗʰ Placeholder Alert RUG IV Special Care High Dx   RUG IV Clinically Complex Dx   RUG IV Special Care Low Dx   Manifestation Code   Other Specified Code ▽Unspecified Code

Other disorders of kidney and ureter (N25-N29)

EXCLUDES 2   *disorders of kidney and ureter with urolithiasis (N20-N23)*

✓4ᵗʰ N25   Disorders resulting from impaired renal tubular function
EXCLUDES 1   *metabolic disorders classifiable to E70-E88*

N25.0   Renal osteodystrophy
Azotemic osteodystrophy
Phosphate-losing tubular disorders
Renal rickets
Renal short stature

N25.1   Nephrogenic diabetes insipidus
EXCLUDES 1   *diabetes insipidus NOS (E23.2)*

✓5ᵗʰ N25.8   Other disorders resulting from impaired renal tubular function

N25.81   Secondary hyperparathyroidism of renal origin
EXCLUDES 1   *secondary hyperparathyroidism, non-renal (E21.1)*

N25.89   Other disorders resulting from impaired renal tubular function
Hypokalemic nephropathy
Lightwood-Albright syndrome
Renal tubular acidosis NOS

N25.9   Disorder resulting from impaired renal tubular function, unspecified ▽

✓4ᵗʰ N26   Unspecified contracted kidney
EXCLUDES 1   *contracted kidney due to hypertension (I12.-)*
diffuse sclerosing glomerulonephritis (N05.8-)
hypertensive nephrosclerosis (arteriolar) (arteriosclerotic) (I12.-)
small kidney of unknown cause (N27.-)

N26.1   Atrophy of kidney (terminal)

N26.2   Page kidney

N26.9   Renal sclerosis, unspecified ▽

✓4ᵗʰ N27   Small kidney of unknown cause
INCLUDES   oligonephronia

N27.0   Small kidney, unilateral

N27.1   Small kidney, bilateral

N27.9   Small kidney, unspecified ▽

✓4ᵗʰ N28   Other disorders of kidney and ureter, not elsewhere classified

N28.0   Ischemia and infarction of kidney
Renal artery embolism   Renal artery thrombosis
Renal artery obstruction   Renal infarct
Renal artery occlusion
EXCLUDES 1   *atherosclerosis of renal artery (extrarenal part) (I70.1)*
congenital stenosis of renal artery (Q27.1)
Goldblatt's kidney (I70.1)

N28.1   Cyst of kidney, acquired
Cyst (multiple)(solitary) of kidney, acquired
EXCLUDES 1   *cystic kidney disease (congenital) (Q61.-)*

✓5ᵗʰ N28.8   Other specified disorders of kidney and ureter
EXCLUDES 1   *hydroureter (N13.4)*
ureteric stricture with hydronephrosis (N13.1)
ureteric stricture without hydronephrosis (N13.5)

N28.81   Hypertrophy of kidney
N28.82   Megaloureter
N28.83   Nephroptosis
N28.84   Pyelitis cystica
N28.85   Pyeloureteritis cystica
N28.86   Ureteritis cystica
N28.89   Other specified disorders of kidney and ureter

N28.9   Disorder of kidney and ureter, unspecified ▽
Nephropathy NOS
Renal disease (acute) NOS
Renal insufficiency (acute)
EXCLUDES 1   *chronic renal insufficiency (N18.9)*
unspecified nephritic syndrome (N05.-)

N29   Other disorders of kidney and ureter in diseases classified elsewhere
Code first underlying disease, such as:
amyloidosis (E85.-)
nephrocalcinosis (E83.5)
schistosomiasis (B65.0-B65.9)
EXCLUDES 1   *disorders of kidney and ureter in:*
cystinosis (E72.0)
gonorrhea (A54.21)
syphilis (A52.75)
tuberculosis (A18.11)

Other diseases of the urinary system (N30-N39)

EXCLUDES 1   *urinary infection (complicating):*
abortion or ectopic or molar pregnancy (O00-O07, O08.8)
pregnancy, childbirth and the puerperium (O23-, O75.3, O86.2-)

✓4ᵗʰ N30   Cystitis
Use additional code to identify infectious agent (B95-B97)
EXCLUDES 1   *prostatocystitis (N41.3)*

✓5ᵗʰ N30.0   Acute cystitis
EXCLUDES 1   *irradiation cystitis (N30.4-)*
trigonitis (N30.3-)

N30.00   Acute cystitis without hematuria
N30.01   Acute cystitis with hematuria

✓5ᵗʰ N30.1   Interstitial cystitis (chronic)
N30.10   Interstitial cystitis (chronic) without hematuria
N30.11   Interstitial cystitis (chronic) with hematuria

✓5ᵗʰ N30.2   Other chronic cystitis
N30.20   Other chronic cystitis without hematuria
N30.21   Other chronic cystitis with hematuria

✓5ᵗʰ N30.3   Trigonitis
Urethrotrigonitis
N30.30   Trigonitis without hematuria
N30.31   Trigonitis with hematuria

✓5ᵗʰ N30.4   Irradiation cystitis
N30.40   Irradiation cystitis without hematuria
N30.41   Irradiation cystitis with hematuria

✓5ᵗʰ N30.8   Other cystitis
Abscess of bladder
N30.80   Other cystitis without hematuria
N30.81   Other cystitis with hematuria

✓5ᵗʰ N30.9   Cystitis, unspecified
N30.90   Cystitis, unspecified without hematuria ▽
N30.91   Cystitis, unspecified with hematuria ▽

✓4ᵗʰ N31   Neuromuscular dysfunction of bladder, not elsewhere classified
Use additional code to identify any associated urinary incontinence (N39.3-N39.4-)
EXCLUDES 1   *cord bladder NOS (G95.89)*
neurogenic bladder due to cauda equina syndrome (G83.4)
neuromuscular dysfunction due to spinal cord lesion (G95.89)

N31.0   Uninhibited neuropathic bladder, not elsewhere classified

N31.1   Reflex neuropathic bladder, not elsewhere classified

N31.2   Flaccid neuropathic bladder, not elsewhere classified
Atonic (motor) (sensory) neuropathic bladder
Autonomous neuropathic bladder
Nonreflex neuropathic bladder

N31.8   Other neuromuscular dysfunction of bladder

N31.9   Neuromuscular dysfunction of bladder, unspecified ▽
Neurogenic bladder dysfunction NOS

✓4ᵗʰ N32   Other disorders of bladder
EXCLUDES 2   *calculus of bladder (N21.0)*
cystocele (N81.1-)
hernia or prolapse of bladder, female (N81.1-)

N32.0   Bladder-neck obstruction
Bladder-neck stenosis (acquired)
EXCLUDES 1   *congenital bladder-neck obstruction (Q64.3-)*

N32.1   Vesicointestinal fistula
Vesicorectal fistula

N32.2   Vesical fistula, not elsewhere classified
EXCLUDES 1   *fistula between bladder and female genital tract (N82.0-N82.1)*

N32.3   Diverticulum of bladder
EXCLUDES 1   *congenital diverticulum of bladder (Q64.6)*
diverticulitis of bladder (N30.8-)

✓5ᵗʰ N32.8   Other specified disorders of bladder
N32.81   Overactive bladder
Detrusor muscle hyperactivity
EXCLUDES 1   *frequent urination due to specified bladder condition—code to condition*

N32.89   Other specified disorders of bladder   CC
Bladder hemorrhage
Bladder hypertrophy
Calcified bladder
Contracted bladder

N32.9   Bladder disorder, unspecified ▽

N Newborn   P Pediatric   M Maternity   A Adult   RIC RIC Dx   NC Dx Noncancer Dx   PDx Primary Dx   CC RIC CC Condition   ►◄ Revised Text   ● New Code   ▲ Revised Code Title

N25–N32.9

762   ICD-10-CM 2016

N33   Bladder disorders in diseases classified elsewhere

Code first underlying disease, such as:
schistosomiasis (B65.0–B65.9)

> EXCLUDES 1   bladder disorder in syphilis (A52.76)
> bladder disorder in tuberculosis (A18.12)
> candidal cystitis (B37.41)
> chlamydial cystitis (A56.01)
> cystitis in gonorrhea (A54.01)
> cystitis in neurogenic bladder (N31.-)
> diphtheritic cystitis (A36.85)
> neurogenic bladder (N31.-)
> syphilitic cystitis (A52.76)
> trichomonal cystitis (A59.03)

✓4th N34   Urethritis and urethral syndrome

Use additional code (B95-B97), to identify infectious agent

> EXCLUDES 2   Reiter's disease (M02.3-)
> urethritis in diseases with a predominantly sexual mode of
> transmission (A50-A64)
> urethrotrigonitis (N30.3-)

N34.0   Urethral abscess

Abscess (of) Cowper's gland
Abscess (of) Littrés gland
Abscess (of) urethral (gland)
Periurethral abscess

> EXCLUDES 1   urethral caruncle (N36.2)

N34.1   Nonspecific urethritis

Nongonococcal urethritis
Nonvenereal urethritis

N34.2   Other urethritis

Meatitis, urethral
Postmenopausal urethritis
Ulcer of urethra (meatus)
Urethritis NOS

N34.3   Urethral syndrome, unspecified   ▽

✓4th N35   Urethral stricture

> EXCLUDES 1   congenital urethral stricture (Q64.3-)
> postprocedural urethral stricture (N99.1-)

✓5th N35.0   Post-traumatic urethral stricture

Urethral stricture due to injury

> EXCLUDES 1   postprocedural urethral stricture (N99.1-)

✓6th N35.01   Post-traumatic urethral stricture, male

N35.010   Post-traumatic urethral stricture,   ♂
male, meatal

N35.011   Post-traumatic bulbous urethral
stricture

N35.012   Post-traumatic membranous urethral
stricture

N35.013   Post-traumatic anterior urethral
stricture

N35.014   Post-traumatic urethral stricture,   ♂ ▽
male, unspecified

✓6th N35.02   Post-traumatic urethral stricture, female

N35.021   Urethral stricture due to childbirth   ♀

N35.028   Other post-traumatic urethral stricture,   ♀
female

✓5th N35.1   Postinfective urethral stricture, not elsewhere classified

> EXCLUDES 1   urethral stricture associated with schistosomiasis (B65-,
> N29)
> gonococcal urethral stricture (A54.01)
> syphilitic urethral stricture (A52.76)

✓6th N35.11   Postinfective urethral stricture, not elsewhere
classified, male

N35.111   Postinfective urethral stricture, not   ♂
elsewhere classified, male, meatal

N35.112   Postinfective bulbous urethral stricture,
not elsewhere classified

N35.113   Postinfective membranous urethral
stricture, not elsewhere classified

N35.114   Postinfective anterior urethral stricture,
not elsewhere classified

N35.119   Postinfective urethral stricture, not   ♂ ▽
elsewhere classified, male, unspecified

N35.12   Postinfective urethral stricture, not elsewhere   ♀
classified, female

N35.8   Other urethral stricture

> EXCLUDES 1   postprocedural urethral stricture (N99.1-)

N35.9   Urethral stricture, unspecified   ▽

✓4th N36   Other disorders of urethra

N36.0   Urethral fistula

Urethroperineal fistula
Urethrorectal fistula
Urinary fistula NOS

> EXCLUDES 1   urethroscrotal fistula (N50.8)
> urethrovaginal fistula (N82.1)
> urethrovesicovaginal fistula (N82.1)

N36.1   Urethral diverticulum

N36.2   Urethral caruncle

✓5th N36.4   Urethral functional and muscular disorders

Use additional code to identify associated urinary stress
incontinence (N39.3)

N36.41   Hypermobility of urethra

N36.42   Intrinsic sphincter deficiency (ISD)

N36.43   Combined hypermobility of urethra and intrinsic
sphincter deficiency

N36.44   Muscular disorders of urethra

Bladder sphincter dyssynergy

N36.5   Urethral false passage

N36.8   Other specified disorders of urethra

N36.9   Urethral disorder, unspecified   ▽

N37   Urethral disorders in diseases classified elsewhere

Code first underlying disease

> EXCLUDES 1   urethritis (in):
> candidal infection (B37.41)
> chlamydial (A56.01)
> gonorrhea (A54.01)
> syphilis (A52.76)
> trichomonal infection (A59.03)
> tuberculosis (A18.13)

✓4th N39   Other disorders of urinary system

> EXCLUDES 2   hematuria NOS (R31.-)
> recurrent or persistent hematuria (N02.-)
> recurrent or persistent hematuria with specified morphological
> lesion (N02.-)
> proteinuria NOS (R80.-)

N39.0   Urinary tract infection, site not specified

Use additional code (B95-B97), to identify infectious agent

> EXCLUDES 1   candidiasis of urinary tract (B37.4-)
> neonatal urinary tract infection (P39.3)
> urinary tract infection of specified site, such as:
> cystitis (N30.-)
> urethritis (N34.-)

AHA: 2012, 4Q, 94

N39.3   Stress incontinence (female) (male)

Code also any associated overactive bladder (N32.81)

> EXCLUDES 1   mixed incontinence (N39.46)

✓5th N39.4   Other specified urinary incontinence

Code also any associated overactive bladder (N32.81)

> EXCLUDES 1   enuresis NOS (R32)
> functional urinary incontinence (R39.81)
> urinary incontinence associated with cognitive
> impairment (R39.81)
> urinary incontinence NOS (R32)
> urinary incontinence of nonorganic origin (F98.0)

N39.41   Urge incontinence

> EXCLUDES 1   mixed incontinence (N39.46)

N39.42   Incontinence without sensory awareness

N39.43   Post-void dribbling

N39.44   Nocturnal enuresis

N39.45   Continuous leakage

N39.46   Mixed incontinence

Urge and stress incontinence

✓6th N39.49   Other specified urinary incontinence

N39.490   Overflow incontinence

N39.498   Other specified urinary incontinence

Reflex incontinence
Total incontinence

N39.8   Other specified disorders of urinary system

N39.9   Disorder of urinary system, unspecified   ▽

☑ Add'l Character Required ✓x7th Placeholder Alert RUG IV Special Care High Dx RUG IV Clinically Complex Dx RUG IV Special Care Low Dx Manifestation Code Other Specified Code ▽ Unspecified Code

CD-10-CM 2016   **763**

Chapter 14. Diseases of the Genitourinary System

Diseases of male genital organs (N40-N53)

✓4ᵗʰ N40 Enlarged prostate
    Adenofibromatous hypertrophy of prostate
    Benign hypertrophy of the prostate
    Benign prostatic hyperplasia
    Benign prostatic hypertrophy
    BPH
    Nodular prostate
    Polyp of prostate
    EXCLUDES 1   benign neoplasms of prostate (adenoma, benign)
        (fibroadenoma) (fibroma) (myoma) (D29.1)
    EXCLUDES 2   malignant neoplasm of prostate (C61)

  N40.0 Enlarged prostate without lower urinary tract symptoms A♂
    Enlarged prostate NOS
    Enlarged prostate without LUTS

  N40.1 Enlarged prostate with lower urinary tract symptoms A♂
    Enlarged prostate with LUTS
    Use additional code for associated symptoms, when specified:
      incomplete bladder emptying (R39.14)
      nocturia (R35.1)
      straining on urination (R39.16)
      urinary frequency (R35.0)
      urinary hesitancy (R39.11)
      urinary incontinence (N39.4-)
      urinary obstruction (N13.8)
      urinary retention (R33.8)
      urinary urgency (R39.15)
      weak urinary stream (R39.12)

  N40.2 Nodular prostate without lower urinary tract symptoms A♂
    Nodular prostate without LUTS

  N40.3 Nodular prostate with lower urinary tract symptoms A♂
    Use additional code for associated symptoms, when specified:
      incomplete bladder emptying (R39.14)
      nocturia (R35.1)
      straining on urination (R39.16)
      urinary frequency (R35.0)
      urinary hesitancy (R39.11)
      urinary incontinence (N39.4-)
      urinary obstruction (N13.8)
      urinary retention (R33.8)
      urinary urgency (R39.15)
      weak urinary stream (R39.12)

✓4ᵗʰ N41 Inflammatory diseases of prostate
    Use additional code (B95-B97), to identify infectious agent

  N41.0 Acute prostatitis A♂
  N41.1 Chronic prostatitis A♂
  N41.2 Abscess of prostate A♂
  N41.3 Prostatocystitis A♂
  N41.4 Granulomatous prostatitis A♂
  N41.8 Other inflammatory diseases of prostate A♂
  N41.9 Inflammatory disease of prostate, unspecified A♂▽
    Prostatitis NOS

✓4ᵗʰ N42 Other and unspecified disorders of prostate

  N42.0 Calculus of prostate A♂
    Prostatic stone

  N42.1 Congestion and hemorrhage of prostate A♂
    EXCLUDES 1   enlarged prostate (N40.-)
        hematuria (R31.-)
        hyperplasia of prostate (N40.-)
        inflammatory diseases of prostate (N41.-)

  N42.3 Dysplasia of prostate ♂
    Prostatic intraepithelial neoplasia I (PIN I)
    Prostatic intraepithelial neoplasia II (PIN II)
    EXCLUDES 1   prostatic intraepithelial neoplasia III (PIN III) (D07.5)

  ✓5ᵗʰ N42.8 Other specified disorders of prostate
    N42.81 Prostatodynia syndrome A♂
      Painful prostate syndrome
    N42.82 Prostatosis syndrome A♂
    N42.83 Cyst of prostate A♂
    N42.89 Other specified disorders of prostate A♂
  N42.9 Disorder of prostate, unspecified A♂▽

✓4ᵗʰ N43 Hydrocele and spermatocele
    INCLUDES   hydrocele of spermatic cord, testis or tunica vaginalis
    EXCLUDES 1   congenital hydrocele (P83.5)

  N43.0 Encysted hydrocele ♂
  N43.1 Infected hydrocele ♂
    Use additional code (B95-B97), to identify infectious agent

  N43.2 Other hydrocele ♂
  N43.3 Hydrocele, unspecified ♂▽
  ✓5ᵗʰ N43.4 Spermatocele of epididymis ♂
    Spermatic cyst
    N43.40 Spermatocele of epididymis, unspecified ♂▽
    N43.41 Spermatocele of epididymis, single ♂
    N43.42 Spermatocele of epididymis, multiple ♂

✓4ᵗʰ N44 Noninflammatory disorders of testis
  ✓5ᵗʰ N44.0 Torsion of testis
    N44.00 Torsion of testis, unspecified ♂▽
    N44.01 Extravaginal torsion of spermatic cord ♂
    N44.02 Intravaginal torsion of spermatic cord ♂
      Torsion of spermatic cord NOS
    N44.03 Torsion of appendix testis ♂
    N44.04 Torsion of appendix epididymis ♂
  N44.1 Cyst of tunica albuginea testis ♂
  N44.2 Benign cyst of testis ♂
  N44.8 Other noninflammatory disorders of the testis ♂

✓4ᵗʰ N45 Orchitis and epididymitis
    Use additional code (B95-B97), to identify infectious agent
  N45.1 Epididymitis ♂
  N45.2 Orchitis ♂
  N45.3 Epididymo-orchitis ♂
  N45.4 Abscess of epididymis or testis ♂

✓4ᵗʰ N46 Male infertility
    EXCLUDES 1   vasectomy status (Z98.52)

  ✓5ᵗʰ N46.0 Azoospermia
    Absolute male infertility
    Male infertility due to germinal (cell) aplasia
    Male infertility due to spermatogenic arrest (complete)
    N46.01 Organic azoospermia A♂
      Azoospermia NOS
    ✓6ᵗʰ N46.02 Azoospermia due to extratesticular causes
      Code also associated cause
      N46.021 Azoospermia due to drug therapy A♂
      N46.022 Azoospermia due to infection A♂
      N46.023 Azoospermia due to obstruction of efferent ducts A♂
      N46.024 Azoospermia due to radiation A♂
      N46.025 Azoospermia due to systemic disease A♂
      N46.029 Azoospermia due to other extratesticular causes A♂

  ✓5ᵗʰ N46.1 Oligospermia
    Male infertility due to germinal cell desquamation
    Male infertility due to hypospermatogenesis
    Male infertility due to incomplete spermatogenic arrest
    N46.11 Organic oligospermia A♂
      Oligospermia NOS
    ✓6ᵗʰ N46.12 Oligospermia due to extratesticular causes
      Code also associated cause
      N46.121 Oligospermia due to drug therapy A♂
      N46.122 Oligospermia due to infection A♂
      N46.123 Oligospermia due to obstruction of efferent ducts A♂
      N46.124 Oligospermia due to radiation A♂
      N46.125 Oligospermia due to systemic disease A♂
      N46.129 Oligospermia due to other extratesticular causes A♂
  N46.8 Other male infertility A♂
  N46.9 Male infertility, unspecified A♂▽

✓4ᵗʰ N47 Disorders of prepuce
  N47.0 Adherent prepuce, newborn N♂
  N47.1 Phimosis ♂
  N47.2 Paraphimosis ♂
  N47.3 Deficient foreskin ♂
  N47.4 Benign cyst of prepuce ♂
  N47.5 Adhesions of prepuce and glans penis ♂
  N47.6 Balanoposthitis
    Use additional code (B95-B97), to identify infectious agent
    EXCLUDES 1   balanitis (N48.1)
  N47.7 Other inflammatory diseases of prepuce ♂
    Use additional code (B95-B97), to identify infectious agent

N40–N47.7

N Newborn   P Pediatric   M Maternity   A Adult   RIC RIC Dx   NC Dx Noncancer Dx   PDx Primary Dx   CC RIC CC Condition   ►◄ Revised Text   ● New Code   ▲ Revised Code Title

764   ICD-10-CM 2016

    N47.8 **Other disorders of prepuce**   ♂

☑4ᵗʰ **N48** **Other disorders of penis**

    N48.0 **Leukoplakia of penis**   ♂
        Balanitis xerotica obliterans
        Kraurosis of penis
        Lichen sclerosus of external male genital organs
        EXCLUDES 1   carcinoma in situ of penis (D07.4)

    N48.1 **Balanitis**   ♂
        Use additional code (B95-B97), to identify infectious agent
        EXCLUDES 1   amebic balanitis (A06.8)
             balanitis xerotica obliterans (N48.0)
             candidal balanitis (B37.42)
             gonococcal balanitis (A54.23)
             herpesviral [herpes simplex] balanitis (A60.01)

    ☑5ᵗʰ **N48.2** **Other inflammatory disorders of penis**
        Use additional code (B95-B97), to identify infectious agent
        EXCLUDES 1   balanitis (N48.1)
             balanitis xerotica obliterans (N48.0)
             balanoposthitis (N47.6)

        N48.21 **Abscess of corpus cavernosum and penis**   ♂
        N48.22 **Cellulitis of corpus cavernosum and penis**   ♂
        N48.29 **Other inflammatory disorders of penis**   ♂

    ☑5ᵗʰ **N48.3** **Priapism**
        Painful erection
        Code first underlying cause

        N48.30 **Priapism, unspecified**   ♂▽
        N48.31 **Priapism** due to trauma   ♂
        N48.32 *Priapism due to disease classified elsewhere*   ♂
        N48.33 **Priapism,** drug-induced   ♂
        N48.39 **Other priapism**   ♂

    N48.5 **Ulcer of penis**   ♂

    N48.6 **Induration penis plastica**   🅰♂
        Peyronie's disease
        Plastic induration of penis

    ☑5ᵗʰ **N48.8** **Other specified disorders of penis**
        N48.81 **Thrombosis of superficial vein of penis**   ♂
        N48.82 **Acquired torsion of penis**   ♂
             Acquired torsion of penis NOS
             EXCLUDES 1   congenital torsion of penis (Q55.63)
        N48.83 **Acquired buried penis**   ♂
             EXCLUDES 1   congenital hidden penis (Q55.64)
        N48.89 **Other specified disorders of penis**   ♂

    N48.9 **Disorder of penis, unspecified**   ♂▽

☑4ᵗʰ **N49** **Inflammatory disorders of male genital organs, not elsewhere classified**
        Use additional code (B95-B97), to identify infectious agent
        EXCLUDES 1   inflammation of penis (N48.1, N48.2-)
             orchitis and epididymitis (N45.-)

    N49.0 **Inflammatory disorders of** seminal vesicle   ♂
        Vesiculitis NOS

    N49.1 **Inflammatory disorders of** spermatic cord, tunica vaginalis and vas deferens   ♂
        Vasitis

    N49.2 **Inflammatory disorders of** scrotum   ♂

    N49.3 Fournier gangrene   ♂

    N49.8 **Inflammatory disorders of other specified male genital organs**   ♂
        Inflammation of multiple sites in male genital organs

    N49.9 **Inflammatory disorder of unspecified male genital organ**   ♂▽
        Abscess of unspecified male genital organ
        Boil of unspecified male genital organ
        Carbuncle of unspecified male genital organ
        Cellulitis of unspecified male genital organ

☑4ᵗʰ **N50** **Other and unspecified disorders of male genital organs**
        EXCLUDES 2   torsion of testis (N44.0-)

    N50.0 **Atrophy of testis**   ♂

    N50.1 **Vascular disorders of male genital organs**   ♂
        Hematocele, NOS, of male genital organs
        Hemorrhage of male genital organs
        Thrombosis of male genital organs

    N50.3 **Cyst of epididymis**   ♂

    N50.8 **Other specified disorders of male genital organs**   ♂
        Atrophy of scrotum, seminal vesicle, spermatic cord, tunica vaginalis and vas deferens
        Chylocele, tunica vaginalis (nonfilarial) NOS
        Edema of scrotum, seminal vesicle, spermatic cord, testis, tunica vaginalis and vas deferens
        Hypertrophy of scrotum, seminal vesicle, spermatic cord, testis, tunica vaginalis and vas deferens
        Stricture of spermatic cord, tunica vaginalis, and vas deferens
        Ulcer of scrotum, seminal vesicle, spermatic cord, testis, tunica vaginalis and vas deferens
        Urethroscrotal fistula

    N50.9 **Disorder of male genital organs, unspecified**   ♂▽

  N51 *Disorders of male genital organs in diseases classified elsewhere*   ♂
        Code first underlying disease, such as:
           filariasis (B74.0-B74.9)
        EXCLUDES 1   amebic balanitis (A06.8)
             candidal balanitis (B37.42)
             gonococcal balanitis (A54.23)
             gonococcal prostatitis (A54.22)
             herpesviral [herpes simplex] balanitis (A60.01)
             trichomonal prostatitis (A59.02)
             tuberculous prostatitis (A18.14)

☑4ᵗʰ **N52** **Male erectile dysfunction**
        EXCLUDES 1   psychogenic impotence (F52.21)

    ☑5ᵗʰ **N52.0** **Vasculogenic** erectile dysfunction
        N52.01 **Erectile dysfunction due to** arterial insufficiency   🅰♂
        N52.02 **Corporo-venous occlusive** erectile dysfunction   🅰♂
        N52.03 **Combined arterial insufficiency and corporo-venous occlusive** erectile dysfunction   🅰♂

    N52.1 *Erectile dysfunction due to diseases classified elsewhere*   🅰♂
        Code first underlying disease

    N52.2 **Drug-induced** erectile dysfunction   🅰♂

    ☑5ᵗʰ **N52.3** **Post-surgical** erectile dysfunction
        N52.31 **Erectile dysfunction following** radical prostatectomy   🅰♂
        N52.32 **Erectile dysfunction following** radical cystectomy   🅰♂
        N52.33 **Erectile dysfunction following** urethral surgery   🅰♂
        N52.34 **Erectile dysfunction following** simple prostatectomy   🅰♂
        N52.39 **Other post-surgical erectile dysfunction**   🅰♂

    N52.8 **Other male erectile dysfunction**   🅰♂

    N52.9 **Male erectile dysfunction, unspecified**   🅰♂▽
        Impotence NOS

☑4ᵗʰ **N53** **Other male sexual dysfunction**
        EXCLUDES 1   psychogenic sexual dysfunction (F52.-)

    ☑5ᵗʰ **N53.1** **Ejaculatory dysfunction**
        EXCLUDES 1   premature ejaculation (F52.4)

        N53.11 **Retarded** ejaculation   🅰♂
        N53.12 **Painful** ejaculation   ♂
        N53.13 **Anejaculatory** orgasm   🅰♂
        N53.14 **Retrograde** ejaculation   🅰♂
        N53.19 **Other ejaculatory dysfunction**   🅰♂
             Ejaculatory dysfunction NOS

    N53.8 **Other male sexual dysfunction**   ♂

    N53.9 **Unspecified male sexual dysfunction**   ♂▽

Disorders of breast (N60-N65)
    EXCLUDES 1   disorders of breast associated with childbirth (O91-O92)

☑4ᵗʰ **N60** **Benign mammary dysplasia**
    INCLUDES fibrocystic mastopathy

    ☑5ᵗʰ **N60.0** **Solitary cyst of breast**
        Cyst of breast

        N60.01 **Solitary cyst of** right **breast**
        N60.02 **Solitary cyst of** left **breast**
        N60.09 **Solitary cyst of unspecified breast**   ▽

    ☑5ᵗʰ **N60.1** **Diffuse cystic mastopathy**
        Cystic breast
        Fibrocystic disease of breast
        EXCLUDES 1   diffuse cystic mastopathy with epithelial proliferation (N60.3-)

        N60.11 **Diffuse cystic mastopathy of** right **breast**   🅰
        N60.12 **Diffuse cystic mastopathy of** left **breast**   🅰

☑ Add'l Character Required ☑x7ᵗʰ Placeholder Alert **RUG IV Special Care High Dx** RUG IV Clinically Complex Dx **RUG IV Special Care Low Dx** Manifestation Code Other Specified Code ▽ Unspecified Code

N60.19   **Diffuse cystic mastopathy of unspecified breast** A ▽

✓5ᵗʰ **N60.2**   **Fibroadenosis of breast**
Adenofibrosis of breast
    EXCLUDES 2   *fibroadenoma of breast (D24.-)*

N60.21   **Fibroadenosis of right breast**
N60.22   **Fibroadenosis of left breast**
N60.29   **Fibroadenosis of unspecified breast** ▽

✓5ᵗʰ **N60.3**   **Fibrosclerosis of breast**
Cystic mastopathy with epithelial proliferation

N60.31   **Fibrosclerosis of right breast**
N60.32   **Fibrosclerosis of left breast**
N60.39   **Fibrosclerosis of unspecified breast** ▽

✓5ᵗʰ **N60.4**   **Mammary duct ectasia**

N60.41   **Mammary duct ectasia of right breast**
N60.42   **Mammary duct ectasia of left breast**
N60.49   **Mammary duct ectasia of unspecified breast** ▽

✓5ᵗʰ **N60.8**   **Other benign mammary dysplasias**

N60.81   **Other benign mammary dysplasias of right breast**
N60.82   **Other benign mammary dysplasias of left breast**
N60.89   **Other benign mammary dysplasias of unspecified breast** ▽

✓5ᵗʰ **N60.9**   **Unspecified benign mammary dysplasia** ▽

N60.91   **Unspecified benign mammary dysplasia of right breast** ▽
N60.92   **Unspecified benign mammary dysplasia of left breast** ▽
N60.99   **Unspecified benign mammary dysplasia of unspecified breast**

N61   **Inflammatory disorders of breast**
Abscess (acute) (chronic) (nonpuerperal) of areola
Abscess (acute) (chronic) (nonpuerperal) of breast
Carbuncle of breast
Infective mastitis (acute) (subacute) (nonpuerperal)
Mastitis (acute) (subacute) (nonpuerperal) NOS
    EXCLUDES 1   *inflammatory carcinoma of breast (C50.9)*
         inflammatory disorder of breast associated with childbirth (O91.-)
         neonatal infective mastitis (P39.0)
         thrombophlebitis of breast [Mondor's disease] (I80.8)

N62   **Hypertrophy of breast**
Gynecomastia
Hypertrophy of breast NOS
Massive pubertal hypertrophy of breast
    EXCLUDES 1   *breast engorgement of newborn (P83.4)*
         disproportion of reconstructed breast (N65.1)

N63   **Unspecified lump in breast** ▽
Nodule(s) NOS in breast

✓4ᵗʰ **N64**   **Other disorders of breast**
    EXCLUDES 2   *mechanical complication of breast prosthesis and implant (T85.4-)*

N64.0   **Fissure and fistula of nipple**
N64.1   **Fat necrosis of breast**
Fat necrosis (segmental) of breast
Code first breast necrosis due to breast graft (T85.89)

N64.2   **Atrophy of breast**
N64.3   **Galactorrhea not associated with childbirth**
N64.4   **Mastodynia**

✓5ᵗʰ **N64.5**   **Other signs and symptoms in breast**
    EXCLUDES 2   *abnormal findings on diagnostic imaging of breast (R92.-)*

N64.51   **Induration of breast**
N64.52   **Nipple discharge**
    EXCLUDES 1   *abnormal findings in nipple discharge (R89.-)*
N64.53   **Retraction of nipple**
N64.59   **Other signs and symptoms in breast**

✓5ᵗʰ **N64.8**   **Other specified disorders of breast**

N64.81   **Ptosis of breast** A
    EXCLUDES 1   *ptosis of native breast in relation to reconstructed breast (N65.1)*

N64.82   **Hypoplasia of breast** A
Micromastia
    EXCLUDES 1   *congenital absence of breast (Q83.0)*
         hypoplasia of native breast in relation to reconstructed breast (N65.1)

N64.89   **Other specified disorders of breast**
Galactocele
Subinvolution of breast (postlactational)

N64.9   **Disorder of breast, unspecified** ▽

✓4ᵗʰ **N65**   **Deformity and disproportion of reconstructed breast** A

N65.0   **Deformity of reconstructed breast** A
Contour irregularity in reconstructed breast
Excess tissue in reconstructed breast
Misshapen reconstructed breast

N65.1   **Disproportion of reconstructed breast** A
Breast asymmetry between native breast and reconstructed breast
Disproportion between native breast and reconstructed breast

Inflammatory diseases of female pelvic organs (N70-N77)

    EXCLUDES 1   *inflammatory diseases of female pelvic organs complicating:*
         abortion or ectopic or molar pregnancy (O00-O07, O08.0)
         pregnancy, childbirth and the puerperium (O23-, O75.3, O85, O86-)

✓4ᵗʰ **N70**   **Salpingitis and oophoritis**
    INCLUDES   abscess (of) fallopian tube
         abscess (of) ovary
         pyosalpinx
         salpingo-oophoritis
         tubo-ovarian abscess
         tubo-ovarian inflammatory disease
Use additional code (B95-B97), to identify infectious agent
    EXCLUDES 1   *gonococcal infection (A54.24)*
         tuberculous infection (A18.17)

✓5ᵗʰ **N70.0**   **Acute salpingitis and oophoritis**

N70.01   **Acute salpingitis** ♀
N70.02   **Acute oophoritis** ♀
N70.03   **Acute salpingitis and oophoritis** ♀

✓5ᵗʰ **N70.1**   **Chronic salpingitis and oophoritis**
Hydrosalpinx

N70.11   **Chronic salpingitis** ♀
N70.12   **Chronic oophoritis** ♀
N70.13   **Chronic salpingitis and oophoritis** ♀

✓5ᵗʰ **N70.9**   **Salpingitis and oophoritis, unspecified**

N70.91   **Salpingitis, unspecified** ♀ ▽
N70.92   **Oophoritis, unspecified** ♀ ▽
N70.93   **Salpingitis and oophoritis, unspecified** ♀ ▽

✓4ᵗʰ **N71**   **Inflammatory disease of uterus, except cervix**
Endo (myo) metritis   Pyometra
Metritis   Uterine abscess
Myometritis
Use additional code (B95-B97), to identify infectious agent
    EXCLUDES 1   *hyperplastic endometritis (N85.0-)*
         infection of uterus following delivery (O85, O86.-)

N71.0   **Acute inflammatory disease of uterus** ♀
N71.1   **Chronic inflammatory disease of uterus** ♀
N71.9   **Inflammatory disease of uterus, unspecified** ♀ ▽

N72   **Inflammatory disease of cervix uteri** ♀
Cervicitis (with or without erosion or ectropion)
Endocervicitis (with or without erosion or ectropion)
Exocervicitis (with or without erosion or ectropion)
Use additional code (B95-B97), to identify infectious agent
    EXCLUDES 1   *erosion and ectropion of cervix without cervicitis (N86)*

✓4ᵗʰ **N73**   **Other female pelvic inflammatory diseases**
Use additional code (B95-B97), to identify infectious agent

N73.0   **Acute parametritis and pelvic cellulitis** ♀
Abscess of broad ligament
Abscess of parametrium
Pelvic cellulitis, female

N73.1   **Chronic parametritis and pelvic cellulitis** ♀
Any condition in N73.0 specified as chronic
    EXCLUDES 1   *tuberculous parametritis and pelvic cellutis (A18.17)*

N73.2   **Unspecified parametritis and pelvic cellulitis** ♀ ▽
Any condition in N73.0 unspecified whether acute or chronic

N73.3   **Female acute pelvic peritonitis** ♀
N73.4   **Female chronic pelvic peritonitis** ♀
    EXCLUDES 1   *tuberculous pelvic (female) peritonitis (A18.17)*

N73.5   **Female pelvic peritonitis, unspecified** ♀ ▽
N73.6   **Female pelvic peritoneal adhesions (postinfective)** ♀
    EXCLUDES 2   *postprocedural pelvic peritoneal adhesions (N99.4)*
AHA: 2014, 1Q, 6

N Newborn   P Pediatric   M Maternity   A Adult   RIC RIC Dx   NC Dx Noncancer Dx   PDx Primary Dx   CC RIC CC Condition   ►◄ Revised Text   ● New Code   ▲ Revised Code Title

ICD-10-CM 2016

766

N73.8   **Other specified female pelvic inflammatory diseases** ♀

N73.9   **Female pelvic inflammatory disease, unspecified** ♀ ▽
　　　　Female pelvic infection or inflammation NOS

N74   *Female pelvic inflammatory disorders in diseases classified elsewhere* ♀
　　　Code first underlying disease
　　　EXCLUDES 1   *chlamydial cervicitis (A56.02)*
　　　　　　　chlamydial pelvic inflammatory disease (A56.11)
　　　　　　　gonococcal cervicitis (A54.03)
　　　　　　　gonococcal pelvic inflammatory disease (A54.24)
　　　　　　　herpesviral [herpes simplex] cervicitis (A60.03)
　　　　　　　herpesviral [herpes simplex] pelvic inflammatory disease (A60.09)
　　　　　　　syphilitic cervicitis (A52.76)
　　　　　　　syphilitic pelvic inflammatory disease (A52.76)
　　　　　　　trichomonal cervicitis (A59.09)
　　　　　　　tuberculous cervicitis (A18.16)
　　　　　　　tuberculous pelvic inflammatory disease (A18.17)

✔4ᵗʰ N75   **Diseases of Bartholin's gland**

N75.0   **Cyst of Bartholin's gland** ♀

N75.1   **Abscess of Bartholin's gland** ♀

N75.8   **Other diseases of Bartholin's gland** ♀
　　　　Bartholinitis

N75.9   **Disease of Bartholin's gland, unspecified** ♀ ▽

✔4ᵗʰ N76   **Other inflammation of vagina and vulva**
　　　Use additional code (B95-B97), to identify infectious agent
　　　EXCLUDES 2   *senile (atrophic) vaginitis (N95.2)*
　　　　　　　vulvar vestibulitis (N94.810)

N76.0   **Acute vaginitis** ♀
　　　　Acute vulvovaginitis
　　　　Vaginitis NOS
　　　　Vulvovaginitis NOS

N76.1   **Subacute and chronic vaginitis** ♀
　　　　Chronic vulvovaginitis
　　　　Subacute vulvovaginitis

N76.2   **Acute vulvitis** ♀
　　　　Vulvitis NOS

N76.3   **Subacute and chronic vulvitis** ♀

N76.4   **Abscess of vulva** ♀
　　　　Furuncle of vulva

N76.5   **Ulceration of vagina** ♀

N76.6   **Ulceration of vulva** ♀

✔5ᵗʰ N76.8   **Other specified inflammation of vagina and vulva**

N76.81   **Mucositis (ulcerative) of vagina and vulva** ♀
　　　　　Code also type of associated therapy, such as:
　　　　　　antineoplastic and immunosuppressive drugs (T45.1X-)
　　　　　　radiological procedure and radiotherapy (Y84.2)
　　　　　EXCLUDES 2   *gastrointestinal mucositis (ulcerative) (K92.81)*
　　　　　　　　nasal mucositis (ulcerative) (J34.81)
　　　　　　　　oral mucositis (ulcerative) (K12.3-)

N76.89   **Other specified inflammation of vagina and vulva** ♀

✔4ᵗʰ N77   **Vulvovaginal ulceration and inflammation in diseases classified elsewhere**

N77.0   *Ulceration of vulva in diseases classified elsewhere* ♀
　　　　Code first underlying disease, such as:
　　　　　Behçet's disease (M35.2)
　　　　EXCLUDES 1   *ulceration of vulva in gonococcal infection (A54.02)*
　　　　　　　ulceration of vulva in herpesviral [herpes simplex] infection (A60.04)
　　　　　　　ulceration of vulva in syphilis (A51.0)
　　　　　　　ulceration of vulva in tuberculosis (A18.18)

N77.1   *Vaginitis, vulvitis and vulvovaginitis in diseases classified elsewhere* ♀
　　　　Code first underlying disease, such as:
　　　　　pinworm (B80)
　　　　EXCLUDES 1   *candidal vulvovaginitis (B37.3)*
　　　　　　　chlamydial vulvovaginitis (A56.02)
　　　　　　　gonococcal vulvovaginitis (A54.02)
　　　　　　　herpesviral [herpes simplex] vulvovaginitis (A60.04)
　　　　　　　trichomonal vulvovaginitis (A59.01)
　　　　　　　tuberculous vulvovaginitis (A18.18)
　　　　　　　vulvovaginitis in early syphilis (A51.0)
　　　　　　　vulvovaginitis in late syphilis (A52.76)

Noninflammatory disorders of female genital tract (N80-N98)

✔4ᵗʰ N80   **Endometriosis**

N80.0   **Endometriosis of uterus** ♀
　　　　Adenomyosis
　　　　EXCLUDES 1   *stromal endometriosis (D39.0)*

N80.1   **Endometriosis of ovary** ♀

N80.2   **Endometriosis of fallopian tube** ♀

N80.3   **Endometriosis of pelvic peritoneum** ♀

N80.4   **Endometriosis of rectovaginal septum and vagina** ♀

N80.5   **Endometriosis of intestine** ♀

N80.6   **Endometriosis in cutaneous scar** ♀

N80.8   **Other endometriosis**

N80.9   **Endometriosis, unspecified** ♀ ▽

✔4ᵗʰ N81   **Female genital prolapse**
　　　EXCLUDES 1   *genital prolapse complicating pregnancy, labor or delivery (O34.5-)*
　　　　　　　prolapse and hernia of ovary and fallopian tube (N83.4)
　　　　　　　prolapse of vaginal vault after hysterectomy (N99.3)

N81.0   **Urethrocele** ♀
　　　　EXCLUDES 1   *urethrocele with cystocele (N81.1-)*
　　　　　　　urethrocele with prolapse of uterus (N81.2-N81.4)

✔5ᵗʰ N81.1   **Cystocele**
　　　　Cystocele with urethrocele
　　　　Cystourethrocele
　　　　EXCLUDES 1   *cystocele with prolapse of uterus (N81.2-N81.4)*

N81.10   **Cystocele, unspecified** ♀ ▽
　　　　　Prolapse of (anterior) vaginal wall NOS

N81.11   **Cystocele, midline** ♀

N81.12   **Cystocele, lateral** ♀
　　　　　Paravaginal cystocele

N81.2   **Incomplete uterovaginal prolapse** ♀
　　　　First degree uterine prolapse
　　　　Prolapse of cervix NOS
　　　　Second degree uterine prolapse
　　　　EXCLUDES 1   *cervical stump prolaspe (N81.85)*

N81.3   **Complete uterovaginal prolapse** ♀
　　　　Procidentia (uteri) NOS
　　　　Third degree uterine prolapse

N81.4   **Uterovaginal prolapse, unspecified** ♀ ▽
　　　　Prolapse of uterus NOS

N81.5   **Vaginal enterocele** ♀
　　　　EXCLUDES 1   *enterocele with prolapse of uterus (N81.2-N81.4)*

N81.6   **Rectocele** ♀
　　　　Prolapse of posterior vaginal wall
　　　　Use additional code for any associated fecal incontinence, if applicable (R15.-)
　　　　EXCLUDES 2   *perineocele (N81.81)*
　　　　　　　rectal prolapse (K62.3)
　　　　　　　rectocele with prolapse of uterus (N81.2-N81.4)

✔5ᵗʰ N81.8   **Other female genital prolapse**

N81.81   **Perineocele** ♀

N81.82   **Incompetence or weakening of pubocervical tissue** ♀

N81.83   **Incompetence or weakening of rectovaginal tissue** ♀

N81.84   **Pelvic muscle wasting** ♀
　　　　　Disuse atrophy of pelvic muscles and anal sphincter

N81.85   **Cervical stump prolapse** ♀

N81.89   **Other female genital prolapse** ♀
　　　　　Deficient perineum
　　　　　Old laceration of muscles of pelvic floor

N81.9   **Female genital prolapse, unspecified** ♀ ▽

✔4ᵗʰ N82   **Fistulae involving female genital tract**
　　　EXCLUDES 1   *vesicointestinal fistulae (N32.1)*

N82.0   **Vesicovaginal fistula** ♀

N82.1   **Other female urinary-genital tract fistulae** ♀
　　　　Cervicovesical fistula
　　　　Ureterovaginal fistula
　　　　Urethrovaginal fistula
　　　　Uteroureteric fistula
　　　　Uterovesical fistula

N82.2   **Fistula of vagina to small intestine** ♀

N82.3   **Fistula of vagina to large intestine** ♀
　　　　Rectovaginal fistula

☑ Add'l Character Required ✔7ᵗʰ Placeholder Alert RUG IV Special Care High Dx   RUG IV Clinically Complex Dx   RUG IV Special Care Low Dx   Manifestation Code   Other Specified Code   ▽ Unspecified Code

Chapter 14. Diseases of the Genitourinary System

N82.4 Other female intestinal-genital tract fistulae ♀
Intestinouterine fistula

N82.5 Female genital tract-skin fistulae ♀
Uterus to abdominal wall fistula
Vaginoperineal fistula

N82.8 Other female genital tract fistulae ♀

N82.9 Female genital tract fistula, unspecified ♀▽

✓4th **N83 Noninflammatory disorders of ovary, fallopian tube and broad ligament**
EXCLUDES 2   hydrosalpinx (N70.1-)

N83.0 Follicular cyst of ovary ♀
Cyst of graafian follicle
Hemorrhagic follicular cyst (of ovary)

N83.1 Corpus luteum cyst ♀
Hemorrhagic corpus luteum cyst

✓5th **N83.2 Other and unspecified ovarian cysts**
EXCLUDES 1   developmental ovarian cyst (Q50.1)
neoplastic ovarian cyst (D27.-)
polycystic ovarian syndrome (E28.2)
Stein-Leventhal syndrome (E28.2)

     N83.20 Unspecified ovarian cysts ♀▽

     N83.29 Other ovarian cysts ♀
Retention cyst of ovary
Simple cyst of ovary

✓5th **N83.3 Acquired atrophy of ovary and fallopian tube**

     N83.31 Acquired atrophy of ovary ♀

     N83.32 Acquired atrophy of fallopian tube ♀

     N83.33 Acquired atrophy of ovary and fallopian tube ♀

N83.4 Prolapse and hernia of ovary and fallopian tube ♀

✓5th **N83.5 Torsion of ovary, ovarian pedicle and fallopian tube**
Torsion of accessory tube

     N83.51 Torsion of ovary and ovarian pedicle ♀

     N83.52 Torsion of fallopian tube ♀
Torsion of hydatid of Morgagni

     N83.53 Torsion of ovary, ovarian pedicle and fallopian tube ♀

N83.6 Hematosalpinx ♀
EXCLUDES 1   hematosalpinx (with) (in):
hematocolpos (N89.7)
hematometra (N85.7)
tubal pregnancy (O00.1)

N83.7 Hematoma of broad ligament ♀

N83.8 Other noninflammatory disorders of ovary, fallopian tube and broad ligament ♀
Broad ligament laceration syndrome [Allen-Masters]

N83.9 Noninflammatory disorder of ovary, fallopian tube and broad ligament, unspecified ♀▽

✓4th **N84 Polyp of female genital tract**
EXCLUDES 1   adenomatous polyp (D28.-)
placental polyp (O90.89)

N84.0 Polyp of corpus uteri ♀
Polyp of endometrium
Polyp of uterus NOS
EXCLUDES 1   polypoid endometrial hyperplasia (N85.0-)

N84.1 Polyp of cervix uteri ♀
Mucous polyp of cervix

N84.2 Polyp of vagina ♀

N84.3 Polyp of vulva ♀
Polyp of labia

N84.8 Polyp of other parts of female genital tract ♀

N84.9 Polyp of female genital tract, unspecified ♀▽

✓4th **N85 Other noninflammatory disorders of uterus, except cervix**
EXCLUDES 1   endometriosis (N80.-)
inflammatory diseases of uterus (N71.-)
noninflammatory disorders of cervix, except malposition (N86-N88)
polyp of corpus uteri (N84.0)
uterine prolapse (N81.-)

✓5th **N85.0 Endometrial hyperplasia**

     N85.00 Endometrial hyperplasia, unspecified ♀▽
Hyperplasia (adenomatous) (cystic) (glandular) of endometrium
Hyperplastic endometritis

     N85.01 Benign endometrial hyperplasia ♀
Endometrial hyperplasia (complex) (simple) without atypia

     N85.02 Endometrial intraepithelial neoplasia [EIN] ♀
Endometrial hyperplasia with atypia
EXCLUDES 1   malignant neoplasm of endometrium (with endometrial intraepithelial neoplasia [EIN]) (C54.1)

N85.2 Hypertrophy of uterus ♀
Bulky or enlarged uterus
EXCLUDES 1   puerperal hypertrophy of uterus (O90.89)

N85.3 Subinvolution of uterus ♀
EXCLUDES 1   puerperal subinvolution of uterus (O90.89)

N85.4 Malposition of uterus ♀
Anteversion of uterus   Retroversion of uterus
Retroflexion of uterus
EXCLUDES 1   malposition of uterus complicating pregnancy, labor or delivery (O34.5-, O65.5)

N85.5 Inversion of uterus ♀
EXCLUDES 1   current obstetric trauma (O71.2)
postpartum inversion of uterus (O71.2)

N85.6 Intrauterine synechiae ♀

N85.7 Hematometra ♀
Hematosalpinx with hematometra
EXCLUDES 1   hematometra with hematocolpos (N89.7)

N85.8 Other specified noninflammatory disorders of uterus ♀
Atrophy of uterus, acquired
Fibrosis of uterus NOS

N85.9 Noninflammatory disorder of uterus, unspecified ♀▽
Disorder of uterus NOS

N86 Erosion and ectropion of cervix uteri ♀
Decubitus (trophic) ulcer of cervix
Eversion of cervix
EXCLUDES 1   erosion and ectropion of cervix with cervicitis (N72)

✓4th **N87 Dysplasia of cervix uteri**
EXCLUDES 1   abnormal results from cervical cytologic examination without histologic confirmation (R87.61-)
carcinoma in situ of cervix uteri (D06.-)
cervical intraepithelial neoplasia III [CIN III] (D06.-)
HGSIL of cervix (R87.613)
severe dysplasia of cervix uteri (D06.-)

N87.0 Mild cervical dysplasia ♀
Cervical intraepithelial neoplasia I [CIN I]

N87.1 Moderate cervical dysplasia ♀
Cervical intraepithelial neoplasia II [CIN II]

N87.9 Dysplasia of cervix uteri, unspecified ♀▽
Anaplasia of cervix   Cervical dysplasia NOS
Cervical atypism

✓4th **N88 Other noninflammatory disorders of cervix uteri**
EXCLUDES 2   inflammatory disease of cervix (N72)
polyp of cervix (N84.1)

N88.0 Leukoplakia of cervix uteri ♀

N88.1 Old laceration of cervix uteri ♀
Adhesions of cervix
EXCLUDES 1   current obstetric trauma (O71.3)

N88.2 Stricture and stenosis of cervix uteri ♀
EXCLUDES 1   stricture and stenosis of cervix uteri complicating labor (O65.5)

N88.3 Incompetence of cervix uteri ♀
Investigation and management of (suspected) cervical incompetence in a nonpregnant woman
EXCLUDES 1   cervical incompetence complicating pregnancy (O34.3-)

N88.4 Hypertrophic elongation of cervix uteri ♀

N88.8 Other specified noninflammatory disorders of cervix uteri ♀
EXCLUDES 1   current obstetric trauma (O71.3)

N88.9 Noninflammatory disorder of cervix uteri, unspecified ♀▽

✓4th **N89 Other noninflammatory disorders of vagina**
EXCLUDES 1   abnormal results from vaginal cytologic examination without histologic confirmation (R87.62-)
carcinoma in situ of vagina (D07.2)
HGSIL of vagina (R87.623)
inflammation of vagina (N76.-)
senile (atrophic) vaginitis (N95.2)
severe dysplasia of vagina (D07.2)
trichomonal leukorrhea (A59.00)
vaginal intraepithelial neoplasia [VAIN], grade III (D07.2)

N89.0 Mild vaginal dysplasia ♀
Vaginal intraepithelial neoplasia [VAIN], grade I

Ⓝ Newborn   Ⓟ Pediatric   Ⓜ Maternity   Ⓐ Adult   RIC RIC Dx   NC Dx Noncancer Dx   PDx Primary Dx   CC RIC CC Condition   ►◄ Revised Text   ● New Code   ▲ Revised Code Title

768   ICD-10-CM 2016

N89.1 Moderate **vaginal dysplasia** ♀
Vaginal intraepithelial neoplasia [VAIN], grade II

N89.3 **Dysplasia of vagina, unspecified** ♀ ▽

N89.4 **Leukoplakia of vagina** ♀

N89.5 **Stricture and atresia of vagina** ♀
Vaginal adhesions
Vaginal stenosis
EXCLUDES 1   *congenital atresia or stricture (Q52.4)*
postprocedural adhesions of vagina (N99.2)

N89.6 **Tight hymenal ring** ♀
Rigid hymen
Tight introitus
EXCLUDES 1   *imperforate hymen (Q52.3)*

N89.7 **Hematocolpos** ♀
Hematocolpos with hematometra or hematosalpinx

N89.8 **Other specified noninflammatory disorders of vagina** ♀
Leukorrhea NOS
Old vaginal laceration
Pessary ulcer of vagina
EXCLUDES 1   *current obstetric trauma (O70-, O71.4, O71.7-O71.8)*
old laceration involving muscles of pelvic floor (N81.8)

N89.9 **Noninflammatory disorder of vagina, unspecified** ♀ ▽

✓4ᵗʰ **N90** **Other noninflammatory disorders of vulva and perineum**
EXCLUDES 1   *anogenital (venereal) warts (A63.0)*
carcinoma in situ of vulva (D07.1)
condyloma acuminatum (A63.0)
current obstetric trauma (O70-, O71.7-O71.8)
inflammation of vulva (N76.-)
severe dysplasia of vulva (D07.1)
vulvar intraepithelial neoplasm III [VIN III] (D07.1)

N90.0 Mild **vulvar dysplasia** ♀
Vulvar intraepithelial neoplasia [VIN], grade I

N90.1 Moderate **vulvar dysplasia** ♀
Vulvar intraepithelial neoplasia [VIN], grade II

N90.3 **Dysplasia of vulva, unspecified** ♀ ▽

N90.4 **Leukoplakia of vulva** ♀
Dystrophy of vulva
Kraurosis of vulva
Lichen sclerosus of external female genital organs

N90.5 **Atrophy of vulva** ♀
Stenosis of vulva

N90.6 **Hypertrophy of vulva** ♀
Hypertrophy of labia

N90.7 **Vulvar cyst** ♀

✓5ᵗʰ **N90.8** **Other specified noninflammatory disorders of vulva and perineum**

✓6ᵗʰ **N90.81** **Female genital mutilation status**
Female genital cutting status

N90.810 **Female genital mutilation status, unspecified** ♀ ▽
Female genital cutting status, unspecified
Female genital mutilation status NOS

N90.811 **Female genital mutilation Type I status** ♀
Clitorectomy status
Female genital cutting Type I status

N90.812 **Female genital mutilation Type II status** ♀
Clitorectomy with excision of labia minora status
Female genital cutting Type II status

N90.813 **Female genital mutilation Type III status** ♀
Female genital cutting Type III status
Infibulation status

N90.818 **Other female genital mutilation status** ♀
Female genital cutting Type IV status
Female genital mutilation Type IV status
Other female genital cutting status

N90.89 **Other specified noninflammatory disorders of vulva and perineum** ♀
Adhesions of vulva   Hypertrophy of clitoris

N90.9 **Noninflammatory disorder of vulva and perineum, unspecified** ♀ ▽

✓4ᵗʰ **N91** **Absent, scanty and rare menstruation**
EXCLUDES 1   *ovarian dysfunction (E28.-)*

N91.0 **Primary amenorrhea** ♀

N91.1 **Secondary amenorrhea** ♀

N91.2 **Amenorrhea, unspecified** ♀ ▽

N91.3 **Primary oligomenorrhea** ♀

N91.4 **Secondary oligomenorrhea** ♀

N91.5 **Oligomenorrhea, unspecified** ♀ ▽
Hypomenorrhea NOS

✓4ᵗʰ **N92** **Excessive, frequent and irregular menstruation**
EXCLUDES 1   *postmenopausal bleeding (N95.0)*
precocious puberty (menstruation) (E30.1)

N92.0 **Excessive and frequent menstruation** with regular cycle ♀
Heavy periods NOS
Menorrhagia NOS
Polymenorrhea

N92.1 **Excessive and frequent menstruation** with irregular cycle ♀
Irregular intermenstrual bleeding
Irregular, shortened intervals between menstrual bleeding
Menometrorrhagia
Metrorrhagia

N92.2 **Excessive menstruation at puberty** ℙ ♀
Excessive bleeding associated with onset of menstrual periods
Pubertal menorrhagia
Puberty bleeding

N92.3 **Ovulation bleeding** ♀
Regular intermenstrual bleeding

N92.4 **Excessive bleeding in the premenopausal period** ♀
Climacteric menorrhagia or metrorrhagia
Menopausal menorrhagia or metrorrhagia
Preclimacteric menorrhagia or metrorrhagia
Premenopausal menorrhagia or metrorrhagia

N92.5 **Other specified irregular menstruation** ♀

N92.6 **Irregular menstruation, unspecified** ♀ ▽
Irregular bleeding NOS
Irregular periods NOS
EXCLUDES 1   *irregular menstruation with:*
lengthened intervals or scanty bleeding (N91.3-N91.5)
shortened intervals or excessive bleeding (N92.1)

✓4ᵗʰ **N93** **Other abnormal uterine and vaginal bleeding**
EXCLUDES 1   *neonatal vaginal hemorrhage (P54.6)*
precocious puberty (menstruation) (E30.1)
pseudomenses (P54.6)

N93.0 **Postcoital and contact bleeding** ♀

N93.8 **Other specified abnormal uterine and vaginal bleeding** ♀
Dysfunctional or functional uterine or vaginal bleeding NOS

N93.9 **Abnormal uterine and vaginal bleeding, unspecified** ♀ ▽

✓4ᵗʰ **N94** **Pain and other conditions associated with female genital organs and menstrual cycle**

N94.0 **Mittelschmerz** ♀

N94.1 **Dyspareunia** ♀
EXCLUDES 1   *psychogenic dyspareunia (F52.6)*

N94.2 **Vaginismus** ♀
EXCLUDES 1   *psychogenic vaginismus (F52.5)*

N94.3 **Premenstrual tension syndrome** ♀
Premenstrual dysphoric disorder
Code also associated menstrual migraine (G43.82-, G43.83-)

N94.4 **Primary dysmenorrhea** ♀

N94.5 **Secondary dysmenorrhea** ♀

N94.6 **Dysmenorrhea, unspecified** ♀ ▽
EXCLUDES 1   *psychogenic dysmenorrhea (F45.8)*

✓5ᵗʰ **N94.8** **Other specified conditions associated with female genital organs and menstrual cycle**

✓6ᵗʰ **N94.81** **Vulvodynia**

N94.810 **Vulvar vestibulitis** ♀

N94.818 **Other vulvodynia** ♀

N94.819 **Vulvodynia, unspecified** ♀ ▽
Vulvodynia NOS

N94.89 **Other specified conditions associated with female genital organs and menstrual cycle** ♀

N94.9 **Unspecified condition associated with female genital organs and menstrual cycle** ♀ ▽

✓4ᵗʰ **N95** **Menopausal and other perimenopausal disorders**
Menopausal and other perimenopausal disorders due to naturally occurring (age-related) menopause and perimenopause
EXCLUDES 1   *excessive bleeding in the premenopausal period (N92.4)*
menopausal and perimenopausal disorders due to artificial or premature menopause (E89.4-, E28.31-)
premature menopause (E28.31-)
EXCLUDES 2   *postmenopausal osteoporosis (M81.0-)*
postmenopausal osteoporosis with current pathological fracture (M80.0-)
postmenopausal urethritis (N34.2)

N95.0 **Postmenopausal bleeding** ♀

N95.1 Menopausal and female climacteric states ♀
Symptoms such as flushing, sleeplessness, headache, lack of concentration, associated with natural (age-related) menopause
Use additional code for associated symptoms
EXCLUDES 1   asymptomatic menopausal state (Z78.0)
symptoms associated with artificial menopause (E89.41)
symptoms associated with premature menopause (E28.310)

N95.2 Postmenopausal atrophic vaginitis ♀
Senile (atrophic) vaginitis

N95.8 Other specified menopausal and perimenopausal disorders ♀

N95.9 Unspecified menopausal and perimenopausal disorder ♀ ▽

N96 Recurrent pregnancy loss ♀
Investigation or care in a nonpregnant woman with history of recurrent pregnancy loss
EXCLUDES 1   recurrent pregnancy loss with current pregnancy (O26.2-)

✓4th N97 Female infertility
INCLUDES   inability to achieve a pregnancy
sterility, female NOS
EXCLUDES 1   female infertility associated with:
hypopituitarism (E23.0)
Stein-Leventhal syndrome (E28.2)
EXCLUDES 2   incompetence of cervix uteri (N88.3)

N97.0 Female infertility associated with anovulation ♀

N97.1 Female infertility of tubal origin ♀
Female infertility associated with congenital anomaly of tube
Female infertility due to tubal block
Female infertility due to tubal occlusion
Female infertility due to tubal stenosis

N97.2 Female infertility of uterine origin ♀
Female infertility associated with congenital anomaly of uterus
Female infertility due to nonimplantation of ovum

N97.8 Female infertility of other origin ♀

N97.9 Female infertility, unspecified ♀ ▽

✓4th N98 Complications associated with artificial fertilization

N98.0 Infection associated with artificial insemination ♀

N98.1 Hyperstimulation of ovaries ♀
Hyperstimulation of ovaries NOS
Hyperstimulation of ovaries associated with induced ovulation

N98.2 Complications of attempted introduction of fertilized ovum following in vitro fertilization ♀

N98.3 Complications of attempted introduction of embryo in embryo transfer ♀

N98.8 Other complications associated with artificial fertilization ♀

N98.9 Complication associated with artificial fertilization, unspecified ♀ ▽

Intraoperative and postprocedural complications and disorders of genitourinary system, not elsewhere classified (N99)

✓4th N99 Intraoperative and postprocedural complications and disorders of genitourinary system, not elsewhere classified
EXCLUDES 2   irradiation cystitis (N30.4-)
postoophorectomy osteoporosis with current pathological fracture (M80.8-)
postoophorectomy osteoporosis without current pathological fracture (M81.8)

N99.0 Postprocedural (acute) (chronic) kidney failure
Use additional code to type of kidney disease

✓5th N99.1 Postprocedural urethral stricture
Postcatheterization urethral stricture

✓6th N99.11 Postprocedural urethral stricture, male
N99.110 Postprocedural urethral stricture, male, meatal ♂
N99.111 Postprocedural bulbous urethral stricture
N99.112 Postprocedural membranous urethral stricture
N99.113 Postprocedural anterior urethral stricture
N99.114 Postprocedural urethral stricture, male unspecified ♂ ▽

N99.12 Postprocedural urethral stricture, female ♀

N99.2 Postprocedural adhesions of vagina ♀

N99.3 Prolapse of vaginal vault after hysterectomy ♀

N99.4 Postprocedural pelvic peritoneal adhesions
EXCLUDES 2   pelvic peritoneal adhesions NOS (N73.6)
postinfective pelvic peritoneal adhesions (N73.6)

✓5th N99.5 Complications of stoma of urinary tract
EXCLUDES 2   mechanical complication of urinary (indwelling) catheter (T83.0-)

✓6th N99.51 Complication of cystostomy
N99.510 Cystostomy hemorrhage
N99.511 Cystostomy infection
N99.512 Cystostomy malfunction
N99.518 Other cystostomy complication

✓6th N99.52 Complication of other external stoma of urinary tract
N99.520 Hemorrhage of other external stoma of urinary tract
N99.521 Infection of other external stoma of urinary tract
N99.522 Malfunction of other external stoma of urinary tract
N99.528 Other complication of other external stoma of urinary tract

✓6th N99.53 Complication of other stoma of urinary tract
N99.530 Hemorrhage of other stoma of urinary tract
N99.531 Infection of other stoma of urinary tract
N99.532 Malfunction of other stoma of urinary tract
N99.538 Other complication of other stoma of urinary tract

✓5th N99.6 Intraoperative hemorrhage and hematoma of a genitourinary system organ or structure complicating a procedure
EXCLUDES 1   intraoperative hemorrhage and hematoma of a genitourinary system organ or structure due to accidental puncture or laceration during a procedure (N99.7-)

N99.61 Intraoperative hemorrhage and hematoma of a genitourinary system organ or structure complicating a genitourinary system procedure

N99.62 Intraoperative hemorrhage and hematoma of a genitourinary system organ or structure complicating other procedure

✓5th N99.7 Accidental puncture and laceration of a genitourinary system organ or structure during a procedure

N99.71 Accidental puncture and laceration of a genitourinary system organ or structure during a genitourinary system procedure

N99.72 Accidental puncture and laceration of a genitourinary system organ or structure during other procedure

✓5th N99.8 Other intraoperative and postprocedural complications and disorders of genitourinary system

N99.81 Other intraoperative complications of genitourinary system

✓6th N99.82 Postprocedural hemorrhage and hematoma of a genitourinary system organ or structure following a procedure
N99.820 Postprocedural hemorrhage and hematoma of a genitourinary system organ or structure following a genitourinary system procedure
N99.821 Postprocedural hemorrhage and hematoma of a genitourinary system organ or structure following other procedure

N99.83 Residual ovary syndrome ♀

N99.89 Other postprocedural complications and disorders of genitourinary system

N95.1–N99.89

Ⓝ Newborn   Ⓟ Pediatric   Ⓜ Maternity   Ⓐ Adult   RIC RIC Dx   NC Dx Noncancer Dx   PDx Primary Dx   CC RIC CC Condition   ►◄ Revised Text   ● New Code   ▲ Revised Code Title

770   ICD-10-CM 2016

Chapter 15. Pregnancy, Childbirth, and the Puerperium (O00–O9A)

Chapter Specific Guidelines with Coding Examples

The chapter specific guidelines from the ICD-10-CM Official Guidelines for Coding and Reporting have been provided below. Along with these guidelines are coding examples, contained in the shaded boxes, that have been developed to help illustrate the coding and/or sequencing guidance found in these guidelines.

a. General rules for obstetric cases

1) Codes from chapter 15 and sequencing priority

Obstetric cases require codes from chapter 15, codes in the range O00-O9A, Pregnancy, Childbirth, and the Puerperium. Chapter 15 codes have sequencing priority over codes from other chapters. Additional codes from other chapters may be used in conjunction with chapter 15 codes to further specify conditions. Should the provider document that the pregnancy is incidental to the encounter, then code Z33.1, Pregnant state, incidental, should be used in place of any chapter 15 codes. It is the provider's responsibility to state that the condition being treated is not affecting the pregnancy.

Bladder abscess in pregnant patient at 25 weeks' gestation	
O23.12	**Infections of bladder in pregnancy, second trimester**
N30.80	**Other cystitis without hematuria**
Z3A.25	**25 weeks gestation of pregnancy**

Explanation: The documentation does not indicate that the pregnancy is incidental or in any way unaffected by the bladder abscess; therefore, an obstetrics code should be sequenced first. An additional code was provided to identify the specific bladder condition as this information is not called out specifically in the obstetrics code.

2) Chapter 15 codes used only on the maternal record

Chapter 15 codes are to be used only on the maternal record, never on the record of the newborn.

3) Final character for trimester

The majority of codes in Chapter 15 have a final character indicating the trimester of pregnancy. The timeframes for the trimesters are indicated at the beginning of the chapter. If trimester is not a component of a code, it is because the condition always occurs in a specific trimester, or the concept of trimester of pregnancy is not applicable. Certain codes have characters for only certain trimesters because the condition does not occur in all trimesters, but it may occur in more than just one.

Assignment of the final character for trimester should be based on the provider's documentation of the trimester (or number of weeks) for the current admission/encounter. This applies to the assignment of trimester for pre-existing conditions as well as those that develop during or are due to the pregnancy. The provider's documentation of the number of weeks may be used to assign the appropriate code identifying the trimester.

Whenever delivery occurs during the current admission, and there is an "in childbirth" option for the obstetric complication being coded, the "in childbirth" code should be assigned.

Pregnant patient at 21 weeks' gestation admitted with excessive vomiting	
O21.2	**Late vomiting of pregnancy**
Z3A.21	**21 weeks gestation of pregnancy**

Explanation: Category O21 classifies vomiting in pregnancy. Although code selection is based on whether the vomiting is before or after 20 completed weeks, these codes are not further classified by trimester. If vomiting only in the second trimester was documented, the provider should be queried for the specific week of gestation, as this will affect code selection.

4) Selection of trimester for inpatient admissions that encompass more than one trimester

In instances when a patient is admitted to a hospital for complications of pregnancy during one trimester and remains in the hospital into a subsequent trimester, the trimester character for the antepartum complication code should be assigned on the basis of the trimester when the complication developed, not the trimester of the discharge. If the condition developed prior to the current admission/encounter or represents a pre-existing condition, the trimester character for the trimester at the time of the admission/encounter should be assigned.

Patient admitted at 27 6/7 weeks' gestation for hemorrhaging from placenta previa; three days after admission at 28 1/7 weeks' gestation, she developed gestational hypertension	
O44.12	**Placenta previa with hemorrhage, second trimester**
O13.3	**Gestational [pregnancy-induced] hypertension without significant proteinuria, third trimester**
Z3A.27	**27 weeks gestation of pregnancy**

Explanation: The patient presented with hemorrhaging from placenta previa while still in her 27th week, which falls within the second trimester. The gestational hypertension did not occur until three days after admission, putting the patient in her 28th week of pregnancy or what is considered to be the third trimester. The weeks of gestation captured by a code from category Z3A should represent only the gestational weeks upon admission.

5) Unspecified trimester

Each category that includes codes for trimester has a code for "unspecified trimester." The "unspecified trimester" code should rarely be used, such as when the documentation in the record is insufficient to determine the trimester and it is not possible to obtain clarification.

6) 7th character for fetus identification

Where applicable, a 7th character is to be assigned for certain categories (O31, O32, O33.3 - O33.6, O35, O36, O40, O41, O60.1, O60.2, O64, and O69) to identify the fetus for which the complication code applies.

Assign 7th character "0":

- For single gestations
- When the documentation in the record is insufficient to determine the fetus affected and it is not possible to obtain clarification.
- When it is not possible to clinically determine which fetus is affected.

Maternal patient with twin gestations is seen after ultrasound identifies fetus B to be in breech presentation	
O32.1XX2	**Maternal care for breech presentation, fetus 2**

Explanation: The documentation indicates that although there are two fetuses, only one fetus is determined to be in breech presentation. Whether fetus 2 or fetus B is used, the coder can assign the seventh character of 2 to identify the second fetus as the one in breech.

b. Selection of OB principal or first-listed diagnosis

1) Routine outpatient prenatal visits

For routine outpatient prenatal visits when no complications are present, a code from category Z34, Encounter for supervision of normal pregnancy, should be used as the first-listed diagnosis. These codes should not be used in conjunction with chapter 15 codes.

2) Prenatal outpatient visits for high-risk patients

For routine prenatal outpatient visits for patients with high-risk pregnancies, a code from category O09, Supervision of high-risk pregnancy, should be used as the first-listed diagnosis. Secondary chapter 15 codes may be used in conjunction with these codes if appropriate.

3) Episodes when no delivery occurs

In episodes when no delivery occurs, the principal diagnosis should correspond to the principal complication of the pregnancy which necessitated the encounter. Should more than one complication exist, all of which are treated or monitored, any of the complications codes may be sequenced first.

4) When a delivery occurs

When a delivery occurs, the principal diagnosis should correspond to the main circumstances or complication of the delivery. In cases of cesarean delivery, the selection of the principal diagnosis should be the condition established after study that was responsible for the patient's admission. If the patient was admitted with a condition that resulted in the performance of a cesarean procedure, that condition should be selected as the principal diagnosis. If the reason for the admission/encounter was unrelated to the condition resulting in the cesarean delivery, the condition related to the reason for the admission/encounter should be selected as the principal diagnosis.

Maternal patient with diet-controlled gestational diabetes was admitted at 38 weeks' gestation in obstructed labor due to footling presentation; cesarean performed for the malpresentation

O64.8XX0	Obstructed labor due to other malposition and malpresentation, fetus not applicable or unspecified
O24.420	Gestational diabetes mellitus in childbirth, diet controlled
Z3A.38	38 weeks gestation of pregnancy
Z37.0	Single live birth

Explanation: The obstructed labor necessitated the cesarean procedure.

At 39 weeks' gestation, a maternal patient presents with hemorrhage with coagulation defect; the next day the patient goes into labor and eventually delivers via cesarean section due to arrested active phase of labor

O46.003	Antepartum hemorrhage with coagulation defect, unspecified, third trimester
O62.1	Secondary uterine inertia
Z3A.39	39 weeks gestation of pregnancy
Z37.0	Single live birth

Explanation: The patient was admitted because of the antepartum hemorrhage with coagulation defect. The arrested active phase, although the reason for the cesarean delivery, did not develop until later into the stay.

5) Outcome of delivery

A code from category Z37, Outcome of delivery, should be included on every maternal record when a delivery has occurred. These codes are not to be used on subsequent records or on the newborn record.

c. Pre-existing conditions versus conditions due to the pregnancy

Certain categories in Chapter 15 distinguish between conditions of the mother that existed prior to pregnancy (pre-existing) and those that are a direct result of pregnancy. When assigning codes from Chapter 15, it is important to assess if a condition was pre-existing prior to pregnancy or developed during or due to the pregnancy in order to assign the correct code.

Categories that do not distinguish between pre-existing and pregnancy-related conditions may be used for either. It is acceptable to use codes specifically for the puerperium with codes complicating pregnancy and childbirth if a condition arises postpartum during the delivery encounter.

d. Pre-existing hypertension in pregnancy

Category O10, Pre-existing hypertension complicating pregnancy, childbirth and the puerperium, includes codes for hypertensive heart and hypertensive chronic kidney disease. When assigning one of the O10 codes that includes hypertensive heart disease or hypertensive chronic kidney disease, it is necessary to add a secondary code from the appropriate hypertension category to specify the type of heart failure or chronic kidney disease.

See Section I.C.9. Hypertension.

e. Fetal conditions affecting the management of the mother

1) Codes from categories O35 and O36

Codes from categories O35, Maternal care for known or suspected fetal abnormality and damage, and O36, Maternal care for other fetal problems, are assigned only when the fetal condition is actually responsible for modifying the management of the mother, i.e., by requiring diagnostic studies, additional observation, special care, or termination of pregnancy. The fact that the fetal condition exists does not justify assigning a code from this series to the mother's record.

A patient is seen for spotting 15 weeks into her pregnancy; the doctors also suspect fetal hydrocephalus

O26.852	Spotting complicating pregnancy
Z3A.15	15 weeks gestation of pregnancy

Explanation: Whether the fetal hydrocephalus was suspected or confirmed, an additional code is not warranted for this condition as the documentation does not indicate that this fetal condition is in any way altering the management of the mother or complicating her pregnancy.

2) In utero surgery

In cases when surgery is performed on the fetus, a diagnosis code from category O35, Maternal care for known or suspected fetal abnormality and damage, should be assigned identifying the fetal condition. Assign the appropriate procedure code for the procedure performed.

No code from Chapter 16, the perinatal codes, should be used on the mother's record to identify fetal conditions. Surgery performed in utero on a fetus is still to be coded as an obstetric encounter.

f. HIV infection in pregnancy, childbirth and the puerperium

During pregnancy, childbirth or the puerperium, a patient admitted because of an HIV-related illness should receive a principal diagnosis from subcategory O98.7-, Human immunodeficiency [HIV] disease complicating pregnancy, childbirth and the puerperium, followed by the code(s) for the HIV-related illness(es).

Patients with asymptomatic HIV infection status admitted during pregnancy, childbirth, or the puerperium should receive codes of O98.7- and Z21, Asymptomatic human immunodeficiency virus [HIV] infection status.

A previously asymptomatic HIV patient who is 13 weeks pregnant is admitted with oral thrush

O98.711	Human immunodeficiency virus [HIV] disease complicating pregnancy, first trimester
B20	Human immunodeficiency virus [HIV] disease
B37.0	Candidal stomatitis
Z3A.13	13 weeks gestation of pregnancy

Explanation: Because oral thrush is an HIV-related condition, this patient is now considered to have HIV disease. An obstetrics code indicating that HIV is complicating the pregnancy is coded first, followed by B20 for HIV disease as well as a code for the oral thrush.

g. Diabetes mellitus in pregnancy

Diabetes mellitus is a significant complicating factor in pregnancy. Pregnant women who are diabetic should be assigned a code from category O24, Diabetes mellitus in pregnancy, childbirth, and the puerperium, first, followed by the appropriate diabetes code(s) (E08-E13) from Chapter 4.

h. Long term use of insulin

Code Z79.4, Long-term (current) use of insulin, should also be assigned if the diabetes mellitus is being treated with insulin.

i. Gestational (pregnancy induced) diabetes

Gestational (pregnancy induced) diabetes can occur during the second and third trimester of pregnancy in women who were not diabetic prior to pregnancy. Gestational diabetes can cause complications in the pregnancy similar to those of pre-existing diabetes mellitus. It also puts the woman at greater risk of developing diabetes after the pregnancy. Codes for gestational diabetes are in subcategory O24.4, Gestational diabetes mellitus. No other code from category O24, Diabetes mellitus in pregnancy, childbirth, and the puerperium, should be used with a code from O24.4.

The codes under subcategory O24.4 include diet controlled and insulin controlled. If a patient with gestational diabetes is treated with both diet and insulin, only the code for insulin-controlled is required.

Code Z79.4, Long-term (current) use of insulin, should not be assigned with codes from subcategory O24.4.

An abnormal glucose tolerance in pregnancy is assigned a code from subcategory O99.81, Abnormal glucose complicating pregnancy, childbirth, and the puerperium.

j. Sepsis and septic shock complicating abortion, pregnancy, childbirth and the puerperium

When assigning a chapter 15 code for sepsis complicating abortion, pregnancy, childbirth, and the puerperium, a code for the specific type of infection should be assigned as an additional diagnosis. If severe sepsis is present, a code from subcategory R65.2, Severe sepsis, and code(s) for associated organ dysfunction(s) should also be assigned as additional diagnoses.

Patient is seen several days after a miscarriage with sepsis; cultures return MSSA

O03.87	Sepsis following complete or unspecified spontaneous abortion
B95.61	Methicillin susceptible Staphylococcus aureus infection as the cause of diseases classified elsewhere

Explanation: The type of infection that caused this patient to become septic was methicillin susceptible *Staphylococcus aureus* (MSSA), which as a secondary code helps capture all aspects related to this patient's septic condition.

k. Puerperal sepsis

Code O85, Puerperal sepsis, should be assigned with a secondary code to identify the causal organism (e.g., for a bacterial infection, assign a code from category B95-B96, Bacterial infections in conditions classified elsewhere). A code from category A40, Streptococcal sepsis, or A41, Other sepsis, should not be used for puerperal sepsis. If applicable, use additional codes to identify severe sepsis (R65.2-) and any associated acute organ dysfunction.

l. Alcohol and tobacco use during pregnancy, childbirth and the puerperium

1) Alcohol use during pregnancy, childbirth and the puerperium

Codes under subcategory O99.31, Alcohol use complicating pregnancy, childbirth, and the puerperium, should be assigned for any pregnancy case when a mother uses alcohol during the pregnancy or postpartum. A secondary code from category F10, Alcohol related disorders, should also be assigned to identify manifestations of the alcohol use.

2) Tobacco use during pregnancy, childbirth and the puerperium

Codes under subcategory O99.33, Smoking (tobacco) complicating pregnancy, childbirth, and the puerperium, should be assigned for any pregnancy case when a mother uses any type of tobacco product during the pregnancy or postpartum. A secondary code from category F17, Nicotine dependence, should also be assigned to identify the type of nicotine dependence.

m. Poisoning, toxic effects, adverse effects and underdosing in a pregnant patient

A code from subcategory O9A.2, Injury, poisoning and certain other consequences of external causes complicating pregnancy, childbirth, and the puerperium, should be sequenced first, followed by the appropriate injury, poisoning, toxic effect, adverse effect or underdosing code, and then the additional code(s) that specifies the condition caused by the poisoning, toxic effect, adverse effect or underdosing.

See Section I.C.19. Adverse effects, poisoning, underdosing and toxic effects.

Patient admitted with accidental carbon monoxide poisoning from a gas heating implement; the patient is 18 weeks' pregnant

O9A.212	Injury, poisoning and certain other consequences of external causes complicating pregnancy, second trimester
T58.11XA	Toxic effect of carbon monoxide from utility gas, accidental (unintentional), initial encounter
Z3A.18	18 weeks gestation of pregnancy

Explanation: Although the carbon monoxide poisoning is the reason the patient was admitted, a code from the obstetrics chapter must be sequenced first. Chapter 15 codes have sequencing priority over codes from other chapters.

n. Normal delivery, code O80

1) Encounter for full term uncomplicated delivery

Code O80 should be assigned when a woman is admitted for a full-term normal delivery and delivers a single, healthy infant without any complications antepartum, during the delivery, or postpartum during the delivery episode. Code O80 is always a principal diagnosis. It is not to be used if any other code from chapter 15 is needed to describe a current complication of the antenatal, delivery, or perinatal period. Additional codes from other chapters may be used with code O80 if they are not related to or are in any way complicating the pregnancy.

2) Uncomplicated delivery with resolved antepartum complication

Code O80 may be used if the patient had a complication at some point during the pregnancy, but the complication is not present at the time of the admission for delivery.

Patient presents in labor at 39 weeks' gestation and delivers a healthy newborn; patient had abnormal glucose levels in her first trimester, which have since resolved

O80	Encounter for full-term uncomplicated delivery
Z37.0	Single live birth

Explanation: The abnormal glucose levels during the first trimester cannot be coded if they are not affecting the patient's current trimester. Without additional complications associated with the pregnancy, fetus, or mother, code O80 is appropriate.

3) Outcome of delivery for O80

Z37.0, Single live birth, is the only outcome of delivery code appropriate for use with O80.

o. The peripartum and postpartum periods

1) Peripartum and postpartum periods

The postpartum period begins immediately after delivery and continues for six weeks following delivery. The peripartum period is defined as the last month of pregnancy to five months postpartum.

2) Peripartum and postpartum complication

A postpartum complication is any complication occurring within the six-week period.

3) Pregnancy-related complications after 6 week period

Chapter 15 codes may also be used to describe pregnancy-related complications after the peripartum or postpartum period if the provider documents that a condition is pregnancy related.

Patient admitted for varicose veins. She had a baby boy three months ago; the varicose veins started to appear one month ago. The doctor attributes the patient's pregnancy as the cause of the varicose veins, which continue to be painful and bother the patient. She is seeking surgical relief.

O87.4	Varicose veins of the lower extremity in the puerperium

Explanation: Although the varicose veins occurred several months after the delivery of the newborn, the doctor attributed the varicose veins to pregnancy and therefore a code from chapter 15 is appropriate.

4) Admission for routine postpartum care following delivery outside hospital

When the mother delivers outside the hospital prior to admission and is admitted for routine postpartum care and no complications are noted, code Z39.0, Encounter for care and examination of mother immediately after delivery, should be assigned as the principal diagnosis.

5) Pregnancy associated cardiomyopathy

Pregnancy associated cardiomyopathy, code O90.3, is unique in that it may be diagnosed in the third trimester of pregnancy but may continue to progress months after delivery. For this reason, it is referred to as peripartum cardiomyopathy. Code O90.3 is only for use when the cardiomyopathy develops as a result of pregnancy in a woman who did not have pre-existing heart disease.

p. Code O94, Sequelae of complication of pregnancy, childbirth, and the puerperium

1) Code O94

Code O94, Sequelae of complication of pregnancy, childbirth, and the puerperium, is for use in those cases when an initial complication of a pregnancy develops a sequelae requiring care or treatment at a future date.

2) After the initial postpartum period

This code may be used at any time after the initial postpartum period.

3) Sequencing of code O94

This code, like all sequela codes, is to be sequenced following the code describing the sequelae of the complication.

q. Termination of pregnancy and spontaneous abortions

1) Abortion with liveborn fetus

When an attempted termination of pregnancy results in a liveborn fetus, assign code Z33.2, Encounter for elective termination of pregnancy and a code from category Z37, Outcome of Delivery.

2) Retained products of conception following an abortion

Subsequent encounters for retained products of conception following a spontaneous abortion or elective termination of pregnancy are assigned the appropriate code from category O03, Spontaneous abortion, or codes O07.4, Failed attempted termination of pregnancy without complication and Z33.2, Encounter for elective termination of pregnancy. This advice is appropriate even when the patient was discharged previously with a discharge diagnosis of complete abortion.

> Patient was seen two days ago for complete spontaneous abortion but returns today for urinary tract infection (UTI) with ultrasound showing retained products of conception
>
> **O03.38   Urinary tract infection following incomplete spontaneous abortion**
>
> *Explanation:* Although the diagnosis from the patient's previous stay indicated that the patient had a complete abortion, it is now determined that there were actually retained products of conception (POC). An abortion with retained POC is considered incomplete and in this case resulted in the patient developing a UTI.

3) Complications leading to abortion

Codes from Chapter 15 may be used as additional codes to identify any documented complications of the pregnancy in conjunction with codes in categories in O07 and O08.

r. Abuse in a pregnant patient

For suspected or confirmed cases of abuse of a pregnant patient, a code(s) from subcategories O9A.3, Physical abuse complicating pregnancy, childbirth, and the puerperium, O9A.4, Sexual abuse complicating pregnancy, childbirth, and the puerperium, and O9A.5, Psychological abuse complicating pregnancy, childbirth, and the puerperium, should be sequenced first, followed by the appropriate codes (if applicable) to identify any associated current injury due to physical abuse, sexual abuse, and the perpetrator of abuse.

See Section I.C.19. Adult and child abuse, neglect and other maltreatment.

Chapter 15. Pregnancy, Childbirth and the Puerperium (O00-O9A)

NOTE   CODES FROM THIS CHAPTER ARE FOR USE ONLY ON MATERNAL RECORDS, NEVER ON NEWBORN RECORDS.

Codes from this chapter are for use for conditions related to or aggravated by the pregnancy, childbirth, or by the puerperium (maternal causes or obstetric causes).

NOTE   Trimesters are counted from the first day of the last menstrual period. They are defined as follows:

1st trimester- less than 14 weeks 0 days
2nd trimester- 14 weeks 0 days to less than 28 weeks 0 days
3rd trimester- 28 weeks 0 days until delivery.

Use additional code from category Z3A, Weeks of gestation, to identify the specific week of the pregnancy

EXCLUDES 1   *supervision of normal pregnancy (Z34.-)*
EXCLUDES 2   *mental and behavioral disorders associated with the puerperium (F53)*
obstetrical tetanus (A34)
postpartum necrosis of pituitary gland (E23.0)
puerperal osteomalacia (M83.0)

AHA: 2014, 3Q, 17

This chapter contains the following blocks:

O00-O08	Pregnancy with abortive outcome
O09	Supervision of high risk pregnancy
O10-O16	Edema, proteinuria and hypertensive disorders in pregnancy, childbirth and the puerperium
O20-O29	Other maternal disorders predominantly related to pregnancy
O30-O48	Maternal care related to the fetus and amniotic cavity and possible delivery problems
O60-O77	Complications of labor and delivery
O80, O82	Encounter for delivery
O85-O92	Complications predominantly related to the puerperium
O94-O9A	Other obstetric conditions, not elsewhere classified

Pregnancy with abortive outcome (O00-O08)

EXCLUDES 1   *continuing pregnancy in multiple gestation after abortion of one fetus or more (O31.1-, O31.3-)*

√4ᵗʰ O00   Ectopic pregnancy
   INCLUDES   ruptured ectopic pregnancy
   Use additional code from category O08 to identify any associated complication
   AHA: 2014, 3Q, 17

   O00.0   Abdominal pregnancy   Ⓜ♀
      EXCLUDES 1   *maternal care for viable fetus in abdominal pregnancy (O36.7-)*

   O00.1   Tubal pregnancy   Ⓜ♀
      Fallopian pregnancy
      Rupture of (fallopian) tube due to pregnancy
      Tubal abortion

   O00.2   Ovarian pregnancy   Ⓜ♀

   O00.8   Other ectopic pregnancy   Ⓜ♀
      Cervical pregnancy
      Cornual pregnancy
      Intraligamentous pregnancy
      Mural pregnancy

   O00.9   Ectopic pregnancy, unspecified   Ⓜ♀▽

√4ᵗʰ O01   Hydatidiform mole
   Use additional code from category O08 to identify any associated complication
      EXCLUDES 1   *chorioadenoma (destruens) (D39.2)*
         malignant hydatidiform mole (D39.2)
   AHA: 2014, 3Q, 17

   O01.0   Classical hydatidiform mole   Ⓜ♀
      Complete hydatidiform mole

   O01.1   Incomplete and partial hydatidiform mole   Ⓜ♀

   O01.9   Hydatidiform mole, unspecified   Ⓜ♀▽
      Trophoblastic disease NOS
      Vesicular mole NOS

√4ᵗʰ O02   Other abnormal products of conception
   Use additional code from category O08 to identify any associated complication
      EXCLUDES 1   *papyraceous fetus (O31.0-)*
   AHA: 2014, 3Q, 17

   O02.0   Blighted ovum and nonhydatidiform mole   Ⓜ♀
      Carneous mole
      Fleshy mole
      Intrauterine mole NOS
      Molar pregnancy NEC
      Pathological ovum

   O02.1   Missed abortion   Ⓜ♀
      Early fetal death, before completion of 20 weeks of gestation, with retention of dead fetus
      EXCLUDES 1   *failed induced abortion (O07.-)*
         fetal death (intrauterine) (late) (O36.4)
         missed abortion with blighted ovum (O02.0)
         missed abortion with hydatidiform mole (O01.-)
         missed abortion with nonhydatidiform (O02.0)
         missed abortion with other abnormal products of conception (O02.8-)
         missed delivery (O36.4)
         stillbirth (P95)

   √5ᵗʰ O02.8   Other specified abnormal products of conception
      EXCLUDES 1   *abnormal products of conception with blighted ovum (O02.0)*
         abnormal products of conception with hydatidiform mole (O01.-)
         abnormal products of conception with nonhydatidiform mole (O02.0)

      O02.81   Inappropriate change in quantitative human chorionic gonadotropin (hCG) in early pregnancy   Ⓜ♀
         Biochemical pregnancy
         Chemical pregnancy
         Inappropriate level of quantitative human chorionic gonadotropin (hCG) for gestational age in early pregnancy

      O02.89   Other abnormal products of conception   Ⓜ♀

   O02.9   Abnormal product of conception, unspecified   Ⓜ♀▽

√4ᵗʰ O03   Spontaneous abortion
   NOTE   Incomplete abortion includes retained products of conception following spontaneous abortion
   INCLUDES   miscarriage

   O03.0   Genital tract and pelvic infection following incomplete spontaneous abortion   Ⓜ♀
      Endometritis following incomplete spontaneous abortion
      Oophoritis following incomplete spontaneous abortion
      Parametritis following incomplete spontaneous abortion
      Pelvic peritonitis following incomplete spontaneous abortion
      Salpingitis following incomplete spontaneous abortion
      Salpingo-oophoritis following incomplete spontaneous abortion
      EXCLUDES 1   *sepsis following incomplete spontaneous abortion (O03.37)*
         urinary tract infection following incomplete spontaneous abortion (O03.38)

   O03.1   Delayed or excessive hemorrhage following incomplete spontaneous abortion   Ⓜ♀
      Afibrinogenemia following incomplete spontaneous abortion
      Defibrination syndrome following incomplete spontaneous abortion
      Hemolysis following incomplete spontaneous abortion
      Intravascular coagulation following incomplete spontaneous abortion

   O03.2   Embolism following incomplete spontaneous abortion   Ⓜ♀
      Air embolism following incomplete spontaneous abortion
      Amniotic fluid embolism following incomplete spontaneous abortion
      Blood-clot embolism following incomplete spontaneous abortion
      Embolism NOS following incomplete spontaneous abortion
      Fat embolism following incomplete spontaneous abortion
      Pulmonary embolism following incomplete spontaneous abortion
      Pyemic embolism following incomplete spontaneous abortion
      Septic or septicopyemic embolism following incomplete spontaneous abortion
      Soap embolism following incomplete spontaneous abortion

   √5ᵗʰ O03.3   Other and unspecified complications following incomplete spontaneous abortion

      O03.30   Unspecified complication following incomplete spontaneous abortion   Ⓜ♀▽

      O03.31   Shock following incomplete spontaneous abortion   Ⓜ♀
         Circulatory collapse following incomplete spontaneous abortion
         Shock (postprocedural) following incomplete spontaneous abortion
         EXCLUDES 1   *shock due to infection following incomplete spontaneous abortion (O03.37)*

☑ Add'l Character Required   ☑x7ᵗʰ Placeholder Alert   RUG IV Special Care High Dx   RUG IV Clinically Complex Dx   RUG IV Special Care Low Dx   Manifestation Code   Other Specified Code   ▽Unspecified Code

ICD-10-CM 2016   775

Chapter 15. Pregnancy, Childbirth and the Puerperium

O03.32   **Renal failure following incomplete spontaneous** Ⓜ♀
   abortion
     Kidney failure (acute) following incomplete
       spontaneous abortion
     Oliguria following incomplete spontaneous abortion
     Renal shutdown following incomplete spontaneous
       abortion
     Renal tubular necrosis following incomplete
       spontaneous abortion
     Uremia following incomplete spontaneous abortion

O03.33   **Metabolic disorder following incomplete** Ⓜ♀
   spontaneous abortion

O03.34   **Damage to pelvic organs following incomplete** Ⓜ♀
   spontaneous abortion
     Laceration, perforation, tear or chemical damage of
       bladder following incomplete spontaneous
       abortion
     Laceration, perforation, tear or chemical damage of
       bowel following incomplete spontaneous
       abortion
     Laceration, perforation, tear or chemical damage of
       broad ligament following incomplete
       spontaneous abortion
     Laceration, perforation, tear or chemical damage of
       cervix following incomplete spontaneous
       abortion
     Laceration, perforation, tear or chemical damage of
       periurethral tissue following incomplete
       spontaneous abortion
     Laceration, perforation, tear or chemical damage of
       uterus following incomplete spontaneous
       abortion
     Laceration, perforation, tear or chemical damage of
       vagina following incomplete spontaneous
       abortion

O03.35   **Other venous complications following** Ⓜ♀
   incomplete spontaneous abortion

O03.36   **Cardiac arrest following incomplete** Ⓜ♀
   spontaneousabortion

O03.37   **Sepsis following incomplete spontaneous** Ⓜ♀
   abortion
     Use additional code to identify infectious agent
       (B95-B97)
     Use additional code to identify severe sepsis, if
       applicable (R65.2-)
     EXCLUDES 1   *septic or septicopyemic embolism following*
       incomplete spontaneous abortion
       (O03.2)

O03.38   **Urinary tract infection following incomplete** Ⓜ♀
   spontaneous abortion
     Cystitis following incomplete spontaneous abortion

O03.39   **Incomplete spontaneous abortion with other** Ⓜ♀
   complications

O03.4   **Incomplete spontaneous abortion without complication** Ⓜ♀

O03.5   **Genital tract and pelvic infection following complete** Ⓜ♀
  or unspecified spontaneous abortion
     Endometritis following complete or unspecified spontaneous
       abortion
     Oophoritis following complete or unspecified spontaneous
       abortion
     Parametritis following complete or unspecified spontaneous
       abortion
     Pelvic peritonitis following complete or unspecified
       spontaneous abortion
     Salpingitis following complete or unspecified spontaneous
       abortion
     Salpingo-oophoritis following complete or unspecified
       spontaneous abortion
     EXCLUDES 1   *sepsis following complete or unspecified spontaneous*
       abortion (O03.87)
       urinary tract infection following complete or
       unspecified spontaneous abortion (O03.88)

O03.6   **Delayed or excessive hemorrhage following complete or** Ⓜ♀
  unspecified spontaneous abortion
     Afibrinogenemia following complete or unspecified
       spontaneous abortion
     Defibrination syndrome following complete or unspecified
       spontaneous abortion
     Hemolysis following complete or unspecified spontaneous
       abortion
     Intravascular coagulation following complete or unspecified
       spontaneous abortion

O03.7   **Embolism following complete or unspecified** Ⓜ♀
  spontaneous abortion
     Air embolism following complete or unspecified spontaneous
       abortion
     Amniotic fluid embolism following complete or unspecified
       spontaneous abortion
     Blood-clot embolism following complete or unspecified
       spontaneous abortion
     Embolism NOS following complete or unspecified spontaneous
       abortion
     Fat embolism following complete or unspecified spontaneous
       abortion
     Pulmonary embolism following complete or unspecified
       spontaneous abortion
     Pyemic embolism following complete or unspecified
       spontaneous abortion
     Septic or septicopyemic embolism following complete or
       unspecified spontaneous abortion
     Soap embolism following complete or unspecified spontaneous
       abortion

✓5ᵗʰ **O03.8**   **Other and unspecified complications following complete**
  or unspecified spontaneous abortion

O03.80   **Unspecified complication following complete** Ⓜ♀▽
   or unspecified spontaneous abortion

O03.81   **Shock following complete or unspecified** Ⓜ♀
   spontaneous abortion
     Circulatory collapse following complete or unspecified
       spontaneous abortion
     Shock (postprocedural) following complete or
       unspecified spontaneous abortion
     EXCLUDES 1   *shock due to infection following complete or*
       unspecified spontaneous abortion
       (O03.87)

O03.82   **Renal failure following complete or** Ⓜ♀
   unspecified spontaneous abortion
     Kidney failure (acute) following complete or
       unspecified spontaneous abortion
     Oliguria following complete or unspecified
       spontaneous abortion
     Renal shutdown following complete or unspecified
       spontaneous abortion
     Renal tubular necrosis following complete or
       unspecified spontaneous abortion
     Uremia following complete or unspecified
       spontaneous abortion

O03.83   **Metabolic disorder following complete or** Ⓜ♀
   unspecified spontaneous abortion

O03.84   **Damage to pelvic organs following complete** Ⓜ♀
   or unspecified spontaneous abortion
     Laceration, perforation, tear or chemical damage of
       bladder following complete or unspecified
       spontaneous abortion
     Laceration, perforation, tear or chemical damage of
       bowel following complete or unspecified
       spontaneous abortion
     Laceration, perforation, tear or chemical damage of
       broad ligament following complete or
       unspecified spontaneous abortion
     Laceration, perforation, tear or chemical damage of
       cervix following complete or unspecified
       spontaneous abortion
     Laceration, perforation, tear or chemical damage of
       periurethral tissue following complete or
       unspecified spontaneous abortion
     Laceration, perforation, tear or chemical damage of
       uterus following complete or unspecified
       spontaneous abortion
     Laceration, perforation, tear or chemical damage of
       vagina following complete or unspecified
       spontaneous abortion

O03.85   **Other venous complications following** Ⓜ♀
   complete or unspecified spontaneous abortion

O03.86   **Cardiac arrest following complete or** Ⓜ♀
   unspecified spontaneous abortion

O03.87   **Sepsis following complete or unspecified** Ⓜ♀
   spontaneous abortion
     Use additional code to identify infectious agent
       (B95-B97)
     Use additional code to identify severe sepsis, if
       applicable (R65.2-)
     EXCLUDES 1   *septic or septicopyemic embolism following*
       complete or unspecified spontaneous
       abortion (O03.7)

Ⓝ Newborn   Ⓟ Pediatric   Ⓜ Maternity   Ⓐ Adult   **RIC** RIC Dx   **NC Dx** Noncancer Dx   **PDx** Primary Dx   **CC** RIC CC Condition   ▶◀ Revised Text   ● New Code   ▲ Revised Code Title

O03.88   Urinary tract infection **following complete or**   Ⓜ♀
unspecified spontaneous abortion
Cystitis following complete or unspecified
spontaneous abortion

O03.89   **Complete or unspecified spontaneous abortion**   Ⓜ♀
with other complications

O03.9   **Complete or unspecified spontaneous abortion**   Ⓜ♀▽
without complication
Miscarriage NOS
Spontaneous abortion NOS

✓4ᵗʰ **O04**   Complications **following (induced)** termination of pregnancy
INCLUDES   complications following (induced) termination of pregnancy
EXCLUDES 1   encounter for elective termination of pregnancy, uncomplicated
(Z33.2)
failed attempted termination of pregnancy (O07.-)

O04.5   Genital tract and pelvic infection **following (induced)**   Ⓜ♀
termination of pregnancy
Endometritis following (induced) termination of pregnancy
Oophoritis following (induced) termination of pregnancy
Parametritis following (induced) termination of pregnancy
Pelvic peritonitis following (induced) termination of pregnancy
Salpingitis following (induced) termination of pregnancy
Salpingo-oophoritis following (induced) termination of
pregnancy
EXCLUDES 1   sepsis following (induced) termination of pregnancy
(O04.87)
urinary tract infection following (induced) termination
of pregnancy (O04.88)

O04.6   Delayed or excessive hemorrhage **following (induced)**   Ⓜ♀
termination of pregnancy
Afibrinogenemia following (induced) termination of pregnancy
Defibrination syndrome following (induced) termination of
pregnancy
Hemolysis following (induced) termination of pregnancy
Intravascular coagulation following (induced) termination of
pregnancy

O04.7   Embolism **following (induced) termination of pregnancy**   Ⓜ♀
Air embolism following (induced) termination of pregnancy
Amniotic fluid embolism following (induced) termination of
pregnancy
Blood-clot embolism following (induced) termination of
pregnancy
Embolism NOS following (induced) termination of pregnancy
Fat embolism following (induced) termination of pregnancy
Pulmonary embolism following (induced) termination of
pregnancy
Pyemic embolism following (induced) termination of pregnancy
Septic or septicopyemic embolism following (induced)
termination of pregnancy
Soap embolism following (induced) termination of pregnancy

✓5ᵗʰ **O04.8**   **(Induced) termination of pregnancy with other and**
unspecified complications

O04.80   **(Induced) termination of pregnancy with**   Ⓜ♀▽
unspecified complications

O04.81   **Shock following (induced) termination of**   Ⓜ♀
pregnancy
Circulatory collapse following (induced) termination of
pregnancy
Shock (postprocedural) following (induced)
termination of pregnancy
EXCLUDES 1   shock due to infection following (induced)
termination of pregnancy (O04.87)

O04.82   **Renal failure following (induced) termination**   Ⓜ♀
of pregnancy
Kidney failure (acute) following (induced) termination
of pregnancy
Oliguria following (induced) termination of pregnancy
Renal shutdown following (induced) termination of
pregnancy
Renal tubular necrosis following (induced) termination
of pregnancy
Uremia following (induced) termination of pregnancy

O04.83   **Metabolic disorder following (induced)**   Ⓜ♀
termination of pregnancy

O04.84   **Damage to pelvic organs following (induced)**   Ⓜ♀
termination of pregnancy
Laceration, perforation, tear or chemical damage of
bladder following (induced) termination of
pregnancy
Laceration, perforation, tear or chemical damage of
bowel following (induced) termination of
pregnancy
Laceration, perforation, tear or chemical damage of
broad ligament following (induced) termination
of pregnancy
Laceration, perforation, tear or chemical damage of
cervix following (induced) termination of
pregnancy
Laceration, perforation, tear or chemical damage of
periurethral tissue following (induced)
termination of pregnLaceration, perforation, tear
or chemical damage of uterus following
(induced) termination of pregnancy
Laceration, perforation, tear or chemical damage of
vagina following (induced) termination of
pregnancy

O04.85   **Other venous complications following**   Ⓜ♀
(induced) termination of pregnancy

O04.86   **Cardiac arrest following (induced) termination**   Ⓜ♀
of pregnancy

O04.87   **Sepsis following (induced) termination of**   Ⓜ♀
pregnancy
Use additional code to identify infectious agent
(B95-B97)
Use additional code to identify severe sepsis, if
applicable (R65.2-)
EXCLUDES 1   septic or septicopyemic embolism following
(induced) termination of pregnancy
(O04.7)

O04.88   **Urinary tract infection following (induced)**   Ⓜ♀
termination of pregnancy
Cystitis following (induced) termination of pregnancy

O04.89   **(Induced) termination of pregnancy with**   Ⓜ♀
other complications

✓4ᵗʰ **O07**   Failed attempted termination **of pregnancy**
INCLUDES   failure of attempted induction of termination of pregnancy
incomplete elective abortion
EXCLUDES 1   incomplete spontaneous abortion (O03.0-)

O07.0   Genital tract and pelvic infection **following failed**   Ⓜ♀
attempted termination of pregnancy
Endometritis following failed attempted termination of
pregnancy
Oophoritis following failed attempted termination of pregnancy
Parametritis following failed attempted termination of
pregnancy
Pelvic peritonitis following failed attempted termination of
pregnancy
Salpingitis following failed attempted termination of pregnancy
Salpingo-oophoritis following failed attempted termination of
pregnancy
EXCLUDES 1   sepsis following failed attempted termination of
pregnancy (O07.37)
urinary tract infection following failed attempted
termination of pregnancy (O07.38)

O07.1   Delayed or excessive hemorrhage **following failed**   Ⓜ♀
attempted termination of pregnancy
Afibrinogenemia following failed attempted termination of
pregnancy
Defibrination syndrome following failed attempted termination
of pregnancy
Hemolysis following failed attempted termination of pregnancy
Intravascular coagulation following failed attempted
termination of pregnancy

✓ Add'l Character Required   ✓x7ᵗʰ Placeholder Alert   RUG IV Special Care High Dx   RUG IV Clinically Complex Dx   RUG IV Special Care Low Dx   Manifestation Code   Other Specified Code   ▽ Unspecified Code

ICD-10-CM 2016   777

Chapter 15. Pregnancy, Childbirth and the Puerperium *(side margin)*

O07.2   **Embolism following failed attempted termination of** Ⓜ♀
    pregnancy
      Air embolism following failed attempted termination of pregnancy
      Amniotic fluid embolism following failed attempted termination of pregnancy
      Blood-clot embolism following failed attempted termination of pregnancy
      Embolism NOS following failed attempted termination of pregnancy
      Fat embolism following failed attempted termination of pregnancy
      Pulmonary embolism following failed attempted termination of pregnancy
      Pyemic embolism following failed attempted termination of pregnancy
      Septic or septicopyemic embolism following failed attempted termination of pregnancy
      Soap embolism following failed attempted termination of pregnancy

✓5ᵗʰ **O07.3**   **Failed attempted termination of pregnancy with other and**
    unspecified complications

    O07.30   **Failed attempted termination of pregnancy** Ⓜ♀▽
          with unspecified complications

    O07.31   **Shock following failed attempted termination** Ⓜ♀
          of pregnancy
            Circulatory collapse following failed attempted termination of pregnancy
            Shock (postprocedural) following failed attempted termination of pregnancy
            EXCLUDES 1 *shock due to infection following failed attempted termination of pregnancy (O07.37)*

    O07.32   **Renal failure following failed attempted** Ⓜ♀
          termination of pregnancy
            Kidney failure (acute) following failed attempted termination of pregnancy
            Oliguria following failed attempted termination of pregnancy
            Renal shutdown following failed attempted termination of pregnancy
            Renal tubular necrosis following failed attempted termination of pregnancy
            Uremia following failed attempted termination of pregnancy

    O07.33   **Metabolic disorder following failed attempted** Ⓜ♀
          termination of pregnancy

    O07.34   **Damage to pelvic organs following failed** Ⓜ♀
          attempted termination of pregnancy
            Laceration, perforation, tear or chemical damage of bladder following failed attempted termination of pregnancy
            Laceration, perforation, tear or chemical damage of bowel following failed attempted termination of pregnancy
            Laceration, perforation, tear or chemical damage of broad ligament following failed attempted termination of pregnancy
            Laceration, perforation, tear or chemical damage of cervix following failed attempted termination of pregnancy
            Laceration, perforation, tear or chemical damage of periurethral tissue following failed attempted termination of pregnancy
            Laceration, perforation, tear or chemical damage of uterus following failed attempted termination of pregnancy
            Laceration, perforation, tear or chemical damage of vagina following failed attempted termination of pregnancy

    O07.35   **Other venous complications following failed** Ⓜ♀
          attempted termination of pregnancy

    O07.36   **Cardiac arrest following failed attempted** Ⓜ♀
          termination of pregnancy

O07.37   **Sepsis following failed attempted termination** Ⓜ♀
    of pregnancy
      Use additional code to identify infectious agent (B95-B97)
      Use additional code to identify severe sepsis, if applicable (R65.2-)
      EXCLUDES 1 *septic or septicopyemic embolism following failed attempted termination of pregnancy (O07.2)*

    O07.38   **Urinary tract infection following failed** Ⓜ♀
          attempted termination of pregnancy
            Cystitis following failed attempted termination of pregnancy

    O07.39   **Failed attempted termination of pregnancy** Ⓜ♀
          with other complications

O07.4   **Failed attempted termination of pregnancy** without Ⓜ♀
    complication

✓4ᵗʰ **O08**   **Complications following ectopic and molar pregnancy**
    This category is for use with categories O00-O02 to identify any associated complications

O08.0   **Genital tract and pelvic infection following ectopic and** Ⓜ♀
    molar pregnancy
      Endometritis following ectopic and molar pregnancy
      Oophoritis following ectopic and molar pregnancy
      Parametritis following ectopic and molar pregnancy
      Pelvic peritonitis following ectopic and molar pregnancy
      Salpingitis following ectopic and molar pregnancy
      Salpingo-oophoritis following ectopic and molar pregnancy
      EXCLUDES 1 *sepsis following ectopic and molar pregnancy (O08.82) urinary tract infection (O08.83)*

O08.1   **Delayed or excessive hemorrhage following ectopic and** Ⓜ♀
    molar pregnancy
      Afibrinogenemia following ectopic and molar pregnancy
      Defibrination syndrome following ectopic and molar pregnancy
      Hemolysis following ectopic and molar pregnancy
      Intravascular coagulation following ectopic and molar pregnancy
      EXCLUDES 1 *delayed or excessive hemorrhage due to incomplete abortion (O03.1)*

O08.2   **Embolism following ectopic and molar pregnancy** Ⓜ♀
      Air embolism following ectopic and molar pregnancy
      Amniotic fluid embolism following ectopic and molar pregnancy
      Blood-clot embolism following ectopic and molar pregnancy
      Embolism NOS following ectopic and molar pregnancy
      Fat embolism following ectopic and molar pregnancy
      Pulmonary embolism following ectopic and molar pregnancy
      Pyemic embolism following ectopic and molar pregnancy
      Septic or septicopyemic embolism following ectopic and molar pregnancy
      Soap embolism following ectopic and molar pregnancy

O08.3   **Shock following ectopic and molar pregnancy** Ⓜ♀
      Circulatory collapse following ectopic and molar pregnancy
      Shock (postprocedural) following ectopic and molar pregnancy
      EXCLUDES 1 *shock due to infection following ectopic and molar pregnancy (O08.82)*

O08.4   **Renal failure following ectopic and molar pregnancy** Ⓜ♀
      Kidney failure (acute) following ectopic and molar pregnancy
      Oliguria following ectopic and molar pregnancy
      Renal shutdown following ectopic and molar pregnancy
      Renal tubular necrosis following ectopic and molar pregnancy
      Uremia following ectopic and molar pregnancy

O08.5   **Metabolic disorders following an ectopic and molar** Ⓜ♀
    pregnancy

O08.6   **Damage to pelvic organs and tissues following an** Ⓜ♀
    ectopic and molar pregnancy
      Laceration, perforation, tear or chemical damage of bladder following an ectopic and molar pregnancy
      Laceration, perforation, tear or chemical damage of bowel following an ectopic and molar pregnancy
      Laceration, perforation, tear or chemical damage of broad ligament following an ectopic and molar pregnancy
      Laceration, perforation, tear or chemical damage of cervix following an ectopic and molar pregnancy
      Laceration, perforation, tear or chemical damage of periurethral tissue following an ectopic and molar pregnancy
      Laceration, perforation, tear or chemical damage of uterus following an ectopic and molar pregnancy
      Laceration, perforation, tear or chemical damage of vagina following an ectopic and molar pregnancy

O08.7   **Other venous complications following an ectopic** Ⓜ♀
    and molar pregnancy

Ⓝ Newborn   Ⓟ Pediatric   Ⓜ Maternity   Ⓐ Adult   **RIC** RIC Dx   **NC Dx** Noncancer Dx   **PDx** Primary Dx   **CC** RIC CC Condition   ►◄ Revised Text   ● New Code   ▲ Revised Code Title

√5ᵗʰ **O08.8** Other complications **following an ectopic and molar pregnancy**

    O08.81 Cardiac arrest **following an ectopic and molar pregnancy** Ⓜ♀

    O08.82 Sepsis **following ectopic and molar pregnancy** Ⓜ♀
       Use additional code to identify infectious agent (B95-B97)
       Use additional code to identify severe sepsis, if applicable (R65.2-)
       EXCLUDES 1 *septic or septicopyemic embolism following ectopic and molar pregnancy (O08.2)*

    O08.83 Urinary tract infection **following an ectopic and molar pregnancy** Ⓜ♀
       Cystitis following an ectopic and molar pregnancy

    O08.89 Other complications following an ectopic and molar pregnancy Ⓜ♀

O08.9 Unspecified complication following an ectopic and molar pregnancy Ⓜ♀▽

Supervision of high risk pregnancy (O09)

√4ᵗʰ **O09** Supervision of high risk **pregnancy**

√5ᵗʰ **O09.0** Supervision of pregnancy with history of infertility

    O09.00 Supervision of pregnancy with history of infertility, unspecified trimester Ⓜ♀▽

    O09.01 Supervision of pregnancy with history of infertility, first trimester Ⓜ♀

    O09.02 Supervision of pregnancy with history of infertility, second trimester Ⓜ♀

    O09.03 Supervision of pregnancy with history of infertility, third trimester Ⓜ♀

√5ᵗʰ **O09.1** Supervision of pregnancy with history of ectopic or molar pregnancy

    O09.10 Supervision of pregnancy with history of ectopic or molar pregnancy, unspecified trimester Ⓜ♀▽

    O09.11 Supervision of pregnancy with history of ectopic or molar pregnancy, first trimester Ⓜ♀

    O09.12 Supervision of pregnancy with history of ectopic or molar pregnancy, second trimester Ⓜ♀

    O09.13 Supervision of pregnancy with history of ectopic or molar pregnancy, third trimester Ⓜ♀

√5ᵗʰ **O09.2** Supervision of pregnancy with other poor reproductive or obstetric history
    EXCLUDES 2 *pregnancy care for patient with history of recurrent pregnancy loss (O26.2-)*

    √6ᵗʰ **O09.21** Supervision of pregnancy with history of pre-term labor

       O09.211 Supervision of pregnancy with history of pre-term labor, first trimester Ⓜ♀

       O09.212 Supervision of pregnancy with history of pre-term labor, second trimester Ⓜ♀

       O09.213 Supervision of pregnancy with history of pre-term labor, third trimester Ⓜ♀

       O09.219 Supervision of pregnancy with history of pre-term labor, unspecified trimester Ⓜ♀▽

    √6ᵗʰ **O09.29** Supervision of pregnancy with other poor reproductive or obstetric history
       Supervision of pregnancy with history of neonatal death
       Supervision of pregnancy with history of stillbirth

       O09.291 Supervision of pregnancy with other poor reproductive or obstetric history, first trimester Ⓜ♀

       O09.292 Supervision of pregnancy with other poor reproductive or obstetric history, second trimester Ⓜ♀

       O09.293 Supervision of pregnancy with other poor reproductive or obstetric history, third trimester Ⓜ♀

       O09.299 Supervision of pregnancy with other poor reproductive or obstetric history, unspecified trimester Ⓜ♀▽

√5ᵗʰ **O09.3** Supervision of pregnancy with insufficient antenatal care
    Supervision of concealed pregnancy
    Supervision of hidden pregnancy

    O09.30 Supervision of pregnancy with insufficient antenatal care, unspecified trimester Ⓜ♀▽

    O09.31 Supervision of pregnancy with insufficient antenatal care, first trimester Ⓜ♀

    O09.32 Supervision of pregnancy with insufficient antenatal care, second trimester Ⓜ♀

    O09.33 Supervision of pregnancy with insufficient antenatal care, third trimester Ⓜ♀

√5ᵗʰ **O09.4** Supervision of pregnancy with grand multiparity

    O09.40 Supervision of pregnancy with grand multiparity, unspecified trimester Ⓜ♀▽

    O09.41 Supervision of pregnancy with grand multiparity, first trimester Ⓜ♀

    O09.42 Supervision of pregnancy with grand multiparity, second trimester Ⓜ♀

    O09.43 Supervision of pregnancy with grand multiparity, third trimester Ⓜ♀

√5ᵗʰ **O09.5** Supervision of elderly primigravida and multigravida
    Pregnancy for a female 35 years and older at expected date of delivery

    √6ᵗʰ **O09.51** Supervision of elderly primigravida

       O09.511 Supervision of elderly primigravida, first trimester Ⓜ♀

       O09.512 Supervision of elderly primigravida, second trimester Ⓜ♀

       O09.513 Supervision of elderly primigravida, third trimester Ⓜ♀

       O09.519 Supervision of elderly primigravida, unspecified trimester Ⓜ♀▽

    √6ᵗʰ **O09.52** Supervision of elderly multigravida

       O09.521 Supervision of elderly multigravida, first trimester Ⓜ♀

       O09.522 Supervision of elderly multigravida, second trimester Ⓜ♀

       O09.523 Supervision of elderly multigravida, third trimester Ⓜ♀

       O09.529 Supervision of elderly multigravida, unspecified trimester Ⓜ♀▽

√5ᵗʰ **O09.6** Supervision of young primigravida and multigravida
    Supervision of pregnancy for a female less than 16 years old at expected date of delivery

    √6ᵗʰ **O09.61** Supervision of young primigravida

       O09.611 Supervision of young primigravida, first trimester Ⓜ♀

       O09.612 Supervision of young primigravida, second trimester Ⓜ♀

       O09.613 Supervision of young primigravida, third trimester Ⓜ♀

       O09.619 Supervision of young primigravida, unspecified trimester Ⓜ♀▽

    √6ᵗʰ **O09.62** Supervision of young multigravida

       O09.621 Supervision of young multigravida, first trimester Ⓜ♀

       O09.622 Supervision of young multigravida, second trimester Ⓜ♀

       O09.623 Supervision of young multigravida, third trimester Ⓜ♀

       O09.629 Supervision of young multigravida, unspecified trimester Ⓜ♀▽

√5ᵗʰ **O09.7** Supervision of high risk pregnancy due to social problems

    O09.70 Supervision of high risk pregnancy due to social problems, unspecified trimester Ⓜ♀▽

    O09.71 Supervision of high risk pregnancy due to social problems, first trimester Ⓜ♀

    O09.72 Supervision of high risk pregnancy due to social problems, second trimester Ⓜ♀

    O09.73 Supervision of high risk pregnancy due to social problems, third trimester Ⓜ♀

√5ᵗʰ **O09.8** Supervision of other high risk pregnancies

    √6ᵗʰ **O09.81** Supervision of pregnancy resulting from assisted reproductive technology
       Supervision of pregnancy resulting from in-vitro fertilization

       O09.811 Supervision of pregnancy resulting from assisted reproductive technology, first trimester Ⓜ♀

       O09.812 Supervision of pregnancy resulting from assisted reproductive technology, second trimester Ⓜ♀

Chapter 15. Pregnancy, Childbirth and the Puerperium

O09.813 Supervision of pregnancy resulting Ⓜ♀ from assisted reproductive technology, **third trimester**

O09.819 Supervision of pregnancy resulting Ⓜ♀▽ from assisted reproductive technology, **unspecified trimester**

✓6ᵗʰ **O09.82** Supervision of pregnancy with history of in utero procedure during previous pregnancy

O09.821 Supervision of pregnancy with history Ⓜ♀ of in utero procedure during previous pregnancy, **first trimester**

O09.822 Supervision of pregnancy with history Ⓜ♀ of in utero procedure during previous pregnancy, **second trimester**

O09.823 Supervision of pregnancy with history Ⓜ♀ of in utero procedure during previous pregnancy, **third trimester**

O09.829 Supervision of pregnancy with Ⓜ♀▽ history of in utero procedure during previous pregnancy, **unspecified trimester**

> **EXCLUDES 1** supervision of pregnancy affected by in utero procedure during current pregnancy (O35.7)

✓6ᵗʰ **O09.89** Supervision of other high risk pregnancies

O09.891 Supervision of other high risk Ⓜ♀ pregnancies, **first trimester**

O09.892 Supervision of other high risk Ⓜ♀ pregnancies, **second trimester**

O09.893 Supervision of other high risk Ⓜ♀ pregnancies, **third trimester**

O09.899 Supervision of other high risk Ⓜ♀▽ pregnancies, **unspecified trimester**

✓5ᵗʰ **O09.9** Supervision of high risk pregnancy, unspecified

O09.90 Supervision of high risk pregnancy, Ⓜ♀▽ unspecified, **unspecified trimester**

O09.91 Supervision of high risk pregnancy, Ⓜ♀▽ unspecified, **first trimester**

O09.92 Supervision of high risk pregnancy, Ⓜ♀▽ unspecified, **second trimester**

O09.93 Supervision of high risk pregnancy, Ⓜ♀▽ unspecified, **third trimester**

Edema, proteinuria and hypertensive disorders in pregnancy, childbirth and the puerperium (O10-O16)

✓4ᵗʰ **O10** Pre-existing hypertension complicating pregnancy, childbirth and the puerperium

Pre-existing hypertension with pre-existing proteinuria complicating pregnancy, childbirth and the puerperium

> **EXCLUDES 2** pre-existing hypertension with superimposed pre-eclampsia complicating pregnancy, childbirth and the puerperium (O11.-)

✓5ᵗʰ **O10.0** Pre-existing essential hypertension complicating pregnancy, childbirth and the puerperium

Any condition in I10 specified as a reason for obstetric care during pregnancy, childbirth or the puerperium

✓6ᵗʰ **O10.01** Pre-existing essential hypertension complicating pregnancy

O10.011 Pre-existing essential hypertension Ⓜ♀ complicating pregnancy, **first trimester**

O10.012 Pre-existing essential hypertension Ⓜ♀ complicating pregnancy, **second trimester**

O10.013 Pre-existing essential hypertension Ⓜ♀ complicating pregnancy, **third trimester**

O10.019 Pre-existing essential hypertension Ⓜ♀▽ complicating pregnancy, **unspecified trimester**

O10.02 Pre-existing essential hypertension Ⓜ♀ complicating childbirth

O10.03 Pre-existing essential hypertension Ⓜ♀ complicating the puerperium

✓5ᵗʰ **O10.1** Pre-existing hypertensive heart disease complicating pregnancy, childbirth and the puerperium

Any condition in I11 specified as a reason for obstetric care during pregnancy, childbirth or the puerperium

Use additional code from I11 to identify the type of hypertensive heart disease

✓6ᵗʰ **O10.11** Pre-existing hypertensive heart disease complicating pregnancy

O10.111 Pre-existing hypertensive heart Ⓜ♀ disease complicating pregnancy, **first trimester**

O10.112 Pre-existing hypertensive heart Ⓜ♀ disease complicating pregnancy, **second trimester**

O10.113 Pre-existing hypertensive heart Ⓜ♀ disease complicating pregnancy, **third trimester**

O10.119 Pre-existing hypertensive heart Ⓜ♀▽ disease complicating pregnancy, **unspecified trimester**

O10.12 Pre-existing hypertensive heart disease Ⓜ♀ complicating childbirth

O10.13 Pre-existing hypertensive heart disease Ⓜ♀ complicating the puerperium

✓5ᵗʰ **O10.2** Pre-existing hypertensive chronic kidney disease complicating pregnancy, childbirth and the puerperium

Any condition in I12 specified as a reason for obstetric care during pregnancy, childbirth or the puerperium

Use additional code from I12 to identify the type of hypertensive chronic kidney disease

✓6ᵗʰ **O10.21** Pre-existing hypertensive chronic kidney disease complicating pregnancy

O10.211 Pre-existing hypertensive chronic Ⓜ♀ kidney disease complicating pregnancy, **first trimester**

O10.212 Pre-existing hypertensive chronic Ⓜ♀ kidney disease complicating pregnancy, **second trimester**

O10.213 Pre-existing hypertensive chronic Ⓜ♀ kidney disease complicating pregnancy, **third trimester**

O10.219 Pre-existing hypertensive chronic Ⓜ♀▽ kidney disease complicating pregnancy, **unspecified trimester**

O10.22 Pre-existing hypertensive chronic kidney Ⓜ♀ disease complicating childbirth

O10.23 Pre-existing hypertensive chronic kidney Ⓜ♀ disease complicating the puerperium

✓5ᵗʰ **O10.3** Pre-existing hypertensive heart and chronic kidney disease complicating pregnancy, childbirth and the puerperium

Any condition in I13 specified as a reason for obstetric care during pregnancy, childbirth or the puerperium

Use additional code from I13 to identify the type of hypertensive heart and chronic kidney disease

✓6ᵗʰ **O10.31** Pre-existing hypertensive heart and chronic kidney disease complicating pregnancy

O10.311 Pre-existing hypertensive heart and Ⓜ♀ chronic kidney disease complicating pregnancy, **first trimester**

O10.312 Pre-existing hypertensive heart and Ⓜ♀ chronic kidney disease complicating pregnancy, **second trimester**

O10.313 Pre-existing hypertensive heart and Ⓜ♀ chronic kidney disease complicating pregnancy, **third trimester**

O10.319 Pre-existing hypertensive heart Ⓜ♀▽ and chronic kidney disease complicating pregnancy, **unspecified trimester**

O10.32 Pre-existing hypertensive heart and chronic Ⓜ♀ kidney disease complicating childbirth

O10.33 Pre-existing hypertensive heart and chronic Ⓜ♀ kidney disease complicating the puerperium

---

Ⓝ Newborn   Ⓟ Pediatric   Ⓜ Maternity   Ⓐ Adult   **RIC** RIC Dx   **NC Dx** Noncancer Dx   **PDx** Primary Dx   **CC** RIC CC Condition   ▶◀ Revised Text   ● New Code   ▲ Revised Code Title

✓5ᵗʰ **O10.4** **Pre-existing** secondary **hypertension complicating pregnancy, childbirth and the puerperium**
Any condition in I15 specified as a reason for obstetric care during pregnancy, childbirth or the puerperium
Use additional code from I15 to identify the type of secondary hypertension

   ✓6ᵗʰ **O10.41** **Pre-existing secondary hypertension complicating** pregnancy

       O10.411 **Pre-existing secondary hypertension** Ⓜ♀ **complicating pregnancy,** first **trimester**

       O10.412 **Pre-existing secondary hypertension** Ⓜ♀ **complicating pregnancy,** second **trimester**

       O10.413 **Pre-existing secondary hypertension** Ⓜ♀ **complicating pregnancy,** third **trimester**

       O10.419 **Pre-existing secondary** Ⓜ♀▽ **hypertension complicating pregnancy, unspecified trimester**

    O10.42 **Pre-existing secondary hypertension** Ⓜ♀ **complicating** childbirth

    O10.43 **Pre-existing secondary hypertension** Ⓜ♀ **complicating the** puerperium

✓5ᵗʰ **O10.9** Unspecified **pre-existing hypertension complicating pregnancy, childbirth and the puerperium**

   ✓6ᵗʰ **O10.91** **Unspecified pre-existing hypertension complicating** pregnancy

       O10.911 **Unspecified pre-existing** Ⓜ♀▽ **hypertension complicating pregnancy,** first trimester

       O10.912 **Unspecified pre-existing** Ⓜ♀▽ **hypertension complicating pregnancy,** second trimester

       O10.913 **Unspecified pre-existing** Ⓜ♀▽ **hypertension complicating pregnancy,** third trimester

       O10.919 **Unspecified pre-existing** Ⓜ♀▽ **hypertension complicating pregnancy, unspecified trimester**

    O10.92 **Unspecified pre-existing hypertension** Ⓜ♀▽ **complicating** childbirth

    O10.93 **Unspecified pre-existing hypertension** Ⓜ♀▽ **complicating the** puerperium

✓4ᵗʰ **O11** Pre-existing **hypertension** with pre-eclampsia
Conditions in O10 complicated by pre-eclampsia
Pre-eclampsia superimposed pre-existing hypertension
Use additional code from O10 to identify the type of hypertension

    O11.1 **Pre-existing hypertension with pre-eclampsia,** Ⓜ♀ first trimester

    O11.2 **Pre-existing hypertension with pre-eclampsia,** Ⓜ♀ second trimester

    O11.3 **Pre-existing hypertension with pre-eclampsia,** Ⓜ♀ third trimester

    O11.9 **Pre-existing hypertension with pre-eclampsia,** Ⓜ♀▽ unspecified trimester

✓4ᵗʰ **O12** Gestational **[pregnancy-induced] edema and proteinuria** without hypertension

   ✓5ᵗʰ **O12.0** Gestational edema

       O12.00 **Gestational edema, unspecified trimester** Ⓜ♀▽

       O12.01 **Gestational edema,** first trimester Ⓜ♀

       O12.02 **Gestational edema,** second trimester Ⓜ♀

       O12.03 **Gestational edema,** third trimester Ⓜ♀

   ✓5ᵗʰ **O12.1** Gestational proteinuria

       O12.10 **Gestational proteinuria, unspecified trimester** Ⓜ♀▽

       O12.11 **Gestational proteinuria,** first trimester Ⓜ♀

       O12.12 **Gestational proteinuria,** second trimester Ⓜ♀

       O12.13 **Gestational proteinuria,** third trimester Ⓜ♀

   ✓5ᵗʰ **O12.2** Gestational edema with proteinuria

       O12.20 **Gestational edema with proteinuria,** Ⓜ♀▽ **unspecified trimester**

       O12.21 **Gestational edema with proteinuria,** Ⓜ♀ first trimester

       O12.22 **Gestational edema with proteinuria,** Ⓜ♀ second trimester

       O12.23 **Gestational edema with proteinuria,** Ⓜ♀ third trimester

✓4ᵗʰ **O13** Gestational **[pregnancy-induced] hypertension without significant proteinuria**
INCLUDES gestational hypertension NOS

    O13.1 **Gestational [pregnancy-induced] hypertension without** Ⓜ♀ **significant proteinuria,** first trimester

    O13.2 **Gestational [pregnancy-induced] hypertension without** Ⓜ♀ **significant proteinuria,** second trimester

    O13.3 **Gestational [pregnancy-induced] hypertension without** Ⓜ♀ **significant proteinuria,** third trimester

    O13.9 **Gestational [pregnancy-induced] hypertension** Ⓜ♀▽ **without significant proteinuria, unspecified trimester**

✓4ᵗʰ **O14** Pre-eclampsia
EXCLUDES 1 pre-existing hypertension with pre-eclampsia (O11)

   ✓5ᵗʰ **O14.0** Mild to moderate **pre-eclampsia**

       O14.00 **Mild to moderate pre-eclampsia, unspecified** Ⓜ♀▽ **trimester**

       O14.02 **Mild to moderate pre-eclampsia,** second Ⓜ♀ **trimester**

       O14.03 **Mild to moderate pre-eclampsia,** third trimester Ⓜ♀

   ✓5ᵗʰ **O14.1** Severe **pre-eclampsia**
EXCLUDES 1 HELLP syndrome (O14.2-)

       O14.10 **Severe pre-eclampsia, unspecified trimester** Ⓜ♀▽

       O14.12 **Severe pre-eclampsia,** second trimester Ⓜ♀

       O14.13 **Severe pre-eclampsia,** third trimester Ⓜ♀

   ✓5ᵗʰ **O14.2** HELLP syndrome
Severe pre-eclampsia with hemolysis, elevated liver enzymes and low platelet count (HELLP)

       O14.20 **HELLP syndrome (HELLP), unspecified** Ⓜ♀▽ **trimester**

       O14.22 **HELLP syndrome (HELLP),** second trimester Ⓜ♀

       O14.23 **HELLP syndrome (HELLP),** third trimester Ⓜ♀

   ✓5ᵗʰ **O14.9** Unspecified **pre-eclampsia**

       O14.90 **Unspecified pre-eclampsia, unspecified** Ⓜ♀▽ **trimester**

       O14.92 **Unspecified pre-eclampsia,** second trimester Ⓜ♀▽

       O14.93 **Unspecified pre-eclampsia,** third trimester Ⓜ♀▽

✓4ᵗʰ **O15** Eclampsia
INCLUDES convulsions following conditions in O10-O14 and O16

   ✓5ᵗʰ **O15.0** Eclampsia in pregnancy

       O15.00 **Eclampsia in pregnancy, unspecified** Ⓜ♀▽ **trimester**

       O15.02 **Eclampsia in pregnancy,** second trimester Ⓜ♀

       O15.03 **Eclampsia in pregnancy,** third trimester Ⓜ♀

    O15.1 **Eclampsia in** labor Ⓜ♀

    O15.2 **Eclampsia in the** puerperium Ⓜ♀

    O15.9 **Eclampsia, unspecified as to time period** Ⓜ♀▽
Eclampsia NOS

✓4ᵗʰ **O16** Unspecified maternal hypertension

    O16.1 **Unspecified maternal hypertension,** first trimester Ⓜ♀▽

    O16.2 **Unspecified maternal hypertension,** second trimester Ⓜ♀▽

    O16.3 **Unspecified maternal hypertension,** third trimester Ⓜ♀▽

    O16.9 **Unspecified maternal hypertension, unspecified** Ⓜ♀▽ **trimester**

Other maternal disorders predominantly related to pregnancy (O20-O29)

EXCLUDES 2 maternal care related to the fetus and amniotic cavity and possible delivery problems (O30-O48)
maternal diseases classifiable elsewhere but complicating pregnancy, labor and delivery, and the puerperium (O98-O99)

✓4ᵗʰ **O20** Hemorrhage in early pregnancy
Hemorrhage before completion of 20 weeks gestation
EXCLUDES 1 pregnancy with abortive outcome (O00-O08)

    O20.0 **Threatened abortion** Ⓜ♀
Hemorrhage specified as due to threatened abortion

    O20.8 **Other hemorrhage in early pregnancy** Ⓜ♀

    O20.9 **Hemorrhage in early pregnancy, unspecified** Ⓜ♀▽

✓4ᵗʰ **O21** Excessive vomiting in pregnancy

    O21.0 Mild hyperemesis gravidarum Ⓜ♀
Hyperemesis gravidarum, mild or unspecified, starting before the end of the 20th week of gestation

---

✓ Add'l Character Required   ✓x7ᵗʰ Placeholder Alert   RUG IV Special Care High Dx   RUG IV Clinically Complex Dx   RUG IV Special Care Low Dx   Manifestation Code   Other Specified Code   ▽ Unspecified Code

ICD-10-CM 2016   **781**

O21.1 Hyperemesis gravidarum with metabolic disturbance   Ⓜ♀
  Hyperemesis gravidarum, starting before the end of the 20th week of gestation, with metabolic disturbance such as carbohydrate depletion
  Hyperemesis gravidarum, starting before the end of the 20th week of gestation, with metabolic disturbance such as dehydration
  Hyperemesis gravidarum, starting before the end of the 20th week of gestation, with metabolic disturbance such as electrolyte imbalance

O21.2 Late vomiting of pregnancy   Ⓜ♀
  Excessive vomiting starting after 20 completed weeks of gestation

O21.8 Other vomiting complicating pregnancy   Ⓜ♀
  Vomiting due to diseases classified elsewhere, complicating pregnancy
  Use additional code, to identify cause

O21.9 Vomiting of pregnancy, unspecified   Ⓜ♀▽

✓4ᵗʰ **O22 Venous complications and hemorrhoids in pregnancy**
  EXCLUDES 1   *venous complications of:*
    abortion NOS (O03.9)
    ectopic or molar pregnancy (O08.7)
    failed attempted abortion (O07.35)
    induced abortion (O04.85)
    spontaneous abortion (O03.89)
  EXCLUDES 2   *obstetric pulmonary embolism (O88.-)*
    venous complications and hemorrhoids of childbirth and the puerperium (O87.-)

✓5ᵗʰ **O22.0** Varicose veins of lower extremity **in pregnancy**
  Varicose veins NOS in pregnancy

  O22.00 Varicose veins of lower extremity in   Ⓜ♀▽
  pregnancy, unspecified trimester

  O22.01 Varicose veins of lower extremity in pregnancy,   Ⓜ♀
  first trimester

  O22.02 Varicose veins of lower extremity in pregnancy,   Ⓜ♀
  second trimester

  O22.03 Varicose veins of lower extremity in pregnancy,   Ⓜ♀
  third trimester

✓5ᵗʰ **O22.1** Genital varices **in pregnancy**
  Perineal varices in pregnancy
  Vaginal varices in pregnancy
  Vulval varices in pregnancy

  O22.10 Genital varices in pregnancy, unspecified   Ⓜ♀▽
  trimester

  O22.11 Genital varices in pregnancy, first trimester   Ⓜ♀

  O22.12 Genital varices in pregnancy, second trimester   Ⓜ♀

  O22.13 Genital varices in pregnancy, third trimester   Ⓜ♀

✓5ᵗʰ **O22.2** Superficial thrombophlebitis **in pregnancy**
  Phlebitis in pregnancy NOS
  Thrombophlebitis of legs in pregnancy
  Thrombosis in pregnancy NOS
  Use additional code to identify the superficial thrombophlebitis (I80.0-)

  O22.20 Superficial thrombophlebitis in pregnancy,   Ⓜ♀▽
  unspecified trimester

  O22.21 Superficial thrombophlebitis in pregnancy,   Ⓜ♀
  first trimester

  O22.22 Superficial thrombophlebitis in pregnancy,   Ⓜ♀
  second trimester

  O22.23 Superficial thrombophlebitis in pregnancy,   Ⓜ♀
  third trimester

✓5ᵗʰ **O22.3** Deep phlebothrombosis **in pregnancy**
  Deep vein thrombosis, antepartum
  Use additional code to identify the deep vein thrombosis (I82.4-, I82.5-, I82.62-. I82.72-)
  Use additional code, if applicable, for associated long-term (current) use of anticoagulants (Z79.01)

  O22.30 Deep phlebothrombosis in pregnancy,   Ⓜ♀▽
  unspecified trimester

  O22.31 Deep phlebothrombosis in pregnancy,   Ⓜ♀
  first trimester

  O22.32 Deep phlebothrombosis in pregnancy,   Ⓜ♀
  second trimester

  O22.33 Deep phlebothrombosis in pregnancy,   Ⓜ♀
  third trimester

✓5ᵗʰ **O22.4 Hemorrhoids in pregnancy**

  O22.40 Hemorrhoids in pregnancy, unspecified   Ⓜ♀▽
  trimester

  O22.41 Hemorrhoids in pregnancy, first trimester   Ⓜ♀

  O22.42 Hemorrhoids in pregnancy, second trimester   Ⓜ♀

  O22.43 Hemorrhoids in pregnancy, third trimester   Ⓜ♀

✓5ᵗʰ **O22.5** Cerebral venous thrombosis **in pregnancy**
  Cerebrovenous sinus thrombosis in pregnancy

  O22.50 Cerebral venous thrombosis in pregnancy,   Ⓜ♀▽
  unspecified trimester

  O22.51 Cerebral venous thrombosis in pregnancy,   Ⓜ♀
  first trimester

  O22.52 Cerebral venous thrombosis in pregnancy,   Ⓜ♀
  second trimester

  O22.53 Cerebral venous thrombosis in pregnancy,   Ⓜ♀
  third trimester

✓5ᵗʰ **O22.8** Other venous complications **in pregnancy**

  ✓6ᵗʰ **O22.8X** Other **venous complications in pregnancy**

    O22.8X1 Other venous complications in   Ⓜ♀
    pregnancy, first trimester

    O22.8X2 Other venous complications in   Ⓜ♀
    pregnancy, second trimester

    O22.8X3 Other venous complications in   Ⓜ♀
    pregnancy, third trimester

    O22.8X9 Other venous complications in   Ⓜ♀▽
    pregnancy, unspecified trimester

✓5ᵗʰ **O22.9** Venous complication **in pregnancy,** unspecified
  Gestational phlebitis NOS
  Gestational phlebopathy NOS
  Gestational thrombosis NOS

  O22.90 Venous complication in pregnancy,   Ⓜ♀▽
  unspecified, unspecified trimester

  O22.91 Venous complication in pregnancy,   Ⓜ♀▽
  unspecified, first trimester

  O22.92 Venous complication in pregnancy,   Ⓜ♀▽
  unspecified, second trimester

  O22.93 Venous complication in pregnancy,   Ⓜ♀▽
  unspecified, third trimester

✓4ᵗʰ **O23 Infections of genitourinary tract in pregnancy**
  Use additional code to identify organism (B95.-, B96.-)
  EXCLUDES 2   *gonococcal infections complicating pregnancy, childbirth and the puerperium (O98.2)*
    infections with a predominantly sexual mode of transmission NOS complicating pregnancy, childbirth and the puerperium (O98.3)
    syphilis complicating pregnancy, childbirth and the puerperium (O98.1)
    tuberculosis of genitourinary system complicating pregnancy, childbirth and the puerperium (O98.0)
    venereal disease NOS complicating pregnancy, childbirth and the puerperium (O98.3)

✓5ᵗʰ **O23.0 Infections of** kidney **in pregnancy**
  Pyelonephritis in pregnancy

  O23.00 Infections of kidney in pregnancy,   Ⓜ♀▽
  unspecified trimester

  O23.01 Infections of kidney in pregnancy, first trimester   Ⓜ♀

  O23.02 Infections of kidney in pregnancy, second   Ⓜ♀
  trimester

  O23.03 Infections of kidney in pregnancy, third   Ⓜ♀
  trimester

✓5ᵗʰ **O23.1 Infections of** bladder **in pregnancy**

  O23.10 Infections of bladder in pregnancy,   Ⓜ♀▽
  unspecified trimester

  O23.11 Infections of bladder in pregnancy,   Ⓜ♀
  first trimester

  O23.12 Infections of bladder in pregnancy,   Ⓜ♀
  second trimester

  O23.13 Infections of bladder in pregnancy,   Ⓜ♀
  third trimester

✓5ᵗʰ **O23.2 Infections of** urethra **in pregnancy**

  O23.20 Infections of urethra in pregnancy,   Ⓜ♀▽
  unspecified trimester

  O23.21 Infections of urethra in pregnancy,   Ⓜ♀
  first trimester

  O23.22 Infections of urethra in pregnancy,   Ⓜ♀
  second trimester

Ⓝ Newborn   Ⓟ Pediatric   Ⓜ Maternity   Ⓐ Adult   RIC RIC Dx   NCDx Noncancer Dx   PDx Primary Dx   CC RIC CC Condition   ►◄ Revised Text   ● New Code   ▲ Revised Code Title

782   ICD-10-CM 2016

O23.23	Infections of urethra in pregnancy, third trimester	Ⓜ♀

✓5ᵗʰ O23.3 Infections of other parts of urinary tract in pregnancy

O23.30	Infections of other parts of urinary tract in pregnancy, unspecified trimester	Ⓜ♀▽
O23.31	Infections of other parts of urinary tract in pregnancy, first trimester	Ⓜ♀
O23.32	Infections of other parts of urinary tract in pregnancy, second trimester	Ⓜ♀
O23.33	Infections of other parts of urinary tract in pregnancy, third trimester	Ⓜ♀

✓5ᵗʰ O23.4 Unspecified infection of urinary tract in pregnancy

O23.40	Unspecified infection of urinary tract in pregnancy, unspecified trimester	Ⓜ♀▽
O23.41	Unspecified infection of urinary tract in pregnancy, first trimester	Ⓜ♀
O23.42	Unspecified infection of urinary tract in pregnancy, second trimester	Ⓜ♀
O23.43	Unspecified infection of urinary tract in pregnancy, third trimester	Ⓜ♀▽

✓5ᵗʰ O23.5 Infections of the genital tract in pregnancy

✓6ᵗʰ O23.51 Infection of cervix in pregnancy

O23.511	Infections of cervix in pregnancy, first trimester	Ⓜ♀
O23.512	Infections of cervix in pregnancy, second trimester	Ⓜ♀
O23.513	Infections of cervix in pregnancy, third trimester	Ⓜ♀
O23.519	Infections of cervix in pregnancy, unspecified trimester	Ⓜ♀▽

✓6ᵗʰ O23.52 Salpingo-oophoritis in pregnancy
Oophoritis in pregnancy
Salpingitis in pregnancy

O23.521	Salpingo-oophoritis in pregnancy, first trimester	Ⓜ♀
O23.522	Salpingo-oophoritis in pregnancy, second trimester	Ⓜ♀
O23.523	Salpingo-oophoritis in pregnancy, third trimester	Ⓜ♀
O23.529	Salpingo-oophoritis in pregnancy, unspecified trimester	Ⓜ♀▽

✓6ᵗʰ O23.59 Infection of other part of genital tract in pregnancy

O23.591	Infection of other part of genital tract in pregnancy, first trimester	Ⓜ♀
O23.592	Infection of other part of genital tract in pregnancy, second trimester	Ⓜ♀
O23.593	Infection of other part of genital tract in pregnancy, third trimester	Ⓜ♀
O23.599	Infection of other part of genital tract in pregnancy, unspecified trimester	Ⓜ♀▽

✓5ᵗʰ O23.9 Unspecified genitourinary tract infection in pregnancy
Genitourinary tract infection in pregnancy NOS

O23.90	Unspecified genitourinary tract infection in pregnancy, unspecified trimester	Ⓜ♀▽
O23.91	Unspecified genitourinary tract infection in pregnancy, first trimester	Ⓜ♀▽
O23.92	Unspecified genitourinary tract infection in pregnancy, second trimester	Ⓜ♀▽
O23.93	Unspecified genitourinary tract infection in pregnancy, third trimester	Ⓜ♀▽

✓4ᵗʰ O24 Diabetes mellitus in pregnancy, childbirth, and the puerperium

✓5ᵗʰ O24.0 Pre-existing diabetes mellitus, type 1, in pregnancy, childbirth and the puerperium
Juvenile onset diabetes mellitus, in pregnancy, childbirth and the puerperium
Ketosis-prone diabetes mellitus in pregnancy, childbirth and the puerperium
Use additional code from category E10 to further identify any manifestations

✓6ᵗʰ O24.01 Pre-existing diabetes mellitus, type 1, in pregnancy

O24.011	Pre-existing diabetes mellitus, type 1, in pregnancy, first trimester	Ⓜ♀
O24.012	Pre-existing diabetes mellitus, type 1, in pregnancy, second trimester	Ⓜ♀
O24.013	Pre-existing diabetes mellitus, type 1, in pregnancy, third trimester	Ⓜ♀

O24.019	Pre-existing diabetes mellitus, type 1 in pregnancy, unspecified trimester	Ⓜ♀▽
O24.02	Pre-existing diabetes mellitus, type 1, in childbirth	Ⓜ♀
O24.03	Pre-existing diabetes mellitus, type 1, in the puerperium	Ⓜ♀

✓5ᵗʰ O24.1 Pre-existing diabetes mellitus, type 2, in pregnancy, childbirth and the puerperium
Insulin-resistant diabetes mellitus in pregnancy, childbirth and the puerperium
Use additional code (for):
from category E11 to further identify any manifestations
long-term (current) use of insulin (Z79.4)

✓6ᵗʰ O24.11 Pre-existing diabetes mellitus, type 2, in pregnancy

O24.111	Pre-existing diabetes mellitus, type 2, in pregnancy, first trimester	Ⓜ♀
O24.112	Pre-existing diabetes mellitus, type 2, in pregnancy, second trimester	Ⓜ♀
O24.113	Pre-existing diabetes mellitus, type 2, in pregnancy, third trimester	Ⓜ♀
O24.119	Pre-existing diabetes mellitus, type 2, in pregnancy, unspecified trimester	Ⓜ♀▽
O24.12	Pre-existing diabetes mellitus, type 2, in childbirth	Ⓜ♀
O24.13	Pre-existing diabetes mellitus, type 2, in the puerperium	Ⓜ♀

✓5ᵗʰ O24.3 Unspecified pre-existing diabetes mellitus in pregnancy, childbirth and the puerperium
Use additional code (for):
from category E11 to further identify any manifestation
long-term (current) use of insulin (Z79.4)

✓6ᵗʰ O24.31 Unspecified pre-existing diabetes mellitus in pregnancy

O24.311	Unspecified pre-existing diabetes mellitus in pregnancy, first trimester	Ⓜ♀▽
O24.312	Unspecified pre-existing diabetes mellitus in pregnancy, second trimester	Ⓜ♀▽
O24.313	Unspecified pre-existing diabetes mellitus in pregnancy, third trimester	Ⓜ♀▽
O24.319	Unspecified pre-existing diabetes mellitus in pregnancy, unspecified trimester	Ⓜ♀▽
O24.32	Unspecified pre-existing diabetes mellitus in childbirth	Ⓜ♀▽
O24.33	Unspecified pre-existing diabetes mellitus in the puerperium	Ⓜ♀▽

✓5ᵗʰ O24.4 Gestational diabetes mellitus
Diabetes mellitus arising in pregnancy
Gestational diabetes mellitus NOS

✓6ᵗʰ O24.41 Gestational diabetes mellitus in pregnancy

O24.410	Gestational diabetes mellitus in pregnancy, diet controlled	Ⓜ♀
O24.414	Gestational diabetes mellitus in pregnancy, insulin controlled	Ⓜ♀
O24.419	Gestational diabetes mellitus in pregnancy, unspecified control	Ⓜ♀▽

✓6ᵗʰ O24.42 Gestational diabetes mellitus in childbirth

O24.420	Gestational diabetes mellitus in childbirth, diet controlled	Ⓜ♀
O24.424	Gestational diabetes mellitus in childbirth, insulin controlled	Ⓜ♀
O24.429	Gestational diabetes mellitus in childbirth, unspecified control	Ⓜ♀▽

✓6ᵗʰ O24.43 Gestational diabetes mellitus in the puerperium

O24.430	Gestational diabetes mellitus in the puerperium, diet controlled	Ⓜ♀
O24.434	Gestational diabetes mellitus in the puerperium, insulin controlled	Ⓜ♀
O24.439	Gestational diabetes mellitus in the puerperium, unspecified control	Ⓜ♀▽

✓5ᵗʰ O24.8 Other pre-existing diabetes mellitus in pregnancy, childbirth, and the puerperium
Use additional code (for):
from categories E08, E09 and E13 to further identify any manifestation
long-term (current) use of insulin (Z79.4)

    ✓6ᵗʰ O24.81 Other pre-existing diabetes mellitus in pregnancy
        O24.811 Other pre-existing diabetes mellitus in pregnancy, first trimester   Ⓜ♀
        O24.812 Other pre-existing diabetes mellitus in pregnancy, second trimester   Ⓜ♀
        O24.813 Other pre-existing diabetes mellitus in pregnancy, third trimester   Ⓜ♀
        O24.819 Other pre-existing diabetes mellitus in pregnancy, unspecified trimester   Ⓜ♀▽

    O24.82 Other pre-existing diabetes mellitus in childbirth   Ⓜ♀
    O24.83 Other pre-existing diabetes mellitus in the puerperium   Ⓜ♀

✓5ᵗʰ O24.9 Unspecified diabetes mellitus in pregnancy, childbirth and the puerperium
Use additional code for long-term (current) use of insulin (Z79.4)

    ✓6ᵗʰ O24.91 Unspecified diabetes mellitus in pregnancy
        O24.911 Unspecified diabetes mellitus in pregnancy, first trimester   Ⓜ♀▽
        O24.912 Unspecified diabetes mellitus in pregnancy, second trimester   Ⓜ♀▽
        O24.913 Unspecified diabetes mellitus in pregnancy, third trimester   Ⓜ♀▽
        O24.919 Unspecified diabetes mellitus in pregnancy, unspecified trimester   Ⓜ♀▽

    O24.92 Unspecified diabetes mellitus in childbirth   Ⓜ♀▽
    O24.93 Unspecified diabetes mellitus in the puerperium   Ⓜ♀▽

✓4ᵗʰ O25 Malnutrition in pregnancy, childbirth and the puerperium

    ✓5ᵗʰ O25.1 Malnutrition in pregnancy
        O25.10 Malnutrition in pregnancy, unspecified trimester   Ⓜ♀▽
        O25.11 Malnutrition in pregnancy, first trimester   Ⓜ♀
        O25.12 Malnutrition in pregnancy, second trimester   Ⓜ♀
        O25.13 Malnutrition in pregnancy, third trimester   Ⓜ♀

    O25.2 Malnutrition in childbirth   Ⓜ♀
    O25.3 Malnutrition in the puerperium   Ⓜ♀

✓4ᵗʰ O26 Maternal care for other conditions predominantly related to pregnancy

    ✓5ᵗʰ O26.0 Excessive weight gain in pregnancy
        EXCLUDES 2 gestational edema (O12.0, O12.2)
        O26.00 Excessive weight gain in pregnancy, unspecified trimester   Ⓜ♀▽
        O26.01 Excessive weight gain in pregnancy, first trimester   Ⓜ♀
        O26.02 Excessive weight gain in pregnancy, second trimester   Ⓜ♀
        O26.03 Excessive weight gain in pregnancy, third trimester   Ⓜ♀

    ✓5ᵗʰ O26.1 Low weight gain in pregnancy
        O26.10 Low weight gain in pregnancy, unspecified trimester   Ⓜ♀▽
        O26.11 Low weight gain in pregnancy, first trimester   Ⓜ♀
        O26.12 Low weight gain in pregnancy, second trimester   Ⓜ♀
        O26.13 Low weight gain in pregnancy, third trimester   Ⓜ♀

    ✓5ᵗʰ O26.2 Pregnancy care for patient with recurrent pregnancy loss
        O26.20 Pregnancy care for patient with recurrent pregnancy loss, unspecified trimester   Ⓜ♀▽
        O26.21 Pregnancy care for patient with recurrent pregnancy loss, first trimester   Ⓜ♀
        O26.22 Pregnancy care for patient with recurrent pregnancy loss, second trimester   Ⓜ♀
        O26.23 Pregnancy care for patient with recurrent pregnancy loss, third trimester   Ⓜ♀

    ✓5ᵗʰ O26.3 Retained intrauterine contraceptive device in pregnancy
        O26.30 Retained intrauterine contraceptive device in pregnancy, unspecified trimester   Ⓜ♀▽

    O26.31 Retained intrauterine contraceptive device in pregnancy, first trimester   Ⓜ♀
    O26.32 Retained intrauterine contraceptive device in pregnancy, second trimester   Ⓜ♀
    O26.33 Retained intrauterine contraceptive device in pregnancy, third trimester   Ⓜ♀

    ✓5ᵗʰ O26.4 Herpes gestationis
        O26.40 Herpes gestationis, unspecified trimester   Ⓜ♀▽
        O26.41 Herpes gestationis, first trimester   Ⓜ♀
        O26.42 Herpes gestationis, second trimester   Ⓜ♀
        O26.43 Herpes gestationis, third trimester   Ⓜ♀

    ✓5ᵗʰ O26.5 Maternal hypotension syndrome
        Supine hypotensive syndrome
        O26.50 Maternal hypotension syndrome, unspecified trimester   Ⓜ♀▽
        O26.51 Maternal hypotension syndrome, first trimester   Ⓜ♀
        O26.52 Maternal hypotension syndrome, second trimester   Ⓜ♀
        O26.53 Maternal hypotension syndrome, third trimester   Ⓜ♀

    ✓5ᵗʰ O26.6 Liver and biliary tract disorders in pregnancy, childbirth and the puerperium
        Use additional code to identify the specific disorder
        EXCLUDES 2 hepatorenal syndrome following labor and delivery (O90.4)

        ✓6ᵗʰ O26.61 Liver and biliary tract disorders in pregnancy
            O26.611 Liver and biliary tract disorders in pregnancy, first trimester   Ⓜ♀
            O26.612 Liver and biliary tract disorders in pregnancy, second trimester   Ⓜ♀
            O26.613 Liver and biliary tract disorders in pregnancy, third trimester   Ⓜ♀
            O26.619 Liver and biliary tract disorders in pregnancy, unspecified trimester   Ⓜ♀▽

        O26.62 Liver and biliary tract disorders in childbirth   Ⓜ♀
        O26.63 Liver and biliary tract disorders in the puerperium   Ⓜ♀

    ✓5ᵗʰ O26.7 Subluxation of symphysis (pubis) in pregnancy, childbirth and the puerperium
        EXCLUDES 1 traumatic separation of symphysis (pubis) during childbirth (O71.6)

        ✓6ᵗʰ O26.71 Subluxation of symphysis (pubis) in pregnancy
            O26.711 Subluxation of symphysis (pubis) in pregnancy, first trimester   Ⓜ♀
            O26.712 Subluxation of symphysis (pubis) in pregnancy, second trimester   Ⓜ♀
            O26.713 Subluxation of symphysis (pubis) in pregnancy, third trimester   Ⓜ♀
            O26.719 Subluxation of symphysis (pubis) in pregnancy, unspecified trimester   Ⓜ♀▽

        O26.72 Subluxation of symphysis (pubis) in childbirth   Ⓜ♀
        O26.73 Subluxation of symphysis (pubis) in the puerperium   Ⓜ♀

    ✓5ᵗʰ O26.8 Other specified pregnancy related conditions
        ✓6ᵗʰ O26.81 Pregnancy related exhaustion and fatigue
            O26.811 Pregnancy related exhaustion and fatigue, first trimester   Ⓜ♀
            O26.812 Pregnancy related exhaustion and fatigue, second trimester   Ⓜ♀
            O26.813 Pregnancy related exhaustion and fatigue, third trimester   Ⓜ♀
            O26.819 Pregnancy related exhaustion and fatigue, unspecified trimester   Ⓜ♀▽

        ✓6ᵗʰ O26.82 Pregnancy related peripheral neuritis
            O26.821 Pregnancy related peripheral neuritis, first trimester   Ⓜ♀
            O26.822 Pregnancy related peripheral neuritis, second trimester   Ⓜ♀
            O26.823 Pregnancy related peripheral neuritis, third trimester   Ⓜ♀
            O26.829 Pregnancy related peripheral neuritis unspecified trimester   Ⓜ♀▽

        ✓6ᵗʰ O26.83 Pregnancy related renal disease
            Use additional code to identify the specific disorder
            O26.831 Pregnancy related renal disease, first trimester   Ⓜ♀

Ⓝ Newborn   Ⓟ Pediatric   Ⓜ Maternity   Ⓐ Adult   RIC RIC Dx   NCDx Noncancer Dx   PDx Primary Dx   CC RIC CC Condition   ►◄ Revised Text   ● New Code   ▲ Revised Code Title

784   ICD-10-CM 2016

    O26.832 Pregnancy related renal disease, Ⓜ♀
second trimester

    O26.833 Pregnancy related renal disease, third Ⓜ♀
trimester

    O26.839 Pregnancy related renal disease, Ⓜ♀▽
unspecified trimester

✓⁶ᵗʰ **O26.84** Uterine size-date discrepancy complicating
pregnancy

    EXCLUDES 1   *encounter for suspected problem with fetal growth ruled out (Z03.74)*

    O26.841 Uterine size-date discrepancy, first Ⓜ♀
trimester

    O26.842 Uterine size-date discrepancy, second Ⓜ♀
trimester

    O26.843 Uterine size-date discrepancy, third Ⓜ♀
trimester

    O26.849 Uterine size-date discrepancy, Ⓜ♀▽
unspecified trimester

✓⁶ᵗʰ **O26.85** Spotting complicating pregnancy

    O26.851 Spotting complicating pregnancy, Ⓜ♀
first trimester

    O26.852 Spotting complicating pregnancy, Ⓜ♀
second trimester

    O26.853 Spotting complicating pregnancy, Ⓜ♀
third trimester

    O26.859 Spotting complicating pregnancy, Ⓜ♀▽
unspecified trimester

    O26.86 Pruritic urticarial papules and plaques of Ⓜ♀
pregnancy (PUPPP)
Polymorphic eruption of pregnancy

✓⁶ᵗʰ **O26.87** Cervical shortening

    EXCLUDES 1   *encounter for suspected cervical shortening ruled out (Z03.75)*

    O26.872 Cervical shortening, second trimester Ⓜ♀

    O26.873 Cervical shortening, third trimester Ⓜ♀

    O26.879 Cervical shortening, unspecified Ⓜ♀▽
trimester

✓⁶ᵗʰ **O26.89** Other specified pregnancy related conditions

    O26.891 Other specified pregnancy related Ⓜ♀
conditions, first trimester

    O26.892 Other specified pregnancy related Ⓜ♀
conditions, second trimester

    O26.893 Other specified pregnancy related Ⓜ♀
conditions, third trimester

    O26.899 Other specified pregnancy related Ⓜ♀▽
conditions, unspecified trimester

✓⁵ᵗʰ **O26.9** Pregnancy related conditions, unspecified

    O26.90 Pregnancy related conditions, Ⓜ♀▽
unspecified trimester

    O26.91 Pregnancy related conditions, Ⓜ♀▽
first trimester

    O26.92 Pregnancy related conditions, Ⓜ♀▽
second trimester

    O26.93 Pregnancy related conditions, Ⓜ♀▽
third trimester

✓⁴ᵗʰ **O28** **Abnormal findings on antenatal screening of mother**

    EXCLUDES 1   *diagnostic findings classified elsewhere—see Alphabetical Index*

    O28.0 Abnormal hematological finding on antenatal screening Ⓜ♀
of mother

    O28.1 Abnormal biochemical finding on antenatal screening Ⓜ♀
of mother

    O28.2 Abnormal cytological finding on antenatal screening Ⓜ♀
of mother

    O28.3 Abnormal ultrasonic finding on antenatal screening Ⓜ♀
of mother

    O28.4 Abnormal radiological finding on antenatal screening Ⓜ♀
of mother

    O28.5 Abnormal chromosomal and genetic finding on Ⓜ♀
antenatal screening of mother

    O28.8 Other abnormal findings on antenatal screening Ⓜ♀
of mother

    O28.9 Unspecified abnormal findings on antenatal Ⓜ♀▽
screening of mother

✓⁴ᵗʰ **O29** **Complications of anesthesia during pregnancy**

    INCLUDES   maternal complications arising from the administration of a general, regional or local anesthetic, analgesic or other sedation during pregnancy

    Use additional code, if necessary, to identify the complication

    EXCLUDES 2   *complications of anesthesia during labor and delivery (O74.-)*
complications of anesthesia during the puerperium (O89.-)

✓⁵ᵗʰ **O29.0** Pulmonary complications of anesthesia during pregnancy

✓⁶ᵗʰ **O29.01** Aspiration pneumonitis due to anesthesia during
pregnancy
Inhalation of stomach contents or secretions NOS due to anesthesia during pregnancy
Mendelson's syndrome due to anesthesia during pregnancy

    O29.011 Aspiration pneumonitis due to Ⓜ♀
anesthesia during pregnancy, first
trimester

    O29.012 Aspiration pneumonitis due to Ⓜ♀
anesthesia during pregnancy, second
trimester

    O29.013 Aspiration pneumonitis due to Ⓜ♀
anesthesia during pregnancy, third
trimester

    O29.019 Aspiration pneumonitis due to Ⓜ♀▽
anesthesia during pregnancy,
unspecified trimester

✓⁶ᵗʰ **O29.02** Pressure collapse of lung due to anesthesia during
pregnancy

    O29.021 Pressure collapse of lung due to Ⓜ♀
anesthesia during pregnancy, first
trimester

    O29.022 Pressure collapse of lung due to Ⓜ♀
anesthesia during pregnancy, second
trimester

    O29.023 Pressure collapse of lung due to Ⓜ♀
anesthesia during pregnancy, third
trimester

    O29.029 Pressure collapse of lung due to Ⓜ♀▽
anesthesia during pregnancy,
unspecified trimester

✓⁶ᵗʰ **O29.09** Other pulmonary complications of anesthesia
during pregnancy

    O29.091 Other pulmonary complications of Ⓜ♀
anesthesia during pregnancy, first
trimester

    O29.092 Other pulmonary complications of Ⓜ♀
anesthesia during pregnancy, second
trimester

    O29.093 Other pulmonary complications of Ⓜ♀
anesthesia during pregnancy, third
trimester

    O29.099 Other pulmonary complications of Ⓜ♀▽
anesthesia during pregnancy,
unspecified trimester

✓⁵ᵗʰ **O29.1** Cardiac complications of anesthesia during pregnancy

✓⁶ᵗʰ **O29.11** Cardiac arrest due to anesthesia during pregnancy

    O29.111 Cardiac arrest due to anesthesia Ⓜ♀
during pregnancy, first trimester

    O29.112 Cardiac arrest due to anesthesia Ⓜ♀
during pregnancy, second trimester

    O29.113 Cardiac arrest due to anesthesia Ⓜ♀
during pregnancy, third trimester

    O29.119 Cardiac arrest due to anesthesia Ⓜ♀▽
during pregnancy, unspecified trimester

✓⁶ᵗʰ **O29.12** Cardiac failure due to anesthesia during pregnancy

    O29.121 Cardiac failure due to anesthesia Ⓜ♀
during pregnancy, first trimester

    O29.122 Cardiac failure due to anesthesia Ⓜ♀
during pregnancy, second trimester

    O29.123 Cardiac failure due to anesthesia Ⓜ♀
during pregnancy, third trimester

    O29.129 Cardiac failure due to anesthesia Ⓜ♀▽
during pregnancy, unspecified trimester

✓⁶ᵗʰ **O29.19** Other cardiac complications of anesthesia during
pregnancy

    O29.191 Other cardiac complications of Ⓜ♀
anesthesia during pregnancy, first
trimester

☑ Add'l Character Required   ☑x7ᵗʰ Placeholder Alert   ▮RUG IV Special Care High Dx   RUG IV Clinically Complex Dx   RUG IV Special Care Low Dx   Manifestation Code   Other Specified Code   ▽ Unspecified Code

O29.192 **Other cardiac complications of anesthesia during pregnancy,** second trimester   Ⓜ♀

O29.193 **Other cardiac complications of anesthesia during pregnancy,** third trimester   Ⓜ♀

O29.199 **Other cardiac complications of anesthesia during pregnancy, unspecified trimester**   Ⓜ♀▽

✓5ᵗʰ O29.2 Central nervous system **complications of anesthesia during pregnancy**

  ✓6ᵗʰ O29.21 Cerebral anoxia **due to anesthesia during pregnancy**

O29.211 **Cerebral anoxia due to anesthesia during pregnancy,** first trimester   Ⓜ♀

O29.212 **Cerebral anoxia due to anesthesia during pregnancy,** second trimester   Ⓜ♀

O29.213 **Cerebral anoxia due to anesthesia during pregnancy,** third trimester   Ⓜ♀

O29.219 **Cerebral anoxia due to anesthesia during pregnancy, unspecified trimester**   Ⓜ♀▽

  ✓6ᵗʰ O29.29 Other central nervous system **complications of anesthesia during pregnancy**

O29.291 **Other central nervous system complications of anesthesia during pregnancy,** first trimester   Ⓜ♀

O29.292 **Other central nervous system complications of anesthesia during pregnancy,** second trimester   Ⓜ♀

O29.293 **Other central nervous system complications of anesthesia during pregnancy,** third trimester   Ⓜ♀

O29.299 **Other central nervous system complications of anesthesia during pregnancy, unspecified trimester**   Ⓜ♀▽

✓5ᵗʰ O29.3 Toxic reaction **to local anesthesia during pregnancy**

  ✓6ᵗʰ O29.3X **Toxic reaction to local anesthesia during pregnancy**

O29.3X1 **Toxic reaction to local anesthesia during pregnancy,** first trimester   Ⓜ♀

O29.3X2 **Toxic reaction to local anesthesia during pregnancy,** second trimester   Ⓜ♀

O29.3X3 **Toxic reaction to local anesthesia during pregnancy,** third trimester   Ⓜ♀

O29.3X9 **Toxic reaction to local anesthesia during pregnancy, unspecified trimester**   Ⓜ♀▽

✓5ᵗʰ O29.4 Spinal and epidural anesthesia induced headache **during pregnancy**

O29.40 **Spinal and epidural anesthesia induced headacheduring pregnancy, unspecified trimester**   Ⓜ♀▽

O29.41 **Spinal and epidural anesthesia induced headache during pregnancy,** first trimester   Ⓜ♀

O29.42 **Spinal and epidural anesthesia induced headache during pregnancy,** second trimester   Ⓜ♀

O29.43 **Spinal and epidural anesthesia induced headache during pregnancy,** third trimester   Ⓜ♀

✓5ᵗʰ O29.5 Other complications of spinal and epidural anesthesia **during pregnancy**

  ✓6ᵗʰ O29.5X **Other complications of spinal and epidural anesthesia during pregnancy**

O29.5X1 **Other complications of spinal and epidural anesthesia during pregnancy,** first trimester   Ⓜ♀

O29.5X2 **Other complications of spinal and epidural anesthesia during pregnancy,** second trimester   Ⓜ♀

O29.5X3 **Other complications of spinal and epidural anesthesia during pregnancy,** third trimester   Ⓜ♀

O29.5X9 **Other complications of spinal and epidural anesthesia during pregnancy, unspecified trimester**   Ⓜ♀▽

✓5ᵗʰ O29.6 Failed or difficult intubation **for anesthesia during pregnancy**

O29.60 **Failed or difficult intubation for anesthesia during pregnancy, unspecified trimester**   Ⓜ♀▽

O29.61 **Failed or difficult intubation for anesthesia during pregnancy,** first trimester   Ⓜ♀

O29.62 **Failed or difficult intubation for anesthesia during pregnancy,** second trimester   Ⓜ♀

O29.63 **Failed or difficult intubation for anesthesia during pregnancy,** third trimester   Ⓜ♀

✓5ᵗʰ O29.8 Other **complications of anesthesia during pregnancy**

  ✓6ᵗʰ O29.8X **Other complications of anesthesia during pregnancy**

O29.8X1 **Other complications of anesthesia during pregnancy,** first trimester   Ⓜ♀

O29.8X2 **Other complications of anesthesia during pregnancy,** second trimester   Ⓜ♀

O29.8X3 **Other complications of anesthesia during pregnancy,** third trimester   Ⓜ♀

O29.8X9 **Other complications of anesthesia during pregnancy, unspecified trimester**   Ⓜ♀▽

✓5ᵗʰ O29.9 Unspecified **complication of anesthesia during pregnancy**

O29.90 **Unspecified complication of anesthesia during pregnancy, unspecified trimester**   Ⓜ♀▽

O29.91 **Unspecified complication of anesthesia during pregnancy,** first trimester   Ⓜ♀▽

O29.92 **Unspecified complication of anesthesia during pregnancy,** second trimester   Ⓜ♀▽

O29.93 **Unspecified complication of anesthesia during pregnancy,** third trimester   Ⓜ♀▽

Maternal care related to the fetus and amniotic cavity and possible delivery problems (O30-O48)

✓4ᵗʰ **O30 Multiple gestation**

Code also any complications specific to multiple gestation

✓5ᵗʰ **O30.0 Twin pregnancy**

  ✓6ᵗʰ O30.00 **Twin pregnancy,** unspecified number **of placenta and** unspecified number **of amniotic sacs**

O30.001 **Twin pregnancy, unspecified number of placenta and unspecified number of amniotic sacs,** first trimester   Ⓜ♀▽

O30.002 **Twin pregnancy, unspecified number of placenta and unspecified number of amniotic sacs,** second trimester   Ⓜ♀▽

O30.003 **Twin pregnancy, unspecified number of placenta and unspecified number of amniotic sacs,** third trimester   Ⓜ♀▽

O30.009 **Twin pregnancy, unspecified number of placenta and unspecified number of amniotic sacs, unspecified trimester**   Ⓜ♀▽

  ✓6ᵗʰ O30.01 **Twin pregnancy,** monochorionic/monoamniotic

Twin pregnancy, one placenta, one amniotic sac

EXCLUDES 1 conjoined twins (O30.02-)

O30.011 **Twin pregnancy, monochorionic/ monoamniotic,** first trimester   Ⓜ♀

O30.012 **Twin pregnancy, monochorionic/ monoamniotic,** second trimester   Ⓜ♀

O30.013 **Twin pregnancy, monochorionic/ monoamniotic,** third trimester   Ⓜ♀

O30.019 **Twin pregnancy, monochorionic/ monoamniotic, unspecified trimester**   Ⓜ♀▽

  ✓6ᵗʰ O30.02 Conjoined **twin pregnancy**

O30.021 **Conjoined twin pregnancy,** first trimester   Ⓜ♀

O30.022 **Conjoined twin pregnancy,** second trimester   Ⓜ♀

O30.023 **Conjoined twin pregnancy,** third trimester   Ⓜ♀

O30.029 **Conjoined twin pregnancy, unspecified trimester**   Ⓜ♀▽

  ✓6ᵗʰ O30.03 **Twin pregnancy,** monochorionic/diamniotic

Twin pregnancy, one placenta, two amniotic sacs

O30.031 **Twin pregnancy, monochorionic/ diamniotic,** first trimester   Ⓜ♀

O30.032 **Twin pregnancy, monochorionic/ diamniotic,** second trimester   Ⓜ♀

O30.033 **Twin pregnancy, monochorionic/ diamniotic,** third trimester   Ⓜ♀

O30.039 **Twin pregnancy, monochorionic/ diamniotic, unspecified trimester**   Ⓜ♀▽

Ⓝ Newborn   Ⓟ Pediatric   Ⓜ Maternity   Ⓐ Adult   **RIC** RIC Dx   **NCDx** Noncancer Dx   **PDx** Primary Dx   **CC** RIC CC Condition   ►◄ Revised Text   ● New Code   ▲ Revised Code Title

786   ICD-10-CM 2016

√6ᵗʰ **O30.04** **Twin pregnancy,** dichorionic/diamniotic
Twin pregnancy, two placentae, two amniotic sacs

O30.041 **Twin pregnancy, dichorionic/** Ⓜ♀
diamniotic, first trimester

O30.042 **Twin pregnancy, dichorionic/** Ⓜ♀
diamniotic, second trimester

O30.043 **Twin pregnancy, dichorionic/** Ⓜ♀
diamniotic, third trimester

O30.049 **Twin pregnancy, dichorionic/** Ⓜ♀▽
diamniotic, unspecified trimester

√6ᵗʰ **O30.09** **Twin pregnancy,** unable to determine number of
placenta and number of amniotic sacs

O30.091 **Twin pregnancy, unable to determine** Ⓜ♀
number of placenta and number of
amniotic sacs, first trimester

O30.092 **Twin pregnancy, unable to determine** Ⓜ♀
number of placenta and number of
amniotic sacs, second trimester

O30.093 **Twin pregnancy, unable to determine** Ⓜ♀
number of placenta and number of
amniotic sacs, third trimester

O30.099 **Twin pregnancy, unable to** Ⓜ♀▽
determine number of placenta and
number of amniotic sacs, unspecified
trimester

√5ᵗʰ **O30.1** Triplet pregnancy

√6ᵗʰ **O30.10** **Triplet pregnancy,** unspecified number of placenta
and unspecified number of amniotic sacs

O30.101 **Triplet pregnancy, unspecified** Ⓜ♀▽
number of placenta and unspecified
number of amniotic sacs, first
trimester

O30.102 **Triplet pregnancy, unspecified** Ⓜ♀▽
number of placenta and unspecified
number of amniotic sacs, second
trimester

O30.103 **Triplet pregnancy, unspecified** Ⓜ♀▽
number of placenta and unspecified
number of amniotic sacs, third
trimester

O30.109 **Triplet pregnancy, unspecified** Ⓜ♀▽
number of placenta and unspecified
number of amniotic sacs, unspecified
trimester

√6ᵗʰ **O30.11** **Triplet pregnancy with** two or more monochorionic
fetuses

O30.111 **Triplet pregnancy with two or more** Ⓜ♀
monochorionic fetuses, first
trimester

O30.112 **Triplet pregnancy with two or more** Ⓜ♀
monochorionic fetuses, second
trimester

O30.113 **Triplet pregnancy with two or more** Ⓜ♀
monochorionic fetuses, third
trimester

O30.119 **Triplet pregnancy with two or** Ⓜ♀▽
more monochorionic fetuses,
unspecified trimester

√6ᵗʰ **O30.12** **Triplet pregnancy with** two or more monoamniotic
fetuses

O30.121 **Triplet pregnancy with two or more** Ⓜ♀
monoamniotic fetuses, first trimester

O30.122 **Triplet pregnancy with two or more** Ⓜ♀
monoamniotic fetuses, second
trimester

O30.123 **Triplet pregnancy with two or more** Ⓜ♀
monoamniotic fetuses, third
trimester

O30.129 **Triplet pregnancy with two or more** Ⓜ♀▽
monoamniotic fetuses, unspecified
trimester

√6ᵗʰ **O30.19** **Triplet pregnancy,** unable to determine number of
placenta and number of amniotic sacs

O30.191 **Triplet pregnancy, unable to** Ⓜ♀
determine number of placenta and
number of amniotic sacs, first
trimester

O30.192 **Triplet pregnancy, unable to** Ⓜ♀
determine number of placenta and
number of amniotic sacs, second
trimester

O30.193 **Triplet pregnancy, unable to** Ⓜ♀
determine number of placenta and
number of amniotic sacs, third
trimester

O30.199 **Triplet pregnancy, unable to** Ⓜ♀▽
determine number of placenta and
number of amniotic sacs, unspecified
trimester

√6ᵗʰ **O30.2** Quadruplet pregnancy

√6ᵗʰ **O30.20** **Quadruplet pregnancy,** unspecified number of
placenta and unspecified number of amniotic sacs

O30.201 **Quadruplet pregnancy,** Ⓜ♀▽
unspecified number of placenta and
unspecified number of amniotic sacs,
first trimester

O30.202 **Quadruplet pregnancy,** Ⓜ♀▽
unspecified number of placenta and
unspecified number of amniotic sacs,
second trimester

O30.203 **Quadruplet pregnancy,** Ⓜ♀▽
unspecified number of placenta and
unspecified number of amniotic sacs,
third trimester

O30.209 **Quadruplet pregnancy, unspecified** Ⓜ♀▽
number of placenta and unspecified
number of amniotic sacs, unspecified
trimester

√6ᵗʰ **O30.21** **Quadruplet pregnancy with** two or more
monochorionic fetuses

O30.211 **Quadruplet pregnancy with two or** Ⓜ♀
more monochorionic fetuses, first
trimester

O30.212 **Quadruplet pregnancy with two or** Ⓜ♀
more monochorionic fetuses, second
trimester

O30.213 **Quadruplet pregnancy with two or** Ⓜ♀
more monochorionic fetuses, third
trimester

O30.219 **Quadruplet pregnancy with two or** Ⓜ♀▽
more monochorionic fetuses,
unspecified trimester

√6ᵗʰ **O30.22** **Quadruplet pregnancy with** two or more
monoamniotic fetuses

O30.221 **Quadruplet pregnancy with two or** Ⓜ♀
more monoamniotic fetuses, first
trimester

O30.222 **Quadruplet pregnancy with two or** Ⓜ♀
more monoamniotic fetuses, second
trimester

O30.223 **Quadruplet pregnancy with two or** Ⓜ♀
more monoamniotic fetuses, third
trimester

O30.229 **Quadruplet pregnancy with two or** Ⓜ♀▽
more monoamniotic fetuses,
unspecified trimester

√6ᵗʰ **O30.29** **Quadruplet pregnancy,** unable to determine number
of placenta and number of amniotic sacs

O30.291 **Quadruplet pregnancy, unable to** Ⓜ♀
determine number of placenta and
number of amniotic sacs, first
trimester

O30.292 **Quadruplet pregnancy, unable to** Ⓜ♀
determine number of placenta and
number of amniotic sacs, second
trimester

O30.293 **Quadruplet pregnancy, unable to** Ⓜ♀
determine number of placenta and
number of amniotic sacs, third
trimester

O30.299 **Quadruplet pregnancy, unable to** Ⓜ♀▽
determine number of placenta and
number of amniotic sacs, unspecified

✅ Add'l Character Required   ✓ₓ7ₜₕ Placeholder Alert   RUG IV Special Care High Dx   RUG IV Clinically Complex Dx   RUG IV Special Care Low Dx   Manifestation Code   Other Specified Code   ▽ Unspecified Code

ICD-10-CM 2016   787

Chapter 15. Pregnancy, Childbirth and the Puerperium

✓5ᵗʰ **O30.8** Other specified multiple gestation
     Multiple gestation pregnancy greater than quadruplets

     ✓6ᵗʰ **O30.80** Other specified multiple gestation, unspecified number of placenta and unspecified number of amniotic sacs

       O30.801 Other specified multiple gestation, unspecified number of placenta and unspecified number of amniotic sacs, first trimester   Ⓜ♀▽

       O30.802 Other specified multiple gestation, unspecified number of placenta and unspecified number of amniotic sacs, second trimester   Ⓜ♀▽

       O30.803 Other specified multiple gestation, unspecified number of placenta and unspecified number of amniotic sacs, third trimester   Ⓜ♀▽

       O30.809 Other specified multiple gestation, unspecified number of placenta and unspecified number of amniotic sacs, unspecified trimester   Ⓜ♀▽

     ✓6ᵗʰ **O30.81** Other specified multiple gestation with two or more monochorionic fetuses

       O30.811 Other specified multiple gestation with two or more monochorionic fetuses, first trimester   Ⓜ♀

       O30.812 Other specified multiple gestation with two or more monochorionic fetuses, second trimester   Ⓜ♀

       O30.813 Other specified multiple gestation with two or more monochorionic fetuses, third trimester   Ⓜ♀

       O30.819 Other specified multiple gestation with two or more monochorionic fetuses, unspecified trimester   Ⓜ♀▽

     ✓6ᵗʰ **O30.82** Other specified multiple gestation with two or more monoamniotic fetuses

       O30.821 Other specified multiple gestation with two or more monoamniotic fetuses, first trimester   Ⓜ♀

       O30.822 Other specified multiple gestation with two or more monoamniotic fetuses, second trimester   Ⓜ♀

       O30.823 Other specified multiple gestation with two or more monoamniotic fetuses, third trimester   Ⓜ♀

       O30.829 Other specified multiple gestation with two or more monoamniotic fetuses, unspecified trimester   Ⓜ♀▽

     ✓6ᵗʰ **O30.89** Other specified multiple gestation, unable to determine number of placenta and number of amniotic sacs

       O30.891 Other specified multiple gestation, unable to determine number of placenta and number of amniotic sacs, first trimester   Ⓜ♀

       O30.892 Other specified multiple gestation, unable to determine number of placenta and number of amniotic sacs, second trimester   Ⓜ♀

       O30.893 Other specified multiple gestation, unable to determine number of placenta and number of amniotic sacs, third trimester   Ⓜ♀

       O30.899 Other specified multiple gestation, unable to determine number of placenta and number of amniotic sacs, unspecified trimester   Ⓜ♀▽

✓5ᵗʰ **O30.9** Multiple gestation, unspecified
     Multiple pregnancy NOS

     O30.90 Multiple gestation, unspecified, unspecified trimester   Ⓜ♀▽

     O30.91 Multiple gestation, unspecified, first trimester   Ⓜ♀▽

     O30.92 Multiple gestation, unspecified, second trimester   Ⓜ♀▽

     O30.93 Multiple gestation, unspecified, third trimester   Ⓜ♀▽

✓4ᵗʰ **O31** Complications specific to multiple gestation

     EXCLUDES 2   delayed delivery of second twin, triplet, etc. (O63.2)
             malpresentation of one fetus or more (O32.9)
             placental transfusion syndromes (O43.0-)

     AHA: 2012, 4Q, 107

> One of the following 7th characters is to be assigned to each code under category O31. 7th character 0 is for single gestations and multiple gestations where the fetus is unspecified. 7th characters 1 through 9 are for cases of multiple gestations to identify the fetus for which the code applies. The appropriate code from category O30, Multiple gestation, must also be assigned when assigning a code from category O31 that has a 7th character of 1 through 9.
>
> 0   not applicable or unspecified   4   fetus 4
> 1   fetus 1   5   fetus 5
> 2   fetus 2   9   other fetus
> 3   fetus 3

     ✓5ᵗʰ **O31.0** Papyraceous fetus
         Fetus compressus

       ✓x7ᵗʰ **O31.00** Papyraceous fetus, unspecified trimester   Ⓜ♀▽

       ✓x7ᵗʰ **O31.01** Papyraceous fetus, first trimester   Ⓜ♀

       ✓x7ᵗʰ **O31.02** Papyraceous fetus, second trimester   Ⓜ♀

       ✓x7ᵗʰ **O31.03** Papyraceous fetus, third trimester   Ⓜ♀

     ✓5ᵗʰ **O31.1** Continuing pregnancy after spontaneous abortion of one fetus or more

       ✓x7ᵗʰ **O31.10** Continuing pregnancy after spontaneous abortion of one fetus or more, unspecified trimester   Ⓜ♀▽

       ✓x7ᵗʰ **O31.11** Continuing pregnancy after spontaneous abortion of one fetus or more, first trimester   Ⓜ♀

       ✓x7ᵗʰ **O31.12** Continuing pregnancy after spontaneous abortion of one fetus or more, second trimester   Ⓜ♀

       ✓x7ᵗʰ **O31.13** Continuing pregnancy after spontaneous abortion of one fetus or more, third trimester   Ⓜ♀

     ✓5ᵗʰ **O31.2** Continuing pregnancy after intrauterine death of one fetus or more

       ✓x7ᵗʰ **O31.20** Continuing pregnancy after intrauterine death of one fetus or more, unspecified trimester   Ⓜ♀▽

       ✓x7ᵗʰ **O31.21** Continuing pregnancy after intrauterine death of one fetus or more, first trimester   Ⓜ♀

       ✓x7ᵗʰ **O31.22** Continuing pregnancy after intrauterine death of one fetus or more, second trimester   Ⓜ♀

       ✓x7ᵗʰ **O31.23** Continuing pregnancy after intrauterine death of one fetus or more, third trimester   Ⓜ♀

     ✓5ᵗʰ **O31.3** Continuing pregnancy after elective fetal reduction of one fetus or more
         Continuing pregnancy after selective termination of one fetus or more

       ✓x7ᵗʰ **O31.30** Continuing pregnancy after elective fetal reduction of one fetus or more, unspecified trimester   Ⓜ♀▽

       ✓x7ᵗʰ **O31.31** Continuing pregnancy after elective fetal reduction of one fetus or more, first trimester   Ⓜ♀

       ✓x7ᵗʰ **O31.32** Continuing pregnancy after elective fetal reduction of one fetus or more, second trimester   Ⓜ♀

       ✓x7ᵗʰ **O31.33** Continuing pregnancy after elective fetal reduction of one fetus or more, third trimester   Ⓜ♀

     ✓5ᵗʰ **O31.8** Other complications specific to multiple gestation

       ✓6ᵗʰ **O31.8X** Other complications specific to multiple gestation

         ✓7ᵗʰ **O31.8X1** Other complications specific to multiple gestation, first trimester   Ⓜ♀

         ✓7ᵗʰ **O31.8X2** Other complications specific to multiple gestation, second trimester   Ⓜ♀

         ✓7ᵗʰ **O31.8X3** Other complications specific to multiple gestation, third trimester   Ⓜ♀

         ✓7ᵗʰ **O31.8X9** Other complications specific to multiple gestation, unspecified trimester   Ⓜ♀▽

Ⓝ Newborn   Ⓟ Pediatric   Ⓜ Maternity   Ⓐ Adult   RIC RIC Dx   NCDx Noncancer Dx   PDx Primary Dx   CC RIC CC Condition   ▶◀ Revised Text   ● New Code   ▲ Revised Code Title

788   ICD-10-CM 2016

✓4ᵗʰ O32 Maternal care for malpresentation of fetus

INCLUDES   the listed conditions as a reason for observation, hospitalization or other obstetric care of the mother, or for cesarean delivery before onset of labor

EXCLUDES 1   malpresentation of fetus with obstructed labor (O64.-)

AHA: 2012, 4Q, 107

One of the following 7th characters is to be assigned to each code under category O32. 7th character Ø is for single gestations and multiple gestations where the fetus is unspecified. 7th characters 1 through 9 are for cases of multiple gestations to identify the fetus for which the code applies. The appropriate code from category O3Ø, Multiple gestation, must also be assigned when assigning a code from category O32 that has a 7th character of 1 through 9.

Ø	not applicable or unspecified	4	fetus 4
1	fetus 1	5	fetus 5
2	fetus 2	9	other fetus
3	fetus 3		

✓x7ᵗʰ **O32.Ø Maternal care for** unstable lie   Ⓜ♀

✓x7ᵗʰ **O32.1 Maternal care for** breech presentation   Ⓜ♀
Maternal care for buttocks presentation
Maternal care for complete breech
Maternal care for frank breech
EXCLUDES 1   footling presentation (O32.8)
incomplete breech (O32.8)

✓x7ᵗʰ **O32.2 Maternal care for** transverse and oblique lie   Ⓜ♀
Maternal care for oblique presentation
Maternal care for transverse presentation

✓x7ᵗʰ **O32.3 Maternal care for** face, brow and chin presentation   Ⓜ♀

✓x7ᵗʰ **O32.4 Maternal care for** high head at term   Ⓜ♀
Maternal care for failure of head to enter pelvic brim

✓x7ᵗʰ **O32.6 Maternal care for** compound presentation   Ⓜ♀

✓x7ᵗʰ **O32.8 Maternal care for other** malpresentation of fetus   Ⓜ♀
Maternal care for footling presentation
Maternal care for incomplete breech

✓x7ᵗʰ **O32.9 Maternal care for malpresentation of fetus, unspecified**   Ⓜ♀▽

✓4ᵗʰ O33 Maternal care for disproportion

INCLUDES   the listed conditions as a reason for observation, hospitalization or other obstetric care of the mother, or for cesarean delivery before onset of labor

EXCLUDES 1   disproportion with obstructed labor (O65-O66)

O33.Ø Maternal care for disproportion due to deformity of maternal pelvic bones   Ⓜ♀
Maternal care for disproportion due to pelvic deformity causing disproportion NOS

O33.1 Maternal care for disproportion due to generally contracted pelvis   Ⓜ♀
Maternal care for disproportion due to contracted pelvis NOS causing disproportion

O33.2 Maternal care for disproportion due to inlet contraction   Ⓜ♀
of pelvis
Maternal care for disproportion due to inlet contraction (pelvis) causing disproportion

✓x7ᵗʰ **O33.3 Maternal care for disproportion due to** outlet contraction   Ⓜ♀
of pelvis
Maternal care for disproportion due to mid-cavity contraction (pelvis)
Maternal care for disproportion due to outlet contraction (pelvis)

One of the following 7th characters is to be assigned to code O33.3. 7th character Ø is for single gestations and multiple gestations where the fetus is unspecified. 7th characters 1 through 9 are for cases of multiple gestations to identify the fetus for which the code applies. The appropriate code from category O3Ø, Multiple gestation, must also be assigned when assigning code O33.3 with a 7th character of 1 through 9.

Ø	not applicable or unspecified	4	fetus 4
1	fetus 1	5	fetus 5
2	fetus 2	9	other fetus
3	fetus 3		

✓x7ᵗʰ **O33.4 Maternal care for disproportion of mixed maternal and**   Ⓜ♀
fetal origin

One of the following 7th characters is to be assigned to code O33.4. 7th character Ø is for single gestations and multiple gestations where the fetus is unspecified. 7th characters 1 through 9 are for cases of multiple gestations to identify the fetus for which the code applies. The appropriate code from category O3Ø, Multiple gestation, must also be assigned when assigning code O33.4 with a 7th character of 1 through 9.

Ø	not applicable or unspecified	4	fetus 4
1	fetus 1	5	fetus 5
2	fetus 2	9	other fetus
3	fetus 3		

✓x7ᵗʰ **O33.5 Maternal care for disproportion due to unusually large**   Ⓜ♀
fetus
Maternal care for disproportion due to disproportion of fetal origin with normally formed fetus
Maternal care for disproportion due to fetal disproportion NOS

One of the following 7th characters is to be assigned to code O33.5. 7th character Ø is for single gestations and multiple gestations where the fetus is unspecified. 7th characters 1 through 9 are for cases of multiple gestations to identify the fetus for which the code applies. The appropriate code from category O3Ø, Multiple gestation, must also be assigned when assigning code O33.5 with a 7th character of 1 through 9.

Ø	not applicable or unspecified	4	fetus 4
1	fetus 1	5	fetus 5
2	fetus 2	9	other fetus
3	fetus 3		

✓x7ᵗʰ **O33.6 Maternal care for disproportion due to hydrocephalic**   Ⓜ♀
fetus

One of the following 7th characters is to be assigned to code O33.6. 7th character Ø is for single gestations and multiple gestations where the fetus is unspecified. 7th characters 1 through 9 are for cases of multiple gestations to identify the fetus for which the code applies. The appropriate code from category O3Ø, Multiple gestation, must also be assigned when assigning code O33.6 with a 7th character of 1 through 9.

Ø	not applicable or unspecified	4	fetus 4
1	fetus 1	5	fetus 5
2	fetus 2	9	other fetus
3	fetus 3		

O33.7 Maternal care for disproportion due to other fetal   Ⓜ♀
deformities
Maternal care for disproportion due to fetal ascites
Maternal care for disproportion due to fetal hydrops
Maternal care for disproportion due to fetal meningomyelocele
Maternal care for disproportion due to fetal sacral teratoma
Maternal care for disproportion due to fetal tumor
EXCLUDES 1   obstructed labor due to other fetal deformities (O66.3)

O33.8 Maternal care for disproportion of other origin   Ⓜ♀

O33.9 Maternal care for disproportion, unspecified   Ⓜ♀▽
Maternal care for disproportion due to cephalopelvic disproportion NOS
Maternal care for disproportion due to fetopelvic disproportion NOS

✓4ᵗʰ O34 Maternal care for abnormality of pelvic organs

INCLUDES   the listed conditions as a reason for hospitalization or other obstetric care of the mother, or for cesarean delivery before onset of labor

Code first any associated obstructed labor (O65.5)
Use additional code for specific condition

✓5ᵗʰ **O34.Ø Maternal care for** congenital malformation of uterus

O34.ØØ Maternal care for unspecified congenital   Ⓜ♀▽
malformation of uterus, unspecified trimester

O34.Ø1 Maternal care for unspecified congenital   Ⓜ♀▽
malformation of uterus, first trimester

O34.Ø2 Maternal care for unspecified congenital   Ⓜ♀▽
malformation of uterus, second trimester

O34.Ø3 Maternal care for unspecified congenital   Ⓜ♀▽
malformation of uterus, third trimester

Chapter 15. Pregnancy, Childbirth and the Puerperium

O32–O34.03

✓5ᵗʰ O34.1 Maternal care for benign tumor of corpus uteri
> EXCLUDES 2 *maternal care for benign tumor of cervix (O34.4-)*
> *maternal care for malignant neoplasm of uterus (O9A.1-)*

O34.10 **Maternal care for benign tumor of corpus uteri, unspecified trimester** Ⓜ♀▽

O34.11 **Maternal care for benign tumor of corpus uteri,** first trimester Ⓜ♀

O34.12 **Maternal care for benign tumor of corpus uteri,** second trimester Ⓜ♀

O34.13 **Maternal care for benign tumor of corpus uteri,** third trimester Ⓜ♀

✓5ᵗʰ O34.2 Maternal care due to uterine scar from previous surgery

O34.21 **Maternal care for scar** from previous cesarean delivery Ⓜ♀

O34.29 **Maternal care due to uterine scar** from other previous surgery Ⓜ♀

✓5ᵗʰ O34.3 Maternal care for cervical incompetence
> Maternal care for cerclage with or without cervical incompetence
> Maternal care for Shirodkar suture with or without cervical incompetence

O34.30 **Maternal care for cervical incompetence, unspecified trimester** Ⓜ♀▽

O34.31 **Maternal care for cervical incompetence,** first trimester Ⓜ♀

O34.32 **Maternal care for cervical incompetence,** second trimester Ⓜ♀

O34.33 **Maternal care for cervical incompetence,** third trimester Ⓜ♀

✓5ᵗʰ O34.4 Maternal care for other abnormalities of cervix

O34.40 **Maternal care for other abnormalities of cervix, unspecified trimester** Ⓜ♀▽

O34.41 **Maternal care for other abnormalities of cervix,** first trimester Ⓜ♀

O34.42 **Maternal care for other abnormalities of cervix,** second trimester Ⓜ♀

O34.43 **Maternal care for other abnormalities of cervix,** third trimester Ⓜ♀

✓5ᵗʰ O34.5 Maternal care for other abnormalities of gravid uterus

✓6ᵗʰ O34.51 Maternal care for incarceration of gravid uterus

O34.511 **Maternal care for incarceration of gravid uterus,** first trimester Ⓜ♀

O34.512 **Maternal care for incarceration of gravid uterus,** second trimester Ⓜ♀

O34.513 **Maternal care for incarceration of gravid uterus,** third trimester Ⓜ♀

O34.519 **Maternal care for incarceration of gravid uterus, unspecified trimester** Ⓜ♀▽

✓6ᵗʰ O34.52 Maternal care for prolapse of gravid uterus

O34.521 **Maternal care for prolapse of gravid uterus,** first trimester Ⓜ♀

O34.522 **Maternal care for prolapse of gravid uterus,** second trimester Ⓜ♀

O34.523 **Maternal care for prolapse of gravid uterus,** third trimester Ⓜ♀

O34.529 **Maternal care for prolapse of gravid uterus, unspecified trimester** Ⓜ♀▽

✓6ᵗʰ O34.53 Maternal care for retroversion of gravid uterus

O34.531 **Maternal care for retroversion of gravid uterus,** first trimester Ⓜ♀

O34.532 **Maternal care for retroversion of gravid uterus,** second trimester Ⓜ♀

O34.533 **Maternal care for retroversion of gravid uterus,** third trimester Ⓜ♀

O34.539 **Maternal care for retroversion of gravid uterus, unspecified trimester** Ⓜ♀▽

✓6ᵗʰ O34.59 Maternal care for other abnormalities of gravid uterus

O34.591 **Maternal care for other abnormalities of gravid uterus,** first trimester Ⓜ♀

O34.592 **Maternal care for other abnormalities of gravid uterus,** second trimester Ⓜ♀

O34.593 **Maternal care for other abnormalities of gravid uterus,** third trimester Ⓜ♀

O34.599 **Maternal care for other abnormalities of gravid uterus, unspecified trimester** Ⓜ♀▽

✓5ᵗʰ O34.6 Maternal care for abnormality of vagina
> EXCLUDES 2 *maternal care for vaginal varices in pregnancy (O22.1-)*

O34.60 **Maternal care for abnormality of vagina, unspecified trimester** Ⓜ♀▽

O34.61 **Maternal care for abnormality of vagina,** first trimester Ⓜ♀

O34.62 **Maternal care for abnormality of vagina,** second trimester Ⓜ♀

O34.63 **Maternal care for abnormality of vagina,** third trimester Ⓜ♀

✓5ᵗʰ O34.7 Maternal care for abnormality of vulva and perineum
> EXCLUDES 2 *maternal care for perineal and vulval varices in pregnancy (O22.1-)*

O34.70 **Maternal care for abnormality of vulva and perineum, unspecified trimester** Ⓜ♀▽

O34.71 **Maternal care for abnormality of vulva and perineum,** first trimester Ⓜ♀

O34.72 **Maternal care for abnormality of vulva and perineum,** second trimester Ⓜ♀

O34.73 **Maternal care for abnormality of vulva and perineum,** third trimester Ⓜ♀

✓5ᵗʰ O34.8 Maternal care for other abnormalities of pelvic organs

O34.80 **Maternal care for other abnormalities of pelvic organs, unspecified trimester** Ⓜ♀▽

O34.81 **Maternal care for other abnormalities of pelvic organs,** first trimester Ⓜ♀

O34.82 **Maternal care for other abnormalities of pelvic organs,** second trimester Ⓜ♀

O34.83 **Maternal care for other abnormalities of pelvic organs,** third trimester Ⓜ♀

✓5ᵗʰ O34.9 Maternal care for abnormality of pelvic organ, unspecified

O34.90 **Maternal care for abnormality of pelvic organ, unspecified, unspecified trimester** Ⓜ♀▽

O34.91 **Maternal care for abnormality of pelvic organ, unspecified,** first trimester Ⓜ♀▽

O34.92 **Maternal care for abnormality of pelvic organ, unspecified,** second trimester Ⓜ♀▽

O34.93 **Maternal care for abnormality of pelvic organ, unspecified,** third trimester Ⓜ♀▽

✓4ᵗʰ O35 Maternal care for known or suspected fetal abnormality and damage
> INCLUDES the listed conditions in the fetus as a reason for hospitalization or other obstetric care to the mother, or for termination of pregnancy
>
> Code also any associated maternal condition
>
> EXCLUDES 1 *encounter for suspected maternal and fetal conditions ruled out (Z03.7-)*

One of the following 7th characters is to be assigned to each code under category O35. 7th character Ø is for single gestations and multiple gestations where the fetus is unspecified. 7th characters 1 through 9 are for cases of multiple gestations to identify the fetus for which the code applies. The appropriate code from category O30, Multiple gestation, must also be assigned when assigning a code from category O35 that has a 7th character of 1 through 9.
Ø not applicable or unspecified
1 fetus 1
2 fetus 2
3 fetus 3
4 fetus 4
5 fetus 5
9 other fetus

✓x7ᵗʰ O35.0 Maternal care for (suspected) central nervous system malformation in fetus Ⓜ♀
> Maternal care for fetal anencephaly
> Maternal care for fetal hydrocephalus
> Maternal care for fetal spina bifida
> EXCLUDES 2 *chromosomal abnormality in fetus (O35.1)*

✓x7ᵗʰ O35.1 Maternal care for (suspected) chromosomal abnormality in fetus Ⓜ♀

✓x7ᵗʰ O35.2 Maternal care for (suspected) hereditary disease in fetus Ⓜ♀
> EXCLUDES 2 *chromosomal abnormality in fetus (O35.1)*

✓x7ᵗʰ O35.3 Maternal care for (suspected) damage to fetus from viral disease in mother Ⓜ♀
> Maternal care for damage to fetus from maternal cytomegalovirus infection
> Maternal care for damage to fetus from maternal rubella

Ⓝ Newborn Ⓟ Pediatric Ⓜ Maternity Ⓐ Adult RIC RIC Dx NCDx Noncancer Dx PDx Primary Dx CC RIC CC Condition ▶◀ Revised Text ● New Code ▲ Revised Code Title

790 ICD-10-CM 2016

√x7ᵗʰ **O35.4 Maternal care for (suspected)** damage to fetus from alcohol Ⓜ♀

√x7ᵗʰ **O35.5 Maternal care for (suspected)** damage to fetus by drugs Ⓜ♀
Maternal care for damage to fetus from drug addiction

√x7ᵗʰ **O35.6 Maternal care for (suspected)** damage to fetus by radiation Ⓜ♀

√x7ᵗʰ **O35.7 Maternal care for (suspected)** damage to fetus by other medical procedures Ⓜ♀
Maternal care for damage to fetus by amniocentesis
Maternal care for damage to fetus by biopsy procedures
Maternal care for damage to fetus by hematological investigation
Maternal care for damage to fetus by intrauterine contraceptive device
Maternal care for damage to fetus by intrauterine surgery

√x7ᵗʰ **O35.8 Maternal care for other (suspected) fetal abnormality and damage** Ⓜ♀
Maternal care for damage to fetus from maternal listeriosis
Maternal care for damage to fetus from maternal toxoplasmosis

√x7ᵗʰ **O35.9 Maternal care for (suspected)** fetal abnormality and damage, **unspecified** Ⓜ♀▽

√4ᵗʰ **O36 Maternal care for other fetal problems**
    INCLUDES   the listed conditions in the fetus as a reason for hospitalization or other obstetric care of the mother, or for termination of pregnancy
    EXCLUDES 1   encounter for suspected maternal and fetal conditions ruled out (Z03.7-)
      placental transfusion syndromes (O43.0-)
    EXCLUDES 2   labor and delivery complicated by fetal stress (O77.-)

> One of the following 7th characters is to be assigned to each code under category O36. 7th character 0 is for single gestations and multiple gestations where the fetus is unspecified. 7th characters 1 through 9 are for cases of multiple gestations to identify the fetus for which the code applies. The appropriate code from category O30, Multiple gestation, must also be assigned when assigning a code from category O36 that has a 7th character of 1 through 9.
> 0   not applicable or unspecified   4   fetus 4
> 1   fetus 1   5   fetus 5
> 2   fetus 2   9   other fetus
> 3   fetus 3

√5ᵗʰ **O36.0 Maternal care for rhesus isoimmunization**
Maternal care for Rh incompatibility (with hydrops fetalis)

    √6ᵗʰ **O36.01 Maternal care for** anti-D [Rh] antibodies
      AHA: 2014, 4Q, 17

      √7ᵗʰ **O36.011 Maternal care for anti-D [Rh] antibodies, first trimester** Ⓜ♀

      √7ᵗʰ **O36.012 Maternal care for anti-D [Rh] antibodies, second trimester** Ⓜ♀

      √7ᵗʰ **O36.013 Maternal care for anti-D [Rh] antibodies, third trimester** Ⓜ♀

      √7ᵗʰ **O36.019 Maternal care for anti-D [Rh] antibodies, unspecified trimester** Ⓜ♀▽

    √6ᵗʰ **O36.09 Maternal care for** other rhesus isoimmunization

      √7ᵗʰ **O36.091 Maternal care for other rhesus isoimmunization, first trimester** Ⓜ♀

      √7ᵗʰ **O36.092 Maternal care for other rhesus isoimmunization, second trimester** Ⓜ♀

      √7ᵗʰ **O36.093 Maternal care for other rhesus isoimmunization, third trimester** Ⓜ♀

      √7ᵗʰ **O36.099 Maternal care for other rhesus isoimmunization, unspecified trimester** Ⓜ♀▽

√5ᵗʰ **O36.1 Maternal care for other isoimmunization**
Maternal care for ABO isoimmunization

    √6ᵗʰ **O36.11 Maternal care for** Anti-A sensitization
Maternal care for isoimmunization NOS (with hydrops fetalis)

      √7ᵗʰ **O36.111 Maternal care for Anti-A sensitization, first trimester** Ⓜ♀

      √7ᵗʰ **O36.112 Maternal care for Anti-A sensitization, second trimester** Ⓜ♀

      √7ᵗʰ **O36.113 Maternal care for Anti-A sensitization, third trimester** Ⓜ♀

      √7ᵗʰ **O36.119 Maternal care for Anti-A sensitization, unspecified trimester** Ⓜ♀▽

√6ᵗʰ **O36.19 Maternal care for** other isoimmunization
Maternal care for Anti-B sensitization

      √7ᵗʰ **O36.191 Maternal care for other isoimmunization, first trimester** Ⓜ♀

      √7ᵗʰ **O36.192 Maternal care for other isoimmunization, second trimester** Ⓜ♀

      √7ᵗʰ **O36.193 Maternal care for other isoimmunization, third trimester** Ⓜ♀

      √7ᵗʰ **O36.199 Maternal care for other isoimmunization, unspecified trimester** Ⓜ♀▽

√5ᵗʰ **O36.2 Maternal care for hydrops fetalis**
Maternal care for hydrops fetalis NOS
Maternal care for hydrops fetalis not associated with isoimmunization
    EXCLUDES 1   hydrops fetalis associated with ABO isoimmunization (O36.1-)
      hydrops fetalis associated with rhesus isoimmunization (O36.0-)

    √x7ᵗʰ **O36.20 Maternal care for hydrops fetalis, unspecified trimester** Ⓜ♀▽

    √x7ᵗʰ **O36.21 Maternal care for hydrops fetalis, first trimester** Ⓜ♀

    √x7ᵗʰ **O36.22 Maternal care for hydrops fetalis, second trimester** Ⓜ♀

    √x7ᵗʰ **O36.23 Maternal care for hydrops fetalis, third trimester** Ⓜ♀

√x7ᵗʰ **O36.4 Maternal care for intrauterine death** Ⓜ♀
Maternal care for intrauterine fetal death NOS
Maternal care for intrauterine fetal death after completion of 20 weeks of gestation
Maternal care for late fetal death
Maternal care for missed delivery
    EXCLUDES 1   missed abortion (O02.1)
      stillbirth (P95)

√5ᵗʰ **O36.5 Maternal care for known or suspected poor fetal growth**

    √6ᵗʰ **O36.51 Maternal care for known or suspected placental insufficiency**

      √7ᵗʰ **O36.511 Maternal care for known or suspected placental insufficiency, first trimester** Ⓜ♀

      √7ᵗʰ **O36.512 Maternal care for known or suspected placental insufficiency, second trimester** Ⓜ♀

      √7ᵗʰ **O36.513 Maternal care for known or suspected placental insufficiency, third trimester** Ⓜ♀

      √7ᵗʰ **O36.519 Maternal care for known or suspected placental insufficiency, unspecified trimester** Ⓜ♀▽

    √6ᵗʰ **O36.59 Maternal care for other known or suspected poor fetal growth**
Maternal care for known or suspected light-for-dates NOS
Maternal care for known or suspected small-for-dates NOS

      √7ᵗʰ **O36.591 Maternal care for other known or suspected poor fetal growth, first trimester** Ⓜ♀

      √7ᵗʰ **O36.592 Maternal care for other known or suspected poor fetal growth, second trimester** Ⓜ♀

      √7ᵗʰ **O36.593 Maternal care for other known or suspected poor fetal growth, third trimester** Ⓜ♀

      √7ᵗʰ **O36.599 Maternal care for other known or suspected poor fetal growth, unspecified trimester** Ⓜ♀▽

√5ᵗʰ **O36.6 Maternal care for excessive fetal growth**
Maternal care for known or suspected large-for-dates

    √x7ᵗʰ **O36.60 Maternal care for excessive fetal growth, unspecified trimester** Ⓜ♀▽

    √x7ᵗʰ **O36.61 Maternal care for excessive fetal growth, first trimester** Ⓜ♀

    √x7ᵗʰ **O36.62 Maternal care for excessive fetal growth, second trimester** Ⓜ♀

    √x7ᵗʰ **O36.63 Maternal care for excessive fetal growth, third trimester** Ⓜ♀

√5ᵗʰ **O36.7 Maternal care for viable fetus in abdominal pregnancy**

√x7ᵗʰ **O36.70 Maternal care for viable fetus in abdominal** Ⓜ♀▽
pregnancy, unspecified trimester

√x7ᵗʰ **O36.71 Maternal care for viable fetus in abdominal** Ⓜ♀
pregnancy, first trimester

√x7ᵗʰ **O36.72 Maternal care for viable fetus in abdominal** Ⓜ♀
pregnancy, second trimester

√x7ᵗʰ **O36.73 Maternal care for viable fetus in abdominal** Ⓜ♀
pregnancy, third trimester

√5ᵗʰ **O36.8 Maternal care for other specified fetal problems**

√x7ᵗʰ **O36.80 Pregnancy with inconclusive fetal viability** Ⓜ♀
Encounter to determine fetal viability of pregnancy

√6ᵗʰ **O36.81 Decreased fetal movements**

√7ᵗʰ **O36.812 Decreased fetal movements, second** Ⓜ♀
trimester

√7ᵗʰ **O36.813 Decreased fetal movements, third** Ⓜ♀
trimester

√7ᵗʰ **O36.819 Decreased fetal movements,** Ⓜ♀▽
unspecified trimester

√6ᵗʰ **O36.82 Fetal anemia and thrombocytopenia**

√7ᵗʰ **O36.821 Fetal anemia and thrombocytopenia,** Ⓜ♀
first trimester

√7ᵗʰ **O36.822 Fetal anemia and thrombocytopenia,** Ⓜ♀
second trimester

√7ᵗʰ **O36.823 Fetal anemia and thrombocytopenia,** Ⓜ♀
third trimester

√7ᵗʰ **O36.829 Fetal anemia and** Ⓜ♀▽
thrombocytopenia, unspecified
trimester

√6ᵗʰ **O36.89 Maternal care for other specified fetal problems**

√7ᵗʰ **O36.891 Maternal care for other specified fetal** Ⓜ♀
problems, first trimester

√7ᵗʰ **O36.892 Maternal care for other specified fetal** Ⓜ♀
problems, second trimester

√7ᵗʰ **O36.893 Maternal care for other specified fetal** Ⓜ♀
problems, third trimester

√7ᵗʰ **O36.899 Maternal care for other specified** Ⓜ♀▽
fetal problems, unspecified trimester

√5ᵗʰ **O36.9 Maternal care for fetal problem, unspecified**

√x7ᵗʰ **O36.90 Maternal care for fetal problem, unspecified,** Ⓜ♀▽
unspecified trimester

√x7ᵗʰ **O36.91 Maternal care for fetal problem, unspecified,** Ⓜ♀▽
first trimester

√x7ᵗʰ **O36.92 Maternal care for fetal problem, unspecified,** Ⓜ♀▽
second trimester

√x7ᵗʰ **O36.93 Maternal care for fetal problem, unspecified,** Ⓜ♀▽
third trimester

√4ᵗʰ **O40 Polyhydramnios**
Hydramnios
EXCLUDES 1 encounter for suspected maternal and fetal conditions ruled out
(Z03.7-)

One of the following 7th characters is to be assigned to each code
under category O40. 7th character Ø is for single gestations and
multiple gestations where the fetus is unspecified. 7th characters 1
through 9 are for cases of multiple gestations to identify the fetus
for which the code applies. The appropriate code from category
O30, Multiple gestation, must also be assigned when assigning a
code from category O40 that has a 7th character of 1 through 9.

Ø   not applicable or unspecified   4   fetus 4
1   fetus 1   5   fetus 5
2   fetus 2   9   other fetus
3   fetus 3

√x7ᵗʰ **O40.1 Polyhydramnios, first trimester** Ⓜ♀

√x7ᵗʰ **O40.2 Polyhydramnios, second trimester** Ⓜ♀

√x7ᵗʰ **O40.3 Polyhydramnios, third trimester** Ⓜ♀

√x7ᵗʰ **O40.9 Polyhydramnios, unspecified trimester** Ⓜ♀▽

√4ᵗʰ **O41 Other disorders of amniotic fluid and membranes**
EXCLUDES 1 encounter for suspected maternal and fetal conditions ruled out
(Z03.7-)

One of the following 7th characters is to be assigned to each code
under category O41. 7th character Ø is for single gestations and
multiple gestations where the fetus is unspecified. 7th characters 1
through 9 are for cases of multiple gestations to identify the fetus
for which the code applies. The appropriate code from category
O30, Multiple gestation, must also be assigned when assigning a
code from category O41 that has a 7th character of 1 through 9.

Ø   not applicable or unspecified   4   fetus 4
1   fetus 1   5   fetus 5
2   fetus 2   9   other fetus
3   fetus 3

√5ᵗʰ **O41.0 Oligohydramnios**
Oligohydramnios without rupture of membranes

√x7ᵗʰ **O41.00 Oligohydramnios, unspecified trimester** Ⓜ♀▽

√x7ᵗʰ **O41.01 Oligohydramnios, first trimester** Ⓜ♀

√x7ᵗʰ **O41.02 Oligohydramnios, second trimester** Ⓜ♀

√x7ᵗʰ **O41.03 Oligohydramnios, third trimester** Ⓜ♀

√5ᵗʰ **O41.1 Infection of amniotic sac and membranes**

√6ᵗʰ **O41.10 Infection of amniotic sac and membranes,**
unspecified

√7ᵗʰ **O41.101 Infection of amniotic sac and** Ⓜ♀▽
membranes, unspecified, first
trimester

√7ᵗʰ **O41.102 Infection of amniotic sac and** Ⓜ♀▽
membranes, unspecified, second
trimester

√7ᵗʰ **O41.103 Infection of amniotic sac and** Ⓜ♀▽
membranes, unspecified, third
trimester

√7ᵗʰ **O41.109 Infection of amniotic sac and** Ⓜ♀▽
membranes, unspecified, unspecified
trimester

√6ᵗʰ **O41.12 Chorioamnionitis**

√7ᵗʰ **O41.121 Chorioamnionitis, first trimester** Ⓜ♀

√7ᵗʰ **O41.122 Chorioamnionitis, second trimester** Ⓜ♀

√7ᵗʰ **O41.123 Chorioamnionitis, third trimester** Ⓜ♀

√7ᵗʰ **O41.129 Chorioamnionitis, unspecified** Ⓜ♀▽
trimester

√6ᵗʰ **O41.14 Placentitis**

√7ᵗʰ **O41.141 Placentitis, first trimester** Ⓜ♀

√7ᵗʰ **O41.142 Placentitis, second trimester** Ⓜ♀

√7ᵗʰ **O41.143 Placentitis, third trimester** Ⓜ♀

√7ᵗʰ **O41.149 Placentitis, unspecified trimester** Ⓜ♀▽

√5ᵗʰ **O41.8 Other specified disorders of amniotic fluid and membranes**

√6ᵗʰ **O41.8X Other specified disorders of amniotic fluid and**
membranes

√7ᵗʰ **O41.8X1 Other specified disorders of amniotic** Ⓜ♀
fluid and membranes, first trimester

√7ᵗʰ **O41.8X2 Other specified disorders of amniotic** Ⓜ♀
fluid and membranes, second trimester

√7ᵗʰ **O41.8X3 Other specified disorders of amniotic** Ⓜ♀
fluid and membranes, third trimester

√7ᵗʰ **O41.8X9 Other specified disorders of** Ⓜ♀▽
amniotic fluid and membranes,
unspecified trimester

√5ᵗʰ **O41.9 Disorder of amniotic fluid and membranes, unspecified**

√x7ᵗʰ **O41.90 Disorder of amniotic fluid and membranes,** Ⓜ♀▽
unspecified, unspecified trimester

√x7ᵗʰ **O41.91 Disorder of amniotic fluid and membranes,** Ⓜ♀▽
unspecified, first trimester

√x7ᵗʰ **O41.92 Disorder of amniotic fluid and membranes,** Ⓜ♀▽
unspecified, second trimester

√x7ᵗʰ **O41.93 Disorder of amniotic fluid and membranes,** Ⓜ♀▽
unspecified, third trimester

√4ᵗʰ **O42 Premature rupture of membranes**

√5ᵗʰ **O42.0 Premature rupture of membranes, onset of labor within 24**
hours of rupture

O42.00 Premature rupture of membranes, onset of Ⓜ♀▽
labor within 24 hours of rupture, unspecified
weeks of gestation

Ⓝ Newborn   Ⓟ Pediatric   Ⓜ Maternity   Ⓐ Adult   RIC RIC Dx   NCDx Noncancer Dx   PDx Primary Dx   CC RIC CC Condition   ▶◀ Revised Text   ● New Code   ▲ Revised Code Title

792   ICD-10-CM 2016

✓6th **O42.01** Preterm **premature rupture of membranes, onset of labor within 24 hours of rupture**
Premature rupture of membranes before 37 completed weeks of gestation

     O42.011 **Preterm premature rupture of membranes, onset of labor within 24 hours of rupture, first trimester** Ⅿ♀

     O42.012 **Preterm premature rupture of membranes, onset of labor within 24 hours of rupture, second trimester** Ⅿ♀

     O42.013 **Preterm premature rupture of membranes, onset of labor within 24 hours of rupture, third trimester** Ⅿ♀

     O42.019 **Preterm premature rupture of membranes, onset of labor within 24 hours of rupture, unspecified trimester** Ⅿ♀▽

O42.02 **Full-term premature rupture of membranes, onset of labor within 24 hours of rupture** Ⅿ♀
Premature rupture of membranes after 37 completed weeks of gestation

✓5th **O42.1** **Premature rupture of membranes, onset of labor more than 24 hours following rupture**

     O42.10 **Premature rupture of membranes, onset of labor more than 24 hours following rupture, unspecified weeks of gestation** Ⅿ♀▽

✓6th **O42.11** **Preterm premature rupture of membranes, onset of labor more than 24 hours following rupture**
Premature rupture of membranes before 37 completed weeks of gestation

     O42.111 **Preterm premature rupture of membranes, onset of labor more than 24 hours following rupture, first trimester** Ⅿ♀

     O42.112 **Preterm premature rupture of membranes, onset of labor more than 24 hours following rupture, second trimester** Ⅿ♀

     O42.113 **Preterm premature rupture of membranes, onset of labor more than 24 hours following rupture, third trimester** Ⅿ♀

     O42.119 **Preterm premature rupture of membranes, onset of labor more than 24 hours following rupture, unspecified trimester** Ⅿ♀▽

O42.12 **Full-term premature rupture of membranes, onset of labor more than 24 hours following rupture** Ⅿ♀
Premature rupture of membranes after 37 completed weeks of gestation

✓5th **O42.9** **Premature rupture of membranes, unspecified as to length of time between rupture and onset of labor**

     O42.90 **Premature rupture of membranes, unspecified as to length of time between rupture and onset of labor, unspecified weeks of gestation** Ⅿ♀▽

✓6th **O42.91** **Preterm premature rupture of membranes, unspecified as to length of time between rupture and onset of labor**
Premature rupture of membranes before 37 completed weeks of gestation

     O42.911 **Preterm premature rupture of membranes, unspecified as to length of time between rupture and onset of labor, first trimester** Ⅿ♀▽

     O42.912 **Preterm premature rupture of membranes, unspecified as to length of time between rupture and onset of labor, second trimester** Ⅿ♀▽

     O42.913 **Preterm premature rupture of membranes, unspecified as to length of time between rupture and onset of labor, third trimester** Ⅿ♀▽

     O42.919 **Preterm premature rupture of membranes, unspecified as to length of time between rupture and onset of labor, unspecified trimester** Ⅿ♀▽

O42.92 **Full-term premature rupture of membranes, unspecified as to length of time between rupture and onset of labor** Ⅿ♀▽
Premature rupture of membranes after 37 completed weeks of gestation

✓4th **O43** **Placental disorders**
     EXCLUDES 2   maternal care for poor fetal growth due to placental insufficiency (O36.5-)
         placenta previa (O44.-)
         placental polyp (O90.89)
         placentitis (O41.14-)
         premature separation of placenta [abruptio placentae] (O45.-)

✓5th **O43.0** **Placental transfusion syndromes**
     ✓6th **O43.01** **Fetomaternal placental transfusion syndrome**
         Maternofetal placental transfusion syndrome

         O43.011 **Fetomaternal placental transfusion syndrome, first trimester** Ⅿ♀

         O43.012 **Fetomaternal placental transfusion syndrome, second trimester** Ⅿ♀

         O43.013 **Fetomaternal placental transfusion syndrome, third trimester** Ⅿ♀

         O43.019 **Fetomaternal placental transfusion syndrome, unspecified trimester** Ⅿ♀▽

     ✓6th **O43.02** **Fetus-to-fetus placental transfusion syndrome**

         O43.021 **Fetus-to-fetus placental transfusion syndrome, first trimester** Ⅿ♀

         O43.022 **Fetus-to-fetus placental transfusion syndrome, second trimester** Ⅿ♀

         O43.023 **Fetus-to-fetus placental transfusion syndrome, third trimester** Ⅿ♀

         O43.029 **Fetus-to-fetus placental transfusion syndrome, unspecified trimester** Ⅿ♀▽

✓5th **O43.1** **Malformation of placenta**
     ✓6th **O43.10** **Malformation of placenta, unspecified**
         Abnormal placenta NOS

         O43.101 **Malformation of placenta, unspecified, first trimester** Ⅿ♀▽

         O43.102 **Malformation of placenta, unspecified, second trimester** Ⅿ♀▽

         O43.103 **Malformation of placenta, unspecified, third trimester** Ⅿ♀▽

         O43.109 **Malformation of placenta, unspecified, unspecified trimester** Ⅿ♀▽

     ✓6th **O43.11** Circumvallate placenta

         O43.111 **Circumvallate placenta, first trimester** Ⅿ♀

         O43.112 **Circumvallate placenta, second trimester** Ⅿ♀

         O43.113 **Circumvallate placenta, third trimester** Ⅿ♀

         O43.119 **Circumvallate placenta, unspecified trimester** Ⅿ♀▽

     ✓6th **O43.12** Velamentous insertion of umbilical cord

         O43.121 **Velamentous insertion of umbilical cord, first trimester** Ⅿ♀

         O43.122 **Velamentous insertion of umbilical cord, second trimester** Ⅿ♀

         O43.123 **Velamentous insertion of umbilical cord, third trimester** Ⅿ♀

         O43.129 **Velamentous insertion of umbilical cord, unspecified trimester** Ⅿ♀▽

     ✓6th **O43.19** Other malformation of placenta

         O43.191 **Other malformation of placenta, first trimester** Ⅿ♀

         O43.192 **Other malformation of placenta, second trimester** Ⅿ♀

         O43.193 **Other malformation of placenta, third trimester** Ⅿ♀

         O43.199 **Other malformation of placenta, unspecified trimester** Ⅿ♀▽

✓5th **O43.2** **Morbidly adherent placenta**
     Code also associated third stage postpartum hemorrhage, if applicable (O72.0)
     EXCLUDES 1   retained placenta (O73.-)

     ✓6th **O43.21** Placenta accreta
         O43.211 **Placenta accreta, first trimester** Ⅿ♀
         O43.212 **Placenta accreta, second trimester** Ⅿ♀
         O43.213 **Placenta accreta, third trimester** Ⅿ♀
         O43.219 **Placenta accreta, unspecified trimester** Ⅿ♀▽

     ✓6th **O43.22** Placenta increta
         O43.221 **Placenta increta, first trimester** Ⅿ♀
         O43.222 **Placenta increta, second trimester** Ⅿ♀

☑ Add'l Character Required   ✓x7th Placeholder Alert   RUG IV Special Care High Dx   RUG IV Clinically Complex Dx   RUG IV Special Care Low Dx   Manifestation Code   Other Specified Code   ▽ Unspecified Code

O43.223 **Placenta increta,** third trimester   Ⓜ♀

O43.229 **Placenta increta, unspecified trimester**   Ⓜ♀▽

✓6ᵗʰ **O43.23 Placenta** percreta

    O43.231 **Placenta percreta,** first trimester   Ⓜ♀

    O43.232 **Placenta percreta,** second trimester   Ⓜ♀

    O43.233 **Placenta percreta,** third trimester   Ⓜ♀

    O43.239 **Placenta percreta, unspecified trimester**   Ⓜ♀▽

✓5ᵗʰ **O43.8 Other placental disorders**

  ✓6ᵗʰ **O43.81 Placental infarction**

    O43.811 **Placental infarction,** first trimester   Ⓜ♀

    O43.812 **Placental infarction,** second trimester   Ⓜ♀

    O43.813 **Placental infarction,** third trimester   Ⓜ♀

    O43.819 **Placental infarction, unspecified trimester**   Ⓜ♀▽

  ✓6ᵗʰ **O43.89 Other placental disorders**
Placental dysfunction

    O43.891 **Other placental disorders,** first trimester   Ⓜ♀

    O43.892 **Other placental disorders,** second trimester   Ⓜ♀

    O43.893 **Other placental disorders,** third trimester   Ⓜ♀

    O43.899 **Other placental disorders, unspecified trimester**   Ⓜ♀▽

✓5ᵗʰ **O43.9 Unspecified placental disorder**

    O43.90 **Unspecified placental disorder, unspecified trimester**   Ⓜ♀▽

    O43.91 **Unspecified placental disorder,** first trimester   Ⓜ♀▽

    O43.92 **Unspecified placental disorder,** second trimester   Ⓜ♀▽

    O43.93 **Unspecified placental disorder,** third trimester   Ⓜ♀▽

✓4ᵗʰ **O44 Placenta previa**

  ✓5ᵗʰ **O44.0 Placenta previa specified as** without hemorrhage
Low implantation of placenta specified as without hemorrhage

    O44.00 **Placenta previa specified as without hemorrhage, unspecified trimester**   Ⓜ♀▽

    O44.01 **Placenta previa specified as without hemorrhage,** first trimester   Ⓜ♀

    O44.02 **Placenta previa specified as without hemorrhage,** second trimester   Ⓜ♀

    O44.03 **Placenta previa specified as without hemorrhage,** third trimester   Ⓜ♀

  ✓5ᵗʰ **O44.1 Placenta previa** with hemorrhage
Low implantation of placenta, NOS or with hemorrhage
Marginal placenta previa, NOS or with hemorrhage
Partial placenta previa, NOS or with hemorrhage
Total placenta previa, NOS or with hemorrhage

    EXCLUDES 1 labor and delivery complicated by hemorrhage from vasa previa (O69.4)

    O44.10 **Placenta previa with hemorrhage, unspecified trimester**   Ⓜ♀▽

    O44.11 **Placenta previa with hemorrhage,** first trimester   Ⓜ♀

    O44.12 **Placenta previa with hemorrhage,** second trimester   Ⓜ♀

    O44.13 **Placenta previa with hemorrhage,** third trimester   Ⓜ♀

✓4ᵗʰ **O45 Premature separation of placenta [abruptio placentae]**

  ✓5ᵗʰ **O45.0 Premature separation of placenta with** coagulation defect

   ✓6ᵗʰ **O45.00 Premature separation of placenta with coagulation defect, unspecified**

    O45.001 **Premature separation of placenta with coagulation defect, unspecified, first trimester**   Ⓜ♀▽

    O45.002 **Premature separation of placenta with coagulation defect, unspecified,** second trimester   Ⓜ♀▽

    O45.003 **Premature separation of placenta with coagulation defect, unspecified,** third trimester   Ⓜ♀▽

    O45.009 **Premature separation of placenta with coagulation defect, unspecified, unspecified trimester**   Ⓜ♀▽

  ✓6ᵗʰ **O45.01 Premature separation of placenta with** afibrinogenemia
Premature separation of placenta with hypofibrinogenemia

    O45.011 **Premature separation of placenta with afibrinogenemia,** first trimester   Ⓜ♀

    O45.012 **Premature separation of placenta with afibrinogenemia,** second trimester   Ⓜ♀

    O45.013 **Premature separation of placenta with afibrinogenemia,** third trimester   Ⓜ♀

    O45.019 **Premature separation of placenta with afibrinogenemia, unspecified trimester**   Ⓜ♀▽

  ✓6ᵗʰ **O45.02 Premature separation of placenta with** disseminated intravascular coagulation

    O45.021 **Premature separation of placenta with disseminated intravascular coagulation,** first trimester   Ⓜ♀

    O45.022 **Premature separation of placenta with disseminated intravascular coagulation,** second trimester   Ⓜ♀

    O45.023 **Premature separation of placenta with disseminated intravascular coagulation,** third trimester   Ⓜ♀

    O45.029 **Premature separation of placenta with disseminated intravascular coagulation, unspecified trimester**   Ⓜ♀▽

  ✓6ᵗʰ **O45.09 Premature separation of placenta with** other coagulation defect

    O45.091 **Premature separation of placenta with other coagulation defect,** first trimester   Ⓜ♀

    O45.092 **Premature separation of placenta with other coagulation defect,** second trimester   Ⓜ♀

    O45.093 **Premature separation of placenta with other coagulation defect,** third trimester   Ⓜ♀

    O45.099 **Premature separation of placenta with other coagulation defect, unspecified trimester**   Ⓜ♀▽

  ✓5ᵗʰ **O45.8 Other premature separation** of placenta

   ✓6ᵗʰ **O45.8X Other premature separation of placenta**

    O45.8X1 **Other premature separation of placenta,** first trimester   Ⓜ♀

    O45.8X2 **Other premature separation of placenta,** second trimester   Ⓜ♀

    O45.8X3 **Other premature separation of placenta,** third trimester   Ⓜ♀

    O45.8X9 **Other premature separation of placenta, unspecified trimester**   Ⓜ♀▽

  ✓5ᵗʰ **O45.9 Premature separation of placenta,** unspecified
Abruptio placentae NOS

    O45.90 **Premature separation of placenta, unspecified, unspecified trimester**   Ⓜ♀▽

    O45.91 **Premature separation of placenta, unspecified,** first trimester   Ⓜ♀▽

    O45.92 **Premature separation of placenta, unspecified,** second trimester   Ⓜ♀▽

    O45.93 **Premature separation of placenta, unspecified,** third trimester   Ⓜ♀▽

✓4ᵗʰ **O46 Antepartum hemorrhage, not elsewhere classified**

    EXCLUDES 1 hemorrhage in early pregnancy (O20.-)
intrapartum hemorrhage NEC (O67.-)
placenta previa (O44.-)
premature separation of placenta [abruptio placentae] (O45.-)

  ✓5ᵗʰ **O46.0 Antepartum hemorrhage with** coagulation defect

   ✓6ᵗʰ **O46.00 Antepartum hemorrhage with coagulation defect, unspecified**

    O46.001 **Antepartum hemorrhage with coagulation defect, unspecified, first trimester**   Ⓜ♀▽

    O46.002 **Antepartum hemorrhage with coagulation defect, unspecified,** second trimester   Ⓜ♀▽

    O46.003 **Antepartum hemorrhage with coagulation defect, unspecified,** third trimester   Ⓜ♀▽

Ⓝ Newborn   Ⓟ Pediatric   Ⓜ Maternity   Ⓐ Adult   **RIC** RIC Dx   **NC Dx** Noncancer Dx   **PDx** Primary Dx   **CC** RIC CC Condition   ▶◀ Revised Text   ● New Code   ▲ Revised Code Title

794   ICD-10-CM 2016

O46.009 **Antepartum hemorrhage with coagulation defect, unspecified, unspecified trimester** Ⓜ♀▽

✓6ᵗʰ O46.01 **Antepartum hemorrhage with afibrinogenemia**
Antepartum hemorrhage with hypofibrinogenemia

O46.011 **Antepartum hemorrhage with afibrinogenemia, first trimester** Ⓜ♀

O46.012 **Antepartum hemorrhage with afibrinogenemia, second trimester** Ⓜ♀

O46.013 **Antepartum hemorrhage with afibrinogenemia, third trimester** Ⓜ♀

O46.019 **Antepartum hemorrhage with afibrinogenemia, unspecified trimester** Ⓜ♀▽

✓6ᵗʰ O46.02 **Antepartum hemorrhage with disseminated intravascular coagulation**

O46.021 **Antepartum hemorrhage with disseminated intravascular coagulation, first trimester** Ⓜ♀

O46.022 **Antepartum hemorrhage with disseminated intravascular coagulation, second trimester** Ⓜ♀

O46.023 **Antepartum hemorrhage with disseminated intravascular coagulation, third trimester** Ⓜ♀

O46.029 **Antepartum hemorrhage with disseminated intravascular coagulation, unspecified trimester** Ⓜ♀▽

✓6ᵗʰ O46.09 **Antepartum hemorrhage with other coagulation defect**

O46.091 **Antepartum hemorrhage with other coagulation defect, first trimester** Ⓜ♀

O46.092 **Antepartum hemorrhage with other coagulation defect, second trimester** Ⓜ♀

O46.093 **Antepartum hemorrhage with other coagulation defect, third trimester** Ⓜ♀

O46.099 **Antepartum hemorrhage with other coagulation defect, unspecified trimester** Ⓜ♀▽

✓5ᵗʰ O46.8 **Other antepartum hemorrhage**

✓6ᵗʰ O46.8X **Other antepartum hemorrhage**

O46.8X1 **Other antepartum hemorrhage, first trimester** Ⓜ♀

O46.8X2 **Other antepartum hemorrhage, second trimester** Ⓜ♀

O46.8X3 **Other antepartum hemorrhage, third trimester** Ⓜ♀

O46.8X9 **Other antepartum hemorrhage, unspecified trimester** Ⓜ♀▽

✓5ᵗʰ O46.9 **Antepartum hemorrhage, unspecified**

O46.90 **Antepartum hemorrhage, unspecified, unspecified trimester** Ⓜ♀▽

O46.91 **Antepartum hemorrhage, unspecified, first trimester** Ⓜ♀▽

O46.92 **Antepartum hemorrhage, unspecified, second trimester** Ⓜ♀▽

O46.93 **Antepartum hemorrhage, unspecified, third trimester** Ⓜ♀▽

✓4ᵗʰ **O47 False labor**
Braxton Hicks contractions
Threatened labor
EXCLUDES 1 preterm labor (O60.-)

✓5ᵗʰ O47.0 **False labor before 37 completed weeks of gestation**

O47.00 **False labor before 37 completed weeks of gestation, unspecified trimester** Ⓜ♀▽

O47.02 **False labor before 37 completed weeks of gestation, second trimester** Ⓜ♀

O47.03 **False labor before 37 completed weeks of gestation, third trimester** Ⓜ♀

O47.1 **False labor at or after 37 completed weeks of gestation** Ⓜ♀

O47.9 **False labor, unspecified** Ⓜ♀▽

✓4ᵗʰ **O48 Late pregnancy**

O48.0 **Post-term pregnancy** Ⓜ♀
Pregnancy over 40 completed weeks to 42 completed weeks gestation

O48.1 **Prolonged pregnancy** Ⓜ♀
Pregnancy which has advanced beyond 42 completed weeks gestation

Complications of labor and delivery (O60-O77)

✓4ᵗʰ **O60 Preterm labor**
INCLUDES onset (spontaneous) of labor before 37 completed weeks of gestation
EXCLUDES 1 false labor (O47.0-)
threatened labor NOS (O47.0-)

✓5ᵗʰ O60.0 **Preterm labor without delivery**

O60.00 **Preterm labor without delivery, unspecified trimester** Ⓜ♀▽

O60.02 **Preterm labor without delivery, second trimester** Ⓜ♀

O60.03 **Preterm labor without delivery, third trimester** Ⓜ♀

✓5ᵗʰ O60.1 **Preterm labor with preterm delivery**

> One of the following 7th characters is to be assigned to each code under subcategory O60.1. 7th character Ø is for single gestations and multiple gestations where the fetus is unspecified. 7th characters 1 through 9 are for cases of multiple gestations to identify the fetus for which the code applies. The appropriate code from category O30, Multiple gestation, must also be assigned when assigning a code from subcategory O60.1 that has a 7th character of 1 through 9.
> Ø not applicable or unspecified   4 fetus 4
> 1 fetus 1   5 fetus 5
> 2 fetus 2   9 other fetus
> 3 fetus 3

✓x7ᵗʰ O60.10 **Preterm labor with preterm delivery, unspecified trimester** Ⓜ♀▽
Preterm labor with delivery NOS

✓x7ᵗʰ O60.12 **Preterm labor second trimester with preterm delivery second trimester** Ⓜ♀

✓x7ᵗʰ O60.13 **Preterm labor second trimester with preterm delivery third trimester** Ⓜ♀

✓x7ᵗʰ O60.14 **Preterm labor third trimester with preterm delivery third trimester** Ⓜ♀

✓5ᵗʰ O60.2 **Term delivery with preterm labor**

> One of the following 7th characters is to be assigned to each code under subcategory O60.2. 7th character Ø is for single gestations and multiple gestations where the fetus is unspecified. 7th characters 1 through 9 are for cases of multiple gestations to identify the fetus for which the code applies. The appropriate code from category O30, Multiple gestation, must also be assigned when assigning a code from subcategory O60.2 that has a 7th character of 1 through 9.
> Ø not applicable or unspecified   4 fetus 4
> 1 fetus 1   5 fetus 5
> 2 fetus 2   9 other fetus
> 3 fetus 3

✓x7ᵗʰ O60.20 **Term delivery with preterm labor, unspecified trimester** Ⓜ♀▽

✓x7ᵗʰ O60.22 **Term delivery with preterm labor, second trimester** Ⓜ♀

✓x7ᵗʰ O60.23 **Term delivery with preterm labor, third trimester** Ⓜ♀

✓4ᵗʰ **O61 Failed induction of labor**

O61.0 **Failed medical induction of labor** Ⓜ♀
Failed induction (of labor) by oxytocin
Failed induction (of labor) by prostaglandins

O61.1 **Failed instrumental induction of labor** Ⓜ♀
Failed mechanical induction (of labor)
Failed surgical induction (of labor)

O61.8 **Other failed induction of labor** Ⓜ♀

O61.9 **Failed induction of labor, unspecified** Ⓜ♀▽

✓4ᵗʰ **O62 Abnormalities of forces of labor**

O62.0 **Primary inadequate contractions** Ⓜ♀
Failure of cervical dilatation
Primary hypotonic uterine dysfunction
Uterine inertia during latent phase of labor

O62.1 **Secondary uterine inertia** Ⓜ♀
Arrested active phase of labor
Secondary hypotonic uterine dysfunction

✓ Add'l Character Required ✓x7ᵗʰ Placeholder Alert RUG IV Special Care High Dx RUG IV Clinically Complex Dx RUG IV Special Care Low Dx Manifestation Code Other Specified Code ▽ Unspecified Code

ICD-10-CM 2016 795

Chapter 15. Pregnancy, Childbirth and the Puerperium

O62.2 Other uterine inertia Ⓜ♀
Atony of uterus without hemorrhage
Atony of uterus NOS
Desultory labor
Hypotonic uterine dysfunction NOS
Irregular labor
Poor contractions
Slow slope active phase of labor
Uterine inertia NOS
     EXCLUDES 1   *atony of uterus with hemorrhage (postpartum) (O72.1)*
           postpartum atony of uterus without hemorrhage (O75.89)

O62.3 Precipitate labor Ⓜ♀

O62.4 Hypertonic, incoordinate, and prolonged uterine contractions Ⓜ♀
Cervical spasm
Contraction ring dystocia
Dyscoordinate labor
Hour-glass contraction of uterus
Hypertonic uterine dysfunction
Incoordinate uterine action
Tetanic contractions
Uterine dystocia NOS
Uterine spasm
     EXCLUDES 1   *dystocia (fetal) (maternal) NOS (O66.9)*

O62.8 Other abnormalities of forces of labor Ⓜ♀

O62.9 Abnormality of forces of labor, unspecified Ⓜ♀▽

✓4ᵗʰ **O63 Long labor**

O63.0 Prolonged first stage (of labor) Ⓜ♀

O63.1 Prolonged second stage (of labor) Ⓜ♀

O63.2 Delayed delivery of second twin, triplet, etc. Ⓜ♀

O63.9 Long labor, unspecified Ⓜ♀▽
Prolonged labor NOS

✓4ᵗʰ **O64 Obstructed labor due to malposition and malpresentation of fetus**

> One of the following 7th characters is to be assigned to each code under category O64. 7th character 0 is for single gestations and multiple gestations where the fetus is unspecified. 7th characters 1 through 9 are for cases of multiple gestations to identify the fetus for which the code applies. The appropriate code from category O30, Multiple gestation, must also be assigned when assigning a code from category O64 that has a 7th character of 1 through 9.
>
> 0   not applicable or unspecified   4   fetus 4
> 1   fetus 1   5   fetus 5
> 2   fetus 2   9   other fetus
> 3   fetus 3

✓x7ᵗʰ **O64.0 Obstructed labor due to incomplete rotation of fetal head** Ⓜ♀
Deep transverse arrest
Obstructed labor due to persistent occipitoiliac (position)
Obstructed labor due to persistent occipitoposterior (position)
Obstructed labor due to persistent occipitosacral (position)
Obstructed labor due to persistent occipitotransverse (position)

✓x7ᵗʰ **O64.1 Obstructed labor due to breech presentation** Ⓜ♀
Obstructed labor due to buttocks presentation
Obstructed labor due to complete breech presentation
Obstructed labor due to frank breech presentation

✓x7ᵗʰ **O64.2 Obstructed labor due to face presentation** Ⓜ♀
Obstructed labor due to chin presentation

✓x7ᵗʰ **O64.3 Obstructed labor due to brow presentation** Ⓜ♀

✓x7ᵗʰ **O64.4 Obstructed labor due to shoulder presentation** Ⓜ♀
Prolapsed arm
     EXCLUDES 1   *impacted shoulders (O66.0)*
            shoulder dystocia (O66.0)

✓x7ᵗʰ **O64.5 Obstructed labor due to compound presentation** Ⓜ♀

✓x7ᵗʰ **O64.8 Obstructed labor due to other malposition and malpresentation** Ⓜ♀
Obstructed labor due to footling presentation
Obstructed labor due to incomplete breech presentation

✓x7ᵗʰ **O64.9 Obstructed labor due to malposition and malpresentation, unspecified** Ⓜ♀▽

✓4ᵗʰ **O65 Obstructed labor due to maternal pelvic abnormality**

O65.0 Obstructed labor due to deformed pelvis Ⓜ♀

O65.1 Obstructed labor due to generally contracted pelvis Ⓜ♀

O65.2 Obstructed labor due to pelvic inlet contraction Ⓜ♀

O65.3 Obstructed labor due to pelvic outlet and mid-cavity contraction Ⓜ♀

O65.4 Obstructed labor due to fetopelvic disproportion, unspecified Ⓜ♀▽
     EXCLUDES 1   *dystocia due to abnormality of fetus (O66.2-O66.3)*

O65.5 Obstructed labor due to abnormality of maternal pelvic organs Ⓜ♀
Obstructed labor due to conditions listed in O34-
Use additional code to identify abnormality of pelvic organs (O34.-)

O65.8 Obstructed labor due to other maternal pelvic abnormalities Ⓜ♀

O65.9 Obstructed labor due to maternal pelvic abnormality, unspecified Ⓜ♀

✓4ᵗʰ **O66 Other obstructed labor**

O66.0 Obstructed labor due to shoulder dystocia Ⓜ♀
Impacted shoulders

O66.1 Obstructed labor due to locked twins Ⓜ♀

O66.2 Obstructed labor due to unusually large fetus Ⓜ♀

O66.3 Obstructed labor due to other abnormalities of fetus Ⓜ♀
Dystocia due to fetal ascites
Dystocia due to fetal hydrops
Dystocia due to fetal meningomyelocele
Dystocia due to fetal sacral teratoma
Dystocia due to fetal tumor
Dystocia due to hydrocephalic fetus
Use additional code to identify cause of obstruction

✓5ᵗʰ **O66.4 Failed trial of labor**

O66.40 Failed trial of labor, unspecified Ⓜ♀▽

O66.41 Failed attempted vaginal birth after previous cesarean delivery Ⓜ♀
Code first rupture of uterus, if applicable (O71.0-, O71.1)

O66.5 Attempted application of vacuum extractor and forceps Ⓜ♀
Attempted application of vacuum or forceps, with subsequent delivery by forceps or cesarean delivery

O66.6 Obstructed labor due to other multiple fetuses Ⓜ♀

O66.8 Other specified obstructed labor Ⓜ♀
Use additional code to identify cause of obstruction

O66.9 Obstructed labor, unspecified Ⓜ♀▽
Dystocia NOS
Fetal dystocia NOS
Maternal dystocia NOS

✓4ᵗʰ **O67 Labor and delivery complicated by intrapartum hemorrhage, not elsewhere classified**
     EXCLUDES 1   *antepartum hemorrhage NEC (O46.-)*
            placenta previa (O44.-)
            premature separation of placenta [abruptio placentae] (O45.-)
     EXCLUDES 2   *postpartum hemorrhage (O72.-)*

O67.0 Intrapartum hemorrhage with coagulation defect Ⓜ♀
Intrapartum hemorrhage (excessive) associated with afibrinogenemia
Intrapartum hemorrhage (excessive) associated with disseminated intravascular coagulation
Intrapartum hemorrhage (excessive) associated with hyperfibrinolysis
Intrapartum hemorrhage (excessive) associated with hypofibrinogenemia

O67.8 Other intrapartum hemorrhage Ⓜ♀
Excessive intrapartum hemorrhage

O67.9 Intrapartum hemorrhage, unspecified Ⓜ♀▽

O68 Labor and delivery complicated by abnormality of fetal acid-base balance Ⓜ♀
Fetal acidemia complicating labor and delivery
Fetal acidosis complicating labor and delivery
Fetal alkalosis complicating labor and delivery
Fetal metabolic acidemia complicating labor and delivery
     EXCLUDES 1   *fetal stress NOS (O77.9)*
            labor and delivery complicated by electrocardiographic evidence of fetal stress (O77.8)
            labor and delivery complicated by ultrasonic evidence of fetal stress (O77.8)
     EXCLUDES 2   *abnormality in fetal heart rate or rhythm (O76)*
            labor and delivery complicated by meconium in amniotic fluid (O77.0)

Ⓝ Newborn   Ⓟ Pediatric   Ⓜ Maternity   Ⓐ Adult   **RIC** RIC Dx   **NC Dx** Noncancer Dx   **PDx** Primary Dx   **CC** RIC CC Condition   ▶◀ Revised Text   ● New Code   ▲ Revised Code Title

796   ICD-10-CM 2016

☑4ᵗʰ O69 Labor and delivery complicated by umbilical cord complications

One of the following 7th characters is to be assigned to each code under category O69. 7th character 0 is for single gestations and multiple gestations where the fetus is unspecified. 7th characters 1 through 9 are for cases of multiple gestations to identify the fetus for which the code applies. The appropriate code from category O30, Multiple gestation, must also be assigned when assigning a code from category O69 that has a 7th character of 1 through 9.

0	not applicable or unspecified	3 fetus 3
1	fetus 1	4 fetus 4
2	fetus 2	5 fetus 5
		9 other fetus

✓x7ᵗʰ **O69.0 Labor and delivery complicated by** prolapse of cord   M♀

✓x7ᵗʰ **O69.1 Labor and delivery complicated by** cord around neck, with compression   M♀

     EXCLUDES 1 *labor and delivery complicated by cord around neck, without compression (O69.81)*

✓x7ᵗʰ **O69.2 Labor and delivery complicated by** other cord entanglement, with compression   M♀

     Labor and delivery complicated by compression of cord NOS

     Labor and delivery complicated by entanglement of cords of twins in monoamniotic sac

     Labor and delivery complicated by knot in cord

     EXCLUDES 1 *labor and delivery complicated by other cord entanglement, without compression (O69.82)*

✓x7ᵗʰ **O69.3 Labor and delivery complicated by** short cord   M♀

✓x7ᵗʰ **O69.4 Labor and delivery complicated by** vasa previa   M♀

     Labor and delivery complicated by hemorrhage from vasa previa

✓x7ᵗʰ **O69.5 Labor and delivery complicated by** vascular lesion of cord M♀

     Labor and delivery complicated by cord bruising

     Labor and delivery complicated by cord hematoma

     Labor and delivery complicated by thrombosis of umbilical vessels

✓5ᵗʰ **O69.8 Labor and delivery complicated by** other cord complications

     ✓x7ᵗʰ **O69.81 Labor and delivery complicated by cord** around neck, without compression   M♀

     ✓x7ᵗʰ **O69.82 Labor and delivery complicated by other cord** entanglement, without compression   M♀

     ✓x7ᵗʰ **O69.89 Labor and delivery complicated by other cord** complications   M♀

✓x7ᵗʰ **O69.9 Labor and delivery complicated by cord complication,** unspecified   M♀▽

☑4ᵗʰ O70 Perineal laceration during delivery

Episiotomy extended by laceration

EXCLUDES 1 *obstetric high vaginal laceration alone (O71.4)*

O70.0 First degree perineal laceration during delivery   M♀

     Perineal laceration, rupture or tear involving fourchette during delivery

     Perineal laceration, rupture or tear involving labia during delivery

     Perineal laceration, rupture or tear involving skin during delivery

     Perineal laceration, rupture or tear involving vagina during delivery

     Perineal laceration, rupture or tear involving vulva during delivery

     Slight perineal laceration, rupture or tear during delivery

O70.1 Second degree perineal laceration during delivery   M♀

     Perineal laceration, rupture or tear during delivery as in O70.0, also involving pelvic floor

     Perineal laceration, rupture or tear during delivery as in O70.0, also involving perineal muscles

     Perineal laceration, rupture or tear during delivery as in O70.0, also involving vaginal muscles

     EXCLUDES 1 *perineal laceration involving anal sphincter (O70.2)*

O70.2 Third degree perineal laceration during delivery   M♀

     Perineal laceration, rupture or tear during delivery as in O70.1, also involving anal sphincter

     Perineal laceration, rupture or tear during delivery as in O70.1, also involving rectovaginal septum

     Perineal laceration, rupture or tear during delivery as in O70.1, also involving sphincter NOS

     EXCLUDES 1 *anal sphincter tear during delivery without third degree perineal laceration (O70.4)*

             perineal laceration involving anal or rectal mucosa (O70.3)

O70.3 Fourth degree perineal laceration during delivery   M♀

     Perineal laceration, rupture or tear during delivery as in O70.2, also involving anal mucosa

     Perineal laceration, rupture or tear during delivery as in O70.2, also involving rectal mucosa

O70.4 Anal sphincter tear complicating delivery, not associated M♀ **with third degree laceration**

     EXCLUDES 1 *anal sphincter tear with third degree perineal laceration (O70.2)*

O70.9 Perineal laceration during delivery, unspecified   M♀▽

☑4ᵗʰ O71 Other obstetric trauma

Obstetric damage from instruments

✓5ᵗʰ **O71.0 Rupture of uterus (spontaneous)** before onset of labor

     EXCLUDES 1 *disruption of (current) cesarean delivery wound (O90.0)*

             laceration of uterus, NEC (O71.81)

     O71.00 Rupture of uterus before onset of labor, CC M♀▽ **unspecified trimester**

     O71.02 Rupture of uterus before onset of labor, CC M♀ **second trimester**

     O71.03 Rupture of uterus before onset of labor, CC M♀ **third trimester**

O71.1 Rupture of uterus during labor   CC M♀

     Rupture of uterus not stated as occurring before onset of labor

     EXCLUDES 1 *disruption of cesarean delivery wound (O90.0)*

             laceration of uterus, NEC (O71.81)

O71.2 Postpartum inversion of uterus   M♀

O71.3 Obstetric laceration of cervix   M♀

     Annular detachment of cervix

O71.4 Obstetric high vaginal laceration alone   M♀

     Laceration of vaginal wall without perineal laceration

     EXCLUDES 1 *obstetric high vaginal laceration with perineal laceration (O70.-)*

O71.5 Other obstetric injury to pelvic organs   M♀

     Obstetric injury to bladder

     Obstetric injury to urethra

     EXCLUDES 2 *obstetric periurethral trauma (O71.82)*

     AHA: 2014, 4Q, 18

O71.6 Obstetric damage to pelvic joints and ligaments   M♀

     Obstetric avulsion of inner symphyseal cartilage

     Obstetric damage to coccyx

     Obstetric traumatic separation of symphysis (pubis)

O71.7 Obstetric hematoma of pelvis   M♀

     Obstetric hematoma of perineum

     Obstetric hematoma of vagina

     Obstetric hematoma of vulva

✓5ᵗʰ **O71.8 Other specified obstetric trauma**

     O71.81 Laceration of uterus, not elsewhere classified   M♀

     O71.82 Other specified trauma to perineum and vulva   M♀

         Obstetric periurethral trauma

         AHA: 2014, 4Q, 18

     O71.89 Other specified obstetric trauma   M♀

O71.9 Obstetric trauma, unspecified   M♀▽

☑4ᵗʰ O72 Postpartum hemorrhage

INCLUDES hemorrhage after delivery of fetus or infant

O72.0 Third-stage hemorrhage   M♀

     Hemorrhage associated with retained, trapped or adherent placenta

     Retained placenta NOS

     Code also type of adherent placenta (O43.2-)

O72.1 Other immediate postpartum hemorrhage   M♀

     Hemorrhage following delivery of placenta

     Postpartum hemorrhage (atonic) NOS

     Uterine atony with hemorrhage

     EXCLUDES 1 *uterine atony NOS (O62.2)*

             uterine atony without hemorrhage (O62.2)

             postpartum atony of uterus without hemorrhage (O75.89)

O72.2 Delayed and secondary postpartum hemorrhage   M♀

     Hemorrhage associated with retained portions of placenta or membranes after the first 24 hours following delivery of placenta

     Retained products of conception NOS, following delivery

O72.3 Postpartum coagulation defects   M♀

     Postpartum afibrinogenemia   Postpartum fibrinolysis

☑ Add'l Character Required   ✓x7ᵗʰ Placeholder Alert   RUG IV Special Care High Dx   RUG IV Clinically Complex Dx   RUG IV Special Care Low Dx   Manifestation Code   Other Specified Code   ▽ Unspecified Code

✓4ᵗʰ O73 Retained placenta and membranes, without hemorrhage

> **EXCLUDES 1**   placenta accreta (O43.21-)
> placenta increta (O43.22-)
> placenta percreta (O43.23-)

O73.0 Retained placenta without hemorrhage   Ⓜ♀
> Adherent placenta, without hemorrhage
> Trapped placenta without hemorrhage

O73.1 Retained portions of placenta and membranes, without hemorrhage   Ⓜ♀
> Retained products of conception following delivery, without hemorrhage

✓4ᵗʰ O74 Complications of anesthesia during labor and delivery

> **INCLUDES**   maternal complications arising from the administration of a general, regional or local anesthetic, analgesic or other sedation during labor and delivery

> Use additional code, if applicable, to identify specific complication

O74.0 Aspiration pneumonitis due to anesthesia during labor and delivery   Ⓜ♀
> Inhalation of stomach contents or secretions NOS due to anesthesia during labor and delivery
> Mendelson's syndrome due to anesthesia during labor and delivery

O74.1 Other pulmonary complications of anesthesia during labor and delivery   Ⓜ♀

O74.2 Cardiac complications of anesthesia during labor and delivery   Ⓜ♀

O74.3 Central nervous system complications of anesthesia during labor and delivery   Ⓜ♀

O74.4 Toxic reaction to local anesthesia during labor and delivery   Ⓜ♀

O74.5 Spinal and epidural anesthesia-induced headache during labor and delivery   Ⓜ♀

O74.6 Other complications of spinal and epidural anesthesia during labor and delivery   Ⓜ♀

O74.7 Failed or difficult intubation for anesthesia during labor and delivery   Ⓜ♀

O74.8 Other complications of anesthesia during labor and delivery   Ⓜ♀

O74.9 Complication of anesthesia during labor and delivery, unspecified   Ⓜ♀▽

✓4ᵗʰ O75 Other complications of labor and delivery, not elsewhere classified

> **EXCLUDES 2**   puerperal (postpartum) infection (O86.-)
> puerperal (postpartum) sepsis (O85)

O75.0 Maternal distress during labor and delivery   Ⓜ♀

O75.1 Shock during or following labor and delivery   cc Ⓜ♀
> Obstetric shock following labor and delivery
> **RIC Excl:** 03 Non-traumatic brain injury

O75.2 Pyrexia during labor, not elsewhere classified   Ⓜ♀

O75.3 Other infection during labor   cc Ⓜ♀
> Sepsis during labor
> Use additional code (B95-B97), to identify infectious agent
> **RIC Excl:** 01 Stroke

O75.4 Other complications of obstetric surgery and procedures   Ⓜ♀
> Cardiac arrest following obstetric surgery or procedures
> Cardiac failure following obstetric surgery or procedures
> Cerebral anoxia following obstetric surgery or procedures
> Pulmonary edema following obstetric surgery or procedures
> Use additional code to identify specific complication
> > **EXCLUDES 2**   complications of anesthesia during labor and delivery (O74.-)
> > disruption of obstetrical (surgical) wound (O90.0-O90.1)
> > hematoma of obstetrical (surgical) wound (O90.2)
> > infection of obstetrical (surgical) wound (O86.0)

O75.5 Delayed delivery after artificial rupture of membranes   Ⓜ♀

✓5ᵗʰ O75.8 Other specified complications of labor and delivery

> **O75.81 Maternal exhaustion complicating labor and delivery**   Ⓜ♀

O75.82 Onset (spontaneous) of labor after 37 completed weeks of gestation but before 39 completed weeks gestation, with delivery by (planned) cesarean section   Ⓜ♀
> Delivery by (planned) cesarean section occurring after 37 completed weeks of gestation but before 39 completed weeks gestation due to (spontaneous) onset of labor
> Code first to specify reason for planned cesarean section such as:
> cephalopelvic disproportion (normally formed fetus) (O33.9)
> previous cesarean delivery (O34.21)

O75.89 Other specified complications of labor and delivery   Ⓜ♀

O75.9 Complication of labor and delivery, unspecified   Ⓜ♀▽

O76 Abnormality in fetal heart rate and rhythm complicating labor and delivery   Ⓜ♀
> Depressed fetal heart rate tones complicating labor and delivery
> Fetal bradycardia complicating labor and delivery
> Fetal heart rate abnormal variability complicating labor and delivery
> Fetal heart rate decelerations complicating labor and delivery
> Fetal heart rate irregularity complicating labor and delivery
> Fetal tachycardia complicating labor and delivery
> Non-reassuring fetal heart rate or rhythm complicating labor and delivery
> > **EXCLUDES 1**   fetal stress NOS (O77.9)
> > labor and delivery complicated by electrocardiographic evidence of fetal stress (O77.8)
> > labor and delivery complicated by ultrasonic evidence of fetal stress (O77.8)
> > **EXCLUDES 2**   fetal metabolic acidemia (O68)
> > other fetal stress (O77.0-O77.1)
> **AHA:** 2013, 4Q, 118

✓4ᵗʰ O77 Other fetal stress complicating labor and delivery

O77.0 Labor and delivery complicated by meconium in amniotic fluid   Ⓜ♀
> **AHA:** 2013, 4Q, 117-118

O77.1 Fetal stress in labor or delivery due to drug administration   Ⓜ♀

O77.8 Labor and delivery complicated by other evidence of fetal stress   Ⓜ♀
> Labor and delivery complicated by electrocardiographic evidence of fetal stress
> Labor and delivery complicated by ultrasonic evidence of fetal stress
> > **EXCLUDES 1**   abnormality in fetal heart rate or rhythm (O76)
> > abnormality of fetal acid-base balance (O68)
> > fetal metabolic acidemia (O68)

O77.9 Labor and delivery complicated by fetal stress, unspecified   Ⓜ♀▽
> > **EXCLUDES 1**   abnormality in fetal heart rate or rhythm (O76)
> > abnormality of fetal acid-base balance (O68)
> > fetal metabolic acidemia (O68)

Encounter for delivery (O80, O82)

O80 Encounter for full-term uncomplicated delivery   Ⓜ♀
> **NOTE**   Delivery requiring minimal or no assistance, with or without episiotomy, without fetal manipulation [e.g., rotation version] or instrumentation [forceps] of a spontaneous, cephalic, vaginal, full-term, single, live-born infant. This code is for use as a single diagnosis code and is not to be used with any other code from chapter 15.
> Use additional code to indicate outcome of delivery (Z37.0)
> **AHA:** 2014, 2Q, 9

O82 Encounter for cesarean delivery without indication   Ⓜ♀
> Use additional code to indicate outcome of delivery (Z37.0)

Ⓝ Newborn   Ⓟ Pediatric   Ⓜ Maternity   Ⓐ Adult   **RIC** RIC Dx   **NC Dx** Noncancer Dx   **PDx** Primary Dx   **CC** RIC CC Condition   ►◄ Revised Text   ● New Code   ▲ Revised Code Title

798   ICD-10-CM 2016

Complications predominantly related to the puerperium (O85-O92)

EXCLUDES 2   *mental and behavioral disorders associated with the puerperium (F53)*
obstetrical tetanus (A34)
puerperal osteomalacia (M83.0)

O85   Puerperal sepsis   M♀
Postpartum sepsis
Puerperal peritonitis
Puerperal pyemia
Use additional code (B95-B97), to identify infectious agent
Use additional code (R65.2-) to identify severe sepsis, if applicable
EXCLUDES 1   *fever of unknown origin following delivery (O86.4)*
genital tract infection following delivery (O86.1-)
obstetric pyemic and septic embolism (O88.3-)
puerperal septic thrombophlebitis (O86.81)
urinary tract infection following delivery (O86.2-)
EXCLUDES 2   *sepsis during labor (O75.3)*

✓4ᵗʰ O86   Other puerperal infections
Use additional code (B95-B97), to identify infectious agent
EXCLUDES 2   *infection during labor (O75.3)*
obstetrical tetanus (A34)

O86.0   Infection of obstetric surgical wound   M♀
Infected cesarean delivery wound following delivery
Infected perineal repair following delivery

✓5ᵗʰ **O86.1   Other infection of genital tract following delivery**
O86.11   Cervicitis following delivery   M♀
O86.12   Endometritis following delivery   M♀
O86.13   Vaginitis following delivery   M♀
O86.19   Other infection of genital tract following delivery   M♀

✓5ᵗʰ **O86.2   Urinary tract infection following delivery**
O86.20   Urinary tract infection following delivery, unspecified   M♀▽
Puerperal urinary tract infection NOS
O86.21   Infection of kidney following delivery   M♀
O86.22   Infection of bladder following delivery   M♀
Infection of urethra following delivery
O86.29   Other urinary tract infection following delivery   M♀

O86.4   Pyrexia of unknown origin following delivery   M♀
Puerperal infection NOS following delivery
Puerperal pyrexia NOS following delivery
EXCLUDES 2   *pyrexia during labor (O75.2)*

✓5ᵗʰ **O86.8   Other specified puerperal infections**
O86.81   Puerperal septic thrombophlebitis   M♀
O86.89   Other specified puerperal infections   M♀

✓4ᵗʰ O87   Venous complications and hemorrhoids in the puerperium
Venous complications in labor, delivery and the puerperium
EXCLUDES 2   *obstetric embolism (O88.-)*
puerperal septic thrombophlebitis (O86.81)
venous complications in pregnancy (O22.-)

O87.0   Superficial thrombophlebitis in the puerperium   M♀
Puerperal phlebitis NOS
Puerperal thrombosis NOS

O87.1   Deep phlebothrombosis in the puerperium   M♀
Deep vein thrombosis, postpartum
Pelvic thrombophlebitis, postpartum
Use additional code to identify the deep vein thrombosis (I82.4-, I82.5-, I82.62-, I82.72-)
Use additional code, if applicable, for associated long-term (current) use of anticoagulants (Z79.01)

O87.2   Hemorrhoids in the puerperium   M♀

O87.3   Cerebral venous thrombosis in the puerperium   M♀
Cerebrovenous sinus thrombosis in the puerperium

O87.4   Varicose veins of lower extremity in the puerperium   M♀

O87.8   Other venous complications in the puerperium   M♀
Genital varices in the puerperium

O87.9   Venous complication in the puerperium, unspecified   M♀▽
Puerperal phlebopathy NOS

✓4ᵗʰ O88   Obstetric embolism
EXCLUDES 1   *embolism complicating abortion NOS (O03.2)*
embolism complicating ectopic or molar pregnancy (O08.2)
embolism complicating failed attempted abortion (O07.2)
embolism complicating induced abortion (O04.7)
embolism complicating spontaneous abortion (O03.2, O03.7)

✓5ᵗʰ **O88.0   Obstetric air embolism**
✓6ᵗʰ **O88.01   Obstetric air embolism in pregnancy**
O88.011   Air embolism in pregnancy, first trimester   cc M♀
RIC Excl: 01 Stroke
O88.012   Air embolism in pregnancy, second trimester   cc M♀
RIC Excl: 01 Stroke
O88.013   Air embolism in pregnancy, third trimester   cc M♀
RIC Excl: 01 Stroke
O88.019   Air embolism in pregnancy, unspecified trimester   cc M♀▽
RIC Excl: 01 Stroke
O88.02   Air embolism in childbirth   cc M♀
RIC Excl: 01 Stroke
O88.03   Air embolism in the puerperium   cc M♀
RIC Excl: 01 Stroke

✓5ᵗʰ **O88.1   Amniotic fluid embolism**
Anaphylactoid syndrome in pregnancy
✓6ᵗʰ **O88.11   Amniotic fluid embolism in pregnancy**
O88.111   Amniotic fluid embolism in pregnancy, first trimester   cc M♀
RIC Excl: 01 Stroke
O88.112   Amniotic fluid embolism in pregnancy, second trimester   cc M♀
RIC Excl: 01 Stroke
O88.113   Amniotic fluid embolism in pregnancy, third trimester   cc M♀
RIC Excl: 01 Stroke
O88.119   Amniotic fluid embolism in pregnancy, unspecified trimester   cc M♀▽
RIC Excl: 01 Stroke
O88.12   Amniotic fluid embolism in childbirth   cc M♀
RIC Excl: 01 Stroke
O88.13   Amniotic fluid embolism in the puerperium   cc M♀
RIC Excl: 01 Stroke

✓5ᵗʰ **O88.2   Obstetric thromboembolism**
✓6ᵗʰ **O88.21   Thromboembolism in pregnancy**
Obstetric (pulmonary) embolism NOS
O88.211   Thromboembolism in pregnancy, first trimester   cc M♀
RIC Excl: 15 Pulmonary
O88.212   Thromboembolism in pregnancy, second trimester   cc M♀
RIC Excl: 15 Pulmonary
O88.213   Thromboembolism in pregnancy, third trimester   cc M♀
RIC Excl: 15 Pulmonary
O88.219   Thromboembolism in pregnancy, unspecified trimester   cc M♀▽
RIC Excl: 15 Pulmonary
O88.22   Thromboembolism in childbirth   cc M♀
RIC Excl: 15 Pulmonary
O88.23   Thromboembolism in the puerperium   cc M♀
RIC Excl: 15 Pulmonary
Puerperal (pulmonary) embolism NOS

✓5ᵗʰ **O88.3   Obstetric pyemic and septic embolism**
✓6ᵗʰ **O88.31   Pyemic and septic embolism in pregnancy**
O88.311   Pyemic and septic embolism in pregnancy, first trimester   cc M♀
RIC Excl: 03 Non-traumatic brain injury
O88.312   Pyemic and septic embolism in pregnancy, second trimester   cc M♀
RIC Excl: 03 Non-traumatic brain injury
O88.313   Pyemic and septic embolism in pregnancy, third trimester   cc M♀
RIC Excl: 03 Non-traumatic brain injury
O88.319   Pyemic and septic embolism in pregnancy, unspecified trimester   cc M♀▽
RIC Excl: 03 Non-traumatic brain injury
O88.32   Pyemic and septic embolism in childbirth   cc M♀
RIC Excl: 03 Non-traumatic brain injury

Chapter 15. Pregnancy, Childbirth and the Puerperium

O88.33 Pyemic and septic embolism in the puerperium   CC M♀
RIC Excl: 03 Non-traumatic brain injury

✓5ᵗʰ **O88.8 Other obstetric embolism**
Obstetric fat embolism

✓6ᵗʰ **O88.81 Other embolism in pregnancy**

O88.811 Other embolism in pregnancy, first trimester   CC M♀
RIC Excl: 15 Pulmonary

O88.812 Other embolism in pregnancy, second trimester   CC M♀
RIC Excl: 15 Pulmonary

O88.813 Other embolism in pregnancy, third trimester   CC M♀
RIC Excl: 15 Pulmonary

O88.819 Other embolism in pregnancy, unspecified trimester   CC M♀▽
RIC Excl: 15 Pulmonary

O88.82 Other embolism in childbirth   CC M♀
RIC Excl: 15 Pulmonary

O88.83 Other embolism in the puerperium   CC M♀
RIC Excl: 15 Pulmonary

✓4ᵗʰ **O89 Complications of anesthesia during the puerperium**
INCLUDES   maternal complications arising from the administration of a general, regional or local anesthetic, analgesic or other sedation during the puerperium
Use additional code, if applicable, to identify specific complication

✓5ᵗʰ **O89.0 Pulmonary complications of anesthesia during the puerperium**

O89.01 Aspiration pneumonitis due to anesthesia during the puerperium   M♀
Inhalation of stomach contents or secretions NOS due to anesthesia during the puerperium
Mendelson's syndrome due to anesthesia during the puerperium

O89.09 Other pulmonary complications of anesthesia during the puerperium   M♀

O89.1 Cardiac complications of anesthesia during the puerperium   M♀

O89.2 Central nervous system complications of anesthesia during the puerperium   M♀

O89.3 Toxic reaction to local anesthesia during the puerperium   M♀

O89.4 Spinal and epidural anesthesia-induced headache during the puerperium   M♀

O89.5 Other complications of spinal and epidural anesthesia during the puerperium   M♀

O89.6 Failed or difficult intubation for anesthesia during the puerperium   M♀

O89.8 Other complications of anesthesia during the puerperium   M♀

O89.9 Complication of anesthesia during the puerperium, unspecified   M♀▽

✓4ᵗʰ **O90 Complications of the puerperium, not elsewhere classified**

O90.0 Disruption of cesarean delivery wound   M♀
Dehiscence of cesarean delivery wound
EXCLUDES 1   rupture of uterus (spontaneous) before onset of labor (O71.0-)
rupture of uterus during labor (O71.1)

O90.1 Disruption of perineal obstetric wound   M♀
Disruption of wound of episiotomy
Disruption of wound of perineal laceration
Secondary perineal tear

O90.2 Hematoma of obstetric wound   M♀

O90.3 Peripartum cardiomyopathy   M♀
Conditions in I42- arising during pregnancy and the puerperium
EXCLUDES 1   pre-existing heart disease complicating pregnancy and the puerperium (O99.4-)

O90.4 Postpartum acute kidney failure   CC M♀
Hepatorenal syndrome following labor and delivery

O90.5 Postpartum thyroiditis   M♀

O90.6 Postpartum mood disturbance   M♀
Postpartum blues
Postpartum dysphoria
Postpartum sadness
EXCLUDES 1   postpartum depression (F53)
puerperal psychosis (F53)

✓5ᵗʰ **O90.8 Other complications of the puerperium, not elsewhere classified**

O90.81 Anemia of the puerperium   M♀
Postpartum anemia NOS
EXCLUDES 1   pre-existing anemia complicating the puerperium (O99.03)

O90.89 Other complications of the puerperium, not elsewhere classified   M♀
Placental polyp

O90.9 Complication of the puerperium, unspecified   M♀▽

✓4ᵗʰ **O91 Infections of breast associated with pregnancy, the puerperium and lactation**
Use additional code to identify infection

✓5ᵗʰ **O91.0 Infection of nipple associated with pregnancy, the puerperium and lactation**

✓6ᵗʰ **O91.01 Infection of nipple associated with pregnancy**
Gestational abscess of nipple

O91.011 Infection of nipple associated with pregnancy, first trimester   M♀

O91.012 Infection of nipple associated with pregnancy, second trimester   M♀

O91.013 Infection of nipple associated with pregnancy, third trimester   M♀

O91.019 Infection of nipple associated with pregnancy, unspecified trimester   M♀▽

O91.02 Infection of nipple associated with the puerperium   M♀
Puerperal abscess of nipple

O91.03 Infection of nipple associated with lactation   M♀
Abscess of nipple associated with lactation

✓5ᵗʰ **O91.1 Abscess of breast associated with pregnancy, the puerperium and lactation**

✓6ᵗʰ **O91.11 Abscess of breast associated with pregnancy**
Gestational mammary abscess
Gestational purulent mastitis
Gestational subareolar abscess

O91.111 Abscess of breast associated with pregnancy, first trimester   M♀

O91.112 Abscess of breast associated with pregnancy, second trimester   M♀

O91.113 Abscess of breast associated with pregnancy, third trimester   M♀

O91.119 Abscess of breast associated with pregnancy, unspecified trimester   M♀▽

O91.12 Abscess of breast associated with the puerperium   M♀
Puerperal mammary abscess
Puerperal purulent mastitis
Puerperal subareolar abscess

O91.13 Abscess of breast associated with lactation   M♀
Mammary abscess associated with lactation
Purulent mastitis associated with lactation
Subareolar abscess associated with lactation

✓5ᵗʰ **O91.2 Nonpurulent mastitis associated with pregnancy, the puerperium and lactation**

✓6ᵗʰ **O91.21 Nonpurulent mastitis associated with pregnancy**
Gestational interstitial mastitis
Gestational lymphangitis of breast
Gestational mastitis NOS
Gestational parenchymatous mastitis

O91.211 Nonpurulent mastitis associated with pregnancy, first trimester   M♀

O91.212 Nonpurulent mastitis associated with pregnancy, second trimester   M♀

O91.213 Nonpurulent mastitis associated with pregnancy, third trimester   M♀

O91.219 Nonpurulent mastitis associated with pregnancy, unspecified trimester   M♀▽

O91.22 Nonpurulent mastitis associated with the puerperium   M♀
Puerperal interstitial mastitis
Puerperal lymphangitis of breast
Puerperal mastitis NOS
Puerperal parenchymatous mastitis

O91.23 Nonpurulent mastitis associated with lactation   M♀
Interstitial mastitis associated with lactation
Lymphangitis of breast associated with lactation
Mastitis NOS associated with lactation
Parenchymatous mastitis associated with lactation

N Newborn   P Pediatric   M Maternity   A Adult   RIC RIC Dx   NC Dx Noncancer Dx   PDx Primary Dx   CC RIC CC Condition   ►◄ Revised Text   ● New Code   ▲ Revised Code Title

800   ICD-10-CM 2016

√4ᵗʰ O92 Other disorders of breast and disorders of lactation associated with pregnancy and the puerperium

√5ᵗʰ O92.0 Retracted nipple associated with pregnancy, the puerperium, and lactation

√6ᵗʰ O92.01 Retracted nipple associated with pregnancy

O92.011 Retracted nipple associated with pregnancy, first trimester   Ⓜ♀

O92.012 Retracted nipple associated with pregnancy, second trimester   Ⓜ♀

O92.013 Retracted nipple associated with pregnancy, third trimester   Ⓜ♀

O92.019 Retracted nipple associated with pregnancy, unspecified trimester   Ⓜ♀▽

O92.02 Retracted nipple associated with the puerperium   Ⓜ♀

O92.03 Retracted nipple associated with lactation   Ⓜ♀

√5ᵗʰ O92.1 Cracked nipple associated with pregnancy, the puerperium, and lactation
Fissure of nipple, gestational or puerperal

√6ᵗʰ O92.11 Cracked nipple associated with pregnancy

O92.111 Cracked nipple associated with pregnancy, first trimester   Ⓜ♀

O92.112 Cracked nipple associated with pregnancy, second trimester   Ⓜ♀

O92.113 Cracked nipple associated with pregnancy, third trimester   Ⓜ♀

O92.119 Cracked nipple associated with pregnancy, unspecified trimester   Ⓜ♀▽

O92.12 Cracked nipple associated with the puerperium   Ⓜ♀

O92.13 Cracked nipple associated with lactation   Ⓜ♀

√5ᵗʰ O92.2 Other and unspecified disorders of breast associated with pregnancy and the puerperium

O92.20 Unspecified disorder of breast associated with pregnancy and the puerperium   Ⓜ♀▽

O92.29 Other disorders of breast associated with pregnancy and the puerperium   Ⓜ♀

O92.3 Agalactia   Ⓜ♀
Primary agalactia
EXCLUDES 1 elective agalactia (O92.5)
secondary agalactia (O92.5)
therapeutic agalactia (O92.5)

O92.4 Hypogalactia   Ⓜ♀

O92.5 Suppressed lactation   Ⓜ♀
Elective agalactia
Secondary agalactia
Therapeutic agalactia
EXCLUDES 1 primary agalactia (O92.3)

O92.6 Galactorrhea   Ⓜ♀

√5ᵗʰ O92.7 Other and unspecified disorders of lactation

O92.70 Unspecified disorders of lactation   Ⓜ♀▽

O92.79 Other disorders of lactation   Ⓜ♀
Puerperal galactocele

Other obstetric conditions, not elsewhere classified (O94-O9A)

O94 Sequelae of complication of pregnancy, childbirth, and the puerperium   Ⓜ♀
NOTE This category is to be used to indicate conditions in O00-O77.-, O85-O94 and O98-O9A.- as the cause of late effects. The sequelae include conditions specified as such, or as late effects, which may occur at any time after the puerperium.
Code first condition resulting from (sequela) of complication of pregnancy, childbirth, and the puerperium

√4ᵗʰ O98 Maternal infectious and parasitic diseases classifiable elsewhere but complicating pregnancy, childbirth and the puerperium
INCLUDES the listed conditions when complicating the pregnant state, when aggravated by the pregnancy, or as a reason for obstetric care
Use additional code (Chapter 1), to identify specific infectious or parasitic disease
EXCLUDES 2 herpes gestationis (O26.4-)
infectious carrier state (O99.82-, O99.83-)
obstetrical tetanus (A34)
puerperal infection (O86.-)
puerperal sepsis (O85)
when the reason for maternal care is that the disease is known or suspected to have affected the fetus (O35-O36)

√5ᵗʰ O98.0 Tuberculosis complicating pregnancy, childbirth and the puerperium
Conditions in A15-A19

√6ᵗʰ O98.01 Tuberculosis complicating pregnancy

O98.011 Tuberculosis complicating pregnancy, first trimester   Ⓜ♀

O98.012 Tuberculosis complicating pregnancy, second trimester   Ⓜ♀

O98.013 Tuberculosis complicating pregnancy, third trimester   Ⓜ♀

O98.019 Tuberculosis complicating pregnancy, unspecified trimester   Ⓜ♀▽

O98.02 Tuberculosis complicating childbirth   Ⓜ♀

O98.03 Tuberculosis complicating the puerperium   Ⓜ♀

√5ᵗʰ O98.1 Syphilis complicating pregnancy, childbirth and the puerperium
Conditions in A50-A53

√6ᵗʰ O98.11 Syphilis complicating pregnancy

O98.111 Syphilis complicating pregnancy, first trimester   Ⓜ♀

O98.112 Syphilis complicating pregnancy, second trimester   Ⓜ♀

O98.113 Syphilis complicating pregnancy, third trimester   Ⓜ♀

O98.119 Syphilis complicating pregnancy, unspecified trimester   Ⓜ♀▽

O98.12 Syphilis complicating childbirth   Ⓜ♀

O98.13 Syphilis complicating the puerperium   Ⓜ♀

√5ᵗʰ O98.2 Gonorrhea complicating pregnancy, childbirth and the puerperium
Conditions in A54-

√6ᵗʰ O98.21 Gonorrhea complicating pregnancy

O98.211 Gonorrhea complicating pregnancy, first trimester   Ⓜ♀

O98.212 Gonorrhea complicating pregnancy, second trimester   Ⓜ♀

O98.213 Gonorrhea complicating pregnancy, third trimester   Ⓜ♀

O98.219 Gonorrhea complicating pregnancy, unspecified trimester   Ⓜ♀▽

O98.22 Gonorrhea complicating childbirth   Ⓜ♀

O98.23 Gonorrhea complicating the puerperium   Ⓜ♀

√5ᵗʰ O98.3 Other infections with a predominantly sexual mode of transmission complicating pregnancy, childbirth and the puerperium
Conditions in A55-A64

√6ᵗʰ O98.31 Other infections with a predominantly sexual mode of transmission complicating pregnancy

O98.311 Other infections with a predominantly sexual mode of transmission complicating pregnancy, first trimester   Ⓜ♀

O98.312 Other infections with a predominantly sexual mode of transmission complicating pregnancy, second trimester   Ⓜ♀

O98.313 Other infections with a predominantly sexual mode of transmission complicating pregnancy, third trimester   Ⓜ♀

O98.319 Other infections with a predominantly sexual mode of transmission complicating pregnancy, unspecified trimester   Ⓜ♀▽

O98.32 Other infections with a predominantly sexual mode of transmission complicating childbirth   Ⓜ♀

O98.33 Other infections with a predominantly sexual mode of transmission complicating the puerperium   Ⓜ♀

√5ᵗʰ O98.4 Viral hepatitis complicating pregnancy, childbirth and the puerperium
Conditions in B15-B19

√6ᵗʰ O98.41 Viral hepatitis complicating pregnancy

O98.411 Viral hepatitis complicating pregnancy, first trimester   Ⓜ♀

O98.412 Viral hepatitis complicating pregnancy, second trimester   Ⓜ♀

O98.413   **Viral hepatitis complicating pregnancy, third trimester**   Ⓜ♀

O98.419   **Viral hepatitis complicating pregnancy, unspecified trimester**   Ⓜ♀▽

O98.42   **Viral hepatitis complicating childbirth**   Ⓜ♀

O98.43   **Viral hepatitis complicating the puerperium**   Ⓜ♀

✓5ᵗʰ O98.5   **Other viral diseases complicating pregnancy, childbirth and the puerperium**
    Conditions in A80-B09, B25-B34, R87.81-, R87.82-
    EXCLUDES 1   *human immunodeficiency virus [HIV] disease complicating pregnancy, childbirth and the puerperium (O98.7-)*

    ✓6ᵗʰ O98.51   **Other viral diseases complicating pregnancy**

       O98.511   **Other viral diseases complicating pregnancy, first trimester**   Ⓜ♀

       O98.512   **Other viral diseases complicating pregnancy, second trimester**   Ⓜ♀

       O98.513   **Other viral diseases complicating pregnancy, third trimester**   Ⓜ♀

       O98.519   **Other viral diseases complicating pregnancy, unspecified trimester**   Ⓜ♀▽

    O98.52   **Other viral diseases complicating childbirth**   Ⓜ♀

    O98.53   **Other viral diseases complicating the puerperium**   Ⓜ♀

✓5ᵗʰ O98.6   **Protozoal diseases complicating pregnancy, childbirth and the puerperium**
    Conditions in B50-B64

    ✓6ᵗʰ O98.61   **Protozoal diseases complicating pregnancy**

       O98.611   **Protozoal diseases complicating pregnancy, first trimester**   Ⓜ♀

       O98.612   **Protozoal diseases complicating pregnancy, second trimester**   Ⓜ♀

       O98.613   **Protozoal diseases complicating pregnancy, third trimester**   Ⓜ♀

       O98.619   **Protozoal diseases complicating pregnancy, unspecified trimester**   Ⓜ♀▽

    O98.62   **Protozoal diseases complicating childbirth**   Ⓜ♀

    O98.63   **Protozoal diseases complicating the puerperium**   Ⓜ♀

✓5ᵗʰ O98.7   **Human immunodeficiency virus [HIV] disease complicating pregnancy, childbirth and the puerperium**
    Use additional code to identify the type of HIV disease:
      acquired immune deficiency syndrome (AIDS) (B20)
      asymptomatic HIV status (Z21)
      HIV positive NOS (Z21)
      symptomatic HIV disease (B20)

    ✓6ᵗʰ O98.71   **Human immunodeficiency virus [HIV] disease complicating pregnancy**

       O98.711   **Human immunodeficiency virus [HIV] disease complicating pregnancy, first trimester**   Ⓜ♀

       O98.712   **Human immunodeficiency virus [HIV] disease complicating pregnancy, second trimester**   Ⓜ♀

       O98.713   **Human immunodeficiency virus [HIV] disease complicating pregnancy, third trimester**   Ⓜ♀

       O98.719   **Human immunodeficiency virus [HIV] disease complicating pregnancy, unspecified trimester**   Ⓜ♀▽

    O98.72   **Human immunodeficiency virus [HIV] disease complicating childbirth**   Ⓜ♀

    O98.73   **Human immunodeficiency virus [HIV] disease complicating the puerperium**   Ⓜ♀

✓5ᵗʰ O98.8   **Other maternal infectious and parasitic diseases complicating pregnancy, childbirth and the puerperium**

    ✓6ᵗʰ O98.81   **Other maternal infectious and parasitic diseases complicating pregnancy**

       O98.811   **Other maternal infectious and parasitic diseases complicating pregnancy, first trimester**   Ⓜ♀

       O98.812   **Other maternal infectious and parasitic diseases complicating pregnancy, second trimester**   Ⓜ♀

       O98.813   **Other maternal infectious and parasitic diseases complicating pregnancy, third trimester**   Ⓜ♀

       O98.819   **Other maternal infectious and parasitic diseases complicating pregnancy, unspecified trimester**   Ⓜ♀▽

    O98.82   **Other maternal infectious and parasitic diseases complicating childbirth**   Ⓜ♀

    O98.83   **Other maternal infectious and parasitic diseases complicating the puerperium**   Ⓜ♀

✓5ᵗʰ O98.9   **Unspecified maternal infectious and parasitic disease complicating pregnancy, childbirth and the puerperium**

    ✓6ᵗʰ O98.91   **Unspecified maternal infectious and parasitic disease complicating pregnancy**

       O98.911   **Unspecified maternal infectious and parasitic disease complicating pregnancy, first trimester**   Ⓜ♀▽

       O98.912   **Unspecified maternal infectious and parasitic disease complicating pregnancy, second trimester**   Ⓜ♀▽

       O98.913   **Unspecified maternal infectious and parasitic disease complicating pregnancy, third trimester**   Ⓜ♀▽

       O98.919   **Unspecified maternal infectious and parasitic disease complicating pregnancy, unspecified trimester**   Ⓜ♀▽

    O98.92   **Unspecified maternal infectious and parasitic disease complicating childbirth**   Ⓜ♀▽

    O98.93   **Unspecified maternal infectious and parasitic disease complicating the puerperium**   Ⓜ♀▽

✓4ᵗʰ **O99**   **Other maternal diseases classifiable elsewhere but complicating pregnancy, childbirth and the puerperium**
    INCLUDES   conditions which complicate the pregnant state, are aggravated by the pregnancy or are a main reason for obstetric care
    Use additional code to identify specific condition
    EXCLUDES 2   *when the reason for maternal care is that the condition is known or suspected to have affected the fetus (O35-O36)*

✓5ᵗʰ O99.0   **Anemia complicating pregnancy, childbirth and the puerperium**
    Conditions in D50-D64
    EXCLUDES 1   *anemia arising in the puerperium (O90.81)*
               postpartum anemia NOS (O90.81)

    ✓6ᵗʰ O99.01   **Anemia complicating pregnancy**

       O99.011   **Anemia complicating pregnancy, first trimester**   Ⓜ♀

       O99.012   **Anemia complicating pregnancy, second trimester**   Ⓜ♀

       O99.013   **Anemia complicating pregnancy, third trimester**   Ⓜ♀

       O99.019   **Anemia complicating pregnancy, unspecified trimester**   Ⓜ♀▽

    O99.02   **Anemia complicating childbirth**   Ⓜ♀

    O99.03   **Anemia complicating the puerperium**   Ⓜ♀
       EXCLUDES 1   *postpartum anemia not pre-existing prior to delivery (O90.81)*

✓5ᵗʰ O99.1   **Other diseases of the blood and blood-forming organs and certain disorders involving the immune mechanism complicating pregnancy, childbirth and the puerperium**
    Conditions in D65-D89
    EXCLUDES 2   *hemorrhage with coagulation defects (O45.-, O46.0-, O67.0, O72.3)*

    ✓6ᵗʰ O99.11   **Other diseases of the blood and blood-forming organs and certain disorders involving the immune mechanism complicating pregnancy**

       O99.111   **Other diseases of the blood and blood-forming organs and certain disorders involving the immune mechanism complicating pregnancy, first trimester**   Ⓜ♀

       O99.112   **Other diseases of the blood and blood-forming organs and certain disorders involving the immune mechanism complicating pregnancy, second trimester**   Ⓜ♀

       O99.113   **Other diseases of the blood and blood-forming organs and certain disorders involving the immune mechanism complicating pregnancy, third trimester**   Ⓜ♀

Ⓝ Newborn   Ⓟ Pediatric   Ⓜ Maternity   Ⓐ Adult   **RIC** RIC Dx   **NC Dx** Noncancer Dx   **PDx** Primary Dx   **CC** RIC CC Condition   ►◄ Revised Text   ● New Code   ▲ Revised Code Title

802   ICD-10-CM 2016

O99.119 Other diseases of the blood and blood-forming organs and certain disorders involving the immune mechanism complicating pregnancy, unspecified trimester Ⓜ♀▽

O99.12 Other diseases of the blood and blood-forming organs and certain disorders involving the immune mechanism complicating childbirth Ⓜ♀

O99.13 Other diseases of the blood and blood-forming organs and certain disorders involving the immune mechanism complicating the puerperium Ⓜ♀

✓5th O99.2 **Endocrine, nutritional and metabolic diseases complicating pregnancy, childbirth and the puerperium**
Conditions in E00-E88
EXCLUDES 2 diabetes mellitus (O24.-)
malnutrition (O25.-)
postpartum thyroiditis (O90.5)

✓6th O99.21 Obesity complicating pregnancy, childbirth, and the puerperium
Use additional code to identify the type of obesity (E66.-)

O99.210 Obesity complicating pregnancy, unspecified trimester Ⓜ♀▽

O99.211 Obesity complicating pregnancy, first trimester Ⓜ♀

O99.212 Obesity complicating pregnancy, second trimester Ⓜ♀

O99.213 Obesity complicating pregnancy, third trimester Ⓜ♀

O99.214 Obesity complicating childbirth Ⓜ♀

O99.215 Obesity complicating the puerperium Ⓜ♀

✓6th O99.28 Other endocrine, nutritional and metabolic diseases complicating pregnancy, childbirth and the puerperium

O99.280 Endocrine, nutritional and metabolic diseases complicating pregnancy, unspecified trimester Ⓜ♀▽

O99.281 Endocrine, nutritional and metabolic diseases complicating pregnancy, first trimester Ⓜ♀

O99.282 Endocrine, nutritional and metabolic diseases complicating pregnancy, second trimester Ⓜ♀

O99.283 Endocrine, nutritional and metabolic diseases complicating pregnancy, third trimester Ⓜ♀

O99.284 Endocrine, nutritional and metabolic diseases complicating childbirth Ⓜ♀

O99.285 Endocrine, nutritional and metabolic diseases complicating the puerperium Ⓜ♀

✓5th O99.3 **Mental disorders and diseases of the nervous system complicating pregnancy, childbirth and the puerperium**

✓6th O99.31 Alcohol use complicating pregnancy, childbirth, and the puerperium
Use additional code(s) from F10 to identify manifestations of the alcohol use

O99.310 Alcohol use complicating pregnanry, unspecified trimester Ⓜ♀▽

O99.311 Alcohol use complicating pregnancy, first trimester Ⓜ♀

O99.312 Alcohol use complicating pregnancy, second trimester Ⓜ♀

O99.313 Alcohol use complicating pregnancy, third trimester Ⓜ♀

O99.314 Alcohol use complicating childbirth Ⓜ♀

O99.315 Alcohol use complicating the puerperium Ⓜ♀

✓6th O99.32 Drug use complicating pregnancy, childbirth, and the puerperium
Use additional code(s) from F11-F16 and F18-F19 to identify manifestations of the drug use

O99.320 Drug use complicating pregnancy, unspecified trimester Ⓜ♀▽

O99.321 Drug use complicating pregnancy, first trimester Ⓜ♀

O99.322 Drug use complicating pregnancy, second trimester Ⓜ♀

O99.323 Drug use complicating pregnancy, third trimester Ⓜ♀

O99.324 Drug use complicating childbirth Ⓜ♀

O99.325 Drug use complicating the puerperium Ⓜ♀

✓6th O99.33 Smoking (tobacco) complicating pregnancy, childbirth, and the puerperium
Use additional code from F17 to identify type of tobacco

O99.330 Smoking (tobacco) complicating pregnancy, unspecified trimester Ⓜ♀▽

O99.331 Smoking (tobacco) complicating pregnancy, first trimester Ⓜ♀

O99.332 Smoking (tobacco) complicating pregnancy, second trimester Ⓜ♀

O99.333 Smoking (tobacco) complicating pregnancy, third trimester Ⓜ♀

O99.334 Smoking (tobacco) complicating childbirth Ⓜ♀

O99.335 Smoking (tobacco) complicating the puerperium Ⓜ♀

✓6th O99.34 Other mental disorders complicating pregnancy, childbirth, and the puerperium
Conditions in F01-F09 and F20-F99
EXCLUDES 2 postpartum mood disturbance (O90.6)
postnatal psychosis (F53)
puerperal psychosis (F53)

O99.340 Other mental disorders complicating pregnancy, unspecified trimester Ⓜ♀▽

O99.341 Other mental disorders complicating pregnancy, first trimester Ⓜ♀

O99.342 Other mental disorders complicating pregnancy, second trimester Ⓜ♀

O99.343 Other mental disorders complicating pregnancy, third trimester Ⓜ♀

O99.344 Other mental disorders complicating childbirth Ⓜ♀

O99.345 Other mental disorders complicating the puerperium Ⓜ♀

✓6th O99.35 Diseases of the nervous system complicating pregnancy, childbirth, and the puerperium
Conditions in G00-G99
EXCLUDES 2 pregnancy related peripheral neuritis (O26.8-)

O99.350 Diseases of the nervous system complicating pregnancy, unspecified trimester Ⓜ♀▽

O99.351 Diseases of the nervous system complicating pregnancy, first trimester Ⓜ♀

O99.352 Diseases of the nervous system complicating pregnancy, second trimester Ⓜ♀

O99.353 Diseases of the nervous system complicating pregnancy, third trimester Ⓜ♀

O99.354 Diseases of the nervous system complicating childbirth Ⓜ♀

O99.355 Diseases of the nervous system complicating the puerperium Ⓜ♀

✓5th O99.4 **Diseases of the circulatory system complicating pregnancy, childbirth and the puerperium**
Conditions in I00-I99
EXCLUDES 1 peripartum cardiomyopathy (O90.3)
EXCLUDES 2 hypertensive disorders (O10-O16)
obstetric embolism (O88.-)
venous complications and cerebrovenous sinus thrombosis in labor, childbirth and the puerperium (O87.-)
venous complications and cerebrovenous sinus thrombosis in pregnancy (O22.-)

✓6th O99.41 Diseases of the circulatory system complicating pregnancy

O99.411 Diseases of the circulatory system complicating pregnancy, first trimester Ⓜ♀

O99.412 Diseases of the circulatory system complicating pregnancy, second trimester Ⓜ♀

O99.413 Diseases of the circulatory system complicating pregnancy, third trimester Ⓜ♀

O99.419   **Diseases of the circulatory system complicating pregnancy, unspecified trimester**   CC M♀▽
RIC Excl: 01 Stroke; 03 Non-traumatic brain injury

O99.42   **Diseases of the circulatory system complicating childbirth**   M♀

O99.43   **Diseases of the circulatory system complicating the puerperium**   M♀

✓5ᵗʰ O99.5   **Diseases of the respiratory system complicating pregnancy, childbirth and the puerperium**
Conditions in J00-J99

✓6ᵗʰ O99.51   **Diseases of the respiratory system complicating pregnancy**

O99.511   **Diseases of the respiratory system complicating pregnancy, first trimester**   M♀

O99.512   **Diseases of the respiratory system complicating pregnancy, second trimester**   M♀

O99.513   **Diseases of the respiratory system complicating pregnancy, third trimester**   M♀

O99.519   **Diseases of the respiratory system complicating pregnancy, unspecified trimester**   M♀▽

O99.52   **Diseases of the respiratory system complicating childbirth**   M♀

O99.53   **Diseases of the respiratory system complicating the puerperium**   M♀

✓5ᵗʰ O99.6   **Diseases of the digestive system complicating pregnancy, childbirth and the puerperium**
Conditions in K00-K93
EXCLUDES 2   liver and biliary tract disorders in pregnancy, childbirth and the puerperium (O26.6-)

✓6ᵗʰ O99.61   **Diseases of the digestive system complicating pregnancy**

O99.611   **Diseases of the digestive system complicating pregnancy, first trimester**   M♀

O99.612   **Diseases of the digestive system complicating pregnancy, second trimester**   M♀

O99.613   **Diseases of the digestive system complicating pregnancy, third trimester**   M♀

O99.619   **Diseases of the digestive system complicating pregnancy, unspecified trimester**   M♀▽

O99.62   **Diseases of the digestive system complicating childbirth**   M♀

O99.63   **Diseases of the digestive system complicating the puerperium**   M♀

✓5ᵗʰ O99.7   **Diseases of the skin and subcutaneous tissue complicating pregnancy, childbirth and the puerperium**
Conditions in L00-L99
EXCLUDES 2   herpes gestationis (O26.4)
pruritic urticarial papules and plaques of pregnancy (PUPPP) (O26.86)

✓6ᵗʰ O99.71   **Diseases of the skin and subcutaneous tissue complicating pregnancy**

O99.711   **Diseases of the skin and subcutaneous tissue complicating pregnancy, first trimester**   M♀

O99.712   **Diseases of the skin and subcutaneous tissue complicating pregnancy, second trimester**   M♀

O99.713   **Diseases of the skin and subcutaneous tissue complicating pregnancy, third trimester**   M♀

O99.719   **Diseases of the skin and subcutaneous tissue complicating pregnancy, unspecified trimester**   M♀▽

O99.72   **Diseases of the skin and subcutaneous tissue complicating childbirth**   M♀

O99.73   **Diseases of the skin and subcutaneous tissue complicating the puerperium**   M♀

✓5ᵗʰ O99.8   **Other specified diseases and conditions complicating pregnancy, childbirth and the puerperium**
Conditions in D00-D48, H00-H95, M00-N99, and Q00-Q99
Use additional code to identify condition
EXCLUDES 2   genitourinary infections in pregnancy (O23.-)
infection of genitourinary tract following delivery (O86.1-O86.3)
malignant neoplasm complicating pregnancy, childbirth and the puerperium (O9A.1-)
maternal care for known or suspected abnormality of maternal pelvic organs (O34.-)
postpartum acute kidney failure (O90.4)
traumatic injuries in pregnancy (O9A.2)

✓6ᵗʰ O99.81   **Abnormal glucose complicating pregnancy, childbirth and the puerperium**
EXCLUDES 1   gestational diabetes (O24.4-)

O99.810   **Abnormal glucose complicating pregnancy**   M♀

O99.814   **Abnormal glucose complicating childbirth**   M♀

O99.815   **Abnormal glucose complicating the puerperium**   M♀

✓6ᵗʰ O99.82   **Streptococcus B carrier state complicating pregnancy, childbirth and the puerperium**

O99.820   **Streptococcus B carrier state complicating pregnancy**   M♀

O99.824   **Streptococcus B carrier state complicating childbirth**   M♀

O99.825   **Streptococcus B carrier state complicating the puerperium**   M♀

✓6ᵗʰ O99.83   **Other infection carrier state complicating pregnancy, childbirth and the puerperium**
Use additional code to identify the carrier state (Z22.-)

O99.830   **Other infection carrier state complicating pregnancy**   M♀

O99.834   **Other infection carrier state complicating childbirth**   M♀

O99.835   **Other infection carrier state complicating the puerperium**   M♀

✓6ᵗʰ O99.84   **Bariatric surgery status complicating pregnancy, childbirth and the puerperium**
Gastric banding status complicating pregnancy, childbirth and the puerperium
Gastric bypass status for obesity complicating pregnancy, childbirth and the puerperium
Obesity surgery status complicating pregnancy, childbirth and the puerperium

O99.840   **Bariatric surgery status complicating pregnancy, unspecified trimester**   M♀▽

O99.841   **Bariatric surgery status complicating pregnancy, first trimester**   M♀

O99.842   **Bariatric surgery status complicating pregnancy, second trimester**   M♀

O99.843   **Bariatric surgery status complicating pregnancy, third trimester**   M♀

O99.844   **Bariatric surgery status complicating childbirth**   M♀

O99.845   **Bariatric surgery status complicating the puerperium**   M♀

O99.89   **Other specified diseases and conditions complicating pregnancy, childbirth and the puerperium**   M♀

✓4ᵗʰ O9A   **Maternal malignant neoplasms, traumatic injuries and abuse classifiable elsewhere but complicating pregnancy, childbirth and the puerperium**

✓5ᵗʰ O9A.1   **Malignant neoplasm complicating pregnancy, childbirth and the puerperium**
Conditions in C00-C96
Use additional code to identify neoplasm
EXCLUDES 2   maternal care for benign tumor of corpus uteri (O34.1-)
maternal care for benign tumor of cervix (O34.4-)

✓6ᵗʰ O9A.11   **Malignant neoplasm complicating pregnancy**

O9A.111   **Malignant neoplasm complicating pregnancy, first trimester**   M♀

O9A.112   **Malignant neoplasm complicating pregnancy, second trimester**   M♀

O9A.113   **Malignant neoplasm complicating pregnancy, third trimester**   M♀

N Newborn   P Pediatric   M Maternity   A Adult   RIC RIC Dx   NC Dx Noncancer Dx   PDx Primary Dx   CC RIC CC Condition   ►◄ Revised Text   ● New Code   ▲ Revised Code Title

804   ICD-10-CM 2016

O9A.119   **Malignant neoplasm complicating**   M♀▽
pregnancy, unspecified trimester

O9A.12   **Malignant neoplasm complicating** childbirth   M♀

O9A.13   **Malignant neoplasm complicating the**   M♀
puerperium

√5ᵗʰ **O9A.2**   Injury, poisoning and **certain other consequences of** external
causes **complicating pregnancy, childbirth and the**
puerperium
> Conditions in S00-T88, except T74 and T76
> Use additional code(s) to identify the injury or poisoning
> EXCLUDES 2   physical, sexual and psychological abuse complicating
> pregnancy, childbirth and the puerperium
> (O9A.3-, O9A.4-, O9A.5-)

√6ᵗʰ **O9A.21**   **Injury, poisoning and certain other consequences of
external causes complicating** pregnancy

O9A.211   **Injury, poisoning and certain other**   M♀
consequences of external causes
complicating pregnancy, first
trimester

O9A.212   **Injury, poisoning and certain other**   M♀
consequences of external causes
complicating pregnancy, second
trimester

O9A.213   **Injury, poisoning and certain other**   M♀
consequences of external causes
complicating pregnancy, third
trimester

O9A.219   **Injury, poisoning and certain other**   M♀▽
consequences of external causes
complicating pregnancy, unspecified
trimester

O9A.22   **Injury, poisoning and certain other**   M♀
consequences of external causes complicating
childbirth

O9A.23   **Injury, poisoning and certain other**   M♀
consequences of external causes complicating
the puerperium

√5ᵗʰ **O9A.3**   Physical abuse **complicating pregnancy, childbirth and the**
puerperium
> Conditions in T74.11 or T76.11
> Use additional code (if applicable):
> to identify any associated current injury due to physical abuse
> to identify the perpetrator of abuse (Y07.-)
> EXCLUDES 2   sexual abuse complicating pregnancy, childbirth and
> the puerperium (O9A.4)

√6ᵗʰ **O9A.31**   **Physical abuse complicating** pregnancy

O9A.311   **Physical abuse complicating**   M♀
pregnancy, first trimester

O9A.312   **Physical abuse complicating**   M♀
pregnancy, second trimester

O9A.313   **Physical abuse complicating**   M♀
pregnancy, third trimester

O9A.319   **Physical abuse complicating**   M♀▽
pregnancy, unspecified trimester

O9A.32   **Physical abuse complicating** childbirth   M♀

O9A.33   **Physical abuse complicating the** puerperium   M♀

√5ᵗʰ **O9A.4**   Sexual abuse **complicating pregnancy, childbirth and the**
puerperium
> Conditions in T74.21 or T76.21
> Use additional code (if applicable):
> to identify any associated current injury due to sexual abuse
> to identify the perpetrator of abuse (Y07.-)

√6ᵗʰ **O9A.41**   **Sexual abuse complicating** pregnancy

O9A.411   **Sexual abuse complicating**   M♀
pregnancy, first trimester

O9A.412   **Sexual abuse complicating**   M♀
pregnancy, second trimester

O9A.413   **Sexual abuse complicating**   M♀
pregnancy, third trimester

O9A.419   **Sexual abuse complicating**   M♀▽
pregnancy, unspecified trimester

O9A.42   **Sexual abuse complicating** childbirth   M♀

O9A.43   **Sexual abuse complicating the** puerperium   M♀

√5ᵗʰ **O9A.5**   Psychological abuse **complicating pregnancy, childbirth and
the puerperium**
> Conditions in T74.31 or T76.31
> Use additional code to identify the perpetrator of abuse (Y07.-)

√6ᵗʰ **O9A.51**   **Psychological abuse complicating** pregnancy

O9A.511   **Psychological abuse complicating**   M♀
pregnancy, first trimester

O9A.512   **Psychological abuse complicating**   M♀
pregnancy, second trimester

O9A.513   **Psychological abuse complicating**   M♀
pregnancy, third trimester

O9A.519   **Psychological abuse complicating**   M♀▽
pregnancy, unspecified trimester

O9A.52   **Psychological abuse complicating** childbirth   M♀

O9A.53   **Psychological abuse complicating the**   M♀
puerperium

Chapter 16. Certain Conditions Originating in the Perinatal Period (P00–P96)

Chapter Specific Guidelines with Coding Examples

The chapter specific guidelines from the ICD-10-CM Official Guidelines for Coding and Reporting have been provided below. Along with these guidelines are coding examples, contained in the shaded boxes, that have been developed to help illustrate the coding and/or sequencing guidance found in these guidelines.

For coding and reporting purposes the perinatal period is defined as before birth through the 28th day following birth. The following guidelines are provided for reporting purposes

a. General Perinatal Rules

1) Use of chapter 16 codes

Codes in this chapter are <u>never</u> for use on the maternal record. Codes from Chapter 15, the obstetric chapter, are never permitted on the newborn record. Chapter 16 codes may be used throughout the life of the patient if the condition is still present.

2) Principal diagnosis for birth record

When coding the birth episode in a newborn record, assign a code from category Z38, Liveborn infants according to place of birth and type of delivery, as the principal diagnosis. A code from category Z38 is assigned only once, to a newborn at the time of birth. If a newborn is transferred to another institution, a code from category Z38 should not be used at the receiving hospital.

A code from category Z38 is used only on the newborn record, not on the mother's record.

> Newborn delivered via vaginal delivery in Rural Hospital A, experienced meconium aspiration resulting in pneumonia. Rural hospital A is not equipped to handle the extensive respiratory therapy this baby needs and transfers the patient to Metropolis Hospital B, where the pneumonia resolves and the newborn is eventually discharged.
>
> *Rural hospital A*
>
> **Z38.00**   **Single liveborn infant, delivered vaginally**
>
> **P24.01**   **Meconium aspiration with respiratory symptoms**
>
> *Metropolis hospital B*
>
> **P24.01**   **Meconium aspiration with respiratory symptoms**
>
> *Explanation:* A code from category Z38 is a one-time use only code. The hospital that actually delivered the newborn, in this case Rural Hospital A, can append a code from category Z38 but for the delivery admission only. Once the patient is transferred or discharged, the Z38 category no longer applies for that patient.
>
> The reason for the transfer to Metropolis Hospital B was for the respiratory symptoms (pneumonia) the newborn was exhibiting secondary to aspirating meconium.

3) Use of codes from other chapters with codes from chapter 16

Codes from other chapters may be used with codes from chapter 16 if the codes from the other chapters provide more specific detail. Codes for signs and symptoms may be assigned when a definitive diagnosis has not been established. If the reason for the encounter is a perinatal condition, the code from chapter 16 should be sequenced first.

4) Use of chapter 16 codes after the perinatal period

Should a condition originate in the perinatal period, and continue throughout the life of the patient, the perinatal code should continue to be used regardless of the patient's age.

> A 7-year-old patient with history of birth injury that resulted in Erb's palsy is seen for subscapularis release
>
> **P14.0**   **Erb's paralysis due to birth injury**
>
> *Explanation:* Although in this instance Erb's palsy is specifically related to a birth injury, it has not resolved and continues to be a health concern. A perinatal code is appropriate even though this patient is beyond the perinatal period.

5) Birth process or community acquired conditions

If a newborn has a condition that may be either due to the birth process or community acquired and the documentation does not indicate which it is, the default is due to the birth process and the code from Chapter 16 should be used. If the condition is community-acquired, a code from Chapter 16 should not be assigned.

6) Code all clinically significant conditions

All clinically significant conditions noted on routine newborn examination should be coded. A condition is clinically significant if it requires:

clinical evaluation; or

therapeutic treatment; or

diagnostic procedures; or

extended length of hospital stay; or

increased nursing care and/or monitoring; or

has implications for future health care needs

Note: The perinatal guidelines listed above are the same as the general coding guidelines for "additional diagnoses", except for the final point regarding implications for future health care needs. Codes should be assigned for conditions that have been specified by the provider as having implications for future health care needs.

b. Observation and evaluation of newborns for suspected conditions not found

Reserved for future expansion

c. Coding additional perinatal diagnoses

1) Assigning codes for conditions that require treatment

Assign codes for conditions that require treatment or further investigation, prolong the length of stay, or require resource utilization.

2) Codes for conditions specified as having implications for future health care needs

Assign codes for conditions that have been specified by the provider as having implications for future health care needs.

Note: This guideline should not be used for adult patients.

> An abnormal noise was heard in the left hip of a post-term newborn during a physical examination. The pediatrician would like to follow the patient after discharge as a hip click can be an early sign of hip dysplasia. The newborn was delivered via cesarean at 41 weeks.
>
> **Z38.01**   **Single liveborn infant, delivered by cesarean**
>
> **P08.21**   **Post-term newborn**
>
> **R29.4**   **Clicking hip**
>
> *Explanation:* The abnormal hip noise or click is appended as a secondary diagnosis not only because it is an abnormal finding upon examination, but also due to its potential to be part of a bigger health issue. The hip dysplasia has not yet been diagnosed and does not warrant a code at this time.

d. Prematurity and fetal growth retardation

Providers utilize different criteria in determining prematurity. A code for prematurity should not be assigned unless it is documented. Assignment of codes in categories P05, Disorders of newborn related to slow fetal growth and fetal malnutrition, and P07, Disorders of newborn related to short gestation and low birth weight, not elsewhere classified, should be based on the recorded birth weight and estimated gestational age. Codes from category P05 should not be assigned with codes from category P07.

When both birth weight and gestational age are available, two codes from category P07 should be assigned, with the code for birth weight sequenced before the code for gestational age.

e. Low birth weight and immaturity status

Codes from category P07, Disorders of newborn related to short gestation and low birth weight, not elsewhere classified, are for use for a child or adult who was premature or had a low birth weight as a newborn and this is affecting the patient's current health status.

See Section I.C.21. Factors influencing health status and contact with health services, Status.

A 35-year-old patient, who weighed 659 grams at birth, is seen for heart disease documented as being a consequence of the low birth weight

I51.9	**Heart disease, unspecified**
P07.02	**Extremely low birth weight newborn, 500–749 grams**

Explanation: A code from subcategories P07.0- and P07.1- is appropriate, regardless of the age of the patient, as long as the documentation provides a clear link between the patient's current illness and the low birth weight.

f. Bacterial Sepsis of Newborn

Category P36, Bacterial sepsis of newborn, includes congenital sepsis. If a perinate is documented as having sepsis without documentation of congenital or community acquired, the default is congenital and a code from category P36 should be assigned. If the P36 code includes the causal organism, an additional code from category B95, Streptococcus, Staphylococcus, and Enterococcus as the cause of diseases classified elsewhere, or B96, Other bacterial agents as the cause of diseases classified elsewhere, should not be assigned. If the P36 code does not include the causal organism, assign an additional code from category B96. If applicable, use additional codes to identify severe sepsis (R65.2-) and any associated acute organ dysfunction.

A full-term infant develops severe sepsis 24 hours after discharge from the hospital and is readmitted; cultures identified *E. coli* as the infective agent

P36.4	**Sepsis of newborn due to Escherichia coli**
R65.20	**Severe sepsis without septic shock**

Explanation: Even though this newborn was discharged and could have acquired *E. coli* from his/her external environment, due to the lack of documentation specifying specifically how this pathogen was acquired, the default is to code the *E. coli* sepsis as congenital. A code from chapter 1, "Certain Infectious and Parasitic Diseases," is not required because the perinatal sepsis code identifies both the sepsis and the bacteria causing the sepsis.

g. Stillbirth

Code P95, Stillbirth, is only for use in institutions that maintain separate records for stillbirths. No other code should be used with P95. Code P95 should not be used on the mother's record.

Chapter 16. Certain Conditions Originating in the Perinatal Period

P00–P02.1

Chapter 16. Certain Conditions Originating in the Perinatal Period (P00-P96)

NOTE   Codes from this chapter are for use on newborn records only, never on maternal records.

INCLUDES   conditions that have their origin in the fetal or perinatal period (before birth through the first 28 days after birth) even if morbidity occurs later

EXCLUDES 2   congenital malformations, deformations and chromosomal abnormalities (Q00-Q99)
endocrine, nutritional and metabolic diseases (E00-E88)
injury, poisoning and certain other consequences of external causes (S00-T88)
neoplasms (C00-D49)
tetanus neonatorum (A33)

This chapter contains the following blocks:

P00-P04	Newborn affected by maternal factors and by complications of pregnancy, labor, and delivery
P05-P08	Disorders of newborn related to length of gestation and fetal growth
P09	Abnormal findings on neonatal screening
P10-P15	Birth trauma
P19-P29	Respiratory and cardiovascular disorders specific to the perinatal period
P35-P39	Infections specific to the perinatal period
P50-P61	Hemorrhagic and hematological disorders of newborn
P70-P74	Transitory endocrine and metabolic disorders specific to newborn
P76-P78	Digestive system disorders of newborn
P80-P83	Conditions involving the integument and temperature regulation of newborn
P84	Other problems with newborn
P90-P96	Other disorders originating in the perinatal period

Newborn affected by maternal factors and by complications of pregnancy, labor, and delivery (P00-P04)

NOTE   These codes are for use when the listed maternal conditions are specified as the cause of confirmed morbidity or potential morbidity which have their origin in the perinatal period (before birth through the first 28 days after birth). Codes from these categories are also for use for newborns who are suspected of having an abnormal condition resulting from exposure from the mother or the birth process, but without signs or symptoms, and, which after examination and observation, is found not to exist. These codes may be used even if treatment is begun for a suspected condition that is ruled out.

✓4ᵗʰ P00   **Newborn (suspected to be) affected by maternal conditions that may be unrelated to present pregnancy**
Code first any current condition in newborn
EXCLUDES 2   newborn (suspected to be) affected by maternal complications of pregnancy (P01.-)
newborn affected by maternal endocrine and metabolic disorders (P70-P74)
newborn affected by noxious substances transmitted via placenta or breast milk (P04.-)

P00.0   **Newborn (suspected to be) affected by maternal hypertensive disorders**   N
Newborn (suspected to be) affected by maternal conditions classifiable to O10-O11, O13-O16

P00.1   **Newborn (suspected to be) affected by maternal renal and urinary tract diseases**   N
Newborn (suspected to be) affected by maternal conditions classifiable to N00-N39

P00.2   **Newborn (suspected to be) affected by maternal infectious and parasitic diseases**   N
Newborn (suspected to be) affected by maternal infectious disease classifiable to A00-B99, J09 and J10
EXCLUDES 1   infections specific to the perinatal period (P35-P39)
maternal genital tract or other localized infections (P00.8)

P00.3   **Newborn (suspected to be) affected by other maternal circulatory and respiratory diseases**   N
Newborn (suspected to be) affected by maternal conditions classifiable to I00-I99, J00-J99, Q20-Q34 and not included in P00.0, P00.2

P00.4   **Newborn (suspected to be) affected by maternal nutritional disorders**   N
Newborn (suspected to be) affected by maternal disorders classifiable to E40-E64
Maternal malnutrition NOS

P00.5   **Newborn (suspected to be) affected by maternal injury**   N
Newborn (suspected to be) affected by maternal conditions classifiable to O9A.2-

P00.6   **Newborn (suspected to be) affected by surgical procedure on mother**   N
Newborn (suspected to be) affected by amniocentesis
EXCLUDES 1   Cesarean delivery for present delivery (P03.4)
damage to placenta from amniocentesis, Cesarean delivery or surgical induction (P02.1)
previous surgery to uterus or pelvic organs (P03.89)
EXCLUDES 2   newborn affected by complication of (fetal) intrauterine procedure (P96.5)

P00.7   **Newborn (suspected to be) affected by other medical procedures on mother, not elsewhere classified**   N
Newborn (suspected to be) affected by radiation to mother
EXCLUDES 1   damage to placenta from amniocentesis, cesarean delivery or surgical induction (P02.1)
newborn affected by other complications of labor and delivery (P03.-)

✓5ᵗʰ P00.8   **Newborn (suspected to be) affected by other maternal conditions**

P00.81   **Newborn (suspected to be) affected by periodontal disease in mother**   N

P00.89   **Newborn (suspected to be) affected by other maternal conditions**   N
Newborn (suspected to be) affected by conditions classifiable to T80-T88
Newborn (suspected to be) affected by maternal genital tract or other localized infections
Newborn (suspected to be) affected by maternal systemic lupus erythematosus

P00.9   **Newborn (suspected to be) affected by unspecified maternal condition**   N▽

✓4ᵗʰ P01   **Newborn (suspected to be) affected by maternal complications of pregnancy**
Code first any current condition in newborn

P01.0   **Newborn (suspected to be) affected by incompetent cervix**   N

P01.1   **Newborn (suspected to be) affected by premature rupture of membranes**   N

P01.2   **Newborn (suspected to be) affected by oligohydramnios**   N
EXCLUDES 1   oligohydramnios due to premature rupture of membranes (P01.1)

P01.3   **Newborn (suspected to be) affected by polyhydramnios**   N
Newborn (suspected to be) affected by hydramnios

P01.4   **Newborn (suspected to be) affected by ectopic pregnancy**   N
Newborn (suspected to be) affected by abdominal pregnancy

P01.5   **Newborn (suspected to be) affected by multiple pregnancy**   N
Newborn (suspected to be) affected by triplet (pregnancy)
Newborn (suspected to be) affected by twin (pregnancy)

P01.6   **Newborn (suspected to be) affected by maternal death**   N

P01.7   **Newborn (suspected to be) affected by malpresentation before labor**   N
Newborn (suspected to be) affected by breech presentation before labor
Newborn (suspected to be) affected by external version before labor
Newborn (suspected to be) affected by face presentation before labor
Newborn (suspected to be) affected by transverse lie before labor
Newborn (suspected to be) affected by unstable lie before labor

P01.8   **Newborn (suspected to be) affected by other maternal complications of pregnancy**   N

P01.9   **Newborn (suspected to be) affected by maternal complication of pregnancy, unspecified**   N▽

✓4ᵗʰ P02   **Newborn (suspected to be) affected by complications of placenta, cord and membranes**
Code first any current condition in newborn

P02.0   **Newborn (suspected to be) affected by placenta previa**   N

P02.1   **Newborn (suspected to be) affected by other forms of placental separation and hemorrhage**   N
Newborn (suspected to be) affected by abruptio placenta
Newborn (suspected to be) affected by accidental hemorrhage
Newborn (suspected to be) affected by antepartum hemorrhage
Newborn (suspected to be) affected by damage to placenta from amniocentesis, cesarean delivery or surgical induction
Newborn (suspected to be) affected by maternal blood loss
Newborn (suspected to be) affected by premature separation of placenta

N Newborn   P Pediatric   M Maternity   A Adult   **RIC** RIC Dx   **NCDx** Noncancer Dx   **PDx** Primary Dx   **CC** RIC CC Condition   ▶◀ Revised Text   ● New Code   ▲ Revised Code Title

808   ICD-10-CM 2016

✓5ᵗʰ **P02.2** **Newborn (suspected to be) affected by other and unspecified morphological and functional abnormalities of placenta**

    P02.20 Newborn (suspected to be) affected by unspecified morphological and functional abnormalities of placenta   N▽

    P02.29 **Newborn (suspected to be) affected by other morphological and functional abnormalities of placenta**   N
        Newborn (suspected to be) affected by placental dysfunction
        Newborn (suspected to be) affected by placental infarction
        Newborn (suspected to be) affected by placental insufficiency

P02.3 **Newborn (suspected to be) affected by placental transfusion syndromes**   N
    Newborn (suspected to be) affected by placental and cord abnormalities resulting in twin-to-twin or other transplacental transfusion

P02.4 **Newborn (suspected to be) affected by prolapsed cord**   N

P02.5 **Newborn (suspected to be) affected by other compression of umbilical cord**   N
    Newborn (suspected to be) affected by umbilical cord (tightly) around neck
    Newborn (suspected to be) affected by entanglement of umbilical cord
    Newborn (suspected to be) affected by knot in umbilical cord

✓5ᵗʰ **P02.6** **Newborn (suspected to be) affected by other and unspecified conditions of umbilical cord**

    P02.60 **Newborn (suspected to be) affected by unspecified conditions of umbilical cord**   N▽

    P02.69 **Newborn (suspected to be) affected by other conditions of umbilical cord**   N
        Newborn (suspected to be) affected by short umbilical cord
        Newborn (suspected to be) affected by vasa previa
        EXCLUDES 1 *newborn affected by single umbilical artery (Q27.0)*

P02.7 **Newborn (suspected to be) affected by chorioamnionitis**   N
    Newborn (suspected to be) affected by amnionitis
    Newborn (suspected to be) affected by membranitis
    Newborn (suspected to be) affected by placentitis

P02.8 **Newborn (suspected to be) affected by other abnormalities of membranes**   N

P02.9 **Newborn (suspected to be) affected by abnormality of membranes, unspecified**   N▽

✓4ᵗʰ **P03** **Newborn (suspected to be) affected by other complications of labor and delivery**
    Code first any current condition in newborn

P03.0 **Newborn (suspected to be) affected by breech delivery and extraction**   N

P03.1 **Newborn (suspected to be) affected by other malpresentation, malposition and disproportion during labor and delivery**   N
    Newborn (suspected to be) affected by contracted pelvis
    Newborn (suspected to be) affected by conditions classifiable to O64-O66
    Newborn (suspected to be) affected by persistent occipitoposterior
    Newborn (suspected to be) affected by transverse lie

P03.2 **Newborn (suspected to be) affected by forceps delivery**   N

P03.3 **Newborn (suspected to be) affected by delivery by vacuum extractor [ventouse]**   N

P03.4 **Newborn (suspected to be) affected by Cesarean delivery**   N

P03.5 **Newborn (suspected to be) affected by precipitate delivery**   N
    Newborn (suspected to be) affected by rapid second stage

P03.6 **Newborn (suspected to be) affected by abnormal uterine contractions**   N
    Newborn (suspected to be) affected by conditions classifiable to O62-, except O62.3
    Newborn (suspected to be) affected by hypertonic labor
    Newborn (suspected to be) affected by uterine inertia

✓5ᵗʰ **P03.8** **Newborn (suspected to be) affected by other specified complications of labor and delivery**

    ✓6ᵗʰ **P03.81** **Newborn (suspected to be) affected by abnormality in fetal (intrauterine) heart rate or rhythm**
        EXCLUDES 1 *neonatal cardiac dysrhythmia (P29.1-)*

        P03.810 **Newborn (suspected to be) affected by abnormality in fetal (intrauterine) heart rate or rhythm before the onset of labor**   N

        P03.811 **Newborn (suspected to be) affected by abnormality in fetal (intrauterine) heart rate or rhythm during labor**   N

        P03.819 **Newborn (suspected to be) affected by abnormality in fetal (intrauterine) heart rate or rhythm, unspecified as to time of onset**   N▽

    P03.82 **Meconium passage during delivery**   N
        EXCLUDES 1 *meconium aspiration (P24.00, P24.01)*
        meconium staining (P96.83)

    P03.89 **Newborn (suspected to be) affected by other specified complications of labor and delivery**   N
        Newborn (suspected to be) affected by abnormality of maternal soft tissues
        Newborn (suspected to be) affected by conditions classifiable to O60-O75 and by procedures used in labor and delivery not included in P02- and P03.0-P03.6
        Newborn (suspected to be) affected by induction of labor

P03.9 **Newborn (suspected to be) affected by complication of labor and delivery, unspecified**   N▽

✓4ᵗʰ **P04** **Newborn (suspected to be) affected by noxious substances transmitted via placenta or breast milk**
    INCLUDES nonteratogenic effects of substances transmitted via placenta
    EXCLUDES 2 *congenital malformations (Q00-Q99)*
    neonatal jaundice from excessive hemolysis due to drugs or toxins transmitted from mother (P58.4)
    newborn in contact with and (suspected) exposures hazardous to health not transmitted via placenta or breast milk (Z77.-)

P04.0 **Newborn (suspected to be) affected by maternal anesthesia and analgesia in pregnancy, labor and delivery**   N
    Newborn (suspected to be) affected by reactions and intoxications from maternal opiates and tranquilizers administered during labor and delivery

P04.1 **Newborn (suspected to be) affected by other maternal medication**   N
    Newborn (suspected to be) affected by cancer chemotherapy
    Newborn (suspected to be) affected by cytotoxic drugs
    EXCLUDES 1 *dysmorphism due to warfarin (Q86.2)*
    fetal hydantoin syndrome (Q86.1)
    maternal use of drugs of addiction (P04.4-)

P04.2 **Newborn (suspected to be) affected by maternal use of tobacco**   N
    Newborn (suspected to be) affected by exposure in utero to tobacco smoke
    EXCLUDES 2 *newborn exposure to environmental tobacco smoke (P96.81)*

P04.3 **Newborn (suspected to be) affected by maternal use of alcohol**   N
    EXCLUDES 1 *fetal alcohol syndrome (Q86.0)*

✓5ᵗʰ **P04.4** **Newborn (suspected to be) affected by maternal use of drugs of addiction**

    P04.41 **Newborn (suspected to be) affected by maternal use of cocaine**   N
        "Crack baby"

    P04.49 **Newborn (suspected to be) affected by maternal use of other drugs of addiction**   N
        EXCLUDES 2 *newborn (suspected to be) affected by maternal anesthesia and analgesia (P04.0)*
        withdrawal symptoms from maternal use of drugs of addiction (P96.1)

P04.5 **Newborn (suspected to be) affected by maternal use of nutritional chemical substances**   N

P04.6 **Newborn (suspected to be) affected by maternal exposure to environmental chemical substances**   N

P04.8 **Newborn (suspected to be) affected by other maternal noxious substances**   N

P04.9 **Newborn (suspected to be) affected by maternal oxious substance, unspecified**   N▽

Chapter 16. Certain Conditions Originating in the Perinatal Period

Disorders of newborn related to length of gestation and fetal growth (P05-P08)

✓4ᵗʰ **P05 Disorders of newborn related to slow fetal growth and fetal malnutrition**

✓5ᵗʰ **P05.0 Newborn light for gestational age**
Newborn light-for-dates

     P05.00 Newborn light for gestational age, unspecified weight Ⓝ ▽

     P05.01 Newborn light for gestational age, less than 500 grams Ⓝ

     P05.02 Newborn light for gestational age, 500-749 grams Ⓝ

     P05.03 Newborn light for gestational age, 750-999 grams Ⓝ

     P05.04 Newborn light for gestational age, 1000-1249 grams Ⓝ

     P05.05 Newborn light for gestational age, 1250-1499 grams Ⓝ

     P05.06 Newborn light for gestational age, 1500-1749 grams Ⓝ

     P05.07 Newborn light for gestational age, 1750-1999 grams Ⓝ

     P05.08 Newborn light for gestational age, 2000-2499 grams Ⓝ

✓5ᵗʰ **P05.1 Newborn small for gestational age**
Newborn small-and-light-for-dates
Newborn small-for-dates

     P05.10 Newborn small for gestational age, unspecified weight Ⓝ ▽

     P05.11 Newborn small for gestational age, less than 500 grams Ⓝ

     P05.12 Newborn small for gestational age, 500-749 grams Ⓝ

     P05.13 Newborn small for gestational age, 750-999 grams Ⓝ

     P05.14 Newborn small for gestational age, 1000-1249 grams Ⓝ

     P05.15 Newborn small for gestational age, 1250-1499 grams Ⓝ

     P05.16 Newborn small for gestational age, 1500-1749 grams Ⓝ

     P05.17 Newborn small for gestational age, 1750-1999 grams Ⓝ

     P05.18 Newborn small for gestational age, 2000-2499 grams Ⓝ

     P05.2 Newborn affected by fetal (intrauterine) malnutrition **not light or small for gestational age** Ⓝ
Infant, not light or small for gestational age, showing signs of fetal malnutrition, such as dry, peeling skin and loss of subcutaneous tissue

        EXCLUDES 1 *newborn affected by fetal malnutrition with light for gestational age (P05.0-)*
newborn affected by fetal malnutrition with small for gestational age (P05.1-)

     P05.9 Newborn affected by slow intrauterine growth, unspecified Ⓝ ▽
Newborn affected by fetal growth retardation NOS

✓4ᵗʰ **P07 Disorders of newborn related to short gestation and low birth weight, not elsewhere classified**

     NOTE   When both birth weight and gestational age of the newborn are available, both should be coded with birth weight sequenced before gestational age

     INCLUDES   The listed conditions, without further specification, as the cause of morbidity or additional care, in newborn

     EXCLUDES 1   *low birth weight due to slow fetal growth and fetal malnutrition (P05.-)*

✓5ᵗʰ **P07.0 Extremely low birth weight newborn**
Newborn birth weight 999 g. or less

     P07.00 Extremely low birth weight newborn, unspecified weight Ⓝ ▽

     P07.01 Extremely low birth weight newborn, less than 500 grams CC Ⓝ

     P07.02 Extremely low birth weight newborn, 500-749 grams CC Ⓝ

     P07.03 Extremely low birth weight newborn, 750-999 grams CC Ⓝ

✓5ᵗʰ **P07.1 Other low birth weight newborn**
Newborn birth weight 1000-2499 g.

     P07.10 Other low birth weight newborn, unspecified weight Ⓝ ▽

     P07.14 Other low birth weight newborn, 1000-1249 grams Ⓝ

     P07.15 Other low birth weight newborn, 1250-1499 grams Ⓝ

     P07.16 Other low birth weight newborn, 1500-1749 grams Ⓝ

     P07.17 Other low birth weight newborn, 1750-1999 grams Ⓝ

     P07.18 Other low birth weight newborn, 2000-2499 grams Ⓝ

✓5ᵗʰ **P07.2 Extreme immaturity of newborn**
Less than 28 completed weeks (less than 196 completed days) of gestation.

     P07.20 Extreme immaturity of newborn, unspecified weeks of gestation Ⓝ ▽
Gestational age less than 28 completed weeks NOS

     P07.21 Extreme immaturity of newborn, gestational age less than 23 completed weeks Ⓝ
Extreme immaturity of newborn, gestational age less than 23 weeks, 0 days

     P07.22 Extreme immaturity of newborn, gestational age 23 completed weeks Ⓝ
Extreme immaturity of newborn, gestational age 23 weeks, 0 days through 23 weeks, 6 days

     P07.23 Extreme immaturity of newborn, gestational age 24 completed weeks Ⓝ
Extreme immaturity of newborn, gestational age 24 weeks, 0 days through 24 weeks, 6 days

     P07.24 Extreme immaturity of newborn, gestational age 25 completed weeks Ⓝ
Extreme immaturity of newborn, gestational age 25 weeks, 0 days through 25 weeks, 6 days

     P07.25 Extreme immaturity of newborn, gestational age 26 completed weeks Ⓝ
Extreme immaturity of newborn, gestational age 26 weeks, 0 days through 26 weeks, 6 days

     P07.26 Extreme immaturity of newborn, gestational age 27 completed weeks Ⓝ
Extreme immaturity of newborn, gestational age 27 weeks, 0 days through 27 weeks, 6 days

✓5ᵗʰ **P07.3 Preterm [premature] newborn [other]**
28 completed weeks or more but less than 37 completed weeks (196 completed days but less than 259 completed days) of gestation
Prematurity NOS

     P07.30 Preterm newborn, unspecified weeks of gestation Ⓝ ▽

     P07.31 Preterm newborn, gestational age 28 completed weeks Ⓝ
Preterm newborn, gestational age 28 weeks, 0 days through 28 weeks, 6 days

     P07.32 Preterm newborn, gestational age 29 completed weeks Ⓝ
Preterm newborn, gestational age 29 weeks, 0 days through 29 weeks, 6 days

     P07.33 Preterm newborn, gestational age 30 completed weeks Ⓝ
Preterm newborn, gestational age 30 weeks, 0 days through 30 weeks, 6 days

     P07.34 Preterm newborn, gestational age 31 completed weeks Ⓝ
Preterm newborn, gestational age 31 weeks, 0 days through 31 weeks, 6 days

     P07.35 Preterm newborn, gestational age 32 completed weeks Ⓝ
Preterm newborn, gestational age 32 weeks, 0 days through 32 weeks, 6 days

     P07.36 Preterm newborn, gestational age 33 completed weeks Ⓝ
Preterm newborn, gestational age 33 weeks, 0 days through 33 weeks, 6 days

     P07.37 Preterm newborn, gestational age 34 completed weeks Ⓝ
Preterm newborn, gestational age 34 weeks, 0 days through 34 weeks, 6 days

Ⓝ Newborn   Ⓟ Pediatric   Ⓜ Maternity   Ⓐ Adult   RIC RIC Dx   NCDx Noncancer Dx   PDx Primary Dx   CC RIC CC Condition   ▶◀ Revised Text   ● New Code   ▲ Revised Code Title

ICD-10-CM 2016

810

P07.38   **Preterm newborn, gestational age** 35 completed   N
weeks
Preterm newborn, gestational age 35 weeks, 0 days
through 35 weeks, 6 days

P07.39   **Preterm newborn, gestational age** 36 completed   N
weeks
Preterm newborn, gestational age 36 weeks, 0 days
through 36 weeks, 6 days

✓4ᵗʰ **P08**   **Disorders of newborn related to long gestation and high birth weight**
> NOTE   When both birth weight and gestational age of the newborn are available, priority of assignment should be given to birth weight
> INCLUDES   the listed conditions, without further specification, as causes of morbidity or additional care, in newborn

P08.0   **Exceptionally large newborn baby**   N
Usually implies a birth weight of 4500 g. or more
> EXCLUDES 1   syndrome of infant of diabetic mother (P70.1)
> syndrome of infant of mother with gestational diabetes (P70.0)

P08.1   **Other heavy for gestational age newborn**   N
Other newborn heavy- or large-for-dates regardless of period of gestation
Usually implies a birth weight of 4000 g. to 4499 g.
> EXCLUDES 1   newborn with a birth weight of 4500 or more (P08.0)
> syndrome of infant of diabetic mother (P70.1)
> syndrome of infant of mother with gestational diabetes (P70.0).

✓5ᵗʰ **P08.2**   **Late newborn, not heavy for gestational age**
AHA: 2014, 1Q, 14

P08.21   **Post-term newborn**   N
Newborn with gestation period over 40 completed weeks to 42 completed weeks

P08.22   **Prolonged gestation of newborn**   N
Newborn with gestation period over 42 completed weeks (294 days or more), not heavy- or large-for-dates.
Postmaturity NOS

Abnormal findings on neonatal screening (P09)

P09   **Abnormal findings on neonatal screening**   N
Use additional code to identify signs, symptoms and conditions associated with the screening
> EXCLUDES 2   nonspecific serologic evidence of human immunodeficiency virus [HIV] (R75)

Birth trauma (P10-P15)

✓4ᵗʰ **P10**   **Intracranial laceration and hemorrhage due to birth injury**
> EXCLUDES 1   intracranial hemorrhage of newborn NOS (P52.9)
> intracranial hemorrhage of newborn due to anoxia or hypoxia (P52.-)
> nontraumatic intracranial hemorrhage of newborn (P52.-)

P10.0   **Subdural hemorrhage due to birth injury**   N
Subdural hematoma (localized) due to birth injury
> EXCLUDES 1   subdural hemorrhage accompanying tentorial tear (P10.4)

P10.1   Cerebral **hemorrhage due to birth injury**   N

P10.2   Intraventricular **hemorrhage due to birth injury**   N

P10.3   Subarachnoid **hemorrhage due to birth injury**   N

P10.4   Tentorial **tear due to birth injury**   N

P10.8   **Other intracranial lacerations and hemorrhages due to birth injury**   N

P10.9   **Unspecified intracranial laceration and hemorrhage due to birth injury**   N ▽

✓4ᵗʰ **P11**   **Other birth injuries to** central nervous system

P11.0   Cerebral **edema due to birth injury**   N

P11.1   **Other specified brain damage due to birth injury**   N

P11.2   **Unspecified brain damage due to birth injury**   N ▽

P11.3   **Birth injury to** facial nerve   N
Facial palsy due to birth injury

P11.4   **Birth injury to other** cranial nerves   N

P11.5   **Birth injury to** spine and spinal cord   N
Fracture of spine due to birth injury

P11.9   **Birth injury to central nervous system, unspecified**   N ▽

✓4ᵗʰ **P12**   **Birth injury to** scalp

P12.0   **Cephalhematoma due to birth injury**   N

P12.1   **Chignon (from vacuum extraction) due to birth injury**   N

P12.2   **Epicranial subaponeurotic hemorrhage due to birth injury**   N
Subgaleal hemorrhage

P12.3   **Bruising of scalp due to birth injury**   N

P12.4   **Injury of scalp of newborn due to** monitoring equipment   N
Sampling incision of scalp of newborn
Scalp clip (electrode) injury of newborn

✓5ᵗʰ **P12.8**   **Other** birth injuries to scalp

P12.81   **Caput succedaneum**   N

P12.89   **Other birth injuries to scalp**   N

P12.9   **Birth injury to scalp, unspecified**   N ▽

✓4ᵗʰ **P13**   **Birth injury to** skeleton
> EXCLUDES 2   birth injury to spine (P11.5)

P13.0   **Fracture of skull due to birth injury**   N

P13.1   **Other birth injuries to** skull   N
> EXCLUDES 1   cephalhematoma (P12.0)

P13.2   **Birth injury to** femur   N

P13.3   **Birth injury to other** long bones   N

P13.4   **Fracture of clavicle due to birth injury**   N

P13.8   **Birth injuries to other** parts of skeleton   N

P13.9   **Birth injury to skeleton, unspecified**   N ▽

✓4ᵗʰ **P14**   **Birth injury to** peripheral nervous system

P14.0   **Erb's paralysis due to birth injury**   N

P14.1   **Klumpke's paralysis due to birth injury**   N

P14.2   **Phrenic nerve paralysis due to birth injury**   N

P14.3   **Other** brachial plexus **birth injuries**   N

P14.8   **Birth injuries to other parts of** peripheral nervous system   N

P14.9   **Birth injury to peripheral nervous system, unspecified**   N ▽

✓4ᵗʰ **P15**   Other **birth injuries**

P15.0   **Birth injury to** liver   N
Rupture of liver due to birth injury

P15.1   **Birth injury to** spleen   N
Rupture of spleen due to birth injury

P15.2   **Sternomastoid injury due to birth injury**   N

P15.3   **Birth injury to** eye   N
Subconjunctival hemorrhage due to birth injury
Traumatic glaucoma due to birth injury

P15.4   **Birth injury to** face   N
Facial congestion due to birth injury

P15.5   **Birth injury to** external genitalia   N

P15.6   **Subcutaneous fat necrosis due to birth injury**   N

P15.8   **Other specified birth injuries**   N

P15.9   **Birth injury, unspecified**   N ▽

Respiratory and cardiovascular disorders specific to the perinatal period (P19-P29)

✓4ᵗʰ **P19**   **Metabolic acidemia in newborn**
Metabolic acidemia in newborn

P19.0   **Metabolic acidemia in newborn first noted** before onset of labor   N

P19.1   **Metabolic acidemia in newborn first noted** during labor   N

P19.2   **Metabolic acidemia noted** at birth   N

P19.9   **Metabolic acidemia, unspecified**   N ▽

✓4ᵗʰ **P22**   **Respiratory distress of newborn**
> EXCLUDES 1   respiratory arrest of newborn (P28.81)
> respiratory failure of newborn NOS (P28.5)

P22.0   **Respiratory distress syndrome of newborn**   N
Cardiorespiratory distress syndrome of newborn
Hyaline membrane disease
Idiopathic respiratory distress syndrome [IRDS or RDS] of newborn
Pulmonary hypoperfusion syndrome
Respiratory distress syndrome, type I

P22.1   **Transient tachypnea of newborn**   N
Idiopathic tachypnea of newborn
Respiratory distress syndrome, type II
Wet lung syndrome

P22.8   **Other respiratory distress of newborn**   N

P22.9   **Respiratory distress of newborn, unspecified**   N ▽

✓ Add'l Character Required   ✓x7ᵗʰ Placeholder Alert   RUG IV Special Care High Dx   RUG IV Clinically Complex Dx   RUG IV Special Care Low Dx   Manifestation Code   Other Specified Code   ▽ Unspecified Code

ICD-10-CM 2016   811

✓4ᵗʰ **P23 Congenital pneumonia**
  INCLUDES infective pneumonia acquired in utero or during birth
  EXCLUDES 1 neonatal pneumonia resulting from aspiration (P24.-)

  P23.Ø Congenital pneumonia due to viral agent N
    Use additional code (B97) to identify organism
    EXCLUDES 1 congenital rubella pneumonitis (P35.Ø)

  P23.1 Congenital pneumonia due to Chlamydia N

  P23.2 Congenital pneumonia due to staphylococcus N

  P23.3 Congenital pneumonia due to streptococcus, group B N

  P23.4 Congenital pneumonia due to Escherichia coli N

  P23.5 Congenital pneumonia due to Pseudomonas N

  P23.6 Congenital pneumonia due to other bacterial agents N
    Congenital pneumonia due to Hemophilus influenzae
    Congenital pneumonia due to Klebsiella pneumoniae
    Congenital pneumonia due to Mycoplasma
    Congenital pneumonia due to Streptococcus, except group B
    Use additional code (B95-B96) to identify organism

  P23.8 Congenital pneumonia due to other organisms N

  P23.9 Congenital pneumonia, unspecified N ▽

✓4ᵗʰ **P24 Neonatal aspiration**
  INCLUDES aspiration in utero and during delivery

  ✓5ᵗʰ **P24.Ø Meconium aspiration**
    EXCLUDES 1 meconium passage (without aspiration) during delivery
      (PØ3.82)
      meconium staining (P96.83)

    P24.ØØ Meconium aspiration without respiratory N
      symptoms
      Meconium aspiration NOS

    P24.Ø1 Meconium aspiration with respiratory symptoms N
      Meconium aspiration pneumonia
      Meconium aspiration pneumonitis
      Meconium aspiration syndrome NOS
      Use additional code to identify any secondary
        pulmonary hypertension, if applicable (I27.2)

  ✓5ᵗʰ **P24.1 Neonatal aspiration of (clear) amniotic fluid and mucus**
    Neonatal aspiration of liquor (amnii)

    P24.1Ø Neonatal aspiration of (clear) amniotic fluid and N
      mucus without respiratory symptoms
      Neonatal aspiration of amniotic fluid and mucus NOS

    P24.11 Neonatal aspiration of (clear) amniotic fluid and N
      mucus with respiratory symptoms
      Neonatal aspiration of amniotic fluid and mucus with
        pneumonia
      Neonatal aspiration of amniotic fluid and mucus with
        pneumonitis
      Use additional code to identify any secondary
        pulmonary hypertension, if applicable (I27.2)

  ✓5ᵗʰ **P24.2 Neonatal aspiration of blood**

    P24.2Ø Neonatal aspiration of blood without respiratory N
      symptoms
      Neonatal aspiration of blood NOS

    P24.21 Neonatal aspiration of blood with respiratory N
      symptoms
      Neonatal aspiration of blood with pneumonia
      Neonatal aspiration of blood with pneumonitis
      Use additional code to identify any secondary
        pulmonary hypertension, if applicable (I27.2)

  ✓5ᵗʰ **P24.3 Neonatal aspiration of milk and regurgitated food**
    Neonatal aspiration of stomach contents

    P24.3Ø Neonatal aspiration of milk and regurgitated N
      food without respiratory symptoms
      Neonatal aspiration of milk and regurgitated food NOS

    P24.31 Neonatal aspiration of milk and regurgitated N
      food with respiratory symptoms
      Neonatal aspiration of milk and regurgitated food with
        pneumonia
      Neonatal aspiration of milk and regurgitated food with
        pneumonitis
      Use additional code to identify any secondary
        pulmonary hypertension, if applicable (I27.2)

  ✓5ᵗʰ **P24.8 Other neonatal aspiration**

    P24.8Ø Other neonatal aspiration without respiratory N
      symptoms
      Neonatal aspiration NEC

    P24.81 Other neonatal aspiration with respiratory N
      symptoms
      Neonatal aspiration pneumonia NEC
      Neonatal aspiration with pneumonitis NEC
      Neonatal aspiration with pneumonia NOS
      Neonatal aspiration with pneumonitis NOS
      Use additional code to identify any secondary
        pulmonary hypertension, if applicable (I27.2)

    P24.9 Neonatal aspiration, unspecified N ▽

✓4ᵗʰ **P25 Interstitial emphysema and related conditions originating in the perinatal period**

  P25.Ø Interstitial emphysema originating in the perinatal period N

  P25.1 Pneumothorax originating in the perinatal period N

  P25.2 Pneumomediastinum originating in the perinatal period N

  P25.3 Pneumopericardium originating in the perinatal period N

  P25.8 Other conditions related to interstitial emphysema originating in the perinatal period N

✓4ᵗʰ **P26 Pulmonary hemorrhage originating in the perinatal period**
  EXCLUDES 1 acute idiopathic hemorrhage in infants over 28 days old
    (RØ4.81)

  P26.Ø Tracheobronchial hemorrhage originating in the N
    perinatal period

  P26.1 Massive pulmonary hemorrhage originating in the N
    perinatal period

  P26.8 Other pulmonary hemorrhages originating in the N
    perinatal period

  P26.9 Unspecified pulmonary hemorrhage originating N ▽
    in the perinatal period

✓4ᵗʰ **P27 Chronic respiratory disease originating in the perinatal period**
  EXCLUDES 1 respiratory distress of newborn (P22.Ø-P22.9)

  P27.Ø Wilson-Mikity syndrome
    Pulmonary dysmaturity

  P27.1 Bronchopulmonary dysplasia originating in the perinatal period

  P27.8 Other chronic respiratory diseases originating in the perinatal period
    Congenital pulmonary fibrosis
    Ventilator lung in newborn

  P27.9 Unspecified chronic respiratory disease originating in the ▽
    perinatal period

✓4ᵗʰ **P28 Other respiratory conditions originating in the perinatal period**
  EXCLUDES 1 congenital malformations of the respiratory system (Q3Ø-Q34)

  P28.Ø Primary atelectasis of newborn N
    Primary failure to expand terminal respiratory units
    Pulmonary hypoplasia associated with short gestation
    Pulmonary immaturity NOS

  ✓5ᵗʰ **P28.1 Other and unspecified atelectasis of newborn**

    P28.1Ø Unspecified atelectasis of newborn N ▽
      Atelectasis of newborn NOS

    P28.11 Resorption atelectasis without respiratory N
      distress syndrome
      EXCLUDES 1 resorption atelectasis with respiratory
        distress syndrome (P22.Ø)

    P28.19 Other atelectasis of newborn N
      Partial atelectasis of newborn
      Secondary atelectasis of newborn

  P28.2 Cyanotic attacks of newborn N
    EXCLUDES 1 apnea of newborn (P28.3-P28.4)

  P28.3 Primary sleep apnea of newborn N
    Central sleep apnea of newborn
    Obstructive sleep apnea of newborn
    Sleep apnea of newborn NOS

  P28.4 Other apnea of newborn N
    Apnea of prematurity
    Obstructive apnea of newborn
    EXCLUDES 1 obstructive sleep apnea of newborn (P28.3)

  P28.5 Respiratory failure of newborn N
    EXCLUDES 1 respiratory arrest of newborn (P28.81)
      respiratory distress of newborn (P22.Ø-)

  ✓5ᵗʰ **P28.8 Other specified respiratory conditions of newborn**

    P28.81 Respiratory arrest of newborn N

    P28.89 Other specified respiratory conditions of N
      newborn
      Congenital laryngeal stridor
      Sniffles in newborn
      Snuffles in newborn
      EXCLUDES 1 early congenital syphilitic rhinitis (A5Ø.Ø5)

N Newborn   P Pediatric   M Maternity   A Adult   RIC RIC Dx   NC Dx Noncancer Dx   PDx Primary Dx   CC RIC CC Condition   ►◄ Revised Text   ● New Code   ▲ Revised Code Title

812   ICD-10-CM 2016

P28.9   **Respiratory condition of newborn, unspecified**   N ▽
Respiratory depression in newborn

☑4ᵗʰ **P29**   **Cardiovascular disorders originating in the perinatal period**
    EXCLUDES 1   *congenital malformations of the circulatory system (Q20–Q28)*

P29.0   **Neonatal cardiac failure**   N

☑5ᵗʰ **P29.1**   **Neonatal cardiac dysrhythmia**
    P29.11   **Neonatal** tachycardia   N
    P29.12   **Neonatal** bradycardia   N

P29.2   **Neonatal hypertension**   N

P29.3   **Persistent fetal circulation**   N
Delayed closure of ductus arteriosus
(Persistent) pulmonary hypertension of newborn

P29.4   **Transient myocardial ischemia in newborn**   N

☑5ᵗʰ **P29.8**   **Other cardiovascular disorders originating in the perinatal period**
    P29.81   **Cardiac arrest of newborn**   N
    P29.89   **Other cardiovascular disorders originating in the perinatal period**   N
      AHA: 2014, 4Q, 23

P29.9   **Cardiovascular disorder originating in the perinatal period, unspecified**   N ▽

Infections specific to the perinatal period (P35-P39)

Infections acquired in utero, during birth via the umbilicus, or during the first 28 days after birth

    EXCLUDES 2   *asymptomatic human immunodeficiency virus [HIV] infection status (Z21)*
      congenital gonococcal infection (A54.-)
      congenital pneumonia (P23.-)
      congenital syphilis (A50.-)
      human immunodeficiency virus [HIV] disease (B20)
      infant botulism (A48.51)
      infectious diseases not specific to the perinatal period (A00-B99, J09, J10-)
      intestinal infectious disease (A00-A09)
      laboratory evidence of human immunodeficiency virus [HIV] (R75)
      tetanus neonatorum (A33)

☑4ᵗʰ **P35**   **Congenital viral diseases**
    INCLUDES   infections acquired in utero or during birth

P35.0   **Congenital** rubella **syndrome**   N
Congenital rubella pneumonitis

P35.1   **Congenital** cytomegalovirus **infection**   N

P35.2   **Congenital** herpesviral **[herpes simplex] infection**   N

P35.3   **Congenital** viral hepatitis   N

P35.8   **Other congenital viral diseases**   N
Congenital varicella [chickenpox]

P35.9   **Congenital viral disease, unspecified**   N ▽

☑4ᵗʰ **P36**   **Bacterial sepsis of newborn**
    INCLUDES   congenital sepsis
    Use additional code(s), if applicable, to identify severe sepsis (R65.2-) and associated acute organ dysfunction(s)

P36.0   **Sepsis of newborn due to** streptococcus, group B   N

☑5ᵗʰ **P36.1**   **Sepsis of newborn due to other and unspecified streptococci**
    P36.10   **Sepsis of newborn due to unspecified streptococci**   N ▽
    P36.19   **Sepsis of newborn due to other streptococci**   N

P36.2   **Sepsis of newborn due to** Staphylococcus aureus   N

☑5ᵗʰ **P36.3**   **Sepsis of newborn due to other and unspecified staphylococci**
    P36.30   **Sepsis of newborn due to unspecified staphylococci**   N ▽
    P36.39   **Sepsis of newborn due to other staphylococci**   N

P36.4   **Sepsis of newborn due to** Escherichia coli   N

P36.5   **Sepsis of newborn due to** anaerobes   N

P36.8   **Other** bacterial sepsis **of newborn**   N
Use additional code from category B96 to identify organism

P36.9   **Bacterial sepsis of newborn, unspecified**   N ▽

☑4ᵗʰ **P37**   **Other congenital infectious and parasitic diseases**
    EXCLUDES 2   *congenital syphilis (A50.-)*
      infectious neonatal diarrhea (A00-A09)
      necrotizing enterocolitis in newborn (P77.-)
      noninfectious neonatal diarrhea (P78.3)
      ophthalmia neonatorum due to gonococcus (A54.31)
      tetanus neonatorum (A33)

P37.0   **Congenital tuberculosis**   N

P37.1   **Congenital** toxoplasmosis   N
Hydrocephalus due to congenital toxoplasmosis

P37.2   **Neonatal (disseminated)** listeriosis   N

P37.3   **Congenital** falciparum malaria   N

P37.4   **Other congenital** malaria   N

P37.5   **Neonatal** candidiasis   N

P37.8   **Other specified congenital infectious and parasitic diseases**   N

P37.9   **Congenital infectious or parasitic disease, unspecified**   N ▽

☑4ᵗʰ **P38**   **Omphalitis of newborn**
    EXCLUDES 1   *omphalitis not of newborn (L08.82)*
      tetanus omphalitis (A33)
      umbilical hemorrhage of newborn (P51.-)

P38.1   **Omphalitis** with mild hemorrhage   N

P38.9   **Omphalitis** without hemorrhage   N
Omphalitis of newborn NOS

☑4ᵗʰ **P39**   **Other infections specific to the perinatal period**
    Use additional code to identify organism or specific infection

P39.0   **Neonatal infective** mastitis   N
    EXCLUDES 1   *breast engorgement of newborn (P83.4)*
      noninfective mastitis of newborn (P83.4)

P39.1   **Neonatal** conjunctivitis and dacryocystitis   N
Neonatal chlamydial conjunctivitis
Ophthalmia neonatorum NOS
    EXCLUDES 1   *gonococcal conjunctivitis (A54.31)*

P39.2   **Intra-amniotic** infection affecting newborn, not elsewhere classified   N

P39.3   **Neonatal** urinary tract **infection**   N

P39.4   **Neonatal** skin **infection**   N
Neonatal pyoderma
    EXCLUDES 1   *pemphigus neonatorum (L00)*
      staphylococcal scalded skin syndrome (L00)

P39.8   **Other specified infections specific to the perinatal period**   N

P39.9   **Infection specific to the perinatal period, unspecified**   N ▽

Hemorrhagic and hematological disorders of newborn (P50-P61)

    EXCLUDES 1   *congenital stenosis and stricture of bile ducts (Q44.3)*
      Crigler-Najjar syndrome (E80.5)
      Dubin-Johnson syndrome (E80.6)
      Gilbert syndrome (E80.4)
      hereditary hemolytic anemias (D55-D58)

☑4ᵗʰ **P50**   **Newborn affected by intrauterine (fetal)** blood loss
    EXCLUDES 1   *congenital anemia from intrauterine (fetal) blood loss (P61.3)*

P50.0   **Newborn affected by intrauterine (fetal) blood loss from vasa previa**   N

P50.1   **Newborn affected by intrauterine (fetal) blood loss from ruptured cord**   N

P50.2   **Newborn affected by intrauterine (fetal) blood loss from placenta**   N

P50.3   **Newborn affected by hemorrhage into** co-twin   N

P50.4   **Newborn affected by hemorrhage into** maternal circulation   N

P50.5   **Newborn affected by intrauterine (fetal) blood loss from cut end of co-twin's cord**   N

P50.8   **Newborn affected by other intrauterine (fetal) blood loss**   N

P50.9   **Newborn affected by intrauterine (fetal) blood loss, unspecified**   N ▽
Newborn affected by fetal hemorrhage NOS

☑4ᵗʰ **P51**   **Umbilical** hemorrhage of newborn
    EXCLUDES 1   *omphalitis with mild hemorrhage (P38.1)*
      umbilical hemorrhage from cut end of co-twins cord (P50.5)

P51.0   **Massive umbilical hemorrhage of newborn**   N

P51.8   **Other umbilical hemorrhages of newborn**   N
Slipped umbilical ligature NOS

P51.9   **Umbilical hemorrhage of newborn, unspecified**   N ▽

☑ Add'l Character Required   ☑x7ᵗʰ Placeholder Alert   RUG IV Special Care High Dx   RUG IV Clinically Complex Dx   RUG IV Special Care Low Dx   Manifestation Code   Other Specified Code   ▽ Unspecified Code

Chapter 16. Certain Conditions Originating in the Perinatal Period

P52–P61.9

✓4ᵗʰ **P52 Intracranial nontraumatic hemorrhage of newborn**
Intracranial hemorrhage due to anoxia or hypoxia
EXCLUDES 1 *intracranial hemorrhage due to birth injury (P10.-)*
intracranial hemorrhage due to other injury (S06.-)

P52.0 Intraventricular (nontraumatic) hemorrhage, grade 1, of newborn Ⓝ
Subependymal hemorrhage (without intraventricular extension)
Bleeding into germinal matrix

P52.1 Intraventricular (nontraumatic) hemorrhage, grade 2, of newborn Ⓝ
Subependymal hemorrhage with intraventricular extension
Bleeding into ventricle

✓5ᵗʰ **P52.2 Intraventricular (nontraumatic) hemorrhage, grade 3 and grade 4, of newborn**

P52.21 Intraventricular (nontraumatic) hemorrhage, grade 3, of newborn Ⓝ
Subependymal hemorrhage with intraventricular extension with enlargement of ventricle

P52.22 Intraventricular (nontraumatic) hemorrhage, grade 4, of newborn Ⓝ
Bleeding into cerebral cortex
Subependymal hemorrhage with intracerebral extension

P52.3 Unspecified intraventricular (nontraumatic) hemorrhage of newborn Ⓝ▽

P52.4 Intracerebral (nontraumatic) hemorrhage of newborn Ⓝ

P52.5 Subarachnoid (nontraumatic) hemorrhage of newborn Ⓝ

P52.6 Cerebellar (nontraumatic) and posterior fossa hemorrhage of newborn Ⓝ

P52.8 Other intracranial (nontraumatic) hemorrhages of newborn Ⓝ

P52.9 Intracranial (nontraumatic) hemorrhage of newborn, unspecified Ⓝ▽

P53 Hemorrhagic disease of newborn Ⓝ
Vitamin K deficiency of newborn

✓4ᵗʰ **P54 Other neonatal hemorrhages**
EXCLUDES 1 *newborn affected by (intrauterine) blood loss (P50.-)*
pulmonary hemorrhage originating in the perinatal period (P26.-)

P54.0 Neonatal hematemesis Ⓝ
EXCLUDES 1 *neonatal hematemesis due to swallowed maternal blood (P78.2)*

P54.1 Neonatal melena Ⓝ
EXCLUDES 1 *neonatal melena due to swallowed maternal blood (P78.2)*

P54.2 Neonatal rectal hemorrhage Ⓝ

P54.3 Other neonatal gastrointestinal hemorrhage Ⓝ

P54.4 Neonatal adrenal hemorrhage Ⓝ

P54.5 Neonatal cutaneous hemorrhage Ⓝ
Neonatal bruising
Neonatal ecchymoses
Neonatal petechiae
Neonatal superficial hematomata
EXCLUDES 2 *bruising of scalp due to birth injury (P12.3)*
cephalhematoma due to birth injury (P12.0)

P54.6 Neonatal vaginal hemorrhage Ⓝ♀
Neonatal pseudomenses

P54.8 Other specified neonatal hemorrhages Ⓝ

P54.9 Neonatal hemorrhage, unspecified Ⓝ▽

✓4ᵗʰ **P55 Hemolytic disease of newborn**

P55.0 Rh isoimmunization of newborn Ⓝ

P55.1 ABO isoimmunization of newborn Ⓝ

P55.8 Other hemolytic diseases of newborn Ⓝ

P55.9 Hemolytic disease of newborn, unspecified Ⓝ▽

✓4ᵗʰ **P56 Hydrops fetalis due to hemolytic disease**
EXCLUDES 1 *hydrops fetalis NOS (P83.2)*

P56.0 Hydrops fetalis due to isoimmunization Ⓝ

✓5ᵗʰ **P56.9 Hydrops fetalis due to other and unspecified hemolytic disease**

P56.90 Hydrops fetalis due to unspecified hemolytic disease Ⓝ▽

P56.99 Hydrops fetalis due to other hemolytic disease Ⓝ

✓4ᵗʰ **P57 Kernicterus**

P57.0 Kernicterus due to isoimmunization Ⓝ

P57.8 Other specified kernicterus Ⓝ
EXCLUDES 1 *Crigler-Najjar syndrome (E80.5)*

P57.9 Kernicterus, unspecified Ⓝ▽

✓4ᵗʰ **P58 Neonatal jaundice due to other excessive hemolysis**
EXCLUDES 1 *jaundice due to isoimmunization (P55-P57)*

P58.0 Neonatal jaundice due to bruising Ⓝ

P58.1 Neonatal jaundice due to bleeding Ⓝ

P58.2 Neonatal jaundice due to infection Ⓝ

P58.3 Neonatal jaundice due to polycythemia Ⓝ

✓5ᵗʰ **P58.4 Neonatal jaundice due to drugs or toxins transmitted from mother or given to newborn**
Code first poisoning due to drug or toxin, if applicable (T36-T65 with fifth or sixth character 1-4 or 6)
Use additional code for adverse effect, if applicable, to identify drug (T36-T50 with fifth or sixth character 5)

P58.41 Neonatal jaundice due to drugs or toxins transmitted from mother Ⓝ

P58.42 Neonatal jaundice due to drugs or toxins given to newborn Ⓝ

P58.5 Neonatal jaundice due to swallowed maternal blood Ⓝ

P58.8 Neonatal jaundice due to other specified excessive hemolysis Ⓝ

P58.9 Neonatal jaundice due to excessive hemolysis, unspecified Ⓝ▽

✓4ᵗʰ **P59 Neonatal jaundice from other and unspecified causes**
EXCLUDES 1 *jaundice due to inborn errors of metabolism (E70-E88)*
kernicterus (P57.-)

P59.0 Neonatal jaundice associated with preterm delivery Ⓝ
Hyperbilirubinemia of prematurity
Jaundice due to delayed conjugation associated with preterm delivery

P59.1 Inspissated bile syndrome Ⓝ

✓5ᵗʰ **P59.2 Neonatal jaundice from other and unspecified hepatocellular damage**
EXCLUDES 1 *congenital viral hepatitis (P35.3)*

P59.20 Neonatal jaundice from unspecified hepatocellular damage Ⓝ▽

P59.29 Neonatal jaundice from other hepatocellular damage Ⓝ
Neonatal giant cell hepatitis
Neonatal (idiopathic) hepatitis

P59.3 Neonatal jaundice from breast milk inhibitor Ⓝ

P59.8 Neonatal jaundice from other specified causes Ⓝ

P59.9 Neonatal jaundice, unspecified Ⓝ▽
Neonatal physiological jaundice (intense)(prolonged) NOS

P60 Disseminated intravascular coagulation of newborn Ⓝ
Defibrination syndrome of newborn

✓4ᵗʰ **P61 Other perinatal hematological disorders**
EXCLUDES 1 *transient hypogammaglobulinemia of infancy (D80.7)*

P61.0 Transient neonatal thrombocytopenia Ⓝ
Neonatal thrombocytopenia due to exchange transfusion
Neonatal thrombocytopenia due to idiopathic maternal thrombocytopenia
Neonatal thrombocytopenia due to isoimmunization

P61.1 Polycythemia neonatorum Ⓝ

P61.2 Anemia of prematurity Ⓝ

P61.3 Congenital anemia from fetal blood loss Ⓝ

P61.4 Other congenital anemias, not elsewhere classified Ⓝ
Congenital anemia NOS

P61.5 Transient neonatal neutropenia Ⓝ
EXCLUDES 1 *congenital neutropenia (nontransient) (D70.0)*

P61.6 Other transient neonatal disorders of coagulation Ⓝ

P61.8 Other specified perinatal hematological disorders Ⓝ

P61.9 Perinatal hematological disorder, unspecified Ⓝ▽

Ⓝ Newborn   Ⓟ Pediatric   Ⓜ Maternity   Ⓐ Adult   **RIC** RIC Dx   **NCDx** Noncancer Dx   **PDx** Primary Dx   **CC** RIC CC Condition   ▶◀ Revised Text   ● New Code   ▲ Revised Code Title

814   ICD-10-CM 2016

Transitory endocrine and metabolic disorders specific to newborn (P70-P74)

INCLUDES   transitory endocrine and metabolic disturbances caused by the infant's response to maternal endocrine and metabolic factors, or its adjustment to extrauterine environment

✓4ᵗʰ **P70** **Transitory disorders of** carbohydrate metabolism **specific to newborn**

  P70.0 **Syndrome of infant of mother with** gestational diabetes   N
     Newborn (with hypoglycemia) affected by maternal gestational diabetes
     EXCLUDES 1   newborn (with hypoglycemia) affected by maternal (pre-existing) diabetes mellitus (P70.1)
        syndrome of infant of a diabetic mother (P70.1)

  P70.1 **Syndrome of infant of a** diabetic mother   N
     Newborn (with hypoglycemia) affected by maternal (pre-existing) diabetes mellitus
     EXCLUDES 1   newborn (with hypoglycemia) affected by maternal gestational diabetes (P70.0)
        syndrome of infant of mother with gestational diabetes (P70.0)

  P70.2 **Neonatal** diabetes mellitus   N

  P70.3 Iatrogenic **neonatal** hypoglycemia   N

  P70.4 **Other neonatal hypoglycemia**   N
     Transitory neonatal hypoglycemia

  P70.8 **Other transitory disorders of carbohydrate metabolism of newborn**   N

  P70.9 **Transitory disorder of carbohydrate metabolism of newborn, unspecified**   N ▽

✓4ᵗʰ **P71** **Transitory neonatal disorders of** calcium and magnesium metabolism

  P71.0 Cow's milk hypocalcemia **in newborn**   N

  P71.1 **Other neonatal hypocalcemia**   N
     EXCLUDES 1   neonatal hypoparathyroidism (P71.4)

  P71.2 **Neonatal** hypomagnesemia   N

  P71.3 **Neonatal** tetany without calcium or magnesium deficiency   N
     Neonatal tetany NOS

  P71.4 **Transitory neonatal** hypoparathyroidism   N

  P71.8 **Other transitory neonatal disorders of calcium and magnesium metabolism**   N

  P71.9 **Transitory neonatal disorder of calcium and magnesium metabolism, unspecified**   N ▽

✓4ᵗʰ **P72** **Other transitory neonatal** endocrine disorders
     EXCLUDES 1   congenital hypothyroidism with or without goiter (E03.0-E03.1)
        dyshormogenetic goiter (E07.1)
        Pendred's syndrome (E07.1)

  P72.0 Neonatal goiter, **not elsewhere classified**   N
     Transitory congenital goiter with normal functioning

  P72.1 Transitory **neonatal** hyperthyroidism   N
     Neonatal thyrotoxicosis

  P72.2 **Other transitory neonatal disorders of** thyroid function, **not elsewhere classified**   N
     Transitory neonatal hypothyroidism

  P72.8 **Other specified transitory neonatal endocrine disorders**   N

  P72.9 **Transitory neonatal endocrine disorder, unspecified**   N ▽

✓4ᵗʰ **P74** **Other transitory neonatal** electrolyte and metabolic disturbances

  P74.0 Late metabolic acidosis **of newborn**   N
     EXCLUDES 1   (fetal) metabolic acidosis of newborn (P19)

  P74.1 Dehydration **of newborn**   N

  P74.2 **Disturbances of** sodium balance **of newborn**   N

  P74.3 **Disturbances of** potassium balance **of newborn**   N

  P74.4 **Other transitory electrolyte disturbances of newborn**   N

  P74.5 **Transitory** tyrosinemia **of newborn**   N

  P74.6 **Transitory** hyperammonemia **of newborn**   N

  P74.8 **Other transitory metabolic disturbances of newborn**   N
     Amino-acid metabolic disorders described as transitory

  P74.9 **Transitory metabolic disturbance of newborn, unspecified**   N ▽

Digestive system disorders of newborn (P76-P78)

✓4ᵗʰ **P76** **Other intestinal obstruction of newborn**

  P76.0 **Meconium plug syndrome**   N
     Meconium ileus NOS
     EXCLUDES 1   meconium ileus in cystic fibrosis (E84.11)

  P76.1 **Transitory ileus of newborn**   N
     EXCLUDES 1   Hirschsprung's disease (Q43.1)

  P76.2 **Intestinal obstruction due to inspissated milk**   N

  P76.8 **Other specified intestinal obstruction of newborn**   N
     EXCLUDES 1   intestinal obstruction classifiable to K56-

  P76.9 **Intestinal obstruction of newborn, unspecified**   N ▽

✓4ᵗʰ **P77** Necrotizing enterocolitis **of newborn**

  P77.1 Stage 1 **necrotizing enterocolitis in newborn**   N
     Necrotizing enterocolitis without pneumatosis, without perforation

  P77.2 Stage 2 **necrotizing enterocolitis in newborn**   N
     Necrotizing enterocolitis with pneumatosis, without perforation

  P77.3 Stage 3 **necrotizing enterocolitis in newborn**   N
     Necrotizing enterocolitis with perforation
     Necrotizing enterocolitis with pneumatosis and perforation

  P77.9 **Necrotizing enterocolitis in newborn, unspecified**   N ▽
     Necrotizing enterocolitis in newborn, NOS

✓4ᵗʰ **P78** **Other perinatal digestive system disorders**
     EXCLUDES 1   cystic fibrosis (E84.0-E84.9)
        neonatal gastrointestinal hemorrhages (P54.0-P54.3)

  P78.0 **Perinatal intestinal perforation**   N
     Meconium peritonitis

  P78.1 **Other neonatal peritonitis**   N
     Neonatal peritonitis NOS

  P78.2 **Neonatal hematemesis and melena due to swallowed maternal blood**   N

  P78.3 **Noninfective neonatal diarrhea**   N
     Neonatal diarrhea NOS

  ✓5ᵗʰ **P78.8** **Other specified perinatal digestive system disorders**

    P78.81 **Congenital cirrhosis (of liver)**   N

    P78.82 **Peptic ulcer of newborn**   N

    P78.83 **Newborn esophageal reflux**   N
       Neonatal esophageal reflux

    P78.89 **Other specified perinatal digestive system disorders**   N

  P78.9 **Perinatal digestive system disorder, unspecified**   N ▽

Conditions involving the integument and temperature regulation of newborn (P80-P83)

✓4ᵗʰ **P80** **Hypothermia of newborn**

  P80.0 **Cold injury syndrome**   N
     Severe and usually chronic hypothermia associated with a pink flushed appearance, edema and neurological and biochemical abnormalities.
     EXCLUDES 1   mild hypothermia of newborn (P80.8)

  P80.8 **Other hypothermia of newborn**   N
     Mild hypothermia of newborn

  P80.9 **Hypothermia of newborn, unspecified**   N

✓4ᵗʰ **P81** **Other disturbances of temperature regulation of newborn**

  P81.0 **Environmental hyperthermia of newborn**   N

  P81.8 **Other specified disturbances of temperature regulation of newborn**   N

  P81.9 **Disturbance of temperature regulation of newborn, unspecified**   N ▽
     Fever of newborn NOS

✓4ᵗʰ **P83** **Other conditions of integument specific to newborn**
     EXCLUDES 1   congenital malformations of skin and integument (Q80-Q84)
        hydrops fetalis due to hemolytic disease (P56.-)
        neonatal skin infection (P39.4)
        staphylococcal scalded skin syndrome (L00)
     EXCLUDES 2   cradle cap (L21.0)
        diaper [napkin] dermatitis (L22)

  P83.0 **Sclerema neonatorum**   N

  P83.1 **Neonatal erythema toxicum**   N

  P83.2 **Hydrops fetalis not due to hemolytic disease**   N
     Hydrops fetalis NOS

☑ Add'l Character Required   ✓x7ᵗʰ Placeholder Alert   RUG IV Special Care High Dx   RUG IV Clinically Complex Dx   RUG IV Special Care Low Dx   Manifestation Code   Other Specified Code   ▽ Unspecified Code

Chapter 16. Certain Conditions Originating in the Perinatal Period

✓5ᵗʰ **P83.3 Other and unspecified edema specific to newborn**

    P83.30 Unspecified edema specific to newborn N ▽

    P83.39 Other edema specific to newborn N

P83.4 Breast engorgement of newborn N
    Noninfective mastitis of newborn

P83.5 Congenital hydrocele ♂

P83.6 Umbilical polyp of newborn

P83.8 Other specified conditions of integument specific N
to newborn
    Bronze baby syndrome
    Neonatal scleroderma
    Urticaria neonatorum

P83.9 Condition of the integument specific to newborn, N ▽
unspecified

Other problems with newborn (P84)

P84 Other problems with newborn N
    Acidemia of newborn
    Acidosis of newborn
    Anoxia of newborn NOS
    Asphyxia of newborn NOS
    Hypercapnia of newborn
    Hypoxemia of newborn
    Hypoxia of newborn NOS
    Mixed metabolic and respiratory acidosis of newborn
    EXCLUDES 1   *intracranial hemorrhage due to anoxia or hypoxia (P52.-)*
         hypoxic ischemic encephalopathy [HIE] (P91.6-)
         late metabolic acidosis of newborn (P74.0)

Other disorders originating in the perinatal period (P90-P96)

P90 Convulsions of newborn N
    EXCLUDES 1   *benign myoclonic epilepsy in infancy (G40.3-)*
         benign neonatal convulsions (familial) (G40.3-)

✓4ᵗʰ **P91 Other disturbances of cerebral status of newborn**

P91.0 Neonatal cerebral ischemia N

P91.1 Acquired periventricular cysts of newborn N

P91.2 Neonatal cerebral leukomalacia N
    Periventricular leukomalacia

P91.3 Neonatal cerebral irritability N

P91.4 Neonatal cerebral depression N

P91.5 Neonatal coma N

✓5ᵗʰ **P91.6 Hypoxic ischemic encephalopathy [HIE]**

    P91.60 Hypoxic ischemic encephalopathy [HIE], N ▽
    unspecified

    P91.61 Mild hypoxic ischemic encephalopathy [HIE] N

    P91.62 Moderate hypoxic ischemic encephalopathy [HIE] N

    P91.63 Severe hypoxic ischemic encephalopathy [HIE] N

P91.8 Other specified disturbances of cerebral status of newborn N

P91.9 Disturbance of cerebral status of newborn, unspecified N ▽

✓4ᵗʰ **P92 Feeding problems of newborn**
    EXCLUDES 1   *feeding problems in child over 28 days old (R63.3)*

✓5ᵗʰ **P92.0 Vomiting of newborn**
    EXCLUDES 1   *vomiting of child over 28 days old (R11.-)*

    P92.01 Bilious vomiting of newborn N
        EXCLUDES 1   *bilious vomiting in child over 28 days old*
             (R11.14)

    P92.09 Other vomiting of newborn N
        EXCLUDES 1   *regurgitation of food in newborn (P92.1)*

P92.1 Regurgitation and rumination of newborn N

P92.2 Slow feeding of newborn N

P92.3 Underfeeding of newborn N

P92.4 Overfeeding of newborn N

P92.5 Neonatal difficulty in feeding at breast N

P92.6 Failure to thrive in newborn N
    EXCLUDES 1   *failure to thrive in child over 28 days old (R62.51)*

P92.8 Other feeding problems of newborn N

P92.9 Feeding problem of newborn, unspecified N ▽

✓4ᵗʰ **P93 Reactions and intoxications due to drugs administered to newborn**
    INCLUDES   reactions and intoxications due to drugs administered to
         fetus affecting newborn
    EXCLUDES 1   *jaundice due to drugs or toxins transmitted from mother or*
         given to newborn (P58.4-)
         reactions and intoxications from maternal opiates, tranquilizers
         and other medication (P04.0-P04.1, P04.4)
         withdrawal symptoms from maternal use of drugs of addiction
         (P96.1)
         withdrawal symptoms from therapeutic use of drugs in
         newborn (P96.2)

P93.0 Grey baby syndrome N
    Grey syndrome from chloramphenicol administration in
    newborn

P93.8 Other reactions and intoxications due to drugs N
administered to newborn
    Use additional code for adverse effect, if applicable, to identify
    drug (T36-T50 with fifth or sixth character 5)

✓4ᵗʰ **P94 Disorders of muscle tone of newborn**

P94.0 Transient neonatal myasthenia gravis N
    EXCLUDES 1   *myasthenia gravis (G70.0)*

P94.1 Congenital hypertonia N

P94.2 Congenital hypotonia N
    Floppy baby syndrome, unspecified

P94.8 Other disorders of muscle tone of newborn N

P94.9 Disorder of muscle tone of newborn, unspecified N ▽

P95 Stillbirth N
    Deadborn fetus NOS
    Fetal death of unspecified cause
    Stillbirth NOS
    EXCLUDES 1   *maternal care for intrauterine death (O36.4)*
         missed abortion (O02.1)
         outcome of delivery, stillbirth (Z37.1, Z37.3, Z37.4, Z37.7)

✓4ᵗʰ **P96 Other conditions originating in the perinatal period**

P96.0 Congenital renal failure N
    Uremia of newborn

P96.1 Neonatal withdrawal symptoms from maternal use N
of drugs of addiction
    Drug withdrawal syndrome in infant of dependent mother
    Neonatal abstinence syndrome
    EXCLUDES 1   *reactions and intoxications from maternal opiates and*
         tranquilizers administered during labor and
         delivery (P04.0)

P96.2 Withdrawal symptoms from therapeutic use of drugs in N
newborn

P96.3 Wide cranial sutures of newborn N
    Neonatal craniotabes

P96.5 Complication to newborn due to (fetal) intrauterine N
procedure
    EXCLUDES 2   *newborn (suspected to be) affected by amniocentesis*
         (P00.6)

✓5ᵗʰ **P96.8 Other specified conditions originating in the perinatal period**

    P96.81 Exposure to (parental) (environmental) tobacco N
    smoke in the perinatal period
        EXCLUDES 2   *newborn affected by in utero exposure to*
             tobacco (P04.2)
             exposure to environmental tobacco smoke
             after the perinatal period (Z77.22)

    P96.82 Delayed separation of umbilical cord N

    P96.83 Meconium staining N
        EXCLUDES 1   *meconium aspiration (P24.00, P24.01)*
             meconium passage during delivery (P03.82)

    P96.89 Other specified conditions originating in the N
    perinatal period
        Use additional code to specify condition

P96.9 Condition originating in the perinatal period, N ▽
unspecified
    Congenital debility NOS

N Newborn   P Pediatric   M Maternity   A Adult   RIC RIC Dx   NC Dx Noncancer Dx   PDx Primary Dx   CC RIC CC Condition   ▶◀ Revised Text   ● New Code   ▲ Revised Code Title

816   ICD-10-CM 2016

Chapter 17. Congenital Malformations, Deformations, and Chromosomal Abnormalities (Q00–Q99)

Chapter Specific Guidelines with Coding Examples

The chapter specific guidelines from the ICD-10-CM Official Guidelines for Coding and Reporting have been provided below. Along with these guidelines are coding examples, contained in the shaded boxes, that have been developed to help illustrate the coding and/or sequencing guidance found in these guidelines.

Assign an appropriate code(s) from categories Q00-Q99, Congenital malformations, deformations, and chromosomal abnormalities when a malformation/deformation or chromosomal abnormality is documented. A malformation/deformation/or chromosomal abnormality may be the principal/first-listed diagnosis on a record or a secondary diagnosis.

When a malformation/deformation/or chromosomal abnormality does not have a unique code assignment, assign additional code(s) for any manifestations that may be present.

When the code assignment specifically identifies the malformation/deformation/or chromosomal abnormality, manifestations that are an inherent component of the anomaly should not be coded separately. Additional codes should be assigned for manifestations that are not an inherent component.

8-day-old infant with tetralogy of Fallot and pulmonary stenosis

Q21.3   **Tetralogy of Fallot**

Explanation: Pulmonary stenosis is inherent in the disease process of tetralogy of Fallot. When the code assignment specifically identifies the malformation/deformation/or chromosomal abnormality, manifestations that are inherent components of the anomaly should not be coded separately.

7-month-old infant with Down syndrome and common atrioventricular canal

Q90.9   **Down syndrome, unspecified**

Q21.2   **Atrioventricular septal defect**

Explanation: While a common atrioventricular canal is often associated with patients with Down syndrome, this manifestation is not an inherent component and may be reported separately. When the code assignment specifically identifies the anomaly, manifestations that are inherent components of the condition should not be coded separately. Additional codes should be assigned for manifestations that are not inherent components.

Codes from Chapter 17 may be used throughout the life of the patient. If a congenital malformation or deformity has been corrected, a personal history code should be used to identify the history of the malformation or deformity. Although present at birth, malformation/deformation/or chromosomal abnormality may not be identified until later in life. Whenever the condition is diagnosed by the physician, it is appropriate to assign a code from codes Q00-Q99. For the birth admission, the appropriate code from category Z38, Liveborn infants, according to place of birth and type of delivery, should be sequenced as the principal diagnosis, followed by any congenital anomaly codes, Q00- Q99.

Three-year-old with history of corrected ventricular septal defect

Z87.74   **Personal history of (corrected) congenital malformations of heart and circulatory system**

Explanation: If a congenital malformation or deformity has been corrected, a personal history code should be used to identify the history of the malformation or deformity.

Forty-year-old man with headaches diagnosed with congenital arteriovenous malformation by brain scan

Q28.2   **Arteriovenous malformation of cerebral vessels**

Explanation: Although present at birth, malformations may not be identified until later in life. Whenever the condition is diagnosed by the physician, it is appropriate to assign a code from the range Q00–Q99.

Newborn with anencephaly delivered vaginally in hospital

Z38.00   **Single liveborn infant, delivered vaginally**

Q00.0   **Anencephaly**

Explanation: For the birth admission, the appropriate code from category Z38 Liveborn infants, according to place of birth and type of delivery, should be sequenced as the principal diagnosis, followed by any congenital anomaly codes, Q00–Q99.

Chapter 17. Congenital Malformations logo in left margin: **Chapter 17. Congenital Malformations, Deformations and Chromosomal Abnormalities**   **Q00–Q07.9**

Chapter 17. Congenital Malformations, Deformations and Chromosomal Abnormalities(Q00-Q99)

NOTE   Codes from this chapter are not for use on maternal or fetal records.

EXCLUDES 2   *inborn errors of metabolism (E70-E88)*

This chapter contains the following blocks:

Q00-Q07   Congenital malformations of the nervous system
Q10-Q18   Congenital malformations of eye, ear, face and neck
Q20-Q28   Congenital malformations of the circulatory system
Q30-Q34   Congenital malformations of the respiratory system
Q35-Q37   Cleft lip and cleft palate
Q38-Q45   Other congenital malformations of the digestive system
Q50-Q56   Congenital malformations of genital organs
Q60-Q64   Congenital malformations of the urinary system
Q65-Q79   Congenital malformations and deformations of the musculoskeletal system
Q80-Q89   Other congenital malformations
Q90-Q99   Chromosomal abnormalities, not elsewhere classified

Congenital malformations of the nervous system (Q00-Q07)

✓4ᵗʰ Q00 Anencephaly and similar malformations

Q00.0 Anencephaly
Acephaly
Acrania
Amyelencephaly
Hemianencephaly
Hemicephaly

Q00.1 Craniorachischisis

Q00.2 Iniencephaly

✓4ᵗʰ Q01 Encephalocele
INCLUDES   Arnold-Chiari syndrome, type III
encephalocystocele
encephalomyelocele
hydroencephalocele
hydromeningocele, cranial
meningocele, cerebral
meningoencephalocele
EXCLUDES 1   *Meckel-Gruber syndrome (Q61.9)*

Q01.0 Frontal encephalocele

Q01.1 Nasofrontal encephalocele

Q01.2 Occipital encephalocele

Q01.8 Encephalocele of other sites

Q01.9 Encephalocele, unspecified   ▽

Q02 Microcephaly
INCLUDES   hydromicrocephaly
micrencephalon
EXCLUDES 1   *Meckel-Gruber syndrome (Q61.9)*

✓4ᵗʰ Q03 Congenital hydrocephalus
INCLUDES   hydrocephalus in newborn
EXCLUDES 1   *Arnold-Chiari syndrome, type II (Q07.0-)*
acquired hydrocephalus (G91.-)
hydrocephalus due to congenital toxoplasmosis (P37.1)
hydrocephalus with spina bifida (Q05.0-Q05.4)

Q03.0 Malformations of aqueduct of Sylvius
Anomaly of aqueduct of Sylvius
Obstruction of aqueduct of Sylvius, congenital
Stenosis of aqueduct of Sylvius

Q03.1 Atresia of foramina of Magendie and Luschka
Dandy-Walker syndrome

Q03.8 Other congenital hydrocephalus

Q03.9 Congenital hydrocephalus, unspecified   ▽

✓4ᵗʰ Q04 Other congenital malformations of brain
EXCLUDES 1   *cyclopia (Q87.0)*
macrocephaly (Q75.3)

Q04.0 Congenital malformations of corpus callosum
Agenesis of corpus callosum

Q04.1 Arhinencephaly

Q04.2 Holoprosencephaly

Q04.3 Other reduction deformities of brain
Absence of part of brain   Hypoplasia of part of brain
Agenesis of part of brain   Lissencephaly
Agyria   Microgyria
Aplasia of part of brain   Pachygyria
Hydranencephaly
EXCLUDES 1   *congenital malformations of corpus callosum (Q04.0)*

Q04.4 Septo-optic dysplasia of brain

Q04.5 Megalencephaly

Q04.6 Congenital cerebral cysts
Porencephaly
Schizencephaly
EXCLUDES 1   *acquired porencephalic cyst (G93.0)*

Q04.8 Other specified congenital malformations of brain
Arnold-Chiari syndrome, type IV
Macrogyria

Q04.9 Congenital malformation of brain, unspecified   ▽
Congenital anomaly NOS of brain
Congenital deformity NOS of brain
Congenital disease or lesion NOS of brain
Multiple anomalies NOS of brain, congenital

✓4ᵗʰ Q05 Spina bifida
Hydromeningocele (spinal)   Myelomeningocele
Meningocele (spinal)   Rachischisis
Meningomyelocele   Spina bifida (aperta)(cystica)
Myelocele   Syringomyelocele
Use additional code for any associated paraplegia (paraparesis) (G82.2-)
EXCLUDES 1   *Arnold-Chiari syndrome, type II (Q07.0-)*
spina bifida occulta (Q76.0)

Q05.0 Cervical spina bifida with hydrocephalus

Q05.1 Thoracic spina bifida with hydrocephalus
Dorsal spina bifida with hydrocephalus
Thoracolumbar spina bifida with hydrocephalus

Q05.2 Lumbar spina bifida with hydrocephalus
Lumbosacral spina bifida with hydrocephalus

Q05.3 Sacral spina bifida with hydrocephalus

Q05.4 Unspecified spina bifida with hydrocephalus   ▽

Q05.5 Cervical spina bifida without hydrocephalus

Q05.6 Thoracic spina bifida without hydrocephalus
Dorsal spina bifida NOS
Thoracolumbar spina bifida NOS

Q05.7 Lumbar spina bifida without hydrocephalus
Lumbosacral spina bifida NOS

Q05.8 Sacral spina bifida without hydrocephalus

Q05.9 Spina bifida, unspecified   ▽

✓4ᵗʰ Q06 Other congenital malformations of spinal cord

Q06.0 Amyelia

Q06.1 Hypoplasia and dysplasia of spinal cord
Atelomyelia
Myelatelia
Myelodysplasia of spinal cord

Q06.2 Diastematomyelia

Q06.3 Other congenital cauda equina malformations

Q06.4 Hydromyelia
Hydrorachis

Q06.8 Other specified congenital malformations of spinal cord

Q06.9 Congenital malformation of spinal cord, unspecified   ▽
Congenital anomaly NOS of spinal cord
Congenital deformity NOS of spinal cord
Congenital disease or lesion NOS of spinal cord

✓4ᵗʰ Q07 Other congenital malformations of nervous system
EXCLUDES 2   *congenital central alveolar hypoventilation syndrome (G47.35)*
familial dysautonomia [Riley-Day] (G90.1)
neurofibromatosis (nonmalignant) (Q85.0-)

✓5ᵗʰ Q07.0 Arnold-Chiari syndrome
Arnold-Chiari syndrome, type II
EXCLUDES 1   *Arnold-Chiari syndrome, type III (Q01.-)*
Arnold-Chiari syndrome, type IV (Q04.8)

Q07.00 Arnold-Chiari syndrome without spina bifida or hydrocephalus

Q07.01 Arnold-Chiari syndrome with spina bifida

Q07.02 Arnold-Chiari syndrome with hydrocephalus

Q07.03 Arnold-Chiari syndrome with spina bifida and hydrocephalus

Q07.8 Other specified congenital malformations of nervous system
Agenesis of nerve
Displacement of brachial plexus
Jaw-winking syndrome
Marcus Gunn's syndrome

Q07.9 Congenital malformation of nervous system, unspecified   ▽
Congenital anomaly NOS of nervous system
Congenital deformity NOS of nervous system
Congenital disease or lesion NOS of nervous system

Ⓝ Newborn   Ⓟ Pediatric   Ⓜ Maternity   Ⓐ Adult   **RIC** RIC Dx   **NCDx** Noncancer Dx   **PDx** Primary Dx   **CC** RIC CC Condition   ▶◀ Revised Text   ● New Code   ▲ Revised Code Title

818   ICD-10-CM 2016

Congenital malformations of eye, ear, face and neck (Q10-Q18)

EXCLUDES 2   cleft lip and cleft palate (Q35-Q37)
     congenital malformation of cervical spine (Q05.0, Q05.5, Q67.5, Q76.0-Q76.4)
     congenital malformation of larynx (Q31.-)
     congenital malformation of lip NEC (Q38.0)
     congenital malformation of nose (Q30.-)
     congenital malformation of parathyroid gland (Q89.2)
     congenital malformation of thyroid gland (Q89.2)

✓4ᵗʰ Q10   Congenital malformations of eyelid, lacrimal apparatus and orbit

EXCLUDES 1   cryptophthalmos NOS (Q11.2)
     cryptophthalmos syndrome (Q87.0)

Q10.0   **Congenital** ptosis

Q10.1   **Congenital** ectropion

Q10.2   **Congenital** entropion

Q10.3   **Other congenital malformations of** eyelid
     Ablepharon
     Blepharophimosis, congenital
     Coloboma of eyelid
     Congenital absence or agenesis of cilia
     Congenital absence or agenesis of eyelid
     Congenital accessory eyelid
     Congenital accessory eye muscle
     Congenital malformation of eyelid NOS

Q10.4   **Absence and agenesis of lacrimal apparatus**
     Congenital absence of punctum lacrimale

Q10.5   **Congenital** stenosis and stricture of lacrimal duct

Q10.6   **Other congenital malformations of** lacrimal apparatus
     Congenital malformation of lacrimal apparatus NOS

Q10.7   **Congenital malformation of** orbit

✓4ᵗʰ Q11   Anophthalmos, microphthalmos and macrophthalmos

Q11.0   **Cystic eyeball**

Q11.1   **Other anophthalmos**
     Anophthalmos NOS
     Agenesis of eye
     Aplasia of eye

Q11.2   **Microphthalmos**
     Cryptophthalmos NOS
     Dysplasia of eye
     Hypoplasia of eye
     Rudimentary eye
     EXCLUDES 1   cryptophthalmos syndrome (Q87.0)

Q11.3   **Macrophthalmos**
     EXCLUDES 1   macrophthalmos in congenital glaucoma (Q15.0)

✓4ᵗʰ Q12   Congenital lens malformations

Q12.0   **Congenital** cataract

Q12.1   **Congenital** displaced lens

Q12.2   **Coloboma of lens**

Q12.3   **Congenital** aphakia

Q12.4   **Spherophakia**

Q12.8   **Other congenital lens malformations**
     Microphakia

Q12.9   **Congenital lens malformation, unspecified**   ▽

✓4ᵗʰ Q13   Congenital malformations of anterior segment of eye

Q13.0   **Coloboma of iris**
     Coloboma NOS

Q13.1   **Absence of iris**
     Aniridia
     Use additional code for associated glaucoma (H42)

Q13.2   **Other congenital malformations of iris**
     Anisocoria, congenital
     Atresia of pupil
     Congenital malformation of iris NOS
     Corectopia

Q13.3   **Congenital** corneal opacity

Q13.4   **Other congenital corneal malformations**
     Congenital malformation of cornea NOS
     Microcornea
     Peter's anomaly

Q13.5   **Blue sclera**

✓5ᵗʰ Q13.8   **Other congenital malformations of anterior segment of eye**

     Q13.81   **Rieger's anomaly**
         Use additional code for associated glaucoma (H42)

     Q13.89   **Other congenital malformations of anterior segment of eye**

Q13.9   **Congenital malformation of anterior segment of eye, unspecified**   ▽

✓4ᵗʰ Q14   Congenital malformations of posterior segment of eye

EXCLUDES 2   optic nerve hypoplasia (H47.03-)

Q14.0   **Congenital malformation of** vitreous humor
     Congenital vitreous opacity

Q14.1   **Congenital malformation of** retina
     Congenital retinal aneurysm

Q14.2   **Congenital malformation of** optic disc
     Coloboma of optic disc

Q14.3   **Congenital malformation of** choroid

Q14.8   **Other congenital malformations of posterior segment of eye**
     Coloboma of the fundus

Q14.9   **Congenital malformation of posterior segment of eye, unspecified**   ▽

✓4ᵗʰ Q15   Other congenital malformations of eye

EXCLUDES 1   congenital nystagmus (H55.01)
     ocular albinism (E70.31-)
     optic nerve hypoplasia (H47.03-)
     retinitis pigmentosa (H35.52)

Q15.0   **Congenital glaucoma**
     Axenfeld's anomaly
     Buphthalmos
     Glaucoma of childhood
     Glaucoma of newborn
     Hydrophthalmos
     Keratoglobus, congenital, with glaucoma
     Macrocornea with glaucoma
     Macrophthalmos in congenital glaucoma
     Megalocornea with glaucoma

Q15.8   **Other specified congenital malformations of eye**

Q15.9   **Congenital malformation of eye, unspecified**   ▽
     Congenital anomaly of eye
     Congenital deformity of eye

✓4ᵗʰ Q16   Congenital malformations of ear causing impairment of hearing

EXCLUDES 1   congenital deafness (H90.-)

Q16.0   **Congenital absence of (ear)** auricle

Q16.1   **Congenital absence, atresia and stricture of auditory canal (external)**
     Congenital atresia or stricture of osseous meatus

Q16.2   **Absence of** eustachian tube

Q16.3   **Congenital malformation of** ear ossicles
     Congenital fusion of ear ossicles

Q16.4   **Other congenital malformations of middle ear**
     Congenital malformation of middle ear NOS

Q16.5   **Congenital malformation of** inner ear
     Congenital anomaly of membranous labyrinth
     Congenital anomaly of organ of Corti

Q16.9   **Congenital malformation of ear causing impairment of hearing, unspecified**   ▽
     Congenital absence of ear NOS

✓4ᵗʰ Q17   Other congenital malformations of ear

EXCLUDES 1   congenital malformations of ear with impairment of hearing (Q16.0- Q16.9)
     preauricular sinus (Q18.1)

Q17.0   **Accessory auricle**
     Accessory tragus
     Polyotia
     Preauricular appendage or tag
     Supernumerary ear
     Supernumerary lobule

Q17.1   **Macrotia**

Q17.2   **Microtia**

Q17.3   **Other misshapen ear**
     Pointed ear

Q17.4   **Misplaced ear**
     Low-set ears
     EXCLUDES 1   cervical auricle (Q18.2)

Q17.5   **Prominent ear**
     Bat ear

Q17.8   **Other specified congenital malformations of ear**
     Congenital absence of lobe of ear

Q17.9   **Congenital malformation of ear, unspecified**   ▽
     Congenital anomaly of ear NOS

☑ Add'l Character Required   ✓x7ᵗʰ Placeholder Alert   RUG IV Special Care High Dx   RUG IV Clinically Complex Dx   RUG IV Special Care Low Dx   Manifestation Code   Other Specified Code   ▽ Unspecified Code

✓4ᵗʰ Q18 Other congenital malformations of face and neck

EXCLUDES 1   cleft lip and cleft palate (Q35-Q37)
conditions classified to Q67.0-Q67.4
congenital malformations of skull and face bones (Q75.-)
cyclopia (Q87.0)
dentofacial anomalies [including malocclusion] (M26.-)
malformation syndromes affecting facial appearance (Q87.0)
persistent thyroglossal duct (Q89.2)

Q18.0 Sinus, fistula and cyst of branchial cleft
Branchial vestige

Q18.1 Preauricular sinus and cyst
Fistula of auricle, congenital
Cervicoaural fistula

Q18.2 Other branchial cleft malformations
Branchial cleft malformation NOS
Cervical auricle
Otocephaly

Q18.3 Webbing of neck
Pterygium colli

Q18.4 Macrostomia

Q18.5 Microstomia

Q18.6 Macrocheilia
Hypertrophy of lip, congenital

Q18.7 Microcheilia

Q18.8 Other specified congenital malformations of face and neck
Medial cyst of face and neck
Medial fistula of face and neck
Medial sinus of face and neck

Q18.9 Congenital malformation of face and neck, unspecified ▽
Congenital anomaly NOS of face and neck

Congenital malformations of the circulatory system (Q20-Q28)

✓4ᵗʰ Q20 Congenital malformations of cardiac chambers and connections

EXCLUDES 1   dextrocardia with situs inversus (Q89.3)
mirror-image atrial arrangement with situs inversus (Q89.3)

Q20.0 Common arterial trunk
Persistent truncus arteriosus
EXCLUDES 1   aortic septal defect (Q21.4)

Q20.1 Double outlet right ventricle
Taussig-Bing syndrome

Q20.2 Double outlet left ventricle

Q20.3 Discordant ventriculoarterial connection
Dextrotransposition of aorta
Transposition of great vessels (complete)

Q20.4 Double inlet ventricle
Common ventricle
Cor triloculare biatriatum
Single ventricle

Q20.5 Discordant atrioventricular connection
Corrected transposition
Levotransposition
Ventricular inversion

Q20.6 Isomerism of atrial appendages
Isomerism of atrial appendages with asplenia or polysplenia

Q20.8 Other congenital malformations of cardiac chambers and connections
Cor binoculare

Q20.9 Congenital malformation of cardiac chambers and connections, unspecified ▽

✓4ᵗʰ Q21 Congenital malformations of cardiac septa

EXCLUDES 1   acquired cardiac septal defect (I51.0)

Q21.0 Ventricular septal defect
Roger's disease

Q21.1 Atrial septal defect
Coronary sinus defect
Patent or persistent foramen ovale
Patent or persistent ostium secundum defect (type II)
Patent or persistent sinus venosus defect

Q21.2 Atrioventricular septal defect
Common atrioventricular canal
Endocardial cushion defect
Ostium primum atrial septal defect (type I)

Q21.3 Tetralogy of Fallot
Ventricular septal defect with pulmonary stenosis or atresia, dextroposition of aorta and hypertrophy of right ventricle.
AHA: 2014, 3Q, 16

Q21.4 Aortopulmonary septal defect
Aortic septal defect
Aortopulmonary window

Q21.8 Other congenital malformations of cardiac septa
Eisenmenger's defect
Pentalogy of Fallot
EXCLUDES 1   Eisenmenger's complex (I27.8)
Eisenmenger's syndrome (I27.8)

Q21.9 Congenital malformation of cardiac septum, unspecified ▽
Septal (heart) defect NOS

✓4ᵗʰ Q22 Congenital malformations of pulmonary and tricuspid valves

Q22.0 Pulmonary valve atresia

Q22.1 Congenital pulmonary valve stenosis

Q22.2 Congenital pulmonary valve insufficiency
Congenital pulmonary valve regurgitation

Q22.3 Other congenital malformations of pulmonary valve
Congenital malformation of pulmonary valve NOS
Supernumerary cusps of pulmonary valve

Q22.4 Congenital tricuspid stenosis
Congenital tricuspid atresia

Q22.5 Ebstein's anomaly

Q22.6 Hypoplastic right heart syndrome

Q22.8 Other congenital malformations of tricuspid valve

Q22.9 Congenital malformation of tricuspid valve, unspecified ▽

✓4ᵗʰ Q23 Congenital malformations of aortic and mitral valves

Q23.0 Congenital stenosis of aortic valve
Congenital aortic atresia
Congenital aortic stenosis NOS
EXCLUDES 1   congenital stenosis of aortic valve in hypoplastic left heart syndrome (Q23.4)
congenital subaortic stenosis (Q24.4)
supravalvular aortic stenosis (congenital) (Q25.3)

Q23.1 Congenital insufficiency of aortic valve
Bicuspid aortic valve
Congenital aortic insufficiency

Q23.2 Congenital mitral stenosis
Congenital mitral atresia

Q23.3 Congenital mitral insufficiency

Q23.4 Hypoplastic left heart syndrome

Q23.8 Other congenital malformations of aortic and mitral valves

Q23.9 Congenital malformation of aortic and mitral valves, unspecified ▽

✓4ᵗʰ Q24 Other congenital malformations of heart

EXCLUDES 1   endocardial fibroelastosis (I42.4)

Q24.0 Dextrocardia
EXCLUDES 1   dextrocardia with situs inversus (Q89.3)
isomerism of atrial appendages (with asplenia or polysplenia) (Q20.6)
mirror-image atrial arrangement with situs inversus (Q89.3)

Q24.1 Levocardia

Q24.2 Cor triatriatum

Q24.3 Pulmonary infundibular stenosis
Subvalvular pulmonic stenosis

Q24.4 Congenital subaortic stenosis

Q24.5 Malformation of coronary vessels
Congenital coronary (artery) aneurysm

Q24.6 Congenital heart block

Q24.8 Other specified congenital malformations of heart
Congenital diverticulum of left ventricle
Congenital malformation of myocardium
Congenital malformation of pericardium
Malposition of heart
Uhl's disease

Q24.9 Congenital malformation of heart, unspecified ▽
Congenital anomaly of heart
Congenital disease of heart

✓4ᵗʰ Q25 Congenital malformations of great arteries

Q25.0 Patent ductus arteriosus
Patent ductus Botallo
Persistent ductus arteriosus

Q25.1 Coarctation of aorta
Coarctation of aorta (preductal) (postductal)

Q25.2 Atresia of aorta

Q25.3 Supravalvular aortic stenosis
EXCLUDES 1   congenital aortic stenosis NOS (Q23.0)
congenital stenosis of aortic valve (Q23.0)

Ⓝ Newborn   Ⓟ Pediatric   Ⓜ Maternity   Ⓐ Adult   RIC RIC Dx   NCDx Noncancer Dx   PDx Primary Dx   CC RIC CC Condition   ▶◀ Revised Text   ● New Code   ▲ Revised Code Title

820   ICD-10-CM 2016

Q25.4 **Other congenital malformations of** aorta
Absence of aorta
Aneurysm of sinus of Valsalva (ruptured)
Aplasia of aorta
Congenital aneurysm of aorta
Congenital malformations of aorta
Congenital dilatation of aorta
Double aortic arch [vascular ring of aorta]
Hypoplasia of aorta
Persistent convolutions of aortic arch
Persistent right aortic arch
EXCLUDES 1 *hypoplasia of aorta in hypoplastic left heart syndrome (Q23.4)*

Q25.5 Atresia **of pulmonary** artery

Q25.6 Stenosis **of pulmonary** artery
Supravalvular pulmonary stenosis

✓5ᵗʰ Q25.7 **Other congenital malformations of** pulmonary artery

Q25.71 Coarctation **of pulmonary artery**

Q25.72 **Congenital pulmonary** arteriovenous malformation
Congenital pulmonary arteriovenous aneurysm

Q25.79 **Other congenital malformations of pulmonary artery**
Aberrant pulmonary artery
Agenesis of pulmonary artery
Congenital aneurysm of pulmonary artery
Congenital anomaly of pulmonary artery
Hypoplasia of pulmonary artery

Q25.8 **Other congenital malformations of other great arteries**

Q25.9 **Congenital malformation of great arteries, unspecified** ▽

✓4ᵗʰ Q26 **Congenital malformations of** great veins

Q26.0 **Congenital** stenosis of **vena cava**
Congenital stenosis of vena cava (inferior)(superior)

Q26.1 **Persistent** left superior vena cava

Q26.2 Total anomalous **pulmonary venous connection**
Total anomalous pulmonary venous return [TAPVR], subdiaphragmatic
Total anomalous pulmonary venous return [TAPVR], supradiaphragmatic

Q26.3 Partial anomalous **pulmonary venous connection**
Partial anomalous pulmonary venous return

Q26.4 **Anomalous pulmonary venous connection, unspecified** ▽

Q26.5 **Anomalous** portal venous connection

Q26.6 **Portal vein-hepatic** artery fistula

Q26.8 **Other congenital malformations of great veins**
Absence of vena cava (inferior) (superior)
Azygos continuation of inferior vena cava
Persistent left posterior cardinal vein
Scimitar syndrome

Q26.9 **Congenital malformation of great vein, unspecified** ▽
Congenital anomaly of vena cava (inferior) (superior) NOS

✓4ᵗʰ Q27 **Other congenital malformations of** peripheral vascular system
EXCLUDES 2 *anomalies of cerebral and precerebral vessels (Q28.0-Q28.3)*
anomalies of coronary vessels (Q24.5)
anomalies of pulmonary artery (Q25.5-Q25.7)
congenital retinal aneurysm (Q14.1)
hemangioma and lymphangioma (D18.-)

Q27.0 **Congenital** absence and hypoplasia **of** umbilical artery
Single umbilical artery

Q27.1 **Congenital** renal artery stenosis

Q27.2 **Other congenital malformations of** renal artery
Congenital malformation of renal artery NOS
Multiple renal arteries

✓5ᵗʰ Q27.3 **Arteriovenous malformation (peripheral)**
Arteriovenous aneurysm
EXCLUDES 1 *acquired arteriovenous aneurysm (I77.0)*
EXCLUDES 2 *arteriovenous malformation of cerebral vessels (Q28.2)*
arteriovenous malformation of precerebral vessels (Q28.0)

Q27.30 **Arteriovenous malformation, site unspecified** ▽

Q27.31 **Arteriovenous malformation of** vessel of upper limb

Q27.32 **Arteriovenous malformation of** vessel of lower limb

Q27.33 **Arteriovenous malformation of** digestive system vessel

Q27.34 **Arteriovenous malformation of** renal vessel

Q27.39 **Arteriovenous malformation, other site**

Q27.4 **Congenital** phlebectasia

Q27.8 **Other specified congenital malformations of peripheral vascular system**
Absence of peripheral vascular system
Atresia of peripheral vascular system
Congenital aneurysm (peripheral)
Congenital stricture, artery
Congenital varix
EXCLUDES 1 *arteriovenous malformation (Q27.3-)*

Q27.9 **Congenital malformation of peripheral vascular system, unspecified** ▽
Anomaly of artery or vein NOS

✓4ᵗʰ Q28 Other **congenital malformations of** circulatory system
EXCLUDES 1 *congenital aneurysm NOS (Q27.8)*
congenital coronary aneurysm (Q24.5)
ruptured cerebral arteriovenous malformation (I60.8)
ruptured malformation of precerebral vessels (I72.0)
EXCLUDES 2 *congenital peripheral aneurysm (Q27.8)*
congenital pulmonary aneurysm (Q25.79)
congenital retinal aneurysm (Q14.1)

Q28.0 Arteriovenous **malformation of** precerebral **vessels**
Congenital arteriovenous precerebral aneurysm (nonruptured)

Q28.1 **Other malformations of** precerebral **vessels**
Congenital malformation of precerebral vessels NOS
Congenital precerebral aneurysm (nonruptured)

Q28.2 Arteriovenous **malformation of** cerebral **vessels**
Arteriovenous malformation of brain NOS
Congenital arteriovenous cerebral aneurysm (nonruptured)

Q28.3 **Other malformations of** cerebral **vessels**
Congenital cerebral aneurysm (nonruptured)
Congenital malformation of cerebral vessels NOS
Developmental venous anomaly

Q28.8 **Other specified congenital malformations of circulatory system**
Congenital aneurysm, specified site NEC
Spinal vessel anomaly

Q28.9 **Congenital malformation of circulatory system, unspecified** ▽

Congenital malformations of the respiratory system (Q30-Q34)

✓4ᵗʰ Q30 **Congenital malformations of** nose
EXCLUDES 1 *congenital deviation of nasal septum (Q67.4)*

Q30.0 **Choanal** atresia
Atresia of nares (anterior) (posterior)
Congenital stenosis of nares (anterior) (posterior)

Q30.1 Agenesis **and underdevelopment of nose**
Congenital absent of nose

Q30.2 **Fissured, notched and cleft** nose

Q30.3 **Congenital** perforated **nasal septum**

Q30.8 **Other congenital malformations of nose**
Accessory nose
Congenital anomaly of nasal sinus wall

Q30.9 **Congenital malformation of nose, unspecified** ▽

✓4ᵗʰ Q31 **Congenital malformations of** larynx
EXCLUDES 1 *congenital laryngeal stridor NOS (P28.89)*

Q31.0 Web **of larynx**
Glottic web of larynx
Subglottic web of larynx
Web of larynx NOS

Q31.1 **Congenital** subglottic stenosis

Q31.2 **Laryngeal** hypoplasia

Q31.3 Laryngocele

Q31.5 **Congenital** laryngomalacia

Q31.8 **Other congenital malformations of larynx**
Absence of larynx
Agenesis of larynx
Atresia of larynx
Congenital cleft thyroid cartilage
Congenital fissure of epiglottis
Congenital stenosis of larynx NEC
Posterior cleft of cricoid cartilage

Q31.9 **Congenital malformation of larynx, unspecified** ▽

✓4ᵗʰ Q32 **Congenital malformations of** trachea and bronchus
EXCLUDES 1 *congenital bronchiectasis (Q33.4)*

Q32.0 **Congenital** tracheomalacia

Q32.1 Other congenital malformations of trachea
Atresia of trachea
Congenital anomaly of tracheal cartilage
Congenital dilatation of trachea
Congenital malformation of trachea
Congenital stenosis of trachea
Congenital tracheocele

Q32.2 Congenital bronchomalacia

Q32.3 Congenital stenosis of bronchus

Q32.4 Other congenital malformations of bronchus
Absence of bronchus
Agenesis of bronchus
Atresia of bronchus
Congenital diverticulum of bronchus
Congenital malformation of bronchus NOS

✓4ᵗʰ Q33 Congenital malformations of lung

Q33.0 Congenital cystic **lung**
Congenital cystic lung disease
Congenital honeycomb lung
Congenital polycystic lung disease
EXCLUDES 1   cystic fibrosis (E84.0)
cystic lung disease, acquired or unspecified (J98.4)

Q33.1 Accessory lobe of lung
Azygos lobe (fissured), lung

Q33.2 Sequestration of lung

Q33.3 Agenesis of lung
Congenital absence of lung (lobe)

Q33.4 Congenital bronchiectasis

Q33.5 Ectopic tissue in lung

Q33.6 Congenital hypoplasia and dysplasia **of lung**
EXCLUDES 1   pulmonary hypoplasia associated with short gestation
(P28.0)

Q33.8 Other congenital malformations of lung

Q33.9 Congenital malformation of lung, unspecified   ▽

✓4ᵗʰ Q34 Other congenital malformations of respiratory system
EXCLUDES 2   congenital central alveolar hypoventilation syndrome (G47.35)

Q34.0 Anomaly of pleura

Q34.1 Congenital cyst of mediastinum

Q34.8 Other specified congenital malformations of respiratory system
Atresia of nasopharynx

Q34.9 Congenital malformation of respiratory system, unspecified   ▽
Congenital absence of respiratory system
Congenital anomaly of respiratory system NOS

Cleft lip and cleft palate (Q35-Q37)

Use additional code to identify associated malformation of the nose (Q30.2)
EXCLUDES 1   Robin's syndrome (Q87.0)

✓4ᵗʰ Q35 Cleft palate
INCLUDES   fissure of palate
palatoschisis
EXCLUDES 1   cleft palate with cleft lip (Q37.-)

Q35.1 Cleft hard **palate**

Q35.3 Cleft soft **palate**

Q35.5 Cleft hard **palate** with cleft soft palate

Q35.7 Cleft uvula

Q35.9 Cleft palate, unspecified   ▽
Cleft palate NOS

✓4ᵗʰ Q36 Cleft lip
Cheiloschisis
Congenital fissure of lip
Harelip
Labium leporinum
EXCLUDES 1   cleft lip with cleft palate (Q37.-)

Q36.0 Cleft lip, bilateral

Q36.1 Cleft lip, median

Q36.9 Cleft lip, unilateral
Cleft lip NOS

✓4ᵗʰ Q37 Cleft palate with cleft lip
Cheilopalatoschisis

Q37.0 Cleft hard **palate with** bilateral **cleft lip**

Q37.1 Cleft hard **palate with** unilateral **cleft lip**
Cleft hard palate with cleft lip NOS

Q37.2 Cleft soft **palate with** bilateral **cleft lip**

Q37.3 Cleft soft **palate with** unilateral **cleft lip**
Cleft soft palate with cleft lip NOS

Q37.4 Cleft hard and soft **palate with** bilateral **cleft lip**

Q37.5 Cleft hard and soft **palate with** unilateral **cleft lip**
Cleft hard and soft palate with cleft lip NOS

Q37.8 Unspecified cleft palate with bilateral cleft lip   ▽

Q37.9 Unspecified cleft palate with unilateral cleft lip   ▽
Cleft palate with cleft lip NOS

Other congenital malformations of the digestive system (Q38-Q45)

✓4ᵗʰ Q38 Other congenital malformations of tongue, mouth and pharynx
EXCLUDES 1   dentofacial anomalies (M26.-)
macrostomia (Q18.4)
microstomia (Q18.5)

Q38.0 Congenital malformations of lips, not elsewhere classified
Congenital fistula of lip
Congenital malformation of lip NOS
Van der Woude's syndrome
EXCLUDES 1   cleft lip (Q36.-)
cleft lip with cleft palate (Q37.-)
macrocheilia (Q18.6)
microcheilia (Q18.7)

Q38.1 Ankyloglossia
Tongue tie

Q38.2 Macroglossia
Congenital hypertrophy of tongue

Q38.3 Other congenital malformations of tongue
Aglossia
Bifid tongue
Congenital adhesion of tongue
Congenital fissure of tongue
Congenital malformation of tongue NOS
Double tongue
Hypoglossia
Hypoplasia of tongue
Microglossia

Q38.4 Congenital malformations of salivary glands and ducts
Atresia of salivary glands and ducts
Congenital absence of salivary glands and ducts
Congenital accessory salivary glands and ducts
Congenital fistula of salivary gland

Q38.5 Congenital malformations of palate, not elsewhere classified
Congenital absence of uvula
Congenital malformation of palate NOS
Congenital high arched palate
EXCLUDES 1   cleft palate (Q35.-)
cleft palate with cleft lip (Q37.-)

Q38.6 Other congenital malformations of mouth
Congenital malformation of mouth NOS

Q38.7 Congenital pharyngeal pouch
Congenital diverticulum of pharynx
EXCLUDES 1   pharyngeal pouch syndrome (D82.1)

Q38.8 Other congenital malformations of pharynx
Congenital malformation of pharynx NOS
Imperforate pharynx

✓4ᵗʰ Q39 Congenital malformations of esophagus

Q39.0 Atresia of esophagus without fistula
Atresia of esophagus NOS

Q39.1 Atresia of esophagus with tracheo-esophageal fistula
Atresia of esophagus with broncho-esophageal fistula

Q39.2 Congenital tracheo-esophageal fistula without atresia
Congenital tracheo-esophageal fistula NOS

Q39.3 Congenital stenosis and stricture **of esophagus**

Q39.4 Esophageal web

Q39.5 Congenital dilatation **of esophagus**
Congenital cardiospasm

Q39.6 Congenital diverticulum **of esophagus**
Congenital esophageal pouch

Q39.8 Other congenital malformations of esophagus
Congenital absence of esophagus
Congenital displacement of esophagus
Congenital duplication of esophagus

Q39.9 Congenital malformation of esophagus, unspecified   ▽

Ⓝ Newborn   Ⓟ Pediatric   Ⓜ Maternity   Ⓐ Adult   RIC RIC Dx   NC Dx Noncancer Dx   PDx Primary Dx   CC RIC CC Condition   ▶◀ Revised Text   ● New Code   ▲ Revised Code Title

822   ICD-10-CM 2016

✓4th Q40   Other congenital malformations of upper alimentary tract

Q40.0 Congenital hypertrophic pyloric stenosis
Congenital or infantile constriction
Congenital or infantile hypertrophy
Congenital or infantile spasm
Congenital or infantile stenosis
Congenital or infantile stricture

Q40.1 Congenital hiatus hernia
Congenital displacement of cardia through esophageal hiatus
EXCLUDES 1   *congenital diaphragmatic hernia (Q79.0)*

Q40.2 Other specified congenital malformations of stomach
Congenital displacement of stomach
Congenital diverticulum of stomach
Congenital hourglass stomach
Congenital duplication of stomach
Megalogastria
Microgastria

Q40.3 Congenital malformation of stomach, unspecified ▽

Q40.8 Other specified congenital malformations of upper alimentary tract

Q40.9 Congenital malformation of upper alimentary tract, unspecified ▽
Congenital anomaly of upper alimentary tract
Congenital deformity of upper alimentary tract

✓4th Q41   Congenital absence, atresia and stenosis of small intestine
Congenital obstruction, occlusion or stricture of small intestine or intestine NOS
EXCLUDES 1   *cystic fibrosis with intestinal manifestation (E84.11)*
meconium ileus NOS (without cystic fibrosis) (P76.0)

Q41.0 Congenital absence, atresia and stenosis of duodenum

Q41.1 Congenital absence, atresia and stenosis of jejunum
Apple peel syndrome
Imperforate jejunum

Q41.2 Congenital absence, atresia and stenosis of ileum

Q41.8 Congenital absence, atresia and stenosis of other specified parts of small intestine

Q41.9 Congenital absence, atresia and stenosis of small intestine, part unspecified ▽
Congenital absence, atresia and stenosis of intestine NOS

✓4th Q42   Congenital absence, atresia and stenosis of large intestine
Congenital obstruction, occlusion and stricture of large intestine

Q42.0 Congenital absence, atresia and stenosis of rectum with fistula

Q42.1 Congenital absence, atresia and stenosis of rectum without fistula
Imperforate rectum

Q42.2 Congenital absence, atresia and stenosis of anus with fistula

Q42.3 Congenital absence, atresia and stenosis of anus without fistula
Imperforate anus

Q42.8 Congenital absence, atresia and stenosis of other parts of large intestine

Q42.9 Congenital absence, atresia and stenosis of large intestine, part unspecified ▽

✓4th Q43   Other congenital malformations of intestine

Q43.0 Meckel's diverticulum (displaced) (hypertrophic)
Persistent omphalomesenteric duct
Persistent vitelline duct

Q43.1 Hirschsprung's disease
Aganglionosis
Congenital (aganglionic) megacolon

Q43.2 Other congenital functional disorders of colon
Congenital dilatation of colon

Q43.3 Congenital malformations of intestinal fixation
Congenital omental, anomalous adhesions [bands]
Congenital peritoneal adhesions [bands]
Incomplete rotation of cecum and colon
Insufficient rotation of cecum and colon
Jackson's membrane
Malrotation of colon
Rotation failure of cecum and colon
Universal mesentery

Q43.4 Duplication of intestine

Q43.5 Ectopic anus

Q43.6 Congenital fistula of rectum and anus
EXCLUDES 1   *congenital fistula of anus with absence, atresia and stenosis (Q42.2)*
congenital fistula of rectum with absence, atresia and stenosis (Q42.0)
congenital rectovaginal fistula (Q52.2)
congenital urethrorectal fistula (Q64.73)
pilonidal fistula or sinus (L05.-)

Q43.7 Persistent cloaca
Cloaca NOS

Q43.8 Other specified congenital malformations of intestine
Congenital blind loop syndrome
Congenital diverticulitis, colon
Congenital diverticulum, intestine
Dolichocolon
Megaloappendix
Megaloduodenum
Microcolon
Transposition of appendix
Transposition of colon
Transposition of intestine
AHA: 2013, 2Q, 31

Q43.9 Congenital malformation of intestine, unspecified ▽

✓4th Q44   Congenital malformations of gallbladder, bile ducts and liver

Q44.0 Agenesis, aplasia and hypoplasia of gallbladder
Congenital absence of gallbladder

Q44.1 Other congenital malformations of gallbladder
Congenital malformation of gallbladder NOS
Intrahepatic gallbladder

Q44.2 Atresia of bile ducts

Q44.3 Congenital stenosis and stricture of bile ducts

Q44.4 Choledochal cyst

Q44.5 Other congenital malformations of bile ducts
Accessory hepatic duct
Biliary duct duplication
Congenital malformation of bile duct NOS
Cystic duct duplication

Q44.6 Cystic disease of liver
Fibrocystic disease of liver

Q44.7 Other congenital malformations of liver
Accessory liver
Alagille's syndrome
Congenital absence of liver
Congenital hepatomegaly
Congenital malformation of liver NOS

✓4th Q45   Other congenital malformations of digestive system
EXCLUDES 2   *congenital diaphragmatic hernia (Q79.0)*
congenital hiatus hernia (Q40.1)

Q45.0 Agenesis, aplasia and hypoplasia of pancreas
Congenital absence of pancreas

Q45.1 Annular pancreas

Q45.2 Congenital pancreatic cyst

Q45.3 Other congenital malformations of pancreas and pancreatic duct
Accessory pancreas
Congenital malformation of pancreas or pancreatic duct NOS
EXCLUDES 1   *congenital diabetes mellitus (E10.-)*
cystic fibrosis (E84.0-E84.9)
fibrocystic disease of pancreas (E84.-)
neonatal diabetes mellitus (P70.2)

Q45.8 Other specified congenital malformations of digestive system
Absence (complete) (partial) of alimentary tract NOS
Duplication of digestive system
Malposition, congenital of digestive system

Q45.9 Congenital malformation of digestive system, unspecified ▽
Congenital anomaly of digestive system
Congenital deformity of digestive system

Congenital malformations of genital organs (Q50-Q56)
EXCLUDES 1   *androgen insensitivity syndrome (E34.5-)*
syndromes associated with anomalies in the number and form of chromosomes (Q90-Q99)

✓4th Q50   Congenital malformations of ovaries, fallopian tubes and broad ligaments

✓5th Q50.0 Congenital absence of ovary
EXCLUDES 1   *Turner's syndrome (Q96.-)*

    Q50.01 Congenital absence of ovary, unilateral ♀

    Q50.02 Congenital absence of ovary, bilateral ♀

☑ Add'l Character Required   ✓x7th Placeholder Alert   RUG IV Special Care High Dx   RUG IV Clinically Complex Dx   RUG IV Special Care Low Dx   Manifestation Code   Other Specified Code   ▽ Unspecified Code

Chapter 17. Congenital Malformations, Deformations and Chromosomal Abnormalities

Q50.1-Q55.61

Q50.1   Developmental ovarian cyst ♀

Q50.2   Congenital torsion of ovary ♀

✓5ᵗʰ **Q50.3**   Other congenital malformations of ovary

     Q50.31   Accessory ovary ♀

     Q50.32   Ovarian streak ♀
         46, XX with streak gonads

     Q50.39   Other congenital malformation of ovary ♀
         Congenital malformation of ovary NOS

Q50.4   Embryonic cyst of fallopian tube ♀
     Fimbrial cyst

Q50.5   Embryonic cyst of broad ligament ♀
     Epoophoron cyst
     Parovarian cyst

Q50.6   Other congenital malformations of fallopian tube and broad ligament ♀
     Absence of fallopian tube and broad ligament
     Accessory fallopian tube and broad ligament
     Atresia of fallopian tube and broad ligament
     Congenital malformation of fallopian tube or broad ligament NOS

✓4ᵗʰ **Q51**   **Congenital malformations of uterus and cervix**

Q51.0   Agenesis and aplasia of uterus ♀
     Congenital absence of uterus

✓5ᵗʰ **Q51.1**   Doubling of uterus with doubling of cervix and vagina

     Q51.10   Doubling of uterus with doubling of cervix and vagina without obstruction ♀
         Doubling of uterus with doubling of cervix and vagina NOS

     Q51.11   Doubling of uterus with doubling of cervix and vagina with obstruction ♀

Q51.2   Other doubling of uterus ♀
     Doubling of uterus NOS
     Septate uterus, complete or partial

Q51.3   Bicornate uterus ♀
     Bicornate uterus, complete or partial

Q51.4   Unicornate uterus ♀
     Unicornate uterus with or without a separate uterine horn
     Uterus with only one functioning horn

Q51.5   Agenesis and aplasia of cervix ♀
     Congenital absence of cervix

Q51.6   Embryonic cyst of cervix ♀

Q51.7   Congenital fistulae between uterus and digestive and urinary tracts ♀

✓5ᵗʰ **Q51.8**   Other congenital malformations of uterus and cervix

     ✓6ᵗʰ **Q51.81**   Other congenital malformations of uterus

         Q51.810   Arcuate uterus ♀
             Arcuatus uterus

         Q51.811   Hypoplasia of uterus ♀

         Q51.818   Other congenital malformations of uterus ♀
             Müllerian anomaly of uterus NEC

     ✓6ᵗʰ **Q51.82**   Other congenital malformations of cervix

         Q51.820   Cervical duplication ♀

         Q51.821   Hypoplasia of cervix ♀

         Q51.828   Other congenital malformations of cervix ♀

Q51.9   Congenital malformation of uterus and cervix, unspecified ♀▽

✓4ᵗʰ **Q52**   **Other congenital malformations of female genitalia**

Q52.0   Congenital absence of vagina ♀
     Vaginal agenesis, total or partial

✓5ᵗʰ **Q52.1**   Doubling of vagina
     EXCLUDES 1   doubling of vagina with doubling of uterus and cervix (Q51.1-)

     Q52.10   Doubling of vagina, unspecified ♀▽
         Septate vagina NOS

     Q52.11   Transverse vaginal septum ♀

     Q52.12   Longitudinal vaginal septum ♀
         Longitudinal vaginal septum with or without obstruction

Q52.2   Congenital rectovaginal fistula ♀
     EXCLUDES 1   cloaca (Q43.7)

Q52.3   Imperforate hymen ♀

Q52.4   Other congenital malformations of vagina ♀
     Canal of Nuck cyst, congenital
     Congenital malformation of vagina NOS
     Embryonic vaginal cyst
     Gartner's duct cyst

Q52.5   Fusion of labia ♀

Q52.6   Congenital malformation of clitoris ♀

✓5ᵗʰ **Q52.7**   Other and unspecified congenital malformations of vulva ♀▽

     Q52.70   Unspecified congenital malformations of vulva ♀▽
         Congenital malformation of vulva NOS

     Q52.71   Congenital absence of vulva ♀

     Q52.79   Other congenital malformations of vulva ♀
         Congenital cyst of vulva

Q52.8   Other specified congenital malformations of female genitalia ♀

Q52.9   Congenital malformation of female genitalia, unspecified ♀▽

✓4ᵗʰ **Q53**   **Undescended and ectopic testicle**

✓5ᵗʰ **Q53.0**   Ectopic testis

     Q53.00   Ectopic testis, unspecified ♂▽

     Q53.01   Ectopic testis, unilateral ♂

     Q53.02   Ectopic testes, bilateral ♂

✓5ᵗʰ **Q53.1**   Undescended testicle, unilateral

     Q53.10   Unspecified undescended testicle, unilateral ♂▽

     Q53.11   Abdominal testis, unilateral ♂

     Q53.12   Ectopic perineal testis, unilateral ♂

✓5ᵗʰ **Q53.2**   Undescended testicle, bilateral

     Q53.20   Undescended testicle, unspecified, bilateral ♂▽

     Q53.21   Abdominal testis, bilateral ♂

     Q53.22   Ectopic perineal testis, bilateral ♂

Q53.9   Undescended testicle, unspecified ♂▽
     Cryptorchism NOS

✓4ᵗʰ **Q54**   **Hypospadias**
     EXCLUDES 1   epispadias (Q64.0)

Q54.0   Hypospadias, balanic ♂
     Hypospadias, coronal
     Hypospadias, glandular

Q54.1   Hypospadias, penile ♂

Q54.2   Hypospadias, penoscrotal ♂

Q54.3   Hypospadias, perineal ♂

Q54.4   Congenital chordee ♂
     Chordee without hypospadias

Q54.8   Other hypospadias ♂
     Hypospadias with intersex state

Q54.9   Hypospadias, unspecified ♂▽

✓4ᵗʰ **Q55**   **Other congenital malformations of male genital organs**
     EXCLUDES 1   congenital hydrocele (P83.5)
                hypospadias (Q54.-)

Q55.0   Absence and aplasia of testis ♂
     Monorchism

Q55.1   Hypoplasia of testis and scrotum ♂
     Fusion of testes

✓5ᵗʰ **Q55.2**   Other and unspecified congenital malformations of testis and scrotum

     Q55.20   Unspecified congenital malformations of testis and scrotum ♂▽
         Congenital malformation of testis or scrotum NOS

     Q55.21   Polyorchism ♂

     Q55.22   Retractile testis ♂

     Q55.23   Scrotal transposition ♂

     Q55.29   Other congenital malformations of testis and scrotum ♂

Q55.3   Atresia of vas deferens ♂
     Code first any associated cystic fibrosis (E84.-)

Q55.4   Other congenital malformations of vas deferens, epididymis, seminal vesicles and prostate ♂
     Absence or aplasia of prostate
     Absence or aplasia of spermatic cord
     Congenital malformation of vas deferens, epididymis, seminal vesicles or prostate NOS

Q55.5   Congenital absence and aplasia of penis ♂

✓5ᵗʰ **Q55.6**   Other congenital malformations of penis

     Q55.61   Curvature of penis (lateral) ♂

Q55.62 Hypoplasia of penis ♂
Micropenis

Q55.63 Congenital torsion of penis ♂
EXCLUDES 1 *acquired torsion of penis (N48.82)*

Q55.64 Hidden penis ♂
Buried penis
Concealed penis
EXCLUDES 1 *acquired buried penis (N48.83)*

Q55.69 Other congenital malformation of penis ♂
Congenital malformation of penis NOS

Q55.7 Congenital vasocutaneous fistula ♂

Q55.8 Other specified congenital malformations of male genital organs ♂

Q55.9 Congenital malformation of male genital organ, unspecified ♂ ▽
Congenital anomaly of male genital organ
Congenital deformity of male genital organ

✓4ᵗʰ Q56 Indeterminate sex and pseudohermaphroditism
EXCLUDES 1 *46, XX true hermaphrodite (Q99.1)*
androgen insensitivity syndrome (E34.5-)
chimera 46, XX/46, XY true hermaphrodite (Q99.0)
female pseudohermaphroditism with adrenocortical disorder (E25.-)
pseudohermaphroditism with specified chromosomal anomaly (Q96-Q99)
pure gonadal dysgenesis (Q99.1)

Q56.0 Hermaphroditism, not elsewhere classified
Ovotestis

Q56.1 Male pseudohermaphroditism, not elsewhere classified ♂
46, XY with streak gonads
Male pseudohermaphroditism NOS

Q56.2 Female pseudohermaphroditism, not elsewhere classified ♀
Female pseudohermaphroditism NOS

Q56.3 Pseudohermaphroditism, unspecified ▽

Q56.4 Indeterminate sex, unspecified ▽
Ambiguous genitalia

Congenital malformations of the urinary system (Q60-Q64)

✓4ᵗʰ Q60 Renal agenesis and other reduction defects of kidney
Congenital absence of kidney
Congenital atrophy of kidney
Infantile atrophy of kidney

Q60.0 Renal agenesis, unilateral

Q60.1 Renal agenesis, bilateral

Q60.2 Renal agenesis, unspecified ▽

Q60.3 Renal hypoplasia, unilateral

Q60.4 Renal hypoplasia, bilateral

Q60.5 Renal hypoplasia, unspecified ▽

Q60.6 Potter's syndrome

✓4ᵗʰ Q61 Cystic kidney disease
EXCLUDES 1 *acquired cyst of kidney (N28.1)*
Potter's syndrome (Q60.6)

✓5ᵗʰ Q61.0 Congenital renal cyst
Q61.00 Congenital renal cyst, unspecified ▽
Cyst of kidney NOS (congenital)
Q61.01 Congenital single renal cyst
Q61.02 Congenital multiple renal cysts

✓5ᵗʰ Q61.1 Polycystic kidney, infantile type
Polycystic kidney, autosomal recessive
Q61.11 Cystic dilatation of collecting ducts
Q61.19 Other polycystic kidney, infantile type

Q61.2 Polycystic kidney, adult type
Polycystic kidney, autosomal dominant

Q61.3 Polycystic kidney, unspecified ▽

Q61.4 Renal dysplasia
Multicystic dysplastic kidney
Multicystic kidney (development)
Multicystic kidney disease
Multicystic renal dysplasia
EXCLUDES 1 *polycystic kidney disease (Q61.11-Q61.3)*

Q61.5 Medullary cystic kidney
Nephronopthisis
Sponge kidney NOS

Q61.8 Other cystic kidney diseases
Fibrocystic kidney
Fibrocystic renal degeneration or disease

Q61.9 Cystic kidney disease, unspecified ▽
Meckel-Gruber syndrome

✓4ᵗʰ Q62 Congenital obstructive defects of renal pelvis and congenital malformations of ureter

Q62.0 Congenital hydronephrosis

✓5ᵗʰ Q62.1 Congenital occlusion of ureter
Atresia and stenosis of ureter
Q62.10 Congenital occlusion of ureter, unspecified ▽
Q62.11 Congenital occlusion of ureteropelvic junction
Q62.12 Congenital occlusion of ureterovesical orifice

Q62.2 Congenital megaureter
Congenital dilatation of ureter

✓5ᵗʰ Q62.3 Other obstructive defects of renal pelvis and ureter
Q62.31 Congenital ureterocele, orthotopic
Q62.32 Cecoureterocele
Ectopic ureterocele
Q62.39 Other obstructive defects of renal pelvis and ureter
Ureteropelvic junction obstruction NOS

Q62.4 Agenesis of ureter
Congenital absence ureter

Q62.5 Duplication of ureter
Accessory ureter
Double ureter

✓5ᵗʰ Q62.6 Malposition of ureter
Q62.60 Malposition of ureter, unspecified ▽
Q62.61 Deviation of ureter
Q62.62 Displacement of ureter
Q62.63 Anomalous implantation of ureter
Ectopia of ureter
Ectopic ureter
Q62.69 Other malposition of ureter

Q62.7 Congenital vesico-uretero-renal reflux

Q62.8 Other congenital malformations of ureter
Anomaly of ureter NOS

✓4ᵗʰ Q63 Other congenital malformations of kidney
EXCLUDES 1 *congenital nephrotic syndrome (N04.-)*

Q63.0 Accessory kidney

Q63.1 Lobulated, fused and horseshoe kidney

Q63.2 Ectopic kidney
Congenital displaced kidney
Malrotation of kidney

Q63.3 Hyperplastic and giant kidney
Compensatory hypertrophy of kidney

Q63.8 Other specified congenital malformations of kidney
Congenital renal calculi

Q63.9 Congenital malformation of kidney, unspecified ▽

✓4ᵗʰ Q64 Other congenital malformations of urinary system

Q64.0 Epispadias ♂
EXCLUDES 1 *hypospadias (Q54.-)*

✓5ᵗʰ Q64.1 Exstrophy of urinary bladder
Q64.10 Exstrophy of urinary bladder, unspecified ▽
Ectopia vesicae
Q64.11 Supravesical fissure of urinary bladder
Q64.12 Cloacal extrophy of urinary bladder
Q64.19 Other exstrophy of urinary bladder
Extroversion of bladder

Q64.2 Congenital posterior urethral valves

✓5ᵗʰ Q64.3 Other atresia and stenosis of urethra and bladder neck
Q64.31 Congenital bladder neck obstruction
Congenital obstruction of vesicourethral orifice
Q64.32 Congenital stricture of urethra
Q64.33 Congenital stricture of urinary meatus
Q64.39 Other atresia and stenosis of urethra and bladder neck
Atresia and stenosis of urethra and bladder neck NOS

Q64.4 Malformation of urachus
Cyst of urachus
Patent urachus
Prolapse of urachus

Q64.5 Congenital absence of bladder and urethra

Q64.6 Congenital diverticulum of bladder

☑ Add'l Character Required   ✓×7ᵗʰ Placeholder Alert   RUG IV Special Care High Dx   RUG IV Clinically Complex Dx   RUG IV Special Care Low Dx   Manifestation Code   Other Specified Code   ▽ Unspecified Code

✓5th **Q64.7** Other and unspecified **congenital malformations of bladder and urethra**
> EXCLUDES 1 *congenital prolapse of bladder (mucosa) (Q79.4)*

Q64.70 **Unspecified congenital malformation of bladder and urethra** ▽
> Malformation of bladder or urethra NOS

Q64.71 **Congenital** prolapse of urethra

Q64.72 **Congenital** prolapse of urinary meatus

Q64.73 **Congenital** urethrorectal fistula

Q64.74 Double urethra

Q64.75 Double urinary meatus

Q64.79 **Other congenital malformations of bladder and urethra**

Q64.8 **Other specified congenital malformations of urinary system**

Q64.9 **Congenital malformation of urinary system, unspecified** ▽
> Congenital anomaly NOS of urinary system
> Congenital deformity NOS of urinary system

Congenital malformations and deformations of the musculoskeletal system (Q65-Q79)

✓4th **Q65** **Congenital deformities of** hip
> EXCLUDES 1 *clicking hip (R29.4)*

✓5th **Q65.0** **Congenital** dislocation of hip, unilateral

Q65.00 **Congenital dislocation of unspecified hip, unilateral** ▽

Q65.01 **Congenital dislocation of** right **hip, unilateral**

Q65.02 **Congenital dislocation of** left **hip, unilateral**

Q65.1 **Congenital** dislocation of hip, bilateral

Q65.2 **Congenital dislocation of hip, unspecified** ▽

✓5th **Q65.3** **Congenital** partial dislocation of hip, unilateral

Q65.30 **Congenital partial dislocation of unspecified hip, unilateral** ▽

Q65.31 **Congenital partial dislocation of** right **hip, unilateral**

Q65.32 **Congenital partial dislocation of** left **hip, unilateral**

Q65.4 **Congenital** partial dislocation of hip, bilateral

Q65.5 **Congenital partial dislocation of hip, unspecified** ▽

Q65.6 **Congenital** unstable **hip**
> Congenital dislocatable hip

✓5th **Q65.8** Other **congenital deformities of hip**

Q65.81 **Congenital** coxa valga

Q65.82 **Congenital** coxa vara

Q65.89 **Other specified congenital deformities of hip**
> Anteversion of femoral neck
> Congenital acetabular dysplasia

Q65.9 **Congenital deformity of hip, unspecified** ▽

✓4th **Q66** **Congenital deformities of** feet
> EXCLUDES 1 *reduction defects of feet (Q72.-)*
> *valgus deformities (acquired) (M21.0-)*
> *varus deformities (acquired) (M21.1-)*

Q66.0 **Congenital** talipes equinovarus

Q66.1 **Congenital** talipes calcaneovarus

Q66.2 **Congenital** metatarsus (primus) varus

Q66.3 **Other congenital varus deformities of feet**
> Hallux varus, congenital

Q66.4 **Congenital** talipes calcaneovalgus

✓5th **Q66.5** **Congenital** pes planus
> Congenital flat foot
> Congenital rigid flat foot
> Congenital spastic (everted) flat foot
> EXCLUDES 1 *pes planus, acquired (M21.4)*

Q66.50 **Congenital pes planus, unspecified foot** ▽

Q66.51 **Congenital pes planus,** right **foot**

Q66.52 **Congenital pes planus,** left **foot**

Q66.6 **Other congenital valgus deformities of feet**
> Congenital metatarsus valgus

Q66.7 **Congenital** pes cavus

✓5th **Q66.8** Other **congenital deformities of feet**

Q66.80 **Congenital vertical talus deformity, unspecified foot** ▽

Q66.81 **Congenital vertical talus deformity,** right **foot**

Q66.82 **Congenital vertical talus deformity,** left **foot**

Q66.89 **Other specified congenital deformities of feet**
> Congenital asymmetric talipes
> Congenital clubfoot NOS
> Congenital talipes NOS
> Congenital tarsal coalition
> Hammer toe, congenital

Q66.9 **Congenital deformity of feet, unspecified** ▽

✓4th **Q67** **Congenital musculoskeletal deformities of** head, face, spine and chest
> EXCLUDES 1 *congenital malformation syndromes classified to Q87-*
> *Potter's syndrome (Q60.6)*

Q67.0 **Congenital** facial asymmetry

Q67.1 **Congenital** compression facies

Q67.2 Dolichocephaly

Q67.3 Plagiocephaly

Q67.4 **Other congenital deformities of skull, face and jaw**
> Congenital depressions in skull
> Congenital hemifacial atrophy or hypertrophy
> Deviation of nasal septum, congenital
> Squashed or bent nose, congenital
> EXCLUDES 1 *dentofacial anomalies [including malocclusion] (M26.-)*
> *syphilitic saddle nose (A50.5)*

Q67.5 **Congenital deformity of** spine
> Congenital postural scoliosis
> Congenital scoliosis NOS
> EXCLUDES 1 *infantile idiopathic scoliosis (M41.0)*
> *scoliosis due to congenital bony malformation (Q76.3)*
> **AHA:** 2014, 4Q, 26

Q67.6 Pectus excavatum
> Congenital funnel chest

Q67.7 Pectus carinatum
> Congenital pigeon chest

Q67.8 **Other congenital deformities of chest**
> Congenital deformity of chest wall NOS

✓4th **Q68** Other **congenital musculoskeletal deformities**
> EXCLUDES 1 *reduction defects of limb(s) (Q71-Q73)*
> EXCLUDES 2 *congenital myotonic chondrodystrophy (G71.13)*

Q68.0 **Congenital deformity of** sternocleidomastoid muscle
> Congenital contracture of sternocleidomastoid (muscle)
> Congenital (sternomastoid) torticollis
> Sternomastoid tumor (congenital)

Q68.1 **Congenital deformity of** finger(s) and hand
> Congenital clubfinger
> Spade-like hand (congenital)

Q68.2 **Congenital deformity of** knee
> Congenital dislocation of knee
> Congenital genu recurvatum

Q68.3 **Congenital bowing of** femur
> EXCLUDES 1 *anteversion of femur (neck) (Q65.89)*

Q68.4 **Congenital bowing of** tibia and fibula

Q68.5 **Congenital bowing of long bones of leg, unspecified** ▽

Q68.6 Discoid meniscus

Q68.8 **Other specified congenital musculoskeletal deformities**
> Congenital deformity of clavicle
> Congenital deformity of elbow
> Congenital deformity of forearm
> Congenital deformity of scapula
> Congenital deformity of wrist
> Congenital dislocation of elbow
> Congenital dislocation of shoulder
> Congenital dislocation of wrist

✓4th **Q69** **Polydactyly**

Q69.0 **Accessory** finger(s)

Q69.1 **Accessory** thumb(s)

Q69.2 **Accessory** toe(s)
> Accessory hallux

Q69.9 **Polydactyly, unspecified** ▽
> Supernumerary digit(s) NOS

✓4th **Q70** **Syndactyly**

✓5th **Q70.0** Fused fingers
> Complex syndactyly of fingers with synostosis

Q70.00 **Fused fingers, unspecified hand** ▽

Q70.01 **Fused fingers,** right **hand**

Q70.02 **Fused fingers,** left **hand**

Q70.03 **Fused fingers, bilateral**

N Newborn   P Pediatric   M Maternity   A Adult   RIC RIC Dx   NC Dx Noncancer Dx   PD Primary Dx   CC RIC CC Condition   ►◄ Revised Text   ● New Code   ▲ Revised Code Title

826

ICD-10-CM 2016

✓5ᵗʰ Q70.1 Webbed fingers
Simple syndactyly of fingers without synostosis
- **Q70.10 Webbed fingers, unspecified hand** ▽
- **Q70.11 Webbed fingers, right hand**
- **Q70.12 Webbed fingers, left hand**
- **Q70.13 Webbed fingers, bilateral**

✓5ᵗʰ Q70.2 Fused toes
Complex syndactyly of toes with synostosis
- **Q70.20 Fused toes, unspecified foot** ▽
- **Q70.21 Fused toes, right foot**
- **Q70.22 Fused toes, left foot**
- **Q70.23 Fused toes, bilateral**

✓5ᵗʰ Q70.3 Webbed toes
Simple syndactyly of toes without synostosis
- **Q70.30 Webbed toes, unspecified foot** ▽
- **Q70.31 Webbed toes, right foot**
- **Q70.32 Webbed toes, left foot**
- **Q70.33 Webbed toes, bilateral**

Q70.4 Polysyndactyly, unspecified ▽
EXCLUDES 1 specified syndactyly of hand and feet—code to specified conditions (Q70.0-Q70.3-)

Q70.9 Syndactyly, unspecified ▽
Symphalangy NOS

✓4ᵗʰ Q71 Reduction defects of upper limb
✓5ᵗʰ Q71.0 Congenital complete absence of upper limb
- **Q71.00 Congenital complete absence of unspecified upper limb** ▽
- **Q71.01 Congenital complete absence of right upper limb**
- **Q71.02 Congenital complete absence of left upper limb**
- **Q71.03 Congenital complete absence of upper limb, bilateral**

✓5ᵗʰ Q71.1 Congenital absence of upper arm and forearm with hand present
- **Q71.10 Congenital absence of unspecified upper arm and forearm with hand present** ▽
- **Q71.11 Congenital absence of right upper arm and forearm with hand present**
- **Q71.12 Congenital absence of left upper arm and forearm with hand present**
- **Q71.13 Congenital absence of upper arm and forearm with hand present, bilateral**

✓5ᵗʰ Q71.2 Congenital absence of both forearm and hand
- **Q71.20 Congenital absence of both forearm and hand, unspecified upper limb** ▽
- **Q71.21 Congenital absence of both forearm and hand, right upper limb**
- **Q71.22 Congenital absence of both forearm and hand, left upper limb**
- **Q71.23 Congenital absence of both forearm and hand, bilateral**

✓5ᵗʰ Q71.3 Congenital absence of hand and finger
- **Q71.30 Congenital absence of unspecified hand and finger** ▽
- **Q71.31 Congenital absence of right hand and finger**
- **Q71.32 Congenital absence of left hand and finger**
- **Q71.33 Congenital absence of hand and finger, bilateral**

✓5ᵗʰ Q71.4 Longitudinal reduction defect of radius
Clubhand (congenital)
Radial clubhand
- **Q71.40 Longitudinal reduction defect of unspecified radius** ▽
- **Q71.41 Longitudinal reduction defect of right radius**
- **Q71.42 Longitudinal reduction defect of left radius**
- **Q71.43 Longitudinal reduction defect of radius, bilateral**

✓5ᵗʰ Q71.5 Longitudinal reduction defect of ulna
- **Q71.50 Longitudinal reduction defect of unspecified ulna** ▽
- **Q71.51 Longitudinal reduction defect of right ulna**
- **Q71.52 Longitudinal reduction defect of left ulna**
- **Q71.53 Longitudinal reduction defect of ulna, bilateral**

✓5ᵗʰ Q71.6 Lobster-claw hand
- **Q71.60 Lobster-claw hand, unspecified hand** ▽
- **Q71.61 Lobster-claw right hand**

- **Q71.62 Lobster-claw left hand**
- **Q71.63 Lobster-claw hand, bilateral**

✓5ᵗʰ Q71.8 Other reduction defects of upper limb
✓6ᵗʰ Q71.81 Congenital shortening of upper limb
- **Q71.811 Congenital shortening of right upper limb**
- **Q71.812 Congenital shortening of left upper limb**
- **Q71.813 Congenital shortening of upper limb, bilateral**
- **Q71.819 Congenital shortening of unspecified upper limb** ▽

✓6ᵗʰ Q71.89 Other reduction defects of upper limb
- **Q71.891 Other reduction defects of right upper limb**
- **Q71.892 Other reduction defects of left upper limb**
- **Q71.893 Other reduction defects of upper limb, bilateral**
- **Q71.899 Other reduction defects of unspecified upper limb** ▽

✓5ᵗʰ Q71.9 Unspecified reduction defect of upper limb
- **Q71.90 Unspecified reduction defect of unspecified upper limb** ▽
- **Q71.91 Unspecified reduction defect of right upper limb** ▽
- **Q71.92 Unspecified reduction defect of left upper limb** ▽
- **Q71.93 Unspecified reduction defect of upper limb, bilateral** ▽

✓4ᵗʰ Q72 Reduction defects of lower limb
✓5ᵗʰ Q72.0 Congenital complete absence of lower limb
- **Q72.00 Congenital complete absence of unspecified lower limb** ▽
- **Q72.01 Congenital complete absence of right lower limb**
- **Q72.02 Congenital complete absence of left lower limb**
- **Q72.03 Congenital complete absence of lower limb, bilateral**

✓5ᵗʰ Q72.1 Congenital absence of thigh and lower leg with foot present
- **Q72.10 Congenital absence of unspecified thigh and lower leg with foot present** ▽
- **Q72.11 Congenital absence of right thigh and lower leg with foot present**
- **Q72.12 Congenital absence of left thigh and lower leg with foot present**
- **Q72.13 Congenital absence of thigh and lower leg with foot present, bilateral**

✓5ᵗʰ Q72.2 Congenital absence of both lower leg and foot
- **Q72.20 Congenital absence of both lower leg and foot, unspecified lower limb** ▽
- **Q72.21 Congenital absence of both lower leg and foot, right lower limb**
- **Q72.22 Congenital absence of both lower leg and foot, left lower limb**
- **Q72.23 Congenital absence of both lower leg and foot, bilateral**

✓5ᵗʰ Q72.3 Congenital absence of foot and toe(s)
- **Q72.30 Congenital absence of unspecified foot and toe(s)** ▽
- **Q72.31 Congenital absence of right foot and toe(s)**
- **Q72.32 Congenital absence of left foot and toe(s)**
- **Q72.33 Congenital absence of foot and toe(s), bilateral**

✓5ᵗʰ Q72.4 Longitudinal reduction defect of femur
Proximal femoral focal deficiency
- **Q72.40 Longitudinal reduction defect of unspecified femur** ▽
- **Q72.41 Longitudinal reduction defect of right femur**
- **Q72.42 Longitudinal reduction defect of left femur**
- **Q72.43 Longitudinal reduction defect of femur, bilateral**

✓5ᵗʰ Q72.5 Longitudinal reduction defect of tibia
- **Q72.50 Longitudinal reduction defect of unspecified tibia** ▽
- **Q72.51 Longitudinal reduction defect of right tibia**
- **Q72.52 Longitudinal reduction defect of left tibia**
- **Q72.53 Longitudinal reduction defect of tibia, bilateral**

✓5ᵗʰ Q72.6 Longitudinal reduction defect of fibula
- **Q72.60 Longitudinal reduction defect of unspecified fibula** ▽
- **Q72.61 Longitudinal reduction defect of right fibula**

✓ Add'l Character Required   ✓⁷ᵗʰ Placeholder Alert   RUG IV Special Care High Dx   RUG IV Clinically Complex Dx   RUG IV Special Care Low Dx   Manifestation Code   Other Specified Code   ▽ Unspecified Code

Chapter 17. Congenital Malformations, Deformations and Chromosomal Abnormalities

Q72.62   **Longitudinal reduction defect of** left **fibula**

Q72.63   **Longitudinal reduction defect of fibula,** bilateral

✓5ᵗʰ **Q72.7   Split foot**

    Q72.70   **Split foot, unspecified lower limb** ▽

    Q72.71   **Split foot,** right **lower limb**

    Q72.72   **Split foot,** left **lower limb**

    Q72.73   **Split foot,** bilateral

✓5ᵗʰ **Q72.8   Other reduction defects of lower limb**

   ✓6ᵗʰ **Q72.81   Congenital** shortening **of lower limb**

     Q72.811   **Congenital shortening of** right **lower limb**

     Q72.812   **Congenital shortening of** left **lower limb**

     Q72.813   **Congenital shortening of lower limb, bilateral**

     Q72.819   **Congenital shortening of unspecified lower limb** ▽

   ✓6ᵗʰ **Q72.89   Other reduction defects of lower limb**

     Q72.891   **Other reduction defects of** right **lower limb**

     Q72.892   **Other reduction defects of** left **lower limb**

     Q72.893   **Other reduction defects of lower limb, bilateral**

     Q72.899   **Other reduction defects of unspecified lower limb** ▽

✓5ᵗʰ **Q72.9   Unspecified reduction defect of lower limb**

    Q72.90   **Unspecified reduction defect of unspecified lower limb** ▽

    Q72.91   **Unspecified reduction defect of** right **lower limb** ▽

    Q72.92   **Unspecified reduction defect of** left **lower limb** ▽

    Q72.93   **Unspecified reduction defect of lower limb, bilateral** ▽

✓4ᵗʰ **Q73   Reduction defects of** unspecified limb

Q73.0   **Congenital** absence **of unspecified limb(s)** ▽

    Amelia NOS

Q73.1   **Phocomelia, unspecified limb(s)** ▽

    Phocomelia NOS

Q73.8   **Other reduction defects of unspecified limb(s)** ▽

    Longitudinal reduction deformity of unspecified limb(s)

    Ectromelia of limb NOS

    Hemimelia of limb NOS

    Reduction defect of limb NOS

✓4ᵗʰ **Q74   Other** congenital malformations of limb(s)

   EXCLUDES 1   polydactyly (Q69.-)

       reduction defect of limb (Q71-Q73)

       syndactyly (Q70.-)

Q74.0   **Other congenital malformations of upper limb(s), including shoulder girdle**

    Accessory carpal bones

    Cleidocranial dysostosis

    Congenital pseudarthrosis of clavicle

    Macrodactylia (fingers)

    Madelung's deformity

    Radioulnar synostosis

    Sprengel's deformity

    Triphalangeal thumb

Q74.1   **Congenital malformation of** knee

    Congenital absence of patella

    Congenital dislocation of patella

    Congenital genu valgum

    Congenital genu varum

    Rudimentary patella

    EXCLUDES 1   congenital dislocation of knee (Q68.2)

       congenital genu recurvatum (Q68.2)

       nail patella syndrome (Q87.2)

Q74.2   **Other congenital malformations of lower limb(s), including pelvic girdle**

    Congenital fusion of sacroiliac joint

    Congenital malformation of ankle joint

    Congenital malformation of sacroiliac joint

    EXCLUDES 1   anteversion of femur (neck) (Q65.89)

Q74.3   **Arthrogryposis multiplex congenita**

Q74.8   **Other specified congenital malformations of limb(s)**

Q74.9   **Unspecified congenital malformation of limb(s)** ▽

    Congenital anomaly of limb(s) NOS

✓4ᵗʰ **Q75   Other congenital malformations of** skull and face bones

   EXCLUDES 1   congenital malformation of face NOS (Q18.-)

       congenital malformation syndromes classified to Q87.-

       dentofacial anomalies [including malocclusion] (M26.-)

       musculoskeletal deformities of head and face (Q67.0-Q67.4)

       skull defects associated with congenital anomalies of brain such as:

         anencephaly (Q00.0)

         encephalocele (Q01.-)

         hydrocephalus (Q03.-)

         microcephaly (Q02)

Q75.0   **Craniosynostosis**

    Acrocephaly

    Imperfect fusion of skull

    Oxycephaly

    Trigonocephaly

Q75.1   **Craniofacial dysostosis**

    Crouzon's disease

Q75.2   **Hypertelorism**

Q75.3   **Macrocephaly**

Q75.4   **Mandibulofacial dysostosis**

    Franceschetti syndrome

    Treacher Collins syndrome

Q75.5   **Oculomandibular dysostosis**

Q75.8   **Other specified congenital malformations of skull and face bones**

    Absence of skull bone, congenital

    Congenital deformity of forehead

    Platybasia

Q75.9   **Congenital malformation of skull and face bones, unspecified** ▽

    Congenital anomaly of face bones NOS

    Congenital anomaly of skull NOS

✓4ᵗʰ **Q76   Congenital malformations of** spine and bony thorax

   EXCLUDES 1   congenital musculoskeletal deformities of spine and chest (Q67.5-Q67.8)

Q76.0   **Spina bifida occulta**

    EXCLUDES 1   meningocele (spinal) (Q05.-)

       spina bifida (aperta) (cystica) (Q05.-)

Q76.1   **Klippel-Feil syndrome**

    Cervical fusion syndrome

Q76.2   **Congenital spondylolisthesis**

    Congenital spondylolysis

    EXCLUDES 1   spondylolisthesis (acquired) (M43.1-)

       spondylolysis (acquired) (M43.0-)

Q76.3   **Congenital scoliosis due to congenital bony malformation**

    Hemivertebra fusion or failure of segmentation with scoliosis

✓5ᵗʰ **Q76.4   Other congenital malformations of spine, not associated with scoliosis**

   ✓6ᵗʰ **Q76.41   Congenital** kyphosis

     Q76.411   **Congenital kyphosis, occipito-atlanto-axial region**

     Q76.412   **Congenital kyphosis, cervical region**

     Q76.413   **Congenital kyphosis, cervicothoracic region**

     Q76.414   **Congenital kyphosis, thoracic region**

     Q76.415   **Congenital kyphosis,** thoracolumbar **region**

     Q76.419   **Congenital kyphosis, unspecified region** ▽

   ✓6ᵗʰ **Q76.42   Congenital** lordosis

     Q76.425   **Congenital lordosis,** thoracolumbar **region**

     Q76.426   **Congenital lordosis,** lumbar **region**

     Q76.427   **Congenital lordosis,** lumbosacral **region**

     Q76.428   **Congenital lordosis,** sacral and sacrococcygeal **region**

     Q76.429   **Congenital lordosis, unspecified region** ▽

Ⓝ Newborn   Ⓟ Pediatric   Ⓜ Maternity   Ⓐ Adult   **RIC** RIC Dx   **NC Dx** Noncancer Dx   **PDx** Primary Dx   **CC** RIC CC Condition   ►◄ Revised Text   ● New Code   ▲ Revised Code Title

Q76.49   **Other congenital malformations of spine, not associated with scoliosis**
    Congenital absence of vertebra NOS
    Congenital fusion of spine NOS
    Congenital malformation of lumbosacral (joint) (region) NOS
    Congenital malformation of spine NOS
    Hemivertebra NOS
    Malformation of spine NOS
    Platyspondylisis NOS
    Supernumerary vertebra NOS

Q76.5   **Cervical rib**
    Supernumerary rib in cervical region

Q76.6   **Other congenital malformations of ribs**
    Accessory rib
    Congenital absence of rib
    Congenital fusion of ribs
    Congenital malformation of ribs NOS
    EXCLUDES 1   short rib syndrome (Q77.2)

Q76.7   **Congenital malformation of sternum**
    Congenital absence of sternum
    Sternum bifidum

Q76.8   **Other congenital malformations of bony thorax**

Q76.9   **Congenital malformation of bony thorax, unspecified**   ▽

✓4ᵗʰ **Q77**   **Osteochondrodysplasia with defects of growth of tubular bones and spine**
    EXCLUDES 1   mucopolysaccharidosis (E76.0-E76.3)
    EXCLUDES 2   congenital myotonic chondrodystrophy (G71.13)

Q77.0   **Achondrogenesis**
    Hypochondrogenesis

Q77.1   **Thanatophoric short stature**

Q77.2   **Short rib syndrome**
    Asphyxiating thoracic dysplasia [Jeune]

Q77.3   **Chondrodysplasia punctata**
    EXCLUDES 1   Rhizomelic chondrodysplasia punctata (E71.43)

Q77.4   **Achondroplasia**
    Hypochondroplasia
    Osteosclerosis congenita

Q77.5   **Diastrophic dysplasia**

Q77.6   **Chondroectodermal dysplasia**
    Ellis-van Creveld syndrome

Q77.7   **Spondyloepiphyseal dysplasia**

Q77.8   **Other osteochondrodysplasia with defects of growth of tubular bones and spine**

Q77.9   **Osteochondrodysplasia with defects of growth of tubular bones and spine, unspecified**   ▽

✓4ᵗʰ **Q78**   **Other osteochondrodysplasias**
    EXCLUDES 2   congenital myotonic chondrodystrophy (G71.13)

Q78.0   **Osteogenesis imperfecta**
    Fragilitas ossium
    Osteopsathyrosis

Q78.1   **Polyostotic fibrous dysplasia**
    Albright(-McCune)(-Sternberg) syndrome

Q78.2   **Osteopetrosis**
    Albers-Schönberg syndrome
    Osteosclerosis NOS

Q78.3   **Progressive diaphyseal dysplasia**
    Camurati-Engelmann syndrome

Q78.4   **Enchondromatosis**
    Maffucci's syndrome
    Ollier's disease

Q78.5   **Metaphyseal dysplasia**
    Pyle's syndrome

Q78.6   **Multiple congenital exostoses**
    Diaphyseal aclasis

Q78.8   **Other specified osteochondrodysplasias**
    Osteopoikilosis

Q78.9   **Osteochondrodysplasia, unspecified**   ▽
    Chondrodystrophy NOS
    Osteodystrophy NOS

✓4ᵗʰ **Q79**   **Congenital malformations of musculoskeletal system, not elsewhere classified**
    EXCLUDES 2   congenital (sternomastoid) torticollis (Q68.0)

Q79.0   **Congenital diaphragmatic hernia**
    EXCLUDES 1   congenital hiatus hernia (Q40.1)

Q79.1   **Other congenital malformations of diaphragm**
    Absence of diaphragm
    Congenital malformation of diaphragm NOS
    Eventration of diaphragm

Q79.2   **Exomphalos**
    Omphalocele
    EXCLUDES 1   umbilical hernia (K42.-)

Q79.3   **Gastroschisis**

Q79.4   **Prune belly syndrome**
    Congenital prolapse of bladder mucosa
    Eagle-Barrett syndrome

✓5ᵗʰ **Q79.5**   **Other congenital malformations of abdominal wall**
    EXCLUDES 1   umbilical hernia (K42.-)

    Q79.51   **Congenital hernia of bladder**

    Q79.59   **Other congenital malformations of abdominal wall**

Q79.6   **Ehlers-Danlos syndrome**

Q79.8   **Other congenital malformations of musculoskeletal system**
    Absence of muscle
    Absence of tendon
    Accessory muscle
    Amyotrophia congenita
    Congenital constricting bands
    Congenital shortening of tendon
    Poland syndrome

Q79.9   **Congenital malformation of musculoskeletal system, unspecified**   ▽
    Congenital anomaly of musculoskeletal system NOS
    Congenital deformity of musculoskeletal system NOS

Other congenital malformations (Q80-Q89)

✓4ᵗʰ **Q80**   **Congenital ichthyosis**
    EXCLUDES 1   Refsum's disease (G60.1)

Q80.0   **Ichthyosis vulgaris**

Q80.1   **X-linked ichthyosis**

Q80.2   **Lamellar ichthyosis**
    Collodion baby

Q80.3   **Congenital bullous ichthyosiform erythroderma**

Q80.4   **Harlequin fetus**

Q80.8   **Other congenital ichthyosis**

Q80.9   **Congenital ichthyosis, unspecified**   ▽

✓4ᵗʰ **Q81**   **Epidermolysis bullosa**

Q81.0   **Epidermolysis bullosa simplex**
    EXCLUDES 1   Cockayne's syndrome (Q87.1)

Q81.1   **Epidermolysis bullosa letalis**
    Herlitz' syndrome

Q81.2   **Epidermolysis bullosa dystrophica**

Q81.8   **Other epidermolysis bullosa**

Q81.9   **Epidermolysis bullosa, unspecified**   ▽

✓4ᵗʰ **Q82**   **Other congenital malformations of skin**
    EXCLUDES 1   acrodermatitis enteropathica (E83.2)
         congenital erythropoietic porphyria (E80.0)
         pilonidal cyst or sinus (L05.-)
         Sturge-Weber (-Dimitri) syndrome (Q85.8)

Q82.0   **Hereditary lymphedema**

Q82.1   **Xeroderma pigmentosum**

Q82.2   **Mastocytosis**
    Urticaria pigmentosa
    EXCLUDES 1   malignant mastocytosis (C96.2)

Q82.3   **Incontinentia pigmenti**

Q82.4   **Ectodermal dysplasia (anhidrotic)**
    EXCLUDES 1   Ellis-van Creveld syndrome (Q77.6)

Q82.5   **Congenital non-neoplastic nevus**

Birthmark NOS	Strawberry Nevus
Flammeus Nevus	Vascular Nevus NOS
Portwine Nevus	Verrucous Nevus
Sanguineous Nevus	

    EXCLUDES 2   araneus nevus (I78.1)
         café au lait spots (L81.3)
         lentigo (L81.4)
         melanocytic nevus (D22.-)
         nevus NOS (D22.-)
         pigmented nevus (D22.-)
         spider nevus (I78.1)
         stellar nevus (I78.1)

☑ Add'l Character Required   ✓x7ᵗʰ Placeholder Alert   RUG IV Special Care High Dx   RUG IV Clinically Complex Dx   RUG IV Special Care Low Dx   Manifestation Code   Other Specified Code   ▽ Unspecified Code

ICD-10-CM 2016   **829**

Q82.8　Other specified congenital malformations of skin
　　　Abnormal palmar creases
　　　Accessory skin tags
　　　Benign familial pemphigus [Hailey-Hailey]
　　　Congenital poikiloderma
　　　Cutis laxa (hyperelastica)
　　　Dermatoglyphic anomalies
　　　Inherited keratosis palmaris et plantaris
　　　Keratosis follicularis [Darier-White]
　　　　EXCLUDES 1　*Ehlers-Danlos syndrome (Q79.6)*

Q82.9　Congenital malformation of skin, unspecified　▽

Q83　Congenital malformations of breast
　　　EXCLUDES 2　*absence of pectoral muscle (Q79.8)*
　　　　　　　　hypoplasia of breast (N64.82)
　　　　　　　　micromastia (N64.82)

Q83.0　Congenital absence of breast with absent nipple

Q83.1　Accessory breast
　　　Supernumerary breast

Q83.2　Absent nipple

Q83.3　Accessory nipple
　　　Supernumerary nipple

Q83.8　Other congenital malformations of breast

Q83.9　Congenital malformation of breast, unspecified　▽

Q84　Other congenital malformations of integument

Q84.0　Congenital alopecia
　　　Congenital atrichosis

Q84.1　Congenital morphological disturbances of hair, not elsewhere classified
　　　Beaded hair　　　　　Pili annulati
　　　Monilethrix
　　　　EXCLUDES 1　*Menkes' kinky hair syndrome (E83.0)*

Q84.2　Other congenital malformations of hair
　　　Congenital hypertrichosis
　　　Congenital malformation of hair NOS
　　　Persistent lanugo

Q84.3　Anonychia
　　　　EXCLUDES 1　*nail patella syndrome (Q87.2)*

Q84.4　Congenital leukonychia

Q84.5　Enlarged and hypertrophic nails
　　　Congenital onychauxis　　　Pachyonychia

Q84.6　Other congenital malformations of nails
　　　Congenital clubnail
　　　Congenital koilonychia
　　　Congenital malformation of nail NOS

Q84.8　Other specified congenital malformations of integument
　　　Aplasia cutis congenita

Q84.9　Congenital malformation of integument, unspecified　▽
　　　Congenital anomaly of integument NOS
　　　Congenital deformity of integument NOS

Q85　Phakomatoses, not elsewhere classified
　　　EXCLUDES 1　*ataxia telangiectasia [Louis-Bar] (G11.3)*
　　　　　　　　familial dysautonomia [Riley-Day] (G90.1)

Q85.0　Neurofibromatosis (nonmalignant)

Q85.00　Neurofibromatosis, unspecified　▽

Q85.01　Neurofibromatosis, type 1
　　　　　Von Recklinghausen disease

Q85.02　Neurofibromatosis, type 2
　　　　　Acoustic neurofibromatosis

Q85.03　Schwannomatosis

Q85.09　Other neurofibromatosis

Q85.1　Tuberous sclerosis
　　　Bourneville's disease
　　　Epiloia

Q85.8　Other phakomatoses, not elsewhere classified
　　　Peutz-Jeghers Syndrome
　　　Sturge-Weber(-Dimitri) syndrome
　　　von Hippel-Lindau syndrome
　　　　EXCLUDES 1　*Meckel-Gruber syndrome (Q61.9)*

Q85.9　Phakomatosis, unspecified　▽
　　　Hamartosis NOS

Q86　Congenital malformation syndromes due to known exogenous causes, not elsewhere classified
　　　EXCLUDES 2　*iodine-deficiency-related hypothyroidism (E00-E02)*
　　　　　　　　nonteratogenic effects of substances transmitted via placenta or breast milk (P04.-)

Q86.0　Fetal alcohol syndrome (dysmorphic)

Q86.1　Fetal hydantoin syndrome　Ⓝ
　　　Meadow's syndrome

Q86.2　Dysmorphism due to warfarin

Q86.8　Other congenital malformation syndromes due to known exogenous causes

Q87　Other specified congenital malformation syndromes affecting multiple systems
　　　Use additional code(s) to identify all associated manifestations

Q87.0　Congenital malformation syndromes predominantly affecting facial appearance
　　　Acrocephalopolysyndactyly
　　　Acrocephalosyndactyly [Apert]　　　Robin syndrome
　　　Cryptophthalmos syndrome　　　　Whistling face
　　　Cyclopia
　　　Goldenhar syndrome
　　　Moebius syndrome
　　　Oro-facial-digital syndrome

Q87.1　Congenital malformation syndromes predominantly associated with short stature
　　　Aarskog syndrome　　　　Robinow-Silverman-Smith
　　　Cockayne syndrome　　　　　syndrome
　　　De Lange syndrome　　　　Russell-Silver syndrome
　　　Dubowitz syndrome　　　　Seckel syndrome
　　　Noonan syndrome
　　　Prader-Willi syndrome
　　　　EXCLUDES 1　*Ellis-van Creveld syndrome (Q77.6)*
　　　　　　　　Smith-Lemli-Opitz syndrome (E78.72)

Q87.2　Congenital malformation syndromes predominantly involving limbs
　　　Holt-Oram syndrome
　　　Klippel-Trenaunay-Weber syndrome
　　　Nail patella syndrome
　　　Rubinstein-Taybi syndrome
　　　Sirenomelia syndrome
　　　Thrombocytopenia with absent radius [TAR] syndrome
　　　VATER syndrome

Q87.3　Congenital malformation syndromes involving early overgrowth
　　　Beckwith-Wiedemann syndrome　　　Weaver syndrome
　　　Sotos syndrome

Q87.4　Marfan's syndrome

Q87.40　Marfan's syndrome, unspecified　▽

Q87.41　Marfan's syndrome with cardiovascular manifestations

Q87.410　Marfan's syndrome with aortic dilation

Q87.418　Marfan's syndrome with other cardiovascular manifestations

Q87.42　Marfan's syndrome with ocular manifestations

Q87.43　Marfan's syndrome with skeletal manifestation

Q87.5　Other congenital malformation syndromes with other skeletal changes

Q87.8　Other specified congenital malformation syndromes, not elsewhere classified
　　　　EXCLUDES 1　*Zellweger syndrome (E71.510)*

Q87.81　Alport syndrome
　　　　　Use additional code to identify stage of chronic kidney disease (N18.1-N18.6)

Q87.89　Other specified congenital malformation syndromes, not elsewhere classified
　　　　　Laurence-Moon (-Bardet)-Biedl syndrome

Q89　Other congenital malformations, not elsewhere classified

Q89.0　Congenital absence and malformations of spleen
　　　　EXCLUDES 1　*isomerism of atrial appendages (with asplenia or polysplenia) (Q20.6)*

Q89.01　Asplenia (congenital)

Q89.09　Congenital malformations of spleen
　　　　　Congenital splenomegaly

Q89.1　Congenital malformations of adrenal gland
　　　　EXCLUDES 1　*adrenogenital disorders (E25.-)*
　　　　　　　　congenital adrenal hyperplasia (E25.0)

Q89.2　Congenital malformations of other endocrine glands
　　　Congenital malformation of parathyroid or thyroid gland
　　　Persistent thyroglossal duct
　　　Thyroglossal cyst
　　　　EXCLUDES 1　*congenital goiter (E03.0)*
　　　　　　　　congenital hypothyroidism (E03.1)

Ⓝ Newborn　Ⓟ Pediatric　Ⓜ Maternity　Ⓐ Adult　**RIC** RIC Dx　**NC Dx** Noncancer Dx　**PDx** Primary Dx　**CC** RIC CC Condition　▶◀ Revised Text　● New Code　▲ Revised Code Title

830　　　　　　　　　　　　　　　　　　　　　　　　　　　　　　　　　ICD-10-CM 2016

Q89.3 Situs inversus
Dextrocardia with situs inversus
Mirror-image atrial arrangement with situs inversus
Situs inversus or transversus abdominalis
Situs inversus or transversus thoracis
Transposition of abdominal viscera
Transposition of thoracic viscera
EXCLUDES 1   dextrocardia NOS (Q24.0)

Q89.4 Conjoined twins
Craniopagus   Pygopagus
Dicephaly   Thoracopagus

Q89.7 Multiple congenital malformations, not elsewhere classified
Multiple congenital anomalies NOS
Multiple congenital deformities NOS
EXCLUDES 1   congenital malformation syndromes affecting multiple systems (Q87.-)

Q89.8 Other specified congenital malformations
Use additional code(s) to identify all associated manifestations

Q89.9 Congenital malformation, unspecified ▽
Congenital anomaly NOS · Congenital deformity NOS

Chromosomal abnormalities, not elsewhere classified (Q90-Q99)

EXCLUDES 2   mitochondrial metabolic disorders (E88.4-)

✓4ᵗʰ **Q90 Down syndrome**
Use additional code(s) to identify any associated physical conditions and degree of intellectual disabilities (F70-F79)

Q90.0 Trisomy 21, nonmosaicism (meiotic nondisjunction)

Q90.1 Trisomy 21, mosaicism (mitotic nondisjunction)

Q90.2 Trisomy 21, translocation

Q90.9 Down syndrome, unspecified ▽
Trisomy 21 NOS

✓4ᵗʰ **Q91 Trisomy 18 and Trisomy 13**

Q91.0 Trisomy 18, nonmosaicism (meiotic nondisjunction)

Q91.1 Trisomy 18, mosaicism (mitotic nondisjunction)

Q91.2 Trisomy 18, translocation

Q91.3 Trisomy 18, unspecified ▽

Q91.4 Trisomy 13, nonmosaicism (meiotic nondisjunction)

Q91.5 Trisomy 13, mosaicism (mitotic nondisjunction)

Q91.6 Trisomy 13, translocation

Q91.7 Trisomy 13, unspecified ▽

✓4ᵗʰ **Q92 Other trisomies and partial trisomies of the autosomes, not elsewhere classified**
INCLUDES   unbalanced translocations and insertions
EXCLUDES 1   trisomies of chromosomes 13, 18, 21 (Q90-Q91)

Q92.0 Whole chromosome trisomy, nonmosaicism (meiotic nondisjunction)

Q92.1 Whole chromosome trisomy, mosaicism (mitotic nondisjunction)

Q92.2 Partial trisomy
Less than whole arm duplicated
Whole arm or more duplicated
EXCLUDES 1   partial trisomy due to unbalanced translocation (Q92.5)

Q92.5 Duplications with other complex rearrangements
Partial trisomy due to unbalanced translocations
Code also any associated deletions due to unbalanced translocations, inversions and insertions (Q93.7)

✓5ᵗʰ **Q92.6 Marker chromosomes**
Trisomies due to dicentrics
Trisomies due to extra rings
Trisomies due to isochromosomes
Individual with marker heterochromatin

Q92.61 Marker chromosomes in normal individual

Q92.62 Marker chromosomes in abnormal individual

Q92.7 Triploidy and polyploidy

Q92.8 Other specified trisomies and partial trisomies of autosomes
Duplications identified by fluorescence in situ hybridization (FISH)
Duplications identified by in situ hybridization (ISH)
Duplications seen only at prometaphase

Q92.9 Trisomy and partial trisomy of autosomes, unspecified ▽

✓4ᵗʰ **Q93 Monosomies and deletions from the autosomes, not elsewhere classified**

Q93.0 Whole chromosome monosomy, nonmosaicism (meiotic nondisjunction)

Q93.1 Whole chromosome monosomy, mosaicism (mitotic nondisjunction)

Q93.2 Chromosome replaced with ring, dicentric or isochromosome

Q93.3 Deletion of short arm of chromosome 4
Wolff-Hirschorn syndrome

Q93.4 Deletion of short arm of chromosome 5
Cri-du-chat syndrome

Q93.5 Other deletions of part of a chromosome
Angelman syndrome

Q93.7 Deletions with other complex rearrangements
Deletions due to unbalanced translocations, inversions and insertions
Code also any associated duplications due to unbalanced translocations, inversions and insertions (Q92.5)

✓5ᵗʰ **Q93.8 Other deletions from the autosomes**

Q93.81 Velo-cardio-facial syndrome
Deletion 22q11.2

Q93.88 Other microdeletions
Miller-Dieker syndrome
Smith-Magenis syndrome

Q93.89 Other deletions from the autosomes
Deletions identified by fluorescence in situ hybridization (FISH)
Deletions identified by in situ hybridization (ISH)
Deletions seen only at prometaphase

Q93.9 Deletion from autosomes, unspecified ▽

✓4ᵗʰ **Q95 Balanced rearrangements and structural markers, not elsewhere classified**
INCLUDES   Robertsonian and balanced reciprocal translocations and insertions

Q95.0 Balanced translocation and insertion in normal individual

Q95.1 Chromosome inversion in normal individual

Q95.2 Balanced autosomal rearrangement in abnormal individual

Q95.3 Balanced sex/autosomal rearrangement in abnormal individual

Q95.5 Individual with autosomal fragile site

Q95.8 Other balanced rearrangements and structural markers

Q95.9 Balanced rearrangement and structural marker, unspecified ▽

✓4ᵗʰ **Q96 Turner's syndrome**
EXCLUDES 1   Noonan syndrome (Q87.1)

Q96.0 Karyotype 45, X ♀

Q96.1 Karyotype 46, X iso (Xq) ♀
Karyotype 46, isochromosome Xq

Q96.2 Karyotype 46, X with abnormal sex chromosome, except iso (Xq) ♀
Karyotype 46, X with abnormal sex chromosome, except isochromosome Xq

Q96.3 Mosaicism, 45, X/46, XX or XY ♀

Q96.4 Mosaicism, 45, X/other cell line(s) with abnormal sex chromosome ♀

Q96.8 Other variants of Turner's syndrome ♀

Q96.9 Turner's syndrome, unspecified ♀ ▽

✓4ᵗʰ **Q97 Other sex chromosome abnormalities, female phenotype, not elsewhere classified**
EXCLUDES 1   Turner's syndrome (Q96.-)

Q97.0 Karyotype 47, XXX ♀

Q97.1 Female with more than three X chromosomes ♀

Q97.2 Mosaicism, lines with various numbers of X chromosomes ♀

Q97.3 Female with 46, XY karyotype ♀

Q97.8 Other specified sex chromosome abnormalities, female phenotype ♀

Q97.9 Sex chromosome abnormality, female phenotype, unspecified ♀ ▽

✓4ᵗʰ **Q98 Other sex chromosome abnormalities, male phenotype, not elsewhere classified**

Q98.0 Klinefelter syndrome karyotype 47, XXY ♂

Q98.1 Klinefelter syndrome, male with more than two X chromosomes ♂

Q98.3 Other male with 46, XX karyotype ♂

Q98.4 Klinefelter syndrome, unspecified ♂ ▽

Q98.5 Karyotype 47, XYY ♂

Q98.6 Male with structurally abnormal sex chromosome ♂

Q98.7 Male with sex chromosome mosaicism ♂

☑ Add'l Character Required ☑7ᵀ Placeholder Alert RUG IV Special Care High Dx   RUG IV Clinically Complex Dx   RUG IV Special Care Low Dx   Manifestation Code   Other Specified Code ▽ Unspecified Code

Q98.8 **Other specified sex chromosome abnormalities, male** ♂
     phenotype

Q98.9 **Sex chromosome abnormality, male phenotype,** ♂▽
     unspecified

✓4ᵗʰ **Q99** **Other chromosome abnormalities, not elsewhere classified**

     Q99.0 **Chimera 46, XX/46, XY**
         Chimera 46, XX/46, XY true hermaphrodite

     Q99.1 **46, XX true hermaphrodite**
         46, XX with streak gonads   Pure gonadal dysgenesis
         46, XY with streak gonads

Q99.2 **Fragile X chromosome**
     Fragile X syndrome

Q99.8 **Other specified chromosome abnormalities**

Q99.9 **Chromosomal abnormality, unspecified** ▽

Ⓝ Newborn   Ⓟ Pediatric   Ⓜ Maternity   Ⓐ Adult   **RIC** RIC Dx   **NCDx** Noncancer Dx   **PDx** Primary Dx   **CC** RIC CC Condition   ▶◀ Revised Text   ● New Code   ▲ Revised Code Title

832   ICD-10-CM 2016

Chapter 18. Symptoms, Signs, and Abnormal Clinical and Laboratory Findings, Not Elsewhere Classified (R00–R99)

Chapter Specific Guidelines with Coding Examples

The chapter specific guidelines from the ICD-10-CM Official Guidelines for Coding and Reporting have been provided below. Along with these guidelines are coding examples, contained in the shaded boxes, that have been developed to help illustrate the coding and/or sequencing guidance found in these guidelines.

Chapter 18 includes symptoms, signs, abnormal results of clinical or other investigative procedures, and ill-defined conditions regarding which no diagnosis classifiable elsewhere is recorded. Signs and symptoms that point to a specific diagnosis have been assigned to a category in other chapters of the classification.

a. Use of symptom codes

Codes that describe symptoms and signs are acceptable for reporting purposes when a related definitive diagnosis has not been established (confirmed) by the provider.

> Chest pain of unknown origin
>
> **R07.9**   **Chest pain, unspecified**
>
> *Explanation:* Codes that describe symptoms such as chest pain are acceptable for reporting purposes when the provider has not established (confirmed) a related definitive diagnosis.

b. Use of a symptom code with a definitive diagnosis code

Codes for signs and symptoms may be reported in addition to a related definitive diagnosis when the sign or symptom is not routinely associated with that diagnosis, such as the various signs and symptoms associated with complex syndromes. The definitive diagnosis code should be sequenced before the symptom code.

Signs or symptoms that are associated routinely with a disease process should not be assigned as additional codes, unless otherwise instructed by the classification.

> Pneumonia with hemoptysis
>
> **J18.9**   **Pneumonia, unspecified organism**
>
> **R04.2**   **Hemoptysis**
>
> *Explanation:* Codes for signs and symptoms may be reported in addition to a related definitive diagnosis when the sign or symptom is not routinely associated with that diagnosis.

> Abdominal pain due to acute appendicitis
>
> **K35.80**   **Unspecified acute appendicitis**
>
> *Explanation:* Codes for signs or symptoms routinely associated with a disease process should not be assigned unless the classification instructs otherwise.

c. Combination codes that include symptoms

ICD-10-CM contains a number of combination codes that identify both the definitive diagnosis and common symptoms of that diagnosis. When using one of these combination codes, an additional code should not be assigned for the symptom.

> Acute gastritis with hemorrhage
>
> **K29.01**   **Acute gastritis with bleeding**
>
> *Explanation:* When a combination code identifies both the definitive diagnosis and the symptom, an additional code should not be assigned for the symptom.

d. Repeated falls

Code R29.6, Repeated falls, is for use for encounters when a patient has recently fallen and the reason for the fall is being investigated.

Code Z91.81, History of falling, is for use when a patient has fallen in the past and is at risk for future falls. When appropriate, both codes R29.6 and Z91.81 may be assigned together.

e. Coma scale

The coma scale codes (R40.2-) can be used in conjunction with traumatic brain injury codes, acute cerebrovascular disease or sequelae of cerebrovascular disease codes. These codes are primarily for use by trauma registries, but they may be used in any setting where this information is collected. The coma scale codes should be sequenced after the diagnosis code(s).

These codes, one from each subcategory, are needed to complete the scale. The 7th character indicates when the scale was recorded. The 7th character should match for all three codes.

At a minimum, report the initial score documented on presentation at your facility. This may be a score from the emergency medicine technician (EMT) or in the emergency department. If desired, a facility may choose to capture multiple coma scale scores.

Assign code R40.24, Glasgow coma scale, total score, when only the total score is documented in the medical record and not the individual score(s).

> 23-year-old man found down after unknown injury with skull fracture and with concussion and loss of consciousness of unknown duration. EMS evaluated the patient in the field and reported the individual Glasgow coma scores:
>
> Eye opening response—3: eyes open to speech
>
> Verbal response—4: confused but coherent speech
>
> Motor response—6: obeys commands fully
>
> **S02.0XXA**   **Fracture of vault of skull, initial encounter for closed fracture**
>
> **S06.0X9A**   **Concussion with loss of consciousness of unspecified duration, initial encounter**
>
> **R40.2131**   **Coma scale, eyes open, to sound, in the field [EMT or ambulance]**
>
> **R40.2241**   **Coma scale, best verbal response, confused conversation, in the field [EMT or ambulance]**
>
> **R40.2361**   **Coma scale, best motor response, obeys commands, in the field [EMT or ambulance]**
>
> *Explanation:* When individual scores for the Glasgow coma scale are documented, one code from each category is needed to complete the scale. The seventh character indicates when the scale was recorded and should match for all three codes. Assign code R40.24 Glasgow coma scale, total score, when only the total and not the individual score(s) is documented in the medical record.

f. Functional quadriplegia

Functional quadriplegia (code R53.2) is the lack of ability to use one's limbs or to ambulate due to extreme debility. It is not associated with neurologic deficit or injury, and code R53.2 should not be used for cases of neurologic quadriplegia. It should only be assigned if functional quadriplegia is specifically documented in the medical record.

g. SIRS due to non-infectious process

The systemic inflammatory response syndrome (SIRS) can develop as a result of certain non-infectious disease processes, such as trauma, malignant neoplasm, or pancreatitis. When SIRS is documented with a noninfectious condition, and no subsequent infection is documented, the code for the underlying condition, such as an injury, should be assigned, followed by code R65.10, Systemic inflammatory response syndrome (SIRS) of non-infectious origin without acute organ dysfunction, or code R65.11, Systemic inflammatory response syndrome (SIRS) of non-infectious origin with acute organ dysfunction. If an associated acute organ dysfunction is documented, the appropriate code(s) for the specific type of organ dysfunction(s) should be assigned in addition to code R65.11. If acute organ dysfunction is documented, but it cannot be determined if the acute organ dysfunction is associated with SIRS or due to another condition (e.g., directly due to the trauma), the provider should be queried.

Systemic inflammatory response syndrome (SIRS) due to acute gallstone pancreatitis

K85.1   **Biliary acute pancreatitis**

R65.10   **Systemic inflammatory response syndrome (SIRS) of noninfectious origin without acute organ dysfunction**

Explanation: When SIRS is documented with a noninfectious condition without subsequent infection documented, the code for the underlying condition such as pancreatitis should be assigned followed by the appropriate code for SIRS of noninfectious origin, either with or without associated organ dysfunction.

h. Death NOS

Code R99, Ill-defined and unknown cause of mortality, is only for use in the very limited circumstance when a patient who has already died is brought into an emergency department or other healthcare facility and is pronounced dead upon arrival. It does not represent the discharge disposition of death.

Chapter 18. Symptoms, Signs and Abnormal Clinical and Laboratory Findings, Not Elsewhere Classified (R00-R99)

NOTE This chapter includes symptoms, signs, abnormal results of clinical or other investigative procedures, and ill-defined conditions regarding which no diagnosis classifiable elsewhere is recorded.

Signs and symptoms that point rather definitely to a given diagnosis have been assigned to a category in other chapters of the classification. In general, categories in this chapter include the less well-defined conditions and symptoms that, without the necessary study of the case to establish a final diagnosis, point perhaps equally to two or more diseases or to two or more systems of the body. Practically all categories in the chapter could be designated "not otherwise specified", "unknown etiology" or "transient". The Alphabetical Index should be consulted to determine which symptoms and signs are to be allocated here and which to other chapters. The residual subcategories, numbered .8, are generally provided for other relevant symptoms that cannot be allocated elsewhere in the classification.

The conditions and signs or symptoms included in categories R00-R94 consist of:

(a) cases for which no more specific diagnosis can be made even after all the facts bearing on the case have been investigated;

(b) signs or symptoms existing at the time of initial encounter that proved to be transient and whose causes could not be determined;

(c) provisional diagnosis in a patient who failed to return for further investigation or care;

(d) cases referred elsewhere for investigation or treatment before the diagnosis was made;

(e) cases in which a more precise diagnosis was not available for any other reason;

(f) certain symptoms, for which supplementary information is provided, that represent important problems in medical care in their own right.

EXCLUDES 2 abnormal findings on antenatal screening of mother (O28.-)
certain conditions originating in the perinatal period (P04-P96)
signs and symptoms classified in the body system chapters
signs and symptoms of breast (N63, N64.5)

This chapter contains the following blocks:

R00-R09 Symptoms and signs involving the circulatory and respiratory systems
R10-R19 Symptoms and signs involving the digestive system and abdomen
R20-R23 Symptoms and signs involving the skin and subcutaneous tissue
R25-R29 Symptoms and signs involving the nervous and musculoskeletal systems
R30-R39 Symptoms and signs involving the genitourinary system
R40-R46 Symptoms and signs involving cognition, perception, emotional state and behavior
R47-R49 Symptoms and signs involving speech and voice
R50-R69 General symptoms and signs
R70-R79 Abnormal findings on examination of blood, without diagnosis
R80-R82 Abnormal findings on examination of urine, without diagnosis
R83-R89 Abnormal findings on examination of other body fluids, substances and tissues, without diagnosis
R90-R94 Abnormal findings on diagnostic imaging and in function studies, without diagnosis
R97 Abnormal tumor markers
R99 Ill-defined and unknown cause of mortality

Symptoms and signs involving the circulatory and respiratory systems (R00-R09)

✓4ᵗʰ R00 Abnormalities of heart beat
EXCLUDES 1 abnormalities originating in the perinatal period (P29.1-)
specified arrhythmias (I47-I49)

R00.0 Tachycardia, unspecified ▽
Rapid heart beat
Sinoauricular tachycardia NOS
Sinus [sinusal] tachycardia NOS
EXCLUDES 1 neonatal tachycardia (P29.11)
paroxysmal tachycardia (I47.-)

R00.1 Bradycardia, unspecified ▽
Sinoatrial bradycardia
Sinus bradycardia
Slow heart beat
Vagal bradycardia
Use additional code for adverse effect, if applicable, to identify drug (T36-T50 with fifth or sixth character 5)
EXCLUDES 1 neonatal bradycardia (P29.12)

R00.2 Palpitations
Awareness of heart beat

R00.8 Other abnormalities of heart beat

R00.9 Unspecified abnormalities of heart beat ▽

✓4ᵗʰ R01 Cardiac murmurs and other cardiac sounds
EXCLUDES 1 cardiac murmurs and sounds originating in the perinatal period (P29.8)

R01.0 Benign and innocent cardiac murmurs
Functional cardiac murmur

R01.1 Cardiac murmur, unspecified ▽
Cardiac bruit NOS
Heart murmur NOS

R01.2 Other cardiac sounds
Cardiac dullness, increased or decreased
Precordial friction

✓4ᵗʰ R03 Abnormal blood-pressure reading, without diagnosis
R03.0 Elevated blood-pressure reading, without diagnosis of hypertension
NOTE This category is to be used to record an episode of elevated blood pressure in a patient in whom no formal diagnosis of hypertension has been made, or as an isolated incidental finding.

R03.1 Nonspecific low blood-pressure reading
EXCLUDES 1 hypotension (I95.-)
maternal hypotension syndrome (O26.5-)
neurogenic orthostatic hypotension (G90.3)

✓4ᵗʰ R04 Hemorrhage from respiratory passages
R04.0 Epistaxis
Hemorrhage from nose
Nosebleed

R04.1 Hemorrhage from throat
EXCLUDES 2 hemoptysis (R04.2)

R04.2 Hemoptysis
Blood-stained sputum
Cough with hemorrhage
AHA: 2013, 4Q, 118

✓5ᵗʰ R04.8 Hemorrhage from other sites in respiratory passages
R04.81 Acute idiopathic pulmonary hemorrhage in infants ℗
AIPHI
Acute idiopathic hemorrhage in infants over 28 days old
EXCLUDES 1 perinatal pulmonary hemorrhage (P26.-)
von Willebrand's disease (D68.0)

R04.89 Hemorrhage from other sites in respiratory passages
Pulmonary hemorrhage NOS

R04.9 Hemorrhage from respiratory passages, unspecified ▽

R05 Cough
EXCLUDES 1 cough with hemorrhage (R04.2)
smoker's cough (J41.0)

✓4ᵗʰ R06 Abnormalities of breathing
EXCLUDES 1 acute respiratory distress syndrome (J80)
respiratory arrest (R09.2)
respiratory arrest of newborn (P28.81)
respiratory distress syndrome of newborn (P22.-)
respiratory failure (J96.-)
respiratory failure of newborn (P28.5)

✓5ᵗʰ R06.0 Dyspnea
EXCLUDES 1 tachypnea NOS (R06.82)
transient tachypnea of newborn (P22.1)

R06.00 Dyspnea, unspecified ▽
R06.01 Orthopnea
R06.02 Shortness of breath
R06.09 Other forms of dyspnea

R06.1 Stridor
EXCLUDES 1 congenital laryngeal stridor (P28.89)
laryngismus (stridulus) (J38.5)

R06.2 Wheezing
EXCLUDES 1 asthma (J45.-)

R06.3 Periodic breathing
Cheyne-Stokes breathing

R06.4 Hyperventilation
EXCLUDES 1 psychogenic hyperventilation (F45.8)

R06.5 Mouth breathing
EXCLUDES 2 dry mouth NOS (R68.2)

☑ Add'l Character Required ✓x7ᵗʰ Placeholder Alert RUG IV Special Care High Dx RUG IV Clinically Complex Dx RUG IV Special Care Low Dx Manifestation Code Other Specified Code ▽ Unspecified Code

Chapter 18. Symptoms, Signs and Abnormal Clinical and Laboratory Findings

R06.6   **Hiccough**
> EXCLUDES 1   *psychogenic hiccough (F45.8)*

R06.7   **Sneezing**

✓5ᵗʰ **R06.8**   **Other abnormalities of breathing**

     R06.81   **Apnea**, not elsewhere classified
       Apnea NOS
> EXCLUDES 1   *apnea (of) newborn (P28.4)*
>   *sleep apnea (G47.3-)*
>   *sleep apnea of newborn (primary) (P28.3)*

     R06.82   **Tachypnea**, not elsewhere classified
       Tachypnea NOS
> EXCLUDES 1   *transitory tachypnea of newborn (P22.1)*

     R06.83   **Snoring**

     R06.89   **Other abnormalities of breathing**
       Breath-holding (spells)
       Sighing

R06.9   **Unspecified abnormalities of breathing**   ▽

✓4ᵗʰ **R07**   **Pain in throat and chest**
> EXCLUDES 1   *epidemic myalgia (B33.0)*
> EXCLUDES 2   *jaw pain (R68.84)*
>   *pain in breast (N64.4)*

R07.0   **Pain in throat**
> EXCLUDES 1   *chronic sore throat (J31.2)*
>   *sore throat (acute) NOS (J02.9)*
> EXCLUDES 2   *dysphagia (R13.1-)*
>   *pain in neck (M54.2)*

R07.1   **Chest pain on breathing**
       Painful respiration

R07.2   **Precordial pain**

✓5ᵗʰ **R07.8**   **Other chest pain**

     R07.81   **Pleurodynia**
       Pleurodynia NOS
> EXCLUDES 1   *epidemic pleurodynia (B33.0)*

     R07.82   **Intercostal pain**

     R07.89   **Other chest pain**
       Anterior chest-wall pain NOS

R07.9   **Chest pain, unspecified**   ▽

✓4ᵗʰ **R09**   **Other symptoms and signs involving the circulatory and respiratory system**
> EXCLUDES 1   *acute respiratory distress syndrome (J80)*
>   *respiratory arrest of newborn (P28.81)*
>   *respiratory distress syndrome of newborn (P22.0)*
>   *respiratory failure (J96.-)*
>   *respiratory failure of newborn (P28.5)*

✓5ᵗʰ **R09.0**   **Asphyxia and hypoxemia**
> EXCLUDES 1   *asphyxia due to carbon monoxide (T58.-)*
>   *asphyxia due to foreign body in respiratory tract (T17.-)*
>   *birth (intrauterine) asphyxia (P84)*
>   *hypercapnia (R06.4)*
>   *hyperventilation (R06.4)*
>   *traumatic asphyxia (T71.-)*

     R09.01   **Asphyxia**

     R09.02   **Hypoxemia**

R09.1   **Pleurisy**
> EXCLUDES 1   *pleurisy with effusion (J90)*

R09.2   **Respiratory arrest**   CC
       Cardiorespiratory failure
> EXCLUDES 1   *cardiac arrest (I46.-)*
>   *respiratory arrest of newborn (P28.81)*
>   *respiratory distress of newborn (P22.0)*
>   *respiratory failure (J96.-)*
>   *respiratory failure of newborn (P28.5)*
>   *respiratory insufficiency (R06.89)*
>   *respiratory insufficiency of newborn (P28.5)*
       RIC Excl: 15 Pulmonary

R09.3   **Abnormal sputum**
       Abnormal amount of sputum
       Abnormal color of sputum
       Abnormal odor of sputum
       Excessive sputum
> EXCLUDES 1   *blood-stained sputum (R04.2)*

✓5ᵗʰ **R09.8**   **Other specified symptoms and signs involving the circulatory and respiratory systems**

     R09.81   **Nasal congestion**

     R09.82   **Postnasal drip**

     R09.89   **Other specified symptoms and signs involving the circulatory and respiratory systems**
       Abnormal chest percussion
       Bruit (arterial)
       Chest tympany
       Choking sensation
       Feeling of foreign body in throat
       Friction sounds in chest
       Rales
       Weak pulse
> EXCLUDES 2   *foreign body in throat (T17.2-)*
>   *wheezing (R06.2)*

Symptoms and signs involving the digestive system and abdomen (R10-R19)

> EXCLUDES 1   *congenital or infantile pylorospasm (Q40.0)*
>   *gastrointestinal hemorrhage (K92.0-K92.2)*
>   *intestinal obstruction (K56.-)*
>   *newborn gastrointestinal hemorrhage (P54.0-P54.3)*
>   *newborn intestinal obstruction (P76.-)*
>   *pylorospasm (K31.3)*
>   *signs and symptoms involving the urinary system (R30-R39)*
>   *symptoms referable to female genital organs (N94.-)*
>   *symptoms referable to male genital organs male (N48-N50)*

✓4ᵗʰ **R10**   **Abdominal and pelvic pain**
> EXCLUDES 1   *renal colic (N23)*
> EXCLUDES 2   *dorsalgia (M54.-)*
>   *flatulence and related conditions (R14.-)*

R10.0   **Acute abdomen**
       Severe abdominal pain (generalized) (with abdominal rigidity)
> EXCLUDES 1   *abdominal rigidity NOS (R19.3)*
>   *generalized abdominal pain NOS (R10.84)*
>   *localized abdominal pain (R10.1-R10.3-)*

✓5ᵗʰ **R10.1**   **Pain localized to upper abdomen**

     R10.10   **Upper abdominal pain, unspecified**   ▽

     R10.11   **Right upper quadrant pain**

     R10.12   **Left upper quadrant pain**

     R10.13   **Epigastric pain**
       Dyspepsia
> EXCLUDES 1   *functional dyspepsia (K30)*

R10.2   **Pelvic and perineal pain**
> EXCLUDES 1   *vulvodynia (N94.81)*

✓5ᵗʰ **R10.3**   **Pain localized to other parts of lower abdomen**

     R10.30   **Lower abdominal pain, unspecified**   ▽

     R10.31   **Right lower quadrant pain**

     R10.32   **Left lower quadrant pain**

     R10.33   **Periumbilical pain**

✓5ᵗʰ **R10.8**   **Other abdominal pain**

     ✓6ᵗʰ **R10.81**   **Abdominal tenderness**
       Abdominal tenderness NOS

         R10.811   **Right upper quadrant abdominal tenderness**

         R10.812   **Left upper quadrant abdominal tenderness**

         R10.813   **Right lower quadrant abdominal tenderness**

         R10.814   **Left lower quadrant abdominal tenderness**

         R10.815   **Periumbilic abdominal tenderness**

         R10.816   **Epigastric abdominal tenderness**

         R10.817   **Generalized abdominal tenderness**

         R10.819   **Abdominal tenderness, unspecified site**   ▽

     ✓6ᵗʰ **R10.82**   **Rebound abdominal tenderness**

         R10.821   **Right upper quadrant rebound abdominal tenderness**

         R10.822   **Left upper quadrant rebound abdominal tenderness**

         R10.823   **Right lower quadrant rebound abdominal tenderness**

         R10.824   **Left lower quadrant rebound abdominal tenderness**

         R10.825   **Periumbilic rebound abdominal tenderness**

         R10.826   **Epigastric rebound abdominal tenderness**

N Newborn   P Pediatric   M Maternity   A Adult   RIC RIC Dx   NC Dx Noncancer Dx   PDx Primary Dx   CC RIC CC Condition   ►◄ Revised Text   ● New Code   ▲ Revised Code Title

836   ICD-10-CM 2016

R06.6–R10.826

R10.827   **Generalized** rebound abdominal tenderness

R10.829   **Rebound abdominal tenderness, unspecified site**   ▽

R10.83   **Colic**   P
Colic NOS
Infantile colic
EXCLUDES 1   *colic in adult and child over 12 months old (R10.84)*

R10.84   **Generalized** abdominal pain
EXCLUDES 1   *generalized abdominal pain associated with acute abdomen (R10.0)*

R10.9   **Unspecified abdominal pain**   ▽

✓4ᵗʰ **R11 Nausea and vomiting**
EXCLUDES 1   *cyclical vomiting associated with migraine (G43.A-)*
excessive vomiting in pregnancy (O21.-)
hematemesis (K92.0)
neonatal hematemesis (P54.0)
newborn vomiting (P92.0-)
psychogenic vomiting (F50.8)
vomiting associated with bulimia nervosa (F50.2)
vomiting following gastrointestinal surgery (K91.0)

R11.0   **Nausea**
Nausea NOS
Nausea without vomiting

✓5ᵗʰ R11.1   **Vomiting**
²R11.10   **Vomiting, unspecified**   ▽
Vomiting NOS

²R11.11   **Vomiting** without nausea
²R11.12   **Projectile** vomiting
²R11.13   **Vomiting** of fecal matter
²R11.14   **Bilious** vomiting
Bilious emesis

² R11.2   **Nausea with vomiting, unspecified**   ▽
Persistent nausea with vomiting NOS

R12   **Heartburn**
EXCLUDES 1   *dyspepsia NOS (R10.13)*
functional dyspepsia (K30)

✓4ᵗʰ **R13 Aphagia and dysphagia**

R13.0   **Aphagia**   CC
Inability to swallow
EXCLUDES 1   *psychogenic aphagia (F50.9)*
RIC Excl: 01 Stroke

✓5ᵗʰ R13.1   **Dysphagia**
Code first, if applicable, dysphagia following cerebrovascular disease (I69. with final characters -91)
EXCLUDES 1   *psychogenic dysphagia (F45.8)*

R13.10   **Dysphagia, unspecified**   CC ▽
Difficulty in swallowing NOS
RIC Excl: 01 Stroke

R13.11   **Dysphagia, oral phase**   CC
RIC Excl: 01 Stroke

R13.12   **Dysphagia, oropharyngeal phase**   CC
RIC Excl: 01 Stroke

R13.13   **Dysphagia, pharyngeal phase**   CC
RIC Excl: 01 Stroke

R13.14   **Dysphagia, pharyngoesophageal phase**   CC
RIC Excl: 01 Stroke

R13.19   **Other dysphagia**   CC
Cervical dysphagia
Neurogenic dysphagia
RIC Excl: 01 Stroke

✓4ᵗʰ **R14 Flatulence and related conditions**
EXCLUDES 1   *psychogenic aerophagy (F45.8)*

R14.0   **Abdominal distension (gaseous)**
Bloating
Tympanites (abdominal) (intestinal)

R14.1   **Gas pain**

R14.2   **Eructation**

R14.3   **Flatulence**

✓4ᵗʰ **R15 Fecal incontinence**
Encopresis NOS
EXCLUDES 1   *fecal incontinence of nonorganic origin (F98.1)*

R15.0   **Incomplete defecation**
EXCLUDES 1   *constipation (K59.0-)*
fecal impaction (K56.41)

R15.1   **Fecal smearing**
Fecal soiling

R15.2   **Fecal urgency**

R15.9   **Full incontinence of feces**
Fecal incontinence NOS

✓4ᵗʰ **R16 Hepatomegaly and splenomegaly, not elsewhere classified**

R16.0   **Hepatomegaly, not elsewhere classified**
Hepatomegaly NOS

R16.1   **Splenomegaly, not elsewhere classified**
Splenomegaly NOS

R16.2   **Hepatomegaly with splenomegaly, not elsewhere classified**
Hepatosplenomegaly NOS

R17   **Unspecified jaundice**   ▽
EXCLUDES 1   *neonatal jaundice (P55, P57-P59)*

✓4ᵗʰ **R18 Ascites**
INCLUDES   fluid in peritoneal cavity
EXCLUDES 1   *ascites in alcoholic cirrhosis (K70.31)*
ascites in alcoholic hepatitis (K70.11)
ascites in toxic liver disease with chronic active hepatitis (K71.51)

R18.0   **Malignant** ascites
Code first malignancy, such as:
malignant neoplasm of ovary (C56.-)
secondary malignant neoplasm of retroperitoneum and peritoneum (C78.6)

R18.8   **Other ascites**
Ascites NOS
Peritoneal effusion (chronic)

✓4ᵗʰ **R19 Other symptoms and signs involving the digestive system and abdomen**
EXCLUDES 1   *acute abdomen (R10.0)*

✓5ᵗʰ R19.0   **Intra-abdominal and pelvic swelling, mass and lump**
EXCLUDES 1   *abdominal distension (gaseous) (R14.-)*
ascites (R18.-)

R19.00   **Intra-abdominal and pelvic swelling, mass and lump, unspecified site**   ▽

R19.01   **Right upper quadrant** abdominal swelling, mass and lump

R19.02   **Left upper quadrant** abdominal swelling, mass and lump

R19.03   **Right lower quadrant** abdominal swelling, mass and lump

R19.04   **Left lower quadrant** abdominal swelling, mass and lump

R19.05   **Periumbilic** swelling, mass or lump
Diffuse or generalized umbilical swelling or mass

R19.06   **Epigastric** swelling, mass or lump

R19.07   **Generalized** intra-abdominal and pelvic swelling, mass and lump
Diffuse or generalized intra-abdominal swelling or mass NOS
Diffuse or generalized pelvic swelling or mass NOS

R19.09   **Other intra-abdominal and pelvic swelling, mass and lump**

✓5ᵗʰ R19.1   **Abnormal bowel sounds**
R19.11   **Absent bowel sounds**
R19.12   **Hyperactive bowel sounds**
R19.15   **Other abnormal bowel sounds**
Abnormal bowel sounds NOS

R19.2   **Visible peristalsis**
Hyperperistalsis

✓5ᵗʰ R19.3   **Abdominal rigidity**
EXCLUDES 1   *abdominal rigidity with severe abdominal pain (R10.0)*

R19.30   **Abdominal rigidity, unspecified site**   ▽
R19.31   **Right upper quadrant** abdominal rigidity
R19.32   **Left upper quadrant** abdominal rigidity
R19.33   **Right lower quadrant** abdominal rigidity
R19.34   **Left lower quadrant** abdominal rigidity
R19.35   **Periumbilic** abdominal rigidity
R19.36   **Epigastric** abdominal rigidity

---

² Special Care High = With fever

✓ Add'l Character Required   ✓ₓ7ᵗʰ Placeholder Alert   RUG IV Special Care High Dx   RUG IV Clinically Complex Dx   RUG IV Special Care Low Dx   Manifestation Code   Other Specified Code   ▽ Unspecified Code

R19.37 Generalized **abdominal rigidity**

R19.4 **Change in bowel habit**
> EXCLUDES 1 *constipation (K59.0-)*
> *functional diarrhea (K59.1)*

R19.5 **Other fecal abnormalities**
Abnormal stool color
Bulky stools
Mucus in stools
Occult blood in feces
Occult blood in stools
> EXCLUDES 1 *melena (K92.1)*
> *neonatal melena (P54.1)*

R19.6 **Halitosis**

R19.7 **Diarrhea, unspecified**   ▽
Diarrhea NOS
> EXCLUDES 1 *functional diarrhea (K59.1)*
> *neonatal diarrhea (P78.3)*
> *psychogenic diarrhea (F45.8)*

R19.8 **Other specified symptoms and signs involving the digestive system and abdomen**

Symptoms and signs involving the skin and subcutaneous tissue (R20-R23)

> EXCLUDES 2 *symptoms relating to breast (N64.4-N64.5)*

✓4ᵗʰ **R20** **Disturbances of skin sensation**
> EXCLUDES 1 *dissociative anesthesia and sensory loss (F44.6)*
> *psychogenic disturbances (F45.8)*

R20.0 **Anesthesia of skin**

R20.1 **Hypoesthesia of skin**

R20.2 **Paresthesia of skin**
Formication
Pins and needles
Tingling skin
> EXCLUDES 1 *acroparesthesia (I73.8)*

R20.3 **Hyperesthesia**

R20.8 **Other disturbances of skin sensation**

R20.9 **Unspecified disturbances of skin sensation**   ▽

R21 **Rash and other nonspecific skin eruption**
Rash NOS
> EXCLUDES 1 *specified type of rash—code to condition*
> *vesicular eruption (R23.8)*

✓4ᵗʰ **R22** **Localized swelling, mass and lump of skin and subcutaneous tissue**
Subcutaneous nodules (localized)(superficial)
> EXCLUDES 1 *abnormal findings on diagnostic imaging (R90-R93)*
> *edema (R60.-)*
> *enlarged lymph nodes (R59.-)*
> *localized adiposity (E65)*
> *swelling of joint (M25.4-)*

R22.0 **Localized swelling, mass and lump, head**

R22.1 **Localized swelling, mass and lump, neck**

R22.2 **Localized swelling, mass and lump, trunk**
> EXCLUDES 1 *intra-abdominal or pelvic mass and lump (R19.0-)*
> *intra-abdominal or pelvic swelling (R19.0-)*
> EXCLUDES 2 *breast mass and lump (N63)*

✓5ᵗʰ **R22.3** **Localized swelling, mass and lump, upper limb**

   R22.30 **Localized swelling, mass and lump, unspecified upper limb**   ▽

   R22.31 **Localized swelling, mass and lump, right upper limb**

   R22.32 **Localized swelling, mass and lump, left upper limb**

   R22.33 **Localized swelling, mass and lump, upper limb, bilateral**

✓5ᵗʰ **R22.4** **Localized swelling, mass and lump, lower limb**

   R22.40 **Localized swelling, mass and lump, unspecified lower limb**   ▽

   R22.41 **Localized swelling, mass and lump, right lower limb**

   R22.42 **Localized swelling, mass and lump, left lower limb**

   R22.43 **Localized swelling, mass and lump, lower limb, bilateral**

R22.9 **Localized swelling, mass and lump, unspecified**   ▽

✓4ᵗʰ **R23** **Other skin changes**

R23.0 **Cyanosis**
> EXCLUDES 1 *acrocyanosis (I73.8)*
> *cyanotic attacks of newborn (P28.2)*

R23.1 **Pallor**
Clammy skin

R23.2 **Flushing**
Excessive blushing
Code first, if applicable, menopausal and female climacteric states (N95.1)

R23.3 **Spontaneous ecchymoses**
Petechiae
> EXCLUDES 1 *ecchymoses of newborn (P54.5)*
> *purpura (D69.-)*

R23.4 **Changes in skin texture**
Desquamation of skin
Induration of skin
Scaling of skin
> EXCLUDES 1 *epidermal thickening NOS (L85.9)*

R23.8 **Other skin changes**

R23.9 **Unspecified skin changes**   ▽

Symptoms and signs involving the nervous and musculoskeletal systems (R25-R29)

✓4ᵗʰ **R25** **Abnormal involuntary movements**
> EXCLUDES 1 *specific movement disorders (G20-G26)*
> *stereotyped movement disorders (F98.4)*
> *tic disorders (F95.-)*

R25.0 **Abnormal head movements**

R25.1 **Tremor, unspecified**   ▽
> EXCLUDES 1 *chorea NOS (G25.5)*
> *essential tremor (G25.0)*
> *hysterical tremor (F44.4)*
> *intention tremor (G25.2)*

R25.2 **Cramp and spasm**
> EXCLUDES 2 *carpopedal spasm (R29.0)*
> *charley-horse (M62.831)*
> *infantile spasms (G40.4-)*
> *muscle spasm of back (M62.830)*
> *muscle spasm of calf (M62.831)*

R25.3 **Fasciculation**
Twitching NOS

R25.8 **Other abnormal involuntary movements**

R25.9 **Unspecified abnormal involuntary movements**   ▽

✓4ᵗʰ **R26** **Abnormalities of gait and mobility**
> EXCLUDES 1 *ataxia NOS (R27.0)*
> *hereditary ataxia (G11.-)*
> *locomotor (syphilitic) ataxia (A52.11)*
> *immobility syndrome (paraplegic) (M62.3)*

R26.0 **Ataxic gait**
Staggering gait

R26.1 **Paralytic gait**
Spastic gait

R26.2 **Difficulty in walking, not elsewhere classified**
> EXCLUDES 1 *falling (R29.6)*
> *unsteadiness on feet (R26.81)*

✓5ᵗʰ **R26.8** **Other abnormalities of gait and mobility**

   R26.81 **Unsteadiness on feet**

   R26.89 **Other abnormalities of gait and mobility**

R26.9 **Unspecified abnormalities of gait and mobility**   ▽

✓4ᵗʰ **R27** **Other lack of coordination**
> EXCLUDES 1 *ataxic gait (R26.0)*
> *hereditary ataxia (G11.-)*
> *vertigo NOS (R42)*

R27.0 **Ataxia, unspecified**   ▽
> EXCLUDES 1 *ataxia following cerebrovascular disease (I69. with final characters -93)*

R27.8 **Other lack of coordination**

R27.9 **Unspecified lack of coordination**   ▽

✓4ᵗʰ **R29** **Other symptoms and signs involving the nervous and musculoskeletal systems**

R29.0 **Tetany**   CC
Carpopedal spasm
> EXCLUDES 1 *hysterical tetany (F44.5)*
> *neonatal tetany (P71.3)*
> *parathyroid tetany (E20.9)*
> *post-thyroidectomy tetany (E89.2)*
> RIC Excl: 06 Neurological

R29.1 **Meningismus**

Ⓝ Newborn   Ⓟ Pediatric   Ⓜ Maternity   Ⓐ Adult   RIC RIC Dx   NCDx Noncancer Dx   PDx Primary Dx   CC RIC CC Condition   ▶◀ Revised Text   ● New Code   ▲ Revised Code Title

838   ICD-10-CM 2016

R29.2 Abnormal reflex
> EXCLUDES 2 *abnormal pupillary reflex (H57.0)*
> *hyperactive gag reflex (J39.2)*
> *vasovagal reaction or syncope (R55)*

R29.3 Abnormal posture

R29.4 Clicking hip
> EXCLUDES 1 *congenital deformities of hip (Q65.-)*

R29.5 Transient paralysis
> Code first any associated spinal cord injury (S14.0, S14.1-, S24.0, S24.1-, S34.0-, S34.1-)
> EXCLUDES 1 *transient ischemic attack (G45.9)*

R29.6 Repeated falls
> Falling
> Tendency to fall
> EXCLUDES 2 *at risk for falling (Z91.81)*
> *history of falling (Z91.81)*

✓5th **R29.8 Other symptoms and signs involving the nervous and musculoskeletal systems**

  ✓6th **R29.81 Other symptoms and signs involving the nervous system**

    R29.810 Facial weakness
> Facial droop
> EXCLUDES 1 *Bell's palsy (G51.0)*
> *facial weakness following cerebrovascular disease (I69. with final characters -92)*

    R29.818 Other symptoms and signs involving the nervous system

  ✓6th **R29.89 Other symptoms and signs involving the musculoskeletal system**
> EXCLUDES 2 *pain in limb (M79.6-)*

    R29.890 Loss of height
> EXCLUDES 1 *osteoporosis (M80-M81)*

    R29.891 Ocular torticollis
> EXCLUDES 1 *congenital (sternomastoid) torticollis Q68.0*
> *psychogenic torticollis (F45.8)*
> *spasmodic torticollis (G24.3)*
> *torticollis due to birth injury (P15.8)*
> *torticollis NOS M43.6*

    R29.898 Other symptoms and signs involving the musculoskeletal system

✓5th **R29.9 Unspecified symptoms and signs involving the nervous and musculoskeletal systems**

  R29.90 Unspecified symptoms and signs involving the nervous system ▽

  R29.91 Unspecified symptoms and signs involving the musculoskeletal system ▽

Symptoms and signs involving the genitourinary system (R30-R39)

✓4th **R30 Pain associated with micturition**
> EXCLUDES 1 *psychogenic pain associated with micturition (F45.8)*

R30.0 Dysuria
> Strangury

R30.1 Vesical tenesmus

R30.9 Painful micturition, unspecified ▽
> Painful urination NOS

✓4th **R31 Hematuria**
> EXCLUDES 1 *hematuria included with underlying conditions, such as:*
> *acute cystitis with hematuria (N30.01)*
> *recurrent and persistent hematuria in glomerular diseases (N02.-)*

R31.0 Gross hematuria

R31.1 Benign essential microscopic hematuria

R31.2 Other microscopic hematuria

R31.9 Hematuria, unspecified ▽

R32 Unspecified urinary incontinence ▽
> Enuresis NOS
> EXCLUDES 1 *functional urinary incontinence (R39.81)*
> *nonorganic enuresis (F98.0)*
> *stress incontinence and other specified urinary incontinence (N39.3-N39.4-)*
> *urinary incontinence associated with cognitive impairment (R39.81)*

✓4th **R33 Retention of urine**
> EXCLUDES 1 *psychogenic retention of urine (F45.8)*

R33.0 Drug induced retention of urine
> Use additional code for adverse effect, if applicable, to identify drug (T36-T50 with fifth or sixth character 5)

R33.8 Other retention of urine
> Code first, if applicable, any causal condition, such as:
> enlarged prostate (N40.1)

R33.9 Retention of urine, unspecified ▽

R34 Anuria and oliguria
> EXCLUDES 1 *anuria and oliguria complicating abortion or ectopic or molar pregnancy (O00-O07, O08.4)*
> *anuria and oliguria complicating pregnancy (O26.83-)*
> *anuria and oliguria complicating the puerperium (O90.4)*

✓4th **R35 Polyuria**
> Code first, if applicable, any causal condition, such as:
> enlarged prostate (N40.1)
> EXCLUDES 1 *psychogenic polyuria (F45.8)*

R35.0 Frequency of micturition

R35.1 Nocturia

R35.8 Other polyuria
> Polyuria NOS

✓4th **R36 Urethral discharge**

R36.0 Urethral discharge without blood

R36.1 Hematospermia ♂

R36.9 Urethral discharge, unspecified ▽
> Penile discharge NOS
> Urethrorrhea

R37 Sexual dysfunction, unspecified ▽

✓4th **R39 Other and unspecified symptoms and signs involving the genitourinary system**

R39.0 Extravasation of urine

✓5th **R39.1 Other difficulties with micturition**
> Code first, if applicable, any causal condition, such as:
> enlarged prostate (N40.1)

  R39.11 Hesitancy of micturition

  R39.12 Poor urinary stream
> Weak urinary steam

  R39.13 Splitting of urinary stream

  R39.14 Feeling of incomplete bladder emptying

  R39.15 Urgency of urination
> EXCLUDES 1 *urge incontinence (N39.41, N39.46)*

  R39.16 Straining to void

  R39.19 Other difficulties with micturition

R39.2 Extrarenal uremia
> Prerenal uremia
> EXCLUDES 1 *uremia NOS (N19)*

✓5th **R39.8 Other symptoms and signs involving the genitourinary system**

  R39.81 Functional urinary incontinence
> Urinary incontinence due to cognitive impairment, or severe physical disability or immobility
> EXCLUDES 1 *stress incontinence and other specified urinary incontinence (N39.3-N39.4-)*
> *urinary incontinence NOS (R32)*

  R39.89 Other symptoms and signs involving the genitourinary system

R39.9 Unspecified symptoms and signs involving the genitourinary system ▽

Symptoms and signs involving cognition, perception, emotional state and behavior (R40-R46)

> EXCLUDES 1 *symptoms and signs constituting part of a pattern of mental disorder (F01-F99)*

✓4th **R40 Somnolence, stupor and coma**
> EXCLUDES 1 *neonatal coma (P91.5)*
> *somnolence, stupor and coma in diabetes (E08-E13)*
> *somnolence, stupor and coma in hepatic failure (K72.-)*
> *somnolence, stupor and coma in hypoglycemia (nondiabetic) (E15)*

R40.0 Somnolence
> Drowsiness
> EXCLUDES 1 *coma (R40.2-)*

☑ Add'l Character Required   ✓x7th Placeholder Alert   **RUG IV Special Care High Dx**   RUG IV Clinically Complex Dx   RUG IV Special Care Low Dx   Manifestation Code   Other Specified Code   ▽ Unspecified Code

Chapter 18. Symptoms, Signs and Abnormal Clinical and Laboratory Findings

R40.1 Stupor
Catatonic stupor
Semicoma
EXCLUDES 1 *catatonic schizophrenia (F20.2)*
coma (R40.2-)
depressive stupor (F31-F33)
dissociative stupor (F44.2)
manic stupor (F30.2)

R40.2 Coma
Code first any associated:
fracture of skull (S02.-)
intracranial injury (S06.-)
NOTE One code from subcategories R40.21-R40.23 is
required to complete the coma scale
AHA: 2014, 1Q, 19

10 R40.20 Unspecified coma ▽
Coma NOS
Unconsciousness NOS

✓6th R40.21 Coma scale, eyes open

The following appropriate 7th character is to be
added to subcategory R40.21-.
0 unspecified time
1 in the field [EMT or ambulance]
2 at arrival to emergency department
3 at hospital admission
4 24 hours or more after hospital admission

✓7th R40.211 Coma scale, eyes open, never
✓7th R40.212 Coma scale, eyes open, to pain
✓7th R40.213 Coma scale, eyes open, to sound
✓7th R40.214 Coma scale, eyes open, spontaneous

✓6th R40.22 Coma scale, best verbal response

The following appropriate 7th character is to be
added to subcategory R40.22-.
0 unspecified time
1 in the field [EMT or ambulance]
2 at arrival to emergency department
3 at hospital admission
4 24 hours or more after hospital admission

✓7th R40.221 Coma scale, best verbal response, none
✓7th R40.222 Coma scale, best verbal response, incomprehensible words
✓7th R40.223 Coma scale, best verbal response, inappropriate words
✓7th R40.224 Coma scale, best verbal response, confused conversation
✓7th R40.225 Coma scale, best verbal response, oriented

✓6th R40.23 Coma scale, best motor response

The following appropriate 7th character is to be
added to subcategory R40.23-.
0 unspecified time
1 in the field [EMT or ambulance]
2 at arrival to emergency department
3 at hospital admission
4 24 hours or more after hospital admission

✓7th R40.231 Coma scale, best motor response, none
✓7th R40.232 Coma scale, best motor response, extension
✓7th R40.233 Coma scale, best motor response, abnormal
✓7th R40.234 Coma scale, best motor response, flexion withdrawal
✓7th R40.235 Coma scale, best motor response, localizes pain
✓7th R40.236 Coma scale, best motor response, obeys commands

✓6th R40.24 Glasgow coma scale, total score
Use codes R40.21- through R40.23- only when the
individual score(s) are documented
R40.241 Glasgow coma scale score 13-15
R40.242 Glasgow coma scale score 9-12
R40.243 Glasgow coma scale score 3-8

R40.244 Other coma, without documented Glasgow coma scale score, or with partial score reported

R40.3 Persistent vegetative state

R40.4 Transient alteration of awareness

✓4th R41 Other symptoms and signs involving cognitive functions and awareness
EXCLUDES 1 *dissociative [conversion] disorders (F44.-)*
mild cognitive impairment, so stated (G31.84)

R41.0 Disorientation, unspecified ▽
Confusion NOS   Delirium NOS

R41.1 Anterograde amnesia

R41.2 Retrograde amnesia

R41.3 Other amnesia
Amnesia NOS
Memory loss NOS
EXCLUDES 1 *amnestic disorder due to known physiologic condition (F04)*
amnestic syndrome due to psychoactive substance use (F10-F19 with 5th character .6)
mild memory disturbance due to known physiological condition (F06.8)
transient global amnesia (G45.4)

R41.4 Neurologic neglect syndrome
Asomatognosia
Hemi-akinesia
Hemi-inattention
Hemispatial neglect
Left-sided neglect
Sensory neglect
Visuospatial neglect
EXCLUDES 1 *visuospatial deficit (R41.842)*

✓5th R41.8 Other symptoms and signs involving cognitive functions and awareness

R41.81 Age-related cognitive decline Ⓐ
Senility NOS

R41.82 Altered mental status, unspecified ▽
Change in mental status NOS
EXCLUDES 1 *altered level of consciousness (R40.-)*
altered mental status due to known condition—code to condition
delirium NOS (R41.0)
AHA: 2012, 4Q, 97

R41.83 Borderline intellectual functioning
IQ level 71 to 84
EXCLUDES 1 *intellectual disabilities (F70-F79)*

✓6th R41.84 Other specified cognitive deficit
R41.840 Attention and concentration deficit
EXCLUDES 1 *attention-deficit hyperactivity disorders (F90.-)*
R41.841 Cognitive communication deficit
R41.842 Visuospatial deficit
R41.843 Psychomotor deficit
R41.844 Frontal lobe and executive function deficit

R41.89 Other symptoms and signs involving cognitive functions and awareness
Anosognosia

R41.9 Unspecified symptoms and signs involving cognitive functions and awareness ▽

R42 Dizziness and giddiness
Light-headedness
Vertigo NOS
EXCLUDES 1 *vertiginous syndromes (H81.-)*
vertigo from infrasound (T75.23)

✓4th R43 Disturbances of smell and taste
R43.0 Anosmia
R43.1 Parosmia
R43.2 Parageusia
R43.8 Other disturbances of smell and taste
Mixed disturbance of smell and taste
R43.9 Unspecified disturbances of smell and taste ▽

---

10 Hospice questionable admission diagnosis

Ⓝ Newborn Ⓟ Pediatric Ⓜ Maternity Ⓐ Adult **RIC** RIC Dx **NC Dx** Noncancer Dx **PDx** Primary Dx **CC** RIC CC Condition ▶◀ Revised Text ● New Code ▲ Revised Code Title

840

ICD-10-CM 2016

R40.1–R43.9

✓4ᵗʰ **R44 Other symptoms and signs involving general sensations and perceptions**
- *EXCLUDES 1*   *alcoholic hallucinations (F1.5)*
  hallucinations in drug psychosis (F11-F19 with .5)
  hallucinations in mood disorders with psychotic symptoms (F30.2, F31.5, F32.3, F33.3)
  hallucinations in schizophrenia, schizotypal and delusional disorders (F20-F29)
- *EXCLUDES 2*   *disturbances of skin sensation (R20.-)*

R44.0 **Auditory** hallucinations

R44.1 **Visual** hallucinations

R44.2 **Other hallucinations**

R44.3 Hallucinations, unspecified ▽

R44.8 **Other symptoms and signs involving general sensations and perceptions**

R44.9 Unspecified symptoms and signs involving general sensations and perceptions ▽

✓4ᵗʰ **R45 Symptoms and signs involving emotional state**

R45.0 **Nervousness**
Nervous tension

R45.1 **Restlessness and agitation**

R45.2 **Unhappiness**

R45.3 **Demoralization and apathy**
- *EXCLUDES 1*   *anhedonia (R45.84)*

R45.4 **Irritability and anger**

R45.5 **Hostility**

R45.6 **Violent behavior**

R45.7 **State of emotional shock and stress, unspecified** ▽

✓5ᵗʰ R45.8 **Other symptoms and signs involving emotional state**

R45.81 **Low self-esteem**

R45.82 **Worries**

R45.83 **Excessive crying of child, adolescent or adult**
- *EXCLUDES 1*   *excessive crying of infant (baby) R68.11*

R45.84 **Anhedonia**

✓6ᵗʰ R45.85 **Homicidal and suicidal ideations**
- *EXCLUDES 1*   *suicide attempt (T14.91)*

R45.850 **Homicidal ideations**

R45.851 **Suicidal ideations**

R45.86 **Emotional lability**

R45.87 **Impulsiveness**

R45.89 **Other symptoms and signs involving emotional state**

✓4ᵗʰ **R46 Symptoms and signs involving appearance and behavior**
- *EXCLUDES 1*   *appearance and behavior in schizophrenia, schizotypal and delusional disorders (F20-F29)*
  mental and behavioral disorders (F01-F99)

R46.0 **Very low level of personal hygiene**

R46.1 **Bizarre personal appearance**

R46.2 **Strange and inexplicable behavior**

R46.3 **Overactivity**

R46.4 **Slowness and poor responsiveness**
- *EXCLUDES 1*   *stupor (R40.1)*

R46.5 **Suspiciousness and marked evasiveness**

R46.6 **Undue concern and preoccupation with stressful events**

R46.7 **Verbosity and circumstantial detail obscuring reason for contact**

✓5ᵗʰ R46.8 **Other symptoms and signs involving appearance and behavior**

R46.81 **Obsessive-compulsive behavior**
- *EXCLUDES 1*   *obsessive-compulsive disorder (F42)*

R46.89 **Other symptoms and signs involving appearance and behavior**

Symptoms and signs involving speech and voice (R47-R49)

✓4ᵗʰ **R47 Speech disturbances, not elsewhere classified**
- *EXCLUDES 1*   *autism (F84.0)*
  cluttering (F80.81)
  specific developmental disorders of speech and language (F80.-)
  stuttering (F80.81)

✓5ᵗʰ R47.0 **Dysphasia and aphasia**

R47.01 **Aphasia**
- *EXCLUDES 1*   *aphasia following cerebrovascular disease (I69. with final characters -20)*
  progressive isolated aphasia (G31.01)

R47.02 **Dysphasia**
- *EXCLUDES 1*   *dysphasia following cerebrovascular disease (I69. with final characters -21)*

R47.1 **Dysarthria and anarthria**
- *EXCLUDES 1*   *dysarthria following cerebrovascular disease (I69. with final characters -22)*

✓5ᵗʰ R47.8 **Other speech disturbances**
- *EXCLUDES 1*   *dysarthria following cerebrovascular disease (I69. with final characters -28)*

R47.81 **Slurred speech**

R47.82 *Fluency disorder in conditions classified elsewhere*
Stuttering in conditions classified elsewhere
Code first underlying disease or condition, such as:
Parkinson's disease (G20)
- *EXCLUDES 1*   *adult onset fluency disorder (F98.5)*
  childhood onset fluency disorder (F80.81)
  fluency disorder (stuttering) following cerebrovascular disease (I69. with final characters-23)

R47.89 **Other speech disturbances**

R47.9 Unspecified speech disturbances ▽

✓4ᵗʰ **R48 Dyslexia and other symbolic dysfunctions, not elsewhere classified**
- *EXCLUDES 1*   *specific developmental disorders of scholastic skills (F81.-)*

R48.0 **Dyslexia and alexia**

R48.1 **Agnosia**
Astereognosia (astereognosis)
Autotopagnosia
- *EXCLUDES 1*   *visual object agnosia (R48.3)*

R48.2 **Apraxia**
- *EXCLUDES 1*   *apraxia following cerebrovascular disease (I69. with final characters -90)*

R48.3 **Visual agnosia**
Prosopagnosia
Simultanagnosia (asimultagnosia)

R48.8 **Other symbolic dysfunctions**
Acalculia
Agraphia

R48.9 Unspecified symbolic dysfunctions ▽

✓4ᵗʰ **R49 Voice and resonance disorders**
- *EXCLUDES 1*   *psychogenic voice and resonance disorders (F44.4)*

R49.0 **Dysphonia**
Hoarseness

R49.1 **Aphonia**
Loss of voice

✓5ᵗʰ R49.2 **Hypernasality and hyponasality**

R49.21 **Hypernasality**

R49.22 **Hyponasality**

R49.8 **Other voice and resonance disorders**

R49.9 **Unspecified voice and resonance disorder** ▽
Change in voice NOS
Resonance disorder NOS

General symptoms and signs (R50-R69)

✓4ᵗʰ **R50 Fever of other and unknown origin**
- *EXCLUDES 1*   *chills without fever (R68.83)*
  febrile convulsions (R56.0-)
  fever of unknown origin during labor (O75.2)
  fever of unknown origin in newborn (P81.9)
  hypothermia due to illness (R68.0)
  malignant hyperthermia due to anesthesia (T88.3)
  puerperal pyrexia NOS (O86.4)

R50.2 **Drug induced fever**
Use additional code for adverse effect, if applicable, to identify drug (T36-T50 with fifth or sixth character 5)
- *EXCLUDES 1*   *postvaccination (postimmunization) fever (R50.83)*

✓ Add'l Character Required   ✓x7ᵗʰ Placeholder Alert   RUG IV Special Care High Dx   RUG IV Clinically Complex Dx   RUG IV Special Care Low Dx   Manifestation Code   Other Specified Code   ▽Unspecified Code

✓5ᵗʰ **R50.8** **Other** specified fever

    R50.81 *Fever presenting with conditions classified elsewhere*
        Code first underlying condition when associated fever is
        present, such as with:
        leukemia (C91-C95)
        neutropenia (D70.-)
        sickle-cell disease (D57.-)
        AHA: 2014, 4Q, 22

    R50.82 **Postprocedural** fever   cc
        EXCLUDES 1   *postprocedural infection (T81.4)*
            posttransfusion fever (R50.84)
            postvaccination (postimmunization) fever
            (R50.83)

    R50.83 **Postvaccination** fever
        Postimmunization fever

    R50.84 **Febrile nonhemolytic transfusion reaction**   cc
        FNHTR
        Posttransfusion fever

³ **R50.9** **Fever, unspecified**   ▽
    Fever NOS
    Fever of unknown origin [FUO]
    Fever with chills
    Fever with rigors
    Hyperpyrexia NOS
    Persistent fever
    Pyrexia NOS

R51 **Headache**
    Facial pain NOS
    EXCLUDES 1   *atypical face pain (G50.1)*
            migraine and other headache syndromes (G43-G44)
            trigeminal neuralgia (G50.0)

R52 **Pain, unspecified**   ▽
    Acute pain NOS
    Generalized pain NOS
    Pain NOS
    EXCLUDES 1   *acute and chronic pain, not elsewhere classified (G89.-)*
            localized pain, unspecified type—code to pain by site, such as:
            abdomen pain (R10.-)
            back pain (M54.9)
            breast pain (N64.4)
            chest pain (R07.1-R07.9)
            ear pain (H92.0-)
            eye pain (H57.1)
            headache (R51)
            joint pain (M25.5-)
            limb pain (M79.6-)
            lumbar region pain (M54.5)
            pelvic and perineal pain (R10.2)
            renal colic (N23)
            shoulder pain (M25.51-)
            spine pain (M54.-)
            throat pain (R07.0)
            tongue pain (K14.6)
            tooth pain (K08.8)
         pain disorders exclusively related to psychological factors
            (F45.41)

✓4ᵗʰ **R53** **Malaise and fatigue**
    R53.0 **Neoplastic (malignant) related fatigue**
        Code first associated neoplasm

    R53.1 **Weakness**
        Asthenia NOS
        EXCLUDES 1   *age-related weakness (R54)*
            muscle weakness (M62.8-)
            senile asthenia (R54)
        AHA: 2015, 1Q, 25

    R53.2 **Functional quadriplegia**
        Complete immobility due to severe physical disability or frailty
        EXCLUDES 1   *frailty NOS (R54)*
            hysterical paralysis (F44.4)
            immobility syndrome (M62.3)
            neurologic quadriplegia (G82.5-)
            quadriplegia (G82.50)

✓5ᵗʰ **R53.8** **Other malaise and fatigue**
    EXCLUDES 1   *combat exhaustion and fatigue (F43.0)*
        congenital debility (P96.9)
        exhaustion and fatigue due to depressive episode
            (F32.-)
        exhaustion and fatigue due to excessive exertion
            (T73.3)
        exhaustion and fatigue due to exposure (T73.2)
        exhaustion and fatigue due to heat (T67.-)
        exhaustion and fatigue due to pregnancy (O26.8-)
        exhaustion and fatigue due to recurrent depressive
            episode (F33)
        exhaustion and fatigue due to senile debility (R54)

    ¹⁰R53.81 **Other malaise**
        Chronic debility
        Debility NOS
        General physical deterioration
        Malaise NOS
        Nervous debility
        EXCLUDES 1   *age-related physical debility (R54)*

    R53.82 **Chronic fatigue, unspecified**   ▽
        Chronic fatigue syndrome NOS
        EXCLUDES 1   *postviral fatigue syndrome (G93.3)*

    R53.83 **Other fatigue**
        Fatigue NOS
        Lack of energy
        Lethargy
        Tiredness

¹⁰ **R54** **Age-related physical debility**   Ⓐ
    Frailty
    Old age
    Senescence
    Senile asthenia
    Senile debility
    EXCLUDES 1   *age-related cognitive decline (R41.81)*
        senile psychosis (F03)
        senility NOS (R41.81)

R55 **Syncope and collapse**
    Blackout
    Fainting
    Vasovagal attack
    EXCLUDES 1   *cardiogenic shock (R57.0)*
        carotid sinus syncope (G90.01)
        heat syncope (T67.1)
        neurocirculatory asthenia (F45.8)
        neurogenic orthostatic hypotension (G90.3)
        orthostatic hypotension (I95.1)
        postprocedural shock (T81.1-)
        psychogenic syncope (F48.8)
        shock NOS (R57.9)
        shock complicating or following abortion or ectopic or molar
            pregnancy (O00-O07, O08.3)
        shock complicating or following labor and delivery (O75.1)
        Stokes-Adams attack (I45.9)
        unconsciousness NOS (R40.2-)

✓4ᵗʰ **R56** **Convulsions, not elsewhere classified**
    EXCLUDES 1   *dissociative convulsions and seizures (F44.5)*
        epileptic convulsions and seizures (G40.-)
        newborn convulsions and seizures (P90)

  ✓5ᵗʰ **R56.0** Febrile convulsions
    R56.00 **Simple febrile convulsions**
        Febrile convulsion NOS
        Febrile seizure NOS

    R56.01 **Complex febrile convulsions**
        Atypical febrile seizure
        Complex febrile seizure
        Complicated febrile seizure
        EXCLUDES 1   *status epilepticus (G40.901)*

    R56.1 **Post traumatic seizures**
        EXCLUDES 1   *post traumatic epilepsy (G40.-)*

    R56.9 **Unspecified convulsions**   ▽
        Convulsion disorder
        Fit NOS
        Recurrent convulsions
        Seizure(s) (convulsive) NOS

---

³ Special Care High = With pneumonia, weight loss, or vomiting

¹⁰ Hospice questionable admission diagnosis

Ⓝ Newborn   Ⓟ Pediatric   Ⓜ Maternity   Ⓐ Adult   **RIC** RIC Dx   **NC Dx** Noncancer Dx   **PDx** Primary Dx   cc RIC CC Condition   ▶◀ Revised Text   ● New Code   ▲ Revised Code Title

☑4ᵗʰ R57 Shock, not elsewhere classified

> **EXCLUDES1**   *anaphylactic shock NOS (T78.2)*
> *anaphylactic reaction or shock due to adverse food reaction (T78.0-)*
> *anaphylactic shock due to adverse effect of correct drug or medicament properly administered (T88.6)*
> *anaphylactic shock due to serum (T80.5-)*
> *anesthetic shock (T88.3)*
> *electric shock (T75.4)*
> *obstetric shock (O75.1)*
> *postprocedural shock (T81.1-)*
> *psychic shock (F43.0)*
> *septic shock (R65.21)*
> *shock complicating or following ectopic or molar pregnancy (O00-O07, O08.3)*
> *shock due to lightning (T75.01)*
> *traumatic shock (T79.4)*
> *toxic shock syndrome (A48.3)*

R57.0 Cardiogenic shock   `CC`
> **RIC Excl:** 14 Cardiac

R57.1 Hypovolemic shock   `CC`

R57.8 Other shock   `CC`

R57.9 Shock, unspecified   ▽
> Failure of peripheral circulation NOS

R58 Hemorrhage, not elsewhere classified
> Hemorrhage NOS
> **EXCLUDES1**   *hemorrhage included with underlying conditions, such as:*
> *acute duodenal ulcer with hemorrhage (K26.0)*
> *acute gastritis with bleeding (K29.01)*
> *ulcerative enterocolitis with rectal bleeding (K51.01)*

☑4ᵗʰ R59 Enlarged lymph nodes
> **INCLUDES**   swollen glands
> **EXCLUDES1**   *acute lymphadenitis (L04.-)*
> *chronic lymphadenitis (I88.1)*
> *lymphadenitis NOS (I88.9)*
> *mesenteric (acute) (chronic) lymphadenitis (I88.0)*

R59.0 Localized enlarged lymph nodes

R59.1 Generalized enlarged lymph nodes
> Lymphadenopathy NOS

R59.9 Enlarged lymph nodes, unspecified   ▽

☑4ᵗʰ R60 Edema, not elsewhere classified
> **EXCLUDES1**   *angioneurotic edema (T78.3)*
> *ascites (R18.-)*
> *cerebral edema (G93.6)*
> *cerebral edema due to birth injury (P11.0)*
> *edema of larynx (J38.4)*
> *edema of nasopharynx (J39.2)*
> *edema of pharynx (J39.2)*
> *gestational edema (O12.0-)*
> *hereditary edema (Q82.0)*
> *hydrops fetalis NOS (P83.2)*
> *hydrothorax (J94.8)*
> *nutritional edema (E40-E46)*
> *hydrops fetalis NOS (P83.2)*
> *newborn edema (P83.3)*
> *pulmonary edema (J81.-)*

R60.0 Localized edema

R60.1 Generalized edema

R60.9 Edema, unspecified   ▽
> Fluid retention NOS

R61 Generalized hyperhidrosis
> Excessive sweating
> Night sweats
> Secondary hyperhidrosis
> Code first, if applicable, menopausal and female climacteric states (N95.1)
> **EXCLUDES1**   *focal (primary) (secondary) hyperhidrosis (L74.5-)*
> *Frey's syndrome (L74.52)*
> *localized (primary) (secondary) hyperhidrosis (L74.5-)*

☑4ᵗʰ R62 Lack of expected normal physiological development in childhood and adults
> **EXCLUDES1**   *delayed puberty (E30.0)*
> *gonadal dysgenesis (Q99.1)*
> *hypopituitarism (E23.0)*

R62.0 Delayed milestone in childhood   `P`
> Delayed attainment of expected physiological developmental stage
> Late talker
> Late walker

☑5ᵗʰ R62.5 Other and unspecified lack of expected normal physiological development in childhood
> **EXCLUDES1**   *HIV disease resulting in failure to thrive (B20)*
> *physical retardation due to malnutrition (E45)*

R62.50 Unspecified lack of expected normal physiological development in childhood   `P` ▽
> Infantilism NOS

R62.51 Failure to thrive (child)   `P`
> Failure to gain weight
> **EXCLUDES1**   *failure to thrive in child under 28 days old (P92.6)*

R62.52 Short stature (child)   `P`
> Lack of growth
> Physical retardation
> Short stature NOS
> **EXCLUDES1**   *short stature due to endocrine disorder (E34.3)*

R62.59 Other lack of expected normal physiological development in childhood   `P`

¹⁰ R62.7 Adult failure to thrive   `A`

☑4ᵗʰ R63 Symptoms and signs concerning food and fluid intake
> **EXCLUDES1**   *bulimia NOS (F50.2)*
> *eating disorders of nonorganic origin (F50.-)*
> *malnutrition (E40-E46)*

R63.0 Anorexia
> Loss of appetite
> **EXCLUDES1**   *anorexia nervosa (F50.0-)*
> *loss of appetite of nonorganic origin (F50.8)*

R63.1 Polydipsia
> Excessive thirst

R63.2 Polyphagia
> Excessive eating
> Hyperalimentation NOS

R63.3 Feeding difficulties
> Feeding problem (elderly) (infant) NOS
> **EXCLUDES1**   *feeding problems of newborn (P92.-)*
> *infant feeding disorder of nonorganic origin (F98.2-)*

² R63.4 Abnormal weight loss

R63.5 Abnormal weight gain
> **EXCLUDES1**   *excessive weight gain in pregnancy (O26.0-)*
> *obesity (E66.-)*

R63.6 Underweight
> Use additional code to identify body mass index (BMI), if known (Z68.-)
> **EXCLUDES1**   *abnormal weight loss (R63.4)*
> *anorexia nervosa (F50.0-)*
> *malnutrition (E40-E46)*

R63.8 Other symptoms and signs concerning food and fluid intake

R64 Cachexia
> Wasting syndrome
> Code first underlying condition, if known
> **EXCLUDES1**   *abnormal weight loss (R63.4)*
> *nutritional marasmus (E41)*

☑4ᵗʰ R65 Symptoms and signs specifically associated with systemic inflammation and infection

☑5ᵗʰ R65.1 Systemic inflammatory response syndrome [SIRS] of non-infectious origin
> Code first underlying condition, such as:
> heatstroke (T67.0)
> injury and trauma (S00-T88)
> **EXCLUDES1**   *sepsis—code to infection*
> *severe sepsis (R65.2)*

R65.10 Systemic inflammatory response syndrome [SIRS] of non-infectious origin without acute organ dysfunction   `CC`
> Systemic inflammatory response syndrome (SIRS) NOS

---

² Special Care High = With fever

¹⁰ Hospice questionable admission diagnosis

☑ Add'l Character Required   ☑ᵡ⁷ᵗʰ Placeholder Alert   RUG IV Special Care High Dx   RUG IV Clinically Complex Dx   RUG IV Special Care Low Dx   Manifestation Code   Other Specified Code   ▽ Unspecified Code

R65.11 **Systemic inflammatory response syndrome [SIRS] of non-infectious origin** with acute organ dysfunction   `CC`
Use additional code to identify specific acute organ dysfunction, such as:
acute kidney failure (N17.-)
acute respiratory failure (J96.0-)
critical illness myopathy (G72.81)
critical illness polyneuropathy (G62.81)
disseminated intravascular coagulopathy [DIC] (D65)
encephalopathy (metabolic) (septic) (G93.41)
hepatic failure (K72.0-)

✓5ᵗʰ **R65.2** **Severe sepsis**
Infection with associated acute organ dysfunction
Sepsis with acute organ dysfunction
Sepsis with multiple organ dysfunction
Systemic inflammatory response syndrome due to infectious process with acute organ dysfunction
Code first underlying infection, such as:
infection following a procedure (T81.4)
infections following infusion, transfusion and therapeutic injection (T80.2-)
puerperal sepsis (O85)
sepsis following complete or unspecified spontaneous abortion (O03.87)
sepsis following ectopic and molar pregnancy (O08.82)
sepsis following incomplete spontaneous abortion (O03.37)
sepsis following (induced) termination of pregnancy (O04.87)
sepsis NOS (A41.9)
Use additional code to identify specific acute organ dysfunction, such as:
acute kidney failure (N17.-)
acute respiratory failure (J96.0-)
critical illness myopathy (G72.81)
critical illness polyneuropathy (G62.81)
disseminated intravascular coagulopathy [DIC] (D65)
encephalopathy (metabolic) (septic) (G93.41)
hepatic failure (K72.0-)

    R65.20 **Severe sepsis** without septic shock   `CC`
Severe sepsis NOS
AHA: 2013, 4Q, 119

    R65.21 **Severe sepsis** with septic shock   `CC`

✓4ᵗʰ **R68** **Other general symptoms and signs**

R68.0 **Hypothermia, not associated with low environmental temperature**
EXCLUDES 1   *hypothermia due to anesthesia (T88.51)*
hypothermia due to low environmental temperature (T68)
hypothermia NOS (accidental) (T68)
newborn hypothermia (P80.-)

✓5ᵗʰ **R68.1** **Nonspecific symptoms peculiar to infancy**
EXCLUDES 1   *colic, infantile (R10.83)*
neonatal cerebral irritability (P91.3)
teething syndrome (K00.7)

    R68.11 **Excessive crying of infant (baby)**   `P`
EXCLUDES 1   *excessive crying of child, adolescent, or adult (R45.83)*

    R68.12 **Fussy infant (baby)**   `P`
Irritable infant

    R68.13 **Apparent life threatening event in infant [ALTE]**   `P`
Apparent life threatening event in newborn
Code first confirmed diagnosis, if known
Use additional code(s) for associated signs and symptoms if no confirmed diagnosis established, or if signs and symptoms are not associated routinely with confirmed diagnosis, or provide additional information for cause of ALTE

    R68.19 **Other nonspecific symptoms peculiar to infancy**   `P`

R68.2 **Dry mouth, unspecified**   ▽
EXCLUDES 1   *dry mouth due to dehydration (E86.0)*
dry mouth due to sicca syndrome [Sjögren] (M35.0-)
salivary gland hyposecretion (K11.7)

R68.3 **Clubbing of fingers**
Clubbing of nails
EXCLUDES 1   *congenital clubfinger (Q68.1)*

✓5ᵗʰ **R68.8** **Other general symptoms and signs**

    R68.81 **Early satiety**

    R68.82 **Decreased libido**   `A`
Decreased sexual desire

R68.83 **Chills (without fever)**
Chills NOS
EXCLUDES 1   *chills with fever (R50.9)*

R68.84 **Jaw pain**
Mandibular pain
Maxilla pain
EXCLUDES 1   *temporomandibular joint arthralgia (M26.62)*

R68.89 **Other general symptoms and signs**

R69 **Illness, unspecified**   ▽
Unknown and unspecified cases of morbidity

Abnormal findings on examination of blood, without diagnosis (R70-R79)

EXCLUDES 1   *abnormalities (of)(on):*
abnormal findings on antenatal screening of mother (O28.-)
coagulation hemorrhagic disorders (D65-D68)
lipids (E78.-)
platelets and thrombocytes (D69.-)
white blood cells classified elsewhere (D70-D72)
diagnostic abnormal findings classified elsewhere—see Alphabetical Index
hemorrhagic and hematological disorders of newborn (P50-P61)

✓4ᵗʰ **R70** **Elevated erythrocyte sedimentation rate and abnormality of plasma viscosity**

R70.0 **Elevated erythrocyte sedimentation rate**

R70.1 **Abnormal plasma viscosity**

✓4ᵗʰ **R71** **Abnormality of red blood cells**
EXCLUDES 1   *anemias (D50-D64)*
anemia of premature infant (P61.2)
benign (familial) polycythemia (D75.0)
congenital anemias (P61.2-P61.4)
newborn anemia due to isoimmunization (P55.-)
polycythemia neonatorum (P61.1)
polycythemia NOS (D75.1)
polycythemia vera (D45)
secondary polycythemia (D75.1)

R71.0 **Precipitous drop in hematocrit**
Drop (precipitous) in hemoglobin
Drop in hematocrit

R71.8 **Other abnormality of red blood cells**
Abnormal red-cell morphology NOS
Abnormal red-cell volume NOS
Anisocytosis
Poikilocytosis

✓4ᵗʰ **R73** **Elevated blood glucose level**
EXCLUDES 1   *diabetes mellitus (E08-E13)*
diabetes mellitus in pregnancy, childbirth and the puerperium (O24.-)
neonatal disorders (P70.0-P70.2)
postsurgical hypoinsulinemia (E89.1)

✓5ᵗʰ **R73.0** **Abnormal glucose**
EXCLUDES 1   *abnormal glucose in pregnancy (O99.81-)*
diabetes mellitus (E08-E13)
dysmetabolic syndrome X (E88.81)
gestational diabetes (O24.4-)
glycosuria (R81)
hypoglycemia (E16.2)

    R73.01 **Impaired fasting glucose**
Elevated fasting glucose

    R73.02 **Impaired glucose tolerance (oral)**
Elevated glucose tolerance

    R73.09 **Other abnormal glucose**
Abnormal glucose NOS
Abnormal non-fasting glucose tolerance
Latent diabetes
Prediabetes

R73.9 **Hyperglycemia, unspecified**   ▽

✓4ᵗʰ **R74** **Abnormal serum enzyme levels**

R74.0 **Nonspecific elevation of levels of transaminase and lactic acid dehydrogenase [LDH]**

R74.8 **Abnormal levels of other serum enzymes**
Abnormal level of acid phosphatase
Abnormal level of alkaline phosphatase
Abnormal level of amylase
Abnormal level of lipase [triacylglycerol lipase]

R74.9 **Abnormal serum enzyme level, unspecified**   ▽

`N` Newborn   `P` Pediatric   `M` Maternity   `A` Adult   `RIC` RIC Dx   `NCDx` Noncancer Dx   `PDx` Primary Dx   `CC` RIC CC Condition   ►◄ Revised Text   ● New Code   ▲ Revised Code Title

844

ICD-10-CM 2016

R75 Inconclusive laboratory evidence of human immunodeficiency virus [HIV]

Nonconclusive HIV-test finding in infants

> EXCLUDES 1   asymptomatic human immunodeficiency virus [HIV] infection status (Z21)
> human immunodeficiency virus [HIV] disease (B20)

✓4ᵗʰ R76 Other abnormal immunological findings in serum

R76.0 Raised antibody titer

> EXCLUDES 1   isoimmunization in pregnancy (O36.0-O36.1)
> isoimmunization affecting newborn (P55.-)

✓5ᵗʰ R76.1 Nonspecific reaction to test for tuberculosis

R76.11 Nonspecific reaction to tuberculin skin test without active tuberculosis

Abnormal result of Mantoux test
PPD positive
Tuberculin (skin test) positive
Tuberculin (skin test) reactor

> EXCLUDES 1   nonspecific reaction to cell mediated immunity measurement of gamma interferon antigen response without active tuberculosis (R76.12)

R76.12 Nonspecific reaction to cell mediated immunity measurement of gamma interferon antigen response without active tuberculosis

Nonspecific reaction to QuantiFERON-TB test (QFT) without active tuberculosis

> EXCLUDES 1   nonspecific reaction to tuberculin skin test without active tuberculosis (R76.11)
> positive tuberculin skin test (R76.11)

R76.8 Other specified abnormal immunological findings in serum

Raised level of immunoglobulins NOS

R76.9 Abnormal immunological finding in serum, unspecified ▽

✓4ᵗʰ R77 Other abnormalities of plasma proteins

> EXCLUDES 1   disorders of plasma-protein metabolism (E88.0)

R77.0 Abnormality of albumin

R77.1 Abnormality of globulin

Hyperglobulinemia NOS

R77.2 Abnormality of alphafetoprotein

R77.8 Other specified abnormalities of plasma proteins

R77.9 Abnormality of plasma protein, unspecified ▽

✓4ᵗʰ R78 Findings of drugs and other substances, not normally found in blood

Use additional code to identify any retained foreign body, if applicable (Z18.-)

> EXCLUDES 1   mental or behavioral disorders due to psychoactive substance use (F10-F19)

R78.0 Finding of alcohol in blood

Use additional external cause code (Y90.-), for detail regarding alcohol level

R78.1 Finding of opiate drug in blood

R78.2 Finding of cocaine in blood

R78.3 Finding of hallucinogen in blood

R78.4 Finding of other drugs of addictive potential in blood

R78.5 Finding of other psychotropic drug in blood

R78.6 Finding of steroid agent in blood

✓5ᵗʰ R78.7 Finding of abnormal level of heavy metals in blood

R78.71 Abnormal lead level in blood

> EXCLUDES 1   lead poisoning (T56.0-)

R78.79 Finding of abnormal level of heavy metals in blood

✓5ᵗʰ R78.8 Finding of other specified substances, not normally found in blood

R78.81 Bacteremia

> EXCLUDES 1   sepsis—code to specified infection (A00-B99)

R78.89 Finding of other specified substances, not normally found in blood

Finding of abnormal level of lithium in blood

R78.9 Finding of unspecified substance, not normally found in blood ▽

✓4ᵗʰ R79 Other abnormal findings of blood chemistry

Use additional code to identify any retained foreign body, if applicable (Z18.-)

> EXCLUDES 1   abnormality of fluid, electrolyte or acid-base balance (E86-E87)
> asymptomatic hyperuricemia (E79.0)
> hyperglycemia NOS (R73.9)
> hypoglycemia NOS (E16.2)
> neonatal hypoglycemia (P70.3-P70.4)
> specific findings indicating disorder of amino-acid metabolism (E70-E72)
> specific findings indicating disorder of carbohydrate metabolism (E73-E74)
> specific findings indicating disorder of lipid metabolism (E75.-)

R79.0 Abnormal level of blood mineral

Abnormal blood level of cobalt
Abnormal blood level of copper
Abnormal blood level of iron
Abnormal blood level of magnesium
Abnormal blood level of mineral NEC
Abnormal blood level of zinc

> EXCLUDES 1   abnormal level of lithium (R78.89)
> disorders of mineral metabolism (E83.-)
> neonatal hypomagnesemia (P71.2)
> nutritional mineral deficiency (E58-E61)

R79.1 Abnormal coagulation profile

Abnormal or prolonged bleeding time
Abnormal or prolonged coagulation time
Abnormal or prolonged partial thromboplastin time [PTT]
Abnormal or prolonged prothrombin time [PT]

> EXCLUDES 1   coagulation defects (D68.-)

✓5ᵗʰ R79.8 Other specified abnormal findings of blood chemistry

R79.81 Abnormal blood-gas level

R79.82 Elevated C-reactive protein [CRP]

R79.89 Other specified abnormal findings of blood chemistry

R79.9 Abnormal finding of blood chemistry, unspecified ▽

Abnormal findings on examination of urine, without diagnosis (R80-R82)

> EXCLUDES 1   abnormal findings on antenatal screening of mother (O28.-)
> diagnostic abnormal findings classified elsewhere—see Alphabetical Index
> specific findings indicating disorder of amino-acid metabolism (E70-E72)
> specific findings indicating disorder of carbohydrate metabolism (E73-E74)

✓4ᵗʰ R80 Proteinuria

> EXCLUDES 1   gestational proteinuria (O12.1-)

R80.0 Isolated proteinuria

Idiopathic proteinuria

> EXCLUDES 1   isolated proteinuria with specific morphological lesion (N06.-)

R80.1 Persistent proteinuria, unspecified ▽

R80.2 Orthostatic proteinuria, unspecified ▽

Postural proteinuria

R80.3 Bence Jones proteinuria

R80.8 Other proteinuria

R80.9 Proteinuria, unspecified ▽

Albuminuria NOS

R81 Glycosuria

> EXCLUDES 1   renal glycosuria (E74.8)

✓4ᵗʰ R82 Other and unspecified abnormal findings in urine

Chromoabnormalities in urine

Use additional code to identify any retained foreign body, if applicable (Z18.-)

> EXCLUDES 2   hematuria (R31.-)

R82.0 Chyluria

> EXCLUDES 1   filarial chyluria (B74.-)

R82.1 Myoglobinuria

R82.2 Biliuria

R82.3 Hemoglobinuria

> EXCLUDES 1   hemoglobinuria due to hemolysis from external causes NEC (D59.6)
> hemoglobinuria due to paroxysmal nocturnal [Marchiafava-Micheli] (D59.5)

R82.4 Acetonuria

Ketonuria

✅ Add'l Character Required   ✅x7ᵗʰ Placeholder Alert   RUG IV Special Care High Dx   RUG IV Clinically Complex Dx   RUG IV Special Care Low Dx   Manifestation Code   Other Specified Code   ▽ Unspecified Code

R82.5 **Elevated urine levels of drugs, medicaments and biological substances**
Elevated urine levels of catecholamines
Elevated urine levels of indoleacetic acid
Elevated urine levels of 17-ketosteroids
Elevated urine levels of steroids

R82.6 **Abnormal urine levels of substances chiefly nonmedicinal as to source**
Abnormal urine level of heavy metals

R82.7 **Abnormal findings on microbiological examination of urine**
Positive culture findings of urine
EXCLUDES 1   *colonization status (Z22.-)*

R82.8 **Abnormal findings on cytological and histological examination of urine**

√5ᵗʰ **R82.9** **Other and unspecified abnormal findings in urine**

R82.90 **Unspecified abnormal findings in urine**   ▽

R82.91 **Other chromoabnormalities of urine**
Chromoconversion (dipstick)
Idiopathic dipstick converts positive for blood with no cellular forms in sediment
EXCLUDES 1   *hemoglobinuria (R82.3)*
            myoglobinuria (R82.1)

R82.99 **Other abnormal findings in urine**
Cells and casts in urine
Crystalluria
Melanuria

Abnormal findings on examination of other body fluids, substances and tissues, without diagnosis (R83-R89)

EXCLUDES 1   *abnormal findings on antenatal screening of mother (O28.-)*
            diagnostic abnormal findings classified elsewhere—see Alphabetical Index
EXCLUDES 2   *abnormal findings on examination of blood, without diagnosis (R70-R79)*
            abnormal findings on examination of urine, without diagnosis (R80-R82)
            abnormal tumor markers (R97.-)

√4ᵗʰ **R83** **Abnormal findings in cerebrospinal fluid**

R83.0 **Abnormal level of enzymes in cerebrospinal fluid**

R83.1 **Abnormal level of hormones in cerebrospinal fluid**

R83.2 **Abnormal level of other drugs, medicaments and biological substances in cerebrospinal fluid**

R83.3 **Abnormal level of substances chiefly nonmedicinal as to source in cerebrospinal fluid**

R83.4 **Abnormal immunological findings in cerebrospinal fluid**

R83.5 **Abnormal microbiological findings in cerebrospinal fluid**
Positive culture findings in cerebrospinal fluid
EXCLUDES 1   *colonization status (Z22.-)*

R83.6 **Abnormal cytological findings in cerebrospinal fluid**

R83.8 **Other abnormal findings in cerebrospinal fluid**
Abnormal chromosomal findings in cerebrospinal fluid

R83.9 **Unspecified abnormal finding in cerebrospinal fluid**   ▽

√4ᵗʰ **R84** **Abnormal findings in specimens from respiratory organs and thorax**
Abnormal findings in bronchial washings
Abnormal findings in nasal secretions
Abnormal findings in pleural fluid
Abnormal findings in sputum
Abnormal findings in throat scrapings
EXCLUDES 1   *blood-stained sputum (R04.2)*

R84.0 **Abnormal level of enzymes in specimens from respiratory organs and thorax**

R84.1 **Abnormal level of hormones in specimens from respiratory organs and thorax**

R84.2 **Abnormal level of other drugs, medicaments and biological substances in specimens from respiratory organs and thorax**

R84.3 **Abnormal level of substances chiefly nonmedicinal as to source in specimens from respiratory organs and thorax**

R84.4 **Abnormal immunological findings in specimens from respiratory organs and thorax**

R84.5 **Abnormal microbiological findings in specimens from respiratory organs and thorax**
Positive culture findings in specimens from respiratory organs and thorax
EXCLUDES 1   *colonization status (Z22.-)*

R84.6 **Abnormal cytological findings in specimens from respiratory organs and thorax**

R84.7 **Abnormal histological findings in specimens from respiratory organs and thorax**

R84.8 **Other abnormal findings in specimens from respiratory organs and thorax**
Abnormal chromosomal findings in specimens from respiratory organs and thorax

R84.9 **Unspecified abnormal finding in specimens from respiratory organs and thorax**   ▽

√4ᵗʰ **R85** **Abnormal findings in specimens from digestive organs and abdominal cavity**
INCLUDES   abnormal findings in peritoneal fluid
            abnormal findings in saliva
EXCLUDES 1   *cloudy peritoneal dialysis effluent (R88.0)*
            fecal abnormalities (R19.5)

R85.0 **Abnormal level of enzymes in specimens from digestive organs and abdominal cavity**

R85.1 **Abnormal level of hormones in specimens from digestive organs and abdominal cavity**

R85.2 **Abnormal level of other drugs, medicaments and biological substances in specimens from digestive organs and abdominal cavity**

R85.3 **Abnormal level of substances chiefly nonmedicinal as to source in specimens from digestive organs and abdominal cavity**

R85.4 **Abnormal immunological findings in specimens from digestive organs and abdominal cavity**

R85.5 **Abnormal microbiological findings in specimens from digestive organs and abdominal cavity**
Positive culture findings in specimens from digestive organs and abdominal cavity
EXCLUDES 1   *colonization status (Z22.-)*

√5ᵗʰ **R85.6** **Abnormal cytological findings in specimens from digestive organs and abdominal cavity**

√6ᵗʰ **R85.61** **Abnormal cytologic smear of anus**
EXCLUDES 1   *abnormal cytological findings in specimens from other digestive organs and abdominal cavity (R85.69)*
            anal intraepithelial neoplasia I [AIN I] (K62.82)
            anal intraepithelial neoplasia II [AIN II] (K62.82)
            anal intraepithelial neoplasia III [AIN III] (D01.3)
            carcinoma in situ of anus (histologically confirmed) (D01.3)
            dysplasia (mild) (moderate) of anus (histologically confirmed) (K62.82)
            severe dysplasia of anus (histologically confirmed) (D01.3)
EXCLUDES 2   *anal high risk human papillomavirus (HPV) DNA test positive (R85.81)*
            anal low risk human papillomavirus (HPV) DNA test positive (R85.82)

R85.610 **Atypical squamous cells of undetermined significance on cytologic smear of anus [ASC-US]**

R85.611 **Atypical squamous cells cannot exclude high grade squamous intraepithelial lesion on cytologic smear of anus [ASC-H]**

R85.612 **Low grade squamous intraepithelial lesion on cytologic smear of anus [LGSIL]**

R85.613 **High grade squamous intraepithelial lesion on cytologic smear of anus [HGSIL]**

R85.614 **Cytologic evidence of malignancy on smear of anus**

R85.615 **Unsatisfactory cytologic smear of anus**
Inadequate sample of cytologic smear of anus

R85.616 **Satisfactory anal smear but lacking transformation zone**

R85.618 **Other abnormal cytological findings on specimens from anus**

R85.619 **Unspecified abnormal cytological findings in specimens from anus**   ▽
Abnormal anal cytology NOS
Atypical glandular cells of anus NOS

R85.69 **Abnormal cytological findings in specimens from other digestive organs and abdominal cavity**

R85.7 **Abnormal histological findings in specimens from digestive organs and abdominal cavity**

Ⓝ Newborn   Ⓟ Pediatric   Ⓜ Maternity   Ⓐ Adult   RIC RIC Dx   NCDx Noncancer Dx   PDx Primary Dx   CC RIC CC Condition   ▶◀ Revised Text   ● New Code   ▲ Revised Code Title

846

ICD-10-CM 2016

✓5ᵗʰ **R85.8** Other abnormal findings in specimens from digestive organs and abdominal cavity

    R85.81 Anal high risk human papillomavirus [HPV] DNA test positive
        EXCLUDES 1　anogenital warts due to human papillomavirus (HPV) (A63.0)
                condyloma acuminatum (A63.0)

    R85.82 Anal low risk human papillomavirus [HPV] DNA test positive
        Use additional code for associated human papillomavirus (B97.7)

    R85.89 Other abnormal findings in specimens from digestive organs and abdominal cavity
        Abnormal chromosomal findings in specimens from digestive organs and abdominal cavity

R85.9 Unspecified abnormal finding in specimens from digestive organs and abdominal cavity　▽

✓4ᵗʰ **R86** Abnormal findings in specimens from male genital organs
    INCLUDES　abnormal findings in prostatic secretions
             abnormal findings in semen, seminal fluid
             abnormal spermatozoa
    EXCLUDES 1　azoospermia (N46.0-)
             oligospermia (N46.1-)

R86.0 Abnormal level of enzymes in specimens from male genital organs　♂

R86.1 Abnormal level of hormones in specimens from male genital organs　♂

R86.2 Abnormal level of other drugs, medicaments and biological substances in specimens from male genital organs　♂

R86.3 Abnormal level of substances chiefly nonmedicinal as to source in specimens from male genital organs　♂

R86.4 Abnormal immunological findings in specimens from male genital organs　♂

R86.5 Abnormal microbiological findings in specimens from male genital organs　♂
    Positive culture findings in specimens from male genital organs
    EXCLUDES 1　colonization status (Z22.-)

R86.6 Abnormal cytological findings in specimens from male genital organs　♂

R86.7 Abnormal histological findings in specimens from male genital organs　♂

R86.8 Other abnormal findings in specimens from male genital organs　♂
    Abnormal chromosomal findings in specimens from male genital organs

R86.9 Unspecified abnormal finding in specimens from male genital organs　♂▽

✓4ᵗʰ **R87** Abnormal findings in specimens from female genital organs
    Abnormal findings in secretion and smears from cervix uteri
    Abnormal findings in secretion and smears from vagina
    Abnormal findings in secretion and smears from vulva

R87.0 Abnormal level of enzymes in specimens from female genital organs　♀

R87.1 Abnormal level of hormones in specimens from female genital organs　♀

R87.2 Abnormal level of other drugs, medicaments and biological substances in specimens from female genital organs　♀

R87.3 Abnormal level of substances chiefly nonmedicinal as to source in specimens from female genital organs　♀

R87.4 Abnormal immunological findings in specimens from female genital organs　♀

R87.5 Abnormal microbiological findings in specimens from female genital organs　♀
    Positive culture findings in specimens from female genital organs
    EXCLUDES 1　colonization status (Z22.-)

✓5ᵗʰ **R87.6** Abnormal cytological findings in specimens from female genital organs

    ✓6ᵗʰ **R87.61** Abnormal cytological findings in specimens from cervix uteri
        EXCLUDES 1　abnormal cytological findings in specimens from other female genital organs (R87.69)
              abnormal cytological findings in specimens from vagina (R87.62-)
              carcinoma in situ of cervix uteri (histologically confirmed) (D06.-)
              cervical intraepithelial neoplasia I [CIN I] (N87.0)
              cervical intraepithelial neoplasia II [CIN II] (N87.1)
              cervical intraepithelial neoplasia III [CIN III] (D06.-)
              dysplasia (mild) (moderate) of cervix uteri (histologically confirmed) (N87.-)
              severe dysplasia of cervix uteri (histologically confirmed) (D06.-)
        EXCLUDES 2　cervical high risk human papillomavirus (HPV) DNA test positive (R87.810)
              cervical low risk human papillomavirus (HPV) DNA test positive (R87.820)

        R87.610 Atypical squamous cells of undetermined significance on cytologic smear of cervix [ASC-US]　♀

        R87.611 Atypical squamous cells cannot exclude high grade squamous intraepithelial lesion on cytologic smear of cervix [ASC-H]　♀

        R87.612 Low grade squamous intraepithelial lesion on cytologic smear of cervix [LGSIL]　♀

        R87.613 High grade squamous intraepithelial lesion on cytologic smear of cervix [HGSIL]　♀

        R87.614 Cytologic evidence of malignancy on smear of cervix　♀

        R87.615 Unsatisfactory cytologic smear of cervix　♀
            Inadequate sample of cytologic smear of cervix

        R87.616 Satisfactory cervical smear but lacking transformation zone　♀

        R87.618 Other abnormal cytological findings on specimens from cervix uteri　♀

        R87.619 Unspecified abnormal cytological findings in specimens from cervix uteri　♀▽
            Abnormal cervical cytology NOS
            Abnormal Papanicolaou smear of cervix NOS
            Abnormal thin preparation smear of cervix NOS
            Atypical endocervial cells of cervix NOS
            Atypical endometrial cells of cervix NOS
            Atypical glandular cells of cervix NOS

Chapter 18. Symptoms, Signs and Abnormal Clinical and Laboratory Findings

✓6ᵗʰ **R87.62 Abnormal cytological findings in specimens from vagina**

Use additional code to identify acquired absence of uterus and cervix, if applicable (Z90.71-)

EXCLUDES 1   *abnormal cytological findings in specimens from cervix uteri (R87.61-)*

abnormal cytological findings in specimens from other female genital organs (R87.69)

carcinoma in situ of vagina (histologically confirmed) (D07.2)

dysplasia (mild) (moderate) of vagina (histologically confirmed) (N89.-)

severe dysplasia of vagina (histologically confirmed) (D07.2)

vaginal intraepithelial neoplasia I [VAIN I] (N89.0)

vaginal intraepithelial neoplasia II [VAIN II] (N89.1)

vaginal intraepithelial neoplasia III [VAIN III] (D07.2)

EXCLUDES 2   *vaginal high risk human papillomavirus (HPV) DNA test positive (R87.811)*

vaginal low risk human papillomavirus (HPV) DNA test positive (R87.821)

R87.620 Atypical squamous cells of undetermined significance on cytologic smear of vagina [ASC-US] ♀

R87.621 Atypical squamous cells cannot exclude high grade squamous intraepithelial lesion on cytologic smear of vagina [ASC-H] ♀

R87.622 Low grade squamous intraepithelial lesion on cytologic smear of vagina [LGSIL] ♀

R87.623 High grade squamous intraepithelial lesion on cytologic smear of vagina [HGSIL] ♀

R87.624 Cytologic evidence of malignancy on smear of vagina ♀

R87.625 Unsatisfactory cytologic smear of vagina ♀

Inadequate sample of cytologic smear of vagina

R87.628 Other abnormal cytological findings on specimens from vagina ♀

R87.629 Unspecified abnormal cytological findings in specimens from vagina ♀▽

Abnormal Papanicolaou smear of vagina NOS

Abnormal thin preparation smear of vagina NOS

Abnormal vaginal cytology NOS

Atypical endocervical cells of vagina NOS

Atypical endometrial cells of vagina NOS

Atypical glandular cells of vagina NOS

R87.69 Abnormal cytological findings in specimens from other female genital organs ♀

Abnormal cytological findings in specimens from female genital organs NOS

EXCLUDES 1   *dysplasia of vulva (histologically confirmed) (N90.0-N90.3)*

R87.7 Abnormal histological findings in specimens from female genital organs ♀

EXCLUDES 1   *carcinoma in situ (histologically confirmed) of female genital organs (D06-D07.3)*

cervical intraepithelial neoplasia I [CIN I] (N87.0)

cervical intraepithelial neoplasia II [CIN II] (N87.1)

cervical intraepithelial neoplasia III [CIN III] (D06.-)

dysplasia (mild) (moderate) of cervix uteri (histologically confirmed) (N87.-)

dysplasia (mild) (moderate) of vagina (histologically confirmed) (N89.-)

severe dysplasia of cervix uteri (histologically confirmed) (D06.-)

severe dysplasia of vagina (histologically confirmed) (D07.2)

vaginal intraepithelial neoplasia I [VAIN I] (N89.0)

vaginal intraepithelial neoplasia II [VAIN II] (N89.1)

vaginal intraepithelial neoplasia III [VAIN III] (D07.2)

✓5ᵗʰ **R87.8 Other abnormal findings in specimens from female genital organs**

✓6ᵗʰ **R87.81 High risk human papillomavirus [HPV] DNA test positive from female genital organs**

EXCLUDES 1   *anogenital warts due to human papillomavirus (HPV) (A63.0)*

condyloma acuminatum (A63.0)

R87.810 Cervical high risk human papillomavirus [HPV] DNA test positive ♀

R87.811 Vaginal high risk human papillomavirus [HPV] DNA test positive ♀

✓6ᵗʰ **R87.82 Low risk human papillomavirus [HPV] DNA test positive from female genital organs**

Use additional code for associated human papillomavirus (B97.7)

R87.820 Cervical low risk human papillomavirus [HPV] DNA test positive ♀

R87.821 Vaginal low risk human papillomavirus [HPV] DNA test positive ♀

R87.89 Other abnormal findings in specimens from female genital organs ♀

Abnormal chromosomal findings in specimens from female genital organs

R87.9 Unspecified abnormal finding in specimens from female genital organs ♀▽

✓4ᵗʰ **R88 Abnormal findings in other body fluids and substances**

R88.0 Cloudy (hemodialysis) (peritoneal) dialysis effluent

R88.8 Abnormal findings in other body fluids and substances

✓4ᵗʰ **R89 Abnormal findings in specimens from other organs, systems and tissues**

INCLUDES   abnormal findings in nipple discharge

abnormal findings in synovial fluid

abnormal findings in wound secretions

R89.0 Abnormal level of enzymes in specimens from other organs, systems and tissues

R89.1 Abnormal level of hormones in specimens from other organs, systems and tissues

R89.2 Abnormal level of other drugs, medicaments and biological substances in specimens from other organs, systems and tissues

R89.3 Abnormal level of substances chiefly nonmedicinal as to source in specimens from other organs, systems and tissues

R89.4 Abnormal immunological findings in specimens from other organs, systems and tissues

R89.5 Abnormal microbiological findings in specimens from other organs, systems and tissues

Positive culture findings in specimens from other organs, systems and tissues

EXCLUDES 1   *colonization status (Z22.-)*

R89.6 Abnormal cytological findings in specimens from other organs, systems and tissues

R89.7 Abnormal histological findings in specimens from other organs, systems and tissues

R89.8 Other abnormal findings in specimens from other organs, systems and tissues

Abnormal chromosomal findings in specimens from other organs, systems and tissues

R89.9 Unspecified abnormal finding in specimens from other organs, systems and tissues ▽

Ⓝ Newborn   Ⓟ Pediatric   Ⓜ Maternity   Ⓐ Adult   RIC RIC Dx   NCDx Noncancer Dx   PDx Primary Dx   CC RIC CC Condition   ▶◀ Revised Text   ● New Code   ▲ Revised Code Title

848   ICD-10-CM 2016

R87.62–R89.9

Abnormal findings on diagnostic imaging and in function studies, without diagnosis (R90-R94)

> **INCLUDES** nonspecific abnormal findings on diagnostic imaging by computerized axial tomography [CAT scan]
> nonspecific abnormal findings on diagnostic imaging by magnetic resonance imaging [MRI][NMR]
> nonspecific abnormal findings on diagnostic imaging by positron emission tomography [PET scan]
> nonspecific abnormal findings on diagnostic imaging by thermography
> nonspecific abnormal findings on diagnostic imaging by ultrasound [echogram]
> nonspecific abnormal findings on diagnostic imaging by X-ray examination
>
> **EXCLUDES 1** abnormal findings on antenatal screening of mother (O28.-)
> diagnostic abnormal findings classified elsewhere—see Alphabetical Index

✓4th R90 Abnormal findings on diagnostic imaging of central nervous system

R90.0 Intracranial space-occupying lesion found on diagnostic imaging of central nervous system

✓5th R90.8 Other abnormal findings on diagnostic imaging of central nervous system

R90.81 Abnormal echoencephalogram

R90.82 White matter disease, unspecified　▽

R90.89 Other abnormal findings on diagnostic imaging of central nervous system
Other cerebrovascular abnormality found on diagnostic imaging of central nervous system

✓4th R91 Abnormal findings on diagnostic imaging of lung

R91.1 Solitary pulmonary nodule
Coin lesion lung
Solitary pulmonary nodule, subsegmental branch of the bronchial tree

R91.8 Other nonspecific abnormal finding of lung field　CC
Lung mass NOS found on diagnostic imaging of lung
Pulmonary infiltrate NOS
Shadow, lung
RIC Excl: 15 Pulmonary

✓4th R92 Abnormal and inconclusive findings on diagnostic imaging of breast

R92.0 Mammographic microcalcification found on diagnostic imaging of breast
EXCLUDES 2 mammographic calcification (calculus) found on diagnostic imaging of breast (R92.1)

R92.1 Mammographic calcification found on diagnostic imaging of breast
Mammographic calculus found on diagnostic imaging of breast

R92.2 Inconclusive mammogram
Dense breasts NOS
Inconclusive mammogram NEC
Inconclusive mammography due to dense breasts
Inconclusive mammography NEC
AHA: 2015, 1Q, 24

R92.8 Other abnormal and inconclusive findings on diagnostic imaging of breast

✓4th R93 Abnormal findings on diagnostic imaging of other body structures

R93.0 Abnormal findings on diagnostic imaging of skull and head, not elsewhere classified
EXCLUDES 1 intracranial space-occupying lesion found on diagnostic imaging (R90.0)

R93.1 Abnormal findings on diagnostic imaging of heart and coronary circulation
Abnormal echocardiogram NOS
Abnormal heart shadow

R93.2 Abnormal findings on diagnostic imaging of liver and biliary tract
Nonvisualization of gallbladder

R93.3 Abnormal findings on diagnostic imaging of other parts of digestive tract

R93.4 Abnormal findings on diagnostic imaging of urinary organs
Filling defect of bladder found on diagnostic imaging
Filling defect of kidney found on diagnostic imaging
Filling defect of ureter found on diagnostic imaging
EXCLUDES 1 hypertrophy of kidney (N28.81)

R93.5 Abnormal findings on diagnostic imaging of other abdominal regions, including retroperitoneum

R93.6 Abnormal findings on diagnostic imaging of limbs
EXCLUDES 2 abnormal finding in skin and subcutaneous tissue (R93.8)

R93.7 Abnormal findings on diagnostic imaging of other parts of musculoskeletal system
EXCLUDES 2 abnormal findings on diagnostic imaging of skull (R93.0)

R93.8 Abnormal findings on diagnostic imaging of other specified body structures
Abnormal finding by radioisotope localization of placenta
Abnormal radiological finding in skin and subcutaneous tissue
Mediastinal shift

R93.9 Diagnostic imaging inconclusive due to excess body fat of patient

✓4th R94 Abnormal results of function studies

> **INCLUDES** abnormal results of radionuclide [radioisotope] uptake studies
> abnormal results of scintigraphy

✓5th R94.0 Abnormal results of function studies of central nervous system

R94.01 Abnormal electroencephalogram [EEG]

R94.02 Abnormal brain scan

R94.09 Abnormal results of other function studies of central nervous system

✓5th R94.1 Abnormal results of function studies of peripheral nervous system and special senses

✓6th R94.11 Abnormal results of function studies of eye

R94.110 Abnormal electro-oculogram [EOG]

R94.111 Abnormal electroretinogram [ERG]
Abnormal retinal function study

R94.112 Abnormal visually evoked potential [VEP]

R94.113 Abnormal oculomotor study

R94.118 Abnormal results of other function studies of eye

✓6th R94.12 Abnormal results of function studies of ear and other special senses

R94.120 Abnormal auditory function study

R94.121 Abnormal vestibular function study

R94.128 Abnormal results of other function studies of ear and other special senses

✓6th R94.13 Abnormal results of function studies of peripheral nervous system

R94.130 Abnormal response to nerve stimulation, unspecified　▽

R94.131 Abnormal electromyogram [EMG]
EXCLUDES 1 electromyogram of eye (R94.113)

R94.138 Abnormal results of other function studies of peripheral nervous system

R94.2 Abnormal results of pulmonary function studies
Reduced ventilatory capacity
Reduced vital capacity

✓5th R94.3 Abnormal results of cardiovascular function studies

R94.30 Abnormal result of cardiovascular function study, unspecified　▽

R94.31 Abnormal electrocardiogram [ECG] [EKG]
EXCLUDES 1 long QT syndrome (I45.81)

R94.39 Abnormal result of other cardiovascular function study
Abnormal electrophysiological intracardiac studies
Abnormal phonocardiogram
Abnormal vectorcardiogram

R94.4 Abnormal results of kidney function studies
Abnormal renal function test

R94.5 Abnormal results of liver function studies

R94.6 Abnormal results of thyroid function studies

R94.7 Abnormal results of other endocrine function studies
EXCLUDES 2 abnormal glucose (R73.0-)

R94.8 Abnormal results of function studies of other organs and systems
Abnormal basal metabolic rate [BMR]
Abnormal bladder function test
Abnormal splenic function test

✓ Add'l Character Required　✓x7th Placeholder Alert　**RUG IV Special Care High Dx**　**RUG IV Clinically Complex Dx**　**RUG IV Special Care Low Dx**　Manifestation Code　Other Specified Code　▽ Unspecified Code

Chapter 18. Symptoms, Signs and Abnormal Clinical and Laboratory Findings

Abnormal tumor markers (R97)

☑4ᵗʰ **R97** **Abnormal tumor markers**
    Elevated tumor associated antigens [TAA]
    Elevated tumor specific antigens [TSA]

  R97.0 **Elevated carcinoembryonic antigen [CEA]**
  R97.1 **Elevated cancer antigen 125 [CA 125]**   ♀
  R97.2 **Elevated prostate specific antigen [PSA]**   Ⓐ♂
  R97.8 **Other abnormal tumor markers**

Ill-defined and unknown cause of mortality (R99)

R99 **Ill-defined and unknown cause of mortality**   ▽
    Death (unexplained) NOS
    Unspecified cause of mortality

Ⓝ Newborn   Ⓟ Pediatric   Ⓜ Maternity   Ⓐ Adult   RIC RIC Dx   NC Dx Noncancer Dx   PDx Primary Dx   CC RIC CC Condition   ►◄ Revised Text   ● New Code   ▲ Revised Code Title

850   ICD-10-CM 2016

Chapter 19. Injury, Poisoning, and Certain Other Consequences of External Causes (S00–T88)

Chapter Specific Guidelines with Coding Examples

The chapter specific guidelines from the ICD-10-CM Official Guidelines for Coding and Reporting have been provided below. Along with these guidelines are coding examples, contained in the shaded boxes, that have been developed to help illustrate the coding and/or sequencing guidance found in these guidelines.

a. Application of 7th Characters in Chapter 19

Most categories in chapter 19 have a 7th character requirement for each applicable code. Most categories in this chapter have three 7th character values (with the exception of fractures): A, initial encounter, D, subsequent encounter and S, sequela. Categories for traumatic fractures have additional 7th character values. While the patient may be seen by a new or different provider over the course of treatment for an injury, assignment of the 7th character is based on whether the patient is undergoing active treatment and not whether the provider is seeing the patient for the first time.

For complication codes, active treatment refers to treatment for the condition described by the code, even though it may be related to an earlier precipitating problem. For example, code T84.50XA, Infection and inflammatory reaction due to unspecified internal joint prosthesis, initial encounter, is used when active treatment is provided for the infection, even though the condition relates to the prosthetic device, implant or graft that was placed at a previous encounter.

7th character "A", initial encounter is used while the patient is receiving active treatment for the condition. Examples of active treatment are: surgical treatment, emergency department encounter, and evaluation and continuing treatment by the same or a different physician.

Patient admitted after fall from a skateboard onto the sidewalk, x-rays identify a nondisplaced fracture to the distal pole of the right scaphoid bone. The patient is placed in a cast.

S62.014A	**Nondisplaced fracture of distal pole of navicular [scaphoid] bone of right wrist, initial encounter for closed fracture**
V00.131A	**Fall from skateboard, initial encounter**
Y92.480	**Sidewalk as the place of occurrence of the external cause**
Y93.51	**Activity, roller skating (inline) and skateboarding**
Y99.8	**Other external cause status**

Explanation: This fracture would be coded with a seventh character A for initial encounter because the patient received x-rays to identify the site of the fracture and treatment was rendered; this would be considered active treatment.

7th character "D" subsequent encounter is used for encounters after the patient has received active treatment of the condition and is receiving routine care for the condition during the healing or recovery phase. Examples of subsequent care are: cast change or removal, an x-ray to check healing status of fracture, removal of external or internal fixation device, medication adjustment, other aftercare and follow up visits following treatment of the injury or condition.

Patient admitted after fall from a skateboard onto the sidewalk resulted in casting of the right arm. X-rays are taken to evaluate how well the nondisplaced fracture to the distal pole of the right scaphoid bone is healing. The physician feels the fracture is healing appropriately; no adjustments to the cast are made.

S62.014D	**Nondisplaced fracture of distal pole of navicular [scaphoid] bone of right wrist, subsequent encounter for fracture with routine healing**
V00.131D	**Fall from skateboard, subsequent encounter**

Explanation: This fracture would be coded with a seventh character D for subsequent encounter, whether the same physician who provided the initial cast application or a different physician is now seeing the patient. Although the patient received x-rays, the intent of the x-rays was to assess how the fracture was healing. There was no active treatment rendered and the visit is therefore considered a subsequent encounter.

The aftercare Z codes should not be used for aftercare for conditions such as injuries or poisonings, where 7th characters are provided to identify subsequent care. For example, for aftercare of an injury, assign the acute injury code with the 7th character "D" (subsequent encounter).

7th character "S", sequela, is for use for complications or conditions that arise as a direct result of a condition, such as scar formation after a burn. The scars are sequelae of the burn. When using 7th character "S", it is necessary to use both the injury code that precipitated the sequela and the code for the sequela itself. The "S" is added only to the injury code, not the sequela code. The 7th character "S" identifies the injury responsible for the sequela. The specific type of sequela (e.g. scar) is sequenced first, followed by the injury code.

See Section I.B.10 Sequelae, (Late Effects)

Patient with a history of a nondisplaced fracture to the distal pole of the right scaphoid bone due to a fall from a skateboard is admitted for evaluation of arthritis to the right wrist that has developed as a consequence of the traumatic fracture.

M12.531	**Traumatic arthropathy, right wrist**
S62.014S	**Nondisplaced fracture of distal pole of navicular [scaphoid] bone of right wrist, sequela**
V00.131S	**Fall from skateboard, sequela**

Explanation: The code identifying the specific sequela condition (traumatic arthritis) should be coded first followed by the injury that instigated the development of the sequela (fracture). The scaphoid fracture injury code is given a 7th character S for sequela to represent its role as the inciting injury. The fracture has healed and is not being managed or treated on this admit and therefore is not applicable as a first listed or principal diagnosis. However, it is directly related to the development of the arthritis and should be appended as a secondary code to signify this cause and effect relationship.

b. Coding of injuries

When coding injuries, assign separate codes for each injury unless a combination code is provided, in which case the combination code is assigned. Code T07, Unspecified multiple injuries should not be assigned in the inpatient setting unless information for a more specific code is not available. Traumatic injury codes (S00-T14.9) are not to be used for normal, healing surgical wounds or to identify complications of surgical wounds.

11-year-old girl fell from her horse, resulting in a laceration to her right forearm with several large pieces of wooden fragments embedded in the wound as well as abrasions to her right ear; in addition, her right shoulder was dislocated

S43.004A	**Unspecified dislocation of right shoulder joint, initial encounter**
S51.821A	**Laceration with foreign body of right forearm, initial encounter**
S00.411A	**Abrasion of right ear, initial encounter**
V80.010A	**Animal-rider injured by fall from or being thrown from horse in noncollision accident, initial encounter**
Y93.52	**Activity, horseback riding**

Explanation: Each separate injury should be reported. The patient's injury to the forearm is reported with one combination code that captures both the laceration and the foreign body.

The code for the most serious injury, as determined by the provider and the focus of treatment, is sequenced first.

1) Superficial injuries

Superficial injuries such as abrasions or contusions are not coded when associated with more severe injuries of the same site.

2) Primary injury with damage to nerves/blood vessels

When a primary injury results in minor damage to peripheral nerves or blood vessels, the primary injury is sequenced first with additional code(s) for injuries to nerves and spinal cord (such as category S04), and/or injury to blood vessels (such as category S15). When the primary injury is to the blood vessels or nerves, that injury should be sequenced first.

c. Coding of traumatic fractures

The principles of multiple coding of injuries should be followed in coding fractures. Fractures of specified sites are coded individually by site in accordance with both the provisions within categories S02, S12, S22, S32, S42, S49, S52, S59, S62, S72, S79, S82, S89, S92 and the level of detail furnished by medical record content.

A fracture not indicated as open or closed should be coded to closed. A fracture not indicated whether displaced or not displaced should be coded to displaced.

More specific guidelines are as follows:

1) Initial vs. Subsequent Encounter for Fractures

Traumatic fractures are coded using the appropriate 7th character for initial encounter (A, B, C) while the patient is receiving active treatment for the fracture. Examples of active treatment are: surgical treatment, emergency department encounter, and evaluation and continuing (ongoing) treatment by the same or different physician. The appropriate 7th character for initial encounter should also be assigned for a patient who delayed seeking treatment for the fracture or nonunion.

Fractures are coded using the appropriate 7th character for subsequent care for encounters after the patient has completed active treatment of the fracture and is receiving routine care for the fracture during the healing or recovery phase. Examples of fracture aftercare are: cast change or removal, an x-ray to check healing status of fracture, removal of external or internal fixation device, medication adjustment, and follow-up visits following fracture treatment.

Care for complications of surgical treatment for fracture repairs during the healing or recovery phase should be coded with the appropriate complication codes.

Care of complications of fractures, such as malunion and nonunion, should be reported with the appropriate 7th character for subsequent care with nonunion (K, M, N,) or subsequent care with malunion (P, Q, R).

Malunion/nonunion: The appropriate 7th character for initial encounter should also be assigned for a patient who delayed seeking treatment for the fracture or nonunion.

Female patient fell during a hiking excursion almost six months ago and until recently did not feel she needed to seek medical attention for her left ankle pain; x-rays show nonunion of lateral malleolus and surgery has been scheduled

S82.862A	**Displaced Maisonneuve's fracture of left leg, initial encounter for closed fracture**
W01.0XXA	**Fall on same level from slipping, tripping and stumbling without subsequent striking against object, initial encounter**
Y92.821	**Forest as place of occurrence of the external cause**
Y93.01	**Activity, walking, marching and hiking**
Y99.8	**Other external cause status**

Explanation: A seventh character of A is used for the lateral malleolus nonunion fracture to signify that the fracture is receiving active treatment. The delayed care for the fracture has resulted in a nonunion, but capturing the nonunion in the seventh character is trumped by the provision of active care.

A code from category M80, not a traumatic fracture code, should be used for any patient with known osteoporosis who suffers a fracture, even if the patient had a minor fall or trauma, if that fall or trauma would not usually break a normal, healthy bone.

See Section I.C.13. Osteoporosis.

The aftercare Z codes should not be used for aftercare for traumatic fractures. For aftercare of a traumatic fracture, assign the acute fracture code with the appropriate 7th character.

2) Multiple fractures sequencing

Multiple fractures are sequenced in accordance with the severity of the fracture.

d. Coding of burns and corrosions

The ICD-10-CM makes a distinction between burns and corrosions. The burn codes are for thermal burns, except sunburns, that come from a heat source, such as a fire or hot appliance. The burn codes are also for burns resulting from electricity and radiation. Corrosions are burns due to chemicals. The guidelines are the same for burns and corrosions.

Current burns (T20-T25) are classified by depth, extent and by agent (X code). Burns are classified by depth as first degree (erythema), second degree (blistering), and third degree (full-thickness involvement). Burns of the eye and internal organs (T26-T28) are classified by site, but not by degree.

1) Sequencing of burn and related condition codes

Sequence first the code that reflects the highest degree of burn when more than one burn is present.

    a.   When the reason for the admission or encounter is for treatment of external multiple burns, sequence first the code that reflects the burn of the highest degree.

    b.   When a patient has both internal and external burns, the circumstances of admission govern the selection of the principal diagnosis or first-listed diagnosis.

    c.   When a patient is admitted for burn injuries and other related conditions such as smoke inhalation and/or respiratory failure, the circumstances of admission govern the selection of the principal or first-listed diagnosis.

Patient admitted with minor first-degree burns to multiple sites of her right and left hands as well as severe smoke inhalation. While she was sleeping at home, a candle on her dresser lit the bedroom curtains on fire.

T59.811A	**Toxic effect of smoke, accidental (unintentional), initial encounter**
J70.5	**Respiratory conditions due to smoke inhalation**
T23.191A	**Burn of first degree of multiple sites of right wrist and hand, initial encounter**
T23.192A	**Burn of first degree of multiple sites of left wrist and hand, initial encounter**
X08.8XXA	**Exposure to other specified smoke, fire and flames, initial encounter**
Y92.003	**Bedroom of unspecified non-institutional (private) residence as the place of occurrence of the external cause**
Y93.84	**Activity, sleeping**

Explanation: Based on the documentation, the inhalation injury is more severe than the first-degree burns and is sequenced first. The burns to the hands are appended as secondary diagnoses.

---

2) Burns of the same local site

Classify burns of the same local site (three-character category level, T20-T28) but of different degrees to the subcategory identifying the highest degree recorded in the diagnosis.

10-year-old male patient is admitted for third-degree burns of his right palm and second-degree burns of multiple right fingers; right thumb not affected

T23.351A	**Burn of third degree of right palm, initial encounter**

Explanation: Although there is a code for second-degree burns of multiple fingers, not including the thumb (T23.131-), this code falls in the same three-digit category that the third-degree burn of the right palm falls under, category T23. Only the subcategory identifying the highest degree is captured when different burn degrees are classified to a single category.

Patient is admitted with third-degree burns of the scalp as well as second-degree burns to the back of the right hand

T20.35XA	**Burn of third degree of scalp [any part], initial encounter**
T23.261A	**Burn of second degree of back of right hand, initial encounter**

Explanation: Since burns to the hand and scalp are classified to two different three-digit categories, both burns may be reported as they represent distinct sites.

---

3) Non-healing burns

Non-healing burns are coded as acute burns.

Necrosis of burned skin should be coded as a non-healed burn.

4) Infected burn

For any documented infected burn site, use an additional code for the infection.

5) **Assign separate codes for each burn site**

When coding burns, assign separate codes for each burn site. Category T30, Burn and corrosion, body region unspecified is extremely vague and should rarely be used.

6) **Burns and Corrosions Classified According to Extent of Body Surface Involved**

Assign codes from category T31, Burns classified according to extent of body surface involved, or T32, Corrosions classified according to extent of body surface involved, when the site of the burn is not specified or when there is a need for additional data. It is advisable to use category T31 as additional coding when needed to provide data for evaluating burn mortality, such as that needed by burn units. It is also advisable to use category T31 as an additional code for reporting purposes when there is mention of a third-degree burn involving 20 percent or more of the body surface.

Categories T31 and T32 are based on the classic "rule of nines" in estimating body surface involved: head and neck are assigned nine percent, each arm nine percent, each leg 18 percent, the anterior trunk 18 percent, posterior trunk 18 percent, and genitalia one percent. Providers may change these percentage assignments where necessary to accommodate infants and children who have proportionately larger heads than adults, and patients who have large buttocks, thighs, or abdomen that involve burns.

> Patient seen for dressing change after he accidentally spilled acetic acid on himself two days ago. The second-degree burns to his right thigh, covering about 3 percent of his body surface, are healing appropriately.
>
> **T54.2X1D**   **Toxic effect of corrosive acids and acid-like substances, accidental (unintentional), subsequent encounter**
>
> **T24.611D**   **Corrosion of second degree of right thigh, subsequent encounter**
>
> **T32.0**   **Corrosions involving less than 10% of body surface**
>
> *Explanation:* Code T32.0 provides additional information as to how much of the patient's body was affected by the corrosive substance.

7) **Encounters for treatment of sequela of burns**

Encounters for the treatment of the late effects of burns or corrosions (i.e., scars or joint contractures) should be coded with a burn or corrosion code with the 7th character "S" for sequela.

8) **Sequelae with a late effect code and current burn**

When appropriate, both a code for a current burn or corrosion with 7th character "A" or "D" and a burn or corrosion code with 7th character "S" may be assigned on the same record (when both a current burn and sequelae of an old burn exist). Burns and corrosions do not heal at the same rate and a current healing wound may still exist with sequela of a healed burn or corrosion.

See Section I.B.10 Sequela (Late Effects)

> Female patient seen for second-degree burn to the left ear; she also has significant scarring on her left elbow from a third-degree burn from childhood
>
> **T20.212A**   **Burn of second degree of left ear [any part, except ear drum], initial encounter**
>
> **L90.5**   **Scar conditions and fibrosis of skin**
>
> **T22.322S**   **Burn of third degree of left elbow, sequela**
>
> *Explanation:* The patient is being seen for management of a current second-degree burn, which is reflected in the code by appending the seventh character of A, indicating active treatment or management of this burn. The elbow scarring is a sequela of a previous third-degree burn. The sequela condition precedes the original burn injury, which is appended with a seventh character of S.

9) **Use of an external cause code with burns and corrosions**

An external cause code should be used with burns and corrosions to identify the source and intent of the burn, as well as the place where it occurred.

e. Adverse effects, poisoning, underdosing and toxic effects

Codes in categories T36-T65 are combination codes that include the substance that was taken as well as the intent. No additional external cause code is required for poisonings, toxic effects, adverse effects and underdosing codes.

1) **Do not code directly from the Table of Drugs**

Do not code directly from the Table of Drugs and Chemicals. Always refer back to the Tabular List.

2) **Use as many codes as necessary to describe**

Use as many codes as necessary to describe completely all drugs, medicinal or biological substances.

3) **If the same code would describe the causative agent**

If the same code would describe the causative agent for more than one adverse reaction, poisoning, toxic effect or underdosing, assign the code only once.

4) **If two or more drugs, medicinal or biological substances**

If two or more drugs, medicinal or biological substances are reported, code each individually unless a combination code is listed in the Table of Drugs and Chemicals.

5) **The occurrence of drug toxicity is classified in ICD-10-CM as follows:**

(a) **Adverse effect**

When coding an adverse effect of a drug that has been correctly prescribed and properly administered, assign the appropriate code for the nature of the adverse effect followed by the appropriate code for the adverse effect of the drug (T36-T50). The code for the drug should have a 5th or 6th character "5" (for example T36.0X5-) Examples of the nature of an adverse effect are tachycardia, delirium, gastrointestinal hemorrhaging, vomiting, hypokalemia, hepatitis, renal failure, or respiratory failure.

> Patient seen for stomach pain and jaundice, indicated by physician as possible side-effects of Inderal, recently started for hypertension. Inderal was discontinued and the patient switched to Atenolol instead.
>
> **R10.9**   **Unspecified abdominal pain**
>
> **R17**   **Unspecified jaundice**
>
> **T44.7X5A**   **Adverse effect of beta-adrenoreceptor antagonists, initial encounter**
>
> **I10**   **Essential (primary) hypertension**
>
> *Explanation:* The side-effects caused by the drug are listed first, followed by the code for the adverse effect of the drug to capture the specific drug that was used.

(b) **Poisoning**

When coding a poisoning or reaction to the improper use of a medication (e.g., overdose, wrong substance given or taken in error, wrong route of administration), first assign the appropriate code from categories T36-T50. The poisoning codes have an associated intent as their 5th or 6th character (accidental, intentional self-harm, assault and undetermined. Use additional code(s) for all manifestations of poisonings.

If there is also a diagnosis of abuse or dependence of the substance, the abuse or dependence is assigned as an additional code.

Examples of poisoning include:

(i) Error was made in drug prescription

Errors made in drug prescription or in the administration of the drug by provider, nurse, patient, or other person.

(ii) Overdose of a drug intentionally taken

If an overdose of a drug was intentionally taken or administered and resulted in drug toxicity, it would be coded as a poisoning.

(iii) Nonprescribed drug taken with correctly prescribed and properly administered drug

If a nonprescribed drug or medicinal agent was taken in combination with a correctly prescribed and properly administered drug, any drug toxicity or other reaction resulting from the interaction of the two drugs would be classified as a poisoning.

(iv) Interaction of drug(s) and alcohol

When a reaction results from the interaction of a drug(s) and alcohol, this would be classified as poisoning.

See Section I.C.4. if poisoning is the result of insulin pump malfunctions.

(c) **Underdosing**

Underdosing refers to taking less of a medication than is prescribed by a provider or a manufacturer's instruction. For underdosing, assign the code from categories T36-T50 (fifth or sixth character "6").

Codes for underdosing should never be assigned as principal or first-listed codes. If a patient has a relapse or exacerbation of the medical condition for which the drug is prescribed because of the reduction in dose, then the medical condition itself should be coded.

Noncompliance (Z91.12-, Z91.13-) or complication of care (Y63.6-Y63.9) codes are to be used with an underdosing code to indicate intent, if known.

> Patient admitted for atrial fibrillation with history of chronic atrial fibrillation for which she is prescribed amiodarone. Financial concerns have left the patient unable to pay for her prescriptions and she has been skipping her amiodarone dose every other day to offset the cost.
>
> | I48.2 | Chronic atrial fibrillation |
> |---|---|
> | T46.2X6A | Underdosing of other antidysrhythmic drugs, initial encounter |
> | Z91.120 | Patient's intentional underdosing of medication regimen due to financial hardship |
>
> *Explanation:* By skipping her amiodarone pill every other day, the patient's atrial fibrillation returned. The condition for which the drug was being taken is reported first, followed by an underdosing code to show that the patient was not adhering to her prescription regiment. The Z code helps elaborate on the patient's social and/or economic circumstances that led to the patient taking less then what she was prescribed.

(d) Toxic effects

When a harmful substance is ingested or comes in contact with a person, this is classified as a toxic effect. The toxic effect codes are in categories T51-T65.

Toxic effect codes have an associated intent: accidental, intentional self-harm, assault and undetermined.

f. Adult and child abuse, neglect and other maltreatment

Sequence first the appropriate code from categories T74.- (Adult and child abuse, neglect and other maltreatment, confirmed) or T76.- (Adult and child abuse, neglect and other maltreatment, suspected) for abuse, neglect and other maltreatment, followed by any accompanying mental health or injury code(s).

If the documentation in the medical record states abuse or neglect it is coded as confirmed (T74.-). It is coded as suspected if it is documented as suspected (T76.-).

For cases of confirmed abuse or neglect an external cause code from the assault section (X92-Y08) should be added to identify the cause of any physical injuries. A perpetrator code (Y07) should be added when the perpetrator of the abuse is known. For suspected cases of abuse or neglect, do not report external cause or perpetrator code.

If a suspected case of abuse, neglect or mistreatment is ruled out during an encounter code Z04.71, Encounter for examination and observation following alleged physical adult abuse, ruled out, or code Z04.72, Encounter for examination and observation following alleged child physical abuse, ruled out, should be used, not a code from T76.

If a suspected case of alleged rape or sexual abuse is ruled out during an encounter code Z04.41, Encounter for examination and observation following alleged physical adult abuse, ruled out, or code Z04.42, Encounter for examination and observation following alleged rape or sexual abuse, ruled out, should be used, not a code from T76.

See Section I.C.15. Abuse in a pregnant patient.

g. Complications of care

1) General guidelines for complications of care

(a) Documentation of complications of care

See Section I.B.16. for information on documentation of complications of care.

2) Pain due to medical devices

Pain associated with devices, implants or grafts left in a surgical site (for example painful hip prosthesis) is assigned to the appropriate code(s) found in Chapter 19, Injury, poisoning, and certain other consequences of external causes. Specific codes for pain due to medical devices are found in the T code section of the ICD-10-CM. Use additional code(s) from category G89 to identify acute or chronic pain due to presence of the device, implant or graft (G89.18 or G89.28).

> Chronic left breast pain secondary to breast implant
>
> | T85.84XA | Pain due to internal prosthetic devices, implants and grafts, not elsewhere classified, initial encounter |
> |---|---|
> | N64.4 | Mastodynia |
> | G89.28 | Other chronic postprocedural pain |
>
> *Explanation:* As the pain is a complication related to the breast implant, the complication code is sequenced first. The T code does not describe the site or type of pain, so additional codes may be appended to indicate that the patient is experiencing chronic pain in the breast.

3) Transplant complications

(a) Transplant complications other than kidney

Codes under category T86, Complications of transplanted organs and tissues, are for use for both complications and rejection of transplanted organs. A transplant complication code is only assigned if the complication affects the function of the transplanted organ. Two codes are required to fully describe a transplant complication: the appropriate code from category T86 and a secondary code that identifies the complication.

Pre-existing conditions or conditions that develop after the transplant are not coded as complications unless they affect the function of the transplanted organs.

See I.C.21. for transplant organ removal status

See I.C.2. for malignant neoplasm associated with transplanted organ.

(b) Kidney transplant complications

Patients who have undergone kidney transplant may still have some form of chronic kidney disease (CKD) because the kidney transplant may not fully restore kidney function. Code T86.1- should be assigned for documented complications of a kidney transplant, such as transplant failure or rejection or other transplant complication. Code T86.1- should not be assigned for post kidney transplant patients who have chronic kidney (CKD) unless a transplant complication such as transplant failure or rejection is documented. If the documentation is unclear as to whether the patient has a complication of the transplant, query the provider.

Conditions that affect the function of the transplanted kidney, other than CKD, should be assigned a code from subcategory T86.1, Complications of transplanted organ, Kidney, and a secondary code that identifies the complication.

For patients with CKD following a kidney transplant, but who do not have a complication such as failure or rejection, *see section I.C.14. Chronic kidney disease and kidney transplant status.*

> Patient seen for chronic kidney disease stage 2; history of successful kidney transplant with no complications identified
>
> | N18.2 | Chronic kidney disease, stage 2 (mild) |
> |---|---|
> | Z94.0 | Kidney transplant status |
>
> *Explanation:* This patient's stage 2 CKD is not indicated as being due to the transplanted kidney but instead is just the residual disease the patient had prior to the transplant.

4) Complication codes that include the external cause

As with certain other T codes, some of the complications of care codes have the external cause included in the code. The code includes the nature of the complication as well as the type of procedure that caused the complication. No external cause code indicating the type of procedure is necessary for these codes.

5) Complications of care codes within the body system chapters

Intraoperative and postprocedural complication codes are found within the body system chapters with codes specific to the organs and structures of that body system. These codes should be sequenced first, followed by a code(s) for the specific complication, if applicable.

> During a spinal fusion procedure, the surgeon inadvertently punctured the dura. The midline durotomy was repaired, and the fusion procedure was completed.
>
> | G97.41 | Accidental puncture or laceration of dura during a procedure |
> |---|---|
>
> *Explanation:* The accidental durotomy is not coded to an injury code in chapter 19 but instead is categorized to the nervous system chapter.

Muscle/Tendon Table

ICD-10-CM categorizes certain muscles and tendons in the upper and lower extremities by their action (e.g., extension, flexion), their anatomical location (e.g., posterior, anterior), and/or whether they are intrinsic or extrinsic to a certain anatomical area. The Muscle/Tendon Table is provided at the beginning of chapters 13 and 19 as a resource to help users when code selection depends on one or more of these characteristics. The categories and/or subcategories that relate to this table are identified by the icon ✦. Please note that this table is not all-inclusive, and proper code assignment should be based on the provider's documentation.

Body Region	Muscle	Extensor Tendon	Flexor Tendon	Other Tendon
Shoulder				
	Deltoid	Posterior deltoid	Anterior deltoid	
	Rotator cuff			
	Infraspinatus			Infraspinatus
	Subscapularis			Subscapularis
	Supraspinatus			Supraspinatus
	Teres minor			Teres minor
	Teres major	Teres major		
Upper arm				
	Anterior muscles			
	Biceps brachii — long head		Biceps brachii — long head	
	Biceps brachii — short head		Biceps brachii — short head	
	Brachialis		Brachialis	
	Coracobrachialis		Coracobrachialis	
	Posterior muscles			
	Triceps brachii	Triceps brachii		
Forearm				
	Anterior muscles			
	Flexors			
	Deep			
	Flexor digitorum profundus		Flexor digitorum profundus	
	Flexor pollicis longus		Flexor pollicis longus	
	Intermediate			
	Flexor digitorum superficialis		Flexor digitorum superficialis	
	Superficial			
	Flexor carpi radialis		Flexor carpi radialis	
	Flexor carpi ulnaris		Flexor carpi ulnaris	
	Palmaris longus		Palmaris longus	
	Pronators			
	Pronator quadratus			Pronator quadratus
	Pronator teres			Pronator teres
	Posterior muscles			
	Extensors			
	Deep			
	Abductor pollicis longus			Abductor pollicis longus
	Extensor indicis	Extensor indicis		
	Extensor pollicis brevis	Extensor pollicis brevis		
	Extensor pollicis longus	Extensor pollicis longus		
	Superficial			
	Brachioradialis			Brachioradialis
	Extensor carpi radialis brevis	Extensor carpi radialis brevis		
	Extensor carpi radialis longus	Extensor carpi radialis longus		
	Extensor carpi ulnaris	Extensor carpi ulnaris		
	Extensor digiti minimi	Extensor digiti minimi		
	Extensor digitorum	Extensor digitorum		
	Anconeus	Anconeus		
	Supinator			Supinator

Body Region	Muscle	Extensor Tendon	Flexor Tendon	Other Tendon
Hand				
Extrinsic — attach to a site in the forearm as well as a site in the hand with action related to hand movement at the wrist				
	Extensor carpi radialis brevis	Extensor carpi radialis brevis		
	Extensor carpi radialis longus	Extensor carpie radialis longus		
	Extensor carpi ulnaris	Extensor carpi ulnaris		
	Flexor carpi radialis		Flexor carpi radialis	
	Flexor carpi ulnaris		Flexor carpi ulnaris	
	Flexor digitorum superficialis		Flexor digitorum superficialis	
	Palmaris longus		Palmaris longus	
Extrinsic — attach to a site in the forearm as well as a site in the hand with action in the hand related to finger movement				
	Adductor pollicis longus			Adductor pollicis longus
	Extensor digiti minimi	Extensor digiti minimi		
	Extensor digitorum	Extensor digitorum		
	Extensor indicis	Extensor indicis		
	Flexor digitorum profundus		Flexor digitorum profundus	
	Flexor digitorum superficialis		Flexor digitorum superficialis	
Extrinsic — attach to a site in the forearm as well as a site in the hand with action in the hand related to thumb movement				
	Extensor pollicis brevis	Extensor pollicis brevis		
	Extensor pollicis longus	Extensor pollicis longus		
	Flexor pollicis longus		Flexor pollicis longus	
Intrinsic — found within the hand only				
	Adductor pollicis			Adductor pollicis
	Dorsal interossei	Dorsal interossei	Dorsal interossei	
	Lumbricals	Lumbricals	Lumbricals	
	Palmaris brevis			Palmaris brevis
	Palmar interossei	Palmar interossei	Palmar interossei	
	Hypothenar muscles			
	Abductor digiti minimi			Abductor digiti minimi
	Flexor digiti minimi brevis		Flexor digiti minimi brevis	
	Oppenens digiti minimi		Oppenens digiti minimi	
	Thenar muscles			
	Abductor pollicis brevis			Abductor pollicis brevis
	Flexor pollicis brevis		Flexor pollicis brevis	
	Oppenens pollicis		Oppenens pollicis	
Thigh				
	Anterior muscles			
	Iliopsoas		Iliopsoas	
	Pectineus		Pectineus	
	Quadriceps	Quadriceps		
	Rectus femoris	Rectus femoris — Extends knee	Rectus femoris — Flexes hip	
	Vastus intermedius	Vastus intermedius		
	Vastus lateralis	Vastus lateralis		
	Vastus medialis	Vastus medialis		
	Sartorius		Sartorius	
	Medial muscles			
	Adductor brevis			Adductor brevis
	Adductor longus			Adductor longus
	Adductor magnus			Adductor magnus
	Gracilis			Gracilis
	Obturator externus			Obturator externus
	Posterior muscles			
	Hamstring	Hamstring — Extends hip	Hamstring — Flexes knee	
	Biceps femoris	Biceps femoris	Biceps femoris	
	Semimembranosus	Semimembranosus	Semimembranosus	
	Semitendinosus	Semitendinosus	Semitendinosus	

Body Region	Muscle	Extensor Tendon	Flexor Tendon	Other Tendon
Lower leg				
	Anterior muscles			
	Extensor digitorum longus	Extensor digitorum longus		
	Extensor hallucis longus	Extensor hallucis longus		
	Fibularis (peroneus) tertius	Fibularis (peroneus) tertius		
	Tibialis anterior	Tibialis anterior		Tibialis anterior
	Lateral muscles			
	Fibularis (peroneus) brevis		Fibularis (peroneus) brevis	
	Fibularis (peroneus) longus		Fibularis (peroneus) longus	
	Posterior muscles			
	Deep			
	Flexor digitorum longus		Flexor digitorum longus	
	Flexor hallucis longus		Flexor hallucis longus	
	Popliteus		Popliteus	
	Tibialis posterior		Tibialis posterior	
	Superficial			
	Gastrocnemius		Gastrocnemius	
	Plantaris		Plantaris	
	Soleus		Soleus	
				Calcaneal (Achilles)
Ankle/Foot				
Extrinsic — attach to a site in the lower leg as well as a site in the foot with action related to foot movement at the ankle				
	Plantaris		Plantaris	
	Soleus		Soleus	
	Tibialis anterior	Tibialis anterior		
	Tibialis posterior		Tibialis posterior	
Extrinsic — attach to a site in the lower leg as well as a site in the foot with action in the foot related to toe movement				
	Extensor digitorum longus	Extensor digitorum longus		
	Extensor hallicus longus	Extensor hallicus longus		
	Flexor digitorum longus		Flexor digitorum longus	
	Flexor hallucis longus		Flexor hallucis longus	
Intrinsic — found within the ankle/foot only				
	Dorsal muscles			
	Extensor digitorum brevis	Extensor digitorum brevis		
	Extensor hallucis brevis	Extensor hallucis brevis		
	Plantar muscles			
	Abductor digiti minimi		Abductor digiti minimi	
	Abductor hallucis		Abductor hallucis	
	Dorsal interossei	Dorsal interossei	Dorsal interossei	
	Flexor digiti minimi brevis		Flexor digiti minimi brevis	
	Flexor digitorum brevis		Flexor digitorum brevis	
	Flexor hallucis brevis		Flexor hallucis brevis	
	Lumbricals	Lumbricals	Lumbricals	
	Quadratus plantae		Quadratus plantae	
	Plantar interossei	Plantar interossei	Plantar interossei	

Chapter 19. Injury, Poisoning and Certain Other Consequences of External Causes (S00-T88)

NOTE   Use secondary code(s) from Chapter 20, External causes of morbidity, to indicate cause of injury. Codes within the T section that include the external cause do not require an additional external cause code.

Use additional code to identify any retained foreign body, if applicable (Z18.-)

EXCLUDES 1   birth trauma (P10-P15)
obstetric trauma (O70-O71)

NOTE   The chapter uses the S-section for coding different types of injuries related to single body regions and the T-section to cover injuries to unspecified body regions as well as poisoning and certain other consequences of external causes.

AHA: 2015, 1Q, 3-21

This chapter contains the following blocks:

S00-S09	Injuries to the head
S10-S19	Injuries to the neck
S20-S29	Injuries to the thorax
S30-S39	Injuries to the abdomen, lower back, lumbar spine, pelvis and external genitals
S40-S49	Injuries to the shoulder and upper arm
S50-S59	Injuries to the elbow and forearm
S60-S69	Injuries to the wrist, hand and fingers
S70-S79	Injuries to the hip and thigh
S80-S89	Injuries to the knee and lower leg
S90-S99	Injuries to the ankle and foot
T07	Injuries involving multiple body regions
T14	Injury of unspecified body region
T15-T19	Effects of foreign body entering through natural orifice
T20-T25	Burns and corrosions of external body surface, specified by site
T26-T28	Burns and corrosions confined to eye and internal organs
T30-T32	Burns and corrosions of multiple and unspecified body regions
T33-T34	Frostbite
T36-T50	Poisoning by, adverse effect of and underdosing of drugs, medicaments and biological substances
T51-T65	Toxic effects of substances chiefly nonmedicinal as to source
T66-T78	Other and unspecified effects of external causes
T79	Certain early complications of trauma
T80-T88	Complications of surgical and medical care, not elsewhere classified

Injuries to the head (S00-S09)

INCLUDES   injuries of ear
injuries of eye
injuries of face [any part]
injuries of gum
injuries of jaw
injuries of oral cavity
injuries of palate
injuries of periocular area
injuries of scalp
injuries of temporomandibular joint area
injuries of tongue
injuries of tooth

Code also for any associated infection

EXCLUDES 2   burns and corrosions (T20-T32)
effects of foreign body in ear (T16)
effects of foreign body in larynx (T17.3)
effects of foreign body in mouth NOS (T18.0)
effects of foreign body in nose (T17.0-T17.1)
effects of foreign body in pharynx (T17.2)
effects of foreign body on external eye (T15.-)
frostbite (T33-T34)
insect bite or sting, venomous (T63.4)

✓4th **S00**   **Superficial injury of head**

    EXCLUDES 1   diffuse cerebral contusion (S06.2-)
focal cerebral contusion (S06.3-)
injury of eye and orbit (S05.-)
open wound of head (S01.-)

> The appropriate 7th character is to be added to each code from category S00.
> A   initial encounter
> D   subsequent encounter
> S   sequela

✓5th **S00.0**   **Superficial injury of scalp**

   ✓x7th **S00.00**   **Unspecified superficial injury of scalp**   ▽

   ✓x7th **S00.01**   Abrasion of scalp

   ✓x7th **S00.02**   Blister (nonthermal) of scalp

   ✓x7th **S00.03**   Contusion of scalp
        Bruise of scalp
        Hematoma of scalp

   ✓x7th **S00.04**   External constriction of part of scalp

   ✓x7th **S00.05**   Superficial foreign body of scalp
        Splinter in the scalp

   ✓x7th **S00.06**   Insect bite (nonvenomous) of scalp

   ✓x7th **S00.07**   **Other superficial bite of scalp**
        EXCLUDES 1   open bite of scalp (S01.05)

✓5th **S00.1**   **Contusion of eyelid and periocular area**
      Black eye
      EXCLUDES 2   contusion of eyeball and orbital tissues (S05.1)

   ✓x7th **S00.10**   **Contusion of unspecified eyelid and periocular area**   ▽

   ✓x7th **S00.11**   **Contusion of right eyelid and periocular area**

   ✓x7th **S00.12**   **Contusion of left eyelid and periocular area**

✓5th **S00.2**   **Other and unspecified superficial injuries of eyelid and periocular area**
      EXCLUDES 2   superficial injury of conjunctiva and cornea (S05.0-)

   ✓6th **S00.20**   Unspecified superficial injury of eyelid and periocular area

     ✓7th **S00.201**   **Unspecified superficial injury of right eyelid and periocular area**   ▽

     ✓7th **S00.202**   **Unspecified superficial injury of left eyelid and periocular area**   ▽

     ✓7th **S00.209**   **Unspecified superficial injury of unspecified eyelid and periocular area**   ▽

   ✓6th **S00.21**   Abrasion of eyelid and periocular area

     ✓7th **S00.211**   **Abrasion of right eyelid and periocular area**

     ✓7th **S00.212**   **Abrasion of left eyelid and periocular area**

     ✓7th **S00.219**   **Abrasion of unspecified eyelid and periocular area**   ▽

   ✓6th **S00.22**   Blister (nonthermal) of eyelid and periocular area

     ✓7th **S00.221**   **Blister (nonthermal) of right eyelid and periocular area**

     ✓7th **S00.222**   **Blister (nonthermal) of left eyelid and periocular area**

     ✓7th **S00.229**   **Blister (nonthermal) of unspecified eyelid and periocular area**   ▽

   ✓6th **S00.24**   External constriction of eyelid and periocular area

     ✓7th **S00.241**   **External constriction of right eyelid and periocular area**

     ✓7th **S00.242**   **External constriction of left eyelid and periocular area**

     ✓7th **S00.249**   **External constriction of unspecified eyelid and periocular area**   ▽

   ✓6th **S00.25**   Superficial foreign body of eyelid and periocular area
       Splinter of eyelid and periocular area
       EXCLUDES 2   retained foreign body in eyelid (H02.81-)

     ✓7th **S00.251**   **Superficial foreign body of right eyelid and periocular area**

     ✓7th **S00.252**   **Superficial foreign body of left eyelid and periocular area**

     ✓7th **S00.259**   **Superficial foreign body of unspecified eyelid and periocular area**   ▽

   ✓6th **S00.26**   Insect bite (nonvenomous) of eyelid and periocular area

     ✓7th **S00.261**   **Insect bite (nonvenomous) of right eyelid and periocular area**

     ✓7th **S00.262**   **Insect bite (nonvenomous) of left eyelid and periocular area**

     ✓7th **S00.269**   **Insect bite (nonvenomous) of unspecified eyelid and periocular area**   ▽

   ✓6th **S00.27**   Other superficial bite of eyelid and periocular area
       EXCLUDES 1   open bite of eyelid and periocular area (S01.15)

     ✓7th **S00.271**   **Other superficial bite of right eyelid and periocular area**

     ✓7th **S00.272**   **Other superficial bite of left eyelid and periocular area**

     ✓7th **S00.279**   **Other superficial bite of unspecified eyelid and periocular area**   ▽

Ⓝ Newborn   Ⓟ Pediatric   Ⓜ Maternity   Ⓐ Adult   **RIC** RIC Dx   **NC Dx** Noncancer Dx   **PDx** Primary Dx   **CC** RIC CC Condition   ▶◀ Revised Text   ● New Code   ▲ Revised Code Title

858   ICD-10-CM 2016

✓5ᵗʰ S00.3 Superficial injury of nose

✓x7ᵗʰ **S00.30** Unspecified superficial injury of nose ▽

✓x7ᵗʰ **S00.31** Abrasion of nose

✓x7ᵗʰ **S00.32** Blister (nonthermal) of nose

✓x7ᵗʰ **S00.33** Contusion of nose
     Bruise of nose
     Hematoma of nose

✓x7ᵗʰ **S00.34** External constriction of nose

✓x7ᵗʰ **S00.35** Superficial foreign body of nose
     Splinter in the nose

✓x7ᵗʰ **S00.36** Insect bite (nonvenomous) of nose

✓x7ᵗʰ **S00.37** Other superficial bite of nose
     EXCLUDES 1 *open bite of nose (S01.25)*

✓5ᵗʰ S00.4 Superficial injury of ear

✓6ᵗʰ **S00.40** Unspecified superficial injury of ear

    ✓7ᵗʰ **S00.401** Unspecified superficial injury of right ear ▽

    ✓7ᵗʰ **S00.402** Unspecified superficial injury of left ear ▽

    ✓7ᵗʰ **S00.409** Unspecified superficial injury of unspecified ear ▽

✓6ᵗʰ **S00.41** Abrasion of ear

    ✓7ᵗʰ **S00.411** Abrasion of right ear

    ✓7ᵗʰ **S00.412** Abrasion of left ear

    ✓7ᵗʰ **S00.419** Abrasion of unspecified ear ▽

✓6ᵗʰ **S00.42** Blister (nonthermal) of ear

    ✓7ᵗʰ **S00.421** Blister (nonthermal) of right ear

    ✓7ᵗʰ **S00.422** Blister (nonthermal) of left ear

    ✓7ᵗʰ **S00.429** Blister (nonthermal) of unspecified ear ▽

✓6ᵗʰ **S00.43** Contusion of ear
     Bruise of ear
     Hematoma of ear

    ✓7ᵗʰ **S00.431** Contusion of right ear

    ✓7ᵗʰ **S00.432** Contusion of left ear

    ✓7ᵗʰ **S00.439** Contusion of unspecified ear ▽

✓6ᵗʰ **S00.44** External constriction of ear

    ✓7ᵗʰ **S00.441** External constriction of right ear

    ✓7ᵗʰ **S00.442** External constriction of left ear

    ✓7ᵗʰ **S00.449** External constriction of unspecified ear ▽

✓6ᵗʰ **S00.45** Superficial foreign body of ear
     Splinter in the ear

    ✓7ᵗʰ **S00.451** Superficial foreign body of right ear

    ✓7ᵗʰ **S00.452** Superficial foreign body of left ear

    ✓7ᵗʰ **S00.459** Superficial foreign body of unspecified ear ▽

✓6ᵗʰ **S00.46** Insect bite (nonvenomous) of ear

    ✓7ᵗʰ **S00.461** Insect bite (nonvenomous) of right ear

    ✓7ᵗʰ **S00.462** Insect bite (nonvenomous) of left ear

    ✓7ᵗʰ **S00.469** Insect bite (nonvenomous) of unspecified ear ▽

✓6ᵗʰ **S00.47** Other superficial bite of ear
     EXCLUDES 1 *open bite of ear (S01.35)*

    ✓7ᵗʰ **S00.471** Other superficial bite of right ear

    ✓7ᵗʰ **S00.472** Other superficial bite of left ear

    ✓7ᵗʰ **S00.479** Other superficial bite of unspecified ear ▽

✓5ᵗʰ S00.5 Superficial injury of lip and oral cavity

✓6ᵗʰ **S00.50** Unspecified superficial injury of lip and oral cavity

    ✓7ᵗʰ **S00.501** Unspecified superficial injury of lip ▽

    ✓7ᵗʰ **S00.502** Unspecified superficial injury of oral cavity ▽

✓6ᵗʰ **S00.51** Abrasion of lip and oral cavity

    ✓7ᵗʰ **S00.511** Abrasion of lip

    ✓7ᵗʰ **S00.512** Abrasion of oral cavity

✓6ᵗʰ **S00.52** Blister (nonthermal) of lip and oral cavity

    ✓7ᵗʰ **S00.521** Blister (nonthermal) of lip

    ✓7ᵗʰ **S00.522** Blister (nonthermal) of oral cavity

✓6ᵗʰ **S00.53** Contusion of lip and oral cavity

    ✓7ᵗʰ **S00.531** Contusion of lip
       Bruise of lip
       Hematoma of oral cavity

    ✓7ᵗʰ **S00.532** Contusion of oral cavity
       Bruise of lip
       Hematoma of oral cavity

✓6ᵗʰ **S00.54** External constriction of lip and oral cavity

    ✓7ᵗʰ **S00.541** External constriction of lip

    ✓7ᵗʰ **S00.542** External constriction of oral cavity

✓6ᵗʰ **S00.55** Superficial foreign body of lip and oral cavity

    ✓7ᵗʰ **S00.551** Superficial foreign body of lip
       Splinter of lip and oral cavity

    ✓7ᵗʰ **S00.552** Superficial foreign body of oral cavity
       Splinter of lip and oral cavity

✓6ᵗʰ **S00.56** Insect bite (nonvenomous) of lip and oral cavity

    ✓7ᵗʰ **S00.561** Insect bite (nonvenomous) of lip

    ✓7ᵗʰ **S00.562** Insect bite (nonvenomous) of oral cavity

✓6ᵗʰ **S00.57** Other superficial bite of lip and oral cavity

    ✓7ᵗʰ **S00.571** Other superficial bite of lip
       EXCLUDES 1 *open bite of lip (S01.551)*

    ✓7ᵗʰ **S00.572** Other superficial bite of oral cavity
       EXCLUDES 1 *open bite of oral cavity (S01.552)*

✓5ᵗʰ S00.8 Superficial injury of other parts of head

✓x7ᵗʰ **S00.80** Unspecified superficial injury of other part of head ▽

✓x7ᵗʰ **S00.81** Abrasion of other part of head

✓x7ᵗʰ **S00.82** Blister (nonthermal) of other part of head

✓x7ᵗʰ **S00.83** Contusion of other part of head
     Bruise of other part of head
     Hematoma of other part of head

✓x7ᵗʰ **S00.84** External constriction of other part of head

✓x7ᵗʰ **S00.85** Superficial foreign body of other part of head
     Splinter in other part of head

✓x7ᵗʰ **S00.86** Insect bite (nonvenomous) of other part of head

✓x7ᵗʰ **S00.87** Other superficial bite of other part of head
     EXCLUDES 1 *open bite of other part of head (S01.85)*

✓5ᵗʰ S00.9 Superficial injury of unspecified part of head

✓x7ᵗʰ **S00.90** Unspecified superficial injury of unspecified part of head ▽

✓x7ᵗʰ **S00.91** Abrasion of unspecified part of head ▽

✓x7ᵗʰ **S00.92** Blister (nonthermal) of unspecified part of head ▽

✓x7ᵗʰ **S00.93** Contusion of unspecified part of head ▽
     Bruise of head
     Hematoma of head

✓x7ᵗʰ **S00.94** External constriction of unspecified part of head ▽

✓x7ᵗʰ **S00.95** Superficial foreign body of unspecified part of head ▽
     Splinter of head

✓x7ᵗʰ **S00.96** Insect bite (nonvenomous) of unspecified part of head ▽

✓x7ᵗʰ **S00.97** Other superficial bite of unspecified part of head ▽
     EXCLUDES 1 *open bite of head (S01.95)*

✓4ᵗʰ S01 Open wound of head

Code also any associated:
     injury of cranial nerve (S04.-)
     injury of muscle and tendon of head (S09.1-)
     intracranial injury (S06.-)
     wound infection
     EXCLUDES 1 *open skull fracture (S02- with 7th character B)*
     EXCLUDES 2 *injury of eye and orbit (S05.-)*
               traumatic amputation of part of head (S08.-)

The appropriate 7th character is to be added to each code from category S01.
A   initial encounter
D   subsequent encounter
S   sequela

✓5ᵗʰ S01.0 Open wound of scalp
     EXCLUDES 1 *avulsion of scalp (S08.0)*

✓x7ᵗʰ **S01.00** Unspecified open wound of scalp ▽

✓x7ᵗʰ **S01.01** Laceration without foreign body of scalp

✓x7ᵗʰ **S01.02** Laceration with foreign body of scalp

✓x7ᵗʰ **S01.03** Puncture wound without foreign body of scalp

✓x7ᵗʰ **S01.04** Puncture wound with foreign body of scalp

☑ Add'l Character Required ✓x7ᵗʰ Placeholder Alert   RUG IV Special Care High Dx   RUG IV Clinically Complex Dx   RUG IV Special Care Low Dx   Manifestation Code   Other Specified Code   ▽ Unspecified Code

ICD-10-CM 2016   859

√x7ᵗʰ **S01.05**   **Open bite of scalp**
Bite of scalp NOS
EXCLUDES 1 *superficial bite of scalp (S00.06, S00.07-)*

√5ᵗʰ **S01.1**   **Open wound of** eyelid and periocular area
Open wound of eyelid and periocular area with or without involvement of lacrimal passages

√6ᵗʰ **S01.10**   Unspecified **open wound of eyelid and periocular area**

√7ᵗʰ **S01.101**   Unspecified open wound of right eyelid and periocular area ▽

√7ᵗʰ **S01.102**   Unspecified open wound of left eyelid and periocular area ▽

√7ᵗʰ **S01.109**   Unspecified open wound of unspecified eyelid and periocular area ▽

√6ᵗʰ **S01.11**   Laceration without foreign body **of eyelid and periocular area**

√7ᵗʰ **S01.111**   Laceration without foreign body of right eyelid and periocular area

√7ᵗʰ **S01.112**   Laceration without foreign body of left eyelid and periocular area

√7ᵗʰ **S01.119**   Laceration without foreign body of unspecified eyelid and periocular area ▽

√6ᵗʰ **S01.12**   Laceration with foreign body **of eyelid and periocular area**

√7ᵗʰ **S01.121**   Laceration with foreign body of right eyelid and periocular area

√7ᵗʰ **S01.122**   Laceration with foreign body of left eyelid and periocular area

√7ᵗʰ **S01.129**   Laceration with foreign body of unspecified eyelid and periocular area ▽

√6ᵗʰ **S01.13**   Puncture wound without foreign body **of eyelid and periocular area**

√7ᵗʰ **S01.131**   Puncture wound without foreign body of right eyelid and periocular area

√7ᵗʰ **S01.132**   Puncture wound without foreign body of left eyelid and periocular area

√7ᵗʰ **S01.139**   Puncture wound without foreign body of unspecified eyelid and periocular area ▽

√6ᵗʰ **S01.14**   Puncture wound with foreign body **of eyelid and periocular area**

√7ᵗʰ **S01.141**   Puncture wound with foreign body of right eyelid and periocular area

√7ᵗʰ **S01.142**   Puncture wound with foreign body of left eyelid and periocular area

√7ᵗʰ **S01.149**   Puncture wound with foreign body of unspecified eyelid and periocular area ▽

√6ᵗʰ **S01.15**   Open bite **of eyelid and periocular area**
Bite of eyelid and periocular area NOS
EXCLUDES 1 *superficial bite of eyelid and periocular area (S00.26, S00.27)*

√7ᵗʰ **S01.151**   Open bite of right eyelid and periocular area

√7ᵗʰ **S01.152**   Open bite of left eyelid and periocular area

√7ᵗʰ **S01.159**   Open bite of unspecified eyelid and periocular area ▽

√5ᵗʰ **S01.2**   **Open wound of** nose

√x7ᵗʰ **S01.20**   Unspecified open wound of nose ▽

√x7ᵗʰ **S01.21**   Laceration without foreign body of nose

√x7ᵗʰ **S01.22**   Laceration with foreign body of nose

√x7ᵗʰ **S01.23**   Puncture wound without foreign body of nose

√x7ᵗʰ **S01.24**   Puncture wound with foreign body of nose

√x7ᵗʰ **S01.25**   Open bite of nose
Bite of nose NOS
EXCLUDES 1 *superficial bite of nose (S00.36, S00.37)*

√5ᵗʰ **S01.3**   **Open wound of** ear

√6ᵗʰ **S01.30**   Unspecified **open wound of ear**

√7ᵗʰ **S01.301**   Unspecified open wound of right ear ▽

√7ᵗʰ **S01.302**   Unspecified open wound of left ear ▽

√7ᵗʰ **S01.309**   Unspecified open wound of unspecified ear ▽

√6ᵗʰ **S01.31**   Laceration without foreign body **of ear**

√7ᵗʰ **S01.311**   Laceration without foreign body of right ear

√7ᵗʰ **S01.312**   Laceration without foreign body of left ear

√7ᵗʰ **S01.319**   Laceration without foreign body of unspecified ear ▽

√6ᵗʰ **S01.32**   Laceration with foreign body **of ear**

√7ᵗʰ **S01.321**   Laceration with foreign body of right ear

√7ᵗʰ **S01.322**   Laceration with foreign body of left ear

√7ᵗʰ **S01.329**   Laceration with foreign body of unspecified ear ▽

√6ᵗʰ **S01.33**   Puncture wound without foreign body **of ear**

√7ᵗʰ **S01.331**   Puncture wound without foreign body of right ear

√7ᵗʰ **S01.332**   Puncture wound without foreign body of left ear

√7ᵗʰ **S01.339**   Puncture wound without foreign body of unspecified ear ▽

√6ᵗʰ **S01.34**   Puncture wound with foreign body **of ear**

√7ᵗʰ **S01.341**   Puncture wound with foreign body of right ear

√7ᵗʰ **S01.342**   Puncture wound with foreign body of left ear

√7ᵗʰ **S01.349**   Puncture wound with foreign body of unspecified ear ▽

√6ᵗʰ **S01.35**   Open bite **of ear**
Bite of ear NOS
EXCLUDES 1 *superficial bite of ear (S00.46, S00.47)*

√7ᵗʰ **S01.351**   Open bite of right ear

√7ᵗʰ **S01.352**   Open bite of left ear

√7ᵗʰ **S01.359**   Open bite of unspecified ear ▽

√5ᵗʰ **S01.4**   **Open wound of** cheek and temporomandibular area

√6ᵗʰ **S01.40**   Unspecified **open wound of cheek and temporomandibular area**

√7ᵗʰ **S01.401**   Unspecified open wound of right cheek and temporomandibular area ▽

√7ᵗʰ **S01.402**   Unspecified open wound of left cheek and temporomandibular area ▽

√7ᵗʰ **S01.409**   Unspecified open wound of unspecified cheek and temporomandibular area ▽

√6ᵗʰ **S01.41**   Laceration without foreign body **of cheek and temporomandibular area**

√7ᵗʰ **S01.411**   Laceration without foreign body of right cheek and temporomandibular area

√7ᵗʰ **S01.412**   Laceration without foreign body of left cheek and temporomandibular area

√7ᵗʰ **S01.419**   Laceration without foreign body of unspecified cheek and temporomandibular area ▽

√6ᵗʰ **S01.42**   Laceration with foreign body **of cheek and temporomandibular area**

√7ᵗʰ **S01.421**   Laceration with foreign body of right cheek and temporomandibular area

√7ᵗʰ **S01.422**   Laceration with foreign body of left cheek and temporomandibular area

√7ᵗʰ **S01.429**   Laceration with foreign body of unspecified cheek and temporomandibular area ▽

√6ᵗʰ **S01.43**   Puncture wound without foreign body **of cheek and temporomandibular area**

√7ᵗʰ **S01.431**   Puncture wound without foreign body of right cheek and temporomandibular area

√7ᵗʰ **S01.432**   Puncture wound without foreign body of left cheek and temporomandibular area

√7ᵗʰ **S01.439**   Puncture wound without foreign body of unspecified cheek and temporomandibular area ▽

√6ᵗʰ **S01.44**   Puncture wound with foreign body **of cheek and temporomandibular area**

√7ᵗʰ **S01.441**   Puncture wound with foreign body of right cheek and temporomandibular area

√7ᵗʰ **S01.442**   Puncture wound with foreign body of left cheek and temporomandibular area

√7ᵗʰ **S01.449**   Puncture wound with foreign body of unspecified cheek and temporomandibular area ▽

Ⓝ Newborn   Ⓟ Pediatric   Ⓜ Maternity   Ⓐ Adult   **RIC** RIC Dx   **NC Dx** Noncancer Dx   **PDx** Primary Dx   **CC** RIC CC Condition   ▶◀ Revised Text   ● New Code   ▲ Revised Code Title

860   ICD-10-CM 2016

✓6ᵗʰ **S01.45** Open bite **of cheek and temporomandibular area**
Bite of cheek and temporomandibular area NOS
EXCLUDES 2 *superficial bite of cheek and temporomandibular area (S00.86, S00.87)*

  ✓7ᵗʰ **S01.451** Open bite **of right cheek and temporomandibular area**

  ✓7ᵗʰ **S01.452** Open bite **of left cheek and temporomandibular area**

  ✓7ᵗʰ **S01.459** Open bite **of unspecified cheek and temporomandibular area** ▽

✓5ᵗʰ **S01.5** Open wound **of lip and oral cavity**
EXCLUDES 2 *tooth dislocation (S03.2)*
tooth fracture (S02.5)

  ✓6ᵗʰ **S01.50** Unspecified open wound **of lip and oral cavity**

    ✓7ᵗʰ **S01.501** Unspecified open wound **of lip** ▽

    ✓7ᵗʰ **S01.502** Unspecified open wound **of oral cavity** ▽

  ✓6ᵗʰ **S01.51** Laceration **of lip and oral cavity without foreign body**

    ✓7ᵗʰ **S01.511** Laceration without foreign body **of lip**

    ✓7ᵗʰ **S01.512** Laceration without foreign body **of oral cavity**

  ✓6ᵗʰ **S01.52** Laceration **of lip and oral cavity with foreign body**

    ✓7ᵗʰ **S01.521** Laceration with foreign body **of lip**

    ✓7ᵗʰ **S01.522** Laceration with foreign body **of oral cavity**

  ✓6ᵗʰ **S01.53** Puncture wound **of lip and oral cavity without foreign body**

    ✓7ᵗʰ **S01.531** Puncture wound without foreign body **of lip**

    ✓7ᵗʰ **S01.532** Puncture wound without foreign body **of oral cavity**

  ✓6ᵗʰ **S01.54** Puncture wound **of lip and oral cavity with foreign body**

    ✓7ᵗʰ **S01.541** Puncture wound with foreign body **of lip**

    ✓7ᵗʰ **S01.542** Puncture wound with foreign body **of oral cavity**

  ✓6ᵗʰ **S01.55** Open bite **of lip and oral cavity**

    ✓7ᵗʰ **S01.551** Open bite **of lip**
Bite of lip NOS
EXCLUDES 1 *superficial bite of lip (S00.571)*

    ✓7ᵗʰ **S01.552** Open bite **of oral cavity**
Bite of oral cavity NOS
EXCLUDES 1 *superficial bite of oral cavity (S00.572)*

✓5ᵗʰ **S01.8** Open wound **of other parts of head**

  ✓x7ᵗʰ **S01.80** Unspecified open wound **of other part of head** ▽

  ✓x7ᵗʰ **S01.81** Laceration without foreign body **of other part of head**

  ✓x7ᵗʰ **S01.82** Laceration with foreign body **of other part of head**

  ✓x7ᵗʰ **S01.83** Puncture wound without foreign body **of other part of head**

  ✓x7ᵗʰ **S01.84** Puncture wound with foreign body **of other part of head**

  ✓x7ᵗʰ **S01.85** Open bite **of other part of head**
Bite of other part of head NOS
EXCLUDES 1 *superficial bite of other part of head (S00.85)*

✓5ᵗʰ **S01.9** Open wound **of unspecified part of head**

  ✓x7ᵗʰ **S01.90** Unspecified open wound **of unspecified part of head** ▽

  ✓x7ᵗʰ **S01.91** Laceration without foreign body **of unspecified part of head** ▽

  ✓x7ᵗʰ **S01.92** Laceration with foreign body **of unspecified part of head** ▽

  ✓x7ᵗʰ **S01.93** Puncture wound without foreign body **of unspecified part of head** ▽

  ✓x7ᵗʰ **S01.94** Puncture wound with foreign body **of unspecified part of head** ▽

  ✓x7ᵗʰ **S01.95** Open bite **of unspecified part of head** ▽
Bite of head NOS
EXCLUDES 1 *superficial bite of head NOS (S00.97)*

✓4ᵗʰ **S02** **Fracture of skull and facial bones**
NOTE   A fracture not indicated as open or closed should be coded to closed.
Code also any associated intracranial injury (S06.-).

The appropriate 7th character is to be added to each code from category S02.
A   initial encounter for closed fracture
B   initial encounter for open fracture
D   subsequent encounter for fracture with routine healing
G   subsequent encounter for fracture with delayed healing
K   subsequent encounter for fracture with nonunion
S   sequela

✓x7ᵗʰ **S02.0** Fracture **of vault of skull**
Fracture of frontal bone
Fracture of parietal bone

✓5ᵗʰ **S02.1** Fracture **of base of skull**
EXCLUDES 1 *orbit NOS (S02.8)*
EXCLUDES 2 *orbital floor (S02.3-)*

  ✓x7ᵗʰ **S02.10** Unspecified fracture of base of skull ▽

  ✓6ᵗʰ **S02.11** Fracture **of occiput**

    ✓7ᵗʰ **S02.110** Type I **occipital condyle fracture**

    ✓7ᵗʰ **S02.111** Type II **occipital condyle fracture**

    ✓7ᵗʰ **S02.112** Type III **occipital condyle fracture**

    ✓7ᵗʰ **S02.113** Unspecified **occipital condyle fracture** ▽

    ✓7ᵗʰ **S02.118** Other fracture of occiput

    ✓7ᵗʰ **S02.119** Unspecified fracture of occiput ▽

  ✓x7ᵗʰ **S02.19** Other fracture of base of skull
Fracture of anterior fossa of base of skull
Fracture of ethmoid sinus
Fracture of frontal sinus
Fracture of middle fossa of base of skull
Fracture of orbital roof
Fracture of posterior fossa of base of skull
Fracture of sphenoid
Fracture of temporal bone

✓x7ᵗʰ **S02.2** Fracture **of nasal bones**

✓x7ᵗʰ **S02.3** Fracture **of orbital floor**
EXCLUDES 1 *orbit NOS (S02.8)*
EXCLUDES 2 *orbital roof (S02.1-)*

✓5ᵗʰ **S02.4** Fracture **of malar, maxillary and zygoma bones**
Fracture of superior maxilla
Fracture of upper jaw (bone)
Fracture of zygomatic process of temporal bone

  ✓6ᵗʰ **S02.40** Fracture **of malar, maxillary and zygoma bones, unspecified**

    ✓7ᵗʰ **S02.400** Malar **fracture unspecified** ▽

    ✓7ᵗʰ **S02.401** Maxillary **fracture, unspecified** ▽

    ✓7ᵗʰ **S02.402** Zygomatic **fracture, unspecified** ▽

  ✓6ᵗʰ **S02.41** LeFort **fracture**

    ✓7ᵗʰ **S02.411** LeFort I **fracture**

    ✓7ᵗʰ **S02.412** LeFort II **fracture**

    ✓7ᵗʰ **S02.413** LeFort III **fracture**

  ✓x7ᵗʰ **S02.42** Fracture **of alveolus of maxilla**

✓x7ᵗʰ **S02.5** Fracture **of tooth (traumatic)**
Broken tooth
EXCLUDES 1 *cracked tooth (nontraumatic) (K03.81)*

✓5ᵗʰ **S02.6** Fracture **of mandible**
Fracture of lower jaw (bone)

  ✓6ᵗʰ **S02.60** Fracture **of mandible, unspecified**

    ✓7ᵗʰ **S02.600** Fracture **of unspecified part of body of mandible** ▽

    ✓7ᵗʰ **S02.609** Fracture **of mandible, unspecified** ▽

  ✓x7ᵗʰ **S02.61** Fracture **of condylar process of mandible**

  ✓x7ᵗʰ **S02.62** Fracture **of subcondylar process of mandible**

  ✓x7ᵗʰ **S02.63** Fracture **of coronoid process of mandible**

  ✓x7ᵗʰ **S02.64** Fracture **of ramus of mandible**

  ✓x7ᵗʰ **S02.65** Fracture **of angle of mandible**

  ✓x7ᵗʰ **S02.66** Fracture **of symphysis of mandible**

  ✓x7ᵗʰ **S02.67** Fracture **of alveolus of mandible**

  ✓x7ᵗʰ **S02.69** Fracture **of mandible of other specified site**

✓ Add'l Character Required   ✓x7ᵗʰ Placeholder Alert   RUG IV Special Care High Dx   RUG IV Clinically Complex Dx   RUG IV Special Care Low Dx   Manifestation Code   Other Specified Code   ▽ Unspecified Code

ICD-10-CM 2016   861

Chapter 19. Injury, Poisoning and Certain Other Consequences of External Causes

√x7ᵗʰ **S02.8 Fractures of other specified skull and facial bones**
Fracture of orbit NOS
Fracture of palate
EXCLUDES 1   *fracture of orbital floor (S02.3-)*
fracture of orbital roof (S02.1-)

√5ᵗʰ **S02.9 Fracture of** unspecified **skull and facial bones**

√x7ᵗʰ **S02.91 Unspecified fracture of** skull ▽

√x7ᵗʰ **S02.92 Unspecified fracture of** facial bones ▽

√4ᵗʰ **S03 Dislocation and sprain of joints and ligaments of head**
INCLUDES   avulsion of joint (capsule) or ligament of head
laceration of cartilage, joint (capsule) or ligament of head
sprain of cartilage, joint (capsule) or ligament of head
traumatic hemarthrosis of joint or ligament of head
traumatic rupture of joint or ligament of head
traumatic subluxation of joint or ligament of head
traumatic tear of joint or ligament of head
Code also any associated open wound
EXCLUDES 2   *strain of muscle or tendon of head (S09.1)*

The appropriate 7th character is to be added to each code from
category S03.
A   initial encounter
D   subsequent encounter
S   sequela

√x7ᵗʰ **S03.0 Dislocation of jaw**
Dislocation of jaw (cartilage) (meniscus)
Dislocation of mandible
Dislocation of temporomandibular (joint)

√x7ᵗʰ **S03.1 Dislocation of septal cartilage of nose**

√x7ᵗʰ **S03.2 Dislocation of tooth**

√x7ᵗʰ **S03.4 Sprain of jaw**
Sprain of temporomandibular (joint) (ligament)

√x7ᵗʰ **S03.8 Sprain of joints and ligaments of other parts of head**

√x7ᵗʰ **S03.9 Sprain of joints and ligaments of unspecified parts of head** ▽

√4ᵗʰ **S04 Injury of cranial nerve**
The selection of side should be based on the side of the body being
affected
Codes first any associated intracranial injury (S06.-)
Code also any associated:
open wound of head (S01.-)
skull fracture (S02.-)

The appropriate 7th character is to be added to each code from
category S04.
A   initial encounter
D   subsequent encounter
S   sequela

√5ᵗʰ **S04.0 Injury of optic nerve and pathways**
Use additional code to identify any visual field defect or
blindness (H53.4-, H54)

√6ᵗʰ **S04.01 Injury of** optic **nerve**
Injury of 2nd cranial nerve

√7ᵗʰ **S04.011 Injury of optic nerve,** right **eye**

√7ᵗʰ **S04.012 Injury of optic nerve,** left **eye**

√7ᵗʰ **S04.019 Injury of optic nerve, unspecified eye** ▽
Injury of optic nerve NOS

√x7ᵗʰ **S04.02 Injury of optic** chiasm

√6ᵗʰ **S04.03 Injury of optic** tract and pathways
Injury of optic radiation

√7ᵗʰ **S04.031 Injury of optic tract and pathways,**
right **eye**

√7ᵗʰ **S04.032 Injury of optic tract and pathways,**
left **eye**

√7ᵗʰ **S04.039 Injury of optic tract and pathways,** ▽
unspecified eye
Injury of optic tract and pathways NOS

√6ᵗʰ **S04.04 Injury of** visual cortex

√7ᵗʰ **S04.041 Injury of visual cortex,** right **eye**

√7ᵗʰ **S04.042 Injury of visual cortex,** left **eye**

√7ᵗʰ **S04.049 Injury of visual cortex, unspecified eye** ▽
Injury of visual cortex NOS

√5ᵗʰ **S04.1 Injury of** oculomotor nerve
Injury of 3rd cranial nerve

√x7ᵗʰ **S04.10 Injury of oculomotor nerve, unspecified side** ▽

√x7ᵗʰ **S04.11 Injury of oculomotor nerve,** right **side**

√x7ᵗʰ **S04.12 Injury of oculomotor nerve,** left **side**

√5ᵗʰ **S04.2 Injury of** trochlear nerve
Injury of 4th cranial nerve

√x7ᵗʰ **S04.20 Injury of trochlear nerve, unspecified side** ▽

√x7ᵗʰ **S04.21 Injury of trochlear nerve,** right **side**

√x7ᵗʰ **S04.22 Injury of trochlear nerve,** left **side**

√5ᵗʰ **S04.3 Injury of** trigeminal nerve
Injury of 5th cranial nerve

√x7ᵗʰ **S04.30 Injury of trigeminal nerve, unspecified side** ▽

√x7ᵗʰ **S04.31 Injury of trigeminal nerve,** right **side**

√x7ᵗʰ **S04.32 Injury of trigeminal nerve,** left **side**

√5ᵗʰ **S04.4 Injury of** abducent nerve
Injury of 6th cranial nerve

√x7ᵗʰ **S04.40 Injury of abducent nerve, unspecified side** ▽

√x7ᵗʰ **S04.41 Injury of abducent nerve,** right **side**

√x7ᵗʰ **S04.42 Injury of abducent nerve,** left **side**

√5ᵗʰ **S04.5 Injury of** facial nerve
Injury of 7th cranial nerve

√x7ᵗʰ **S04.50 Injury of facial nerve, unspecified side** ▽

√x7ᵗʰ **S04.51 Injury of facial nerve,** right **side**

√x7ᵗʰ **S04.52 Injury of facial nerve,** left **side**

√5ᵗʰ **S04.6 Injury of** acoustic nerve
Injury of auditory nerve
Injury of 8th cranial nerve

√x7ᵗʰ **S04.60 Injury of acoustic nerve, unspecified side** ▽

√x7ᵗʰ **S04.61 Injury of acoustic nerve,** right **side**

√x7ᵗʰ **S04.62 Injury of acoustic nerve,** left **side**

√5ᵗʰ **S04.7 Injury of** accessory nerve
Injury of 11th cranial nerve

√x7ᵗʰ **S04.70 Injury of accessory nerve, unspecified side** ▽

√x7ᵗʰ **S04.71 Injury of accessory nerve,** right **side**

√x7ᵗʰ **S04.72 Injury of accessory nerve,** left **side**

√5ᵗʰ **S04.8 Injury of** other cranial nerves

√6ᵗʰ **S04.81 Injury of** olfactory [1st] **nerve**

√7ᵗʰ **S04.811 Injury of olfactory [1st] nerve,** right **side**

√7ᵗʰ **S04.812 Injury of olfactory [1st] nerve,** left **side**

√7ᵗʰ **S04.819 Injury of olfactory [1st] nerve,** ▽
unspecified side

√6ᵗʰ **S04.89 Injury of** other cranial nerves
Injury of vagus [10th] nerve

√7ᵗʰ **S04.891 Injury of other cranial nerves,** right **side**

√7ᵗʰ **S04.892 Injury of other cranial nerves,** left **side**

√7ᵗʰ **S04.899 Injury of other cranial nerves,** ▽
unspecified side

√x7ᵗʰ **S04.9 Injury of unspecified cranial nerve** ▽

√4ᵗʰ **S05 Injury of eye and orbit**
Open wound of eye and orbit
EXCLUDES 2   *2nd cranial [optic] nerve injury (S04.0-)*
3rd cranial [oculomotor] nerve injury (S04.1-)
open wound of eyelid and periocular area (S01.1-)
orbital bone fracture (S02.1-, S02.3-, S02.8-)
superficial injury of eyelid (S00.1-S00.2)

The appropriate 7th character is to be added to each code from
category S05.
A   initial encounter
D   subsequent encounter
S   sequela

√5ᵗʰ **S05.0 Injury of conjunctiva and corneal abrasion** without foreign
body
EXCLUDES 1   *foreign body in conjunctival sac (T15.1)*
foreign body in cornea (T15.0)

√x7ᵗʰ **S05.00 Injury of conjunctiva and corneal abrasion** ▽
without foreign body, unspecified eye

√x7ᵗʰ **S05.01 Injury of conjunctiva and corneal abrasion without**
foreign body, right **eye**

√x7ᵗʰ **S05.02 Injury of conjunctiva and corneal abrasion without**
foreign body, left **eye**

Ⓝ Newborn   Ⓟ Pediatric   Ⓜ Maternity   Ⓐ Adult   **RIC** RIC Dx   **NCDx** Noncancer Dx   **PDx** Primary Dx   **CC** RIC CC Condition   ▶◀ Revised Text   ● New Code   ▲ Revised Code Title

862   ICD-10-CM 2016

✓5ᵗʰ **S05.1 Contusion** of eyeball and orbital tissues
Traumatic hyphema
EXCLUDES 2 *black eye NOS (S00.1)*
contusion of eyelid and periocular area (S00.1)

✓x7ᵗʰ **S05.10 Contusion of eyeball and orbital tissues, unspecified eye** ▽

✓x7ᵗʰ **S05.11 Contusion of eyeball and orbital tissues, right eye**

✓x7ᵗʰ **S05.12 Contusion of eyeball and orbital tissues, left eye**

✓5ᵗʰ **S05.2 Ocular laceration and rupture** with prolapse or loss of intraocular tissue

✓x7ᵗʰ **S05.20 Ocular laceration and rupture with prolapse or loss of intraocular tissue, unspecified eye** ▽

✓x7ᵗʰ **S05.21 Ocular laceration and rupture with prolapse or loss of intraocular tissue, right eye**

✓x7ᵗʰ **S05.22 Ocular laceration and rupture with prolapse or loss of intraocular tissue, left eye**

✓5ᵗʰ **S05.3 Ocular laceration** without prolapse or loss of intraocular tissue
Laceration of eye NOS

✓x7ᵗʰ **S05.30 Ocular laceration without prolapse or loss of intraocular tissue, unspecified eye** ▽

✓x7ᵗʰ **S05.31 Ocular laceration without prolapse or loss of intraocular tissue, right eye**

✓x7ᵗʰ **S05.32 Ocular laceration without prolapse or loss of intraocular tissue, left eye**

✓5ᵗʰ **S05.4 Penetrating wound** of orbit with or without foreign body
EXCLUDES 2 *retained (old) foreign body following penetrating wound in orbit (H05.5-)*

✓x7ᵗʰ **S05.40 Penetrating wound of orbit with or without foreign body, unspecified eye** ▽

✓x7ᵗʰ **S05.41 Penetrating wound of orbit with or without foreign body, right eye**

✓x7ᵗʰ **S05.42 Penetrating wound of orbit with or without foreign body, left eye**

✓5ᵗʰ **S05.5 Penetrating wound with foreign body** of eyeball
EXCLUDES 2 *retained (old) intraocular foreign body (H44.6-, H44.7)*

✓x7ᵗʰ **S05.50 Penetrating wound with foreign body of unspecified eyeball** ▽

✓x7ᵗʰ **S05.51 Penetrating wound with foreign body of right eyeball**

✓x7ᵗʰ **S05.52 Penetrating wound with foreign body of left eyeball**

✓5ᵗʰ **S05.6 Penetrating wound without foreign body** of eyeball
Ocular penetration NOS

✓x7ᵗʰ **S05.60 Penetrating wound without foreign body of unspecified eyeball** ▽

✓x7ᵗʰ **S05.61 Penetrating wound without foreign body of right eyeball**

✓x7ᵗʰ **S05.62 Penetrating wound without foreign body of left eyeball**

✓5ᵗʰ **S05.7 Avulsion of eye**
Traumatic enucleation

✓x7ᵗʰ **S05.70 Avulsion of unspecified eye** ▽

✓x7ᵗʰ **S05.71 Avulsion of right eye**

✓x7ᵗʰ **S05.72 Avulsion of left eye**

✓5ᵗʰ **S05.8 Other injuries of eye and orbit**
Lacrimal duct injury

✓6ᵗʰ **S05.8X Other injuries of eye and orbit**

✓7ᵗʰ **S05.8X1 Other injuries of right eye and orbit**

✓7ᵗʰ **S05.8X2 Other injuries of left eye and orbit**

✓7ᵗʰ **S05.8X9 Other injuries of unspecified eye and orbit** ▽

✓5ᵗʰ **S05.9 Unspecified injury of eye and orbit**
Injury of eye NOS

✓x7ᵗʰ **S05.90 Unspecified injury of unspecified eye and orbit** ▽

✓x7ᵗʰ **S05.91 Unspecified injury of right eye and orbit** ▽

✓x7ᵗʰ **S05.92 Unspecified injury of left eye and orbit** ▽

✓4ᵗʰ **S06 Intracranial injury**
Traumatic brain injury
Code also any associated:
open wound of head (S01.-)
skull fracture (S02.-)
EXCLUDES 1 *head injury NOS (S09.90)*

The appropriate 7th character is to be added to each code from category S06.
A   initial encounter
D   subsequent encounter
S   sequela

✓5ᵗʰ **S06.0 Concussion**
Commotio cerebri
EXCLUDES 1 *concussion with other intracranial injuries classified in category S06—code to specified intracranial injury*

✓6ᵗʰ **S06.0X Concussion**

✓7ᵗʰ **S06.0X0 Concussion** without loss of consciousness

✓7ᵗʰ **S06.0X1 Concussion with loss of consciousness of 30 minutes or less**

✓7ᵗʰ **S06.0X2 Concussion with loss of consciousness of 31 minutes to 59 minutes**

✓7ᵗʰ **S06.0X3 Concussion with loss of consciousness of 1 hour to 5 hours 59 minutes**

✓7ᵗʰ **S06.0X4 Concussion with loss of consciousness of 6 hours to 24 hours**

✓7ᵗʰ **S06.0X5 Concussion with loss of consciousness greater than 24 hours with return to pre-existing conscious level**

4,9 ✓7ᵗʰ **S06.0X6 Concussion with loss of consciousness greater than 24 hours without return to pre-existing conscious level with patient surviving** NC Dx

✓7ᵗʰ **S06.0X7 Concussion with loss of consciousness of any duration with death due to brain injury prior to regaining consciousness**

✓7ᵗʰ **S06.0X8 Concussion with loss of consciousness of any duration with death due to other cause prior to regaining consciousness**

✓7ᵗʰ **S06.0X9 Concussion with loss of consciousness of unspecified duration** ▽
Concussion NOS

✓5ᵗʰ **S06.1 Traumatic cerebral edema**
Diffuse traumatic cerebral edema
Focal traumatic cerebral edema

✓6ᵗʰ **S06.1X Traumatic cerebral edema**

✓7ᵗʰ **S06.1X0 Traumatic cerebral edema without loss of consciousness**

✓7ᵗʰ **S06.1X1 Traumatic cerebral edema with loss of consciousness of 30 minutes or less**

✓7ᵗʰ **S06.1X2 Traumatic cerebral edema with loss of consciousness of 31 minutes to 59 minutes**

✓7ᵗʰ **S06.1X3 Traumatic cerebral edema with loss of consciousness of 1 hour to 5 hours 59 minutes**

✓7ᵗʰ **S06.1X4 Traumatic cerebral edema with loss of consciousness of 6 hours to 24 hours**

✓7ᵗʰ **S06.1X5 Traumatic cerebral edema with loss of consciousness greater than 24 hours with return to pre-existing conscious level**

4,9 ✓7ᵗʰ **S06.1X6 Traumatic cerebral edema with loss of consciousness greater than 24 hours without return to pre-existing conscious level with patient surviving** NC Dx

✓7ᵗʰ **S06.1X7 Traumatic cerebral edema with loss of consciousness of any duration with death due to brain injury prior to regaining consciousness**

✓7ᵗʰ **S06.1X8 Traumatic cerebral edema with loss of consciousness of any duration with death due to other cause prior to regaining consciousness**

✓7ᵗʰ **S06.1X9 Traumatic cerebral edema with loss of consciousness of unspecified duration** ▽
Traumatic cerebral edema NOS

---

4 Special Care High = With 7th character indicating a subsequent encounter

9 Hospice Noncancer Diagnosis only when reported using an appropriate 7th character indicating a subsequent encounter or sequela

---

☑ Add'l Character Required ✓x7ᵗʰ Placeholder Alert RUG IV Special Care High Dx RUG IV Clinically Complex Dx RUG IV Special Care Low Dx Manifestation Code Other Specified Code ▽Unspecified Code

✓5ᵗʰ **S06.2** **Diffuse traumatic brain injury**
Diffuse axonal brain injury
EXCLUDES 1 *traumatic diffuse cerebral edema (S06.1X-)*

     ✓6ᵗʰ **S06.2X** Diffuse traumatic brain injury

       ✓7ᵗʰ **S06.2X0** **Diffuse traumatic brain injury** without loss of consciousness

       ✓7ᵗʰ **S06.2X1** **Diffuse traumatic brain injury with loss of consciousness of** 30 minutes or less

       ✓7ᵗʰ **S06.2X2** **Diffuse traumatic brain injury with loss of consciousness of** 31 minutes to 59 minutes

       ✓7ᵗʰ **S06.2X3** **Diffuse traumatic brain injury with loss of consciousness of** 1 hour to 5 hours 59 minutes

       ✓7ᵗʰ **S06.2X4** **Diffuse traumatic brain injury with loss of consciousness of** 6 hours to 24 hours

       ✓7ᵗʰ **S06.2X5** **Diffuse traumatic brain injury with loss of consciousness** greater than 24 hours with return to pre-existing conscious levels

       4,9 ✓7ᵗʰ **S06.2X6** **Diffuse traumatic brain injury with loss of consciousness** greater than 24 hours without return to pre-existing conscious level with patient surviving   **NC Dx**

       ✓7ᵗʰ **S06.2X7** **Diffuse traumatic brain injury with loss of consciousness of** any duration with death due to brain injury prior to regaining consciousness

       ✓7ᵗʰ **S06.2X8** **Diffuse traumatic brain injury with loss of consciousness of** any duration with death due to **other** cause prior to regaining consciousness

       ✓7ᵗʰ **S06.2X9** **Diffuse traumatic brain injury with loss of consciousness of unspecified duration** ▽
Diffuse traumatic brain injury NOS

✓5ᵗʰ **S06.3** Focal traumatic brain injury
EXCLUDES 1 *any condition classifiable to S06.4-S06.6 focal cerebral edema (S06.1)*

     ✓6ᵗʰ **S06.30** Unspecified focal traumatic brain injury

       ✓7ᵗʰ **S06.300** **Unspecified focal traumatic brain injury** ▽ without loss of consciousness

       ✓7ᵗʰ **S06.301** **Unspecified focal traumatic brain injury** ▽ with loss of consciousness of 30 minutes or less

       ✓7ᵗʰ **S06.302** **Unspecified focal traumatic brain injury** ▽ with loss of consciousness of 31 minutes to 59 minutes

       ✓7ᵗʰ **S06.303** **Unspecified focal traumatic brain injury** ▽ with loss of consciousness of 1 hour to 5 hours 59 minutes

       ✓7ᵗʰ **S06.304** **Unspecified focal traumatic brain injury** ▽ with loss of consciousness of 6 hours to 24 hours

       ✓7ᵗʰ **S06.305** **Unspecified focal traumatic brain injury** ▽ with loss of consciousness greater than 24 hours with return to pre-existing conscious level

       4,9 ✓7ᵗʰ **S06.306** **Unspecified focal traumatic brain injury with loss of consciousness** greater than 24 hours without return to pre-existing conscious level with patient surviving   **NC Dx** ▽

       ✓7ᵗʰ **S06.307** **Unspecified focal traumatic brain injury** ▽ with loss of consciousness of any duration with death due to brain injury prior to regaining consciousness

       ✓7ᵗʰ **S06.308** **Unspecified focal traumatic brain injury** ▽ with loss of consciousness of any duration with death due to **other** cause prior to regaining consciousness

       ✓7ᵗʰ **S06.309** **Unspecified focal traumatic brain injury** ▽ with loss of consciousness of unspecified duration
Unspecified focal traumatic brain injury NOS

✓6ᵗʰ **S06.31** Contusion and laceration of right cerebrum

     ✓7ᵗʰ **S06.310** **Contusion and laceration of right cerebrum** without loss of consciousness

     ✓7ᵗʰ **S06.311** **Contusion and laceration of right cerebrum with loss of consciousness of** 30 minutes or less

     ✓7ᵗʰ **S06.312** **Contusion and laceration of right cerebrum with loss of consciousness of** 31 minutes to 59 minutes

     ✓7ᵗʰ **S06.313** **Contusion and laceration of right cerebrum with loss of consciousness of** 1 hour to 5 hours 59 minutes

     ✓7ᵗʰ **S06.314** **Contusion and laceration of right cerebrum with loss of consciousness of** 6 hours to 24 hours

     ✓7ᵗʰ **S06.315** **Contusion and laceration of right cerebrum with loss of consciousness** greater than 24 hours with return to pre-existing conscious level

     4,9 ✓7ᵗʰ **S06.316** **Contusion and laceration of right cerebrum with loss of consciousness** greater than 24 hours without return to pre-existing conscious level with patient surviving   **NC Dx**

     ✓7ᵗʰ **S06.317** **Contusion and laceration of right cerebrum with loss of consciousness of** any duration with death due to brain injury prior to regaining consciousness

     ✓7ᵗʰ **S06.318** **Contusion and laceration of right cerebrum with loss of consciousness of** any duration with death due to **other** cause prior to regaining consciousness

     ✓7ᵗʰ **S06.319** **Contusion and laceration of right cerebrum with loss of consciousness of unspecified duration** ▽
Contusion and laceration of right cerebrum NOS

✓6ᵗʰ **S06.32** Contusion and laceration of left cerebrum

     ✓7ᵗʰ **S06.320** **Contusion and laceration of left cerebrum** without loss of consciousness

     ✓7ᵗʰ **S06.321** **Contusion and laceration of left cerebrum with loss of consciousness of** 30 minutes or less

     ✓7ᵗʰ **S06.322** **Contusion and laceration of left cerebrum with loss of consciousness of** 31 minutes to 59 minutes

     ✓7ᵗʰ **S06.323** **Contusion and laceration of left cerebrum with loss of consciousness of** 1 hour to 5 hours 59 minutes

     ✓7ᵗʰ **S06.324** **Contusion and laceration of left cerebrum with loss of consciousness of** 6 hours to 24 hours

     ✓7ᵗʰ **S06.325** **Contusion and laceration of left cerebrum with loss of consciousness** greater than 24 hours with return to pre-existing conscious level

     4,9 ✓7ᵗʰ **S06.326** **Contusion and laceration of left cerebrum with loss of consciousness** greater than 24 hours without return to pre-existing conscious level with patient surviving   **NC Dx**

     ✓7ᵗʰ **S06.327** **Contusion and laceration of left cerebrum with loss of consciousness of** any duration with death due to brain injury prior to regaining consciousness

     ✓7ᵗʰ **S06.328** **Contusion and laceration of left cerebrum with loss of consciousness of** any duration with death due to **other** cause prior to regaining consciousness

     ✓7ᵗʰ **S06.329** **Contusion and laceration of left cerebrum with loss of consciousness of unspecified duration** ▽
Contusion and laceration of left cerebrum NOS

---

⁴ Special Care High = With 7th character indicating a subsequent encounter

⁹ Hospice Noncancer Diagnosis only when reported using an appropriate 7th character indicating a subsequent encounter or sequela

N Newborn   P Pediatric   M Maternity   A Adult   **RIC** RIC Dx   **NC Dx** Noncancer Dx   **PDx** Primary Dx   **CC** RIC CC Condition   ▶◀ Revised Text   ● New Code   ▲ Revised Code Title

✓6ᵗʰ **S06.33 Contusion and laceration of** cerebrum, unspecified

    ✓7ᵗʰ **S06.330 Contusion and laceration of cerebrum,** ▽
    unspecified, without loss of consciousness

    ✓7ᵗʰ **S06.331 Contusion and laceration of cerebrum,** ▽
    unspecified, with loss of consciousness of 30 minutes or less

    ✓7ᵗʰ **S06.332 Contusion and laceration of cerebrum,** ▽
    unspecified, with loss of consciousness of 31 minutes to 59 minutes

    ✓7ᵗʰ **S06.333 Contusion and laceration of cerebrum,** ▽
    unspecified, with loss of consciousness of 1 hour to 5 hours 59 minutes

    ✓7ᵗʰ **S06.334 Contusion and laceration of cerebrum,** ▽
    unspecified, with loss of consciousness of 6 hours to 24 hours

    ✓7ᵗʰ **S06.335 Contusion and laceration of cerebrum,** ▽
    unspecified, with loss of consciousness greater than 24 hours with return to pre-existing conscious level

    4,9 ✓7ᵗʰ **S06.336 Contusion and laceration of** NC Dx ▽
    cerebrum, unspecified, with loss of consciousness greater than 24 hours without return to pre-existing conscious level with patient surviving

    ✓7ᵗʰ **S06.337 Contusion and laceration of cerebrum,** ▽
    unspecified, with loss of consciousness of any duration with death due to brain injury prior to regaining consciousness

    ✓7ᵗʰ **S06.338 Contusion and laceration of cerebrum,** ▽
    unspecified, with loss of consciousness of any duration with death due to **other cause prior to regaining consciousness**

    ✓7ᵗʰ **S06.339 Contusion and laceration of cerebrum,** ▽
    unspecified, with loss of consciousness of unspecified duration
        Contusion and laceration of cerebrum NOS

✓6ᵗʰ **S06.34 Traumatic hemorrhage of** right cerebrum
    Traumatic intracerebral hemorrhage and hematoma of right cerebrum

    ✓7ᵗʰ **S06.340 Traumatic hemorrhage of right cerebrum** without loss of consciousness

    ✓7ᵗʰ **S06.341 Traumatic hemorrhage of right cerebrum with loss of consciousness of** 30 minutes or less

    ✓7ᵗʰ **S06.342 Traumatic hemorrhage of right cerebrum with loss of consciousness of** 31 minutes to 59 minutes

    ✓7ᵗʰ **S06.343 Traumatic hemorrhage of right cerebrum with loss of consciousness of** 1 hours to 5 hours 59 minutes

    ✓7ᵗʰ **S06.344 Traumatic hemorrhage of right cerebrum with loss of consciousness of** 6 hours to 24 hours

    ✓7ᵗʰ **S06.345 Traumatic hemorrhage of right cerebrum with loss of consciousness** greater than 24 hours with return to pre-existing conscious level

    4,9 ✓7ᵗʰ **S06.346 Traumatic hemorrhage of right** NC Dx
    cerebrum with loss of consciousness greater than 24 hours without return to pre-existing conscious level with patient surviving

    ✓7ᵗʰ **S06.347 Traumatic hemorrhage of right cerebrum with loss of consciousness of** any duration with death due to brain injury prior to regaining consciousness

    ✓7ᵗʰ **S06.348 Traumatic hemorrhage of right cerebrum with loss of consciousness of** any duration with death due to **other** cause prior to regaining consciousness

    ✓7ᵗʰ **S06.349 Traumatic hemorrhage of right** ▽
    cerebrum with loss of consciousness of unspecified duration
        Traumatic hemorrhage of right cerebrum NOS

✓6ᵗʰ **S06.35 Traumatic hemorrhage of** left cerebrum
    Traumatic intracerebral hemorrhage and hematoma of left cerebrum

    ✓7ᵗʰ **S06.350 Traumatic hemorrhage of left cerebrum** without loss of consciousness

    ✓7ᵗʰ **S06.351 Traumatic hemorrhage of left cerebrum with loss of consciousness of** 30 minutes or less

    ✓7ᵗʰ **S06.352 Traumatic hemorrhage of left cerebrum with loss of consciousness of** 31 minutes to 59 minutes

    ✓7ᵗʰ **S06.353 Traumatic hemorrhage of left cerebrum with loss of consciousness of** 1 hours to 5 hours 59 minutes

    ✓7ᵗʰ **S06.354 Traumatic hemorrhage of left cerebrum with loss of consciousness of** 6 hours to 24 hours

    ✓7ᵗʰ **S06.355 Traumatic hemorrhage of left cerebrum with loss of consciousness** greater than 24 hours with return to pre-existing conscious level

    4,9 ✓7ᵗʰ **S06.356 Traumatic hemorrhage of left** NC Dx
    cerebrum with loss of consciousness greater than 24 hours without return to pre-existing conscious level with patient surviving

    ✓7ᵗʰ **S06.357 Traumatic hemorrhage of left cerebrum with loss of consciousness of** any duration with death due to brain injury prior to regaining consciousness

    ✓7ᵗʰ **S06.358 Traumatic hemorrhage of left cerebrum with loss of consciousness of** any duration with death due to **other** cause prior to regaining consciousness

    ✓7ᵗʰ **S06.359 Traumatic hemorrhage of left cerebrum** ▽
    with loss of consciousness of unspecified duration
        Traumatic hemorrhage of left cerebrum NOS

✓6ᵗʰ **S06.36 Traumatic hemorrhage of** cerebrum, unspecified
    Traumatic intracerebral hemorrhage and hematoma, unspecified

    ✓7ᵗʰ **S06.360 Traumatic hemorrhage of cerebrum,** ▽
    unspecified, without loss of consciousness

    ✓7ᵗʰ **S06.361 Traumatic hemorrhage of cerebrum,** ▽
    unspecified, with loss of consciousness of 30 minutes or less

    ✓7ᵗʰ **S06.362 Traumatic hemorrhage of cerebrum,** ▽
    unspecified, with loss of consciousness of 31 minutes to 59 minutes

    ✓7ᵗʰ **S06.363 Traumatic hemorrhage of cerebrum,** ▽
    unspecified, with loss of consciousness of 1 hours to 5 hours 59 minutes

    ✓7ᵗʰ **S06.364 Traumatic hemorrhage of cerebrum,** ▽
    unspecified, with loss of consciousness of 6 hours to 24 hours

    ✓7ᵗʰ **S06.365 Traumatic hemorrhage of cerebrum,** ▽
    unspecified, with loss of consciousness greater than 24 hours with return to pre-existing conscious level

    4,9 ✓7ᵗʰ **S06.366 Traumatic hemorrhage of** NC Dx ▽
    cerebrum, unspecified, with loss of consciousness greater than 24 hours without return to pre-existing conscious level with patient surviving

    ✓7ᵗʰ **S06.367 Traumatic hemorrhage of cerebrum,** ▽
    unspecified, with loss of consciousness of any duration with death due to brain injury prior to regaining consciousness

    ✓7ᵗʰ **S06.368 Traumatic hemorrhage of cerebrum,** ▽
    unspecified, with loss of consciousness of any duration with death due to **other** cause prior to regaining consciousness

---

⁴ Special Care High = With 7th character indicating a subsequent encounter

⁹ Hospice Noncancer Diagnosis only when reported using an appropriate 7th character indicating a subsequent encounter or sequela

---

☑ Add'l Character Required   ✓ₓ7ᵗʰ Placeholder Alert   RUG IV Special Care High Dx   RUG IV Clinically Complex Dx   RUG IV Special Care Low Dx   Manifestation Code   Other Specified Code   ▽ Unspecified Code

ICD-10-CM 2016   **865**

Chapter 19. Injury, Poisoning and Certain Other Consequences of External Causes

✓6th **S06.37** **Contusion, laceration, and hemorrhage of cerebellum**

    ✓7th **S06.370** Contusion, laceration, and hemorrhage of cerebellum without loss of consciousness

    ✓7th **S06.371** Contusion, laceration, and hemorrhage of cerebellum with loss of consciousness of 30 minutes or less

    ✓7th **S06.372** Contusion, laceration, and hemorrhage of cerebellum with loss of consciousness of 31 minutes to 59 minutes

    ✓7th **S06.373** Contusion, laceration, and hemorrhage of cerebellum with loss of consciousness of 1 hour to 5 hours 59 minutes

    ✓7th **S06.374** Contusion, laceration, and hemorrhage of cerebellum with loss of consciousness of 6 hours to 24 hours

    ✓7th **S06.375** Contusion, laceration, and hemorrhage of cerebellum with loss of consciousness greater than 24 hours with return to pre-existing conscious level

    4,9 ✓7th **S06.376** **Contusion, laceration, and hemorrhage of cerebellum with loss of consciousness greater than 24 hours without return to pre-existing conscious level with patient surviving** NC Dx

    ✓7th **S06.377** Contusion, laceration, and hemorrhage of cerebellum with loss of consciousness of any duration with death due to brain injury prior to regaining consciousness

    ✓7th **S06.378** **Contusion, laceration, and hemorrhage of cerebellum with loss of consciousness of any duration with death due to other cause prior to regaining consciousness**

    ✓7th **S06.379** Contusion, laceration, and hemorrhage of cerebellum with loss of consciousness of unspecified duration ▽
       Contusion, laceration, and hemorrhage of cerebellum NOS

✓6th **S06.38** **Contusion, laceration, and hemorrhage of brainstem**

    ✓7th **S06.380** Contusion, laceration, and hemorrhage of brainstem without loss of consciousness

    ✓7th **S06.381** Contusion, laceration, and hemorrhage of brainstem with loss of consciousness of 30 minutes or less

    ✓7th **S06.382** Contusion, laceration, and hemorrhage of brainstem with loss of consciousness of 31 minutes to 59 minutes

    ✓7th **S06.383** Contusion, laceration, and hemorrhage of brainstem with loss of consciousness of 1 hour to 5 hours 59 minutes

    ✓7th **S06.384** Contusion, laceration, and hemorrhage of brainstem with loss of consciousness of 6 hours to 24 hours

    ✓7th **S06.385** Contusion, laceration, and hemorrhage of brainstem with loss of consciousness greater than 24 hours with return to pre-existing conscious level

    4,9 ✓7th **S06.386** **Contusion, laceration, and hemorrhage of brainstem with loss of consciousness greater than 24 hours without return to pre-existing conscious level with patient surviving** NC Dx

    ✓7th **S06.387** Contusion, laceration, and hemorrhage of brainstem with loss of consciousness of any duration with death due to brain injury prior to regaining consciousness

    ✓7th **S06.388** **Contusion, laceration, and hemorrhage of brainstem with loss of consciousness of any duration with death due to other cause prior to regaining consciousness**

    ✓7th **S06.389** Contusion, laceration, and hemorrhage of brainstem with loss of consciousness of unspecified duration ▽
       Contusion, laceration, and hemorrhage of brainstem NOS

✓5th **S06.4** **Epidural hemorrhage**
    Extradural hemorrhage NOS
    Extradural hemorrhage (traumatic)

    ✓6th **S06.4X** **Epidural hemorrhage**

      ✓7th **S06.4X0** Epidural hemorrhage without loss of consciousness

      ✓7th **S06.4X1** Epidural hemorrhage with loss of consciousness of 30 minutes or less

      ✓7th **S06.4X2** Epidural hemorrhage with loss of consciousness of 31 minutes to 59 minutes

      ✓7th **S06.4X3** Epidural hemorrhage with loss of consciousness of 1 hour to 5 hours 59 minutes

      ✓7th **S06.4X4** Epidural hemorrhage with loss of consciousness of 6 hours to 24 hours

      ✓7th **S06.4X5** Epidural hemorrhage with loss of consciousness greater than 24 hours with return to pre-existing conscious level

      4,9 ✓7th **S06.4X6** **Epidural hemorrhage with loss of consciousness greater than 24 hours without return to pre-existing conscious level with patient surviving** NC Dx

      ✓7th **S06.4X7** Epidural hemorrhage with loss of consciousness of any duration with death due to brain injury prior to regaining consciousness

      ✓7th **S06.4X8** Epidural hemorrhage with loss of consciousness of any duration with death due to other causes prior to regaining consciousness

      ✓7th **S06.4X9** Epidural hemorrhage with loss of consciousness of unspecified duration ▽
         Epidural hemorrhage NOS

✓5th **S06.5** **Traumatic subdural hemorrhage**

    ✓6th **S06.5X** **Traumatic subdural hemorrhage**

      ✓7th **S06.5X0** Traumatic subdural hemorrhage without loss of consciousness

      ✓7th **S06.5X1** Traumatic subdural hemorrhage with loss of consciousness of 30 minutes or less

      ✓7th **S06.5X2** Traumatic subdural hemorrhage with loss of consciousness of 31 minutes to 59 minutes

      ✓7th **S06.5X3** Traumatic subdural hemorrhage with loss of consciousness of 1 hour to 5 hours 59 minutes

      ✓7th **S06.5X4** Traumatic subdural hemorrhage with loss of consciousness of 6 hours to 24 hours

      ✓7th **S06.5X5** Traumatic subdural hemorrhage with loss of consciousness greater than 24 hours with return to pre-existing conscious level

      4,9 ✓7th **S06.5X6** **Traumatic subdural hemorrhage with loss of consciousness greater than 24 hours without return to pre-existing conscious level with patient surviving** NC Dx

      ✓7th **S06.5X7** Traumatic subdural hemorrhage with loss of consciousness of any duration with death due to brain injury before regaining consciousness

      ✓7th **S06.5X8** **Traumatic subdural hemorrhage with loss of consciousness of any duration with death due to other cause before regaining consciousness**

      ✓7th **S06.5X9** Traumatic subdural hemorrhage with loss of consciousness of unspecified duration ▽
         Traumatic subdural hemorrhage NOS

✓5th **S06.6** **Traumatic subarachnoid hemorrhage**

    ✓6th **S06.6X** **Traumatic subarachnoid hemorrhage**

      ✓7th **S06.6X0** Traumatic subarachnoid hemorrhage without loss of consciousness

      ✓7th **S06.6X1** Traumatic subarachnoid hemorrhage with loss of consciousness of 30 minutes or less

      ✓7th **S06.6X2** Traumatic subarachnoid hemorrhage with loss of consciousness of 31 minutes to 59 minutes

---

4 Special Care High = With 7th character indicating a subsequent encounter

9 Hospice Noncancer Diagnosis only when reported using an appropriate 7th character indicating a subsequent encounter or sequela

N Newborn   P Pediatric   M Maternity   A Adult   RIC RIC Dx   NC Dx Noncancer Dx   PDx Primary Dx   CC RIC CC Condition   ▶◀ Revised Text   ● New Code   ▲ Revised Code Title

866   ICD-10-CM 2016

✓7ᵗʰ **S06.6X3 Traumatic subarachnoid hemorrhage with loss of consciousness of** 1 hour to 5 hours 59 minutes

✓7ᵗʰ **S06.6X4 Traumatic subarachnoid hemorrhage with loss of consciousness of** 6 hours to 24 hours

✓7ᵗʰ **S06.6X5 Traumatic subarachnoid hemorrhage with loss of consciousness** greater than 24 hours with return to pre-existing conscious level

4,9 ✓7ᵗʰ **S06.6X6 Traumatic subarachnoid hemorrhage** NC Dx **with loss of consciousness** greater than 24 hours without return to pre-existing conscious level with patient surviving

✓7ᵗʰ **S06.6X7 Traumatic subarachnoid hemorrhage with loss of consciousness of** any duration with death due to brain injury prior to regaining consciousness

✓7ᵗʰ **S06.6X8 Traumatic subarachnoid hemorrhage with loss of consciousness of** any duration with death due to **other** cause prior to regaining consciousness

✓7ᵗʰ **S06.6X9 Traumatic subarachnoid hemorrhage** ▽ **with loss of consciousness of unspecified duration**
Traumatic subarachnoid hemorrhage NOS

✓5ᵗʰ **S06.8 Other specified intracranial injuries**

✓6ᵗʰ **S06.81 Injury of** right internal carotid artery, **intracranial portion, not elsewhere classified**

✓7ᵗʰ **S06.810 Injury of right internal carotid artery, intracranial portion, not elsewhere classified** without loss of consciousness

✓7ᵗʰ **S06.811 Injury of right internal carotid artery, intracranial portion, not elsewhere classified with loss of consciousness of** 30 minutes or less

✓7ᵗʰ **S06.812 Injury of right internal carotid artery, intracranial portion, not elsewhere classified with loss of consciousness of** 31 minutes to 59 minutes

✓7ᵗʰ **S06.813 Injury of right internal carotid artery, intracranial portion, not elsewhere classified with loss of consciousness of** 1 hour to 5 hours 59 minutes

✓7ᵗʰ **S06.814 Injury of right internal carotid artery, intracranial portion, not elsewhere classified with loss of consciousness of** 6 hours to 24 hours

✓7ᵗʰ **S06.815 Injury of right internal carotid artery, intracranial portion, not elsewhere classified with loss of consciousness** greater than 24 hours with return to pre-existing conscious level

4,9 ✓7ᵗʰ **S06.816 Injury of right internal carotid artery,** NC Dx **intracranial portion, not elsewhere classified with loss of consciousness** greater than 24 hours without return to pre-existing conscious level with patient surviving

✓7ᵗʰ **S06.817 Injury of right internal carotid artery, intracranial portion, not elsewhere classified with loss of consciousness of** any duration with death due to brain injury prior to regaining consciousness

✓7ᵗʰ **S06.818 Injury of right internal carotid artery, intracranial portion, not elsewhere classified with loss of consciousness of** any duration with death due to **other** cause prior to regaining consciousness

✓7ᵗʰ **S06.819 Injury of right internal carotid artery,** ▽ **intracranial portion, not elsewhere classified with loss of consciousness of unspecified duration**
Injury of right internal carotid artery, intracranial portion, not elsewhere classified NOS

✓6ᵗʰ **S06.82 Injury of** left internal carotid artery, **intracranial portion, not elsewhere classified**

✓7ᵗʰ **S06.820 Injury of left internal carotid artery, intracranial portion, not elsewhere classified** without loss of consciousness
30

✓7ᵗʰ **S06.821 Injury of left internal carotid artery, intracranial portion, not elsewhere classified with loss of consciousness of** minutes or less
31

✓7ᵗʰ **S06.822 Injury of left internal carotid artery, intracranial portion, not elsewhere classified with loss of consciousness of** minutes to 59 minutes
1

✓7ᵗʰ **S06.823 Injury of left internal carotid artery, intracranial portion, not elsewhere classified with loss of consciousness of** hour to 5 hours 59 minutes
6

✓7ᵗʰ **S06.824 Injury of left internal carotid artery, intracranial portion, not elsewhere classified with loss of consciousness of** hours to 24 hours

✓7ᵗʰ **S06.825 Injury of left internal carotid artery, intracranial portion, not elsewhere classified with loss of consciousness** NC Dx greater than 24 hours with return to pre-existing conscious level

4,9 ✓7ᵗʰ **S06.826 Injury of left internal carotid artery, intracranial portion, not elsewhere classified with loss of consciousness** greater than 24 hours without return to pre-existing conscious level with patient surviving
any

✓7ᵗʰ **S06.827 Injury of left internal carotid artery, intracranial portion, not elsewhere classified with loss of consciousness of** duration with death due to brain injury prior to regaining consciousness
any

✓7ᵗʰ **S06.828 Injury of left internal carotid artery, intracranial portion, not elsewhere classified with loss of consciousness of** duration with death due to **other** cause ▽ prior to regaining consciousness

✓7ᵗʰ **S06.829 Injury of left internal carotid artery, intracranial portion, not elsewhere classified with loss of consciousness of unspecified duration**
Injury of left internal carotid artery, intracranial portion, not elsewhere classified NOS

✓6ᵗʰ **S06.89 Other** specified intracranial injury

✓7ᵗʰ **S06.890 Other specified intracranial injury** without loss of consciousness

✓7ᵗʰ **S06.891 Other specified intracranial injury with loss of consciousness of** 30 minutes or less

✓7ᵗʰ **S06.892 Other specified intracranial injury with loss of consciousness of** 31 minutes to 59 minutes

✓7ᵗʰ **S06.893 Other specified intracranial injury with loss of consciousness of** 1 hour to 5 hours 59 minutes

✓7ᵗʰ **S06.894 Other specified intracranial injury with loss of consciousness of** 6 hours to 24 hours

✓7ᵗʰ **S06.895 Other specified intracranial injury with loss of consciousness** greater than 24 NC Dx hours with return to pre-existing conscious level

4,9 ✓7ᵗʰ **S06.896 Other specified intracranial injury with loss of consciousness** greater than 24 hours without return to pre-existing conscious level with patient surviving

✓7ᵗʰ **S06.897 Other specified intracranial injury with loss of consciousness of** any duration with death due to brain injury prior to regaining consciousness

✓7ᵗʰ **S06.898 Other specified intracranial injury with loss of consciousness of** any duration with death due to **other** cause prior to regaining consciousness

---

⁴ Special Care High = With 7th character indicating a subsequent encounter

⁹ Hospice Noncancer Diagnosis only when reported using an appropriate 7th character indicating a subsequent encounter or sequela

☑ Add'l Character Required   ✓x7ᵗʰ Placeholder Alert   RUG IV Special Care High Dx   RUG IV Clinically Complex Dx   RUG IV Special Care Low Dx   Manifestation Code   Other Specified Code   ▽ Unspecified Code

✓7ᵗʰ **S06.899** **Other specified intracranial injury with loss of consciousness of unspecified duration** ▽

✓5ᵗʰ **S06.9** **Unspecified intracranial injury**
Brain injury NOS
Head injury NOS with loss of consciousness
EXCLUDES 1 head injury NOS (S09.90)

✓6ᵗʰ **S06.9X** **Unspecified intracranial injury**

✓7ᵗʰ **S06.9X0** **Unspecified intracranial injury** without ▽ loss of consciousness

✓7ᵗʰ **S06.9X1** **Unspecified intracranial injury with loss of consciousness of** 30 minutes or less ▽

✓7ᵗʰ **S06.9X2** **Unspecified intracranial injury with loss of consciousness of** 31 minutes to 59 minutes ▽

✓7ᵗʰ **S06.9X3** **Unspecified intracranial injury with loss of consciousness of** 1 hour to 5 hours 59 minutes ▽

✓7ᵗʰ **S06.9X4** **Unspecified intracranial injury with loss of consciousness of** 6 hours to 24 hours ▽

✓7ᵗʰ **S06.9X5** **Unspecified intracranial injury with loss of consciousness** greater than 24 hours with return to pre-existing conscious level ▽

4,9 ✓7ᵗʰ **S06.9X6** **Unspecified intracranial injury with** NCDx ▽ **loss of consciousness** greater than 24 hours without return to pre-existing conscious level with patient surviving

✓7ᵗʰ **S06.9X7** **Unspecified intracranial injury with loss of consciousness of** any duration with death due to brain injury prior to regaining consciousness ▽

✓7ᵗʰ **S06.9X8** **Unspecified intracranial injury with loss of consciousness of** any duration with death due to other cause prior to regaining consciousness ▽

✓7ᵗʰ **S06.9X9** **Unspecified intracranial injury with loss of consciousness of unspecified duration** ▽

✓4ᵗʰ **S07** **Crushing injury of head**
Use additional code for all associated injuries, such as:
intracranial injuries (S06.-)
skull fractures (S02.-)

The appropriate 7th character is to be added to each code from category S07.
A   initial encounter
D   subsequent encounter
S   sequela

✓x7ᵗʰ **S07.0** **Crushing injury of** face

✓x7ᵗʰ **S07.1** **Crushing injury of** skull

✓x7ᵗʰ **S07.8** **Crushing injury of other parts of head**

✓x7ᵗʰ **S07.9** **Crushing injury of** head, part unspecified ▽

✓4ᵗʰ **S08** **Avulsion and traumatic amputation of part of head**
NOTE An amputation not identified as partial or complete should be coded to complete

The appropriate 7th character is to be added to each code from category S08.
A   initial encounter
D   subsequent encounter
S   sequela

✓x7ᵗʰ **S08.0** **Avulsion of** scalp

✓5ᵗʰ **S08.1** **Traumatic amputation of** ear

✓6ᵗʰ **S08.11** Complete **traumatic amputation of** ear

✓7ᵗʰ **S08.111** **Complete traumatic amputation of** right ear

✓7ᵗʰ **S08.112** **Complete traumatic amputation of** left ear

✓7ᵗʰ **S08.119** **Complete traumatic amputation of unspecified ear** ▽

✓6ᵗʰ **S08.12** Partial **traumatic amputation of** ear

✓7ᵗʰ **S08.121** **Partial traumatic amputation of** right ear

✓7ᵗʰ **S08.122** **Partial traumatic amputation of** left ear

---

✓7ᵗʰ **S08.129** **Partial traumatic amputation of unspecified ear** ▽

✓5ᵗʰ **S08.8** **Traumatic amputation of** other parts of head

✓6ᵗʰ **S08.81** **Traumatic amputation of** nose

✓7ᵗʰ **S08.811** Complete **traumatic amputation of nose**

✓7ᵗʰ **S08.812** Partial **traumatic amputation of nose**

✓x7ᵗʰ **S08.89** **Traumatic amputation of other parts of head**

✓4ᵗʰ **S09** **Other and unspecified injuries of head**

The appropriate 7th character is to be added to each code from category S09.
A   initial encounter
D   subsequent encounter
S   sequela

✓x7ᵗʰ **S09.0** **Injury of** blood vessels **of head, not elsewhere classified**
EXCLUDES 1 injury of cerebral blood vessels (S06.-)
injury of precerebral blood vessels (S15.-)

✓5ᵗʰ **S09.1** **Injury of** muscle and tendon **of head**
Code also any associated open wound (S01.-)
EXCLUDES 2 sprain to joints and ligament of head (S03.9)

✓x7ᵗʰ **S09.10** **Unspecified injury of muscle and tendon of head** ▽
Injury of muscle and tendon of head NOS

✓x7ᵗʰ **S09.11** Strain **of muscle and tendon of head**

✓x7ᵗʰ **S09.12** Laceration **of muscle and tendon of head**

✓x7ᵗʰ **S09.19** **Other specified injury of muscle and tendon of head**

✓5ᵗʰ **S09.2** **Traumatic rupture of** ear drum
EXCLUDES 1 traumatic rupture of ear drum due to blast injury (S09.31-)

✓x7ᵗʰ **S09.20** **Traumatic rupture of unspecified ear drum** ▽

✓x7ᵗʰ **S09.21** **Traumatic rupture of** right ear drum

✓x7ᵗʰ **S09.22** **Traumatic rupture of** left ear drum

✓5ᵗʰ **S09.3** **Other specified and unspecified injury of middle and inner ear**
EXCLUDES 1 injury to ear NOS (S09.91-)
EXCLUDES 2 injury to external ear (S00.4-, S01.3-, S08.1-)

✓6ᵗʰ **S09.30** **Unspecified injury of** middle and inner ear

✓7ᵗʰ **S09.301** **Unspecified injury of** right middle and inner ear ▽

✓7ᵗʰ **S09.302** **Unspecified injury of** left middle and inner ear ▽

✓7ᵗʰ **S09.309** **Unspecified injury of unspecified middle and inner ear** ▽

✓6ᵗʰ **S09.31** **Primary** blast injury **of ear**
Blast injury of ear NOS

✓7ᵗʰ **S09.311** **Primary blast injury of** right ear

✓7ᵗʰ **S09.312** **Primary blast injury of** left ear

✓7ᵗʰ **S09.313** **Primary blast injury of ear,** bilateral

✓7ᵗʰ **S09.319** **Primary blast injury of unspecified ear** ▽

✓6ᵗʰ **S09.39** Other **specified injury of middle and inner ear**
Secondary blast injury to ear

✓7ᵗʰ **S09.391** **Other specified injury of** right middle and inner ear

✓7ᵗʰ **S09.392** **Other specified injury of** left middle and inner ear

✓7ᵗʰ **S09.399** **Other specified injury of unspecified middle and inner ear** ▽

✓x7ᵗʰ **S09.8** **Other specified injuries of head**

✓5ᵗʰ **S09.9** **Unspecified injury of face and head**

✓x7ᵗʰ **S09.90** **Unspecified injury of** head ▽
Head injury NOS
EXCLUDES 1 brain injury NOS (S06.9-)
head injury NOS with loss of consciousness (S06.9-)
intracranial injury NOS (S06.9-)

✓x7ᵗʰ **S09.91** **Unspecified injury of** ear ▽
Injury of ear NOS

✓x7ᵗʰ **S09.92** **Unspecified injury of** nose ▽
Injury of nose NOS

✓x7ᵗʰ **S09.93** **Unspecified injury of** face ▽
Injury of face NOS

---

[4] Special Care High = With 7th character indicating a subsequent encounter

[9] Hospice Noncancer Diagnosis only when reported using an appropriate 7th character indicating a subsequent encounter or sequela

Injuries to the neck (S10-S19)

INCLUDES injuries of nape
injuries of supraclavicular region
injuries of throat

EXCLUDES 2 burns and corrosions (T20-T32)
effects of foreign body in esophagus (T18.1)
effects of foreign body in larynx (T17.3)
effects of foreign body in pharynx (T17.2)
effects of foreign body in trachea (T17.4)
frostbite (T33-T34)
insect bite or sting, venomous (T63.4)

✓4th S10 Superficial injury of neck

The appropriate 7th character is to be added to each code from category S10.
A   initial encounter
D   subsequent encounter
S   sequela

✓x7th **S10.0 Contusion of throat**
Contusion of cervical esophagus
Contusion of larynx
Contusion of pharynx
Contusion of trachea

✓5th **S10.1 Other and unspecified superficial injuries of throat**
- ✓x7th **S10.10 Unspecified superficial injuries of throat** ▽
- ✓x7th **S10.11 Abrasion of throat**
- ✓x7th **S10.12 Blister (nonthermal) of throat**
- ✓x7th **S10.14 External constriction of part of throat**
- ✓x7th **S10.15 Superficial foreign body of throat**
  Splinter in the throat
- ✓x7th **S10.16 Insect bite (nonvenomous) of throat**
- ✓x7th **S10.17 Other superficial bite of throat**
  EXCLUDES 1 open bite of throat (S11.85)

✓5th **S10.8 Superficial injury of other specified parts of neck**
- ✓x7th **S10.80 Unspecified superficial injury of other specified part of neck** ▽
- ✓x7th **S10.81 Abrasion of other specified part of neck**
- ✓x7th **S10.82 Blister (nonthermal) of other specified part of neck**
- ✓x7th **S10.83 Contusion of other specified part of neck**
- ✓x7th **S10.84 External constriction of other specified part of neck**
- ✓x7th **S10.85 Superficial foreign body of other specified part of neck**
  Splinter in other specified part of neck
- ✓x7th **S10.86 Insect bite of other specified part of neck**
- ✓x7th **S10.87 Other superficial bite of other specified part of neck**
  EXCLUDES 1 open bite of other specified parts of neck (S11.85)

✓5th **S10.9 Superficial injury of unspecified part of neck**
- ✓x7th **S10.90 Unspecified superficial injury of unspecified part of neck** ▽
- ✓x7th **S10.91 Abrasion of unspecified part of neck** ▽
- ✓x7th **S10.92 Blister (nonthermal) of unspecified part of neck** ▽
- ✓x7th **S10.93 Contusion of unspecified part of neck** ▽
- ✓x7th **S10.94 External constriction of unspecified part of neck** ▽
- ✓x7th **S10.95 Superficial foreign body of unspecified part of neck** ▽
- ✓x7th **S10.96 Insect bite of unspecified part of neck** ▽
- ✓x7th **S10.97 Other superficial bite of unspecified part of neck** ▽

✓4th S11 Open wound of neck

Code also any associated:
spinal cord injury (S14.0, S14.1-)
wound infection

EXCLUDES 2 open fracture of vertebra (S12- with 7th character B)

The appropriate 7th character is to be added to each code from category S11.
A   initial encounter
D   subsequent encounter
S   sequela

✓5th **S11.0 Open wound of larynx and trachea**
- ✓6th **S11.01 Open wound of larynx**
  EXCLUDES 2 open wound of vocal cord (S11.03)
  - ✓7th **S11.011 Laceration without foreign body of larynx**
  - ✓7th **S11.012 Laceration with foreign body of larynx**
  - ✓7th **S11.013 Puncture wound without foreign body of larynx**
  - ✓7th **S11.014 Puncture wound with foreign body of larynx**
  - ✓7th **S11.015 Open bite of larynx**
    Bite of larynx NOS
  - ✓7th **S11.019 Unspecified open wound of larynx** ▽
- ✓6th **S11.02 Open wound of trachea**
  Open wound of cervical trachea
  Open wound of trachea NOS
  EXCLUDES 2 open wound of thoracic trachea (S27.5-)
  - ✓7th **S11.021 Laceration without foreign body of trachea**
  - ✓7th **S11.022 Laceration with foreign body of trachea**
  - ✓7th **S11.023 Puncture wound without foreign body of trachea**
  - ✓7th **S11.024 Puncture wound with foreign body of trachea**
  - ✓7th **S11.025 Open bite of trachea**
    Bite of trachea NOS
  - ✓7th **S11.029 Unspecified open wound of trachea** ▽
- ✓6th **S11.03 Open wound of vocal cord**
  - ✓7th **S11.031 Laceration without foreign body of vocal cord**
  - ✓7th **S11.032 Laceration with foreign body of vocal cord**
  - ✓7th **S11.033 Puncture wound without foreign body of vocal cord**
  - ✓7th **S11.034 Puncture wound with foreign body of vocal cord**
  - ✓7th **S11.035 Open bite of vocal cord**
    Bite of vocal cord NOS
  - ✓7th **S11.039 Unspecified open wound of vocal cord** ▽

✓5th **S11.1 Open wound of thyroid gland**
- ✓x7th **S11.10 Unspecified open wound of thyroid gland** ▽
- ✓x7th **S11.11 Laceration without foreign body of thyroid gland**
- ✓x7th **S11.12 Laceration with foreign body of thyroid gland**
- ✓x7th **S11.13 Puncture wound without foreign body of thyroid gland**
- ✓x7th **S11.14 Puncture wound with foreign body of thyroid gland**
- ✓x7th **S11.15 Open bite of thyroid gland**
  Bite of thyroid gland NOS

✓5th **S11.2 Open wound of pharynx and cervical esophagus**
EXCLUDES 1 open wound of esophagus NOS (S27.8-)
- ✓x7th **S11.20 Unspecified open wound of pharynx and cervical esophagus** ▽
- ✓x7th **S11.21 Laceration without foreign body of pharynx and cervical esophagus**
- ✓x7th **S11.22 Laceration with foreign body of pharynx and cervical esophagus**
- ✓x7th **S11.23 Puncture wound without foreign body of pharynx and cervical esophagus**
- ✓x7th **S11.24 Puncture wound with foreign body of pharynx and cervical esophagus**
- ✓x7th **S11.25 Open bite of pharynx and cervical esophagus**
  Bite of pharynx and cervical esophagus NOS

✓5th **S11.8 Open wound of other specified parts of neck**
- ✓x7th **S11.80 Unspecified open wound of other specified part of neck** ▽
- ✓x7th **S11.81 Laceration without foreign body of other specified part of neck**
- ✓x7th **S11.82 Laceration with foreign body of other specified part of neck**
- ✓x7th **S11.83 Puncture wound without foreign body of other specified part of neck**
- ✓x7th **S11.84 Puncture wound with foreign body of other specified part of neck**
- ✓x7th **S11.85 Open bite of other specified part of neck**
  Bite of other specified part of neck NOS
  EXCLUDES 1 superficial bite of other specified part of neck (S10.87)
- ✓x7th **S11.89 Other open wound of other specified part of neck**

√5ᵗʰ **S11.9** **Open wound of** unspecified **part of neck**

  √ₓ7ᵗʰ **S11.90** **Unspecified open wound of unspecified part of neck** ▽

  √ₓ7ᵗʰ **S11.91** **Laceration without foreign body of unspecified part of neck** ▽

  √ₓ7ᵗʰ **S11.92** **Laceration with foreign body of unspecified part of neck** ▽

  √ₓ7ᵗʰ **S11.93** **Puncture wound without foreign body of unspecified part of neck** ▽

  √ₓ7ᵗʰ **S11.94** **Puncture wound with foreign body of unspecified part of neck** ▽

  √ₓ7ᵗʰ **S11.95** **Open bite of unspecified part of neck** ▽
    Bite of neck NOS
    EXCLUDES 1 superficial bite of neck (S10.97)

√4ᵗʰ **S12** **Fracture of cervical vertebra and other parts of neck**
  NOTE A fracture not indicated as nondisplaced or displaced should be coded to displaced.
    A fracture not indicated as open or closed should be coded to closed.
  INCLUDES fracture of cervical neural arch
    fracture of cervical spine
    fracture of cervical spinous process
    fracture of cervical transverse process
    fracture of cervical vertebral arch
    fracture of neck
  Code first any associated cervical spinal cord injury (S14.0, S14.1-)

  The appropriate 7th character is to be added to all codes from subcategories S12.0–S12.6.
  A   initial encounter for closed fracture
  B   initial encounter for open fracture
  D   subsequent encounter for fracture with routine healing
  G   subsequent encounter for fracture with delayed healing
  K   subsequent encounter for fracture with nonunion
  S   sequela

√5ᵗʰ **S12.0** **Fracture of** first **cervical vertebra**
    Atlas

  √6ᵗʰ **S12.00** **Unspecified fracture of first cervical vertebra**

    √7ᵗʰ **S12.000** **Unspecified** displaced **fracture of first cervical vertebra** ▽

    √7ᵗʰ **S12.001** **Unspecified** nondisplaced **fracture of first cervical vertebra** ▽

  √ₓ7ᵗʰ **S12.01** **Stable burst fracture of first cervical vertebra**

  √ₓ7ᵗʰ **S12.02** **Unstable burst fracture of first cervical vertebra**

  √6ᵗʰ **S12.03** **Posterior arch fracture of first cervical vertebra**

    √7ᵗʰ **S12.030** **Displaced posterior arch fracture of first cervical vertebra**

    √7ᵗʰ **S12.031** **Nondisplaced posterior arch fracture of first cervical vertebra**

  √6ᵗʰ **S12.04** **Lateral mass fracture of first cervical vertebra**

    √7ᵗʰ **S12.040** **Displaced lateral mass fracture of first cervical vertebra**

    √7ᵗʰ **S12.041** **Nondisplaced lateral mass fracture of first cervical vertebra**

  √6ᵗʰ **S12.09** **Other fracture of first cervical vertebra**

    √7ᵗʰ **S12.090** **Other** displaced **fracture of first cervical vertebra**

    √7ᵗʰ **S12.091** **Other** nondisplaced **fracture of first cervical vertebra**

√5ᵗʰ **S12.1** **Fracture of** second **cervical vertebra**
    Axis

  √6ᵗʰ **S12.10** **Unspecified fracture of second cervical vertebra**

    √7ᵗʰ **S12.100** **Unspecified** displaced **fracture of second cervical vertebra** ▽

    √7ᵗʰ **S12.101** **Unspecified** nondisplaced **fracture of second cervical vertebra** ▽

  √6ᵗʰ **S12.11** **Type II dens fracture**

    √7ᵗʰ **S12.110** **Anterior displaced Type II dens fracture**

    √7ᵗʰ **S12.111** **Posterior displaced Type II dens fracture**

    √7ᵗʰ **S12.112** **Nondisplaced Type II dens fracture**

  √6ᵗʰ **S12.12** **Other dens fracture**

    √7ᵗʰ **S12.120** **Other** displaced **dens fracture**

    √7ᵗʰ **S12.121** **Other** nondisplaced **dens fracture**

√6ᵗʰ **S12.13** **Unspecified** traumatic spondylolisthesis **of second cervical vertebra**

    √7ᵗʰ **S12.130** **Unspecified traumatic** displaced **spondylolisthesis of second cervical vertebra** ▽

    √7ᵗʰ **S12.131** **Unspecified traumatic** nondisplaced **spondylolisthesis of second cervical vertebra**

√ₓ7ᵗʰ **S12.14** **Type III** traumatic spondylolisthesis **of second cervical vertebra**

√6ᵗʰ **S12.15** **Other** traumatic spondylolisthesis **of second cervical vertebra**

    √7ᵗʰ **S12.150** **Other traumatic** displaced **spondylolisthesis of second cervical vertebra**

    √7ᵗʰ **S12.151** **Other traumatic** nondisplaced **spondylolisthesis of second cervical vertebra**

  √6ᵗʰ **S12.19** **Other fracture of second cervical vertebra**

    √7ᵗʰ **S12.190** **Other** displaced **fracture of second cervical vertebra**

    √7ᵗʰ **S12.191** **Other** nondisplaced **fracture of second cervical vertebra**

√5ᵗʰ **S12.2** **Fracture of** third **cervical vertebra**

  √6ᵗʰ **S12.20** **Unspecified fracture of third cervical vertebra**

    √7ᵗʰ **S12.200** **Unspecified** displaced **fracture of third cervical vertebra** ▽

    √7ᵗʰ **S12.201** **Unspecified** nondisplaced **fracture of third cervical vertebra** ▽

  √6ᵗʰ **S12.23** **Unspecified** traumatic spondylolisthesis **of third cervical vertebra**

    √7ᵗʰ **S12.230** **Unspecified traumatic** displaced **spondylolisthesis of third cervical vertebra** ▽

    √7ᵗʰ **S12.231** **Unspecified traumatic** nondisplaced **spondylolisthesis of third cervical vertebra** ▽

  √ₓ7ᵗʰ **S12.24** **Type III** traumatic spondylolisthesis **of third cervical vertebra**

  √6ᵗʰ **S12.25** **Other** traumatic spondylolisthesis **of third cervical vertebra**

    √7ᵗʰ **S12.250** **Other traumatic** displaced **spondylolisthesis of third cervical vertebra**

    √7ᵗʰ **S12.251** **Other traumatic** nondisplaced **spondylolisthesis of third cervical vertebra**

  √6ᵗʰ **S12.29** **Other fracture of third cervical vertebra**

    √7ᵗʰ **S12.290** **Other** displaced **fracture of third cervical vertebra**

    √7ᵗʰ **S12.291** **Other** nondisplaced **fracture of third cervical vertebra**

√5ᵗʰ **S12.3** **Fracture of** fourth **cervical vertebra**

  √6ᵗʰ **S12.30** **Unspecified fracture of fourth cervical vertebra**

    √7ᵗʰ **S12.300** **Unspecified** displaced **fracture of fourth cervical vertebra** ▽

    √7ᵗʰ **S12.301** **Unspecified** nondisplaced **fracture of fourth cervical vertebra** ▽

  √6ᵗʰ **S12.33** **Unspecified** traumatic spondylolisthesis **of fourth cervical vertebra**

    √7ᵗʰ **S12.330** **Unspecified traumatic** displaced **spondylolisthesis of fourth cervical vertebra** ▽

    √7ᵗʰ **S12.331** **Unspecified traumatic** nondisplaced **spondylolisthesis of fourth cervical vertebra** ▽

  √ₓ7ᵗʰ **S12.34** **Type III** traumatic spondylolisthesis **of fourth cervical vertebra**

  √6ᵗʰ **S12.35** **Other** traumatic spondylolisthesis **of fourth cervical vertebra**

    √7ᵗʰ **S12.350** **Other traumatic** displaced **spondylolisthesis of fourth cervical vertebra**

    √7ᵗʰ **S12.351** **Other traumatic** nondisplaced **spondylolisthesis of fourth cervical vertebra**

Ⓝ Newborn   🄿 Pediatric   Ⓜ Maternity   🄰 Adult   **RIC** RIC Dx   **NCDx** Noncancer Dx   **PDx** Primary Dx   **CC** RIC CC Condition   ▶◀ Revised Text   ● New Code   ▲ Revised Code Title

870   ICD-10-CM 2016

☑6ᵗʰ **S12.39** Other fracture of fourth cervical vertebra

     ☑7ᵗʰ **S12.390** Other displaced fracture of fourth cervical vertebra

     ☑7ᵗʰ **S12.391** Other nondisplaced fracture of fourth cervical vertebra

☑5ᵗʰ **S12.4** Fracture of fifth cervical vertebra

   ☑6ᵗʰ **S12.40** Unspecified fracture of fifth cervical vertebra

     ☑7ᵗʰ **S12.400** Unspecified displaced fracture of fifth cervical vertebra ▽

     ☑7ᵗʰ **S12.401** Unspecified nondisplaced fracture of fifth cervical vertebra ▽

   ☑6ᵗʰ **S12.43** Unspecified traumatic spondylolisthesis of fifth cervical vertebra

     ☑7ᵗʰ **S12.430** Unspecified traumatic displaced spondylolisthesis of fifth cervical vertebra ▽

     ☑7ᵗʰ **S12.431** Unspecified traumatic nondisplaced spondylolisthesis of fifth cervical vertebra ▽

   ☑x7ᵗʰ **S12.44** Type III traumatic spondylolisthesis of fifth cervical vertebra

   ☑6ᵗʰ **S12.45** Other traumatic spondylolisthesis of fifth cervical vertebra

     ☑7ᵗʰ **S12.450** Other traumatic displaced spondylolisthesis of fifth cervical vertebra

     ☑7ᵗʰ **S12.451** Other traumatic nondisplaced spondylolisthesis of fifth cervical vertebra

   ☑6ᵗʰ **S12.49** Other fracture of fifth cervical vertebra

     ☑7ᵗʰ **S12.490** Other displaced fracture of fifth cervical vertebra

     ☑7ᵗʰ **S12.491** Other nondisplaced fracture of fifth cervical vertebra

☑5ᵗʰ **S12.5** Fracture of sixth cervical vertebra

   ☑6ᵗʰ **S12.50** Unspecified fracture of sixth cervical vertebra

     ☑7ᵗʰ **S12.500** Unspecified displaced fracture of sixth cervical vertebra ▽

     ☑7ᵗʰ **S12.501** Unspecified nondisplaced fracture of sixth cervical vertebra ▽

   ☑6ᵗʰ **S12.53** Unspecified traumatic spondylolisthesis of sixth cervical vertebra

     ☑7ᵗʰ **S12.530** Unspecified traumatic displaced spondylolisthesis of sixth cervical vertebra ▽

     ☑7ᵗʰ **S12.531** Unspecified traumatic nondisplaced spondylolisthesis of sixth cervical vertebra ▽

   ☑x7ᵗʰ **S12.54** Type III traumatic spondylolisthesis of sixth cervical vertebra

   ☑6ᵗʰ **S12.55** Other traumatic spondylolisthesis of sixth cervical vertebra

     ☑7ᵗʰ **S12.550** Other traumatic displaced spondylolisthesis of sixth cervical vertebra

     ☑7ᵗʰ **S12.551** Other traumatic nondisplaced spondylolisthesis of sixth cervical vertebra

   ☑6ᵗʰ **S12.59** Other fracture of sixth cervical vertebra

     ☑7ᵗʰ **S12.590** Other displaced fracture of sixth cervical vertebra

     ☑7ᵗʰ **S12.591** Other nondisplaced fracture of sixth cervical vertebra

☑5ᵗʰ **S12.6** Fracture of seventh cervical vertebra

   ☑6ᵗʰ **S12.60** Unspecified fracture of seventh cervical vertebra

     ☑7ᵗʰ **S12.600** Unspecified displaced fracture of seventh cervical vertebra ▽

     ☑7ᵗʰ **S12.601** Unspecified nondisplaced fracture of seventh cervical vertebra ▽

   ☑6ᵗʰ **S12.63** Unspecified traumatic spondylolisthesis of seventh cervical vertebra

     ☑7ᵗʰ **S12.630** Unspecified traumatic displaced spondylolisthesis of seventh cervical vertebra ▽

     ☑7ᵗʰ **S12.631** Unspecified traumatic nondisplaced spondylolisthesis of seventh cervical vertebra ▽

   ☑x7ᵗʰ **S12.64** Type III traumatic spondylolisthesis of seventh cervical vertebra

   ☑6ᵗʰ **S12.65** Other traumatic spondylolisthesis of seventh cervical vertebra

     ☑7ᵗʰ **S12.650** Other traumatic displaced spondylolisthesis of seventh cervical vertebra

     ☑7ᵗʰ **S12.651** Other traumatic nondisplaced spondylolisthesis of seventh cervical vertebra

   ☑6ᵗʰ **S12.69** Other fracture of seventh cervical vertebra

     ☑7ᵗʰ **S12.690** Other displaced fracture of seventh cervical vertebra

     ☑7ᵗʰ **S12.691** Other nondisplaced fracture of seventh cervical vertebra

☑x7ᵗʰ **S12.8** **Fracture of other parts of neck**
Hyoid bone
Larynx
Thyroid cartilage
Trachea

> The appropriate 7th character is to be added to code S12.8.
> A   initial encounter
> D   subsequent encounter
> S   sequela

☑x7ᵗʰ **S12.9** **Fracture of neck, unspecified** ▽
Fracture of cervical spine NOS
Fracture of cervical vertebra NOS
Fracture of neck NOS

> The appropriate 7th character is to be added to code S12.9.
> A   initial encounter
> D   subsequent encounter
> S   sequela

☑4ᵗʰ **S13** **Dislocation and sprain of joints and ligaments at neck level**
    INCLUDES   avulsion of joint or ligament at neck level
              laceration of cartilage, joint or ligament at neck level
              sprain of cartilage, joint or ligament at neck level
              traumatic hemarthrosis of joint or ligament at neck level
              traumatic rupture of joint or ligament at neck level
              traumatic subluxation of joint or ligament at neck level
              traumatic tear of joint or ligament at neck level

Code also any associated open wound
EXCLUDES 2   strain of muscle or tendon at neck level (S16.1)

> The appropriate 7th character is to be added to each code from category S13.
> A   initial encounter
> D   subsequent encounter
> S   sequela

☑x7ᵗʰ **S13.0** **Traumatic rupture of cervical intervertebral disc**
     EXCLUDES 1   rupture or displacement (nontraumatic) of cervical intervertebral disc NOS (M50.-)

☑5ᵗʰ **S13.1** **Subluxation and dislocation of cervical vertebrae**
Code also any associated:
   open wound of neck (S11.-)
   spinal cord injury (S14.1-)
EXCLUDES 2   fracture of cervical vertebrae (S12.0--S12.3-)

   ☑6ᵗʰ **S13.10** Subluxation and dislocation of unspecified cervical vertebrae

     ☑7ᵗʰ **S13.100** Subluxation of unspecified cervical vertebrae ▽

     ☑7ᵗʰ **S13.101** Dislocation of unspecified cervical vertebrae ▽

   ☑6ᵗʰ **S13.11** Subluxation and dislocation of C0/C1 cervical vertebrae
Subluxation and dislocation of atlantooccipital joint
Subluxation and dislocation of atloidooccipital joint
Subluxation and dislocation of occipitoatloid joint

     ☑7ᵗʰ **S13.110** Subluxation of C0/C1 cervical vertebrae

     ☑7ᵗʰ **S13.111** Dislocation of C0/C1 cervical vertebrae

   ☑6ᵗʰ **S13.12** Subluxation and dislocation of C1/C2 cervical vertebrae
Subluxation and dislocation of atlantoaxial joint

     ☑7ᵗʰ **S13.120** Subluxation of C1/C2 cervical vertebrae

     ☑7ᵗʰ **S13.121** Dislocation of C1/C2 cervical vertebrae

---

☑ Add'l Character Required   ☑x7ᵗʰ Placeholder Alert   RUG IV Special Care High Dx   RUG IV Clinically Complex Dx   RUG IV Special Care Low Dx   Manifestation Code   Other Specified Code   ▽ Unspecified Code

√6ᵗʰ **S13.13** **Subluxation and dislocation of** C2/C3 **cervical vertebrae**

    √7ᵗʰ **S13.130** Subluxation of C2/C3 cervical vertebrae

    √7ᵗʰ **S13.131** Dislocation of C2/C3 cervical vertebrae

√6ᵗʰ **S13.14** **Subluxation and dislocation of** C3/C4 **cervical vertebrae**

    √7ᵗʰ **S13.140** Subluxation of C3/C4 cervical vertebrae

    √7ᵗʰ **S13.141** Dislocation of C3/C4 cervical vertebrae

√6ᵗʰ **S13.15** **Subluxation and dislocation of** C4/C5 **cervical vertebrae**

    √7ᵗʰ **S13.150** Subluxation of C4/C5 cervical vertebrae

    √7ᵗʰ **S13.151** Dislocation of C4/C5 cervical vertebrae

√6ᵗʰ **S13.16** **Subluxation and dislocation of** C5/C6 **cervical vertebrae**

    √7ᵗʰ **S13.160** Subluxation of C5/C6 cervical vertebrae

    √7ᵗʰ **S13.161** Dislocation of C5/C6 cervical vertebrae

√6ᵗʰ **S13.17** **Subluxation and dislocation of** C6/C7 **cervical vertebrae**

    √7ᵗʰ **S13.170** Subluxation of C6/C7 cervical vertebrae

    √7ᵗʰ **S13.171** Dislocation of C6/C7 cervical vertebrae

√6ᵗʰ **S13.18** **Subluxation and dislocation of** C7/T1 **cervical vertebrae**

    √7ᵗʰ **S13.180** Subluxation of C7/T1 cervical vertebrae

    √7ᵗʰ **S13.181** Dislocation of C7/T1 cervical vertebrae

√5ᵗʰ **S13.2** **Dislocation of other and unspecified parts of neck**

    √x7ᵗʰ **S13.20** **Dislocation of unspecified parts of neck** ▽

    √x7ᵗʰ **S13.29** **Dislocation of other parts of neck**

√x7ᵗʰ **S13.4** **Sprain of ligaments of cervical spine**

    Sprain of anterior longitudinal (ligament), cervical
    Sprain of atlanto-axial (joints)
    Sprain of atlanto-occipital (joints)
    Whiplash injury of cervical spine

√x7ᵗʰ **S13.5** **Sprain of thyroid region**

    Sprain of cricoarytenoid (joint) (ligament)
    Sprain of cricothyroid (joint) (ligament)
    Sprain of thyroid cartilage

√x7ᵗʰ **S13.8** **Sprain of joints and ligaments of other parts of neck**

√x7ᵗʰ **S13.9** **Sprain of joints and ligaments of unspecified parts of neck** ▽

√4ᵗʰ **S14** **Injury of nerves and spinal cord at neck level**

    NOTE Code to highest level of cervical cord injury.

    Code also any associated:
      fracture of cervical vertebra (S12.0- -S12.6-)
      open wound of neck (S11.-)
      transient paralysis (R29.5)

    The appropriate 7th character is to be added to each code from category S14.
    A   initial encounter
    D   subsequent encounter
    S   sequela

√x7ᵗʰ **S14.0** **Concussion and edema of cervical spinal cord**

√5ᵗʰ **S14.1** **Other and unspecified injuries of cervical spinal cord**

  √6ᵗʰ **S14.10** Unspecified injury of cervical spinal cord

    √7ᵗʰ **S14.101** **Unspecified injury at** C1 **level of cervical spinal cord** ▽

    √7ᵗʰ **S14.102** **Unspecified injury at** C2 **level of cervical spinal cord** ▽

    √7ᵗʰ **S14.103** **Unspecified injury at** C3 **level of cervical spinal cord** ▽

    √7ᵗʰ **S14.104** **Unspecified injury at** C4 **level of cervical spinal cord** ▽

    √7ᵗʰ **S14.105** **Unspecified injury at** C5 **level of cervical spinal cord** ▽

    √7ᵗʰ **S14.106** **Unspecified injury at** C6 **level of cervical spinal cord** ▽

    √7ᵗʰ **S14.107** **Unspecified injury at** C7 **level of cervical spinal cord** ▽

    √7ᵗʰ **S14.108** **Unspecified injury at** C8 **level of cervical spinal cord** ▽

    √7ᵗʰ **S14.109** **Unspecified injury at unspecified level of cervical spinal cord** ▽
      Injury of cervical spinal cord NOS

√6ᵗʰ **S14.11** Complete lesion of cervical spinal cord

    √7ᵗʰ **S14.111** **Complete lesion at** C1 **level of cervical spinal cord**

    √7ᵗʰ **S14.112** **Complete lesion at** C2 **level of cervical spinal cord**

    √7ᵗʰ **S14.113** **Complete lesion at** C3 **level of cervical spinal cord**

    √7ᵗʰ **S14.114** **Complete lesion at** C4 **level of cervical spinal cord**

    √7ᵗʰ **S14.115** **Complete lesion at** C5 **level of cervical spinal cord**

    √7ᵗʰ **S14.116** **Complete lesion at** C6 **level of cervical spinal cord**

    √7ᵗʰ **S14.117** **Complete lesion at** C7 **level of cervical spinal cord**

    √7ᵗʰ **S14.118** **Complete lesion at** C8 **level of cervical spinal cord**

    √7ᵗʰ **S14.119** **Complete lesion at unspecified level of cervical spinal cord** ▽

√6ᵗʰ **S14.12** Central cord syndrome of cervical spinal cord

    √7ᵗʰ **S14.121** **Central cord syndrome at** C1 **level of cervical spinal cord**

    √7ᵗʰ **S14.122** **Central cord syndrome at** C2 **level of cervical spinal cord**

    √7ᵗʰ **S14.123** **Central cord syndrome at** C3 **level of cervical spinal cord**

    √7ᵗʰ **S14.124** **Central cord syndrome at** C4 **level of cervical spinal cord**

    √7ᵗʰ **S14.125** **Central cord syndrome at** C5 **level of cervical spinal cord**

    √7ᵗʰ **S14.126** **Central cord syndrome at** C6 **level of cervical spinal cord**

    √7ᵗʰ **S14.127** **Central cord syndrome at** C7 **level of cervical spinal cord**

    √7ᵗʰ **S14.128** **Central cord syndrome at** C8 **level of cervical spinal cord**

    √7ᵗʰ **S14.129** **Central cord syndrome at unspecified level of cervical spinal cord** ▽

√6ᵗʰ **S14.13** Anterior cord syndrome of cervical spinal cord

    √7ᵗʰ **S14.131** **Anterior cord syndrome at** C1 **level of cervical spinal cord**

    √7ᵗʰ **S14.132** **Anterior cord syndrome at** C2 **level of cervical spinal cord**

    √7ᵗʰ **S14.133** **Anterior cord syndrome at** C3 **level of cervical spinal cord**

    √7ᵗʰ **S14.134** **Anterior cord syndrome at** C4 **level of cervical spinal cord**

    √7ᵗʰ **S14.135** **Anterior cord syndrome at** C5 **level of cervical spinal cord**

    √7ᵗʰ **S14.136** **Anterior cord syndrome at** C6 **level of cervical spinal cord**

    √7ᵗʰ **S14.137** **Anterior cord syndrome at** C7 **level of cervical spinal cord**

    √7ᵗʰ **S14.138** **Anterior cord syndrome at** C8 **level of cervical spinal cord**

    √7ᵗʰ **S14.139** **Anterior cord syndrome at unspecified level of cervical spinal cord** ▽

√6ᵗʰ **S14.14** Brown-Séquard syndrome of cervical spinal cord

    √7ᵗʰ **S14.141** **Brown-Séquard syndrome at** C1 **level of cervical spinal cord**

    √7ᵗʰ **S14.142** **Brown-Séquard syndrome at** C2 **level of cervical spinal cord**

    √7ᵗʰ **S14.143** **Brown-Séquard syndrome at** C3 **level of cervical spinal cord**

    √7ᵗʰ **S14.144** **Brown-Séquard syndrome at** C4 **level of cervical spinal cord**

    √7ᵗʰ **S14.145** **Brown-Séquard syndrome at** C5 **level of cervical spinal cord**

    √7ᵗʰ **S14.146** **Brown-Séquard syndrome at** C6 **level of cervical spinal cord**

    √7ᵗʰ **S14.147** **Brown-Séquard syndrome at** C7 **level of cervical spinal cord**

Ⓝ Newborn Ⓟ Pediatric Ⓜ Maternity Ⓐ Adult **RIC** RIC Dx **NC Dx** Noncancer Dx **PDx** Primary Dx **CC** RIC CC Condition ▶◀ Revised Text ● New Code ▲ Revised Code Title

872   ICD-10-CM 2016

✓7ᵗʰ	**S14.148**	**Brown-Séquard syndrome at C8 level of cervical spinal cord**
✓7ᵗʰ	**S14.149**	**Brown-Séquard syndrome at unspecified level of cervical spinal cord** ▽
✓6ᵗʰ	**S14.15**	Other incomplete lesions of cervical spinal cord

              Incomplete lesion of cervical spinal cord NOS
              Posterior cord syndrome of cervical spinal cord

✓7ᵗʰ	**S14.151**	**Other incomplete lesion at C1 level of cervical spinal cord**
✓7ᵗʰ	**S14.152**	**Other incomplete lesion at C2 level of cervical spinal cord**
✓7ᵗʰ	**S14.153**	**Other incomplete lesion at C3 level of cervical spinal cord**
✓7ᵗʰ	**S14.154**	**Other incomplete lesion at C4 level of cervical spinal cord**
✓7ᵗʰ	**S14.155**	**Other incomplete lesion at C5 level of cervical spinal cord**
✓7ᵗʰ	**S14.156**	**Other incomplete lesion at C6 level of cervical spinal cord**
✓7ᵗʰ	**S14.157**	**Other incomplete lesion at C7 level of cervical spinal cord**
✓7ᵗʰ	**S14.158**	**Other incomplete lesion at C8 level of cervical spinal cord**
✓7ᵗʰ	**S14.159**	**Other incomplete lesion at unspecified level of cervical spinal cord** ▽
✓x7ᵗʰ	**S14.2**	**Injury of nerve root of cervical spine**
✓x7ᵗʰ	**S14.3**	**Injury of brachial plexus**
✓x7ᵗʰ	**S14.4**	**Injury of peripheral nerves of neck**
✓x7ᵗʰ	**S14.5**	**Injury of cervical sympathetic nerves**
✓x7ᵗʰ	**S14.8**	**Injury of other specified nerves of neck**
✓x7ᵗʰ	**S14.9**	**Injury of unspecified nerves of neck** ▽

✓4ᵗʰ	**S15**	**Injury of blood vessels at neck level**

    Code also any associated open wound (S11.-)

> The appropriate 7th character is to be added to each code from category S15.
> A   initial encounter
> D   subsequent encounter
> S   sequela

✓5ᵗʰ	**S15.0**	**Injury of carotid artery of neck**

    Injury of carotid artery (common) (external) (internal, extracranial portion)
    Injury of carotid artery NOS
    EXCLUDES 1 injury of internal carotid artery, intracranial portion (S06.8)

✓6ᵗʰ	**S15.00**	Unspecified injury of carotid artery
✓7ᵗʰ	**S15.001**	**Unspecified injury of right carotid artery** ▽
✓7ᵗʰ	**S15.002**	**Unspecified injury of left carotid artery** ▽
✓7ᵗʰ	**S15.009**	**Unspecified injury of unspecified carotid artery** ▽
✓6ᵗʰ	**S15.01**	Minor laceration of carotid artery

              Incomplete transection of carotid artery
              Laceration of carotid artery NOS
              Superficial laceration of carotid artery

✓7ᵗʰ	**S15.011**	**Minor laceration of right carotid artery**
✓7ᵗʰ	**S15.012**	**Minor laceration of left carotid artery**
✓7ᵗʰ	**S15.019**	**Minor laceration of unspecified carotid artery** ▽
✓6ᵗʰ	**S15.02**	Major laceration of carotid artery

              Complete transection of carotid artery
              Traumatic rupture of carotid artery

✓7ᵗʰ	**S15.021**	**Major laceration of right carotid artery**
✓7ᵗʰ	**S15.022**	**Major laceration of left carotid artery**
✓7ᵗʰ	**S15.029**	**Major laceration of unspecified carotid artery** ▽
✓6ᵗʰ	**S15.09**	Other specified injury of carotid artery
✓7ᵗʰ	**S15.091**	**Other specified injury of right carotid artery**
✓7ᵗʰ	**S15.092**	**Other specified injury of left carotid artery**
✓7ᵗʰ	**S15.099**	**Other specified injury of unspecified carotid artery** ▽

✓5ᵗʰ	**S15.1**	**Injury of vertebral artery**
✓6ᵗʰ	**S15.10**	Unspecified injury of vertebral artery
✓7ᵗʰ	**S15.101**	**Unspecified injury of right vertebral artery** ▽
✓7ᵗʰ	**S15.102**	**Unspecified injury of left vertebral artery** ▽
✓7ᵗʰ	**S15.109**	**Unspecified injury of unspecified vertebral artery** ▽
✓6ᵗʰ	**S15.11**	Minor laceration of vertebral artery

              Incomplete transection of vertebral artery
              Laceration of vertebral artery NOS
              Superficial laceration of vertebral artery

✓7ᵗʰ	**S15.111**	**Minor laceration of right vertebral artery**
✓7ᵗʰ	**S15.112**	**Minor laceration of left vertebral artery**
✓7ᵗʰ	**S15.119**	**Minor laceration of unspecified vertebral artery** ▽
✓6ᵗʰ	**S15.12**	Major laceration of vertebral artery

              Complete transection of vertebral artery
              Traumatic rupture of vertebral artery

✓7ᵗʰ	**S15.121**	**Major laceration of right vertebral artery**
✓7ᵗʰ	**S15.122**	**Major laceration of left vertebral artery**
✓7ᵗʰ	**S15.129**	**Major laceration of unspecified vertebral artery** ▽
✓6ᵗʰ	**S15.19**	Other specified injury of vertebral artery
✓7ᵗʰ	**S15.191**	**Other specified injury of right vertebral artery**
✓7ᵗʰ	**S15.192**	**Other specified injury of left vertebral artery**
✓7ᵗʰ	**S15.199**	**Other specified injury of unspecified vertebral artery** ▽

✓5ᵗʰ	**S15.2**	**Injury of external jugular vein**
✓6ᵗʰ	**S15.20**	Unspecified injury of external jugular vein
✓7ᵗʰ	**S15.201**	**Unspecified injury of right external jugular vein** ▽
✓7ᵗʰ	**S15.202**	**Unspecified injury of left external jugular vein** ▽
✓7ᵗʰ	**S15.209**	**Unspecified injury of unspecified external jugular vein** ▽
✓6ᵗʰ	**S15.21**	Minor laceration of external jugular vein

              Incomplete transection of external jugular vein
              Laceration of external jugular vein NOS
              Superficial laceration of external jugular vein

✓7ᵗʰ	**S15.211**	**Minor laceration of right external jugular vein**
✓7ᵗʰ	**S15.212**	**Minor laceration of left external jugular vein**
✓7ᵗʰ	**S15.219**	**Minor laceration of unspecified external jugular vein** ▽
✓6ᵗʰ	**S15.22**	Major laceration of external jugular vein

              Complete transection of external jugular vein
              Traumatic rupture of external jugular vein

✓7ᵗʰ	**S15.221**	**Major laceration of right external jugular vein**
✓7ᵗʰ	**S15.222**	**Major laceration of left external jugular vein**
✓7ᵗʰ	**S15.229**	**Major laceration of unspecified external jugular vein** ▽
✓6ᵗʰ	**S15.29**	Other specified injury of external jugular vein
✓7ᵗʰ	**S15.291**	**Other specified injury of right external jugular vein**
✓7ᵗʰ	**S15.292**	**Other specified injury of left external jugular vein**
✓7ᵗʰ	**S15.299**	**Other specified injury of unspecified external jugular vein** ▽

✓5ᵗʰ	**S15.3**	**Injury of internal jugular vein**
✓6ᵗʰ	**S15.30**	Unspecified injury of internal jugular vein
✓7ᵗʰ	**S15.301**	**Unspecified injury of right internal jugular vein** ▽
✓7ᵗʰ	**S15.302**	**Unspecified injury of left internal jugular vein** ▽
✓7ᵗʰ	**S15.309**	**Unspecified injury of unspecified internal jugular vein** ▽

✓ Add'l Character Required   ✓x7ᵗʰ Placeholder Alert   RUG IV Special Care High Dx   RUG IV Clinically Complex Dx   RUG IV Special Care Low Dx   Manifestation Code   Other Specified Code   ▽ Unspecified Code

ICD-10-CM 2016   873

Chapter 19. Injury, Poisoning and Certain Other Consequences of External Causes

S15.31–S20.171

✓6ᵗʰ **S15.31** Minor laceration of internal jugular vein
Incomplete transection of internal jugular vein
Laceration of internal jugular vein NOS
Superficial laceration of internal jugular vein

✓7ᵗʰ **S15.311** Minor laceration of right internal jugular vein

✓7ᵗʰ **S15.312** Minor laceration of left internal jugular vein

✓7ᵗʰ **S15.319** Minor laceration of unspecified internal jugular vein ▽

✓6ᵗʰ **S15.32** Major laceration of internal jugular vein
Complete transection of internal jugular vein
Traumatic rupture of internal jugular vein

✓7ᵗʰ **S15.321** Major laceration of right internal jugular vein

✓7ᵗʰ **S15.322** Major laceration of left internal jugular vein

✓7ᵗʰ **S15.329** Major laceration of unspecified internal ▽ jugular vein

✓6ᵗʰ **S15.39** Other specified injury of internal jugular vein

✓7ᵗʰ **S15.391** Other specified injury of right internal jugular vein

✓7ᵗʰ **S15.392** Other specified injury of left internal jugular vein

✓7ᵗʰ **S15.399** Other specified injury of unspecified ▽ internal jugular vein

✓x7ᵗʰ **S15.8** Injury of other specified blood vessels at neck level

✓x7ᵗʰ **S15.9** Injury of unspecified blood vessel at neck level ▽

✓4ᵗʰ **S16** Injury of muscle, fascia and tendon at neck level
Code also any associated open wound (S11.-)
EXCLUDES 2 sprain of joint or ligament at neck level (S13.9)

The appropriate 7th character is to be added to each code from category S16.
A   initial encounter
D   subsequent encounter
S   sequela

✓x7ᵗʰ **S16.1** Strain of muscle, fascia and tendon at neck level

✓x7ᵗʰ **S16.2** Laceration of muscle, fascia and tendon at neck level

✓x7ᵗʰ **S16.8** Other specified injury of muscle, fascia and tendon at neck level

✓x7ᵗʰ **S16.9** Unspecified injury of muscle, fascia and tendon at neck level ▽

✓4ᵗʰ **S17** Crushing injury of neck
Use additional code for all associated injuries, such as:
injury of blood vessels (S15.-)
open wound of neck (S11.-)
spinal cord injury (S14.0, S14.1-)
vertebral fracture (S12.0- -S12.3-)

The appropriate 7th character is to be added to each code from category S17.
A   initial encounter
D   subsequent encounter
S   sequela

✓x7ᵗʰ **S17.0** Crushing injury of larynx and trachea

✓x7ᵗʰ **S17.8** Crushing injury of other specified parts of neck

✓x7ᵗʰ **S17.9** Crushing injury of neck, part unspecified ▽

✓4ᵗʰ **S19** Other specified and unspecified injuries of neck

The appropriate 7th character is to be added to each code from category S19.
A   initial encounter
D   subsequent encounter
S   sequela

✓5ᵗʰ **S19.8** Other specified injuries of neck

✓x7ᵗʰ **S19.80** Other specified injuries of unspecified part of ▽ neck

✓x7ᵗʰ **S19.81** Other specified injuries of larynx

✓x7ᵗʰ **S19.82** Other specified injuries of cervical trachea
EXCLUDES 2 other specified injury of thoracic trachea (S27.5-)

✓x7ᵗʰ **S19.83** Other specified injuries of vocal cord

✓x7ᵗʰ **S19.84** Other specified injuries of thyroid gland

✓x7ᵗʰ **S19.85** Other specified injuries of pharynx and cervical esophagus

✓x7ᵗʰ **S19.89** Other specified injuries of other specified part of neck

✓x7ᵗʰ **S19.9** Unspecified injury of neck ▽

Injuries to the thorax (S20-S29)

INCLUDES injuries of breast
injuries of chest (wall)
injuries of interscapular area
EXCLUDES 2 burns and corrosions (T20-T32)
effects of foreign body in bronchus (T17.5)
effects of foreign body in esophagus (T18.1)
effects of foreign body in lung (T17.8)
effects of foreign body in trachea (T17.4)
frostbite (T33-T34)
injuries of axilla
injuries of clavicle
injuries of scapular region
injuries of shoulder
insect bite or sting, venomous (T63.4)

✓4ᵗʰ **S20** Superficial injury of thorax

The appropriate 7th character is to be added to each code from category S20.
A   initial encounter
D   subsequent encounter
S   sequela

✓5ᵗʰ **S20.0** Contusion of breast

✓x7ᵗʰ **S20.00** Contusion of breast, unspecified breast ▽

✓x7ᵗʰ **S20.01** Contusion of right breast

✓x7ᵗʰ **S20.02** Contusion of left breast

✓5ᵗʰ **S20.1** Other and unspecified superficial injuries of breast

✓6ᵗʰ **S20.10** Unspecified superficial injuries of breast

✓7ᵗʰ **S20.101** Unspecified superficial injuries of ▽ breast, right breast

✓7ᵗʰ **S20.102** Unspecified superficial injuries of ▽ breast, left breast

✓7ᵗʰ **S20.109** Unspecified superficial injuries of ▽ breast, unspecified breast

✓6ᵗʰ **S20.11** Abrasion of breast

✓7ᵗʰ **S20.111** Abrasion of breast, right breast

✓7ᵗʰ **S20.112** Abrasion of breast, left breast

✓7ᵗʰ **S20.119** Abrasion of breast, unspecified breast ▽

✓6ᵗʰ **S20.12** Blister (nonthermal) of breast

✓7ᵗʰ **S20.121** Blister (nonthermal) of breast, right breast

✓7ᵗʰ **S20.122** Blister (nonthermal) of breast, left breast

✓7ᵗʰ **S20.129** Blister (nonthermal) of breast, ▽ unspecified breast

✓6ᵗʰ **S20.14** External constriction of part of breast

✓7ᵗʰ **S20.141** External constriction of part of breast, right breast

✓7ᵗʰ **S20.142** External constriction of part of breast, left breast

✓7ᵗʰ **S20.149** External constriction of part of breast, ▽ unspecified breast

✓6ᵗʰ **S20.15** Superficial foreign body of breast
Splinter in the breast

✓7ᵗʰ **S20.151** Superficial foreign body of breast, right breast

✓7ᵗʰ **S20.152** Superficial foreign body of breast, left breast

✓7ᵗʰ **S20.159** Superficial foreign body of breast, ▽ unspecified breast

✓6ᵗʰ **S20.16** Insect bite (nonvenomous) of breast

✓7ᵗʰ **S20.161** Insect bite (nonvenomous) of breast, right breast

✓7ᵗʰ **S20.162** Insect bite (nonvenomous) of breast, left breast

✓7ᵗʰ **S20.169** Insect bite (nonvenomous) of breast, ▽ unspecified breast

✓6ᵗʰ **S20.17** Other superficial bite of breast
EXCLUDES 1 open bite of breast (S21.05-)

✓7ᵗʰ **S20.171** Other superficial bite of breast, right breast

N Newborn   P Pediatric   M Maternity   A Adult   **RIC** RIC Dx   **NCDx** Noncancer Dx   **PDx** Primary Dx   **CC** RIC CC Condition   ▶◀ Revised Text   ● New Code   ▲ Revised Code Title

874   ICD-10-CM 2016

√7ᵗʰ **S20.172** Other superficial bite of breast, left breast

√7ᵗʰ **S20.179** Other superficial bite of breast, unspecified breast ▽

√5ᵗʰ **S20.2 Contusion of thorax**

  √x7ᵗʰ **S20.20** Contusion of thorax, unspecified ▽

  √6ᵗʰ **S20.21** Contusion of front wall of thorax

    √7ᵗʰ **S20.211** Contusion of right front wall of thorax

    √7ᵗʰ **S20.212** Contusion of left front wall of thorax

    √7ᵗʰ **S20.219** Contusion of unspecified front wall of thorax ▽

  √6ᵗʰ **S20.22** Contusion of back wall of thorax

    √7ᵗʰ **S20.221** Contusion of right back wall of thorax

    √7ᵗʰ **S20.222** Contusion of left back wall of thorax

    √7ᵗʰ **S20.229** Contusion of unspecified back wall of thorax ▽

√5ᵗʰ **S20.3 Other and unspecified superficial injuries of front wall of thorax**

  √6ᵗʰ **S20.30** Unspecified superficial injuries of front wall of thorax

    √7ᵗʰ **S20.301** Unspecified superficial injuries of right front wall of thorax ▽

    √7ᵗʰ **S20.302** Unspecified superficial injuries of left front wall of thorax ▽

    √7ᵗʰ **S20.309** Unspecified superficial injuries of unspecified front wall of thorax ▽

  √6ᵗʰ **S20.31** Abrasion of front wall of thorax

    √7ᵗʰ **S20.311** Abrasion of right front wall of thorax

    √7ᵗʰ **S20.312** Abrasion of left front wall of thorax

    √7ᵗʰ **S20.319** Abrasion of unspecified front wall of thorax ▽

  √6ᵗʰ **S20.32** Blister (nonthermal) of front wall of thorax

    √7ᵗʰ **S20.321** Blister (nonthermal) of right front wall of thorax

    √7ᵗʰ **S20.322** Blister (nonthermal) of left front wall of thorax

    √7ᵗʰ **S20.329** Blister (nonthermal) of unspecified front wall of thorax ▽

  √6ᵗʰ **S20.34** External constriction of front wall of thorax

    √7ᵗʰ **S20.341** External constriction of right front wall of thorax

    √7ᵗʰ **S20.342** External constriction of left front wall of thorax

    √7ᵗʰ **S20.349** External constriction of unspecified front wall of thorax ▽

  √6ᵗʰ **S20.35** Superficial foreign body of front wall of thorax
    Splinter in front wall of thorax

    √7ᵗʰ **S20.351** Superficial foreign body of right front wall of thorax

    √7ᵗʰ **S20.352** Superficial foreign body of left front wall of thorax

    √7ᵗʰ **S20.359** Superficial foreign body of unspecified front wall of thorax ▽

  √6ᵗʰ **S20.36** Insect bite (nonvenomous) of front wall of thorax

    √7ᵗʰ **S20.361** Insect bite (nonvenomous) of right front wall of thorax

    √7ᵗʰ **S20.362** Insect bite (nonvenomous) of left front wall of thorax

    √7ᵗʰ **S20.369** Insect bite (nonvenomous) of unspecified front wall of thorax ▽

  √6ᵗʰ **S20.37** Other superficial bite of front wall of thorax
    EXCLUDES 1 open bite of front wall of thorax (S21.14)

    √7ᵗʰ **S20.371** Other superficial bite of right front wall of thorax

    √7ᵗʰ **S20.372** Other superficial bite of left front wall of thorax

    √7ᵗʰ **S20.379** Other superficial bite of unspecified front wall of thorax ▽

√5ᵗʰ **S20.4 Other and unspecified superficial injuries of back wall of thorax**

  √6ᵗʰ **S20.40** Unspecified superficial injuries of back wall of thorax

    √7ᵗʰ **S20.401** Unspecified superficial injuries of right back wall of thorax ▽

    √7ᵗʰ **S20.402** Unspecified superficial injuries of left back wall of thorax ▽

    √7ᵗʰ **S20.409** Unspecified superficial injuries of unspecified back wall of thorax ▽

  √6ᵗʰ **S20.41** Abrasion of back wall of thorax

    √7ᵗʰ **S20.411** Abrasion of right back wall of thorax

    √7ᵗʰ **S20.412** Abrasion of left back wall of thorax

    √7ᵗʰ **S20.419** Abrasion of unspecified back wall of thorax ▽

  √6ᵗʰ **S20.42** Blister (nonthermal) of back wall of thorax

    √7ᵗʰ **S20.421** Blister (nonthermal) of right back wall of thorax

    √7ᵗʰ **S20.422** Blister (nonthermal) of left back wall of thorax

    √7ᵗʰ **S20.429** Blister (nonthermal) of unspecified back wall of thorax ▽

  √6ᵗʰ **S20.44** External constriction of back wall of thorax

    √7ᵗʰ **S20.441** External constriction of right back wall of thorax

    √7ᵗʰ **S20.442** External constriction of left back wall of thorax

    √7ᵗʰ **S20.449** External constriction of unspecified back wall of thorax ▽

  √6ᵗʰ **S20.45** Superficial foreign body of back wall of thorax
    Splinter of back wall of thorax

    √7ᵗʰ **S20.451** Superficial foreign body of right back wall of thorax

    √7ᵗʰ **S20.452** Superficial foreign body of left back wall of thorax

    √7ᵗʰ **S20.459** Superficial foreign body of unspecified back wall of thorax ▽

  √6ᵗʰ **S20.46** Insect bite (nonvenomous) of back wall of thorax

    √7ᵗʰ **S20.461** Insect bite (nonvenomous) of right back wall of thorax

    √7ᵗʰ **S20.462** Insect bite (nonvenomous) of left back wall of thorax

    √7ᵗʰ **S20.469** Insect bite (nonvenomous) of unspecified back wall of thorax ▽

  √6ᵗʰ **S20.47** Other superficial bite of back wall of thorax
    EXCLUDES 1 open bite of back wall of thorax (S21.24)

    √7ᵗʰ **S20.471** Other superficial bite of right back wall of thorax

    √7ᵗʰ **S20.472** Other superficial bite of left back wall of thorax

    √7ᵗʰ **S20.479** Other superficial bite of unspecified back wall of thorax ▽

√5ᵗʰ **S20.9 Superficial injury of unspecified parts of thorax**
  EXCLUDES 1 contusion of thorax NOS (S20.20)

  √x7ᵗʰ **S20.90** Unspecified superficial injury of unspecified parts of thorax ▽
    Superficial injury of thoracic wall NOS

  √x7ᵗʰ **S20.91** Abrasion of unspecified parts of thorax ▽

  √x7ᵗʰ **S20.92** Blister (nonthermal) of unspecified parts of thorax ▽

  √x7ᵗʰ **S20.94** External constriction of unspecified parts of thorax ▽

  √x7ᵗʰ **S20.95** Superficial foreign body of unspecified parts of thorax ▽
    Splinter in thorax NOS

  √x7ᵗʰ **S20.96** Insect bite (nonvenomous) of unspecified parts of thorax ▽

  √x7ᵗʰ **S20.97** Other superficial bite of unspecified parts of thorax ▽
    EXCLUDES 1 open bite of thorax NOS (S21.95)

☑ Add'l Character Required   √x7ᵗʰ Placeholder Alert   RUG IV Special Care High Dx   RUG IV Clinically Complex Dx   RUG IV Special Care Low Dx   Manifestation Code   Other Specified Code   ▽ Unspecified Code

ICD-10-CM 2016   **875**

Chapter 19. Injury, Poisoning and Certain Other Consequences of External Causes

√4th S21 Open wound of thorax

Code also any associated injury, such as:
injury of heart (S26.-)
injury of intrathoracic organs (S27.-)
rib fracture (S22.3-, S22.4-)
spinal cord injury (S24.0-, S24.1-)
traumatic hemopneumothorax (S27.3)
traumatic hemothorax (S27.1)
traumatic pneumothorax (S27.0)
wound infection

EXCLUDES 1 *traumatic amputation (partial) of thorax (S28.1)*

The appropriate 7th character is to be added to each code from category S21.
A   initial encounter
D   subsequent encounter
S   sequela

√5th S21.0 Open wound of breast

√6th S21.00 Unspecified open wound of breast
   √7th S21.001 Unspecified open wound of right breast ▽
   √7th S21.002 Unspecified open wound of left breast ▽
   √7th S21.009 Unspecified open wound of unspecified ▽ breast

√6th S21.01 Laceration without foreign body of breast
   √7th S21.011 Laceration without foreign body of right breast
   √7th S21.012 Laceration without foreign body of left breast
   √7th S21.019 Laceration without foreign body of ▽ unspecified breast

√6th S21.02 Laceration with foreign body of breast
   √7th S21.021 Laceration with foreign body of right breast
   √7th S21.022 Laceration with foreign body of left breast
   √7th S21.029 Laceration with foreign body of ▽ unspecified breast

√6th S21.03 Puncture wound without foreign body of breast
   √7th S21.031 Puncture wound without foreign body of right breast
   √7th S21.032 Puncture wound without foreign body of left breast
   √7th S21.039 Puncture wound without foreign body ▽ of unspecified breast

√6th S21.04 Puncture wound with foreign body of breast
   √7th S21.041 Puncture wound with foreign body of right breast
   √7th S21.042 Puncture wound with foreign body of left breast
   √7th S21.049 Puncture wound with foreign body of ▽ unspecified breast

√6th S21.05 Open bite of breast
Bite of breast NOS
EXCLUDES 1 *superficial bite of breast (S20.17)*
   √7th S21.051 Open bite of right breast
   √7th S21.052 Open bite of left breast
   √7th S21.059 Open bite of unspecified breast ▽

√5th S21.1 Open wound of front wall of thorax without penetration into thoracic cavity
Open wound of chest without penetration into thoracic cavity

√6th S21.10 Unspecified open wound of front wall of thorax without penetration into thoracic cavity
   √7th S21.101 Unspecified open wound of right front ▽ wall of thorax without penetration into thoracic cavity
   √7th S21.102 Unspecified open wound of left front ▽ wall of thorax without penetration into thoracic cavity
   √7th S21.109 Unspecified open wound of unspecified ▽ front wall of thorax without penetration into thoracic cavity

√6th S21.11 Laceration without foreign body of front wall of thorax without penetration into thoracic cavity
   √7th S21.111 Laceration without foreign body of right front wall of thorax without penetration into thoracic cavity

   √7th S21.112 Laceration without foreign body of left front wall of thorax without penetration into thoracic cavity
   √7th S21.119 Laceration without foreign body of ▽ unspecified front wall of thorax without penetration into thoracic cavity

√6th S21.12 Laceration with foreign body of front wall of thorax without penetration into thoracic cavity
   √7th S21.121 Laceration with foreign body of right front wall of thorax without penetration into thoracic cavity
   √7th S21.122 Laceration with foreign body of left front wall of thorax without penetration into thoracic cavity
   √7th S21.129 Laceration with foreign body of ▽ unspecified front wall of thorax without penetration into thoracic cavity

√6th S21.13 Puncture wound without foreign body of front wall of thorax without penetration into thoracic cavity
   √7th S21.131 Puncture wound without foreign body of right front wall of thorax without penetration into thoracic cavity
   √7th S21.132 Puncture wound without foreign body of left front wall of thorax without penetration into thoracic cavity
   √7th S21.139 Puncture wound without foreign body ▽ of unspecified front wall of thorax without penetration into thoracic cavity

√6th S21.14 Puncture wound with foreign body of front wall of thorax without penetration into thoracic cavity
   √7th S21.141 Puncture wound with foreign body of right front wall of thorax without penetration into thoracic cavity
   √7th S21.142 Puncture wound with foreign body of left front wall of thorax without penetration into thoracic cavity
   √7th S21.149 Puncture wound with foreign body of ▽ unspecified front wall of thorax without penetration into thoracic cavity

√6th S21.15 Open bite of front wall of thorax without penetration into thoracic cavity
Bite of front wall of thorax NOS
EXCLUDES 1 *superficial bite of front wall of thorax (S20.37)*
   √7th S21.151 Open bite of right front wall of thorax without penetration into thoracic cavity
   √7th S21.152 Open bite of left front wall of thorax without penetration into thoracic cavity
   √7th S21.159 Open bite of unspecified front wall of ▽ thorax without penetration into thoracic cavity

√5th S21.2 Open wound of back wall of thorax without penetration into thoracic cavity

√6th S21.20 Unspecified open wound of back wall of thorax without penetration into thoracic cavity
   √7th S21.201 Unspecified open wound of right back ▽ wall of thorax without penetration into thoracic cavity
   √7th S21.202 Unspecified open wound of left back ▽ wall of thorax without penetration into thoracic cavity
   √7th S21.209 Unspecified open wound of unspecified ▽ back wall of thorax without penetration into thoracic cavity

√6th S21.21 Laceration without foreign body of back wall of thorax without penetration into thoracic cavity
   √7th S21.211 Laceration without foreign body of right back wall of thorax without penetration into thoracic cavity
   √7th S21.212 Laceration without foreign body of left back wall of thorax without penetration into thoracic cavity
   √7th S21.219 Laceration without foreign body of ▽ unspecified back wall of thorax without penetration into thoracic cavity

N Newborn   P Pediatric   M Maternity   A Adult   RIC RIC Dx   NC Dx Noncancer Dx   PDx Primary Dx   CC RIC CC Condition   ►◄ Revised Text   ● New Code   ▲ Revised Code Title

876

ICD-10-CM 2016

S21–S21.219

✓6ᵗʰ **S21.22** Laceration with foreign body of back wall of thorax without penetration into thoracic cavity

    ✓7ᵗʰ **S21.221** Laceration with foreign body of right back wall of thorax without penetration into thoracic cavity

    ✓7ᵗʰ **S21.222** Laceration with foreign body of left back wall of thorax without penetration into thoracic cavity

    ✓7ᵗʰ **S21.229** Laceration with foreign body of ▽ unspecified back wall of thorax without penetration into thoracic cavity

✓6ᵗʰ **S21.23** Puncture wound without foreign body of back wall of thorax without penetration into thoracic cavity

    ✓7ᵗʰ **S21.231** Puncture wound without foreign body of right back wall of thorax without penetration into thoracic cavity

    ✓7ᵗʰ **S21.232** Puncture wound without foreign body of left back wall of thorax without penetration into thoracic cavity

    ✓7ᵗʰ **S21.239** Puncture wound without foreign body ▽ of unspecified back wall of thorax without penetration into thoracic cavity

✓6ᵗʰ **S21.24** Puncture wound with foreign body of back wall of thorax without penetration into thoracic cavity

    ✓7ᵗʰ **S21.241** Puncture wound with foreign body of right back wall of thorax without penetration into thoracic cavity

    ✓7ᵗʰ **S21.242** Puncture wound with foreign body of left back wall of thorax without penetration into thoracic cavity

    ✓7ᵗʰ **S21.249** Puncture wound with foreign body of ▽ unspecified back wall of thorax without penetration into thoracic cavity

✓6ᵗʰ **S21.25** Open bite of back wall of thorax without penetration into thoracic cavity

    Bite of back wall of thorax NOS

    EXCLUDES 1 *superficial bite of back wall of thorax (S20.47)*

    ✓7ᵗʰ **S21.251** Open bite of right back wall of thorax without penetration into thoracic cavity

    ✓7ᵗʰ **S21.252** Open bite of left back wall of thorax without penetration into thoracic cavity

    ✓7ᵗʰ **S21.259** Open bite of unspecified back wall of ▽ thorax without penetration into thoracic cavity

✓5ᵗʰ **S21.3** Open wound of front wall of thorax with penetration into thoracic cavity

    Open wound of chest with penetration into thoracic cavity

    ✓6ᵗʰ **S21.30** Unspecified open wound of front wall of thorax with penetration into thoracic cavity

      ✓7ᵗʰ **S21.301** Unspecified open wound of right front ▽ wall of thorax with penetration into thoracic cavity

      ✓7ᵗʰ **S21.302** Unspecified open wound of left front ▽ wall of thorax with penetration into thoracic cavity

      ✓7ᵗʰ **S21.309** Unspecified open wound of ▽ unspecified front wall of thorax with penetration into thoracic cavity

    ✓6ᵗʰ **S21.31** Laceration without foreign body of front wall of thorax with penetration into thoracic cavity

      ✓7ᵗʰ **S21.311** Laceration without foreign body of right front wall of thorax with penetration into thoracic cavity

      ✓7ᵗʰ **S21.312** Laceration without foreign body of left front wall of thorax with penetration into thoracic cavity

      ✓7ᵗʰ **S21.319** Laceration without foreign body of ▽ unspecified front wall of thorax with penetration into thoracic cavity

    ✓6ᵗʰ **S21.32** Laceration with foreign body of front wall of thorax with penetration into thoracic cavity

      ✓7ᵗʰ **S21.321** Laceration with foreign body of right front wall of thorax with penetration into thoracic cavity

      ✓7ᵗʰ **S21.322** Laceration with foreign body of left front wall of thorax with penetration into thoracic cavity

      ✓7ᵗʰ **S21.329** Laceration with foreign body of ▽ unspecified front wall of thorax with penetration into thoracic cavity

✓6ᵗʰ **S21.33** Puncture wound without foreign body of front wall of thorax with penetration into thoracic cavity

    ✓7ᵗʰ **S21.331** Puncture wound without foreign body of right front wall of thorax with penetration into thoracic cavity

    ✓7ᵗʰ **S21.332** Puncture wound without foreign body of left front wall of thorax with penetration into thoracic cavity

    ✓7ᵗʰ **S21.339** Puncture wound without foreign body ▽ of unspecified front wall of thorax with penetration into thoracic cavity

✓6ᵗʰ **S21.34** Puncture wound with foreign body of front wall of thorax with penetration into thoracic cavity

    ✓7ᵗʰ **S21.341** Puncture wound with foreign body of right front wall of thorax with penetration into thoracic cavity

    ✓7ᵗʰ **S21.342** Puncture wound with foreign body of left front wall of thorax with penetration into thoracic cavity

    ✓7ᵗʰ **S21.349** Puncture wound with foreign body of ▽ unspecified front wall of thorax with penetration into thoracic cavity

✓6ᵗʰ **S21.35** Open bite of front wall of thorax with penetration into thoracic cavity

    EXCLUDES 1 *superficial bite of front wall of thorax (S20.37)*

    ✓7ᵗʰ **S21.351** Open bite of right front wall of thorax with penetration into thoracic cavity

    ✓7ᵗʰ **S21.352** Open bite of left front wall of thorax with penetration into thoracic cavity

    ✓7ᵗʰ **S21.359** Open bite of unspecified front wall of ▽ thorax with penetration into thoracic cavity

✓5ᵗʰ **S21.4** Open wound of back wall of thorax with penetration into thoracic cavity

    ✓6ᵗʰ **S21.40** Unspecified open wound of back wall of thorax with penetration into thoracic cavity

      ✓7ᵗʰ **S21.401** Unspecified open wound of right back ▽ wall of thorax with penetration into thoracic cavity

      ✓7ᵗʰ **S21.402** Unspecified open wound of left back ▽ wall of thorax with penetration into thoracic cavity

      ✓7ᵗʰ **S21.409** Unspecified open wound of ▽ unspecified back wall of thorax with penetration into thoracic cavity

    ✓6ᵗʰ **S21.41** Laceration without foreign body of back wall of thorax with penetration into thoracic cavity

      ✓7ᵗʰ **S21.411** Laceration without foreign body of right back wall of thorax with penetration into thoracic cavity

      ✓7ᵗʰ **S21.412** Laceration without foreign body of left back wall of thorax with penetration into thoracic cavity

      ✓7ᵗʰ **S21.419** Laceration without foreign body of ▽ unspecified back wall of thorax with penetration into thoracic cavity

    ✓6ᵗʰ **S21.42** Laceration with foreign body of back wall of thorax with penetration into thoracic cavity

      ✓7ᵗʰ **S21.421** Laceration with foreign body of right back wall of thorax with penetration into thoracic cavity

      ✓7ᵗʰ **S21.422** Laceration with foreign body of left back wall of thorax with penetration into thoracic cavity

      ✓7ᵗʰ **S21.429** Laceration with foreign body of ▽ unspecified back wall of thorax with penetration into thoracic cavity

---

☑ Add'l Character Required   ☑x7ᵗʰ Placeholder Alert   RUG IV Special Care High Dx   RUG IV Clinically Complex Dx   RUG IV Special Care Low Dx   Manifestation Code   Other Specified Code   ▽ Unspecified Code

ICD-10-CM 2016   877

√6th S21.43 Puncture wound without foreign body of back wall of thorax with penetration into thoracic cavity

     √7th S21.431 Puncture wound without foreign body of **right** back wall of thorax with penetration into thoracic cavity

     √7th S21.432 Puncture wound without foreign body of **left** back wall of thorax with penetration into thoracic cavity

     √7th S21.439 Puncture wound without foreign body of unspecified back wall of thorax with penetration into thoracic cavity   ▽

√6th S21.44 Puncture wound with foreign body of back wall of thorax with penetration into thoracic cavity

     √7th S21.441 Puncture wound with foreign body of **right** back wall of thorax with penetration into thoracic cavity

     √7th S21.442 Puncture wound with foreign body of **left** back wall of thorax with penetration into thoracic cavity

     √7th S21.449 Puncture wound with foreign body of unspecified back wall of thorax with penetration into thoracic cavity   ▽

√6th S21.45 Open bite of back wall of thorax with penetration into thoracic cavity
     Bite of back wall of thorax NOS
     EXCLUDES 1   superficial bite of back wall of thorax (S20.47)

     √7th S21.451 Open bite of **right** back wall of thorax with penetration into thoracic cavity

     √7th S21.452 Open bite of **left** back wall of thorax with penetration into thoracic cavity

     √7th S21.459 Open bite of unspecified back wall of thorax with penetration into thoracic cavity   ▽

√5th S21.9 Open wound of unspecified part of thorax
     Open wound of thoracic wall NOS

     √x7th S21.90 Unspecified open wound of unspecified part of thorax   ▽

     √x7th S21.91 Laceration without foreign body of unspecified part of thorax   ▽

     √x7th S21.92 Laceration with foreign body of unspecified part of thorax   ▽

     √x7th S21.93 Puncture wound without foreign body of unspecified part of thorax   ▽

     √x7th S21.94 Puncture wound with foreign body of unspecified part of thorax   ▽

     √x7th S21.95 Open bite of unspecified part of thorax   ▽
         EXCLUDES 1   superficial bite of thorax (S20.97)

√4th S22 Fracture of rib(s), sternum and thoracic spine
     NOTE   A fracture not indicated as nondisplaced or displaced should be coded to displaced.
         A fracture not indicated as open or closed should be coded to closed.
     INCLUDES   fracture of thoracic neural arch
         fracture of thoracic spinous process
         fracture of thoracic transverse process
         fracture of thoracic vertebra
         fracture of thoracic vertebral arch
     Code first any associated:
         injury of intrathoracic organ (S27.-)
         spinal cord injury (S24.0-, S24.1-)
     EXCLUDES 1   transection of thorax (S28.1)
     EXCLUDES 2   fracture of clavicle (S42.0-)
         fracture of scapula (S42.1-)

> The appropriate 7th character is to be added to each code from category S22.
> A   initial encounter for closed fracture
> B   initial encounter for open fracture
> D   subsequent encounter for fracture with routine healing
> G   subsequent encounter for fracture with delayed healing
> K   subsequent encounter for fracture with nonunion
> S   sequela

√5th S22.0 Fracture of thoracic vertebra

     √6th S22.00 Fracture of unspecified thoracic vertebra

         √7th S22.000 Wedge compression fracture of unspecified thoracic vertebra   ▽

         √7th S22.001 Stable burst fracture of unspecified thoracic vertebra   ▽

         √7th S22.002 Unstable burst fracture of unspecified thoracic vertebra   ▽

         √7th S22.008 Other fracture of unspecified thoracic vertebra   ▽

         √7th S22.009 Unspecified fracture of unspecified thoracic vertebra   ▽

     √6th S22.01 Fracture of first thoracic vertebra

         √7th S22.010 Wedge compression fracture of first thoracic vertebra

         √7th S22.011 Stable burst fracture of first thoracic vertebra

         √7th S22.012 Unstable burst fracture of first thoracic vertebra

         √7th S22.018 Other fracture of first thoracic vertebra

         √7th S22.019 Unspecified fracture of first thoracic vertebra   ▽

     √6th S22.02 Fracture of second thoracic vertebra

         √7th S22.020 Wedge compression fracture of second thoracic vertebra

         √7th S22.021 Stable burst fracture of second thoracic vertebra

         √7th S22.022 Unstable burst fracture of second thoracic vertebra

         √7th S22.028 Other fracture of second thoracic vertebra

         √7th S22.029 Unspecified fracture of second thoracic vertebra   ▽

     √6th S22.03 Fracture of third thoracic vertebra

         √7th S22.030 Wedge compression fracture of third thoracic vertebra

         √7th S22.031 Stable burst fracture of third thoracic vertebra

         √7th S22.032 Unstable burst fracture of third thoracic vertebra

         √7th S22.038 Other fracture of third thoracic vertebra

         √7th S22.039 Unspecified fracture of third thoracic vertebra   ▽

     √6th S22.04 Fracture of fourth thoracic vertebra

         √7th S22.040 Wedge compression fracture of fourth thoracic vertebra

         √7th S22.041 Stable burst fracture of fourth thoracic vertebra

         √7th S22.042 Unstable burst fracture of fourth thoracic vertebra

         √7th S22.048 Other fracture of fourth thoracic vertebra

         √7th S22.049 Unspecified fracture of fourth thoracic vertebra   ▽

     √6th S22.05 Fracture of T5-T6 vertebra

         √7th S22.050 Wedge compression fracture of T5-T6 vertebra

         √7th S22.051 Stable burst fracture of T5-T6 vertebra

         √7th S22.052 Unstable burst fracture of T5-T6 vertebra

         √7th S22.058 Other fracture of T5-T6 vertebra

         √7th S22.059 Unspecified fracture of T5-T6 vertebra   ▽

     √6th S22.06 Fracture of T7-T8 vertebra

         √7th S22.060 Wedge compression fracture of T7-T8 vertebra

         √7th S22.061 Stable burst fracture of T7-T8 vertebra

         √7th S22.062 Unstable burst fracture of T7-T8 vertebra

         √7th S22.068 Other fracture of T7-T8 thoracic vertebra

         √7th S22.069 Unspecified fracture of T7-T8 vertebra   ▽

     √6th S22.07 Fracture of T9-T10 vertebra

         √7th S22.070 Wedge compression fracture of T9-T10 vertebra

         √7th S22.071 Stable burst fracture of T9-T10 vertebra

         √7th S22.072 Unstable burst fracture of T9-T10 vertebra

         √7th S22.078 Other fracture of T9-T10 vertebra

         √7th S22.079 Unspecified fracture of T9-T10 vertebra   ▽

     √6th S22.08 Fracture of T11-T12 vertebra

         √7th S22.080 Wedge compression fracture of T11-T12 vertebra

         √7th S22.081 Stable burst fracture of T11-T12 vertebra

N Newborn   P Pediatric   M Maternity   A Adult   **RIC** RIC Dx   **NC Dx** Noncancer Dx   **PDx** Primary Dx   **CC** RIC CC Condition   ►◄ Revised Text   ● New Code   ▲ Revised Code Title

878   ICD-10-CM 2016

✓7ᵗʰ **S22.082** Unstable burst fracture of T11-T12 vertebra

✓7ᵗʰ **S22.088** Other fracture of T11-T12 vertebra

✓7ᵗʰ **S22.089** Unspecified fracture of T11-T12 vertebra ▽

✓5ᵗʰ **S22.2 Fracture of sternum**

✓x7ᵗʰ **S22.20** Unspecified fracture of sternum ▽

✓x7ᵗʰ **S22.21** Fracture of manubrium

✓x7ᵗʰ **S22.22** Fracture of body of sternum

✓x7ᵗʰ **S22.23** Sternal manubrial dissociation

✓x7ᵗʰ **S22.24** Fracture of xiphoid process

✓5ᵗʰ **S22.3 Fracture of one rib**

✓x7ᵗʰ **S22.31** Fracture of one rib, right side

✓x7ᵗʰ **S22.32** Fracture of one rib, left side

✓x7ᵗʰ **S22.39** Fracture of one rib, unspecified side ▽

✓5ᵗʰ **S22.4 Multiple fractures of ribs**
Fractures of two or more ribs
EXCLUDES 1 flail chest (S22.5-)

✓x7ᵗʰ **S22.41** Multiple fractures of ribs, right side

✓x7ᵗʰ **S22.42** Multiple fractures of ribs, left side

✓x7ᵗʰ **S22.43** Multiple fractures of ribs, bilateral

✓x7ᵗʰ **S22.49** Multiple fractures of ribs, unspecified side ▽

✓x7ᵗʰ **S22.5 Flail chest**

✓x7ᵗʰ **S22.9 Fracture of bony thorax, part unspecified** ▽

✓4ᵗʰ **S23 Dislocation and sprain of joints and ligaments of thorax**
INCLUDES avulsion of joint or ligament of thorax
laceration of cartilage, joint or ligament of thorax
sprain of cartilage, joint or ligament of thorax
traumatic hemarthrosis of joint or ligament of thorax
traumatic rupture of joint or ligament of thorax
traumatic subluxation of joint or ligament of thorax
traumatic tear of joint or ligament of thorax
Code also any associated open wound
EXCLUDES 2 dislocation, sprain of sternoclavicular joint (S43.2, S43.6)
strain of muscle or tendon of thorax (S29.01-)

The appropriate 7th character is to be added to each code from
category S23.
A   initial encounter
D   subsequent encounter
S   sequela

✓x7ᵗʰ **S23.0 Traumatic rupture of thoracic intervertebral disc**
EXCLUDES 1 rupture or displacement (nontraumatic) of thoracic
intervertebral disc NOS (M51- with fifth
character 4)

✓5ᵗʰ **S23.1 Subluxation and dislocation of thoracic vertebra**
Code also any associated
open wound of thorax (S21.-)
spinal cord injury (S24.0-, S24.1-)
EXCLUDES 2 fracture of thoracic vertebrae (S22.0-)

✓6ᵗʰ **S23.10** Subluxation and dislocation of unspecified thoracic vertebra

✓7ᵗʰ **S23.100** Subluxation of unspecified thoracic vertebra ▽

✓7ᵗʰ **S23.101** Dislocation of unspecified thoracic vertebra ▽

✓6ᵗʰ **S23.11** Subluxation and dislocation of T1/T2 thoracic vertebra

✓7ᵗʰ **S23.110** Subluxation of T1/T2 thoracic vertebra

✓7ᵗʰ **S23.111** Dislocation of T1/T2 thoracic vertebra

✓6ᵗʰ **S23.12** Subluxation and dislocation of T2/T3-T3/T4 thoracic vertebra

✓7ᵗʰ **S23.120** Subluxation of T2/T3 thoracic vertebra

✓7ᵗʰ **S23.121** Dislocation of T2/T3 thoracic vertebra

✓7ᵗʰ **S23.122** Subluxation of T3/T4 thoracic vertebra

✓7ᵗʰ **S23.123** Dislocation of T3/T4 thoracic vertebra

✓6ᵗʰ **S23.13** Subluxation and dislocation of T4/T5-T5/T6 thoracic vertebra

✓7ᵗʰ **S23.130** Subluxation of T4/T5 thoracic vertebra

✓7ᵗʰ **S23.131** Dislocation of T4/T5 thoracic vertebra

✓7ᵗʰ **S23.132** Subluxation of T5/T6 thoracic vertebra

✓7ᵗʰ **S23.133** Dislocation of T5/T6 thoracic vertebra

✓6ᵗʰ **S23.14** Subluxation and dislocation of T6/T7-T7/T8 thoracic vertebra

✓7ᵗʰ **S23.140** Subluxation of T6/T7 thoracic vertebra

✓7ᵗʰ **S23.141** Dislocation of T6/T7 thoracic vertebra

✓7ᵗʰ **S23.142** Subluxation of T7/T8 thoracic vertebra

✓7ᵗʰ **S23.143** Dislocation of T7/T8 thoracic vertebra

✓6ᵗʰ **S23.15** Subluxation and dislocation of T8/T9-T9/T10 thoracic vertebra

✓7ᵗʰ **S23.150** Subluxation of T8/T9 thoracic vertebra

✓7ᵗʰ **S23.151** Dislocation of T8/T9 thoracic vertebra

✓7ᵗʰ **S23.152** Subluxation of T9/T10 thoracic vertebra

✓7ᵗʰ **S23.153** Dislocation of T9/T10 thoracic vertebra

✓6ᵗʰ **S23.16** Subluxation and dislocation of T10/T11-T11/T12 thoracic vertebra

✓7ᵗʰ **S23.160** Subluxation of T10/T11 thoracic vertebra

✓7ᵗʰ **S23.161** Dislocation of T10/T11 thoracic vertebra

✓7ᵗʰ **S23.162** Subluxation of T11/T12 thoracic vertebra

✓7ᵗʰ **S23.163** Dislocation of T11/T12 thoracic vertebra

✓6ᵗʰ **S23.17** Subluxation and dislocation of T12/L1 thoracic vertebra

✓7ᵗʰ **S23.170** Subluxation of T12/L1 thoracic vertebra

✓7ᵗʰ **S23.171** Dislocation of T12/L1 thoracic vertebra

✓5ᵗʰ **S23.2 Dislocation of other and unspecified parts of thorax**

✓x7ᵗʰ **S23.20** Dislocation of unspecified part of thorax ▽

✓x7ᵗʰ **S23.29** Dislocation of other parts of thorax

✓x7ᵗʰ **S23.3 Sprain of ligaments of thoracic spine**

✓5ᵗʰ **S23.4 Sprain of ribs and sternum**

✓x7ᵗʰ **S23.41** Sprain of ribs

✓6ᵗʰ **S23.42** Sprain of sternum

✓7ᵗʰ **S23.420** Sprain of sternoclavicular (joint) (ligament)

✓7ᵗʰ **S23.421** Sprain of chondrosternal joint

✓7ᵗʰ **S23.428** Other sprain of sternum

✓7ᵗʰ **S23.429** Unspecified sprain of sternum ▽

✓x7ᵗʰ **S23.8 Sprain of other specified parts of thorax**

✓x7ᵗʰ **S23.9 Sprain of unspecified parts of thorax** ▽

✓4ᵗʰ **S24 Injury of nerves and spinal cord at thorax level**
NOTE Code to highest level of thoracic spinal cord injury.
Injuries to the spinal cord (S24.0 and S24.1) refer to the cord
level and not bone level injury, and can affect nerve roots at
and below the level given.
Code also any associated:
fracture of thoracic vertebra (S22.0-)
open wound of thorax (S21.-)
transient paralysis (R29.5)
EXCLUDES 2 injury of brachial plexus (S14.3)

The appropriate 7th character is to be added to each code from
category S24.
A   initial encounter
D   subsequent encounter
S   sequela

✓x7ᵗʰ **S24.0 Concussion and edema of thoracic spinal cord**

✓5ᵗʰ **S24.1 Other and unspecified injuries of thoracic spinal cord**

✓6ᵗʰ **S24.10** Unspecified injury of thoracic spinal cord

✓7ᵗʰ **S24.101** Unspecified injury at T1 level of thoracic spinal cord ▽

✓7ᵗʰ **S24.102** Unspecified injury at T2-T6 level of thoracic spinal cord ▽

✓7ᵗʰ **S24.103** Unspecified injury at T7-T10 level of thoracic spinal cord ▽

✓7ᵗʰ **S24.104** Unspecified injury at T11-T12 level of thoracic spinal cord ▽

✓7ᵗʰ **S24.109** Unspecified injury at unspecified level of thoracic spinal cord ▽
Injury of thoracic spinal cord NOS

✓6ᵗʰ **S24.11** Complete lesion of thoracic spinal cord

✓7ᵗʰ **S24.111** Complete lesion at T1 level of thoracic spinal cord

✓7ᵗʰ **S24.112** Complete lesion at T2-T6 level of thoracic spinal cord

✓ Add'l Character Required   ✓x7ᵗʰ Placeholder Alert   **RUG IV Special Care High Dx**   **RUG IV Clinically Complex Dx**   **RUG IV Special Care Low Dx**   Manifestation Code   Other Specified Code   ▽ Unspecified Code

ICD-10-CM 2016   **879**

     ✓7ᵗʰ **S24.113** **Complete lesion at** T7-T10 **level of thoracic spinal cord**

     ✓7ᵗʰ **S24.114** **Complete lesion at** T11-T12 **level of thoracic spinal cord**

     ✓7ᵗʰ **S24.119** **Complete lesion at unspecified level of** ▽ **thoracic spinal cord**

✓6ᵗʰ **S24.13** Anterior cord syndrome **of thoracic spinal cord**

     ✓7ᵗʰ **S24.131** **Anterior cord syndrome at** T1 **level of thoracic spinal cord**

     ✓7ᵗʰ **S24.132** **Anterior cord syndrome at** T2-T6 **level of thoracic spinal cord**

     ✓7ᵗʰ **S24.133** **Anterior cord syndrome at** T7-T10 **level of thoracic spinal cord**

     ✓7ᵗʰ **S24.134** **Anterior cord syndrome at** T11-T12 **level of thoracic spinal cord**

     ✓7ᵗʰ **S24.139** **Anterior cord syndrome at unspecified** ▽ **level of thoracic spinal cord**

✓6ᵗʰ **S24.14** Brown-Séquard syndrome **of thoracic spinal cord**

     ✓7ᵗʰ **S24.141** **Brown-Séquard syndrome at** T1 **level of thoracic spinal cord**

     ✓7ᵗʰ **S24.142** **Brown-Séquard syndrome at** T2-T6 **level of thoracic spinal cord**

     ✓7ᵗʰ **S24.143** **Brown-Séquard syndrome at** T7-T10 **level of thoracic spinal cord**

     ✓7ᵗʰ **S24.144** **Brown-Séquard syndrome at** T11-T12 **level of thoracic spinal cord**

     ✓7ᵗʰ **S24.149** **Brown-Séquard syndrome at** ▽ **unspecified level of thoracic spinal cord**

✓6ᵗʰ **S24.15** Other incomplete **lesions of thoracic spinal cord**
Incomplete lesion of thoracic spinal cord NOS
Posterior cord syndrome of thoracic spinal cord

     ✓7ᵗʰ **S24.151** **Other incomplete lesion at** T1 **level of thoracic spinal cord**

     ✓7ᵗʰ **S24.152** **Other incomplete lesion at** T2-T6 **level of thoracic spinal cord**

     ✓7ᵗʰ **S24.153** **Other incomplete lesion at** T7-T10 **level of thoracic spinal cord**

     ✓7ᵗʰ **S24.154** **Other incomplete lesion at** T11-T12 **level of thoracic spinal cord**

     ✓7ᵗʰ **S24.159** **Other incomplete lesion at** ▽ **unspecified level of thoracic spinal cord**

✓x7ᵗʰ **S24.2** **Injury of nerve root of thoracic spine**

✓x7ᵗʰ **S24.3** **Injury of peripheral nerves of thorax**

✓x7ᵗʰ **S24.4** **Injury of thoracic sympathetic nervous system**
Injury of cardiac plexus
Injury of esophageal plexus
Injury of pulmonary plexus
Injury of stellate ganglion
Injury of thoracic sympathetic ganglion

✓x7ᵗʰ **S24.8** **Injury of other specified nerves of thorax**

✓x7ᵗʰ **S24.9** **Injury of unspecified nerve of thorax** ▽

✓4ᵗʰ **S25** **Injury of blood vessels of thorax**
Code also any associated open wound (S21.-)

> The appropriate 7th character is to be added to each code from category S25.
> A   initial encounter
> D   subsequent encounter
> S   sequela

✓5ᵗʰ **S25.0** **Injury of** thoracic aorta
Injury of aorta NOS

   ✓x7ᵗʰ **S25.00** **Unspecified injury of thoracic aorta** ▽

   ✓x7ᵗʰ **S25.01** Minor laceration **of thoracic aorta**
Incomplete transection of thoracic aorta
Laceration of thoracic aorta NOS
Superficial laceration of thoracic aorta

   ✓x7ᵗʰ **S25.02** Major laceration **of thoracic aorta**
Complete transection of thoracic aorta
Traumatic rupture of thoracic aorta

   ✓x7ᵗʰ **S25.09** **Other specified injury of thoracic aorta**

✓5ᵗʰ **S25.1** **Injury of** innominate or subclavian artery

   ✓6ᵗʰ **S25.10** Unspecified **injury of innominate or subclavian artery**

     ✓7ᵗʰ **S25.101** **Unspecified injury of** right **innominate** ▽ **or subclavian artery**

     ✓7ᵗʰ **S25.102** **Unspecified injury of** left **innominate** ▽ **or subclavian artery**

     ✓7ᵗʰ **S25.109** **Unspecified injury of unspecified innominate or subclavian artery**

   ✓6ᵗʰ **S25.11** Minor laceration **of innominate or subclavian artery**
Incomplete transection of innominate or subclavian artery
Laceration of innominate or subclavian artery NOS
Superficial laceration of innominate or subclavian artery

     ✓7ᵗʰ **S25.111** **Minor laceration of** right **innominate or subclavian artery**

     ✓7ᵗʰ **S25.112** **Minor laceration of** left **innominate or subclavian artery**

     ✓7ᵗʰ **S25.119** **Minor laceration of unspecified** ▽ **innominate or subclavian artery**

   ✓6ᵗʰ **S25.12** Major laceration **of innominate or subclavian artery**
Complete transection of innominate or subclavian artery
Traumatic rupture of innominate or subclavian artery

     ✓7ᵗʰ **S25.121** **Major laceration of** right **innominate or subclavian artery**

     ✓7ᵗʰ **S25.122** **Major laceration of** left **innominate or subclavian artery**

     ✓7ᵗʰ **S25.129** **Major laceration of unspecified** ▽ **innominate or subclavian artery**

   ✓6ᵗʰ **S25.19** Other **specified injury of innominate or subclavian artery**

     ✓7ᵗʰ **S25.191** **Other specified injury of** right **innominate or subclavian artery**

     ✓7ᵗʰ **S25.192** **Other specified injury of** left **innominate or subclavian artery**

     ✓7ᵗʰ **S25.199** **Other specified injury of unspecified** ▽ **innominate or subclavian artery**

✓5ᵗʰ **S25.2** **Injury of** superior vena cava
Injury of vena cava NOS

   ✓x7ᵗʰ **S25.20** **Unspecified injury of superior vena cava** ▽

   ✓x7ᵗʰ **S25.21** Minor laceration **of superior vena cava**
Incomplete transection of superior vena cava
Laceration of superior vena cava NOS
Superficial laceration of superior vena cava

   ✓x7ᵗʰ **S25.22** Major laceration **of superior vena cava**
Complete transection of superior vena cava
Traumatic rupture of superior vena cava

   ✓x7ᵗʰ **S25.29** **Other specified injury of superior vena cava**

✓5ᵗʰ **S25.3** **Injury of** innominate or subclavian vein

   ✓6ᵗʰ **S25.30** Unspecified **injury of innominate or subclavian vein**

     ✓7ᵗʰ **S25.301** **Unspecified injury of** right **innominate** ▽ **or subclavian vein**

     ✓7ᵗʰ **S25.302** **Unspecified injury of** left **innominate** ▽ **or subclavian vein**

     ✓7ᵗʰ **S25.309** **Unspecified injury of unspecified** ▽ **innominate or subclavian vein**

   ✓6ᵗʰ **S25.31** Minor laceration **of innominate or subclavian vein**
Incomplete transection of innominate or subclavian vein
Laceration of innominate or subclavian vein NOS
Superficial laceration of innominate or subclavian vein

     ✓7ᵗʰ **S25.311** **Minor laceration of** right **innominate or subclavian vein**

     ✓7ᵗʰ **S25.312** **Minor laceration of** left **innominate or subclavian vein**

     ✓7ᵗʰ **S25.319** **Minor laceration of unspecified** ▽ **innominate or subclavian vein**

   ✓6ᵗʰ **S25.32** Major laceration **of innominate or subclavian vein**
Complete transection of innominate or subclavian vein
Traumatic rupture of innominate or subclavian vein

     ✓7ᵗʰ **S25.321** **Major laceration of** right **innominate or subclavian vein**

     ✓7ᵗʰ **S25.322** **Major laceration of** left **innominate or subclavian vein**

     ✓7ᵗʰ **S25.329** **Major laceration of unspecified** ▽ **innominate or subclavian vein**

Ⓝ Newborn   Ⓟ Pediatric   Ⓜ Maternity   Ⓐ Adult   **RIC** RIC Dx   **NCDx** Noncancer Dx   **PDx** Primary Dx   **CC** RIC CC Condition   ▶◀ Revised Text   ● New Code   ▲ Revised Code Title

880   ICD-10-CM 2016

✓6th **S25.39** Other specified injury of innominate or subclavian vein

    ✓7th **S25.391** Other specified injury of right innominate or subclavian vein

    ✓7th **S25.392** Other specified injury of left innominate or subclavian vein

    ✓7th **S25.399** Other specified injury of unspecified innominate or subclavian vein ▽

✓5th **S25.4** Injury of pulmonary blood vessels

    ✓6th **S25.40** Unspecified injury of pulmonary blood vessels

      ✓7th **S25.401** Unspecified injury of right pulmonary blood vessels ▽

      ✓7th **S25.402** Unspecified injury of left pulmonary blood vessels ▽

      ✓7th **S25.409** Unspecified injury of unspecified pulmonary blood vessels ▽

    ✓6th **S25.41** Minor laceration of pulmonary blood vessels
      Incomplete transection of pulmonary blood vessels
      Laceration of pulmonary blood vessels NOS
      Superficial laceration of pulmonary blood vessels

      ✓7th **S25.411** Minor laceration of right pulmonary blood vessels

      ✓7th **S25.412** Minor laceration of left pulmonary blood vessels

      ✓7th **S25.419** Minor laceration of unspecified pulmonary blood vessels ▽

    ✓6th **S25.42** Major laceration of pulmonary blood vessels
      Complete transection of pulmonary blood vessels
      Traumatic rupture of pulmonary blood vessels

      ✓7th **S25.421** Major laceration of right pulmonary blood vessels

      ✓7th **S25.422** Major laceration of left pulmonary blood vessels

      ✓7th **S25.429** Major laceration of unspecified pulmonary blood vessels ▽

    ✓6th **S25.49** Other specified injury of pulmonary blood vessels

      ✓7th **S25.491** Other specified injury of right pulmonary blood vessels

      ✓7th **S25.492** Other specified injury of left pulmonary blood vessels

      ✓7th **S25.499** Other specified injury of unspecified pulmonary blood vessels ▽

✓5th **S25.5** Injury of intercostal blood vessels

    ✓6th **S25.50** Unspecified injury of intercostal blood vessels

      ✓7th **S25.501** Unspecified injury of intercostal blood vessels, right side ▽

      ✓7th **S25.502** Unspecified injury of intercostal blood vessels, left side ▽

      ✓7th **S25.509** Unspecified injury of intercostal blood vessels, unspecified side ▽

    ✓6th **S25.51** Laceration of intercostal blood vessels

      ✓7th **S25.511** Laceration of intercostal blood vessels, right side

      ✓7th **S25.512** Laceration of intercostal blood vessels, left side

      ✓7th **S25.519** Laceration of intercostal blood vessels, unspecified side ▽

    ✓6th **S25.59** Other specified injury of intercostal blood vessels

      ✓7th **S25.591** Other specified injury of intercostal blood vessels, right side

      ✓7th **S25.592** Other specified injury of intercostal blood vessels, left side

      ✓7th **S25.599** Other specified injury of intercostal blood vessels, unspecified side ▽

✓5th **S25.8** Injury of other blood vessels of thorax
    Injury of azygos vein   Injury of mammary artery or vein

    ✓6th **S25.80** Unspecified injury of other blood vessels of thorax

      ✓7th **S25.801** Unspecified injury of other blood vessels of thorax, right side ▽

      ✓7th **S25.802** Unspecified injury of other blood vessels of thorax, left side ▽

      ✓7th **S25.809** Unspecified injury of other blood vessels of thorax, unspecified side ▽

✓6th **S25.81** Laceration of other blood vessels of thorax

    ✓7th **S25.811** Laceration of other blood vessels of thorax, right side

    ✓7th **S25.812** Laceration of other blood vessels of thorax, left side

    ✓7th **S25.819** Laceration of other blood vessels of thorax, unspecified side ▽

✓6th **S25.89** Other specified injury of other blood vessels of thorax

    ✓7th **S25.891** Other specified injury of other blood vessels of thorax, right side

    ✓7th **S25.892** Other specified injury of other blood vessels of thorax, left side

    ✓7th **S25.899** Other specified injury of other blood vessels of thorax, unspecified side ▽

✓5th **S25.9** Injury of unspecified blood vessel of thorax

    ✓x7th **S25.90** Unspecified injury of unspecified blood vessel of thorax ▽

    ✓x7th **S25.91** Laceration of unspecified blood vessel of thorax ▽

    ✓x7th **S25.99** Other specified injury of unspecified blood vessel of thorax ▽

✓4th **S26** Injury of heart
    Code also any associated:
      open wound of thorax (S21.-)
      traumatic hemopneumothorax (S27.2)
      traumatic hemothorax (S27.1)
      traumatic pneumothorax (S27.0)

> The appropriate 7th character is to be added to each code from category S26.
> A   initial encounter
> D   subsequent encounter
> S   sequela

✓5th **S26.0** Injury of heart with hemopericardium

    ✓x7th **S26.00** Unspecified injury of heart with hemopericardium ▽

    ✓x7th **S26.01** Contusion of heart with hemopericardium

    ✓6th **S26.02** Laceration of heart with hemopericardium

      ✓7th **S26.020** Mild laceration of heart with hemopericardium
        Laceration of heart without penetration of heart chamber

      ✓7th **S26.021** Moderate laceration of heart with hemopericardium
        Laceration of heart with penetration of heart chamber

      ✓7th **S26.022** Major laceration of heart with hemopericardium
        Laceration of heart with penetration of multiple heart chambers

    ✓x7th **S26.09** Other injury of heart with hemopericardium

✓5th **S26.1** Injury of heart without hemopericardium

    ✓x7th **S26.10** Unspecified injury of heart without hemopericardium ▽

    ✓x7th **S26.11** Contusion of heart without hemopericardium

    ✓x7th **S26.12** Laceration of heart without hemopericardium

    ✓x7th **S26.19** Other injury of heart without hemopericardium

✓5th **S26.9** Injury of heart, unspecified with or without hemopericardium

    ✓x7th **S26.90** Unspecified injury of heart, unspecified with or without hemopericardium ▽

    ✓x7th **S26.91** Contusion of heart, unspecified with or without hemopericardium ▽

    ✓x7th **S26.92** Laceration of heart, unspecified with or without hemopericardium ▽
      Laceration of heart NOS

    ✓x7th **S26.99** Other injury of heart, unspecified with or without hemopericardium ▽

☑ Add'l Character Required   ✓x7th Placeholder Alert   RUG IV Special Care High Dx   RUG IV Clinically Complex Dx   RUG IV Special Care Low Dx   Manifestation Code   Other Specified Code   ▽ Unspecified Code

Chapter 19. Injury, Poisoning and Certain Other Consequences of External Causes

☑4ᵗʰ **S27 Injury of other and unspecified intrathoracic organs**
Code also any associated open wound of thorax (S21.-)
EXCLUDES 2   injury of cervical esophagus (S10-S19)
          injury of trachea (cervical) (S10-S19)

> The appropriate 7th character is to be added to each code from category S27.
> A   initial encounter
> D   subsequent encounter
> S   sequela

☑x7ᵗʰ **S27.0 Traumatic pneumothorax**
     EXCLUDES 1   spontaneous pneumothorax (J93.-)

☑x7ᵗʰ **S27.1 Traumatic hemothorax**

☑x7ᵗʰ **S27.2 Traumatic hemopneumothorax**

☑5ᵗʰ **S27.3 Other and unspecified injuries of lung**

    ☑6ᵗʰ **S27.30 Unspecified injury of lung**
       ☑7ᵗʰ **S27.301 Unspecified injury of lung, unilateral** ▽
       ☑7ᵗʰ **S27.302 Unspecified injury of lung, bilateral** ▽
       ☑7ᵗʰ **S27.309 Unspecified injury of lung, unspecified** ▽

    ☑6ᵗʰ **S27.31 Primary blast injury of lung**
         Blast injury of lung NOS
       ☑7ᵗʰ **S27.311 Primary blast injury of lung, unilateral**
       ☑7ᵗʰ **S27.312 Primary blast injury of lung, bilateral**
       ☑7ᵗʰ **S27.319 Primary blast injury of lung, unspecified** ▽

    ☑6ᵗʰ **S27.32 Contusion of lung**
       ☑7ᵗʰ **S27.321 Contusion of lung, unilateral**
       ☑7ᵗʰ **S27.322 Contusion of lung, bilateral**
       ☑7ᵗʰ **S27.329 Contusion of lung, unspecified** ▽

    ☑6ᵗʰ **S27.33 Laceration of lung**
       ☑7ᵗʰ **S27.331 Laceration of lung, unilateral**
       ☑7ᵗʰ **S27.332 Laceration of lung, bilateral**
       ☑7ᵗʰ **S27.339 Laceration of lung, unspecified** ▽

    ☑6ᵗʰ **S27.39 Other injuries of lung**
         Secondary blast injury of lung
       ☑7ᵗʰ **S27.391 Other injuries of lung, unilateral**
       ☑7ᵗʰ **S27.392 Other injuries of lung, bilateral**
       ☑7ᵗʰ **S27.399 Other injuries of lung, unspecified** ▽

☑5ᵗʰ **S27.4 Injury of bronchus**

    ☑6ᵗʰ **S27.40 Unspecified injury of bronchus**
       ☑7ᵗʰ **S27.401 Unspecified injury of bronchus, unilateral** ▽
       ☑7ᵗʰ **S27.402 Unspecified injury of bronchus, bilateral** ▽
       ☑7ᵗʰ **S27.409 Unspecified injury of bronchus, unspecified** ▽

    ☑6ᵗʰ **S27.41 Primary blast injury of bronchus**
         Blast injury of bronchus NOS
       ☑7ᵗʰ **S27.411 Primary blast injury of bronchus, unilateral**
       ☑7ᵗʰ **S27.412 Primary blast injury of bronchus, bilateral**
       ☑7ᵗʰ **S27.419 Primary blast injury of bronchus, unspecified** ▽

    ☑6ᵗʰ **S27.42 Contusion of bronchus**
       ☑7ᵗʰ **S27.421 Contusion of bronchus, unilateral**
       ☑7ᵗʰ **S27.422 Contusion of bronchus, bilateral**
       ☑7ᵗʰ **S27.429 Contusion of bronchus, unspecified** ▽

    ☑6ᵗʰ **S27.43 Laceration of bronchus**
       ☑7ᵗʰ **S27.431 Laceration of bronchus, unilateral**
       ☑7ᵗʰ **S27.432 Laceration of bronchus, bilateral**
       ☑7ᵗʰ **S27.439 Laceration of bronchus, unspecified** ▽

    ☑6ᵗʰ **S27.49 Other injury of bronchus**
         Secondary blast injury of bronchus
       ☑7ᵗʰ **S27.491 Other injury of bronchus, unilateral**
       ☑7ᵗʰ **S27.492 Other injury of bronchus, bilateral**
       ☑7ᵗʰ **S27.499 Other injury of bronchus, unspecified** ▽

☑5ᵗʰ **S27.5 Injury of thoracic trachea**

    ☑x7ᵗʰ **S27.50 Unspecified injury of thoracic trachea** ▽

    ☑x7ᵗʰ **S27.51 Primary blast injury of thoracic trachea**
         Blast injury of thoracic trachea NOS

☑x7ᵗʰ **S27.52 Contusion of thoracic trachea**

☑x7ᵗʰ **S27.53 Laceration of thoracic trachea**

☑x7ᵗʰ **S27.59 Other injury of thoracic trachea**
         Secondary blast injury of thoracic trachea

☑5ᵗʰ **S27.6 Injury of pleura**

    ☑x7ᵗʰ **S27.60 Unspecified injury of pleura** ▽

    ☑x7ᵗʰ **S27.63 Laceration of pleura**

    ☑x7ᵗʰ **S27.69 Other injury of pleura**

☑5ᵗʰ **S27.8 Injury of other specified intrathoracic organs**

    ☑6ᵗʰ **S27.80 Injury of diaphragm**
       ☑7ᵗʰ **S27.802 Contusion of diaphragm**
       ☑7ᵗʰ **S27.803 Laceration of diaphragm**
       ☑7ᵗʰ **S27.808 Other injury of diaphragm**
       ☑7ᵗʰ **S27.809 Unspecified injury of diaphragm** ▽

    ☑6ᵗʰ **S27.81 Injury of esophagus (thoracic part)**
       ☑7ᵗʰ **S27.812 Contusion of esophagus (thoracic part)**
       ☑7ᵗʰ **S27.813 Laceration of esophagus (thoracic part)**
       ☑7ᵗʰ **S27.818 Other injury of esophagus (thoracic part)**
       ☑7ᵗʰ **S27.819 Unspecified injury of esophagus (thoracic part)** ▽

    ☑6ᵗʰ **S27.89 Injury of other specified intrathoracic organs**
         Injury of lymphatic thoracic duct
         Injury of thymus gland
       ☑7ᵗʰ **S27.892 Contusion of other specified intrathoracic organs**
       ☑7ᵗʰ **S27.893 Laceration of other specified intrathoracic organs**
       ☑7ᵗʰ **S27.898 Other injury of other specified intrathoracic organs**
       ☑7ᵗʰ **S27.899 Unspecified injury of other specified intrathoracic organs** ▽

☑x7ᵗʰ **S27.9 Injury of unspecified intrathoracic organ** ▽

☑4ᵗʰ **S28 Crushing injury of thorax, and traumatic amputation of part of thorax**

> The appropriate 7th character is to be added to each code from category S28.
> A   initial encounter
> D   subsequent encounter
> S   sequela

☑x7ᵗʰ **S28.0 Crushed chest**
     Use additional code for all associated injuries
     EXCLUDES 1   flail chest (S22.5)

☑x7ᵗʰ **S28.1 Traumatic amputation (partial) of part of thorax, except breast**

☑5ᵗʰ **S28.2 Traumatic amputation of breast**

    ☑6ᵗʰ **S28.21 Complete traumatic amputation of breast**
         Traumatic amputation of breast NOS
       ☑7ᵗʰ **S28.211 Complete traumatic amputation of right breast**
       ☑7ᵗʰ **S28.212 Complete traumatic amputation of left breast**
       ☑7ᵗʰ **S28.219 Complete traumatic amputation of unspecified breast** ▽

    ☑6ᵗʰ **S28.22 Partial traumatic amputation of breast**
       ☑7ᵗʰ **S28.221 Partial traumatic amputation of right breast**
       ☑7ᵗʰ **S28.222 Partial traumatic amputation of left breast**
       ☑7ᵗʰ **S28.229 Partial traumatic amputation of unspecified breast** ▽

☑4ᵗʰ **S29 Other and unspecified injuries of thorax**
Code also any associated open wound (S21.-)

> The appropriate 7th character is to be added to each code from category S29.
> A   initial encounter
> D   subsequent encounter
> S   sequela

☑5ᵗʰ **S29.0 Injury of muscle and tendon at thorax level**

    ☑6ᵗʰ **S29.00 Unspecified injury of muscle and tendon of thorax**
       ☑7ᵗʰ **S29.001 Unspecified injury of muscle and tendon of front wall of thorax** ▽

Ⓝ Newborn   Ⓟ Pediatric   Ⓜ Maternity   Ⓐ Adult   RIC RIC Dx   NCDx Noncancer Dx   PDx Primary Dx   CC RIC CC Condition   ►◄ Revised Text   ● New Code   ▲ Revised Code Title

882   ICD-10-CM 2016

✓7ᵗʰ **S29.002** Unspecified injury of muscle and tendon of back wall of thorax ▽

✓7ᵗʰ **S29.009** Unspecified injury of muscle and tendon of unspecified wall of thorax ▽

✓6ᵗʰ **S29.01** Strain of muscle and tendon of thorax

    ✓7ᵗʰ **S29.011** Strain of muscle and tendon of front wall of thorax

    ✓7ᵗʰ **S29.012** Strain of muscle and tendon of back wall of thorax

    ✓7ᵗʰ **S29.019** Strain of muscle and tendon of unspecified wall of thorax ▽

✓6ᵗʰ **S29.02** Laceration of muscle and tendon of thorax

    ✓7ᵗʰ **S29.021** Laceration of muscle and tendon of front wall of thorax

    ✓7ᵗʰ **S29.022** Laceration of muscle and tendon of back wall of thorax

    ✓7ᵗʰ **S29.029** Laceration of muscle and tendon of unspecified wall of thorax ▽

✓6ᵗʰ **S29.09** Other injury of muscle and tendon of thorax

    ✓7ᵗʰ **S29.091** Other injury of muscle and tendon of front wall of thorax

    ✓7ᵗʰ **S29.092** Other injury of muscle and tendon of back wall of thorax

    ✓7ᵗʰ **S29.099** Other injury of muscle and tendon of unspecified wall of thorax ▽

✓x7ᵗʰ **S29.8** Other specified injuries of thorax

✓x7ᵗʰ **S29.9** Unspecified injury of thorax ▽

Injuries to the abdomen, lower back, lumbar spine, pelvis and external genitals (S30-S39)

INCLUDES injuries to the abdominal wall
injuries to the anus
injuries to the buttock
injuries to the external genitalia
injuries to the flank
injuries to the groin

EXCLUDES 2 *burns and corrosions (T20-T32)*
effects of foreign body in anus and rectum (T18.5)
effects of foreign body in genitourinary tract (T19.-)
effects of foreign body in stomach, small intestine and colon (T18.2-T18.4)
frostbite (T33-T34)
insect bite or sting, venomous (T63.4)

✓4ᵗʰ **S30** Superficial injury of abdomen, lower back, pelvis and external genitals

    EXCLUDES 2 *superficial injury of hip (S70.-)*

The appropriate 7th character is to be added to each code from category S30.
A   initial encounter
D   subsequent encounter
S   sequela

✓x7ᵗʰ **S30.0** Contusion of lower back and pelvis
    Contusion of buttock

✓x7ᵗʰ **S30.1** Contusion of abdominal wall
    Contusion of flank   Contusion of groin

✓5ᵗʰ **S30.2** Contusion of external genital organs

  ✓6ᵗʰ **S30.20** Contusion of unspecified external genital organ

    ✓7ᵗʰ **S30.201** Contusion of unspecified external genital organ, male ♂▽

    ✓7ᵗʰ **S30.202** Contusion of unspecified external genital organ, female ♀▽

  ✓x7ᵗʰ **S30.21** Contusion of penis ♂

  ✓x7ᵗʰ **S30.22** Contusion of scrotum and testes ♂

  ✓x7ᵗʰ **S30.23** Contusion of vagina and vulva ♀

✓x7ᵗʰ **S30.3** Contusion of anus

✓5ᵗʰ **S30.8** Other superficial injuries of abdomen, lower back, pelvis and external genitals

  ✓6ᵗʰ **S30.81** Abrasion of abdomen, lower back, pelvis and external genitals

    ✓7ᵗʰ **S30.810** Abrasion of lower back and pelvis

    ✓7ᵗʰ **S30.811** Abrasion of abdominal wall

    ✓7ᵗʰ **S30.812** Abrasion of penis ♂

    ✓7ᵗʰ **S30.813** Abrasion of scrotum and testes ♂

    ✓7ᵗʰ **S30.814** Abrasion of vagina and vulva ♀

    ✓7ᵗʰ **S30.815** Abrasion of unspecified external genital organs, male ♂▽

    ✓7ᵗʰ **S30.816** Abrasion of unspecified external genital organs, female ♀▽

    ✓7ᵗʰ **S30.817** Abrasion of anus

  ✓6ᵗʰ **S30.82** Blister (nonthermal) of abdomen, lower back, pelvis and external genitals

    ✓7ᵗʰ **S30.820** Blister (nonthermal) of lower back and pelvis

    ✓7ᵗʰ **S30.821** Blister (nonthermal) of abdominal wall

    ✓7ᵗʰ **S30.822** Blister (nonthermal) of penis ♂

    ✓7ᵗʰ **S30.823** Blister (nonthermal) of scrotum and testes ♂

    ✓7ᵗʰ **S30.824** Blister (nonthermal) of vagina and vulva ♀

    ✓7ᵗʰ **S30.825** Blister (nonthermal) of unspecified external genital organs, male ♂▽

    ✓7ᵗʰ **S30.826** Blister (nonthermal) of unspecified external genital organs, female ♀▽

    ✓7ᵗʰ **S30.827** Blister (nonthermal) of anus

  ✓6ᵗʰ **S30.84** External constriction of abdomen, lower back, pelvis and external genitals

    ✓7ᵗʰ **S30.840** External constriction of lower back and pelvis

    ✓7ᵗʰ **S30.841** External constriction of abdominal wall

    ✓7ᵗʰ **S30.842** External constriction of penis ♂
        Hair tourniquet syndrome of penis
        Use additional cause code to identify the constricting item (W49.0-)

    ✓7ᵗʰ **S30.843** External constriction of scrotum and testes ♂

    ✓7ᵗʰ **S30.844** External constriction of vagina and vulva ♀

    ✓7ᵗʰ **S30.845** External constriction of unspecified external genital organs, male ♂▽

    ✓7ᵗʰ **S30.846** External constriction of unspecified external genital organs, female ♀▽

  ✓6ᵗʰ **S30.85** Superficial foreign body of abdomen, lower back, pelvis and external genitals
    Splinter in the abdomen, lower back, pelvis and external genitals

    ✓7ᵗʰ **S30.850** Superficial foreign body of lower back and pelvis

    ✓7ᵗʰ **S30.851** Superficial foreign body of abdominal wall

    ✓7ᵗʰ **S30.852** Superficial foreign body of penis ♂

    ✓7ᵗʰ **S30.853** Superficial foreign body of scrotum and testes ♂

    ✓7ᵗʰ **S30.854** Superficial foreign body of vagina and vulva ♀

    ✓7ᵗʰ **S30.855** Superficial foreign body of unspecified external genital organs, male ♂▽

    ✓7ᵗʰ **S30.856** Superficial foreign body of unspecified external genital organs, female ♀▽

    ✓7ᵗʰ **S30.857** Superficial foreign body of anus

  ✓6ᵗʰ **S30.86** Insect bite (nonvenomous) of abdomen, lower back, pelvis and external genitals

    ✓7ᵗʰ **S30.860** Insect bite (nonvenomous) of lower back and pelvis

    ✓7ᵗʰ **S30.861** Insect bite (nonvenomous) of abdominal wall

    ✓7ᵗʰ **S30.862** Insect bite (nonvenomous) of penis ♂

    ✓7ᵗʰ **S30.863** Insect bite (nonvenomous) of scrotum and testes ♂

    ✓7ᵗʰ **S30.864** Insect bite (nonvenomous) of vagina and vulva ♀

    ✓7ᵗʰ **S30.865** Insect bite (nonvenomous) of unspecified external genital organs, male ♂▽

    ✓7ᵗʰ **S30.866** Insect bite (nonvenomous) of unspecified external genital organs, female ♀▽

    ✓7ᵗʰ **S30.867** Insect bite (nonvenomous) of anus

✓ Add'l Character Required ✓x7ᵗʰ Placeholder Alert RUG IV Special Care High Dx RUG IV Clinically Complex Dx RUG IV Special Care Low Dx Manifestation Code Other Specified Code ▽ Unspecified Code

√6ᵗʰ **S30.87** Other superficial bite of abdomen, lower back, pelvis and external genitals
> **EXCLUDES 1**   open bite of abdomen, lower back, pelvis and external genitals (S31.05, S31.15, S31.25, S31.35, S31.45, S31.55)

√7ᵗʰ **S30.870** Other superficial bite of lower back and pelvis

√7ᵗʰ **S30.871** Other superficial bite of abdominal wall

√7ᵗʰ **S30.872** Other superficial bite of penis   ♂

√7ᵗʰ **S30.873** Other superficial bite of scrotum and testes   ♂

√7ᵗʰ **S30.874** Other superficial bite of vagina and vulva   ♀

√7ᵗʰ **S30.875** Other superficial bite of unspecified external genital organs, male   ♂▽

√7ᵗʰ **S30.876** Other superficial bite of unspecified external genital organs, female   ♀▽

√7ᵗʰ **S30.877** Other superficial bite of anus

√5ᵗʰ **S30.9** Unspecified superficial injury of abdomen, lower back, pelvis and external genitals

√x7ᵗʰ **S30.91** Unspecified superficial injury of lower back and pelvis   ▽

√x7ᵗʰ **S30.92** Unspecified superficial injury of abdominal wall   ▽

√x7ᵗʰ **S30.93** Unspecified superficial injury of penis   ♂▽

√x7ᵗʰ **S30.94** Unspecified superficial injury of scrotum and testes   ♂▽

√x7ᵗʰ **S30.95** Unspecified superficial injury of vagina and vulva   ♀▽

√x7ᵗʰ **S30.96** Unspecified superficial injury of unspecified external genital organs, male   ♂▽

√x7ᵗʰ **S30.97** Unspecified superficial injury of unspecified external genital organs, female   ♀▽

√x7ᵗʰ **S30.98** Unspecified superficial injury of anus   ▽

√4ᵗʰ **S31** Open wound of abdomen, lower back, pelvis and external genitals
> Code also any associated:
>   spinal cord injury (S24.0, S24.1-, S34.0-, S34.1-)
>   wound infection
> **EXCLUDES 1**   traumatic amputation of part of abdomen, lower back and pelvis (S38.2-, S38.3)
> **EXCLUDES 2**   open wound of hip (S71.00-S71.02)
>   open fracture of pelvis (S32.1- -S32.9 with 7th character B)

> The appropriate 7th character is to be added to each code from category S31.
> A   initial encounter
> D   subsequent encounter
> S   sequela

√5ᵗʰ **S31.0** Open wound of lower back and pelvis

√6ᵗʰ **S31.00** Unspecified open wound of lower back and pelvis

√7ᵗʰ **S31.000** Unspecified open wound of lower back and pelvis without penetration into retroperitoneum   ▽
> Unspecified open wound of lower back and pelvis NOS

√7ᵗʰ **S31.001** Unspecified open wound of lower back and pelvis with penetration into retroperitoneum   ▽

√6ᵗʰ **S31.01** Laceration without foreign body of lower back and pelvis

√7ᵗʰ **S31.010** Laceration without foreign body of lower back and pelvis without penetration into retroperitoneum
> Laceration without foreign body of lower back and pelvis NOS

√7ᵗʰ **S31.011** Laceration without foreign body of lower back and pelvis with penetration into retroperitoneum

√6ᵗʰ **S31.02** Laceration with foreign body of lower back and pelvis

√7ᵗʰ **S31.020** Laceration with foreign body of lower back and pelvis without penetration into retroperitoneum
> Laceration with foreign body of lower back and pelvis NOS

√7ᵗʰ **S31.021** Laceration with foreign body of lower back and pelvis with penetration into retroperitoneum

√6ᵗʰ **S31.03** Puncture wound without foreign body of lower back and pelvis

√7ᵗʰ **S31.030** Puncture wound without foreign body of lower back and pelvis without penetration into retroperitoneum
> Puncture wound without foreign body of lower back and pelvis NOS

√7ᵗʰ **S31.031** Puncture wound without foreign body of lower back and pelvis with penetration into retroperitoneum

√6ᵗʰ **S31.04** Puncture wound with foreign body of lower back and pelvis

√7ᵗʰ **S31.040** Puncture wound with foreign body of lower back and pelvis without penetration into retroperitoneum
> Puncture wound with foreign body of lower back and pelvis NOS

√7ᵗʰ **S31.041** Puncture wound with foreign body of lower back and pelvis with penetration into retroperitoneum

√6ᵗʰ **S31.05** Open bite of lower back and pelvis
> Bite of lower back and pelvis NOS
> **EXCLUDES 1**   superficial bite of lower back and pelvis (S30.860, S30.870)

√7ᵗʰ **S31.050** Open bite of lower back and pelvis without penetration into retroperitoneum
> Open bite of lower back and pelvis NOS

√7ᵗʰ **S31.051** Open bite of lower back and pelvis with penetration into retroperitoneum

√5ᵗʰ **S31.1** Open wound of abdominal wall without penetration into peritoneal cavity
> Open wound of abdominal wall NOS
> **EXCLUDES 2**   open wound of abdominal wall with penetration into peritoneal cavity (S31.6-)

√6ᵗʰ **S31.10** Unspecified open wound of abdominal wall without penetration into peritoneal cavity

√7ᵗʰ **S31.100** Unspecified open wound of abdominal wall, right upper quadrant without penetration into peritoneal cavity   ▽

√7ᵗʰ **S31.101** Unspecified open wound of abdominal wall, left upper quadrant without penetration into peritoneal cavity   ▽

√7ᵗʰ **S31.102** Unspecified open wound of abdominal wall, epigastric region without penetration into peritoneal cavity   ▽

√7ᵗʰ **S31.103** Unspecified open wound of abdominal wall, right lower quadrant without penetration into peritoneal cavity   ▽

√7ᵗʰ **S31.104** Unspecified open wound of abdominal wall, left lower quadrant without penetration into peritoneal cavity   ▽

√7ᵗʰ **S31.105** Unspecified open wound of abdominal wall, periumbilic region without penetration into peritoneal cavity   ▽

√7ᵗʰ **S31.109** Unspecified open wound of abdominal wall, unspecified quadrant without penetration into peritoneal cavity   ▽
> Unspecified open wound of abdominal wall NOS

√6ᵗʰ **S31.11** Laceration without foreign body of abdominal wall without penetration into peritoneal cavity

√7ᵗʰ **S31.110** Laceration without foreign body of abdominal wall, right upper quadrant without penetration into peritoneal cavity

√7ᵗʰ **S31.111** Laceration without foreign body of abdominal wall, left upper quadrant without penetration into peritoneal cavity

√7ᵗʰ **S31.112** Laceration without foreign body of abdominal wall, epigastric region without penetration into peritoneal cavity

√7ᵗʰ **S31.113** Laceration without foreign body of abdominal wall, right lower quadrant without penetration into peritoneal cavity

√7ᵗʰ **S31.114** Laceration without foreign body of abdominal wall, left lower quadrant without penetration into peritoneal cavity

√7ᵗʰ **S31.115** **Laceration without foreign body of abdominal wall,** periumbilic region **without penetration into peritoneal cavity**

√7ᵗʰ **S31.119** **Laceration without foreign body of** ▽ **abdominal wall, unspecified quadrant without penetration into peritoneal cavity**

√6ᵗʰ **S31.12** Laceration with foreign body of abdominal wall without penetration into peritoneal cavity

√7ᵗʰ **S31.120** **Laceration of abdominal wall with foreign body,** right upper quadrant **without penetration into peritoneal cavity**

√7ᵗʰ **S31.121** **Laceration of abdominal wall with foreign body,** left upper quadrant **without penetration into peritoneal cavity**

√7ᵗʰ **S31.122** **Laceration of abdominal wall with foreign body,** epigastric region **without penetration into peritoneal cavity**

√7ᵗʰ **S31.123** **Laceration of abdominal wall with foreign body,** right lower quadrant **without penetration into peritoneal cavity**

√7ᵗʰ **S31.124** **Laceration of abdominal wall with foreign body,** left lower quadrant **without penetration into peritoneal cavity**

√7ᵗʰ **S31.125** **Laceration of abdominal wall with foreign body,** periumbilic region **without penetration into peritoneal cavity**

√7ᵗʰ **S31.129** **Laceration of abdominal wall with** ▽ **foreign body, unspecified quadrant without penetration into peritoneal cavity**

√6ᵗʰ **S31.13** Puncture wound of abdominal wall without foreign body without penetration into peritoneal cavity

√7ᵗʰ **S31.130** **Puncture wound of abdominal wall without foreign body,** right upper quadrant **without penetration into peritoneal cavity**

√7ᵗʰ **S31.131** **Puncture wound of abdominal wall without foreign body,** left upper quadrant **without penetration into peritoneal cavity**

√7ᵗʰ **S31.132** **Puncture wound of abdominal wall without foreign body,** epigastric region **without penetration into peritoneal cavity**

√7ᵗʰ **S31.133** **Puncture wound of abdominal wall without foreign body,** right lower quadrant **without penetration into peritoneal cavity**

√7ᵗʰ **S31.134** **Puncture wound of abdominal wall without foreign body,** left lower quadrant **without penetration into peritoneal cavity**

√7ᵗʰ **S31.135** **Puncture wound of abdominal wall without foreign body,** periumbilic region **without penetration into peritoneal cavity**

√7ᵗʰ **S31.139** **Puncture wound of abdominal wall** ▽ **without foreign body, unspecified quadrant without penetration into peritoneal cavity**

√6ᵗʰ **S31.14** Puncture wound of abdominal wall with foreign body without penetration into peritoneal cavity

√7ᵗʰ **S31.140** **Puncture wound of abdominal wall with foreign body,** right upper quadrant **without penetration into peritoneal cavity**

√7ᵗʰ **S31.141** **Puncture wound of abdominal wall with foreign body,** left upper quadrant **without penetration into peritoneal cavity**

√7ᵗʰ **S31.142** **Puncture wound of abdominal wall with foreign body,** epigastric region **without penetration into peritoneal cavity**

√7ᵗʰ **S31.143** **Puncture wound of abdominal wall with foreign body,** right lower quadrant **without penetration into peritoneal cavity**

√7ᵗʰ **S31.144** **Puncture wound of abdominal wall with foreign body,** left lower quadrant **without penetration into peritoneal cavity**

√7ᵗʰ **S31.145** **Puncture wound of abdominal wall with foreign body,** periumbilic region **without penetration into peritoneal cavity**

√7ᵗʰ **S31.149** **Puncture wound of abdominal wall** ▽ **with foreign body, unspecified quadrant without penetration into peritoneal cavity**

√6ᵗʰ **S31.15** Open bite of abdominal wall without penetration into peritoneal cavity
Bite of abdominal wall NOS
EXCLUDES 1 *superficial bite of abdominal wall (S30.871)*

√7ᵗʰ **S31.150** **Open bite of abdominal wall,** right upper quadrant **without penetration into peritoneal cavity**

√7ᵗʰ **S31.151** **Open bite of abdominal wall,** left upper quadrant **without penetration into peritoneal cavity**

√7ᵗʰ **S31.152** **Open bite of abdominal wall,** epigastric region **without penetration into peritoneal cavity**

√7ᵗʰ **S31.153** **Open bite of abdominal wall,** right lower quadrant **without penetration into peritoneal cavity**

√7ᵗʰ **S31.154** **Open bite of abdominal wall,** left lower quadrant **without penetration into peritoneal cavity**

√7ᵗʰ **S31.155** **Open bite of abdominal wall,** periumbilic region **without penetration into peritoneal cavity**

√7ᵗʰ **S31.159** **Open bite of abdominal wall,** ▽ **unspecified quadrant without penetration into peritoneal cavity**

√5ᵗʰ **S31.2** Open wound of penis

√x7ᵗʰ **S31.20** **Unspecified open wound of penis** ♂▽

√x7ᵗʰ **S31.21** Laceration without foreign body **of penis** ♂

√x7ᵗʰ **S31.22** Laceration with foreign body **of penis** ♂

√x7ᵗʰ **S31.23** Puncture wound without foreign body **of penis** ♂

√x7ᵗʰ **S31.24** Puncture wound with foreign body **of penis** ♂

√x7ᵗʰ **S31.25** Open bite **of penis** ♂
Bite of penis NOS
EXCLUDES 1 *superficial bite of penis (S30.862, S30.872)*

√5ᵗʰ **S31.3** Open wound of scrotum and testes

√x7ᵗʰ **S31.30** **Unspecified open wound of scrotum and testes** ♂▽

√x7ᵗʰ **S31.31** Laceration without foreign body **of scrotum** ♂ **and testes**

√x7ᵗʰ **S31.32** Laceration with foreign body **of scrotum and** ♂ **testes**

√x7ᵗʰ **S31.33** Puncture wound without foreign body **of** ♂ **scrotum and testes**

√x7ᵗʰ **S31.34** Puncture wound with foreign body **of scrotum** ♂ **and testes**

√x7ᵗʰ **S31.35** Open bite **of scrotum and testes** ♂
Bite of scrotum and testes NOS
EXCLUDES 1 *superficial bite of scrotum and testes (S30.863, S30.873)*

√5ᵗʰ **S31.4** Open wound of vagina and vulva
EXCLUDES 1 *injury to vagina and vulva during delivery (O70-, O71.4)*

√x7ᵗʰ **S31.40** **Unspecified open wound of vagina and vulva** ♀▽

√x7ᵗʰ **S31.41** Laceration without foreign body **of vagina** ♀ **and vulva**

√x7ᵗʰ **S31.42** Laceration with foreign body **of vagina and** ♀ **vulva**

√x7ᵗʰ **S31.43** Puncture wound without foreign body **of** ♀ **vagina and vulva**

√x7ᵗʰ **S31.44** Puncture wound with foreign body **of vagina** ♀ **and vulva**

√x7ᵗʰ **S31.45** Open bite **of vagina and vulva** ♀
Bite of vagina and vulva NOS
EXCLUDES 1 *superficial bite of vagina and vulva (S30.864, S30.874)*

√5ᵗʰ **S31.5** Open wound of unspecified external genital organs
EXCLUDES 1 *traumatic amputation of external genital organs (S38.21, S38.22)*

√6ᵗʰ **S31.50** Unspecified open wound of unspecified external genital organs

√7ᵗʰ **S31.501** **Unspecified open wound of** ♂▽ **unspecified external genital organs,** male

√7ᵗʰ **S31.502** **Unspecified open wound of** ♀▽ **unspecified external genital organs,** female

---

☑ Add'l Character Required   √x7ᵗʰ Placeholder Alert   RUG IV Special Care High Dx   RUG IV Clinically Complex Dx   RUG IV Special Care Low Dx   Manifestation Code   Other Specified Code   ▽ Unspecified Code

✓6ᵗʰ **S31.51** Laceration without foreign body of unspecified external genital organs

  ✓7ᵗʰ **S31.511** Laceration without foreign body of unspecified external genital organs, male ♂▽

  ✓7ᵗʰ **S31.512** Laceration without foreign body of unspecified external genital organs, female ♀▽

✓6ᵗʰ **S31.52** Laceration with foreign body of unspecified external genital organs

  ✓7ᵗʰ **S31.521** Laceration with foreign body of unspecified external genital organs, male ♂▽

  ✓7ᵗʰ **S31.522** Laceration with foreign body of unspecified external genital organs, female ♀▽

✓6ᵗʰ **S31.53** Puncture wound without foreign body of unspecified external genital organs

  ✓7ᵗʰ **S31.531** Puncture wound without foreign body of unspecified external genital organs, male ♂▽

  ✓7ᵗʰ **S31.532** Puncture wound without foreign body of unspecified external genital organs, female ♀▽

✓6ᵗʰ **S31.54** Puncture wound with foreign body of unspecified external genital organs

  ✓7ᵗʰ **S31.541** Puncture wound with foreign body of unspecified external genital organs, male ♂▽

  ✓7ᵗʰ **S31.542** Puncture wound with foreign body of unspecified external genital organs, female ♀▽

✓6ᵗʰ **S31.55** Open bite of unspecified external genital organs
Bite of unspecified external genital organs NOS
  EXCLUDES 1 superficial bite of unspecified external genital organs (S30.865, S30.866, S30.875, S30.876)

  ✓7ᵗʰ **S31.551** Open bite of unspecified external genital organs, male ♂▽

  ✓7ᵗʰ **S31.552** Open bite of unspecified external genital organs, female ♀▽

✓5ᵗʰ **S31.6** Open wound of abdominal wall with penetration into peritoneal cavity

  ✓6ᵗʰ **S31.60** Unspecified open wound of abdominal wall with penetration into peritoneal cavity

    ✓7ᵗʰ **S31.600** Unspecified open wound of abdominal wall, right upper quadrant with penetration into peritoneal cavity ▽

    ✓7ᵗʰ **S31.601** Unspecified open wound of abdominal wall, left upper quadrant with penetration into peritoneal cavity ▽

    ✓7ᵗʰ **S31.602** Unspecified open wound of abdominal wall, epigastric region with penetration into peritoneal cavity ▽

    ✓7ᵗʰ **S31.603** Unspecified open wound of abdominal wall, right lower quadrant with penetration into peritoneal cavity ▽

    ✓7ᵗʰ **S31.604** Unspecified open wound of abdominal wall, left lower quadrant with penetration into peritoneal cavity ▽

    ✓7ᵗʰ **S31.605** Unspecified open wound of abdominal wall, periumbilic region with penetration into peritoneal cavity ▽

    ✓7ᵗʰ **S31.609** Unspecified open wound of abdominal wall, unspecified quadrant with penetration into peritoneal cavity ▽

  ✓6ᵗʰ **S31.61** Laceration without foreign body of abdominal wall with penetration into peritoneal cavity

    ✓7ᵗʰ **S31.610** Laceration without foreign body of abdominal wall, right upper quadrant with penetration into peritoneal cavity

    ✓7ᵗʰ **S31.611** Laceration without foreign body of abdominal wall, left upper quadrant with penetration into peritoneal cavity

    ✓7ᵗʰ **S31.612** Laceration without foreign body of abdominal wall, epigastric region with penetration into peritoneal cavity

    ✓7ᵗʰ **S31.613** Laceration without foreign body of abdominal wall, right lower quadrant with penetration into peritoneal cavity

    ✓7ᵗʰ **S31.614** Laceration without foreign body of abdominal wall, left lower quadrant with penetration into peritoneal cavity

    ✓7ᵗʰ **S31.615** Laceration without foreign body of abdominal wall, periumbilic region with penetration into peritoneal cavity

    ✓7ᵗʰ **S31.619** Laceration without foreign body of abdominal wall, unspecified quadrant with penetration into peritoneal cavity ▽

  ✓6ᵗʰ **S31.62** Laceration with foreign body of abdominal wall with penetration into peritoneal cavity

    ✓7ᵗʰ **S31.620** Laceration with foreign body of abdominal wall, right upper quadrant with penetration into peritoneal cavity

    ✓7ᵗʰ **S31.621** Laceration with foreign body of abdominal wall, left upper quadrant with penetration into peritoneal cavity

    ✓7ᵗʰ **S31.622** Laceration with foreign body of abdominal wall, epigastric region with penetration into peritoneal cavity

    ✓7ᵗʰ **S31.623** Laceration with foreign body of abdominal wall, right lower quadrant with penetration into peritoneal cavity

    ✓7ᵗʰ **S31.624** Laceration with foreign body of abdominal wall, left lower quadrant with penetration into peritoneal cavity

    ✓7ᵗʰ **S31.625** Laceration with foreign body of abdominal wall, periumbilic region with penetration into peritoneal cavity

    ✓7ᵗʰ **S31.629** Laceration with foreign body of abdominal wall, unspecified quadrant with penetration into peritoneal cavity ▽

  ✓6ᵗʰ **S31.63** Puncture wound without foreign body of abdominal wall with penetration into peritoneal cavity

    ✓7ᵗʰ **S31.630** Puncture wound without foreign body of abdominal wall, right upper quadrant with penetration into peritoneal cavity

    ✓7ᵗʰ **S31.631** Puncture wound without foreign body of abdominal wall, left upper quadrant with penetration into peritoneal cavity

    ✓7ᵗʰ **S31.632** Puncture wound without foreign body of abdominal wall, epigastric region with penetration into peritoneal cavity

    ✓7ᵗʰ **S31.633** Puncture wound without foreign body of abdominal wall, right lower quadrant with penetration into peritoneal cavity

    ✓7ᵗʰ **S31.634** Puncture wound without foreign body of abdominal wall, left lower quadrant with penetration into peritoneal cavity

    ✓7ᵗʰ **S31.635** Puncture wound without foreign body of abdominal wall, periumbilic region with penetration into peritoneal cavity

    ✓7ᵗʰ **S31.639** Puncture wound without foreign body of abdominal wall, unspecified quadrant with penetration into peritoneal cavity ▽

  ✓6ᵗʰ **S31.64** Puncture wound with foreign body of abdominal wall with penetration into peritoneal cavity

    ✓7ᵗʰ **S31.640** Puncture wound with foreign body of abdominal wall, right upper quadrant with penetration into peritoneal cavity

    ✓7ᵗʰ **S31.641** Puncture wound with foreign body of abdominal wall, left upper quadrant with penetration into peritoneal cavity

    ✓7ᵗʰ **S31.642** Puncture wound with foreign body of abdominal wall, epigastric region with penetration into peritoneal cavity

    ✓7ᵗʰ **S31.643** Puncture wound with foreign body of abdominal wall, right lower quadrant with penetration into peritoneal cavity

    ✓7ᵗʰ **S31.644** Puncture wound with foreign body of abdominal wall, left lower quadrant with penetration into peritoneal cavity

√7ᵗʰ **S31.645   Puncture wound with foreign body of abdominal wall, periumbilic region with penetration into peritoneal cavity**

√7ᵗʰ **S31.649   Puncture wound with foreign body of abdominal wall, unspecified quadrant with penetration into peritoneal cavity** ▽

√6ᵗʰ **S31.65   Open bite of abdominal wall with penetration into peritoneal cavity**
> *EXCLUDES✚*   superficial bite of abdominal wall (S30.861, S30.871)

√7ᵗʰ **S31.650   Open bite of abdominal wall, right upper quadrant with penetration into peritoneal cavity**

√7ᵗʰ **S31.651   Open bite of abdominal wall, left upper quadrant with penetration into peritoneal cavity**

√7ᵗʰ **S31.652   Open bite of abdominal wall, epigastric region with penetration into peritoneal cavity**

√7ᵗʰ **S31.653   Open bite of abdominal wall, right lower quadrant with penetration into peritoneal cavity**

√7ᵗʰ **S31.654   Open bite of abdominal wall, left lower quadrant with penetration into peritoneal cavity**

√7ᵗʰ **S31.655   Open bite of abdominal wall, periumbilic region with penetration into peritoneal cavity**

√7ᵗʰ **S31.659   Open bite of abdominal wall, unspecified quadrant with penetration into peritoneal cavity** ▽

√5ᵗʰ **S31.8   Open wound of other parts of abdomen, lower back and pelvis**

√6ᵗʰ **S31.80   Open wound of unspecified buttock**

√7ᵗʰ **S31.801   Laceration without foreign body of unspecified buttock** ▽

√7ᵗʰ **S31.802   Laceration with foreign body of unspecified buttock** ▽

√7ᵗʰ **S31.803   Puncture wound without foreign body of unspecified buttock** ▽

√7ᵗʰ **S31.804   Puncture wound with foreign body of unspecified buttock** ▽

√7ᵗʰ **S31.805   Open bite of unspecified buttock** ▽
> Bite of buttock NOS
> *EXCLUDES 1*   superficial bite of buttock (S30.870)

√7ᵗʰ **S31.809   Unspecified open wound of unspecified buttock** ▽

√6ᵗʰ **S31.81   Open wound of right buttock**

√7ᵗʰ **S31.811   Laceration without foreign body of right buttock**

√7ᵗʰ **S31.812   Laceration with foreign body of right buttock**

√7ᵗʰ **S31.813   Puncture wound without foreign body of right buttock**

√7ᵗʰ **S31.814   Puncture wound with foreign body of right buttock**

√7ᵗʰ **S31.815   Open bite of right buttock**
> Bite of right buttock NOS
> *EXCLUDES 1*   superficial bite of buttock (S30.870)

√7ᵗʰ **S31.819   Unspecified open wound of right buttock** ▽

√6ᵗʰ **S31.82   Open wound of left buttock**

√7ᵗʰ **S31.821   Laceration without foreign body of left buttock**

√7ᵗʰ **S31.822   Laceration with foreign body of left buttock**

√7ᵗʰ **S31.823   Puncture wound without foreign body of left buttock**

√7ᵗʰ **S31.824   Puncture wound with foreign body of left buttock**

√7ᵗʰ **S31.825   Open bite of left buttock**
> Bite of left buttock NOS
> *EXCLUDES 1*   superficial bite of buttock (S30.870)

√7ᵗʰ **S31.829   Unspecified open wound of left buttock** ▽

√6ᵗʰ **S31.83   Open wound of anus**

√7ᵗʰ **S31.831   Laceration without foreign body of anus**

√7ᵗʰ **S31.832   Laceration with foreign body of anus**

√7ᵗʰ **S31.833   Puncture wound without foreign body of anus**

√7ᵗʰ **S31.834   Puncture wound with foreign body of anus**

√7ᵗʰ **S31.835   Open bite of anus**
> Bite of anus NOS
> *EXCLUDES 1*   superficial bite of anus (S30.877)

√7ᵗʰ **S31.839   Unspecified open wound of anus** ▽

√4ᵗʰ **S32   Fracture of lumbar spine and pelvis**
> **NOTE**   A fracture not indicated as displaced or nondisplaced should be coded to displaced.
> A fracture not indicated as opened or closed should be coded to closed.
> **INCLUDES**   fracture of lumbosacral neural arch
> fracture of lumbosacral spinous process
> fracture of lumbosacral transverse process
> fracture of lumbosacral vertebra
> fracture of lumbosacral vertebral arch

Code first any associated spinal cord and spinal nerve injury (S34.-)
> *EXCLUDES 1*   transection of abdomen (S38.3)
> *EXCLUDES 2*   fracture of hip NOS (S72.0-)
AHA: 2012, 4Q, 93

The appropriate 7th character is to be added to each code from category S32.
A   initial encounter for closed fracture
B   initial encounter for open fracture
D   subsequent encounter for fracture with routine healing
G   subsequent encounter for fracture with delayed healing
K   subsequent encounter for fracture with nonunion
S   sequela

√5ᵗʰ **S32.0   Fracture of lumbar vertebra**
> Fracture of lumbar spine NOS

√6ᵗʰ **S32.00   Fracture of unspecified lumbar vertebra**

√7ᵗʰ **S32.000   Wedge compression fracture of unspecified lumbar vertebra** ▽

√7ᵗʰ **S32.001   Stable burst fracture of unspecified lumbar vertebra** ▽

√7ᵗʰ **S32.002   Unstable burst fracture of unspecified lumbar vertebra** ▽

√7ᵗʰ **S32.008   Other fracture of unspecified lumbar vertebra** ▽

√7ᵗʰ **S32.009   Unspecified fracture of unspecified lumbar vertebra** ▽

√6ᵗʰ **S32.01   Fracture of first lumbar vertebra**

√7ᵗʰ **S32.010   Wedge compression fracture of first lumbar vertebra**

√7ᵗʰ **S32.011   Stable burst fracture of first lumbar vertebra**

√7ᵗʰ **S32.012   Unstable burst fracture of first lumbar vertebra**

√7ᵗʰ **S32.018   Other fracture of first lumbar vertebra**

√7ᵗʰ **S32.019   Unspecified fracture of first lumbar vertebra** ▽

√6ᵗʰ **S32.02   Fracture of second lumbar vertebra**

√7ᵗʰ **S32.020   Wedge compression fracture of second lumbar vertebra**

√7ᵗʰ **S32.021   Stable burst fracture of second lumbar vertebra**

√7ᵗʰ **S32.022   Unstable burst fracture of second lumbar vertebra**

√7ᵗʰ **S32.028   Other fracture of second lumbar vertebra**

√7ᵗʰ **S32.029   Unspecified fracture of second lumbar vertebra** ▽

√6ᵗʰ **S32.03   Fracture of third lumbar vertebra**

√7ᵗʰ **S32.030   Wedge compression fracture of third lumbar vertebra**

√7ᵗʰ **S32.031   Stable burst fracture of third lumbar vertebra**

√7ᵗʰ **S32.032   Unstable burst fracture of third lumbar vertebra**

☑ Add'l Character Required   √x7ᵗʰ Placeholder Alert   RUG IV Special Care High Dx   RUG IV Clinically Complex Dx   RUG IV Special Care Low Dx   Manifestation Code   Other Specified Code   ▽ Unspecified Code

ICD-10-CM 2016   887

√7ᵗʰ **S32.038** Other fracture of third lumbar vertebra

√7ᵗʰ **S32.039** Unspecified fracture of third lumbar vertebra ▽

√6ᵗʰ **S32.04** Fracture of fourth lumbar vertebra

√7ᵗʰ **S32.040** Wedge compression fracture of fourth lumbar vertebra

√7ᵗʰ **S32.041** Stable burst fracture of fourth lumbar vertebra

√7ᵗʰ **S32.042** Unstable burst fracture of fourth lumbar vertebra

√7ᵗʰ **S32.048** Other fracture of fourth lumbar vertebra

√7ᵗʰ **S32.049** Unspecified fracture of fourth lumbar vertebra ▽

√6ᵗʰ **S32.05** Fracture of fifth lumbar vertebra

√7ᵗʰ **S32.050** Wedge compression fracture of fifth lumbar vertebra

√7ᵗʰ **S32.051** Stable burst fracture of fifth lumbar vertebra

√7ᵗʰ **S32.052** Unstable burst fracture of fifth lumbar vertebra

√7ᵗʰ **S32.058** Other fracture of fifth lumbar vertebra

√7ᵗʰ **S32.059** Unspecified fracture of fifth lumbar vertebra ▽

√5ᵗʰ **S32.1** Fracture of sacrum

    NOTE For vertical fractures, code to most medial fracture extension.
    Use two codes if both a vertical and transverse fracture are present.

    Code also any associated fracture of pelvic ring (S32.8-)

√x7ᵗʰ **S32.10** Unspecified fracture of sacrum ▽

√6ᵗʰ **S32.11** Zone I fracture of sacrum
    Vertical sacral ala fracture of sacrum

√7ᵗʰ **S32.110** Nondisplaced Zone I fracture of sacrum

√7ᵗʰ **S32.111** Minimally displaced Zone I fracture of sacrum

√7ᵗʰ **S32.112** Severely displaced Zone I fracture of sacrum

√7ᵗʰ **S32.119** Unspecified Zone I fracture of sacrum ▽

√6ᵗʰ **S32.12** Zone II fracture of sacrum
    Vertical foraminal region fracture of sacrum

√7ᵗʰ **S32.120** Nondisplaced Zone II fracture of sacrum

√7ᵗʰ **S32.121** Minimally displaced Zone II fracture of sacrum

√7ᵗʰ **S32.122** Severely displaced Zone II fracture of sacrum

√7ᵗʰ **S32.129** Unspecified Zone II fracture of sacrum ▽

√6ᵗʰ **S32.13** Zone III fracture of sacrum
    Vertical fracture into spinal canal region of sacrum

√7ᵗʰ **S32.130** Nondisplaced Zone III fracture of sacrum

√7ᵗʰ **S32.131** Minimally displaced Zone III fracture of sacrum

√7ᵗʰ **S32.132** Severely displaced Zone III fracture of sacrum

√7ᵗʰ **S32.139** Unspecified Zone III fracture of sacrum ▽

√x7ᵗʰ **S32.14** Type 1 fracture of sacrum
    Transverse flexion fracture of sacrum without displacement

√x7ᵗʰ **S32.15** Type 2 fracture of sacrum
    Transverse flexion fracture of sacrum with posterior displacement

√x7ᵗʰ **S32.16** Type 3 fracture of sacrum
    Transverse extension fracture of sacrum with anterior displacement

√x7ᵗʰ **S32.17** Type 4 fracture of sacrum
    Transverse segmental comminution of upper sacrum

√x7ᵗʰ **S32.19** Other fracture of sacrum

√x7ᵗʰ **S32.2** Fracture of coccyx

√5ᵗʰ **S32.3** Fracture of ilium

    EXCLUDES 1 fracture of ilium with associated disruption of pelvic ring (S32.8-)

√6ᵗʰ **S32.30** Unspecified fracture of ilium

√7ᵗʰ **S32.301** Unspecified fracture of right ilium ▽

√7ᵗʰ **S32.302** Unspecified fracture of left ilium ▽

√7ᵗʰ **S32.309** Unspecified fracture of unspecified ilium ▽

√6ᵗʰ **S32.31** Avulsion fracture of ilium

√7ᵗʰ **S32.311** Displaced avulsion fracture of right ilium

√7ᵗʰ **S32.312** Displaced avulsion fracture of left ilium

√7ᵗʰ **S32.313** Displaced avulsion fracture of unspecified ilium ▽

√7ᵗʰ **S32.314** Nondisplaced avulsion fracture of right ilium

√7ᵗʰ **S32.315** Nondisplaced avulsion fracture of left ilium

√7ᵗʰ **S32.316** Nondisplaced avulsion fracture of unspecified ilium ▽

√6ᵗʰ **S32.39** Other fracture of ilium

√7ᵗʰ **S32.391** Other fracture of right ilium

√7ᵗʰ **S32.392** Other fracture of left ilium

√7ᵗʰ **S32.399** Other fracture of unspecified ilium ▽

√5ᵗʰ **S32.4** Fracture of acetabulum
    Code also any associated fracture of pelvic ring (S32.8-)

√6ᵗʰ **S32.40** Unspecified fracture of acetabulum

√7ᵗʰ **S32.401** Unspecified fracture of right acetabulum ▽

√7ᵗʰ **S32.402** Unspecified fracture of left acetabulum ▽

√7ᵗʰ **S32.409** Unspecified fracture of unspecified acetabulum ▽

√6ᵗʰ **S32.41** Fracture of anterior wall of acetabulum

√7ᵗʰ **S32.411** Displaced fracture of anterior wall of right acetabulum

√7ᵗʰ **S32.412** Displaced fracture of anterior wall of left acetabulum

√7ᵗʰ **S32.413** Displaced fracture of anterior wall of unspecified acetabulum ▽

√7ᵗʰ **S32.414** Nondisplaced fracture of anterior wall of right acetabulum

√7ᵗʰ **S32.415** Nondisplaced fracture of anterior wall of left acetabulum

√7ᵗʰ **S32.416** Nondisplaced fracture of anterior wall of unspecified acetabulum ▽

√6ᵗʰ **S32.42** Fracture of posterior wall of acetabulum

√7ᵗʰ **S32.421** Displaced fracture of posterior wall of right acetabulum

√7ᵗʰ **S32.422** Displaced fracture of posterior wall of left acetabulum

√7ᵗʰ **S32.423** Displaced fracture of posterior wall of unspecified acetabulum ▽

√7ᵗʰ **S32.424** Nondisplaced fracture of posterior wall of right acetabulum

√7ᵗʰ **S32.425** Nondisplaced fracture of posterior wall of left acetabulum

√7ᵗʰ **S32.426** Nondisplaced fracture of posterior wall of unspecified acetabulum ▽

√6ᵗʰ **S32.43** Fracture of anterior column [iliopubic] of acetabulum

√7ᵗʰ **S32.431** Displaced fracture of anterior column [iliopubic] of right acetabulum

√7ᵗʰ **S32.432** Displaced fracture of anterior column [iliopubic] of left acetabulum

√7ᵗʰ **S32.433** Displaced fracture of anterior column [iliopubic] of unspecified acetabulum ▽

√7ᵗʰ **S32.434** Nondisplaced fracture of anterior column [iliopubic] of right acetabulum

√7ᵗʰ **S32.435** Nondisplaced fracture of anterior column [iliopubic] of left acetabulum

√7ᵗʰ **S32.436** Nondisplaced fracture of anterior column [iliopubic] of unspecified acetabulum ▽

√6ᵗʰ **S32.44** Fracture of posterior column [ilioischial] of acetabulum

√7ᵗʰ **S32.441** Displaced fracture of posterior column [ilioischial] of right acetabulum

√7ᵗʰ **S32.442** Displaced fracture of posterior column [ilioischial] of left acetabulum

Ⓝ Newborn   Ⓟ Pediatric   Ⓜ Maternity   Ⓐ Adult   **RIC** RIC Dx   **NC Dx** Noncancer Dx   **PDx** Primary Dx   **CC** RIC CC Condition   ▶◀ Revised Text   ● New Code   ▲ Revised Code Title

888   ICD-10-CM 2016

☑7ᵗʰ **S32.443** Displaced fracture of posterior column [ilioischial] of unspecified acetabulum ▽

☑7ᵗʰ **S32.444** Nondisplaced fracture of posterior column [ilioischial] of right acetabulum

☑7ᵗʰ **S32.445** Nondisplaced fracture of posterior column [ilioischial] of left acetabulum

☑7ᵗʰ **S32.446** Nondisplaced fracture of posterior column [ilioischial] of unspecified acetabulum ▽

☑6ᵗʰ **S32.45** Transverse fracture of acetabulum

☑7ᵗʰ **S32.451** Displaced transverse fracture of right acetabulum

☑7ᵗʰ **S32.452** Displaced transverse fracture of left acetabulum

☑7ᵗʰ **S32.453** Displaced transverse fracture of unspecified acetabulum ▽

☑7ᵗʰ **S32.454** Nondisplaced transverse fracture of right acetabulum

☑7ᵗʰ **S32.455** Nondisplaced transverse fracture of left acetabulum

☑7ᵗʰ **S32.456** Nondisplaced transverse fracture of unspecified acetabulum ▽

☑6ᵗʰ **S32.46** Associated transverse-posterior fracture of acetabulum

☑7ᵗʰ **S32.461** Displaced associated transverse-posterior fracture of right acetabulum

☑7ᵗʰ **S32.462** Displaced associated transverse-posterior fracture of left acetabulum

☑7ᵗʰ **S32.463** Displaced associated transverse-posterior fracture of unspecified acetabulum ▽

☑7ᵗʰ **S32.464** Nondisplaced associated transverse-posterior fracture of right acetabulum

☑7ᵗʰ **S32.465** Nondisplaced associated transverse-posterior fracture of left acetabulum

☑7ᵗʰ **S32.466** Nondisplaced associated transverse-posterior fracture of unspecified acetabulum ▽

☑6ᵗʰ **S32.47** Fracture of medial wall of acetabulum

☑7ᵗʰ **S32.471** Displaced fracture of medial wall of right acetabulum

☑7ᵗʰ **S32.472** Displaced fracture of medial wall of left acetabulum

☑7ᵗʰ **S32.473** Displaced fracture of medial wall of unspecified acetabulum ▽

☑7ᵗʰ **S32.474** Nondisplaced fracture of medial wall of right acetabulum

☑7ᵗʰ **S32.475** Nondisplaced fracture of medial wall of left acetabulum

☑7ᵗʰ **S32.476** Nondisplaced fracture of medial wall of unspecified acetabulum ▽

☑6ᵗʰ **S32.48** Dome fracture of acetabulum

☑7ᵗʰ **S32.481** Displaced dome fracture of right acetabulum

☑7ᵗʰ **S32.482** Displaced dome fracture of left acetabulum

☑7ᵗʰ **S32.483** Displaced dome fracture of unspecified acetabulum ▽

☑7ᵗʰ **S32.484** Nondisplaced dome fracture of right acetabulum

☑7ᵗʰ **S32.485** Nondisplaced dome fracture of left acetabulum

☑7ᵗʰ **S32.486** Nondisplaced dome fracture of unspecified acetabulum ▽

☑6ᵗʰ **S32.49** Other specified fracture of acetabulum

☑7ᵗʰ **S32.491** Other specified fracture of right acetabulum

☑7ᵗʰ **S32.492** Other specified fracture of left acetabulum

☑7ᵗʰ **S32.499** Other specified fracture of unspecified acetabulum ▽

☑5ᵗʰ **S32.5** Fracture of pubis

EXCLUDES 1   *fracture of pubis with associated disruption of pelvic ring (S32.8-)*

☑6ᵗʰ **S32.50** Unspecified fracture of pubis

☑7ᵗʰ **S32.501** Unspecified fracture of right pubis ▽

☑7ᵗʰ **S32.502** Unspecified fracture of left pubis ▽

☑7ᵗʰ **S32.509** Unspecified fracture of unspecified pubis ▽

☑6ᵗʰ **S32.51** Fracture of superior rim of pubis

☑7ᵗʰ **S32.511** Fracture of superior rim of right pubis

☑7ᵗʰ **S32.512** Fracture of superior rim of left pubis

☑7ᵗʰ **S32.519** Fracture of superior rim of unspecified pubis ▽

☑6ᵗʰ **S32.59** Other specified fracture of pubis

☑7ᵗʰ **S32.591** Other specified fracture of right pubis

☑7ᵗʰ **S32.592** Other specified fracture of left pubis

☑7ᵗʰ **S32.599** Other specified fracture of unspecified pubis ▽

☑5ᵗʰ **S32.6** Fracture of ischium

EXCLUDES 1   *fracture of ischium with associated disruption of pelvic ring (S32.8-)*

☑6ᵗʰ **S32.60** Unspecified fracture of ischium

☑7ᵗʰ **S32.601** Unspecified fracture of right ischium ▽

☑7ᵗʰ **S32.602** Unspecified fracture of left ischium ▽

☑7ᵗʰ **S32.609** Unspecified fracture of unspecified ischium ▽

☑6ᵗʰ **S32.61** Avulsion fracture of ischium

☑7ᵗʰ **S32.611** Displaced avulsion fracture of right ischium

☑7ᵗʰ **S32.612** Displaced avulsion fracture of left ischium

☑7ᵗʰ **S32.613** Displaced avulsion fracture of unspecified ischium ▽

☑7ᵗʰ **S32.614** Nondisplaced avulsion fracture of right ischium

☑7ᵗʰ **S32.615** Nondisplaced avulsion fracture of left ischium

☑7ᵗʰ **S32.616** Nondisplaced avulsion fracture of unspecified ischium ▽

☑6ᵗʰ **S32.69** Other specified fracture of ischium

☑7ᵗʰ **S32.691** Other specified fracture of right ischium

☑7ᵗʰ **S32.692** Other specified fracture of left ischium

☑7ᵗʰ **S32.699** Other specified fracture of unspecified ischium ▽

☑5ᵗʰ **S32.8** Fracture of other parts of pelvis

Code also any associated:
    fracture of acetabulum (S32.4-)
    sacral fracture (S32.1-)

☑6ᵗʰ **S32.81** Multiple fractures of pelvis with disruption of pelvic ring

    Multiple pelvic fractures with disruption of pelvic circle

☑7ᵗʰ **S32.810** Multiple fractures of pelvis with stable disruption of pelvic ring

☑7ᵗʰ **S32.811** Multiple fractures of pelvis with unstable disruption of pelvic ring

☑x7ᵗʰ **S32.82** Multiple fractures of pelvis without disruption of pelvic ring

    Multiple pelvic fractures without disruption of pelvic circle

☑x7ᵗʰ **S32.89** Fracture of other parts of pelvis

☑x7ᵗʰ **S32.9** Fracture of unspecified parts of lumbosacral spine and pelvis ▽

    Fracture of lumbosacral spine NOS
    Fracture of pelvis NOS
    AHA: 2012, 4Q, 93

☑ Add'l Character Required   ☑x7ᵗʰ Placeholder Alert   RUG IV Special Care High Dx   RUG IV Clinically Complex Dx   RUG IV Special Care Low Dx   Manifestation Code   Other Specified Code   ▽ Unspecified Code

✓4ᵗʰ S33 Dislocation and sprain of joints and ligaments of lumbar spine and pelvis

INCLUDES avulsion of joint or ligament of lumbar spine and pelvis
laceration of cartilage, joint or ligament of lumbar spine and pelvis
sprain of cartilage, joint or ligament of lumbar spine and pelvis
traumatic hemarthrosis of joint or ligament of lumbar spine and pelvis
traumatic rupture of joint or ligament of lumbar spine and pelvis
traumatic subluxation of joint or ligament of lumbar spine and pelvis
traumatic tear of joint or ligament of lumbar spine and pelvis

Code also any associated open wound

EXCLUDES 1 nontraumatic rupture or displacement of lumbar intervertebral disc NOS (M51.-)
obstetric damage to pelvic joints and ligaments (O71.6)

EXCLUDES 2 dislocation and sprain of joints and ligaments of hip (S73.-)
strain of muscle of lower back and pelvis (S39.01-)

The appropriate 7th character is to be added to each code from category S33.
A   initial encounter
D   subsequent encounter
S   sequela

✓x7ᵗʰ S33.0 Traumatic rupture of lumbar intervertebral disc

EXCLUDES 1 rupture or displacement (nontraumatic) of lumbar intervertebral disc NOS (M51- with fifth character 6)

✓5ᵗʰ S33.1 Subluxation and dislocation of lumbar vertebra

Code also any associated:
open wound of abdomen, lower back and pelvis (S31)
spinal cord injury (S24.0, S24.1-, S34.0-, S34.1-)

EXCLUDES 2 fracture of lumbar vertebrae (S32.0-)

✓6ᵗʰ S33.10 Subluxation and dislocation of unspecified lumbar vertebra

   ✓7ᵗʰ S33.100 Subluxation of unspecified lumbar vertebra ▽

   ✓7ᵗʰ S33.101 Dislocation of unspecified lumbar vertebra ▽

✓6ᵗʰ S33.11 Subluxation and dislocation of L1/L2 lumbar vertebra

   ✓7ᵗʰ S33.110 Subluxation of L1/L2 lumbar vertebra

   ✓7ᵗʰ S33.111 Dislocation of L1/L2 lumbar vertebra

✓6ᵗʰ S33.12 Subluxation and dislocation of L2/L3 lumbar vertebra

   ✓7ᵗʰ S33.120 Subluxation of L2/L3 lumbar vertebra

   ✓7ᵗʰ S33.121 Dislocation of L2/L3 lumbar vertebra

✓6ᵗʰ S33.13 Subluxation and dislocation of L3/L4 lumbar vertebra

   ✓7ᵗʰ S33.130 Subluxation of L3/L4 lumbar vertebra

   ✓7ᵗʰ S33.131 Dislocation of L3/L4 lumbar vertebra

✓6ᵗʰ S33.14 Subluxation and dislocation of L4/L5 lumbar vertebra

   ✓7ᵗʰ S33.140 Subluxation of L4/L5 lumbar vertebra

   ✓7ᵗʰ S33.141 Dislocation of L4/L5 lumbar vertebra

✓x7ᵗʰ S33.2 Dislocation of sacroiliac and sacrococcygeal joint

✓5ᵗʰ S33.3 Dislocation of other and unspecified parts of lumbar spine and pelvis

   ✓x7ᵗʰ S33.30 Dislocation of unspecified parts of lumbar spine and pelvis ▽

   ✓x7ᵗʰ S33.39 Dislocation of other parts of lumbar spine and pelvis

✓x7ᵗʰ S33.4 Traumatic rupture of symphysis pubis

✓x7ᵗʰ S33.5 Sprain of ligaments of lumbar spine

✓x7ᵗʰ S33.6 Sprain of sacroiliac joint

✓x7ᵗʰ S33.8 Sprain of other parts of lumbar spine and pelvis

✓x7ᵗʰ S33.9 Sprain of unspecified parts of lumbar spine and pelvis ▽

✓4ᵗʰ S34 Injury of lumbar and sacral spinal cord and nerves at abdomen, lower back and pelvis level

NOTE Code to highest level of lumbar cord injury.
Injuries to the spinal cord (S34.0 and S34.1) refer to the cord level and not bone level injury, and can affect nerve roots at and below the level given.

Code also any associated:
fracture of vertebra (S22.0-, S32.0-)
open wound of abdomen, lower back and pelvis (S31.-)
transient paralysis (R29.5)

The appropriate 7th character is to be added to each code from category S34.
A   initial encounter
D   subsequent encounter
S   sequela

✓5ᵗʰ S34.0 Concussion and edema of lumbar and sacral spinal cord

   ✓x7ᵗʰ S34.01 Concussion and edema of lumbar spinal cord

   ✓x7ᵗʰ S34.02 Concussion and edema of sacral spinal cord
   Concussion and edema of conus medullaris

✓5ᵗʰ S34.1 Other and unspecified injury of lumbar and sacral spinal cord

   ✓6ᵗʰ S34.10 Unspecified injury to lumbar spinal cord

      ✓7ᵗʰ S34.101 Unspecified injury to L1 level of lumbar spinal cord ▽

      ✓7ᵗʰ S34.102 Unspecified injury to L2 level of lumbar spinal cord ▽

      ✓7ᵗʰ S34.103 Unspecified injury to L3 level of lumbar spinal cord ▽

      ✓7ᵗʰ S34.104 Unspecified injury to L4 level of lumbar spinal cord ▽

      ✓7ᵗʰ S34.105 Unspecified injury to L5 level of lumbar spinal cord ▽

      ✓7ᵗʰ S34.109 Unspecified injury to unspecified level of lumbar spinal cord ▽

   ✓6ᵗʰ S34.11 Complete lesion of lumbar spinal cord

      ✓7ᵗʰ S34.111 Complete lesion of L1 level of lumbar spinal cord

      ✓7ᵗʰ S34.112 Complete lesion of L2 level of lumbar spinal cord

      ✓7ᵗʰ S34.113 Complete lesion of L3 level of lumbar spinal cord

      ✓7ᵗʰ S34.114 Complete lesion of L4 level of lumbar spinal cord

      ✓7ᵗʰ S34.115 Complete lesion of L5 level of lumbar spinal cord

      ✓7ᵗʰ S34.119 Complete lesion of unspecified level of lumbar spinal cord ▽

   ✓6ᵗʰ S34.12 Incomplete lesion of lumbar spinal cord

      ✓7ᵗʰ S34.121 Incomplete lesion of L1 level of lumbar spinal cord

      ✓7ᵗʰ S34.122 Incomplete lesion of L2 level of lumbar spinal cord

      ✓7ᵗʰ S34.123 Incomplete lesion of L3 level of lumbar spinal cord

      ✓7ᵗʰ S34.124 Incomplete lesion of L4 level of lumbar spinal cord

      ✓7ᵗʰ S34.125 Incomplete lesion of L5 level of lumbar spinal cord

      ✓7ᵗʰ S34.129 Incomplete lesion of unspecified level of lumbar spinal cord ▽

   ✓6ᵗʰ S34.13 Other and unspecified injury to sacral spinal cord
   Other injury to conus medullaris

      ✓7ᵗʰ S34.131 Complete lesion of sacral spinal cord
      Complete lesion of conus medullaris

      ✓7ᵗʰ S34.132 Incomplete lesion of sacral spinal cord
      Incomplete lesion of conus medullaris

      ✓7ᵗʰ S34.139 Unspecified injury to sacral spinal cord ▽
      Unspecified injury of conus medullaris

✓5ᵗʰ S34.2 Injury of nerve root of lumbar and sacral spine

   ✓x7ᵗʰ S34.21 Injury of nerve root of lumbar spine

   ✓x7ᵗʰ S34.22 Injury of nerve root of sacral spine

✓x7ᵗʰ S34.3 Injury of cauda equina

✓x7ᵗʰ S34.4 Injury of lumbosacral plexus

N Newborn   P Pediatric   M Maternity   A Adult   RIC RIC Dx   NCx Noncancer Dx   PDx Primary Dx   CC RIC CC Condition   ►◄ Revised Text   ● New Code   ▲ Revised Code Title

890   ICD-10-CM 2016

√x7ᵗʰ **S34.5 Injury of lumbar, sacral and pelvic sympathetic nerves**
Injury of celiac ganglion or plexus
Injury of hypogastric plexus
Injury of mesenteric plexus (inferior) (superior)
Injury of splanchnic nerve

√x7ᵗʰ **S34.6 Injury of peripheral nerve(s) at abdomen, lower back and pelvis level**

√x7ᵗʰ **S34.8 Injury of other nerves at abdomen, lower back and pelvis level**

√x7ᵗʰ **S34.9 Injury of unspecified nerves at abdomen, lower back and pelvis level** ▽

√4ᵗʰ **S35 Injury of blood vessels at abdomen, lower back and pelvis level**
Code also any associated open wound (S31.-)

> The appropriate 7th character is to be added to each code from category S35.
> A   initial encounter
> D   subsequent encounter
> S   sequela

√5ᵗʰ **S35.0 Injury of abdominal aorta**
EXCLUDES 1   injury of aorta NOS (S25.0)

√x7ᵗʰ **S35.00 Unspecified injury of abdominal aorta** ▽

√x7ᵗʰ **S35.01 Minor laceration of abdominal aorta**
Incomplete transection of abdominal aorta
Laceration of abdominal aorta NOS
Superficial laceration of abdominal aorta

√x7ᵗʰ **S35.02 Major laceration of abdominal aorta**
Complete transection of abdominal aorta
Traumatic rupture of abdominal aorta

√x7ᵗʰ **S35.09 Other injury of abdominal aorta**

√5ᵗʰ **S35.1 Injury of inferior vena cava**
Injury of hepatic vein
EXCLUDES 1   injury of vena cava NOS (S25.2)

√x7ᵗʰ **S35.10 Unspecified injury of inferior vena cava** ▽

√x7ᵗʰ **S35.11 Minor laceration of inferior vena cava**
Incomplete transection of inferior vena cava
Laceration of inferior vena cava NOS
Superficial laceration of inferior vena cava

√x7ᵗʰ **S35.12 Major laceration of inferior vena cava**
Complete transection of inferior vena cava
Traumatic rupture of inferior vena cava

√x7ᵗʰ **S35.19 Other injury of inferior vena cava**

√5ᵗʰ **S35.2 Injury of celiac or mesenteric artery and branches**

√6ᵗʰ **S35.21 Injury of celiac artery**

√7ᵗʰ **S35.211 Minor laceration of celiac artery**
Incomplete transection of celiac artery
Laceration of celiac artery NOS
Superficial laceration of celiac artery

√7ᵗʰ **S35.212 Major laceration of celiac artery**
Complete transection of celiac artery
Traumatic rupture of celiac artery

√7ᵗʰ **S35.218 Other injury of celiac artery**

√7ᵗʰ **S35.219 Unspecified injury of celiac artery** ▽

√6ᵗʰ **S35.22 Injury of superior mesenteric artery**

√7ᵗʰ **S35.221 Minor laceration of superior mesenteric artery**
Incomplete transection of superior mesenteric artery
Laceration of superior mesenteric artery NOS
Superficial laceration of superior mesenteric artery

√7ᵗʰ **S35.222 Major laceration of superior mesenteric artery**
Complete transection of superior mesenteric artery
Traumatic rupture of superior mesenteric artery

√7ᵗʰ **S35.228 Other injury of superior mesenteric artery**

√7ᵗʰ **S35.229 Unspecified injury of superior mesenteric artery** ▽

√6ᵗʰ **S35.23 Injury of inferior mesenteric artery**

√7ᵗʰ **S35.231 Minor laceration of inferior mesenteric artery**
Incomplete transection of inferior mesenteric artery
Laceration of inferior mesenteric artery NOS
Superficial laceration of inferior mesenteric artery

√7ᵗʰ **S35.232 Major laceration of inferior mesenteric artery**
Complete transection of inferior mesenteric artery
Traumatic rupture of inferior mesenteric artery

√7ᵗʰ **S35.238 Other injury of inferior mesenteric artery**

√7ᵗʰ **S35.239 Unspecified injury of inferior mesenteric artery** ▽

√6ᵗʰ **S35.29 Injury of branches of celiac and mesenteric artery**
Injury of gastric artery
Injury of gastroduodenal artery
Injury of hepatic artery
Injury of splenic artery

√7ᵗʰ **S35.291 Minor laceration of branches of celiac and mesenteric artery**
Incomplete transection of branches of celiac and mesenteric artery
Laceration of branches of celiac and mesenteric artery NOS
Superficial laceration of branches of celiac and mesenteric artery

√7ᵗʰ **S35.292 Major laceration of branches of celiac and mesenteric artery**
Complete transection of branches of celiac and mesenteric artery
Traumatic rupture of branches of celiac and mesenteric artery

√7ᵗʰ **S35.298 Other injury of branches of celiac and mesenteric artery**

√7ᵗʰ **S35.299 Unspecified injury of branches of celiac and mesenteric artery** ▽

√5ᵗʰ **S35.3 Injury of portal or splenic vein and branches**

√6ᵗʰ **S35.31 Injury of portal vein**

√7ᵗʰ **S35.311 Laceration of portal vein**

√7ᵗʰ **S35.318 Other specified injury of portal vein**

√7ᵗʰ **S35.319 Unspecified injury of portal vein** ▽

√6ᵗʰ **S35.32 Injury of splenic vein**

√7ᵗʰ **S35.321 Laceration of splenic vein**

√7ᵗʰ **S35.328 Other specified injury of splenic vein**

√7ᵗʰ **S35.329 Unspecified injury of splenic vein** ▽

√6ᵗʰ **S35.33 Injury of superior mesenteric vein**

√7ᵗʰ **S35.331 Laceration of superior mesenteric vein**

√7ᵗʰ **S35.338 Other specified injury of superior mesenteric vein**

√7ᵗʰ **S35.339 Unspecified injury of superior mesenteric vein** ▽

√6ᵗʰ **S35.34 Injury of inferior mesenteric vein**

√7ᵗʰ **S35.341 Laceration of inferior mesenteric vein**

√7ᵗʰ **S35.348 Other specified injury of inferior mesenteric vein**

√7ᵗʰ **S35.349 Unspecified injury of inferior mesenteric vein** ▽

√5ᵗʰ **S35.4 Injury of renal blood vessels**

√6ᵗʰ **S35.40 Unspecified injury of renal blood vessel**

√7ᵗʰ **S35.401 Unspecified injury of right renal artery** ▽

√7ᵗʰ **S35.402 Unspecified injury of left renal artery** ▽

√7ᵗʰ **S35.403 Unspecified injury of unspecified renal artery** ▽

√7ᵗʰ **S35.404 Unspecified injury of right renal vein** ▽

√7ᵗʰ **S35.405 Unspecified injury of left renal vein** ▽

√7ᵗʰ **S35.406 Unspecified injury of unspecified renal vein** ▽

√6ᵗʰ **S35.41 Laceration of renal blood vessel**

√7ᵗʰ **S35.411 Laceration of right renal artery**

√7ᵗʰ **S35.412 Laceration of left renal artery**

✓ Add'l Character Required   √x7ᵗʰ Placeholder Alert   RUG IV Special Care High Dx   RUG IV Clinically Complex Dx   RUG IV Special Care Low Dx   Manifestation Code   Other Specified Code   ▽ Unspecified Code

ICD-10-CM 2016   891

✓7ᵗʰ **S35.413** **Laceration of unspecified renal artery** ▽

✓7ᵗʰ **S35.414** **Laceration of right renal vein**

✓7ᵗʰ **S35.415** **Laceration of left renal vein**

✓7ᵗʰ **S35.416** **Laceration of unspecified renal vein** ▽

✓6ᵗʰ **S35.49** **Other specified injury of renal blood vessel**

✓7ᵗʰ **S35.491** **Other specified injury of right renal artery**

✓7ᵗʰ **S35.492** **Other specified injury of left renal artery**

✓7ᵗʰ **S35.493** **Other specified injury of unspecified** ▽
renal artery

✓7ᵗʰ **S35.494** **Other specified injury of right renal vein**

✓7ᵗʰ **S35.495** **Other specified injury of left renal vein**

✓7ᵗʰ **S35.496** **Other specified injury of unspecified** ▽
renal vein

✓5ᵗʰ **S35.5** **Injury of iliac blood vessels**

✓x7ᵗʰ **S35.50** **Injury of unspecified iliac blood vessel(s)** ▽

✓6ᵗʰ **S35.51** **Injury of iliac artery or vein**
Injury of hypogastric artery or vein

✓7ᵗʰ **S35.511** **Injury of right iliac artery**

✓7ᵗʰ **S35.512** **Injury of left iliac artery**

✓7ᵗʰ **S35.513** **Injury of unspecified iliac artery** ▽

✓7ᵗʰ **S35.514** **Injury of right iliac vein**

✓7ᵗʰ **S35.515** **Injury of left iliac vein**

✓7ᵗʰ **S35.516** **Injury of unspecified iliac vein** ▽

✓6ᵗʰ **S35.53** **Injury of uterine artery or vein**

✓7ᵗʰ **S35.531** **Injury of right uterine artery** ♀

✓7ᵗʰ **S35.532** **Injury of left uterine artery** ♀

✓7ᵗʰ **S35.533** **Injury of unspecified uterine artery** ♀▽

✓7ᵗʰ **S35.534** **Injury of right uterine vein** ♀

✓7ᵗʰ **S35.535** **Injury of left uterine vein** ♀

✓7ᵗʰ **S35.536** **Injury of unspecified uterine vein** ♀▽

✓x7ᵗʰ **S35.59** **Injury of other iliac blood vessels**

✓5ᵗʰ **S35.8** **Injury of other blood vessels at abdomen, lower back and pelvis level**
Injury of ovarian artery or vein

✓6ᵗʰ **S35.8X** **Injury of other blood vessels at abdomen, lower back and pelvis level**

✓7ᵗʰ **S35.8X1** **Laceration of other blood vessels at abdomen, lower back and pelvis level**

✓7ᵗʰ **S35.8X8** **Other specified injury of other blood vessels at abdomen, lower back and pelvis level**

✓7ᵗʰ **S35.8X9** **Unspecified injury of other blood** ▽
vessels at abdomen, lower back and pelvis level

✓5ᵗʰ **S35.9** **Injury of unspecified blood vessel at abdomen, lower back and pelvis level**

✓x7ᵗʰ **S35.90** **Unspecified injury of unspecified blood vessel at** ▽
abdomen, lower back and pelvis level

✓x7ᵗʰ **S35.91** **Laceration of unspecified blood vessel at** ▽
abdomen, lower back and pelvis level

✓x7ᵗʰ **S35.99** **Other specified injury of unspecified blood vessel** ▽
at abdomen, lower back and pelvis level

✓4ᵗʰ **S36** **Injury of intra-abdominal organs**
Code also any associated open wound (S31.-)

The appropriate 7th character is to be added to each code from category S36.
A　　initial encounter
D　　subsequent encounter
S　　sequela

✓5ᵗʰ **S36.0** **Injury of spleen**

✓x7ᵗʰ **S36.00** **Unspecified injury of spleen** ▽

✓6ᵗʰ **S36.02** **Contusion of spleen**

✓7ᵗʰ **S36.020** **Minor contusion of spleen**
Contusion of spleen less than 2 cm

✓7ᵗʰ **S36.021** **Major contusion of spleen**
Contusion of spleen greater than 2 cm

✓7ᵗʰ **S36.029** **Unspecified contusion of spleen** ▽

✓6ᵗʰ **S36.03** **Laceration of spleen**

✓7ᵗʰ **S36.030** **Superficial (capsular) laceration of spleen**
Laceration of spleen less than 1cm
Minor laceration of spleen

✓7ᵗʰ **S36.031** **Moderate laceration of spleen**
Laceration of spleen 1 to 3 cm

✓7ᵗʰ **S36.032** **Major laceration of spleen**
Avulsion of spleen
Laceration of spleen greater than 3 cm
Massive laceration of spleen
Multiple moderate lacerations of spleen
Stellate laceration of spleen

✓7ᵗʰ **S36.039** **Unspecified laceration of spleen** ▽

✓x7ᵗʰ **S36.09** **Other injury of spleen**

✓5ᵗʰ **S36.1** **Injury of liver and gallbladder and bile duct**

✓6ᵗʰ **S36.11** **Injury of liver**

✓7ᵗʰ **S36.112** **Contusion of liver**

✓7ᵗʰ **S36.113** **Laceration of liver, unspecified degree** ▽

✓7ᵗʰ **S36.114** **Minor laceration of liver**
Laceration involving capsule only, or, without significant involvement of hepatic parenchyma [i.e., less than 1cm deep]

✓7ᵗʰ **S36.115** **Moderate laceration of liver**
Laceration involving parenchyma but without major disruption of parenchyma [i.e., less than 10 cm long and less than 3 cm deep]

✓7ᵗʰ **S36.116** **Major laceration of liver**
Laceration with significant disruption of hepatic parenchyma [i.e., greater than 10 cm long and 3 cm deep]
Multiple moderate lacerations, with or without hematoma
Stellate laceration of liver

✓7ᵗʰ **S36.118** **Other injury of liver**

✓7ᵗʰ **S36.119** **Unspecified injury of liver** ▽

✓6ᵗʰ **S36.12** **Injury of gallbladder**

✓7ᵗʰ **S36.122** **Contusion of gallbladder**

✓7ᵗʰ **S36.123** **Laceration of gallbladder**

✓7ᵗʰ **S36.128** **Other injury of gallbladder**

✓7ᵗʰ **S36.129** **Unspecified injury of gallbladder** ▽

✓x7ᵗʰ **S36.13** **Injury of bile duct**

✓5ᵗʰ **S36.2** **Injury of pancreas**

✓6ᵗʰ **S36.20** **Unspecified injury of pancreas**

✓7ᵗʰ **S36.200** **Unspecified injury of head of pancreas** ▽

✓7ᵗʰ **S36.201** **Unspecified injury of body of pancreas** ▽

✓7ᵗʰ **S36.202** **Unspecified injury of tail of pancreas** ▽

✓7ᵗʰ **S36.209** **Unspecified injury of unspecified part** ▽
of pancreas

✓6ᵗʰ **S36.22** **Contusion of pancreas**

✓7ᵗʰ **S36.220** **Contusion of head of pancreas**

✓7ᵗʰ **S36.221** **Contusion of body of pancreas**

✓7ᵗʰ **S36.222** **Contusion of tail of pancreas**

✓7ᵗʰ **S36.229** **Contusion of unspecified part of** ▽
pancreas

✓6ᵗʰ **S36.23** **Laceration of pancreas, unspecified degree**

✓7ᵗʰ **S36.230** **Laceration of head of pancreas,** ▽
unspecified degree

✓7ᵗʰ **S36.231** **Laceration of body of pancreas,** ▽
unspecified degree

✓7ᵗʰ **S36.232** **Laceration of tail of pancreas,** ▽
unspecified degree

✓7ᵗʰ **S36.239** **Laceration of unspecified part of** ▽
pancreas, unspecified degree

✓6ᵗʰ **S36.24** **Minor laceration of pancreas**

✓7ᵗʰ **S36.240** **Minor laceration of head of pancreas**

✓7ᵗʰ **S36.241** **Minor laceration of body of pancreas**

✓7ᵗʰ **S36.242** **Minor laceration of tail of pancreas**

✓7ᵗʰ **S36.249** **Minor laceration of unspecified part of** ▽
pancreas

Ⓝ Newborn　　Ⓟ Pediatric　　Ⓜ Maternity　　Ⓐ Adult　　RIC RIC Dx　　NCDx Noncancer Dx　　PDx Primary Dx　　CC RIC CC Condition　　▶◀ Revised Text　　● New Code　　▲ Revised Code Title

892　　　ICD-10-CM 2016

✓6th **S36.25** Moderate laceration of pancreas
- ✓7th **S36.250** Moderate laceration of head of pancreas
- ✓7th **S36.251** Moderate laceration of body of pancreas
- ✓7th **S36.252** Moderate laceration of tail of pancreas
- ✓7th **S36.259** Moderate laceration of unspecified part of pancreas ▽

✓6th **S36.26** Major laceration of pancreas
- ✓7th **S36.260** Major laceration of head of pancreas
- ✓7th **S36.261** Major laceration of body of pancreas
- ✓7th **S36.262** Major laceration of tail of pancreas
- ✓7th **S36.269** Major laceration of unspecified part of pancreas ▽

✓6th **S36.29** Other injury of pancreas
- ✓7th **S36.290** Other injury of head of pancreas
- ✓7th **S36.291** Other injury of body of pancreas
- ✓7th **S36.292** Other injury of tail of pancreas
- ✓7th **S36.299** Other injury of unspecified part of pancreas ▽

✓5th **S36.3** Injury of stomach
- ✓x7th **S36.30** Unspecified injury of stomach ▽
- ✓x7th **S36.32** Contusion of stomach
- ✓x7th **S36.33** Laceration of stomach
- ✓x7th **S36.39** Other injury of stomach

✓5th **S36.4** Injury of small intestine
- ✓6th **S36.40** Unspecified injury of small intestine
  - ✓7th **S36.400** Unspecified injury of duodenum ▽
  - ✓7th **S36.408** Unspecified injury of other part of small intestine ▽
  - ✓7th **S36.409** Unspecified injury of unspecified part of small intestine ▽
- ✓6th **S36.41** Primary blast injury of small intestine
  Blast injury of small intestine NOS
  - ✓7th **S36.410** Primary blast injury of duodenum
  - ✓7th **S36.418** Primary blast injury of other part of small intestine
  - ✓7th **S36.419** Primary blast injury of unspecified part of small intestine ▽
- ✓6th **S36.42** Contusion of small intestine
  - ✓7th **S36.420** Contusion of duodenum
  - ✓7th **S36.428** Contusion of other part of small intestine
  - ✓7th **S36.429** Contusion of unspecified part of small intestine ▽
- ✓6th **S36.43** Laceration of small intestine
  - ✓7th **S36.430** Laceration of duodenum
  - ✓7th **S36.438** Laceration of other part of small intestine
  - ✓7th **S36.439** Laceration of unspecified part of small intestine ▽
- ✓6th **S36.49** Other injury of small intestine
  - ✓7th **S36.490** Other injury of duodenum
  - ✓7th **S36.498** Other injury of other part of small intestine
  - ✓7th **S36.499** Other injury of unspecified part of small intestine ▽

✓5th **S36.5** Injury of colon
  EXCLUDES 2 injury of rectum (S36.6-)
- ✓6th **S36.50** Unspecified injury of colon
  - ✓7th **S36.500** Unspecified injury of ascending [right] colon ▽
  - ✓7th **S36.501** Unspecified injury of transverse colon ▽
  - ✓7th **S36.502** Unspecified injury of descending [left] colon ▽
  - ✓7th **S36.503** Unspecified injury of sigmoid colon ▽
  - ✓7th **S36.508** Unspecified injury of other part of colon ▽
  - ✓7th **S36.509** Unspecified injury of unspecified part of colon ▽
- ✓6th **S36.51** Primary blast injury of colon
  Blast injury of colon NOS
  - ✓7th **S36.510** Primary blast injury of ascending [right] colon
  - ✓7th **S36.511** Primary blast injury of transverse colon

- ✓7th **S36.512** Primary blast injury of descending [left] colon
- ✓7th **S36.513** Primary blast injury of sigmoid colon
- ✓7th **S36.518** Primary blast injury of other part of colon
- ✓7th **S36.519** Primary blast injury of unspecified part of colon ▽

✓6th **S36.52** Contusion of colon
- ✓7th **S36.520** Contusion of ascending [right] colon
- ✓7th **S36.521** Contusion of transverse colon
- ✓7th **S36.522** Contusion of descending [left] colon
- ✓7th **S36.523** Contusion of sigmoid colon
- ✓7th **S36.528** Contusion of other part of colon
- ✓7th **S36.529** Contusion of unspecified part of colon ▽

✓6th **S36.53** Laceration of colon
- ✓7th **S36.530** Laceration of ascending [right] colon
- ✓7th **S36.531** Laceration of transverse colon
- ✓7th **S36.532** Laceration of descending [left] colon
- ✓7th **S36.533** Laceration of sigmoid colon
- ✓7th **S36.538** Laceration of other part of colon
- ✓7th **S36.539** Laceration of unspecified part of colon ▽

✓6th **S36.59** Other injury of colon
  Secondary blast injury of colon
- ✓7th **S36.590** Other injury of ascending [right] colon
- ✓7th **S36.591** Other injury of transverse colon
- ✓7th **S36.592** Other injury of descending [left] colon
- ✓7th **S36.593** Other injury of sigmoid colon
- ✓7th **S36.598** Other injury of other part of colon
- ✓7th **S36.599** Other injury of unspecified part of colon ▽

✓5th **S36.6** Injury of rectum
- ✓x7th **S36.60** Unspecified injury of rectum ▽
- ✓x7th **S36.61** Primary blast injury of rectum
  Blast injury of rectum NOS
- ✓x7th **S36.62** Contusion of rectum
- ✓x7th **S36.63** Laceration of rectum
- ✓x7th **S36.69** Other injury of rectum
  Secondary blast injury of rectum

✓5th **S36.8** Injury of other intra-abdominal organs
- ✓x7th **S36.81** Injury of peritoneum
- ✓6th **S36.89** Injury of other intra-abdominal organs
  Injury of retroperitoneum
  - ✓7th **S36.892** Contusion of other intra-abdominal organs
  - ✓7th **S36.893** Laceration of other intra-abdominal organs
  - ✓7th **S36.898** Other injury of other intra-abdominal organs
  - ✓7th **S36.899** Unspecified injury of other intra-abdominal organs ▽

✓5th **S36.9** Injury of unspecified intra-abdominal organ
- ✓x7th **S36.90** Unspecified injury of unspecified intra-abdominal organ ▽
- ✓x7th **S36.92** Contusion of unspecified intra-abdominal organ ▽
- ✓x7th **S36.93** Laceration of unspecified intra-abdominal organ ▽
- ✓x7th **S36.99** Other injury of unspecified intra-abdominal organ ▽

✓4th **S37** Injury of urinary and pelvic organs
  Code also any associated open wound (S31.-)
  EXCLUDES 1 obstetric trauma to pelvic organs (O71.-)
  EXCLUDES 2 injury of peritoneum (S36.81)
  injury of retroperitoneum (S36.89-)

  The appropriate 7th character is to be added to each code from category S37.
  A   initial encounter
  D   subsequent encounter
  S   sequela

✓5th **S37.0** Injury of kidney
  EXCLUDES 2 acute kidney injury (nontraumatic) (N17.9)
- ✓6th **S37.00** Unspecified injury of kidney
  - ✓7th **S37.001** Unspecified injury of right kidney ▽

✔ Add'l Character Required   ✓x7th Placeholder Alert   RUG IV Special Care High Dx   RUG IV Clinically Complex Dx   RUG IV Special Care Low Dx   Manifestation Code   Other Specified Code   ▽ Unspecified Code

ICD-10-CM 2016   893

   ✓7ᵗʰ **S37.002**   Unspecified injury of left kidney ▽
   ✓7ᵗʰ **S37.009**   Unspecified injury of unspecified kidney ▽

✓6ᵗʰ **S37.01**   Minor contusion of kidney
   Contusion of kidney less than 2 cm
   Contusion of kidney NOS
   ✓7ᵗʰ **S37.011**   Minor contusion of right kidney
   ✓7ᵗʰ **S37.012**   Minor contusion of left kidney
   ✓7ᵗʰ **S37.019**   Minor contusion of unspecified kidney ▽

✓6ᵗʰ **S37.02**   Major contusion of kidney
   Contusion of kidney greater than 2 cm
   ✓7ᵗʰ **S37.021**   Major contusion of right kidney
   ✓7ᵗʰ **S37.022**   Major contusion of left kidney
   ✓7ᵗʰ **S37.029**   Major contusion of unspecified kidney ▽

✓6ᵗʰ **S37.03**   Laceration of kidney, unspecified degree
   ✓7ᵗʰ **S37.031**   Laceration of right kidney, unspecified degree ▽
   ✓7ᵗʰ **S37.032**   Laceration of left kidney, unspecified degree ▽
   ✓7ᵗʰ **S37.039**   Laceration of unspecified kidney, unspecified degree ▽

✓6ᵗʰ **S37.04**   Minor laceration of kidney
   Laceration of kidney less than 1 cm
   ✓7ᵗʰ **S37.041**   Minor laceration of right kidney
   ✓7ᵗʰ **S37.042**   Minor laceration of left kidney
   ✓7ᵗʰ **S37.049**   Minor laceration of unspecified kidney ▽

✓6ᵗʰ **S37.05**   Moderate laceration of kidney
   Laceration of kidney 1 to 3 cm
   ✓7ᵗʰ **S37.051**   Moderate laceration of right kidney
   ✓7ᵗʰ **S37.052**   Moderate laceration of left kidney
   ✓7ᵗʰ **S37.059**   Moderate laceration of unspecified kidney ▽

✓6ᵗʰ **S37.06**   Major laceration of kidney
   Avulsion of kidney
   Laceration of kidney greater than 3 cm
   Massive laceration of kidney
   Multiple moderate lacerations of kidney
   Stellate laceration of kidney
   ✓7ᵗʰ **S37.061**   Major laceration of right kidney
   ✓7ᵗʰ **S37.062**   Major laceration of left kidney
   ✓7ᵗʰ **S37.069**   Major laceration of unspecified kidney ▽

✓6ᵗʰ **S37.09**   Other injury of kidney
   ✓7ᵗʰ **S37.091**   Other injury of right kidney
   ✓7ᵗʰ **S37.092**   Other injury of left kidney
   ✓7ᵗʰ **S37.099**   Other injury of unspecified kidney ▽

✓5ᵗʰ **S37.1**   Injury of ureter
  ✓x7ᵗʰ **S37.10**   Unspecified injury of ureter ▽
  ✓x7ᵗʰ **S37.12**   Contusion of ureter
  ✓x7ᵗʰ **S37.13**   Laceration of ureter
  ✓x7ᵗʰ **S37.19**   Other injury of ureter

✓5ᵗʰ **S37.2**   Injury of bladder
  ✓x7ᵗʰ **S37.20**   Unspecified injury of bladder ▽
  ✓x7ᵗʰ **S37.22**   Contusion of bladder
  ✓x7ᵗʰ **S37.23**   Laceration of bladder
  ✓x7ᵗʰ **S37.29**   Other injury of bladder

✓5ᵗʰ **S37.3**   Injury of urethra
  ✓x7ᵗʰ **S37.30**   Unspecified injury of urethra ▽
  ✓x7ᵗʰ **S37.32**   Contusion of urethra
  ✓x7ᵗʰ **S37.33**   Laceration of urethra
  ✓x7ᵗʰ **S37.39**   Other injury of urethra

✓5ᵗʰ **S37.4**   Injury of ovary
  ✓6ᵗʰ **S37.40**   Unspecified injury of ovary
   ✓7ᵗʰ **S37.401**   Unspecified injury of ovary, unilateral ♀▽
   ✓7ᵗʰ **S37.402**   Unspecified injury of ovary, bilateral ♀▽
   ✓7ᵗʰ **S37.409**   Unspecified injury of ovary, unspecified ♀▽
  ✓6ᵗʰ **S37.42**   Contusion of ovary
   ✓7ᵗʰ **S37.421**   Contusion of ovary, unilateral ♀
   ✓7ᵗʰ **S37.422**   Contusion of ovary, bilateral ♀
   ✓7ᵗʰ **S37.429**   Contusion of ovary, unspecified ♀▽

✓6ᵗʰ **S37.43**   Laceration of ovary
   ✓7ᵗʰ **S37.431**   Laceration of ovary, unilateral ♀
   ✓7ᵗʰ **S37.432**   Laceration of ovary, bilateral ♀
   ✓7ᵗʰ **S37.439**   Laceration of ovary, unspecified ♀▽

✓6ᵗʰ **S37.49**   Other injury of ovary
   ✓7ᵗʰ **S37.491**   Other injury of ovary, unilateral ♀
   ✓7ᵗʰ **S37.492**   Other injury of ovary, bilateral ♀
   ✓7ᵗʰ **S37.499**   Other injury of ovary, unspecified ♀▽

✓5ᵗʰ **S37.5**   Injury of fallopian tube
  S37.50   Unspecified injury of fallopian tube
   ✓7ᵗʰ **S37.501**   Unspecified injury of fallopian tube, unilateral ♀▽
   ✓7ᵗʰ **S37.502**   Unspecified injury of fallopian tube, bilateral ♀▽
   ✓7ᵗʰ **S37.509**   Unspecified injury of fallopian tube, unspecified ♀▽

✓6ᵗʰ **S37.51**   Primary blast injury of fallopian tube
   Blast injury of fallopian tube NOS
   ✓7ᵗʰ **S37.511**   Primary blast injury of fallopian tube, unilateral ♀
   ✓7ᵗʰ **S37.512**   Primary blast injury of fallopian tube, bilateral ♀
   ✓7ᵗʰ **S37.519**   Primary blast injury of fallopian tube, unspecified ♀▽

✓6ᵗʰ **S37.52**   Contusion of fallopian tube
   ✓7ᵗʰ **S37.521**   Contusion of fallopian tube, unilateral ♀
   ✓7ᵗʰ **S37.522**   Contusion of fallopian tube, bilateral ♀
   ✓7ᵗʰ **S37.529**   Contusion of fallopian tube, unspecified ♀▽

✓6ᵗʰ **S37.53**   Laceration of fallopian tube
   ✓7ᵗʰ **S37.531**   Laceration of fallopian tube, unilateral ♀
   ✓7ᵗʰ **S37.532**   Laceration of fallopian tube, bilateral ♀
   ✓7ᵗʰ **S37.539**   Laceration of fallopian tube, unspecified ♀▽

✓6ᵗʰ **S37.59**   Other injury of fallopian tube
   Secondary blast injury of fallopian tube
   ✓7ᵗʰ **S37.591**   Other injury of fallopian tube, unilateral ♀
   ✓7ᵗʰ **S37.592**   Other injury of fallopian tube, bilateral ♀
   ✓7ᵗʰ **S37.599**   Other injury of fallopian tube, unspecified ♀▽

✓5ᵗʰ **S37.6**   Injury of uterus
  EXCLUDES1   injury to gravid uterus (O9A.2-)
          injury to uterus during delivery (O71.-)
  ✓x7ᵗʰ **S37.60**   Unspecified injury of uterus ♀▽
  ✓x7ᵗʰ **S37.62**   Contusion of uterus ♀
  ✓x7ᵗʰ **S37.63**   Laceration of uterus ♀
  ✓x7ᵗʰ **S37.69**   Other injury of uterus ♀

✓5ᵗʰ **S37.8**   Injury of other urinary and pelvic organs
  ✓6ᵗʰ **S37.81**   Injury of adrenal gland
   ✓7ᵗʰ **S37.812**   Contusion of adrenal gland
   ✓7ᵗʰ **S37.813**   Laceration of adrenal gland
   ✓7ᵗʰ **S37.818**   Other injury of adrenal gland
   ✓7ᵗʰ **S37.819**   Unspecified injury of adrenal gland ▽
  ✓6ᵗʰ **S37.82**   Injury of prostate
   ✓7ᵗʰ **S37.822**   Contusion of prostate ♂
   ✓7ᵗʰ **S37.823**   Laceration of prostate ♂
   ✓7ᵗʰ **S37.828**   Other injury of prostate ♂
   ✓7ᵗʰ **S37.829**   Unspecified injury of prostate ♂▽
  ✓6ᵗʰ **S37.89**   Injury of other urinary and pelvic organ
   ✓7ᵗʰ **S37.892**   Contusion of other urinary and pelvic organ
   ✓7ᵗʰ **S37.893**   Laceration of other urinary and pelvic organ
   ✓7ᵗʰ **S37.898**   Other injury of other urinary and pelvic organ
   ✓7ᵗʰ **S37.899**   Unspecified injury of other urinary and pelvic organ ▽

✓5ᵗʰ **S37.9**   Injury of unspecified urinary and pelvic organ
  ✓x7ᵗʰ **S37.90**   Unspecified injury of unspecified urinary and pelvic organ ▽

Ⓝ Newborn   Ⓟ Pediatric   Ⓜ Maternity   Ⓐ Adult   **RIC** RIC Dx   **NC Dx** Noncancer Dx   **PDx** Primary Dx   **CC** RIC CC Condition   ►◄ Revised Text   ● New Code   ▲ Revised Code Title

√x7ᵗʰ **S37.92** Contusion of unspecified urinary and pelvic organ ▽

√x7ᵗʰ **S37.93** Laceration of unspecified urinary and pelvic organ ▽

√x7ᵗʰ **S37.99** Other injury of unspecified urinary and pelvic organ ▽

√4ᵗʰ **S38** **Crushing injury and traumatic amputation of abdomen, lower back, pelvis and external genitals**
> **NOTE** An amputation not identified as partial or complete should be coded to complete.

> The appropriate 7th character is to be added to each code from category S38.
> A   initial encounter
> D   subsequent encounter
> S   sequela

√5ᵗʰ **S38.0** **Crushing injury of** external genital organs
> Use additional code for any associated injuries

  √6ᵗʰ **S38.00** **Crushing injury of** unspecified **external genital organs**

    √7ᵗʰ **S38.001** **Crushing injury of unspecified external genital organs,** male ♂▽

    √7ᵗʰ **S38.002** **Crushing injury of unspecified external genital organs,** female ♀▽

  √x7ᵗʰ **S38.01** **Crushing injury of** penis ♂

  √x7ᵗʰ **S38.02** **Crushing injury of** scrotum and testis ♂

  √x7ᵗʰ **S38.03** **Crushing injury of** vulva ♀

√x7ᵗʰ **S38.1** **Crushing injury of abdomen, lower back, and pelvis**
> Use additional code for all associated injuries, such as:
> fracture of thoracic or lumbar spine and pelvis (S22.0-, S32-)
> injury to intra-abdominal organs (S36.-)
> injury to urinary and pelvic organs (S37.-)
> open wound of abdominal wall (S31.-)
> spinal cord injury (S34.0, S34.1-)
> **EXCLUDES 2** crushing injury of external genital organs (S38.0-)

√5ᵗʰ **S38.2** **Traumatic amputation** of external genital organs

  √6ᵗʰ **S38.21** **Traumatic amputation of** female **external genital organs**
> Traumatic amputation of clitoris
> Traumatic amputation of labium (majus) (minus)
> Traumatic amputation of vulva

    √7ᵗʰ **S38.211** **Complete traumatic amputation of female external genital organs** ♀

    √7ᵗʰ **S38.212** **Partial traumatic amputation of female external genital organs** ♀

  √6ᵗʰ **S38.22** **Traumatic amputation of** penis

    √7ᵗʰ **S38.221** **Complete traumatic amputation of penis** ♂

    √7ᵗʰ **S38.222** **Partial traumatic amputation of penis** ♂

  √6ᵗʰ **S38.23** **Traumatic amputation of** scrotum and testis

    √7ᵗʰ **S38.231** **Complete traumatic amputation of scrotum and testis** ♂

    √7ᵗʰ **S38.232** **Partial traumatic amputation of scrotum and testis** ♂

√x7ᵗʰ **S38.3** **Transection (partial) of abdomen**

√4ᵗʰ **S39** **Other and unspecified injuries of abdomen, lower back, pelvis and external genitals**
> Code also any associated open wound (S31.-)
> **EXCLUDES 2** sprain of joints and ligaments of lumbar spine and pelvis (S33.-)

> The appropriate 7th character is to be added to each code from category S39.
> A   initial encounter
> D   subsequent encounter
> S   sequela

√5ᵗʰ **S39.0** **Injury of muscle, fascia and tendon of abdomen, lower back and pelvis**

  √6ᵗʰ **S39.00** Unspecified **injury of muscle, fascia and tendon of abdomen, lower back and pelvis**

    √7ᵗʰ **S39.001** **Unspecified injury of muscle, fascia and tendon of** abdomen ▽

    √7ᵗʰ **S39.002** **Unspecified injury of muscle, fascia and tendon of** lower back ▽

    √7ᵗʰ **S39.003** **Unspecified injury of muscle, fascia and tendon of** pelvis ▽

√6ᵗʰ **S39.01** Strain **of muscle, fascia and tendon of abdomen, lower back and pelvis**

  √7ᵗʰ **S39.011** **Strain of muscle, fascia and tendon of** abdomen

  √7ᵗʰ **S39.012** **Strain of muscle, fascia and tendon of** lower back

  √7ᵗʰ **S39.013** **Strain of muscle, fascia and tendon of** pelvis

√6ᵗʰ **S39.02** Laceration **of muscle, fascia and tendon of abdomen, lower back and pelvis**

  √7ᵗʰ **S39.021** **Laceration of muscle, fascia and tendon of** abdomen

  √7ᵗʰ **S39.022** **Laceration of muscle, fascia and tendon of** lower back

  √7ᵗʰ **S39.023** **Laceration of muscle, fascia and tendon of** pelvis

√6ᵗʰ **S39.09** Other **injury of muscle, fascia and tendon of abdomen, lower back and pelvis**

  √7ᵗʰ **S39.091** **Other injury of muscle, fascia and tendon of** abdomen

  √7ᵗʰ **S39.092** **Other injury of muscle, fascia and tendon of** lower back

  √7ᵗʰ **S39.093** **Other injury of muscle, fascia and tendon of** pelvis

√5ᵗʰ **S39.8** Other **specified injuries of abdomen, lower back, pelvis and external genitals**

  √x7ᵗʰ **S39.81** **Other specified injuries of** abdomen

  √x7ᵗʰ **S39.82** **Other specified injuries of** lower back

  √x7ᵗʰ **S39.83** **Other specified injuries of** pelvis

  √6ᵗʰ **S39.84** **Other specified injuries of** external genitals

    √7ᵗʰ **S39.840** **Fracture of** corpus cavernosum penis ♂

    √7ᵗʰ **S39.848** **Other specified injuries of external genitals**

√5ᵗʰ **S39.9** Unspecified **injury of abdomen, lower back, pelvis and external genitals**

  √x7ᵗʰ **S39.91** **Unspecified injury of** abdomen ▽

  √x7ᵗʰ **S39.92** **Unspecified injury of** lower back ▽

  √x7ᵗʰ **S39.93** **Unspecified injury of** pelvis ▽

  √x7ᵗʰ **S39.94** **Unspecified injury of** external genitals ▽

Injuries to the shoulder and upper arm (S40-S49)

INCLUDES injuries of axilla
injuries of scapular region
EXCLUDES 2 burns and corrosions (T20-T32)
frostbite (T33-T34)
injuries of elbow (S50-S59)
insect bite or sting, venomous (T63.4)

√4ᵗʰ **S40** **Superficial injury of shoulder and upper arm**

> The appropriate 7th character is to be added to each code from category S40.
> A   initial encounter
> D   subsequent encounter
> S   sequela

√5ᵗʰ **S40.0** Contusion **of shoulder and upper arm**

  √6ᵗʰ **S40.01** **Contusion of** shoulder

    √7ᵗʰ **S40.011** **Contusion of** right **shoulder**

    √7ᵗʰ **S40.012** **Contusion of** left **shoulder**

    √7ᵗʰ **S40.019** **Contusion of unspecified shoulder** ▽

  √6ᵗʰ **S40.02** **Contusion of** upper arm

    √7ᵗʰ **S40.021** **Contusion of** right **upper arm**

    √7ᵗʰ **S40.022** **Contusion of** left **upper arm**

    √7ᵗʰ **S40.029** **Contusion of unspecified upper arm** ▽

√5ᵗʰ **S40.2** Other **superficial injuries of shoulder**

  √6ᵗʰ **S40.21** Abrasion **of shoulder**

    √7ᵗʰ **S40.211** **Abrasion of** right **shoulder**

    √7ᵗʰ **S40.212** **Abrasion of** left **shoulder**

    √7ᵗʰ **S40.219** **Abrasion of unspecified shoulder** ▽

  √6ᵗʰ **S40.22** Blister **(nonthermal) of shoulder**

    √7ᵗʰ **S40.221** **Blister (nonthermal) of** right **shoulder**

☑ Add'l Character Required   √x7ᵗʰ Placeholder Alert   RUG IV Special Care High Dx   RUG IV Clinically Complex Dx   RUG IV Special Care Low Dx   Manifestation Code   Other Specified Code   ▽Unspecified Code

√7th **S40.222**   Blister (nonthermal) of left shoulder

√7th **S40.229**   Blister (nonthermal) of unspecified shoulder ▽

√6th **S40.24**   External constriction of shoulder

    √7th **S40.241**   External constriction of right shoulder

    √7th **S40.242**   External constriction of left shoulder

    √7th **S40.249**   External constriction of unspecified shoulder ▽

√6th **S40.25**   Superficial foreign body of shoulder
    Splinter in the shoulder

    √7th **S40.251**   Superficial foreign body of right shoulder

    √7th **S40.252**   Superficial foreign body of left shoulder

    √7th **S40.259**   Superficial foreign body of unspecified shoulder ▽

√6th **S40.26**   Insect bite (nonvenomous) of shoulder

    √7th **S40.261**   Insect bite (nonvenomous) of right shoulder

    √7th **S40.262**   Insect bite (nonvenomous) of left shoulder

    √7th **S40.269**   Insect bite (nonvenomous) of unspecified shoulder ▽

√6th **S40.27**   Other superficial bite of shoulder
    EXCLUDES 1   *open bite of shoulder (S41.05)*

    √7th **S40.271**   **Other superficial bite of right shoulder**

    √7th **S40.272**   **Other superficial bite of left shoulder**

    √7th **S40.279**   **Other superficial bite of unspecified shoulder** ▽

√5th **S40.8**   Other superficial injuries of upper arm

√6th **S40.81**   Abrasion of upper arm

    √7th **S40.811**   Abrasion of right upper arm

    √7th **S40.812**   Abrasion of left upper arm

    √7th **S40.819**   Abrasion of unspecified upper arm ▽

√6th **S40.82**   Blister (nonthermal) of upper arm

    √7th **S40.821**   Blister (nonthermal) of right upper arm

    √7th **S40.822**   Blister (nonthermal) of left upper arm

    √7th **S40.829**   Blister (nonthermal) of unspecified upper arm ▽

√6th **S40.84**   External constriction of upper arm

    √7th **S40.841**   External constriction of right upper arm

    √7th **S40.842**   External constriction of left upper arm

    √7th **S40.849**   External constriction of unspecified upper arm ▽

√6th **S40.85**   Superficial foreign body of upper arm
    Splinter in the upper arm

    √7th **S40.851**   Superficial foreign body of right upper arm

    √7th **S40.852**   Superficial foreign body of left upper arm

    √7th **S40.859**   Superficial foreign body of unspecified upper arm ▽

√6th **S40.86**   Insect bite (nonvenomous) of upper arm

    √7th **S40.861**   Insect bite (nonvenomous) of right upper arm

    √7th **S40.862**   Insect bite (nonvenomous) of left upper arm

    √7th **S40.869**   Insect bite (nonvenomous) of unspecified upper arm ▽

√6th **S40.87**   Other superficial bite of upper arm
    EXCLUDES 1   *open bite of upper arm (S41.14)*
    EXCLUDES 2   *other superficial bite of shoulder (S40.27-)*

    √7th **S40.871**   **Other superficial bite of right upper arm**

    √7th **S40.872**   **Other superficial bite of left upper arm**

    √7th **S40.879**   **Other superficial bite of unspecified upper arm** ▽

√5th **S40.9**   Unspecified superficial injury of shoulder and upper arm

√6th **S40.91**   Unspecified superficial injury of shoulder

    √7th **S40.911**   Unspecified superficial injury of right shoulder ▽

    √7th **S40.912**   Unspecified superficial injury of left shoulder ▽

    √7th **S40.919**   Unspecified superficial injury of unspecified shoulder ▽

√6th **S40.92**   Unspecified superficial injury of upper arm

    √7th **S40.921**   Unspecified superficial injury of right upper arm ▽

    √7th **S40.922**   Unspecified superficial injury of left upper arm ▽

    √7th **S40.929**   Unspecified superficial injury of unspecified upper arm ▽

√4th **S41**   **Open wound of shoulder and upper arm**
    Code also any associated wound infection
    EXCLUDES 1   *traumatic amputation of shoulder and upper arm (S48.-)*
    EXCLUDES 2   *open fracture of shoulder and upper arm (S42.- with 7th character B or C)*

    The appropriate 7th character is to be added to each code from category S41.
    A   initial encounter
    D   subsequent encounter
    S   sequela

√5th **S41.0**   Open wound of shoulder

√6th **S41.00**   Unspecified open wound of shoulder

    √7th **S41.001**   Unspecified open wound of right shoulder ▽

    √7th **S41.002**   Unspecified open wound of left shoulder ▽

    √7th **S41.009**   Unspecified open wound of unspecified shoulder ▽

√6th **S41.01**   Laceration without foreign body of shoulder

    √7th **S41.011**   Laceration without foreign body of right shoulder

    √7th **S41.012**   Laceration without foreign body of left shoulder

    √7th **S41.019**   Laceration without foreign body of unspecified shoulder ▽

√6th **S41.02**   Laceration with foreign body of shoulder

    √7th **S41.021**   Laceration with foreign body of right shoulder

    √7th **S41.022**   Laceration with foreign body of left shoulder

    √7th **S41.029**   Laceration with foreign body of unspecified shoulder ▽

√6th **S41.03**   Puncture wound without foreign body of shoulder

    √7th **S41.031**   Puncture wound without foreign body of right shoulder

    √7th **S41.032**   Puncture wound without foreign body of left shoulder

    √7th **S41.039**   Puncture wound without foreign body of unspecified shoulder ▽

√6th **S41.04**   Puncture wound with foreign body of shoulder

    √7th **S41.041**   Puncture wound with foreign body of right shoulder

    √7th **S41.042**   Puncture wound with foreign body of left shoulder

    √7th **S41.049**   Puncture wound with foreign body of unspecified shoulder ▽

√6th **S41.05**   Open bite of shoulder
    Bite of shoulder NOS
    EXCLUDES 1   *superficial bite of shoulder (S40.27)*

    √7th **S41.051**   Open bite of right shoulder

    √7th **S41.052**   Open bite of left shoulder

    √7th **S41.059**   Open bite of unspecified shoulder ▽

√5th **S41.1**   Open wound of upper arm

√6th **S41.10**   Unspecified open wound of upper arm

    √7th **S41.101**   Unspecified open wound of right upper arm ▽

    √7th **S41.102**   Unspecified open wound of left upper arm ▽

    √7th **S41.109**   Unspecified open wound of unspecified upper arm ▽

√6th **S41.11**   Laceration without foreign body of upper arm

    √7th **S41.111**   Laceration without foreign body of right upper arm

Ⓝ Newborn   Ⓟ Pediatric   Ⓜ Maternity   Ⓐ Adult   **RIC** RIC Dx   **NCDx** Noncancer Dx   **PDx** Primary Dx   **CC** RIC CC Condition   ►◄ Revised Text   ● New Code   ▲ Revised Code Title

896   ICD-10-CM 2016

✓7ᵗʰ **S41.112** **Laceration without foreign body of** left **upper arm**

✓7ᵗʰ **S41.119** **Laceration without foreign body of** ▽ **unspecified upper arm**

✓6ᵗʰ **S41.12** Laceration with foreign body **of upper arm**

✓7ᵗʰ **S41.121** **Laceration with foreign body of** right **upper arm**

✓7ᵗʰ **S41.122** **Laceration with foreign body of** left **upper arm**

✓7ᵗʰ **S41.129** **Laceration with foreign body of** ▽ **unspecified upper arm**

✓6ᵗʰ **S41.13** Puncture wound without foreign body **of upper arm**

✓7ᵗʰ **S41.131** **Puncture wound without foreign body of** right **upper arm**

✓7ᵗʰ **S41.132** **Puncture wound without foreign body of** left **upper arm**

✓7ᵗʰ **S41.139** **Puncture wound without foreign body** ▽ **of unspecified upper arm**

✓6ᵗʰ **S41.14** Puncture wound with foreign body **of upper arm**

✓7ᵗʰ **S41.141** **Puncture wound with foreign body of** right **upper arm**

✓7ᵗʰ **S41.142** **Puncture wound with foreign body of** left **upper arm**

✓7ᵗʰ **S41.149** **Puncture wound with foreign body of** ▽ **unspecified upper arm**

✓6ᵗʰ **S41.15** Open bite **of upper arm**
Bite of upper arm NOS
EXCLUDES 1 *superficial bite of upper arm (S40.87)*

✓7ᵗʰ **S41.151** **Open bite of** right **upper arm**

✓7ᵗʰ **S41.152** **Open bite of** left **upper arm**

✓7ᵗʰ **S41.159** **Open bite of unspecified upper arm** ▽

✓4ᵗʰ **S42** **Fracture of shoulder and upper arm**
NOTE A fracture not indicated as displaced or nondisplaced should be coded to displaced.
A fracture not indicated as open or closed should be coded to closed.
EXCLUDES 1 *traumatic amputation of shoulder and upper arm (S48.-)*

The appropriate 7th character is to be added to all codes from category S42 [unless otherwise indicated].
A initial encounter for closed fracture
B initial encounter for open fracture
D subsequent encounter for fracture with routine healing
G subsequent encounter for fracture with delayed healing
K subsequent encounter for fracture with nonunion
P subsequent encounter for fracture with malunion
S sequela

✓5ᵗʰ **S42.0** **Fracture of** clavicle

✓6ᵗʰ **S42.00** **Fracture of** unspecified **part of clavicle**

✓7ᵗʰ **S42.001** **Fracture of unspecified part of** right ▽ **clavicle**

✓7ᵗʰ **S42.002** **Fracture of unspecified part of** left ▽ **clavicle**

✓7ᵗʰ **S42.009** **Fracture of unspecified part of** ▽ **unspecified clavicle**
AHA: 2012, 4Q, 93

✓6ᵗʰ **S42.01** **Fracture of** sternal end **of clavicle**

✓7ᵗʰ **S42.011** Anterior displaced **fracture of sternal end of** right **clavicle**

✓7ᵗʰ **S42.012** Anterior displaced **fracture of sternal end of** left **clavicle**

✓7ᵗʰ **S42.013** Anterior displaced **fracture of sternal** ▽ **end of unspecified clavicle**
Displaced fracture of sternal end of clavicle NOS

✓7ᵗʰ **S42.014** Posterior displaced **fracture of sternal end of** right **clavicle**

✓7ᵗʰ **S42.015** Posterior displaced **fracture of sternal end of** left **clavicle**

✓7ᵗʰ **S42.016** Posterior displaced **fracture of sternal** ▽ **end of unspecified clavicle**

✓7ᵗʰ **S42.017** Nondisplaced **fracture of sternal end of** right **clavicle**

✓7ᵗʰ **S42.018** Nondisplaced **fracture of sternal end of** left **clavicle**

✓7ᵗʰ **S42.019** Nondisplaced **fracture of sternal end** ▽ **of unspecified clavicle**

✓6ᵗʰ **S42.02** **Fracture of** shaft **of clavicle**

✓7ᵗʰ **S42.021** Displaced **fracture of shaft of** right **clavicle**

✓7ᵗʰ **S42.022** Displaced **fracture of shaft of** left **clavicle**

✓7ᵗʰ **S42.023** Displaced **fracture of shaft of** ▽ **unspecified clavicle**

✓7ᵗʰ **S42.024** Nondisplaced **fracture of shaft of** right **clavicle**

✓7ᵗʰ **S42.025** Nondisplaced **fracture of shaft of** left **clavicle**

✓7ᵗʰ **S42.026** Nondisplaced **fracture of shaft of** ▽ **unspecified clavicle**

✓6ᵗʰ **S42.03** **Fracture of** lateral end **of clavicle**
Fracture of acromial end of clavicle

✓7ᵗʰ **S42.031** Displaced **fracture of lateral end of** right **clavicle**

✓7ᵗʰ **S42.032** Displaced **fracture of lateral end of** left **clavicle**

✓7ᵗʰ **S42.033** Displaced **fracture of lateral end of** ▽ **unspecified clavicle**

✓7ᵗʰ **S42.034** Nondisplaced **fracture of lateral end of** right **clavicle**

✓7ᵗʰ **S42.035** Nondisplaced **fracture of lateral end of** left **clavicle**

✓7ᵗʰ **S42.036** Nondisplaced **fracture of lateral end** ▽ **of unspecified clavicle**

✓5ᵗʰ **S42.1** **Fracture of** scapula

✓6ᵗʰ **S42.10** **Fracture of** unspecified **part of scapula**

✓7ᵗʰ **S42.101** **Fracture of unspecified part of scapula,** ▽ right **shoulder**

✓7ᵗʰ **S42.102** **Fracture of unspecified part of scapula,** ▽ left **shoulder**

✓7ᵗʰ **S42.109** **Fracture of unspecified part of scapula,** ▽ **unspecified shoulder**

✓6ᵗʰ **S42.11** **Fracture of** body **of scapula**

✓7ᵗʰ **S42.111** Displaced **fracture of body of scapula,** right **shoulder**

✓7ᵗʰ **S42.112** Displaced **fracture of body of scapula,** left **shoulder**

✓7ᵗʰ **S42.113** Displaced **fracture of body of scapula,** ▽ **unspecified shoulder**

✓7ᵗʰ **S42.114** Nondisplaced **fracture of body of scapula,** right **shoulder**

✓7ᵗʰ **S42.115** Nondisplaced **fracture of body of scapula,** left **shoulder**

✓7ᵗʰ **S42.116** Nondisplaced **fracture of body of** ▽ **scapula, unspecified shoulder**

✓6ᵗʰ **S42.12** **Fracture of** acromial process

✓7ᵗʰ **S42.121** Displaced **fracture of acromial process,** right **shoulder**

✓7ᵗʰ **S42.122** Displaced **fracture of acromial process,** left **shoulder**

✓7ᵗʰ **S42.123** Displaced **fracture of acromial process,** ▽ **unspecified shoulder**

✓7ᵗʰ **S42.124** Nondisplaced **fracture of acromial process,** right **shoulder**

✓7ᵗʰ **S42.125** Nondisplaced **fracture of acromial process,** left **shoulder**

✓7ᵗʰ **S42.126** Nondisplaced **fracture of acromial** ▽ **process, unspecified shoulder**

✓6ᵗʰ **S42.13** **Fracture of** coracoid process

✓7ᵗʰ **S42.131** Displaced **fracture of coracoid process,** right **shoulder**

✓7ᵗʰ **S42.132** Displaced **fracture of coracoid process,** left **shoulder**

✓7ᵗʰ **S42.133** Displaced **fracture of coracoid process,** ▽ **unspecified shoulder**

✓7ᵗʰ **S42.134** Nondisplaced **fracture of coracoid process,** right **shoulder**

✓7ᵗʰ **S42.135** Nondisplaced fracture of coracoid process, left shoulder

✓7ᵗʰ **S42.136** Nondisplaced fracture of coracoid process, unspecified shoulder ▽

✓6ᵗʰ **S42.14** Fracture of glenoid cavity of scapula

✓7ᵗʰ **S42.141** Displaced fracture of glenoid cavity of scapula, right shoulder

✓7ᵗʰ **S42.142** Displaced fracture of glenoid cavity of scapula, left shoulder

✓7ᵗʰ **S42.143** Displaced fracture of glenoid cavity of scapula, unspecified shoulder ▽

✓7ᵗʰ **S42.144** Nondisplaced fracture of glenoid cavity of scapula, right shoulder

✓7ᵗʰ **S42.145** Nondisplaced fracture of glenoid cavity of scapula, left shoulder

✓7ᵗʰ **S42.146** Nondisplaced fracture of glenoid cavity of scapula, unspecified shoulder ▽

✓6ᵗʰ **S42.15** Fracture of neck of scapula

✓7ᵗʰ **S42.151** Displaced fracture of neck of scapula, right shoulder

✓7ᵗʰ **S42.152** Displaced fracture of neck of scapula, left shoulder

✓7ᵗʰ **S42.153** Displaced fracture of neck of scapula, unspecified shoulder ▽

✓7ᵗʰ **S42.154** Nondisplaced fracture of neck of scapula, right shoulder

✓7ᵗʰ **S42.155** Nondisplaced fracture of neck of scapula, left shoulder

✓7ᵗʰ **S42.156** Nondisplaced fracture of neck of scapula, unspecified shoulder ▽

✓6ᵗʰ **S42.19** Fracture of other part of scapula

✓7ᵗʰ **S42.191** Fracture of other part of scapula, right shoulder

✓7ᵗʰ **S42.192** Fracture of other part of scapula, left shoulder

✓7ᵗʰ **S42.199** Fracture of other part of scapula, unspecified shoulder ▽

✓5ᵗʰ **S42.2** Fracture of upper end of humerus
Fracture of proximal end of humerus
EXCLUDES 2   fracture of shaft of humerus (S42.3-)
physeal fracture of upper end of humerus (S49.0-)

✓6ᵗʰ **S42.20** Unspecified fracture of upper end of humerus

✓7ᵗʰ **S42.201** Unspecified fracture of upper end of right humerus ▽

✓7ᵗʰ **S42.202** Unspecified fracture of upper end of left humerus ▽

✓7ᵗʰ **S42.209** Unspecified fracture of upper end of unspecified humerus ▽

✓6ᵗʰ **S42.21** Unspecified fracture of surgical neck of humerus
Fracture of neck of humerus NOS

✓7ᵗʰ **S42.211** Unspecified displaced fracture of surgical neck of right humerus ▽

✓7ᵗʰ **S42.212** Unspecified displaced fracture of surgical neck of left humerus ▽

✓7ᵗʰ **S42.213** Unspecified displaced fracture of surgical neck of unspecified humerus ▽

✓7ᵗʰ **S42.214** Unspecified nondisplaced fracture of surgical neck of right humerus ▽

✓7ᵗʰ **S42.215** Unspecified nondisplaced fracture of surgical neck of left humerus ▽

✓7ᵗʰ **S42.216** Unspecified nondisplaced fracture of surgical neck of unspecified humerus ▽

✓6ᵗʰ **S42.22** 2-part fracture of surgical neck of humerus

✓7ᵗʰ **S42.221** 2-part displaced fracture of surgical neck of right humerus

✓7ᵗʰ **S42.222** 2-part displaced fracture of surgical neck of left humerus

✓7ᵗʰ **S42.223** 2-part displaced fracture of surgical neck of unspecified humerus ▽

✓7ᵗʰ **S42.224** 2-part nondisplaced fracture of surgical neck of right humerus

✓7ᵗʰ **S42.225** 2-part nondisplaced fracture of surgical neck of left humerus

✓7ᵗʰ **S42.226** 2-part nondisplaced fracture of surgical neck of unspecified humerus ▽

✓6ᵗʰ **S42.23** 3-part fracture of surgical neck of humerus

✓7ᵗʰ **S42.231** 3-part fracture of surgical neck of right humerus

✓7ᵗʰ **S42.232** 3-part fracture of surgical neck of left humerus

✓7ᵗʰ **S42.239** 3-part fracture of surgical neck of unspecified humerus ▽

✓6ᵗʰ **S42.24** 4-part fracture of surgical neck of humerus

✓7ᵗʰ **S42.241** 4-part fracture of surgical neck of right humerus

✓7ᵗʰ **S42.242** 4-part fracture of surgical neck of left humerus

✓7ᵗʰ **S42.249** 4-part fracture of surgical neck of unspecified humerus ▽

✓6ᵗʰ **S42.25** Fracture of greater tuberosity of humerus

✓7ᵗʰ **S42.251** Displaced fracture of greater tuberosity of right humerus

✓7ᵗʰ **S42.252** Displaced fracture of greater tuberosity of left humerus

✓7ᵗʰ **S42.253** Displaced fracture of greater tuberosity of unspecified humerus ▽

✓7ᵗʰ **S42.254** Nondisplaced fracture of greater tuberosity of right humerus

✓7ᵗʰ **S42.255** Nondisplaced fracture of greater tuberosity of left humerus

✓7ᵗʰ **S42.256** Nondisplaced fracture of greater tuberosity of unspecified humerus ▽

✓6ᵗʰ **S42.26** Fracture of lesser tuberosity of humerus

✓7ᵗʰ **S42.261** Displaced fracture of lesser tuberosity of right humerus

✓7ᵗʰ **S42.262** Displaced fracture of lesser tuberosity of left humerus

✓7ᵗʰ **S42.263** Displaced fracture of lesser tuberosity of unspecified humerus ▽

✓7ᵗʰ **S42.264** Nondisplaced fracture of lesser tuberosity of right humerus

✓7ᵗʰ **S42.265** Nondisplaced fracture of lesser tuberosity of left humerus

✓7ᵗʰ **S42.266** Nondisplaced fracture of lesser tuberosity of unspecified humerus ▽

✓6ᵗʰ **S42.27** Torus fracture of upper end of humerus

> The appropriate 7th character is to be added to all codes in subcategory S42.27.
> A   initial encounter for closed fracture
> D   subsequent encounter for fracture with routine healing
> G   subsequent encounter for fracture with delayed healing
> K   subsequent encounter for fracture with nonunion
> P   subsequent encounter for fracture with malunion
> S   sequela

✓7ᵗʰ **S42.271** Torus fracture of upper end of right humerus

✓7ᵗʰ **S42.272** Torus fracture of upper end of left humerus

✓7ᵗʰ **S42.279** Torus fracture of upper end of unspecified humerus ▽

✓6ᵗʰ **S42.29** Other fracture of upper end of humerus
Fracture of anatomical neck of humerus
Fracture of articular head of humerus

✓7ᵗʰ **S42.291** Other displaced fracture of upper end of right humerus

✓7ᵗʰ **S42.292** Other displaced fracture of upper end of left humerus

✓7ᵗʰ **S42.293** Other displaced fracture of upper end of unspecified humerus ▽

✓7ᵗʰ **S42.294** Other nondisplaced fracture of upper end of right humerus

✓7ᵗʰ **S42.295** Other nondisplaced fracture of upper end of left humerus

✓7ᵗʰ **S42.296** Other nondisplaced fracture of upper end of unspecified humerus ▽

✓5th **S42.3 Fracture of shaft of humerus**
Fracture of humerus NOS
Fracture of upper arm NOS
EXCLUDES 2   physeal fractures of upper end of humerus (S49.0-)
physeal fractures of lower end of humerus (S49.1-)

✓6th **S42.30 Unspecified fracture of shaft of humerus**

✓7th **S42.301 Unspecified fracture of shaft of humerus, right arm** ▽

✓7th **S42.302 Unspecified fracture of shaft of humerus, left arm** ▽

✓7th **S42.309 Unspecified fracture of shaft of humerus, unspecified arm** ▽

✓6th **S42.31 Greenstick fracture of shaft of humerus**

> The appropriate 7th character is to be added to all codes in subcategory S42.31.
> A   initial encounter for closed fracture
> D   subsequent encounter for fracture with routine healing
> G   subsequent encounter for fracture with delayed healing
> K   subsequent encounter for fracture with nonunion
> P   subsequent encounter for fracture with malunion
> S   sequela

✓7th **S42.311 Greenstick fracture of shaft of humerus, right arm**

✓7th **S42.312 Greenstick fracture of shaft of humerus, left arm**

✓7th **S42.319 Greenstick fracture of shaft of humerus, unspecified arm** ▽

✓6th **S42.32 Transverse fracture of shaft of humerus**

✓7th **S42.321 Displaced transverse fracture of shaft of humerus, right arm**

✓7th **S42.322 Displaced transverse fracture of shaft of humerus, left arm**

✓7th **S42.323 Displaced transverse fracture of shaft of humerus, unspecified arm** ▽

✓7th **S42.324 Nondisplaced transverse fracture of shaft of humerus, right arm**

✓7th **S42.325 Nondisplaced transverse fracture of shaft of humerus, left arm**

✓7th **S42.326 Nondisplaced transverse fracture of shaft of humerus, unspecified arm** ▽

✓6th **S42.33 Oblique fracture of shaft of humerus**

✓7th **S42.331 Displaced oblique fracture of shaft of humerus, right arm**

✓7th **S42.332 Displaced oblique fracture of shaft of humerus, left arm**

✓7th **S42.333 Displaced oblique fracture of shaft of humerus, unspecified arm** ▽

✓7th **S42.334 Nondisplaced oblique fracture of shaft of humerus, right arm**

✓7th **S42.335 Nondisplaced oblique fracture of shaft of humerus, left arm**

✓7th **S42.336 Nondisplaced oblique fracture of shaft of humerus, unspecified arm** ▽

✓6th **S42.34 Spiral fracture of shaft of humerus**

✓7th **S42.341 Displaced spiral fracture of shaft of humerus, right arm**

✓7th **S42.342 Displaced spiral fracture of shaft of humerus, left arm**

✓7th **S42.343 Displaced spiral fracture of shaft of humerus, unspecified arm** ▽

✓7th **S42.344 Nondisplaced spiral fracture of shaft of humerus, right arm**

✓7th **S42.345 Nondisplaced spiral fracture of shaft of humerus, left arm**

✓7th **S42.346 Nondisplaced spiral fracture of shaft of humerus, unspecified arm** ▽

✓6th **S42.35 Comminuted fracture of shaft of humerus**

✓7th **S42.351 Displaced comminuted fracture of shaft of humerus, right arm**

✓7th **S42.352 Displaced comminuted fracture of shaft of humerus, left arm**

✓7th **S42.353 Displaced comminuted fracture of shaft of humerus, unspecified arm** ▽

✓7th **S42.354 Nondisplaced comminuted fracture of shaft of humerus, right arm**

✓7th **S42.355 Nondisplaced comminuted fracture of shaft of humerus, left arm**

✓7th **S42.356 Nondisplaced comminuted fracture of shaft of humerus, unspecified arm** ▽

✓6th **S42.36 Segmental fracture of shaft of humerus**

✓7th **S42.361 Displaced segmental fracture of shaft of humerus, right arm**

✓7th **S42.362 Displaced segmental fracture of shaft of humerus, left arm**

✓7th **S42.363 Displaced segmental fracture of shaft of humerus, unspecified arm** ▽

✓7th **S42.364 Nondisplaced segmental fracture of shaft of humerus, right arm**

✓7th **S42.365 Nondisplaced segmental fracture of shaft of humerus, left arm**

✓7th **S42.366 Nondisplaced segmental fracture of shaft of humerus, unspecified arm** ▽

✓6th **S42.39 Other fracture of shaft of humerus**

✓7th **S42.391 Other fracture of shaft of right humerus**

✓7th **S42.392 Other fracture of shaft of left humerus**

✓7th **S42.399 Other fracture of shaft of unspecified humerus** ▽

✓5th **S42.4 Fracture of lower end of humerus**
Fracture of distal end of humerus
EXCLUDES 2   fracture of shaft of humerus (S42.3-)
physeal fracture of lower end of humerus (S49.1-)

✓6th **S42.40 Unspecified fracture of lower end of humerus**
Fracture of elbow NOS

✓7th **S42.401 Unspecified fracture of lower end of right humerus** ▽

✓7th **S42.402 Unspecified fracture of lower end of left humerus** ▽

✓7th **S42.409 Unspecified fracture of lower end of unspecified humerus** ▽

✓6th **S42.41 Simple supracondylar fracture without intercondylar fracture of humerus**

✓7th **S42.411 Displaced simple supracondylar fracture without intercondylar fracture of right humerus**

✓7th **S42.412 Displaced simple supracondylar fracture without intercondylar fracture of left humerus**

✓7th **S42.413 Displaced simple supracondylar fracture without intercondylar fracture of unspecified humerus** ▽

✓7th **S42.414 Nondisplaced simple supracondylar fracture without intercondylar fracture of right humerus**

✓7th **S42.415 Nondisplaced simple supracondylar fracture without intercondylar fracture of left humerus**

✓7th **S42.416 Nondisplaced simple supracondylar fracture without intercondylar fracture of unspecified humerus** ▽

✓6th **S42.42 Comminuted supracondylar fracture without intercondylar fracture of humerus**

✓7th **S42.421 Displaced comminuted supracondylar fracture without intercondylar fracture of right humerus**

✓7th **S42.422 Displaced comminuted supracondylar fracture without intercondylar fracture of left humerus**

✓7th **S42.423 Displaced comminuted supracondylar fracture without intercondylar fracture of unspecified humerus** ▽

✓7th **S42.424 Nondisplaced comminuted supracondylar fracture without intercondylar fracture of right humerus**

✓7th **S42.425 Nondisplaced comminuted supracondylar fracture without intercondylar fracture of left humerus**

✓7th **S42.426** Nondisplaced comminuted ▽
supracondylar fracture without
intercondylar fracture of unspecified
humerus

✓6th **S42.43** Fracture (avulsion) of lateral epicondyle of humerus

✓7th **S42.431** Displaced fracture (avulsion) of lateral
epicondyle of right humerus

✓7th **S42.432** Displaced fracture (avulsion) of lateral
epicondyle of left humerus

✓7th **S42.433** Displaced fracture (avulsion) of lateral ▽
epicondyle of unspecified humerus

✓7th **S42.434** Nondisplaced fracture (avulsion) of lateral
epicondyle of right humerus

✓7th **S42.435** Nondisplaced fracture (avulsion) of lateral
epicondyle of left humerus

✓7th **S42.436** Nondisplaced fracture (avulsion) of ▽
lateral epicondyle of unspecified humerus

✓6th **S42.44** Fracture (avulsion) of medial epicondyle of humerus

S42.441 Displaced fracture (avulsion) of medial
epicondyle of right humerus

✓7th **S42.442** Displaced fracture (avulsion) of medial
epicondyle of left humerus

✓7th **S42.443** Displaced fracture (avulsion) of medial ▽
epicondyle of unspecified humerus

✓7th **S42.444** Nondisplaced fracture (avulsion) of
medial epicondyle of right humerus

✓7th **S42.445** Nondisplaced fracture (avulsion) of
medial epicondyle of left humerus

✓7th **S42.446** Nondisplaced fracture (avulsion) of ▽
medial epicondyle of unspecified
humerus

✓7th **S42.447** Incarcerated fracture (avulsion) of
medial epicondyle of right humerus

✓7th **S42.448** Incarcerated fracture (avulsion) of
medial epicondyle of left humerus

✓7th **S42.449** Incarcerated fracture (avulsion) of ▽
medial epicondyle of unspecified humerus

✓6th **S42.45** Fracture of lateral condyle of humerus
Fracture of capitellum of humerus

✓7th **S42.451** Displaced fracture of lateral condyle of
right humerus

✓7th **S42.452** Displaced fracture of lateral condyle of
left humerus

✓7th **S42.453** Displaced fracture of lateral condyle of ▽
unspecified humerus

✓7th **S42.454** Nondisplaced fracture of lateral condyle
of right humerus

✓7th **S42.455** Nondisplaced fracture of lateral condyle
of left humerus

✓7th **S42.456** Nondisplaced fracture of lateral ▽
condyle of unspecified humerus

✓6th **S42.46** Fracture of medial condyle of humerus
Trochlea fracture of humerus

✓7th **S42.461** Displaced fracture of medial condyle of
right humerus

✓7th **S42.462** Displaced fracture of medial condyle of
left humerus

✓7th **S42.463** Displaced fracture of medial condyle ▽
of unspecified humerus

✓7th **S42.464** Nondisplaced fracture of medial condyle
of right humerus

✓7th **S42.465** Nondisplaced fracture of medial condyle
of left humerus

✓7th **S42.466** Nondisplaced fracture of medial ▽
condyle of unspecified humerus

✓6th **S42.47** Transcondylar fracture of humerus

✓7th **S42.471** Displaced transcondylar fracture of right
humerus

✓7th **S42.472** Displaced transcondylar fracture of left
humerus

✓7th **S42.473** Displaced transcondylar fracture of ▽
unspecified humerus

✓7th **S42.474** Nondisplaced transcondylar fracture of
right humerus

✓7th **S42.475** Nondisplaced transcondylar fracture of
left humerus

✓7th **S42.476** Nondisplaced transcondylar fracture ▽
of unspecified humerus

✓6th **S42.48** Torus fracture of lower end of humerus

The appropriate 7th character is to be added to all
codes in subcategory S42.48.
A   initial encounter for closed fracture
D   subsequent encounter for fracture with
    routine healing
G   subsequent encounter for fracture with
    delayed healing
K   subsequent encounter for fracture with
    nonunion
P   subsequent encounter for fracture with
    malunion
S   sequela

✓7th **S42.481** Torus fracture of lower end of right
humerus

✓7th **S42.482** Torus fracture of lower end of left
humerus

✓7th **S42.489** Torus fracture of lower end of ▽
unspecified humerus

✓6th **S42.49** Other fracture of lower end of humerus

✓7th **S42.491** Other displaced fracture of lower end of
right humerus

✓7th **S42.492** Other displaced fracture of lower end of
left humerus

✓7th **S42.493** Other displaced fracture of lower end ▽
of unspecified humerus

✓7th **S42.494** Other nondisplaced fracture of lower end
of right humerus

✓7th **S42.495** Other nondisplaced fracture of lower end
of left humerus

✓7th **S42.496** Other nondisplaced fracture of lower ▽
end of unspecified humerus

✓5th **S42.9** Fracture of shoulder girdle, part unspecified
Fracture of shoulder NOS

✓x7th **S42.90** Fracture of unspecified shoulder girdle, part ▽
unspecified

✓x7th **S42.91** Fracture of right shoulder girdle, part unspecified ▽

✓x7th **S42.92** Fracture of left shoulder girdle, part unspecified ▽

✓4th **S43** **Dislocation and sprain of joints and ligaments of shoulder girdle**
INCLUDES   avulsion of joint or ligament of shoulder girdle
laceration of cartilage, joint or ligament of shoulder girdle
sprain of cartilage, joint or ligament of shoulder girdle
traumatic hemarthrosis of joint or ligament of shoulder girdle
traumatic rupture of joint or ligament of shoulder girdle
traumatic subluxation of joint or ligament of shoulder girdle
traumatic tear of joint or ligament of shoulder girdle

Code also any associated open wound
EXCLUDES 2 strain of muscle, fascia and tendon of shoulder and upper arm
(S46.-)

The appropriate 7th character is to be added to each code from
category S43.
A   initial encounter
D   subsequent encounter
S   sequela

✓5th **S43.0** Subluxation and dislocation of shoulder joint
Dislocation of glenohumeral joint
Subluxation of glenohumeral joint

✓6th **S43.00** Unspecified subluxation and dislocation of shoulder
joint
Dislocation of humerus NOS
Subluxation of humerus NOS

✓7th **S43.001** Unspecified subluxation of right ▽
shoulder joint

✓7th **S43.002** Unspecified subluxation of left ▽
shoulder joint

✓7th **S43.003** Unspecified subluxation of ▽
unspecified shoulder joint

✓7th **S43.004** Unspecified dislocation of right ▽
shoulder joint

✓7th **S43.005** Unspecified dislocation of left ▽
shoulder joint

✓7th **S43.006** Unspecified dislocation of unspecified ▽
shoulder joint

√6ᵗʰ S43.01 Anterior subluxation and dislocation of humerus
- **√7ᵗʰ S43.011** Anterior subluxation of right humerus
- **√7ᵗʰ S43.012** Anterior subluxation of left humerus
- **√7ᵗʰ S43.013** Anterior subluxation of unspecified humerus ▽
- **√7ᵗʰ S43.014** Anterior dislocation of right humerus
- **√7ᵗʰ S43.015** Anterior dislocation of left humerus
- **√7ᵗʰ S43.016** Anterior dislocation of unspecified humerus ▽

√6ᵗʰ S43.02 Posterior subluxation and dislocation of humerus
- **√7ᵗʰ S43.021** Posterior subluxation of right humerus
- **√7ᵗʰ S43.022** Posterior subluxation of left humerus
- **√7ᵗʰ S43.023** Posterior subluxation of unspecified humerus ▽
- **√7ᵗʰ S43.024** Posterior dislocation of right humerus
- **√7ᵗʰ S43.025** Posterior dislocation of left humerus
- **√7ᵗʰ S43.026** Posterior dislocation of unspecified humerus ▽

√6ᵗʰ S43.03 Inferior subluxation and dislocation of humerus
- **√7ᵗʰ S43.031** Inferior subluxation of right humerus
- **√7ᵗʰ S43.032** Inferior subluxation of left humerus
- **√7ᵗʰ S43.033** Inferior subluxation of unspecified humerus ▽
- **√7ᵗʰ S43.034** Inferior dislocation of right humerus
- **√7ᵗʰ S43.035** Inferior dislocation of left humerus
- **√7ᵗʰ S43.036** Inferior dislocation of unspecified humerus ▽

√6ᵗʰ S43.08 Other subluxation and dislocation of shoulder joint
- **√7ᵗʰ S43.081** Other subluxation of right shoulder joint
- **√7ᵗʰ S43.082** Other subluxation of left shoulder joint
- **√7ᵗʰ S43.083** Other subluxation of unspecified shoulder joint ▽
- **√7ᵗʰ S43.084** Other dislocation of right shoulder joint
- **√7ᵗʰ S43.085** Other dislocation of left shoulder joint
- **√7ᵗʰ S43.086** Other dislocation of unspecified shoulder joint ▽

√5ᵗʰ S43.1 Subluxation and dislocation of acromioclavicular joint
√6ᵗʰ S43.10 Unspecified dislocation of acromioclavicular joint
- **√7ᵗʰ S43.101** Unspecified dislocation of right acromioclavicular joint ▽
- **√7ᵗʰ S43.102** Unspecified dislocation of left acromioclavicular joint ▽
- **√7ᵗʰ S43.109** Unspecified dislocation of unspecified acromioclavicular joint ▽

√6ᵗʰ S43.11 Subluxation of acromioclavicular joint
- **√7ᵗʰ S43.111** Subluxation of right acromioclavicular joint
- **√7ᵗʰ S43.112** Subluxation of left acromioclavicular joint
- **√7ᵗʰ S43.119** Subluxation of unspecified acromioclavicular joint ▽

√6ᵗʰ S43.12 Dislocation of acromioclavicular joint, 100%-200% displacement
- **√7ᵗʰ S43.121** Dislocation of right acromioclavicular joint, 100%-200% displacement
- **√7ᵗʰ S43.122** Dislocation of left acromioclavicular joint, 100%-200% displacement
- **√7ᵗʰ S43.129** Dislocation of unspecified acromioclavicular joint, 100%-200% displacement ▽

√6ᵗʰ S43.13 Dislocation of acromioclavicular joint, greater than 200% displacement
- **√7ᵗʰ S43.131** Dislocation of right acromioclavicular joint, greater than 200% displacement
- **√7ᵗʰ S43.132** Dislocation of left acromioclavicular joint, greater than 200% displacement
- **√7ᵗʰ S43.139** Dislocation of unspecified acromioclavicular joint, greater than 200% displacement ▽

√6ᵗʰ S43.14 Inferior dislocation of acromioclavicular joint
- **√7ᵗʰ S43.141** Inferior dislocation of right acromioclavicular joint

- **√7ᵗʰ S43.142** Inferior dislocation of left acromioclavicular joint
- **√7ᵗʰ S43.149** Inferior dislocation of unspecified acromioclavicular joint ▽

√6ᵗʰ S43.15 Posterior dislocation of acromioclavicular joint
- **√7ᵗʰ S43.151** Posterior dislocation of right acromioclavicular joint
- **√7ᵗʰ S43.152** Posterior dislocation of left acromioclavicular joint
- **√7ᵗʰ S43.159** Posterior dislocation of unspecified acromioclavicular joint ▽

√5ᵗʰ S43.2 Subluxation and dislocation of sternoclavicular joint
√6ᵗʰ S43.20 Unspecified subluxation and dislocation of sternoclavicular joint
- **√7ᵗʰ S43.201** Unspecified subluxation of right sternoclavicular joint ▽
- **√7ᵗʰ S43.202** Unspecified subluxation of left sternoclavicular joint ▽
- **√7ᵗʰ S43.203** Unspecified subluxation of unspecified sternoclavicular joint ▽
- **√7ᵗʰ S43.204** Unspecified dislocation of right sternoclavicular joint ▽
- **√7ᵗʰ S43.205** Unspecified dislocation of left sternoclavicular joint ▽
- **√7ᵗʰ S43.206** Unspecified dislocation of unspecified sternoclavicular joint ▽

√6ᵗʰ S43.21 Anterior subluxation and dislocation of sternoclavicular joint
- **√7ᵗʰ S43.211** Anterior subluxation of right sternoclavicular joint
- **√7ᵗʰ S43.212** Anterior subluxation of left sternoclavicular joint
- **√7ᵗʰ S43.213** Anterior subluxation of unspecified sternoclavicular joint ▽
- **√7ᵗʰ S43.214** Anterior dislocation of right sternoclavicular joint
- **√7ᵗʰ S43.215** Anterior dislocation of left sternoclavicular joint
- **√7ᵗʰ S43.216** Anterior dislocation of unspecified sternoclavicular joint ▽

√6ᵗʰ S43.22 Posterior subluxation and dislocation of sternoclavicular joint
- **√7ᵗʰ S43.221** Posterior subluxation of right sternoclavicular joint
- **√7ᵗʰ S43.222** Posterior subluxation of left sternoclavicular joint
- **√7ᵗʰ S43.223** Posterior subluxation of unspecified sternoclavicular joint ▽
- **√7ᵗʰ S43.224** Posterior dislocation of right sternoclavicular joint
- **√7ᵗʰ S43.225** Posterior dislocation of left sternoclavicular joint
- **√7ᵗʰ S43.226** Posterior dislocation of unspecified sternoclavicular joint ▽

√5ᵗʰ S43.3 Subluxation and dislocation of other and unspecified parts of shoulder girdle
√6ᵗʰ S43.30 Subluxation and dislocation of unspecified parts of shoulder girdle
    Dislocation of shoulder girdle NOS
    Subluxation of shoulder girdle NOS
- **√7ᵗʰ S43.301** Subluxation of unspecified parts of right shoulder girdle ▽
- **√7ᵗʰ S43.302** Subluxation of unspecified parts of left shoulder girdle ▽
- **√7ᵗʰ S43.303** Subluxation of unspecified parts of unspecified shoulder girdle ▽
- **√7ᵗʰ S43.304** Dislocation of unspecified parts of right shoulder girdle ▽
- **√7ᵗʰ S43.305** Dislocation of unspecified parts of left shoulder girdle ▽
- **√7ᵗʰ S43.306** Dislocation of unspecified parts of unspecified shoulder girdle ▽

√6ᵗʰ S43.31 Subluxation and dislocation of scapula
- **√7ᵗʰ S43.311** Subluxation of right scapula
- **√7ᵗʰ S43.312** Subluxation of left scapula

☑ Add'l Character Required   √ˣ⁷ᵗʰ Placeholder Alert   RUG IV Special Care High Dx   RUG IV Clinically Complex Dx   RUG IV Special Care Low Dx   Manifestation Code   Other Specified Code   ▽ Unspecified Code

√7ᵗʰ **S43.313** Subluxation of unspecified scapula ▽

√7ᵗʰ **S43.314** Dislocation of right scapula

√7ᵗʰ **S43.315** Dislocation of left scapula

√7ᵗʰ **S43.316** Dislocation of unspecified scapula ▽

√6ᵗʰ **S43.39** Subluxation and dislocation of other parts of shoulder girdle

√7ᵗʰ **S43.391** Subluxation of other parts of right shoulder girdle

√7ᵗʰ **S43.392** Subluxation of other parts of left shoulder girdle

√7ᵗʰ **S43.393** Subluxation of other parts of unspecified shoulder girdle ▽

√7ᵗʰ **S43.394** Dislocation of other parts of right shoulder girdle

√7ᵗʰ **S43.395** Dislocation of other parts of left shoulder girdle

√7ᵗʰ **S43.396** Dislocation of other parts of unspecified shoulder girdle ▽

√5ᵗʰ **S43.4** Sprain of shoulder joint

√6ᵗʰ **S43.40** Unspecified sprain of shoulder joint

√7ᵗʰ **S43.401** Unspecified sprain of right shoulder joint ▽

√7ᵗʰ **S43.402** Unspecified sprain of left shoulder joint ▽

√7ᵗʰ **S43.409** Unspecified sprain of unspecified shoulder joint ▽

√6ᵗʰ **S43.41** Sprain of coracohumeral (ligament)

√7ᵗʰ **S43.411** Sprain of right coracohumeral (ligament)

√7ᵗʰ **S43.412** Sprain of left coracohumeral (ligament)

√7ᵗʰ **S43.419** Sprain of unspecified coracohumeral (ligament) ▽

√6ᵗʰ **S43.42** Sprain of rotator cuff capsule

EXCLUDES 1 rotator cuff syndrome (complete) (incomplete), not specified as traumatic (M75.1-)

EXCLUDES 2 injury of tendon of rotator cuff (S46.0-)

√7ᵗʰ **S43.421** Sprain of right rotator cuff capsule

√7ᵗʰ **S43.422** Sprain of left rotator cuff capsule

√7ᵗʰ **S43.429** Sprain of unspecified rotator cuff capsule ▽

√6ᵗʰ **S43.43** Superior glenoid labrum lesion
SLAP lesion

√7ᵗʰ **S43.431** Superior glenoid labrum lesion of right shoulder

√7ᵗʰ **S43.432** Superior glenoid labrum lesion of left shoulder

√7ᵗʰ **S43.439** Superior glenoid labrum lesion of unspecified shoulder ▽

√6ᵗʰ **S43.49** Other sprain of shoulder joint

√7ᵗʰ **S43.491** Other sprain of right shoulder joint

√7ᵗʰ **S43.492** Other sprain of left shoulder joint

√7ᵗʰ **S43.499** Other sprain of unspecified shoulder joint ▽

√5ᵗʰ **S43.5** Sprain of acromioclavicular joint
Sprain of acromioclavicular ligament

√x7ᵗʰ **S43.50** Sprain of unspecified acromioclavicular joint ▽

√x7ᵗʰ **S43.51** Sprain of right acromioclavicular joint

√x7ᵗʰ **S43.52** Sprain of left acromioclavicular joint

√5ᵗʰ **S43.6** Sprain of sternoclavicular joint

√x7ᵗʰ **S43.60** Sprain of unspecified sternoclavicular joint ▽

√x7ᵗʰ **S43.61** Sprain of right sternoclavicular joint

√x7ᵗʰ **S43.62** Sprain of left sternoclavicular joint

√5ᵗʰ **S43.8** Sprain of other specified parts of shoulder girdle

√x7ᵗʰ **S43.80** Sprain of other specified parts of unspecified shoulder girdle ▽

√x7ᵗʰ **S43.81** Sprain of other specified parts of right shoulder girdle

√x7ᵗʰ **S43.82** Sprain of other specified parts of left shoulder girdle

√5ᵗʰ **S43.9** Sprain of unspecified parts of shoulder girdle

√x7ᵗʰ **S43.90** Sprain of unspecified parts of unspecified shoulder girdle ▽
Sprain of shoulder girdle NOS

√x7ᵗʰ **S43.91** Sprain of unspecified parts of right shoulder girdle ▽

√x7ᵗʰ **S43.92** Sprain of unspecified parts of left shoulder girdle ▽

√4ᵗʰ **S44** Injury of nerves at shoulder and upper arm level
Code also any associated open wound (S41.-)
EXCLUDES 2 injury of brachial plexus (S14.3-)

The appropriate 7th character is to be added to each code from category S44.
A   initial encounter
D   subsequent encounter
S   sequela

√5ᵗʰ **S44.0** Injury of ulnar nerve at upper arm level
EXCLUDES 1 ulnar nerve NOS (S54.0)

√x7ᵗʰ **S44.00** Injury of ulnar nerve at upper arm level, unspecified arm ▽

√x7ᵗʰ **S44.01** Injury of ulnar nerve at upper arm level, right arm

√x7ᵗʰ **S44.02** Injury of ulnar nerve at upper arm level, left arm

√5ᵗʰ **S44.1** Injury of median nerve at upper arm level
EXCLUDES 1 median nerve NOS (S54.1)

√x7ᵗʰ **S44.10** Injury of median nerve at upper arm level, unspecified arm ▽

√x7ᵗʰ **S44.11** Injury of median nerve at upper arm level, right arm

√x7ᵗʰ **S44.12** Injury of median nerve at upper arm level, left arm

√5ᵗʰ **S44.2** Injury of radial nerve at upper arm level
EXCLUDES 1 radial nerve NOS (S54.2)

√x7ᵗʰ **S44.20** Injury of radial nerve at upper arm level, unspecified arm ▽

√x7ᵗʰ **S44.21** Injury of radial nerve at upper arm level, right arm

√x7ᵗʰ **S44.22** Injury of radial nerve at upper arm level, left arm

√5ᵗʰ **S44.3** Injury of axillary nerve

√x7ᵗʰ **S44.30** Injury of axillary nerve, unspecified arm ▽

√x7ᵗʰ **S44.31** Injury of axillary nerve, right arm

√x7ᵗʰ **S44.32** Injury of axillary nerve, left arm

√5ᵗʰ **S44.4** Injury of musculocutaneous nerve

√x7ᵗʰ **S44.40** Injury of musculocutaneous nerve, unspecified arm ▽

√x7ᵗʰ **S44.41** Injury of musculocutaneous nerve, right arm

√x7ᵗʰ **S44.42** Injury of musculocutaneous nerve, left arm

√5ᵗʰ **S44.5** Injury of cutaneous sensory nerve at shoulder and upper arm level

√x7ᵗʰ **S44.50** Injury of cutaneous sensory nerve at shoulder and upper arm level, unspecified arm ▽

√x7ᵗʰ **S44.51** Injury of cutaneous sensory nerve at shoulder and upper arm level, right arm

√x7ᵗʰ **S44.52** Injury of cutaneous sensory nerve at shoulder and upper arm level, left arm

√5ᵗʰ **S44.8** Injury of other nerves at shoulder and upper arm level

√6ᵗʰ **S44.8X** Injury of other nerves at shoulder and upper arm level

√7ᵗʰ **S44.8X1** Injury of other nerves at shoulder and upper arm level, right arm

√7ᵗʰ **S44.8X2** Injury of other nerves at shoulder and upper arm level, left arm

√7ᵗʰ **S44.8X9** Injury of other nerves at shoulder and upper arm level, unspecified arm ▽

√5ᵗʰ **S44.9** Injury of unspecified nerve at shoulder and upper arm level

√x7ᵗʰ **S44.90** Injury of unspecified nerve at shoulder and upper arm level, unspecified arm ▽

√x7ᵗʰ **S44.91** Injury of unspecified nerve at shoulder and upper arm level, right arm ▽

√x7ᵗʰ **S44.92** Injury of unspecified nerve at shoulder and upper arm level, left arm ▽

Ⓝ Newborn   Ⓟ Pediatric   Ⓜ Maternity   Ⓐ Adult   **RIC** RIC Dx   **NC Dx** Noncancer Dx   **PDx** Primary Dx   **CC** RIC CC Condition   ▶◀ Revised Text   ● New Code   ▲ Revised Code Title

902
ICD-10-CM 2016

✓4ᵗʰ S45 Injury of blood vessels at shoulder and upper arm level

Code also any associated open wound (S41.-)

EXCLUDES 2   injury of subclavian artery (S25.1)
          injury of subclavian vein (S25.3)

The appropriate 7th character is to be added to each code from category S45.
A   initial encounter
D   subsequent encounter
S   sequela

✓5ᵗʰ S45.0 Injury of axillary artery

✓6ᵗʰ S45.00 Unspecified injury of axillary artery

- ✓7ᵗʰ **S45.001** Unspecified injury of axillary artery, right side ▽
- ✓7ᵗʰ **S45.002** Unspecified injury of axillary artery, left side ▽
- ✓7ᵗʰ **S45.009** Unspecified injury of axillary artery, unspecified side ▽

✓6ᵗʰ S45.01 Laceration of axillary artery

- ✓7ᵗʰ **S45.011** Laceration of axillary artery, right side
- ✓7ᵗʰ **S45.012** Laceration of axillary artery, left side
- ✓7ᵗʰ **S45.019** Laceration of axillary artery, unspecified side ▽

✓6ᵗʰ S45.09 Other specified injury of axillary artery

- ✓7ᵗʰ **S45.091** Other specified injury of axillary artery, right side
- ✓7ᵗʰ **S45.092** Other specified injury of axillary artery, left side
- ✓7ᵗʰ **S45.099** Other specified injury of axillary artery, unspecified side ▽

✓5ᵗʰ S45.1 Injury of brachial artery

✓6ᵗʰ S45.10 Unspecified injury of brachial artery

- ✓7ᵗʰ **S45.101** Unspecified injury of brachial artery, right side ▽
- ✓7ᵗʰ **S45.102** Unspecified injury of brachial artery, left side ▽
- ✓7ᵗʰ **S45.109** Unspecified injury of brachial artery, unspecified side ▽

✓6ᵗʰ S45.11 Laceration of brachial artery

- ✓7ᵗʰ **S45.111** Laceration of brachial artery, right side
- ✓7ᵗʰ **S45.112** Laceration of brachial artery, left side
- ✓7ᵗʰ **S45.119** Laceration of brachial artery, unspecified side ▽

✓6ᵗʰ S45.19 Other specified injury of brachial artery

- ✓7ᵗʰ **S45.191** Other specified injury of brachial artery, right side
- ✓7ᵗʰ **S45.192** Other specified injury of brachial artery, left side
- ✓7ᵗʰ **S45.199** Other specified injury of brachial artery, unspecified side ▽

✓5ᵗʰ S45.2 Injury of axillary or brachial vein

✓6ᵗʰ S45.20 Unspecified injury of axillary or brachial vein

- ✓7ᵗʰ **S45.201** Unspecified injury of axillary or brachial vein, right side ▽
- ✓7ᵗʰ **S45.202** Unspecified injury of axillary or brachial vein, left side ▽
- ✓7ᵗʰ **S45.209** Unspecified injury of axillary or brachial vein, unspecified side ▽

✓6ᵗʰ S45.21 Laceration of axillary or brachial vein

- ✓7ᵗʰ **S45.211** Laceration of axillary or brachial vein, right side
- ✓7ᵗʰ **S45.212** Laceration of axillary or brachial vein, left side
- ✓7ᵗʰ **S45.219** Laceration of axillary or brachial vein, unspecified side ▽

✓6ᵗʰ S45.29 Other specified injury of axillary or brachial vein

- ✓7ᵗʰ **S45.291** Other specified injury of axillary or brachial vein, right side
- ✓7ᵗʰ **S45.292** Other specified injury of axillary or brachial vein, left side
- ✓7ᵗʰ **S45.299** Other specified injury of axillary or brachial vein, unspecified side ▽

✓5ᵗʰ S45.3 Injury of superficial vein at shoulder and upper arm level

✓6ᵗʰ S45.30 Unspecified injury of superficial vein at shoulder and upper arm level

- ✓7ᵗʰ **S45.301** Unspecified injury of superficial vein at shoulder and upper arm level, right arm ▽
- ✓7ᵗʰ **S45.302** Unspecified injury of superficial vein at shoulder and upper arm level, left arm ▽
- ✓7ᵗʰ **S45.309** Unspecified injury of superficial vein at shoulder and upper arm level, unspecified arm ▽

✓6ᵗʰ S45.31 Laceration of superficial vein at shoulder and upper arm level

- ✓7ᵗʰ **S45.311** Laceration of superficial vein at shoulder and upper arm level, right arm
- ✓7ᵗʰ **S45.312** Laceration of superficial vein at shoulder and upper arm level, left arm
- ✓7ᵗʰ **S45.319** Laceration of superficial vein at shoulder and upper arm level, unspecified arm ▽

✓6ᵗʰ S45.39 Other specified injury of superficial vein at shoulder and upper arm level

- ✓7ᵗʰ **S45.391** Other specified injury of superficial vein at shoulder and upper arm level, right arm
- ✓7ᵗʰ **S45.392** Other specified injury of superficial vein at shoulder and upper arm level, left arm
- ✓7ᵗʰ **S45.399** Other specified injury of superficial vein at shoulder and upper arm level, unspecified arm ▽

✓5ᵗʰ S45.8 Injury of other specified blood vessels at shoulder and upper arm level

✓6ᵗʰ S45.80 Unspecified injury of other specified blood vessels at shoulder and upper arm level

- ✓7ᵗʰ **S45.801** Unspecified injury of other specified blood vessels at shoulder and upper arm level, right arm ▽
- ✓7ᵗʰ **S45.802** Unspecified injury of other specified blood vessels at shoulder and upper arm level, left arm ▽
- ✓7ᵗʰ **S45.809** Unspecified injury of other specified blood vessels at shoulder and upper arm level, unspecified arm ▽

✓6ᵗʰ S45.81 Laceration of other specified blood vessels at shoulder and upper arm level

- ✓7ᵗʰ **S45.811** Laceration of other specified blood vessels at shoulder and upper arm level, right arm
- ✓7ᵗʰ **S45.812** Laceration of other specified blood vessels at shoulder and upper arm level, left arm
- ✓7ᵗʰ **S45.819** Laceration of other specified blood vessels at shoulder and upper arm level, unspecified arm ▽

✓6ᵗʰ S45.89 Other specified injury of other specified blood vessels at shoulder and upper arm level

- ✓7ᵗʰ **S45.891** Other specified injury of other specified blood vessels at shoulder and upper arm level, right arm
- ✓7ᵗʰ **S45.892** Other specified injury of other specified blood vessels at shoulder and upper arm level, left arm
- ✓7ᵗʰ **S45.899** Other specified injury of other specified blood vessels at shoulder and upper arm level, unspecified arm ▽

✓5ᵗʰ S45.9 Injury of unspecified blood vessel at shoulder and upper arm level

✓6ᵗʰ S45.90 Unspecified injury of unspecified blood vessel at shoulder and upper arm level

- ✓7ᵗʰ **S45.901** Unspecified injury of unspecified blood vessel at shoulder and upper arm level, right arm ▽
- ✓7ᵗʰ **S45.902** Unspecified injury of unspecified blood vessel at shoulder and upper arm level, left arm ▽
- ✓7ᵗʰ **S45.909** Unspecified injury of unspecified blood vessel at shoulder and upper arm level, unspecified arm ▽

☑ Add'l Character Required   ✓ₓ7ᵗʰ Placeholder Alert   RUG IV Special Care High Dx   RUG IV Clinically Complex Dx   RUG IV Special Care Low Dx   Manifestation Code   Other Specified Code   ▽ Unspecified Code

Chapter 19. Injury, Poisoning and Certain Other Consequences of External Causes

S45.91–S46.309

√6ᵗʰ **S45.91** Laceration of unspecified blood vessel at shoulder and upper arm level

    √7ᵗʰ **S45.911** Laceration of unspecified blood vessel ▽ at shoulder and upper arm level, right arm

    √7ᵗʰ **S45.912** Laceration of unspecified blood vessel ▽ at shoulder and upper arm level, left arm

    √7ᵗʰ **S45.919** Laceration of unspecified blood vessel ▽ at shoulder and upper arm level, unspecified arm

√6ᵗʰ **S45.99** Other specified injury of unspecified blood vessel at shoulder and upper arm level

    √7ᵗʰ **S45.991** Other specified injury of unspecified ▽ blood vessel at shoulder and upper arm level, right arm

    √7ᵗʰ **S45.992** Other specified injury of unspecified ▽ blood vessel at shoulder and upper arm level, left arm

    √7ᵗʰ **S45.999** Other specified injury of unspecified ▽ blood vessel at shoulder and upper arm level, unspecified arm

✦ √4ᵗʰ **S46 Injury of muscle, fascia and tendon at shoulder and upper arm level**

Code also any associated open wound (S41.-)

EXCLUDES 2   injury of muscle, fascia and tendon at elbow (S56.-)
       sprain of joints and ligaments of shoulder girdle (S43.9)

The appropriate 7th character is to be added to each code from category S46.
A   initial encounter
D   subsequent encounter
S   sequela

√5ᵗʰ **S46.0** Injury of muscle(s) and tendon(s) of the rotator cuff of shoulder

    √6ᵗʰ **S46.00** Unspecified injury of muscle(s) and tendon(s) of the rotator cuff of shoulder

       √7ᵗʰ **S46.001** Unspecified injury of muscle(s) and ▽ tendon(s) of the rotator cuff of right shoulder

       √7ᵗʰ **S46.002** Unspecified injury of muscle(s) and ▽ tendon(s) of the rotator cuff of left shoulder

       √7ᵗʰ **S46.009** Unspecified injury of muscle(s) and ▽ tendon(s) of the rotator cuff of unspecified shoulder

    √6ᵗʰ **S46.01** Strain of muscle(s) and tendon(s) of the rotator cuff of shoulder

       √7ᵗʰ **S46.011** Strain of muscle(s) and tendon(s) of the rotator cuff of right shoulder

       √7ᵗʰ **S46.012** Strain of muscle(s) and tendon(s) of the rotator cuff of left shoulder

       √7ᵗʰ **S46.019** Strain of muscle(s) and tendon(s) of the ▽ rotator cuff of unspecified shoulder

    √6ᵗʰ **S46.02** Laceration of muscle(s) and tendon(s) of the rotator cuff of shoulder

       √7ᵗʰ **S46.021** Laceration of muscle(s) and tendon(s) of the rotator cuff of right shoulder

       √7ᵗʰ **S46.022** Laceration of muscle(s) and tendon(s) of the rotator cuff of left shoulder

       √7ᵗʰ **S46.029** Laceration of muscle(s) and tendon(s) ▽ of the rotator cuff of unspecified shoulder

    √6ᵗʰ **S46.09** Other injury of muscle(s) and tendon(s) of the rotator cuff of shoulder

       √7ᵗʰ **S46.091** Other injury of muscle(s) and tendon(s) of the rotator cuff of right shoulder

       √7ᵗʰ **S46.092** Other injury of muscle(s) and tendon(s) of the rotator cuff of left shoulder

       √7ᵗʰ **S46.099** Other injury of muscle(s) and tendon(s) ▽ of the rotator cuff of unspecified shoulder

√5ᵗʰ **S46.1** Injury of muscle, fascia and tendon of long head of biceps

    √6ᵗʰ **S46.10** Unspecified injury of muscle, fascia and tendon of long head of biceps

       √7ᵗʰ **S46.101** Unspecified injury of muscle, fascia and ▽ tendon of long head of biceps, right arm

√7ᵗʰ **S46.102** Unspecified injury of muscle, fascia and ▽ tendon of long head of biceps, left arm

√7ᵗʰ **S46.109** Unspecified injury of muscle, fascia and ▽ tendon of long head of biceps, unspecified arm

√6ᵗʰ **S46.11** Strain of muscle, fascia and tendon of long head of biceps

    √7ᵗʰ **S46.111** Strain of muscle, fascia and tendon of long head of biceps, right arm

    √7ᵗʰ **S46.112** Strain of muscle, fascia and tendon of long head of biceps, left arm

    √7ᵗʰ **S46.119** Strain of muscle, fascia and tendon of ▽ long head of biceps, unspecified arm

√6ᵗʰ **S46.12** Laceration of muscle, fascia and tendon of long head of biceps

    √7ᵗʰ **S46.121** Laceration of muscle, fascia and tendon of long head of biceps, right arm

    √7ᵗʰ **S46.122** Laceration of muscle, fascia and tendon of long head of biceps, left arm

    √7ᵗʰ **S46.129** Laceration of muscle, fascia and tendon ▽ of long head of biceps, unspecified arm

√6ᵗʰ **S46.19** Other injury of muscle, fascia and tendon of long head of biceps

    √7ᵗʰ **S46.191** Other injury of muscle, fascia and tendon of long head of biceps, right arm

    √7ᵗʰ **S46.192** Other injury of muscle, fascia and tendon of long head of biceps, left arm

    √7ᵗʰ **S46.199** Other injury of muscle, fascia and ▽ tendon of long head of biceps, unspecified arm

√5ᵗʰ **S46.2** Injury of muscle, fascia and tendon of other parts of biceps

    √6ᵗʰ **S46.20** Unspecified injury of muscle, fascia and tendon of other parts of biceps

       √7ᵗʰ **S46.201** Unspecified injury of muscle, fascia and ▽ tendon of other parts of biceps, right arm

       √7ᵗʰ **S46.202** Unspecified injury of muscle, fascia and ▽ tendon of other parts of biceps, left arm

       √7ᵗʰ **S46.209** Unspecified injury of muscle, fascia and ▽ tendon of other parts of biceps, unspecified arm

    √6ᵗʰ **S46.21** Strain of muscle, fascia and tendon of other parts of biceps

       √7ᵗʰ **S46.211** Strain of muscle, fascia and tendon of other parts of biceps, right arm

       √7ᵗʰ **S46.212** Strain of muscle, fascia and tendon of other parts of biceps, left arm

       √7ᵗʰ **S46.219** Strain of muscle, fascia and tendon of ▽ other parts of biceps, unspecified arm

    √6ᵗʰ **S46.22** Laceration of muscle, fascia and tendon of other parts of biceps

       √7ᵗʰ **S46.221** Laceration of muscle, fascia and tendon of other parts of biceps, right arm

       √7ᵗʰ **S46.222** Laceration of muscle, fascia and tendon of other parts of biceps, left arm

       √7ᵗʰ **S46.229** Laceration of muscle, fascia and tendon ▽ of other parts of biceps, unspecified arm

    √6ᵗʰ **S46.29** Other injury of muscle, fascia and tendon of other parts of biceps

       √7ᵗʰ **S46.291** Other injury of muscle, fascia and tendon of other parts of biceps, right arm

       √7ᵗʰ **S46.292** Other injury of muscle, fascia and tendon of other parts of biceps, left arm

       √7ᵗʰ **S46.299** Other injury of muscle, fascia and ▽ tendon of other parts of biceps, unspecified arm

√5ᵗʰ **S46.3** Injury of muscle, fascia and tendon of triceps

    √6ᵗʰ **S46.30** Unspecified injury of muscle, fascia and tendon of triceps

       √7ᵗʰ **S46.301** Unspecified injury of muscle, fascia and ▽ tendon of triceps, right arm

       √7ᵗʰ **S46.302** Unspecified injury of muscle, fascia and ▽ tendon of triceps, left arm

       √7ᵗʰ **S46.309** Unspecified injury of muscle, fascia and ▽ tendon of triceps, unspecified arm

✦   Refer to the Muscle/Tendon Table at beginning of this chapter.

Ⓝ Newborn   Ⓟ Pediatric   Ⓜ Maternity   Ⓐ Adult   **RIC** RIC Dx   **NC Dx** Noncancer Dx   **PDx** Primary Dx   **CC** RIC CC Condition   ▶◀ Revised Text   ● New Code   ▲ Revised Code Title

904   ICD-10-CM 2016

✓6ᵗʰ **S46.31** Strain of muscle, fascia and tendon of triceps
- ✓7ᵗʰ **S46.311** Strain of muscle, fascia and tendon of triceps, right arm
- ✓7ᵗʰ **S46.312** Strain of muscle, fascia and tendon of triceps, left arm
- ✓7ᵗʰ **S46.319** Strain of muscle, fascia and tendon of triceps, unspecified arm ▽

✓6ᵗʰ **S46.32** Laceration of muscle, fascia and tendon of triceps
- ✓7ᵗʰ **S46.321** Laceration of muscle, fascia and tendon of triceps, right arm
- ✓7ᵗʰ **S46.322** Laceration of muscle, fascia and tendon of triceps, left arm
- ✓7ᵗʰ **S46.329** Laceration of muscle, fascia and tendon of triceps, unspecified arm ▽

✓6ᵗʰ **S46.39** Other injury of muscle, fascia and tendon of triceps
- ✓7ᵗʰ **S46.391** Other injury of muscle, fascia and tendon of triceps, right arm
- ✓7ᵗʰ **S46.392** Other injury of muscle, fascia and tendon of triceps, left arm
- ✓7ᵗʰ **S46.399** Other injury of muscle, fascia and tendon of triceps, unspecified arm ▽

✓5ᵗʰ **S46.8** Injury of other muscles, fascia and tendons at shoulder and upper arm level
✓6ᵗʰ **S46.80** Unspecified injury of other muscles, fascia and tendons at shoulder and upper arm level
- ✓7ᵗʰ **S46.801** Unspecified injury of other muscles, fascia and tendons at shoulder and upper arm level, right arm ▽
- ✓7ᵗʰ **S46.802** Unspecified injury of other muscles, fascia and tendons at shoulder and upper arm level, left arm ▽
- ✓7ᵗʰ **S46.809** Unspecified injury of other muscles, fascia and tendons at shoulder and upper arm level, unspecified arm ▽

✓6ᵗʰ **S46.81** Strain of other muscles, fascia and tendons at shoulder and upper arm level
- ✓7ᵗʰ **S46.811** Strain of other muscles, fascia and tendons at shoulder and upper arm level, right arm
- ✓7ᵗʰ **S46.812** Strain of other muscles, fascia and tendons at shoulder and upper arm level, left arm
- ✓7ᵗʰ **S46.819** Strain of other muscles, fascia and tendons at shoulder and upper arm level, unspecified arm ▽

✓6ᵗʰ **S46.82** Laceration of other muscles, fascia and tendons at shoulder and upper arm level
- ✓7ᵗʰ **S46.821** Laceration of other muscles, fascia and tendons at shoulder and upper arm level, right arm
- ✓7ᵗʰ **S46.822** Laceration of other muscles, fascia and tendons at shoulder and upper arm level, left arm
- ✓7ᵗʰ **S46.829** Laceration of other muscles, fascia and tendons at shoulder and upper arm level, unspecified arm ▽

✓6ᵗʰ **S46.89** Other injury of other muscles, fascia and tendons at shoulder and upper arm level
- ✓7ᵗʰ **S46.891** Other injury of other muscles, fascia and tendons at shoulder and upper arm level, right arm
- ✓7ᵗʰ **S46.892** Other injury of other muscles, fascia and tendons at shoulder and upper arm level, left arm
- ✓7ᵗʰ **S46.899** Other injury of other muscles, fascia and tendons at shoulder and upper arm level, unspecified arm ▽

✓5ᵗʰ **S46.9** Injury of unspecified muscle, fascia and tendon at shoulder and upper arm level
✓6ᵗʰ **S46.90** Unspecified injury of unspecified muscle, fascia and tendon at shoulder and upper arm level
- ✓7ᵗʰ **S46.901** Unspecified injury of unspecified muscle, fascia and tendon at shoulder and upper arm level, right arm ▽

- ✓7ᵗʰ **S46.902** Unspecified injury of unspecified muscle, fascia and tendon at shoulder and upper arm level, left arm ▽
- ✓7ᵗʰ **S46.909** Unspecified injury of unspecified muscle, fascia and tendon at shoulder and upper arm level, unspecified arm ▽

✓6ᵗʰ **S46.91** Strain of unspecified muscle, fascia and tendon at shoulder and upper arm level
- ✓7ᵗʰ **S46.911** Strain of unspecified muscle, fascia and tendon at shoulder and upper arm level, right arm ▽
- ✓7ᵗʰ **S46.912** Strain of unspecified muscle, fascia and tendon at shoulder and upper arm level, left arm ▽
- ✓7ᵗʰ **S46.919** Strain of unspecified muscle, fascia and tendon at shoulder and upper arm level, unspecified arm ▽

✓6ᵗʰ **S46.92** Laceration of unspecified muscle, fascia and tendon at shoulder and upper arm level
- ✓7ᵗʰ **S46.921** Laceration of unspecified muscle, fascia and tendon at shoulder and upper arm level, right arm ▽
- ✓7ᵗʰ **S46.922** Laceration of unspecified muscle, fascia and tendon at shoulder and upper arm level, left arm ▽
- ✓7ᵗʰ **S46.929** Laceration of unspecified muscle, fascia and tendon at shoulder and upper arm level, unspecified arm ▽

✓6ᵗʰ **S46.99** Other injury of unspecified muscle, fascia and tendon at shoulder and upper arm level
- ✓7ᵗʰ **S46.991** Other injury of unspecified muscle, fascia and tendon at shoulder and upper arm level, right arm ▽
- ✓7ᵗʰ **S46.992** Other injury of unspecified muscle, fascia and tendon at shoulder and upper arm level, left arm ▽
- ✓7ᵗʰ **S46.999** Other injury of unspecified muscle, fascia and tendon at shoulder and upper arm level, unspecified arm ▽

✓4ᵗʰ **S47** Crushing injury of shoulder and upper arm
Use additional code for all associated injuries
EXCLUDES 2   crushing injury of elbow (S57.0-)

The appropriate 7th character is to be added to each code from category S47.
A   initial encounter
D   subsequent encounter
S   sequela

✓×7ᵗʰ **S47.1** Crushing injury of right shoulder and upper arm
✓×7ᵗʰ **S47.2** Crushing injury of left shoulder and upper arm
✓×7ᵗʰ **S47.9** Crushing injury of shoulder and upper arm, unspecified arm ▽

✓4ᵗʰ **S48** Traumatic amputation of shoulder and upper arm
NOTE   An amputation not identified as partial or complete should be coded to complete.
EXCLUDES 1   traumatic amputation at elbow level (S58.0)

The appropriate 7th character is to be added to each code from category S48.
A   initial encounter
D   subsequent encounter
S   sequela

✓5ᵗʰ **S48.0** Traumatic amputation at shoulder joint
✓6ᵗʰ **S48.01** Complete traumatic amputation at shoulder joint
- ✓7ᵗʰ **S48.011** Complete traumatic amputation at right shoulder joint
- ✓7ᵗʰ **S48.012** Complete traumatic amputation at left shoulder joint
- ✓7ᵗʰ **S48.019** Complete traumatic amputation at unspecified shoulder joint ▽

✓6ᵗʰ **S48.02** Partial traumatic amputation at shoulder joint
- ✓7ᵗʰ **S48.021** Partial traumatic amputation at right shoulder joint
- ✓7ᵗʰ **S48.022** Partial traumatic amputation at left shoulder joint
- ✓7ᵗʰ **S48.029** Partial traumatic amputation at unspecified shoulder joint ▽

✓ Add'l Character Required   ✓×7ᵗʰ Placeholder Alert   RUG IV Special Care High Dx   RUG IV Clinically Complex Dx   RUG IV Special Care Low Dx   Manifestation Code   Other Specified Code   ▽Unspecified Code

ICD-10-CM 2016   905

√5ᵗʰ **S48.1 Traumatic amputation at** level between shoulder and elbow

  √6ᵗʰ **S48.11** Complete **traumatic amputation at level between shoulder and elbow**

    √7ᵗʰ **S48.111** **Complete traumatic amputation at level between** right **shoulder and elbow**

    √7ᵗʰ **S48.112** **Complete traumatic amputation at level between** left **shoulder and elbow**

    √7ᵗʰ **S48.119** **Complete traumatic amputation at level between unspecified shoulder and elbow** ▽

  √6ᵗʰ **S48.12** Partial **traumatic amputation at level between shoulder and elbow**

    √7ᵗʰ **S48.121** **Partial traumatic amputation at level between** right **shoulder and elbow**

    √7ᵗʰ **S48.122** **Partial traumatic amputation at level between** left **shoulder and elbow**

    √7ᵗʰ **S48.129** **Partial traumatic amputation at level between unspecified shoulder and elbow** ▽

√5ᵗʰ **S48.9 Traumatic amputation of shoulder and upper arm,** level unspecified

  √6ᵗʰ **S48.91** Complete **traumatic amputation of shoulder and upper arm, level unspecified**

    √7ᵗʰ **S48.911** **Complete traumatic amputation of** right **shoulder and upper arm, level unspecified** ▽

    √7ᵗʰ **S48.912** **Complete traumatic amputation of** left **shoulder and upper arm, level unspecified** ▽

    √7ᵗʰ **S48.919** **Complete traumatic amputation of unspecified shoulder and upper arm, level unspecified** ▽

  √6ᵗʰ **S48.92** Partial **traumatic amputation of shoulder and upper arm, level unspecified**

    √7ᵗʰ **S48.921** **Partial traumatic amputation of** right **shoulder and upper arm, level unspecified** ▽

    √7ᵗʰ **S48.922** **Partial traumatic amputation of** left **shoulder and upper arm, level unspecified** ▽

    √7ᵗʰ **S48.929** **Partial traumatic amputation of unspecified shoulder and upper arm, level unspecified** ▽

√4ᵗʰ **S49 Other and unspecified injuries of shoulder and upper arm**

> The appropriate 7th character is to be added to each code from subcategories S49.0 and S49.1.
> A   initial encounter for closed fracture
> D   subsequent encounter for fracture with routine healing
> G   subsequent encounter for fracture with delayed healing
> K   subsequent encounter for fracture with nonunion
> P   subsequent encounter for fracture with malunion
> S   sequela

√5ᵗʰ **S49.0** Physeal **fracture of** upper end of humerus

  √6ᵗʰ **S49.00** Unspecified **physeal fracture of upper end of humerus**

    √7ᵗʰ **S49.001** **Unspecified physeal fracture of upper end of humerus,** right **arm** ▽

    √7ᵗʰ **S49.002** **Unspecified physeal fracture of upper end of humerus,** left **arm** ▽

    √7ᵗʰ **S49.009** **Unspecified physeal fracture of upper end of humerus, unspecified arm** ▽

  √6ᵗʰ **S49.01** Salter-Harris Type I **physeal fracture of upper end of humerus**

    √7ᵗʰ **S49.011** **Salter-Harris Type I physeal fracture of upper end of humerus,** right **arm**

    √7ᵗʰ **S49.012** **Salter-Harris Type I physeal fracture of upper end of humerus,** left **arm**

    √7ᵗʰ **S49.019** **Salter-Harris Type I physeal fracture of upper end of humerus, unspecified arm** ▽

  √6ᵗʰ **S49.02** Salter-Harris Type II **physeal fracture of upper end of humerus**

    √7ᵗʰ **S49.021** **Salter-Harris Type II physeal fracture of upper end of humerus,** right **arm**

    √7ᵗʰ **S49.022** **Salter-Harris Type II physeal fracture of upper end of humerus,** left **arm**

    √7ᵗʰ **S49.029** **Salter-Harris Type II physeal fracture of upper end of humerus, unspecified arm** ▽

  √6ᵗʰ **S49.03** Salter-Harris Type III **physeal fracture of upper end of humerus**

    √7ᵗʰ **S49.031** **Salter Harris Type III physeal fracture of upper end of humerus,** right **arm**

    √7ᵗʰ **S49.032** **Salter Harris Type III physeal fracture of upper end of humerus,** left **arm**

    √7ᵗʰ **S49.039** **Salter Harris Type III physeal fracture of upper end of humerus, unspecified arm** ▽

  √6ᵗʰ **S49.04** Salter-Harris Type IV **physeal fracture of upper end of humerus**

    √7ᵗʰ **S49.041** **Salter-Harris Type IV physeal fracture of upper end of humerus,** right **arm**

    √7ᵗʰ **S49.042** **Salter-Harris Type IV physeal fracture of upper end of humerus,** left **arm**

    √7ᵗʰ **S49.049** **Salter-Harris Type IV physeal fracture of upper end of humerus, unspecified arm** ▽

  √6ᵗʰ **S49.09** Other **physeal fracture of upper end of humerus**

    √7ᵗʰ **S49.091** **Other physeal fracture of upper end of humerus,** left **arm**

    √7ᵗʰ **S49.092** **Other physeal fracture of upper end of humerus,** left **arm**

    √7ᵗʰ **S49.099** **Other physeal fracture of upper end of humerus, unspecified arm** ▽

√5ᵗʰ **S49.1 Physeal fracture of** lower end of humerus

  √6ᵗʰ **S49.10** Unspecified **physeal fracture of lower end of humerus**

    √7ᵗʰ **S49.101** **Unspecified physeal fracture of lower end of humerus,** right **arm** ▽

    √7ᵗʰ **S49.102** **Unspecified physeal fracture of lower end of humerus,** left **arm** ▽

    √7ᵗʰ **S49.109** **Unspecified physeal fracture of lower end of humerus, unspecified arm** ▽

  √6ᵗʰ **S49.11** Salter-Harris Type I **physeal fracture of lower end of humerus**

    √7ᵗʰ **S49.111** **Salter-Harris Type I physeal fracture of lower end of humerus,** right **arm**

    √7ᵗʰ **S49.112** **Salter-Harris Type I physeal fracture of lower end of humerus,** left **arm**

    √7ᵗʰ **S49.119** **Salter-Harris Type I physeal fracture of lower end of humerus, unspecified arm** ▽

  √6ᵗʰ **S49.12** Salter-Harris Type II **physeal fracture of lower end of humerus**

    √7ᵗʰ **S49.121** **Salter-Harris Type II physeal fracture of lower end of humerus,** right **arm**

    √7ᵗʰ **S49.122** **Salter-Harris Type II physeal fracture of lower end of humerus,** left **arm**

    √7ᵗʰ **S49.129** **Salter-Harris Type II physeal fracture of lower end of humerus, unspecified arm** ▽

  √6ᵗʰ **S49.13** Salter Harris Type III **physeal fracture of lower end of humerus**

    √7ᵗʰ **S49.131** **Salter Harris Type III physeal fracture of lower end of humerus,** right **arm**

    √7ᵗʰ **S49.132** **Salter Harris Type III physeal fracture of lower end of humerus,** left **arm**

    √7ᵗʰ **S49.139** **Salter Harris Type III physeal fracture of lower end of humerus, unspecified arm** ▽

  √6ᵗʰ **S49.14** Salter-Harris Type IV **physeal fracture of lower end of humerus**

    √7ᵗʰ **S49.141** **Salter-Harris Type IV physeal fracture of lower end of humerus,** right **arm**

    √7ᵗʰ **S49.142** **Salter-Harris Type IV physeal fracture of lower end of humerus,** left **arm**

    √7ᵗʰ **S49.149** **Salter-Harris Type IV physeal fracture of lower end of humerus, unspecified arm** ▽

  √6ᵗʰ **S49.19** Other **physeal fracture of lower end of humerus**

    √7ᵗʰ **S49.191** **Other physeal fracture of lower end of humerus,** right **arm**

    √7ᵗʰ **S49.192** **Other physeal fracture of lower end of humerus,** left **arm**

    √7ᵗʰ **S49.199** **Other physeal fracture of lower end of humerus, unspecified arm** ▽

Ⓝ Newborn   Ⓟ Pediatric   Ⓜ Maternity   Ⓐ Adult   **RIC Dx** RIC Dx   **NC Dx** Noncancer Dx   **PDx** Primary Dx   **CC** RIC CC Condition   ►◄ Revised Text   ● New Code   ▲ Revised Code Title

906   ICD-10-CM 2016

√5ᵗʰ **S49.8 Other specified injuries of shoulder and upper arm**

> The appropriate 7th character is to be added to each code in subcategory S49.8.
> A   initial encounter
> D   subsequent encounter
> S   sequela

√x7ᵗʰ **S49.80 Other specified injuries of shoulder and upper arm, unspecified arm** ▽

√x7ᵗʰ **S49.81 Other specified injuries of right shoulder and upper arm**

√x7ᵗʰ **S49.82 Other specified injuries of left shoulder and upper arm**

√5ᵗʰ **S49.9 Unspecified injury of shoulder and upper arm**

> The appropriate 7th character is to be added to each code in subcategory S49.9.
> A   initial encounter
> D   subsequent encounter
> S   sequela

√x7ᵗʰ **S49.90 Unspecified injury of shoulder and upper arm, unspecified arm** ▽

√x7ᵗʰ **S49.91 Unspecified injury of right shoulder and upper arm** ▽

√x7ᵗʰ **S49.92 Unspecified injury of left shoulder and upper arm** ▽

Injuries to the elbow and forearm (S50-S59)

EXCLUDES 2   *burns and corrosions (T20-T32)*
frostbite (T33-T34)
injuries of wrist and hand (S60-S69)
insect bite or sting, venomous (T63.4)

√4ᵗʰ **S50 Superficial injury of elbow and forearm**
EXCLUDES 2   *superficial injury of wrist and hand (S60.-)*

> The appropriate 7th character is to be added to each code from category S50.
> A   initial encounter
> D   subsequent encounter
> S   sequela

√5ᵗʰ **S50.0 Contusion of elbow**

√x7ᵗʰ **S50.00 Contusion of unspecified elbow** ▽

√x7ᵗʰ **S50.01 Contusion of right elbow**

√x7ᵗʰ **S50.02 Contusion of left elbow**

√5ᵗʰ **S50.1 Contusion of forearm**

√x7ᵗʰ **S50.10 Contusion of unspecified forearm** ▽

√x7ᵗʰ **S50.11 Contusion of right forearm**

√x7ᵗʰ **S50.12 Contusion of left forearm**

√5ᵗʰ **S50.3 Other superficial injuries of elbow**

√6ᵗʰ **S50.31 Abrasion of elbow**

√7ᵗʰ **S50.311 Abrasion of right elbow**

√7ᵗʰ **S50.312 Abrasion of left elbow**

√7ᵗʰ **S50.319 Abrasion of unspecified elbow** ▽

√6ᵗʰ **S50.32 Blister (nonthermal) of elbow**

√7ᵗʰ **S50.321 Blister (nonthermal) of right elbow**

√7ᵗʰ **S50.322 Blister (nonthermal) of left elbow**

√7ᵗʰ **S50.329 Blister (nonthermal) of unspecified elbow** ▽

√6ᵗʰ **S50.34 External constriction of elbow**

√7ᵗʰ **S50.341 External constriction of right elbow**

√7ᵗʰ **S50.342 External constriction of left elbow**

√7ᵗʰ **S50.349 External constriction of unspecified elbow** ▽

√6ᵗʰ **S50.35 Superficial foreign body of elbow**
Splinter in the elbow

√7ᵗʰ **S50.351 Superficial foreign body of right elbow**

√7ᵗʰ **S50.352 Superficial foreign body of left elbow**

√7ᵗʰ **S50.359 Superficial foreign body of unspecified elbow** ▽

√6ᵗʰ **S50.36 Insect bite (nonvenomous) of elbow**

√7ᵗʰ **S50.361 Insect bite (nonvenomous) of right elbow**

√7ᵗʰ **S50.362 Insect bite (nonvenomous) of left elbow**

√7ᵗʰ **S50.369 Insect bite (nonvenomous) of unspecified elbow** ▽

√6ᵗʰ **S50.37 Other superficial bite of elbow**
EXCLUDES 1   *open bite of elbow (S51.05)*

√7ᵗʰ **S50.371 Other superficial bite of right elbow**

√7ᵗʰ **S50.372 Other superficial bite of left elbow**

√7ᵗʰ **S50.379 Other superficial bite of unspecified elbow** ▽

√5ᵗʰ **S50.8 Other superficial injuries of forearm**

√6ᵗʰ **S50.81 Abrasion of forearm**

√7ᵗʰ **S50.811 Abrasion of right forearm**

√7ᵗʰ **S50.812 Abrasion of left forearm**

√7ᵗʰ **S50.819 Abrasion of unspecified forearm** ▽

√6ᵗʰ **S50.82 Blister (nonthermal) of forearm**

√7ᵗʰ **S50.821 Blister (nonthermal) of right forearm**

√7ᵗʰ **S50.822 Blister (nonthermal) of left forearm**

√7ᵗʰ **S50.829 Blister (nonthermal) of unspecified forearm** ▽

√6ᵗʰ **S50.84 External constriction of forearm**

√7ᵗʰ **S50.841 External constriction of right forearm**

√7ᵗʰ **S50.842 External constriction of left forearm**

√7ᵗʰ **S50.849 External constriction of unspecified forearm** ▽

√6ᵗʰ **S50.85 Superficial foreign body of forearm**
Splinter in the forearm

√7ᵗʰ **S50.851 Superficial foreign body of right forearm**

√7ᵗʰ **S50.852 Superficial foreign body of left forearm**

√7ᵗʰ **S50.859 Superficial foreign body of unspecified forearm** ▽

√6ᵗʰ **S50.86 Insect bite (nonvenomous) of forearm**

√7ᵗʰ **S50.861 Insect bite (nonvenomous) of right forearm**

√7ᵗʰ **S50.862 Insect bite (nonvenomous) of left forearm**

√7ᵗʰ **S50.869 Insect bite (nonvenomous) of unspecified forearm** ▽

√6ᵗʰ **S50.87 Other superficial bite of forearm**
EXCLUDES 1   *open bite of forearm (S51.85)*

√7ᵗʰ **S50.871 Other superficial bite of right forearm**

√7ᵗʰ **S50.872 Other superficial bite of left forearm**

√7ᵗʰ **S50.879 Other superficial bite of unspecified forearm** ▽

√5ᵗʰ **S50.9 Unspecified superficial injury of elbow and forearm**

√6ᵗʰ **S50.90 Unspecified superficial injury of elbow**

√7ᵗʰ **S50.901 Unspecified superficial injury of right elbow** ▽

√7ᵗʰ **S50.902 Unspecified superficial injury of left elbow** ▽

√7ᵗʰ **S50.909 Unspecified superficial injury of unspecified elbow** ▽

√6ᵗʰ **S50.91 Unspecified superficial injury of forearm**

√7ᵗʰ **S50.911 Unspecified superficial injury of right forearm** ▽

√7ᵗʰ **S50.912 Unspecified superficial injury of left forearm** ▽

√7ᵗʰ **S50.919 Unspecified superficial injury of unspecified forearm** ▽

√4ᵗʰ **S51 Open wound of elbow and forearm**
Code also any associated wound infection
EXCLUDES 1   *open fracture of elbow and forearm (S52- with open fracture 7th character)*
traumatic amputation of elbow and forearm (S58.-)
EXCLUDES 2   *open wound of wrist and hand (S61.-)*

> The appropriate 7th character is to be added to each code from category S51.
> A   initial encounter
> D   subsequent encounter
> S   sequela

√5ᵗʰ **S51.0 Open wound of elbow**

√6ᵗʰ **S51.00 Unspecified open wound of elbow**

√7ᵗʰ **S51.001 Unspecified open wound of right elbow** ▽
AHA: 2012, 4Q, 108

☑ Add'l Character Required √x7ᵗʰ Placeholder Alert   RUG IV Special Care High Dx   RUG IV Clinically Complex Dx   RUG IV Special Care Low Dx   Manifestation Code   Other Specified Code   ▽ Unspecified Code

CD-10-CM 2016   907

√7ᵗʰ **S51.002** **Unspecified open wound of** left **elbow** ▽

√7ᵗʰ **S51.009** **Unspecified open wound of unspecified** ▽ **elbow**
Open wound of elbow NOS

√6ᵗʰ **S51.01** Laceration without foreign body **of elbow**

√7ᵗʰ **S51.011** **Laceration without foreign body of** right **elbow**

√7ᵗʰ **S51.012** **Laceration without foreign body of** left **elbow**

√7ᵗʰ **S51.019** **Laceration without foreign body of** ▽ **unspecified elbow**

√6ᵗʰ **S51.02** Laceration with foreign body **of elbow**

√7ᵗʰ **S51.021** **Laceration with foreign body of** right **elbow**

√7ᵗʰ **S51.022** **Laceration with foreign body of** left **elbow**

√7ᵗʰ **S51.029** **Laceration with foreign body of** ▽ **unspecified elbow**

√6ᵗʰ **S51.03** Puncture wound without foreign body **of elbow**

√7ᵗʰ **S51.031** **Puncture wound without foreign body of** right **elbow**

√7ᵗʰ **S51.032** **Puncture wound without foreign body of** left **elbow**

√7ᵗʰ **S51.039** **Puncture wound without foreign body** ▽ **of unspecified elbow**

√6ᵗʰ **S51.04** Puncture wound with foreign body **of elbow**

√7ᵗʰ **S51.041** **Puncture wound with foreign body of** right **elbow**

√7ᵗʰ **S51.042** **Puncture wound with foreign body of** left **elbow**

√7ᵗʰ **S51.049** **Puncture wound with foreign body of** ▽ **unspecified elbow**

√6ᵗʰ **S51.05** Open bite **of elbow**
Bite of elbow NOS
EXCLUDES 1 superficial bite of elbow (S50.36, S50.37)

√7ᵗʰ **S51.051** **Open bite,** right **elbow**

√7ᵗʰ **S51.052** **Open bite,** left **elbow**

√7ᵗʰ **S51.059** **Open bite, unspecified elbow** ▽

√5ᵗʰ **S51.8** **Open wound of** forearm
EXCLUDES 2 open wound of elbow (S51.0-)

√6ᵗʰ **S51.80** Unspecified **open wound of forearm**

√7ᵗʰ **S51.801** **Unspecified open wound of** right **forearm** ▽

√7ᵗʰ **S51.802** **Unspecified open wound of** left **forearm** ▽

√7ᵗʰ **S51.809** **Unspecified open wound of** ▽ **unspecified forearm**
Open wound of forearm NOS

√6ᵗʰ **S51.81** Laceration without foreign body **of forearm**

√7ᵗʰ **S51.811** **Laceration without foreign body of** right **forearm**

√7ᵗʰ **S51.812** **Laceration without foreign body of** left **forearm**

√7ᵗʰ **S51.819** **Laceration without foreign body of** ▽ **unspecified forearm**

√6ᵗʰ **S51.82** Laceration with foreign body **of forearm**

√7ᵗʰ **S51.821** **Laceration with foreign body of** right **forearm**

√7ᵗʰ **S51.822** **Laceration with foreign body of** left **forearm**

√7ᵗʰ **S51.829** **Laceration with foreign body of** ▽ **unspecified forearm**

√6ᵗʰ **S51.83** Puncture wound without foreign body **of forearm**

√7ᵗʰ **S51.831** **Puncture wound without foreign body of** right **forearm**

√7ᵗʰ **S51.832** **Puncture wound without foreign body of** left **forearm**

√7ᵗʰ **S51.839** **Puncture wound without foreign body** ▽ **of unspecified forearm**

√6ᵗʰ **S51.84** Puncture wound with foreign body **of forearm**

√7ᵗʰ **S51.841** **Puncture wound with foreign body of** right **forearm**

√7ᵗʰ **S51.842** **Puncture wound with foreign body of** left **forearm**

√7ᵗʰ **S51.849** **Puncture wound with foreign body of** ▽ **unspecified forearm**

√6ᵗʰ **S51.85** Open bite **of forearm**
Bite of forearm NOS
EXCLUDES 1 superficial bite of forearm (S50.86, S50.87)

√7ᵗʰ **S51.851** **Open bite of** right **forearm**

√7ᵗʰ **S51.852** **Open bite of** left **forearm**

√7ᵗʰ **S51.859** **Open bite of unspecified forearm** ▽

√4ᵗʰ **S52** **Fracture of forearm**
NOTE A fracture not indicated as displaced or nondisplaced should be coded to displaced.
A fracture not indicated as open or closed should be coded to closed.
The open fracture designations are based on the Gustilo open fracture classification.
EXCLUDES 1 traumatic amputation of forearm (S58.-)
EXCLUDES 2 fracture at wrist and hand level (S62.-)

The appropriate 7th character is to be added to all codes from category S52 [unless otherwise indicated].
A   initial encounter for closed fracture
B   initial encounter for open fracture type I or II
      initial encounter for open fracture NOS
C   initial encounter for open fracture type IIIA, IIIB, or IIIC
D   subsequent encounter for closed fracture with routine healing
E   subsequent encounter for open fracture type I or II with routine healing
F   subsequent encounter for open fracture type IIIA, IIIB, or IIIC with routine healing
G   subsequent encounter for closed fracture with delayed healing
H   subsequent encounter for open fracture type I or II with delayed healing
J   subsequent encounter for open fracture type IIIA, IIIB, or IIIC with delayed healing
K   subsequent encounter for closed fracture with nonunion
M   subsequent encounter for open fracture type I or II with nonunion
N   subsequent encounter for open fracture type IIIA, IIIB, or IIIC with nonunion
P   subsequent encounter for closed fracture with malunion
Q   subsequent encounter for open fracture type I or II with malunion
R   subsequent encounter for open fracture type IIIA, IIIB, or IIIC with malunion
S   sequela

√5ᵗʰ **S52.0** **Fracture of** upper end of ulna
Fracture of proximal end of ulna
EXCLUDES 2 fracture of elbow NOS (S42.40-)
fractures of shaft of ulna (S52.2-)

√6ᵗʰ **S52.00** Unspecified **fracture of upper end of ulna**

√7ᵗʰ **S52.001** **Unspecified fracture of upper end of** ▽ right **ulna**

√7ᵗʰ **S52.002** **Unspecified fracture of upper end of** ▽ left **ulna**

√7ᵗʰ **S52.009** **Unspecified fracture of upper end of** ▽ **unspecified ulna**

√6ᵗʰ **S52.01** Torus **fracture of upper end of ulna**

The appropriate 7th character is to be added to all codes in subcategory S52.01.
A   initial encounter for closed fracture
D   subsequent encounter for fracture with routine healing
G   subsequent encounter for fracture with delayed healing
K   subsequent encounter for fracture with nonunion
P   subsequent encounter for fracture with malunion
S   sequela

√7ᵗʰ **S52.011** **Torus fracture of upper end of** right **ulna**

√7ᵗʰ **S52.012** **Torus fracture of upper end of** left **ulna**

√7ᵗʰ **S52.019** **Torus fracture of upper end of** ▽ **unspecified ulna**

Ⓝ Newborn   Ⓟ Pediatric   Ⓜ Maternity   Ⓐ Adult   **RIC** RIC Dx   **NC Dx** Noncancer Dx   **PDx** Primary Dx   **CC** RIC CC Condition   ▶◀ Revised Text   ● New Code   ▲ Revised Code Title

908   ICD-10-CM 2016

√6ᵗʰ **S52.02** **Fracture of** olecranon process without intraarticular extension **of ulna**

　√7ᵗʰ **S52.021** Displaced **fracture of olecranon process without intraarticular extension of** right **ulna**

　√7ᵗʰ **S52.022** Displaced **fracture of olecranon process without intraarticular extension of** left **ulna**

　√7ᵗʰ **S52.023** Displaced **fracture of olecranon process without intraarticular extension of unspecified ulna** ▽

　√7ᵗʰ **S52.024** Nondisplaced **fracture of olecranon process without intraarticular extension of** right **ulna**

　√7ᵗʰ **S52.025** Nondisplaced **fracture of olecranon process without intraarticular extension of** left **ulna**

　√7ᵗʰ **S52.026** Nondisplaced **fracture of olecranon process without intraarticular extension of unspecified ulna** ▽

√6ᵗʰ **S52.03** **Fracture of** olecranon process with intraarticular extension **of ulna**

　√7ᵗʰ **S52.031** Displaced **fracture of olecranon process with intraarticular extension of** right **ulna**

　√7ᵗʰ **S52.032** Displaced **fracture of olecranon process with intraarticular extension of** left **ulna**

　√7ᵗʰ **S52.033** Displaced **fracture of olecranon process** ▽ **with intraarticular extension of unspecified ulna**

　√7ᵗʰ **S52.034** Nondisplaced **fracture of olecranon process with intraarticular extension of** right **ulna**

　√7ᵗʰ **S52.035** Nondisplaced **fracture of olecranon process with intraarticular extension of** left **ulna**

　√7ᵗʰ **S52.036** Nondisplaced **fracture of olecranon process with intraarticular extension of unspecified ulna** ▽

√6ᵗʰ **S52.04** **Fracture of** coronoid process **of ulna**

　√7ᵗʰ **S52.041** Displaced **fracture of coronoid process of** right **ulna**

　√7ᵗʰ **S52.042** Displaced **fracture of coronoid process of** left **ulna**

　√7ᵗʰ **S52.043** Displaced **fracture of coronoid process** ▽ **of unspecified ulna**

　√7ᵗʰ **S52.044** Nondisplaced **fracture of coronoid process of** right **ulna**

　√7ᵗʰ **S52.045** Nondisplaced **fracture of coronoid process of** left **ulna**

　√7ᵗʰ **S52.046** Nondisplaced **fracture of coronoid process of unspecified ulna** ▽

√6ᵗʰ **S52.09** Other **fracture of upper end of ulna**

　√7ᵗʰ **S52.091** Other fracture of upper end of right ulna

　√7ᵗʰ **S52.092** Other fracture of upper end of left ulna

　√7ᵗʰ **S52.099** Other fracture of upper end of unspecified ulna ▽

√5ᵗʰ **S52.1** **Fracture of** upper end of radius

　　Fracture of proximal end of radius

　　EXCLUDES 2　physeal fractures of upper end of radius (S59.2-)
　　　　　　　fracture of shaft of radius (S52.3-)

√6ᵗʰ **S52.10** Unspecified **fracture of upper end of radius**

　√7ᵗʰ **S52.101** Unspecified **fracture of upper end of** ▽ right **radius**

　√7ᵗʰ **S52.102** Unspecified **fracture of upper end of** ▽ left **radius**

　√7ᵗʰ **S52.109** Unspecified **fracture of upper end of unspecified radius** ▽

√6ᵗʰ **S52.11** Torus **fracture of upper end of radius**

The appropriate 7th character is to be added to all codes in subcategory S52.11.
A　initial encounter for closed fracture
D　subsequent encounter for fracture with routine healing
G　subsequent encounter for fracture with delayed healing
K　subsequent encounter for fracture with nonunion
P　subsequent encounter for fracture with malunion
S　sequela

　√7ᵗʰ **S52.111** Torus **fracture of upper end of** right **radius**

　√7ᵗʰ **S52.112** Torus **fracture of upper end of** left **radius**

　√7ᵗʰ **S52.119** Torus **fracture of upper end of unspecified radius** ▽

√6ᵗʰ **S52.12** **Fracture of** head **of radius**

　√7ᵗʰ **S52.121** Displaced **fracture of head of** right **radius**

　√7ᵗʰ **S52.122** Displaced **fracture of head of** left **radius**

　√7ᵗʰ **S52.123** Displaced **fracture of head of unspecified radius** ▽

　√7ᵗʰ **S52.124** Nondisplaced **fracture of head of** right **radius**

　√7ᵗʰ **S52.125** Nondisplaced **fracture of head of** left **radius**

　√7ᵗʰ **S52.126** Nondisplaced **fracture of head of unspecified radius** ▽

√6ᵗʰ **S52.13** **Fracture of** neck **of radius**

　√7ᵗʰ **S52.131** Displaced **fracture of neck of** right **radius**

　√7ᵗʰ **S52.132** Displaced **fracture of neck of** left **radius**

　√7ᵗʰ **S52.133** Displaced **fracture of neck of unspecified radius** ▽

　√7ᵗʰ **S52.134** Nondisplaced **fracture of neck of** right **radius**

　√7ᵗʰ **S52.135** Nondisplaced **fracture of neck of** left **radius**

　√7ᵗʰ **S52.136** Nondisplaced **fracture of neck of unspecified radius** ▽

√6ᵗʰ **S52.18** Other **fracture of upper end of radius**

　√7ᵗʰ **S52.181** Other fracture of upper end of right radius

　√7ᵗʰ **S52.182** Other fracture of upper end of left radius

　√7ᵗʰ **S52.189** Other fracture of upper end of unspecified radius ▽

√5ᵗʰ **S52.2** **Fracture of** shaft of ulna

√6ᵗʰ **S52.20** Unspecified **fracture of shaft of ulna**

　　Fracture of ulna NOS

　√7ᵗʰ **S52.201** Unspecified **fracture of shaft of** right **ulna** ▽

　√7ᵗʰ **S52.202** Unspecified **fracture of shaft of** left **ulna** ▽

　√7ᵗʰ **S52.209** Unspecified **fracture of shaft of unspecified ulna** ▽

√6ᵗʰ **S52.21** Greenstick **fracture of shaft of ulna**

The appropriate 7th character is to be added to all codes in subcategory S52.21.
A　initial encounter for closed fracture
D　subsequent encounter for fracture with routine healing
G　subsequent encounter for fracture with delayed healing
K　subsequent encounter for fracture with nonunion
P　subsequent encounter for fracture with malunion
S　sequela

　√7ᵗʰ **S52.211** Greenstick **fracture of shaft of** right **ulna**

　√7ᵗʰ **S52.212** Greenstick **fracture of shaft of** left **ulna**

　√7ᵗʰ **S52.219** Greenstick **fracture of shaft of unspecified ulna** ▽

☑ Add'l Character Required　√ₓ7ᵗʰ Placeholder Alert　RUG IV Special Care High Dx　RUG IV Clinically Complex Dx　RUG IV Special Care Low Dx　Manifestation Code　Other Specified Code　▽Unspecified Code

ICD-10-CM 2016　　　909

Chapter 19. Injury, Poisoning and Certain Other Consequences of External Causes

S52.22–S52.346

✓6ᵗʰ **S52.22** Transverse fracture of shaft of ulna
- ✓7ᵗʰ **S52.221** Displaced transverse fracture of shaft of right ulna
- ✓7ᵗʰ **S52.222** Displaced transverse fracture of shaft of left ulna
- ✓7ᵗʰ **S52.223** Displaced transverse fracture of shaft of unspecified ulna ▽
- ✓7ᵗʰ **S52.224** Nondisplaced transverse fracture of shaft of right ulna
- ✓7ᵗʰ **S52.225** Nondisplaced transverse fracture of shaft of left ulna
- ✓7ᵗʰ **S52.226** Nondisplaced transverse fracture of shaft of unspecified ulna ▽

✓6ᵗʰ **S52.23** Oblique fracture of shaft of ulna
- ✓7ᵗʰ **S52.231** Displaced oblique fracture of shaft of right ulna
- ✓7ᵗʰ **S52.232** Displaced oblique fracture of shaft of left ulna
- ✓7ᵗʰ **S52.233** Displaced oblique fracture of shaft of unspecified ulna ▽
- ✓7ᵗʰ **S52.234** Nondisplaced oblique fracture of shaft of right ulna
- ✓7ᵗʰ **S52.235** Nondisplaced oblique fracture of shaft of left ulna
- ✓7ᵗʰ **S52.236** Nondisplaced oblique fracture of shaft of unspecified ulna ▽

✓6ᵗʰ **S52.24** Spiral fracture of shaft of ulna
- ✓7ᵗʰ **S52.241** Displaced spiral fracture of shaft of ulna, right arm
- ✓7ᵗʰ **S52.242** Displaced spiral fracture of shaft of ulna, left arm
- ✓7ᵗʰ **S52.243** Displaced spiral fracture of shaft of ulna, unspecified arm ▽
- ✓7ᵗʰ **S52.244** Nondisplaced spiral fracture of shaft of ulna, right arm
- ✓7ᵗʰ **S52.245** Nondisplaced spiral fracture of shaft of ulna, left arm
- ✓7ᵗʰ **S52.246** Nondisplaced spiral fracture of shaft of ulna, unspecified arm ▽

✓6ᵗʰ **S52.25** Comminuted fracture of shaft of ulna
- ✓7ᵗʰ **S52.251** Displaced comminuted fracture of shaft of ulna, right arm
- ✓7ᵗʰ **S52.252** Displaced comminuted fracture of shaft of ulna, left arm
- ✓7ᵗʰ **S52.253** Displaced comminuted fracture of shaft of ulna, unspecified arm ▽
- ✓7ᵗʰ **S52.254** Nondisplaced comminuted fracture of shaft of ulna, right arm
- ✓7ᵗʰ **S52.255** Nondisplaced comminuted fracture of shaft of ulna, left arm
- ✓7ᵗʰ **S52.256** Nondisplaced comminuted fracture of shaft of ulna, unspecified arm ▽

✓6ᵗʰ **S52.26** Segmental fracture of shaft of ulna
- ✓7ᵗʰ **S52.261** Displaced segmental fracture of shaft of ulna, right arm
- ✓7ᵗʰ **S52.262** Displaced segmental fracture of shaft of ulna, left arm
- ✓7ᵗʰ **S52.263** Displaced segmental fracture of shaft of ulna, unspecified arm ▽
- ✓7ᵗʰ **S52.264** Nondisplaced segmental fracture of shaft of ulna, right arm
- ✓7ᵗʰ **S52.265** Nondisplaced segmental fracture of shaft of ulna, left arm
- ✓7ᵗʰ **S52.266** Nondisplaced segmental fracture of shaft of ulna, unspecified arm ▽

✓6ᵗʰ **S52.27** Monteggia's fracture of ulna
     Fracture of upper shaft of ulna with dislocation of radial head
- ✓7ᵗʰ **S52.271** Monteggia's fracture of right ulna
- ✓7ᵗʰ **S52.272** Monteggia's fracture of left ulna
- ✓7ᵗʰ **S52.279** Monteggia's fracture of unspecified ulna ▽

✓6ᵗʰ **S52.28** Bent bone of ulna
- ✓7ᵗʰ **S52.281** Bent bone of right ulna
- ✓7ᵗʰ **S52.282** Bent bone of left ulna
- ✓7ᵗʰ **S52.283** Bent bone of unspecified ulna ▽

✓6ᵗʰ **S52.29** Other fracture of shaft of ulna
- ✓7ᵗʰ **S52.291** Other fracture of shaft of right ulna
- ✓7ᵗʰ **S52.292** Other fracture of shaft of left ulna
- ✓7ᵗʰ **S52.299** Other fracture of shaft of unspecified ulna ▽

✓5ᵗʰ **S52.3** Fracture of shaft of radius
✓6ᵗʰ **S52.30** Unspecified fracture of shaft of radius
- ✓7ᵗʰ **S52.301** Unspecified fracture of shaft of right radius ▽
- ✓7ᵗʰ **S52.302** Unspecified fracture of shaft of left radius ▽
- ✓7ᵗʰ **S52.309** Unspecified fracture of shaft of unspecified radius ▽

✓6ᵗʰ **S52.31** Greenstick fracture of shaft of radius

> The appropriate 7th character is to be added to all codes in subcategory S52.31.
> A   initial encounter for closed fracture
> D   subsequent encounter for fracture with routine healing
> G   subsequent encounter for fracture with delayed healing
> K   subsequent encounter for fracture with nonunion
> P   subsequent encounter for fracture with malunion
> S   sequela

- ✓7ᵗʰ **S52.311** Greenstick fracture of shaft of radius, right arm
- ✓7ᵗʰ **S52.312** Greenstick fracture of shaft of radius, left arm
- ✓7ᵗʰ **S52.319** Greenstick fracture of shaft of radius, unspecified arm ▽

✓6ᵗʰ **S52.32** Transverse fracture of shaft of radius
- ✓7ᵗʰ **S52.321** Displaced transverse fracture of shaft of right radius
- ✓7ᵗʰ **S52.322** Displaced transverse fracture of shaft of left radius
- ✓7ᵗʰ **S52.323** Displaced transverse fracture of shaft of unspecified radius ▽
- ✓7ᵗʰ **S52.324** Nondisplaced transverse fracture of shaft of right radius
- ✓7ᵗʰ **S52.325** Nondisplaced transverse fracture of shaft of left radius
- ✓7ᵗʰ **S52.326** Nondisplaced transverse fracture of shaft of unspecified radius ▽

✓6ᵗʰ **S52.33** Oblique fracture of shaft of radius
- ✓7ᵗʰ **S52.331** Displaced oblique fracture of shaft of right radius
- ✓7ᵗʰ **S52.332** Displaced oblique fracture of shaft of left radius
- ✓7ᵗʰ **S52.333** Displaced oblique fracture of shaft of unspecified radius ▽
- ✓7ᵗʰ **S52.334** Nondisplaced oblique fracture of shaft of right radius
- ✓7ᵗʰ **S52.335** Nondisplaced oblique fracture of shaft of left radius
- ✓7ᵗʰ **S52.336** Nondisplaced oblique fracture of shaft of unspecified radius ▽

✓6ᵗʰ **S52.34** Spiral fracture of shaft of radius
- ✓7ᵗʰ **S52.341** Displaced spiral fracture of shaft of radius, right arm
- ✓7ᵗʰ **S52.342** Displaced spiral fracture of shaft of radius, left arm
- ✓7ᵗʰ **S52.343** Displaced spiral fracture of shaft of radius, unspecified arm ▽
- ✓7ᵗʰ **S52.344** Nondisplaced spiral fracture of shaft of radius, right arm
- ✓7ᵗʰ **S52.345** Nondisplaced spiral fracture of shaft of radius, left arm
- ✓7ᵗʰ **S52.346** Nondisplaced spiral fracture of shaft of radius, unspecified arm ▽

N Newborn   P Pediatric   M Maternity   A Adult   RIC RIC Dx   NCDx Noncancer Dx   PDx Primary Dx   CC RIC CC Condition   ►◄ Revised Text   ● New Code   ▲ Revised Code Title

910   ICD-10-CM 2016

√6ᵗʰ **S52.35** Comminuted fracture of shaft of radius
- √7ᵗʰ **S52.351** Displaced comminuted fracture of shaft of radius, right arm
- √7ᵗʰ **S52.352** Displaced comminuted fracture of shaft of radius, left arm
- √7ᵗʰ **S52.353** Displaced comminuted fracture of shaft of radius, unspecified arm ▽
- √7ᵗʰ **S52.354** Nondisplaced comminuted fracture of shaft of radius, right arm
- √7ᵗʰ **S52.355** Nondisplaced comminuted fracture of shaft of radius, left arm
- √7ᵗʰ **S52.356** Nondisplaced comminuted fracture of shaft of radius, unspecified arm ▽

√6ᵗʰ **S52.36** Segmental fracture of shaft of radius
- √7ᵗʰ **S52.361** Displaced segmental fracture of shaft of radius, right arm
- √7ᵗʰ **S52.362** Displaced segmental fracture of shaft of radius, left arm
- √7ᵗʰ **S52.363** Displaced segmental fracture of shaft of radius, unspecified arm ▽
- √7ᵗʰ **S52.364** Nondisplaced segmental fracture of shaft of radius, right arm
- √7ᵗʰ **S52.365** Nondisplaced segmental fracture of shaft of radius, left arm
- √7ᵗʰ **S52.366** Nondisplaced segmental fracture of shaft of radius, unspecified arm ▽

√6ᵗʰ **S52.37** Galeazzi's fracture
    Fracture of lower shaft of radius with radioulnar joint dislocation
- √7ᵗʰ **S52.371** Galeazzi's fracture of right radius
- √7ᵗʰ **S52.372** Galeazzi's fracture of left radius
- √7ᵗʰ **S52.379** Galeazzi's fracture of unspecified radius ▽

√6ᵗʰ **S52.38** Bent bone of radius
- √7ᵗʰ **S52.381** Bent bone of right radius
- √7ᵗʰ **S52.382** Bent bone of left radius
- √7ᵗʰ **S52.389** Bent bone of unspecified radius ▽

√6ᵗʰ **S52.39** Other fracture of shaft of radius
- √7ᵗʰ **S52.391** Other fracture of shaft of radius, right arm
- √7ᵗʰ **S52.392** Other fracture of shaft of radius, left arm
- √7ᵗʰ **S52.399** Other fracture of shaft of radius, unspecified arm ▽

√5ᵗʰ **S52.5** Fracture of lower end of radius
    Fracture of distal end of radius
    EXCLUDES 2 physeal fractures of lower end of radius (S59.2-)

√6ᵗʰ **S52.50** Unspecified fracture of the lower end of radius
- √7ᵗʰ **S52.501** Unspecified fracture of the lower end of right radius ▽
- √7ᵗʰ **S52.502** Unspecified fracture of the lower end of left radius ▽
- √7ᵗʰ **S52.509** Unspecified fracture of the lower end of unspecified radius ▽

√6ᵗʰ **S52.51** Fracture of radial styloid process
- √7ᵗʰ **S52.511** Displaced fracture of right radial styloid process
- √7ᵗʰ **S52.512** Displaced fracture of left radial styloid process
- √7ᵗʰ **S52.513** Displaced fracture of unspecified radial styloid process ▽
- √7ᵗʰ **S52.514** Nondisplaced fracture of right radial styloid process
- √7ᵗʰ **S52.515** Nondisplaced fracture of left radial styloid process
- √7ᵗʰ **S52.516** Nondisplaced fracture of unspecified radial styloid process

√6ᵗʰ **S52.52** Torus fracture of lower end of radius

> The appropriate 7th character is to be added to all codes in subcategory S52.52.
> A   initial encounter for closed fracture
> D   subsequent encounter for fracture with routine healing
> G   subsequent encounter for fracture with delayed healing
> K   subsequent encounter for fracture with nonunion
> P   subsequent encounter for fracture with malunion
> S   sequela

- √7ᵗʰ **S52.521** Torus fracture of lower end of right radius
- √7ᵗʰ **S52.522** Torus fracture of lower end of left radius
- √7ᵗʰ **S52.529** Torus fracture of lower end of unspecified radius ▽

√6ᵗʰ **S52.53** Colles' fracture
- √7ᵗʰ **S52.531** Colles' fracture of right radius
- √7ᵗʰ **S52.532** Colles' fracture of left radius
- √7ᵗʰ **S52.539** Colles' fracture of unspecified radius ▽

√6ᵗʰ **S52.54** Smith's fracture
- √7ᵗʰ **S52.541** Smith's fracture of right radius
- √7ᵗʰ **S52.542** Smith's fracture of left radius
- √7ᵗʰ **S52.549** Smith's fracture of unspecified radius ▽

√6ᵗʰ **S52.55** Other extraarticular fracture of lower end of radius
- √7ᵗʰ **S52.551** Other extraarticular fracture of lower end of right radius
- √7ᵗʰ **S52.552** Other extraarticular fracture of lower end of left radius
- √7ᵗʰ **S52.559** Other extraarticular fracture of lower end of unspecified radius ▽

√6ᵗʰ **S52.56** Barton's fracture
- √7ᵗʰ **S52.561** Barton's fracture of right radius
- √7ᵗʰ **S52.562** Barton's fracture of left radius
- √7ᵗʰ **S52.569** Barton's fracture of unspecified radius ▽

√6ᵗʰ **S52.57** Other intraarticular fracture of lower end of radius
- √7ᵗʰ **S52.571** Other intraarticular fracture of lower end of right radius
- √7ᵗʰ **S52.572** Other intraarticular fracture of lower end of left radius
- √7ᵗʰ **S52.579** Other intraarticular fracture of lower end of unspecified radius ▽

√6ᵗʰ **S52.59** Other fractures of lower end of radius
- √7ᵗʰ **S52.591** Other fractures of lower end of right radius
- √7ᵗʰ **S52.592** Other fractures of lower end of left radius
- √7ᵗʰ **S52.599** Other fractures of lower end of unspecified radius ▽

√5ᵗʰ **S52.6** Fracture of lower end of ulna

√6ᵗʰ **S52.60** Unspecified fracture of lower end of ulna
- √7ᵗʰ **S52.601** Unspecified fracture of lower end of right ulna ▽
- √7ᵗʰ **S52.602** Unspecified fracture of lower end of left ulna ▽
- √7ᵗʰ **S52.609** Unspecified fracture of lower end of unspecified ulna ▽

√6ᵗʰ **S52.61** Fracture of ulna styloid process
- √7ᵗʰ **S52.611** Displaced fracture of right ulna styloid process
- √7ᵗʰ **S52.612** Displaced fracture of left ulna styloid process
- √7ᵗʰ **S52.613** Displaced fracture of unspecified ulna styloid process ▽
- √7ᵗʰ **S52.614** Nondisplaced fracture of right ulna styloid process
- √7ᵗʰ **S52.615** Nondisplaced fracture of left ulna styloid process
- √7ᵗʰ **S52.616** Nondisplaced fracture of unspecified ulna styloid process ▽

☑ Add'l Character Required   √×7ᵗʰ Placeholder Alert   RUG IV Special Care High Dx   RUG IV Clinically Complex Dx   RUG IV Special Care Low Dx   Manifestation Code   Other Specified Code   ▽ Unspecified Code

Chapter 19. Injury, Poisoning and Certain Other Consequences of External Causes

√6ᵗʰ **S52.62** Torus **fracture of lower end of ulna**

> The appropriate 7th character is to be added to all codes in subcategory S52.62.
> A   initial encounter for closed fracture
> D   subsequent encounter for fracture with routine healing
> G   subsequent encounter for fracture with delayed healing
> K   subsequent encounter for fracture with nonunion
> P   subsequent encounter for fracture with malunion
> S   sequela

> √7ᵗʰ **S52.621** Torus fracture of lower end of right ulna
> √7ᵗʰ **S52.622** Torus fracture of lower end of left ulna
> √7ᵗʰ **S52.629** Torus fracture of lower end of unspecified ulna ▽

√6ᵗʰ **S52.69** Other **fracture of lower end of ulna**

> √7ᵗʰ **S52.691** Other fracture of lower end of right ulna
> √7ᵗʰ **S52.692** Other fracture of lower end of left ulna
> √7ᵗʰ **S52.699** Other fracture of lower end of unspecified ulna ▽

√5ᵗʰ **S52.9** Unspecified fracture of forearm

> √ˣ7ᵗʰ **S52.90** Unspecified fracture of unspecified forearm ▽
> √ˣ7ᵗʰ **S52.91** Unspecified fracture of right forearm ▽
> √ˣ7ᵗʰ **S52.92** Unspecified fracture of left forearm ▽

√4ᵗʰ **S53** Dislocation and sprain of joints and ligaments of elbow

> **INCLUDES**   avulsion of joint or ligament of elbow
> laceration of cartilage, joint or ligament of elbow
> sprain of cartilage, joint or ligament of elbow
> traumatic hemarthrosis of joint or ligament of elbow
> traumatic rupture of joint or ligament of elbow
> traumatic subluxation of joint or ligament of elbow
> traumatic tear of joint or ligament of elbow

> Code also any associated open wound
> **EXCLUDES 2** strain of muscle, fascia and tendon at forearm level (S56.-)

> The appropriate 7th character is to be added to each code from category S53.
> A   initial encounter
> D   subsequent encounter
> S   sequela

√5ᵗʰ **S53.0** Subluxation and dislocation of radial head

> Dislocation of radiohumeral joint
> Subluxation of radiohumeral joint
> **EXCLUDES 1** Monteggia's fracture-dislocation (S52.27-)

> √6ᵗʰ **S53.00** Unspecified **subluxation and dislocation of radial head**

>> √7ᵗʰ **S53.001** Unspecified subluxation of right radial head ▽
>> √7ᵗʰ **S53.002** Unspecified subluxation of left radial head ▽
>> √7ᵗʰ **S53.003** Unspecified subluxation of unspecified radial head ▽
>> √7ᵗʰ **S53.004** Unspecified dislocation of right radial head ▽
>> √7ᵗʰ **S53.005** Unspecified dislocation of left radial head ▽
>> √7ᵗʰ **S53.006** Unspecified dislocation of unspecified radial head ▽

> √6ᵗʰ **S53.01** Anterior **subluxation and dislocation of radial head**
> Anteriomedial subluxation and dislocation of radial head

>> √7ᵗʰ **S53.011** Anterior subluxation of right radial head
>> √7ᵗʰ **S53.012** Anterior subluxation of left radial head
>> √7ᵗʰ **S53.013** Anterior subluxation of unspecified radial head ▽
>> √7ᵗʰ **S53.014** Anterior dislocation of right radial head
>> √7ᵗʰ **S53.015** Anterior dislocation of left radial head
>> √7ᵗʰ **S53.016** Anterior dislocation of unspecified radial head ▽

> √6ᵗʰ **S53.02** Posterior **subluxation and dislocation of radial head**
> Posteriolateral subluxation and dislocation of radial head

>> √7ᵗʰ **S53.021** Posterior subluxation of right radial head

√7ᵗʰ **S53.022** Posterior subluxation of left radial head
√7ᵗʰ **S53.023** Posterior subluxation of unspecified radial head ▽
√7ᵗʰ **S53.024** Posterior dislocation of right radial head
√7ᵗʰ **S53.025** Posterior dislocation of left radial head
√7ᵗʰ **S53.026** Posterior dislocation of unspecified radial head

√6ᵗʰ **S53.03** Nursemaid's **elbow**

> √7ᵗʰ **S53.031** Nursemaid's elbow, right elbow
> √7ᵗʰ **S53.032** Nursemaid's elbow, left elbow
> √7ᵗʰ **S53.033** Nursemaid's elbow, unspecified elbow ▽

√6ᵗʰ **S53.09** Other **subluxation and dislocation of radial head**

> √7ᵗʰ **S53.091** Other subluxation of right radial head
> √7ᵗʰ **S53.092** Other subluxation of left radial head
> √7ᵗʰ **S53.093** Other subluxation of unspecified radial head ▽
> √7ᵗʰ **S53.094** Other dislocation of right radial head
> √7ᵗʰ **S53.095** Other dislocation of left radial head
> √7ᵗʰ **S53.096** Other dislocation of unspecified radial head ▽

√5ᵗʰ **S53.1** Subluxation and dislocation of ulnohumeral joint

> Subluxation and dislocation of elbow NOS
> **EXCLUDES 1** dislocation of radial head alone (S53.0-)

> √6ᵗʰ **S53.10** Unspecified **subluxation and dislocation of ulnohumeral joint**

>> √7ᵗʰ **S53.101** Unspecified subluxation of right ulnohumeral joint ▽
>> √7ᵗʰ **S53.102** Unspecified subluxation of left ulnohumeral joint ▽
>> √7ᵗʰ **S53.103** Unspecified subluxation of unspecified ulnohumeral joint ▽
>> √7ᵗʰ **S53.104** Unspecified dislocation of right ulnohumeral joint ▽
>> √7ᵗʰ **S53.105** Unspecified dislocation of left ulnohumeral joint ▽
>> √7ᵗʰ **S53.106** Unspecified dislocation of unspecified ulnohumeral joint ▽

> √6ᵗʰ **S53.11** Anterior **subluxation and dislocation of ulnohumeral joint**

>> √7ᵗʰ **S53.111** Anterior subluxation of right ulnohumeral joint
>> √7ᵗʰ **S53.112** Anterior subluxation of left ulnohumeral joint
>> √7ᵗʰ **S53.113** Anterior subluxation of unspecified ulnohumeral joint ▽
>> √7ᵗʰ **S53.114** Anterior dislocation of right ulnohumeral joint
>>   **AHA:** 2012, 4Q, 108
>> √7ᵗʰ **S53.115** Anterior dislocation of left ulnohumeral joint
>> √7ᵗʰ **S53.116** Anterior dislocation of unspecified ulnohumeral joint ▽

> √6ᵗʰ **S53.12** Posterior **subluxation and dislocation of ulnohumeral joint**

>> √7ᵗʰ **S53.121** Posterior subluxation of right ulnohumeral joint
>> √7ᵗʰ **S53.122** Posterior subluxation of left ulnohumeral joint
>> √7ᵗʰ **S53.123** Posterior subluxation of unspecified ulnohumeral joint ▽
>> √7ᵗʰ **S53.124** Posterior dislocation of right ulnohumeral joint
>> √7ᵗʰ **S53.125** Posterior dislocation of left ulnohumeral joint
>> √7ᵗʰ **S53.126** Posterior dislocation of unspecified ulnohumeral joint ▽

> √6ᵗʰ **S53.13** Medial **subluxation and dislocation of ulnohumeral joint**

>> √7ᵗʰ **S53.131** Medial subluxation of right ulnohumeral joint
>> √7ᵗʰ **S53.132** Medial subluxation of left ulnohumeral joint
>> √7ᵗʰ **S53.133** Medial subluxation of unspecified ulnohumeral joint ▽

Ⓝ Newborn   Ⓟ Pediatric   Ⓜ Maternity   Ⓐ Adult   **RIC** RIC Dx   **NCDx** Noncancer Dx   **PDx** Primary Dx   **CC** RIC CC Condition   ▶◀ Revised Text   ● New Code   ▲ Revised Code Title

912   ICD-10-CM 2016

☑7ᵗʰ **S53.134** Medial dislocation of right ulnohumeral joint

☑7ᵗʰ **S53.135** Medial dislocation of left ulnohumeral joint

☑7ᵗʰ **S53.136** Medial dislocation of unspecified ulnohumeral joint ▽

☑6ᵗʰ **S53.14** Lateral subluxation and dislocation of ulnohumeral joint

    ☑7ᵗʰ **S53.141** Lateral subluxation of right ulnohumeral joint

    ☑7ᵗʰ **S53.142** Lateral subluxation of left ulnohumeral joint

    ☑7ᵗʰ **S53.143** Lateral subluxation of unspecified ulnohumeral joint ▽

    ☑7ᵗʰ **S53.144** Lateral dislocation of right ulnohumeral joint

    ☑7ᵗʰ **S53.145** Lateral dislocation of left ulnohumeral joint

    ☑7ᵗʰ **S53.146** Lateral dislocation of unspecified ulnohumeral joint ▽

☑6ᵗʰ **S53.19** Other subluxation and dislocation of ulnohumeral joint

    ☑7ᵗʰ **S53.191** Other subluxation of right ulnohumeral joint

    ☑7ᵗʰ **S53.192** Other subluxation of left ulnohumeral joint

    ☑7ᵗʰ **S53.193** Other subluxation of unspecified ulnohumeral joint ▽

    ☑7ᵗʰ **S53.194** Other dislocation of right ulnohumeral joint

    ☑7ᵗʰ **S53.195** Other dislocation of left ulnohumeral joint

    ☑7ᵗʰ **S53.196** Other dislocation of unspecified ulnohumeral joint ▽

☑5ᵗʰ **S53.2 Traumatic rupture of** radial collateral ligament
    EXCLUDES 1   sprain of radial collateral ligament NOS (S53.43-)

☑x7ᵗʰ **S53.20 Traumatic rupture of** unspecified radial collateral ligament ▽

☑x7ᵗʰ **S53.21 Traumatic rupture of** right radial collateral ligament

☑x7ᵗʰ **S53.22 Traumatic rupture of** left radial collateral ligament

☑5ᵗʰ **S53.3 Traumatic rupture of** ulnar collateral ligament
    EXCLUDES 1   sprain of ulnar collateral ligament (S53.44-)

☑x7ᵗʰ **S53.30 Traumatic rupture of** unspecified ulnar collateral ligament ▽

☑x7ᵗʰ **S53.31 Traumatic rupture of** right ulnar collateral ligament

☑x7ᵗʰ **S53.32 Traumatic rupture of** left ulnar collateral ligament

☑5ᵗʰ **S53.4 Sprain of** elbow
    EXCLUDES 2   traumatic rupture of radial collateral ligament (S53.2-)
                traumatic rupture of ulnar collateral ligament (S53.3-)

☑6ᵗʰ **S53.40 Unspecified sprain of** elbow

    ☑7ᵗʰ **S53.401 Unspecified sprain of** right elbow ▽

    ☑7ᵗʰ **S53.402 Unspecified sprain of** left elbow ▽

    ☑7ᵗʰ **S53.409 Unspecified sprain of** unspecified elbow ▽
          Sprain of elbow NOS

☑6ᵗʰ **S53.41** Radiohumeral (joint) sprain

    ☑7ᵗʰ **S53.411** Radiohumeral (joint) sprain of right elbow

    ☑7ᵗʰ **S53.412** Radiohumeral (joint) sprain of left elbow

    ☑7ᵗʰ **S53.419** Radiohumeral (joint) sprain of unspecified elbow ▽

☑6ᵗʰ **S53.42** Ulnohumeral (joint) sprain

    ☑7ᵗʰ **S53.421** Ulnohumeral (joint) sprain of right elbow

    ☑7ᵗʰ **S53.422** Ulnohumeral (joint) sprain of left elbow

    ☑7ᵗʰ **S53.429** Ulnohumeral (joint) sprain of unspecified elbow ▽

☑6ᵗʰ **S53.43** Radial collateral ligament sprain

    ☑7ᵗʰ **S53.431** Radial collateral ligament sprain of right elbow

    ☑7ᵗʰ **S53.432** Radial collateral ligament sprain of left elbow

    ☑7ᵗʰ **S53.439** Radial collateral ligament sprain of unspecified elbow ▽

☑6ᵗʰ **S53.44** Ulnar collateral ligament sprain

    ☑7ᵗʰ **S53.441** Ulnar collateral ligament sprain of right elbow

    ☑7ᵗʰ **S53.442** Ulnar collateral ligament sprain of left elbow

    ☑7ᵗʰ **S53.449** Ulnar collateral ligament sprain of unspecified elbow ▽

☑6ᵗʰ **S53.49** Other sprain of elbow

    ☑7ᵗʰ **S53.491** Other sprain of right elbow

    ☑7ᵗʰ **S53.492** Other sprain of left elbow

    ☑7ᵗʰ **S53.499** Other sprain of unspecified elbow ▽

☑4ᵗʰ **S54 Injury of nerves at forearm level**
     Code also any associated open wound (S51.-)
    EXCLUDES 2   injury of nerves at wrist and hand level (S64.-)

> The appropriate 7th character is to be added to each code from category S54.
> A   initial encounter
> D   subsequent encounter
> S   sequela

☑5ᵗʰ **S54.0 Injury of** ulnar nerve at forearm level
     Injury of ulnar nerve NOS

    ☑x7ᵗʰ **S54.00 Injury of ulnar nerve at forearm level, unspecified** ▽ **arm**

    ☑x7ᵗʰ **S54.01 Injury of ulnar nerve at forearm level,** right **arm**

    ☑x7ᵗʰ **S54.02 Injury of ulnar nerve at forearm level,** left **arm**

☑5ᵗʰ **S54.1 Injury of** median nerve at forearm level
     Injury of median nerve NOS

    ☑x7ᵗʰ **S54.10 Injury of median nerve at forearm level,** ▽ **unspecified arm**

    ☑x7ᵗʰ **S54.11 Injury of median nerve at forearm level,** right **arm**

    ☑x7ᵗʰ **S54.12 Injury of median nerve at forearm level,** left **arm**

☑5ᵗʰ **S54.2 Injury of** radial nerve at forearm level
     Injury of radial nerve NOS

    ☑x7ᵗʰ **S54.20 Injury of radial nerve at forearm level,** ▽ **unspecified arm**

    ☑x7ᵗʰ **S54.21 Injury of radial nerve at forearm level,** right **arm**

    ☑x7ᵗʰ **S54.22 Injury of radial nerve at forearm level,** left **arm**

☑5ᵗʰ **S54.3 Injury of** cutaneous sensory nerve at forearm level

    ☑x7ᵗʰ **S54.30 Injury of cutaneous sensory nerve at forearm** ▽ **level, unspecified arm**

    ☑x7ᵗʰ **S54.31 Injury of cutaneous sensory nerve at forearm level,** right **arm**

    ☑x7ᵗʰ **S54.32 Injury of cutaneous sensory nerve at forearm level,** left **arm**

☑5ᵗʰ **S54.8 Injury of** other nerves at forearm level

    ☑6ᵗʰ **S54.8X Unspecified injury of other nerves at forearm level**

        ☑7ᵗʰ **S54.8X1 Unspecified injury of other nerves at** ▽ **forearm level,** right **arm**

        ☑7ᵗʰ **S54.8X2 Unspecified injury of other nerves at** ▽ **forearm level,** left **arm**

        ☑7ᵗʰ **S54.8X9 Unspecified injury of other nerves at** ▽ **forearm level, unspecified arm**

☑5ᵗʰ **S54.9 Injury of** unspecified nerve at forearm level

    ☑x7ᵗʰ **S54.90 Injury of unspecified nerve at forearm level,** ▽ **unspecified arm**

    ☑x7ᵗʰ **S54.91 Injury of unspecified nerve at forearm level,** ▽ **right arm**

    ☑x7ᵗʰ **S54.92 Injury of unspecified nerve at forearm level,** ▽ **left arm**

☑4ᵗʰ **S55 Injury of blood vessels at forearm level**
     Code also any associated open wound (S51.-)
    EXCLUDES 2   injury of blood vessels at wrist and hand level (S65.-)
                injury of brachial vessels (S45.1-S45.2)

> The appropriate 7th character is to be added to each code from category S55.
> A   initial encounter
> D   subsequent encounter
> S   sequela

☑5ᵗʰ **S55.0 Injury of** ulnar artery at forearm level

    ☑6ᵗʰ **S55.00 Unspecified injury of ulnar artery at forearm level**

☑ Add'l Character Required   ☑x7ᵗʰ Placeholder Alert   **RUG IV Special Care High Dx**   **RUG IV Clinically Complex Dx**   **RUG IV Special Care Low Dx**   Manifestation Code   Other Specified Code   ▽ Unspecified Code

ICD-10-CM 2016   **913**

✓7ᵗʰ **S55.001** Unspecified injury of ulnar artery at forearm level, right arm ▽

✓7ᵗʰ **S55.002** Unspecified injury of ulnar artery at forearm level, left arm ▽

✓7ᵗʰ **S55.009** Unspecified injury of ulnar artery at forearm level, unspecified arm ▽

✓6ᵗʰ **S55.01** Laceration of ulnar artery at forearm level

✓7ᵗʰ **S55.011** Laceration of ulnar artery at forearm level, right arm

✓7ᵗʰ **S55.012** Laceration of ulnar artery at forearm level, left arm

✓7ᵗʰ **S55.019** Laceration of ulnar artery at forearm level, unspecified arm ▽

✓6ᵗʰ **S55.09** Other specified injury of ulnar artery at forearm level

✓7ᵗʰ **S55.091** Other specified injury of ulnar artery at forearm level, right arm

✓7ᵗʰ **S55.092** Other specified injury of ulnar artery at forearm level, left arm

✓7ᵗʰ **S55.099** Other specified injury of ulnar artery at forearm level, unspecified arm ▽

✓5ᵗʰ **S55.1** Injury of radial artery at forearm level

✓6ᵗʰ **S55.10** Unspecified injury of radial artery at forearm level

✓7ᵗʰ **S55.101** Unspecified injury of radial artery at forearm level, right arm ▽

✓7ᵗʰ **S55.102** Unspecified injury of radial artery at forearm level, left arm ▽

✓7ᵗʰ **S55.109** Unspecified injury of radial artery at forearm level, unspecified arm ▽

✓6ᵗʰ **S55.11** Laceration of radial artery at forearm level

✓7ᵗʰ **S55.111** Laceration of radial artery at forearm level, right arm

✓7ᵗʰ **S55.112** Laceration of radial artery at forearm level, left arm

✓7ᵗʰ **S55.119** Laceration of radial artery at forearm level, unspecified arm ▽

✓6ᵗʰ **S55.19** Other specified injury of radial artery at forearm level

✓7ᵗʰ **S55.191** Other specified injury of radial artery at forearm level, right arm

✓7ᵗʰ **S55.192** Other specified injury of radial artery at forearm level, left arm

✓7ᵗʰ **S55.199** Other specified injury of radial artery at forearm level, unspecified arm ▽

✓5ᵗʰ **S55.2** Injury of vein at forearm level

✓6ᵗʰ **S55.20** Unspecified injury of vein at forearm level

✓7ᵗʰ **S55.201** Unspecified injury of vein at forearm level, right arm ▽

✓7ᵗʰ **S55.202** Unspecified injury of vein at forearm level, left arm ▽

✓7ᵗʰ **S55.209** Unspecified injury of vein at forearm level, unspecified arm ▽

✓6ᵗʰ **S55.21** Laceration of vein at forearm level

✓7ᵗʰ **S55.211** Laceration of vein at forearm level, right arm

✓7ᵗʰ **S55.212** Laceration of vein at forearm level, left arm

✓7ᵗʰ **S55.219** Laceration of vein at forearm level, unspecified arm ▽

✓6ᵗʰ **S55.29** Other specified injury of vein at forearm level

✓7ᵗʰ **S55.291** Other specified injury of vein at forearm level, right arm

✓7ᵗʰ **S55.292** Other specified injury of vein at forearm level, left arm

✓7ᵗʰ **S55.299** Other specified injury of vein at forearm level, unspecified arm ▽

✓5ᵗʰ **S55.8** Injury of other blood vessels at forearm level

✓6ᵗʰ **S55.80** Unspecified injury of other blood vessels at forearm level

✓7ᵗʰ **S55.801** Unspecified injury of other blood vessels at forearm level, right arm ▽

✓7ᵗʰ **S55.802** Unspecified injury of other blood vessels at forearm level, left arm ▽

✓7ᵗʰ **S55.809** Unspecified injury of other blood vessels at forearm level, unspecified arm ▽

✓6ᵗʰ **S55.81** Laceration of other blood vessels at forearm level

✓7ᵗʰ **S55.811** Laceration of other blood vessels at forearm level, right arm

✓7ᵗʰ **S55.812** Laceration of other blood vessels at forearm level, left arm

✓7ᵗʰ **S55.819** Laceration of other blood vessels at forearm level, unspecified arm ▽

✓6ᵗʰ **S55.89** Other specified injury of other blood vessels at forearm level

✓7ᵗʰ **S55.891** Other specified injury of other blood vessels at forearm level, right arm

✓7ᵗʰ **S55.892** Other specified injury of other blood vessels at forearm level, left arm

✓7ᵗʰ **S55.899** Other specified injury of other blood vessels at forearm level, unspecified arm ▽

✓5ᵗʰ **S55.9** Injury of unspecified blood vessel at forearm level

✓6ᵗʰ **S55.90** Unspecified injury of unspecified blood vessel at forearm level

✓7ᵗʰ **S55.901** Unspecified injury of unspecified blood vessel at forearm level, right arm ▽

✓7ᵗʰ **S55.902** Unspecified injury of unspecified blood vessel at forearm level, left arm ▽

✓7ᵗʰ **S55.909** Unspecified injury of unspecified blood vessel at forearm level, unspecified arm ▽

✓6ᵗʰ **S55.91** Laceration of unspecified blood vessel at forearm level

✓7ᵗʰ **S55.911** Laceration of unspecified blood vessel at forearm level, right arm ▽

✓7ᵗʰ **S55.912** Laceration of unspecified blood vessel at forearm level, left arm ▽

✓7ᵗʰ **S55.919** Laceration of unspecified blood vessel at forearm level, unspecified arm ▽

✓6ᵗʰ **S55.99** Other specified injury of unspecified blood vessel at forearm level

✓7ᵗʰ **S55.991** Other specified injury of unspecified blood vessel at forearm level, right arm ▽

✓7ᵗʰ **S55.992** Other specified injury of unspecified blood vessel at forearm level, left arm ▽

✓7ᵗʰ **S55.999** Other specified injury of unspecified blood vessel at forearm level, unspecified arm ▽

✦ ✓4ᵗʰ **S56 Injury of muscle, fascia and tendon at forearm level**

Code also any associated open wound (S51.-)

EXCLUDES 2 injury of muscle, fascia and tendon at or below wrist (S66.-)
sprain of joints and ligaments of elbow (S53.4-)

The appropriate 7th character is to be added to each code from category S56.
A   initial encounter
D   subsequent encounter
S   sequela

✓5ᵗʰ **S56.0** Injury of flexor muscle, fascia and tendon of thumb at forearm level

✓6ᵗʰ **S56.00** Unspecified injury of flexor muscle, fascia and tendon of thumb at forearm level

✓7ᵗʰ **S56.001** Unspecified injury of flexor muscle, fascia and tendon of right thumb at forearm level ▽

✓7ᵗʰ **S56.002** Unspecified injury of flexor muscle, fascia and tendon of left thumb at forearm level ▽

✓7ᵗʰ **S56.009** Unspecified injury of flexor muscle, fascia and tendon of unspecified thumb at forearm level ▽

✓6ᵗʰ **S56.01** Strain of flexor muscle, fascia and tendon of thumb at forearm level

✓7ᵗʰ **S56.011** Strain of flexor muscle, fascia and tendon of right thumb at forearm level

---

✦ Refer to the Muscle/Tendon Table at beginning of this chapter.

Ⓝ Newborn   Ⓟ Pediatric   Ⓜ Maternity   Ⓐ Adult   **RIC** RIC Dx   **NCDx** Noncancer Dx   **PDx** Primary Dx   **CC** RIC CC Condition   ►◄ Revised Text   ● New Code   ▲ Revised Code Title

914   ICD-10-CM 2016

☑7ᵗʰ **S56.012** Strain of flexor muscle, fascia and tendon of left thumb at forearm level

☑7ᵗʰ **S56.019** Strain of flexor muscle, fascia and tendon of unspecified thumb at forearm level ▽

✓6ᵗʰ **S56.02** Laceration of flexor muscle, fascia and tendon of thumb at forearm level

☑7ᵗʰ **S56.021** Laceration of flexor muscle, fascia and tendon of right thumb at forearm level

☑7ᵗʰ **S56.022** Laceration of flexor muscle, fascia and tendon of left thumb at forearm level

☑7ᵗʰ **S56.029** Laceration of flexor muscle, fascia and tendon of unspecified thumb at forearm level ▽

✓6ᵗʰ **S56.09** Other injury of flexor muscle, fascia and tendon of thumb at forearm level

☑7ᵗʰ **S56.091** Other injury of flexor muscle, fascia and tendon of right thumb at forearm level

☑7ᵗʰ **S56.092** Other injury of flexor muscle, fascia and tendon of left thumb at forearm level

☑7ᵗʰ **S56.099** Other injury of flexor muscle, fascia and tendon of unspecified thumb at forearm level ▽

✓5ᵗʰ **S56.1** Injury of flexor muscle, fascia and tendon of other and unspecified finger at forearm level

✓6ᵗʰ **S56.10** Unspecified injury of flexor muscle, fascia and tendon of other and unspecified finger at forearm level

☑7ᵗʰ **S56.101** Unspecified injury of flexor muscle, fascia and tendon of right index finger at forearm level ▽

☑7ᵗʰ **S56.102** Unspecified injury of flexor muscle, fascia and tendon of left index finger at forearm level ▽

☑7ᵗʰ **S56.103** Unspecified injury of flexor muscle, fascia and tendon of right middle finger at forearm level ▽

☑7ᵗʰ **S56.104** Unspecified injury of flexor muscle, fascia and tendon of left middle finger at forearm level ▽

☑7ᵗʰ **S56.105** Unspecified injury of flexor muscle, fascia and tendon of right ring finger at forearm level ▽

☑7ᵗʰ **S56.106** Unspecified injury of flexor muscle, fascia and tendon of left ring finger at forearm level ▽

☑7ᵗʰ **S56.107** Unspecified injury of flexor muscle, fascia and tendon of right little finger at forearm level ▽

☑7ᵗʰ **S56.108** Unspecified injury of flexor muscle, fascia and tendon of left little finger at forearm level ▽

☑7ᵗʰ **S56.109** Unspecified injury of flexor muscle, fascia and tendon of unspecified finger at forearm level ▽

✓6ᵗʰ **S56.11** Strain of flexor muscle, fascia and tendon of other and unspecified finger at forearm level

☑7ᵗʰ **S56.111** Strain of flexor muscle, fascia and tendon of right index finger at forearm level

☑7ᵗʰ **S56.112** Strain of flexor muscle, fascia and tendon of left index finger at forearm level

☑7ᵗʰ **S56.113** Strain of flexor muscle, fascia and tendon of right middle finger at forearm level

☑7ᵗʰ **S56.114** Strain of flexor muscle, fascia and tendon of left middle finger at forearm level

☑7ᵗʰ **S56.115** Strain of flexor muscle, fascia and tendon of right ring finger at forearm level

☑7ᵗʰ **S56.116** Strain of flexor muscle, fascia and tendon of left ring finger at forearm level

☑7ᵗʰ **S56.117** Strain of flexor muscle, fascia and tendon of right little finger at forearm level

☑7ᵗʰ **S56.118** Strain of flexor muscle, fascia and tendon of left little finger at forearm level

☑7ᵗʰ **S56.119** Strain of flexor muscle, fascia and tendon of finger of unspecified finger at forearm level ▽

✓6ᵗʰ **S56.12** Laceration of flexor muscle, fascia and tendon of other and unspecified finger at forearm level

☑7ᵗʰ **S56.121** Laceration of flexor muscle, fascia and tendon of right index finger at forearm level

☑7ᵗʰ **S56.122** Laceration of flexor muscle, fascia and tendon of left index finger at forearm level

☑7ᵗʰ **S56.123** Laceration of flexor muscle, fascia and tendon of right middle finger at forearm level

☑7ᵗʰ **S56.124** Laceration of flexor muscle, fascia and tendon of left middle finger at forearm level

☑7ᵗʰ **S56.125** Laceration of flexor muscle, fascia and tendon of right ring finger at forearm level

☑7ᵗʰ **S56.126** Laceration of flexor muscle, fascia and tendon of left ring finger at forearm level

☑7ᵗʰ **S56.127** Laceration of flexor muscle, fascia and tendon of right little finger at forearm level

☑7ᵗʰ **S56.128** Laceration of flexor muscle, fascia and tendon of left little finger at forearm level

☑7ᵗʰ **S56.129** Laceration of flexor muscle, fascia and tendon of unspecified finger at forearm level ▽

✓6ᵗʰ **S56.19** Other injury of flexor muscle, fascia and tendon of other and unspecified finger at forearm level

☑7ᵗʰ **S56.191** Other injury of flexor muscle, fascia and tendon of right index finger at forearm level

☑7ᵗʰ **S56.192** Other injury of flexor muscle, fascia and tendon of left index finger at forearm level

☑7ᵗʰ **S56.193** Other injury of flexor muscle, fascia and tendon of right middle finger at forearm level

☑7ᵗʰ **S56.194** Other injury of flexor muscle, fascia and tendon of left middle finger at forearm level

☑7ᵗʰ **S56.195** Other injury of flexor muscle, fascia and tendon of right ring finger at forearm level

☑7ᵗʰ **S56.196** Other injury of flexor muscle, fascia and tendon of left ring finger at forearm level

☑7ᵗʰ **S56.197** Other injury of flexor muscle, fascia and tendon of right little finger at forearm level

☑7ᵗʰ **S56.198** Other injury of flexor muscle, fascia and tendon of left little finger at forearm level

☑7ᵗʰ **S56.199** Other injury of flexor muscle, fascia and tendon of unspecified finger at forearm level ▽

✓5ᵗʰ **S56.2** Injury of other flexor muscle, fascia and tendon at forearm level

✓6ᵗʰ **S56.20** Unspecified injury of other flexor muscle, fascia and tendon at forearm level

☑7ᵗʰ **S56.201** Unspecified injury of other flexor muscle, fascia and tendon at forearm level, right arm ▽

☑7ᵗʰ **S56.202** Unspecified injury of other flexor muscle, fascia and tendon at forearm level, left arm ▽

☑7ᵗʰ **S56.209** Unspecified injury of other flexor muscle, fascia and tendon at forearm level, unspecified arm ▽

✓6ᵗʰ **S56.21** Strain of other flexor muscle, fascia and tendon at forearm level

☑7ᵗʰ **S56.211** Strain of other flexor muscle, fascia and tendon at forearm level, right arm

☑7ᵗʰ **S56.212** Strain of other flexor muscle, fascia and tendon at forearm level, left arm

☑7ᵗʰ **S56.219** Strain of other flexor muscle, fascia and tendon at forearm level, unspecified arm ▽

✓6ᵗʰ **S56.22** Laceration of other flexor muscle, fascia and tendon at forearm level

☑7ᵗʰ **S56.221** Laceration of other flexor muscle, fascia and tendon at forearm level, right arm

---

☑ Add'l Character Required   ✓×7ᵗʰ Placeholder Alert   RUG IV Special Care High Dx   RUG IV Clinically Complex Dx   RUG IV Special Care Low Dx   Manifestation Code   Other Specified Code   ▽Unspecified Code

☑7ᵗʰ **S56.222** **Laceration of other flexor muscle, fascia and tendon at forearm level,** left arm

☑7ᵗʰ **S56.229** **Laceration of other flexor muscle, fascia and tendon at forearm level, unspecified arm** ▽

☑6ᵗʰ **S56.29** Other injury **of other flexor muscle, fascia and tendon at forearm level**

    ☑7ᵗʰ **S56.291** **Other injury of other flexor muscle, fascia and tendon at forearm level,** right arm

    ☑7ᵗʰ **S56.292** **Other injury of other flexor muscle, fascia and tendon at forearm level,** left arm

    ☑7ᵗʰ **S56.299** **Other injury of other flexor muscle, fascia and tendon at forearm level, unspecified arm** ▽

☑5ᵗʰ **S56.3** **Injury of** extensor or abductor **muscles, fascia and tendons of** thumb **at forearm level**

    ☑6ᵗʰ **S56.30** Unspecified injury **of extensor or abductor muscles, fascia and tendons of thumb at forearm level**

        ☑7ᵗʰ **S56.301** **Unspecified injury of extensor or abductor muscles, fascia and tendons of** right thumb **at forearm level** ▽

        ☑7ᵗʰ **S56.302** **Unspecified injury of extensor or abductor muscles, fascia and tendons of** left thumb **at forearm level** ▽

        ☑7ᵗʰ **S56.309** **Unspecified injury of extensor or abductor muscles, fascia and tendons of unspecified thumb at forearm level** ▽

    ☑6ᵗʰ **S56.31** Strain **of extensor or abductor muscles, fascia and tendons of thumb at forearm level**

        ☑7ᵗʰ **S56.311** **Strain of extensor or abductor muscles, fascia and tendons of** right thumb **at forearm level**

        ☑7ᵗʰ **S56.312** **Strain of extensor or abductor muscles, fascia and tendons of** left thumb **at forearm level**

        ☑7ᵗʰ **S56.319** **Strain of extensor or abductor muscles, fascia and tendons of unspecified thumb at forearm level** ▽

    ☑6ᵗʰ **S56.32** Laceration **of extensor or abductor muscles, fascia and tendons of thumb at forearm level**

        ☑7ᵗʰ **S56.321** **Laceration of extensor or abductor muscles, fascia and tendons of** right thumb **at forearm level**

        ☑7ᵗʰ **S56.322** **Laceration of extensor or abductor muscles, fascia and tendons of** left thumb **at forearm level**

        ☑7ᵗʰ **S56.329** **Laceration of extensor or abductor muscles, fascia and tendons of unspecified thumb at forearm level** ▽

    ☑6ᵗʰ **S56.39** Other injury **of extensor or abductor muscles, fascia and tendons of thumb at forearm level**

        ☑7ᵗʰ **S56.391** **Other injury of extensor or abductor muscles, fascia and tendons of** right thumb **at forearm level**

        ☑7ᵗʰ **S56.392** **Other injury of extensor or abductor muscles, fascia and tendons of** left thumb **at forearm level**

        ☑7ᵗʰ **S56.399** **Other injury of extensor or abductor muscles, fascia and tendons of unspecified thumb at forearm level** ▽

☑5ᵗʰ **S56.4** **Injury of** extensor **muscle, fascia and tendon of other and unspecified** finger **at forearm level**

    ☑6ᵗʰ **S56.40** Unspecified injury **of extensor muscle, fascia and tendon of other and unspecified finger at forearm level**

        ☑7ᵗʰ **S56.401** **Unspecified injury of extensor muscle, fascia and tendon of** right index finger **at forearm level** ▽

        ☑7ᵗʰ **S56.402** **Unspecified injury of extensor muscle, fascia and tendon of** left index finger **at forearm level** ▽

        ☑7ᵗʰ **S56.403** **Unspecified injury of extensor muscle, fascia and tendon of** right middle finger **at forearm level** ▽

        ☑7ᵗʰ **S56.404** **Unspecified injury of extensor muscle, fascia and tendon of** left middle finger **at forearm level** ▽

☑7ᵗʰ **S56.405** **Unspecified injury of extensor muscle, fascia and tendon of** right ring finger **at forearm level** ▽

☑7ᵗʰ **S56.406** **Unspecified injury of extensor muscle, fascia and tendon of** left ring finger **at forearm level** ▽

☑7ᵗʰ **S56.407** **Unspecified injury of extensor muscle, fascia and tendon of** right little finger **at forearm level** ▽

☑7ᵗʰ **S56.408** **Unspecified injury of extensor muscle, fascia and tendon of** left little finger **at forearm level** ▽

☑7ᵗʰ **S56.409** **Unspecified injury of extensor muscle, fascia and tendon of unspecified finger at forearm level** ▽

☑6ᵗʰ **S56.41** Strain **of extensor muscle, fascia and tendon of other and unspecified** finger **at forearm level**

    ☑7ᵗʰ **S56.411** **Strain of extensor muscle, fascia and tendon of** right index finger **at forearm level**

    ☑7ᵗʰ **S56.412** **Strain of extensor muscle, fascia and tendon of** left index finger **at forearm level**

    ☑7ᵗʰ **S56.413** **Strain of extensor muscle, fascia and tendon of** right middle finger **at forearm level**

    ☑7ᵗʰ **S56.414** **Strain of extensor muscle, fascia and tendon of** left middle finger **at forearm level**

    ☑7ᵗʰ **S56.415** **Strain of extensor muscle, fascia and tendon of** right ring finger **at forearm level**

    ☑7ᵗʰ **S56.416** **Strain of extensor muscle, fascia and tendon of** left ring finger **at forearm level**

    ☑7ᵗʰ **S56.417** **Strain of extensor muscle, fascia and tendon of** right little finger **at forearm level**

    ☑7ᵗʰ **S56.418** **Strain of extensor muscle, fascia and tendon of** left little finger **at forearm level**

    ☑7ᵗʰ **S56.419** **Strain of extensor muscle, fascia and tendon of finger, unspecified finger at forearm level** ▽

☑6ᵗʰ **S56.42** Laceration **of extensor muscle, fascia and tendon of other and unspecified** finger **at forearm level**

    ☑7ᵗʰ **S56.421** **Laceration of extensor muscle, fascia and tendon of** right index finger **at forearm level**

    ☑7ᵗʰ **S56.422** **Laceration of extensor muscle, fascia and tendon of** left index finger **at forearm level**

    ☑7ᵗʰ **S56.423** **Laceration of extensor muscle, fascia and tendon of** right middle finger **at forearm level**

    ☑7ᵗʰ **S56.424** **Laceration of extensor muscle, fascia and tendon of** left middle finger **at forearm level**

    ☑7ᵗʰ **S56.425** **Laceration of extensor muscle, fascia and tendon of** right ring finger **at forearm level**

    ☑7ᵗʰ **S56.426** **Laceration of extensor muscle, fascia and tendon of** left ring finger **at forearm level**

    ☑7ᵗʰ **S56.427** **Laceration of extensor muscle, fascia and tendon of** right little finger **at forearm level**

    ☑7ᵗʰ **S56.428** **Laceration of extensor muscle, fascia and tendon of** left little finger **at forearm level**

    ☑7ᵗʰ **S56.429** **Laceration of extensor muscle, fascia and tendon of unspecified finger at forearm level** ▽

☑6ᵗʰ **S56.49** Other injury **of extensor muscle, fascia and tendon of other and unspecified** finger **at forearm level**

    ☑7ᵗʰ **S56.491** **Other injury of extensor muscle, fascia and tendon of** right index finger **at forearm level**

    ☑7ᵗʰ **S56.492** **Other injury of extensor muscle, fascia and tendon of** left index finger **at forearm level**

    ☑7ᵗʰ **S56.493** **Other injury of extensor muscle, fascia and tendon of** right middle finger **at forearm level**

Ⓝ Newborn   Ⓟ Pediatric   Ⓜ Maternity   Ⓐ Adult   **RIC** RIC Dx   **NCDx** Noncancer Dx   **PDx** Primary Dx   **CC** RIC CC Condition   ▶◀ Revised Text   ● New Code   ▲ Revised Code Title

916   ICD-10-CM 2016

√7ᵗʰ **S56.494** Other injury of extensor muscle, fascia and tendon of left middle finger at forearm level

√7ᵗʰ **S56.495** Other injury of extensor muscle, fascia and tendon of right ring finger at forearm level

√7ᵗʰ **S56.496** Other injury of extensor muscle, fascia and tendon of left ring finger at forearm level

√7ᵗʰ **S56.497** Other injury of extensor muscle, fascia and tendon of right little finger at forearm level

√7ᵗʰ **S56.498** Other injury of extensor muscle, fascia and tendon of left little finger at forearm level

√7ᵗʰ **S56.499** Other injury of extensor muscle, fascia and tendon of unspecified finger at forearm level ▽

√5ᵗʰ **S56.5** Injury of other extensor muscle, fascia and tendon at forearm level

     √6ᵗʰ **S56.50** Unspecified injury of other extensor muscle, fascia and tendon at forearm level

       √7ᵗʰ **S56.501** Unspecified injury of other extensor muscle, fascia and tendon at forearm level, right arm ▽

       √7ᵗʰ **S56.502** Unspecified injury of other extensor muscle, fascia and tendon at forearm level, left arm ▽

       √7ᵗʰ **S56.509** Unspecified injury of other extensor muscle, fascia and tendon at forearm level, unspecified arm ▽

     √6ᵗʰ **S56.51** Strain of other extensor muscle, fascia and tendon at forearm level

       √7ᵗʰ **S56.511** Strain of other extensor muscle, fascia and tendon at forearm level, right arm

       √7ᵗʰ **S56.512** Strain of other extensor muscle, fascia and tendon at forearm level, left arm

       √7ᵗʰ **S56.519** Strain of other extensor muscle, fascia and tendon at forearm level, unspecified arm ▽

     √6ᵗʰ **S56.52** Laceration of other extensor muscle, fascia and tendon at forearm level

       √7ᵗʰ **S56.521** Laceration of other extensor muscle, fascia and tendon at forearm level, right arm

       √7ᵗʰ **S56.522** Laceration of other extensor muscle, fascia and tendon at forearm level, left arm

       √7ᵗʰ **S56.529** Laceration of other extensor muscle, fascia and tendon at forearm level, unspecified arm ▽

     √6ᵗʰ **S56.59** Other injury of other extensor muscle, fascia and tendon at forearm level

       √7ᵗʰ **S56.591** Other injury of other extensor muscle, fascia and tendon at forearm level, right arm

       √7ᵗʰ **S56.592** Other injury of other extensor muscle, fascia and tendon at forearm level, left arm

       √7ᵗʰ **S56.599** Other injury of other extensor muscle, fascia and tendon at forearm level, unspecified arm ▽

√5ᵗʰ **S56.8** Injury of other muscles, fascia and tendons at forearm level

     √6ᵗʰ **S56.80** Unspecified injury of other muscles, fascia and tendons at forearm level

       √7ᵗʰ **S56.801** Unspecified injury of other muscles, fascia and tendons at forearm level, right arm ▽

       √7ᵗʰ **S56.802** Unspecified injury of other muscles, fascia and tendons at forearm level, left arm ▽

       √7ᵗʰ **S56.809** Unspecified injury of other muscles, fascia and tendons at forearm level, unspecified arm ▽

     √6ᵗʰ **S56.81** Strain of other muscles, fascia and tendons at forearm level

       √7ᵗʰ **S56.811** Strain of other muscles, fascia and tendons at forearm level, right arm

       √7ᵗʰ **S56.812** Strain of other muscles, fascia and tendons at forearm level, left arm

       √7ᵗʰ **S56.819** Strain of other muscles, fascia and tendons at forearm level, unspecified arm ▽

     √6ᵗʰ **S56.82** Laceration of other muscles, fascia and tendons at forearm level

       √7ᵗʰ **S56.821** Laceration of other muscles, fascia and tendons at forearm level, right arm

       √7ᵗʰ **S56.822** Laceration of other muscles, fascia and tendons at forearm level, left arm

       √7ᵗʰ **S56.829** Laceration of other muscles, fascia and tendons at forearm level, unspecified arm ▽

     √6ᵗʰ **S56.89** Other injury of other muscles, fascia and tendons at forearm level

       √7ᵗʰ **S56.891** Other injury of other muscles, fascia and tendons at forearm level, right arm

       √7ᵗʰ **S56.892** Other injury of other muscles, fascia and tendons at forearm level, left arm

       √7ᵗʰ **S56.899** Other injury of other muscles, fascia and tendons at forearm level, unspecified arm ▽

√5ᵗʰ **S56.9** Injury of unspecified muscles, fascia and tendons at forearm level

     √6ᵗʰ **S56.90** Unspecified injury of unspecified muscles, fascia and tendons at forearm level

       √7ᵗʰ **S56.901** Unspecified injury of unspecified muscles, fascia and tendons at forearm level, right arm ▽

       √7ᵗʰ **S56.902** Unspecified injury of unspecified muscles, fascia and tendons at forearm level, left arm ▽

       √7ᵗʰ **S56.909** Unspecified injury of unspecified muscles, fascia and tendons at forearm level, unspecified arm ▽

     √6ᵗʰ **S56.91** Strain of unspecified muscles, fascia and tendons at forearm level

       √7ᵗʰ **S56.911** Strain of unspecified muscles, fascia and tendons at forearm level, right arm ▽

       √7ᵗʰ **S56.912** Strain of unspecified muscles, fascia and tendons at forearm level, left arm ▽

       √7ᵗʰ **S56.919** Strain of unspecified muscles, fascia and tendons at forearm level, unspecified arm ▽

     √6ᵗʰ **S56.92** Laceration of unspecified muscles, fascia and tendons at forearm level

       √7ᵗʰ **S56.921** Laceration of unspecified muscles, fascia and tendons at forearm level, right arm ▽

       √7ᵗʰ **S56.922** Laceration of unspecified muscles, fascia and tendons at forearm level, left arm ▽

       √7ᵗʰ **S56.929** Laceration of unspecified muscles, fascia and tendons at forearm level, unspecified arm ▽

     √6ᵗʰ **S56.99** Other injury of unspecified muscles, fascia and tendons at forearm level

       √7ᵗʰ **S56.991** Other injury of unspecified muscles, fascia and tendons at forearm level, right arm ▽

       √7ᵗʰ **S56.992** Other injury of unspecified muscles, fascia and tendons at forearm level, left arm ▽

       √7ᵗʰ **S56.999** Other injury of unspecified muscles, fascia and tendons at forearm level, unspecified arm ▽

√4ᵗʰ **S57** Crushing injury of elbow and forearm

     Use additional code(s) for all associated injuries

     EXCLUDES 2 crushing injury of wrist and hand (S67.-)

     The appropriate 7th character is to be added to each code from category S57.
     A   initial encounter
     D   subsequent encounter
     S   sequela

√5ᵗʰ **S57.0** Crushing injury of elbow

     √x7ᵗʰ **S57.00** Crushing injury of unspecified elbow ▽

☑ Add'l Character Required   √x7ᵗʰ Placeholder Alert   RUG IV Special Care High Dx   RUG IV Clinically Complex Dx   RUG IV Special Care Low Dx   Manifestation Code   Other Specified Code   ▽ Unspecified Code

ICD-10-CM 2016   917

Chapter 19. Injury, Poisoning and Certain Other Consequences of External Causes

S56.494–S57.00

✓x7ᵗʰ **S57.01**   Crushing injury of right elbow

✓x7ᵗʰ **S57.02**   Crushing injury of left elbow

✓5ᵗʰ **S57.8**   Crushing injury of forearm

    ✓x7ᵗʰ **S57.80**   Crushing injury of unspecified forearm   ▽

    ✓x7ᵗʰ **S57.81**   Crushing injury of right forearm

    ✓x7ᵗʰ **S57.82**   Crushing injury of left forearm

✓4ᵗʰ **S58**   **Traumatic amputation of elbow and forearm**

    NOTE   An amputation not identified as partial or complete should be coded to complete.

    EXCLUDES 1   traumatic amputation of wrist and hand (S68.-)

> The appropriate 7th character is to be added to each code from category S58.
> A   initial encounter
> D   subsequent encounter
> S   sequela

✓5ᵗʰ **S58.0**   Traumatic amputation at elbow level

    ✓6ᵗʰ **S58.01**   Complete traumatic amputation at elbow level

      ✓7ᵗʰ **S58.011**   Complete traumatic amputation at elbow level, right arm

      ✓7ᵗʰ **S58.012**   Complete traumatic amputation at elbow level, left arm

      ✓7ᵗʰ **S58.019**   Complete traumatic amputation at elbow level, unspecified arm   ▽

    ✓6ᵗʰ **S58.02**   Partial traumatic amputation at elbow level

      ✓7ᵗʰ **S58.021**   Partial traumatic amputation at elbow level, right arm

      ✓7ᵗʰ **S58.022**   Partial traumatic amputation at elbow level, left arm

      ✓7ᵗʰ **S58.029**   Partial traumatic amputation at elbow level, unspecified arm   ▽

✓5ᵗʰ **S58.1**   Traumatic amputation at level between elbow and wrist

    ✓6ᵗʰ **S58.11**   Complete traumatic amputation at level between elbow and wrist

      ✓7ᵗʰ **S58.111**   Complete traumatic amputation at level between elbow and wrist, right arm

      ✓7ᵗʰ **S58.112**   Complete traumatic amputation at level between elbow and wrist, left arm

      ✓7ᵗʰ **S58.119**   Complete traumatic amputation at level between elbow and wrist, unspecified arm   ▽

    ✓6ᵗʰ **S58.12**   Partial traumatic amputation at level between elbow and wrist

      ✓7ᵗʰ **S58.121**   Partial traumatic amputation at level between elbow and wrist, right arm

      ✓7ᵗʰ **S58.122**   Partial traumatic amputation at level between elbow and wrist, left arm

      ✓7ᵗʰ **S58.129**   Partial traumatic amputation at level between elbow and wrist, unspecified arm   ▽

✓5ᵗʰ **S58.9**   Traumatic amputation of forearm, level unspecified

    EXCLUDES 1   traumatic amputation of wrist (S68.-)

    ✓6ᵗʰ **S58.91**   Complete traumatic amputation of forearm, level unspecified

      ✓7ᵗʰ **S58.911**   Complete traumatic amputation of right forearm, level unspecified   ▽

      ✓7ᵗʰ **S58.912**   Complete traumatic amputation of left forearm, level unspecified   ▽

      ✓7ᵗʰ **S58.919**   Complete traumatic amputation of unspecified forearm, level unspecified   ▽

    ✓6ᵗʰ **S58.92**   Partial traumatic amputation of forearm, level unspecified

      ✓7ᵗʰ **S58.921**   Partial traumatic amputation of right forearm, level unspecified   ▽

      ✓7ᵗʰ **S58.922**   Partial traumatic amputation of left forearm, level unspecified   ▽

      ✓7ᵗʰ **S58.929**   Partial traumatic amputation of unspecified forearm, level unspecified   ▽

✓4ᵗʰ **S59**   **Other and unspecified injuries of elbow and forearm**

    EXCLUDES 2   other and unspecified injuries of wrist and hand (S69.-)

> The appropriate 7th character is to be added to each code from subcategories S59.0, S59.1, and S59.2.
> A   initial encounter for closed fracture
> D   subsequent encounter for fracture with routine healing
> G   subsequent encounter for fracture with delayed healing
> K   subsequent encounter for fracture with nonunion
> P   subsequent encounter for fracture with malunion
> S   sequela

✓5ᵗʰ **S59.0**   Physeal fracture of lower end of ulna

    ✓6ᵗʰ **S59.00**   Unspecified physeal fracture of lower end of ulna

      ✓7ᵗʰ **S59.001**   Unspecified physeal fracture of lower end of ulna, right arm   ▽

      ✓7ᵗʰ **S59.002**   Unspecified physeal fracture of lower end of ulna, left arm   ▽

      ✓7ᵗʰ **S59.009**   Unspecified physeal fracture of lower end of ulna, unspecified arm   ▽

    ✓6ᵗʰ **S59.01**   Salter-Harris Type I physeal fracture of lower end of ulna

      ✓7ᵗʰ **S59.011**   Salter-Harris Type I physeal fracture of lower end of ulna, right arm

      ✓7ᵗʰ **S59.012**   Salter-Harris Type I physeal fracture of lower end of ulna, left arm

      ✓7ᵗʰ **S59.019**   Salter-Harris Type I physeal fracture of lower end of ulna, unspecified arm   ▽

    ✓6ᵗʰ **S59.02**   Salter-Harris Type II physeal fracture of lower end of ulna

      ✓7ᵗʰ **S59.021**   Salter-Harris Type II physeal fracture of lower end of ulna, right arm

      ✓7ᵗʰ **S59.022**   Salter-Harris Type II physeal fracture of lower end of ulna, left arm

      ✓7ᵗʰ **S59.029**   Salter-Harris Type II physeal fracture of lower end of ulna, unspecified arm   ▽

    ✓6ᵗʰ **S59.03**   Salter-Harris Type III physeal fracture of lower end of ulna

      ✓7ᵗʰ **S59.031**   Salter-Harris Type III physeal fracture of lower end of ulna, right arm

      ✓7ᵗʰ **S59.032**   Salter-Harris Type III physeal fracture of lower end of ulna, left arm

      ✓7ᵗʰ **S59.039**   Salter-Harris Type III physeal fracture of lower end of ulna, unspecified arm   ▽

    ✓6ᵗʰ **S59.04**   Salter-Harris Type IV physeal fracture of lower end of ulna

      ✓7ᵗʰ **S59.041**   Salter-Harris Type IV physeal fracture of lower end of ulna, right arm

      ✓7ᵗʰ **S59.042**   Salter-Harris Type IV physeal fracture of lower end of ulna, left arm

      ✓7ᵗʰ **S59.049**   Salter-Harris Type IV physeal fracture of lower end of ulna, unspecified arm   ▽

    ✓6ᵗʰ **S59.09**   Other physeal fracture of lower end of ulna

      ✓7ᵗʰ **S59.091**   Other physeal fracture of lower end of ulna, right arm

      ✓7ᵗʰ **S59.092**   Other physeal fracture of lower end of ulna, left arm

      ✓7ᵗʰ **S59.099**   Other physeal fracture of lower end of ulna, unspecified arm   ▽

✓5ᵗʰ **S59.1**   Physeal fracture of upper end of radius

    ✓6ᵗʰ **S59.10**   Unspecified physeal fracture of upper end of radius

      ✓7ᵗʰ **S59.101**   Unspecified physeal fracture of upper end of radius, right arm   ▽

      ✓7ᵗʰ **S59.102**   Unspecified physeal fracture of upper end of radius, left arm   ▽

      ✓7ᵗʰ **S59.109**   Unspecified physeal fracture of upper end of radius, unspecified arm   ▽

    ✓6ᵗʰ **S59.11**   Salter-Harris Type I physeal fracture of upper end of radius

      ✓7ᵗʰ **S59.111**   Salter-Harris Type I physeal fracture of upper end of radius, right arm

      ✓7ᵗʰ **S59.112**   Salter-Harris Type I physeal fracture of upper end of radius, left arm

      ✓7ᵗʰ **S59.119**   Salter-Harris Type I physeal fracture of upper end of radius, unspecified arm   ▽

Ⓝ Newborn   Ⓟ Pediatric   Ⓜ Maternity   Ⓐ Adult   **RIC** RIC Dx   **NCDx** Noncancer Dx   **PDx** Primary Dx   **CC** RIC CC Condition   ►◄ Revised Text   ● New Code   ▲ Revised Code Title

918   ICD-10-CM 2016

√6ᵗʰ **S59.12** Salter-Harris Type II physeal fracture of upper end of radius

    √7ᵗʰ **S59.121** Salter-Harris Type II physeal fracture of upper end of radius, right arm

    √7ᵗʰ **S59.122** Salter-Harris Type II physeal fracture of upper end of radius, left arm

    √7ᵗʰ **S59.129** Salter-Harris Type II physeal fracture of upper end of radius, unspecified arm ▽

√6ᵗʰ **S59.13** Salter-Harris Type III physeal fracture of upper end of radius

    √7ᵗʰ **S59.131** Salter-Harris Type III physeal fracture of upper end of radius, right arm

    √7ᵗʰ **S59.132** Salter-Harris Type III physeal fracture of upper end of radius, left arm

    √7ᵗʰ **S59.139** Salter-Harris Type III physeal fracture of upper end of radius, unspecified arm ▽

√6ᵗʰ **S59.14** Salter-Harris Type IV physeal fracture of upper end of radius

    √7ᵗʰ **S59.141** Salter-Harris Type IV physeal fracture of upper end of radius, right arm

    √7ᵗʰ **S59.142** Salter-Harris Type IV physeal fracture of upper end of radius, left arm

    √7ᵗʰ **S59.149** Salter-Harris Type IV physeal fracture of upper end of radius, unspecified arm ▽

√6ᵗʰ **S59.19** Other physeal fracture of upper end of radius

    √7ᵗʰ **S59.191** Other physeal fracture of upper end of radius, right arm

    √7ᵗʰ **S59.192** Other physeal fracture of upper end of radius, left arm

    √7ᵗʰ **S59.199** Other physeal fracture of upper end of radius, unspecified arm ▽

√5ᵗʰ **S59.2** Physeal fracture of lower end of radius

√6ᵗʰ **S59.20** Unspecified physeal fracture of lower end of radius

    √7ᵗʰ **S59.201** Unspecified physeal fracture of lower end of radius, right arm ▽

    √7ᵗʰ **S59.202** Unspecified physeal fracture of lower end of radius, left arm ▽

    √7ᵗʰ **S59.209** Unspecified physeal fracture of lower end of radius, unspecified arm ▽

√6ᵗʰ **S59.21** Salter-Harris Type I physeal fracture of lower end of radius

    √7ᵗʰ **S59.211** Salter-Harris Type I physeal fracture of lower end of radius, right arm

    √7ᵗʰ **S59.212** Salter-Harris Type I physeal fracture of lower end of radius, left arm

    √7ᵗʰ **S59.219** Salter-Harris Type I physeal fracture of lower end of radius, unspecified arm ▽

√6ᵗʰ **S59.22** Salter-Harris Type II physeal fracture of lower end of radius

    √7ᵗʰ **S59.221** Salter-Harris Type II physeal fracture of lower end of radius, right arm

    √7ᵗʰ **S59.222** Salter-Harris Type II physeal fracture of lower end of radius, left arm

    √7ᵗʰ **S59.229** Salter-Harris Type II physeal fracture of lower end of radius, unspecified arm ▽

√6ᵗʰ **S59.23** Salter-Harris Type III physeal fracture of lower end of radius

    √7ᵗʰ **S59.231** Salter-Harris Type III physeal fracture of lower end of radius, right arm

    √7ᵗʰ **S59.232** Salter-Harris Type III physeal fracture of lower end of radius, left arm

    √7ᵗʰ **S59.239** Salter-Harris Type III physeal fracture of lower end of radius, unspecified arm ▽

√6ᵗʰ **S59.24** Salter-Harris Type IV physeal fracture of lower end of radius

    √7ᵗʰ **S59.241** Salter-Harris Type IV physeal fracture of lower end of radius, right arm

    √7ᵗʰ **S59.242** Salter-Harris Type IV physeal fracture of lower end of radius, left arm

    √7ᵗʰ **S59.249** Salter-Harris Type IV physeal fracture of lower end of radius, unspecified arm ▽

√6ᵗʰ **S59.29** Other physeal fracture of lower end of radius

    √7ᵗʰ **S59.291** Other physeal fracture of lower end of radius, right arm

    √7ᵗʰ **S59.292** Other physeal fracture of lower end of radius, left arm

    √7ᵗʰ **S59.299** Other physeal fracture of lower end of radius, unspecified arm ▽

√5ᵗʰ **S59.8** Other specified injuries of elbow and forearm

> The appropriate 7th character is to be added to each code in subcategory S59.8.
> A   initial encounter
> D   subsequent encounter
> S   sequela

√6ᵗʰ **S59.80** Other specified injuries of elbow

    √7ᵗʰ **S59.801** Other specified injuries of right elbow

    √7ᵗʰ **S59.802** Other specified injuries of left elbow

    √7ᵗʰ **S59.809** Other specified injuries of unspecified elbow ▽

√6ᵗʰ **S59.81** Other specified injuries of forearm

    √7ᵗʰ **S59.811** Other specified injuries right forearm

    √7ᵗʰ **S59.812** Other specified injuries left forearm

    √7ᵗʰ **S59.819** Other specified injuries unspecified forearm ▽

√5ᵗʰ **S59.9** Unspecified injury of elbow and forearm

> The appropriate 7th character is to be added to each code in subcategory S59.9.
> A   initial encounter
> D   subsequent encounter
> S   sequela

√6ᵗʰ **S59.90** Unspecified injury of elbow

    √7ᵗʰ **S59.901** Unspecified injury of right elbow ▽

    √7ᵗʰ **S59.902** Unspecified injury of left elbow ▽

    √7ᵗʰ **S59.909** Unspecified injury of unspecified elbow ▽

√6ᵗʰ **S59.91** Unspecified injury of forearm

    √7ᵗʰ **S59.911** Unspecified injury of right forearm ▽

    √7ᵗʰ **S59.912** Unspecified injury of left forearm ▽

    √7ᵗʰ **S59.919** Unspecified injury of unspecified forearm ▽

Injuries to the wrist, hand and fingers (S60-S69)

EXCLUDES 2   burns and corrosions (T20-T32)
      frostbite (T33-T34)
      insect bite or sting, venomous (T63.4)

√4ᵗʰ **S60** Superficial injury of wrist, hand and fingers

> The appropriate 7th character is to be added to each code from category S60.
> A   initial encounter
> D   subsequent encounter
> S   sequela

√5ᵗʰ **S60.0** Contusion of finger without damage to nail

    EXCLUDES 1   contusion involving nail (matrix) (S60.1)

√×7ᵗʰ **S60.00** Contusion of unspecified finger without damage to nail ▽

      Contusion of finger(s) NOS

√6ᵗʰ **S60.01** Contusion of thumb without damage to nail

    √7ᵗʰ **S60.011** Contusion of right thumb without damage to nail

    √7ᵗʰ **S60.012** Contusion of left thumb without damage to nail

    √7ᵗʰ **S60.019** Contusion of unspecified thumb without damage to nail ▽

√6ᵗʰ **S60.02** Contusion of index finger without damage to nail

    √7ᵗʰ **S60.021** Contusion of right index finger without damage to nail

    √7ᵗʰ **S60.022** Contusion of left index finger without damage to nail

    √7ᵗʰ **S60.029** Contusion of unspecified index finger without damage to nail ▽

√6ᵗʰ **S60.03** Contusion of middle finger without damage to nail

    √7ᵗʰ **S60.031** Contusion of right middle finger without damage to nail

    √7ᵗʰ **S60.032** Contusion of left middle finger without damage to nail

√7ᵗʰ **S60.039** Contusion of unspecified middle finger without damage to nail ▽

√6ᵗʰ **S60.04** Contusion of ring finger without damage to nail

√7ᵗʰ **S60.041** Contusion of right ring finger without damage to nail

√7ᵗʰ **S60.042** Contusion of left ring finger without damage to nail

√7ᵗʰ **S60.049** Contusion of unspecified ring finger without damage to nail ▽

√6ᵗʰ **S60.05** Contusion of little finger without damage to nail

√7ᵗʰ **S60.051** Contusion of right little finger without damage to nail

√7ᵗʰ **S60.052** Contusion of left little finger without damage to nail

√7ᵗʰ **S60.059** Contusion of unspecified little finger without damage to nail ▽

√5ᵗʰ **S60.1** Contusion of finger with damage to nail

√x7ᵗʰ **S60.10** Contusion of unspecified finger with damage to nail ▽

√6ᵗʰ **S60.11** Contusion of thumb with damage to nail

√7ᵗʰ **S60.111** Contusion of right thumb with damage to nail

√7ᵗʰ **S60.112** Contusion of left thumb with damage to nail

√7ᵗʰ **S60.119** Contusion of unspecified thumb with damage to nail ▽

√6ᵗʰ **S60.12** Contusion of index finger with damage to nail

√7ᵗʰ **S60.121** Contusion of right index finger with damage to nail

√7ᵗʰ **S60.122** Contusion of left index finger with damage to nail

√7ᵗʰ **S60.129** Contusion of unspecified index finger with damage to nail ▽

√6ᵗʰ **S60.13** Contusion of middle finger with damage to nail

√7ᵗʰ **S60.131** Contusion of right middle finger with damage to nail

√7ᵗʰ **S60.132** Contusion of left middle finger with damage to nail

√7ᵗʰ **S60.139** Contusion of unspecified middle finger with damage to nail ▽

√6ᵗʰ **S60.14** Contusion of ring finger with damage to nail

√7ᵗʰ **S60.141** Contusion of right ring finger with damage to nail

√7ᵗʰ **S60.142** Contusion of left ring finger with damage to nail

√7ᵗʰ **S60.149** Contusion of unspecified ring finger with damage to nail ▽

√6ᵗʰ **S60.15** Contusion of little finger with damage to nail

√7ᵗʰ **S60.151** Contusion of right little finger with damage to nail

√7ᵗʰ **S60.152** Contusion of left little finger with damage to nail

√7ᵗʰ **S60.159** Contusion of unspecified little finger with damage to nail ▽

√5ᵗʰ **S60.2** Contusion of wrist and hand

EXCLUDES 2 contusion of fingers (S60.0-, S60.1-)

√6ᵗʰ **S60.21** Contusion of wrist

√7ᵗʰ **S60.211** Contusion of right wrist

√7ᵗʰ **S60.212** Contusion of left wrist

√7ᵗʰ **S60.219** Contusion of unspecified wrist ▽

√6ᵗʰ **S60.22** Contusion of hand

√7ᵗʰ **S60.221** Contusion of right hand

√7ᵗʰ **S60.222** Contusion of left hand

√7ᵗʰ **S60.229** Contusion of unspecified hand ▽

√5ᵗʰ **S60.3** Other superficial injuries of thumb

√6ᵗʰ **S60.31** Abrasion of thumb

√7ᵗʰ **S60.311** Abrasion of right thumb

√7ᵗʰ **S60.312** Abrasion of left thumb

√7ᵗʰ **S60.319** Abrasion of unspecified thumb ▽

√6ᵗʰ **S60.32** Blister (nonthermal) of thumb

√7ᵗʰ **S60.321** Blister (nonthermal) of right thumb

√7ᵗʰ **S60.322** Blister (nonthermal) of left thumb

√7ᵗʰ **S60.329** Blister (nonthermal) of unspecified thumb ▽

√6ᵗʰ **S60.34** External constriction of thumb
Hair tourniquet syndrome of thumb
Use additional cause code to identify the constricting item (W49.0-)

√7ᵗʰ **S60.341** External constriction of right thumb

√7ᵗʰ **S60.342** External constriction of left thumb

√7ᵗʰ **S60.349** External constriction of unspecified thumb ▽

√6ᵗʰ **S60.35** Superficial foreign body of thumb
Splinter in the thumb

√7ᵗʰ **S60.351** Superficial foreign body of right thumb

√7ᵗʰ **S60.352** Superficial foreign body of left thumb

√7ᵗʰ **S60.359** Superficial foreign body of unspecified ▽ thumb

√6ᵗʰ **S60.36** Insect bite (nonvenomous) of thumb

√7ᵗʰ **S60.361** Insect bite (nonvenomous) of right thumb

√7ᵗʰ **S60.362** Insect bite (nonvenomous) of left thumb

√7ᵗʰ **S60.369** Insect bite (nonvenomous) of ▽ unspecified thumb

√6ᵗʰ **S60.37** Other superficial bite of thumb
EXCLUDES 1 open bite of thumb (S61.05-, S61.15-)

√7ᵗʰ **S60.371** Other superficial bite of right thumb

√7ᵗʰ **S60.372** Other superficial bite of left thumb

√7ᵗʰ **S60.379** Other superficial bite of unspecified ▽ thumb

√6ᵗʰ **S60.39** Other superficial injuries of thumb

√7ᵗʰ **S60.391** Other superficial injuries of right thumb

√7ᵗʰ **S60.392** Other superficial injuries of left thumb

√7ᵗʰ **S60.399** Other superficial injuries of ▽ unspecified thumb

√5ᵗʰ **S60.4** Other superficial injuries of other fingers

√6ᵗʰ **S60.41** Abrasion of fingers

√7ᵗʰ **S60.410** Abrasion of right index finger

√7ᵗʰ **S60.411** Abrasion of left index finger

√7ᵗʰ **S60.412** Abrasion of right middle finger

√7ᵗʰ **S60.413** Abrasion of left middle finger

√7ᵗʰ **S60.414** Abrasion of right ring finger

√7ᵗʰ **S60.415** Abrasion of left ring finger

√7ᵗʰ **S60.416** Abrasion of right little finger

√7ᵗʰ **S60.417** Abrasion of left little finger

√7ᵗʰ **S60.418** Abrasion of other finger
Abrasion of specified finger with unspecified laterality

√7ᵗʰ **S60.419** Abrasion of unspecified finger ▽

√6ᵗʰ **S60.42** Blister (nonthermal) of fingers

√7ᵗʰ **S60.420** Blister (nonthermal) of right index finger

√7ᵗʰ **S60.421** Blister (nonthermal) of left index finger

√7ᵗʰ **S60.422** Blister (nonthermal) of right middle finger

√7ᵗʰ **S60.423** Blister (nonthermal) of left middle finger

√7ᵗʰ **S60.424** Blister (nonthermal) of right ring finger

√7ᵗʰ **S60.425** Blister (nonthermal) of left ring finger

√7ᵗʰ **S60.426** Blister (nonthermal) of right little finger

√7ᵗʰ **S60.427** Blister (nonthermal) of left little finger

√7ᵗʰ **S60.428** Blister (nonthermal) of other finger
Blister (nonthermal) of specified finger with unspecified laterality

√7ᵗʰ **S60.429** Blister (nonthermal) of unspecified ▽ finger

√6ᵗʰ **S60.44** External constriction of fingers
Hair tourniquet syndrome of finger
Use additional cause code to identify the constricting item (W49.0-)

√7ᵗʰ **S60.440** External constriction of right index finger

√7ᵗʰ **S60.441** External constriction of left index finger

√7ᵗʰ **S60.442** External constriction of right middle finger

√7ᵗʰ **S60.443** External constriction of left middle finger

√7ᵗʰ **S60.444** External constriction of right ring finger

√7ᵗʰ **S60.445** External constriction of left ring finger

Ⓝ Newborn　Ⓟ Pediatric　Ⓜ Maternity　Ⓐ Adult　RIC Dx RIC Dx　NCDx Noncancer Dx　PDx Primary Dx　CC RIC CC Condition　►◄ Revised Text　● New Code　▲ Revised Code Title

920

ICD-10-CM 2016

✓7ᵗʰ **S60.446**   External constriction of right little finger

✓7ᵗʰ **S60.447**   External constriction of left little finger

✓7ᵗʰ **S60.448**   External constriction of other finger
External constriction of specified finger with unspecified laterality

✓7ᵗʰ **S60.449**   External constriction of unspecified finger ▽

✓6ᵗʰ **S60.45**   **Superficial foreign body of fingers**
Splinter in the finger(s)

✓7ᵗʰ **S60.450**   Superficial foreign body of right index finger

✓7ᵗʰ **S60.451**   Superficial foreign body of left index finger

✓7ᵗʰ **S60.452**   Superficial foreign body of right middle finger

✓7ᵗʰ **S60.453**   Superficial foreign body of left middle finger

✓7ᵗʰ **S60.454**   Superficial foreign body of right ring finger

✓7ᵗʰ **S60.455**   Superficial foreign body of left ring finger

✓7ᵗʰ **S60.456**   Superficial foreign body of right little finger

✓7ᵗʰ **S60.457**   Superficial foreign body of left little finger

✓7ᵗʰ **S60.458**   Superficial foreign body of other finger
Superficial foreign body of specified finger with unspecified laterality

✓7ᵗʰ **S60.459**   Superficial foreign body of unspecified finger ▽

✓6ᵗʰ **S60.46**   **Insect bite (nonvenomous) of fingers**

✓7ᵗʰ **S60.460**   Insect bite (nonvenomous) of right index finger

✓7ᵗʰ **S60.461**   Insect bite (nonvenomous) of left index finger

✓7ᵗʰ **S60.462**   Insect bite (nonvenomous) of right middle finger

✓7ᵗʰ **S60.463**   Insect bite (nonvenomous) of left middle finger

✓7ᵗʰ **S60.464**   Insect bite (nonvenomous) of right ring finger

✓7ᵗʰ **S60.465**   Insect bite (nonvenomous) of left ring finger

✓7ᵗʰ **S60.466**   Insect bite (nonvenomous) of right little finger

✓7ᵗʰ **S60.467**   Insect bite (nonvenomous) of left little finger

✓7ᵗʰ **S60.468**   Insect bite (nonvenomous) of other finger
Insect bite (nonvenomous) of specified finger with unspecified laterality

✓7ᵗʰ **S60.469**   Insect bite (nonvenomous) of unspecified finger ▽

✓6ᵗʰ **S60.47**   **Other superficial bite of fingers**
EXCLUDES 1   open bite of fingers (S61.25-, S61.35-)

✓7ᵗʰ **S60.470**   Other superficial bite of right index finger

✓7ᵗʰ **S60.471**   Other superficial bite of left index finger

✓7ᵗʰ **S60.472**   Other superficial bite of right middle finger

✓7ᵗʰ **S60.473**   Other superficial bite of left middle finger

✓7ᵗʰ **S60.474**   Other superficial bite of right ring finger

✓7ᵗʰ **S60.475**   Other superficial bite of left ring finger

✓7ᵗʰ **S60.476**   Other superficial bite of right little finger

✓7ᵗʰ **S60.477**   Other superficial bite of left little finger

✓7ᵗʰ **S60.478**   Other superficial bite of other finger
Other superficial bite of specified finger with unspecified laterality

✓7ᵗʰ **S60.479**   Other superficial bite of unspecified finger ▽

✓5ᵗʰ **S60.5**   **Other superficial injuries of hand**
EXCLUDES 2   superficial injuries of fingers (S60.3-, S60.4-)

✓6ᵗʰ **S60.51**   **Abrasion of hand**

✓7ᵗʰ **S60.511**   Abrasion of right hand

✓7ᵗʰ **S60.512**   Abrasion of left hand

✓7ᵗʰ **S60.519**   Abrasion of unspecified hand ▽

✓6ᵗʰ **S60.52**   **Blister (nonthermal) of hand**

✓7ᵗʰ **S60.521**   Blister (nonthermal) of right hand

✓7ᵗʰ **S60.522**   Blister (nonthermal) of left hand

✓7ᵗʰ **S60.529**   Blister (nonthermal) of unspecified hand ▽

✓6ᵗʰ **S60.54**   **External constriction of hand**

✓7ᵗʰ **S60.541**   External constriction of right hand

✓7ᵗʰ **S60.542**   External constriction of left hand

✓7ᵗʰ **S60.549**   External constriction of unspecified hand ▽

✓6ᵗʰ **S60.55**   **Superficial foreign body of hand**
Splinter in the hand

✓7ᵗʰ **S60.551**   Superficial foreign body of right hand

✓7ᵗʰ **S60.552**   Superficial foreign body of left hand

✓7ᵗʰ **S60.559**   Superficial foreign body of unspecified hand ▽

✓6ᵗʰ **S60.56**   **Insect bite (nonvenomous) of hand**

✓7ᵗʰ **S60.561**   Insect bite (nonvenomous) of right hand

✓7ᵗʰ **S60.562**   Insect bite (nonvenomous) of left hand

✓7ᵗʰ **S60.569**   Insect bite (nonvenomous) of unspecified hand ▽

✓6ᵗʰ **S60.57**   **Other superficial bite of hand**
EXCLUDES 1   open bite of hand (S61.45-)

✓7ᵗʰ **S60.571**   Other superficial bite of hand of right hand

✓7ᵗʰ **S60.572**   Other superficial bite of hand of left hand

✓7ᵗʰ **S60.579**   Other superficial bite of hand of unspecified hand ▽

✓5ᵗʰ **S60.8**   **Other superficial injuries of wrist**

✓6ᵗʰ **S60.81**   **Abrasion of wrist**

✓7ᵗʰ **S60.811**   Abrasion of right wrist

✓7ᵗʰ **S60.812**   Abrasion of left wrist

✓7ᵗʰ **S60.819**   Abrasion of unspecified wrist ▽

✓6ᵗʰ **S60.82**   **Blister (nonthermal) of wrist**

✓7ᵗʰ **S60.821**   Blister (nonthermal) of right wrist

✓7ᵗʰ **S60.822**   Blister (nonthermal) of left wrist

✓7ᵗʰ **S60.829**   Blister (nonthermal) of unspecified wrist ▽

✓6ᵗʰ **S60.84**   **External constriction of wrist**

✓7ᵗʰ **S60.841**   External constriction of right wrist

✓7ᵗʰ **S60.842**   External constriction of left wrist

✓7ᵗʰ **S60.849**   External constriction of unspecified wrist ▽

✓6ᵗʰ **S60.85**   **Superficial foreign body of wrist**
Splinter in the wrist

✓7ᵗʰ **S60.851**   Superficial foreign body of right wrist

✓7ᵗʰ **S60.852**   Superficial foreign body of left wrist

✓7ᵗʰ **S60.859**   Superficial foreign body of unspecified wrist ▽

✓6ᵗʰ **S60.86**   **Insect bite (nonvenomous) of wrist**

✓7ᵗʰ **S60.861**   Insect bite (nonvenomous) of right wrist

✓7ᵗʰ **S60.862**   Insect bite (nonvenomous) of left wrist

✓7ᵗʰ **S60.869**   Insect bite (nonvenomous) of unspecified wrist ▽

✓6ᵗʰ **S60.87**   **Other superficial bite of wrist**
EXCLUDES 1   open bite of wrist (S61.55)

✓7ᵗʰ **S60.871**   Other superficial bite of right wrist

✓7ᵗʰ **S60.872**   Other superficial bite of left wrist

✓7ᵗʰ **S60.879**   Other superficial bite of unspecified wrist ▽

✓5ᵗʰ **S60.9**   **Unspecified superficial injury of wrist, hand and fingers**

✓6ᵗʰ **S60.91**   **Unspecified superficial injury of wrist**

✓7ᵗʰ **S60.911**   Unspecified superficial injury of right wrist ▽

✓7ᵗʰ **S60.912**   Unspecified superficial injury of left wrist ▽

✓7ᵗʰ **S60.919**   Unspecified superficial injury of unspecified wrist ▽

☑ Add'l Character Required   ✓ˣ7ᵗʰ Placeholder Alert   RUG IV Special Care High Dx   RUG IV Clinically Complex Dx   RUG IV Special Care Low Dx   Manifestation Code   Other Specified Code   ▽ Unspecified Code

√6ᵗʰ **S60.92** Unspecified superficial injury of hand

    √7ᵗʰ **S60.921** Unspecified superficial injury of right hand ▽

    √7ᵗʰ **S60.922** Unspecified superficial injury of left hand ▽

    √7ᵗʰ **S60.929** Unspecified superficial injury of unspecified hand ▽

√6ᵗʰ **S60.93** Unspecified superficial injury of thumb

    √7ᵗʰ **S60.931** Unspecified superficial injury of right thumb ▽

    √7ᵗʰ **S60.932** Unspecified superficial injury of left thumb ▽

    √7ᵗʰ **S60.939** Unspecified superficial injury of unspecified thumb ▽

√6ᵗʰ **S60.94** Unspecified superficial injury of other fingers

    √7ᵗʰ **S60.940** Unspecified superficial injury of right index finger ▽

    √7ᵗʰ **S60.941** Unspecified superficial injury of left index finger ▽

    √7ᵗʰ **S60.942** Unspecified superficial injury of right middle finger ▽

    √7ᵗʰ **S60.943** Unspecified superficial injury of left middle finger ▽

    √7ᵗʰ **S60.944** Unspecified superficial injury of right ring finger ▽

    √7ᵗʰ **S60.945** Unspecified superficial injury of left ring finger ▽

    √7ᵗʰ **S60.946** Unspecified superficial injury of right little finger ▽

    √7ᵗʰ **S60.947** Unspecified superficial injury of left little finger ▽

    √7ᵗʰ **S60.948** Unspecified superficial injury of other finger ▽
        Unspecified superficial injury of specified finger with unspecified laterality

    √7ᵗʰ **S60.949** Unspecified superficial injury of unspecified finger ▽

√4ᵗʰ **S61** **Open wound of wrist, hand and fingers**
    Code also any associated wound infection
    EXCLUDES 1   open fracture of wrist, hand and finger (S62- with 7th character B)
        traumatic amputation of wrist and hand (S68.-)

    The appropriate 7th character is to be added to each code from category S61.
    A   initial encounter
    D   subsequent encounter
    S   sequela

√5ᵗʰ **S61.0** **Open wound of** thumb without damage to nail
    EXCLUDES 1   open wound of thumb with damage to nail (S61.1-)

    √6ᵗʰ **S61.00** Unspecified open wound of thumb without damage to nail

       √7ᵗʰ **S61.001** Unspecified open wound of right thumb without damage to nail ▽

       √7ᵗʰ **S61.002** Unspecified open wound of left thumb without damage to nail ▽

       √7ᵗʰ **S61.009** Unspecified open wound of unspecified thumb without damage to nail ▽

    √6ᵗʰ **S61.01** Laceration without foreign body of thumb without damage to nail

       √7ᵗʰ **S61.011** Laceration without foreign body of right thumb without damage to nail

       √7ᵗʰ **S61.012** Laceration without foreign body of left thumb without damage to nail

       √7ᵗʰ **S61.019** Laceration without foreign body of unspecified thumb without damage to nail ▽

    √6ᵗʰ **S61.02** Laceration with foreign body of thumb without damage to nail

       √7ᵗʰ **S61.021** Laceration with foreign body of right thumb without damage to nail

       √7ᵗʰ **S61.022** Laceration with foreign body of left thumb without damage to nail

       √7ᵗʰ **S61.029** Laceration with foreign body of unspecified thumb without damage to nail ▽

√6ᵗʰ **S61.03** Puncture wound without foreign body of thumb without damage to nail

    √7ᵗʰ **S61.031** Puncture wound without foreign body of right thumb without damage to nail

    √7ᵗʰ **S61.032** Puncture wound without foreign body of left thumb without damage to nail

    √7ᵗʰ **S61.039** Puncture wound without foreign body of unspecified thumb without damage to nail ▽

√6ᵗʰ **S61.04** Puncture wound with foreign body of thumb without damage to nail

    √7ᵗʰ **S61.041** Puncture wound with foreign body of right thumb without damage to nail

    √7ᵗʰ **S61.042** Puncture wound with foreign body of left thumb without damage to nail

    √7ᵗʰ **S61.049** Puncture wound with foreign body of unspecified thumb without damage to nail ▽

√6ᵗʰ **S61.05** Open bite of thumb without damage to nail
    Bite of thumb NOS
    EXCLUDES 1   superficial bite of thumb (S60.36-, S60.37-)

    √7ᵗʰ **S61.051** Open bite of right thumb without damage to nail

    √7ᵗʰ **S61.052** Open bite of left thumb without damage to nail

    √7ᵗʰ **S61.059** Open bite of unspecified thumb without damage to nail ▽

√5ᵗʰ **S61.1** **Open wound of** thumb with damage to nail

    √6ᵗʰ **S61.10** Unspecified open wound of thumb with damage to nail

       √7ᵗʰ **S61.101** Unspecified open wound of right thumb with damage to nail ▽

       √7ᵗʰ **S61.102** Unspecified open wound of left thumb with damage to nail ▽

       √7ᵗʰ **S61.109** Unspecified open wound of unspecified thumb with damage to nail ▽

    √6ᵗʰ **S61.11** Laceration without foreign body of thumb with damage to nail

       √7ᵗʰ **S61.111** Laceration without foreign body of right thumb with damage to nail

       √7ᵗʰ **S61.112** Laceration without foreign body of left thumb with damage to nail

       √7ᵗʰ **S61.119** Laceration without foreign body of unspecified thumb with damage to nail ▽

    √6ᵗʰ **S61.12** Laceration with foreign body of thumb with damage to nail

       √7ᵗʰ **S61.121** Laceration with foreign body of right thumb with damage to nail

       √7ᵗʰ **S61.122** Laceration with foreign body of left thumb with damage to nail

       √7ᵗʰ **S61.129** Laceration with foreign body of unspecified thumb with damage to nail ▽

    √6ᵗʰ **S61.13** Puncture wound without foreign body of thumb with damage to nail

       √7ᵗʰ **S61.131** Puncture wound without foreign body of right thumb with damage to nail

       √7ᵗʰ **S61.132** Puncture wound without foreign body of left thumb with damage to nail

       √7ᵗʰ **S61.139** Puncture wound without foreign body of unspecified thumb with damage to nail ▽

    √6ᵗʰ **S61.14** Puncture wound with foreign body of thumb with damage to nail

       √7ᵗʰ **S61.141** Puncture wound with foreign body of right thumb with damage to nail

       √7ᵗʰ **S61.142** Puncture wound with foreign body of left thumb with damage to nail

       √7ᵗʰ **S61.149** Puncture wound with foreign body of unspecified thumb with damage to nail ▽

Ⓝ Newborn   Ⓟ Pediatric   Ⓜ Maternity   Ⓐ Adult   **RIC** RIC Dx   **NCDx** Noncancer Dx   **PDx** Primary Dx   **CC** RIC CC Condition   ►◄ Revised Text   ● New Code   ▲ Revised Code Title

922   ICD-10-CM 2016

✓6ᵗʰ **S61.15** Open bite **of thumb** with damage to nail
Bite of thumb with damage to nail NOS
EXCLUDES 1 *superficial bite of thumb (S60.36-, S60.37-)*

    ✓7ᵗʰ **S61.151** Open bite of **right** thumb with damage to nail

    ✓7ᵗʰ **S61.152** Open bite of **left** thumb with damage to nail

    ✓7ᵗʰ **S61.159** Open bite of unspecified thumb with damage to nail ▽

✓5ᵗʰ **S61.2** Open wound of **other finger without damage to nail**
EXCLUDES 1 *open wound of finger involving nail (matrix) (S61.3-)*
EXCLUDES 2 *open wound of thumb without damage to nail (S61.0-)*

✓6ᵗʰ **S61.20** Unspecified **open wound of other finger without damage to nail**

    ✓7ᵗʰ **S61.200** Unspecified open wound of **right index** ▽ finger without damage to nail

    ✓7ᵗʰ **S61.201** Unspecified open wound of **left index** ▽ finger without damage to nail

    ✓7ᵗʰ **S61.202** Unspecified open wound of **right** ▽ **middle** finger without damage to nail

    ✓7ᵗʰ **S61.203** Unspecified open wound of **left middle** ▽ finger without damage to nail

    ✓7ᵗʰ **S61.204** Unspecified open wound of **right ring** ▽ finger without damage to nail

    ✓7ᵗʰ **S61.205** Unspecified open wound of **left ring** ▽ finger without damage to nail

    ✓7ᵗʰ **S61.206** Unspecified open wound of **right little** ▽ finger without damage to nail

    ✓7ᵗʰ **S61.207** Unspecified open wound of **left little** ▽ finger without damage to nail

    ✓7ᵗʰ **S61.208** Unspecified open wound of other ▽ finger without damage to nail
Unspecified open wound of specified finger with unspecified laterality without damage to nail

    ✓7ᵗʰ **S61.209** Unspecified open wound of unspecified ▽ finger without damage to nail

✓6ᵗʰ **S61.21** Laceration **without foreign body** of finger without damage to nail

    ✓7ᵗʰ **S61.210** Laceration without foreign body of **right index** finger without damage to nail

    ✓7ᵗʰ **S61.211** Laceration without foreign body of **left index** finger without damage to nail

    ✓7ᵗʰ **S61.212** Laceration without foreign body of **right middle** finger without damage to nail

    ✓7ᵗʰ **S61.213** Laceration without foreign body of **left middle** finger without damage to nail

    ✓7ᵗʰ **S61.214** Laceration without foreign body of **right ring** finger without damage to nail

    ✓7ᵗʰ **S61.215** Laceration without foreign body of **left ring** finger without damage to nail

    ✓7ᵗʰ **S61.216** Laceration without foreign body of **right little** finger without damage to nail

    ✓7ᵗʰ **S61.217** Laceration without foreign body of **left little** finger without damage to nail

    ✓7ᵗʰ **S61.218** Laceration without foreign body of other finger without damage to nail
Laceration without foreign body of specified finger with unspecified laterality without damage to nail

    ✓7ᵗʰ **S61.219** Laceration without foreign body of ▽ unspecified finger without damage to nail

✓6ᵗʰ **S61.22** Laceration **with foreign body** of finger without damage to nail

    ✓7ᵗʰ **S61.220** Laceration with foreign body of **right index** finger without damage to nail

    ✓7ᵗʰ **S61.221** Laceration with foreign body of **left index** finger without damage to nail

    ✓7ᵗʰ **S61.222** Laceration with foreign body of **right middle** finger without damage to nail

    ✓7ᵗʰ **S61.223** Laceration with foreign body of **left middle** finger without damage to nail

    ✓7ᵗʰ **S61.224** Laceration with foreign body of **right ring** finger without damage to nail

    ✓7ᵗʰ **S61.225** Laceration with foreign body of **left ring** finger without damage to nail

    ✓7ᵗʰ **S61.226** Laceration with foreign body of **right little** finger without damage to nail

    ✓7ᵗʰ **S61.227** Laceration with foreign body of **left little** finger without damage to nail

    ✓7ᵗʰ **S61.228** Laceration with foreign body of other finger without damage to nail
Laceration with foreign body of specified finger with unspecified laterality without damage to nail

    ✓7ᵗʰ **S61.229** Laceration with foreign body of ▽ unspecified finger without damage to nail

✓6ᵗʰ **S61.23** Puncture wound **without foreign body** of finger without damage to nail

    ✓7ᵗʰ **S61.230** Puncture wound without foreign body of **right index** finger without damage to nail

    ✓7ᵗʰ **S61.231** Puncture wound without foreign body of **left index** finger without damage to nail

    ✓7ᵗʰ **S61.232** Puncture wound without foreign body of **right middle** finger without damage to nail

    ✓7ᵗʰ **S61.233** Puncture wound without foreign body of **left middle** finger without damage to nail

    ✓7ᵗʰ **S61.234** Puncture wound without foreign body of **right ring** finger without damage to nail

    ✓7ᵗʰ **S61.235** Puncture wound without foreign body of **left ring** finger without damage to nail

    ✓7ᵗʰ **S61.236** Puncture wound without foreign body of **right little** finger without damage to nail

    ✓7ᵗʰ **S61.237** Puncture wound without foreign body of **left little** finger without damage to nail

    ✓7ᵗʰ **S61.238** Puncture wound without foreign body of other finger without damage to nail
Puncture wound without foreign body of specified finger with unspecified laterality without damage to nail

    ✓7ᵗʰ **S61.239** Puncture wound without foreign body ▽ of unspecified finger without damage to nail

✓6ᵗʰ **S61.24** Puncture wound **with foreign body** of finger without damage to nail

    ✓7ᵗʰ **S61.240** Puncture wound with foreign body of **right index** finger without damage to nail

    ✓7ᵗʰ **S61.241** Puncture wound with foreign body of **left index** finger without damage to nail

    ✓7ᵗʰ **S61.242** Puncture wound with foreign body of **right middle** finger without damage to nail

    ✓7ᵗʰ **S61.243** Puncture wound with foreign body of **left middle** finger without damage to nail

    ✓7ᵗʰ **S61.244** Puncture wound with foreign body of **right ring** finger without damage to nail

    ✓7ᵗʰ **S61.245** Puncture wound with foreign body of **left ring** finger without damage to nail

    ✓7ᵗʰ **S61.246** Puncture wound with foreign body of **right little** finger without damage to nail

    ✓7ᵗʰ **S61.247** Puncture wound with foreign body of **left little** finger without damage to nail

    ✓7ᵗʰ **S61.248** Puncture wound with foreign body of other finger without damage to nail
Puncture wound with foreign body of specified finger with unspecified laterality without damage to nail

    ✓7ᵗʰ **S61.249** Puncture wound with foreign body of ▽ unspecified finger without damage to nail

✓6ᵗʰ **S61.25** Open bite **of finger without damage to nail**
Bite of finger without damage to nail NOS
EXCLUDES 1 *superficial bite of finger (S60.46-, S60.47-)*

    ✓7ᵗʰ **S61.250** Open bite of **right index** finger without damage to nail

    ✓7ᵗʰ **S61.251** Open bite of **left index** finger without damage to nail

    ✓7ᵗʰ **S61.252** Open bite of **right middle** finger without damage to nail

    ✓7ᵗʰ **S61.253** Open bite of **left middle** finger without damage to nail

    ✓7ᵗʰ **S61.254** Open bite of **right ring** finger without damage to nail

---

☑ Add'l Character Required   ✓x7ᵗʰ Placeholder Alert   RUG IV Special Care High Dx   RUG IV Clinically Complex Dx   RUG IV Special Care Low Dx   Manifestation Code   Other Specified Code   ▽ Unspecified Code

✓7ᵗʰ **S61.255** Open bite of left ring finger without damage to nail

✓7ᵗʰ **S61.256** Open bite of right little finger without damage to nail

✓7ᵗʰ **S61.257** Open bite of left little finger without damage to nail

✓7ᵗʰ **S61.258** Open bite of other finger without damage to nail
Open bite of specified finger with unspecified laterality without damage to nail

✓7ᵗʰ **S61.259** Open bite of unspecified finger without ▽ damage to nail

✓5ᵗʰ **S61.3** Open wound of other finger with damage to nail

✓6ᵗʰ **S61.30** Unspecified open wound of finger with damage to nail

✓7ᵗʰ **S61.300** Unspecified open wound of right index ▽ finger with damage to nail

✓7ᵗʰ **S61.301** Unspecified open wound of left index ▽ finger with damage to nail

✓7ᵗʰ **S61.302** Unspecified open wound of right ▽ middle finger with damage to nail

✓7ᵗʰ **S61.303** Unspecified open wound of left middle ▽ finger with damage to nail

✓7ᵗʰ **S61.304** Unspecified open wound of right ring ▽ finger with damage to nail

✓7ᵗʰ **S61.305** Unspecified open wound of left ring ▽ finger with damage to nail

✓7ᵗʰ **S61.306** Unspecified open wound of right little ▽ finger with damage to nail

✓7ᵗʰ **S61.307** Unspecified open wound of left little ▽ finger with damage to nail

✓7ᵗʰ **S61.308** Unspecified open wound of other ▽ finger with damage to nail
Unspecified open wound of specified finger with unspecified laterality with damage to nail

✓7ᵗʰ **S61.309** Unspecified open wound of ▽ unspecified finger with damage to nail

✓6ᵗʰ **S61.31** Laceration without foreign body of finger with damage to nail

✓7ᵗʰ **S61.310** Laceration without foreign body of right index finger with damage to nail

✓7ᵗʰ **S61.311** Laceration without foreign body of left index finger with damage to nail

✓7ᵗʰ **S61.312** Laceration without foreign body of right middle finger with damage to nail

✓7ᵗʰ **S61.313** Laceration without foreign body of left middle finger with damage to nail

✓7ᵗʰ **S61.314** Laceration without foreign body of right ring finger with damage to nail

✓7ᵗʰ **S61.315** Laceration without foreign body of left ring finger with damage to nail

✓7ᵗʰ **S61.316** Laceration without foreign body of right little finger with damage to nail

✓7ᵗʰ **S61.317** Laceration without foreign body of left little finger with damage to nail

✓7ᵗʰ **S61.318** Laceration without foreign body of other finger with damage to nail
Laceration without foreign body of specified finger with unspecified laterality with damage to nail

✓7ᵗʰ **S61.319** Laceration without foreign body of ▽ unspecified finger with damage to nail

✓6ᵗʰ **S61.32** Laceration with foreign body of finger with damage to nail

✓7ᵗʰ **S61.320** Laceration with foreign body of right index finger with damage to nail

✓7ᵗʰ **S61.321** Laceration with foreign body of left index finger with damage to nail

✓7ᵗʰ **S61.322** Laceration with foreign body of right middle finger with damage to nail

✓7ᵗʰ **S61.323** Laceration with foreign body of left middle finger with damage to nail

✓7ᵗʰ **S61.324** Laceration with foreign body of right ring finger with damage to nail

✓7ᵗʰ **S61.325** Laceration with foreign body of left ring finger with damage to nail

✓7ᵗʰ **S61.326** Laceration with foreign body of right little finger with damage to nail

✓7ᵗʰ **S61.327** Laceration with foreign body of left little finger with damage to nail

✓7ᵗʰ **S61.328** Laceration with foreign body of other finger with damage to nail
Laceration with foreign body of specified finger with unspecified laterality with damage to nail

✓7ᵗʰ **S61.329** Laceration with foreign body of ▽ unspecified finger with damage to nail

✓6ᵗʰ **S61.33** Puncture wound without foreign body of finger with damage to nail

✓7ᵗʰ **S61.330** Puncture wound without foreign body of right index finger with damage to nail

✓7ᵗʰ **S61.331** Puncture wound without foreign body of left index finger with damage to nail

✓7ᵗʰ **S61.332** Puncture wound without foreign body of right middle finger with damage to nail

✓7ᵗʰ **S61.333** Puncture wound without foreign body of left middle finger with damage to nail

✓7ᵗʰ **S61.334** Puncture wound without foreign body of right ring finger with damage to nail

✓7ᵗʰ **S61.335** Puncture wound without foreign body of left ring finger with damage to nail

✓7ᵗʰ **S61.336** Puncture wound without foreign body of right little finger with damage to nail

✓7ᵗʰ **S61.337** Puncture wound without foreign body of left little finger with damage to nail

✓7ᵗʰ **S61.338** Puncture wound without foreign body of other finger with damage to nail
Puncture wound without foreign body of specified finger with unspecified laterality with damage to nail

✓7ᵗʰ **S61.339** Puncture wound without foreign body ▽ of unspecified finger with damage to nail

✓6ᵗʰ **S61.34** Puncture wound with foreign body of finger with damage to nail

✓7ᵗʰ **S61.340** Puncture wound with foreign body of right index finger with damage to nail

✓7ᵗʰ **S61.341** Puncture wound with foreign body of left index finger with damage to nail

✓7ᵗʰ **S61.342** Puncture wound with foreign body of right middle finger with damage to nail

✓7ᵗʰ **S61.343** Puncture wound with foreign body of left middle finger with damage to nail

✓7ᵗʰ **S61.344** Puncture wound with foreign body of right ring finger with damage to nail

✓7ᵗʰ **S61.345** Puncture wound with foreign body of left ring finger with damage to nail

✓7ᵗʰ **S61.346** Puncture wound with foreign body of right little finger with damage to nail

✓7ᵗʰ **S61.347** Puncture wound with foreign body of left little finger with damage to nail

✓7ᵗʰ **S61.348** Puncture wound with foreign body of other finger with damage to nail
Puncture wound with foreign body of specified finger with unspecified laterality with damage to nail

✓7ᵗʰ **S61.349** Puncture wound with foreign body of ▽ unspecified finger with damage to nail

✓6ᵗʰ **S61.35** Open bite of finger with damage to nail
Bite of finger with damage to nail NOS
EXCLUDES 1 superficial bite of finger (S60.46-, S60.47-)

✓7ᵗʰ **S61.350** Open bite of right index finger with damage to nail

✓7ᵗʰ **S61.351** Open bite of left index finger with damage to nail

✓7ᵗʰ **S61.352** Open bite of right middle finger with damage to nail

✓7ᵗʰ **S61.353** Open bite of left middle finger with damage to nail

✓7ᵗʰ **S61.354** Open bite of right ring finger with damage to nail

√7ᵗʰ **S61.355** **Open bite of** left ring **finger with damage to nail**

√7ᵗʰ **S61.356** **Open bite of** right little **finger with damage to nail**

√7ᵗʰ **S61.357** **Open bite of** left little **finger with damage to nail**

√7ᵗʰ **S61.358** **Open bite of other finger with damage to nail**
    Open bite of specified finger with unspecified laterality with damage to nail

√7ᵗʰ **S61.359** **Open bite of unspecified finger with damage to nail** ▽

√5ᵗʰ **S61.4** **Open wound of** hand

  √6ᵗʰ **S61.40** Unspecified **open wound of hand**

    √7ᵗʰ **S61.401** **Unspecified open wound of** right **hand** ▽

    √7ᵗʰ **S61.402** **Unspecified open wound of** left **hand** ▽

    √7ᵗʰ **S61.409** **Unspecified open wound of unspecified hand** ▽

  √6ᵗʰ **S61.41** Laceration without foreign body **of hand**

    √7ᵗʰ **S61.411** **Laceration without foreign body of** right **hand**

    √7ᵗʰ **S61.412** **Laceration without foreign body of** left **hand**

    √7ᵗʰ **S61.419** **Laceration without foreign body of unspecified hand** ▽

  √6ᵗʰ **S61.42** Laceration with foreign body **of hand**

    √7ᵗʰ **S61.421** **Laceration with foreign body of** right **hand**

    √7ᵗʰ **S61.422** **Laceration with foreign body of** left **hand**

    √7ᵗʰ **S61.429** **Laceration with foreign body of unspecified hand** ▽

  √6ᵗʰ **S61.43** Puncture wound without foreign body **of hand**

    √7ᵗʰ **S61.431** **Puncture wound without foreign body of** right **hand**

    √7ᵗʰ **S61.432** **Puncture wound without foreign body of** left **hand**

    √7ᵗʰ **S61.439** **Puncture wound without foreign body of unspecified hand** ▽

  √6ᵗʰ **S61.44** Puncture wound with foreign body **of hand**

    √7ᵗʰ **S61.441** **Puncture wound with foreign body of** right **hand**

    √7ᵗʰ **S61.442** **Puncture wound with foreign body of** left **hand**

    √7ᵗʰ **S61.449** **Puncture wound with foreign body of unspecified hand** ▽

  √6ᵗʰ **S61.45** Open bite **of hand**
     Bite of hand NOS
     EXCLUDES 1 superficial bite of hand (S60.56-, S60.57-)

    √7ᵗʰ **S61.451** **Open bite of** right **hand**

    √7ᵗʰ **S61.452** **Open bite of** left **hand**

    √7ᵗʰ **S61.459** **Open bite of unspecified hand** ▽

√5ᵗʰ **S61.5** **Open wound of** wrist

  √6ᵗʰ **S61.50** Unspecified **open wound of wrist**

    √7ᵗʰ **S61.501** **Unspecified open wound of** right **wrist** ▽

    √7ᵗʰ **S61.502** **Unspecified open wound of** left **wrist** ▽

    √7ᵗʰ **S61.509** **Unspecified open wound of unspecified wrist** ▽

  √6ᵗʰ **S61.51** Laceration without foreign body **of wrist**

    √7ᵗʰ **S61.511** **Laceration without foreign body of** right **wrist**

    √7ᵗʰ **S61.512** **Laceration without foreign body of** left **wrist**

    √7ᵗʰ **S61.519** **Laceration without foreign body of unspecified wrist** ▽

  √6ᵗʰ **S61.52** Laceration with foreign body **of wrist**

    √7ᵗʰ **S61.521** **Laceration with foreign body of** right **wrist**

    √7ᵗʰ **S61.522** **Laceration with foreign body of** left **wrist**

    √7ᵗʰ **S61.529** **Laceration with foreign body of unspecified wrist** ▽

  √6ᵗʰ **S61.53** Puncture wound without foreign body **of wrist**

    √7ᵗʰ **S61.531** **Puncture wound without foreign body of** right **wrist**

    √7ᵗʰ **S61.532** **Puncture wound without foreign body of** left **wrist**

    √7ᵗʰ **S61.539** **Puncture wound without foreign body of unspecified wrist** ▽

  √6ᵗʰ **S61.54** Puncture wound with foreign body **of wrist**

    √7ᵗʰ **S61.541** **Puncture wound with foreign body of** right **wrist**

    √7ᵗʰ **S61.542** **Puncture wound with foreign body of** left **wrist**

    √7ᵗʰ **S61.549** **Puncture wound with foreign body of unspecified wrist** ▽

  √6ᵗʰ **S61.55** Open bite **of wrist**
     Bite of wrist NOS
     EXCLUDES 1 superficial bite of wrist (S60.86-, S60.87-)

    √7ᵗʰ **S61.551** **Open bite of** right **wrist**

    √7ᵗʰ **S61.552** **Open bite of** left **wrist**

    √7ᵗʰ **S61.559** **Open bite of unspecified wrist** ▽

√4ᵗʰ **S62** **Fracture at wrist and hand level**
   NOTE A fracture not indicated as displaced or nondisplaced should be coded to displaced.
      A fracture not indicated as open or closed should be coded to closed.
   EXCLUDES 1 traumatic amputation of wrist and hand (S68.-)
   EXCLUDES 2 fracture of distal parts of ulna and radius (S52.-)

> The appropriate 7th character is to be added to each code from category S62.
> A   initial encounter for closed fracture
> B   initial encounter for open fracture
> D   subsequent encounter for fracture with routine healing
> G   subsequent encounter for fracture with delayed healing
> K   subsequent encounter for fracture with nonunion
> P   subsequent encounter for fracture with malunion
> S   sequela

√5ᵗʰ **S62.0** **Fracture of** navicular [scaphoid] bone of wrist

  √6ᵗʰ **S62.00** Unspecified **fracture of navicular [scaphoid] bone of wrist**

    √7ᵗʰ **S62.001** **Unspecified fracture of navicular [scaphoid] bone of** right **wrist** ▽

    √7ᵗʰ **S62.002** **Unspecified fracture of navicular [scaphoid] bone of** left **wrist** ▽
      AHA: 2012, 4Q, 106

    √7ᵗʰ **S62.009** **Unspecified fracture of navicular [scaphoid] bone of unspecified wrist** ▽

  √6ᵗʰ **S62.01** Fracture of distal pole of navicular [scaphoid] bone of wrist
     Fracture of volar tuberosity of navicular [scaphoid] bone of wrist

    √7ᵗʰ **S62.011** **Displaced fracture of distal pole of navicular [scaphoid] bone of** right **wrist**

    √7ᵗʰ **S62.012** **Displaced fracture of distal pole of navicular [scaphoid] bone of** left **wrist**

    √7ᵗʰ **S62.013** **Displaced fracture of distal pole of navicular [scaphoid] bone of unspecified wrist** ▽

    √7ᵗʰ **S62.014** **Nondisplaced fracture of distal pole of navicular [scaphoid] bone of** right **wrist**

    √7ᵗʰ **S62.015** **Nondisplaced fracture of distal pole of navicular [scaphoid] bone of** left **wrist**

    √7ᵗʰ **S62.016** **Nondisplaced fracture of distal pole of navicular [scaphoid] bone of unspecified wrist** ▽

  √6ᵗʰ **S62.02** Fracture of middle third of navicular [scaphoid] bone of wrist

    √7ᵗʰ **S62.021** **Displaced fracture of middle third of navicular [scaphoid] bone of** right **wrist**

    √7ᵗʰ **S62.022** **Displaced fracture of middle third of navicular [scaphoid] bone of** left **wrist**

    √7ᵗʰ **S62.023** **Displaced fracture of middle third of navicular [scaphoid] bone of unspecified wrist** ▽

    √7ᵗʰ **S62.024** **Nondisplaced fracture of middle third of navicular [scaphoid] bone of** right **wrist**

    √7ᵗʰ **S62.025** **Nondisplaced fracture of middle third of navicular [scaphoid] bone of** left **wrist**

✓ Add'l Character Required   ✓ₓ7ᵗʰ Placeholder Alert   ▨ RUG IV Special Care High Dx   RUG IV Clinically Complex Dx   ▨ RUG IV Special Care Low Dx   Manifestation Code   Other Specified Code   ▽ Unspecified Code

ICD-10-CM 2016   925

√7ᵗʰ **S62.026** Nondisplaced fracture of middle third of navicular [scaphoid] bone of unspecified wrist ▽

√6ᵗʰ **S62.03** Fracture of proximal third of navicular [scaphoid] bone of wrist

     √7ᵗʰ **S62.031** Displaced fracture of proximal third of navicular [scaphoid] bone of right wrist

     √7ᵗʰ **S62.032** Displaced fracture of proximal third of navicular [scaphoid] bone of left wrist

     √7ᵗʰ **S62.033** Displaced fracture of proximal third of navicular [scaphoid] bone of unspecified wrist ▽

     √7ᵗʰ **S62.034** Nondisplaced fracture of proximal third of navicular [scaphoid] bone of right wrist

     √7ᵗʰ **S62.035** Nondisplaced fracture of proximal third of navicular [scaphoid] bone of left wrist

     √7ᵗʰ **S62.036** Nondisplaced fracture of proximal third of navicular [scaphoid] bone of unspecified wrist ▽

√5ᵗʰ **S62.1** Fracture of other and unspecified carpal bone(s)
     EXCLUDES 2 *fracture of scaphoid of wrist (S62.0-)*

     √6ᵗʰ **S62.10** Fracture of unspecified carpal bone
         Fracture of wrist NOS

         √7ᵗʰ **S62.101** Fracture of unspecified carpal bone, right wrist ▽

         √7ᵗʰ **S62.102** Fracture of unspecified carpal bone, left wrist ▽
             AHA: 2012, 4Q, 95

         √7ᵗʰ **S62.109** Fracture of unspecified carpal bone, unspecified wrist ▽

     √6ᵗʰ **S62.11** Fracture of triquetrum [cuneiform] bone of wrist

         √7ᵗʰ **S62.111** Displaced fracture of triquetrum [cuneiform] bone, right wrist

         √7ᵗʰ **S62.112** Displaced fracture of triquetrum [cuneiform] bone, left wrist

         √7ᵗʰ **S62.113** Displaced fracture of triquetrum [cuneiform] bone, unspecified wrist ▽

         √7ᵗʰ **S62.114** Nondisplaced fracture of triquetrum [cuneiform] bone, right wrist

         √7ᵗʰ **S62.115** Nondisplaced fracture of triquetrum [cuneiform] bone, left wrist

         √7ᵗʰ **S62.116** Nondisplaced fracture of triquetrum [cuneiform] bone, unspecified wrist ▽

     √6ᵗʰ **S62.12** Fracture of lunate [semilunar]

         √7ᵗʰ **S62.121** Displaced fracture of lunate [semilunar], right wrist

         √7ᵗʰ **S62.122** Displaced fracture of lunate [semilunar], left wrist

         √7ᵗʰ **S62.123** Displaced fracture of lunate [semilunar], unspecified wrist ▽

         √7ᵗʰ **S62.124** Nondisplaced fracture of lunate [semilunar], right wrist

         √7ᵗʰ **S62.125** Nondisplaced fracture of lunate [semilunar], left wrist

         √7ᵗʰ **S62.126** Nondisplaced fracture of lunate [semilunar], unspecified wrist ▽

     √6ᵗʰ **S62.13** Fracture of capitate [os magnum] bone

         √7ᵗʰ **S62.131** Displaced fracture of capitate [os magnum] bone, right wrist

         √7ᵗʰ **S62.132** Displaced fracture of capitate [os magnum] bone, left wrist

         √7ᵗʰ **S62.133** Displaced fracture of capitate [os magnum] bone, unspecified wrist ▽

         √7ᵗʰ **S62.134** Nondisplaced fracture of capitate [os magnum] bone, right wrist

         √7ᵗʰ **S62.135** Nondisplaced fracture of capitate [os magnum] bone, left wrist

         √7ᵗʰ **S62.136** Nondisplaced fracture of capitate [os magnum] bone, unspecified wrist ▽

     √6ᵗʰ **S62.14** Fracture of body of hamate [unciform] bone
         Fracture of hamate [unciform] bone NOS

         √7ᵗʰ **S62.141** Displaced fracture of body of hamate [unciform] bone, right wrist

         √7ᵗʰ **S62.142** Displaced fracture of body of hamate [unciform] bone, left wrist

√7ᵗʰ **S62.143** Displaced fracture of body of hamate [unciform] bone, unspecified wrist ▽

√7ᵗʰ **S62.144** Nondisplaced fracture of body of hamate [unciform] bone, right wrist

√7ᵗʰ **S62.145** Nondisplaced fracture of body of hamate [unciform] bone, left wrist

√7ᵗʰ **S62.146** Nondisplaced fracture of body of hamate [unciform] bone, unspecified wrist ▽

√6ᵗʰ **S62.15** Fracture of hook process of hamate [unciform] bone
     Fracture of unciform process of hamate [unciform] bone

     √7ᵗʰ **S62.151** Displaced fracture of hook process of hamate [unciform] bone, right wrist

     √7ᵗʰ **S62.152** Displaced fracture of hook process of hamate [unciform] bone, left wrist

     √7ᵗʰ **S62.153** Displaced fracture of hook process of hamate [unciform] bone, unspecified wrist ▽

     √7ᵗʰ **S62.154** Nondisplaced fracture of hook process of hamate [unciform] bone, right wrist

     √7ᵗʰ **S62.155** Nondisplaced fracture of hook process of hamate [unciform] bone, left wrist

     √7ᵗʰ **S62.156** Nondisplaced fracture of hook process of hamate [unciform] bone, unspecified wrist ▽

√6ᵗʰ **S62.16** Fracture of pisiform

     √7ᵗʰ **S62.161** Displaced fracture of pisiform, right wrist

     √7ᵗʰ **S62.162** Displaced fracture of pisiform, left wrist

     √7ᵗʰ **S62.163** Displaced fracture of pisiform, unspecified wrist ▽

     √7ᵗʰ **S62.164** Nondisplaced fracture of pisiform, right wrist

     √7ᵗʰ **S62.165** Nondisplaced fracture of pisiform, left wrist

     √7ᵗʰ **S62.166** Nondisplaced fracture of pisiform, unspecified wrist ▽

√6ᵗʰ **S62.17** Fracture of trapezium [larger multangular]

     √7ᵗʰ **S62.171** Displaced fracture of trapezium [larger multangular], right wrist

     √7ᵗʰ **S62.172** Displaced fracture of trapezium [larger multangular], left wrist

     √7ᵗʰ **S62.173** Displaced fracture of trapezium [larger multangular], unspecified wrist ▽

     √7ᵗʰ **S62.174** Nondisplaced fracture of trapezium [larger multangular], right wrist

     √7ᵗʰ **S62.175** Nondisplaced fracture of trapezium [larger multangular], left wrist

     √7ᵗʰ **S62.176** Nondisplaced fracture of trapezium [larger multangular], unspecified wrist ▽

√6ᵗʰ **S62.18** Fracture of trapezoid [smaller multangular]

     √7ᵗʰ **S62.181** Displaced fracture of trapezoid [smaller multangular], right wrist

     √7ᵗʰ **S62.182** Displaced fracture of trapezoid [smaller multangular], left wrist

     √7ᵗʰ **S62.183** Displaced fracture of trapezoid [smaller multangular], unspecified wrist ▽

     √7ᵗʰ **S62.184** Nondisplaced fracture of trapezoid [smaller multangular], right wrist

     √7ᵗʰ **S62.185** Nondisplaced fracture of trapezoid [smaller multangular], left wrist

     √7ᵗʰ **S62.186** Nondisplaced fracture of trapezoid [smaller multangular], unspecified wrist ▽

√5ᵗʰ **S62.2** Fracture of first metacarpal bone

     √6ᵗʰ **S62.20** Unspecified fracture of first metacarpal bone

         √7ᵗʰ **S62.201** Unspecified fracture of first metacarpal bone, right hand ▽

         √7ᵗʰ **S62.202** Unspecified fracture of first metacarpal bone, left hand ▽

         √7ᵗʰ **S62.209** Unspecified fracture of first metacarpal bone, unspecified hand ▽

     √6ᵗʰ **S62.21** Bennett's fracture

         √7ᵗʰ **S62.211** Bennett's fracture, right hand

         √7ᵗʰ **S62.212** Bennett's fracture, left hand

         √7ᵗʰ **S62.213** Bennett's fracture, unspecified hand ▽

N Newborn   P Pediatric   M Maternity   A Adult   **RIC** RIC Dx   **NC Dx** Noncancer Dx   **PDx** Primary Dx   **CC** RIC CC Condition   ►◄ Revised Text   ● New Code   ▲ Revised Code Title

✓6ᵗʰ **S62.22** Rolando's fracture

✓7ᵗʰ **S62.221** Displaced Rolando's fracture, right hand

✓7ᵗʰ **S62.222** Displaced Rolando's fracture, left hand

✓7ᵗʰ **S62.223** Displaced Rolando's fracture, unspecified hand ▽

✓7ᵗʰ **S62.224** Nondisplaced Rolando's fracture, right hand

✓7ᵗʰ **S62.225** Nondisplaced Rolando's fracture, left hand

✓7ᵗʰ **S62.226** Nondisplaced Rolando's fracture, unspecified hand ▽

✓6ᵗʰ **S62.23** Other fracture of base of first metacarpal bone

✓7ᵗʰ **S62.231** Other displaced fracture of base of first metacarpal bone, right hand

✓7ᵗʰ **S62.232** Other displaced fracture of base of first metacarpal bone, left hand

✓7ᵗʰ **S62.233** Other displaced fracture of base of first metacarpal bone, unspecified hand ▽

✓7ᵗʰ **S62.234** Other nondisplaced fracture of base of first metacarpal bone, right hand

✓7ᵗʰ **S62.235** Other nondisplaced fracture of base of first metacarpal bone, left hand

✓7ᵗʰ **S62.236** Other nondisplaced fracture of base of first metacarpal bone, unspecified hand ▽

✓6ᵗʰ **S62.24** Fracture of shaft of first metacarpal bone

✓7ᵗʰ **S62.241** Displaced fracture of shaft of first metacarpal bone, right hand

✓7ᵗʰ **S62.242** Displaced fracture of shaft of first metacarpal bone, left hand

✓7ᵗʰ **S62.243** Displaced fracture of shaft of first metacarpal bone, unspecified hand ▽

✓7ᵗʰ **S62.244** Nondisplaced fracture of shaft of first metacarpal bone, right hand

✓7ᵗʰ **S62.245** Nondisplaced fracture of shaft of first metacarpal bone, left hand

✓7ᵗʰ **S62.246** Nondisplaced fracture of shaft of first metacarpal bone, unspecified hand ▽

✓6ᵗʰ **S62.25** Fracture of neck of first metacarpal bone

✓7ᵗʰ **S62.251** Displaced fracture of neck of first metacarpal bone, right hand

✓7ᵗʰ **S62.252** Displaced fracture of neck of first metacarpal bone, left hand

✓7ᵗʰ **S62.253** Displaced fracture of neck of first metacarpal bone, unspecified hand ▽

✓7ᵗʰ **S62.254** Nondisplaced fracture of neck of first metacarpal bone, right hand

✓7ᵗʰ **S62.255** Nondisplaced fracture of neck of first metacarpal bone, left hand

✓7ᵗʰ **S62.256** Nondisplaced fracture of neck of first metacarpal bone, unspecified hand ▽

✓6ᵗʰ **S62.29** Other fracture of first metacarpal bone

✓7ᵗʰ **S62.291** Other fracture of first metacarpal bone, right hand

✓7ᵗʰ **S62.292** Other fracture of first metacarpal bone, left hand

✓7ᵗʰ **S62.299** Other fracture of first metacarpal bone, unspecified hand ▽

✓5ᵗʰ **S62.3** Fracture of other and unspecified metacarpal bone

EXCLUDES 2 fracture of first metacarpal bone (S62.2-)

✓6ᵗʰ **S62.30** Unspecified fracture of other metacarpal bone

✓7ᵗʰ **S62.300** Unspecified fracture of second metacarpal bone, right hand ▽

✓7ᵗʰ **S62.301** Unspecified fracture of second metacarpal bone, left hand ▽

✓7ᵗʰ **S62.302** Unspecified fracture of third metacarpal bone, right hand ▽

✓7ᵗʰ **S62.303** Unspecified fracture of third metacarpal bone, left hand ▽

✓7ᵗʰ **S62.304** Unspecified fracture of fourth metacarpal bone, right hand ▽

✓7ᵗʰ **S62.305** Unspecified fracture of fourth metacarpal bone, left hand ▽

✓7ᵗʰ **S62.306** Unspecified fracture of fifth metacarpal bone, right hand ▽

✓7ᵗʰ **S62.307** Unspecified fracture of fifth metacarpal bone, left hand ▽

✓7ᵗʰ **S62.308** Unspecified fracture of other metacarpal bone ▽
Unspecified fracture of specified metacarpal bone with unspecified laterality

✓7ᵗʰ **S62.309** Unspecified fracture of unspecified metacarpal bone ▽

✓6ᵗʰ **S62.31** Displaced fracture of base of other metacarpal bone

✓7ᵗʰ **S62.310** Displaced fracture of base of second metacarpal bone, right hand

✓7ᵗʰ **S62.311** Displaced fracture of base of second metacarpal bone, left hand

✓7ᵗʰ **S62.312** Displaced fracture of base of third metacarpal bone, right hand

✓7ᵗʰ **S62.313** Displaced fracture of base of third metacarpal bone, left hand

✓7ᵗʰ **S62.314** Displaced fracture of base of fourth metacarpal bone, right hand

✓7ᵗʰ **S62.315** Displaced fracture of base of fourth metacarpal bone, left hand

✓7ᵗʰ **S62.316** Displaced fracture of base of fifth metacarpal bone, right hand

✓7ᵗʰ **S62.317** Displaced fracture of base of fifth metacarpal bone, left hand

✓7ᵗʰ **S62.318** Displaced fracture of base of other metacarpal bone
Displaced fracture of base of specified metacarpal bone with unspecified laterality

✓7ᵗʰ **S62.319** Displaced fracture of base of unspecified metacarpal bone ▽

✓6ᵗʰ **S62.32** Displaced fracture of shaft of other metacarpal bone

✓7ᵗʰ **S62.320** Displaced fracture of shaft of second metacarpal bone, right hand

✓7ᵗʰ **S62.321** Displaced fracture of shaft of second metacarpal bone, left hand

✓7ᵗʰ **S62.322** Displaced fracture of shaft of third metacarpal bone, right hand

✓7ᵗʰ **S62.323** Displaced fracture of shaft of third metacarpal bone, left hand

✓7ᵗʰ **S62.324** Displaced fracture of shaft of fourth metacarpal bone, right hand

✓7ᵗʰ **S62.325** Displaced fracture of shaft of fourth metacarpal bone, left hand

✓7ᵗʰ **S62.326** Displaced fracture of shaft of fifth metacarpal bone, right hand

✓7ᵗʰ **S62.327** Displaced fracture of shaft of fifth metacarpal bone, left hand

✓7ᵗʰ **S62.328** Displaced fracture of shaft of other metacarpal bone
Displaced fracture of shaft of specified metacarpal bone with unspecified laterality

✓7ᵗʰ **S62.329** Displaced fracture of shaft of unspecified metacarpal bone ▽

✓6ᵗʰ **S62.33** Displaced fracture of neck of other metacarpal bone

✓7ᵗʰ **S62.330** Displaced fracture of neck of second metacarpal bone, right hand

✓7ᵗʰ **S62.331** Displaced fracture of neck of second metacarpal bone, left hand

✓7ᵗʰ **S62.332** Displaced fracture of neck of third metacarpal bone, right hand

✓7ᵗʰ **S62.333** Displaced fracture of neck of third metacarpal bone, left hand

✓7ᵗʰ **S62.334** Displaced fracture of neck of fourth metacarpal bone, right hand

✓7ᵗʰ **S62.335** Displaced fracture of neck of fourth metacarpal bone, left hand

✓7ᵗʰ **S62.336** Displaced fracture of neck of fifth metacarpal bone, right hand

✓7ᵗʰ **S62.337** Displaced fracture of neck of fifth metacarpal bone, left hand

☑ Add'l Character Required ✓x7ᵗʰ Placeholder Alert RUG IV Special Care High Dx RUG IV Clinically Complex Dx RUG IV Special Care Low Dx Manifestation Code Other Specified Code ▽ Unspecified Code

ICD-10-CM 2016   927

√7ᵗʰ **S62.338 Displaced fracture of neck of other metacarpal bone**
Displaced fracture of neck of specified metacarpal bone with unspecified laterality

√7ᵗʰ **S62.339 Displaced fracture of neck of unspecified metacarpal bone** ▽

√6ᵗʰ **S62.34 Nondisplaced fracture of base of other metacarpal bone**

√7ᵗʰ **S62.340 Nondisplaced fracture of base of second metacarpal bone, right hand**

√7ᵗʰ **S62.341 Nondisplaced fracture of base of second metacarpal bone, left hand**

√7ᵗʰ **S62.342 Nondisplaced fracture of base of third metacarpal bone, right hand**

√7ᵗʰ **S62.343 Nondisplaced fracture of base of third metacarpal bone, left hand**

√7ᵗʰ **S62.344 Nondisplaced fracture of base of fourth metacarpal bone, right hand**

√7ᵗʰ **S62.345 Nondisplaced fracture of base of fourth metacarpal bone, left hand**

√7ᵗʰ **S62.346 Nondisplaced fracture of base of fifth metacarpal bone, right hand**

√7ᵗʰ **S62.347 Nondisplaced fracture of base of fifth metacarpal bone, left hand**

√7ᵗʰ **S62.348 Nondisplaced fracture of base of other metacarpal bone**
Nondisplaced fracture of base of specified metacarpal bone with unspecified laterality

√7ᵗʰ **S62.349 Nondisplaced fracture of base of unspecified metacarpal bone** ▽

√6ᵗʰ **S62.35 Nondisplaced fracture of shaft of other metacarpal bone**

√7ᵗʰ **S62.350 Nondisplaced fracture of shaft of second metacarpal bone, right hand**

√7ᵗʰ **S62.351 Nondisplaced fracture of shaft of second metacarpal bone, left hand**

√7ᵗʰ **S62.352 Nondisplaced fracture of shaft of third metacarpal bone, right hand**

√7ᵗʰ **S62.353 Nondisplaced fracture of shaft of third metacarpal bone, left hand**

√7ᵗʰ **S62.354 Nondisplaced fracture of shaft of fourth metacarpal bone, right hand**

√7ᵗʰ **S62.355 Nondisplaced fracture of shaft of fourth metacarpal bone, left hand**

√7ᵗʰ **S62.356 Nondisplaced fracture of shaft of fifth metacarpal bone, right hand**

√7ᵗʰ **S62.357 Nondisplaced fracture of shaft of fifth metacarpal bone, left hand**

√7ᵗʰ **S62.358 Nondisplaced fracture of shaft of other metacarpal bone**
Nondisplaced fracture of shaft of specified metacarpal bone with unspecified laterality

√7ᵗʰ **S62.359 Nondisplaced fracture of shaft of unspecified metacarpal bone** ▽

√6ᵗʰ **S62.36 Nondisplaced fracture of neck of other metacarpal bone**

√7ᵗʰ **S62.360 Nondisplaced fracture of neck of second metacarpal bone, right hand**

√7ᵗʰ **S62.361 Nondisplaced fracture of neck of second metacarpal bone, left hand**

√7ᵗʰ **S62.362 Nondisplaced fracture of neck of third metacarpal bone, right hand**

√7ᵗʰ **S62.363 Nondisplaced fracture of neck of third metacarpal bone, left hand**

√7ᵗʰ **S62.364 Nondisplaced fracture of neck of fourth metacarpal bone, right hand**

√7ᵗʰ **S62.365 Nondisplaced fracture of neck of fourth metacarpal bone, left hand**

√7ᵗʰ **S62.366 Nondisplaced fracture of neck of fifth metacarpal bone, right hand**

√7ᵗʰ **S62.367 Nondisplaced fracture of neck of fifth metacarpal bone, left hand**

√7ᵗʰ **S62.368 Nondisplaced fracture of neck of other metacarpal bone**
Nondisplaced fracture of neck of specified metacarpal bone with unspecified laterality

√7ᵗʰ **S62.369 Nondisplaced fracture of neck of unspecified metacarpal bone** ▽

√6ᵗʰ **S62.39 Other fracture of other metacarpal bone**

√7ᵗʰ **S62.390 Other fracture of second metacarpal bone, right hand**

√7ᵗʰ **S62.391 Other fracture of second metacarpal bone, left hand**

√7ᵗʰ **S62.392 Other fracture of third metacarpal bone, right hand**

√7ᵗʰ **S62.393 Other fracture of third metacarpal bone, left hand**

√7ᵗʰ **S62.394 Other fracture of fourth metacarpal bone, right hand**

√7ᵗʰ **S62.395 Other fracture of fourth metacarpal bone, left hand**

√7ᵗʰ **S62.396 Other fracture of fifth metacarpal bone, right hand**

√7ᵗʰ **S62.397 Other fracture of fifth metacarpal bone, left hand**

√7ᵗʰ **S62.398 Other fracture of other metacarpal bone**
Other fracture of specified metacarpal bone with unspecified laterality

√7ᵗʰ **S62.399 Other fracture of unspecified metacarpal bone** ▽

√5ᵗʰ **S62.5 Fracture of thumb**

√6ᵗʰ **S62.50 Fracture of unspecified phalanx of thumb**

√7ᵗʰ **S62.501 Fracture of unspecified phalanx of right thumb** ▽

√7ᵗʰ **S62.502 Fracture of unspecified phalanx of left thumb** ▽

√7ᵗʰ **S62.509 Fracture of unspecified phalanx of unspecified thumb** ▽

√6ᵗʰ **S62.51 Fracture of proximal phalanx of thumb**

√7ᵗʰ **S62.511 Displaced fracture of proximal phalanx of right thumb**

√7ᵗʰ **S62.512 Displaced fracture of proximal phalanx of left thumb**

√7ᵗʰ **S62.513 Displaced fracture of proximal phalanx of unspecified thumb** ▽

√7ᵗʰ **S62.514 Nondisplaced fracture of proximal phalanx of right thumb**

√7ᵗʰ **S62.515 Nondisplaced fracture of proximal phalanx of left thumb**

√7ᵗʰ **S62.516 Nondisplaced fracture of proximal phalanx of unspecified thumb** ▽

√6ᵗʰ **S62.52 Fracture of distal phalanx of thumb**

√7ᵗʰ **S62.521 Displaced fracture of distal phalanx of right thumb**

√7ᵗʰ **S62.522 Displaced fracture of distal phalanx of left thumb**

√7ᵗʰ **S62.523 Displaced fracture of distal phalanx of unspecified thumb** ▽

√7ᵗʰ **S62.524 Nondisplaced fracture of distal phalanx of right thumb**

√7ᵗʰ **S62.525 Nondisplaced fracture of distal phalanx of left thumb**

√7ᵗʰ **S62.526 Nondisplaced fracture of distal phalanx of unspecified thumb** ▽

√5ᵗʰ **S62.6 Fracture of other and unspecified finger(s)**
EXCLUDES 2 fracture of thumb (S62.5-)

√6ᵗʰ **S62.60 Fracture of unspecified phalanx of finger**

√7ᵗʰ **S62.600 Fracture of unspecified phalanx of right index finger** ▽

√7ᵗʰ **S62.601 Fracture of unspecified phalanx of left index finger** ▽

√7ᵗʰ **S62.602 Fracture of unspecified phalanx of right middle finger** ▽

√7ᵗʰ **S62.603 Fracture of unspecified phalanx of left middle finger** ▽

Ⓝ Newborn   Ⓟ Pediatric   Ⓜ Maternity   Ⓐ Adult   **RIC** RIC Dx   **NC Dx** Noncancer Dx   **PDx** Primary Dx   **CC** RIC CC Condition   ►◄ Revised Text   ● New Code   ▲ Revised Code Title

928   ICD-10-CM 2016

✓7ᵗʰ **S62.604** Fracture of unspecified phalanx of right ▽ ring finger

✓7ᵗʰ **S62.605** Fracture of unspecified phalanx of left ▽ ring finger

✓7ᵗʰ **S62.606** Fracture of unspecified phalanx of right ▽ little finger

✓7ᵗʰ **S62.607** Fracture of unspecified phalanx of left ▽ little finger

✓7ᵗʰ **S62.608** Fracture of unspecified phalanx of ▽ other finger
    Fracture of unspecified phalanx of specified finger with unspecified laterality

✓7ᵗʰ **S62.609** Fracture of unspecified phalanx of ▽ unspecified finger

✓6ᵗʰ **S62.61** Displaced fracture of proximal phalanx of finger

✓7ᵗʰ **S62.610** Displaced fracture of proximal phalanx of right index finger

✓7ᵗʰ **S62.611** Displaced fracture of proximal phalanx of left index finger

✓7ᵗʰ **S62.612** Displaced fracture of proximal phalanx of right middle finger

✓7ᵗʰ **S62.613** Displaced fracture of proximal phalanx of left middle finger

✓7ᵗʰ **S62.614** Displaced fracture of proximal phalanx of right ring finger

✓7ᵗʰ **S62.615** Displaced fracture of proximal phalanx of left ring finger

✓7ᵗʰ **S62.616** Displaced fracture of proximal phalanx of right little finger

✓7ᵗʰ **S62.617** Displaced fracture of proximal phalanx of left little finger

✓7ᵗʰ **S62.618** Displaced fracture of proximal phalanx of other finger
    Displaced fracture of proximal phalanx of specified finger with unspecified laterality

✓7ᵗʰ **S62.619** Displaced fracture of proximal ▽ phalanx of unspecified finger

✓6ᵗʰ **S62.62** Displaced fracture of medial phalanx of finger

✓7ᵗʰ **S62.620** Displaced fracture of medial phalanx of right index finger

✓7ᵗʰ **S62.621** Displaced fracture of medial phalanx of left index finger

✓7ᵗʰ **S62.622** Displaced fracture of medial phalanx of right middle finger

✓7ᵗʰ **S62.623** Displaced fracture of medial phalanx of left middle finger

✓7ᵗʰ **S62.624** Displaced fracture of medial phalanx of right ring finger

✓7ᵗʰ **S62.625** Displaced fracture of medial phalanx of left ring finger

✓7ᵗʰ **S62.626** Displaced fracture of medial phalanx of right little finger

✓7ᵗʰ **S62.627** Displaced fracture of medial phalanx of left little finger

✓7ᵗʰ **S62.628** Displaced fracture of medial phalanx of other finger
    Displaced fracture of medial phalanx of specified finger with unspecified laterality

✓7ᵗʰ **S62.629** Displaced fracture of medial phalanx ▽ of unspecified finger

✓6ᵗʰ **S62.63** Displaced fracture of distal phalanx of finger

✓7ᵗʰ **S62.630** Displaced fracture of distal phalanx of right index finger

✓7ᵗʰ **S62.631** Displaced fracture of distal phalanx of left index finger

✓7ᵗʰ **S62.632** Displaced fracture of distal phalanx of right middle finger

✓7ᵗʰ **S62.633** Displaced fracture of distal phalanx of left middle finger

✓7ᵗʰ **S62.634** Displaced fracture of distal phalanx of right ring finger

✓7ᵗʰ **S62.635** Displaced fracture of distal phalanx of left ring finger

✓7ᵗʰ **S62.636** Displaced fracture of distal phalanx of right little finger

✓7ᵗʰ **S62.637** Displaced fracture of distal phalanx of left little finger

✓7ᵗʰ **S62.638** Displaced fracture of distal phalanx of other finger
    Displaced fracture of distal phalanx of specified finger with unspecified laterality

✓7ᵗʰ **S62.639** Displaced fracture of distal phalanx of ▽ unspecified finger

✓6ᵗʰ **S62.64** Nondisplaced fracture of proximal phalanx of finger

✓7ᵗʰ **S62.640** Nondisplaced fracture of proximal phalanx of right index finger

✓7ᵗʰ **S62.641** Nondisplaced fracture of proximal phalanx of left index finger

✓7ᵗʰ **S62.642** Nondisplaced fracture of proximal phalanx of right middle finger

✓7ᵗʰ **S62.643** Nondisplaced fracture of proximal phalanx of left middle finger

✓7ᵗʰ **S62.644** Nondisplaced fracture of proximal phalanx of right ring finger

✓7ᵗʰ **S62.645** Nondisplaced fracture of proximal phalanx of left ring finger

✓7ᵗʰ **S62.646** Nondisplaced fracture of proximal phalanx of right little finger

✓7ᵗʰ **S62.647** Nondisplaced fracture of proximal phalanx of left little finger

✓7ᵗʰ **S62.648** Nondisplaced fracture of proximal phalanx of other finger
    Nondisplaced fracture of proximal phalanx of specified finger with unspecified laterality

✓7ᵗʰ **S62.649** Nondisplaced fracture of proximal ▽ phalanx of unspecified finger

✓6ᵗʰ **S62.65** Nondisplaced fracture of medial phalanx of finger

✓7ᵗʰ **S62.650** Nondisplaced fracture of medial phalanx of right index finger

✓7ᵗʰ **S62.651** Nondisplaced fracture of medial phalanx of left index finger

✓7ᵗʰ **S62.652** Nondisplaced fracture of medial phalanx of right middle finger

✓7ᵗʰ **S62.653** Nondisplaced fracture of medial phalanx of left middle finger

✓7ᵗʰ **S62.654** Nondisplaced fracture of medial phalanx of right ring finger

✓7ᵗʰ **S62.655** Nondisplaced fracture of medial phalanx of left ring finger

✓7ᵗʰ **S62.656** Nondisplaced fracture of medial phalanx of right little finger

✓7ᵗʰ **S62.657** Nondisplaced fracture of medial phalanx of left little finger

✓7ᵗʰ **S62.658** Nondisplaced fracture of medial phalanx of other finger
    Nondisplaced fracture of medial phalanx of specified finger with unspecified laterality

✓7ᵗʰ **S62.659** Nondisplaced fracture of medial ▽ phalanx of unspecified finger

✓6ᵗʰ **S62.66** Nondisplaced fracture of distal phalanx of finger

✓7ᵗʰ **S62.660** Nondisplaced fracture of distal phalanx of right index finger

✓7ᵗʰ **S62.661** Nondisplaced fracture of distal phalanx of left index finger

✓7ᵗʰ **S62.662** Nondisplaced fracture of distal phalanx of right middle finger

✓7ᵗʰ **S62.663** Nondisplaced fracture of distal phalanx of left middle finger

✓7ᵗʰ **S62.664** Nondisplaced fracture of distal phalanx of right ring finger

✓7ᵗʰ **S62.665** Nondisplaced fracture of distal phalanx of left ring finger

✓7ᵗʰ **S62.666** Nondisplaced fracture of distal phalanx of right little finger

---

√7ᵗʰ **S62.667** **Nondisplaced fracture of distal phalanx of left little finger**

√7ᵗʰ **S62.668** **Nondisplaced fracture of distal phalanx of other finger**
Nondisplaced fracture of distal phalanx of specified finger with unspecified laterality

√7ᵗʰ **S62.669** **Nondisplaced fracture of distal phalanx of unspecified finger** ▽

√5ᵗʰ **S62.9** **Unspecified fracture of wrist and hand**

√x7ᵗʰ **S62.90** **Unspecified fracture of unspecified wrist and hand** ▽

√x7ᵗʰ **S62.91** **Unspecified fracture of right wrist and hand** ▽

√x7ᵗʰ **S62.92** **Unspecified fracture of left wrist and hand** ▽

√4ᵗʰ **S63** **Dislocation and sprain of joints and ligaments at wrist and hand level**

INCLUDES avulsion of joint or ligament at wrist and hand level
laceration of cartilage, joint or ligament at wrist and hand level
sprain of cartilage, joint or ligament at wrist and hand level
traumatic hemarthrosis of joint or ligament at wrist and hand level
traumatic rupture of joint or ligament at wrist and hand level
traumatic subluxation of joint or ligament at wrist and hand level
traumatic tear of joint or ligament at wrist and hand level

Code also any associated open wound
EXCLUDES 2 strain of muscle, fascia and tendon of wrist and hand (S66.-)

The appropriate 7th character is to be added to each code from category S63.
A   initial encounter
D   subsequent encounter
S   sequela

√5ᵗʰ **S63.0** **Subluxation and dislocation of wrist and hand joints**

√6ᵗʰ **S63.00** **Unspecified subluxation and dislocation of wrist and hand**
Dislocation of carpal bone NOS
Dislocation of distal end of radius NOS
Subluxation of carpal bone NOS
Subluxation of distal end of radius NOS

√7ᵗʰ **S63.001** **Unspecified subluxation of right wrist and hand** ▽

√7ᵗʰ **S63.002** **Unspecified subluxation of left wrist and hand** ▽

√7ᵗʰ **S63.003** **Unspecified subluxation of unspecified wrist and hand** ▽

√7ᵗʰ **S63.004** **Unspecified dislocation of right wrist and hand** ▽

√7ᵗʰ **S63.005** **Unspecified dislocation of left wrist and hand** ▽

√7ᵗʰ **S63.006** **Unspecified dislocation of unspecified wrist and hand** ▽

√6ᵗʰ **S63.01** **Subluxation and dislocation of distal radioulnar joint**

√7ᵗʰ **S63.011** Subluxation of distal radioulnar joint of right wrist

√7ᵗʰ **S63.012** Subluxation of distal radioulnar joint of left wrist

√7ᵗʰ **S63.013** Subluxation of distal radioulnar joint of unspecified wrist ▽

√7ᵗʰ **S63.014** Dislocation of distal radioulnar joint of right wrist

√7ᵗʰ **S63.015** Dislocation of distal radioulnar joint of left wrist

√7ᵗʰ **S63.016** Dislocation of distal radioulnar joint of unspecified wrist ▽

√6ᵗʰ **S63.02** **Subluxation and dislocation of radiocarpal joint**

√7ᵗʰ **S63.021** Subluxation of radiocarpal joint of right wrist

√7ᵗʰ **S63.022** Subluxation of radiocarpal joint of left wrist

√7ᵗʰ **S63.023** Subluxation of radiocarpal joint of unspecified wrist ▽

√7ᵗʰ **S63.024** Dislocation of radiocarpal joint of right wrist

√7ᵗʰ **S63.025** Dislocation of radiocarpal joint of left wrist

√7ᵗʰ **S63.026** Dislocation of radiocarpal joint of unspecified wrist ▽

√6ᵗʰ **S63.03** **Subluxation and dislocation of midcarpal joint**

√7ᵗʰ **S63.031** Subluxation of midcarpal joint of right wrist

√7ᵗʰ **S63.032** Subluxation of midcarpal joint of left wrist

√7ᵗʰ **S63.033** Subluxation of midcarpal joint of unspecified wrist ▽

√7ᵗʰ **S63.034** Dislocation of midcarpal joint of right wrist

√7ᵗʰ **S63.035** Dislocation of midcarpal joint of left wrist

√7ᵗʰ **S63.036** Dislocation of midcarpal joint of unspecified wrist ▽

√6ᵗʰ **S63.04** **Subluxation and dislocation of carpometacarpal joint of thumb**
EXCLUDES 2 interphalangeal subluxation and dislocation of thumb (S63.1-)

√7ᵗʰ **S63.041** Subluxation of carpometacarpal joint of right thumb

√7ᵗʰ **S63.042** Subluxation of carpometacarpal joint of left thumb

√7ᵗʰ **S63.043** Subluxation of carpometacarpal joint of unspecified thumb ▽

√7ᵗʰ **S63.044** Dislocation of carpometacarpal joint of right thumb

√7ᵗʰ **S63.045** Dislocation of carpometacarpal joint of left thumb

√7ᵗʰ **S63.046** Dislocation of carpometacarpal joint of unspecified thumb ▽

√6ᵗʰ **S63.05** **Subluxation and dislocation of other carpometacarpal joint**
EXCLUDES 2 subluxation and dislocation of carpometacarpal joint of thumb (S63.04-)

√7ᵗʰ **S63.051** Subluxation of other carpometacarpal joint of right hand

√7ᵗʰ **S63.052** Subluxation of other carpometacarpal joint of left hand

√7ᵗʰ **S63.053** Subluxation of other carpometacarpal joint of unspecified hand ▽

√7ᵗʰ **S63.054** Dislocation of other carpometacarpal joint of right hand

√7ᵗʰ **S63.055** Dislocation of other carpometacarpal joint of left hand

√7ᵗʰ **S63.056** Dislocation of other carpometacarpal joint of unspecified hand ▽

√6ᵗʰ **S63.06** **Subluxation and dislocation of metacarpal (bone), proximal end**

√7ᵗʰ **S63.061** Subluxation of metacarpal (bone), proximal end of right hand

√7ᵗʰ **S63.062** Subluxation of metacarpal (bone), proximal end of left hand

√7ᵗʰ **S63.063** Subluxation of metacarpal (bone), proximal end of unspecified hand ▽

√7ᵗʰ **S63.064** Dislocation of metacarpal (bone), proximal end of right hand

√7ᵗʰ **S63.065** Dislocation of metacarpal (bone), proximal end of left hand

√7ᵗʰ **S63.066** Dislocation of metacarpal (bone), proximal end of unspecified hand ▽

√6ᵗʰ **S63.07** **Subluxation and dislocation of distal end of ulna**

√7ᵗʰ **S63.071** Subluxation of distal end of right ulna

√7ᵗʰ **S63.072** Subluxation of distal end of left ulna

√7ᵗʰ **S63.073** Subluxation of distal end of unspecified ulna ▽

√7ᵗʰ **S63.074** Dislocation of distal end of right ulna

√7ᵗʰ **S63.075** Dislocation of distal end of left ulna

√7ᵗʰ **S63.076** Dislocation of distal end of unspecified ulna ▽

√6ᵗʰ **S63.09** **Other subluxation and dislocation of wrist and hand**

√7ᵗʰ **S63.091** **Other subluxation of right wrist and hand**

√7ᵗʰ **S63.092** **Other subluxation of left wrist and hand**

Ⓝ Newborn　Ⓟ Pediatric　Ⓜ Maternity　Ⓐ Adult　RIC RIC Dx　NCDx Noncancer Dx　PDx Primary Dx　CC RIC CC Condition　▶◀ Revised Text　● New Code　▲ Revised Code Title

☑7ᵗʰ **S63.093** **Other subluxation of unspecified wrist and hand** ▽

☑7ᵗʰ **S63.094** **Other dislocation of right wrist and hand**

☑7ᵗʰ **S63.095** **Other dislocation of left wrist and hand**

☑7ᵗʰ **S63.096** **Other dislocation of unspecified wrist and hand** ▽

√5ᵗʰ **S63.1** **Subluxation and dislocation of thumb**

√6ᵗʰ **S63.10** **Unspecified subluxation and dislocation of thumb**

☑7ᵗʰ **S63.101** **Unspecified subluxation of right thumb** ▽

☑7ᵗʰ **S63.102** **Unspecified subluxation of left thumb** ▽

☑7ᵗʰ **S63.103** **Unspecified subluxation of unspecified thumb** ▽

☑7ᵗʰ **S63.104** **Unspecified dislocation of right thumb** ▽

☑7ᵗʰ **S63.105** **Unspecified dislocation of left thumb** ▽

☑7ᵗʰ **S63.106** **Unspecified dislocation of unspecified thumb** ▽

√6ᵗʰ **S63.11** **Subluxation and dislocation of metacarpophalangeal joint of thumb**

☑7ᵗʰ **S63.111** **Subluxation of metacarpophalangeal joint of right thumb**

☑7ᵗʰ **S63.112** **Subluxation of metacarpophalangeal joint of left thumb**

☑7ᵗʰ **S63.113** **Subluxation of metacarpophalangeal joint of unspecified thumb** ▽

☑7ᵗʰ **S63.114** **Dislocation of metacarpophalangeal joint of right thumb**

☑7ᵗʰ **S63.115** **Dislocation of metacarpophalangeal joint of left thumb**

☑7ᵗʰ **S63.116** **Dislocation of metacarpophalangeal joint of unspecified thumb** ▽

√6ᵗʰ **S63.12** **Subluxation and dislocation of unspecified interphalangeal joint of thumb**

☑7ᵗʰ **S63.121** **Subluxation of unspecified interphalangeal joint of right thumb** ▽

☑7ᵗʰ **S63.122** **Subluxation of unspecified interphalangeal joint of left thumb** ▽

☑7ᵗʰ **S63.123** **Subluxation of unspecified interphalangeal joint of unspecified thumb** ▽

☑7ᵗʰ **S63.124** **Dislocation of unspecified interphalangeal joint of right thumb** ▽

☑7ᵗʰ **S63.125** **Dislocation of unspecified interphalangeal joint of left thumb** ▽

☑7ᵗʰ **S63.126** **Dislocation of unspecified interphalangeal joint of unspecified thumb** ▽

√6ᵗʰ **S63.13** **Subluxation and dislocation of proximal interphalangeal joint of thumb**

☑7ᵗʰ **S63.131** **Subluxation of proximal interphalangeal joint of right thumb**

☑7ᵗʰ **S63.132** **Subluxation of proximal interphalangeal joint of left thumb**

☑7ᵗʰ **S63.133** **Subluxation of proximal interphalangeal joint of unspecified thumb** ▽

☑7ᵗʰ **S63.134** **Dislocation of proximal interphalangeal joint of right thumb**

☑7ᵗʰ **S63.135** **Dislocation of proximal interphalangeal joint of left thumb**

☑7ᵗʰ **S63.136** **Dislocation of proximal interphalangeal joint of unspecified thumb** ▽

√6ᵗʰ **S63.14** **Subluxation and dislocation of distal interphalangeal joint of thumb**

☑7ᵗʰ **S63.141** **Subluxation of distal interphalangeal joint of right thumb**

☑7ᵗʰ **S63.142** **Subluxation of distal interphalangeal joint of left thumb**

☑7ᵗʰ **S63.143** **Subluxation of distal interphalangeal joint of unspecified thumb** ▽

☑7ᵗʰ **S63.144** **Dislocation of distal interphalangeal joint of right thumb**

☑7ᵗʰ **S63.145** **Dislocation of distal interphalangeal joint of left thumb**

☑7ᵗʰ **S63.146** **Dislocation of distal interphalangeal joint of unspecified thumb** ▽

√5ᵗʰ **S63.2** **Subluxation and dislocation of other finger(s)**

EXCLUDES 2 subluxation and dislocation of thumb (S63.1-)

√6ᵗʰ **S63.20** **Unspecified subluxation of other finger**

☑7ᵗʰ **S63.200** **Unspecified subluxation of right index finger** ▽

☑7ᵗʰ **S63.201** **Unspecified subluxation of left index finger** ▽

☑7ᵗʰ **S63.202** **Unspecified subluxation of right middle finger** ▽

☑7ᵗʰ **S63.203** **Unspecified subluxation of left middle finger** ▽

☑7ᵗʰ **S63.204** **Unspecified subluxation of right ring finger** ▽

☑7ᵗʰ **S63.205** **Unspecified subluxation of left ring finger** ▽

☑7ᵗʰ **S63.206** **Unspecified subluxation of right little finger** ▽

☑7ᵗʰ **S63.207** **Unspecified subluxation of left little finger** ▽

☑7ᵗʰ **S63.208** **Unspecified subluxation of other finger** ▽
Unspecified subluxation of specified finger with unspecified laterality

☑7ᵗʰ **S63.209** **Unspecified subluxation of unspecified finger** ▽

√6ᵗʰ **S63.21** **Subluxation of metacarpophalangeal joint of finger**

☑7ᵗʰ **S63.210** **Subluxation of metacarpophalangeal joint of right index finger**

☑7ᵗʰ **S63.211** **Subluxation of metacarpophalangeal joint of left index finger**

☑7ᵗʰ **S63.212** **Subluxation of metacarpophalangeal joint of right middle finger**

☑7ᵗʰ **S63.213** **Subluxation of metacarpophalangeal joint of left middle finger**

☑7ᵗʰ **S63.214** **Subluxation of metacarpophalangeal joint of right ring finger**

☑7ᵗʰ **S63.215** **Subluxation of metacarpophalangeal joint of left ring finger**

☑7ᵗʰ **S63.216** **Subluxation of metacarpophalangeal joint of right little finger**

☑7ᵗʰ **S63.217** **Subluxation of metacarpophalangeal joint of left little finger**

☑7ᵗʰ **S63.218** **Subluxation of metacarpophalangeal joint of other finger**
Subluxation of metacarpophalangeal joint of specified finger with unspecified laterality

☑7ᵗʰ **S63.219** **Subluxation of metacarpophalangeal joint of unspecified finger** ▽

√6ᵗʰ **S63.22** **Subluxation of unspecified interphalangeal joint of finger**

☑7ᵗʰ **S63.220** **Subluxation of unspecified interphalangeal joint of right index finger** ▽

☑7ᵗʰ **S63.221** **Subluxation of unspecified interphalangeal joint of left index finger** ▽

☑7ᵗʰ **S63.222** **Subluxation of unspecified interphalangeal joint of right middle finger** ▽

☑7ᵗʰ **S63.223** **Subluxation of unspecified interphalangeal joint of left middle finger** ▽

☑7ᵗʰ **S63.224** **Subluxation of unspecified interphalangeal joint of right ring finger** ▽

☑7ᵗʰ **S63.225** **Subluxation of unspecified interphalangeal joint of left ring finger** ▽

☑7ᵗʰ **S63.226** **Subluxation of unspecified interphalangeal joint of right little finger** ▽

☑7ᵗʰ **S63.227** **Subluxation of unspecified interphalangeal joint of left little finger** ▽

☑ Add'l Character Required   ☑7ᵗʰ Placeholder Alert   RUG IV Special Care High Dx   RUG IV Clinically Complex Dx   RUG IV Special Care Low Dx   Manifestation Code   Other Specified Code   ▽Unspecified Code

ICD-10-CM 2016   931

√7ᵗʰ **S63.228 Subluxation of unspecified** ▽
interphalangeal joint of other finger
Subluxation of unspecified interphalangeal
joint of specified finger with
unspecified laterality

√7ᵗʰ **S63.229 Subluxation of unspecified inter-** ▽
phalangeal joint of unspecified finger

√6ᵗʰ **S63.23 Subluxation of proximal interphalangeal joint of**
finger

√7ᵗʰ **S63.230 Subluxation of proximal interphalangeal**
joint of right index finger

√7ᵗʰ **S63.231 Subluxation of proximal interphalangeal**
joint of left index finger

√7ᵗʰ **S63.232 Subluxation of proximal interphalangeal**
joint of right middle finger

√7ᵗʰ **S63.233 Subluxation of proximal interphalangeal**
joint of left middle finger

√7ᵗʰ **S63.234 Subluxation of proximal interphalangeal**
joint of right ring finger

√7ᵗʰ **S63.235 Subluxation of proximal interphalangeal**
joint of left ring finger

√7ᵗʰ **S63.236 Subluxation of proximal interphalangeal**
joint of right little finger

√7ᵗʰ **S63.237 Subluxation of proximal interphalangeal**
joint of left little finger

√7ᵗʰ **S63.238 Subluxation of proximal interphalangeal**
joint of other finger
Subluxation of proximal interphalangeal
joint of specified finger with
unspecified laterality

√7ᵗʰ **S63.239 Subluxation of proximal** ▽
interphalangeal joint of unspecified finger

√6ᵗʰ **S63.24 Subluxation of distal interphalangeal joint of finger**

√7ᵗʰ **S63.240 Subluxation of distal interphalangeal**
joint of right index finger

√7ᵗʰ **S63.241 Subluxation of distal interphalangeal**
joint of left index finger

√7ᵗʰ **S63.242 Subluxation of distal interphalangeal**
joint of right middle finger

√7ᵗʰ **S63.243 Subluxation of distal interphalangeal**
joint of left middle finger

√7ᵗʰ **S63.244 Subluxation of distal interphalangeal**
joint of right ring finger

√7ᵗʰ **S63.245 Subluxation of distal interphalangeal**
joint of left ring finger

√7ᵗʰ **S63.246 Subluxation of distal interphalangeal**
joint of right little finger

√7ᵗʰ **S63.247 Subluxation of distal interphalangeal**
joint of left little finger

√7ᵗʰ **S63.248 Subluxation of distal interphalangeal**
joint of other finger
Subluxation of distal interphalangeal joint
of specified finger with unspecified
laterality

√7ᵗʰ **S63.249 Subluxation of distal interphalangeal** ▽
joint of unspecified finger

√6ᵗʰ **S63.25 Unspecified dislocation of other finger**

√7ᵗʰ **S63.250 Unspecified dislocation of right index** ▽
finger

√7ᵗʰ **S63.251 Unspecified dislocation of left index** ▽
finger

√7ᵗʰ **S63.252 Unspecified dislocation of right middle** ▽
finger

√7ᵗʰ **S63.253 Unspecified dislocation of left middle** ▽
finger

√7ᵗʰ **S63.254 Unspecified dislocation of right ring** ▽
finger

√7ᵗʰ **S63.255 Unspecified dislocation of left ring** ▽
finger

√7ᵗʰ **S63.256 Unspecified dislocation of right little** ▽
finger

√7ᵗʰ **S63.257 Unspecified dislocation of left little** ▽
finger

√7ᵗʰ **S63.258 Unspecified dislocation of other finger** ▽
Unspecified dislocation of specified finger
with unspecified laterality

√7ᵗʰ **S63.259 Unspecified dislocation of unspecified** ▽
finger
Unspecified dislocation of specified finger
with unspecified laterality

√6ᵗʰ **S63.26 Dislocation of metacarpophalangeal joint of finger**

√7ᵗʰ **S63.260 Dislocation of metacarpophalangeal joint**
of right index finger

√7ᵗʰ **S63.261 Dislocation of metacarpophalangeal joint**
of left index finger

√7ᵗʰ **S63.262 Dislocation of metacarpophalangeal joint**
of right middle finger

√7ᵗʰ **S63.263 Dislocation of metacarpophalangeal joint**
of left middle finger

√7ᵗʰ **S63.264 Dislocation of metacarpophalangeal joint**
of right ring finger

√7ᵗʰ **S63.265 Dislocation of metacarpophalangeal joint**
of left ring finger

√7ᵗʰ **S63.266 Dislocation of metacarpophalangeal joint**
of right little finger

√7ᵗʰ **S63.267 Dislocation of metacarpophalangeal joint**
of left little finger

√7ᵗʰ **S63.268 Dislocation of metacarpophalangeal joint**
of other finger
Dislocation of metacarpophalangeal joint
of specified finger with unspecified
laterality

√7ᵗʰ **S63.269 Dislocation of metacarpophalangeal** ▽
joint of unspecified finger

√6ᵗʰ **S63.27 Dislocation of unspecified interphalangeal joint of**
finger

√7ᵗʰ **S63.270 Dislocation of unspecified** ▽
interphalangeal joint of right index finger

√7ᵗʰ **S63.271 Dislocation of unspecified** ▽
interphalangeal joint of left index finger

√7ᵗʰ **S63.272 Dislocation of unspecified** ▽
interphalangeal joint of right middle
finger

√7ᵗʰ **S63.273 Dislocation of unspecified** ▽
interphalangeal joint of left middle finger

√7ᵗʰ **S63.274 Dislocation of unspecified** ▽
interphalangeal joint of right ring finger

√7ᵗʰ **S63.275 Dislocation of unspecified** ▽
interphalangeal joint of left ring finger

√7ᵗʰ **S63.276 Dislocation of unspecified** ▽
interphalangeal joint of right little finger

√7ᵗʰ **S63.277 Dislocation of unspecified** ▽
interphalangeal joint of left little finger

√7ᵗʰ **S63.278 Dislocation of unspecified** ▽
interphalangeal joint of other finger
Dislocation of unspecified interphalangeal
joint of specified finger with
unspecified laterality

√7ᵗʰ **S63.279 Dislocation of unspecified** ▽
interphalangeal joint of unspecified finger
Dislocation of unspecified interphalangeal
joint of specified finger without
specified laterality

√6ᵗʰ **S63.28 Dislocation of proximal interphalangeal joint of**
finger

√7ᵗʰ **S63.280 Dislocation of proximal interphalangeal**
joint of right index finger

√7ᵗʰ **S63.281 Dislocation of proximal interphalangeal**
joint of left index finger

√7ᵗʰ **S63.282 Dislocation of proximal interphalangeal**
joint of right middle finger

√7ᵗʰ **S63.283 Dislocation of proximal interphalangeal**
joint of left middle finger

√7ᵗʰ **S63.284 Dislocation of proximal interphalangeal**
joint of right ring finger

√7ᵗʰ **S63.285 Dislocation of proximal interphalangeal**
joint of left ring finger

N Newborn P Pediatric M Maternity A Adult RIC RIC Dx NCDx Noncancer Dx PDx Primary Dx CC RIC CC Condition ►◄ Revised Text ● New Code ▲ Revised Code Title

√7ᵗʰ **S63.286** Dislocation of proximal interphalangeal joint of right little finger

√7ᵗʰ **S63.287** Dislocation of proximal interphalangeal joint of left little finger

√7ᵗʰ **S63.288** Dislocation of proximal interphalangeal joint of other finger
Dislocation of proximal interphalangeal joint of specified finger with unspecified laterality

√7ᵗʰ **S63.289** Dislocation of proximal interphalangeal joint of unspecified finger ▽

√6ᵗʰ **S63.29** Dislocation of distal interphalangeal joint of finger

√7ᵗʰ **S63.290** Dislocation of distal interphalangeal joint of right index finger

√7ᵗʰ **S63.291** Dislocation of distal interphalangeal joint of left index finger

√7ᵗʰ **S63.292** Dislocation of distal interphalangeal joint of right middle finger

√7ᵗʰ **S63.293** Dislocation of distal interphalangeal joint of left middle finger

√7ᵗʰ **S63.294** Dislocation of distal interphalangeal joint of right ring finger

√7ᵗʰ **S63.295** Dislocation of distal interphalangeal joint of left ring finger

√7ᵗʰ **S63.296** Dislocation of distal interphalangeal joint of right little finger

√7ᵗʰ **S63.297** Dislocation of distal interphalangeal joint of left little finger

√7ᵗʰ **S63.298** Dislocation of distal interphalangeal joint of other finger
Dislocation of distal interphalangeal joint of specified finger with unspecified laterality

√7ᵗʰ **S63.299** Dislocation of distal interphalangeal joint of unspecified finger ▽

√5ᵗʰ **S63.3** Traumatic rupture of ligament of wrist

√6ᵗʰ **S63.30** Traumatic rupture of unspecified ligament of wrist

√7ᵗʰ **S63.301** Traumatic rupture of unspecified ligament of right wrist ▽

√7ᵗʰ **S63.302** Traumatic rupture of unspecified ligament of left wrist ▽

√7ᵗʰ **S63.309** Traumatic rupture of unspecified ligament of unspecified wrist ▽

√6ᵗʰ **S63.31** Traumatic rupture of collateral ligament of wrist

√7ᵗʰ **S63.311** Traumatic rupture of collateral ligament of right wrist

√7ᵗʰ **S63.312** Traumatic rupture of collateral ligament of left wrist

√7ᵗʰ **S63.319** Traumatic rupture of collateral ligament of unspecified wrist ▽

√6ᵗʰ **S63.32** Traumatic rupture of radiocarpal ligament

√7ᵗʰ **S63.321** Traumatic rupture of right radiocarpal ligament

√7ᵗʰ **S63.322** Traumatic rupture of left radiocarpal ligament

√7ᵗʰ **S63.329** Traumatic rupture of unspecified radiocarpal ligament ▽

√6ᵗʰ **S63.33** Traumatic rupture of ulnocarpal (palmar) ligament

√7ᵗʰ **S63.331** Traumatic rupture of right ulnocarpal (palmar) ligament

√7ᵗʰ **S63.332** Traumatic rupture of left ulnocarpal (palmar) ligament

√7ᵗʰ **S63.339** Traumatic rupture of unspecified ulnocarpal (palmar) ligament ▽

√6ᵗʰ **S63.39** Traumatic rupture of other ligament of wrist

√7ᵗʰ **S63.391** Traumatic rupture of other ligament of right wrist

√7ᵗʰ **S63.392** Traumatic rupture of other ligament of left wrist

√7ᵗʰ **S63.399** Traumatic rupture of other ligament of unspecified wrist ▽

√5ᵗʰ **S63.4** Traumatic rupture of ligament of finger at metacarpophalangeal and interphalangeal joint(s)

√6ᵗʰ **S63.40** Traumatic rupture of unspecified ligament of finger at metacarpophalangeal and interphalangeal joint

√7ᵗʰ **S63.400** Traumatic rupture of unspecified ligament of right index finger at metacarpo- phalangeal and interphalangeal joint ▽

√7ᵗʰ **S63.401** Traumatic rupture of unspecified ligament of left index finger at metacarpo-phalangeal and interphalangeal joint ▽

√7ᵗʰ **S63.402** Traumatic rupture of unspecified ligament of right middle finger at metacarpo- phalangeal and interphalangeal joint ▽

√7ᵗʰ **S63.403** Traumatic rupture of unspecified ligament of left middle finger at metacarpo- phalangeal and interphalangeal joint ▽

√7ᵗʰ **S63.404** Traumatic rupture of unspecified ligament of right ring finger at metacarpo-phalangeal and interphalangeal joint ▽

√7ᵗʰ **S63.405** Traumatic rupture of unspecified ligament of left ring finger at metacarpophalangeal and interphalangeal joint ▽

√7ᵗʰ **S63.406** Traumatic rupture of unspecified ligament of right little finger at metacarpo- phalangeal and interphalangeal joint ▽

√7ᵗʰ **S63.407** Traumatic rupture of unspecified ligament of left little finger at metacarpo-phalangeal and interphalangeal joint ▽

√7ᵗʰ **S63.408** Traumatic rupture of unspecified ligament of other finger at metacarpophalangeal and interphalangeal joint ▽
Traumatic rupture of unspecified ligament of specified finger with unspecified laterality at metacarpophalangeal and interphalangeal joint

√7ᵗʰ **S63.409** Traumatic rupture of unspecified ligament of unspecified finger at metacarpo- phalangeal and interphalangeal joint ▽

√6ᵗʰ **S63.41** Traumatic rupture of collateral ligament of finger at metacarpophalangeal and interphalangeal joint

√7ᵗʰ **S63.410** Traumatic rupture of collateral ligament of right index finger at metacarpo-phalangeal and interphalangeal joint

√7ᵗʰ **S63.411** Traumatic rupture of collateral ligament of left index finger at metacarpo-phalangeal and interphalangeal joint

√7ᵗʰ **S63.412** Traumatic rupture of collateral ligament of right middle finger at metacarpo-phalangeal and interphalangeal joint

√7ᵗʰ **S63.413** Traumatic rupture of collateral ligament of left middle finger at metacarpo-phalangeal and interphalangeal joint

√7ᵗʰ **S63.414** Traumatic rupture of collateral ligament of right ring finger at metacarpo-phalangeal and interphalangeal joint

√7ᵗʰ **S63.415** Traumatic rupture of collateral ligament of left ring finger at metacarpophalangeal and interphalangeal joint

√7ᵗʰ **S63.416** Traumatic rupture of collateral ligament of right little finger at metacarpo-phalangeal and interphalangeal joint

√7ᵗʰ **S63.417** Traumatic rupture of collateral ligament of left little finger at metacarpo-phalangeal and interphalangeal joint

√7ᵗʰ **S63.418 Traumatic rupture of collateral ligament of other finger at metacarpophalangeal and interphalangeal joint**
Traumatic rupture of collateral ligament of specified finger with unspecified laterality at metacarpophalangeal and interphalangeal joint

√7ᵗʰ **S63.419 Traumatic rupture of collateral ligament of unspecified finger at metacarpo- phalangeal and interphalangeal joint** ▽

√6ᵗʰ **S63.42 Traumatic rupture of palmar ligament of finger at metacarpophalangeal and interphalangeal joint**

√7ᵗʰ **S63.420 Traumatic rupture of palmar ligament of right index finger at metacarpo- phalangeal and interphalangeal joint**

√7ᵗʰ **S63.421 Traumatic rupture of palmar ligament of left index finger at metacarpophalangeal and interphalangeal joint**

√7ᵗʰ **S63.422 Traumatic rupture of palmar ligament of right middle finger at metacarpo- phalangeal and interphalangeal joint**

√7ᵗʰ **S63.423 Traumatic rupture of palmar ligament of left middle finger at metacarpo- phalangeal and interphalangeal joint**

√7ᵗʰ **S63.424 Traumatic rupture of palmar ligament of right ring finger at metacarpophalangeal and interphalangeal joint**

√7ᵗʰ **S63.425 Traumatic rupture of palmar ligament of left ring finger at metacarpophalangeal and interphalangeal joint**

√7ᵗʰ **S63.426 Traumatic rupture of palmar ligament of right little finger at metacarpophalangeal and interphalangeal joint**

√7ᵗʰ **S63.427 Traumatic rupture of palmar ligament of left little finger at metacarpophalangeal and interphalangeal joint**

√7ᵗʰ **S63.428 Traumatic rupture of palmar ligament of other finger at metacarpophalangeal and interphalangeal joint**
Traumatic rupture of palmar ligament of specified finger with unspecified laterality at metacarpophalangeal and interphalangeal joint

√7ᵗʰ **S63.429 Traumatic rupture of palmar ligament of unspecified finger at metacarpo- phalangeal and interphalangeal joint** ▽

√6ᵗʰ **S63.43 Traumatic rupture of volar plate of finger at metacarpophalangeal and interphalangeal joint**

√7ᵗʰ **S63.430 Traumatic rupture of volar plate of right index finger at metacarpophalangeal and interphalangeal joint**

√7ᵗʰ **S63.431 Traumatic rupture of volar plate of left index finger at metacarpophalangeal and interphalangeal joint**

√7ᵗʰ **S63.432 Traumatic rupture of volar plate of right middle finger at metacarpophalangeal and interphalangeal joint**

√7ᵗʰ **S63.433 Traumatic rupture of volar plate of left middle finger at metacarpophalangeal and interphalangeal joint**

√7ᵗʰ **S63.434 Traumatic rupture of volar plate of right ring finger at metacarpophalangeal and interphalangeal joint**

√7ᵗʰ **S63.435 Traumatic rupture of volar plate of left ring finger at metacarpophalangeal and interphalangeal joint**

√7ᵗʰ **S63.436 Traumatic rupture of volar plate of right little finger at metacarpophalangeal and interphalangeal joint**

√7ᵗʰ **S63.437 Traumatic rupture of volar plate of left little finger at metacarpophalangeal and interphalangeal joint**

√7ᵗʰ **S63.438 Traumatic rupture of volar plate of other finger at metacarpophalangeal and interphalangeal joint**
Traumatic rupture of volar plate of specified finger with unspecified laterality at metacarpophalangeal and interphalangeal joint

√7ᵗʰ **S63.439 Traumatic rupture of volar plate of unspecified finger at metacarpo- phalangeal and interphalangeal joint** ▽

√6ᵗʰ **S63.49 Traumatic rupture of other ligament of finger at metacarpophalangeal and interphalangeal joint**

√7ᵗʰ **S63.490 Traumatic rupture of other ligament of right index finger at metacarpo- phalangeal and interphalangeal joint**

√7ᵗʰ **S63.491 Traumatic rupture of other ligament of left index finger at metacarpophalangeal and interphalangeal joint**

√7ᵗʰ **S63.492 Traumatic rupture of other ligament of right middle finger at metacarpo- phalangeal and interphalangeal joint**

√7ᵗʰ **S63.493 Traumatic rupture of other ligament of left middle finger at metacarpo- phalangeal and interphalangeal joint**

√7ᵗʰ **S63.494 Traumatic rupture of other ligament of right ring finger at metacarpophalangeal and interphalangeal joint**

√7ᵗʰ **S63.495 Traumatic rupture of other ligament of left ring finger at metacarpophalangeal and interphalangeal joint**

√7ᵗʰ **S63.496 Traumatic rupture of other ligament of right little finger at metacarpophalangeal and interphalangeal joint**

√7ᵗʰ **S63.497 Traumatic rupture of other ligament of left little finger at metacarpophalangeal and interphalangeal joint**

√7ᵗʰ **S63.498 Traumatic rupture of other ligament of other finger at metacarpophalangeal and interphalangeal joint**
Traumatic rupture of ligament of specified finger with unspecified laterality at metacarpophalangeal and interphalangeal joint

√7ᵗʰ **S63.499 Traumatic rupture of other ligament of unspecified finger at metacarpo- phalangeal and interphalangeal joint** ▽

√5ᵗʰ **S63.5 Other and unspecified sprain of wrist**

√6ᵗʰ **S63.50 Unspecified sprain of wrist**

√7ᵗʰ **S63.501 Unspecified sprain of right wrist** ▽
√7ᵗʰ **S63.502 Unspecified sprain of left wrist** ▽
√7ᵗʰ **S63.509 Unspecified sprain of unspecified wrist** ▽

√6ᵗʰ **S63.51 Sprain of carpal (joint)**

√7ᵗʰ **S63.511 Sprain of carpal joint of right wrist**
√7ᵗʰ **S63.512 Sprain of carpal joint of left wrist**
√7ᵗʰ **S63.519 Sprain of carpal joint of unspecified wrist** ▽

√6ᵗʰ **S63.52 Sprain of radiocarpal joint**
EXCLUDES 1 *traumatic rupture of radiocarpal ligament (S63.32-)*

√7ᵗʰ **S63.521 Sprain of radiocarpal joint of right wrist**
√7ᵗʰ **S63.522 Sprain of radiocarpal joint of left wrist**
√7ᵗʰ **S63.529 Sprain of radiocarpal joint of unspecified wrist** ▽

√6ᵗʰ **S63.59 Other specified sprain of wrist**

√7ᵗʰ **S63.591 Other specified sprain of right wrist**
√7ᵗʰ **S63.592 Other specified sprain of left wrist**
√7ᵗʰ **S63.599 Other specified sprain of unspecified wrist** ▽

√5ᵗʰ **S63.6 Other and unspecified sprain of finger(s)**
EXCLUDES 1 *traumatic rupture of ligament of finger at metacarpophalangeal and interphalangeal joint(s) (S63.4-)*

√6ᵗʰ **S63.60 Unspecified sprain of thumb**

√7ᵗʰ **S63.601 Unspecified sprain of right thumb** ▽
√7ᵗʰ **S63.602 Unspecified sprain of left thumb** ▽

Ⓝ Newborn   Ⓟ Pediatric   Ⓜ Maternity   Ⓐ Adult   **RIC** RIC Dx   **NCDx** Noncancer Dx   **PDx** Primary Dx   **CC** RIC CC Condition   ►◄ Revised Text   ● New Code   ▲ Revised Code Title

934   ICD-10-CM 2016

☑7ᵗʰ **S63.609** Unspecified sprain of unspecified thumb ▽

☑6ᵗʰ **S63.61** Unspecified sprain of other and unspecified finger(s)

    ☑7ᵗʰ **S63.610** Unspecified sprain of right index finger ▽

    ☑7ᵗʰ **S63.611** Unspecified sprain of left index finger ▽

    ☑7ᵗʰ **S63.612** Unspecified sprain of right middle finger ▽

    ☑7ᵗʰ **S63.613** Unspecified sprain of left middle finger ▽

    ☑7ᵗʰ **S63.614** Unspecified sprain of right ring finger ▽

    ☑7ᵗʰ **S63.615** Unspecified sprain of left ring finger ▽

    ☑7ᵗʰ **S63.616** Unspecified sprain of right little finger ▽

    ☑7ᵗʰ **S63.617** Unspecified sprain of left little finger ▽

    ☑7ᵗʰ **S63.618** Unspecified sprain of other finger
       Unspecified sprain of specified finger with unspecified laterality

    ☑7ᵗʰ **S63.619** Unspecified sprain of unspecified finger ▽

☑6ᵗʰ **S63.62** Sprain of interphalangeal joint of thumb

    ☑7ᵗʰ **S63.621** Sprain of interphalangeal joint of right thumb

    ☑7ᵗʰ **S63.622** Sprain of interphalangeal joint of left thumb

    ☑7ᵗʰ **S63.629** Sprain of interphalangeal joint of unspecified thumb ▽

☑6ᵗʰ **S63.63** Sprain of interphalangeal joint of other and unspecified finger(s)

    ☑7ᵗʰ **S63.630** Sprain of interphalangeal joint of right index finger

    ☑7ᵗʰ **S63.631** Sprain of interphalangeal joint of left index finger

    ☑7ᵗʰ **S63.632** Sprain of interphalangeal joint of right middle finger

    ☑7ᵗʰ **S63.633** Sprain of interphalangeal joint of left middle finger

    ☑7ᵗʰ **S63.634** Sprain of interphalangeal joint of right ring finger

    ☑7ᵗʰ **S63.635** Sprain of interphalangeal joint of left ring finger

    ☑7ᵗʰ **S63.636** Sprain of interphalangeal joint of right little finger

    ☑7ᵗʰ **S63.637** Sprain of interphalangeal joint of left little finger

    ☑7ᵗʰ **S63.638** Sprain of interphalangeal joint of other finger

    ☑7ᵗʰ **S63.639** Sprain of interphalangeal joint of unspecified finger ▽

☑6ᵗʰ **S63.64** Sprain of metacarpophalangeal joint of thumb

    ☑7ᵗʰ **S63.641** Sprain of metacarpophalangeal joint of right thumb

    ☑7ᵗʰ **S63.642** Sprain of metacarpophalangeal joint of left thumb

    ☑7ᵗʰ **S63.649** Sprain of metacarpophalangeal joint of unspecified thumb ▽

☑6ᵗʰ **S63.65** Sprain of metacarpophalangeal joint of other and unspecified finger(s)

    ☑7ᵗʰ **S63.650** Sprain of metacarpophalangeal joint of right index finger

    ☑7ᵗʰ **S63.651** Sprain of metacarpophalangeal joint of left index finger

    ☑7ᵗʰ **S63.652** Sprain of metacarpophalangeal joint of right middle finger

    ☑7ᵗʰ **S63.653** Sprain of metacarpophalangeal joint of left middle finger

    ☑7ᵗʰ **S63.654** Sprain of metacarpophalangeal joint of right ring finger

    ☑7ᵗʰ **S63.655** Sprain of metacarpophalangeal joint of left ring finger

    ☑7ᵗʰ **S63.656** Sprain of metacarpophalangeal joint of right little finger

    ☑7ᵗʰ **S63.657** Sprain of metacarpophalangeal joint of left little finger

☑7ᵗʰ **S63.658** Sprain of metacarpophalangeal joint of other finger
       Sprain of metacarpophalangeal joint of specified finger with unspecified laterality

☑7ᵗʰ **S63.659** Sprain of metacarpophalangeal joint of unspecified finger ▽

☑6ᵗʰ **S63.68** Other sprain of thumb

    ☑7ᵗʰ **S63.681** Other sprain of right thumb

    ☑7ᵗʰ **S63.682** Other sprain of left thumb

    ☑7ᵗʰ **S63.689** Other sprain of unspecified thumb ▽

☑6ᵗʰ **S63.69** Other sprain of other and unspecified finger(s)

    ☑7ᵗʰ **S63.690** Other sprain of right index finger

    ☑7ᵗʰ **S63.691** Other sprain of left index finger

    ☑7ᵗʰ **S63.692** Other sprain of right middle finger

    ☑7ᵗʰ **S63.693** Other sprain of left middle finger

    ☑7ᵗʰ **S63.694** Other sprain of right ring finger

    ☑7ᵗʰ **S63.695** Other sprain of left ring finger

    ☑7ᵗʰ **S63.696** Other sprain of right little finger

    ☑7ᵗʰ **S63.697** Other sprain of left little finger

    ☑7ᵗʰ **S63.698** Other sprain of other finger
       Other sprain of specified finger with unspecified laterality

    ☑7ᵗʰ **S63.699** Other sprain of unspecified finger ▽

☑5ᵗʰ **S63.8** Sprain of other part of wrist and hand

    ☑6ᵗʰ **S63.8X** Sprain of other part of wrist and hand

       ☑7ᵗʰ **S63.8X1** Sprain of other part of right wrist and hand

       ☑7ᵗʰ **S63.8X2** Sprain of other part of left wrist and hand

       ☑7ᵗʰ **S63.8X9** Sprain of other part of unspecified wrist and hand ▽

☑5ᵗʰ **S63.9** Sprain of unspecified part of wrist and hand

    ☑x7ᵗʰ **S63.90** Sprain of unspecified part of unspecified wrist and hand ▽

    ☑x7ᵗʰ **S63.91** Sprain of unspecified part of right wrist and hand ▽

    ☑x7ᵗʰ **S63.92** Sprain of unspecified part of left wrist and hand ▽

☑4ᵗʰ **S64** **Injury of nerves at wrist and hand level**
    Code also any associated open wound (S61.-)

> The appropriate 7th character is to be added to each code from category S64.
> A   initial encounter
> D   subsequent encounter
> S   sequela

☑5ᵗʰ **S64.0** Injury of ulnar nerve at wrist and hand level

    ☑x7ᵗʰ **S64.00** Injury of ulnar nerve at wrist and hand level of unspecified arm ▽

    ☑x7ᵗʰ **S64.01** Injury of ulnar nerve at wrist and hand level of right arm

    ☑x7ᵗʰ **S64.02** Injury of ulnar nerve at wrist and hand level of left arm

☑5ᵗʰ **S64.1** Injury of median nerve at wrist and hand level

    ☑x7ᵗʰ **S64.10** Injury of median nerve at wrist and hand level of unspecified arm ▽

    ☑x7ᵗʰ **S64.11** Injury of median nerve at wrist and hand level of right arm

    ☑x7ᵗʰ **S64.12** Injury of median nerve at wrist and hand level of left arm

☑5ᵗʰ **S64.2** Injury of radial nerve at wrist and hand level

    ☑x7ᵗʰ **S64.20** Injury of radial nerve at wrist and hand level of unspecified arm ▽

    ☑x7ᵗʰ **S64.21** Injury of radial nerve at wrist and hand level of right arm

    ☑x7ᵗʰ **S64.22** Injury of radial nerve at wrist and hand level of left arm

☑5ᵗʰ **S64.3** Injury of digital nerve of thumb

    ☑x7ᵗʰ **S64.30** Injury of digital nerve of unspecified thumb ▽

    ☑x7ᵗʰ **S64.31** Injury of digital nerve of right thumb

    ☑x7ᵗʰ **S64.32** Injury of digital nerve of left thumb

☑5ᵗʰ **S64.4** Injury of digital nerve of other and unspecified finger

    ☑x7ᵗʰ **S64.40** Injury of digital nerve of unspecified finger ▽

☑ Add'l Character Required   ☑x7ᵗʰ Placeholder Alert   RUG IV Special Care High Dx   RUG IV Clinically Complex Dx   RUG IV Special Care Low Dx   Manifestation Code   Other Specified Code   ▽ Unspecified Code

✓6th **S64.49** Injury of digital nerve of other finger
- ✓7th **S64.490** Injury of digital nerve of right index finger
- ✓7th **S64.491** Injury of digital nerve of left index finger
- ✓7th **S64.492** Injury of digital nerve of right middle finger
- ✓7th **S64.493** Injury of digital nerve of left middle finger
- ✓7th **S64.494** Injury of digital nerve of right ring finger
- ✓7th **S64.495** Injury of digital nerve of left ring finger
- ✓7th **S64.496** Injury of digital nerve of right little finger
- ✓7th **S64.497** Injury of digital nerve of left little finger
- ✓7th **S64.498** Injury of digital nerve of other finger
  Injury of digital nerve of specified finger with unspecified laterality

✓5th **S64.8** Injury of other nerves at wrist and hand level
- ✓6th **S64.8X** Injury of other nerves at wrist and hand level
  - ✓7th **S64.8X1** Injury of other nerves at wrist and hand level of right arm
  - ✓7th **S64.8X2** Injury of other nerves at wrist and hand level of left arm
  - ✓7th **S64.8X9** Injury of other nerves at wrist and hand level of unspecified arm ▽

✓5th **S64.9** Injury of unspecified nerve at wrist and hand level
- ✓x7th **S64.90** Injury of unspecified nerve at wrist and hand level of unspecified arm ▽
- ✓x7th **S64.91** Injury of unspecified nerve at wrist and hand level of right arm ▽
- ✓x7th **S64.92** Injury of unspecified nerve at wrist and hand level of left arm ▽

✓4th **S65 Injury of blood vessels at wrist and hand level**
Code also any associated open wound (S61.-)

The appropriate 7th character is to be added to each code from category S65.
A   initial encounter
D   subsequent encounter
S   sequela

✓5th **S65.0** Injury of ulnar artery at wrist and hand level
- ✓6th **S65.00** Unspecified injury of ulnar artery at wrist and hand level
  - ✓7th **S65.001** Unspecified injury of ulnar artery at wrist and hand level of right arm ▽
  - ✓7th **S65.002** Unspecified injury of ulnar artery at wrist and hand level of left arm ▽
  - ✓7th **S65.009** Unspecified injury of ulnar artery at wrist and hand level of unspecified arm ▽
- ✓6th **S65.01** Laceration of ulnar artery at wrist and hand level
  - ✓7th **S65.011** Laceration of ulnar artery at wrist and hand level of right arm
  - ✓7th **S65.012** Laceration of ulnar artery at wrist and hand level of left arm
  - ✓7th **S65.019** Laceration of ulnar artery at wrist and hand level of unspecified arm ▽
- ✓6th **S65.09** Other specified injury of ulnar artery at wrist and hand level
  - ✓7th **S65.091** Other specified injury of ulnar artery at wrist and hand level of right arm
  - ✓7th **S65.092** Other specified injury of ulnar artery at wrist and hand level of left arm
  - ✓7th **S65.099** Other specified injury of ulnar artery at wrist and hand level of unspecified arm ▽

✓5th **S65.1** Injury of radial artery at wrist and hand level
- ✓6th **S65.10** Unspecified injury of radial artery at wrist and hand level
  - ✓7th **S65.101** Unspecified injury of radial artery at wrist and hand level of right arm ▽
  - ✓7th **S65.102** Unspecified injury of radial artery at wrist and hand level of left arm ▽
  - ✓7th **S65.109** Unspecified injury of radial artery at wrist and hand level of unspecified arm ▽
- ✓6th **S65.11** Laceration of radial artery at wrist and hand level
  - ✓7th **S65.111** Laceration of radial artery at wrist and hand level of right arm
  - ✓7th **S65.112** Laceration of radial artery at wrist and hand level of left arm

- ✓7th **S65.119** Laceration of radial artery at wrist and hand level of unspecified arm ▽
- ✓6th **S65.19** Other specified injury of radial artery at wrist and hand level
  - ✓7th **S65.191** Other specified injury of radial artery at wrist and hand level of right arm
  - ✓7th **S65.192** Other specified injury of radial artery at wrist and hand level of left arm
  - ✓7th **S65.199** Other specified injury of radial artery at wrist and hand level of unspecified arm ▽

✓5th **S65.2** Injury of superficial palmar arch
- ✓6th **S65.20** Unspecified injury of superficial palmar arch
  - ✓7th **S65.201** Unspecified injury of superficial palmar arch of right hand ▽
  - ✓7th **S65.202** Unspecified injury of superficial palmar arch of left hand ▽
  - ✓7th **S65.209** Unspecified injury of superficial palmar arch of unspecified hand ▽
- ✓6th **S65.21** Laceration of superficial palmar arch
  - ✓7th **S65.211** Laceration of superficial palmar arch of right hand
  - ✓7th **S65.212** Laceration of superficial palmar arch of left hand
  - ✓7th **S65.219** Laceration of superficial palmar arch of unspecified hand ▽
- ✓6th **S65.29** Other specified injury of superficial palmar arch
  - ✓7th **S65.291** Other specified injury of superficial palmar arch of right hand
  - ✓7th **S65.292** Other specified injury of superficial palmar arch of left hand
  - ✓7th **S65.299** Other specified injury of superficial palmar arch of unspecified hand ▽

✓5th **S65.3** Injury of deep palmar arch
- ✓6th **S65.30** Unspecified injury of deep palmar arch
  - ✓7th **S65.301** Unspecified injury of deep palmar arch of right hand ▽
  - ✓7th **S65.302** Unspecified injury of deep palmar arch of left hand ▽
  - ✓7th **S65.309** Unspecified injury of deep palmar arch of unspecified hand ▽
- ✓6th **S65.31** Laceration of deep palmar arch
  - ✓7th **S65.311** Laceration of deep palmar arch of right hand
  - ✓7th **S65.312** Laceration of deep palmar arch of left hand
  - ✓7th **S65.319** Laceration of deep palmar arch of unspecified hand ▽
- ✓6th **S65.39** Other specified injury of deep palmar arch
  - ✓7th **S65.391** Other specified injury of deep palmar arch of right hand
  - ✓7th **S65.392** Other specified injury of deep palmar arch of left hand
  - ✓7th **S65.399** Other specified injury of deep palmar arch of unspecified hand ▽

✓5th **S65.4** Injury of blood vessel of thumb
- ✓6th **S65.40** Unspecified injury of blood vessel of thumb
  - ✓7th **S65.401** Unspecified injury of blood vessel of right thumb ▽
  - ✓7th **S65.402** Unspecified injury of blood vessel of left thumb ▽
  - ✓7th **S65.409** Unspecified injury of blood vessel of unspecified thumb ▽
- ✓6th **S65.41** Laceration of blood vessel of thumb
  - ✓7th **S65.411** Laceration of blood vessel of right thumb
  - ✓7th **S65.412** Laceration of blood vessel of left thumb
  - ✓7th **S65.419** Laceration of blood vessel of unspecified thumb ▽
- ✓6th **S65.49** Other specified injury of blood vessel of thumb
  - ✓7th **S65.491** Other specified injury of blood vessel of right thumb
  - ✓7th **S65.492** Other specified injury of blood vessel of left thumb

N Newborn   P Pediatric   M Maternity   A Adult   RIC RIC Dx   NCDx Noncancer Dx   PDx Primary Dx   CC RIC CC Condition   ▶◀ Revised Text   ● New Code   ▲ Revised Code Title

936   ICD-10-CM 2016

√7ᵗʰ **S65.499** **Other specified injury of blood vessel of unspecified thumb** ▽

√5ᵗʰ **S65.5** Injury of blood vessel of other and unspecified finger

  √6ᵗʰ **S65.50** Unspecified injury of blood vessel of other and unspecified finger

    √7ᵗʰ **S65.500** **Unspecified injury of blood vessel of** right index **finger** ▽

    √7ᵗʰ **S65.501** **Unspecified injury of blood vessel of** left index **finger** ▽

    √7ᵗʰ **S65.502** **Unspecified injury of blood vessel of** right middle **finger** ▽

    √7ᵗʰ **S65.503** **Unspecified injury of blood vessel of** left middle **finger** ▽

    √7ᵗʰ **S65.504** **Unspecified injury of blood vessel of** right ring **finger** ▽

    √7ᵗʰ **S65.505** **Unspecified injury of blood vessel of** left ring **finger** ▽

    √7ᵗʰ **S65.506** **Unspecified injury of blood vessel of** right little **finger** ▽

    √7ᵗʰ **S65.507** **Unspecified injury of blood vessel of** left little **finger** ▽

    √7ᵗʰ **S65.508** **Unspecified injury of blood vessel of other finger** ▽
         Unspecified injury of blood vessel of specified finger with unspecified laterality

    √7ᵗʰ **S65.509** **Unspecified injury of blood vessel of unspecified finger** ▽

  √6ᵗʰ **S65.51** Laceration of blood vessel of other and unspecified finger

    √7ᵗʰ **S65.510** **Laceration of blood vessel of** right index **finger**

    √7ᵗʰ **S65.511** **Laceration of blood vessel of** left index **finger**

    √7ᵗʰ **S65.512** **Laceration of blood vessel of** right middle **finger**

    √7ᵗʰ **S65.513** **Laceration of blood vessel of** left middle **finger**

    √7ᵗʰ **S65.514** **Laceration of blood vessel of** right ring **finger**

    √7ᵗʰ **S65.515** **Laceration of blood vessel of** left ring **finger**

    √7ᵗʰ **S65.516** **Laceration of blood vessel of** right little **finger**

    √7ᵗʰ **S65.517** **Laceration of blood vessel of** left little **finger**

    √7ᵗʰ **S65.518** **Laceration of blood vessel of other finger**
         Laceration of blood vessel of specified finger with unspecified laterality

    √7ᵗʰ **S65.519** **Laceration of blood vessel of unspecified finger** ▽

  √6ᵗʰ **S65.59** Other specified injury of blood vessel of other and unspecified finger

    √7ᵗʰ **S65.590** **Other specified injury of blood vessel of** right index **finger**

    √7ᵗʰ **S65.591** **Other specified injury of blood vessel of** left index **finger**

    √7ᵗʰ **S65.592** **Other specified injury of blood vessel of** right middle **finger**

    √7ᵗʰ **S65.593** **Other specified injury of blood vessel of** left middle **finger**

    √7ᵗʰ **S65.594** **Other specified injury of blood vessel of** right ring **finger**

    √7ᵗʰ **S65.595** **Other specified injury of blood vessel of** left ring **finger**

    √7ᵗʰ **S65.596** **Other specified injury of blood vessel of** right little **finger**

    √7ᵗʰ **S65.597** **Other specified injury of blood vessel of** left little **finger**

    √7ᵗʰ **S65.598** **Other specified injury of blood vessel of other finger**
         Other specified injury of blood vessel of specified finger with unspecified laterality

    √7ᵗʰ **S65.599** **Other specified injury of blood vessel of unspecified finger** ▽

√5ᵗʰ **S65.8** Injury of other blood vessels at wrist and hand level

  √6ᵗʰ **S65.80** Unspecified injury of other blood vessels at wrist and hand level

    √7ᵗʰ **S65.801** **Unspecified injury of other blood vessels at wrist and hand level of** right arm ▽

    √7ᵗʰ **S65.802** **Unspecified injury of other blood vessels at wrist and hand level of** left arm ▽

    √7ᵗʰ **S65.809** **Unspecified injury of other blood vessels at wrist and hand level of unspecified arm** ▽

  √6ᵗʰ **S65.81** Laceration of other blood vessels at wrist and hand level

    √7ᵗʰ **S65.811** **Laceration of other blood vessels at wrist and hand level of** right arm

    √7ᵗʰ **S65.812** **Laceration of other blood vessels at wrist and hand level of** left arm

    √7ᵗʰ **S65.819** **Laceration of other blood vessels at wrist and hand level of unspecified arm** ▽

  √6ᵗʰ **S65.89** Other specified injury of other blood vessels at wrist and hand level

    √7ᵗʰ **S65.891** **Other specified injury of other blood vessels at wrist and hand level of** right arm

    √7ᵗʰ **S65.892** **Other specified injury of other blood vessels at wrist and hand level of** left arm

    √7ᵗʰ **S65.899** **Other specified injury of other blood vessels at wrist and hand level of unspecified arm** ▽

√5ᵗʰ **S65.9** Injury of unspecified blood vessel at wrist and hand level

  √6ᵗʰ **S65.90** Unspecified injury of unspecified blood vessel at wrist and hand level

    √7ᵗʰ **S65.901** **Unspecified injury of unspecified blood vessel at wrist and hand level of** right arm ▽

    √7ᵗʰ **S65.902** **Unspecified injury of unspecified blood vessel at wrist and hand level of** left arm ▽

    √7ᵗʰ **S65.909** **Unspecified injury of unspecified blood vessel at wrist and hand level of unspecified arm** ▽

  √6ᵗʰ **S65.91** Laceration of unspecified blood vessel at wrist and hand level

    √7ᵗʰ **S65.911** **Laceration of unspecified blood vessel at wrist and hand level of** right arm ▽

    √7ᵗʰ **S65.912** **Laceration of unspecified blood vessel at wrist and hand level of** left arm ▽

    √7ᵗʰ **S65.919** **Laceration of unspecified blood vessel at wrist and hand level of unspecified arm** ▽

  √6ᵗʰ **S65.99** Other specified injury of unspecified blood vessel at wrist and hand level

    √7ᵗʰ **S65.991** **Other specified injury of unspecified blood vessel at wrist and hand of** right arm ▽

    √7ᵗʰ **S65.992** **Other specified injury of unspecified blood vessel at wrist and hand of** left arm ▽

    √7ᵗʰ **S65.999** **Other specified injury of unspecified blood vessel at wrist and hand of unspecified arm** ▽

☑ Add'l Character Required   ☑x7ᵗʰ Placeholder Alert   RUG IV Special Care High Dx   RUG IV Clinically Complex Dx   RUG IV Special Care Low Dx   Manifestation Code   Other Specified Code   ▽Unspecified Code

ICD-10-CM 2016   937

Chapter 19. Injury, Poisoning and Certain Other Consequences of External Causes

S65.499–S65.999

✦ ✓4ᵗʰ S66 Injury of muscle, fascia and tendon at wrist and hand level

Code also any associated open wound (S61.-)

EXCLUDES 2   sprain of joints and ligaments of wrist and hand (S63.-)

> The appropriate 7th character is to be added to each code from category S66.
> A   initial encounter
> D   subsequent encounter
> S   sequela

✓5ᵗʰ **S66.0 Injury of long flexor muscle, fascia and tendon of thumb at wrist and hand level**

✓6ᵗʰ **S66.00 Unspecified injury of long flexor muscle, fascia and tendon of thumb at wrist and hand level**

     ✓7ᵗʰ **S66.001 Unspecified injury of long flexor muscle, fascia and tendon of right thumb at wrist and hand level** ▽

     ✓7ᵗʰ **S66.002 Unspecified injury of long flexor muscle, fascia and tendon of left thumb at wrist and hand level** ▽

     ✓7ᵗʰ **S66.009 Unspecified injury of long flexor muscle, fascia and tendon of unspecified thumb at wrist and hand level** ▽

✓6ᵗʰ **S66.01 Strain of long flexor muscle, fascia and tendon of thumb at wrist and hand level**

     ✓7ᵗʰ **S66.011 Strain of long flexor muscle, fascia and tendon of right thumb at wrist and hand level**

     ✓7ᵗʰ **S66.012 Strain of long flexor muscle, fascia and tendon of left thumb at wrist and hand level**

     ✓7ᵗʰ **S66.019 Strain of long flexor muscle, fascia and tendon of unspecified thumb at wrist and hand level** ▽

✓6ᵗʰ **S66.02 Laceration of long flexor muscle, fascia and tendon of thumb at wrist and hand level**

     ✓7ᵗʰ **S66.021 Laceration of long flexor muscle, fascia and tendon of right thumb at wrist and hand level**

     ✓7ᵗʰ **S66.022 Laceration of long flexor muscle, fascia and tendon of left thumb at wrist and hand level**

     ✓7ᵗʰ **S66.029 Laceration of long flexor muscle, fascia and tendon of unspecified thumb at wrist and hand level** ▽

✓6ᵗʰ **S66.09 Other specified injury of long flexor muscle, fascia and tendon of thumb at wrist and hand level**

     ✓7ᵗʰ **S66.091 Other specified injury of long flexor muscle, fascia and tendon of right thumb at wrist and hand level**

     ✓7ᵗʰ **S66.092 Other specified injury of long flexor muscle, fascia and tendon of left thumb at wrist and hand level**

     ✓7ᵗʰ **S66.099 Other specified injury of long flexor muscle, fascia and tendon of unspecified thumb at wrist and hand level** ▽

✓5ᵗʰ **S66.1 Injury of flexor muscle, fascia and tendon of other and unspecified finger at wrist and hand level**

EXCLUDES 2   Injury of long flexor muscle, fascia and tendon of thumb at wrist and hand level (S66.0-)

✓6ᵗʰ **S66.10 Unspecified injury of flexor muscle, fascia and tendon of other and unspecified finger at wrist and hand level**

     ✓7ᵗʰ **S66.100 Unspecified injury of flexor muscle, fascia and tendon of right index finger at wrist and hand level** ▽

     ✓7ᵗʰ **S66.101 Unspecified injury of flexor muscle, fascia and tendon of left index finger at wrist and hand level** ▽

     ✓7ᵗʰ **S66.102 Unspecified injury of flexor muscle, fascia and tendon of right middle finger at wrist and hand level** ▽

     ✓7ᵗʰ **S66.103 Unspecified injury of flexor muscle, fascia and tendon of left middle finger at wrist and hand level** ▽

     ✓7ᵗʰ **S66.104 Unspecified injury of flexor muscle, fascia and tendon of right ring finger at wrist and hand level** ▽

     ✓7ᵗʰ **S66.105 Unspecified injury of flexor muscle, fascia and tendon of left ring finger at wrist and hand level** ▽

     ✓7ᵗʰ **S66.106 Unspecified injury of flexor muscle, fascia and tendon of right little finger at wrist and hand level** ▽

     ✓7ᵗʰ **S66.107 Unspecified injury of flexor muscle, fascia and tendon of left little finger at wrist and hand level** ▽

     ✓7ᵗʰ **S66.108 Unspecified injury of flexor muscle, fascia and tendon of other finger at wrist and hand level**

> Unspecified injury of flexor muscle, fascia and tendon of specified finger with unspecified laterality at wrist and hand level

     ✓7ᵗʰ **S66.109 Unspecified injury of flexor muscle, fascia and tendon of unspecified finger at wrist and hand level** ▽

✓6ᵗʰ **S66.11 Strain of flexor muscle, fascia and tendon of other and unspecified finger at wrist and hand level**

     ✓7ᵗʰ **S66.110 Strain of flexor muscle, fascia and tendon of right index finger at wrist and hand level**

     ✓7ᵗʰ **S66.111 Strain of flexor muscle, fascia and tendon of left index finger at wrist and hand level**

     ✓7ᵗʰ **S66.112 Strain of flexor muscle, fascia and tendon of right middle finger at wrist and hand level**

     ✓7ᵗʰ **S66.113 Strain of flexor muscle, fascia and tendon of left middle finger at wrist and hand level**

     ✓7ᵗʰ **S66.114 Strain of flexor muscle, fascia and tendon of right ring finger at wrist and hand level**

     ✓7ᵗʰ **S66.115 Strain of flexor muscle, fascia and tendon of left ring finger at wrist and hand level**

     ✓7ᵗʰ **S66.116 Strain of flexor muscle, fascia and tendon of right little finger at wrist and hand level**

     ✓7ᵗʰ **S66.117 Strain of flexor muscle, fascia and tendon of left little finger at wrist and hand level**

     ✓7ᵗʰ **S66.118 Strain of flexor muscle, fascia and tendon of other finger at wrist and hand level**

> Strain of flexor muscle, fascia and tendon of specified finger with unspecified laterality at wrist and hand level

     ✓7ᵗʰ **S66.119 Strain of flexor muscle, fascia and tendon of unspecified finger at wrist and hand level** ▽

✓6ᵗʰ **S66.12 Laceration of flexor muscle, fascia and tendon of other and unspecified finger at wrist and hand level**

     ✓7ᵗʰ **S66.120 Laceration of flexor muscle, fascia and tendon of right index finger at wrist and hand level**

     ✓7ᵗʰ **S66.121 Laceration of flexor muscle, fascia and tendon of left index finger at wrist and hand level**

     ✓7ᵗʰ **S66.122 Laceration of flexor muscle, fascia and tendon of right middle finger at wrist and hand level**

     ✓7ᵗʰ **S66.123 Laceration of flexor muscle, fascia and tendon of left middle finger at wrist and hand level**

     ✓7ᵗʰ **S66.124 Laceration of flexor muscle, fascia and tendon of right ring finger at wrist and hand level**

     ✓7ᵗʰ **S66.125 Laceration of flexor muscle, fascia and tendon of left ring finger at wrist and hand level**

     ✓7ᵗʰ **S66.126 Laceration of flexor muscle, fascia and tendon of right little finger at wrist and hand level**

     ✓7ᵗʰ **S66.127 Laceration of flexor muscle, fascia and tendon of left little finger at wrist and hand level**

✦ Refer to the Muscle/Tendon Table at beginning of this chapter.

N Newborn   P Pediatric   M Maternity   A Adult   RIC RIC Dx   NCDx Noncancer Dx   PDx Primary Dx   CC RIC CC Condition   ▶◀ Revised Text   ● New Code   ▲ Revised Code Title

938

ICD-10-CM 2016

√7ᵗʰ **S66.128** **Laceration of flexor muscle, fascia and tendon of other finger at wrist and hand level**

Laceration of flexor muscle, fascia and tendon of specified finger with unspecified laterality at wrist and hand level

√7ᵗʰ **S66.129** **Laceration of flexor muscle, fascia and tendon of unspecified finger at wrist and hand level** ▽

√6ᵗʰ **S66.19** Other injury of flexor muscle, fascia and tendon of other and unspecified finger at wrist and hand level

√7ᵗʰ **S66.190** **Other injury of flexor muscle, fascia and tendon of right index finger at wrist and hand level**

√7ᵗʰ **S66.191** **Other injury of flexor muscle, fascia and tendon of left index finger at wrist and hand level**

√7ᵗʰ **S66.192** **Other injury of flexor muscle, fascia and tendon of right middle finger at wrist and hand level**

√7ᵗʰ **S66.193** **Other injury of flexor muscle, fascia and tendon of left middle finger at wrist and hand level**

√7ᵗʰ **S66.194** **Other injury of flexor muscle, fascia and tendon of right ring finger at wrist and hand level**

√7ᵗʰ **S66.195** **Other injury of flexor muscle, fascia and tendon of left ring finger at wrist and hand level**

√7ᵗʰ **S66.196** **Other injury of flexor muscle, fascia and tendon of right little finger at wrist and hand level**

√7ᵗʰ **S66.197** **Other injury of flexor muscle, fascia and tendon of left little finger at wrist and hand level**

√7ᵗʰ **S66.198** **Other injury of flexor muscle, fascia and tendon of other finger at wrist and hand level**

Other injury of flexor muscle, fascia and tendon of specified finger with unspecified laterality at wrist and hand level

√7ᵗʰ **S66.199** **Other injury of flexor muscle, fascia and tendon of unspecified finger at wrist and hand level** ▽

√5ᵗʰ **S66.2** Injury of extensor muscle, fascia and tendon of thumb at wrist and hand level

√6ᵗʰ **S66.20** Unspecified injury of extensor muscle, fascia and tendon of thumb at wrist and hand level

√7ᵗʰ **S66.201** **Unspecified injury of extensor muscle, fascia and tendon of right thumb at wrist and hand level** ▽

√7ᵗʰ **S66.202** **Unspecified injury of extensor muscle, fascia and tendon of left thumb at wrist and hand level** ▽

√7ᵗʰ **S66.209** **Unspecified injury of extensor muscle, fascia and tendon of unspecified thumb at wrist and hand level** ▽

√6ᵗʰ **S66.21** Strain of extensor muscle, fascia and tendon of thumb at wrist and hand level

√7ᵗʰ **S66.211** **Strain of extensor muscle, fascia and tendon of right thumb at wrist and hand level**

√7ᵗʰ **S66.212** **Strain of extensor muscle, fascia and tendon of left thumb at wrist and hand level**

√7ᵗʰ **S66.219** **Strain of extensor muscle, fascia and tendon of unspecified thumb at wrist and hand level** ▽

√6ᵗʰ **S66.22** Laceration of extensor muscle, fascia and tendon of thumb at wrist and hand level

√7ᵗʰ **S66.221** **Laceration of extensor muscle, fascia and tendon of right thumb at wrist and hand level**

√7ᵗʰ **S66.222** **Laceration of extensor muscle, fascia and tendon of left thumb at wrist and hand level**

√7ᵗʰ **S66.229** **Laceration of extensor muscle, fascia and tendon of unspecified thumb at wrist and hand level** ▽

√6ᵗʰ **S66.29** Other specified injury of extensor muscle, fascia and tendon of thumb at wrist and hand level

√7ᵗʰ **S66.291** **Other specified injury of extensor muscle, fascia and tendon of right thumb at wrist and hand level**

√7ᵗʰ **S66.292** **Other specified injury of extensor muscle, fascia and tendon of left thumb at wrist and hand level**

√7ᵗʰ **S66.299** **Other specified injury of extensor muscle, fascia and tendon of unspecified thumb at wrist and hand level** ▽

√5ᵗʰ **S66.3** Injury of extensor muscle, fascia and tendon of other and unspecified finger at wrist and hand level

EXCLUDES 2   Injury of extensor muscle, fascia and tendon of thumb at wrist and hand level (S66.2-)

√6ᵗʰ **S66.30** Unspecified injury of extensor muscle, fascia and tendon of other and unspecified finger at wrist and hand level

√7ᵗʰ **S66.300** **Unspecified injury of extensor muscle, fascia and tendon of right index finger at wrist and hand level** ▽

√7ᵗʰ **S66.301** **Unspecified injury of extensor muscle, fascia and tendon of left index finger at wrist and hand level** ▽

√7ᵗʰ **S66.302** **Unspecified injury of extensor muscle, fascia and tendon of right middle finger at wrist and hand level** ▽

√7ᵗʰ **S66.303** **Unspecified injury of extensor muscle, fascia and tendon of left middle finger at wrist and hand level** ▽

√7ᵗʰ **S66.304** **Unspecified injury of extensor muscle, fascia and tendon of right ring finger at wrist and hand level** ▽

√7ᵗʰ **S66.305** **Unspecified injury of extensor muscle, fascia and tendon of left ring finger at wrist and hand level** ▽

√7ᵗʰ **S66.306** **Unspecified injury of extensor muscle, fascia and tendon of right little finger at wrist and hand level** ▽

√7ᵗʰ **S66.307** **Unspecified injury of extensor muscle, fascia and tendon of left little finger at wrist and hand level** ▽

√7ᵗʰ **S66.308** **Unspecified injury of extensor muscle, fascia and tendon of other finger at wrist and hand level** ▽

Unspecified injury of extensor muscle, fascia and tendon of specified finger with unspecified laterality at wrist and hand level

√7ᵗʰ **S66.309** **Unspecified injury of extensor muscle, fascia and tendon of unspecified finger at wrist and hand level** ▽

√6ᵗʰ **S66.31** Strain of extensor muscle, fascia and tendon of other and unspecified finger at wrist and hand level

√7ᵗʰ **S66.310** **Strain of extensor muscle, fascia and tendon of right index finger at wrist and hand level**

√7ᵗʰ **S66.311** **Strain of extensor muscle, fascia and tendon of left index finger at wrist and hand level**

√7ᵗʰ **S66.312** **Strain of extensor muscle, fascia and tendon of right middle finger at wrist and hand level**

√7ᵗʰ **S66.313** **Strain of extensor muscle, fascia and tendon of left middle finger at wrist and hand level**

√7ᵗʰ **S66.314** **Strain of extensor muscle, fascia and tendon of right ring finger at wrist and hand level**

√7ᵗʰ **S66.315** **Strain of extensor muscle, fascia and tendon of left ring finger at wrist and hand level**

√7ᵗʰ **S66.316** **Strain of extensor muscle, fascia and tendon of right little finger at wrist and hand level**

✔ Add'l Character Required   √x7ᵗʰ Placeholder Alert   RUG IV Special Care High Dx   RUG IV Clinically Complex Dx   RUG IV Special Care Low Dx   Manifestation Code   Other Specified Code   ▽ Unspecified Code

ICD-10-CM 2016   939

Chapter 19. Injury, Poisoning and Certain Other Consequences of External Causes

S66.317–S66.503

√7ᵗʰ **S66.317** Strain of extensor muscle, fascia and tendon of **left little** finger at wrist and hand level

√7ᵗʰ **S66.318** Strain of extensor muscle, fascia and tendon of **other** finger at wrist and hand level
Strain of extensor muscle, fascia and tendon of specified finger with unspecified laterality at wrist and hand level

√7ᵗʰ **S66.319** Strain of extensor muscle, fascia and tendon of unspecified finger at wrist and hand level ▽

√6ᵗʰ **S66.32** Laceration of extensor muscle, fascia and tendon of other and unspecified finger at wrist and hand level

√7ᵗʰ **S66.320** Laceration of extensor muscle, fascia and tendon of **right index** finger at wrist and hand level

√7ᵗʰ **S66.321** Laceration of extensor muscle, fascia and tendon of **left index** finger at wrist and hand level

√7ᵗʰ **S66.322** Laceration of extensor muscle, fascia and tendon of **right middle** finger at wrist and hand level

√7ᵗʰ **S66.323** Laceration of extensor muscle, fascia and tendon of **left middle** finger at wrist and hand level

√7ᵗʰ **S66.324** Laceration of extensor muscle, fascia and tendon of **right ring** finger at wrist and hand level

√7ᵗʰ **S66.325** Laceration of extensor muscle, fascia and tendon of **left ring** finger at wrist and hand level

√7ᵗʰ **S66.326** Laceration of extensor muscle, fascia and tendon of **right little** finger at wrist and hand level

√7ᵗʰ **S66.327** Laceration of extensor muscle, fascia and tendon of **left little** finger at wrist and hand level

√7ᵗʰ **S66.328** Laceration of extensor muscle, fascia and tendon of **other** finger at wrist and hand level
Laceration of extensor muscle, fascia and tendon of specified finger with unspecified laterality at wrist and hand level

√7ᵗʰ **S66.329** Laceration of extensor muscle, fascia and tendon of unspecified finger at wrist and hand level ▽

√6ᵗʰ **S66.39** Other injury of extensor muscle, fascia and tendon of other and unspecified finger at wrist and hand level

√7ᵗʰ **S66.390** Other injury of extensor muscle, fascia and tendon of **right index** finger at wrist and hand level

√7ᵗʰ **S66.391** Other injury of extensor muscle, fascia and tendon of **left index** finger at wrist and hand level

√7ᵗʰ **S66.392** Other injury of extensor muscle, fascia and tendon of **right middle** finger at wrist and hand level

√7ᵗʰ **S66.393** Other injury of extensor muscle, fascia and tendon of **left middle** finger at wrist and hand level

√7ᵗʰ **S66.394** Other injury of extensor muscle, fascia and tendon of **right ring** finger at wrist and hand level

√7ᵗʰ **S66.395** Other injury of extensor muscle, fascia and tendon of **left ring** finger at wrist and hand level

√7ᵗʰ **S66.396** Other injury of extensor muscle, fascia and tendon of **right little** finger at wrist and hand level

√7ᵗʰ **S66.397** Other injury of extensor muscle, fascia and tendon of **left little** finger at wrist and hand level

√7ᵗʰ **S66.398** Other injury of extensor muscle, fascia and tendon of **other** finger at wrist and hand level
Other injury of extensor muscle, fascia and tendon of specified finger with unspecified laterality at wrist and hand level

√7ᵗʰ **S66.399** Other injury of extensor muscle, fascia and tendon of unspecified finger at wrist and hand level ▽

√5ᵗʰ **S66.4** Injury of **intrinsic muscle**, fascia and tendon of **thumb** at wrist and hand level

√6ᵗʰ **S66.40** **Unspecified** injury of intrinsic muscle, fascia and tendon of thumb at wrist and hand level

√7ᵗʰ **S66.401** Unspecified injury of intrinsic muscle, fascia and tendon of **right** thumb at wrist and hand level ▽

√7ᵗʰ **S66.402** Unspecified injury of intrinsic muscle, fascia and tendon of **left** thumb at wrist and hand level ▽

√7ᵗʰ **S66.409** Unspecified injury of intrinsic muscle, fascia and tendon of unspecified thumb at wrist and hand level ▽

√6ᵗʰ **S66.41** **Strain** of intrinsic muscle, fascia and tendon of thumb at wrist and hand level

√7ᵗʰ **S66.411** Strain of intrinsic muscle, fascia and tendon of **right** thumb at wrist and hand level

√7ᵗʰ **S66.412** Strain of intrinsic muscle, fascia and tendon of **left** thumb at wrist and hand level

√7ᵗʰ **S66.419** Strain of intrinsic muscle, fascia and tendon of unspecified thumb at wrist and hand level ▽

√6ᵗʰ **S66.42** **Laceration** of intrinsic muscle, fascia and tendon of thumb at wrist and hand level

√7ᵗʰ **S66.421** Laceration of intrinsic muscle, fascia and tendon of **right** thumb at wrist and hand level

√7ᵗʰ **S66.422** Laceration of intrinsic muscle, fascia and tendon of **left** thumb at wrist and hand level

√7ᵗʰ **S66.429** Laceration of intrinsic muscle, fascia and tendon of unspecified thumb at wrist and hand level ▽

√6ᵗʰ **S66.49** **Other** specified injury of intrinsic muscle, fascia and tendon of thumb at wrist and hand level

√7ᵗʰ **S66.491** Other specified injury of intrinsic muscle, fascia and tendon of **right** thumb at wrist and hand level

√7ᵗʰ **S66.492** Other specified injury of intrinsic muscle, fascia and tendon of **left** thumb at wrist and hand level

√7ᵗʰ **S66.499** Other specified injury of intrinsic muscle, fascia and tendon of unspecified thumb at wrist and hand level ▽

√5ᵗʰ **S66.5** Injury of **intrinsic muscle**, fascia and tendon of **other and unspecified finger** at wrist and hand level
EXCLUDES 2 injury of intrinsic muscle, fascia and tendon of thumb at wrist and hand level (S66.4-)

√6ᵗʰ **S66.50** **Unspecified** injury of intrinsic muscle, fascia and tendon of other and unspecified finger at wrist and hand level

√7ᵗʰ **S66.500** Unspecified injury of intrinsic muscle, fascia and tendon of **right index** finger at wrist and hand level ▽

√7ᵗʰ **S66.501** Unspecified injury of intrinsic muscle, fascia and tendon of **left index** finger at wrist and hand level ▽

√7ᵗʰ **S66.502** Unspecified injury of intrinsic muscle, fascia and tendon of **right middle** finger at wrist and hand level ▽

√7ᵗʰ **S66.503** Unspecified injury of intrinsic muscle, fascia and tendon of **left middle** finger at wrist and hand level ▽

Ⓝ Newborn   Ⓟ Pediatric   Ⓜ Maternity   Ⓐ Adult   **RIC** RIC Dx   **NC Dx** Noncancer Dx   **PDx** Primary Dx   **CC** RIC CC Condition   ►◄ Revised Text   ● New Code   ▲ Revised Code Title

√7ᵗʰ **S66.504** Unspecified injury of intrinsic muscle, ▽
fascia and tendon of right ring
finger at wrist and hand level

√7ᵗʰ **S66.505** Unspecified injury of intrinsic muscle, ▽
fascia and tendon of left ring
finger at wrist and hand level

√7ᵗʰ **S66.506** Unspecified injury of intrinsic muscle, ▽
fascia and tendon of right little
finger at wrist and hand level

√7ᵗʰ **S66.507** Unspecified injury of intrinsic muscle, ▽
fascia and tendon of left little
finger at wrist and hand level

√7ᵗʰ **S66.508** Unspecified injury of intrinsic muscle, ▽
fascia and tendon of other finger at
wrist and hand level
     Unspecified injury of intrinsic muscle, fascia
and tendon of specified finger with
unspecified laterality at wrist and
hand level

√7ᵗʰ **S66.509** Unspecified injury of intrinsic muscle, ▽
fascia and tendon of unspecified finger
at wrist and hand level

√6ᵗʰ **S66.51** Strain of intrinsic muscle, fascia and tendon of other
and unspecified finger at wrist and hand level

√7ᵗʰ **S66.510** Strain of intrinsic muscle, fascia and
tendon of right index finger at wrist
and hand level

√7ᵗʰ **S66.511** Strain of intrinsic muscle, fascia and
tendon of left index finger at wrist
and hand level

√7ᵗʰ **S66.512** Strain of intrinsic muscle, fascia and
tendon of right middle finger at wrist
and hand level

√7ᵗʰ **S66.513** Strain of intrinsic muscle, fascia and
tendon of left middle finger at wrist
and hand level

√7ᵗʰ **S66.514** Strain of intrinsic muscle, fascia and
tendon of right ring finger at wrist
and hand level

√7ᵗʰ **S66.515** Strain of intrinsic muscle, fascia and
tendon of left ring finger at wrist and
hand level

√7ᵗʰ **S66.516** Strain of intrinsic muscle, fascia and
tendon of right little finger at wrist
and hand level

√7ᵗʰ **S66.517** Strain of intrinsic muscle, fascia and
tendon of left little finger at wrist
and hand level

√7ᵗʰ **S66.518** Strain of intrinsic muscle, fascia and
tendon of other finger at wrist and
hand level
     Strain of intrinsic muscle, fascia and tendon
of specified finger with unspecified
laterality at wrist and hand level

√7ᵗʰ **S66.519** Strain of intrinsic muscle, fascia and ▽
tendon of unspecified finger at wrist
and hand level

√6ᵗʰ **S66.52** Laceration of intrinsic muscle, fascia and tendon of
other and unspecified finger at wrist and hand level

√7ᵗʰ **S66.520** Laceration of intrinsic muscle, fascia
and tendon of right index finger at
wrist and hand level

√7ᵗʰ **S66.521** Laceration of intrinsic muscle, fascia
and tendon of left index finger at
wrist and hand level

√7ᵗʰ **S66.522** Laceration of intrinsic muscle, fascia
and tendon of right middle finger at
wrist and hand level

√7ᵗʰ **S66.523** Laceration of intrinsic muscle, fascia
and tendon of left middle finger at
wrist and hand level

√7ᵗʰ **S66.524** Laceration of intrinsic muscle, fascia
and tendon of right ring finger at
wrist and hand level

√7ᵗʰ **S66.525** Laceration of intrinsic muscle, fascia
and tendon of left ring finger at wrist
and hand level

√7ᵗʰ **S66.526** Laceration of intrinsic muscle, fascia
and tendon of right little finger at wrist
and hand level

√7ᵗʰ **S66.527** Laceration of intrinsic muscle, fascia and
tendon of left little finger at wrist and
hand level

√7ᵗʰ **S66.528** Laceration of intrinsic muscle, fascia and
tendon of other finger at wrist and hand
level
     Laceration of intrinsic muscle, fascia and
tendon of specified finger with
unspecified laterality at wrist and
hand level

√7ᵗʰ **S66.529** Laceration of intrinsic muscle, fascia ▽
and tendon of unspecified finger at
wrist and hand level

√6ᵗʰ **S66.59** Other injury of intrinsic muscle, fascia and tendon of
other and unspecified finger at wrist and hand level

√7ᵗʰ **S66.590** Other injury of intrinsic muscle, fascia
and tendon of right index finger at wrist
and hand level

√7ᵗʰ **S66.591** Other injury of intrinsic muscle, fascia
and tendon of left index finger at wrist
and hand level

√7ᵗʰ **S66.592** Other injury of intrinsic muscle, fascia
and tendon of right middle finger at wrist
and hand level

√7ᵗʰ **S66.593** Other injury of intrinsic muscle, fascia
and tendon of left middle finger at wrist
and hand level

√7ᵗʰ **S66.594** Other injury of intrinsic muscle, fascia
and tendon of right ring finger at wrist
and hand level

√7ᵗʰ **S66.595** Other injury of intrinsic muscle, fascia
and tendon of left ring finger at wrist and
hand level

√7ᵗʰ **S66.596** Other injury of intrinsic muscle, fascia
and tendon of right little finger at wrist
and hand level

√7ᵗʰ **S66.597** Other injury of intrinsic muscle, fascia
and tendon of left little finger at wrist and
hand level

√7ᵗʰ **S66.598** Other injury of intrinsic muscle, fascia
and tendon of other finger at wrist and
hand level
     Other injury of intrinsic muscle, fascia and
tendon of specified finger with
unspecified laterality at wrist and
hand level

√7ᵗʰ **S66.599** Other injury of intrinsic muscle, fascia ▽
and tendon of unspecified finger at
wrist and hand level

√5ᵗʰ **S66.8** Injury of other specified muscles, fascia and tendons at wrist
and hand level

√6ᵗʰ **S66.80** Unspecified injury of other specified muscles, fascia
and tendons at wrist and hand level

√7ᵗʰ **S66.801** Unspecified injury of other specified ▽
muscles, fascia and tendons at wrist
and hand level, right hand

√7ᵗʰ **S66.802** Unspecified injury of other specified ▽
muscles, fascia and tendons at wrist
and hand level, left hand

√7ᵗʰ **S66.809** Unspecified injury of other specified ▽
muscles, fascia and tendons at wrist
and hand level, unspecified hand

√6ᵗʰ **S66.81** Strain of other specified muscles, fascia and tendons
at wrist and hand level

√7ᵗʰ **S66.811** Strain of other specified muscles, fascia
and tendons at wrist and hand level, right
hand

√7ᵗʰ **S66.812** Strain of other specified muscles, fascia
and tendons at wrist and hand level, left
hand

√7ᵗʰ **S66.819** Strain of other specified muscles, ▽
fascia and tendons at wrist and hand
level, unspecified hand

√6ᵗʰ **S66.82** Laceration of other specified muscles, fascia and
tendons at wrist and hand level

√7ᵗʰ **S66.821** Laceration of other specified muscles,
fascia and tendons at wrist and hand
level, right hand

☑ Add'l Character Required   √x7ᵗʰ Placeholder Alert   RUG IV Special Care High Dx   RUG IV Clinically Complex Dx   RUG IV Special Care Low Dx   Manifestation Code   Other Specified Code   ▽ Unspecified Code

ICD-10-CM 2016   **941**

√7ᵗʰ **S66.822** **Laceration of other specified muscles, fascia and tendons at wrist and hand level, left hand**

√7ᵗʰ **S66.829** **Laceration of other specified muscles, fascia and tendons at wrist and hand level, unspecified hand** ▽

√6ᵗʰ **S66.89** Other injury of other specified muscles, fascia and tendons at wrist and hand level

√7ᵗʰ **S66.891** **Other injury of other specified muscles, fascia and tendons at wrist and hand level, right hand**

√7ᵗʰ **S66.892** **Other injury of other specified muscles, fascia and tendons at wrist and hand level, left hand**

√7ᵗʰ **S66.899** **Other injury of other specified muscles, fascia and tendons at wrist and hand level, unspecified hand** ▽

√5ᵗʰ **S66.9** Injury of unspecified muscle, fascia and tendon at wrist and hand level

√6ᵗʰ **S66.90** Unspecified injury of unspecified muscle, fascia and tendon at wrist and hand level

√7ᵗʰ **S66.901** **Unspecified injury of unspecified muscle, fascia and tendon at wrist and hand level, right hand** ▽

√7ᵗʰ **S66.902** **Unspecified injury of unspecified muscle, fascia and tendon at wrist and hand level, left hand** ▽

√7ᵗʰ **S66.909** **Unspecified injury of unspecified muscle, fascia and tendon at wrist and hand level, unspecified hand** ▽

√6ᵗʰ **S66.91** Strain of unspecified muscle, fascia and tendon at wrist and hand level

√7ᵗʰ **S66.911** **Strain of unspecified muscle, fascia and tendon at wrist and hand level, right hand** ▽

√7ᵗʰ **S66.912** **Strain of unspecified muscle, fascia and tendon at wrist and hand level, left hand** ▽

√7ᵗʰ **S66.919** **Strain of unspecified muscle, fascia and tendon at wrist and hand level, unspecified hand** ▽

√6ᵗʰ **S66.92** Laceration of unspecified muscle, fascia and tendon at wrist and hand level

√7ᵗʰ **S66.921** **Laceration of unspecified muscle, fascia and tendon at wrist and hand level, right hand** ▽

√7ᵗʰ **S66.922** **Laceration of unspecified muscle, fascia and tendon at wrist and hand level, left hand** ▽

√7ᵗʰ **S66.929** **Laceration of unspecified muscle, fascia and tendon at wrist and hand level, unspecified hand** ▽

√6ᵗʰ **S66.99** Other injury of unspecified muscle, fascia and tendon at wrist and hand level

√7ᵗʰ **S66.991** **Other injury of unspecified muscle, fascia and tendon at wrist and hand level, right hand** ▽

√7ᵗʰ **S66.992** **Other injury of unspecified muscle, fascia and tendon at wrist and hand level, left hand** ▽

√7ᵗʰ **S66.999** **Other injury of unspecified muscle, fascia and tendon at wrist and hand level, unspecified hand** ▽

√4ᵗʰ **S67** Crushing injury of wrist, hand and fingers

Use additional code for all associated injuries, such as:
  fracture of wrist and hand (S62.-)
  open wound of wrist and hand (S61.-)

> The appropriate 7th character is to be added to each code from category S67.
> A   initial encounter
> D   subsequent encounter
> S   sequela

√5ᵗʰ **S67.0** Crushing injury of thumb

√x7ᵗʰ **S67.00** **Crushing injury of unspecified thumb** ▽

√x7ᵗʰ **S67.01** **Crushing injury of right thumb**

√x7ᵗʰ **S67.02** **Crushing injury of left thumb**

√5ᵗʰ **S67.1** Crushing injury of other and unspecified finger(s)

  EXCLUDES 2   crushing injury of thumb (S67.0-)

√x7ᵗʰ **S67.10** **Crushing injury of unspecified finger(s)** ▽

√6ᵗʰ **S67.19** **Crushing injury of other finger(s)**

√7ᵗʰ **S67.190** **Crushing injury of right index finger**

√7ᵗʰ **S67.191** **Crushing injury of left index finger**

√7ᵗʰ **S67.192** **Crushing injury of right middle finger**

√7ᵗʰ **S67.193** **Crushing injury of left middle finger**

√7ᵗʰ **S67.194** **Crushing injury of right ring finger**

√7ᵗʰ **S67.195** **Crushing injury of left ring finger**

√7ᵗʰ **S67.196** **Crushing injury of right little finger**

√7ᵗʰ **S67.197** **Crushing injury of left little finger**

√7ᵗʰ **S67.198** **Crushing injury of other finger**
    Crushing injury of specified finger with unspecified laterality

√5ᵗʰ **S67.2** Crushing injury of hand

  EXCLUDES 2   crushing injury of fingers (S67.1-)
             crushing injury of thumb (S67.0-)

√x7ᵗʰ **S67.20** **Crushing injury of unspecified hand** ▽

√x7ᵗʰ **S67.21** **Crushing injury of right hand**

√x7ᵗʰ **S67.22** **Crushing injury of left hand**

√5ᵗʰ **S67.3** Crushing injury of wrist

√x7ᵗʰ **S67.30** **Crushing injury of unspecified wrist** ▽

√x7ᵗʰ **S67.31** **Crushing injury of right wrist**

√x7ᵗʰ **S67.32** **Crushing injury of left wrist**

√5ᵗʰ **S67.4** Crushing injury of wrist and hand

  EXCLUDES 1   crushing injury of hand alone (S67.2-)
             crushing injury of wrist alone (S67.3-)
  EXCLUDES 2   crushing injury of fingers (S67.1-)
             crushing injury of thumb (S67.0-)

√x7ᵗʰ **S67.40** **Crushing injury of unspecified wrist and hand** ▽

√x7ᵗʰ **S67.41** **Crushing injury of right wrist and hand**

√x7ᵗʰ **S67.42** **Crushing injury of left wrist and hand**

√5ᵗʰ **S67.9** Crushing injury of unspecified part(s) of wrist, hand and fingers

√x7ᵗʰ **S67.90** **Crushing injury of unspecified part(s) of unspecified wrist, hand and fingers** ▽

√x7ᵗʰ **S67.91** **Crushing injury of unspecified part(s) of right wrist, hand and fingers** ▽

√x7ᵗʰ **S67.92** **Crushing injury of unspecified part(s) of left wrist, hand and fingers** ▽

√4ᵗʰ **S68** Traumatic amputation of wrist, hand and fingers

  NOTE   An amputation not identified as partial or complete should be coded to complete.

> The appropriate 7th character is to be added to each code from category S68.
> A   initial encounter
> D   subsequent encounter
> S   sequela

√5ᵗʰ **S68.0** Traumatic metacarpophalangeal amputation of thumb
    Traumatic amputation of thumb NOS

√6ᵗʰ **S68.01** Complete traumatic metacarpophalangeal amputation of thumb

√7ᵗʰ **S68.011** **Complete traumatic metacarpophalangeal amputation of right thumb**

√7ᵗʰ **S68.012** **Complete traumatic metacarpophalangeal amputation of left thumb**

√7ᵗʰ **S68.019** **Complete traumatic metacarpophalangeal amputation of unspecified thumb** ▽

√6ᵗʰ **S68.02** Partial traumatic metacarpophalangeal amputation of thumb

√7ᵗʰ **S68.021** **Partial traumatic metacarpophalangeal amputation of right thumb**

√7ᵗʰ **S68.022** **Partial traumatic metacarpophalangeal amputation of left thumb**

√7ᵗʰ **S68.029** **Partial traumatic metacarpophalangeal amputation of unspecified thumb** ▽

Ⓝ Newborn   Ⓟ Pediatric   Ⓜ Maternity   Ⓐ Adult   **RIC** RIC Dx   **NC Dx** Noncancer Dx   **PDx** Primary Dx   **CC** RIC CC Condition   ►◄ Revised Text   ● New Code   ▲ Revised Code Title

942   ICD-10-CM 2016

✓5ᵗʰ **S68.1 Traumatic** metacarpophalangeal **amputation of** other and unspecified finger

Traumatic amputation of finger NOS

EXCLUDES 2   *traumatic metacarpophalangeal amputation of thumb (S68.0-)*

✓6ᵗʰ **S68.11 Complete traumatic metacarpophalangeal amputation of other and unspecified finger**

✓7ᵗʰ **S68.110 Complete traumatic metacarpophalangeal amputation of** right index **finger**

✓7ᵗʰ **S68.111 Complete traumatic metacarpophalangeal amputation of** left index **finger**

✓7ᵗʰ **S68.112 Complete traumatic metacarpophalangeal amputation of** right middle **finger**

✓7ᵗʰ **S68.113 Complete traumatic metacarpophalangeal amputation of** left middle **finger**

✓7ᵗʰ **S68.114 Complete traumatic metacarpophalangeal amputation of** right ring **finger**

✓7ᵗʰ **S68.115 Complete traumatic metacarpophalangeal amputation of** left ring **finger**

✓7ᵗʰ **S68.116 Complete traumatic metacarpophalangeal amputation of** right little **finger**

✓7ᵗʰ **S68.117 Complete traumatic metacarpophalangeal amputation of** left little **finger**

✓7ᵗʰ **S68.118 Complete traumatic metacarpophalangeal amputation of other finger**

Complete traumatic metacarpophalangeal amputation of specified finger with unspecified laterality

✓7ᵗʰ **S68.119 Complete traumatic metacarpophalangeal amputation of unspecified finger** ▽

✓6ᵗʰ **S68.12 Partial traumatic metacarpophalangeal amputation of other and unspecified finger**

✓7ᵗʰ **S68.120 Partial traumatic metacarpophalangeal amputation of** right index **finger**

✓7ᵗʰ **S68.121 Partial traumatic metacarpophalangeal amputation of** left index **finger**

✓7ᵗʰ **S68.122 Partial traumatic metacarpophalangeal amputation of** right middle **finger**

✓7ᵗʰ **S68.123 Partial traumatic metacarpophalangeal amputation of** left middle **finger**

✓7ᵗʰ **S68.124 Partial traumatic metacarpophalangeal amputation of** right ring **finger**

✓7ᵗʰ **S68.125 Partial traumatic metacarpophalangeal amputation of** left ring **finger**

✓7ᵗʰ **S68.126 Partial traumatic metacarpophalangeal amputation of** right little **finger**

✓7ᵗʰ **S68.127 Partial traumatic metacarpophalangeal amputation of** left little **finger**

✓7ᵗʰ **S68.128 Partial traumatic metacarpophalangeal amputation of other finger**

Partial traumatic metacarpophalangeal amputation of specified finger with unspecified laterality

✓7ᵗʰ **S68.129 Partial traumatic metacarpophalangeal** ▽ **amputation of unspecified finger**

✓5ᵗʰ **S68.4 Traumatic amputation of** hand at wrist level

Traumatic amputation of hand NOS

Traumatic amputation of wrist

✓6ᵗʰ **S68.41 Complete traumatic amputation of hand at wrist level**

✓7ᵗʰ **S68.411 Complete traumatic amputation of** right **hand at wrist level**

✓7ᵗʰ **S68.412 Complete traumatic amputation of** left **hand at wrist level**

✓7ᵗʰ **S68.419 Complete traumatic amputation of** ▽ **unspecified hand at wrist level**

✓6ᵗʰ **S68.42 Partial traumatic amputation of hand at wrist level**

✓7ᵗʰ **S68.421 Partial traumatic amputation of** right **hand at wrist level**

✓7ᵗʰ **S68.422 Partial traumatic amputation of** left **hand at wrist level**

✓7ᵗʰ **S68.429 Partial traumatic amputation of** ▽ **unspecified hand at wrist level**

✓5ᵗʰ **S68.5 Traumatic** transphalangeal **amputation of** thumb

Traumatic interphalangeal joint amputation of thumb

✓6ᵗʰ **S68.51 Complete traumatic transphalangeal amputation of thumb**

✓7ᵗʰ **S68.511 Complete traumatic transphalangeal amputation of** right **thumb**

✓7ᵗʰ **S68.512 Complete traumatic transphalangeal amputation of** left **thumb**

✓7ᵗʰ **S68.519 Complete traumatic transphalangeal** ▽ **amputation of unspecified thumb**

✓6ᵗʰ **S68.52 Partial traumatic transphalangeal amputation of thumb**

✓7ᵗʰ **S68.521 Partial traumatic transphalangeal amputation of** right **thumb**

✓7ᵗʰ **S68.522 Partial traumatic transphalangeal amputation of** left **thumb**

✓7ᵗʰ **S68.529 Partial traumatic transphalangeal** ▽ **amputation of unspecified thumb**

✓5ᵗʰ **S68.6 Traumatic** transphalangeal **amputation of** other and unspecified finger

✓6ᵗʰ **S68.61 Complete traumatic transphalangeal amputation of other and unspecified finger(s)**

✓7ᵗʰ **S68.610 Complete traumatic transphalangeal amputation of** right index **finger**

✓7ᵗʰ **S68.611 Complete traumatic transphalangeal amputation of** left index **finger**

✓7ᵗʰ **S68.612 Complete traumatic transphalangeal amputation of** right middle **finger**

✓7ᵗʰ **S68.613 Complete traumatic transphalangeal amputation of** left middle **finger**

✓7ᵗʰ **S68.614 Complete traumatic transphalangeal amputation of** right ring **finger**

✓7ᵗʰ **S68.615 Complete traumatic transphalangeal amputation of** left ring **finger**

✓7ᵗʰ **S68.616 Complete traumatic transphalangeal amputation of** right little **finger**

✓7ᵗʰ **S68.617 Complete traumatic transphalangeal amputation of** left little **finger**

✓7ᵗʰ **S68.618 Complete traumatic transphalangeal amputation of other finger**

Complete traumatic transphalangeal amputation of specified finger with unspecified laterality

✓7ᵗʰ **S68.619 Complete traumatic transphalangeal** ▽ **amputation of unspecified finger**

✓6ᵗʰ **S68.62 Partial traumatic transphalangeal amputation of other and unspecified finger**

✓7ᵗʰ **S68.620 Partial traumatic transphalangeal amputation of** right index **finger**

✓7ᵗʰ **S68.621 Partial traumatic transphalangeal amputation of** left index **finger**

✓7ᵗʰ **S68.622 Partial traumatic transphalangeal amputation of** right middle **finger**

✓7ᵗʰ **S68.623 Partial traumatic transphalangeal amputation of** left middle **finger**

✓7ᵗʰ **S68.624 Partial traumatic transphalangeal amputation of** right ring **finger**

✓7ᵗʰ **S68.625 Partial traumatic transphalangeal amputation of** left ring **finger**

✓7ᵗʰ **S68.626 Partial traumatic transphalangeal amputation of** right little **finger**

✓7ᵗʰ **S68.627 Partial traumatic transphalangeal amputation of** left little **finger**

✓7ᵗʰ **S68.628 Partial traumatic transphalangeal amputation of other finger**

Partial traumatic transphalangeal amputation of specified finger with unspecified laterality

✓7ᵗʰ **S68.629 Partial traumatic transphalangeal** ▽ **amputation of unspecified finger**

✅ Add'l Character Required   ✓ₓ7ᵗʰ Placeholder Alert   RUG IV Special Care High Dx   RUG IV Clinically Complex Dx   RUG IV Special Care Low Dx   Manifestation Code   Other Specified Code   ▽ Unspecified Code

Chapter 19. Injury, Poisoning and Certain Other Consequences of External Causes

S68.7   ✓5ᵗʰ   **S68.7**   Traumatic transmetacarpal amputation of hand

    ✓6ᵗʰ   **S68.71**   Complete traumatic transmetacarpal amputation of hand

       ✓7ᵗʰ   **S68.711**   **Complete traumatic transmetacarpal amputation of right hand**

       ✓7ᵗʰ   **S68.712**   **Complete traumatic transmetacarpal amputation of left hand**

       ✓7ᵗʰ   **S68.719**   **Complete traumatic transmetacarpal amputation of unspecified hand** ▽

    ✓6ᵗʰ   **S68.72**   Partial traumatic transmetacarpal amputation of hand

       ✓7ᵗʰ   **S68.721**   **Partial traumatic transmetacarpal amputation of right hand**

       ✓7ᵗʰ   **S68.722**   **Partial traumatic transmetacarpal amputation of left hand**

       ✓7ᵗʰ   **S68.729**   **Partial traumatic transmetacarpal amputation of unspecified hand** ▽

✓4ᵗʰ   **S69**   **Other and unspecified injuries of wrist, hand and finger(s)**

> The appropriate 7th character is to be added to each code from category S69.
> A   initial encounter
> D   subsequent encounter
> S   sequela

  ✓5ᵗʰ   **S69.8**   **Other specified injuries of wrist, hand and finger(s)**

    ✓x7ᵗʰ   **S69.80**   **Other specified injuries of unspecified wrist, hand and finger(s)** ▽

    ✓x7ᵗʰ   **S69.81**   **Other specified injuries of right wrist, hand and finger(s)**

    ✓x7ᵗʰ   **S69.82**   **Other specified injuries of left wrist, hand and finger(s)**

  ✓5ᵗʰ   **S69.9**   **Unspecified injury of wrist, hand and finger(s)**

    ✓x7ᵗʰ   **S69.90**   **Unspecified injury of unspecified wrist, hand and finger(s)** ▽

    ✓x7ᵗʰ   **S69.91**   **Unspecified injury of right wrist, hand and finger(s)** ▽

    ✓x7ᵗʰ   **S69.92**   **Unspecified injury of left wrist, hand and finger(s)** ▽

Injuries to the hip and thigh (S70-S79)

> **EXCLUDES 2**   burns and corrosions (T20-T32)
> frostbite (T33-T34)
> snake bite (T63.0-)
> venomous insect bite or sting (T63.4-)

✓4ᵗʰ   **S70**   **Superficial injury of hip and thigh**

> The appropriate 7th character is to be added to each code from category S70.
> A   initial encounter
> D   subsequent encounter
> S   sequela

  ✓5ᵗʰ   **S70.0**   **Contusion of hip**

    ✓x7ᵗʰ   **S70.00**   **Contusion of unspecified hip** ▽

    ✓x7ᵗʰ   **S70.01**   **Contusion of right hip**

    ✓x7ᵗʰ   **S70.02**   **Contusion of left hip**

  ✓5ᵗʰ   **S70.1**   **Contusion of thigh**

    ✓x7ᵗʰ   **S70.10**   **Contusion of unspecified thigh** ▽

    ✓x7ᵗʰ   **S70.11**   **Contusion of right thigh**

    ✓x7ᵗʰ   **S70.12**   **Contusion of left thigh**

  ✓5ᵗʰ   **S70.2**   Other superficial injuries of hip

    ✓6ᵗʰ   **S70.21**   Abrasion of hip

       ✓7ᵗʰ   **S70.211**   **Abrasion, right hip**

       ✓7ᵗʰ   **S70.212**   **Abrasion, left hip**

       ✓7ᵗʰ   **S70.219**   **Abrasion, unspecified hip** ▽

    ✓6ᵗʰ   **S70.22**   Blister (nonthermal) of hip

       ✓7ᵗʰ   **S70.221**   **Blister (nonthermal), right hip**

       ✓7ᵗʰ   **S70.222**   **Blister (nonthermal), left hip**

       ✓7ᵗʰ   **S70.229**   **Blister (nonthermal), unspecified hip** ▽

    ✓6ᵗʰ   **S70.24**   External constriction of hip

       ✓7ᵗʰ   **S70.241**   **External constriction, right hip**

       ✓7ᵗʰ   **S70.242**   **External constriction, left hip**

       ✓7ᵗʰ   **S70.249**   **External constriction, unspecified hip** ▽

    ✓6ᵗʰ   **S70.25**   Superficial foreign body of hip
> Splinter in the hip

       ✓7ᵗʰ   **S70.251**   **Superficial foreign body, right hip**

       ✓7ᵗʰ   **S70.252**   **Superficial foreign body, left hip**

       ✓7ᵗʰ   **S70.259**   **Superficial foreign body, unspecified hip** ▽

    ✓6ᵗʰ   **S70.26**   Insect bite (nonvenomous) of hip

       ✓7ᵗʰ   **S70.261**   **Insect bite (nonvenomous), right hip**

       ✓7ᵗʰ   **S70.262**   **Insect bite (nonvenomous), left hip**

       ✓7ᵗʰ   **S70.269**   **Insect bite (nonvenomous), unspecified hip** ▽

    ✓6ᵗʰ   **S70.27**   Other superficial bite of hip
> **EXCLUDES 1**   open bite of hip (S71.05-)

       ✓7ᵗʰ   **S70.271**   **Other superficial bite of hip, right hip**

       ✓7ᵗʰ   **S70.272**   **Other superficial bite of hip, left hip**

       ✓7ᵗʰ   **S70.279**   **Other superficial bite of hip, unspecified hip** ▽

  ✓5ᵗʰ   **S70.3**   **Other superficial injuries of thigh**

    ✓6ᵗʰ   **S70.31**   Abrasion of thigh

       ✓7ᵗʰ   **S70.311**   **Abrasion, right thigh**

       ✓7ᵗʰ   **S70.312**   **Abrasion, left thigh**

       ✓7ᵗʰ   **S70.319**   **Abrasion, unspecified thigh** ▽

    ✓6ᵗʰ   **S70.32**   Blister (nonthermal) of thigh

       ✓7ᵗʰ   **S70.321**   **Blister (nonthermal), right thigh**

       ✓7ᵗʰ   **S70.322**   **Blister (nonthermal), left thigh**

       ✓7ᵗʰ   **S70.329**   **Blister (nonthermal), unspecified thigh** ▽

    ✓6ᵗʰ   **S70.34**   External constriction of thigh

       ✓7ᵗʰ   **S70.341**   **External constriction, right thigh**

       ✓7ᵗʰ   **S70.342**   **External constriction, left thigh**

       ✓7ᵗʰ   **S70.349**   **External constriction, unspecified thigh** ▽

    ✓6ᵗʰ   **S70.35**   Superficial foreign body of thigh
> Splinter in the thigh

       ✓7ᵗʰ   **S70.351**   **Superficial foreign body, right thigh**

       ✓7ᵗʰ   **S70.352**   **Superficial foreign body, left thigh**

       ✓7ᵗʰ   **S70.359**   **Superficial foreign body, unspecified thigh** ▽

    ✓6ᵗʰ   **S70.36**   Insect bite (nonvenomous) of thigh

       ✓7ᵗʰ   **S70.361**   **Insect bite (nonvenomous), right thigh**

       ✓7ᵗʰ   **S70.362**   **Insect bite (nonvenomous), left thigh**

       ✓7ᵗʰ   **S70.369**   **Insect bite (nonvenomous), unspecified thigh** ▽

    ✓6ᵗʰ   **S70.37**   Other superficial bite of thigh
> **EXCLUDES 1**   open bite of thigh (S71.15-)

       ✓7ᵗʰ   **S70.371**   **Other superficial bite of right thigh**

       ✓7ᵗʰ   **S70.372**   **Other superficial bite of left thigh**

       ✓7ᵗʰ   **S70.379**   **Other superficial bite of unspecified thigh** ▽

  ✓5ᵗʰ   **S70.9**   **Unspecified superficial injury of hip and thigh**

    ✓6ᵗʰ   **S70.91**   Unspecified superficial injury of hip

       ✓7ᵗʰ   **S70.911**   **Unspecified superficial injury of right hip**

       ✓7ᵗʰ   **S70.912**   **Unspecified superficial injury of left hip** ▽

       ✓7ᵗʰ   **S70.919**   **Unspecified superficial injury of unspecified hip** ▽

    ✓6ᵗʰ   **S70.92**   Unspecified superficial injury of thigh

       ✓7ᵗʰ   **S70.921**   **Unspecified superficial injury of right thigh** ▽

       ✓7ᵗʰ   **S70.922**   **Unspecified superficial injury of left thigh** ▽

       ✓7ᵗʰ   **S70.929**   **Unspecified superficial injury of unspecified thigh** ▽

Ⓝ Newborn   Ⓟ Pediatric   Ⓜ Maternity   Ⓐ Adult   **RIC** RIC Dx   **NC Dx** Noncancer Dx   **PDx** Primary Dx   **CC** RIC CC Condition   ▶◀ Revised Text   ● New Code   ▲ Revised Code Title

944   ICD-10-CM 2016

✓4ᵗʰ S71 Open wound of hip and thigh
Code also any associated wound infection
EXCLUDES 1 *open fracture of hip and thigh (S72.-)*
traumatic amputation of hip and thigh (S78.-)
EXCLUDES 2 *bite of venomous animal (T63.-)*
open wound of ankle, foot and toes (S91.-)
open wound of knee and lower leg (S81.-)

The appropriate 7th character is to be added to each code from category S71.
A   initial encounter
D   subsequent encounter
S   sequela

✓5ᵗʰ S71.0 Open wound of hip
   ✓6ᵗʰ S71.00 Unspecified open wound of hip
     ✓7ᵗʰ S71.001 Unspecified open wound, right hip ▽
     ✓7ᵗʰ S71.002 Unspecified open wound, left hip ▽
     ✓7ᵗʰ S71.009 Unspecified open wound, unspecified hip ▽

   ✓6ᵗʰ S71.01 Laceration without foreign body of hip
     ✓7ᵗʰ S71.011 Laceration without foreign body, right hip
     ✓7ᵗʰ S71.012 Laceration without foreign body, left hip
     ✓7ᵗʰ S71.019 Laceration without foreign body, unspecified hip ▽

   ✓6ᵗʰ S71.02 Laceration with foreign body of hip
     ✓7ᵗʰ S71.021 Laceration with foreign body, right hip
     ✓7ᵗʰ S71.022 Laceration with foreign body, left hip
     ✓7ᵗʰ S71.029 Laceration with foreign body, unspecified hip ▽

   ✓6ᵗʰ S71.03 Puncture wound without foreign body of hip
     ✓7ᵗʰ S71.031 Puncture wound without foreign body, right hip
     ✓7ᵗʰ S71.032 Puncture wound without foreign body, left hip
     ✓7ᵗʰ S71.039 Puncture wound without foreign body, unspecified hip ▽

   ✓6ᵗʰ S71.04 Puncture wound with foreign body of hip
     ✓7ᵗʰ S71.041 Puncture wound with foreign body, right hip
     ✓7ᵗʰ S71.042 Puncture wound with foreign body, left hip
     ✓7ᵗʰ S71.049 Puncture wound with foreign body, unspecified hip ▽

   ✓6ᵗʰ S71.05 Open bite of hip
     Bite of hip NOS
     EXCLUDES 1 *superficial bite of hip (S70.26, S70.27)*
     ✓7ᵗʰ S71.051 Open bite, right hip
     ✓7ᵗʰ S71.052 Open bite, left hip
     ✓7ᵗʰ S71.059 Open bite, unspecified hip ▽

✓5ᵗʰ S71.1 Open wound of thigh
   ✓6ᵗʰ S71.10 Unspecified open wound of thigh
     ✓7ᵗʰ S71.101 Unspecified open wound, right thigh ▽
     ✓7ᵗʰ S71.102 Unspecified open wound, left thigh ▽
     ✓7ᵗʰ S71.109 Unspecified open wound, unspecified thigh ▽

   ✓6ᵗʰ S71.11 Laceration without foreign body of thigh
     ✓7ᵗʰ S71.111 Laceration without foreign body, right thigh
     ✓7ᵗʰ S71.112 Laceration without foreign body, left thigh
     ✓7ᵗʰ S71.119 Laceration without foreign body, unspecified thigh ▽

   ✓6ᵗʰ S71.12 Laceration with foreign body of thigh
     ✓7ᵗʰ S71.121 Laceration with foreign body, right thigh
     ✓7ᵗʰ S71.122 Laceration with foreign body, left thigh
     ✓7ᵗʰ S71.129 Laceration with foreign body, unspecified thigh ▽

   ✓6ᵗʰ S71.13 Puncture wound without foreign body of thigh
     ✓7ᵗʰ S71.131 Puncture wound without foreign body, right thigh
     ✓7ᵗʰ S71.132 Puncture wound without foreign body, left thigh

     ✓7ᵗʰ S71.139 Puncture wound without foreign body, unspecified thigh ▽

   ✓6ᵗʰ S71.14 Puncture wound with foreign body of thigh
     ✓7ᵗʰ S71.141 Puncture wound with foreign body, right thigh
     ✓7ᵗʰ S71.142 Puncture wound with foreign body, left thigh
     ✓7ᵗʰ S71.149 Puncture wound with foreign body, unspecified thigh ▽

   ✓6ᵗʰ S71.15 Open bite of thigh
     Bite of thigh NOS
     EXCLUDES 1 *superficial bite of thigh (S70.37-)*
     ✓7ᵗʰ S71.151 Open bite, right thigh
     ✓7ᵗʰ S71.152 Open bite, left thigh
     ✓7ᵗʰ S71.159 Open bite, unspecified thigh ▽

✓4ᵗʰ S72 Fracture of femur
NOTE A fracture not indicated as displaced or nondisplaced should be coded to displaced.
The open fracture designations are based on the Gustilo open fracture classification.
A fracture not indicated as open or closed should be coded to closed.
EXCLUDES 1 *traumatic amputation of hip and thigh (S78.-)*
EXCLUDES 2 *fracture of foot (S92.-)*
fracture of lower leg and ankle (S82.-)
periprosthetic fracture of prosthetic implant of hip (T84.040, T84.041)
AHA: 2015, 1Q, 17; 2013, 4Q, 128

The appropriate 7th character is to be added to all codes from category S72 [unless otherwise indicated].
A   initial encounter for closed fracture
B   initial encounter for open fracture type I or II
     initial encounter for open fracture NOS
C   initial encounter for open fracture type IIIA, IIIB, or IIIC
D   subsequent encounter for closed fracture with routine healing
E   subsequent encounter for open fracture type I or II with routine healing
F   subsequent encounter for open fracture type IIIA, IIIB, or IIIC with routine healing
G   subsequent encounter for closed fracture with delayed healing
H   subsequent encounter for open fracture type I or II with delayed healing
J   subsequent encounter for open fracture type IIIA, IIIB, or IIIC with delayed healing
K   subsequent encounter for closed fracture with nonunion
M   subsequent encounter for open fracture type I or II with nonunion
N   subsequent encounter for open fracture type IIIA, IIIB, or IIIC with nonunion
P   subsequent encounter for closed fracture with malunion
Q   subsequent encounter for open fracture type I or II with malunion
R   subsequent encounter for open fracture type IIIA, IIIB, or IIIC with malunion
S   sequela

✓5ᵗʰ S72.0 Fracture of head and neck of femur
   EXCLUDES 2 *physeal fracture of upper end of femur (S79.0-)*

   ✓6ᵗʰ S72.00 Fracture of unspecified part of neck of femur
     Fracture of hip NOS Fracture of neck of femur NOS
     ✓7ᵗʰ S72.001 Fracture of unspecified part of neck of right femur ▽
     ✓7ᵗʰ S72.002 Fracture of unspecified part of neck of left femur ▽
     ✓7ᵗʰ S72.009 Fracture of unspecified part of neck of unspecified femur ▽

   ✓6ᵗʰ S72.01 Unspecified intracapsular fracture of femur
     Subcapital fracture of femur
     ✓7ᵗʰ S72.011 Unspecified intracapsular fracture of right femur ▽
     ✓7ᵗʰ S72.012 Unspecified intracapsular fracture of left femur ▽
     ✓7ᵗʰ S72.019 Unspecified intracapsular fracture of unspecified femur ▽

☑ Add'l Character Required   ✓x7ᵗʰ Placeholder Alert   RUG IV Special Care High Dx   RUG IV Clinically Complex Dx   RUG IV Special Care Low Dx   Manifestation Code   Other Specified Code   ▽ Unspecified Code

ICD-10-CM 2016   945

√6ᵗʰ S72.02   **Fracture of epiphysis (separation) (upper) of femur**
Transepiphyseal fracture of femur
EXCLUDES 1   capital femoral epiphyseal fracture (pediatric) of femur (S79.01-)
Salter-Harris Type I physeal fracture of upper end of femur (S79.01-)

    √7ᵗʰ S72.021   **Displaced fracture of epiphysis (separation) (upper) of right femur**

    √7ᵗʰ S72.022   **Displaced fracture of epiphysis (separation) (upper) of left femur**

    √7ᵗʰ S72.023   **Displaced fracture of epiphysis (separation) (upper) of unspecified femur** ▽

    √7ᵗʰ S72.024   **Nondisplaced fracture of epiphysis (separation) (upper) of right femur**

    √7ᵗʰ S72.025   **Nondisplaced fracture of epiphysis (separation) (upper) of left femur**

    √7ᵗʰ S72.026   **Nondisplaced fracture of epiphysis (separation) (upper) of unspecified femur** ▽

√6ᵗʰ S72.03   **Midcervical fracture of femur**
Transcervical fracture of femur NOS

    √7ᵗʰ S72.031   **Displaced midcervical fracture of right femur**

    √7ᵗʰ S72.032   **Displaced midcervical fracture of left femur**

    √7ᵗʰ S72.033   **Displaced midcervical fracture of unspecified femur** ▽

    √7ᵗʰ S72.034   **Nondisplaced midcervical fracture of right femur**

    √7ᵗʰ S72.035   **Nondisplaced midcervical fracture of left femur**

    √7ᵗʰ S72.036   **Nondisplaced midcervical fracture of unspecified femur** ▽

√6ᵗʰ S72.04   **Fracture of base of neck of femur**
Cervicotrochanteric fracture of femur

    √7ᵗʰ S72.041   **Displaced fracture of base of neck of right femur**

    √7ᵗʰ S72.042   **Displaced fracture of base of neck of left femur**

    √7ᵗʰ S72.043   **Displaced fracture of base of neck of unspecified femur** ▽

    √7ᵗʰ S72.044   **Nondisplaced fracture of base of neck of right femur**

    √7ᵗʰ S72.045   **Nondisplaced fracture of base of neck of left femur**

    √7ᵗʰ S72.046   **Nondisplaced fracture of base of neck of unspecified femur** ▽

√6ᵗʰ S72.05   **Unspecified fracture of head of femur**
Fracture of head of femur NOS

    √7ᵗʰ S72.051   **Unspecified fracture of head of right femur** ▽

    √7ᵗʰ S72.052   **Unspecified fracture of head of left femur** ▽

    √7ᵗʰ S72.059   **Unspecified fracture of head of unspecified femur** ▽

√6ᵗʰ S72.06   **Articular fracture of head of femur**

    √7ᵗʰ S72.061   **Displaced articular fracture of head of right femur**

    √7ᵗʰ S72.062   **Displaced articular fracture of head of left femur**

    √7ᵗʰ S72.063   **Displaced articular fracture of head of unspecified femur** ▽

    √7ᵗʰ S72.064   **Nondisplaced articular fracture of head of right femur**

    √7ᵗʰ S72.065   **Nondisplaced articular fracture of head of left femur**

    √7ᵗʰ S72.066   **Nondisplaced articular fracture of head of unspecified femur** ▽

√6ᵗʰ S72.09   **Other fracture of head and neck of femur**

    √7ᵗʰ S72.091   **Other fracture of head and neck of right femur**

    √7ᵗʰ S72.092   **Other fracture of head and neck of left femur**

    √7ᵗʰ S72.099   **Other fracture of head and neck of unspecified femur** ▽

√5ᵗʰ S72.1   **Pertrochanteric fracture**

    √6ᵗʰ S72.10   **Unspecified trochanteric fracture of femur**
Fracture of trochanter NOS

      √7ᵗʰ S72.101   **Unspecified trochanteric fracture of right femur** ▽

      √7ᵗʰ S72.102   **Unspecified trochanteric fracture of left femur** ▽

      √7ᵗʰ S72.109   **Unspecified trochanteric fracture of unspecified femur** ▽

    √6ᵗʰ S72.11   **Fracture of greater trochanter of femur**

      √7ᵗʰ S72.111   **Displaced fracture of greater trochanter of right femur**

      √7ᵗʰ S72.112   **Displaced fracture of greater trochanter of left femur**

      √7ᵗʰ S72.113   **Displaced fracture of greater trochanter of unspecified femur** ▽

      √7ᵗʰ S72.114   **Nondisplaced fracture of greater trochanter of right femur**

      √7ᵗʰ S72.115   **Nondisplaced fracture of greater trochanter of left femur**

      √7ᵗʰ S72.116   **Nondisplaced fracture of greater trochanter of unspecified femur** ▽

    √6ᵗʰ S72.12   **Fracture of lesser trochanter of femur**

      √7ᵗʰ S72.121   **Displaced fracture of lesser trochanter of right femur**

      √7ᵗʰ S72.122   **Displaced fracture of lesser trochanter of left femur**

      √7ᵗʰ S72.123   **Displaced fracture of lesser trochanter of unspecified femur** ▽

      √7ᵗʰ S72.124   **Nondisplaced fracture of lesser trochanter of right femur**

      √7ᵗʰ S72.125   **Nondisplaced fracture of lesser trochanter of left femur**

      √7ᵗʰ S72.126   **Nondisplaced fracture of lesser trochanter of unspecified femur** ▽

    √6ᵗʰ S72.13   **Apophyseal fracture of femur**
EXCLUDES 1   chronic (nontraumatic) slipped upper femoral epiphysis (M93.0-)

      √7ᵗʰ S72.131   **Displaced apophyseal fracture of right femur**

      √7ᵗʰ S72.132   **Displaced apophyseal fracture of left femur**

      √7ᵗʰ S72.133   **Displaced apophyseal fracture of unspecified femur** ▽

      √7ᵗʰ S72.134   **Nondisplaced apophyseal fracture of right femur**

      √7ᵗʰ S72.135   **Nondisplaced apophyseal fracture of left femur**

      √7ᵗʰ S72.136   **Nondisplaced apophyseal fracture of unspecified femur** ▽

    √6ᵗʰ S72.14   **Intertrochanteric fracture of femur**

      √7ᵗʰ S72.141   **Displaced intertrochanteric fracture of right femur**

      √7ᵗʰ S72.142   **Displaced intertrochanteric fracture of left femur**

      √7ᵗʰ S72.143   **Displaced intertrochanteric fracture of unspecified femur** ▽

      √7ᵗʰ S72.144   **Nondisplaced intertrochanteric fracture of right femur**

      √7ᵗʰ S72.145   **Nondisplaced intertrochanteric fracture of left femur**

      √7ᵗʰ S72.146   **Nondisplaced intertrochanteric fracture of unspecified femur** ▽

√5ᵗʰ S72.2   **Subtrochanteric fracture of femur**

    √x7ᵗʰ S72.21   **Displaced subtrochanteric fracture of right femur**

    √x7ᵗʰ S72.22   **Displaced subtrochanteric fracture of left femur**

    √x7ᵗʰ S72.23   **Displaced subtrochanteric fracture of unspecified femur** ▽

    √x7ᵗʰ S72.24   **Nondisplaced subtrochanteric fracture of right femur**

    √x7ᵗʰ S72.25   **Nondisplaced subtrochanteric fracture of left femur**

    √x7ᵗʰ S72.26   **Nondisplaced subtrochanteric fracture of unspecified femur** ▽

Ⓝ Newborn   Ⓟ Pediatric   Ⓜ Maternity   Ⓐ Adult   RIC RIC Dx   NCDx Noncancer Dx   PDx Primary Dx   CC RIC CC Condition   ►◄ Revised Text   ● New Code   ▲ Revised Code Title

946   ICD-10-CM 2016

√5ᵗʰ **S72.3　Fracture of shaft of femur**

　√6ᵗʰ **S72.30　Unspecified fracture of shaft of femur**

　　√7ᵗʰ **S72.301　Unspecified fracture of shaft of right femur** ▽

　　√7ᵗʰ **S72.302　Unspecified fracture of shaft of left femur** ▽

　　√7ᵗʰ **S72.309　Unspecified fracture of shaft of unspecified femur** ▽

　√6ᵗʰ **S72.32　Transverse fracture of shaft of femur**

　　√7ᵗʰ **S72.321　Displaced transverse fracture of shaft of right femur**

　　√7ᵗʰ **S72.322　Displaced transverse fracture of shaft of left femur**

　　√7ᵗʰ **S72.323　Displaced transverse fracture of shaft of unspecified femur** ▽

　　√7ᵗʰ **S72.324　Nondisplaced transverse fracture of shaft of right femur**

　　√7ᵗʰ **S72.325　Nondisplaced transverse fracture of shaft of left femur**

　　√7ᵗʰ **S72.326　Nondisplaced transverse fracture of shaft of unspecified femur** ▽

　√6ᵗʰ **S72.33　Oblique fracture of shaft of femur**

　　√7ᵗʰ **S72.331　Displaced oblique fracture of shaft of right femur**

　　√7ᵗʰ **S72.332　Displaced oblique fracture of shaft of left femur**

　　√7ᵗʰ **S72.333　Displaced oblique fracture of shaft of unspecified femur** ▽

　　√7ᵗʰ **S72.334　Nondisplaced oblique fracture of shaft of right femur**

　　√7ᵗʰ **S72.335　Nondisplaced oblique fracture of shaft of left femur**

　　√7ᵗʰ **S72.336　Nondisplaced oblique fracture of shaft of unspecified femur** ▽

　√6ᵗʰ **S72.34　Spiral fracture of shaft of femur**

　　√7ᵗʰ **S72.341　Displaced spiral fracture of shaft of right femur**

　　√7ᵗʰ **S72.342　Displaced spiral fracture of shaft of left femur**

　　√7ᵗʰ **S72.343　Displaced spiral fracture of shaft of unspecified femur** ▽

　　√7ᵗʰ **S72.344　Nondisplaced spiral fracture of shaft of right femur**

　　√7ᵗʰ **S72.345　Nondisplaced spiral fracture of shaft of left femur**

　　√7ᵗʰ **S72.346　Nondisplaced spiral fracture of shaft of unspecified femur** ▽

　√6ᵗʰ **S72.35　Comminuted fracture of shaft of femur**

　　√7ᵗʰ **S72.351　Displaced comminuted fracture of shaft of right femur**

　　√7ᵗʰ **S72.352　Displaced comminuted fracture of shaft of left femur**

　　√7ᵗʰ **S72.353　Displaced comminuted fracture of shaft of unspecified femur** ▽

　　√7ᵗʰ **S72.354　Nondisplaced comminuted fracture of shaft of right femur**

　　√7ᵗʰ **S72.355　Nondisplaced comminuted fracture of shaft of left femur**

　　√7ᵗʰ **S72.356　Nondisplaced comminuted fracture of shaft of unspecified femur** ▽

　√6ᵗʰ **S72.36　Segmental fracture of shaft of femur**

　　√7ᵗʰ **S72.361　Displaced segmental fracture of shaft of right femur**

　　√7ᵗʰ **S72.362　Displaced segmental fracture of shaft of left femur**

　　√7ᵗʰ **S72.363　Displaced segmental fracture of shaft of unspecified femur** ▽

　　√7ᵗʰ **S72.364　Nondisplaced segmental fracture of shaft of right femur**

　　√7ᵗʰ **S72.365　Nondisplaced segmental fracture of shaft of left femur**

　　√7ᵗʰ **S72.366　Nondisplaced segmental fracture of shaft of unspecified femur** ▽

　√6ᵗʰ **S72.39　Other fracture of shaft of femur**

　　√7ᵗʰ **S72.391　Other fracture of shaft of right femur**

　　√7ᵗʰ **S72.392　Other fracture of shaft of left femur**

　　√7ᵗʰ **S72.399　Other fracture of shaft of unspecified femur** ▽

√5ᵗʰ **S72.4　Fracture of lower end of femur**
　　　Fracture of distal end of femur
　　　EXCLUDES 2 *fracture of shaft of femur (S72.3-)*
　　　　　　　　　physeal fracture of lower end of femur (S79.1-)

　√6ᵗʰ **S72.40　Unspecified fracture of lower end of femur**

　　√7ᵗʰ **S72.401　Unspecified fracture of lower end of right femur** ▽

　　√7ᵗʰ **S72.402　Unspecified fracture of lower end of left femur** ▽

　　√7ᵗʰ **S72.409　Unspecified fracture of lower end of unspecified femur** ▽

　√6ᵗʰ **S72.41　Unspecified condyle fracture of lower end of femur**
　　　　Condyle fracture of femur NOS

　　√7ᵗʰ **S72.411　Displaced unspecified condyle fracture of lower end of right femur** ▽

　　√7ᵗʰ **S72.412　Displaced unspecified condyle fracture of lower end of left femur** ▽

　　√7ᵗʰ **S72.413　Displaced unspecified condyle fracture of lower end of unspecified femur** ▽

　　√7ᵗʰ **S72.414　Nondisplaced unspecified condyle fracture of lower end of right femur** ▽

　　√7ᵗʰ **S72.415　Nondisplaced unspecified condyle fracture of lower end of left femur** ▽

　　√7ᵗʰ **S72.416　Nondisplaced unspecified condyle fracture of lower end of unspecified femur** ▽

　√6ᵗʰ **S72.42　Fracture of lateral condyle of femur**

　　√7ᵗʰ **S72.421　Displaced fracture of lateral condyle of right femur**

　　√7ᵗʰ **S72.422　Displaced fracture of lateral condyle of left femur**

　　√7ᵗʰ **S72.423　Displaced fracture of lateral condyle of unspecified femur** ▽

　　√7ᵗʰ **S72.424　Nondisplaced fracture of lateral condyle of right femur**

　　√7ᵗʰ **S72.425　Nondisplaced fracture of lateral condyle of left femur**

　　√7ᵗʰ **S72.426　Nondisplaced fracture of lateral condyle of unspecified femur** ▽

　√6ᵗʰ **S72.43　Fracture of medial condyle of femur**

　　√7ᵗʰ **S72.431　Displaced fracture of medial condyle of right femur**

　　√7ᵗʰ **S72.432　Displaced fracture of medial condyle of left femur**

　　√7ᵗʰ **S72.433　Displaced fracture of medial condyle of unspecified femur** ▽

　　√7ᵗʰ **S72.434　Nondisplaced fracture of medial condyle of right femur**

　　√7ᵗʰ **S72.435　Nondisplaced fracture of medial condyle of left femur**

　　√7ᵗʰ **S72.436　Nondisplaced fracture of medial condyle of unspecified femur** ▽

　√6ᵗʰ **S72.44　Fracture of lower epiphysis (separation) of femur**
　　　　EXCLUDES 1 *Salter-Harris Type I physeal fracture of lower end of femur (S79.11-)*

　　√7ᵗʰ **S72.441　Displaced fracture of lower epiphysis (separation) of right femur**

　　√7ᵗʰ **S72.442　Displaced fracture of lower epiphysis (separation) of left femur**

　　√7ᵗʰ **S72.443　Displaced fracture of lower epiphysis (separation) of unspecified femur** ▽

　　√7ᵗʰ **S72.444　Nondisplaced fracture of lower epiphysis (separation) of right femur**

　　√7ᵗʰ **S72.445　Nondisplaced fracture of lower epiphysis (separation) of left femur**

　　√7ᵗʰ **S72.446　Nondisplaced fracture of lower epiphysis (separation) of unspecified femur** ▽

☑ Add'l Character Required　█x7ᵗʰ Placeholder Alert　RUG IV Special Care High Dx　RUG IV Clinically Complex Dx　RUG IV Special Care Low Dx　Manifestation Code　Other Specified Code　▽ Unspecified Code

✓6ᵗʰ S72.45 Supracondylar fracture without intracondylar extension of lower end of femur
Supracondylar fracture of lower end of femur NOS
> *EXCLUDES 1* supracondylar fracture with intracondylar extension of lower end of femur (S72.46-)

    ✓7ᵗʰ S72.451 Displaced supracondylar fracture without intracondylar extension of lower end of right femur

    ✓7ᵗʰ S72.452 Displaced supracondylar fracture without intracondylar extension of lower end of left femur

    ✓7ᵗʰ S72.453 Displaced supracondylar fracture without intracondylar extension of lower end of unspecified femur ▽

    ✓7ᵗʰ S72.454 Nondisplaced supracondylar fracture without intracondylar extension of lower end of right femur

    ✓7ᵗʰ S72.455 Nondisplaced supracondylar fracture without intracondylar extension of lower end of left femur

    ✓7ᵗʰ S72.456 Nondisplaced supracondylar fracture without intracondylar extension of lower end of unspecified femur ▽

✓6ᵗʰ S72.46 Supracondylar fracture with intracondylar extension of lower end of femur
> *EXCLUDES 1* supracondylar fracture without intracondylar extension of lower end of femur (S72.45-)

    ✓7ᵗʰ S72.461 Displaced supracondylar fracture with intracondylar extension of lower end of right femur

    ✓7ᵗʰ S72.462 Displaced supracondylar fracture with intracondylar extension of lower end of left femur

    ✓7ᵗʰ S72.463 Displaced supracondylar fracture with intracondylar extension of lower end of unspecified femur ▽

    ✓7ᵗʰ S72.464 Nondisplaced supracondylar fracture with intracondylar extension of lower end of right femur

    ✓7ᵗʰ S72.465 Nondisplaced supracondylar fracture with intracondylar extension of lower end of left femur

    ✓7ᵗʰ S72.466 Nondisplaced supracondylar fracture with intracondylar extension of lower end of unspecified femur ▽

✓6ᵗʰ S72.47 Torus fracture of lower end of femur

> The appropriate 7th character is to be added to all codes in subcategory S72.47.
> A initial encounter for closed fracture
> D subsequent encounter for fracture with routine healing
> G subsequent encounter for fracture with delayed healing
> K subsequent encounter for fracture with nonunion
> P subsequent encounter for fracture with malunion
> S sequela

    ✓7ᵗʰ S72.471 Torus fracture of lower end of right femur

    ✓7ᵗʰ S72.472 Torus fracture of lower end of left femur

    ✓7ᵗʰ S72.479 Torus fracture of lower end of unspecified femur ▽

✓6ᵗʰ S72.49 Other fracture of lower end of femur

    ✓7ᵗʰ S72.491 Other fracture of lower end of right femur

    ✓7ᵗʰ S72.492 Other fracture of lower end of left femur

    ✓7ᵗʰ S72.499 Other fracture of lower end of unspecified femur ▽

✓5ᵗʰ S72.8 Other fracture of femur

    ✓6ᵗʰ S72.8X Other fracture of femur

      ✓7ᵗʰ S72.8X1 Other fracture of right femur

      ✓7ᵗʰ S72.8X2 Other fracture of left femur

      ✓7ᵗʰ S72.8X9 Other fracture of unspecified femur ▽

✓5ᵗʰ S72.9 Unspecified fracture of femur
Fracture of thigh NOS
Fracture of upper leg NOS
> *EXCLUDES 1* fracture of hip NOS (S72.00-, S72.01-)

    ✓x7ᵗʰ S72.90 Unspecified fracture of unspecified femur ▽
      AHA: 2012, 4Q, 93

    ✓x7ᵗʰ S72.91 Unspecified fracture of right femur ▽

    ✓x7ᵗʰ S72.92 Unspecified fracture of left femur ▽

✓4ᵗʰ S73 Dislocation and sprain of joint and ligaments of hip
> *INCLUDES* avulsion of joint or ligament of hip
> laceration of cartilage, joint or ligament of hip
> sprain of cartilage, joint or ligament of hip
> traumatic hemarthrosis of joint or ligament of hip
> traumatic rupture of joint or ligament of hip
> traumatic subluxation of joint or ligament of hip
> traumatic tear of joint or ligament of hip

Code also any associated open wound
> *EXCLUDES 2* strain of muscle, fascia and tendon of hip and thigh (S76.-)

> The appropriate 7th character is to be added to each code from category S73.
> A initial encounter
> D subsequent encounter
> S sequela

✓5ᵗʰ S73.0 Subluxation and dislocation of hip
> *EXCLUDES 2* dislocation and subluxation of hip prosthesis (T84.020, T84.021)

    ✓6ᵗʰ S73.00 Unspecified subluxation and dislocation of hip
    Dislocation of hip NOS
    Subluxation of hip NOS

      ✓7ᵗʰ S73.001 Unspecified subluxation of right hip ▽

      ✓7ᵗʰ S73.002 Unspecified subluxation of left hip ▽

      ✓7ᵗʰ S73.003 Unspecified subluxation of unspecified hip ▽

      ✓7ᵗʰ S73.004 Unspecified dislocation of right hip ▽

      ✓7ᵗʰ S73.005 Unspecified dislocation of left hip ▽

      ✓7ᵗʰ S73.006 Unspecified dislocation of unspecified hip ▽

    ✓6ᵗʰ S73.01 Posterior subluxation and dislocation of hip

      ✓7ᵗʰ S73.011 Posterior subluxation of right hip

      ✓7ᵗʰ S73.012 Posterior subluxation of left hip

      ✓7ᵗʰ S73.013 Posterior subluxation of unspecified hip ▽

      ✓7ᵗʰ S73.014 Posterior dislocation of right hip

      ✓7ᵗʰ S73.015 Posterior dislocation of left hip

      ✓7ᵗʰ S73.016 Posterior dislocation of unspecified hip ▽

    ✓6ᵗʰ S73.02 Obturator subluxation and dislocation of hip

      ✓7ᵗʰ S73.021 Obturator subluxation of right hip

      ✓7ᵗʰ S73.022 Obturator subluxation of left hip

      ✓7ᵗʰ S73.023 Obturator subluxation of unspecified hip ▽

      ✓7ᵗʰ S73.024 Obturator dislocation of right hip

      ✓7ᵗʰ S73.025 Obturator dislocation of left hip

      ✓7ᵗʰ S73.026 Obturator dislocation of unspecified hip ▽

    ✓6ᵗʰ S73.03 Other anterior dislocation of hip

      ✓7ᵗʰ S73.031 Other anterior subluxation of right hip

      ✓7ᵗʰ S73.032 Other anterior subluxation of left hip

      ✓7ᵗʰ S73.033 Other anterior subluxation of unspecified hip ▽

      ✓7ᵗʰ S73.034 Other anterior dislocation of right hip

      ✓7ᵗʰ S73.035 Other anterior dislocation of left hip

      ✓7ᵗʰ S73.036 Other anterior dislocation of unspecified hip ▽

    ✓6ᵗʰ S73.04 Central dislocation of hip

      ✓7ᵗʰ S73.041 Central subluxation of right hip

      ✓7ᵗʰ S73.042 Central subluxation of left hip

      ✓7ᵗʰ S73.043 Central subluxation of unspecified hip ▽

      ✓7ᵗʰ S73.044 Central dislocation of right hip

      ✓7ᵗʰ S73.045 Central dislocation of left hip

      ✓7ᵗʰ S73.046 Central dislocation of unspecified hip ▽

✓5ᵗʰ **S73.1** Sprain of hip
    AHA: 2014, 4Q, 25

  ✓6ᵗʰ **S73.10** Unspecified sprain of hip

    ✓7ᵗʰ **S73.101** Unspecified sprain of right hip ▽

    ✓7ᵗʰ **S73.102** Unspecified sprain of left hip ▽

    ✓7ᵗʰ **S73.109** Unspecified sprain of unspecified hip ▽

  ✓6ᵗʰ **S73.11** Iliofemoral ligament sprain of hip

    ✓7ᵗʰ **S73.111** Iliofemoral ligament sprain of right hip

    ✓7ᵗʰ **S73.112** Iliofemoral ligament sprain of left hip

    ✓7ᵗʰ **S73.119** Iliofemoral ligament sprain of unspecified hip ▽

  ✓6ᵗʰ **S73.12** Ischiocapsular (ligament) sprain of hip

    ✓7ᵗʰ **S73.121** Ischiocapsular ligament sprain of right hip

    ✓7ᵗʰ **S73.122** Ischiocapsular ligament sprain of left hip

    ✓7ᵗʰ **S73.129** Ischiocapsular ligament sprain of unspecified hip ▽

  ✓6ᵗʰ **S73.19** Other sprain of hip

    ✓7ᵗʰ **S73.191** Other sprain of right hip

    ✓7ᵗʰ **S73.192** Other sprain of left hip

    ✓7ᵗʰ **S73.199** Other sprain of unspecified hip ▽

✓4ᵗʰ **S74** Injury of nerves at hip and thigh level
    Code also any associated open wound (S71.-)
    EXCLUDES 2 injury of nerves at ankle and foot level (S94.-)
              injury of nerves at lower leg level (S84.-)

    The appropriate 7th character is to be added to each code from category S74.
    A   initial encounter
    D   subsequent encounter
    S   sequela

  ✓5ᵗʰ **S74.0** Injury of sciatic nerve at hip and thigh level

    ✓x7ᵗʰ **S74.00** Injury of sciatic nerve at hip and thigh level, unspecified leg ▽

    ✓x7ᵗʰ **S74.01** Injury of sciatic nerve at hip and thigh level, right leg

    ✓x7ᵗʰ **S74.02** Injury of sciatic nerve at hip and thigh level, left leg

  ✓5ᵗʰ **S74.1** Injury of femoral nerve at hip and thigh level

    ✓x7ᵗʰ **S74.10** Injury of femoral nerve at hip and thigh level, unspecified leg ▽

    ✓x7ᵗʰ **S74.11** Injury of femoral nerve at hip and thigh level, right leg

    ✓x7ᵗʰ **S74.12** Injury of femoral nerve at hip and thigh level, left leg

  ✓5ᵗʰ **S74.2** Injury of cutaneous sensory nerve at hip and thigh level

    ✓x7ᵗʰ **S74.20** Injury of cutaneous sensory nerve at hip and thigh level, unspecified leg ▽

    ✓x7ᵗʰ **S74.21** Injury of cutaneous sensory nerve at hip and high level, right leg

    ✓x7ᵗʰ **S74.22** Injury of cutaneous sensory nerve at hip and thigh level, left leg

  ✓5ᵗʰ **S74.8** Injury of other nerves at hip and thigh level

    ✓6ᵗʰ **S74.8X** Injury of other nerves at hip and thigh level

      ✓7ᵗʰ **S74.8X1** Injury of other nerves at hip and thigh level, right leg

      ✓7ᵗʰ **S74.8X2** Injury of other nerves at hip and thigh level, left leg

      ✓7ᵗʰ **S74.8X9** Injury of other nerves at hip and thigh level, unspecified leg ▽

  ✓5ᵗʰ **S74.9** Injury of unspecified nerve at hip and thigh level

    ✓x7ᵗʰ **S74.90** Injury of unspecified nerve at hip and thigh level, unspecified leg ▽

    ✓x7ᵗʰ **S74.91** Injury of unspecified nerve at hip and thigh level, right leg ▽

    ✓x7ᵗʰ **S74.92** Injury of unspecified nerve at hip and thigh level, left leg ▽

✓4ᵗʰ **S75** Injury of blood vessels at hip and thigh level
    Code also any associated open wound (S71.-)
    EXCLUDES 2 injury of blood vessels at lower leg level (S85.-)
              injury of popliteal artery (S85.0)

    The appropriate 7th character is to be added to each code from category S75.
    A   initial encounter
    D   subsequent encounter
    S   sequela

  ✓5ᵗʰ **S75.0** Injury of femoral artery

    ✓6ᵗʰ **S75.00** Unspecified injury of femoral artery

      ✓7ᵗʰ **S75.001** Unspecified injury of femoral artery, right leg ▽

      ✓7ᵗʰ **S75.002** Unspecified injury of femoral artery, left leg ▽

      ✓7ᵗʰ **S75.009** Unspecified injury of femoral artery, unspecified leg ▽

    ✓6ᵗʰ **S75.01** Minor laceration of femoral artery
        Incomplete transection of femoral artery
        Laceration of femoral artery NOS
        Superficial laceration of femoral artery

      ✓7ᵗʰ **S75.011** Minor laceration of femoral artery, right leg

      ✓7ᵗʰ **S75.012** Minor laceration of femoral artery, left leg

      ✓7ᵗʰ **S75.019** Minor laceration of femoral artery, unspecified leg ▽

    ✓6ᵗʰ **S75.02** Major laceration of femoral artery
        Complete transection of femoral artery
        Traumatic rupture of femoral artery

      ✓7ᵗʰ **S75.021** Major laceration of femoral artery, right leg

      ✓7ᵗʰ **S75.022** Major laceration of femoral artery, left leg

      ✓7ᵗʰ **S75.029** Major laceration of femoral artery, unspecified leg ▽

    ✓6ᵗʰ **S75.09** Other specified injury of femoral artery

      ✓7ᵗʰ **S75.091** Other specified injury of femoral artery, right leg

      ✓7ᵗʰ **S75.092** Other specified injury of femoral artery, left leg

      ✓7ᵗʰ **S75.099** Other specified injury of femoral artery, unspecified leg ▽

  ✓5ᵗʰ **S75.1** Injury of femoral vein at hip and thigh level

    ✓6ᵗʰ **S75.10** Unspecified injury of femoral vein at hip and thigh level

      ✓7ᵗʰ **S75.101** Unspecified injury of femoral vein at hip and thigh level, right leg ▽

      ✓7ᵗʰ **S75.102** Unspecified injury of femoral vein at hip and thigh level, left leg ▽

      ✓7ᵗʰ **S75.109** Unspecified injury of femoral vein at hip and thigh level, unspecified leg ▽

    ✓6ᵗʰ **S75.11** Minor laceration of femoral vein at hip and thigh level
        Incomplete transection of femoral vein at hip and thigh level
        Laceration of femoral vein at hip and thigh level NOS
        Superficial laceration of femoral vein at hip and thigh level

      ✓7ᵗʰ **S75.111** Minor laceration of femoral vein at hip and thigh level, right leg

      ✓7ᵗʰ **S75.112** Minor laceration of femoral vein at hip and thigh level, left leg

      ✓7ᵗʰ **S75.119** Minor laceration of femoral vein at hip and thigh level, unspecified leg ▽

    ✓6ᵗʰ **S75.12** Major laceration of femoral vein at hip and thigh level
        Complete transection of femoral vein at hip and thigh level
        Traumatic rupture of femoral vein at hip and thigh level

      ✓7ᵗʰ **S75.121** Major laceration of femoral vein at hip and thigh level, right leg

      ✓7ᵗʰ **S75.122** Major laceration of femoral vein at hip and thigh level, left leg

      ✓7ᵗʰ **S75.129** Major laceration of femoral vein at hip and thigh level, unspecified leg ▽

☑ Add'l Character Required   ✓x7ᵗʰ Placeholder Alert   **RUG IV Special Care High Dx**   RUG IV Clinically Complex Dx   RUG IV Special Care Low Dx   Manifestation Code   Other Specified Code   ▽ Unspecified Code

√6ᵗʰ **S75.19** Other specified injury of femoral vein at hip and thigh level

     √7ᵗʰ **S75.191** Other specified injury of femoral vein at hip and thigh level, right leg

     √7ᵗʰ **S75.192** Other specified injury of femoral vein at hip and thigh level, left leg

     √7ᵗʰ **S75.199** Other specified injury of femoral vein at hip and thigh level, unspecified leg ▽

√5ᵗʰ **S75.2** Injury of greater saphenous vein at hip and thigh level

     EXCLUDES 1 greater saphenous vein NOS (S85.3)

   √6ᵗʰ **S75.20** Unspecified injury of greater saphenous vein at hip and thigh level

     √7ᵗʰ **S75.201** Unspecified injury of greater saphenous vein at hip and thigh level, right leg ▽

     √7ᵗʰ **S75.202** Unspecified injury of greater saphenous vein at hip and thigh level, left leg ▽

     √7ᵗʰ **S75.209** Unspecified injury of greater saphenous vein at hip and thigh level, unspecified leg ▽

   √6ᵗʰ **S75.21** Minor laceration of greater saphenous vein at hip and thigh level

     Incomplete transection of greater saphenous vein at hip and thigh level

     Laceration of greater saphenous vein at hip and thigh level NOS

     Superficial laceration of greater saphenous vein at hip and thigh level

     √7ᵗʰ **S75.211** Minor laceration of greater saphenous vein at hip and thigh level, right leg

     √7ᵗʰ **S75.212** Minor laceration of greater saphenous vein at hip and thigh level, left leg

     √7ᵗʰ **S75.219** Minor laceration of greater saphenous vein at hip and thigh level, unspecified leg ▽

   √6ᵗʰ **S75.22** Major laceration of greater saphenous vein at hip and thigh level

     Complete transection of greater saphenous vein at hip and thigh level

     Traumatic rupture of greater saphenous vein at hip and thigh level

     √7ᵗʰ **S75.221** Major laceration of greater saphenous vein at hip and thigh level, right leg

     √7ᵗʰ **S75.222** Major laceration of greater saphenous vein at hip and thigh level, left leg

     √7ᵗʰ **S75.229** Major laceration of greater saphenous vein at hip and thigh level, unspecified leg ▽

   √6ᵗʰ **S75.29** Other specified injury of greater saphenous vein at hip and thigh level

     √7ᵗʰ **S75.291** Other specified injury of greater saphenous vein at hip and thigh level, right leg

     √7ᵗʰ **S75.292** Other specified injury of greater saphenous vein at hip and thigh level, left leg

     √7ᵗʰ **S75.299** Other specified injury of greater saphenous vein at hip and thigh level, unspecified leg ▽

√5ᵗʰ **S75.8** Injury of other blood vessels at hip and thigh level

   √6ᵗʰ **S75.80** Unspecified injury of other blood vessels at hip and thigh level

     √7ᵗʰ **S75.801** Unspecified injury of other blood vessels at hip and thigh level, right leg ▽

     √7ᵗʰ **S75.802** Unspecified injury of other blood vessels at hip and thigh level, left leg ▽

     √7ᵗʰ **S75.809** Unspecified injury of other blood vessels at hip and thigh level, unspecified leg ▽

   √6ᵗʰ **S75.81** Laceration of other blood vessels at hip and thigh level

     √7ᵗʰ **S75.811** Laceration of other blood vessels at hip and thigh level, right leg

     √7ᵗʰ **S75.812** Laceration of other blood vessels at hip and thigh level, left leg

     √7ᵗʰ **S75.819** Laceration of other blood vessels at hip and thigh level, unspecified leg ▽

√6ᵗʰ **S75.89** Other specified injury of other blood vessels at hip and thigh level

     √7ᵗʰ **S75.891** Other specified injury of other blood vessels at hip and thigh level, right leg

     √7ᵗʰ **S75.892** Other specified injury of other blood vessels at hip and thigh level, left leg

     √7ᵗʰ **S75.899** Other specified injury of other blood vessels at hip and thigh level, unspecified leg ▽

√5ᵗʰ **S75.9** Injury of unspecified blood vessel at hip and thigh level

   √6ᵗʰ **S75.90** Unspecified injury of unspecified blood vessel at hip and thigh level

     √7ᵗʰ **S75.901** Unspecified injury of unspecified blood vessel at hip and thigh level, right leg ▽

     √7ᵗʰ **S75.902** Unspecified injury of unspecified blood vessel at hip and thigh level, left leg ▽

     √7ᵗʰ **S75.909** Unspecified injury of unspecified blood vessel at hip and thigh level, unspecified leg ▽

   √6ᵗʰ **S75.91** Laceration of unspecified blood vessel at hip and thigh level

     √7ᵗʰ **S75.911** Laceration of unspecified blood vessel at hip and thigh level, right leg ▽

     √7ᵗʰ **S75.912** Laceration of unspecified blood vessel at hip and thigh level, left leg ▽

     √7ᵗʰ **S75.919** Laceration of unspecified blood vessel at hip and thigh level, unspecified leg ▽

   √6ᵗʰ **S75.99** Other specified injury of unspecified blood vessel at hip and thigh level

     √7ᵗʰ **S75.991** Other specified injury of unspecified blood vessel at hip and thigh level, right leg ▽

     √7ᵗʰ **S75.992** Other specified injury of unspecified blood vessel at hip and thigh level, left leg ▽

     √7ᵗʰ **S75.999** Other specified injury of unspecified blood vessel at hip and thigh level, unspecified leg ▽

✦ √4ᵗʰ **S76 Injury of muscle, fascia and tendon at hip and thigh level**

   Code also any associated open wound (S71.-)

   EXCLUDES 2 injury of muscle, fascia and tendon at lower leg level (S86) sprain of joint and ligament of hip (S73.1)

   The appropriate 7th character is to be added to each code from category S76.
   A   initial encounter
   D   subsequent encounter
   S   sequela

√5ᵗʰ **S76.0** Injury of muscle, fascia and tendon of hip

   √6ᵗʰ **S76.00** Unspecified injury of muscle, fascia and tendon of hip

     √7ᵗʰ **S76.001** Unspecified injury of muscle, fascia and tendon of right hip ▽

     √7ᵗʰ **S76.002** Unspecified injury of muscle, fascia and tendon of left hip ▽

     √7ᵗʰ **S76.009** Unspecified injury of muscle, fascia and tendon of unspecified hip ▽

   √6ᵗʰ **S76.01** Strain of muscle, fascia and tendon of hip

     √7ᵗʰ **S76.011** Strain of muscle, fascia and tendon of right hip

     √7ᵗʰ **S76.012** Strain of muscle, fascia and tendon of left hip

     √7ᵗʰ **S76.019** Strain of muscle, fascia and tendon of unspecified hip ▽

   √6ᵗʰ **S76.02** Laceration of muscle, fascia and tendon of hip

     √7ᵗʰ **S76.021** Laceration of muscle, fascia and tendon of right hip

     √7ᵗʰ **S76.022** Laceration of muscle, fascia and tendon of left hip

     √7ᵗʰ **S76.029** Laceration of muscle, fascia and tendon of unspecified hip ▽

   √6ᵗʰ **S76.09** Other specified injury of muscle, fascia and tendon of hip

     √7ᵗʰ **S76.091** Other specified injury of muscle, fascia and tendon of right hip

---

✦   Refer to the Muscle/Tendon Table at beginning of this chapter.

Ⓝ Newborn   Ⓟ Pediatric   Ⓜ Maternity   Ⓐ Adult   **RIC** RIC Dx   **NC Dx** Noncancer Dx   **PDx** Primary Dx   **CC** RIC CC Condition   ▶◀ Revised Text   ● New Code   ▲ Revised Code Title

950   ICD-10-CM 2016

☑7ᵗʰ **S76.092** Other specified injury of muscle, fascia and tendon of left hip

☑7ᵗʰ **S76.099** Other specified injury of muscle, fascia and tendon of unspecified hip ▽

☑5ᵗʰ **S76.1** Injury of quadriceps muscle, fascia and tendon
Injury of patellar ligament (tendon)

☑6ᵗʰ **S76.10** Unspecified injury of quadriceps muscle, fascia and tendon

☑7ᵗʰ **S76.101** Unspecified injury of right quadriceps muscle, fascia and tendon ▽

☑7ᵗʰ **S76.102** Unspecified injury of left quadriceps muscle, fascia and tendon ▽

☑7ᵗʰ **S76.109** Unspecified injury of unspecified quadriceps muscle, fascia and tendon ▽

☑6ᵗʰ **S76.11** Strain of quadriceps muscle, fascia and tendon

☑7ᵗʰ **S76.111** Strain of right quadriceps muscle, fascia and tendon

☑7ᵗʰ **S76.112** Strain of left quadriceps muscle, fascia and tendon

☑7ᵗʰ **S76.119** Strain of unspecified quadriceps muscle, fascia and tendon ▽

☑6ᵗʰ **S76.12** Laceration of quadriceps muscle, fascia and tendon

☑7ᵗʰ **S76.121** Laceration of right quadriceps muscle, fascia and tendon

☑7ᵗʰ **S76.122** Laceration of left quadriceps muscle, fascia and tendon

☑7ᵗʰ **S76.129** Laceration of unspecified quadriceps muscle, fascia and tendon ▽

☑6ᵗʰ **S76.19** Other specified injury of quadriceps muscle, fascia and tendon

☑7ᵗʰ **S76.191** Other specified injury of right quadriceps muscle, fascia and tendon

☑7ᵗʰ **S76.192** Other specified injury of left quadriceps muscle, fascia and tendon

☑7ᵗʰ **S76.199** Other specified injury of unspecified quadriceps muscle, fascia and tendon ▽

☑5ᵗʰ **S76.2** Injury of adductor muscle, fascia and tendon of thigh

☑6ᵗʰ **S76.20** Unspecified injury of adductor muscle, fascia and tendon of thigh

☑7ᵗʰ **S76.201** Unspecified injury of adductor muscle, fascia and tendon of right thigh ▽

☑7ᵗʰ **S76.202** Unspecified injury of adductor muscle, fascia and tendon of left thigh ▽

☑7ᵗʰ **S76.209** Unspecified injury of adductor muscle, fascia and tendon of unspecified thigh ▽

☑6ᵗʰ **S76.21** Strain of adductor muscle, fascia and tendon of thigh

☑7ᵗʰ **S76.211** Strain of adductor muscle, fascia and tendon of right thigh

☑7ᵗʰ **S76.212** Strain of adductor muscle, fascia and tendon of left thigh

☑7ᵗʰ **S76.219** Strain of adductor muscle, fascia and tendon of unspecified thigh ▽

☑6ᵗʰ **S76.22** Laceration of adductor muscle, fascia and tendon of thigh

☑7ᵗʰ **S76.221** Laceration of adductor muscle, fascia and tendon of right thigh

☑7ᵗʰ **S76.222** Laceration of adductor muscle, fascia and tendon of left thigh

☑7ᵗʰ **S76.229** Laceration of adductor muscle, fascia and tendon of unspecified thigh ▽

☑6ᵗʰ **S76.29** Other injury of adductor muscle, fascia and tendon of thigh

☑7ᵗʰ **S76.291** Other injury of adductor muscle, fascia and tendon of right thigh

☑7ᵗʰ **S76.292** Other injury of adductor muscle, fascia and tendon of left thigh

☑7ᵗʰ **S76.299** Other injury of adductor muscle, fascia and tendon of unspecified thigh ▽

☑5ᵗʰ **S76.3** Injury of muscle, fascia and tendon of the posterior muscle group at thigh level

☑6ᵗʰ **S76.30** Unspecified injury of muscle, fascia and tendon of the posterior muscle group at thigh level

☑7ᵗʰ **S76.301** Unspecified injury of muscle, fascia and tendon of the posterior muscle group at thigh level, right thigh ▽

☑7ᵗʰ **S76.302** Unspecified injury of muscle, fascia and tendon of the posterior muscle group at thigh level, left thigh ▽

☑7ᵗʰ **S76.309** Unspecified injury of muscle, fascia and tendon of the posterior muscle group at thigh level, unspecified thigh ▽

☑6ᵗʰ **S76.31** Strain of muscle, fascia and tendon of the posterior muscle group at thigh level

☑7ᵗʰ **S76.311** Strain of muscle, fascia and tendon of the posterior muscle group at thigh level, right thigh

☑7ᵗʰ **S76.312** Strain of muscle, fascia and tendon of the posterior muscle group at thigh level, left thigh

☑7ᵗʰ **S76.319** Strain of muscle, fascia and tendon of the posterior muscle group at thigh level, unspecified thigh ▽

☑6ᵗʰ **S76.32** Laceration of muscle, fascia and tendon of the posterior muscle group at thigh level

☑7ᵗʰ **S76.321** Laceration of muscle, fascia and tendon of the posterior muscle group at thigh level, right thigh

☑7ᵗʰ **S76.322** Laceration of muscle, fascia and tendon of the posterior muscle group at thigh level, left thigh

☑7ᵗʰ **S76.329** Laceration of muscle, fascia and tendon of the posterior muscle group at thigh level, unspecified thigh ▽

☑6ᵗʰ **S76.39** Other specified injury of muscle, fascia and tendon of the posterior muscle group at thigh level

☑7ᵗʰ **S76.391** Other specified injury of muscle, fascia and tendon of the posterior muscle group at thigh level, right thigh

☑7ᵗʰ **S76.392** Other specified injury of muscle, fascia and tendon of the posterior muscle group at thigh level, left thigh

☑7ᵗʰ **S76.399** Other specified injury of muscle, ascia and tendon of the posterior muscle group at thigh level, unspecified thigh ▽

☑5ᵗʰ **S76.8** Injury of other specified muscles, fascia and tendons at thigh level

☑6ᵗʰ **S76.80** Unspecified injury of other specified muscles, fascia and tendons at thigh level

☑7ᵗʰ **S76.801** Unspecified injury of other specified muscles, fascia and tendons at thigh level, right thigh ▽

☑7ᵗʰ **S76.802** Unspecified injury of other specified muscles, fascia and tendons at thigh level, left thigh ▽

☑7ᵗʰ **S76.809** Unspecified injury of other specified muscles, fascia and tendons at thigh level, unspecified thigh ▽

☑6ᵗʰ **S76.81** Strain of other specified muscles, fascia and tendons at thigh level

☑7ᵗʰ **S76.811** Strain of other specified muscles, fascia and tendons at thigh level, right thigh

☑7ᵗʰ **S76.812** Strain of other specified muscles, fascia and tendons at thigh level, left thigh

☑7ᵗʰ **S76.819** Strain of other specified muscles, fascia and tendons at thigh level, unspecified thigh ▽

☑6ᵗʰ **S76.82** Laceration of other specified muscles, fascia and tendons at thigh level

☑7ᵗʰ **S76.821** Laceration of other specified muscles, fascia and tendons at thigh level, right thigh

---

☑ Add'l Character Required ☑✗7ᵗʰ Placeholder Alert **RUG IV Special Care High Dx** RUG IV Clinically Complex Dx RUG IV Special Care Low Dx Manifestation Code Other Specified Code ▽Unspecified Code

ICD-10-CM 2016

951

☑7ᵗʰ **S76.822** Laceration of other specified muscles, fascia and tendons at thigh level, left thigh

☑7ᵗʰ **S76.829** Laceration of other specified muscles, fascia and tendons at thigh level, unspecified thigh ▽

✓6ᵗʰ **S76.89** Other injury of other specified muscles, fascia and tendons at thigh level

     ☑7ᵗʰ **S76.891** Other injury of other specified muscles, fascia and tendons at thigh level, right thigh

     ☑7ᵗʰ **S76.892** Other injury of other specified muscles, fascia and tendons at thigh level, left thigh

     ☑7ᵗʰ **S76.899** Other injury of other specified muscles, fascia and tendons at thigh level, unspecified thigh ▽

✓5ᵗʰ **S76.9** Injury of unspecified muscles, fascia and tendons at thigh level

   ✓6ᵗʰ **S76.90** Unspecified injury of unspecified muscles, fascia and tendons at thigh level

     ☑7ᵗʰ **S76.901** Unspecified injury of unspecified muscles, fascia and tendons at thigh level, right thigh ▽

     ☑7ᵗʰ **S76.902** Unspecified injury of unspecified muscles, fascia and tendons at thigh level, left thigh ▽

     ☑7ᵗʰ **S76.909** Unspecified injury of unspecified muscles, fascia and tendons at thigh level, unspecified thigh ▽

   ✓6ᵗʰ **S76.91** Strain of unspecified muscles, fascia and tendons at thigh level

     ☑7ᵗʰ **S76.911** Strain of unspecified muscles, fascia and tendons at thigh level, right thigh ▽

     ☑7ᵗʰ **S76.912** Strain of unspecified muscles, fascia and tendons at thigh level, left thigh ▽

     ☑7ᵗʰ **S76.919** Strain of unspecified muscles, fascia and tendons at thigh level, unspecified thigh ▽

   ✓6ᵗʰ **S76.92** Laceration of unspecified muscles, fascia and tendons at thigh level

     ☑7ᵗʰ **S76.921** Laceration of unspecified muscles, fascia and tendons at thigh level, right thigh ▽

     ☑7ᵗʰ **S76.922** Laceration of unspecified muscles, fascia and tendons at thigh level, left thigh ▽

     ☑7ᵗʰ **S76.929** Laceration of unspecified muscles, fascia and tendons at thigh level, unspecified thigh ▽

   ✓6ᵗʰ **S76.99** Other specified injury of unspecified muscles, fascia and tendons at thigh level

     ☑7ᵗʰ **S76.991** Other specified injury of unspecified muscles, fascia and tendons at thigh level, right thigh ▽

     ☑7ᵗʰ **S76.992** Other specified injury of unspecified muscles, fascia and tendons at thigh level, left thigh ▽

     ☑7ᵗʰ **S76.999** Other specified injury of unspecified muscles, fascia and tendons at thigh level, unspecified thigh ▽

✓4ᵗʰ **S77** Crushing injury of hip and thigh

   Use additional code(s) for all associated injuries

   EXCLUDES 2   crushing injury of ankle and foot (S97.-)
              crushing injury of lower leg (S87.-)

   The appropriate 7th character is to be added to each code from category S77.
   A   initial encounter
   D   subsequent encounter
   S   sequela

   ✓5ᵗʰ **S77.0** Crushing injury of hip

     ✓x7ᵗʰ **S77.00** Crushing injury of unspecified hip ▽

     ✓x7ᵗʰ **S77.01** Crushing injury of right hip

     ✓x7ᵗʰ **S77.02** Crushing injury of left hip

   ✓5ᵗʰ **S77.1** Crushing injury of thigh

     ✓x7ᵗʰ **S77.10** Crushing injury of unspecified thigh ▽

     ✓x7ᵗʰ **S77.11** Crushing injury of right thigh

     ✓x7ᵗʰ **S77.12** Crushing injury of left thigh

   ✓5ᵗʰ **S77.2** Crushing injury of hip with thigh

     ✓x7ᵗʰ **S77.20** Crushing injury of unspecified hip with thigh ▽

     ✓x7ᵗʰ **S77.21** Crushing injury of right hip with thigh

     ✓x7ᵗʰ **S77.22** Crushing injury of left hip with thigh

✓4ᵗʰ **S78** Traumatic amputation of hip and thigh

   NOTE   An amputation not identified as partial or complete should be coded to complete.

   EXCLUDES 1   traumatic amputation of knee (S88.0-)

   The appropriate 7th character is to be added to each code from category S78.
   A   initial encounter
   D   subsequent encounter
   S   sequela

   ✓5ᵗʰ **S78.0** Traumatic amputation at hip joint

     ✓6ᵗʰ **S78.01** Complete traumatic amputation at hip joint

       ☑7ᵗʰ **S78.011** Complete traumatic amputation at right hip joint

       ☑7ᵗʰ **S78.012** Complete traumatic amputation at left hip joint

       ☑7ᵗʰ **S78.019** Complete traumatic amputation at unspecified hip joint ▽

     ✓6ᵗʰ **S78.02** Partial traumatic amputation at hip joint

       ☑7ᵗʰ **S78.021** Partial traumatic amputation at right hip joint

       ☑7ᵗʰ **S78.022** Partial traumatic amputation at left hip joint

       ☑7ᵗʰ **S78.029** Partial traumatic amputation at unspecified hip joint ▽

   ✓5ᵗʰ **S78.1** Traumatic amputation at level between hip and knee

     EXCLUDES 1   traumatic amputation of knee (S88.0-)

     ✓6ᵗʰ **S78.11** Complete traumatic amputation at level between hip and knee

       ☑7ᵗʰ **S78.111** Complete traumatic amputation at level between right hip and knee

       ☑7ᵗʰ **S78.112** Complete traumatic amputation at level between left hip and knee

       ☑7ᵗʰ **S78.119** Complete traumatic amputation at level between unspecified hip and knee ▽

     ✓6ᵗʰ **S78.12** Partial traumatic amputation at level between hip and knee

       ☑7ᵗʰ **S78.121** Partial traumatic amputation at level between right hip and knee

       ☑7ᵗʰ **S78.122** Partial traumatic amputation at level between left hip and knee

       ☑7ᵗʰ **S78.129** Partial traumatic amputation at level between unspecified hip and knee ▽

   ✓5ᵗʰ **S78.9** Traumatic amputation of hip and thigh, level unspecified

     ✓6ᵗʰ **S78.91** Complete traumatic amputation of hip and thigh, level unspecified

       ☑7ᵗʰ **S78.911** Complete traumatic amputation of right hip and thigh, level unspecified ▽

       ☑7ᵗʰ **S78.912** Complete traumatic amputation of left hip and thigh, level unspecified ▽

       ☑7ᵗʰ **S78.919** Complete traumatic amputation of unspecified hip and thigh, level unspecified ▽

     ✓6ᵗʰ **S78.92** Partial traumatic amputation of hip and thigh, level unspecified

       ☑7ᵗʰ **S78.921** Partial traumatic amputation of right hip and thigh, level unspecified ▽

       ☑7ᵗʰ **S78.922** Partial traumatic amputation of left hip and thigh, level unspecified ▽

       ☑7ᵗʰ **S78.929** Partial traumatic amputation of unspecified hip and thigh, level unspecified ▽

Ⓝ Newborn   Ⓟ Pediatric   Ⓜ Maternity   Ⓐ Adult   **RIC** RIC Dx   **NC Dx** Noncancer Dx   **PDx** Primary Dx   **CC** RIC CC Condition   ▶◀ Revised Text   ● New Code   ▲ Revised Code Title

952   ICD-10-CM 2016

✓4th **S79** **Other and unspecified injuries of hip and thigh**

✓5th **S79.0** **Physeal fracture of upper end of femur**

NOTE A fracture not indicated as open or closed should be coded to closed.

EXCLUDES 1 *apophyseal fracture of upper end of femur (S72.13-)*
nontraumatic slipped upper femoral epiphysis (M93.0-)

The appropriate 7th character is to be added to each code from subcategory S79.0.
A initial encounter for closed fracture
D subsequent encounter for fracture with routine healing
G subsequent encounter for fracture with delayed healing
K subsequent encounter for fracture with nonunion
P subsequent encounter for fracture with malunion
S sequela

✓6th **S79.00** Unspecified physeal fracture of upper end of femur

✓7th **S79.001** Unspecified physeal fracture of upper end of right femur ▽

✓7th **S79.002** Unspecified physeal fracture of upper end of left femur ▽

✓7th **S79.009** Unspecified physeal fracture of upper end of unspecified femur ▽

✓6th **S79.01** Salter-Harris Type I physeal fracture of upper end of femur

Acute on chronic slipped capital femoral epiphysis (traumatic)
Acute slipped capital femoral epiphysis (traumatic)
Capital femoral epiphyseal fracture

EXCLUDES 1 *chronic slipped upper femoral epiphysis (nontraumatic) (M93.02-)*

✓7th **S79.011** Salter-Harris Type I physeal fracture of upper end of right femur

✓7th **S79.012** Salter-Harris Type I physeal fracture of upper end of left femur

✓7th **S79.019** Salter-Harris Type I physeal fracture of upper end of unspecified femur ▽

✓6th **S79.09** Other physeal fracture of upper end of femur

✓7th **S79.091** Other physeal fracture of upper end of right femur

✓7th **S79.092** Other physeal fracture of upper end of left femur

✓7th **S79.099** Other physeal fracture of upper end of unspecified femur ▽

✓5th **S79.1** **Physeal fracture of lower end of femur**

NOTE A fracture not indicated as open or closed should be coded to closed.

The appropriate 7th character is to be added to each code from subcategory S79.1.
A initial encounter for closed fracture
D subsequent encounter for fracture with routine healing
G subsequent encounter for fracture with delayed healing
K subsequent encounter for fracture with nonunion
P subsequent encounter for fracture with malunion
S sequela

✓6th **S79.10** Unspecified physeal fracture of lower end of femur

✓7th **S79.101** Unspecified physeal fracture of lower end of right femur ▽

✓7th **S79.102** Unspecified physeal fracture of lower end of left femur ▽

✓7th **S79.109** Unspecified physeal fracture of lower end of unspecified femur ▽

✓6th **S79.11** Salter-Harris Type I physeal fracture of lower end of femur

✓7th **S79.111** Salter-Harris Type I physeal fracture of lower end of right femur

✓7th **S79.112** Salter-Harris Type I physeal fracture of lower end of left femur

✓7th **S79.119** Salter-Harris Type I physeal fracture of lower end of unspecified femur ▽

✓6th **S79.12** Salter-Harris Type II physeal fracture of lower end of femur

✓7th **S79.121** Salter-Harris Type II physeal fracture of lower end of right femur

✓7th **S79.122** Salter-Harris Type II physeal fracture of lower end of left femur

✓7th **S79.129** Salter-Harris Type II physeal fracture of lower end of unspecified femur ▽

✓6th **S79.13** Salter-Harris Type III physeal fracture of lower end of femur

✓7th **S79.131** Salter-Harris Type III physeal fracture of lower end of right femur

✓7th **S79.132** Salter-Harris Type III physeal fracture of lower end of left femur

✓7th **S79.139** Salter-Harris Type III physeal fracture of lower end of unspecified femur ▽

✓6th **S79.14** Salter-Harris Type IV physeal fracture of lower end of femur

✓7th **S79.141** Salter-Harris Type IV physeal fracture of lower end of right femur

✓7th **S79.142** Salter-Harris Type IV physeal fracture of lower end of left femur

✓7th **S79.149** Salter-Harris Type IV physeal fracture of lower end of unspecified femur ▽

✓6th **S79.19** Other physeal fracture of lower end of femur

✓7th **S79.191** Other physeal fracture of lower end of right femur

✓7th **S79.192** Other physeal fracture of lower end of left femur

✓7th **S79.199** Other physeal fracture of lower end of unspecified femur ▽

✓5th **S79.8** **Other specified injuries of hip and thigh**

The appropriate 7th character is to be added to each code in subcategory S79.8.
A initial encounter
D subsequent encounter
S sequela

✓6th **S79.81** Other specified injuries of hip

✓7th **S79.811** Other specified injuries of right hip

✓7th **S79.812** Other specified injuries of left hip

✓7th **S79.819** Other specified injuries of unspecified hip ▽

✓6th **S79.82** Other specified injuries of thigh

✓7th **S79.821** Other specified injuries of right thigh

✓7th **S79.822** Other specified injuries of left thigh

✓7th **S79.829** Other specified injuries of unspecified thigh ▽

✓5th **S79.9** **Unspecified injury of hip and thigh**

The appropriate 7th character is to be added to each code in subcategory S79.9.
A initial encounter
D subsequent encounter
S sequela

✓6th **S79.91** Unspecified injury of hip

✓7th **S79.911** Unspecified injury of right hip ▽

✓7th **S79.912** Unspecified injury of left hip ▽

✓7th **S79.919** Unspecified injury of unspecified hip ▽

✓6th **S79.92** Unspecified injury of thigh

✓7th **S79.921** Unspecified injury of right thigh ▽

✓7th **S79.922** Unspecified injury of left thigh ▽

✓7th **S79.929** Unspecified injury of unspecified thigh ▽

✔ Add'l Character Required ✔x7th Placeholder Alert RUG IV Special Care High Dx RUG IV Clinically Complex Dx RUG IV Special Care Low Dx Manifestation Code Other Specified Code ▽ Unspecified Code

Injuries to the knee and lower leg (S80-S89)

EXCLUDES 2   burns and corrosions (T20-T32)
frostbite (T33-T34)
injuries of ankle and foot, except fracture of ankle and malleolus
(S90-S99)
insect bite or sting, venomous (T63.4)

✓4th S80   Superficial injury of knee and lower leg

EXCLUDES 2   superficial injury of ankle and foot (S90.-)

The appropriate 7th character is to be added to each code from
category S80.
A   initial encounter
D   subsequent encounter
S   sequela

✓5th S80.0   Contusion of knee
- **✓x7th S80.00   Contusion of unspecified knee** ▽
- **✓x7th S80.01   Contusion of right knee**
- **✓x7th S80.02   Contusion of left knee**

✓5th S80.1   Contusion of lower leg
- **✓x7th S80.10   Contusion of unspecified lower leg** ▽
- **✓x7th S80.11   Contusion of right lower leg**
- **✓x7th S80.12   Contusion of left lower leg**

✓5th S80.2   Other superficial injuries of knee
- **✓6th S80.21   Abrasion of knee**
  - **✓7th S80.211   Abrasion, right knee**
  - **✓7th S80.212   Abrasion, left knee**
  - **✓7th S80.219   Abrasion, unspecified knee** ▽
- **✓6th S80.22   Blister (nonthermal) of knee**
  - **✓7th S80.221   Blister (nonthermal), right knee**
  - **✓7th S80.222   Blister (nonthermal), left knee**
  - **✓7th S80.229   Blister (nonthermal), unspecified knee** ▽
- **✓6th S80.24   External constriction of knee**
  - **✓7th S80.241   External constriction, right knee**
  - **✓7th S80.242   External constriction, left knee**
  - **✓7th S80.249   External constriction, unspecified knee** ▽
- **✓6th S80.25   Superficial foreign body of knee**
  Splinter in the knee
  - **✓7th S80.251   Superficial foreign body, right knee**
  - **✓7th S80.252   Superficial foreign body, left knee**
  - **✓7th S80.259   Superficial foreign body, unspecified knee** ▽
- **✓6th S80.26   Insect bite (nonvenomous) of knee**
  - **✓7th S80.261   Insect bite (nonvenomous), right knee**
  - **✓7th S80.262   Insect bite (nonvenomous), left knee**
  - **✓7th S80.269   Insect bite (nonvenomous), unspecified knee** ▽
- **✓6th S80.27   Other superficial bite of knee**
  EXCLUDES 1   open bite of knee (S81.05-)
  - **✓7th S80.271   Other superficial bite of right knee**
  - **✓7th S80.272   Other superficial bite of left knee**
  - **✓7th S80.279   Other superficial bite of unspecified knee** ▽

✓5th S80.8   Other superficial injuries of lower leg
- **✓6th S80.81   Abrasion of lower leg**
  - **✓7th S80.811   Abrasion, right lower leg**
  - **✓7th S80.812   Abrasion, left lower leg**
  - **✓7th S80.819   Abrasion, unspecified lower leg** ▽
- **✓6th S80.82   Blister (nonthermal) of lower leg**
  - **✓7th S80.821   Blister (nonthermal), right lower leg**
  - **✓7th S80.822   Blister (nonthermal), left lower leg**
  - **✓7th S80.829   Blister (nonthermal), unspecified lower leg** ▽
- **✓6th S80.84   External constriction of lower leg**
  - **✓7th S80.841   External constriction, right lower leg**
  - **✓7th S80.842   External constriction, left lower leg**
  - **✓7th S80.849   External constriction, unspecified lower leg** ▽

- **✓6th S80.85   Superficial foreign body of lower leg**
  Splinter in the lower leg
  - **✓7th S80.851   Superficial foreign body, right lower leg**
  - **✓7th S80.852   Superficial foreign body, left lower leg**
  - **✓7th S80.859   Superficial foreign body, unspecified lower leg** ▽
- **✓6th S80.86   Insect bite (nonvenomous) of lower leg**
  - **✓7th S80.861   Insect bite (nonvenomous), right lower leg**
  - **✓7th S80.862   Insect bite (nonvenomous), left lower leg**
  - **✓7th S80.869   Insect bite (nonvenomous), unspecified lower leg**
- **✓6th S80.87   Other superficial bite of lower leg**
  EXCLUDES 1   open bite of lower leg (S81.85-)
  - **✓7th S80.871   Other superficial bite, right lower leg**
  - **✓7th S80.872   Other superficial bite, left lower leg**
  - **✓7th S80.879   Other superficial bite, unspecified lower leg** ▽

✓5th S80.9   Unspecified superficial injury of knee and lower leg
- **✓6th S80.91   Unspecified superficial injury of knee**
  - **✓7th S80.911   Unspecified superficial injury of right knee** ▽
  - **✓7th S80.912   Unspecified superficial injury of left knee** ▽
  - **✓7th S80.919   Unspecified superficial injury of unspecified knee** ▽
- **✓6th S80.92   Unspecified superficial injury of lower leg**
  - **✓7th S80.921   Unspecified superficial injury of right lower leg** ▽
  - **✓7th S80.922   Unspecified superficial injury of left lower leg** ▽
  - **✓7th S80.929   Unspecified superficial injury of unspecified lower leg** ▽

✓4th S81   Open wound of knee and lower leg
Code also any associated wound infection
EXCLUDES 1   open fracture of knee and lower leg (S82.-)
traumatic amputation of lower leg (S88.-)
EXCLUDES 2   open wound of ankle and foot (S91.-)

The appropriate 7th character is to be added to each code from
category S81.
A   initial encounter
D   subsequent encounter
S   sequela

✓5th S81.0   Open wound of knee
- **✓6th S81.00   Unspecified open wound of knee**
  - **✓7th S81.001   Unspecified open wound, right knee** ▽
  - **✓7th S81.002   Unspecified open wound, left knee** ▽
  - **✓7th S81.009   Unspecified open wound, unspecified knee** ▽
- **✓6th S81.01   Laceration without foreign body of knee**
  - **✓7th S81.011   Laceration without foreign body, right knee**
  - **✓7th S81.012   Laceration without foreign body, left knee**
  - **✓7th S81.019   Laceration without foreign body, unspecified knee** ▽
- **✓6th S81.02   Laceration with foreign body of knee**
  - **✓7th S81.021   Laceration with foreign body, right knee**
  - **✓7th S81.022   Laceration with foreign body, left knee**
  - **✓7th S81.029   Laceration with foreign body, unspecified knee** ▽
- **✓6th S81.03   Puncture wound without foreign body of knee**
  - **✓7th S81.031   Puncture wound without foreign body, right knee**
  - **✓7th S81.032   Puncture wound without foreign body, left knee**
  - **✓7th S81.039   Puncture wound without foreign body, unspecified knee** ▽
- **✓6th S81.04   Puncture wound with foreign body of knee**
  - **✓7th S81.041   Puncture wound with foreign body, right knee**
  - **✓7th S81.042   Puncture wound with foreign body, left knee**

N Newborn   P Pediatric   M Maternity   A Adult   RIC RIC Dx   NCDx Noncancer Dx   PDx Primary Dx   CC RIC CC Condition   ▶◀ Revised Text   ● New Code   ▲ Revised Code Title

954   ICD-10-CM 2016

✓7ᵗʰ **S81.049**   **Puncture wound with foreign body, unspecified knee** ▽

✓6ᵗʰ **S81.05**   **Open bite** of knee
     Bite of knee NOS
     EXCLUDES 1   superficial bite of knee (S80.27-)

   ✓7ᵗʰ **S81.051**   **Open bite, right knee**
   ✓7ᵗʰ **S81.052**   **Open bite, left knee**
   ✓7ᵗʰ **S81.059**   **Open bite, unspecified knee** ▽

✓5ᵗʰ **S81.8**   **Open wound of lower leg**

✓6ᵗʰ **S81.80**   **Unspecified open wound of lower leg**

   ✓7ᵗʰ **S81.801**   **Unspecified open wound, right lower leg** ▽
   ✓7ᵗʰ **S81.802**   **Unspecified open wound, left lower leg** ▽
   ✓7ᵗʰ **S81.809**   **Unspecified open wound, unspecified lower leg** ▽

✓6ᵗʰ **S81.81**   **Laceration without foreign body of lower leg**

   ✓7ᵗʰ **S81.811**   **Laceration without foreign body, right lower leg**
   ✓7ᵗʰ **S81.812**   **Laceration without foreign body, left lower leg**
   ✓7ᵗʰ **S81.819**   **Laceration without foreign body, unspecified lower leg** ▽

✓6ᵗʰ **S81.82**   **Laceration with foreign body of lower leg**

   ✓7ᵗʰ **S81.821**   **Laceration with foreign body, right lower leg**
   ✓7ᵗʰ **S81.822**   **Laceration with foreign body, left lower leg**
   ✓7ᵗʰ **S81.829**   **Laceration with foreign body, unspecified lower leg** ▽

✓6ᵗʰ **S81.83**   **Puncture wound without foreign body of lower leg**

   ✓7ᵗʰ **S81.831**   **Puncture wound without foreign body, right lower leg**
   ✓7ᵗʰ **S81.832**   **Puncture wound without foreign body, left lower leg**
   ✓7ᵗʰ **S81.839**   **Puncture wound without foreign body, unspecified lower leg** ▽

✓6ᵗʰ **S81.84**   **Puncture wound with foreign body of lower leg**

   ✓7ᵗʰ **S81.841**   **Puncture wound with foreign body, right lower leg**
   ✓7ᵗʰ **S81.842**   **Puncture wound with foreign body, left lower leg**
   ✓7ᵗʰ **S81.849**   **Puncture wound with foreign body, unspecified lower leg** ▽

✓6ᵗʰ **S81.85**   **Open bite of lower leg**
     Bite of lower leg NOS
     EXCLUDES 1   superficial bite of lower leg (S80.86-, S80.87-)

   ✓7ᵗʰ **S81.851**   **Open bite, right lower leg**
   ✓7ᵗʰ **S81.852**   **Open bite, left lower leg**
   ✓7ᵗʰ **S81.859**   **Open bite, unspecified lower leg** ▽

✓4ᵗʰ **S82**   **Fracture of lower leg, including ankle**
     NOTE   A fracture not indicated as displaced or nondisplaced should be coded to displaced.
     A fracture not designated as open or closed should be coded to closed.
     The open fracture designations are based on the Gustilo open fracture classification.
     INCLUDES   fracture of malleolus
     EXCLUDES 1   traumatic amputation of lower leg (S88.-)
     EXCLUDES 2   fracture of foot, except ankle (S92.-)
     periprosthetic fracture of prosthetic implant of knee (T84.042, T84.043)

The appropriate 7th character is to be added to all codes from category S82 [unless otherwise indicated].
A   initial encounter for closed fracture
B   initial encounter for open fracture type I or II
     initial encounter for open fracture NOS
C   initial encounter for open fracture type IIIA, IIIB, or IIIC
D   subsequent encounter for closed fracture with routine healing
E   subsequent encounter for open fracture type I or II with routine healing
F   subsequent encounter for open fracture type IIIA, IIIB, or IIIC with routine healing
G   subsequent encounter for closed fracture with delayed healing
H   subsequent encounter for open fracture type I or II with delayed healing
J   subsequent encounter for open fracture type IIIA, IIIB or IIIC with delayed healing
K   subsequent encounter for closed fracture with nonunion
M   subsequent encounter for open fracture type I or II with nonunion
N   subsequent encounter for open fracture type IIIA, IIIB or IIIC with nonunion
P   subsequent encounter for closed fracture with malunion
Q   subsequent encounter for open fracture type I or II with malunion
R   subsequent encounter for open fracture type IIIA, IIIB or IIIC with malunion
S   sequela

✓5ᵗʰ **S82.0**   **Fracture of patella**
     Knee cap

✓6ᵗʰ **S82.00**   **Unspecified fracture of patella**

   ✓7ᵗʰ **S82.001**   **Unspecified fracture of right patella** ▽
   ✓7ᵗʰ **S82.002**   **Unspecified fracture of left patella** ▽
   ✓7ᵗʰ **S82.009**   **Unspecified fracture of unspecified patella** ▽

✓6ᵗʰ **S82.01**   **Osteochondral fracture of patella**

   ✓7ᵗʰ **S82.011**   **Displaced osteochondral fracture of right patella**
   ✓7ᵗʰ **S82.012**   **Displaced osteochondral fracture of left patella**
   ✓7ᵗʰ **S82.013**   **Displaced osteochondral fracture of unspecified patella** ▽
   ✓7ᵗʰ **S82.014**   **Nondisplaced osteochondral fracture of right patella**
   ✓7ᵗʰ **S82.015**   **Nondisplaced osteochondral fracture of left patella**
   ✓7ᵗʰ **S82.016**   **Nondisplaced osteochondral fracture of unspecified patella** ▽

✓6ᵗʰ **S82.02**   **Longitudinal fracture of patella**

   ✓7ᵗʰ **S82.021**   **Displaced longitudinal fracture of right patella**
   ✓7ᵗʰ **S82.022**   **Displaced longitudinal fracture of left patella**
   ✓7ᵗʰ **S82.023**   **Displaced longitudinal fracture of unspecified patella** ▽
   ✓7ᵗʰ **S82.024**   **Nondisplaced longitudinal fracture of right patella**
   ✓7ᵗʰ **S82.025**   **Nondisplaced longitudinal fracture of left patella**
   ✓7ᵗʰ **S82.026**   **Nondisplaced longitudinal fracture of unspecified patella** ▽

✓6ᵗʰ **S82.03**   **Transverse fracture of patella**

   ✓7ᵗʰ **S82.031**   **Displaced transverse fracture of right patella**

✓ Add'l Character Required   ✓×7ᵗʰ Placeholder Alert   RUG IV Special Care High Dx   RUG IV Clinically Complex Dx   RUG IV Special Care Low Dx   Manifestation Code   Other Specified Code   ▽ Unspecified Code

ICD-10-CM 2016   955

☑7ᵗʰ **S82.032** Displaced **transverse fracture of** left **patella**

☑7ᵗʰ **S82.033** Displaced **transverse fracture of** unspecified **patella** ▽

☑7ᵗʰ **S82.034** Nondisplaced **transverse fracture of** right **patella**

☑7ᵗʰ **S82.035** Nondisplaced **transverse fracture of** left **patella**

☑7ᵗʰ **S82.036** Nondisplaced **transverse fracture of** unspecified **patella** ▽

✓6ᵗʰ **S82.04** Comminuted **fracture of patella**

☑7ᵗʰ **S82.041** Displaced **comminuted fracture of** right **patella**

☑7ᵗʰ **S82.042** Displaced **comminuted fracture of** left **patella**

☑7ᵗʰ **S82.043** Displaced **comminuted fracture of** unspecified **patella** ▽

☑7ᵗʰ **S82.044** Nondisplaced **comminuted fracture of** right **patella**

☑7ᵗʰ **S82.045** Nondisplaced **comminuted fracture of** left **patella**

☑7ᵗʰ **S82.046** Nondisplaced **comminuted fracture of** unspecified **patella** ▽

✓6ᵗʰ **S82.09** Other **fracture of patella**

☑7ᵗʰ **S82.091** Other fracture of right patella

☑7ᵗʰ **S82.092** Other fracture of left patella

☑7ᵗʰ **S82.099** Other fracture of unspecified patella ▽

✓5ᵗʰ **S82.1** **Fracture of** upper end of tibia
Fracture of proximal end of tibia
EXCLUDES 2 *fracture of shaft of tibia (S82.2-)*
physeal fracture of upper end of tibia (S89.0-)

✓6ᵗʰ **S82.10** Unspecified **fracture of upper end of tibia**

☑7ᵗʰ **S82.101** Unspecified **fracture of upper end of** right **tibia** ▽

☑7ᵗʰ **S82.102** Unspecified **fracture of upper end of** left **tibia** ▽

☑7ᵗʰ **S82.109** Unspecified **fracture of upper end of** unspecified **tibia** ▽

✓6ᵗʰ **S82.11** Fracture of tibial spine

☑7ᵗʰ **S82.111** Displaced **fracture of** right **tibial spine**

☑7ᵗʰ **S82.112** Displaced **fracture of** left **tibial spine**

☑7ᵗʰ **S82.113** Displaced **fracture of** unspecified **tibial spine** ▽

☑7ᵗʰ **S82.114** Nondisplaced **fracture of** right **tibial spine**

☑7ᵗʰ **S82.115** Nondisplaced **fracture of** left **tibial spine**

☑7ᵗʰ **S82.116** Nondisplaced **fracture of** unspecified **tibial spine** ▽

✓6ᵗʰ **S82.12** Fracture of lateral condyle of tibia

☑7ᵗʰ **S82.121** Displaced **fracture of lateral condyle of** right **tibia**

☑7ᵗʰ **S82.122** Displaced **fracture of lateral condyle of** left **tibia**

☑7ᵗʰ **S82.123** Displaced **fracture of lateral condyle of** unspecified **tibia** ▽

☑7ᵗʰ **S82.124** Nondisplaced **fracture of lateral condyle of** right **tibia**

☑7ᵗʰ **S82.125** Nondisplaced **fracture of lateral condyle of** left **tibia**

☑7ᵗʰ **S82.126** Nondisplaced **fracture of lateral condyle of** unspecified **tibia** ▽

✓6ᵗʰ **S82.13** Fracture of medial condyle of tibia

☑7ᵗʰ **S82.131** Displaced **fracture of medial condyle of** right **tibia**

☑7ᵗʰ **S82.132** Displaced **fracture of medial condyle of** left **tibia**

☑7ᵗʰ **S82.133** Displaced **fracture of medial condyle of** unspecified **tibia** ▽

☑7ᵗʰ **S82.134** Nondisplaced **fracture of medial condyle of** right **tibia**

☑7ᵗʰ **S82.135** Nondisplaced **fracture of medial condyle of** left **tibia**

☑7ᵗʰ **S82.136** Nondisplaced **fracture of medial condyle of** unspecified **tibia** ▽

✓6ᵗʰ **S82.14** Bicondylar **fracture of tibia**
Fracture of tibial plateau NOS

☑7ᵗʰ **S82.141** Displaced **bicondylar fracture of** right **tibia**

☑7ᵗʰ **S82.142** Displaced **bicondylar fracture of** left **tibia**

☑7ᵗʰ **S82.143** Displaced **bicondylar fracture of** unspecified **tibia** ▽

☑7ᵗʰ **S82.144** Nondisplaced **bicondylar fracture of** right **tibia**

☑7ᵗʰ **S82.145** Nondisplaced **bicondylar fracture of** left **tibia**

☑7ᵗʰ **S82.146** Nondisplaced **bicondylar fracture of** unspecified **tibia** ▽

✓6ᵗʰ **S82.15** Fracture of tibial tuberosity

☑7ᵗʰ **S82.151** Displaced **fracture of** right **tibial tuberosity**

☑7ᵗʰ **S82.152** Displaced **fracture of** left **tibial tuberosity**

☑7ᵗʰ **S82.153** Displaced **fracture of** unspecified **tibial tuberosity** ▽

☑7ᵗʰ **S82.154** Nondisplaced **fracture of** right **tibial tuberosity**

☑7ᵗʰ **S82.155** Nondisplaced **fracture of** left **tibial tuberosity**

☑7ᵗʰ **S82.156** Nondisplaced **fracture of** unspecified **tibial tuberosity** ▽

✓6ᵗʰ **S82.16** Torus **fracture of upper end of tibia**

> The appropriate 7th character is to be added to all codes in subcategory S82.16.
> A   initial encounter for closed fracture
> D   subsequent encounter for fracture with routine healing
> G   subsequent encounter for fracture with delayed healing
> K   subsequent encounter for fracture with nonunion
> P   subsequent encounter for fracture with malunion
> S   sequela

☑7ᵗʰ **S82.161** Torus **fracture of upper end of** right **tibia**

☑7ᵗʰ **S82.162** Torus **fracture of upper end of** left **tibia**

☑7ᵗʰ **S82.169** Torus **fracture of upper end of** unspecified **tibia** ▽

✓6ᵗʰ **S82.19** Other **fracture of upper end of tibia**

☑7ᵗʰ **S82.191** Other fracture of upper end of right tibia

☑7ᵗʰ **S82.192** Other fracture of upper end of left tibia

☑7ᵗʰ **S82.199** Other fracture of upper end of unspecified tibia ▽

✓5ᵗʰ **S82.2** **Fracture of** shaft of tibia

✓6ᵗʰ **S82.20** Unspecified **fracture of shaft of tibia**
Fracture of tibia NOS

☑7ᵗʰ **S82.201** Unspecified **fracture of shaft of** right **tibia** ▽

☑7ᵗʰ **S82.202** Unspecified **fracture of shaft of** left **tibia** ▽

☑7ᵗʰ **S82.209** Unspecified **fracture of shaft of** unspecified **tibia** ▽

✓6ᵗʰ **S82.22** Transverse **fracture of shaft of tibia**

☑7ᵗʰ **S82.221** Displaced **transverse fracture of shaft of** right **tibia**

☑7ᵗʰ **S82.222** Displaced **transverse fracture of shaft of** left **tibia**

☑7ᵗʰ **S82.223** Displaced **transverse fracture of shaft of** unspecified **tibia** ▽

☑7ᵗʰ **S82.224** Nondisplaced **transverse fracture of shaft of** right **tibia**

☑7ᵗʰ **S82.225** Nondisplaced **transverse fracture of shaft of** left **tibia**

☑7ᵗʰ **S82.226** Nondisplaced **transverse fracture of shaft of** unspecified **tibia** ▽

✓6ᵗʰ **S82.23** Oblique **fracture of shaft of tibia**

☑7ᵗʰ **S82.231** Displaced **oblique fracture of shaft of** right **tibia**

☑7ᵗʰ **S82.232** Displaced **oblique fracture of shaft of** left **tibia**

Ⓝ Newborn   Ⓟ Pediatric   Ⓜ Maternity   Ⓐ Adult   **RIC** RIC Dx   **NC Dx** Noncancer Dx   **PDx** Primary Dx   **CC** RIC CC Condition   ▶◀ Revised Text   ● New Code   ▲ Revised Code Title

956   ICD-10-CM 2016

✔7ᵗʰ **S82.233** Displaced **oblique** fracture of shaft of unspecified **tibia** ▽

✔7ᵗʰ **S82.234** Nondisplaced **oblique** fracture of shaft of right **tibia**

✔7ᵗʰ **S82.235** Nondisplaced **oblique** fracture of shaft of left **tibia**

✔7ᵗʰ **S82.236** Nondisplaced **oblique** fracture of shaft of unspecified **tibia** ▽

✔6ᵗʰ **S82.24** Spiral **fracture of shaft of tibia**
Toddler fracture

✔7ᵗʰ **S82.241** Displaced **spiral** fracture of shaft of right **tibia**

✔7ᵗʰ **S82.242** Displaced **spiral** fracture of shaft of left **tibia**

✔7ᵗʰ **S82.243** Displaced **spiral** fracture of shaft of unspecified **tibia** ▽

✔7ᵗʰ **S82.244** Nondisplaced **spiral** fracture of shaft of right **tibia**

✔7ᵗʰ **S82.245** Nondisplaced **spiral** fracture of shaft of left **tibia**

✔7ᵗʰ **S82.246** Nondisplaced **spiral** fracture of shaft of unspecified **tibia** ▽

✔6ᵗʰ **S82.25** Comminuted **fracture of shaft of tibia**

✔7ᵗʰ **S82.251** Displaced **comminuted** fracture of shaft of right **tibia**

✔7ᵗʰ **S82.252** Displaced **comminuted** fracture of shaft of left **tibia**

✔7ᵗʰ **S82.253** Displaced **comminuted** fracture of shaft of unspecified **tibia** ▽

✔7ᵗʰ **S82.254** Nondisplaced **comminuted** fracture of shaft of right **tibia**

✔7ᵗʰ **S82.255** Nondisplaced **comminuted** fracture of shaft of left **tibia**

✔7ᵗʰ **S82.256** Nondisplaced **comminuted** fracture of shaft of unspecified **tibia** ▽

✔6ᵗʰ **S82.26** Segmental **fracture of shaft of tibia**

✔7ᵗʰ **S82.261** Displaced **segmental** fracture of shaft of right **tibia**

✔7ᵗʰ **S82.262** Displaced **segmental** fracture of shaft of left **tibia**

✔7ᵗʰ **S82.263** Displaced **segmental** fracture of shaft of unspecified **tibia** ▽

✔7ᵗʰ **S82.264** Nondisplaced **segmental** fracture of shaft of right **tibia**

✔7ᵗʰ **S82.265** Nondisplaced **segmental** fracture of shaft of left **tibia**

✔7ᵗʰ **S82.266** Nondisplaced **segmental** fracture of shaft of unspecified **tibia** ▽

✔6ᵗʰ **S82.29** Other **fracture of shaft of tibia**

✔7ᵗʰ **S82.291** Other fracture of shaft of right **tibia**

✔7ᵗʰ **S82.292** Other fracture of shaft of left **tibia**

✔7ᵗʰ **S82.299** Other fracture of shaft of unspecified **tibia** ▽

✔5ᵗʰ **S82.3** Fracture of lower end of tibia
EXCLUDES 1   bimalleolar fracture of lower leg (S82.84-)
     fracture of medial malleolus alone (S82.5-)
     Maisonneuve's fracture (S82.86-)
     pilon fracture of distal tibia (S82.87-)
     trimalleolar fractures of lower leg (S82.85-)

✔6ᵗʰ **S82.30** Unspecified **fracture of lower end of tibia**

✔7ᵗʰ **S82.301** Unspecified fracture of lower end of right **tibia** ▽

✔7ᵗʰ **S82.302** Unspecified fracture of lower end of left **tibia** ▽

✔7ᵗʰ **S82.309** Unspecified fracture of lower end of unspecified **tibia** ▽

✔6ᵗʰ **S82.31** Torus **fracture of lower end of tibia**

> The appropriate 7th character is to be added to all codes in subcategory S82.31.
> A   initial encounter for closed fracture
> D   subsequent encounter for fracture with routine healing
> G   subsequent encounter for fracture with delayed healing
> K   subsequent encounter for fracture with nonunion
> P   subsequent encounter for fracture with malunion
> S   sequela

✔7ᵗʰ **S82.311** Torus fracture of lower end of right **tibia**

✔7ᵗʰ **S82.312** Torus fracture of lower end of left **tibia**

✔7ᵗʰ **S82.319** Torus fracture of lower end of unspecified **tibia** ▽

✔6ᵗʰ **S82.39** Other **fracture of lower end of tibia**
AHA: 2015, 1Q, 25

✔7ᵗʰ **S82.391** Other fracture of lower end of right **tibia**

✔7ᵗʰ **S82.392** Other fracture of lower end of left **tibia**

✔7ᵗʰ **S82.399** Other fracture of lower end of unspecified **tibia** ▽

✔5ᵗʰ **S82.4** Fracture of shaft of fibula
EXCLUDES 2   fracture of lateral malleolus alone (S82.6-)

✔6ᵗʰ **S82.40** Unspecified **fracture of shaft of fibula**

✔7ᵗʰ **S82.401** Unspecified fracture of shaft of right **fibula** ▽

✔7ᵗʰ **S82.402** Unspecified fracture of shaft of left **fibula** ▽

✔7ᵗʰ **S82.409** Unspecified fracture of shaft of unspecified **fibula** ▽

✔6ᵗʰ **S82.42** Transverse **fracture of shaft of fibula**

✔7ᵗʰ **S82.421** Displaced **transverse** fracture of shaft of right **fibula**

✔7ᵗʰ **S82.422** Displaced **transverse** fracture of shaft of left **fibula**

✔7ᵗʰ **S82.423** Displaced **transverse** fracture of shaft of unspecified **fibula** ▽

✔7ᵗʰ **S82.424** Nondisplaced **transverse** fracture of shaft of right **fibula**

✔7ᵗʰ **S82.425** Nondisplaced **transverse** fracture of shaft of left **fibula**

✔7ᵗʰ **S82.426** Nondisplaced **transverse** fracture of shaft of unspecified **fibula** ▽

✔6ᵗʰ **S82.43** Oblique **fracture of shaft of fibula**

✔7ᵗʰ **S82.431** Displaced **oblique** fracture of shaft of right **fibula**

✔7ᵗʰ **S82.432** Displaced **oblique** fracture of shaft of left **fibula**

✔7ᵗʰ **S82.433** Displaced **oblique** fracture of shaft of unspecified **fibula** ▽

✔7ᵗʰ **S82.434** Nondisplaced **oblique** fracture of shaft of right **fibula**

✔7ᵗʰ **S82.435** Nondisplaced **oblique** fracture of shaft of left **fibula**

✔7ᵗʰ **S82.436** Nondisplaced **oblique** fracture of shaft of unspecified **fibula** ▽

✔6ᵗʰ **S82.44** Spiral **fracture of shaft of fibula**

✔7ᵗʰ **S82.441** Displaced **spiral** fracture of shaft of right **fibula**

✔7ᵗʰ **S82.442** Displaced **spiral** fracture of shaft of left **fibula**

✔7ᵗʰ **S82.443** Displaced **spiral** fracture of shaft of unspecified **fibula** ▽

✔7ᵗʰ **S82.444** Nondisplaced **spiral** fracture of shaft of right **fibula**

✔7ᵗʰ **S82.445** Nondisplaced **spiral** fracture of shaft of left **fibula**

✔7ᵗʰ **S82.446** Nondisplaced **spiral** fracture of shaft of unspecified **fibula** ▽

Chapter 19. Injury, Poisoning and Certain Other Consequences of External Causes

S82.45–S82.875

✓6ᵗʰ **S82.45** Comminuted fracture of shaft of fibula

  ✓7ᵗʰ **S82.451** Displaced comminuted fracture of shaft of right fibula

  ✓7ᵗʰ **S82.452** Displaced comminuted fracture of shaft of left fibula

  ✓7ᵗʰ **S82.453** Displaced comminuted fracture of shaft of unspecified fibula ▽

  ✓7ᵗʰ **S82.454** Nondisplaced comminuted fracture of shaft of right fibula

  ✓7ᵗʰ **S82.455** Nondisplaced comminuted fracture of shaft of left fibula

  ✓7ᵗʰ **S82.456** Nondisplaced comminuted fracture of shaft of unspecified fibula ▽

✓6ᵗʰ **S82.46** Segmental fracture of shaft of fibula

  ✓7ᵗʰ **S82.461** Displaced segmental fracture of shaft of right fibula

  ✓7ᵗʰ **S82.462** Displaced segmental fracture of shaft of left fibula

  ✓7ᵗʰ **S82.463** Displaced segmental fracture of shaft of unspecified fibula ▽

  ✓7ᵗʰ **S82.464** Nondisplaced segmental fracture of shaft of right fibula

  ✓7ᵗʰ **S82.465** Nondisplaced segmental fracture of shaft of left fibula

  ✓7ᵗʰ **S82.466** Nondisplaced segmental fracture of shaft of unspecified fibula ▽

✓6ᵗʰ **S82.49** Other fracture of shaft of fibula

  ✓7ᵗʰ **S82.491** Other fracture of shaft of right fibula

  ✓7ᵗʰ **S82.492** Other fracture of shaft of left fibula

  ✓7ᵗʰ **S82.499** Other fracture of shaft of unspecified fibula ▽

✓5ᵗʰ **S82.5** Fracture of medial malleolus

  EXCLUDES 1 pilon fracture of distal tibia (S82.87-)
    Salter-Harris type III of lower end of tibia (S89.13-)
    Salter-Harris type IV of lower end of tibia (S89.14-)

  ✓x7ᵗʰ **S82.51** Displaced fracture of medial malleolus of right tibia

  ✓x7ᵗʰ **S82.52** Displaced fracture of medial malleolus of left tibia

  ✓x7ᵗʰ **S82.53** Displaced fracture of medial malleolus of unspecified tibia ▽

  ✓x7ᵗʰ **S82.54** Nondisplaced fracture of medial malleolus of right tibia

  ✓x7ᵗʰ **S82.55** Nondisplaced fracture of medial malleolus of left tibia

  ✓x7ᵗʰ **S82.56** Nondisplaced fracture of medial malleolus of unspecified tibia ▽

✓5ᵗʰ **S82.6** Fracture of lateral malleolus

  EXCLUDES 1 pilon fracture of distal tibia (S82.87-)

  ✓x7ᵗʰ **S82.61** Displaced fracture of lateral malleolus of right fibula

  ✓x7ᵗʰ **S82.62** Displaced fracture of lateral malleolus of left fibula

  ✓x7ᵗʰ **S82.63** Displaced fracture of lateral malleolus of unspecified fibula ▽

  ✓x7ᵗʰ **S82.64** Nondisplaced fracture of lateral malleolus of right fibula

  ✓x7ᵗʰ **S82.65** Nondisplaced fracture of lateral malleolus of left fibula

  ✓x7ᵗʰ **S82.66** Nondisplaced fracture of lateral malleolus of unspecified fibula ▽

✓5ᵗʰ **S82.8** Other fractures of lower leg

  ✓6ᵗʰ **S82.81** Torus fracture of upper end of fibula

> The appropriate 7th character is to be added to all codes in subcategory S82.81.
> A   initial encounter for closed fracture
> D   subsequent encounter for fracture with routine healing
> G   subsequent encounter for fracture with delayed healing
> K   subsequent encounter for fracture with nonunion
> P   subsequent encounter for fracture with malunion
> S   sequela

  ✓7ᵗʰ **S82.811** Torus fracture of upper end of right fibula

  ✓7ᵗʰ **S82.812** Torus fracture of upper end of left fibula

  ✓7ᵗʰ **S82.819** Torus fracture of upper end of unspecified fibula ▽

✓6ᵗʰ **S82.82** Torus fracture of lower end of fibula

> The appropriate 7th character is to be added to all codes in subcategory S82.82.
> A   initial encounter for closed fracture
> D   subsequent encounter for fracture with routine healing
> G   subsequent encounter for fracture with delayed healing
> K   subsequent encounter for fracture with nonunion
> P   subsequent encounter for fracture with malunion
> S   sequela

  ✓7ᵗʰ **S82.821** Torus fracture of lower end of right fibula

  ✓7ᵗʰ **S82.822** Torus fracture of lower end of left fibula

  ✓7ᵗʰ **S82.829** Torus fracture of lower end of unspecified fibula ▽

✓6ᵗʰ **S82.83** Other fracture of upper and lower end of fibula
  AHA: 2015, 1Q, 25

  ✓7ᵗʰ **S82.831** Other fracture of upper and lower end of right fibula

  ✓7ᵗʰ **S82.832** Other fracture of upper and lower end of left fibula

  ✓7ᵗʰ **S82.839** Other fracture of upper and lower end of unspecified fibula ▽

✓6ᵗʰ **S82.84** Bimalleolar fracture of lower leg

  ✓7ᵗʰ **S82.841** Displaced bimalleolar fracture of right lower leg

  ✓7ᵗʰ **S82.842** Displaced bimalleolar fracture of left lower leg

  ✓7ᵗʰ **S82.843** Displaced bimalleolar fracture of unspecified lower leg ▽

  ✓7ᵗʰ **S82.844** Nondisplaced bimalleolar fracture of right lower leg

  ✓7ᵗʰ **S82.845** Nondisplaced bimalleolar fracture of left lower leg

  ✓7ᵗʰ **S82.846** Nondisplaced bimalleolar fracture of unspecified lower leg ▽

✓6ᵗʰ **S82.85** Trimalleolar fracture of lower leg

  ✓7ᵗʰ **S82.851** Displaced trimalleolar fracture of right lower leg

  ✓7ᵗʰ **S82.852** Displaced trimalleolar fracture of left lower leg

  ✓7ᵗʰ **S82.853** Displaced trimalleolar fracture of unspecified lower leg ▽

  ✓7ᵗʰ **S82.854** Nondisplaced trimalleolar fracture of right lower leg

  ✓7ᵗʰ **S82.855** Nondisplaced trimalleolar fracture of left lower leg

  ✓7ᵗʰ **S82.856** Nondisplaced trimalleolar fracture of unspecified lower leg ▽

✓6ᵗʰ **S82.86** Maisonneuve's fracture

  ✓7ᵗʰ **S82.861** Displaced Maisonneuve's fracture of right leg

  ✓7ᵗʰ **S82.862** Displaced Maisonneuve's fracture of left leg

  ✓7ᵗʰ **S82.863** Displaced Maisonneuve's fracture of unspecified leg ▽

  ✓7ᵗʰ **S82.864** Nondisplaced Maisonneuve's fracture of right leg

  ✓7ᵗʰ **S82.865** Nondisplaced Maisonneuve's fracture of left leg

  ✓7ᵗʰ **S82.866** Nondisplaced Maisonneuve's fracture of unspecified leg ▽

✓6ᵗʰ **S82.87** Pilon fracture of tibia

  ✓7ᵗʰ **S82.871** Displaced pilon fracture of right tibia

  ✓7ᵗʰ **S82.872** Displaced pilon fracture of left tibia

  ✓7ᵗʰ **S82.873** Displaced pilon fracture of unspecified tibia ▽

  ✓7ᵗʰ **S82.874** Nondisplaced pilon fracture of right tibia

  ✓7ᵗʰ **S82.875** Nondisplaced pilon fracture of left tibia

Ⓝ Newborn   Ⓟ Pediatric   Ⓜ Maternity   Ⓐ Adult   **RIC** RIC Dx   **NC Dx** Noncancer Dx   **PDx** Primary Dx   **CC** RIC CC Condition   ►◄ Revised Text   ● New Code   ▲ Revised Code Title

958   ICD-10-CM 2016

✓7ᵗʰ **S82.876**   Nondisplaced pilon fracture of unspecified tibia   ▽

✓6ᵗʰ **S82.89**   Other fractures of lower leg
Fracture of ankle NOS

    ✓7ᵗʰ **S82.891**   Other fracture of right lower leg

    ✓7ᵗʰ **S82.892**   Other fracture of left lower leg

    ✓7ᵗʰ **S82.899**   Other fracture of unspecified lower leg   ▽

✓5ᵗʰ **S82.9**   Unspecified fracture of lower leg

    ✓ₓ7ᵗʰ **S82.90**   Unspecified fracture of unspecified lower leg   ▽

    ✓ₓ7ᵗʰ **S82.91**   Unspecified fracture of right lower leg   ▽

    ✓ₓ7ᵗʰ **S82.92**   Unspecified fracture of left lower leg   ▽

✓4ᵗʰ **S83**   **Dislocation and sprain of joints and ligaments of knee**

    INCLUDES   avulsion of joint or ligament of knee
laceration of cartilage, joint or ligament of knee
sprain of cartilage, joint or ligament of knee
traumatic hemarthrosis of joint or ligament of knee
traumatic rupture of joint or ligament of knee
traumatic subluxation of joint or ligament of knee
traumatic tear of joint or ligament of knee

Code also any associated open wound

    EXCLUDES 1   derangement of patella (M22.0-M22.3)
injury of patellar ligament (tendon) (S76.1-)
internal derangement of knee (M23.-)
old dislocation of knee (M24.36)
pathological dislocation of knee (M24.36)
recurrent dislocation of knee (M22.0)

    EXCLUDES 2   strain of muscle, fascia and tendon of lower leg (S86.-)

> The appropriate 7th character is to be added to each code from category S83.
> A   initial encounter
> D   subsequent encounter
> S   sequela

✓5ᵗʰ **S83.0**   Subluxation and dislocation of patella

    ✓6ᵗʰ **S83.00**   Unspecified subluxation and dislocation of patella

       ✓7ᵗʰ **S83.001**   Unspecified subluxation of right patella   ▽

       ✓7ᵗʰ **S83.002**   Unspecified subluxation of left patella   ▽

       ✓7ᵗʰ **S83.003**   Unspecified subluxation of unspecified patella   ▽

       ✓7ᵗʰ **S83.004**   Unspecified dislocation of right patella   ▽

       ✓7ᵗʰ **S83.005**   Unspecified dislocation of left patella   ▽

       ✓7ᵗʰ **S83.006**   Unspecified dislocation of unspecified patella   ▽

    ✓6ᵗʰ **S83.01**   Lateral subluxation and dislocation of patella

       ✓7ᵗʰ **S83.011**   Lateral subluxation of right patella

       ✓7ᵗʰ **S83.012**   Lateral subluxation of left patella

       ✓7ᵗʰ **S83.013**   Lateral subluxation of unspecified patella   ▽

       ✓7ᵗʰ **S83.014**   Lateral dislocation of right patella

       ✓7ᵗʰ **S83.015**   Lateral dislocation of left patella

       ✓7ᵗʰ **S83.016**   Lateral dislocation of unspecified patella   ▽

    ✓6ᵗʰ **S83.09**   Other subluxation and dislocation of patella

       ✓7ᵗʰ **S83.091**   Other subluxation of right patella

       ✓7ᵗʰ **S83.092**   Other subluxation of left patella

       ✓7ᵗʰ **S83.093**   Other subluxation of unspecified patella   ▽

       ✓7ᵗʰ **S83.094**   Other dislocation of right patella

       ✓7ᵗʰ **S83.095**   Other dislocation of left patella

       ✓7ᵗʰ **S83.096**   Other dislocation of unspecified patella   ▽

✓5ᵗʰ **S83.1**   Subluxation and dislocation of knee

    EXCLUDES 2   instability of knee prosthesis (T84.022, T84.023)

    ✓6ᵗʰ **S83.10**   Unspecified subluxation and dislocation of knee

       ✓7ᵗʰ **S83.101**   Unspecified subluxation of right knee   ▽

       ✓7ᵗʰ **S83.102**   Unspecified subluxation of left knee   ▽

       ✓7ᵗʰ **S83.103**   Unspecified subluxation of unspecified knee   ▽

       ✓7ᵗʰ **S83.104**   Unspecified dislocation of right knee   ▽

       ✓7ᵗʰ **S83.105**   Unspecified dislocation of left knee   ▽

       ✓7ᵗʰ **S83.106**   Unspecified dislocation of unspecified knee   ▽

    ✓6ᵗʰ **S83.11**   Anterior subluxation and dislocation of proximal end of tibia
Posterior subluxation and dislocation of distal end of femur

       ✓7ᵗʰ **S83.111**   Anterior subluxation of proximal end of tibia, right knee

       ✓7ᵗʰ **S83.112**   Anterior subluxation of proximal end of tibia, left knee

       ✓7ᵗʰ **S83.113**   Anterior subluxation of proximal end of tibia, unspecified knee   ▽

       ✓7ᵗʰ **S83.114**   Anterior dislocation of proximal end of tibia, right knee

       ✓7ᵗʰ **S83.115**   Anterior dislocation of proximal end of tibia, left knee

       ✓7ᵗʰ **S83.116**   Anterior dislocation of proximal end of tibia, unspecified knee   ▽

    ✓6ᵗʰ **S83.12**   Posterior subluxation and dislocation of proximal end of tibia
Anterior dislocation of distal end of femur

       ✓7ᵗʰ **S83.121**   Posterior subluxation of proximal end of tibia, right knee

       ✓7ᵗʰ **S83.122**   Posterior subluxation of proximal end of tibia, left knee

       ✓7ᵗʰ **S83.123**   Posterior subluxation of proximal end of tibia, unspecified knee   ▽

       ✓7ᵗʰ **S83.124**   Posterior dislocation of proximal end of tibia, right knee

       ✓7ᵗʰ **S83.125**   Posterior dislocation of proximal end of tibia, left knee

       ✓7ᵗʰ **S83.126**   Posterior dislocation of proximal end of tibia, unspecified knee   ▽

    ✓6ᵗʰ **S83.13**   Medial subluxation and dislocation of proximal end of tibia

       ✓7ᵗʰ **S83.131**   Medial subluxation of proximal end of tibia, right knee

       ✓7ᵗʰ **S83.132**   Medial subluxation of proximal end of tibia, left knee

       ✓7ᵗʰ **S83.133**   Medial subluxation of proximal end of tibia, unspecified knee   ▽

       ✓7ᵗʰ **S83.134**   Medial dislocation of proximal end of tibia, right knee

       ✓7ᵗʰ **S83.135**   Medial dislocation of proximal end of tibia, left knee

       ✓7ᵗʰ **S83.136**   Medial dislocation of proximal end of tibia, unspecified knee   ▽

    ✓6ᵗʰ **S83.14**   Lateral subluxation and dislocation of proximal end of tibia

       ✓7ᵗʰ **S83.141**   Lateral subluxation of proximal end of tibia, right knee

       ✓7ᵗʰ **S83.142**   Lateral subluxation of proximal end of tibia, left knee

       ✓7ᵗʰ **S83.143**   Lateral subluxation of proximal end of tibia, unspecified knee   ▽

       ✓7ᵗʰ **S83.144**   Lateral dislocation of proximal end of tibia, right knee

       ✓7ᵗʰ **S83.145**   Lateral dislocation of proximal end of tibia, left knee

       ✓7ᵗʰ **S83.146**   Lateral dislocation of proximal end of tibia, unspecified knee   ▽

    ✓6ᵗʰ **S83.19**   Other subluxation and dislocation of knee

       ✓7ᵗʰ **S83.191**   Other subluxation of right knee

       ✓7ᵗʰ **S83.192**   Other subluxation of left knee

       ✓7ᵗʰ **S83.193**   Other subluxation of unspecified knee   ▽

       ✓7ᵗʰ **S83.194**   Other dislocation of right knee

       ✓7ᵗʰ **S83.195**   Other dislocation of left knee

       ✓7ᵗʰ **S83.196**   Other dislocation of unspecified knee   ▽

✓5ᵗʰ **S83.2**   Tear of meniscus, current injury

    EXCLUDES 1   old bucket-handle tear (M23.2)

    ✓6ᵗʰ **S83.20**   Tear of unspecified meniscus, current injury
Tear of meniscus of knee NOS

       ✓7ᵗʰ **S83.200**   Bucket-handle tear of unspecified meniscus, current injury, right knee   ▽

       ✓7ᵗʰ **S83.201**   Bucket-handle tear of unspecified meniscus, current injury, left knee

---

✓ Add'l Character Required   ✓ₓ7ᵗʰ Placeholder Alert   RUG IV Special Care High Dx   RUG IV Clinically Complex Dx   RUG IV Special Care Low Dx   Manifestation Code   Other Specified Code   ▽ Unspecified Code

√7th **S83.202** Bucket-handle tear of unspecified meniscus, current injury, unspecified knee ▽

√7th **S83.203** Other tear of unspecified meniscus, current injury, right knee ▽

√7th **S83.204** Other tear of unspecified meniscus, current injury, left knee ▽

√7th **S83.205** Other tear of unspecified meniscus, current injury, unspecified knee ▽

√7th **S83.206** Unspecified tear of unspecified meniscus, current injury, right knee ▽

√7th **S83.207** Unspecified tear of unspecified meniscus, current injury, left knee ▽

√7th **S83.209** Unspecified tear of unspecified meniscus, current injury, unspecified knee ▽

√6th **S83.21** Bucket-handle tear of medial meniscus, current injury

√7th **S83.211** Bucket-handle tear of medial meniscus, current injury, right knee

√7th **S83.212** Bucket-handle tear of medial meniscus, current injury, left knee

√7th **S83.219** Bucket-handle tear of medial meniscus, current injury, unspecified knee ▽

√6th **S83.22** Peripheral tear of medial meniscus, current injury

√7th **S83.221** Peripheral tear of medial meniscus, current injury, right knee

√7th **S83.222** Peripheral tear of medial meniscus, current injury, left knee

√7th **S83.229** Peripheral tear of medial meniscus, current injury, unspecified knee ▽

√6th **S83.23** Complex tear of medial meniscus, current injury

√7th **S83.231** Complex tear of medial meniscus, current injury, right knee

√7th **S83.232** Complex tear of medial meniscus, current injury, left knee

√7th **S83.239** Complex tear of medial meniscus, current injury, unspecified knee ▽

√6th **S83.24** Other tear of medial meniscus, current injury

√7th **S83.241** Other tear of medial meniscus, current injury, right knee

√7th **S83.242** Other tear of medial meniscus, current injury, left knee

√7th **S83.249** Other tear of medial meniscus, current injury, unspecified knee ▽

√6th **S83.25** Bucket-handle tear of lateral meniscus, current injury

√7th **S83.251** Bucket-handle tear of lateral meniscus, current injury, right knee

√7th **S83.252** Bucket-handle tear of lateral meniscus, current injury, left knee

√7th **S83.259** Bucket-handle tear of lateral meniscus, current injury, unspecified knee ▽

√6th **S83.26** Peripheral tear of lateral meniscus, current injury

√7th **S83.261** Peripheral tear of lateral meniscus, current injury, right knee

√7th **S83.262** Peripheral tear of lateral meniscus, current injury, left knee

√7th **S83.269** Peripheral tear of lateral meniscus, current injury, unspecified knee ▽

√6th **S83.27** Complex tear of lateral meniscus, current injury

√7th **S83.271** Complex tear of lateral meniscus, current injury, right knee

√7th **S83.272** Complex tear of lateral meniscus, current injury, left knee

√7th **S83.279** Complex tear of lateral meniscus, current injury, unspecified knee ▽

√6th **S83.28** Other tear of lateral meniscus, current injury

√7th **S83.281** Other tear of lateral meniscus, current injury, right knee

√7th **S83.282** Other tear of lateral meniscus, current injury, left knee

√7th **S83.289** Other tear of lateral meniscus, current injury, unspecified knee ▽

√5th **S83.3** Tear of articular cartilage of knee, current

√x7th **S83.30** Tear of articular cartilage of unspecified knee, current

√x7th **S83.31** Tear of articular cartilage of right knee, current

√x7th **S83.32** Tear of articular cartilage of left knee, current

√5th **S83.4** Sprain of collateral ligament of knee

√6th **S83.40** Sprain of unspecified collateral ligament of knee

√7th **S83.401** Sprain of unspecified collateral ligament of right knee ▽

√7th **S83.402** Sprain of unspecified collateral ligament of left knee ▽

√7th **S83.409** Sprain of unspecified collateral ligament of unspecified knee ▽

√6th **S83.41** Sprain of medial collateral ligament of knee
Sprain of tibial collateral ligament

√7th **S83.411** Sprain of medial collateral ligament of right knee

√7th **S83.412** Sprain of medial collateral ligament of left knee

√7th **S83.419** Sprain of medial collateral ligament of unspecified knee ▽

√6th **S83.42** Sprain of lateral collateral ligament of knee
Sprain of fibular collateral ligament

√7th **S83.421** Sprain of lateral collateral ligament of right knee

√7th **S83.422** Sprain of lateral collateral ligament of left knee

√7th **S83.429** Sprain of lateral collateral ligament of unspecified knee ▽

√5th **S83.5** Sprain of cruciate ligament of knee

√6th **S83.50** Sprain of unspecified cruciate ligament of knee

√7th **S83.501** Sprain of unspecified cruciate ligament of right knee ▽

√7th **S83.502** Sprain of unspecified cruciate ligament of left knee ▽

√7th **S83.509** Sprain of unspecified cruciate ligament of unspecified knee ▽

√6th **S83.51** Sprain of anterior cruciate ligament of knee

√7th **S83.511** Sprain of anterior cruciate ligament of right knee

√7th **S83.512** Sprain of anterior cruciate ligament of 0left knee

√7th **S83.519** Sprain of anterior cruciate ligament of unspecified knee ▽

√6th **S83.52** Sprain of posterior cruciate ligament of knee

√7th **S83.521** Sprain of posterior cruciate ligament of right knee

√7th **S83.522** Sprain of posterior cruciate ligament of left knee

√7th **S83.529** Sprain of posterior cruciate ligament of unspecified knee ▽

√5th **S83.6** Sprain of the superior tibiofibular joint and ligament

√x7th **S83.60** Sprain of the superior tibiofibular joint and ligament, unspecified knee ▽

√x7th **S83.61** Sprain of the superior tibiofibular joint and ligament, right knee

√x7th **S83.62** Sprain of the superior tibiofibular joint and ligament, left knee

√5th **S83.8** Sprain of other specified parts of knee

√6th **S83.8X** Sprain of other specified parts of knee

√7th **S83.8X1** Sprain of other specified parts of right knee

√7th **S83.8X2** Sprain of other specified parts of left knee

√7th **S83.8X9** Sprain of other specified parts of unspecified knee ▽

√5th **S83.9** Sprain of unspecified site of knee

√x7th **S83.90** Sprain of unspecified site of unspecified knee ▽

√x7th **S83.91** Sprain of unspecified site of right knee ▽

N Newborn P Pediatric M Maternity A Adult RIC RIC Dx NC Dx Noncancer Dx PDx Primary Dx CC RIC CC Condition ►◄ Revised Text ● New Code ▲ Revised Code Title

960 ICD-10-CM 2016

√x7ᵗʰ **S83.92**   Sprain of unspecified site of left knee   ▽

✓4ᵗʰ **S84**   **Injury of nerves at lower leg level**
Code also any associated open wound (S81.-)
EXCLUDES 2   injury of nerves at ankle and foot level (S94.-)

> The appropriate 7th character is to be added to each code from category S84.
> A   initial encounter
> D   subsequent encounter
> S   sequela

✓5ᵗʰ **S84.0**   Injury of tibial nerve at lower leg level
   √x7ᵗʰ **S84.00**   Injury of tibial nerve at lower leg level, unspecified leg
   √x7ᵗʰ **S84.01**   Injury of tibial nerve at lower leg level, right leg
   √x7ᵗʰ **S84.02**   Injury of tibial nerve at lower leg level, left leg

✓5ᵗʰ **S84.1**   Injury of peroneal nerve at lower leg level
   √x7ᵗʰ **S84.10**   Injury of peroneal nerve at lower leg level, unspecified leg
   √x7ᵗʰ **S84.11**   Injury of peroneal nerve at lower leg level, right leg
   √x7ᵗʰ **S84.12**   Injury of peroneal nerve at lower leg level, left leg

✓5ᵗʰ **S84.2**   Injury of cutaneous sensory nerve at lower leg level
   √x7ᵗʰ **S84.20**   Injury of cutaneous sensory nerve at lower leg level, unspecified leg
   √x7ᵗʰ **S84.21**   Injury of cutaneous sensory nerve at lower leg level, right leg
   √x7ᵗʰ **S84.22**   Injury of cutaneous sensory nerve at lower leg level, left leg

✓5ᵗʰ **S84.8**   Injury of other nerves at lower leg level
   ✓6ᵗʰ **S84.80**   Injury of other nerves at lower leg level
     √7ᵗʰ **S84.801**   Injury of other nerves at lower leg level, right leg
     √7ᵗʰ **S84.802**   Injury of other nerves at lower leg level, left leg
     √7ᵗʰ **S84.809**   Injury of other nerves at lower leg level, unspecified leg   ▽

✓5ᵗʰ **S84.9**   Injury of unspecified nerve at lower leg level
   √x7ᵗʰ **S84.90**   Injury of unspecified nerve at lower leg level, unspecified leg   ▽
   √x7ᵗʰ **S84.91**   Injury of unspecified nerve at lower leg level, right leg   ▽
   √x7ᵗʰ **S84.92**   Injury of unspecified nerve at lower leg level, left leg   ▽

✓4ᵗʰ **S85**   **Injury of blood vessels at lower leg level**
Code also any associated open wound (S81.-)
EXCLUDES 2   injury of blood vessels at ankle and foot level (S95.-)

> The appropriate 7th character is to be added to each code from category S85.
> A   initial encounter
> D   subsequent encounter
> S   sequela

✓5ᵗʰ **S85.0**   Injury of popliteal artery
   ✓6ᵗʰ **S85.00**   Unspecified injury of popliteal artery
     √7ᵗʰ **S85.001**   Unspecified injury of popliteal artery, right leg   ▽
     √7ᵗʰ **S85.002**   Unspecified injury of popliteal artery, left leg   ▽
     √7ᵗʰ **S85.009**   Unspecified injury of popliteal artery, unspecified leg   ▽
   ✓6ᵗʰ **S85.01**   Laceration of popliteal artery
     √7ᵗʰ **S85.011**   Laceration of popliteal artery, right leg
     √7ᵗʰ **S85.012**   Laceration of popliteal artery, left leg
     √7ᵗʰ **S85.019**   Laceration of popliteal artery, unspecified leg   ▽
   ✓6ᵗʰ **S85.09**   Other specified injury of popliteal artery
     √7ᵗʰ **S85.091**   Other specified injury of popliteal artery, right leg
     √7ᵗʰ **S85.092**   Other specified injury of popliteal artery, left leg
     √7ᵗʰ **S85.099**   Other specified injury of popliteal artery, unspecified leg   ▽

✓5ᵗʰ **S85.1**   Injury of tibial artery
   ✓6ᵗʰ **S85.10**   Unspecified injury of unspecified tibial artery
     Injury of tibial artery NOS
     √7ᵗʰ **S85.101**   Unspecified injury of unspecified tibial artery, right leg   ▽
     √7ᵗʰ **S85.102**   Unspecified injury of unspecified tibial artery, left leg   ▽
     √7ᵗʰ **S85.109**   Unspecified injury of unspecified tibial artery, unspecified leg   ▽
   ✓6ᵗʰ **S85.11**   Laceration of unspecified tibial artery
     √7ᵗʰ **S85.111**   Laceration of unspecified tibial artery, right leg   ▽
     √7ᵗʰ **S85.112**   Laceration of unspecified tibial artery, left leg   ▽
     √7ᵗʰ **S85.119**   Laceration of unspecified tibial artery, unspecified leg   ▽
   ✓6ᵗʰ **S85.12**   Other specified injury of unspecified tibial artery
     √7ᵗʰ **S85.121**   Other specified injury of unspecified tibial artery, right leg   ▽
     √7ᵗʰ **S85.122**   Other specified injury of unspecified tibial artery, left leg   ▽
     √7ᵗʰ **S85.129**   Other specified injury of unspecified tibial artery, unspecified leg   ▽
   ✓6ᵗʰ **S85.13**   Unspecified injury of anterior tibial artery
     √7ᵗʰ **S85.131**   Unspecified injury of anterior tibial artery, right leg   ▽
     √7ᵗʰ **S85.132**   Unspecified injury of anterior tibial artery, left leg   ▽
     √7ᵗʰ **S85.139**   Unspecified injury of anterior tibial artery, unspecified leg   ▽
   ✓6ᵗʰ **S85.14**   Laceration of anterior tibial artery
     √7ᵗʰ **S85.141**   Laceration of anterior tibial artery, right leg
     √7ᵗʰ **S85.142**   Laceration of anterior tibial artery, left leg
     √7ᵗʰ **S85.149**   Laceration of anterior tibial artery, unspecified leg   ▽
   ✓6ᵗʰ **S85.15**   Other specified injury of anterior tibial artery
     √7ᵗʰ **S85.151**   Other specified injury of anterior tibial artery, right leg
     √7ᵗʰ **S85.152**   Other specified injury of anterior tibial artery, left leg
     √7ᵗʰ **S85.159**   Other specified injury of anterior tibial artery, unspecified leg   ▽
   ✓6ᵗʰ **S85.16**   Unspecified injury of posterior tibial artery
     √7ᵗʰ **S85.161**   Unspecified injury of posterior tibial artery, right leg   ▽
     √7ᵗʰ **S85.162**   Unspecified injury of posterior tibial artery, left leg   ▽
     √7ᵗʰ **S85.169**   Unspecified injury of posterior tibial artery, unspecified leg   ▽
   ✓6ᵗʰ **S85.17**   Laceration of posterior tibial artery
     √7ᵗʰ **S85.171**   Laceration of posterior tibial artery, right leg
     √7ᵗʰ **S85.172**   Laceration of posterior tibial artery, left leg
     √7ᵗʰ **S85.179**   Laceration of posterior tibial artery, unspecified leg   ▽
   ✓6ᵗʰ **S85.18**   Other specified injury of posterior tibial artery
     √7ᵗʰ **S85.181**   Other specified injury of posterior tibial artery, right leg
     √7ᵗʰ **S85.182**   Other specified injury of posterior tibial artery, left leg
     √7ᵗʰ **S85.189**   Other specified injury of posterior tibial artery, unspecified leg   ▽

✓5ᵗʰ **S85.2**   Injury of peroneal artery
   ✓6ᵗʰ **S85.20**   Unspecified injury of peroneal artery
     √7ᵗʰ **S85.201**   Unspecified injury of peroneal artery, right leg   ▽
     √7ᵗʰ **S85.202**   Unspecified injury of peroneal artery, left leg   ▽
     √7ᵗʰ **S85.209**   Unspecified injury of peroneal artery, unspecified leg   ▽

√6ᵗʰ **S85.21** Laceration of peroneal artery
- √7ᵗʰ **S85.211** Laceration of peroneal artery, right leg
- √7ᵗʰ **S85.212** Laceration of peroneal artery, left leg
- √7ᵗʰ **S85.219** Laceration of peroneal artery, unspecified leg ▽

√6ᵗʰ **S85.29** Other specified injury of peroneal artery
- √7ᵗʰ **S85.291** Other specified injury of peroneal artery, right leg
- √7ᵗʰ **S85.292** Other specified injury of peroneal artery, left leg
- √7ᵗʰ **S85.299** Other specified injury of peroneal artery, unspecified leg ▽

√5ᵗʰ **S85.3** Injury of greater saphenous vein at lower leg level
Injury of greater saphenous vein NOS
Injury of saphenous vein NOS

√6ᵗʰ **S85.30** Unspecified injury of greater saphenous vein at lower leg level
- √7ᵗʰ **S85.301** Unspecified injury of greater saphenous vein at lower leg level, right leg ▽
- √7ᵗʰ **S85.302** Unspecified injury of greater saphenous vein at lower leg level, left leg ▽
- √7ᵗʰ **S85.309** Unspecified injury of greater saphenous vein at lower leg level, unspecified leg ▽

√6ᵗʰ **S85.31** Laceration of greater saphenous vein at lower leg level
- √7ᵗʰ **S85.311** Laceration of greater saphenous vein at lower leg level, right leg
- √7ᵗʰ **S85.312** Laceration of greater saphenous vein at lower leg level, left leg
- √7ᵗʰ **S85.319** Laceration of greater saphenous vein at lower leg level, unspecified leg ▽

√6ᵗʰ **S85.39** Other specified injury of greater saphenous vein at lower leg level
- √7ᵗʰ **S85.391** Other specified injury of greater saphenous vein at lower leg level, right leg
- √7ᵗʰ **S85.392** Other specified injury of greater saphenous vein at lower leg level, left leg
- √7ᵗʰ **S85.399** Other specified injury of greater saphenous vein at lower leg level, unspecified leg ▽

√5ᵗʰ **S85.4** Injury of lesser saphenous vein at lower leg level

√6ᵗʰ **S85.40** Unspecified injury of lesser saphenous vein at lower leg level
- √7ᵗʰ **S85.401** Unspecified injury of lesser saphenous vein at lower leg level, right leg ▽
- √7ᵗʰ **S85.402** Unspecified injury of lesser saphenous vein at lower leg level, left leg ▽
- √7ᵗʰ **S85.409** Unspecified injury of lesser saphenous vein at lower leg level, unspecified leg ▽

√6ᵗʰ **S85.41** Laceration of lesser saphenous vein at lower leg level
- √7ᵗʰ **S85.411** Laceration of lesser saphenous vein at lower leg level, right leg
- √7ᵗʰ **S85.412** Laceration of lesser saphenous vein at lower leg level, left leg
- √7ᵗʰ **S85.419** Laceration of lesser saphenous vein at lower leg level, unspecified leg ▽

√6ᵗʰ **S85.49** Other specified injury of lesser saphenous vein at lower leg level
- √7ᵗʰ **S85.491** Other specified injury of lesser saphenous vein at lower leg level, right leg
- √7ᵗʰ **S85.492** Other specified injury of lesser saphenous vein at lower leg level, left leg
- √7ᵗʰ **S85.499** Other specified injury of lesser saphenous vein at lower leg level, unspecified leg ▽

√5ᵗʰ **S85.5** Injury of popliteal vein

√6ᵗʰ **S85.50** Unspecified injury of popliteal vein
- √7ᵗʰ **S85.501** Unspecified injury of popliteal vein, right leg ▽
- √7ᵗʰ **S85.502** Unspecified injury of popliteal vein, left leg ▽
- √7ᵗʰ **S85.509** Unspecified injury of popliteal vein, unspecified leg ▽

√6ᵗʰ **S85.51** Laceration of popliteal vein
- √7ᵗʰ **S85.511** Laceration of popliteal vein, right leg
- √7ᵗʰ **S85.512** Laceration of popliteal vein, left leg
- √7ᵗʰ **S85.519** Laceration of popliteal vein, unspecified leg ▽

√6ᵗʰ **S85.59** Other specified injury of popliteal vein
- √7ᵗʰ **S85.591** Other specified injury of popliteal vein, right leg
- √7ᵗʰ **S85.592** Other specified injury of popliteal vein, left leg
- √7ᵗʰ **S85.599** Other specified injury of popliteal vein, unspecified leg ▽

√5ᵗʰ **S85.8** Injury of other blood vessels at lower leg level

√6ᵗʰ **S85.80** Unspecified injury of other blood vessels at lower leg level
- √7ᵗʰ **S85.801** Unspecified injury of other blood vessels at lower leg level, right leg ▽
- √7ᵗʰ **S85.802** Unspecified injury of other blood vessels at lower leg level, left leg ▽
- √7ᵗʰ **S85.809** Unspecified injury of other blood vessels at lower leg level, unspecified leg ▽

√6ᵗʰ **S85.81** Laceration of other blood vessels at lower leg level
- √7ᵗʰ **S85.811** Laceration of other blood vessels at lower leg level, right leg
- √7ᵗʰ **S85.812** Laceration of other blood vessels at lower leg level, left leg
- √7ᵗʰ **S85.819** Laceration of other blood vessels at lower leg level, unspecified leg ▽

√6ᵗʰ **S85.89** Other specified injury of other blood vessels at lower leg level
- √7ᵗʰ **S85.891** Other specified injury of other blood vessels at lower leg level, right leg
- √7ᵗʰ **S85.892** Other specified injury of other blood vessels at lower leg level, left leg
- √7ᵗʰ **S85.899** Other specified injury of other blood vessels at lower leg level, unspecified leg ▽

√5ᵗʰ **S85.9** Injury of unspecified blood vessel at lower leg level

√6ᵗʰ **S85.90** Unspecified injury of unspecified blood vessel at lower leg level
- √7ᵗʰ **S85.901** Unspecified injury of unspecified blood vessel at lower leg level, right leg ▽
- √7ᵗʰ **S85.902** Unspecified injury of unspecified blood vessel at lower leg level, left leg ▽
- √7ᵗʰ **S85.909** Unspecified injury of unspecified blood vessel at lower leg level, unspecified leg ▽

√6ᵗʰ **S85.91** Laceration of unspecified blood vessel at lower leg level
- √7ᵗʰ **S85.911** Laceration of unspecified blood vessel at lower leg level, right leg ▽
- √7ᵗʰ **S85.912** Laceration of unspecified blood vessel at lower leg level, left leg ▽
- √7ᵗʰ **S85.919** Laceration of unspecified blood vessel at lower leg level, unspecified leg ▽

√6ᵗʰ **S85.99** Other specified injury of unspecified blood vessel at lower leg level
- √7ᵗʰ **S85.991** Other specified injury of unspecified blood vessel at lower leg level, right leg ▽
- √7ᵗʰ **S85.992** Other specified injury of unspecified blood vessel at lower leg level, left leg ▽
- √7ᵗʰ **S85.999** Other specified injury of unspecified blood vessel at lower leg level, unspecified leg ▽

Ⓝ Newborn   Ⓟ Pediatric   Ⓜ Maternity   Ⓐ Adult   **RIC** RIC Dx   **NCDx** Noncancer Dx   **PDx** Primary Dx   **CC** RIC CC Condition   ►◄ Revised Text   ● New Code   ▲ Revised Code Title

962   ICD-10-CM 2016

✚ ✓4ᵗʰ S86 Injury of muscle, fascia and tendon at lower leg level

Code also any associated open wound (S81.-)

EXCLUDES 2   injury of muscle, fascia and tendon at ankle (S96.-)
injury of patellar ligament (tendon) (S76.1-)
sprain of joints and ligaments of knee (S83.-)

The appropriate 7th character is to be added to each code from category S86.
A   initial encounter
D   subsequent encounter
S   sequela

✓5ᵗʰ S86.0 Injury of Achilles tendon

✓6ᵗʰ S86.00 Unspecified injury of Achilles tendon

    ✓7ᵗʰ S86.001 Unspecified injury of right Achilles tendon ▽

    ✓7ᵗʰ S86.002 Unspecified injury of left Achilles tendon ▽

    ✓7ᵗʰ S86.009 Unspecified injury of unspecified Achilles tendon ▽

✓6ᵗʰ S86.01 Strain of Achilles tendon

    ✓7ᵗʰ S86.011 Strain of right Achilles tendon

    ✓7ᵗʰ S86.012 Strain of left Achilles tendon

    ✓7ᵗʰ S86.019 Strain of unspecified Achilles tendon ▽

✓6ᵗʰ S86.02 Laceration of Achilles tendon

    ✓7ᵗʰ S86.021 Laceration of right Achilles tendon

    ✓7ᵗʰ S86.022 Laceration of left Achilles tendon

    ✓7ᵗʰ S86.029 Laceration of unspecified Achilles tendon ▽

✓6ᵗʰ S86.09 Other specified injury of Achilles tendon

    ✓7ᵗʰ S86.091 Other specified injury of right Achilles tendon

    ✓7ᵗʰ S86.092 Other specified injury of left Achilles tendon

    ✓7ᵗʰ S86.099 Other specified injury of unspecified Achilles tendon ▽

✓5ᵗʰ S86.1 Injury of other muscle(s) and tendon(s) of posterior muscle group at lower leg level

✓6ᵗʰ S86.10 Unspecified injury of other muscle(s) and tendon(s) of posterior muscle group at lower leg level

    ✓7ᵗʰ S86.101 Unspecified injury of other muscle(s) and tendon(s) of posterior muscle group at lower leg level, right leg ▽

    ✓7ᵗʰ S86.102 Unspecified injury of other muscle(s) and tendon(s) of posterior muscle group at lower leg level, left leg ▽

    ✓7ᵗʰ S86.109 Unspecified injury of other muscle(s) and tendon(s) of posterior muscle group at lower leg level, unspecified leg ▽

✓6ᵗʰ S86.11 Strain of other muscle(s) and tendon(s) of posterior muscle group at lower leg level

    ✓7ᵗʰ S86.111 Strain of other muscle(s) and tendon(s) of posterior muscle group at lower leg level, right leg

    ✓7ᵗʰ S86.112 Strain of other muscle(s) and tendon(s) of posterior muscle group at lower leg level, left leg

    ✓7ᵗʰ S86.119 Strain of other muscle(s) and tendon(s) of posterior muscle group at lower leg level, unspecified leg ▽

✓6ᵗʰ S86.12 Laceration of other muscle(s) and tendon(s) of posterior muscle group at lower leg level

    ✓7ᵗʰ S86.121 Laceration of other muscle(s) and tendon(s) of posterior muscle group at lower leg level, right leg

    ✓7ᵗʰ S86.122 Laceration of other muscle(s) and tendon(s) of posterior muscle group at lower leg level, left leg

    ✓7ᵗʰ S86.129 Laceration of other muscle(s) and tendon(s) of posterior muscle group at lower leg level, unspecified leg ▽

✓6ᵗʰ S86.19 Other injury of other muscle(s) and tendon(s) of posterior muscle group at lower leg level

    ✓7ᵗʰ S86.191 Other injury of other muscle(s) and tendon(s) of posterior muscle group at lower leg level, right leg

    ✓7ᵗʰ S86.192 Other injury of other muscle(s) and tendon(s) of posterior muscle group at lower leg level, left leg

    ✓7ᵗʰ S86.199 Other injury of other muscle(s) and tendon(s) of posterior muscle group at lower leg level, unspecified leg ▽

✓5ᵗʰ S86.2 Injury of muscle(s) and tendon(s) of anterior muscle group at lower leg level

✓6ᵗʰ S86.20 Unspecified injury of muscle(s) and tendon(s) of anterior muscle group at lower leg level

    ✓7ᵗʰ S86.201 Unspecified injury of muscle(s) and tendon(s) of anterior muscle group at lower leg level, right leg ▽

    ✓7ᵗʰ S86.202 Unspecified injury of muscle(s) and tendon(s) of anterior muscle group at lower leg level, left leg ▽

    ✓7ᵗʰ S86.209 Unspecified injury of muscle(s) and tendon(s) of anterior muscle group at lower leg level, unspecified leg ▽

✓6ᵗʰ S86.21 Strain of muscle(s) and tendon(s) of anterior muscle group at lower leg level

    ✓7ᵗʰ S86.211 Strain of muscle(s) and tendon(s) of anterior muscle group at lower leg level, right leg

    ✓7ᵗʰ S86.212 Strain of muscle(s) and tendon(s) of anterior muscle group at lower leg level, left leg

    ✓7ᵗʰ S86.219 Strain of muscle(s) and tendon(s) of anterior muscle group at lower leg level, unspecified leg ▽

✓6ᵗʰ S86.22 Laceration of muscle(s) and tendon(s) of anterior muscle group at lower leg level

    ✓7ᵗʰ S86.221 Laceration of muscle(s) and tendon(s) of anterior muscle group at lower leg level, right leg

    ✓7ᵗʰ S86.222 Laceration of muscle(s) and tendon(s) of anterior muscle group at lower leg level, left leg

    ✓7ᵗʰ S86.229 Laceration of muscle(s) and tendon(s) of anterior muscle group at lower leg level, unspecified leg ▽

✓6ᵗʰ S86.29 Other injury of muscle(s) and tendon(s) of anterior muscle group at lower leg level

    ✓7ᵗʰ S86.291 Other injury of muscle(s) and tendon(s) of anterior muscle group at lower leg level, right leg

    ✓7ᵗʰ S86.292 Other injury of muscle(s) and tendon(s) of anterior muscle group at lower leg level, left leg

    ✓7ᵗʰ S86.299 Other injury of muscle(s) and tendon(s) of anterior muscle group at lower leg level, unspecified leg ▽

✓5ᵗʰ S86.3 Injury of muscle(s) and tendon(s) of peroneal muscle group at lower leg level

✓6ᵗʰ S86.30 Unspecified injury of muscle(s) and tendon(s) of peroneal muscle group at lower leg level

    ✓7ᵗʰ S86.301 Unspecified injury of muscle(s) and tendon(s) of peroneal muscle group at lower leg level, right leg ▽

    ✓7ᵗʰ S86.302 Unspecified injury of muscle(s) and tendon(s) of peroneal muscle group at lower leg level, left leg ▽

    ✓7ᵗʰ S86.309 Unspecified injury of muscle(s) and tendon(s) of peroneal muscle group at lower leg level, unspecified leg ▽

✓6ᵗʰ S86.31 Strain of muscle(s) and tendon(s) of peroneal muscle group at lower leg level

    ✓7ᵗʰ S86.311 Strain of muscle(s) and tendon(s) of peroneal muscle group at lower leg level, right leg

    ✓7ᵗʰ S86.312 Strain of muscle(s) and tendon(s) of peroneal muscle group at lower leg level, left leg

    ✓7ᵗʰ S86.319 Strain of muscle(s) and tendon(s) of peroneal muscle group at lower leg level, unspecified leg ▽

✚ Refer to the Muscle/Tendon Table at beginning of this chapter.

☑ Add'l Character Required   ✓ₓ7ᵗʰ Placeholder Alert   RUG IV Special Care High Dx   RUG IV Clinically Complex Dx   RUG IV Special Care Low Dx   Manifestation Code   Other Specified Code   ▽ Unspecified Code

ICD-10-CM 2016   963

✓6ᵗʰ **S86.32** Laceration of muscle(s) and tendon(s) of peroneal muscle group at lower leg level

　✓7ᵗʰ **S86.321** Laceration of muscle(s) and tendon(s) of peroneal muscle group at lower leg level, right leg

　✓7ᵗʰ **S86.322** Laceration of muscle(s) and tendon(s) of peroneal muscle group at lower leg level, left leg

　✓7ᵗʰ **S86.329** Laceration of muscle(s) and tendon(s) of peroneal muscle group at lower leg level, unspecified leg ▽

✓6ᵗʰ **S86.39** Other injury of muscle(s) and tendon(s) of peroneal muscle group at lower leg level

　✓7ᵗʰ **S86.391** Other injury of muscle(s) and tendon(s) of peroneal muscle group at lower leg level, right leg

　✓7ᵗʰ **S86.392** Other injury of muscle(s) and tendon(s) of peroneal muscle group at lower leg level, left leg

　✓7ᵗʰ **S86.399** Other injury of muscle(s) and tendon(s) of peroneal muscle group at lower leg level, unspecified leg ▽

✓5ᵗʰ **S86.8** Injury of other muscles and tendons at lower leg level

✓6ᵗʰ **S86.80** Unspecified injury of other muscles and tendons at lower leg level

　✓7ᵗʰ **S86.801** Unspecified injury of other muscle(s) and tendon(s) at lower leg level, right leg ▽

　✓7ᵗʰ **S86.802** Unspecified injury of other muscle(s) and tendon(s) at lower leg level, left leg ▽

　✓7ᵗʰ **S86.809** Unspecified injury of other muscle(s) and tendon(s) at lower leg level, unspecified leg ▽

✓6ᵗʰ **S86.81** Strain of other muscles and tendons at lower leg level

　✓7ᵗʰ **S86.811** Strain of other muscle(s) and tendon(s) at lower leg level, right leg

　✓7ᵗʰ **S86.812** Strain of other muscle(s) and tendon(s) at lower leg level, left leg

　✓7ᵗʰ **S86.819** Strain of other muscle(s) and tendon(s) at lower leg level, unspecified leg ▽

✓6ᵗʰ **S86.82** Laceration of other muscles and tendons at lower leg level

　✓7ᵗʰ **S86.821** Laceration of other muscle(s) and tendon(s) at lower leg level, right leg

　✓7ᵗʰ **S86.822** Laceration of other muscle(s) and tendon(s) at lower leg level, left leg

　✓7ᵗʰ **S86.829** Laceration of other muscle(s) and tendon(s) at lower leg level, unspecified leg ▽

✓6ᵗʰ **S86.89** Other injury of other muscles and tendons at lower leg level

　✓7ᵗʰ **S86.891** Other injury of other muscle(s) and tendon(s) at lower leg level, right leg

　✓7ᵗʰ **S86.892** Other injury of other muscle(s) and tendon(s) at lower leg level, left leg

　✓7ᵗʰ **S86.899** Other injury of other muscle(s) and tendon(s) at lower leg level, unspecified leg ▽

✓5ᵗʰ **S86.9** Injury of unspecified muscle and tendon at lower leg level

✓6ᵗʰ **S86.90** Unspecified injury of unspecified muscle and tendon at lower leg level

　✓7ᵗʰ **S86.901** Unspecified injury of unspecified muscle(s) and tendon(s) at lower leg level, right leg ▽

　✓7ᵗʰ **S86.902** Unspecified injury of unspecified muscle(s) and tendon(s) at lower leg level, left leg ▽

　✓7ᵗʰ **S86.909** Unspecified injury of unspecified muscle(s) and tendon(s) at lower leg level, unspecified leg ▽

✓6ᵗʰ **S86.91** Strain of unspecified muscle and tendon at lower leg level

　✓7ᵗʰ **S86.911** Strain of unspecified muscle(s) and tendon(s) at lower leg level, right leg ▽

　✓7ᵗʰ **S86.912** Strain of unspecified muscle(s) and tendon(s) at lower leg level, left leg ▽

　✓7ᵗʰ **S86.919** Strain of unspecified muscle(s) and tendon(s) at lower leg level, unspecified leg ▽

✓6ᵗʰ **S86.92** Laceration of unspecified muscle and tendon at lower leg level

　✓7ᵗʰ **S86.921** Laceration of unspecified muscle(s) and tendon(s) at lower leg level, right leg ▽

　✓7ᵗʰ **S86.922** Laceration of unspecified muscle(s) and tendon(s) at lower leg level, left leg ▽

　✓7ᵗʰ **S86.929** Laceration of unspecified muscle(s) and tendon(s) at lower leg level, unspecified leg ▽

✓6ᵗʰ **S86.99** Other injury of unspecified muscle and tendon at lower leg level

　✓7ᵗʰ **S86.991** Other injury of unspecified muscle(s) and tendon(s) at lower leg level, right leg ▽

　✓7ᵗʰ **S86.992** Other injury of unspecified muscle(s) and tendon(s) at lower leg level, left leg ▽

　✓7ᵗʰ **S86.999** Other injury of unspecified muscle(s) and tendon(s) at lower leg level, unspecified leg ▽

✓4ᵗʰ **S87** **Crushing injury of lower leg**

Use additional code(s) for all associated injuries

EXCLUDES 2　crushing injury of ankle and foot (S97.-)

The appropriate 7th character is to be added to each code from category S87.
A　initial encounter
D　subsequent encounter
S　sequela

✓5ᵗʰ **S87.0** Crushing injury of knee

　✓x7ᵗʰ **S87.00** Crushing injury of unspecified knee ▽

　✓x7ᵗʰ **S87.01** Crushing injury of right knee

　✓x7ᵗʰ **S87.02** Crushing injury of left knee

✓5ᵗʰ **S87.8** Crushing injury of lower leg

　✓x7ᵗʰ **S87.80** Crushing injury of unspecified lower leg ▽

　✓x7ᵗʰ **S87.81** Crushing injury of right lower leg

　✓x7ᵗʰ **S87.82** Crushing injury of left lower leg

✓4ᵗʰ **S88** **Traumatic amputation of lower leg**

NOTE　An amputation not identified as partial or complete should be coded to complete.

EXCLUDES 1　traumatic amputation of ankle and foot (S98.-)

The appropriate 7th character is to be added to each code from category S88.
A　initial encounter
D　subsequent encounter
S　sequela

✓5ᵗʰ **S88.0** Traumatic amputation at knee level

✓6ᵗʰ **S88.01** Complete traumatic amputation at knee level

　✓7ᵗʰ **S88.011** Complete traumatic amputation at knee level, right lower leg

　✓7ᵗʰ **S88.012** Complete traumatic amputation at knee level, left lower leg

　✓7ᵗʰ **S88.019** Complete traumatic amputation at knee level, unspecified lower leg ▽

✓6ᵗʰ **S88.02** Partial traumatic amputation at knee level

　✓7ᵗʰ **S88.021** Partial traumatic amputation at knee level, right lower leg

　✓7ᵗʰ **S88.022** Partial traumatic amputation at knee level, left lower leg

　✓7ᵗʰ **S88.029** Partial traumatic amputation at knee level, unspecified lower leg ▽

✓6ᵗʰ **S88.1** Traumatic amputation at level between knee and ankle

✓6ᵗʰ **S88.11** Complete traumatic amputation at level between knee and ankle

　✓7ᵗʰ **S88.111** Complete traumatic amputation at level between knee and ankle, right lower leg

　✓7ᵗʰ **S88.112** Complete traumatic amputation at level between knee and ankle, left lower leg

Ⓝ Newborn　　Ⓟ Pediatric　　Ⓜ Maternity　　Ⓐ Adult　　**RIC** RIC Dx　　**NC Dx** Noncancer Dx　　**PDx** Primary Dx　　**CC** RIC CC Condition　　►◄ Revised Text　　● New Code　　▲ Revised Code Title

964　　　　　　　　　　　　　　　　　　　　　　　　　　　　　　　　　　　　　　　ICD-10-CM 2016

✓7ᵗʰ **S88.119** Complete traumatic amputation at level between knee and ankle, unspecified lower leg ▽

✓6ᵗʰ **S88.12** Partial traumatic amputation at level between knee and ankle

    ✓7ᵗʰ **S88.121** Partial traumatic amputation at level between knee and ankle, right lower leg

    ✓7ᵗʰ **S88.122** Partial traumatic amputation at level between knee and ankle, left lower leg

    ✓7ᵗʰ **S88.129** Partial traumatic amputation at level between knee and ankle, unspecified lower leg

✓5ᵗʰ **S88.9** Traumatic amputation of lower leg, level unspecified

    ✓6ᵗʰ **S88.91** Complete traumatic amputation of lower leg, level unspecified

      ✓7ᵗʰ **S88.911** Complete traumatic amputation of right lower leg, level unspecified ▽

      ✓7ᵗʰ **S88.912** Complete traumatic amputation of left lower leg, level unspecified ▽

      ✓7ᵗʰ **S88.919** Complete traumatic amputation of unspecified lower leg, level unspecified ▽

    ✓6ᵗʰ **S88.92** Partial traumatic amputation of lower leg, level unspecified

      ✓7ᵗʰ **S88.921** Partial traumatic amputation of right lower leg, level unspecified ▽

      ✓7ᵗʰ **S88.922** Partial traumatic amputation of left lower leg, level unspecified ▽

      ✓7ᵗʰ **S88.929** Partial traumatic amputation of unspecified lower leg, level unspecified ▽

✓4ᵗʰ **S89** **Other and unspecified injuries of lower leg**

    NOTE A fracture not indicated as open or closed should be coded to closed.

    EXCLUDES 2 other and unspecified injuries of ankle and foot (S99.-)

    The appropriate 7th character is to be added to each code from subcategories S89.0, S89.1, S89.2, and S89.3.
    A   initial encounter for closed fracture
    D   subsequent encounter for fracture with routine healing
    G   subsequent encounter for fracture with delayed healing
    K   subsequent encounter for fracture with nonunion
    P   subsequent encounter for fracture with malunion
    S   sequela

✓5ᵗʰ **S89.0** Physeal fracture of upper end of tibia

    ✓6ᵗʰ **S89.00** Unspecified physeal fracture of upper end of tibia

      ✓7ᵗʰ **S89.001** Unspecified physeal fracture of upper end of right tibia ▽

      ✓7ᵗʰ **S89.002** Unspecified physeal fracture of upper end of left tibia ▽

      ✓7ᵗʰ **S89.009** Unspecified physeal fracture of upper end of unspecified tibia ▽

    ✓6ᵗʰ **S89.01** Salter-Harris Type I physeal fracture of upper end of tibia

      ✓7ᵗʰ **S89.011** Salter-Harris Type I physeal fracture of upper end of right tibia

      ✓7ᵗʰ **S89.012** Salter-Harris Type I physeal fracture of upper end of left tibia

      ✓7ᵗʰ **S89.019** Salter-Harris Type I physeal fracture of upper end of unspecified tibia ▽

    ✓6ᵗʰ **S89.02** Salter-Harris Type II physeal fracture of upper end of tibia

      ✓7ᵗʰ **S89.021** Salter-Harris Type II physeal fracture of upper end of right tibia

      ✓7ᵗʰ **S89.022** Salter-Harris Type II physeal fracture of upper end of left tibia

      ✓7ᵗʰ **S89.029** Salter-Harris Type II physeal fracture of upper end of unspecified tibia ▽

    ✓6ᵗʰ **S89.03** Salter-Harris Type III physeal fracture of upper end of tibia

      ✓7ᵗʰ **S89.031** Salter-Harris Type III physeal fracture of upper end of right tibia

      ✓7ᵗʰ **S89.032** Salter-Harris Type III physeal fracture of upper end of left tibia

      ✓7ᵗʰ **S89.039** Salter-Harris Type III physeal fracture of upper end of unspecified tibia ▽

    ✓6ᵗʰ **S89.04** Salter-Harris Type IV physeal fracture of upper end of tibia

      ✓7ᵗʰ **S89.041** Salter-Harris Type IV physeal fracture of upper end of right tibia

      ✓7ᵗʰ **S89.042** Salter-Harris Type IV physeal fracture of upper end of left tibia

      ✓7ᵗʰ **S89.049** Salter-Harris Type IV physeal fracture of upper end of unspecified tibia ▽

    ✓6ᵗʰ **S89.09** Other physeal fracture of upper end of tibia

      ✓7ᵗʰ **S89.091** Other physeal fracture of upper end of right tibia

      ✓7ᵗʰ **S89.092** Other physeal fracture of upper end of left tibia

      ✓7ᵗʰ **S89.099** Other physeal fracture of upper end of unspecified tibia ▽

✓5ᵗʰ **S89.1** Physeal fracture of lower end of tibia

    ✓6ᵗʰ **S89.10** Unspecified physeal fracture of lower end of tibia

      ✓7ᵗʰ **S89.101** Unspecified physeal fracture of lower end of right tibia

      ✓7ᵗʰ **S89.102** Unspecified physeal fracture of lower end of left tibia

      ✓7ᵗʰ **S89.109** Unspecified physeal fracture of lower end of unspecified tibia ▽

    ✓6ᵗʰ **S89.11** Salter-Harris Type I physeal fracture of ower end of tibia

      ✓7ᵗʰ **S89.111** Salter-Harris Type I physeal fracture of lower end of right tibia

      ✓7ᵗʰ **S89.112** Salter-Harris Type I physeal fracture of lower end of left tibia

      ✓7ᵗʰ **S89.119** Salter-Harris Type I physeal fracture of lower end of unspecified tibia ▽

    ✓6ᵗʰ **S89.12** Salter-Harris Type II physeal fracture of lower end of tibia

      ✓7ᵗʰ **S89.121** Salter-Harris Type II physeal fracture of lower end of right tibia

      ✓7ᵗʰ **S89.122** Salter-Harris Type II physeal fracture of lower end of left tibia

      ✓7ᵗʰ **S89.129** Salter-Harris Type II physeal fracture of lower end of unspecified tibia ▽

    ✓6ᵗʰ **S89.13** Salter-Harris Type III physeal fracture of lower end of tibia

      EXCLUDES 1 fracture of medial malleolus (adult) (S82.5-)

      ✓7ᵗʰ **S89.131** Salter-Harris Type III physeal fracture of lower end of right tibia

      ✓7ᵗʰ **S89.132** Salter-Harris Type III physeal fracture of lower end of left tibia

      ✓7ᵗʰ **S89.139** Salter-Harris Type III physeal fracture of lower end of unspecified tibia ▽

    ✓6ᵗʰ **S89.14** Salter-Harris Type IV physeal fracture of lower end of tibia

      EXCLUDES 1 fracture of medial malleolus (adult) (S82.5-)

      ✓7ᵗʰ **S89.141** Salter-Harris Type IV physeal fracture of lower end of right tibia

      ✓7ᵗʰ **S89.142** Salter-Harris Type IV physeal fracture of lower end of left tibia

      ✓7ᵗʰ **S89.149** Salter-Harris Type IV physeal fracture of lower end of unspecified tibia ▽

    ✓6ᵗʰ **S89.19** Other physeal fracture of lower end of tibia

      ✓7ᵗʰ **S89.191** Other physeal fracture of lower end of right tibia

      ✓7ᵗʰ **S89.192** Other physeal fracture of lower end of left tibia

      ✓7ᵗʰ **S89.199** Other physeal fracture of lower end of unspecified tibia ▽

✓5ᵗʰ **S89.2** Physeal fracture of upper end of fibula

    ✓6ᵗʰ **S89.20** Unspecified physeal fracture of upper end of fibula

      ✓7ᵗʰ **S89.201** Unspecified physeal fracture of upper end of right fibula

      ✓7ᵗʰ **S89.202** Unspecified physeal fracture of upper end of left fibula

      ✓7ᵗʰ **S89.209** Unspecified physeal fracture of upper end of unspecified fibula ▽

✓6th **S89.21** Salter-Harris Type I physeal fracture of upper end of fibula

    ✓7th **S89.211** Salter-Harris Type I physeal fracture of upper end of right fibula

    ✓7th **S89.212** Salter-Harris Type I physeal fracture of upper end of left fibula

    ✓7th **S89.219** Salter-Harris Type I physeal fracture of upper end of unspecified fibula ▽

✓6th **S89.22** Salter-Harris Type II physeal fracture of upper end of fibula

    ✓7th **S89.221** Salter-Harris Type II physeal fracture of upper end of right fibula

    ✓7th **S89.222** Salter-Harris Type II physeal fracture of upper end of left fibula

    ✓7th **S89.229** Salter-Harris Type II physeal fracture of upper end of unspecified fibula ▽

✓6th **S89.29** Other physeal fracture of upper end of fibula

    ✓7th **S89.291** Other physeal fracture of upper end of right fibula

    ✓7th **S89.292** Other physeal fracture of upper end of left fibula

    ✓7th **S89.299** Other physeal fracture of upper end of unspecified fibula ▽

✓5th **S89.3** Physeal fracture of lower end of fibula

    ✓6th **S89.30** Unspecified physeal fracture of lower end of fibula

       ✓7th **S89.301** Unspecified physeal fracture of lower end of right fibula ▽

       ✓7th **S89.302** Unspecified physeal fracture of lower end of left fibula ▽

       ✓7th **S89.309** Unspecified physeal fracture of lower end of unspecified fibula ▽

    ✓6th **S89.31** Salter-Harris Type I physeal fracture of lower end of fibula

       ✓7th **S89.311** Salter-Harris Type I physeal fracture of lower end of right fibula

       ✓7th **S89.312** Salter-Harris Type I physeal fracture of lower end of left fibula

       ✓7th **S89.319** Salter-Harris Type I physeal fracture of lower end of unspecified fibula ▽

    ✓6th **S89.32** Salter-Harris Type II physeal fracture of lower end of fibula

       ✓7th **S89.321** Salter-Harris Type II physeal fracture of lower end of right fibula

       ✓7th **S89.322** Salter-Harris Type II physeal fracture of lower end of left fibula

       ✓7th **S89.329** Salter-Harris Type II physeal fracture of lower end of unspecified fibula ▽

    ✓6th **S89.39** Other physeal fracture of lower end of fibula

       ✓7th **S89.391** Other physeal fracture of lower end of right fibula

       ✓7th **S89.392** Other physeal fracture of lower end of left fibula

       ✓7th **S89.399** Other physeal fracture of lower end of unspecified fibula ▽

✓5th **S89.8** Other specified injuries of lower leg

> The appropriate 7th character is to be added to each code in subcategory S89.8.
> A   initial encounter
> D   subsequent encounter
> S   sequela

    ✓x7th **S89.80** Other specified injuries of unspecified lower leg ▽

    ✓x7th **S89.81** Other specified injuries of right lower leg

    ✓x7th **S89.82** Other specified injuries of left lower leg

✓5th **S89.9** Unspecified injury of lower leg

> The appropriate 7th character is to be added to each code in subcategory S89.9.
> A   initial encounter
> D   subsequent encounter
> S   sequela

    ✓x7th **S89.90** Unspecified injury of unspecified lower leg ▽

    ✓x7th **S89.91** Unspecified injury of right lower leg ▽

    ✓x7th **S89.92** Unspecified injury of left lower leg ▽

Injuries to the ankle and foot (S90-S99)

EXCLUDES 2   burns and corrosions (T20-T32)
    fracture of ankle and malleolus (S82.-)
    frostbite (T33-T34)
    insect bite or sting, venomous (T63.4)

✓4th **S90** Superficial injury of ankle, foot and toes

> The appropriate 7th character is to be added to each code from category S90.
> A   initial encounter
> D   subsequent encounter
> S   sequela

✓5th **S90.0** Contusion of ankle

    ✓x7th **S90.00** Contusion of unspecified ankle ▽

    ✓x7th **S90.01** Contusion of right ankle

    ✓x7th **S90.02** Contusion of left ankle

✓5th **S90.1** Contusion of toe without damage to nail

    ✓6th **S90.11** Contusion of great toe without damage to nail

       ✓7th **S90.111** Contusion of right great toe without damage to nail

       ✓7th **S90.112** Contusion of left great toe without damage to nail

       ✓7th **S90.119** Contusion of unspecified great toe without damage to nail ▽

    ✓6th **S90.12** Contusion of lesser toe without damage to nail

       ✓7th **S90.121** Contusion of right lesser toe(s) without damage to nail

       ✓7th **S90.122** Contusion of left lesser toe(s) without damage to nail

       ✓7th **S90.129** Contusion of unspecified lesser toe(s) without damage to nail ▽
         Contusion of toe NOS

✓5th **S90.2** Contusion of toe with damage to nail

    ✓6th **S90.21** Contusion of great toe with damage to nail

       ✓7th **S90.211** Contusion of right great toe with damage to nail

       ✓7th **S90.212** Contusion of left great toe with damage to nail

       ✓7th **S90.219** Contusion of unspecified great toe with damage to nail ▽

    ✓6th **S90.22** Contusion of lesser toe with damage to nail

       ✓7th **S90.221** Contusion of right lesser toe(s) with damage to nail

       ✓7th **S90.222** Contusion of left lesser toe(s) with damage to nail

       ✓7th **S90.229** Contusion of unspecified lesser toe(s) with damage to nail ▽

✓5th **S90.3** Contusion of foot

    EXCLUDES 2   contusion of toes (S90.1-, S90.2-)

    ✓x7th **S90.30** Contusion of unspecified foot ▽
       Contusion of foot NOS

    ✓x7th **S90.31** Contusion of right foot

    ✓x7th **S90.32** Contusion of left foot

✓5th **S90.4** Other superficial injuries of toe

    ✓6th **S90.41** Abrasion of toe

       ✓7th **S90.411** Abrasion, right great toe

       ✓7th **S90.412** Abrasion, left great toe

       ✓7th **S90.413** Abrasion, unspecified great toe ▽

       ✓7th **S90.414** Abrasion, right lesser toe(s)

       ✓7th **S90.415** Abrasion, left lesser toe(s)

       ✓7th **S90.416** Abrasion, unspecified lesser toe(s) ▽

    ✓6th **S90.42** Blister (nonthermal) of toe

       ✓7th **S90.421** Blister (nonthermal), right great toe

       ✓7th **S90.422** Blister (nonthermal), left great toe

       ✓7th **S90.423** Blister (nonthermal), unspecified great toe ▽

       ✓7th **S90.424** Blister (nonthermal), right lesser toe(s)

       ✓7th **S90.425** Blister (nonthermal), left lesser toe(s)

       ✓7th **S90.426** Blister (nonthermal), unspecified lesser toe(s) ▽

Ⓝ Newborn   Ⓟ Pediatric   Ⓜ Maternity   Ⓐ Adult   **RIC** RIC Dx   **NCDx** Noncancer Dx   **PDx** Primary Dx   **CC** RIC CC Condition   ▶◀ Revised Text   ● New Code   ▲ Revised Code Title

✓6ᵗʰ **S90.44** External constriction of toe
    Hair tourniquet syndrome of toe

  ✓7ᵗʰ **S90.441** External constriction, right great toe

  ✓7ᵗʰ **S90.442** External constriction, left great toe

  ✓7ᵗʰ **S90.443** External constriction, unspecified great toe ▽

  ✓7ᵗʰ **S90.444** External constriction, right lesser toe(s)

  ✓7ᵗʰ **S90.445** External constriction, left lesser toe(s)

  ✓7ᵗʰ **S90.446** External constriction, unspecified lesser toe(s) ▽

✓6ᵗʰ **S90.45** Superficial foreign body of toe
    Splinter in the toe

  ✓7ᵗʰ **S90.451** Superficial foreign body, right great toe

  ✓7ᵗʰ **S90.452** Superficial foreign body, left great toe

  ✓7ᵗʰ **S90.453** Superficial foreign body, unspecified great toe ▽

  ✓7ᵗʰ **S90.454** Superficial foreign body, right lesser toe(s)

  ✓7ᵗʰ **S90.455** Superficial foreign body, left lesser toe(s)

  ✓7ᵗʰ **S90.456** Superficial foreign body, unspecified lesser toe(s) ▽

✓6ᵗʰ **S90.46** Insect bite (nonvenomous) of toe

  ✓7ᵗʰ **S90.461** Insect bite (nonvenomous), right great toe

  ✓7ᵗʰ **S90.462** Insect bite (nonvenomous), left great toe

  ✓7ᵗʰ **S90.463** Insect bite (nonvenomous), unspecified great toe ▽

  ✓7ᵗʰ **S90.464** Insect bite (nonvenomous), right lesser toe(s)

  ✓7ᵗʰ **S90.465** Insect bite (nonvenomous), left lesser toe(s)

  ✓7ᵗʰ **S90.466** Insect bite (nonvenomous), unspecified lesser toe(s) ▽

✓6ᵗʰ **S90.47** Other superficial bite of toe
    EXCLUDES 1 open bite of toe (S91.15-, S91.25-)

  ✓7ᵗʰ **S90.471** Other superficial bite of right great toe

  ✓7ᵗʰ **S90.472** Other superficial bite of left great toe

  ✓7ᵗʰ **S90.473** Other superficial bite of unspecified great toe ▽

  ✓7ᵗʰ **S90.474** Other superficial bite of right lesser toe(s)

  ✓7ᵗʰ **S90.475** Other superficial bite of left lesser toe(s)

  ✓7ᵗʰ **S90.476** Other superficial bite of unspecified lesser toe(s) ▽

✓5ᵗʰ **S90.5** Other superficial injuries of ankle

 ✓6ᵗʰ **S90.51** Abrasion of ankle

  ✓7ᵗʰ **S90.511** Abrasion, right ankle

  ✓7ᵗʰ **S90.512** Abrasion, left ankle

  ✓7ᵗʰ **S90.519** Abrasion, unspecified ankle ▽

 ✓6ᵗʰ **S90.52** Blister (nonthermal) of ankle

  ✓7ᵗʰ **S90.521** Blister (nonthermal), right ankle

  ✓7ᵗʰ **S90.522** Blister (nonthermal), left ankle

  ✓7ᵗʰ **S90.529** Blister (nonthermal), unspecified ankle ▽

 ✓6ᵗʰ **S90.54** External constriction of ankle

  ✓7ᵗʰ **S90.541** External constriction, right ankle

  ✓7ᵗʰ **S90.542** External constriction, left ankle

  ✓7ᵗʰ **S90.549** External constriction, unspecified ankle ▽

 ✓6ᵗʰ **S90.55** Superficial foreign body of ankle
    Splinter in the ankle

  ✓7ᵗʰ **S90.551** Superficial foreign body, right ankle

  ✓7ᵗʰ **S90.552** Superficial foreign body, left ankle

  ✓7ᵗʰ **S90.559** Superficial foreign body, unspecified ankle ▽

 ✓6ᵗʰ **S90.56** Insect bite (nonvenomous) of ankle

  ✓7ᵗʰ **S90.561** Insect bite (nonvenomous), right ankle

  ✓7ᵗʰ **S90.562** Insect bite (nonvenomous), left ankle

  ✓7ᵗʰ **S90.569** Insect bite (nonvenomous), unspecified ankle ▽

 ✓6ᵗʰ **S90.57** Other superficial bite of ankle
    EXCLUDES 1 open bite of ankle (S91.05-)

  ✓7ᵗʰ **S90.571** Other superficial bite of ankle, right ankle

  ✓7ᵗʰ **S90.572** Other superficial bite of ankle, left ankle

  ✓7ᵗʰ **S90.579** Other superficial bite of ankle, unspecified ankle ▽

✓5ᵗʰ **S90.8** Other superficial injuries of foot

 ✓6ᵗʰ **S90.81** Abrasion of foot

  ✓7ᵗʰ **S90.811** Abrasion, right foot

  ✓7ᵗʰ **S90.812** Abrasion, left foot

  ✓7ᵗʰ **S90.819** Abrasion, unspecified foot ▽

 ✓6ᵗʰ **S90.82** Blister (nonthermal) of foot

  ✓7ᵗʰ **S90.821** Blister (nonthermal), right foot

  ✓7ᵗʰ **S90.822** Blister (nonthermal), left foot

  ✓7ᵗʰ **S90.829** Blister (nonthermal), unspecified foot ▽

 ✓6ᵗʰ **S90.84** External constriction of foot

  ✓7ᵗʰ **S90.841** External constriction, right foot

  ✓7ᵗʰ **S90.842** External constriction, left foot

  ✓7ᵗʰ **S90.849** External constriction, unspecified foot ▽

 ✓6ᵗʰ **S90.85** Superficial foreign body of foot
    Splinter in the foot

  ✓7ᵗʰ **S90.851** Superficial foreign body, right foot

  ✓7ᵗʰ **S90.852** Superficial foreign body, left foot

  ✓7ᵗʰ **S90.859** Superficial foreign body, unspecified foot ▽

 ✓6ᵗʰ **S90.86** Insect bite (nonvenomous) of foot

  ✓7ᵗʰ **S90.861** Insect bite (nonvenomous), right foot

  ✓7ᵗʰ **S90.862** Insect bite (nonvenomous), left foot

  ✓7ᵗʰ **S90.869** Insect bite (nonvenomous), unspecified foot ▽

 ✓6ᵗʰ **S90.87** Other superficial bite of foot
    EXCLUDES 1 open bite of foot (S91.35-)

  ✓7ᵗʰ **S90.871** Other superficial bite of right foot

  ✓7ᵗʰ **S90.872** Other superficial bite of left foot

  ✓7ᵗʰ **S90.879** Other superficial bite of unspecified foot ▽

✓5ᵗʰ **S90.9** Unspecified superficial injury of ankle, foot and toe

 ✓6ᵗʰ **S90.91** Unspecified superficial injury of ankle

  ✓7ᵗʰ **S90.911** Unspecified superficial injury of right ankle

  ✓7ᵗʰ **S90.912** Unspecified superficial injury of left ankle

  ✓7ᵗʰ **S90.919** Unspecified superficial injury of unspecified ankle ▽

 ✓6ᵗʰ **S90.92** Unspecified superficial injury of foot

  ✓7ᵗʰ **S90.921** Unspecified superficial injury of right foot ▽

  ✓7ᵗʰ **S90.922** Unspecified superficial injury of left foot ▽

  ✓7ᵗʰ **S90.929** Unspecified superficial injury of unspecified foot ▽

 ✓6ᵗʰ **S90.93** Unspecified superficial injury of toes

  ✓7ᵗʰ **S90.931** Unspecified superficial injury of right great toe ▽

  ✓7ᵗʰ **S90.932** Unspecified superficial injury of left great toe ▽

  ✓7ᵗʰ **S90.933** Unspecified superficial injury of unspecified great toe ▽

  ✓7ᵗʰ **S90.934** Unspecified superficial injury of right lesser toe(s) ▽

  ✓7ᵗʰ **S90.935** Unspecified superficial injury of left lesser toe(s) ▽

  ✓7ᵗʰ **S90.936** Unspecified superficial injury of unspecified lesser toe(s) ▽

✓4ᵗʰ **S91** Open wound of ankle, foot and toes
    Code also any associated wound infection
    EXCLUDES 1 open fracture of ankle, foot and toes (S92-with 7th character B)
          traumatic amputation of ankle and foot (S98.-)

    The appropriate 7th character is to be added to each code from category S91.
    A   initial encounter
    D   subsequent encounter
    S   sequela

 ✓5ᵗʰ **S91.0** Open wound of ankle

  ✓6ᵗʰ **S91.00** Unspecified open wound of ankle

   ✓7ᵗʰ **S91.001** Unspecified open wound, right ankle ▽

   ✓7ᵗʰ **S91.002** Unspecified open wound, left ankle ▽

✓7ᵗʰ **S91.009**   **Unspecified open wound, unspecified ankle** ▽

✓6ᵗʰ **S91.01**   Laceration without foreign body of ankle

    ✓7ᵗʰ **S91.011**   **Laceration without foreign body, right ankle**

    ✓7ᵗʰ **S91.012**   **Laceration without foreign body, left ankle**

    ✓7ᵗʰ **S91.019**   **Laceration without foreign body, unspecified ankle** ▽

✓6ᵗʰ **S91.02**   Laceration with foreign body of ankle

    ✓7ᵗʰ **S91.021**   **Laceration with foreign body, right ankle**

    ✓7ᵗʰ **S91.022**   **Laceration with foreign body, left ankle**

    ✓7ᵗʰ **S91.029**   **Laceration with foreign body, unspecified ankle** ▽

✓6ᵗʰ **S91.03**   Puncture wound without foreign body of ankle

    ✓7ᵗʰ **S91.031**   **Puncture wound without foreign body, right ankle**

    ✓7ᵗʰ **S91.032**   **Puncture wound without foreign body, left ankle**

    ✓7ᵗʰ **S91.039**   **Puncture wound without foreign body, unspecified ankle** ▽

✓6ᵗʰ **S91.04**   Puncture wound with foreign body of ankle

    ✓7ᵗʰ **S91.041**   **Puncture wound with foreign body, right ankle**

    ✓7ᵗʰ **S91.042**   **Puncture wound with foreign body, left ankle**

    ✓7ᵗʰ **S91.049**   **Puncture wound with foreign body, unspecified ankle** ▽

✓6ᵗʰ **S91.05**   Open bite of ankle

    EXCLUDES 1   *superficial bite of ankle (S90.56-, S90.57-)*

    ✓7ᵗʰ **S91.051**   **Open bite, right ankle**

    ✓7ᵗʰ **S91.052**   **Open bite, left ankle**

    ✓7ᵗʰ **S91.059**   **Open bite, unspecified ankle** ▽

✓5ᵗʰ **S91.1**   Open wound of toe without damage to nail

  ✓6ᵗʰ **S91.10**   Unspecified open wound of toe without damage to nail

    ✓7ᵗʰ **S91.101**   **Unspecified open wound of right great toe without damage to nail** ▽

    ✓7ᵗʰ **S91.102**   **Unspecified open wound of left great toe without damage to nail** ▽

    ✓7ᵗʰ **S91.103**   **Unspecified open wound of unspecified great toe without damage to nail** ▽

    ✓7ᵗʰ **S91.104**   **Unspecified open wound of right lesser toe(s) without damage to nail** ▽

    ✓7ᵗʰ **S91.105**   **Unspecified open wound of left lesser toe(s) without damage to nail** ▽

    ✓7ᵗʰ **S91.106**   **Unspecified open wound of unspecified lesser toe(s) without damage to nail** ▽

    ✓7ᵗʰ **S91.109**   **Unspecified open wound of unspecified toe(s) without damage to nail** ▽

  ✓6ᵗʰ **S91.11**   Laceration without foreign body of toe without damage to nail

    ✓7ᵗʰ **S91.111**   **Laceration without foreign body of right great toe without damage to nail**

    ✓7ᵗʰ **S91.112**   **Laceration without foreign body of left great toe without damage to nail**

    ✓7ᵗʰ **S91.113**   **Laceration without foreign body of unspecified great toe without damage to nail** ▽

    ✓7ᵗʰ **S91.114**   **Laceration without foreign body of right lesser toe(s) without damage to nail**

    ✓7ᵗʰ **S91.115**   **Laceration without foreign body of left lesser toe(s) without damage to nail**

    ✓7ᵗʰ **S91.116**   **Laceration without foreign body of unspecified lesser toe(s) without damage to nail** ▽

    ✓7ᵗʰ **S91.119**   **Laceration without foreign body of unspecified toe without damage to nail** ▽

  ✓6ᵗʰ **S91.12**   Laceration with foreign body of toe without damage to nail

    ✓7ᵗʰ **S91.121**   **Laceration with foreign body of right great toe without damage to nail**

✓7ᵗʰ **S91.122**   **Laceration with foreign body of left great toe without damage to nail**

✓7ᵗʰ **S91.123**   **Laceration with foreign body of unspecified great toe without damage to nail** ▽

✓7ᵗʰ **S91.124**   **Laceration with foreign body of right lesser toe(s) without damage to nail**

✓7ᵗʰ **S91.125**   **Laceration with foreign body of left lesser toe(s) without damage to nail**

✓7ᵗʰ **S91.126**   **Laceration with foreign body of unspecified lesser toe(s) without damage to nail** ▽

✓7ᵗʰ **S91.129**   **Laceration with foreign body of unspecified toe(s) without damage to nail** ▽

✓6ᵗʰ **S91.13**   Puncture wound without foreign body of toe without damage to nail

    ✓7ᵗʰ **S91.131**   **Puncture wound without foreign body of right great toe without damage to nail**

    ✓7ᵗʰ **S91.132**   **Puncture wound without foreign body of left great toe without damage to nail**

    ✓7ᵗʰ **S91.133**   **Puncture wound without foreign body of unspecified great toe without damage to nail** ▽

    ✓7ᵗʰ **S91.134**   **Puncture wound without foreign body of right lesser toe(s) without damage to nail**

    ✓7ᵗʰ **S91.135**   **Puncture wound without foreign body of left lesser toe(s) without damage to nail**

    ✓7ᵗʰ **S91.136**   **Puncture wound without foreign body of unspecified lesser toe(s) without damage to nail** ▽

    ✓7ᵗʰ **S91.139**   **Puncture wound without foreign body of unspecified toe(s) without damage to nail** ▽

✓6ᵗʰ **S91.14**   Puncture wound with foreign body of toe without damage to nail

    ✓7ᵗʰ **S91.141**   **Puncture wound with foreign body of right great toe without damage to nail**

    ✓7ᵗʰ **S91.142**   **Puncture wound with foreign body of left great toe without damage to nail**

    ✓7ᵗʰ **S91.143**   **Puncture wound with foreign body of unspecified great toe without damage to nail** ▽

    ✓7ᵗʰ **S91.144**   **Puncture wound with foreign body of right lesser toe(s) without damage to nail**

    ✓7ᵗʰ **S91.145**   **Puncture wound with foreign body of left lesser toe(s) without damage to nail**

    ✓7ᵗʰ **S91.146**   **Puncture wound with foreign body of unspecified lesser toe(s) without damage to nail** ▽

    ✓7ᵗʰ **S91.149**   **Puncture wound with foreign body of unspecified toe(s) without damage to nail** ▽

✓6ᵗʰ **S91.15**   Open bite of toe without damage to nail

    Bite of toe NOS

    EXCLUDES 1   *superficial bite of toe (S90.46-, S90.47-)*

    ✓7ᵗʰ **S91.151**   **Open bite of right great toe without damage to nail**

    ✓7ᵗʰ **S91.152**   **Open bite of left great toe without damage to nail**

    ✓7ᵗʰ **S91.153**   **Open bite of unspecified great toe without damage to nail** ▽

    ✓7ᵗʰ **S91.154**   **Open bite of right lesser toe(s) without damage to nail**

    ✓7ᵗʰ **S91.155**   **Open bite of left lesser toe(s) without damage to nail**

    ✓7ᵗʰ **S91.156**   **Open bite of unspecified lesser toe(s) without damage to nail** ▽

    ✓7ᵗʰ **S91.159**   **Open bite of unspecified toe(s) without damage to nail** ▽

✓5ᵗʰ **S91.2**   Open wound of toe with damage to nail

  ✓6ᵗʰ **S91.20**   Unspecified open wound of toe with damage to nail

    ✓7ᵗʰ **S91.201**   **Unspecified open wound of right great toe with damage to nail** ▽

    ✓7ᵗʰ **S91.202**   **Unspecified open wound of left great toe with damage to nail** ▽

Ⓝ Newborn   Ⓟ Pediatric   Ⓜ Maternity   Ⓐ Adult   **RIC** RIC Dx   **NC Dx** Noncancer Dx   **PDx** Primary Dx   **CC** RIC CC Condition   ▶◀ Revised Text   ● New Code   ▲ Revised Code Title

968   ICD-10-CM 2016

√7ᵗʰ **S91.203** **Unspecified open wound of unspecified great toe with damage to nail** ▽

√7ᵗʰ **S91.204** **Unspecified open wound of right lesser toe(s) with damage to nail** ▽

√7ᵗʰ **S91.205** **Unspecified open wound of left lesser toe(s) with damage to nail** ▽

√7ᵗʰ **S91.206** **Unspecified open wound of unspecified lesser toe(s) with damage to nail** ▽

√7ᵗʰ **S91.209** **Unspecified open wound of unspecified toe(s) with damage to nail** ▽

√6ᵗʰ **S91.21** Laceration without foreign body of toe with damage to nail

√7ᵗʰ **S91.211** **Laceration without foreign body of right great toe with damage to nail**

√7ᵗʰ **S91.212** **Laceration without foreign body of left great toe with damage to nail**

√7ᵗʰ **S91.213** **Laceration without foreign body of unspecified great toe with damage to nail** ▽

√7ᵗʰ **S91.214** **Laceration without foreign body of right lesser toe(s) with damage to nail**

√7ᵗʰ **S91.215** **Laceration without foreign body of left lesser toe(s) with damage to nail**

√7ᵗʰ **S91.216** **Laceration without foreign body of unspecified lesser toe(s) with damage to nail** ▽

√7ᵗʰ **S91.219** **Laceration without foreign body of unspecified toe(s) with damage to nail** ▽

√6ᵗʰ **S91.22** Laceration with foreign body of toe with damage to nail

√7ᵗʰ **S91.221** **Laceration with foreign body of right great toe with damage to nail**

√7ᵗʰ **S91.222** **Laceration with foreign body of left great toe with damage to nail**

√7ᵗʰ **S91.223** **Laceration with foreign body of unspecified great toe with damage to nail** ▽

√7ᵗʰ **S91.224** **Laceration with foreign body of right lesser toe(s) with damage to nail**

√7ᵗʰ **S91.225** **Laceration with foreign body of left lesser toe(s) with damage to nail**

√7ᵗʰ **S91.226** **Laceration with foreign body of unspecified lesser toe(s) with damage to nail** ▽

√7ᵗʰ **S91.229** **Laceration with foreign body of unspecified toe(s) with damage to nail** ▽

√6ᵗʰ **S91.23** Puncture wound without foreign body of toe with damage to nail

√7ᵗʰ **S91.231** **Puncture wound without foreign body of right great toe with damage to nail**

√7ᵗʰ **S91.232** **Puncture wound without foreign body of left great toe with damage to nail**

√7ᵗʰ **S91.233** **Puncture wound without foreign body of unspecified great toe with damage to nail** ▽

√7ᵗʰ **S91.234** **Puncture wound without foreign body of right lesser toe(s) with damage to nail**

√7ᵗʰ **S91.235** **Puncture wound without foreign body of left lesser toe(s) with damage to nail**

√7ᵗʰ **S91.236** **Puncture wound without foreign body of unspecified lesser toe(s) with damage to nail** ▽

√7ᵗʰ **S91.239** **Puncture wound without foreign body of unspecified toe(s) with damage to nail** ▽

√6ᵗʰ **S91.24** Puncture wound with foreign body of toe with damage to nail

√7ᵗʰ **S91.241** **Puncture wound with foreign body of right great toe with damage to nail**

√7ᵗʰ **S91.242** **Puncture wound with foreign body of left great toe with damage to nail**

√7ᵗʰ **S91.243** **Puncture wound with foreign body of unspecified great toe with damage to nail** ▽

√7ᵗʰ **S91.244** **Puncture wound with foreign body of right lesser toe(s) with damage to nail**

√7ᵗʰ **S91.245** **Puncture wound with foreign body of left lesser toe(s) with damage to nail**

√7ᵗʰ **S91.246** **Puncture wound with foreign body of unspecified lesser toe(s) with damage to nail** ▽

√7ᵗʰ **S91.249** **Puncture wound with foreign body of unspecified toe(s) with damage to nail** ▽

√6ᵗʰ **S91.25** Open bite of toe with damage to nail
Bite of toe with damage to nail NOS
EXCLUDES 1 superficial bite of toe (S90.46-, S90.47-)

√7ᵗʰ **S91.251** **Open bite of right great toe with damage to nail**

√7ᵗʰ **S91.252** **Open bite of left great toe with damage to nail**

√7ᵗʰ **S91.253** **Open bite of unspecified great toe with damage to nail** ▽

√7ᵗʰ **S91.254** **Open bite of right lesser toe(s) with damage to nail**

√7ᵗʰ **S91.255** **Open bite of left lesser toe(s) with damage to nail**

√7ᵗʰ **S91.256** **Open bite of unspecified lesser toe(s) with damage to nail** ▽

√7ᵗʰ **S91.259** **Open bite of unspecified toe(s) with damage to nail** ▽

√5ᵗʰ **S91.3** Open wound of foot

√6ᵗʰ **S91.30** Unspecified open wound of foot

√7ᵗʰ **S91.301** **Unspecified open wound, right foot** ▽

√7ᵗʰ **S91.302** **Unspecified open wound, left foot** ▽

√7ᵗʰ **S91.309** **Unspecified open wound, unspecified foot** ▽

√6ᵗʰ **S91.31** Laceration without foreign body of foot

√7ᵗʰ **S91.311** **Laceration without foreign body, right foot**

√7ᵗʰ **S91.312** **Laceration without foreign body, left foot**

√7ᵗʰ **S91.319** **Laceration without foreign body, unspecified foot** ▽

√6ᵗʰ **S91.32** Laceration with foreign body of foot

√7ᵗʰ **S91.321** **Laceration with foreign body, right foot**

√7ᵗʰ **S91.322** **Laceration with foreign body, left foot**

√7ᵗʰ **S91.329** **Laceration with foreign body, unspecified foot** ▽

√6ᵗʰ **S91.33** Puncture wound without foreign body of foot

√7ᵗʰ **S91.331** **Puncture wound without foreign body, right foot**

√7ᵗʰ **S91.332** **Puncture wound without foreign body, left foot**

√7ᵗʰ **S91.339** **Puncture wound without foreign body, unspecified foot** ▽

√6ᵗʰ **S91.34** Puncture wound with foreign body of foot

√7ᵗʰ **S91.341** **Puncture wound with foreign body, right foot**

√7ᵗʰ **S91.342** **Puncture wound with foreign body, left foot**

√7ᵗʰ **S91.349** **Puncture wound with foreign body, unspecified foot** ▽

√6ᵗʰ **S91.35** Open bite of foot
EXCLUDES 1 superficial bite of foot (S90.86-, S90.87-)

√7ᵗʰ **S91.351** **Open bite, right foot**

√7ᵗʰ **S91.352** **Open bite, left foot**

√7ᵗʰ **S91.359** **Open bite, unspecified foot** ▽

☑ Add'l Character Required   √x7ᵗʰ Placeholder Alert   RUG IV Special Care High Dx   RUG IV Clinically Complex Dx   RUG IV Special Care Low Dx   Manifestation Code   Other Specified Code   ▽ Unspecified Code

ICD-10-CM 2016   **969**

☑4ᵗʰ **S92** **Fracture of foot and toe, except ankle**

> **NOTE**   A fracture not indicated as displaced or nondisplaced should be coded to displaced.
> A fracture not indicated as open or closed should be coded to closed.

EXCLUDES 1   traumatic amputation of ankle and foot (S98.-)

EXCLUDES 2   fracture of ankle (S82.-)
                 fracture of malleolus (S82.-)

> The appropriate 7th character is to be added to each code from category S92.
> A   initial encounter for closed fracture
> B   initial encounter for open fracture
> D   subsequent encounter for fracture with routine healing
> G   subsequent encounter for fracture with delayed healing
> K   subsequent encounter for fracture with nonunion
> P   subsequent encounter for fracture with malunion
> S   sequela

☑5ᵗʰ **S92.0** **Fracture of calcaneus**
     Heel bone
     Os calcis

☑6ᵗʰ   **S92.00**   **Unspecified fracture of calcaneus**

☑7ᵗʰ   **S92.001**   Unspecified fracture of right calcaneus ▽

☑7ᵗʰ   **S92.002**   Unspecified fracture of left calcaneus ▽

☑7ᵗʰ   **S92.009**   Unspecified fracture of unspecified calcaneus ▽

☑6ᵗʰ   **S92.01**   **Fracture of body of calcaneus**

☑7ᵗʰ   **S92.011**   Displaced fracture of body of right calcaneus

☑7ᵗʰ   **S92.012**   Displaced fracture of body of left calcaneus

☑7ᵗʰ   **S92.013**   Displaced fracture of body of unspecified calcaneus ▽

☑7ᵗʰ   **S92.014**   Nondisplaced fracture of body of right calcaneus

☑7ᵗʰ   **S92.015**   Nondisplaced fracture of body of left calcaneus

☑7ᵗʰ   **S92.016**   Nondisplaced fracture of body of unspecified calcaneus ▽

☑6ᵗʰ   **S92.02**   **Fracture of anterior process of calcaneus**

☑7ᵗʰ   **S92.021**   Displaced fracture of anterior process of right calcaneus

☑7ᵗʰ   **S92.022**   Displaced fracture of anterior process of left calcaneus

☑7ᵗʰ   **S92.023**   Displaced fracture of anterior process of unspecified calcaneus ▽

☑7ᵗʰ   **S92.024**   Nondisplaced fracture of anterior process of right calcaneus

☑7ᵗʰ   **S92.025**   Nondisplaced fracture of anterior process of left calcaneus

☑7ᵗʰ   **S92.026**   Nondisplaced fracture of anterior process of unspecified calcaneus ▽

☑6ᵗʰ   **S92.03**   **Avulsion fracture of tuberosity of calcaneus**

☑7ᵗʰ   **S92.031**   Displaced avulsion fracture of tuberosity of right calcaneus

☑7ᵗʰ   **S92.032**   Displaced avulsion fracture of tuberosity of left calcaneus

☑7ᵗʰ   **S92.033**   Displaced avulsion fracture of tuberosity of unspecified calcaneus ▽

☑7ᵗʰ   **S92.034**   Nondisplaced avulsion fracture of tuberosity of right calcaneus

☑7ᵗʰ   **S92.035**   Nondisplaced avulsion fracture of tuberosity of left calcaneus

☑7ᵗʰ   **S92.036**   Nondisplaced avulsion fracture of tuberosity of unspecified calcaneus ▽

☑6ᵗʰ   **S92.04**   **Other fracture of tuberosity of calcaneus**

☑7ᵗʰ   **S92.041**   Displaced other fracture of tuberosity of right calcaneus

☑7ᵗʰ   **S92.042**   Displaced other fracture of tuberosity of left calcaneus

☑7ᵗʰ   **S92.043**   Displaced other fracture of tuberosity of unspecified calcaneus ▽

☑7ᵗʰ   **S92.044**   Nondisplaced other fracture of tuberosity of right calcaneus

☑7ᵗʰ   **S92.045**   Nondisplaced other fracture of tuberosity of left calcaneus

☑7ᵗʰ   **S92.046**   Nondisplaced other fracture of tuberosity of unspecified calcaneus ▽

☑6ᵗʰ   **S92.05**   **Other extraarticular fracture of calcaneus**

☑7ᵗʰ   **S92.051**   Displaced other extraarticular fracture of right calcaneus

☑7ᵗʰ   **S92.052**   Displaced other extraarticular fracture of left calcaneus

☑7ᵗʰ   **S92.053**   Displaced other extraarticular fracture of unspecified calcaneus ▽

☑7ᵗʰ   **S92.054**   Nondisplaced other extraarticular fracture of right calcaneus

☑7ᵗʰ   **S92.055**   Nondisplaced other extraarticular fracture of left calcaneus

☑7ᵗʰ   **S92.056**   Nondisplaced other extraarticular fracture of unspecified calcaneus ▽

☑6ᵗʰ   **S92.06**   **Intraarticular fracture of calcaneus**

☑7ᵗʰ   **S92.061**   Displaced intraarticular fracture of right calcaneus

☑7ᵗʰ   **S92.062**   Displaced intraarticular fracture of left calcaneus

☑7ᵗʰ   **S92.063**   Displaced intraarticular fracture of unspecified calcaneus ▽

☑7ᵗʰ   **S92.064**   Nondisplaced intraarticular fracture of right calcaneus

☑7ᵗʰ   **S92.065**   Nondisplaced intraarticular fracture of left calcaneus

☑7ᵗʰ   **S92.066**   Nondisplaced intraarticular fracture of unspecified calcaneus ▽

☑5ᵗʰ **S92.1** **Fracture of talus**
     Astragalus

☑6ᵗʰ   **S92.10**   **Unspecified fracture of talus**

☑7ᵗʰ   **S92.101**   Unspecified fracture of right talus ▽

☑7ᵗʰ   **S92.102**   Unspecified fracture of left talus ▽

☑7ᵗʰ   **S92.109**   Unspecified fracture of unspecified talus ▽

☑6ᵗʰ   **S92.11**   **Fracture of neck of talus**

☑7ᵗʰ   **S92.111**   Displaced fracture of neck of right talus

☑7ᵗʰ   **S92.112**   Displaced fracture of neck of left talus

☑7ᵗʰ   **S92.113**   Displaced fracture of neck of unspecified talus ▽

☑7ᵗʰ   **S92.114**   Nondisplaced fracture of neck of right talus

☑7ᵗʰ   **S92.115**   Nondisplaced fracture of neck of left talus

☑7ᵗʰ   **S92.116**   Nondisplaced fracture of neck of unspecified talus ▽

☑6ᵗʰ   **S92.12**   **Fracture of body of talus**

☑7ᵗʰ   **S92.121**   Displaced fracture of body of right talus

☑7ᵗʰ   **S92.122**   Displaced fracture of body of left talus

☑7ᵗʰ   **S92.123**   Displaced fracture of body of unspecified talus ▽

☑7ᵗʰ   **S92.124**   Nondisplaced fracture of body of right talus

☑7ᵗʰ   **S92.125**   Nondisplaced fracture of body of left talus

☑7ᵗʰ   **S92.126**   Nondisplaced fracture of body of unspecified talus ▽

☑6ᵗʰ   **S92.13**   **Fracture of posterior process of talus**

☑7ᵗʰ   **S92.131**   Displaced fracture of posterior process of right talus

☑7ᵗʰ   **S92.132**   Displaced fracture of posterior process of left talus

☑7ᵗʰ   **S92.133**   Displaced fracture of posterior process of unspecified talus ▽

☑7ᵗʰ   **S92.134**   Nondisplaced fracture of posterior process of right talus

☑7ᵗʰ   **S92.135**   Nondisplaced fracture of posterior process of left talus

☑7ᵗʰ   **S92.136**   Nondisplaced fracture of posterior process of unspecified talus ▽

☑6ᵗʰ   **S92.14**   **Dome fracture of talus**

> *EXCLUDES 1*   osteochondritis dissecans (M93.2)

☑7ᵗʰ   **S92.141**   Displaced dome fracture of right talus

☑7ᵗʰ   **S92.142**   Displaced dome fracture of left talus

Ⓝ Newborn   Ⓟ Pediatric   Ⓜ Maternity   Ⓐ Adult   **RIC** RIC Dx   **NC Dx** Noncancer Dx   **PDx** Primary Dx   **CC** RIC CC Condition   ►◄ Revised Text   ● New Code   ▲ Revised Code Title

970   ICD-10-CM 2016

☑7ᵗʰ **S92.143** Displaced dome fracture of unspecified ▽
talus

☑7ᵗʰ **S92.144** Nondisplaced dome fracture of right talus

☑7ᵗʰ **S92.145** Nondisplaced dome fracture of left talus

☑7ᵗʰ **S92.146** Nondisplaced dome fracture of ▽
unspecified talus

☑6ᵗʰ **S92.15** Avulsion fracture (chip fracture) of talus

☑7ᵗʰ **S92.151** Displaced avulsion fracture (chip fracture)
of right talus

☑7ᵗʰ **S92.152** Displaced avulsion fracture (chip fracture)
of left talus

☑7ᵗʰ **S92.153** Displaced avulsion fracture (chip ▽
fracture) of unspecified talus

☑7ᵗʰ **S92.154** Nondisplaced avulsion fracture (chip
fracture) of right talus

☑7ᵗʰ **S92.155** Nondisplaced avulsion fracture (chip
fracture) of left talus

☑7ᵗʰ **S92.156** Nondisplaced avulsion fracture (chip ▽
fracture) of unspecified talus

☑6ᵗʰ **S92.19** Other fracture of talus

☑7ᵗʰ **S92.191** Other fracture of right talus

☑7ᵗʰ **S92.192** Other fracture of left talus

☑7ᵗʰ **S92.199** Other fracture of unspecified talus ▽

☑5ᵗʰ **S92.2** Fracture of other and unspecified tarsal bone(s)

☑6ᵗʰ **S92.20** Fracture of unspecified tarsal bone(s)

☑7ᵗʰ **S92.201** Fracture of unspecified tarsal bone(s) ▽
of right foot

☑7ᵗʰ **S92.202** Fracture of unspecified tarsal bone(s) ▽
of left foot

☑7ᵗʰ **S92.209** Fracture of unspecified tarsal bone(s) ▽
of unspecified foot

☑6ᵗʰ **S92.21** Fracture of cuboid bone

☑7ᵗʰ **S92.211** Displaced fracture of cuboid bone of right
foot

☑7ᵗʰ **S92.212** Displaced fracture of cuboid bone of left
foot

☑7ᵗʰ **S92.213** Displaced fracture of cuboid bone of ▽
unspecified foot

☑7ᵗʰ **S92.214** Nondisplaced fracture of cuboid bone of
right foot

☑7ᵗʰ **S92.215** Nondisplaced fracture of cuboid bone of
left foot

☑7ᵗʰ **S92.216** Nondisplaced fracture of cuboid bone ▽
of unspecified foot

☑6ᵗʰ **S92.22** Fracture of lateral cuneiform

☑7ᵗʰ **S92.221** Displaced fracture of lateral cuneiform of
right foot

☑7ᵗʰ **S92.222** Displaced fracture of lateral cuneiform of
left foot

☑7ᵗʰ **S92.223** Displaced fracture of lateral cuneiform ▽
of unspecified foot

☑7ᵗʰ **S92.224** Nondisplaced fracture of lateral
cuneiform of right foot

☑7ᵗʰ **S92.225** Nondisplaced fracture of lateral
cuneiform of left foot

☑7ᵗʰ **S92.226** Nondisplaced fracture of lateral ▽
cuneiform of unspecified foot

☑6ᵗʰ **S92.23** Fracture of intermediate cuneiform

☑7ᵗʰ **S92.231** Displaced fracture of intermediate
cuneiform of right foot

☑7ᵗʰ **S92.232** Displaced fracture of intermediate
cuneiform of left foot

☑7ᵗʰ **S92.233** Displaced fracture of intermediate ▽
cuneiform of unspecified foot

☑7ᵗʰ **S92.234** Nondisplaced fracture of intermediate
cuneiform of right foot

☑7ᵗʰ **S92.235** Nondisplaced fracture of intermediate
cuneiform of left foot

☑7ᵗʰ **S92.236** Nondisplaced fracture of intermediate ▽
cuneiform of unspecified foot

☑6ᵗʰ **S92.24** Fracture of medial cuneiform

☑7ᵗʰ **S92.241** Displaced fracture of medial cuneiform
of right foot

☑7ᵗʰ **S92.242** Displaced fracture of medial cuneiform
of left foot

☑7ᵗʰ **S92.243** Displaced fracture of medial cuneiform ▽
of unspecified foot

☑7ᵗʰ **S92.244** Nondisplaced fracture of medial
cuneiform of right foot

☑7ᵗʰ **S92.245** Nondisplaced fracture of medial
cuneiform of left foot

☑7ᵗʰ **S92.246** Nondisplaced fracture of medial ▽
cuneiform of unspecified foot

☑6ᵗʰ **S92.25** Fracture of navicular [scaphoid] of foot

☑7ᵗʰ **S92.251** Displaced fracture of navicular
[scaphoid] of right foot

☑7ᵗʰ **S92.252** Displaced fracture of navicular
[scaphoid] of left foot

☑7ᵗʰ **S92.253** Displaced fracture of navicular ▽
[scaphoid] of unspecified foot

☑7ᵗʰ **S92.254** Nondisplaced fracture of navicular
[scaphoid] of right foot

☑7ᵗʰ **S92.255** Nondisplaced fracture of navicular
[scaphoid] of left foot

☑7ᵗʰ **S92.256** Nondisplaced fracture of navicular ▽
[scaphoid] of unspecified foot

☑5ᵗʰ **S92.3** Fracture of metatarsal bone(s)

☑6ᵗʰ **S92.30** Fracture of unspecified metatarsal bone(s)

☑7ᵗʰ **S92.301** Fracture of unspecified metatarsal ▽
bone(s), right foot

☑7ᵗʰ **S92.302** Fracture of unspecified metatarsal ▽
bone(s), left foot

☑7ᵗʰ **S92.309** Fracture of unspecified metatarsal ▽
bone(s), unspecified foot

☑6ᵗʰ **S92.31** Fracture of first metatarsal bone

☑7ᵗʰ **S92.311** Displaced fracture of first metatarsal
bone, right foot

☑7ᵗʰ **S92.312** Displaced fracture of first metatarsal
bone, left foot

☑7ᵗʰ **S92.313** Displaced fracture of first metatarsal ▽
bone, unspecified foot

☑7ᵗʰ **S92.314** Nondisplaced fracture of first metatarsal
bone, right foot

☑7ᵗʰ **S92.315** Nondisplaced fracture of first metatarsal
bone, left foot

☑7ᵗʰ **S92.316** Nondisplaced fracture of first ▽
metatarsal bone, unspecified foot

☑6ᵗʰ **S92.32** Fracture of second metatarsal bone

☑7ᵗʰ **S92.321** Displaced fracture of second metatarsal
bone, right foot

☑7ᵗʰ **S92.322** Displaced fracture of second metatarsal
bone, left foot

☑7ᵗʰ **S92.323** Displaced fracture of second ▽
metatarsal bone, unspecified foot

☑7ᵗʰ **S92.324** Nondisplaced fracture of second
metatarsal bone, right foot

☑7ᵗʰ **S92.325** Nondisplaced fracture of second
metatarsal bone, left foot

☑7ᵗʰ **S92.326** Nondisplaced fracture of second ▽
metatarsal bone, unspecified foot

☑6ᵗʰ **S92.33** Fracture of third metatarsal bone

☑7ᵗʰ **S92.331** Displaced fracture of third metatarsal
bone, right foot

☑7ᵗʰ **S92.332** Displaced fracture of third metatarsal
bone, left foot

☑7ᵗʰ **S92.333** Displaced fracture of third metatarsal ▽
bone, unspecified foot

☑7ᵗʰ **S92.334** Nondisplaced fracture of third
metatarsal bone, right foot

☑7ᵗʰ **S92.335** Nondisplaced fracture of third
metatarsal bone, left foot

☑7ᵗʰ **S92.336** Nondisplaced fracture of third ▽
metatarsal bone, unspecified foot

✓6ᵗʰ **S92.34 Fracture of fourth metatarsal bone**

✓7ᵗʰ S92.341 Displaced fracture of fourth metatarsal bone, right foot

✓7ᵗʰ S92.342 Displaced fracture of fourth metatarsal bone, left foot

✓7ᵗʰ S92.343 Displaced fracture of fourth metatarsal bone, unspecified foot ▽

✓7ᵗʰ S92.344 Nondisplaced fracture of fourth metatarsal bone, right foot

✓7ᵗʰ S92.345 Nondisplaced fracture of fourth metatarsal bone, left foot

✓7ᵗʰ S92.346 Nondisplaced fracture of fourth metatarsal bone, unspecified foot ▽

✓6ᵗʰ **S92.35 Fracture of fifth metatarsal bone**

✓7ᵗʰ S92.351 Displaced fracture of fifth metatarsal bone, right foot

✓7ᵗʰ S92.352 Displaced fracture of fifth metatarsal bone, left foot

✓7ᵗʰ S92.353 Displaced fracture of fifth metatarsal bone, unspecified foot ▽

✓7ᵗʰ S92.354 Nondisplaced fracture of fifth metatarsal bone, right foot

✓7ᵗʰ S92.355 Nondisplaced fracture of fifth metatarsal bone, left foot

✓7ᵗʰ S92.356 Nondisplaced fracture of fifth metatarsal bone, unspecified foot ▽

✓5ᵗʰ **S92.4 Fracture of great toe**

✓6ᵗʰ **S92.40 Unspecified fracture of great toe**

✓7ᵗʰ S92.401 Displaced unspecified fracture of right great toe ▽

✓7ᵗʰ S92.402 Displaced unspecified fracture of left great toe ▽

✓7ᵗʰ S92.403 Displaced unspecified fracture of unspecified great toe ▽

✓7ᵗʰ S92.404 Nondisplaced unspecified fracture of right great toe ▽

✓7ᵗʰ S92.405 Nondisplaced unspecified fracture of left great toe ▽

✓7ᵗʰ S92.406 Nondisplaced unspecified fracture of unspecified great toe ▽

✓6ᵗʰ **S92.41 Fracture of proximal phalanx of great toe**

✓7ᵗʰ S92.411 Displaced fracture of proximal phalanx of right great toe

✓7ᵗʰ S92.412 Displaced fracture of proximal phalanx of left great toe

✓7ᵗʰ S92.413 Displaced fracture of proximal phalanx of unspecified great toe ▽

✓7ᵗʰ S92.414 Nondisplaced fracture of proximal phalanx of right great toe

✓7ᵗʰ S92.415 Nondisplaced fracture of proximal phalanx of left great toe

✓7ᵗʰ S92.416 Nondisplaced fracture of proximal phalanx of unspecified great toe ▽

✓6ᵗʰ **S92.42 Fracture of distal phalanx of great toe**

✓7ᵗʰ S92.421 Displaced fracture of distal phalanx of right great toe

✓7ᵗʰ S92.422 Displaced fracture of distal phalanx of left great toe

✓7ᵗʰ S92.423 Displaced fracture of distal phalanx of unspecified great toe ▽

✓7ᵗʰ S92.424 Nondisplaced fracture of distal phalanx of right great toe

✓7ᵗʰ S92.425 Nondisplaced fracture of distal phalanx of left great toe

✓7ᵗʰ S92.426 Nondisplaced fracture of distal phalanx of unspecified great toe ▽

✓6ᵗʰ **S92.49 Other fracture of great toe**

✓7ᵗʰ S92.491 Other fracture of right great toe

✓7ᵗʰ S92.492 Other fracture of left great toe

✓7ᵗʰ S92.499 Other fracture of unspecified great toe ▽

✓5ᵗʰ **S92.5 Fracture of lesser toe(s)**

✓6ᵗʰ **S92.50 Unspecified fracture of lesser toe(s)**

✓7ᵗʰ S92.501 Displaced unspecified fracture of right lesser toe(s) ▽

✓7ᵗʰ S92.502 Displaced unspecified fracture of left lesser toe(s) ▽

✓7ᵗʰ S92.503 Displaced unspecified fracture of unspecified lesser toe(s) ▽

✓7ᵗʰ S92.504 Nondisplaced unspecified fracture of right lesser toe(s) ▽

✓7ᵗʰ S92.505 Nondisplaced unspecified fracture of left lesser toe(s) ▽

✓7ᵗʰ S92.506 Nondisplaced unspecified fracture of unspecified lesser toe(s) ▽

✓6ᵗʰ **S92.51 Fracture of proximal phalanx of lesser toe(s)**

✓7ᵗʰ S92.511 Displaced fracture of proximal phalanx of right lesser toe(s)

✓7ᵗʰ S92.512 Displaced fracture of proximal phalanx of left lesser toe(s)

✓7ᵗʰ S92.513 Displaced fracture of proximal phalanx of unspecified lesser toe(s) ▽

✓7ᵗʰ S92.514 Nondisplaced fracture of proximal phalanx of right lesser toe(s)

✓7ᵗʰ S92.515 Nondisplaced fracture of proximal phalanx of left lesser toe(s)

✓7ᵗʰ S92.516 Nondisplaced fracture of proximal phalanx of unspecified lesser toe(s) ▽

✓6ᵗʰ **S92.52 Fracture of medial phalanx of lesser toe(s)**

✓7ᵗʰ S92.521 Displaced fracture of medial phalanx of right lesser toe(s)

✓7ᵗʰ S92.522 Displaced fracture of medial phalanx of left lesser toe(s)

✓7ᵗʰ S92.523 Displaced fracture of medial phalanx of unspecified lesser toe(s) ▽

✓7ᵗʰ S92.524 Nondisplaced fracture of medial phalanx of right lesser toe(s)

✓7ᵗʰ S92.525 Nondisplaced fracture of medial phalanx of left lesser toe(s)

✓7ᵗʰ S92.526 Nondisplaced fracture of medial phalanx of unspecified lesser toe(s) ▽

✓6ᵗʰ **S92.53 Fracture of distal phalanx of lesser toe(s)**

✓7ᵗʰ S92.531 Displaced fracture of distal phalanx of right lesser toe(s)

✓7ᵗʰ S92.532 Displaced fracture of distal phalanx of left lesser toe(s)

✓7ᵗʰ S92.533 Displaced fracture of distal phalanx of unspecified lesser toe(s) ▽

✓7ᵗʰ S92.534 Nondisplaced fracture of distal phalanx of right lesser toe(s)

✓7ᵗʰ S92.535 Nondisplaced fracture of distal phalanx of left lesser toe(s)

✓7ᵗʰ S92.536 Nondisplaced fracture of distal phalanx of unspecified lesser toe(s) ▽

✓6ᵗʰ **S92.59 Other fracture of lesser toe(s)**

✓7ᵗʰ S92.591 Other fracture of right lesser toe(s)

✓7ᵗʰ S92.592 Other fracture of left lesser toe(s)

✓7ᵗʰ S92.599 Other fracture of unspecified lesser toe(s) ▽

✓5ᵗʰ **S92.9 Unspecified fracture of foot and toe**

✓6ᵗʰ **S92.90 Unspecified fracture of foot**

✓7ᵗʰ S92.901 Unspecified fracture of right foot ▽

✓7ᵗʰ S92.902 Unspecified fracture of left foot ▽

✓7ᵗʰ S92.909 Unspecified fracture of unspecified foot ▽

✓6ᵗʰ **S92.91 Unspecified fracture of toe**

✓7ᵗʰ S92.911 Unspecified fracture of right toe(s) ▽

✓7ᵗʰ S92.912 Unspecified fracture of left toe(s) ▽

✓7ᵗʰ S92.919 Unspecified fracture of unspecified toe(s) ▽

Ⓝ Newborn Ⓟ Pediatric Ⓜ Maternity Ⓐ Adult **RIC** RIC Dx **NCDx** Noncancer Dx **PDx** Primary Dx **CC** RIC CC Condition ▶◀ Revised Text ● New Code ▲ Revised Code Title

✓4ᵗʰ **S93 Dislocation and sprain of joints and ligaments at ankle, foot and toe level**

INCLUDES   avulsion of joint or ligament of ankle, foot and toe
laceration of cartilage, joint or ligament of ankle, foot and toe
sprain of cartilage, joint or ligament of ankle, foot and toe
traumatic hemarthrosis of joint or ligament of ankle, foot and toe
traumatic rupture of joint or ligament of ankle, foot and toe
traumatic subluxation of joint or ligament of ankle, foot and toe
traumatic tear of joint or ligament of ankle, foot and toe

Code also any associated open wound

EXCLUDES 2   *strain of muscle and tendon of ankle and foot (S96.-)*

> The appropriate 7th character is to be added to each code from category S93.
> A   initial encounter
> D   subsequent encounter
> S   sequela

✓5ᵗʰ **S93.0 Subluxation and dislocation of** ankle joint
Subluxation and dislocation of astragalus
Subluxation and dislocation of fibula, lower end
Subluxation and dislocation of talus
Subluxation and dislocation of tibia, lower end

   ✓x7ᵗʰ **S93.01 Subluxation of** right **ankle joint**
   ✓x7ᵗʰ **S93.02 Subluxation of** left **ankle joint**
   ✓x7ᵗʰ **S93.03 Subluxation of unspecified ankle joint** ▽
   ✓x7ᵗʰ **S93.04 Dislocation of** right **ankle joint**
   ✓x7ᵗʰ **S93.05 Dislocation of** left **ankle joint**
   ✓x7ᵗʰ **S93.06 Dislocation of unspecified ankle joint** ▽

✓5ᵗʰ **S93.1 Subluxation and dislocation of** toe

   ✓6ᵗʰ **S93.10 Unspecified subluxation and dislocation of toe**
     Dislocation of toe NOS
     Subluxation of toe NOS

     ✓7ᵗʰ **S93.101 Unspecified subluxation of** right **toe(s)** ▽
     ✓7ᵗʰ **S93.102 Unspecified subluxation of** left **toe(s)** ▽
     ✓7ᵗʰ **S93.103 Unspecified subluxation of unspecified toe(s)** ▽
     ✓7ᵗʰ **S93.104 Unspecified dislocation of** right **toe(s)** ▽
     ✓7ᵗʰ **S93.105 Unspecified dislocation of** left **toe(s)** ▽
     ✓7ᵗʰ **S93.106 Unspecified dislocation of unspecified toe(s)** ▽

   ✓6ᵗʰ **S93.11 Dislocation of** interphalangeal joint

     ✓7ᵗʰ **S93.111 Dislocation of interphalangeal joint of** right great **toe**
     ✓7ᵗʰ **S93.112 Dislocation of interphalangeal joint of** left great **toe**
     ✓7ᵗʰ **S93.113 Dislocation of interphalangeal joint of unspecified great toe** ▽
     ✓7ᵗʰ **S93.114 Dislocation of interphalangeal joint of** right lesser **toe(s)**
     ✓7ᵗʰ **S93.115 Dislocation of interphalangeal joint of** left lesser **toe(s)**
     ✓7ᵗʰ **S93.116 Dislocation of interphalangeal joint of unspecified lesser toe(s)** ▽
     ✓7ᵗʰ **S93.119 Dislocation of interphalangeal joint of unspecified toe(s)** ▽

   ✓6ᵗʰ **S93.12 Dislocation of** metatarsophalangeal joint

     ✓7ᵗʰ **S93.121 Dislocation of metatarsophalangeal joint of** right great **toe**
     ✓7ᵗʰ **S93.122 Dislocation of metatarsophalangeal joint of** left great **toe**
     ✓7ᵗʰ **S93.123 Dislocation of metatarsophalangeal joint of unspecified great toe** ▽
     ✓7ᵗʰ **S93.124 Dislocation of metatarsophalangeal joint of** right lesser **toe(s)**
     ✓7ᵗʰ **S93.125 Dislocation of metatarsophalangeal joint of** left lesser **toe(s)**
     ✓7ᵗʰ **S93.126 Dislocation of metatarsophalangeal joint of unspecified lesser toe(s)** ▽
     ✓7ᵗʰ **S93.129 Dislocation of metatarsophalangeal joint of unspecified toe(s)** ▽

   ✓6ᵗʰ **S93.13 Subluxation of** interphalangeal joint

     ✓7ᵗʰ **S93.131 Subluxation of interphalangeal joint of** right great **toe**
     ✓7ᵗʰ **S93.132 Subluxation of interphalangeal joint of** left great **toe**
     ✓7ᵗʰ **S93.133 Subluxation of interphalangeal joint of unspecified great toe** ▽
     ✓7ᵗʰ **S93.134 Subluxation of interphalangeal joint of** right lesser **toe(s)**
     ✓7ᵗʰ **S93.135 Subluxation of interphalangeal joint of** left lesser **toe(s)**
     ✓7ᵗʰ **S93.136 Subluxation of interphalangeal joint of unspecified lesser toe(s)** ▽
     ✓7ᵗʰ **S93.139 Subluxation of interphalangeal joint of unspecified toe(s)** ▽

   ✓6ᵗʰ **S93.14 Subluxation of** metatarsophalangeal joint

     ✓7ᵗʰ **S93.141 Subluxation of metatarsophalangeal joint of** right great **toe**
     ✓7ᵗʰ **S93.142 Subluxation of metatarsophalangeal joint of** left great **toe**
     ✓7ᵗʰ **S93.143 Subluxation of metatarsophalangeal joint of unspecified great toe** ▽
     ✓7ᵗʰ **S93.144 Subluxation of metatarsophalangeal joint of** right lesser **toe(s)**
     ✓7ᵗʰ **S93.145 Subluxation of metatarsophalangeal joint of** left lesser **toe(s)**
     ✓7ᵗʰ **S93.146 Subluxation of metatarsophalangeal joint of unspecified lesser toe(s)** ▽
     ✓7ᵗʰ **S93.149 Subluxation of metatarsophalangeal joint of unspecified toe(s)**

✓5ᵗʰ **S93.3 Subluxation and dislocation of** foot

   EXCLUDES 2   *dislocation of toe (S93.1-)*

   ✓6ᵗʰ **S93.30 Unspecified subluxation and dislocation of foot**
     Dislocation of foot NOS
     Subluxation of foot NOS

     ✓7ᵗʰ **S93.301 Unspecified subluxation of** right **foot** ▽
     ✓7ᵗʰ **S93.302 Unspecified subluxation of** left **foot** ▽
     ✓7ᵗʰ **S93.303 Unspecified subluxation of unspecified foot** ▽
     ✓7ᵗʰ **S93.304 Unspecified dislocation of** right **foot** ▽
     ✓7ᵗʰ **S93.305 Unspecified dislocation of** left **foot** ▽
     ✓7ᵗʰ **S93.306 Unspecified dislocation of unspecified foot** ▽

   ✓6ᵗʰ **S93.31 Subluxation and dislocation of** tarsal joint

     ✓7ᵗʰ **S93.311 Subluxation of tarsal joint of** right **foot**
     ✓7ᵗʰ **S93.312 Subluxation of tarsal joint of** left **foot**
     ✓7ᵗʰ **S93.313 Subluxation of tarsal joint of unspecified foot** ▽
     ✓7ᵗʰ **S93.314 Dislocation of tarsal joint of** right **foot**
     ✓7ᵗʰ **S93.315 Dislocation of tarsal joint of** left **foot**
     ✓7ᵗʰ **S93.316 Dislocation of tarsal joint of unspecified foot** ▽

   ✓6ᵗʰ **S93.32 Subluxation and dislocation of** tarsometatarsal **joint**

     ✓7ᵗʰ **S93.321 Subluxation of tarsometatarsal joint of** right **foot**
     ✓7ᵗʰ **S93.322 Subluxation of tarsometatarsal joint of** left **foot**
     ✓7ᵗʰ **S93.323 Subluxation of tarsometatarsal joint of unspecified foot** ▽
     ✓7ᵗʰ **S93.324 Dislocation of tarsometatarsal joint of** right **foot**
     ✓7ᵗʰ **S93.325 Dislocation of tarsometatarsal joint of** left **foot**
     ✓7ᵗʰ **S93.326 Dislocation of tarsometatarsal joint of unspecified foot** ▽

   ✓6ᵗʰ **S93.33 Other subluxation and dislocation of foot**

     ✓7ᵗʰ **S93.331 Other subluxation of** right **foot**
     ✓7ᵗʰ **S93.332 Other subluxation of** left **foot**
     ✓7ᵗʰ **S93.333 Other subluxation of unspecified foot** ▽
     ✓7ᵗʰ **S93.334 Other dislocation of** right **foot**
     ✓7ᵗʰ **S93.335 Other dislocation of** left **foot**
     ✓7ᵗʰ **S93.336 Other dislocation of unspecified foot** ▽

✓ Add'l Character Required   ✓x7ᵗʰ Placeholder Alert   RUG IV Special Care High Dx   RUG IV Clinically Complex Dx   RUG IV Special Care Low Dx   Manifestation Code   Other Specified Code   ▽Unspecified Code

√5ᵗʰ **S93.4 Sprain of ankle**

> EXCLUDES 2   injury of Achilles tendon (S86.0-)

√6ᵗʰ   **S93.40 Sprain of unspecified ligament of ankle**
Sprain of ankle NOS
Sprained ankle NOS

√7ᵗʰ   S93.401   Sprain of unspecified ligament of right ankle ▽

√7ᵗʰ   S93.402   Sprain of unspecified ligament of left ankle ▽

√7ᵗʰ   S93.409   Sprain of unspecified ligament of unspecified ankle ▽

√6ᵗʰ   **S93.41 Sprain of calcaneofibular ligament**

√7ᵗʰ   S93.411   Sprain of calcaneofibular ligament of right ankle

√7ᵗʰ   S93.412   Sprain of calcaneofibular ligament of left ankle

√7ᵗʰ   S93.419   Sprain of calcaneofibular ligament of unspecified ankle ▽

√6ᵗʰ   **S93.42 Sprain of deltoid ligament**

√7ᵗʰ   S93.421   Sprain of deltoid ligament of right ankle

√7ᵗʰ   S93.422   Sprain of deltoid ligament of left ankle

√7ᵗʰ   S93.429   Sprain of deltoid ligament of unspecified ankle ▽

√6ᵗʰ   **S93.43 Sprain of tibiofibular ligament**

√7ᵗʰ   S93.431   Sprain of tibiofibular ligament of right ankle

√7ᵗʰ   S93.432   Sprain of tibiofibular ligament of left ankle

√7ᵗʰ   S93.439   Sprain of tibiofibular ligament of unspecified ankle ▽

√6ᵗʰ   **S93.49 Sprain of other ligament of ankle**
Sprain of internal collateral ligament
Sprain of talofibular ligament

√7ᵗʰ   S93.491   **Sprain of other ligament of right ankle**

√7ᵗʰ   S93.492   **Sprain of other ligament of left ankle**

√7ᵗʰ   S93.499   **Sprain of other ligament of unspecified ankle** ▽

√5ᵗʰ **S93.5 Sprain of toe**

√6ᵗʰ   **S93.50 Unspecified sprain of toe**

√7ᵗʰ   S93.501   Unspecified sprain of right great toe ▽

√7ᵗʰ   S93.502   Unspecified sprain of left great toe ▽

√7ᵗʰ   S93.503   Unspecified sprain of unspecified great toe ▽

√7ᵗʰ   S93.504   Unspecified sprain of right lesser toe(s) ▽

√7ᵗʰ   S93.505   Unspecified sprain of left lesser toe(s) ▽

√7ᵗʰ   S93.506   Unspecified sprain of unspecified lesser toe(s) ▽

√7ᵗʰ   S93.509   Unspecified sprain of unspecified toe(s) ▽

√6ᵗʰ   **S93.51 Sprain of interphalangeal joint of toe**

√7ᵗʰ   S93.511   Sprain of interphalangeal joint of right great toe

√7ᵗʰ   S93.512   Sprain of interphalangeal joint of left great toe

√7ᵗʰ   S93.513   Sprain of interphalangeal joint of unspecified great toe ▽

√7ᵗʰ   S93.514   Sprain of interphalangeal joint of right lesser toe(s)

√7ᵗʰ   S93.515   Sprain of interphalangeal joint of left lesser toe(s)

√7ᵗʰ   S93.516   Sprain of interphalangeal joint of unspecified lesser toe(s) ▽

√7ᵗʰ   S93.519   Sprain of interphalangeal joint of unspecified toe(s) ▽

√6ᵗʰ   **S93.52 Sprain of metatarsophalangeal joint of toe**

√7ᵗʰ   S93.521   Sprain of metatarsophalangeal joint of right great toe

√7ᵗʰ   S93.522   Sprain of metatarsophalangeal joint of left great toe

√7ᵗʰ   S93.523   Sprain of metatarsophalangeal joint of unspecified great toe ▽

√7ᵗʰ   S93.524   Sprain of metatarsophalangeal joint of right lesser toe(s)

√7ᵗʰ   S93.525   Sprain of metatarsophalangeal joint of left lesser toe(s)

√7ᵗʰ   S93.526   Sprain of metatarsophalangeal joint of unspecified lesser toe(s) ▽

√7ᵗʰ   S93.529   Sprain of metatarsophalangeal joint of unspecified toe(s) ▽

√5ᵗʰ **S93.6 Sprain of foot**

> EXCLUDES 2   sprain of metatarsophalangeal joint of toe (S93.52-)
> sprain of toe (S93.5-)

√6ᵗʰ   **S93.60 Unspecified sprain of foot**

√7ᵗʰ   S93.601   Unspecified sprain of right foot ▽

√7ᵗʰ   S93.602   Unspecified sprain of left foot ▽

√7ᵗʰ   S93.609   Unspecified sprain of unspecified foot ▽

√6ᵗʰ   **S93.61 Sprain of tarsal ligament of foot**

√7ᵗʰ   S93.611   Sprain of tarsal ligament of right foot

√7ᵗʰ   S93.612   Sprain of tarsal ligament of left foot

√7ᵗʰ   S93.619   Sprain of tarsal ligament of unspecified foot ▽

√6ᵗʰ   **S93.62 Sprain of tarsometatarsal ligament of foot**

√7ᵗʰ   S93.621   Sprain of tarsometatarsal ligament of right foot

√7ᵗʰ   S93.622   Sprain of tarsometatarsal ligament of left foot

√7ᵗʰ   S93.629   Sprain of tarsometatarsal ligament of unspecified foot ▽

√6ᵗʰ   **S93.69 Other sprain of foot**

√7ᵗʰ   S93.691   **Other sprain of right foot**

√7ᵗʰ   S93.692   **Other sprain of left foot**

√7ᵗʰ   S93.699   **Other sprain of unspecified foot** ▽

√4ᵗʰ **S94 Injury of nerves at ankle and foot level**
Code also any associated open wound (S91.-)

> The appropriate 7th character is to be added to each code from category S94.
> A   initial encounter
> D   subsequent encounter
> S   sequela

√5ᵗʰ **S94.0 Injury of lateral plantar nerve**

√x7ᵗʰ   S94.00   Injury of lateral plantar nerve, unspecified leg ▽

√x7ᵗʰ   S94.01   Injury of lateral plantar nerve, right leg

√x7ᵗʰ   S94.02   Injury of lateral plantar nerve, left leg

√5ᵗʰ **S94.1 Injury of medial plantar nerve**

√x7ᵗʰ   S94.10   Injury of medial plantar nerve, unspecified leg ▽

√x7ᵗʰ   S94.11   Injury of medial plantar nerve, right leg

√x7ᵗʰ   S94.12   Injury of medial plantar nerve, left leg

√5ᵗʰ **S94.2 Injury of deep peroneal nerve at ankle and foot level**
Injury of terminal, lateral branch of deep peroneal nerve

√x7ᵗʰ   S94.20   Injury of deep peroneal nerve at ankle and foot level, unspecified leg ▽

√x7ᵗʰ   S94.21   Injury of deep peroneal nerve at ankle and foot level, right leg

√x7ᵗʰ   S94.22   Injury of deep peroneal nerve at ankle and foot level, left leg

√5ᵗʰ **S94.3 Injury of cutaneous sensory nerve at ankle and foot level**

√x7ᵗʰ   S94.30   Injury of cutaneous sensory nerve at ankle and foot level, unspecified leg ▽

√x7ᵗʰ   S94.31   Injury of cutaneous sensory nerve at ankle and foot level, right leg

√x7ᵗʰ   S94.32   Injury of cutaneous sensory nerve at ankle and foot level, left leg

√5ᵗʰ **S94.8 Injury of other nerves at ankle and foot level**

√6ᵗʰ   **S94.8X Injury of other nerves at ankle and foot level**

√7ᵗʰ   S94.8X1   **Injury of other nerves at ankle and foot level, right leg**

√7ᵗʰ   S94.8X2   **Injury of other nerves at ankle and foot level, left leg**

√7ᵗʰ   S94.8X9   **Injury of other nerves at ankle and foot level, unspecified leg** ▽

√5ᵗʰ **S94.9 Injury of unspecified nerve at ankle and foot level**

√x7ᵗʰ   S94.90   Injury of unspecified nerve at ankle and foot level, unspecified leg ▽

Ⓝ Newborn   Ⓟ Pediatric   Ⓜ Maternity   Ⓐ Adult   **RIC** RIC Dx   **NC Dx** Noncancer Dx   **PDx** Primary Dx   **CC** RIC CC Condition   ►◄ Revised Text   ● New Code   ▲ Revised Code Title

974   ICD-10-CM 2016

✔x7ᵗʰ **S94.91**   Injury of unspecified nerve at ankle and foot level, right leg ▽

✔x7ᵗʰ **S94.92**   Injury of unspecified nerve at ankle and foot level, left leg ▽

✔4ᵗʰ **S95   Injury of blood vessels at ankle and foot level**
Code also any associated open wound (S91.-)
EXCLUDES 2   injury of posterior tibial artery and vein (S85.1-, S85.8-)

The appropriate 7th character is to be added to each code from category S95.
A   initial encounter
D   subsequent encounter
S   sequela

✔5ᵗʰ **S95.0   Injury of dorsal artery of foot**
  ✔6ᵗʰ **S95.00   Unspecified injury of dorsal artery of foot**
      ✔7ᵗʰ **S95.001**   Unspecified injury of dorsal artery of right foot ▽
      ✔7ᵗʰ **S95.002**   Unspecified injury of dorsal artery of left foot ▽
      ✔7ᵗʰ **S95.009**   Unspecified injury of dorsal artery of unspecified foot ▽
  ✔6ᵗʰ **S95.01   Laceration of dorsal artery of foot**
      ✔7ᵗʰ **S95.011**   Laceration of dorsal artery of right foot
      ✔7ᵗʰ **S95.012**   Laceration of dorsal artery of left foot
      ✔7ᵗʰ **S95.019**   Laceration of dorsal artery of unspecified foot ▽
  ✔6ᵗʰ **S95.09   Other specified injury of dorsal artery of foot**
      ✔7ᵗʰ **S95.091**   Other specified injury of dorsal artery of right foot
      ✔7ᵗʰ **S95.092**   Other specified injury of dorsal artery of left foot
      ✔7ᵗʰ **S95.099**   Other specified injury of dorsal artery of unspecified foot ▽

✔5ᵗʰ **S95.1   Injury of plantar artery of foot**
  ✔6ᵗʰ **S95.10   Unspecified injury of plantar artery of foot**
      ✔7ᵗʰ **S95.101**   Unspecified injury of plantar artery of right foot ▽
      ✔7ᵗʰ **S95.102**   Unspecified injury of plantar artery of left foot ▽
      ✔7ᵗʰ **S95.109**   Unspecified injury of plantar artery of unspecified foot ▽
  ✔6ᵗʰ **S95.11   Laceration of plantar artery of foot**
      ✔7ᵗʰ **S95.111**   Laceration of plantar artery of right foot
      ✔7ᵗʰ **S95.112**   Laceration of plantar artery of left foot
      ✔7ᵗʰ **S95.119**   Laceration of plantar artery of unspecified foot
  ✔6ᵗʰ **S95.19   Other specified injury of plantar artery of foot**
      ✔7ᵗʰ **S95.191**   Other specified injury of plantar artery of right foot
      ✔7ᵗʰ **S95.192**   Other specified injury of plantar artery of left foot
      ✔7ᵗʰ **S95.199**   Other specified injury of plantar artery of unspecified foot ▽

✔5ᵗʰ **S95.2   Injury of dorsal vein of foot**
  ✔6ᵗʰ **S95.20   Unspecified injury of dorsal vein of foot**
      ✔7ᵗʰ **S95.201**   Unspecified injury of dorsal vein of right foot ▽
      ✔7ᵗʰ **S95.202**   Unspecified injury of dorsal vein of left foot ▽
      ✔7ᵗʰ **S95.209**   Unspecified injury of dorsal vein of unspecified foot ▽
  ✔6ᵗʰ **S95.21   Laceration of dorsal vein of foot**
      ✔7ᵗʰ **S95.211**   Laceration of dorsal vein of right foot
      ✔7ᵗʰ **S95.212**   Laceration of dorsal vein of left foot
      ✔7ᵗʰ **S95.219**   Laceration of dorsal vein of unspecified foot ▽
  ✔6ᵗʰ **S95.29   Other specified injury of dorsal vein of foot**
      ✔7ᵗʰ **S95.291**   Other specified injury of dorsal vein of right foot
      ✔7ᵗʰ **S95.292**   Other specified injury of dorsal vein of left foot

✔7ᵗʰ **S95.299**   Other specified injury of dorsal vein of unspecified foot ▽

✔5ᵗʰ **S95.8   Injury of other blood vessels at ankle and foot level**
  ✔6ᵗʰ **S95.80   Unspecified injury of other blood vessels at ankle and foot level**
      ✔7ᵗʰ **S95.801**   Unspecified injury of other blood vessels at ankle and foot level, right leg ▽
      ✔7ᵗʰ **S95.802**   Unspecified injury of other blood vessels at ankle and foot level, left leg ▽
      ✔7ᵗʰ **S95.809**   Unspecified injury of other blood vessels at ankle and foot level, unspecified leg ▽
  ✔6ᵗʰ **S95.81   Laceration of other blood vessels at ankle and foot level**
      ✔7ᵗʰ **S95.811**   Laceration of other blood vessels at ankle and foot level, right leg
      ✔7ᵗʰ **S95.812**   Laceration of other blood vessels at ankle and foot level, left leg
      ✔7ᵗʰ **S95.819**   Laceration of other blood vessels at ankle and foot level, unspecified leg ▽
  ✔6ᵗʰ **S95.89   Other specified injury of other blood vessels at ankle and foot level**
      ✔7ᵗʰ **S95.891**   Other specified injury of other blood vessels at ankle and foot level, right leg
      ✔7ᵗʰ **S95.892**   Other specified injury of other blood vessels at ankle and foot level, left leg
      ✔7ᵗʰ **S95.899**   Other specified injury of other blood vessels at ankle and foot level, unspecified leg ▽

✔5ᵗʰ **S95.9   Injury of unspecified blood vessel at ankle and foot level**
  ✔6ᵗʰ **S95.90   Unspecified injury of unspecified blood vessel at ankle and foot level**
      ✔7ᵗʰ **S95.901**   Unspecified injury of unspecified blood vessel at ankle and foot level, right leg ▽
      ✔7ᵗʰ **S95.902**   Unspecified injury of unspecified blood vessel at ankle and foot level, left leg ▽
      ✔7ᵗʰ **S95.909**   Unspecified injury of unspecified blood vessel at ankle and foot level, unspecified leg ▽
  ✔6ᵗʰ **S95.91   Laceration of unspecified blood vessel at ankle and foot level**
      ✔7ᵗʰ **S95.911**   Laceration of unspecified blood vessel at ankle and foot level, right leg ▽
      ✔7ᵗʰ **S95.912**   Laceration of unspecified blood vessel at ankle and foot level, left leg ▽
      ✔7ᵗʰ **S95.919**   Laceration of unspecified blood vessel at ankle and foot level, unspecified leg ▽
  ✔6ᵗʰ **S95.99   Other specified injury of unspecified blood vessel at ankle and foot level**
      ✔7ᵗʰ **S95.991**   Other specified injury of unspecified blood vessel at ankle and foot level, right leg
      ✔7ᵗʰ **S95.992**   Other specified injury of unspecified blood vessel at ankle and foot level, left leg
      ✔7ᵗʰ **S95.999**   Other specified injury of unspecified blood vessel at ankle and foot level, unspecified leg ▽

✦ ✔4ᵗʰ **S96   Injury of muscle and tendon at ankle and foot level**
Code also any associated open wound (S91.-)
EXCLUDES 2   injury of Achilles tendon (S86.0-)
                    sprain of joints and ligaments of ankle and foot (S93.-)

The appropriate 7th character is to be added to each code from category S96.
A   initial encounter
D   subsequent encounter
S   sequela

✔5ᵗʰ **S96.0   Injury of muscle and tendon of long flexor muscle of toe at ankle and foot level**
  ✔6ᵗʰ **S96.00   Unspecified injury of muscle and tendon of long flexor muscle of toe at ankle and foot level**
      ✔7ᵗʰ **S96.001**   Unspecified injury of muscle and tendon of long flexor muscle of toe at ankle and foot level, right foot ▽

✦   Refer to the Muscle/Tendon Table at beginning of this chapter.

☑ Add'l Character Required   ✔x7ᵗʰ Placeholder Alert   RUG IV Special Care High Dx   RUG IV Clinically Complex Dx   RUG IV Special Care Low Dx   Manifestation Code   Other Specified Code   ▽Unspecified Code

☑7ᵗʰ **S96.002** Unspecified injury of muscle and tendon of long flexor muscle of toe at ankle and foot level, left foot ▽

☑7ᵗʰ **S96.009** Unspecified injury of muscle and tendon of long flexor muscle of toe at ankle and foot level, unspecified foot ▽

☑6ᵗʰ **S96.01** Strain of muscle and tendon of long flexor muscle of toe at ankle and foot level

☑7ᵗʰ **S96.011** Strain of muscle and tendon of long flexor muscle of toe at ankle and foot level, right foot

☑7ᵗʰ **S96.012** Strain of muscle and tendon of long flexor muscle of toe at ankle and foot level, left foot

☑7ᵗʰ **S96.019** Strain of muscle and tendon of long flexor muscle of toe at ankle and foot level, unspecified foot ▽

☑6ᵗʰ **S96.02** Laceration of muscle and tendon of long flexor muscle of toe at ankle and foot level

☑7ᵗʰ **S96.021** Laceration of muscle and tendon of long flexor muscle of toe at ankle and foot level, right foot

☑7ᵗʰ **S96.022** Laceration of muscle and tendon of long flexor muscle of toe at ankle and foot level, left foot

☑7ᵗʰ **S96.029** Laceration of muscle and tendon of long flexor muscle of toe at ankle and foot level, unspecified foot ▽

☑6ᵗʰ **S96.09** Other injury of muscle and tendon of long flexor muscle of toe at ankle and foot level

☑7ᵗʰ **S96.091** Other injury of muscle and tendon of long flexor muscle of toe at ankle and foot level, right foot

☑7ᵗʰ **S96.092** Other injury of muscle and tendon of long flexor muscle of toe at ankle and foot level, left foot

☑7ᵗʰ **S96.099** Other injury of muscle and tendon of long flexor muscle of toe at ankle and foot level, unspecified foot ▽

☑5ᵗʰ **S96.1** Injury of muscle and tendon of long extensor muscle of toe at ankle and foot level

☑6ᵗʰ **S96.10** Unspecified injury of muscle and tendon of long extensor muscle of toe at ankle and foot level

☑7ᵗʰ **S96.101** Unspecified injury of muscle and tendon of long extensor muscle of toe at ankle and foot level, right foot ▽

☑7ᵗʰ **S96.102** Unspecified injury of muscle and tendon of long extensor muscle of toe at ankle and foot level, left foot ▽

☑7ᵗʰ **S96.109** Unspecified injury of muscle and tendon of long extensor muscle of toe at ankle and foot level, unspecified foot ▽

☑6ᵗʰ **S96.11** Strain of muscle and tendon of long extensor muscle of toe at ankle and foot level

☑7ᵗʰ **S96.111** Strain of muscle and tendon of long extensor muscle of toe at ankle and foot level, right foot

☑7ᵗʰ **S96.112** Strain of muscle and tendon of long extensor muscle of toe at ankle and foot level, left foot

☑7ᵗʰ **S96.119** Strain of muscle and tendon of long extensor muscle of toe at ankle and foot level, unspecified foot ▽

☑6ᵗʰ **S96.12** Laceration of muscle and tendon of long extensor muscle of toe at ankle and foot level

☑7ᵗʰ **S96.121** Laceration of muscle and tendon of long extensor muscle of toe at ankle and foot level, right foot

☑7ᵗʰ **S96.122** Laceration of muscle and tendon of long extensor muscle of toe at ankle and foot level, left foot

☑7ᵗʰ **S96.129** Laceration of muscle and tendon of long extensor muscle of toe at ankle and foot level, unspecified foot ▽

☑6ᵗʰ **S96.19** Other specified injury of muscle and tendon of long extensor muscle of toe at ankle and foot level

☑7ᵗʰ **S96.191** Other specified injury of muscle and tendon of long extensor muscle of toe at ankle and foot level, right foot

☑7ᵗʰ **S96.192** Other specified injury of muscle and tendon of long extensor muscle of toe at ankle and foot level, left foot

☑7ᵗʰ **S96.199** Other specified injury of muscle and tendon of long extensor muscle of toe at ankle and foot level, unspecified foot

☑5ᵗʰ **S96.2** Injury of intrinsic muscle and tendon at ankle and foot level

☑6ᵗʰ **S96.20** Unspecified injury of intrinsic muscle and tendon at ankle and foot level

☑7ᵗʰ **S96.201** Unspecified injury of intrinsic muscle and tendon at ankle and foot level, right foot ▽

☑7ᵗʰ **S96.202** Unspecified injury of intrinsic muscle and tendon at ankle and foot level, left foot ▽

☑7ᵗʰ **S96.209** Unspecified injury of intrinsic muscle and tendon at ankle and foot level, unspecified foot ▽

☑6ᵗʰ **S96.21** Strain of intrinsic muscle and tendon at ankle and foot level

☑7ᵗʰ **S96.211** Strain of intrinsic muscle and tendon at ankle and foot level, right foot

☑7ᵗʰ **S96.212** Strain of intrinsic muscle and tendon at ankle and foot level, left foot

☑7ᵗʰ **S96.219** Strain of intrinsic muscle and tendon at ankle and foot level, unspecified foot ▽

☑6ᵗʰ **S96.22** Laceration of intrinsic muscle and tendon at ankle and foot level

☑7ᵗʰ **S96.221** Laceration of intrinsic muscle and tendon at ankle and foot level, right foot

☑7ᵗʰ **S96.222** Laceration of intrinsic muscle and tendon at ankle and foot level, left foot

☑7ᵗʰ **S96.229** Laceration of intrinsic muscle and tendon at ankle and foot level, unspecified foot ▽

☑6ᵗʰ **S96.29** Other specified injury of intrinsic muscle and tendon at ankle and foot level

☑7ᵗʰ **S96.291** Other specified injury of intrinsic muscle and tendon at ankle and foot level, right foot

☑7ᵗʰ **S96.292** Other specified injury of intrinsic muscle and tendon at ankle and foot level, left foot

☑7ᵗʰ **S96.299** Other specified injury of intrinsic muscle and tendon at ankle and foot level, unspecified foot ▽

☑5ᵗʰ **S96.8** Injury of other specified muscles and tendons at ankle and foot level

☑6ᵗʰ **S96.80** Unspecified injury of other specified muscles and tendons at ankle and foot level

☑7ᵗʰ **S96.801** Unspecified injury of other specified muscles and tendons at ankle and foot level, right foot ▽

☑7ᵗʰ **S96.802** Unspecified injury of other specified muscles and tendons at ankle and foot level, left foot ▽

☑7ᵗʰ **S96.809** Unspecified injury of other specified muscles and tendons at ankle and foot level, unspecified foot ▽

☑6ᵗʰ **S96.81** Strain of other specified muscles and tendons at ankle and foot level

☑7ᵗʰ **S96.811** Strain of other specified muscles and tendons at ankle and foot level, right foot

☑7ᵗʰ **S96.812** Strain of other specified muscles and tendons at ankle and foot level, left foot

☑7ᵗʰ **S96.819** Strain of other specified muscles and tendons at ankle and foot level, unspecified foot ▽

☑6ᵗʰ **S96.82** Laceration of other specified muscles and tendons at ankle and foot level

☑7ᵗʰ **S96.821** Laceration of other specified muscles and tendons at ankle and foot level, right foot

☑7ᵗʰ **S96.822** Laceration of other specified muscles and tendons at ankle and foot level, left foot

Ⓝ Newborn   Ⓟ Pediatric   Ⓜ Maternity   Ⓐ Adult   **RIC** RIC Dx   **NCDx** Noncancer Dx   **PDx** Primary Dx   **CC** RIC CC Condition   ▶◀ Revised Text   ● New Code   ▲ Revised Code Title

976   ICD-10-CM 2016

✓6ᵗʰ **S96.829** **Laceration of other specified muscles and tendons at ankle and foot level, unspecified foot** ▽

✓6ᵗʰ **S96.89** Other specified injury of other specified muscles and tendons at ankle and foot level

  ✓7ᵗʰ **S96.891** **Other specified injury of other specified muscles and tendons at ankle and foot level, right foot**

  ✓7ᵗʰ **S96.892** **Other specified injury of other specified muscles and tendons at ankle and foot level, left foot**

  ✓7ᵗʰ **S96.899** **Other specified injury of other specified muscles and tendons at ankle and foot level, unspecified foot** ▽

✓5ᵗʰ **S96.9** Injury of unspecified muscle and tendon at ankle and foot level

  ✓6ᵗʰ **S96.90** Unspecified injury of unspecified muscle and tendon at ankle and foot level

    ✓7ᵗʰ **S96.901** **Unspecified injury of unspecified muscle and tendon at ankle and foot level, right foot** ▽

    ✓7ᵗʰ **S96.902** **Unspecified injury of unspecified muscle and tendon at ankle and foot level, left foot** ▽

    ✓7ᵗʰ **S96.909** **Unspecified injury of unspecified muscle and tendon at ankle and foot level, unspecified foot** ▽

  ✓6ᵗʰ **S96.91** Strain of unspecified muscle and tendon at ankle and foot level

    ✓7ᵗʰ **S96.911** **Strain of unspecified muscle and tendon at ankle and foot level, right foot** ▽

    ✓7ᵗʰ **S96.912** **Strain of unspecified muscle and tendon at ankle and foot level, left foot** ▽

    ✓7ᵗʰ **S96.919** **Strain of unspecified muscle and tendon at ankle and foot level, unspecified foot** ▽

  ✓6ᵗʰ **S96.92** Laceration of unspecified muscle and tendon at ankle and foot level

    ✓7ᵗʰ **S96.921** **Laceration of unspecified muscle and tendon at ankle and foot level, right foot** ▽

    ✓7ᵗʰ **S96.922** **Laceration of unspecified muscle and tendon at ankle and foot level, left foot** ▽

    ✓7ᵗʰ **S96.929** **Laceration of unspecified muscle and tendon at ankle and foot level, unspecified foot** ▽

  ✓6ᵗʰ **S96.99** Other specified injury of unspecified muscle and tendon at ankle and foot level

    ✓7ᵗʰ **S96.991** **Other specified injury of unspecified muscle and tendon at ankle and foot level, right foot** ▽

    ✓7ᵗʰ **S96.992** **Other specified injury of unspecified muscle and tendon at ankle and foot level, left foot** ▽

    ✓7ᵗʰ **S96.999** **Other specified injury of unspecified muscle and tendon at ankle and foot level, unspecified foot** ▽

✓4ᵗʰ **S97** Crushing injury of ankle and foot

Use additional code(s) for all associated injuries

The appropriate 7th character is to be added to each code from category S97.
A   initial encounter
D   subsequent encounter
S   sequela

✓5ᵗʰ **S97.0** Crushing injury of ankle

  ✓x7ᵗʰ **S97.00** **Crushing injury of unspecified ankle** ▽

  ✓x7ᵗʰ **S97.01** **Crushing injury of right ankle**

  ✓x7ᵗʰ **S97.02** **Crushing injury of left ankle**

✓5ᵗʰ **S97.1** Crushing injury of toe

  ✓6ᵗʰ **S97.10** Crushing injury of unspecified toe(s)

    ✓7ᵗʰ **S97.101** **Crushing injury of unspecified right toe(s)** ▽

    ✓7ᵗʰ **S97.102** **Crushing injury of unspecified left toe(s)** ▽

    ✓7ᵗʰ **S97.109** **Crushing injury of unspecified toe(s)** ▽
         Crushing injury of toe NOS

  ✓7ᵗʰ **S97.11** **Crushing injury of great toe**

    ✓7ᵗʰ **S97.111** **Crushing injury of right great toe**

    ✓7ᵗʰ **S97.112** **Crushing injury of left great toe**

    ✓7ᵗʰ **S97.119** **Crushing injury of unspecified great toe** ▽

  ✓6ᵗʰ **S97.12** Crushing injury of lesser toe(s)

    ✓7ᵗʰ **S97.121** **Crushing injury of right lesser toe(s)**

    ✓7ᵗʰ **S97.122** **Crushing injury of left lesser toe(s)**

    ✓7ᵗʰ **S97.129** **Crushing injury of unspecified lesser toe(s)** ▽

✓5ᵗʰ **S97.8** Crushing injury of foot

  ✓x7ᵗʰ **S97.80** **Crushing injury of unspecified foot** ▽
      Crushing injury of foot NOS

  ✓x7ᵗʰ **S97.81** **Crushing injury of right foot**

  ✓x7ᵗʰ **S97.82** **Crushing injury of left foot**

✓4ᵗʰ **S98** Traumatic amputation of ankle and foot

An amputation not identified as partial or complete should be coded to complete

The appropriate 7th character is to be added to each code from category S98.
A   initial encounter
D   subsequent encounter
S   sequela

✓5ᵗʰ **S98.0** Traumatic amputation of foot at ankle level

  ✓6ᵗʰ **S98.01** Complete traumatic amputation of foot at ankle level

    ✓7ᵗʰ **S98.011** **Complete traumatic amputation of right foot at ankle level**

    ✓7ᵗʰ **S98.012** **Complete traumatic amputation of left foot at ankle level**

    ✓7ᵗʰ **S98.019** **Complete traumatic amputation of unspecified foot at ankle level** ▽

  ✓6ᵗʰ **S98.02** Partial traumatic amputation of foot at ankle level

    ✓7ᵗʰ **S98.021** **Partial traumatic amputation of right foot at ankle level**

    ✓7ᵗʰ **S98.022** **Partial traumatic amputation of left foot at ankle level**

    ✓7ᵗʰ **S98.029** **Partial traumatic amputation of unspecified foot at ankle level** ▽

✓5ᵗʰ **S98.1** Traumatic amputation of one toe

  ✓6ᵗʰ **S98.11** Complete traumatic amputation of great toe

    ✓7ᵗʰ **S98.111** **Complete traumatic amputation of right great toe**

    ✓7ᵗʰ **S98.112** **Complete traumatic amputation of left great toe**

    ✓7ᵗʰ **S98.119** **Complete traumatic amputation of unspecified great toe** ▽

  ✓6ᵗʰ **S98.12** Partial traumatic amputation of great toe

    ✓7ᵗʰ **S98.121** **Partial traumatic amputation of right great toe**

    ✓7ᵗʰ **S98.122** **Partial traumatic amputation of left great toe**

    ✓7ᵗʰ **S98.129** **Partial traumatic amputation of unspecified great toe** ▽

  ✓6ᵗʰ **S98.13** Complete traumatic amputation of one lesser toe
      Traumatic amputation of toe NOS

    ✓7ᵗʰ **S98.131** **Complete traumatic amputation of one right lesser toe**

    ✓7ᵗʰ **S98.132** **Complete traumatic amputation of one left lesser toe**

    ✓7ᵗʰ **S98.139** **Complete traumatic amputation of one unspecified lesser toe** ▽

  ✓6ᵗʰ **S98.14** Partial traumatic amputation of one lesser toe

    ✓7ᵗʰ **S98.141** **Partial traumatic amputation of one right lesser toe**

    ✓7ᵗʰ **S98.142** **Partial traumatic amputation of one left lesser toe**

    ✓7ᵗʰ **S98.149** **Partial traumatic amputation of one unspecified lesser toe** ▽

✓5ᵗʰ **S98.2** Traumatic amputation of two or more lesser toes

  ✓6ᵗʰ **S98.21** Complete traumatic amputation of two or more lesser toes

✓ Add'l Character Required ✓x7ᵗʰ Placeholder Alert RUG IV Special Care High Dx RUG IV Clinically Complex Dx RUG IV Special Care Low Dx Manifestation Code Other Specified Code ▽ Unspecified Code

ICD-10-CM 2016   **977**

√7ᵗʰ **S98.211** **Complete traumatic amputation of two or more right lesser toes**

√7ᵗʰ **S98.212** **Complete traumatic amputation of two or more left lesser toes**

√7ᵗʰ **S98.219** **Complete traumatic amputation of two or more unspecified lesser toes** ▽

√6ᵗʰ **S98.22** **Partial traumatic amputation of two or more lesser toes**

√7ᵗʰ **S98.221** **Partial traumatic amputation of two or more right lesser toes**

√7ᵗʰ **S98.222** **Partial traumatic amputation of two or more left lesser toes**

√7ᵗʰ **S98.229** **Partial traumatic amputation of two or more unspecified lesser toes** ▽

√5ᵗʰ **S98.3** **Traumatic amputation of midfoot**

√6ᵗʰ **S98.31** **Complete traumatic amputation of midfoot**

√7ᵗʰ **S98.311** **Complete traumatic amputation of right midfoot**

√7ᵗʰ **S98.312** **Complete traumatic amputation of left midfoot**

√7ᵗʰ **S98.319** **Complete traumatic amputation of unspecified midfoot** ▽

√6ᵗʰ **S98.32** **Partial traumatic amputation of midfoot**

√7ᵗʰ **S98.321** **Partial traumatic amputation of right midfoot**

√7ᵗʰ **S98.322** **Partial traumatic amputation of left midfoot**

√7ᵗʰ **S98.329** **Partial traumatic amputation of unspecified midfoot** ▽

√5ᵗʰ **S98.9** **Traumatic amputation of foot, level unspecified**

√6ᵗʰ **S98.91** **Complete traumatic amputation of foot, level unspecified**

√7ᵗʰ **S98.911** **Complete traumatic amputation of right foot, level unspecified** ▽

√7ᵗʰ **S98.912** **Complete traumatic amputation of left foot, level unspecified** ▽

√7ᵗʰ **S98.919** **Complete traumatic amputation of unspecified foot, level unspecified** ▽

√6ᵗʰ **S98.92** **Partial traumatic amputation of foot, level unspecified**

√7ᵗʰ **S98.921** **Partial traumatic amputation of right foot, level unspecified** ▽

√7ᵗʰ **S98.922** **Partial traumatic amputation of left foot, level unspecified** ▽

√7ᵗʰ **S98.929** **Partial traumatic amputation of unspecified foot, level unspecified** ▽

√4ᵗʰ **S99** **Other and unspecified injuries of ankle and foot**

> The appropriate 7th character is to be added to each code from category S99.
> A   initial encounter
> D   subsequent encounter
> S   sequela

√5ᵗʰ **S99.8** **Other specified injuries of ankle and foot**

√6ᵗʰ **S99.81** **Other specified injuries of ankle**

√7ᵗʰ **S99.811** **Other specified injuries of right ankle**

√7ᵗʰ **S99.812** **Other specified injuries of left ankle**

√7ᵗʰ **S99.819** **Other specified injuries of unspecified ankle** ▽

√6ᵗʰ **S99.82** **Other specified injuries of foot**

√7ᵗʰ **S99.821** **Other specified injuries of right foot**

√7ᵗʰ **S99.822** **Other specified injuries of left foot**

√7ᵗʰ **S99.829** **Other specified injuries of unspecified foot** ▽

√5ᵗʰ **S99.9** **Unspecified injury of ankle and foot**

√6ᵗʰ **S99.91** **Unspecified injury of ankle**

√7ᵗʰ **S99.911** **Unspecified injury of right ankle** ▽

√7ᵗʰ **S99.912** **Unspecified injury of left ankle** ▽

√7ᵗʰ **S99.919** **Unspecified injury of unspecified ankle** ▽

√6ᵗʰ **S99.92** **Unspecified injury of foot**

√7ᵗʰ **S99.921** **Unspecified injury of right foot** ▽

√7ᵗʰ **S99.922** **Unspecified injury of left foot** ▽

√7ᵗʰ **S99.929** **Unspecified injury of unspecified foot** ▽

Injury, Poisoning And Certain Other Consequences Of External Causes (T07-T88)

Injuries involving multiple body regions (T07)

EXCLUDES 1   burns and corrosions (T20-T32)
frostbite (T33-T34)
insect bite or sting, venomous (T63.4)
sunburn (L55.-)

T07 **Unspecified multiple injuries** ▽
EXCLUDES 1   injury NOS (T14)

Injury of unspecified body region (T14)

√4ᵗʰ **T14** **Injury of unspecified body region**
EXCLUDES 1   multiple unspecified injuries (T07)

T14.8 **Other injury of unspecified body region** ▽
Abrasion NOS
Contusion NOS
Crush injury NOS
Fracture NOS
Skin injury NOS
Vascular injury NOS

√5ᵗʰ **T14.9** **Unspecified injury**

T14.90 **Injury, unspecified** ▽
Injury NOS

T14.91 **Suicide attempt**
Attempted suicide NOS

Effects of foreign body entering through natural orifice (T15-T19)

EXCLUDES 2   foreign body accidentally left in operation wound (T81.5-)
foreign body in penetrating wound—See open wound by body region
residual foreign body in soft tissue (M79.5)
splinter, without open wound—See superficial injury by body region

√4ᵗʰ **T15** **Foreign body on external eye**
EXCLUDES 2   foreign body in penetrating wound of orbit and eye ball (S05.4-, S05.5-)
open wound of eyelid and periocular area (S01.1-)
retained foreign body in eyelid (H02.8-)
retained (old) foreign body in penetrating wound of orbit and eye ball (H05.5-, H44.6-, H44.7-)
superficial foreign body of eyelid and periocular area (S00.25-)

> The appropriate 7th character is to be added to each code from category T15.
> A   initial encounter
> D   subsequent encounter
> S   sequela

√5ᵗʰ **T15.0** **Foreign body in cornea**

√x7ᵗʰ **T15.00** **Foreign body in cornea, unspecified eye** ▽

√x7ᵗʰ **T15.01** **Foreign body in cornea, right eye**

√x7ᵗʰ **T15.02** **Foreign body in cornea, left eye**

√5ᵗʰ **T15.1** **Foreign body in conjunctival sac**

√x7ᵗʰ **T15.10** **Foreign body in conjunctival sac, unspecified eye** ▽

√x7ᵗʰ **T15.11** **Foreign body in conjunctival sac, right eye**

√x7ᵗʰ **T15.12** **Foreign body in conjunctival sac, left eye**

√5ᵗʰ **T15.8** **Foreign body in other and multiple parts of external eye**
Foreign body in lacrimal punctum

√x7ᵗʰ **T15.80** **Foreign body in other and multiple parts of external eye, unspecified eye** ▽

√x7ᵗʰ **T15.81** **Foreign body in other and multiple parts of external eye, right eye**

√x7ᵗʰ **T15.82** **Foreign body in other and multiple parts of external eye, left eye**

√5ᵗʰ **T15.9** **Foreign body on external eye, part unspecified**

√x7ᵗʰ **T15.90** **Foreign body on external eye, part unspecified, unspecified eye** ▽

√x7ᵗʰ **T15.91** **Foreign body on external eye, part unspecified, right eye** ▽

√x7ᵗʰ **T15.92** **Foreign body on external eye, part unspecified, left eye** ▽

Ⓝ Newborn   Ⓟ Pediatric   Ⓜ Maternity   Ⓐ Adult   **RIC** RIC Dx   **NC Dx** Noncancer Dx   **PD▸** Primary Dx   **CC** RIC CC Condition   ▸◂ Revised Text   ● New Code   ▲ Revised Code Title

978   ICD-10-CM 2016

✓4ᵗʰ T16　Foreign body in ear
　　Foreign body in auditory canal

> The appropriate 7th character is to be added to each code from category T16.
> A　　initial encounter
> D　　subsequent encounter
> S　　sequela

✓x7ᵗʰ T16.1　Foreign body in right ear

✓x7ᵗʰ T16.2　Foreign body in left ear

✓x7ᵗʰ T16.9　Foreign body in ear, unspecified ear ▽

✓4ᵗʰ T17　Foreign body in respiratory tract

> The appropriate 7th character is to be added to each code from category T17.
> A　　initial encounter
> D　　subsequent encounter
> S　　sequela

✓x7ᵗʰ T17.0　Foreign body in nasal sinus

✓x7ᵗʰ T17.1　Foreign body in nostril
　　Foreign body in nose NOS

✓5ᵗʰ T17.2　Foreign body in pharynx
　　Foreign body in nasopharynx
　　Foreign body in throat NOS

　✓6ᵗʰ T17.20　Unspecified foreign body in pharynx

　　　✓7ᵗʰ T17.200　Unspecified foreign body in pharynx causing asphyxiation ▽

　　　✓7ᵗʰ T17.208　Unspecified foreign body in pharynx causing other injury ▽

　✓6ᵗʰ T17.21　Gastric contents in pharynx
　　　Aspiration of gastric contents into pharynx
　　　Vomitus in pharynx

　　　✓7ᵗʰ T17.210　Gastric contents in pharynx causing asphyxiation

　　　✓7ᵗʰ T17.218　Gastric contents in pharynx causing other injury

　✓6ᵗʰ T17.22　Food in pharynx
　　　Bones in pharynx
　　　Seeds in pharynx

　　　✓7ᵗʰ T17.220　Food in pharynx causing asphyxiation

　　　✓7ᵗʰ T17.228　Food in pharynx causing other injury

　✓6ᵗʰ T17.29　Other foreign object in pharynx

　　　✓7ᵗʰ T17.290　Other foreign object in pharynx causing asphyxiation

　　　✓7ᵗʰ T17.298　Other foreign object in pharynx causing other injury

✓5ᵗʰ T17.3　Foreign body in larynx

　✓6ᵗʰ T17.30　Unspecified foreign body in larynx

　　　✓7ᵗʰ T17.300　Unspecified foreign body in larynx causing asphyxiation ▽

　　　✓7ᵗʰ T17.308　Unspecified foreign body in larynx causing other injury ▽

　✓6ᵗʰ T17.31　Gastric contents in larynx
　　　Aspiration of gastric contents into larynx
　　　Vomitus in larynx

　　　✓7ᵗʰ T17.310　Gastric contents in larynx causing asphyxiation

　　　✓7ᵗʰ T17.318　Gastric contents in larynx causing other injury

　✓6ᵗʰ T17.32　Food in larynx
　　　Bones in larynx
　　　Seeds in larynx

　　　✓7ᵗʰ T17.320　Food in larynx causing asphyxiation

　　　✓7ᵗʰ T17.328　Food in larynx causing other injury

　✓6ᵗʰ T17.39　Other foreign object in larynx

　　　✓7ᵗʰ T17.390　Other foreign object in larynx causing asphyxiation

　　　✓7ᵗʰ T17.398　Other foreign object in larynx causing other injury

✓5ᵗʰ T17.4　Foreign body in trachea

　✓6ᵗʰ T17.40　Unspecified foreign body in trachea

　　　✓7ᵗʰ T17.400　Unspecified foreign body in trachea causing asphyxiation ▽

　　　✓7ᵗʰ T17.408　Unspecified foreign body in trachea causing other injury ▽

　✓6ᵗʰ T17.41　Gastric contents in trachea
　　　Aspiration of gastric contents into trachea
　　　Vomitus in trachea

　　　✓7ᵗʰ T17.410　Gastric contents in trachea causing asphyxiation

　　　✓7ᵗʰ T17.418　Gastric contents in trachea causing other injury

　✓6ᵗʰ T17.42　Food in trachea
　　　Bones in trachea
　　　Seeds in trachea

　　　✓7ᵗʰ T17.420　Food in trachea causing asphyxiation

　　　✓7ᵗʰ T17.428　Food in trachea causing other injury

　✓6ᵗʰ T17.49　Other foreign object in trachea

　　　✓7ᵗʰ T17.490　Other foreign object in trachea causing asphyxiation

　　　✓7ᵗʰ T17.498　Other foreign object in trachea causing other injury

✓5ᵗʰ T17.5　Foreign body in bronchus

　✓6ᵗʰ T17.50　Unspecified foreign body in bronchus

　　　✓7ᵗʰ T17.500　Unspecified foreign body in bronchus causing asphyxiation ▽

　　　✓7ᵗʰ T17.508　Unspecified foreign body in bronchus causing other injury ▽

　✓6ᵗʰ T17.51　Gastric contents in bronchus
　　　Aspiration of gastric contents into bronchus
　　　Vomitus in bronchus

　　　✓7ᵗʰ T17.510　Gastric contents in bronchus causing asphyxiation

　　　✓7ᵗʰ T17.518　Gastric contents in bronchus causing other injury

　✓6ᵗʰ T17.52　Food in bronchus
　　　Bones in bronchusSeeds in bronchus

　　　✓7ᵗʰ T17.520　Food in bronchus causing asphyxiation

　　　✓7ᵗʰ T17.528　Food in bronchus causing other injury

　✓6ᵗʰ T17.59　Other foreign object in bronchus

　　　✓7ᵗʰ T17.590　Other foreign object in bronchus causing asphyxiation

　　　✓7ᵗʰ T17.598　Other foreign object in bronchus causing other injury

✓5ᵗʰ T17.8　Foreign body in other parts of respiratory tract
　　Foreign body in bronchioles
　　Foreign body in lung

　✓6ᵗʰ T17.80　Unspecified foreign body in other parts of respiratory tract

　　　✓7ᵗʰ T17.800　Unspecified foreign body in other parts of respiratory tract causing asphyxiation ▽

　　　✓7ᵗʰ T17.808　Unspecified foreign body in other parts of respiratory tract causing other injury ▽

　✓6ᵗʰ T17.81　Gastric contents in other parts of respiratory tract
　　　Aspiration of gastric contents into other parts of respiratory tract
　　　Vomitus in other parts of respiratory tract

　　　✓7ᵗʰ T17.810　Gastric contents in other parts of respiratory tract causing asphyxiation

　　　✓7ᵗʰ T17.818　Gastric contents in other parts of respiratory tract causing other injury

　✓6ᵗʰ T17.82　Food in other parts of respiratory tract
　　　Bones in other parts of respiratory tract
　　　Seeds in other parts of respiratory tract

　　　✓7ᵗʰ T17.820　Food in other parts of respiratory tract causing asphyxiation

　　　✓7ᵗʰ T17.828　Food in other parts of respiratory tract causing other injury

　✓6ᵗʰ T17.89　Other foreign object in other parts of respiratory tract

　　　✓7ᵗʰ T17.890　Other foreign object in other parts of respiratory tract causing asphyxiation

　　　✓7ᵗʰ T17.898　Other foreign object in other parts of respiratory tract causing other injury

✓5ᵗʰ T17.9　Foreign body in respiratory tract, part unspecified

　✓6ᵗʰ T17.90　Unspecified foreign body in respiratory tract, part unspecified

　　　✓7ᵗʰ T17.900　Unspecified foreign body in respiratory tract, part unspecified causing asphyxiation ▽

✓ Add'l Character Required　✓x7ᵗʰ Placeholder Alert　RUG IV Special Care High Dx　RUG IV Clinically Complex Dx　RUG IV Special Care Low Dx　Manifestation Code　Other Specified Code　▽ Unspecified Code

✓7th **T17.908** **Unspecified foreign body in respiratory tract, part unspecified** causing other injury ▽

✓6th **T17.91** Gastric contents in respiratory tract, part unspecified
Aspiration of gastric contents into respiratory tract, part unspecified
Vomitus in trachea respiratory tract, part unspecified

  ✓7th **T17.910** **Gastric contents in respiratory tract, part unspecified** causing asphyxiation ▽

  ✓7th **T17.918** **Gastric contents in respiratory tract, part unspecified** causing other injury ▽

✓6th **T17.92** Food in respiratory tract, part unspecified
Bones in respiratory tract, part unspecified
Seeds in respiratory tract, part unspecified

  ✓7th **T17.920** **Food in respiratory tract, part unspecified** causing asphyxiation ▽

  ✓7th **T17.928** **Food in respiratory tract, part unspecified** causing other injury ▽

✓6th **T17.99** Other foreign object in respiratory tract, part unspecified

  ✓7th **T17.990** **Other foreign object in respiratory tract, part unspecified in** causing asphyxiation ▽

  ✓7th **T17.998** **Other foreign object in respiratory tract, part unspecified** causing other injury ▽

✓4th **T18** **Foreign body in alimentary tract**
  EXCLUDES 2 foreign body in pharynx (T17.2-)

> The appropriate 7th character is to be added to each code from category T18.
> A   initial encounter
> D   subsequent encounter
> S   sequela

✓x7th **T18.0** **Foreign body in** mouth

✓5th **T18.1** **Foreign body in** esophagus
  EXCLUDES 2 foreign body in respiratory tract (T17.-)

✓6th **T18.10** Unspecified foreign body in esophagus

  ✓7th **T18.100** **Unspecified foreign body in esophagus** causing compression of trachea ▽
Unspecified foreign body in esophagus causing obstruction of respiration

  ✓7th **T18.108** **Unspecified foreign body in esophagus** causing other injury ▽

✓6th **T18.11** Gastric contents in esophagus
Vomitus in esophagus

  ✓7th **T18.110** **Gastric contents in esophagus** causing compression of trachea
Gastric contents in esophagus causing obstruction of respiration

  ✓7th **T18.118** **Gastric contents in esophagus** causing other injury

✓6th **T18.12** Food in esophagus
Bones in esophagus
Seeds in esophagus

  ✓7th **T18.120** **Food in esophagus** causing compression of trachea
Food in esophagus causing obstruction of respiration

  ✓7th **T18.128** **Food in esophagus** causing other injury

✓6th **T18.19** Other foreign object in esophagus
AHA: 2015, 1Q, 23

  ✓7th **T18.190** **Other foreign object in esophagus** causing compression of trachea
Other foreign body in esophagus causing obstruction of respiration

  ✓7th **T18.198** **Other foreign object in esophagus** causing other injury

✓x7th **T18.2** **Foreign body in** stomach

✓x7th **T18.3** **Foreign body in** small intestine

✓x7th **T18.4** **Foreign body in** colon

✓x7th **T18.5** **Foreign body in** anus and rectum
Foreign body in rectosigmoid (junction)

✓x7th **T18.8** **Foreign body in other** parts of alimentary tract

✓x7th **T18.9** **Foreign body of alimentary tract, part unspecified** ▽
Foreign body in digestive system NOS
Swallowed foreign body NOS

✓4th **T19** **Foreign body in genitourinary tract**
  EXCLUDES 2 complications due to implanted mesh (T83.7-)
    mechanical complications of contraceptive device (intrauterine) (vaginal) (T83.3-)
    presence of contraceptive device (intrauterine) (vaginal) (Z97.5)

> The appropriate 7th character is to be added to each code from category T19.
> A   initial encounter
> D   subsequent encounter
> S   sequela

✓x7th **T19.0** **Foreign body in** urethra

✓x7th **T19.1** **Foreign body in** bladder

✓x7th **T19.2** **Foreign body in** vulva and vagina ♀

✓x7th **T19.3** **Foreign body in** uterus ♀

✓x7th **T19.4** **Foreign body in** penis ♂

✓x7th **T19.8** **Foreign body in other parts of genitourinary tract**

✓x7th **T19.9** **Foreign body in genitourinary tract, part unspecified** ▽

Burns and corrosions (T20-T32)

INCLUDES burns (thermal) from electrical heating appliances
burns (thermal) from electricity
burns (thermal) from flame
burns (thermal) from friction
burns (thermal) from hot air and hot gases
burns (thermal) from hot objects
burns (thermal) from lightning
burns (thermal) from radiation
chemical burn [corrosion] (external) (internal)
scalds

EXCLUDES 2 erythema [dermatitis] ab igne (L59.0)
radiation-related disorders of the skin and subcutaneous tissue (L55-L59)
sunburn (L55.-)

Burns and corrosions of external body surface, specified by site (T20-T25)

INCLUDES burns and corrosions of first degree [erythema]
burns and corrosions of second degree [blisters] [epidermal loss]
burns and corrosions of third degree [deep necrosis of underlying tissue] [full-thickness skin loss]

Use additional code from category T31 or T32 to identify extent of body surface involved

✓4th **T20** **Burn and corrosion of head, face, and neck**
  EXCLUDES 2 burn and corrosion of ear drum (T28.41, T28.91)
    burn and corrosion of eye and adnexa (T26.-)
    burn and corrosion of mouth and pharynx (T28.0)
  AHA: 2015, 1Q, 18-19

> The appropriate 7th character is to be added to each code from category T20.
> A   initial encounter
> D   subsequent encounter
> S   sequela

✓5th **T20.0** Burn of unspecified degree of head, face, and neck
Use additional external cause code to identify the source, place and intent of the burn (X00-X19, X75-X77, X96-X98, Y92)

✓x7th **T20.00** **Burn of unspecified degree of head, face, and neck, unspecified site** ▽

✓6th **T20.01** **Burn of unspecified degree of ear [any part, except ear drum]**
  EXCLUDES 2 burn of ear drum (T28.41-)

  ✓7th **T20.011** **Burn of unspecified degree of right ear [any part, except ear drum]** ▽

  ✓7th **T20.012** **Burn of unspecified degree of left ear [any part, except ear drum]** ▽

  ✓7th **T20.019** **Burn of unspecified degree of unspecified ear [any part, except ear drum]** ▽

✓x7th **T20.02** **Burn of unspecified degree of** lip(s) ▽

✓x7th **T20.03** **Burn of unspecified degree of** chin ▽

✓x7th **T20.04** **Burn of unspecified degree of** nose (septum) ▽

✓x7th **T20.05** **Burn of unspecified degree of** scalp [any part] ▽

✓x7th **T20.06** **Burn of unspecified degree of** forehead and cheek ▽

√x7ᵗʰ **T20.07** Burn of unspecified degree of neck ▽

√x7ᵗʰ **T20.09** Burn of unspecified degree of multiple sites of head, face, and neck ▽

√5ᵗʰ **T20.1** Burn of first degree of head, face, and neck
Use additional external cause code to identify the source, place and intent of the burn (X00-X19, X75-X77, X96-X98, Y92)

√x7ᵗʰ **T20.10** Burn of first degree of head, face, and neck, unspecified site ▽

√6ᵗʰ **T20.11** Burn of first degree of ear [any part, except ear drum]
EXCLUDES 2 burn of ear drum (T28.41-)

√7ᵗʰ **T20.111** Burn of first degree of right ear [any part, except ear drum]

√7ᵗʰ **T20.112** Burn of first degree of left ear [any part, except ear drum]

√7ᵗʰ **T20.119** Burn of first degree of unspecified ear [any part, except ear drum] ▽

√x7ᵗʰ **T20.12** Burn of first degree of lip(s)

√x7ᵗʰ **T20.13** Burn of first degree of chin

√x7ᵗʰ **T20.14** Burn of first degree of nose (septum)

√x7ᵗʰ **T20.15** Burn of first degree of scalp [any part]

√x7ᵗʰ **T20.16** Burn of first degree of forehead and cheek

√x7ᵗʰ **T20.17** Burn of first degree of neck

√x7ᵗʰ **T20.19** Burn of first degree of multiple sites of head, face, and neck

√5ᵗʰ **T20.2** Burn of second degree of head, face, and neck
Use additional external cause code to identify the source, place and intent of the burn (X00-X19, X75-X77, X96-X98, Y92)

7 √x7ᵗʰ **T20.20** Burn of second degree of head, face, and neck, unspecified site ▽

√6ᵗʰ **T20.21** Burn of second degree of ear [any part, except ear drum]
EXCLUDES 2 burn of ear drum (T28.41-)

7 √7ᵗʰ **T20.211** Burn of second degree of right ear [any part, except ear drum]

7 √7ᵗʰ **T20.212** Burn of second degree of left ear [any part, except ear drum]

7 √7ᵗʰ **T20.219** Burn of second degree of unspecified ear [any part, except ear drum] ▽

7 √x7ᵗʰ **T20.22** Burn of second degree of lip(s)

7 √x7ᵗʰ **T20.23** Burn of second degree of chin

7 √x7ᵗʰ **T20.24** Burn of second degree of nose (septum)

7 √x7ᵗʰ **T20.25** Burn of second degree of scalp [any part]

7 √x7ᵗʰ **T20.26** Burn of second degree of forehead and cheek

7 √x7ᵗʰ **T20.27** Burn of second degree of neck

7 √x7ᵗʰ **T20.29** Burn of second degree of multiple sites of head, face, and neck

√5ᵗʰ **T20.3** Burn of third degree of head, face, and neck
Use additional external cause code to identify the source, place and intent of the burn (X00-X19, X75-X77, X96-X98, Y92)

7 √x7ᵗʰ **T20.30** Burn of third degree of head, face, and neck, unspecified site ▽

√6ᵗʰ **T20.31** Burn of third degree of ear [any part, except ear drum]
EXCLUDES 2 burn of ear drum (T28.41-)
AHA: 2015, 1Q, 18

7 √7ᵗʰ **T20.311** Burn of third degree of right ear [any part, except ear drum]

7 √7ᵗʰ **T20.312** Burn of third degree of left ear [any part, except ear drum]

7 √7ᵗʰ **T20.319** Burn of third degree of unspecified ear [any part, except ear drum] ▽

7 √x7ᵗʰ **T20.32** Burn of third degree of lip(s)

7 √x7ᵗʰ **T20.33** Burn of third degree of chin

7 √x7ᵗʰ **T20.34** Burn of third degree of nose (septum)

7 √x7ᵗʰ **T20.35** Burn of third degree of scalp [any part]

7 √x7ᵗʰ **T20.36** Burn of third degree of forehead and cheek

7 √x7ᵗʰ **T20.37** Burn of third degree of neck

7 √x7ᵗʰ **T20.39** Burn of third degree of multiple sites of head, face, and neck

√5ᵗʰ **T20.4** Corrosion of unspecified degree of head, face, and neck
Code first (T51-T65) to identify chemical and intent
Use additional external cause code to identify place (Y92)

√x7ᵗʰ **T20.40** Corrosion of unspecified degree of head, face, and neck, unspecified site ▽

√6ᵗʰ **T20.41** Corrosion of unspecified degree of ear [any part, except ear drum]
EXCLUDES 2 corrosion of ear drum (T28.91-)

√7ᵗʰ **T20.411** Corrosion of unspecified degree of right ear [any part, except ear drum] ▽

√7ᵗʰ **T20.412** Corrosion of unspecified degree of left ear [any part, except ear drum] ▽

√7ᵗʰ **T20.419** Corrosion of unspecified degree of unspecified ear [any part, except ear drum] ▽

√x7ᵗʰ **T20.42** Corrosion of unspecified degree of lip(s) ▽

√x7ᵗʰ **T20.43** Corrosion of unspecified degree of chin ▽

√x7ᵗʰ **T20.44** Corrosion of unspecified degree of nose (septum) ▽

√x7ᵗʰ **T20.45** Corrosion of unspecified degree of scalp [any part] ▽

√x7ᵗʰ **T20.46** Corrosion of unspecified degree of forehead and cheek ▽

√x7ᵗʰ **T20.47** Corrosion of unspecified degree of neck ▽

√x7ᵗʰ **T20.49** Corrosion of unspecified degree of multiple sites of head, face, and neck ▽

√5ᵗʰ **T20.5** Corrosion of first degree of head, face, and neck
Code first (T51-T65) to identify chemical and intent
Use additional external cause code to identify place (Y92)

√x7ᵗʰ **T20.50** Corrosion of first degree of head, face, and neck, unspecified site ▽

√6ᵗʰ **T20.51** Corrosion of first degree of ear [any part, except ear drum]
EXCLUDES 2 corrosion of ear drum (T28.91-)

√7ᵗʰ **T20.511** Corrosion of first degree of right ear [any part, except ear drum]

√7ᵗʰ **T20.512** Corrosion of first degree of left ear [any part, except ear drum]

√7ᵗʰ **T20.519** Corrosion of first degree of unspecified ear [any part, except ear drum] ▽

√x7ᵗʰ **T20.52** Corrosion of first degree of lip(s)

√x7ᵗʰ **T20.53** Corrosion of first degree of chin

√x7ᵗʰ **T20.54** Corrosion of first degree of nose (septum)

√x7ᵗʰ **T20.55** Corrosion of first degree of scalp [any part]

√x7ᵗʰ **T20.56** Corrosion of first degree of forehead and cheek

√x7ᵗʰ **T20.57** Corrosion of first degree of neck

√x7ᵗʰ **T20.59** Corrosion of first degree of multiple sites of head, face, and neck

√5ᵗʰ **T20.6** Corrosion of second degree of head, face, and neck
Code first (T51-T65) to identify chemical and intent
Use additional external cause code to identify place (Y92)

√x7ᵗʰ **T20.60** Corrosion of second degree of head, face, and neck, unspecified site ▽

√6ᵗʰ **T20.61** Corrosion of second degree of ear [any part, except ear drum]
EXCLUDES 2 corrosion of ear drum (T28.91-)

√7ᵗʰ **T20.611** Corrosion of second degree of right ear [any part, except ear drum]

√7ᵗʰ **T20.612** Corrosion of second degree of left ear [any part, except ear drum]

√7ᵗʰ **T20.619** Corrosion of second degree of unspecified ear [any part, except ear drum] ▽

√x7ᵗʰ **T20.62** Corrosion of second degree of lip(s)

√x7ᵗʰ **T20.63** Corrosion of second degree of chin

√x7ᵗʰ **T20.64** Corrosion of second degree of nose (septum)

√x7ᵗʰ **T20.65** Corrosion of second degree of scalp [any part]

√x7ᵗʰ **T20.66** Corrosion of second degree of forehead and cheek

√x7ᵗʰ **T20.67** Corrosion of second degree of neck

√x7ᵗʰ **T20.69** Corrosion of second degree of multiple sites of head, face, and neck

---

7 Clinically Complex = With 7th character indicating a subsequent encounter

☑ Add'l Character Required   √x7ᵗʰ Placeholder Alert   RUG IV Special Care High Dx   RUG IV Clinically Complex Dx   RUG IV Special Care Low Dx   Manifestation Code   Other Specified Code   ▽Unspecified Code

ICD-10-CM 2016   981

✓5ᵗʰ **T20.7** **Corrosion of** third degree **of head, face, and neck**
Code first (T51-T65) to identify chemical and intent
Use additional external cause code to identify place (Y92)

✓x7ᵗʰ **T20.70** **Corrosion of third degree of head, face, and neck, unspecified site** ▽

✓6ᵗʰ **T20.71** **Corrosion of third degree of** ear **[any part, except ear drum]**
EXCLUDES 2 corrosion of ear drum (T28.91-)

✓7ᵗʰ **T20.711** **Corrosion of third degree of** right ear **[any part, except ear drum]**

✓7ᵗʰ **T20.712** **Corrosion of third degree of** left ear **[any part, except ear drum]**

✓7ᵗʰ **T20.719** **Corrosion of third degree of unspecified ear [any part, except ear drum]** ▽

✓x7ᵗʰ **T20.72** **Corrosion of third degree of** lip(s)

✓x7ᵗʰ **T20.73** **Corrosion of third degree of** chin

✓x7ᵗʰ **T20.74** **Corrosion of third degree of** nose **(septum)**

✓x7ᵗʰ **T20.75** **Corrosion of third degree of** scalp **[any part]**

✓x7ᵗʰ **T20.76** **Corrosion of third degree of** forehead and cheek

✓x7ᵗʰ **T20.77** **Corrosion of third degree of** neck

✓x7ᵗʰ **T20.79** **Corrosion of third degree of** multiple sites **of head, face, and neck**

✓4ᵗʰ **T21** **Burn and corrosion of trunk**
Burns and corrosion of hip region
EXCLUDES 2 burns and corrosion of axilla (T22.- with fifth character 4)
burns and corrosion of scapular region (T22.- with fifth character 6)
burns and corrosion of shoulder (T22.- with fifth character 5)

The appropriate 7th character is to be added to each code from category T21.
A   initial encounter
D   subsequent encounter
S   sequela

✓5ᵗʰ **T21.0** **Burn of** unspecified degree **of trunk**
Use additional external cause code to identify the source, place and intent of the burn (X00-X19, X75-X77, X96-X98, Y92)

✓x7ᵗʰ **T21.00** **Burn of unspecified degree of trunk, unspecified site** ▽

✓x7ᵗʰ **T21.01** **Burn of unspecified degree of** chest wall ▽
Burn of of unspecified degree of breast

✓x7ᵗʰ **T21.02** **Burn of unspecified degree of** abdominal wall ▽
Burn of unspecified degree of flank
Burn of unspecified degree of groin

✓x7ᵗʰ **T21.03** **Burn of unspecified degree of** upper back ▽
Burn of unspecified degree of interscapular region

✓x7ᵗʰ **T21.04** **Burn of unspecified degree of** lower back ▽

✓x7ᵗʰ **T21.05** **Burn of unspecified degree of** buttock ▽
Burn of unspecified degree of anus

✓x7ᵗʰ **T21.06** **Burn of unspecified degree of** male genital region ♂▽
Burn of unspecified degree of penis
Burn of unspecified degree of scrotum
Burn of unspecified degree of testis

✓x7ᵗʰ **T21.07** **Burn of unspecified degree of** female genital region ♀▽
Burn of unspecified degree of labium (majus) (minus)
Burn of unspecified degree of perineum
Burn of unspecified degree of vulva
EXCLUDES 2 burn of vagina (T28.3)

✓x7ᵗʰ **T21.09** **Burn of unspecified degree of other site of trunk** ▽

✓5ᵗʰ **T21.1** **Burn of** first degree **of trunk**
Use additional external cause code to identify the source, place and intent of the burn (X00-X19, X75-X77, X96-X98, Y92)

✓x7ᵗʰ **T21.10** **Burn of first degree of trunk, unspecified site** ▽

✓x7ᵗʰ **T21.11** **Burn of first degree of** chest wall
Burn of first degree of breast

✓x7ᵗʰ **T21.12** **Burn of first degree of** abdominal wall
Burn of first degree of flank
Burn of first degree of groin

✓x7ᵗʰ **T21.13** **Burn of first degree of** upper back
Burn of first degree of interscapular region

✓x7ᵗʰ **T21.14** **Burn of first degree of** lower back

✓x7ᵗʰ **T21.15** **Burn of first degree of** buttock
Burn of first degree of anus

✓x7ᵗʰ **T21.16** **Burn of first degree of** male genital region ♂
Burn of first degree of penis
Burn of first degree of scrotum
Burn of first degree of testis

✓x7ᵗʰ **T21.17** **Burn of first degree of** female genital region ♀
Burn of first degree of labium (majus) (minus)
Burn of first degree of perineum
Burn of first degree of vulva
EXCLUDES 2 burn of vagina (T28.3)

✓x7ᵗʰ **T21.19** **Burn of first degree of other site of trunk**

✓5ᵗʰ **T21.2** **Burn of** second degree **of trunk**
Use additional external cause code to identify the source, place and intent of the burn (X00-X19, X75-X77, X96-X98, Y92)

7 ✓x7ᵗʰ **T21.20** **Burn of second degree of trunk, unspecified site** ▽

7 ✓x7ᵗʰ **T21.21** **Burn of second degree of** chest wall
Burn of second degree of breast

7 ✓x7ᵗʰ **T21.22** **Burn of second degree of** abdominal wall
Burn of second degree of flank
Burn of second degree of groin

7 ✓x7ᵗʰ **T21.23** **Burn of second degree of** upper back
Burn of second degree of interscapular region

7 ✓x7ᵗʰ **T21.24** **Burn of second degree of** lower back

7 ✓x7ᵗʰ **T21.25** **Burn of second degree of** buttock
Burn of second degree of anus

7 ✓x7ᵗʰ **T21.26** **Burn of second degree of** male genital region ♂
Burn of second degree of penis
Burn of second degree of scrotum
Burn of second degree of testis

7 ✓x7ᵗʰ **T21.27** **Burn of second degree of** female genital region ♀
Burn of second degree of labium (majus) (minus)
Burn of second degree of perineum
Burn of second degree of vulva
EXCLUDES 2 burn of vagina (T28.3)

7 ✓x7ᵗʰ **T21.29** **Burn of second degree of other site of trunk**

✓5ᵗʰ **T21.3** **Burn of** third degree **of trunk**
Use additional external cause code to identify the source, place and intent of the burn (X00-X19, X75-X77, X96-X98, Y92)

7 ✓x7ᵗʰ **T21.30** **Burn of third degree of trunk, unspecified site** ▽

7 ✓x7ᵗʰ **T21.31** **Burn of third degree of** chest wall
Burn of third degree of breast

7 ✓x7ᵗʰ **T21.32** **Burn of third degree of** abdominal wall
Burn of third degree of flank
Burn of third degree of groin

7 ✓x7ᵗʰ **T21.33** **Burn of third degree of** upper back
Burn of third degree of interscapular region

7 ✓x7ᵗʰ **T21.34** **Burn of third degree of** lower back

7 ✓x7ᵗʰ **T21.35** **Burn of third degree of** buttock
Burn of third degree of anus

7 ✓x7ᵗʰ **T21.36** **Burn of third degree of** male genital region ♂
Burn of third degree of penis
Burn of third degree of scrotum
Burn of third degree of testis

7 ✓x7ᵗʰ **T21.37** **Burn of third degree of** female genital region ♀
Burn of third degree of labium (majus) (minus)
Burn of third degree of perineum
Burn of third degree of vulva
EXCLUDES 2 burn of vagina (T28.3)

7 ✓x7ᵗʰ **T21.39** **Burn of third degree of other site of trunk**

✓5ᵗʰ **T21.4** **Corrosion of** unspecified degree **of trunk**
Code first (T51-T65) to identify chemical and intent
Use additional external cause code to identify place (Y92)

✓x7ᵗʰ **T21.40** **Corrosion of unspecified degree of trunk, unspecified site** ▽

✓x7ᵗʰ **T21.41** **Corrosion of unspecified degree of** chest wall ▽
Corrosion of unspecified degree of breast

✓x7ᵗʰ **T21.42** **Corrosion of unspecified degree of** abdominal wall ▽
Corrosion of unspecified degree of flank
Corrosion of unspecified degree of groin

✓x7ᵗʰ **T21.43** **Corrosion of unspecified degree of** upper back ▽
Corrosion of unspecified degree of interscapular region

✓x7ᵗʰ **T21.44** **Corrosion of unspecified degree of** lower back ▽

---

⁷ Clinically Complex = With 7th character indicating a subsequent encounter

√x7ᵗʰ **T21.45** **Corrosion of unspecified degree of** buttock ▽
Corrosion of unspecified degree of anus

√x7ᵗʰ **T21.46** **Corrosion of unspecified degree of** male genital ♂▽ **region**
Corrosion of unspecified degree of penis
Corrosion of unspecified degree of scrotum
Corrosion of unspecified degree of testis

√x7ᵗʰ **T21.47** **Corrosion of unspecified degree of** female ♀▽ **genital region**
Corrosion of unspecified degree of labium (majus) (minus)
Corrosion of unspecified degree of perineum
Corrosion of unspecified degree of vulva
EXCLUDES 2   corrosion of vagina (T28.8)

√x7ᵗʰ **T21.49** **Corrosion of unspecified degree of other site of** ▽ **trunk**

√5ᵗʰ **T21.5** **Corrosion of** first degree **of trunk**
Code first (T51-T65) to identify chemical and intent
Use additional external cause code to identify place (Y92)

√x7ᵗʰ **T21.50** **Corrosion of first degree of trunk, unspecified site** ▽

√x7ᵗʰ **T21.51** **Corrosion of first degree of** chest wall
Corrosion of first degree of breast

√x7ᵗʰ **T21.52** **Corrosion of first degree of** abdominal wall
Corrosion of first degree of flank
Corrosion of first degree of groin

√x7ᵗʰ **T21.53** **Corrosion of first degree of** upper back
Corrosion of first degree of interscapular region

√x7ᵗʰ **T21.54** **Corrosion of first degree of** lower back

√x7ᵗʰ **T21.55** **Corrosion of first degree of** buttock
Corrosion of first degree of anus

√x7ᵗʰ **T21.56** **Corrosion of first degree of** male genital region ♂
Corrosion of first degree of penis
Corrosion of first degree of scrotum
Corrosion of first degree of testis

√x7ᵗʰ **T21.57** **Corrosion of first degree of** female genital region ♀
Corrosion of first degree of labium (majus) (minus)
Corrosion of first degree of perineum
Corrosion of first degree of vulva
EXCLUDES 2   corrosion of vagina (T28.8)

√x7ᵗʰ **T21.59** **Corrosion of first degree of other site of trunk**

√5ᵗʰ **T21.6** **Corrosion of** second degree **of trunk**
Code first (T51-T65) to identify chemical and intent
Use additional external cause code to identify place (Y92)

√x7ᵗʰ **T21.60** **Corrosion of second degree of trunk, unspecified site** ▽

√x7ᵗʰ **T21.61** **Corrosion of second degree of** chest wall
Corrosion of second degree of breast

√x7ᵗʰ **T21.62** **Corrosion of second degree of** abdominal wall
Corrosion of second degree of flank
Corrosion of second degree of groin

√x7ᵗʰ **T21.63** **Corrosion of second degree of** upper back
Corrosion of second degree of interscapular region

√x7ᵗʰ **T21.64** **Corrosion of second degree of** lower back

√x7ᵗʰ **T21.65** **Corrosion of second degree of** buttock
Corrosion of second degree of anus

√x7ᵗʰ **T21.66** **Corrosion of second degree of** male genital region ♂
Corrosion of second degree of penis
Corrosion of second degree of scrotum
Corrosion of second degree of testis

√x7ᵗʰ **T21.67** **Corrosion of second degree of** female genital ♀ **region**
Corrosion of second degree of labium (majus) (minus)
Corrosion of second degree of perineum
Corrosion of second degree of vulva
EXCLUDES 2   corrosion of vagina (T28.8)

√x7ᵗʰ **T21.69** **Corrosion of second degree of other site of trunk**

√5ᵗʰ **T21.7** **Corrosion of** third degree **of trunk**
Code first (T51-T65) to identify chemical and intent
Use additional external cause code to identify place (Y92)

√x7ᵗʰ **T21.70** **Corrosion of third degree of trunk, unspecified site** ▽

√x7ᵗʰ **T21.71** **Corrosion of third degree of** chest wall
Corrosion of third degree of breast

√x7ᵗʰ **T21.72** **Corrosion of third degree of** abdominal wall
Corrosion of third degree of flank
Corrosion of third degree of groin

√x7ᵗʰ **T21.73** **Corrosion of third degree of** upper back
Corrosion of third degree of interscapular region

√x7ᵗʰ **T21.74** **Corrosion of third degree of** lower back

√x7ᵗʰ **T21.75** **Corrosion of third degree of** buttock
Corrosion of third degree of anus

√x7ᵗʰ **T21.76** **Corrosion of third degree of** male genital region ♂
Corrosion of third degree of penis
Corrosion of third degree of scrotum
Corrosion of third degree of testis

√x7ᵗʰ **T21.77** **Corrosion of third degree of** female genital region ♀
Corrosion of third degree of labium (majus) (minus)
Corrosion of third degree of perineum
Corrosion of third degree of vulva
EXCLUDES 2   corrosion of vagina (T28.8)

√x7ᵗʰ **T21.79** **Corrosion of third degree of other site of trunk**

√4ᵗʰ **T22** **Burn and corrosion of shoulder and upper limb, except wrist and hand**
EXCLUDES 2   burn and corrosion of interscapular region (T21.-)
burn and corrosion of wrist and hand (T23.-)

The appropriate 7th character is to be added to each code from category T22.
A   initial encounter
D   subsequent encounter
S   sequela

√5ᵗʰ **T22.0** **Burn of** unspecified degree **of shoulder and upper limb, except wrist and hand**
Use additional external cause code to identify the source, place and intent of the burn (X00-X19, X75-X77, X96-X98, Y92)

√x7ᵗʰ **T22.00** **Burn of unspecified degree of shoulder and upper limb, except wrist and hand, unspecified site** ▽

√6ᵗʰ **T22.01** **Burn of unspecified degree of** forearm

√7ᵗʰ **T22.011** **Burn of unspecified degree of** right **forearm** ▽

√7ᵗʰ **T22.012** **Burn of unspecified degree of** left **forearm** ▽

√7ᵗʰ **T22.019** **Burn of unspecified degree of unspecified forearm** ▽

√6ᵗʰ **T22.02** **Burn of unspecified degree of** elbow

√7ᵗʰ **T22.021** **Burn of unspecified degree of** right **elbow** ▽

√7ᵗʰ **T22.022** **Burn of unspecified degree of** left **elbow** ▽

√7ᵗʰ **T22.029** **Burn of unspecified degree of unspecified elbow** ▽

√6ᵗʰ **T22.03** **Burn of unspecified degree of** upper arm

√7ᵗʰ **T22.031** **Burn of unspecified degree of** right **upper arm** ▽

√7ᵗʰ **T22.032** **Burn of unspecified degree of** left **upper arm** ▽

√7ᵗʰ **T22.039** **Burn of unspecified degree of unspecified upper arm** ▽

√6ᵗʰ **T22.04** **Burn of unspecified degree of** axilla

√7ᵗʰ **T22.041** **Burn of unspecified degree of** right **axilla** ▽

√7ᵗʰ **T22.042** **Burn of unspecified degree of** left **axilla** ▽

√7ᵗʰ **T22.049** **Burn of unspecified degree of unspecified axilla** ▽

√6ᵗʰ **T22.05** **Burn of unspecified degree of** shoulder

√7ᵗʰ **T22.051** **Burn of unspecified degree of** right **shoulder** ▽

√7ᵗʰ **T22.052** **Burn of unspecified degree of** left **shoulder** ▽

√7ᵗʰ **T22.059** **Burn of unspecified degree of unspecified shoulder** ▽

√6ᵗʰ **T22.06** **Burn of unspecified degree of** scapular region

√7ᵗʰ **T22.061** **Burn of unspecified degree of** right **scapular region** ▽

√7ᵗʰ **T22.062** **Burn of unspecified degree of** left **scapular region** ▽

√7ᵗʰ **T22.069** **Burn of unspecified degree of unspecified scapular region** ▽

✓6th **T22.09** Burn of unspecified degree of multiple sites of shoulder and upper limb, except wrist and hand

    ✓7th **T22.091** Burn of unspecified degree of multiple sites of right shoulder and upper limb, except wrist and hand ▽

    ✓7th **T22.092** Burn of unspecified degree of multiple sites of left shoulder and upper limb, except wrist and hand ▽

    ✓7th **T22.099** Burn of unspecified degree of multiple sites of unspecified shoulder and upper limb, except wrist and hand ▽

✓5th **T22.1** Burn of first degree of shoulder and upper limb, except wrist and hand

    Use additional external cause code to identify the source, place and intent of the burn (X00-X19, X75-X77, X96-X98, Y92)

    ✓x7th **T22.10** Burn of first degree of shoulder and upper limb, except wrist and hand, unspecified site ▽

    ✓6th **T22.11** Burn of first degree of forearm

        ✓7th **T22.111** Burn of first degree of right forearm

        ✓7th **T22.112** Burn of first degree of left forearm

        ✓7th **T22.119** Burn of first degree of unspecified forearm ▽

    ✓6th **T22.12** Burn of first degree of elbow

        ✓7th **T22.121** Burn of first degree of right elbow

        ✓7th **T22.122** Burn of first degree of left elbow

        ✓7th **T22.129** Burn of first degree of unspecified elbow ▽

    ✓6th **T22.13** Burn of first degree of upper arm

        ✓7th **T22.131** Burn of first degree of right upper arm

        ✓7th **T22.132** Burn of first degree of left upper arm

        ✓7th **T22.139** Burn of first degree of unspecified upper arm ▽

    ✓6th **T22.14** Burn of first degree of axilla

        ✓7th **T22.141** Burn of first degree of right axilla

        ✓7th **T22.142** Burn of first degree of left axilla

        ✓7th **T22.149** Burn of first degree of unspecified axilla ▽

    ✓6th **T22.15** Burn of first degree of shoulder

        ✓7th **T22.151** Burn of first degree of right shoulder

        ✓7th **T22.152** Burn of first degree of left shoulder

        ✓7th **T22.159** Burn of first degree of unspecified shoulder ▽

    ✓6th **T22.16** Burn of first degree of scapular region

        ✓7th **T22.161** Burn of first degree of right scapular region

        ✓7th **T22.162** Burn of first degree of left scapular region

        ✓7th **T22.169** Burn of first degree of unspecified scapular region ▽

    ✓6th **T22.19** Burn of first degree of multiple sites of shoulder and upper limb, except wrist and hand

        ✓7th **T22.191** Burn of first degree of multiple sites of right shoulder and upper limb, except wrist and hand

        ✓7th **T22.192** Burn of first degree of multiple sites of left shoulder and upper limb, except wrist and hand

        ✓7th **T22.199** Burn of first degree of multiple sites of unspecified shoulder and upper limb, except wrist and hand ▽

✓5th **T22.2** Burn of second degree of shoulder and upper limb, except wrist and hand

    Use additional external cause code to identify the source, place and intent of the burn (X00-X19, X75-X77, X96-X98, Y92)

    7 ✓x7th **T22.20** Burn of second degree of shoulder and upper limb, except wrist and hand, unspecified site ▽

    ✓6th **T22.21** Burn of second degree of forearm

        7 ✓7th **T22.211** Burn of second degree of right forearm

        7 ✓7th **T22.212** Burn of second degree of left forearm

        7 ✓7th **T22.219** Burn of second degree of unspecified forearm ▽

    ✓6th **T22.22** Burn of second degree of elbow

        7 ✓7th **T22.221** Burn of second degree of right elbow

        7 ✓7th **T22.222** Burn of second degree of left elbow

        7 ✓7th **T22.229** Burn of second degree of unspecified elbow ▽

    ✓6th **T22.23** Burn of second degree of upper arm

        7 ✓7th **T22.231** Burn of second degree of right upper arm

        7 ✓7th **T22.232** Burn of second degree of left upper arm

        7 ✓7th **T22.239** Burn of second degree of unspecified upper arm

    ✓6th **T22.24** Burn of second degree of axilla

        7 ✓7th **T22.241** Burn of second degree of right axilla

        7 ✓7th **T22.242** Burn of second degree of left axilla

        7 ✓7th **T22.249** Burn of second degree of unspecified axilla ▽

    ✓6th **T22.25** Burn of second degree of shoulder

        7 ✓7th **T22.251** Burn of second degree of right shoulder

        7 ✓7th **T22.252** Burn of second degree of left shoulder

        7 ✓7th **T22.259** Burn of second degree of unspecified shoulder ▽

    ✓6th **T22.26** Burn of second degree of scapular region

        7 ✓7th **T22.261** Burn of second degree of right scapular region

        7 ✓7th **T22.262** Burn of second degree of left scapular region

        7 ✓7th **T22.269** Burn of second degree of unspecified scapular region ▽

    ✓6th **T22.29** Burn of second degree of multiple sites of shoulder and upper limb, except wrist and hand

        7 ✓7th **T22.291** Burn of second degree of multiple sites of right shoulder and upper limb, except wrist and hand

        7 ✓7th **T22.292** Burn of second degree of multiple sites of left shoulder and upper limb, except wrist and hand

        7 ✓7th **T22.299** Burn of second degree of multiple sites ▽ of unspecified shoulder and upper limb, except wrist and hand

✓5th **T22.3** Burn of third degree of shoulder and upper limb, except wrist and hand

    Use additional external cause code to identify the source, place and intent of the burn (X00-X19, X75-X77, X96-X98, Y92)

    7 ✓x7th **T22.30** Burn of third degree of shoulder and upper limb, ▽ except wrist and hand, unspecified site

    ✓6th **T22.31** Burn of third degree of forearm

        7 ✓7th **T22.311** Burn of third degree of right forearm

        7 ✓7th **T22.312** Burn of third degree of left forearm

        7 ✓7th **T22.319** Burn of third degree of unspecified forearm ▽

    ✓6th **T22.32** Burn of third degree of elbow

        7 ✓7th **T22.321** Burn of third degree of right elbow

        7 ✓7th **T22.322** Burn of third degree of left elbow

        7 ✓7th **T22.329** Burn of third degree of unspecified elbow ▽

    ✓6th **T22.33** Burn of third degree of upper arm

        7 ✓7th **T22.331** Burn of third degree of right upper arm

        7 ✓7th **T22.332** Burn of third degree of left upper arm

        7 ✓7th **T22.339** Burn of third degree of unspecified upper arm ▽

    ✓6th **T22.34** Burn of third degree of axilla

        7 ✓7th **T22.341** Burn of third degree of right axilla

        7 ✓7th **T22.342** Burn of third degree of left axilla

        7 ✓7th **T22.349** Burn of third degree of unspecified axilla ▽

    ✓6th **T22.35** Burn of third degree of shoulder

        7 ✓7th **T22.351** Burn of third degree of right shoulder

        7 ✓7th **T22.352** Burn of third degree of left shoulder

        7 ✓7th **T22.359** Burn of third degree of unspecified shoulder ▽

    ✓6th **T22.36** Burn of third degree of scapular region

        7 ✓7th **T22.361** Burn of third degree of right scapular region

---

7 Clinically Complex = With 7th character indicating a subsequent encounter

Ⓝ Newborn   Ⓟ Pediatric   Ⓜ Maternity   Ⓐ Adult   **RIC** RIC Dx   **NCDx** Noncancer Dx   **PDx** Primary Dx   **CC** RIC CC Condition   ►◄ Revised Text   ● New Code   ▲ Revised Code Title

984   ICD-10-CM 2016

⁷ ✓7ᵗʰ **T22.362** Burn of third degree of left scapular region

⁷ ✓7ᵗʰ **T22.369** Burn of third degree of unspecified scapular region ▽

✓6ᵗʰ **T22.39** Burn of third degree of multiple sites of shoulder and upper limb, except wrist and hand

⁷ ✓7ᵗʰ **T22.391** Burn of third degree of multiple sites of right shoulder and upper limb, except wrist and hand

⁷ ✓7ᵗʰ **T22.392** Burn of third degree of multiple sites of left shoulder and upper limb, except wrist and hand

⁷ ✓7ᵗʰ **T22.399** Burn of third degree of multiple sites of unspecified shoulder and upper limb, except wrist and hand ▽

✓5ᵗʰ **T22.4** Corrosion of unspecified degree of shoulder and upper limb, except wrist and hand

Code first (T51-T65) to identify chemical and intent
Use additional external cause code to identify place (Y92)

✓ₓ7ᵗʰ **T22.40** Corrosion of unspecified degree of shoulder and upper limb, except wrist and hand, unspecified site ▽

✓6ᵗʰ **T22.41** Corrosion of unspecified degree of forearm

✓7ᵗʰ **T22.411** Corrosion of unspecified degree of right forearm ▽

✓7ᵗʰ **T22.412** Corrosion of unspecified degree of left forearm ▽

✓7ᵗʰ **T22.419** Corrosion of unspecified degree of unspecified forearm ▽

✓6ᵗʰ **T22.42** Corrosion of unspecified degree of elbow

✓7ᵗʰ **T22.421** Corrosion of unspecified degree of right elbow ▽

✓7ᵗʰ **T22.422** Corrosion of unspecified degree of left elbow ▽

✓7ᵗʰ **T22.429** Corrosion of unspecified degree of unspecified elbow ▽

✓6ᵗʰ **T22.43** Corrosion of unspecified degree of upper arm

✓7ᵗʰ **T22.431** Corrosion of unspecified degree of right upper arm ▽

✓7ᵗʰ **T22.432** Corrosion of unspecified degree of left upper arm ▽

✓7ᵗʰ **T22.439** Corrosion of unspecified degree of unspecified upper arm ▽

✓6ᵗʰ **T22.44** Corrosion of unspecified degree of axilla

✓7ᵗʰ **T22.441** Corrosion of unspecified degree of right axilla ▽

✓7ᵗʰ **T22.442** Corrosion of unspecified degree of left axilla ▽

✓7ᵗʰ **T22.449** Corrosion of unspecified degree of unspecified axilla ▽

✓6ᵗʰ **T22.45** Corrosion of unspecified degree of shoulder

✓7ᵗʰ **T22.451** Corrosion of unspecified degree of right shoulder ▽

✓7ᵗʰ **T22.452** Corrosion of unspecified degree of left shoulder ▽

✓7ᵗʰ **T22.459** Corrosion of unspecified degree of unspecified shoulder ▽

✓6ᵗʰ **T22.46** Corrosion of unspecified degree of scapular region

✓7ᵗʰ **T22.461** Corrosion of unspecified degree of right scapular region ▽

✓7ᵗʰ **T22.462** Corrosion of unspecified degree of left scapular region ▽

✓7ᵗʰ **T22.469** Corrosion of unspecified degree of unspecified scapular region ▽

✓6ᵗʰ **T22.49** Corrosion of unspecified degree of multiple sites of shoulder and upper limb, except wrist and hand

✓7ᵗʰ **T22.491** Corrosion of unspecified degree of multiple sites of right shoulder and upper limb, except wrist and hand ▽

✓7ᵗʰ **T22.492** Corrosion of unspecified degree of multiple sites of left shoulder and upper limb, except wrist and hand ▽

✓7ᵗʰ **T22.499** Corrosion of unspecified degree of multiple sites of unspecified shoulder and upper limb, except wrist and hand ▽

✓5ᵗʰ **T22.5** Corrosion of first degree of shoulder and upper limb, except wrist and hand

Code first (T51-T65) to identify chemical and intent
Use additional external cause code to identify place (Y92)

✓ₓ7ᵗʰ **T22.50** Corrosion of first degree of shoulder and upper limb, except wrist and hand unspecified site ▽

✓6ᵗʰ **T22.51** Corrosion of first degree of forearm

✓7ᵗʰ **T22.511** Corrosion of first degree of right forearm

✓7ᵗʰ **T22.512** Corrosion of first degree of left forearm

✓7ᵗʰ **T22.519** Corrosion of first degree of unspecified forearm ▽

✓6ᵗʰ **T22.52** Corrosion of first degree of elbow

✓7ᵗʰ **T22.521** Corrosion of first degree of right elbow

✓7ᵗʰ **T22.522** Corrosion of first degree of left elbow

✓7ᵗʰ **T22.529** Corrosion of first degree of unspecified elbow ▽

✓6ᵗʰ **T22.53** Corrosion of first degree of upper arm

✓7ᵗʰ **T22.531** Corrosion of first degree of right upper arm

✓7ᵗʰ **T22.532** Corrosion of first degree of left upper arm

✓7ᵗʰ **T22.539** Corrosion of first degree of unspecified upper arm ▽

✓6ᵗʰ **T22.54** Corrosion of first degree of axilla

✓7ᵗʰ **T22.541** Corrosion of first degree of right axilla

✓7ᵗʰ **T22.542** Corrosion of first degree of left axilla

✓7ᵗʰ **T22.549** Corrosion of first degree of unspecified axilla ▽

✓6ᵗʰ **T22.55** Corrosion of first degree of shoulder

✓7ᵗʰ **T22.551** Corrosion of first degree of right shoulder

✓7ᵗʰ **T22.552** Corrosion of first degree of left shoulder

✓7ᵗʰ **T22.559** Corrosion of first degree of unspecified shoulder ▽

✓6ᵗʰ **T22.56** Corrosion of first degree of scapular region

✓7ᵗʰ **T22.561** Corrosion of first degree of right scapular region

✓7ᵗʰ **T22.562** Corrosion of first degree of left scapular region

✓7ᵗʰ **T22.569** Corrosion of first degree of unspecified scapular region ▽

✓6ᵗʰ **T22.59** Corrosion of first degree of multiple sites of shoulder and upper limb, except wrist and hand

✓7ᵗʰ **T22.591** Corrosion of first degree of multiple sites of right shoulder and upper limb, except wrist and hand

✓7ᵗʰ **T22.592** Corrosion of first degree of multiple sites of left shoulder and upper limb, except wrist and hand

✓7ᵗʰ **T22.599** Corrosion of first degree of multiple sites of unspecified shoulder and upper limb, except wrist and hand ▽

✓5ᵗʰ **T22.6** Corrosion of second degree of shoulder and upper limb, except wrist and hand

Code first (T51-T65) to identify chemical and intent
Use additional external cause code to identify place (Y92)

✓ₓ7ᵗʰ **T22.60** Corrosion of second degree of shoulder and upper limb, except wrist and hand, unspecified site ▽

✓6ᵗʰ **T22.61** Corrosion of second degree of forearm

✓7ᵗʰ **T22.611** Corrosion of second degree of right forearm

✓7ᵗʰ **T22.612** Corrosion of second degree of left forearm

✓7ᵗʰ **T22.619** Corrosion of second degree of unspecified forearm ▽

✓6ᵗʰ **T22.62** Corrosion of second degree of elbow

✓7ᵗʰ **T22.621** Corrosion of second degree of right elbow

✓7ᵗʰ **T22.622** Corrosion of second degree of left elbow

✓7ᵗʰ **T22.629** Corrosion of second degree of unspecified elbow ▽

✓6ᵗʰ **T22.63** Corrosion of second degree of upper arm

✓7ᵗʰ **T22.631** Corrosion of second degree of right upper arm

---

⁷ Clinically Complex = With 7th character indicating a subsequent encounter

✓ Add'l Character Required   ✓ₓ7ᵗʰ Placeholder Alert   RUG IV Special Care High Dx   RUG IV Clinically Complex Dx   RUG IV Special Care Low Dx   Manifestation Code   Other Specified Code   ▽ Unspecified Code

☑7ᵗʰ **T22.632** Corrosion of second degree of left upper arm

☑7ᵗʰ **T22.639** Corrosion of second degree of unspecified upper arm ▽

✓6ᵗʰ **T22.64** Corrosion of second degree of axilla

　☑7ᵗʰ **T22.641** Corrosion of second degree of right axilla

　☑7ᵗʰ **T22.642** Corrosion of second degree of left axilla

　☑7ᵗʰ **T22.649** Corrosion of second degree of unspecified axilla ▽

✓6ᵗʰ **T22.65** Corrosion of second degree of shoulder

　☑7ᵗʰ **T22.651** Corrosion of second degree of right shoulder

　☑7ᵗʰ **T22.652** Corrosion of second degree of left shoulder

　☑7ᵗʰ **T22.659** Corrosion of second degree of unspecified shoulder ▽

✓6ᵗʰ **T22.66** Corrosion of second degree of scapular region

　☑7ᵗʰ **T22.661** Corrosion of second degree of right scapular region

　☑7ᵗʰ **T22.662** Corrosion of second degree of left scapular region

　☑7ᵗʰ **T22.669** Corrosion of second degree of unspecified scapular region ▽

✓6ᵗʰ **T22.69** Corrosion of second degree of multiple sites of shoulder and upper limb, except wrist and hand

　☑7ᵗʰ **T22.691** Corrosion of second degree of multiple sites of right shoulder and upper limb, except wrist and hand

　☑7ᵗʰ **T22.692** Corrosion of second degree of multiple sites of left shoulder and upper limb, except wrist and hand

　☑7ᵗʰ **T22.699** Corrosion of second degree of multiple sites of unspecified shoulder and upper limb, except wrist and hand ▽

✓5ᵗʰ **T22.7** Corrosion of third degree of shoulder and upper limb, except wrist and hand

　Code first (T51-T65) to identify chemical and intent
　Use additional external cause code to identify place (Y92)

✓x7ᵗʰ **T22.70** Corrosion of third degree of shoulder and upper limb, except wrist and hand, unspecified site ▽

✓6ᵗʰ **T22.71** Corrosion of third degree of forearm

　☑7ᵗʰ **T22.711** Corrosion of third degree of right forearm

　☑7ᵗʰ **T22.712** Corrosion of third degree of left forearm

　☑7ᵗʰ **T22.719** Corrosion of third degree of unspecified forearm ▽

✓6ᵗʰ **T22.72** Corrosion of third degree of elbow

　☑7ᵗʰ **T22.721** Corrosion of third degree of right elbow

　☑7ᵗʰ **T22.722** Corrosion of third degree of left elbow

　☑7ᵗʰ **T22.729** Corrosion of third degree of unspecified elbow ▽

✓6ᵗʰ **T22.73** Corrosion of third degree of upper arm

　☑7ᵗʰ **T22.731** Corrosion of third degree of right upper arm

　☑7ᵗʰ **T22.732** Corrosion of third degree of left upper arm

　☑7ᵗʰ **T22.739** Corrosion of third degree of unspecified upper arm ▽

✓6ᵗʰ **T22.74** Corrosion of third degree of axilla

　☑7ᵗʰ **T22.741** Corrosion of third degree of right axilla

　☑7ᵗʰ **T22.742** Corrosion of third degree of left axilla

　☑7ᵗʰ **T22.749** Corrosion of third degree of unspecified axilla ▽

✓6ᵗʰ **T22.75** Corrosion of third degree of shoulder

　☑7ᵗʰ **T22.751** Corrosion of third degree of right shoulder

　☑7ᵗʰ **T22.752** Corrosion of third degree of left shoulder

　☑7ᵗʰ **T22.759** Corrosion of third degree of unspecified shoulder ▽

✓6ᵗʰ **T22.76** Corrosion of third degree of scapular region

　☑7ᵗʰ **T22.761** Corrosion of third degree of right scapular region

　☑7ᵗʰ **T22.762** Corrosion of third degree of left scapular region

　☑7ᵗʰ **T22.769** Corrosion of third degree of unspecified scapular region ▽

☑6ᵗʰ **T22.79** Corrosion of third degree of multiple sites of shoulder and upper limb, except wrist and hand

　☑7ᵗʰ **T22.791** Corrosion of third degree of multiple sites of right shoulder and upper limb, except wrist and hand

　☑7ᵗʰ **T22.792** Corrosion of third degree of multiple sites of left shoulder and upper limb, except wrist and hand

　☑7ᵗʰ **T22.799** Corrosion of third degree of multiple sites of unspecified shoulder and upper limb, except wrist and hand ▽

✓4ᵗʰ **T23** **Burn and corrosion of wrist and hand**

　AHA: 2015, 1Q, 19

　The appropriate 7th character is to be added to each code from category T23.
　A　initial encounter
　D　subsequent encounter
　S　sequela

✓5ᵗʰ **T23.0** Burn of unspecified degree of wrist and hand

　Use additional external cause code to identify the source, place and intent of the burn (X00-X19, X75-X77, X96-X98, Y92)

✓6ᵗʰ **T23.00** Burn of unspecified degree of hand, unspecified site

　☑7ᵗʰ **T23.001** Burn of unspecified degree of right hand, unspecified site ▽

　☑7ᵗʰ **T23.002** Burn of unspecified degree of left hand, unspecified site ▽

　☑7ᵗʰ **T23.009** Burn of unspecified degree of unspecified hand, unspecified site ▽

✓6ᵗʰ **T23.01** Burn of unspecified degree of thumb (nail)

　☑7ᵗʰ **T23.011** Burn of unspecified degree of right thumb (nail) ▽

　☑7ᵗʰ **T23.012** Burn of unspecified degree of left thumb (nail) ▽

　☑7ᵗʰ **T23.019** Burn of unspecified degree of unspecified thumb (nail) ▽

✓6ᵗʰ **T23.02** Burn of unspecified degree of single finger (nail) except thumb

　☑7ᵗʰ **T23.021** Burn of unspecified degree of single right finger (nail) except thumb ▽

　☑7ᵗʰ **T23.022** Burn of unspecified degree of single left finger (nail) except thumb ▽

　☑7ᵗʰ **T23.029** Burn of unspecified degree of unspecified single finger (nail) except thumb ▽

✓6ᵗʰ **T23.03** Burn of unspecified degree of multiple fingers (nail), not including thumb

　☑7ᵗʰ **T23.031** Burn of unspecified degree of multiple right fingers (nail), not including thumb ▽

　☑7ᵗʰ **T23.032** Burn of unspecified degree of multiple left fingers (nail), not including thumb ▽

　☑7ᵗʰ **T23.039** Burn of unspecified degree of unspecified multiple fingers (nail), not including thumb ▽

✓6ᵗʰ **T23.04** Burn of unspecified degree of multiple fingers (nail), including thumb

　☑7ᵗʰ **T23.041** Burn of unspecified degree of multiple right fingers (nail), including thumb ▽

　☑7ᵗʰ **T23.042** Burn of unspecified degree of multiple left fingers (nail), including thumb ▽

　☑7ᵗʰ **T23.049** Burn of unspecified degree of unspecified multiple fingers (nail), including thumb ▽

✓6ᵗʰ **T23.05** Burn of unspecified degree of palm

　☑7ᵗʰ **T23.051** Burn of unspecified degree of right palm ▽

　☑7ᵗʰ **T23.052** Burn of unspecified degree of left palm ▽

　☑7ᵗʰ **T23.059** Burn of unspecified degree of unspecified palm ▽

✓6ᵗʰ **T23.06** Burn of unspecified degree of back of hand

　☑7ᵗʰ **T23.061** Burn of unspecified degree of back of right hand ▽

　☑7ᵗʰ **T23.062** Burn of unspecified degree of back of left hand ▽

√7th   **T23.069**   Burn of unspecified degree of back of unspecified hand   ▽

√6th   **T23.07**   **Burn of unspecified degree of wrist**

    √7th   **T23.071**   Burn of unspecified degree of right wrist   ▽

    √7th   **T23.072**   Burn of unspecified degree of left wrist   ▽

    √7th   **T23.079**   Burn of unspecified degree of unspecified wrist   ▽

√6th   **T23.09**   **Burn of unspecified degree of multiple sites of wrist and hand**

    √7th   **T23.091**   Burn of unspecified degree of multiple sites of right wrist and hand   ▽

    √7th   **T23.092**   Burn of unspecified degree of multiple sites of left wrist and hand   ▽

    √7th   **T23.099**   Burn of unspecified degree of multiple sites of unspecified wrist and hand   ▽

√5th   **T23.1**   **Burn of first degree of wrist and hand**

    Use additional external cause code to identify the source, place and intent of the burn (X00-X19, X75-X77, X96-X98, Y92)

√6th   **T23.10**   **Burn of first degree of hand, unspecified site**

    √7th   **T23.101**   Burn of first degree of right hand, unspecified site   ▽

    √7th   **T23.102**   Burn of first degree of left hand, unspecified site   ▽

    √7th   **T23.109**   Burn of first degree of unspecified hand, unspecified site   ▽

√6th   **T23.11**   **Burn of first degree of thumb (nail)**

    √7th   **T23.111**   Burn of first degree of right thumb (nail)

    √7th   **T23.112**   Burn of first degree of left thumb (nail)

    √7th   **T23.119**   Burn of first degree of unspecified thumb (nail)   ▽

√6th   **T23.12**   **Burn of first degree of single finger (nail) except thumb**

    √7th   **T23.121**   Burn of first degree of single right finger (nail) except thumb

    √7th   **T23.122**   Burn of first degree of single left finger (nail) except thumb

    √7th   **T23.129**   Burn of first degree of unspecified single finger (nail) except thumb   ▽

√6th   **T23.13**   **Burn of first degree of multiple fingers (nail), not including thumb**

    √7th   **T23.131**   Burn of first degree of multiple right fingers (nail), not including thumb

    √7th   **T23.132**   Burn of first degree of multiple left fingers (nail), not including thumb

    √7th   **T23.139**   Burn of first degree of unspecified multiple fingers (nail), not including thumb   ▽

√6th   **T23.14**   **Burn of first degree of multiple fingers (nail), including thumb**

    √7th   **T23.141**   Burn of first degree of multiple right fingers (nail), including thumb

    √7th   **T23.142**   Burn of first degree of multiple left fingers (nail), including thumb

    √7th   **T23.149**   Burn of first degree of unspecified multiple fingers (nail), including thumb   ▽

√6th   **T23.15**   **Burn of first degree of palm**

    √7th   **T23.151**   Burn of first degree of right palm

    √7th   **T23.152**   Burn of first degree of left palm

    √7th   **T23.159**   Burn of first degree of unspecified palm   ▽

√6th   **T23.16**   **Burn of first degree of back of hand**

    √7th   **T23.161**   Burn of first degree of back of right hand

    √7th   **T23.162**   Burn of first degree of back of left hand

    √7th   **T23.169**   Burn of first degree of back of unspecified hand   ▽

√6th   **T23.17**   **Burn of first degree of wrist**

    √7th   **T23.171**   Burn of first degree of right wrist

    √7th   **T23.172**   Burn of first degree of left wrist

√7th   **T23.179**   Burn of first degree of unspecified wrist   ▽

√6th   **T23.19**   **Burn of first degree of multiple sites of wrist and hand**

    √7th   **T23.191**   Burn of first degree of multiple sites of right wrist and hand

    √7th   **T23.192**   Burn of first degree of multiple sites of left wrist and hand

    √7th   **T23.199**   Burn of first degree of multiple sites of unspecified wrist and hand   ▽

√5th   **T23.2**   **Burn of second degree of wrist and hand**

    Use additional external cause code to identify the source, place and intent of the burn (X00-X19, X75-X77, X96-X98, Y92)

√6th   **T23.20**   **Burn of second degree of hand, unspecified site**

    7 √7th   **T23.201**   Burn of second degree of right hand, unspecified site   ▽

    7 √7th   **T23.202**   Burn of second degree of left hand, unspecified site   ▽

    7 √7th   **T23.209**   Burn of second degree of unspecified hand, unspecified site   ▽

√6th   **T23.21**   **Burn of second degree of thumb (nail)**

    7 √7th   **T23.211**   Burn of second degree of right thumb (nail)

    7 √7th   **T23.212**   Burn of second degree of left thumb (nail)

    7 √7th   **T23.219**   Burn of second degree of unspecified thumb (nail)   ▽

√6th   **T23.22**   **Burn of second degree of single finger (nail) except thumb**

    7 √7th   **T23.221**   Burn of second degree of single right finger (nail) except thumb

    7 √7th   **T23.222**   Burn of second degree of single left finger (nail) except thumb

    7 √7th   **T23.229**   Burn of second degree of unspecified single finger (nail) except thumb   ▽

√6th   **T23.23**   **Burn of second degree of multiple fingers (nail), not including thumb**

    7 √7th   **T23.231**   Burn of second degree of multiple right fingers (nail), not including thumb

    7 √7th   **T23.232**   Burn of second degree of multiple left fingers (nail), not including thumb

    7 √7th   **T23.239**   Burn of second degree of unspecified multiple fingers (nail), not including thumb   ▽

√6th   **T23.24**   **Burn of second degree of multiple fingers (nail), including thumb**

    7 √7th   **T23.241**   Burn of second degree of multiple right fingers (nail), including thumb

    7 √7th   **T23.242**   Burn of second degree of multiple left fingers (nail), including thumb

    7 √7th   **T23.249**   Burn of second degree of unspecified multiple fingers (nail), including thumb   ▽

√6th   **T23.25**   **Burn of second degree of palm**

    7 √7th   **T23.251**   Burn of second degree of right palm

    7 √7th   **T23.252**   Burn of second degree of left palm

    7 √7th   **T23.259**   Burn of second degree of unspecified palm   ▽

√6th   **T23.26**   **Burn of second degree of back of hand**

    7 √7th   **T23.261**   Burn of second degree of back of right hand

    7 √7th   **T23.262**   Burn of second degree of back of left hand

    7 √7th   **T23.269**   Burn of second degree of back of unspecified hand   ▽

√6th   **T23.27**   **Burn of second degree of wrist**

    7 √7th   **T23.271**   Burn of second degree of right wrist

    7 √7th   **T23.272**   Burn of second degree of left wrist

    7 √7th   **T23.279**   Burn of second degree of unspecified wrist   ▽

√6th   **T23.29**   **Burn of second degree of multiple sites of wrist and hand**

    7 √7th   **T23.291**   Burn of second degree of multiple sites of right wrist and hand

    7 √7th   **T23.292**   Burn of second degree of multiple sites of left wrist and hand

---

7 Clinically Complex = With 7th character indicating a subsequent encounter

☑ Add'l Character Required   √x7th Placeholder Alert   RUG IV Special Care High Dx   RUG IV Clinically Complex Dx   RUG IV Special Care Low Dx   Manifestation Code   Other Specified Code   ▽ Unspecified Code

ICD-10-CM 2016   **987**

⁷ ✓7ᵗʰ **T23.299 Burn of second degree of multiple sites** ▽
of unspecified wrist and hand

✓5ᵗʰ **T23.3 Burn of third degree of wrist and hand**
Use additional external cause code to identify the source, place
and intent of the burn (X00-X19, X75-X77, X96-X98, Y92)

✓6ᵗʰ **T23.30 Burn of third degree of hand, unspecified site**
⁷ ✓7ᵗʰ **T23.301 Burn of third degree of right hand,** ▽
unspecified site
⁷ ✓7ᵗʰ **T23.302 Burn of third degree of left hand,** ▽
unspecified site
⁷ ✓7ᵗʰ **T23.309 Burn of third degree of unspecified** ▽
hand, unspecified site

✓6ᵗʰ **T23.31 Burn of third degree of thumb (nail)**
⁷ ✓7ᵗʰ **T23.311 Burn of third degree of right thumb (nail)**
⁷ ✓7ᵗʰ **T23.312 Burn of third degree of left thumb (nail)**
⁷ ✓7ᵗʰ **T23.319 Burn of third degree of unspecified** ▽
thumb (nail)

✓6ᵗʰ **T23.32 Burn of third degree of single finger (nail) except**
thumb
⁷ ✓7ᵗʰ **T23.321 Burn of third degree of single right**
finger (nail) except thumb
⁷ ✓7ᵗʰ **T23.322 Burn of third degree of single left**
finger (nail) except thumb
⁷ ✓7ᵗʰ **T23.329 Burn of third degree of unspecified** ▽
single finger (nail) except thumb

✓6ᵗʰ **T23.33 Burn of third degree of multiple fingers (nail), not**
including thumb
⁷ ✓7ᵗʰ **T23.331 Burn of third degree of multiple right**
fingers (nail), not including thumb
⁷ ✓7ᵗʰ **T23.332 Burn of third degree of multiple left**
fingers (nail), not including thumb
⁷ ✓7ᵗʰ **T23.339 Burn of third degree of unspecified** ▽
multiple fingers (nail), not including
thumb

✓6ᵗʰ **T23.34 Burn of third degree of multiple fingers (nail),**
including thumb
⁷ ✓7ᵗʰ **T23.341 Burn of third degree of multiple right**
fingers (nail), including thumb
⁷ ✓7ᵗʰ **T23.342 Burn of third degree of multiple left**
fingers (nail), including thumb
⁷ ✓7ᵗʰ **T23.349 Burn of third degree of unspecified** ▽
multiple fingers (nail), including thumb

✓6ᵗʰ **T23.35 Burn of third degree of palm**
⁷ ✓7ᵗʰ **T23.351 Burn of third degree of right palm**
⁷ ✓7ᵗʰ **T23.352 Burn of third degree of left palm**
⁷ ✓7ᵗʰ **T23.359 Burn of third degree of unspecified** ▽
palm

✓6ᵗʰ **T23.36 Burn of third degree of back of hand**
⁷ ✓7ᵗʰ **T23.361 Burn of third degree of back of right hand**
⁷ ✓7ᵗʰ **T23.362 Burn of third degree of back of left hand**
⁷ ✓7ᵗʰ **T23.369 Burn of third degree of back of** ▽
unspecified hand

✓6ᵗʰ **T23.37 Burn of third degree of wrist**
⁷ ✓7ᵗʰ **T23.371 Burn of third degree of right wrist**
⁷ ✓7ᵗʰ **T23.372 Burn of third degree of left wrist**
⁷ ✓7ᵗʰ **T23.379 Burn of third degree of unspecified** ▽
wrist

✓6ᵗʰ **T23.39 Burn of third degree of multiple sites of wrist and**
hand
⁷ ✓7ᵗʰ **T23.391 Burn of third degree of multiple sites of**
right wrist and hand
⁷ ✓7ᵗʰ **T23.392 Burn of third degree of multiple sites of**
left wrist and hand
⁷ ✓7ᵗʰ **T23.399 Burn of third degree of multiple sites** ▽
of unspecified wrist and hand

✓5ᵗʰ **T23.4 Corrosion of unspecified degree of wrist and hand**
Code first (T51-T65) to identify chemical and intent
Use additional external cause code to identify place (Y92)

✓6ᵗʰ **T23.40 Corrosion of unspecified degree of hand,**
unspecified site
✓7ᵗʰ **T23.401 Corrosion of unspecified degree of** ▽
right hand, unspecified site

✓7ᵗʰ **T23.402 Corrosion of unspecified degree of** ▽
left hand, unspecified site
✓7ᵗʰ **T23.409 Corrosion of unspecified degree of** ▽
unspecified hand, unspecified site

✓6ᵗʰ **T23.41 Corrosion of unspecified degree of thumb (nail)**
✓7ᵗʰ **T23.411 Corrosion of unspecified degree of** ▽
right thumb (nail)
✓7ᵗʰ **T23.412 Corrosion of unspecified degree of** ▽
left thumb (nail)
✓7ᵗʰ **T23.419 Corrosion of unspecified degree of** ▽
unspecified thumb (nail)

✓6ᵗʰ **T23.42 Corrosion of unspecified degree of single finger**
(nail) except thumb
✓7ᵗʰ **T23.421 Corrosion of unspecified degree of** ▽
single right finger (nail) except thumb
✓7ᵗʰ **T23.422 Corrosion of unspecified degree of** ▽
single left finger (nail) except thumb
✓7ᵗʰ **T23.429 Corrosion of unspecified degree of** ▽
unspecified single finger (nail) except
thumb

✓6ᵗʰ **T23.43 Corrosion of unspecified degree of multiple fingers**
(nail), not including thumb
✓7ᵗʰ **T23.431 Corrosion of unspecified degree of** ▽
multiple right fingers (nail), not including
thumb
✓7ᵗʰ **T23.432 Corrosion of unspecified degree of** ▽
multiple left fingers (nail), not including
thumb
✓7ᵗʰ **T23.439 Corrosion of unspecified degree of** ▽
unspecified multiple fingers (nail), not
including thumb

✓6ᵗʰ **T23.44 Corrosion of unspecified degree of multiple fingers**
(nail), including thumb
✓7ᵗʰ **T23.441 Corrosion of unspecified degree of** ▽
multiple right fingers (nail), including
thumb
✓7ᵗʰ **T23.442 Corrosion of unspecified degree of** ▽
multiple left fingers (nail), including
thumb
✓7ᵗʰ **T23.449 Corrosion of unspecified degree of** ▽
unspecified multiple fingers (nail),
including thumb

✓6ᵗʰ **T23.45 Corrosion of unspecified degree of palm**
✓7ᵗʰ **T23.451 Corrosion of unspecified degree of** ▽
right palm
✓7ᵗʰ **T23.452 Corrosion of unspecified degree of** ▽
left palm
✓7ᵗʰ **T23.459 Corrosion of unspecified degree of** ▽
unspecified palm

✓6ᵗʰ **T23.46 Corrosion of unspecified degree of back of hand**
✓7ᵗʰ **T23.461 Corrosion of unspecified degree of** ▽
back of right hand
✓7ᵗʰ **T23.462 Corrosion of unspecified degree of** ▽
back of left hand
✓7ᵗʰ **T23.469 Corrosion of unspecified degree of** ▽
back of unspecified hand

✓6ᵗʰ **T23.47 Corrosion of unspecified degree of wrist**
✓7ᵗʰ **T23.471 Corrosion of unspecified degree of** ▽
right wrist
✓7ᵗʰ **T23.472 Corrosion of unspecified degree of** ▽
left wrist
✓7ᵗʰ **T23.479 Corrosion of unspecified degree of** ▽
unspecified wrist

✓6ᵗʰ **T23.49 Corrosion of unspecified degree of multiple sites of**
wrist and hand
✓7ᵗʰ **T23.491 Corrosion of unspecified degree of** ▽
multiple sites of right wrist and hand
✓7ᵗʰ **T23.492 Corrosion of unspecified degree of** ▽
multiple sites of left wrist and hand
✓7ᵗʰ **T23.499 Corrosion of unspecified degree of** ▽
multiple sites of unspecified wrist and
hand

---

⁷ Clinically Complex = With 7th character indicating a subsequent encounter

☑5ᵗʰ **T23.5 Corrosion of first degree of wrist and hand**
Code first (T51-T65) to identify chemical and intent
Use additional external cause code to identify place (Y92)

☑6ᵗʰ **T23.50 Corrosion of first degree of hand, unspecified site**
☑7ᵗʰ **T23.501** Corrosion of first degree of right hand, ▽ unspecified site
☑7ᵗʰ **T23.502** Corrosion of first degree of left hand, ▽ unspecified site
☑7ᵗʰ **T23.509** Corrosion of first degree of unspecified ▽ hand, unspecified site

☑6ᵗʰ **T23.51 Corrosion of first degree of thumb (nail)**
☑7ᵗʰ **T23.511** Corrosion of first degree of right thumb (nail)
☑7ᵗʰ **T23.512** Corrosion of first degree of left thumb (nail)
☑7ᵗʰ **T23.519** Corrosion of first degree of unspecified ▽ thumb (nail)

☑6ᵗʰ **T23.52 Corrosion of first degree of single finger (nail) except thumb**
☑7ᵗʰ **T23.521** Corrosion of first degree of single right finger (nail) except thumb
☑7ᵗʰ **T23.522** Corrosion of first degree of single left finger (nail) except thumb
☑7ᵗʰ **T23.529** Corrosion of first degree of unspecified ▽ single finger (nail) except thumb

☑6ᵗʰ **T23.53 Corrosion of first degree of multiple fingers (nail), not including thumb**
☑7ᵗʰ **T23.531** Corrosion of first degree of multiple right fingers (nail), not including thumb
☑7ᵗʰ **T23.532** Corrosion of first degree of multiple left fingers (nail), not including thumb
☑7ᵗʰ **T23.539** Corrosion of first degree of unspecified ▽ multiple fingers (nail), not including thumb

☑6ᵗʰ **T23.54 Corrosion of first degree of multiple fingers (nail), including thumb**
☑7ᵗʰ **T23.541** Corrosion of first degree of multiple right fingers (nail), including thumb
☑7ᵗʰ **T23.542** Corrosion of first degree of multiple left fingers (nail), including thumb
☑7ᵗʰ **T23.549** Corrosion of first degree of unspecified ▽ multiple fingers (nail), including thumb

☑6ᵗʰ **T23.55 Corrosion of first degree of palm**
☑7ᵗʰ **T23.551** Corrosion of first degree of right palm
☑7ᵗʰ **T23.552** Corrosion of first degree of left palm
☑7ᵗʰ **T23.559** Corrosion of first degree of unspecified ▽ palm

☑6ᵗʰ **T23.56 Corrosion of first degree of back of hand**
☑7ᵗʰ **T23.561** Corrosion of first degree of back of right hand
☑7ᵗʰ **T23.562** Corrosion of first degree of back of left hand
☑7ᵗʰ **T23.569** Corrosion of first degree of back of ▽ unspecified hand

☑6ᵗʰ **T23.57 Corrosion of first degree of wrist**
☑7ᵗʰ **T23.571** Corrosion of first degree of right wrist
☑7ᵗʰ **T23.572** Corrosion of first degree of left wrist
☑7ᵗʰ **T23.579** Corrosion of first degree of unspecified ▽ wrist

☑6ᵗʰ **T23.59 Corrosion of first degree of multiple sites of wrist and hand**
☑7ᵗʰ **T23.591** Corrosion of first degree of multiple sites of right wrist and hand
☑7ᵗʰ **T23.592** Corrosion of first degree of multiple sites of left wrist and hand
☑7ᵗʰ **T23.599** Corrosion of first degree of multiple ▽ sites of unspecified wrist and hand

☑5ᵗʰ **T23.6 Corrosion of second degree of wrist and hand**
Code first (T51-T65) to identify chemical and intent
Use additional external cause code to identify place (Y92)

☑6ᵗʰ **T23.60 Corrosion of second degree of hand, unspecified site**
☑7ᵗʰ **T23.601** Corrosion of second degree of right ▽ hand, unspecified site

☑7ᵗʰ **T23.602** Corrosion of second degree of left ▽ hand, unspecified site
☑7ᵗʰ **T23.609** Corrosion of second degree of ▽ unspecified hand, unspecified site

☑6ᵗʰ **T23.61 Corrosion of second degree of thumb (nail)**
☑7ᵗʰ **T23.611** Corrosion of second degree of right thumb (nail)
☑7ᵗʰ **T23.612** Corrosion of second degree of left thumb (nail)
☑7ᵗʰ **T23.619** Corrosion of second degree of ▽ unspecified thumb (nail)

☑6ᵗʰ **T23.62 Corrosion of second degree of single finger (nail) except thumb**
☑7ᵗʰ **T23.621** Corrosion of second degree of single right finger (nail) except thumb
☑7ᵗʰ **T23.622** Corrosion of second degree of single left finger (nail) except thumb
☑7ᵗʰ **T23.629** Corrosion of second degree of ▽ unspecified single finger (nail) except thumb

☑6ᵗʰ **T23.63 Corrosion of second degree of multiple fingers (nail), not including thumb**
☑7ᵗʰ **T23.631** Corrosion of second degree of multiple right fingers (nail), not including thumb
☑7ᵗʰ **T23.632** Corrosion of second degree of multiple left fingers (nail), not including thumb
☑7ᵗʰ **T23.639** Corrosion of second degree of ▽ unspecified multiple fingers (nail), not including thumb

☑6ᵗʰ **T23.64 Corrosion of second degree of multiple fingers (nail), including thumb**
☑7ᵗʰ **T23.641** Corrosion of second degree of multiple right fingers (nail), including thumb
☑7ᵗʰ **T23.642** Corrosion of second degree of multiple left fingers (nail), including thumb
☑7ᵗʰ **T23.649** Corrosion of second degree of ▽ unspecified multiple fingers (nail), including thumb

☑6ᵗʰ **T23.65 Corrosion of second degree of palm**
☑7ᵗʰ **T23.651** Corrosion of second degree of right palm
☑7ᵗʰ **T23.652** Corrosion of second degree of left palm
☑7ᵗʰ **T23.659** Corrosion of second degree of ▽ unspecified palm

☑6ᵗʰ **T23.66 Corrosion of second degree of back of hand**
☑7ᵗʰ **T23.661** Corrosion of second degree back of right hand
☑7ᵗʰ **T23.662** Corrosion of second degree back of left hand
☑7ᵗʰ **T23.669** Corrosion of second degree back of ▽ unspecified hand

☑6ᵗʰ **T23.67 Corrosion of second degree of wrist**
☑7ᵗʰ **T23.671** Corrosion of second degree of right wrist
☑7ᵗʰ **T23.672** Corrosion of second degree of left wrist
☑7ᵗʰ **T23.679** Corrosion of second degree of ▽ unspecified wrist

☑6ᵗʰ **T23.69 Corrosion of second degree of multiple sites of wrist and hand**
☑7ᵗʰ **T23.691** Corrosion of second degree of multiple sites of right wrist and hand
☑7ᵗʰ **T23.692** Corrosion of second degree of multiple sites of left wrist and hand
☑7ᵗʰ **T23.699** Corrosion of second degree of multiple ▽ sites of unspecified wrist and hand

☑5ᵗʰ **T23.7 Corrosion of third degree of wrist and hand**
Code first (T51-T65) to identify chemical and intent
Use additional external cause code to identify place (Y92)

☑6ᵗʰ **T23.70 Corrosion of third degree of hand, unspecified site**
☑7ᵗʰ **T23.701** Corrosion of third degree of right hand, ▽ unspecified site
☑7ᵗʰ **T23.702** Corrosion of third degree of left hand, ▽ unspecified site
☑7ᵗʰ **T23.709** Corrosion of third degree of unspecified ▽ hand, unspecified site

☑6ᵗʰ **T23.71 Corrosion of third degree of thumb (nail)**

✓7ᵗʰ **T23.711** Corrosion of third degree of right thumb (nail)

✓7ᵗʰ **T23.712** Corrosion of third degree of left thumb (nail)

✓7ᵗʰ **T23.719** Corrosion of third degree of unspecified thumb (nail) ▽

✓6ᵗʰ **T23.72** Corrosion of third degree of single finger (nail) except thumb

✓7ᵗʰ **T23.721** Corrosion of third degree of single right finger (nail) except thumb

✓7ᵗʰ **T23.722** Corrosion of third degree of single left finger (nail) except thumb

✓7ᵗʰ **T23.729** Corrosion of third degree of unspecified ▽ single finger (nail) except thumb

✓6ᵗʰ **T23.73** Corrosion of third degree of multiple fingers (nail), not including thumb

✓7ᵗʰ **T23.731** Corrosion of third degree of multiple right fingers (nail), not including thumb

✓7ᵗʰ **T23.732** Corrosion of third degree of multiple left fingers (nail), not including thumb

✓7ᵗʰ **T23.739** Corrosion of third degree of ▽ unspecified multiple fingers (nail), not including thumb

✓6ᵗʰ **T23.74** Corrosion of third degree of multiple fingers (nail), including thumb

✓7ᵗʰ **T23.741** Corrosion of third degree of multiple right fingers (nail), including thumb

✓7ᵗʰ **T23.742** Corrosion of third degree of multiple left fingers (nail), including thumb

✓7ᵗʰ **T23.749** Corrosion of third degree of ▽ unspecified multiple fingers (nail), including thumb

✓6ᵗʰ **T23.75** Corrosion of third degree of palm

✓7ᵗʰ **T23.751** Corrosion of third degree of right palm

✓7ᵗʰ **T23.752** Corrosion of third degree of left palm

✓7ᵗʰ **T23.759** Corrosion of third degree of ▽ unspecified palm

✓6ᵗʰ **T23.76** Corrosion of third degree of back of hand

✓7ᵗʰ **T23.761** Corrosion of third degree of back of right hand

✓7ᵗʰ **T23.762** Corrosion of third degree of back of left hand

✓7ᵗʰ **T23.769** Corrosion of third degree back of ▽ unspecified hand

✓6ᵗʰ **T23.77** Corrosion of third degree of wrist

✓7ᵗʰ **T23.771** Corrosion of third degree of right wrist

✓7ᵗʰ **T23.772** Corrosion of third degree of left wrist

✓7ᵗʰ **T23.779** Corrosion of third degree of ▽ unspecified wrist

✓6ᵗʰ **T23.79** Corrosion of third degree of multiple sites of wrist and hand

✓7ᵗʰ **T23.791** Corrosion of third degree of multiple sites of right wrist and hand

✓7ᵗʰ **T23.792** Corrosion of third degree of multiple sites of left wrist and hand

✓7ᵗʰ **T23.799** Corrosion of third degree of multiple ▽ sites of unspecified wrist and hand

✓4ᵗʰ **T24** **Burn and corrosion of lower limb, except ankle and foot**

EXCLUDES 2 *burn and corrosion of ankle and foot (T25.-)*
burn and corrosion of hip region (T21.-)

The appropriate 7th character is to be added to each code from category T24.
A   initial encounter
D   subsequent encounter
S   sequela

✓5ᵗʰ **T24.0** **Burn of unspecified degree of lower limb, except ankle and foot**

Use additional external cause code to identify the source, place and intent of the burn (X00-X19, X75-X77, X96-X98, Y92)

✓6ᵗʰ **T24.00** Burn of unspecified degree of unspecified site of lower limb, except ankle and foot

✓7ᵗʰ **T24.001** Burn of unspecified degree of ▽ unspecified site of right lower limb, except ankle and foot

✓7ᵗʰ **T24.002** Burn of unspecified degree of ▽ unspecified site of left lower limb, except ankle and foot

✓7ᵗʰ **T24.009** Burn of unspecified degree of ▽ unspecified site of unspecified lower limb, except ankle and foot

✓6ᵗʰ **T24.01** Burn of unspecified degree of thigh

✓7ᵗʰ **T24.011** Burn of unspecified degree of right ▽ thigh

✓7ᵗʰ **T24.012** Burn of unspecified degree of left ▽ thigh

✓7ᵗʰ **T24.019** Burn of unspecified degree of ▽ unspecified thigh

✓6ᵗʰ **T24.02** Burn of unspecified degree of knee

✓7ᵗʰ **T24.021** Burn of unspecified degree of right ▽ knee

✓7ᵗʰ **T24.022** Burn of unspecified degree of left ▽ knee

✓7ᵗʰ **T24.029** Burn of unspecified degree of ▽ unspecified knee

✓6ᵗʰ **T24.03** Burn of unspecified degree of lower leg

✓7ᵗʰ **T24.031** Burn of unspecified degree of right ▽ lower leg

✓7ᵗʰ **T24.032** Burn of unspecified degree of left ▽ lower leg

✓7ᵗʰ **T24.039** Burn of unspecified degree of ▽ unspecified lower leg

✓6ᵗʰ **T24.09** Burn of unspecified degree of multiple sites of lower limb, except ankle and foot

✓7ᵗʰ **T24.091** Burn of unspecified degree of multiple ▽ sites of right lower limb, except ankle and foot

✓7ᵗʰ **T24.092** Burn of unspecified degree of multiple ▽ sites of left lower limb, except ankle and foot

✓7ᵗʰ **T24.099** Burn of unspecified degree of multiple ▽ sites of unspecified lower limb, except ankle and foot

✓5ᵗʰ **T24.1** **Burn of first degree of lower limb, except ankle and foot**

Use additional external cause code to identify the source, place and intent of the burn (X00-X19, X75-X77, X96-X98, Y92)

✓6ᵗʰ **T24.10** Burn of first degree of unspecified site of lower limb, except ankle and foot

✓7ᵗʰ **T24.101** Burn of first degree of unspecified site ▽ of right lower limb, except ankle and foot

✓7ᵗʰ **T24.102** Burn of first degree of unspecified site ▽ of left lower limb, except ankle and foot

✓7ᵗʰ **T24.109** Burn of first degree of unspecified site ▽ of unspecified lower limb, except ankle and foot

✓6ᵗʰ **T24.11** Burn of first degree of thigh

✓7ᵗʰ **T24.111** Burn of first degree of right thigh

✓7ᵗʰ **T24.112** Burn of first degree of left thigh

✓7ᵗʰ **T24.119** Burn of first degree of unspecified ▽ thigh

✓6ᵗʰ **T24.12** Burn of first degree of knee

✓7ᵗʰ **T24.121** Burn of first degree of right knee

✓7ᵗʰ **T24.122** Burn of first degree of left knee

✓7ᵗʰ **T24.129** Burn of first degree of unspecified ▽ knee

✓6ᵗʰ **T24.13** Burn of first degree of lower leg

✓7ᵗʰ **T24.131** Burn of first degree of right lower leg

✓7ᵗʰ **T24.132** Burn of first degree of left lower leg

✓7ᵗʰ **T24.139** Burn of first degree of unspecified ▽ lower leg

✓6ᵗʰ **T24.19** Burn of first degree of multiple sites of lower limb, except ankle and foot

✓7ᵗʰ **T24.191** Burn of first degree of multiple sites of right lower limb, except ankle and foot

✓7ᵗʰ **T24.192** Burn of first degree of multiple sites of left lower limb, except ankle and foot

✓7ᵗʰ **T24.199** Burn of first degree of multiple sites ▽ of unspecified lower limb, except ankle and foot

Ⓝ Newborn   Ⓟ Pediatric   Ⓜ Maternity   Ⓐ Adult   RIC RIC Dx   NCDx Noncancer Dx   PDx Primary Dx   CC RIC CC Condition   ▶◀ Revised Text   ● New Code   ▲ Revised Code Title

990   ICD-10-CM 2016

√5ᵗʰ **T24.2 Burn of second degree of lower limb, except ankle and foot**
Use additional external cause code to identify the source, place and intent of the burn (X00-X19, X75-X77, X96-X98, Y92)

  √6ᵗʰ **T24.20 Burn of** unspecified site **of lower limb, except ankle and foot**

    7 √7ᵗʰ **T24.201 Burn of second degree of unspecified** ▽
      site of right **lower limb, except ankle and foot**

    7 √7ᵗʰ **T24.202 Burn of second degree of unspecified** ▽
      site of left **lower limb, except ankle and foot**

    7 √7ᵗʰ **T24.209 Burn of second degree of unspecified** ▽
      site of unspecified lower limb, except ankle and foot

  √6ᵗʰ **T24.21 Burn of second degree of** thigh
    7 √7ᵗʰ **T24.211 Burn of second degree of** right **thigh**
    7 √7ᵗʰ **T24.212 Burn of second degree of** left **thigh**
    7 √7ᵗʰ **T24.219 Burn of second degree of unspecified** ▽
      thigh

  √6ᵗʰ **T24.22 Burn of second degree of** knee
    7 √7ᵗʰ **T24.221 Burn of second degree of** right **knee**
    7 √7ᵗʰ **T24.222 Burn of second degree of** left **knee**
    7 √7ᵗʰ **T24.229 Burn of second degree of unspecified** ▽
      knee

  √6ᵗʰ **T24.23 Burn of second degree of** lower leg
    7 √7ᵗʰ **T24.231 Burn of second degree of** right **lower leg**
    7 √7ᵗʰ **T24.232 Burn of second degree of** left **lower leg**
    7 √7ᵗʰ **T24.239 Burn of second degree of unspecified** ▽
      lower leg

  √6ᵗʰ **T24.29 Burn of second degree of** multiple sites **of lower limb, except ankle and foot**
    7 √7ᵗʰ **T24.291 Burn of second degree of multiple sites of** right **lower limb, except ankle and foot**
    7 √7ᵗʰ **T24.292 Burn of second degree of multiple sites of** left **lower limb, except ankle and foot**
    7 √7ᵗʰ **T24.299 Burn of second degree of multiple sites** ▽ **of unspecified lower limb, except ankle and foot**

√5ᵗʰ **T24.3 Burn of** third degree **of lower limb, except ankle and foot**
Use additional external cause code to identify the source, place and intent of the burn (X00-X19, X75-X77, X96-X98, Y92)

  √6ᵗʰ **T24.30 Burn of third degree of** unspecified site **of lower limb, except ankle and foot**
    7 √7ᵗʰ **T24.301 Burn of third degree of unspecified site** ▽ **of** right **lower limb, except ankle and foot**
    7 √7ᵗʰ **T24.302 Burn of third degree of unspecified site** ▽ **of** left **lower limb, except ankle and foot**
    7 √7ᵗʰ **T24.309 Burn of third degree of unspecified site** ▽ **of unspecified lower limb, except ankle and foot**

  √6ᵗʰ **T24.31 Burn of third degree of** thigh
    7 √7ᵗʰ **T24.311 Burn of third degree of** right **thigh**
    7 √7ᵗʰ **T24.312 Burn of third degree of** left **thigh**
    7 √7ᵗʰ **T24.319 Burn of third degree of unspecified** ▽ **thigh**

  √6ᵗʰ **T24.32 Burn of third degree of** knee
    7 √7ᵗʰ **T24.321 Burn of third degree of** right **knee**
    7 √7ᵗʰ **T24.322 Burn of third degree of** left **knee**
    7 √7ᵗʰ **T24.329 Burn of third degree of unspecified** ▽ **knee**

  √6ᵗʰ **T24.33 Burn of third degree of** lower leg
    7 √7ᵗʰ **T24.331 Burn of third degree of** right **lower leg**
    7 √7ᵗʰ **T24.332 Burn of third degree of** left **lower leg**
    7 √7ᵗʰ **T24.339 Burn of third degree of unspecified** ▽ **lower leg**

  √6ᵗʰ **T24.39 Burn of third degree of** multiple sites **of lower limb, except ankle and foot**
    7 √7ᵗʰ **T24.391 Burn of third degree of multiple sites of** right **lower limb, except ankle and foot**
    7 √7ᵗʰ **T24.392 Burn of third degree of multiple sites of** left **lower limb, except ankle and foot**

    7 √7ᵗʰ **T24.399 Burn of third degree of multiple sites** ▽ **of unspecified lower limb, except ankle and foot**

√5ᵗʰ **T24.4 Corrosion of** unspecified degree **of lower limb, except ankle and foot**
Code first (T51-T65) to identify chemical and intent
Use additional external cause code to identify place (Y92)

  √6ᵗʰ **T24.40 Corrosion of unspecified degree of** unspecified site **of lower limb, except ankle and foot**
    √7ᵗʰ **T24.401 Corrosion of unspecified degree of** ▽ **unspecified site of** right **lower limb, except ankle and foot**
    √7ᵗʰ **T24.402 Corrosion of unspecified degree of** ▽ **unspecified site of** left **lower limb, except ankle and foot**
    √7ᵗʰ **T24.409 Corrosion of unspecified degree of** ▽ **unspecified site of unspecified lower limb, except ankle and foot**

  √6ᵗʰ **T24.41 Corrosion of unspecified degree of** thigh
    √7ᵗʰ **T24.411 Corrosion of unspecified degree of** ▽ **right thigh**
    √7ᵗʰ **T24.412 Corrosion of unspecified degree of** ▽ **left thigh**
    √7ᵗʰ **T24.419 Corrosion of unspecified degree of** ▽ **unspecified thigh**

  √6ᵗʰ **T24.42 Corrosion of unspecified degree of** knee
    √7ᵗʰ **T24.421 Corrosion of unspecified degree of** ▽ **right knee**
    √7ᵗʰ **T24.422 Corrosion of unspecified degree of** ▽ **left knee**
    √7ᵗʰ **T24.429 Corrosion of unspecified degree of** ▽ **unspecified knee**

  √6ᵗʰ **T24.43 Corrosion of unspecified degree of** lower leg
    √7ᵗʰ **T24.431 Corrosion of unspecified degree of** ▽ **right lower leg**
    √7ᵗʰ **T24.432 Corrosion of unspecified degree of** ▽ **left lower leg**
    √7ᵗʰ **T24.439 Corrosion of unspecified degree of** ▽ **unspecified lower leg**

  √6ᵗʰ **T24.49 Corrosion of unspecified degree of** multiple sites **of lower limb, except ankle and foot**
    √7ᵗʰ **T24.491 Corrosion of unspecified degree of** ▽ **multiple sites of** right **lower limb, except ankle and foot**
    √7ᵗʰ **T24.492 Corrosion of unspecified degree of** ▽ **multiple sites of** left **lower limb, except ankle and foot**
    √7ᵗʰ **T24.499 Corrosion of unspecified degree of** ▽ **multiple sites of unspecified lower limb, except ankle and foot**

√5ᵗʰ **T24.5 Corrosion of** first degree **of lower limb, except ankle and foot**
Code first (T51-T65) to identify chemical and intent
Use additional external cause code to identify place (Y92)

  √6ᵗʰ **T24.50 Corrosion of first degree of** unspecified site **of lower limb, except ankle and foot**
    √7ᵗʰ **T24.501 Corrosion of first degree of** ▽ **unspecified site of** right **lower limb, except ankle and foot**
    √7ᵗʰ **T24.502 Corrosion of first degree of unspecified** ▽ **site of** left **lower limb, except ankle and foot**
    √7ᵗʰ **T24.509 Corrosion of first degree of unspecified** ▽ **site of unspecified lower limb, except ankle and foot**

  √6ᵗʰ **T24.51 Corrosion of first degree of** thigh
    √7ᵗʰ **T24.511 Corrosion of first degree of** right **thigh**
    √7ᵗʰ **T24.512 Corrosion of first degree of** left **thigh**
    √7ᵗʰ **T24.519 Corrosion of first degree of unspecified** ▽ **thigh**

  √6ᵗʰ **T24.52 Corrosion of first degree of** knee
    √7ᵗʰ **T24.521 Corrosion of first degree of** right **knee**
    √7ᵗʰ **T24.522 Corrosion of first degree of** left **knee**
    √7ᵗʰ **T24.529 Corrosion of first degree of unspecified** ▽ **knee**

---

⁷ Clinically Complex = With 7th character indicating a subsequent encounter

☑ Add'l Character Required   √7ᵗʰ Placeholder Alert   RUG IV Special Care High Dx   RUG IV Clinically Complex Dx   RUG IV Special Care Low Dx   Manifestation Code   Other Specified Code   ▽ Unspecified Code

√6ᵗʰ **T24.53** Corrosion of first degree of lower leg

     √7ᵗʰ **T24.531** Corrosion of first degree of right lower leg

     √7ᵗʰ **T24.532** Corrosion of first degree of left lower leg

     √7ᵗʰ **T24.539** Corrosion of first degree of unspecified ▽ lower leg

√6ᵗʰ **T24.59** Corrosion of first degree of multiple sites of lower limb, except ankle and foot

     √7ᵗʰ **T24.591** Corrosion of first degree of multiple sites of right lower limb, except ankle and foot

     √7ᵗʰ **T24.592** Corrosion of first degree of multiple sites of left lower limb, except ankle and foot

     √7ᵗʰ **T24.599** Corrosion of first degree of multiple ▽ sites of unspecified lower limb, except ankle and foot

√5ᵗʰ **T24.6** Corrosion of second degree of lower limb, except ankle and foot

     Code first (T51-T65) to identify chemical and intent

     Use additional external cause code to identify place (Y92)

   √6ᵗʰ **T24.60** Corrosion of second degree of unspecified site of lower limb, except ankle and foot

     √7ᵗʰ **T24.601** Corrosion of second degree of ▽ unspecified site of right lower limb, except ankle and foot

     √7ᵗʰ **T24.602** Corrosion of second degree of ▽ unspecified site of left lower limb, except ankle and foot

     √7ᵗʰ **T24.609** Corrosion of second degree of ▽ unspecified site of unspecified lower limb, except ankle and foot

   √6ᵗʰ **T24.61** Corrosion of second degree of thigh

     √7ᵗʰ **T24.611** Corrosion of second degree of right thigh

     √7ᵗʰ **T24.612** Corrosion of second degree of left thigh

     √7ᵗʰ **T24.619** Corrosion of second degree of ▽ unspecified thigh

   √6ᵗʰ **T24.62** Corrosion of second degree of knee

     √7ᵗʰ **T24.621** Corrosion of second degree of right knee

     √7ᵗʰ **T24.622** Corrosion of second degree of left knee

     √7ᵗʰ **T24.629** Corrosion of second degree of ▽ unspecified knee

   √6ᵗʰ **T24.63** Corrosion of second degree of lower leg

     √7ᵗʰ **T24.631** Corrosion of second degree of right lower leg

     √7ᵗʰ **T24.632** Corrosion of second degree of left lower leg

     √7ᵗʰ **T24.639** Corrosion of second degree of ▽ unspecified lower leg

   √6ᵗʰ **T24.69** Corrosion of second degree of multiple sites of lower limb, except ankle and foot

     √7ᵗʰ **T24.691** Corrosion of second degree of multiple sites of right lower limb, except ankle and foot

     √7ᵗʰ **T24.692** Corrosion of second degree of multiple sites of left lower limb, except ankle and foot

     √7ᵗʰ **T24.699** Corrosion of second degree of multiple ▽ sites of unspecified lower limb, except ankle and foot

√5ᵗʰ **T24.7** Corrosion of third degree of lower limb, except ankle and foot

     Code first (T51-T65) to identify chemical and intent

     Use additional external cause code to identify place (Y92)

   √6ᵗʰ **T24.70** Corrosion of third degree of unspecified site of lower limb, except ankle and foot

     √7ᵗʰ **T24.701** Corrosion of third degree of ▽ unspecified site of right lower limb, except ankle and foot

     √7ᵗʰ **T24.702** Corrosion of third degree of ▽ unspecified site of left lower limb, except ankle and foot

     √7ᵗʰ **T24.709** Corrosion of third degree of ▽ unspecified site of unspecified lower limb, except ankle and foot

   √6ᵗʰ **T24.71** Corrosion of third degree of thigh

     √7ᵗʰ **T24.711** Corrosion of third degree of right thigh

     √7ᵗʰ **T24.712** Corrosion of third degree of left thigh

     √7ᵗʰ **T24.719** Corrosion of third degree of ▽ unspecified thigh

   √6ᵗʰ **T24.72** Corrosion of third degree of knee

     √7ᵗʰ **T24.721** Corrosion of third degree of right knee

     √7ᵗʰ **T24.722** Corrosion of third degree of left knee

     √7ᵗʰ **T24.729** Corrosion of third degree of ▽ unspecified knee

   √6ᵗʰ **T24.73** Corrosion of third degree of lower leg

     √7ᵗʰ **T24.731** Corrosion of third degree of right lower leg

     √7ᵗʰ **T24.732** Corrosion of third degree of left lower leg

     √7ᵗʰ **T24.739** Corrosion of third degree of ▽ unspecified lower leg

   √6ᵗʰ **T24.79** Corrosion of third degree of multiple sites of lower limb, except ankle and foot

     √7ᵗʰ **T24.791** Corrosion of third degree of multiple sites of right lower limb, except ankle and foot

     √7ᵗʰ **T24.792** Corrosion of third degree of multiple sites of left lower limb, except ankle and foot

     √7ᵗʰ **T24.799** Corrosion of third degree of multiple ▽ sites of unspecified lower limb, except ankle and foot

√4ᵗʰ **T25** **Burn and corrosion of ankle and foot**

     The appropriate 7th character is to be added to each code from category T25.

     A   initial encounter

     D   subsequent encounter

     S   sequela

√5ᵗʰ **T25.0** Burn of unspecified degree of ankle and foot

     Use additional external cause code to identify the source, place and intent of the burn (X00-X19, X75-X77, X96-X98, Y92)

   √6ᵗʰ **T25.01** Burn of unspecified degree of ankle

     √7ᵗʰ **T25.011** Burn of unspecified degree of right ▽ ankle

     √7ᵗʰ **T25.012** Burn of unspecified degree of left ▽ ankle

     √7ᵗʰ **T25.019** Burn of unspecified degree of ▽ unspecified ankle

   √6ᵗʰ **T25.02** Burn of unspecified degree of foot

     EXCLUDES 2   burn of unspecified degree of toe(s) (nail) (T25.03-)

     √7ᵗʰ **T25.021** Burn of unspecified degree of right foot ▽

     √7ᵗʰ **T25.022** Burn of unspecified degree of left foot ▽

     √7ᵗʰ **T25.029** Burn of unspecified degree of ▽ unspecified foot

   √6ᵗʰ **T25.03** Burn of unspecified degree of toe(s) (nail)

     √7ᵗʰ **T25.031** Burn of unspecified degree of right ▽ toe(s) (nail)

     √7ᵗʰ **T25.032** Burn of unspecified degree of left ▽ toe(s) (nail)

     √7ᵗʰ **T25.039** Burn of unspecified degree of ▽ unspecified toe(s) (nail)

   √6ᵗʰ **T25.09** Burn of unspecified degree of multiple sites of ankle and foot

     √7ᵗʰ **T25.091** Burn of unspecified degree of multiple ▽ sites of right ankle and foot

     √7ᵗʰ **T25.092** Burn of unspecified degree of multiple ▽ sites of left ankle and foot

     √7ᵗʰ **T25.099** Burn of unspecified degree of multiple ▽ sites of unspecified ankle and foot

√5ᵗʰ **T25.1** Burn of first degree of ankle and foot

     Use additional external cause code to identify the source, place and intent of the burn (X00-X19, X75-X77, X96-X98, Y92)

   √6ᵗʰ **T25.11** Burn of first degree of ankle

     √7ᵗʰ **T25.111** Burn of first degree of right ankle

     √7ᵗʰ **T25.112** Burn of first degree of left ankle

     √7ᵗʰ **T25.119** Burn of first degree of unspecified ▽ ankle

   √6ᵗʰ **T25.12** Burn of first degree of foot

     EXCLUDES 2   burn of first degree of toe(s) (nail) (T25.13-)

     √7ᵗʰ **T25.121** Burn of first degree of right foot

     √7ᵗʰ **T25.122** Burn of first degree of left foot

Ⓝ Newborn   Ⓟ Pediatric   Ⓜ Maternity   Ⓐ Adult   **RIC** RIC Dx   **NCDx** Noncancer Dx   **PDx** Primary Dx   **CC** RIC CC Condition   ▶◀ Revised Text   ● New Code   ▲ Revised Code Title

992   ICD-10-CM 2016

✓7ᵗʰ **T25.129** Burn of first degree of unspecified foot ▽

✓6ᵗʰ **T25.13** Burn of first degree of toe(s) (nail)

  ✓7ᵗʰ **T25.131** Burn of first degree of right toe(s) (nail)

  ✓7ᵗʰ **T25.132** Burn of first degree of left toe(s) (nail)

  ✓7ᵗʰ **T25.139** Burn of first degree of unspecified toe(s) (nail) ▽

✓6ᵗʰ **T25.19** Burn of first degree of multiple sites of ankle and foot

  ✓7ᵗʰ **T25.191** Burn of first degree of multiple sites of right ankle and foot

  ✓7ᵗʰ **T25.192** Burn of first degree of multiple sites of left ankle and foot

  ✓7ᵗʰ **T25.199** Burn of first degree of multiple sites of unspecified ankle and foot ▽

✓5ᵗʰ **T25.2** Burn of second degree of ankle and foot
Use additional external cause code to identify the source, place and intent of the burn (X00-X19, X75-X77, X96-X98, Y92)

✓6ᵗʰ **T25.21** Burn of second degree of ankle

  7 ✓7ᵗʰ **T25.211** Burn of second degree of right ankle

  7 ✓7ᵗʰ **T25.212** Burn of second degree of left ankle

  7 ✓7ᵗʰ **T25.219** Burn of second degree of unspecified ankle ▽

✓6ᵗʰ **T25.22** Burn of second degree of foot
EXCLUDES 2 burn of second degree of toe(s) (nail) (T25.23-)

  7 ✓7ᵗʰ **T25.221** Burn of second degree of right foot

  7 ✓7ᵗʰ **T25.222** Burn of second degree of left foot

  7 ✓7ᵗʰ **T25.229** Burn of second degree of unspecified foot ▽

✓6ᵗʰ **T25.23** Burn of second degree of toe(s) (nail)

  7 ✓7ᵗʰ **T25.231** Burn of second degree of right toe(s) (nail)

  7 ✓7ᵗʰ **T25.232** Burn of second degree of left toe(s) (nail)

  7 ✓7ᵗʰ **T25.239** Burn of second degree of unspecified toe(s) (nail) ▽

✓6ᵗʰ **T25.29** Burn of second degree of multiple sites of ankle and foot

  7 ✓7ᵗʰ **T25.291** Burn of second degree of multiple sites of right ankle and foot

  7 ✓7ᵗʰ **T25.292** Burn of second degree of multiple sites of left ankle and foot

  7 ✓7ᵗʰ **T25.299** Burn of second degree of multiple sites of unspecified ankle and foot ▽

✓5ᵗʰ **T25.3** Burn of third degree of ankle and foot
Use additional external cause code to identify the source, place and intent of the burn (X00-X19, X75-X77, X96-X98, Y92)

✓6ᵗʰ **T25.31** Burn of third degree of ankle

  7 ✓7ᵗʰ **T25.311** Burn of third degree of right ankle

  7 ✓7ᵗʰ **T25.312** Burn of third degree of left ankle

  7 ✓7ᵗʰ **T25.319** Burn of third degree of unspecified ankle ▽

✓6ᵗʰ **T25.32** Burn of third degree of foot
EXCLUDES 2 burn of third degree of toe(s) (nail) (T25.33-)

  7 ✓7ᵗʰ **T25.321** Burn of third degree of right foot

  7 ✓7ᵗʰ **T25.322** Burn of third degree of left foot

  7 ✓7ᵗʰ **T25.329** Burn of third degree of unspecified foot ▽

✓6ᵗʰ **T25.33** Burn of third degree of toe(s) (nail)

  7 ✓7ᵗʰ **T25.331** Burn of third degree of right toe(s) (nail)

  7 ✓7ᵗʰ **T25.332** Burn of third degree of left toe(s) (nail)

  7 ✓7ᵗʰ **T25.339** Burn of third degree of unspecified toe(s) (nail) ▽

✓6ᵗʰ **T25.39** Burn of third degree of multiple sites of ankle and foot

  7 ✓7ᵗʰ **T25.391** Burn of third degree of multiple sites of right ankle and foot

  7 ✓7ᵗʰ **T25.392** Burn of third degree of multiple sites of left ankle and foot

  7 ✓7ᵗʰ **T25.399** Burn of third degree of multiple sites of unspecified ankle and foot ▽

✓5ᵗʰ **T25.4** Corrosion of unspecified degree of ankle and foot
Code first (T51-T65) to identify chemical and intent
Use additional external cause code to identify place (Y92)

✓6ᵗʰ **T25.41** Corrosion of unspecified degree of ankle

  ✓7ᵗʰ **T25.411** Corrosion of unspecified degree of right ankle ▽

  ✓7ᵗʰ **T25.412** Corrosion of unspecified degree of left ankle ▽

  ✓7ᵗʰ **T25.419** Corrosion of unspecified degree of unspecified ankle ▽

✓6ᵗʰ **T25.42** Corrosion of unspecified degree of foot
EXCLUDES 2 corrosion of unspecified degree of toe(s) (nail) (T25.43-)

  ✓7ᵗʰ **T25.421** Corrosion of unspecified degree of right foot ▽

  ✓7ᵗʰ **T25.422** Corrosion of unspecified degree of left foot ▽

  ✓7ᵗʰ **T25.429** Corrosion of unspecified degree of unspecified foot ▽

✓6ᵗʰ **T25.43** Corrosion of unspecified degree of toe(s) (nail)

  ✓7ᵗʰ **T25.431** Corrosion of unspecified degree of right toe(s) (nail) ▽

  ✓7ᵗʰ **T25.432** Corrosion of unspecified degree of left toe(s) (nail) ▽

  ✓7ᵗʰ **T25.439** Corrosion of unspecified degree of unspecified toe(s) (nail) ▽

✓6ᵗʰ **T25.49** Corrosion of unspecified degree of multiple sites of ankle and foot

  ✓7ᵗʰ **T25.491** Corrosion of unspecified degree of multiple sites of right ankle and foot ▽

  ✓7ᵗʰ **T25.492** Corrosion of unspecified degree of multiple sites of left ankle and foot ▽

  ✓7ᵗʰ **T25.499** Corrosion of unspecified degree of multiple sites of unspecified ankle and foot ▽

✓5ᵗʰ **T25.5** Corrosion of first degree of ankle and foot
Code first (T51-T65) to identify chemical and intent
Use additional external cause code to identify place (Y92)

✓6ᵗʰ **T25.51** Corrosion of first degree of ankle

  ✓7ᵗʰ **T25.511** Corrosion of first degree of right ankle

  ✓7ᵗʰ **T25.512** Corrosion of first degree of left ankle

  ✓7ᵗʰ **T25.519** Corrosion of first degree of unspecified ankle ▽

✓6ᵗʰ **T25.52** Corrosion of first degree of foot
EXCLUDES 2 corrosion of first degree of toe(s) (nail) (T25.53-)

  ✓7ᵗʰ **T25.521** Corrosion of first degree of right foot

  ✓7ᵗʰ **T25.522** Corrosion of first degree of left foot

  ✓7ᵗʰ **T25.529** Corrosion of first degree of unspecified foot ▽

✓6ᵗʰ **T25.53** Corrosion of first degree of toe(s) (nail)

  ✓7ᵗʰ **T25.531** Corrosion of first degree of right toe(s) (nail)

  ✓7ᵗʰ **T25.532** Corrosion of first degree of left toe(s) (nail)

  ✓7ᵗʰ **T25.539** Corrosion of first degree of unspecified toe(s) (nail) ▽

✓6ᵗʰ **T25.59** Corrosion of first degree of multiple sites of ankle and foot

  ✓7ᵗʰ **T25.591** Corrosion of first degree of multiple sites of right ankle and foot

  ✓7ᵗʰ **T25.592** Corrosion of first degree of multiple sites of left ankle and foot

  ✓7ᵗʰ **T25.599** Corrosion of first degree of multiple sites of unspecified ankle and foot ▽

✓5ᵗʰ **T25.6** Corrosion of second degree of ankle and foot
Code first (T51-T65) to identify chemical and intent
Use additional external cause code to identify place (Y92)

✓6ᵗʰ **T25.61** Corrosion of second degree of ankle

  ✓7ᵗʰ **T25.611** Corrosion of second degree of right ankle

  ✓7ᵗʰ **T25.612** Corrosion of second degree of left ankle

  ✓7ᵗʰ **T25.619** Corrosion of second degree of unspecified ankle ▽

---

7 Clinically Complex = With 7th character indicating a subsequent encounter

☑ Add'l Character Required   ✓x7ᵗʰ Placeholder Alert   RUG IV Special Care High Dx   RUG IV Clinically Complex Dx   RUG IV Special Care Low Dx   Manifestation Code   Other Specified Code   ▽ Unspecified Code

✓6ᵗʰ **T25.62 Corrosion of second degree of foot**
    EXCLUDES 2 *corrosion of second degree of toe(s) (nail) (T25.63-)*

     ✓7ᵗʰ **T25.621 Corrosion of second degree of right foot**
     ✓7ᵗʰ **T25.622 Corrosion of second degree of left foot**
     ✓7ᵗʰ **T25.629 Corrosion of second degree of unspecified foot** ▽

✓6ᵗʰ **T25.63 Corrosion of second degree of toe(s) (nail)**
     ✓7ᵗʰ **T25.631 Corrosion of second degree of right toe(s) (nail)**
     ✓7ᵗʰ **T25.632 Corrosion of second degree of left toe(s) (nail)**
     ✓7ᵗʰ **T25.639 Corrosion of second degree of unspecified toe(s) (nail)** ▽

✓6ᵗʰ **T25.69 Corrosion of second degree of multiple sites of ankle and foot**
     ✓7ᵗʰ **T25.691 Corrosion of second degree of right ankle and foot**
     ✓7ᵗʰ **T25.692 Corrosion of second degree of left ankle and foot**
     ✓7ᵗʰ **T25.699 Corrosion of second degree of unspecified ankle and foot** ▽

✓5ᵗʰ **T25.7 Corrosion of third degree of ankle and foot**
    Code first (T51-T65) to identify chemical and intent
    Use additional external cause code to identify place (Y92)

✓6ᵗʰ **T25.71 Corrosion of third degree of ankle**
     ✓7ᵗʰ **T25.711 Corrosion of third degree of right ankle**
     ✓7ᵗʰ **T25.712 Corrosion of third degree of left ankle**
     ✓7ᵗʰ **T25.719 Corrosion of third degree of unspecified ankle** ▽

✓6ᵗʰ **T25.72 Corrosion of third degree of foot**
    EXCLUDES 2 *corrosion of third degree of toe(s) (nail) (T25.73-)*
     ✓7ᵗʰ **T25.721 Corrosion of third degree of right foot**
     ✓7ᵗʰ **T25.722 Corrosion of third degree of left foot**
     ✓7ᵗʰ **T25.729 Corrosion of third degree of unspecified foot** ▽

✓6ᵗʰ **T25.73 Corrosion of third degree of toe(s) (nail)**
     ✓7ᵗʰ **T25.731 Corrosion of third degree of right toe(s) (nail)**
     ✓7ᵗʰ **T25.732 Corrosion of third degree of left toe(s) (nail)**
     ✓7ᵗʰ **T25.739 Corrosion of third degree of unspecified toe(s) (nail)** ▽

✓6ᵗʰ **T25.79 Corrosion of third degree of multiple sites of ankle and foot**
     ✓7ᵗʰ **T25.791 Corrosion of third degree of multiple sites of right ankle and foot**
     ✓7ᵗʰ **T25.792 Corrosion of third degree of multiple sites of left ankle and foot**
     ✓7ᵗʰ **T25.799 Corrosion of third degree of multiple sites of unspecified ankle and foot** ▽

Burns and corrosions confined to eye and internal organs (T26-T28)

✓4ᵗʰ **T26 Burn and corrosion confined to eye and adnexa**

> The appropriate 7th character is to be added to each code from category T26.
> A   initial encounter
> D   subsequent encounter
> S   sequela

✓5ᵗʰ **T26.0 Burn of eyelid and periocular area**
    Use additional external cause code to identify the source, place and intent of the burn (X00-X19, X75-X77, X96-X98, Y92)
    7 ✓x7ᵗʰ **T26.00 Burn of unspecified eyelid and periocular area** ▽
    7 ✓x7ᵗʰ **T26.01 Burn of right eyelid and periocular area**
    7 ✓x7ᵗʰ **T26.02 Burn of left eyelid and periocular area**

✓5ᵗʰ **T26.1 Burn of cornea and conjunctival sac**
    Use additional external cause code to identify the source, place and intent of the burn (X00-X19, X75-X77, X96-X98, Y92)
    7 ✓x7ᵗʰ **T26.10 Burn of cornea and conjunctival sac, unspecified eye** ▽

    7 ✓x7ᵗʰ **T26.11 Burn of cornea and conjunctival sac, right eye**
    7 ✓x7ᵗʰ **T26.12 Burn of cornea and conjunctival sac, left eye**

✓5ᵗʰ **T26.2 Burn with resulting rupture and destruction of eyeball**
    Use additional external cause code to identify the source, place and intent of the burn (X00-X19, X75-X77, X96-X98, Y92)
    7 ✓x7ᵗʰ **T26.20 Burn with resulting rupture and destruction of unspecified eyeball**
    7 ✓x7ᵗʰ **T26.21 Burn with resulting rupture and destruction of right eyeball**
    7 ✓x7ᵗʰ **T26.22 Burn with resulting rupture and destruction of left eyeball**

✓5ᵗʰ **T26.3 Burns of other specified parts of eye and adnexa**
    Use additional external cause code to identify the source, place and intent of the burn (X00-X19, X75-X77, X96-X98, Y92)
    7 ✓x7ᵗʰ **T26.30 Burns of other specified parts of unspecified eye and adnexa** ▽
    7 ✓x7ᵗʰ **T26.31 Burns of other specified parts of right eye and adnexa**
    7 ✓x7ᵗʰ **T26.32 Burns of other specified parts of left eye and adnexa**

✓5ᵗʰ **T26.4 Burn of eye and adnexa, part unspecified**
    Use additional external cause code to identify the source, place and intent of the burn (X00-X19, X75-X77, X96-X98, Y92)
    7 ✓x7ᵗʰ **T26.40 Burn of unspecified eye and adnexa, part unspecified** ▽
    7 ✓x7ᵗʰ **T26.41 Burn of right eye and adnexa, part unspecified** ▽
    7 ✓x7ᵗʰ **T26.42 Burn of left eye and adnexa, part unspecified** ▽

✓5ᵗʰ **T26.5 Corrosion of eyelid and periocular area**
    Code first (T51-T65) to identify chemical and intent
    Use additional external cause code to identify place (Y92)
    ✓x7ᵗʰ **T26.50 Corrosion of unspecified eyelid and periocular area** ▽
    ✓x7ᵗʰ **T26.51 Corrosion of right eyelid and periocular area**
    ✓x7ᵗʰ **T26.52 Corrosion of left eyelid and periocular area**

✓5ᵗʰ **T26.6 Corrosion of cornea and conjunctival sac**
    Code first (T51-T65) to identify chemical and intent
    Use additional external cause code to identify place (Y92)
    ✓x7ᵗʰ **T26.60 Corrosion of cornea and conjunctival sac, unspecified eye** ▽
    ✓x7ᵗʰ **T26.61 Corrosion of cornea and conjunctival sac, right eye**
    ✓x7ᵗʰ **T26.62 Corrosion of cornea and conjunctival sac, left eye**

✓5ᵗʰ **T26.7 Corrosion with resulting rupture and destruction of eyeball**
    Code first (T51-T65) to identify chemical and intent
    Use additional external cause code to identify place (Y92)
    ✓x7ᵗʰ **T26.70 Corrosion with resulting rupture and destruction of unspecified eyeball** ▽
    ✓x7ᵗʰ **T26.71 Corrosion with resulting rupture and destruction of right eyeball**
    ✓x7ᵗʰ **T26.72 Corrosion with resulting rupture and destruction of left eyeball**

✓5ᵗʰ **T26.8 Corrosions of other specified parts of eye and adnexa**
    Code first (T51-T65) to identify chemical and intent
    Use additional external cause code to identify place (Y92)
    ✓x7ᵗʰ **T26.80 Corrosions of other specified parts of unspecified eye and adnexa** ▽
    ✓x7ᵗʰ **T26.81 Corrosions of other specified parts of right eye and adnexa**
    ✓x7ᵗʰ **T26.82 Corrosions of other specified parts of left eye and adnexa**

✓5ᵗʰ **T26.9 Corrosion of eye and adnexa, part unspecified**
    Code first (T51-T65) to identify chemical and intent
    Use additional external cause code to identify place (Y92)
    ✓x7ᵗʰ **T26.90 Corrosion of unspecified eye and adnexa, part unspecified** ▽
    ✓x7ᵗʰ **T26.91 Corrosion of right eye and adnexa, part unspecified** ▽
    ✓x7ᵗʰ **T26.92 Corrosion of left eye and adnexa, part unspecified** ▽

---

7 Clinically Complex = With 7th character indicating a subsequent encounter

✓4ᵗʰ T27 Burn and corrosion of respiratory tract

Use additional external cause code to identify the source and intent of the burn (X00-X19, X75-X77, X96-X98)

Use additional external cause code to identify place (Y92)

> The appropriate 7th character is to be added to each code from category T27.
> A   initial encounter
> D   subsequent encounter
> S   sequela

✓x7ᵗʰ **T27.0**   Burn of larynx and trachea

✓x7ᵗʰ **T27.1**   Burn involving larynx and trachea with lung

✓x7ᵗʰ **T27.2**   Burn of other parts of respiratory tract
> Burn of thoracic cavity

✓x7ᵗʰ **T27.3**   Burn of respiratory tract, part unspecified   ▽
> Code first (T51-T65) to identify chemical and intent for codes T27.4-T27.7

✓x7ᵗʰ **T27.4**   Corrosion of larynx and trachea

✓x7ᵗʰ **T27.5**   Corrosion involving larynx and trachea with lung

✓x7ᵗʰ **T27.6**   Corrosion of other parts of respiratory tract

✓x7ᵗʰ **T27.7**   Corrosion of respiratory tract, part unspecified   ▽

✓4ᵗʰ T28 Burn and corrosion of other internal organs

Use additional external cause code to identify the source and intent of the burn (X00- X19, X75-X77, X96-X98)

Use additional external cause code to identify place (Y92)

> The appropriate 7th character is to be added to each code from category T28.
> A   initial encounter
> D   subsequent encounter
> S   sequela

✓x7ᵗʰ **T28.0**   Burn of mouth and pharynx

✓x7ᵗʰ **T28.1**   Burn of esophagus

✓x7ᵗʰ **T28.2**   Burn of other parts of alimentary tract

✓x7ᵗʰ **T28.3**   Burn of internal genitourinary organs

✓5ᵗʰ **T28.4**   Burns of other and unspecified internal organs

    ✓x7ᵗʰ **T28.40**   Burn of unspecified internal organ   ▽

    ✓6ᵗʰ **T28.41**   Burn of ear drum

        ✓7ᵗʰ **T28.411**   Burn of right ear drum

        ✓7ᵗʰ **T28.412**   Burn of left ear drum

        ✓7ᵗʰ **T28.419**   Burn of unspecified ear drum   ▽

    ✓x7ᵗʰ **T28.49**   Burn of other internal organ
> Code first (T51-T65) to identify chemical and intent for T28.5-T28.9-

✓x7ᵗʰ **T28.5**   Corrosion of mouth and pharynx

✓x7ᵗʰ **T28.6**   Corrosion of esophagus

✓x7ᵗʰ **T28.7**   Corrosion of other parts of alimentary tract

✓x7ᵗʰ **T28.8**   Corrosion of internal genitourinary organs

✓5ᵗʰ **T28.9**   Corrosions of other and unspecified internal organs

    ✓x7ᵗʰ **T28.90**   Corrosions of unspecified internal organs   ▽

    ✓6ᵗʰ **T28.91**   Corrosions of ear drum

        ✓7ᵗʰ **T28.911**   Corrosions of right ear drum

        ✓7ᵗʰ **T28.912**   Corrosions of left ear drum

        ✓7ᵗʰ **T28.919**   Corrosions of unspecified ear drum   ▽

    ✓x7ᵗʰ **T28.99**   Corrosions of other internal organs

Burns and corrosions of multiple and unspecified body regions (T30-T32)

✓4ᵗʰ T30 Burn and corrosion, body region unspecified

T30.0   Burn of unspecified body region, unspecified degree   ▽
> **NOTE**   This code is not for inpatient use. Code to specified site and degree of burns.
> Burn NOS
> Multiple burns NOS

T30.4   Corrosion of unspecified body region, unspecified degree   ▽
> **NOTE**   This code is not for inpatient use. Code to specified site and degree of corrosion.
> Corrosion NOS
> Multiple corrosion NOS

✓4ᵗʰ T31 Burns classified according to extent of body surface involved

> **NOTE**   This category is to be used as the primary code only when the site of the burn is unspecified. It should be used as a supplementary code with categories T20-T25 when the site is specified.

T31.0   Burns involving less than 10% of body surface

✓5ᵗʰ **T31.1**   Burns involving 10-19% of body surface

    T31.10   Burns involving 10-19% of body surface with 0% to 9% third degree burns
> Burns involving 10-19% of body surface NOS

    T31.11   Burns involving 10-19% of body surface with 10-19% third degree burns

✓5ᵗʰ **T31.2**   Burns involving 20-29% of body surface

    T31.20   Burns involving 20-29% of body surface with 0% to 9% third degree burns
> Burns involving 20-29% of body surface NOS

    T31.21   Burns involving 20-29% of body surface with 10-19% third degree burns

    T31.22   Burns involving 20-29% of body surface with 20-29% third degree burns

✓5ᵗʰ **T31.3**   Burns involving 30-39% of body surface

    T31.30   Burns involving 30-39% of body surface with 0% to 9% third degree burns
> Burns involving 30-39% of body surface NOS

    T31.31   Burns involving 30-39% of body surface with 10-19% third degree burns

    T31.32   Burns involving 30-39% of body surface with 20-29% third degree burns

    T31.33   Burns involving 30-39% of body surface with 30-39% third degree burns

✓5ᵗʰ **T31.4**   Burns involving 40-49% of body surface

    T31.40   Burns involving 40-49% of body surface with 0% to 9% third degree burns
> Burns involving 40-49% of body surface NOS

    T31.41   Burns involving 40-49% of body surface with 10-19% third degree burns

    T31.42   Burns involving 40-49% of body surface with 20-29% third degree burns

    T31.43   Burns involving 40-49% of body surface with 30-39% third degree burns

    T31.44   Burns involving 40-49% of body surface with 40-49% third degree burns

✓5ᵗʰ **T31.5**   Burns involving 50-59% of body surface

    T31.50   Burns involving 50-59% of body surface with 0% to 9% third degree burns
> Burns involving 50-59% of body surface NOS

    T31.51   Burns involving 50-59% of body surface with 10-19% third degree burns

    T31.52   Burns involving 50-59% of body surface with 20-29% third degree burns

    T31.53   Burns involving 50-59% of body surface with 30-39% third degree burns

    T31.54   Burns involving 50-59% of body surface with 40-49% third degree burns

    T31.55   Burns involving 50-59% of body surface with 50-59% third degree burns

✓5ᵗʰ **T31.6**   Burns involving 60-69% of body surface

    T31.60   Burns involving 60-69% of body surface with 0% to 9% third degree burns
> Burns involving 60-69% of body surface NOS

    T31.61   Burns involving 60-69% of body surface with 10-19% third degree burns

    T31.62   Burns involving 60-69% of body surface with 20-29% third degree burns

    T31.63   Burns involving 60-69% of body surface with 30-39% third degree burns

    T31.64   Burns involving 60-69% of body surface with 40-49% third degree burns

    T31.65   Burns involving 60-69% of body surface with 50-59% third degree burns

    T31.66   Burns involving 60-69% of body surface with 60-69% third degree burns

✓5ᵗʰ **T31.7**   Burns involving 70-79% of body surface

    T31.70   Burns involving 70-79% of body surface with 0% to 9% third degree burns
> Burns involving 70-79% of body surface NOS

✓ Add'l Character Required   ✓x7ᵗʰ Placeholder Alert   RUG IV Special Care High Dx   RUG IV Clinically Complex Dx   RUG IV Special Care Low Dx   Manifestation Code   Other Specified Code   ▽ Unspecified Code
ICD-10-CM 2016   995

T27–T31.70

T31.71 Burns involving 70-79% of body surface with 10-19% third degree **burns**

T31.72 Burns involving 70-79% of body surface with 20-29% third degree **burns**

T31.73 Burns involving 70-79% of body surface with 30-39% third degree **burns**

T31.74 Burns involving 70-79% of body surface with 40-49% third degree **burns**

T31.75 Burns involving 70-79% of body surface with 50-59% third degree **burns**

T31.76 Burns involving 70-79% of body surface with 60-69% third degree **burns**

T31.77 Burns involving 70-79% of body surface with 70-79% third degree **burns**

✓5ᵗʰ **T31.8** Burns involving 80-89% of body surface

T31.80 Burns involving 80-89% of body surface with 0% to 9% third degree **burns**
Burns involving 80-89% of body surface NOS

T31.81 Burns involving 80-89% of body surface with 10-19% third degree **burns**

T31.82 Burns involving 80-89% of body surface with 20-29% third degree **burns**

T31.83 Burns involving 80-89% of body surface with 30-39% third degree **burns**

T31.84 Burns involving 80-89% of body surface with 40-49% third degree **burns**

T31.85 Burns involving 80-89% of body surface with 50-59% third degree **burns**

T31.86 Burns involving 80-89% of body surface with 60-69% third degree **burns**

T31.87 Burns involving 80-89% of body surface with 70-79% third degree **burns**

T31.88 Burns involving 80-89% of body surface with 80-89% third degree **burns**

✓5ᵗʰ **T31.9** Burns involving 90% or more of body surface

T31.90 Burns involving 90% or more of body surface with 0% to 9% third degree **burns**
Burns involving 90% or more of body surface NOS

T31.91 Burns involving 90% or more of body surface with 10-19% third degree **burns**

T31.92 Burns involving 90% or more of body surface with 20-29% third degree **burns**

T31.93 Burns involving 90% or more of body surface with 30-39% third degree **burns**

T31.94 Burns involving 90% or more of body surface with 40-49% third degree **burns**

T31.95 Burns involving 90% or more of body surface with 50-59% third degree **burns**

T31.96 Burns involving 90% or more of body surface with 60-69% third degree **burns**

T31.97 Burns involving 90% or more of body surface with 70-79% third degree **burns**

T31.98 Burns involving 90% or more of body surface with 80-89% third degree **burns**

T31.99 Burns involving 90% or more of body surface with 90% or more third degree **burns**

✓4ᵗʰ **T32** Corrosions classified according to extent of body surface involved

> **NOTE** This category is to be used as the primary code only when the site of the corrosion is unspecified. It may be used as a supplementary code with categories T20-T25 when the site is specified.

T32.0 Corrosions involving less than 10% of body surface

✓5ᵗʰ **T32.1** Corrosions involving 10-19% of body surface

T32.10 Corrosions involving 10-19% of body surface with 0% to 9% third degree **corrosion**
Corrosions involving 10-19% of body surface NOS

T32.11 Corrosions involving 10-19% of body surface with 10-19% third degree **corrosion**

✓5ᵗʰ **T32.2** Corrosions involving 20-29% of body surface

T32.20 Corrosions involving 20-29% of body surface with 0% to 9% third degree **corrosion**

T32.21 Corrosions involving 20-29% of body surface with 10-19% third degree **corrosion**

T32.22 Corrosions involving 20-29% of body surface with 20-29% third degree **corrosion**

✓5ᵗʰ **T32.3** Corrosions involving 30-39% of body surface

T32.30 Corrosions involving 30-39% of body surface with 0% to 9% third degree **corrosion**

T32.31 Corrosions involving 30-39% of body surface with 10-19% third degree **corrosion**

T32.32 Corrosions involving 30-39% of body surface with 20-29% third degree **corrosion**

T32.33 Corrosions involving 30-39% of body surface with 30-39% third degree **corrosion**

✓5ᵗʰ **T32.4** Corrosions involving 40-49% of body surface

T32.40 Corrosions involving 40-49% of body surface with 0% to 9% third degree **corrosion**

T32.41 Corrosions involving 40-49% of body surface with 10-19% third degree **corrosion**

T32.42 Corrosions involving 40-49% of body surface with 20-29% third degree **corrosion**

T32.43 Corrosions involving 40-49% of body surface with 30-39% third degree **corrosion**

T32.44 Corrosions involving 40-49% of body surface with 40-49% third degree **corrosion**

✓5ᵗʰ **T32.5** Corrosions involving 50-59% of body surface

T32.50 Corrosions involving 50-59% of body surface with 0% to 9% third degree **corrosion**

T32.51 Corrosions involving 50-59% of body surface with 10-19% third degree **corrosion**

T32.52 Corrosions involving 50-59% of body surface with 20-29% third degree **corrosion**

T32.53 Corrosions involving 50-59% of body surface with 30-39% third degree **corrosion**

T32.54 Corrosions involving 50-59% of body surface with 40-49% third degree **corrosion**

T32.55 Corrosions involving 50-59% of body surface with 50-59% third degree **corrosion**

✓5ᵗʰ **T32.6** Corrosions involving 60-69% of body surface

T32.60 Corrosions involving 60-69% of body surface with 0% to 9% third degree **corrosion**

T32.61 Corrosions involving 60-69% of body surface with 10-19% third degree **corrosion**

T32.62 Corrosions involving 60-69% of body surface with 20-29% third degree **corrosion**

T32.63 Corrosions involving 60-69% of body surface with 30-39% third degree **corrosion**

T32.64 Corrosions involving 60-69% of body surface with 40-49% third degree **corrosion**

T32.65 Corrosions involving 60-69% of body surface with 50-59% third degree **corrosion**

T32.66 Corrosions involving 60-69% of body surface with 60-69% third degree **corrosion**

✓5ᵗʰ **T32.7** Corrosions involving 70-79% of body surface

T32.70 Corrosions involving 70-79% of body surface with 0% to 9% third degree **corrosion**

T32.71 Corrosions involving 70-79% of body surface with 10-19% third degree **corrosion**

T32.72 Corrosions involving 70-79% of body surface with 20-29% third degree **corrosion**

T32.73 Corrosions involving 70-79% of body surface with 30-39% third degree **corrosion**

T32.74 Corrosions involving 70-79% of body surface with 40-49% third degree **corrosion**

T32.75 Corrosions involving 70-79% of body surface with 50-59% third degree **corrosion**

T32.76 Corrosions involving 70-79% of body surface with 60-69% third degree **corrosion**

T32.77 Corrosions involving 70-79% of body surface with 70-79% third degree **corrosion**

✓5ᵗʰ **T32.8** Corrosions involving 80-89% of body surface

T32.80 Corrosions involving 80-89% of body surface with 0% to 9% third degree **corrosion**

T32.81 Corrosions involving 80-89% of body surface with 10-19% third degree **corrosion**

T32.82 Corrosions involving 80-89% of body surface with 20-29% third degree **corrosion**

T32.83 Corrosions involving 80-89% of body surface with 30-39% third degree **corrosion**

T32.84 Corrosions involving 80-89% of body surface with 40-49% third degree **corrosion**

Ⓝ Newborn   Ⓟ Pediatric   Ⓜ Maternity   Ⓐ Adult   **RIC** RIC Dx   **NC Dx** Noncancer Dx   **PDx** Primary Dx   **CC** RIC CC Condition   ▶◀ Revised Text   ● New Code   ▲ Revised Code Title

996   ICD-10-CM 2016

T32.85   Corrosions involving 80-89% of body surface with 50-59% third degree **corrosion**

T32.86   Corrosions involving 80-89% of body surface with 60-69% third degree **corrosion**

T32.87   Corrosions involving 80-89% of body surface with 70-79% third degree **corrosion**

T32.88   Corrosions involving 80-89% of body surface with 80-89% third degree **corrosion**

√5ᵗʰ **T32.9**   **Corrosions involving** 90% or more **of body surface**

T32.90   Corrosions involving 90% or more of body surface with 0% to 9% third degree **corrosion**

T32.91   Corrosions involving 90% or more of body surface with 10-19% third degree **corrosion**

T32.92   Corrosions involving 90% or more of body surface with 20-29% third degree **corrosion**

T32.93   Corrosions involving 90% or more of body surface with 30-39% third degree **corrosion**

T32.94   Corrosions involving 90% or more of body surface with 40-49% third degree **corrosion**

T32.95   Corrosions involving 90% or more of body surface with 50-59% third degree **corrosion**

T32.96   Corrosions involving 90% or more of body surface with 60-69% third degree **corrosion**

T32.97   Corrosions involving 90% or more of body surface with 70-79% third degree **corrosion**

T32.98   Corrosions involving 90% or more of body surface with 80-89% third degree **corrosion**

T32.99   Corrosions involving 90% or more of body surface with 90% or more third degree **corrosion**

Frostbite (T33-T34)

EXCLUDES 2   *hypothermia and other effects of reduced temperature (T68, T69-)*

√4ᵗʰ **T33**   **Superficial frostbite**

INCLUDES   frostbite with partial thickness skin loss

The appropriate 7th character is to be added to each code from category T33.
A   initial encounter
D   subsequent encounter
S   sequela

√5ᵗʰ **T33.0**   **Superficial frostbite of** head

√6ᵗʰ **T33.01**   **Superficial frostbite of** ear

√7ᵗʰ **T33.011**   Superficial frostbite of right ear

√7ᵗʰ **T33.012**   Superficial frostbite of left ear

√7ᵗʰ **T33.019**   Superficial frostbite of unspecified ear ▽

√x7ᵗʰ **T33.02**   Superficial frostbite of nose

√x7ᵗʰ **T33.09**   **Superficial frostbite of other** part of head

√x7ᵗʰ **T33.1**   **Superficial frostbite of** neck

√x7ᵗʰ **T33.2**   **Superficial frostbite of** thorax

√x7ᵗʰ **T33.3**   **Superficial frostbite of** abdominal wall, lower back and pelvis

√5ᵗʰ **T33.4**   **Superficial frostbite of** arm

EXCLUDES 2   *superficial frostbite of wrist and hand (T33.5-)*

√x7ᵗʰ **T33.40**   Superficial frostbite of unspecified arm ▽

√x7ᵗʰ **T33.41**   Superficial frostbite of right arm

√x7ᵗʰ **T33.42**   Superficial frostbite of left arm

√5ᵗʰ **T33.5**   **Superficial frostbite of** wrist, hand, and fingers

√6ᵗʰ **T33.51**   **Superficial frostbite of** wrist

√7ᵗʰ **T33.511**   Superficial frostbite of right wrist

√7ᵗʰ **T33.512**   Superficial frostbite of left wrist

√7ᵗʰ **T33.519**   Superficial frostbite of unspecified wrist ▽

√6ᵗʰ **T33.52**   **Superficial frostbite of** hand

EXCLUDES 2   *superficial frostbite of fingers (T33.53-)*

√7ᵗʰ **T33.521**   Superficial frostbite of right hand

√7ᵗʰ **T33.522**   Superficial frostbite of left hand

√7ᵗʰ **T33.529**   Superficial frostbite of unspecified hand ▽

√6ᵗʰ **T33.53**   **Superficial frostbite of** finger(s)

√7ᵗʰ **T33.531**   Superficial frostbite of right finger(s)

√7ᵗʰ **T33.532**   Superficial frostbite of left finger(s)

√7ᵗʰ **T33.539**   Superficial frostbite of unspecified finger(s) ▽

√5ᵗʰ **T33.6**   **Superficial frostbite of** hip and thigh

√x7ᵗʰ **T33.60**   Superficial frostbite of unspecified hip and thigh ▽

√x7ᵗʰ **T33.61**   Superficial frostbite of right hip and thigh

√x7ᵗʰ **T33.62**   Superficial frostbite of left hip and thigh

√5ᵗʰ **T33.7**   **Superficial frostbite of** knee and lower leg

EXCLUDES 2   *superficial frostbite of ankle and foot (T33.8-)*

√x7ᵗʰ **T33.70**   Superficial frostbite of unspecified knee and lower leg ▽

√x7ᵗʰ **T33.71**   Superficial frostbite of right knee and lower leg

√x7ᵗʰ **T33.72**   Superficial frostbite of left knee and lower leg

√5ᵗʰ **T33.8**   **Superficial frostbite of** ankle, foot, and toe(s)

√6ᵗʰ **T33.81**   **Superficial frostbite of** ankle

√7ᵗʰ **T33.811**   Superficial frostbite of right ankle

√7ᵗʰ **T33.812**   Superficial frostbite of left ankle

√7ᵗʰ **T33.819**   Superficial frostbite of unspecified ankle ▽

√6ᵗʰ **T33.82**   **Superficial frostbite of** foot

√7ᵗʰ **T33.821**   Superficial frostbite of right foot

√7ᵗʰ **T33.822**   Superficial frostbite of left foot

√7ᵗʰ **T33.829**   Superficial frostbite of unspecified foot ▽

√6ᵗʰ **T33.83**   **Superficial frostbite of** toe(s)

√7ᵗʰ **T33.831**   Superficial frostbite of right toe(s)

√7ᵗʰ **T33.832**   Superficial frostbite of left toe(s)

√7ᵗʰ **T33.839**   Superficial frostbite of unspecified toe(s) ▽

√5ᵗʰ **T33.9**   **Superficial frostbite of other and unspecified sites**

√x7ᵗʰ **T33.90**   Superficial frostbite of unspecified sites ▽
Superficial frostbite NOS

√x7ᵗʰ **T33.99**   **Superficial frostbite of other sites**
Superficial frostbite of leg NOS
Superficial frostbite of trunk NOS

√4ᵗʰ **T34**   **Frostbite** with tissue necrosis

The appropriate 7th character is to be added to each code from category T34.
A   initial encounter
D   subsequent encounter
S   sequela

√5ᵗʰ **T34.0**   **Frostbite with tissue necrosis of** head

√6ᵗʰ **T34.01**   **Frostbite with tissue necrosis of** ear

√7ᵗʰ **T34.011**   Frostbite with tissue necrosis of right ear

√7ᵗʰ **T34.012**   Frostbite with tissue necrosis of left ear

√7ᵗʰ **T34.019**   Frostbite with tissue necrosis of unspecified ear ▽

√x7ᵗʰ **T34.02**   Frostbite with tissue necrosis of nose

√x7ᵗʰ **T34.09**   **Frostbite with tissue necrosis of other part of head**

√x7ᵗʰ **T34.1**   **Frostbite with tissue necrosis of** neck

√x7ᵗʰ **T34.2**   **Frostbite with tissue necrosis of** thorax

√x7ᵗʰ **T34.3**   **Frostbite with tissue necrosis of** abdominal wall, lower back and pelvis

√5ᵗʰ **T34.4**   **Frostbite with tissue necrosis of** arm

EXCLUDES 2   *frostbite with tissue necrosis of wrist and hand (T34.5-)*

√x7ᵗʰ **T34.40**   Frostbite with tissue necrosis of unspecified arm ▽

√x7ᵗʰ **T34.41**   Frostbite with tissue necrosis of right arm

√x7ᵗʰ **T34.42**   Frostbite with tissue necrosis of left arm

√5ᵗʰ **T34.5**   **Frostbite with tissue necrosis of** wrist, hand, and finger(s)

√6ᵗʰ **T34.51**   **Frostbite with tissue necrosis of** wrist

√7ᵗʰ **T34.511**   Frostbite with tissue necrosis of right wrist

√7ᵗʰ **T34.512**   Frostbite with tissue necrosis of left wrist

√7ᵗʰ **T34.519**   Frostbite with tissue necrosis of unspecified wrist ▽

√6ᵗʰ **T34.52**   **Frostbite with tissue necrosis of** hand

EXCLUDES 2   *frostbite with tissue necrosis of finger(s) (T34.53-)*

√7ᵗʰ **T34.521**   Frostbite with tissue necrosis of right hand

√7ᵗʰ **T34.522**   Frostbite with tissue necrosis of left hand

✔ Add'l Character Required   √x7ᵗʰ Placeholder Alert   ▨ RUG IV Special Care High Dx   ▨ RUG IV Clinically Complex Dx   ▨ RUG IV Special Care Low Dx   ▨ Manifestation Code   ▨ Other Specified Code   ▽ Unspecified Code

ICD-10-CM 2016   **997**

✓7ᵗʰ **T34.529** **Frostbite with tissue necrosis of** unspecified hand

✓6ᵗʰ **T34.53** **Frostbite with tissue necrosis of** finger(s)

     ✓7ᵗʰ **T34.531** **Frostbite with tissue necrosis of** right finger(s)

     ✓7ᵗʰ **T34.532** **Frostbite with tissue necrosis of** left finger(s)

     ✓7ᵗʰ **T34.539** **Frostbite with tissue necrosis of** unspecified finger(s)

✓5ᵗʰ **T34.6** **Frostbite with tissue necrosis of** hip and thigh

     ✓x7ᵗʰ **T34.60** **Frostbite with tissue necrosis of unspecified hip and thigh**

     ✓x7ᵗʰ **T34.61** **Frostbite with tissue necrosis of** right **hip and thigh**

     ✓x7ᵗʰ **T34.62** **Frostbite with tissue necrosis of** left **hip and thigh**

✓5ᵗʰ **T34.7** **Frostbite with tissue necrosis of** knee and lower leg

     EXCLUDES 2   *frostbite with tissue necrosis of ankle and foot (T34.8-)*

     ✓x7ᵗʰ **T34.70** **Frostbite with tissue necrosis of unspecified knee and lower leg**

     ✓x7ᵗʰ **T34.71** **Frostbite with tissue necrosis of** right **knee and lower leg**

     ✓x7ᵗʰ **T34.72** **Frostbite with tissue necrosis of** left **knee and lower leg**

✓5ᵗʰ **T34.8** **Frostbite with tissue necrosis of** ankle, foot, and toe(s)

     ✓6ᵗʰ **T34.81** **Frostbite with tissue necrosis of** ankle

       ✓7ᵗʰ **T34.811** **Frostbite with tissue necrosis of** right ankle

       ✓7ᵗʰ **T34.812** **Frostbite with tissue necrosis of** left ankle

       ✓7ᵗʰ **T34.819** **Frostbite with tissue necrosis of** unspecified ankle

     ✓6ᵗʰ **T34.82** **Frostbite with tissue necrosis of** foot

       ✓7ᵗʰ **T34.821** **Frostbite with tissue necrosis of** right foot

       ✓7ᵗʰ **T34.822** **Frostbite with tissue necrosis of** left foot

       ✓7ᵗʰ **T34.829** **Frostbite with tissue necrosis of** unspecified foot

     ✓6ᵗʰ **T34.83** **Frostbite with tissue necrosis of** toe(s)

       ✓7ᵗʰ **T34.831** **Frostbite with tissue necrosis of** right toe(s)

       ✓7ᵗʰ **T34.832** **Frostbite with tissue necrosis of** left **toe(s)**

       ✓7ᵗʰ **T34.839** **Frostbite with tissue necrosis of** unspecified toe(s)

✓5ᵗʰ **T34.9** **Frostbite with tissue necrosis of other and unspecified sites**

     ✓x7ᵗʰ **T34.90** **Frostbite with tissue necrosis of unspecified sites**
       Frostbite with tissue necrosis NOS

     ✓x7ᵗʰ **T34.99** **Frostbite with tissue necrosis of other sites**
       Frostbite with tissue necrosis of leg NOS
       Frostbite with tissue necrosis of trunk NOS

Poisoning by, adverse effects of and underdosing of drugs, medicaments and biological substances (T36-T50)

INCLUDES   adverse effect of correct substance properly administered
     poisoning by overdose of substance
     poisoning by wrong substance given or taken in error
     underdosing by (inadvertently) (deliberately) taking less substance than prescribed or instructed

Code first, for adverse effects, the nature of the adverse effect, such as:
     adverse effect NOS (T88.7)
     aspirin gastritis (K29.-)
     blood disorders (D56-D76)
     contact dermatitis (L23-L25)
     dermatitis due to substances taken internally (L27.-)
     nephropathy (N14.0-N14.2)

NOTE   The drug giving rise to the adverse effect should be identified by use of codes from categories T36-T50 with fifth or sixth character 5.

Use additional code(s) to specify:
     manifestations of poisoning
     underdosing or failure in dosage during medical and surgical care (Y63.6, Y63.8-Y63.9)
     underdosing of medication regimen (Z91.12-, Z91.13-)

EXCLUDES 1   *toxic reaction to local anesthesia in pregnancy (O29.3-)*

EXCLUDES 2   *abuse and dependence of psychoactive substances (F10-F19)*
     abuse of non-dependence-producing substances (F55.-)
     drug reaction and poisoning affecting newborn (P00-P96)
     pathological drug intoxication (inebriation) (F10-F19)

✓4ᵗʰ **T36** **Poisoning by, adverse effect of and underdosing of systemic antibiotics**

     EXCLUDES 1   *antineoplastic antibiotics (T45.1-)*
       locally applied antibiotic NEC (T49.0)
       topically used antibiotic for ear, nose and throat (T49.6)
       topically used antibiotic for eye (T49.5)

> The appropriate 7th character is to be added to each code from category T36.
> A   initial encounter
> D   subsequent encounter
> S   sequela

✓5ᵗʰ **T36.0** **Poisoning by, adverse effect of and underdosing of penicillins**

     ✓6ᵗʰ **T36.0X** **Poisoning by, adverse effect of and underdosing of** penicillins

       ✓7ᵗʰ **T36.0X1** **Poisoning by penicillins,** accidental **(unintentional)**
         Poisoning by penicillins NOS

       ✓7ᵗʰ **T36.0X2** **Poisoning by penicillins,** intentional self-harm

       ✓7ᵗʰ **T36.0X3** **Poisoning by penicillins,** assault

       ✓7ᵗʰ **T36.0X4** **Poisoning by penicillins,** undetermined

       ✓7ᵗʰ **T36.0X5** Adverse effect **of penicillins**

       ✓7ᵗʰ **T36.0X6** Underdosing **of penicillins**

✓5ᵗʰ **T36.1** **Poisoning by, adverse effect of and underdosing of cephalosporins and other beta-lactam antibiotics**

     ✓6ᵗʰ **T36.1X** **Poisoning by, adverse effect of and underdosing of** cephalosporins and other beta-lactam antibiotics

       ✓7ᵗʰ **T36.1X1** **Poisoning by cephalosporins and other beta-lactam antibiotics,** accidental **(unintentional)**
         Poisoning by cephalosporins and other beta-lactam antibiotics NOS

       ✓7ᵗʰ **T36.1X2** **Poisoning by cephalosporins and other beta-lactam antibiotics,** intentional self-harm

       ✓7ᵗʰ **T36.1X3** **Poisoning by cephalosporins and other beta-lactam antibiotics,** assault

       ✓7ᵗʰ **T36.1X4** **Poisoning by cephalosporins and other beta-lactam antibiotics,** undetermined

       ✓7ᵗʰ **T36.1X5** Adverse effect **of cephalosporins and other beta-lactam antibiotics**

       ✓7ᵗʰ **T36.1X6** Underdosing **of cephalosporins and other beta-lactam antibiotics**

✓5ᵗʰ **T36.2** **Poisoning by, adverse effect of and underdosing of chloramphenicol group**

     ✓6ᵗʰ **T36.2X** **Poisoning by, adverse effect of and underdosing of** chloramphenicol group

       ✓7ᵗʰ **T36.2X1** **Poisoning by chloramphenicol group,** accidental **(unintentional)**
         Poisoning by chloramphenicol group NOS

       ✓7ᵗʰ **T36.2X2** **Poisoning by chloramphenicol group,** intentional self-harm

       ✓7ᵗʰ **T36.2X3** **Poisoning by chloramphenicol group,** assault

       ✓7ᵗʰ **T36.2X4** **Poisoning by chloramphenicol group,** undetermined

       ✓7ᵗʰ **T36.2X5** Adverse effect **of chloramphenicol group**

       ✓7ᵗʰ **T36.2X6** Underdosing **of chloramphenicol group**

✓5ᵗʰ **T36.3** **Poisoning by, adverse effect of and underdosing of macrolides**

     ✓6ᵗʰ **T36.3X** **Poisoning by, adverse effect of and underdosing of** macrolides

       ✓7ᵗʰ **T36.3X1** **Poisoning by macrolides,** accidental **(unintentional)**
         Poisoning by macrolides NOS

       ✓7ᵗʰ **T36.3X2** **Poisoning by macrolides,** intentional self-harm

       ✓7ᵗʰ **T36.3X3** **Poisoning by macrolides,** assault

       ✓7ᵗʰ **T36.3X4** **Poisoning by macrolides,** undetermined

       ✓7ᵗʰ **T36.3X5** Adverse effect **of macrolides**

       ✓7ᵗʰ **T36.3X6** Underdosing **of macrolides**

✓5ᵗʰ **T36.4** **Poisoning by, adverse effect of and underdosing of tetracyclines**

     ✓6ᵗʰ **T36.4X** **Poisoning by, adverse effect of and underdosing of** tetracyclines

---

N Newborn   P Pediatric   M Maternity   A Adult   RIC RIC Dx   NC Dx Noncancer Dx   PDx Primary Dx   CC RIC CC Condition   ►◄ Revised Text   ● New Code   ▲ Revised Code Title

998   ICD-10-CM 2016

√7ᵗʰ **T36.4X1** **Poisoning by tetracyclines,** accidental (unintentional)
Poisoning by tetracyclines NOS

√7ᵗʰ **T36.4X2** **Poisoning by tetracyclines,** intentional self-harm

√7ᵗʰ **T36.4X3** **Poisoning by tetracyclines,** assault

√7ᵗʰ **T36.4X4** **Poisoning by tetracyclines,** undetermined

√7ᵗʰ **T36.4X5** Adverse effect of tetracyclines

√7ᵗʰ **T36.4X6** Underdosing of tetracyclines

√5ᵗʰ **T36.5** **Poisoning by, adverse effect of and underdosing of aminoglycosides**
Poisoning by, adverse effect of and underdosing of streptomycin

√6ᵗʰ **T36.5X** **Poisoning by, adverse effect of and underdosing of** aminoglycosides

√7ᵗʰ **T36.5X1** **Poisoning by aminoglycosides,** accidental (unintentional)
Poisoning by aminoglycosides NOS

√7ᵗʰ **T36.5X2** **Poisoning by aminoglycosides,** intentional self-harm

√7ᵗʰ **T36.5X3** **Poisoning by aminoglycosides,** assault

√7ᵗʰ **T36.5X4** **Poisoning by aminoglycosides,** undetermined

√7ᵗʰ **T36.5X5** Adverse effect of aminoglycosides

√7ᵗʰ **T36.5X6** Underdosing of aminoglycosides

√5ᵗʰ **T36.6** **Poisoning by, adverse effect of and underdosing of rifampicins**

√6ᵗʰ **T36.6X** **Poisoning by, adverse effect of and underdosing of** rifampicins

√7ᵗʰ **T36.6X1** **Poisoning by rifampicins,** accidental (unintentional)
Poisoning by rifampicins NOS

√7ᵗʰ **T36.6X2** **Poisoning by rifampicins,** intentional self-harm

√7ᵗʰ **T36.6X3** **Poisoning by rifampicins,** assault

√7ᵗʰ **T36.6X4** **Poisoning by rifampicins,** undetermined

√7ᵗʰ **T36.6X5** Adverse effect of rifampicins

√7ᵗʰ **T36.6X6** Underdosing of rifampicins

√5ᵗʰ **T36.7** **Poisoning by, adverse effect of and underdosing of antifungal antibiotics, systemically used**

√6ᵗʰ **T36.7X** **Poisoning by, adverse effect of and underdosing of** antifungal antibiotics, systemically used

√7ᵗʰ **T36.7X1** **Poisoning by antifungal antibiotics, systemically used,** accidental (unintentional)
Poisoning by antifungal antibiotics, systemically used NOS

√7ᵗʰ **T36.7X2** **Poisoning by antifungal antibiotics, systemically used,** intentional self-harm

√7ᵗʰ **T36.7X3** **Poisoning by antifungal antibiotics, systemically used,** assault

√7ᵗʰ **T36.7X4** **Poisoning by antifungal antibiotics, systemically used,** undetermined

√7ᵗʰ **T36.7X5** Adverse effect of antifungal antibiotics, systemically used

√7ᵗʰ **T36.7X6** Underdosing of antifungal antibiotics, systemically used

√5ᵗʰ **T36.8** **Poisoning by, adverse effect of and underdosing of other systemic antibiotics**

√6ᵗʰ **T36.8X** **Poisoning by, adverse effect of and underdosing of** other systemic antibiotics

√7ᵗʰ **T36.8X1** **Poisoning by other systemic antibiotics,** accidental (unintentional)
Poisoning by other systemic antibiotics NOS

√7ᵗʰ **T36.8X2** **Poisoning by other systemic antibiotics,** intentional self-harm

√7ᵗʰ **T36.8X3** **Poisoning by other systemic antibiotics,** assault

√7ᵗʰ **T36.8X4** **Poisoning by other systemic antibiotics,** undetermined

√7ᵗʰ **T36.8X5** Adverse effect of other systemic antibiotics

√7ᵗʰ **T36.8X6** Underdosing of other systemic antibiotics

√5ᵗʰ **T36.9** **Poisoning by, adverse effect of and underdosing of** unspecified systemic antibiotic

√x7ᵗʰ **T36.91** **Poisoning by unspecified systemic antibiotic,** accidental (unintentional) ▽
Poisoning by systemic antibiotic NOS

√x7ᵗʰ **T36.92** **Poisoning by unspecified systemic antibiotic,** intentional self-harm ▽

√x7ᵗʰ **T36.93** **Poisoning by unspecified systemic antibiotic,** assault ▽

√x7ᵗʰ **T36.94** **Poisoning by unspecified systemic antibiotic,** undetermined ▽

√x7ᵗʰ **T36.95** Adverse effect of unspecified systemic antibiotic ▽

√x7ᵗʰ **T36.96** Underdosing of unspecified systemic antibiotic ▽

√4ᵗʰ **T37** **Poisoning by, adverse effect of and underdosing of other systemic anti-infectives and antiparasitics**
EXCLUDES 1 *anti-infectives topically used for ear, nose and throat (T49.6-)*
anti-infectives topically used for eye (T49.5-)
locally applied anti-infectives NEC (T49.0-)

The appropriate 7th character is to be added to each code from category T37.
A   initial encounter
D   subsequent encounter
S   sequela

√5ᵗʰ **T37.0** **Poisoning by, adverse effect of and underdosing of sulfonamides**

√6ᵗʰ **T37.0X** **Poisoning by, adverse effect of and underdosing of** sulfonamides

√7ᵗʰ **T37.0X1** **Poisoning by sulfonamides,** accidental (unintentional)
Poisoning by sulfonamides NOS

√7ᵗʰ **T37.0X2** **Poisoning by sulfonamides,** intentional self-harm

√7ᵗʰ **T37.0X3** **Poisoning by sulfonamides,** assault

√7ᵗʰ **T37.0X4** **Poisoning by sulfonamides,** undetermined

√7ᵗʰ **T37.0X5** Adverse effect of sulfonamides

√7ᵗʰ **T37.0X6** Underdosing of sulfonamides

√5ᵗʰ **T37.1** **Poisoning by, adverse effect of and underdosing of antimycobacterial drugs**
EXCLUDES 1 *rifampicins (T36.6-)*
streptomycin (T36.5-)

√6ᵗʰ **T37.1X** **Poisoning by, adverse effect of and underdosing of** antimycobacterial drugs

√7ᵗʰ **T37.1X1** **Poisoning by antimycobacterial drugs,** accidental (unintentional)
Poisoning by antimycobacterial drugs NOS

√7ᵗʰ **T37.1X2** **Poisoning by antimycobacterial drugs,** intentional self-harm

√7ᵗʰ **T37.1X3** **Poisoning by antimycobacterial drugs,** assault

√7ᵗʰ **T37.1X4** **Poisoning by antimycobacterial drugs,** undetermined

√7ᵗʰ **T37.1X5** Adverse effect of antimycobacterial drugs

√7ᵗʰ **T37.1X6** Underdosing of antimycobacterial drugs

√5ᵗʰ **T37.2** **Poisoning by, adverse effect of and underdosing of antimalarials and drugs acting on other blood protozoa**
EXCLUDES 1 *hydroxyquinoline derivatives (T37.8-)*

√6ᵗʰ **T37.2X** **Poisoning by, adverse effect of and underdosing of** antimalarials and drugs acting on other blood protozoa

√7ᵗʰ **T37.2X1** **Poisoning by antimalarials and drugs acting on other blood protozoa,** accidental (unintentional)
Poisoning by antimalarials and drugs acting on other blood protozoa NOS

√7ᵗʰ **T37.2X2** **Poisoning by antimalarials and drugs acting on other blood protozoa,** intentional self-harm

√7ᵗʰ **T37.2X3** **Poisoning by antimalarials and drugs acting on other blood protozoa,** assault

√7ᵗʰ **T37.2X4** **Poisoning by antimalarials and drugs acting on other blood protozoa,** undetermined

√7ᵗʰ **T37.2X5** Adverse effect of antimalarials and drugs acting on other blood protozoa

☑7ᵗʰ **T37.2X6**   Underdosing of antimalarials and drugs acting on other blood protozoa

☑5ᵗʰ **T37.3**   Poisoning by, adverse effect of and underdosing of other antiprotozoal drugs

  ☑6ᵗʰ **T37.3X**   Poisoning by, adverse effect of and underdosing of other antiprotozoal drugs

    ☑7ᵗʰ **T37.3X1**   **Poisoning by other antiprotozoal drugs, accidental (unintentional)**
        Poisoning by other antiprotozoal drugs NOS

    ☑7ᵗʰ **T37.3X2**   **Poisoning by other antiprotozoal drugs, intentional self-harm**

    ☑7ᵗʰ **T37.3X3**   **Poisoning by other antiprotozoal drugs, assault**

    ☑7ᵗʰ **T37.3X4**   **Poisoning by other antiprotozoal drugs, undetermined**

    ☑7ᵗʰ **T37.3X5**   Adverse effect of other antiprotozoal drugs

    ☑7ᵗʰ **T37.3X6**   Underdosing of other antiprotozoal drugs

☑5ᵗʰ **T37.4**   Poisoning by, adverse effect of and underdosing of anthelminthics

  ☑6ᵗʰ **T37.4X**   Poisoning by, adverse effect of and underdosing of anthelminthics

    ☑7ᵗʰ **T37.4X1**   **Poisoning by anthelminthics, accidental (unintentional)**
        Poisoning by anthelminthics NOS

    ☑7ᵗʰ **T37.4X2**   **Poisoning by anthelminthics, intentional self-harm**

    ☑7ᵗʰ **T37.4X3**   **Poisoning by anthelminthics, assault**

    ☑7ᵗʰ **T37.4X4**   **Poisoning by anthelminthics, undetermined**

    ☑7ᵗʰ **T37.4X5**   Adverse effect of anthelminthics

    ☑7ᵗʰ **T37.4X6**   Underdosing of anthelminthics

☑5ᵗʰ **T37.5**   Poisoning by, adverse effect of and underdosing of antiviral drugs
  EXCLUDES 1   amantadine (T42.8-)
        cytarabine (T45.1-)

  ☑6ᵗʰ **T37.5X**   Poisoning by, adverse effect of and underdosing of antiviral drugs

    ☑7ᵗʰ **T37.5X1**   **Poisoning by antiviral drugs, accidental (unintentional)**
        Poisoning by antiviral drugs NOS

    ☑7ᵗʰ **T37.5X2**   **Poisoning by antiviral drugs, intentional self-harm**

    ☑7ᵗʰ **T37.5X3**   **Poisoning by antiviral drugs, assault**

    ☑7ᵗʰ **T37.5X4**   **Poisoning by antiviral drugs, undetermined**

    ☑7ᵗʰ **T37.5X5**   Adverse effect of antiviral drugs

    ☑7ᵗʰ **T37.5X6**   Underdosing of antiviral drugs

☑5ᵗʰ **T37.8**   Poisoning by, adverse effect of and underdosing of other specified systemic anti-infectives and antiparasitics
  Poisoning by, adverse effect of and underdosing of hydroxyquinoline derivatives
  EXCLUDES 1   antimalarial drugs (T37.2-)

  ☑6ᵗʰ **T37.8X**   Poisoning by, adverse effect of and underdosing of other specified systemic anti-infectives and antiparasitics

    ☑7ᵗʰ **T37.8X1**   **Poisoning by other specified systemic anti-infectives and antiparasitics, accidental (unintentional)**
        Poisoning by other specified systemic anti-infectives and antiparasitics NOS

    ☑7ᵗʰ **T37.8X2**   **Poisoning by other specified systemic anti-infectives and antiparasitics, intentional self-harm**

    ☑7ᵗʰ **T37.8X3**   **Poisoning by other specified systemic anti-infectives and antiparasitics, assault**

    ☑7ᵗʰ **T37.8X4**   **Poisoning by other specified systemic anti-infectives and antiparasitics, undetermined**

    ☑7ᵗʰ **T37.8X5**   Adverse effect of other specified systemic anti-infectives and antiparasitics

    ☑7ᵗʰ **T37.8X6**   Underdosing of other specified systemic anti-infectives and antiparasitics

☑5ᵗʰ **T37.9**   Poisoning by, adverse effect of and underdosing of unspecified systemic anti-infective and antiparasitics

  ☑x7ᵗʰ **T37.91**   **Poisoning by unspecified systemic anti-infective and antiparasitics, accidental (unintentional)** ▽
    Poisoning by, adverse effect of and underdosing of systemic anti-infective and antiparasitics NOS

  ☑x7ᵗʰ **T37.92**   **Poisoning by unspecified systemic anti-infective and antiparasitics, intentional self-harm** ▽

  ☑x7ᵗʰ **T37.93**   **Poisoning by unspecified systemic anti-infective and antiparasitics, assault** ▽

  ☑x7ᵗʰ **T37.94**   **Poisoning by unspecified systemic anti-infective and antiparasitics, undetermined** ▽

  ☑x7ᵗʰ **T37.95**   Adverse effect of unspecified systemic anti-infective and antiparasitic ▽

  ☑x7ᵗʰ **T37.96**   Underdosing of unspecified systemic anti-infectives and antiparasitics ▽

☑4ᵗʰ **T38**   **Poisoning by, adverse effect of and underdosing of hormones and their synthetic substitutes and antagonists, not elsewhere classified**
  EXCLUDES 1   mineralocorticoids and their antagonists (T50.0-)
        oxytocic hormones (T48.0-)
        parathyroid hormones and derivatives (T50.9-)

> The appropriate 7th character is to be added to each code from category T38.
> A   initial encounter
> D   subsequent encounter
> S   sequela

☑5ᵗʰ **T38.0**   Poisoning by, adverse effect of and underdosing of glucocorticoids and synthetic analogues
  EXCLUDES 1   glucocorticoids, topically used (T49.-)

  ☑6ᵗʰ **T38.0X**   Poisoning by, adverse effect of and underdosing of glucocorticoids and synthetic analogues

    ☑7ᵗʰ **T38.0X1**   **Poisoning by glucocorticoids and synthetic analogues, accidental (unintentional)**
        Poisoning by glucocorticoids and synthetic analogues NOS

    ☑7ᵗʰ **T38.0X2**   **Poisoning by glucocorticoids and synthetic analogues, intentional self-harm**

    ☑7ᵗʰ **T38.0X3**   **Poisoning by glucocorticoids and synthetic analogues, assault**

    ☑7ᵗʰ **T38.0X4**   **Poisoning by glucocorticoids and synthetic analogues, undetermined**

    ☑7ᵗʰ **T38.0X5**   Adverse effect of glucocorticoids and synthetic analogues

    ☑7ᵗʰ **T38.0X6**   Underdosing of glucocorticoids and synthetic analogues

☑5ᵗʰ **T38.1**   Poisoning by, adverse effect of and underdosing of thyroid hormones and substitutes

  ☑6ᵗʰ **T38.1X**   Poisoning by, adverse effect of and underdosing of thyroid hormones and substitutes

    ☑7ᵗʰ **T38.1X1**   **Poisoning by thyroid hormones and substitutes, accidental (unintentional)**
        Poisoning by thyroid hormones and substitutes NOS

    ☑7ᵗʰ **T38.1X2**   **Poisoning by thyroid hormones and substitutes, intentional self-harm**

    ☑7ᵗʰ **T38.1X3**   **Poisoning by thyroid hormones and substitutes, assault**

    ☑7ᵗʰ **T38.1X4**   **Poisoning by thyroid hormones and substitutes, undetermined**

    ☑7ᵗʰ **T38.1X5**   Adverse effect of thyroid hormones and substitutes

    ☑7ᵗʰ **T38.1X6**   Underdosing of thyroid hormones and substitutes

☑5ᵗʰ **T38.2**   Poisoning by, adverse effect of and underdosing of antithyroid drugs

  ☑6ᵗʰ **T38.2X**   Poisoning by, adverse effect of and underdosing of antithyroid drugs

    ☑7ᵗʰ **T38.2X1**   **Poisoning by antithyroid drugs, accidental (unintentional)**
        Poisoning by antithyroid drugs NOS

    ☑7ᵗʰ **T38.2X2**   **Poisoning by antithyroid drugs, intentional self-harm**

    ☑7ᵗʰ **T38.2X3**   **Poisoning by antithyroid drugs, assault**

Ⓝ Newborn   Ⓟ Pediatric   Ⓜ Maternity   Ⓐ Adult   **RIC** RIC Dx   **NCDx** Noncancer Dx   **PDx** Primary Dx   **CC** RIC CC Condition   ►◄ Revised Text   ● New Code   ▲ Revised Code Title

√7ᵗʰ **T38.2X4** **Poisoning by antithyroid drugs,** undetermined

√7ᵗʰ **T38.2X5** Adverse effect **of antithyroid drugs**

√7ᵗʰ **T38.2X6** Underdosing **of antithyroid drugs**

√5ᵗʰ **T38.3** **Poisoning by, adverse effect of and underdosing of insulin and oral hypoglycemic [antidiabetic] drugs**

√6ᵗʰ **T38.3X** **Poisoning by, adverse effect of and underdosing of** insulin and oral hypoglycemic [antidiabetic] drugs

√7ᵗʰ **T38.3X1** **Poisoning by insulin and oral hypoglycemic [antidiabetic] drugs,** accidental (unintentional)
Poisoning by insulin and oral hypoglycemic [antidiabetic] drugs NOS

√7ᵗʰ **T38.3X2** **Poisoning by insulin and oral hypoglycemic [antidiabetic] drugs,** intentional self-harm

√7ᵗʰ **T38.3X3** **Poisoning by insulin and oral hypoglycemic [antidiabetic] drugs,** assault

√7ᵗʰ **T38.3X4** **Poisoning by insulin and oral hypoglycemic [antidiabetic] drugs,** undetermined

√7ᵗʰ **T38.3X5** Adverse effect **of insulin and oral hypoglycemic [antidiabetic] drugs**

√7ᵗʰ **T38.3X6** Underdosing **of insulin and oral hypoglycemic [antidiabetic] drugs**

√5ᵗʰ **T38.4** **Poisoning by, adverse effect of and underdosing of oral contraceptives**
Poisoning by, adverse effect of and underdosing of multiple- and single-ingredient oral contraceptive preparations

√6ᵗʰ **T38.4X** **Poisoning by, adverse effect of and underdosing of** oral contraceptives

√7ᵗʰ **T38.4X1** **Poisoning by oral contraceptives,** accidental (unintentional)
Poisoning by oral contraceptives NOS

√7ᵗʰ **T38.4X2** **Poisoning by oral contraceptives,** intentional self-harm

√7ᵗʰ **T38.4X3** **Poisoning by oral contraceptives,** assault

√7ᵗʰ **T38.4X4** **Poisoning by oral contraceptives,** undetermined

√7ᵗʰ **T38.4X5** Adverse effect **of oral contraceptives**

√7ᵗʰ **T38.4X6** Underdosing **of oral contraceptives**

√5ᵗʰ **T38.5** **Poisoning by, adverse effect of and underdosing of other estrogens and progestogens**
Poisoning by, adverse effect of and underdosing of estrogens and progestogens mixtures and substitutes

√6ᵗʰ **T38.5X** **Poisoning by, adverse effect of and underdosing of** other estrogens and progestogens

√7ᵗʰ **T38.5X1** **Poisoning by other estrogens and progestogens,** accidental (unintentional)
Poisoning by other estrogens and progestogens NOS

√7ᵗʰ **T38.5X2** **Poisoning by other estrogens and progestogens,** intentional self-harm

√7ᵗʰ **T38.5X3** **Poisoning by other estrogens and progestogens,** assault

√7ᵗʰ **T38.5X4** **Poisoning by other estrogens and progestogens,** undetermined

√7ᵗʰ **T38.5X5** Adverse effect **of other estrogens and progestogens**

√7ᵗʰ **T38.5X6** Underdosing **of other estrogens and progestogens**

√5ᵗʰ **T38.6** **Poisoning by, adverse effect of and underdosing of antigonadotrophins, antiestrogens, antiandrogens, not elsewhere classified**
Poisoning by, adverse effect of and underdosing of tamoxifen

√6ᵗʰ **T38.6X** **Poisoning by, adverse effect of and underdosing of** antigonadotrophins, antiestrogens, antiandrogens, not elsewhere classified

√7ᵗʰ **T38.6X1** **Poisoning by antigonadotrophins, antiestrogens, antiandrogens, not elsewhere classified,** accidental (unintentional)
Poisoning by antigonadotrophins, antiestrogens, antiandrogens, not elsewhere classified NOS

√7ᵗʰ **T38.6X2** **Poisoning by antigonadotrophins, antiestrogens, antiandrogens, not elsewhere classified,** intentional self-harm

√7ᵗʰ **T38.6X3** **Poisoning by antigonadotrophins, antiestrogens, antiandrogens, not elsewhere classified,** assault

√7ᵗʰ **T38.6X4** **Poisoning by antigonadotrophins, antiestrogens, antiandrogens, not elsewhere classified,** undetermined

√7ᵗʰ **T38.6X5** Adverse effect **of antigonadotrophins, antiestrogens, antiandrogens, not elsewhere classified**

√7ᵗʰ **T38.6X6** Underdosing **of antigonadotrophins, antiestrogens, antiandrogens, not elsewhere classified**

√5ᵗʰ **T38.7** **Poisoning by, adverse effect of and underdosing of androgens and anabolic congeners**

√6ᵗʰ **T38.7X** **Poisoning by, adverse effect of and underdosing of** androgens and anabolic congeners

√7ᵗʰ **T38.7X1** **Poisoning by androgens and anabolic congeners,** accidental (unintentional)
Poisoning by androgens and anabolic congeners NOS

√7ᵗʰ **T38.7X2** **Poisoning by androgens and anabolic congeners,** intentional self-harm

√7ᵗʰ **T38.7X3** **Poisoning by androgens and anabolic congeners,** assault

√7ᵗʰ **T38.7X4** **Poisoning by androgens and anabolic congeners,** undetermined

√7ᵗʰ **T38.7X5** Adverse effect **of androgens and anabolic congeners**

√7ᵗʰ **T38.7X6** Underdosing **of androgens and anabolic congeners**

√5ᵗʰ **T38.8** **Poisoning by, adverse effect of and underdosing of other and unspecified hormones and synthetic substitutes**

√6ᵗʰ **T38.80** **Poisoning by, adverse effect of and underdosing of** unspecified hormones and synthetic substitutes

√7ᵗʰ **T38.801** **Poisoning by unspecified hormones and synthetic substitutes,** accidental (unintentional) ▽
Poisoning by unspecified hormones and synthetic substitutes NOS

√7ᵗʰ **T38.802** **Poisoning by unspecified hormones and synthetic substitutes,** intentional self-harm ▽

√7ᵗʰ **T38.803** **Poisoning by unspecified hormones and synthetic substitutes,** assault ▽

√7ᵗʰ **T38.804** **Poisoning by unspecified hormones and synthetic substitutes,** undetermined ▽

√7ᵗʰ **T38.805** Adverse effect **of unspecified hormones and synthetic substitutes** ▽

√7ᵗʰ **T38.806** Underdosing **of unspecified hormones and synthetic substitutes** ▽

√6ᵗʰ **T38.81** **Poisoning by, adverse effect of and underdosing of** anterior pituitary [adenohypophyseal] hormones

√7ᵗʰ **T38.811** **Poisoning by anterior pituitary [adenohypophyseal] hormones,** accidental (unintentional)
Poisoning by anterior pituitary [adenohypophyseal] hormones NOS

√7ᵗʰ **T38.812** **Poisoning by anterior pituitary [adenohypophyseal] hormones,** intentional self-harm

√7ᵗʰ **T38.813** **Poisoning by anterior pituitary [adenohypophyseal] hormones,** assault

√7ᵗʰ **T38.814** **Poisoning by anterior pituitary [adenohypophyseal] hormones,** undetermined

√7ᵗʰ **T38.815** Adverse effect **of anterior pituitary [adenohypophyseal] hormones**

√7ᵗʰ **T38.816** Underdosing **of anterior pituitary [adenohypophyseal] hormones**

✔ Add'l Character Required   ✔x7ᵗʰ Placeholder Alert   RUG IV Special Care High Dx   RUG IV Clinically Complex Dx   RUG IV Special Care Low Dx   Manifestation Code   Other Specified Code   ▽Unspecified Code

✓6ᵗʰ **T38.89** Poisoning by, adverse effect of and underdosing of other hormones and synthetic substitutes

  ✓7ᵗʰ **T38.891** **Poisoning by other hormones and synthetic substitutes, accidental (unintentional)**
      Poisoning by other hormones and synthetic substitutes NOS

  ✓7ᵗʰ **T38.892** **Poisoning by other hormones and synthetic substitutes, intentional self-harm**

  ✓7ᵗʰ **T38.893** **Poisoning by other hormones and synthetic substitutes, assault**

  ✓7ᵗʰ **T38.894** **Poisoning by other hormones and synthetic substitutes, undetermined**

  ✓7ᵗʰ **T38.895** **Adverse effect of other hormones and synthetic substitutes**

  ✓7ᵗʰ **T38.896** **Underdosing of other hormones and synthetic substitutes**

✓5ᵗʰ **T38.9** Poisoning by, adverse effect of and underdosing of other and unspecified hormone antagonists

  ✓6ᵗʰ **T38.90** Poisoning by, adverse effect of and underdosing of unspecified hormone antagonists

    ✓7ᵗʰ **T38.901** **Poisoning by unspecified hormone antagonists, accidental (unintentional)** ▽
      Poisoning by unspecified hormone antagonists NOS

    ✓7ᵗʰ **T38.902** **Poisoning by unspecified hormone antagonists, intentional self-harm** ▽

    ✓7ᵗʰ **T38.903** **Poisoning by unspecified hormone antagonists, assault** ▽

    ✓7ᵗʰ **T38.904** **Poisoning by unspecified hormone antagonists, undetermined** ▽

    ✓7ᵗʰ **T38.905** **Adverse effect of unspecified hormone antagonists** ▽

    ✓7ᵗʰ **T38.906** **Underdosing of unspecified hormone antagonists** ▽

  ✓6ᵗʰ **T38.99** Poisoning by, adverse effect of and underdosing of other hormone antagonists

    ✓7ᵗʰ **T38.991** **Poisoning by other hormone antagonists, accidental (unintentional)**
      Poisoning by other hormone antagonists NOS

    ✓7ᵗʰ **T38.992** **Poisoning by other hormone antagonists, intentional self-harm**

    ✓7ᵗʰ **T38.993** **Poisoning by other hormone antagonists, assault**

    ✓7ᵗʰ **T38.994** **Poisoning by other hormone antagonists, undetermined**

    ✓7ᵗʰ **T38.995** **Adverse effect of other hormone antagonists**

    ✓7ᵗʰ **T38.996** **Underdosing of other hormone antagonists**

✓4ᵗʰ **T39** **Poisoning by, adverse effect of and underdosing of nonopioid analgesics, antipyretics and antirheumatics**

> The appropriate 7th character is to be added to each code from category T39.
> A   initial encounter
> D   subsequent encounter
> S   sequela

✓5ᵗʰ **T39.0** Poisoning by, adverse effect of and underdosing of salicylates

  ✓6ᵗʰ **T39.01** Poisoning by, adverse effect of and underdosing of aspirin
    Poisoning by, adverse effect of and underdosing of acetylsalicylic acid

    ✓7ᵗʰ **T39.011** **Poisoning by aspirin, accidental (unintentional)**

    ✓7ᵗʰ **T39.012** **Poisoning by aspirin, intentional self-harm**

    ✓7ᵗʰ **T39.013** **Poisoning by aspirin, assault**

    ✓7ᵗʰ **T39.014** **Poisoning by aspirin, undetermined**

    ✓7ᵗʰ **T39.015** **Adverse effect of aspirin**

    ✓7ᵗʰ **T39.016** **Underdosing of aspirin**

  ✓6ᵗʰ **T39.09** Poisoning by, adverse effect of and underdosing of other salicylates

    ✓7ᵗʰ **T39.091** **Poisoning by salicylates, accidental (unintentional)**
      Poisoning by salicylates NOS

    ✓7ᵗʰ **T39.092** **Poisoning by salicylates, intentional self-harm**

    ✓7ᵗʰ **T39.093** **Poisoning by salicylates, assault**

    ✓7ᵗʰ **T39.094** **Poisoning by salicylates, undetermined**

    ✓7ᵗʰ **T39.095** **Adverse effect of salicylates**

    ✓7ᵗʰ **T39.096** **Underdosing of salicylates**

✓5ᵗʰ **T39.1** Poisoning by, adverse effect of and underdosing of 4-Aminophenol derivatives

  ✓6ᵗʰ **T39.1X** Poisoning by, adverse effect of and underdosing of 4-Aminophenol derivatives

    ✓7ᵗʰ **T39.1X1** **Poisoning by 4-Aminophenol derivatives, accidental (unintentional)**
      Poisoning by 4-Aminophenol derivatives NOS

    ✓7ᵗʰ **T39.1X2** **Poisoning by 4-Aminophenol derivatives, intentional self-harm**

    ✓7ᵗʰ **T39.1X3** **Poisoning by 4-Aminophenol derivatives, assault**

    ✓7ᵗʰ **T39.1X4** **Poisoning by 4-Aminophenol derivatives, undetermined**

    ✓7ᵗʰ **T39.1X5** **Adverse effect of 4-Aminophenol derivatives**

    ✓7ᵗʰ **T39.1X6** **Underdosing of 4-Aminophenol derivatives**

✓5ᵗʰ **T39.2** Poisoning by, adverse effect of and underdosing of pyrazolone derivatives

  ✓6ᵗʰ **T39.2X** Poisoning by, adverse effect of and underdosing of pyrazolone derivatives

    ✓7ᵗʰ **T39.2X1** **Poisoning by pyrazolone derivatives, accidental (unintentional)**
      Poisoning by pyrazolone derivatives NOS

    ✓7ᵗʰ **T39.2X2** **Poisoning by pyrazolone derivatives, intentional self-harm**

    ✓7ᵗʰ **T39.2X3** **Poisoning by pyrazolone derivatives, assault**

    ✓7ᵗʰ **T39.2X4** **Poisoning by pyrazolone derivatives, undetermined**

    ✓7ᵗʰ **T39.2X5** **Adverse effect of pyrazolone derivatives**

    ✓7ᵗʰ **T39.2X6** **Underdosing of pyrazolone derivatives**

✓5ᵗʰ **T39.3** Poisoning by, adverse effect of and underdosing of other nonsteroidal anti-inflammatory drugs [NSAID]

  ✓6ᵗʰ **T39.31** Poisoning by, adverse effect of and underdosing of propionic acid derivatives
    Poisoning by, adverse effect of and underdosing of fenoprofen
    Poisoning by, adverse effect of and underdosing of flurbiprofen
    Poisoning by, adverse effect of and underdosing of ibuprofen
    Poisoning by, adverse effect of and underdosing of ketoprofen
    Poisoning by, adverse effect of and underdosing of naproxen
    Poisoning by, adverse effect of and underdosing of oxaprozin

    ✓7ᵗʰ **T39.311** **Poisoning by propionic acid derivatives, accidental (unintentional)**

    ✓7ᵗʰ **T39.312** **Poisoning by propionic acid derivatives, intentional self-harm**

    ✓7ᵗʰ **T39.313** **Poisoning by propionic acid derivatives, assault**

    ✓7ᵗʰ **T39.314** **Poisoning by propionic acid derivatives, undetermined**

    ✓7ᵗʰ **T39.315** **Adverse effect of propionic acid derivatives**

    ✓7ᵗʰ **T39.316** **Underdosing of propionic acid derivatives**

  ✓6ᵗʰ **T39.39** Poisoning by, adverse effect of and underdosing of other nonsteroidal anti-inflammatory drugs [NSAID]

    ✓7ᵗʰ **T39.391** **Poisoning by other nonsteroidal anti-inflammatory drugs [NSAID], accidental (unintentional)**
      Poisoning by other nonsteroidal anti-inflammatory drugs NOS

Ⓝ Newborn   Ⓟ Pediatric   Ⓜ Maternity   Ⓐ Adult   **RIC** RIC Dx   **NCDx** Noncancer Dx   **PDx** Primary Dx   **CC** RIC CC Condition   ►◄ Revised Text   ● New Code   ▲ Revised Code Title

1002   ICD-10-CM 2016

☑7ᵗʰ **T39.392** Poisoning by other nonsteroidal anti-inflammatory drugs [NSAID], intentional self-harm

☑7ᵗʰ **T39.393** Poisoning by other nonsteroidal anti-inflammatory drugs [NSAID], assault

☑7ᵗʰ **T39.394** Poisoning by other nonsteroidal anti-inflammatory drugs [NSAID], undetermined

☑7ᵗʰ **T39.395** Adverse effect of other nonsteroidal anti-inflammatory drugs [NSAID]

☑7ᵗʰ **T39.396** Underdosing of other nonsteroidal anti-inflammatory drugs [NSAID]

☑5ᵗʰ **T39.4** Poisoning by, adverse effect of and underdosing of antirheumatics, not elsewhere classified

> EXCLUDES 1   poisoning by, adverse effect of and underdosing of glucocorticoids (T38.0-)
> poisoning by, adverse effect of and underdosing of salicylates (T39.0-)

☑6ᵗʰ **T39.4X** Poisoning by, adverse effect of and underdosing of antirheumatics, not elsewhere classified

☑7ᵗʰ **T39.4X1** Poisoning by antirheumatics, not elsewhere classified, accidental (unintentional)
> Poisoning by antirheumatics, not elsewhere classified NOS

☑7ᵗʰ **T39.4X2** Poisoning by antirheumatics, not elsewhere classified, intentional self-harm

☑7ᵗʰ **T39.4X3** Poisoning by antirheumatics, not elsewhere classified, assault

☑7ᵗʰ **T39.4X4** Poisoning by antirheumatics, not elsewhere classified, undetermined

☑7ᵗʰ **T39.4X5** Adverse effect of antirheumatics, not elsewhere classified

☑7ᵗʰ **T39.4X6** Underdosing of antirheumatics, not elsewhere classified

☑5ᵗʰ **T39.8** Poisoning by, adverse effect of and underdosing of other nonopioid analgesics and antipyretics, not elsewhere classified

☑6ᵗʰ **T39.8X** Poisoning by, adverse effect of and underdosing of other nonopioid analgesics and antipyretics, not elsewhere classified

☑7ᵗʰ **T39.8X1** Poisoning by other nonopioid analgesics and antipyretics, not elsewhere classified, accidental (unintentional)
> Poisoning by other nonopioid analgesics and antipyretics, not elsewhere classified NOS

☑7ᵗʰ **T39.8X2** Poisoning by other nonopioid analgesics and antipyretics, not elsewhere classified, intentional self-harm

☑7ᵗʰ **T39.8X3** Poisoning by other nonopioid analgesics and antipyretics, not elsewhere classified, assault

☑7ᵗʰ **T39.8X4** Poisoning by other nonopioid analgesics and antipyretics, not elsewhere classified, undetermined

☑7ᵗʰ **T39.8X5** Adverse effect of other nonopioid analgesics and antipyretics, not elsewhere classified

☑7ᵗʰ **T39.8X6** Underdosing of other nonopioid analgesics and antipyretics, not elsewhere classified

☑5ᵗʰ **T39.9** Poisoning by, adverse effect of and underdosing of unspecified nonopioid analgesic, antipyretic and antirheumatic

☑x7ᵗʰ **T39.91** Poisoning by unspecified nonopioid analgesic, antipyretic and antirheumatic, accidental (unintentional) ▽
> Poisoning by nonopioid analgesic, antipyretic and antirheumatic NOS

☑x7ᵗʰ **T39.92** Poisoning by unspecified nonopioid analgesic, antipyretic and antirheumatic, intentional self-harm ▽

☑x7ᵗʰ **T39.93** Poisoning by unspecified nonopioid analgesic, antipyretic and antirheumatic, assault ▽

☑x7ᵗʰ **T39.94** Poisoning by unspecified nonopioid analgesic, antipyretic and antirheumatic, undetermined ▽

☑x7ᵗʰ **T39.95** Adverse effect of unspecified nonopioid analgesic, antipyretic and antirheumatic ▽

☑x7ᵗʰ **T39.96** Underdosing of unspecified nonopioid analgesic, antipyretic and antirheumatic ▽

☑4ᵗʰ **T40** Poisoning by, adverse effect of and underdosing of narcotics and psychodysleptics [hallucinogens]

> EXCLUDES 2   drug dependence and related mental and behavioral disorders due to psychoactive substance use (F10-F19-)

> The appropriate 7th character is to be added to each code from category T40.
> A   initial encounter
> D   subsequent encounter
> S   sequela

☑5ᵗʰ **T40.0** Poisoning by, adverse effect of and underdosing of opium

☑6ᵗʰ **T40.0X** Poisoning by, adverse effect of and underdosing of opium

☑7ᵗʰ **T40.0X1** Poisoning by opium, accidental (unintentional)
> Poisoning by opium NOS

☑7ᵗʰ **T40.0X2** Poisoning by opium, intentional self-harm

☑7ᵗʰ **T40.0X3** Poisoning by opium, assault

☑7ᵗʰ **T40.0X4** Poisoning by opium, undetermined

☑7ᵗʰ **T40.0X5** Adverse effect of opium

☑7ᵗʰ **T40.0X6** Underdosing of opium

☑5ᵗʰ **T40.1** Poisoning by and adverse effect of heroin

☑6ᵗʰ **T40.1X** Poisoning by and adverse effect of heroin

☑7ᵗʰ **T40.1X1** Poisoning by heroin, accidental (unintentional)
> Poisoning by heroin NOS

☑7ᵗʰ **T40.1X2** Poisoning by heroin, intentional self-harm

☑7ᵗʰ **T40.1X3** Poisoning by heroin, assault

☑7ᵗʰ **T40.1X4** Poisoning by heroin, undetermined

☑5ᵗʰ **T40.2** Poisoning by, adverse effect of and underdosing of other opioids

☑6ᵗʰ **T40.2X** Poisoning by, adverse effect of and underdosing of other opioids

☑7ᵗʰ **T40.2X1** Poisoning by other opioids, accidental (unintentional)
> Poisoning by other opioids NOS

☑7ᵗʰ **T40.2X2** Poisoning by other opioids, intentional self-harm

☑7ᵗʰ **T40.2X3** Poisoning by other opioids, assault

☑7ᵗʰ **T40.2X4** Poisoning by other opioids, undetermined

☑7ᵗʰ **T40.2X5** Adverse effect of other opioids

☑7ᵗʰ **T40.2X6** Underdosing of other opioids

☑5ᵗʰ **T40.3** Poisoning by, adverse effect of and underdosing of methadone

☑6ᵗʰ **T40.3X** Poisoning by, adverse effect of and underdosing of methadone

☑7ᵗʰ **T40.3X1** Poisoning by methadone, accidental (unintentional)
> Poisoning by methadone NOS

☑7ᵗʰ **T40.3X2** Poisoning by methadone, intentional self-harm

☑7ᵗʰ **T40.3X3** Poisoning by methadone, assault

☑7ᵗʰ **T40.3X4** Poisoning by methadone, undetermined

☑7ᵗʰ **T40.3X5** Adverse effect of methadone

☑7ᵗʰ **T40.3X6** Underdosing of methadone

☑5ᵗʰ **T40.4** Poisoning by, adverse effect of and underdosing of other synthetic narcotics

☑6ᵗʰ **T40.4X** Poisoning by, adverse effect of and underdosing of other synthetic narcotics

☑7ᵗʰ **T40.4X1** Poisoning by other synthetic narcotics, accidental (unintentional)
> Poisoning by other synthetic narcotics NOS

☑7ᵗʰ **T40.4X2** Poisoning by other synthetic narcotics, intentional self-harm

☑7ᵗʰ **T40.4X3** Poisoning by other synthetic narcotics, assault

☑7ᵗʰ **T40.4X4** Poisoning by other synthetic narcotics, undetermined

☑7ᵗʰ **T40.4X5** Adverse effect of other synthetic narcotics

☑7ᵗʰ **T40.4X6** Underdosing of other synthetic narcotics

☑ Add'l Character Required   ☑x7ᵗʰ Placeholder Alert   RUG IV Special Care High Dx   RUG IV Clinically Complex Dx   RUG IV Special Care Low Dx   Manifestation Code   Other Specified Code   ▽ Unspecified Code

CD-10-CM 2016   **1003**

Chapter 19. Injury, Poisoning and Certain Other Consequences of External Causes

T40.5–T41.1X6

√5th **T40.5** Poisoning by, adverse effect of and underdosing of cocaine

    √6th **T40.5X** Poisoning by, adverse effect of and underdosing of cocaine

        √7th **T40.5X1** Poisoning by cocaine, accidental (unintentional)
                Poisoning by cocaine NOS

        √7th **T40.5X2** Poisoning by cocaine, intentional self-harm

        √7th **T40.5X3** Poisoning by cocaine, assault

        √7th **T40.5X4** Poisoning by cocaine, undetermined

        √7th **T40.5X5** Adverse effect of cocaine

        √7th **T40.5X6** Underdosing of cocaine

√5th **T40.6** Poisoning by, adverse effect of and underdosing of other and unspecified narcotics

    √6th **T40.60** Poisoning by, adverse effect of and underdosing of unspecified narcotics

        √7th **T40.601** Poisoning by unspecified narcotics, accidental (unintentional) ▽
                Poisoning by narcotics NOS

        √7th **T40.602** Poisoning by unspecified narcotics, intentional self-harm ▽

        √7th **T40.603** Poisoning by unspecified narcotics, assault ▽

        √7th **T40.604** Poisoning by unspecified narcotics, undetermined ▽

        √7th **T40.605** Adverse effect of unspecified narcotics ▽

        √7th **T40.606** Underdosing of unspecified narcotics ▽

    √6th **T40.69** Poisoning by, adverse effect of and underdosing of other narcotics

        √7th **T40.691** Poisoning by other narcotics, accidental (unintentional)
                Poisoning by other narcotics NOS

        √7th **T40.692** Poisoning by other narcotics, intentional self-harm

        √7th **T40.693** Poisoning by other narcotics, assault

        √7th **T40.694** Poisoning by other narcotics, undetermined

        √7th **T40.695** Adverse effect of other narcotics

        √7th **T40.696** Underdosing of other narcotics

√5th **T40.7** Poisoning by, adverse effect of and underdosing of cannabis (derivatives)

    √6th **T40.7X** Poisoning by, adverse effect of and underdosing of cannabis (derivatives)

        √7th **T40.7X1** Poisoning by cannabis (derivatives), accidental (unintentional)
                Poisoning by cannabis NOS

        √7th **T40.7X2** Poisoning by cannabis (derivatives), intentional self-harm

        √7th **T40.7X3** Poisoning by cannabis (derivatives), assault

        √7th **T40.7X4** Poisoning by cannabis (derivatives), undetermined

        √7th **T40.7X5** Adverse effect of cannabis (derivatives)

        √7th **T40.7X6** Underdosing of cannabis (derivatives)

√5th **T40.8** Poisoning by and adverse effect of lysergide [LSD]

    √6th **T40.8X** Poisoning by and adverse effect of lysergide [LSD]

        √7th **T40.8X1** Poisoning by lysergide [LSD], accidental (unintentional)
                Poisoning by lysergide [LSD]NOS

        √7th **T40.8X2** Poisoning by lysergide [LSD], intentional self-harm

        √7th **T40.8X3** Poisoning by lysergide [LSD], assault

        √7th **T40.8X4** Poisoning by lysergide [LSD], undetermined

√5th **T40.9** Poisoning by, adverse effect of and underdosing of other and unspecified psychodysleptics [hallucinogens]

    √6th **T40.90** Poisoning by, adverse effect of and underdosing of unspecified psychodysleptics [hallucinogens]

        √7th **T40.901** Poisoning by unspecified psychodysleptics [hallucinogens], accidental (unintentional) ▽

        √7th **T40.902** Poisoning by unspecified psychodysleptics [hallucinogens], intentional self-harm ▽

        √7th **T40.903** Poisoning by unspecified psychodysleptics [hallucinogens], assault ▽

        √7th **T40.904** Poisoning by unspecified psychodysleptics [hallucinogens], undetermined ▽

        √7th **T40.905** Adverse effect of unspecified psychodysleptics [hallucinogens] ▽

        √7th **T40.906** Underdosing of unspecified psychodysleptics ▽

    √6th **T40.99** Poisoning by, adverse effect of and underdosing of other psychodysleptics [hallucinogens]

        √7th **T40.991** Poisoning by other psychodysleptics [hallucinogens], accidental (unintentional)
                Poisoning by other psychodysleptics [hallucinogens] NOS

        √7th **T40.992** Poisoning by other psychodysleptics [hallucinogens], intentional self-harm

        √7th **T40.993** Poisoning by other psychodysleptics [hallucinogens], assault

        √7th **T40.994** Poisoning by other psychodysleptics [hallucinogens], undetermined

        √7th **T40.995** Adverse effect of other psychodysleptics [hallucinogens]

        √7th **T40.996** Underdosing of other psychodysleptics

√4th **T41** Poisoning by, adverse effect of and underdosing of anesthetics and therapeutic gases

    EXCLUDES 1   benzodiazepines (T42.4-)
          cocaine (T40.5-)
          complications of anesthesia during labor and delivery (O74.-)
          complications of anesthesia during pregnancy (O29.-)
          complications of anesthesia during the puerperium (O89.-)
          opioids (T40.0-T40.2-)

    The appropriate 7th character is to be added to each code from category T41.
    A   initial encounter
    D   subsequent encounter
    S   sequela

√5th **T41.0** Poisoning by, adverse effect of and underdosing of inhaled anesthetics

    EXCLUDES 1   oxygen (T41.5-)

    √6th **T41.0X** Poisoning by, adverse effect of and underdosing of inhaled anesthetics

        √7th **T41.0X1** Poisoning by inhaled anesthetics, accidental (unintentional)
                Poisoning by inhaled anesthetics NOS

        √7th **T41.0X2** Poisoning by inhaled anesthetics, intentional self-harm

        √7th **T41.0X3** Poisoning by inhaled anesthetics, assault

        √7th **T41.0X4** Poisoning by inhaled anesthetics, undetermined

        √7th **T41.0X5** Adverse effect of inhaled anesthetics

        √7th **T41.0X6** Underdosing of inhaled anesthetics

√5th **T41.1** Poisoning by, adverse effect of and underdosing of intravenous anesthetics
    Poisoning by, adverse effect of and underdosing of thiobarbiturates

    √6th **T41.1X** Poisoning by, adverse effect of and underdosing of intravenous anesthetics

        √7th **T41.1X1** Poisoning by intravenous anesthetics, accidental (unintentional)
                Poisoning by intravenous anesthetics NOS

        √7th **T41.1X2** Poisoning by intravenous anesthetics, intentional self-harm

        √7th **T41.1X3** Poisoning by intravenous anesthetics, assault

        √7th **T41.1X4** Poisoning by intravenous anesthetics, undetermined

        √7th **T41.1X5** Adverse effect of intravenous anesthetics

        √7th **T41.1X6** Underdosing of intravenous anesthetics

N Newborn   P Pediatric   M Maternity   A Adult   RIC RIC Dx   NCDx Noncancer Dx   PDx Primary Dx   CC RIC CC Condition   ►◄ Revised Text   ● New Code   ▲ Revised Code Title

1004   ICD-10-CM 2016

✓5ᵗʰ **T41.2** **Poisoning by, adverse effect of and underdosing of other and unspecified general anesthetics**

  ✓6ᵗʰ **T41.20** **Poisoning by, adverse effect of and underdosing of** unspecified general anesthetics

    ✓7ᵗʰ **T41.201** **Poisoning by unspecified general anesthetics, accidental (unintentional)** ▽
      Poisoning by general anesthetics NOS

    ✓7ᵗʰ **T41.202** **Poisoning by unspecified general anesthetics, intentional self-harm** ▽

    ✓7ᵗʰ **T41.203** **Poisoning by unspecified general anesthetics, assault** ▽

    ✓7ᵗʰ **T41.204** **Poisoning by unspecified general anesthetics, undetermined** ▽

    ✓7ᵗʰ **T41.205** Adverse effect of unspecified general anesthetics ▽

    ✓7ᵗʰ **T41.206** Underdosing of unspecified general anesthetics ▽

  ✓6ᵗʰ **T41.29** **Poisoning by, adverse effect of and underdosing of** other general anesthetics

    ✓7ᵗʰ **T41.291** **Poisoning by other general anesthetics, accidental (unintentional)**
      Poisoning by other general anesthetics NOS

    ✓7ᵗʰ **T41.292** **Poisoning by other general anesthetics, intentional self-harm**

    ✓7ᵗʰ **T41.293** **Poisoning by other general anesthetics, assault**

    ✓7ᵗʰ **T41.294** **Poisoning by other general anesthetics, undetermined**

    ✓7ᵗʰ **T41.295** Adverse effect of other general anesthetics

    ✓7ᵗʰ **T41.296** Underdosing of other general anesthetics

✓5ᵗʰ **T41.3** **Poisoning by, adverse effect of and underdosing of local anesthetics**
  Cocaine (topical)
  EXCLUDES 2 *poisoning by cocaine used as a central nervous system stimulant (T40.5X1-T40.5X4)*

  ✓6ᵗʰ **T41.3X** **Poisoning by, adverse effect of and underdosing of** local anesthetics

    ✓7ᵗʰ **T41.3X1** **Poisoning by local anesthetics, accidental (unintentional)**
      Poisoning by local anesthetics NOS

    ✓7ᵗʰ **T41.3X2** **Poisoning by local anesthetics, intentional self-harm**

    ✓7ᵗʰ **T41.3X3** **Poisoning by local anesthetics, assault**

    ✓7ᵗʰ **T41.3X4** **Poisoning by local anesthetics, undetermined**

    ✓7ᵗʰ **T41.3X5** Adverse effect of local anesthetics

    ✓7ᵗʰ **T41.3X6** Underdosing of local anesthetics

✓5ᵗʰ **T41.4** **Poisoning by, adverse effect of and underdosing of** unspecified anesthetic

  ✓x7ᵗʰ **T41.41** **Poisoning by unspecified anesthetic, accidental (unintentional)** ▽
    Poisoning by anesthetic NOS

  ✓x7ᵗʰ **T41.42** **Poisoning by unspecified anesthetic, intentional self-harm** ▽

  ✓x7ᵗʰ **T41.43** **Poisoning by unspecified anesthetic, assault** ▽

  ✓x7ᵗʰ **T41.44** **Poisoning by unspecified anesthetic, undetermined** ▽

  ✓x7ᵗʰ **T41.45** Adverse effect of unspecified anesthetic ▽

  ✓x7ᵗʰ **T41.46** Underdosing of unspecified anesthetics ▽

✓5ᵗʰ **T41.5** **Poisoning by, adverse effect of and underdosing of therapeutic gases**

  ✓6ᵗʰ **T41.5X** **Poisoning by, adverse effect of and underdosing of** therapeutic gases

    ✓7ᵗʰ **T41.5X1** **Poisoning by therapeutic gases, accidental (unintentional)**
      Poisoning by therapeutic gases NOS

    ✓7ᵗʰ **T41.5X2** **Poisoning by therapeutic gases, intentional self-harm**

    ✓7ᵗʰ **T41.5X3** **Poisoning by therapeutic gases, assault**

    ✓7ᵗʰ **T41.5X4** **Poisoning by therapeutic gases, undetermined**

    ✓7ᵗʰ **T41.5X5** Adverse effect of therapeutic gases

    ✓7ᵗʰ **T41.5X6** Underdosing of therapeutic gases

✓4ᵗʰ **T42** **Poisoning by, adverse effect of and underdosing of antiepileptic, sedative- hypnotic and antiparkinsonism drugs**
  EXCLUDES 2 *drug dependence and related mental and behavioral disorders due to psychoactive substance use (F10.- -F19.-)*

> The appropriate 7th character is to be added to each code from category T42.
> A   initial encounter
> D   subsequent encounter
> S   sequela

✓5ᵗʰ **T42.0** **Poisoning by, adverse effect of and underdosing of hydantoin derivatives**

  ✓6ᵗʰ **T42.0X** **Poisoning by, adverse effect of and underdosing of** hydantoin derivatives

    ✓7ᵗʰ **T42.0X1** **Poisoning by hydantoin derivatives, accidental (unintentional)**
      Poisoning by hydantoin derivatives NOS

    ✓7ᵗʰ **T42.0X2** **Poisoning by hydantoin derivatives, intentional self-harm**

    ✓7ᵗʰ **T42.0X3** **Poisoning by hydantoin derivatives, assault**

    ✓7ᵗʰ **T42.0X4** **Poisoning by hydantoin derivatives, undetermined**

    ✓7ᵗʰ **T42.0X5** Adverse effect of hydantoin derivatives

    ✓7ᵗʰ **T42.0X6** Underdosing of hydantoin derivatives

✓5ᵗʰ **T42.1** **Poisoning by, adverse effect of and underdosing of iminostilbenes**
  Poisoning by, adverse effect of and underdosing of carbamazepine

  ✓6ᵗʰ **T42.1X** **Poisoning by, adverse effect of and underdosing of** iminostilbenes

    ✓7ᵗʰ **T42.1X1** **Poisoning by iminostilbenes, accidental (unintentional)**
      Poisoning by iminostilbenes NOS

    ✓7ᵗʰ **T42.1X2** **Poisoning by iminostilbenes, intentional self-harm**

    ✓7ᵗʰ **T42.1X3** **Poisoning by iminostilbenes, assault**

    ✓7ᵗʰ **T42.1X4** **Poisoning by iminostilbenes, undetermined**

    ✓7ᵗʰ **T42.1X5** Adverse effect of iminostilbenes

    ✓7ᵗʰ **T42.1X6** Underdosing of iminostilbenes

✓5ᵗʰ **T42.2** **Poisoning by, adverse effect of and underdosing of succinimides and oxazolidinediones**

  ✓6ᵗʰ **T42.2X** **Poisoning by, adverse effect of and underdosing of** succinimides and oxazolidinediones

    ✓7ᵗʰ **T42.2X1** **Poisoning by succinimides and oxazolidinediones, accidental (unintentional)**
      Poisoning by succinimides and oxazolidinediones NOS

    ✓7ᵗʰ **T42.2X2** **Poisoning by succinimides and oxazolidinediones, intentional self-harm**

    ✓7ᵗʰ **T42.2X3** **Poisoning by succinimides and oxazolidinediones, assault**

    ✓7ᵗʰ **T42.2X4** **Poisoning by succinimides and oxazolidinediones, undetermined**

    ✓7ᵗʰ **T42.2X5** Adverse effect of succinimides and oxazolidinediones

    ✓7ᵗʰ **T42.2X6** Underdosing of succinimides and oxazolidinediones

✓5ᵗʰ **T42.3** **Poisoning by, adverse effect of and underdosing of barbiturates**
  EXCLUDES 1 *poisoning by, adverse effect of and underdosing of thiobarbiturates (T41.1-)*

  ✓6ᵗʰ **T42.3X** **Poisoning by, adverse effect of and underdosing of** barbiturates

    ✓7ᵗʰ **T42.3X1** **Poisoning by barbiturates, accidental (unintentional)**
      Poisoning by barbiturates NOS

    ✓7ᵗʰ **T42.3X2** **Poisoning by barbiturates, intentional self-harm**

    ✓7ᵗʰ **T42.3X3** **Poisoning by barbiturates, assault**

    ✓7ᵗʰ **T42.3X4** **Poisoning by barbiturates, undetermined**

    ✓7ᵗʰ **T42.3X5** Adverse effect of barbiturates

    ✓7ᵗʰ **T42.3X6** Underdosing of barbiturates

✔ Add'l Character Required   ✓x7ᵗʰ Placeholder Alert   RUG IV Special Care High Dx   RUG IV Clinically Complex Dx   RUG IV Special Care Low Dx   Manifestation Code   Other Specified Code   ▽Unspecified Code

ICD-10-CM 2016   **1005**

☑5th **T42.4 Poisoning by, adverse effect of and underdosing of benzodiazepines**

  ☑6th **T42.4X Poisoning by, adverse effect of and underdosing of benzodiazepines**

    ☑7th **T42.4X1 Poisoning by benzodiazepines, accidental (unintentional)**
      Poisoning by benzodiazepines NOS

    ☑7th **T42.4X2 Poisoning by benzodiazepines, intentional self-harm**

    ☑7th **T42.4X3 Poisoning by benzodiazepines, assault**

    ☑7th **T42.4X4 Poisoning by benzodiazepines, undetermined**

    ☑7th **T42.4X5 Adverse effect of benzodiazepines**

    ☑7th **T42.4X6 Underdosing of benzodiazepines**

☑5th **T42.5 Poisoning by, adverse effect of and underdosing of mixed antiepileptics**

  ☑6th **T42.5X Poisoning by, adverse effect of and underdosing of antiepileptics**

    ☑7th **T42.5X1 Poisoning by mixed antiepileptics, accidental (unintentional)**
      Poisoning by mixed antiepileptics NOS

    ☑7th **T42.5X2 Poisoning by mixed antiepileptics, intentional self-harm**

    ☑7th **T42.5X3 Poisoning by mixed antiepileptics, assault**

    ☑7th **T42.5X4 Poisoning by mixed antiepileptics, undetermined**

    ☑7th **T42.5X5 Adverse effect of mixed antiepileptics**

    ☑7th **T42.5X6 Underdosing of mixed antiepileptics**

☑5th **T42.6 Poisoning by, adverse effect of and underdosing of other antiepileptic and sedative-hypnotic drugs**
  Poisoning by, adverse effect of and underdosing of methaqualone
  Poisoning by, adverse effect of and underdosing of valproic acid
  EXCLUDES 1 *poisoning by, adverse effect of and underdosing of carbamazepine (T42.1-)*

  ☑6th **T42.6X Poisoning by, adverse effect of and underdosing of other antiepileptic and sedative-hypnotic drugs**

    ☑7th **T42.6X1 Poisoning by other antiepileptic and sedative-hypnotic drugs, accidental (unintentional)**
      Poisoning by other antiepileptic and sedative-hypnotic drugs NOS

    ☑7th **T42.6X2 Poisoning by other antiepileptic and sedative-hypnotic drugs, intentional self-harm**

    ☑7th **T42.6X3 Poisoning by other antiepileptic and sedative-hypnotic drugs, assault**

    ☑7th **T42.6X4 Poisoning by other antiepileptic and sedative-hypnotic drugs, undetermined**

    ☑7th **T42.6X5 Adverse effect of other antiepileptic and sedative-hypnotic drugs**

    ☑7th **T42.6X6 Underdosing of other antiepileptic and sedative-hypnotic drugs**

☑5th **T42.7 Poisoning by, adverse effect of and underdosing of unspecified antiepileptic and sedative-hypnotic drugs**

  ☑x7th **T42.71 Poisoning by unspecified antiepileptic and sedative-hypnotic drugs, accidental (unintentional)** ▽
    Poisoning by antiepileptic and sedative-hypnotic drugs NOS

  ☑x7th **T42.72 Poisoning by unspecified antiepileptic and sedative-hypnotic drugs, intentional self-harm** ▽

  ☑x7th **T42.73 Poisoning by unspecified antiepileptic and sedative-hypnotic drugs, assault** ▽

  ☑x7th **T42.74 Poisoning by unspecified antiepileptic and sedative-hypnotic drugs, undetermined** ▽

  ☑x7th **T42.75 Adverse effect of unspecified antiepileptic and sedative-hypnotic drugs** ▽

  ☑x7th **T42.76 Underdosing of unspecified antiepileptic and sedative-hypnotic drugs** ▽

☑5th **T42.8 Poisoning by, adverse effect of and underdosing of antiparkinsonism drugs and other central muscle-tone depressants**
  Poisoning by, adverse effect of and underdosing of amantadine

  ☑6th **T42.8X Poisoning by, adverse effect of and underdosing of antiparkinsonism drugs and other central muscle-tone depressants**

    ☑7th **T42.8X1 Poisoning by antiparkinsonism drugs and other central muscle-tone depressants, accidental (unintentional)**
      Poisoning by antiparkinsonism drugs and other central muscle-tone depressants NOS

    ☑7th **T42.8X2 Poisoning by antiparkinsonism drugs and other central muscle-tone depressants, intentional self-harm**

    ☑7th **T42.8X3 Poisoning by antiparkinsonism drugs and other central muscle-tone depressants, assault**

    ☑7th **T42.8X4 Poisoning by antiparkinsonism drugs and other central muscle-tone depressants, undetermined**

    ☑7th **T42.8X5 Adverse effect of antiparkinsonism drugs and other central muscle-tone depressants**

    ☑7th **T42.8X6 Underdosing of antiparkinsonism drugs and other central muscle-tone depressants**

☑4th **T43 Poisoning by, adverse effect of and underdosing of psychotropic drugs, not elsewhere classified**
  EXCLUDES 1 *appetite depressants (T50.5-)*
    barbiturates (T42.3-)
    benzodiazepines (T42.4-)
    methaqualone (T42.6-)
    psychodysleptics [hallucinogens] (T40.7-T40.9-)
  EXCLUDES 2 *drug dependence and related mental and behavioral disorders due to psychoactive substance use (F10.- -F19.-)*

  The appropriate 7th character is to be added to each code from category T43.
  A   initial encounter
  D   subsequent encounter
  S   sequela

  ☑5th **T43.0 Poisoning by, adverse effect of and underdosing of tricyclic and tetracyclic antidepressants**

    ☑6th **T43.01 Poisoning by, adverse effect of and underdosing of tricyclic antidepressants**

      ☑7th **T43.011 Poisoning by tricyclic antidepressants, accidental (unintentional)**
        Poisoning by tricyclic antidepressants NOS

      ☑7th **T43.012 Poisoning by tricyclic antidepressants, intentional self-harm**

      ☑7th **T43.013 Poisoning by tricyclic antidepressants, assault**

      ☑7th **T43.014 Poisoning by tricyclic antidepressants, undetermined**

      ☑7th **T43.015 Adverse effect of tricyclic antidepressants**

      ☑7th **T43.016 Underdosing of tricyclic antidepressants**

    ☑6th **T43.02 Poisoning by, adverse effect of and underdosing of tetracyclic antidepressants**

      ☑7th **T43.021 Poisoning by tetracyclic antidepressants, accidental (unintentional)**
        Poisoning by tetracyclic antidepressants NOS

      ☑7th **T43.022 Poisoning by tetracyclic antidepressants, intentional self-harm**

      ☑7th **T43.023 Poisoning by tetracyclic antidepressants, assault**

      ☑7th **T43.024 Poisoning by tetracyclic antidepressants, undetermined**

      ☑7th **T43.025 Adverse effect of tetracyclic antidepressants**

      ☑7th **T43.026 Underdosing of tetracyclic antidepressants**

✓5ᵗʰ **T43.1 Poisoning by, adverse effect of and underdosing of monoamine-oxidase-inhibitor antidepressants**

✓6ᵗʰ **T43.1X Poisoning by, adverse effect of and underdosing of monoamine-oxidase-inhibitor antidepressants**

✓7ᵗʰ **T43.1X1 Poisoning by monoamine-oxidase-inhibitor antidepressants, accidental (unintentional)**
Poisoning by monoamine-oxidase-inhibitor antidepressants NOS

✓7ᵗʰ **T43.1X2 Poisoning by monoamine-oxidase-inhibitor antidepressants, intentional self-harm**

✓7ᵗʰ **T43.1X3 Poisoning by monoamine-oxidase-inhibitor antidepressants, assault**

✓7ᵗʰ **T43.1X4 Poisoning by monoamine-oxidase-inhibitor antidepressants, undetermined**

✓7ᵗʰ **T43.1X5 Adverse effect of monoamine-oxidase-inhibitor antidepressants**

✓7ᵗʰ **T43.1X6 Underdosing of monoamine-oxidase-inhibitor antidepressants**

✓5ᵗʰ **T43.2 Poisoning by, adverse effect of and underdosing of other and unspecified antidepressants**

✓6ᵗʰ **T43.20 Poisoning by, adverse effect of and underdosing of unspecified antidepressants**

✓7ᵗʰ **T43.201 Poisoning by unspecified antidepressants, accidental (unintentional)** ▽
Poisoning by antidepressants NOS

✓7ᵗʰ **T43.202 Poisoning by unspecified antidepressants, intentional self-harm** ▽

✓7ᵗʰ **T43.203 Poisoning by unspecified antidepressants, assault** ▽

✓7ᵗʰ **T43.204 Poisoning by unspecified antidepressants, undetermined** ▽

✓7ᵗʰ **T43.205 Adverse effect of unspecified antidepressants** ▽

✓7ᵗʰ **T43.206 Underdosing of unspecified antidepressants** ▽

✓6ᵗʰ **T43.21 Poisoning by, adverse effect of and underdosing of selective serotonin and norepinephrine reuptake inhibitors**
Poisoning by, adverse effect of and underdosing of SSNRI antidepressants

✓7ᵗʰ **T43.211 Poisoning by selective serotonin and norepinephrine reuptake inhibitors, accidental (unintentional)**

✓7ᵗʰ **T43.212 Poisoning by selective serotonin and norepinephrine reuptake inhibitors, intentional self-harm**

✓7ᵗʰ **T43.213 Poisoning by selective serotonin and norepinephrine reuptake inhibitors, assault**

✓7ᵗʰ **T43.214 Poisoning by selective serotonin and norepinephrine reuptake inhibitors, undetermined**

✓7ᵗʰ **T43.215 Adverse effect of selective serotonin and norepinephrine reuptake inhibitors**

✓7ᵗʰ **T43.216 Underdosing of selective serotonin and norepinephrine reuptake inhibitors**

✓6ᵗʰ **T43.22 Poisoning by, adverse effect of and underdosing of selective serotonin reuptake inhibitors**
Poisoning by, adverse effect of and underdosing of SSRI antidepressants

✓7ᵗʰ **T43.221 Poisoning by selective serotonin reuptake inhibitors, accidental (unintentional)**

✓7ᵗʰ **T43.222 Poisoning by selective serotonin reuptake inhibitors, intentional self-harm**

✓7ᵗʰ **T43.223 Poisoning by selective serotonin reuptake inhibitors, assault**

✓7ᵗʰ **T43.224 Poisoning by selective serotonin reuptake inhibitors, undetermined**

✓7ᵗʰ **T43.225 Adverse effect of selective serotonin reuptake inhibitors**

✓7ᵗʰ **T43.226 Underdosing of selective serotonin reuptake inhibitors**

✓6ᵗʰ **T43.29 Poisoning by, adverse effect of and underdosing of other antidepressants**

✓7ᵗʰ **T43.291 Poisoning by other antidepressants, accidental (unintentional)**
Poisoning by other antidepressants NOS

✓7ᵗʰ **T43.292 Poisoning by other antidepressants, intentional self-harm**

✓7ᵗʰ **T43.293 Poisoning by other antidepressants, assault**

✓7ᵗʰ **T43.294 Poisoning by other antidepressants, undetermined**

✓7ᵗʰ **T43.295 Adverse effect of other antidepressants**

✓7ᵗʰ **T43.296 Underdosing of other antidepressants**

✓5ᵗʰ **T43.3 Poisoning by, adverse effect of and underdosing of phenothiazine antipsychotics and neuroleptics**

✓6ᵗʰ **T43.3X Poisoning by, adverse effect of and underdosing of phenothiazine antipsychotics and neuroleptics**

✓7ᵗʰ **T43.3X1 Poisoning by phenothiazine antipsychotics and neuroleptics, accidental (unintentional)**
Poisoning by phenothiazine antipsychotics and neuroleptics NOS

✓7ᵗʰ **T43.3X2 Poisoning by phenothiazine antipsychotics and neuroleptics, intentional self-harm**

✓7ᵗʰ **T43.3X3 Poisoning by phenothiazine antipsychotics and neuroleptics, assault**

✓7ᵗʰ **T43.3X4 Poisoning by phenothiazine antipsychotics and neuroleptics, undetermined**

✓7ᵗʰ **T43.3X5 Adverse effect of phenothiazine antipsychotics and neuroleptics**

✓7ᵗʰ **T43.3X6 Underdosing of phenothiazine antipsychotics and neuroleptics**

✓5ᵗʰ **T43.4 Poisoning by, adverse effect of and underdosing of butyrophenone and thiothixene neuroleptics**

✓6ᵗʰ **T43.4X Poisoning by, adverse effect of and underdosing of butyrophenone and thiothixene neuroleptics**

✓7ᵗʰ **T43.4X1 Poisoning by butyrophenone and thiothixene neuroleptics, accidental (unintentional)**
Poisoning by butyrophenone and thiothixene neuroleptics NOS

✓7ᵗʰ **T43.4X2 Poisoning by butyrophenone and thiothixene neuroleptics, intentional self-harm**

✓7ᵗʰ **T43.4X3 Poisoning by butyrophenone and thiothixene neuroleptics, assault**

✓7ᵗʰ **T43.4X4 Poisoning by butyrophenone and thiothixene neuroleptics, undetermined**

✓7ᵗʰ **T43.4X5 Adverse effect of butyrophenone and thiothixene neuroleptics**

✓7ᵗʰ **T43.4X6 Underdosing of butyrophenone and thiothixene neuroleptics**

✓5ᵗʰ **T43.5 Poisoning by, adverse effect of and underdosing of other and unspecified antipsychotics and neuroleptics**
EXCLUDES 1 poisoning by, adverse effect of and underdosing of rauwolfia (T46.5-)

✓6ᵗʰ **T43.50 Poisoning by, adverse effect of and underdosing of unspecified antipsychotics and neuroleptics**

✓7ᵗʰ **T43.501 Poisoning by unspecified antipsychotics and neuroleptics, accidental (unintentional)** ▽
Poisoning by antipsychotics and neuroleptics NOS

✓7ᵗʰ **T43.502 Poisoning by unspecified antipsychotics and neuroleptics, intentional self-harm** ▽

✓7ᵗʰ **T43.503 Poisoning by unspecified antipsychotics and neuroleptics, assault** ▽

✓7ᵗʰ **T43.504 Poisoning by unspecified antipsychotics and neuroleptics, undetermined** ▽

✓7ᵗʰ **T43.505 Adverse effect of unspecified antipsychotics and neuroleptics** ▽

✓7ᵗʰ **T43.506 Underdosing of unspecified antipsychotics and neuroleptics** ▽

☑ Add'l Character Required ✓ₓ7ᵗʰ Placeholder Alert **RUG IV Special Care High Dx** **RUG IV Clinically Complex Dx** **RUG IV Special Care Low Dx** **Manifestation Code** Other Specified Code ▽ Unspecified Code

ICD-10-CM 2016 **1007**

☑6ᵗʰ **T43.59** **Poisoning by, adverse effect of and underdosing of** other antipsychotics and neuroleptics

     ☑7ᵗʰ **T43.591** **Poisoning by other antipsychotics and neuroleptics, accidental (unintentional)**
         Poisoning by other antipsychotics and neuroleptics NOS

     ☑7ᵗʰ **T43.592** **Poisoning by other antipsychotics and neuroleptics, intentional self-harm**

     ☑7ᵗʰ **T43.593** **Poisoning by other antipsychotics and neuroleptics, assault**

     ☑7ᵗʰ **T43.594** **Poisoning by other antipsychotics and neuroleptics, undetermined**

     ☑7ᵗʰ **T43.595** **Adverse effect of other antipsychotics and neuroleptics**

     ☑7ᵗʰ **T43.596** **Underdosing of other antipsychotics and neuroleptics**

☑5ᵗʰ **T43.6** **Poisoning by, adverse effect of and underdosing of psychostimulants**
     EXCLUDES 1   poisoning by, adverse effect of and underdosing of cocaine (T40.5-)

☑6ᵗʰ **T43.60** **Poisoning by, adverse effect of and underdosing of** unspecified psychostimulant

     ☑7ᵗʰ **T43.601** **Poisoning by unspecified psychostimulants, accidental (unintentional)** ▽
         Poisoning by psychostimulants NOS

     ☑7ᵗʰ **T43.602** **Poisoning by unspecified psychostimulants, intentional self-harm** ▽

     ☑7ᵗʰ **T43.603** **Poisoning by unspecified psychostimulants, assault** ▽

     ☑7ᵗʰ **T43.604** **Poisoning by unspecified psychostimulants, undetermined** ▽

     ☑7ᵗʰ **T43.605** **Adverse effect of unspecified psychostimulants** ▽

     ☑7ᵗʰ **T43.606** **Underdosing of unspecified psychostimulants** ▽

☑6ᵗʰ **T43.61** **Poisoning by, adverse effect of and underdosing of** caffeine

     ☑7ᵗʰ **T43.611** **Poisoning by caffeine, accidental (unintentional)**
         Poisoning by caffeine NOS

     ☑7ᵗʰ **T43.612** **Poisoning by caffeine, intentional self-harm**

     ☑7ᵗʰ **T43.613** **Poisoning by caffeine, assault**

     ☑7ᵗʰ **T43.614** **Poisoning by caffeine, undetermined**

     ☑7ᵗʰ **T43.615** **Adverse effect of caffeine**

     ☑7ᵗʰ **T43.616** **Underdosing of caffeine**

☑6ᵗʰ **T43.62** **Poisoning by, adverse effect of and underdosing of** amphetamines
     Poisoning by, adverse effect of and underdosing of methamphetamines

     ☑7ᵗʰ **T43.621** **Poisoning by amphetamines, accidental (unintentional)**
         Poisoning by amphetamines NOS

     ☑7ᵗʰ **T43.622** **Poisoning by amphetamines, intentional self-harm**

     ☑7ᵗʰ **T43.623** **Poisoning by amphetamines, assault**

     ☑7ᵗʰ **T43.624** **Poisoning by amphetamines, undetermined**

     ☑7ᵗʰ **T43.625** **Adverse effect of amphetamines**

     ☑7ᵗʰ **T43.626** **Underdosing of amphetamines**

☑6ᵗʰ **T43.63** **Poisoning by, adverse effect of and underdosing of** methylphenidate

     ☑7ᵗʰ **T43.631** **Poisoning by methylphenidate, accidental (unintentional)**
         Poisoning by methylphenidate NOS

     ☑7ᵗʰ **T43.632** **Poisoning by methylphenidate, intentional self-harm**

     ☑7ᵗʰ **T43.633** **Poisoning by methylphenidate, assault**

     ☑7ᵗʰ **T43.634** **Poisoning by methylphenidate, undetermined**

     ☑7ᵗʰ **T43.635** **Adverse effect of methylphenidate**

     ☑7ᵗʰ **T43.636** **Underdosing of methylphenidate**

☑6ᵗʰ **T43.69** **Poisoning by, adverse effect of and underdosing of** other psychostimulants

     ☑7ᵗʰ **T43.691** **Poisoning by other psychostimulants, accidental (unintentional)**
         Poisoning by other psychostimulants NOS

     ☑7ᵗʰ **T43.692** **Poisoning by other psychostimulants, intentional self-harm**

     ☑7ᵗʰ **T43.693** **Poisoning by other psychostimulants, assault**

     ☑7ᵗʰ **T43.694** **Poisoning by other psychostimulants, undetermined**

     ☑7ᵗʰ **T43.695** **Adverse effect of other psychostimulants**

     ☑7ᵗʰ **T43.696** **Underdosing of other psychostimulants**

☑5ᵗʰ **T43.8** **Poisoning by, adverse effect of and underdosing of other psychotropic drugs**

☑6ᵗʰ **T43.8X** **Poisoning by, adverse effect of and underdosing of** other psychotropic drugs

     ☑7ᵗʰ **T43.8X1** **Poisoning by other psychotropic drugs, accidental (unintentional)**
         Poisoning by other psychotropic drugs NOS

     ☑7ᵗʰ **T43.8X2** **Poisoning by other psychotropic drugs, intentional self-harm**

     ☑7ᵗʰ **T43.8X3** **Poisoning by other psychotropic drugs, assault**

     ☑7ᵗʰ **T43.8X4** **Poisoning by other psychotropic drugs, undetermined**

     ☑7ᵗʰ **T43.8X5** **Adverse effect of other psychotropic drugs**

     ☑7ᵗʰ **T43.8X6** **Underdosing of other psychotropic drugs**

☑5ᵗʰ **T43.9** **Poisoning by, adverse effect of and underdosing of** unspecified psychotropic drug

     ☑x7ᵗʰ **T43.91** **Poisoning by unspecified psychotropic drug, accidental (unintentional)** ▽
         Poisoning by psychotropic drug NOS

     ☑x7ᵗʰ **T43.92** **Poisoning by unspecified psychotropic drug, intentional self-harm** ▽

     ☑x7ᵗʰ **T43.93** **Poisoning by unspecified psychotropic drug, assault** ▽

     ☑x7ᵗʰ **T43.94** **Poisoning by unspecified psychotropic drug, undetermined** ▽

     ☑x7ᵗʰ **T43.95** **Adverse effect of unspecified psychotropic drug** ▽

     ☑x7ᵗʰ **T43.96** **Underdosing of unspecified psychotropic drug** ▽

☑4ᵗʰ **T44** **Poisoning by, adverse effect of and underdosing of drugs primarily affecting the autonomic nervous system**

     The appropriate 7th character is to be added to each code from category T44.
     A   initial encounter
     D   subsequent encounter
     S   sequela

☑5ᵗʰ **T44.0** **Poisoning by, adverse effect of and underdosing of anticholinesterase agents**

☑6ᵗʰ **T44.0X** **Poisoning by, adverse effect of and underdosing of** anticholinesterase agents

     ☑7ᵗʰ **T44.0X1** **Poisoning by anticholinesterase agents, accidental (unintentional)**
         Poisoning by anticholinesterase agents NOS

     ☑7ᵗʰ **T44.0X2** **Poisoning by anticholinesterase agents, intentional self-harm**

     ☑7ᵗʰ **T44.0X3** **Poisoning by anticholinesterase agents, assault**

     ☑7ᵗʰ **T44.0X4** **Poisoning by anticholinesterase agents, undetermined**

     ☑7ᵗʰ **T44.0X5** **Adverse effect of anticholinesterase agents**

     ☑7ᵗʰ **T44.0X6** **Underdosing of anticholinesterase agents**

☑5ᵗʰ **T44.1** **Poisoning by, adverse effect of and underdosing of other parasympathomimetics [cholinergics]**

☑6ᵗʰ **T44.1X** **Poisoning by, adverse effect of and underdosing of** other parasympathomimetics [cholinergics]

     ☑7ᵗʰ **T44.1X1** **Poisoning by other parasympathomimetics [cholinergics], accidental (unintentional)**
         Poisoning by other parasympathomimetics [cholinergics] NOS

Ⓝ Newborn   Ⓟ Pediatric   Ⓜ Maternity   Ⓐ Adult   **RIC** RIC Dx   **NCDx** Noncancer Dx   **PDx** Primary Dx   **CC** RIC CC Condition   ▶◀ Revised Text   ● New Code   ▲ Revised Code Title

1008   ICD-10-CM 2016

√7ᵗʰ **T44.1X2** **Poisoning by other parasympathomimetics [cholinergics], intentional self-harm**

√7ᵗʰ **T44.1X3** **Poisoning by other parasympathomimetics [cholinergics], assault**

√7ᵗʰ **T44.1X4** **Poisoning by other parasympathomimetics [cholinergics], undetermined**

√7ᵗʰ **T44.1X5** Adverse effect of other parasympathomimetics [cholinergics]

√7ᵗʰ **T44.1X6** Underdosing of other parasympathomimetics

√5ᵗʰ **T44.2** **Poisoning by, adverse effect of and underdosing of ganglionic blocking drugs**

√6ᵗʰ **T44.2X** **Poisoning by, adverse effect of and underdosing of ganglionic blocking drugs**

√7ᵗʰ **T44.2X1** **Poisoning by ganglionic blocking drugs, accidental (unintentional)**
Poisoning by ganglionic blocking drugs NOS

√7ᵗʰ **T44.2X2** **Poisoning by ganglionic blocking drugs, intentional self-harm**

√7ᵗʰ **T44.2X3** **Poisoning by ganglionic blocking drugs, assault**

√7ᵗʰ **T44.2X4** **Poisoning by ganglionic blocking drugs, undetermined**

√7ᵗʰ **T44.2X5** Adverse effect of ganglionic blocking drugs

√7ᵗʰ **T44.2X6** Underdosing of ganglionic blocking drugs

√5ᵗʰ **T44.3** **Poisoning by, adverse effect of and underdosing of other parasympatholytics [anticholinergics and antimuscarinics] and spasmolytics**
Poisoning by, adverse effect of and underdosing of papaverine

√6ᵗʰ **T44.3X** **Poisoning by, adverse effect of and underdosing of other parasympatholytics [anticholinergics and antimuscarinics] and spasmolytics**

√7ᵗʰ **T44.3X1** **Poisoning by other parasympatholytics [anticholinergics and antimuscarinics] and spasmolytics, accidental (unintentional)**
Poisoning by other parasympatholytics [anticholinergics and antimuscarinics] and spasmolytics NOS

√7ᵗʰ **T44.3X2** **Poisoning by other parasympatholytics [anticholinergics and antimuscarinics] and spasmolytics, intentional self-harm**

√7ᵗʰ **T44.3X3** **Poisoning by other parasympatholytics [anticholinergics and antimuscarinics] and spasmolytics, assault**

√7ᵗʰ **T44.3X4** **Poisoning by other parasympatholytics [anticholinergics and antimuscarinics] and spasmolytics, undetermined**

√7ᵗʰ **T44.3X5** Adverse effect of other parasympatholytics [anticholinergics and antimuscarinics] and spasmolytics

√7ᵗʰ **T44.3X6** Underdosing of other parasympatholytics [anticholinergics and antimuscarinics] and spasmolytics

√5ᵗʰ **T44.4** **Poisoning by, adverse effect of and underdosing of predominantly alpha-adrenoreceptor agonists**
Poisoning by, adverse effect of and underdosing of metaraminol

√6ᵗʰ **T44.4X** **Poisoning by, adverse effect of and underdosing of predominantly alpha-adrenoreceptor agonists**

√7ᵗʰ **T44.4X1** **Poisoning by predominantly alpha-adrenoreceptor agonists, accidental (unintentional)**
Poisoning by predominantly alpha-adrenoreceptor agonists NOS

√7ᵗʰ **T44.4X2** **Poisoning by predominantly alpha-adrenoreceptor agonists, intentional self-harm**

√7ᵗʰ **T44.4X3** **Poisoning by predominantly alpha-adrenoreceptor agonists, assault**

√7ᵗʰ **T44.4X4** **Poisoning by predominantly alpha-adrenoreceptor agonists, undetermined**

√7ᵗʰ **T44.4X5** Adverse effect of predominantly alpha-adrenoreceptor agonists

√7ᵗʰ **T44.4X6** Underdosing of predominantly alpha-adrenoreceptor agonists

√5ᵗʰ **T44.5** **Poisoning by, adverse effect of and underdosing of predominantly beta-adrenoreceptor agonists**
EXCLUDES 1 *poisoning by, adverse effect of and underdosing of beta-adrenoreceptor agonists used in asthma therapy (T48.6-)*

√6ᵗʰ **T44.5X** **Poisoning by, adverse effect of and underdosing of predominantly beta-adrenoreceptor agonists**

√7ᵗʰ **T44.5X1** **Poisoning by predominantly beta-adrenoreceptor agonists, accidental (unintentional)**
Poisoning by predominantly beta-adrenoreceptor agonists NOS

√7ᵗʰ **T44.5X2** **Poisoning by predominantly beta-adrenoreceptor agonists, intentional self-harm**

√7ᵗʰ **T44.5X3** **Poisoning by predominantly beta-adrenoreceptor agonists, assault**

√7ᵗʰ **T44.5X4** **Poisoning by predominantly beta-adrenoreceptor agonists, undetermined**

√7ᵗʰ **T44.5X5** Adverse effect of predominantly beta-adrenoreceptor agonists

√7ᵗʰ **T44.5X6** Underdosing of predominantly beta-adrenoreceptor agonists

√5ᵗʰ **T44.6** **Poisoning by, adverse effect of and underdosing of alpha-adrenoreceptor antagonists**
EXCLUDES 1 *poisoning by, adverse effect of and underdosing of ergot alkaloids (T48.0)*

√6ᵗʰ **T44.6X** **Poisoning by, adverse effect of and underdosing of alpha-adrenoreceptor antagonists**

√7ᵗʰ **T44.6X1** **Poisoning by alpha-adrenoreceptor antagonists, accidental (unintentional)**
Poisoning by alpha-adrenoreceptor antagonists NOS

√7ᵗʰ **T44.6X2** **Poisoning by alpha-adrenoreceptor antagonists, intentional self-harm**

√7ᵗʰ **T44.6X3** **Poisoning by alpha-adrenoreceptor antagonists, assault**

√7ᵗʰ **T44.6X4** **Poisoning by alpha-adrenoreceptor antagonists, undetermined**

√7ᵗʰ **T44.6X5** Adverse effect of alpha-adrenoreceptor antagonists

√7ᵗʰ **T44.6X6** Underdosing of alpha-adrenoreceptor antagonists

√5ᵗʰ **T44.7** **Poisoning by, adverse effect of and underdosing of beta-adrenoreceptor antagonists**

√6ᵗʰ **T44.7X** **Poisoning by, adverse effect of and underdosing of beta-adrenoreceptor antagonists**

√7ᵗʰ **T44.7X1** **Poisoning by beta-adrenoreceptor antagonists, accidental (unintentional)**
Poisoning by beta-adrenoreceptor antagonists NOS

√7ᵗʰ **T44.7X2** **Poisoning by beta-adrenoreceptor antagonists, intentional self-harm**

√7ᵗʰ **T44.7X3** **Poisoning by beta-adrenoreceptor antagonists, assault**

√7ᵗʰ **T44.7X4** **Poisoning by beta-adrenoreceptor antagonists, undetermined**

√7ᵗʰ **T44.7X5** Adverse effect of beta-adrenoreceptor antagonists

√7ᵗʰ **T44.7X6** Underdosing of beta-adrenoreceptor antagonists

☑5ᵗʰ **T44.8** **Poisoning by, adverse effect of and underdosing of centrally-acting and adrenergic-neuron- blocking agents**

     EXCLUDES 1   *poisoning by, adverse effect of and underdosing of clonidine (T46.5)*
        poisoning by, adverse effect of and underdosing of guanethidine (T46.5)

   ☑6ᵗʰ **T44.8X** **Poisoning by, adverse effect of and underdosing of centrally-acting and adrenergic-neuron-blocking agents**

     ☑7ᵗʰ **T44.8X1** **Poisoning by centrally-acting and adrenergic-neuron-blocking agents, accidental (unintentional)**
         Poisoning by centrally-acting and adrenergic-neuron-blocking agents NOS

     ☑7ᵗʰ **T44.8X2** **Poisoning by centrally-acting and adrenergic-neuron-blocking agents, intentional self-harm**

     ☑7ᵗʰ **T44.8X3** **Poisoning by centrally-acting and adrenergic-neuron-blocking agents, assault**

     ☑7ᵗʰ **T44.8X4** **Poisoning by centrally-acting and adrenergic-neuron-blocking agents, undetermined**

     ☑7ᵗʰ **T44.8X5** **Adverse effect of centrally-acting and adrenergic-neuron-blocking agents**

     ☑7ᵗʰ **T44.8X6** **Underdosing of centrally-acting and adrenergic-neuron-blocking agents**

☑5ᵗʰ **T44.9** **Poisoning by, adverse effect of and underdosing of other and unspecified drugs** primarily affecting the autonomic nervous system

     Poisoning by, adverse effect of and underdosing of drug stimulating both alpha and beta-adrenoreceptors

   ☑6ᵗʰ **T44.90** **Poisoning by, adverse effect of and underdosing of unspecified drugs primarily affecting the autonomic nervous system**

     ☑7ᵗʰ **T44.901** **Poisoning by unspecified drugs primarily affecting the autonomic nervous system, accidental (unintentional)** ▽
         Poisoning by unspecified drugs primarily affecting the autonomic nervous system NOS

     ☑7ᵗʰ **T44.902** **Poisoning by unspecified drugs primarily affecting the autonomic nervous system, intentional self-harm** ▽

     ☑7ᵗʰ **T44.903** **Poisoning by unspecified drugs primarily affecting the autonomic nervous system, assault** ▽

     ☑7ᵗʰ **T44.904** **Poisoning by unspecified drugs primarily affecting the autonomic nervous system, undetermined** ▽

     ☑7ᵗʰ **T44.905** **Adverse effect of unspecified drugs primarily affecting the autonomic nervous system** ▽

     ☑7ᵗʰ **T44.906** **Underdosing of unspecified drugs primarily affecting the autonomic nervous system** ▽

   ☑6ᵗʰ **T44.99** **Poisoning by, adverse effect of and underdosing of other drugs primarily affecting the autonomic nervous system**

     ☑7ᵗʰ **T44.991** **Poisoning by other drug primarily affecting the autonomic nervous system, accidental (unintentional)**
         Poisoning by other drugs primarily affecting the autonomic nervous system NOS

     ☑7ᵗʰ **T44.992** **Poisoning by other drug primarily affecting the autonomic nervous system, intentional self-harm**

     ☑7ᵗʰ **T44.993** **Poisoning by other drug primarily affecting the autonomic nervous system, assault**

     ☑7ᵗʰ **T44.994** **Poisoning by other drug primarily affecting the autonomic nervous system, undetermined**

     ☑7ᵗʰ **T44.995** **Adverse effect of other drug primarily affecting the autonomic nervous system**

     ☑7ᵗʰ **T44.996** **Underdosing of other drug primarily affecting the autonomic nervous system**

☑4ᵗʰ **T45** **Poisoning by, adverse effect of and underdosing of primarily systemic and hematological agents, not elsewhere classified**

     The appropriate 7th character is to be added to each code from category T45.
     A   initial encounter
     D   subsequent encounter
     S   sequela

☑5ᵗʰ **T45.Ø** **Poisoning by, adverse effect of and underdosing of antiallergic and antiemetic drugs**

     EXCLUDES 1   *poisoning by, adverse effect of and underdosing of phenothiazine-based neuroleptics (T43.3)*

   ☑6ᵗʰ **T45.ØX** **Poisoning by, adverse effect of and underdosing of antiallergic and antiemetic drugs**

     ☑7ᵗʰ **T45.ØX1** **Poisoning by antiallergic and antiemetic drugs, accidental (unintentional)**
         Poisoning by antiallergic and antiemetic drugs NOS

     ☑7ᵗʰ **T45.ØX2** **Poisoning by antiallergic and antiemetic drugs, intentional self-harm**

     ☑7ᵗʰ **T45.ØX3** **Poisoning by antiallergic and antiemetic drugs, assault**

     ☑7ᵗʰ **T45.ØX4** **Poisoning by antiallergic and antiemetic drugs, undetermined**

     ☑7ᵗʰ **T45.ØX5** **Adverse effect of antiallergic and antiemetic drugs**

     ☑7ᵗʰ **T45.ØX6** **Underdosing of antiallergic and antiemetic drugs**

☑5ᵗʰ **T45.1** **Poisoning by, adverse effect of and underdosing of antineoplastic and immunosuppressive drugs**

     EXCLUDES 1   *poisoning by, adverse effect of and underdosing of tamoxifen (T38.6)*

     AHA: 2014, 4Q, 22

   ☑6ᵗʰ **T45.1X** **Poisoning by, adverse effect of and underdosing of antineoplastic and immunosuppressive drugs**

     ☑7ᵗʰ **T45.1X1** **Poisoning by antineoplastic and immunosuppressive drugs, accidental (unintentional)**
         Poisoning by antineoplastic and immunosuppressive drugs NOS

     ☑7ᵗʰ **T45.1X2** **Poisoning by antineoplastic and immunosuppressive drugs, intentional self-harm**

     ☑7ᵗʰ **T45.1X3** **Poisoning by antineoplastic and immunosuppressive drugs, assault**

     ☑7ᵗʰ **T45.1X4** **Poisoning by antineoplastic and immunosuppressive drugs, undetermined**

     ☑7ᵗʰ **T45.1X5** **Adverse effect of antineoplastic and immunosuppressive drugs**

     ☑7ᵗʰ **T45.1X6** **Underdosing of antineoplastic and immunosuppressive drugs**

☑5ᵗʰ **T45.2** **Poisoning by, adverse effect of and underdosing of vitamins**

     EXCLUDES 2   *poisoning by, adverse effect of and underdosing of iron (T45.4)*
        poisoning by, adverse effect of and underdosing of nicotinic acid (derivatives) (T46.7)
        poisoning by, adverse effect of and underdosing of vitamin K (T45.7)

   ☑6ᵗʰ **T45.2X** **Poisoning by, adverse effect of and underdosing of vitamins**

     ☑7ᵗʰ **T45.2X1** **Poisoning by vitamins, accidental (unintentional)**
         Poisoning by vitamins NOS

     ☑7ᵗʰ **T45.2X2** **Poisoning by vitamins, intentional self-harm**

     ☑7ᵗʰ **T45.2X3** **Poisoning by vitamins, assault**

     ☑7ᵗʰ **T45.2X4** **Poisoning by vitamins, undetermined**

     ☑7ᵗʰ **T45.2X5** **Adverse effect of vitamins**

     ☑7ᵗʰ **T45.2X6** **Underdosing of vitamins**
         EXCLUDES 1   *vitamin deficiencies (E5Ø-E56)*

☑5ᵗʰ **T45.3** **Poisoning by, adverse effect of and underdosing of enzymes**

   ☑6ᵗʰ **T45.3X** **Poisoning by, adverse effect of and underdosing of enzymes**

     ☑7ᵗʰ **T45.3X1** **Poisoning by enzymes, accidental (unintentional)**
         Poisoning by enzymes NOS

     ☑7ᵗʰ **T45.3X2** **Poisoning by enzymes, intentional self-harm**

Ⓝ Newborn   Ⓟ Pediatric   Ⓜ Maternity   Ⓐ Adult   **RIC** RIC Dx   **NC Dx** Noncancer Dx   **PDx** Primary Dx   **CC** RIC CC Condition   ▶◀ Revised Text   ● New Code   ▲ Revised Code Title

1010   ICD-10-CM 2016

☑7ᵗʰ   **T45.3X3**   Poisoning by enzymes, assault

☑7ᵗʰ   **T45.3X4**   Poisoning by enzymes, undetermined

☑7ᵗʰ   **T45.3X5**   Adverse effect of enzymes

☑7ᵗʰ   **T45.3X6**   Underdosing of enzymes

☑5ᵗʰ   **T45.4**   **Poisoning by, adverse effect of and underdosing of iron and its compounds**

    ☑6ᵗʰ   **T45.4X**   **Poisoning by, adverse effect of and underdosing of iron and its compounds**

       T45.4X1   **Poisoning by iron and its compounds, accidental (unintentional)**
           Poisoning by iron and its compounds NOS

       ☑7ᵗʰ   **T45.4X2**   **Poisoning by iron and its compounds, intentional self-harm**

       ☑7ᵗʰ   **T45.4X3**   **Poisoning by iron and its compounds, assault**

       ☑7ᵗʰ   **T45.4X4**   **Poisoning by iron and its compounds, undetermined**

       ☑7ᵗʰ   **T45.4X5**   Adverse effect of iron and its compounds

       ☑7ᵗʰ   **T45.4X6**   Underdosing of iron and its compounds
           EXCLUDES 1   iron deficiency (E61.1)

☑5ᵗʰ   **T45.5**   **Poisoning by, adverse effect of and underdosing of anticoagulants and antithrombotic drugs**

    ☑6ᵗʰ   **T45.51**   **Poisoning by, adverse effect of and underdosing of anticoagulants**

       ☑7ᵗʰ   **T45.511**   **Poisoning by anticoagulants, accidental (unintentional)**
           Poisoning by anticoagulants NOS

       ☑7ᵗʰ   **T45.512**   **Poisoning by anticoagulants, intentional self-harm**

       ☑7ᵗʰ   **T45.513**   **Poisoning by anticoagulants, assault**

       ☑7ᵗʰ   **T45.514**   **Poisoning by anticoagulants, undetermined**

       ☑7ᵗʰ   **T45.515**   Adverse effect of anticoagulants
           AHA: 2013, 2Q, 34

       ☑7ᵗʰ   **T45.516**   Underdosing of anticoagulants

    ☑6ᵗʰ   **T45.52**   **Poisoning by, adverse effect of and underdosing of antithrombotic drugs**
       Poisoning by, adverse effect of and underdosing of antiplatelet drugs
         EXCLUDES 2   poisoning by, adverse effect of and underdosing of aspirin (T39.01-)
                 poisoning by, adverse effect of and underdosing of acetylsalicylic acid (T39.01-)

       ☑7ᵗʰ   **T45.521**   **Poisoning by antithrombotic drugs, accidental (unintentional)**
           Poisoning by antithrombotic drug NOS

       ☑7ᵗʰ   **T45.522**   **Poisoning by antithrombotic drugs, intentional self-harm**

       ☑7ᵗʰ   **T45.523**   **Poisoning by antithrombotic drugs, assault**

       ☑7ᵗʰ   **T45.524**   **Poisoning by antithrombotic drugs, undetermined**

       ☑7ᵗʰ   **T45.525**   Adverse effect of antithrombotic drugs

       ☑7ᵗʰ   **T45.526**   Underdosing of antithrombotic drugs

☑5ᵗʰ   **T45.6**   **Poisoning by, adverse effect of and underdosing of fibrinolysis-affecting drugs**

    ☑6ᵗʰ   **T45.60**   **Poisoning by, adverse effect of and underdosing of unspecified fibrinolysis-affecting drugs**

       ☑7ᵗʰ   **T45.601**   **Poisoning by unspecified fibrinolysis-affecting drugs, accidental (unintentional)**   ▽
           Poisoning by fibrinolysis-affecting drug NOS

       ☑7ᵗʰ   **T45.602**   **Poisoning by unspecified fibrinolysis-affecting drugs, intentional self-harm**   ▽

       ☑7ᵗʰ   **T45.603**   **Poisoning by unspecified fibrinolysis-affecting drugs, assault**   ▽

       ☑7ᵗʰ   **T45.604**   **Poisoning by unspecified fibrinolysis-affecting drugs, undetermined**   ▽

       ☑7ᵗʰ   **T45.605**   Adverse effect of unspecified fibrinolysis- affecting drugs   ▽

       ☑7ᵗʰ   **T45.606**   Underdosing of unspecified fibrinolysis- affecting drugs   ▽

    ☑6ᵗʰ   **T45.61**   **Poisoning by, adverse effect of and underdosing of thrombolytic drugs**

       ☑7ᵗʰ   **T45.611**   **Poisoning by thrombolytic drug, accidental (unintentional)**
           Poisoning by thrombolytic drug NOS

       ☑7ᵗʰ   **T45.612**   **Poisoning by thrombolytic drug, intentional self-harm**

       ☑7ᵗʰ   **T45.613**   **Poisoning by thrombolytic drug, assault**

       ☑7ᵗʰ   **T45.614**   **Poisoning by thrombolytic drug, undetermined**

       ☑7ᵗʰ   **T45.615**   Adverse effect of thrombolytic drugs

       ☑7ᵗʰ   **T45.616**   Underdosing of thrombolytic drugs

    ☑6ᵗʰ   **T45.62**   **Poisoning by, adverse effect of and underdosing of hemostatic drugs**

       ☑7ᵗʰ   **T45.621**   **Poisoning by hemostatic drug, accidental (unintentional)**
           Poisoning by hemostatic drug NOS

       ☑7ᵗʰ   **T45.622**   **Poisoning by hemostatic drug, intentional self-harm**

       ☑7ᵗʰ   **T45.623**   **Poisoning by hemostatic drug, assault**

       ☑7ᵗʰ   **T45.624**   **Poisoning by hemostatic drug, undetermined**

       ☑7ᵗʰ   **T45.625**   Adverse effect of hemostatic drug

       ☑7ᵗʰ   **T45.626**   Underdosing of hemostatic drugs

    ☑6ᵗʰ   **T45.69**   **Poisoning by, adverse effect of and underdosing of other fibrinolysis-affecting drugs**

       ☑7ᵗʰ   **T45.691**   **Poisoning by other fibrinolysis-affecting drugs, accidental (unintentional)**
           Poisoning by other fibrinolysis-affecting drug NOS

       ☑7ᵗʰ   **T45.692**   **Poisoning by other fibrinolysis-affecting drugs, intentional self-harm**

       ☑7ᵗʰ   **T45.693**   **Poisoning by other fibrinolysis-affecting drugs, assault**

       ☑7ᵗʰ   **T45.694**   **Poisoning by other fibrinolysis-affecting drugs, undetermined**

       ☑7ᵗʰ   **T45.695**   Adverse effect of other fibrinolysis-affecting drugs

       ☑7ᵗʰ   **T45.696**   Underdosing of other fibrinolysis-affecting drugs

☑5ᵗʰ   **T45.7**   **Poisoning by, adverse effect of and underdosing of anticoagulant antagonists, vitamin K and other coagulants**

    ☑6ᵗʰ   **T45.7X**   **Poisoning by, adverse effect of and underdosing of anticoagulant antagonists, vitamin K and other coagulants**

       ☑7ᵗʰ   **T45.7X1**   **Poisoning by anticoagulant antagonists, vitamin K and other coagulants, accidental (unintentional)**
           Poisoning by anticoagulant antagonists, vitamin K and other coagulants NOS

       ☑7ᵗʰ   **T45.7X2**   **Poisoning by anticoagulant antagonists, vitamin K and other coagulants, intentional self-harm**

       ☑7ᵗʰ   **T45.7X3**   **Poisoning by anticoagulant antagonists, vitamin K and other coagulants, assault**

       ☑7ᵗʰ   **T45.7X4**   **Poisoning by anticoagulant antagonists, vitamin K and other coagulants, undetermined**

       ☑7ᵗʰ   **T45.7X5**   Adverse effect of anticoagulant antagonists, vitamin K and other coagulants

       ☑7ᵗʰ   **T45.7X6**   Underdosing of anticoagulant antagonist, vitamin K and other coagulants
           EXCLUDES 1   vitamin K deficiency (E56.1)

☑ Add'l Character Required   ☑x7ᵗʰ Placeholder Alert   RUG IV Special Care High Dx   RUG IV Clinically Complex Dx   RUG IV Special Care Low Dx   Manifestation Code   Other Specified Code   ▽ Unspecified Code

✓5ᵗʰ **T45.8** **Poisoning by, adverse effect of and underdosing of other** primarily systemic and hematological agents

    Poisoning by, adverse effect of and underdosing of liver preparations and other antianemic agents

    Poisoning by, adverse effect of and underdosing of natural blood and blood products

    Poisoning by, adverse effect of and underdosing of plasma substitute

    EXCLUDES 2 *poisoning by, adverse effect of and underdosing of immunoglobulin (T50.Z1)*
    poisoning by, adverse effect of and underdosing of iron (T45.4)
    transfusion reactions (T80.-)

  ✓6ᵗʰ **T45.8X** **Poisoning by, adverse effect of and underdosing of** other primarily systemic and hematological agents

    ✓7ᵗʰ **T45.8X1** **Poisoning by other primarily systemic and hematological agents,** accidental (unintentional)
      Poisoning by other primarily systemic and hematological agents NOS

    ✓7ᵗʰ **T45.8X2** **Poisoning by other primarily systemic and hematological agents,** intentional self-harm

    ✓7ᵗʰ **T45.8X3** **Poisoning by other primarily systemic and hematological agents,** assault

    ✓7ᵗʰ **T45.8X4** **Poisoning by other primarily systemic and hematological agents,** undetermined

    ✓7ᵗʰ **T45.8X5** **Adverse effect of other primarily systemic and hematological agents**

    ✓7ᵗʰ **T45.8X6** **Underdosing of other primarily systemic and hematological agents**

✓5ᵗʰ **T45.9** **Poisoning by, adverse effect of and underdosing of** unspecified primarily systemic and hematological agent

  ✓x7ᵗʰ **T45.91** **Poisoning by unspecified primarily systemic and hematological agent,** accidental (unintentional) ▽
    Poisoning by primarily systemic and hematological agent NOS

  ✓x7ᵗʰ **T45.92** **Poisoning by unspecified primarily systemic and hematological agent,** intentional self-harm ▽

  ✓x7ᵗʰ **T45.93** **Poisoning by unspecified primarily systemic and hematological agent,** assault ▽

  ✓x7ᵗʰ **T45.94** **Poisoning by unspecified primarily systemic and hematological agent,** undetermined ▽

  ✓x7ᵗʰ **T45.95** **Adverse effect of unspecified primarily systemic and hematological agent** ▽

  ✓x7ᵗʰ **T45.96** **Underdosing of unspecified primarily systemic and hematological agent** ▽

✓4ᵗʰ **T46** **Poisoning by, adverse effect of and underdosing of agents primarily affecting the cardiovascular system**

  EXCLUDES 1 *poisoning by, adverse effect of and underdosing of metaraminol (T44.4)*

  The appropriate 7th character is to be added to each code from category T46.
  A   initial encounter
  D   subsequent encounter
  S   sequela

✓5ᵗʰ **T46.0** **Poisoning by, adverse effect of and underdosing of cardiac-stimulant glycosides and drugs of similar action**

  ✓6ᵗʰ **T46.0X** **Poisoning by, adverse effect of and underdosing of** cardiac-stimulant glycosides and drugs of similar action

    ✓7ᵗʰ **T46.0X1** **Poisoning by cardiac-stimulant glycosides and drugs of similar action,** accidental (unintentional)
      Poisoning by cardiac-stimulant glycosides and drugs of similar action NOS

    ✓7ᵗʰ **T46.0X2** **Poisoning by cardiac-stimulant glycosides and drugs of similar action,** intentional self-harm

    ✓7ᵗʰ **T46.0X3** **Poisoning by cardiac-stimulant glycosides and drugs of similar action,** assault

    ✓7ᵗʰ **T46.0X4** **Poisoning by cardiac-stimulant glycosides and drugs of similar action,** undetermined

    ✓7ᵗʰ **T46.0X5** **Adverse effect of cardiac-stimulant glycosides and drugs of similar action**

    ✓7ᵗʰ **T46.0X6** **Underdosing of cardiac-stimulant glycosides and drugs of similar action**

✓5ᵗʰ **T46.1** **Poisoning by, adverse effect of and underdosing of calcium-channel blockers**

  ✓6ᵗʰ **T46.1X** **Poisoning by, adverse effect of and underdosing of** calcium-channel blockers

    ✓7ᵗʰ **T46.1X1** **Poisoning by calcium-channel blockers,** accidental (unintentional)
      Poisoning by calcium-channel blockers NOS

    ✓7ᵗʰ **T46.1X2** **Poisoning by calcium-channel blockers,** intentional self-harm

    ✓7ᵗʰ **T46.1X3** **Poisoning by calcium-channel blockers,** assault

    ✓7ᵗʰ **T46.1X4** **Poisoning by calcium-channel blockers,** undetermined

    ✓7ᵗʰ **T46.1X5** **Adverse effect of calcium-channel blockers**

    ✓7ᵗʰ **T46.1X6** **Underdosing of calcium-channel blockers**

✓5ᵗʰ **T46.2** **Poisoning by, adverse effect of and underdosing of other antidysrhythmic drugs, not elsewhere classified**

  EXCLUDES 1 *poisoning by, adverse effect of and underdosing of beta-adrenoreceptor antagonists (T44.7-)*

  ✓6ᵗʰ **T46.2X** **Poisoning by, adverse effect of and underdosing of** other antidysrhythmic drugs

    ✓7ᵗʰ **T46.2X1** **Poisoning by other antidysrhythmic drugs,** accidental (unintentional)
      Poisoning by other antidysrhythmic drugs NOS

    ✓7ᵗʰ **T46.2X2** **Poisoning by other antidysrhythmic drugs,** intentional self-harm

    ✓7ᵗʰ **T46.2X3** **Poisoning by other antidysrhythmic drugs,** assault

    ✓7ᵗʰ **T46.2X4** **Poisoning by other antidysrhythmic drugs,** undetermined

    ✓7ᵗʰ **T46.2X5** **Adverse effect of other antidysrhythmic drugs**

    ✓7ᵗʰ **T46.2X6** **Underdosing of other antidysrhythmic drugs**

✓5ᵗʰ **T46.3** **Poisoning by, adverse effect of and underdosing of coronary vasodilators**

  Poisoning by, adverse effect of and underdosing of dipyridamole

  EXCLUDES 1 *poisoning by, adverse effect of and underdosing of calcium-channel blockers (T46.1)*

  ✓6ᵗʰ **T46.3X** **Poisoning by, adverse effect of and underdosing of** coronary vasodilators

    ✓7ᵗʰ **T46.3X1** **Poisoning by coronary vasodilators,** accidental (unintentional)
      Poisoning by coronary vasodilators NOS

    ✓7ᵗʰ **T46.3X2** **Poisoning by coronary vasodilators,** intentional self-harm

    ✓7ᵗʰ **T46.3X3** **Poisoning by coronary vasodilators,** assault

    ✓7ᵗʰ **T46.3X4** **Poisoning by coronary vasodilators,** undetermined

    ✓7ᵗʰ **T46.3X5** **Adverse effect of coronary vasodilators**

    ✓7ᵗʰ **T46.3X6** **Underdosing of coronary vasodilators**

✓5ᵗʰ **T46.4** **Poisoning by, adverse effect of and underdosing of angiotensin-converting-enzyme inhibitors**

  ✓6ᵗʰ **T46.4X** **Poisoning by, adverse effect of and underdosing of** angiotensin-converting-enzyme inhibitors

    ✓7ᵗʰ **T46.4X1** **Poisoning by angiotensin-converting-enzyme inhibitors,** accidental (unintentional)
      Poisoning by angiotensin-converting-enzyme inhibitors NOS

    ✓7ᵗʰ **T46.4X2** **Poisoning by angiotensin-converting-enzyme inhibitors,** intentional self-harm

    ✓7ᵗʰ **T46.4X3** **Poisoning by angiotensin-converting-enzyme inhibitors,** assault

    ✓7ᵗʰ **T46.4X4** **Poisoning by angiotensin-converting-enzyme inhibitors,** undetermined

    ✓7ᵗʰ **T46.4X5** **Adverse effect of angiotensin-converting-enzyme inhibitors**

    ✓7ᵗʰ **T46.4X6** **Underdosing of angiotensin-converting-enzyme inhibitors**

🅝 Newborn   🅟 Pediatric   🅜 Maternity   🅐 Adult   **RIC** RIC Dx   **NCDx** Noncancer Dx   **PDx** Primary Dx   **CC** RIC CC Condition   ▶◀ Revised Text   ● New Code   ▲ Revised Code Title

1012   ICD-10-CM 2016

☑5ᵗʰ **T46.5 Poisoning by, adverse effect of and underdosing of other antihypertensive drugs**

  EXCLUDES 2   *poisoning by, adverse effect of and underdosing of beta-adrenoreceptor antagonists (T44.7)*
            poisoning by, adverse effect of and underdosing of calcium-channel blockers (T46.1)
            poisoning by, adverse effect of and underdosing of diuretics (T50.0-T50.2)

  ☑6ᵗʰ **T46.5X Poisoning by, adverse effect of and underdosing of other antihypertensive drugs**

    ☑7ᵗʰ **T46.5X1 Poisoning by other antihypertensive drugs, accidental (unintentional)**
           Poisoning by other antihypertensive drugs NOS

    ☑7ᵗʰ **T46.5X2 Poisoning by other antihypertensive drugs, intentional self-harm**

    ☑7ᵗʰ **T46.5X3 Poisoning by other antihypertensive drugs, assault**

    ☑7ᵗʰ **T46.5X4 Poisoning by other antihypertensive drugs, undetermined**

    ☑7ᵗʰ **T46.5X5 Adverse effect of other antihypertensive drugs**

    ☑7ᵗʰ **T46.5X6 Underdosing of other antihypertensive drugs**

☑5ᵗʰ **T46.6 Poisoning by, adverse effect of and underdosing of antihyperlipidemic and antiarteriosclerotic drugs**

  ☑6ᵗʰ **T46.6X Poisoning by, adverse effect of and underdosing of antihyperlipidemic and antiarteriosclerotic drugs**

    ☑7ᵗʰ **T46.6X1 Poisoning by antihyperlipidemic and antiarteriosclerotic drugs, accidental (unintentional)**
           Poisoning by antihyperlipidemic and antiarteriosclerotic drugs NOS

    ☑7ᵗʰ **T46.6X2 Poisoning by antihyperlipidemic and antiarteriosclerotic drugs, intentional self-harm**

    ☑7ᵗʰ **T46.6X3 Poisoning by antihyperlipidemic and antiarteriosclerotic drugs, assault**

    ☑7ᵗʰ **T46.6X4 Poisoning by antihyperlipidemic and antiarteriosclerotic drugs, undetermined**

    ☑7ᵗʰ **T46.6X5 Adverse effect of antihyperlipidemic and antiarteriosclerotic drugs**

    ☑7ᵗʰ **T46.6X6 Underdosing of antihyperlipidemic and antiarteriosclerotic drugs**

☑5ᵗʰ **T46.7 Poisoning by, adverse effect of and underdosing of peripheral vasodilators**
     Poisoning by, adverse effect of and underdosing of nicotinic acid (derivatives)

  EXCLUDES 1   *poisoning by, adverse effect of and underdosing of papaverine (T44.3)*

  ☑6ᵗʰ **T46.7X Poisoning by, adverse effect of and underdosing of peripheral vasodilators**

    ☑7ᵗʰ **T46.7X1 Poisoning by peripheral vasodilators, accidental (unintentional)**
           Poisoning by peripheral vasodilators NOS

    ☑7ᵗʰ **T46.7X2 Poisoning by peripheral vasodilators, intentional self-harm**

    ☑7ᵗʰ **T46.7X3 Poisoning by peripheral vasodilators, assault**

    ☑7ᵗʰ **T46.7X4 Poisoning by peripheral vasodilators, undetermined**

    ☑7ᵗʰ **T46.7X5 Adverse effect of peripheral vasodilators**

    ☑7ᵗʰ **T46.7X6 Underdosing of peripheral vasodilators**

☑5ᵗʰ **T46.8 Poisoning by, adverse effect of and underdosing of antivaricose drugs, including sclerosing agents**

  ☑6ᵗʰ **T46.8X Poisoning by, adverse effect of and underdosing of antivaricose drugs, including sclerosing agents**

    ☑7ᵗʰ **T46.8X1 Poisoning by antivaricose drugs, including sclerosing agents, accidental (unintentional)**
           Poisoning by antivaricose drugs, including sclerosing agents NOS

    ☑7ᵗʰ **T46.8X2 Poisoning by antivaricose drugs, including sclerosing agents, intentional self-harm**

    ☑7ᵗʰ **T46.8X3 Poisoning by antivaricose drugs, including sclerosing agents, assault**

    ☑7ᵗʰ **T46.8X4 Poisoning by antivaricose drugs, including sclerosing agents, undetermined**

    ☑7ᵗʰ **T46.8X5 Adverse effect of antivaricose drugs, including sclerosing agents**

    ☑7ᵗʰ **T46.8X6 Underdosing of antivaricose drugs, including sclerosing agents**

☑5ᵗʰ **T46.9 Poisoning by, adverse effect of and underdosing of other and unspecified agents primarily affecting the cardiovascular system**

  ☑6ᵗʰ **T46.90 Poisoning by, adverse effect of and underdosing of unspecified agents primarily affecting the cardiovascular system**

    ☑7ᵗʰ **T46.901 Poisoning by unspecified agents primarily affecting the cardiovascular system, accidental (unintentional)** ▽

    ☑7ᵗʰ **T46.902 Poisoning by unspecified agents primarily affecting the cardiovascular system, intentional self-harm** ▽

    ☑7ᵗʰ **T46.903 Poisoning by unspecified agents primarily affecting the cardiovascular system, assault** ▽

    ☑7ᵗʰ **T46.904 Poisoning by unspecified agents primarily affecting the cardiovascular system, undetermined** ▽

    ☑7ᵗʰ **T46.905 Adverse effect of unspecified agents primarily affecting the cardiovascular system** ▽

    ☑7ᵗʰ **T46.906 Underdosing of unspecified agents primarily affecting the cardiovascular system** ▽

  ☑6ᵗʰ **T46.99 Poisoning by, adverse effect of and underdosing of other agents primarily affecting the cardiovascular system**

    ☑7ᵗʰ **T46.991 Poisoning by other agents primarily affecting the cardiovascular system, accidental (unintentional)**

    ☑7ᵗʰ **T46.992 Poisoning by other agents primarily affecting the cardiovascular system, intentional self-harm**

    ☑7ᵗʰ **T46.993 Poisoning by other agents primarily affecting the cardiovascular system, assault**

    ☑7ᵗʰ **T46.994 Poisoning by other agents primarily affecting the cardiovascular system, undetermined**

    ☑7ᵗʰ **T46.995 Adverse effect of other agents primarily affecting the cardiovascular system**

    ☑7ᵗʰ **T46.996 Underdosing of other agents primarily affecting the cardiovascular system**

☑4ᵗʰ **T47 Poisoning by, adverse effect of and underdosing of agents primarily affecting the gastrointestinal system**

  The appropriate 7th character is to be added to each code from category T47.
  A   initial encounter
  D   subsequent encounter
  S   sequela

☑5ᵗʰ **T47.0 Poisoning by, adverse effect of and underdosing of histamine H2-receptor blockers**

  ☑6ᵗʰ **T47.0X Poisoning by, adverse effect of and underdosing of histamine H2-receptor blockers**

    ☑7ᵗʰ **T47.0X1 Poisoning by histamine H2-receptor blockers, accidental (unintentional)**
           Poisoning by histamine H2-receptor blockers NOS

    ☑7ᵗʰ **T47.0X2 Poisoning by histamine H2-receptor blockers, intentional self-harm**

    ☑7ᵗʰ **T47.0X3 Poisoning by histamine H2-receptor blockers, assault**

    ☑7ᵗʰ **T47.0X4 Poisoning by histamine H2-receptor blockers, undetermined**

    ☑7ᵗʰ **T47.0X5 Adverse effect of histamine H2-receptor blockers**

    ☑7ᵗʰ **T47.0X6 Underdosing of histamine H2-receptor blockers**

☑ Add'l Character Required   ✗ᵥ₇ᵗʰ Placeholder Alert   RUG IV Special Care High Dx   RUG IV Clinically Complex Dx   RUG IV Special Care Low Dx   Manifestation Code   Other Specified Code   ▽ Unspecified Code

√5ᵗʰ **T47.1** **Poisoning by, adverse effect of and underdosing of other antacids and anti-gastric-secretion drugs**

√6ᵗʰ **T47.1X** **Poisoning by, adverse effect of and underdosing of** other antacids and anti-gastric-secretion **drugs**

√7ᵗʰ **T47.1X1** **Poisoning by other antacids and anti-gastric-secretion drugs,** accidental **(unintentional)**
Poisoning by other antacids and anti-gastric-secretion drugs NOS

√7ᵗʰ **T47.1X2** **Poisoning by other antacids and anti-gastric-secretion drugs,** intentional **self-harm**

√7ᵗʰ **T47.1X3** **Poisoning by other antacids and anti-gastric-secretion drugs,** assault

√7ᵗʰ **T47.1X4** **Poisoning by other antacids and anti-gastric-secretion drugs, undetermined**

√7ᵗʰ **T47.1X5** Adverse effect **of other antacids and anti-gastric-secretion drugs**

√7ᵗʰ **T47.1X6** Underdosing **of other antacids and anti-gastric-secretion drugs**

√5ᵗʰ **T47.2** **Poisoning by, adverse effect of and underdosing of stimulant laxatives**

√6ᵗʰ **T47.2X** **Poisoning by, adverse effect of and underdosing of** stimulant laxatives

√7ᵗʰ **T47.2X1** **Poisoning by stimulant laxatives,** accidental **(unintentional)**
Poisoning by stimulant laxatives NOS

√7ᵗʰ **T47.2X2** **Poisoning by stimulant laxatives,** intentional self-harm

√7ᵗʰ **T47.2X3** **Poisoning by stimulant laxatives,** assault

√7ᵗʰ **T47.2X4** **Poisoning by stimulant laxatives, undetermined**

√7ᵗʰ **T47.2X5** Adverse effect **of stimulant laxatives**

√7ᵗʰ **T47.2X6** Underdosing **of stimulant laxatives**

√5ᵗʰ **T47.3** **Poisoning by, adverse effect of and underdosing of saline and osmotic laxatives**

√6ᵗʰ **T47.3X** **Poisoning by and adverse effect of** saline and osmotic laxatives

√7ᵗʰ **T47.3X1** **Poisoning by saline and osmotic laxatives,** accidental **(unintentional)**
Poisoning by saline and osmotic laxatives NOS

√7ᵗʰ **T47.3X2** **Poisoning by saline and osmotic laxatives,** intentional self-harm

√7ᵗʰ **T47.3X3** **Poisoning by saline and osmotic laxatives,** assault

√7ᵗʰ **T47.3X4** **Poisoning by saline and osmotic laxatives, undetermined**

√7ᵗʰ **T47.3X5** Adverse effect **of saline and osmotic laxatives**

√7ᵗʰ **T47.3X6** Underdosing **of saline and osmotic laxatives**

√5ᵗʰ **T47.4** **Poisoning by, adverse effect of and underdosing of other laxatives**

√6ᵗʰ **T47.4X** **Poisoning by, adverse effect of and underdosing of** other laxatives

√7ᵗʰ **T47.4X1** **Poisoning by other laxatives,** accidental **(unintentional)**
Poisoning by other laxatives NOS

√7ᵗʰ **T47.4X2** **Poisoning by other laxatives,** intentional self-harm

√7ᵗʰ **T47.4X3** **Poisoning by other laxatives,** assault

√7ᵗʰ **T47.4X4** **Poisoning by other laxatives, undetermined**

√7ᵗʰ **T47.4X5** Adverse effect **of other laxatives**

√7ᵗʰ **T47.4X6** Underdosing **of other laxatives**

√5ᵗʰ **T47.5** **Poisoning by, adverse effect of and underdosing of digestants**

√6ᵗʰ **T47.5X** **Poisoning by, adverse effect of and underdosing of** digestants

√7ᵗʰ **T47.5X1** **Poisoning by digestants,** accidental **(unintentional)**
Poisoning by digestants NOS

√7ᵗʰ **T47.5X2** **Poisoning by digestants,** intentional self-harm

√7ᵗʰ **T47.5X3** **Poisoning by digestants,** assault

√7ᵗʰ **T47.5X4** **Poisoning by digestants,** undetermined

√7ᵗʰ **T47.5X5** Adverse effect **of digestants**

√7ᵗʰ **T47.5X6** Underdosing **of digestants**

√5ᵗʰ **T47.6** **Poisoning by, adverse effect of and underdosing of antidiarrheal drugs**

EXCLUDES 2 *poisoning by, adverse effect of and underdosing of systemic antibiotics and other anti-infectives (T36-T37)*

√6ᵗʰ **T47.6X** **Poisoning by, adverse effect of and underdosing of** antidiarrheal **drugs**

√7ᵗʰ **T47.6X1** **Poisoning by antidiarrheal drugs,** accidental **(unintentional)**
Poisoning by antidiarrheal drugs NOS

√7ᵗʰ **T47.6X2** **Poisoning by antidiarrheal drugs,** intentional self-harm

√7ᵗʰ **T47.6X3** **Poisoning by antidiarrheal drugs,** assault

√7ᵗʰ **T47.6X4** **Poisoning by antidiarrheal drugs, undetermined**

√7ᵗʰ **T47.6X5** Adverse effect **of antidiarrheal drugs**

√7ᵗʰ **T47.6X6** Underdosing **of antidiarrheal drugs**

√5ᵗʰ **T47.7** **Poisoning by, adverse effect of and underdosing of emetics**

√6ᵗʰ **T47.7X** **Poisoning by, adverse effect of and underdosing of** emetics

√7ᵗʰ **T47.7X1** **Poisoning by emetics,** accidental **(unintentional)**
Poisoning by emetics NOS

√7ᵗʰ **T47.7X2** **Poisoning by emetics,** intentional self-harm

√7ᵗʰ **T47.7X3** **Poisoning by emetics,** assault

√7ᵗʰ **T47.7X4** **Poisoning by emetics,** undetermined

√7ᵗʰ **T47.7X5** Adverse effect **of emetics**

√7ᵗʰ **T47.7X6** Underdosing **of emetics**

√5ᵗʰ **T47.8** **Poisoning by, adverse effect of and underdosing of other** agents primarily affecting gastrointestinal system

√6ᵗʰ **T47.8X** **Poisoning by, adverse effect of and underdosing of** other **agents primarily affecting gastrointestinal system**

√7ᵗʰ **T47.8X1** **Poisoning by other agents primarily affecting gastrointestinal system,** accidental **(unintentional)**
Poisoning by other agents primarily affecting gastrointestinal system NOS

√7ᵗʰ **T47.8X2** **Poisoning by other agents primarily affecting gastrointestinal system,** intentional self-harm

√7ᵗʰ **T47.8X3** **Poisoning by other agents primarily affecting gastrointestinal system,** assault

√7ᵗʰ **T47.8X4** **Poisoning by other agents primarily affecting gastrointestinal system, undetermined**

√7ᵗʰ **T47.8X5** Adverse effect **of other agents primarily affecting gastrointestinal system**

√7ᵗʰ **T47.8X6** Underdosing **of other agents primarily affecting gastrointestinal system**

√5ᵗʰ **T47.9** **Poisoning by, adverse effect of and underdosing of** unspecified **agents primarily affecting the gastrointestinal system**

√x7ᵗʰ **T47.91** **Poisoning by unspecified agents primarily affecting the gastrointestinal system,** accidental **(unintentional)** ▽
Poisoning by agents primarily affecting the gastrointestinal system NOS

√x7ᵗʰ **T47.92** **Poisoning by unspecified agents primarily affecting the gastrointestinal system,** intentional self-harm ▽

√x7ᵗʰ **T47.93** **Poisoning by unspecified agents primarily affecting the gastrointestinal system,** assault ▽

√x7ᵗʰ **T47.94** **Poisoning by unspecified agents primarily affecting the gastrointestinal system, undetermined** ▽

√x7ᵗʰ **T47.95** Adverse effect **of unspecified agents primarily affecting the gastrointestinal system** ▽

√x7ᵗʰ **T47.96** Underdosing **of unspecified agents primarily affecting the gastrointestinal system** ▽

🅿 Pediatric   Ⓜ Maternity   🄰 Adult   **RIC** RIC Dx   **NC Dx** Noncancer Dx   **PDx** Primary Dx   **CC** RIC CC Condition   ►◄ Revised Text   ● New Code   ▲ Revised Code Title

ICD-10-CM 2016

✓4ᵗʰ **T48** **Poisoning by, adverse effect of and underdosing of agents primarily acting on smooth and skeletal muscles and the respiratory system**

> The appropriate 7th character is to be added to each code from category T48.
> A   initial encounter
> D   subsequent encounter
> S   sequela

✓5ᵗʰ **T48.0** **Poisoning by, adverse effect of and underdosing of oxytocic drugs**
> EXCLUDES 1   poisoning by, adverse effect of and underdosing of estrogens, progestogens and antagonists (T38.4-T38.6)

✓6ᵗʰ **T48.0X** **Poisoning by, adverse effect of and underdosing of oxytocic drugs**

   ✓7ᵗʰ **T48.0X1** **Poisoning by oxytocic drugs, accidental (unintentional)**
      Poisoning by oxytocic drugs NOS

   ✓7ᵗʰ **T48.0X2** **Poisoning by oxytocic drugs, intentional self-harm**

   ✓7ᵗʰ **T48.0X3** **Poisoning by oxytocic drugs, assault**

   ✓7ᵗʰ **T48.0X4** **Poisoning by oxytocic drugs, undetermined**

   ✓7ᵗʰ **T48.0X5** **Adverse effect of oxytocic drugs**

   ✓7ᵗʰ **T48.0X6** **Underdosing of oxytocic drugs**

✓5ᵗʰ **T48.1** **Poisoning by, adverse effect of and underdosing of skeletal muscle relaxants [neuromuscular blocking agents]**

✓6ᵗʰ **T48.1X** **Poisoning by, adverse effect of and underdosing of skeletal muscle relaxants [neuromuscular blocking agents]**

   ✓7ᵗʰ **T48.1X1** **Poisoning by skeletal muscle relaxants [neuromuscular blocking agents], accidental (unintentional)**
      Poisoning by skeletal muscle relaxants [neuromuscular blocking agents] NOS

   ✓7ᵗʰ **T48.1X2** **Poisoning by skeletal muscle relaxants [neuromuscular blocking agents], intentional self-harm**

   ✓7ᵗʰ **T48.1X3** **Poisoning by skeletal muscle relaxants [neuromuscular blocking agents], assault**

   ✓7ᵗʰ **T48.1X4** **Poisoning by skeletal muscle relaxants [neuromuscular blocking agents], undetermined**

   ✓7ᵗʰ **T48.1X5** **Adverse effect of skeletal muscle relaxants [neuromuscular blocking agents]**

   ✓7ᵗʰ **T48.1X6** **Underdosing of skeletal muscle relaxants [neuromuscular blocking agents]**

✓5ᵗʰ **T48.2** **Poisoning by, adverse effect of and underdosing of other and unspecified drugs acting on muscles**

✓6ᵗʰ **T48.20** **Poisoning by, adverse effect of and underdosing of unspecified drugs acting on muscles**

   ✓7ᵗʰ **T48.201** **Poisoning by unspecified drugs acting on muscles, accidental (unintentional)** ▽
      Poisoning by unspecified drugs acting on muscles NOS

   ✓7ᵗʰ **T48.202** **Poisoning by unspecified drugs acting on muscles, intentional self-harm** ▽

   ✓7ᵗʰ **T48.203** **Poisoning by unspecified drugs acting on muscles, assault** ▽

   ✓7ᵗʰ **T48.204** **Poisoning by unspecified drugs acting on muscles, undetermined** ▽

   ✓7ᵗʰ **T48.205** **Adverse effect of unspecified drugs acting on muscles** ▽

   ✓7ᵗʰ **T48.206** **Underdosing of unspecified drugs acting on muscles** ▽

✓6ᵗʰ **T48.29** **Poisoning by, adverse effect of and underdosing of other drugs acting on muscles**

   ✓7ᵗʰ **T48.291** **Poisoning by other drugs acting on muscles, accidental (unintentional)**
      Poisoning by other drugs acting on muscles NOS

   ✓7ᵗʰ **T48.292** **Poisoning by other drugs acting on muscles, intentional self-harm**

   ✓7ᵗʰ **T48.293** **Poisoning by other drugs acting on muscles, assault**

   ✓7ᵗʰ **T48.294** **Poisoning by other drugs acting on muscles, undetermined**

   ✓7ᵗʰ **T48.295** **Adverse effect of other drugs acting on muscles**

   ✓7ᵗʰ **T48.296** **Underdosing of other drugs acting on muscles**

✓5ᵗʰ **T48.3** **Poisoning by, adverse effect of and underdosing of antitussives**

✓6ᵗʰ **T48.3X** **Poisoning by, adverse effect of and underdosing of antitussives**

   ✓7ᵗʰ **T48.3X1** **Poisoning by antitussives, accidental (unintentional)**
      Poisoning by antitussives NOS

   ✓7ᵗʰ **T48.3X2** **Poisoning by antitussives, intentional self-harm**

   ✓7ᵗʰ **T48.3X3** **Poisoning by antitussives, assault**

   ✓7ᵗʰ **T48.3X4** **Poisoning by antitussives, undetermined**

   ✓7ᵗʰ **T48.3X5** **Adverse effect of antitussives**

   ✓7ᵗʰ **T48.3X6** **Underdosing of antitussives**

✓5ᵗʰ **T48.4** **Poisoning by, adverse effect of and underdosing of expectorants**

✓6ᵗʰ **T48.4X** **Poisoning by, adverse effect of and underdosing of expectorants**

   ✓7ᵗʰ **T48.4X1** **Poisoning by expectorants, accidental (unintentional)**
      Poisoning by expectorants NOS

   ✓7ᵗʰ **T48.4X2** **Poisoning by expectorants, intentional self-harm**

   ✓7ᵗʰ **T48.4X3** **Poisoning by expectorants, assault**

   ✓7ᵗʰ **T48.4X4** **Poisoning by expectorants, undetermined**

   ✓7ᵗʰ **T48.4X5** **Adverse effect of expectorants**

   ✓7ᵗʰ **T48.4X6** **Underdosing of expectorants**

✓5ᵗʰ **T48.5** **Poisoning by, adverse effect of and underdosing of other anti-common-cold drugs**
> Poisoning by, adverse effect of and underdosing of decongestants
> EXCLUDES 2   poisoning by, adverse effect of and underdosing of antipyretics, NEC (T39.9-)
> poisoning by, adverse effect of and underdosing of non-steroidal antiinflammatory drugs (T39.3-)
> poisoning by, adverse effect of and underdosing of salicylates (T39.0-)

✓6ᵗʰ **T48.5X** **Poisoning by, adverse effect of and underdosing of other anti-common-cold drugs**

   ✓7ᵗʰ **T48.5X1** **Poisoning by other anti-common-cold drugs, accidental (unintentional)**
      Poisoning by other anti-common-cold drugs NOS

   ✓7ᵗʰ **T48.5X2** **Poisoning by other anti-common-cold drugs, intentional self-harm**

   ✓7ᵗʰ **T48.5X3** **Poisoning by other anti-common-cold drugs, assault**

   ✓7ᵗʰ **T48.5X4** **Poisoning by other anti-common-cold drugs, undetermined**

   ✓7ᵗʰ **T48.5X5** **Adverse effect of other anti-common-cold drugs**

   ✓7ᵗʰ **T48.5X6** **Underdosing of other anti-common-cold drugs**

✓5ᵗʰ **T48.6** **Poisoning by, adverse effect of and underdosing of antiasthmatics, not elsewhere classified**
> Poisoning by, adverse effect of and underdosing of beta-adrenoreceptor agonists used in asthma therapy
> EXCLUDES 1   poisoning by, adverse effect of and underdosing of anterior pituitary [adenohypophyseal] hormones (T38.8)
> poisoning by, adverse effect of and underdosing of beta-adrenoreceptor agonists not used in asthma therapy (T44.5)

✓6ᵗʰ **T48.6X** **Poisoning by, adverse effect of and underdosing of antiasthmatics**

   ✓7ᵗʰ **T48.6X1** **Poisoning by antiasthmatics, accidental (unintentional)**
      Poisoning by antiasthmatics NOS

   ✓7ᵗʰ **T48.6X2** **Poisoning by antiasthmatics, intentional self-harm**

   ✓7ᵗʰ **T48.6X3** **Poisoning by antiasthmatics, assault**

✓ Add'l Character Required ✓×7ᵗʰ Placeholder Alert RUG IV Special Care High Dx RUG IV Clinically Complex Dx RUG IV Special Care Low Dx Manifestation Code Other Specified Code ▽ Unspecified Code

✓7ᵗ **T48.6X4** **Poisoning by antiasthmatics,** undetermined

✓7ᵗ **T48.6X5** Adverse effect **of antiasthmatics**

✓7ᵗ **T48.6X6** Underdosing **of antiasthmatics**

✓5ᵗ **T48.9** **Poisoning by, adverse effect of and underdosing of other and unspecified** agents primarily acting on the respiratory system

    ✓6ᵗ **T48.90** **Poisoning by, adverse effect of and underdosing of unspecified** agents primarily acting on the respiratory system

        ✓7ᵗ **T48.901** **Poisoning by unspecified agents primarily acting on the respiratory system,** accidental (unintentional) ▽

        ✓7ᵗ **T48.902** **Poisoning by unspecified agents primarily acting on the respiratory system,** intentional self-harm ▽

        ✓7ᵗ **T48.903** **Poisoning by unspecified agents primarily acting on the respiratory system,** assault ▽

        ✓7ᵗ **T48.904** **Poisoning by unspecified agents primarily acting on the respiratory system,** undetermined ▽

        ✓7ᵗ **T48.905** Adverse effect **of unspecified agents primarily acting on the respiratory system** ▽

        ✓7ᵗ **T48.906** Underdosing **of unspecified agents primarily acting on the respiratory system** ▽

    ✓6ᵗ **T48.99** **Poisoning by, adverse effect of and underdosing of other** agents primarily acting on the respiratory system

        ✓7ᵗ **T48.991** **Poisoning by other agents primarily acting on the respiratory system,** accidental (unintentional)

        ✓7ᵗ **T48.992** **Poisoning by other agents primarily acting on the respiratory system,** intentional self-harm

        ✓7ᵗ **T48.993** **Poisoning by other agents primarily acting on the respiratory system,** assault

        ✓7ᵗ **T48.994** **Poisoning by other agents primarily acting on the respiratory system,** undetermined

        ✓7ᵗ **T48.995** Adverse effect **of other agents primarily acting on the respiratory system**

        ✓7ᵗ **T48.996** Underdosing **of other agents primarily acting on the respiratory system**

✓4ᵗ **T49** **Poisoning by, adverse effect of and underdosing of topical agents primarily affecting skin and mucous membrane and by ophthalmological, otorhinolaryngological and dental drugs**
Poisoning by, adverse effect of and underdosing of glucocorticoids, topically used

> The appropriate 7th character is to be added to each code from category T49.
> A   initial encounter
> D   subsequent encounter
> S   sequela

✓5ᵗ **T49.0** **Poisoning by, adverse effect of and underdosing of local antifungal, anti-infective and anti-inflammatory drugs**

    ✓6ᵗ **T49.0X** **Poisoning by, adverse effect of and underdosing of** local antifungal, anti-infective and anti-inflammatory **drugs**

        ✓7ᵗ **T49.0X1** **Poisoning by local antifungal, anti-infective and anti-inflammatory drugs,** accidental (unintentional)
Poisoning by local antifungal, anti-infective and anti-inflammatory drugs NOS

        ✓7ᵗ **T49.0X2** **Poisoning by local antifungal, anti-infective and anti-inflammatory drugs,** intentional self-harm

        ✓7ᵗ **T49.0X3** **Poisoning by local antifungal, anti-infective and anti-inflammatory drugs,** assault

        ✓7ᵗ **T49.0X4** **Poisoning by local antifungal, anti-infective and anti-inflammatory drugs,** undetermined

        ✓7ᵗ **T49.0X5** Adverse effect **of local antifungal, anti-infective and anti-inflammatory drugs**

        ✓7ᵗ **T49.0X6** Underdosing **of local antifungal, anti-infective and anti-inflammatory drugs**

✓5ᵗ **T49.1** **Poisoning by, adverse effect of and underdosing of antipruritics**

    ✓6ᵗ **T49.1X** **Poisoning by, adverse effect of and underdosing of** antipruritics

        ✓7ᵗ **T49.1X1** **Poisoning by antipruritics,** accidental (unintentional)
Poisoning by antipruritics NOS

        ✓7ᵗ **T49.1X2** **Poisoning by antipruritics,** intentional self-harm

        ✓7ᵗ **T49.1X3** **Poisoning by antipruritics,** assault

        ✓7ᵗ **T49.1X4** **Poisoning by antipruritics,** undetermined

        ✓7ᵗ **T49.1X5** Adverse effect **of antipruritics**

        ✓7ᵗ **T49.1X6** Underdosing **of antipruritics**

✓5ᵗ **T49.2** **Poisoning by, adverse effect of and underdosing of local astringents and local detergents**

    ✓6ᵗ **T49.2X** **Poisoning by, adverse effect of and underdosing of** local astringents and local detergents

        ✓7ᵗ **T49.2X1** **Poisoning by local astringents and local detergents,** accidental (unintentional)
Poisoning by local astringents and local detergents NOS

        ✓7ᵗ **T49.2X2** **Poisoning by local astringents and local detergents,** intentional self-harm

        ✓7ᵗ **T49.2X3** **Poisoning by local astringents and local detergents,** assault

        ✓7ᵗ **T49.2X4** **Poisoning by local astringents and local detergents,** undetermined

        ✓7ᵗ **T49.2X5** Adverse effect **of local astringents and local detergents**

        ✓7ᵗ **T49.2X6** Underdosing **of local astringents and local detergents**

✓5ᵗ **T49.3** **Poisoning by, adverse effect of and underdosing of emollients, demulcents and protectants**

    ✓6ᵗ **T49.3X** **Poisoning by, adverse effect of and underdosing of** emollients, demulcents and protectants

        ✓7ᵗ **T49.3X1** **Poisoning by emollients, demulcents and protectants,** accidental (unintentional)
Poisoning by emollients, demulcents and protectants NOS

        ✓7ᵗ **T49.3X2** **Poisoning by emollients, demulcents and protectants,** intentional self-harm

        ✓7ᵗ **T49.3X3** **Poisoning by emollients, demulcents and protectants,** assault

        ✓7ᵗ **T49.3X4** **Poisoning by emollients, demulcents and protectants,** undetermined

        ✓7ᵗ **T49.3X5** Adverse effect **of emollients, demulcents and protectants**

        ✓7ᵗ **T49.3X6** Underdosing **of emollients, demulcents and protectants**

✓5ᵗ **T49.4** **Poisoning by, adverse effect of and underdosing of keratolytics, keratoplastics, and other hair treatment drugs and preparations**

    ✓6ᵗ **T49.4X** **Poisoning by, adverse effect of and underdosing of** keratolytics, keratoplastics, and other hair treatment drugs and preparations

        ✓7ᵗ **T49.4X1** **Poisoning by keratolytics, keratoplastics, and other hair treatment drugs and preparations,** accidental (unintentional)
Poisoning by keratolytics, keratoplastics, and other hair treatment drugs and preparations NOS

        ✓7ᵗ **T49.4X2** **Poisoning by keratolytics, keratoplastics, and other hair treatment drugs and preparations,** intentional self-harm

        ✓7ᵗ **T49.4X3** **Poisoning by keratolytics, keratoplastics, and other hair treatment drugs and preparations,** assault

        ✓7ᵗ **T49.4X4** **Poisoning by keratolytics, keratoplastics, and other hair treatment drugs and preparations,** undetermined

        ✓7ᵗ **T49.4X5** Adverse effect **of keratolytics, keratoplastics, and other hair treatment drugs and preparations**

N Newborn   P Pediatric   M Maternity   A Adult   RIC RIC Dx   NC Dx Noncancer Dx   PDx Primary Dx   CC RIC CC Condition   ►◄ Revised Text   ● New Code   ▲ Revised Code Title

1016   ICD-10-CM 2016

✓7ᵗʰ **T49.4X6** Underdosing of keratolytics, keratoplastics, and other hair treatment drugs and preparations

✓5ᵗʰ **T49.5** Poisoning by, adverse effect of and underdosing of ophthalmological drugs and preparations

  ✓6ᵗʰ **T49.5X** Poisoning by, adverse effect of and underdosing of ophthalmological drugs and preparations

    ✓7ᵗʰ **T49.5X1** Poisoning by ophthalmological drugs and preparations, accidental (unintentional)
        Poisoning by ophthalmological drugs and preparations NOS

    ✓7ᵗʰ **T49.5X2** Poisoning by ophthalmological drugs and preparations, intentional self-harm

    ✓7ᵗʰ **T49.5X3** Poisoning by ophthalmological drugs and preparations, assault

    ✓7ᵗʰ **T49.5X4** Poisoning by ophthalmological drugs and preparations, undetermined

    ✓7ᵗʰ **T49.5X5** Adverse effect of ophthalmological drugs and preparations

    ✓7ᵗʰ **T49.5X6** Underdosing of ophthalmological drugs and preparations

✓5ᵗʰ **T49.6** Poisoning by, adverse effect of and underdosing of otorhinolaryngological drugs and preparations

  ✓6ᵗʰ **T49.6X** Poisoning by, adverse effect of and underdosing of otorhinolaryngological drugs and preparations

    ✓7ᵗʰ **T49.6X1** Poisoning by otorhinolaryngological drugs and preparations, accidental (unintentional)
        Poisoning by otorhinolaryngological drugs and preparations NOS

    ✓7ᵗʰ **T49.6X2** Poisoning by otorhinolaryngological drugs and preparations, intentional self-harm

    ✓7ᵗʰ **T49.6X3** Poisoning by otorhinolaryngological drugs and preparations, assault

    ✓7ᵗʰ **T49.6X4** Poisoning by otorhinolaryngological drugs and preparations, undetermined

    ✓7ᵗʰ **T49.6X5** Adverse effect of otorhinolaryngological drugs and preparations

    ✓7ᵗʰ **T49.6X6** Underdosing of otorhinolaryngological drugs and preparations

✓5ᵗʰ **T49.7** Poisoning by, adverse effect of and underdosing of dental drugs, topically applied

  ✓6ᵗʰ **T49.7X** Poisoning by, adverse effect of and underdosing of dental drugs, topically applied

    ✓7ᵗʰ **T49.7X1** Poisoning by dental drugs, topically applied, accidental (unintentional)
        Poisoning by dental drugs, topically applied NOS

    ✓7ᵗʰ **T49.7X2** Poisoning by dental drugs, topically applied, intentional self-harm

    ✓7ᵗʰ **T49.7X3** Poisoning by dental drugs, topically applied, assault

    ✓7ᵗʰ **T49.7X4** Poisoning by dental drugs, topically applied, undetermined

    ✓7ᵗʰ **T49.7X5** Adverse effect of dental drugs, topically applied

    ✓7ᵗʰ **T49.7X6** Underdosing of dental drugs, topically applied

✓5ᵗʰ **T49.8** Poisoning by, adverse effect of and underdosing of other topical agents
    Poisoning by, adverse effect of and underdosing of spermicides

  ✓6ᵗʰ **T49.8X** Poisoning by, adverse effect of and underdosing of other topical agents

    ✓7ᵗʰ **T49.8X1** Poisoning by other topical agents, accidental (unintentional)
        Poisoning by other topical agents NOS

    ✓7ᵗʰ **T49.8X2** Poisoning by other topical agents, intentional self-harm

    ✓7ᵗʰ **T49.8X3** Poisoning by other topical agents, assault

    ✓7ᵗʰ **T49.8X4** Poisoning by other topical agents, undetermined

    ✓7ᵗʰ **T49.8X5** Adverse effect of other topical agents

    ✓7ᵗʰ **T49.8X6** Underdosing of other topical agents

✓5ᵗʰ **T49.9** Poisoning by, adverse effect of and underdosing of unspecified topical agent

  ✓x7ᵗʰ **T49.91** Poisoning by unspecified topical agent, accidental (unintentional) ▽

  ✓x7ᵗʰ **T49.92** Poisoning by unspecified topical agent, intentional self-harm ▽

  ✓x7ᵗʰ **T49.93** Poisoning by unspecified topical agent, assault ▽

  ✓x7ᵗʰ **T49.94** Poisoning by unspecified topical agent, undetermined ▽

  ✓x7ᵗʰ **T49.95** Adverse effect of unspecified topical agent ▽

  ✓x7ᵗʰ **T49.96** Underdosing of unspecified topical agent ▽

✓4ᵗʰ **T50** Poisoning by, adverse effect of and underdosing of diuretics and other and unspecified drugs, medicaments and biological substances

> The appropriate 7th character is to be added to each code from category T50.
> A   initial encounter
> D   subsequent encounter
> S   sequela

✓5ᵗʰ **T50.0** Poisoning by, adverse effect of and underdosing of mineralocorticoids and their antagonists

  ✓6ᵗʰ **T50.0X** Poisoning by, adverse effect of and underdosing of mineralocorticoids and their antagonists

    ✓7ᵗʰ **T50.0X1** Poisoning by mineralocorticoids and their antagonists, accidental (unintentional)
        Poisoning by mineralocorticoids and their antagonists NOS

    ✓7ᵗʰ **T50.0X2** Poisoning by mineralocorticoids and their antagonists, intentional self-harm

    ✓7ᵗʰ **T50.0X3** Poisoning by mineralocorticoids and their antagonists, assault

    ✓7ᵗʰ **T50.0X4** Poisoning by mineralocorticoids and their antagonists, undetermined

    ✓7ᵗʰ **T50.0X5** Adverse effect of mineralocorticoids and their antagonists

    ✓7ᵗʰ **T50.0X6** Underdosing of mineralocorticoids and their antagonists

✓5ᵗʰ **T50.1** Poisoning by, adverse effect of and underdosing of loop [high-ceiling] diuretics

  ✓6ᵗʰ **T50.1X** Poisoning by, adverse effect of and underdosing of loop [high-ceiling] diuretics

    ✓7ᵗʰ **T50.1X1** Poisoning by loop [high-ceiling] diuretics, accidental (unintentional)
        Poisoning by loop [high-ceiling] diuretics NOS

    ✓7ᵗʰ **T50.1X2** Poisoning by loop [high-ceiling] diuretics, intentional self-harm

    ✓7ᵗʰ **T50.1X3** Poisoning by loop [high-ceiling] diuretics, assault

    ✓7ᵗʰ **T50.1X4** Poisoning by loop [high-ceiling] diuretics, undetermined

    ✓7ᵗʰ **T50.1X5** Adverse effect of loop [high-ceiling] diuretics

    ✓7ᵗʰ **T50.1X6** Underdosing of loop [high-ceiling] diuretics

✓5ᵗʰ **T50.2** Poisoning by, adverse effect of and underdosing of carbonic-anhydrase inhibitors, benzothiadiazides and other diuretics
    Poisoning by, adverse effect of and underdosing of acetazolamide

  ✓6ᵗʰ **T50.2X** Poisoning by, adverse effect of and underdosing of carbonic-anhydrase inhibitors, benzothiadiazides and other diuretics

    ✓7ᵗʰ **T50.2X1** Poisoning by carbonic-anhydrase inhibitors, benzothiadiazides and other diuretics, accidental (unintentional)
        Poisoning by carbonic-anhydrase inhibitors, benzothiadiazides and other diuretics NOS

    ✓7ᵗʰ **T50.2X2** Poisoning by carbonic-anhydrase inhibitors, benzothiadiazides and other diuretics, intentional self-harm

    ✓7ᵗʰ **T50.2X3** Poisoning by carbonic-anhydrase inhibitors, benzothiadiazides and other diuretics, assault

√7ᵗʰ **T50.2X4** **Poisoning by carbonic-anhydrase inhibitors, benzothiadiazides and other diuretics,** undetermined

√7ᵗʰ **T50.2X5** Adverse effect **of carbonic-anhydrase inhibitors, benzothiadiazides and other diuretics**

√7ᵗʰ **T50.2X6** Underdosing **of carbonic-anhydrase inhibitors, benzothiadiazides and other diuretics**

√5ᵗʰ **T50.3** **Poisoning by, adverse effect of and underdosing of electrolytic, caloric and water-balance agents**
Poisoning by, adverse effect of and underdosing of oral rehydration salts

√6ᵗʰ **T50.3X** **Poisoning by, adverse effect of and underdosing of** electrolytic, caloric and water-balance agents

√7ᵗʰ **T50.3X1** **Poisoning by electrolytic, caloric and water-balance agents,** accidental **(unintentional)**
Poisoning by electrolytic, caloric and water-balance agents NOS

√7ᵗʰ **T50.3X2** **Poisoning by electrolytic, caloric and water-balance agents,** intentional self-harm

√7ᵗʰ **T50.3X3** **Poisoning by electrolytic, caloric and water-balance agents,** assault

√7ᵗʰ **T50.3X4** **Poisoning by electrolytic, caloric and water-balance agents,** undetermined

√7ᵗʰ **T50.3X5** Adverse effect **of electrolytic, caloric and water-balance agents**

√7ᵗʰ **T50.3X6** Underdosing **of electrolytic, caloric and water-balance agents**

√5ᵗʰ **T50.4** **Poisoning by, adverse effect of and underdosing of drugs affecting uric acid metabolism**

√6ᵗʰ **T50.4X** **Poisoning by, adverse effect of and underdosing of drugs** affecting uric acid metabolism

√7ᵗʰ **T50.4X1** **Poisoning by drugs affecting uric acid metabolism,** accidental **(unintentional)**
Poisoning by drugs affecting uric acid metabolism NOS

√7ᵗʰ **T50.4X2** **Poisoning by drugs affecting uric acid metabolism,** intentional self-harm

√7ᵗʰ **T50.4X3** **Poisoning by drugs affecting uric acid metabolism,** assault

√7ᵗʰ **T50.4X4** **Poisoning by drugs affecting uric acid metabolism,** undetermined

√7ᵗʰ **T50.4X5** Adverse effect **of drugs affecting uric acid metabolism**

√7ᵗʰ **T50.4X6** Underdosing **of drugs affecting uric acid metabolism**

√5ᵗʰ **T50.5** **Poisoning by, adverse effect of and underdosing of appetite depressants**

√6ᵗʰ **T50.5X** **Poisoning by, adverse effect of and underdosing of** appetite depressants

√7ᵗʰ **T50.5X1** **Poisoning by appetite depressants,** accidental **(unintentional)**
Poisoning by appetite depressants NOS

√7ᵗʰ **T50.5X2** **Poisoning by appetite depressants,** intentional self-harm

√7ᵗʰ **T50.5X3** **Poisoning by appetite depressants,** assault

√7ᵗʰ **T50.5X4** **Poisoning by appetite depressants,** undetermined

√7ᵗʰ **T50.5X5** Adverse effect **of appetite depressants**

√7ᵗʰ **T50.5X6** Underdosing **of appetite depressants**

√5ᵗʰ **T50.6** **Poisoning by, adverse effect of and underdosing of antidotes and chelating agents**
Poisoning by, adverse effect of and underdosing of alcohol deterrents

√6ᵗʰ **T50.6X** **Poisoning by, adverse effect of and underdosing of** antidotes and chelating agents

√7ᵗʰ **T50.6X1** **Poisoning by antidotes and chelating agents,** accidental **(unintentional)**
Poisoning by antidotes and chelating agents NOS

√7ᵗʰ **T50.6X2** **Poisoning by antidotes and chelating agents,** intentional self-harm

√7ᵗʰ **T50.6X3** **Poisoning by antidotes and chelating agents,** assault

√7ᵗʰ **T50.6X4** **Poisoning by antidotes and chelating agents,** undetermined

√7ᵗʰ **T50.6X5** Adverse effect **of antidotes and chelating agents**

√7ᵗʰ **T50.6X6** Underdosing **of antidotes and chelating agents**

√5ᵗʰ **T50.7** **Poisoning by, adverse effect of and underdosing of analeptics and opioid receptor antagonists**

√6ᵗʰ **T50.7X** **Poisoning by, adverse effect of and underdosing of** analeptics and opioid receptor antagonists

√7ᵗʰ **T50.7X1** **Poisoning by analeptics and opioid receptor antagonists,** accidental **(unintentional)**
Poisoning by analeptics and opioid receptor antagonists NOS

√7ᵗʰ **T50.7X2** **Poisoning by analeptics and opioid receptor antagonists,** intentional self-harm

√7ᵗʰ **T50.7X3** **Poisoning by analeptics and opioid receptor antagonists,** assault

√7ᵗʰ **T50.7X4** **Poisoning by analeptics and opioid receptor antagonists,** undetermined

√7ᵗʰ **T50.7X5** Adverse effect **of analeptics and opioid receptor antagonists**

√7ᵗʰ **T50.7X6** Underdosing **of analeptics and opioid receptor antagonists**

√5ᵗʰ **T50.8** **Poisoning by, adverse effect of and underdosing of diagnostic agents**

√6ᵗʰ **T50.8X** **Poisoning by, adverse effect of and underdosing of** diagnostic agents

√7ᵗʰ **T50.8X1** **Poisoning by diagnostic agents,** accidental **(unintentional)**
Poisoning by diagnostic agents NOS

√7ᵗʰ **T50.8X2** **Poisoning by diagnostic agents,** intentional self-harm

√7ᵗʰ **T50.8X3** **Poisoning by diagnostic agents,** assault

√7ᵗʰ **T50.8X4** **Poisoning by diagnostic agents,** undetermined

√7ᵗʰ **T50.8X5** Adverse effect **of diagnostic agents**

√7ᵗʰ **T50.8X6** Underdosing **of diagnostic agents**

√5ᵗʰ **T50.A** **Poisoning by, adverse effect of and underdosing of bacterial vaccines**

√6ᵗʰ **T50.A1** **Poisoning by, adverse effect of and underdosing of** pertussis vaccine, including combinations with a pertussis component

√7ᵗʰ **T50.A11** **Poisoning by pertussis vaccine, including combinations with a pertussis component,** accidental **(unintentional)**

√7ᵗʰ **T50.A12** **Poisoning by pertussis vaccine, including combinations with a pertussis component,** intentional self-harm

√7ᵗʰ **T50.A13** **Poisoning by pertussis vaccine, including combinations with a pertussis component,** assault

√7ᵗʰ **T50.A14** **Poisoning by pertussis vaccine, including combinations with a pertussis component,** undetermined

√7ᵗʰ **T50.A15** Adverse effect **of pertussis vaccine, including combinations with a pertussis component**

√7ᵗʰ **T50.A16** Underdosing **of pertussis vaccine, including combinations with a pertussis component**

√6ᵗʰ **T50.A2** **Poisoning by, adverse effect of and underdosing of** mixed bacterial vaccines without a pertussis component

√7ᵗʰ **T50.A21** **Poisoning by mixed bacterial vaccines without a pertussis component,** accidental **(unintentional)**

√7ᵗʰ **T50.A22** **Poisoning by mixed bacterial vaccines without a pertussis component,** intentional self-harm

√7ᵗʰ **T50.A23** **Poisoning by mixed bacterial vaccines without a pertussis component,** assault

Ⓝ Newborn Ⓟ Pediatric Ⓜ Maternity Ⓐ Adult **RIC** RIC Dx **NC Dx** Noncancer Dx **PDx** Primary Dx **CC** RIC CC Condition ►◄ Revised Text ● New Code ▲ Revised Code Title

1018 ICD-10-CM 2016

☑7ᵗʰ **T50.A24** Poisoning by mixed bacterial vaccines without a pertussis component, undetermined

☑7ᵗʰ **T50.A25** Adverse effect of mixed bacterial vaccines without a pertussis component

☑7ᵗʰ **T50.A26** Underdosing of mixed bacterial vaccines without a pertussis component

☑6ᵗʰ **T50.A9** Poisoning by, adverse effect of and underdosing of other bacterial vaccines

☑7ᵗʰ **T50.A91** Poisoning by other bacterial vaccines, accidental (unintentional)

☑7ᵗʰ **T50.A92** Poisoning by other bacterial vaccines, intentional self-harm

☑7ᵗʰ **T50.A93** Poisoning by other bacterial vaccines, assault

☑7ᵗʰ **T50.A94** Poisoning by other bacterial vaccines, undetermined

☑7ᵗʰ **T50.A95** Adverse effect of other bacterial vaccines

☑7ᵗʰ **T50.A96** Underdosing of other bacterial vaccines

☑5ᵗʰ **T50.B** Poisoning by, adverse effect of and underdosing of viral vaccines

☑6ᵗʰ **T50.B1** Poisoning by, adverse effect of and underdosing of smallpox vaccines

☑7ᵗʰ **T50.B11** Poisoning by smallpox vaccines, accidental (unintentional)

☑7ᵗʰ **T50.B12** Poisoning by smallpox vaccines, intentional self-harm

☑7ᵗʰ **T50.B13** Poisoning by smallpox vaccines, assault

☑7ᵗʰ **T50.B14** Poisoning by smallpox vaccines, undetermined

☑7ᵗʰ **T50.B15** Adverse effect of smallpox vaccines

☑7ᵗʰ **T50.B16** Underdosing of smallpox vaccines

☑6ᵗʰ **T50.B9** Poisoning by, adverse effect of and underdosing of other viral vaccines

☑7ᵗʰ **T50.B91** Poisoning by other viral vaccines, accidental (unintentional)

☑7ᵗʰ **T50.B92** Poisoning by other viral vaccines, intentional self-harm

☑7ᵗʰ **T50.B93** Poisoning by other viral vaccines, assault

☑7ᵗʰ **T50.B94** Poisoning by other viral vaccines, undetermined

☑7ᵗʰ **T50.B95** Adverse effect of other viral vaccines

☑7ᵗʰ **T50.B96** Underdosing of other viral vaccines

☑5ᵗʰ **T50.Z** Poisoning by, adverse effect of and underdosing of other vaccines and biological substances

☑6ᵗʰ **T50.Z1** Poisoning by, adverse effect of and underdosing of immunoglobulin

☑7ᵗʰ **T50.Z11** Poisoning by immunoglobulin, accidental (unintentional)

☑7ᵗʰ **T50.Z12** Poisoning by immunoglobulin, intentional self-harm

☑7ᵗʰ **T50.Z13** Poisoning by immunoglobulin, assault

☑7ᵗʰ **T50.Z14** Poisoning by immunoglobulin, undetermined

☑7ᵗʰ **T50.Z15** Adverse effect of immunoglobulin

☑7ᵗʰ **T50.Z16** Underdosing of immunoglobulin

☑6ᵗʰ **T50.Z9** Poisoning by, adverse effect of and underdosing of other vaccines and biological substances

☑7ᵗʰ **T50.Z91** Poisoning by other vaccines and biological substances, accidental (unintentional)

☑7ᵗʰ **T50.Z92** Poisoning by other vaccines and biological substances, intentional self-harm

☑7ᵗʰ **T50.Z93** Poisoning by other vaccines and biological substances, assault

☑7ᵗʰ **T50.Z94** Poisoning by other vaccines and biological substances, undetermined

☑7ᵗʰ **T50.Z95** Adverse effect of other vaccines and biological substances

☑7ᵗʰ **T50.Z96** Underdosing of other vaccines and biological substances

☑5ᵗʰ **T50.9** Poisoning by, adverse effect of and underdosing of other and unspecified drugs, medicaments and biological substances
AHA: 2015, 1Q, 21

☑6ᵗʰ **T50.90** Poisoning by, adverse effect of and underdosing of unspecified drugs, medicaments and biological substances

☑7ᵗʰ **T50.901** Poisoning by unspecified drugs, medicaments and biological substances, accidental (unintentional) ▽

☑7ᵗʰ **T50.902** Poisoning by unspecified drugs, medicaments and biological substances, intentional self-harm ▽

☑7ᵗʰ **T50.903** Poisoning by unspecified drugs, medicaments and biological substances, assault ▽

☑7ᵗʰ **T50.904** Poisoning by unspecified drugs, medicaments and biological substances, undetermined ▽

☑7ᵗʰ **T50.905** Adverse effect of unspecified drugs, medicaments and biological substances ▽

☑7ᵗʰ **T50.906** Underdosing of unspecified drugs, medicaments and biological substances ▽

☑6ᵗʰ **T50.99** Poisoning by, adverse effect of and underdosing of other drugs, medicaments and biological substances

☑7ᵗʰ **T50.991** Poisoning by other drugs, medicaments and biological substances, accidental (unintentional)

☑7ᵗʰ **T50.992** Poisoning by other drugs, medicaments and biological substances, intentional self-harm

☑7ᵗʰ **T50.993** Poisoning by other drugs, medicaments and biological substances, assault

☑7ᵗʰ **T50.994** Poisoning by other drugs, medicaments and biological substances, undetermined

☑7ᵗʰ **T50.995** Adverse effect of other drugs, medicaments and biological substances

☑7ᵗʰ **T50.996** Underdosing of other drugs, medicaments and biological substances

Toxic effects of substances chiefly nonmedicinal as to source (T51-T65)

NOTE   When no intent is indicated code to accidental. Undetermined intent is only for use when there is specific documentation in the record that the intent of the toxic effect cannot be determined.

Use additional code(s) for all associated manifestations of toxic effect, such as:
personal history of foreign body fully removed (Z87.821)
respiratory conditions due to external agents (J60-J70)
to identify any retained foreign body, if applicable (Z18.-)
EXCLUDES 1   contact with and (suspected) exposure to toxic substances (Z77.-)

☑4ᵗʰ **T51**   **Toxic effect of alcohol**

The appropriate 7th character is to be added to each code from category T51.
A   initial encounter
D   subsequent encounter
S   sequela

☑5ᵗʰ **T51.0**   **Toxic effect of ethanol**
Toxic effect of ethyl alcohol
EXCLUDES 2   acute alcohol intoxication or 'hangover' effects (F10.129, F10.229, F10.929)
drunkenness (F10.129, F10.229, F10.929)
pathological alcohol intoxication (F10.129, F10.229, F10.929)

☑6ᵗʰ **T51.0X**   **Toxic effect of ethanol**

☑7ᵗʰ **T51.0X1** Toxic effect of ethanol, accidental (unintentional)
Toxic effect of ethanol NOS

☑7ᵗʰ **T51.0X2** Toxic effect of ethanol, intentional self-harm

☑7ᵗʰ **T51.0X3** Toxic effect of ethanol, assault

☑7ᵗʰ **T51.0X4** Toxic effect of ethanol, undetermined

☑5ᵗʰ **T51.1**   **Toxic effect of methanol**
Toxic effect of methyl alcohol

☑6ᵗʰ **T51.1X**   **Toxic effect of methanol**

☑7ᵗʰ **T51.1X1** Toxic effect of methanol, accidental (unintentional)
Toxic effect of methanol NOS

☑ Add'l Character Required   ✓ₓ7ᵗʰ Placeholder Alert   RUG IV Special Care High Dx   RUG IV Clinically Complex Dx   RUG IV Special Care Low Dx   Manifestation Code   Other Specified Code   ▽ Unspecified Code

√7ᵗʰ **T51.1X2** **Toxic effect of methanol,** intentional self-harm

√7ᵗʰ **T51.1X3** **Toxic effect of methanol,** assault

√7ᵗʰ **T51.1X4** **Toxic effect of methanol,** undetermined

√5ᵗʰ **T51.2** **Toxic effect of 2-Propanol**
Toxic effect of isopropyl alcohol

√6ᵗʰ **T51.2X** **Toxic effect of** 2-Propanol

√7ᵗʰ **T51.2X1** **Toxic effect of 2-Propanol,** accidental (unintentional)
Toxic effect of 2-Propanol NOS

√7ᵗʰ **T51.2X2** **Toxic effect of 2-Propanol,** intentional self-harm

√7ᵗʰ **T51.2X3** **Toxic effect of 2-Propanol,** assault

√7ᵗʰ **T51.2X4** **Toxic effect of 2-Propanol,** undetermined

√5ᵗʰ **T51.3** **Toxic effect of fusel oil**
Toxic effect of amyl alcohol
Toxic effect of butyl [1-butanol] alcohol
Toxic effect of propyl [1-propanol] alcohol

√6ᵗʰ **T51.3X** **Toxic effect of** fusel oil

√7ᵗʰ **T51.3X1** **Toxic effect of fusel oil,** accidental (unintentional)
Toxic effect of fusel oil NOS

√7ᵗʰ **T51.3X2** **Toxic effect of fusel oil,** intentional self-harm

√7ᵗʰ **T51.3X3** **Toxic effect of fusel oil,** assault

√7ᵗʰ **T51.3X4** **Toxic effect of fusel oil,** undetermined

√5ᵗʰ **T51.8** **Toxic effect of other alcohols**

√6ᵗʰ **T51.8X** **Toxic effect of** other alcohols

√7ᵗʰ **T51.8X1** **Toxic effect of other alcohols,** accidental (unintentional)
Toxic effect of other alcohols NOS

√7ᵗʰ **T51.8X2** **Toxic effect of other alcohols, intentional self-harm**

√7ᵗʰ **T51.8X3** **Toxic effect of other alcohols, assault**

√7ᵗʰ **T51.8X4** **Toxic effect of other alcohols, undetermined**

√5ᵗʰ **T51.9** **Toxic effect of** unspecified alcohol

√x7ᵗʰ **T51.91** **Toxic effect of unspecified alcohol,** accidental (unintentional)   ▽

√x7ᵗʰ **T51.92** **Toxic effect of unspecified alcohol,** intentional self-harm   ▽

√x7ᵗʰ **T51.93** **Toxic effect of unspecified alcohol,** assault   ▽

√x7ᵗʰ **T51.94** **Toxic effect of unspecified alcohol,** undetermined ▽

√4ᵗʰ **T52** **Toxic effect of organic solvents**

EXCLUDES 1 *halogen derivatives of aliphatic and aromatic hydrocarbons (T53.-)*

The appropriate 7th character is to be added to each code from category T52.
A   initial encounter
D   subsequent encounter
S   sequela

√5ᵗʰ **T52.0** **Toxic effects of petroleum products**
Toxic effects of ether petroleum
Toxic effects of gasoline [petrol]
Toxic effects of kerosene [paraffin oil]
Toxic effects of naphtha petroleum
Toxic effects of paraffin wax
Toxic effects of spirit petroleum

√6ᵗʰ **T52.0X** **Toxic effects of** petroleum products

√7ᵗʰ **T52.0X1** **Toxic effect of petroleum products,** accidental (unintentional)
Toxic effects of petroleum products NOS

√7ᵗʰ **T52.0X2** **Toxic effect of petroleum products,** intentional self-harm

√7ᵗʰ **T52.0X3** **Toxic effect of petroleum products,** assault

√7ᵗʰ **T52.0X4** **Toxic effect of petroleum products,** undetermined

√5ᵗʰ **T52.1** **Toxic effects of benzene**

EXCLUDES 1 *homologues of benzene (T52.2)*
nitroderivatives and aminoderivatives of benzene and its homologues (T65.3)

√6ᵗʰ **T52.1X** **Toxic effects of** benzene

√7ᵗʰ **T52.1X1** **Toxic effect of benzene,** accidental (unintentional)
Toxic effects of benzene NOS

√7ᵗʰ **T52.1X2** **Toxic effect of benzene,** intentional self-harm

√7ᵗʰ **T52.1X3** **Toxic effect of benzene,** assault

√7ᵗʰ **T52.1X4** **Toxic effect of benzene,** undetermined

√5ᵗʰ **T52.2** **Toxic effects of homologues of benzene**
Toxic effects of toluene [methylbenzene]
Toxic effects of xylene [dimethylbenzene]

√6ᵗʰ **T52.2X** **Toxic effects of** homologues of benzene

√7ᵗʰ **T52.2X1** **Toxic effect of homologues of benzene,** accidental (unintentional)
Toxic effects of homologues of benzene NOS

√7ᵗʰ **T52.2X2** **Toxic effect of homologues of benzene,** intentional self-harm

√7ᵗʰ **T52.2X3** **Toxic effect of homologues of benzene,** assault

√7ᵗʰ **T52.2X4** **Toxic effect of homologues of benzene,** undetermined

√5ᵗʰ **T52.3** **Toxic effects of glycols**

√6ᵗʰ **T52.3X** **Toxic effects of** glycols

√7ᵗʰ **T52.3X1** **Toxic effect of glycols,** accidental (unintentional)
Toxic effects of glycols NOS

√7ᵗʰ **T52.3X2** **Toxic effect of glycols,** intentional self-harm

√7ᵗʰ **T52.3X3** **Toxic effect of glycols,** assault

√7ᵗʰ **T52.3X4** **Toxic effect of glycols,** undetermined

√5ᵗʰ **T52.4** **Toxic effects of ketones**

√6ᵗʰ **T52.4X** **Toxic effects of** ketones

√7ᵗʰ **T52.4X1** **Toxic effect of ketones,** accidental (unintentional)
Toxic effects of ketones NOS

√7ᵗʰ **T52.4X2** **Toxic effect of ketones,** intentional self-harm

√7ᵗʰ **T52.4X3** **Toxic effect of ketones,** assault

√7ᵗʰ **T52.4X4** **Toxic effect of ketones,** undetermined

√5ᵗʰ **T52.8** **Toxic effects of other organic solvents**

√6ᵗʰ **T52.8X** **Toxic effects of** other organic solvents

√7ᵗʰ **T52.8X1** **Toxic effect of other organic solvents, accidental (unintentional)**
Toxic effects of other organic solvents NOS

√7ᵗʰ **T52.8X2** **Toxic effect of other organic solvents, intentional self-harm**

√7ᵗʰ **T52.8X3** **Toxic effect of other organic solvents, assault**

√7ᵗʰ **T52.8X4** **Toxic effect of other organic solvents,** undetermined

√5ᵗʰ **T52.9** **Toxic effects of** unspecified organic solvent

√x7ᵗʰ **T52.91** **Toxic effect of unspecified organic solvent,** accidental (unintentional)   ▽

√x7ᵗʰ **T52.92** **Toxic effect of unspecified organic solvent,** intentional self-harm   ▽

√x7ᵗʰ **T52.93** **Toxic effect of unspecified organic solvent,** assault   ▽

√x7ᵗʰ **T52.94** **Toxic effect of unspecified organic solvent,** undetermined   ▽

Ⓝ Newborn   Ⓟ Pediatric   Ⓜ Maternity   Ⓐ Adult   **RIC** RIC Dx   **NC Dx** Noncancer Dx   **PDx** Primary Dx   **CC** RIC CC Condition   ►◄ Revised Text   ● New Code   ▲ Revised Code Title

1020   ICD-10-CM 2016

☑4ᵗʰ **T53** **Toxic effect of halogen derivatives of aliphatic and aromatic hydrocarbons**

> The appropriate 7th character is to be added to each code from category T53.
> A   initial encounter
> D   subsequent encounter
> S   sequela

☑5ᵗʰ **T53.0** **Toxic effects of carbon tetrachloride**
Toxic effects of tetrachloromethane

  ☑6ᵗʰ **T53.0X** **Toxic effects of** carbon tetrachloride

    ☑7ᵗʰ **T53.0X1** **Toxic effect of carbon tetrachloride, accidental (unintentional)**
Toxic effects of carbon tetrachloride NOS

    ☑7ᵗʰ **T53.0X2** **Toxic effect of carbon tetrachloride, intentional self-harm**

    ☑7ᵗʰ **T53.0X3** **Toxic effect of carbon tetrachloride, assault**

    ☑7ᵗʰ **T53.0X4** **Toxic effect of carbon tetrachloride, undetermined**

☑5ᵗʰ **T53.1** **Toxic effects of chloroform**
Toxic effects of trichloromethane

  ☑6ᵗʰ **T53.1X** **Toxic effects of** chloroform

    ☑7ᵗʰ **T53.1X1** **Toxic effect of chloroform, accidental (unintentional)**
Toxic effects of chloroform NOS

    ☑7ᵗʰ **T53.1X2** **Toxic effect of chloroform, intentional self-harm**

    ☑7ᵗʰ **T53.1X3** **Toxic effect of chloroform, assault**

    ☑7ᵗʰ **T53.1X4** **Toxic effect of chloroform, undetermined**

☑5ᵗʰ **T53.2** **Toxic effects of trichloroethylene**
Toxic effects of trichloroethene

  ☑6ᵗʰ **T53.2X** **Toxic effects of** trichloroethylene

    ☑7ᵗʰ **T53.2X1** **Toxic effect of trichloroethylene, accidental (unintentional)**
Toxic effects of trichloroethylene NOS

    ☑7ᵗʰ **T53.2X2** **Toxic effect of trichloroethylene, intentional self-harm**

    ☑7ᵗʰ **T53.2X3** **Toxic effect of trichloroethylene, assault**

    ☑7ᵗʰ **T53.2X4** **Toxic effect of trichloroethylene, undetermined**

☑5ᵗʰ **T53.3** **Toxic effects of tetrachloroethylene**
Toxic effects of perchloroethylene
Toxic effect of tetrachloroethene

  ☑6ᵗʰ **T53.3X** **Toxic effects of** tetrachloroethylene

    ☑7ᵗʰ **T53.3X1** **Toxic effect of tetrachloroethylene, accidental (unintentional)**
Toxic effects of tetrachloroethylene NOS

    ☑7ᵗʰ **T53.3X2** **Toxic effect of tetrachloroethylene, intentional self-harm**

    ☑7ᵗʰ **T53.3X3** **Toxic effect of tetrachloroethylene, assault**

    ☑7ᵗʰ **T53.3X4** **Toxic effect of tetrachloroethylene, undetermined**

☑5ᵗʰ **T53.4** **Toxic effects of dichloromethane**
Toxic effects of methylene chloride

  ☑6ᵗʰ **T53.4X** **Toxic effects of** dichloromethane

    ☑7ᵗʰ **T53.4X1** **Toxic effect of dichloromethane, accidental (unintentional)**
Toxic effects of dichloromethane NOS

    ☑7ᵗʰ **T53.4X2** **Toxic effect of dichloromethane, intentional self-harm**

    ☑7ᵗʰ **T53.4X3** **Toxic effect of dichloromethane, assault**

    ☑7ᵗʰ **T53.4X4** **Toxic effect of dichloromethane, undetermined**

☑5ᵗʰ **T53.5** **Toxic effects of chlorofluorocarbons**

  ☑6ᵗʰ **T53.5X** **Toxic effects of** chlorofluorocarbons

    ☑7ᵗʰ **T53.5X1** **Toxic effect of chlorofluorocarbons, accidental (unintentional)**
Toxic effects of chlorofluorocarbons NOS

    ☑7ᵗʰ **T53.5X2** **Toxic effect of chlorofluorocarbons, intentional self-harm**

    ☑7ᵗʰ **T53.5X3** **Toxic effect of chlorofluorocarbons, assault**

    ☑7ᵗʰ **T53.5X4** **Toxic effect of chlorofluorocarbons, undetermined**

☑5ᵗʰ **T53.6** **Toxic effects of other halogen derivatives of aliphatic hydrocarbons**

  ☑6ᵗʰ **T53.6X** **Toxic effects of other** halogen derivatives of aliphatic hydrocarbons

    ☑7ᵗʰ **T53.6X1** **Toxic effect of other halogen derivatives of aliphatic hydrocarbons, accidental (unintentional)**
Toxic effect of other halogen derivatives of aliphatic hydrocarbons NOS

    ☑7ᵗʰ **T53.6X2** **Toxic effect of other halogen derivatives of aliphatic hydrocarbons, intentional self-harm**

    ☑7ᵗʰ **T53.6X3** **Toxic effect of other halogen derivatives of aliphatic hydrocarbons, assault**

    ☑7ᵗʰ **T53.6X4** **Toxic effect of other halogen derivatives of aliphatic hydrocarbons, undetermined**

☑5ᵗʰ **T53.7** **Toxic effects of other halogen derivatives of aromatic hydrocarbons**

  ☑6ᵗʰ **T53.7X** **Toxic effects of other** halogen derivatives of aromatic hydrocarbons

    ☑7ᵗʰ **T53.7X1** **Toxic effect of other halogen derivatives of aromatic hydrocarbons, accidental (unintentional)**
Toxic effect of other halogen derivatives of aromatic hydrocarbons NOS

    ☑7ᵗʰ **T53.7X2** **Toxic effect of other halogen derivatives of aromatic hydrocarbons, intentional self-harm**

    ☑7ᵗʰ **T53.7X3** **Toxic effect of other halogen derivatives of aromatic hydrocarbons, assault**

    ☑7ᵗʰ **T53.7X4** **Toxic effect of other halogen derivatives of aromatic hydrocarbons, undetermined**

☑5ᵗʰ **T53.9** **Toxic effects of** unspecified halogen derivatives of aliphatic and aromatic hydrocarbons

  ☑x7ᵗʰ **T53.91** **Toxic effect of unspecified halogen derivatives of ▽ aliphatic and aromatic hydrocarbons, accidental (unintentional)**

  ☑x7ᵗʰ **T53.92** **Toxic effect of unspecified halogen derivatives of ▽ aliphatic and aromatic hydrocarbons, intentional self-harm**

  ☑x7ᵗʰ **T53.93** **Toxic effect of unspecified halogen derivatives of ▽ aliphatic and aromatic hydrocarbons, assault**

  ☑x7ᵗʰ **T53.94** **Toxic effect of unspecified halogen derivatives of ▽ aliphatic and aromatic hydrocarbons, undetermined**

☑4ᵗʰ **T54** **Toxic effect of corrosive substances**

> The appropriate 7th character is to be added to each code from category T54.
> A   initial encounter
> D   subsequent encounter
> S   sequela

☑5ᵗʰ **T54.0** **Toxic effects of phenol and phenol homologues**

  ☑6ᵗʰ **T54.0X** **Toxic effects of** phenol and phenol homologues

    ☑7ᵗʰ **T54.0X1** **Toxic effect of phenol and phenol homologues, accidental (unintentional)**
Toxic effects of phenol and phenol homologues NOS

    ☑7ᵗʰ **T54.0X2** **Toxic effect of phenol and phenol homologues, intentional self-harm**

    ☑7ᵗʰ **T54.0X3** **Toxic effect of phenol and phenol homologues, assault**

    ☑7ᵗʰ **T54.0X4** **Toxic effect of phenol and phenol homologues, undetermined**

☑5ᵗʰ **T54.1** **Toxic effects of other corrosive organic compounds**

  ☑6ᵗʰ **T54.1X** **Toxic effects of other** corrosive organic compounds

    ☑7ᵗʰ **T54.1X1** **Toxic effect of other corrosive organic compounds, accidental (unintentional)**
Toxic effects of other corrosive organic compounds NOS

    ☑7ᵗʰ **T54.1X2** **Toxic effect of other corrosive organic compounds, intentional self-harm**

    ☑7ᵗʰ **T54.1X3** **Toxic effect of other corrosive organic compounds, assault**

    ☑7ᵗʰ **T54.1X4** **Toxic effect of other corrosive organic compounds, undetermined**

☑ Add'l Character Required   ☑x7ᵗʰ Placeholder Alert   RUG IV Special Care High Dx   RUG IV Clinically Complex Dx   RUG IV Special Care Low Dx   Manifestation Code   Other Specified Code   ▽ Unspecified Code

✓5ᵗʰ **T54.2 Toxic effects of corrosive acids and acid-like substances**
Toxic effects of hydrochloric acid
Toxic effects of sulfuric acid

   ✓6ᵗʰ **T54.2X Toxic effects of corrosive** acids and acid-like substances

      ✓7ᵗʰ **T54.2X1 Toxic effect of corrosive acids and acid-like substances, accidental (unintentional)**
Toxic effects of corrosive acids and acid-like substances NOS

      ✓7ᵗʰ **T54.2X2 Toxic effect of corrosive acids and acid-like substances, intentional self-harm**

      ✓7ᵗʰ **T54.2X3 Toxic effect of corrosive acids and acid-like substances, assault**

      ✓7ᵗʰ **T54.2X4 Toxic effect of corrosive acids and acid-like substances, undetermined**

✓5ᵗʰ **T54.3 Toxic effects of corrosive alkalis and alkali-like substances**
Toxic effects of potassium hydroxide
Toxic effects of sodium hydroxide

   ✓6ᵗʰ **T54.3X Toxic effects of corrosive** alkalis and alkali-like substances

      ✓7ᵗʰ **T54.3X1 Toxic effect of corrosive alkalis and alkali-like substances, accidental (unintentional)**
Toxic effects of corrosive alkalis and alkali-like substances NOS

      ✓7ᵗʰ **T54.3X2 Toxic effect of corrosive alkalis and alkali-like substances, intentional self-harm**

      ✓7ᵗʰ **T54.3X3 Toxic effect of corrosive alkalis and alkali-like substances, assault**

      ✓7ᵗʰ **T54.3X4 Toxic effect of corrosive alkalis and alkali-like substances, undetermined**

✓5ᵗʰ **T54.9 Toxic effects of** unspecified **corrosive substance**

   ✓x7ᵗʰ **T54.91 Toxic effect of unspecified corrosive substance, accidental (unintentional)** ▽

   ✓x7ᵗʰ **T54.92 Toxic effect of unspecified corrosive substance, intentional self-harm** ▽

   ✓x7ᵗʰ **T54.93 Toxic effect of unspecified corrosive substance, assault** ▽

   ✓x7ᵗʰ **T54.94 Toxic effect of unspecified corrosive substance, undetermined** ▽

✓4ᵗʰ **T55 Toxic effect of soaps and detergents**

> The appropriate 7th character is to be added to each code from category T55.
> A   initial encounter
> D   subsequent encounter
> S   sequela

✓5ᵗʰ **T55.0 Toxic effect of soaps**

   ✓6ᵗʰ **T55.0X Toxic effect of** soaps

      ✓7ᵗʰ **T55.0X1 Toxic effect of soaps, accidental (unintentional)**
Toxic effect of soaps NOS

      ✓7ᵗʰ **T55.0X2 Toxic effect of soaps, intentional self-harm**

      ✓7ᵗʰ **T55.0X3 Toxic effect of soaps, assault**

      ✓7ᵗʰ **T55.0X4 Toxic effect of soaps,** undetermined

✓5ᵗʰ **T55.1 Toxic effect of detergents**

   ✓6ᵗʰ **T55.1X Toxic effect of** detergents

      ✓7ᵗʰ **T55.1X1 Toxic effect of detergents, accidental (unintentional)**
Toxic effect of detergents NOS

      ✓7ᵗʰ **T55.1X2 Toxic effect of detergents, intentional self-harm**

      ✓7ᵗʰ **T55.1X3 Toxic effect of detergents, assault**

      ✓7ᵗʰ **T55.1X4 Toxic effect of detergents, undetermined**

✓4ᵗʰ **T56 Toxic effect of metals**
   INCLUDES toxic effects of fumes and vapors of metals
         toxic effects of metals from all sources, except medicinal substances
Use additional code to identify any retained metal foreign body, if applicable (Z18.0-, T18.1-)
   EXCLUDES 1 arsenic and its compounds (T57.0)
          manganese and its compounds (T57.2)

> The appropriate 7th character is to be added to each code from category T56.
> A   initial encounter
> D   subsequent encounter
> S   sequela

✓5ᵗʰ **T56.0 Toxic effects of lead and its compounds**

   ✓6ᵗʰ **T56.0X Toxic effects of** lead **and its compounds**

      ✓7ᵗʰ **T56.0X1 Toxic effect of lead and its compounds, accidental (unintentional)**
Toxic effects of lead and its compounds NOS

      ✓7ᵗʰ **T56.0X2 Toxic effect of lead and its compounds, intentional self-harm**

      ✓7ᵗʰ **T56.0X3 Toxic effect of lead and its compounds, assault**

      ✓7ᵗʰ **T56.0X4 Toxic effect of lead and its compounds, undetermined**

✓5ᵗʰ **T56.1 Toxic effects of mercury and its compounds**

   ✓6ᵗʰ **T56.1X Toxic effects of** mercury **and its compounds**

      ✓7ᵗʰ **T56.1X1 Toxic effect of mercury and its compounds, accidental (unintentional)**
Toxic effects of mercury and its compounds NOS

      ✓7ᵗʰ **T56.1X2 Toxic effect of mercury and its compounds, intentional self-harm**

      ✓7ᵗʰ **T56.1X3 Toxic effect of mercury and its compounds, assault**

      ✓7ᵗʰ **T56.1X4 Toxic effect of mercury and its compounds, undetermined**

✓5ᵗʰ **T56.2 Toxic effects of chromium and its compounds**

   ✓6ᵗʰ **T56.2X Toxic effects of** chromium **and its compounds**

      ✓7ᵗʰ **T56.2X1 Toxic effect of chromium and its compounds, accidental (unintentional)**
Toxic effects of chromium and its compounds NOS

      ✓7ᵗʰ **T56.2X2 Toxic effect of chromium and its compounds, intentional self-harm**

      ✓7ᵗʰ **T56.2X3 Toxic effect of chromium and its compounds, assault**

      ✓7ᵗʰ **T56.2X4 Toxic effect of chromium and its compounds, undetermined**

✓5ᵗʰ **T56.3 Toxic effects of** cadmium **and its compounds**

   ✓6ᵗʰ **T56.3X Toxic effects of cadmium and its compounds**

      ✓7ᵗʰ **T56.3X1 Toxic effect of cadmium and its compounds, accidental (unintentional)**
Toxic effects of cadmium and its compounds NOS

      ✓7ᵗʰ **T56.3X2 Toxic effect of cadmium and its compounds, intentional self-harm**

      ✓7ᵗʰ **T56.3X3 Toxic effect of cadmium and its compounds, assault**

      ✓7ᵗʰ **T56.3X4 Toxic effect of cadmium and its compounds, undetermined**

✓5ᵗʰ **T56.4 Toxic effects of copper and its compounds**

   ✓6ᵗʰ **T56.4X Toxic effects of** copper **and its compounds**

      ✓7ᵗʰ **T56.4X1 Toxic effect of copper and its compounds, accidental (unintentional)**
Toxic effects of copper and its compounds NOS

      ✓7ᵗʰ **T56.4X2 Toxic effect of copper and its compounds, intentional self-harm**

      ✓7ᵗʰ **T56.4X3 Toxic effect of copper and its compounds, assault**

      ✓7ᵗʰ **T56.4X4 Toxic effect of copper and its compounds, undetermined**

Ⓝ Newborn   Ⓟ Pediatric   Ⓜ Maternity   Ⓐ Adult   **RIC** RIC Dx   **NC Dx** Noncancer Dx   **PDx** Primary Dx   **CC** RIC CC Condition   ►◄ Revised Text   ● New Code   ▲ Revised Code Title

1022
ICD-10-CM 2016

√5ᵗʰ T56.5 Toxic effects of zinc and its compounds

   √6ᵗʰ T56.5X Toxic effects of zinc and its compounds

      √7ᵗʰ T56.5X1 Toxic effect of zinc and its compounds, accidental (unintentional)
         Toxic effects of zinc and its compounds NOS

      √7ᵗʰ T56.5X2 Toxic effect of zinc and its compounds, intentional self-harm

      √7ᵗʰ T56.5X3 Toxic effect of zinc and its compounds, assault

      √7ᵗʰ T56.5X4 Toxic effect of zinc and its compounds, undetermined

√5ᵗʰ T56.6 Toxic effects of tin and its compounds

   √6ᵗʰ T56.6X Toxic effects of tin and its compounds

      √7ᵗʰ T56.6X1 Toxic effect of tin and its compounds, accidental (unintentional)
         Toxic effects of tin and its compounds NOS

      √7ᵗʰ T56.6X2 Toxic effect of tin and its compounds, intentional self-harm

      √7ᵗʰ T56.6X3 Toxic effect of tin and its compounds, assault

      √7ᵗʰ T56.6X4 Toxic effect of tin and its compounds, undetermined

√5ᵗʰ T56.7 Toxic effects of beryllium and its compounds

   √6ᵗʰ T56.7X Toxic effects of beryllium and its compounds

      √7ᵗʰ T56.7X1 Toxic effect of beryllium and its compounds, accidental (unintentional)
         Toxic effects of beryllium and its compounds NOS

      √7ᵗʰ T56.7X2 Toxic effect of beryllium and its compounds, intentional self-harm

      √7ᵗʰ T56.7X3 Toxic effect of beryllium and its compounds, assault

      √7ᵗʰ T56.7X4 Toxic effect of beryllium and its compounds, undetermined

√5ᵗʰ T56.8 Toxic effects of other metals

   √6ᵗʰ T56.81 Toxic effect of thallium

      √7ᵗʰ T56.811 Toxic effect of thallium, accidental (unintentional)
         Toxic effect of thallium NOS

      √7ᵗʰ T56.812 Toxic effect of thallium, intentional self-harm

      √7ᵗʰ T56.813 Toxic effect of thallium, assault

      √7ᵗʰ T56.814 Toxic effect of thallium, undetermined

   √6ᵗʰ T56.89 Toxic effects of other metals

      √7ᵗʰ T56.891 Toxic effect of other metals, accidental (unintentional)
         Toxic effects of other metals NOS

      √7ᵗʰ T56.892 Toxic effect of other metals, intentional self-harm

      √7ᵗʰ T56.893 Toxic effect of other metals, assault

      √7ᵗʰ T56.894 Toxic effect of other metals, undetermined

√5ᵗʰ T56.9 Toxic effects of unspecified metal

   √x7ᵗʰ T56.91 Toxic effect of unspecified metal, accidental (unintentional) ▽

   √x7ᵗʰ T56.92 Toxic effect of unspecified metal, intentional self-harm ▽

   √x7ᵗʰ T56.93 Toxic effect of unspecified metal, assault ▽

   √x7ᵗʰ T56.94 Toxic effect of unspecified metal, undetermined ▽

√4ᵗʰ T57 Toxic effect of other inorganic substances

> The appropriate 7th character is to be added to each code from category T57.
> A   initial encounter
> D   subsequent encounter
> S   sequela

   √5ᵗʰ T57.Ø Toxic effect of arsenic and its compounds

      √6ᵗʰ T57.ØX Toxic effect of arsenic and its compounds

         √7ᵗʰ T57.ØX1 Toxic effect of arsenic and its compounds, accidental (unintentional)
            Toxic effect of arsenic and its compounds NOS

         √7ᵗʰ T57.ØX2 Toxic effect of arsenic and its compounds, intentional self-harm

         √7ᵗʰ T57.ØX3 Toxic effect of arsenic and its compounds, assault

         √7ᵗʰ T57.ØX4 Toxic effect of arsenic and its compounds, undetermined

   √5ᵗʰ T57.1 Toxic effect of phosphorus and its compounds
      EXCLUDES 1   organophosphate insecticides (T60.Ø)

      √6ᵗʰ T57.1X Toxic effect of phosphorus and its compounds

         √7ᵗʰ T57.1X1 Toxic effect of phosphorus and its compounds, accidental (unintentional)
            Toxic effect of phosphorus and its compounds NOS

         √7ᵗʰ T57.1X2 Toxic effect of phosphorus and its compounds, intentional self-harm

         √7ᵗʰ T57.1X3 Toxic effect of phosphorus and its compounds, assault

         √7ᵗʰ T57.1X4 Toxic effect of phosphorus and its compounds, undetermined

   √5ᵗʰ T57.2 Toxic effect of manganese and its compounds

      √6ᵗʰ T57.2X Toxic effect of manganese and its compounds

         √7ᵗʰ T57.2X1 Toxic effect of manganese and its compounds, accidental (unintentional)
            Toxic effect of manganese and its compounds NOS

         √7ᵗʰ T57.2X2 Toxic effect of manganese and its compounds, intentional self-harm

         √7ᵗʰ T57.2X3 Toxic effect of manganese and its compounds, assault

         √7ᵗʰ T57.2X4 Toxic effect of manganese and its compounds, undetermined

   √5ᵗʰ T57.3 Toxic effect of hydrogen cyanide

      √6ᵗʰ T57.3X Toxic effect of hydrogen cyanide

         √7ᵗʰ T57.3X1 Toxic effect of hydrogen cyanide, accidental (unintentional)
            Toxic effect of hydrogen cyanide NOS

         √7ᵗʰ T57.3X2 Toxic effect of hydrogen cyanide, intentional self-harm

         √7ᵗʰ T57.3X3 Toxic effect of hydrogen cyanide, assault

         √7ᵗʰ T57.3X4 Toxic effect of hydrogen cyanide, undetermined

   √5ᵗʰ T57.8 Toxic effect of other specified inorganic substances

      √6ᵗʰ T57.8X Toxic effect of other specified inorganic substances

         √7ᵗʰ T57.8X1 Toxic effect of other specified inorganic substances, accidental (unintentional)
            Toxic effect of other specified inorganic substances NOS

         √7ᵗʰ T57.8X2 Toxic effect of other specified inorganic substances, intentional self-harm

         √7ᵗʰ T57.8X3 Toxic effect of other specified inorganic substances, assault

         √7ᵗʰ T57.8X4 Toxic effect of other specified inorganic substances, undetermined

   √5ᵗʰ T57.9 Toxic effect of unspecified inorganic substance

      √x7ᵗʰ T57.91 Toxic effect of unspecified inorganic substance, accidental (unintentional) ▽

      √x7ᵗʰ T57.92 Toxic effect of unspecified inorganic substance, intentional self-harm ▽

      √x7ᵗʰ T57.93 Toxic effect of unspecified inorganic substance, assault ▽

      √x7ᵗʰ T57.94 Toxic effect of unspecified inorganic substance, undetermined ▽

☑ Add'l Character Required   √x7ᵗʰ Placeholder Alert   RUG IV Special Care High Dx   RUG IV Clinically Complex Dx   RUG IV Special Care Low Dx   Manifestation Code   Other Specified Code   ▽ Unspecified Code

☑4ᵗʰ **T58 Toxic effect of carbon monoxide**

> **INCLUDES** asphyxiation from carbon monoxide
> toxic effect of carbon monoxide from all sources

> The appropriate 7th character is to be added to each code from category T58.
> A   initial encounter
> D   subsequent encounter
> S   sequela

☑5ᵗʰ **T58.0 Toxic effect of carbon monoxide** from motor vehicle exhaust
> Toxic effect of exhaust gas from gas engine
> Toxic effect of exhaust gas from motor pump

☑ₓ7ᵗʰ **T58.01 Toxic effect of carbon monoxide from motor vehicle exhaust,** accidental (unintentional)

☑ₓ7ᵗʰ **T58.02 Toxic effect of carbon monoxide from motor vehicle exhaust,** intentional self-harm

☑ₓ7ᵗʰ **T58.03 Toxic effect of carbon monoxide from motor vehicle exhaust,** assault

☑ₓ7ᵗʰ **T58.04 Toxic effect of carbon monoxide from motor vehicle exhaust,** undetermined

☑5ᵗʰ **T58.1 Toxic effect of carbon monoxide** from utility gas
> Toxic effect of acetylene
> Toxic effect of gas NOS used for lighting, heating, cooking
> Toxic effect of water gas

☑ₓ7ᵗʰ **T58.11 Toxic effect of carbon monoxide from utility gas,** accidental (unintentional)

☑ₓ7ᵗʰ **T58.12 Toxic effect of carbon monoxide from utility gas,** intentional self-harm

☑ₓ7ᵗʰ **T58.13 Toxic effect of carbon monoxide from utility gas,** assault

☑ₓ7ᵗʰ **T58.14 Toxic effect of carbon monoxide from utility gas,** undetermined

☑5ᵗʰ **T58.2 Toxic effect of carbon monoxide** from incomplete combustion of other domestic fuels
> Toxic effect of carbon monoxide from incomplete combustion of coal, coke, kerosene, wood

☑6ᵗʰ **T58.2X Toxic effect of carbon monoxide from incomplete combustion of other domestic fuels**

☑7ᵗʰ **T58.2X1 Toxic effect of carbon monoxide from incomplete combustion of other domestic fuels,** accidental (unintentional)

☑7ᵗʰ **T58.2X2 Toxic effect of carbon monoxide from incomplete combustion of other domestic fuels,** intentional self-harm

☑7ᵗʰ **T58.2X3 Toxic effect of carbon monoxide from incomplete combustion of other domestic fuels,** assault

☑7ᵗʰ **T58.2X4 Toxic effect of carbon monoxide from incomplete combustion of other domestic fuels,** undetermined

☑5ᵗʰ **T58.8 Toxic effect of carbon monoxide** from other source
> Toxic effect of carbon monoxide from blast furnace gas
> Toxic effect of carbon monoxide from fuels in industrial use
> Toxic effect of carbon monoxide from kiln vapor

☑6ᵗʰ **T58.8X Toxic effect of carbon monoxide from other source**

☑7ᵗʰ **T58.8X1 Toxic effect of carbon monoxide from other source,** accidental (unintentional)

☑7ᵗʰ **T58.8X2 Toxic effect of carbon monoxide from other source,** intentional self-harm

☑7ᵗʰ **T58.8X3 Toxic effect of carbon monoxide from other source,** assault

☑7ᵗʰ **T58.8X4 Toxic effect of carbon monoxide from other source,** undetermined

☑5ᵗʰ **T58.9 Toxic effect of carbon monoxide** from unspecified source

☑ₓ7ᵗʰ **T58.91 Toxic effect of carbon monoxide from unspecified ▽ source,** accidental (unintentional)

☑ₓ7ᵗʰ **T58.92 Toxic effect of carbon monoxide from unspecified ▽ source,** intentional self-harm

☑ₓ7ᵗʰ **T58.93 Toxic effect of carbon monoxide from unspecified ▽ source,** assault

☑ₓ7ᵗʰ **T58.94 Toxic effect of carbon monoxide from unspecified ▽ source,** undetermined

☑4ᵗʰ **T59 Toxic effect of other gases, fumes and vapors**

> **INCLUDES** aerosol propellants
> **EXCLUDES 1** chlorofluorocarbons (T53.5)

> The appropriate 7th character is to be added to each code from category T59.
> A   initial encounter
> D   subsequent encounter
> S   sequela

☑5ᵗʰ **T59.0 Toxic effect of nitrogen oxides**

☑6ᵗʰ **T59.0X Toxic effect of** nitrogen oxides

☑7ᵗʰ **T59.0X1 Toxic effect of nitrogen oxides,** accidental (unintentional)
> Toxic effect of nitrogen oxides NOS

☑7ᵗʰ **T59.0X2 Toxic effect of nitrogen oxides,** intentional self-harm

☑7ᵗʰ **T59.0X3 Toxic effect of nitrogen oxides,** assault

☑7ᵗʰ **T59.0X4 Toxic effect of nitrogen oxides,** undetermined

☑5ᵗʰ **T59.1 Toxic effect of sulfur dioxide**

☑6ᵗʰ **T59.1X Toxic effect of** sulfur dioxide

☑7ᵗʰ **T59.1X1 Toxic effect of sulfur dioxide,** accidental (unintentional)
> Toxic effect of sulfur dioxide NOS

☑7ᵗʰ **T59.1X2 Toxic effect of sulfur dioxide,** intentional self-harm

☑7ᵗʰ **T59.1X3 Toxic effect of sulfur dioxide,** assault

☑7ᵗʰ **T59.1X4 Toxic effect of sulfur dioxide,** undetermined

☑5ᵗʰ **T59.2 Toxic effect of formaldehyde**

☑6ᵗʰ **T59.2X Toxic effect of** formaldehyde

☑7ᵗʰ **T59.2X1 Toxic effect of formaldehyde,** accidental (unintentional)
> Toxic effect of formaldehyde NOS

☑7ᵗʰ **T59.2X2 Toxic effect of formaldehyde,** intentional self-harm

☑7ᵗʰ **T59.2X3 Toxic effect of formaldehyde,** assault

☑7ᵗʰ **T59.2X4 Toxic effect of formaldehyde,** undetermined

☑5ᵗʰ **T59.3 Toxic effect of lacrimogenic gas**
> Toxic effect of tear gas

☑6ᵗʰ **T59.3X Toxic effect of** lacrimogenic gas

☑7ᵗʰ **T59.3X1 Toxic effect of lacrimogenic gas,** accidental (unintentional)
> Toxic effect of lacrimogenic gas NOS

☑7ᵗʰ **T59.3X2 Toxic effect of lacrimogenic gas,** intentional self-harm

☑7ᵗʰ **T59.3X3 Toxic effect of lacrimogenic gas,** assault

☑7ᵗʰ **T59.3X4 Toxic effect of lacrimogenic gas,** undetermined

☑5ᵗʰ **T59.4 Toxic effect of chlorine gas**

☑6ᵗʰ **T59.4X Toxic effect of** chlorine gas

☑7ᵗʰ **T59.4X1 Toxic effect of chlorine gas,** accidental (unintentional)
> Toxic effect of chlorine gas NOS

☑7ᵗʰ **T59.4X2 Toxic effect of chlorine gas,** intentional self-harm

☑7ᵗʰ **T59.4X3 Toxic effect of chlorine gas,** assault

☑7ᵗʰ **T59.4X4 Toxic effect of chlorine gas,** undetermined

☑5ᵗʰ **T59.5 Toxic effect of fluorine gas and hydrogen fluoride**

☑6ᵗʰ **T59.5X Toxic effect of** fluorine gas and hydrogen fluoride

☑7ᵗʰ **T59.5X1 Toxic effect of fluorine gas and hydrogen fluoride,** accidental (unintentional)
> Toxic effect of fluorine gas and hydrogen fluoride NOS

☑7ᵗʰ **T59.5X2 Toxic effect of fluorine gas and hydrogen fluoride,** intentional self-harm

☑7ᵗʰ **T59.5X3 Toxic effect of fluorine gas and hydrogen fluoride,** assault

☑7ᵗʰ **T59.5X4 Toxic effect of fluorine gas and hydrogen fluoride,** undetermined

Ⓝ Newborn   Ⓟ Pediatric   Ⓜ Maternity   Ⓐ Adult   **RIC** RIC Dx   **NCDx** Noncancer Dx   **PDx** Primary Dx   **CC** RIC CC Condition   ►◄ Revised Text   ● New Code   ▲ Revised Code Title

1024   ICD-10-CM 2016

✓5ᵗʰ **T59.6 Toxic effect of hydrogen sulfide**

  ✓6ᵗʰ **T59.6X Toxic effect of** hydrogen sulfide

    ✓7ᵗʰ **T59.6X1 Toxic effect of hydrogen sulfide, accidental (unintentional)**
      Toxic effect of hydrogen sulfide NOS

    ✓7ᵗʰ **T59.6X2 Toxic effect of hydrogen sulfide, intentional self-harm**

    ✓7ᵗʰ **T59.6X3 Toxic effect of hydrogen sulfide, assault**

    ✓7ᵗʰ **T59.6X4 Toxic effect of hydrogen sulfide, undetermined**

✓5ᵗʰ **T59.7 Toxic effect of carbon dioxide**

  ✓6ᵗʰ **T59.7X Toxic effect of** carbon dioxide

    ✓7ᵗʰ **T59.7X1 Toxic effect of carbon dioxide, accidental (unintentional)**
      Toxic effect of carbon dioxide NOS

    ✓7ᵗʰ **T59.7X2 Toxic effect of carbon dioxide, intentional self-harm**

    ✓7ᵗʰ **T59.7X3 Toxic effect of carbon dioxide, assault**

    ✓7ᵗʰ **T59.7X4 Toxic effect of carbon dioxide, undetermined**

✓5ᵗʰ **T59.8 Toxic effect of** other **specified gases, fumes and vapors**

  ✓6ᵗʰ **T59.81 Toxic effect of** smoke
    Smoke inhalation
    EXCLUDES 2 *toxic effect of cigarette (tobacco) smoke (T65.22-)*

    ✓7ᵗʰ **T59.811 Toxic effect of smoke, accidental (unintentional)**
      Toxic effect of smoke NOS
      AHA: 2013, 4Q, 121

    ✓7ᵗʰ **T59.812 Toxic effect of smoke, intentional self-harm**

    ✓7ᵗʰ **T59.813 Toxic effect of smoke, assault**

    ✓7ᵗʰ **T59.814 Toxic effect of smoke, undetermined**

  ✓6ᵗʰ **T59.89 Toxic effect of** other **specified gases, fumes and vapors**

    ✓7ᵗʰ **T59.891 Toxic effect of other specified gases, fumes and vapors, accidental (unintentional)**

    ✓7ᵗʰ **T59.892 Toxic effect of other specified gases, fumes and vapors, intentional self-harm**

    ✓7ᵗʰ **T59.893 Toxic effect of other specified gases, fumes and vapors, assault**

    ✓7ᵗʰ **T59.894 Toxic effect of other specified gases, fumes and vapors, undetermined**

✓5ᵗʰ **T59.9 Toxic effect of** unspecified **gases, fumes and vapors**

  ✓×7ᵗʰ **T59.91 Toxic effect of unspecified gases, fumes and vapors, accidental (unintentional)** ▽

  ✓×7ᵗʰ **T59.92 Toxic effect of unspecified gases, fumes and vapors, intentional self-harm** ▽

  ✓×7ᵗʰ **T59.93 Toxic effect of unspecified gases, fumes and vapors, assault** ▽

  ✓×7ᵗʰ **T59.94 Toxic effect of unspecified gases, fumes and vapors, undetermined** ▽

✓4ᵗʰ **T60 Toxic effect of pesticides**
  INCLUDES   toxic effect of wood preservatives

> The appropriate 7th character is to be added to each code from category T60.
> A   initial encounter
> D   subsequent encounter
> S   sequela

✓5ᵗʰ **T60.0 Toxic effect of organophosphate and carbamate insecticides**

  ✓6ᵗʰ **T60.0X Toxic effect of** organophosphate and carbamate insecticides

    ✓7ᵗʰ **T60.0X1 Toxic effect of organophosphate and carbamate insecticides, accidental (unintentional)**
      Toxic effect of organophosphate and carbamate insecticides NOS

    ✓7ᵗʰ **T60.0X2 Toxic effect of organophosphate and carbamate insecticides, intentional self-harm**

    ✓7ᵗʰ **T60.0X3 Toxic effect of organophosphate and carbamate insecticides, assault**

    ✓7ᵗʰ **T60.0X4 Toxic effect of organophosphate and carbamate insecticides, undetermined**

✓5ᵗʰ **T60.1 Toxic effect of halogenated insecticides**
  EXCLUDES 1 *chlorinated hydrocarbon (T53.-)*

  ✓6ᵗʰ **T60.1X Toxic effect of** halogenated insecticides

    ✓7ᵗʰ **T60.1X1 Toxic effect of halogenated insecticides, accidental (unintentional)**
      Toxic effect of halogenated insecticides NOS

    ✓7ᵗʰ **T60.1X2 Toxic effect of halogenated insecticides, intentional self-harm**

    ✓7ᵗʰ **T60.1X3 Toxic effect of halogenated insecticides, assault**

    ✓7ᵗʰ **T60.1X4 Toxic effect of halogenated insecticides, undetermined**

✓5ᵗʰ **T60.2 Toxic effect of other insecticides**

  ✓6ᵗʰ **T60.2X Toxic effect of** other insecticides

    ✓7ᵗʰ **T60.2X1 Toxic effect of other insecticides, accidental (unintentional)**
      Toxic effect of other insecticides NOS

    ✓7ᵗʰ **T60.2X2 Toxic effect of other insecticides, intentional self-harm**

    ✓7ᵗʰ **T60.2X3 Toxic effect of other insecticides, assault**

    ✓7ᵗʰ **T60.2X4 Toxic effect of other insecticides, undetermined**

✓5ᵗʰ **T60.3 Toxic effect of herbicides and fungicides**

  ✓6ᵗʰ **T60.3X Toxic effect of** herbicides and fungicides

    ✓7ᵗʰ **T60.3X1 Toxic effect of herbicides and fungicides, accidental (unintentional)**
      Toxic effect of herbicides and fungicides NOS

    ✓7ᵗʰ **T60.3X2 Toxic effect of herbicides and fungicides, intentional self-harm**

    ✓7ᵗʰ **T60.3X3 Toxic effect of herbicides and fungicides, assault**

    ✓7ᵗʰ **T60.3X4 Toxic effect of herbicides and fungicides, undetermined**

✓5ᵗʰ **T60.4 Toxic effect of rodenticides**
  EXCLUDES 1 *strychnine and its salts (T65.1)*
            thallium (T56.81-)

  ✓6ᵗʰ **T60.4X Toxic effect of** rodenticides

    ✓7ᵗʰ **T60.4X1 Toxic effect of rodenticides, accidental (unintentional)**
      Toxic effect of rodenticides NOS

    ✓7ᵗʰ **T60.4X2 Toxic effect of rodenticides, intentional self-harm**

    ✓7ᵗʰ **T60.4X3 Toxic effect of rodenticides, assault**

    ✓7ᵗʰ **T60.4X4 Toxic effect of rodenticides, undetermined**

✓5ᵗʰ **T60.8 Toxic effect of other pesticides**

  ✓6ᵗʰ **T60.8X Toxic effect of** other pesticides

    ✓7ᵗʰ **T60.8X1 Toxic effect of other pesticides, accidental (unintentional)**
      Toxic effect of other pesticides NOS

    ✓7ᵗʰ **T60.8X2 Toxic effect of other pesticides, intentional self-harm**

    ✓7ᵗʰ **T60.8X3 Toxic effect of other pesticides, assault**

    ✓7ᵗʰ **T60.8X4 Toxic effect of other pesticides, undetermined**

✓5ᵗʰ **T60.9 Toxic effect of** unspecified **pesticide**

  ✓×7ᵗʰ **T60.91 Toxic effect of unspecified pesticide, accidental (unintentional)** ▽

  ✓×7ᵗʰ **T60.92 Toxic effect of unspecified pesticide, intentional self-harm** ▽

  ✓×7ᵗʰ **T60.93 Toxic effect of unspecified pesticide, assault** ▽

  ✓×7ᵗʰ **T60.94 Toxic effect of unspecified pesticide, undetermined** ▽

☑ Add'l Character Required   ✓×7ᵗʰ Placeholder Alert   RUG IV Special Care High Dx   RUG IV Clinically Complex Dx   RUG IV Special Care Low Dx   Manifestation Code   Other Specified Code   ▽ Unspecified Code

✓4ᵗʰ **T61 Toxic effect of noxious substances eaten as seafood**

EXCLUDES 1 *allergic reaction to food, such as:*
anaphylactic reaction or shock due to adverse food reaction (T78.0-)
dermatitis (L23.6, L25.4, L27.2)
gastroenteritis (noninfective) (K52.2)
bacterial foodborne intoxications (A05.-)
toxic effect of aflatoxin and other mycotoxins (T64)
toxic effect of cyanides (T65.0-)
toxic effect of harmful algae bloom (T65.82-)
toxic effect of hydrogen cyanide (T57.3-)
toxic effect of mercury (T56.1-)
toxic effect of red tide (T65.82-)

The appropriate 7th character is to be added to each code from category T61.
A   initial encounter
D   subsequent encounter
S   sequela

✓5ᵗʰ **T61.0 Ciguatera fish poisoning**

✓x7ᵗʰ **T61.01 Ciguatera fish poisoning,** accidental (unintentional)

✓x7ᵗʰ **T61.02 Ciguatera fish poisoning,** intentional self-harm

✓x7ᵗʰ **T61.03 Ciguatera fish poisoning,** assault

✓x7ᵗʰ **T61.04 Ciguatera fish poisoning,** undetermined

✓5ᵗʰ **T61.1 Scombroid fish poisoning**
Histamine-like syndrome

✓x7ᵗʰ **T61.11 Scombroid fish poisoning,** accidental (unintentional)

✓x7ᵗʰ **T61.12 Scombroid fish poisoning,** intentional self-harm

✓x7ᵗʰ **T61.13 Scombroid fish poisoning,** assault

✓x7ᵗʰ **T61.14 Scombroid fish poisoning,** undetermined

✓5ᵗʰ **T61.7 Other fish and shellfish poisoning**

✓6ᵗʰ **T61.77 Other fish poisoning**

✓7ᵗʰ **T61.771 Other fish poisoning,** accidental (unintentional)

✓7ᵗʰ **T61.772 Other fish poisoning,** intentional self-harm

✓7ᵗʰ **T61.773 Other fish poisoning,** assault

✓7ᵗʰ **T61.774 Other fish poisoning,** undetermined

✓6ᵗʰ **T61.78 Other shellfish poisoning**

✓7ᵗʰ **T61.781 Other shellfish poisoning,** accidental (unintentional)

✓7ᵗʰ **T61.782 Other shellfish poisoning,** intentional self-harm

✓7ᵗʰ **T61.783 Other shellfish poisoning,** assault

✓7ᵗʰ **T61.784 Other shellfish poisoning,** undetermined

✓5ᵗʰ **T61.8 Toxic effect of other seafood**

✓6ᵗʰ **T61.8X Toxic effect of** other seafood

✓7ᵗʰ **T61.8X1 Toxic effect of other seafood,** accidental (unintentional)

✓7ᵗʰ **T61.8X2 Toxic effect of other seafood,** intentional self-harm

✓7ᵗʰ **T61.8X3 Toxic effect of other seafood,** assault

✓7ᵗʰ **T61.8X4 Toxic effect of other seafood,** undetermined

✓5ᵗʰ **T61.9 Toxic effect of** unspecified seafood

✓x7ᵗʰ **T61.91 Toxic effect of unspecified seafood,** accidental (unintentional) ▽

✓x7ᵗʰ **T61.92 Toxic effect of unspecified seafood,** intentional self-harm ▽

✓x7ᵗʰ **T61.93 Toxic effect of unspecified seafood,** assault ▽

✓x7ᵗʰ **T61.94 Toxic effect of unspecified seafood,** undetermined ▽

✓4ᵗʰ **T62 Toxic effect of other noxious substances eaten as food**

EXCLUDES 1 *allergic reaction to food, such as:*
anaphylactic shock (reaction) due to adverse food reaction (T78.0-)
dermatitis (L23.6, L25.4, L27.2)
gastroenteritis (noninfective) (K52.2)
bacterial food borne intoxications (A05.-)
toxic effect of aflatoxin and other mycotoxins (T64)
toxic effect of cyanides (T65.0-)
toxic effect of hydrogen cyanide (T57.3-)
toxic effect of mercury (T56.1-)

The appropriate 7th character is to be added to each code from category T62.
A   initial encounter
D   subsequent encounter
S   sequela

✓5ᵗʰ **T62.0 Toxic effect of ingested mushrooms**

✓6ᵗʰ **T62.0X Toxic effect of** ingested mushrooms

✓7ᵗʰ **T62.0X1 Toxic effect of ingested mushrooms,** accidental (unintentional)
Toxic effect of ingested mushrooms NOS

✓7ᵗʰ **T62.0X2 Toxic effect of ingested mushrooms,** intentional self-harm

✓7ᵗʰ **T62.0X3 Toxic effect of ingested mushrooms,** assault

✓7ᵗʰ **T62.0X4 Toxic effect of ingested mushrooms,** undetermined

✓5ᵗʰ **T62.1 Toxic effect of ingested berries**

✓6ᵗʰ **T62.1X Toxic effect of** ingested berries

✓7ᵗʰ **T62.1X1 Toxic effect of ingested berries,** accidental (unintentional)
Toxic effect of ingested berries NOS

✓7ᵗʰ **T62.1X2 Toxic effect of ingested berries,** intentional self-harm

✓7ᵗʰ **T62.1X3 Toxic effect of ingested berries,** assault

✓7ᵗʰ **T62.1X4 Toxic effect of ingested berries,** undetermined

✓5ᵗʰ **T62.2 Toxic effect of other ingested (parts of) plant(s)**

✓6ᵗʰ **T62.2X Toxic effect of** other ingested (parts of) plant(s)

✓7ᵗʰ **T62.2X1 Toxic effect of other ingested (parts of) plant(s),** accidental (unintentional)
Toxic effect of other ingested (parts of) plant(s) NOS

✓7ᵗʰ **T62.2X2 Toxic effect of other ingested (parts of) plant(s),** intentional self-harm

✓7ᵗʰ **T62.2X3 Toxic effect of other ingested (parts of) plant(s),** assault

✓7ᵗʰ **T62.2X4 Toxic effect of other ingested (parts of) plant(s),** undetermined

✓5ᵗʰ **T62.8 Toxic effect of other specified** noxious substances eaten as food

✓6ᵗʰ **T62.8X Toxic effect of** other specified noxious substances eaten as food

✓7ᵗʰ **T62.8X1 Toxic effect of other specified noxious substances eaten as food,** accidental (unintentional)
Toxic effect of other specified noxious substances eaten as food NOS

✓7ᵗʰ **T62.8X2 Toxic effect of other specified noxious substances eaten as food,** intentional self-harm

✓7ᵗʰ **T62.8X3 Toxic effect of other specified noxious substances eaten as food,** assault

✓7ᵗʰ **T62.8X4 Toxic effect of other specified noxious substances eaten as food,** undetermined

✓5ᵗʰ **T62.9 Toxic effect of** unspecified noxious substance eaten as food

✓x7ᵗʰ **T62.91 Toxic effect of unspecified noxious substance eaten as food,** accidental (unintentional) ▽
Toxic effect of unspecified noxious substance eaten as food NOS

✓x7ᵗʰ **T62.92 Toxic effect of unspecified noxious substance eaten as food,** intentional self-harm ▽

√x7ʰ T62.93   **Toxic effect of unspecified noxious substance eaten as food, assault** ▽

√x7ʰ T62.94   **Toxic effect of unspecified noxious substance eaten as food, undetermined** ▽

√4ʰ T63   **Toxic effect of contact with venomous animals and plants**

INCLUDES   bite or touch of venomous animal
pricked or stuck by thorn or leaf

EXCLUDES 2   *ingestion of toxic animal or plant (T61.-, T62.-)*

The appropriate 7th character is to be added to each code from category T63.
A   initial encounter
D   subsequent encounter
S   sequela

√5ʰ T63.0   **Toxic effect of snake venom**

√6ʰ T63.00   **Toxic effect of unspecified snake venom**

    √7ʰ T63.001   **Toxic effect of unspecified snake venom, accidental (unintentional)** ▽
Toxic effect of unspecified snake venom NOS

    √7ʰ T63.002   **Toxic effect of unspecified snake venom, intentional self-harm** ▽

    √7ʰ T63.003   **Toxic effect of unspecified snake venom, assault** ▽

    √7ʰ T63.004   **Toxic effect of unspecified snake venom, undetermined** ▽

√6ʰ T63.01   **Toxic effect of rattlesnake venom**

    √7ʰ T63.011   **Toxic effect of rattlesnake venom, accidental (unintentional)**
Toxic effect of rattlesnake venom NOS

    √7ʰ T63.012   **Toxic effect of rattlesnake venom, intentional self-harm**

    √7ʰ T63.013   **Toxic effect of rattlesnake venom, assault**

    √7ʰ T63.014   **Toxic effect of rattlesnake venom, undetermined**

√6ʰ T63.02   **Toxic effect of coral snake venom**

    √7ʰ T63.021   **Toxic effect of coral snake venom, accidental (unintentional)**
Toxic effect of coral snake venom NOS

    √7ʰ T63.022   **Toxic effect of coral snake venom, intentional self-harm**

    √7ʰ T63.023   **Toxic effect of coral snake venom, assault**

    √7ʰ T63.024   **Toxic effect of coral snake venom, undetermined**

√6ʰ T63.03   **Toxic effect of taipan venom**

    √7ʰ T63.031   **Toxic effect of taipan venom, accidental (unintentional)**
Toxic effect of taipan venom NOS

    √7ʰ T63.032   **Toxic effect of taipan venom, intentional self-harm**

    √7ʰ T63.033   **Toxic effect of taipan venom, assault**

    √7ʰ T63.034   **Toxic effect of taipan venom, undetermined**

√6ʰ T63.04   **Toxic effect of cobra venom**

    √7ʰ T63.041   **Toxic effect of cobra venom, accidental (unintentional)**
Toxic effect of cobra venom NOS

    √7ʰ T63.042   **Toxic effect of cobra venom, intentional self-harm**

    √7ʰ T63.043   **Toxic effect of cobra venom, assault**

    √7ʰ T63.044   **Toxic effect of cobra venom, undetermined**

√6ʰ T63.06   **Toxic effect of venom of other North and South American snake**

    √7ʰ T63.061   **Toxic effect of venom of other North and South American snake, accidental (unintentional)**
Toxic effect of venom of other North and South American snake NOS

    √7ʰ T63.062   **Toxic effect of venom of other North and South American snake, intentional self-harm**

    √7ʰ T63.063   **Toxic effect of venom of other North and South American snake, assault**

    √7ʰ T63.064   **Toxic effect of venom of other North and South American snake, undetermined**

√6ʰ T63.07   **Toxic effect of venom of other Australian snake**

    √7ʰ T63.071   **Toxic effect of venom of other Australian snake, accidental (unintentional)**
Toxic effect of venom of other Australian snake NOS

    √7ʰ T63.072   **Toxic effect of venom of other Australian snake, intentional self-harm**

    √7ʰ T63.073   **Toxic effect of venom of other Australian snake, assault**

    √7ʰ T63.074   **Toxic effect of venom of other Australian snake, undetermined**

√6ʰ T63.08   **Toxic effect of venom of other African and Asian snake**

    √7ʰ T63.081   **Toxic effect of venom of other African and Asian snake, accidental (unintentional)**
Toxic effect of venom of other African and Asian snake NOS

    √7ʰ T63.082   **Toxic effect of venom of other African and Asian snake, intentional self-harm**

    √7ʰ T63.083   **Toxic effect of venom of other African and Asian snake, assault**

    √7ʰ T63.084   **Toxic effect of venom of other African and Asian snake, undetermined**

√6ʰ T63.09   **Toxic effect of venom of other snake**

    √7ʰ T63.091   **Toxic effect of venom of other snake, accidental (unintentional)**
Toxic effect of venom of other snake NOS

    √7ʰ T63.092   **Toxic effect of venom of other snake, intentional self-harm**

    √7ʰ T63.093   **Toxic effect of venom of other snake, assault**

    √7ʰ T63.094   **Toxic effect of venom of other snake, undetermined**

√5ʰ T63.1   **Toxic effect of venom of other reptiles**

√6ʰ T63.11   **Toxic effect of venom of gila monster**

    √7ʰ T63.111   **Toxic effect of venom of gila monster, accidental (unintentional)**
Toxic effect of venom of gila monster NOS

    √7ʰ T63.112   **Toxic effect of venom of gila monster, intentional self-harm**

    √7ʰ T63.113   **Toxic effect of venom of gila monster, assault**

    √7ʰ T63.114   **Toxic effect of venom of gila monster, undetermined**

√6ʰ T63.12   **Toxic effect of venom of other venomous lizard**

    √7ʰ T63.121   **Toxic effect of venom of other venomous lizard, accidental (unintentional)**
Toxic effect of venom of other venomous lizard NOS

    √7ʰ T63.122   **Toxic effect of venom of other venomous lizard, intentional self-harm**

    √7ʰ T63.123   **Toxic effect of venom of other venomous lizard, assault**

    √7ʰ T63.124   **Toxic effect of venom of other venomous lizard, undetermined**

√6ʰ T63.19   **Toxic effect of venom of other reptiles**

    √7ʰ T63.191   **Toxic effect of venom of other reptiles, accidental (unintentional)**
Toxic effect of venom of other reptiles NOS

    √7ʰ T63.192   **Toxic effect of venom of other reptiles, intentional self-harm**

    √7ʰ T63.193   **Toxic effect of venom of other reptiles, assault**

    √7ʰ T63.194   **Toxic effect of venom of other reptiles, undetermined**

√5ʰ T63.2   **Toxic effect of venom of scorpion**

√6ʰ T63.2X   **Toxic effect of venom of scorpion**

    √7ʰ T63.2X1   **Toxic effect of venom of scorpion, accidental (unintentional)**
Toxic effect of venom of scorpion NOS

    √7ʰ T63.2X2   **Toxic effect of venom of scorpion, intentional self-harm**

    √7ʰ T63.2X3   **Toxic effect of venom of scorpion, assault**

    √7ʰ T63.2X4   **Toxic effect of venom of scorpion, undetermined**

☑ Add'l Character Required   √x7ʰ Placeholder Alert   RUG IV Special Care High Dx   RUG IV Clinically Complex Dx   RUG IV Special Care Low Dx   Manifestation Code   Other Specified Code   ▽ Unspecified Code

√5ᵗʰ **T63.3** **Toxic effect of venom of** spider
  √6ᵗʰ **T63.30** **Toxic effect of** unspecified **spider venom**
    √7ᵗʰ **T63.301** **Toxic effect of unspecified spider venom,** accidental (unintentional) ▽
    √7ᵗʰ **T63.302** **Toxic effect of unspecified spider venom,** intentional self-harm ▽
    √7ᵗʰ **T63.303** **Toxic effect of unspecified spider venom,** assault ▽
    √7ᵗʰ **T63.304** **Toxic effect of unspecified spider venom,** undetermined ▽
  √6ᵗʰ **T63.31** **Toxic effect of venom of** black widow **spider**
    √7ᵗʰ **T63.311** **Toxic effect of venom of black widow spider,** accidental (unintentional)
    √7ᵗʰ **T63.312** **Toxic effect of venom of black widow spider,** intentional self-harm
    √7ᵗʰ **T63.313** **Toxic effect of venom of black widow spider,** assault
    √7ᵗʰ **T63.314** **Toxic effect of venom of black widow spider,** undetermined
  √6ᵗʰ **T63.32** **Toxic effect of venom of** tarantula
    √7ᵗʰ **T63.321** **Toxic effect of venom of tarantula,** accidental (unintentional)
    √7ᵗʰ **T63.322** **Toxic effect of venom of tarantula,** intentional self-harm
    √7ᵗʰ **T63.323** **Toxic effect of venom of tarantula,** assault
    √7ᵗʰ **T63.324** **Toxic effect of venom of tarantula,** undetermined
  √6ᵗʰ **T63.33** **Toxic effect of venom of** brown recluse **spider**
    √7ᵗʰ **T63.331** **Toxic effect of venom of brown recluse spider,** accidental (unintentional)
    √7ᵗʰ **T63.332** **Toxic effect of venom of brown recluse spider,** intentional self-harm
    √7ᵗʰ **T63.333** **Toxic effect of venom of brown recluse spider,** assault
    √7ᵗʰ **T63.334** **Toxic effect of venom of brown recluse spider,** undetermined
  √6ᵗʰ **T63.39** **Toxic effect of venom of** other **spider**
    √7ᵗʰ **T63.391** **Toxic effect of venom of other spider, accidental (unintentional)**
    √7ᵗʰ **T63.392** **Toxic effect of venom of other spider, intentional self-harm**
    √7ᵗʰ **T63.393** **Toxic effect of venom of other spider, assault**
    √7ᵗʰ **T63.394** **Toxic effect of venom of other spider, undetermined**
√5ᵗʰ **T63.4** **Toxic effect of venom of** other arthropods
  √6ᵗʰ **T63.41** **Toxic effect of venom of** centipedes and venomous millipedes
    √7ᵗʰ **T63.411** **Toxic effect of venom of centipedes and venomous millipedes,** accidental (unintentional)
    √7ᵗʰ **T63.412** **Toxic effect of venom of centipedes and venomous millipedes,** intentional self-harm
    √7ᵗʰ **T63.413** **Toxic effect of venom of centipedes and venomous millipedes,** assault
    √7ᵗʰ **T63.414** **Toxic effect of venom of centipedes and venomous millipedes,** undetermined
  √6ᵗʰ **T63.42** **Toxic effect of venom of** ants
    √7ᵗʰ **T63.421** **Toxic effect of venom of ants,** accidental (unintentional)
    √7ᵗʰ **T63.422** **Toxic effect of venom of ants,** intentional self-harm
    √7ᵗʰ **T63.423** **Toxic effect of venom of ants,** assault
    √7ᵗʰ **T63.424** **Toxic effect of venom of ants,** undetermined
  √6ᵗʰ **T63.43** **Toxic effect of venom of** caterpillars
    √7ᵗʰ **T63.431** **Toxic effect of venom of caterpillars,** accidental (unintentional)
    √7ᵗʰ **T63.432** **Toxic effect of venom of caterpillars,** intentional self-harm
    √7ᵗʰ **T63.433** **Toxic effect of venom of caterpillars,** assault

    √7ᵗʰ **T63.434** **Toxic effect of venom of caterpillars,** undetermined
  √6ᵗʰ **T63.44** **Toxic effect of venom of** bees
    √7ᵗʰ **T63.441** **Toxic effect of venom of bees,** accidental (unintentional)
    √7ᵗʰ **T63.442** **Toxic effect of venom of bees,** intentional self-harm
    √7ᵗʰ **T63.443** **Toxic effect of venom of bees,** assault
    √7ᵗʰ **T63.444** **Toxic effect of venom of bees,** undetermined
  √6ᵗʰ **T63.45** **Toxic effect of venom of** hornets
    √7ᵗʰ **T63.451** **Toxic effect of venom of hornets,** accidental (unintentional)
    √7ᵗʰ **T63.452** **Toxic effect of venom of hornets,** intentional self-harm
    √7ᵗʰ **T63.453** **Toxic effect of venom of hornets,** assault
    √7ᵗʰ **T63.454** **Toxic effect of venom of hornets,** undetermined
  √6ᵗʰ **T63.46** **Toxic effect of venom of** wasps
    Toxic effect of yellow jacket
    √7ᵗʰ **T63.461** **Toxic effect of venom of wasps,** accidental (unintentional)
    √7ᵗʰ **T63.462** **Toxic effect of venom of wasps,** intentional self-harm
    √7ᵗʰ **T63.463** **Toxic effect of venom of wasps,** assault
    √7ᵗʰ **T63.464** **Toxic effect of venom of wasps,** undetermined
  √6ᵗʰ **T63.48** **Toxic effect of venom of** other arthropod
    √7ᵗʰ **T63.481** **Toxic effect of venom of other arthropod, accidental (unintentional)**
    √7ᵗʰ **T63.482** **Toxic effect of venom of other arthropod, intentional self-harm**
    √7ᵗʰ **T63.483** **Toxic effect of venom of other arthropod, assault**
    √7ᵗʰ **T63.484** **Toxic effect of venom of other arthropod, undetermined**
√5ᵗʰ **T63.5** **Toxic effect of contact with** venomous fish
  EXCLUDES 2 poisoning by ingestion of fish (T61.-)
  √6ᵗʰ **T63.51** **Toxic effect of contact with** stingray
    √7ᵗʰ **T63.511** **Toxic effect of contact with stingray,** accidental (unintentional)
    √7ᵗʰ **T63.512** **Toxic effect of contact with stingray,** intentional self-harm
    √7ᵗʰ **T63.513** **Toxic effect of contact with stingray,** assault
    √7ᵗʰ **T63.514** **Toxic effect of contact with stingray,** undetermined
  √6ᵗʰ **T63.59** **Toxic effect of contact with** other **venomous fish**
    √7ᵗʰ **T63.591** **Toxic effect of contact with other venomous fish, accidental (unintentional)**
    √7ᵗʰ **T63.592** **Toxic effect of contact with other venomous fish, intentional self-harm**
    √7ᵗʰ **T63.593** **Toxic effect of contact with other venomous fish, assault**
    √7ᵗʰ **T63.594** **Toxic effect of contact with other venomous fish, undetermined**
√5ᵗʰ **T63.6** **Toxic effect of contact with other** venomous marine animals
  EXCLUDES 1 sea-snake venom (T63.09)
  EXCLUDES 2 poisoning by ingestion of shellfish (T61.78-)
  √6ᵗʰ **T63.61** **Toxic effect of contact with** Portugese Man-o-war
    Toxic effect of contact with bluebottle
    √7ᵗʰ **T63.611** **Toxic effect of contact with Portugese Man-o-war,** accidental (unintentional)
    √7ᵗʰ **T63.612** **Toxic effect of contact with Portugese Man-o-war,** intentional self-harm
    √7ᵗʰ **T63.613** **Toxic effect of contact with Portugese Man-o-war,** assault
    √7ᵗʰ **T63.614** **Toxic effect of contact with Portugese Man-o-war,** undetermined
  √6ᵗʰ **T63.62** **Toxic effect of contact with** other jellyfish
    √7ᵗʰ **T63.621** **Toxic effect of contact with other jellyfish,** accidental (unintentional)
    √7ᵗʰ **T63.622** **Toxic effect of contact with other jellyfish,** intentional self-harm

N Newborn   P Pediatric   M Maternity   A Adult   RIC RIC Dx   NC Dx Noncancer Dx   PDx Primary Dx   CC RIC CC Condition   ►◄ Revised Text   ● New Code   ▲ Revised Code Title

1028   ICD-10-CM 2016

✓7ᵗʰ **T63.623** Toxic effect of contact with other jellyfish, assault

✓7ᵗʰ **T63.624** Toxic effect of contact with other jellyfish, undetermined

✓6ᵗʰ **T63.63** Toxic effect of contact with sea anemone

✓7ᵗʰ **T63.631** Toxic effect of contact with sea anemone, accidental (unintentional)

✓7ᵗʰ **T63.632** Toxic effect of contact with sea anemone, intentional self-harm

✓7ᵗʰ **T63.633** Toxic effect of contact with sea anemone, assault

✓7ᵗʰ **T63.634** Toxic effect of contact with sea anemone, undetermined

✓6ᵗʰ **T63.69** Toxic effect of contact with other venomous marine animals

✓7ᵗʰ **T63.691** Toxic effect of contact with other venomous marine animals, accidental (unintentional)

✓7ᵗʰ **T63.692** Toxic effect of contact with other venomous marine animals, intentional self-harm

✓7ᵗʰ **T63.693** Toxic effect of contact with other venomous marine animals, assault

✓7ᵗʰ **T63.694** Toxic effect of contact with other venomous marine animals, undetermined

✓5ᵗʰ **T63.7** Toxic effect of contact with venomous plant

✓6ᵗʰ **T63.71** Toxic effect of contact with venomous marine plant

✓7ᵗʰ **T63.711** Toxic effect of contact with venomous marine plant, accidental (unintentional)

✓7ᵗʰ **T63.712** Toxic effect of contact with venomous marine plant, intentional self-harm

✓7ᵗʰ **T63.713** Toxic effect of contact with venomous marine plant, assault

✓7ᵗʰ **T63.714** Toxic effect of contact with venomous marine plant, undetermined

✓6ᵗʰ **T63.79** Toxic effect of contact with other venomous plant

✓7ᵗʰ **T63.791** Toxic effect of contact with other venomous plant, accidental (unintentional)

✓7ᵗʰ **T63.792** Toxic effect of contact with other venomous plant, intentional self-harm

✓7ᵗʰ **T63.793** Toxic effect of contact with other venomous plant, assault

✓7ᵗʰ **T63.794** Toxic effect of contact with other venomous plant, undetermined

✓5ᵗʰ **T63.8** Toxic effect of contact with other venomous animals

✓6ᵗʰ **T63.81** Toxic effect of contact with venomous frog

    EXCLUDES 1   contact with nonvenomous frog (W62.0)

✓7ᵗʰ **T63.811** Toxic effect of contact with venomous frog, accidental (unintentional)

✓7ᵗʰ **T63.812** Toxic effect of contact with venomous frog, intentional self-harm

✓7ᵗʰ **T63.813** Toxic effect of contact with venomous frog, assault

✓7ᵗʰ **T63.814** Toxic effect of contact with venomous frog, undetermined

✓6ᵗʰ **T63.82** Toxic effect of contact with venomous toad

    EXCLUDES 1   contact with nonvenomous toad (W62.1)

✓7ᵗʰ **T63.821** Toxic effect of contact with venomous toad, accidental (unintentional)

✓7ᵗʰ **T63.822** Toxic effect of contact with venomous toad, intentional self-harm

✓7ᵗʰ **T63.823** Toxic effect of contact with venomous toad, assault

✓7ᵗʰ **T63.824** Toxic effect of contact with venomous toad, undetermined

✓6ᵗʰ **T63.83** Toxic effect of contact with other venomous amphibian

    EXCLUDES 1   contact with nonvenomous amphibian (W62.9)

✓7ᵗʰ **T63.831** Toxic effect of contact with other venomous amphibian, accidental (unintentional)

✓7ᵗʰ **T63.832** Toxic effect of contact with other venomous amphibian, intentional self-harm

✓7ᵗʰ **T63.833** Toxic effect of contact with other venomous amphibian, assault

✓7ᵗʰ **T63.834** Toxic effect of contact with other venomous amphibian, undetermined

✓6ᵗʰ **T63.89** Toxic effect of contact with other venomous animals

✓7ᵗʰ **T63.891** Toxic effect of contact with other venomous animals, accidental (unintentional)

✓7ᵗʰ **T63.892** Toxic effect of contact with other venomous animals, intentional self-harm

✓7ᵗʰ **T63.893** Toxic effect of contact with other venomous animals, assault

✓7ᵗʰ **T63.894** Toxic effect of contact with other venomous animals, undetermined

✓5ᵗʰ **T63.9** Toxic effect of contact with unspecified venomous animal

✓x7ᵗʰ **T63.91** Toxic effect of contact with unspecified venomous animal, accidental (unintentional) ▽

✓x7ᵗʰ **T63.92** Toxic effect of contact with unspecified venomous animal, intentional self-harm ▽

✓x7ᵗʰ **T63.93** Toxic effect of contact with unspecified venomous animal, assault ▽

✓x7ᵗʰ **T63.94** Toxic effect of contact with unspecified venomous animal, undetermined ▽

✓4ᵗʰ **T64** Toxic effect of aflatoxin and other mycotoxin food contaminants

> The appropriate 7th character is to be added to each code from category T64.
> A   initial encounter
> D   subsequent encounter
> S   sequela

✓5ᵗʰ **T64.0** Toxic effect of aflatoxin

✓x7ᵗʰ **T64.01** Toxic effect of aflatoxin, accidental (unintentional)

✓x7ᵗʰ **T64.02** Toxic effect of aflatoxin, intentional self-harm

✓x7ᵗʰ **T64.03** Toxic effect of aflatoxin, assault

✓x7ᵗʰ **T64.04** Toxic effect of aflatoxin, undetermined

✓5ᵗʰ **T64.8** Toxic effect of other mycotoxin food contaminants

✓x7ᵗʰ **T64.81** Toxic effect of other mycotoxin food contaminants, accidental (unintentional)

✓x7ᵗʰ **T64.82** Toxic effect of other mycotoxin food contaminants, intentional self-harm

✓x7ᵗʰ **T64.83** Toxic effect of other mycotoxin food contaminants, assault

✓x7ᵗʰ **T64.84** Toxic effect of other mycotoxin food contaminants, undetermined

✓4ᵗʰ **T65** Toxic effect of other and unspecified substances

> The appropriate 7th character is to be added to each code from category T65.
> A   initial encounter
> D   subsequent encounter
> S   sequela

✓5ᵗʰ **T65.0** Toxic effect of cyanides

    EXCLUDES 1   hydrogen cyanide (T57.3-)

✓6ᵗʰ **T65.0X** Toxic effect of cyanides

✓7ᵗʰ **T65.0X1** Toxic effect of cyanides, accidental (unintentional)

    Toxic effect of cyanides NOS

✓7ᵗʰ **T65.0X2** Toxic effect of cyanides, intentional self-harm

✓7ᵗʰ **T65.0X3** Toxic effect of cyanides, assault

✓7ᵗʰ **T65.0X4** Toxic effect of cyanides, undetermined

✓5ᵗʰ **T65.1** Toxic effect of strychnine and its salts

✓6ᵗʰ **T65.1X** Toxic effect of strychnine and its salts

✓7ᵗʰ **T65.1X1** Toxic effect of strychnine and its salts, accidental (unintentional)

    Toxic effect of strychnine and its salts NOS

✓7ᵗʰ **T65.1X2** Toxic effect of strychnine and its salts, intentional self-harm

☑ Add'l Character Required   ✓x7ᵗʰ Placeholder Alert   RUG IV Special Care High Dx   RUG IV Clinically Complex Dx   RUG IV Special Care Low Dx   Manifestation Code   Other Specified Code   ▽ Unspecified Code

ICD-10-CM 2016   1029

Chapter 19. Injury, Poisoning and Certain Other Consequences of External Causes

T65.1X3–T65.894

✓7ᵗʰ **T65.1X3** **Toxic effect of strychnine and its salts,** assault

✓7ᵗʰ **T65.1X4** **Toxic effect of strychnine and its salts,** undetermined

✓5ᵗʰ **T65.2** **Toxic effect of** tobacco and nicotine
EXCLUDES 2 *nicotine dependence (F17.-)*

✓6ᵗʰ **T65.21** **Toxic effect of** chewing tobacco

✓7ᵗʰ **T65.211** **Toxic effect of chewing tobacco,** accidental **(unintentional)**
Toxic effect of chewing tobacco NOS

✓7ᵗʰ **T65.212** **Toxic effect of chewing tobacco,** intentional self-harm

✓7ᵗʰ **T65.213** **Toxic effect of chewing tobacco,** assault

✓7ᵗʰ **T65.214** **Toxic effect of chewing tobacco,** undetermined

✓6ᵗʰ **T65.22** **Toxic effect of** tobacco cigarettes
Toxic effect of tobacco smoke
Use additional code for exposure to second hand tobacco smoke (Z57.31, Z77.22)

✓7ᵗʰ **T65.221** **Toxic effect of tobacco cigarettes,** accidental **(unintentional)**
Toxic effect of tobacco cigarettes NOS

✓7ᵗʰ **T65.222** **Toxic effect of tobacco cigarettes,** intentional self-harm

✓7ᵗʰ **T65.223** **Toxic effect of tobacco cigarettes,** assault

✓7ᵗʰ **T65.224** **Toxic effect of tobacco cigarettes,** undetermined

✓6ᵗʰ **T65.29** **Toxic effect of** other tobacco and nicotine

✓7ᵗʰ **T65.291** **Toxic effect of other tobacco and nicotine,** accidental **(unintentional)**
Toxic effect of other tobacco and nicotine NOS

✓7ᵗʰ **T65.292** **Toxic effect of other tobacco and nicotine,** intentional self-harm

✓7ᵗʰ **T65.293** **Toxic effect of other tobacco and nicotine,** assault

✓7ᵗʰ **T65.294** **Toxic effect of other tobacco and nicotine,** undetermined

✓5ᵗʰ **T65.3** **Toxic effect of** nitroderivatives and aminoderivatives of benzene and its homologues
Toxic effect of anilin [benzenamine]
Toxic effect of nitrobenzene
Toxic effect of trinitrotoluene

✓6ᵗʰ **T65.3X** **Toxic effect of nitroderivatives and aminoderivatives of benzene and its homologues**

✓7ᵗʰ **T65.3X1** **Toxic effect of nitroderivatives and aminoderivatives of benzene and its homologues,** accidental **(unintentional)**
Toxic effect of nitroderivatives and aminoderivatives of benzene and its homologues NOS

✓7ᵗʰ **T65.3X2** **Toxic effect of nitroderivatives and aminoderivatives of benzene and its homologues,** intentional self-harm

✓7ᵗʰ **T65.3X3** **Toxic effect of nitroderivatives and aminoderivatives of benzene and its homologues,** assault

✓7ᵗʰ **T65.3X4** **Toxic effect of nitroderivatives and aminoderivatives of benzene and its homologues,** undetermined

✓5ᵗʰ **T65.4** **Toxic effect of** carbon disulfide

✓6ᵗʰ **T65.4X** **Toxic effect of carbon disulfide**

✓7ᵗʰ **T65.4X1** **Toxic effect of carbon disulfide,** accidental **(unintentional)**
Toxic effect of carbon disulfide NOS

✓7ᵗʰ **T65.4X2** **Toxic effect of carbon disulfide,** intentional self-harm

✓7ᵗʰ **T65.4X3** **Toxic effect of carbon disulfide,** assault

✓7ᵗʰ **T65.4X4** **Toxic effect of carbon disulfide,** undetermined

✓5ᵗʰ **T65.5** **Toxic effect of** nitroglycerin and other nitric acids and esters
Toxic effect of 1,2,3-Propanetriol trinitrate

✓6ᵗʰ **T65.5X** **Toxic effect of nitroglycerin and other nitric acids and esters**

✓7ᵗʰ **T65.5X1** **Toxic effect of nitroglycerin and other nitric acids and esters,** accidental **(unintentional)**
Toxic effect of nitroglycerin and other nitric acids and esters NOS

✓7ᵗʰ **T65.5X2** **Toxic effect of nitroglycerin and other nitric acids and esters,** intentional self-harm

✓7ᵗʰ **T65.5X3** **Toxic effect of nitroglycerin and other nitric acids and esters,** assault

✓7ᵗʰ **T65.5X4** **Toxic effect of nitroglycerin and other nitric acids and esters,** undetermined

✓5ᵗʰ **T65.6** **Toxic effect of** paints and dyes, **not elsewhere classified**

✓6ᵗʰ **T65.6X** **Toxic effect of paints and dyes, not elsewhere classified**

✓7ᵗʰ **T65.6X1** **Toxic effect of paints and dyes, not elsewhere classified,** accidental **(unintentional)**
Toxic effect of paints and dyes NOS

✓7ᵗʰ **T65.6X2** **Toxic effect of paints and dyes, not elsewhere classified,** intentional self-harm

✓7ᵗʰ **T65.6X3** **Toxic effect of paints and dyes, not elsewhere classified,** assault

✓7ᵗʰ **T65.6X4** **Toxic effect of paints and dyes, not elsewhere classified,** undetermined

✓5ᵗʰ **T65.8** **Toxic effect of** other specified substances

✓6ᵗʰ **T65.81** **Toxic effect of** latex

✓7ᵗʰ **T65.811** **Toxic effect of latex,** accidental **(unintentional)**
Toxic effect of latex NOS

✓7ᵗʰ **T65.812** **Toxic effect of latex,** intentional self-harm

✓7ᵗʰ **T65.813** **Toxic effect of latex,** assault

✓7ᵗʰ **T65.814** **Toxic effect of latex,** undetermined

✓6ᵗʰ **T65.82** **Toxic effect of harmful** algae and algae toxins
Toxic effect of (harmful) algae bloom NOS
Toxic effect of blue-green algae bloom
Toxic effect of brown tide
Toxic effect of cyanobacteria bloom
Toxic effect of Florida red tide
Toxic effect of pfiesteria piscicida
Toxic effect of red tide

✓7ᵗʰ **T65.821** **Toxic effect of harmful algae and algae toxins,** accidental **(unintentional)**
Toxic effect of harmful algae and algae toxins NOS

✓7ᵗʰ **T65.822** **Toxic effect of harmful algae and algae toxins,** intentional self-harm

✓7ᵗʰ **T65.823** **Toxic effect of harmful algae and algae toxins,** assault

✓7ᵗʰ **T65.824** **Toxic effect of harmful algae and algae toxins,** undetermined

✓6ᵗʰ **T65.83** **Toxic effect of** fiberglass

✓7ᵗʰ **T65.831** **Toxic effect of fiberglass,** accidental **(unintentional)**
Toxic effect of fiberglass NOS

✓7ᵗʰ **T65.832** **Toxic effect of fiberglass,** intentional self-harm

✓7ᵗʰ **T65.833** **Toxic effect of fiberglass,** assault

✓7ᵗʰ **T65.834** **Toxic effect of fiberglass,** undetermined

✓6ᵗʰ **T65.89** **Toxic effect of** other specified substances

✓7ᵗʰ **T65.891** **Toxic effect of other specified substances,** accidental **(unintentional)**
Toxic effect of other specified substances NOS

✓7ᵗʰ **T65.892** **Toxic effect of other specified substances,** intentional self-harm

✓7ᵗʰ **T65.893** **Toxic effect of other specified substances,** assault

✓7ᵗʰ **T65.894** **Toxic effect of other specified substances,** undetermined

N Newborn   P Pediatric   M Maternity   A Adult   RIC RIC Dx   NC Dx Noncancer Dx   PDx Primary Dx   CC RIC CC Condition   ▶◀ Revised Text   ● New Code   ▲ Revised Code Title

1030   ICD-10-CM 2016

✓5ᵗʰ **T65.9 Toxic effect of unspecified substance**

   ✓x7ᵗʰ **T65.91 Toxic effect of unspecified substance, accidental** ▽
     (unintentional)
       Poisoning NOS

   ✓x7ᵗʰ **T65.92 Toxic effect of unspecified substance, intentional** ▽
     self-harm

   ✓x7ᵗʰ **T65.93 Toxic effect of unspecified substance, assault** ▽

   ✓x7ᵗʰ **T65.94 Toxic effect of unspecified substance,** ▽
     undetermined

Other and unspecified effects of external causes (T66-T78)

✓x7ᵗʰ **T66 Radiation sickness, unspecified** ▽
   EXCLUDES 1   specified adverse effects of radiation, such as:
      burns (T20-T31)
      leukemia (C91-C95)
      radiation gastroenteritis and colitis (K52.0)
      radiation pneumonitis (J70.0)
      radiation related disorders of the skin and subcutaneous tissue
        (L55-L59)
      radiation sunburn (L55.-)

> The appropriate 7th character is to be added to code T66.
> A   initial encounter
> D   subsequent encounter
> S   sequela

✓4ᵗʰ **T67 Effects of heat and light**
   EXCLUDES 1   erythema [dermatitis] ab igne (L59.0)
      malignant hyperpyrexia due to anesthesia (T88.3)
      radiation-related disorders of the skin and subcutaneous tissue
        (L55-L59)
   EXCLUDES 2   burns (T20-T31)
      sunburn (L55.-)
      sweat disorder due to heat (L74-L75)

> The appropriate 7th character is to be added to each code from
> category T67.
> A   initial encounter
> D   subsequent encounter
> S   sequela

  ✓x7ᵗʰ **T67.0 Heatstroke and sunstroke**
     Heat apoplexy   Siriasis
     Heat pyrexia   Thermoplegia
     Use additional code(s) to identify any associated complications
       of heatstroke, such as:
        coma and stupor (R40.-)
        systemic inflammatory response syndrome (R65.1-)

  ✓x7ᵗʰ **T67.1 Heat syncope**
     Heat collapse

  ✓x7ᵗʰ **T67.2 Heat cramp**

  ✓x7ᵗʰ **T67.3 Heat exhaustion, anhydrotic**
     Heat prostration due to water depletion
    EXCLUDES 1   heat exhaustion due to salt depletion (T67.4)

  ✓x7ᵗʰ **T67.4 Heat exhaustion due to salt depletion**
     Heat prostration due to salt (and water) depletion ▽

  ✓x7ᵗʰ **T67.5 Heat exhaustion, unspecified**
     Heat prostration NOS

  ✓x7ᵗʰ **T67.6 Heat fatigue, transient**

  ✓x7ᵗʰ **T67.7 Heat edema**

  ✓x7ᵗʰ **T67.8 Other effects of heat and light**

  ✓x7ᵗʰ **T67.9 Effect of heat and light, unspecified** ▽

✓x7ᵗʰ **T68 Hypothermia**
     Accidental hypothermia   Hypothermia NOS
     Use additional code to identify source of exposure:
      exposure to excessive cold of man-made origin (W93)
      exposure to excessive cold of natural origin (X31)
   EXCLUDES 1   hypothermia following anesthesia (T88.51)
      hypothermia not associated with low environmental
        temperature (R68.0)
      hypothermia of newborn (P80.-)
   EXCLUDES 2   frostbite (T33-T34)

> The appropriate 7th character is to be added to code T68.
> A   initial encounter
> D   subsequent encounter
> S   sequela

✓4ᵗʰ **T69 Other effects of reduced temperature**
     Use additional code to identify source of exposure:
      exposure to excessive cold of man-made origin (W93)
      exposure to excessive cold of natural origin (X31)
   EXCLUDES 2   frostbite (T33-T34)

> The appropriate 7th character is to be added to each code from
> category T69.
> A   initial encounter
> D   subsequent encounter
> S   sequela

  ✓5ᵗʰ **T69.0 Immersion hand and foot**

    ✓6ᵗʰ **T69.01 Immersion hand**

      ✓7ᵗʰ **T69.011 Immersion hand, right hand**

      ✓7ᵗʰ **T69.012 Immersion hand, left hand**

      ✓7ᵗʰ **T69.019 Immersion hand, unspecified hand** ▽

    ✓6ᵗʰ **T69.02 Immersion foot**
       Trench foot

      ✓7ᵗʰ **T69.021 Immersion foot, right foot**

      ✓7ᵗʰ **T69.022 Immersion foot, left foot**

      ✓7ᵗʰ **T69.029 Immersion foot, unspecified foot** ▽

  ✓x7ᵗʰ **T69.1 Chilblains**

  ✓x7ᵗʰ **T69.8 Other specified effects of reduced temperature**

  ✓x7ᵗʰ **T69.9 Effect of reduced temperature, unspecified** ▽

✓4ᵗʰ **T70 Effects of air pressure and water pressure**

> The appropriate 7th character is to be added to each code from
> category T70.
> A   initial encounter
> D   subsequent encounter
> S   sequela

  ✓x7ᵗʰ **T70.0 Otitic barotrauma**
     Aero-otitis media
     Effects of change in ambient atmospheric pressure or water
       pressure on ears

  ✓x7ᵗʰ **T70.1 Sinus barotrauma**
     Aerosinusitis
     Effects of change in ambient atmospheric pressure on sinuses

  ✓5ᵗʰ **T70.2 Other and unspecified effects of high altitude**
    EXCLUDES 2   polycythemia due to high altitude (D75.1)

    ✓x7ᵗʰ **T70.20 Unspecified effects of high altitude** ▽

    ✓x7ᵗʰ **T70.29 Other effects of high altitude**
      Alpine sickness
      Anoxia due to high altitude
      Barotrauma NOS
      Hypobaropathy
      Mountain sickness

  ✓x7ᵗʰ **T70.3 Caisson disease [decompression sickness]**
     Compressed-air disease
     Diver's palsy or paralysis

  ✓x7ᵗʰ **T70.4 Effects of high-pressure fluids**
     Hydraulic jet injection (industrial)
     Pneumatic jet injection (industrial)
     Traumatic jet injection (industrial)

  ✓x7ᵗʰ **T70.8 Other effects of air pressure and water pressure**

  ✓x7ᵗʰ **T70.9 Effect of air pressure and water pressure, unspecified** ▽

☑ Add'l Character Required   ✓x7ᵗʰ Placeholder Alert   RUG IV Special Care High Dx   RUG IV Clinically Complex Dx   RUG IV Special Care Low Dx   Manifestation Code   Other Specified Code   ▽ Unspecified Code

ICD-10-CM 2016   **1031**

√4ᵗʰ **T71 Asphyxiation**
Mechanical suffocation
Traumatic suffocation
EXCLUDES 1   acute respiratory distress (syndrome) (J80)
anoxia due to high altitude (T70.2)
asphyxia NOS (R09.01)
asphyxia from carbon monoxide (T58.-)
asphyxia from inhalation of food or foreign body (T17.-)
asphyxia from other gases, fumes and vapors (T59.-)
respiratory distress (syndrome) in newborn (P22.-)

The appropriate 7th character is to be added to each code from
category T71.
A   initial encounter
D   subsequent encounter
S   sequela

√5ᵗʰ **T71.1 Asphyxiation due to** mechanical threat to breathing
Suffocation due to mechanical threat to breathing

√6ᵗʰ **T71.11 Asphyxiation due to** smothering under pillow

√7ᵗʰ **T71.111 Asphyxiation due to smothering under
pillow,** accidental
Asphyxiation due to smothering under
pillow NOS

√7ᵗʰ **T71.112 Asphyxiation due to smothering under
pillow,** intentional self-harm

√7ᵗʰ **T71.113 Asphyxiation due to smothering under
pillow,** assault

√7ᵗʰ **T71.114 Asphyxiation due to smothering under
pillow,** undetermined

√6ᵗʰ **T71.12 Asphyxiation due to** plastic bag

√7ᵗʰ **T71.121 Asphyxiation due to plastic bag,**
accidental
Asphyxiation due to plastic bag NOS

√7ᵗʰ **T71.122 Asphyxiation due to plastic bag,**
intentional self-harm

√7ᵗʰ **T71.123 Asphyxiation due to plastic bag,** assault

√7ᵗʰ **T71.124 Asphyxiation due to plastic bag,**
undetermined

√6ᵗʰ **T71.13 Asphyxiation due to being** trapped in bed linens

√7ᵗʰ **T71.131 Asphyxiation due to being trapped in bed
linens,** accidental
Asphyxiation due to being trapped in bed
linens NOS

√7ᵗʰ **T71.132 Asphyxiation due to being trapped in bed
linens,** intentional self-harm

√7ᵗʰ **T71.133 Asphyxiation due to being trapped in bed
linens,** assault

√7ᵗʰ **T71.134 Asphyxiation due to being trapped in bed
linens,** undetermined

√6ᵗʰ **T71.14 Asphyxiation due to** smothering under another
person's body (in bed)

√7ᵗʰ **T71.141 Asphyxiation due to smothering under
another person's body (in bed),** accidental
Asphyxiation due to smothering under
another person's body (in bed) NOS

√7ᵗʰ **T71.143 Asphyxiation due to smothering under
another person's body (in bed),** assault

√7ᵗʰ **T71.144 Asphyxiation due to smothering under
another person's body (in bed),**
undetermined

√6ᵗʰ **T71.15 Asphyxiation due to** smothering in furniture

√7ᵗʰ **T71.151 Asphyxiation due to smothering in
furniture,** accidental
Asphyxiation due to smothering in
furniture NOS

√7ᵗʰ **T71.152 Asphyxiation due to smothering in
furniture,** intentional self-harm

√7ᵗʰ **T71.153 Asphyxiation due to smothering in
furniture,** assault

√7ᵗʰ **T71.154 Asphyxiation due to smothering in
furniture,** undetermined

√6ᵗʰ **T71.16 Asphyxiation due to** hanging
Hanging by window shade cord
Use additional code for any associated injuries, such
as:
crushing injury of neck (S17.-)
fracture of cervical vertebrae (S12.0-S12.2-)
open wound of neck (S11.-)

√7ᵗʰ **T71.161 Asphyxiation due to hanging,** accidental
Asphyxiation due to hanging NOS
Hanging NOS

√7ᵗʰ **T71.162 Asphyxiation due to hanging,** intentional
self-harm

√7ᵗʰ **T71.163 Asphyxiation due to hanging,** assault

√7ᵗʰ **T71.164 Asphyxiation due to hanging,**
undetermined

√6ᵗʰ **T71.19 Asphyxiation due to mechanical threat to breathing
due to other causes**

√7ᵗʰ **T71.191 Asphyxiation due to mechanical threat to
breathing due to other causes,** accidental
Asphyxiation due to other causes NOS

√7ᵗʰ **T71.192 Asphyxiation due to mechanical threat to
breathing due to other causes,** intentional
self-harm

√7ᵗʰ **T71.193 Asphyxiation due to mechanical threat to
breathing due to other causes,** assault

√7ᵗʰ **T71.194 Asphyxiation due to mechanical threat to
breathing due to other causes,**
undetermined

√5ᵗʰ **T71.2 Asphyxiation due to** systemic oxygen deficiency due to low
oxygen content in ambient air
Suffocation due to systemic oxygen deficiency due to low
oxygen content in ambient air

√x7ᵗʰ **T71.20 Asphyxiation due to systemic oxygen deficiency** ▽
**due to low oxygen content in ambient air due to
unspecified cause**

√x7ᵗʰ **T71.21 Asphyxiation due to** cave-in or falling earth
Use additional code for any associated cataclysm
(X34-X38)

√6ᵗʰ **T71.22 Asphyxiation due to** being trapped in a car trunk

√7ᵗʰ **T71.221 Asphyxiation due to being trapped in a car
trunk,** accidental

√7ᵗʰ **T71.222 Asphyxiation due to being trapped in a car
trunk,** intentional self-harm

√7ᵗʰ **T71.223 Asphyxiation due to being trapped in a car
trunk,** assault

√7ᵗʰ **T71.224 Asphyxiation due to being trapped in a car
trunk,** undetermined

√6ᵗʰ **T71.23 Asphyxiation due to being** trapped in a (discarded)
refrigerator

√7ᵗʰ **T71.231 Asphyxiation due to being trapped in a
(discarded) refrigerator,** accidental

√7ᵗʰ **T71.232 Asphyxiation due to being trapped in a
(discarded) refrigerator,** intentional
self-harm

√7ᵗʰ **T71.233 Asphyxiation due to being trapped in a
(discarded) refrigerator,** assault

√7ᵗʰ **T71.234 Asphyxiation due to being trapped in a
(discarded) refrigerator,** undetermined

√x7ᵗʰ **T71.29 Asphyxiation due to being trapped in other low
oxygen environment**

√x7ᵗʰ **T71.9 Asphyxiation due to unspecified cause** ▽
Suffocation (by strangulation) due to unspecified cause
Suffocation NOS
Systemic oxygen deficiency due to low oxygen content in
ambient air due to unspecified cause
Systemic oxygen deficiency due to mechanical threat to
breathing due to unspecified cause
Traumatic asphyxia NOS

√4ᵗʰ **T73 Effects of other deprivation**

The appropriate 7th character is to be added to each code from
category T73.
A   initial encounter
D   subsequent encounter
S   sequela

√x7ᵗʰ **T73.0 Starvation**
Deprivation of food

Ⓝ Newborn   Ⓟ Pediatric   Ⓜ Maternity   Ⓐ Adult   **RIC** RIC Dx   **NC Dx** Noncancer Dx   **PDx** Primary Dx   **CC** RIC CC Condition   ▶◀ Revised Text   ● New Code   ▲ Revised Code Title

1032   ICD-10-CM 2016

√x7ᵗʰ **T73.1** Deprivation of water

√x7ᵗʰ **T73.2** Exhaustion due to exposure

√x7ᵗʰ **T73.3** Exhaustion due to excessive exertion
Exhaustion due to overexertion

√x7ᵗʰ **T73.8** **Other effects of deprivation**

√x7ᵗʰ **T73.9** Effect of deprivation, unspecified ▽

√4ᵗʰ **T74** **Adult and child abuse, neglect and other maltreatment, confirmed**
Use additional code, if applicable, to identify any associated current injury
Use additional external cause code to identify perpetrator, if known (Y07.-)
EXCLUDES 1 abuse and maltreatment in pregnancy (O9A.3-, O9A.4-, O9A.5-)
adult and child maltreatment, suspected (T76.-)

The appropriate 7th character is to be added to each code from category T74.
A   initial encounter
D   subsequent encounter
S   sequela

√5ᵗʰ **T74.0** **Neglect or abandonment, confirmed**

√x7ᵗʰ **T74.01** Adult neglect or abandonment, confirmed 🅐

√x7ᵗʰ **T74.02** Child neglect or abandonment, confirmed 🅟

√5ᵗʰ **T74.1** Physical abuse, confirmed
EXCLUDES 2 sexual abuse (T74.2-)

√x7ᵗʰ **T74.11** Adult physical abuse, confirmed 🅐

√x7ᵗʰ **T74.12** Child physical abuse, confirmed 🅟
EXCLUDES 2 shaken infant syndrome (T74.4)

√5ᵗʰ **T74.2** Sexual abuse, confirmed
Rape, confirmed
Sexual assault, confirmed

√x7ᵗʰ **T74.21** Adult sexual abuse, confirmed 🅐

√x7ᵗʰ **T74.22** Child sexual abuse, confirmed 🅟

√5ᵗʰ **T74.3** Psychological abuse, confirmed

√x7ᵗʰ **T74.31** Adult psychological abuse, confirmed 🅐

√x7ᵗʰ **T74.32** Child psychological abuse, confirmed 🅟

√x7ᵗʰ **T74.4** Shaken infant syndrome 🅟

√5ᵗʰ **T74.9** Unspecified maltreatment, confirmed

√x7ᵗʰ **T74.91** Unspecified adult maltreatment, confirmed 🅐▽

√x7ᵗʰ **T74.92** Unspecified child maltreatment, confirmed 🅟▽

√4ᵗʰ **T75** **Other and unspecified effects of other external causes**
EXCLUDES 1 adverse effects NEC (T78.-)
EXCLUDES 2 burns (electric) (T20-T31)

The appropriate 7th character is to be added to each code from category T75.
A   initial encounter
D   subsequent encounter
S   sequela

√5ᵗʰ **T75.0** **Effects of lightning**
Struck by lightning

√x7ᵗʰ **T75.00** **Unspecified effects of lightning** ▽
Struck by lightning NOS

√x7ᵗʰ **T75.01** **Shock due to being struck by lightning**

√x7ᵗʰ **T75.09** **Other effects of lightning**
Use additional code for other effects of lightning

√x7ᵗʰ **T75.1** Unspecified effects of drowning and nonfatal submersion ▽
Immersion
EXCLUDES 1 specified effects of drowning—code to effects

√5ᵗʰ **T75.2** Effects of vibration

√x7ᵗʰ **T75.20** **Unspecified effects of vibration** ▽

√x7ᵗʰ **T75.21** **Pneumatic hammer syndrome**

√x7ᵗʰ **T75.22** **Traumatic vasospastic syndrome**

√x7ᵗʰ **T75.23** **Vertigo from infrasound**
EXCLUDES 1 vertigo NOS (R42)

√x7ᵗʰ **T75.29** **Other effects of vibration**

√x7ᵗʰ **T75.3** Motion sickness
Airsickness
Seasickness
Travel sickness
Use additional external cause code to identify vehicle or type of motion (Y92.81-, Y93.5-)

√x7ᵗʰ **T75.4** **Electrocution**
Shock from electric current
Shock from electroshock gun (taser)

√5ᵗʰ **T75.8** Other specified effects of external causes

√x7ᵗʰ **T75.81** **Effects of abnormal gravitation [G] forces**

√x7ᵗʰ **T75.82** **Effects of weightlessness**

√x7ᵗʰ **T75.89** **Other specified effects of external causes**

√4ᵗʰ **T76** **Adult and child abuse, neglect and other maltreatment, suspected**
Use additional code, if applicable, to identify any associated current injury
EXCLUDES 1 adult and child maltreatment, confirmed (T74.-)
suspected abuse and maltreatment in pregnancy (O9A.3-, O9A.4-, O9A.5-)
suspected adult physical abuse, ruled out (Z04.71)
suspected adult sexual abuse, ruled out (Z04.41)
suspected child physical abuse, ruled out (Z04.72)
suspected child sexual abuse, ruled out (Z04.42)

The appropriate 7th character is to be added to each code from category T76.
A   initial encounter
D   subsequent encounter
S   sequela

√5ᵗʰ **T76.0** Neglect or abandonment, suspected

√x7ᵗʰ **T76.01** Adult neglect or abandonment, suspected 🅐

√x7ᵗʰ **T76.02** Child neglect or abandonment, suspected 🅟

√5ᵗʰ **T76.1** Physical abuse, suspected

√x7ᵗʰ **T76.11** Adult physical abuse, suspected 🅐

√x7ᵗʰ **T76.12** Child physical abuse, suspected 🅟

√5ᵗʰ **T76.2** Sexual abuse, suspected
Rape, suspected
Sexual abuse, suspected
EXCLUDES 1 alleged abuse, ruled out (Z04.7)

√x7ᵗʰ **T76.21** Adult sexual abuse, suspected 🅐

√x7ᵗʰ **T76.22** Child sexual abuse, suspected 🅟

√5ᵗʰ **T76.3** Psychological abuse, suspected

√x7ᵗʰ **T76.31** Adult psychological abuse, suspected 🅐

√x7ᵗʰ **T76.32** Child psychological abuse, suspected 🅟

√5ᵗʰ **T76.9** Unspecified maltreatment, suspected

√x7ᵗʰ **T76.91** Unspecified adult maltreatment, suspected 🅐▽

√x7ᵗʰ **T76.92** Unspecified child maltreatment, suspected 🅟▽

√4ᵗʰ **T78** **Adverse effects, not elsewhere classified**
EXCLUDES 2 complications of surgical and medical care NEC (T80-T88)

The appropriate 7th character is to be added to each code from category T78.
A   initial encounter
D   subsequent encounter
S   sequela

√5ᵗʰ **T78.0** Anaphylactic reaction due to food
Anaphylactic reaction due to adverse food reaction
Anaphylactic shock or reaction due to nonpoisonous foods
Anaphylactoid reaction due to food

√x7ᵗʰ **T78.00** **Anaphylactic reaction due to unspecified food** ▽

√x7ᵗʰ **T78.01** **Anaphylactic reaction due to** peanuts

√x7ᵗʰ **T78.02** **Anaphylactic reaction due to** shellfish (crustaceans)

√x7ᵗʰ **T78.03** **Anaphylactic reaction due to** other fish

√x7ᵗʰ **T78.04** **Anaphylactic reaction due to** fruits and vegetables

√x7ᵗʰ **T78.05** **Anaphylactic reaction due to** tree nuts and seeds
EXCLUDES 1 anaphylactic reaction due to peanuts (T78.01)

√x7ᵗʰ **T78.06** **Anaphylactic reaction due to** food additives

√x7ᵗʰ **T78.07** **Anaphylactic reaction due to** milk and dairy products

√x7ᵗʰ **T78.08** **Anaphylactic reaction due to** eggs

√x7ᵗʰ **T78.09** **Anaphylactic reaction due to other** food products

√x 7ᵗʰ **T78.1** **Other adverse food reactions, not elsewhere classified**
Use additional code to identify the type of reaction
  EXCLUDES 1　anaphylactic reaction or shock due to adverse food
　　　　　　　reaction (T78.0-)
　　　　　　anaphylactic reaction due to food (T78.0-)
　　　　　　bacterial food borne intoxications (A05.-)
  EXCLUDES 2　allergic and dietetic gastroenteritis and colitis (K52.2)
　　　　　　allergic rhinitis due to food (J30.5)
　　　　　　dermatitis due to food in contact with skin (L23.6, L24.6,
　　　　　　　L25.4)
　　　　　　dermatitis due to ingested food (L27.2)

√x 7ᵗʰ **T78.2** **Anaphylactic shock, unspecified**　　　　　　　　　▽
Allergic shock
Anaphylactic reaction
Anaphylaxis
  EXCLUDES 1　anaphylactic reaction or shock due to adverse effect of
　　　　　　correct medicinal substance properly
　　　　　　administered (T88.6)
　　　　　　anaphylactic reaction or shock due to adverse food
　　　　　　reaction (T78.0-)
　　　　　　anaphylactic reaction or shock due to serum (T80.5-)

√x 7ᵗʰ **T78.3** **Angioneurotic edema**
Allergic angioedema
Giant urticaria
Quincke's edema
  EXCLUDES 1　serum urticaria (T80.6-)
　　　　　　urticaria (L50.-)

√ 5ᵗʰ **T78.4** **Other and unspecified allergy**
  EXCLUDES 1　specified types of allergic reaction such as:
　　　　　　allergic diarrhea (K52.2)
　　　　　　allergic gastroenteritis and colitis (K52.2)
　　　　　　dermatitis (L23-L25, L27-)
　　　　　　hay fever (J30.1)

　√x 7ᵗʰ **T78.40** **Allergy, unspecified**　　　　　　　　　　　▽
　　　　Allergic reaction NOS
　　　　Hypersensitivity NOS

　√x 7ᵗʰ **T78.41** **Arthus phenomenon**
　　　　Arthus reaction

　√x 7ᵗʰ **T78.49** **Other allergy**

√x 7ᵗʰ **T78.8** **Other adverse effects, not elsewhere classified**

Certain early complications of trauma (T79)

√ 4ᵗʰ **T79** **Certain early complications of trauma, not elsewhere classified**
  EXCLUDES 2　acute respiratory distress syndrome (J80)
　　　　　　complications occurring during or following medical procedures
　　　　　　　(T80-T88)
　　　　　　complications of surgical and medical care NEC (T80-T88)
　　　　　　newborn respiratory distress syndrome (P22.0)

　The appropriate 7th character is to be added to each code from
　category T79.
　A　　initial encounter
　D　　subsequent encounter
　S　　sequela

√x 7ᵗʰ **T79.0** **Air embolism (traumatic)**　　　　　　　　　　CC
  EXCLUDES 1　air embolism complicating abortion or ectopic or molar
　　　　　　　pregnancy (O00-O07, O08.2)
　　　　　　air embolism complicating pregnancy, childbirth and
　　　　　　　the puerperium (O88.0)
　　　　　　air embolism following infusion, transfusion, and
　　　　　　　therapeutic injection (T80.0)
　　　　　　air embolism following procedure NEC (T81.7-)
　RIC Excl 7th Character A: 02 Traumatic brain injury; 03
　Non-traumatic brain injury

√x 7ᵗʰ **T79.1** **Fat embolism (traumatic)**　　　　　　　　　　CC
  EXCLUDES 1　fat embolism complicating:
　　　　　　abortion or ectopic or molar pregnancy (O00-O07,
　　　　　　　O08.2)
　　　　　　pregnancy, childbirth and the puerperium (O88.8)
　RIC Excl 7th Character A: 02 Traumatic brain injury; 03
　Non-traumatic brain injury

√x 7ᵗʰ **T79.2** **Traumatic secondary and recurrent hemorrhage and seroma**

√x 7ᵗʰ **T79.4** **Traumatic shock**
Shock (immediate) (delayed) following injury
  EXCLUDES 1　anaphylactic shock due to adverse food reaction
　　　　　　　(T78.0-)
　　　　　　anaphylactic shock due to correct medicinal substance
　　　　　　　properly administered (T88.6)
　　　　　　anaphylactic shock due to serum (T80.5-)
　　　　　　anaphylactic shock NOS (T78.2)
　　　　　　anesthetic shock (T88.2)
　　　　　　electric shock (T75.4)
　　　　　　nontraumatic shock NEC (R57.-)
　　　　　　obstetric shock (O75.1)
　　　　　　postprocedural shock (T81.1-)
　　　　　　septic shock (R65.21)
　　　　　　shock complicating abortion or ectopic or molar
　　　　　　　pregnancy (O00-O07, O08.3)
　　　　　　shock due to lightning (T75.01)
　　　　　　shock NOS (R57.9)

√x 7ᵗʰ **T79.5** **Traumatic anuria**　　　　　　　　　　　　　CC
Crush syndrome
Renal failure following crushing

√x 7ᵗʰ **T79.6** **Traumatic ischemia of muscle**
Traumatic rhabdomyolysis
Volkmann's ischemic contracture
  EXCLUDES 2　anterior tibial syndrome (M76.8)
　　　　　　compartment syndrome (traumatic) (T79.A-)
　　　　　　nontraumatic ischemia of muscle (M62.2-)

√x 7ᵗʰ **T79.7** **Traumatic subcutaneous emphysema**
  EXCLUDES 1　emphysema NOS (J43)
　　　　　　emphysema (subcutaneous) resulting from a procedure
　　　　　　　(T81.82)

√ 5ᵗʰ **T79.A** **Traumatic compartment syndrome**
  EXCLUDES 1　fibromyalgia (M79.7)
　　　　　　nontraumatic compartment syndrome (M79.A-)
　　　　　　traumatic ischemic infarction of muscle (T79.6)

　√x 7ᵗʰ **T79.A0** **Compartment syndrome, unspecified**　　　▽
　　　　Compartment syndrome NOS

　√ 6ᵗʰ **T79.A1** **Traumatic compartment syndrome of upper
　　　　extremity**
　　　　Traumatic compartment syndrome of shoulder, arm,
　　　　　forearm, wrist, hand, and fingers

　　√ 7ᵗʰ **T79.A11** **Traumatic compartment syndrome of
　　　　　right upper extremity**

　　√ 7ᵗʰ **T79.A12** **Traumatic compartment syndrome of left
　　　　　upper extremity**

　　√ 7ᵗʰ **T79.A19** **Traumatic compartment syndrome of　▽
　　　　　unspecified upper extremity**

　√ 6ᵗʰ **T79.A2** **Traumatic compartment syndrome of lower
　　　　extremity**
　　　　Traumatic compartment syndrome of hip, buttock,
　　　　　thigh, leg, foot, and toes

　　√ 7ᵗʰ **T79.A21** **Traumatic compartment syndrome of
　　　　　right lower extremity**

　　√ 7ᵗʰ **T79.A22** **Traumatic compartment syndrome of left
　　　　　lower extremity**

　　√ 7ᵗʰ **T79.A29** **Traumatic compartment syndrome of　▽
　　　　　unspecified lower extremity**

　√x 7ᵗʰ **T79.A3** **Traumatic compartment syndrome of abdomen**

　√x 7ᵗʰ **T79.A9** **Traumatic compartment syndrome of other sites**

√x 7ᵗʰ **T79.8** **Other early complications of trauma**

√x 7ᵗʰ **T79.9** **Unspecified early complication of trauma**　　　　▽

N Newborn　　P Pediatric　　M Maternity　　A Adult　　RIC RIC Dx　　NCDx Noncancer Dx　　PDx Primary Dx　　CC RIC CC Condition　　▶◀ Revised Text　　● New Code　　▲ Revised Code Title

1034　　ICD-10-CM 2016

Complications of surgical and medical care, not elsewhere classified (T80-T88)

Use additional code for adverse effect, if applicable, to identify drug (T36-T50 with fifth or sixth character 5)

Use additional code(s) to identify the specified condition resulting from the complication

Use additional code to identify devices involved and details of circumstances (Y62-Y82)

EXCLUDES 2 *any encounters with medical care for postprocedural conditions in which no complications are present, such as:*
    artificial opening status (Z93.-)
    closure of external stoma (Z43.-)
    fitting and adjustment of external prosthetic device (Z44.-)
  burns and corrosions from local applications and irradiation (T20-T32)
  complications of surgical procedures during pregnancy, childbirth and the puerperium (O00-O9A)
  mechanical complication of respirator [ventilator] (J95.850)
  poisoning and toxic effects of drugs and chemicals (T36-T65 with fifth or sixth character 1-4 or 6)
  postprocedural fever (R50.82)
  specified complications classified elsewhere, such as:
    cerebrospinal fluid leak from spinal puncture (G97.0)
    colostomy malfunction (K94.0-)
    disorders of fluid and electrolyte imbalance (E86-E87)
    functional disturbances following cardiac surgery (I97.0-I97.1)
    intraoperative and postprocedural complications of specified body systems (D78.-, E36.-, E89.-, G97.3-, G97.4, H59.3-, H59.-, H95.2-, H95.3, I97.4-, I97.5, J95.6-, J95.7, K91.6-, L76.-, M96.-, N99.-)
    ostomy complications (J95.0-, K94.-, N99.5-)
    postgastric surgery syndromes (K91.1)
    postlaminectomy syndrome NEC (M96.1)
    postmastectomy lymphedema syndrome (I97.2)
    postsurgical blind-loop syndrome (K91.2)
    ventilator associated pneumonia (J95.851)

  AHA: 2015, 1Q, 15

✓4ᵗʰ T80 Complications following infusion, transfusion and therapeutic injection

INCLUDES complications following perfusion

EXCLUDES 2 *bone marrow transplant rejection (T86.01)*
  febrile nonhemolytic transfusion reaction (R50.84)
  fluid overload due to transfusion (E87.71)
  posttransfusion purpura (D69.51)
  transfusion associated circulatory overload (TACO) (E87.71)
  transfusion (red blood cell) associated hemochromatosis (E83.111)
  transfusion related acute lung injury (TRALI) (J95.84)

> The appropriate 7th character is to be added to each code from category T80.
> A   initial encounter
> D   subsequent encounter
> S   sequela

[9] ✓x7ᵗʰ **T80.0 Air embolism following infusion, transfusion and therapeutic injection** CC NC Dx
  RIC Excl 7th Character A: 03 Non-traumatic brain injury

✓x7ᵗʰ **T80.1 Vascular complications following infusion, transfusion and therapeutic injection**
  Use additional code to identify the vascular complication
  EXCLUDES 2 *extravasation of vesicant agent (T80.81-)*
    infiltration of vesicant agent (T80.81-)
    postprocedural vascular complications (T81.7-)
    vascular complications specified as due to prosthetic devices, implants and grafts (T82.8-, T83.8, T84.8-, T85.8)

✓5ᵗʰ **T80.2 Infections following infusion, transfusion and therapeutic injection**
  Use additional code to identify the specific infection, such as: sepsis (A41.9)
  Use additional code (R65.2-) to identify severe sepsis, if applicable
  EXCLUDES 2 *infections specified as due to prosthetic devices, implants and grafts (T82.6-T82.7, T83.5-T83.6, T84.5-T84.7, T85.7)*
    postprocedural infections (T81.4)

  ✓6ᵗʰ **T80.21 Infection due to central venous catheter**

✓7ᵗʰ **T80.211 Bloodstream infection due to central venous catheter** CC
  Catheter-related bloodstream infection (CRBSI) NOS
  Central line-associated bloodstream infection (CLABSI)
  Bloodstream infection due to Hickman catheter
  Bloodstream infection due to peripherally inserted central catheter (PICC)
  Bloodstream infection due to portacath (port-a-cath)
  Bloodstream infection due to triple lumen catheter
  Bloodstream infection due to umbilical venous catheter

✓7ᵗʰ **T80.212 Local infection due to central venous catheter** CC
  Exit or insertion site infection
  Local infection due to Hickman catheter
  Local infection due to peripherally inserted central catheter (PICC)
  Local infection due to portacath (port-a-cath)
  Local infection due to triple lumen catheter
  Local infection due to umbilical venous catheter
  Port or reservoir infection
  Tunnel infection

✓7ᵗʰ **T80.218 Other infection due to central venous catheter** CC
  Other central line-associated infection
  Other infection due to Hickman catheter
  Other infection due to peripherally inserted central catheter (PICC)
  Other infection due to portacath (port-a-cath)
  Other infection due to triple lumen catheter
  Other infection due to umbilical venous catheter

✓7ᵗʰ **T80.219 Unspecified infection due to central venous catheter** CC ▽
  Central line-associated infection NOS
  Unspecified infection due to Hickman catheter
  Unspecified infection due to peripherally inserted central catheter (PICC)
  Unspecified infection due to portacath (port-a-cath)
  Unspecified infection due to triple lumen catheter
  Unspecified infection due to umbilical venous catheter

✓x7ᵗʰ **T80.22 Acute infection following transfusion, infusion, or injection of blood and blood products**

✓x7ᵗʰ **T80.29 Infection following other infusion, transfusion and therapeutic injection**

✓5ᵗʰ **T80.3 ABO incompatibility reaction due to transfusion of blood or blood products**
  EXCLUDES 1 *minor blood group antigens reactions (Duffy) (E) (K(ell)) (Kidd) (Lewis) (M) (N) (P) (S) (T80.A)*

✓x7ᵗʰ **T80.30 ABO incompatibility reaction due to transfusion of blood or blood products, unspecified** ▽
  ABO incompatibility blood transfusion NOS
  Reaction to ABO incompatibility from transfusion NOS

✓6ᵗʰ **T80.31 ABO incompatibility with hemolytic transfusion reaction**

✓7ᵗʰ **T80.310 ABO incompatibility with acute hemolytic transfusion reaction**
  ABO incompatibility with hemolytic transfusion reaction less than 24 hours after transfusion
  Acute hemolytic transfusion reaction (AHTR) due to ABO incompatibility

✓7ᵗʰ **T80.311 ABO incompatibility with delayed hemolytic transfusion reaction**
  ABO incompatibility with hemolytic transfusion reaction 24 hours or more after transfusion
  Delayed hemolytic transfusion reaction (DHTR) due to ABO incompatibility

---

[9] Hospice Noncancer Diagnosis only when reported using an appropriate 7th character indicating a subsequent encounter or sequela

☑ Add'l Character Required ✓x7ᵗʰ Placeholder Alert RUG IV Special Care High Dx RUG IV Clinically Complex Dx RUG IV Special Care Low Dx Manifestation Code Other Specified Code ▽ Unspecified Code

Chapter 19. Injury, Poisoning and Certain Other Consequences of External Causes

T80.319–T80.92

☑7ᵗʰ **T80.319 ABO incompatibility with hemolytic transfusion reaction, unspecified** ▽
ABO incompatibility with hemolytic transfusion reaction at unspecified time after transfusion
Hemolytic transfusion reaction (HTR) due to ABO incompatibility NOS

☑x7ᵗʰ **T80.39 Other ABO incompatibility reaction due to transfusion of blood or blood products**
Delayed serologic transfusion reaction (DSTR) from ABO incompatibility
Other ABO incompatible blood transfusion
Other reaction to ABO incompatible blood transfusion

☑x7ᵗʰ **T80.4 Rh incompatibility reaction due to transfusion of blood or blood products**
Reaction due to incompatibility of Rh antigens (C) (c) (D) (E) (e)

☑x7ᵗʰ **T80.40 Rh incompatibility reaction due to transfusion of blood or blood products, unspecified** ▽
Reaction due to Rh factor in transfusion NOS
Rh incompatible blood transfusion NOS

☑6ᵗʰ **T80.41 Rh incompatibility with hemolytic transfusion reaction**

☑7ᵗʰ **T80.410 Rh incompatibility with acute hemolytic transfusion reaction**
Acute hemolytic transfusion reaction (AHTR) due to Rh incompatibility
Rh incompatibility with hemolytic transfusion reaction less than 24 hours after transfusion

☑7ᵗʰ **T80.411 Rh incompatibility with delayed hemolytic transfusion reaction**
Delayed hemolytic transfusion reaction (DHTR) due to Rh incompatibility
Rh incompatibility with hemolytic transfusion reaction 24 hours or more after transfusion

☑7ᵗʰ **T80.419 Rh incompatibility with hemolytic transfusion reaction, unspecified** ▽
Hemolytic transfusion reaction (HTR) due to Rh incompatibility NOS
Rh incompatibility with hemolytic transfusion reaction at unspecified time after transfusion

☑x7ᵗʰ **T80.49 Other Rh incompatibility reaction due to transfusion of blood or blood products**
Delayed serologic transfusion reaction (DSTR) from Rh incompatibility
Other reaction to Rh incompatible blood transfusion

☑5ᵗʰ **T80.A Non-ABO incompatibility reaction due to transfusion of blood or blood products**
Reaction due to incompatibility of minor antigens (Duffy) (Kell) (Kidd) (Lewis) (M) (N) (P) (S)

☑x7ᵗʰ **T80.A0 Non-ABO incompatibility reaction due to transfusion of blood or blood products, unspecified** ▽
Non-ABO antigen incompatibility reaction from transfusion NOS

☑6ᵗʰ **T80.A1 Non-ABO incompatibility with hemolytic transfusion reaction**

☑7ᵗʰ **T80.A10 Non-ABO incompatibility with acute hemolytic transfusion reaction**
Acute hemolytic transfusion reaction (AHTR) due to non-ABO incompatibility
Non-ABO incompatibility with hemolytic transfusion reaction less than 24 hours after transfusion

☑7ᵗʰ **T80.A11 Non-ABO incompatibility with delayed hemolytic transfusion reaction**
Delayed hemolytic transfusion reaction (DHTR) due to non-ABO incompatibility
Non-ABO incompatibility with hemolytic transfusion reaction 24 or more hours after transfusion

☑7ᵗʰ **T80.A19 Non-ABO incompatibility with hemolytic transfusion reaction, unspecified** ▽
Hemolytic transfusion reaction (HTR) due to non-ABO incompatibility NOS
Non-ABO incompatibility with hemolytic transfusion reaction at unspecified time after transfusion

☑x7ᵗʰ **T80.A9 Other non-ABO incompatibility reaction due to transfusion of blood or blood products**
Delayed serologic transfusion reaction (DSTR) from non-ABO incompatibility
Other reaction to non-ABO incompatible blood transfusion

☑5ᵗʰ **T80.5 Anaphylactic reaction due to serum**
Allergic shock due to serum
Anaphylactic shock due to serum
Anaphylactoid reaction due to serum
Anaphylaxis due to serum
EXCLUDES 1 *ABO incompatibility reaction due to transfusion of blood or blood products (T80.3-)*
allergic reaction or shock NOS (T78.2)
anaphylactic reaction or shock NOS (T78.2)
anaphylactic reaction or shock due to adverse effect of correct medicinal substance properly administered (T88.6)
other serum reaction (T80.6-)

☑x7ᵗʰ **T80.51 Anaphylactic reaction due to administration of blood and blood products**

☑x7ᵗʰ **T80.52 Anaphylactic reaction due to vaccination**

☑x7ᵗʰ **T80.59 Anaphylactic reaction due to other serum**

☑5ᵗʰ **T80.6 Other serum reactions**
Intoxication by serum
Protein sickness
Serum rash
Serum sickness
Serum urticaria
EXCLUDES 2 *serum hepatitis (B16.-)*

☑x7ᵗʰ **T80.61 Other serum reaction due to administration of blood and blood products**

☑x7ᵗʰ **T80.62 Other serum reaction due to vaccination**

☑x7ᵗʰ **T80.69 Other serum reaction due to other serum**

☑5ᵗʰ **T80.8 Other complications following infusion, transfusion and therapeutic injection**

☑6ᵗʰ **T80.81 Extravasation of vesicant agent**
Infiltration of vesicant agent

☑7ᵗʰ **T80.810 Extravasation of vesicant antineoplastic chemotherapy**
Infiltration of vesicant antineoplastic chemotherapy

☑7ᵗʰ **T80.818 Extravasation of other vesicant agent**
Infiltration of other vesicant agent

☑x7ᵗʰ **T80.89 Other complications following infusion, transfusion and therapeutic injection**
Delayed serologic transfusion reaction (DSTR), unspecified incompatibility
Use additional code to identify graft-versus-host reaction, if applicable, (D89.81-)

☑5ᵗʰ **T80.9 Unspecified complication following infusion, transfusion and therapeutic injection**

☑x7ᵗʰ **T80.90 Unspecified complication following infusion and therapeutic injection** ▽

☑6ᵗʰ **T80.91 Hemolytic transfusion reaction, unspecified incompatibility**
EXCLUDES 1 *ABO incompatibility with hemolytic transfusion reaction (T80.31-)*
Non-ABO incompatibility with hemolytic transfusion reaction (T80.A1-)
Rh incompatibility with hemolytic transfusion reaction (T80.41-)

☑7ᵗʰ **T80.910 Acute hemolytic transfusion reaction, unspecified incompatibility** ▽

☑7ᵗʰ **T80.911 Delayed hemolytic transfusion reaction, unspecified incompatibility** ▽

☑7ᵗʰ **T80.919 Hemolytic transfusion reaction, unspecified incompatibility, unspecified as acute or delayed** ▽
Hemolytic transfusion reaction NOS

☑x7ᵗʰ **T80.92 Unspecified transfusion reaction** ▽
Transfusion reaction NOS

N Newborn   P Pediatric   M Maternity   A Adult   **RIC** RIC Dx   **NCDx** Noncancer Dx   **PDx** Primary Dx   **CC** RIC CC Condition   ►◄ Revised Text   ● New Code   ▲ Revised Code Title

1036   ICD-10-CM 2016

☑4ᵗʰ **T81** **Complications of procedures, not elsewhere classified**

Use additional code for adverse effect, if applicable, to identify drug (T36-T50 with fifth or sixth character 5)

EXCLUDES 2 *complications following immunization (T88.0-T88.1)*
complications following infusion, transfusion and therapeutic injection (T80.-)
complications of transplanted organs and tissue (T86.-)
specified complications classified elsewhere, such as:
  complication of prosthetic devices, implants and grafts (T82-T85)
  dermatitis due to drugs and medicaments (L23.3, L24.4, L25.1, L27.0-L27.1)
  endosseous dental implant failure (M27.6-)
  floppy iris syndrome (IFIS) (intraoperative) (H21.81)
  intraoperative and postprocedural complications of specific body system (D78.-, E36.-, E89.-, G97.3-, G97.4, H59.3-, H59.-, H95.2-, H95.3, I97.4-, I97.5, J95, K91.-, L76.-, M96.-, N99.-)
  ostomy complications (J95.0-, K94.-, N99.5-)
  plateau iris syndrome (post-iridectomy) (postprocedural) (H21.82)
  poisoning and toxic effects of drugs and chemicals (T36-T65 with fifth or sixth character 1-4 or 6)

> The appropriate 7th character is to be added to each code from category T81.
> A   initial encounter
> D   subsequent encounter
> S   sequela

☑5ᵗʰ **T81.1** **Postprocedural shock**

Shock during or resulting from a procedure, not elsewhere classified

EXCLUDES 1 *anaphylactic shock due to correct substance properly administered (T88.6)*
anaphylactic shock due to serum (T80.5-)
anaphylactic shock NOS (T78.2)
anesthetic shock (T88.2)
electric shock (T75.4)
obstetric shock (O75.1)
septic shock (R65.21)
shock following abortion or ectopic or molar pregnancy (O00-O07, O08.3)
traumatic shock (T79.4)

  ☑x7ᵗʰ **T81.10** **Postprocedural shock unspecified**   cc ▽

Collapse NOS during or resulting from a procedure, not elsewhere classified
Postprocedural failure of peripheral circulation
Postprocedural shock NOS

  ☑x7ᵗʰ **T81.11** **Postprocedural cardiogenic shock**   cc

  ☑x7ᵗʰ **T81.12** **Postprocedural septic shock**   cc

Postprocedural endotoxic shock during or resulting from a procedure, not elsewhere classified
Postprocedural gram-negative shock during or resulting from a procedure, not elsewhere classified
Code first underlying infection
Use additional code, to identify any associated acute organ dysfunction, if applicable

  ☑x7ᵗʰ **T81.19** **Other postprocedural shock**   cc

Postprocedural hypovolemic shock

☑5ᵗʰ **T81.3** **Disruption of wound, not elsewhere classified**

Disruption of any suture materials or other closure methods

EXCLUDES 1 *breakdown (mechanical) of permanent sutures (T85.612)*
displacement of permanent sutures (T85.622)
disruption of cesarean delivery wound (O90.0)
disruption of perineal obstetric wound (O90.1)
mechanical complication of permanent sutures NEC (T85.692)

AHA: 2014, 1Q, 23

7 ☑x7ᵗʰ **T81.30** **Disruption of wound, unspecified**   cc ▽

Disruption of wound NOS

7 ☑x7ᵗʰ **T81.31** **Disruption of external operation (surgical) wound, not elsewhere classified**   cc

Dehiscence of operation wound NOS
Disruption of operation wound NOS
Disruption or dehiscence of closure of cornea
Disruption or dehiscence of closure of mucosa
Disruption or dehiscence of closure of skin and subcutaneous tissue
Full-thickness skin disruption or dehiscence
Superficial disruption or dehiscence of operation wound

EXCLUDES 1 *dehiscence of amputation stump (T87.81)*

☑x7ᵗʰ **T81.32** **Disruption of internal operation (surgical) wound, not elsewhere classified**   cc

Deep disruption or dehiscence of operation wound NOS
Disruption or dehiscence of closure of internal organ or other internal tissue
Disruption or dehiscence of closure of muscle or muscle flap
Disruption or dehiscence of closure of ribs or rib cage
Disruption or dehiscence of closure of skull or craniotomy
Disruption or dehiscence of closure of sternum or sternotomy
Disruption or dehiscence of closure of tendon or ligament
Disruption or dehiscence of closure of superficial or muscular fascia

7 ☑x7ᵗʰ **T81.33** **Disruption of traumatic injury wound repair**   cc

Disruption or dehiscence of closure of traumatic laceration (external) (internal)

7 ☑x7ᵗʰ **T81.4** **Infection following a procedure**   cc

Intra-abdominal abscess following a procedure
Postprocedural infection, not elsewhere classified
Sepsis following a procedure
Stitch abscess following a procedure
Subphrenic abscess following a procedure
Wound abscess following a procedure
Use additional code to identify infection
Use additional code (R65.2-) to identify severe sepsis, if applicable

EXCLUDES 1 *obstetric surgical wound infection (O86.0)*
postprocedural fever NOS (R50.82)
postprocedural retroperitoneal abscess (K68.11)

EXCLUDES 2 *bleb associated endophthalmitis (H59.4-)*
infection due to infusion, transfusion and therapeutic injection (T80.2-)
infection due to prosthetic devices, implants and grafts (T82.6-T82.7, T83.5-T83.6, T84.5-T84.7, T85.7)

AHA: 2014, 1Q, 23

☑5ᵗʰ **T81.5** **Complications of foreign body accidentally left in body following procedure**

AHA: 2014, 4Q, 24

☑6ᵗʰ **T81.50** **Unspecified complication of foreign body accidentally left in body following procedure**

  ☑7ᵗʰ **T81.500** **Unspecified complication of foreign body accidentally left in body following surgical operation** ▽

  ☑7ᵗʰ **T81.501** **Unspecified complication of foreign body accidentally left in body following infusion or transfusion** ▽

  ☑7ᵗʰ **T81.502** **Unspecified complication of foreign body accidentally left in body following kidney dialysis** ▽

  ☑7ᵗʰ **T81.503** **Unspecified complication of foreign body accidentally left in body following injection or immunization** ▽

  ☑7ᵗʰ **T81.504** **Unspecified complication of foreign body accidentally left in body following endoscopic examination** ▽

  ☑7ᵗʰ **T81.505** **Unspecified complication of foreign body accidentally left in body following heart catheterization** ▽

  ☑7ᵗʰ **T81.506** **Unspecified complication of foreign body accidentally left in body following aspiration, puncture or other catheterization** ▽

---

⁷ Clinically Complex = With 7th character indicating a subsequent encounter

Chapter 19. Injury, Poisoning and Certain Other Consequences of External Causes

✓7ᵗʰ **T81.507 Unspecified complication of foreign body accidentally left in body following** removal of catheter or packing ▽

✓7ᵗʰ **T81.508 Unspecified complication of foreign body accidentally left in body following other procedure** ▽

✓7ᵗʰ **T81.509 Unspecified complication of foreign body accidentally left in body following unspecified procedure** ▽

✓6ᵗʰ **T81.51** Adhesions **due to foreign body accidentally left in body following procedure**

     ✓7ᵗʰ **T81.510 Adhesions due to foreign body accidentally left in body following** surgical operation

     ✓7ᵗʰ **T81.511 Adhesions due to foreign body accidentally left in body following** infusion or transfusion

     ✓7ᵗʰ **T81.512 Adhesions due to foreign body accidentally left in body following** kidney dialysis

     ✓7ᵗʰ **T81.513 Adhesions due to foreign body accidentally left in body following** injection or immunization

     ✓7ᵗʰ **T81.514 Adhesions due to foreign body accidentally left in body following** endoscopic examination

     ✓7ᵗʰ **T81.515 Adhesions due to foreign body accidentally left in body following** heart catheterization

     ✓7ᵗʰ **T81.516 Adhesions due to foreign body accidentally left in body following** aspiration, puncture or other catheterization

     ✓7ᵗʰ **T81.517 Adhesions due to foreign body accidentally left in body following** removal of catheter or packing

     ✓7ᵗʰ **T81.518 Adhesions due to foreign body accidentally left in body following other procedure**

     ✓7ᵗʰ **T81.519 Adhesions due to foreign body accidentally left in body following unspecified procedure** ▽

✓6ᵗʰ **T81.52** Obstruction **due to foreign body accidentally left in body following procedure**

     ✓7ᵗʰ **T81.520 Obstruction due to foreign body accidentally left in body following** surgical operation

     ✓7ᵗʰ **T81.521 Obstruction due to foreign body accidentally left in body following** infusion or transfusion

     ✓7ᵗʰ **T81.522 Obstruction due to foreign body accidentally left in body following** kidney dialysis

     ✓7ᵗʰ **T81.523 Obstruction due to foreign body accidentally left in body following** injection or immunization

     ✓7ᵗʰ **T81.524 Obstruction due to foreign body accidentally left in body following** endoscopic examination

     ✓7ᵗʰ **T81.525 Obstruction due to foreign body accidentally left in body following** heart catheterization

     ✓7ᵗʰ **T81.526 Obstruction due to foreign body accidentally left in body following** aspiration, puncture or other catheterization

     ✓7ᵗʰ **T81.527 Obstruction due to foreign body accidentally left in body following** removal of catheter or packing

     ✓7ᵗʰ **T81.528 Obstruction due to foreign body accidentally left in body following other procedure**

     ✓7ᵗʰ **T81.529 Obstruction due to foreign body accidentally left in body following unspecified procedure** ▽

✓6ᵗʰ **T81.53** Perforation **due to foreign body accidentally left in body following procedure**

     ✓7ᵗʰ **T81.530 Perforation due to foreign body accidentally left in body following** surgical operation

     ✓7ᵗʰ **T81.531 Perforation due to foreign body accidentally left in body following** infusion or transfusion

     ✓7ᵗʰ **T81.532 Perforation due to foreign body accidentally left in body following** kidney dialysis

     ✓7ᵗʰ **T81.533 Perforation due to foreign body accidentally left in body following** injection or immunization

     ✓7ᵗʰ **T81.534 Perforation due to foreign body accidentally left in body following** endoscopic examination

     ✓7ᵗʰ **T81.535 Perforation due to foreign body accidentally left in body following** heart catheterization

     ✓7ᵗʰ **T81.536 Perforation due to foreign body accidentally left in body following** aspiration, puncture or other catheterization

     ✓7ᵗʰ **T81.537 Perforation due to foreign body accidentally left in body following** removal of catheter or packing

     ✓7ᵗʰ **T81.538 Perforation due to foreign body accidentally left in body following other procedure**

     ✓7ᵗʰ **T81.539 Perforation due to foreign body accidentally left in body following unspecified procedure** ▽

✓6ᵗʰ **T81.59** Other **complications of foreign body accidentally left in body following procedure**

     EXCLUDES 2   *obstruction or perforation due to prosthetic devices and implants intentionally left in body (T82.0-T82.5, T83.0-T83.4, T83.7, T84.0-T84.4, T85.0-T85.6)*

     ✓7ᵗʰ **T81.590 Other complications of foreign body accidentally left in body following** surgical operation

     ✓7ᵗʰ **T81.591 Other complications of foreign body accidentally left in body following** infusion or transfusion

     ✓7ᵗʰ **T81.592 Other complications of foreign body accidentally left in body following** kidney dialysis

     ✓7ᵗʰ **T81.593 Other complications of foreign body accidentally left in body following** injection or immunization

     ✓7ᵗʰ **T81.594 Other complications of foreign body accidentally left in body following** endoscopic examination

     ✓7ᵗʰ **T81.595 Other complications of foreign body accidentally left in body following** heart catheterization

     ✓7ᵗʰ **T81.596 Other complications of foreign body accidentally left in body following** aspiration, puncture or other catheterization

     ✓7ᵗʰ **T81.597 Other complications of foreign body accidentally left in body following** removal of catheter or packing

     ✓7ᵗʰ **T81.598 Other complications of foreign body accidentally left in body following other procedure**

     ✓7ᵗʰ **T81.599 Other complications of foreign body accidentally left in body following unspecified procedure** ▽

✓5ᵗʰ **T81.6 Acute reaction to foreign substance accidentally left during a procedure**

     EXCLUDES 2   *complications of foreign body accidentally left in body cavity or operation wound following procedure (T81.5-)*

     ✓x7ᵗʰ **T81.60 Unspecified acute reaction to foreign substance accidentally left during a procedure** ▽

Ⓝ Newborn   Ⓟ Pediatric   Ⓜ Maternity   Ⓐ Adult   RIC RIC Dx   NCDx Noncancer Dx   PDx Primary Dx   CC RIC CC Condition   ▶◀ Revised Text   ● New Code   ▲ Revised Code Title

1038   ICD-10-CM 2016

√x7ᵗʰ **T81.61** Aseptic peritonitis **due to foreign substance accidentally left during a procedure**
    Chemical peritonitis

√x7ᵗʰ **T81.69 Other acute reaction to foreign substance accidentally left during a procedure**

√5ᵗʰ **T81.7 Vascular complications following a procedure, not elsewhere classified**
    Air embolism following procedure NEC
    Phlebitis or thrombophlebitis resulting from a procedure

    EXCLUDES 1 *embolism complicating abortion or ectopic or molar pregnancy (O00–O07, O08.2)*
       embolism complicating pregnancy, childbirth and the puerperium (O88.-)
       traumatic embolism (T79.0)

    EXCLUDES 2 *embolism due to prosthetic devices, implants and grafts (T82.8-, T83.8, T84.8-, T85.8)*
       embolism following infusion, transfusion and therapeutic injection (T80.0)

√6ᵗʰ **T81.71 Complication of artery following a procedure, not elsewhere classified**

    √7ᵗʰ **T81.710 Complication of** mesenteric **artery following a procedure, not elsewhere classified**

    √7ᵗʰ **T81.711 Complication of** renal **artery following a procedure, not elsewhere classified**

    9 √7ᵗʰ **T81.718 Complication of other artery following a procedure, not elsewhere classified**   NC Dx

    √7ᵗʰ **T81.719 Complication of unspecified artery following a procedure, not elsewhere classified** ▽

    9 √x7ᵗʰ **T81.72 Complication of** vein **following a procedure, not elsewhere classified**   NC Dx

√5ᵗʰ **T81.8 Other complications of procedures, not elsewhere classified**

    EXCLUDES 2 *hypothermia following anesthesia (T88.51)*
       malignant hyperpyrexia due to anesthesia (T88.3)

    √x7ᵗʰ **T81.81 Complication of inhalation therapy**

    √x7ᵗʰ **T81.82 Emphysema (subcutaneous) resulting from a procedure**

    √x7ᵗʰ **T81.83 Persistent postprocedural fistula**   CC

    √x7ᵗʰ **T81.89 Other complications of procedures, not elsewhere classified**
       Use additional code to specify complication, such as:
       postprocedural delirium (F05)
       AHA: 2014, 1Q, 23

√x7ᵗʰ **T81.9 Unspecified complication of procedure** ▽

√4ᵗʰ **T82 Complications of cardiac and vascular prosthetic devices, implants and grafts**

    EXCLUDES 2 *failure and rejection of transplanted organs and tissue (T86.-)*

    The appropriate 7th character is to be added to each code from category T82.
    A   initial encounter
    D   subsequent encounter
    S   sequela

√5ᵗʰ **T82.0 Mechanical complication of** heart valve prosthesis
    Mechanical complication of artificial heart valve

    EXCLUDES 1 *mechanical complication of biological heart valve graft (T82.22-)*

    √x7ᵗʰ **T82.01** Breakdown **(mechanical) of heart valve prosthesis**   CC
       RIC Excl 7th Character A: 14 Cardiac

    √x7ᵗʰ **T82.02** Displacement **of heart valve prosthesis**   CC
       Malposition of heart valve prosthesis
       RIC Excl 7th Character A: 14 Cardiac

    √x7ᵗʰ **T82.03** Leakage **of heart valve prosthesis**   CC
       RIC Excl 7th Character A: 14 Cardiac

    √x7ᵗʰ **T82.09 Other mechanical complication of heart valve prosthesis**   CC
       Obstruction (mechanical) of heart valve prosthesis
       Perforation of heart valve prosthesis
       Protrusion of heart valve prosthesis
       RIC Excl 7th Character A: 14 Cardiac

√5ᵗʰ **T82.1 Mechanical complication of** cardiac electronic device

    √6ᵗʰ **T82.11** Breakdown **(mechanical) of cardiac electronic device**

       √7ᵗʰ **T82.110 Breakdown (mechanical) of cardiac** electrode

       √7ᵗʰ **T82.111 Breakdown (mechanical) of cardiac** pulse generator (battery)

       √7ᵗʰ **T82.118 Breakdown (mechanical) of other cardiac** electronic device

       √7ᵗʰ **T82.119 Breakdown (mechanical) of unspecified cardiac electronic device** ▽

    √6ᵗʰ **T82.12** Displacement **of cardiac electronic device**
       Malposition of cardiac electronic device

       √7ᵗʰ **T82.120 Displacement of** cardiac electrode

       √7ᵗʰ **T82.121 Displacement of cardiac** pulse generator (battery)

       √7ᵗʰ **T82.128 Displacement of other cardiac** electronic device

       √7ᵗʰ **T82.129 Displacement of unspecified cardiac electronic device** ▽

    √6ᵗʰ **T82.19** Other **mechanical complication of cardiac electronic device**
       Leakage of cardiac electronic device
       Obstruction of cardiac electronic device
       Perforation of cardiac electronic device
       Protrusion of cardiac electronic device

       √7ᵗʰ **T82.190 Other mechanical complication of cardiac electrode**

       √7ᵗʰ **T82.191 Other mechanical complication of cardiac pulse generator (battery)**

       √7ᵗʰ **T82.198 Other mechanical complication of other cardiac electronic device**

       √7ᵗʰ **T82.199 Other mechanical complication of unspecified cardiac device** ▽

√5ᵗʰ **T82.2 Mechanical complication of** coronary artery bypass graft **and** biological heart valve graft

    EXCLUDES 1 *mechanical complication of artificial heart valve prosthesis (T82.0-)*

    √6ᵗʰ **T82.21 Mechanical complication of** coronary artery bypass graft

       √7ᵗʰ **T82.211** Breakdown **(mechanical) of coronary artery bypass graft**

       √7ᵗʰ **T82.212** Displacement **of coronary artery bypass graft**
          Malposition of coronary artery bypass graft

       √7ᵗʰ **T82.213** Leakage **of coronary artery bypass graft**

       √7ᵗʰ **T82.218 Other mechanical complication of coronary artery bypass graft**
          Obstruction, mechanical of coronary artery bypass graft
          Perforation of coronary artery bypass graft
          Protrusion of coronary artery bypass graft

    √6ᵗʰ **T82.22 Mechanical complication of** biological heart valve graft

       √7ᵗʰ **T82.221** Breakdown **(mechanical) of biological heart valve graft**

       √7ᵗʰ **T82.222** Displacement **of biological heart valve graft**
          Malposition of biological heart valve graft

       √7ᵗʰ **T82.223** Leakage **of biological heart valve graft**

       √7ᵗʰ **T82.228 Other mechanical complication of biological heart valve graft**
          Obstruction of biological heart valve graft
          Perforation of biological heart valve graft
          Protrusion of biological heart valve graft

√5ᵗʰ **T82.3 Mechanical complication of** other vascular grafts

    √6ᵗʰ **T82.31** Breakdown **(mechanical) of other vascular grafts**

       √7ᵗʰ **T82.310 Breakdown (mechanical) of** aortic (bifurcation) graft (replacement)

       √7ᵗʰ **T82.311 Breakdown (mechanical) of** carotid arterial graft (bypass)

       √7ᵗʰ **T82.312 Breakdown (mechanical) of** femoral arterial graft (bypass)

       √7ᵗʰ **T82.318 Breakdown (mechanical) of other vascular grafts**

       √7ᵗʰ **T82.319 Breakdown (mechanical) of unspecified vascular grafts** ▽

    √6ᵗʰ **T82.32** Displacement **of other vascular grafts**
       Malposition of other vascular grafts

---

9   Hospice Noncancer Diagnosis only when reported using an appropriate 7th character indicating a subsequent encounter or sequela

☑ Add'l Character Required   √x7ᵗʰ Placeholder Alert   RUG IV Special Care High Dx   RUG IV Clinically Complex Dx   RUG IV Special Care Low Dx   Manifestation Code   Other Specified Code   ▽ Unspecified Code

√7ᵗʰ **T82.320** Displacement of aortic (bifurcation) graft (replacement)

√7ᵗʰ **T82.321** Displacement of carotid arterial graft (bypass)

√7ᵗʰ **T82.322** Displacement of femoral arterial graft (bypass)

√7ᵗʰ **T82.328** Displacement of other vascular grafts

√7ᵗʰ **T82.329** Displacement of unspecified vascular grafts ▽

√6ᵗʰ **T82.33** Leakage of other vascular grafts

√7ᵗʰ **T82.330** Leakage of aortic (bifurcation) graft (replacement)

√7ᵗʰ **T82.331** Leakage of carotid arterial graft (bypass)

√7ᵗʰ **T82.332** Leakage of femoral arterial graft (bypass)

√7ᵗʰ **T82.338** Leakage of other vascular grafts

√7ᵗʰ **T82.339** Leakage of unspecified vascular graft ▽

√6ᵗʰ **T82.39** Other mechanical complication of other vascular grafts
Obstruction (mechanical) of other vascular grafts
Perforation of other vascular grafts
Protrusion of other vascular grafts

√7ᵗʰ **T82.390** Other mechanical complication of aortic (bifurcation) graft (replacement)

√7ᵗʰ **T82.391** Other mechanical complication of carotid arterial graft (bypass)

√7ᵗʰ **T82.392** Other mechanical complication of femoral arterial graft (bypass)

√7ᵗʰ **T82.398** Other mechanical complication of other vascular grafts

√7ᵗʰ **T82.399** Other mechanical complication of unspecified vascular grafts ▽

√5ᵗʰ **T82.4** Mechanical complication of vascular dialysis catheter
Mechanical complication of hemodialysis catheter
EXCLUDES 1   mechanical complication of intraperitoneal dialysis catheter (T85.62)

√x7ᵗʰ **T82.41** Breakdown (mechanical) of vascular dialysis catheter

√x7ᵗʰ **T82.42** Displacement of vascular dialysis catheter
Malposition of vascular dialysis catheter

√x7ᵗʰ **T82.43** Leakage of vascular dialysis catheter

√x7ᵗʰ **T82.49** Other complication of vascular dialysis catheter
Obstruction (mechanical) of vascular dialysis catheter
Perforation of vascular dialysis catheter
Protrusion of vascular dialysis catheter

√5ᵗʰ **T82.5** Mechanical complication of other cardiac and vascular devices and implants
EXCLUDES 2   mechanical complication of epidural and subdural infusion catheter (T85.61)

√6ᵗʰ **T82.51** Breakdown (mechanical) of other cardiac and vascular devices and implants

√7ᵗʰ **T82.510** Breakdown (mechanical) of surgically created arteriovenous fistula

√7ᵗʰ **T82.511** Breakdown (mechanical) of surgically created arteriovenous shunt

√7ᵗʰ **T82.512** Breakdown (mechanical) of artificial heart

√7ᵗʰ **T82.513** Breakdown (mechanical) of balloon (counterpulsation) device

√7ᵗʰ **T82.514** Breakdown (mechanical) of infusion catheter

√7ᵗʰ **T82.515** Breakdown (mechanical) of umbrella device

√7ᵗʰ **T82.518** Breakdown (mechanical) of other cardiac and vascular devices and implants

√7ᵗʰ **T82.519** Breakdown (mechanical) of unspecified ▽ cardiac and vascular devices and implants

√6ᵗʰ **T82.52** Displacement of other cardiac and vascular devices and implants
Malposition of other cardiac and vascular devices and implants

√7ᵗʰ **T82.520** Displacement of surgically created arteriovenous fistula

√7ᵗʰ **T82.521** Displacement of surgically created arteriovenous shunt

√7ᵗʰ **T82.522** Displacement of artificial heart

√7ᵗʰ **T82.523** Displacement of balloon (counterpulsation) device

√7ᵗʰ **T82.524** Displacement of infusion catheter

√7ᵗʰ **T82.525** Displacement of umbrella device

√7ᵗʰ **T82.528** Displacement of other cardiac and vascular devices and implants

√7ᵗʰ **T82.529** Displacement of unspecified cardiac ▽ and vascular devices and implants

√6ᵗʰ **T82.53** Leakage of other cardiac and vascular devices and implants

√7ᵗʰ **T82.530** Leakage of surgically created arteriovenous fistula

√7ᵗʰ **T82.531** Leakage of surgically created arteriovenous shunt

√7ᵗʰ **T82.532** Leakage of artificial heart

√7ᵗʰ **T82.533** Leakage of balloon (counterpulsation) device

√7ᵗʰ **T82.534** Leakage of infusion catheter

√7ᵗʰ **T82.535** Leakage of umbrella device

√7ᵗʰ **T82.538** Leakage of other cardiac and vascular devices and implants

√7ᵗʰ **T82.539** Leakage of unspecified cardiac and ▽ vascular devices and implants

√6ᵗʰ **T82.59** Other mechanical complication of other cardiac and vascular devices and implants
Obstruction (mechanical) of other cardiac and vascular devices and implants
Perforation of other cardiac and vascular devices and implants
Protrusion of other cardiac and vascular devices and implants

√7ᵗʰ **T82.590** Other mechanical complication of surgically created arteriovenous fistula

√7ᵗʰ **T82.591** Other mechanical complication of surgically created arteriovenous shunt

√7ᵗʰ **T82.592** Other mechanical complication of artificial heart

√7ᵗʰ **T82.593** Other mechanical complication of balloon (counterpulsation) device

√7ᵗʰ **T82.594** Other mechanical complication of infusion catheter

√7ᵗʰ **T82.595** Other mechanical complication of umbrella device

√7ᵗʰ **T82.598** Other mechanical complication of other cardiac and vascular devices and implants

√7ᵗʰ **T82.599** Other mechanical complication of ▽ unspecified cardiac and vascular devices and implants

√x7ᵗʰ **T82.6** Infection and inflammatory reaction due to cardiac valve **CC** prosthesis
Use additional code to identify infection
RIC Excl 7th Character A: 14 Cardiac

√x7ᵗʰ **T82.7** Infection and inflammatory reaction due to other cardiac **CC** and vascular devices, implants and grafts
Use additional code to identify infection

√5ᵗʰ **T82.8** Other specified complications of cardiac and vascular prosthetic devices, implants and grafts

√6ᵗʰ **T82.81** Embolism of cardiac and vascular prosthetic devices, implants and grafts

⁹ √7ᵗʰ **T82.817** Embolism of cardiac prosthetic **NC Dx** devices, implants and grafts

⁹ √7ᵗʰ **T82.818** Embolism of vascular prosthetic **NC Dx** devices, implants and grafts

√6ᵗʰ **T82.82** Fibrosis of cardiac and vascular prosthetic devices, implants and grafts

√7ᵗʰ **T82.827** Fibrosis of cardiac prosthetic devices, implants and grafts

√7ᵗʰ **T82.828** Fibrosis of vascular prosthetic devices, implants and grafts

√6ᵗʰ **T82.83** Hemorrhage of cardiac and vascular prosthetic devices, implants and grafts

√7ᵗʰ **T82.837** Hemorrhage of cardiac prosthetic devices, implants and grafts

---

⁹ Hospice Noncancer Diagnosis only when reported using an appropriate 7th character indicating a subsequent encounter

Ⓝ Newborn   Ⓟ Pediatric   Ⓜ Maternity   Ⓐ Adult   **RIC** RIC Dx   **NC Dx** Noncancer Dx   **PDx** Primary Dx   **CC** RIC CC Condition   ►◄ Revised Text   ● New Code   ▲ Revised Code Title

1040   ICD-10-CM 2016

√7ᵗʰ **T82.838** Hemorrhage of vascular prosthetic devices, implants and grafts

√6ᵗʰ **T82.84** Pain from cardiac and vascular prosthetic devices, implants and grafts

  √7ᵗʰ **T82.847** Pain from cardiac prosthetic devices, implants and grafts

  √7ᵗʰ **T82.848** Pain from vascular prosthetic devices, implants and grafts

√6ᵗʰ **T82.85** Stenosis of cardiac and vascular prosthetic devices, implants and grafts

  √7ᵗʰ **T82.857** Stenosis of cardiac prosthetic devices, implants and grafts

  √7ᵗʰ **T82.858** Stenosis of vascular prosthetic devices, implants and grafts

√6ᵗʰ **T82.86** Thrombosis of cardiac and vascular prosthetic devices, implants and grafts

  √7ᵗʰ **T82.867** Thrombosis of cardiac prosthetic devices, implants and grafts

  √7ᵗʰ **T82.868** Thrombosis of vascular prosthetic devices, implants and grafts

√6ᵗʰ **T82.89** Other specified complication of cardiac and vascular prosthetic devices, implants and grafts

  √7ᵗʰ **T82.897** Other specified complication of cardiac prosthetic devices, implants and grafts

  √7ᵗʰ **T82.898** Other specified complication of vascular prosthetic devices, implants and grafts

√x7ᵗʰ **T82.9** Unspecified complication of cardiac and vascular prosthetic device, implant and graft ▽

√4ᵗʰ **T83** **Complications of genitourinary prosthetic devices, implants and grafts**

EXCLUDES 2   failure and rejection of transplanted organs and tissue (T86.-)

The appropriate 7th character is to be added to each code from category T83.
A   initial encounter
D   subsequent encounter
S   sequela

√5ᵗʰ **T83.0** Mechanical complication of urinary (indwelling) catheter

EXCLUDES 2   complications of stoma of urinary tract (N99.5-)

√6ᵗʰ **T83.01** Breakdown (mechanical) of urinary (indwelling) catheter

  √7ᵗʰ **T83.010** Breakdown (mechanical) of cystostomy catheter

  √7ᵗʰ **T83.018** Breakdown (mechanical) of other indwelling urethral catheter

√6ᵗʰ **T83.02** Displacement of urinary (indwelling) catheter
Malposition of urinary (indwelling) catheter

  √7ᵗʰ **T83.020** Displacement of cystostomy catheter

  √7ᵗʰ **T83.028** Displacement of other indwelling urethral catheter

√6ᵗʰ **T83.03** Leakage of urinary (indwelling) catheter

  √7ᵗʰ **T83.030** Leakage of cystostomy catheter

  √7ᵗʰ **T83.038** Leakage of other indwelling urethral catheter

√6ᵗʰ **T83.09** Other mechanical complication of urinary (indwelling) catheter
Obstruction (mechanical) of urinary (indwelling) catheter
Perforation of urinary (indwelling) catheter
Protrusion of urinary (indwelling) catheter

  √7ᵗʰ **T83.090** Other mechanical complication of cystostomy catheter

  √7ᵗʰ **T83.098** Other mechanical complication of other indwelling urethral catheter

√5ᵗʰ **T83.1** Mechanical complication of other urinary devices and implants

√6ᵗʰ **T83.11** Breakdown (mechanical) of other urinary devices and implants

  √7ᵗʰ **T83.110** Breakdown (mechanical) of urinary electronic stimulator device

  √7ᵗʰ **T83.111** Breakdown (mechanical) of urinary sphincter implant

  √7ᵗʰ **T83.112** Breakdown (mechanical) of urinary stent

  √7ᵗʰ **T83.118** Breakdown (mechanical) of other urinary devices and implants

√6ᵗʰ **T83.12** Displacement of other urinary devices and implants
Malposition of other urinary devices and implants

  √7ᵗʰ **T83.120** Displacement of urinary electronic stimulator device

  √7ᵗʰ **T83.121** Displacement of urinary sphincter implant

  √7ᵗʰ **T83.122** Displacement of urinary stent

  √7ᵗʰ **T83.128** Displacement of other urinary devices and implants

√6ᵗʰ **T83.19** Other mechanical complication of other urinary devices and implants
Leakage of other urinary devices and implants
Obstruction (mechanical) of other urinary devices and implants
Perforation of other urinary devices and implants
Protrusion of other urinary devices and implants

  √7ᵗʰ **T83.190** Other mechanical complication of urinary electronic stimulator device

  √7ᵗʰ **T83.191** Other mechanical complication of urinary sphincter implant

  √7ᵗʰ **T83.192** Other mechanical complication of urinary stent

  √7ᵗʰ **T83.198** Other mechanical complication of other urinary devices and implants

√5ᵗʰ **T83.2** Mechanical complication of graft of urinary organ

√x7ᵗʰ **T83.21** Breakdown (mechanical) of graft of urinary organ

√x7ᵗʰ **T83.22** Displacement of graft of urinary organ
Malposition of graft of urinary organ

√x7ᵗʰ **T83.23** Leakage of graft of urinary organ

√x7ᵗʰ **T83.29** Other mechanical complication of graft of urinary organ
Obstruction (mechanical) of graft of urinary organ
Perforation of graft of urinary organ
Protrusion of graft of urinary organ

√5ᵗʰ **T83.3** Mechanical complication of intrauterine contraceptive device

[11] √x7ᵗʰ **T83.31** Breakdown (mechanical) of intrauterine contraceptive device Ⓜ♀

[11] √x7ᵗʰ **T83.32** Displacement of intrauterine contraceptive device Ⓜ♀
Malposition of intrauterine contraceptive device

[11] √x7ᵗʰ **T83.39** Other mechanical complication of intrauterine contraceptive device Ⓜ♀
Leakage of intrauterine contraceptive device
Obstruction (mechanical) of intrauterine contraceptive device
Perforation of intrauterine contraceptive device
Protrusion of intrauterine contraceptive device

√5ᵗʰ **T83.4** Mechanical complication of other prosthetic devices, implants and grafts of genital tract

√6ᵗʰ **T83.41** Breakdown (mechanical) of other prosthetic devices, implants and grafts of genital tract

  √7ᵗʰ **T83.410** Breakdown (mechanical) of penile (implanted) prosthesis ♂

  √7ᵗʰ **T83.418** Breakdown (mechanical) of other prosthetic devices, implants and grafts of genital tract

√6ᵗʰ **T83.42** Displacement of other prosthetic devices, implants and grafts of genital tract
Malposition of other prosthetic devices, implants and grafts of genital tract

  √7ᵗʰ **T83.420** Displacement of penile (implanted) prosthesis ♂

  √7ᵗʰ **T83.428** Displacement of other prosthetic devices, implants and grafts of genital tract

√6ᵗʰ **T83.49** Other mechanical complication of other prosthetic devices, implants and grafts of genital tract
Leakage of other prosthetic devices, implants and grafts of genital tract
Obstruction, mechanical of other prosthetic devices, implants and grafts of genital tract
Perforation of other prosthetic devices, implants and grafts of genital tract
Protrusion of other prosthetic devices, implants and grafts of genital tract

---

[11] Maternity diagnosis only when code is reported using 7th character A for initial encounter.

☑ Add'l Character Required   √x7ᵗʰ Placeholder Alert   RUG IV Special Care High Dx   RUG IV Clinically Complex Dx   RUG IV Special Care Low Dx   Manifestation Code   Other Specified Code   ▽ Unspecified Code

ICD-10-CM 2016   1041

☑7ᵗʰ **T83.490 Other mechanical complication of** ♂
penile (implanted) prosthesis

☑7ᵗʰ **T83.498 Other mechanical complication of other**
prosthetic devices, implants and grafts of
genital tract

☑5ᵗʰ **T83.5 Infection and inflammatory reaction due to prosthetic device,**
implant and graft in urinary system
Use additional code to identify infection

☑x7ᵗʰ **T83.51 Infection and inflammatory reaction due to**
indwelling urinary catheter
EXCLUDES 2 *complications of stoma of urinary tract*
(N99.5-)

☑x7ᵗʰ **T83.59 Infection and inflammatory reaction due to**
prosthetic device, implant and graft in urinary
system

☑x7ᵗʰ **T83.6 Infection and inflammatory reaction due to prosthetic device,**
implant and graft in genital tract
Use additional code to identify infection

☑5ᵗʰ **T83.7 Complications due to implanted mesh and other prosthetic**
materials

☑6ᵗʰ **T83.71 Erosion of implanted mesh and other prosthetic**
materials to surrounding organ or tissue

☑7ᵗʰ **T83.711 Erosion of implanted vaginal mesh and** ♀
other prosthetic materials to
surrounding organ or tissue
Erosion of implanted vaginal mesh and
other prosthetic materials into pelvic
floor muscles

☑7ᵗʰ **T83.718 Erosion of other implanted mesh and**
other prosthetic materials to surrounding
organ or tissue

☑6ᵗʰ **T83.72 Exposure of implanted mesh and other prosthetic**
materials into surrounding organ or tissue

☑7ᵗʰ **T83.721 Exposure of implanted vaginal mesh** ♀
and other prosthetic materials into
vagina
Exposure of implanted vaginal mesh and
other prosthetic materials through
vaginal wall

☑7ᵗʰ **T83.728 Exposure of other implanted mesh and**
other prosthetic materials to surrounding
organ or tissue

☑5ᵗʰ **T83.8 Other specified complications of genitourinary prosthetic**
devices, implants and grafts

☑x7ᵗʰ **T83.81 Embolism of genitourinary prosthetic devices,**
implants and grafts

☑x7ᵗʰ **T83.82 Fibrosis of genitourinary prosthetic devices,**
implants and grafts

☑x7ᵗʰ **T83.83 Hemorrhage of genitourinary prosthetic devices,**
implants and grafts

☑x7ᵗʰ **T83.84 Pain from genitourinary prosthetic devices,**
implants and grafts

☑x7ᵗʰ **T83.85 Stenosis of genitourinary prosthetic devices,**
implants and grafts

☑x7ᵗʰ **T83.86 Thrombosis of genitourinary prosthetic devices,**
implants and grafts

☑x7ᵗʰ **T83.89 Other specified complication of genitourinary**
prosthetic devices, implants and grafts

☑x7ᵗʰ **T83.9 Unspecified complication of genitourinary prosthetic** ▽
device, implant and graft

☑4ᵗʰ **T84 Complications of internal orthopedic prosthetic devices,**
implants and grafts
EXCLUDES 2 *failure and rejection of transplanted organs and tissues (T86.-)*
fracture of bone following insertion of orthopedic implant, joint
prosthesis or bone plate (M96.6)

The appropriate 7th character is to be added to each code from
category T84.
A   initial encounter
D   subsequent encounter
S   sequela

☑5ᵗʰ **T84.0 Mechanical complication of internal joint prosthesis**

☑6ᵗʰ **T84.01 Broken internal joint prosthesis**
Breakage (fracture) of prosthetic joint
Broken prosthetic joint implant
EXCLUDES 1 *periprosthetic joint implant fracture (T84.04)*

☑7ᵗʰ **T84.010 Broken internal right hip prosthesis**

☑7ᵗʰ **T84.011 Broken internal left hip prosthesis**

☑7ᵗʰ **T84.012 Broken internal right knee prosthesis**

☑7ᵗʰ **T84.013 Broken internal left knee prosthesis**

☑7ᵗʰ **T84.018 Broken internal joint prosthesis, other site**
Use additional code to identify the joint
(Z96.6-)

☑7ᵗʰ **T84.019 Broken internal joint prosthesis,** ▽
unspecified site

☑6ᵗʰ **T84.02 Dislocation of internal joint prosthesis**
Instability of internal joint prosthesis
Subluxation of internal joint prosthesis

☑7ᵗʰ **T84.020 Dislocation of internal right hip prosthesis**

☑7ᵗʰ **T84.021 Dislocation of internal left hip prosthesis**

☑7ᵗʰ **T84.022 Instability of internal right knee**
prosthesis

☑7ᵗʰ **T84.023 Instability of internal left knee prosthesis**

☑7ᵗʰ **T84.028 Dislocation of other internal joint**
prosthesis
Use additional code to identify the joint
(Z96.6-)

☑7ᵗʰ **T84.029 Dislocation of unspecified internal** ▽
joint prosthesis

☑6ᵗʰ **T84.03 Mechanical loosening of internal prosthetic joint**
Aseptic loosening of prosthetic joint

☑7ᵗʰ **T84.030 Mechanical loosening of internal right hip**
prosthetic joint

☑7ᵗʰ **T84.031 Mechanical loosening of internal left hip**
prosthetic joint

☑7ᵗʰ **T84.032 Mechanical loosening of internal right**
knee prosthetic joint

☑7ᵗʰ **T84.033 Mechanical loosening of internal left knee**
prosthetic joint

☑7ᵗʰ **T84.038 Mechanical loosening of other internal**
prosthetic joint
Use additional code to identify the joint
(Z96.6-)

☑7ᵗʰ **T84.039 Mechanical loosening of unspecified** ▽
internal prosthetic joint

☑6ᵗʰ **T84.04 Periprosthetic fracture around internal prosthetic**
joint
EXCLUDES 2 *breakage (fracture) of prosthetic joint*
(T84.01)

☑7ᵗʰ **T84.040 Periprosthetic fracture around internal**
prosthetic right hip joint

☑7ᵗʰ **T84.041 Periprosthetic fracture around internal**
prosthetic left hip joint

☑7ᵗʰ **T84.042 Periprosthetic fracture around internal**
prosthetic right knee joint

☑7ᵗʰ **T84.043 Periprosthetic fracture around internal**
prosthetic left knee joint

☑7ᵗʰ **T84.048 Periprosthetic fracture around other**
internal prosthetic joint
Use additional code to identify the joint
(Z96.6-)

☑7ᵗʰ **T84.049 Periprosthetic fracture around** ▽
unspecified internal prosthetic joint

☑6ᵗʰ **T84.05 Periprosthetic osteolysis of internal prosthetic joint**
Use additional code to identify major osseous defect, if
applicable (M89.7-)

☑7ᵗʰ **T84.050 Periprosthetic osteolysis of internal**
prosthetic right hip joint

☑7ᵗʰ **T84.051 Periprosthetic osteolysis of internal**
prosthetic left hip joint

☑7ᵗʰ **T84.052 Periprosthetic osteolysis of internal**
prosthetic right knee joint

☑7ᵗʰ **T84.053 Periprosthetic osteolysis of internal**
prosthetic left knee joint

☑7ᵗʰ **T84.058 Periprosthetic osteolysis of other internal**
prosthetic joint
Use additional code to identify the joint
(Z96.6-)

☑7ᵗʰ **T84.059 Periprosthetic osteolysis of** ▽
unspecified internal prosthetic joint

Ⓝ Newborn   Ⓟ Pediatric   Ⓜ Maternity   Ⓐ Adult   RIC RIC Dx   NC Dx Noncancer Dx   PDx Primary Dx   CC RIC CC Condition   ▶◀ Revised Text   ● New Code   ▲ Revised Code Title

1042   ICD-10-CM 2016

✓6ᵗʰ **T84.06** **Wear of articular bearing surface** of internal prosthetic joint

  ✓7ᵗʰ **T84.060** **Wear of articular bearing surface of internal prosthetic** right hip joint

  ✓7ᵗʰ **T84.061** **Wear of articular bearing surface of internal prosthetic** left hip joint

  ✓7ᵗʰ **T84.062** **Wear of articular bearing surface of internal prosthetic** right knee joint

  ✓7ᵗʰ **T84.063** **Wear of articular bearing surface of internal prosthetic** left knee joint

  ✓7ᵗʰ **T84.068** **Wear of articular bearing surface of other internal prosthetic joint**
      Use additional code to identify the joint (Z96.6-)

  ✓7ᵗʰ **T84.069** **Wear of articular bearing surface of unspecified internal prosthetic joint** ▽

✓6ᵗʰ **T84.09** **Other** mechanical complication of internal joint prosthesis
    Prosthetic joint implant failure NOS

  ✓7ᵗʰ **T84.090** **Other mechanical complication of internal** right hip prosthesis

  ✓7ᵗʰ **T84.091** **Other mechanical complication of internal** left hip prosthesis

  ✓7ᵗʰ **T84.092** **Other mechanical complication of internal** right knee prosthesis

  ✓7ᵗʰ **T84.093** **Other mechanical complication of internal** left knee prosthesis

  ✓7ᵗʰ **T84.098** **Other mechanical complication of other internal joint prosthesis**
      Use additional code to identify the joint (Z96.6-)

  ✓7ᵗʰ **T84.099** **Other mechanical complication of unspecified internal joint prosthesis** ▽

✓5ᵗʰ **T84.1** Mechanical complication of **internal fixation device** of bones of limb
  EXCLUDES 2   *mechanical complication of internal fixation device of bones of feet (T84.2-)*
    mechanical complication of internal fixation device of bones of fingers (T84.2-)
    mechanical complication of internal fixation device of bones of hands (T84.2-)
    mechanical complication of internal fixation device of toes (T84.2-)

 ✓6ᵗʰ **T84.11** **Breakdown (mechanical)** of internal fixation device of bones of limb

  ✓7ᵗʰ **T84.110** **Breakdown (mechanical) of internal fixation device of** right humerus

  ✓7ᵗʰ **T84.111** **Breakdown (mechanical) of internal fixation device of** left humerus

  ✓7ᵗʰ **T84.112** **Breakdown (mechanical) of internal fixation device of bone of** right forearm

  ✓7ᵗʰ **T84.113** **Breakdown (mechanical) of internal fixation device of bone of** left forearm

  ✓7ᵗʰ **T84.114** **Breakdown (mechanical) of internal fixation device of** right femur

  ✓7ᵗʰ **T84.115** **Breakdown (mechanical) of internal fixation device of** left femur

  ✓7ᵗʰ **T84.116** **Breakdown (mechanical) of internal fixation device of bone of** right lower leg

  ✓7ᵗʰ **T84.117** **Breakdown (mechanical) of internal fixation device of bone of** left lower leg

  ✓7ᵗʰ **T84.119** **Breakdown (mechanical) of internal fixation device of unspecified bone of limb** ▽

 ✓6ᵗʰ **T84.12** **Displacement** of internal fixation device of bones of limb
    Malposition of internal fixation device of bones of limb

  ✓7ᵗʰ **T84.120** **Displacement of internal fixation device of** right humerus

  ✓7ᵗʰ **T84.121** **Displacement of internal fixation device of** left humerus

  ✓7ᵗʰ **T84.122** **Displacement of internal fixation device of bone of** right forearm

  ✓7ᵗʰ **T84.123** **Displacement of internal fixation device of bone of** left forearm

  ✓7ᵗʰ **T84.124** **Displacement of internal fixation device of** right femur

  ✓7ᵗʰ **T84.125** **Displacement of internal fixation device of** left femur

  ✓7ᵗʰ **T84.126** **Displacement of internal fixation device of bone of** right lower leg

  ✓7ᵗʰ **T84.127** **Displacement of internal fixation device of bone of** left lower leg

  ✓7ᵗʰ **T84.129** **Displacement of internal fixation device of unspecified bone of limb** ▽

 ✓6ᵗʰ **T84.19** **Other** mechanical complication of internal fixation device of bones of limb
    Obstruction (mechanical) of internal fixation device of bones of limb
    Perforation of internal fixation device of bones of limb
    Protrusion of internal fixation device of bones of limb

  ✓7ᵗʰ **T84.190** **Other mechanical complication of internal fixation device of** right humerus

  ✓7ᵗʰ **T84.191** **Other mechanical complication of internal fixation device of** left humerus

  ✓7ᵗʰ **T84.192** **Other mechanical complication of internal fixation device of bone of** right forearm

  ✓7ᵗʰ **T84.193** **Other mechanical complication of internal fixation device of bone of** left forearm

  ✓7ᵗʰ **T84.194** **Other mechanical complication of internal fixation device of** right femur

  ✓7ᵗʰ **T84.195** **Other mechanical complication of internal fixation device of** left femur

  ✓7ᵗʰ **T84.196** **Other mechanical complication of internal fixation device of bone of** right lower leg

  ✓7ᵗʰ **T84.197** **Other mechanical complication of internal fixation device of bone of** left lower leg

  ✓7ᵗʰ **T84.199** **Other mechanical complication of internal fixation device of unspecified bone of limb** ▽

✓5ᵗʰ **T84.2** Mechanical complication of **internal fixation device** of other bones

 ✓6ᵗʰ **T84.21** **Breakdown (mechanical)** of internal fixation device of other bones

  ✓7ᵗʰ **T84.210** **Breakdown (mechanical) of internal fixation device of bones of** hand and fingers

  ✓7ᵗʰ **T84.213** **Breakdown (mechanical) of internal fixation device of bones of** foot and toes

  ✓7ᵗʰ **T84.216** **Breakdown (mechanical) of internal fixation device of** vertebrae

  ✓7ᵗʰ **T84.218** **Breakdown (mechanical) of internal fixation device of other bones**

 ✓6ᵗʰ **T84.22** **Displacement** of internal fixation device of other bones
    Malposition of internal fixation device of other bones

  ✓7ᵗʰ **T84.220** **Displacement of internal fixation device of bones of** hand and fingers

  ✓7ᵗʰ **T84.223** **Displacement of internal fixation device of bones of** foot and toes

  ✓7ᵗʰ **T84.226** **Displacement of internal fixation device of** vertebrae

  ✓7ᵗʰ **T84.228** **Displacement of internal fixation device of other bones**

 ✓6ᵗʰ **T84.29** **Other** mechanical complication of internal fixation device of other bones
    Obstruction (mechanical) of internal fixation device of other bones
    Perforation of internal fixation device of other bones
    Protrusion of internal fixation device of other bones

  ✓7ᵗʰ **T84.290** **Other mechanical complication of internal fixation device of bones of** hand and fingers

  ✓7ᵗʰ **T84.293** **Other mechanical complication of internal fixation device of bones of** foot and toes

  ✓7ᵗʰ **T84.296** **Other mechanical complication of internal fixation device of** vertebrae

  ✓7ᵗʰ **T84.298** **Other mechanical complication of internal fixation device of other bones**

✓5ᵗʰ **T84.3** Mechanical complication of **other bone devices, implants and grafts**
  EXCLUDES 2   *other complications of bone graft (T86.83-)*

 ✓6ᵗʰ **T84.31** **Breakdown (mechanical)** of other bone devices, implants and grafts

Chapter 19. Injury, Poisoning and Certain Other Consequences of External Causes

T84.310–T84.63

✓7th **T84.310** **Breakdown (mechanical) of** electronic bone stimulator

✓7th **T84.318** **Breakdown (mechanical) of other bone devices, implants and grafts**

✓6th **T84.32** Displacement **of other bone devices, implants and grafts**
Malposition of other bone devices, implants and grafts

    ✓7th **T84.320** **Displacement of** electronic bone stimulator

    ✓7th **T84.328** **Displacement of other bone devices, implants and grafts**
AHA: 2014, 4Q, 28

✓6th **T84.39** Other **mechanical complication of other bone devices, implants and grafts**
Obstruction (mechanical) of other bone devices, implants and grafts
Perforation of other bone devices, implants and grafts
Protrusion of other bone devices, implants and grafts

    ✓7th **T84.390** **Other mechanical complication of** electronic bone stimulator

    ✓7th **T84.398** **Other mechanical complication of other bone devices, implants and grafts**

✓5th **T84.4** **Mechanical complication of** other internal orthopedic devices, implants and grafts

✓6th **T84.41** Breakdown **(mechanical) of other internal orthopedic devices, implants and grafts**

    ✓7th **T84.410** **Breakdown (mechanical) of** muscle and tendon graft

    ✓7th **T84.418** **Breakdown (mechanical) of other internal orthopedic devices, implants and grafts**

✓6th **T84.42** Displacement **of other internal orthopedic devices, implants and grafts**
Malposition of other internal orthopedic devices, implants and grafts

    ✓7th **T84.420** **Displacement of** muscle and tendon graft

    ✓7th **T84.428** **Displacement of other internal orthopedic devices, implants and grafts**

✓6th **T84.49** Other **mechanical complication of other internal orthopedic devices, implants and grafts**
Mechanical complication of other internal orthopedic devices, implants and grafts NOS
Obstruction (mechanical) of other internal orthopedic devices, implants and grafts
Perforation of other internal orthopedic devices, implants and grafts
Protrusion of other internal orthopedic devices, implants and grafts

    ✓7th **T84.490** **Other mechanical complication of** muscle and tendon graft

    ✓7th **T84.498** **Other mechanical complication of other internal orthopedic devices, implants and grafts**

✓5th **T84.5** **Infection and inflammatory reaction due to** internal joint prosthesis
Use additional code to identify infection
AHA: 2015, 1Q, 16

✓x7th **T84.50** **Infection and inflammatory reaction due to unspecified internal joint prosthesis** OGG ▽
RIC Excl 7th Character A: 08 Replacement of lower extremity joint

✓x7th **T84.51** **Infection and inflammatory reaction due to internal** right hip **prosthesis** CC
RIC Excl 7th Character A: 08 Replacement of lower extremity joint

✓x7th **T84.52** **Infection and inflammatory reaction due to internal** left hip **prosthesis** CC
RIC Excl 7th Character A: 08 Replacement of lower extremity joint

✓x7th **T84.53** **Infection and inflammatory reaction due to internal** right knee **prosthesis** CC
RIC Excl 7th Character A: 08 Replacement of lower extremity joint

✓x7th **T84.54** **Infection and inflammatory reaction due to internal** left knee **prosthesis** CC
RIC Excl 7th Character A: 08 Replacement of lower extremity joint

✓x7th **T84.59** **Infection and inflammatory reaction due to other internal joint prosthesis** CC
RIC Excl 7th Character A: 08 Replacement of lower extremity joint

✓5th **T84.6** **Infection and inflammatory reaction due to** internal fixation device
Use additional code to identify infection

✓x7th **T84.60** **Infection and inflammatory reaction due to internal fixation device of unspecified site** CC ▽
RIC Excl 7th Character A: 09 Other orthopedic

✓6th **T84.61** **Infection and inflammatory reaction due to internal fixation device of** arm

    ✓7th **T84.610** **Infection and inflammatory reaction due to internal fixation device of** right humerus   CC
RIC Excl 7th Character A: 09 Other orthopedic

    ✓7th **T84.611** **Infection and inflammatory reaction due to internal fixation device of** left humerus   CC
RIC Excl 7th Character A: 09 Other orthopedic

    ✓7th **T84.612** **Infection and inflammatory reaction due to internal fixation device of** right radius   CC
RIC Excl 7th Character A: 09 Other orthopedic

    ✓7th **T84.613** **Infection and inflammatory reaction due to internal fixation device of** left radius   CC
RIC Excl 7th Character A: 09 Other orthopedic

    ✓7th **T84.614** **Infection and inflammatory reaction due to internal fixation device of** right ulna   CC
RIC Excl 7th Character A: 09 Other orthopedic

    ✓7th **T84.615** **Infection and inflammatory reaction due to internal fixation device of** left ulna   CC
RIC Excl 7th Character A: 09 Other orthopedic

    ✓7th **T84.619** **Infection and inflammatory reaction due to internal fixation device of unspecified** bone **of arm** CC ▽
RIC Excl 7th Character A: 09 Other orthopedic

✓6th **T84.62** **Infection and inflammatory reaction due to internal fixation device of** leg

    ✓7th **T84.620** **Infection and inflammatory reaction due to internal fixation device of** right femur   CC
RIC Excl 7th Character A: 09 Other orthopedic

    ✓7th **T84.621** **Infection and inflammatory reaction due to internal fixation device of** left femur   CC
RIC Excl 7th Character A: 09 Other orthopedic

    ✓7th **T84.622** **Infection and inflammatory reaction due to internal fixation device of** right tibia   CC
RIC Excl 7th Character A: 09 Other orthopedic

    ✓7th **T84.623** **Infection and inflammatory reaction due to internal fixation device of** left tibia   CC
RIC Excl 7th Character A: 09 Other orthopedic

    ✓7th **T84.624** **Infection and inflammatory reaction due to internal fixation device of** right fibula   CC
RIC Excl 7th Character A: 09 Other orthopedic

    ✓7th **T84.625** **Infection and inflammatory reaction due to internal fixation device of** left fibula   CC
RIC Excl 7th Character A: 09 Other orthopedic

    ✓7th **T84.629** **Infection and inflammatory reaction due to internal fixation device of unspecified** bone **of leg** CC ▽
RIC Excl 7th Character A: 09 Other orthopedic

✓x7th **T84.63** **Infection and inflammatory reaction due to internal fixation device of** spine   CC
RIC Excl 7th Character A: 09 Other orthopedic

N Newborn   P Pediatric   M Maternity   A Adult   RIC RIC Dx   NCDx Noncancer Dx   PDx Primary Dx   CC RIC CC Condition   ►◄ Revised Text   ● New Code   ▲ Revised Code Title

1044   ICD-10-CM 2016

✓x7th **T84.69 Infection and inflammatory reaction due to internal fixation device of other site** `CC`
RIC Excl 7th Character A: 09 Other orthopedic

✓x7th **T84.7 Infection and inflammatory reaction due to other internal orthopedic prosthetic devices, implants and grafts** `CC`
Use additional code to identify infection
RIC Excl 7th Character A: 09 Other orthopedic

✓5th **T84.8 Other specified complications of internal orthopedic prosthetic devices, implants and grafts**

✓x7th **T84.81 Embolism due to internal orthopedic prosthetic devices, implants and grafts**

✓x7th **T84.82 Fibrosis due to internal orthopedic prosthetic devices, implants and grafts**

✓x7th **T84.83 Hemorrhage due to internal orthopedic prosthetic devices, implants and grafts**

✓x7th **T84.84 Pain due to internal orthopedic prosthetic devices, implants and grafts**

✓x7th **T84.85 Stenosis due to internal orthopedic prosthetic devices, implants and grafts**

✓x7th **T84.86 Thrombosis due to internal orthopedic prosthetic devices, implants and grafts**

✓x7th **T84.89 Other specified complication of internal orthopedic prosthetic devices, implants and grafts**

✓x7th **T84.9 Unspecified complication of internal orthopedic prosthetic device, implant and graft** ▽

✓4th **T85 Complications of other internal prosthetic devices, implants and grafts**
EXCLUDES 2 failure and rejection of transplanted organs and tissue (T86.-)

The appropriate 7th character is to be added to each code from category T85.
A   initial encounter
D   subsequent encounter
S   sequela

✓5th **T85.0 Mechanical complication of ventricular intracranial (communicating) shunt**

✓x7th **T85.01 Breakdown (mechanical) of ventricular intracranial (communicating) shunt**

✓x7th **T85.02 Displacement of ventricular intracranial (communicating) shunt**
Malposition of ventricular intracranial (communicating) shunt

✓x7th **T85.03 Leakage of ventricular intracranial (communicating) shunt**

✓x7th **T85.09 Other mechanical complication of ventricular intracranial (communicating) shunt**
Obstruction (mechanical) of ventricular intracranial (communicating) shunt
Perforation of ventricular intracranial (communicating) shunt
Protrusion of ventricular intracranial (communicating) shunt

✓5th **T85.1 Mechanical complication of implanted electronic stimulator of nervous system**

✓6th **T85.11 Breakdown (mechanical) of implanted electronic stimulator of nervous system**

✓7th **T85.110 Breakdown (mechanical) of implanted electronic neurostimulator (electrode) of brain**

✓7th **T85.111 Breakdown (mechanical) of implanted electronic neurostimulator (electrode) of peripheral nerve**

✓7th **T85.112 Breakdown (mechanical) of implanted electronic neurostimulator (electrode) of spinal cord**

✓7th **T85.118 Breakdown (mechanical) of other implanted electronic stimulator of nervous system**

✓6th **T85.12 Displacement of implanted electronic stimulator of nervous system**
Malposition of implanted electronic stimulator of nervous system

✓7th **T85.120 Displacement of implanted electronic neurostimulator (electrode) of brain**

✓7th **T85.121 Displacement of implanted electronic neurostimulator (electrode) of peripheral nerve**

✓7th **T85.122 Displacement of implanted electronic neurostimulator (electrode) of spinal cord**

✓7th **T85.128 Displacement of other implanted electronic stimulator of nervous system**

✓6th **T85.19 Other mechanical complication of implanted electronic stimulator of nervous system**
Leakage of implanted electronic stimulator of nervous system
Obstruction (mechanical) of implanted electronic stimulator of nervous system
Perforation of implanted electronic stimulator of nervous system
Protrusion of implanted electronic stimulator of nervous system

✓7th **T85.190 Other mechanical complication of implanted electronic neurostimulator (electrode) of brain**

✓7th **T85.191 Other mechanical complication of implanted electronic neurostimulator (electrode) of peripheral nerve**

✓7th **T85.192 Other mechanical complication of implanted electronic neurostimulator (electrode) of spinal cord**

✓7th **T85.199 Other mechanical complication of other implanted electronic stimulator of nervous system**

✓5th **T85.2 Mechanical complication of intraocular lens**

✓x7th **T85.21 Breakdown (mechanical) of intraocular lens**

✓x7th **T85.22 Displacement of intraocular lens**
Malposition of intraocular lens

✓x7th **T85.29 Other mechanical complication of intraocular lens**
Obstruction (mechanical) of intraocular lens
Perforation of intraocular lens
Protrusion of intraocular lens

✓5th **T85.3 Mechanical complication of other ocular prosthetic devices, implants and grafts**
EXCLUDES 2 other complications of corneal graft (T86.84-)

✓6th **T85.31 Breakdown (mechanical) of other ocular prosthetic devices, implants and grafts**

✓7th **T85.310 Breakdown (mechanical) of prosthetic orbit of right eye**

✓7th **T85.311 Breakdown (mechanical) of prosthetic orbit of left eye**

✓7th **T85.318 Breakdown (mechanical) of other ocular prosthetic devices, implants and grafts**

✓6th **T85.32 Displacement of other ocular prosthetic devices, implants and grafts**
Malposition of other ocular prosthetic devices, implants and grafts

✓7th **T85.320 Displacement of prosthetic orbit of right eye**

✓7th **T85.321 Displacement of prosthetic orbit of left eye**

✓7th **T85.328 Displacement of other ocular prosthetic devices, implants and grafts**

✓6th **T85.39 Other mechanical complication of other ocular prosthetic devices, implants and grafts**
Obstruction (mechanical) of other ocular prosthetic devices, implants and grafts
Perforation of other ocular prosthetic devices, implants and grafts
Protrusion of other ocular prosthetic devices, implants and grafts

✓7th **T85.390 Other mechanical complication of prosthetic orbit of right eye**

✓7th **T85.391 Other mechanical complication of prosthetic orbit of left eye**

✓7th **T85.398 Other mechanical complication of other ocular prosthetic devices, implants and grafts**

✓5th **T85.4 Mechanical complication of breast prosthesis and implant**

✓x7th **T85.41 Breakdown (mechanical) of breast prosthesis and implant**

✓x7th **T85.42 Displacement of breast prosthesis and implant**
Malposition of breast prosthesis and implant

✓x7th **T85.43 Leakage of breast prosthesis and implant**

✓x7th **T85.44 Capsular contracture of breast implant**

√x7ᵗʰ T85.49 Other mechanical complication of breast prosthesis and implant
Obstruction (mechanical) of breast prosthesis and implant
Perforation of breast prosthesis and implant
Protrusion of breast prosthesis and implant

√5ᵗʰ T85.5 Mechanical complication of gastrointestinal prosthetic devices, implants and grafts

√6ᵗʰ T85.51 Breakdown (mechanical) of gastrointestinal prosthetic devices, implants and grafts

√7ᵗʰ T85.510 Breakdown (mechanical) of bile duct prosthesis

√7ᵗʰ T85.511 Breakdown (mechanical) of esophageal anti-reflux **device**

√7ᵗʰ T85.518 Breakdown (mechanical) of other gastrointestinal prosthetic devices, implants and grafts

√6ᵗʰ T85.52 Displacement of gastrointestinal prosthetic devices, implants and grafts
Malposition of gastrointestinal prosthetic devices, implants and grafts

√7ᵗʰ T85.520 Displacement of bile duct **prosthesis**

√7ᵗʰ T85.521 Displacement of esophageal anti-reflux **device**

√7ᵗʰ T85.528 Displacement of other gastrointestinal prosthetic devices, implants and grafts

√6ᵗʰ T85.59 Other **mechanical complication of gastrointestinal prosthetic devices, implants and grafts**
Obstruction, mechanical of gastrointestinal prosthetic devices, implants and grafts
Perforation of gastrointestinal prosthetic devices, implants and grafts
Protrusion of gastrointestinal prosthetic devices, implants and grafts

√7ᵗʰ T85.590 Other mechanical complication of bile duct **prosthesis**

√7ᵗʰ T85.591 Other mechanical complication of esophageal anti-reflux **device**

√7ᵗʰ T85.598 Other mechanical complication of other gastrointestinal prosthetic devices, implants and grafts

√5ᵗʰ T85.6 Mechanical complication of other **specified internal and external prosthetic** devices, implants and grafts

√6ᵗʰ T85.61 Breakdown (mechanical) of other specified internal prosthetic devices, implants and grafts

√7ᵗʰ T85.610 Breakdown (mechanical) of epidural and subdural infusion catheter

√7ᵗʰ T85.611 Breakdown (mechanical) of intraperitoneal dialysis catheter
EXCLUDES 1   mechanical complication of vascular dialysis catheter (T82.4-)

√7ᵗʰ T85.612 Breakdown (mechanical) of permanent sutures
EXCLUDES 1   mechanical complication of permanent (wire) suture used in bone repair (T84.1-T84.2)

√7ᵗʰ T85.613 Breakdown (mechanical) of artificial skin graft and decellularized allodermis
Failure of artificial skin graft and decellularized allodermis
Non-adherence of artificial skin graft and decellularized allodermis
Poor incorporation of artificial skin graft and decellularized allodermis
Shearing of artificial skin graft and decellularized allodermis

√7ᵗʰ T85.614 Breakdown (mechanical) of insulin pump

√7ᵗʰ T85.618 Breakdown (mechanical) of other specified internal prosthetic devices, implants and grafts

√6ᵗʰ T85.62 Displacement of other specified internal prosthetic devices, implants and grafts
Malposition of other specified internal prosthetic devices, implants and grafts

√7ᵗʰ T85.620 Displacement of epidural and subdural infusion catheter

√7ᵗʰ T85.621 Displacement of intraperitoneal dialysis catheter
EXCLUDES 1   mechanical complication of vascular dialysis catheter (T82.4-)

√7ᵗʰ T85.622 Displacement of permanent sutures
EXCLUDES 1   mechanical complication of permanent (wire) suture used in bone repair (T84.1-T84.2)

√7ᵗʰ T85.623 Displacement of artificial skin graft and decellularized allodermis
Dislodgement of artificial skin graft and decellularized allodermis
Displacement of artificial skin graft and decellularized allodermis

√7ᵗʰ T85.624 Displacement of insulin pump

√7ᵗʰ T85.628 Displacement of other specified internal prosthetic devices, implants and grafts

√6ᵗʰ T85.63 Leakage of other specified internal prosthetic devices, implants and grafts

√7ᵗʰ T85.630 Leakage of epidural and subdural infusion catheter

√7ᵗʰ T85.631 Leakage of intraperitoneal dialysis catheter
EXCLUDES 1   mechanical complication of vascular dialysis catheter (T82.4)

√7ᵗʰ T85.633 Leakage of insulin pump

√7ᵗʰ T85.638 Leakage of other specified internal prosthetic devices, implants and grafts

√6ᵗʰ T85.69 Other **mechanical complication of other specified internal prosthetic devices, implants and grafts**
Obstruction, mechanical of other specified internal prosthetic devices, implants and grafts
Perforation of other specified internal prosthetic devices, implants and grafts
Protrusion of other specified internal prosthetic devices, implants and grafts

√7ᵗʰ T85.690 Other mechanical complication of epidural and subdural infusion catheter

√7ᵗʰ T85.691 Other mechanical complication of intraperitoneal dialysis catheter
EXCLUDES 1   mechanical complication of vascular dialysis catheter (T82.4)

√7ᵗʰ T85.692 Other mechanical complication of permanent sutures
EXCLUDES 1   mechanical complication of permanent (wire) suture used in bone repair (T84.1-T84.2)

√7ᵗʰ T85.693 Other mechanical complication of artificial skin graft and decellularized allodermis

√7ᵗʰ T85.694 Other mechanical complication of insulin pump

√7ᵗʰ T85.698 Other mechanical complication of other specified internal prosthetic devices, implants and grafts
Mechanical complication of nonabsorbable surgical material NOS

√5ᵗʰ T85.7 Infection and inflammatory reaction due to other internal prosthetic devices, implants and grafts
Use additional code to identify infection

√x7ᵗʰ T85.71 Infection and inflammatory reaction due to peritoneal dialysis catheter   [CC]
RIC Excl 7th Character A: 09 Other orthopedic

√x7ᵗʰ T85.72 Infection and inflammatory reaction due to insulin pump   [CC]
RIC Excl 7th Character A: 09 Other orthopedic

√x7ᵗʰ T85.79 Infection and inflammatory reaction due to other internal prosthetic devices, implants and grafts   [CC]
RIC Excl 7th Character A: 09 Other orthopedic

√5ᵗʰ T85.8 Other specified complications of internal prosthetic devices, implants and grafts, not elsewhere classified

√x7ᵗʰ T85.81 Embolism **due to internal prosthetic devices, implants and grafts, not elsewhere classified**

√x7ᵗʰ T85.82 Fibrosis **due to internal prosthetic devices, implants and grafts, not elsewhere classified**

[N] Newborn   [P] Pediatric   [M] Maternity   [A] Adult   [RIC] RIC Dx   [NCDx] Noncancer Dx   [PDx] Primary Dx   [CC] RIC CC Condition   ▶◀ Revised Text   ● New Code   ▲ Revised Code Title

√x7ᵗʰ **T85.83** Hemorrhage due to internal prosthetic devices, implants and grafts, not elsewhere classified

√x7ᵗʰ **T85.84** Pain due to internal prosthetic devices, implants and grafts, not elsewhere classified

√x7ᵗʰ **T85.85** Stenosis due to internal prosthetic devices, implants and grafts, not elsewhere classified

√x7ᵗʰ **T85.86** Thrombosis due to internal prosthetic devices, implants and grafts, not elsewhere classified

√x7ᵗʰ **T85.89** Other specified complication of internal prosthetic devices, implants and grafts, not elsewhere classified

√x7ᵗʰ **T85.9** Unspecified complication of internal prosthetic device, implant and graft ▽
     Complication of internal prosthetic device, implant and graft NOS

√4ᵗʰ **T86 Complications of transplanted organs and tissue**
     Use additional code to identify other transplant complications, such as:
     graft-versus-host disease (D89.81-)
     malignancy associated with organ transplant (C80.2)
     post-transplant lymphoproliferative disorders (PTLD) (D47.Z1)

√5ᵗʰ **T86.0** Complications of bone marrow transplant
     T86.00 Unspecified complication of bone marrow transplant ▽
     T86.01 Bone marrow transplant rejection
     T86.02 Bone marrow transplant failure
     T86.03 Bone marrow transplant infection
     T86.09 Other complications of bone marrow transplant

√5ᵗʰ **T86.1** Complications of kidney transplant
     T86.10 Unspecified complication of kidney transplant ▽
     T86.11 Kidney transplant rejection
     T86.12 Kidney transplant failure
        AHA: 2013, 1Q, 24
     T86.13 Kidney transplant infection
        Use additional code to specify infection
     T86.19 Other complication of kidney transplant

√5ᵗʰ **T86.2** Complications of heart transplant
     EXCLUDES 1 complication of:
        artificial heart device (T82.5)
        heart-lung transplant (T86.3)
     T86.20 Unspecified complication of heart transplant ▽
     T86.21 Heart transplant rejection
     T86.22 Heart transplant failure
     T86.23 Heart transplant infection
        Use additional code to specify infection
     √6ᵗʰ **T86.29** Other complications of heart transplant
        T86.290 Cardiac allograft vasculopathy
           EXCLUDES 1 atherosclerosis of coronary arteries (I25.75-, I25.76-, I25.81-)
        T86.298 Other complications of heart transplant

√5ᵗʰ **T86.3** Complications of heart-lung transplant
     T86.30 Unspecified complication of heart-lung transplant ▽
     T86.31 Heart-lung transplant rejection
     T86.32 Heart-lung transplant failure
     T86.33 Heart-lung transplant infection
        Use additional code to specify infection
     T86.39 Other complications of heart-lung transplant

√5ᵗʰ **T86.4** Complications of liver transplant
     T86.40 Unspecified complication of liver transplant ▽
     T86.41 Liver transplant rejection
     T86.42 Liver transplant failure
     T86.43 Liver transplant infection
        Use additional code to identify infection, such as:
           cytomegalovirus (CMV) infection (B25.-)
     T86.49 Other complications of liver transplant

T86.5 Complications of stem cell transplant
     Complications from stem cells from peripheral blood
     Complications from stem cells from umbilical cord

√5ᵗʰ **T86.8** Complications of other transplanted organs and tissues
     √6ᵗʰ **T86.81** Complications of lung transplant
        EXCLUDES 1 complication of heart-lung transplant (T86.3-)
        T86.810 Lung transplant rejection

        T86.811 Lung transplant failure
        T86.812 Lung transplant infection
           Use additional code to specify infection
        T86.818 Other complications of lung transplant
        T86.819 Unspecified complication of lung transplant ▽

     √6ᵗʰ **T86.82** Complications of skin graft (allograft) (autograft)
        EXCLUDES 2 complication of artificial skin graft (T85.693)
        T86.820 Skin graft (allograft) rejection
        T86.821 Skin graft (allograft) (autograft) failure
        T86.822 Skin graft (allograft) (autograft) infection
           Use additional code to specify infection
        T86.828 Other complications of skin graft (allograft) (autograft)
        T86.829 Unspecified complication of skin graft (allograft) (autograft) ▽

     √6ᵗʰ **T86.83** Complications of bone graft
        EXCLUDES 2 mechanical complications of bone graft (T84.3-)
        T86.830 Bone graft rejection
        T86.831 Bone graft failure
        T86.832 Bone graft infection
           Use additional code to specify infection
        T86.838 Other complications of bone graft
        T86.839 Unspecified complication of bone graft ▽

     √6ᵗʰ **T86.84** Complications of corneal transplant
        EXCLUDES 2 mechanical complications of corneal graft (T85.3-)
        T86.840 Corneal transplant rejection
        T86.841 Corneal transplant failure
        T86.842 Corneal transplant infection   CC
           Use additional code to specify infection
           RIC Excl 7th Character A: 09 Other orthopedic
        T86.848 Other complications of corneal transplant
        T86.849 Unspecified complication of corneal transplant ▽

     √6ᵗʰ **T86.85** Complication of intestine transplant
        T86.850 Intestine transplant rejection
        T86.851 Intestine transplant failure
        T86.852 Intestine transplant infection
           Use additional code to specify infection
        T86.858 Other complications of intestine transplant
        T86.859 Unspecified complication of intestine transplant ▽

     √6ᵗʰ **T86.89** Complications of other transplanted tissue
        Transplant failure or rejection of pancreas
        T86.890 Other transplanted tissue rejection
        T86.891 Other transplanted tissue failure
        T86.892 Other transplanted tissue infection
           Use additional code to specify infection
        T86.898 Other complications of other transplanted tissue
        T86.899 Unspecified complication of other transplanted tissue ▽

     √5ᵗʰ **T86.9** Complication of unspecified transplanted organ and tissue
        T86.90 Unspecified complication of unspecified transplanted organ and tissue ▽
        T86.91 Unspecified transplanted organ and tissue rejection ▽
        T86.92 Unspecified transplanted organ and tissue failure ▽
        T86.93 Unspecified transplanted organ and tissue infection ▽
           Use additional code to specify infection
        T86.99 Other complications of unspecified transplanted organ and tissue ▽

√4ᵗʰ **T87 Complications peculiar to reattachment and amputation**
     √5ᵗʰ **T87.0** Complications of reattached (part of) upper extremity
        √6ᵗʰ **T87.0X** Complications of reattached (part of) upper extremity
        T87.0X1 Complications of reattached (part of) right upper extremity
        T87.0X2 Complications of reattached (part of) left upper extremity

---

✓ Add'l Character Required   √x7ᵗʰ Placeholder Alert   RUG IV Special Care High Dx   RUG IV Clinically Complex Dx   RUG IV Special Care Low Dx   Manifestation Code   Other Specified Code   ▽ Unspecified Code

Chapter 19. Injury, Poisoning and Certain Other Consequences of External Causes

T87.0X9   **Complications of reattached (part of) unspecified upper extremity**   ▽

✓5ᵗʰ **T87.1**   **Complications of reattached (part of) lower extremity**

   ✓6ᵗʰ **T87.1X**   **Complications of reattached (part of) lower extremity**

     T87.1X1   **Complications of reattached (part of) right lower extremity**

     T87.1X2   **Complications of reattached (part of) left lower extremity**

     T87.1X9   **Complications of reattached (part of) unspecified lower extremity**   ▽

T87.2   **Complications of other reattached body part**

✓5ᵗʰ **T87.3**   **Neuroma of amputation stump**

   T87.30   **Neuroma of amputation stump, unspecified extremity**   ▽

   T87.31   **Neuroma of amputation stump, right upper extremity**

   T87.32   **Neuroma of amputation stump, left upper extremity**

   T87.33   **Neuroma of amputation stump, right lower extremity**

   T87.34   **Neuroma of amputation stump, left lower extremity**

✓5ᵗʰ **T87.4**   **Infection of amputation stump**

   T87.40   **Infection of amputation stump, unspecified extremity**   CC ▽
     RIC Excl 7th Character A: 09 Other orthopedic; 10 Amputation, lower extremity; 11 Amputation, non-lower extremity

   T87.41   **Infection of amputation stump, right upper extremity**   CC
     RIC Excl 7th Character A: 09 Other orthopedic; 10 Amputation, lower extremity; 11 Amputation, non-lower extremity

   T87.42   **Infection of amputation stump, left upper extremity**   CC
     RIC Excl 7th Character A: 09 Other orthopedic; 10 Amputation, lower extremity; 11 Amputation, non-lower extremity

   T87.43   **Infection of amputation stump, right lower extremity**   CC
     RIC Excl 7th Character A: 09 Other orthopedic; 10 Amputation, lower extremity; 11 Amputation, non-lower extremity

   T87.44   **Infection of amputation stump, left lower extremity**   CC
     RIC Excl 7th Character A: 09 Other orthopedic; 10 Amputation, lower extremity; 11 Amputation, non-lower extremity

✓5ᵗʰ **T87.5**   **Necrosis of amputation stump**

   T87.50   **Necrosis of amputation stump, unspecified extremity**   ▽

   T87.51   **Necrosis of amputation stump, right upper extremity**

   T87.52   **Necrosis of amputation stump, left upper extremity**

   T87.53   **Necrosis of amputation stump, right lower extremity**

   T87.54   **Necrosis of amputation stump, left lower extremity**

✓5ᵗʰ **T87.8**   **Other complications of amputation stump**

   T87.81   ~~**Dehiscence**~~ **of amputation stump**

   T87.89   **Other complications of amputation stump**
     Amputation stump contracture
     Amputation stump contracture of next proximal joint
     Amputation stump flexion
     Amputation stump edema
     Amputation stump hematoma
     EXCLUDES 2   *phantom limb syndrome (G54.6-G54.7)*

T87.9   **Unspecified complications of amputation stump**   ▽

✓4ᵗʰ **T88**   **Other complications of surgical and medical care, not elsewhere classified**

   EXCLUDES 2   *complication following infusion, transfusion and therapeutic injection (T80.-)*
     complication following procedure NEC (T81.-)
     complications of anesthesia in labor and delivery (O74.-)
     complications of anesthesia in pregnancy (O29.-)
     complications of anesthesia in puerperium (O89.-)
     complications of devices, implants and grafts (T82-T85)
     complications of obstetric surgery and procedure (O75.4)
     dermatitis due to drugs and medicaments (L23.3, L24.4, L25.1, L27.0-L27.1)
     poisoning and toxic effects of drugs and chemicals (T36-T65 with fifth or sixth character 1-4 or 6)
     specified complications classified elsewhere

> The appropriate 7th character is to be added to each code from category T88.
> A   initial encounter
> D   subsequent encounter
> S   sequela

✓x7ᵗʰ **T88.0**   **Infection following immunization**
   Sepsis following immunization

✓x7ᵗʰ **T88.1**   **Other complications following immunization, not elsewhere classified**
   Generalized vaccinia
   Rash following immunization
   EXCLUDES 1   *vaccinia not from vaccine (B08.011)*
   EXCLUDES 2   *anaphylactic shock due to serum (T80.5-)*
     other serum reactions (T80.6-)
     postimmunization arthropathy (M02.2)
     postimmunization encephalitis (G04.02)
     postimmunization fever (R50.83)

✓x7ᵗʰ **T88.2**   **Shock due to anesthesia**
   Use additional code for adverse effect, if applicable, to identify drug (T41.- with fifth or sixth character 5)
   EXCLUDES 1   *complications of anesthesia (in):*
     labor and delivery (O74.-)
     postprocedural shock NOS (T81.1-)
     pregnancy (O29.-)
     puerperium (O89.-)

✓x7ᵗʰ **T88.3**   **Malignant hyperthermia due to anesthesia**
   Use additional code for adverse effect, if applicable, to identify drug (T41.- with fifth or sixth character 5)

✓x7ᵗʰ **T88.4**   **Failed or difficult intubation**

✓5ᵗʰ **T88.5**   **Other complications of anesthesia**
   Use additional code for adverse effect, if applicable, to identify drug (T41.- with fifth or sixth character 5)

   ✓x7ᵗʰ **T88.51**   **Hypothermia following anesthesia**

   ✓x7ᵗʰ **T88.52**   **Failed moderate sedation during procedure**
     Failed conscious sedation during procedure
     EXCLUDES 2   *personal history of failed moderate sedation (Z92.83)*

   ✓x7ᵗʰ **T88.59**   **Other complications of anesthesia**

✓x7ᵗʰ **T88.6**   **Anaphylactic reaction due to adverse effect of correct drug or medicament properly administered**
   Anaphylactic shock due to adverse effect of correct drug or medicament properly administered
   Anaphylactoid reaction NOS
   Use additional code for adverse effect, if applicable, to identify drug (T36-T50 with fifth or sixth character 5)
   EXCLUDES 1   *anaphylactic reaction due to serum (T80.5-)*
     anaphylactic shock or reaction due to adverse food reaction (T78.0-)

✓x7ᵗʰ **T88.7**   **Unspecified adverse effect of drug or medicament**   ▽
   Drug hypersensitivity NOS
   Drug reaction NOS
   Use additional code for adverse effect, if applicable, to identify drug (T36-T50 with fifth or sixth character 5)
   EXCLUDES 1   *specified adverse effects of drugs and medicaments (A00-R94 and T80-T88.6, T88.8)*

✓x7ᵗʰ **T88.8**   **Other specified complications of surgical and medical care, not elsewhere classified**
   Use additional code to identify the complication

✓x7ᵗʰ **T88.9**   **Complication of surgical and medical care, unspecified**   ▽

Ⓝ Newborn   Ⓟ Pediatric   Ⓜ Maternity   Ⓐ Adult   **RIC** RIC Dx   **NC Dx** Noncancer Dx   **PDx** Primary Dx   **CC** RIC CC Condition   ▶◀ Revised Text   ● New Code   ▲ Revised Code Titl

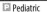

1048   ICD-10-CM 2016

Chapter 20. External Causes of Morbidity (VØØ–Y99)

Chapter Specific Guidelines with Coding Examples

The chapter specific guidelines from the ICD-10-CM Official Guidelines for Coding and Reporting have been provided below. Along with these guidelines are coding examples, contained in the shaded boxes, that have been developed to help illustrate the coding and/or sequencing guidance found in these guidelines.

The external causes of morbidity codes should never be sequenced as the first-listed or principal diagnosis.

External cause codes are intended to provide data for injury research and evaluation of injury prevention strategies. These codes capture how the injury or health condition happened (cause), the intent (unintentional or accidental; or intentional, such as suicide or assault), the place where the event occurred, the activity of the patient at the time of the event, and the person's status (e.g., civilian, military).

There is no national requirement for mandatory ICD-10-CM external cause code reporting. Unless a provider is subject to a state-based external cause code reporting mandate or these codes are required by a particular payer, reporting of ICD-10-CM codes in Chapter 20, External Causes of Morbidity, is not required. In the absence of a mandatory reporting requirement, providers are encouraged to voluntarily report external cause codes, as they provide valuable data for injury research and evaluation of injury prevention strategies.

a. General external cause coding guidelines

1) Used with any code in the range of A00.0–T88.9, Z00–Z99

An external cause code may be used with any code in the range of A00.0–T88.9, Z00–Z99, classification that is a health condition due to an external cause. Though they are most applicable to injuries, they are also valid for use with such things as infections or diseases due to an external source, and other health conditions, such as a heart attack that occurs during strenuous physical activity.

> Actinic reticuloid due to tanning bed use
>
> **L57.1**   **Actinic reticuloid**
>
> **W89.1XXA**   **Exposure to tanning bed, initial encounter**
>
> *Explanation:* An external cause code may be used with any code in the range of A00.0–T88.9, Z00–Z99, classifications that describe health conditions due to an external cause. Code W89.1 Exposure to tanning bed requires a seventh character of A to report this initial encounter, with a placeholder X for the fifth and sixth characters.

2) External cause code used for length of treatment

Assign the external cause code, with the appropriate 7th character (initial encounter, subsequent encounter or sequela) for each encounter for which the injury or condition is being treated.

Most categories in chapter 20 have a 7th character requirement for each applicable code. Most categories in this chapter have three 7th character values: A, initial encounter, D, subsequent encounter and S, sequela. While the patient may be seen by a new or different provider over the course of treatment for an injury or condition, assignment of the 7th character for external cause should match the 7th character of the code assigned for the associated injury or condition for the encounter.

3) Use the full range of external cause codes

Use the full range of external cause codes to completely describe the cause, the intent, the place of occurrence, and if applicable, the activity of the patient at the time of the event, and the patient's status, for all injuries, and other health conditions due to an external cause.

4) Assign as many external cause codes as necessary

Assign as many external cause codes as necessary to fully explain each cause. If only one external code can be recorded, assign the code most related to the principal diagnosis.

5) The selection of the appropriate external cause code

The selection of the appropriate external cause code is guided by the Alphabetic Index of External Causes and by Inclusion and Exclusion notes in the Tabular List.

6) External cause code can never be a principal diagnosis

An external cause code can never be a principal (first-listed) diagnosis.

7) Combination external cause codes

Certain of the external cause codes are combination codes that identify sequential events that result in an injury, such as a fall which results in striking against an object. The injury may be due to either event or both.

The combination external cause code used should correspond to the sequence of events regardless of which caused the most serious injury.

> Toddler tripped and fell while walking and struck his head on an end table, sustaining a scalp contusion
>
> **S00.03XA**   **Contusion of scalp, initial encounter**
>
> **W01.190A**   **Fall on same level from slipping, tripping and stumbling with subsequent striking against furniture, initial encounter**
>
> *Explanation:* Combination external cause codes identify sequential events that result in an injury, such as a fall resulting in striking against an object. The injury may be due to either or both events.

8) No external cause code needed in certain circumstances

No external cause code from Chapter 20 is needed if the external cause and intent are included in a code from another chapter (e.g. T36.0X1- Poisoning by penicillins, accidental (unintentional)).

b. Place of occurrence guideline

Codes from category Y92, Place of occurrence of the external cause, are secondary codes for use after other external cause codes to identify the location of the patient at the time of injury or other condition.

Generally, a place of occurrence code is assigned only once, at the initial encounter for treatment. However, in the rare instance that a new injury occurs during hospitalization, an additional place of occurrence code may be assigned. No 7th characters are used for Y92.

Do not use place of occurrence code Y92.9 if the place is not stated or is not applicable.

> A farmer was working in his barn and sustained a foot contusion when the horse stepped on his left foot
>
> **S90.32XA**   **Contusion of left foot, initial encounter**
>
> **W55.19XA**   **Other contact with horse, initial encounter**
>
> **Y92.71**   **Barn as the place of occurrence of the external cause**
>
> *Explanation:* A place-of-occurrence code from category Y92 is assigned at the initial encounter to identify the location of the patient at the time the injury occurred.

c. Activity code

Assign a code from category Y93, Activity code, to describe the activity of the patient at the time the injury or other health condition occurred.

An activity code is used only once, at the initial encounter for treatment. Only one code from Y93 should be recorded on a medical record.

The activity codes are not applicable to poisonings, adverse effects, misadventures or sequela.

Do not assign Y93.9, Unspecified activity, if the activity is not stated.

A code from category Y93 is appropriate for use with external cause and intent codes if identifying the activity provides additional information about the event.

> Ranch hand who was grooming a horse sustained a foot contusion when the horse stepped on his left foot
>
> **S90.32XA**   **Contusion of left foot, initial encounter**
>
> **W55.19XA**   **Other contact with horse, initial encounter**
>
> **Y93.K3**   **Activity, grooming and shearing an animal**
>
> *Explanation:* One activity code from category Y93 is assigned at the initial encounter only to describe the activity of the patient at the time the injury occurred.

d. Place of occurrence, activity, and status codes used with other external cause code

When applicable, place of occurrence, activity, and external cause status codes are sequenced after the main external cause code(s). Regardless of the number of external cause codes assigned, there should be only one place of occurrence code, one activity code, and one external cause status code assigned to an encounter.

e. If the reporting format limits the number of external cause codes

If the reporting format limits the number of external cause codes that can be used in reporting clinical data, report the code for the cause/intent most related to the principal diagnosis. If the format permits, capture of additional external cause codes, the cause/intent, including medical misadventures, of the additional events should be reported rather than the codes for place, activity, or external status.

f. Multiple external cause coding guidelines

More than one external cause code is required to fully describe the external cause of an illness or injury. The assignment of external cause codes should be sequenced in the following priority:

If two or more events cause separate injuries, an external cause code should be assigned for each cause. The first-listed external cause code will be selected in the following order:

External codes for child and adult abuse take priority over all other external cause codes.

See Section I.C.19., Child and Adult abuse guidelines.

External cause codes for terrorism events take priority over all other external cause codes except child and adult abuse.

External cause codes for cataclysmic events take priority over all other external cause codes except child and adult abuse and terrorism.

External cause codes for transport accidents take priority over all other external cause codes except cataclysmic events, child and adult abuse and terrorism.

Activity and external cause status codes are assigned following all causal (intent) external cause codes.

The first-listed external cause code should correspond to the cause of the most serious diagnosis due to an assault, accident, or self-harm, following the order of hierarchy listed above..

30-year-old man accidentally discharged his hunting rifle, sustaining an open gunshot wound to the right thigh, which caused him to fall down the stairs, resulting in closed displaced comminuted fracture of his left radial shaft

S71.101A	**Unspecified open wound, right thigh, initial encounter**
W33.02XA	**Accidental discharge of hunting rifle, initial encounter**
S52.352A	**Displaced comminuted fracture of shaft of radius, left arm, initial encounter for closed fracture**
W10.9XXA	**Fall (on) (from) unspecified stairs and steps, initial encounter**

Explanation: If two or more events cause separate injuries, an external cause code should be assigned for each cause.

---

g. Child and adult abuse guideline

Adult and child abuse, neglect and maltreatment are classified as assault. Any of the assault codes may be used to indicate the external cause of any injury resulting from the confirmed abuse.

For confirmed cases of abuse, neglect and maltreatment, when the perpetrator is known, a code from Y07, Perpetrator of maltreatment and neglect, should accompany any other assault codes.

See Section I.C.19. Adult and child abuse, neglect and other maltreatment

h. Unknown or Undetermined Intent Guideline

If the intent (accident, self-harm, assault) of the cause of an injury or other condition is unknown or unspecified, code the intent as accidental intent. All transport accident categories assume accidental intent.

1) Use of undetermined intent

External cause codes for events of undetermined intent are only for use if the documentation in the record specifies that the intent cannot be determined.

i. Sequelae (late effects) of external cause guidelines

1) Sequelae external cause codes

Sequela are reported using the external cause code with the 7th character "S" for sequela. These codes should be used with any report of a late effect or sequela resulting from a previous injury.

See Section I.B.10 Sequela (Late Effects)

2) Sequela external cause code with a related current injury

A sequela external cause code should never be used with a related current nature of injury code.

3) Use of sequela external cause codes for subsequent visits

Use a late effect external cause code for subsequent visits when a late effect of the initial injury is being treated. Do not use a late effect external cause code for subsequent visits for follow-up care (e.g., to assess healing, to receive rehabilitative therapy) of the injury when no late effect of the injury has been documented.

j. Terrorism guidelines

1) Cause of injury identified by the Federal Government (FBI) as terrorism

When the cause of an injury is identified by the Federal Government (FBI) as terrorism, the first-listed external cause code should be a code from category Y38, Terrorism. The definition of terrorism employed by the FBI is found at the inclusion note at the beginning of category Y38. Use additional code for place of occurrence (Y92.-). More than one Y38 code may be assigned if the injury is the result of more than one mechanism of terrorism.

2) Cause of an injury is suspected to be the result of terrorism

When the cause of an injury is suspected to be the result of terrorism a code from category Y38 should not be assigned. Suspected cases should be classified as assault.

3) Code Y38.9, Terrorism, secondary effects

Assign code Y38.9, Terrorism, secondary effects, for conditions occurring subsequent to the terrorist event. This code should not be assigned for conditions that are due to the initial terrorist act.

It is acceptable to assign code Y38.9 with another code from Y38 if there is an injury due to the initial terrorist event and an injury that is a subsequent result of the terrorist event.

k. External cause status

A code from category Y99, External cause status, should be assigned whenever any other external cause code is assigned for an encounter, including an Activity code, except for the events noted below. Assign a code from category Y99, External cause status, to indicate the work status of the person at the time the event occurred. The status code indicates whether the event occurred during military activity, whether a non-military person was at work, whether an individual including a student or volunteer was involved in a non-work activity at the time of the causal event.

A code from Y99, External cause status, should be assigned, when applicable, with other external cause codes, such as transport accidents and falls. The external cause status codes are not applicable to poisonings, adverse effects, misadventures or late effects.

Do not assign a code from category Y99 if no other external cause codes (cause, activity) are applicable for the encounter.

An external cause status code is used only once, at the initial encounter for treatment. Only one code from Y99 should be recorded on a medical record.

Do not assign code Y99.9, Unspecified external cause status, if the status is not stated.

Chapter 20. External Causes of Morbidity (V00-Y99)

NOTE This chapter permits the classification of environmental events and circumstances as the cause of injury, and other adverse effects. Where a code from this section is applicable, it is intended that it shall be used secondary to a code from another chapter of the Classification indicating the nature of the condition. Most often, the condition will be classifiable to Chapter 19, Injury, poisoning and certain other consequences of external causes (S00-T88). Other conditions that may be stated to be due to external causes are classified in Chapters I to XVIII. For these conditions, codes from Chapter 20 should be used to provide additional information as to the cause of the condition.

This chapter contains the following blocks:

V00-X58	Accidents
V00-V99	Transport accidents
V00-V09	Pedestrian injured in transport accident
V10-V19	Pedal cycle rider injured in transport accident
V20-V29	Motorcycle rider injured in transport accident
V30-V39	Occupant of three-wheeled motor vehicle injured in transport accident
V40-V49	Car occupant injured in transport accident
V50-V59	Occupant of pick-up truck or van injured in transport accident
V60-V69	Occupant of heavy transport vehicle injured in transport accident
V70-V79	Bus occupant injured in transport accident
V80-V89	Other land transport accidents
V90-V94	Water transport accidents
V95-V97	Air and space transport accidents
V98-V99	Other and unspecified transport accidents
W00-X58	Other external causes of accidental injury
W00-W19	Slipping, tripping, stumbling and falls
W20-W49	Exposure to inanimate mechanical forces
W50-W64	Exposure to animate mechanical forces
W65-W74	Accidental non-transport drowning and submersion
W85-W99	Exposure to electric current, radiation and extreme ambient air temperature and pressure
X00-X08	Exposure to smoke, fire and flames
X10-X19	Contact with heat and hot substances
X30-X39	Exposure to forces of nature
X52-X58	Accidental exposure to other specified factors
X71-X83	Intentional self-harm
X92-Y08	Assault
Y21-Y33	Event of undetermined intent
Y35-Y38	Legal intervention, operations of war, military operations, and terrorism
Y62-Y84	Complications of medical and surgical care
Y62-Y69	Misadventures to patients during surgical and medical care
Y70-Y82	Medical devices associated with adverse incidents in diagnostic and therapeutic use
Y83-Y84	Surgical and other medical procedures as the cause of abnormal reaction of the patient, or of later complication, without mention of misadventure at the time of the procedure
Y90-Y99	Supplementary factors related to causes of morbidity classified elsewhere

Accidents (V00-X58)

Transport accidents (V00-V99)

NOTE This section is structured in 12 groups. Those relating to land transport accidents (V01-V89) reflect the victim's mode of transport and are subdivided to identify the victim's 'counterpart' or the type of event. The vehicle of which the injured person is an occupant is identified in the first two characters since it is seen as the most important factor to identify for prevention purposes. A transport accident is one in which the vehicle involved must be moving or running or in use for transport purposes at the time of the accident.

Use additional code to identify:
  airbag injury (W22.1)
  type of street or road (Y92.4-)
  use of cellular telephone and other electronic equipment at the time of the transport accident (Y93.C-)

EXCLUDES 1 *agricultural vehicles in stationary use or maintenance (W31.-)*
  assault by crashing of motor vehicle (Y03.-)
  automobile or motor cycle in stationary use or maintenance—code to type of accident
  crashing of motor vehicle, undetermined intent (Y32)
  intentional self-harm by crashing of motor vehicle (X82)

EXCLUDES 2 *transport accidents due to cataclysm (X34-X38)*

NOTE Definitions of transport vehicles:

(a) A transport accident is any accident involving a device designed primarily for, or used at the time primarily for, conveying persons or good from one place to another.

(b) A public highway [trafficway] or street is the entire width between property lines (or other boundary lines) of land open to the public as a matter of right or custom for purposes of moving persons or property from one place to another. A roadway is that part of the public highway designed, improved and customarily used for vehicular traffic.

(c) A traffic accident is any vehicle accident occurring on the public highway [i.e. originating on, terminating on, or involving a vehicle partially on the highway]. A vehicle accident is assumed to have occurred on the public highway unless another place is specified, except in the case of accidents involving only off-road motor vehicles, which are classified as nontraffic accidents unless the contrary is stated.

(d) A nontraffic accident is any vehicle accident that occurs entirely in any place other than a public highway.

(e) A pedestrian is any person involved in an accident who was not at the time of the accident riding in or on a motor vehicle, railway train, streetcar or animal-drawn or other vehicle, or on a pedal cycle or animal. This includes, a person changing a tire or working on a parked car. It also includes the use of a pedestrian conveyance such as a baby carriage, ice-skates, roller skates, a skateboard, nonmotorized or motorized wheelchair, motorized mobility scooter, or nonmotorized scooter.

(f) A driver is an occupant of a transport vehicle who is operating or intending to operate it.

(g) A passenger is any occupant of a transport vehicle other than the driver, except a person traveling on the outside of the vehicle.

(h) A person on the outside of a vehicle is any person being transported by a vehicle but not occupying the space normally reserved for the driver or passengers, or the space intended for the transport of property. This includes the body, bumper, fender, roof, running board or step of a vehicle.

(i) A pedal cycle is any land transport vehicle operated solely by nonmotorized pedals including a bicycle or tricycle.

(j) A pedal cyclist is any person riding a pedal cycle or in a sidecar or trailer attached to a pedal cycle.

(k) A motorcycle is a two-wheeled motor vehicle with one or two riding saddles and sometimes with a third wheel for the support of a sidecar. The sidecar is considered part of the motorcycle.

(l) A motorcycle rider is any person riding a motorcycle or in a sidecar or trailer attached to the motorcycle.

(m) A three-wheeled motor vehicle is a motorized tricycle designed primarily for on-road use. This includes a motor-driven tricycle, a motorized rickshaw, or a three-wheeled motor car.

(n) A car [automobile] is a four-wheeled motor vehicle designed primarily for carrying up to 7 persons. A trailer being towed by the car is considered part of the car.

(o) A pick-up truck or van is a four or six-wheeled motor vehicle designed for carrying passengers as well as property or cargo weighing less than the local limit for classification as a heavy goods vehicle, and not requiring a special driver's license. This includes a minivan and a sport-utility vehicle (SUV).

(p) A heavy transport vehicle is a motor vehicle designed primarily for carrying property, meeting local criteria for classification as a heavy goods vehicle in terms of weight and requiring a special driver's license.

(q) A bus (coach) is a motor vehicle designed or adapted primarily for carrying more than 10 passengers, and requiring a special driver's license.

(r) A railway train or railway vehicle is any device, with or without freight or passenger cars couple to it, designed for traffic on a railway track. This includes subterranean (subways) or elevated trains.

(s) A streetcar, is a device designed and used primarily for transporting passengers within a municipality, running on rails, usually subject to normal traffic control signals, and operated principally on a right-of-way that forms part of the roadway. This includes a tram or trolley that runs on rails. A trailer being towed by a streetcar is considered part of the streetcar.

(t) A special vehicle mainly used on industrial premises is a motor vehicle designed primarily for use within the buildings and premises of industrial or commercial establishments. This includes battery-powered trucks, forklifts, coal-cars in a coal mine, logging cars and trucks used in mines or quarries.

(u) A special vehicle mainly used in agriculture is a motor vehicle designed specifically for use in farming and agriculture (horticulture), to work the land, tend and harvest crops and transport materials on the farm. This includes harvesters, farm machinery and tractor and trailers.

(v) A special construction vehicle is a motor vehicle designed specifically for use on construction and demolition sites. This includes bulldozers, diggers, earth levellers, dump trucks, backhoes, front-end loaders, pavers, and mechanical shovels.

(w) A special all-terrain vehicle is a motor vehicle of special design to enable it to negotiate over rough or soft terrain, snow or sand. This includes snow mobiles, All-terrain vehicles (ATV), and dune buggies. It does not include passenger vehicle designated as Sport Utility Vehicles. (SUV)

(x) A watercraft is any device designed for transporting passengers or goods on water. This includes motor or sailboats, ships, and hovercraft.

(y) An aircraft is any device for transporting passengers or goods in the air. This includes hot-air balloons, gliders, helicopters and airplanes.

(z) A military vehicle is any motorized vehicle operating on a public roadway owned by the military and being operated by a member of the military.

Pedestrian injured in transport accident (V00-V09)

INCLUDES person changing tire on transport vehicle
person examining engine of vehicle broken down in (on side of) road

EXCLUDES 1 *fall due to non-transport collision with other person (W03)*
pedestrian on foot falling (slipping) on ice and snow (W00.-)
struck or bumped by another person (W51)

✓4ᵗʰ **V00 Pedestrian conveyance accident**

Use additional place of occurrence and activity external cause codes, if known (Y92-, Y93-)

EXCLUDES 1 *collision with another person without fall (W51)*
fall due to person on foot colliding with another person on foot (W03)
fall from non-moving wheelchair, nonmotorized scooter and motorized mobility scooter without collision (W05.-)
pedestrian (conveyance) collision with other land transport vehicle (V01-V09)
pedestrian on foot falling (slipping) on ice and snow (W00.-)

> The appropriate 7th character is to be added to each code from category V00.
> A   initial encounter
> D   subsequent encounter
> S   sequela

✓5ᵗʰ **V00.0 Pedestrian on foot injured in collision with pedestrian conveyance**

  ✓x7ᵗʰ **V00.01 Pedestrian on foot injured in collision with roller-skater**

  ✓x7ᵗʰ **V00.02 Pedestrian on foot injured in collision with skateboarder**

  ✓x7ᵗʰ **V00.09 Pedestrian on foot injured in collision with other pedestrian conveyance**

✓5ᵗʰ **V00.1 Rolling-type pedestrian conveyance accident**

  EXCLUDES 1 *accident with babystroller (V00.82-)*
accident with motorized mobility scooter (V00.83-)
accident with wheelchair (powered) (V00.81-)

  ✓6ᵗʰ **V00.11 In-line roller-skate accident**

    ✓7ᵗʰ **V00.111 Fall from in-line roller-skates**

    ✓7ᵗʰ **V00.112 In-line roller-skater colliding with stationary object**

    ✓7ᵗʰ **V00.118 Other in-line roller-skate accident**
      EXCLUDES 1 *roller-skater collision with other land transport vehicle (V01-V09 with 5th character 1)*

  ✓6ᵗʰ **V00.12 Non-in-line roller-skate accident**

    ✓7ᵗʰ **V00.121 Fall from non-in-line roller-skates**

    ✓7ᵗʰ **V00.122 Non-in-line roller-skater colliding with stationary object**

    ✓7ᵗʰ **V00.128 Other non-in-line roller-skating accident**
      EXCLUDES 1 *roller-skater collision with other land transport vehicle (V01-V09 with 5th character 1)*

  ✓6ᵗʰ **V00.13 Skateboard accident**

    ✓7ᵗʰ **V00.131 Fall from skateboard**

    ✓7ᵗʰ **V00.132 Skateboarder colliding with stationary object**

    ✓7ᵗʰ **V00.138 Other skateboard accident**
      EXCLUDES 1 *skateboarder collision with other land transport vehicle (V01-V09 with 5th character 2)*

  ✓6ᵗʰ **V00.14 Scooter (nonmotorized) accident**
    EXCLUDES 1 *motorscooter accident (V20-V29)*

    ✓7ᵗʰ **V00.141 Fall from scooter (nonmotorized)**

    ✓7ᵗʰ **V00.142 Scooter (nonmotorized) colliding with stationary object**

    ✓7ᵗʰ **V00.148 Other scooter (nonmotorized) accident**
      EXCLUDES 1 *scooter (nonmotorized) collision with other land transport vehicle (V01-V09 with fifth character 9)*

  ✓6ᵗʰ **V00.15 Heelies accident**
    Rolling shoe
    Wheeled shoe
    Wheelies accident

    ✓7ᵗʰ **V00.151 Fall from heelies**

    ✓7ᵗʰ **V00.152 Heelies colliding with stationary object**

    ✓7ᵗʰ **V00.158 Other heelies accident**

  ✓6ᵗʰ **V00.18 Accident on other rolling-type pedestrian conveyance**

    ✓7ᵗʰ **V00.181 Fall from other rolling-type pedestrian conveyance**

    ✓7ᵗʰ **V00.182 Pedestrian on other rolling-type pedestrian conveyance colliding with stationary object**

    ✓7ᵗʰ **V00.188 Other accident on other rolling-type pedestrian conveyance**

✓5ᵗʰ **V00.2 Gliding-type pedestrian conveyance accident**

  ✓6ᵗʰ **V00.21 Ice-skates accident**

    ✓7ᵗʰ **V00.211 Fall from ice-skates**

    ✓7ᵗʰ **V00.212 Ice-skater colliding with stationary object**

    ✓7ᵗʰ **V00.218 Other ice-skates accident**
      EXCLUDES 1 *ice-skater collision with other land transport vehicle (V01-V09 with 5th digit 9)*

  ✓6ᵗʰ **V00.22 Sled accident**

    ✓7ᵗʰ **V00.221 Fall from sled**

    ✓7ᵗʰ **V00.222 Sledder colliding with stationary object**

    ✓7ᵗʰ **V00.228 Other sled accident**
      EXCLUDES 1 *sled collision with other land transport vehicle (V01-V09 with 5th digit 9)*

  ✓6ᵗʰ **V00.28 Other gliding-type pedestrian conveyance accident**

    ✓7ᵗʰ **V00.281 Fall from other gliding-type pedestrian conveyance**

    ✓7ᵗʰ **V00.282 Pedestrian on other gliding-type pedestrian conveyance colliding with stationary object**

    ✓7ᵗʰ **V00.288 Other accident on other gliding-type pedestrian conveyance**
      EXCLUDES 1 *gliding-type pedestrian conveyance collision with other land transport vehicle (V01-V09 with 5th digit 9)*

✓5ᵗʰ **V00.3 Flat-bottomed pedestrian conveyance accident**

  ✓6ᵗʰ **V00.31 Snowboard accident**

    ✓7ᵗʰ **V00.311 Fall from snowboard**

    ✓7ᵗʰ **V00.312 Snowboarder colliding with stationary object**

    ✓7ᵗʰ **V00.318 Other snowboard accident**
      EXCLUDES 1 *snowboarder collision with other land transport vehicle (V01-V09 with 5th digit 9)*

  ✓6ᵗʰ **V00.32 Snow-ski accident**

    ✓7ᵗʰ **V00.321 Fall from snow-skis**

    ✓7ᵗʰ **V00.322 Snow-skier colliding with stationary object**

    ✓7ᵗʰ **V00.328 Other snow-ski accident**
      EXCLUDES 1 *snow-skier collision with other land transport vehicle (V01-V09 with 5th digit 9)*

  ✓6ᵗʰ **V00.38 Other flat-bottomed pedestrian conveyance accident**

    ✓7ᵗʰ **V00.381 Fall from other flat-bottomed pedestrian conveyance**

☑7ᵗʰ **V00.382** **Pedestrian on other flat-bottomed pedestrian conveyance** colliding with stationary object

☑7ᵗʰ **V00.388** Other accident on other flat-bottomed pedestrian conveyance

☑5ᵗʰ **V00.8** **Accident on other pedestrian conveyance**

  ☑6ᵗʰ **V00.81** **Accident with** wheelchair (powered)

    ☑7ᵗʰ **V00.811** Fall from **moving wheelchair (powered)**
        EXCLUDES 1 *fall from non-moving wheelchair (W05.0)*

    ☑7ᵗʰ **V00.812** **Wheelchair (powered)** colliding with stationary object

    ☑7ᵗʰ **V00.818** Other accident with wheelchair (powered)

  ☑6ᵗʰ **V00.82** **Accident with** babystroller

    ☑7ᵗʰ **V00.821** Fall from **babystroller**

    ☑7ᵗʰ **V00.822** **Babystroller** colliding with stationary object

    ☑7ᵗʰ **V00.828** Other accident with babystroller

  ☑6ᵗʰ **V00.83** **Accident with motorized** mobility scooter

    V00.831 Fall from **motorized mobility scooter**
        EXCLUDES 1 *fall from non-moving motorized mobility scooter (W05.2)*

    V00.832 **Motorized mobility scooter** colliding with stationary object

    V00.838 Other accident with motorized mobility scooter

  ☑6ᵗʰ **V00.89** **Accident on** other pedestrian conveyance

    ☑7ᵗʰ **V00.891** Fall from **other pedestrian conveyance**

    ☑7ᵗʰ **V00.892** **Pedestrian on other pedestrian conveyance** colliding with stationary object

    ☑7ᵗʰ **V00.898** Other accident on other pedestrian conveyance
        EXCLUDES 1 *other pedestrian (conveyance) collision with other land transport vehicle (V01-V09 with 5th digit 9)*

☑4ᵗʰ **V01** **Pedestrian injured in collision with pedal cycle**

The appropriate 7th character is to be added to each code from category V01.
A   initial encounter
D   subsequent encounter
S   sequela

☑5ᵗʰ **V01.0** **Pedestrian injured in collision with pedal cycle in** nontraffic accident

  ☑x7ᵗʰ **V01.00** **Pedestrian** on foot **injured in collision with pedal cycle in nontraffic accident**
    Pedestrian NOS injured in collision with pedal cycle in nontraffic accident

  ☑x7ᵗʰ **V01.01** **Pedestrian** on roller-skates **injured in collision with pedal cycle in nontraffic accident**

  ☑x7ᵗʰ **V01.02** **Pedestrian** on skateboard **injured in collision with pedal cycle in nontraffic accident**

  ☑x7ᵗʰ **V01.09** **Pedestrian with other** conveyance **injured in collision with pedal cycle in nontraffic accident**
    Pedestrian with babystroller injured in collision with pedal cycle in nontraffic accident
    Pedestrian on ice-skates injured in collision with pedal cycle in nontraffic accident
    Pedestrian on nonmotorized scooter injured in collision with pedal cycle in nontraffic accident
    Pedestrian on sled injured in collision with pedal cycle in nontraffic accident
    Pedestrian on snowboard injured in collision with pedal cycle in nontraffic accident
    Pedestrian on snow-skis injured in collision with pedal cycle in nontraffic accident
    Pedestrian in wheelchair (powered) injured in collision with pedal cycle in nontraffic accident
    Pedestrian in motorized mobility scooter injured in collision with pedal cycle in nontraffic accident

☑5ᵗʰ **V01.1** **Pedestrian injured in collision with pedal cycle in** traffic accident

  ☑x7ᵗʰ **V01.10** **Pedestrian** on foot **injured in collision with pedal cycle in traffic accident**
    Pedestrian NOS injured in collision with pedal cycle in traffic accident

☑x7ᵗʰ **V01.11** **Pedestrian** on roller-skates **injured in collision with pedal cycle in traffic accident**

☑x7ᵗʰ **V01.12** **Pedestrian** on skateboard **injured in collision with pedal cycle in traffic accident**

☑x7ᵗʰ **V01.19** **Pedestrian with other** conveyance **injured in collision with pedal cycle in traffic accident**
  Pedestrian with babystroller injured in collision with pedal cycle in traffic accident
  Pedestrian on ice-skates injured in collision with pedal cycle in traffic accident
  Pedestrian on nonmotorized scooter injured in collision with pedal cycle in traffic accident
  Pedestrian on sled injured in collision with pedal cycle in traffic accident
  Pedestrian on snowboard injured in collision with pedal cycle in traffic accident
  Pedestrian on snow-skis injured in collision with pedal cycle in traffic accident
  Pedestrian in wheelchair (powered) injured in collision with pedal cycle in traffic accident
  Pedestrian in motorized mobility scooter injured in collision with pedal cycle in traffic accident

☑5ᵗʰ **V01.9** **Pedestrian injured in collision with pedal cycle,** unspecified whether traffic or nontraffic accident

  ☑x7ᵗʰ **V01.90** **Pedestrian** on foot **injured in collision with pedal cycle, unspecified whether traffic or nontraffic accident** ▽
    Pedestrian NOS injured in collision with pedal cycle, unspecified whether traffic or nontraffic accident

  ☑x7ᵗʰ **V01.91** **Pedestrian** on roller-skates **injured in collision with pedal cycle, unspecified whether traffic or nontraffic accident** ▽

  ☑x7ᵗʰ **V01.92** **Pedestrian** on skateboard **injured in collision with pedal cycle, unspecified whether traffic or nontraffic accident** ▽

  ☑x7ᵗʰ **V01.99** **Pedestrian with other** conveyance **injured in collision with pedal cycle, unspecified whether traffic or nontraffic accident** ▽
    Pedestrian with babystroller injured in collision with pedal cycle, unspecified whether traffic or nontraffic accident
    Pedestrian on ice-skates injured in collision with pedal cycle unspecified, whether traffic or nontraffic accident
    Pedestrian on nonmotorized scooter injured in collision with pedal cycle, unspecified whether traffic or nontraffic accident
    Pedestrian on sled injured in collision with pedal cycle unspecified, whether traffic or nontraffic accident
    Pedestrian on snowboard injured in collision with pedal cycle, unspecified whether traffic or nontraffic accident
    Pedestrian on snow-skis injured in collision with pedal cycle, unspecified whether traffic or nontraffic accident
    Pedestrian in wheelchair (powered) injured in collision with pedal cycle, unspecified whether traffic or nontraffic accident
    Pedestrian in motorized mobility scooter injured in collision with pedal cycle, unspecified whether traffic or nontraffic accident

☑4ᵗʰ **V02** **Pedestrian injured in collision with two- or three-wheeled motor vehicle**

The appropriate 7th character is to be added to each code from category V02.
A   initial encounter
D   subsequent encounter
S   sequela

☑5ᵗʰ **V02.0** **Pedestrian injured in collision with two- or three-wheeled motor vehicle in** nontraffic accident

  ☑x7ᵗʰ **V02.00** **Pedestrian** on foot **injured in collision with two- or three-wheeled motor vehicle in nontraffic accident**
    Pedestrian NOS injured in collision with two- or three-wheeled motor vehicle in nontraffic accident

  ☑x7ᵗʰ **V02.01** **Pedestrian** on roller-skates **injured in collision with two- or three-wheeled motor vehicle in nontraffic accident**

  ☑x7ᵗʰ **V02.02** **Pedestrian** on skateboard **injured in collision with two- or three-wheeled motor vehicle in nontraffic accident**

√x7ᵗʰ **V02.09** **Pedestrian with other conveyance injured in collision with two- or three-wheeled motor vehicle in nontraffic accident**
    Pedestrian with babystroller injured in collision with two- or three-wheeled motor vehicle in nontraffic accident
    Pedestrian on ice-skates injured in collision with two- or three-wheeled motor vehicle in nontraffic accident
    Pedestrian on nonmotorized scooter injured in collision with two- or three-wheeled motor vehicle in nontraffic accident
    Pedestrian on sled injured in collision with two- or three-wheeled motor vehicle in nontraffic accident
    Pedestrian on snowboard injured in collision with two- or three-wheeled motor vehicle in nontraffic accident
    Pedestrian on snow-skis injured in collision with two- or three-wheeled motor vehicle in nontraffic accident
    Pedestrian in wheelchair (powered) injured in collision with two- or three-wheeled motor vehicle in nontraffic accident
    Pedestrian in motorized mobility scooter injured in collision with two- or three-wheeled motor vehicle in nontraffic accident

√5ᵗʰ **V02.1** **Pedestrian injured in collision with two- or three-wheeled motor vehicle in traffic accident**

√x7ᵗʰ **V02.10** **Pedestrian on foot injured in collision with two- or three-wheeled motor vehicle in traffic accident**
    Pedestrian NOS injured in collision with two- or three-wheeled motor vehicle in traffic accident

√x7ᵗʰ **V02.11** **Pedestrian on roller-skates injured in collision with two- or three-wheeled motor vehicle in traffic accident**

√x7ᵗʰ **V02.12** **Pedestrian on skateboard injured in collision with two- or three-wheeled motor vehicle in traffic accident**

√x7ᵗʰ **V02.19** **Pedestrian with other conveyance injured in collision with two- or three-wheeled motor vehicle in traffic accident**
    Pedestrian with babystroller injured in collision with two- or three-wheeled motor vehicle in traffic accident
    Pedestrian on ice-skates injured in collision with two- or three-wheeled motor vehicle in traffic accident
    Pedestrian on nonmotorized scooter injured in collision with two- or three-wheeled motor vehicle in traffic accident
    Pedestrian on sled injured in collision with two- or three-wheeled motor vehicle in traffic accident
    Pedestrian on snowboard injured in collision with two- or three-wheeled motor vehicle in traffic accident
    Pedestrian on snow-skis injured in collision with two- or three-wheeled motor vehicle in traffic accident
    Pedestrian in wheelchair (powered) injured in collision with two- or three-wheeled motor vehicle in traffic accident
    Pedestrian in motorized mobility scooter injured in collision with two- or three-wheeled motor vehicle in traffic accident

√5ᵗʰ **V02.9** **Pedestrian injured in collision with two- or three-wheeled motor vehicle, unspecified whether traffic or nontraffic accident**

√x7ᵗʰ **V02.90** **Pedestrian on foot injured in collision with two- or three-wheeled motor vehicle, unspecified whether traffic or nontraffic accident** ▽
    Pedestrian NOS injured in collision with two- or three-wheeled motor vehicle, unspecified whether traffic or nontraffic accident

√x7ᵗʰ **V02.91** **Pedestrian on roller-skates injured in collision with two- or three-wheeled motor vehicle, unspecified whether traffic or nontraffic accident** ▽

√x7ᵗʰ **V02.92** **Pedestrian on skateboard injured in collision with two- or three-wheeled motor vehicle, unspecified whether traffic or nontraffic accident** ▽

√x7ᵗʰ **V02.99** **Pedestrian with other conveyance injured in collision with two- or three-wheeled motor vehicle, unspecified whether traffic or nontraffic accident** ▽
    Pedestrian with babystroller injured in collision with two- or three-wheeled motor vehicle, unspecified whether traffic or nontraffic accident
    Pedestrian on ice-skates injured in collision with two- or three-wheeled motor vehicle, unspecified whether traffic or nontraffic accident
    Pedestrian on nonmotorized scooter injured in collision with two- or three-wheeled motor vehicle, unspecified whether traffic or nontraffic accident
    Pedestrian on sled injured in collision with two- or three-wheeled motor vehicle, unspecified whether traffic or nontraffic accident
    Pedestrian on snowboard injured in collision with two- or three-wheeled motor vehicle, unspecified whether traffic or nontraffic accident
    Pedestrian on snow-skis injured in collision with two- or three-wheeled motor vehicle, unspecified whether traffic or nontraffic accident
    Pedestrian in wheelchair (powered) injured in collision with two- or three-wheeled motor vehicle, unspecified whether traffic or nontraffic accident
    Pedestrian in motorized mobility scooter injured in collision with two- or three-wheeled motor vehicle, unspecified whether traffic or nontraffic accident

√4ᵗʰ **V03** **Pedestrian injured in collision with car, pick-up truck or van**

The appropriate 7th character is to be added to each code from category V03.
A   initial encounter
D   subsequent encounter
S   sequela

√5ᵗʰ **V03.0** **Pedestrian injured in collision with car, pick-up truck or van in nontraffic accident**

√x7ᵗʰ **V03.00** **Pedestrian on foot injured in collision with car, pick-up truck or van in nontraffic accident**
    Pedestrian NOS injured in collision with car, pick-up truck or van in nontraffic accident

√x7ᵗʰ **V03.01** **Pedestrian on roller-skates injured in collision with car, pick-up truck or van in nontraffic accident**

√x7ᵗʰ **V03.02** **Pedestrian on skateboard injured in collision with car, pick-up truck or van in nontraffic accident**

√x7ᵗʰ **V03.09** **Pedestrian with other conveyance injured in collision with car, pick-up truck or van in nontraffic accident**
    Pedestrian with babystroller injured in collision with car, pick-up truck or van in nontraffic accident
    Pedestrian on ice-skates injured in collision with car, pick-up truck or van in nontraffic accident
    Pedestrian on nonmotorized scooter injured in collision with car, pick-up truck or van in nontraffic accident
    Pedestrian on sled injured in collision with car, pick-up truck or van in nontraffic accident
    Pedestrian on snowboard injured in collision with car, pick-up truck or van in nontraffic accident
    Pedestrian on snow-skis injured in collision with car, pick-up truck or van in nontraffic accident
    Pedestrian in wheelchair (powered) injured in collision with car, pick-up truck or van in nontraffic accident
    Pedestrian in motorized mobility scooter injured in collision with car, pick-up truck or van in nontraffic accident

√5ᵗʰ **V03.1** **Pedestrian injured in collision with car, pick-up truck or van in traffic accident**

√x7ᵗʰ **V03.10** **Pedestrian on foot injured in collision with car, pick-up truck or van in traffic accident**
    Pedestrian NOS injured in collision with car, pick-up truck or van in traffic accident

√x7ᵗʰ **V03.11** **Pedestrian on roller-skates injured in collision with car, pick-up truck or van in traffic accident**

√x7ᵗʰ **V03.12** **Pedestrian on skateboard injured in collision with car, pick-up truck or van in traffic accident**

Ⓝ Newborn   Ⓟ Pediatric   Ⓜ Maternity   Ⓐ Adult   RIC RIC Dx   NCDx Noncancer Dx   PDx Primary Dx   CC RIC CC Condition   ▶◀ Revised Text   ● New Code   ▲ Revised Code Title

1054   ICD-10-CM 2016

√7ᵗʰ V03.19 **Pedestrian with other** conveyance **injured in collision with car, pick-up truck or van in traffic accident**
> Pedestrian with babystroller injured in collision with car, pick-up truck or van in traffic accident
> Pedestrian on ice-skates injured in collision with car, pick-up truck or van in traffic accident
> Pedestrian on nonmotorized scooter injured in collision with car, pick-up truck or van in traffic accident
> Pedestrian on sled injured in collision with car, pick-up truck or van in traffic accident
> Pedestrian on snowboard injured in collision with car, pick-up truck or van in traffic accident
> Pedestrian on snow-skis injured in collision with car, pick-up truck or van in traffic accident
> Pedestrian in wheelchair (powered) injured in collision with car, pick-up truck or van in traffic accident
> Pedestrian in motorized mobility scooter injured in collision with car, pick-up truck or van in traffic accident

√5ᵗʰ V03.9 **Pedestrian injured in collision with car, pick-up truck or van,** unspecified whether traffic or nontraffic accident

√7ᵗʰ V03.90 **Pedestrian** on foot **injured in collision with car, pick-up truck or van, unspecified whether traffic or nontraffic accident** ▽
> Pedestrian NOS injured in collision with car, pick-up truck or van, unspecified whether traffic or nontraffic accident

√7ᵗʰ V03.91 **Pedestrian** on roller-skates **injured in collision with car, pick-up truck or van, unspecified whether traffic or nontraffic accident** ▽

√7ᵗʰ V03.92 **Pedestrian** on skateboard **injured in collision with car, pick-up truck or van, unspecified whether traffic or nontraffic accident** ▽

√7ᵗʰ V03.99 **Pedestrian with other** conveyance **injured in collision with car, pick-up truck or van, unspecified whether traffic or nontraffic accident** ▽
> Pedestrian with babystroller injured in collision with car, pick-up truck or van, unspecified whether traffic or nontraffic accident
> Pedestrian on ice-skates injured in collision with car, pick-up truck or van, unspecified whether traffic or nontraffic accident
> Pedestrian on nonmotorized scooter injured in collision with car, pick-up truck or van, unspecified whether traffic or nontraffic accident
> Pedestrian on sled injured in collision with car, pick-up truck or van in nontraffic accident
> Pedestrian on snowboard injured in collision with car, pick-up truck or van, unspecified whether traffic or nontraffic accident
> Pedestrian on snow-skis injured in collision with car, pick-up truck or van, unspecified whether traffic or nontraffic accident
> Pedestrian in wheelchair (powered) injured in collision with car, pick-up truck or van, unspecified whether traffic or nontraffic accident
> Pedestrian in motorized mobility scooter injured in collision with car, pick-up truck or van, unspecified whether traffic or nontraffic accident

√4ᵗʰ V04 **Pedestrian injured in collision with heavy transport vehicle or bus**
> **EXCLUDES 1** *pedestrian injured in collision with military vehicle (V09.01, V09.21)*

> The appropriate 7th character is to be added to each code from category V04.
> A   initial encounter
> D   subsequent encounter
> S   sequela

√5ᵗʰ V04.0 **Pedestrian injured in collision with heavy transport vehicle or bus** in nontraffic accident

√7ᵗʰ V04.00 **Pedestrian** on foot **injured in collision with heavy transport vehicle or bus in nontraffic accident**
> Pedestrian NOS injured in collision with heavy transport vehicle or bus in nontraffic accident

√7ᵗʰ V04.01 **Pedestrian** on roller-skates **injured in collision with heavy transport vehicle or bus in nontraffic accident**

√7ᵗʰ V04.02 **Pedestrian** on skateboard **injured in collision with heavy transport vehicle or bus in nontraffic accident**

√7ᵗʰ V04.09 **Pedestrian with other** conveyance **injured in collision with heavy transport vehicle or bus in nontraffic accident**
> Pedestrian with babystroller injured in collision with heavy transport vehicle or bus in nontraffic accident
> Pedestrian on ice-skates injured in collision with heavy transport vehicle or bus in nontraffic accident
> Pedestrian on nonmotorized scooter injured in collision with heavy transport vehicle or bus in nontraffic accident
> Pedestrian on sled injured in collision with heavy transport vehicle or bus in nontraffic accident
> Pedestrian on snowboard injured in collision with heavy transport vehicle or bus in nontraffic accident
> Pedestrian on snow-skis injured in collision with heavy transport vehicle or bus in nontraffic accident
> Pedestrian in wheelchair (powered) injured in collision with heavy transport vehicle or bus in nontraffic accident
> Pedestrian in motorized mobility scooter injured in collision with heavy transport vehicle or bus in nontraffic accident

√5ᵗʰ V04.1 **Pedestrian injured in collision with heavy transport vehicle or bus** in traffic accident

√7ᵗʰ V04.10 **Pedestrian** on foot **injured in collision with heavy transport vehicle or bus in traffic accident**
> Pedestrian NOS injured in collision with heavy transport vehicle or bus in traffic accident

√7ᵗʰ V04.11 **Pedestrian** on roller-skates **injured in collision with heavy transport vehicle or bus in traffic accident**

√7ᵗʰ V04.12 **Pedestrian** on skateboard **injured in collision with heavy transport vehicle or bus in traffic accident**

√7ᵗʰ V04.19 **Pedestrian with other** conveyance **injured in collision with heavy transport vehicle or bus in traffic accident**
> Pedestrian with babystroller injured in collision with heavy transport vehicle or bus in traffic accident
> Pedestrian on ice-skates injured in collision with heavy transport vehicle or bus in traffic accident
> Pedestrian on nonmotorized scooter injured in collision with heavy transport vehicle or bus in traffic accident
> Pedestrian on sled injured in collision with heavy transport vehicle or bus in traffic accident
> Pedestrian on snowboard injured in collision with heavy transport vehicle or bus in traffic accident
> Pedestrian on snow-skis injured in collision with heavy transport vehicle or bus in traffic accident
> Pedestrian in wheelchair (powered) injured in collision with heavy transport vehicle or bus in traffic accident
> Pedestrian in motorized mobility scooter injured in collision with heavy transport vehicle or bus in traffic accident

√5ᵗʰ V04.9 **Pedestrian injured in collision with heavy transport vehicle or bus,** unspecified whether traffic or nontraffic accident

√7ᵗʰ V04.90 **Pedestrian** on foot **injured in collision with heavy transport vehicle or bus, unspecified whether traffic or nontraffic accident** ▽
> Pedestrian NOS injured in collision with heavy transport vehicle or bus, unspecified whether traffic or nontraffic accident

√7ᵗʰ V04.91 **Pedestrian** on roller-skates **injured in collision with heavy transport vehicle or bus, unspecified whether traffic or nontraffic accident** ▽

√7ᵗʰ V04.92 **Pedestrian** on skateboard **injured in collision with heavy transport vehicle or bus, unspecified whether traffic or nontraffic accident** ▽

☑ Add'l Character Required   √7ᵗʰ Placeholder Alert   RUG IV Special Care High Dx   RUG IV Clinically Complex Dx   RUG IV Special Care Low Dx   Manifestation Code   Other Specified Code   ▽ Unspecified Code

√x7ᵗʰ **V04.99** **Pedestrian with other** conveyance **injured in collision with heavy transport vehicle or bus, unspecified whether traffic or nontraffic accident** ▽

Pedestrian with babystroller injured in collision with heavy transport vehicle or bus, unspecified whether traffic or nontraffic accident

Pedestrian on ice-skates injured in collision with heavy transport vehicle or bus, unspecified whether traffic or nontraffic accident

Pedestrian on nonmotorized scooter injured in collision with heavy transport vehicle or bus, unspecified whether traffic or nontraffic accident

Pedestrian on sled injured in collision with heavy transport vehicle or bus, unspecified whether traffic or nontraffic accident

Pedestrian on snowboard injured in collision with heavy transport vehicle or bus, unspecified whether traffic or nontraffic accident

Pedestrian on snow-skis injured in collision with heavy transport vehicle or bus, unspecified whether traffic or nontraffic accident

Pedestrian in wheelchair (powered) injured in collision with heavy transport vehicle or bus, unspecified whether traffic or nontraffic accident

Pedestrian in motorized mobility scooter injured in collision with heavy transport vehicle or bus, unspecified whether traffic or nontraffic accident

√4ᵗʰ **V05** **Pedestrian injured in collision with railway train or railway vehicle**

The appropriate 7th character is to be added to each code from category V05.
A initial encounter
D subsequent encounter
S sequela

√5ᵗʰ **V05.0** **Pedestrian injured in collision with railway train or railway vehicle** in nontraffic accident

√x7ᵗʰ **V05.00** **Pedestrian** on foot **injured in collision with railway train or railway vehicle in nontraffic accident**

Pedestrian NOS injured in collision with railway train or railway vehicle in nontraffic accident

√x7ᵗʰ **V05.01** **Pedestrian** on roller-skates **injured in collision with railway train or railway vehicle in nontraffic accident**

√x7ᵗʰ **V05.02** **Pedestrian** on skateboard **injured in collision with railway train or railway vehicle in nontraffic accident**

√x7ᵗʰ **V05.09** **Pedestrian with other** conveyance **injured in collision with railway train or railway vehicle in nontraffic accident**

Pedestrian with babystroller injured in collision with railway train or railway vehicle in nontraffic accident

Pedestrian on ice-skates injured in collision with railway train or railway vehicle in nontraffic accident

Pedestrian on nonmotorized scooter injured in collision with railway train or railway vehicle in nontraffic accident

Pedestrian on sled injured in collision with railway train or railway vehicle in nontraffic accident

Pedestrian on snowboard injured in collision with railway train or railway vehicle in nontraffic accident

Pedestrian on snow-skis injured in collision with railway train or railway vehicle in nontraffic accident

Pedestrian in wheelchair (powered) injured in collision with railway train or railway vehicle in nontraffic accident

Pedestrian in motorized mobility scooter injured in collision with railway train or railway vehicle in nontraffic accident

√5ᵗʰ **V05.1** **Pedestrian injured in collision with railway train or railway vehicle** in traffic accident

√x7ᵗʰ **V05.10** **Pedestrian** on foot **injured in collision with railway train or railway vehicle in traffic accident**

Pedestrian NOS injured in collision with railway train or railway vehicle in traffic accident

√x7ᵗʰ **V05.11** **Pedestrian** on roller-skates **injured in collision with railway train or railway vehicle in traffic accident**

√x7ᵗʰ **V05.12** **Pedestrian** on skateboard **injured in collision with railway train or railway vehicle in traffic accident**

√x7ᵗʰ **V05.19** **Pedestrian with other** conveyance **injured in collision with railway train or railway vehicle in traffic accident**

Pedestrian with babystroller injured in collision with railway train or railway vehicle in traffic accident

Pedestrian on ice-skates injured in collision with railway train or railway vehicle in traffic accident

Pedestrian on nonmotorized scooter injured in collision with railway train or railway vehicle in traffic accident

Pedestrian on sled injured in collision with railway train or railway vehicle in traffic accident

Pedestrian on snowboard injured in collision with railway train or railway vehicle in traffic accident

Pedestrian on snow-skis injured in collision with railway train or railway vehicle in traffic accident

Pedestrian in wheelchair (powered) injured in collision with railway train or railway vehicle in traffic accident

Pedestrian in motorized mobility scooter injured in collision with railway train or railway vehicle in traffic accident

√5ᵗʰ **V05.9** **Pedestrian injured in collision with railway train or railway vehicle,** unspecified whether traffic or nontraffic accident

√x7ᵗʰ **V05.90** **Pedestrian** on foot **injured in collision with railway train or railway vehicle, unspecified whether traffic or nontraffic accident** ▽

Pedestrian NOS injured in collision with railway train or railway vehicle, unspecified whether traffic or nontraffic accident

√x7ᵗʰ **V05.91** **Pedestrian** on roller-skates **injured in collision with railway train or railway vehicle, unspecified whether traffic or nontraffic accident** ▽

√x7ᵗʰ **V05.92** **Pedestrian** on skateboard **injured in collision with railway train or railway vehicle, unspecified whether traffic or nontraffic accident** ▽

√x7ᵗʰ **V05.99** **Pedestrian with other** conveyance **injured in collision with railway train or railway vehicle, unspecified whether traffic or nontraffic accident** ▽

Pedestrian with babystroller injured in collision with railway train or railway vehicle, unspecified whether traffic or nontraffic

Pedestrian on ice-skates injured in collision with railway train or railway vehicle, unspecified whether traffic or nontraffic

Pedestrian on nonmotorized scooter injured in collision with railway train or railway vehicle, unspecified whether traffic or nontraffic

Pedestrian on sled injured in collision with railway train or railway vehicle, unspecified whether traffic or nontraffic

Pedestrian on snowboard injured in collision with railway train or railway vehicle, unspecified whether traffic or nontraffic

Pedestrian on snow-skis injured in collision with railway train or railway vehicle, unspecified whether traffic or nontraffic

Pedestrian in wheelchair (powered) injured in collision with railway train or railway vehicle, unspecified whether traffic or nontraffic

Pedestrian in motorized mobility scooter injured in collision with railway train or railway vehicle, unspecified whether traffic or nontraffic

√4ᵗʰ **V06** **Pedestrian injured in collision with other nonmotor vehicle**

INCLUDES collision with animal-drawn vehicle, animal being ridden, nonpowered streetcar

EXCLUDES 1 pedestrian injured in collision with pedestrian conveyance (V00.0-)

The appropriate 7th character is to be added to each code from category V06.
A initial encounter
D subsequent encounter
S sequela

√5ᵗʰ **V06.0** **Pedestrian injured in collision with other nonmotor vehicle** in nontraffic accident

√x7ᵗʰ **V06.00** **Pedestrian** on foot **injured in collision with other nonmotor vehicle in nontraffic accident**

Pedestrian NOS injured in collision with other nonmotor vehicle in nontraffic accident

√x7ᵗʰ **V06.01** **Pedestrian** on roller-skates **injured in collision with other nonmotor vehicle in nontraffic accident**

Ⓝ Newborn Ⓟ Pediatric Ⓜ Maternity Ⓐ Adult RIC RIC Dx NCDx Noncancer Dx PDx Primary Dx CC RIC CC Condition ►◄ Revised Text ● New Code ▲ Revised Code Title

1056

ICD-10-CM 2016

✓x7ᵗʰ **V06.02** Pedestrian on skateboard injured in collision with other nonmotor vehicle in nontraffic accident

✓x7ᵗʰ **V06.09** Pedestrian with other conveyance injured in collision with other nonmotor vehicle in nontraffic accident

     Pedestrian with babystroller injured in collision with other nonmotor vehicle in nontraffic accident

     Pedestrian on ice-skates injured in collision with other nonmotor vehicle in nontraffic accident

     Pedestrian on nonmotorized scooter injured in collision with other nonmotor vehicle in nontraffic accident

     Pedestrian on sled injured in collision with other nonmotor vehicle in nontraffic accident

     Pedestrian on snowboard injured in collision with other nonmotor vehicle in nontraffic accident

     Pedestrian on snow-skis injured in collision with other nonmotor vehicle in nontraffic accident

     Pedestrian in wheelchair (powered) injured in collision with other nonmotor vehicle in nontraffic accident

     Pedestrian in motorized mobility scooter injured in collision with other nonmotor vehicle in nontraffic accident

✓5ᵗʰ **V06.1** Pedestrian injured in collision with other nonmotor vehicle in traffic accident

✓x7ᵗʰ **V06.10** Pedestrian on foot injured in collision with other nonmotor vehicle in traffic accident

     Pedestrian NOS injured in collision with other nonmotor vehicle in traffic accident

✓x7ᵗʰ **V06.11** Pedestrian on roller-skates injured in collision with other nonmotor vehicle in traffic accident

✓x7ᵗʰ **V06.12** Pedestrian on skateboard injured in collision with other nonmotor vehicle in traffic accident

✓x7ᵗʰ **V06.19** Pedestrian with other conveyance injured in collision with other nonmotor vehicle in traffic accident

     Pedestrian with babystroller injured in collision with other nonmotor vehicle in nontraffic accident

     Pedestrian on ice-skates injured in collision with other nonmotor vehicle in traffic accident

     Pedestrian on nonmotorized scooter injured in collision with other nonmotor vehicle in traffic accident

     Pedestrian on sled injured in collision with other nonmotor vehicle in traffic accident

     Pedestrian on snowboard injured in collision with other nonmotor vehicle in traffic accident

     Pedestrian on snow-skis injured in collision with other nonmotor vehicle in traffic accident

     Pedestrian in wheelchair (powered) injured in collision with other nonmotor vehicle in traffic accident

     Pedestrian in motorized mobility scooter injured in collision with other nonmotor vehicle in traffic accident

✓5ᵗʰ **V06.9** Pedestrian injured in collision with other nonmotor vehicle, unspecified whether traffic or nontraffic accident

✓x7ᵗʰ **V06.90** Pedestrian on foot injured in collision with other nonmotor vehicle, unspecified whether traffic or nontraffic accident ▽

     Pedestrian NOS injured in collision with other nonmotor vehicle, unspecified whether traffic or nontraffic accident

✓x7ᵗʰ **V06.91** Pedestrian on roller-skates injured in collision with other nonmotor vehicle, unspecified whether traffic or nontraffic accident ▽

✓x7ᵗʰ **V06.92** Pedestrian on skateboard injured in collision with other nonmotor vehicle, unspecified whether traffic or nontraffic accident ▽

✓x7ᵗʰ **V06.99** Pedestrian with other conveyance injured in collision with other nonmotor vehicle, unspecifiedwhether traffic or nontraffic accident ▽

     Pedestrian with babystroller injured in collision with other nonmotor vehicle, unspecified whether traffic or nontraffic accident

     Pedestrian on ice-skates injured in collision with other nonmotor vehicle, unspecified whether traffic or nontraffic accident

     Pedestrian on nonmotorized scooter injured in collision with other nonmotor vehicle, unspecified whether traffic or nontraffic accident

     Pedestrian on sled injured in collision with other nonmotor vehicle, unspecified whether traffic or nontraffic accident

     Pedestrian on snowboard injured in collision with other nonmotor vehicle, unspecified whether traffic or nontraffic accident

     Pedestrian on snow-skis injured in collision with other nonmotor vehicle, unspecified whether traffic or nontraffic accident

     Pedestrian in wheelchair (powered) injured in collision with other nonmotor vehicle, unspecified whether traffic or nontraffic accident

     Pedestrian in motorized mobility scooter injured in collision with other nonmotor vehicle, unspecified whether traffic or nontraffic accident

✓4ᵗʰ **V09** Pedestrian injured in other and unspecified transport accidents

     The appropriate 7th character is to be added to each code from category V09.
     A   initial encounter
     D   subsequent encounter
     S   sequela

✓5ᵗʰ **V09.0** Pedestrian injured in nontraffic accident involving other and unspecified motor vehicles

✓x7ᵗʰ **V09.00** Pedestrian injured in nontraffic accident involving unspecified motor vehicles ▽

✓x7ᵗʰ **V09.01** Pedestrian injured in nontraffic accident involving military vehicle

✓x7ᵗʰ **V09.09** Pedestrian injured in nontraffic accident involving other motor vehicles

     Pedestrian injured in nontraffic accident by special vehicle

✓x7ᵗʰ **V09.1** Pedestrian injured in unspecified nontraffic accident ▽

✓5ᵗʰ **V09.2** Pedestrian injured in traffic accident involving other and unspecified motor vehicles

✓x7ᵗʰ **V09.20** Pedestrian injured in traffic accident involving unspecified motor vehicles ▽

✓x7ᵗʰ **V09.21** Pedestrian injured in traffic accident involving military vehicle

✓x7ᵗʰ **V09.29** Pedestrian injured in traffic accident involving other motor vehicles

✓x7ᵗʰ **V09.3** Pedestrian injured in unspecified traffic accident ▽

✓x7ᵗʰ **V09.9** Pedestrian injured in unspecified transport accident ▽

Pedal cycle rider injured in transport accident (V10-V19)

INCLUDES   any non-motorized vehicle, excluding an animal-drawn vehicle, or a sidecar or trailer attached to the pedal cycle
EXCLUDES 2   *rupture of pedal cycle tire (W37.0)*

✓4ᵗʰ **V10** Pedal cycle rider injured in collision with pedestrian or animal

     EXCLUDES 1   *pedal cycle rider collision with animal-drawn vehicle or animal being ridden (V16.-)*

     The appropriate 7th character is to be added to each code from category V10.
     A   initial encounter
     D   subsequent encounter
     S   sequela

✓x7ᵗʰ **V10.0** Pedal cycle driver injured in collision with pedestrian or animal in nontraffic accident

✓x7ᵗʰ **V10.1** Pedal cycle passenger injured in collision with pedestrian or animal in nontraffic accident

✓x7ᵗʰ **V10.2** Unspecified pedal cyclist injured in collision with pedestrian or animal in nontraffic accident ▽

✓x7ᵗʰ **V10.3** Person boarding or alighting a pedal cycle injured in collision with pedestrian or animal

☑ Add'l Character Required   ✓x7ᵗʰ Placeholder Alert   **RUG IV Special Care High Dx**   RUG IV Clinically Complex Dx   RUG IV Special Care Low Dx   Manifestation Code   Other Specified Code   ▽ Unspecified Code

ICD-10-CM 2016   1057

Chapter 20. External Causes of Morbidity

✓x7ᵗʰ **V10.4** Pedal cycle driver injured in collision with pedestrian or animal in traffic accident

✓x7ᵗʰ **V10.5** Pedal cycle passenger injured in collision with pedestrian or animal in traffic accident

✓x7ᵗʰ **V10.9** Unspecified pedal cyclist injured in collision with pedestrian or animal in traffic accident ▽

✓4ᵗʰ **V11** Pedal cycle rider injured in collision with other pedal cycle

> The appropriate 7th character is to be added to each code from category V11.
> A   initial encounter
> D   subsequent encounter
> S   sequela

✓x7ᵗʰ **V11.0** Pedal cycle driver injured in collision with other pedal cycle in nontraffic accident

✓x7ᵗʰ **V11.1** Pedal cycle passenger injured in collision with other pedal cycle in nontraffic accident

✓x7ᵗʰ **V11.2** Unspecified pedal cyclist injured in collision with other pedal cycle in nontraffic accident ▽

✓x7ᵗʰ **V11.3** Person boarding or alighting a pedal cycle injured in collision with other pedal cycle

✓x7ᵗʰ **V11.4** Pedal cycle driver injured in collision with other pedal cycle in traffic accident

✓x7ᵗʰ **V11.5** Pedal cycle passenger injured in collision with other pedal cycle in traffic accident

✓x7ᵗʰ **V11.9** Unspecified pedal cyclist injured in collision with other pedal cycle in traffic accident ▽

✓4ᵗʰ **V12** Pedal cycle rider injured in collision with two- or three-wheeled motor vehicle

> The appropriate 7th character is to be added to each code from category V12.
> A   initial encounter
> D   subsequent encounter
> S   sequela

✓x7ᵗʰ **V12.0** Pedal cycle driver injured in collision with two- or three-wheeled motor vehicle in nontraffic accident

✓x7ᵗʰ **V12.1** Pedal cycle passenger injured in collision with two- or three-wheeled motor vehicle in nontraffic accident

✓x7ᵗʰ **V12.2** Unspecified pedal cyclist injured in collision with two- or three-wheeled motor vehicle in nontraffic accident ▽

✓x7ᵗʰ **V12.3** Person boarding or alighting a pedal cycle injured in collision with two- or three-wheeled motor vehicle

✓x7ᵗʰ **V12.4** Pedal cycle driver injured in collision with two- or three-wheeled motor vehicle in traffic accident

✓x7ᵗʰ **V12.5** Pedal cycle passenger injured in collision with two- or three-wheeled motor vehicle in traffic accident

✓x7ᵗʰ **V12.9** Unspecified pedal cyclist injured in collision with two- or three-wheeled motor vehicle in traffic accident ▽

✓4ᵗʰ **V13** Pedal cycle rider injured in collision with car, pick-up truck or van

> The appropriate 7th character is to be added to each code from category V13.
> A   initial encounter
> D   subsequent encounter
> S   sequela

✓x7ᵗʰ **V13.0** Pedal cycle driver injured in collision with car, pick-up truck or van in nontraffic accident

✓x7ᵗʰ **V13.1** Pedal cycle passenger injured in collision with car, pick-up truck or van in nontraffic accident

✓x7ᵗʰ **V13.2** Unspecified pedal cyclist injured in collision with car, pick-up truck or van in nontraffic accident ▽

✓x7ᵗʰ **V13.3** Person boarding or alighting a pedal cycle injured in collision with car, pick-up truck or van

✓x7ᵗʰ **V13.4** Pedal cycle driver injured in collision with car, pick-up truck or van in traffic accident

✓x7ᵗʰ **V13.5** Pedal cycle passenger injured in collision with car, pick-up truck or van in traffic accident

✓x7ᵗʰ **V13.9** Unspecified pedal cyclist injured in collision with car, pick-up truck or van in traffic accident ▽

✓4ᵗʰ **V14** Pedal cycle rider injured in collision with heavy transport vehicle or bus

> **EXCLUDES 1**   pedal cycle rider injured in collision with military vehicle (V19.81)

> The appropriate 7th character is to be added to each code from category V14.
> A   initial encounter
> D   subsequent encounter
> S   sequela

✓x7ᵗʰ **V14.0** Pedal cycle driver injured in collision with heavy transport vehicle or bus in nontraffic accident

✓x7ᵗʰ **V14.1** Pedal cycle passenger injured in collision with heavy transport vehicle or bus in nontraffic accident

✓x7ᵗʰ **V14.2** Unspecified pedal cyclist injured in collision with heavy transport vehicle or bus in nontraffic accident ▽

✓x7ᵗʰ **V14.3** Person boarding or alighting a pedal cycle injured in collision with heavy transport vehicle or bus

✓x7ᵗʰ **V14.4** Pedal cycle driver injured in collision with heavy transport vehicle or bus in traffic accident

✓x7ᵗʰ **V14.5** Pedal cycle passenger injured in collision with heavy transport vehicle or bus in traffic accident

✓x7ᵗʰ **V14.9** Unspecified pedal cyclist injured in collision with heavy transport vehicle or bus in traffic accident ▽

✓4ᵗʰ **V15** Pedal cycle rider injured in collision with railway train or railway vehicle

> The appropriate 7th character is to be added to each code from category V15.
> A   initial encounter
> D   subsequent encounter
> S   sequela

✓x7ᵗʰ **V15.0** Pedal cycle driver injured in collision with railway train or railway vehicle in nontraffic accident

✓x7ᵗʰ **V15.1** Pedal cycle passenger injured in collision with railway train or railway vehicle in nontraffic accident

✓x7ᵗʰ **V15.2** Unspecified pedal cyclist injured in collision with railway train or railway vehicle in nontraffic accident ▽

✓x7ᵗʰ **V15.3** Person boarding or alighting a pedal cycle injured in collision with railway train or railway vehicle

✓x7ᵗʰ **V15.4** Pedal cycle driver injured in collision with railway train or railway vehicle in traffic accident

✓x7ᵗʰ **V15.5** Pedal cycle passenger injured in collision with railway train or railway vehicle in traffic accident

✓x7ᵗʰ **V15.9** Unspecified pedal cyclist injured in collision with railway train or railway vehicle in traffic accident ▽

✓4ᵗʰ **V16** Pedal cycle rider injured in collision with other nonmotor vehicle

> **INCLUDES**   collision with animal-drawn vehicle, animal being ridden, streetcar

> The appropriate 7th character is to be added to each code from category V16.
> A   initial encounter
> D   subsequent encounter
> S   sequela

✓x7ᵗʰ **V16.0** Pedal cycle driver injured in collision with other nonmotor vehicle in nontraffic accident

✓x7ᵗʰ **V16.1** Pedal cycle passenger injured in collision with other nonmotor vehicle in nontraffic accident

✓x7ᵗʰ **V16.2** Unspecified pedal cyclist injured in collision with other nonmotor vehicle in nontraffic accident ▽

✓x7ᵗʰ **V16.3** Person boarding or alighting a pedal cycle injured in collision with other nonmotor vehicle in nontraffic accident

✓x7ᵗʰ **V16.4** Pedal cycle driver injured in collision with other nonmotor vehicle in traffic accident

✓x7ᵗʰ **V16.5** Pedal cycle passenger injured in collision with other nonmotor vehicle in traffic accident

✓x7ᵗʰ **V16.9** Unspecified pedal cyclist injured in collision with other nonmotor vehicle in traffic accident ▽

Ⓝ Newborn   Ⓟ Pediatric   Ⓜ Maternity   Ⓐ Adult   **RIC** RIC Dx   **NCDx** Noncancer Dx   **PDx** Primary Dx   **CC** RIC CC Condition   ▶◀ Revised Text   ● New Code   ▲ Revised Code Title

1058

ICD-10-CM 2016

√4ᵗʰ **V17** **Pedal cycle rider injured in collision with fixed or stationary object**

> The appropriate 7th character is to be added to each code from category V17.
> A   initial encounter
> D   subsequent encounter
> S   sequela

√x7ᵗʰ **V17.0** **Pedal cycle** driver **injured in collision with fixed or stationary object** in nontraffic accident

√x7ᵗʰ **V17.1** **Pedal cycle** passenger **injured in collision with fixed or stationary object** in nontraffic accident

√x7ᵗʰ **V17.2** **Unspecified pedal cyclist injured in collision with fixed or stationary object** in nontraffic accident ▽

√x7ᵗʰ **V17.3** Person boarding or alighting **a pedal cycle injured in collision with fixed or stationary object**

√x7ᵗʰ **V17.4** **Pedal cycle** driver **injured in collision with fixed or stationary object** in traffic accident

√x7ᵗʰ **V17.5** **Pedal cycle** passenger **injured in collision with fixed or stationary object** in traffic accident

√x7ᵗʰ **V17.9** **Unspecified pedal cyclist injured in collision with fixed or stationary object** in traffic accident ▽

√4ᵗʰ **V18** **Pedal cycle rider injured in noncollision transport accident**

> INCLUDES   fall or thrown from pedal cycle (without antecedent collision)
> overturning pedal cycle NOS
> overturning pedal cycle without collision

> The appropriate 7th character is to be added to each code from category V18.
> A   initial encounter
> D   subsequent encounter
> S   sequela

√x7ᵗʰ **V18.0** **Pedal cycle** driver **injured in noncollision transport accident** in nontraffic accident

√x7ᵗʰ **V18.1** **Pedal cycle** passenger **injured in noncollision transport accident** in nontraffic accident

√x7ᵗʰ **V18.2** **Unspecified pedal cyclist injured in noncollision transport accident** in nontraffic accident ▽

√x7ᵗʰ **V18.3** Person boarding or alighting **a pedal cycle injured in noncollision transport accident**

√x7ᵗʰ **V18.4** **Pedal cycle** driver **injured in noncollision transport accident** in traffic accident

√x7ᵗʰ **V18.5** **Pedal cycle** passenger **injured in noncollision transport accident** in traffic accident

√x7ᵗʰ **V18.9** **Unspecified pedal cyclist injured in noncollision transport accident** in traffic accident ▽

√4ᵗʰ **V19** **Pedal cycle rider injured in other and unspecified transport accidents**

> The appropriate 7th character is to be added to each code from category V19.
> A   initial encounter
> D   subsequent encounter
> S   sequela

√5ᵗʰ **V19.0** **Pedal cycle** driver **injured in collision with other and unspecified motor vehicles in nontraffic accident**

√x7ᵗʰ **V19.00** **Pedal cycle driver injured in collision with unspecified motor vehicles in nontraffic accident** ▽

√x7ᵗʰ **V19.09** **Pedal cycle driver injured in collision with other motor vehicles in nontraffic accident**

√5ᵗʰ **V19.1** **Pedal cycle** passenger **injured in collision with other and unspecified motor vehicles in nontraffic accident**

√x7ᵗʰ **V19.10** **Pedal cycle passenger injured in collision with unspecified motor vehicles in nontraffic accident** ▽

√x7ᵗʰ **V19.19** **Pedal cycle passenger injured in collision with other motor vehicles in nontraffic accident**

√5ᵗʰ **V19.2** **Unspecified pedal cyclist injured in collision with** other and unspecified motor vehicles in traffic accident

√x7ᵗʰ **V19.20** **Unspecified pedal cyclist injured in collision with unspecified motor vehicles in nontraffic accident** ▽
Pedal cycle collision NOS, nontraffic

√x7ᵗʰ **V19.29** **Unspecified pedal cyclist injured in collision with other motor vehicles in nontraffic accident** ▽

√5ᵗʰ **V19.3** **Pedal cyclist (driver) (passenger) injured in unspecified nontraffic accident** ▽
Pedal cycle accident NOS, nontraffic
Pedal cyclist injured in nontraffic accident NOS

√5ᵗʰ **V19.4** **Pedal cycle** driver **injured in collision with other and unspecified motor vehicles in traffic accident**

√x7ᵗʰ **V19.40** **Pedal cycle driver injured in collision with unspecified motor vehicles in traffic accident** ▽

√x7ᵗʰ **V19.49** **Pedal cycle driver injured in collision with other motor vehicles in traffic accident**

√5ᵗʰ **V19.5** **Pedal cycle** passenger **injured in collision with other and unspecified motor vehicles in traffic accident**

√x7ᵗʰ **V19.50** **Pedal cycle passenger injured in collision with unspecified motor vehicles in traffic accident** ▽

√x7ᵗʰ **V19.59** **Pedal cycle passenger injured in collision with other motor vehicles in traffic accident**

√5ᵗʰ **V19.6** Unspecified **pedal cyclist injured in collision with** other and unspecified motor vehicles in traffic accident

√x7ᵗʰ **V19.60** **Unspecified pedal cyclist injured in collision with unspecified motor vehicles in traffic accident** ▽
Pedal cycle collision NOS (traffic)

√x7ᵗʰ **V19.69** **Unspecified pedal cyclist injured in collision with other motor vehicles in traffic accident** ▽

√5ᵗʰ **V19.8** **Pedal cyclist (driver) (passenger) injured in** other specified transport accidents

√x7ᵗʰ **V19.81** **Pedal cyclist (driver) (passenger) injured in transport accident with** military vehicle

√x7ᵗʰ **V19.88** **Pedal cyclist (driver) (passenger) injured in other specified transport accidents**

√x7ᵗʰ **V19.9** **Pedal cyclist (driver) (passenger) injured in unspecified traffic accident** ▽
Pedal cycle accident NOS

Motorcycle rider injured in transport accident (V20-V29)

> INCLUDES   moped
> motorcycle with sidecar
> motorized bicycle
> motor scooter
> EXCLUDES 1   three-wheeled motor vehicle (V30-V39)

√4ᵗʰ **V20** **Motorcycle rider injured in collision with pedestrian or animal**

> EXCLUDES 1   motorcycle rider collision with animal-drawn vehicle or animal being ridden (V26.-)

> The appropriate 7th character is to be added to each code from category V20.
> A   initial encounter
> D   subsequent encounter
> S   sequela

√x7ᵗʰ **V20.0** **Motorcycle** driver **injured in collision with pedestrian or animal** in nontraffic accident

√x7ᵗʰ **V20.1** **Motorcycle** passenger **injured in collision with pedestrian or animal** in nontraffic accident

√x7ᵗʰ **V20.2** **Unspecified motorcycle rider injured in collision with pedestrian or animal** in nontraffic accident ▽

√x7ᵗʰ **V20.3** Person boarding or alighting **a motorcycle injured in collision with pedestrian or animal**

√x7ᵗʰ **V20.4** **Motorcycle** driver **injured in collision with pedestrian or animal** in traffic accident

√x7ᵗʰ **V20.5** **Motorcycle** passenger **injured in collision with pedestrian or animal** in traffic accident

√x7ᵗʰ **V20.9** **Unspecified motorcycle rider injured in collision with pedestrian or animal** in traffic accident ▽

√4ᵗʰ **V21** **Motorcycle rider injured in collision with pedal cycle**

> The appropriate 7th character is to be added to each code from category V21.
> A   initial encounter
> D   subsequent encounter
> S   sequela

√x7ᵗʰ **V21.0** **Motorcycle** driver **injured in collision with pedal cycle** in nontraffic accident

√x7ᵗʰ **V21.1** **Motorcycle** passenger **injured in collision with pedal cycle** in nontraffic accident

√x7ᵗʰ **V21.2** **Unspecified motorcycle rider injured in collision with pedal cycle** in nontraffic accident ▽

☑ Add'l Character Required √x7ᵗʰ Placeholder Alert RUG IV Special Care High Dx RUG IV Clinically Complex Dx RUG IV Special Care Low Dx Manifestation Code Other Specified Code ▽Unspecified Code

√x7ᵗʰ **V21.3** Person boarding or alighting a motorcycle injured in collision with pedal cycle

√x7ᵗʰ **V21.4** Motorcycle driver injured in collision with pedal cycle in traffic accident

√x7ᵗʰ **V21.5** Motorcycle passenger injured in collision with pedal cycle in traffic accident

√x7ᵗʰ **V21.9** Unspecified motorcycle rider injured in collision with ▽ pedal cycle in traffic accident

√4ᵗʰ **V22** Motorcycle rider injured in collision with two- or three-wheeled motor vehicle

The appropriate 7th character is to be added to each code from category V22.
A   initial encounter
D   subsequent encounter
S   sequela

√x7ᵗʰ **V22.0** Motorcycle driver injured in collision with two- or three-wheeled motor vehicle in nontraffic accident

√x7ᵗʰ **V22.1** Motorcycle passenger injured in collision with two- or three-wheeled motor vehicle in nontraffic accident

√x7ᵗʰ **V22.2** Unspecified motorcycle rider injured in collision with ▽ two- or three-wheeled motor vehicle in nontraffic accident

√x7ᵗʰ **V22.3** Person boarding or alighting a motorcycle injured in collision with two- or three-wheeled motor vehicle

√x7ᵗʰ **V22.4** Motorcycle driver injured in collision with two- or three-wheeled motor vehicle in traffic accident

√x7ᵗʰ **V22.5** Motorcycle passenger injured in collision with two- or three-wheeled motor vehicle in traffic accident

√x7ᵗʰ **V22.9** Unspecified motorcycle rider injured in collision with ▽ two- or three-wheeled motor vehicle in traffic accident

√4ᵗʰ **V23** Motorcycle rider injured in collision with car, pick-up truck or van

The appropriate 7th character is to be added to each code from category V23.
A   initial encounter
D   subsequent encounter
S   sequela

√x7ᵗʰ **V23.0** Motorcycle driver injured in collision with car, pick-up truck or van in nontraffic accident

√x7ᵗʰ **V23.1** Motorcycle passenger injured in collision with car, pick-up truck or van in nontraffic accident

√x7ᵗʰ **V23.2** Unspecified motorcycle rider injured in collision with car, ▽ pick-up truck or van in nontraffic accident

√x7ᵗʰ **V23.3** Person boarding or alighting a motorcycle injured in collision with car, pick-up truck or van

√x7ᵗʰ **V23.4** Motorcycle driver injured in collision with car, pick-up truck or van in traffic accident

√x7ᵗʰ **V23.5** Motorcycle passenger injured in collision with car, pick-up truck or van in traffic accident

√x7ᵗʰ **V23.9** Unspecified motorcycle rider injured in collision with car, ▽ pick-up truck or van in traffic accident

√4ᵗʰ **V24** Motorcycle rider injured in collision with heavy transport vehicle or bus

EXCLUDES 1   motorcycle rider injured in collision with military vehicle (V29.81)

The appropriate 7th character is to be added to each code from category V24.
A   initial encounter
D   subsequent encounter
S   sequela

√x7ᵗʰ **V24.0** Motorcycle driver injured in collision with heavy transport vehicle or bus in nontraffic accident

√x7ᵗʰ **V24.1** Motorcycle passenger injured in collision with heavy transport vehicle or bus in nontraffic accident

√x7ᵗʰ **V24.2** Unspecified motorcycle rider injured in collision with ▽ heavy transport vehicle or bus in nontraffic accident

√x7ᵗʰ **V24.3** Person boarding or alighting a motorcycle injured in collision with heavy transport vehicle or bus

√x7ᵗʰ **V24.4** Motorcycle driver injured in collision with heavy transport vehicle or bus in traffic accident

√x7ᵗʰ **V24.5** Motorcycle passenger injured in collision with heavy transport vehicle or bus in traffic accident

√x7ᵗʰ **V24.9** Unspecified motorcycle rider injured in collision with ▽ heavy transport vehicle or bus in traffic accident

√4ᵗʰ **V25** Motorcycle rider injured in collision with railway train or railway vehicle

The appropriate 7th character is to be added to each code from category V25.
A   initial encounter
D   subsequent encounter
S   sequela

√x7ᵗʰ **V25.0** Motorcycle driver injured in collision with railway train or railway vehicle in nontraffic accident

√x7ᵗʰ **V25.1** Motorcycle passenger injured in collision with railway train or railway vehicle in nontraffic accident

√x7ᵗʰ **V25.2** Unspecified motorcycle rider injured in collision with ▽ railway train or railway vehicle in nontraffic accident

√x7ᵗʰ **V25.3** Person boarding or alighting a motorcycle injured in collision with railway train or railway vehicle

√x7ᵗʰ **V25.4** Motorcycle driver injured in collision with railway train or railway vehicle in traffic accident

√x7ᵗʰ **V25.5** Motorcycle passenger injured in collision with railway train or railway vehicle in traffic accident

√x7ᵗʰ **V25.9** Unspecified motorcycle rider injured in collision with ▽ railway train or railway vehicle in traffic accident

√4ᵗʰ **V26** Motorcycle rider injured in collision with other nonmotor vehicle
INCLUDES   collision with animal-drawn vehicle, animal being ridden, streetcar

The appropriate 7th character is to be added to each code from category V26.
A   initial encounter
D   subsequent encounter
S   sequela

√x7ᵗʰ **V26.0** Motorcycle driver injured in collision with other nonmotor vehicle in nontraffic accident

√x7ᵗʰ **V26.1** Motorcycle passenger injured in collision with other nonmotor vehicle in nontraffic accident

√x7ᵗʰ **V26.2** Unspecified motorcycle rider injured in collision with ▽ other nonmotor vehicle in nontraffic accident

√x7ᵗʰ **V26.3** Person boarding or alighting a motorcycle injured in collision with other nonmotor vehicle

√x7ᵗʰ **V26.4** Motorcycle driver injured in collision with other nonmotor vehicle in traffic accident

√x7ᵗʰ **V26.5** Motorcycle passenger injured in collision with other nonmotor vehicle in traffic accident

√x7ᵗʰ **V26.9** Unspecified motorcycle rider injured in collision with ▽ other nonmotor vehicle in traffic accident

√4ᵗʰ **V27** Motorcycle rider injured in collision with fixed or stationary object

The appropriate 7th character is to be added to each code from category V27.
A   initial encounter
D   subsequent encounter
S   sequela

√x7ᵗʰ **V27.0** Motorcycle driver injured in collision with fixed or stationary object in nontraffic accident

√x7ᵗʰ **V27.1** Motorcycle passenger injured in collision with fixed or stationary object in nontraffic accident

√x7ᵗʰ **V27.2** Unspecified motorcycle rider injured in collision with ▽ fixed or stationary object in nontraffic accident

√x7ᵗʰ **V27.3** Person boarding or alighting a motorcycle injured in collision with fixed or stationary object

√x7ᵗʰ **V27.4** Motorcycle driver injured in collision with fixed or stationary object in traffic accident

√x7ᵗʰ **V27.5** Motorcycle passenger injured in collision with fixed or stationary object in traffic accident

√x7ᵗʰ **V27.9** Unspecified motorcycle rider injured in collision with ▽ fixed or stationary object in traffic accident

✓4ᵗʰ **V28 Motorcycle rider injured in noncollision transport accident**

INCLUDES   fall or thrown from motorcycle (without antecedent collision)
overturning motorcycle NOS
overturning motorcycle without collision

The appropriate 7th character is to be added to each code from category V28.
A   initial encounter
D   subsequent encounter
S   sequela

✓x7ᵗʰ **V28.0 Motorcycle** driver **injured in noncollision transport accident in nontraffic accident**

✓x7ᵗʰ **V28.1 Motorcycle** passenger **injured in noncollision transport accident in nontraffic accident**

✓x7ᵗʰ **V28.2 Unspecified motorcycle rider injured in noncollision** ▽ **transport accident in nontraffic accident**

✓x7ᵗʰ **V28.3** Person boarding or alighting **a motorcycle injured in noncollision transport accident**

✓x7ᵗʰ **V28.4 Motorcycle** driver **injured in noncollision transport accident in traffic accident**

✓x7ᵗʰ **V28.5 Motorcycle** passenger **injured in noncollision transport accident in traffic accident**

✓x7ᵗʰ **V28.9 Unspecified motorcycle rider injured in noncollision** ▽ **transport accident in traffic accident**

✓4ᵗʰ **V29 Motorcycle rider injured in other and unspecified transport accidents**

The appropriate 7th character is to be added to each code from category V29.
A   initial encounter
D   subsequent encounter
S   sequela

✓5ᵗʰ **V29.0 Motorcycle** driver **injured in collision with other and unspecified motor vehicles** in nontraffic accident

    ✓x7ᵗʰ **V29.00 Motorcycle driver injured in collision with** ▽ **unspecified motor vehicles in nontraffic accident**

    ✓x7ᵗʰ **V29.09 Motorcycle driver injured in collision with other motor vehicles in nontraffic accident**

✓5ᵗʰ **V29.1 Motorcycle** passenger **injured in collision with other and unspecified motor vehicles** in nontraffic accident

    ✓x7ᵗʰ **V29.10 Motorcycle passenger injured in collision with** ▽ **unspecified motor vehicles in nontraffic accident**

    ✓x7ᵗʰ **V29.19 Motorcycle passenger injured in collision with other motor vehicles in nontraffic accident**

✓5ᵗʰ **V29.2** Unspecified motorcycle rider injured in collision with other and unspecified motor vehicles in nontraffic accident

    ✓x7ᵗʰ **V29.20 Unspecified motorcycle rider injured in collision** ▽ **with unspecified motor vehicles in nontraffic accident**
       Motorcycle collision NOS, nontraffic

    ✓x7ᵗʰ **V29.29 Unspecified motorcycle rider injured in collision** ▽ **with other motor vehicles in nontraffic accident**

✓x7ᵗʰ **V29.3 Motorcycle rider (driver) (passenger) injured in** **unspecified nontraffic accident** ▽
      Motorcycle accident NOS, nontraffic
      Motorcycle rider injured in nontraffic accident NOS

✓5ᵗʰ **V29.4 Motorcycle** driver **injured in collision with other and unspecified motor vehicles** in traffic accident

    ✓x7ᵗʰ **V29.40 Motorcycle driver injured in collision with** ▽ **unspecified motor vehicles in traffic accident**

    ✓x7ᵗʰ **V29.49 Motorcycle driver injured in collision with other motor vehicles in traffic accident**

✓5ᵗʰ **V29.5 Motorcycle** passenger **injured in collision with other and unspecified motor vehicles** in traffic accident

    ✓x7ᵗʰ **V29.50 Motorcycle passenger injured in collision with** ▽ **unspecified motor vehicles in traffic accident**

    ✓x7ᵗʰ **V29.59 Motorcycle passenger injured in collision with other motor vehicles in traffic accident**

✓5ᵗʰ **V29.6** Unspecified motorcycle rider injured in collision with other and unspecified motor vehicles in traffic accident

    ✓x7ᵗʰ **V29.60 Unspecified motorcycle rider injured in collision** ▽ **with unspecified motor vehicles in traffic accident**
       Motorcycle collision NOS (traffic)

    ✓x7ᵗʰ **V29.69 Unspecified motorcycle rider injured in collision** ▽ **with other motor vehicles in traffic accident**

✓5ᵗʰ **V29.8 Motorcycle rider (driver) (passenger) injured in** other **specified transport accidents**

    ✓x7ᵗʰ **V29.81 Motorcycle rider (driver) (passenger) injured in transport accident with** military vehicle

    ✓x7ᵗʰ **V29.88 Motorcycle rider (driver) (passenger) injured in other specified transport accidents**

✓x7ᵗʰ **V29.9 Motorcycle rider (driver) (passenger) injured in** ▽ **unspecified traffic accident**
      Motorcycle accident NOS

Occupant of three-wheeled motor vehicle injured in transport accident (V30-V39)

INCLUDES   motorized tricycle
motorized rickshaw
three-wheeled motor car
EXCLUDES 1   all-terrain vehicles (V86.-)
motorcycle with sidecar (V20-V29)
vehicle designed primarily for off-road use (V86.-)

✓4ᵗʰ **V30 Occupant of three-wheeled motor vehicle injured in collision with pedestrian or animal**

EXCLUDES 1   three-wheeled motor vehicle collision with animal-drawn vehicle or animal being ridden (V36.-)

The appropriate 7th character is to be added to each code from category V30.
A   initial encounter
D   subsequent encounter
S   sequela

✓x7ᵗʰ **V30.0** Driver **of three-wheeled motor vehicle injured in collision with pedestrian or animal** in nontraffic accident

✓x7ᵗʰ **V30.1** Passenger **in three-wheeled motor vehicle injured in collision with pedestrian or animal** in nontraffic accident

✓x7ᵗʰ **V30.2** Person on outside **of three-wheeled motor vehicle injured in collision with pedestrian or animal** in nontraffic accident

✓x7ᵗʰ **V30.3** Unspecified occupant of three-wheeled motor vehicle ▽ injured in collision with pedestrian or animal in nontraffic accident

✓x7ᵗʰ **V30.4** Person boarding or alighting **a three-wheeled motor vehicle injured in collision with pedestrian or animal**

✓x7ᵗʰ **V30.5** Driver **of three-wheeled motor vehicle injured in collision with pedestrian or animal** in traffic accident

✓x7ᵗʰ **V30.6** Passenger **in three-wheeled motor vehicle injured in collision with pedestrian or animal** in traffic accident

✓x7ᵗʰ **V30.7** Person on outside **of three-wheeled motor vehicle injured in collision with pedestrian or animal** in traffic accident

✓x7ᵗʰ **V30.9** Unspecified occupant of three-wheeled motor vehicle ▽ injured in collision with pedestrian or animal in traffic accident

✓4ᵗʰ **V31 Occupant of three-wheeled motor vehicle injured in collision with pedal cycle**

The appropriate 7th character is to be added to each code from category V31.
A   initial encounter
D   subsequent encounter
S   sequela

✓x7ᵗʰ **V31.0** Driver **of three-wheeled motor vehicle injured in collision with pedal cycle** in nontraffic accident

✓x7ᵗʰ **V31.1** Passenger **in three-wheeled motor vehicle injured in collision with pedal cycle** in nontraffic accident

✓x7ᵗʰ **V31.2** Person on outside **of three-wheeled motor vehicle injured in collision with pedal cycle** in nontraffic accident

✓x7ᵗʰ **V31.3** Unspecified occupant of three-wheeled motor vehicle ▽ injured in collision with pedal cycle in nontraffic accident

✓x7ᵗʰ **V31.4** Person boarding or alighting **a three-wheeled motor vehicle injured in collision with pedal cycle**

✓x7ᵗʰ **V31.5** Driver **of three-wheeled motor vehicle injured in collision with pedal cycle** in traffic accident

✓x7ᵗʰ **V31.6** Passenger **in three-wheeled motor vehicle injured in collision with pedal cycle** in traffic accident

✓x7ᵗʰ **V31.7** Person on outside **of three-wheeled motor vehicle injured in collision with pedal cycle** in traffic accident

✓x7ᵗʰ **V31.9** Unspecified occupant of three-wheeled motor vehicle ▽ injured in collision with pedal cycle in traffic accident

✓4ᵗʰ **V32** **Occupant of three-wheeled motor vehicle injured in collision with two- or three-wheeled motor vehicle**

The appropriate 7th character is to be added to each code from category V32.
A   initial encounter
D   subsequent encounter
S   sequela

✓x7ᵗʰ **V32.0** Driver of three-wheeled motor vehicle injured in collision with two- or three-wheeled motor vehicle in nontraffic accident

✓x7ᵗʰ **V32.1** Passenger in three-wheeled motor vehicle injured in collision with two- or three-wheeled motor vehicle in nontraffic accident

✓x7ᵗʰ **V32.2** Person on outside of three-wheeled motor vehicle injured in collision with two- or three-wheeled motor vehicle in nontraffic accident

✓x7ᵗʰ **V32.3** Unspecified occupant of three-wheeled motor vehicle injured in collision with two- or three-wheeled motor vehicle in nontraffic accident ▽

✓x7ᵗʰ **V32.4** Person boarding or alighting a three-wheeled motor vehicle injured in collision with two- or three-wheeled motor vehicle

✓x7ᵗʰ **V32.5** Driver of three-wheeled motor vehicle injured in collision with two- or three-wheeled motor vehicle in traffic accident

✓x7ᵗʰ **V32.6** Passenger in three-wheeled motor vehicle injured in collision with two- or three-wheeled motor vehicle in traffic accident

✓x7ᵗʰ **V32.7** Person on outside of three-wheeled motor vehicle injured in collision with two- or three-wheeled motor vehicle in traffic accident

✓x7ᵗʰ **V32.9** Unspecified occupant of three-wheeled motor vehicle injured in collision with two- or three-wheeled motor vehicle in traffic accident ▽

✓4ᵗʰ **V33** **Occupant of three-wheeled motor vehicle injured in collision with car, pick-up truck or van**

The appropriate 7th character is to be added to each code from category V33.
A   initial encounter
D   subsequent encounter
S   sequela

✓x7ᵗʰ **V33.0** Driver of three-wheeled motor vehicle injured in collision with car, pick-up truck or van in nontraffic accident

✓x7ᵗʰ **V33.1** Passenger in three-wheeled motor vehicle injured in collision with car, pick-up truck or van in nontraffic accident

✓x7ᵗʰ **V33.2** Person on outside of three-wheeled motor vehicle injured in collision with car, pick-up truck or van in nontraffic accident

✓x7ᵗʰ **V33.3** Unspecified occupant of three-wheeled motor vehicle injured in collision with car, pick-up truck or van in nontraffic accident ▽

✓x7ᵗʰ **V33.4** Person boarding or alighting a three-wheeled motor vehicle injured in collision with car, pick-up truck or van

✓x7ᵗʰ **V33.5** Driver of three-wheeled motor vehicle injured in collision with car, pick-up truck or van in traffic accident

✓x7ᵗʰ **V33.6** Passenger in three-wheeled motor vehicle injured in collision with car, pick-up truck or van in traffic accident

✓x7ᵗʰ **V33.7** Person on outside of three-wheeled motor vehicle injured in collision with car, pick-up truck or van in traffic accident

✓x7ᵗʰ **V33.9** Unspecified occupant of three-wheeled motor vehicle injured in collision with car, pick-up truck or van in traffic accident ▽

✓4ᵗʰ **V34** **Occupant of three-wheeled motor vehicle injured in collision with heavy transport vehicle or bus**

EXCLUDES 1   occupant of three-wheeled motor vehicle injured in collision with military vehicle (V39.81)

The appropriate 7th character is to be added to each code from category V34.
A   initial encounter
D   subsequent encounter
S   sequela

✓x7ᵗʰ **V34.0** Driver of three-wheeled motor vehicle injured in collision with heavy transport vehicle or bus in nontraffic accident

✓x7ᵗʰ **V34.1** Passenger in three-wheeled motor vehicle injured in collision with heavy transport vehicle or bus in nontraffic accident

✓x7ᵗʰ **V34.2** Person on outside of three-wheeled motor vehicle injured in collision with heavy transport vehicle or bus in nontraffic accident

✓x7ᵗʰ **V34.3** Unspecified occupant of three-wheeled motor vehicle injured in collision with heavy transport vehicle or bus in nontraffic accident ▽

✓x7ᵗʰ **V34.4** Person boarding or alighting a three-wheeled motor vehicle injured in collision with heavy transport vehicle or bus

✓x7ᵗʰ **V34.5** Driver of three-wheeled motor vehicle injured in collision with heavy transport vehicle or bus in traffic accident

✓x7ᵗʰ **V34.6** Passenger in three-wheeled motor vehicle injured in collision with heavy transport vehicle or bus in traffic accident

✓x7ᵗʰ **V34.7** Person on outside of three-wheeled motor vehicle injured in collision with heavy transport vehicle or bus in traffic accident

✓x7ᵗʰ **V34.9** Unspecified occupant of three-wheeled motor vehicle injured in collision with heavy transport vehicle or bus in traffic accident ▽

✓4ᵗʰ **V35** **Occupant of three-wheeled motor vehicle injured in collision with railway train or railway vehicle**

The appropriate 7th character is to be added to each code from category V35.
A   initial encounter
D   subsequent encounter
S   sequela

✓x7ᵗʰ **V35.0** Driver of three-wheeled motor vehicle injured in collision with railway train or railway vehicle in nontraffic accident

✓x7ᵗʰ **V35.1** Passenger in three-wheeled motor vehicle injured in collision with railway train or railway vehicle in nontraffic accident

✓x7ᵗʰ **V35.2** Person on outside of three-wheeled motor vehicle injured in collision with railway train or railway vehicle in nontraffic accident

✓x7ᵗʰ **V35.3** Unspecified occupant of three-wheeled motor vehicle injured in collision with railway train or railway vehicle in nontraffic accident ▽

✓x7ᵗʰ **V35.4** Person boarding or alighting a three-wheeled motor vehicle injured in collision with railway train or railway vehicle

✓x7ᵗʰ **V35.5** Driver of three-wheeled motor vehicle injured in collision with railway train or railway vehicle in traffic accident

✓x7ᵗʰ **V35.6** Passenger in three-wheeled motor vehicle injured in collision with railway train or railway vehicle in traffic accident

✓x7ᵗʰ **V35.7** Person on outside of three-wheeled motor vehicle injured in collision with railway train or railway vehicle in traffic accident

✓x7ᵗʰ **V35.9** Unspecified occupant of three-wheeled motor vehicle injured in collision with railway train or railway vehicle in traffic accident ▽

✓4ᵗʰ **V36** **Occupant of three-wheeled motor vehicle injured in collision with other nonmotor vehicle**

INCLUDES   collision with animal-drawn vehicle, animal being ridden, streetcar

The appropriate 7th character is to be added to each code from category V36.
A   initial encounter
D   subsequent encounter
S   sequela

✓x7ᵗʰ **V36.0** Driver of three-wheeled motor vehicle injured in collision with other nonmotor vehicle in nontraffic accident

✓x7ᵗʰ **V36.1** Passenger in three-wheeled motor vehicle injured in collision with other nonmotor vehicle in nontraffic accident

✓x7ᵗʰ **V36.2** Person on outside of three-wheeled motor vehicle injured in collision with other nonmotor vehicle in nontraffic accident

✓x7ᵗʰ **V36.3** Unspecified occupant of three-wheeled motor vehicle injured in collision with other nonmotor vehicle in nontraffic accident ▽

✓x7ᵗʰ **V36.4** Person boarding or alighting a three-wheeled motor vehicle injured in collision with other nonmotor vehicle

✓x7ᵗʰ **V36.5** Driver of three-wheeled motor vehicle injured in collision with other nonmotor vehicle in traffic accident

✓x7ᵗʰ **V36.6** Passenger in three-wheeled motor vehicle injured in collision with other nonmotor vehicle in traffic accident

✓x7ᵗʰ **V36.7** Person on outside of three-wheeled motor vehicle injured in collision with other nonmotor vehicle in traffic accident

✓x7ᵗʰ **V36.9** Unspecified occupant of three-wheeled motor vehicle injured in collision with other nonmotor vehicle in traffic accident ▽

N Newborn   P Pediatric   M Maternity   A Adult   RIC RIC Dx   NC Dx Noncancer Dx   PDx Primary Dx   CC RIC CC Condition   ►◄ Revised Text   ● New Code   ▲ Revised Code Title

1062   ICD-10-CM 2016

✓4ᵗʰ **V37 Occupant of three-wheeled motor vehicle injured in collision with fixed or stationary object**

> The appropriate 7th character is to be added to each code from category V37.
> A   initial encounter
> D   subsequent encounter
> S   sequela

✓x7ᵗʰ **V37.0** Driver of three-wheeled motor vehicle injured in collision with fixed or stationary object in nontraffic accident

✓x7ᵗʰ **V37.1** Passenger in three-wheeled motor vehicle injured in collision with fixed or stationary object in nontraffic accident

✓x7ᵗʰ **V37.2** Person on outside of three-wheeled motor vehicle injured in collision with fixed or stationary object in nontraffic accident

✓x7ᵗʰ **V37.3** Unspecified occupant of three-wheeled motor vehicle   ▽ injured in collision with fixed or stationary object in nontraffic accident

✓x7ᵗʰ **V37.4** Person boarding or alighting a three-wheeled motor vehicle injured in collision with fixed or stationary object

✓x7ᵗʰ **V37.5** Driver of three-wheeled motor vehicle injured in collision with fixed or stationary object in traffic accident

✓x7ᵗʰ **V37.6** Passenger in three-wheeled motor vehicle injured in collision with fixed or stationary object in traffic accident

✓x7ᵗʰ **V37.7** Person on outside of three-wheeled motor vehicle injured in collision with fixed or stationary object in traffic accident

✓x7ᵗʰ **V37.9** Unspecified occupant of three-wheeled motor vehicle   ▽ injured in collision with fixed or stationary object in traffic accident

✓4ᵗʰ **V38 Occupant of three-wheeled motor vehicle injured in noncollision transport accident**

> INCLUDES fall or thrown from three-wheeled motor vehicle
> overturning of three-wheeled motor vehicle NOS
> overturning of three-wheeled motor vehicle without collision

> The appropriate 7th character is to be added to each code from category V38.
> A   initial encounter
> D   subsequent encounter
> S   sequela

✓x7ᵗʰ **V38.0** Driver of three-wheeled motor vehicle injured in noncollision transport accident in nontraffic accident

✓x7ᵗʰ **V38.1** Passenger in three-wheeled motor vehicle injured in noncollision transport accident in nontraffic accident

✓x7ᵗʰ **V38.2** Person on outside of three-wheeled motor vehicle injured in noncollision transport accident in nontraffic accident

✓x7ᵗʰ **V38.3** Unspecified occupant of three-wheeled motor vehicle   ▽ injured in noncollision transport accident in nontraffic accident

✓x7ᵗʰ **V38.4** Person boarding or alighting a three-wheeled motor vehicle injured in noncollision transport accident

✓x7ᵗʰ **V38.5** Driver of three-wheeled motor vehicle injured in noncollision transport accident in traffic accident

✓x7ᵗʰ **V38.6** Passenger in three-wheeled motor vehicle injured in noncollision transport accident in traffic accident

✓x7ᵗʰ **V38.7** Person on outside of three-wheeled motor vehicle injured in noncollision transport accident in traffic accident

✓x7ᵗʰ **V38.9** Unspecified occupant of three-wheeled motor vehicle   ▽ injured in noncollision transport accident in traffic accident

✓4ᵗʰ **V39 Occupant of three-wheeled motor vehicle injured in other and unspecified transport accidents**

> The appropriate 7th character is to be added to each code from category V39.
> A   initial encounter
> D   subsequent encounter
> S   sequela

✓5ᵗʰ **V39.0** Driver of three-wheeled motor vehicle injured in collision with other and unspecified motor vehicles in nontraffic accident

    ✓x7ᵗʰ **V39.00** Driver of three-wheeled motor vehicle injured in   ▽ collision with unspecified motor vehicles in nontraffic accident

    ✓x7ᵗʰ **V39.09** Driver of three-wheeled motor vehicle injured in collision with other motor vehicles in nontraffic accident

✓5ᵗʰ **V39.1** Passenger in three-wheeled motor vehicle injured in collision with other and unspecified motor vehicles in nontraffic accident

    ✓x7ᵗʰ **V39.10** Passenger in three-wheeled motor vehicle   ▽ injured in collision with unspecified motor vehicles in nontraffic accident

    ✓x7ᵗʰ **V39.19** Passenger in three-wheeled motor vehicle injured in collision with other motor vehicles in nontraffic accident

✓5ᵗʰ **V39.2** Unspecified occupant of three-wheeled motor vehicle injured in collision with other and unspecified motor vehicles in nontraffic accident

    ✓x7ᵗʰ **V39.20** Unspecified occupant of three-wheeled motor   ▽ vehicle injured in collision with unspecified motor vehicles in nontraffic accident
          Collision NOS involving three-wheeled motor vehicle, nontraffic

    ✓x7ᵗʰ **V39.29** Unspecified occupant of three-wheeled motor   ▽ vehicle injured in collision with other motor vehicles in nontraffic accident

✓x7ᵗʰ **V39.3** Occupant (driver) (passenger) of three-wheeled motor   ▽ vehicle injured in unspecified nontraffic accident
        Accident NOS involving three-wheeled motor vehicle, nontraffic
        Occupant of three-wheeled motor vehicle injured in nontraffic accident NOS

✓5ᵗʰ **V39.4** Driver of three-wheeled motor vehicle injured in collision with other and unspecified motor vehicles in traffic accident

    ✓x7ᵗʰ **V39.40** Driver of three-wheeled motor vehicle injured in   ▽ collision with unspecified motor vehicles in traffic accident

    ✓x7ᵗʰ **V39.49** Driver of three-wheeled motor vehicle injured in collision with other motor vehicles in traffic accident

✓5ᵗʰ **V39.5** Passenger in three-wheeled motor vehicle injured in collision with other and unspecified motor vehicles in traffic accident

    ✓x7ᵗʰ **V39.50** Passenger in three-wheeled motor vehicle   ▽ injured in collision with unspecified motor vehicles in traffic accident

    ✓x7ᵗʰ **V39.59** Passenger in three-wheeled motor vehicle injured in collision with other motor vehicles in traffic accident

✓5ᵗʰ **V39.6** Unspecified occupant of three-wheeled motor vehicle injured in collision with other and unspecified motor vehicles in traffic accident

    ✓x7ᵗʰ **V39.60** Unspecified occupant of three-wheeled motor   ▽ vehicle injured in collision with unspecified motor vehicles in traffic accident
          Collision NOS involving three-wheeled motor vehicle (traffic)

    ✓x7ᵗʰ **V39.69** Unspecified occupant of three-wheeled motor   ▽ vehicle injured in collision with other motor vehicles in traffic accident

✓5ᵗʰ **V39.8** Occupant (driver) (passenger) of three-wheeled motor vehicle injured in other specified transport accidents

    ✓x7ᵗʰ **V39.81** Occupant (driver) (passenger) of three-wheeled motor vehicle injured in transport accident with military vehicle

    ✓x7ᵗʰ **V39.89** Occupant (driver) (passenger) of three-wheeled motor vehicle injured in other specified transport accidents

✓x7ᵗʰ **V39.9** Occupant (driver) (passenger) of three-wheeled motor   ▽ vehicle injured in unspecified traffic accident
        Accident NOS involving three-wheeled motor vehicle

✓ Add'l Character Required   ✓x7ᵗʰ Placeholder Alert   RUG IV Special Care High Dx   RUG IV Clinically Complex Dx   RUG IV Special Care Low Dx   Manifestation Code   Other Specified Code   ▽ Unspecified Code

Car occupant injured in transport accident (V40-V49)

INCLUDES a four-wheeled motor vehicle designed primarily for carrying passengers
automobile (pulling a trailer or camper)

EXCLUDES 1 bus (V50-V59)
minibus (V50-V59)
minivan (V50-V59)
motorcoach (V70-V79)
pick-up truck (V50-V59)
sport utility vehicle (SUV) (V50-V59)

✓4ᵗʰ V40   Car occupant injured in collision with pedestrian or animal

EXCLUDES 1 car collision with animal-drawn vehicle or animal being ridden (V46.-)

The appropriate 7th character is to be added to each code from category V40.
A   initial encounter
D   subsequent encounter
S   sequela

✓x7ᵗʰ **V40.0** Car driver injured in collision with pedestrian or animal in nontraffic accident

✓x7ᵗʰ **V40.1** Car passenger injured in collision with pedestrian or animal in nontraffic accident

✓x7ᵗʰ **V40.2** Person on outside of car injured in collision with pedestrian or animal in nontraffic accident

✓x7ᵗʰ **V40.3** Unspecified car occupant injured in collision with pedestrian or animal in nontraffic accident ▽

✓x7ᵗʰ **V40.4** Person boarding or alighting a car injured in collision with pedestrian or animal

✓x7ᵗʰ **V40.5** Car driver injured in collision with pedestrian or animal in traffic accident

✓x7ᵗʰ **V40.6** Car passenger injured in collision with pedestrian or animal in traffic accident

✓x7ᵗʰ **V40.7** Person on outside of car injured in collision with pedestrian or animal in traffic accident

✓x7ᵗʰ **V40.9** Unspecified car occupant injured in collision with pedestrian or animal in traffic accident ▽

✓4ᵗʰ V41   Car occupant injured in collision with pedal cycle

The appropriate 7th character is to be added to each code from category V41.
A   initial encounter
D   subsequent encounter
S   sequela

✓x7ᵗʰ **V41.0** Car driver injured in collision with pedal cycle in nontraffic accident

✓x7ᵗʰ **V41.1** Car passenger injured in collision with pedal cycle in nontraffic accident

✓x7ᵗʰ **V41.2** Person on outside of car injured in collision with pedal cycle in nontraffic accident

✓x7ᵗʰ **V41.3** Unspecified car occupant injured in collision with pedal cycle in nontraffic accident ▽

✓x7ᵗʰ **V41.4** Person boarding or alighting a car injured in collision with pedal cycle

✓x7ᵗʰ **V41.5** Car driver injured in collision with pedal cycle in traffic accident

✓x7ᵗʰ **V41.6** Car passenger injured in collision with pedal cycle in traffic accident

✓x7ᵗʰ **V41.7** Person on outside of car injured in collision with pedal cycle in traffic accident

✓x7ᵗʰ **V41.9** Unspecified car occupant injured in collision with pedal cycle in traffic accident ▽

✓4ᵗʰ V42   Car occupant injured in collision with two- or three-wheeled motor vehicle

The appropriate 7th character is to be added to each code from category V42.
A   initial encounter
D   subsequent encounter
S   sequela

✓x7ᵗʰ **V42.0** Car driver injured in collision with two- or three-wheeled motor vehicle in nontraffic accident

✓x7ᵗʰ **V42.1** Car passenger injured in collision with two- or three-wheeled motor vehicle in nontraffic accident

✓x7ᵗʰ **V42.2** Person on outside of car injured in collision with two- or three-wheeled motor vehicle in nontraffic accident

✓x7ᵗʰ **V42.3** Unspecified car occupant injured in collision with two- or three-wheeled motor vehicle in nontraffic accident ▽

✓x7ᵗʰ **V42.4** Person boarding or alighting a car injured in collision with two- or three-wheeled motor vehicle

✓x7ᵗʰ **V42.5** Car driver injured in collision with two- or three-wheeled motor vehicle in traffic accident

✓x7ᵗʰ **V42.6** Car passenger injured in collision with two- or three-wheeled motor vehicle in traffic accident

✓x7ᵗʰ **V42.7** Person on outside of car injured in collision with two- or three-wheeled motor vehicle in traffic accident

✓x7ᵗʰ **V42.9** Unspecified car occupant injured in collision with two- or three-wheeled motor vehicle in traffic accident ▽

✓4ᵗʰ V43   Car occupant injured in collision with car, pick-up truck or van

The appropriate 7th character is to be added to each code from category V43.
A   initial encounter
D   subsequent encounter
S   sequela

✓5ᵗʰ **V43.0** Car driver injured in collision with car, pick-up truck or van in nontraffic accident

    ✓x7ᵗʰ **V43.01** Car driver injured in collision with sport utility vehicle in nontraffic accident

    ✓x7ᵗʰ **V43.02** Car driver injured in collision with other type car in nontraffic accident

    ✓x7ᵗʰ **V43.03** Car driver injured in collision with pick-up truck in nontraffic accident

    ✓x7ᵗʰ **V43.04** Car driver injured in collision with van in nontraffic accident

✓5ᵗʰ **V43.1** Car passenger injured in collision with car, pick-up truck or van in nontraffic accident

    ✓x7ᵗʰ **V43.11** Car passenger injured in collision with sport utility vehicle in nontraffic accident

    ✓x7ᵗʰ **V43.12** Car passenger injured in collision with other type car in nontraffic accident

    ✓x7ᵗʰ **V43.13** Car passenger injured in collision with pick-up in nontraffic accident

    ✓x7ᵗʰ **V43.14** Car passenger injured in collision with van in nontraffic accident

✓5ᵗʰ **V43.2** Person on outside of car injured in collision with car, pick-up truck or van in nontraffic accident

    ✓x7ᵗʰ **V43.21** Person on outside of car injured in collision with sport utility vehicle in nontraffic accident

    ✓x7ᵗʰ **V43.22** Person on outside of car injured in collision with other type car in nontraffic accident

    ✓x7ᵗʰ **V43.23** Person on outside of car injured in collision with pick-up truck in nontraffic accident

    ✓x7ᵗʰ **V43.24** Person on outside of car injured in collision with van in nontraffic accident

✓5ᵗʰ **V43.3** Unspecified car occupant injured in collision with car, pick-up truck or van in nontraffic accident

    ✓x7ᵗʰ **V43.31** Unspecified car occupant injured in collision with sport utility vehicle in nontraffic accident ▽

    ✓x7ᵗʰ **V43.32** Unspecified car occupant injured in collision with other type car in nontraffic accident ▽

    ✓x7ᵗʰ **V43.33** Unspecified car occupant injured in collision with pick-up truck in nontraffic accident ▽

    ✓x7ᵗʰ **V43.34** Unspecified car occupant injured in collision with van in nontraffic accident ▽

✓5ᵗʰ **V43.4** Person boarding or alighting a car injured in collision with car, pick-up truck or van

    ✓x7ᵗʰ **V43.41** Person boarding or alighting a car injured in collision with sport utility vehicle

    ✓x7ᵗʰ **V43.42** Person boarding or alighting a car injured in collision with other type car

    ✓x7ᵗʰ **V43.43** Person boarding or alighting a car injured in collision with pick-up truck

    ✓x7ᵗʰ **V43.44** Person boarding or alighting a car injured in collision with van

✓5ᵗʰ **V43.5** Car driver injured in collision with car, pick-up truck or van in traffic accident

    ✓x7ᵗʰ **V43.51** Car driver injured in collision with sport utility vehicle in traffic accident

---

☒ Newborn   ☒ Pediatric   ☒ Maternity   ☒ Adult   **RIC** RIC Dx   **NC Dx** Noncancer Dx   **PDx** Primary Dx   **CC** RIC CC Condition   ►◄ Revised Text   ● New Code   ▲ Revised Code Title

✓x7ᵗʰ **V43.52** **Car driver injured in collision with other type car in traffic accident**

✓x7ᵗʰ **V43.53** Car driver injured in collision with pick-up truck in traffic accident

✓x7ᵗʰ **V43.54** Car driver injured in collision with van in traffic accident

✓5ᵗʰ **V43.6** Car passenger injured in collision with car, pick-up truck or van in traffic accident

✓x7ᵗʰ **V43.61** Car passenger injured in collision with sport utility vehicle in traffic accident

✓x7ᵗʰ **V43.62** **Car passenger injured in collision with other type car in traffic accident**

✓x7ᵗʰ **V43.63** Car passenger injured in collision with pick-up truck in traffic accident

✓x7ᵗʰ **V43.64** Car passenger injured in collision with van in traffic accident

✓5ᵗʰ **V43.7** Person on outside of car injured in collision with car, pick-up truck or van in traffic accident

✓x7ᵗʰ **V43.71** Person on outside of car injured in collision with sport utility vehicle in traffic accident

✓x7ᵗʰ **V43.72** **Person on outside of car injured in collision with other type car in traffic accident**

✓x7ᵗʰ **V43.73** Person on outside of car injured in collision with pick-up truck in traffic accident

✓x7ᵗʰ **V43.74** Person on outside of car injured in collision with van in traffic accident

✓5ᵗʰ **V43.9** Unspecified car occupant injured in collision with car, pick-up truck or van in traffic accident

✓x7ᵗʰ **V43.91** Unspecified car occupant injured in collision with sport utility vehicle in traffic accident ▽

✓x7ᵗʰ **V43.92** **Unspecified car occupant injured in collision with other type car in traffic accident** ▽

✓x7ᵗʰ **V43.93** Unspecified car occupant injured in collision with pick-up truck in traffic accident ▽

✓x7ᵗʰ **V43.94** Unspecified car occupant injured in collision with van in traffic accident ▽

✓4ᵗʰ **V44** **Car occupant injured in collision with heavy transport vehicle or bus**

     EXCLUDES 1   *car occupant injured in collision with military vehicle (V49.81)*

     The appropriate 7th character is to be added to each code from category V44.
     A   initial encounter
     D   subsequent encounter
     S   sequela

✓x7ᵗʰ **V44.0** Car driver injured in collision with heavy transport vehicle or bus in nontraffic accident

✓x7ᵗʰ **V44.1** Car passenger injured in collision with heavy transport vehicle or bus in nontraffic accident

✓x7ᵗʰ **V44.2** Person on outside of car injured in collision with heavy transport vehicle or bus in nontraffic accident

✓x7ᵗʰ **V44.3** Unspecified car occupant injured in collision with heavy transport vehicle or bus in nontraffic accident ▽

✓x7ᵗʰ **V44.4** Person boarding or alighting a car injured in collision with heavy transport vehicle or bus

✓x7ᵗʰ **V44.5** Car driver injured in collision with heavy transport vehicle or bus in traffic accident

✓x7ᵗʰ **V44.6** Car passenger injured in collision with heavy transport vehicle or bus in traffic accident

✓x7ᵗʰ **V44.7** Person on outside of car injured in collision with heavy transport vehicle or bus in traffic accident

✓x7ᵗʰ **V44.9** Unspecified car occupant injured in collision with heavy transport vehicle or bus in traffic accident ▽

✓4ᵗʰ **V45** **Car occupant injured in collision with railway train or railway vehicle**

     The appropriate 7th character is to be added to each code from category V45.
     A   initial encounter
     D   subsequent encounter
     S   sequela

✓x7ᵗʰ **V45.0** Car driver injured in collision with railway train or railway vehicle in nontraffic accident

✓x7ᵗʰ **V45.1** Car passenger injured in collision with railway train or railway vehicle in nontraffic accident

✓x7ᵗʰ **V45.2** Person on outside of car injured in collision with railway train or railway vehicle in nontraffic accident

✓x7ᵗʰ **V45.3** Unspecified car occupant injured in collision with railway train or railway vehicle in nontraffic accident ▽

✓x7ᵗʰ **V45.4** Person boarding or alighting a car injured in collision with railway train or railway vehicle

✓x7ᵗʰ **V45.5** Car driver injured in collision with railway train or railway vehicle in traffic accident

✓x7ᵗʰ **V45.6** Car passenger injured in collision with railway train or railway vehicle in traffic accident

✓x7ᵗʰ **V45.7** Person on outside of car injured in collision with railway train or railway vehicle in traffic accident

✓x7ᵗʰ **V45.9** Unspecified car occupant injured in collision with railway train or railway vehicle in traffic accident ▽

✓4ᵗʰ **V46** **Car occupant injured in collision with other nonmotor vehicle**

     INCLUDES   collision with animal-drawn vehicle, animal being ridden, streetcar

     The appropriate 7th character is to be added to each code from category V46.
     A   initial encounter
     D   subsequent encounter
     S   sequela

✓x7ᵗʰ **V46.0** Car driver injured in collision with other nonmotor vehicle in nontraffic accident

✓x7ᵗʰ **V46.1** Car passenger injured in collision with other nonmotor vehicle in nontraffic accident

✓x7ᵗʰ **V46.2** Person on outside of car injured in collision with other nonmotor vehicle in nontraffic accident

✓x7ᵗʰ **V46.3** Unspecified car occupant injured in collision with other nonmotor vehicle in nontraffic accident ▽

✓x7ᵗʰ **V46.4** Person boarding or alighting a car injured in collision with other nonmotor vehicle

✓x7ᵗʰ **V46.5** Car driver injured in collision with other nonmotor vehicle in traffic accident

✓x7ᵗʰ **V46.6** Car passenger injured in collision with other nonmotor vehicle in traffic accident

✓x7ᵗʰ **V46.7** Person on outside of car injured in collision with other nonmotor vehicle in traffic accident

✓x7ᵗʰ **V46.9** Unspecified car occupant injured in collision with other nonmotor vehicle in traffic accident ▽

✓4ᵗʰ **V47** **Car occupant injured in collision with fixed or stationary object**

     The appropriate 7th character is to be added to each code from category V47.
     A   initial encounter
     D   subsequent encounter
     S   sequela

✓5ᵗʰ **V47.0** Car driver injured in collision with fixed or stationary object in nontraffic accident

✓x7ᵗʰ **V47.01** Driver of sport utility vehicle injured in collision with fixed or stationary object in nontraffic accident

✓x7ᵗʰ **V47.02** **Driver of other type car injured in collision with fixed or stationary object in nontraffic accident**

✓5ᵗʰ **V47.1** Car passenger injured in collision with fixed or stationary object in nontraffic accident

✓x7ᵗʰ **V47.11** Passenger of sport utility vehicle injured in collision with fixed or stationary object in nontraffic accident

✓x7ᵗʰ **V47.12** **Passenger of other type car injured in collision with fixed or stationary object in nontraffic accident**

✓x7ᵗʰ **V47.2** Person on outside of car injured in collision with fixed or stationary object in nontraffic accident

✓5ᵗʰ **V47.3** Unspecified car occupant injured in collision with fixed or stationary object in nontraffic accident

✓x7ᵗʰ **V47.31** Unspecified occupant of sport utility vehicle injured in collision with fixed or stationary object in nontraffic accident ▽

✓x7ᵗʰ **V47.32** **Unspecified occupant of other type car injured in collision with fixed or stationary object in nontraffic accident** ▽

✓x7ᵗʰ **V47.4** Person boarding or alighting a car injured in collision with fixed or stationary object

✓5ᵗʰ **V47.5** Car driver injured in collision with fixed or stationary object in traffic accident

✓x7ᵗʰ **V47.51** Driver of sport utility vehicle injured in collision with fixed or stationary object in traffic accident

---

☑ Add'l Character Required   ✓x7ᵗʰ Placeholder Alert   RUG IV Special Care High Dx   RUG IV Clinically Complex Dx   RUG IV Special Care Low Dx   Manifestation Code   Other Specified Code   ▽ Unspecified Code

√x7th V47.52 **Driver of other type car injured in collision with fixed or stationary object in traffic accident**

√5th V47.6 **Car** passenger **injured in collision with fixed or stationary object in traffic accident**

     √x7th V47.61 **Passenger of** sport utility vehicle **injured in collision with fixed or stationary object in traffic accident**

     √x7th V47.62 **Passenger of other type car injured in collision with fixed or stationary object in traffic accident**

√x7th V47.7 Person on outside **of car injured in collision with fixed or stationary object** in traffic accident

√5th V47.9 Unspecified **car occupant injured in collision with fixed or stationary object** in traffic accident

     √x7th V47.91 **Unspecified occupant of** sport utility vehicle **injured in collision with fixed or stationary object in traffic accident** ▽

     √x7th V47.92 **Unspecified occupant of other type car injured in collision with fixed or stationary object in traffic accident** ▽

√4th V48 Car occupant injured in noncollision transport accident
     INCLUDES overturning car NOS
                 overturning car without collision

> The appropriate 7th character is to be added to each code from category V48.
> A   initial encounter
> D   subsequent encounter
> S   sequela

√x7th V48.0 Car driver **injured in noncollision transport accident in** nontraffic accident

√x7th V48.1 Car passenger **injured in noncollision transport accident in** nontraffic accident

√x7th V48.2 Person on outside **of car injured in noncollision transport accident in nontraffic accident**

√x7th V48.3 Unspecified car occupant injured in noncollision transport **accident in nontraffic accident** ▽

√x7th V48.4 Person boarding or alighting **a car injured in noncollision transport accident**

√x7th V48.5 Car driver **injured in noncollision transport accident in traffic accident**

√x7th V48.6 Car passenger **injured in noncollision transport accident in traffic accident**

√x7th V48.7 Person on outside **of car injured in noncollision transport accident in traffic accident**

√x7th V48.9 Unspecified car occupant injured in noncollision **transport accident in traffic accident** ▽

√4th V49 Car occupant injured in other and unspecified transport accidents

> The appropriate 7th character is to be added to each code from category V49.
> A   initial encounter
> D   subsequent encounter
> S   sequela

√5th V49.0 Driver **injured in collision with other and unspecified motor vehicles** in nontraffic accident

     √x7th V49.00 **Driver injured in collision with unspecified motor vehicles in nontraffic accident** ▽

     √x7th V49.09 **Driver injured in collision with other motor vehicles in nontraffic accident**

√5th V49.1 Passenger **injured in collision with other and unspecified motor vehicles** in nontraffic accident

     √x7th V49.10 **Passenger injured in collision with unspecified motor vehicles in nontraffic accident** ▽

     √x7th V49.19 **Passenger injured in collision with other motor vehicles in nontraffic accident**

√5th V49.2 Unspecified **car occupant injured in collision with other and unspecified motor vehicles** in nontraffic accident

     √x7th V49.20 **Unspecified car occupant injured in collision with unspecified motor vehicles in nontraffic accident** ▽
            Car collision NOS, nontraffic

     √x7th V49.29 **Unspecified car occupant injured in collision with other motor vehicles in nontraffic accident** ▽

√x7th V49.3 Car occupant (driver) (passenger) injured in unspecified nontraffic accident ▽
     Car accident NOS, nontraffic
     Car occupant injured in nontraffic accident NOS

√5th V49.4 Driver **injured in collision with other and unspecified motor vehicles** in traffic accident

     √x7th V49.40 **Driver injured in collision with unspecified motor vehicles in traffic accident** ▽

     √x7th V49.49 **Driver injured in collision with other motor vehicles in traffic accident**

√5th V49.5 Passenger **injured in collision with other and unspecified motor vehicles** in traffic accident

     √x7th V49.50 **Passenger injured in collision with unspecified motor vehicles in traffic accident** ▽

     √x7th V49.59 **Passenger injured in collision with other motor vehicles in traffic accident**

√5th V49.6 Unspecified **car occupant injured in collision with other and unspecified motor vehicles** in traffic accident

     √x7th V49.60 **Unspecified car occupant injured in collision with unspecified motor vehicles in traffic accident** ▽
            Car collision NOS (traffic)

     √x7th V49.69 **Unspecified car occupant injured in collision with other motor vehicles in traffic accident** ▽

√5th V49.8 Car occupant (driver) (passenger) injured in other specified **transport accidents**

     √x7th V49.81 **Car occupant (driver) (passenger) injured in transport accident with** military vehicle

     √x7th V49.88 **Car occupant (driver) (passenger) injured in other** specified **transport accidents**

√x7th V49.9 Car occupant (driver) (passenger) injured in unspecified traffic accident ▽
     Car accident NOS

Occupant of pick-up truck or van injured in transport accident (V50-V59)

     INCLUDES a four or six wheel motor vehicle designed primarily for carrying passengers and property but weighing less than the local limit for classification as a heavy goods vehicle
     minibus
     minivan
     sport utility vehicle (SUV)
     truck
     van
     EXCLUDES1 heavy transport vehicle (V60-V69)

√4th V50 Occupant of pick-up truck or van injured in collision with pedestrian or animal
     EXCLUDES1 pick-up truck or van collision with animal-drawn vehicle or animal being ridden (V56.-)

> The appropriate 7th character is to be added to each code from category V50.
> A   initial encounter
> D   subsequent encounter
> S   sequela

√x7th V50.0 Driver **of pick-up truck or van injured in collision with pedestrian or animal** in nontraffic accident

√x7th V50.1 Passenger **in pick-up truck or van injured in collision with pedestrian or animal** in nontraffic accident

√x7th V50.2 Person on outside **of pick-up truck or van injured in collision with pedestrian or animal** in nontraffic accident

√x7th V50.3 Unspecified occupant of pick-up truck or van injured in **collision with pedestrian or animal** in nontraffic accident ▽

√x7th V50.4 Person boarding or alighting **a pick-up truck or van injured in collision with pedestrian or animal**

√x7th V50.5 Driver **of pick-up truck or van injured in collision with pedestrian or animal** in traffic accident

√x7th V50.6 Passenger **in pick-up truck or van injured in collision with pedestrian or animal** in traffic accident

√x7th V50.7 Person on outside **of pick-up truck or van injured in collision with pedestrian or animal** in traffic accident

√x7th V50.9 Unspecified occupant of pick-up truck or van injured in **collision with pedestrian or animal** in traffic accident ▽

◻N Newborn   ◻P Pediatric   ◻M Maternity   ◻A Adult   RIC RIC Dx   NCDx Noncancer Dx   PDx Primary Dx   CC RIC CC Condition   ►◄ Revised Text   ● New Code   ▲ Revised Code Title

1066   ICD-10-CM 2016

☑4ᵗʰ **V51 Occupant of pick-up truck or van injured in collision with pedal cycle**

> The appropriate 7th character is to be added to each code from category V51.
> A   initial encounter
> D   subsequent encounter
> S   sequela

√x7ᵗʰ **V51.0** Driver of pick-up truck or van injured in collision with pedal cycle in nontraffic accident

√x7ᵗʰ **V51.1** Passenger in pick-up truck or van injured in collision with pedal cycle in nontraffic accident

√x7ᵗʰ **V51.2** Person on outside of pick-up truck or van injured in collision with pedal cycle in nontraffic accident

√x7ᵗʰ **V51.3** Unspecified occupant of pick-up truck or van injured in ▽ collision with pedal cycle in nontraffic accident

√x7ᵗʰ **V51.4** Person boarding or alighting a pick-up truck or van injured in collision with pedal cycle

√x7ᵗʰ **V51.5** Driver of pick-up truck or van injured in collision with pedal cycle in traffic accident

√x7ᵗʰ **V51.6** Passenger in pick-up truck or van injured in collision with pedal cycle in traffic accident

√x7ᵗʰ **V51.7** Person on outside of pick-up truck or van injured in collision with pedal cycle in traffic accident

√x7ᵗʰ **V51.9** Unspecified occupant of pick-up truck or van injured in ▽ collision with pedal cycle in traffic accident

☑4ᵗʰ **V52 Occupant of pick-up truck or van injured in collision with two- or three-wheeled motor vehicle**

> The appropriate 7th character is to be added to each code from category V52.
> A   initial encounter
> D   subsequent encounter
> S   sequela

√x7ᵗʰ **V52.0** Driver of pick-up truck or van injured in collision with two- or three-wheeled motor vehicle in nontraffic accident

√x7ᵗʰ **V52.1** Passenger in pick-up truck or van injured in collision with two- or three-wheeled motor vehicle in nontraffic accident

√x7ᵗʰ **V52.2** Person on outside of pick-up truck or van injured in collision with two- or three-wheeled motor vehicle in nontraffic accident

√x7ᵗʰ **V52.3** Unspecified occupant of pick-up truck or van injured in ▽ collision with two- or three-wheeled motor vehicle in nontraffic accident

√x7ᵗʰ **V52.4** Person boarding or alighting a pick-up truck or van injured in collision with two- or three-wheeled motor vehicle

√x7ᵗʰ **V52.5** Driver of pick-up truck or van injured in collision with two- or three-wheeled motor vehicle in traffic accident

√x7ᵗʰ **V52.6** Passenger in pick-up truck or van injured in collision with two- or three-wheeled motor vehicle in traffic accident

√x7ᵗʰ **V52.7** Person on outside of pick-up truck or van injured in collision with two- or three-wheeled motor vehicle in traffic accident

√x7ᵗʰ **V52.9** Unspecified occupant of pick-up truck or van injured in ▽ collision with two- or three-wheeled motor vehicle in traffic accident

☑4ᵗʰ **V53 Occupant of pick-up truck or van injured in collision with car, pick-up truck or van**

> The appropriate 7th character is to be added to each code from category V53.
> A   initial encounter
> D   subsequent encounter
> S   sequela

√x7ᵗʰ **V53.0** Driver of pick-up truck or van injured in collision with car, pick-up truck or van in nontraffic accident

√x7ᵗʰ **V53.1** Passenger in pick-up truck or van injured in collision with car, pick-up truck or van in nontraffic accident

√x7ᵗʰ **V53.2** Person on outside of pick-up truck or van injured in collision with car, pick-up truck or van in nontraffic accident

√x7ᵗʰ **V53.3** Unspecified occupant of pick-up truck or van injured in ▽ collision with car, pick-up truck or van in nontraffic accident

√x7ᵗʰ **V53.4** Person boarding or alighting a pick-up truck or van injured in collision with car, pick-up truck or van

√x7ᵗʰ **V53.5** Driver of pick-up truck or van injured in collision with car, pick-up truck or van in traffic accident

√x7ᵗʰ **V53.6** Passenger in pick-up truck or van injured in collision with car, pick-up truck or van in traffic accident

√x7ᵗʰ **V53.7** Person on outside of pick-up truck or van injured in collision with car, pick-up truck or van in traffic accident

√x7ᵗʰ **V53.9** Unspecified occupant of pick-up truck or van injured in ▽ collision with car, pick-up truck or van in traffic accident

☑4ᵗʰ **V54 Occupant of pick-up truck or van injured in collision with heavy transport vehicle or bus**

> **EXCLUDES 1**   occupant of pick-up truck or van injured in collision with military vehicle (V59.81)

> The appropriate 7th character is to be added to each code from category V54.
> A   initial encounter
> D   subsequent encounter
> S   sequela

√x7ᵗʰ **V54.0** Driver of pick-up truck or van injured in collision with heavy transport vehicle or bus in nontraffic accident

√x7ᵗʰ **V54.1** Passenger in pick-up truck or van injured in collision with heavy transport vehicle or bus in nontraffic accident

√x7ᵗʰ **V54.2** Person on outside of pick-up truck or van injured in collision with heavy transport vehicle or bus in nontraffic accident

√x7ᵗʰ **V54.3** Unspecified occupant of pick-up truck or van injured in ▽ collision with heavy transport vehicle or bus in nontraffic accident

√x7ᵗʰ **V54.4** Person boarding or alighting a pick-up truck or van injured in collision with heavy transport vehicle or bus

√x7ᵗʰ **V54.5** Driver of pick-up truck or van injured in collision with heavy transport vehicle or bus in traffic accident

√x7ᵗʰ **V54.6** Passenger in pick-up truck or van injured in collision with heavy transport vehicle or bus in traffic accident

√x7ᵗʰ **V54.7** Person on outside of pick-up truck or van injured in collision with heavy transport vehicle or bus in traffic accident

√x7ᵗʰ **V54.9** Unspecified occupant of pick-up truck or van injured in ▽ collision with heavy transport vehicle or bus in traffic accident

☑4ᵗʰ **V55 Occupant of pick-up truck or van injured in collision with railway train or railway vehicle**

> The appropriate 7th character is to be added to each code from category V55.
> A   initial encounter
> D   subsequent encounter
> S   sequela

√x7ᵗʰ **V55.0** Driver of pick-up truck or van injured in collision with railway train or railway vehicle in nontraffic accident

√x7ᵗʰ **V55.1** Passenger in pick-up truck or van injured in collision with railway train or railway vehicle in nontraffic accident

√x7ᵗʰ **V55.2** Person on outside of pick-up truck or van injured in collision with railway train or railway vehicle in nontraffic accident

√x7ᵗʰ **V55.3** Unspecified occupant of pick-up truck or van injured in ▽ collision with railway train or railway vehicle in nontraffic accident

√x7ᵗʰ **V55.4** Person boarding or alighting a pick-up truck or van injured in collision with railway train or railway vehicle

√x7ᵗʰ **V55.5** Driver of pick-up truck or van injured in collision with railway train or railway vehicle in traffic accident

√x7ᵗʰ **V55.6** Passenger in pick-up truck or van injured in collision with railway train or railway vehicle in traffic accident

√x7ᵗʰ **V55.7** Person on outside of pick-up truck or van injured in collision with railway train or railway vehicle in traffic accident

√x7ᵗʰ **V55.9** Unspecified occupant of pick-up truck or van injured in ▽ collision with railway train or railway vehicle in traffic accident

☑4ᵗʰ **V56 Occupant of pick-up truck or van injured in collision with other nonmotor vehicle**

> **INCLUDES**   collision with animal-drawn vehicle, animal being ridden, streetcar

> The appropriate 7th character is to be added to each code from category V56.
> A   initial encounter
> D   subsequent encounter
> S   sequela

√x7ᵗʰ **V56.0** Driver of pick-up truck or van injured in collision with other nonmotor vehicle in nontraffic accident

√x7ᵗʰ **V56.1** Passenger in pick-up truck or van injured in collision with other nonmotor vehicle in nontraffic accident

---

✓x7ᵗʰ **V56.2** Person on outside of pick-up truck or van injured in collision with other nonmotor vehicle in nontraffic accident

✓x7ᵗʰ **V56.3** Unspecified occupant of pick-up truck or van injured in collision with other nonmotor vehicle in nontraffic accident ▽

✓x7ᵗʰ **V56.4** Person boarding or alighting a pick-up truck or van injured in collision with other nonmotor vehicle

✓x7ᵗʰ **V56.5** Driver of pick-up truck or van injured in collision with other nonmotor vehicle in traffic accident

✓x7ᵗʰ **V56.6** Passenger in pick-up truck or van injured in collision with other nonmotor vehicle in traffic accident

✓x7ᵗʰ **V56.7** Person on outside of pick-up truck or van injured in collision with other nonmotor vehicle in traffic accident

✓x7ᵗʰ **V56.9** Unspecified occupant of pick-up truck or van injured in collision with other nonmotor vehicle in traffic accident ▽

✓4ᵗʰ **V57** Occupant of pick-up truck or van injured in collision with fixed or stationary object

The appropriate 7th character is to be added to each code from category V57.
A   initial encounter
D   subsequent encounter
S   sequela

✓x7ᵗʰ **V57.0** Driver of pick-up truck or van injured in collision with fixed or stationary object in nontraffic accident

✓x7ᵗʰ **V57.1** Passenger in pick-up truck or van injured in collision with fixed or stationary object in nontraffic accident

✓x7ᵗʰ **V57.2** Person on outside of pick-up truck or van injured in collision with fixed or stationary object in nontraffic accident

✓x7ᵗʰ **V57.3** Unspecified occupant of pick-up truck or van injured in collision with fixed or stationary object in nontraffic accident ▽

✓x7ᵗʰ **V57.4** Person boarding or alighting a pick-up truck or van injured in collision with fixed or stationary object

✓x7ᵗʰ **V57.5** Driver of pick-up truck or van injured in collision with fixed or stationary object in traffic accident

✓x7ᵗʰ **V57.6** Passenger in pick-up truck or van injured in collision with fixed or stationary object in traffic accident

✓x7ᵗʰ **V57.7** Person on outside of pick-up truck or van injured in collision with fixed or stationary object in traffic accident

✓x7ᵗʰ **V57.9** Unspecified occupant of pick-up truck or van injured in collision with fixed or stationary object in traffic accident ▽

✓4ᵗʰ **V58** Occupant of pick-up truck or van injured in noncollision transport accident
INCLUDES   overturning pick-up truck or van NOS
overturning pick-up truck or van without collision

The appropriate 7th character is to be added to each code from category V58.
A   initial encounter
D   subsequent encounter
S   sequela

✓x7ᵗʰ **V58.0** Driver of pick-up truck or van injured in noncollision transport accident in nontraffic accident

✓x7ᵗʰ **V58.1** Passenger in pick-up truck or van injured in noncollision transport accident in nontraffic accident

✓x7ᵗʰ **V58.2** Person on outside of pick-up truck or van injured in noncollision transport accident in nontraffic accident

✓x7ᵗʰ **V58.3** Unspecified occupant of pick-up truck or van injured in noncollision transport accident in nontraffic accident ▽

✓x7ᵗʰ **V58.4** Person boarding or alighting a pick-up truck or van injured in noncollision transport accident

✓x7ᵗʰ **V58.5** Driver of pick-up truck or van injured in noncollision transport accident in traffic accident

✓x7ᵗʰ **V58.6** Passenger in pick-up truck or van injured in noncollision transport accident in traffic accident

✓x7ᵗʰ **V58.7** Person on outside of pick-up truck or van injured in noncollision transport accident in traffic accident

✓x7ᵗʰ **V58.9** Unspecified occupant of pick-up truck or van injured in noncollision transport accident in traffic accident ▽

✓4ᵗʰ **V59** Occupant of pick-up truck or van injured in other and unspecified transport accidents

The appropriate 7th character is to be added to each code from category V59.
A   initial encounter
D   subsequent encounter
S   sequela

✓5ᵗʰ **V59.0** Driver of pick-up truck or van injured in collision with other and unspecified motor vehicles in nontraffic accident

✓x7ᵗʰ **V59.00** Driver of pick-up truck or van injured in collision with unspecified motor vehicles in nontraffic accident ▽

✓x7ᵗʰ **V59.09** Driver of pick-up truck or van injured in collision with other motor vehicles in nontraffic accident

✓5ᵗʰ **V59.1** Passenger in pick-up truck or van injured in collision with other and unspecified motor vehicles in nontraffic accident

✓x7ᵗʰ **V59.10** Passenger in pick-up truck or van injured in collision with unspecified motor vehicles in nontraffic accident ▽

✓x7ᵗʰ **V59.19** Passenger in pick-up truck or van injured in collision with other motor vehicles in nontraffic accident

✓5ᵗʰ **V59.2** Unspecified occupant of pick-up truck or van injured in collision with other and unspecified motor vehicles in nontraffic accident

✓x7ᵗʰ **V59.20** Unspecified occupant of pick-up truck or van injured in collision with unspecified motor vehicles in nontraffic accident ▽
Collision NOS involving pick-up truck or van, nontraffic

✓x7ᵗʰ **V59.29** Unspecified occupant of pick-up truck or van injured in collision with other motor vehicles in nontraffic accident ▽

✓x7ᵗʰ **V59.3** Occupant (driver) (passenger) of pick-up truck or van injured in unspecified nontraffic accident ▽
Accident NOS involving pick-up truck or van, nontraffic
Occupant of pick-up truck or van injured in nontraffic accident NOS

✓5ᵗʰ **V59.4** Driver of pick-up truck or van injured in collision with other and unspecified motor vehicles in traffic accident

✓x7ᵗʰ **V59.40** Driver of pick-up truck or van injured in collision with unspecified motor vehicles in traffic accident ▽

✓x7ᵗʰ **V59.49** Driver of pick-up truck or van injured in collision with other motor vehicles in traffic accident

✓5ᵗʰ **V59.5** Passenger in pick-up truck or van injured in collision with other and unspecified motor vehicles in traffic accident

✓x7ᵗʰ **V59.50** Passenger in pick-up truck or van injured in collision with unspecified motor vehicles in traffic accident ▽

✓x7ᵗʰ **V59.59** Passenger in pick-up truck or van injured in collision with other motor vehicles in traffic accident

✓5ᵗʰ **V59.6** Unspecified occupant of pick-up truck or van injured in collision with other and unspecified motor vehicles in traffic accident

✓x7ᵗʰ **V59.60** Unspecified occupant of pick-up truck or van injured in collision with unspecified motor vehicles in traffic accident ▽
Collision NOS involving pick-up truck or van (traffic)

✓x7ᵗʰ **V59.69** Unspecified occupant of pick-up truck or van injured in collision with other motor vehicles in traffic accident ▽

✓5ᵗʰ **V59.8** Occupant (driver) (passenger) of pick-up truck or van injured in other specified transport accidents

✓x7ᵗʰ **V59.81** Occupant (driver) (passenger) of pick-up truck or van injured in transport accident with military vehicle

✓x7ᵗʰ **V59.88** Occupant (driver) (passenger) of pick-up truck or van injured in other specified transport accidents

✓x7ᵗʰ **V59.9** Occupant (driver) (passenger) of pick-up truck or van injured in unspecified traffic accident ▽
Accident NOS involving pick-up truck or van

Occupant of heavy transport vehicle injured in transport accident (V60-V69)

> **INCLUDES**   18 wheeler
> armored car
> panel truck
> **EXCLUDES 1**   bus
> motorcoach

✓4ᵗʰ V60   Occupant of heavy transport vehicle injured in collision with pedestrian or animal

> **EXCLUDES 1**   heavy transport vehicle collision with animal-drawn vehicle or animal being ridden (V66.-)

> The appropriate 7th character is to be added to each code from category V60.
> A   initial encounter
> D   subsequent encounter
> S   sequela

- ✓x7ᵗʰ **V60.0   Driver** of heavy transport vehicle injured in collision with pedestrian or animal in nontraffic accident
- ✓x7ᵗʰ **V60.1   Passenger** in heavy transport vehicle injured in collision with pedestrian or animal in nontraffic accident
- ✓x7ᵗʰ **V60.2   Person on outside** of heavy transport vehicle injured in collision with pedestrian or animal in nontraffic accident
- ✓x7ᵗʰ **V60.3   Unspecified occupant** of heavy transport vehicle injured in collision with pedestrian or animal in nontraffic accident ▽
- ✓x7ᵗʰ **V60.4   Person boarding or alighting** a heavy transport vehicle injured in collision with pedestrian or animal
- ✓x7ᵗʰ **V60.5   Driver** of heavy transport vehicle injured in collision with pedestrian or animal in traffic accident
- ✓x7ᵗʰ **V60.6   Passenger** in heavy transport vehicle injured in collision with pedestrian or animal in traffic accident
- ✓x7ᵗʰ **V60.7   Person on outside** of heavy transport vehicle injured in collision with pedestrian or animal in traffic accident
- ✓x7ᵗʰ **V60.9   Unspecified occupant** of heavy transport vehicle injured in collision with pedestrian or animal in traffic accident ▽

✓4ᵗʰ V61   Occupant of heavy transport vehicle injured in collision with pedal cycle

> The appropriate 7th character is to be added to each code from category V61.
> A   initial encounter
> D   subsequent encounter
> S   sequela

- ✓x7ᵗʰ **V61.0   Driver** of heavy transport vehicle injured in collision with pedal cycle in nontraffic accident
- ✓x7ᵗʰ **V61.1   Passenger** in heavy transport vehicle injured in collision with pedal cycle in nontraffic accident
- ✓x7ᵗʰ **V61.2   Person on outside** of heavy transport vehicle injured in collision with pedal cycle in nontraffic accident
- ✓x7ᵗʰ **V61.3   Unspecified occupant** of heavy transport vehicle injured in collision with pedal cycle in nontraffic accident ▽
- ✓x7ᵗʰ **V61.4   Person boarding or alighting** a heavy transport vehicle injured in collision with pedal cycle while boarding or alighting
- ✓x7ᵗʰ **V61.5   Driver** of heavy transport vehicle injured in collision with pedal cycle in traffic accident
- ✓x7ᵗʰ **V61.6   Passenger** in heavy transport vehicle injured in collision with pedal cycle in traffic accident
- ✓x7ᵗʰ **V61.7   Person on outside** of heavy transport vehicle injured in collision with pedal cycle in traffic accident
- ✓x7ᵗʰ **V61.9   Unspecified occupant** of heavy transport vehicle injured in collision with pedal cycle in traffic accident ▽

✓4ᵗʰ V62   Occupant of heavy transport vehicle injured in collision with two- or three-wheeled motor vehicle

> The appropriate 7th character is to be added to each code from category V62.
> A   initial encounter
> D   subsequent encounter
> S   sequela

- ✓x7ᵗʰ **V62.0   Driver** of heavy transport vehicle injured in collision with two- or three-wheeled motor vehicle in nontraffic accident
- ✓x7ᵗʰ **V62.1   Passenger** in heavy transport vehicle injured in collision with two- or three-wheeled motor vehicle in nontraffic accident
- ✓x7ᵗʰ **V62.2   Person on outside** of heavy transport vehicle injured in collision with two- or three-wheeled motor vehicle in nontraffic accident
- ✓x7ᵗʰ **V62.3   Unspecified occupant** of heavy transport vehicle injured in collision with two- or three-wheeled motor vehicle in nontraffic accident ▽
- ✓x7ᵗʰ **V62.4   Person boarding or alighting** a heavy transport vehicle injured in collision with two- or three-wheeled motor vehicle
- ✓x7ᵗʰ **V62.5   Driver** of heavy transport vehicle injured in collision with two- or three-wheeled motor vehicle in traffic accident
- ✓x7ᵗʰ **V62.6   Passenger** in heavy transport vehicle injured in collision with two- or three-wheeled motor vehicle in traffic accident
- ✓x7ᵗʰ **V62.7   Person on outside** of heavy transport vehicle injured in collision with two- or three-wheeled motor vehicle in traffic accident
- ✓x7ᵗʰ **V62.9   Unspecified occupant** of heavy transport vehicle injured in collision with two- or three-wheeled motor vehicle in traffic accident ▽

✓4ᵗʰ V63   Occupant of heavy transport vehicle injured in collision with car, pick-up truck or van

> The appropriate 7th character is to be added to each code from category V63.
> A   initial encounter
> D   subsequent encounter
> S   sequela

- ✓x7ᵗʰ **V63.0   Driver** of heavy transport vehicle injured in collision with car, pick-up truck or van in nontraffic accident
- ✓x7ᵗʰ **V63.1   Passenger** in heavy transport vehicle injured in collision with car, pick-up truck or van in nontraffic accident
- ✓x7ᵗʰ **V63.2   Person on outside** of heavy transport vehicle injured in collision with car, pick-up truck or van in nontraffic accident
- ✓x7ᵗʰ **V63.3   Unspecified occupant** of heavy transport vehicle injured in collision with car, pick-up truck or van in nontraffic accident ▽
- ✓x7ᵗʰ **V63.4   Person boarding or alighting** a heavy transport vehicle injured in collision with car, pick-up truck or van
- ✓x7ᵗʰ **V63.5   Driver** of heavy transport vehicle injured in collision with car, pick-up truck or van in traffic accident
- ✓x7ᵗʰ **V63.6   Passenger** in heavy transport vehicle injured in collision with car, pick-up truck or van in traffic accident
- ✓x7ᵗʰ **V63.7   Person on outside** of heavy transport vehicle injured in collision with car, pick-up truck or van in traffic accident
- ✓x7ᵗʰ **V63.9   Unspecified occupant** of heavy transport vehicle injured in collision with car, pick-up truck or van in traffic accident ▽

✓4ᵗʰ V64   Occupant of heavy transport vehicle injured in collision with heavy transport vehicle or bus

> **EXCLUDES 1**   occupant of heavy transport vehicle injured in collision with military vehicle (V69.81)

> The appropriate 7th character is to be added to each code from category V64.
> A   initial encounter
> D   subsequent encounter
> S   sequela

- ✓x7ᵗʰ **V64.0   Driver** of heavy transport vehicle injured in collision with heavy transport vehicle or bus in nontraffic accident
- ✓x7ᵗʰ **V64.1   Passenger** in heavy transport vehicle injured in collision with heavy transport vehicle or bus in nontraffic accident
- ✓x7ᵗʰ **V64.2   Person on outside** of heavy transport vehicle injured in collision with heavy transport vehicle or bus in nontraffic accident
- ✓x7ᵗʰ **V64.3   Unspecified occupant** of heavy transport vehicle injured in collision with heavy transport vehicle or bus in nontraffic accident ▽
- ✓x7ᵗʰ **V64.4   Person boarding or alighting** a heavy transport vehicle injured in collision with heavy transport vehicle or bus while boarding or alighting
- ✓x7ᵗʰ **V64.5   Driver** of heavy transport vehicle injured in collision with heavy transport vehicle or bus in traffic accident
- ✓x7ᵗʰ **V64.6   Passenger** in heavy transport vehicle injured in collision with heavy transport vehicle or bus in traffic accident
- ✓x7ᵗʰ **V64.7   Person on outside** of heavy transport vehicle injured in collision with heavy transport vehicle or bus in traffic accident
- ✓x7ᵗʰ **V64.9   Unspecified occupant** of heavy transport vehicle injured in collision with heavy transport vehicle or bus in traffic accident ▽

✅ Add'l Character Required   ✓x7ᵗʰ Placeholder Alert   RUG IV Special Care High Dx   RUG IV Clinically Complex Dx   RUG IV Special Care Low Dx   Manifestation Code   Other Specified Code   ▽ Unspecified Code

☑4ᵗʰ **V65 Occupant of heavy transport vehicle injured in collision with railway train or railway vehicle**

> The appropriate 7th character is to be added to each code from category V65.
> A   initial encounter
> D   subsequent encounter
> S   sequela

√x7ᵗʰ **V65.0** Driver of heavy transport vehicle injured in collision with railway train or railway vehicle in nontraffic accident

√x7ᵗʰ **V65.1** Passenger in heavy transport vehicle injured in collision with railway train or railway vehicle in nontraffic accident

√x7ᵗʰ **V65.2** Person on outside of heavy transport vehicle injured in collision with railway train or railway vehicle in nontraffic accident

√x7ᵗʰ **V65.3** Unspecified occupant of heavy transport vehicle injured in ▽ collision with railway train or railway vehicle in nontraffic accident

√x7ᵗʰ **V65.4** Person boarding or alighting a heavy transport vehicle injured in collision with railway train or railway vehicle

√x7ᵗʰ **V65.5** Driver of heavy transport vehicle injured in collision with railway train or railway vehicle in traffic accident

√x7ᵗʰ **V65.6** Passenger in heavy transport vehicle injured in collision with railway train or railway vehicle in traffic accident

√x7ᵗʰ **V65.7** Person on outside of heavy transport vehicle injured in collision with railway train or railway vehicle in traffic accident

√x7ᵗʰ **V65.9** Unspecified occupant of heavy transport vehicle injured in ▽ collision with railway train or railway vehicle in traffic accident

☑4ᵗʰ **V66 Occupant of heavy transport vehicle injured in collision with other nonmotor vehicle**

> INCLUDES collision with animal-drawn vehicle, animal being ridden, streetcar

> The appropriate 7th character is to be added to each code from category V66.
> A   initial encounter
> D   subsequent encounter
> S   sequela

√x7ᵗʰ **V66.0** Driver of heavy transport vehicle injured in collision with other nonmotor vehicle in nontraffic accident

√x7ᵗʰ **V66.1** Passenger in heavy transport vehicle injured in collision with other nonmotor vehicle in nontraffic accident

√x7ᵗʰ **V66.2** Person on outside of heavy transport vehicle injured in collision with other nonmotor vehicle in nontraffic accident

√x7ᵗʰ **V66.3** Unspecified occupant of heavy transport vehicle injured in ▽ collision with other nonmotor vehicle in nontraffic accident

√x7ᵗʰ **V66.4** Person boarding or alighting a heavy transport vehicle injured in collision with other nonmotor vehicle

√x7ᵗʰ **V66.5** Driver of heavy transport vehicle injured in collision with other nonmotor vehicle in traffic accident

√x7ᵗʰ **V66.6** Passenger in heavy transport vehicle injured in collision with other nonmotor vehicle in traffic accident

√x7ᵗʰ **V66.7** Person on outside of heavy transport vehicle injured in collision with other nonmotor vehicle in traffic accident

√x7ᵗʰ **V66.9** Unspecified occupant of heavy transport vehicle injured in ▽ collision with other nonmotor vehicle in traffic accident

☑4ᵗʰ **V67 Occupant of heavy transport vehicle injured in collision with fixed or stationary object**

> The appropriate 7th character is to be added to each code from category V67.
> A   initial encounter
> D   subsequent encounter
> S   sequela

√x7ᵗʰ **V67.0** Driver of heavy transport vehicle injured in collision with fixed or stationary object in nontraffic accident

√x7ᵗʰ **V67.1** Passenger in heavy transport vehicle injured in collision with fixed or stationary object in nontraffic accident

√x7ᵗʰ **V67.2** Person on outside of heavy transport vehicle injured in collision with fixed or stationary object in nontraffic accident

√x7ᵗʰ **V67.3** Unspecified occupant of heavy transport vehicle injured in ▽ collision with fixed or stationary object in nontraffic accident

√x7ᵗʰ **V67.4** Person boarding or alighting a heavy transport vehicle injured in collision with fixed or stationary object

√x7ᵗʰ **V67.5** Driver of heavy transport vehicle injured in collision with fixed or stationary object in traffic accident

√x7ᵗʰ **V67.6** Passenger in heavy transport vehicle injured in collision with fixed or stationary object in traffic accident

√x7ᵗʰ **V67.7** Person on outside of heavy transport vehicle injured in collision with fixed or stationary object in traffic accident

√x7ᵗʰ **V67.9** Unspecified occupant of heavy transport vehicle injured in ▽ collision with fixed or stationary object in traffic accident

☑4ᵗʰ **V68 Occupant of heavy transport vehicle injured in noncollision transport accident**

> INCLUDES overturning heavy transport vehicle NOS
> overturning heavy transport vehicle without collision

> The appropriate 7th character is to be added to each code from category V68.
> A   initial encounter
> D   subsequent encounter
> S   sequela

√x7ᵗʰ **V68.0** Driver of heavy transport vehicle injured in noncollision transport accident in nontraffic accident

√x7ᵗʰ **V68.1** Passenger in heavy transport vehicle injured in noncollision transport accident in nontraffic accident

√x7ᵗʰ **V68.2** Person on outside of heavy transport vehicle injured in noncollision transport accident in nontraffic accident

√x7ᵗʰ **V68.3** Unspecified occupant of heavy transport vehicle injured ▽ in noncollision transport accident in nontraffic accident

√x7ᵗʰ **V68.4** Person boarding or alighting a heavy transport vehicle injured in noncollision transport accident

√x7ᵗʰ **V68.5** Driver of heavy transport vehicle injured in noncollision transport accident in traffic accident

√x7ᵗʰ **V68.6** Passenger in heavy transport vehicle injured in noncollision transport accident in traffic accident

√x7ᵗʰ **V68.7** Person on outside of heavy transport vehicle injured in noncollision transport accident in traffic accident

√x7ᵗʰ **V68.9** Unspecified occupant of heavy transport vehicle injured in ▽ noncollision transport accident in traffic accident

☑4ᵗʰ **V69 Occupant of heavy transport vehicle injured in other and unspecified transport accidents**

> The appropriate 7th character is to be added to each code from category V69.
> A   initial encounter
> D   subsequent encounter
> S   sequela

√5ᵗʰ **V69.0** Driver of heavy transport vehicle injured in collision with other and unspecified motor vehicles in nontraffic accident

√x7ᵗʰ **V69.00** Driver of heavy transport vehicle injured in ▽ collision with unspecified motor vehicles in nontraffic accident

√x7ᵗʰ **V69.09** Driver of heavy transport vehicle injured in collision with other motor vehicles in nontraffic accident

√5ᵗʰ **V69.1** Passenger in heavy transport vehicle injured in collision with other and unspecified motor vehicles in nontraffic accident

√x7ᵗʰ **V69.10** Passenger in heavy transport vehicle injured ▽ in collision with unspecified motor vehicles in nontraffic accident

√x7ᵗʰ **V69.19** Passenger in heavy transport vehicle injured in collision with other motor vehicles in nontraffic accident

√5ᵗʰ **V69.2** Unspecified occupant of heavy transport vehicle injured in collision with other and unspecified motor vehicles in nontraffic accident

√x7ᵗʰ **V69.20** Unspecified occupant of heavy transport vehicle ▽ injured in collision with unspecified motor vehicles in nontraffic accident
> Collision NOS involving heavy transport vehicle, nontraffic

√x7ᵗʰ **V69.29** Unspecified occupant of heavy transport vehicle ▽ injured in collision with   other motor vehicles in nontraffic accident

√x7ᵗʰ **V69.3** Occupant (driver) (passenger) of heavy transport vehicle ▽ injured in unspecified nontraffic accident
> Accident NOS involving heavy transport vehicle, nontraffic
> Occupant of heavy transport vehicle injured in nontraffic accident NOS

Ⓝ Newborn   Ⓟ Pediatric   Ⓜ Maternity   Ⓐ Adult   **RIC Dx** RIC Dx   **NC Dx** Noncancer Dx   **PDx** Primary Dx   **CC** RIC CC Condition   ►◄ Revised Text   ● New Code   ▲ Revised Code Title

✓5ᵗʰ **V69.4** Driver of heavy transport vehicle injured in collision with other and unspecified motor vehicles in traffic accident

     ✓x7ᵗʰ **V69.40** Driver of heavy transport vehicle injured in collision with unspecified motor vehicles in traffic accident ▽

     ✓x7ᵗʰ **V69.49** Driver of heavy transport vehicle injured in collision with other motor vehicles in traffic accident

✓5ᵗʰ **V69.5** Passenger in heavy transport vehicle injured in collision with other and unspecified motor vehicles in traffic accident

     ✓x7ᵗʰ **V69.50** Passenger in heavy transport vehicle injured in collision with unspecified motor vehicles in traffic accident ▽

     ✓x7ᵗʰ **V69.59** Passenger in heavy transport vehicle injured in collision with other motor vehicles in traffic accident

✓5ᵗʰ **V69.6** Unspecified occupant of heavy transport vehicle injured in collision with other and unspecified motor vehicles in traffic accident

     ✓x7ᵗʰ **V69.60** Unspecified occupant of heavy transport vehicle injured in collision with unspecified motor vehicles in traffic accident ▽
            Collision NOS involving heavy transport vehicle (traffic)

     ✓x7ᵗʰ **V69.69** Unspecified occupant of heavy transport vehicle injured in collision with other motor vehicles in traffic accident ▽

✓5ᵗʰ **V69.8** Occupant (driver) (passenger) of heavy transport vehicle injured in other specified transport accidents

     ✓x7ᵗʰ **V69.81** Occupant (driver) (passenger) of heavy transport vehicle injured in transport accidents with military vehicle

     ✓x7ᵗʰ **V69.88** Occupant (driver) (passenger) of heavy transport vehicle injured in other specified transport accidents

✓x7ᵗʰ **V69.9** Occupant (driver) (passenger) of heavy transport vehicle injured in unspecified traffic accident ▽
     Accident NOS involving heavy transport vehicle

Bus occupant injured in transport accident (V70-V79)

INCLUDES   motorcoach
EXCLUDES 1   minibus (V50-V59)

✓4ᵗʰ **V70** Bus occupant injured in collision with pedestrian or animal
     EXCLUDES 1   bus collision with animal-drawn vehicle or animal being ridden (V76.-)

     The appropriate 7th character is to be added to each code from category V70.
     A   initial encounter
     D   subsequent encounter
     S   sequela

     ✓x7ᵗʰ **V70.0** Driver of bus injured in collision with pedestrian or animal in nontraffic accident

     ✓x7ᵗʰ **V70.1** Passenger on bus injured in collision with pedestrian or animal in nontraffic accident

     ✓x7ᵗʰ **V70.2** Person on outside of bus injured in collision with pedestrian or animal in nontraffic accident

     ✓x7ᵗʰ **V70.3** Unspecified occupant of bus injured in collision with pedestrian or animal in nontraffic accident ▽

     ✓x7ᵗʰ **V70.4** Person boarding or alighting from bus injured in collision with pedestrian or animal

     ✓x7ᵗʰ **V70.5** Driver of bus injured in collision with pedestrian or animal in traffic accident

     ✓x7ᵗʰ **V70.6** Passenger on bus injured in collision with pedestrian or animal in traffic accident

     ✓x7ᵗʰ **V70.7** Person on outside of bus injured in collision with pedestrian or animal in traffic accident

     ✓x7ᵗʰ **V70.9** Unspecified occupant of bus injured in collision with pedestrian or animal in traffic accident ▽

✓4ᵗʰ **V71** Bus occupant injured in collision with pedal cycle

     The appropriate 7th character is to be added to each code from category V71.
     A   initial encounter
     D   subsequent encounter
     S   sequela

     ✓x7ᵗʰ **V71.0** Driver of bus injured in collision with pedal cycle in nontraffic accident

     ✓x7ᵗʰ **V71.1** Passenger on bus injured in collision with pedal cycle in nontraffic accident

     ✓x7ᵗʰ **V71.2** Person on outside of bus injured in collision with pedal cycle in nontraffic accident

     ✓x7ᵗʰ **V71.3** Unspecified occupant of bus injured in collision with pedal cycle in nontraffic accident ▽

     ✓x7ᵗʰ **V71.4** Person boarding or alighting from bus injured in collision with pedal cycle

     ✓x7ᵗʰ **V71.5** Driver of bus injured in collision with pedal cycle in traffic accident

     ✓x7ᵗʰ **V71.6** Passenger on bus injured in collision with pedal cycle in traffic accident

     ✓x7ᵗʰ **V71.7** Person on outside of bus injured in collision with pedal cycle in traffic accident

     ✓x7ᵗʰ **V71.9** Unspecified occupant of bus injured in collision with pedal cycle in traffic accident ▽

✓4ᵗʰ **V72** Bus occupant injured in collision with two- or three-wheeled motor vehicle

     The appropriate 7th character is to be added to each code from category V72.
     A   initial encounter
     D   subsequent encounter
     S   sequela

     ✓x7ᵗʰ **V72.0** Driver of bus injured in collision with two- or three-wheeled motor vehicle in nontraffic accident

     ✓x7ᵗʰ **V72.1** Passenger on bus injured in collision with two- or three-wheeled motor vehicle in nontraffic accident

     ✓x7ᵗʰ **V72.2** Person on outside of bus injured in collision with two- or three-wheeled motor vehicle in nontraffic accident

     ✓x7ᵗʰ **V72.3** Unspecified occupant of bus injured in collision with two- or three-wheeled motor vehicle in nontraffic accident ▽

     ✓x7ᵗʰ **V72.4** Person boarding or alighting from bus injured in collision with two- or three-wheeled motor vehicle

     ✓x7ᵗʰ **V72.5** Driver of bus injured in collision with two- or three-wheeled motor vehicle in traffic accident

     ✓x7ᵗʰ **V72.6** Passenger on bus injured in collision with two- or three-wheeled motor vehicle in traffic accident

     ✓x7ᵗʰ **V72.7** Person on outside of bus injured in collision with two- or three-wheeled motor vehicle in traffic accident

     ✓x7ᵗʰ **V72.9** Unspecified occupant of bus injured in collision with two- or three-wheeled motor vehicle in traffic accident ▽

✓4ᵗʰ **V73** Bus occupant injured in collision with car, pick-up truck or van

     The appropriate 7th character is to be added to each code from category V73.
     A   initial encounter
     D   subsequent encounter
     S   sequela

     ✓x7ᵗʰ **V73.0** Driver of bus injured in collision with car, pick-up truck or van in nontraffic accident

     ✓x7ᵗʰ **V73.1** Passenger on bus injured in collision with car, pick-up truck or van in nontraffic accident

     ✓x7ᵗʰ **V73.2** Person on outside of bus injured in collision with car, pick-up truck or van in nontraffic accident

     ✓x7ᵗʰ **V73.3** Unspecified occupant of bus injured in collision with car, pick-up truck or van in nontraffic accident ▽

     ✓x7ᵗʰ **V73.4** Person boarding or alighting from bus injured in collision with car, pick-up truck or van

     ✓x7ᵗʰ **V73.5** Driver of bus injured in collision with car, pick-up truck or van in traffic accident

     ✓x7ᵗʰ **V73.6** Passenger on bus injured in collision with car, pick-up truck or van in traffic accident

     ✓x7ᵗʰ **V73.7** Person on outside of bus injured in collision with car, pick-up truck or van in traffic accident

     ✓x7ᵗʰ **V73.9** Unspecified occupant of bus injured in collision with car, pick-up truck or van in traffic accident ▽

✓4ᵗʰ **V74** Bus occupant injured in collision with heavy transport vehicle or bus
     EXCLUDES 1   bus occupant injured in collision with military vehicle (V79.81)

     The appropriate 7th character is to be added to each code from category V74.
     A   initial encounter
     D   subsequent encounter
     S   sequela

     ✓x7ᵗʰ **V74.0** Driver of bus injured in collision with heavy transport vehicle or bus in nontraffic accident

✓x7ᵗʰ **V74.1** Passenger on bus injured in collision with heavy transport vehicle or bus in nontraffic accident

✓x7ᵗʰ **V74.2** Person on outside of bus injured in collision with heavy transport vehicle or bus in nontraffic accident

✓x7ᵗʰ **V74.3** Unspecified occupant of bus injured in collision with heavy transport vehicle or bus in nontraffic accident ▽

✓x7ᵗʰ **V74.4** Person boarding or alighting from bus injured in collision with heavy transport vehicle or bus

✓x7ᵗʰ **V74.5** Driver of bus injured in collision with heavy transport vehicle or bus in traffic accident

✓x7ᵗʰ **V74.6** Passenger on bus injured in collision with heavy transport vehicle or bus in traffic accident

✓x7ᵗʰ **V74.7** Person on outside of bus injured in collision with heavy transport vehicle or bus in traffic accident

✓x7ᵗʰ **V74.9** Unspecified occupant of bus injured in collision with heavy transport vehicle or bus in traffic accident ▽

✓4ᵗʰ **V75** **Bus occupant injured in collision with railway train or railway vehicle**

> The appropriate 7th character is to be added to each code from category V75.
> A   initial encounter
> D   subsequent encounter
> S   sequela

✓x7ᵗʰ **V75.0** Driver of bus injured in collision with railway train or railway vehicle in nontraffic accident

✓x7ᵗʰ **V75.1** Passenger on bus injured in collision with railway train or railway vehicle in nontraffic accident

✓x7ᵗʰ **V75.2** Person on outside of bus injured in collision with railway train or railway vehicle in nontraffic accident

✓x7ᵗʰ **V75.3** Unspecified occupant of bus injured in collision with railway train or railway vehicle in nontraffic accident ▽

✓x7ᵗʰ **V75.4** Person boarding or alighting from bus injured in collision with railway train or railway vehicle

✓x7ᵗʰ **V75.5** Driver of bus injured in collision with railway train or railway vehicle in traffic accident

✓x7ᵗʰ **V75.6** Passenger on bus injured in collision with railway train or railway vehicle in traffic accident

✓x7ᵗʰ **V75.7** Person on outside of bus injured in collision with railway train or railway vehicle in traffic accident

✓x7ᵗʰ **V75.9** Unspecified occupant of bus injured in collision with railway train or railway vehicle in traffic accident ▽

✓4ᵗʰ **V76** **Bus occupant injured in collision with other nonmotor vehicle**
> INCLUDES   collision with animal-drawn vehicle, animal being ridden, streetcar

> The appropriate 7th character is to be added to each code from category V76.
> A   initial encounter
> D   subsequent encounter
> S   sequela

✓x7ᵗʰ **V76.0** Driver of bus injured in collision with other nonmotor vehicle in nontraffic accident

✓x7ᵗʰ **V76.1** Passenger on bus injured in collision with other nonmotor vehicle in nontraffic accident

✓x7ᵗʰ **V76.2** Person on outside of bus injured in collision with other nonmotor vehicle in nontraffic accident

✓x7ᵗʰ **V76.3** Unspecified occupant of bus injured in collision with other nonmotor vehicle in nontraffic accident ▽

✓x7ᵗʰ **V76.4** Person boarding or alighting from bus injured in collision with other nonmotor vehicle

✓x7ᵗʰ **V76.5** Driver of bus injured in collision with other nonmotor vehicle in traffic accident

✓x7ᵗʰ **V76.6** Passenger on bus injured in collision with other nonmotor vehicle in traffic accident

✓x7ᵗʰ **V76.7** Person on outside of bus injured in collision with other nonmotor vehicle in traffic accident

✓x7ᵗʰ **V76.9** Unspecified occupant of bus injured in collision with other nonmotor vehicle in traffic accident ▽

✓4ᵗʰ **V77** **Bus occupant injured in collision with fixed or stationary object**

> The appropriate 7th character is to be added to each code from category V77.
> A   initial encounter
> D   subsequent encounter
> S   sequela

✓x7ᵗʰ **V77.0** Driver of bus injured in collision with fixed or stationary object in nontraffic accident

✓x7ᵗʰ **V77.1** Passenger on bus injured in collision with fixed or stationary object in nontraffic accident

✓x7ᵗʰ **V77.2** Person on outside of bus injured in collision with fixed or stationary object in nontraffic accident

✓x7ᵗʰ **V77.3** Unspecified occupant of bus injured in collision with fixed ▽ or stationary object in nontraffic accident

✓x7ᵗʰ **V77.4** Person boarding or alighting from bus injured in collision with fixed or stationary object

✓x7ᵗʰ **V77.5** Driver of bus injured in collision with fixed or stationary object in traffic accident

✓x7ᵗʰ **V77.6** Passenger on bus injured in collision with fixed or stationary object in traffic accident

✓x7ᵗʰ **V77.7** Person on outside of bus injured in collision with fixed or stationary object in traffic accident

✓x7ᵗʰ **V77.9** Unspecified occupant of bus injured in collision with fixed ▽ or stationary object in traffic accident

✓4ᵗʰ **V78** **Bus occupant injured in noncollision transport accident**
> INCLUDES   overturning bus NOS
> overturning bus without collision

> The appropriate 7th character is to be added to each code from category V78.
> A   initial encounter
> D   subsequent encounter
> S   sequela

✓x7ᵗʰ **V78.0** Driver of bus injured in noncollision transport accident in nontraffic accident

✓x7ᵗʰ **V78.1** Passenger on bus injured in noncollision transport accident in nontraffic accident

✓x7ᵗʰ **V78.2** Person on outside of bus injured in noncollision transport accident in nontraffic accident

✓x7ᵗʰ **V78.3** Unspecified occupant of bus injured in noncollision ▽ transport accident in nontraffic accident

✓x7ᵗʰ **V78.4** Person boarding or alighting from bus injured in noncollision transport accident

✓x7ᵗʰ **V78.5** Driver of bus injured in noncollision transport accident in traffic accident

✓x7ᵗʰ **V78.6** Passenger on bus injured in noncollision transport accident in traffic accident

✓x7ᵗʰ **V78.7** Person on outside of bus injured in noncollision transport accident in traffic accident

✓x7ᵗʰ **V78.9** Unspecified occupant of bus injured in noncollision ▽ transport accident in traffic accident

✓4ᵗʰ **V79** **Bus occupant injured in other and unspecified transport accidents**

> The appropriate 7th character is to be added to each code from category V79.
> A   initial encounter
> D   subsequent encounter
> S   sequela

✓5ᵗʰ **V79.0** Driver of bus injured in collision with other and unspecified motor vehicles in nontraffic accident

 ✓x7ᵗʰ **V79.00** Driver of bus injured in collision with unspecified ▽ motor vehicles in nontraffic accident

 ✓x7ᵗʰ **V79.09** Driver of bus injured in collision with other motor vehicles in nontraffic accident

✓5ᵗʰ **V79.1** Passenger on bus injured in collision with other and unspecified motor vehicles in nontraffic accident

 ✓x7ᵗʰ **V79.10** Passenger on bus injured in collision with ▽ unspecified motor vehicles in nontraffic accident

 ✓x7ᵗʰ **V79.19** Passenger on bus injured in collision with other motor vehicles in nontraffic accident

Ⓝ Newborn   Ⓟ Pediatric   Ⓜ Maternity   Ⓐ Adult   **RIC** RIC Dx   **NCDx** Noncancer Dx   **PDx** Primary Dx   **CC** RIC CC Condition   ▶◀ Revised Text   ● New Code   ▲ Revised Code Title

1072   ICD-10-CM 2016

☑5ᵗʰ **V79.2** Unspecified **bus occupant injured in collision with other and unspecified** motor vehicles in nontraffic accident

   ☑x7ᵗʰ **V79.20** **Unspecified bus occupant injured in collision with unspecified** motor vehicles **in nontraffic accident** ▽
       Bus collision NOS, nontraffic

   ☑x7ᵗʰ **V79.29** **Unspecified bus occupant injured in collision with** ▽ **other** motor vehicles **in nontraffic accident**

☑x7ᵗʰ **V79.3** **Bus** occupant (driver) (passenger) **injured in unspecified** ▽ nontraffic accident
     Bus accident NOS, nontraffic
     Bus occupant injured in nontraffic accident NOS

☑5ᵗʰ **V79.4** Driver of bus injured in collision with other and unspecified motor vehicles in traffic accident

   ☑x7ᵗʰ **V79.40** **Driver of bus injured in collision with unspecified** ▽ motor vehicles **in traffic accident**

   ☑x7ᵗʰ **V79.49** **Driver of bus injured in collision with other** motor vehicles **in traffic accident**

☑5ᵗʰ **V79.5** Passenger **on bus injured in collision with other and unspecified motor vehicles** in traffic accident

   ☑x7ᵗʰ **V79.50** **Passenger on bus injured in collision with unspecified** motor vehicles **in traffic accident** ▽

   ☑x7ᵗʰ **V79.59** **Passenger on bus injured in collision with other** motor vehicles **in traffic accident**

☑5ᵗʰ **V79.6** Unspecified **bus occupant injured in collision with other and unspecified motor vehicles** in traffic accident

   ☑x7ᵗʰ **V79.60** **Unspecified bus occupant injured in collision** ▽ **with unspecified** motor vehicles **in traffic accident**
       Bus collision NOS (traffic)

   ☑x7ᵗʰ **V79.69** **Unspecified bus occupant injured in collision** ▽ **with other** motor vehicles **in traffic accident**

☑5ᵗʰ **V79.8** **Bus** occupant (driver) (passenger) **injured in** other **specified transport accidents**

   ☑x7ᵗʰ **V79.81** **Bus occupant (driver) (passenger) injured in transport accidents with** military vehicle

   ☑x7ᵗʰ **V79.88** **Bus occupant (driver) (passenger) injured in other specified transport accidents**

☑x7ᵗʰ **V79.9** **Bus** occupant (driver) (passenger) **injured in unspecified** ▽ traffic accident
     Bus accident NOS

Other land transport accidents (V80-V89)

☑4ᵗʰ **V80** **Animal-rider or occupant of animal-drawn vehicle injured in transport accident**

    The appropriate 7th character is to be added to each code from category V80.
    A   initial encounter
    D   subsequent encounter
    S   sequela

☑5ᵗʰ **V80.0** **Animal-rider or occupant of animal drawn vehicle injured by fall from or being thrown from animal or animal-drawn vehicle in** noncollision accident

   ☑6ᵗʰ **V80.01** Animal-rider **injured by fall from or being thrown from animal in noncollision accident**

      ☑7ᵗʰ **V80.010** **Animal-rider injured by fall from or being thrown from** horse **in noncollision accident**

      ☑7ᵗʰ **V80.018** **Animal-rider injured by fall from or being thrown from other** animal **in noncollision accident**

   ☑x7ᵗʰ **V80.02** Occupant **of animal-drawn vehicle injured by fall from or being thrown from animal-drawn vehicle in noncollision accident**
       Overturning animal-drawn vehicle NOS
       Overturning animal-drawn vehicle without collision

☑5ᵗʰ **V80.1** **Animal-rider or occupant of animal-drawn vehicle injured in collision with** pedestrian or animal
     EXCLUDES 1   animal-rider or animal-drawn vehicle collision with animal-drawn vehicle or animal being ridden (V80.7)

   ☑x7ᵗʰ **V80.11** Animal-rider **injured in collision with pedestrian or animal**

   ☑x7ᵗʰ **V80.12** Occupant **of animal-drawn vehicle injured in collision with pedestrian or animal**

☑5ᵗʰ **V80.2** **Animal-rider or occupant of animal-drawn vehicle injured in collision with** pedal cycle

   ☑x7ᵗʰ **V80.21** Animal-rider **injured in collision with pedal cycle**

   ☑x7ᵗʰ **V80.22** Occupant **of animal-drawn vehicle injured in collision with pedal cycle**

☑5ᵗʰ **V80.3** **Animal-rider or occupant of animal-drawn vehicle injured in collision with** two- or three-wheeled motor vehicle

   ☑x7ᵗʰ **V80.31** Animal-rider **injured in collision with two- or three-wheeled motor vehicle**

   ☑x7ᵗʰ **V80.32** Occupant **of animal-drawn vehicle injured in collision with two- or three-wheeled motor vehicle**

☑5ᵗʰ **V80.4** **Animal-rider or occupant of animal-drawn vehicle injured in collision with** car, pick-up truck, van, heavy transport vehicle or bus
     EXCLUDES 1   animal-rider injured in collision with military vehicle (V80.910)
       occupant of animal-drawn vehicle injured in collision with military vehicle (V80.920)

   ☑x7ᵗʰ **V80.41** Animal-rider **injured in collision with car, pick-up truck, van, heavy transport vehicle or bus**

   ☑x7ᵗʰ **V80.42** Occupant **of animal-drawn vehicle injured in collision with car, pick-up truck, van, heavy transport vehicle or bus**

☑5ᵗʰ **V80.5** **Animal-rider or occupant of animal-drawn vehicle injured in collision with** other specified motor vehicle

   ☑x7ᵗʰ **V80.51** Animal-rider **injured in collision with other specified motor vehicle**

   ☑x7ᵗʰ **V80.52** Occupant **of animal-drawn vehicle injured in collision with other specified motor vehicle**

☑5ᵗʰ **V80.6** **Animal-rider or occupant of animal-drawn vehicle injured in collision with** railway train or railway vehicle

   ☑x7ᵗʰ **V80.61** Animal-rider **injured in collision with railway train or railway vehicle**

   ☑x7ᵗʰ **V80.62** Occupant **of animal-drawn vehicle injured in collision with railway train or railway vehicle**

☑5ᵗʰ **V80.7** **Animal-rider or occupant of animal-drawn vehicle injured in collision with** other nonmotor vehicles

   ☑6ᵗʰ **V80.71** **Animal-rider or occupant of animal-drawn vehicle injured in collision with** animal being ridden

      ☑7ᵗʰ **V80.710** Animal-rider **injured in collision with other animal being ridden**

      ☑7ᵗʰ **V80.711** Occupant **of animal-drawn vehicle injured in collision with animal being ridden**

   ☑6ᵗʰ **V80.72** **Animal-rider or occupant of animal-drawn vehicle injured in collision with** other animal-drawn vehicle

      ☑7ᵗʰ **V80.720** Animal-rider **injured in collision with animal-drawn vehicle**

      ☑7ᵗʰ **V80.721** Occupant **of animal-drawn vehicle injured in collision with other animal-drawn vehicle**

   ☑6ᵗʰ **V80.73** **Animal-rider or occupant of animal-drawn vehicle injured in collision with** streetcar

      ☑7ᵗʰ **V80.730** Animal-rider **injured in collision with streetcar**

      ☑7ᵗʰ **V80.731** Occupant **of animal-drawn vehicle injured in collision with streetcar**

   ☑6ᵗʰ **V80.79** **Animal-rider or occupant of animal-drawn vehicle injured in collision with** other nonmotor vehicles

      ☑7ᵗʰ **V80.790** Animal-rider **injured in collision with other nonmotor vehicles**

      ☑7ᵗʰ **V80.791** Occupant **of animal-drawn vehicle injured in collision with other nonmotor vehicles**

☑5ᵗʰ **V80.8** **Animal-rider or occupant of animal-drawn vehicle injured in collision with** fixed or stationary object

   ☑x7ᵗʰ **V80.81** Animal-rider **injured in collision with fixed or stationary object**

   ☑x7ᵗʰ **V80.82** Occupant **of animal-drawn vehicle injured in collision with fixed or stationary object**

☑5ᵗʰ **V80.9** **Animal-rider or occupant of animal-drawn vehicle injured in** other and unspecified transport accidents

   ☑6ᵗʰ **V80.91** Animal-rider **injured in other and unspecified transport accidents**

      ☑7ᵗʰ **V80.910** **Animal-rider injured in transport accident with** military vehicle

---

☑ Add'l Character Required   ☑x7ᵗʰ Placeholder Alert   RUG IV Special Care High Dx   RUG IV Clinically Complex Dx   RUG IV Special Care Low Dx   Manifestation Code   Other Specified Code   ▽ Unspecified Code

Chapter 20. External Causes of Morbidity

V80.918–V83.7

√7ᵗʰ **V80.918** **Animal-rider injured in other transport accident**

√7ᵗʰ **V80.919** **Animal-rider injured in unspecified transport accident** ▽
Animal rider accident NOS

√6ᵗʰ **V80.92** Occupant of animal-drawn vehicle injured in other and unspecified transport accidents

√7ᵗʰ **V80.920** **Occupant of animal-drawn vehicle injured in transport accident with** military vehicle

√7ᵗʰ **V80.928** **Occupant of animal-drawn vehicle injured in other transport accident**

√7ᵗʰ **V80.929** **Occupant of animal-drawn vehicle injured in unspecified transport accident** ▽
Animal-drawn vehicle accident NOS

√4ᵗʰ **V81** **Occupant of railway train or railway vehicle injured in transport accident**
INCLUDES   derailment of railway train or railway vehicle
person on outside of train
EXCLUDES 1   streetcar (V82.-)

The appropriate 7th character is to be added to each code from category V81.
A   initial encounter
D   subsequent encounter
S   sequela

√x7ᵗʰ **V81.0** **Occupant of railway train or railway vehicle injured in collision with motor vehicle** in nontraffic accident
EXCLUDES 1   occupant of railway train or railway vehicle injured due to collision with military vehicle (V81.83)

√x7ᵗʰ **V81.1** **Occupant of railway train or railway vehicle injured in collision with motor vehicle** in traffic accident
EXCLUDES 1   occupant of railway train or railway vehicle injured due to collision with military vehicle (V81.83)

√x7ᵗʰ **V81.2** **Occupant of railway train or railway vehicle injured in collision with or** hit by rolling stock

√x7ᵗʰ **V81.3** **Occupant of railway train or railway vehicle injured in collision with other** object
Railway collision NOS

√x7ᵗʰ **V81.4** **Person injured** while boarding or alighting **from railway train or railway vehicle**

√x7ᵗʰ **V81.5** **Occupant of railway train or railway vehicle injured** by fall in railway train **or railway vehicle**

√x7ᵗʰ **V81.6** **Occupant of railway train or railway vehicle injured by** fall from railway train **or railway vehicle**

√x7ᵗʰ **V81.7** **Occupant of railway train or railway vehicle injured in** derailment without antecedent collision

√5ᵗʰ **V81.8** **Occupant of railway train or railway vehicle injured in** other specified railway accidents

√x7ᵗʰ **V81.81** **Occupant of railway train or railway vehicle injured due to** explosion or fire **on train**

√x7ᵗʰ **V81.82** **Occupant of railway train or railway vehicle injured due to** object falling onto **train**
Occupant of railway train or railway vehicle injured due to falling earth onto train
Occupant of railway train or railway vehicle injured due to falling rocks onto train
Occupant of railway train or railway vehicle injured due to falling snow onto train
Occupant of railway train or railway vehicle injured due to falling trees onto train

√x7ᵗʰ **V81.83** **Occupant of railway train or railway vehicle injured due to** collision with military vehicle

√x7ᵗʰ **V81.89** **Occupant of railway train or railway vehicle injured due to other** specified railway accident

√x7ᵗʰ **V81.9** **Occupant of railway train or railway vehicle injured in** unspecified railway accident ▽
Railway accident NOS

√4ᵗʰ **V82** **Occupant of powered streetcar injured in transport accident**
INCLUDES   interurban electric car
person on outside of streetcar
tram (car)
trolley (car)
EXCLUDES 1   bus (V70-V79)
motorcoach (V70-V79)
nonpowered streetcar (V76.-)
train (V81.-)

The appropriate 7th character is to be added to each code from category V82.
A   initial encounter
D   subsequent encounter
S   sequela

√x7ᵗʰ **V82.0** **Occupant of streetcar injured in collision with motor vehicle in nontraffic accident**

√x7ᵗʰ **V82.1** **Occupant of streetcar injured in collision with motor vehicle in traffic accident**

√x7ᵗʰ **V82.2** **Occupant of streetcar injured in collision with or** hit by rolling stock

√x7ᵗʰ **V82.3** **Occupant of streetcar injured in collision with other** object
EXCLUDES 1   collision with animal-drawn vehicle or animal being ridden (V82.8)

√x7ᵗʰ **V82.4** **Person injured** while boarding or alighting **from streetcar**

√x7ᵗʰ **V82.5** **Occupant of streetcar injured by** fall in streetcar
EXCLUDES 1   fall in streetcar:
while boarding or alighting (V82.4)
with antecedent collision (V82.0-V82.3)

√x7ᵗʰ **V82.6** **Occupant of streetcar injured by** fall from streetcar
EXCLUDES 1   fall from streetcar:
while boarding or alighting (V82.4)\
with antecedent collision (V82.0-V82.3)

√x7ᵗʰ **V82.7** **Occupant of streetcar injured in** derailment without antecedent collision
EXCLUDES 1   occupant of streetcar injured in derailment with antecedent collision (V82.0-V82.3)

√x7ᵗʰ **V82.8** **Occupant of streetcar injured in other** specified transport accidents
Streetcar collision with military vehicle
Streetcar collision with train or nonmotor vehicles

√x7ᵗʰ **V82.9** **Occupant of streetcar injured in unspecified** traffic accident ▽
Streetcar accident NOS

√4ᵗʰ **V83** **Occupant of special vehicle mainly used on industrial premises injured in transport accident**
INCLUDES   battery-powered airport passenger vehicle
battery-powered truck (baggage) (mail)
coal-car in mine
forklift (truck)
logging car
self-propelled industrial truck
station baggage truck (powered)
tram, truck, or tub (powered) in mine or quarry
EXCLUDES 1   special construction vehicles (V85.-)
special industrial vehicle in stationary use or maintenance (W31.-)

The appropriate 7th character is to be added to each code from category V83.
A   initial encounter
D   subsequent encounter
S   sequela

√x7ᵗʰ **V83.0** Driver of special industrial vehicle injured in traffic accident

√x7ᵗʰ **V83.1** Passenger of special industrial vehicle injured in traffic accident

√x7ᵗʰ **V83.2** Person on outside of special industrial vehicle injured in traffic accident

√x7ᵗʰ **V83.3** **Unspecified occupant of special industrial vehicle injured** in traffic accident ▽

√x7ᵗʰ **V83.4** **Person injured while** boarding or alighting **from special industrial vehicle**

√x7ᵗʰ **V83.5** Driver of special industrial vehicle injured in nontraffic accident

√x7ᵗʰ **V83.6** Passenger of special industrial vehicle injured in nontraffic accident

√x7ᵗʰ **V83.7** Person on outside of special industrial vehicle injured in nontraffic accident

N Newborn   P Pediatric   M Maternity   A Adult   RIC RIC Dx   NCDx Noncancer Dx   PDx Primary Dx   CC RIC CC Condition   ►◄ Revised Text   ● New Code   ▲ Revised Code Title

1074   ICD-10-CM 2016

√x7ᵗʰ **V83.9** **Unspecified occupant of special industrial vehicle injured** ▽
in nontraffic accident
Special-industrial-vehicle accident NOS

✓4ᵗʰ **V84** **Occupant of special vehicle mainly used in agriculture injured in transport accident**
INCLUDES   self-propelled farm machinery
tractor (and trailer)
EXCLUDES1   animal-powered farm machinery accident (W30.8-)
contact with combine harvester (W30.0)
special agricultural vehicle in stationary use or maintenance (W30.-)

The appropriate 7th character is to be added to each code from category V84.
A   initial encounter
D   subsequent encounter
S   sequela

√x7ᵗʰ **V84.0** **Driver** of special agricultural vehicle injured in traffic accident

√x7ᵗʰ **V84.1** **Passenger** of special agricultural vehicle injured in traffic accident

√x7ᵗʰ **V84.2** **Person on outside** of special agricultural vehicle injured in traffic accident

√x7ᵗʰ **V84.3** **Unspecified occupant of special agricultural vehicle** ▽
injured in traffic accident

√x7ᵗʰ **V84.4** **Person injured while** boarding or alighting **from special agricultural vehicle**

√x7ᵗʰ **V84.5** **Driver** of special agricultural vehicle injured in nontraffic accident

√x7ᵗʰ **V84.6** **Passenger** of special agricultural vehicle injured in nontraffic accident

√x7ᵗʰ **V84.7** **Person on outside** of special agricultural vehicle injured in nontraffic accident

√x7ᵗʰ **V84.9** **Unspecified occupant of special agricultural vehicle** ▽
injured in nontraffic accident
Special-agricultural vehicle accident NOS

✓4ᵗʰ **V85** **Occupant of special construction vehicle injured in transport accident**
INCLUDES   bulldozer
digger
dump truck
earth-leveller
mechanical shovel
road-roller
EXCLUDES1   special industrial vehicle (V83.-)
special construction vehicle in stationary use or maintenance (W31.-)

The appropriate 7th character is to be added to each code from category V85.
A   initial encounter
D   subsequent encounter
S   sequela

√x7ᵗʰ **V85.0** **Driver** of special construction vehicle injured in traffic accident

√x7ᵗʰ **V85.1** **Passenger** of special construction vehicle injured in traffic accident

√x7ᵗʰ **V85.2** **Person on outside** of special construction vehicle injured in traffic accident

√x7ᵗʰ **V85.3** **Unspecified occupant of special construction vehicle** ▽
injured in traffic accident

√x7ᵗʰ **V85.4** **Person injured while** boarding or alighting **from special construction vehicle**

√x7ᵗʰ **V85.5** **Driver** of special construction vehicle injured in nontraffic accident

√x7ᵗʰ **V85.6** **Passenger** of special construction vehicle injured in nontraffic accident

√x7ᵗʰ **V85.7** **Person on outside** of special construction vehicle injured in nontraffic accident

√x7ᵗʰ **V85.9** **Unspecified occupant of special construction vehicle** ▽
injured in nontraffic accident
Special-construction-vehicle accident NOS

✓4ᵗʰ **V86** **Occupant of special all-terrain or other off-road motor vehicle, injured in transport accident**
EXCLUDES1   special all-terrain vehicle in stationary use or maintenance (W31.-)
sport-utility vehicle (V50-V59)
three-wheeled motor vehicle designed for on-road use (V30-V39)

The appropriate 7th character is to be added to each code from category V86.
A   initial encounter
D   subsequent encounter
S   sequela

√5ᵗʰ **V86.0** **Driver** of special all-terrain or other off-road motor vehicle injured in traffic accident

√x7ᵗʰ **V86.01** **Driver of** ambulance **or** fire engine **injured in traffic accident**

√x7ᵗʰ **V86.02** **Driver of** snowmobile **injured in traffic accident**

√x7ᵗʰ **V86.03** **Driver of** dune buggy **injured in traffic accident**

√x7ᵗʰ **V86.04** **Driver of** military vehicle **injured in traffic accident**

√x7ᵗʰ **V86.09** **Driver of other special all-terrain or other off-road motor vehicle injured in traffic accident**
Driver of dirt bike injured in traffic accident
Driver of go cart injured in traffic accident
Driver of golf cart injured in traffic accident

√5ᵗʰ **V86.1** **Passenger** of special all-terrain or other off-road motor vehicle injured in traffic accident

√x7ᵗʰ **V86.11** **Passenger of** ambulance **or** fire engine **injured in traffic accident**

√x7ᵗʰ **V86.12** **Passenger of** snowmobile **injured in traffic accident**

√x7ᵗʰ **V86.13** **Passenger of** dune buggy **injured in traffic accident**

√x7ᵗʰ **V86.14** **Passenger of** military vehicle **injured in traffic accident**

√x7ᵗʰ **V86.19** **Passenger of other special all-terrain or other off-road motor vehicle injured in traffic accident**
Passenger of dirt bike injured in traffic accident
Passenger of go cart injured in traffic accident
Passenger of golf cart injured in traffic accident

√5ᵗʰ **V86.2** **Person on outside** of special all-terrain or other off-road motor vehicle injured in traffic accident

√x7ᵗʰ **V86.21** **Person on outside of** ambulance **or** fire engine **injured in traffic accident**

√x7ᵗʰ **V86.22** **Person on outside of** snowmobile **injured in traffic accident**

√x7ᵗʰ **V86.23** **Person on outside of** dune buggy **injured in traffic accident**

√x7ᵗʰ **V86.24** **Person on outside of** military vehicle **injured in traffic accident**

√x7ᵗʰ **V86.29** **Person on outside of other special all-terrain or other off-road motor vehicle injured in traffic accident**
Person on outside of dirt bike injured in traffic accident
Person on outside of go cart injured in traffic accident
Person on outside of golf cart injured in traffic accident

√5ᵗʰ **V86.3** **Unspecified occupant** of special all-terrain or other off-road motor vehicle injured in traffic accident

√x7ᵗʰ **V86.31** **Unspecified occupant of** ambulance **or** fire engine ▽
injured in traffic accident

√x7ᵗʰ **V86.32** **Unspecified occupant of** snowmobile **injured in** ▽
traffic accident

√x7ᵗʰ **V86.33** **Unspecified occupant of** dune buggy **injured in** ▽
traffic accident

√x7ᵗʰ **V86.34** **Unspecified occupant of** military vehicle **injured** ▽
in traffic accident

√x7ᵗʰ **V86.39** **Unspecified occupant of other special all-terrain** ▽
or other off-road motor vehicle injured in traffic accident
Unspecified occupant of dirt bike injured in traffic accident
Unspecified occupant of go cart injured in traffic accident
Unspecified occupant of golf cart injured in traffic accident

√5ᵗʰ **V86.4** **Person injured while** boarding or alighting **from special all-terrain or other off-road motor vehicle**

√x7ᵗʰ **V86.41** **Person injured while boarding or alighting from** ambulance **or** fire engine

---

☑ Add'l Character Required √x7ᵗʰ Placeholder Alert RUG IV Special Care High Dx RUG IV Clinically Complex Dx RUG IV Special Care Low Dx Manifestation Code Other Specified Code ▽Unspecified Code

✓x7ᵗʰ **V86.42** **Person injured while boarding or alighting from** snowmobile

✓x7ᵗʰ **V86.43** **Person injured while boarding or alighting from** dune buggy

✓x7ᵗʰ **V86.44** **Person injured while boarding or alighting from** military vehicle

✓x7ᵗʰ **V86.49** **Person injured while boarding or alighting from other special all-terrain or other off-road motor vehicle**
Person injured while boarding or alighting from dirt bike
Person injured while boarding or alighting from go cart
Person injured while boarding or alighting from golf cart

✓5ᵗʰ **V86.5** **Driver** of special all-terrain or other off-road motor vehicle injured in nontraffic accident

✓x7ᵗʰ **V86.51** **Driver of** ambulance **or** fire engine **injured in** nontraffic accident

✓x7ᵗʰ **V86.52** **Driver of** snowmobile **injured in nontraffic accident**

✓x7ᵗʰ **V86.53** **Driver of** dune buggy **injured in nontraffic accident**

✓x7ᵗʰ **V86.54** **Driver of** military vehicle **injured in nontraffic accident**

✓x7ᵗʰ **V86.59** **Driver of other special all-terrain or other off-road motor vehicle injured in nontraffic accident**
Driver of dirt bike injured in nontraffic accident
Driver of go cart injured in nontraffic accident
Driver of golf cart injured in nontraffic accident

✓5ᵗʰ **V86.6** **Passenger** of special all-terrain or other off-road motor vehicle injured in nontraffic accident

✓x7ᵗʰ **V86.61** **Passenger of** ambulance **or** fire engine **injured in** nontraffic accident

✓x7ᵗʰ **V86.62** **Passenger of** snowmobile **injured in nontraffic accident**

✓x7ᵗʰ **V86.63** **Passenger of** dune buggy **injured in nontraffic accident**

✓x7ᵗʰ **V86.64** **Passenger of** military vehicle **injured in nontraffic accident**

✓x7ᵗʰ **V86.69** **Passenger of other special all-terrain or other off-road motor vehicle injured in nontraffic accident**
Passenger of dirt bike injured in nontraffic accident
Passenger of go cart injured in nontraffic accident
Passenger of golf cart injured in nontraffic accident

✓5ᵗʰ **V86.7** **Person on outside** of special all-terrain or other off-road motor vehicle injured in nontraffic accident

✓x7ᵗʰ **V86.71** **Person on outside of** ambulance **or** fire engine **injured in nontraffic accident**

✓x7ᵗʰ **V86.72** **Person on outside of** snowmobile **injured in** nontraffic accident

✓x7ᵗʰ **V86.73** **Person on outside of** dune buggy **injured in** nontraffic accident

✓x7ᵗʰ **V86.74** **Person on outside of** military vehicle **injured in** nontraffic accident

✓x7ᵗʰ **V86.79** **Person on outside of other special all-terrain or other off-road motor vehicles injured in nontraffic accident**
Person on outside of dirt bike injured in nontraffic accident
Person on outside of go cart injured in nontraffic accident
Person on outside of golf cart injured in nontraffic accident

✓5ᵗʰ **V86.9** **Unspecified occupant** of special all-terrain or other off-road motor vehicle injured in nontraffic accident

✓x7ᵗʰ **V86.91** **Unspecified occupant of** ambulance **or** fire engine ▽ **injured in nontraffic accident**

✓x7ᵗʰ **V86.92** **Unspecified occupant of** snowmobile **injured in** ▽ **nontraffic accident**

✓x7ᵗʰ **V86.93** **Unspecified occupant of** dune buggy **injured in** ▽ **nontraffic accident**

✓x7ᵗʰ **V86.94** **Unspecified occupant of** military vehicle **injured** ▽ **in nontraffic accident**

✓x7ᵗʰ **V86.99** **Unspecified occupant of other special all-terrain** ▽ **or other off-road motor vehicle injured in nontraffic accident**
All-terrain motor-vehicle accident NOS
Off-road motor-vehicle accident NOS
Other motor-vehicle accident NOS
Unspecified occupant of dirt bike injured in nontraffic accident
Unspecified occupant of go cart injured in nontraffic accident
Unspecified occupant of golf cart injured in nontraffic accident

✓4ᵗʰ **V87** **Traffic accident of specified type but victim's mode of transport unknown**
EXCLUDES 1 collision involving:
pedal cycle (V10-V19)
pedestrian (V01-V09)

The appropriate 7th character is to be added to each code from category V87.
A   initial encounter
D   subsequent encounter
S   sequela

✓x7ᵗʰ **V87.0** **Person injured in collision between** car and two- or three-wheeled powered vehicle **(traffic)**

✓x7ᵗʰ **V87.1** **Person injured in collision between other** motor vehicle and two- or three-wheeled motor vehicle **(traffic)**

✓x7ᵗʰ **V87.2** **Person injured in collision between** car and pick-up truck or van **(traffic)**

✓x7ᵗʰ **V87.3** **Person injured in collision between** car and bus **(traffic)**

✓x7ᵗʰ **V87.4** **Person injured in collision between** car and heavy transport vehicle **(traffic)**

✓x7ᵗʰ **V87.5** **Person injured in collision between** heavy transport vehicle and bus **(traffic)**

✓x7ᵗʰ **V87.6** **Person injured in collision between** railway train or railway vehicle and car **(traffic)**

✓x7ᵗʰ **V87.7** **Person injured in collision between other** specified motor vehicles **(traffic)**

✓x7ᵗʰ **V87.8** **Person injured in other** specified noncollision transport accidents involving motor vehicle **(traffic)**

✓x7ᵗʰ **V87.9** **Person injured in other** specified (collision)(noncollision) transport accidents involving nonmotor vehicle **(traffic)**

✓4ᵗʰ **V88** **Nontraffic accident of specified type but victim's mode of transport unknown**
EXCLUDES 1 collision involving:
pedal cycle (V10-V19)
pedestrian (V01-V09)

The appropriate 7th character is to be added to each code from category V88.
A   initial encounter
D   subsequent encounter
S   sequela

✓x7ᵗʰ **V88.0** **Person injured in collision between** car and two- or three-wheeled motor vehicle, **nontraffic**

✓x7ᵗʰ **V88.1** **Person injured in collision between other** motor vehicle and two- or three-wheeled motor vehicle, **nontraffic**

✓x7ᵗʰ **V88.2** **Person injured in collision between** car and pick-up truck or van, **nontraffic**

✓x7ᵗʰ **V88.3** **Person injured in collision between** car and bus, **nontraffic**

✓x7ᵗʰ **V88.4** **Person injured in collision between** car and heavy transport vehicle, **nontraffic**

✓x7ᵗʰ **V88.5** **Person injured in collision between** heavy transport vehicle and bus, **nontraffic**

✓x7ᵗʰ **V88.6** **Person injured in collision between** railway train or railway vehicle and car, **nontraffic**

✓x7ᵗʰ **V88.7** **Person injured in collision between other** specified motor vehicle, **nontraffic**

✓x7ᵗʰ **V88.8** **Person injured in other** specified noncollision transport accidents involving motor vehicle, **nontraffic**

✓x7ᵗʰ **V88.9** **Person injured in** other specified (collision)(noncollision) transport accidents involving nonmotor vehicle, **nontraffic**

✓4ᵗʰ V89   Motor- or nonmotor-vehicle accident, type of vehicle unspecified

> The appropriate 7th character is to be added to each code from category V89.
> A   initial encounter
> D   subsequent encounter
> S   sequela

✓x7ᵗʰ **V89.0**   **Person injured in unspecified motor-vehicle accident, nontraffic**   ▽
  Motor-vehicle accident NOS, nontraffic

✓x7ᵗʰ **V89.1**   **Person injured in unspecified nonmotor-vehicle accident, nontraffic**   ▽
  Nonmotor-vehicle accident NOS (nontraffic)

✓x7ᵗʰ **V89.2**   **Person injured in unspecified motor-vehicle accident, traffic**   ▽
  Motor-vehicle accident [MVA] NOS
  Road (traffic) accident [RTA] NOS

✓x7ᵗʰ **V89.3**   **Person injured in unspecified nonmotor-vehicle accident, traffic**   ▽
  Nonmotor-vehicle traffic accident NOS

✓x7ᵗʰ **V89.9**   **Person injured in unspecified vehicle accident**   ▽
  Collision NOS

Water transport accidents (V90-V94)

✓4ᵗʰ V90   Drowning and submersion due to accident to watercraft

> EXCLUDES 1   civilian water transport accident involving military watercraft (V94.81-)
> fall into water not from watercraft (W16.-)
> military watercraft accident in military or war operations (Y36.0-, Y37.0-)
> water-transport-related drowning or submersion without accident to watercraft (V92.-)

> The appropriate 7th character is to be added to each code from category V90.
> A   initial encounter
> D   subsequent encounter
> S   sequela

✓5ᵗʰ **V90.0**   **Drowning and submersion due to watercraft overturning**

  ✓x7ᵗʰ **V90.00**   **Drowning and submersion due to merchant ship overturning**

  ✓x7ᵗʰ **V90.01**   **Drowning and submersion due to passenger ship overturning**
  Drowning and submersion due to Ferry-boat overturning
  Drowning and submersion due to Liner overturning

  ✓x7ᵗʰ **V90.02**   **Drowning and submersion due to fishing boat overturning**

  ✓x7ᵗʰ **V90.03**   **Drowning and submersion due to other powered watercraft overturning**
  Drowning and submersion due to Hovercraft (on open water) overturning
  Drowning and submersion due to Jet ski overturning

  ✓x7ᵗʰ **V90.04**   **Drowning and submersion due to sailboat overturning**

  ✓x7ᵗʰ **V90.05**   **Drowning and submersion due to canoe or kayak overturning**

  ✓x7ᵗʰ **V90.06**   **Drowning and submersion due to (nonpowered) inflatable craft overturning**

  ✓x7ᵗʰ **V90.08**   **Drowning and submersion due to other unpowered watercraft overturning**
  Drowning and submersion due to windsurfer overturning

  ✓x7ᵗʰ **V90.09**   **Drowning and submersion due to unspecified watercraft overturning**   ▽
  Drowning and submersion due to boat NOS overturning
  Drowning and submersion due to ship NOS overturning
  Drowning and submersion due to watercraft NOS overturning

✓5ᵗʰ **V90.1**   **Drowning and submersion due to watercraft sinking**

  ✓x7ᵗʰ **V90.10**   **Drowning and submersion due to merchant ship sinking**

  ✓x7ᵗʰ **V90.11**   **Drowning and submersion due to passenger ship sinking**
  Drowning and submersion due to Ferry-boat sinking
  Drowning and submersion due to Liner sinking

  ✓x7ᵗʰ **V90.12**   **Drowning and submersion due to fishing boat sinking**

  ✓x7ᵗʰ **V90.13**   **Drowning and submersion due to other powered watercraft sinking**
  Drowning and submersion due to Hovercraft (on open water) sinking
  Drowning and submersion due to Jet ski sinking

  ✓x7ᵗʰ **V90.14**   **Drowning and submersion due to sailboat sinking**

  ✓x7ᵗʰ **V90.15**   **Drowning and submersion due to canoe or kayak sinking**

  ✓x7ᵗʰ **V90.16**   **Drowning and submersion due to (nonpowered) inflatable craft sinking**

  ✓x7ᵗʰ **V90.18**   **Drowning and submersion due to other unpowered watercraft sinking**

  ✓x7ᵗʰ **V90.19**   **Drowning and submersion due to unspecified watercraft sinking**   ▽
  Drowning and submersion due to boat NOS sinking
  Drowning and submersion due to ship NOS sinking
  Drowning and submersion due to watercraft NOS sinking

✓5ᵗʰ **V90.2**   **Drowning and submersion due to falling or jumping from burning watercraft**

  ✓x7ᵗʰ **V90.20**   **Drowning and submersion due to falling or jumping from burning merchant ship**

  ✓x7ᵗʰ **V90.21**   **Drowning and submersion due to falling or jumping from burning passenger ship**
  Drowning and submersion due to falling or jumping from burning Ferry-boat
  Drowning and submersion due to falling or jumping from burning Liner

  ✓x7ᵗʰ **V90.22**   **Drowning and submersion due to falling or jumping from burning fishing boat**

  ✓x7ᵗʰ **V90.23**   **Drowning and submersion due to falling or jumping from other burning powered watercraft**
  Drowning and submersion due to falling and jumping from burning Hovercraft (on open water)
  Drowning and submersion due to falling and jumping from burning Jet ski

  ✓x7ᵗʰ **V90.24**   **Drowning and submersion due to falling or jumping from burning sailboat**

  ✓x7ᵗʰ **V90.25**   **Drowning and submersion due to falling or jumping from burning canoe or kayak**

  ✓x7ᵗʰ **V90.26**   **Drowning and submersion due to falling or jumping from burning (nonpowered) inflatable craft**

  ✓x7ᵗʰ **V90.27**   **Drowning and submersion due to falling or jumping from burning water-skis**

  ✓x7ᵗʰ **V90.28**   **Drowning and submersion due to falling or jumping from other burning unpowered watercraft**
  Drowning and submersion due to falling and jumping from burning surf-board
  Drowning and submersion due to falling and jumping from burning windsurfer

  ✓x7ᵗʰ **V90.29**   **Drowning and submersion due to falling or jumping from unspecified burning watercraft**   ▽
  Drowning and submersion due to falling or jumping from burning boat NOS
  Drowning and submersion due to falling or jumping from burning ship NOS
  Drowning and submersion due to falling or jumping from burning watercraft NOS

✓5ᵗʰ **V90.3**   **Drowning and submersion due to falling or jumping from crushed watercraft**

  ✓x7ᵗʰ **V90.30**   **Drowning and submersion due to falling or jumping from crushed merchant ship**

  ✓x7ᵗʰ **V90.31**   **Drowning and submersion due to falling or jumping from crushed passenger ship**
  Drowning and submersion due to falling and jumping from crushed Ferry boat
  Drowning and submersion due to falling and jumping from crushed Liner

  ✓x7ᵗʰ **V90.32**   **Drowning and submersion due to falling or jumping from crushed fishing boat**

  ✓x7ᵗʰ **V90.33**   **Drowning and submersion due to falling or jumping from other crushed powered watercraft**
  Drowning and submersion due to falling and jumping from crushed Hovercraft
  Drowning and submersion due to falling and jumping from crushed Jet ski

---

☑ Add'l Character Required   ✓x7ᵗʰ Placeholder Alert   RUG IV Special Care High Dx   RUG IV Clinically Complex Dx   RUG IV Special Care Low Dx   Manifestation Code   Other Specified Code   ▽ Unspecified Code

Chapter 20. External Causes of Morbidity

√x7ᵗʰ **V90.34** **Drowning and submersion due to falling or jumping from crushed sailboat**

√x7ᵗʰ **V90.35** **Drowning and submersion due to falling or jumping from crushed canoe or kayak**

√x7ᵗʰ **V90.36** **Drowning and submersion due to falling or jumping from crushed (nonpowered) inflatable craft**

√x7ᵗʰ **V90.37** **Drowning and submersion due to falling or jumping from crushed water-skis**

√x7ᵗʰ **V90.38** **Drowning and submersion due to falling or jumping from other crushed unpowered watercraft**
Drowning and submersion due to falling and jumping from crushed surf-board
Drowning and submersion due to falling and jumping from crushed windsurfer

√x7ᵗʰ **V90.39** **Drowning and submersion due to falling or jumping from crushed unspecified watercraft** ▽
Drowning and submersion due to falling and jumping from crushed boat NOS
Drowning and submersion due to falling and jumping from crushed ship NOS
Drowning and submersion due to falling and jumping from crushed watercraft NOS

√5ᵗʰ **V90.8** **Drowning and submersion due to other accident to watercraft**

√x7ᵗʰ **V90.80** **Drowning and submersion due to other accident to merchant ship**

√x7ᵗʰ **V90.81** **Drowning and submersion due to other accident to passenger ship**
Drowning and submersion due to other accident to Ferry-boat
Drowning and submersion due to other accident to Liner

√x7ᵗʰ **V90.82** **Drowning and submersion due to other accident to fishing boat**

√x7ᵗʰ **V90.83** **Drowning and submersion due to other accident to other powered watercraft**
Drowning and submersion due to other accident to Hovercraft (on open water)
Drowning and submersion due to other accident to Jet ski

√x7ᵗʰ **V90.84** **Drowning and submersion due to other accident to sailboat**

√x7ᵗʰ **V90.85** **Drowning and submersion due to other accident to canoe or kayak**

√x7ᵗʰ **V90.86** **Drowning and submersion due to other accident to (nonpowered) inflatable craft**

√x7ᵗʰ **V90.87** **Drowning and submersion due to other accident to water-skis**

√x7ᵗʰ **V90.88** **Drowning and submersion due to other accident to other unpowered watercraft**
Drowning and submersion due to other accident to surf-board
Drowning and submersion due to other accident to windsurfer

√x7ᵗʰ **V90.89** **Drowning and submersion due to other accident to unspecified watercraft** ▽
Drowning and submersion due to other accident to boat NOS
Drowning and submersion due to other accident to ship NOS
Drowning and submersion due to other accident to watercraft NOS

√4ᵗʰ **V91** **Other injury due to accident to watercraft**
INCLUDES   any injury except drowning and submersion as a result of an accident to watercraft
EXCLUDES 1   civilian water transport accident involving military watercraft (V94.81-)
military watercraft accident in military or war operations (Y36, Y37.-)
EXCLUDES 2   drowning and submersion due to accident to watercraft (V90.-)

The appropriate 7th character is to be added to each code from category V91.
A   initial encounter
D   subsequent encounter
S   sequela

√5ᵗʰ **V91.0** **Burn due to watercraft on fire**
EXCLUDES 1   burn from localized fire or explosion on board ship without accident to watercraft (V93.-)

√x7ᵗʰ **V91.00** **Burn due to merchant ship on fire**

√x7ᵗʰ **V91.01** **Burn due to passenger ship on fire**
Burn due to Ferry-boat on fire
Burn due to Liner on fire

√x7ᵗʰ **V91.02** **Burn due to fishing boat on fire**

√x7ᵗʰ **V91.03** **Burn due to other powered watercraft on fire**
Burn due to Hovercraft (on open water) on fire
Burn due to Jet ski on fire

√x7ᵗʰ **V91.04** **Burn due to sailboat on fire**

√x7ᵗʰ **V91.05** **Burn due to canoe or kayak on fire**

√x7ᵗʰ **V91.06** **Burn due to (nonpowered) inflatable craft on fire**

√x7ᵗʰ **V91.07** **Burn due to water-skis on fire**

√x7ᵗʰ **V91.08** **Burn due to other unpowered watercraft on fire**

√x7ᵗʰ **V91.09** **Burn due to unspecified watercraft on fire** ▽
Burn due to boat NOS on fire
Burn due to ship NOS on fire
Burn due to watercraft NOS on fire

√5ᵗʰ **V91.1** **Crushed between watercraft and other watercraft or other object due to collision**
Crushed by lifeboat after abandoning ship in a collision
NOTE   Select the specified type of watercraft that the victim was on at the time of the collision

√x7ᵗʰ **V91.10** **Crushed between merchant ship and other watercraft or other object due to collision**

√x7ᵗʰ **V91.11** **Crushed between passenger ship and other watercraft or other object due to collision**
Crushed between Ferry-boat and other watercraft or other object due to collision
Crushed between Liner and other watercraft or other object due to collision

√x7ᵗʰ **V91.12** **Crushed between fishing boat and other watercraft or other object due to collision**

√x7ᵗʰ **V91.13** **Crushed between other powered watercraft and other watercraft or other object due to collision**
Crushed between Hovercraft (on open water) and other watercraft or other object due to collision
Crushed between Jet ski and other watercraft or other object due to collision

√x7ᵗʰ **V91.14** **Crushed between sailboat and other watercraft or other object due to collision**

√x7ᵗʰ **V91.15** **Crushed between canoe or kayak and other watercraft or other object due to collision**

√x7ᵗʰ **V91.16** **Crushed between (nonpowered) inflatable craft and other watercraft or other object due to collision**

√x7ᵗʰ **V91.18** **Crushed between other unpowered watercraft and other watercraft or other object due to collision**
Crushed between surfboard and other watercraft or other object due to collision
Crushed between windsurfer and other watercraft or other object due to collision

√x7ᵗʰ **V91.19** **Crushed between unspecified watercraft and other watercraft or other object due to collision** ▽
Crushed between boat NOS and other watercraft or other object due to collision
Crushed between ship NOS and other watercraft or other object due to collision
Crushed between watercraft NOS and other watercraft or other object due to collision

√5ᵗʰ **V91.2** **Fall due to collision between watercraft and other watercraft or other object**
Fall while remaining on watercraft after collision
NOTE   Select the specified type of watercraft that the victim was on at the time of the collision.
EXCLUDES 1   crushed between watercraft and other watercraft and other object due to collision (V91.1-)
drowning and submersion due to falling from crushed watercraft (V90.3-)

√x7ᵗʰ **V91.20** **Fall due to collision between merchant ship and other watercraft or other object**

√x7ᵗʰ **V91.21** **Fall due to collision between passenger ship and other watercraft or other object**
Fall due to collision between Ferry-boat and other watercraft or other object
Fall due to collision between Liner and other watercraft or other object

☑x7ᵗʰ **V91.22** **Fall due to collision between** fishing boat **and other watercraft or other object**

☑x7ᵗʰ **V91.23** **Fall due to collision between other** powered **watercraft and other watercraft or other object**
Fall due to collision between Hovercraft (on open water) and other watercraft or other object
Fall due to collision between Jet ski and other watercraft or other object

☑x7ᵗʰ **V91.24** **Fall due to collision between** sailboat **and other watercraft or other object**

☑x7ᵗʰ **V91.25** **Fall due to collision between** canoe or kayak **and other watercraft or other object**

☑x7ᵗʰ **V91.26** **Fall due to collision between (nonpowered)** inflatable craft **and other watercraft or other object**

☑x7ᵗʰ **V91.29** **Fall due to collision between unspecified watercraft and other watercraft or other object** ▽
Fall due to collision between boat NOS and other watercraft or other object
Fall due to collision between ship NOS and other watercraft or other object
Fall due to collision between watercraft NOS and other watercraft or other object

☑5ᵗʰ **V91.3** **Hit or struck by falling object due to accident to watercraft**
Hit or struck by falling object (part of damaged watercraft or other object) after falling or jumping from damaged watercraft
EXCLUDES 2   drowning or submersion due to fall or jumping from damaged watercraft (V90.2-, V90.3-)

☑x7ᵗʰ **V91.30** **Hit or struck by falling object due to accident to** merchant ship

☑x7ᵗʰ **V91.31** **Hit or struck by falling object due to accident to** passenger ship
Hit or struck by falling object due to accident to Ferry-boat
Hit or struck by falling object due to accident to Liner

☑x7ᵗʰ **V91.32** **Hit or struck by falling object due to accident to** fishing boat

☑x7ᵗʰ **V91.33** **Hit or struck by falling object due to accident to other** powered **watercraft**
Hit or struck by falling object due to accident to Hovercraft (on open water)
Hit or struck by falling object due to accident to Jet ski

☑x7ᵗʰ **V91.34** **Hit or struck by falling object due to accident to** sailboat

☑x7ᵗʰ **V91.35** **Hit or struck by falling object due to accident to** canoe or kayak

☑x7ᵗʰ **V91.36** **Hit or struck by falling object due to accident to (nonpowered)** inflatable craft

☑x7ᵗʰ **V91.37** **Hit or struck by falling object due to accident to** water-skis
Hit by water-skis after jumping off of waterskis

☑x7ᵗʰ **V91.38** **Hit or struck by falling object due to accident to other** unpowered **watercraft**
Hit or struck by surf-board after falling off damaged surf-board
Hit or struck by object after falling off damaged windsurfer

☑x7ᵗʰ **V91.39** **Hit or struck by falling object due to accident to unspecified watercraft** ▽
Hit or struck by falling object due to accident to boat NOS
Hit or struck by falling object due to accident to ship NOS
Hit or struck by falling object due to accident to watercraft NOS

☑5ᵗʰ **V91.8** **Other injury due to other accident to watercraft**

☑x7ᵗʰ **V91.80** **Other injury due to other accident to** merchant ship

☑x7ᵗʰ **V91.81** **Other injury due to other accident to** passenger ship
Other injury due to other accident to Ferry-boat
Other injury due to other accident to Liner

☑x7ᵗʰ **V91.82** **Other injury due to other accident to** fishing boat

☑x7ᵗʰ **V91.83** **Other injury due to other accident to other** powered **watercraft**
Other injury due to other accident to Hovercraft (on open water)
Other injury due to other accident to Jet ski

☑x7ᵗʰ **V91.84** **Other injury due to other accident to** sailboat

☑x7ᵗʰ **V91.85** **Other injury due to other accident to** canoe or kayak

☑x7ᵗʰ **V91.86** **Other injury due to other accident to (nonpowered)** inflatable craft

☑x7ᵗʰ **V91.87** **Other injury due to other accident to** water-skis

☑x7ᵗʰ **V91.88** **Other injury due to other accident to other** unpowered **watercraft**
Other injury due to other accident to surf-board
Other injury due to other accident to windsurfer

☑x7ᵗʰ **V91.89** **Other injury due to other accident to unspecified watercraft** ▽
Other injury due to other accident to boat NOS
Other injury due to other accident to ship NOS
Other injury due to other accident to watercraft NOS

☑4ᵗʰ **V92** **Drowning and submersion due to accident on board watercraft, without accident to watercraft**
EXCLUDES 1   civilian water transport accident involving military watercraft (V94.81-)
drowning or submersion due to accident to watercraft (V90-V91)
drowning or submersion of diver who voluntarily jumps from boat not involved in an accident (W16.711, W16.721)
fall into water without watercraft (W16.-)
military watercraft accident in military or war operations (Y36, Y37)

The appropriate 7th character is to be added to each code from category V92.
A   initial encounter
D   subsequent encounter
S   sequela

☑5ᵗʰ **V92.0** **Drowning and submersion due to** fall off **watercraft**
Drowning and submersion due to fall from gangplank of watercraft
Drowning and submersion due to fall overboard watercraft
EXCLUDES 2   hitting head on object or bottom of body of water due to fall from watercraft (V94.0-)

☑x7ᵗʰ **V92.00** **Drowning and submersion due to fall off** merchant ship

☑x7ᵗʰ **V92.01** **Drowning and submersion due to fall off** passenger ship
Drowning and submersion due to fall off Ferry-boat
Drowning and submersion due to fall off Liner

☑x7ᵗʰ **V92.02** **Drowning and submersion due to fall off** fishing boat

☑x7ᵗʰ **V92.03** **Drowning and submersion due to fall off other** powered **watercraft**
Drowning and submersion due to fall off Hovercraft (on open water)
Drowning and submersion due to fall off Jet ski

☑x7ᵗʰ **V92.04** **Drowning and submersion due to fall off** sailboat

☑x7ᵗʰ **V92.05** **Drowning and submersion due to fall off** canoe or kayak

☑x7ᵗʰ **V92.06** **Drowning and submersion due to fall off (nonpowered)** inflatable craft

☑x7ᵗʰ **V92.07** **Drowning and submersion due to fall off** water-skis
EXCLUDES 1   drowning and submersion due to falling off burning water-skis (V90.27)
drowning and submersion due to falling off crushed water-skis (V90.37)
hit by boat while water-skiing NOS (V94.X)

☑x7ᵗʰ **V92.08** **Drowning and submersion due to fall off other** unpowered **watercraft**
Drowning and submersion due to fall off surf-board
Drowning and submersion due to fall off windsurfer
EXCLUDES 1   drowning and submersion due to fall off burning unpowered watercraft (V90.28)
drowning and submersion due to fall off crushed unpowered watercraft (V90.38)
drowning and submersion due to fall off damaged unpowered watercraft (V90.88)
drowning and submersion due to rider of nonpowered watercraft being hit by other watercraft (V94.-)
other injury due to rider of nonpowered watercraft being hit by other watercraft (V94.-)

✓x7ᵗʰ **V92.09** **Drowning and submersion due to fall off**   ▽
unspecified watercraft
Drowning and submersion due to fall off boat NOS
Drowning and submersion due to fall off ship
Drowning and submersion due to fall off watercraft NOS

✓5ᵗʰ **V92.1** **Drowning and submersion due to being** thrown overboard
by motion of watercraft

> EXCLUDES 1   drowning and submersion due to fall off surf-board (V92.08)
> drowning and submersion due to fall off water-skis (V92.07)
> drowning and submersion due to fall off windsurfer (V92.08)

✓x7ᵗʰ **V92.10** **Drowning and submersion due to being thrown overboard by motion of** merchant ship

✓x7ᵗʰ **V92.11** **Drowning and submersion due to being thrown overboard by motion of** passenger ship
Drowning and submersion due to being thrown overboard by motion of Ferry-boat
Drowning and submersion due to being thrown overboard by motion of Liner

✓x7ᵗʰ **V92.12** **Drowning and submersion due to being thrown overboard by motion of** fishing boat

✓x7ᵗʰ **V92.13** **Drowning and submersion due to being thrown overboard by motion of other** powered **watercraft**
Drowning and submersion due to being thrown overboard by motion of Hovercraft

✓x7ᵗʰ **V92.14** **Drowning and submersion due to being thrown overboard by motion of** sailboat

✓x7ᵗʰ **V92.15** **Drowning and submersion due to being thrown overboard by motion of** canoe or kayak

✓x7ᵗʰ **V92.16** **Drowning and submersion due to being thrown overboard by motion of (nonpowered)** inflatable craft

✓x7ᵗʰ **V92.19** **Drowning and submersion due to being thrown** ▽
overboard by motion of unspecified watercraft
Drowning and submersion due to being thrown overboard by motion of boat NOS
Drowning and submersion due to being thrown overboard by motion of ship NOS
Drowning and submersion due to being thrown overboard by motion of watercraft NOS

✓5ᵗʰ **V92.2** **Drowning and submersion due to being** washed overboard
from watercraft
Code first any associated cataclysm (X37.0-)

✓x7ᵗʰ **V92.20** **Drowning and submersion due to being washed overboard from** merchant ship

✓x7ᵗʰ **V92.21** **Drowning and submersion due to being washed overboard from** passenger ship
Drowning and submersion due to being washed overboard from Ferry-boat
Drowning and submersion due to being washed overboard from Liner

✓x7ᵗʰ **V92.22** **Drowning and submersion due to being washed overboard from** fishing boat

✓x7ᵗʰ **V92.23** **Drowning and submersion due to being washed overboard from other** powered **watercraft**
Drowning and submersion due to being washed overboard from Hovercraft (on open water)
Drowning and submersion due to being washed overboard from Jet ski

✓x7ᵗʰ **V92.24** **Drowning and submersion due to being washed overboard from** sailboat

✓x7ᵗʰ **V92.25** **Drowning and submersion due to being washed overboard from** canoe or kayak

✓x7ᵗʰ **V92.26** **Drowning and submersion due to being washed overboard from (nonpowered)** inflatable craft

✓x7ᵗʰ **V92.27** **Drowning and submersion due to being washed overboard from** water-skis

> EXCLUDES 1   drowning and submersion due to fall off water-skis (V92.07)

✓x7ᵗʰ **V92.28** **Drowning and submersion due to being washed overboard from other** unpowered **watercraft**
Drowning and submersion due to being washed overboard from surf-board
Drowning and submersion due to being washed overboard from windsurfer

✓x7ᵗʰ **V92.29** **Drowning and submersion due to being washed** ▽
overboard from unspecified watercraft
Drowning and submersion due to being washed overboard from boat NOS
Drowning and submersion due to being washed overboard from ship NOS
Drowning and submersion due to being washed overboard from watercraft NOS

✓4ᵗʰ **V93** **Other injury due to accident on board watercraft, without accident to watercraft**

> EXCLUDES 1   civilian water transport accident involving military watercraft (V94.81-)
> other injury due to accident to watercraft (V91.-)
> military watercraft accident in military or war operations (Y36, Y37.-)

> EXCLUDES 2   drowning and submersion due to accident on board watercraft, without accident to watercraft (V92.-)

The appropriate 7th character is to be added to each code from category V93.
A   initial encounter
D   subsequent encounter
S   sequela

✓5ᵗʰ **V93.0** **Burn due to localized fire on board watercraft**

> EXCLUDES 1   burn due to watercraft on fire (V91.0-)

✓x7ᵗʰ **V93.00** **Burn due to localized fire on board** merchant vessel

✓x7ᵗʰ **V93.01** **Burn due to localized fire on board** passenger vessel
Burn due to localized fire on board Ferry-boat
Burn due to localized fire on board Liner

✓x7ᵗʰ **V93.02** **Burn due to localized fire on board** fishing boat

✓x7ᵗʰ **V93.03** **Burn due to localized fire on board other** powered **watercraft**
Burn due to localized fire on board Hovercraft
Burn due to localized fire on board Jet ski

✓x7ᵗʰ **V93.04** **Burn due to localized fire on board** sailboat

✓x7ᵗʰ **V93.09** **Burn due to localized fire on board unspecified** ▽
watercraft
Burn due to localized fire on board boat NOS
Burn due to localized fire on board ship NOS
Burn due to localized fire on board watercraft NOS

✓5ᵗʰ **V93.1** **Other burn on board watercraft**
Burn due to source other than fire on board watercraft

> EXCLUDES 1   burn due to watercraft on fire (V91.0-)

✓x7ᵗʰ **V93.10** **Other burn on board** merchant vessel

✓x7ᵗʰ **V93.11** **Other burn on board** passenger vessel
Other burn on board Ferry-boat
Other burn on board Liner

✓x7ᵗʰ **V93.12** **Other burn on board** fishing boat

✓x7ᵗʰ **V93.13** **Other burn on board other** powered **watercraft**
Other burn on board Hovercraft
Other burn on board Jet ski

✓x7ᵗʰ **V93.14** **Other burn on board** sailboat

✓x7ᵗʰ **V93.19** **Other burn on board unspecified watercraft** ▽
Other burn on board boat NOS
Other burn on board ship NOS
Other burn on board watercraft NOS

✓5ᵗʰ **V93.2** **Heat exposure on board watercraft**

> EXCLUDES 1   exposure to man-made heat not aboard watercraft (W92)
> exposure to natural heat while on board watercraft (X30)
> exposure to sunlight while on board watercraft (X32)

> EXCLUDES 2   burn due to fire on board watercraft (V93.0-)

✓x7ᵗʰ **V93.20** **Heat exposure on board** merchant ship

✓x7ᵗʰ **V93.21** **Heat exposure on board** passenger ship
Heat exposure on board Ferry-boat
Heat exposure on board Liner

✓x7ᵗʰ **V93.22** **Heat exposure on board** fishing boat

✓x7ᵗʰ **V93.23** **Heat exposure on board other** powered **watercraft**
Heat exposure on board hovercraft

✓x7ᵗʰ **V93.24** **Heat exposure on board** sailboat

✓x7ᵗʰ **V93.29** **Heat exposure on board unspecified watercraft** ▽
Heat exposure on board boat NOS
Heat exposure on board ship NOS
Heat exposure on board watercraft NOS

Ⓝ Newborn   Ⓟ Pediatric   Ⓜ Maternity   Ⓐ Adult   RIC RIC Dx   NC Dx Noncancer Dx   PDx Primary Dx   CC RIC CC Condition   ►◄ Revised Text   ● New Code   ▲ Revised Code Title

1080   ICD-10-CM 2016

☑5ᵗʰ **V93.3 Fall on board watercraft**
> **EXCLUDES 1**   *fall due to collision of watercraft (V91.2-)*

  √x7ᵗʰ **V93.30 Fall on board** merchant ship

  √x7ᵗʰ **V93.31 Fall on board** passenger ship
> Fall on board Ferry-boat
> Fall on board Liner

  √x7ᵗʰ **V93.32 Fall on board** fishing boat

  √x7ᵗʰ **V93.33 Fall on board other** powered **watercraft**
> Fall on board Hovercraft (on open water)
> Fall on board Jet ski

  √x7ᵗʰ **V93.34 Fall on board** sailboat

  √x7ᵗʰ **V93.35 Fall on board** canoe or kayak

  √x7ᵗʰ **V93.36 Fall on board (nonpowered)** inflatable craft

  √x7ᵗʰ **V93.38 Fall on board other** unpowered **watercraft**

  √x7ᵗʰ **V93.39 Fall on board unspecified watercraft** ▽
> Fall on board boat NOS
> Fall on board ship NOS
> Fall on board watercraft NOS

☑5ᵗʰ **V93.4 Struck by falling object on board watercraft**
> Hit by falling object on board watercraft
> **EXCLUDES 1**   *struck by falling object due to accident to watercraft (V91.3)*

  √x7ᵗʰ **V93.40 Struck by falling object on** merchant ship

  √x7ᵗʰ **V93.41 Struck by falling object on** passenger ship
> Struck by falling object on Ferry-boat
> Struck by falling object on Liner

  √x7ᵗʰ **V93.42 Struck by falling object on** fishing boat

  √x7ᵗʰ **V93.43 Struck by falling object on other** powered **watercraft**
> Struck by falling object on Hovercraft

  √x7ᵗʰ **V93.44 Struck by falling object on** sailboat

  √x7ᵗʰ **V93.48 Struck by falling object on other** unpowered **watercraft**

  √x7ᵗʰ **V93.49 Struck by falling object on unspecified watercraft** ▽

☑5ᵗʰ **V93.5 Explosion on board watercraft**
> Boiler explosion on steamship
> **EXCLUDES 2**   *fire on board watercraft (V93.0-)*

  √x7ᵗʰ **V93.50 Explosion on board** merchant ship

  √x7ᵗʰ **V93.51 Explosion on board** passenger ship
> Explosion on board Ferry-boat
> Explosion on board Liner

  √x7ᵗʰ **V93.52 Explosion on board** fishing boat

  √x7ᵗʰ **V93.53 Explosion on board other** powered **watercraft**
> Explosion on board Hovercraft
> Explosion on board Jet ski

  √x7ᵗʰ **V93.54 Explosion on board** sailboat

  √x7ᵗʰ **V93.59 Explosion on board unspecified watercraft** ▽
> Explosion on board boat NOS
> Explosion on board ship NOS
> Explosion on board watercraft NOS

☑5ᵗʰ **V93.6 Machinery accident on board watercraft**
> **EXCLUDES 1**   *machinery explosion on board watercraft (V93.4-)*
> *machinery fire on board watercraft (V93.0-)*

  √x7ᵗʰ **V93.60 Machinery accident on board** merchant ship

  √x7ᵗʰ **V93.61 Machinery accident on board** passenger ship
> Machinery accident on board Ferry-boat
> Machinery accident on board Liner

  √x7ᵗʰ **V93.62 Machinery accident on board** fishing boat

  √x7ᵗʰ **V93.63 Machinery accident on board other** powered **watercraft**
> Machinery accident on board Hovercraft

  √x7ᵗʰ **V93.64 Machinery accident on board** sailboat

  √x7ᵗʰ **V93.69 Machinery accident on board unspecified watercraft** ▽
> Machinery accident on board boat NOS
> Machinery accident on board ship NOS
> Machinery accident on board watercraft NOS

☑5ᵗʰ **V93.8 Other injury due to other accident on board watercraft**
> Accidental poisoning by gases or fumes on watercraft

  √x7ᵗʰ **V93.80 Other injury due to other accident on board** merchant ship

  √x7ᵗʰ **V93.81 Other injury due to other accident on board** passenger ship
> Other injury due to other accident on board Ferry-boat
> Other injury due to other accident on board Liner

  √x7ᵗʰ **V93.82 Other injury due to other accident on board** fishing boat

  √x7ᵗʰ **V93.83 Other injury due to other accident on board other** powered **watercraft**
> Other injury due to other accident on board Hovercraft
> Other injury due to other accident on board Jet ski

  √x7ᵗʰ **V93.84 Other injury due to other accident on board** sailboat

  √x7ᵗʰ **V93.85 Other injury due to other accident on board** canoe or kayak

  √x7ᵗʰ **V93.86 Other injury due to other accident on board (nonpowered)** inflatable craft

  √x7ᵗʰ **V93.87 Other injury due to other accident on board** water-skis
> Hit or struck by object while waterskiing

  √x7ᵗʰ **V93.88 Other injury due to other accident on board other** unpowered **watercraft**
> Hit or struck by object while surfing
> Hit or struck by object while on board windsurfer

  √x7ᵗʰ **V93.89 Other injury due to other accident on board unspecified watercraft** ▽
> Other injury due to other accident on board boat NOS
> Other injury due to other accident on board ship NOS
> Other injury due to other accident on board watercraft NOS

☑4ᵗʰ **V94 Other and unspecified water transport accidents**
> **EXCLUDES 1**   *military watercraft accidents in military or war operations (Y36, Y37)*

> The appropriate 7th character is to be added to each code from category V94.
> A   initial encounter
> D   subsequent encounter
> S   sequela

  √x7ᵗʰ **V94.0 Hitting object or bottom of body of water due to fall from watercraft**
> **EXCLUDES 2**   *drowning and submersion due to fall from watercraft (V92.0-)*

☑5ᵗʰ **V94.1 Bather struck by watercraft**
> Swimmer hit by watercraft

  √x7ᵗʰ **V94.11 Bather struck by** powered **watercraft**

  √x7ᵗʰ **V94.12 Bather struck by** nonpowered **watercraft**

☑5ᵗʰ **V94.2 Rider of nonpowered watercraft struck by other watercraft**

  √x7ᵗʰ **V94.21 Rider of nonpowered watercraft struck by other** nonpowered **watercraft**
> Canoer hit by other nonpowered watercraft
> Surfer hit by other nonpowered watercraft
> Windsurfer hit by other nonpowered watercraft

  √x7ᵗʰ **V94.22 Rider of nonpowered watercraft struck by** powered **watercraft**
> Canoer hit by motorboat
> Surfer hit by motorboat
> Windsurfer hit by motorboat

☑5ᵗʰ **V94.3 Injury to rider of (inflatable) watercraft being pulled behind other watercraft**

  √x7ᵗʰ **V94.31 Injury to rider of (inflatable)** recreational **watercraft being pulled behind other watercraft**
> Injury to rider of inner-tube pulled behind motor boat

  √x7ᵗʰ **V94.32 Injury to rider of** non-recreational **watercraft being pulled behind other watercraft**
> Injury to occupant of dingy being pulled behind boat or ship
> Injury to occupant of life-raft being pulled behind boat or ship

  √x7ᵗʰ **V94.4 Injury to barefoot water-skier**
> Injury to person being pulled behind boat or ship

☑5ᵗʰ **V94.8 Other water transport accident**

  √6ᵗʰ **V94.81 Water transport accident involving military watercraft**

    √7ᵗʰ **V94.810 Civilian watercraft involved in water transport accident with military watercraft**
> Passenger on civilian watercraft injured due to accident with military watercraft

---

☑ Add'l Character Required   √x7ᵗʰ Placeholder Alert   RUG IV Special Care High Dx   RUG IV Clinically Complex Dx   RUG IV Special Care Low Dx   Manifestation Code   Other Specified Code   ▽ Unspecified Code

√7ᵗʰ **V94.811** **Civilian in water injured by military watercraft**

√7ᵗʰ **V94.818** **Other water transport accident involving military watercraft**

√x7ᵗʰ **V94.89** **Other water transport accident**

√x7ᵗʰ **V94.9** **Unspecified water transport accident** ▽
Water transport accident NOS

Air and space transport accidents (V95-V97)

EXCLUDES 1 *military aircraft accidents in military or war operations (Y36, Y37)*

√4ᵗʰ **V95** **Accident to powered aircraft causing injury to occupant**

The appropriate 7th character is to be added to each code from category V95.
A   initial encounter
D   subsequent encounter
S   sequela

√5ᵗʰ **V95.0** Helicopter **accident injuring occupant**

√x7ᵗʰ **V95.00** **Unspecified helicopter accident injuring occupant** ▽

√x7ᵗʰ **V95.01** **Helicopter** crash **injuring occupant**

√x7ᵗʰ **V95.02** Forced landing **of helicopter injuring occupant**

√x7ᵗʰ **V95.03** **Helicopter** collision **injuring occupant**
Helicopter collision with any object, fixed, movable or moving

√x7ᵗʰ **V95.04** **Helicopter** fire **injuring occupant**

√x7ᵗʰ **V95.05** **Helicopter** explosion **injuring occupant**

√x7ᵗʰ **V95.09** **Other helicopter accident injuring occupant**

√5ᵗʰ **V95.1** Ultralight, microlight or powered-glider **accident injuring occupant**

√x7ᵗʰ **V95.10** **Unspecified ultralight, microlight or powered-glider accident injuring occupant** ▽

√x7ᵗʰ **V95.11** **Ultralight, microlight or powered-glider** crash **injuring occupant**

√x7ᵗʰ **V95.12** Forced landing **of ultralight, microlight or powered-glider injuring occupant**

√x7ᵗʰ **V95.13** **Ultralight, microlight or powered-glider** collision **injuring occupant**
Ultralight, microlight or powered-glider collision with any object, fixed, movable or moving

√x7ᵗʰ **V95.14** **Ultralight, microlight or powered-glider** fire **injuring occupant**

√x7ᵗʰ **V95.15** **Ultralight, microlight or powered-glider** explosion **injuring occupant**

√x7ᵗʰ **V95.19** **Other ultralight, microlight or powered-glider accident injuring occupant**

√5ᵗʰ **V95.2** Other private fixed-wing **aircraft accident injuring occupant**

√x7ᵗʰ **V95.20** **Unspecified accident to other private fixed-wing aircraft, injuring occupant** ▽

√x7ᵗʰ **V95.21** **Other private fixed-wing aircraft crash injuring occupant**

√x7ᵗʰ **V95.22** Forced landing **of other private fixed-wing aircraft injuring occupant**

√x7ᵗʰ **V95.23** **Other private fixed-wing aircraft** collision **injuring occupant**
Other private fixed-wing aircraft collision with any object, fixed, movable or moving

√x7ᵗʰ **V95.24** **Other private fixed-wing aircraft** fire **injuring occupant**

√x7ᵗʰ **V95.25** **Other private fixed-wing aircraft** explosion **injuring occupant**

√x7ᵗʰ **V95.29** **Other accident to other private fixed-wing aircraft injuring occupant**

√5ᵗʰ **V95.3** Commercial fixed-wing **aircraft accident injuring occupant**

√x7ᵗʰ **V95.30** **Unspecified accident to commercial fixed-wing aircraft injuring occupant** ▽

√x7ᵗʰ **V95.31** **Commercial fixed-wing aircraft** crash **injuring occupant**

√x7ᵗʰ **V95.32** Forced landing **of commercial fixed-wing aircraft injuring occupant**

√x7ᵗʰ **V95.33** **Commercial fixed-wing aircraft** collision **injuring occupant**
Commercial fixed-wing aircraft collision with any object, fixed, movable or moving

√x7ᵗʰ **V95.34** **Commercial fixed-wing aircraft** fire **injuring occupant**

√x7ᵗʰ **V95.35** **Commercial fixed-wing aircraft** explosion **injuring occupant**

√x7ᵗʰ **V95.39** **Other accident to commercial fixed-wing aircraft injuring occupant**

√5ᵗʰ **V95.4** Spacecraft **accident injuring occupant**

√x7ᵗʰ **V95.40** **Unspecified spacecraft accident injuring occupant** ▽

√x7ᵗʰ **V95.41** **Spacecraft** crash **injuring occupant**

√x7ᵗʰ **V95.42** Forced landing **of spacecraft injuring occupant**

√x7ᵗʰ **V95.43** **Spacecraft** collision **injuring occupant**
Spacecraft collision with any object, fixed, moveable or moving

√x7ᵗʰ **V95.44** **Spacecraft** fire **injuring occupant**

√x7ᵗʰ **V95.45** **Spacecraft** explosion **injuring occupant**

√x7ᵗʰ **V95.49** **Other spacecraft accident injuring occupant**

√x7ᵗʰ **V95.8** **Other** powered **aircraft accidents injuring occupant**

√x7ᵗʰ **V95.9** **Unspecified aircraft accident injuring occupant** ▽
Aircraft accident NOS
Air transport accident NOS

√4ᵗʰ **V96** **Accident to nonpowered aircraft causing injury to occupant**

The appropriate 7th character is to be added to each code from category V96.
A   initial encounter
D   subsequent encounter
S   sequela

√5ᵗʰ **V96.0** Balloon **accident injuring occupant**

√x7ᵗʰ **V96.00** **Unspecified balloon accident injuring occupant** ▽

√x7ᵗʰ **V96.01** **Balloon** crash **injuring occupant**

√x7ᵗʰ **V96.02** Forced landing **of balloon injuring occupant**

√x7ᵗʰ **V96.03** **Balloon** collision **injuring occupant**
Balloon collision with any object, fixed, moveable or moving

√x7ᵗʰ **V96.04** **Balloon** fire **injuring occupant**

√x7ᵗʰ **V96.05** **Balloon** explosion **injuring occupant**

√x7ᵗʰ **V96.09** **Other balloon accident injuring occupant**

√5ᵗʰ **V96.1** Hang-glider **accident injuring occupant**

√x7ᵗʰ **V96.10** **Unspecified hang-glider accident injuring occupant** ▽

√x7ᵗʰ **V96.11** **Hang-glider** crash **injuring occupant**

√x7ᵗʰ **V96.12** Forced landing **of hang-glider injuring occupant**

√x7ᵗʰ **V96.13** **Hang-glider** collision **injuring occupant**
Hang-glider collision with any object, fixed, moveable or moving

√x7ᵗʰ **V96.14** **Hang-glider** fire **injuring occupant**

√x7ᵗʰ **V96.15** **Hang-glider** explosion **injuring occupant**

√x7ᵗʰ **V96.19** **Other hang-glider accident injuring occupant**

√5ᵗʰ **V96.2** Glider (nonpowered) **accident injuring occupant**

√x7ᵗʰ **V96.20** **Unspecified glider (nonpowered) accident injuring occupant** ▽

√x7ᵗʰ **V96.21** **Glider (nonpowered)** crash **injuring occupant**

√x7ᵗʰ **V96.22** Forced landing **of glider (nonpowered) injuring occupant**

√x7ᵗʰ **V96.23** **Glider (nonpowered)** collision **injuring occupant**
Glider (nonpowered) collision with any object, fixed, moveable or moving

√x7ᵗʰ **V96.24** **Glider (nonpowered)** fire **injuring occupant**

√x7ᵗʰ **V96.25** **Glider (nonpowered)** explosion **injuring occupant**

√x7ᵗʰ **V96.29** **Other glider (nonpowered) accident injuring occupant**

√x7ᵗʰ **V96.8** **Other** nonpowered-aircraft **accidents injuring occupant**
Kite carrying a person accident injuring occupant

√x7ᵗʰ **V96.9** **Unspecified nonpowered-aircraft accident injuring occupant** ▽
Nonpowered-aircraft accident NOS

Ⓝ Newborn   🅟 Pediatric   🅜 Maternity   🅐 Adult   RIC RIC Dx   NC Dx Noncancer Dx   PDx Primary Dx   CC RIC CC Condition   ►◄ Revised Text   ● New Code   ▲ Revised Code Title

1082

ICD-10-CM 2016

✓4ᵗʰ **V97 Other specified air transport accidents**

> The appropriate 7th character is to be added to each code from category V97.
> A   initial encounter
> D   subsequent encounter
> S   sequela

✓x7ᵗʰ **V97.0 Occupant of aircraft injured in other specified air transport accidents**
> Fall in, on or from aircraft in air transport accident
> *EXCLUDES 1*   *accident while boarding or alighting aircraft (V97.1)*

✓x7ᵗʰ **V97.1 Person injured while boarding or alighting from aircraft**

✓5ᵗʰ **V97.2 Parachutist accident**

    ✓x7ᵗʰ **V97.21 Parachutist entangled in object**
> Parachutist landing in tree

    ✓x7ᵗʰ **V97.22 Parachutist injured on landing**

    ✓x7ᵗʰ **V97.29 Other parachutist accident**

✓5ᵗʰ **V97.3 Person on ground injured in air transport accident**

    ✓x7ᵗʰ **V97.31 Hit by object falling from aircraft**
> Hit by crashing aircraft
> Injured by aircraft hitting house
> Injured by aircraft hitting car

    ✓x7ᵗʰ **V97.32 Injured by rotating propeller**

    ✓x7ᵗʰ **V97.33 Sucked into jet engine**

    ✓x7ᵗʰ **V97.39 Other injury to person on ground due to air transport accident**

✓5ᵗʰ **V97.8 Other air transport accidents, not elsewhere classified**
> *EXCLUDES 1*   *aircraft accident NOS (V95.9)*
> *exposure to changes in air pressure during ascent or descent (W94.-)*

    ✓6ᵗʰ **V97.81 Air transport accident involving military aircraft**

      ✓7ᵗʰ **V97.810 Civilian aircraft involved in air transport accident with military aircraft**
> Passenger in civilian aircraft injured due to accident with military aircraft

      ✓7ᵗʰ **V97.811 Civilian injured by military aircraft**

      ✓7ᵗʰ **V97.818 Other air transport accident involving military aircraft**

    ✓x7ᵗʰ **V97.89 Other air transport accidents, not elsewhere classified**
> Injury from machinery on aircraft

Other and unspecified transport accidents (V98-V99)
> *EXCLUDES 1*   *vehicle accident, type of vehicle unspecified (V89.-)*

✓4ᵗʰ **V98 Other specified transport accidents**

> The appropriate 7th character is to be added to each code from category V98.
> A   initial encounter
> D   subsequent encounter
> S   sequela

✓x7ᵗʰ **V98.0 Accident to, on or involving cable-car, not on rails**
> Caught or dragged by cable-car, not on rails
> Fall or jump from cable-car, not on rails
> Object thrown from or in cable-car, not on rails

✓x7ᵗʰ **V98.1 Accident to, on or involving land-yacht**

✓x7ᵗʰ **V98.2 Accident to, on or involving ice yacht**

✓x7ᵗʰ **V98.3 Accident to, on or involving ski lift**
> Accident to, on or involving ski chair-lift
> Accident to, on or involving ski-lift with gondola

✓x7ᵗʰ **V98.8 Other specified transport accidents**

✓x7ᵗʰ **V99 Unspecified transport accident**   ▽

> The appropriate 7th character is to be added to code V99.
> A   initial encounter
> D   subsequent encounter
> S   sequela

OTHER EXTERNAL CAUSES OF ACCIDENTAL INJURY (W00-X58)

Slipping, tripping, stumbling and falls (W00-W19)
> *EXCLUDES 1*   *assault involving a fall (Y01-Y02)*
> *fall from animal (V80.-)*
> *fall (in) (from) machinery (in operation) (W28-W31)*
> *fall (in) (from) transport vehicle (V01-V99)*
> *intentional self-harm involving a fall (X80-X81)*
> *EXCLUDES 2*   *at risk for fall (history of fall) (Z91.81)*
> *fall (in) (from) burning building (X00.-)*
> *fall into fire (X00-X04, X08-X09)*

✓4ᵗʰ **W00 Fall due to ice and snow**
> *INCLUDES*   pedestrian on foot falling (slipping) on ice and snow
> *EXCLUDES 1*   *fall on (from) ice and snow involving pedestrian conveyance (V00.-)*
> *fall from stairs and steps not due to ice and snow (W10.-)*

> The appropriate 7th character is to be added to each code from category W00.
> A   initial encounter
> D   subsequent encounter
> S   sequela

✓x7ᵗʰ **W00.0 Fall on same level due to ice and snow**

✓x7ᵗʰ **W00.1 Fall from stairs and steps due to ice and snow**

✓x7ᵗʰ **W00.2 Other fall from one level to another due to ice and snow**

✓x7ᵗʰ **W00.9 Unspecified fall due to ice and snow**   ▽

✓4ᵗʰ **W01 Fall on same level from slipping, tripping and stumbling**
> *INCLUDES*   fall on moving sidewalk
> *EXCLUDES 1*   *fall due to bumping (striking) against object (W18.0-)*
> *fall in shower or bathtub (W18.2-)*
> *fall on same level NOS (W18.30)*
> *fall on same level from slipping, tripping and stumbling due to ice or snow (W00.0)*
> *fall off or from toilet (W18.1-)*
> *slipping, tripping and stumbling NOS (W18.40)*
> *slipping, tripping and stumbling without falling (W18.4-)*

> The appropriate 7th character is to be added to each code from category W01.
> A   initial encounter
> D   subsequent encounter
> S   sequela

✓x7ᵗʰ **W01.0 Fall on same level from slipping, tripping and stumbling without subsequent striking against object**
> Falling over animal

✓5ᵗʰ **W01.1 Fall on same level from slipping, tripping and stumbling with subsequent striking against object**

    ✓x7ᵗʰ **W01.10 Fall on same level from slipping, tripping and stumbling with subsequent striking against unspecified object**   ▽

    ✓6ᵗʰ **W01.11 Fall on same level from slipping, tripping and stumbling with subsequent striking against sharp object**

      ✓7ᵗʰ **W01.110 Fall on same level from slipping, tripping and stumbling with subsequent striking against sharp glass**

      ✓7ᵗʰ **W01.111 Fall on same level from slipping, tripping and stumbling with subsequent striking against power tool or machine**

      ✓7ᵗʰ **W01.118 Fall on same level from slipping, tripping and stumbling with subsequent striking against other sharp object**

      ✓7ᵗʰ **W01.119 Fall on same level from slipping, tripping and stumbling with subsequent striking against unspecified sharp object**   ▽

    ✓6ᵗʰ **W01.19 Fall on same level from slipping, tripping and stumbling with subsequent striking against other object**

      ✓7ᵗʰ **W01.190 Fall on same level from slipping, tripping and stumbling with subsequent striking against furniture**

      ✓7ᵗʰ **W01.198 Fall on same level from slipping, tripping and stumbling with subsequent striking against other object**

✓ Add'l Character Required   ✓x7ᵗʰ Placeholder Alert   RUG IV Special Care High Dx   RUG IV Clinically Complex Dx   RUG IV Special Care Low Dx   Manifestation Code   Other Specified Code   ▽ Unspecified Code

ICD-10-CM 2016   1083

Chapter 20. External Causes of Morbidity

W03–W16.022

✓x7ᵗʰ W03 Other fall on same level due to collision with another person
Fall due to non-transport collision with other person
EXCLUDES 1   collision with another person without fall (W51)
crushed or pushed by a crowd or human stampede (W52)
fall involving pedestrian conveyance (V00-V09)
fall due to ice or snow (W00)
fall on same level NOS (W18.30)
AHA: 2012, 4Q, 108

The appropriate 7th character is to be added to code W03.
A   initial encounter
D   subsequent encounter
S   sequela

✓x7ᵗʰ W04 Fall while being carried or supported by other persons
Accidentally dropped while being carried

The appropriate 7th character is to be added to code W04.
A   initial encounter
D   subsequent encounter
S   sequela

✓4ᵗʰ W05 Fall from non-moving wheelchair, nonmotorized scooter and motorized mobility scooter
EXCLUDES 1   fall from moving wheelchair (powered) (V00.811)
fall from moving motorized mobility scooter (V00.831)
fall from nonmotorized scooter (V00.141)

The appropriate 7th character is to be added to each code from category W05.
A   initial encounter
D   subsequent encounter
S   sequela

   ✓x7ᵗʰ W05.0 Fall from non-moving wheelchair
   ✓x7ᵗʰ W05.1 Fall from non-moving nonmotorized scooter
   ✓x7ᵗʰ W05.2 Fall from non-moving motorized mobility scooter

✓x7ᵗʰ W06 Fall from bed

The appropriate 7th character is to be added to code W06.
A   initial encounter
D   subsequent encounter
S   sequela

✓x7ᵗʰ W07 Fall from chair

The appropriate 7th character is to be added to code W07.
A   initial encounter
D   subsequent encounter
S   sequela

✓x7ᵗʰ W08 Fall from other furniture

The appropriate 7th character is to be added to code W08.
A   initial encounter
D   subsequent encounter
S   sequela

✓4ᵗʰ W09 Fall on and from playground equipment
EXCLUDES 1   fall involving recreational machinery (W31)

The appropriate 7th character is to be added to each code from category W09.
A   initial encounter
D   subsequent encounter
S   sequela

   ✓x7ᵗʰ W09.0 Fall on or from playground slide
   ✓x7ᵗʰ W09.1 Fall from playground swing
   ✓x7ᵗʰ W09.2 Fall on or from jungle gym
   ✓x7ᵗʰ W09.8 Fall on or from other playground equipment

✓4ᵗʰ W10 Fall on and from stairs and steps
EXCLUDES 1   Fall from stairs and steps due to ice and snow (W00.1)

The appropriate 7th character is to be added to each code from category W10.
A   initial encounter
D   subsequent encounter
S   sequela

   ✓x7ᵗʰ W10.0 Fall (on)(from) escalator
   ✓x7ᵗʰ W10.1 Fall (on)(from) sidewalk curb
   ✓x7ᵗʰ W10.2 Fall (on)(from) incline
     Fall (on) (from) ramp
   ✓x7ᵗʰ W10.8 Fall (on) (from) other stairs and steps
   ✓x7ᵗʰ W10.9 Fall (on) (from) unspecified stairs and steps   ▽

✓x7ᵗʰ W11 Fall on and from ladder

The appropriate 7th character is to be added code W11.
A   initial encounter
D   subsequent encounter
S   sequela

✓x7ᵗʰ W12 Fall on and from scaffolding

The appropriate 7th character is to be added to code W12.
A   initial encounter
D   subsequent encounter
S   sequela

✓4ᵗʰ W13 Fall from, out of or through building or structure

The appropriate 7th character is to be added to each code from category W13.
A   initial encounter
D   subsequent encounter
S   sequela

   ✓x7ᵗʰ W13.0 Fall from, out of or through balcony
     Fall from, out of or through railing
   ✓x7ᵗʰ W13.1 Fall from, out of or through bridge
   ✓x7ᵗʰ W13.2 Fall from, out of or through roof
   ✓x7ᵗʰ W13.3 Fall through floor
   ✓x7ᵗʰ W13.4 Fall from, out of or through window
     EXCLUDES 2   fall with subsequent striking against sharp glass (W01.110)
   ✓x7ᵗʰ W13.8 Fall from, out of or through other building or structure
     Fall from, out of or through viaduct
     Fall from, out of or through wall
     Fall from, out of or through flag-pole
   ✓x7ᵗʰ W13.9 Fall from, out of or through building, not otherwise specified
     EXCLUDES 1   collapse of a building or structure (W20.-)
       fall or jump from burning building or structure (X00.-)

✓x7ᵗʰ W14 Fall from tree

The appropriate 7th character is to be added to code W14.
A   initial encounter
D   subsequent encounter
S   sequela

✓x7ᵗʰ W15 Fall from cliff

The appropriate 7th character is to be added to code W15.
A   initial encounter
D   subsequent encounter
S   sequela

✓4ᵗʰ W16 Fall, jump or diving into water
EXCLUDES 1   accidental non-watercraft drowning and submersion not involving fall (W65-W74)
effects of air pressure from diving (W94.-)
fall into water from watercraft (V90-V94)
hitting an object or against bottom when falling from watercraft (V94.0)
EXCLUDES 2   striking or hitting diving board (W21.4)

The appropriate 7th character is to be added to each code from category W16.
A   initial encounter
D   subsequent encounter
S   sequela

   ✓5ᵗʰ W16.0 Fall into swimming pool
     Fall into swimming pool NOS
     EXCLUDES 1   fall into empty swimming pool (W17.3)

     ✓6ᵗʰ W16.01 Fall into swimming pool striking water surface
       ✓7ᵗʰ W16.011 Fall into swimming pool striking water surface causing drowning and submersion
         EXCLUDES 1   drowning and submersion while in swimming pool without fall (W67)
       ✓7ᵗʰ W16.012 Fall into swimming pool striking water surface causing other injury
     ✓6ᵗʰ W16.02 Fall into swimming pool striking bottom
       ✓7ᵗʰ W16.021 Fall into swimming pool striking bottom causing drowning and submersion
         EXCLUDES 1   drowning and submersion while in swimming pool without fall (W67)
       ✓7ᵗʰ W16.022 Fall into swimming pool striking bottom causing other injury

✓6ᵗʰ **W16.03**   Fall into swimming pool striking wall

     ✓7ᵗʰ **W16.031**   **Fall into swimming pool striking wall causing** drowning **and submersion**
         EXCLUDES 1   *drowning and submersion while in swimming pool without fall (W67)*

     ✓7ᵗʰ **W16.032**   **Fall into swimming pool striking wall causing other injury**

✓5ᵗʰ **W16.1**   **Fall into natural body of water**
     Fall into lake
     Fall into open sea
     Fall into river
     Fall into stream

     ✓6ᵗʰ **W16.11**   **Fall into natural body of water** striking water surface

         ✓7ᵗʰ **W16.111**   **Fall into natural body of water striking water surface causing** drowning **and submersion**
             EXCLUDES 1   *drowning and submersion while in natural body of water without fall (W69)*

         ✓7ᵗʰ **W16.112**   **Fall into natural body of water striking water surface causing other injury**

     ✓6ᵗʰ **W16.12**   **Fall into natural body of water** striking bottom

         ✓7ᵗʰ **W16.121**   **Fall into natural body of water striking bottom causing** drowning **and submersion**
             EXCLUDES 1   *drowning and submersion while in natural body of water without fall (W69)*

         ✓7ᵗʰ **W16.122**   **Fall into natural body of water striking bottom causing other injury**

     ✓6ᵗʰ **W16.13**   **Fall into natural body of water** striking side

         ✓7ᵗʰ **W16.131**   **Fall into natural body of water striking side causing** drowning **and submersion**
             EXCLUDES 1   *drowning and submersion while in natural body of water without fall (W69)*

         ✓7ᵗʰ **W16.132**   **Fall into natural body of water striking side causing other injury**

✓5ᵗʰ **W16.2**   **Fall in (into) filled bathtub or bucket of water**

     ✓6ᵗʰ **W16.21**   **Fall in (into)** filled bathtub
         EXCLUDES 1   *fall into empty bathtub (W18.2)*

         ✓7ᵗʰ **W16.211**   **Fall in (into) filled bathtub causing** drowning **and submersion**
             EXCLUDES 1   *drowning and submersion while in filled bathtub without fall (W65)*

         ✓7ᵗʰ **W16.212**   **Fall in (into) filled bathtub causing other injury**

     ✓6ᵗʰ **W16.22**   **Fall in (into)** bucket of water

         ✓7ᵗʰ **W16.221**   **Fall in (into) bucket of water causing** drowning **and submersion**

         ✓7ᵗʰ **W16.222**   **Fall in (into) bucket of water causing other injury**

✓5ᵗʰ **W16.3**   **Fall into other water**
     Fall into fountain
     Fall into reservoir

     ✓6ᵗʰ **W16.31**   **Fall into other water** striking water surface

         ✓7ᵗʰ **W16.311**   **Fall into other water striking water surface causing** drowning **and submersion**
             EXCLUDES 1   *drowning and submersion while in other water without fall (W73)*

         ✓7ᵗʰ **W16.312**   **Fall into other water striking water surface causing other injury**

     ✓6ᵗʰ **W16.32**   **Fall into other water** striking bottom

         ✓7ᵗʰ **W16.321**   **Fall into other water striking bottom causing** drowning **and submersion**
             EXCLUDES 1   *drowning and submersion while in other water without fall (W73)*

         ✓7ᵗʰ **W16.322**   **Fall into other water striking bottom causing other injury**

     ✓6ᵗʰ **W16.33**   **Fall into other water** striking wall

         ✓7ᵗʰ **W16.331**   **Fall into other water striking wall causing** drowning **and submersion**
             EXCLUDES 1   *drowning and submersion while in other water without fall (W73)*

         ✓7ᵗʰ **W16.332**   **Fall into other water striking wall causing other injury**

✓5ᵗʰ **W16.4**   **Fall into unspecified water**

     ✓x7ᵗʰ **W16.41**   **Fall into unspecified water causing drowning and** ▽ **submersion**

     ✓x7ᵗʰ **W16.42**   **Fall into unspecified water causing other injury** ▽

✓5ᵗʰ **W16.5**   **Jumping or diving into swimming pool**

     ✓6ᵗʰ **W16.51**   **Jumping or diving into swimming pool** striking water surface

         ✓7ᵗʰ **W16.511**   **Jumping or diving into swimming pool striking water surface causing** drowning **and submersion**
             EXCLUDES 1   *drowning and submersion while in swimming pool without jumping or diving (W67)*

         ✓7ᵗʰ **W16.512**   **Jumping or diving into swimming pool striking water surface causing other injury**

     ✓6ᵗʰ **W16.52**   **Jumping or diving into swimming pool** striking bottom

         ✓7ᵗʰ **W16.521**   **Jumping or diving into swimming pool striking bottom causing** drowning **and submersion**
             EXCLUDES 1   *drowning and submersion while in swimming pool without jumping or diving (W67)*

         ✓7ᵗʰ **W16.522**   **Jumping or diving into swimming pool striking bottom causing other injury**

     ✓6ᵗʰ **W16.53**   **Jumping or diving into swimming pool** striking wall

         ✓7ᵗʰ **W16.531**   **Jumping or diving into swimming pool striking wall causing** drowning **and submersion**
             EXCLUDES 1   *drowning and submersion while in swimming pool without jumping or diving (W67)*

         ✓7ᵗʰ **W16.532**   **Jumping or diving into swimming pool striking wall causing other injury**

✓5ᵗʰ **W16.6**   **Jumping or diving into** natural body of water
     Jumping or diving into lake
     Jumping or diving into open sea
     Jumping or diving into river
     Jumping or diving into stream

     ✓6ᵗʰ **W16.61**   **Jumping or diving into natural body of water** striking water surface

         ✓7ᵗʰ **W16.611**   **Jumping or diving into natural body of water striking water surface causing** drowning **and submersion**
             EXCLUDES 1   *drowning and submersion while in natural body of water without jumping or diving (W69)*

         ✓7ᵗʰ **W16.612**   **Jumping or diving into natural body of water striking water surface causing other injury**

     ✓6ᵗʰ **W16.62**   **Jumping or diving into natural body of water** striking bottom

         ✓7ᵗʰ **W16.621**   **Jumping or diving into natural body of water striking bottom causing** drowning **and submersion**
             EXCLUDES 1   *drowning and submersion while in natural body of water without jumping or diving (W69)*

         ✓7ᵗʰ **W16.622**   **Jumping or diving into natural body of water striking bottom causing other injury**

✓5ᵗʰ **W16.7**   **Jumping or diving** from boat
     EXCLUDES 1   *Fall from boat into water—see watercraft accident (V90–V94)*

     ✓6ᵗʰ **W16.71**   **Jumping or diving from boat** striking water surface

         ✓7ᵗʰ **W16.711**   **Jumping or diving from boat striking water surface causing** drowning **and submersion**

         ✓7ᵗʰ **W16.712**   **Jumping or diving from boat striking water surface causing other injury**

     ✓6ᵗʰ **W16.72**   **Jumping or diving from boat** striking bottom

         ✓7ᵗʰ **W16.721**   **Jumping or diving from boat striking bottom causing** drowning **and submersion**

         ✓7ᵗʰ **W16.722**   **Jumping or diving from boat striking bottom causing other injury**

☑ Add'l Character Required   ✓x7ᵗʰ Placeholder Alert   RUG IV Special Care High Dx   RUG IV Clinically Complex Dx   RUG IV Special Care Low Dx   Manifestation Code   Other Specified Code   ▽ Unspecified Code

Chapter 20. External Causes of Morbidity (side margin)

W16.8–W20.8 (side margin)

√5ᵗʰ **W16.8 Jumping or diving** into other water
Jumping or diving into fountain
Jumping or diving into reservoir

  √6ᵗʰ **W16.81 Jumping or diving into other water** striking water surface

    √7ᵗʰ **W16.811 Jumping or diving into other water striking water surface causing** drowning **and submersion**
      EXCLUDES 1   drowning and submersion while in other water without jumping or diving (W73)

    √7ᵗʰ **W16.812 Jumping or diving into other water striking water surface causing other injury**

  √6ᵗʰ **W16.82 Jumping or diving into other water** striking bottom

    √7ᵗʰ **W16.821 Jumping or diving into other water striking bottom causing** drowning **and submersion**
      EXCLUDES 1   drowning and submersion while in other water without jumping or diving (W73)

    √7ᵗʰ **W16.822 Jumping or diving into other water striking bottom causing other injury**

  √6ᵗʰ **W16.83 Jumping or diving into other water** striking wall

    √7ᵗʰ **W16.831 Jumping or diving into other water striking wall causing** drowning **and submersion**
      EXCLUDES 1   drowning and submersion while in other water without jumping or diving (W73)

    √7ᵗʰ **W16.832 Jumping or diving into other water striking wall causing other injury**

√5ᵗʰ **W16.9 Jumping or diving into** unspecified **water**

  √x7ᵗʰ **W16.91 Jumping or diving into unspecified water causing** drowning **and submersion** ▽

  √x7ᵗʰ **W16.92 Jumping or diving into unspecified water causing other injury** ▽

√4ᵗʰ **W17 Other fall from one level to another**

The appropriate 7th character is to be added to each code from category W17.
A   initial encounter
D   subsequent encounter
S   sequela

√x7ᵗʰ **W17.0 Fall into well**

√x7ᵗʰ **W17.1 Fall into storm drain or manhole**

√x7ᵗʰ **W17.2 Fall into hole**
Fall into pit

√x7ᵗʰ **W17.3 Fall into empty swimming pool**
  EXCLUDES 1   fall into filled swimming pool (W16.0-)

√x7ᵗʰ **W17.4 Fall from dock**

√5ᵗʰ **W17.8 Other fall from one level to another**

  √x7ᵗʰ **W17.81 Fall down embankment (hill)**

  √x7ᵗʰ **W17.82 Fall from (out of) grocery cart**
Fall due to grocery cart tipping over

  √x7ᵗʰ **W17.89 Other fall from one level to another**
Fall from cherry picker
Fall from lifting device
Fall from mobile elevated work platform [MEWP]
Fall from sky lift

√4ᵗʰ **W18 Other slipping, tripping and stumbling and falls**

The appropriate 7th character is to be added to each code from category W18.
A   initial encounter
D   subsequent encounter
S   sequela

√5ᵗʰ **W18.0 Fall due to bumping against object**
Striking against object with subsequent fall
  EXCLUDES 1   fall on same level due to slipping, tripping, or stumbling with subsequent striking against object (W01.1-)

  √x7ᵗʰ **W18.00 Striking against unspecified object with subsequent fall** ▽

  √x7ᵗʰ **W18.01 Striking against** sports equipment **with subsequent fall**

  √x7ᵗʰ **W18.02 Striking against** glass **with subsequent fall**

  √x7ᵗʰ **W18.09 Striking against other object with subsequent fall**

√5ᵗʰ **W18.1 Fall from or off toilet**

  √x7ᵗʰ **W18.11 Fall from or off toilet** without subsequent striking against object
Fall from (off) toilet NOS

  √x7ᵗʰ **W18.12 Fall from or off toilet** with subsequent striking against object

√x7ᵗʰ **W18.2 Fall in (into) shower or empty bathtub**
  EXCLUDES 1   fall in full bathtub causing drowning or submersion (W16.21-)

√5ᵗʰ **W18.3 Other and unspecified fall on same level**

  √x7ᵗʰ **W18.30 Fall on same level, unspecified** ▽

  √x7ᵗʰ **W18.31 Fall on same level due to stepping on an object**
Fall on same level due to stepping on an animal
  EXCLUDES 1   slipping, tripping and stumbling without fall due to stepping on animal (W18.41)

  √x7ᵗʰ **W18.39 Other fall on same level**

√5ᵗʰ **W18.4 Slipping, tripping and stumbling without falling**
  EXCLUDES 1   collision with another person without fall (W51)

  √x7ᵗʰ **W18.40 Slipping, tripping and stumbling without falling, unspecified** ▽

  √x7ᵗʰ **W18.41 Slipping, tripping and stumbling without falling due to** stepping on object
Slipping, tripping and stumbling without falling due to stepping on animal
  EXCLUDES 1   slipping, tripping and stumbling with fall due to stepping on animal (W18.31)

  √x7ᵗʰ **W18.42 Slipping, tripping and stumbling without falling due to** stepping into hole or opening

  √x7ᵗʰ **W18.43 Slipping, tripping and stumbling without falling due to** stepping from one level to another

  √x7ᵗʰ **W18.49 Other slipping, tripping and stumbling without falling**

√x7ᵗʰ **W19 Unspecified fall** ▽
Accidental fall NOS
AHA: 2012, 4Q, 95

The appropriate 7th character is to be added to code W19.
A   initial encounter
D   subsequent encounter
S   sequela

Exposure to inanimate mechanical forces (W20-W49)

EXCLUDES 1   assault (X92-Y08)
  contact or collision with animals or persons (W50-W64)
  exposure to inanimate mechanical forces involving military or war operations (Y36-, Y37-)
  intentional self-harm (X71-X83)

√4ᵗʰ **W20 Struck by thrown, projected or falling object**
Code first any associated:
  cataclysm (X34-X39)
  lightning strike (T75.00)
  EXCLUDES 1   falling object in machinery accident (W24, W28-W31)
  falling object in transport accident (V01-V99)
  object set in motion by explosion (W35-W40)
  object set in motion by firearm (W32-W34)
  struck by thrown sports equipment (W21.-)

The appropriate 7th character is to be added to each code from category W20.
A   initial encounter
D   subsequent encounter
S   sequela

√x7ᵗʰ **W20.0 Struck by falling object in cave-in**
  EXCLUDES 2   asphyxiation due to cave-in (T71.21)

√x7ᵗʰ **W20.1 Struck by object due to collapse of building**
  EXCLUDES 1   struck by object due to collapse of burning building (X00.2, X02.2)

√x7ᵗʰ **W20.8 Other cause of strike by thrown, projected or falling object**
  EXCLUDES 1   struck by thrown sports equipment (W21.-)

Ⓝ Newborn   Ⓟ Pediatric   Ⓜ Maternity   Ⓐ Adult   **RIC** RIC Dx   **NC Dx** Noncancer Dx   **PDx** Primary Dx   **CC** RIC CC Condition   ▶◀ Revised Text   ● New Code   ▲ Revised Code Title

1086   ICD-10-CM 2016

✓4ᵗʰ W21 Striking against or struck by sports equipment

EXCLUDES 1 assault with sports equipment (YØ8.Ø-)
striking against or struck by sports equipment with subsequent fall (W18.Ø1)

The appropriate 7th character is to be added to each code from category W21.
A   initial encounter
D   subsequent encounter
S   sequela

✓5ᵗʰ W21.Ø Struck by hit or thrown ball

- ✓ₓ7ᵗʰ **W21.ØØ** Struck by hit or thrown ball, unspecified type ▽
- ✓ₓ7ᵗʰ **W21.Ø1** Struck by football
- ✓ₓ7ᵗʰ **W21.Ø2** Struck by soccer ball
- ✓ₓ7ᵗʰ **W21.Ø3** Struck by baseball
- ✓ₓ7ᵗʰ **W21.Ø4** Struck by golf ball
- ✓ₓ7ᵗʰ **W21.Ø5** Struck by basketball
- ✓ₓ7ᵗʰ **W21.Ø6** Struck by volleyball
- ✓ₓ7ᵗʰ **W21.Ø7** Struck by softball
- ✓ₓ7ᵗʰ **W21.Ø9** Struck by other hit or thrown ball

✓5ᵗʰ W21.1 Struck by bat, racquet or club

- ✓ₓ7ᵗʰ **W21.11** Struck by baseball bat
- ✓ₓ7ᵗʰ **W21.12** Struck by tennis racquet
- ✓ₓ7ᵗʰ **W21.13** Struck by golf club
- ✓ₓ7ᵗʰ **W21.19** Struck by other bat, racquet or club

✓5ᵗʰ W21.2 Struck by hockey stick or puck

- ✓6ᵗʰ **W21.21** Struck by hockey stick
  - ✓7ᵗʰ **W21.21Ø** Struck by ice hockey stick
  - ✓7ᵗʰ **W21.211** Struck by field hockey stick
- ✓6ᵗʰ **W21.22** Struck by hockey puck
  - ✓7ᵗʰ **W21.22Ø** Struck by ice hockey puck
  - ✓7ᵗʰ **W21.221** Struck by field hockey puck

✓5ᵗʰ W21.3 Struck by sports foot wear

- ✓ₓ7ᵗʰ **W21.31** Struck by shoe cleats
  Stepped on by shoe cleats
- ✓ₓ7ᵗʰ **W21.32** Struck by skate blades
  Skated over by skate blades
- ✓ₓ7ᵗʰ **W21.39** Struck by other sports foot wear

✓ₓ7ᵗʰ W21.4 Striking against diving board

Use additional code for subsequent falling into water, if applicable (W16.-)

✓5ᵗʰ W21.8 Striking against or struck by other sports equipment

- ✓ₓ7ᵗʰ **W21.81** Striking against or struck by football helmet
- ✓ₓ7ᵗʰ **W21.89** Striking against or struck by other sports equipment

✓ₓ7ᵗʰ W21.9 Striking against or struck by unspecified sports equipment ▽

✓4ᵗʰ W22 Striking against or struck by other objects

EXCLUDES 1 striking against or struck by object with subsequent fall (W18.Ø9)

The appropriate 7th character is to be added to each code from category W22.
A   initial encounter
D   subsequent encounter
S   sequela

✓5ᵗʰ W22.Ø Striking against stationary object

EXCLUDES 1 striking against stationary sports equipment (W21.8)

- ✓ₓ7ᵗʰ **W22.Ø1** Walked into wall
- ✓ₓ7ᵗʰ **W22.Ø2** Walked into lamppost
- ✓ₓ7ᵗʰ **W22.Ø3** Walked into furniture
- ✓6ᵗʰ **W22.Ø4** Striking against wall of swimming pool
  - ✓7ᵗʰ **W22.Ø41** Striking against wall of swimming pool causing drowning and submersion
    EXCLUDES 1 drowning and submersion while swimming without striking against wall (W67)
  - ✓7ᵗʰ **W22.Ø42** Striking against wall of swimming pool causing other injury
- ✓ₓ7ᵗʰ **W22.Ø9** Striking against other stationary object

✓5ᵗʰ W22.1 Striking against or struck by automobile airbag

- ✓ₓ7ᵗʰ **W22.1Ø** Striking against or struck by unspecified automobile airbag ▽
- ✓ₓ7ᵗʰ **W22.11** Striking against or struck by driver side automobile airbag
- ✓ₓ7ᵗʰ **W22.12** Striking against or struck by front passenger side automobile airbag
- ✓ₓ7ᵗʰ **W22.19** Striking against or struck by other automobile airbag

✓ₓ7ᵗʰ W22.8 Striking against or struck by other objects

Striking against or struck by object NOS
EXCLUDES 1 struck by thrown, projected or falling object (W2Ø.-)

✓4ᵗʰ W23 Caught, crushed, jammed or pinched in or between objects

EXCLUDES 1 injury caused by cutting or piercing instruments (W25-W27)
injury caused by firearms malfunction (W32.1, W33.1-, W34.1-)
injury caused by lifting and transmission devices (W24.-)
injury caused by machinery (W28-W31)
injury caused by nonpowered hand tools (W27.-)
injury caused by transport vehicle being used as a means of transportation (VØ1-V99)
injury caused by struck by thrown, projected or falling object (W2Ø.-)

The appropriate 7th character is to be added to each code from category W23.
A   initial encounter
D   subsequent encounter
S   sequela

✓ₓ7ᵗʰ W23.Ø Caught, crushed, jammed, or pinched between moving objects

✓ₓ7ᵗʰ W23.1 Caught, crushed, jammed, or pinched between stationary objects

✓4ᵗʰ W24 Contact with lifting and transmission devices, not elsewhere classified

EXCLUDES 1 transport accidents (VØ1-V99)

The appropriate 7th character is to be added to each code from category W24.
A   initial encounter
D   subsequent encounter
S   sequela

✓ₓ7ᵗʰ W24.Ø Contact with lifting devices, not elsewhere classified

Contact with chain hoist
Contact with drive belt
Contact with pulley (block)

✓ₓ7ᵗʰ W24.1 Contact with transmission devices, not elsewhere classified

Contact with transmission belt or cable

✓ₓ7ᵗʰ W25 Contact with sharp glass

Code first any associated:
injury due to flying glass from explosion or firearm discharge (W32-W4Ø)
transport accident (VØØ-V99)
EXCLUDES 1 fall on same level due to slipping, tripping and stumbling with subsequent striking against sharp glass (WØ1.1Ø)
striking against sharp glass with subsequent fall (W18.Ø2)

The appropriate 7th character is to be added to code W25.
A   initial encounter
D   subsequent encounter
S   sequela

✓4ᵗʰ W26 Contact with knife, sword or dagger

The appropriate 7th character is to be added to each code from category W26.
A   initial encounter
D   subsequent encounter
S   sequela

✓ₓ7ᵗʰ W26.Ø Contact with knife

EXCLUDES 1 contact with electric knife (W29.1)

✓ₓ7ᵗʰ W26.1 Contact with sword or dagger

✓4ᵗʰ W27 Contact with nonpowered hand tool

The appropriate 7th character is to be added to each code from category W27.
A   initial encounter
D   subsequent encounter
S   sequela

✓ₓ7ᵗʰ W27.Ø Contact with workbench tool

Contact with auger
Contact with axe
Contact with chisel
Contact with handsaw
Contact with screwdriver

√x7ᵗʰ W27.1 Contact with garden tool
Contact with hoe
Contact with nonpowered lawn mower
Contact with pitchfork
Contact with rake

√x7ᵗʰ W27.2 Contact with scissors

√x7ᵗʰ W27.3 Contact with needle (sewing)
EXCLUDES 1 contact with hypodermic needle (W46.-)

√x7ᵗʰ W27.4 Contact with kitchen utensil
Contact with fork
Contact with ice-pick
Contact with can-opener NOS

√x7ᵗʰ W27.5 Contact with paper-cutter

√x7ᵗʰ W27.8 Contact with other nonpowered hand tool
Contact with nonpowered sewing machine
Contact with shovel

√x7ᵗʰ W28 Contact with powered lawn mower
Powered lawn mower (commercial) (residential)
EXCLUDES 1 contact with nonpowered lawn mower (W27.1)
EXCLUDES 2 exposure to electric current (W86.-)

The appropriate 7th character is to be added to code W28.
A   initial encounter
D   subsequent encounter
S   sequela

√4ᵗʰ W29 Contact with other powered hand tools and household machinery
EXCLUDES 1 contact with commercial machinery (W31.82)
contact with hot household appliance (X15)
contact with nonpowered hand tool (W27.-)
exposure to electric current (W86)

The appropriate 7th character is to be added to each code from category W29.
A   initial encounter
D   subsequent encounter
S   sequela

√x7ᵗʰ W29.0 Contact with powered kitchen appliance
Contact with blender
Contact with can-opener
Contact with garbage disposal
Contact with mixer

√x7ᵗʰ W29.1 Contact with electric knife

√x7ᵗʰ W29.2 Contact with other powered household machinery
Contact with electric fan
Contact with powered dryer (clothes) (powered) (spin)
Contact with washing-machine
Contact with sewing machine

√x7ᵗʰ W29.3 Contact with powered garden and outdoor hand tools and machinery
Contact with chainsaw
Contact with edger
Contact with garden cultivator (tiller)
Contact with hedge trimmer
Contact with other powered garden tool
EXCLUDES 1 contact with powered lawn mower (W28)

√x7ᵗʰ W29.4 Contact with nail gun

√x7ᵗʰ W29.8 Contact with other powered hand tools and household machinery
Contact with do-it-yourself tool NOS

√4ᵗʰ W30 Contact with agricultural machinery
INCLUDES animal-powered farm machine
EXCLUDES 1 agricultural transport vehicle accident (V01-V99)
explosion of grain store (W40.8)
exposure to electric current (W86.-)

The appropriate 7th character is to be added to each code from category W30.
A   initial encounter
D   subsequent encounter
S   sequela

√x7ᵗʰ W30.0 Contact with combine harvester
Contact with reaper
Contact with thresher

√x7ᵗʰ W30.1 Contact with power take-off devices (PTO)

√x7ᵗʰ W30.2 Contact with hay derrick

√x7ᵗʰ W30.3 Contact with grain storage elevator
EXCLUDES 1 explosion of grain store (W40.8)

√5ᵗʰ W30.8 Contact with other specified agricultural machinery

√x7ᵗʰ W30.81 Contact with agricultural transport vehicle in stationary use
Contact with agricultural transport vehicle under repair, not on public roadway
EXCLUDES 1 agricultural transport vehicle accident (V01-V99)

√x7ᵗʰ W30.89 Contact with other specified agricultural machinery

√x7ᵗʰ W30.9 Contact with unspecified agricultural machinery ▽
Contact with farm machinery NOS

√4ᵗʰ W31 Contact with other and unspecified machinery
EXCLUDES 1 contact with agricultural machinery (W30.-)
contact with machinery in transport under own power or being towed by a vehicle (V01-V99)
exposure to electric current (W86)

The appropriate 7th character is to be added to each code from category W31.
A   initial encounter
D   subsequent encounter
S   sequela

√x7ᵗʰ W31.0 Contact with mining and earth-drilling machinery
Contact with bore or drill (land) (seabed)
Contact with shaft hoist
Contact with shaft lift
Contact with undercutter

√x7ᵗʰ W31.1 Contact with metalworking machines
Contact with abrasive wheel
Contact with forging machine
Contact with lathe
Contact with mechanical shears
Contact with metal drilling machine
Contact with milling machine
Contact with power press
Contact with rolling-mill
Contact with metal sawing machine

√x7ᵗʰ W31.2 Contact with powered woodworking and forming machines
Contact with band saw
Contact with bench saw
Contact with circular saw
Contact with molding machine
Contact with overhead plane
Contact with powered saw
Contact with radial saw
Contact with sander
EXCLUDES 1 nonpowered woodworking tools (W27.0)

√x7ᵗʰ W31.3 Contact with prime movers
Contact with gas turbine
Contact with internal combustion engine
Contact with steam engine
Contact with water driven turbine

√5ᵗʰ W31.8 Contact with other specified machinery

√x7ᵗʰ W31.81 Contact with recreational machinery
Contact with roller coaster

√x7ᵗʰ W31.82 Contact with other commercial machinery
Contact with commercial electric fan
Contact with commercial kitchen appliances
Contact with commercial powered dryer (clothes) (powered) (spin)
Contact with commercial washing-machine
Contact with commercial sewing machine
EXCLUDES 1 contact with household machinery (W29.-)
contact with powered lawn mower (W28)

√x7ᵗʰ W31.83 Contact with special construction vehicle in stationary use
Contact with special construction vehicle under repair, not on public roadway
EXCLUDES 1 special construction vehicle accident (V01-V99)

√x7ᵗʰ W31.89 Contact with other specified machinery

√x7ᵗʰ W31.9 Contact with unspecified machinery ▽
Contact with machinery NOS

N Newborn   P Pediatric   M Maternity   A Adult   RIC RIC Dx   NC Dx Noncancer Dx   PDx Primary Dx   CC RIC CC Condition   ►◄ Revised Text   ● New Code   ▲ Revised Code Title

1088   ICD-10-CM 2016

☑4ᵗʰ **W32 Accidental handgun discharge and malfunction**

INCLUDES   accidental discharge and malfunction of gun for single hand use
accidental discharge and malfunction of pistol
accidental discharge and malfunction of revolver
handgun discharge and malfunction NOS

EXCLUDES1   *accidental airgun discharge and malfunction (W34.010, W34.110)*
accidental BB gun discharge and malfunction (W34.010, W34.110)
accidental pellet gun discharge and malfunction (W34.010, W34.110)
accidental shotgun discharge and malfunction (W33.01, W33.11)
assault by handgun discharge (X93)
handgun discharge involving legal intervention (Y35.0-)
handgun discharge involving military or war operations (Y36.4-)
intentional self-harm by handgun discharge (X72)
Very pistol discharge and malfunction (W34.09, W34.19)

The appropriate 7th character is to be added to each code from category W32.
A   initial encounter
D   subsequent encounter
S   sequela

✓x7ᵗʰ **W32.0 Accidental handgun discharge**

✓x7ᵗʰ **W32.1 Accidental handgun malfunction**
Injury due to explosion of handgun (parts)
Injury due to malfunction of mechanism or component of handgun
Injury due to recoil of handgun
Powder burn from handgun

☑4ᵗʰ **W33 Accidental rifle, shotgun and larger firearm discharge and malfunction**

INCLUDES   rifle, shotgun and larger firearm discharge and malfunction NOS

EXCLUDES1   *accidental airgun discharge and malfunction (W34.010, W34.110)*
accidental BB gun discharge and malfunction (W34.010, W34.110)
accidental handgun discharge and malfunction (W32.-)
accidental pellet gun discharge and malfunction (W34.010, W34.110)
assault by rifle, shotgun and larger firearm discharge (X94)
firearm discharge involving legal intervention (Y35.0-)
firearm discharge involving military or war operations (Y36.4-)
intentional self-harm by rifle, shotgun and larger firearm discharge (X73)

The appropriate 7th character is to be added to each code from category W33.
A   initial encounter
D   subsequent encounter
S   sequela

✓5ᵗʰ **W33.0 Accidental rifle, shotgun and larger firearm discharge**

✓x7ᵗʰ **W33.00 Accidental discharge of unspecified larger firearm** ▽
Discharge of unspecified larger firearm NOS

✓x7ᵗʰ **W33.01 Accidental discharge of shotgun**
Discharge of shotgun NOS

✓x7ᵗʰ **W33.02 Accidental discharge of hunting rifle**
Discharge of hunting rifle NOS

✓x7ᵗʰ **W33.03 Accidental discharge of machine gun**
Discharge of machine gun NOS

✓x7ᵗʰ **W33.09 Accidental discharge of other larger firearm**
Discharge of other larger firearm NOS

✓5ᵗʰ **W33.1 Accidental rifle, shotgun and larger firearm malfunction**
Injury due to explosion of rifle, shotgun and larger firearm (parts)
Injury due to malfunction of mechanism or component of rifle, shotgun and larger firearm
Injury due to piercing, cutting, crushing or pinching due to (by) slide trigger mechanism, scope or other gun part
Injury due to recoil of rifle, shotgun and larger firearm
Powder burn from rifle, shotgun and larger firearm

✓x7ᵗʰ **W33.10 Accidental malfunction of unspecified larger firearm** ▽
Malfunction of unspecified larger firearm NOS

✓x7ᵗʰ **W33.11 Accidental malfunction of shotgun**
Malfunction of shotgun NOS

✓x7ᵗʰ **W33.12 Accidental malfunction of hunting rifle**
Malfunction of hunting rifle NOS

✓x7ᵗʰ **W33.13 Accidental malfunction of machine gun**
Malfunction of machine gun NOS

✓x7ᵗʰ **W33.19 Accidental malfunction of other larger firearm**
Malfunction of other larger firearm NOS

☑4ᵗʰ **W34 Accidental discharge and malfunction from other and unspecified firearms and guns**

The appropriate 7th character is to be added to each code from category W34.
A   initial encounter
D   subsequent encounter
S   sequela

✓5ᵗʰ **W34.0 Accidental discharge from other and unspecified firearms and guns**

✓x7ᵗʰ **W34.00 Accidental discharge from unspecified firearms or gun** ▽
Discharge from firearm NOS
Gunshot wound NOS
Shot NOS

✓6ᵗʰ **W34.01 Accidental discharge of gas, air or spring-operated guns**

✓7ᵗʰ **W34.010 Accidental discharge of airgun**
Accidental discharge of BB gun
Accidental discharge of pellet gun

✓7ᵗʰ **W34.011 Accidental discharge of paintball gun**
Accidental injury due to paintball discharge

✓7ᵗʰ **W34.018 Accidental discharge of other gas, air or spring-operated gun**

✓x7ᵗʰ **W34.09 Accidental discharge from other specified firearms**
Accidental discharge from Very pistol [flare]

✓5ᵗʰ **W34.1 Accidental malfunction from other and unspecified firearms and guns**

✓x7ᵗʰ **W34.10 Accidental malfunction from unspecified firearms or gun** ▽
Firearm malfunction NOS

✓6ᵗʰ **W34.11 Accidental malfunction of gas, air or spring-operated guns**

✓7ᵗʰ **W34.110 Accidental malfunction of airgun**
Accidental malfunction of BB gun
Accidental malfunction of pellet gun

✓7ᵗʰ **W34.111 Accidental malfunction of paintball gun**
Accidental injury due to paintball gun malfunction

✓7ᵗʰ **W34.118 Accidental malfunction of other gas, air or spring-operated gun**

✓x7ᵗʰ **W34.19 Accidental malfunction from other specified firearms**
Accidental malfunction from Very pistol [flare]

✓x7ᵗʰ **W35 Explosion and rupture of boiler**
EXCLUDES1   *explosion and rupture of boiler on watercraft (V93.4)*

The appropriate 7th character is to be added to code W35.
A   initial encounter
D   subsequent encounter
S   sequela

☑4ᵗʰ **W36 Explosion and rupture of gas cylinder**

The appropriate 7th character is to be added to each code from category W36.
A   initial encounter
D   subsequent encounter
S   sequela

✓x7ᵗʰ **W36.1 Explosion and rupture of aerosol can**

✓x7ᵗʰ **W36.2 Explosion and rupture of air tank**

✓x7ᵗʰ **W36.3 Explosion and rupture of pressurized-gas tank**

✓x7ᵗʰ **W36.8 Explosion and rupture of other gas cylinder**

✓x7ᵗʰ **W36.9 Explosion and rupture of unspecified gas cylinder** ▽

☑4ᵗʰ **W37 Explosion and rupture of pressurized tire, pipe or hose**

The appropriate 7th character is to be added to each code from category W37.
A   initial encounter
D   subsequent encounter
S   sequela

✓x7ᵗʰ **W37.0 Explosion of bicycle tire**

☑ Add'l Character Required   ✓x7ᵗʰ Placeholder Alert   RUG IV Special Care High Dx   RUG IV Clinically Complex Dx   RUG IV Special Care Low Dx   Manifestation Code   Other Specified Code   ▽ Unspecified Code

Chapter 20. External Causes of Morbidity

W37.8 Explosion and rupture of other pressurized tire, pipe or hose

W38 Explosion and rupture of other specified pressurized devices

The appropriate 7th character is to be added to code W38.
A   initial encounter
D   subsequent encounter
S   sequela

W39 Discharge of firework

The appropriate 7th character is to be added to code W39.
A   initial encounter
D   subsequent encounter
S   sequela

W40 Explosion of other materials
    EXCLUDES 1   *assault by explosive material (X96)*
            explosion involving legal intervention (Y35.1-)
            explosion involving military or war operations (Y36.0-, Y36.2-)
            intentional self-harm by explosive material (X75)

The appropriate 7th character is to be added to each code from category W40.
A   initial encounter
D   subsequent encounter
S   sequela

    W40.0 Explosion of blasting material
       Explosion of blasting cap
       Explosion of detonator
       Explosion of dynamite
       Explosion of explosive (any) used in blasting operations

    W40.1 Explosion of explosive gases
       Explosion of acetylene
       Explosion of butane
       Explosion of coal gas
       Explosion in mine NOS
       Explosion of explosive gas
       Explosion of fire damp
       Explosion of gasoline fumes
       Explosion of methane
       Explosion of propane

    W40.8 Explosion of other specified explosive materials
       Explosion in dump NOS
       Explosion in factory NOS
       Explosion in grain store
       Explosion in munitions
       EXCLUDES 1   *explosion involving legal intervention (Y35.1-)*
               explosion involving military or war operations (Y36.0-, Y36.2-)

    W40.9 Explosion of unspecified explosive materials   ▽
       Explosion NOS

W42 Exposure to noise

The appropriate 7th character is to be added to each code from category W42.
A   initial encounter
D   subsequent encounter
S   sequela

    W42.0 Exposure to supersonic waves
    W42.9 Exposure to other noise
       Exposure to sound waves NOS

W45 Foreign body or object entering through skin
    EXCLUDES 2   *contact with hand tools (nonpowered) (powered) (W27-W29)*
            contact with knife, sword or dagger (W26.-)
            contact with sharp glass (W25.-)
            struck by objects (W20-W22)

The appropriate 7th character is to be added to each code from category W45.
A   initial encounter
D   subsequent encounter
S   sequela

    W45.0 Nail entering through skin
    W45.1 Paper entering through skin
       Paper cut
    W45.2 Lid of can entering through skin
    W45.8 Other foreign body or object entering through skin
       Splinter in skin NOS

W46 Contact with hypodermic needle

The appropriate 7th character is to be added to each code from category W46.
A   initial encounter
D   subsequent encounter
S   sequela

    W46.0 Contact with hypodermic needle
       Hypodermic needle stick NOS
    W46.1 Contact with contaminated hypodermic needle

W49 Exposure to other inanimate mechanical forces
    INCLUDES   exposure to abnormal gravitational [G] forces
           exposure to inanimate mechanical forces NEC
    EXCLUDES 1   *exposure to inanimate mechanical forces involving military or war operations (Y36.-, Y37.-)*

The appropriate 7th character is to be added to each code from category W49.
A   initial encounter
D   subsequent encounter
S   sequela

    W49.0 Item causing external constriction
       W49.01 Hair causing external constriction
       W49.02 String or thread causing external constriction
       W49.03 Rubber band causing external constriction
       W49.04 Ring or other jewelry causing external constriction
       W49.09 Other specified item causing external constriction
    W49.9 Exposure to other inanimate mechanical forces

Exposure to animate mechanical forces (W50-W64)
    EXCLUDES 1   *Toxic effect of contact with venomous animals and plants (T63.-)*

W50 Accidental hit, strike, kick, twist, bite or scratch by another person
       Hit, strike, kick, twist, bite, or scratch by another person NOS
    EXCLUDES 1   *assault by bodily force (Y04)*
            struck by objects (W20-W22)

The appropriate 7th character is to be added to each code from category W50.
A   initial encounter
D   subsequent encounter
S   sequela

    W50.0 Accidental hit or strike by another person
       Hit or strike by another person NOS
    W50.1 Accidental kick by another person
       Kick by another person NOS
    W50.2 Accidental twist by another person
       Twist by another person NOS
    W50.3 Accidental bite by another person
       Human bite
       Bite by another person NOS
    W50.4 Accidental scratch by another person
       Scratch by another person NOS

W51 Accidental striking against or bumped into by another person
    EXCLUDES 1   *assault by striking against or bumping into by another person (Y04.2)*
            fall due to collision with another person (W03)

The appropriate 7th character is to be added to code W51.
A   initial encounter
D   subsequent encounter
S   sequela

W52 Crushed, pushed or stepped on by crowd or human stampede
       Crushed, pushed or stepped on by crowd or human stampede with or without fall

The appropriate 7th character is to be added to code W52.
A   initial encounter
D   subsequent encounter
S   sequela

N Newborn   P Pediatric   M Maternity   A Adult   RIC RIC Dx   NC Dx Noncancer Dx   PDx Primary Dx   CC RIC CC Condition   ►◄ Revised Text   ● New Code   ▲ Revised Code Title

1090   ICD-10-CM 2016

✓4th W53 Contact with rodent

INCLUDES   contact with saliva, feces or urine of rodent

The appropriate 7th character is to be added to each code from category W53.
A   initial encounter
D   subsequent encounter
S   sequela

✓5th **W53.0 Contact with** mouse

   ✓x7th **W53.01 Bitten by mouse**

   ✓x7th **W53.09 Other contact with mouse**

✓5th **W53.1 Contact with** rat

   ✓x7th **W53.11 Bitten by rat**

   ✓x7th **W53.19 Other contact with rat**

✓5th **W53.2 Contact with** squirrel

   ✓x7th **W53.21 Bitten by squirrel**

   ✓x7th **W53.29 Other contact with squirrel**

✓5th **W53.8 Contact with** other **rodent**

   ✓x7th **W53.81 Bitten by other rodent**

   ✓x7th **W53.89 Other contact with other rodent**

✓4th W54 Contact with dog

INCLUDES   contact with saliva, feces or urine of dog

The appropriate 7th character is to be added to each code from category W54.
A   initial encounter
D   subsequent encounter
S   sequela

✓x7th **W54.0 Bitten by dog**

✓x7th **W54.1 Struck by dog**
       Knocked over by dog

✓x7th **W54.8 Other contact with dog**

✓4th W55 Contact with other mammals

INCLUDES   contact with saliva, feces or urine of mammal
EXCLUDES 1   animal being ridden—see transport accidents
            bitten or struck by dog (W54)
            bitten or struck by rodent (W53.-)
            contact with marine mammals (W56.-)

The appropriate 7th character is to be added to each code from category W55.
A   initial encounter
D   subsequent encounter
S   sequela

✓5th **W55.0 Contact with** cat

   ✓x7th **W55.01 Bitten by cat**

   ✓x7th **W55.03 Scratched by cat**

   ✓x7th **W55.09 Other contact with cat**

✓5th **W55.1 Contact with** horse

   ✓x7th **W55.11 Bitten by horse**

   ✓x7th **W55.12 Struck by horse**

   ✓x7th **W55.19 Other contact with horse**

✓5th **W55.2 Contact with** cow
       Contact with bull

   ✓x7th **W55.21 Bitten by cow**

   ✓x7th **W55.22 Struck by cow**
           Gored by bull

   ✓x7th **W55.29 Other contact with cow**

✓5th **W55.3 Contact with other** hoof stock
       Contact with goats
       Contact with sheep

   ✓x7th **W55.31 Bitten by other hoof stock**

   ✓x7th **W55.32 Struck by other hoof stock**
           Gored by goat
           Gored by ram

   ✓x7th **W55.39 Other contact with other hoof stock**

✓5th **W55.4 Contact with** pig

   ✓x7th **W55.41 Bitten by pig**

   ✓x7th **W55.42 Struck by pig**

   ✓x7th **W55.49 Other contact with pig**

✓5th **W55.5 Contact with** raccoon

   ✓x7th **W55.51 Bitten by raccoon**

   ✓x7th **W55.52 Struck by raccoon**

   ✓x7th **W55.59 Other contact with raccoon**

✓5th **W55.8 Contact with** other mammals

   ✓x7th **W55.81 Bitten by other mammals**

   ✓x7th **W55.82 Struck by other mammals**

   ✓x7th **W55.89 Other contact with other mammals**

✓4th W56 Contact with nonvenomous marine animal

EXCLUDES 1   contact with venomous marine animal (T63.-)

The appropriate 7th character is to be added to each code from category W56.
A   initial encounter
D   subsequent encounter
S   sequela

✓5th **W56.0 Contact with** dolphin

   ✓x7th **W56.01 Bitten by dolphin**

   ✓x7th **W56.02 Struck by dolphin**

   ✓x7th **W56.09 Other contact with dolphin**

✓5th **W56.1 Contact with** sea lion

   ✓x7th **W56.11 Bitten by sea lion**

   ✓x7th **W56.12 Struck by sea lion**

   ✓x7th **W56.19 Other contact with sea lion**

✓5th **W56.2 Contact with** orca
       Contact with killer whale

   ✓x7th **W56.21 Bitten by orca**

   ✓x7th **W56.22 Struck by orca**

   ✓x7th **W56.29 Other contact with orca**

✓5th **W56.3 Contact with** other marine mammals

   ✓x7th **W56.31 Bitten by other marine mammals**

   ✓x7th **W56.32 Struck by other marine mammals**

   ✓x7th **W56.39 Other contact with other marine mammals**

✓5th **W56.4 Contact with** shark

   ✓x7th **W56.41 Bitten by shark**

   ✓x7th **W56.42 Struck by shark**

   ✓x7th **W56.49 Other contact with shark**

✓5th **W56.5 Contact with other** fish

   ✓x7th **W56.51 Bitten by other fish**

   ✓x7th **W56.52 Struck by other fish**

   ✓x7th **W56.59 Other contact with other fish**

✓5th **W56.8 Contact with** other nonvenomous marine animals

   ✓x7th **W56.81 Bitten by other nonvenomous marine animals**

   ✓x7th **W56.82 Struck by other nonvenomous marine animals**

   ✓x7th **W56.89 Other contact with other nonvenomous marine animals**

✓x7th W57 Bitten or stung by nonvenomous insect and other nonvenomous arthropods

EXCLUDES 1   contact with venomous insects and arthropods (T63.2-, T63.3-, T63.4-)

The appropriate 7th character is to be added to code W57.
A   initial encounter
D   subsequent encounter
S   sequela

✓4th W58 Contact with crocodile or alligator

The appropriate 7th character is to be added to each code from category W58.
A   initial encounter
D   subsequent encounter
S   sequela

✓5th **W58.0 Contact with** alligator

   ✓x7th **W58.01 Bitten by alligator**

   ✓x7th **W58.02 Struck by alligator**

   ✓x7th **W58.03 Crushed by alligator**

   ✓x7th **W58.09 Other contact with alligator**

✓5th **W58.1 Contact with** crocodile

   ✓x7th **W58.11 Bitten by crocodile**

   ✓x7th **W58.12 Struck by crocodile**

   ✓x7th **W58.13 Crushed by crocodile**

   ✓x7th **W58.19 Other contact with crocodile**

✓ Add'l Character Required   ✓x7th Placeholder Alert   ■ RUG IV Special Care High Dx   ■ RUG IV Clinically Complex Dx   ■ RUG IV Special Care Low Dx   ■ Manifestation Code   Other Specified Code   ▽ Unspecified Code

Chapter 20. External Causes of Morbidity

W59–W73

☑4ᵗʰ **W59 Contact with other nonvenomous reptiles**
> EXCLUDES 1   contact with venomous reptile (T63.0-, T63.1-)

> The appropriate 7th character is to be added to each code from category W59.
> A   initial encounter
> D   subsequent encounter
> S   sequela

☑5ᵗʰ **W59.0 Contact with nonvenomous lizards**
   ☑x7ᵗʰ **W59.01 Bitten by nonvenomous lizards**
   ☑x7ᵗʰ **W59.02 Struck by nonvenomous lizards**
   ☑x7ᵗʰ **W59.09 Other contact with nonvenomous lizards**
       Exposure to nonvenomous lizards

☑5ᵗʰ **W59.1 Contact with nonvenomous snakes**
   ☑x7ᵗʰ **W59.11 Bitten by nonvenomous snake**
   ☑x7ᵗʰ **W59.12 Struck by nonvenomous snake**
   ☑x7ᵗʰ **W59.13 Crushed by nonvenomous snake**
   ☑x7ᵗʰ **W59.19 Other contact with nonvenomous snake**

☑5ᵗʰ **W59.2 Contact with turtles**
> EXCLUDES 1   contact with tortoises (W59.8-)

   ☑x7ᵗʰ **W59.21 Bitten by turtle**
   ☑x7ᵗʰ **W59.22 Struck by turtle**
   ☑x7ᵗʰ **W59.29 Other contact with turtle**
       Exposure to turtles

☑5ᵗʰ **W59.8 Contact with other nonvenomous reptiles**
   ☑x7ᵗʰ **W59.81 Bitten by other nonvenomous reptiles**
   ☑x7ᵗʰ **W59.82 Struck by other nonvenomous reptiles**
   ☑x7ᵗʰ **W59.83 Crushed by other nonvenomous reptiles**
   ☑x7ᵗʰ **W59.89 Other contact with other nonvenomous reptiles**

☑x7ᵗʰ **W60 Contact with nonvenomous plant thorns and spines and sharp leaves**
> EXCLUDES 1   contact with venomous plants (T63.7-)

> The appropriate 7th character is to be added to code W60.
> A   initial encounter
> D   subsequent encounter
> S   sequela

☑4ᵗʰ **W61 Contact with birds (domestic) (wild)**
> INCLUDES   contact with excreta of birds

> The appropriate 7th character is to be added to each code from category W61.
> A   initial encounter
> D   subsequent encounter
> S   sequela

☑5ᵗʰ **W61.0 Contact with parrot**
   ☑x7ᵗʰ **W61.01 Bitten by parrot**
   ☑x7ᵗʰ **W61.02 Struck by parrot**
   ☑x7ᵗʰ **W61.09 Other contact with parrot**
       Exposure to parrots

☑5ᵗʰ **W61.1 Contact with macaw**
   ☑x7ᵗʰ **W61.11 Bitten by macaw**
   ☑x7ᵗʰ **W61.12 Struck by macaw**
   ☑x7ᵗʰ **W61.19 Other contact with macaw**
       Exposure to macaws

☑5ᵗʰ **W61.2 Contact with other psittacines**
   ☑x7ᵗʰ **W61.21 Bitten by other psittacines**
   ☑x7ᵗʰ **W61.22 Struck by other psittacines**
   ☑x7ᵗʰ **W61.29 Other contact with other psittacines**
       Exposure to other psittacines

☑5ᵗʰ **W61.3 Contact with chicken**
   ☑x7ᵗʰ **W61.32 Struck by chicken**
   ☑x7ᵗʰ **W61.33 Pecked by chicken**
   ☑x7ᵗʰ **W61.39 Other contact with chicken**
       Exposure to chickens

☑5ᵗʰ **W61.4 Contact with turkey**
   ☑x7ᵗʰ **W61.42 Struck by turkey**
   ☑x7ᵗʰ **W61.43 Pecked by turkey**
   ☑x7ᵗʰ **W61.49 Other contact with turkey**

☑5ᵗʰ **W61.5 Contact with goose**
   ☑x7ᵗʰ **W61.51 Bitten by goose**

   ☑x7ᵗʰ **W61.52 Struck by goose**
   ☑x7ᵗʰ **W61.59 Other contact with goose**

☑5ᵗʰ **W61.6 Contact with duck**
   ☑x7ᵗʰ **W61.61 Bitten by duck**
   ☑x7ᵗʰ **W61.62 Struck by duck**
   ☑x7ᵗʰ **W61.69 Other contact with duck**

☑5ᵗʰ **W61.9 Contact with other birds**
   ☑x7ᵗʰ **W61.91 Bitten by other birds**
   ☑x7ᵗʰ **W61.92 Struck by other birds**
   ☑x7ᵗʰ **W61.99 Other contact with other birds**
       Contact with bird NOS

☑4ᵗʰ **W62 Contact with nonvenomous amphibians**
> EXCLUDES 1   contact with venomous amphibians (T63.81-R63.83)

> The appropriate 7th character is to be added to each code from category W62.
> A   initial encounter
> D   subsequent encounter
> S   sequela

☑x7ᵗʰ **W62.0 Contact with nonvenomous frogs**
☑x7ᵗʰ **W62.1 Contact with nonvenomous toads**
☑x7ᵗʰ **W62.9 Contact with other nonvenomous amphibians**

☑x7ᵗʰ **W64 Exposure to other animate mechanical forces**
> INCLUDES   exposure to nonvenomous animal NOS
> EXCLUDES 1   contact with venomous animal (T63.-)

> The appropriate 7th character is to be added to code W64.
> A   initial encounter
> D   subsequent encounter
> S   sequela

Accidental non-transport drowning and submersion (W65-W74)

> EXCLUDES 1   accidental drowning and submersion due to fall into water (W16.-)
>   accidental drowning and submersion due to water transport accident (V90.-, V92.-)
> EXCLUDES 2   accidental drowning and submersion due to cataclysm (X34-X39)

☑x7ᵗʰ **W65 Accidental drowning and submersion while in bath-tub**
> EXCLUDES 1   accidental drowning and submersion due to fall in (into) bathtub (W16.211)

> The appropriate 7th character is to be added to code W65.
> A   initial encounter
> D   subsequent encounter
> S   sequela

☑x7ᵗʰ **W67 Accidental drowning and submersion while in swimming-pool**
> EXCLUDES 1   accidental drowning and submersion due to fall into swimming pool (W16.011, W16.021, W16.031)
>   accidental drowning and submersion due to striking into wall of swimming pool (W22.041)

> The appropriate 7th character is to be added to code W67.
> A   initial encounter
> D   subsequent encounter
> S   sequela

☑x7ᵗʰ **W69 Accidental drowning and submersion while in natural water**
   Accidental drowning and submersion while in lake
   Accidental drowning and submersion while in open sea
   Accidental drowning and submersion while in river
   Accidental drowning and submersion while in stream
> EXCLUDES 1   accidental drowning and submersion due to fall into natural body of water (W16.111, W16.121, W16.131)

> The appropriate 7th character is to be added to code W69.
> A   initial encounter
> D   subsequent encounter
> S   sequela

☑x7ᵗʰ **W73 Other specified cause of accidental non-transport drowning and submersion**
   Accidental drowning and submersion while in quenching tank
   Accidental drowning and submersion while in reservoir
> EXCLUDES 1   accidental drowning and submersion due to fall into other water (W16.311, W16.321, W16.331)

> The appropriate 7th character is to be added to code W73.
> A   initial encounter
> D   subsequent encounter
> S   sequela

N Newborn   P Pediatric   M Maternity   A Adult   RIC RIC Dx   NC Dx Noncancer Dx   PDx Primary Dx   CC RIC CC Condition   ►◄ Revised Text   ● New Code   ▲ Revised Code Title

1092   ICD-10-CM 2016

√x7ᵗʰ **W74 Unspecified cause of accidental drowning and submersion** ▽
Drowning NOS

The appropriate 7th character is to be added to code W74.
A   initial encounter
D   subsequent encounter
S   sequela

Exposure to electric current, radiation and extreme ambient air temperature and pressure (W85-W99)

EXCLUDES1   exposure to:
     failure in dosage of radiation or temperature during surgical and
         medical care (Y63.2-Y63.5)
     lightning (T75.0-)
     natural cold (X31)
     natural heat (X30)
     natural radiation NOS (X39)
     radiological procedure and radiotherapy (Y84.2)
     sunlight (X32)

√x7ᵗʰ **W85 Exposure to electric transmission lines**
Broken power line

The appropriate 7th character is to be added to code W85.
A   initial encounter
D   subsequent encounter
S   sequela

√4ᵗʰ **W86 Exposure to other specified electric current**

The appropriate 7th character is to be added to each code from
category W86.
A   initial encounter
D   subsequent encounter
S   sequela

√x7ᵗʰ **W86.0 Exposure to domestic wiring and appliances**
√x7ᵗʰ **W86.1 Exposure to industrial wiring, appliances and electrical machinery**
Exposure to conductors
Exposure to control apparatus
Exposure to electrical equipment and machinery
Exposure to transformers

√x7ᵗʰ **W86.8 Exposure to other electric current**
Exposure to wiring and appliances in or on farm (not farmhouse)
Exposure to wiring and appliances outdoors
Exposure to wiring and appliances in or on public building
Exposure to wiring and appliances in or on residential
     institutions
Exposure to wiring and appliances in or on schools

√4ᵗʰ **W88 Exposure to ionizing radiation**
EXCLUDES1   exposure to sunlight (X32)

The appropriate 7th character is to be added to each code from
category W88.
A   initial encounter
D   subsequent encounter
S   sequela

√x7ᵗʰ **W88.0 Exposure to X-rays**
√x7ᵗʰ **W88.1 Exposure to radioactive isotopes**
√x7ᵗʰ **W88.8 Exposure to other ionizing radiation**

√4ᵗʰ **W89 Exposure to man-made visible and ultraviolet light**
INCLUDES   exposure to welding light (arc)
EXCLUDES2   exposure to sunlight (X32)

The appropriate 7th character is to be added to each code from
category W89.
A   initial encounter
D   subsequent encounter
S   sequela

√x7ᵗʰ **W89.0 Exposure to welding light (arc)**
√x7ᵗʰ **W89.1 Exposure to tanning bed**
√x7ᵗʰ **W89.8 Exposure to other man-made visible and ultraviolet light**
√x7ᵗʰ **W89.9 Exposure to unspecified man-made visible and ultraviolet light** ▽

√4ᵗʰ **W90 Exposure to other nonionizing radiation**
EXCLUDES1   exposure to sunlight (X32)

The appropriate 7th character is to be added to each code from
category W90.
A   initial encounter
D   subsequent encounter
S   sequela

√x7ᵗʰ **W90.0 Exposure to radiofrequency**
√x7ᵗʰ **W90.1 Exposure to infrared radiation**
√x7ᵗʰ **W90.2 Exposure to laser radiation**
√x7ᵗʰ **W90.8 Exposure to other nonionizing radiation**

√x7ᵗʰ **W92 Exposure to excessive heat of man-made origin**

The appropriate 7th character is to be added to code W92.
A   initial encounter
D   subsequent encounter
S   sequela

√4ᵗʰ **W93 Exposure to excessive cold of man-made origin**

The appropriate 7th character is to be added to each code from
category W93.
A   initial encounter
D   subsequent encounter
S   sequela

√5ᵗʰ **W93.0 Contact with or inhalation of dry ice**
√x7ᵗʰ **W93.01 Contact with dry ice**
√x7ᵗʰ **W93.02 Inhalation of dry ice**

√5ᵗʰ **W93.1 Contact with or inhalation of liquid air**
√x7ᵗʰ **W93.11 Contact with liquid air**
Contact with liquid hydrogen
Contact with liquid nitrogen
√x7ᵗʰ **W93.12 Inhalation of liquid air**
Inhalation of liquid hydrogen
Inhalation of liquid nitrogen

√x7ᵗʰ **W93.2 Prolonged exposure in deep freeze unit or refrigerator**
√x7ᵗʰ **W93.8 Exposure to other excessive cold of man-made origin**

√4ᵗʰ **W94 Exposure to high and low air pressure and changes in air pressure**

The appropriate 7th character is to be added to each code from
category W94.
A   initial encounter
D   subsequent encounter
S   sequela

√x7ᵗʰ **W94.0 Exposure to prolonged high air pressure**
√5ᵗʰ **W94.1 Exposure to prolonged low air pressure**
√x7ᵗʰ **W94.11 Exposure to residence or prolonged visit at high altitude**
√x7ᵗʰ **W94.12 Exposure to other prolonged low air pressure**
√5ᵗʰ **W94.2 Exposure to rapid changes in air pressure during ascent**
√x7ᵗʰ **W94.21 Exposure to reduction in atmospheric pressure while surfacing from deep-water diving**
√x7ᵗʰ **W94.22 Exposure to reduction in atmospheric pressure while surfacing from underground**
√x7ᵗʰ **W94.23 Exposure to sudden change in air pressure in aircraft during ascent**
√x7ᵗʰ **W94.29 Exposure to other rapid changes in air pressure during ascent**
√5ᵗʰ **W94.3 Exposure to rapid changes in air pressure during descent**
√x7ᵗʰ **W94.31 Exposure to sudden change in air pressure in aircraft during descent**
√x7ᵗʰ **W94.32 Exposure to high air pressure from rapid descent in water**
√x7ᵗʰ **W94.39 Exposure to other rapid changes in air pressure during descent**

√x7ᵗʰ **W99 Exposure to other man-made environmental factors**

The appropriate 7th character is to be added to code W99.
A   initial encounter
D   subsequent encounter
S   sequela

Chapter 20. External Causes of Morbidity

X00–X08.19

Exposure to smoke, fire and flames (X00-X08)

EXCLUDES1   arson (X97)
EXCLUDES2   explosions (W35-W40)
     lightning (T75.0-)
     transport accident (V01-V99)

✓4ᵗʰ X00   **Exposure to uncontrolled fire in building or structure**
     INCLUDES   conflagration in building or structure
     Code first any associated cataclysm
     EXCLUDES2   exposure to ignition or melting of nightwear (X05)
             exposure to ignition or melting of other clothing and apparel (X06.-)
             exposure to other specified smoke, fire and flames (X08.-)

     The appropriate 7th character is to be added to each code from category X00.
     A   initial encounter
     D   subsequent encounter
     S   sequela

   ✓x7ᵗʰ X00.0   **Exposure to flames in uncontrolled fire in building or structure**

   ✓x7ᵗʰ X00.1   **Exposure to smoke in uncontrolled fire in building or structure**

   ✓x7ᵗʰ X00.2   **Injury due to collapse of burning building or structure in uncontrolled fire**
       EXCLUDES1   injury due to collapse of building not on fire (W20.1)

   ✓x7ᵗʰ X00.3   **Fall from burning building or structure in uncontrolled fire**

   ✓x7ᵗʰ X00.4   **Hit by object from burning building or structure in uncontrolled fire**

   ✓x7ᵗʰ X00.5   **Jump from burning building or structure in uncontrolled fire**

   ✓x7ᵗʰ X00.8   **Other exposure to uncontrolled fire in building or structure**

✓4ᵗʰ X01   **Exposure to uncontrolled fire, not in building or structure**
     INCLUDES   exposure to forest fire

     The appropriate 7th character is to be added to each code from category X01.
     A   initial encounter
     D   subsequent encounter
     S   sequela

   ✓x7ᵗʰ X01.0   **Exposure to flames in uncontrolled fire, not in building or structure**

   ✓x7ᵗʰ X01.1   **Exposure to smoke in uncontrolled fire, not in building or structure**

   ✓x7ᵗʰ X01.3   **Fall due to uncontrolled fire, not in building or structure**

   ✓x7ᵗʰ X01.4   **Hit by object due to uncontrolled fire, not in building or structure**

   ✓x7ᵗʰ X01.8   **Other exposure to uncontrolled fire, not in building or structure**

✓4ᵗʰ X02   **Exposure to controlled fire in building or structure**
     INCLUDES   exposure to fire in fireplace
             exposure to fire in stove

     The appropriate 7th character is to be added to each code from category X02.
     A   initial encounter
     D   subsequent encounter
     S   sequela

   ✓x7ᵗʰ X02.0   **Exposure to flames in controlled fire in building or structure**

   ✓x7ᵗʰ X02.1   **Exposure to smoke in controlled fire in building or structure**

   ✓x7ᵗʰ X02.2   **Injury due to collapse of burning building or structure in controlled fire**
       EXCLUDES1   injury due to collapse of building not on fire (W20.1)

   ✓x7ᵗʰ X02.3   **Fall from burning building or structure in controlled fire**

   ✓x7ᵗʰ X02.4   **Hit by object from burning building or structure in controlled fire**

   ✓x7ᵗʰ X02.5   **Jump from burning building or structure in controlled fire**

   ✓x7ᵗʰ X02.8   **Other exposure to controlled fire in building or structure**

✓4ᵗʰ X03   **Exposure to controlled fire, not in building or structure**
     INCLUDES   exposure to bon fire
             exposure to camp-fire
             exposure to trash fire

     The appropriate 7th character is to be added to each code from category X03.
     A   initial encounter
     D   subsequent encounter
     S   sequela

   ✓x7ᵗʰ X03.0   **Exposure to flames in controlled fire, not in building or structure**

   ✓x7ᵗʰ X03.1   **Exposure to smoke in controlled fire, not in building or structure**

   ✓x7ᵗʰ X03.3   **Fall due to controlled fire, not in building or structure**

   ✓x7ᵗʰ X03.4   **Hit by object due to controlled fire, not in building or structure**

   ✓x7ᵗʰ X03.8   **Other exposure to controlled fire, not in building or structure**

✓x7ᵗʰ X04   **Exposure to ignition of highly flammable material**
     Exposure to ignition of gasoline
     Exposure to ignition of kerosene
     Exposure to ignition of petrol
     EXCLUDES2   exposure to ignition or melting of nightwear (X05)
             exposure to ignition or melting of other clothing and apparel (X06)

     The appropriate 7th character is to be added to code X04.
     A   initial encounter
     D   subsequent encounter
     S   sequela

✓x7ᵗʰ X05   **Exposure to ignition or melting of nightwear**
     EXCLUDES2   exposure to uncontrolled fire in building or structure (X00.-)
             exposure to uncontrolled fire, not in building or structure (X01.-)
             exposure to controlled fire in building or structure (X02.-)
             exposure to controlled fire, not in building or structure (X03.-)
             exposure to ignition of highly flammable materials (X04.-)

     The appropriate 7th character is to be added to code X05.
     A   initial encounter
     D   subsequent encounter
     S   sequela

✓4ᵗʰ X06   **Exposure to ignition or melting of other clothing and apparel**
     EXCLUDES2   exposure to uncontrolled fire in building or structure (X00.-)
             exposure to uncontrolled fire, not in building or structure (X01.-)
             exposure to controlled fire in building or structure (X02.-)
             exposure to controlled fire, not in building or structure (X03.-)
             exposure to ignition of highly flammable materials (X04.-)

     The appropriate 7th character is to be added to each code from category X06.
     A   initial encounter
     D   subsequent encounter
     S   sequela

   ✓x7ᵗʰ X06.0   **Exposure to ignition of plastic jewelry**

   ✓x7ᵗʰ X06.1   **Exposure to melting of plastic jewelry**

   ✓x7ᵗʰ X06.2   **Exposure to ignition of other clothing and apparel**

   ✓x7ᵗʰ X06.3   **Exposure to melting of other clothing and apparel**

✓4ᵗʰ X08   **Exposure to other specified smoke, fire and flames**

     The appropriate 7th character is to be added to each code from category X08.
     A   initial encounter
     D   subsequent encounter
     S   sequela

   ✓5ᵗʰ X08.0   **Exposure to bed fire**
       Exposure to mattress fire

     ✓x7ᵗʰ X08.00   **Exposure to bed fire due to unspecified burning material** ▽

     ✓x7ᵗʰ X08.01   **Exposure to bed fire due to burning cigarette**

     ✓x7ᵗʰ X08.09   **Exposure to bed fire due to other burning material**

   ✓5ᵗʰ X08.1   **Exposure to sofa fire**

     ✓x7ᵗʰ X08.10   **Exposure to sofa fire due to unspecified burning material** ▽

     ✓x7ᵗʰ X08.11   **Exposure to sofa fire due to burning cigarette**

     ✓x7ᵗʰ X08.19   **Exposure to sofa fire due to other burning material**

 Newborn   Pediatric   Maternity   Adult   **RIC** RIC Dx   **NCDx** Noncancer Dx   **PDx** Primary Dx   **CC** RIC CC Condition   ▶◀ Revised Text   ● New Code   ▲ Revised Code Title

1094   ICD-10-CM 2016

✓5th **X08.2 Exposure to** other furniture **fire**

  ✓x7th **X08.20 Exposure to other furniture fire due to unspecified burning material** ▽

  ✓x7th **X08.21 Exposure to other furniture fire due to** burning cigarette

  ✓x7th **X08.29 Exposure to other furniture fire due to other burning material**

✓x7th **X08.8 Exposure to other specified smoke, fire and flames**

Contact with heat and hot substances (X10-X19)

EXCLUDES 1   exposure to excessive natural heat (X30)
exposure to fire and flames (X00-X09)

✓4th **X10 Contact with hot drinks, food, fats and cooking oils**

The appropriate 7th character is to be added to each code from category X10.
A   initial encounter
D   subsequent encounter
S   sequela

✓x7th **X10.0 Contact with hot** drinks

✓x7th **X10.1 Contact with hot** food

✓x7th **X10.2 Contact with** fats and cooking oils

✓4th **X11 Contact with hot tap-water**

  INCLUDES   contact with boiling tap-water
contact with boiling water NOS

  EXCLUDES 1   contact with water heated on stove (X12)

The appropriate 7th character is to be added to each code from category X11.
A   initial encounter
D   subsequent encounter
S   sequela

✓x7th **X11.0 Contact with hot water** in bath or tub

  EXCLUDES 1   contact with running hot water in bath or tub (X11.1)

✓x7th **X11.1 Contact with** running **hot water**

Contact with hot water running out of hose
Contact with hot water running out of tap

✓x7th **X11.8 Contact with other hot tap-water**

Contact with hot water in bucket
Contact with hot tap-water NOS

✓x7th **X12 Contact with other hot fluids**

Contact with water heated on stove

  EXCLUDES 1   hot (liquid) metals (X18)

The appropriate 7th character is to be added to code X12.
A   initial encounter
D   subsequent encounter
S   sequela

✓4th **X13 Contact with steam and other hot vapors**

The appropriate 7th character is to be added to each code from category X13.
A   initial encounter
D   subsequent encounter
S   sequela

✓x7th **X13.0 Inhalation of steam and other hot vapors**

✓x7th **X13.1 Other contact with steam and other hot vapors**

✓4th **X14 Contact with hot air and other hot gases**

The appropriate 7th character is to be added to each code from category X14.
A   initial encounter
D   subsequent encounter
S   sequela

✓x7th **X14.0 Inhalation of hot air and gases**

✓x7th **X14.1 Other contact with hot air and other hot gases**

✓4th **X15 Contact with hot household appliances**

  EXCLUDES 1   contact with heating appliances (X16)
contact with powered household appliances (W29.-)
exposure to controlled fire in building or structure due to household appliance (X02.8)
exposure to household appliances electrical current (W86.0)

The appropriate 7th character is to be added to each code from category X15.
A   initial encounter
D   subsequent encounter
S   sequela

✓x7th **X15.0 Contact with hot** stove (kitchen)

✓x7th **X15.1 Contact with hot** toaster

✓x7th **X15.2 Contact with** hotplate

✓x7th **X15.3 Contact with hot** saucepan or skillet

✓x7th **X15.8 Contact with other hot household appliances**

Contact with cooker   Contact with light bulbs
Contact with kettle

✓x7th **X16 Contact with hot heating appliances, radiators and pipes**

  EXCLUDES 1   contact with powered appliances (W29.-)
exposure to controlled fire in building or structure due to appliance (X02.8)
exposure to industrial appliances electrical current (W86.1)

The appropriate 7th character is to be added to code X16.
A   initial encounter
D   subsequent encounter
S   sequela

✓x7th **X17 Contact with hot engines, machinery and tools**

  EXCLUDES 1   contact with hot heating appliances, radiators and pipes (X16)
contact with hot household appliances (X15)

The appropriate 7th character is to be added to code X17.
A   initial encounter
D   subsequent encounter
S   sequela

✓x7th **X18 Contact with other hot metals**

Contact with liquid metal

The appropriate 7th character is to be added to code X18.
A   initial encounter
D   subsequent encounter
S   sequela

✓x7th **X19 Contact with other heat and hot substances**

  EXCLUDES 1   objects that are not normally hot, e.g., an object made hot by a house fire (X00-X09)

The appropriate 7th character is to be added to code X19.
A   initial encounter
D   subsequent encounter
S   sequela

Exposure to forces of nature (X30-X39)

✓x7th **X30 Exposure to excessive** natural heat

Exposure to excessive heat as the cause of sunstroke
Exposure to heat NOS

  EXCLUDES 1   excessive heat of man-made origin (W92)
exposure to man-made radiation (W89)
exposure to sunlight (X32)
exposure to tanning bed (W89)

The appropriate 7th character is to be added to code X30.
A   initial encounter
D   subsequent encounter
S   sequela

✓x7th **X31 Exposure to excessive** natural cold

Excessive cold as the cause of chilblains NOS
Excessive cold as the cause of immersion foot or hand
Exposure to cold NOS
Exposure to weather conditions

  EXCLUDES 1   cold of man-made origin (W93.-)
contact with or inhalation of dry ice (W93.-)
contact with or inhalation of liquefied gas (W93.-)

The appropriate 7th character is to be added to code X31.
A   initial encounter
D   subsequent encounter
S   sequela

√x7ᵗʰ **X32 Exposure to sunlight**
> EXCLUDES 1 *radiation-related disorders of the skin and subcutaneous tissue (L55-L59)*
> *man-made radiation (tanning bed) (W89)*

> The appropriate 7th character is to be added to code X32.
> A   initial encounter
> D   subsequent encounter
> S   sequela

√x7ᵗʰ **X34 Earthquake**
> EXCLUDES 2 *tidal wave (tsunami) due to earthquake (X37.41)*

> The appropriate 7th character is to be added to code X34.
> A   initial encounter
> D   subsequent encounter
> S   sequela

√x7ᵗʰ **X35 Volcanic eruption**
> EXCLUDES 2 *tidal wave (tsunami) due to volcanic eruption (X37.41)*

> The appropriate 7th character is to be added to code X35.
> A   initial encounter
> D   subsequent encounter
> S   sequela

√4ᵗʰ **X36 Avalanche, landslide and other earth movements**
> INCLUDES victim of mudslide of cataclysmic nature
> EXCLUDES 1 *earthquake (X34)*
> EXCLUDES 2 *transport accident involving collision with avalanche or landslide not in motion (V01-V99)*

> The appropriate 7th character is to be added to each code from category X36.
> A   initial encounter
> D   subsequent encounter
> S   sequela

√x7ᵗʰ **X36.0 Collapse of dam or man-made structure causing earth movement**

√x7ᵗʰ **X36.1 Avalanche, landslide, or mudslide**

√4ᵗʰ **X37 Cataclysmic storm**
> The appropriate 7th character is to be added to each code from category X37.
> A   initial encounter
> D   subsequent encounter
> S   sequela

√x7ᵗʰ **X37.0 Hurricane**
> Storm surge
> Typhoon

√x7ᵗʰ **X37.1 Tornado**
> Cyclone
> Twister

√x7ᵗʰ **X37.2 Blizzard (snow)(ice)**

√x7ᵗʰ **X37.3 Dust storm**

√5ᵗʰ **X37.4 Tidalwave**

> √x7ᵗʰ **X37.41 Tidal wave due to earthquake or volcanic eruption**
> Tidal wave NOS
> Tsunami

> √x7ᵗʰ **X37.42 Tidal wave due to storm**

> √x7ᵗʰ **X37.43 Tidal wave due to landslide**

√x7ᵗʰ **X37.8 Other cataclysmic storms**
> Cloudburst
> Torrential rain
> EXCLUDES 2 *flood (X38)*

√x7ᵗʰ **X37.9 Unspecified cataclysmic storm**   ▽
> Storm NOS
> EXCLUDES 1 *collapse of dam or man-made structure causing earth movement (X39.0)*

√x7ᵗʰ **X38 Flood**
> Flood arising from remote storm
> Flood of cataclysmic nature arising from melting snow
> Flood resulting directly from storm
> EXCLUDES 1 *collapse of dam or man-made structure causing earth movement (X39.0)*
> *tidal wave NOS (X37.41)*
> *tidal wave caused by storm (X37.2)*

> The appropriate 7th character is to be added to code X38.
> A   initial encounter
> D   subsequent encounter
> S   sequela

√4ᵗʰ **X39 Exposure to other forces of nature**
> The appropriate 7th character is to be added to each code from category X39.
> A   initial encounter
> D   subsequent encounter
> S   sequela

√5ᵗʰ **X39.0 Exposure to natural radiation**
> EXCLUDES 1 *contact with and (suspected) exposure to radon and other naturally occuring radiation (Z77.122)*
> *exposure to man-made radiation (W88-W90)*
> *exposure to sunlight (X32)*

> √x7ᵗʰ **X39.01 Exposure to radon**
> √x7ᵗʰ **X39.08 Exposure to other natural radiation**
√x7ᵗʰ **X39.8 Other exposure to forces of nature**

Accidental exposure to other specified factors (X52, X58)

√x7ᵗʰ **X52 Prolonged stay in weightless environment**
> Weightlessness in spacecraft (simulator)

> The appropriate 7th character is to be added to code X52.
> A   initial encounter
> D   subsequent encounter
> S   sequela

√x7ᵗʰ **X58 Exposure to other specified factors**
> Accident NOS
> Exposure NOS

> The appropriate 7th character is to be added to code X58.
> A   initial encounter
> D   subsequent encounter
> S   sequela

Intentional self-harm (X71-X83)
Purposely self-inflicted injury
Suicide (attempted)

√4ᵗʰ **X71 Intentional self-harm by drowning and submersion**
> The appropriate 7th character is to be added to each code from category X71.
> A   initial encounter
> D   subsequent encounter
> S   sequela

√x7ᵗʰ **X71.0 Intentional self-harm by drowning and submersion while in bathtub**

√x7ᵗʰ **X71.1 Intentional self-harm by drowning and submersion while in swimming pool**

√x7ᵗʰ **X71.2 Intentional self-harm by drowning and submersion after jump into swimming pool**

√x7ᵗʰ **X71.3 Intentional self-harm by drowning and submersion in natural water**

√x7ᵗʰ **X71.8 Other intentional self-harm by drowning and submersion**

√x7ᵗʰ **X71.9 Intentional self-harm by drowning and submersion, unspecified**   ▽

√x7ᵗʰ **X72 Intentional self-harm by handgun discharge**
> Intentional self-harm by gun for single hand use
> Intentional self-harm by pistol
> Intentional self-harm by revolver
> EXCLUDES 1 *Very pistol (X74.8)*

> The appropriate 7th character is to be added to code X72.
> A   initial encounter
> D   subsequent encounter
> S   sequela

√4ᵗʰ **X73 Intentional self-harm by rifle, shotgun and larger firearm discharge**
> EXCLUDES 1 *airgun (X74.01)*

> The appropriate 7th character is to be added to each code from category X73.
> A   initial encounter
> D   subsequent encounter
> S   sequela

√x7ᵗʰ **X73.0 Intentional self-harm by shotgun discharge**
√x7ᵗʰ **X73.1 Intentional self-harm by hunting rifle discharge**
√x7ᵗʰ **X73.2 Intentional self-harm by machine gun discharge**
√x7ᵗʰ **X73.8 Intentional self-harm by other larger firearm discharge**

N Newborn   P Pediatric   M Maternity   A Adult   RIC RIC Dx   NCDx Noncancer Dx   PDx Primary Dx   CC RIC CC Condition   ►◄ Revised Text   ● New Code   ▲ Revised Code Title

1096   ICD-10-CM 2016

✓x7ᵗʰ **X73.9**   Intentional self-harm by unspecified larger firearm discharge ▽

✓4ᵗʰ **X74**   **Intentional self-harm by other and unspecified firearm and gun discharge**

> The appropriate 7th character is to be added to each code from category X74.
> A   initial encounter
> D   subsequent encounter
> S   sequela

   ✓5ᵗʰ **X74.0**   Intentional self-harm by **gas, air or spring-operated guns**

     ✓x7ᵗʰ **X74.01**   **Intentional self-harm by airgun**
       Intentional self-harm by BB gun discharge
       Intentional self-harm by pellet gun discharge

     ✓x7ᵗʰ **X74.02**   **Intentional self-harm by paintball gun**

     ✓x7ᵗʰ **X74.09**   **Intentional self-harm by other gas, air or spring-operated gun**

   ✓x7ᵗʰ **X74.8**   **Intentional self-harm by other firearm discharge**
     Intentional self-harm by Very pistol [flare] discharge

   ✓x7ᵗʰ **X74.9**   Intentional self-harm by unspecified firearm discharge ▽

✓x7ᵗʰ **X75**   **Intentional self-harm by explosive material**

> The appropriate 7th character is to be added to code X75.
> A   initial encounter
> D   subsequent encounter
> S   sequela

✓x7ᵗʰ **X76**   **Intentional self-harm by smoke, fire and flames**

> The appropriate 7th character is to be added to code X76.
> A   initial encounter
> D   subsequent encounter
> S   sequela

✓4ᵗʰ **X77**   **Intentional self-harm by steam, hot vapors and hot objects**

> The appropriate 7th character is to be added to each code from category X77.
> A   initial encounter
> D   subsequent encounter
> S   sequela

   ✓x7ᵗʰ **X77.0**   Intentional self-harm by **steam** or hot **vapors**

   ✓x7ᵗʰ **X77.1**   Intentional self-harm by hot **tap water**

   ✓x7ᵗʰ **X77.2**   Intentional self-harm by other hot **fluids**

   ✓x7ᵗʰ **X77.3**   Intentional self-harm by hot **household appliances**

   ✓x7ᵗʰ **X77.8**   Intentional self-harm by other hot **objects**

   ✓x7ᵗʰ **X77.9**   Intentional self-harm by unspecified hot objects ▽

✓4ᵗʰ **X78**   **Intentional self-harm by sharp object**

> The appropriate 7th character is to be added to each code from category X78.
> A   initial encounter
> D   subsequent encounter
> S   sequela

   ✓x7ᵗʰ **X78.0**   Intentional self-harm by sharp **glass**

   ✓x7ᵗʰ **X78.1**   Intentional self-harm by **knife**

   ✓x7ᵗʰ **X78.2**   Intentional self-harm by **sword or dagger**

   ✓x7ᵗʰ **X78.8**   **Intentional self-harm by other sharp object**

   ✓x7ᵗʰ **X78.9**   Intentional self-harm by unspecified sharp object ▽

✓x7ᵗʰ **X79**   **Intentional self-harm by blunt object**

> The appropriate 7th character is to be added to code X79.
> A   initial encounter
> D   subsequent encounter
> S   sequela

✓x7ᵗʰ **X80**   **Intentional self-harm by jumping from a high place**
   Intentional fall from one level to another

> The appropriate 7th character is to be added to code X80.
> A   initial encounter
> D   subsequent encounter
> S   sequela

✓4ᵗʰ **X81**   **Intentional self-harm by jumping or lying in front of moving object**

> The appropriate 7th character is to be added to each code from category X81.
> A   initial encounter
> D   subsequent encounter
> S   sequela

   ✓x7ᵗʰ **X81.0**   Intentional self-harm by jumping or lying in front of **motor vehicle**

   ✓x7ᵗʰ **X81.1**   Intentional self-harm by jumping or lying in front of (subway) **train**

   ✓x7ᵗʰ **X81.8**   **Intentional self-harm by jumping or lying in front of other moving object**

✓4ᵗʰ **X82**   **Intentional self-harm by crashing of motor vehicle**

> The appropriate 7th character is to be added to each code from category X82.
> A   initial encounter
> D   subsequent encounter
> S   sequela

   ✓x7ᵗʰ **X82.0**   Intentional collision of motor vehicle with other motor vehicle

   ✓x7ᵗʰ **X82.1**   Intentional collision of motor vehicle with **train**

   ✓x7ᵗʰ **X82.2**   Intentional collision of motor vehicle with **tree**

   ✓x7ᵗʰ **X82.8**   **Other intentional self-harm by crashing of motor vehicle**

✓4ᵗʰ **X83**   **Intentional self-harm by other specified means**
   EXCLUDES1   *intentional self-harm by poisoning or contact with toxic substance—see Table of Drugs and Chemicals*

> The appropriate 7th character is to be added to each code from category X83.
> A   initial encounter
> D   subsequent encounter
> S   sequela

   ✓x7ᵗʰ **X83.0**   Intentional self-harm by **crashing of aircraft**

   ✓x7ᵗʰ **X83.1**   Intentional self-harm by **electrocution**

   ✓x7ᵗʰ **X83.2**   Intentional self-harm by **exposure to extremes of cold**

   ✓x7ᵗʰ **X83.8**   **Intentional self-harm by other specified means**

Assault (X92-Y08)

INCLUDES   homicide
     injuries inflicted by another person with intent to injure or kill, by any means
EXCLUDES1   *injuries due to legal intervention (Y35.-)*
     injuries due to operations of war (Y36.-)
     injuries due to terrorism (Y38.-)

✓4ᵗʰ **X92**   **Assault by drowning and submersion**

> The appropriate 7th character is to be added to each code from category X92.
> A   initial encounter
> D   subsequent encounter
> S   sequela

   ✓x7ᵗʰ **X92.0**   Assault by drowning and submersion while in **bathtub**

   ✓x7ᵗʰ **X92.1**   Assault by drowning and submersion while in **swimming pool**

   ✓x7ᵗʰ **X92.2**   Assault by drowning and submersion **after push into** swimming pool

   ✓x7ᵗʰ **X92.3**   Assault by drowning and submersion **in natural water**

   ✓x7ᵗʰ **X92.8**   **Other assault by drowning and submersion**

   ✓x7ᵗʰ **X92.9**   Assault by drowning and submersion, unspecified ▽

✓x7ᵗʰ **X93**   **Assault by handgun discharge**
   Assault by discharge of gun for single hand use
   Assault by discharge of pistol
   Assault by discharge of revolver
   EXCLUDES1   *Very pistol (X95.8)*

> The appropriate 7th character is to be added to code X93.
> A   initial encounter
> D   subsequent encounter
> S   sequela

✓ Add'l Character Required   ✓x7ᵗʰ Placeholder Alert   RUG IV Special Care High Dx   RUG IV Clinically Complex Dx   RUG IV Special Care Low Dx   Manifestation Code   Other Specified Code   ▽Unspecified Code

Chapter 20. External Causes of Morbidity

X94–Y04.8

☑4ᵗʰ **X94** **Assault by rifle, shotgun and larger firearm discharge**
    EXCLUDES 1   airgun (X95.01)

The appropriate 7th character is to be added to each code from category X94.
- A   initial encounter
- D   subsequent encounter
- S   sequela

✓x7ᵗʰ **X94.0**   **Assault by shotgun**
✓x7ᵗʰ **X94.1**   **Assault by hunting rifle**
✓x7ᵗʰ **X94.2**   **Assault by machine gun**
✓x7ᵗʰ **X94.8**   **Assault by other larger firearm discharge**
✓x7ᵗʰ **X94.9**   **Assault by unspecified larger firearm discharge**   ▽

☑4ᵗʰ **X95** **Assault by other and unspecified firearm and gun discharge**

The appropriate 7th character is to be added to each code from category X95.
- A   initial encounter
- D   subsequent encounter
- S   sequela

✓5ᵗʰ **X95.0**   **Assault by gas, air or spring-operated guns**

✓x7ᵗʰ   **X95.01**   **Assault by airgun discharge**
      Assault by BB gun discharge
      Assault by pellet gun discharge

✓x7ᵗʰ   **X95.02**   **Assault by paintball gun discharge**

✓x7ᵗʰ   **X95.09**   **Assault by other gas, air or spring-operated gun**

✓x7ᵗʰ **X95.8**   **Assault by other firearm discharge**
      Assault by Very pistol [flare] discharge

✓x7ᵗʰ **X95.9**   **Assault by unspecified firearm discharge**   ▽

☑4ᵗʰ **X96** **Assault by explosive material**
    EXCLUDES 1   incendiary device (X97)
               terrorism involving explosive material (Y38.2-)

The appropriate 7th character is to be added to each code from category X96.
- A   initial encounter
- D   subsequent encounter
- S   sequela

✓x7ᵗʰ **X96.0**   **Assault by antipersonnel bomb**
    EXCLUDES 1   antipersonnel bomb use in military or war (Y36.2-)

✓x7ᵗʰ **X96.1**   **Assault by gasoline bomb**
✓x7ᵗʰ **X96.2**   **Assault by letter bomb**
✓x7ᵗʰ **X96.3**   **Assault by fertilizer bomb**
✓x7ᵗʰ **X96.4**   **Assault by pipe bomb**
✓x7ᵗʰ **X96.8**   **Assault by other specified explosive**
✓x7ᵗʰ **X96.9**   **Assault by unspecified explosive**   ▽

✓x7ᵗʰ **X97** **Assault by smoke, fire and flames**
      Assault by arson
      Assault by cigarettes
      Assault by incendiary device

The appropriate 7th character is to be added to code X97.
- A   initial encounter
- D   subsequent encounter
- S   sequela

☑4ᵗʰ **X98** **Assault by steam, hot vapors and hot objects**

The appropriate 7th character is to be added to each code from category X98.
- A   initial encounter
- D   subsequent encounter
- S   sequela

✓x7ᵗʰ **X98.0**   **Assault by steam or hot vapors**
✓x7ᵗʰ **X98.1**   **Assault by hot tap water**
✓x7ᵗʰ **X98.2**   **Assault by hot fluids**
✓x7ᵗʰ **X98.3**   **Assault by hot household appliances**
✓x7ᵗʰ **X98.8**   **Assault by other hot objects**
✓x7ᵗʰ **X98.9**   **Assault by unspecified hot objects**   ▽

☑4ᵗʰ **X99** **Assault by sharp object**
    EXCLUDES 1   assault by strike by sports equipment (Y08.0-)

The appropriate 7th character is to be added to each code from category X99.
- A   initial encounter
- D   subsequent encounter
- S   sequela

✓x7ᵗʰ **X99.0**   **Assault by sharp glass**
✓x7ᵗʰ **X99.1**   **Assault by knife**
✓x7ᵗʰ **X99.2**   **Assault by sword or dagger**
✓x7ᵗʰ **X99.8**   **Assault by other sharp object**
✓x7ᵗʰ **X99.9**   **Assault by unspecified sharp object**   ▽
      Assault by stabbing NOS

✓x7ᵗʰ **Y00** **Assault by blunt object**
    EXCLUDES 1   assault by strike by sports equipment (Y08.0-)

The appropriate 7th character is to be added to code Y00.
- A   initial encounter
- D   subsequent encounter
- S   sequela

✓x7ᵗʰ **Y01** **Assault by pushing from high place**

The appropriate 7th character is to be added to code Y01.
- A   initial encounter
- D   subsequent encounter
- S   sequela

☑4ᵗʰ **Y02** **Assault by pushing or placing victim in front of moving object**

The appropriate 7th character is to be added to each code from category Y02.
- A   initial encounter
- D   subsequent encounter
- S   sequela

✓x7ᵗʰ **Y02.0**   **Assault by pushing or placing victim in front of motor vehicle**
✓x7ᵗʰ **Y02.1**   **Assault by pushing or placing victim in front of (subway) train**
✓x7ᵗʰ **Y02.8**   **Assault by pushing or placing victim in front of other moving object**

☑4ᵗʰ **Y03** **Assault by crashing of motor vehicle**

The appropriate 7th character is to be added to each code from category Y03.
- A   initial encounter
- D   subsequent encounter
- S   sequela

✓x7ᵗʰ **Y03.0**   **Assault by being hit or run over by motor vehicle**
✓x7ᵗʰ **Y03.8**   **Other assault by crashing of motor vehicle**

☑4ᵗʰ **Y04** **Assault by bodily force**
    EXCLUDES 1   assault by:
               submersion (X92.-)
               use of weapon (X93-X95, X99, Y00)

The appropriate 7th character is to be added to each code from category Y04.
- A   initial encounter
- D   subsequent encounter
- S   sequela

✓x7ᵗʰ **Y04.0**   **Assault by unarmed brawl or fight**
✓x7ᵗʰ **Y04.1**   **Assault by human bite**
✓x7ᵗʰ **Y04.2**   **Assault by strike against or bumped into by another person**
✓x7ᵗʰ **Y04.8**   **Assault by other bodily force**
      Assault by bodily force NOS

Ⓝ Newborn   Ⓟ Pediatric   Ⓜ Maternity   Ⓐ Adult   **RIC** RIC Dx   **HCDx** Noncancer Dx   **PDx** Primary Dx   **CC** RIC CC Condition   ►◄ Revised Text   ● New Code   ▲ Revised Code Title

1098   ICD-10-CM 2016

✓4ᵗʰ Y07 Perpetrator of assault, maltreatment and neglect

NOTE   Codes from this category are for use only in cases of confirmed abuse (T74.-)

Selection of the correct perpetrator code is based on the relationship between the perpetrator and the victim

INCLUDES   perpetrator of abandonment
perpetrator of emotional neglect
perpetrator of mental cruelty
perpetrator of physical abuse
perpetrator of physical neglect
perpetrator of sexual abuse
perpetrator of torture

✓5ᵗʰ Y07.0 Spouse or partner, perpetrator of maltreatment and neglect

NOTE   Spouse or partner, perpetrator of maltreatment and neglect against spouse or partner

     Y07.01 Husband, perpetrator of maltreatment and neglect

     Y07.02 Wife, perpetrator of maltreatment and neglect

     Y07.03 Male partner, perpetrator of maltreatment and neglect

     Y07.04 Female partner, perpetrator of maltreatment and neglect

✓5ᵗʰ Y07.1 Parent (adoptive) (biological), perpetrator of maltreatment and neglect

     Y07.11 Biological father, perpetrator of maltreatment and neglect

     Y07.12 Biological mother, perpetrator of maltreatment and neglect

     Y07.13 Adoptive father, perpetrator of maltreatment and neglect

     Y07.14 Adoptive mother, perpetrator of maltreatment and neglect

✓5ᵗʰ Y07.4 Other family member, perpetrator of maltreatment and neglect

   ✓6ᵗʰ Y07.41 Sibling, perpetrator of maltreatment and neglect

      EXCLUDES 1   stepsibling, perpetrator of maltreatment and neglect (Y07.435, Y07.436)

      Y07.410 Brother, perpetrator of maltreatment and neglect

      Y07.411 Sister, perpetrator of maltreatment and neglect

   ✓6ᵗʰ Y07.42 Foster parent, perpetrator of maltreatment and neglect

      Y07.420 Foster father, perpetrator of maltreatment and neglect

      Y07.421 Foster mother, perpetrator of maltreatment and neglect

   ✓6ᵗʰ Y07.43 Stepparent or stepsibling, perpetrator of maltreatment and neglect

      Y07.430 Stepfather, perpetrator of maltreatment and neglect

      Y07.432 Male friend of parent (co-residing in household), perpetrator of maltreatment and neglect

      Y07.433 Stepmother, perpetrator of maltreatment and neglect

      Y07.434 Female friend of parent (co-residing in household), perpetrator of maltreatment and neglect

      Y07.435 Stepbrother, perpetrator or maltreatment and neglect

      Y07.436 Stepsister, perpetrator of maltreatment and neglect

   ✓6ᵗʰ Y07.49 Other family member, perpetrator of maltreatment and neglect

      Y07.490 Male cousin, perpetrator of maltreatment and neglect

      Y07.491 Female cousin, perpetrator of maltreatment and neglect

      Y07.499 Other family member, perpetrator of maltreatment and neglect

✓5ᵗʰ Y07.5 Non-family member, perpetrator of maltreatment and neglect

     Y07.50 Unspecified non-family member, perpetrator of maltreatment and neglect ▽

   ✓6ᵗʰ Y07.51 Daycare provider, perpetrator of maltreatment and neglect

      Y07.510 At-home childcare provider, perpetrator of maltreatment and neglect

      Y07.511 Daycare center childcare provider, perpetrator of maltreatment and neglect

      Y07.512 At-home adultcare provider, perpetrator of maltreatment and neglect

      Y07.513 Adultcare center provider, perpetrator of maltreatment and neglect

      Y07.519 Unspecified daycare provider, perpetrator of maltreatment and neglect ▽

   ✓6ᵗʰ Y07.52 Healthcare provider, perpetrator of maltreatment and neglect

      Y07.521 Mental health provider, perpetrator of maltreatment and neglect

      Y07.528 Other therapist or healthcare provider, perpetrator of maltreatment and neglect
        Nurse, perpetrator of maltreatment and neglect
        Occupational therapist, perpetrator of maltreatment and neglect
        Physical therapist, perpetrator of maltreatment and neglect
        Speech therapist, perpetrator of maltreatment and neglect

      Y07.529 Unspecified healthcare provider, perpetrator of maltreatment and neglect ▽

     Y07.53 Teacher or instructor, perpetrator of maltreatment and neglect
       Coach, perpetrator of maltreatment and neglect

     Y07.59 Other non-family member, perpetrator of maltreatment and neglect

   Y07.9 Unspecified perpetrator of maltreatment and neglect ▽

✓4ᵗʰ Y08 Assault by other specified means

The appropriate 7th character is to be added to each code from category Y08.
A   initial encounter
D   subsequent encounter
S   sequela

   ✓5ᵗʰ Y08.0 Assault by strike by sport equipment

     ✓x7ᵗʰ Y08.01 Assault by strike by hockey stick

     ✓x7ᵗʰ Y08.02 Assault by strike by baseball bat

     ✓x7ᵗʰ Y08.09 Assault by strike by other specified type of sport equipment

   ✓5ᵗʰ Y08.8 Assault by other specified means

     ✓x7ᵗʰ Y08.81 Assault by crashing of aircraft

     ✓x7ᵗʰ Y08.89 Assault by other specified means

Y09 Assault by unspecified means ▽
Assassination (attempted) NOS
Homicide (attempted) NOS
Manslaughter (attempted) NOS
Murder (attempted) NOS

Event of undetermined intent (Y21-Y33)

Undetermined intent is only for use when there is specific documentation in the record that the intent of the injury cannot be determined. If no such documentation is present, code to accidental (unintentional)

✓4ᵗʰ Y21 Drowning and submersion, undetermined intent

The appropriate 7th character is to be added to each code from category Y21.
A   initial encounter
D   subsequent encounter
S   sequela

   ✓x7ᵗʰ Y21.0 Drowning and submersion while in bathtub, undetermined intent

   ✓x7ᵗʰ Y21.1 Drowning and submersion after fall into bathtub, undetermined intent

✓ Add'l Character Required   ✓x7ᵗʰ Placeholder Alert   RUG IV Special Care High Dx   RUG IV Clinically Complex Dx   RUG IV Special Care Low Dx   Manifestation Code   Other Specified Code   ▽ Unspecified Code

ICD-10-CM 2016   1099

Chapter 20. External Causes of Morbidity

Y21.2–Y35.013

✓x7th **Y21.2** **Drowning and submersion** while in swimming pool, undetermined intent

✓x7th **Y21.3** **Drowning and submersion** after fall into swimming pool, undetermined intent

✓x7th **Y21.4** **Drowning and submersion** in natural water, **undetermined intent**

✓x7th **Y21.8** **Other drowning and submersion, undetermined intent**

✓x7th **Y21.9** **Unspecified drowning and submersion, undetermined intent** ▽

✓x7th **Y22** **Handgun discharge, undetermined intent**
Discharge of gun for single hand use, undetermined intent
Discharge of pistol, undetermined intent
Discharge of revolver, undetermined intent
EXCLUDES 2   Very pistol (Y24.8)

The appropriate 7th character is to be added to code Y22.
A   initial encounter
D   subsequent encounter
S   sequela

✓4th **Y23** **Rifle, shotgun and larger firearm discharge, undetermined intent**
EXCLUDES 2   airgun (Y24.0)

The appropriate 7th character is to be added to each code from category Y23.
A   initial encounter
D   subsequent encounter
S   sequela

✓x7th **Y23.0** Shotgun **discharge, undetermined intent**

✓x7th **Y23.1** Hunting rifle **discharge, undetermined intent**

✓x7th **Y23.2** Military firearm **discharge, undetermined intent**

✓x7th **Y23.3** Machine gun **discharge, undetermined intent**

✓x7th **Y23.8** **Other larger firearm discharge, undetermined intent**

✓x7th **Y23.9** **Unspecified larger firearm discharge, undetermined intent** ▽

✓4th **Y24** **Other and unspecified firearm discharge, undetermined intent**

The appropriate 7th character is to be added to each code from category Y24.
A   initial encounter
D   subsequent encounter
S   sequela

✓x7th **Y24.0** Airgun **discharge, undetermined intent**
BB gun discharge, undetermined intent
Pellet gun discharge, undetermined intent

✓x7th **Y24.8** **Other firearm discharge, undetermined intent**
Paintball gun discharge, undetermined intent
Very pistol [flare] discharge, undetermined intent

✓x7th **Y24.9** **Unspecified firearm discharge, undetermined intent** ▽

✓x7th **Y25** **Contact with explosive material, undetermined intent**

The appropriate 7th character is to be added to code Y25.
A   initial encounter
D   subsequent encounter
S   sequela

✓x7th **Y26** **Exposure to smoke, fire and flames, undetermined intent**

The appropriate 7th character is to be added to code Y26.
A   initial encounter
D   subsequent encounter
S   sequela

✓4th **Y27** **Contact with steam, hot vapors and hot objects, undetermined intent**

The appropriate 7th character is to be added to each code from category Y27.
A   initial encounter
D   subsequent encounter
S   sequela

✓x7th **Y27.0** **Contact with steam and hot** vapors, **undetermined intent**

✓x7th **Y27.1** **Contact with hot** tap water, **undetermined intent**

✓x7th **Y27.2** **Contact with hot** fluids, **undetermined intent**

✓x7th **Y27.3** **Contact with hot household** appliance, **undetermined intent**

✓x7th **Y27.8** **Contact with other hot objects, undetermined intent**

✓x7th **Y27.9** **Contact with unspecified hot objects, undetermined intent** ▽

Y28 **Contact with sharp object, undetermined intent**

The appropriate 7th character is to be added to each code from category Y28.
A   initial encounter
D   subsequent encounter
S   sequela

✓x7th **Y28.0** **Contact with sharp** glass, **undetermined intent**

✓x7th **Y28.1** **Contact with** knife, **undetermined intent**

✓x7th **Y28.2** **Contact with** sword or dagger, **undetermined intent**

✓x7th **Y28.8** **Contact with other sharp object, undetermined intent**

✓x7th **Y28.9** **Contact with unspecified hot objects, undetermined intent** ▽

✓x7th **Y29** **Contact with blunt object, undetermined intent**

The appropriate 7th character is to be added to code Y29.
A   initial encounter
D   subsequent encounter
S   sequela

✓x7th **Y30** **Falling, jumping or pushed from a high place, undetermined intent**
Victim falling from one level to another, undetermined intent

The appropriate 7th character is to be added to code Y30.
A   initial encounter
D   subsequent encounter
S   sequela

✓x7th **Y31** **Falling, lying or running before or into moving object, undetermined intent**

The appropriate 7th character is to be added to code Y31.
A   initial encounter
D   subsequent encounter
S   sequela

✓x7th **Y32** **Crashing of motor vehicle, undetermined intent**

The appropriate 7th character is to be added to code Y32.
A   initial encounter
D   subsequent encounter
S   sequela

✓x7th **Y33** **Other specified events, undetermined intent**

The appropriate 7th character is to be added to code Y33.
A   initial encounter
D   subsequent encounter
S   sequela

Legal intervention, operations of war, military operations, and terrorism (Y35-Y38)

✓4th **Y35** **Legal intervention**
INCLUDES   any injury sustained as a result of an encounter with any law enforcement official, serving in any capacity at the time of the encounter, whether on-duty or off-duty. Includes: injury to law enforcement official, suspect and bystander

✓5th **Y35.0** **Legal intervention involving** firearm discharge

✓6th **Y35.00** **Legal intervention involving** unspecified **firearm discharge**
Legal intervention involving gunshot wound
Legal intervention involving shot NOS

✓7th **Y35.001** **Legal intervention involving unspecified firearm discharge,** law enforcement **official injured** ▽

✓7th **Y35.002** **Legal intervention involving unspecified firearm discharge,** bystander **injured** ▽

✓7th **Y35.003** **Legal intervention involving unspecified firearm discharge,** suspect **injured** ▽

✓6th **Y35.01** **Legal intervention involving injury by** machine gun

✓7th **Y35.011** **Legal intervention involving injury by machine gun,** law enforcement **official injured**

✓7th **Y35.012** **Legal intervention involving injury by machine gun,** bystander **injured**

✓7th **Y35.013** **Legal intervention involving injury by machine gun,** suspect **injured**

N Newborn   P Pediatric   M Maternity   A Adult   **RIC** RIC Dx   **NCDx** Noncancer Dx   **PDx** Primary Dx   **CC** RIC CC Condition   ▶◀ Revised Text   ● New Code   ▲ Revised Code Title

✓6ᵗʰ **Y35.02** Legal intervention involving injury by handgun

   ✓7ᵗʰ **Y35.021** Legal intervention involving injury by handgun, law enforcement official injured

   ✓7ᵗʰ **Y35.022** Legal intervention involving injury by handgun, bystander injured

   ✓7ᵗʰ **Y35.023** Legal intervention involving injury by handgun, suspect injured

✓6ᵗʰ **Y35.03** Legal intervention involving injury by rifle pellet

   ✓7ᵗʰ **Y35.031** Legal intervention involving injury by rifle pellet, law enforcement official injured

   ✓7ᵗʰ **Y35.032** Legal intervention involving injury by rifle pellet, bystander injured

   ✓7ᵗʰ **Y35.033** Legal intervention involving injury by rifle pellet, suspect injured

✓6ᵗʰ **Y35.04** Legal intervention involving injury by rubber bullet

   ✓7ᵗʰ **Y35.041** Legal intervention involving injury by rubber bullet, law enforcement official injured

   ✓7ᵗʰ **Y35.042** Legal intervention involving injury by rubber bullet, bystander injured

   ✓7ᵗʰ **Y35.043** Legal intervention involving injury by rubber bullet, suspect injured

✓6ᵗʰ **Y35.09** Legal intervention involving other firearm discharge

   ✓7ᵗʰ **Y35.091** Legal intervention involving other firearm discharge, law enforcement official injured

   ✓7ᵗʰ **Y35.092** Legal intervention involving other firearm discharge, bystander injured

   ✓7ᵗʰ **Y35.093** Legal intervention involving other firearm discharge, suspect injured

✓5ᵗʰ **Y35.1** Legal intervention involving explosives

  ✓6ᵗʰ **Y35.10** Legal intervention involving unspecified explosives

   ✓7ᵗʰ **Y35.101** Legal intervention involving unspecified explosives, law enforcement official injured ▽

   ✓7ᵗʰ **Y35.102** Legal intervention involving unspecified explosives, bystander injured ▽

   ✓7ᵗʰ **Y35.103** Legal intervention involving unspecified explosives, suspect injured ▽

  ✓6ᵗʰ **Y35.11** Legal intervention involving injury by dynamite

   ✓7ᵗʰ **Y35.111** Legal intervention involving injury by dynamite, law enforcement official injured

   ✓7ᵗʰ **Y35.112** Legal intervention involving injury by dynamite, bystander injured

   ✓7ᵗʰ **Y35.113** Legal intervention involving injury by dynamite, suspect injured

  ✓6ᵗʰ **Y35.12** Legal intervention involving injury by explosive shell

   ✓7ᵗʰ **Y35.121** Legal intervention involving injury by explosive shell, law enforcement official injured

   ✓7ᵗʰ **Y35.122** Legal intervention involving injury by explosive shell, bystander injured

   ✓7ᵗʰ **Y35.123** Legal intervention involving injury by explosive shell, suspect injured

  ✓6ᵗʰ **Y35.19** Legal intervention involving other explosives
        Legal intervention involving injury by grenade
        Legal intervention involving injury by mortar bomb

   ✓7ᵗʰ **Y35.191** Legal intervention involving other explosives, law enforcement official injured

   ✓7ᵗʰ **Y35.192** Legal intervention involving other explosives, bystander injured

   ✓7ᵗʰ **Y35.193** Legal intervention involving other explosives, suspect injured

✓5ᵗʰ **Y35.2** Legal intervention involving gas
     Legal intervention involving asphyxiation by gas
     Legal intervention involving poisoning by gas

  ✓6ᵗʰ **Y35.20** Legal intervention involving unspecified gas

   ✓7ᵗʰ **Y35.201** Legal intervention involving unspecified gas, law enforcement official injured ▽

   ✓7ᵗʰ **Y35.202** Legal intervention involving unspecified gas, bystander injured ▽

   ✓7ᵗʰ **Y35.203** Legal intervention involving unspecified gas, suspect injured ▽

  ✓6ᵗʰ **Y35.21** Legal intervention involving injury by tear gas

   ✓7ᵗʰ **Y35.211** Legal intervention involving injury by tear gas, law enforcement official injured

   ✓7ᵗʰ **Y35.212** Legal intervention involving injury by tear gas, bystander injured

   ✓7ᵗʰ **Y35.213** Legal intervention involving injury by tear gas, suspect injured

  ✓6ᵗʰ **Y35.29** Legal intervention involving other gas

   ✓7ᵗʰ **Y35.291** Legal intervention involving other gas, law enforcement official injured

   ✓7ᵗʰ **Y35.292** Legal intervention involving other gas, bystander injured

   ✓7ᵗʰ **Y35.293** Legal intervention involving other gas, suspect injured

✓5ᵗʰ **Y35.3** Legal intervention involving blunt objects
     Legal intervention involving being hit or struck by blunt object

  ✓6ᵗʰ **Y35.30** Legal intervention involving unspecified blunt objects

   ✓7ᵗʰ **Y35.301** Legal intervention involving unspecified blunt objects, law enforcement official injured ▽

   ✓7ᵗʰ **Y35.302** Legal intervention involving unspecified blunt objects, bystander injured ▽

   ✓7ᵗʰ **Y35.303** Legal intervention involving unspecified blunt objects, suspect injured ▽

  ✓6ᵗʰ **Y35.31** Legal intervention involving baton

   ✓7ᵗʰ **Y35.311** Legal intervention involving baton, law enforcement official injured

   ✓7ᵗʰ **Y35.312** Legal intervention involving baton, bystander injured

   ✓7ᵗʰ **Y35.313** Legal intervention involving baton, suspect injured

  ✓6ᵗʰ **Y35.39** Legal intervention involving other blunt objects

   ✓7ᵗʰ **Y35.391** Legal intervention involving other blunt objects, law enforcement official injured

   ✓7ᵗʰ **Y35.392** Legal intervention involving other blunt objects, bystander injured

   ✓7ᵗʰ **Y35.393** Legal intervention involving other blunt objects, suspect injured

✓5ᵗʰ **Y35.4** Legal intervention involving sharp objects
     Legal intervention involving being cut by sharp objects
     Legal intervention involving being stabbed by sharp objects

  ✓6ᵗʰ **Y35.40** Legal intervention involving unspecified sharp objects

   ✓7ᵗʰ **Y35.401** Legal intervention involving unspecified sharp objects, law enforcement official injured ▽

   ✓7ᵗʰ **Y35.402** Legal intervention involving unspecified sharp objects, bystander injured ▽

   ✓7ᵗʰ **Y35.403** Legal intervention involving unspecified sharp objects, suspect injured ▽

  ✓6ᵗʰ **Y35.41** Legal intervention involving bayonet

   ✓7ᵗʰ **Y35.411** Legal intervention involving bayonet, law enforcement official injured

   ✓7ᵗʰ **Y35.412** Legal intervention involving bayonet, bystander injured

   ✓7ᵗʰ **Y35.413** Legal intervention involving bayonet, suspect injured

  ✓6ᵗʰ **Y35.49** Legal intervention involving other sharp objects

   ✓7ᵗʰ **Y35.491** Legal intervention involving other sharp objects, law enforcement official injured

   ✓7ᵗʰ **Y35.492** Legal intervention involving other sharp objects, bystander injured

   ✓7ᵗʰ **Y35.493** Legal intervention involving other sharp objects, suspect injured

---

✓5th Y35.8 Legal intervention involving other specified means

✓6th Y35.81 Legal intervention involving manhandling

✓7th Y35.811 Legal intervention involving manhandling, law enforcement **official injured**

✓7th Y35.812 Legal intervention involving manhandling, bystander **injured**

✓7th Y35.813 Legal intervention involving manhandling, suspect **injured**

✓6th Y35.89 Legal intervention involving other specified means

✓7th Y35.891 Legal intervention involving other specified means, law enforcement **official injured**

✓7th Y35.892 Legal intervention involving other specified means, bystander **injured**

✓7th Y35.893 Legal intervention involving other specified means, suspect **injured**

✓5th Y35.9 Legal intervention, means unspecified

✓x7th Y35.91 Legal intervention, means unspecified, law enforcement **official injured** ▽

✓x7th Y35.92 Legal intervention, means unspecified, bystander **injured** ▽

✓x7th Y35.93 Legal intervention, means unspecified, suspect **injured** ▽

✓4th Y36 Operations of war

INCLUDES injuries to military personnel and civilians caused by war, civil insurrection, and peacekeeping missions

EXCLUDES 1 *injury to military personnel occurring during peacetime military operations (Y37.-)*
military vehicles involved in transport accidents with non-military vehicle during peacetime (V09.01, V09.21, V19.81, V29.81, V39.81, V49.81, V59.81, V69.81, V79.81)

AHA: 2014, 3Q, 4

The appropriate 7th character is to be added to each code from category Y36.
A   initial encounter
D   subsequent encounter
S   sequela

✓5th Y36.0 War operations involving explosion of marine weapons

✓6th Y36.00 War operations involving explosion of unspecified **marine weapon**

War operations involving underwater blast NOS

✓7th Y36.000 War operations involving explosion of unspecified marine weapon, military **personnel** ▽

✓7th Y36.001 War operations involving explosion of unspecified marine weapon, civilian ▽

✓6th Y36.01 War operations involving explosion of depth-charge

✓7th Y36.010 War operations involving explosion of depth-charge, military personnel

✓7th Y36.011 War operations involving explosion of depth-charge, civilian

✓6th Y36.02 War operations involving explosion of marine mine

War operations involving explosion of marine mine, at sea or in harbor

✓7th Y36.020 War operations involving explosion of marine mine, military personnel

✓7th Y36.021 War operations involving explosion of marine mine, civilian

✓6th Y36.03 War operations involving explosion of sea-based artillery shell

✓7th Y36.030 War operations involving explosion of sea-based artillery shell, military personnel

✓7th Y36.031 War operations involving explosion of sea-based artillery shell, civilian

✓6th Y36.04 War operations involving explosion of torpedo

✓7th Y36.040 War operations involving explosion of torpedo, military personnel

✓7th Y36.041 War operations involving explosion of torpedo, civilian

✓6th Y36.05 War operations involving accidental detonation of onboard marine weapons

✓7th Y36.050 War operations involving accidental detonation of onboard marine weapons, military personnel

✓7th Y36.051 War operations involving accidental detonation of onboard marine weapons, civilian

✓6th Y36.09 War operations involving explosion of other marine weapons

✓7th Y36.090 War operations involving explosion of other marine weapons, military personnel

✓7th Y36.091 War operations involving explosion of other marine weapons, civilian

✓5th Y36.1 War operations involving destruction of aircraft

✓6th Y36.10 War operations involving unspecified **destruction of aircraft**

✓7th Y36.100 War operations involving unspecified destruction of aircraft, military personnel ▽

✓7th Y36.101 War operations involving unspecified destruction of aircraft, civilian ▽

✓6th Y36.11 War operations involving destruction of aircraft due to enemy fire or explosives

War operations involving destruction of aircraft due to air to air missile

War operations involving destruction of aircraft due to explosive placed on aircraft

War operations involving destruction of aircraft due to rocket propelled grenade [RPG]

War operations involving destruction of aircraft due to small arms fire

War operations involving destruction of aircraft due to surface to air missile

✓7th Y36.110 War operations involving destruction of aircraft due to enemy fire or explosives, military personnel

✓7th Y36.111 War operations involving destruction of aircraft due to enemy fire or explosives, civilian

✓6th Y36.12 War operations involving destruction of aircraft due to collision with other aircraft

✓7th Y36.120 War operations involving destruction of aircraft due to collision with other aircraft, military personnel

✓7th Y36.121 War operations involving destruction of aircraft due to collision with other aircraft, civilian

✓6th Y36.13 War operations involving destruction of aircraft due to onboard fire

✓7th Y36.130 War operations involving destruction of aircraft due to onboard fire, military personnel

✓7th Y36.131 War operations involving destruction of aircraft due to onboard fire, civilian

✓6th Y36.14 War operations involving destruction of aircraft due to accidental detonation of onboard munitions and explosives

✓7th Y36.140 War operations involving destruction of aircraft due to accidental detonation of onboard munitions and explosives, military personnel

✓7th Y36.141 War operations involving destruction of aircraft due to accidental detonation of onboard munitions and explosives, civilian

✓6th Y36.19 War operations involving other destruction of aircraft

✓7th Y36.190 War operations involving other destruction of aircraft, military personnel

✓7th Y36.191 War operations involving other destruction of aircraft, civilian

N Newborn   P Pediatric   M Maternity   A Adult   RIC RIC Dx   NCDx Noncancer Dx   PDx Primary Dx   CC RIC CC Condition   ►◄ Revised Text   ● New Code   ▲ Revised Code Title

1102   ICD-10-CM 2016

✓5ᵗʰ Y36.2 War operations involving other explosions and fragments

> *EXCLUDES 1*   *war operations involving explosion of aircraft (Y36.1-)*
> *war operations involving explosion of marine weapons (Y36.0-)*
> *war operations involving explosion of nuclear weapons (Y36.5-)*
> *war operations involving explosion occurring after cessation of hostilities (Y36.8-)*

✓6ᵗʰ Y36.20 War operations involving unspecified explosion and fragments
War operations involving air blast NOS
War operations involving blast NOS
War operations involving blast fragments NOS
War operations involving blast wave NOS
War operations involving blast wind NOS
War operations involving explosion NOS
War operations involving explosion of bomb NOS

    ✓7ᵗʰ Y36.200 War operations involving unspecified explosion and fragments, military personnel ▽

    ✓7ᵗʰ Y36.201 War operations involving unspecified explosion and fragments, civilian ▽

✓6ᵗʰ Y36.21 War operations involving explosion of aerial bomb

    ✓7ᵗʰ Y36.210 War operations involving explosion of aerial bomb, military personnel

    ✓7ᵗʰ Y36.211 War operations involving explosion of aerial bomb, civilian

✓6ᵗʰ Y36.22 War operations involving explosion of guided missile

    ✓7ᵗʰ Y36.220 War operations involving explosion of guided missile, military personnel

    ✓7ᵗʰ Y36.221 War operations involving explosion of guided missile, civilian

✓6ᵗʰ Y36.23 War operations involving explosion of improvised explosive device [IED]
War operations involving explosion of person-borne improvised explosive device [IED]
War operations involving explosion of vehicle-borne improvised explosive device [IED]
War operations involving explosion of roadside improvised explosive device [IED]

    ✓7ᵗʰ Y36.230 War operations involving explosion of improvised explosive device [IED], military personnel

    ✓7ᵗʰ Y36.231 War operations involving explosion of improvised explosive device [IED], civilian

✓6ᵗʰ Y36.24 War operations involving explosion due to accidental detonation and discharge of own munitions or munitions launch device

    ✓7ᵗʰ Y36.240 War operations involving explosion due to accidental detonation and discharge of own munitions or munitions launch device, military personnel

    ✓7ᵗʰ Y36.241 War operations involving explosion due to accidental detonation and discharge of own munitions or munitions launch device, civilian

✓6ᵗʰ Y36.25 War operations involving fragments from munitions

    ✓7ᵗʰ Y36.250 War operations involving fragments from munitions, military personnel

    ✓7ᵗʰ Y36.251 War operations involving fragments from munitions, civilian

✓6ᵗʰ Y36.26 War operations involving fragments of improvised explosive device [IED]
War operations involving fragments of person-borne improvised explosive device [IED]
War operations involving fragments of vehicle-borne improvised explosive device [IED]
War operations involving fragments of roadside improvised explosive device [IED]

    ✓7ᵗʰ Y36.260 War operations involving fragments of improvised explosive device [IED], military personnel

    ✓7ᵗʰ Y36.261 War operations involving fragments of improvised explosive device [IED], civilian

✓6ᵗʰ Y36.27 War operations involving fragments from weapons

    ✓7ᵗʰ Y36.270 War operations involving fragments from weapons, military personnel

    ✓7ᵗʰ Y36.271 War operations involving fragments from weapons, civilian

✓6ᵗʰ Y36.29 War operations involving other explosions and fragments
War operations involving explosion of grenade
War operations involving explosions of land mine
War operations involving shrapnel NOS

    ✓7ᵗʰ Y36.290 War operations involving other explosions and fragments, military personnel

    ✓7ᵗʰ Y36.291 War operations involving other explosions and fragments, civilian

✓5ᵗʰ Y36.3 War operations involving fires, conflagrations and hot substances
War operations involving smoke, fumes, and heat from fires, conflagrations and hot substances

> *EXCLUDES 1*   *war operations involving fires and conflagrations aboard military aircraft (Y36.1-)*
> *war operations involving fires and conflagrations aboard military watercraft (Y36.0-)*
> *war operations involving fires and conflagrations caused indirectly by conventional weapons (Y36.2-)*
> *war operations involving fires and thermal effects of nuclear weapons (Y36.53-)*

✓6ᵗʰ Y36.30 War operations involving unspecified fire, conflagration and hot substance

    ✓7ᵗʰ Y36.300 War operations involving unspecified fire, conflagration and hot substance, military personnel ▽

    ✓7ᵗʰ Y36.301 War operations involving unspecified fire, conflagration and hot substance, civilian ▽

✓6ᵗʰ Y36.31 War operations involving gasoline bomb
War operations involving incendiary bomb
War operations involving petrol bomb

    ✓7ᵗʰ Y36.310 War operations involving gasoline bomb, military personnel

    ✓7ᵗʰ Y36.311 War operations involving gasoline bomb, civilian

✓6ᵗʰ Y36.32 War operations involving incendiary bullet

    ✓7ᵗʰ Y36.320 War operations involving incendiary bullet, military personnel

    ✓7ᵗʰ Y36.321 War operations involving incendiary bullet, civilian

✓6ᵗʰ Y36.33 War operations involving flamethrower

    ✓7ᵗʰ Y36.330 War operations involving flamethrower, military personnel

    ✓7ᵗʰ Y36.331 War operations involving flamethrower, civilian

✓6ᵗʰ Y36.39 War operations involving other fires, conflagrations and hot substances

    ✓7ᵗʰ Y36.390 War operations involving other fires, conflagrations and hot substances, military personnel

    ✓7ᵗʰ Y36.391 War operations involving other fires, conflagrations and hot substances, civilian

✓5ᵗʰ Y36.4 War operations involving firearm discharge and other forms of conventional warfare

✓6ᵗʰ Y36.41 War operations involving rubber bullets

    ✓7ᵗʰ Y36.410 War operations involving rubber bullets, military personnel

    ✓7ᵗʰ Y36.411 War operations involving rubber bullets, civilian

✓6ᵗʰ Y36.42 War operations involving firearms pellets

    ✓7ᵗʰ Y36.420 War operations involving firearms pellets, military personnel

    ✓7ᵗʰ Y36.421 War operations involving firearms pellets, civilian

✓6ᵗʰ Y36.43 War operations involving other firearms discharge
War operations involving bullets NOS

> *EXCLUDES 1*   *war operations involving munitions fragments (Y36.25-)*
> *war operations involving incendiary bullets (Y36.32-)*

    ✓7ᵗʰ Y36.430 War operations involving other firearms discharge, military personnel

---

✓7th **Y36.431** **War operations involving other firearms discharge, civilian**

✓6th **Y36.44** **War operations involving** unarmed hand to hand combat

EXCLUDES 1 *war operations involving combat using blunt or piercing object (Y36.45-)*
war operations involving intentional restriction of air and airway (Y36.46-)
war operations involving unintentional restriction of air and airway (Y36.47-)

✓7th **Y36.440** **War operations involving unarmed hand to hand combat, military personnel**

✓7th **Y36.441** **War operations involving unarmed hand to hand combat, civilian**

✓6th **Y36.45** **War operations involving combat using blunt or** piercing object

✓7th **Y36.450** **War operations involving combat using blunt or piercing object, military personnel**

✓7th **Y36.451** **War operations involving combat using blunt or piercing object, civilian**

✓6th **Y36.46** **War operations involving** intentional restriction of air and airway

✓7th **Y36.460** **War operations involving intentional restriction of air and airway, military personnel**

✓7th **Y36.461** **War operations involving intentional restriction of air and airway, civilian**

✓6th **Y36.47** **War operations involving** unintentional restriction of air and airway

✓7th **Y36.470** **War operations involving unintentional restriction of air and airway, military personnel**

✓7th **Y36.471** **War operations involving unintentional restriction of air and airway, civilian**

✓6th **Y36.49** **War operations involving** other forms of conventional warfare

✓7th **Y36.490** **War operations involving other forms of conventional warfare, military personnel**

✓7th **Y36.491** **War operations involving other forms of conventional warfare, civilian**

✓5th **Y36.5** **War operations involving** nuclear weapons
War operations involving dirty bomb NOS

✓6th **Y36.50** **War operations involving** unspecified effect of nuclear weapon

✓7th **Y36.500** **War operations involving unspecified effect of nuclear weapon, military personnel** ▽

✓7th **Y36.501** **War operations involving unspecified effect of nuclear weapon, civilian** ▽

✓6th **Y36.51** **War operations involving** direct blast effect of nuclear weapon
War operations involving blast pressure of nuclear weapon

✓7th **Y36.510** **War operations involving direct blast effect of nuclear weapon, military personnel**

✓7th **Y36.511** **War operations involving direct blast effect of nuclear weapon, civilian**

✓6th **Y36.52** **War operations involving** indirect blast effect of nuclear weapon
War operations involving being thrown by blast of nuclear weapon
War operations involving being struck or crushed by blast debris of nuclear weapon

✓7th **Y36.520** **War operations involving indirect blast effect of nuclear weapon, military personnel**

✓7th **Y36.521** **War operations involving indirect blast effect of nuclear weapon, civilian**

✓6th **Y36.53** **War operations involving** thermal radiation **effect of** nuclear weapon
War operations involving direct heat from nuclear weapon
War operation involving fireball effects from nuclear weapon

✓7th **Y36.530** **War operations involving thermal radiation effect of nuclear weapon, military personnel**

✓7th **Y36.531** **War operations involving thermal radiation effect of nuclear weapon, civilian**

✓6th **Y36.54** **War operation involving** nuclear radiation **effects of** nuclear weapon
War operation involving acute radiation exposure from nuclear weapon
War operation involving exposure to immediate ionizing radiation from nuclear weapon
War operation involving fallout exposure from nuclear weapon
War operation involving secondary effects of nuclear weapons

✓7th **Y36.540** **War operation involving nuclear radiation effects of nuclear weapon, military personnel**

✓7th **Y36.541** **War operation involving nuclear radiation effects of nuclear weapon, civilian**

✓6th **Y36.59** **War operation involving** other effects of nuclear weapons

✓7th **Y36.590** **War operation involving other effects of nuclear weapons, military personnel**

✓7th **Y36.591** **War operation involving other effects of nuclear weapons, civilian**

✓5th **Y36.6** **War operations involving biological weapons**

✓6th **Y36.6X** **War operations involving** biological weapons

✓7th **Y36.6X0** **War operations involving biological weapons, military personnel**

✓7th **Y36.6X1** **War operations involving biological weapons, civilian**

✓5th **Y36.7** **War operations involving chemical weapons and other forms of unconventional warfare**

EXCLUDES 1 *war operations involving incendiary devices (Y36.3-, Y36.5-)*

✓6th **Y36.7X** **War operations involving** chemical weapons **and** other **forms of** unconventional warfare

✓7th **Y36.7X0** **War operations involving chemical weapons and other forms of unconventional warfare, military personnel**

✓7th **Y36.7X1** **War operations involving chemical weapons and other forms of unconventional warfare, civilian**

✓5th **Y36.8** **War operations occurring** after cessation of hostilities
War operations classifiable to categories Y36.0-Y36.8 but occurring after cessation of hostilities

✓6th **Y36.81** **Explosion of** mine placed during war operations but exploding after cessation of hostilities

✓7th **Y36.810** **Explosion of mine placed during war operations but exploding after cessation of hostilities, military personnel**

✓7th **Y36.811** **Explosion of mine placed during war operations but exploding after cessation of hostilities, civilian**

✓6th **Y36.82** **Explosion of** bomb placed during war operations but exploding after cessation of hostilities

✓7th **Y36.820** **Explosion of bomb placed during war operations but exploding after cessation of hostilities, military personnel**

✓7th **Y36.821** **Explosion of bomb placed during war operations but exploding after cessation of hostilities, civilian**

✓6th **Y36.88** Other **war operations occurring after cessation of** hostilities

✓7th **Y36.880** **Other war operations occurring after cessation of hostilities, military personnel**

✓7th **Y36.881** **Other war operations occurring after cessation of hostilities, civilian**

☑6ᵗʰ **Y36.89** Unspecified war operations occurring after cessation of hostilities

    ☑7ᵗʰ **Y36.890** Unspecified war operations occurring after cessation of hostilities, military personnel ▽

    ☑7ᵗʰ **Y36.891** Unspecified war operations occurring after cessation of hostilities, civilian ▽

☑5ᵗʰ **Y36.9 Other and unspecified war operations**

    ☑x7ᵗʰ **Y36.90** War operations, unspecified ▽

    ☑x7ᵗʰ **Y36.91** War operations involving unspecified weapon of mass destruction [WMD] ▽

    ☑x7ᵗʰ **Y36.92** War operations involving friendly fire

☑4ᵗʰ **Y37 Military operations**

    INCLUDES   injuries to military personnel and civilians occurring during peacetime on military property and during routine military exercises and operations

    EXCLUDES 1   military aircraft involved in aircraft accident with civilian aircraft (V97.81-)
         military vehicles involved in transport accident with civilian vehicle (V09.01, V09.21, V19.81, V29.81, V39.81, V49.81, V59.81, V69.81, V79.81)
         military watercraft involved in water transport accident with civilian watercraft (V94.81-)
         war operations (Y36.-)

> The appropriate 7th character is to be added to each code from category Y37.
> A   initial encounter
> D   subsequent encounter
> S   sequela

☑5ᵗʰ **Y37.0 Military operations involving explosion of marine weapons**

    ☑6ᵗʰ **Y37.00 Military operations involving explosion of unspecified marine weapon**
         Military operations involving underwater blast NOS

        ☑7ᵗʰ **Y37.000** Military operations involving explosion of unspecified marine weapon, military personnel ▽

        ☑7ᵗʰ **Y37.001** Military operations involving explosion of unspecified marine weapon, civilian ▽

    ☑6ᵗʰ **Y37.01 Military operations involving explosion of depth-charge**

        ☑7ᵗʰ **Y37.010** Military operations involving explosion of depth-charge, military personnel

        ☑7ᵗʰ **Y37.011** Military operations involving explosion of depth-charge, civilian

    ☑6ᵗʰ **Y37.02 Military operations involving explosion of marine mine**
         Military operations involving explosion of marine mine, at sea or in harbor

        ☑7ᵗʰ **Y37.020** Military operations involving explosion of marine mine, military personnel

        ☑7ᵗʰ **Y37.021** Military operations involving explosion of marine mine, civilian

    ☑6ᵗʰ **Y37.03 Military operations involving explosion of sea-based artillery shell**

        ☑7ᵗʰ **Y37.030** Military operations involving explosion of sea-based artillery shell, military personnel

        ☑7ᵗʰ **Y37.031** Military operations involving explosion of sea-based artillery shell, civilian

    ☑6ᵗʰ **Y37.04 Military operations involving explosion of torpedo**

        ☑7ᵗʰ **Y37.040** Military operations involving explosion of torpedo, military personnel

        ☑7ᵗʰ **Y37.041** Military operations involving explosion of torpedo, civilian

    ☑6ᵗʰ **Y37.05 Military operations involving accidental detonation of onboard marine weapons**

        ☑7ᵗʰ **Y37.050** Military operations involving accidental detonation of onboard marine weapons, military personnel

        ☑7ᵗʰ **Y37.051** Military operations involving accidental detonation of onboard marine weapons, civilian

    ☑6ᵗʰ **Y37.09 Military operations involving explosion of other marine weapons**

        ☑7ᵗʰ **Y37.090** Military operations involving explosion of other marine weapons, military personnel

        ☑7ᵗʰ **Y37.091** Military operations involving explosion of other marine weapons, civilian

☑5ᵗʰ **Y37.1 Military operations involving destruction of aircraft**

    ☑6ᵗʰ **Y37.10 Military operations involving unspecified destruction of aircraft**

        ☑7ᵗʰ **Y37.100** Military operations involving unspecified destruction of aircraft, military personnel ▽

        ☑7ᵗʰ **Y37.101** Military operations involving unspecified destruction of aircraft, civilian ▽

    ☑6ᵗʰ **Y37.11 Military operations involving destruction of aircraft due to enemy fire or explosives**
         Military operations involving destruction of aircraft due to air to air missile
         Military operations involving destruction of aircraft due to explosive placed on aircraft
         Military operations involving destruction of aircraft due to rocket propelled grenade [RPG]
         Military operations involving destruction of aircraft due to small arms fire
         Military operations involving destruction of aircraft due to surface to air missile

        ☑7ᵗʰ **Y37.110** Military operations involving destruction of aircraft due to enemy fire or explosives, military personnel

        ☑7ᵗʰ **Y37.111** Military operations involving destruction of aircraft due to enemy fire or explosives, civilian

    ☑6ᵗʰ **Y37.12 Military operations involving destruction of aircraft due to collision with other aircraft**

        ☑7ᵗʰ **Y37.120** Military operations involving destruction of aircraft due to collision with other aircraft, military personnel

        ☑7ᵗʰ **Y37.121** Military operations involving destruction of aircraft due to collision with other aircraft, civilian

    ☑6ᵗʰ **Y37.13 Military operations involving destruction of aircraft due to onboard fire**

        ☑7ᵗʰ **Y37.130** Military operations involving destruction of aircraft due to onboard fire, military personnel

        ☑7ᵗʰ **Y37.131** Military operations involving destruction of aircraft due to onboard fire, civilian

    ☑6ᵗʰ **Y37.14 Military operations involving destruction of aircraft due to accidental detonation of onboard munitions and explosives**

        ☑7ᵗʰ **Y37.140** Military operations involving destruction of aircraft due to accidental detonation of onboard munitions and explosives, military personnel

        ☑7ᵗʰ **Y37.141** Military operations involving destruction of aircraft due to accidental detonation of onboard munitions and explosives, civilian

    ☑6ᵗʰ **Y37.19 Military operations involving other destruction of aircraft**

        ☑7ᵗʰ **Y37.190** Military operations involving other destruction of aircraft, military personnel

        ☑7ᵗʰ **Y37.191** Military operations involving other destruction of aircraft, civilian

☑5ᵗʰ **Y37.2 Military operations involving other explosions and fragments**

    EXCLUDES 1   military operations involving explosion of aircraft (Y37.1-)
         military operations involving explosion of marine weapons (Y37.0-)
         military operations involving explosion of nuclear weapons (Y37.5-)

    ☑6ᵗʰ **Y37.20 Military operations involving unspecified explosion and fragments**
         Military operations involving air blast NOS
         Military operations involving blast NOS
         Military operations involving blast fragments NOS
         Military operations involving blast wave NOS
         Military operations involving blast wind NOS
         Military operations involving explosion NOS
         Military operations involving explosion of bomb NOS

        ☑7ᵗʰ **Y37.200** Military operations involving unspecified explosion and fragments, military personnel ▽

✓7ᵗʰ **Y37.201** **Military operations involving unspecified explosion and fragments, civilian** ▽

✓6ᵗʰ **Y37.21** **Military operations involving explosion of aerial bomb**

✓7ᵗʰ **Y37.210** **Military operations involving explosion of aerial bomb, military personnel**

✓7ᵗʰ **Y37.211** **Military operations involving explosion of aerial bomb, civilian**

✓6ᵗʰ **Y37.22** **Military operations involving explosion of guided missile**

✓7ᵗʰ **Y37.220** **Military operations involving explosion of guided missile, military personnel**

✓7ᵗʰ **Y37.221** **Military operations involving explosion of guided missile, civilian**

✓6ᵗʰ **Y37.23** **Military operations involving explosion of improvised explosive device [IED]**
Military operations involving explosion of person-borne improvised explosive device [IED]
Military operations involving explosion of vehicle-borne improvised explosive device [IED]
Military operations involving explosion of roadside improvised explosive device [IED]

✓7ᵗʰ **Y37.230** **Military operations involving explosion of improvised explosive device [IED], military personnel**

✓7ᵗʰ **Y37.231** **Military operations involving explosion of improvised explosive device [IED], civilian**

✓6ᵗʰ **Y37.24** **Military operations involving explosion due to accidental detonation and discharge of own munitions or munitions launch device**

✓7ᵗʰ **Y37.240** **Military operations involving explosion due to accidental detonation and discharge of own munitions or munitions launch device, military personnel**

✓7ᵗʰ **Y37.241** **Military operations involving explosion due to accidental detonation and discharge of own munitions or munitions launch device, civilian**

✓6ᵗʰ **Y37.25** **Military operations involving fragments from munitions**

✓7ᵗʰ **Y37.250** **Military operations involving fragments from munitions, military personnel**

✓7ᵗʰ **Y37.251** **Military operations involving fragments from munitions, civilian**

✓6ᵗʰ **Y37.26** **Military operations involving fragments of improvised explosive device [IED]**
Military operations involving fragments of person-borne improvised explosive device [IED]
Military operations involving fragments of vehicle-borne improvised explosive device [IED]
Military operations involving fragments of roadside improvised explosive device [IED]

✓7ᵗʰ **Y37.260** **Military operations involving fragments of improvised explosive device [IED], military personnel**

✓7ᵗʰ **Y37.261** **Military operations involving fragments of improvised explosive device [IED], civilian**

✓6ᵗʰ **Y37.27** **Military operations involving fragments from weapons**

✓7ᵗʰ **Y37.270** **Military operations involving fragments from weapons, military personnel**

✓7ᵗʰ **Y37.271** **Military operations involving fragments from weapons, civilian**

✓6ᵗʰ **Y37.29** **Military operations involving other explosions and fragments**
Military operations involving explosion of grenade
Military operations involving explosions of land mine
Military operations involving shrapnel NOS

✓7ᵗʰ **Y37.290** **Military operations involving other explosions and fragments, military personnel**

✓7ᵗʰ **Y37.291** **Military operations involving other explosions and fragments, civilian**

✓5ᵗʰ **Y37.3** **Military operations involving fires, conflagrations and hot substances**
Military operations involving smoke, fumes, and heat from fires, conflagrations and hot substances

EXCLUDES 1 *military operations involving fires and conflagrations aboard military aircraft (Y37.1-)*
military operations involving fires and conflagrations aboard military watercraft (Y37.0-)
military operations involving fires and conflagrations caused indirectly by conventional weapons (Y37.2-)
military operations involving fires and thermal effects of nuclear weapons (Y36.53-)

✓6ᵗʰ **Y37.30** **Military operations involving unspecified fire, conflagration and hot substance**

✓7ᵗʰ **Y37.300** **Military operations involving unspecified fire, conflagration and hot substance, military personnel** ▽

✓7ᵗʰ **Y37.301** **Military operations involving unspecified fire, conflagration and hot substance, civilian** ▽

✓6ᵗʰ **Y37.31** **Military operations involving gasoline bomb**
Military operations involving incendiary bomb
Military operations involving petrol bomb

✓7ᵗʰ **Y37.310** **Military operations involving gasoline bomb, military personnel**

✓7ᵗʰ **Y37.311** **Military operations involving gasoline bomb, civilian**

✓6ᵗʰ **Y37.32** **Military operations involving incendiary bullet**

✓7ᵗʰ **Y37.320** **Military operations involving incendiary bullet, military personnel**

✓7ᵗʰ **Y37.321** **Military operations involving incendiary bullet, civilian**

✓6ᵗʰ **Y37.33** **Military operations involving flamethrower**

✓7ᵗʰ **Y37.330** **Military operations involving flamethrower, military personnel**

✓7ᵗʰ **Y37.331** **Military operations involving flamethrower, civilian**

✓6ᵗʰ **Y37.39** **Military operations involving other fires, conflagrations and hot substances**

✓7ᵗʰ **Y37.390** **Military operations involving other fires, conflagrations and hot substances, military personnel**

✓7ᵗʰ **Y37.391** **Military operations involving other fires, conflagrations and hot substances, civilian**

✓5ᵗʰ **Y37.4** **Military operations involving firearm discharge and other forms of conventional warfare**

✓6ᵗʰ **Y37.41** **Military operations involving rubber bullets**

✓7ᵗʰ **Y37.410** **Military operations involving rubber bullets, military personnel**

✓7ᵗʰ **Y37.411** **Military operations involving rubber bullets, civilian**

✓6ᵗʰ **Y37.42** **Military operations involving firearms pellets**

✓7ᵗʰ **Y37.420** **Military operations involving firearms pellets, military personnel**

✓7ᵗʰ **Y37.421** **Military operations involving firearms pellets, civilian**

✓6ᵗʰ **Y37.43** **Military operations involving other firearms discharge**
Military operations involving bullets NOS

EXCLUDES 1 *military operations involving munitions fragments (Y37.25-)*
military operations involving incendiary bullets (Y37.32-)

✓7ᵗʰ **Y37.430** **Military operations involving other firearms discharge, military personnel**

✓7ᵗʰ **Y37.431** **Military operations involving other firearms discharge, civilian**

☑6ᵗʰ **Y37.44 Military operations involving** unarmed hand to hand combat

> **EXCLUDES 1**   *military operations involving combat using blunt or piercing object (Y37.45-)*
> *military operations involving intentional restriction of air and airway (Y37.46-)*
> *military operations involving unintentional restriction of air and airway (Y37.47-)*

     ☑7ᵗʰ **Y37.440 Military operations involving unarmed hand to hand combat,** military personnel

     ☑7ᵗʰ **Y37.441 Military operations involving unarmed hand to hand combat,** civilian

☑6ᵗʰ **Y37.45 Military operations involving** combat using blunt or piercing object

     ☑7ᵗʰ **Y37.450 Military operations involving combat using blunt or piercing object,** military personnel

     ☑7ᵗʰ **Y37.451 Military operations involving combat using blunt or piercing object,** civilian

☑6ᵗʰ **Y37.46 Military operations involving** intentional restriction of air and airway

     ☑7ᵗʰ **Y37.460 Military operations involving intentional restriction of air and airway,** military personnel

     ☑7ᵗʰ **Y37.461 Military operations involving intentional restriction of air and airway,** civilian

☑6ᵗʰ **Y37.47 Military operations involving** unintentional restriction of air and airway

     ☑7ᵗʰ **Y37.470 Military operations involving unintentional restriction of air and airway,** military personnel

     ☑7ᵗʰ **Y37.471 Military operations involving unintentional restriction of air and airway,** civilian

☑6ᵗʰ **Y37.49 Military operations involving** other forms of conventional warfare

     ☑7ᵗʰ **Y37.490 Military operations involving other forms of conventional warfare,** military personnel

     ☑7ᵗʰ **Y37.491 Military operations involving other forms of conventional warfare,** civilian

☑5ᵗʰ **Y37.5 Military operations involving** nuclear weapons
     Military operation involving dirty bomb NOS

☑6ᵗʰ **Y37.50 Military operations involving** unspecified effect of nuclear weapon

     ☑7ᵗʰ **Y37.500 Military operations involving unspecified effect of nuclear weapon,** military personnel   ▽

     ☑7ᵗʰ **Y37.501 Military operations involving unspecified effect of nuclear weapon,** civilian   ▽

☑6ᵗʰ **Y37.51 Military operations involving** direct blast effect of nuclear weapon
     Military operations involving blast pressure of nuclear weapon

     ☑7ᵗʰ **Y37.510 Military operations involving direct blast effect of nuclear weapon,** military personnel

     ☑7ᵗʰ **Y37.511 Military operations involving direct blast effect of nuclear weapon,** civilian

☑6ᵗʰ **Y37.52 Military operations involving** indirect blast effect of nuclear weapon
     Military operations involving being thrown by blast of nuclear weapon
     Military operations involving being struck or crushed by blast debris of nuclear weapon

     ☑7ᵗʰ **Y37.520 Military operations involving indirect blast effect of nuclear weapon,** military personnel

     ☑7ᵗʰ **Y37.521 Military operations involving indirect blast effect of nuclear weapon,** civilian

☑6ᵗʰ **Y37.53 Military operations involving** thermal radiation effect of nuclear weapon
     Military operations involving direct heat from nuclear weapon
     Military operation involving fireball effects from nuclear weapon

     ☑7ᵗʰ **Y37.530 Military operations involving thermal radiation effect of nuclear weapon,** military personnel

     ☑7ᵗʰ **Y37.531 Military operations involving thermal radiation effect of nuclear weapon,** civilian

☑6ᵗʰ **Y37.54 Military operation involving** nuclear radiation effects of nuclear weapon
     Military operation involving acute radiation exposure from nuclear weapon
     Military operation involving exposure to immediate ionizing radiation from nuclear weapon
     Military operation involving fallout exposure from nuclear weapon
     Military operation involving secondary effects of nuclear weapons

     ☑7ᵗʰ **Y37.540 Military operation involving nuclear radiation effects of nuclear weapon,** military personnel

     ☑7ᵗʰ **Y37.541 Military operation involving nuclear radiation effects of nuclear weapon,** civilian

☑6ᵗʰ **Y37.59 Military operation involving** other effects of nuclear weapons

     ☑7ᵗʰ **Y37.590 Military operation involving other effects of nuclear weapons,** military personnel

     ☑7ᵗʰ **Y37.591 Military operation involving other effects of nuclear weapons,** civilian

☑5ᵗʰ **Y37.6 Military operations involving** biological weapons

☑6ᵗʰ **Y37.6X Military operations involving** biological weapons

     ☑7ᵗʰ **Y37.6X0 Military operations involving biological weapons,** military personnel

     ☑7ᵗʰ **Y37.6X1 Military operations involving biological weapons,** civilian

☑5ᵗʰ **Y37.7 Military operations involving** chemical weapons and other forms of unconventional warfare

> **EXCLUDES 1**   *military operations involving incendiary devices (Y36.3-, Y36.5-)*

☑6ᵗʰ **Y37.7X Military operations involving** chemical weapons and other forms of unconventional warfare

     ☑7ᵗʰ **Y37.7X0 Military operations involving chemical weapons and other forms of unconventional warfare,** military personnel

     ☑7ᵗʰ **Y37.7X1 Military operations involving chemical weapons and other forms of unconventional warfare,** civilian

☑5ᵗʰ **Y37.9 Other and unspecified military operations**

     ☑x7ᵗʰ **Y37.90 Military operations, unspecified**   ▽

     ☑x7ᵗʰ **Y37.91 Military operations involving unspecified weapon of mass destruction [WMD]**   ▽

     ☑x7ᵗʰ **Y37.92 Military operations involving** friendly fire

---

☑ Add'l Character Required   ☑x7ᵗʰ Placeholder Alert   RUG IV Special Care High Dx   RUG IV Clinically Complex Dx   RUG IV Special Care Low Dx   Manifestation Code   Other Specified Code   ▽ Unspecified Code

Chapter 20. External Causes of Morbidity

✓4ᵗʰ **Y38 Terrorism**

NOTE These codes are for use to identify injuries resulting from the unlawful use of force or violence against persons or property to intimidate or coerce a Government, the civilian population, or any segment thereof, in furtherance of political or social objective.

Use additional code for place of occurrence (Y92.-)

The appropriate 7th character is to be added to each code from category Y38.
A   initial encounter
D   subsequent encounter
S   sequela

✓5ᵗʰ **Y38.0 Terrorism involving explosion of marine weapons**
Terrorism involving depth-charge
Terrorism involving marine mine
Terrorism involving mine NOS, at sea or in harbor
Terrorism involving sea-based artillery shell
Terrorism involving torpedo
Terrorism involving underwater blast

   ✓6ᵗʰ **Y38.0X Terrorism involving explosion of marine weapons**

     ✓7ᵗʰ **Y38.0X1 Terrorism involving explosion of marine weapons, public safety official injured**

     ✓7ᵗʰ **Y38.0X2 Terrorism involving explosion of marine weapons, civilian injured**

     ✓7ᵗʰ **Y38.0X3 Terrorism involving explosion of marine weapons, terrorist injured**

✓5ᵗʰ **Y38.1 Terrorism involving destruction of aircraft**
Terrorism involving aircraft burned
Terrorism involving aircraft exploded
Terrorism involving aircraft being shot down
Terrorism involving aircraft used as a weapon

   ✓6ᵗʰ **Y38.1X Terrorism involving destruction of aircraft**

     ✓7ᵗʰ **Y38.1X1 Terrorism involving destruction of aircraft, public safety official injured**

     ✓7ᵗʰ **Y38.1X2 Terrorism involving destruction of aircraft, civilian injured**

     ✓7ᵗʰ **Y38.1X3 Terrorism involving destruction of aircraft, terrorist injured**

✓5ᵗʰ **Y38.2 Terrorism involving other explosions and fragments**
Terrorism involving antipersonnel (fragments) bomb
Terrorism involving blast NOS
Terrorism involving explosion NOS
Terrorism involving explosion of breech block
Terrorism involving explosion of cannon block
Terrorism involving explosion (fragments) of artillery shell
Terrorism involving explosion (fragments) of bomb
Terrorism involving explosion (fragments) of grenade
Terrorism involving explosion (fragments) of guided missile
Terrorism involving explosion (fragments) of land mine
Terrorism involving explosion of mortar bomb
Terrorism involving explosion of munitions
Terrorism involving explosion (fragments) of rocket
Terrorism involving explosion (fragments) of shell
Terrorism involving shrapnel
Terrorism involving mine NOS, on land
EXCLUDES 1 *terrorism involving explosion of nuclear weapon (Y38.5)*
terrorism involving suicide bomber (Y38.81)

   ✓6ᵗʰ **Y38.2X Terrorism involving other explosions and fragments**

     ✓7ᵗʰ **Y38.2X1 Terrorism involving other explosions and fragments, public safety official injured**

     ✓7ᵗʰ **Y38.2X2 Terrorism involving other explosions and fragments, civilian injured**

     ✓7ᵗʰ **Y38.2X3 Terrorism involving other explosions and fragments, terrorist injured**

✓5ᵗʰ **Y38.3 Terrorism involving fires, conflagration and hot substances**
Terrorism involving conflagration NOS
Terrorism involving fire NOS
Terrorism involving petrol bomb
EXCLUDES 1 *terrorism involving fire or heat of nuclear weapon (Y38.5)*

   ✓6ᵗʰ **Y38.3X Terrorism involving fires, conflagration and hot substances**

     ✓7ᵗʰ **Y38.3X1 Terrorism involving fires, conflagration and hot substances, public safety official injured**

     ✓7ᵗʰ **Y38.3X2 Terrorism involving fires, conflagration and hot substances, civilian injured**

     ✓7ᵗʰ **Y38.3X3 Terrorism involving fires, conflagration and hot substances, terrorist injured**

✓5ᵗʰ **Y38.4 Terrorism involving firearms**
Terrorism involving carbine bullet
Terrorism involving machine gun bullet
Terrorism involving pellets (shotgun)
Terrorism involving pistol bullet
Terrorism involving rifle bullet
Terrorism involving rubber (rifle) bullet

   ✓6ᵗʰ **Y38.4X Terrorism involving firearms**

     ✓7ᵗʰ **Y38.4X1 Terrorism involving firearms, public safety official injured**

     ✓7ᵗʰ **Y38.4X2 Terrorism involving firearms, civilian injured**

     ✓7ᵗʰ **Y38.4X3 Terrorism involving firearms, terrorist injured**

✓5ᵗʰ **Y38.5 Terrorism involving nuclear weapons**
Terrorism involving blast effects of nuclear weapon
Terrorism involving exposure to ionizing radiation from nuclear weapon
Terrorism involving fireball effect of nuclear weapon
Terrorism involving heat from nuclear weapon

   ✓6ᵗʰ **Y38.5X Terrorism involving nuclear weapons**

     ✓7ᵗʰ **Y38.5X1 Terrorism involving nuclear weapons, public safety official injured**

     ✓7ᵗʰ **Y38.5X2 Terrorism involving nuclear weapons, civilian injured**

     ✓7ᵗʰ **Y38.5X3 Terrorism involving nuclear weapons, terrorist injured**

✓5ᵗʰ **Y38.6 Terrorism involving biological weapons**
Terrorism involving anthrax
Terrorism involving cholera
Terrorism involving smallpox

   ✓6ᵗʰ **Y38.6X Terrorism involving biological weapons**

     ✓7ᵗʰ **Y38.6X1 Terrorism involving biological weapons, public safety official injured**

     ✓7ᵗʰ **Y38.6X2 Terrorism involving biological weapons, civilian injured**

     ✓7ᵗʰ **Y38.6X3 Terrorism involving biological weapons, terrorist injured**

✓5ᵗʰ **Y38.7 Terrorism involving chemical weapons**
Terrorism involving gases, fumes, chemicals
Terrorism involving hydrogen cyanide
Terrorism involving phosgene
Terrorism involving sarin

   ✓6ᵗʰ **Y38.7X Terrorism involving chemical weapons**

     ✓7ᵗʰ **Y38.7X1 Terrorism involving chemical weapons, public safety official injured**

     ✓7ᵗʰ **Y38.7X2 Terrorism involving chemical weapons, civilian injured**

     ✓7ᵗʰ **Y38.7X3 Terrorism involving chemical weapons, terrorist injured**

✓5ᵗʰ **Y38.8 Terrorism involving other and unspecified means**

   Y38.80 Terrorism involving unspecified means ▽
Terrorism NOS

   ✓6ᵗʰ **Y38.81 Terrorism involving suicide bomber**

     ✓7ᵗʰ **Y38.811 Terrorism involving suicide bomber, public safety official injured**

     ✓7ᵗʰ **Y38.812 Terrorism involving suicide bomber, civilian injured**

   ✓6ᵗʰ **Y38.89 Terrorism involving other means**
Terrorism involving drowning and submersion
Terrorism involving lasers
Terrorism involving piercing or stabbing instruments

     ✓7ᵗʰ **Y38.891 Terrorism involving other means, public safety official injured**

     ✓7ᵗʰ **Y38.892 Terrorism involving other means, civilian injured**

     ✓7ᵗʰ **Y38.893 Terrorism involving other means, terrorist injured**

Ⓝ Newborn   Ⓟ Pediatric   Ⓜ Maternity   Ⓐ Adult   **RIC** RIC Dx   **NC Dx** Noncancer Dx   **PDx** Primary Dx   **CC** RIC CC Condition   ▶◀ Revised Text   ● New Code   ▲ Revised Code Title

1108   ICD-10-CM 2016

☑5ᵗʰ **Y38.9 Terrorism, secondary effects**
> **NOTE** This code is for use to identify injuries occurring subsequent to a terrorist attack, not those that are due to the initial terrorist attack.

　　☑6ᵗʰ **Y38.9X Terrorism,** secondary effects

　　　　☑7ᵗʰ **Y38.9X1 Terrorism, secondary effects,** public safety official **injured**

　　　　☑7ᵗʰ **Y38.9X2 Terrorism, secondary effects,** civilian **injured**

Complications of medical and surgical care (Y62-Y84)
> **INCLUDES** complications of medical devices
> surgical and medical procedures as the cause of abnormal reaction of the patient, or of later complication, without mention of misadventure at the time of the procedure

Misadventures to patients during surgical and medical care (Y62-Y69)
> **EXCLUDES 2** breakdown or malfunctioning of medical device (during procedure) (after implantation) (ongoing use) (Y70-Y82)
> surgical and medical procedures as the cause of abnormal reaction of the patient, without mention of misadventure at the time of the procedure (Y83-Y84)

☑4ᵗʰ **Y62 Failure of** sterile precautions **during surgical and medical care**

　Y62.0 Failure of sterile precautions during surgical operation

　Y62.1 Failure of sterile precautions during infusion or transfusion

　Y62.2 Failure of sterile precautions during kidney dialysis and other perfusion

　Y62.3 Failure of sterile precautions during injection or immunization

　Y62.4 Failure of sterile precautions during endoscopic examination

　Y62.5 Failure of sterile precautions during heart catheterization

　Y62.6 Failure of sterile precautions during aspiration, puncture and other catheterization

　Y62.8 Failure of sterile precautions during other surgical and medical care

　Y62.9 Failure of sterile precautions during unspecified surgical and medical care ▽

☑4ᵗʰ **Y63 Failure in** dosage **during surgical and medical care**
> **EXCLUDES 2** accidental overdose of drug or wrong drug given in error (T36-T50)

　Y63.0 Excessive amount of blood or other fluid given during transfusion or infusion

　Y63.1 Incorrect dilution of fluid used during infusion

　Y63.2 Overdose of radiation given during therapy

　Y63.3 Inadvertent exposure of patient to radiation during medical care

　Y63.4 Failure in dosage in electroshock or insulin-shock therapy

　Y63.5 Inappropriate temperature in local application and packing

　Y63.6 Underdosing and nonadministration of necessary drug, medicament or biological substance

　Y63.8 Failure in dosage during other surgical and medical care

　Y63.9 Failure in dosage during unspecified surgical and medical care ▽

☑4ᵗʰ **Y64 Contaminated medical or biological** substances

　Y64.0 Contaminated medical or biological substance, transfused or infused

　Y64.1 Contaminated medical or biological substance, injected or used for immunization

　Y64.8 Contaminated medical or biological substance administered by other means

　Y64.9 Contaminated medical or biological substance administered by unspecified means ▽
> Administered contaminated medical or biological substance NOS

☑4ᵗʰ **Y65 Other misadventures during surgical and medical care**

　Y65.0 Mismatched blood in transfusion

　Y65.1 Wrong fluid used in infusion

　Y65.2 Failure in suture or ligature during surgical operation

　Y65.3 Endotracheal tube wrongly placed during anesthetic procedure

　Y65.4 Failure to introduce or to remove other tube or instrument

☑5ᵗʰ **Y65.5 Performance of** wrong procedure (operation)

　　Y65.51 Performance of wrong procedure (operation) on correct patient
> Wrong device implanted into correct surgical site
> **EXCLUDES 1** performance of correct procedure (operation) on wrong side or body part (Y65.53)

　　Y65.52 Performance of procedure (operation) on patient not scheduled for surgery
> Performance of procedure (operation) intended for another patient
> Performance of procedure (operation) on wrong patient

　　Y65.53 Performance of correct procedure (operation) on wrong side or body part
> Performance of correct procedure (operation) on wrong side
> Performance of correct procedure (operation) on wrong site

　Y65.8 Other specified misadventures **during surgical and medical care**

Y66 Nonadministration of surgical and medical care
> Premature cessation of surgical and medical care
> **EXCLUDES 1** DNR status (Z66)
> palliative care (Z51.5)

Y69 Unspecified misadventure during surgical and medical care ▽

Medical devices associated with adverse incidents in diagnostic and therapeutic use (Y70-Y82)
> **INCLUDES** breakdown or malfunction of medical devices (during use) (after implantation) (ongoing use)
> **EXCLUDES 1** misadventure to patients during surgical and medical care, classifiable to (Y62-Y69)
> later complications following use of medical devices without breakdown or malfunctioning of device (Y83-Y84)

☑4ᵗʰ **Y70 Anesthesiology devices associated with adverse incidents**

　Y70.0 Diagnostic and monitoring anesthesiology devices associated with adverse incidents

　Y70.1 Therapeutic (nonsurgical) and rehabilitative anesthesiology devices associated with adverse incidents

　Y70.2 Prosthetic and other implants, materials and accessory anesthesiology devices associated with adverse incidents

　Y70.3 Surgical instruments, materials and anesthesiology devices (including sutures) associated with adverse incidents

　Y70.8 Miscellaneous anesthesiology devices associated with adverse incidents, not elsewhere classified

☑4ᵗʰ **Y71 Cardiovascular devices associated with adverse incidents**

　Y71.0 Diagnostic and monitoring cardiovascular devices associated with adverse incidents

　Y71.1 Therapeutic (nonsurgical) and rehabilitative cardiovascular devices associated with adverse incidents

　Y71.2 Prosthetic and other implants, materials and accessory cardiovascular devices associated with adverse incidents

　Y71.3 Surgical instruments, materials and cardiovascular devices (including sutures) associated with adverse incidents

　Y71.8 Miscellaneous cardiovascular devices associated with adverse incidents, not elsewhere classified

☑4ᵗʰ **Y72 Otorhinolaryngological devices associated with adverse incidents**

　Y72.0 Diagnostic and monitoring otorhinolaryngological devices associated with adverse incidents

　Y72.1 Therapeutic (nonsurgical) and rehabilitative otorhinolaryngological devices associated with adverse incidents

　Y72.2 Prosthetic and other implants, materials and accessory otorhinolaryngological devices associated with adverse incidents

　Y72.3 Surgical instruments, materials and otorhinolaryngological devices (including sutures) associated with adverse incidents

　Y72.8 Miscellaneous otorhinolaryngological devices associated with adverse incidents, not elsewhere classified

☑4ᵗʰ **Y73 Gastroenterology and urology devices associated with adverse incidents**

　Y73.0 Diagnostic and monitoring gastroenterology and urology devices associated with adverse incidents

　Y73.1 Therapeutic (nonsurgical) and rehabilitative gastroenterology and urology devices associated with adverse incidents

Y73.2 Prosthetic and other implants, materials and accessory gastroenterology and urology devices associated with adverse incidents

Y73.3 Surgical instruments, materials and gastroenterology and urology devices (including sutures) associated with adverse incidents

Y73.8 Miscellaneous gastroenterology and urology devices associated with adverse incidents, not elsewhere classified

✓4ᵗʰ **Y74** General hospital and personal-use devices associated with adverse incidents

Y74.0 Diagnostic and monitoring general hospital and personal-use devices associated with adverse incidents

Y74.1 Therapeutic (nonsurgical) and rehabilitative general hospital and personal-use devices associated with adverse incidents

Y74.2 Prosthetic and other implants, materials and accessory general hospital and personal-use devices associated with adverse incidents

Y74.3 Surgical instruments, materials and general hospital and personal-use devices (including sutures) associated with adverse incidents

Y74.8 Miscellaneous general hospital and personal-use devices associated with adverse incidents, not elsewhere classified

✓4ᵗʰ **Y75** Neurological devices associated with adverse incidents

Y75.0 Diagnostic and monitoring neurological devices associated with adverse incidents

Y75.1 Therapeutic (nonsurgical) and rehabilitative neurological devices associated with adverse incidents

Y75.2 Prosthetic and other implants, materials and neurological devices associated with adverse incidents

Y75.3 Surgical instruments, materials and neurological devices (including sutures) associated with adverse incidents

Y75.8 Miscellaneous neurological devices associated with adverse incidents, not elsewhere classified

✓4ᵗʰ **Y76** Obstetric and gynecological devices associated with adverse incidents

Y76.0 Diagnostic and monitoring obstetric and gynecological devices associated with adverse incidents ♀

Y76.1 Therapeutic (nonsurgical) and rehabilitative obstetric and gynecological devices associated with adverse incidents ♀

Y76.2 Prosthetic and other implants, materials and accessory obstetric and gynecological devices associated with adverse incidents ♀

Y76.3 Surgical instruments, materials and obstetric and gynecological devices (including sutures) associated with adverse incidents ♀

Y76.8 Miscellaneous obstetric and gynecological devices associated with adverse incidents, not elsewhere classified ♀

✓4ᵗʰ **Y77** Ophthalmic devices associated with adverse incidents

Y77.0 Diagnostic and monitoring ophthalmic devices associated with adverse incidents

Y77.1 Therapeutic (nonsurgical) and rehabilitative ophthalmic devices associated with adverse incidents

Y77.2 Prosthetic and other implants, materials and accessory ophthalmic devices associated with adverse incidents

Y77.3 Surgical instruments, materials and ophthalmic devices (including sutures) associated with adverse incidents

Y77.8 Miscellaneous ophthalmic devices associated with adverse incidents, not elsewhere classified

✓4ᵗʰ **Y78** Radiological devices associated with adverse incidents

Y78.0 Diagnostic and monitoring radiological devices associated with adverse incidents

Y78.1 Therapeutic (nonsurgical) and rehabilitative radiological devices associated with adverse incidents

Y78.2 Prosthetic and other implants, materials and accessory radiological devices associated with adverse incidents

Y78.3 Surgical instruments, materials and radiological devices (including sutures) associated with adverse incidents

Y78.8 Miscellaneous radiological devices associated with adverse incidents, not elsewhere classified

✓4ᵗʰ **Y79** Orthopedic devices associated with adverse incidents

Y79.0 Diagnostic and monitoring orthopedic devices associated with adverse incidents

Y79.1 Therapeutic (nonsurgical) and rehabilitative orthopedic devices associated with adverse incidents

Y79.2 Prosthetic and other implants, materials and accessory orthopedic devices associated with adverse incidents

Y79.3 Surgical instruments, materials and orthopedic devices (including sutures) associated with adverse incidents

Y79.8 Miscellaneous orthopedic devices associated with adverse incidents, not elsewhere classified

✓4ᵗʰ **Y80** Physical medicine devices associated with adverse incidents

Y80.0 Diagnostic and monitoring physical medicine devices associated with adverse incidents

Y80.1 Therapeutic (nonsurgical) and rehabilitative physical medicine devices associated with adverse incidents

Y80.2 Prosthetic and other implants, materials and accessory physical medicine devices associated with adverse incidents

Y80.3 Surgical instruments, materials and physical medicine devices (including sutures) associated with adverse incidents

Y80.8 Miscellaneous physical medicine devices associated with adverse incidents, not elsewhere classified

✓4ᵗʰ **Y81** General- and plastic-surgery devices associated with adverse incidents

Y81.0 Diagnostic and monitoring general- and plastic-surgery devices associated with adverse incidents

Y81.1 Therapeutic (nonsurgical) and rehabilitative general- and plastic-surgery devices associated with adverse incidents

Y81.2 Prosthetic and other implants, materials and accessory general- and plastic-surgery devices associated with adverse incidents

Y81.3 Surgical instruments, materials and general- and plastic-surgery devices (including sutures) associated with adverse incidents

Y81.8 Miscellaneous general- and plastic-surgery devices associated with adverse incidents, not elsewhere classified

✓4ᵗʰ **Y82** Other and unspecified medical devices associated with adverse incidents

Y82.8 Other medical devices associated with adverse incidents

Y82.9 Unspecified medical devices associated with adverse ▽ incidents

Surgical and other medical procedures as the cause of abnormal reaction of the patient, or of later complication, without mention of misadventure at the time of the procedure (Y83-Y84)

EXCLUDES 1 misadventures to patients during surgical and medical care, classifiable to (Y62-Y69)

✓4ᵗʰ **Y83** Surgical operation and other surgical procedures as the cause of abnormal reaction of the patient, or of later complication, without mention of misadventure at the time of the procedure

Y83.0 Surgical operation with transplant of whole organ as the cause of abnormal reaction of the patient, or of later complication, without mention of misadventure at the time of the procedure

Y83.1 Surgical operation with implant of artificial internal device as the cause of abnormal reaction of the patient, or of later complication, without mention of misadventure at the time of the procedure

Y83.2 Surgical operation with anastomosis, bypass or graft as the cause of abnormal reaction of the patient, or of later complication, without mention of misadventure at the time of the procedure

Y83.3 Surgical operation with formation of external stoma as the cause of abnormal reaction of the patient, or of later complication, without mention of misadventure at the time of the procedure

Y83.4 Other reconstructive surgery as the cause of abnormal reaction of the patient, or of later complication, without mention of misadventure at the time of the procedure

Y83.5 Amputation of limb(s) as the cause of abnormal reaction of the patient, or of later complication, without mention of misadventure at the time of the procedure

Y83.6 Removal of other organ (partial) (total) as the cause of abnormal reaction of the patient, or of later complication, without mention of misadventure at the time of the procedure

Y83.8 Other surgical procedures as the cause of abnormal reaction of the patient, or of later complication, without mention of misadventure at the time of the procedure

Y83.9 Surgical procedure, unspecified as the cause of abnormal ▽ reaction of the patient, or of later complication, without mention of misadventure at the time of the procedure

Ⓝ Newborn   Ⓟ Pediatric   Ⓜ Maternity   Ⓐ Adult   **RIC** RIC Dx   **NCDx** Noncancer Dx   **PDx** Primary Dx   **CC** RIC CC Condition   ►◄ Revised Text   ● New Code   ▲ Revised Code Title

1110   ICD-10-CM 2016

☑4ᵗʰ **Y84** Other medical procedures as the cause of abnormal reaction of the patient, or of later complication, without mention of misadventure at the time of the procedure

    Y84.0 Cardiac catheterization as the cause of abnormal reaction of the patient, or of later complication, without mention of misadventure at the time of the procedure

    Y84.1 Kidney dialysis as the cause of abnormal reaction of the patient, or of later complication, without mention of misadventure at the time of the procedure

    Y84.2 Radiological procedure and radiotherapy as the cause of abnormal reaction of the patient, or of later complication, without mention of misadventure at the time of the procedure

    Y84.3 Shock therapy as the cause of abnormal reaction of the patient, or of later complication, without mention of misadventure at the time of the procedure

    Y84.4 Aspiration of fluid as the cause of abnormal reaction of the patient, or of later complication, without mention of misadventure at the time of the procedure

    Y84.5 Insertion of gastric or duodenal sound as the cause of abnormal reaction of the patient, or of later complication, without mention of misadventure at the time of the procedure

    Y84.6 Urinary catheterization as the cause of abnormal reaction of the patient, or of later complication, without mention of misadventure at the time of the procedure

    Y84.7 Blood-sampling as the cause of abnormal reaction of the patient, or of later complication, without mention of misadventure at the time of the procedure

    Y84.8 Other medical procedures as the cause of abnormal reaction of the patient, or of later complication, without mention of misadventure at the time of the procedure
        AHA: 2014, 4Q, 24

    Y84.9 Medical procedure, unspecified as the cause of abnormal ▽ reaction of the patient, or of later complication, without mention of misadventure at the time of the procedure

Supplementary factors related to causes of morbidity classified elsewhere (Y90-Y99)

    NOTE   These categories may be used to provide supplementary information concerning causes of morbidity. They are not to be used for single-condition coding.

☑4ᵗʰ **Y90** Evidence of alcohol involvement determined by blood alcohol level
    Code first any associated alcohol related disorders (F10)

    Y90.0 Blood alcohol level of less than 20 mg/100 ml
    Y90.1 Blood alcohol level of 20-39 mg/100 ml
    Y90.2 Blood alcohol level of 40-59 mg/100 ml
    Y90.3 Blood alcohol level of 60-79 mg/100 ml
    Y90.4 Blood alcohol level of 80-99 mg/100 ml
    Y90.5 Blood alcohol level of 100-119 mg/100 ml
    Y90.6 Blood alcohol level of 120-199 mg/100 ml
    Y90.7 Blood alcohol level of 200-239 mg/100 ml
    Y90.8 Blood alcohol level of 240 mg/100 ml or more
    Y90.9 Presence of alcohol in blood, level not specified   ▽

☑4ᵗʰ **Y92** Place of occurrence of the external cause
    The following category is for use, when relevant, to identify the place of occurrence of the external cause. Use in conjunction with an activity code.
    Place of occurrence should be recorded only at the initial encounter for treatment

    ☑5ᵗʰ **Y92.0** Non-institutional (private) residence as the place of occurrence of the external cause
        EXCLUDES 1 abandoned or derelict house (Y92.89)
             home under construction but not yet occupied (Y92.6-)
             institutional place of residence (Y92.1-)

        ☑6ᵗʰ **Y92.00** Unspecified non-institutional (private) residence as the place of occurrence of the external cause
            Y92.000 Kitchen of unspecified non-institutional ▽ (private) residence as the place of occurrence of the external cause
            Y92.001 Dining room of unspecified ▽ non-institutional (private) residence as the place of occurrence of the external cause

            Y92.002 Bathroom of unspecified ▽ non-institutional (private) residence single-family (private) house as the place of occurrence of the external cause
            Y92.003 Bedroom of unspecified ▽ non-institutional (private) residence as the place of occurrence of the external cause
            Y92.007 Garden or yard of unspecified non- ▽ institutional (private) residence as the place of occurrence of the external cause
            Y92.008 Other place in unspecified non- ▽ institutional (private) residence as the place of occurrence of the external cause
            Y92.009 Unspecified place in unspecified non- ▽ institutional (private) residence as the place of occurrence of the external cause
                Home (NOS) as the place of occurrence of the external cause

        ☑6ᵗʰ **Y92.01** Single-family non-institutional (private) house as the place of occurrence of the external cause
            Farmhouse as the place of occurrence of the external cause
            EXCLUDES 1 barn (Y92.71)
                chicken coop or hen house (Y92.72)
                farm field (Y92.73)
                orchard (Y92.74)
                single family mobile home or trailer (Y92.02-)
                slaughter house (Y92.86)
            Y92.010 Kitchen of single-family (private) house as the place of occurrence of the external cause
            Y92.011 Dining room of single-family (private) house as the place of occurrence of the external cause
            Y92.012 Bathroom of single-family (private) house as the place of occurrence of the external cause
            Y92.013 Bedroom of single-family (private) house as the place of occurrence of the external cause
            Y92.014 Private driveway to single-family (private) house as the place of occurrence of the external cause
            Y92.015 Private garage of single-family (private) house as the place of occurrence of the external cause
            Y92.016 Swimming-pool in single-family (private) house or garden as the place of occurrence of the external cause
            Y92.017 Garden or yard in single-family (private) house as the place of occurrence of the external cause
            Y92.018 Other place in single-family (private) house as the place of occurrence of the external cause
            Y92.019 Unspecified place in single-family ▽ (private) house as the place of occurrence of the external cause

        ☑6ᵗʰ **Y92.02** Mobile home as the place of occurrence of the external cause
            Y92.020 Kitchen in mobile home as the place of occurrence of the external cause
            Y92.021 Dining room in mobile home as the place of occurrence of the external cause
            Y92.022 Bathroom in mobile home as the place of occurrence of the external cause
            Y92.023 Bedroom in mobile home as the place of occurrence of the external cause
            Y92.024 Driveway of mobile home as the place of occurrence of the external cause
            Y92.025 Garage of mobile home as the place of occurrence of the external cause
            Y92.026 Swimming-pool of mobile home as the place of occurrence of the external cause
            Y92.027 Garden or yard of mobile home as the place of occurrence of the external cause
            Y92.028 Other place in mobile home as the place of occurrence of the external cause

Y92.029   Unspecified place in mobile home as the place of occurrence of the external cause ▽

✓6ᵗʰ **Y92.03**   **Apartment as the place of occurrence of the external cause**
     Condominium as the place of occurrence of the external cause
     Co-op apartment as the place of occurrence of the external cause

Y92.030   Kitchen in apartment as the place of occurrence of the external cause

Y92.031   Bathroom in apartment as the place of occurrence of the external cause

Y92.032   Bedroom in apartment as the place of occurrence of the external cause

Y92.038   Other place in apartment as the place of occurrence of the external cause

Y92.039   Unspecified place in apartment as the place of occurrence of the external cause ▽

✓6ᵗʰ **Y92.04**   **Boarding-house as the place of occurrence of the external cause**

Y92.040   Kitchen in boarding-house as the place of occurrence of the external cause

Y92.041   Bathroom in boarding-house as the place of occurrence of the external cause

Y92.042   Bedroom in boarding-house as the place of occurrence of the external cause

Y92.043   Driveway of boarding-house as the place of occurrence of the external cause

Y92.044   Garage of boarding-house as the place of occurrence of the external cause

Y92.045   Swimming-pool of boarding-house as the place of occurrence of the external cause

Y92.046   Garden or yard of boarding-house as the place of occurrence of the external cause

Y92.048   Other place in boarding-house as the place of occurrence of the external cause

Y92.049   Unspecified place in boarding-house as the place of occurrence of the external cause ▽

✓6ᵗʰ **Y92.09**   **Other non-institutional residence as the place of occurrence of the external cause**

Y92.090   Kitchen in other non-institutional residence as the place of occurrence of the external cause

Y92.091   Bathroom in other non-institutional residence as the place of occurrence of the external cause

Y92.092   Bedroom in other non-institutional residence as the place of occurrence of the external cause

Y92.093   Driveway of other non-institutional residence as the place of occurrence of the external cause

Y92.094   Garage of other non-institutional residence as the place of occurrence of the external cause

Y92.095   Swimming-pool of other non-institutional residence as the place of occurrence of the external cause

Y92.096   Garden or yard of other non-institutional residence as the place of occurrence of the external cause

Y92.098   Other place in other non-institutional residence as the place of occurrence of the external cause

Y92.099   Unspecified place in other non-institutional residence as the place of occurrence of the external cause ▽

✓5ᵗʰ **Y92.1**   **Institutional (nonprivate) residence as the place of occurrence of the external cause**

Y92.10   Unspecified residential institution as the place of occurrence of the external cause ▽

✓6ᵗʰ **Y92.11**   **Children's home and orphanage as the place of occurrence of the external cause**

Y92.110   Kitchen in children's home and orphanage as the place of occurrence of the external cause

Y92.111   Bathroom in children's home and orphanage as the place of occurrence of the external cause

Y92.112   Bedroom in children's home and orphanage as the place of occurrence of the external cause

Y92.113   Driveway of children's home and orphanage as the place of occurrence of the external cause

Y92.114   Garage of children's home and orphanage as the place of occurrence of the external cause

Y92.115   Swimming-pool of children's home and orphanage as the place of occurrence of the external cause

Y92.116   Garden or yard of children's home and orphanage as the place of occurrence of the external cause

Y92.118   Other place in children's home and orphanage as the place of occurrence of the external cause

Y92.119   Unspecified place in children's home and orphanage as the place of occurrence of the external cause ▽

✓6ᵗʰ **Y92.12**   **Nursing home as the place of occurrence of the external cause**
     Home for the sick as the place of occurrence of the external cause
     Hospice as the place of occurrence of the external cause

Y92.120   Kitchen in nursing home as the place of occurrence of the external cause

Y92.121   Bathroom in nursing home as the place of occurrence of the external cause

Y92.122   Bedroom in nursing home as the place of occurrence of the external cause

Y92.123   Driveway of nursing home as the place of occurrence of the external cause

Y92.124   Garage of nursing home as the place of occurrence of the external cause

Y92.125   Swimming-pool of nursing home as the place of occurrence of the external cause

Y92.126   Garden or yard of nursing home as the place of occurrence of the external cause

Y92.128   Other place in nursing home as the place of occurrence of the external cause

Y92.129   Unspecified place in nursing home as the place of occurrence of the external cause ▽

✓6ᵗʰ **Y92.13**   **Military base as the place of occurrence of the external cause**
     EXCLUDES 1   *military training grounds (Y92.83)*

Y92.130   Kitchen on military base as the place of occurrence of the external cause

Y92.131   Mess hall on military base as the place of occurrence of the external cause

Y92.133   Barracks on military base as the place of occurrence of the external cause

Y92.135   Garage on military base as the place of occurrence of the external cause

Y92.136   Swimming-pool on military base as the place of occurrence of the external cause

Y92.137   Garden or yard on military base as the place of occurrence of the external cause

Y92.138   Other place on military base as the place of occurrence of the external cause

Y92.139   Unspecified place military base as the place of occurrence of the external cause ▽

✓6ᵗʰ **Y92.14**   **Prison as the place of occurrence of the external cause**

Y92.140   Kitchen in prison as the place of occurrence of the external cause

Y92.141   Dining room in prison as the place of occurrence of the external cause

Y92.142   Bathroom in prison as the place of occurrence of the external cause

Y92.143   Cell of prison as the place of occurrence of the external cause

Y92.146   Swimming-pool of prison as the place of occurrence of the external cause

Y92.147   Courtyard of prison as the place of occurrence of the external cause

Y92.148   **Other place in prison as the place of occurrence of the external cause**

Y92.149   Unspecified place in prison as the place ▽ of occurrence of the external cause

✓6ᵗʰ   **Y92.15**   Reform school as the place of occurrence of the external cause

Y92.150   Kitchen in reform school as the place of occurrence of the external cause

Y92.151   Dining room in reform school as the place of occurrence of the external cause

Y92.152   Bathroom in reform school as the place of occurrence of the external cause

Y92.153   Bedroom in reform school as the place of occurrence of the external cause

Y92.154   Driveway of reform school as the place of occurrence of the external cause

Y92.155   Garage of reform school as the place of occurrence of the external cause

Y92.156   Swimming-pool of reform school as the place of occurrence of the external cause

Y92.157   Garden or yard of reform school as the place of occurrence of the external cause

Y92.158   **Other place in reform school as the place of occurrence of the external cause**

Y92.159   Unspecified place in reform school as ▽ the place of occurrence of the external cause

✓6ᵗʰ   **Y92.16**   School dormitory as the place of occurrence of the external cause

> _EXCLUDES 1_   reform school as the place of occurrence of the external cause (Y92.15-)
> school buildings and grounds as the place of occurrence of the external cause (Y92.2-)
> school sports and athletic areas as the place of occurrence of the external cause (Y92.3-)

Y92.160   Kitchen in school dormitory as the place of occurrence of the external cause

Y92.161   Dining room in school dormitory as the place of occurrence of the external cause

Y92.162   Bathroom in school dormitory as the place of occurrence of the external cause

Y92.163   Bedroom in school dormitory as the place of occurrence of the external cause

Y92.168   **Other place in school dormitory as the place of occurrence of the external cause**

Y92.169   Unspecified place in school dormitory ▽ as the place of occurrence of the external cause

✓6ᵗʰ   **Y92.19**   Other specified residential institution as the place of occurrence of the external cause

Y92.190   **Kitchen in other specified residential institution as the place of occurrence of the external cause**

Y92.191   **Dining room in other specified residential institution as the place of occurrence of the external cause**

Y92.192   **Bathroom in other specified residential institution as the place of occurrence of the external cause**

Y92.193   **Bedroom in other specified residential institution as the place of occurrence of the external cause**

Y92.194   **Driveway of other specified residential institution as the place of occurrence of the external cause**

Y92.195   **Garage of other specified residential institution as the place of occurrence of the external cause**

Y92.196   **Pool of other specified residential institution as the place of occurrence of the external cause**

Y92.197   **Garden or yard of other specified residential institution as the place of occurrence of the external cause**

Y92.198   **Other place in other specified residential institution as the place of occurrence of the external cause**

Y92.199   **Unspecified place in other specified ▽ residential institution as the place of occurrence of the external cause**

✓5ᵗʰ   **Y92.2**   School, other institution and public administrative area as the place of occurrence of the external cause
Building and adjacent grounds used by the general public or by a particular group of the public

> _EXCLUDES 1_   building under construction as the place of occurrence of the external cause (Y92.6)
> residential institution as the place of occurrence of the external cause (Y92.1)
> school dormitory as the place of occurrence of the external cause (Y92.16-)
> sports and athletics area of schools as the place of occurrence of the external cause (Y92.3-)

✓6ᵗʰ   **Y92.21**   School (private) (public) (state) as the place of occurrence of the external cause

Y92.210   Daycare center as the place of occurrence of the external cause

Y92.211   Elementary school as the place of occurrence of the external cause
Kindergarten as the place of occurrence of the external cause

Y92.212   Middle school as the place of occurrence of the external cause

Y92.213   High school as the place of occurrence of the external cause
AHA: 2012, 4Q, 108

Y92.214   College as the place of occurrence of the external cause
University as the place of occurrence of the external cause

Y92.215   Trade school as the place of occurrence of the external cause

Y92.218   **Other school as the place of occurrence of the external cause**

Y92.219   Unspecified school as the place of ▽ occurrence of the external cause

Y92.22   Religious institution as the place of occurrence of the external cause
Church as the place of occurrence of the external cause
Mosque as the place of occurrence of the external cause
Synagogue as the place of occurrence of the external cause

✓6ᵗʰ   **Y92.23**   Hospital as the place of occurrence of the external cause

> _EXCLUDES 1_   ambulatory (outpatient) health services establishments (Y92.53-)
> home for the sick as the place of occurrence of the external cause (Y92.12-)
> hospice as the place of occurrence of the external cause (Y92.12-)
> nursing home as the place of occurrence of the external cause (Y92.12-)

Y92.230   Patient room in hospital as the place of occurrence of the external cause

Y92.231   Patient bathroom in hospital as the place of occurrence of the external cause

Y92.232   Corridor of hospital as the place of occurrence of the external cause

Y92.233   Cafeteria of hospital as the place of occurrence of the external cause

Y92.234   Operating room of hospital as the place of occurrence of the external cause

Y92.238   **Other place in hospital as the place of occurrence of the external cause**

Y92.239   Unspecified place in hospital as the ▽ place of occurrence of the external cause

✓6ᵗʰ   **Y92.24**   Public administrative building as the place of occurrence of the external cause

Y92.240   Courthouse as the place of occurrence of the external cause

Y92.241   Library as the place of occurrence of the external cause

Y92.242   Post office as the place of occurrence of the external cause

Y92.243   City hall as the place of occurrence of the external cause

---

☑ Add'l Character Required   ✓x7ᵗʰ Placeholder Alert   RUG IV Special Care High Dx   RUG IV Clinically Complex Dx   RUG IV Special Care Low Dx   Manifestation Code   Other Specified Code   ▽ Unspecified Code

        Y92.248   **Other public administrative building as the place of occurrence of the external cause**

✓6ᵗʰ   **Y92.25**   Cultural building **as the place of occurrence of the external cause**

        Y92.250   Art Gallery **as the place of occurrence of the external cause**

        Y92.251   Museum **as the place of occurrence of the external cause**

        Y92.252   Music hall **as the place of occurrence of the external cause**

        Y92.253   Opera house **as the place of occurrence of the external cause**

        Y92.254   Theater (live) **as the place of occurrence of the external cause**

        Y92.258   **Other cultural public building as the place of occurrence of the external cause**

    Y92.26   Movie house or cinema **as the place of occurrence of the external cause**

    Y92.29   **Other specified public building as the place of occurrence of the external cause**

        Assembly hall as the place of occurrence of the external cause

        Clubhouse as the place of occurrence of the external cause

✓5ᵗʰ   **Y92.3**   Sports and athletics area **as the place of occurrence of the external cause**

✓6ᵗʰ   **Y92.31**   Athletic court **as the place of occurrence of the external cause**

        EXCLUDES 1   *tennis court in private home or garden (Y92.09)*

        Y92.310   Basketball **court as the place of occurrence of the external cause**

        Y92.311   Squash **court as the place of occurrence of the external cause**

        Y92.312   Tennis **court as the place of occurrence of the external cause**

        Y92.318   **Other athletic court as the place of occurrence of the external cause**

✓6ᵗʰ   **Y92.32**   Athletic field **as the place of occurrence of the external cause**

        Y92.320   Baseball **field as the place of occurrence of the external cause**

        Y92.321   Football **field as the place of occurrence of the external cause**

        Y92.322   Soccer **field as the place of occurrence of the external cause**

        Y92.328   **Other athletic field as the place of occurrence of the external cause**

            Cricket field as the place of occurrence of the external cause

            Hockey field as the place of occurrence of the external cause

✓6ᵗʰ   **Y92.33**   Skating rink **as the place of occurrence of the external cause**

        Y92.330   Ice skating **rink (indoor) (outdoor) as the place of occurrence of the external cause**

        Y92.331   Roller skating **rink as the place of occurrence of the external cause**

    Y92.34   Swimming pool (public) **as the place of occurrence of the external cause**

        EXCLUDES 1   *swimming pool in private home or garden (Y92.016)*

    Y92.39   **Other specified sports and athletic area as the place of occurrence of the external cause**

        Golf-course as the place of occurrence of the external cause

        Gymnasium as the place of occurrence of the external cause

        Riding-school as the place of occurrence of the external cause

        Stadium as the place of occurrence of the external cause

---

✓5ᵗʰ   **Y92.4**   Street, highway and other paved roadways as the place of occurrence of the external cause

    EXCLUDES 1   *private driveway of residence (Y92.014, Y92.024, Y92.043, Y92.093, Y92.113, Y92.123, Y92.154, Y92.194)*

✓6ᵗʰ   **Y92.41**   Street and highway **as the place of occurrence of the external cause**

        Y92.410   **Unspecified street and highway as the place of occurrence of the external cause** ▽

            Road NOS as the place of occurrence of the external cause

        Y92.411   Interstate **highway as the place of occurrence of the external cause**

            Freeway as the place of occurrence of the external cause

            Motorway as the place of occurrence of the external cause

        Y92.412   Parkway **as the place of occurrence of the external cause**

        Y92.413   State road **as the place of occurrence of the external cause**

        Y92.414   Local residential or business street **as the place of occurrence of the external cause**

        Y92.415   Exit ramp or entrance ramp **of street or highway as the place of occurrence of the external cause**

✓6ᵗʰ   **Y92.48**   Other paved roadways **as the place of occurrence of the external cause**

        Y92.480   Sidewalk **as the place of occurrence of the external cause**

        Y92.481   Parking lot **as the place of occurrence of the external cause**

        Y92.482   Bike path **as the place of occurrence of the external cause**

        Y92.488   **Other paved roadways as the place of occurrence of the external cause**

✓5ᵗʰ   **Y92.5**   Trade and service area **as the place of occurrence of the external cause**

    EXCLUDES 1   *garage in private home (Y92.015)*

          schools and other public administration buildings (Y92.2-)

✓6ᵗʰ   **Y92.51**   Private commercial establishments **as the place of occurrence of the external cause**

        Y92.510   Bank **as the place of occurrence of the external cause**

        Y92.511   Restaurant or café **as the place of occurrence of the external cause**

        Y92.512   Supermarket, store or market **as the place of occurrence of the external cause**

        Y92.513   Shop (commercial) **as the place of occurrence of the external cause**

✓6ᵗʰ   **Y92.52**   Service areas **as the place of occurrence of the external cause**

        Y92.520   Airport **as the place of occurrence of the external cause**

        Y92.521   Bus station **as the place of occurrence of the external cause**

        Y92.522   Railway station **as the place of occurrence of the external cause**

        Y92.523   Highway rest stop **as the place of occurrence of the external cause**

        Y92.524   Gas station **as the place of occurrence of the external cause**

            Petroleum station as the place of occurrence of the external cause

            Service station as the place of occurrence of the external cause

---

Ⓝ Newborn   Ⓟ Pediatric   Ⓜ Maternity   Ⓐ Adult   **RIC** RIC Dx   **NCDx** Noncancer Dx   **PDx** Primary Dx   **CC** RIC CC Condition   ►◄ Revised Text   ● New Code   ▲ Revised Code Title

1114   ICD-10-CM 2016

✓6ᵗʰ **Y92.53**   Ambulatory health services establishments **as the place of occurrence of the external cause**

     Y92.530   Ambulatory surgery center **as the place of occurrence of the external cause**
         Outpatient surgery center, including that connected with a hospital as the place of occurrence of the external cause
         Same day surgery center, including that connected with a hospital as the place of occurrence of the external cause

     Y92.531   Health care provider office **as the place of occurrence of the external cause**
         Physician office as the place of occurrence of the external cause

     Y92.532   Urgent care center **as the place of occurrence of the external cause**

     Y92.538   Other ambulatory health services establishments as the place of occurrence of the external cause

Y92.59   Other trade areas **as the place of occurrence of the external cause**
     Office building as the place of occurrence of the external cause
     Casino as the place of occurrence of the external cause
     Garage (commercial) as the place of occurrence of the external cause
     Hotel as the place of occurrence of the external cause
     Radio or television station as the place of occurrence of the external cause
     Shopping mall as the place of occurrence of the external cause
     Warehouse as the place of occurrence of the external cause

✓5ᵗʰ **Y92.6**   Industrial and construction area **as the place of occurrence of the external cause**

Y92.61   Building [any] under construction **as the place of occurrence of the external cause**

Y92.62   Dock or shipyard **as the place of occurrence of the external cause**
     Dockyard as the place of occurrence of the external cause
     Dry dock as the place of occurrence of the external cause
     Shipyard as the place of occurrence of the external cause

Y92.63   Factory **as the place of occurrence of the external cause**
     Factory building as the place of occurrence of the external cause
     Factory premises as the place of occurrence of the external cause
     Industrial yard as the place of occurrence of the external cause

Y92.64   Mine or pit **as the place of occurrence of the external cause**
     Mine as the place of occurrence of the external cause

Y92.65   Oil rig **as the place of occurrence of the external cause**
     Pit (coal) (gravel) (sand) as the place of occurrence of the external cause

Y92.69   Other specified industrial and construction area as the place of occurrence of the external cause
     Gasworks as the place of occurrence of the external cause
     Power-station (coal) (nuclear) (oil) as the place of occurrence of the external cause
     Tunnel under construction as the place of occurrence of the external cause
     Workshop as the place of occurrence of the external cause

✓5ᵗʰ **Y92.7**   Farm **as the place of occurrence of the external cause**
     Ranch as the place of occurrence of the external cause
     EXCLUDES 1   farmhouse and home premises of farm (Y92.01-)

Y92.71   Barn **as the place of occurrence of the external cause**

Y92.72   Chicken coop **as the place of occurrence of the external cause**
     Hen house as the place of occurrence of the external cause

Y92.73   Farm field **as the place of occurrence of the external cause**

Y92.74   Orchard **as the place of occurrence of the external cause**

Y92.79   Other farm location **as the place of occurrence of the external cause**

✓5ᵗʰ **Y92.8**   Other places **as the place of occurrence of the external cause**

✓6ᵗʰ **Y92.81**   Transport vehicle **as the place of occurrence of the external cause**
     EXCLUDES 1   transport accidents (V00-V99)

     Y92.810   Car **as the place of occurrence of the external cause**

     Y92.811   Bus **as the place of occurrence of the external cause**

     Y92.812   Truck **as the place of occurrence of the external cause**

     Y92.813   Airplane **as the place of occurrence of the external cause**

     Y92.814   Boat **as the place of occurrence of the external cause**

     Y92.815   Train **as the place of occurrence of the external cause**

     Y92.816   Subway car **as the place of occurrence of the external cause**

     Y92.818   Other transport vehicle as the place of occurrence of the external cause

✓6ᵗʰ **Y92.82**   Wilderness area

     Y92.820   Desert **as the place of occurrence of the external cause**

     Y92.821   Forest **as the place of occurrence of the external cause**

     Y92.828   Other wilderness area as the place of occurrence of the external cause
         Swamp as the place of occurrence of the external cause
         Mountain as the place of occurrence of the external cause
         Marsh as the place of occurrence of the external cause
         Prairie as the place of occurrence of the external cause

✓6ᵗʰ **Y92.83**   Recreation area **as the place of occurrence of the external cause**

     Y92.830   Public park **as the place of occurrence of the external cause**

     Y92.831   Amusement park **as the place of occurrence of the external cause**

     Y92.832   Beach **as the place of occurrence of the external cause**
         Seashore as the place of occurrence of the external cause

     Y92.833   Campsite **as the place of occurrence of the external cause**

     Y92.834   Zoological garden (Zoo) **as the place of occurrence of the external cause**

     Y92.838   Other recreation area as the place of occurrence of the external cause

Y92.84   Military training ground **as the place of occurrence of the external cause**

Y92.85   Railroad track **as the place of occurrence of the external cause**

Y92.86   Slaughter house **as the place of occurrence of the external cause**

Y92.89   Other specified places as the place of occurrence of the external cause
     Derelict house as the place of occurrence of the external cause

Y92.9   Unspecified place or not applicable   ▽

✓ Add'l Character Required   ✓x7ᵗʰ Placeholder Alert   RUG IV Special Care High Dx   RUG IV Clinically Complex Dx   RUG IV Special Care Low Dx   Manifestation Code   Other Specified Code   ▽ Unspecified Code

✓4ᵗʰ **Y93** **Activity codes**

> **NOTE**   Category Y93 is provided for use to indicate the activity of the person seeking healthcare for an injury or health condition, such as a heart attack while shoveling snow, which resulted from, or was contributed to, by the activity. These codes are appropriate for use for both acute injuries, such as those from chapter 19, and conditions that are due to the long-term, cumulative effects of an activity, such as those from chapter 13. They are also appropriate for use with external cause codes for cause and intent if identifying the activity provides additional information on the event. These codes should be used in conjunction with codes for external cause status (Y99) and place of occurrence (Y92).

This section contains the following broad activity categories:
- Y93.0   Activities involving walking and running
- Y93.1   Activities involving water and water craft
- Y93.2   Activities involving ice and snow
- Y93.3   Activities involving climbing, rappelling, and jumping off
- Y93.4   Activities involving dancing and other rhythmic movement
- Y93.5   Activities involving other sports and athletics played individually
- Y93.6   Activities involving other sports and athletics played as a team or group
- Y93.7   Activities involving other specified sports and athletics
- Y93.A   Activities involving other cardiorespiratory exercise
- Y93.B   Activities involving other muscle strengthening exercises
- Y93.C   Activities involving computer technology and electronic devices
- Y93.D   Activities involving arts and handcrafts
- Y93.E   Activities involving personal hygiene and interior property and clothing maintenance
- Y93.F   Activities involving caregiving
- Y93.G   Activities involving food preparation, cooking and grilling
- Y93.H   Activities involving exterior property and land maintenance, building and construction
- Y93.I   Activities involving roller coasters and other types of external motion
- Y93.J   Activities involving playing musical instrument
- Y93.K   Activities involving animal care
- Y93.8   Activities, other specified
- Y93.9   Activity, unspecified

✓5ᵗʰ **Y93.0** **Activities involving walking and running**

> **EXCLUDES 1**   activity, walking an animal (Y93.K1)
> activity, walking or running on a treadmill (Y93.A1)

Y93.01 **Activity, walking, marching and hiking**
Activity, walking, marching and hiking on level or elevated terrain
> **EXCLUDES 1**   activity, mountain climbing (Y93.31)

Y93.02 **Activity, running**

✓5ᵗʰ **Y93.1** **Activities involving water and water craft**

> **EXCLUDES 1**   activities involving ice (Y93.2-)

Y93.11 **Activity, swimming**

Y93.12 **Activity, springboard and platform diving**

Y93.13 **Activity, water polo**

Y93.14 **Activity, water aerobics and water exercise**

Y93.15 **Activity, underwater diving and snorkeling**
Activity, SCUBA diving

Y93.16 **Activity, rowing, canoeing, kayaking, rafting and tubing**
Activity, canoeing, kayaking, rafting and tubing in calm and turbulent water

Y93.17 **Activity, water skiing and wake boarding**

Y93.18 **Activity, surfing, windsurfing and boogie boarding**
Activity, water sliding

Y93.19 **Activity, other involving water and watercraft**
Activity involving water NOS
Activity, parasailing
Activity, water survival training and testing

✓5ᵗʰ **Y93.2** **Activities involving ice and snow**

> **EXCLUDES 1**   activity, shoveling ice and snow (Y93.H1)

Y93.21 **Activity, ice skating**
Activity, figure skating (singles) (pairs)
Activity, ice dancing
> **EXCLUDES 1**   activity, ice hockey (Y93.22)

Y93.22 **Activity, ice hockey**

Y93.23 **Activity, snow (alpine) (downhill) skiing, snow boarding, sledding, tobogganing and snow tubing**
> **EXCLUDES 1**   activity, cross country skiing (Y93.24)

Y93.24 **Activity, cross country skiing**
Activity, nordic skiing

Y93.29 **Activity, other involving ice and snow**
Activity involving ice and snow NOS

✓5ᵗʰ **Y93.3** **Activities involving climbing, rappelling and jumping off**

> **EXCLUDES 1**   activity, hiking on level or elevated terrain (Y93.01)
> activity, jumping rope (Y93.56)
> activity, trampoline jumping (Y93.44)

Y93.31 **Activity, mountain climbing, rock climbing and wall climbing**

Y93.32 **Activity, rappelling**

Y93.33 **Activity, BASE jumping**
Activity, Building, Antenna, Span, Earth jumping

Y93.34 **Activity, bungee jumping**

Y93.35 **Activity, hang gliding**

Y93.39 **Activity, other involving climbing, rappelling and jumping off**

✓5ᵗʰ **Y93.4** **Activities involving dancing and other rhythmic movement**

> **EXCLUDES 1**   activity, martial arts (Y93.75)

Y93.41 **Activity, dancing**
AHA: 2012, 4Q, 108

Y93.42 **Activity, yoga**

Y93.43 **Activity, gymnastics**
Activity, rhythmic gymnastics
> **EXCLUDES 1**   activity, trampolining (Y93.44)

Y93.44 **Activity, trampolining**

Y93.45 **Activity, cheerleading**

Y93.49 **Activity, other involving dancing and other rhythmic movements**

✓5ᵗʰ **Y93.5** **Activities involving other sports and athletics played individually**

> **EXCLUDES 1**   activity, dancing (Y93.41)
> activity, gymnastic (Y93.43)
> activity, trampolining (Y93.44)
> activity, yoga (Y93.42)

Y93.51 **Activity, roller skating (inline) and skateboarding**

Y93.52 **Activity, horseback riding**

Y93.53 **Activity, golf**

Y93.54 **Activity, bowling**

Y93.55 **Activity, bike riding**

Y93.56 **Activity, jumping rope**

Y93.57 **Activity, non-running track and field events**
> **EXCLUDES 1**   activity, running (any form) (Y93.02)

Y93.59 **Activity, other involving other sports and athletics played individually**
> **EXCLUDES 1**   activities involving climbing, rappelling, and jumping (Y93.3-)
> activities involving ice and snow (Y93.2-)
> activities involving walking and running (Y93.0-)
> activities involving water and watercraft (Y93.1-)

✓5ᵗʰ **Y93.6** **Activities involving other sports and athletics played as a team or group**

> **EXCLUDES 1**   activity, ice hockey (Y93.22)
> activity, water polo (Y93.13)

Y93.61 **Activity, American tackle football**
Activity, football NOS

Y93.62 **Activity, American flag or touch football**

Y93.63 **Activity, rugby**

Y93.64 **Activity, baseball**
Activity, softball

Y93.65 **Activity, lacrosse and field hockey**

Y93.66 **Activity, soccer**

Y93.67 **Activity, basketball**

Y93.68 **Activity, volleyball (beach) (court)**

Y93.6A **Activity, physical games generally associated with school recess, summer camp and children**   🅿
Activity, capture the flag
Activity, dodge ball
Activity, four square
Activity, kickball

Y93.69 **Activity, other involving other sports and athletics played as a team or group**
Activity, cricket

✓5ᵗʰ **Y93.7** **Activities involving other specified sports and athletics**

Y93.71 **Activity, boxing**

Y93.72 **Activity, wrestling**

🅽 Newborn   🅿 Pediatric   🅼 Maternity   🅰 Adult   **RIC** RIC Dx   **NC Dx** Noncancer Dx   **PDx** Primary Dx   **CC** RIC CC Condition   ▶◀ Revised Text   ● New Code   ▲ Revised Code Title

1116   ICD-10-CM 2016

Y93.73   **Activity, racquet and hand sports**
     Activity, handball
     Activity, racquetball
     Activity, squash
     Activity, tennis

Y93.74   **Activity, frisbee**
     Activity, ultimate frisbee

Y93.75   **Activity, martial arts**
     Activity, combatives

Y93.79   **Activity, other specified sports and athletics**
     EXCLUDES 1   sports and athletics activities specified in
          categories Y93.0-Y93.6

✓5ᵗʰ **Y93.A**   **Activities involving other cardiorespiratory exercise**
     Activities involving physical training

Y93.A1   **Activity, exercise machines primarily for cardiorespiratory conditioning**
     Activity, elliptical and stepper machines
     Activity, stationary bike
     Activity, treadmill

Y93.A2   **Activity, calisthenics**
     Activity, jumping jacks
     Activity, warm up and cool down

Y93.A3   **Activity, aerobic and step exercise**

Y93.A4   **Activity, circuit training**

Y93.A5   **Activity, obstacle course**
     Activity, challenge course
     Activity, confidence course

Y93.A6   **Activity, grass drills**
     Activity, guerilla drills

Y93.A9   **Activity, other involving cardiorespiratory exercise**
     EXCLUDES 1   activities involving cardiorespiratory exercise
          specified in categories Y93.0-Y93.7

✓5ᵗʰ **Y93.B**   **Activities involving other muscle strengthening exercises**

Y93.B1   **Activity, exercise machines primarily for muscle strengthening**

Y93.B2   **Activity, push-ups, pull-ups, sit-ups**

Y93.B3   **Activity, free weights**
     Activity, barbells
     Activity, dumbbells

Y93.B4   **Activity, pilates**

Y93.B9   **Activity, other involving muscle strengthening exercises**
     EXCLUDES 1   activities involving muscle strengthening
          specified in categories Y93.0-Y93.A

✓5ᵗʰ **Y93.C**   **Activities involving computer technology and electronic devices**
     EXCLUDES 1   activity, electronic musical keyboard or instruments
          (Y93.J-)

Y93.C1   **Activity, computer keyboarding**
     Activity, electronic game playing using keyboard or other stationary device

Y93.C2   **Activity, hand held interactive electronic device**
     Activity, cellular telephone and communication device
     Activity, electronic game playing using interactive device
     EXCLUDES 1   activity, electronic game playing using
          keyboard or other stationary device
          (Y93.C1)

Y93.C9   **Activity, other involving computer technology and electronic devices**

✓5ᵗʰ **Y93.D**   **Activities involving arts and handcrafts**
     EXCLUDES 1   activities involving playing musical instrument (Y93.J-)

Y93.D1   **Activity, knitting and crocheting**

Y93.D2   **Activity, sewing**

Y93.D3   **Activity, furniture building and finishing**
     Activity, furniture repair

Y93.D9   **Activity, other involving arts and handcrafts**

✓5ᵗʰ **Y93.E**   **Activities involving personal hygiene and interior property and clothing maintenance**
     EXCLUDES 1   activities involving cooking and grilling (Y93.G-)
          activities involving exterior property and land
             maintenance, building and construction (Y93.H-)
          activities involving caregiving (Y93.F-)
          activity, dishwashing (Y93.G1)
          activity, food preparation (Y93.G1)
          activity, gardening (Y93.H2)

Y93.E1   **Activity, personal bathing and showering**

Y93.E2   **Activity, laundry**

Y93.E3   **Activity, vacuuming**

Y93.E4   **Activity, ironing**

Y93.E5   **Activity, floor mopping and cleaning**

Y93.E6   **Activity, residential relocation**
     Activity, packing up and unpacking involved in moving to a new residence

Y93.E8   **Activity, other personal hygiene**

Y93.E9   **Activity, other interior property and clothing maintenance**

✓5ᵗʰ **Y93.F**   **Activities involving caregiving**
     Activity involving the provider of caregiving

Y93.F1   **Activity, caregiving, bathing**

Y93.F2   **Activity, caregiving, lifting**

Y93.F9   **Activity, other caregiving**

✓5ᵗʰ **Y93.G**   **Activities involving food preparation, cooking and grilling**

Y93.G1   **Activity, food preparation and clean up**
     Activity, dishwashing

Y93.G2   **Activity, grilling and smoking food**

Y93.G3   **Activity, cooking and baking**
     Activity, use of stove, oven and microwave oven

Y93.G9   **Activity, other involving cooking and grilling**

✓5ᵗʰ **Y93.H**   **Activities involving exterior property and land maintenance, building and construction**

Y93.H1   **Activity, digging, shoveling and raking**
     Activity, dirt digging
     Activity, raking leaves
     Activity, snow shoveling

Y93.H2   **Activity, gardening and landscaping**
     Activity, pruning, trimming shrubs, weeding

Y93.H3   **Activity, building and construction**

Y93.H9   **Activity, other involving exterior property and land maintenance, building and construction**

✓5ᵗʰ **Y93.I**   **Activities involving roller coasters and other types of external motion**

Y93.I1   **Activity, rollercoaster riding**

Y93.I9   **Activity, other involving external motion**

✓5ᵗʰ **Y93.J**   **Activities involving playing musical instrument**
     Activity involving playing electric musical instrument

Y93.J1   **Activity, piano playing**
     Activity, musical keyboard (electronic) playing

Y93.J2   **Activity, drum and other percussion instrument playing**

Y93.J3   **Activity, string instrument playing**

Y93.J4   **Activity, winds and brass instrument playing**

✓5ᵗʰ **Y93.K**   **Activities involving animal care**
     EXCLUDES 1   activity, horseback riding (Y93.52)

Y93.K1   **Activity, walking an animal**

Y93.K2   **Activity, milking an animal**

Y93.K3   **Activity, grooming and shearing an animal**

Y93.K9   **Activity, other involving animal care**

✓5ᵗʰ **Y93.8**   **Activities, other specified**

Y93.81   **Activity, refereeing a sports activity**

Y93.82   **Activity, spectator at an event**

Y93.83   **Activity, rough housing and horseplay**

Y93.84   **Activity, sleeping**

Y93.89   **Activity, other specified**

Y93.9   **Activity, unspecified**   ▽

Y95   **Nosocomial condition**
     AHA: 2013, 4Q, 119

☑ Add'l Character Required   ✓x7ᵗʰ Placeholder Alert   RUG IV Special Care High Dx   RUG IV Clinically Complex Dx   RUG IV Special Care Low Dx   Manifestation Code   Other Specified Code   ▽ Unspecified Code

ICD-10-CM 2016   **1117**

☑4ᵗʰ Y99   External cause status

> **NOTE**   A single code from category Y99 should be used in conjunction with the external cause code(s) assigned to a record to indicate the status of the person at the time the event occurred.

Y99.0   Civilian activity done for income or pay
> Civilian activity done for financial or other compensation
> **EXCLUDES 1**   military activity (Y99.1)
>   volunteer activity (Y99.2)

Y99.1   Military activity
> **EXCLUDES 1**   activity of off duty military personnel (Y99.8)

Y99.2   Volunteer activity
> **EXCLUDES 1**   activity of child or other family member assisting in compensated work of other family member (Y99.8)

Y99.8   Other external cause status
> Activity NEC
> Activity of child or other family member assisting in compensated work of other family member
> Hobby not done for income
> Leisure activity
> Off-duty activity of military personnel
> Recreation or sport not for income or while a student
> Student activity
> **EXCLUDES 1**   civilian activity done for income or compensation (Y99.0)
>   military activity (Y99.1)
> **AHA:** 2012, 4Q, 108

Y99.9   Unspecified external cause status   ▽

☒ Newborn   ☒ Pediatric   ☒ Maternity   ☒ Adult   **RIC** RIC Dx   **NCDx** Noncancer Dx   **PDx** Primary Dx   **CC** RIC CC Condition   ▶◀ Revised Text   ● New Code   ▲ Revised Code Title

1118   ICD-10-CM 2016

Chapter 21. Factors Influencing Health Status and Contact with Health Services (Z00–Z99)

Chapter Specific Guidelines with Coding Examples

The chapter specific guidelines from the ICD-10-CM Official Guidelines for Coding and Reporting have been provided below. Along with these guidelines are coding examples, contained in the shaded boxes, that have been developed to help illustrate the coding and/or sequencing guidance found in these guidelines.

Note: The chapter specific guidelines provide additional information about the use of Z codes for specified encounters.

a. Use of Z codes in any healthcare setting

Z codes are for use in any healthcare setting. Z codes may be used as either a first-listed (principal diagnosis code in the inpatient setting) or secondary code, depending on the circumstances of the encounter. Certain Z codes may only be used as first-listed or principal diagnosis.

> Patient with middle lobe lung cancer admitted for initiation of chemotherapy
>
> **Z51.11**   **Encounter for antineoplastic chemotherapy**
>
> **C34.2**   **Malignant neoplasm of middle lobe, bronchus or lung**
>
> *Explanation:* A Z code can be used as first-listed in this situation based on guidelines in this chapter as well as chapter 2, "Neoplasms."

> Patient has chronic lymphocytic leukemia for which the patient had previous chemotherapy and is now in remission
>
> **C91.11**   **Chronic lymphocytic leukemia of B-cell type in remission**
>
> **Z92.21**   **Personal history of antineoplastic chemotherapy**
>
> *Explanation:*The personal history Z code is used to describe a secondary (supplementary) diagnosis to identify that this patient has had chemotherapy in the past.

b. Z Codes indicate a reason for an encounter

Z codes are not procedure codes. A corresponding procedure code must accompany a Z code to describe any procedure performed.

c. Categories of Z codes

1) Contact/exposure

Category Z20 indicates contact with, and suspected exposure to, communicable diseases. These codes are for patients who do not show any sign or symptom of a disease but are suspected to have been exposed to it by close personal contact with an infected individual or are in an area where a disease is epidemic.

Category Z77, Other contact with and (suspected) exposures hazardous to health, indicates contact with and suspected exposures hazardous to health.

Contact/exposure codes may be used as a first-listed code to explain an encounter for testing, or, more commonly, as a secondary code to identify a potential risk.

2) Inoculations and vaccinations

Code Z23 is for encounters for inoculations and vaccinations. It indicates that a patient is being seen to receive a prophylactic inoculation against a disease. Procedure codes are required to identify the actual administration of the injection and the type(s) of immunizations given. Code Z23 may be used as a secondary code if the inoculation is given as a routine part of preventive health care, such as a well-baby visit.

3) Status

Status codes indicate that a patient is either a carrier of a disease or has the sequelae or residual of a past disease or condition. This includes such things as the presence of prosthetic or mechanical devices resulting from past treatment. A status code is informative, because the status may affect the course of treatment and its outcome. A status code is distinct from a history code. The history code indicates that the patient no longer has the condition.

A status code should not be used with a diagnosis code from one of the body system chapters, if the diagnosis code includes the information provided by the status code. For example, code Z94.1, Heart transplant status, should not be used with a code from subcategory T86.2, Complications of heart transplant. The status code does not provide additional information. The complication code indicates that the patient is a heart transplant patient.

For encounters for weaning from a mechanical ventilator, assign a code from subcategory J96.1, Chronic respiratory failure, followed by code Z99.11, Dependence on respirator [ventilator] status.

The status Z codes/categories are:

Z14   Genetic carrier

    Genetic carrier status indicates that a person carries a gene, associated with a particular disease, which may be passed to offspring who may develop that disease. The person does not have the disease and is not at risk of developing the disease.

Z15   Genetic susceptibility to disease

    Genetic susceptibility indicates that a person has a gene that increases the risk of that person developing the disease.

    Codes from category Z15 should not be used as principal or first-listed codes. If the patient has the condition to which he/she is susceptible, and that condition is the reason for the encounter, the code for the current condition should be sequenced first. If the patient is being seen for follow-up after completed treatment for this condition, and the condition no longer exists, a follow-up code should be sequenced first, followed by the appropriate personal history and genetic susceptibility codes. If the purpose of the encounter is genetic counseling associated with procreative management, code Z31.5, Encounter for genetic counseling, should be assigned as the first-listed code, followed by a code from category Z15. Additional codes should be assigned for any applicable family or personal history.

Z16   Resistance to antimicrobial drugs

    This code indicates that a patient has a condition that is resistant to antimicrobial drug treatment. Sequence the infection code first.

Z17   Estrogen receptor status

Z18   Retained foreign body fragments

Z21   Asymptomatic HIV infection status

    This code indicates that a patient has tested positive for HIV but has manifested no signs or symptoms of the disease.

Z22   Carrier of infectious disease

    Carrier status indicates that a person harbors the specific organisms of a disease without manifest symptoms and is capable of transmitting the infection.

Z28.3   Underimmunization status

Z33.1   Pregnant state, incidental

    This code is a secondary code only for use when the pregnancy is in no way complicating the reason for visit. Otherwise, a code from the obstetric chapter is required.

Z66   Do not resuscitate

    This code may be used when it is documented by the provider that a patient is on do not resuscitate status at any time during the stay.

Z67   Blood type

Z68   Body mass index (BMI)

Z74.01   Bed confinement status

Z76.82   Awaiting organ transplant status

Z78   Other specified health status

    Code Z78.1, Physical restraint status, may be used when it is documented by the provider that a patient has been put in restraints during the current encounter. Please note that this code should not be reported when it is documented by the provider that a patient is temporarily restrained during a procedure.

Z79   Long-term (current) drug therapy

    Codes from this category indicate a patient's continuous use of a prescribed drug (including such things as aspirin therapy) for the long-term treatment of a condition or for prophylactic use. It is not for use for patients who have addictions to drugs. This subcategory is not for use of medications for detoxification or maintenance programs to prevent withdrawal symptoms in patients with drug dependence (e.g., methadone maintenance for opiate dependence). Assign the appropriate code for the drug dependence instead.

Assign a code from Z79 if the patient is receiving a medication for an extended period as a prophylactic measure (such as for the prevention of deep vein thrombosis) or as treatment of a chronic condition (such as arthritis) or a disease requiring a lengthy course of treatment (such as cancer). Do not assign a code from category Z79 for medication being administered for a brief period of time to treat an acute illness or injury (such as a course of antibiotics to treat acute bronchitis).

Z88	Allergy status to drugs, medicaments and biological substances

Except: Z88.9, Allergy status to unspecified drugs, medicaments and biological substances status

Z89	Acquired absence of limb
Z90	Acquired absence of organs, not elsewhere classified
Z91.0-	Allergy status, other than to drugs and biological substances
Z92.82	Status post administration of tPA (rtPA) in a different facility within the last 24 hours prior to admission to a current facility

Assign code Z92.82, Status post administration of tPA (rtPA) in a different facility within the last 24 hours prior to admission to current facility, as a secondary diagnosis when a patient is received by transfer into a facility and documentation indicates they were administered tissue plasminogen activator (tPA) within the last 24 hours prior to admission to the current facility.

This guideline applies even if the patient is still receiving the tPA at the time they are received into the current facility.

The appropriate code for the condition for which the tPA was administered (such as cerebrovascular disease or myocardial infarction) should be assigned first.

Code Z92.82 is only applicable to the receiving facility record and not to the transferring facility record.

Z93	Artificial opening status
Z94	Transplanted organ and tissue status
Z95	Presence of cardiac and vascular implants and grafts
Z96	Presence of other functional implants
Z97	Presence of other devices
Z98	Other postprocedural states

Assign code Z98.85, Transplanted organ removal status, to indicate that a transplanted organ has been previously removed. This code should not be assigned for the encounter in which the transplanted organ is removed. The complication necessitating removal of the transplant organ should be assigned for that encounter.

See section I.C19. for information on the coding of organ transplant complications.

Z99	Dependence on enabling machines and devices, not elsewhere classified

Note: Categories Z89-Z90 and Z93-Z99 are for use only if there are no complications or malfunctions of the organ or tissue replaced, the amputation site or the equipment on which the patient is dependent..

4) History (of)

There are two types of history Z codes, personal and family. Personal history codes explain a patient's past medical condition that no longer exists and is not receiving any treatment, but that has the potential for recurrence, and therefore may require continued monitoring.

Family history codes are for use when a patient has a family member(s) who has had a particular disease that causes the patient to be at higher risk of also contracting the disease.

Personal history codes may be used in conjunction with follow-up codes and family history codes may be used in conjunction with screening codes to explain the need for a test or procedure. History codes are also acceptable on any medical record regardless of the reason for visit. A history of an illness, even if no longer present, is important information that may alter the type of treatment ordered.

The history Z code categories are:

Z80	Family history of primary malignant neoplasm
Z81	Family history of mental and behavioral disorders
Z82	Family history of certain disabilities and chronic diseases (leading to disablement)
Z83	Family history of other specific disorders
Z84	Family history of other conditions
Z85	Personal history of malignant neoplasm

Z86	Personal history of certain other diseases
Z87	Personal history of other diseases and conditions
Z91.4-	Personal history of psychological trauma, not elsewhere classified
Z91.5	Personal history of self-harm
Z91.8-	Other specified personal risk factors, not elsewhere classified

Except: Z91.83, Wandering in diseases classified elsewhere

Z92	Personal history of medical treatment

Except: Z92.0, Personal history of contraception

Except: Z92.82, Status post administration of tPA (rtPA) in a different facility within the last 24 hours prior to admission to a current facility

5) Screening

Screening is the testing for disease or disease precursors in seemingly well individuals so that early detection and treatment can be provided for those who test positive for the disease (e.g., screening mammogram).

The testing of a person to rule out or confirm a suspected diagnosis because the patient has some sign or symptom is a diagnostic examination, not a screening. In these cases, the sign or symptom is used to explain the reason for the test.

A screening code may be a first-listed code if the reason for the visit is specifically the screening exam. It may also be used as an additional code if the screening is done during an office visit for other health problems. A screening code is not necessary if the screening is inherent to a routine examination, such as a pap smear done during a routine pelvic examination.

Should a condition be discovered during the screening then the code for the condition may be assigned as an additional diagnosis.

Prostate screening of healthy 50-year-old male patient; PSA noted to be elevated but normal digital rectal exam

Z12.5   **Encounter for screening for malignant neoplasm of prostate**

R97.2   **Elevated prostate specific antigen [PSA]**

Explanation: The patient had no signs or symptoms of any prostate-related illness prior to coming in for the screening. The screening code is appropriately used as the first-listed code to signify that this was for routine screening. The elevated PSA is reported as a secondary diagnosis to reflect that an abnormal lab value was found as a result of the screening procedure(s).

The Z code indicates that a screening exam is planned. A procedure code is required to confirm that the screening was performed.

The screening Z codes/categories:

Z11	Encounter for screening for infectious and parasitic diseases
Z12	Encounter for screening for malignant neoplasms
Z13	Encounter for screening for other diseases and disorders

Except: Z13.9, Encounter for screening, unspecified

Z36	Encounter for antenatal screening for mother

6) Observation

There are two observation Z code categories. They are for use in very limited circumstances when a person is being observed for a suspected condition that is ruled out. The observation codes are not for use if an injury or illness or any signs or symptoms related to the suspected condition are present. In such cases the diagnosis/symptom code is used with the corresponding external cause code.

The observation codes are to be used as principal diagnosis only. Additional codes may be used in addition to the observation code but only if they are unrelated to the suspected condition being observed.

Codes from subcategory Z03.7, Encounter for suspected maternal and fetal conditions ruled out, may either be used as a first-listed or as an additional code assignment depending on the case. They are for use in very limited circumstances on a maternal record when an encounter is for a suspected maternal or fetal condition that is ruled out during that encounter (for example, a maternal or fetal condition may be suspected due to an abnormal test result). These codes should not be used when the condition is confirmed. In those cases, the confirmed condition should be coded. In addition, these codes are not for use if an illness or any signs or symptoms related to the suspected condition or problem are present. In such cases the diagnosis/symptom code is used.

Additional codes may be used in addition to the code from subcategory Z03.7, but only if they are unrelated to the suspected condition being evaluated.

Codes from subcategory Z03.7 may not be used for encounters for antenatal screening of mother. *See Section I.C.21. Screening.*

For encounters for suspected fetal condition that are inconclusive following testing and evaluation, assign the appropriate code from category O35, O36, O40 or O41.

The observation Z code categories:

Z03	Encounter for medical observation for suspected diseases and conditions ruled out
Z04	Encounter for examination and observation for other reasons
	Except: Z04.9, Encounter for examination and observation for unspecified reason

7) Aftercare

Aftercare visit codes cover situations when the initial treatment of a disease has been performed and the patient requires continued care during the healing or recovery phase, or for the long-term consequences of the disease. The aftercare Z code should not be used if treatment is directed at a current, acute disease. The diagnosis code is to be used in these cases. Exceptions to this rule are codes Z51.0, Encounter for antineoplastic radiation therapy, and codes from subcategory Z51.1, Encounter for antineoplastic chemotherapy and immunotherapy. These codes are to be first-listed, followed by the diagnosis code when a patient's encounter is solely to receive radiation therapy, chemotherapy, or immunotherapy for the treatment of a neoplasm. If the reason for the encounter is more than one type of antineoplastic therapy, code Z51.0 and a code from subcategory Z51.1 may be assigned together, in which case one of these codes would be reported as a secondary diagnosis.

The aftercare Z codes should also not be used for aftercare for injuries. For aftercare of an injury, assign the acute injury code with the appropriate 7th character (for subsequent encounter).

The aftercare codes are generally first-listed to explain the specific reason for the encounter. An aftercare code may be used as an additional code when some type of aftercare is provided in addition to the reason for admission and no diagnosis code is applicable. An example of this would be the closure of a colostomy during an encounter for treatment of another condition.

Aftercare codes should be used in conjunction with other aftercare codes or diagnosis codes to provide better detail on the specifics of an aftercare encounter visit, unless otherwise directed by the classification. Should a patient receive multiple types of antineoplastic therapy during the same encounter, code Z51.0, Encounter for antineoplastic radiation therapy, and codes from subcategory Z51.1, Encounter for antineoplastic chemotherapy and immunotherapy, may be used together on a record. The sequencing of multiple aftercare codes depends on the circumstances of the encounter.

Certain aftercare Z code categories need a secondary diagnosis code to describe the resolving condition or sequelae. For others, the condition is included in the code title.

Additional Z code aftercare category terms include fitting and adjustment, and attention to artificial openings.

Status Z codes may be used with aftercare Z codes to indicate the nature of the aftercare. For example code Z95.1, Presence of aortocoronary bypass graft, may be used with code Z48.812, Encounter for surgical aftercare following surgery on the circulatory system, to indicate the surgery for which the aftercare is being performed. A status code should not be used when the aftercare code indicates the type of status, such as using Z43.0, Encounter for attention to tracheostomy, with Z93.0, Tracheostomy status.

The aftercare Z category/codes:

Z42	Encounter for plastic and reconstructive surgery following medical procedure or healed injury
Z43	Encounter for attention to artificial openings
Z44	Encounter for fitting and adjustment of external prosthetic device
Z45	Encounter for adjustment and management of implanted device
Z46	Encounter for fitting and adjustment of other devices
Z47	Orthopedic aftercare
Z48	Encounter for other postprocedural aftercare
Z49	Encounter for care involving renal dialysis
Z51	Encounter for other aftercare

8) Follow-up

The follow-up codes are used to explain continuing surveillance following completed treatment of a disease, condition, or injury. They imply that the condition has been fully treated and no longer exists. They should not be confused with aftercare codes, or injury codes with a 7th character for subsequent encounter, that explain ongoing care of a healing condition

or its sequelae. Follow-up codes may be used in conjunction with history codes to provide the full picture of the healed condition and its treatment. The follow-up code is sequenced first, followed by the history code.

A follow-up code may be used to explain multiple visits. Should a condition be found to have recurred on the follow-up visit, then the diagnosis code for the condition should be assigned in place of the follow-up code.

The follow-up Z code categories:

Z08	Encounter for follow-up examination after completed treatment for malignant neoplasm
Z09	Encounter for follow-up examination after completed treatment for conditions other than malignant neoplasm
Z39	Encounter for maternal postpartum care and examination

Follow-up for patient several months after completing a regime of IV antibiotics for recurrent pneumonia; lungs are clear and pneumonia is resolved

Z09	**Encounter for follow-up examination after completed treatment for conditions other than malignant neoplasm**
Z87.01	**Personal history of pneumonia (recurrent)**

Explanation: Code Z09 identifies the follow-up visit as being unrelated to a malignant neoplasm, and code Z87 describes the condition that has now resolved.

Follow-up for patient several months after completing a regime of IV antibiotics for recurrent pneumonia; pneumonia has recurred, and a new antibiotic regimen has been prescribed

J18.9	**Pneumonia, unspecified organism**

Explanation: Since the follow-up exam for pneumonia determined that the pneumonia was not resolved or recurred, code Z09 Encounter for follow-up examination after completed treatment for conditions other than malignant neoplasm, no longer applies. Instead the first-listed code describes the pneumonia.

---

9) Donor

Codes in category Z52, Donors of organs and tissues, are used for living individuals who are donating blood or other body tissue. These codes are only for individuals donating for others, not for self-donations. They are not used to identify cadaveric donations.

10) Counseling

Counseling Z codes are used when a patient or family member receives assistance in the aftermath of an illness or injury, or when support is required in coping with family or social problems. They are not used in conjunction with a diagnosis code when the counseling component of care is considered integral to standard treatment.

The counseling Z codes/categories:

Z30.0-	Encounter for general counseling and advice on contraception
Z31.5	Encounter for genetic counseling
Z31.6-	Encounter for general counseling and advice on procreation
Z32.2	Encounter for childbirth instruction
Z32.3	Encounter for childcare instruction
Z69	Encounter for mental health services for victim and perpetrator of abuse
Z70	Counseling related to sexual attitude, behavior and orientation
Z71	Persons encountering health services for other counseling and medical advice, not elsewhere classified
Z76.81	Expectant mother prebirth pediatrician visit

11) Encounters for obstetrical and reproductive services

See Section I.C.15. Pregnancy, Childbirth, and the Puerperium, for further instruction on the use of these codes.

Z codes for pregnancy are for use in those circumstances when none of the problems or complications included in the codes from the Obstetrics chapter exist (a routine prenatal visit or postpartum care). Codes in category Z34, Encounter for supervision of normal pregnancy, are always first-listed and are not to be used with any other code from the OB chapter.

Codes in category Z3A, Weeks of gestation, may be assigned to provide additional information about the pregnancy. The date of the admission should be used to determine weeks of gestation for inpatient admissions that encompass more than one gestational week.

The outcome of delivery, category Z37, should be included on all maternal delivery records. It is always a secondary code. Codes in category Z37 should not be used on the newborn record.

Z codes for family planning (contraceptive) or procreative management and counseling should be included on an obstetric record either during the pregnancy or the postpartum stage, if applicable.

Z codes/categories for obstetrical and reproductive services:

Z30	Encounter for contraceptive management
Z31	Encounter for procreative management
Z32.2	Encounter for childbirth instruction
Z32.3	Encounter for childcare instruction
Z33	Pregnant state
Z34	Encounter for supervision of normal pregnancy
Z36	Encounter for antenatal screening of mother
Z3A	Weeks of gestation
Z37	Outcome of delivery
Z39	Encounter for maternal postpartum care and examination
Z76.81	Expectant mother prebirth pediatrician visit

12) Newborns and infants

See Section I.C.16. Newborn (Perinatal) Guidelines, for further instruction on the use of these codes.

Newborn Z codes/categories:

Z76.1	Encounter for health supervision and care of foundling
Z00.1-	Encounter for routine child health examination
Z38	Liveborn infants according to place of birth and type of delivery

13) Routine and administrative examinations

The Z codes allow for the description of encounters for routine examinations, such as, a general check-up, or, examinations for administrative purposes, such as, a pre-employment physical. The codes are not to be used if the examination is for diagnosis of a suspected condition or for treatment purposes. In such cases the diagnosis code is used. During a routine exam, should a diagnosis or condition be discovered, it should be coded as an additional code. Pre-existing and chronic conditions and history codes may also be included as additional codes as long as the examination is for administrative purposes and not focused on any particular condition.

Some of the codes for routine health examinations distinguish between "with" and "without" abnormal findings. Code assignment depends on the information that is known at the time the encounter is being coded. For example, if no abnormal findings were found during the examination, but the encounter is being coded before test results are back, it is acceptable to assign the code for "without abnormal findings." When assigning a code for "with abnormal findings," additional code(s) should be assigned to identify the specific abnormal finding(s).

12-month-old boy admitted for well-child visit; pediatrician notices some eczema on the child's scalp and back of the knees

Z00.121   Encounter for routine child health examination with abnormal findings

L30.9   Dermatitis, unspecified

Explanation: The Z code identifying that this is a routine well-child visit is reported first. Because an abnormal finding (eczema) was documented, a code for this condition may also be appended.

Pre-operative examination and pre-procedural laboratory examination Z codes are for use only in those situations when a patient is being cleared for a procedure or surgery and no treatment is given.

The Z codes/categories for routine and administrative examinations:

Z00	Encounter for general examination without complaint, suspected or reported diagnosis
Z01	Encounter for other special examination without complaint, suspected or reported diagnosis
Z02	Encounter for administrative examination
	Except: Z02.9, Encounter for administrative examinations, unspecified
Z32.0-	Encounter for pregnancy test

14) Miscellaneous Z codes

The miscellaneous Z codes capture a number of other health care encounters that do not fall into one of the other categories. Certain of these codes identify the reason for the encounter; others are for use as additional codes that provide useful information on circumstances that may affect a patient's care and treatment.

Prophylactic Organ Removal

For encounters specifically for prophylactic removal of an organ (such as prophylactic removal of breasts due to a genetic susceptibility to cancer or a family history of cancer), the principal or first-listed code should be a code from category Z40, Encounter for prophylactic surgery, followed by the appropriate codes to identify the associated risk factor (such as genetic susceptibility or family history).

If the patient has a malignancy of one site and is having prophylactic removal at another site to prevent either a new primary malignancy or metastatic disease, a code for the malignancy should also be assigned in addition to a code from subcategory Z40.0, Encounter for prophylactic surgery for risk factors related to malignant neoplasms. A Z40.0 code should not be assigned if the patient is having organ removal for treatment of a malignancy, such as the removal of the testes for the treatment of prostate cancer.

Miscellaneous Z codes/categories:

Z28	Immunization not carried out
	Except: Z28.3, Underimmunization status
Z40	Encounter for prophylactic surgery
Z41	Encounter for procedures for purposes other than remedying health state
	Except: Z41.9, Encounter for procedure for purposes other than remedying health state, unspecified
Z53	Persons encountering health services for specific procedures and treatment, not carried out
Z55	Problems related to education and literacy
Z56	Problems related to employment and unemployment
Z57	Occupational exposure to risk factors
Z58	Problems related to physical environment
Z59	Problems related to housing and economic circumstances
Z60	Problems related to social environment
Z62	Problems related to upbringing
Z63	Other problems related to primary support group, including family circumstances
Z64	Problems related to certain psychosocial circumstances
Z65	Problems related to other psychosocial circumstances
Z72	Problems related to lifestyle
Z73	Problems related to life management difficulty
Z74	Problems related to care provider dependency
	Except: Z74.01, Bed confinement status
Z75	Problems related to medical facilities and other health care
Z76.0	Encounter for issue of repeat prescription
Z76.3	Healthy person accompanying sick person
Z76.4	Other boarder to healthcare facility
Z76.5	Malingerer [conscious simulation]
Z91.1-	Patient's noncompliance with medical treatment and regimen
Z91.83	Wandering in diseases classified elsewhere
Z91.89	Other specified personal risk factors, not elsewhere classified

15) Nonspecific Z codes

Certain Z codes are so non-specific, or potentially redundant with other codes in the classification, that there can be little justification for their use in the inpatient setting. Their use in the outpatient setting should be limited to those instances when there is no further documentation to permit more precise coding. Otherwise, any sign or symptom or any other reason for visit that is captured in another code should be used.

Nonspecific Z codes/categories:

Z02.9	Encounter for administrative examinations, unspecified
Z04.9	Encounter for examination and observation for unspecified reason
Z13.9	Encounter for screening, unspecified
Z41.9	Encounter for procedure for purposes other than remedying health state, unspecified
Z52.9	Donor of unspecified organ or tissue
Z86.59	Personal history of other mental and behavioral disorders
Z88.9	Allergy status to unspecified drugs, medicaments and biological substances status
Z92.0	Personal history of contraception

16) Z codes that may only be principal/first-listed diagnosis

The following Z codes/categories may only be reported as the principal/first-listed diagnosis, except when there are multiple encounters on the same day and the medical records for the encounters are combined:

Z00   Encounter for general examination without complaint, suspected or reported diagnosis

     Except: Z00.6

Z01   Encounter for other special examination without complaint, suspected or reported diagnosis

Z02   Encounter for administrative examination

Z03   Encounter for medical observation for suspected diseases and conditions ruled out

Z04   Encounter for examination and observation for other reasons

Z33.2   Encounter for elective termination of pregnancy

Z31.81   Encounter for male factor infertility in female patient

Z31.82   Encounter for Rh incompatibility status

Z31.83   Encounter for assisted reproductive fertility procedure cycle

Z31.84   Encounter for fertility preservation procedure

Z34   Encounter for supervision of normal pregnancy

Z39   Encounter for maternal postpartum care and examination

Z38   Liveborn infants according to place of birth and type of delivery

Z42   Encounter for plastic and reconstructive surgery following medical procedure or healed injury

Z51.0   Encounter for antineoplastic radiation therapy

Z51.1-   Encounter for antineoplastic chemotherapy and immunotherapy

Z52   Donors of organs and tissues

     Except: Z52.9, Donor of unspecified organ or tissue

Z76.1   Encounter for health supervision and care of foundling

Z76.2   Encounter for health supervision and care of other healthy infant and child

Z99.12   Encounter for respirator [ventilator] dependence during power failure

---

Female patient seen at 32 weeks' gestation to check the progress of her first pregnancy

Z34.03   **Encounter for supervision of normal first pregnancy, third trimester**

Z3A.32   **32 weeks gestation of pregnancy**

Explanation: Category Z34 is appropriate as a first-listed diagnosis. Category Z3A helps to clarify at which point in the pregnancy the patient was provided supervision.

Chapter 21. Factors Influencing Health Status and Contact With Health Services (Z00-Z99)

NOTE   Z codes represent reasons for encounters. A corresponding procedure code must accompany a Z code if a procedure is performed. Categories Z00-Z99 are provided for occasions when circumstances other than a disease, injury or external cause classifiable to categories A00-Y89 are recorded as "diagnoses" or "problems". This can arise in two main ways:

(a) When a person who may or may not be sick encounters the health services for some specific purpose, such as to receive limited care or service for a current condition, to donate an organ or tissue, to receive prophylactic vaccination (immunization), or to discuss a problem which is in itself not a disease or injury.

(b) When some circumstance or problem is present which influences the person's health status but is not in itself a current illness or injury.

This chapter contains the following blocks:

Z00-Z13	Persons encountering health services for examinations
Z14-Z15	Genetic carrier and genetic susceptibility to disease
Z16	Resistance to antimicrobial drugs
Z17	Estrogen receptor status
Z18	Retained foreign body fragments
Z20-Z28	Persons with potential health hazards related to communicable diseases
Z30-Z39	Persons encountering health services in circumstances related to reproduction
Z40-Z53	Encounters for other specific health care
Z55-Z65	Persons with potential health hazards related to socioeconomic and psychosocial circumstances
Z66	Do not resuscitate status
Z67	Blood type
Z68	Body mass index (BMI)
Z69-Z76	Persons encountering health services in other circumstances
Z77-Z99	Persons with potential health hazards related to family and personal history and certain conditions influencing health status

Persons encountering health services for examinations (Z00-Z13)

NOTE   Nonspecific abnormal findings disclosed at the time of these examinations are classified to categories R70-R94.

EXCLUDES 1   examinations related to pregnancy and reproduction (Z30-Z36, Z39-)

✓4ᵗʰ **Z00**   **Encounter for general examination without complaint, suspected or reported diagnosis**

    EXCLUDES 1   encounter for examination for administrative purposes (Z02.-)
    EXCLUDES 2   encounter for pre-procedural examinations (Z01.81-)
          special screening examinations (Z11-Z13)

    ✓5ᵗʰ **Z00.0**   **Encounter for general adult medical examination**
       Encounter for adult periodic examination (annual) (physical) and any associated laboratory and radiologic examinations
       EXCLUDES 1   encounter for examination of sign or symptom—code to sign or symptom
            general health check-up of infant or child (Z00.12-)

       Z00.00   **Encounter for general adult medical examination without abnormal findings**   PDx A
          Encounter for adult health check-up NOS

       Z00.01   **Encounter for general adult medical examination with abnormal findings**   PDx A
          Use additional code to identify abnormal findings

    ✓5ᵗʰ **Z00.1**   **Encounter for newborn, infant and child health examinations**

       ✓6ᵗʰ **Z00.11**   **Newborn health examination**
          Health check for child under 29 days old
          Use additional code to identify any abnormal findings
          EXCLUDES 1   health check for child over 28 days old (Z00.12-)

          Z00.110   **Health examination for newborn under 8 days old**   PDx N
             Health check for newborn under 8 days old

          Z00.111   **Health examination for newborn 8 to 28 days old**   PDx N
             Health check for newborn 8 to 28 days old
             Newborn weight check

       ✓6ᵗʰ **Z00.12**   **Encounter for routine child health examination**
          Encounter for development testing of infant or child
          Health check (routine) for child over 28 days old
          EXCLUDES 1   health check for child under 29 days old (Z00.11-)
             health supervision of foundling or other healthy infant or child (Z76.1-Z76.2)
             newborn health examination (Z00.11-)

          Z00.121   **Encounter for routine child health examination with abnormal findings**   PDx P
             Use additional code to identify abnormal findings

          Z00.129   **Encounter for routine child health examination without abnormal findings**   PDx P
             Encounter for routine child health examination NOS

    Z00.2   **Encounter for examination for period of rapid growth in childhood**   PDx P

    Z00.3   **Encounter for examination for adolescent development state**   PDx P
       Encounter for puberty development state

    Z00.5   **Encounter for examination of potential donor of organ and tissue**   PDx

    Z00.6   **Encounter for examination for normal comparison and control in clinical research program**
       Examination of participant or control in clinical research program

    ✓5ᵗʰ **Z00.7**   **Encounter for examination for period of delayed growth in childhood**

       Z00.70   **Encounter for examination for period of delayed growth in childhood without abnormal findings**   PDx P

       Z00.71   **Encounter for examination for period of delayed growth in childhood with abnormal findings**   PDx P
          Use additional code to identify abnormal findings

    Z00.8   **Encounter for other general examination**   PDx
       Encounter for health examination in population surveys

✓4ᵗʰ **Z01**   **Encounter for other special examination without complaint, suspected or reported diagnosis**

    INCLUDES   routine examination of specific system
    NOTE   Codes from category Z01 represent the reason for the encounter. A separate procedure code is required to identify any examinations or procedures performed.
    EXCLUDES 1   encounter for examination for administrative purposes (Z02.-)
          encounter for examination for suspected conditions, proven not to exist (Z03.-)
          encounter for laboratory and radiologic examinations as a component of general medical examinations (Z00.0-)
          encounter for laboratory, radiologic and imaging examinations for sign(s) and symptom(s)—code to the sign(s) or symptom(s)
    EXCLUDES 2   screening examinations (Z11-Z13)

    ✓5ᵗʰ **Z01.0**   **Encounter for examination of eyes and vision**
       EXCLUDES 1   examination for driving license (Z02.4)

       Z01.00   **Encounter for examination of eyes and vision without abnormal findings**   PDx
          Encounter for examination of eyes and vision NOS

       Z01.01   **Encounter for examination of eyes and vision with abnormal findings**   PDx
          Use additional code to identify abnormal findings

    ✓5ᵗʰ **Z01.1**   **Encounter for examination of ears and hearing**

       Z01.10   **Encounter for examination of ears and hearing without abnormal findings**   PDx
          Encounter for examination of ears and hearing NOS

       ✓6ᵗʰ **Z01.11**   **Encounter for examination of ears and hearing with abnormal findings**

          Z01.110   **Encounter for hearing examination following failed hearing screening**   PDx

          Z01.118   **Encounter for examination of ears and hearing with other abnormal findings**   PDx
             Use additional code to identify abnormal findings

       Z01.12   **Encounter for hearing conservation and treatment**   PDx

---

N Newborn   P Pediatric   M Maternity   A Adult   RIC RIC Dx   NC Dx Noncancer Dx   PDx Primary Dx   CC RIC CC Condition   ►◄ Revised Text   ● New Code   ▲ Revised Code Title

✓5ᵗʰ **Z01.2** Encounter for dental examination and cleaning

Z01.20 **Encounter for dental examination and cleaning without abnormal findings** 〔PDx〕
Encounter for dental examination and cleaning NOS

Z01.21 **Encounter for dental examination and cleaning with abnormal findings** 〔PDx〕
Use additional code to identify abnormal findings

✓5ᵗʰ **Z01.3** Encounter for examination of blood pressure

Z01.30 **Encounter for examination of blood pressure without abnormal findings** 〔PDx〕
Encounter for examination of blood pressure NOS

Z01.31 **Encounter for examination of blood pressure with abnormal findings** 〔PDx〕
Use additional code to identify abnormal findings

✓5ᵗʰ **Z01.4** Encounter for gynecological examination

EXCLUDES 2　pregnancy examination or test (Z32.0-)
routine examination for contraceptive maintenance (Z30.4-)

✓6ᵗʰ **Z01.41** **Encounter for routine gynecological examination**
Encounter for general gynecological examination with or without cervical smear
Encounter for gynecological examination (general) (routine) NOS
Encounter for pelvic examination (annual) (periodic)
Use additional code:
for screening for human papillomavirus, if applicable, (Z11.51)
for screening vaginal pap smear, if applicable (Z12.72)
to identify acquired absence of uterus, if applicable (Z90.71-)

EXCLUDES 1　gynecologic examination status-post hysterectomy for malignant condition (Z08)
screening cervical pap smear not a part of a routine gynecological examination (Z12.4)

Z01.411 **Encounter for gynecological examination (general) (routine) with abnormal findings** 〔PDx〕♀

Z01.419 **Encounter for gynecological examination (general) (routine) without abnormal findings** 〔PDx〕♀
Use additional code to identify abnormal findings

Z01.42 **Encounter for cervical smear to confirm findings of recent normal smear following initial abnormal smear** 〔PDx〕♀

✓5ᵗʰ **Z01.8** Encounter for other specified special examinations

✓6ᵗʰ **Z01.81** **Encounter for preprocedural examinations**
Encounter for preoperative examinations
Encounter for radiological and imaging examinations as part of preprocedural examination

Z01.810 **Encounter for preprocedural cardiovascular examination** 〔PDx〕

Z01.811 **Encounter for preprocedural respiratory examination** 〔PDx〕

Z01.812 **Encounter for preprocedural laboratory examination** 〔PDx〕
Blood and urine tests prior to treatment or procedure

Z01.818 **Encounter for other preprocedural examination** 〔PDx〕
Encounter for preprocedural examination NOS
Encounter for examinations prior to antineoplastic chemotherapy

Z01.82 **Encounter for allergy testing** 〔PDx〕
EXCLUDES 1　encounter for antibody response examination (Z01.84)

Z01.83 **Encounter for blood typing** 〔PDx〕
Encounter for Rh typing

Z01.84 **Encounter for antibody response examination** 〔PDx〕
Encounter for immunity status testing
EXCLUDES 1　encounter for allergy testing (Z01.82)

Z01.89 **Encounter for other specified special examinations** 〔PDx〕

✓4ᵗʰ **Z02** Encounter for administrative examination

Z02.0 **Encounter for examination for admission to educational institution** 〔PDx〕
Encounter for examination for admission to preschool (education)
Encounter for examination for re-admission to school following illness or medical treatment

Z02.1 **Encounter for pre-employment examination** 〔PDx〕

Z02.2 **Encounter for examination for admission to residential institution** 〔PDx〕
EXCLUDES 1　examination for admission to prison (Z02.89)

Z02.3 **Encounter for examination for recruitment to armed forces** 〔PDx〕

Z02.4 **Encounter for examination for driving license** 〔PDx〕

Z02.5 **Encounter for examination for participation in sport** 〔PDx〕
EXCLUDES 1　blood-alcohol and blood-drug test (Z02.83)

Z02.6 **Encounter for examination for insurance purposes** 〔PDx〕

✓5ᵗʰ **Z02.7** Encounter for issue of medical certificate
EXCLUDES 1　encounter for general medical examination (Z00-Z01, Z02.0-Z02.6, Z02.8-Z02.9)

Z02.71 **Encounter for disability determination** 〔PDx〕
Encounter for issue of medical certificate of incapacity
Encounter for issue of medical certificate of invalidity

Z02.79 **Encounter for issue of other medical certificate** 〔PDx〕

✓5ᵗʰ **Z02.8** Encounter for other administrative examinations

Z02.81 **Encounter for paternity testing** 〔PDx〕

Z02.82 **Encounter for adoption services** 〔PDx〕

Z02.83 **Encounter for blood-alcohol and blood-drug test** 〔PDx〕
Use additional code for findings of alcohol or drugs in blood (R78.-)

Z02.89 **Encounter for other administrative examinations** 〔PDx〕
Encounter for examination for admission to prison
Encounter for examination for admission to summer camp
Encounter for immigration examination
Encounter for naturalization examination
Encounter for premarital examination
EXCLUDES 1　health supervision of foundling or other healthy infant or child (Z76.1-Z76.2)

Z02.9 **Encounter for administrative examinations, unspecified** 〔PDx〕▽

✓4ᵗʰ **Z03** Encounter for medical observation for suspected diseases and conditions ruled out
NOTE　This category is to be used when a person without a diagnosis is suspected of having an abnormal condition, without signs or symptoms, which requires study, but after examination and observation, is ruled out. This category is also for use for administrative and legal observation status.
EXCLUDES 1　contact with and (suspected) exposures hazardous to health (Z77.-)
newborn observation for suspected condition, ruled out (P00-P04)
person with feared complaint in whom no diagnosis is made (Z71.1)
signs or symptoms under study—code to signs or symptoms

Z03.6 **Encounter for observation for suspected toxic effect from ingested substance ruled out** 〔PDx〕
Encounter for observation for suspected adverse effect from drug
Encounter for observation for suspected poisoning

✓5ᵗʰ **Z03.7** Encounter for suspected maternal and fetal conditions ruled out
Encounter for suspected maternal and fetal conditions not found
EXCLUDES 1　known or suspected fetal anomalies affecting management of mother, not ruled out (O26-, O35-, O36-, O40-, O41-)

Z03.71 **Encounter for suspected problem with amniotic cavity and membrane ruled out** 〔PDx〕 Ⓜ ♀
Encounter for suspected oligohydramnios ruled out
Encounter for suspected polyhydramnios ruled out

Z03.72 **Encounter for suspected placental problem ruled out** 〔PDx〕 Ⓜ ♀

Z03.73 **Encounter for suspected fetal anomaly ruled out** 〔PDx〕 Ⓜ ♀

Z03.74 **Encounter for suspected problem with fetal growth ruled out** 〔PDx〕 Ⓜ ♀

Z03.75   **Encounter for suspected** cervical shortening **ruled out** `PDx` `M` ♀

Z03.79   **Encounter for other suspected maternal and fetal conditions ruled out** `PDx` `M` ♀

✓5ᵗʰ **Z03.8**   **Encounter for** observation **for other suspected diseases and conditions ruled out**

     ✓6ᵗʰ **Z03.81**   **Encounter for observation for suspected** exposure to biological agents **ruled out**

        Z03.810   **Encounter for observation for suspected exposure to** anthrax **ruled out** `PDx`

        Z03.818   **Encounter for observation for suspected exposure to other biological agents ruled out** `PDx`

     Z03.89   **Encounter for observation for other suspected diseases and conditions ruled out** `PDx`

✓4ᵗʰ **Z04**   **Encounter for examination and observation for other reasons**
     `INCLUDES`   encounter for examination for medicolegal reasons
     `NOTE`   This category is to be used when a person without a diagnosis is suspected of having an abnormal condition, without signs or symptoms, which requires study, but after examination and observation, is ruled-out. This category is also for use for administrative and legal observation status.

     Z04.1   **Encounter for examination and observation following** transport accident `PDx`
        `EXCLUDES 1`   *encounter for examination and observation following work accident (Z04.2)*

     Z04.2   **Encounter for examination and observation following** work accident `PDx`

     Z04.3   **Encounter for examination and observation following other accident** `PDx`

   ✓5ᵗʰ **Z04.4**   **Encounter for examination and observation following** alleged rape
     Encounter for examination and observation of victim following alleged rape
     Encounter for examination and observation of victim following alleged sexual abuse

     Z04.41   **Encounter for examination and observation following alleged** adult rape `PDx` `A`
        Suspected adult rape, ruled out
        Suspected adult sexual abuse, ruled out

     Z04.42   **Encounter for examination and observation following alleged** child rape `PDx` `P`
        Suspected child rape, ruled out
        Suspected child sexual abuse, ruled out

     Z04.6   **Encounter for** general psychiatric examination, requested by authority `PDx`

   ✓5ᵗʰ **Z04.7**   **Encounter for examination and observation following** alleged physical abuse

     Z04.71   **Encounter for examination and observation following alleged** adult **physical abuse** `PDx` `A`
        Suspected adult physical abuse, ruled out
        `EXCLUDES 1`   *confirmed case of adult physical abuse (T74.-)*
        encounter for examination and observation following alleged adult sexual abuse (Z04.41)
        suspected case of adult physical abuse, not ruled out (T76.-)

     Z04.72   **Encounter for examination and observation following alleged** child **physical abuse** `PDx` `P`
        Suspected child physical abuse, ruled out
        `EXCLUDES 1`   *confirmed case of child physical abuse (T74.-)*
        encounter for examination and observation following alleged child sexual abuse (Z04.42)
        suspected case of child physical abuse, not ruled out (T76.-)

     Z04.8   **Encounter for examination and observation for other specified reasons** `PDx`
        Encounter for examination and observation for request for expert evidence

     Z04.9   **Encounter for examination and observation for unspecified reason** `PDx` ▽
        Encounter for observation NOS

Z08   **Encounter for** follow-up **examination** after completed treatment **for** malignant neoplasm
     Medical surveillance following completed treatment
     Use additional code to identify any acquired absence of organs (Z90.-)
     Use additional code to identify the personal history of malignant neoplasm (Z85.-)
     `EXCLUDES 1`   *aftercare following medical care (Z43-Z49, Z51)*

Z09   **Encounter for** follow-up **examination** after completed treatment **for conditions** other than malignant neoplasm
     Medical surveillance following completed treatment
     Use additional code to identify any applicable history of disease code (Z86-. Z87-)
     `EXCLUDES 1`   *aftercare following medical care (Z43-Z49, Z51)*
     surveillance of contraception (Z30.4-)
     surveillance of prosthetic and other medical devices (Z44-Z46)
     AHA: 2015, 1Q, 8

✓4ᵗʰ **Z11**   **Encounter for** screening **for** infectious and parasitic diseases
     `NOTE`   Screening is the testing for disease or disease precursors in asymptomatic individuals so that early detection and treatment can be provided for those who test positive for the disease.
     `EXCLUDES 1`   *encounter for diagnostic examination—code to sign or symptom*

     Z11.0   **Encounter for screening for** intestinal **infectious diseases**

     Z11.1   **Encounter for screening for** respiratory tuberculosis

     Z11.2   **Encounter for screening for other** bacterial **diseases**

     Z11.3   **Encounter for screening for infections with a** predominantly sexual mode of transmission
        `EXCLUDES 2`   *encounter for screening for human immunodeficiency virus [HIV] (Z11.4)*
        encounter for screening for human papillomavirus (Z11.51)

     Z11.4   **Encounter for screening for** human immunodeficiency virus [HIV]

   ✓5ᵗʰ **Z11.5**   **Encounter for screening for** other viral **diseases**
        `EXCLUDES 2`   *encounter for screening for viral intestinal disease (Z11.0)*

     Z11.51   **Encounter for screening for** human papillomavirus (HPV)

     Z11.59   **Encounter for screening for other** viral **diseases**

     Z11.6   **Encounter for screening for other** protozoal diseases and helminthiases
        `EXCLUDES 2`   *encounter for screening for protozoal intestinal disease (Z11.0)*

     Z11.8   **Encounter for screening for other infectious and parasitic diseases**
        Encounter for screening for chlamydia
        Encounter for screening for rickettsial
        Encounter for screening for spirochetal
        Encounter for screening for mycoses

     Z11.9   **Encounter for screening for infectious and parasitic diseases, unspecified** ▽

✓4ᵗʰ **Z12**   **Encounter for** screening **for** malignant neoplasms
     `NOTE`   Screening is the testing for disease or disease precursors in asymptomatic individuals so that early detection and treatment can be provided for those who test positive for the disease.
     Use additional code to identify any family history of malignant neoplasm (Z80.-)
     `EXCLUDES 1`   *encounter for diagnostic examination—code to sign or symptom*

     Z12.0   **Encounter for screening for malignant neoplasm of** stomach

   ✓5ᵗʰ **Z12.1**   **Encounter for screening for malignant neoplasm of** intestinal tract

     Z12.10   **Encounter for screening for malignant neoplasm of intestinal tract, unspecified** ▽

     Z12.11   **Encounter for screening for malignant neoplasm of** colon
        Encounter for screening colonoscopy NOS

     Z12.12   **Encounter for screening for malignant neoplasm of** rectum

     Z12.13   **Encounter for screening for malignant neoplasm of** small intestine

     Z12.2   **Encounter for screening for malignant neoplasm of** respiratory organs

---

`N` Newborn   `P` Pediatric   `M` Maternity   `A` Adult   `RIC` RIC Dx   `NCDx` Noncancer Dx   `PDx` Primary Dx   `CC` RIC CC Condition   ▶◀ Revised Text   ● New Code   ▲ Revised Code Title

1126   ICD-10-CM 2016

✓5ᵗʰ **Z12.3** Encounter for screening for malignant neoplasm of breast

    Z12.31 Encounter for screening mammogram for malignant neoplasm of breast
      EXCLUDES 1   *inconclusive mammogram (R92.2)*
      AHA: 2015, 1Q, 24

    Z12.39 Encounter for other screening for malignant neoplasm of breast

Z12.4 Encounter for screening for malignant neoplasm of cervix ♀
    Encounter for screening pap smear for malignant neoplasm of cervix
      EXCLUDES 1   *encounter for screening for human papillomavirus (Z11.51)*
      when screening is part of general gynecological examination (Z01.4-)

Z12.5 Encounter for screening for malignant neoplasm of prostate ♂

Z12.6 Encounter for screening for malignant neoplasm of bladder

✓5ᵗʰ **Z12.7** Encounter for screening for malignant neoplasm of other genitourinary organs

    Z12.71 Encounter for screening for malignant neoplasm of testis ♂

    Z12.72 Encounter for screening for malignant neoplasm of vagina ♀
      Vaginal pap smear status-post hysterectomy for non-malignant condition
      Use additional code to identify acquired absence of uterus (Z90.71-)
      EXCLUDES 1   *vaginal pap smear status-post hysterectomy for malignant conditions (Z08)*

    Z12.73 Encounter for screening for malignant neoplasm of ovary ♀

    Z12.79 Encounter for screening for malignant neoplasm of other genitourinary organs

✓5ᵗʰ **Z12.8** Encounter for screening for malignant neoplasm of other sites

    Z12.81 Encounter for screening for malignant neoplasm of oral cavity

    Z12.82 Encounter for screening for malignant neoplasm of nervous system

    Z12.83 Encounter for screening for malignant neoplasm of skin

    Z12.89 Encounter for screening for malignant neoplasm of other sites

Z12.9 Encounter for screening for malignant neoplasm, site unspecified   ▽

✓4ᵗʰ **Z13** Encounter for screening for other diseases and disorders
    NOTE   Screening is the testing for disease or disease precursors in asymptomatic individuals so that early detection and treatment can be provided for those who test positive for the disease.
    EXCLUDES 1   *encounter for diagnostic examination—code to sign or symptom*

Z13.0 Encounter for screening for diseases of the blood and blood-forming organs and certain disorders involving the immune mechanism

Z13.1 Encounter for screening for diabetes mellitus

✓5ᵗʰ **Z13.2** Encounter for screening for nutritional, metabolic and other endocrine disorders

    Z13.21 Encounter for screening for nutritional disorder

    ✓6ᵗʰ **Z13.22** Encounter for screening for metabolic disorder

      Z13.220 Encounter for screening for lipoid disorders
        Encounter for screening for cholesterol level
        Encounter for screening for hypercholesterolemia
        Encounter for screening for hyperlipidemia

      Z13.228 Encounter for screening for other metabolic disorders

    Z13.29 Encounter for screening for other suspected endocrine disorder
      EXCLUDES 1   *encounter for screening for diabetes mellitus (Z13.1)*

Z13.4 Encounter for screening for certain developmental disorders in childhood   P
    Encounter for screening for developmental handicaps in early childhood
    EXCLUDES 1   *routine development testing of infant or child (Z00.1-)*

Z13.5 Encounter for screening for eye and ear disorders
    EXCLUDES 2   *encounter for general hearing examination (Z01.1-)*
      encounter for general vision examination (Z01.0-)

Z13.6 Encounter for screening for cardiovascular disorders

✓5ᵗʰ **Z13.7** Encounter for screening for genetic and chromosomal anomalies
    EXCLUDES 1   *genetic testing for procreative management (Z31.4-)*

    Z13.71 Encounter for nonprocreative screening for genetic disease carrier status

    Z13.79 Encounter for other screening for genetic and chromosomal anomalies

✓5ᵗʰ **Z13.8** Encounter for screening for other specified diseases and disorders
    EXCLUDES 2   *screening for malignant neoplasms (Z12.-)*

    ✓6ᵗʰ **Z13.81** Encounter for screening for digestive system disorders

      Z13.810 Encounter for screening for upper gastrointestinal disorder

      Z13.811 Encounter for screening for lower gastrointestinal disorder
        EXCLUDES 1   *encounter for screening for intestinal infectious disease (Z11.0)*

      Z13.818 Encounter for screening for other digestive system disorders

    ✓6ᵗʰ **Z13.82** Encounter for screening for musculoskeletal disorder

      Z13.820 Encounter for screening for osteoporosis

      Z13.828 Encounter for screening for other musculoskeletal disorder

    Z13.83 Encounter for screening for respiratory disorder NEC
      EXCLUDES 1   *encounter for screening for respiratory tuberculosis (Z11.1)*

    Z13.84 Encounter for screening for dental disorders

    ✓6ᵗʰ **Z13.85** Encounter for screening for nervous system disorders

      Z13.850 Encounter for screening for traumatic brain injury

      Z13.858 Encounter for screening for other nervous system disorders

    Z13.88 Encounter for screening for disorder due to exposure to contaminants
      EXCLUDES 1   *those exposed to contaminants without suspected disorders (Z57-Z77-)*

    Z13.89 Encounter for screening for other disorder   M
      Encounter for screening for genitourinary disorders

Z13.9 Encounter for screening, unspecified   ▽

Genetic carrier and genetic susceptibility to disease (Z14-Z15)

✓4ᵗʰ **Z14** Genetic carrier

    ✓5ᵗʰ **Z14.0** Hemophilia A carrier

      Z14.01 Asymptomatic hemophilia A carrier

      Z14.02 Symptomatic hemophilia A carrier

    Z14.1 Cystic fibrosis carrier

    Z14.8 Genetic carrier of other disease

✓4ᵗʰ **Z15** Genetic susceptibility to disease
    Confirmed abnormal gene
    Use additional code, if applicable, for any associated family history of the disease (Z80-Z84)
    EXCLUDES 1   *chromosomal anomalies (Q90-Q99)*

    ✓5ᵗʰ **Z15.0** Genetic susceptibility to malignant neoplasm
      Code first, if applicable, any current malignant neoplasm (C00-C75, C81-C96)
      Use additional code, if applicable, for any personal history of malignant neoplasm (Z85.-)

      Z15.01 Genetic susceptibility to malignant neoplasm of breast

      Z15.02 Genetic susceptibility to malignant neoplasm of ovary ♀

      Z15.03 Genetic susceptibility to malignant neoplasm of prostate ♂

      Z15.04 Genetic susceptibility to malignant neoplasm of endometrium ♀

      Z15.09 Genetic susceptibility to other malignant neoplasm

---

Chapter 21. Factors Influencing Health Status and Contact With Health Services

✓5ᵗʰ **Z15.8 Genetic susceptibility to other disease**

Z15.81 Genetic susceptibility to multiple endocrine neoplasia **[MEN]**

EXCLUDES 1   *multiple endocrine neoplasia [MEN] syndromes (E31.2-)*

Z15.89 Genetic susceptibility to other disease

Resistance to antimicrobial drugs (Z16)

✓4ᵗʰ **Z16 Resistance to antimicrobial drugs**

NOTE   The codes in this category are provided for use as additional codes to identify the resistance and non-responsiveness of a condition to antimicrobial drugs.

Code first the infection

EXCLUDES 1   *Methicillin resistant Staphylococcus aureus infection (A49.02)*
Methicillin resistant Staphylococcus aureus infection in diseases classified elsewhere (B95.62)
Methicillin resistant Staphylococcus aureus pneumonia (J15.212)
Sepsis due to Methicillin resistant Staphylococcus aureus (A41.02)

✓5ᵗʰ **Z16.1 Resistance to** beta lactam **antibiotics**

Z16.10 Resistance to unspecified beta lactam antibiotics ▽

Z16.11 Resistance to penicillins
Resistance to amoxicillin
Resistance to ampicillin

Z16.12 Extended spectrum beta lactamase (ESBL) resistance

Z16.19 Resistance to other specified beta lactam antibiotics
Resistance to cephalosporins

✓5ᵗʰ **Z16.2 Resistance to** other **antibiotics**

Z16.20 Resistance to unspecified antibiotic ▽
Resistance to antibiotics NOS

Z16.21 Resistance to vancomycin

Z16.22 Resistance to vancomycin related **antibiotics**

Z16.23 Resistance to quinolones and fluoroquinolones

Z16.24 Resistance to multiple antibiotics

Z16.29 Resistance to other single specified **antibiotic**
Resistance to aminoglycosides
Resistance to macrolides
Resistance to sulfonamides
Resistance to tetracyclines

✓5ᵗʰ **Z16.3 Resistance to** other antimicrobial **drugs**

EXCLUDES 1   *resistance to antibiotics (Z16.1-, Z16.2-)*

Z16.30 Resistance to unspecified antimicrobial drugs ▽
Drug resistance NOS

Z16.31 Resistance to antiparasitic **drug(s)**
Resistance to quinine and related compounds

Z16.32 Resistance to antifungal **drug(s)**

Z16.33 Resistance to antiviral **drug(s)**

✓6ᵗʰ **Z16.34 Resistance to** antimycobacterial **drug(s)**
Resistance to tuberculostatics

Z16.341 Resistance to single **antimycobacterial drug**
Resistance to antimycobacterial drug NOS

Z16.342 Resistance to multiple **antimycobacterial drugs**

Z16.35 Resistance to multiple **antimicrobial drugs**
EXCLUDES 1   *Resistance to multiple antibiotics only (Z16.24)*

Z16.39 Resistance to other specified antimicrobial drug

Estrogen receptor status (Z17)

✓4ᵗʰ **Z17 Estrogen receptor status**
Code first malignant neoplasm of breast (C50.-)

Z17.0 Estrogen receptor positive **status [ER+]**

Z17.1 Estrogen receptor negative **status [ER-]**

Retained foreign body fragment (Z18)

✓4ᵗʰ **Z18 Retained foreign body fragments**
Embedded fragment (status)
Embedded splinter (status)
Retained foreign body status

EXCLUDES 1   *artificial joint prosthesis status (Z96.6-)*
foreign body accidentally left during a procedure (T81.5-)
foreign body entering through orifice (T15-T19)
in situ cardiac device (Z95.-)
organ or tissue replaced by means other than transplant (Z96.-, Z97.-)
organ or tissue replaced by transplant (Z94.-)
personal history of retained foreign body fully removed (Z87.821)
superficial foreign body (non-embedded splinter)—code to superficial foreign body, by site

✓5ᵗʰ **Z18.0 Retained** radioactive **fragments**

Z18.01 Retained depleted **uranium fragments**

Z18.09 Other retained radioactive fragments
Other retained depleted isotope fragments
Retained nontherapeutic radioactive fragments

✓5ᵗʰ **Z18.1 Retained** metal **fragments**

EXCLUDES 1   *retained radioactive metal fragments (Z18.01-Z18.09)*

Z18.10 Retained metal fragments, unspecified ▽
Retained metal fragment NOS

Z18.11 Retained magnetic **metal fragments**

Z18.12 Retained nonmagnetic **metal fragments**

Z18.2 Retained plastic **fragments**
Acrylics fragments
Diethylhexylphthalates fragments
Isocyanate fragments

✓5ᵗʰ **Z18.3 Retained** organic **fragments**

Z18.31 Retained animal quills or spines

Z18.32 Retained tooth

Z18.33 Retained wood **fragments**

Z18.39 Other retained organic fragments

✓5ᵗʰ **Z18.8 Other** specified retained foreign body

Z18.81 Retained glass **fragments**

Z18.83 Retained stone or crystalline **fragments**
Retained concrete or cement fragments

Z18.89 Other specified retained foreign body fragments

Z18.9 Retained foreign body fragments, unspecified material ▽

Persons with potential health hazards related to communicable diseases (Z20-Z28)

✓4ᵗʰ **Z20 Contact with and (suspected) exposure to communicable diseases**

EXCLUDES 1   *carrier of infectious disease (Z22.-)*
diagnosed current infectious or parasitic disease—see Alphabetic Index

EXCLUDES 2   *personal history of infectious and parasitic diseases (Z86.1-)*

✓5ᵗʰ **Z20.0 Contact with and (suspected) exposure to** intestinal infectious diseases

Z20.01 Contact with and (suspected) exposure to intestinal infectious diseases due to Escherichia coli (E. coli)

Z20.09 Contact with and (suspected) exposure to other intestinal infectious diseases

Z20.1 Contact with and (suspected) exposure to tuberculosis

Z20.2 Contact with and (suspected) exposure to infections with a predominantly sexual mode of transmission

Z20.3 Contact with and (suspected) exposure to rabies

Z20.4 Contact with and (suspected) exposure to rubella

Z20.5 Contact with and (suspected) exposure to viral hepatitis

Z20.6 Contact with and (suspected) exposure to human immunodeficiency virus **[HIV]**

EXCLUDES 1   *asymptomatic human immunodeficiency virus [HIV] HIV infection status (Z21)*

Z20.7 Contact with and (suspected) exposure to pediculosis, acariasis **and** other **infestations**

ℕ Newborn   ℙ Pediatric   𝕄 Maternity   𝔸 Adult   **RIC** RIC Dx   **NC Dx** Noncancer Dx   **PDx** Primary Dx   **CC** RIC CC Condition   ▶◀ Revised Text   ● New Code   ▲ Revised Code Title

1128   ICD-10-CM 2016

☑5ᵗʰ Z20.8 Contact with and (suspected) exposure to other communicable **diseases**

  ☑6ᵗʰ Z20.81 Contact with and (suspected) exposure to other bacterial **communicable diseases**

    Z20.810 Contact with and (suspected) exposure to anthrax

    Z20.811 Contact with and (suspected) exposure to meningococcus

    Z20.818 Contact with and (suspected) exposure to other bacterial communicable diseases

  ☑6ᵗʰ Z20.82 Contact with and (suspected) exposure to other viral **communicable diseases**

    Z20.820 Contact with and (suspected) exposure to varicella

    Z20.828 Contact with and (suspected) exposure to other viral communicable diseases

  Z20.89 Contact with and (suspected) exposure to other communicable diseases

Z20.9 Contact with and (suspected) exposure to unspecified communicable disease ▽

Z21 Asymptomatic human immunodeficiency virus [HIV] infection status

  HIV positive NOS

  Code first human immunodeficiency virus [HIV] disease complicating pregnancy, childbirth and the puerperium, if applicable (O98.7-)

    EXCLUDES 1   acquired immunodeficiency syndrome (B20)
         contact with human immunodeficiency virus [HIV] (Z20.6)
         exposure to human immunodeficiency virus [HIV] (Z20.6)
         human immunodeficiency virus [HIV] disease (B20)
         inconclusive laboratory evidence of human immunodeficiency virus [HIV] (R75)

☑4ᵗʰ Z22 Carrier of infectious disease

  Colonization status
  Suspected carrier

Z22.0 Carrier of typhoid

Z22.1 Carrier of other intestinal **infectious diseases**

Z22.2 Carrier of diphtheria

☑5ᵗʰ Z22.3 Carrier of other **specified bacterial diseases**

  Z22.31 Carrier of bacterial disease due to meningococci

  ☑6ᵗʰ Z22.32 Carrier of bacterial disease due to staphylococci

    Z22.321 Carrier or suspected carrier of Methicillin susceptible **Staphylococcus aureus**
      MSSA colonization

    Z22.322 Carrier or suspected carrier of Methicillin resistant **Staphylococcus aureus**
      MRSA colonization

  ☑6ᵗʰ Z22.33 Carrier of bacterial disease due to streptococci

    Z22.330 Carrier of Group B **streptococcus**

    Z22.338 Carrier of other streptococcus

  Z22.39 Carrier of other specified bacterial diseases

Z22.4 Carrier of infections with a predominantly sexual mode of transmission

☑5ᵗʰ Z22.5 Carrier of viral hepatitis

  Z22.50 Carrier of unspecified viral hepatitis ▽

  Z22.51 Carrier of viral hepatitis B
    Hepatitis B surface antigen [HBsAg] carrier

  Z22.52 Carrier of viral hepatitis C

  Z22.59 Carrier of other viral hepatitis

Z22.6 Carrier of human T-lymphotropic virus type-1 [HTLV-1] **infection**

Z22.8 Carrier of other infectious diseases

Z22.9 Carrier of infectious disease, unspecified ▽

Z23 Encounter for immunization

  Code first any routine childhood examination
    NOTE   Procedure codes are required to identify the types of immunizations given

☑4ᵗʰ Z28 Immunization not carried out and underimmunization status

  Vaccination not carried out

☑5ᵗʰ Z28.0 Immunization not carried out because of contraindication

  Z28.01 Immunization not carried out because of acute illness **of patient**

  Z28.02 Immunization not carried out because of chronic illness **or condition of patient**

  Z28.03 Immunization not carried out because of immune compromised state **of patient**

  Z28.04 Immunization not carried out because of patient allergy to vaccine or component

  Z28.09 Immunization not carried out because of other contraindication

Z28.1 Immunization not carried out because of patient decision for reasons of belief or group pressure
  Immunization not carried out because of religious belief

☑5ᵗʰ Z28.2 Immunization not carried out because of patient decision for other and unspecified **reason**

  Z28.20 Immunization not carried out because of patient ▽ **decision for unspecified reason**

  Z28.21 Immunization not carried out because of patient refusal

  Z28.29 Immunization not carried out because of patient decision for other reason

Z28.3 Underimmunization status
  Delinquent immunization status
  Lapsed immunization schedule status

☑5ᵗʰ Z28.8 Immunization not carried out for other reason

  Z28.81 Immunization not carried out due to patient having had the disease

  Z28.82 Immunization not carried out because of caregiver refusal
    Immunization not carried out because of guardian refusal
    Immunization not carried out because of parent refusal
    EXCLUDES 1   immunization not carried out because of caregiver refusal because of religious belief (Z28.1)

  Z28.89 Immunization not carried out for other reason

Z28.9 Immunization not carried out for unspecified reason ▽

Persons encountering health services in circumstances related to reproduction (Z30-Z39)

☑4ᵗʰ Z30 Encounter for contraceptive management

  ☑5ᵗʰ Z30.0 Encounter for general counseling and advice on contraception

    ☑6ᵗʰ Z30.01 Encounter for initial prescription **of contraceptives**
      EXCLUDES 1   encounter for surveillance of contraceptives (Z30.4-)

      Z30.011 Encounter for initial prescription **of** Ⓜ♀ **contraceptive pills**

      Z30.012 Encounter for prescription of ♀ emergency **contraception**
        Encounter for postcoital contraception

      Z30.013 Encounter for initial prescription of ♀ injectable **contraceptive**

      Z30.014 Encounter for initial prescription of ♀ intrauterine **contraceptive device**
        EXCLUDES 1   encounter for insertion of intrauterine contraceptive device (Z30.430, Z30.432)

      Z30.018 Encounter for initial prescription of ♀ **other contraceptives**

      Z30.019 Encounter for initial prescription of ♀▽ **contraceptives, unspecified**

    Z30.02 Counseling and instruction in natural family planning **to avoid pregnancy**

    Z30.09 Encounter for other general counseling and advice on contraception
      Encounter for family planning advice NOS

  Z30.2 Encounter for sterilization

  ☑5ᵗʰ Z30.4 Encounter for surveillance **of contraceptives**

    Z30.40 Encounter for surveillance of contraceptives, ▽ **unspecified**

    Z30.41 Encounter for surveillance of contraceptive pills Ⓜ ♀
      Encounter for repeat prescription for contraceptive pill

    Z30.42 Encounter for surveillance of injectable ♀ **contraceptive**

Chapter 21. Factors Influencing Health Status and Contact With Health Services

✓6ᵗʰ Z30.43 Encounter for surveillance of intrauterine contraceptive device

Z30.430 Encounter for insertion of intrauterine contraceptive device ♀

Z30.431 Encounter for routine checking of intrauterine contraceptive device Ⓜ♀

Z30.432 Encounter for removal of intrauterine contraceptive device ♀

Z30.433 Encounter for removal and reinsertion of intrauterine contraceptive device ♀
Encounter for replacement of intrauterine contraceptive device

Z30.49 Encounter for surveillance of other contraceptives Ⓜ♀

Z30.8 Encounter for other contraceptive management
Encounter for postvasectomy sperm count
Encounter for routine examination for contraceptive maintenance
EXCLUDES 1   sperm count following sterilization reversal (Z31.42)
     sperm count for fertility testing (Z31.41)

Z30.9 Encounter for contraceptive management, unspecified ▽

✓4ᵗʰ Z31 Encounter for procreative management
EXCLUDES 1   complications associated with artificial fertilization (N98.-)
     female infertility (N97.-)
     male infertility (N46.-)

Z31.0 Encounter for reversal of previous sterilization

✓5ᵗʰ Z31.4 Encounter for procreative investigation and testing
EXCLUDES 1   postvasectomy sperm count (Z30.8)

Z31.41 Encounter for fertility testing
Encounter for fallopian tube patency testing
Encounter for sperm count for fertility testing

Z31.42 Aftercare following sterilization reversal
Sperm count following sterilization reversal

✓6ᵗʰ Z31.43 Encounter for genetic testing of female for procreative management
Use additional code for recurrent pregnancy loss, if applicable (N96, O26.2-)
EXCLUDES 1   nonprocreative genetic testing (Z13.7-)

Z31.430 Encounter of female for testing for genetic disease carrier status for procreative management ♀

Z31.438 Encounter for other genetic testing of female for procreative management ♀

✓6ᵗʰ Z31.44 Encounter for genetic testing of male for procreative management
EXCLUDES 1   nonprocreative genetic testing (Z13.7-)

Z31.440 Encounter of male for testing for genetic disease carrier status for procreative management ♂

Z31.441 Encounter for testing of male partner patient with recurrent pregnancy loss Ⓐ♂

Z31.448 Encounter for other genetic testing of male for procreative management Ⓐ♂

Z31.49 Encounter for other procreative investigation and testing

Z31.5 Encounter for genetic counseling

✓5ᵗʰ Z31.6 Encounter for general counseling and advice on procreation

Z31.61 Procreative counseling and advice using natural family planning

Z31.62 Encounter for fertility preservation counseling
Encounter for fertility preservation counseling prior to cancer therapy
Encounter for fertility preservation counseling prior to surgical removal of gonads

Z31.69 Encounter for other general counseling and advice on procreation

✓5ᵗʰ Z31.8 Encounter for other procreative management

Z31.81 Encounter for male factor infertility in female patient PDx ♀

Z31.82 Encounter for Rh incompatibility status PDx ♀
AHA: 2014, 4Q, 17

Z31.83 Encounter for assisted reproductive fertility procedure cycle PDx ♀
Patient undergoing in vitro fertilization cycle
Use additional code to identify the type of infertility
EXCLUDES 1   pre-cycle diagnosis and testing—code to reason for encounter

Z31.84 Encounter for fertility preservation procedure PDx
Encounter for fertility preservation procedure prior to cancer therapy
Encounter for fertility preservation procedure prior to surgical removal of gonads

Z31.89 Encounter for other procreative management Ⓜ

Z31.9 Encounter for procreative management, unspecified ▽

✓4ᵗʰ Z32 Encounter for pregnancy test and childbirth and childcare instruction

✓5ᵗʰ Z32.0 Encounter for pregnancy test

Z32.00 Encounter for pregnancy test, result unknown ♀
Encounter for pregnancy test NOS

Z32.01 Encounter for pregnancy test, result positive Ⓜ♀

Z32.02 Encounter for pregnancy test, result negative ♀

Z32.2 Encounter for childbirth instruction

Z32.3 Encounter for childcare instruction
Encounter for prenatal or postpartum childcare instruction

✓4ᵗʰ Z33 Pregnant state

Z33.1 Pregnant state, incidental Ⓜ♀
Pregnant state NOS
EXCLUDES 1   complications of pregnancy (O00-O9A)

Z33.2 Encounter for elective termination of pregnancy PDx Ⓜ♀
EXCLUDES 1   early fetal death with retention of dead fetus (O02.1)
     late fetal death (O36.4)
     spontaneous abortion (O03)

✓4ᵗʰ Z34 Encounter for supervision of normal pregnancy
EXCLUDES 1   any complication of pregnancy (O00-O9A)
     encounter for pregnancy test (Z32.0-)
     encounter for supervision of high risk pregnancy (O09.-)
AHA: 2014, 4Q, 17

✓5ᵗʰ Z34.0 Encounter for supervision of normal first pregnancy

Z34.00 Encounter for supervision of normal first pregnancy, unspecified trimester PDx Ⓜ♀▽

Z34.01 Encounter for supervision of normal first pregnancy, first trimester PDx Ⓜ♀

Z34.02 Encounter for supervision of normal first pregnancy, second trimester PDx Ⓜ♀

Z34.03 Encounter for supervision of normal first pregnancy, third trimester PDx Ⓜ♀

✓5ᵗʰ Z34.8 Encounter for supervision of other normal pregnancy

Z34.80 Encounter for supervision of other normal pregnancy, unspecified trimester PDx Ⓜ♀▽

Z34.81 Encounter for supervision of other normal pregnancy, first trimester PDx Ⓜ♀

Z34.82 Encounter for supervision of other normal pregnancy, second trimester PDx Ⓜ♀

Z34.83 Encounter for supervision of other normal pregnancy, third trimester PDx Ⓜ♀

✓5ᵗʰ Z34.9 Encounter for supervision of normal pregnancy, unspecified

Z34.90 Encounter for supervision of normal pregnancy, unspecified, unspecified trimester PDx Ⓜ♀▽

Z34.91 Encounter for supervision of normal pregnancy, unspecified, first trimester PDx Ⓜ♀▽

Z34.92 Encounter for supervision of normal pregnancy, unspecified, second trimester PDx Ⓜ♀▽

Z34.93 Encounter for supervision of normal pregnancy, unspecified, third trimester PDx Ⓜ♀▽

Z36 Encounter for antenatal screening of mother Ⓜ♀
EXCLUDES 1   abnormal findings on antenatal screening of mother (O28.-)
     diagnostic examination—code to sign or symptom
     encounter for suspected maternal and fetal conditions ruled out (Z03.7-)
     suspected fetal condition affecting management of pregnancy—code to condition in Chapter 15
EXCLUDES 2   genetic counseling and testing (Z31.43-, Z31.5)
     routine prenatal care (Z34)

Ⓝ Newborn   Ⓟ Pediatric   Ⓜ Maternity   Ⓐ Adult   RIC RIC Dx   NCDx Noncancer Dx   PDx Primary Dx   CC RIC CC Condition   ▶◀ Revised Text   ● New Code   ▲ Revised Code Title
1130   ICD-10-CM 2016

Z30.43–Z36

✓4ᵗʰ **Z3A Weeks of gestation**
> **NOTE** Codes from category Z3A are for use, only on the maternal record, to indicate the weeks of gestation of the pregnancy.
> Code first complications of pregnancy, childbirth and the puerperium (O00-O9A)
> AHA: 2014, 3Q, 17; 2014, 2Q, 9; 2013, 2Q, 33

✓5ᵗʰ **Z3A.0 Weeks of gestation of pregnancy,** unspecified or less than 10 weeks
- **Z3A.00** Weeks of gestation of pregnancy not specified   Ⓜ♀
- **Z3A.01** Less than 8 weeks gestation of pregnancy   Ⓜ♀
- **Z3A.08** 8 weeks gestation of pregnancy   Ⓜ♀
- **Z3A.09** 9 weeks gestation of pregnancy   Ⓜ♀

✓5ᵗʰ **Z3A.1 Weeks of gestation of pregnancy,** weeks 10-19
- **Z3A.10** 10 weeks gestation of pregnancy   Ⓜ♀
- **Z3A.11** 11 weeks gestation of pregnancy   Ⓜ♀
- **Z3A.12** 12 weeks gestation of pregnancy   Ⓜ♀
- **Z3A.13** 13 weeks gestation of pregnancy   Ⓜ♀
- **Z3A.14** 14 weeks gestation of pregnancy   Ⓜ♀
- **Z3A.15** 15 weeks gestation of pregnancy   Ⓜ♀
- **Z3A.16** 16 weeks gestation of pregnancy   Ⓜ♀
- **Z3A.17** 17 weeks gestation of pregnancy   Ⓜ♀
- **Z3A.18** 18 weeks gestation of pregnancy   Ⓜ♀
- **Z3A.19** 19 weeks gestation of pregnancy   Ⓜ♀

✓5ᵗʰ **Z3A.2 Weeks of gestation of pregnancy,** weeks 20-29
- **Z3A.20** 20 weeks gestation of pregnancy   Ⓜ♀
- **Z3A.21** 21 weeks gestation of pregnancy   Ⓜ♀
- **Z3A.22** 22 weeks gestation of pregnancy   Ⓜ♀
- **Z3A.23** 23 weeks gestation of pregnancy   Ⓜ♀
- **Z3A.24** 24 weeks gestation of pregnancy   Ⓜ♀
- **Z3A.25** 25 weeks gestation of pregnancy   Ⓜ♀
- **Z3A.26** 26 weeks gestation of pregnancy   Ⓜ♀
- **Z3A.27** 27 weeks gestation of pregnancy   Ⓜ♀
- **Z3A.28** 28 weeks gestation of pregnancy   Ⓜ♀
- **Z3A.29** 29 weeks gestation of pregnancy   Ⓜ♀

✓5ᵗʰ **Z3A.3 Weeks of gestation of pregnancy,** weeks 30-39
- **Z3A.30** 30 weeks gestation of pregnancy   Ⓜ♀
- **Z3A.31** 31 weeks gestation of pregnancy   Ⓜ♀
- **Z3A.32** 32 weeks gestation of pregnancy   Ⓜ♀
- **Z3A.33** 33 weeks gestation of pregnancy   Ⓜ♀
- **Z3A.34** 34 weeks gestation of pregnancy   Ⓜ♀
- **Z3A.35** 35 weeks gestation of pregnancy   Ⓜ♀
- **Z3A.36** 36 weeks gestation of pregnancy   Ⓜ♀
- **Z3A.37** 37 weeks gestation of pregnancy   Ⓜ♀
- **Z3A.38** 38 weeks gestation of pregnancy   Ⓜ♀
- **Z3A.39** 39 weeks gestation of pregnancy   Ⓜ♀

✓5ᵗʰ **Z3A.4 Weeks of gestation of pregnancy,** weeks 40 or greater
> AHA: 2014, 4Q, 23
- **Z3A.40** 40 weeks gestation of pregnancy   Ⓜ♀
- **Z3A.41** 41 weeks gestation of pregnancy   Ⓜ♀
- **Z3A.42** 42 weeks gestation of pregnancy   Ⓜ♀
- **Z3A.49** Greater than 42 weeks gestation of pregnancy   Ⓜ♀

✓4ᵗʰ **Z37 Outcome of delivery**
> **NOTE** This category is intended for use as an additional code to identify the outcome of delivery on the mother's record. It is not for use on the newborn record.
> **EXCLUDES 1** stillbirth (P95)

- **Z37.0 Single live birth**   Ⓜ♀
  > AHA: 2014, 2Q, 9
- **Z37.1 Single stillbirth**   Ⓜ♀
- **Z37.2 Twins, both liveborn**   Ⓜ♀
- **Z37.3 Twins, one liveborn and one stillborn**   Ⓜ♀
- **Z37.4 Twins, both stillborn**   Ⓜ♀

✓5ᵗʰ **Z37.5 Other multiple births, all liveborn**
- **Z37.50** Multiple births, unspecified, all liveborn   Ⓜ♀ ▽
- **Z37.51** Triplets, all liveborn   Ⓜ♀
- **Z37.52** Quadruplets, all liveborn   Ⓜ♀
- **Z37.53** Quintuplets, all liveborn   Ⓜ♀
- **Z37.54** Sextuplets, all liveborn   Ⓜ♀
- **Z37.59** Other multiple births, all liveborn   Ⓜ♀

✓5ᵗʰ **Z37.6 Other multiple births, some liveborn**
- **Z37.60** Multiple births, unspecified, some liveborn   Ⓜ♀ ▽
- **Z37.61** Triplets, some liveborn   Ⓜ♀
- **Z37.62** Quadruplets, some liveborn   Ⓜ♀
- **Z37.63** Quintuplets, some liveborn   Ⓜ♀
- **Z37.64** Sextuplets, some liveborn   Ⓜ♀
- **Z37.69** Other multiple births, some liveborn   Ⓜ♀

- **Z37.7 Other multiple births, all stillborn**   Ⓜ♀
- **Z37.9 Outcome of delivery, unspecified**   Ⓜ♀ ▽
  Multiple birth NOS
  Single birth NOS

✓4ᵗʰ **Z38 Liveborn infants according to place of birth and type of delivery**
> **NOTE** This category is for use as the principal code on the initial record of a newborn baby. It is to be used for the initial birth record only. It is not to be used on the mother's record.

✓5ᵗʰ **Z38.0 Single liveborn infant,** born in hospital
> Single liveborn infant, born in birthing center or other health care facility
- **Z38.00** Single liveborn infant, delivered vaginally   PDx Ⓝ
- **Z38.01** Single liveborn infant, delivered by cesarean   PDx Ⓝ

- **Z38.1 Single liveborn infant, born** outside hospital   PDx Ⓝ
- **Z38.2 Single liveborn infant, unspecified as to place of birth**   PDx Ⓝ ▽
  Single liveborn infant NOS

✓5ᵗʰ **Z38.3 Twin liveborn infant,** born in hospital
- **Z38.30** Twin liveborn infant, delivered vaginally   PDx Ⓝ
- **Z38.31** Twin liveborn infant, delivered by cesarean   PDx Ⓝ

- **Z38.4 Twin liveborn infant, born** outside hospital   PDx Ⓝ
- **Z38.5 Twin liveborn infant, unspecified as to place of birth**   PDx Ⓝ ▽

✓5ᵗʰ **Z38.6 Other multiple liveborn infant, born in hospital**
- **Z38.61** Triplet liveborn infant, delivered vaginally   PDx Ⓝ
- **Z38.62** Triplet liveborn infant, delivered by cesarean   PDx Ⓝ
- **Z38.63** Quadruplet liveborn infant, delivered vaginally   PDx Ⓝ
- **Z38.64** Quadruplet liveborn infant, delivered by cesarean   PDx Ⓝ
- **Z38.65** Quintuplet liveborn infant, delivered vaginally   PDx Ⓝ
- **Z38.66** Quintuplet liveborn infant, delivered by cesarean   PDx Ⓝ
- **Z38.68** Other multiple liveborn infant, delivered vaginally   PDx Ⓝ
- **Z38.69** Other multiple liveborn infant, delivered by cesarean   PDx Ⓝ

- **Z38.7 Other multiple liveborn infant, born** outside hospital   PDx Ⓝ
- **Z38.8 Other multiple liveborn infant, unspecified as to place of birth**   PDx Ⓝ ▽

✓4ᵗʰ **Z39 Encounter for maternal postpartum care and examination**
- **Z39.0 Encounter for care and examination of mother immediately after delivery**   PDx Ⓜ♀
  > Care and observation in uncomplicated cases when the delivery occurs outside a healthcare facility
  > **EXCLUDES 1** care for postpartum complication—see Alphabetic index
- **Z39.1 Encounter for care and examination of lactating mother**   PDx Ⓜ♀
  > Encounter for supervision of lactation
  > **EXCLUDES 1** disorders of lactation (O92.-)
- **Z39.2 Encounter for routine postpartum follow-up**   PDx Ⓜ♀

✅ Add'l Character Required   ✓x7ᵗʰ Placeholder Alert   RUG IV Special Care High Dx   RUG IV Clinically Complex Dx   RUG IV Special Care Low Dx   Manifestation Code   Other Specified Code   ▽ Unspecified Code

Chapter 21. Factors Influencing Health Status and Contact With Health Services

Z40–Z44.30

Encounters for other specific health care (Z40-Z53)

NOTE   Categories Z40-Z53 are intended for use to indicate a reason for care. They may be used for patients who have already been treated for a disease or injury, but who are receiving aftercare or prophylactic care, or care to consolidate the treatment, or to deal with a residual state.

EXCLUDES 2   *follow-up examination for medical surveillance after treatment (Z08-Z09)*

☑4ᵗʰ **Z40**   **Encounter for prophylactic surgery**

EXCLUDES 1   *organ donations (Z52.-)*
therapeutic organ removal—code to condition

☑5ᵗʰ **Z40.0**   **Encounter for prophylactic surgery for risk factors related to malignant neoplasms**
Admission for prophylactic organ removal
Use additional code to identify risk factor

     Z40.00   **Encounter for prophylactic removal of unspecified organ** ▽

     Z40.01   **Encounter for prophylactic removal of breast**

     Z40.02   **Encounter for prophylactic removal of ovary** ♀

     Z40.09   **Encounter for prophylactic removal of other organ**

   Z40.8   **Encounter for other prophylactic surgery**

   Z40.9   **Encounter for prophylactic surgery, unspecified** ▽

☑4ᵗʰ **Z41**   **Encounter for procedures for purposes other than remedying health state**

   Z41.1   **Encounter for cosmetic surgery**
Encounter for cosmetic breast implant
Encounter for cosmetic procedure

EXCLUDES 1   *encounter for plastic and reconstructive surgery following medical procedure or healed injury (Z42.-)*
encounter for post-mastectomy breast implantation (Z42.1)

   Z41.2   **Encounter for routine and ritual male circumcision** ♂

   Z41.3   **Encounter for ear piercing**

   Z41.8   **Encounter for other procedures for purposes other than remedying health state**

   Z41.9   **Encounter for procedure for purposes other than remedying health state, unspecified** ▽

☑4ᵗʰ **Z42**   **Encounter for plastic and reconstructive surgery following medical procedure or healed injury**

EXCLUDES 1   *encounter for cosmetic plastic surgery (Z41.1)*
encounter for plastic surgery for treatment of current injury—code to relevent injury

   Z42.1   **Encounter for breast reconstruction following mastectomy**   **PDx** **A**

EXCLUDES 1   *deformity and disproportion of reconstructed breast (N65.1-)*

   Z42.8   **Encounter for other plastic and reconstructive surgery following medical procedure or healed injury**   **PDx**

☑4ᵗʰ **Z43**   **Encounter for attention to artificial openings**

INCLUDES   closure of artificial openings
passage of sounds or bougies through artificial openings
reforming artificial openings
removal of catheter from artificial openings
toilet or cleansing of artificial openings

EXCLUDES 1   *artificial opening status only, without need for care (Z93.-)*
complications of external stoma (J95.0-, K94.-, N99.5-)

EXCLUDES 2   *fitting and adjustment of prosthetic and other devices (Z44-Z46)*

   Z43.0   **Encounter for attention to tracheostomy**   **CC**

   Z43.1   **Encounter for attention to gastrostomy**

   Z43.2   **Encounter for attention to ileostomy**

   Z43.3   **Encounter for attention to colostomy**

   Z43.4   **Encounter for attention to other artificial openings of digestive tract**

   Z43.5   **Encounter for attention to cystostomy**

   Z43.6   **Encounter for attention to other artificial openings of urinary tract**
Encounter for attention to nephrostomy
Encounter for attention to ureterostomy
Encounter for attention to urethrostomy

   Z43.7   **Encounter for attention to artificial vagina**

   Z43.8   **Encounter for attention to other artificial openings**

   Z43.9   **Encounter for attention to unspecified artificial opening** ▽

☑4ᵗʰ **Z44**   **Encounter for fitting and adjustment of external prosthetic device**

INCLUDES   removal or replacement of external prosthetic device

EXCLUDES 1   *malfunction or other complications of device—see Alphabetical Index*
presence of prosthetic device (Z97.-)

☑5ᵗʰ **Z44.0**   **Encounter for fitting and adjustment of artificial arm**

☑6ᵗʰ **Z44.00**   **Encounter for fitting and adjustment of unspecified artificial arm**

     Z44.001   **Encounter for fitting and adjustment of unspecified right artificial arm** ▽

     Z44.002   **Encounter for fitting and adjustment of unspecified left artificial arm** ▽

     Z44.009   **Encounter for fitting and adjustment of unspecified artificial arm, unspecified arm** ▽

☑6ᵗʰ **Z44.01**   **Encounter for fitting and adjustment of complete artificial arm**

     Z44.011   **Encounter for fitting and adjustment of complete right artificial arm**

     Z44.012   **Encounter for fitting and adjustment of complete left artificial arm**

     Z44.019   **Encounter for fitting and adjustment of complete artificial arm, unspecified arm** ▽

☑6ᵗʰ **Z44.02**   **Encounter for fitting and adjustment of partial artificial arm**

     Z44.021   **Encounter for fitting and adjustment of partial artificial right arm**

     Z44.022   **Encounter for fitting and adjustment of partial artificial left arm**

     Z44.029   **Encounter for fitting and adjustment of partial artificial arm, unspecified arm** ▽

☑5ᵗʰ **Z44.1**   **Encounter for fitting and adjustment of artificial leg**

☑6ᵗʰ **Z44.10**   **Encounter for fitting and adjustment of unspecified artificial leg**

     Z44.101   **Encounter for fitting and adjustment of unspecified right artificial leg** ▽

     Z44.102   **Encounter for fitting and adjustment of unspecified left artificial leg** ▽

     Z44.109   **Encounter for fitting and adjustment of unspecified artificial leg, unspecified leg** ▽

☑6ᵗʰ **Z44.11**   **Encounter for fitting and adjustment of complete artificial leg**

     Z44.111   **Encounter for fitting and adjustment of complete right artificial leg**

     Z44.112   **Encounter for fitting and adjustment of complete left artificial leg**

     Z44.119   **Encounter for fitting and adjustment of complete artificial leg, unspecified leg** ▽

☑6ᵗʰ **Z44.12**   **Encounter for fitting and adjustment of partial artificial leg**

     Z44.121   **Encounter for fitting and adjustment of partial artificial right leg**

     Z44.122   **Encounter for fitting and adjustment of partial artificial left leg**

     Z44.129   **Encounter for fitting and adjustment of partial artificial leg, unspecified leg** ▽

☑5ᵗʰ **Z44.2**   **Encounter for fitting and adjustment of artificial eye**

EXCLUDES 1   *mechanical complication of ocular prosthesis (T85.3)*

     Z44.20   **Encounter for fitting and adjustment of artificial eye, unspecified** ▽

     Z44.21   **Encounter for fitting and adjustment of artificial right eye**

     Z44.22   **Encounter for fitting and adjustment of artificial left eye**

☑5ᵗʰ **Z44.3**   **Encounter for fitting and adjustment of external breast prosthesis**

EXCLUDES 1   *complications of breast implant (T85.4-)*
encounter for adjustment or removal of breast implant (Z45.81-)
encounter for initial breast implant insertion for cosmetic breast augmentation (Z41.1)
encounter for breast reconstruction following mastectomy (Z42.1)

     Z44.30   **Encounter for fitting and adjustment of external breast prosthesis, unspecified breast** ♀▽

N Newborn   **P** Pediatric   **M** Maternity   **A** Adult   **RIC** RIC Dx   **NCDx** Noncancer Dx   **PDx** Primary Dx   **CC** RIC CC Condition   ▶◀ Revised Text   ● New Code   ▲ Revised Code Title

1132   ICD-10-CM 2016

Z44.31 Encounter for fitting and adjustment of external ♀
right breast prosthesis

Z44.32 Encounter for fitting and adjustment of ruf external ♀
left breast prosthesis

Z44.8 Encounter for fitting and adjustment of other external
prosthetic devices

Z44.9 Encounter for fitting and adjustment of unspecified ▽
external prosthetic device

✓4th **Z45** **Encounter for adjustment and management of implanted device**
INCLUDES removal or replacement of implanted device
EXCLUDES 1 malfunction or other complications of device—see Alphabetical
Index
presence of prosthetic and other devices (Z95-Z97)
EXCLUDES 2 encounter for fitting and adjustment of non-implanted device
(Z46.-)

✓5th **Z45.0** **Encounter for adjustment and management of cardiac device**

✓6th **Z45.01** **Encounter for adjustment and management of
cardiac pacemaker**
EXCLUDES 1 encounter for adjustment and management
of automatic implantable cardiac
defibrillator with synchronous cardiac
pacemaker (Z45.02)

Z45.010 **Encounter for checking and testing of
cardiac pacemaker pulse generator
[battery]**
Encounter for replacing cardiac pacemaker
pulse generator [battery]

Z45.018 **Encounter for adjustment and
management of other part of cardiac
pacemaker**

Z45.02 **Encounter for adjustment and management of
automatic implantable cardiac defibrillator**
Encounter for adjustment and management of
automatic implantable cardiac defibrillator with
synchronous cardiac pacemaker

Z45.09 **Encounter for adjustment and management of other
cardiac device**

Z45.1 **Encounter for adjustment and management of infusion pump**

Z45.2 **Encounter for adjustment and management of vascular
access device**
Encounter for adjustment and management of vascular
catheters
EXCLUDES 1 encounter for adjustment and management of renal
dialysis catheter (Z49.01)

✓5th **Z45.3** **Encounter for adjustment and management of implanted
devices of the special senses**

Z45.31 **Encounter for adjustment and management of
implanted visual substitution device**

✓6th **Z45.32** **Encounter for adjustment and management of
implanted hearing device**
EXCLUDES 1 Encounter for fitting and adjustment of
hearing aide (Z46.1)

Z45.320 **Encounter for adjustment and
management of bone conduction device**

Z45.321 **Encounter for adjustment and
management of cochlear device**

Z45.328 **Encounter for adjustment and
management of other implanted hearing
device**

✓5th **Z45.4** **Encounter for adjustment and management of implanted
nervous system device**

Z45.41 **Encounter for adjustment and management of
cerebrospinal fluid drainage device**
Encounter for adjustment and management of
cerebral ventricular (communicating) shunt

Z45.42 **Encounter for adjustment and management of
neuropacemaker (brain) (peripheral nerve) (spinal
cord)**

Z45.49 **Encounter for adjustment and management of other
implanted nervous system device**
AHA: 2014, 3Q, 19

✓5th **Z45.8** **Encounter for adjustment and management of other
implanted devices**

✓6th **Z45.81** **Encounter for adjustment or removal of breast
implant**
Encounter for elective implant exchange (different
material) (different size)
Encounter for removal of tissue expander without
synchronous insertion of permanent implant
EXCLUDES 1 complications of breast implant (T85.4-)
encounter for initial breast implant insertion
for cosmetic breast augmentation
(Z41.1)
encounter for breast reconstruction following
mastectomy (Z42.1)

Z45.811 **Encounter for adjustment or removal of ♀
right breast implant**

Z45.812 **Encounter for adjustment or removal of ♀
left breast implant**

Z45.819 **Encounter for adjustment or removal ♀▽
of unspecified breast implant**

Z45.82 **Encounter for adjustment or removal of
myringotomy device (stent) (tube)**

Z45.89 **Encounter for adjustment and management of other
implanted devices**
AHA: 2014, 4Q, 26-28

Z45.9 **Encounter for adjustment and management of unspecified ▽
implanted device**

✓4th **Z46** **Encounter for fitting and adjustment of other devices**
INCLUDES removal or replacement of other device
EXCLUDES 1 malfunction or other complications of device—see Alphabetical
Index
EXCLUDES 2 encounter for fitting and management of implanted devices
(Z45.-)
issue of repeat prescription only (Z76.0)
presence of prosthetic and other devices (Z95-Z97)

Z46.0 **Encounter for fitting and adjustment of spectacles and
contact lenses**

Z46.1 **Encounter for fitting and adjustment of hearing aid**
EXCLUDES 1 encounter for adjustment and management of
implanted hearing device (Z45.32-)

Z46.2 **Encounter for fitting and adjustment of other devices related
to nervous system and special senses**
EXCLUDES 2 encounter for adjustment and management of
implanted nervous system device (Z45.4-)
encounter for adjustment and management of
implanted visual substitution device (Z45.31)

Z46.3 **Encounter for fitting and adjustment of dental prosthetic
device**
Encounter for fitting and adjustment of dentures

Z46.4 **Encounter for fitting and adjustment of orthodontic device**

✓5th **Z46.5** **Encounter for fitting and adjustment of other
gastrointestinal appliance and device**
EXCLUDES 1 encounter for attention to artificial openings of
digestive tract (Z43.1-Z43.4)

Z46.51 **Encounter for fitting and adjustment of gastric lap
band**

Z46.59 **Encounter for fitting and adjustment of other
gastrointestinal appliance and device**

Z46.6 **Encounter for fitting and adjustment of urinary device**
EXCLUDES 2 attention to artificial openings of urinary tract (Z43.5,
Z43.6)

✓5th **Z46.8** **Encounter for fitting and adjustment of other specified
devices**

Z46.81 **Encounter for fitting and adjustment of insulin
pump**
Encounter for insulin pump instruction and training
Encounter for insulin pump titration

Z46.82 **Encounter for fitting and adjustment of
non-vascular catheter**

Z46.89 **Encounter for fitting and adjustment of other
specified devices**
Encounter for fitting and adjustment of wheelchair

Z46.9 **Encounter for fitting and adjustment of unspecified device** ▽

✓ Add'l Character Required ✓x7th Placeholder Alert RUG IV Special Care High Dx RUG IV Clinically Complex Dx RUG IV Special Care Low Dx Manifestation Code Other Specified Code ▽ Unspecified Code

Chapter 21. Factors Influencing Health Status and Contact With Health Services

☑4ᵗʰ **Z47** **Orthopedic aftercare**
> EXCLUDES 1 *aftercare for healing fracture—code to fracture with 7th character D*

Z47.1 **Aftercare following** joint replacement surgery
> Use additional code to identify the joint (Z96.6-)

Z47.2 **Encounter for removal of** internal fixation device
> EXCLUDES 1 *encounter for adjustment of internal fixation device for fracture treatment—code to fracture with appropriate 7th character*
> *encounter for removal of external fixation device—code to fracture with 7th character D*
> *infection or inflammatory reaction to internal fixation device (T84.6-)*
> *mechanical complication of internal fixation device (T84.1-)*

☑5ᵗʰ **Z47.3** **Aftercare following explantation of** joint prosthesis
> Aftercare following explantation of joint prosthesis, staged procedure
> Encounter for joint prosthesis insertion following prior explantation of joint prosthesis
> **AHA:** 2015, 1Q, 16

Z47.31 **Aftercare following explantation of** shoulder **joint prosthesis**
> EXCLUDES 1 *acquired absence of shoulder joint following prior explantation of shoulder joint prosthesis (Z89.23-)*
> *shoulder joint prosthesis explantation status (Z89.23-)*

Z47.32 **Aftercare following explantation of** hip **joint prosthesis**
> EXCLUDES 1 *acquired absence of hip joint following prior explantation of hip joint prosthesis (Z89.62-)*
> *hip joint prosthesis explantation status (Z89.62-)*

Z47.33 **Aftercare following explantation of** knee **joint prosthesis**
> EXCLUDES 1 *acquired absence of knee joint following prior explantation of knee prosthesis (Z89.52-)*
> *knee joint prosthesis explantation status (Z89.52-)*

☑5ᵗʰ **Z47.8** **Encounter for** other **orthopedic aftercare**

Z47.81 **Encounter for orthopedic aftercare** following surgical amputation
> Use additional code to identify the limb amputated (Z89.-)

Z47.82 **Encounter for orthopedic aftercare** following scoliosis surgery

Z47.89 **Encounter for other orthopedic aftercare**
> **AHA:** 2015, 1Q, 8

☑4ᵗʰ **Z48** **Encounter for other postprocedural aftercare**
> EXCLUDES 1 *encounter for follow-up examination after completed treatment (Z08-Z09)*
> EXCLUDES 2 *encounter for attention to artificial openings (Z43.-)*
> *encounter for fitting and adjustment of prosthetic and other devices (Z44-Z46)*
> **AHA:** 2015, 1Q, 6-7

☑5ᵗʰ **Z48.0** **Encounter for** attention to dressings, sutures and drains
> EXCLUDES 1 *encounter for planned postprocedural wound closure (Z48.1)*

Z48.00 **Encounter for change or removal of** nonsurgical **wound** dressing
> Encounter for change or removal of wound dressing NOS

Z48.01 **Encounter for change or removal of** surgical **wound** dressing

Z48.02 **Encounter for removal of** sutures
> Encounter for removal of staples

Z48.03 **Encounter for change or removal of** drains

Z48.1 **Encounter for planned** postprocedural **wound closure**
> EXCLUDES 1 *encounter for attention to dressings and sutures (Z48.0-)*

☑5ᵗʰ **Z48.2** **Encounter for aftercare following** organ transplant

Z48.21 **Encounter for aftercare following** heart **transplant**

Z48.22 **Encounter for aftercare following** kidney **transplant**

Z48.23 **Encounter for aftercare following** liver **transplant**

Z48.24 **Encounter for aftercare following** lung **transplant**

☑6ᵗʰ **Z48.28** **Encounter for aftercare following** multiple **organ transplant**

Z48.280 **Encounter for aftercare following** heart-lung **transplant**

Z48.288 **Encounter for aftercare following** multiple **organ transplant**

☑6ᵗʰ **Z48.29** **Encounter for aftercare following** other **organ transplant**

Z48.290 **Encounter for aftercare following** bone marrow **transplant**

Z48.298 **Encounter for aftercare following other organ transplant**

Z48.3 **Aftercare following** surgery for neoplasm
> Use additional code to identify the neoplasm

☑5ᵗʰ **Z48.8** **Encounter for other specified postprocedural aftercare**

☑6ᵗʰ **Z48.81** **Encounter for surgical aftercare following** surgery on specified body systems
> NOTE These codes identify the body system requiring aftercare. They are for use in conjunction with other aftercare codes to fully explain the aftercare encounter. The condition treated should also be coded if still present.
> EXCLUDES 1 *aftercare for injury—code the injury with 7th character D*
> *aftercare following surgery for neoplasm (Z48.3)*
> EXCLUDES 2 *aftercare following organ transplant (Z48.2-)*
> *orthopedic aftercare (Z47.-)*

Z48.810 **Encounter for surgical aftercare following surgery on the** sense organs

Z48.811 **Encounter for surgical aftercare following surgery on the** nervous system
> EXCLUDES 2 *encounter for surgical aftercare following surgery on the sense organs (Z48.810)*

Z48.812 **Encounter for surgical aftercare following surgery on the** circulatory system
> **AHA:** 2012, 4Q, 96

Z48.813 **Encounter for surgical aftercare following surgery on the** respiratory system

Z48.814 **Encounter for surgical aftercare following surgery on the** teeth or oral cavity

Z48.815 **Encounter for surgical aftercare following surgery on the** digestive system

Z48.816 **Encounter for surgical aftercare following surgery on the** genitourinary system
> EXCLUDES 1 *encounter for aftercare following sterilization reversal (Z31.42)*

Z48.817 **Encounter for surgical aftercare following surgery on the** skin and subcutaneous tissue

Z48.89 **Encounter for other specified surgical aftercare**

☑4ᵗʰ **Z49** **Encounter for care involving renal dialysis**
> Code also associated end stage renal disease (N18.6)

☑5ᵗʰ **Z49.0** Preparatory care **for renal dialysis**
> Encounter for dialysis instruction and training

Z49.01 **Encounter for fitting and adjustment of** extracorporeal dialysis catheter
> Removal or replacement of renal dialysis catheter
> Toilet or cleansing of renal dialysis catheter

Z49.02 **Encounter for fitting and adjustment of** peritoneal dialysis catheter

☑5ᵗʰ **Z49.3** **Encounter for** adequacy testing for dialysis

Z49.31 **Encounter for adequacy testing for** hemodialysis

Z49.32 **Encounter for adequacy testing for** peritoneal dialysis
> Encounter for peritoneal equilibration test

Ⓝ Newborn   Ⓟ Pediatric   Ⓜ Maternity   Ⓐ Adult   **RIC** RIC Dx   **NC Dx** Noncancer Dx   **PDx** Primary Dx   **CC** RIC CC Condition   ▶◀ Revised Text   ● New Code   ▲ Revised Code Title

1134   ICD-10-CM 2016

Z51 ☑4ᵗʰ **Encounter for other aftercare**
Code also condition requiring care
EXCLUDES 1   follow-up examination after treatment (Z08-Z09)

Z51.0 Encounter for antineoplastic radiation therapy   PDx

☑5ᵗʰ **Z51.1** **Encounter for antineoplastic chemotherapy and immunotherapy**
EXCLUDES 2   encounter for chemotherapy and immunotherapy for nonneoplastic condition—code to condition

Z51.11 Encounter for antineoplastic chemotherapy   PDx
Z51.12 Encounter for antineoplastic immunotherapy   PDx

Z51.5 **Encounter for** palliative care

☑5ᵗʰ **Z51.8** **Encounter for** other specified aftercare
EXCLUDES 1   holiday relief care (Z75.5)

Z51.81 Encounter for therapeutic drug level monitoring
Code also any long-term (current) drug therapy (Z79.-)
EXCLUDES 1   encounter for blood-drug test for administrative or medicolegal reasons (Z02.83)

Z51.89 Encounter for other specified aftercare
AHA: 2012, 4Q, 95-97

Z52 ☑4ᵗʰ **Donors of organs and tissues**
INCLUDES   autologous and other living donors
EXCLUDES 1   cadaveric donor—omit code
examination of potential donor (Z00.5)
AHA: 2012, 4Q, 99

☑5ᵗʰ **Z52.0** Blood donor
☑6ᵗʰ **Z52.00** Unspecified blood donor
Z52.000 Unspecified donor, whole blood   PDx ▽
Z52.001 Unspecified donor, stem cells   PDx ▽
Z52.008 Unspecified donor, other blood   PDx ▽

☑6ᵗʰ **Z52.01** Autologous blood donor
Z52.010 Autologous donor, whole blood   PDx
Z52.011 Autologous donor, stem cells   PDx
Z52.018 Autologous donor, other blood   PDx

☑6ᵗʰ **Z52.09** Other blood donor
Volunteer donor
Z52.090 Other blood donor, whole blood   PDx
Z52.091 Other blood donor, stem cells   PDx
Z52.098 Other blood donor, other blood   PDx

☑5ᵗʰ **Z52.1** Skin donor
Z52.10 Skin donor, unspecified   PDx ▽
Z52.11 Skin donor, autologous   PDx
Z52.19 Skin donor, other   PDx

☑5ᵗʰ **Z52.2** Bone donor
Z52.20 Bone donor, unspecified   PDx ▽
Z52.21 Bone donor, autologous   PDx
Z52.29 Bone donor, other   PDx

Z52.3 Bone marrow donor   PDx
Z52.4 Kidney donor   PDx
Z52.5 Cornea donor   PDx
Z52.6 Liver donor   PDx

☑5ᵗʰ **Z52.8** Donor of other specified organs or tissues
☑6ᵗʰ **Z52.81** Egg (Oocyte) donor
Z52.810 Egg (Oocyte) donor under age 35, anonymous recipient   PDx M♀
Egg donor under age 35 NOS
Z52.811 Egg (Oocyte) donor under age 35, designated recipient   PDx M♀
Z52.812 Egg (Oocyte) donor age 35 and over, anonymous recipient   PDx M♀
Egg donor age 35 and over NOS
Z52.813 Egg (Oocyte) donor age 35 and over, designated recipient   PDx M♀
Z52.819 Egg (Oocyte) donor, unspecified   PDx M♀ ▽
Z52.89 Donor of other specified organs or tissues   PDx

Z52.9 Donor of unspecified organ or tissue   ▽
Donor NOS

Z53 ☑4ᵗʰ **Persons encountering health services for specific procedures and treatment, not carried out**
☑5ᵗʰ **Z53.0** **Procedure and treatment not carried out because of** contraindication
Z53.01 Procedure and treatment not carried out due to patient smoking

Z53.09 Procedure and treatment not carried out because of other contraindication

Z53.1 Procedure and treatment not carried out because of patient's decision for reasons of belief and group pressure

☑5ᵗʰ **Z53.2** Procedure and treatment not carried out because of patient's decision for other and unspecified reasons
Z53.20 Procedure and treatment not carried out because of patient's decision for unspecified reasons   ▽
Z53.21 Procedure and treatment not carried out due to patient leaving prior to being seen by health care provider
Z53.29 Procedure and treatment not carried out because of patient's decision for other reasons

Z53.8 Procedure and treatment not carried out for other reasons
Z53.9 Procedure and treatment not carried out, unspecified reason   ▽

Persons with potential health hazards related to socioeconomic and psychosocial circumstances (Z55-Z65)

Z55 ☑4ᵗʰ **Problems related to education and literacy**
EXCLUDES 1   disorders of psychological development (F80-F89)

Z55.0 Illiteracy and low-level literacy
Z55.1 Schooling unavailable and unattainable
Z55.2 Failed school examinations
Z55.3 Underachievement in school
Z55.4 Educational maladjustment and discord with teachers and classmates
Z55.8 Other problems related to education and literacy
Problems related to inadequate teaching
Z55.9 Problems related to education and literacy, unspecified   ▽
Academic problems NOS

Z56 ☑4ᵗʰ **Problems related to employment and unemployment**
EXCLUDES 2   occupational exposure to risk factors (Z57.-)
problems related to housing and economic circumstances (Z59.-)

Z56.0 Unemployment, unspecified   ▽
Z56.1 Change of job   A
Z56.2 Threat of job loss
Z56.3 Stressful work schedule
Z56.4 Discord with boss and workmates
Z56.5 Uncongenial work environment
Difficult conditions at work
Z56.6 Other physical and mental strain related to work
☑5ᵗʰ **Z56.8** Other problems related to employment
Z56.81 Sexual harassment on the job
Z56.82 Military deployment status   A
Individual (civilian or military) currently deployed in theater or in support of military war, peacekeeping and humanitarian operations
Z56.89 Other problems related to employment
Z56.9 Unspecified problems related to employment   ▽
Occupational problems NOS

Z57 ☑4ᵗʰ **Occupational exposure to risk factors**
Z57.0 Occupational exposure to noise
Z57.1 Occupational exposure to radiation
Z57.2 Occupational exposure to dust
☑5ᵗʰ **Z57.3** Occupational exposure to other air contaminants
Z57.31 Occupational exposure to environmental tobacco smoke
EXCLUDES 2   exposure to environmental tobacco smoke (Z77.22)
Z57.39 Occupational exposure to other air contaminants
Z57.4 Occupational exposure to toxic agents in agriculture
Occupational exposure to solids, liquids, gases or vapors in agriculture
Z57.5 Occupational exposure to toxic agents in other industries
Occupational exposure to solids, liquids, gases or vapors in other industries
Z57.6 Occupational exposure to extreme temperature
Z57.7 Occupational exposure to vibration
Z57.8 Occupational exposure to other risk factors
Z57.9 Occupational exposure to unspecified risk factor   ▽

☑ Add'l Character Required   ☑7ᵗʰ Placeholder Alert   RUG IV Special Care High Dx   RUG IV Clinically Complex Dx   RUG IV Special Care Low Dx   Manifestation Code   Other Specified Code   ▽ Unspecified Code

Chapter 21. Factors Influencing Health Status and Contact With Health Services

☑4ᵗʰ Z59 Problems related to housing and economic circumstances
EXCLUDES 2   *problems related to upbringing (Z62.-)*

Z59.0 Homelessness

Z59.1 Inadequate housing
Lack of heating
Restriction of space
Technical defects in home preventing adequate care
Unsatisfactory surroundings
EXCLUDES 1   *problems related to the natural and physical environment (Z77.1-)*

Z59.2 Discord with neighbors, lodgers and landlord

Z59.3 Problems related to living in residential institution
Boarding-school resident
EXCLUDES 1   *institutional upbringing (Z62.2)*

Z59.4 Lack of adequate food and safe drinking water
Inadequate drinking water supply
EXCLUDES 1   *effects of hunger (T73.0)*
        inappropriate diet or eating habits (Z72.4)
        malnutrition (E40-E46)

Z59.5 Extreme poverty

Z59.6 Low income

Z59.7 Insufficient social insurance and welfare support

Z59.8 Other problems related to housing and economic circumstances
Foreclosure on loan
Isolated dwelling
Problems with creditors

Z59.9 Problem related to housing and economic circumstances, unspecified ▽

☑4ᵗʰ Z60 Problems related to social environment

Z60.0 Problems of adjustment to life-cycle transitions
Empty nest syndrome
Phase of life problem
Problem with adjustment to retirement [pension]

Z60.2 Problems related to living alone

Z60.3 Acculturation difficulty
Problem with migration
Problem with social transplantation

Z60.4 Social exclusion and rejection
Exclusion and rejection on the basis of personal characteristics, such as unusual physical appearance, illness or behavior.
EXCLUDES 1   *target of adverse discrimination such as for racial or religious reasons (Z60.5)*

Z60.5 Target of (perceived) adverse discrimination and persecution
EXCLUDES 1   *social exclusion and rejection (Z60.4)*

Z60.8 Other problems related to social environment

Z60.9 Problem related to social environment, unspecified ▽

☑4ᵗʰ Z62 Problems related to upbringing
Current and past negative life events in childhood
Current and past problems of a child related to upbringing
EXCLUDES 2   *maltreatment syndrome (T74.-)*
        problems related to housing and economic circumstances (Z59.-)

Z62.0 Inadequate parental supervision and control

Z62.1 Parental overprotection

☑5ᵗʰ Z62.2 Upbringing away from parents
EXCLUDES 1   *problems with boarding school (Z59.3)*

Z62.21 Child in welfare custody   P
Child in care of non-parental family member
Child in foster care
EXCLUDES 2   *problem for parent due to child in welfare custody (Z63.5)*

Z62.22 Institutional upbringing
Child living in orphanage or group home

Z62.29 Other upbringing away from parents

Z62.3 Hostility towards and scapegoating of child   P

Z62.6 Inappropriate (excessive) parental pressure

☑5ᵗʰ Z62.8 Other specified problems related to upbringing

☑6ᵗʰ Z62.81 Personal history of abuse in childhood

Z62.810 Personal history of physical and sexual abuse in childhood
EXCLUDES 1   *current child physical abuse (T74.12, T76.12)*
        current child sexual abuse (T74.22, T76.22)

Z62.811 Personal history of psychological abuse in childhood
EXCLUDES 1   *current child psychological abuse (T74.32, T76.32)*

Z62.812 Personal history of neglect in childhood
EXCLUDES 1   *current child neglect (T74.02, T76.02)*

Z62.819 Personal history of unspecified abuse in childhood ▽
EXCLUDES 1   *current child abuse NOS (T74.92, T76.92)*

☑6ᵗʰ Z62.82 Parent-child conflict

Z62.820 Parent-biological child conflict
Parent-child problem NOS

Z62.821 Parent-adopted child conflict

Z62.822 Parent-foster child conflict

☑6ᵗʰ Z62.89 Other specified problems related to upbringing

Z62.890 Parent-child estrangement NEC

Z62.891 Sibling rivalry

Z62.898 Other specified problems related to upbringing

Z62.9 Problem related to upbringing, unspecified ▽

☑4ᵗʰ Z63 Other problems related to primary support group, including family circumstances
EXCLUDES 2   *maltreatment syndrome (T74-, T76)*
        parent-child problems (Z62.-)
        problems related to negative life events in childhood (Z62.-)
        problems related to upbringing (Z62.-)

Z63.0 Problems in relationship with spouse or partner
EXCLUDES 1   *counseling for spousal or partner abuse problems (Z69.1)*
        counseling related to sexual attitude, behavior, and orientation (Z70.-)

Z63.1 Problems in relationship with in-laws

☑5ᵗʰ Z63.3 Absence of family member
EXCLUDES 1   *absence of family member due to disappearance and death (Z63.4)*
        absence of family member due to separation and divorce (Z63.5)

Z63.31 Absence of family member due to military deployment
Individual or family affected by other family member being on military deployment
EXCLUDES 1   *family disruption due to return of family member from military deployment (Z63.71)*

Z63.32 Other absence of family member

Z63.4 Disappearance and death of family member
Assumed death of family member
Bereavement
AHA: 2014, 1Q, 25

Z63.5 Disruption of family by separation and divorce
Marital estrangement

Z63.6 Dependent relative needing care at home

☑5ᵗʰ Z63.7 Other stressful life events affecting family and household

Z63.71 Stress on family due to return of family member from military deployment
Individual or family affected by family member having returned from military deployment (current or past conflict)

Z63.72 Alcoholism and drug addiction in family

Z63.79 Other stressful life events affecting family and household
Anxiety (normal) about sick person in family
Health problems within family
Ill or disturbed family member
Isolated family

N Newborn   P Pediatric   M Maternity   A Adult   RIC RIC Dx   NC Dx Noncancer Dx   PDx Primary Dx   CC RIC CC Condition   ►◄ Revised Text   ● New Code   ▲ Revised Code Title

1136   ICD-10-CM 2016

Z63.8 **Other specified problems related to primary support group**
Family discord NOS
Family estrangement NOS
High expressed emotional level within family
Inadequate family support NOS
Inadequate or distorted communication within family

Z63.9 **Problem related to primary support group, unspecified** ▽
Relationship disorder NOS

✓4ᵗʰ **Z64** **Problems related to certain psychosocial circumstances**

Z64.0 **Problems related to unwanted pregnancy** Ⓜ♀

Z64.1 **Problems related to multiparity** ♀

Z64.4 **Discord with counselors**
Discord with probation officer
Discord with social worker

✓4ᵗʰ **Z65** **Problems related to other psychosocial circumstances**

Z65.0 **Conviction in civil and criminal proceedings without imprisonment**

Z65.1 **Imprisonment and other incarceration**

Z65.2 **Problems related to release from prison**

Z65.3 **Problems related to other legal circumstances**
Arrest
Child custody or support proceedings
Litigation
Prosecution

Z65.4 **Victim of crime and terrorism**
Victim of torture

Z65.5 **Exposure to disaster, war and other hostilities** Ⓐ
EXCLUDES 1 *target of perceived discrimination or persecution (Z60.5)*

Z65.8 **Other specified problems related to psychosocial circumstances**

Z65.9 **Problem related to unspecified psychosocial circumstances** ▽

Do not resuscitate status (Z66)

Z66 **Do not resuscitate**
DNR status

Blood type (Z67)

✓4ᵗʰ **Z67** **Blood type**

✓5ᵗʰ **Z67.1** Type A blood
Z67.10 **Type A blood,** Rh positive
Z67.11 **Type A blood,** Rh negative

✓5ᵗʰ **Z67.2** Type B blood
Z67.20 **Type B blood,** Rh positive
Z67.21 **Type B blood,** Rh negative

✓5ᵗʰ **Z67.3** Type AB blood
Z67.30 **Type AB blood,** Rh positive
Z67.31 **Type AB blood,** Rh negative

✓5ᵗʰ **Z67.4** Type O blood
Z67.40 **Type O blood,** Rh positive
Z67.41 **Type O blood,** Rh negative

✓5ᵗʰ **Z67.9** Unspecified blood type
Z67.90 **Unspecified blood type,** Rh positive ▽
Z67.91 **Unspecified blood type,** Rh negative ▽

Body mass index [BMI] (Z68)

✓4ᵗʰ **Z68** **Body mass index [BMI]**
Kilograms per meters squared
NOTE BMI adult codes are for use for persons 21 years of age or older.
BMI pediatric codes are for use for persons 2-20 years of age. These percentiles are based on the growth charts published by the Centers for Disease Control and Prevention (CDC).

Z68.1 **Body mass index [BMI]** 19 or less, adult Ⓐ

✓5ᵗʰ **Z68.2** Body mass index [BMI] 20-29, adult
Z68.20 **Body mass index [BMI]** 20.0-20.9, adult Ⓐ
Z68.21 **Body mass index [BMI]** 21.0-21.9, adult Ⓐ
Z68.22 **Body mass index [BMI]** 22.0-22.9, adult Ⓐ
Z68.23 **Body mass index [BMI]** 23.0-23.9, adult Ⓐ
Z68.24 **Body mass index [BMI]** 24.0-24.9, adult Ⓐ
Z68.25 **Body mass index [BMI]** 25.0-25.9, adult Ⓐ
Z68.26 **Body mass index [BMI]** 26.0-26.9, adult Ⓐ

Z68.27 **Body mass index [BMI]** 27.0-27.9, adult Ⓐ
Z68.28 **Body mass index [BMI]** 28.0-28.9, adult Ⓐ
Z68.29 **Body mass index [BMI]** 29.0-29.9, adult Ⓐ

✓5ᵗʰ **Z68.3** Body mass index [BMI] 30-39, adult
Z68.30 **Body mass index [BMI]** 30.0-30.9, adult Ⓐ
Z68.31 **Body mass index [BMI]** 31.0-31.9, adult Ⓐ
Z68.32 **Body mass index [BMI]** 32.0-32.9, adult Ⓐ
Z68.33 **Body mass index [BMI]** 33.0-33.9, adult Ⓐ
Z68.34 **Body mass index [BMI]** 34.0-34.9, adult Ⓐ
Z68.35 **Body mass index [BMI]** 35.0-35.9, adult Ⓐ
Z68.36 **Body mass index [BMI]** 36.0-36.9, adult Ⓐ
Z68.37 **Body mass index [BMI]** 37.0-37.9, adult Ⓐ
Z68.38 **Body mass index [BMI]** 38.0-38.9, adult Ⓐ
Z68.39 **Body mass index [BMI]** 39.0-39.9, adult Ⓐ

✓5ᵗʰ **Z68.4** Body mass index [BMI] 40 or greater, adult
Z68.41 **Body mass index [BMI]** 40.0-44.9, adult Ⓐ
Z68.42 **Body mass index [BMI]** 45.0-49.9, adult Ⓐ
Z68.43 **Body mass index [BMI]** 50-59.9, adult Ⓐ
Z68.44 **Body mass index [BMI]** 60.0-69.9, adult Ⓐ
Z68.45 **Body mass index [BMI]** 70 or greater, adult Ⓐ

✓5ᵗʰ **Z68.5** Body mass index [BMI] pediatric
Z68.51 **Body mass index [BMI] pediatric,** less than 5th percentile for age Ⓟ
Z68.52 **Body mass index [BMI] pediatric,** 5th percentile to less than 85th percentile for age Ⓟ
Z68.53 **Body mass index [BMI] pediatric,** 85th percentile to less than 95th percentile for age Ⓟ
Z68.54 **Body mass index [BMI] pediatric,** greater than or equal to 95th percentile for age Ⓟ

Persons encountering health services in other circumstances (Z69-Z76)

✓4ᵗʰ **Z69** **Encounter for mental health services for victim and perpetrator of abuse**
Counseling for victims and perpetrators of abuse

✓5ᵗʰ **Z69.0** **Encounter for mental health services for** child abuse problems

✓6ᵗʰ **Z69.01** **Encounter for mental health services for** parental child abuse

Z69.010 **Encounter for mental health services for** victim of parental child abuse Ⓟ

Z69.011 **Encounter for mental health services for** perpetrator of parental child abuse
EXCLUDES 1 *encounter for mental health services for non-parental child abuse (Z69.02-)*

✓6ᵗʰ **Z69.02** **Encounter for mental health services for** non-parental child abuse

Z69.020 **Encounter for mental health services for** victim of non-parental child abuse Ⓟ

Z69.021 **Encounter for mental health services for** perpetrator of non-parental child abuse

✓5ᵗʰ **Z69.1** **Encounter for mental health services for** spousal or partner abuse problems

Z69.11 **Encounter for mental health services for** victim of spousal or partner abuse

Z69.12 **Encounter for mental health services for** perpetrator of spousal or partner abuse

✓5ᵗʰ **Z69.8** **Encounter for mental health services for victim or perpetrator of** other abuse

Z69.81 **Encounter for mental health services for** victim of other abuse
Encounter for rape victim counseling

Z69.82 **Encounter for mental health services for** perpetrator of other abuse

☑ Add'l Character Required ✓7ᵗʰ Placeholder Alert RUG IV Special Care High Dx RUG IV Clinically Complex Dx RUG IV Special Care Low Dx Manifestation Code Other Specified Code ▽ Unspecified Code

ICD-10-CM 2016 **1137**

✓4ᵗʰ Z70   Counseling related to sexual attitude, behavior and orientation
Encounter for mental health services for sexual attitude, behavior and orientation
EXCLUDES 2   contraceptive or procreative counseling (Z30-Z31)

Z70.0   Counseling related to sexual attitude

Z70.1   Counseling related to patient's sexual behavior and orientation
Patient concerned regarding impotence
Patient concerned regarding non-responsiveness
Patient concerned regarding promiscuity
Patient concerned regarding sexual orientation

Z70.2   Counseling related to sexual behavior and orientation of third party
Advice sought regarding sexual behavior and orientation of child
Advice sought regarding sexual behavior and orientation of partner
Advice sought regarding sexual behavior and orientation of spouse

Z70.3   Counseling related to combined concerns regarding sexual attitude, behavior and orientation

Z70.8   Other sex counseling
Encounter for sex education

Z70.9   Sex counseling, unspecified   ▽

✓4ᵗʰ Z71   Persons encountering health services for other counseling and medical advice, not elsewhere classified
EXCLUDES 2   contraceptive or procreation counseling (Z30-Z31)
sex counseling (Z70.-)

Z71.0   Person encountering health services to consult on behalf of another person
Person encountering health services to seek advice or treatment for non-attending third party
EXCLUDES 2   anxiety (normal) about sick person in family (Z63.7)
expectant (adoptive) parent(s) pre-birth pediatrician visit (Z76.81)

Z71.1   Person with feared health complaint in whom no diagnosis is made
Person encountering health services with feared condition which was not demonstrated
Person encountering health services in which problem was normal state
"Worried well"
EXCLUDES 1   medical observation for suspected diseases and conditions proven not to exist (Z03.-)

Z71.2   Person consulting for explanation of examination or test findings

Z71.3   Dietary counseling and surveillance
Use additional code for any associated underlying medical condition
Use additional code to identify body mass index (BMI), if known (Z68.-)

✓5ᵗʰ Z71.4   Alcohol abuse counseling and surveillance
Use additional code for alcohol abuse or dependence (F10.-)

Z71.41   Alcohol abuse counseling and surveillance of alcoholic

Z71.42   Counseling for family member of alcoholic
Counseling for significant other, partner, or friend of alcoholic

✓5ᵗʰ Z71.5   Drug abuse counseling and surveillance
Use additional code for drug abuse or dependence (F11-F16, F18-F19)

Z71.51   Drug abuse counseling and surveillance of drug abuser

Z71.52   Counseling for family member of drug abuser
Counseling for significant other, partner, or friend of drug abuser

Z71.6   Tobacco abuse counseling
Use additional code for nicotine dependence (F17.-)

Z71.7   Human immunodeficiency virus [HIV] counseling

✓5ᵗʰ Z71.8   Other specified counseling
EXCLUDES 2   counseling for contraception (Z30.0-)
counseling for genetics (Z31.5)
counseling for procreative management (Z31.6-)

Z71.81   Spiritual or religious counseling

Z71.89   Other specified counseling

Z71.9   Counseling, unspecified   ▽
Encounter for medical advice NOS

✓4ᵗʰ Z72   Problems related to lifestyle
EXCLUDES 2   problems related to life-management difficulty (Z73.-)
problems related to socioeconomic and psychosocial circumstances (Z55-Z65)

Z72.0   Tobacco use
Tobacco use NOS
EXCLUDES 1   history of tobacco dependence (Z87.891)
nicotine dependence (F17.2-)
tobacco dependence (F17.2-)
tobacco use during pregnancy (O99.33-)

Z72.3   Lack of physical exercise

Z72.4   Inappropriate diet and eating habits
EXCLUDES 1   behavioral eating disorders of infancy or childhood (F98.2- F98.3)
eating disorders (F50.-)
lack of adequate food (Z59.4)
malnutrition and other nutritional deficiencies (E40-E64)

✓5ᵗʰ Z72.5   High risk sexual behavior
Promiscuity
EXCLUDES 1   paraphilias (F65)

Z72.51   High risk heterosexual behavior

Z72.52   High risk homosexual behavior

Z72.53   High risk bisexual behavior

Z72.6   Gambling and betting
EXCLUDES 1   compulsive or pathological gambling (F63.0)

✓5ᵗʰ Z72.8   Other problems related to lifestyle

✓6ᵗʰ Z72.81   Antisocial behavior
EXCLUDES 1   conduct disorders (F91.-)

Z72.810   Child and adolescent antisocial behavior   P
Antisocial behavior (child) (adolescent) without manifest psychiatric disorder
Delinquency NOS
Group delinquency
Offenses in the context of gang membership
Stealing in company with others
Truancy from school

Z72.811   Adult antisocial behavior   A
Adult antisocial behavior without manifest psychiatric disorder

✓6ᵗʰ Z72.82   Problems related to sleep

Z72.820   Sleep deprivation
Lack of adequate sleep
EXCLUDES 1   insomnia (G47.0-)

Z72.821   Inadequate sleep hygiene
Bad sleep habits
Irregular sleep habits
Unhealthy sleep wake schedule
EXCLUDES 1   insomnia (F51.0-, G47.0-)

Z72.89   Other problems related to lifestyle
Self-damaging behavior

Z72.9   Problem related to lifestyle, unspecified   ▽

✓4ᵗʰ Z73   Problems related to life management difficulty
EXCLUDES 2   problems related to socioeconomic and psychosocial circumstances (Z55-Z65)

Z73.0   Burn-out

Z73.1   Type A behavior pattern

Z73.2   Lack of relaxation and leisure

Z73.3   Stress, not elsewhere classified
Physical and mental strain NOS
EXCLUDES 1   stress related to employment or unemployment (Z56.-)

Z73.4   Inadequate social skills, not elsewhere classified

Z73.5   Social role conflict, not elsewhere classified

Z73.6   Limitation of activities due to disability
EXCLUDES 1   care-provider dependency (Z74.-)

✓5ᵗʰ Z73.8   Other problems related to life management difficulty

✓6ᵗʰ Z73.81   Behavioral insomnia of childhood

Z73.810   Behavioral insomnia of childhood, sleep-onset association type   P

Z73.811   Behavioral insomnia of childhood, limit setting type   P

Z73.812   Behavioral insomnia of childhood, combined type   P

Z73.819   Behavioral insomnia of childhood, unspecified type   P▽

Ⓝ Newborn   Ⓟ Pediatric   Ⓜ Maternity   Ⓐ Adult   RIC RIC Dx   NCDx Noncancer Dx   PDx Primary Dx   CC RIC CC Condition   ▶◀ Revised Text   ● New Code   ▲ Revised Code Title

1138   ICD-10-CM 2016

Z73.82   **Dual sensory impairment**

Z73.89   **Other problems related to life management difficulty**

Z73.9   **Problem related to life management difficulty, unspecified** ▽

☑4ᵗʰ **Z74   Problems related to care provider dependency**
   EXCLUDES 2   *dependence on enabling machines or devices NEC (Z99.-)*

   ☑5ᵗʰ **Z74.0   Reduced mobility**

   Z74.01   **Bed confinement status**
      Bedridden

   Z74.09   **Other reduced mobility**
      Chair ridden
      Reduced mobility NOS
      EXCLUDES 2   *wheelchair dependence (Z99.3)*

   Z74.1   **Need for assistance with** personal care

   Z74.2   **Need for assistance at home and** no other household member able to render care

   Z74.3   **Need for** continuous supervision

   Z74.8   **Other problems related to care provider dependency**

   Z74.9   **Problem related to care provider dependency, unspecified** ▽

☑4ᵗʰ **Z75   Problems related to medical facilities and other health care**

   Z75.0   **Medical services** not available in home
      EXCLUDES 1   *no other household member able to render care (Z74.2)*

   Z75.1   **Person** awaiting admission **to adequate facility elsewhere**

   Z75.2   **Other** waiting period for investigation **and treatment**

   Z75.3   **Unavailability** and inaccessibility of health-care facilities
      EXCLUDES 1   *bed unavailable (Z75.1)*

   Z75.4   **Unavailability** and inaccessibility of other helping agencies

   Z75.5   **Holiday relief care**

   Z75.8   **Other problems related to medical facilities and other health care**

   Z75.9   **Unspecified problem related to medical facilities and** ▽ **other health care**

☑4ᵗʰ **Z76   Persons encountering health services in other circumstances**

   Z76.0   **Encounter for issue of repeat prescription**
      Encounter for issue of repeat prescription for appliance
      Encounter for issue of repeat prescription for medicaments
      Encounter for issue of repeat prescription for spectacles
      EXCLUDES 2   *issue of medical certificate (Z02.7)*
            repeat prescription for contraceptive (Z30.4-)

   Z76.1   **Encounter for health supervision and care of foundling**   PDx

   Z76.2   **Encounter for health supervision and care of other**   PDx P **healthy infant and child**
      Encounter for medical or nursing care or supervision of healthy infant under circumstances such as adverse socioeconomic conditions at home
      Encounter for medical or nursing care or supervision of healthy infant under circumstances such as awaiting foster or adoptive placement
      Encounter for medical or nursing care or supervision of healthy infant under circumstances such as maternal illness
      Encounter for medical or nursing care or supervision of healthy infant under circumstances such as number of children at home preventing or interfering with normal care

   Z76.3   **Healthy person accompanying sick person**

   Z76.4   **Other boarder to healthcare facility**
      EXCLUDES 1   *homelessness (Z59.0)*

   Z76.5   **Malingerer [conscious simulation]**
      Person feigning illness (with obvious motivation)
      EXCLUDES 1   *factitious disorder (F68.1-)*
            peregrinating patient (F68.1-)

   ☑5ᵗʰ **Z76.8   Persons encountering health services in other specified circumstances**

   Z76.81   **Expectant parent(s) prebirth pediatrician visit**
      Pre-adoption pediatrician visit for adoptive parent(s)

   Z76.82   **Awaiting organ transplant status**
      Patient waiting for organ availability

   Z76.89   **Persons encountering health services in other specified circumstances**
      Persons encountering health services NOS
      AHA: 2014, 2Q, 10

Persons with potential health hazards related to family and personal history and certain conditions influencing health status (Z77-Z99)
Code also any follow-up examination (Z08-Z09)

☑4ᵗʰ **Z77   Other contact with and (suspected) exposures hazardous to health**
   INCLUDES   contact with and (suspected) exposures to potential hazards to health
   EXCLUDES 2   *contact with and (suspected) exposure to communicable diseases (Z20.-)*
      exposure to (parental) (environmental) tobacco smoke in the perinatal period (P96.81)
      newborn (suspected to be) affected by noxious substances transmitted via placenta or breast milk (P04.-)
      occupational exposure to risk factors (Z57.-)
      retained foreign body (Z18.-)
      retained foreign body fully removed (Z87.821)
      toxic effects of substances chiefly nonmedicinal as to source (T51-T65)

   ☑5ᵗʰ **Z77.0   Contact with and (suspected) exposure to** hazardous, chiefly nonmedicinal, chemicals

   ☑6ᵗʰ **Z77.01   Contact with and (suspected) exposure to hazardous metals**

   Z77.010   **Contact with and (suspected) exposure to** arsenic

   Z77.011   **Contact with and (suspected) exposure to** lead

   Z77.012   **Contact with and (suspected) exposure to** uranium
      EXCLUDES 1   *retained depleted uranium fragments (Z18.01)*

   Z77.018   **Contact with and (suspected) exposure to other hazardous metals**
      Contact with and (suspected) exposure to chromium compounds
      Contact with and (suspected) exposure to nickel dust

   ☑6ᵗʰ **Z77.02   Contact with and (suspected) exposure to hazardous aromatic compounds**

   Z77.020   **Contact with and (suspected) exposure to** aromatic amines

   Z77.021   **Contact with and (suspected) exposure to** benzene

   Z77.028   **Contact with and (suspected) exposure to other hazardous aromatic compounds**
      Aromatic dyes NOS
      Polycyclic aromatic hydrocarbons

   ☑6ᵗʰ **Z77.09   Contact with and (suspected) exposure to other hazardous, chiefly** nonmedicinal, chemicals

   Z77.090   **Contact with and (suspected) exposure to** asbestos

   Z77.098   **Contact with and (suspected) exposure to other hazardous, chiefly nonmedicinal, chemicals**
      Dyes NOS

   ☑5ᵗʰ **Z77.1   Contact with and (suspected) exposure to environmental pollution and** hazards in the physical environment

   ☑6ᵗʰ **Z77.11   Contact with and (suspected) exposure to** environmental pollution

   Z77.110   **Contact with and (suspected) exposure to** air **pollution**

   Z77.111   **Contact with and (suspected) exposure to** water **pollution**

   Z77.112   **Contact with and (suspected) exposure to** soil **pollution**

   Z77.118   **Contact with and (suspected) exposure to other environmental pollution**

   ☑6ᵗʰ **Z77.12   Contact with and (suspected) exposure to hazards in the physical environment**

   Z77.120   **Contact with and (suspected) exposure to** mold **(toxic)**

Z77.121　Contact with and (suspected) exposure to harmful algae and algae toxins
　　Contact with and (suspected) exposure to (harmful) algae bloom NOS
　　Contact with and (suspected) exposure to blue-green algae bloom
　　Contact with and (suspected) exposure to brown tide
　　Contact with and (suspected) exposure to cyanobacteria bloom
　　Contact with and (suspected) exposure to Florida red tide
　　Contact with and (suspected) exposure to pfiesteria piscicida
　　Contact with and (suspected) exposure to red tide

Z77.122　Contact with and (suspected) exposure to noise

Z77.123　Contact with and (suspected) exposure to radon and other naturally occuring radiation
　　　EXCLUDES 2　radiation exposure as the cause of a confirmed condition (W88-W90, X39.0-)
　　　　radiation sickness NOS (T66)

Z77.128　Contact with and (suspected) exposure to other hazards in the physical environment

✓5ᵗʰ　Z77.2　Contact with and (suspected) exposure to other hazardous substances

Z77.21　Contact with and (suspected) exposure to potentially hazardous body fluids

Z77.22　Contact with and (suspected) exposure to environmental tobacco smoke (acute) (chronic)
　　Exposure to second hand tobacco smoke (acute) (chronic)
　　Passive smoking (acute) (chronic)
　　　EXCLUDES 1　nicotine dependence (F17.-)
　　　　tobacco use (Z72.0)
　　　EXCLUDES 2　occupational exposure to environmental tobacco smoke (Z57.31)

Z77.29　Contact with and (suspected) exposure to other hazardous substances

Z77.9　Other contact with and (suspected) exposures hazardous to health

✓4ᵗʰ　Z78　Other specified health status
　　EXCLUDES 2　asymptomatic human immunodeficiency virus [HIV] infection status (Z21)
　　　postprocedural status (Z93- Z99)
　　　sex reassignment status (Z87.890)

Z78.0　Asymptomatic menopausal state　　Ⓐ♀
　　Menopausal state NOS
　　Postmenopausal status NOS
　　　EXCLUDES 2　symptomatic menopausal state (N95.1)

Z78.1　Physical restraint status
　　　EXCLUDES 1　physical restraint due to a procedure - omit code

Z78.9　Other specified health status

✓4ᵗʰ　Z79　Long term (current) drug therapy
　　INCLUDES　long term (current) drug use for prophylactic purposes
　　Code also any therapeutic drug level monitoring (Z51.81)
　　EXCLUDES 2　drug abuse and dependence (F11-F19)
　　　drug use complicating pregnancy, childbirth, and the puerperium (O99.32-)

✓5ᵗʰ　Z79.0　Long term (current) use of anticoagulants and antithrombotics/antiplatelets
　　　EXCLUDES 2　long term (current) use of aspirin (Z79.82)

Z79.01　Long term (current) use of anticoagulants

Z79.02　Long term (current) use of antithrombotics/antiplatelets

Z79.1　Long term (current) use of non-steroidal anti-inflammatories (NSAID)
　　　EXCLUDES 2　long term (current) use of aspirin (Z79.82)

Z79.2　Long term (current) use of antibiotics

Z79.3　Long term (current) use of hormonal contraceptives
　　Long term (current) use of birth control pill or patch

Z79.4　Long term (current) use of insulin

✓5ᵗʰ　Z79.5　Long term (current) use of steroids

Z79.51　Long term (current) use of inhaled steroids

Z79.52　Long term (current) use of systemic steroids

✓5ᵗʰ　Z79.8　Other long term (current) drug therapy

✓6ᵗʰ　Z79.81　Long term (current) use of agents affecting estrogen receptors and estrogen levels
　　Code first, if applicable:
　　　malignant neoplasm of breast (C50.-)
　　　malignant neoplasm of prostate (C61)
　　Use additional code, if applicable, to identify:
　　　estrogen receptor positive status (Z17.0)
　　　family history of breast cancer (Z80.3)
　　　genetic susceptibility to malignant neoplasm (cancer) (Z15.0-)
　　　personal history of breast cancer (Z85.3)
　　　personal history of prostate cancer (Z85.46)
　　　postmenopausal status (Z78.0)
　　　EXCLUDES 1　hormone replacement therapy (postmenopausal) (Z79.890)

Z79.810　Long term (current) use of selective estrogen receptor modulators (SERMs)
　　Long term (current) use of raloxifene (Evista)
　　Long term (current) use of tamoxifen (Nolvadex)
　　Long term (current) use of toremifene (Fareston)

Z79.811　Long term (current) use of aromatase inhibitors
　　Long term (current) use of anastrozole (Arimidex)
　　Long term (current) use of exemestane (Aromasin)
　　Long term (current) use of letrozole (Femara)

Z79.818　Long term (current) use of other agents affecting estrogen receptors and estrogen levels
　　Long term (current) use of estrogen receptor downregulators
　　Long term (current) use of fulvestrant (Faslodex)
　　Long term (current) use of gonadotropin-releasing hormone (GnRH) agonist
　　Long term (current) use of goserelin acetate (Zoladex)
　　Long term (current) use of leuprolide acetate (leuprorelin) (Lupron)
　　Long term (current) use of megestrol acetate (Megace)

Z79.82　Long term (current) use of aspirin

Z79.83　Long term (current) use of bisphosphonates

✓6ᵗʰ　Z79.89　Other long term (current) drug therapy

Z79.890　Hormone replacement therapy (postmenopausal)　　♀

Z79.891　Long term (current) use of opiate analgesic
　　Long term (current) use of methadone for pain management
　　　EXCLUDES 1　methadone use NOS (F11.2-)
　　　　use of methadone for treatment of heroin addiction (F11.2-)

Z79.899　Other long term (current) drug therapy

✓4ᵗʰ　Z80　Family history of primary malignant neoplasm

Z80.0　Family history of malignant neoplasm of digestive organs
　　Conditions classifiable to C15-C26

Z80.1　Family history of malignant neoplasm of trachea, bronchus and lung
　　Conditions classifiable to C33-C34

Z80.2　Family history of malignant neoplasm of other respiratory and intrathoracic organs
　　Conditions classifiable to C30-C32, C37-C39

Z80.3　Family history of malignant neoplasm of breast
　　Conditions classifiable to C50-

✓5ᵗʰ **Z80.4 Family history of malignant neoplasm of genital organs**
Conditions classifiable to C51-C63

    Z80.41 Family history of malignant neoplasm of ovary ♀

    Z80.42 Family history of malignant neoplasm of prostate ♂

    Z80.43 Family history of malignant neoplasm of testis ♂

    Z80.49 Family history of malignant neoplasm of other genital organs

✓5ᵗʰ **Z80.5 Family history of malignant neoplasm of urinary tract**
Conditions classifiable to C64-C68

    Z80.51 Family history of malignant neoplasm of kidney

    Z80.52 Family history of malignant neoplasm of bladder

    Z80.59 Family history of malignant neoplasm of other urinary tract organ

Z80.6 Family history of leukemia
Conditions classifiable to C91-C95

Z80.7 Family history of other malignant neoplasms of lymphoid, hematopoietic and related tissues
Conditions classifiable to C81-C90, C96-

Z80.8 Family history of malignant neoplasm of other organs or systems
Conditions classifiable to C00-C14, C40-C49, C69-C79

Z80.9 Family history of malignant neoplasm, unspecified ▽
Conditions classifiable to C80.1

✓4ᵗʰ **Z81 Family history of mental and behavioral disorders**

Z81.0 Family history of intellectual disabilities
Conditions classifiable to F70-F79

Z81.1 Family history of alcohol abuse and dependence
Conditions classifiable to F10-

Z81.2 Family history of tobacco abuse and dependence
Conditions classifiable to F17-

Z81.3 Family history of other psychoactive substance abuse and dependence
Conditions classifiable to F11-F16, F18-F19

Z81.4 Family history of other substance abuse and dependence
Conditions classifiable to F55

Z81.8 Family history of other mental and behavioral **disorders**
Conditions classifiable elsewhere in F01-F99

✓4ᵗʰ **Z82 Family history of certain disabilities and chronic diseases (leading to disablement)**

Z82.0 Family history of epilepsy **and other diseases of the nervous system**
Conditions classifiable to G00-G99

Z82.1 Family history of blindness and visual loss
Conditions classifiable to H54-

Z82.2 Family history of deafness and hearing loss
Conditions classifiable to H90-H91

Z82.3 Family history of stroke
Conditions classifiable to I60-I64

✓5ᵗʰ **Z82.4 Family history of ischemic heart disease and other diseases of the circulatory system**
Conditions classifiable to I00-I52, I65-I99

    Z82.41 Family history of sudden cardiac death

    Z82.49 Family history of ischemic heart disease **and other diseases of the circulatory system**

Z82.5 Family history of asthma **and other chronic lower respiratory diseases**
Conditions classifiable to J40-J47
EXCLUDES 2 *family history of other diseases of the respiratory system (Z83.6)*

✓5ᵗʰ **Z82.6 Family history of arthritis and other diseases of the musculoskeletal system and connective tissue**
Conditions classifiable to M00-M99

    Z82.61 Family history of arthritis

    Z82.62 Family history of osteoporosis

    Z82.69 Family history of other diseases of the musculoskeletal system and connective tissue

✓5ᵗʰ **Z82.7 Family history of congenital malformations, deformations and chromosomal abnormalities**
Conditions classifiable to Q00-Q99

    Z82.71 Family history of polycystic kidney

    Z82.79 Family history of other congenital malformations, deformations and chromosomal abnormalities

Z82.8 Family history of other disabilities and chronic diseases leading to disablement, **not elsewhere classified**

✓4ᵗʰ **Z83 Family history of other specific disorders**
EXCLUDES 2 *contact with and (suspected) exposure to communicable disease in the family (Z20.-)*

Z83.0 Family history of human immunodeficiency virus [HIV] **disease**
Conditions classifiable to B20

Z83.1 Family history of other infectious and parasitic diseases
Conditions classifiable to A00-B19, B25-B94, B99

Z83.2 Family history of diseases of the blood and blood-forming organs **and certain disorders involving the immune mechanism**
Conditions classifiable to D50-D89

Z83.3 Family history of diabetes mellitus
Conditions classifiable to E08-E13

✓5ᵗʰ **Z83.4 Family history of other endocrine, nutritional and metabolic diseases**
Conditions classifiable to E00-E07, E15-E88

    Z83.41 Family history of multiple endocrine neoplasia [MEN] syndrome

    Z83.49 Family history of other endocrine, nutritional and metabolic diseases

✓5ᵗʰ **Z83.5 Family history of eye and ear disorders**

    ✓6ᵗʰ **Z83.51 Family history of** eye disorders
Conditions classifiable to H00-H53, H55-H59
EXCLUDES 2 *family history of blindness and visual loss (Z82.1)*

      Z83.511 Family history of glaucoma

      Z83.518 Family history of other specified eye disorder

    Z83.52 Family history of ear disorders
Conditions classifiable to H60-H83, H92-H95
EXCLUDES 2 *family history of deafness and hearing loss (Z82.2)*

Z83.6 Family history of other diseases of the respiratory system
Conditions classifiable to J00-J39, J60-J99
EXCLUDES 2 *family history of asthma and other chronic lower respiratory diseases (Z82.5)*

✓5ᵗʰ **Z83.7 Family history of diseases of the digestive system**
Conditions classifiable to K00-K93

    Z83.71 Family history of colonic polyps
EXCLUDES 1 *family history of malignant neoplasm of digestive organs (Z80.0)*

    Z83.79 Family history of other diseases of the digestive system

✓4ᵗʰ **Z84 Family history of other conditions**

Z84.0 Family history of diseases of the skin and subcutaneous tissue
Conditions classifiable to L00-L99

Z84.1 Family history of disorders of kidney and ureter
Conditions classifiable to N00-N29

Z84.2 Family history of other diseases of the genitourinary system
Conditions classifiable to N30-N99

Z84.3 Family history of consanguinity

✓5ᵗʰ **Z84.8 Family history of other specified conditions**

    Z84.81 Family history of carrier of genetic disease

    Z84.89 Family history of other specified conditions

✓4ᵗʰ **Z85 Personal history of malignant neoplasm**
Code first any follow-up examination after treatment of malignant neoplasm (Z08)
Use additional code to identify:
alcohol use and dependence (F10.-)
exposure to environmental tobacco smoke (Z77.22)
history of tobacco use (Z87.891)
occupational exposure to environmental tobacco smoke (Z57.31)
tobacco dependence (F17.-)
tobacco use (Z72.0)
EXCLUDES 2 *personal history of benign neoplasm (Z86.01-)*
personal history of carcinoma-in-situ (Z86.00-)

✓5ᵗʰ **Z85.0 Personal history of malignant neoplasm of** digestive organs

    Z85.00 Personal history of malignant neoplasm of unspecified digestive organ ▽

    Z85.01 Personal history of malignant neoplasm of esophagus
Conditions classifiable to C15

Chapter 21. Factors Influencing Health Status and Contact With Health Services

Z85.02–Z85.828

✓6th **Z85.02** **Personal history of malignant neoplasm of** stomach

Z85.020 **Personal history of malignant** carcinoid **tumor of stomach**
Conditions classifiable to C7A.092

Z85.028 **Personal history of other malignant neoplasm of stomach**
Conditions classifiable to C16

✓6th **Z85.03** **Personal history of malignant neoplasm of** large intestine

Z85.030 **Personal history of** malignant carcinoid tumor of large intestine
Conditions classifiable to C7A.022-C7A.025, C7A.029

Z85.038 **Personal history of other malignant neoplasm of large intestine**
Conditions classifiable to C18

✓6th **Z85.04** **Personal history of malignant neoplasm of** rectum, rectosigmoid junction, and anus

Z85.040 **Personal history of malignant** carcinoid **tumor of rectum**
Conditions classifiable to C7A.026

Z85.048 **Personal history of other malignant neoplasm of rectum, rectosigmoid junction, and anus**
Conditions classifiable to C19-C21

Z85.05 **Personal history of malignant neoplasm of** liver
Conditions classifiable to C22

✓6th **Z85.06** **Personal history of malignant neoplasm of** small intestine

Z85.060 **Personal history of malignant** carcinoid **tumor of small intestine**
Conditions classifiable to C7A.01-

Z85.068 **Personal history of other malignant neoplasm of small intestine**
Conditions classifiable to C17

Z85.07 **Personal history of malignant neoplasm of** pancreas
Conditions classifiable to C25

Z85.09 **Personal history of malignant neoplasm of other digestive organs**

✓5th **Z85.1** **Personal history of malignant neoplasm of** trachea, bronchus and lung

✓6th **Z85.11** **Personal history of malignant neoplasm of** bronchus and lung

Z85.110 **Personal history of malignant** carcinoid **tumor of bronchus and lung**
Conditions classifiable to C7A.090

Z85.118 **Personal history of other malignant neoplasm of bronchus and lung**
Conditions classifiable to C34

Z85.12 **Personal history of malignant neoplasm of** trachea
Conditions classifiable to C33

✓5th **Z85.2** **Personal history of malignant neoplasm of other** respiratory and intrathoracic organs

Z85.20 **Personal history of malignant neoplasm of** unspecified respiratory organ   ▽

Z85.21 **Personal history of malignant neoplasm of** larynx
Conditions classifiable to C32

Z85.22 **Personal history of malignant neoplasm of** nasal cavities, middle ear, and accessory sinuses
Conditions classifiable to C30-C31

✓6th **Z85.23** **Personal history of malignant neoplasm of** thymus

Z85.230 **Personal history of malignant** carcinoid **tumor of thymus**
Conditions classifiable to C7A.091

Z85.238 **Personal history of other malignant neoplasm of thymus**
Conditions classifiable to C37

Z85.29 **Personal history of malignant neoplasm of other respiratory and intrathoracic organs**

Z85.3 **Personal history of malignant neoplasm of** breast
Conditions classifiable to C50.-

✓5th **Z85.4** **Personal history of malignant neoplasm of** genital organs
Conditions classifiable to C51-C63

Z85.40 **Personal history of malignant neoplasm of unspecified female genital organ**   ♀▽

Z85.41 **Personal history of malignant neoplasm of** cervix uteri   ♀

Z85.42 **Personal history of malignant neoplasm of other parts of uterus**   ♀

Z85.43 **Personal history of malignant neoplasm of** ovary   ♀

Z85.44 **Personal history of malignant neoplasm of other female genital organs**   ♀

Z85.45 **Personal history of malignant neoplasm of unspecified male genital organ**   ♂▽

Z85.46 **Personal history of malignant neoplasm of** prostate   ♂

Z85.47 **Personal history of malignant neoplasm of** testis   ♂

Z85.48 **Personal history of malignant neoplasm of epididymis**   ♂

Z85.49 **Personal history of malignant neoplasm of other male genital organs**   ♂

✓5th **Z85.5** **Personal history of malignant neoplasm of** urinary tract
Conditions classifiable to C64-C68

Z85.50 **Personal history of malignant neoplasm of unspecified urinary tract organ**   ▽

Z85.51 **Personal history of malignant neoplasm of** bladder

✓6th **Z85.52** **Personal history of malignant neoplasm of** kidney

EXCLUDES 1 *personal history of malignant neoplasm of renal pelvis (Z85.53)*

Z85.520 **Personal history of malignant** carcinoid **tumor of kidney**
Conditions classifiable to C7A.093

Z85.528 **Personal history of other malignant neoplasm of kidney**
Conditions classifiable to C64

Z85.53 **Personal history of malignant neoplasm of** renal pelvis

Z85.54 **Personal history of malignant neoplasm of** ureter

Z85.59 **Personal history of malignant neoplasm of other urinary tract organ**

Z85.6 **Personal history of** leukemia
Conditions classifiable to C91-C95

EXCLUDES 1 *leukemia in remission C91.0-C95.9 with 5th character 1*

✓5th **Z85.7** **Personal history of other malignant neoplasms of lymphoid, hematopoietic and related tissues**

Z85.71 **Personal history of** Hodgkin lymphoma
Conditions classifiable to C81

Z85.72 **Personal history of** non-Hodgkin lymphomas
Conditions classifiable to C82-C85

Z85.79 **Personal history of other malignant neoplasms of lymphoid, hematopoietic and related tissues**
Conditions classifiable to C88-C90, C96

EXCLUDES 1 *multiple myeloma in remission (C90.01) plasma cell leukemia in remission (C90.11) plasmacytoma in remission (C90.21)*

✓5th **Z85.8** **Personal history of malignant neoplasms of other organs and systems**
Conditions classifiable to C00-C14, C40-C49, C69-C79, C7A.098

✓6th **Z85.81** **Personal history of malignant neoplasm of** lip, oral cavity, and pharynx

Z85.810 **Personal history of malignant neoplasm of** tongue

Z85.818 **Personal history of malignant neoplasm of other sites of** lip, oral cavity, and pharynx

Z85.819 **Personal history of malignant neoplasm of unspecified site of** lip, oral cavity, and pharynx   ▽

✓6th **Z85.82** **Personal history of malignant neoplasm of** skin

Z85.820 **Personal history of malignant** melanoma **of skin**
Conditions classifiable to C43

Z85.821 **Personal history of** Merkel cell carcinoma
Conditions classifiable to C4A

Z85.828 **Personal history of other malignant neoplasm of skin**
Conditions classifiable to C44

N Newborn   P Pediatric   M Maternity   A Adult   RIC RIC Dx   NCDx Noncancer Dx   PDx Primary Dx   CC RIC CC Condition   ▶◀ Revised Text   ● New Code   ▲ Revised Code Title

1142   ICD-10-CM 2016

✓6ᵗʰ **Z85.83** **Personal history of malignant neoplasm of** bone and soft tissue

    Z85.830 **Personal history of malignant neoplasm of** bone

    Z85.831 **Personal history of malignant neoplasm of** soft tissue
        EXCLUDES 2   *personal history of malignant neoplasm of skin (Z85.82-)*

✓6ᵗʰ **Z85.84** **Personal history of malignant neoplasm of** eye and nervous tissue

    Z85.840 **Personal history of malignant neoplasm of** eye

    Z85.841 **Personal history of malignant neoplasm of** brain

    Z85.848 **Personal history of malignant neoplasm of other parts of nervous tissue**

✓6ᵗʰ **Z85.85** **Personal history of malignant neoplasm of** endocrine glands

    Z85.850 **Personal history of malignant neoplasm of thyroid**

    Z85.858 **Personal history of malignant neoplasm of other endocrine glands**

  Z85.89 **Personal history of malignant neoplasm of other organs and systems**

Z85.9 **Personal history of malignant neoplasm, unspecified** ▽
    Conditions classifiable to C7A.00, C80.1

✓4ᵗʰ **Z86** **Personal history of certain other diseases**
    Code first any follow-up examination after treatment (Z09)

✓5ᵗʰ **Z86.0** **Personal history of in-situ and benign neoplasms and neoplasms of uncertain behavior**
    EXCLUDES 2   *personal history of malignant neoplasms (Z85.-)*

✓6ᵗʰ **Z86.00** **Personal history of** in-situ neoplasm

    Z86.000 **Personal history of in-situ neoplasm of breast**

    Z86.001 **Personal history of in-situ neoplasm of** cervix uteri ♀

    Z86.008 **Personal history of in-situ neoplasm of other site**

✓6ᵗʰ **Z86.01** **Personal history of** benign neoplasm

    Z86.010 **Personal history of** colonic polyps

    Z86.011 **Personal history of benign neoplasm of the** brain

    Z86.012 **Personal history of benign** carcinoid tumor

    Z86.018 **Personal history of other benign neoplasm**

  Z86.03 **Personal history of** neoplasm of uncertain behavior

✓5ᵗʰ **Z86.1** **Personal history of** infectious and parasitic diseases
    Conditions classifiable to A00-B89, B99
    EXCLUDES 1   *personal history of infectious diseases specific to a body system*
        sequelae of infectious and parasitic diseases (B90-B94)

  Z86.11 **Personal history of** tuberculosis

  Z86.12 **Personal history of** poliomyelitis

  Z86.13 **Personal history of** malaria

  Z86.14 **Personal history of** Methicillin resistant Staphylococcus aureus **infection**
    Personal history of MRSA infection

  Z86.19 **Personal history of other infectious and parasitic diseases**

  Z86.2 **Personal history of diseases of the** blood and blood-forming organs **and certain disorders involving the** immune mechanism
    Conditions classifiable to D50-D89

✓5ᵗʰ **Z86.3** **Personal history of** endocrine, nutritional and metabolic diseases
    Conditions classifiable to E00-E88

  Z86.31 **Personal history of** diabetic foot ulcer
    EXCLUDES 2   *current diabetic foot ulcer (E08.621, E09.621, E10.621, E11.621, E13.621)*

  Z86.32 **Personal history of** gestational diabetes ♀
    Personal history of conditions classifiable to O24.4-
    EXCLUDES 1   *gestational diabetes mellitus in current pregnancy (O24.4-)*

  Z86.39 **Personal history of other endocrine, nutritional and metabolic disease**

✓5ᵗʰ **Z86.5** **Personal history of** mental and behavioral disorders
    Conditions classifiable to F40-F59

  Z86.51 **Personal history of combat and operational stress reaction** A

  Z86.59 **Personal history of other mental and behavioral disorders**

✓5ᵗʰ **Z86.6** **Personal history of diseases of the** nervous system and sense organs
    Conditions classifiable to G00-G99, H00-H95
    EXCLUDES 2   *personal history of anaphylactic shock (Z87.892)*

  Z86.61 **Personal history of infections of the central nervous system**
    Personal history of encephalitis
    Personal history of meningitis

  Z86.69 **Personal history of other diseases of the nervous system and sense organs**

✓5ᵗʰ **Z86.7** **Personal history of diseases of the** circulatory system
    Conditions classifiable to I00-I99
    EXCLUDES 2   *old myocardial infarction (I25.2)*
        personal history of anaphylactic shock (Z87.892)
        postmyocardial infarction syndrome (I24.1)

✓6ᵗʰ **Z86.71** **Personal history of** venous thrombosis and embolism

    Z86.711 **Personal history of** pulmonary **embolism**

    Z86.718 **Personal history of other venous thrombosis and embolism**

  Z86.72 **Personal history of** thrombophlebitis

  Z86.73 **Personal history of** transient ischemic attack **(TIA), and cerebral infarction without residual deficits**
    Personal history of prolonged reversible ischemic neurological deficit (PRIND)
    Personal history of stroke NOS without residual deficits
    EXCLUDES 1   *personal history of traumatic brain injury (Z87.820)*
        sequelae of cerebrovascular disease (I69.-)
    AHA: 2012, 4Q, 92

  Z86.74 **Personal history of** sudden cardiac arrest
    Personal history of sudden cardiac death successfully resuscitated

  Z86.79 **Personal history of other diseases of the circulatory system**

✓4ᵗʰ **Z87** **Personal history of other diseases and conditions**
    Code first any follow-up examination after treatment (Z09)

✓5ᵗʰ **Z87.0** **Personal history of diseases of the** respiratory system
    Conditions classifiable to J00-J99

  Z87.01 **Personal history of** pneumonia **(recurrent)**

  Z87.09 **Personal history of other diseases of the respiratory system**

✓5ᵗʰ **Z87.1** **Personal history of diseases of the** digestive system
    Conditions classifiable to K00-K93

  Z87.11 **Personal history of** peptic ulcer **disease**

  Z87.19 **Personal history of other diseases of the digestive system**

  Z87.2 **Personal history of diseases of the** skin and subcutaneous tissue
    Conditions classifiable to L00-L99
    EXCLUDES 2   *personal history of diabetic foot ulcer (Z86.31)*

✓5ᵗʰ **Z87.3** **Personal history of diseases of the** musculoskeletal system and connective tissue
    Conditions classifiable to M00-M99
    EXCLUDES 2   *personal history of (healed) traumatic fracture (Z87.81)*

✓6ᵗʰ **Z87.31** **Personal history of (healed)** nontraumatic fracture

    Z87.310 **Personal history of (healed)** osteoporosis **fracture**
        Personal history of (healed) fragility fracture
        Personal history of (healed) collapsed vertebra due to osteoporosis

    Z87.311 **Personal history of (healed) other pathological fracture**
        Personal history of (healed) collapsed vertebra NOS
        EXCLUDES 2   *personal history of osteoporosis fracture (Z87.310)*

    Z87.312 **Personal history of (healed)** stress fracture
        Personal history of (healed) fatigue fracture

  Z87.39 **Personal history of other diseases of the musculoskeletal system and connective tissue**

✅ Add'l Character Required   ✓7ᵗʰ Placeholder Alert   RUG IV Special Care High Dx   RUG IV Clinically Complex Dx   RUG IV Special Care Low Dx   Manifestation Code   Other Specified Code   ▽ Unspecified Code

✓5ᵗʰ **Z87.4 Personal history of diseases of** genitourinary system
Conditions classifiable to N00-N99

✓6ᵗʰ **Z87.41 Personal history of** dysplasia of the female genital tract
    EXCLUDES 1 *personal history of malignant neoplasm of female genital tract (Z85.40-Z85.44)*

    Z87.410 Personal history of cervical **dysplasia** ♀
    Z87.411 Personal history of vaginal **dysplasia** ♀
    Z87.412 Personal history of vulvar **dysplasia** ♀

   Z87.42 Personal history of other diseases of the female genital tract ♀

✓6ᵗʰ **Z87.43 Personal history of diseases of the** male genital organs
    Z87.430 Personal history of prostatic dysplasia ♂
      EXCLUDES 1 *personal history of malignant neoplasm of prostate (Z85.46)*

    Z87.438 Personal history of other diseases of male **genital organs** ♂

✓6ᵗʰ **Z87.44 Personal history of diseases of the** urinary system
    EXCLUDES 1 *personal history of malignant neoplasm of cervix uteri (Z85.41)*

    Z87.440 Personal history of urinary (tract) infections
    Z87.441 Personal history of nephrotic syndrome
    Z87.442 Personal history of urinary calculi
      Personal history of kidney stones
    Z87.448 Personal history of other diseases of urinary system

✓5ᵗʰ **Z87.5 Personal history of complications of** pregnancy, childbirth and the puerperium
Conditions classifiable to O00-O9A
    EXCLUDES 2 *recurrent pregnancy loss (N96)*

   Z87.51 Personal history of pre-term labor Ⓜ♀
    EXCLUDES 1 *current pregnancy with history of pre-term labor (O09.21-)*

   Z87.59 Personal history of other complications of pregnancy, childbirth and the puerperium ♀
    Personal history of trophoblastic disease

✓5ᵗʰ **Z87.7 Personal history of (corrected)** congenital malformations
Conditions classifiable to Q00-Q89 that have been repaired or corrected
    EXCLUDES 1 *congenital malformations that have been partially corrected or repaired but which still require medical treatment—code to condition*
    EXCLUDES 2 *other postprocedural states (Z98.-)*
      personal history of medical treatment (Z92.-)
      presence of cardiac and vascular implants and grafts (Z95.-)
      presence of other devices (Z97.-)
      presence of other functional implants (Z96.-)
      transplanted organ and tissue status (Z94.-)

✓6ᵗʰ **Z87.71 Personal history of (corrected) congenital malformations of** genitourinary system
    Z87.710 Personal history of (corrected) hypospadias ♂
    Z87.718 Personal history of other specified (corrected) congenital malformations of genitourinary system

✓6ᵗʰ **Z87.72 Personal history of (corrected) congenital malformations of** nervous system and sense organs
    Z87.720 Personal history of (corrected) congenital malformations of eye
    Z87.721 Personal history of (corrected) congenital malformations of ear
    Z87.728 Personal history of other specified (corrected) congenital malformations of nervous system and sense organs

✓6ᵗʰ **Z87.73 Personal history of (corrected) congenital malformations of** digestive system
    Z87.730 Personal history of (corrected) cleft lip and palate
    Z87.738 Personal history of other specified (corrected) congenital malformations of digestive system

Z87.74 Personal history of (corrected) congenital malformations of heart and circulatory system

Z87.75 Personal history of (corrected) congenital malformations of respiratory system

Z87.76 Personal history of (corrected) congenital malformations of integument, limbs and musculoskeletal system

✓6ᵗʰ **Z87.79 Personal history of** other (corrected) congenital malformations
    Z87.790 Personal history of (corrected) congenital malformations of face and neck
    Z87.798 Personal history of other (corrected) congenital malformations

✓5ᵗʰ **Z87.8 Personal history of other specified conditions**
    EXCLUDES 2 *personal history of self harm (Z91.5)*

   Z87.81 Personal history of (healed) traumatic fracture
    EXCLUDES 2 *personal history of (healed) nontraumatic fracture (Z87.31-)*

✓6ᵗʰ **Z87.82 Personal history of other (healed)** physical injury and trauma
    Conditions classifiable to S00-T88, except traumatic fractures
    Z87.820 Personal history of traumatic brain injury
      EXCLUDES 1 *personal history of transient ischemic attack (TIA), and cerebral infarction without residual deficits (Z86.73)*

    Z87.821 Personal history of retained foreign body fully removed
    Z87.828 Personal history of other (healed) physical injury and trauma

✓6ᵗʰ **Z87.89 Personal history of** other **specified conditions**
    Z87.890 Personal history of sex reassignment
    Z87.891 Personal history of nicotine dependence
      EXCLUDES 1 *current nicotine dependence (F17.2-)*

    Z87.892 Personal history of anaphylaxis
      Code also allergy status such as:
       allergy status to drugs, medicaments and biological substances (Z88.-)
       allergy status, other than to drugs and biological substances (Z91.0-)

    Z87.898 Personal history of other specified conditions
      AHA: 2013, 1Q, 21

✓4ᵗʰ **Z88 Allergy status to drugs, medicaments and biological substances**
    EXCLUDES 2 *allergy status, other than to drugs and biological substances (Z91.0-)*

   Z88.0 Allergy status to penicillin
   Z88.1 Allergy status to other antibiotic **agents status**
   Z88.2 Allergy status to sulfonamides **status**
   Z88.3 Allergy status to other anti-infective **agents status**
   Z88.4 Allergy status to anesthetic **agent status**
   Z88.5 Allergy status to narcotic **agent status**
   Z88.6 Allergy status to analgesic **agent status**
   Z88.7 Allergy status to serum and vaccine **status**
   Z88.8 Allergy status to other drugs, medicaments and biological substances status
   Z88.9 Allergy status to unspecified drugs, medicaments and biological substances status ▽

✓4ᵗʰ **Z89 Acquired absence of limb**
    INCLUDES amputation status
      postprocedural loss of limb
      post-traumatic loss of limb
    EXCLUDES 1 *acquired deformities of limbs (M20-M21)*
      congenital absence of limbs (Q71-Q73)

✓5ᵗʰ **Z89.0 Acquired absence of** thumb and other finger(s)

✓6ᵗʰ **Z89.01 Acquired absence of** thumb
    Z89.011 Acquired absence of right **thumb**
    Z89.012 Acquired absence of left **thumb**
    Z89.019 Acquired absence of unspecified thumb ▽

✓6ᵗʰ **Z89.02** **Acquired absence of** other finger(s)
     EXCLUDES 2   *acquired absence of thumb (Z89.01-)*
     Z89.021 **Acquired absence of** right finger(s)
     Z89.022 **Acquired absence of** left finger(s)
     Z89.029 **Acquired absence of unspecified** ▽
             finger(s)

✓5ᵗʰ **Z89.1** **Acquired absence of** hand and wrist
     ✓6ᵗʰ **Z89.11** **Acquired absence of** hand
         Z89.111 **Acquired absence of** right hand
         Z89.112 **Acquired absence of** left hand
         Z89.119 **Acquired absence of unspecified hand** ▽
     ✓6ᵗʰ **Z89.12** **Acquired absence of** wrist
         Disarticulation at wrist
         Z89.121 **Acquired absence of** right wrist
         Z89.122 **Acquired absence of** left wrist
         Z89.129 **Acquired absence of unspecified wrist** ▽

✓5ᵗʰ **Z89.2** **Acquired absence of** upper limb above wrist
     ✓6ᵗʰ **Z89.20** **Acquired absence of** upper limb, unspecified level
         Z89.201 **Acquired absence of** right upper limb, ▽
               unspecified level
         Z89.202 **Acquired absence of** left upper limb, ▽
               unspecified level
         Z89.209 **Acquired absence of unspecified upper** ▽
               limb, unspecified level
               Acquired absence of arm NOS
     ✓6ᵗʰ **Z89.21** **Acquired absence of** upper limb below elbow
         Z89.211 **Acquired absence of** right upper limb
               below elbow
         Z89.212 **Acquired absence of** left upper limb below
               elbow
         Z89.219 **Acquired absence of unspecified upper** ▽
               limb below elbow
     ✓6ᵗʰ **Z89.22** **Acquired absence of** upper limb above elbow
         Disarticulation at elbow
         Z89.221 **Acquired absence of** right upper limb
               above elbow
         Z89.222 **Acquired absence of** left upper limb above
               elbow
         Z89.229 **Acquired absence of unspecified upper** ▽
               limb above elbow
     ✓6ᵗʰ **Z89.23** **Acquired absence of** shoulder
         Acquired absence of shoulder joint following
             explantation of shoulder joint prosthesis, with or
             without presence of antibiotic-impregnated
             cement spacer
         Z89.231 **Acquired absence of** right shoulder
         Z89.232 **Acquired absence of** left shoulder
         Z89.239 **Acquired absence of unspecified** ▽
               shoulder

✓5ᵗʰ **Z89.4** **Acquired absence of** toe(s), foot, and ankle
     ✓6ᵗʰ **Z89.41** **Acquired absence of** great toe
         Z89.411 **Acquired absence of** right great toe
         Z89.412 **Acquired absence of** left great toe
         Z89.419 **Acquired absence of unspecified great** ▽
               toe
     ✓6ᵗʰ **Z89.42** **Acquired absence of** other toe(s)
         EXCLUDES 2   *acquired absence of great toe (Z89.41-)*
         Z89.421 **Acquired absence of** other right toe(s)
         Z89.422 **Acquired absence of** other left toe(s)
         Z89.429 **Acquired absence of** other toe(s), ▽
               unspecified side
     ✓6ᵗʰ **Z89.43** **Acquired absence of** foot
         Z89.431 **Acquired absence of** right foot
         Z89.432 **Acquired absence of** left foot
         Z89.439 **Acquired absence of unspecified foot** ▽
     ✓6ᵗʰ **Z89.44** **Acquired absence of** ankle
         Disarticulation of ankle
         Z89.441 **Acquired absence of** right ankle
         Z89.442 **Acquired absence of** left ankle
         Z89.449 **Acquired absence of unspecified ankle** ▽

✓5ᵗʰ **Z89.5** **Acquired absence of** leg below knee
     ✓6ᵗʰ **Z89.51** **Acquired absence of** leg below knee
         Z89.511 **Acquired absence of** right leg below knee
         Z89.512 **Acquired absence of** left leg below knee
         Z89.519 **Acquired absence of unspecified leg** ▽
               below knee
     ✓6ᵗʰ **Z89.52** **Acquired absence of** knee
         Acquired absence of knee joint following explantation
             of knee joint prosthesis, with or without presence
             of antibiotic-impregnated cement spacer
         Z89.521 **Acquired absence of** right knee
         Z89.522 **Acquired absence of** left knee
         Z89.529 **Acquired absence of unspecified knee** ▽

✓5ᵗʰ **Z89.6** **Acquired absence of** leg above knee
     ✓6ᵗʰ **Z89.61** **Acquired absence of** leg above knee
         Acquired absence of leg NOS
         Disarticulation at knee
         Z89.611 **Acquired absence of** right leg above knee
         Z89.612 **Acquired absence of** left leg above knee
         Z89.619 **Acquired absence of unspecified leg** ▽
               above knee
     ✓6ᵗʰ **Z89.62** **Acquired absence of** hip
         Acquired absence of hip joint following explantation
             of hip joint prosthesis, with or without presence
             of antibiotic-impregnated cement spacer
         Disarticulation at hip
         Z89.621 **Acquired absence of** right hip joint
         Z89.622 **Acquired absence of** left hip joint
         Z89.629 **Acquired absence of unspecified hip** ▽
               joint
     Z89.9 **Acquired absence of limb, unspecified** ▽

✓4ᵗʰ **Z90** **Acquired absence of organs, not elsewhere classified**
     INCLUDES   postprocedural or post-traumatic loss of body part NEC
     EXCLUDES 1   *congenital absence—see Alphabetical Index*
     EXCLUDES 2   *postprocedural absence of endocrine glands (E89.-)*
     ✓5ᵗʰ **Z90.0** **Acquired absence of** part of head and neck
         Z90.01 **Acquired absence of** eye
         Z90.02 **Acquired absence of** larynx
         Z90.09 **Acquired absence of other part of head and neck**
             Acquired absence of nose
             EXCLUDES 2   *teeth (K08.1)*
     ✓5ᵗʰ **Z90.1** **Acquired absence of** breast and nipple
         Z90.10 **Acquired absence of unspecified breast and** ▽
             nipple
         Z90.11 **Acquired absence of** right breast and nipple
         Z90.12 **Acquired absence of** left breast and nipple
         Z90.13 **Acquired absence of** bilateral breasts and nipples
     Z90.2 **Acquired absence of** lung [part of]
     Z90.3 **Acquired absence of** stomach [part of]
     ✓5ᵗʰ **Z90.4** **Acquired absence of** other specified parts of digestive tract
         ✓6ᵗʰ **Z90.41** **Acquired absence of** pancreas
             Use additional code to identify any associated:
               insulin use (Z79.4)
               diabetes mellitus, postpancreatectomy (E13.-)
             Z90.410 **Acquired total absence of pancreas**
                Acquired absence of pancreas NOS
             Z90.411 **Acquired partial absence of pancreas**
         Z90.49 **Acquired absence of other specified parts of**
             digestive tract
     Z90.5 **Acquired absence of** kidney
     Z90.6 **Acquired absence of other** parts of urinary tract
         Acquired absence of bladder
     ✓5ᵗʰ **Z90.7** **Acquired absence of** genital organ(s)
         EXCLUDES 1   *personal history of sex reassignment (Z87.890)*
         EXCLUDES 2   *female genital mutilation status (N90.81-)*
         ✓6ᵗʰ **Z90.71** **Acquired absence of** cervix and uterus
             Z90.710 **Acquired absence of** both cervix and ♀
                uterus
                   Acquired absence of uterus NOS
                   Status post total hysterectomy
             Z90.711 **Acquired absence of uterus with** ♀
                remaining cervical stump
                   Status post partial hysterectomy with
                   remaining cervical stump

Chapter 21. Factors Influencing Health Status and Contact With Health Services

Z89.02–Z90.711

Chapter 21. Factors Influencing Health Status and Contact With Health Services

Z90.712 Acquired absence of cervix with remaining uterus ♀

☑6th **Z90.72** Acquired absence of **ovaries**

Z90.721 Acquired absence of ovaries, **unilateral** ♀

Z90.722 Acquired absence of ovaries, **bilateral** ♀

Z90.79 Acquired absence of other genital organ(s)

☑5th **Z90.8** Acquired absence of **other** organs

Z90.81 Acquired absence of **spleen**

Z90.89 Acquired absence of other organs

☑4th **Z91 Personal risk factors, not elsewhere classified**

     EXCLUDES 2 *contact with and (suspected) exposures hazardous to health (Z77.-)*
         exposure to pollution and other problems related to physical environment (Z77.1-)
         personal history of physical injury and trauma (Z87.81, Z87.82-)
         occupational exposure to risk factors (Z57.-)

☑5th **Z91.0 Allergy status, other than to drugs and biological substances**

     EXCLUDES 2 *allergy status to drugs, medicaments, and biological substances (Z88.-)*

☑6th **Z91.01** Food allergy status

     EXCLUDES 2 *food additives allergy status (Z91.02)*

Z91.010 **Allergy to peanuts**

Z91.011 **Allergy to milk products**
     EXCLUDES 1 *lactose intolerance (E73.-)*

Z91.012 **Allergy to eggs**

Z91.013 **Allergy to seafood**
     Allergy to shellfish
     Allergy to octopus or squid ink

Z91.018 **Allergy to other foods**
     Allergy to nuts other than peanuts

Z91.02 Food additives allergy status

☑6th **Z91.03** **Insect** allergy status

Z91.030 **Bee** allergy status

Z91.038 **Other insect** allergy status

☑6th **Z91.04** Nonmedicinal substance allergy status

Z91.040 **Latex** allergy status
     Latex sensitivity status

Z91.041 **Radiographic dye** allergy status
     Allergy status to contrast media used for diagnostic X-ray procedure

Z91.048 **Other nonmedicinal substance allergy status**

Z91.09 **Other allergy status, other than to drugs and biological substances**

☑5th **Z91.1** Patient's noncompliance with medical treatment and regimen

Z91.11 Patient's noncompliance with **dietary regimen**

☑6th **Z91.12** Patient's **intentional underdosing of medication regimen**
     Code first underdosing of medication (T36-T50) with fifth or sixth character 6
     EXCLUDES 1 *adverse effect of prescribed drug taken as directed—code to adverse effect*
         poisoning (overdose)—code to poisoning

Z91.120 **Patient's intentional underdosing of medication regimen due to financial hardship**

Z91.128 **Patient's intentional underdosing of medication regimen for other reason**

☑6th **Z91.13** Patient's **unintentional underdosing of medication regimen**
     Code first underdosing of medication (T36-T50) with fifth or sixth character 6
     EXCLUDES 1 *adverse effect of prescribed drug taken as directed—code to adverse effect*
         poisoning (overdose)—code to poisoning

Z91.130 **Patient's unintentional underdosing of medication regimen due to age-related debility**

Z91.138 **Patient's unintentional underdosing of medication regimen for other reason**

Z91.14 Patient's **other noncompliance with medication regimen**
     Patient's underdosing of medication NOS

Z91.15 Patient's noncompliance with **renal dialysis**

Z91.19 Patient's noncompliance with other medical treatment and regimen

☑5th **Z91.4** Personal history of psychological trauma, not elsewhere classified

☑6th **Z91.41** **Personal history of adult abuse**
     EXCLUDES 2 *personal history of abuse in childhood (Z62.81-)*

Z91.410 **Personal history of adult physical and sexual abuse** 🅰
     EXCLUDES 1 *current adult physical abuse (T74.11, T76.11)*
         current adult sexual abuse (T74.21, T76.11)

Z91.411 **Personal history of adult psychological abuse** 🅰

Z91.412 **Personal history of adult neglect** 🅰
     EXCLUDES 1 *current adult neglect (T74.01, T76.01)*

Z91.419 **Personal history of unspecified adult abuse** 🅰▽

Z91.49 **Other personal history of psychological trauma, not elsewhere classified**

Z91.5 Personal history of self-harm
     Personal history of parasuicide
     Personal history of self-poisoning
     Personal history of suicide attempt

☑5th **Z91.8** Other specified personal risk factors, not elsewhere classified

Z91.81 **History of falling**
     At risk for falling

Z91.82 Personal history of military deployment
     Individual (civilian or military) with past history of military war, peacekeeping and humanitarian deployment (current or past conflict)
     Returned from military deployment

Z91.83 *Wandering in diseases classified elsewhere*
     Code first underlying disorder such as:
     Alzheimer's disease (G30.-)
     autism or pervasive developmental disorder (F84.-)
     intellectual disabilities (F70-F79)
     unspecified dementia with behavioral disturbance (F03.9-)

Z91.89 **Other specified personal risk factors, not elsewhere classified**

☑4th **Z92 Personal history of medical treatment**
     EXCLUDES 2 *postprocedural states (Z98.-)*

Z92.0 Personal history of **contraception**
     EXCLUDES 1 *counseling or management of current contraceptive practices (Z30.-)*
         long term (current) use of contraception (Z79.3)
         presence of (intrauterine) contraceptive device (Z97.5)

☑5th **Z92.2** Personal history of **drug therapy**
     EXCLUDES 2 *long term (current) drug therapy (Z79.-)*

Z92.21 Personal history of **antineoplastic chemotherapy**

Z92.22 Personal history of **monoclonal drug therapy**

Z92.23 Personal history of **estrogen therapy**

☑6th **Z92.24** Personal history of **steroid therapy**

Z92.240 **Personal history of inhaled steroid therapy**

Z92.241 **Personal history of systemic steroid therapy**
     Personal history of steroid therapy NOS

Z92.25 Personal history of **immunosupression therapy**
     EXCLUDES 2 *personal history of steroid therapy (Z92.24)*

Z92.29 **Personal history of other drug therapy**

Z92.3 Personal history of **irradiation**
     Personal history of exposure to therapeutic radiation
     EXCLUDES 1 *exposure to radiation in the physical environment (Z77.12)*
         occupational exposure to radiation (Z57.1)

☑5th **Z92.8** Personal history of other medical treatment

Z92.81 Personal history of extracorporeal membrane oxygenation (ECMO)

Z92.82 Status post administration of tPA (rtPA) in a different facility within the last 24 hours prior to admission to current facility
     Code first condition requiring tPA administration, such as:
     acute cerebral infarction (I63.-)
     acute myocardial infarction (I21-, I22-)
     AHA: 2013, 4Q, 124

Ⓝ Newborn   Ⓟ Pediatric   Ⓜ Maternity   🅰 Adult   **RIC** RIC Dx   **NC Dx** Noncancer Dx   **PDx** Primary Dx   **CC** RIC CC Condition   ▶◀ Revised Text   ● New Code   ▲ Revised Code Title

1146   ICD-10-CM 2016

Z92.83   **Personal history of failed moderate sedation**
Personal history of failed conscious sedation
EXCLUDES 2   *failed moderate sedation during procedure (T88.52)*

Z92.89   **Personal history of other medical treatment**

✓4ᵗʰ **Z93   Artificial opening status**
EXCLUDES 1   *artificial openings requiring attention or management (Z43.-)*
complications of external stoma (J95.0-, K94.-, N99.5-)

Z93.0   **Tracheostomy status**   CC
AHA: 2013, 4Q, 129

Z93.1   **Gastrostomy status**

Z93.2   **Ileostomy status**

Z93.3   **Colostomy status**

Z93.4   **Other artificial openings of gastrointestinal tract status**

✓5ᵗʰ Z93.5   **Cystostomy status**

Z93.50   **Unspecified cystostomy status**   ▽

Z93.51   **Cutaneous-vesicostomy status**

Z93.52   **Appendico-vesicostomy status**

Z93.59   **Other cystostomy status**

Z93.6   **Other artificial openings of urinary tract status**
Nephrostomy status
Ureterostomy status
Urethrostomy status

Z93.8   **Other artificial opening status**

Z93.9   **Artificial opening status, unspecified**   ▽

✓4ᵗʰ **Z94   Transplanted organ and tissue status**
INCLUDES   organ or tissue replaced by heterogenous or homogenous transplant
EXCLUDES 1   *complications of transplanted organ or tissue—see Alphabetical Index*
EXCLUDES 2   *presence of vascular grafts (Z95.-)*

Z94.0   **Kidney transplant status**

Z94.1   **Heart transplant status**
EXCLUDES 1   *artificial heart status (Z95.812)*
heart-valve replacement status (Z95.2-Z95.4)

Z94.2   **Lung transplant status**

Z94.3   **Heart and lungs transplant status**

Z94.4   **Liver transplant status**

Z94.5   **Skin transplant status**
Autogenous skin transplant status

Z94.6   **Bone transplant status**

Z94.7   **Corneal transplant status**

✓5ᵗʰ Z94.8   **Other transplanted organ and tissue status**

Z94.81   **Bone marrow transplant status**

Z94.82   **Intestine transplant status**

Z94.83   **Pancreas transplant status**

Z94.84   **Stem cells transplant status**

Z94.89   **Other transplanted organ and tissue status**

Z94.9   **Transplanted organ and tissue status, unspecified**   ▽

✓4ᵗʰ **Z95   Presence of cardiac and vascular implants and grafts**
EXCLUDES 1   *complications of cardiac and vascular devices, implants and grafts (T82.-)*

Z95.0   **Presence of cardiac pacemaker**
EXCLUDES 1   *adjustment or management of cardiac pacemaker (Z45.0)*
presence of automatic (implantable) cardiac defibrillator with synchronous cardiac pacemaker (Z95.810)

Z95.1   **Presence of aortocoronary bypass graft**

Z95.2   **Presence of prosthetic heart valve**
Presence of heart valve NOS

Z95.3   **Presence of xenogenic heart valve**

Z95.4   **Presence of other heart-valve replacement**

Z95.5   **Presence of coronary angioplasty implant and graft**
EXCLUDES 1   *coronary angioplasty status without implant and graft (Z98.61)*

✓5ᵗʰ Z95.8   **Presence of other cardiac and vascular implants and grafts**

✓6ᵗʰ Z95.81   **Presence of other cardiac implants and grafts**

Z95.810   **Presence of automatic (implantable) cardiac defibrillator**
Presence of automatic (implantable) cardiac defibrillator with synchronous cardiac pacemaker

Z95.811   **Presence of heart assist device**

Z95.812   **Presence of fully implantable artificial heart**

Z95.818   **Presence of other cardiac implants and grafts**

✓6ᵗʰ Z95.82   **Presence of other vascular implants and grafts**

Z95.820   **Peripheral vascular angioplasty status with implants and grafts**
EXCLUDES 1   *peripheral vascular angioplasty without implant and graft (Z98.62)*

Z95.828   **Presence of other vascular implants and grafts**
Presence of intravascular prosthesis NEC

Z95.9   **Presence of cardiac and vascular implant and graft, unspecified**   ▽

✓4ᵗʰ **Z96   Presence of other functional implants**
EXCLUDES 2   *complications of internal prosthetic devices, implants and grafts (T82-T85)*
fitting and adjustment of prosthetic and other devices (Z44-Z46)

Z96.0   **Presence of urogenital implants**

Z96.1   **Presence of intraocular lens**
Presence of pseudophakia

✓5ᵗʰ Z96.2   **Presence of otological and audiological implants**

Z96.20   **Presence of otological and audiological implant, unspecified**   ▽

Z96.21   **Cochlear implant status**

Z96.22   **Myringotomy tube(s) status**

Z96.29   **Presence of other otological and audiological implants**
Presence of bone-conduction hearing device
Presence of eustachian tube stent
Stapes replacement

Z96.3   **Presence of artificial larynx**

✓5ᵗʰ Z96.4   **Presence of endocrine implants**

Z96.41   **Presence of insulin pump (external) (internal)**

Z96.49   **Presence of other endocrine implants**

Z96.5   **Presence of tooth-root and mandibular implants**

✓5ᵗʰ Z96.6   **Presence of orthopedic joint implants**

Z96.60   **Presence of unspecified orthopedic joint implant**   ▽

✓6ᵗʰ Z96.61   **Presence of artificial shoulder joint**

Z96.611   **Presence of right artificial shoulder joint**

Z96.612   **Presence of left artificial shoulder joint**

Z96.619   **Presence of unspecified artificial shoulder joint**   ▽

✓6ᵗʰ Z96.62   **Presence of artificial elbow joint**

Z96.621   **Presence of right artificial elbow joint**

Z96.622   **Presence of left artificial elbow joint**

Z96.629   **Presence of unspecified artificial elbow joint**   ▽

✓6ᵗʰ Z96.63   **Presence of artificial wrist joint**

Z96.631   **Presence of right artificial wrist joint**

Z96.632   **Presence of left artificial wrist joint**

Z96.639   **Presence of unspecified artificial wrist joint**   ▽

✓6ᵗʰ Z96.64   **Presence of artificial hip joint**
Hip-joint replacement (partial) (total)

Z96.641   **Presence of right artificial hip joint**

Z96.642   **Presence of left artificial hip joint**

Z96.643   **Presence of artificial hip joint, bilateral**

Z96.649   **Presence of unspecified artificial hip joint**   ▽

✓6ᵗʰ Z96.65   **Presence of artificial knee joint**

Z96.651   **Presence of right artificial knee joint**

Z96.652   **Presence of left artificial knee joint**

Z96.653   **Presence of artificial knee joint, bilateral**

Z96.659   **Presence of unspecified artificial knee joint**   ▽

☑ Add'l Character Required   ✓x7ᵗʰ Placeholder Alert   RUG IV Special Care High Dx   RUG IV Clinically Complex Dx   RUG IV Special Care Low Dx   Manifestation Code   Other Specified Code   ▽ Unspecified Code

CD-10-CM 2016

1147

Chapter 21. Factors Influencing Health Status and Contact With Health Services

Z92.83–Z96.659

☑6ᵗʰ **Z96.66** Presence of artificial ankle joint
    Z96.661 Presence of right artificial ankle joint
    Z96.662 Presence of left artificial ankle joint
    Z96.669 Presence of unspecified artificial ankle joint ▽

☑6ᵗʰ **Z96.69** Presence of other orthopedic joint implants
    Z96.691 Finger-joint replacement of right hand
    Z96.692 Finger-joint replacement of left hand
    Z96.693 Finger-joint replacement, bilateral
    Z96.698 Presence of other orthopedic joint implants

Z96.7 Presence of other bone and tendon implants
    Presence of skull plate

☑5ᵗʰ **Z96.8** Presence of other specified functional implants
    Z96.81 Presence of artificial skin
    Z96.89 Presence of other specified functional implants

Z96.9 Presence of functional implant, unspecified ▽

☑4ᵗʰ **Z97** **Presence of other devices**
    EXCLUDES 1 complications of internal prosthetic devices, implants and grafts (T82-T85)
    fitting and adjustment of prosthetic and other devices (Z44-Z46)
    EXCLUDES 2 presence of cerebrospinal fluid drainage device (Z98.2)

Z97.0 Presence of artificial eye

☑5ᵗʰ **Z97.1** Presence of artificial limb (complete) (partial)
    Z97.10 Presence of artificial limb (complete) (partial), unspecified ▽
    Z97.11 Presence of artificial right arm (complete) (partial)
    Z97.12 Presence of artificial left arm (complete) (partial)
    Z97.13 Presence of artificial right leg (complete) (partial)
    Z97.14 Presence of artificial left leg (complete) (partial)
    Z97.15 Presence of artificial arms, bilateral (complete) (partial)
    Z97.16 Presence of artificial legs, bilateral (complete) (partial)

Z97.2 Presence of dental prosthetic device (complete) (partial)
    Presence of dentures (complete) (partial)

Z97.3 Presence of spectacles and contact lenses

Z97.4 Presence of external hearing-aid

Z97.5 Presence of (intrauterine) contraceptive device Ⓜ♀
    EXCLUDES 1 checking, reinsertion or removal of contraceptive device (Z30.43)

Z97.8 Presence of other specified devices

☑4ᵗʰ **Z98** **Other postprocedural states**
    EXCLUDES 2 aftercare (Z43-Z49, Z51)
    follow-up medical care (Z08- Z09)
    postprocedural complication—see Alphabetical Index

Z98.0 Intestinal bypass and anastomosis status
    EXCLUDES 2 bariatric surgery status (Z98.84)
    gastric bypass status (Z98.84)
    obesity surgery status (Z98.84)

Z98.1 Arthrodesis status

Z98.2 Presence of cerebrospinal fluid drainage device
    Presence of CSF shunt

Z98.3 Post therapeutic collapse of lung status
    Code first underlying disease

☑5ᵗʰ **Z98.4** Cataract extraction status
    Use additional code to identify intraocular lens implant status (Z96.1)
    EXCLUDES 1 aphakia (H27.0)
    Z98.41 Cataract extraction status, right eye
    Z98.42 Cataract extraction status, left eye
    Z98.49 Cataract extraction status, unspecified eye ▽

☑5ᵗʰ **Z98.5** Sterilization status
    EXCLUDES 1 female infertility (N97.-)
    male infertility (N46.-)
    Z98.51 Tubal ligation status ♀
    Z98.52 Vasectomy status Ⓐ♂

☑5ᵗʰ **Z98.6** Angioplasty status
    Z98.61 Coronary angioplasty status
        EXCLUDES 1 coronary angioplasty status with implant and graft (Z95.5)
    Z98.62 Peripheral vascular angioplasty status
        EXCLUDES 1 peripheral vascular angioplasty status with implant and graft (Z95.820)

☑5ᵗʰ **Z98.8** Other specified postprocedural states
    ☑6ᵗʰ **Z98.81** Dental procedure status
        Z98.810 Dental sealant status
        Z98.811 Dental restoration status
            Dental crown status
            Dental fillings status
        Z98.818 Other dental procedure status
    Z98.82 Breast implant status
        EXCLUDES 1 breast implant removal status (Z98.86)
    Z98.83 Filtering (vitreous) bleb after glaucoma surgery status
        EXCLUDES 1 inflammation (infection) of postprocedural bleb (H59.4-)
    Z98.84 Bariatric surgery status
        Gastric banding status
        Gastric bypass status for obesity
        Obesity surgery status
        EXCLUDES 1 bariatric surgery status complicating pregnancy, childbirth, or the puerperium (O99.84)
        EXCLUDES 2 intestinal bypass and anastomosis status (Z98.0)
    Z98.85 Transplanted organ removal status
        Transplanted organ previously removed due to complication, failure, rejection or infection
        EXCLUDES 1 encounter for removal of transplanted organ—code to complication of transplanted organ (T86.-)
    Z98.86 Personal history of breast implant removal
    ☑6ᵗʰ **Z98.87** Personal history of in utero procedure
        Z98.870 Personal history of in utero procedure during pregnancy ♀
            EXCLUDES 2 complications from in utero procedure for current pregnancy (O35.7)
                supervision of current pregnancy with history of in utero procedure during previous pregnancy (O09.82-)
        Z98.871 Personal history of in utero procedure while a fetus
    Z98.89 Other specified postprocedural states
        Personal history of surgery, not elsewhere classified

☑4ᵗʰ **Z99** **Dependence on enabling machines and devices, not elsewhere classified**
    EXCLUDES 1 cardiac pacemaker status (Z95.0)

Z99.0 Dependence on aspirator

☑5ᵗʰ **Z99.1** Dependence on respirator
    Dependence on ventilator
    Z99.11 Dependence on respirator [ventilator] status
        AHA: 2015, 1Q, 21
    Z99.12 Encounter for respirator [ventilator] dependence during power failure PDx
        EXCLUDES 1 mechanical complication of respirator [ventilator] (J95.850)

Z99.2 Dependence on renal dialysis CC
    Hemodialysis status
    Peritoneal dialysis status
    Presence of arteriovenous shunt for dialysis
    Renal dialysis status NOS
    EXCLUDES 1 encounter for fitting and adjustment of dialysis catheter (Z49.0-)
    noncompliance with renal dialysis (Z91.15)
    AHA: 2013, 4Q, 125

Z99.3 Dependence on wheelchair
    Wheelchair confinement status
    Code first cause of dependence, such as:
        muscular dystrophy (G71.0)
        obesity (E66.-)

Ⓝ Newborn   Ⓟ Pediatric   Ⓜ Maternity   Ⓐ Adult   **RIC** RIC Dx   **NCDx** Noncancer Dx   **PDx** Primary Dx   **CC** RIC CC Condition   ▶◀ Revised Text   ● New Code   ▲ Revised Code Title

1148   ICD-10-CM 2016

✓5ᵗʰ **Z99.8** **Dependence on other enabling machines and devices**

    Z99.81 **Dependence on** supplemental oxygen
         Dependence on long-term oxygen
         AHA: 2013, 4Q, 129

    Z99.89 **Dependence on other enabling machines and devices**
         Dependence on machine or device NOS

Appendixes

Appendix A: 10 Steps to Correct Coding

Follow the 10 steps below to correctly code encounters for health care services.

Step 1: Identify the reason for the visit or encounter (i.e., a sign, symptom, diagnosis and/or condition).

The medical record documentation should accurately reflect the patient's condition, using terminology that includes specific diagnoses and symptoms or clearly states the reasons for the encounter.

Choosing the main term that best describes the reason chiefly responsible for the service provided is the most important step in coding. If symptoms are present and documented but a definitive diagnosis has not yet been determined, code the symptoms. **For outpatient cases, do not code conditions that are referred to as "rule out," "suspected," "probable," or "questionable."** Diagnoses often are not established at the time of the initial encounter/visit and may require two or more visits to be established. Code only what is documented in the available records and only to the highest degree of certainty known at the time of the patient's visit, unless it is an inpatient medical record, in which case uncertain diagnoses may be reported if documented at the time of discharge.

Step 2: After selecting the reason for the encounter, always consult the alphabetic index before verifying code selection in the tabular section.

The most critical rule is to begin code selection in the *alphabetic index*. Never turn first to the tabular list. The index provides cross-references, essential and nonessential modifiers, and inclusion terms not found in the tabular list. To prevent coding errors, always use both the alphabetic index (to identify a code) and the tabular list (to verify a code), as the index does not include the important instructional notes found in the tabular list. An added benefit of using the tabular list, which groups like things together, is that while looking at one code in the list, a coder might see a more specific one that would have been missed had the coder relied solely on the alphabetic index. Additionally, many of the codes require a fourth, fifth, sixth, or seventh, character to be valid, and many of these characters can be found only in the tabular list.

Step 3: Locate the main term entry.

The alphabetic index is a listing of conditions, which may be expressed as nouns or eponyms, with critical use of adjectives. Some conditions known by several names have multiple main entries. Reasons for encounters may be located under general terms such as admission, encounter, and examination. Other general terms such as history of, status post, or presence (of) are used to locate factors influencing health.

Step 4: Read cross-references listed with the main term or the subterm.

Cross-references such as *"see"* and *"see also"* are identified by italicized type and should always be checked to ensure that all alternative terms are researched.

Step 5: Review entries for modifiers.

Nonessential modifiers are the terms in parentheses following the main term entry. These parenthetical terms are supplementary words or explanatory information that may or may not appear in the diagnostic statement and do not affect code selection. The subterms listed under the main term are essential modifiers that do affect coding assignment. Each line of indent represents a more specific code entry. The nonessential modifiers apply to the subterms following a main term except when they are mutually exclusive, in which case the subterm takes precedence. For example, if "acute" is listed as a nonessential modifier but there is a subentry for "chronic," then the nonessential modifier of "acute" does not apply.

Step 6: Interpret abbreviations, cross-references, default codes, additional characters, and brackets.

The abbreviation NEC (not elsewhere classified) that follows some main terms or subterms indicates that there is no specific code for the condition even though the medical documentation may be very specific. The code next to the main term is called the default code. It represents the condition most commonly associated with the main term or the unspecified code for the main term. Additional characters may be required to construct the code; the tabular list must be referenced to determine what those specific characters should be. The alphabetic index uses brackets [] to enclose manifestation codes that can be used only as secondary codes to the underlying condition code immediately preceding it. Both codes must be reported in this multiple-coding situation.

Step 7: Choose a potential code and locate it in the tabular list.

The coder must follow any Includes, Excludes 1 and Excludes 2 notes, and other instructional notes, such as "Code first" and "Use additional code," listed in the tabular list for the chapter, category, subcategory, and subclassification level of code selection that direct the coder to use a different or additional code. Any codes in the tabular range, A00.0- through T88.9-, may be used to identify the diagnostic reason for the encounter. The tabular list encompasses many codes describing disease and injury classifications (e.g., infectious and parasitic diseases, neoplasms, symptoms, nervous and circulatory system etc.).

Codes that describe symptoms and signs, as opposed to definitive diagnoses, should be used for reporting purposes when an established diagnosis has not been made (confirmed) by the physician. Chapter 18 of the ICD-10-CM code book, "Symptoms, Signs, and Abnormal Clinical and Laboratory Findings" (codes R00.--R99), contains many, but not all, codes for symptoms.

ICD-10-CM classifies encounters with health care providers for circumstances other than a disease or injury using codes in chapter 21, "Factors Influencing Health Status and Contact with Health Services" (codes Z00–Z99.8). Circumstances other than a disease or injury often are recorded as chiefly responsible for the encounter.

Step 8: Determine whether the code is at the highest level of specificity.

A code is invalid if it has not been coded to the full number of characters (greatest level of specificity) required. Codes in ICD-10-CM can contain from three up to seven alphanumeric characters. A three-character code is to be used only if the category is not further subdivided into four-, five-, or six-character codes. Placeholder character X is used both to allow for future expansion and as a placeholder for empty characters in a code that requires a seventh character but has no fourth, fifth, or sixth character. Certain categories require seventh characters that apply to all codes in that category. Always check the category level for applicable seventh characters for that category.

Step 9: Assign the code.

Having reviewed all relevant information concerning the possible code choices, assign the code that most completely describes the condition.

Repeat steps one through nine for all additional documented conditions that meet the following criteria:

- Conditions that currently exist at the time of the visit
- Conditions that require or affect patient care, treatment, or management

Step 10: Sequence codes correctly.

Sequencing is the order in which the codes are listed on the claim. List first the ICD-10-CM code for the diagnosis, condition, problem, or other reason for the encounter/visit, which is shown in the medical record to be chiefly responsible for the services provided. List additional codes that describe any coexisting conditions. Follow the official coding guidelines (see section II, "Selection of Principal Diagnosis"; section III, "Reporting Additional Diagnoses"; and section IV, "Diagnostic Coding and Reporting Guidelines for Outpatient Services") on proper sequencing of codes.

Coding Examples

Diagnosis: Anorexia

Step 1: The reason for the encounter was the condition, anorexia.

Step 2: Consult the alphabetic index.

Step 3: Locate the main term "Anorexia."

Step 4: There are no cross-references to check.

Step 5: Note that there are two possible subterms (essential modifiers), "hysterical" and "nervosa," neither of which is documented in this instance and therefore cannot be used in code selection. The code listed next to the main term is called the default code selection.

Step 6: There are no abbreviations, cross-references, additional character icons, or brackets.

Step 7: Turn to code R63.0 in the tabular list and read the instructional notes. In this case the Excludes 1 note indicates that anorexia nervosa and loss of appetite determined to be of nonorganic origin should be coded to a code from chapter 5. The diagnostic statement does not indicate nonorganic origin.

Step 8: There is no further division of the category past the fourth character subcategory. Therefore, the subcategory code level is the highest level of specificity.

Step 9: The default code, R63.0 Anorexia, is the correct code selection

Step 10: Since anorexia is listed as the chief reason for the health care encounter, the first-listed, or principal, diagnosis is R63.0. Note that this is a chapter 18 symptom code but can be assigned since the provider did not establish a more definitive diagnosis.

Diagnosis: Acute bronchitis

Step 1: The reason for the encounter was the condition, acute bronchitis.

Step 2: Consult the alphabetic index.

Step 3: Locate the main term "Bronchitis."

Step 4: There are cross-references to interpret.

Step 5: Review entries for modifiers. Since "acute" is not listed as a nonessential modifier, read past the "with" modifier until you find the subterm "acute or subacute" with a nonessential modifier of "with bronchospasm or obstruction," code J20.9.

Step 6: There are no abbreviations, cross-references, additional character icons, or brackets.

Step 7: Since there are no more appropriate subterms, turn to code J20.9 in the tabular list. The Includes note under category J20 does refer to other alternative terms for acute bronchitis. Note that the inclusion term list is not exhaustive but is only a representative selection of diagnoses that are included in the subcategory. The Excludes 1 note refers bronchitis and tracheobronchitis NOS to category J40. There are several Excludes 2 notes that, if applicable, can be coded in addition to this code.

Step 8: Note that the subcategories included in J20 represent acute bronchitis due to various infectious organisms that would be selected if identified in the documentation. In this case, the organism was not identified and there is no further division of the category past the fourth character subcategory. Therefore, the subcategory code level is the highest level of specificity.

Step 9: Assign code J20.9 Acute bronchitis, unspecified.

Step 10: Repeat steps 1-9 for any additional code assignments.

Diagnosis: Infectious diarrhea

Step 1: The reason for the encounter was the condition, infectious diarrhea.

Step 2: Consult the alphabetic index.

Step 3: Locate the main term "Diarrhea" in the alphabetic index.

Step 4: There are no cross-references to check.

Step 5: Review entries for modifiers. Note that the nonessential modifiers (in parentheses) after the main term do not include the term "infectious," which means that the coder should search the subterms for the term "infectious." The subterm "infectious" refers to code A09.

Step 6: There are no abbreviations, cross-references, additional character icons, or brackets.

Step 7: Locate code A09 in the tabular list, and read all instructional notes under the main category and subcategories. The Includes notes does not list the term "infectious diarrhea" under code A09; however, as instructed by the alphabetic index, you should code the condition to A09. The ICD-10-CM code book implies that infectious diarrhea is the same as infectious gastroenteritis, enteritis, and colitis.

Step 8: There is no further division of the category past the third-character category level. Therefore, the category code level is the highest level of specificity. The final code assignment would be A09.

Step 9: Assign code A09 Infectious gastroenteritis and colitis, unspecified.

Step 10: Since infectious diarrhea is listed as the chief reason for the health care encounter, the first-listed, or principal, diagnosis is A09.

Diagnosis: Decubitus ulcer of right elbow with skin loss and necrosis of subcutaneous tissue

Step 1: The reason for the encounter was the condition, decubitus ulcer.

Step 2: Consult the alphabetic index.

Step 3: Locate the main term "Ulcer" in the alphabetic index.

Step 4: There are no cross-references to check.

Step 5: This entry does not have any important nonessential modifiers; however, there are other terms such as ulcerated, ulcerating, etc., that are included as main terms. Locate the subterm "decubitus" and note that there is an italicized cross-reference to "see Ulcer, pressure, by site." Go to the subterm "pressure" and locate "elbow," which refers to code L89.0-.

Step 6: Note that the code L89.0 is followed by a dash and an additional character icon, which indicate that more characters are required. From here, the tabular list can be consulted at code L89.0-.

Step 7: Locate code L89.0 in the tabular list, and check the category level L89 for any instructional, Includes, and Excludes 1 and 2 notes. Note that "decubitus" is an Includes note under L89 Pressure ulcer. Excludes 2 notes indicate that if this were documented as a diabetic pressure ulcer, it would be necessary to use a code from chapter 4.

Step 8: Read through the subcategory codes under L89.0 and note that the fifth character describes laterality. Locate the right elbow at subcategory L89.01. See that an additional sixth character is now needed to complete the code. The sixth character specifies the stage of the ulcer, which can be determined either by the specific documentation of the stage (e.g., stage 1, stage 2) or in this case, a description that matches one of the Includes notes that follow each stage code. For example, the description in this case of "skin loss and necrosis of the subcutaneous tissue" matches the Includes notes under L89.013 Pressure ulcer of right elbow, stage 3.

Step 9: Assign code L89.013 Pressure ulcer of right elbow, stage 3

Step 10: Since the decubitus ulcer is listed as the chief reason for the health care encounter, the first-listed, or principal, diagnosis is L89.013. However, according to the Code first instructional note at the L89 category level, gangrene would be sequenced before the pressure ulcer if it were documented.

Diagnosis: First visit for bimalleolar fracture of the right ankle due to trauma

Step 1: The reason for the encounter was the condition, bimalleolar fracture of the right ankle.

Step 2: Consult the alphabetic index.

Step 3: Locate the main term "Fracture" in the alphabetic index.

Step 4: Note that the first main term for Fracture is pathological with cross-reference to "see also Fracture, traumatic." Locate the main term "Fracture, traumatic."

Step 5: Review entries for nonessential modifiers. Locate the subterms "ankle," "bimalleolar." Note that "displaced" is a nonessential modifier following "bimalleolar," indicating that S82.84- is the default code unless the fracture is specified as nondisplaced.

Step 6: Note that code S82.84- is followed by a dash and an additional character icon, both of which indicate that more characters are required. From here, the tabular list can be consulted at code S82.84.

Step 7: Locate code S82.84 Bimalleolar fracture of lower leg, in the tabular list and check the category level S82 for any instructional, Includes, and Excludes 1 and 2 notes. See the instructional notes indicating that fractures not specified as displaced or nondisplaced default to displaced, and fractures not designated as open or closed default to closed. See also the list of appropriate seventh characters to be added to all codes from category S82.

Step 8: Read through the subcategory codes under S82.84, and note that the sixth character specifies displaced or nondisplaced and laterality. Locate the displaced bimalleolar fracture of the right lower leg at code S82.841. See that an additional seventh character is still needed to complete the code. The seventh character specifies the type of encounter and whether the fracture is open or closed. Use character A listed in the box at the category level to describe initial encounter, closed fracture.

Step 9: Assign code S82.841A Displaced bimalleolar fracture of right lower leg, initial encounter for closed fracture.

Step 10: Since this is an injury code, code additionally any external cause, place of occurrence, and activity codes, with the injury (fracture) sequenced first.

Appendix B: Valid 3-character ICD-10-CM Codes

A09	Infectious gastroenteritis and colitis, unspecified
A33	Tetanus neonatorum
A34	Obstetrical tetanus
A35	Other tetanus
A46	Erysipelas
A55	Chlamydial lymphogranuloma (venereum)
A57	Chancroid
A58	Granuloma inguinale
A64	Unspecified sexually transmitted disease
A65	Nonvenereal syphilis
A70	Chlamydia psittaci infections
A78	Q fever
A86	Unspecified viral encephalitis
A89	Unspecified viral infection of central nervous system
A90	Dengue fever [classical dengue]
A91	Dengue hemorrhagic fever
A94	Unspecified arthropod-borne viral fever
A99	Unspecified viral hemorrhagic fever
B03	Smallpox
B04	Monkeypox
B09	Unspecified viral infection characterized by skin and mucous membrane lesions
B20	Human immunodeficiency virus [HIV] disease
B49	Unspecified mycosis
B54	Unspecified malaria
B59	Pneumocystosis
B64	Unspecified protozoal disease
B72	Dracunculiasis
B75	Trichinellosis
B79	Trichuriasis
B80	Enterobiasis
B86	Scabies
B89	Unspecified parasitic disease
B91	Sequelae of poliomyelitis
B92	Sequelae of leprosy
C01	Malignant neoplasm of base of tongue
C07	Malignant neoplasm of parotid gland
C12	Malignant neoplasm of pyriform sinus
C19	Malignant neoplasm of rectosigmoid junction
C20	Malignant neoplasm of rectum
C23	Malignant neoplasm of gallbladder
C33	Malignant neoplasm of trachea
C37	Malignant neoplasm of thymus
C52	Malignant neoplasm of vagina
C55	Malignant neoplasm of uterus, part unspecified
C58	Malignant neoplasm of placenta
C61	Malignant neoplasm of prostate
C73	Malignant neoplasm of thyroid gland
D34	Benign neoplasm of thyroid gland
D45	Polycythemia vera
D62	Acute posthemorrhagic anemia
D65	Disseminated intravascular coagulation [defibrination A syndrome]
D66	Hereditary factor VIII deficiency
D67	Hereditary factor IX deficiency
D71	Functional disorders of polymorphonuclear neutrophils
D77	Other disorders of blood and blood-forming organs in diseases classified elsewhere
E02	Subclinical iodine-deficiency hypothyroidism
E15	Nondiabetic hypoglycemic coma
E35	Disorders of endocrine glands in diseases classified elsewhere
E40	Kwashiorkor
E41	Nutritional marasmus
E42	Marasmic kwashiorkor

E43	Unspecified severe protein-calorie malnutrition
E45	Retarded development following protein-calorie malnutrition
E46	Unspecified protein-calorie malnutrition
E52	Niacin deficiency [pellagra]
E54	Ascorbic acid deficiency
E58	Dietary calcium deficiency
E59	Dietary selenium deficiency
E60	Dietary zinc deficiency
E65	Localized adiposity
E68	Sequelae of hyperalimentation
F04	Amnestic disorder due to known physiological condition
F05	Delirium due to known physiological condition
F09	Unspecified mental disorder due to known physiological condition
F21	Schizotypal disorder
F22	Delusional disorders
F23	Brief psychotic disorder
F24	Shared psychotic disorder
F28	Other psychotic disorder not due to a substance or known physiological condition
F29	Unspecified psychosis not due to a substance or known physiological condition
F39	Unspecified mood [affective] disorder
F42	Obsessive-compulsive disorder
F53	Puerperal psychosis
F54	Psychological and behavioral factors associated with disorders or diseases classified elsewhere
F59	Unspecified behavioral syndromes associated with physiological disturbances and physical factors
F66	Other sexual disorders
F69	Unspecified disorder of adult personality and behavior
F70	Mild intellectual disabilities
F71	Moderate intellectual disabilities
F72	Severe intellectual disabilities
F73	Profound intellectual disabilities
F78	Other intellectual disabilities
F79	Unspecified intellectual disabilities
F82	Specific developmental disorder of motor function
F88	Other disorders of psychological development
F89	Unspecified disorder of psychological development
F99	Mental disorder, not otherwise specified
G01	Meningitis in bacterial diseases classified elsewhere
G02	Meningitis in other infectious and parasitic diseases classified elsewhere
G07	Intracranial and intraspinal abscess and granuloma in diseases classified elsewhere
G08	Intracranial and intraspinal phlebitis and thrombophlebitis
G09	Sequelae of inflammatory diseases of central nervous system
G10	Huntington's disease
G14	Postpolio syndrome
G20	Parkinson's disease
G26	Extrapyramidal and movement disorders in diseases classified elsewhere
G35	Multiple sclerosis
G53	Cranial nerve disorders in diseases classified elsewhere
G55	Nerve root and plexus compressions in diseases classified elsewhere
G59	Mononeuropathy in diseases classified elsewhere
G63	Polyneuropathy in diseases classified elsewhere
G64	Other disorders of peripheral nervous system
G92	Toxic encephalopathy
G94	Other disorders of brain in diseases classified elsewhere
H22	Disorders of iris and ciliary body in diseases classified elsewhere
H28	Cataract in diseases classified elsewhere
H32	Chorioretinal disorders in diseases classified elsewhere
H36	Retinal disorders in diseases classified elsewhere

H42	Glaucoma in diseases classified elsewhere		N72	Inflammatory disease of cervix uteri
I00	Rheumatic fever without heart involvement		N74	Female pelvic inflammatory disorders in diseases classified elsewhere
I10	Essential (primary) hypertension		N86	Erosion and ectropion of cervix uteri
I32	Pericarditis in diseases classified elsewhere		N96	Recurrent pregnancy loss
I38	Endocarditis, valve unspecified		O68	Labor and delivery complicated by abnormality of fetal acid-base balance
I39	Endocarditis and heart valve disorders in diseases classified elsewhere		O76	Abnormality in fetal heart rate and rhythm complicating labor and delivery
I41	Myocarditis in diseases classified elsewhere		O80	Encounter for full-term uncomplicated delivery
I43	Cardiomyopathy in diseases classified elsewhere		O82	Encounter for cesarean delivery without indication
I52	Other heart disorders in diseases classified elsewhere		O85	Puerperal sepsis
I76	Septic arterial embolism		O94	Sequelae of complication of pregnancy, childbirth, and the puerperium
I81	Portal vein thrombosis		P09	Abnormal findings on neonatal screening
I96	Gangrene, not elsewhere classified		P53	Hemorrhagic disease of newborn
J00	Acute nasopharyngitis (common cold)		P60	Disseminated intravascular coagulation of newborn
J13	Pneumonia due to Streptococcus pneumoniae		P84	Other problems with newborn
J14	Pneumonia due to Hemophilus influenzae		P90	Convulsions of newborn
J17	Pneumonia in diseases classified elsewhere		P95	Stillbirth
J22	Unspecified acute lower respiratory infection		Q02	Microcephaly
J36	Peritonsillar abscess		R05	Cough
J40	Bronchitis, not specified as acute or chronic		R12	Heartburn
J42	Unspecified chronic bronchitis		R17	Unspecified jaundice
J60	Coalworker's pneumoconiosis		R21	Rash and other nonspecific skin eruption
J61	Pneumoconiosis due to asbestos and other mineral fibers		R32	Unspecified urinary incontinence
J64	Unspecified pneumoconiosis		R34	Anuria and oliguria
J65	Pneumoconiosis associated with tuberculosis		R37	Sexual dysfunction, unspecified
J80	Acute respiratory distress syndrome		R42	Dizziness and giddiness
J82	Pulmonary eosinophilia, not elsewhere classified		R51	Headache
J90	Pleural effusion, not elsewhere classified		R52	Pain, unspecified
J99	Respiratory disorders in diseases classified elsewhere		R54	Age-related physical debility
K23	Disorders of esophagus in diseases classified elsewhere		R55	Syncope and collapse
K30	Functional dyspepsia		R58	Hemorrhage, not elsewhere classified
K36	Other appendicitis		R61	Generalized hyperhidrosis
K37	Unspecified appendicitis		R64	Cachexia
K67	Disorders of peritoneum in infectious diseases classified elsewhere		R69	Illness, unspecified
K77	Liver disorders in diseases classified elsewhere		R75	Inconclusive laboratory evidence of human immunodeficiency virus [HIV]
K87	Disorders of gallbladder, biliary tract and pancreas in diseases classified elsewhere		R81	Glycosuria
L00	Staphylococcal scalded skin syndrome		R99	Ill-defined and unknown cause of mortality
L14	Bullous disorders in diseases classified elsewhere		T07	Unspecified multiple injuries
L22	Diaper dermatitis		Y09	Assault by unspecified means
L26	Exfoliative dermatitis		Y66	Nonadministration of surgical and medical care
L42	Pityriasis rosea		Y69	Unspecified misadventure during surgical and medical care
L45	Papulosquamous disorders in diseases classified elsewhere		Y95	Nosocomial condition
L52	Erythema nodosum		Z08	Encounter for follow-up examination after completed treatment for malignant neoplasm
L54	Erythema in diseases classified elsewhere		Z09	Encounter for follow-up examination after completed treatment for conditions other than malignant neoplasm
L62	Nail disorders in diseases classified elsewhere			
L80	Vitiligo		Z21	Asymptomatic human immunodeficiency virus [HIV] infection status
L83	Acanthosis nigricans		Z23	Encounter for immunization
L84	Corns and callosities		Z36	Encounter for antenatal screening of mother
L86	Keratoderma in diseases classified elsewhere		Z66	Do not resuscitate
L88	Pyoderma gangrenosum			
L99	Other disorders of skin and subcutaneous tissue in diseases classified elsewhere			
N08	Glomerular disorders in diseases classified elsewhere			
N10	Acute tubulo-interstitial nephritis			
N12	Tubulo-interstitial nephritis, not specified as acute or chronic			
N16	Renal tubulo-interstitial disorders in diseases classified elsewhere			
N19	Unspecified kidney failure			
N22	Calculus of urinary tract in diseases classified elsewhere			
N23	Unspecified renal colic			
N29	Other disorders of kidney and ureter in diseases classified elsewhere			
N33	Bladder disorders in diseases classified elsewhere			
N37	Urethral disorders in diseases classified elsewhere			
N51	Disorders of male genital organs in diseases classified elsewhere			
N61	Inflammatory disorders of breast			
N62	Hypertrophy of breast			
N63	Unspecified lump in breast			

Appendix C: Pharmacology List 2016

This section enables the coder to quickly review drugs, drug actions, and indications that are often associated with overlooked or undocumented diagnoses. The coder should review the patient's medication record and know what condition the physician is treating with the prescribed medication based on documentation in the medical record. When documentation is lacking, the coder can reference this section to locate the drug, determine the drug action, confirm drug indications, and when necessary query the physician.

Drug	Drug Action	Indications
Accupril [quinapril]	ACE inhibitor; antihypertensive	Congestive heart failure; essential hypertension
Acetaminophen and codeine [acetominophen/codeine phosphate]	Analgesic	Pain, moderate to severe
Actemra [tocilizumab]	Antirheumatic	Rheumatoid arthritis
Actonel [risedronate]	Electrolytic and renal agent; bone resorption inhibitor	Decrease bone loss in multiple myeloma patients; Paget's disease; hyperparathyroidism; osteoporosis
Adalat CC [nifedipine]	Calcium channel blocker	Vasospastic angina; chronic stable angina; essential hypertension
Aldactone [spironolactone]	Cardiovascular agent; antihypertensive agent; diuretic; electrolytic and renal agent	Treatment of severe heart failure; ascites associated with cirrhosis; hypokalemia
Allegra [fexofenadine/ hydrochloride pseudoephedrine]	Antihistamine	Seasonal allergic rhinitis
Allopurinol [allopurinol]	Antigout	Gouty arthritis, renal calculus, hyperuricemia, hyperuricemia secondary to leukemia, hyperuricemia secondary to lymphoma
Alphagan P [brimonidine]	Antiglaucoma agent (ophthalmic) antihypertensive, ocular	Open angle glaucoma or another condition in which pressure in the eye is too high (ocular hypertension)
Alprazolam [alprazolam]	Antianxiety; sedative/hypnotic	
Altace [ramipril]	ACE inhibitor; antihypertensive	Congestive heart failure, essential hypertension
Amaryl [glimepiride]	Blood glucose regulator	Diabetes mellitus
Ambien [zolpidem]	Sedative/hypnotic	Insomnia
Abilify [aripiprazole]	Antipsychotic	Depression, bipolar disorder, schizophrenia, autism symptoms
Amikacin [amikacin sulfate]	Aminoglycoside antibiotic	Active in treatment of gram-negative bacterial infections such as *Pseudomonas, Escherichia coli (E. coli), Proteus, Klebsiella-Enterobacter-Serratia*
Aminophylline [aminophylline]	Bronchodilator, pulmonary vasodilator, smooth muscle relaxant	Relief and/or prevention of symptoms from asthma and reversible bronchospasms in bronchitis and emphysema
Amitriptyline hydrochloride [amitriptyline hydrochloride]	Anorexiant/CNS stimulant; antidepressant	Depression
Amoxicillin, Amoxil [amoxicillin]	Penicillin	Effective for infections with a broad spectrum of bactericidal activity against many gram-positive and gram-negative micro-organisms; otitis media, gonorrhea, skin, respiratory, gastrointestinal, and genitourinary infections
Amrix [cyclobenzaprine hydrochloride]	Muscle relaxant	Adjunct to rest and physical therapy for muscle spasms
Ancef [cefazoline sodium]	Semisynthetic cephalosporin antibiotic	Respiratory tract infections due to *Streptococcus pneumoniae, Klebsiella species, Haemophilus influenzae (H. influenzae), Staphylococcus aureus*, and group A betahemolytic streptococci; urinary tract infections due to *E. coli, Proteus mirabilis, Klebsiella* species and some strains of Enterobacter and enterococci; skin and skin structure infections, biliary tract infections, bone and joint infections, genital infections, septicemia, and endocarditis
Antabuse [disulfiram]	Alcohol treatment	Alcoholism
Anzemet [dolasetron mesylate]	Antiemetic/ antinauseant	Management of nausea/vomiting following surgery or from effects of chemotherapy or cancer
Aranesp [darbepoetin alfa]	Erythropoiesis-stimulating agent (ESA)	Treat lower than normal blood cells (anemia) from disorders such as CKD and neoplasms
Aricept [donepezil hydrochloride]	Acetylcholine sterase inhibitor	Symptoms of mild to moderate Alzheimer's disease; can improve thinking ability in some patients
Arthrotec [diclofenac/misoprostol]	Analgesic	Treatment of patients with arthritis who may develop stomach ulcers from taking nonsteroidal anti-inflammatory drugs (NSAIDs) alone; used to help relieve some symptoms of arthritis, such as inflammation, swelling, stiffness, and joint pain
Atenolol [atenolol]	Antianginal; antihypertensive; beta blocker	Chronic stable angina pectoris; essential hypertension; reduces cardiovascular mortality in those with definite or suspected acute myocardial infarction

Drug	Drug Action	Indications
Ativan [lorazepam]	Antianxiety; sedative/hypnotic	Anxiety disorder associated with depressive symptoms; controls tension, agitation, irritability, and insomnia
Atrovent [ipratropium bromide]	Antiasthmatic/bronchodilator	Chronic bronchitis, emphysema; bronchial asthma
Augmentin [amoxicillin/clavulanate]	Antibacterial	Middle ear, lower respiratory, sinus, skin and skin structures, and urinary tract infections
Avapro [irbesartan]	Antihypertensive	Hypertension
Axid [nizatidine]	Histamine H2-receptor antagonist	Acid/peptic disorder; gastroesophageal reflux; duodenal, gastric, and peptic ulcers
Bactrim [sulfamethoxazole trimethoprim]	Antibacterial	Treatment of urinary tract infections, acute otitis media, acute exacerbation of chronic bronchitis, shigellosis, and pneumocystis carinii
Bactroban [mupirocin]	Dermatologic; topical anti-infective	Topical treatment of impetigo
Beconase AQ [beclomethasone dipropionate monohydrate]	Corticosteroids; antiasthmatic	Bronchial asthma, prevention of nasal polyps, perennial allergies, seasonal allergies and vasomotor rhinitis
Betoptic [betaxolol hydrochloride]	Cardioselective beta-adrenergic receptor blocking agent	Lowers intraocular pressure; also used for treatment of ocular hypertension and chronic open-angle glaucoma
Biaxin [clarithromycin]	Macrolide	Acid/peptic disorder or ulcer, acute exacerbation chronic bronchitis, human immunodeficiency virus, lower and upper respiratory tract infection, sinus infection, prophylaxis mycobacterium avium complex, pharyngitis, pneumonia, tonsillitis
Buspirone [buspirone hydrochloride]	Antianxiety	Generalized anxiety disorder
Butorphanol Tartrate [butorphanol tartrate]	Narcotic analgesic	Moderate to severe postsurgical pain
Calan [verapamil hydrochloride]	Antianginal; antiarrhythmic, antiarthritic, antihypertensive, calcium channel blocker	Angina pectoris at rest and chronic stable, arrhythmia, atrial fibrillation, atrial flutter, paroxysmal supraventricular tachycardia, ventricular arrhythmia, essential hypertension
Cardizem CD, Tiazac [diltiazem hydrochloride]	Antianginal, antiarrhythmic, antihypertensive, channel blocker, coronary vasodilator	Chronic stable angina, atrial fibrillation, atrial flutter, essential hypertension, paroxysmal supraventricular tachycardia
Cardura [doxazosin mesylate]	Antihypertensive	Benign prostatic hyperplasia, essential hypertension
Catapres, Clonidine [clonidine]	Antihypertensive	Hypertension
Ceftin [cefuroxime axetil]	Antibiotic: second generation cephalosporins	Acute exacerbation and chronic bronchitis, middle ear infection, sexually transmitted gonorrhea infection, upper respiratory tract infection, urinary tract infection, pharyngitis, tonsillitis
Cefprozil [cefprozil]	Antibiotic: second generation cephalosporins	Acute exacerbation and chronic bronchitis, lower respiratory tract infection, upper respiratory tract infection, pharyngitis, tonsillitis
Celebrex [celecoxib]	Antirheumatic, nonsteroidal anti-inflammatory	Relief of some symptoms caused by arthritis, such as inflammation, swelling, stiffness, and joint pain
Celexa [citalopram hydrobromide]	Antidepressant	Depression
Chantix [varenicline]	Smoking cessation aid	Nicotine addiction, smoking
Cipro [ciprofloxacin]	Anti-infective; quinolone	Cystitis, infectious diarrhea, gonorrhea, bone and joint infection, gastrointestinal tract infection, lower and upper respiratory tract infection, sinus infection, urinary tract infection, nosocomial pneumonia, chronic prostatitis
Claritin [loratadine/ pseudoephedrine sulfate]	Antihistamine	Seasonal allergic rhinitis, chronic idiopathic urticaria
Clonazepam, Klonopin [clonazepam]	Anticonvulsant	Absence, akinetic and myoclonic epilepsy, Lennox-Gastaut syndrome
Cogentin [benztropine mesylate]	Antiparkinsonism	Parkinson's disease
Colace [docusate sodium]	Gastrointestinal agent; laxative, stool softener	Constipation
Combivent [ipratropium bromide/albuterol sulfate]	Antiasthmatic/bronchodilator	Chronic bronchitis, emphysema; bronchial asthma
Compro [prochlorperazine] suppository form only	Antiemetic, antipsychotic	Nausea, vomiting, and manic phase of bipolar syndrome or schizophrenia
Cortisporin [hydrocortisone acetate/neomycin sulfate]	Topical anti-infective, topical steroid	Dermatosis
Coumadin [warfarin sodium]	Thrombolytic agent/anticoagulant	Prophylaxis and treatment of venous thrombosis, treatment of atrial fibrillation with embolization (pulmonary embolism), arrhythmias, myocardial infarction, and stroke prevention

Drug	Drug Action	Indications
Cozaar [losartan]	Antihypertensive	Essential hypertension
Crestor [rosuvastatin calcium]	HMG-CoA reductase inhibitor (statin)	Hypercholesterolemia, hyperlipidemia, hyperproteinemia
Crixivan [indinavir sulfate]	HIV inhibitor	HIV, asymptomatic HIV
Cytomel [liothyronine sodium]	Thyroid hormone	Treatment of hypothyroidism or prevention of euthyroid goiters
Daypro [oxaprozin]	Nonsteroidal anti-inflammatory drug (NSAID)	Osteoarthritis and rheumatoid arthritis
Depakote [divalproex]	Anticonvulsant	Bipolar affective disorder; complex absence, complex partial and mixed pattern epilepsy; migraine headache
Desogen [desogestrel/ethinyl estradiol]	Contraceptive; estrogen/progestin	Contraception
Detrol [tolterodine tartrate]	Muscarinic receptor antagonist	Overactive bladders in patients with urinary frequency, urgency, or urge incontinence
Diflucan [fluconazole]	Antifungal agent	Oropharyngeal and esophageal candidiasis and cryptococcal meningitis in AIDS patients
Digoxin [digoxin]	Cardiotonic glycoside	Heart failure, atrial flutter, atrial fibrillation, and supraventricular tachycardia
Dilantin [phenytoin sodium]	Anticonvulsant	Control of grand mal and psychomotor seizures
Diovan [valsartan]	Ace inhibitor	Essential hypertension
Effexor XR [venlafaxine]	Antidepressant	Depression
Epinephrine [epinephrine]	Bronchodilator, cardiotonic	Most commonly used to relieve respiratory distress due to bronchospasm and to restore cardiac rhythm in cardiac arrest
Epivir, Epivir-HBV [lamivudine]	HIV and HBV inhibitor	HIV, hepatitis B (HBV), asymptomatic HIV
ERY-TAB [erythromycin]	Acne product; macrolide; ocular anti-infective; topical anti-infective	Acne vulgaris, intestinal amebiasis, infectious conjunctivitis, diphtheria, endocarditis, prevention, erythrasma treatment of infections: endocervical, gynecologic, lower and upper respiratory tract, ophthalmic, rectal; skin and skin structures, and urethral; Legionnaires' disease, pelvic inflammatory disease, pertussis, pneumonia, rheumatic fever, prophylaxis, syphilis
Estrace [estradiol]	Estrogen therapy	Vaginal cream used to treat vaginal and vulvar atrophy
Estraderm, Climara [estradiol]	Estrogen therapy	Osteoporosis prevention and to treat menopausal symptoms, vaginal and vulvar atrophy, hypoestrogenism, ovarian failure
Evista [raloxifene hydrochloride]	Estrogen receptor modulator, selective osteoporosis prophylactic	Prevention of thinning of the bones (osteoporosis) only in postmenopausal women
Flavoxate hydrochloride [flavoxate hydrochloride]	Urinary tract spasmolytic	Relief of dysuria, urgency, nocturia, suprapubic pain, frequency, and incontinence associated with cystitis, prostatitis, urethritis, and urethrocystitis/urethrotrigonitis
Flomax [tamsulosin hydrochloride]	Benign prostatic hypertrophy therapy agent	Signs and symptoms of benign enlargement of the prostate (benign prostatic hyperplasia or BPH)
Flonase [fluticasone propionate]	Corticosteroid-inhalation/nasal; topical steroid	Corticosteroid-responsive dermatosis; perennial allergic and seasonal allergic rhinitis
Flovent HFA [fluticasone propionate]	Corticosteroid-inhalation/nasal; topical steroid	Corticosteroid-responsive dermatosis, perennial allergic and seasonal allergic rhinitis
Fosamax [alendronate sodium]	Calcium metabolism	Osteoporosis; Paget's disease
Fosinopril sodium [fosinopril sodium]	ACE inhibitor; antihypertensive	Essential hypertension
Glucophage [metformin hydrochloride]	Blood glucose regulator	Diabetes mellitus antihyperglycemic drug used in the management of non-insulin-dependent diabetes mellitus (NIDDM)
Glucotrol [glipizide]	Oral blood-glucose-lowering agent	Adjunct to diet for the control of hyperglycemia in patients with noninsulin dependent diabetes mellitus (NIDDM, type II)
Glyburide (micronized) [glyburide]	Blood glucose regulator	Diabetes mellitus
Heparin sodium [heparin sodium]	Anticoagulant	Prophylaxis and treatment of venous thrombosis, pulmonary embolism; prevention of cerebral thrombosis, and treatment of consumptive coagulopathies
Hydrochlorothiazide [hydrochlorothiazide]	Diuretic, antihypertensive	Management of hypertension and in adjunctive therapy for edema associated with congestive heart failure, hepatic cirrhosis, corticosteroid, and estrogen therapy
Hydrocodone bitartrate and acetaminophen [acetaminophen/hydrocodone bitartrate]	Analgesic, general; analgesic-narcotic; antitussive/expectorant	Pain, moderate to severe

Drug	Drug Action	Indications
Hyzaar [hydrochlorothiazide/losartan/potassium]	Antihypertensive	Hypertension
Imitrex [sumatriptan succinate]	Antimigraine	Migraine headache
Inderal [propranolol hydrochloride]	Beta-adrenergic blocking agent	Management of hypertension, long-term management of angina pectoris due to coronary atherosclerosis, cardiac arrhythmias
Isordil [isosorbide dinitrate]	Smooth muscle relaxant	Acute anginal attacks
Isuprel [isoproterenol hydrochloride]	Adrenergic agent	Bronchodilator for asthma, chronic pulmonary emphysema, bronchitis, and other conditions accompanied by bronchospasm; can be used in cardiogenic shock cases
K-Tab, Klor-Con [potassium chloride]	Replaces potassium and maintains potassium level	Hypokalemia
Keflex [cephalexin]	Antibacterial	Bone, middle ear, skin and skin structures, upper respiratory tract and urinary tract infections; acute prostatitis
Klonopin [clonazepam]	Anticonvulsant, anxiolytic - benzodiazepine	Epilepsy, seizures, panic disorder
Lamisil [terbinafine hydrochloride]	Antifungal	*Tinea cruris* (jock itch), *T. pedis* (athlete's foot), *T. corporis* (ringworm)
Lanoxin [digoxin]	Cardiotonic glycoside	Congestive heart failure
Lasix [furosemide]	Antihypertensive; diuretic	Management of edema associated with congestive heart failure, renal disease, including nephrotic syndrome and hypertension
Lescol [fluvastatin]	HMG-CoA reductase inhibitor (statin)	Hypercholesterolemia; hyperlipidemia; hyperlipoproteinemia
Levaquin [levofloxacin]	Fluoroquinolone antibacterial	Acute exacerbation chronic bronchitis; cellulitis; furuncle; impetigo; infections of the lower and upper respiratory tract, sinus, skin and skin structures, and urinary tract; pneumonia, community-acquired; pyoderma
Levoxyl [levothyroxine sodium]	Synthetic thyroid hormone	Euthyroid goiter; hypothyroidism
Lexapro [escitalopram oxalate]	Antidepressant—selective serotonin reuptake inhibitor (SSRI)	Depression, anxiety
Librium [chlordiazepoxide hydrochloride]	Antianxiety agent	Acute withdrawal symptoms, especially from alcohol, or for other anxiety-producing conditions
Lidocaine [lidocaine hydrochloride]	Antiarrhythmic	Management of ventricular arrhythmias or during cardiac manipulation, such as cardiac surgery
Lipitor [atorvastatin calcium]	HMG-CoA reductase inhibitor (statin)	Hypercholesterolemia, hyperlipidemia, hyperproteinemia
Lithium [lithium carbonate]	Antimanic	Control of manic episodes in bipolar disorders
Lomotil [diphenoxylate hydrochloride with atropine]	Antidiarrheal	Treatment of symptoms of chronic and functional diarrhea
Lopid [gemfibrozil]	Lipid regulating agent	Hypercholesterolemia, hyperlipidemia, hyperlipoproteinemia, hypertriglyceridemia
Lopressor [metoprolol tartrate]	Antihypertensive, betablocker antianginal; antihypertensive; betablocker	Essential hypertension therapy, angina pectoris, and myocardial infarction
Lorazepam [lorazepam]	Antianxiety; sedative/hypnotic	Anxiety disorder associated with depressive symptoms; controls tension, agitation, irritability, and insomnia
Lotensin [benazepril]	ACE inhibitor; antihypertensive	Essential hypertension
Lotrel [amlodipine/benazepril]	Antihypertensive	Hypertension
Lotrisone [clotrimazole/betamethasone]	Antifungal-corticosteroid	Relief of redness, swelling, itching, and other discomfort of fungus infections
Lovastatin [lovastatin]	HMG-CoA reductase inhibitor (statin)	Hypercholesterolemia; hyperlipidemia, hyperlipoproteinemia
Macrodantin [nitrofurantoin]	Antibacterial	Urinary tract infection; prophylaxis
Meclinzine hydrochloride [meclizine hydrochloride]	Antihistamine	Management of nausea and vomiting, and dizziness associated with motion sickness
Medrol [methylprednisolone]	Glucocorticoid; anti-inflammatory	Acute/chronic adrenal insufficiency, congenital adrenal hyperplasia, adrenal insufficiency secondary to pituitary insufficiency; nonendocrine disorders include arthritis, rheumatic carditis, bronchial asthma, cerebral edema, and allergic, collagen, intestinal tract, liver, ocular, renal, and skin diseases
Methergine [methylergonovine maleate]	Oxytocic agent	Routine management of postpartum hemorrhage after delivery of placenta
Miacalcin [calcitonin salmon]	Calcitonin; a peptide hormone	Hypercalcemia, osteoporosis, postmenopausal symptoms, Paget's disease

Drug	Drug Action	Indications
Monoket [isosorbide mononitrate]	Antianginal; coronary vasodilator, nitrate	Angina pectoris
Motrin [ibuprofen]	Analgesic, general; analgesic, non-narcotic; antiarthritic; antigout; antipyretic; NSAID	Osteoarthritis and rheumatoid arthritis, dysmenorrhea, fever; pain, mild to moderate
Multaq [dronedarone]	Cardiac rhythm regulator	Treatment of patients with recent episodes of atrial fibrillation or atrial flutter
Nabumetone [nabumetone]	Non-steroidal anti-inflammatory drug (NSAID)	Osteoarthritis and rheumatoid arthritis
Naprosyn [naproxen]	Anti-inflammatory analgesic, general; analgesic, non-narcotic; antiarthritic; antigout; NSAID	Rheumatoid, gouty arthritis and osteoarthritis; ankylosing spondylitis; bursitis; dysmenorrhea; pain, mild to moderate; tendonitis
Nefazodone hydrochloride [nefazodone hydrochloride]	Antidepressant	Depression
Nembutal sodium [pentobarbital sodium]	Sedative; hypnotic	Adjunct medication in diagnostic procedures or for emergency use with convulsive disorders
Neurontin [gabapentin]	Anticonvulsant	Epilepsy, partial
Nexium [esomeprazole magnesium]	Proton pump inhibitor	Gastroesophageal reflux disease (GERD), erosive esophagitis
Nitropress [sodium nitroprusside]	Vasodilator	Potent, rapid action in reducing blood pressure in hypertensive crisis or for controlling bleeding during anesthesia by producing controlled hypotension
Nitrostat [nitroglycerin]	Muscle relaxant antianginal; antihypertensive; coronary vasodilator	Prophylaxis and treatment of angina pectoris; heart failure associated with myocardial infarction; hypertension, perioperative; surgery, adjunct
Norpace [disopyramide]	Antiarrhythmic	Coronary artery disease, for prevention, recurrence and control of unifocal, multifocal, and paired PVCs
Norvasc [amlodipine besylate]	Calcium channel blocker	Hypertension, chronic stable angina, and vasospastic angina
Onglyza [saxagliptin]	Blood glucose regulator	Adjunct to diet and exercise for the control of hyperglycemia in patients with noninsulin-dependent diabetes mellitus (NIDDM, type II)
Orphenadrine citrate [orphenadrine citrate]	Muscle relaxant	Acute spasms, tension, and post-trauma cases
Ortho-Novum [norethindrone/ethinyl estradiol]	Contraceptive; estrogen/progestin	Contraception
Oxazepam [oxazepam]	Antianxiety	Anxiety, tension, and alcohol withdrawal
Pavabid [papaverine hydrochloride]	Vasodilator	Relief of cerebral and peripheral ischemia
Paxil [paroxetine]	Antidepressant	Anxiety with panic disorder and depression; obsessive-compulsive disorder
Penicillin-VK [penicillin V potassium]	Natural penicillin	Chorea, prevention; endocarditis, prevention, secondary to tooth extraction; erysipelas; infections of the skin and skin structures, upper respiratory tract; rheumatic fever, prophylaxis; scarlet fever; Vincent's gingivitis; Vincent's pharyngitis
Pepcid [famotidine]	Histamine H2-receptor inhibitor	Acid/peptic disorder; adenoma, secretory; gastroesophageal reflux; duodenal and gastric ulcer; Zollinger-Ellison syndrome
Percocet, Roxicet [oxycodone and acetaminophen]	Analgesic, general; analgesic-narcotic	Pain, moderate to severe
Persantine [dipyridamole]	Platelet inhibitor	Therapy for chronic angina pectoris, preventing clots post heart valve surgery
Phenobarbital [phenobarbital sodium]	Barbiturate	Grand mal epilepsy
Pitocin [oxytocin]	Synthetic oxytocin	Induction or stimulation of labor at term
Plasmanate [plasma, plasma protein fraction]	Blood volume expander	Hypovolemic shock, burn patients, and hemorrhages when whole blood is unavailable
Plavix [clopidogrel bisulfate]	Antithrombotic platelet aggregation inhibitor	Lessening of the chance of heart attack or stroke
Plendil [felodipine]	Antihypertensive; calcium channel blocker	Essential hypertension
Pravachol [pravastatin]	HMG-CoA reductase inhibitor (statin)	Hypercholesterolemia, hyperlipidemia, hyperlipoproteinemia
Prednisone [prednisone]	Adrenocorticoid, corticosteroid	Used for its immunosuppressant effects and for relief of inflammations; used in arthritis, polymyositis and other systemic diseases
Pregnyl [chorionic gonadotropin]	Gonadotropic hormone	Prepubertal cryptorchidism, hypogonadism, corpus luteum insufficiency and infertility
Premarin [conjugated estrogens]	Antineoplastic; estrogen	Vasomotor symptoms associated with menopause; atrophic vaginitis; kraurosis vulvae, female hypogonadism; primary ovarian failure

Drug	Drug Action	Indications
Prempro [conjugated estrogens/medroxyproges- terone]	Estrogen/progestin	Menopause, osteoporosis, atrophic vaginitis
Prevacid [lansoprazole]	Proton pump inhibitor (PPI)	Acid/peptic disorder, erosive esophagitis, duodenal ulcer, Zollinger-Ellison syndrome
Prinivil [lisinopril]	Synthetic peptide derivative, long-acting angiotensin converting enzyme inhibitor	Congestive heart failure, essential hypertension
Prilosec [omeprazole]	Proton pump inhibitor	Acid/peptic disorder; endocrine adenoma; erosive esophagitis; systemic mastocytosis; gastroesophageal reflux; duodenal, peptic and gastric ulcer; Zollinger-Ellison syndrome
Procardia [nifedipine]	Antianginal agent; calcium channel blocker	Management of vasospastic angina and chronic stable angina, essential hypertension
Promethazine hydrochloride [promethazine hydrochloride]	Anesthesia, adjunct to; antiemetic; antihistamine; antitussive/expectorant; sedative/hypnotic; vertigo/motion sickness/vomiting	Anesthesia; adjunct; angioedema; conjunctivitis; dermographism; hypersensitivity, motion sickness; pain; perennial, seasonal, and allergic rhinitis; sedation, obstetrical; urticaria
Protonix [pantoprazole]	Proton pump inhibitor (PPI)	Short-term treatment and maintenance therapy of erosive esophagitis associated with gastroesophageal reflux disease (GERD)
Proventil-HFA [albuterol sulfate]	Antiasthmatic/bronchodilator	Asthma
Provera/Depo-Provera [medroxyprogesterone acetate]	Antineoplastic; contraceptive; progestin	Amenorrhea; carcinoma, endometrium, adjunct; carcinoma, renal; contraception; hemorrhage
Prozac [fluoxetine hydrochloride]	Serotonin reuptake inhibitor	Bulimia nervosa; depression; obsessive-compulsive disorder
Qnasl [beclomethasone dipropionate]	Corticosteroid	Perennial allergies, seasonal allergies, and vasomotor rhinitis
Quinidine gluconate [quinidine gluconate]	Antiarrhythmic	Management of cardiac arrhythmias
Qvar [beclomethasone dipropionate]	Corticosteroids; antiasthmatic	Prevention and control of symptoms related to asthma
Restoril [temazepam]	Sedative/hypnotic	Insomnia
Retrovir [zidovudine]	Antiretroviral agent	Indicated in symptomatic HIV infection
Risperdal [risperidone]	Antipsychotic/antimanic	Schizophrenia; bipolar I disorder
Ritalin [methylphenidate hydrochloride]	Central nervous system (CNS) stimulant	Treatment of depression and hyperkinetic activity in children
Sabril [vigabatrin]	Anticonvulsant	Refractory complex partial seizures
Septra [sulfamethoxazole trimethoprim]	Antibacterial	Treatment of urinary tract infections, acute otitis media, acute exacerbations of chronic bronchitis, and shigellosis
Serevent [salmeterol xinafoate]	Bronchodilator	Asthma
Sinemet [carbidopa, levodopa]	Antiparkinsonian	Parkinson's disease
Singulair [montelukast]	Antiasthmatic, leukotriene receptor antagonist	Treatment of mild to moderate asthma to decrease the symptoms of asthma and the number of acute asthma attacks
Soltamox [tamoxifen citrate]	Antineoplastic; hormonal/biological response modifier	Breast cancer
Solu-Medrol [methylprednisolone sodium succinate]	Adrenocorticosteroid	Anti-inflammatory and antiallergenic for shock and ulcerative colitis
Synthroid, Levothroid [levothyroxine sodium]	Thyroid hormone	Treatment of hypothyroidism
Tagamet [cimetidine]	Acid reducer	Treatment of active duodenal ulcer, short-term treatment of active, benign gastric ulcer, and treatment of pathological hypersecretory conditions
Tegretol [carbamazepine]	Anticonvulsant; analgesic	Epilepsy, especially with complex symptomatology; specific analgesic for trigeminal neuralgia
Tenormin [atenolol]	Antianginal; antihypertensive; beta blocker	Treatment of hypertension; lowering blood pressure lowers the risk of fatal and nonfatal cardiovascular events, primarily strokes and myocardial infarctions
Terazosin hydrochloride [terazosin hydrochloride]	Alphablocker; antihypertensive; diuretic	Benign prostatic hypertrophy; essential hypertension
Tobradex [tobramycin and dexamethasone]	Aminoglycoside ocular anti-infective; anti-inflammatory	Infectious conjunctivitis; dermatosis, corticosteroid-responsive with secondary infection; foreign body in eye; corneal inflammation; uveitis
Toprol-XL [metoprolol succinate]	Antianginal antihypertensive beta blocker	Angina pectoris, essential hypertension

Drug	Drug Action	Indications
Trazodone hydrochloride [trazodone hydrochloride]	Antidepressant	Depression
Triamterene and hydrochlorothiazide [triamterene/ hydrochlorothiazide]	Antihypertensive, diuretic	Edema; essential hypertension
Trimethoprim [trimethoprim]	Antibacterial	Acute exacerbation chronic bronchitis; travelers' diarrhea; infections of the middle, lower respiratory tract, and urinary tract; pneumonia, pneumocystis; shigellosis
Trivora-28 [ethinyl estradiol/ levonorgestrel]	Contraceptive, estrogen/progestin	Contraception
Ultram [tramadol]	Analgesic, non-narcotic	Pain, moderate to moderately severe
Uniphyl [theophylline]	Bronchodilator, pulmonary vasodilator, smooth muscle relaxant	Treatment of bronchial obstruction in asthma and chronic obstructive pulmonary disease
Valium [diazepam]	Antianxiety, muscle relaxant, anticonvulsant	Anxiety, tension, withdrawal from alcohol, muscle spasms and anticonvulsant therapy; epilepsy, generalized tonic-clonic; status epilepticus; stiff-man syndrome; tetanus
Vasotec [enalaprilat]	ACE inhibitor, antihypertensive	Congestive heart failure; essential hypertension
Ventolin HFA [albuterol, albuterol sulfate]	Antiasthmatic/bronchodilator	Asthma
Verapamil HCL, Calan [verapamil hydrochloride]	Antianginal, antiarrhythmic, antiarthritic, antihypertensive, calcium channel blocker	Angina pectoris, chronic stable angina, atrial fibrillation, atrial flutter, paroxysmal supraventricular tachycardia, ventricular arrhythmia, essential hypertension
Viagra [sildenafil citrate]	Phosphodiesterase-5 (PDE5) inhibitor	Erectile dysfunction
Victoza [liraglutide recombinant]	Glucagon-like peptide-1 (GLP-1) receptor agonist	Adjunct to diet and exercise for the control of hyperglycemia in patients with noninsulin-dependent diabetes mellitus (NIDDM, type II)
Vistaril [hydroxyzine pamoate]	Antianxiety agent, antiemetic	Treatment of nausea and vomiting, for reducing narcotic requirement in surgery and as tranquilizer for tension, anxiety, or agitation states
Wellbutrin SR, Welbutrin XL [bupropion hydrochloride]	Antidepressant; CNS	Depression; smoking cessation
Xalatan [latanoprost]	Prostaglandin F2α analogue	Glaucoma, open-angle; ocular hypertension
Xanax, Xanax XR [alprazolam]	Antianxiety; sedative/hypnotic	Anxiety disorders with panic disorder and depression
Xigris [drotrecogin alfa]	Biologic response modifier	Severe sepsis
Zantac [ranitidine hydrochloride]	Histamine H2-receptors inhibitor	Acid/peptic disorder, erosive esophagitis, gastrointestinal hypersecretion, mastocytosis, gastroesophageal reflux, peptic ulcer, Zollinger-Ellison syndrome
Zestoretic [lisinopril and hydrochlorothiazide]	ACE inhibitor; antihypertensive	Congestive heart failure; essential hypertension
Zestril [lisinopril]	ACE inhibitor; antihypertensive	Congestive heart failure; essential hypertension
Ziac [bisoprolol fumarate/ hydrochlorothiazide]	Antihypertensive	Essential hypertension
Zithromax [azithromycin]	Macrolide	Infections of the cervix, lower respiratory tract, skin and skin structures, urethra, nongonococcal; mycobacterium avium complex; pharyngitis; streptococcal pneumonia; tonsillitis
Zocor [simvastatin]	HMG-CoA reductase inhibitor (statin)	Hypercholesterolemia, hyperlipidemia, hyperlipoproteinemia, hypertriglyceridemia
Zoloft [sertraline hydrochloride]	Antidepressant	Anxiety with panic disorder and depression; obsessive-compulsive disorder
Zovirax [acyclovir]	Antiviral	Genital herpes and herpes zoster infections
Zyloprim [allopurinol]	Antigout	Gouty arthritis, renal calculus, hyperuricemia, hyperuricemia secondary to leukemia, hyperuricemia secondary to lymphoma
Zyprexa [olanzapine]	Antipsychotic/antimanic	Psychotic disorders; schizophrenia
Zyrtec [cetirizine hydrochloride]	Antihistamine	Perennial allergic and seasonal allergic rhinitis; chronic urticaria

Appendix D: Z Codes for Long-Term Drug Use with Associated Drugs

Z79.01 Long term (current) use of anticoagulants
Arixtra
Coumadin
Eliquis
Heparin
Jantoven
Lovenox
Pradaxa
Warfarin
Xarelto

Z79.02 Long term (current) use of antithrombotics/antiplatelets
Aggrenox
Aggrastat
Clopidogrel
Clopidogrel bisulfate
Effient
Persantine
Plavix
Pletal
Pradaxa
Ticlid

Z79.1 Long term (current) use of non-steroidal anti-inflammatories (NSAID)
Advil
Aleve
Anaprox
Celebrex
Clinoril
Daypro
Feldene
Ibuprofen
Indocin
Lodine
Motrin
Nalfon
Naprosyn
Orudis
Ponstel
Relafen
Tolectin
Toradol
Voltaren

Z79.2 Long term (current) use of antibiotics
Amikin
Amoxicillin
Amoxil
Ampicillin
Ancef
Augmentin
Azactam
Azithromycin
Bactrim
Cefaclor
Ceftriaxone
Cephalexin
Cephalosporin
Cipro
Ciprofloxacin
Clarithromycin
Cleocin
Clindamycin
Co-trimoxazole
Daptomycin
Dificid
Doxycycline
Ertapenem
ERYC
Erythromycin
Factive
Flagyl
Flucloxacillin
Gentamicin
Isoniazid
Invanz
Keflex
Levaquin
Macrobid
Merrem
Metronidazole
Minocin
Nitrofurantoin
Omnipen
Ornidazole
Penicillin G
Penicillin V
Polycillin
Primaxin
Rifampicin
Rocephin
Septra
Streptomycin
Tazicef
Tazocin
Tetracycline HCl
Timentin
Trimethoprim
Tobramycin
Unipen
Vancocin
Vancomycin
Vibramycin
Zinacef
Zithromax
Zosyn
Zyvox

Z79.3 Long term (current) use of hormonal contraceptives
Oral
   Combined oral contraceptive
   Progestin-only pills
Patch
   Ortho Evra
   Injectable
   DMPA—depo medroxyprogesterone acetate
Vaginal Ring
   NuvaRing
Implantable rods
   Implanon

Z79.4 Long term (current) use of insulin
Apidra
Humalog
Humulin
Lantus
Levemir
Novolin
NovoLog
Velosulin

Z79.51 Long term (current) use of inhaled steroids
Advair
Aerospan
Alvesco
Asmanex Twisthaler
Dulera
Flovent
Pulmicort
Qvar
Symbicort

Z79.52 Long term (current) use of systemic steroids
Cortef
Cortisone acetate
Depo-Medrol
Dexamethasone
Hydrocortisone
Kenalog
Medrol
Methylprednisolone
Prednisolone
Prednisone
Solu-Medrol

Z79.810 Long term (current) use of selective estrogen receptor modulators (SERMs)
Evista
Fareston
Nolvadex
Osphena
Raloxifene
Soltamox
Tamoxifen
Toremifene

Z79.811 Long term (current) use of aromatase inhibitors
Anastrozole
Arimidex
Aromasin
Exemestane
Femara
Letrozole

Z79.818 Long term (current) use of other agents affecting estrogen receptors and estrogen levels
Eligard
Faslodex
Fulvestrant
Lupron
Megace

Supprelin La
Synarel
Trelstar
Vantas
Viadur
Zoladex

Z79.82   Long term (current) use of aspirin
Bayer
Ecotrin
Bufferin

Z79.83   Long term (current) use of bisphosphonates
Actonel
Aredia
Atelvia
Binosto
Boniva
Didronel
Fosamax
Reclast
Zometa

Z79.890 Hormone replacement therapy (postmenopausal)
Activella
Alora
Angeliq
Climara
Enjuvia
Estrace
Estratest
EstroGel
Femring

Femtrace
Menostar
Premarin
Provera
Vivelle

Z79.891 Long term (current) use of opiate analgesic
Astramorph
Avinza
Buprenex
Buprenorphine
Codeine
Demerol
Dilaudid
Duragesic
Duramorph
Fentanyl
Fentora
Fioricet with codeine
Hydrocodone
Hydromorphone
Kadian
Lorcet
Lortab
Methadone HCL
Methadose
Morphine
MS Contin
Norco
Oxycodone
OxyContin
Percocet
Roxicodone

Sublimaze
Tylenol with codeine
Ultram

Z79.899 Other long term (current) drug therapy]
Actimmune
Antineoplastic/chemotherapy
Astagraf XL
Avonex
Cellcept
Cyclosporin
Envarsus XR
Gengraf
Imuran
Interferon
Monoclonal antibodies
Neoral
Orthoclone OKT3
Peginterferon
Prograf
Protopic
Rapamune
Rebif
Sandimmune
Simulect
Sirolimus
Sylatron
Tacrolimus
Torisel
Zenapax

Appendix E: Z Code Only as Principal Diagnosis

Z00.00	Z01.21	Z02.5	Z04.1	Z34.80	Z38.64	Z52.011	Z52.819
Z00.01	Z01.30	Z02.6	Z04.2	Z34.81	Z38.65	Z52.018	Z52.89
Z00.110	Z01.31	Z02.71	Z04.3	Z34.82	Z38.66	Z52.090	Z76.1
Z00.111	Z01.411	Z02.79	Z04.41	Z34.83	Z38.68	Z52.091	Z76.2
Z00.121	Z01.419	Z02.81	Z04.42	Z34.90	Z38.69	Z52.098	Z99.12
Z00.129	Z01.42	Z02.82	Z04.6	Z34.91	Z38.7	Z52.10	
Z00.2	Z01.810	Z02.83	Z04.71	Z34.92	Z38.8	Z52.11	
Z00.3	Z01.811	Z02.89	Z04.72	Z34.93	Z39.0	Z52.19	
Z00.5	Z01.812	Z02.9	Z04.8	Z38.00	Z39.1	Z52.20	
Z00.70	Z01.818	Z03.6	Z04.9	Z38.01	Z39.2	Z52.21	
Z00.71	Z01.82	Z03.71	Z31.81	Z38.1	Z42.1	Z52.29	
Z00.8	Z01.83	Z03.72	Z31.82	Z38.2	Z42.8	Z52.3	
Z01.00	Z01.84	Z03.73	Z31.83	Z38.30	Z51.0	Z52.4	
Z01.01	Z01.89	Z03.74	Z31.84	Z38.31	Z51.11	Z52.5	
Z01.10	Z02.0	Z03.75	Z33.2	Z38.4	Z51.12	Z52.6	
Z01.110	Z02.1	Z03.79	Z34.00	Z38.5	Z52.000	Z52.810	
Z01.118	Z02.2	Z03.810	Z34.01	Z38.61	Z52.001	Z52.811	
Z01.12	Z02.3	Z03.818	Z34.02	Z38.62	Z52.008	Z52.812	
Z01.20	Z02.4	Z03.89	Z34.03	Z38.63	Z52.010	Z52.813	

Appendix F: Hospice Criteria for Medicare Coverage of Noncancer Hospice Care

Coverage of Hospice Services Under Hospital Insurance

CMS Manual Publication Number 100-04, *Medicare Claims Processing Manual*, Chapter 11

CMS Manual Publication 100-2, Medicare Benefits Policy Chapter 9

Requirements – General

Hospice care is a benefit under the hospital insurance program. To be eligible to elect hospice care under Medicare, an individual must be entitled to Part A of Medicare and be certified as being terminally ill. An individual is considered to be terminally ill if the medical prognosis is that the individual's life expectancy is six months or less if the illness runs its normal course.

Section §1814(a)(7) of the Social Security Act (the Act) specifies that certification of terminal illness for hospice benefits shall be based on the hospice's physician's and the individual's attending physician if he/she has one or medical director's clinical judgment regarding the normal course of the individual's illness. No one other than a medical doctor or doctor of osteopathy can certify or re-certify a terminal illness. Predicting of life expectancy is not always exact. The fact that a beneficiary lives longer than expected in itself is not cause to terminate benefits. "Attending physician" is further defined in Section 20.1 and 40.2.5. Making medical prognostication of life expectancy is not always exact. If a beneficiary lives longer than expected this in itself is not cause to terminate benefits.

An individual (or his authorized representative) must elect hospice care to receive it. The first election is for a 90-day period. An individual may elect to receive Medicare coverage for an unlimited number of election periods of hospice care. The periods consist of two 90-day periods, and an unlimited number of 60-day periods. If the individual (or authorized representative) elects to receive hospice care, he or she must file an election statement with a particular hospice. Hospices obtain elections from the individual and forward them to the intermediary, which transmits them to the Common Working File (CWF) in electronic format. Once the initial election is processed, CWF maintains the beneficiary in hospice status until death or until an election termination is received.

An individual must waive all rights to Medicare payments for the duration of the election/revocation of hospice care for the following services:

- Hospice care provided by a hospice other than the hospice designated by the individual (unless provided under arrangements made by the designated hospice); and
- Any Medicare services that are related to the treatment of the terminal condition for which hospice care was elected or a related condition or services that are equivalent to hospice care, except for services provided by:
    1. The designated hospice (either directly or under arrangement);
    2. Another hospice under arrangements made by the designated hospice; or
    3. The individual's attending physician, if that physician is not an employee of the designated hospice or receiving compensation from the hospice for those services.

Medicare services for a condition completely unrelated to the terminal condition for which hospice was elected remain available to the patient if he or she is eligible for such care.

Noncancer Hospice Care Eligibility Criteria

Medicare coverage of hospice care depends upon a physician's certification of an individual's prognosis of a life expectancy of six months or less if the terminal illness runs its normal course. Recognizing that determination of life expectancy during the course of a terminal illness is difficult, the following policies were originally developed by the Medicare home health and hospice administrative contractors (HHH MACs) and are included in the resource for guidance only. These medical criteria form a reasonable approach to the determination of prognosis for certain noncancer diagnoses and were found not to be in conflict with any existing CMS national coverage rules and/or regulations. However, some patients may not meet the criteria, yet still be appropriate for hospice care, because of other comorbidities or rapid decline. Coverage for these patients may be approved on an individual consideration basis.

The criteria in each of these policies are considered to be the most accurate parameters to determine Medicare coverage for these specific noncancer diagnoses. As of April 2015, there were four HHH areas handled by three HHH MACs.

As this book goes to press, these local coverage decisions (LCDs) still contained ICD-9-CM diagnosis codes. The editors have replaced the codes with ICD-10-CM diagnosis codes, but these may not match the codes in the LCDs. When the codes have been updated in the LCDs, Optum360 will publish the updated codes on its product website.

Physician Recertification Changes

The Affordable Care Act required hospice physicians or hospice nurse practitioners to have a face-to-face encounter with Medicare hospice patients prior to the 180th-day recertification and every recertification thereafter, and to attest that the encounter occurred. This face-to-face encounter requirement became effective on January 1, 2011.

A hospice physician or hospice nurse practitioner must have a face-to-face encounter with the patient prior to the third benefit period recertification and each subsequent recertification. This encounter can occur up to 30 calendar days prior to recertification, and the hospice physician or nurse practitioner must attest that the visit occurred. The certification or recertification must include the benefit period dates to which it applies, and be signed and dated by the certifying or recertifying physician. Initial certifications may be prepared no more than 15 calendar days prior to the effective date of election. Recertifications may be prepared no more than 15 calendar days prior to the start of the subsequent benefit period.

Hospice certifications and recertifications must include a brief narrative explanation of the clinical findings that support a life expectancy of six months or less. This may be part of the form or as an addendum. Physicians must briefly describe the clinical information supporting the terminal diagnosis and attest that they composed the narrative after reviewing the clinical information and, where applicable, after examining the patient. The narrative must reflect the patient's individual clinical circumstances. Narratives associated with the third and later benefit period must also include an explanation of why the clinical findings of the face-to-face encounter support a life expectancy of six months or less.

The written certification must be on file in the hospice patient's record prior to submission of a claim to the Medicare contractor. A failure to meet the face-to-face encounter requirement would prohibit the hospice from recertifying the patient as being terminally ill, and the patient would cease to be eligible for the Medicare hospice benefit. In such instances, the hospice must discharge the patient from the Medicare hospice benefit because he or she is not considered terminally ill for Medicare purposes. When a discharge from the Medicare hospice benefit occurs due to failure to perform a required face-to-face encounter in a timely way, the claim should include the most appropriate patient discharge status code. The patient can be readmitted when the required encounter is completed if the patient continues to meet all of the eligibility requirements and if the patient files an election statement. When the only reason the patient ceases to be eligible for the Medicare hospice benefit is the hospice's failure to meet the face-to-face requirement, CMS has stated that it expects the hospice to continue to care for the patient at its own expense until the required encounter occurs, enabling the hospice to reestablish Medicare eligibility. Note that occurrence span code 77 does not apply to the above-described situations when the face-to-face encounter has not occurred in a timely manner.

A patient will be considered to have a life expectancy of six months or less if he/she meets the non-disease specific decline in clinical status guidelines described in Part I. Alternatively, the baseline non-disease specific guidelines described in Part II plus the applicable disease specific guidelines listed in the appendix will establish the necessary expectancy.

Part I. Decline in clinical status guidelines

Patients will be considered to have a life expectancy of six months or less if there is documented evidence of decline in clinical status based on the guidelines listed below. Since determination of decline presumes assessment of the patient's status over time, it is essential that both baseline and follow-up determinations be reported where appropriate. Baseline data may be established on admission to hospice or by using existing information from records. Other clinical variables not on this list may support a six-month or less life expectancy. These should be documented in the clinical record.

These changes in clinical variables apply to patients whose decline is not considered to be reversible. They are listed in order of their likelihood to predict poor survival, the most predictive first and the least predictive last. No specific number of variables must be met, but fewer of those listed first (more predictive) and more of those listed last (least predictive) would be expected to predict longevity of six months or less.

Progression of disease as documented by worsening clinical status, symptoms, signs and laboratory results.

1. Clinical Status

   a. Recurrent or intractable infections such as pneumonia, sepsis or upper urinary tract. National Government Services (NGS) adds: or pyelonephritis in place of upper urinary tract)

   b. Progressive inanition as documented by:

      1) Weight loss (NGS states weight loss of at least 10% body weight in the prior six months) not due to reversible causes such as depression or use of diuretics

      2) Decreasing anthropomorphic measurements (mid-arm circumference, abdominal girth), not due to reversible causes such as depression or use of diuretics

      3) Decreasing serum albumin or cholesterol

   c. Dysphagia leading to recurrent aspiration and/or inadequate oral intake documented by decreasing food portion consumption

2. Symptoms

   a. Dyspnea with increasing respiratory rate

   b. Cough, intractable

   c. Nausea/vomiting poorly responsive to treatment

   d. Diarrhea, intractable

   e. Pain requiring increasing doses of major analgesics more than briefly

3. Signs

   a. Decline in systolic blood pressure to below 90 or progressive postural hypotension

   b. Ascites

   c. Venous, arterial or lymphatic obstruction due to local progression or metastatic disease

   d. Edema

   e. Pleural/pericardial effusion

   f. Weakness

   g. Change in level of consciousness

4. Laboratory (When available. Lab testing is not required to establish hospice eligibility.)

   a. Increasing pCO2 or decreasing pO2 or decreasing SaO2

   b. Increasing calcium, creatinine or liver function studies

   c. Increasing tumor markers (e.g. CEA, PSA)

   d. Progressively decreasing or increasing serum sodium or increasing serum potassium

5. Decline in Karnofsky Performance Status (KPS) or Palliative Performance Score (PPS) from < 70% due to progression of disease

6. Progressive decline in Functional Assessment Staging (FAST) for dementia (from ≥ 7A on the FAST)

7. Progression to dependence on assistance with additional activities of daily living. See Part II, Section B

8. Progressive stage 3-4 pressure ulcers in spite of optimal care

9. Increasing emergency room visits, hospitalizations, or physician's visits related to hospice primary diagnosis

Part II. Non-disease specific baseline guidelines (both of these should be met)

A. Physiologic impairment of functional status as demonstrated by: Karnofsky Performance Status (KPS) or Palliative Performance Score (PPS) < 70%. Note that two of the disease specific guidelines (HIV Disease, Stroke and Coma) establish a lower qualifying KPS or PPS.

B. Dependence on assistance for two or more activities of daily living (ADLs)

   1. Ambulation
   2. Continence
   3. Transfer
   4. Dressing
   5. Feeding
   6. Bathing

Part III. Co-morbidities

Although not the primary hospice diagnosis, the presence of disease such as the following, the severity of which is likely to contribute to a life expectancy of six months or less, should be considered in determining hospice eligibility.

   A. Chronic obstructive pulmonary disease
   B. Congestive heart failure
   C. Ischemic heart disease
   D. Diabetes mellitus
   E. Neurologic disease (CVA, ALS, MS, Parkinson's)
   F. Renal failure
   G. Liver Disease
   H. Neoplasia
   I. Acquired immune deficiency syndrome
   J. Dementia

(NGS adds: Refractory severe autoimmune disease [e.g., lupus or rheumatoid arthritis])

Hospice HIV Disease

L31535, Palmetto GBA (PGBA); L32015, CGS Administrators, LLC (CGS); L25678, National Government Services (NGS)

Indications and limitations of coverage and/or medical necessity:

Patients will be considered to be in the terminal stage of their illness (life expectancy of six months or less) if they meet the following criteria (1 and 2 must be present; factors from 3 will add supporting documentation):

1. CD4+ Count < 25 cells/mcL or persistent viral load > l00,000 copies/ml, plus one of the following:

   • CNS lymphoma

   • Untreated, or not responsive to treatment, wasting (loss of 33% lean body mass per Palmetto; loss of at least 10% lean body mass per NGS and CGS)

   • Mycobacterium avium complex (MAC) bacteremia, untreated, unresponsive to treatment, or treatment refused

   • Progressive multifocal leukoencephalopathy

   • Systemic lymphoma, with advanced HIV disease and partial response to chemotherapy

   • Visceral Kaposi's sarcoma unresponsive to therapy

   • Renal failure in the absence of dialysis

   • Cryptosporidium infection

   • Toxoplasmosis, unresponsive to therapy

2. Decreased performance status, as measured by the Karnofsky Performance Status (KPS) scale, of less than 50%

3. Documentation of the following factors will support eligibility for hospice care:

   • Chronic persistent diarrhea for one year

   • Persistent serum albumin <2.5

   • Concomitant, active substance abuse

   • Age > 50 years

   • Absence of (CGS and NGS add "or resistance to effective") antiretroviral, chemotherapeutic and prophylactic drug therapy related specifically to HIV disease

   • Advanced AIDS dementia complex

   • Toxoplasmosis

   • Congestive heart failure, symptomatic at rest

   • Advanced liver disease (per CGS and NGS)

ICD-10-CM codes that support medical necessity

   B20 Human immunodeficiency virus (HIV) disease

Hospice Pulmonary Disease

L32015, CGS Administrators, LLC(CGS); L25678, National Government Services (NGS)

Indications and limitations of coverage and/or medical necessity:

Patients will be considered to be in the terminal stage of pulmonary disease (life expectancy of six months or less) if they meet the following criteria. The criteria refer to patients with various forms of advanced pulmonary disease who eventually follow a final common pathway for end stage pulmonary disease. (1 and 2 must be present. Documentation of 3, 4, and/or 5 will lend supporting documentation.):

1. Severe chronic lung disease as documented by both a and b:

   a. Disabling dyspnea at rest, poorly or unresponsive to bronchodilators, resulting in decreased functional capacity, e.g., bed to chair existence, fatigue, and cough: (Documentation of Forced Expiratory Volume in one second (FEV1), after bronchodilator, less than 30% of predicated is objective evidence for disabling dyspnea, but is not necessary to obtain.)

   b. Progression of end stage pulmonary disease, as evidenced by prior increasing visits to the emergency department or hospitalizations for pulmonary infections and/or respiratory failure. (Documentation of serial decrease of FEV1 >40 ml/year is objective evidence for disease progression, but is not necessary to obtain.)

2. Hypoxemia at rest on room air, as evidenced by $p0_2 \leq 55$ mmHg or oxygen saturation $\leq 88\%$. (These values may be obtained from recent hospital records.) Or hypercapnia, as evidenced by $pCO_2 \geq 50$ mmHg. (This value may be obtained from recent hospital records.)

3. Cor pulmonale and right heart failure (RHF) secondary to pulmonary disease (e.g., not secondary to left heart disease or valvulopathy).

4. Unintentional progressive weight loss of greater than 10% of body weight over the preceding six months.

5. Resting tachycardia >100 beats/min.

There is no ICD-10-CM code for end stage pulmonary disease. Diagnoses for pulmonary disease which lead to end stage pulmonary disease will be accepted.

Hospice Stroke and Coma

L32015, CGS Administrators, LLC(CGS); L25678, National Government Services (NGS)

Indications and limitations of coverage and/or medical necessity: Patients will be considered to be in the terminal stage of stroke or coma (life expectancy of six months or less) if they meet the following criteria.

Stroke:

1. Poor functional status with Karnofsky score 40% or less;

2. Inability to maintain hydration and caloric intake with one of the following:

   - Weight loss > 10% in the last 6 months or > 7.5% in the last 3 months

   - Serum albumin < 2.5 gm/dl

   - Current history of pulmonary aspiration not responsive to speech language pathology intervention; Sequential calorie counts documenting inadequate caloric/fluid intake

   - Dysphagia severe enough to prevent patient from continuing fluids/foods necessary to sustain life and patient does not receive artificial nutrition and hydration

Coma (any etiology):

1. Comatose patients with any three of the following on day three of coma:

   - Abnormal brain stem response

   - Absent verbal response

   - Absent withdrawal response to pain

   - Serum creatinine >1.5 mg/dl

Documentation of the following factors will support eligibility for hospice care:

1. Documentation of medical complications, in the context of progressive clinical decline, within the previous 12 months, which support a terminal prognosis:

   - Aspiration pneumonia

   - Upper urinary tract infection (pyelonephritis)

   - Sepsis

   - Refractory stage 3-4 decubitus ulcers

   - Fever recurrent after antibiotics

Documentation of diagnostic imaging factors which support poor prognosis after stroke include:

A. For non-traumatic hemorrhagic stroke:

   - Large-volume hemorrhage on CT:

     – Infratentorial: 20 ml.

     – Supratentorial: 50 ml.

   - Ventricular extension of hemorrhage

   - Surface area of involvement of hemorrhage ≥30% of cerebrum.

   - Midline shift ≥1.5 cm.

   - Obstructive hydrocephalus in patient who declines, or is not a candidate for, ventriculoperitoneal shunt.

B. For thrombotic/embolic stroke:

   - Large anterior infarcts with both cortical and subcortical involvement.

   - Large bihemispheric infarcts.

   - Basilar artery occlusion.

   - Bilateral vertebral artery occlusion.

ICD-10-CM codes that support medical necessity:

I60.00–I60.9	Nontraumatic subarachnoid hemorrhage
I61.0–I61.9	Nontraumatic intercerebral hemorrhage
I62.00–I62.9	Other and unspecified nontraumatic intracranial hemorrhage
I63.00–I63.9	Cerebral infarction due to occlusion and stenosis of cerebral and precerebral arteries
I65.01–I65.9	Occlusion and stenosis of precerebral arteries not resulting in cerebral infarction
I66.01–I66.9	Occlusion and stenosis of cerebral arteries not resulting in cerebral infarction
R40.20–R40.244	Coma

Hospice Alzheimer's Disease and Related Disorders

L32015, CGS Administrators, LLC (CGS); L25678, National Government Services (NGS); L31539, Palmetto GBA (PGBA)

The following criteria based on the FAST scale is from the PGBA local coverage determination.

The Reisberg Functional Assessment Staging (FAST) Scale has been used for many years to describe Medicare beneficiaries with Alzheimer's disease and a prognosis of six months or less. The FAST Scale is a 16-item scale designed to parallel the progressive activity limitations associated with Alzheimer's disease. Stage 7 identifies the threshold of activity limitation that would support a six-month prognosis. The FAST Scale does not address the impact of comorbid and secondary conditions. These two variables are thus considered separately by this policy.

FAST Scale Items:

Stage #1: No difficulty, either subjectively or objectively

Stage #2: Complains of forgetting location of objects; subjective work difficulties

Stage #3: Decreased job functioning evident to coworkers; difficulty in traveling to new locations

Stage #4: Decreased ability to perform complex tasks (e.g., planning dinner for guests; handling finances)

Stage #5: Requires assistance in choosing proper clothing

Stage #6: Decreased ability to dress, bathe, and toilet independently:

   - Sub-stage 6a: Difficulty putting clothing on properly

   - Sub-stage 6b: Unable to bathe properly; may develop fear of bathing

   - Sub-stage 6c: Inability to handle mechanics of toileting (i.e., forgets to flush, does not wipe properly)

   - Sub-stage 6d: Urinary incontinence

   - Sub-stage 6e: Fecal incontinence

Stage #7: Loss of speech, locomotion, and consciousness:

   - Sub-stage 7a: Ability to speak limited (1 to 5 words a day)

   - Sub-stage 7b: All intelligible vocabulary lost

   - Sub-stage 7c: Non-ambulatory

   - Sub-stage 7d: Unable to sit up independently

   - Sub-stage 7e: Unable to smile

   - Sub-stage 7f: Unable to hold head up

Comorbid Conditions:

The significance of a given comorbid condition is best described by defining the structural/functional impairments - together with any limitation in activity - related to the comorbid condition. For example, a beneficiary with Alzheimer's disease and clinically significant CHD or COPD would have specific impairments of cardiorespiratory function (e.g., dyspnea, orthopnea, wheezing, chest pain) which may or may not respond/be amenable to treatment. The identified impairments in cardiorespiratory function would be associated with both specific structural impairments of the coronary arteries or bronchial tree and may be associated with activity limitations (e.g., mobility, self-care). Ultimately, the combined effects of the Alzheimer's disease (stage 7) and any comorbid condition should be such that most beneficiaries with Alzheimer's disease and similar impairments would have a prognosis of six months or less.

Secondary Conditions:

Alzheimer's disease may be complicated by secondary conditions. The significance of a given secondary condition is best described by defining the structural/functional impairments - together with any limitation in activity related to the secondary condition. The occurrence of secondary conditions in beneficiaries with Alzheimer's disease is facilitated by the presence of impairments in such body functions as mental functioning and movement functions. Such functional impairments contribute to the increased incidence of secondary conditions such as delirium and pressure ulcers observed in Medicare beneficiaries with Alzheimer's Disease. Secondary conditions themselves may be associated with a new set of structural/functional impairments that may or may not respond/be amenable to treatment. Ultimately, the combined effects of the Alzheimer's disease (stage 7) and any secondary condition should be such that most beneficiaries with Alzheimer's disease and similar impairments would have a prognosis of six months or less.

The documentation of structural/functional impairments and activity limitations facilitate the selection of intervention strategies (palliative vs. curative) and provide objective criteria for determining the effects of such interventions. The documentation of these variables is thus essential in the determination of reasonable and necessary Medicare Hospice Services.

For beneficiaries with Alzheimer's disease to be eligible for hospice the individual should have a FAST level of greater than or equal to 7 and specific comorbid or secondary conditions meeting the above criteria.

ICD-10-CM codes that support medical necessity:

F03.90–F03.91	Unspecified dementia
G30.0–G30.9	Alzheimer's disease
G31.01–G31.09	Pick's disease and other frontotemporal dementia
G31.1	Senile degeneration of brain, not elsewhere classified

The following criteria are from the CGS and NGS local coverage determinations.

Patients will be considered to be in the terminal stage of dementia (life expectancy of six months or less) if they meet the following criteria. This section is specific for Alzheimer's disease and related disorders and is not appropriate for other types of dementia.

1. Patients with dementia should show all the following characteristics:
   a. Stage seven or beyond according to the Functional Assessment Staging Scale;
   b. Unable to ambulate without assistance;
   c. Unable to dress without assistance;
   d. Unable to bathe without assistance;
   e. Urinary and fecal incontinence, intermittent or constant;
   f. No consistently meaningful verbal communication: stereotypical phrases only or the ability to speak is limited to six or fewer intelligible words.

2. Patients should have had one of the following within the past 12 months:
   a. Aspiration pneumonia;
   b. Pyelonephritis (NGS adds "or other upper urinary tract infection");
   c. Septicemia;
   d. Decubitus ulcers, multiple, stage 3-4;
   e. Fever, recurrent after antibiotics;
   f. Inability to maintain sufficient fluid and calorie intake with 10% weight loss during the previous six months or serum albumin < 2.5 gm/dl.

ICD-10 Codes That Support Medical Necessity

F03.90–F03.91	Unspecified dementia
G30.0–G30.9	Alzheimer's disease
G31.01–G31.09	Pick's disease and other frontotemporal dementia
G31.1	Senile degeneration of brain, not elsewhere classified
G31.85	Corticobasal degeneration

Hospice Amyotrophic Lateral Sclerosis (ALS)

L32015, CGS Administrators, LLC (CGS); L25678, National Government Services (NGS); L31536, Palmetto GBA (PGBA)

Indications and limitations of coverage and/or medical necessity:

General Considerations:

1. ALS tends to progress in a linear fashion over time. Thus the overall rate of decline in each patient is fairly constant and predictable, unlike many other non-cancer diseases.

2. However, no single variable deteriorates at a uniform rate in all patients. Therefore, multiple clinical parameters are required to judge the progression of ALS.

3. Although ALS usually presents in a localized anatomical area, the location of initial presentation does not correlate with survival time. By the time patients become end-stage, muscle denervation has become widespread, affecting all areas of the body, and initial predominance patterns do not persist.

4. Progression of disease differs markedly from patient to patient. Some patients decline rapidly and die quickly; others progress more slowly. For this reason, the history of the rate of progression in individual patients is important to obtain to predict prognosis.

5. In end-stage ALS, two factors are critical in determining prognosis: ability to breathe, and to a lesser extent ability to swallow. The former can be managed by artificial ventilation, and the latter by gastrostomy or other artificial feeding, unless the patient has recurrent aspiration pneumonia. While not necessarily a contraindication to hospice care, the decision to institute either artificial ventilation or artificial feeding will significantly alter six month prognosis.

6. Examination by a neurologist within three months of assessment for hospice is advised, both to confirm the diagnosis and to assist with prognosis.

CGS specifics:

Patients will be considered to be in the terminal stage of ALS (life expectancy of six months or less) if they meet the following criteria: (Must fulfill 1, 2, or 3.)

1. The patient must demonstrate critically impaired breathing capacity.
   a. Critically impaired breathing capacity as demonstrated by all the following characteristics occurring within the 12 months preceding initial hospice certification:
      – Vital capacity (VC) less than 30% of normal
      – Significant dyspnea at rest
      – Requiring supplemental oxygen at rest
      – Patient declines invasive artificial ventilation.

2. Patient must demonstrate both rapid progression of ALS and critical nutritional impairment.
   a. Rapid progression of ALS as demonstrated by all the following characteristics occurring within the 12 months preceding initial hospice certification:
      – Progression from independent ambulation to wheelchair or bed-bound status;
      – Progression from normal to barely intelligible or unintelligible speech;
      – Progression from normal to pureed diet;
      – Progression from independence in most or all activities of daily living (ADLs) to needing major assistance by caretaker in all ADLs.
   b. Critical nutritional impairment as demonstrated by all the following characteristics occurring within the 12 months preceding initial hospice certification:
      – Oral intake of nutrients and fluids insufficient to sustain life;
      – Continuing weight loss;
      – Dehydration or hypovolemia;
      – Absence of artificial feeding methods.

3. Patient must demonstrate both rapid progression of ALS and life-threatening complications
   a. Rapid progression of ALS, see 2.a. above.
   b. Life-threatening complications as demonstrated by one of the following characteristics occurring within the 12 months preceding initial hospice certification:
      – Recurrent aspiration pneumonia (with or without tube feedings);
      – Upper urinary tract infection, e.g., pyelonephritis;
      – Sepsis;
      – Recurrent fever after antibiotic therapy.

NGS specifics:

Patients are considered eligible for Hospice care if they do not elect tracheostomy and invasive ventilation and display evidence of critically impaired respiratory function (with or without use of NIPPV) and/or severe nutritional insufficiency (with or without use of a gastrostomy tube).

Critically impaired respiratory function is as defined by:

1. FVC < 40% predicted (seated or supine) and 2 or more of the following symptoms and/or signs:

Dyspnea at rest

Orthopnea

Use of accessory respiratory musculature

Paradoxical abdominal motion

Respiratory rate > 20

Reduced speech/vocal volume

Weakened cough

Symptoms of sleep disordered breathing

Frequent awakening

Daytime somnolence / excessive daytime sleepiness

Unexplained headaches

Unexplained confusion

Unexplained anxiety

Unexplained nausea

2. If unable to perform the FVC test, patients meet this criterion if they manifest 3 or more of the above symptoms/signs.

    Severe nutritional insufficiency is defined as:

    Dysphagia with progressive weight loss of at least 5% of body weight with or without election for gastrostomy tube insertion.

    These revised criteria rely less on the measured FVC, and as such reflect the reality that not all patients with ALS can or will undertake regular pulmonary function tests.

ICD-10-CM codes that support medical necessity:

G12.21   Amyotrophic lateral sclerosis

Hospice Liver Disease

L32015, CGS Administrators, LLC (CGS); L25678, National Government Services (NGS); L31536,] Palmetto GBA (PGBA)

Indications and limitations of coverage and/or medical necessity:

Patients will be considered to be in the terminal stage of liver disease (life expectancy of six months or less) if they meet the following criteria: (1 and 2 must be present, factors from 3 will lend supporting documentation.)

1. The patient should show both a and b:

    a. Prothrombin time prolonged more than 5 seconds over control, or International Normalized Ration (INR) >1.5;

    b. Serum albumin < 2.5 gm/dl.

2. End stage liver disease is present and the patient shows at least one of the following:

    a. Ascites, refractory to treatment or patient noncompliant;

    b. Spontaneous bacterial peritonitis;

    c. Hepatorenal syndrome (elevated creatinine and BUN with oliguria (< 400 ml/day) and urine sodium concentration <10 mEq/l);

    d. Hepatic encephalopathy, refractory to treatment, or patient noncompliant;

    e. Recurrent variceal bleeding, despite intensive therapy.

3. Documentation of the following factors will support eligibility for hospice care:

    a. Progressive malnutrition

    b. Muscle wasting with reduced strength and endurance

    c. Continued active alcoholism (>80 gm ethanol/day)

    d. Hepatocellular carcinoma

    e. HBsAg (Hepatitis B) positivity

    f. Hepatitis C refractory to interferon treatment.

CGS and PGBA add:

Patients awaiting liver transplant who otherwise fit the above criteria may be certified for the Medicare hospice benefit, but if a donor organ is procured, the patient must be discharged from hospice.

ICD-10-CM codes that support medical necessity:

B15.0	Hepatitis A with hepatic coma
B15.2, B16.0	Hepatitis B with hepatic coma
B17.11	Hepatitis C with hepatic coma
B18.0–B18.9	Chronic viral hepatitis
B19.0	Unspecified viral hepatitis with hepatic coma
B19.11	Unspecified viral hepatitis B with hepatic coma
B19.21	Unspecified viral hepatitis C with hepatic coma

K70.30–K70.31	Alcoholic cirrhosis of liver
K72.10–K72.11	Chronic hepatic failure
K73.0–K73.9	Chronic hepatitis not elsewhere classified
K74.3–K74.5	Biliary cirrhosis
K74.60–K74.69	Other and unspecified cirrhosis of liver
K75.81	Hepatopulmonary syndrome

Hospice Renal Disease

L32015, CGS Administrators, LLC (CGS); L25678, National Government Services (NGS); L31538, Palmetto GBA (PGBA)

Indications and limitations of coverage and/or medical necessity:

Patients will be considered to be in the terminal stage of renal disease (life expectancy of six months or less) if they meet the following criteria:

CGS criteria:

Acute renal failure (1, 2, and 3 must be present; factors from 4 will lend supporting documentation):

1. The patient is not seeking dialysis or renal transplant;

2. Creatinine clearance <10 cc/min (<15 cc/min. for diabetes); based on measurement or calculation; or <15cc/min (<20cc/min for diabetics) with comorbidity of congestive heart failure;

3. Serum creatinine >8.0 mg/dl (>6.0 mg/dl for diabetes)

4. Comorbid conditions:

    *   Mechanical ventilation;

    *   Malignancy (other organ system);

    *   Chronic lung disease;

    *   Advanced cardiac disease;

    *   Advanced liver disease;

    *   Sepsis;

    *   Immunosuppression/AIDS;

    *   Albumin < 3.5 gm/dl;

    *   Cachexia;

    *   Platelet count < 25,000;

    *   Disseminated intravascular coagulation;

    *   Gastrointestinal bleeding.

Chronic renal failure (1, 2, and 3 must be present; factors from 4 will lend supporting documentation):

1. The patient is not seeking dialysis or renal transplant or is discontinuing dialysis;

2. Creatinine clearance <10 cc/min (<15 cc/min for diabetics) based on measurement or calculation; or < 15cc/min (< 20cc/min for diabetics) with co-morbidity of congestive heart failure

3. Serum creatinine > 8.0 mg/dl (> 6.0 mg/dl for diabetes);

4. Signs and symptoms of renal failure:

    *   Uremia;

    *   Oliguria (< 400 cc/24 hours);

    *   Intractable hyperkalemia (> 7.0) not responsive to treatment;

    *   Uremic pericarditis;

    *   Hepatorenal syndrome;

    *   Intractable fluid overload, not responsive to treatment.

NGS criteria:

Patients will be considered to be in the terminal stage of renal disease (life expectancy of six months or less) if they meet the following criteria.

Acute Renal Failure (1 and either 2, 3 or 4 should be present. Factors from 5 will lend supporting documentation.)

1. The patient is not seeking dialysis or renal transplant, or is discontinuing dialysis. As with any other condition, an individual with renal disease is eligible for the Hospice benefit if that individual has a prognosis of six months or less, if the illness runs its normal course. There is no regulation precluding patients on dialysis from electing Hospice care. However, the continuation of dialysis will significantly alter a patient's prognosis, and thus potentially impact that individual's eligibility.

    When an individual elects Hospice care for end stage renal disease (ESRD) or for a condition to which the need for dialysis is related, the Hospice agency is financially responsible for the dialysis. In such cases, there is no additional reimbursement beyond the per diem rate. The only situation in which a beneficiary may access both the Hospice benefit and the ESRD benefit is when the need for dialysis is not related to the patient's terminal illness.

2. Creatinine clearance <10 cc/min (<15 cc/min. for diabetics); or <15cc/min (<20cc/min for diabetics) with comorbidity of congestive heart failure.

3. Serum creatinine > 8.0 mg/dl (>6.0 mg/dl for diabetics).

4. Estimated glomerular filtration rate (GFR) <10 ml/min.

5. Comorbid conditions:

   a. Mechanical ventilation;

   b. Malignancy (other organ system);

   c. Chronic lung disease;

   d. Advanced cardiac disease;

   e. Advanced liver disease;

   f. Immunosuppression/AIDS;

   g. Albumin < 3.5 gm/dl;

   h. Platelet count < 25,000;

   i. Disseminated intravascular coagulation;

   j. Gastrointestinal bleeding.

Chronic Kidney Disease (1 and either 2, 3 or 4 should be present. Factors from 5 will lend supporting documentation.)

1. The patient is not seeking dialysis or renal transplant, or is discontinuing dialysis; As with any other condition, an individual with renal disease is eligible for the Hospice benefit if that individual has a prognosis of six months or less, if the illness runs its normal course. There is no regulation precluding patients on dialysis from electing Hospice care. However, the continuation of dialysis will significantly alter a patient's prognosis, and thus potentially impact that individual's eligibility.

   When an individual elects hospice care for end stage renal disease (ESRD) or for a condition to which the need for dialysis is related, the Hospice agency is financially responsible for the dialysis. In such cases, there is no additional reimbursement beyond the per diem rate. The only situation in which a beneficiary may access both the Hospice benefit and the ESRD benefit is when the need for dialysis is not related to the patient's terminal illness.

2. Creatinine clearance <10 cc/min (<15 cc/min for diabetics); or <15cc/min (<20cc/min for diabetics) with comorbidity of congestive heart failure.

3. Serum creatinine >8.0 mg/dl (>6.0 mg/dl for diabetics).

4. Signs and symptoms of renal failure:

   a. Uremia;

   b. Oliguria (<400 cc/24 hours);

   c. Intractable hyperkalemia (> 7.0) not responsive to treatment;

   d. Uremic pericarditis;

   e. Hepatorenal syndrome;

   f. Intractable fluid overload, not responsive to treatment.

5. Estimated glomerular filtration rate (GFR) <10 ml/min.

ICD-10-CM codes that support medical necessity:

I12.0	Hypertensive chronic kidney disease with stage 5 chronic kidney disease or end stage renal disease
N17.0	Acute kidney failure with tubular necrosis
N17.1	Acute kidney failure with acute cortical necrosis
N17.2	Acute kidney failure with medullary necrosis
N17.8	Other acute kidney failure
N17.9	Acute kidney failure, unspecified
N18.6	End stage renal disease
N18.9	Chronic renal; disease, unspecified
N19	Unspecified kidney failure

Hospice Heart Disease

L32015, CGS Administrators, LLC (CGS); L25678, National Government Services (NGS); L31540, Palmetto GBA (PGBA)

Indications and limitations of coverage and/or medical necessity:

NGS and CGS criteria:

Patients will be considered to be in the terminal stage of heart disease (life expectancy of six months or less) if they meet the following criteria (I and 2 mus be present. Factors from 3 will add supporting documentation.):

1. At the time of initial certification or recertification for hospice, the patient is or has been already optimally treated for heart disease or is not a candidate for a surgical procedure or has declined a procedure. (Optimally treated means that patients who are not on vasodilators have a medical reason for refusing these drugs, e.g., hypotension or renal disease.)

2. The patient is classified as New York Heart Association (NYHA) Class IV and may have significant symptoms of heart failure or angina at rest. (Class IV Patients with heart disease have an inability to carry on any physical activity without discomfort. Symptoms of heart failure or of the anginal syndrome may be present even at rest. If any physical activity is undertaken, discomfor is increased.) Significant congestive heart failure may be documented by an ejection fraction of ≤20%, but is not required if not already available.

3. Documentation of the following factors will support eligibility for hospice care:

   • Treatment-resistant symptomatic supraventricular or ventricular arrhythmias;

   • History of cardiac arrest or resuscitation;

   • History of unexplained syncope;

   • Brain embolism of cardiac origin;

   • Concomitant HIV disease.

ICD-10-CM codes that support medical necessity:

I09.81	Rheumatic heart failure
I11.0	Hypertensive heart disease with heart failure
I13.0	Hypertensive heart and chronic kidney disease with heart failure and stage 1 through 4 chronic kidney disease or unspecified chronic kidney disease
I13.2	Hypertensive heart and chronic kidney disease with heart failure and with stage 5 chronic kidney disease or end stage renal disease
I50.1	Left ventricular failure
I50.20–I50.23	Systolic (congestive) heart failure
I50.30–I50.33	Diastolic (congestive) heart failure
I50.40–I50.43	Combined systolic (congestive) and diastolic (congestive) hear failure
I50.9	Heart failure, unspecified

Source of Information

Social Security Act, Sections, 1102, 1812 (a)(4)and (d);1813 (a) (4); 1814 (a)(7) and (I); 1862 (a)(1),(6), and (9); 1861 (dd), 1871

42 CFR Part 418

CMS Manual Publication 100-2, Medicare Benefits Policy Chapter 9 Coverage of Hospice Services under Hospital Insurance, §10 Requirements

CMS Manual Publication 100-3, Medicare National Coverage Determinations

CMS Medicare Coverage Database:

http://www.cms.hhs.gov/mcd/search.asp? Search: Local Coverage, policies (LMRP/LCD); Final policies only Geographic area: all states Coverage topics: Hospice

Appendix G: Hospice Diagnosis and Quality Reporting Guidance

Highlights of the 2015 Hospice Final Rule

Hospice Cap Determinations and Overpayment Remittances

Effective for the 2016 cap year (November 1, 2015, through October 31, 2016), the IMPACT Act requires that the cap amount for the previous year be updated by the hospice payment update percentage, rather than the original $6,500 being annually adjusted by the change in the CPI–U for medical care expenditures since 1984. This new provision will sunset for cap years ending after September 30, 2025, at which time the annual update to the cap amount will revert back to the original methodology. This provision is expected to result in $540 million in savings over 10 years starting in 2017.

The hospice aggregate cap amount for the 2015 cap year, starting on November 1, 2014, and ending on October 31, 2015, will be $27,135.96. This amount was calculated by multiplying the original cap amount of $6,500 by the change in the CPI–U medical care expenditure category, from the fifth month of the 1984 accounting year (March 1984) to the fifth month of the current accounting year (in this case, March 2015). The CPI–U for medical care expenditures for 1984 to present is available from the Bureau of Labor Statistics (BLS) web site.

The hospice aggregate cap amount for the 2016 cap year, starting on November 1, 2015, and ending on October 31, 2016, will be the 2015 cap amount updated by the FY 2016 hospice payment update percentage. As such, the 2016 cap amount will be $27,624.41 ($27,135.96 * 1.018 = $27,624.41).

When the Medicare hospice benefit was implemented, the Congress included two limits on payments to hospices: an aggregate cap and an inpatient cap. The intent of the hospice aggregate cap was to protect Medicare from spending more for hospice care than it would for conventional care at the end-of-life. If a hospice's total Medicare payments for the cap year exceed such hospice's aggregate cap amount, then the hospice must repay the excess back to Medicare. The intent of the inpatient cap was to ensure that hospice remained a home-based benefit. If a hospice's inpatient days (GIP and respite) exceed 20 percent of all hospice days then, for inpatient care, the hospice is paid: (1) the sum of the total reimbursement for inpatient care multiplied by the ratio of the maximum number of allowable inpatient days to actual number of all inpatient days; and (2) the sum of the actual number of inpatient days in excess of the limitation by the routine home care rate.

The aggregate cap amount for any given hospice is established by multiplying the cap amount by the number of Medicare beneficiaries who received hospice services during the year. Originally, the number of Medicare beneficiaries who received hospice services during the year was determined using a "streamlined" methodology whereby each beneficiary is counted as one in the initial cap year of the hospice election and is not counted in subsequent cap years. Specifically, the hospice includes in its number of Medicare beneficiaries those Medicare beneficiaries who have not previously been included in the calculation of any hospice cap, and who have filed an election to receive hospice care during the period beginning on September 28th (34 days before the beginning of the cap year) and ending on September 27th (35 days before the end of the cap year), using the best data available at the time of the calculation. This is applicable for cases in which a beneficiary received care from only one hospice. If a beneficiary received care from more than one hospice, each hospice includes in its number of Medicare beneficiaries only that fraction which represents the portion of a patient's total days of care with that hospice in that cap year, using the best data available at the time of the calculation. Using the streamlined method, a different timeframe from the cap year is used to count the number of Medicare beneficiaries because it allows those beneficiaries who elected hospice near the end of the cap year to be counted in the year when most of the services were provided.

During FY 2012 rule making, CMS added a "patient-by-patient proportional" method as a way of calculating the number of Medicare beneficiaries who received hospice services during the year in determining the aggregate cap amount for any given hospice. This method specifies that a hospice should include in its number of Medicare beneficiaries only that fraction which represents the portion of a patient's total days of care in all hospices and all years that was spent in that hospice in that cap year, using the best data available at the time of the calculation. The total number of Medicare beneficiaries for a given hospice's cap year is determined by summing the whole or fractional share of each Medicare beneficiary that received hospice care during the cap year, from that hospice. Under the patient-by-patient proportional methodology, the timeframe for counting the number of Medicare beneficiaries is the same as the cap accounting year (November 1 through October 31). The aggregate cap amount for each hospice is now calculated using the patient-by-patient proportional method, except for those hospices that had their cap determination calculated under the streamlined method prior to the 2012 cap year, did not

appeal the streamlined method used to determine the number of Medicare beneficiaries used in the aggregate cap calculation, and opted to continue to have their hospice aggregate cap calculated using the streamlined method no later than 60 days after receipt of its 2012 cap determination.

The cap accounting year is currently November 1 to October 31. In the past, CMS has considered changing the cap accounting year to coincide with the hospice rate update year. The majority of providers now use the patient-by-patient proportional method; there is no longer an advantage to defining the cap accounting year differently from the hospice rate update year and maintaining a cap accounting year (as well as the period for counting beneficiaries under the streamlined method) that is different from the federal fiscal year creates an added layer of complexity that can lead to hospices unintentionally calculating their aggregate cap determinations incorrectly. In addition, shifting the cap accounting year timeframes to coincide with the hospice rate update year (the federal fiscal year) would better align with the intent of the new cap calculation methodology required by the IMPACT Act of 2014.

CMS is proposing to align the cap accounting year for both the inpatient cap and the hospice aggregate cap with the federal fiscal year for FYs 2017 and later. Under this proposal, in addition to aligning the cap accounting year with the federal fiscal year, the agency would also align the timeframe for counting the number of beneficiaries with the federal fiscal year. This proposal would eliminate timeframe complexities associated with counting payments and beneficiaries differently from the federal fiscal year and would help hospices avoid mistakes in calculating their aggregate cap determinations. IMPACT Act requires the cap amount for 2016 to be updated by the hospice payment update percentage in effect "during the FY beginning on the October 1 preceding the beginning of the accounting year." In other words, this means that the statute requires the 2016 cap amount to be updated using the most current hospice payment update percentage in effect at the start of that cap year. For the 2016 cap year, the 2015 cap amount would be updated by the FY 2016 hospice payment update percentage. For the 2017 cap year through the 2025 cap year, CMS would update the previous year's cap amount by the hospice payment update percentage for that current federal fiscal year. For the 2026 cap year and beyond, changing the cap accounting year to coincide with the federal fiscal year will require CMS to use the CPI–U for February when updating the cap amount, instead of the current process which uses the March CPI–U to update the cap amount.

CMS is required to update the cap amount by the same percentage as the percentage increase or decrease in the medical care expenditure category of the CPI–U from March 1984 to the "fifth month of the accounting year" for all years except those accounting years that end after September 30, 2016, and before October 1, 2025. In shifting the cap year to match the federal fiscal year, CMS proposes to also align the timeframes in which beneficiaries and payments are counted for the purposes of determining each individual hospice's aggregate cap amount as well as the timeframes in which days of hospice care are counted for the purposes of determining whether a given hospice exceeded the inpatient cap. In the year of transition (2017 cap year), for the inpatient cap, CMS proposes to calculate the percentage of all hospice days of care that were provided as inpatient days (GIP care and respite care) from November 1, 2016, through September 30, 2017 (11 months). For those hospices using the patient-by-patient proportional method for their aggregate cap determinations, for the 2017 cap year, CMS would count beneficiaries from November 1, 2016, to September 30, 2017. For those hospices using the streamlined method for their aggregate cap determinations, CMS proposes to allow three extra days to count beneficiaries in the year of transition. Specifically, for the 2017 cap year (October 1, 2016, to September 30, 2017), CMS would count beneficiaries from September 28, 2016, to September 30, 2017, which is 12 months plus 3 days, in that cap year's calculation. For hospices using either the streamlined method or the patient-by- patient proportional method, CMS proposes to count 11 months of payments from November 1, 2016, to September 30, 2017, for the 2017 cap year. For the 2018 cap year (October 1, 2017, to September 30, 2018), CMS would count both beneficiaries and payments for hospices using the streamlined or the patient-by-patient proportional methods from October 1, 2017, to September 30, 2018. Likewise, for the 2018 cap year CMS would calculate the percentage of all hospice days of care that were provided as inpatient days (GIP care or respite care) from October 1, 2017, to September 30, 2018. Because of the nondiscretionary language used by Congress in determining the cap for a year, the actual cap amount for the adjustment year would not be prorated for a shorter time frame.

Filing the Notice of Election and Notice of Termination/Revocation

The Medicare hospice benefit requires a patient (or representative) to intentionally choose hospice care through a notice of election (NOE). As part of that election, patients (or their representative) acknowledge that they fully understand the palliative, rather than curative, nature of hospice care. Another important aspect of the election is a waiver of beneficiary rights to Medicare payment for any Medicare services related to the terminal illness and related conditions during a hospice election except when provided by, or under arrangement by, the designated hospice, or by the individual's attending physician if he/she is not employed by the designated hospice. This waiver prevents providers other than the designated hospice or attending physician from receiving payment for services to a hospice beneficiary unless those services are unrelated to the terminal illness and related conditions. In order to properly enforce this waiver, it is necessary that the hospice election be recorded in the claims processing system as soon as possible after the election occurs.

The fiscal 2015 hospice rate update final rule mandated that the notice of election (NOE) be filed within five calendar days after the effective date of hospice election.

Previously, payment for hospice services began on the effective date of the hospice election, regardless of when the NOE was filed. CMS applies a consequence for failing to file NOEs in a timely way. For those hospices that do not file the NOE in a timely way, Medicare would not cover and pay for days of hospice care from the effective date of election to the date of filing of the NOE. These days would be considered the financial responsibility of the hospice and could not be billed to the beneficiary.

Upon discharge from the hospice or revocation by the beneficiary, Medicare coverage resumes. It is imperative that hospices record the discharge or revocation in the claims processing system in a timely manner. It is critical for beneficiary revocations and live discharges from hospice to be recorded as soon as possible within CMS claims processing systems to ensure that the beneficiary is able to access needed items or services, and to ensure that payment for the item or service is from the appropriate source. Even though a hospice is not prepared to file a claim quickly, it should file a notice of termination or revocation of election (NOTR), so that the claims processing systems are updated to no longer show the beneficiary as being under a hospice election.

CMS requires hospices to file a NOTR within five calendar days after the effective date of a beneficiary's discharge or revocation if they have not already filed a final claim. This would safeguard beneficiaries from any delays or difficulties in accessing needed drugs, items, or services that could occur if the CWF or DTRR erroneously continued to show a hospice election in place.

For the Medicare hospice benefit, "attending physician" means, with respect to an individual, the physician who may be employed by a hospice program, whom the individual identifies as having the most significant role in the determination and delivery of medical care to the individual at the time the individual makes an election to receive hospice care. The patient is required to identify the attending physician at the time he or she elects to receive hospice care, as having the most significant role in the determination and delivery of the individual's medical care. The National Provider Identifier (NPI) of the attending physician must be included on the NOE and on each claim. The hospice patient (or his or her representative), not the hospice, chooses the attending physician. This requirement is included as part of the CoPs at §418.52(c)(4), which states that the patient has the right to choose his or her attending physician. If a beneficiary has designated an attending physician, that physician must sign the initial certification for Medicare to cover and pay for hospice services, unless the attending is an NP.

CMS requires that the election statement include the patient's choice of attending physician to ensure the attending physician of record is properly documented in the patient's medical record. The information identifying the attending physician should be recorded on the election statement in enough detail that it is clear which physician or NP was designated as the attending physician. The language on the election form should include an acknowledgment by the patient (or representative) that the designated attending physician was the patient's (or representative's) choice.

If a patient (or representative) wants to change his or her designated attending physician, he or she must follow a procedure similar to that which currently exists for changing the designated hospice. The patient (or representative) would be required to file a signed statement, with the hospice, that identifies the new attending physician in enough detail that it is clear which physician or NP was designated as the new attending physician. This statement must include the date the change is to be effective, the date that the statement is signed, and the patient's (or representative's) signature, along with an acknowledgment that this change in the attending physician is the patient's (or representative's) choice. The effective date of the change in attending physician cannot be earlier than the date the statement is signed.

FY 2016 Proposed Wage Index and Annual Payment Updates

Improving Medicare Post-Acute Care Transformation Act

The Improving Medicare Post-Acute Care Transformation Act (IMPACT Act) of 2014 became law on October 6, 2014 (Pub. L. 113–185). Since it was found that surveys of hospices were being performed on an infrequent basis, this law mandates that all Medicare certified hospices be surveyed every three years beginning April 6, 2015, and ending September 30, 2025.

Additionally, the IMPACT Act implemented a provision set forth in the Affordable Care Act that requires medical review of hospice cases involving patients receiving more than 180 days of care in select hospices that show a preponderance of such patients. The IMPACT Act also contains a new provision mandating that the aggregate cap amount for accounting years that end after September 30, 2016, and before October 1, 2025, be updated by the hospice payment update rather than using the consumer price index for urban consumers (CPI–U) for medical care expenditures. Specifically, the 2016 cap year, which starts on November 1, 2015, and ends on October 31, 2016, will be updated by the FY 2016 payment update percentage for hospice care. This will continue through any cap year ending before October 1, 2025 (through cap year 2025).

Summary of the Major Provisions Regarding Diagnosis Reporting

Trends in Diagnosis Reporting on Hospice Claims

Since the implementation of the hospice benefit in 1983 there has been substantial growth in hospice utilization. The number of Medicare beneficiaries receiving hospice services has grown from 513,000 in FY 2000 to over 1.3 million in FY 2013. There have also been noted changes in the diagnosis patterns among Medicare hospice enrollees, with a growing percentage of beneficiaries with non-cancer diagnoses. Specifically, there were notable increases in neurologically-based diagnoses, including various dementia diagnoses. Additionally, there have been significant increases in the use of non-specific, symptom-classified diagnoses, such as debility and adult failure to thrive.

The diagnosis of adult failure to thrive is often used interchangeably with "debility" as a primary hospice diagnosis. However, adult failure to thrive is defined as undefined weight loss, decreasing anthromorphic measurements, and a Palliative Performance Scale < 40 percent. This condition is also associated with multiple primary conditions contributing to the physical and functional decline of the individual. Claims with a principal hospice diagnosis of adult failure to thrive included secondary diagnoses, such as pneumonia, cerebral vascular accident (stroke), atrial fibrillation, heart disease, Alzheimer's disease, congestive heart failure and Parkinson's disease.

A comprehensive hospice plan of care starts with accurate and thorough assessment and identification of the conditions contributing to the terminal illness and decline. "Debility" and "adult failure to thrive" are not appropriate principal diagnoses in the terminally ill population as these diagnoses are incongruous to the comprehensive nature of the hospice assessment. When "debility" and "adult failure to thrive" are reported as a principal diagnosis, these would be considered questionable encounters for hospice care, and the claim would be returned to the provider for a more definitive principal diagnosis. "Debility" and "adult failure to thrive" may be listed on the hospice claim as other, additional, or coexisting diagnoses.

Effective October 1, 2014, for those claims submitted on and after October 1, 2014, claims with "debility" and "adult failure to thrive" coded in the principal diagnosis field will be returned to the provider unprocessed for more definitive coding.

Effective October 1, 2014, for all hospice claims submitted on and after October 1, 2014, CMS will implement certain edits from the Medicare Code Editor (MCE), which detect and report errors in the coding of claims data. These edits are being implemented to ensure additional compliance with ICD-9-CM coding guidelines. Hospice claims containing inappropriate principal or secondary diagnosis codes, per ICD-9-CM coding conventions and guidelines, will be returned to the provider unprocessed. The claim will have to be corrected and resubmitted to be processed and paid. These edits include the etiology/manifestation code pairs.

In a recent report, the Office of Inspector General (OIG) identified instances in which Medicare may be paying under Part D for drugs that should be provided by the hospice as part of the plan of care. Acumen, LLC developed case studies that were reviewed and evaluated by CMS clinical staff in an effort to assist CMS in identifying and evaluating instances where drugs, supplies, durable medical equipment (DME), and Part B services provided to hospice patients appear to be related to the principal diagnosis reported on the hospice claim but were billed separately to other parts of the Medicare program.

Hospice patients with hospice claims-reported principal diagnoses of chronic airway obstruction, congestive heart failure, cerebral degeneration, and lung cancer were receiving services clinically indicated and recommended for these conditions outside of the hospice benefit, which is in violation of requirements regarding the Medicare hospice benefit. This could be attributed to hospices incorrectly classifying conditions as unrelated and referring patients to nonhospice providers, not communicating and coordinating the care and services needed to manage the needs of the hospice beneficiary, or deliberately avoiding costs. The following studies are focused on four of the most commonly reported principal hospice diagnoses on hospice claims based on evidence-based clinical guidelines as described for each principal hospice diagnosis.

Malignant Neoplasm of the Trachea, Bronchus, and Lung

Malignant neoplasm of the trachea, bronchus, and lung (or lung cancer) is reported using ICD-9-CM diagnosis codes beginning with 162; and ICD-10-CM diagnosis codes C33 and C34.00–C34.92. These codes describe pulmonary system cancers. Symptoms for these conditions may include chronic and worsening cough, shortness of breath, chest pain, metastatic bone pain, and anorexia and weight loss. Clinical practice guidelines for end-stage cancer recommend treatment and management of refractory symptoms, including pain, mucositis, dyspnea, fatigue, depression, and anorexia through the use of pharmacological interventions including nonsteroidal anti-inflammatories, corticosteroids, opioids and antidepressants. Additionally, evidence shows that palliative chemotherapy and radiotherapy can provide symptom relief from bone and brain metastasis.

Recommended interventions for dyspnea include treatment of the underlying reason, such as thoracentesis for pleural effusion, bronchodilators and systemic corticosteroids for inflammation and secretions, and supportive measures such as supplemental oxygen, opioids, and anxiolytics to decrease the sensation of breathlessness.

CMS assessed concurrently billed Part D drugs included 89,925 stays for beneficiaries with ICD-9 code 162 listed as a primary diagnosis on the hospice claim. CMS's assessment of concurrently billed Part B services included 153,199 stays. In CY 2013, concurrent billing for all services related to this terminal condition comprised $3.4 million. Part D drugs that should have been covered under the hospice benefit for the treatment of this condition accounted for $2.1 million. DME services that were billed during hospice stays related to this condition during the same time cost $640,166. Concurrent services provided in Part B institutional settings accounted for $591,772.

Chronic Airway Obstruction

Chronic airway obstruction, also known as chronic obstructive pulmonary disease (or COPD) is reported with ICD-9-CM diagnosis codes beginning with 496 and ICD-10-CM diagnosis codes J44.0–J44.9. It includes chronic lung disease with unspecified cause and is characterized by inflammation of the lungs and airways. Symptoms of these pulmonary diseases typically include increasing and disabling shortness of breath, labored breathing, increased coughing, increased heart rate, decreased functional reserve, increased infections, and unintentional, progressive weight loss.

Evidence-based practice supports the benefits of oral opioids, neuromuscular electrical stimulation, chest wall vibration, walking aids, respiratory assist devices, and pursed-lip breathing in the management of dyspnea in the individual patient with advanced COPD. Oxygen is recommended for COPD patients with resting hypoxemia for symptomatic benefit. Additionally, guidelines recommend inhaled bronchodilators, systemic corticosteroids, and pulmonary physiotherapy for the management of COPD exacerbations.

An analysis shows concurrently billed Part D drugs included 130,283 stays for beneficiaries with ICD-9 code 496 listed as a primary diagnosis on the hospice claim. Additionally, concurrently billed Part B services included 198,098 such stays. In CY 2013, concurrent billing for all services related to this terminal condition comprised $10.4 million. Part D drugs that should have been covered under the hospice benefit for the treatment of this condition accounted for $8.6 million. DME services that were billed during hospice stays related to this condition during the same time amounted to $1.2 million dollars. Finally, concurrent services provided in Part B institutional settings accounted for $605,110.

Cerebral Degeneration

Cerebral degeneration is reporting using ICD-9-CM diagnosis codes beginning with 331 and ICD-10-CM diagnosis codes G30, G31, and G32. It includes conditions such as Alzheimer's disease and Reye's syndrome. These conditions usually encompass a progressive loss of cognitive function with symptoms including the loss of memory and changes in language ability, behavior, and personality. As these cerebral degenerations progress, other clinical manifestations occur such as dysphagia, motor dysfunction, impaired mobility, increased need for activities of daily living assistance, urinary and fecal incontinence, weight loss and muscle wasting. Individuals with these conditions

are also at increased risk for aspiration, falls, pneumonias, decubitus ulcers, and urinary tract infections.

Clinical practice guidelines for the treatment of cerebral degenerative conditions includes pharmacological interventions, including angiotensin converting enzyme inhibitors, memantine or combination therapy depending on severity of disease, as well as antidepressants, antipsychotics, psychostimulants, mood stabilizers, benzodiazepines, and neuroleptics, depending on behavioral manifestations. Nonpharmacological interventions recommended include mental, behavioral, and cognitive therapy, speech language pathology to address swallowing issues, and other interventions to treat and manage manifestations, including pressure ulcers, cachexia, and infections.

CMS's assessment of concurrently billed Part D drugs included 208,346 stays for beneficiaries with ICD-9 code 331 listed as a primary diagnosis on the hospice claim. An assessment of concurrently billed Part B services included 318,044 stays. In CY 2013, concurrent billing for all services related to this principal diagnosis comprised $11.2 million. Part D drugs that should have been covered under the hospice benefit for the treatment of this condition accounted for $10.3 million. Concurrently billed DME products that were related to this condition cost Medicare an additional $390,476. Concurrent services provided in Part B institutional settings accounted for $496,790.

Congestive Heart Failure

Congestive heart failure (CHF) is defined by ICD-9 diagnosis codes beginning with 428 and ICD-10-CM diagnosis codes beginning with I09, I11, I13, and I50. CHF is characterized by symptoms such as shortness of breath, edema, diminished endurance, angina, productive cough, and fatigue. For the management of congestive heart failure, clinical practice guidelines recommend pharmacological interventions, including beta blockers, angiotensin converting enzyme inhibitors, angiotensin receptor blockers, diuretics, antiplatelets, anticoagulants, and digoxin, depending on symptomology and response or nonresponse to other treatments. Nonpharmacological interventions recommended include continuous positive airway pressure and supplemental oxygen for those with coexisting pulmonary disease.

CMS's assessment of concurrently billed Part D drugs included 158,220 stays for beneficiaries with ICD-9 code 428 listed as a primary diagnosis on the hospice claim. An assessment of concurrently billed Part B services included 256,236 stays. In CY 2013, concurrent billing for all services related to this terminal condition comprised $5.8 million. Part D drugs that should have been covered under the hospice benefit for the treatment of this condition accounted for $3.8 million. DME services that were billed during hospice stays related to this condition during this time cost $843,534. Concurrent services provided in Part B institutional settings accounted for $1.2 million.

Regulations at §418.56(c) require that hospices provide all services necessary for the palliation and management of the terminal illness and related conditions. CMS feels that it has discussed recommended evidence-based practice clinical guidelines for the hospice claims-reported principal diagnoses mentioned in this section. The HHH MACs have local coverage determinations on these subjects. However, this analysis reveals that these recommended practices are not being covered under the Medicare hospice benefit. The case studies in this section offer evidence of the potential systematic unbundling of the Medicare hospice benefit.

Proposed Routine Home Care Rates

Routine home care (RHC) is the basic level of care when a patient receives hospice care but remains at home. This level of care allows hospice providers to be reimbursed per day regardless of the volume or intensity of services provided to a patient on any given day. As CMS has stated in prior updates, it is CMS's intent to ensure that hospice reimbursement rates align as closely as possible with the average costs hospices incur when efficiently providing covered services to patients. However, there is evidence of a misalignment between the current RHC per diem payment rate and the cost of providing RHC.

An analysis of FY 2013 hospice claims data continues to demonstrate a U-shaped pattern of resource use. There is increased utilization at both the beginning and end of a stay. FY 2013 resource costs (as captured by wage-weighted minutes) are significantly higher in the first two days of a hospice election and once again in the six days preceding the date of death and on the date of death itself.

CMS is using authority granted under section 3132(a) of the Affordable Care Act to propose a revision to the current RHC per diem payment rate to more accurately align the per diem payments with visit intensity (the cost of providing care for the clinical service [labor] components of the RHC rate). In conjunction with a proposed service intensity add-on (SIA) payment, CMS proposes two different RHC rates that would result in a higher base payment rate for the first 60 days of hospice care and a reduced base payment rate for days 61 or over of hospice care. The two proposed rates for RHC are based on an extensive body of research concerning visit intensity during a hospice episode.

CMS considers a hospice episode of care to be a hospice election period or series of election periods. Visit intensity is commonly measured in terms of wage-weighted minutes and reflects variation in the provision of care for the clinical service (labor) components of the RHC rate. The labor components of the RHC rate make up nearly 70 percent of the RHC rate. Therefore, visit intensity is a close proxy for the reasonable cost of providing hospice care absent data on the nonlabor components of the RHC rate, such as drugs and DME.

As data demonstrate, the daily cost of care, as measured in wage-weighted minutes, declines quickly for individual patients during their hospice episodes. It remains low for long-episode patients, making long-episode patients potentially more profitable than shorter-episode patients under the current per diem payment system. Since the percentage of patients who enter hospice less than seven days prior to death has remained relatively constant (approximately 30 percent) over this time period, the increase in the average episode length can be attributed to an increasing number of long-stay patients. CMS found that the percentage of episodes that are more than six months in length has nearly doubled from about 7 percent in 1999 to 13 percent in 2013.

Visit intensity declines rapidly after seven days and then at a slower rate until 60 days, when it becomes flat throughout the remainder of episodes (excluding the last seven days prior to death). For this reason CMS is proposing to pay the higher rate for the first 60 days and a lower rate thereafter. The most important reason for proposing a different RHC rate for the first 60 days versus days 61 and beyond is that CMS must account for differences in average visit intensity between episodes that will end within 60 days and those that will go on for longer episodes.

The SIA payments, which are based on actual visits provided, would be added to the applicable rate during the last seven days to reflect the rapid increase in visit intensity during that time period.

The current labor-related share of the hospice payment rate for RHC is 68.71 percent. The nonlabor share is 31.29 percent. Given the current base rate for RHC for FY 2015 of $159.34, the labor and nonlabor components are as follows: the labor share portion is $159.34 multiplied by 68.71 percent, or $109.48; the nonlabor share portion is $159.34 multiplied by 31.29 percent, or $49.86.

Applying these same percentages, the proposed RHC rates would need to be adjusted by a ratio of the total labor payments for RHC using the current single rate for RHC, to the estimated total labor payments for RHC using the two proposed rates for RHC. This ratio results in a budget neutrality adjustment of 0.9985. Adding the revised labor portion with budget neutrality to the nonlabor portion results in revised FY 2015 RHC proposed payment rates of $187.63 for days one through 60 and $145.21 for days 61 and over. The proposed RHC rates for days one through 60 and days 61 and over would replace the current single RHC per diem payment rate with two new RHC per diem rates for patients who require RHC level of care during a hospice election.

CMS further proposes that the count of days follow the patient. This is intended to mitigate potential high rates of discharge and readmissions. For hospice patients who are discharged and readmitted to hospice within 60 days of that discharge, his or her prior hospice days will continue to follow the patient and count toward his or her patient days for the receiving hospice upon hospice election. The hospice days would continue to follow the patient solely to determine whether the receiving hospice may bill at the one through 60 or 61+ RHC rate. This then defines an episode of care to be a hospice election period or series of election periods separated by no more than a 60-day gap.

Proposed Service Intensity Add-On Payment

Regulations including those for the Affordable Care Act, require revisions to the methodology for determining the payment rates for RHCs and other services included in hospice care under Medicare Part A. CMS believes that implementing revisions to the payment system that align with the concept of a U-shaped cost pattern supports the requirements of reasonable cost.

CMS considered implementing a tiered payment to better align payments with observed resource use over the length of a hospice stay. The concept of an SAI that could be implemented with minimal systems changes that limit reprocessing of hospice claims due to sequential billing requirements seemed to have less operational concerns and programmatic complexity.

As one of the first steps in addressing the observed misalignment between resource use and associated Medicare payments and in improving patient care through the promotion of skilled visits at end of life with minimal claims processing systems changes, CMS proposes to implement an SIA payment if the criteria outlined below are met.

Proposed qualifications for the SIA payment, include:

1. The day is billed as an RHC level of care day.
2. The day occurs during the last seven days of life (and the patient is discharged dead).
3. Direct patient care is provided by an RN or a social worker that day.

4. The service is not provided in a skilled nursing facility/nursing facility (SNF/NF).

The proposed SIA payment would be equal to the continuous home care (CHC) hourly payment rate (the current FY 2015 CHC rate is $38.75 per hour), multiplied by the amount of direct patient care provided by an RN or social worker for up to four hours total, per day, as long as the four criteria listed above are met. The proposed SIA payment would be paid in addition to the current per diem rate for the RHC level of care.

CMS would create two separate HCPCS Level II G codes for use when billing skilled nursing visits (revenue code 055X), one for an RN and one for a Licensed Practical Nurse (LPN). During periods of crisis, such as the precipitous decline before death. RNs are more highly trained clinicians with commensurately higher payment rates. Medicare rules require the RN member of the hospice interdisciplinary group to be responsible for ensuring that the needs of the patient and family are continually assessed. CMS expects that at end of life, the needs of the patient and family would be frequently assessed; thus the skills of the interdisciplinary group RN are required.

Social workers also often play a crucial role in providing support for the patient and family when a patient is at end of life. CMS proposes to pay an SIA only for those social work services provided by means of in-person visits. The SIA payment would be in addition to the RHC payment amount, and the costs associated with social work phone conversations; visits by LPNs, aides, and therapists; counseling; drugs; medical supplies; DME; and any other item or service usually covered by Medicare would still be covered by the existing RHC payment amount.

As required by law, any changes to the hospice payment system must be made in a budget-neutral manner in the first year of implementation. CMS wants to improve patient care by promoting skilled visits at end of life, regardless of the patient's lifetime length of stay, and it is proposing to make the SIA payments budget neutral through a reduction to the overall RHC rate. The SIA payment budget neutrality factor (SBNF) used to reduce the overall RHC rate is outlined below and is reflected in the proposed RHC payment rate tables.

The SIA payments are budget neutral through an annual determination of the SBNF, which will then be applied to the RHC payment rate. The SBNF for the SIA payments would be calculated for each FY using the most current and complete fiscal year utilization data available at the time of rule making.

Proposed FY 2016 Hospice Wage Index

The hospice wage index is used to adjust payment rates for hospice agencies under the Medicare program to reflect local differences in area wage levels based on the location where services are furnished. The hospice wage index utilizes the wage adjustment factors used for hospital wage adjustments.

CMS uses the previous fiscal year's hospital wage index data to calculate the hospice wage index values. For FY 2016, the hospice wage index will be based on the FY 2015 hospital prefloor, prereclassified wage index. This means that the hospital wage data used for the hospice wage index is not adjusted to take into account any geographic reclassification of hospitals.

The appropriate wage index value is applied to the labor portion of the payment rate based on the geographic area in which the patient resides when receiving RHC or CHC. The appropriate wage index value is applied to the labor portion of the payment rate based on the geographic location of the facility for patients receiving general inpatient care (GIP) or inpatient respite care (IRC).

In FY 2016, the only CBSA without a hospital from which hospital wage data could be derived is 25980, Hinesville-Fort Stewart, Georgia. For this, CMS implemented a new methodology to update the hospice wage index for rural areas without a hospital, and thus no hospital wage data. In this situation, CMS used the average prefloor, prereclassified hospital wage index data from all contiguous CBSAs to represent a reasonable proxy for the rural area.

Currently, the only rural area without a hospital from which hospital wage data could be derived is Puerto Rico. However, the CMS policy does not recognize the unique circumstances of Puerto Rico. In this proposed rule, for FY 2016, CMS proposes to continue to use the most recent prefloor, prereclassified hospital wage index value available for Puerto Rico, which is 0.4047.

Elimination of the Wage Index Budget Neutrality Factor

This proposed rule would update the hospice wage index values for FY 2016 using the FY 2015 prefloor, prereclassified hospital wage index. These raw wage index values were then subject to either a budget neutrality adjustment or application of the hospice floor to compute the hospice wage index used to determine payments to hospices.

Prefloor, prereclassified hospital wage index values below 0.8 were adjusted by either: (1) The hospice BNAF; or (2) the hospice floor—a 15 percent increase subject to a maximum wage index value of 0.8; whichever results in the greater value. The BNAF was being phased out over seven years, with a complete phase-out in FY 2016.

In the FY 2015 inpatient prospective payment system (IPPS) final rule, CMS finalized the proposal to use OMB's new area delineations, based on the 2010 census, in the FY 2015 hospital wage index. Although the revisions OMB published on February 28, 2013, are not as sweeping as the changes made when CMS adopted the CBSA geographic designations for FY 2006, there are a number of significant changes. For example, there are new CBSAs, urban counties that have become rural, rural counties that have become urban, and existing CBSAs that have been split apart. CMS proposes to implement the new OMB delineations as described in the February 28, 2013, OMB Bulletin No. 13–01 for the hospice wage index effective beginning in FY 2016.

The OMB defines a "micropolitan statistical area" as a CBSA "associated with at least one urban cluster that has a population of at least 10,000, but less than 50,000." After extensive impact analysis, consistent with the treatment of these areas under the IPPS, CMS determined the best course of action would be to treat micropolitan areas as "rural" and include them in the calculation of each state's hospice rural wage index. Thus, the hospice statewide rural wage index is determined using IPPS hospital data from hospitals located in non-MSA areas.

If CMS adopts the new OMB delineations (based upon the 2010 decennial census data), a total of 37 counties (and county equivalents) that are currently considered urban would be considered rural beginning in FY 2016. A total of 105 counties (and county equivalents) that are currently designated rural would be considered urban beginning in FY 2016. In addition to rural counties becoming urban and urban counties becoming rural, several urban counties would shift from one urban CBSA to another urban CBSA under the proposal to adopt the new OMB delineations.

CMS believes that implementing the new OMB delineations would result in wage index values being more representative of the actual costs of labor in a given area. Among the 458 total CBSA and statewide rural areas, 20 (4 percent) would have a higher wage index using the newer delineations. However, 34 (7.4 percent) would have a lower wage index using the newer delineations. Therefore, to remain consistent with the manner in which CMS ultimately adopted the revised OMB delineations for FY 2006, CMS proposes to implement a one-year transition to the new OMB delineations.

Specifically, a blended wage index would be applied for one year (FY 2016) for all geographic areas that would consist of a 50/50 blend of the wage index values using OMB's old area delineations and the wage index values using OMB's new area delineations. That is, for each county, a blended wage index would be calculated equal to 50 percent of the FY 2016 wage index using the old labor market area delineation and 50 percent of the FY 2016 wage index using the new labor market area delineation. This results in an average of the two values. This blended wage index will be referred to as the FY 2016 hospice transition wage index. This transition policy would be for a one-year period, going into effect on October 1, 2015, and continuing through September 30, 2016. Beginning October 1, 2016, the wage index for all hospice payments would be fully based on the new OMB delineations.

Due to the way that the transition wage index is calculated, some CBSAs and statewide rural areas may have more than one transition wage index value associated with that CBSA or rural area. However, each county will have only one transition wage index. For counties located in CBSAs and rural areas that correspond to more than one transition wage index value, the CBSA number will not be able to be used for FY 2016 claims. In these cases, a number other than the CBSA number would be necessary to identify the appropriate wage index value on claims for hospice care provided in FY 2016. These numbers are five digits in length and begin with "50."

Proposed Hospice Payment Update
Hospice rates were to be updated by a factor equal to the market basket index, minus 1 percentage point. CMS is required to use the inpatient hospital market basket to determine the hospice payment rate update. In addition, the Affordable Care Act mandates that, starting with FY 2013 (and in subsequent FYs), the hospice payment update percentage will be annually reduced by changes in economy-wide productivity. The statute defines the productivity adjustment to be equal to the 10-year moving average of changes in annual economy-wide private nonfarm business multifactor productivity (MFP) (as projected by the Secretary for the 10-year period ending with the applicable FY, year, cost reporting period, or other annual period).

In addition to the MFP adjustment, the Affordable Care Act also mandates that in FY 2013 through FY 2019, the hospice payment update percentage will be reduced by an additional 0.3 percentage point (although for FY 2014 to FY 2019, the potential 0.3 percentage point reduction is subject to suspension under conditions specified in the Act). The proposed hospice payment update percentage for FY 2016 is based on the estimated inpatient hospital market

basket update of 2.7 percent (based on IHS Global Insight, Inc.'s first quarter 2015 forecast with historical data through the fourth quarter of 2014).

The estimated inpatient hospital market basket update for FY 2016 of 2.7 percent must be reduced by an MFP adjustment as mandated by Affordable Care Act (currently estimated to be a 0.6 percentage point for FY 2016). The estimated inpatient hospital market basket update for FY 2016 is reduced further by a 0.3 percentage point, as mandated by the Affordable Care Act. In effect, the proposed hospice payment update percentage for FY 2016 is 1.8 percent. If more recent data are subsequently available, CMS may use such data, if appropriate, to determine the FY 2016 market basket update and the MFP adjustment in the FY 2016 Hospice Rate Update final rule.

Currently, breakdown of the hospice payment rate percentages is as follows:

Service	Labor	Nonlabor
RHC	68.71	31.29
CHC	68.71	31.29
General Inpatient care	64.01	35.99
Respite care	54.43	45.87

There are four payment categories that are distinguished by the location and intensity of the services provided. The base payments are adjusted for geographic differences in wages by multiplying the labor share, which varies by category, of each base rate by the applicable hospice wage index. A hospice is paid the RHC rate for each day the beneficiary is enrolled in hospice, unless the hospice provides continuous home care, IRC, or general inpatient care. CHC is provided during a period of patient crisis to maintain the patient at home; IRC is short-term care to allow the usual caregiver to rest; and GIP is to treat symptoms that cannot be managed in another setting.

This proposed rule proposes two different RHC payment rates, one RHC rate for the first 60 days and a second for days 60 and beyond. CMS also proposes to make an SIA payment, in addition to the daily RHC payment, when direct patient care is provided by an RN or social worker during the last seven days of the patient's life. The SIA payment would be equal to the CHC hourly rate multiplied by the hours of nursing or social work provided (up to four hours total) that occurred on the day of service. The SIA payment would also be adjusted by the appropriate wage index. In order to maintain budget neutrality, for the proposed SIA payment, the proposed RHC rates would need to be adjusted by a budget neutrality factor. The budget neutrality adjustment that would apply to days one through 60 is equal to 1 minus the ratio of SIA payments for days one through 60 to the total payments for days one through 60 and is calculated to be 0.9853. The budget neutrality adjustment that would apply to days 61 and beyond is equal to 1 minus the ratio of SIA payments for days 61 and beyond to the total payments for days 61 and beyond and is calculated to be 0.9967.

Lastly, the RHC rates would be increased by the proposed FY 2016 hospice payment update percentage of 1.8 percent. The proposed FY 2016 payment rates for CHC, IRC, and GIP would be the FY 2015 payment rates increased by 1.8 percent. The proposed FY 2016 rates for hospices that do not submit the required quality data are the update minus 2 percent (1.8 – 2.0) or –0.2%. The proposed FY 2016 hospice payment rates would be effective for care and services furnished on or after October 1, 2015, through September 30, 2016.

Guidance on Coding of Principal and Other, Additional, and/or Co-existing Diagnoses

Clarification Regarding Diagnosis Reporting on Hospice Claims
As mentioned previously, there are data suggesting a significant amount of "unbundling" is occurring for services that should be included in the hospice bundled payment. Data analysis shows that $1.3 billion is being paid outside of the Medicare hospice benefit for those under an active hospice election. With such a significant amount of services being provided outside of the Medicare hospice benefit, it raises questions about whether hospices are providing full disclosure of the nature of hospice care, which focuses on improving quality of life as one is approaching the end of life while eliminating the need for unnecessary, futile, and possibly harmful diagnostics, treatments, and therapies.

Additionally, CMS has received anecdotal reports from nonhospice providers who have rendered care and services to hospice beneficiaries in which the nonhospice provider states that the care given was related to the terminal prognosis of the individual. These reports go on to say that they have contacted hospices to coordinate the care of the hospice beneficiary only to be told by those hospices that they disagreed with the nonhospice providers' clinical judgment that the care was related to the terminal prognosis. CMS has been told that hospices are refusing to reimburse the nonhospice provider for care related to the terminal prognosis. These nonhospice providers also informed CMS that the hospices told them to code the claim with a different diagnosis or to code condition code 07 (Treatment of non-terminal condition for hospice) or the modifier GW (service not related to the hospice patient's terminal condition) on their claims to ensure that the nonhospice provider would consequently get paid through Medicare. These nonhospice providers stated that they disagreed with this practice and considered it fraudulent. As such, they were unable to be reimbursed by the hospice or by Medicare for services provided that they felt were the responsibility of hospice.

CMS is concerned that some hospices are making determinations of hospice coverage based solely on cost and reimbursement as opposed to being based on patient-centered needs, preferences, and goals for those approaching the end of life. CMS feels that this is counter to the holistic, comprehensive, and coordinated hospice care model promoted during the development of the Medicare hospice benefit.

The Medicare hospice regulations state that in reaching a decision to certify that a patient is terminally ill, meaning that the patient has a medical prognosis of a life expectancy of six months or less, the certifying physician(s) must consider at least the following information:

- Diagnosis of the terminal condition of the patient.

- Other health conditions, whether related or unrelated to the terminal condition.

- Current clinically relevant information supporting all diagnoses.

Eligibility for the Medicare hospice benefit has always been based on the prognosis of the individual. Prognosis is not necessarily established through just a single diagnosis or even multiple diagnoses. Rather, it is based on the totality of the individual and everything that affects life expectancy.

CMS has reminded providers that there are multiple public sources available to assist in determining whether a patient meets Medicare hospice prognosis eligibility criteria (that is, industry-specific clinical and functional assessment tools and information on MAC web sites, including local coverage determinations [LCDs]). There are prognostication tools available for hospices to assist in thoughtful evaluation of Medicare beneficiaries for determining eligibility for the Medicare hospice benefit.

The hospice industry has come under increased media scrutiny, much of it related to hospices enrolling patients who may not be eligible for the benefit because they are not terminally ill and enrolling patients with certain diagnoses that typically have a longer length of stay, mainly noncancer diagnoses.

To address some of these noted hospice vulnerabilities, the recent IMPACT Act legislation requires increased hospice program oversight through more frequent hospice surveys and medical review efforts. All of these efforts seek to protect the Medicare hospice beneficiaries, as well as the integrity of the Medicare hospice benefit.

CMS recognizes that the total person is to be assessed, including acute and chronic conditions, as well as controlled and uncontrolled conditions and comorbidities in order to determine an individual's terminal prognosis.

CMS regulations at §418.54(c) require that the comprehensive assessment must take into consideration the following factors:

- The nature and condition causing admission (including the presence or lack of objective data and subjective complaints).

- Complications and risk factors that affect care planning.

- Functional status, including the patient's ability to understand and participate in his or her own care.

- Imminence of death.

- Severity of symptoms.

- Drug profile. A review of all of the patient's prescription and over-the-counter drugs, herbal remedies, and other alternative treatments that could affect drug therapy.

- Bereavement. An initial bereavement assessment of the needs of the patient's family and other individuals focusing on the social, spiritual, and cultural factors that may impact their ability to cope with the patient's death. Information gathered from the initial bereavement assessment must be incorporated into the plan of care and considered in the bereavement plan of care.

- The need for referrals and further evaluation by appropriate health professionals.

The hospice CoPs at §418.56(c) require that the hospice plan of care reflect patient and family goals and have measurable outcomes. Furthermore, the plan of care is a dynamic and fluid document that will change as the individual's condition changes throughout the course of a hospice election. A

comprehensive, holistic, integrated, and coordinated approach to service delivery is the hallmark of hospice care and a valued service for Medicare beneficiaries and families as the individual approaches the end of life.

CMS believes that many hospices practice this comprehensive approach as they recognize that it is the hospices' responsibility to provide all medical, emotional, psychosocial, and spiritual services for all component conditions of the terminal prognosis along the continuum of care.

Diagnosis Reporting on Hospice Claims

International Classification of Diseases, Tenth Revision, Clinical Modification (ICD-10-CM) Coding Guidelines state the following regarding the selection of the principal diagnosis:

The principal diagnosis is defined in the Uniform Hospital Discharge Data Set (UHDDS) as that condition established after study to be chiefly responsible for occasioning the admission of the patient to the hospital for care. In the case of selection of a principal diagnosis for hospice care, this would mean the diagnosis most contributory to the terminal prognosis of the individual. In the instance where two or more diagnoses equally meet the criteria for principal diagnosis, ICD-10-CM coding guidelines do not provide sequencing direction, and thus, any one of the diagnoses may be sequenced first, meaning to report all of those diagnoses meeting the criteria as a principal diagnosis. Per ICD-10-CM coding guidelines, for diagnosis reporting purposes, the definition for "other diagnoses" is interpreted as additional conditions that affect patient care in terms of requiring:

- Clinical evaluation; or

- Therapeutic treatment; or

- Diagnostic procedures; or

- Extended length of hospital stay; or

- Increased nursing care and/or monitoring.

The UHDDS item #11–b defines other diagnoses as all conditions that coexist at the time of admission, that develop subsequently, or that affect the treatment received and/or the length of stay. ICD-10-CM coding guidelines are clear that all diagnoses affecting the management and treatment of the individual within the health care setting are required to be reported. This has been longstanding existing policy. Adherence to coding guidelines when assigning ICD-9-CM and ICD-10-CM diagnosis and procedure codes is required under the Health Insurance Portability and Accountability Act (HIPAA) as well as in CMS regulations.

However, though established coding guidelines are required, it does not appear that all hospices are coding on hospice claims per these guidelines. In 2010, over 77 percent of hospice claims reported only one diagnosis. Previous rules have discussed requirements for hospice diagnosis reporting on claims and the importance of complete and accurate coding. Preliminary analysis of FY 2014 claims data demonstrates that hospice diagnosis coding is improving; however, challenges remain. Analysis of FY 2014 claims data indicate that 49 percent of hospice claims listed only one diagnosis. Additional analysis on instances where only one diagnosis was reported on the FY 2014 hospice claim revealed that 50 percent of these beneficiaries had, on average, eight or more chronic conditions and 75 percent had, on average, five or more chronic conditions. These chronic, comorbid conditions include hypertension, anemia, congestive heart failure, chronic obstructive pulmonary disease, ischemic heart disease, depression, diabetes, and atrial fibrillation, to name a few.

CMS has stated that hospices should report on hospice claims all coexisting or additional diagnoses that are related to the terminal illness; they should not report coexisting or additional diagnoses that are unrelated to the terminal illness, even though coding guidelines required the reporting of all diagnoses that affect patient assessment and planning. There is widely varying interpretation as to what factors influence the terminal prognosis of the individual (that is, what conditions render the individual terminally ill and which conditions are related). CMS is further concerned that hospices may not be conducting a comprehensive assessment nor updating the plan of care as articulated by the CoPs to recognize the conditions that affect an individual's terminal prognosis.

Therefore, CMS is clarifying that hospices will report all diagnoses identified in the initial and comprehensive assessments on hospice claims, whether related or unrelated to the terminal prognosis of the individual. This is in keeping with the requirements of determining whether an individual is terminally ill. This would also include the reporting of any mental health disorders and conditions that would affect the plan of care as hospices are to assess and provide care for identified psychosocial and emotional needs, as well as for physical and spiritual needs.

Update to the Hospice Quality Reporting Program

Quality Measures for Hospice Quality Reporting Program and Data Submission Requirements

Beginning with the FY 2018 payment determination, CMS proposes that when measures are adopted for the hospice quality reporting program (HQRP) beginning with a payment determination year, these measures are automatically adopted for all subsequent years' payment determinations, unless the measures are proposed for removal, suspension, or replacement.

Quality measures may be considered for removal by CMS if:

- Measure performance among hospices is so high and unvarying that meaningful distinctions in improvements in performance can no longer be made.

- Performance or improvement on a measure does not result in better patient outcomes.

- A measure does not align with current clinical guidelines or practice.

- A more broadly applicable measure (across settings, populations, or conditions) for the particular topic is available.

- A measure that is more proximal in time to desired patient outcomes for the particular topic. is available.

- A measure that is more strongly associated with desired patient outcomes for the particular topic. is available.

- Collection or public reporting of a measure leads to negative unintended consequences.

For any such removal, the public will be given an opportunity to comment through the annual rule-making process. If CMS feels there is reason to believe continued collection of a measure raises potential safety concerns, the agency will take immediate action to remove the measure from the HQRP and will not wait for the annual rule-making cycle. The measures will be promptly removed and the agency will immediately notify hospices and the public of such a decision through the usual HQRP communication channels, including listening sessions, memos, email notification, and web postings. In such instances, the removal of a measure will be formally announced in the next annual rule-making cycle.

CMS is not proposing to remove any measures for the FY 2017 reporting cycle.

CMS developed and tested a hospice patient-level item set, the HIS. Hospices are required to submit an HIS-Admission record and an HIS-Discharge record for each patient admission to hospice on or after July 1, 2014. In developing the standardized HIS, CMS considered comments offered in response to the CY 2013 proposed rule. In the FY 2014 Hospice Wage Index final rule CMS finalized the specific collection of data items that support the following six NQF-endorsed measures and one modified measure for hospice:

- NQF #1617 Patients Treated with an Opioid Who Are Given a Bowel Regimen
- NQF #1634 Pain Screening
- NQF #1637 Pain Assessment
- NQF #1638 Dyspnea Treatment
- NQF #1639 Dyspnea Screening
- NQF #1641 Treatment Preferences
- NQF #1647 Beliefs/Values Addressed (if desired by the patient) (modified)

CMS finalized the HIS effective July 1, 2014, to achieve a comprehensive set of hospice quality measures available for widespread use for quality improvement and informed decision making, and to carry out its commitment to develop a quality reporting program for hospices that uses standardized methods to collect data needed to calculate quality measures. CMS requires regular and ongoing electronic submission of the HIS data for each patient admission to hospice on or after July 1, 2014, regardless of payer or patient age, in order to meet the quality reporting requirements for hospices for the FY 2016 payment determination and each subsequent year.

CMS collects quality data necessary to calculate the adopted measures on all patients so that the agency has the data on all patients provides the most robust, accurate reflection of the quality of care delivered to Medicare beneficiaries as compared with non-Medicare patients.

In FY 2014, CMS finalized that hospice providers collect data on all patients in order to ensure that all patients, regardless of payer or patient age, are receiving the same care and that provider metrics measure performance across the spectrum of patients.

Hospices are required to complete and submit an HIS-Admission and an HIS-discharge record for each patient admission. Hospices failing to report

quality data via the HIS in FY 2015 will have their market basket update reduced by 2 percentage points in FY 2017 beginning October 1, 2016.

CMS is not currently proposing any new measures for FY 2017. However, the agency is working with their measure development and maintenance contractor to identify measure concepts for future implementation in the HQRP. In identifying priority areas for future measure enhancement and development, CMS takes into consideration input from numerous stakeholders, including the Measures Application Partnership (MAP), the Medicare Payment Advisory Commission (MedPAC), technical expert panels, and national priorities, such as those established by the National Priorities Partnership, the HHS Strategic Plan, the National Strategy for Quality Improvement in Healthcare, and the CMS Quality Strategy.

Based on input from stakeholders, CMS has identified several high-priority concept areas for future measure development:

- Patient-reported pain outcome measure that incorporates patient and/or proxy report regarding pain management.

- Claims-based measures focused on care practice patterns, including skilled visits in the last days of life, burdensome transitions of care for patients in and out of the hospice benefit, and rates of live discharges from hospice.

- Responsiveness of hospice to patient and family care needs.

- Hospice team communication and care coordination.

These measure concepts are under development, and details regarding for implementation will be communicated in future rule making. CMS invites comments about these four high-priority concept areas for future measure development.

Each hospice is required to submit data to the Secretary on quality measures specified by the Secretary. Such data must be submitted in a form and manner, and at a time specified by the Secretary. Beginning with the FY 2014 and for each subsequent FY, the Secretary shall reduce the market basket update by 2 percentage points for any hospice that does not comply with the quality data submission requirements with respect to that FY.

Any hospice that receives its CCN notification letter on or after November 1 of the preceding year is excluded from any payment penalty for quality reporting purposes for the following fiscal year. For example, if a hospice provider receives their CCN notification letter on November 2, 2015, they would not be required to submit quality data for the current reporting period ending December 31, 2015 (which would affect the FY 2017 APU). In this instance, the hospice would begin with the next reporting period beginning January 1, 2016, and all subsequent years.

CMS proposes that beginning with the FY 2018 payment determination and for each subsequent payment determination, a new hospice will be responsible for HQRP quality data reporting beginning on the date they receive their certification number (CCN) (also known as the Medicare provider number) notification letter from CMS. Currently, new hospices may experience a lag between Medicare certification and receipt of their actual CCN. Since hospices cannot submit data to the Quality Improvement and Evaluation System (QIES) Assessment Submission and Processing (ASAP) system without a valid CCN, CMS proposes that new hospices begin collecting HIS quality data beginning on the date they receive their CCN notification letter by CMS.

In the FY 15 Hospice Wage Index final rule, CMS finalized the policy requiring that, for the FY 2017 reporting requirements, hospices must complete and submit HIS records for all patient admissions to hospice on or after July 1, 2014. Electronic submission is required for all HIS records. Although electronic submission of HIS records is required, hospices do not need to have an electronic medical record to complete or submit HIS data. Providers can use either the Hospice Abstraction Reporting Tool (HART) software, which is free to download and use, or a vendor-designed software. HART provides an alternative option for hospice providers to collect and maintain facility, patient, and HIS Record information for subsequent submission to the QIES ASAP system to complete HIS records. Once HIS records are complete, electronic HIS files must be submitted to CMS via the QIES ASAP system. Electronic data submission via the QIES ASAP system is required for all HIS submissions; there are no other data submission methods available. Hospices have 30 days from a patient admission or discharge to submit the appropriate HIS record for that patient through the QIES ASAP system. CMS will continue to make HIS completion and submission software available to hospices at no cost.

Details on data collection and submission timing are at http://www.cms.gov/Medicare/Quality-Initiatives-Patient-Assessment Instruments/Hospice-Quality-Reporting/Hospice-Item-Set-HIS.html.

The QIES ASAP system provides reports upon successful submission and processing of the HIS records. The final validation report may serve as evidence of submission. This is the same data submission system used by nursing homes, inpatient rehabilitation facilities, home health agencies, and long-term care hospitals for the submission of Minimum Data Set Version 3.0 (MDS 3.0), Inpatient Rehabilitation Facility—Patient Assessment Instrument (IRF–PAI), Outcome Assessment Information Set (OASIS), and Long-Term Care Hospital Continuity Assessment Record & Evaluation Data Set (LTCH CARE), respectively.

Beginning with the FY 2018 payment determination, CMS proposes that hospices must submit all HIS records within 30 days of the event date, which is the patient's admission date for HIS-Admission records or discharge date for HIS-Discharge records.

For HIS-Admission records, the submission date should be no later than the admission date plus 30 calendar days. The submission date can be equal to the admission date, or no greater than 30 days later. The QIES ASAP system will issue a warning on the Final Validation Report if the submission date is more than 30 days after the patient's admission date.

For HIS-Discharge records, the submission date should be no later than the discharge date plus 30 calendar days. The submission date can be equal to the discharge date, or no greater than 30 days later. The QIES ASAP system will issue a warning on the Final Validation Report if the submission date is more than 30 days after the patient's discharge date.

The QIES ASAP system validation edits are designed to monitor the timeliness and ensure that providers submitted records that conform to the HIS data submission specifications. Providers are notified when timing criteria have not been met by warnings that appear on their Final Validation Reports. A standardized data collection approach that coincides with timely submission of data is essential in order to establish a robust quality reporting program and ensure the scientific reliability of the data received.

CMS is proposing to set specific HQRP thresholds for timeliness of submission of hospice quality data beginning with data affecting the FY 2018 payment determination and subsequent years. Beginning with the FY 2018 payment determination and subsequent FY payment determinations, the agency proposes that all HIS records must be submitted within 30 days of the Event Date, which is the patient's admission date or discharge date. The agency also proposes to establish an incremental threshold for compliance with this timeliness requirement; the proposed threshold would be implemented over a three-year period. CMS proposes that for timeliness compliance, hospices would have to submit no less than 70 percent of their total number of HIS-Admission and HIS-Discharge records by no later than 30 days from the Event Date for the FY 2018 APU determination. The timeliness threshold would be set at 80 percent for FY 2019 and at 90 percent for FY 2020 and subsequent years.

The proposed timeliness threshold beginning with all HIS-Admission and HIS-Discharge records that occur on or after January 1, 2016, will be:

- Beginning on or after January 1, 2016, to December 31, 2016, at least 70 percent of all required HIS records must be received within the 30-day submission timeframe for the year or be subject to a 2 percentage point reduction to their market basket update for FY 2018.

- Beginning on or after January 1, 2017, to December 31, 2017, at least 80 percent of all HIS records must be received within the 30-day submission timeframe for the year or be subject to a 2 percentage point reduction to their market basket update for FY 2019.

- Beginning on or after January 1, 2018, to December 31, 2018, at least 90 percent of all HIS records must be received within the 30-day submission timeframe for the year or be subject to a 2 percentage point reduction to their market basket update for FY 2020.

In the FY 2015 Update final rule, CMS finalized a proposal to allow hospices to request and for CMS to grant exemptions/extensions with respect to the reporting of required quality data when there are extraordinary circumstances beyond the control of the provider. When an extension/exception is granted, a hospice will not incur payment reduction penalties for failure to comply with the requirements of the HQRP.

For the FY 2016 payment determination and subsequent payment determinations, a hospice may request an extension/exception of the requirement to submit quality data for a specified time period. In the event that a hospice requests an extension/exception for quality reporting purposes, the hospice would submit a written request to CMS. In general, exceptions and extensions will not be granted for hospice vendor issues, fatal error messages preventing record submission, or staff error.

In the event that a hospice seeks to request an exception or extension for quality reporting purposes, the hospice must request an exception or extension within 30 days of the date that the extraordinary circumstances occurred by submitting the request to CMS via email to the HQRP mailbox at HQRPReconsiderations@cms.hhs.gov. Exception or extension requests sent to CMS through any other channel would not be considered as a valid request for an exception or extension from the HQRP's reporting requirements for any payment determination. In order to be considered, a request for an exception or extension must contain all of the finalized requirements as outlined on the CMS web site at http://www.cms.gov/Medicare/Quality-Initiatives-Patient-Assessment-Instruments/HospiceQuality-Reporting/index.html.

Adoption of the CAHPS® Hospice Survey for the FY 2017 Payment Determination and That of Subsequent Fiscal Years

CMS began national implementation of the Consumer Assessment of Healthcare Providers and Systems (CAHPS) hospice survey as of January 1, 2015. This CAHPS Hospice Survey is a component of CMS's Hospice Quality Reporting Program that emphasizes the experiences of hospice patients and their primary caregivers listed in the hospice patients' records. Measures from the survey will be submitted to the National Quality Forum (NQF) for endorsement as hospice quality measures.

CMS developed the CAHPS Hospice Survey with input from many stakeholders, including other government agencies, industry stakeholders, consumer groups and other key individuals and organizations involved in hospice care. The survey was designed to measure and assess the experiences of patients who died while receiving hospice care as well as the experiences of their informal caregivers.

The CAHPS Hospice Survey treats the dying patient and his or her informal caregivers (family members or friends) as the unit of care. The Survey seeks information from the informal caregivers of patients who died while enrolled in hospices. Survey-eligible patients and caregivers are identified using hospice records. During national implementation of this survey, hospices are required to conduct the survey to meet the Hospice Quality Reporting requirements, but individual caregivers will respond only if they voluntarily choose to do so.

Hospices with fewer than 50 survey eligible decedents/caregivers during the prior calendar year are exempt from the hospice survey data collection and reporting requirements for payment determination. Hospices with 50 to 699 survey-eligible decedents/caregivers in the prior year will be required to survey all cases. For hospices with 700 or more survey-eligible decedents/caregivers in the prior year, a sample of 700 will be drawn under an equal-probability design. Medicare-certified hospices are required to contract with a third-party vendor that is CMS-trained and approved to administer the survey on their behalf. A list of approved vendors can be found at this web site: www.hospicecahpssurvey.org.

Consistent with many other CMS CAHPS surveys that are publicly reported on CMS web sites, CMS will publicly report hospice data when at least 12 months of data are available, so that valid comparisons can be made across hospice providers in the United States, to help patients, family, and friends choose a hospice program for themselves or their loved ones.

Hospices that have fewer than 50 survey-eligible decedents/caregivers in the period from January 1, 2015, through December 31, 2015, are exempt from CAHPS Hospice Survey data collection and reporting requirements for the 2018 APU. Hospices must request a survey exemption for the FY 2018 APU by submitting an exemption request form. This form will be available on the CAHPS Hospice Survey web site www.hospicecahpssurvey.org.

In accordance with the Affordable Care Act, beginning with FY 2014 and each subsequent fiscal year, the market basket update will be reduced by 2 percentage points for any hospice that does not comply with the quality data submission requirements with respect to that fiscal year, unless covered by specific exemptions. Any such reduction will not be cumulative and will not be taken into account in computing the payment amount for subsequent fiscal years.

Appendix H: Skilled Nursing Facility Resource Utilization Groups (RUG-IV) Classification System

The Balanced Budget Act of 1997 required the implementation of a Medicare skilled nursing facility (SNF) prospective payment system (PPS). Part of the PPS for skilled nursing facilities is the resource utilization groups (RUG-IV) classification system.

Note: This classification system employs a two-stage process involving a clinical qualification stage followed by a classification stage. The clinical qualification stage includes the patient diagnoses, conditions and comorbidities, treatments, and services. The classification stage involves the levels of assistance used in performing activities of daily living (ADLs) and skilled services rendered. Assignment of a resident to a specific clinical category must be based upon the patient's meeting all the required qualifications for that category level.

Each of the categories of the RUG-IV classification system is covered in detail in the following excerpts from the *Federal Register*. Please note that the diagnosis and procedure codes identified by Optum's exclusive color-coding system represent only the clinical qualification stage of the classification process. All other qualifications referred to in the explanation of the categories must be addressed. The color-coding system provided is meant only as an alert to the coder that there is the potential to assign a resident to a particular category, provided other qualifications are met. Also, the diagnoses identified are representative and not all-inclusive of the clinical conditions considered to qualify a case for assignment to a specific RUG-IV category.

A comprehensive discussion regarding the original provisions of the SNF prospective payment system can be found in the Medicare Program: Prospective Payment System and Consolidated Billing for Skilled Nursing Facilities; Final Rule (*Federal Register*: May 12, 1998 [volume 63, number 91]), 42 CFR Parts 409, 410, 411, 413, 424, 483, and 489.

Annual updates to the PPS rates are required by section 1888(e) of the Social Security Act as amended by the Medicare, Medicaid, and SCHIP Balanced Budget Refinement Act of 1999 (BBRA), the Medicare, Medicaid, and SCHIP Benefits Improvement and Protection Act of 2000 (BIPA), and the Medicare Prescription Drug, Improvement, and Modernization Act of 2003 (MMA), relating to Medicare payments and consolidated billing for SNFs. The Prospective Payment System and Consolidated Billing for Skilled Nursing Facilities-Update; Final Rule, was published in the *Federal Register* July 31, 2001 (volume 66, number 147), CFR Parts 410, 411, 413, 424, and 489. In the final rule effective October 1, 2001, the Centers for Medicare and Medicaid Services (CMS) rebased and revised the routine market basket, modified certain variables for some of the cost categories, and implemented the transition of swing-bed facilities to the SNF PPS.

On August 4, 2005, the Prospective Payment System and Consolidated Billing for Skilled Nursing Facilities for FY 2006; Final Rule, was published in the *Federal Register* (volume 70, number 149), CFR Parts 409, 411, 424, and 489. In the final rule effective October 1, 2005, CMS made significant revisions to SNF PPS to included refinements to the case-mix classification system. The revisions included the creation of nine new RUG-III categories to better account for medically complex patients. These additional groups were intended to capture residents receiving both rehabilitation services and extensive services. This expanded the classification system from 44 groups to 53 groups, effective with dates of service on or after January 1, 2006.

The following list includes the added RUG-III groups:

- RUX Rehabilitation, Ultra High, Plus Extensive Services, High, ADL Index 16–18
- RUL Rehabilitation, Ultra High, Plus Extensive Services, Low, ADL Index 7–15
- RVX Rehabilitation, Very High, Plus Extensive Services, High, ADL Index 16–18
- RVL Rehabilitation, Very High, Plus Extensive Services, Low, ADL Index 7–15
- RHX Rehabilitation, High, plus Extensive Services, High, ADL Index 13–18
- RHL Rehabilitation, High, plus Extensive Services, Low, ADL Index 7–12
- RMX Rehabilitation, Medium, Plus Extensive Services, High, ADL Index 15–18
- RML Rehabilitation, Medium, Plus Extensive Services, Low, ADL Index 7–14
- RLX Rehabilitation, Low, Plus Extensive Services, ADL Index 7–18

The five-digit HIPPS code that is reported includes two components: the three-digit classification code assigned to each RUG version 3 (RUG-III) group, and a two-digit assessment indicator that specifies the type of Medicare-required assessment used to support billing.

RUG IV Classification System and MDS 3.0

Section 10325 of the Patient Protection and Affordable Care Act (ACA) includes a provision addressing Medicare payments for SNFs in fiscal 2011. This section mandates a delay in the introduction of the RUG-IV case-mix classification system until fiscal 2012. However, On December 15, 2010, President Obama singed into law the Medicare and Medicaid Extenders Act of 2010 (MMEA). Section 202 of the MMEA repeals the delay of the SNF PPS RUG-IV classification system. Therefore, RUG-IV continues to remain in effect from October 1, 2010, as previously implemented by the FY 2011 final SNF payment regulation.

The incentives created by the SNF prospective payment system, quality measures reporting, advances in technology, and a changing SNF resident population necessitate modifications to the current case-mix classification system.

Modifications to the RUG Model

a. Concurrent Therapy

Concurrent therapy is the practice of one professional therapist treating multiple patients at the same time while the patients are performing different activities. Concurrent therapy is distinct from group therapy, in which one therapist provides the same services to everyone in the group. Effective with the introduction of RUG-IV, concurrent therapy time provided in a Part A SNF setting would no longer be counted as individual therapy time for each of the patients involved. For each discipline, concurrent therapy minutes must be allocated before reporting total therapy minutes on the MDS 3.0. Concurrent therapy should never be the sole mode of delivering therapy care to any individual in a SNF setting. Concurrent therapy should be used as an adjunct to individual therapy when clinically appropriate, as determined by the individual's current medical and physical status based on a therapist's clinical judgment.

b. Adjustments to Therapy Minutes

The steps for making the therapy time adjustment included:

- Totaling each resident's time for each discipline by adding times across the several practitioners of that discipline (for example, for physical therapy, there could be time reported for therapists, assistants, and aides).
- Computing the resident's average therapy session time for each separate discipline. There had to be 15 minutes or more of therapy for inclusion in the computation.
- Estimating the total adjusted number of days the resident received that therapy discipline. A day of therapy is considered 15 minutes or more of therapy time.

c. ADL Adjustments

The RUG-IV ADL index is intended to reflect both clinical and statistical considerations, with the aim of scoring similarly those residents with similar function. Component scores have been adjusted to make the scale more proportional to physical function. In addition, CMS increased the range of the RUG-IV ADL index (17 points), as compared with the RUG-III ADL index (15 points), to allow somewhat greater distinction in physical function. To compute the RUG-IV ADL index, CMS summed the component ADL scores for bed mobility, transfer, eating, and toilet use.

d. "Look-Back" Period

CMS proposes to modify the look-back period under RUG-IV for those items in section P.1.a. of the MDS 2.0, Special Treatments and Procedures, to include only these services that are provided after admission (or readmission) to the SNF.

e. Organizing the Nursing and Therapy Minutes

The proposed RUG-IV model uses the same basic methodology that was used to develop the RUG-III model that is in use today. The current RUG-III model was created as a hierarchy from highest to lowest resource use. Clinical conditions and services were assigned to a hierarchy level based on similarity of staff time required to treat a beneficiary with that condition. For RUG-IV, the ADL scale remains a critical part of the model. CMS is proposing two modifications to the existing ADL methodology. First, in RUG-IV, the ADL categories will be standardized across the various levels of the hierarchy. Second, the ADL scale will be revised to make it more sensitive to differences in functional levels.

f. RUG Classification System Modification

In developing the RUG-IV system, several modifications were made to the RUG-III system to better reflect current medical practice and staff resources. The major changes in the classification system are discussed in the next section.

In the RUG-IV classification system, patient characteristics and health status information from the proposed MDS 3.0 would be used to assign the patient to a resource group for payment. The new RUG-IV system is a hierarchy of major patient types and reflects current medical practice and staff resource use in SNFs. In the RUG-IV model, CMS proposes to modify the eight levels of the hierarchy and increase the number of case-mix groups from 53 to 66. Functional status is a key component of both the existing RUG-III model and the proposed RUG-IV and is used to distinguish the level of resource need between patients with similar conditions. RUG-IV, like RUG-III, uses a scale measuring ADLs to identify residents with similar levels of physical function. This scale is used to subdivide ("split") each of the major hierarchical categories except Extensive Services.

Since the case-mix index (CMI) assigned to each RUG group is based on average resource time for the conditions and services included in that RUG group, the individual RUG groups are as homogeneous as possible with respect to the resource times associated with the conditions and services included in each group.

The RUG-IV classification model is an iterative process whereby patients are assigned first to one of eight major categories that indicate the primary patient nursing and/or therapy needs. Each case is assigned to the highest major category for which it qualifies. In hierarchical order, from highest to lowest, the categories are:

- Rehabilitation plus Extensive Services
- Rehabilitation
- Extensive Services
- Special Care High
- Special Care Low
- Clinically Complex
- Behavioral Symptoms and Cognitive Performance
- Reduced Physical Function

These major categories are further differentiated into more specific patient groupings or secondary splits. Except for the Extensive Services category, CMS uses a secondary split based on the resident's ADL score discussed earlier in this section. The RUG-IV groups may be further differentiated based on nursing rehabilitation services and signs of depression. Thus, a record for a patient who is admitted to a SNF for treatment that qualifies for the Special Care High major category will be further evaluated to assign the most appropriate of the eight Special Care High groups. The final group selection will be made based on the patient's ADL level and on the existence of signs/symptoms of depression.

More detailed description of the eight RUG-IV classification categories follows the SNF PPS discussion follows.

Prospective Payment System for Skilled Nursing Facilities

1. Background on the Resource Utilization Groups (RUGs) Patient Classification System

As part of the Nursing Home Case-Mix and Quality demonstration project, version III of the resource utilization groups (RUG-III) case-mix classification system was developed to capture resource use of nursing home patients and to provide an improved method of tracking the quality of care.

RUG-III was a 44-group model for classifying nursing home patients into homogeneous groups according to the amount and type of resources they use. The RUG groups are the basis for the payment indexes used to establish equitable prospective payment levels for patients with different service use. Care provided directly to, or for, a patient is represented by an index score that is based on the amount of staff time, weighted by salary levels, associated with each group. That is, each RUG-III group was assigned an index score that represents the amount of nursing time and rehabilitation treatment time associated with caring for the patients who qualify for the group. The nursing weight includes both patient-specific time spent daily on behalf of each patient type by registered nurses, licensed practical nurses, and aides, as well as patient nonspecific time spent by these staff members on other necessary functions such as staff education, administrative duties, and other tasks associated with maintenance of the care-giving environment.

The principal goal of case-mix measurement is to identify patient characteristics associated with measured resource use. In nursing homes, no adequate models have been found for using length of stay or episode cost to explain resource use. Thus, the RUG nursing home case-mix system explains patient resource use on a daily basis.

The classification system was designed using resident characteristic information and measures of wage-weighted staff time. Information regarding a patient's characteristics and care needs is derived from the MDS, a set of core screening

and assessment items and item definitions. The MDS is part of a standardized, comprehensive patient assessment instrument (the Resident Assessment Instrument or RAI) that all long-term care facilities that are certified to participate in Medicare or Medicaid are required to use to develop individualized plans of care for each individual in the facility. The staff time measure (STM) study captured the amount of nursing staff time required to care for groups of residents over a 24-hour period and over the span of a week for therapy services.

Patient assessment and staff time data used to develop the initial version of the RUG-III classification system were collected from March to December 1990 for 7,648 patients in 202 nursing facilities in Kansas, Maine, Mississippi, South Dakota, Nebraska, Texas, and New York. Since then, two more staff time data collections have been performed on 154 Medicare certified units of hospital and freestanding facilities in 12 states (California, Colorado, Florida, Kansas, Maine, Maryland, Mississippi, New York, Ohio, South Dakota, Texas, and Washington). Only units that were judged to be providing adequate care were considered for participation in the study. Of these, the states were asked to select facilities that included 35 percent Medicare certified units, 25 percent hospital units, and two Alzheimer's units. "Unit" was defined as a nursing center such as a corridor or a floor, controlled from one nursing station. The remainder of the sample was selected by the state's demonstration project staff to represent the characteristics of the state's nursing homes.

The sample was purposefully targeted toward residents needing complex care and/or with cognitive impairments. This ensured that sufficient numbers of patients with rare types of complex care needs were included in the sample. Facilities with special care units (for example, Alzheimer's or rehabilitation units) that participated in the study were also asked to provide data from a nonspecialized unit.

During the data collection, personnel on the study units electronically recorded all of the time in their work days: time providing services directly to patients; in activities related to specific patients, such as charting or consultation with family members or other members of the patient care team; as well as time that is not attributable to any particular patient, like that spent in meetings, in training, on breaks, etc. The time was allocated according to whether or not it was directly related to a particular patient and was categorized as either patient-specific time or nonpatient specific time.

Those data have been used to modify the classification system to create the current RUG-IV and establish updated average staff times to be salary-weighted. Analyses of the staff time data in conjunction with the patient MDS information identified three main predictors of a patient's resource utilization: 1) clinical characteristics; 2) limitations in the ADLs; and 3) skilled services received. The RUG-IV classification system uses these three types of variables to describe SNF patients for the purposes of determining the relative cost of caring for different types of patients (case-mix).

Analysis of the data indicated that patients with serious clinical conditions such as ventilator care, IV feeding, and respiratory infections, as well as patients who were very dependent in ADLs, require more nursing time than do patients without complicating conditions. The RUG-IV classification system resulting from the analyses is hierarchical. The clinical characteristics of patients, as identified by the MDS, that were associated with the greatest utilization of nursing time and rehabilitative therapy time were used to categorize patients into the highest case-mix classification groups.

Similarly, the clinical characteristics associated with the lowest utilization of nursing time were used to categorize patients into the lowest case-mix classification group. Not all clinical characteristics are recognized separately by the classification system. Only those characteristics that were predictive of resource use and that would not introduce incentives that are considered to be negative, or not compatible with high-quality patient care, are used to classify patients into RUG-III groups.

The mutually exclusive, layered categories of the RUG-IV classification system describe which patient clinical characteristics, levels of assistance used in performing ADLs, and services are used to assign the patient to a RUGs group. Clinical characteristics include the patient diagnoses, conditions, and comorbidities. ADLs include bed mobility, toilet use, transfer from bed to chair, and eating. Patients receive a single RUG-IV ADL score that measures the patient's ability to perform these activities (scores range from 2–16; higher scores represent greater functional dependence and a need for more assistance). Finally, treatments and services include respiratory therapy, amount of rehabilitation received, and treatments such as parenteral feeding and intravenous medication administration.

2. The RUG-IV Classification System

In the RUG-IV classification system, patient characteristics and health status information from the MDS, such as "diagnoses," "ability to perform ADLs," and "treatments received," will be used to assign the patient to a resource group for payment. The RUG-IV system is a hierarchy of major patient types. RUG-IV consists of eight major categories that are the first level of patient classification. The eight major categories, in hierarchical order, are Rehabilitation Plus Extensive Services, Rehabilitation, Extensive Services, Special Care High, Special Care Low, Clinically Complex, Behavior Symptoms and Cognitive Performance, and Reduced Physical Function. These major categories are further differentiated into 66 more specific patient groupings. Except for Rehabilitation and Extensive Services, these categories are first subdivided into groups based on the patient's ADL score. The next level of subdivision is based on nursing rehabilitation services and signs of depression.

The initial subdivision of the Rehabilitation category is based on minutes per week of rehabilitative therapy services. The second level of subdivision uses the ADL score. The Extensive Services category does not use ADL limitations except as a threshold for assignment into the category. Rather, services that require more technical clinical knowledge and skill are the variables used for assigning patients into this category. Examples of these services are ventilator care, tracheostomy care, or isolation for active infectious disease.

For example, the Special Care High category includes patients:

- With quadriplegia
- With septicemia
- In a coma
- With diabetes with daily injections
- With COPD
- Receiving respiratory therapy
- With fever with pneumonia, or vomiting weight loss, or tube feedings
- Requiring parenteral /IV feeding

Any patient with one or more of these conditions who is not receiving rehabilitation services will be assigned to this category. The patient's assignment to one of the three groups within this category is dependent on the patient's ADL score.

The Rehabilitation category is organized differently from the clinical categories that follow in the hierarchy. Within this category, there are five subcategories (Ultra High, Very High, High, Medium, and Low) that are then further split into the individual groups for payment. The subcategories are defined by minutes per week of rehabilitation received by the patient, number of rehabilitation disciplines providing service, and the number of days per week on which rehabilitation services were provided. Assignment into a specific payment group is based on the patient's ability to perform certain of the activities of daily living as represented by his ADL score. As stated elsewhere, the patient is assessed on his ability to perform independently all of the activities of daily living and is assigned an ADL sum score that represents performance of the four "late loss" ADLs. The "late loss" ADLs used in the MDS ADL sum score are eating; toileting; bed mobility; and transferring.

A brief description of the respective RUG-IV categories below.

Rehabilitation plus Extensive Services: This category includes residents who qualify for both the Extensive Services group and Rehabilitation Services groups with an ADL score greater than 2. Residents classified to this category are receiving physical, speech, or occupational therapy AND IV feeding or tracheostomy care, and are ventilation/respirator dependent or in isolation for an active infectious disease. In addition residents are stratified according to ADL scores into two levels; low with ADL scores of 7–15 and high with ADL scores 16–18.

Rehabilitation: This category includes patients who, if they were not receiving rehabilitation therapy, would qualify for one of the other RUG-IV skilled care categories. This category is divided into subcategories based on the number of minutes of physical, occupational, or speech-language services received in a week, combinations of rehabilitation disciplines providing services, receipt of nursing rehabilitative services, and the patient ADL scores. The range of rehabilitation therapy minutes per day represented in the Rehabilitation category varies from a low of 45 minutes per week to a high of more than 720 minutes per week. Patients who qualify for assignment to the Ultra High Rehabilitation subcategory receive at least 720 minutes per week of rehabilitation therapies. At least two disciplines must be providing services: one of the disciplines must provide services five days each week, and the other at least three days each week. In contrast, patients assigned to the lowest rehabilitation sub-category, Low Rehabilitation, must receive at least 45 minutes of rehabilitative therapy services across at least three days each week, in addition to six days per week of nursing rehabilitation in two activities.

Extensive Services: To qualify for this category, patients must have, in the past 14 days, received tracheostomy care, required a ventilator/respirator, or been put in isolation for active infectious disease. In addition, the patients assigned to this category will have an ADL score that is at least 2. There are three levels of care in

the Extensive Services category: ES3 for tracheostomy AND ventilator/respirator care; ES2 for tracheostomy OR ventilator/respirator care; and ES3 for isolation for infectious disease.

Special Care High: Patients who are assigned to this category have at least one of the following: they must be in a coma, have septicemia, diabetes with daily injections, quadriplegia (with ADL = 5), COPD, or fever with pneumonia or vomiting or weight loss or tube feeding, or be undergoing parenteral feeding or respiratory therapy for seven days and an ADL score = 2. Signs of depression are used as an end split.

Special Care Low: Patients who are assigned to this category have at least one of the following: they must have multiple sclerosis (ADL = 5), cerebral palsy (ADL = 5), Parkinson's disease (ADL = 5), or respiratory failure with oxygen therapy, be receiving treatment for pressure or stasis ulcers on two or more body sites, or radiation therapy; or suffer from foot infections (diabetic foot ulcers, open lesions) and have an ADL = 2. Signs of depression are used as an end split.

Clinically Complex: Patients qualify for this category if they are comatose, have burns, pneumonia, hemiplegia in combination with an ADL = 5, or surgical wounds with treatment, or are receiving chemotherapy, oxygen therapy, IV medications, or transfusions.

Behavioral Symptoms and Cognition Performance: Patients in this category and the following two categories frequently will not qualify for Medicare coverage although some may, due to specific circumstances. The patients in this category will have scores on the MDS 3.0 Cognition Performance Scale (CPS) = 3 or BIMS score = 9, or hallucinations or delusions. Residents also qualify for this category if they have four or more of the following symptoms: physical or verbal behavioral symptoms towards others, rejection of care, wandering, or other behavioral symptoms and an ADL = 5. Under the SNF coverage guidelines, these patients could qualify based on the need for skilled nursing rehabilitation.

Physical Function Reduced: The patients in this category are those who do not have any of the conditions or characteristics identified above. However, some have been documented as receiving "skilled nursing" and have been covered by Medicare in the past. With proper documentation and justification regarding the need for skilled care, Medicare may continue to cover skilled nursing services. No clinical variables are used for this category.

Proposed FY 2016 Changes

There is no FY 2015 forecast error adjustment. In FY 2014, the estimated increase in the market basket index was 2.3 percentage points, while the actual increase for FY 2014 was 1.7 percentage points, resulting in the actual increase being 0.6 percentage points lower than the estimated increase. Proposed changes for FY 2015 currently project an increase in payments to SNFs of $500 million, or 1.4 percent, from payments in FY 2015. This estimated increase is attributable to a 2.6 percent market basket increase, reduced by a 0.6 percentage point forecast error adjustment and further reduced by a 0.6 percentage point, in accordance with the multifactor productivity adjustment required by law.

Statutes define the productivity adjustment to be equal to "the 10-year moving average of changes in annual economy-wide private nonfarm business multi-factor productivity (as projected by the Secretary for the 10-year period ending with the applicable fiscal year, year, cost-reporting period, or other annual period)" (the MFP adjustment). For the FY 2016 update, the MFP adjustment is calculated as the 10-year moving average of changes in MFP for the period ending September 30, 2016, which is 0.4 percent.

Each RUG–IV category has a case-mix adjusted federal rate with unique labor-related and non-labor-related components. CMS proposes to continue to use hospital inpatient wage data, exclusive of the occupational mix adjustment, in developing a wage index to be applied to SNFs.

The budget neutrality factor for FY 2016 would be 0.9989.

Proposed Wage Index Changes

The Office of Management and Budget (OMB) published revisions on February 28, 2013, that contain a number of significant changes. For example, there are new CBSAs, urban counties that become rural, rural counties that become urban, and existing CBSAs that are being split apart.

CMS assessed these changes and is proposing changes to the SNF PPS wage index beginning in FY 2015. This change includes a proposed one-year transition with a blended wage index for FY 2015.

CMS applied a one-year transition with a 50/50 blended wage index for all providers in FY 2015. The agency calculated the FY 2015 wage indexes using both the current FY 2014 and proposed new labor market delineations. Providers received 50 percent of their FY 2015 wage index based on the new OMB delineations, and 50 percent of their FY 2015 wage index based on the labor market area delineations for FY 2014. CMS notes that this ultimately results in an average of the two values.

Appendix H: Skilled Nursing Facility Resource Utilization Groups (RUG-IV) Classification System

This blended wage index will be referred to as the FY 2015 SNF PPS transition wage index. This transition policy was for a one-year period, from October 1, 2014, and continuing through September 30, 2015. Beginning October 1, 2015, the wage index for all SNFs would be fully based on the new OMB delineations.

Quality Reporting

The Improving Medicare Post-Acute Care Transformation Act of 2014 (P.L. 113-185, IMPACT Act), of October 6, 2014, required the implementation of a quality reporting program for SNFs. Beginning with FY 2018, the act requires SNFs that fail to submit required quality data to CMS under the SNF Quality Reporting Program (QRP) to have their annual updates reduced by two percentage points.

CMS is proposing to adopt three measures addressing three quality domains identified in the IMPACT Act:

- Skin integrity and changes in skin integrity
- Incidence of major falls
- Functional status, cognitive function, and changes in function and cognitive function

These measures will be in place for the FY 2018 SNF QRP and subsequent years. The proposed measures satisfy the IMPACT Act requirement of standardized data reporting across four post-acute care settings, including home health agencies, inpatient rehabilitation facilities, skilled nursing facilities, and long-term care hospitals.

Below is a table summarizing domains and proposed measures for the SNF QPR:

Domain	Proposed Measures
Skin Integrity and Changes in Skin Integrity	Outcome Measure: Percent of Residents or Patients with Pressure Ulcers That Are New or Worsened (Short-Stay) (NQF #0678; Measure Steward: CMS)
Incidence of Major Falls	Outcome Measure: Application of Percent of Residents Experiencing One or More Falls with Major Injury (Long Stay) (NQF #0674; Measure Steward: CMS)
Functional Status, Cognitive Function, and Changes in Function and Cognitive Function	Process Measure: Application of Percent of Patients or Residents with an Admission and Discharge Functional Assessment and a Care Plan that Addresses Function (NQF#2631) (Under NQF review Measure Steward: CMS)

Skilled Nursing Facility Value-Based Purchasing Program

The Protecting Access to Medicare Act (PAMA) of 2014 establishes a Skilled Nursing Facility Value-Based Purchasing (SNF VBP) Program beginning with FY 2019. This program will provide value-based incentive payments to SNFs in a fiscal year based on performance.

CMS is proposing to adopt the Skilled Nursing Facility 30-Day All-Cause Readmission Measure, (SNFRM) (NQF #2510), to be used in the SNF VBP Program. The Skilled Nursing Facility 30-Day All-Cause Readmission Measure estimates the risk-standardized rate of all-cause, unplanned, hospital readmissions for SNF Medicare beneficiaries within 30 days of their prior proximal short-stay acute hospital discharge. This proposed measure is claims-based and its adoption would not result in any increased costs to SNFs.

In the proposed rule, CMS seeks public comments on numerous SNF VBP policies. CMS intends to propose additional details of the SNF VBP in the FY 2017 SNF PPS proposed and final rules, and is currently seeking comments on:

- Performance standards
- Measuring improvement
- Appropriate baseline and performance periods
- Performance scoring methodology
- Public reporting of performance information
- Feedback reports

Staffing Data Collection

The Affordable Care Act of 2010 (Pub. L. 111-148, March 23, 2010) added new mandates that aim to promote greater accountability for long-term care (LTC) facilities (defined as skilled nursing facilities and nursing facilities). The act allows the collection of staffing data for LTC facilities. It requires that a facility electronically submit to the Secretary direct care staffing information (including information with respect to agency and contract staff) based on payroll and other verifiable and auditable data in a uniform format (according to specifications established by the Secretary in consultation with such programs, groups, and parties). These specifications require that the information submitted specify the category of work a certified employee performs (such as whether the employee is a registered nurse, licensed practical nurse, licensed vocational nurse, certified nursing assistant, therapist, or other medical personnel), include resident census data and information on resident case mix, be reported on a regular schedule, and include information on employee turnover and tenure and on the hours of care provided by each category of certified employee per resident per day.

New MDS Data

New items will be required on the MDS 3.0 to support data collection and reporting for these three proposed measures. New items will be included on the following assessments:

SNF PPS 5-Day; Swing Bed PPS 5-Day; OMRA—Start of Therapy Discharge; OMRA—Other Discharge, OBRA Discharge; Swing Bed OMRA—Start of Therapy, Discharge; Swing Bed OMRA—Other Discharge;, and Swing Bed Discharge on the MDS 3.0.

The SNF QRP will also require the addition of a SNF PPS Part A Discharge Assessment, which will also include new items. These new required data elements are to identify whether pressure ulcers were present on admission, to inform future development of the Percent of Residents or Patients with Pressure Ulcers That Are New or Worsened (Short Stay) (NQF #0678), as well as to indicate changes in function and occurrence of falls with major injury.

Appendix I: Skilled Nursing Facility Active Diagnosis List

The following list includes disease processes that can have a significant adverse effect on an individual's health status and quality of life. This list identifies the active diseases and infections that have been determined to drive the current plan of care for a resident and should be reported on the MDS form. Active diagnoses have a direct relationship with the resident's functional status, cognitive status, mood or behavior, medical treatments, nursing monitoring, or risk of death during the look–back period.

NOTE: The list is not all–inclusive and includes primary examples of the conditions that affect resident care. Please be advised that it is the responsibility of the health care professional to determine all active conditions currently affecting treatment decisions or health status.

MDS Data Element	Diagnoses	ICD–10–CM Codes
Cancer		
I0100	Cancer (with or without metastasis)	Categories C00–D49
Heart/Circulation		
I0200	Anemia:	
	• aplastic	Category D60, D61.9
	• iron deficiency	D50.8, D50.9
	• pernicious	D51.0
	• sickle cell	Category D57
I0300	Atrial dysrhythmia:	
	• fibrillation	I48.0–I48.2, I48.91
	• flutter	I48.3–I48.4, I48.92
	Other dysrhythmias:	I49.8, I49.9
	• sick sinus syndrome	I49.5
	• bradycardia NOS	R00.1
	• tachycardia NOS	R00.0
	• tachycardia, atrial	I47.1
I0400	Coronary artery disease [CAD]:	
	• CAD without angina	I25.10, I25.810–I25.812
	• CAD with angina	I25.110–I25.119, I25.700–I25.799
	Myocardial infarction	Categories I21 and I22
	Angina	I20.0–I20.9
I0500	Deep venous thrombosis [DVT] (lower extremity):	
	• acute	I82.401–I82.4Z9
	• chronic	I82.501–I82.5Z9
	Pulmonary embolus [PE]	Category I26
	Pulmonary thromboembolism [PTE]	Category I26
I0600	Heart failure:	
	• congestive heart failure [CHF]	Category I50
	• pulmonary edema	Category J81
I0700	Hypertension	I10
	• with heart disease	Category I11
	• with CKD	Category I12
	• with heart disease and CKD	Category I13
I0800	Orthostatic hypotension	I95.1
I0900	Peripheral vascular disease NOS	I73.9
	Peripheral arterial disease	I73.9
Gastrointestinal		
I1100	Cirrhosis	K74.3–K74.69
I1200	Gastroesophageal reflux disease [GERD]	Category K21
	Ulcer:	
	• esophageal	K22.10–K22.11
	• gastric	Category K25
	• peptic ulcers NOS	Category K27

MDS Data Element	Diagnoses	ICD–10–CM Codes
I1300	Ulcerative colitis NOS	Category K51
	Crohn's disease	Category K50
	Inflammatory bowel disease	Category K58
Genitourinary		
I1400	Benign prostatic hyperplasia [BPH]	Category N40
I1500	Renal insufficiency (acute):	N28.9
	• chronic	N18.9
	Renal failure NOS:	N19
	• acute	Category N17
	• chronic	Category N18
	End stage renal disease [ESRD]	N18.6
I1550	Neurogenic bladder	Category N31
I1650	Obstructive uropathy	N13.8–N13.9
Infections		
I1700	Multidrug resistant organism [MDRO]	Category Z16
I2000	Pneumonia	Categories J12–J18, J69
I2100	Septicemia	Categories A40, A41
I2200	Tuberculosis	Categories A15, A17, A18, A19
I2300	Urinary tract infection [UTI] (last 30 days)	N39.0
I2400	Viral hepatitis:	
	• hepatitis A	
	acute	Category B15
	chronic	B18.8
	• hepatitis B	
	acute	Category B16
	chronic	B18.0–B18.1
	NOS	B19.10–B19.11
	• hepatitis C	
	acute	B17.10–B17.11
	chronic	B18.2
	NOS	B19.20–B19.21
	• hepatitis D	
	acute	B17.8
	chronic	B18.8
	• hepatitis E	
	acute	B17.2
	chronic	B18.8
	• NOS	B19.0, B19.9
	acute	B17.9
	chronic	B18.9
I2500	Wound infection (other than foot)	

MDS Data Element	Diagnoses	ICD–10–CM Codes	MDS Data Element	Diagnoses	ICD–10–CM Codes
Metabolic			I4800	Non–Alzheimer's Dementia:	
I2900	Diabetes mellitus (DM):	Categories E08–E13		• Lewy body dementia	
	• diabetic retinopathy	E08.311–E08.359, E09.311–E09.359, E10.311–E10.359, E11.311–E11.359, E13.311–E13.359		• vascular dementia	
				• multi–infarct dementia	
				• frontotemporal dementia	
	• nephropathy	E08.21–E08.29, E09.21–E09.29, E10.21–E10.29, E11.21–E11.29, E13.21–E13.29		Pick's disease dementia related to stroke	
				• Parkinson's disease	
				• Parkinsonism	
				• Creutzfeldt–Jakob diseases	
	• neuropathy (peripheral autonomic)(polyneuropathy)	E08.40–E08.49, E09.40–E09.49, E10.40–E10.49, E11.40–E11.49, E13.40–E13.49	I4900	Hemiplegia, hemiparesis late effect of CVA	Category G81 I69.05, I69.15, I69.25, I69.35, I69.85, I69.95
I3100	Hyponatremia	E87.1	I5000	Paraplegia	G82.20–G82.22
I3200	Hyperkalemia	E87.5	I5100	Quadriplegia	G82.50–G82.54
I3300	Hyperlipidemia	E78.4–E78.5	I5200	Multiple sclerosis (MS)	G35
	Hypercholesterolemia	E78.0	I5250	Huntington's disease	G10
I3400	Thyroid disorder:		I5300	Parkinson's disease	G20
	• hypothyroidism (primary) NOS	E03.9	I5350	Tourette's syndrome	F95.2
	• hyperthyroidism NOS	Category E05	I5400	Seizure disorder NOS	G40.909
	• Hashimoto's thyroiditis	E06.3		Epilepsy	Category G40
Musculoskeletal			I5500	Traumatic brain injury (TBI)	Category S06
I3700	Arthritis:		**Nutritional**		
	• degenerative joint disease [DJD]	See osteoarthritis categories	I5600	Malnutrition (protein or calorie) or at risk for malnutrition:	E44.0, E44.1, E46
	• osteoarthritis	Categories M15–M19 Categories M05, M06		• calorie (protein–calorie), severe	E43
	• rheumatoid arthritis [RA]	M08.00–M08.09, M08.20–M08.48		• protein	E46
I3800	Osteoporosis	Categories M80, M81	**Psychiatric/Mood Disorder**		
I3900	Hip fracture – any hip fracture		I5700	Anxiety disorder	F41.9
	that has a relationship to current		I5800	Depression (other than bipolar)	F32.9
	status, treatments, monitoring (e.g., sub–capital fractures, and fractures of the trochanter and femoral neck):		I5900	Manic depression (bipolar disease)	F31.9
			I5950	Psychotic disorder (other than schizophrenia)	Categories F23, F24, F28, F29
	• traumatic	S72.001–S72.26	I6000	Schizophrenia:	Category F20
	• pathological	M84.451–M84.459, M84.550–84.559, M84.650–M84.659		• schizoaffective	Category F25
				• schizophreniform disorders	F20.81
I4000	Other fracture		I6100	Posttraumatic stress disorder (PTSD)	F43.10–F43.12
	• traumatic	Categories S02, S22, S32, S42, S52, S62, S72, S82	**Pulmonary**		
			I6200	Asthma	Category J45
	• pathological	Category M84		Chronic obstructive pulmonary disease [COPD]	Category J44
Neurological				Chronic bronchitis	Categories J40, J41, J42
I4200	Alzheimer's disease	Category G30		Asbestosis	J61
I4300	Aphasia	R47.01	I6300	Respiratory Failure	Category J96
	d/t CVA	I69.020, I69.120, I69.220, I69.320, I69.820, I69.920	**Vision**		
I4400	Cerebral palsy	Category G80	I6200	Cataracts	Categories H25–H26, H28
I4500	Cerebrovascular accident (CVA) (stroke)			Glaucoma	Categories H40–H42
	• cerebral hemorrhage	Category I61		Macular Degeneration	H35.30–H35.389
	• cerebral infarction	Category I63			
	Transient ischemic attack (TIA)	G45.9			

Appendix J: Coding Issues for Long-Term Care (LTC)

The Uniform Hospital Discharge Data Set (UHDDS) definition of principal diagnosis, "that condition established after study to be chiefly responsible for occasioning the admission of the patient to the hospital for care," is applied across all nonoutpatient settings, including long-term care.

In a long-term care setting, the principal diagnosis is regarded as the "first-listed diagnosis" and is the diagnosis that is chiefly responsible for the admission to the facility, or the diagnosis that is chiefly responsible for continued residence in the facility and should be sequenced first. In addition, chronic conditions that affect a resident's care are also coded. The diagnoses present and the sequencing of these diagnoses depend on the point in time the coding is done as ICD-10-CM codes can be assigned upon admission; concurrently as diagnoses arise; or at the time of discharge, transfer, or death of the resident.

The following guidelines and examples have been developed and approved by the Cooperating Parties in conjunction with the Editorial Advisory Board of *Coding Clinic*, to standardize the process of data collection for LTC and to assist the coder in coding and reporting these cases using ICD-10-CM. This guidance appeared in *Coding Clinic for ICD-10-CM*, published by the American Hospital Association, 4Q, '12, 90-98.

Example 1:

The patient is discharged from the acute care hospital and admitted to the LTC facility with a diagnosis of acute cerebrovascular accident (CVA) with left-sided hemiparesis and dysphasia.

First listed diagnosis:
I69.354, Hemiplegia and hemiparesis following cerebral infarction affecting left non-dominant side

Additional diagnosis:
I69.321, Dysphasia following cerebral infarction

The hemiparesis and dysphasia are considered sequelae of the acute CVA for this LTC admission. Coding guidelines state that these "late effects" include neurologic deficits that persist after initial onset of conditions classifiable to categories I60-I67. Codes from I60-I67 are reserved for the initial (first) episode of care for the acute cerebrovascular disease. Coding guidelines also provide guidance as to the use of dominant/nondominant side for codes from category I69.

There is no time limit on when a late effect code may be used since the neurologic deficit caused by cerebrovascular disease may be present from the onset or may arise at any time after the onset of the condition classifiable to I60-I67. When the patient is admitted to LTC following treatment of an acute CVA, a code from subcategory I69.3, Sequelae of cerebral infarction, is assigned for the LTC admission.

Example 2:

A patient with progressive senile dementia, coronary artery disease, and congestive heart failure is admitted to a LTC facility after suffering a CVA and receiving treatment elsewhere. The patient has made a complete recovery from the CVA prior to admission to the LTC facility. She is admitted for long-term care because of her chronic illnesses and her deteriorating mental status.

First listed diagnosis:
F03.90, Unspecified dementia without behavioral disturbance

Additional diagnoses:
I50.9, Heart failure, unspecified

I25.10, Atherosclerotic heart disease of native coronary artery without angina pectoris

Z86.73, Personal history of transient ischemic attack (TIA), and cerebral infarction without residual deficits

Any of the patient's chronic diseases can be listed first, since each one could be considered chiefly responsible for LTC facility admission. Since this patient has no residuals from the CVA, a code from category I69, Sequelae of cerebrovascular disease, is inappropriate. Instead, code Z86.73, Personal history of transient ischemic attack (TIA), and cerebral infarction without residual deficits, may be assigned to identify the history of CVA without residual deficits.

Example 3:

A patient is admitted to the LTC facility for physical therapy from an acute care setting after treatment for acute pelvic and clavicular fractures.

First listed diagnosis:
S32.9XXD, Fracture of unspecified parts of lumbosacral spine and pelvis, subsequent encounter for fracture with routine healing

Additional diagnoses:
S42.009D, Fracture of unspecified part of unspecified clavicle, subsequent encounter for fracture with routine healing

The first-listed diagnosis for a patient admitted to LTC specifically for physical therapy following an injury should be the acute injury code with the appropriate 7th character for subsequent encounter. Assigning a Z code for any aftercare provided for traumatic fractures is inappropriate in ICD-10-CM. For further guidance on the application of the 7th characters for Chapter 19, refer to Section I.C.19.c., of the Official Guidelines for Coding and Reporting.

Either of these fractures could be the reason for the LTC admission and therefore either one could be assigned as the "first-listed" diagnosis. The appropriate ICD-10-PCS procedure code(s) should also be assigned to show that physical therapy was provided.

Example 4:

A patient is admitted to LTC following hospital treatment of a traumatic fracture of the right femur in order to heal the fracture and regain strength.

First listed diagnosis:
S72.90XD, Unspecified fracture of right femur, subsequent encounter for closed fracture with routine healing

Additional diagnoses:
Code any other existing conditions that require treatment.

The patient is no longer receiving active treatment for the fracture and instead is receiving routine care while the fracture heals. The acute injury is still coded but with a 7th character of "D" signifying a subsequent encounter for fracture with routine healing. Do not assign an aftercare Z code.

Example 5:

A LTC patient develops a urinary tract infection during the LTC stay that was subsequently treated and resolved.

First listed diagnosis:
N39.0, Urinary tract infection, site not specified

Additional diagnoses:
Code any other existing conditions that require treatment.

The urinary tract infection would remain on the active problem list until resolution of the infection, after which it would no longer be correct to code or report it.

Example 6:

A patient returns to the LTC facility after hospitalization for pneumonia. The admission orders request "IV antibiotic continuation for three days, and then repeat x-ray to determine pneumonia status."

First listed diagnosis:
J18.9, Pneumonia, unspecified organism

Additional diagnoses:
Code any other existing conditions that require treatment.

Code the pneumonia until it is resolved, after which it should no longer be coded and reported.

Example 7:

After hospitalization for pneumonia, a nursing home resident is readmitted with orders for continued antibiotic regimen for pneumonia. Other specified residuals from a CVA several years ago are the chief reason for her original admission and continued residence in the LTC facility.

First listed diagnosis:
I69.30, Unspecified sequelae of cerebral infarction

Additional diagnoses:
J18.9, Pneumonia, unspecified organism

Assign the appropriate code from subcategory I69.3, Sequelae of cerebral infarction, as the first-listed diagnosis to identify the residual neurologic deficits from the acute CVA. It is also appropriate to assign the code for the pneumonia as an additional diagnosis for as long as the patient receives treatment for the condition.

Example 8:

After surgical treatment in the acute care setting for a left wrist fracture sustained while a resident in a nursing home, the patient returns to the nursing home. The patient was admitted several years ago and has received continued care for Alzheimer's disease. Occupational therapy is ordered for the wrist, but the therapy is not the primary reason for the patient's admission.

First listed diagnosis:
G30.9, Alzheimer's disease, unspecified

Additional diagnoses:
S62.102D, Fracture of unspecified carpal bone, left wrist, subsequent encounter for fracture with routine healing

W19.XXXD, Unspecified fall, subsequent encounter

Although the patient is receiving therapy for the wrist fracture, it is the Alzheimer's disease that is the reason the patient is continuing care in the nursing home and should be reported as the first-listed diagnosis, over the wrist fracture. However, the appropriate ICD-10-PCS procedure code should still be assigned to show that the patient received occupational therapy.

Example 9:
A patient is admitted to the LTC facility for convalescence following an acute illness or injury.

First listed diagnosis:
Z51.89, Encounter for other specified aftercare

Additional diagnoses:
Code any other existing conditions that require treatment.

Use only if the patient is admitted solely for convalescence and there is no information in the medical record identifying a more definitive diagnosis.

Selection of codes in all cases is based on documentation in the medical record of conditions treated. Codes for any late effects, signs, and symptoms present are assigned if documented.

Example 10:
A patient is transferred to a nursing home for convalescence and strengthening following coronary artery bypass surgery. The patient's degree of debility and inability to care for himself at home are the reasons for the nursing home admission.

First listed diagnosis:
Z48.812, Encounter for surgical aftercare following surgery on the circulatory system

Additional diagnoses:
Code any other existing conditions that require treatment.

Code any symptoms such as gait disturbance, weakness, or pain.

The condition that was treated surgically if still present would be coded.

Example 11:
A patient is transferred to a nursing home for convalescence following a hospitalization for an acute inferior wall myocardial infarction.

First listed diagnosis:
I21.19, ST elevation (STEMI) myocardial infarction involving other coronary artery of inferior wall

Additional diagnoses:
Code any other existing conditions that require treatment.

If the patient is in the recovery phase and requires continued care for the acute myocardial infarction, and is within the four-week time frame for the acute myocardial infarction (AMI), assign a code from category I21. This includes transfers to another acute setting or a postacute setting. If, however, the acute myocardial infarction occurred more than four weeks prior, assign instead code Z51.89, Encounter for other specified aftercare.

It would be inappropriate to assign code I22.1, Subsequent ST elevation (STEMI) myocardial infarction of inferior wall, for the long-term care admission. The codes in category (I22) are reserved for patients who have suffered an acute MI and experience a new acute MI within the four week time frame of the initial AMI. It is not for subsequent episodes of care.

Example 12:
The reason for admission to a nursing home is stated as "deconditioning".

First listed diagnosis:
Code whatever symptoms for deconditioning that the patient manifests, such as weakness, gait disturbance, etc.

Additional diagnoses:
Code any other existing conditions that require treatment.

Example 13:
A LTC facility patients' record has "mental status change" as a current condition.

First listed diagnosis:
R41.82, Altered mental status, unspecified

Additional diagnoses:
Code any other existing conditions that require treatment.

Example 14:
A patient does not have a specific diagnosis, but is admitted to a LTC facility for symptoms such as weakness, debility, deterioration, or old age.

First listed diagnosis:
The correct approach is to code the symptoms related to the admission.

Additional diagnoses:
Code any other existing conditions that require treatment.

Appendix K: Inpatient Rehabilitation Facility Prospective Payment System (PPS) Overview

The inpatient rehabilitation facility (IRF) prospective payment system (PPS) system has been in place since January 1, 2002. Rehabilitation facilities provide post-acute care for patients discharged from acute care short-term general hospitals that require additional services. The goal of post-acute services is to provide care that restores a person's ability to live and work as normally as possible after a disabling injury or illness. The PPS payment rates include all costs of furnishing covered IRF services, such as routine, ancillary, and capital-related costs. Excluded are costs associated with operating approved educational activities, bad debts, and other costs not covered under PPS.

FY 2014 Inpatient Rehabilitation Facility Prospective Payment System Update

In the final rule (*Federal Register*, August 6, 2013, CMS-1448-F) the Centers for Medicare and Medicaid Services (CMS) proposed to revise the list of diagnosis codes used to determine presumptive compliance under the "60 percent rule," update the inpatient rehabilitation facility (IRF) facility-level adjustment factors, revise sections of the IRF-Patient Assessment Instrument, revise requirements for acute care hospitals that have IRF units, clarify the IRF regulation text regarding limitation of review, update references to previously changed sections in the regulations text, and revise and update quality measures and reporting requirements under the IRF quality reporting program.

The following excerpt from the final rule outlines the revisions to the list of diagnosis codes used to determine presumptive compliance under the "60 percent rule," the revisions to sections of the IRF-PAI, and the revisions and update to the quality measures and reporting requirements. For complete coverage of all other issues discussed in the final rule, visit the CMS website at: http://www.cms.gov/Medicare/Medicare-Fee-for-Service-Payment/InpatientRehabFacPPS/index.html.

Proposed Changes to the ICD-10-CM Codes That Meet the Presumptive Compliance Criteria

The IRF must serve an inpatient population of whom at least 60 percent required intensive rehabilitation services for treatment of one or more of the conditions specified under the presumptive compliance criteria and the specific conditions under which a comorbidity may be used has caused significant decline in functional ability in the individual that, even in the absence of the admitting condition, the individual would require the intensive rehabilitation treatment that is unique to inpatient rehabilitation facilities.

To meet the required compliance criteria under the 60 percent rule, the IRF PAI assessments from the most recently completed 12 month compliance review period must contain any of the codes listed on the presumptive compliance list. Each selected assessment is categorized as either meeting or not meeting the IRF 60 percent rule requirements based upon the impairment group representing the primary reason for the patient to be treated in the IRF and the ICD-10-CM codes listed as either the etiologic or one of 10 comorbidities on the assessment. The ICD-10-CM diagnosis codes used to categorize a patient as meeting the 60 percent rule criteria are listed in "Appendix C: ICD-10-CM Codes That Meet Presumptive Compliance Criteria" from the IRF Compliance Rule Specification Files found on the CMS web site.

The ICD-10-CM diagnosis codes that meet presumptive compliance criteria are available at: http://www.cms.gov/Medicare/Medicare-Fee-for-Service-Payment/InpatientRehabFacPPS/Data-Files.html.

Proposed FY 2016 IRF—PAI Changes

Upon the admission and discharge of a Medicare Part A fee-for-service patient, the IRF is required to complete the appropriate sections of a patient assessment instrument (PAI), designated as the IRF-PAI. The IRF is also required to complete the appropriate sections of the IRF-PAI upon the admission and discharge of each Medicare Part C (Medicare Advantage) patient.

All required data must be electronically encoded into the IRF-PAI software product. Generally, the software product includes patient classification programming called the grouper software. The grouper software uses specific IRF-PAI data elements to classify (or group) patients into distinct case-mix groups (CMGs) and account for the existence of any relevant comorbidities. The software assigns a five-character CMG number. The first character is an alphabetic character that indicates the comorbidity tier. The last four characters are numeric and represent the distinct CMG number.

For IRF discharges occurring on or after October 1, 2015, CMS proposes to add a new Therapy Information Section to the IRF–PAI to record the amount and mode of therapy (individual, group, cotreatment) patients receive in each therapy

discipline (physical therapy, occupational therapy, and speech-language pathology) to better understand the ways in which therapy services are currently being provided in IRFs.

For purposes of recording therapy services in IRFs, CMS proposes the following definitions:

- Individual Therapy: the provision of therapy services by one licensed or certified therapist (or licensed therapy assistant, under the appropriate direction of a licensed or certified therapist) to one patient at a time (this is sometimes referred to as "one-on-one" therapy).

- Group Therapy: the provision of therapy services by one licensed or certified therapist (or licensed therapy assistant, under the appropriate direction of a licensed or certified therapist) to between 2 and 6 IRF patients at one time, regardless of whether those 2 to 6 IRF patients are performing the same activity or different activities.

- Cotreatment: the provision of therapy services by more than one licensed or certified therapist (or licensed therapy assistant, under the appropriate direction of a licensed therapist) from different therapy disciplines to one patient at the same time. For example, cotreatment could involve one physical therapist and one occupational therapist working with one patient at the same time to achieve the patient's goals.

This information would be collected in a new Therapy Information Section on the IRF–PAI, which would be effective for IRF discharges beginning on or after October 1, 2015. The proposed new Therapy Information Section would be completed as part of the patient's discharge assessment. In this new proposed section, the IRF would record how many minutes of individual, group, and cotreatment therapies the patient received, according to each therapy discipline (physical therapy, occupational therapy, and speech-language pathology), during the first week (seven calendar day period) of the IRF stay; how many minutes of individual, group, and cotreatment therapies the patient received, according to each therapy discipline, during the second week (seven calendar day period) of the IRF stay; and the average number of minutes of individual, group, and cotreatment therapies the patient received, according to each therapy discipline, during all subsequent weeks (seven calendar day periods) of the IRF stay, beginning with the third week.

For cotreatment, each therapist would record the amount of time spent with the patient. CMS proposes to use this data to analyze the types of therapy services Medicare is currently paying for under the IRF prospective payment system and to monitor the amount of therapy given and the use of different therapy modes in IRFs to support future rulemaking in this area.

In the FY 2014 IRF PPS final rule, the list of ICD-9-CM diagnosis codes that are used to determine presumptive compliance were revised, effective for compliance review periods beginning on or after October 1, 2014. As part of these revisions, all of the ICD-9-CM codes for arthritis conditions were removed as CMS found that such codes did not provide any information as to whether the patients met the severity and prior treatment requirement portions of the criteria for the medical conditions that may be counted toward an IRF's compliance percentage under the presumptive compliance method.

An additional new proposed item would be added to the IRF–PAI form for IRF discharges occurring on or after October 1, 2015. This proposed new item would record the specific arthritis diagnosis code(s) for each patient that meets the severity and prior treatment requirements outlined in the regulation. Coding arthritis diagnosis codes in this section would allow the IRF to indicate that the patient's arthritis conditions have met all of the severity and prior treatment requirements to be counted toward an IRF's compliance percentage under the presumptive compliance method.

This new proposed item would provide CMS with additional severity and prior treatment information necessary for it to identify the arthritis diagnoses that are appropriate to count toward an IRF's compliance percentage under the presumptive compliance method, thus reducing the medical review burden. If an IRF's presumptive compliance percentage is below the compliance threshold (currently, 60 percent) but inclusion of the arthritis codes reported in this new proposed data item would result in the IRF's presumptive compliance percentage meeting or exceeding the compliance threshold, CMS proposes to perform a "limited" medical review on a statistically valid random sample of the cases documented under this new item to ensure that the severity and prior treatment requirements were actually met. The number of cases from the valid sample that are found to meet the severity and prior treatment requirements will be extrapolated to the total number of cases documented under this new item.

The draft of the proposed IRF–PAI for FY 2016 that would include this new proposed section is available for download from the IRF PPS website at http://www.cms.gov/Medicare/Medicare-Fee-for-Service-Payment/InpatientRehabFacPPS/IRFPAI.html.

Revisions and Updates to the Quality Reporting Program

The Affordable Care Act required the HHS secretary to establish the Inpatient Rehabilitation Facility Quality Reporting Program (IRF QRP). This program applies to freestanding IRFs, as well as IRF units affiliated with either acute care facilities or critical access hospitals (CAHs).

Beginning with the FY 2014 payment determination and subsequent years, the annual update to the standard federal rate for discharges occurring during such fiscal year will be reduced by 2 percentage points for any IRF that does not comply with the established requirements.

CMS is directed to specify measures that relate to at least five IRF-PAI stated quality domains and three stated resource use and other measure domains. The specified quality measures must be with respect to at least the following domains:

- Functional status, cognitive function, and changes in function and cognitive function

- Skin integrity and changes in skin integrity

- Medication reconciliation

- Incidence of major falls

- Accurately communicating the existence of and providing for the transfer of health information and care references of an individual to the individual, family caregiver of the individual, and providers of services furnishing items and services to the individual when the individual transitions (1) from a hospital or CAH to another applicable setting, including a PAC provider or the home of the individual, or (2) from a PAC provider to another applicable setting, including a different PAC provider, hospital, CAH, or the home of the individual.

The resource use and other measures must be with respect to at least the following domains:

- Resource use measures, including total estimated Medicare spending per beneficiary

- Discharge to community

- Measures to reflect all-condition risk-adjusted potentially preventable hospital readmissions rates

The Affordable Care Act indicates that data satisfying the eight measure domains in the IMPACT Act are the minimum data reporting requirement.

When CMS adopts a measure for the IRF QRP that satisfies an IMPACT Act measure domain, the agency intends to require IRFs to report data on the measure for the fiscal year that begins two years after the specified application date for that measure. Similarly CMS will require IRFs to begin reporting any other data specifically required under the IMPACT Act for the fiscal year that begins two years after the adoption of the requirements that would govern the submission of those data.

The totality of the measures considered to meet the requirements of the IMPACT Act will evolve, and additional measures will be proposed over time as they become available.

The first specified application date applicable to IRFs is October 1, 2016, and CMS has focused on measures that:

- Correspond to a measure domain in sections 1899B(c)(1) or (d)(1) of the Act and are setting-agnostic for example, falls with major injury and the incidence of pressure ulcers

- Are currently adopted for one or more of PAC quality reporting programs, are already either NQF-endorsed and in use or finalized for use, or already previewed by the Measure Applications Partnership (MAP) with support

- Minimize added burden on IRFs

- Minimize or avoid, to the extent feasible, revisions to the existing items in assessment tools currently in use (for example, the IRF-PAI)

- Where possible, avoid duplication of existing assessment items

CMS initiated an ad hoc Measure Applications Partnership (MAP) process for the review of the quality measures under consideration for proposal, in preparation for adoption of those quality measures into the IRF QRP that are required by the IMPACT Act and that must be implemented by October 1, 2016. Under the IMPACT Act, these measures must be standardized so they can be applied across PAC settings and must correspond to measure domains specified in sections 1899B(c)(1) and (d)(1) of the IMPACT Act. The MAP reviewed each IMPACT

Act-related quality measure proposed for the IRF QRP, in light of its intended cross-setting use. The MAP's final report, MAP Off-Cycle Deliberations 2015: Measures Under Consideration to Implement Provisions of the IMPACT Act: Final Report, is available at http://www.qualityforum.org/Setting_Priorities/Partnership/MAP_Final_Reports.aspx.

CMS allows for stakeholder input, such as through town halls, open door forums, and mailbox submissions, before the initial rule-making process to implement section 1899B. For measures that do not have NQF endorsement, or that are not fully supported by the MAP for the IRF QRP, the agency is proposing the measure domains required under the IMPACT Act that most closely align with the national priorities identified in the National Quality Strategy (http://www.ahrq.gov/workingforquality/) and for which the MAP supports the measure concept.

Additionally, for measures not endorsed by the NQF, CMS has sought to adopt measures that have been endorsed or adopted by a national consensus organization, recommended by multi-stakeholder organizations, and/or developed with the input of providers, purchasers/payers, and other stakeholders.

Quality Measures Previously Finalized for and Currently Used in the IRF QRP

In FY 2012, CMS adopted applications of two quality measures for use in the first data reporting cycle of the IRF QRP: (1) An application of Catheter-Associated Urinary Tract Infection (CAUTI) for Intensive Care Unit Patients (NQF#0138); and (2) an application of Percent of Residents with Pressure Ulcers That Are New or Worsened (Short-Stay) (NQF #0678).

In CY 2013 OPPS/ASC final rule, CMS adopted the National Healthcare Safety Network (NHSN) Catheter Associated Urinary Tract Infection (CAUTI) Outcome Measure (NQF #0138). In the same rule, CMS adopted the NHSN CAUTI Outcome Measure (NQF #0138) to replace an application of this measure that was initially adopted in the FY 2012 IRF PPS. Data submission for the NQF-endorsed measure applies to the FY 2015 adjustments to the IRF PPS annual increase factor and for all subsequent annual increase IRFs must submit their CAUTI measure data to the Centers for Disease Control and Prevention (CDC) NHSN.

In CY 2013 OPPS/ASC final rule, CMS adopted a non-risk-adjusted application of the measure of the percentage of residents or patients with pressure ulcers that are new or worsened (short-stay) (NQF #0678).

For the FY 2016 adjustments to the IRF PPS annual increase factor, CMS finalized the adoption of one additional measure: Influenza Vaccination Coverage Among Healthcare Personnel (NQF #0431). For the FY 2017 adjustments to the IRF PPS annual increase factor, CMS finalized the adoption of three additional quality measures: (1) All-Cause Unplanned Readmission Measure for 30 Days Post-Discharge from Inpatient Rehabilitation Facilities; (2) Percent of Residents or Patients Who Were Assessed and Appropriately Given the Seasonal Influenza Vaccine (Short-Stay) (NQF #0680); and (3) the Percent of Residents or Patients with Pressure Ulcers That Are New or Worsened (Short-Stay) (NQF #0678).

A revised version of the IRF-PAI (Version 1.2) was adopted and providers began using it as of October 1, 2014. This revised version will be included in the FY 2017 adjustments to the IRF PPS annual increase factor and subsequent year annual increase factors.

Influenza Vaccination Coverage Among Healthcare Personnel (NQF #0431)

In FY 2014 IRF PPS final rule, CMS adopted the CDC-developed Influenza Vaccination Coverage among Healthcare Personnel (NQF #0431) quality measure that is collected by the CDC via the NHSN. This measure will have its own reporting period to align with the influenza vaccination season, which is defined by the CDC as October 1 (or when the vaccine becomes available) through March 31. IRFs submit their data for this measure to the NHSN (http://www.cdc.gov/nhsn/). Data submission is required only once per influenza vaccination season. The final deadline for data submission associated with this quality measure is May 15th of each year.

FY 2016 adjustments to the IRF PPS annual increase factor data collection will cover the period from October 1, 2014 (or when the vaccine becomes available) through March 31, 2015.

In the FY 2014 IRF PPS final rule, the measure for All-Cause Unplanned Readmission Measure for 30 Days Post-Discharge From Inpatient Rehabilitation Facilities (NQF #2502) was adopted. This quality measure estimates the risk-standardized rate of unplanned, all-cause hospital readmissions for cases discharged from an IRF who were readmitted to a short-stay acute care hospital or LTCH within 30 days of an IRF discharge. This is a claims-based measure that will not require reporting of new data by IRFs and thus will not be used to determine IRF reporting compliance for the IRF QRP.

In the FY 2014 IRF PPS final rule, the measure for Percent of Residents or Patients Who Were Assessed and Appropriately Given the Seasonal Influenza Vaccine (Short-Stay) (NQF #0680) was adopted. The data elements needed for this measure were added to the "Quality Indicator" section of the IRF-PAI Version 1.2, which became effective on October 1, 2014. These data elements are harmonized with data elements (O0250: Influenza Vaccination Status) from the Minimum Data Set (MDS) 3.0 and the LTCH CARE Data Set Version 2.01, and the specifications and data elements for this measure are available at http://www.cms.gov/Medicare/Medicare-Fee-for-Service-Payment/InpatientRehabFacPPS/IRFPAI.html. For purposes of this quality measure, the influenza vaccination season is October 1 (or when the vaccine becomes available) through March 31 each year.

Percent of Residents or Patients with Pressure Ulcers That Are New or Worsened (Short-Stay) (NQF #0678)

In FY 2014, CMS adopted the NQF-endorsed version of the Percent of Residents or Patients with Pressure Ulcers That Are New or Worsened (Short-Stay) (NQF #0678). Data collection began October 1, 2014, using the IRF-PAI Version 1.2, for quality reporting affecting the FY 2017 adjustments to the IRF PPS annual increase factor and subsequent year annual increase factors.

Two additional quality measures were adopted in FY 2015. The first was the National Healthcare Safety Network (NHSN) Facility-Wide Inpatient Hospital-Onset Methicillin-Resistant *Staphylococcus aureus* (MRSA) Bacteremia Outcome Measure (NQF #1716). This is a measure of hospital-onset unique blood source MRSA laboratory-identified events among all patients in the inpatient rehabilitation facility. This measure was developed by the CDC and is NQF-endorsed. Data submission would start on January 1, 2015, and adjustments to the IRF PPS annual increase factor would begin with FY 2017. Data are submitted via the CDC's NHSN.

The second quality measure was the National Healthcare Safety Network (NHSN) Facility-Wide Inpatient Hospital-Onset Clostridium difficile Infection (CDI) Outcome Measure (NQF #1717). This is a measure of hospital onset CDI laboratory-identified events among all inpatients in the facility. This measure was developed by the CDC and is NQF-endorsed. Data started being submitted starting January 1, 2015, and adjustments to the IRF PPS annual increase factor would begin with FY 2017. Providers will use the CDC/NHSN data collection and submission framework for reporting of the proposed NHSN Facility-Wide Inpatient Hospital-Onset CDI Outcome Measure (NQF #1717).

Quality Measures Previously Finalized and Currently Used in the IRF QRP

NQF #0138	National Health Safety Network (NHSN) Catheter-Associated Urinary Tract Infection (CAUTI) Outcome Measure.
NQF #0431	Influenza Vaccination Coverage Among Healthcare Personnel. CDC NHSN.
NQF #0680	Percent of Residents or Patients Who Were Assessed and Appropriately Given the Seasonal Influenza Vaccine (Short-Stay). IRF-PAI
NQF #0678	Percent of Residents or Patients with Pressure Ulcers That Are New or Worsened (Short-Stay). IRF-PAI
NQF #2502	All-Cause Unplanned Readmission Measure for 30 Days Post-Discharge from Inpatient Rehabilitation Facilities*. Claims-based
NQF #1716	National Healthcare Safety Network (NHSN) Facility-Wide Inpatient Hospital-Onset Methicillin-Resistant [ital]Staphylococcus aureus[end ital] (MRSA) Bacteremia Outcome Measure. CDC NHSN.
NQF #1717	National Healthcare Safety Network (NHSN) Facility-Wide Inpatient Hospital-Onset [ital]Clostridium difficile[end ital] Infection (CDI) Outcome Measure. CDC NHSN.

* Claims-based measure; no additional data submission required by IRFs.

For the FY 2018 adjustments to the IRF PPS annual increase factor, CMS is retaining the previously discussed measures:

NQF #0138	NHSN CAUTI Outcome Measure
NQF #0680	Percent of Residents or Patients Who Were Assessed and Appropriately Given the Seasonal Influenza Vaccine (Short-Stay)
NQF #0678	Percent of Residents or Patients with Pressure Ulcers That Are New or Worsened (Short-Stay)
NQF #2502	All-Cause Unplanned Readmission Measure for 30 Days Post-Discharge from IRFs
NQF #0431	Influenza Vaccination Coverage among Healthcare Personnel
NQF #1716	NHSN Facility-Wide Inpatient Hospital- Onset MRSA Bacteremia Outcome Measure
NQF #1717	NHSN Facility-Wide Inpatient Hospital-Onset CDI Outcome Measure

For the FY 2018 payment determination and subsequent years, CMS proposes to adopt two quality measures to reflect NQF endorsement or to meet the requirements of the IMPACT Act: All-Cause Unplanned Readmission Measure for

30 Days Post-Discharge from IRFs (NQF #2502) and Percent of Residents or Patients with Pressure Ulcers That Are New or Worsened (NQF #0678).

The All-Cause Unplanned Readmission Measure for 30 Days Post Discharge from IRFs (NQF #2502) measure was adopted for use in the IRF QRP in the FY 2014 IRF PPS final rule. CMS is proposing to adopt this measure for the FY 2018 payment determination and subsequent years to reflect that it is NQF-endorsed for use in the IRF setting as of December 2014. For current specifications of this measure, please visit http://www.qualityforum.org/QPS/2502.

This is a Medicare fee-for-service (FFS) claims-based measure. IRFs would not be required to report any additional data to CMS because CMS would calculate this measure based on claims data that are already reported to the Medicare program for payment purposes. There would be no additional data collection burden on providers resulting from this implementation.

Percent of Residents or Patients with Pressure Ulcers That Are New or Worsened (NQF #0678) corresponds to one of the top five quality domains highlighted in the IMPACT Act. CMS has already adopted it for the IRF QRP as a cross-setting quality measure that satisfies the domain of skin integrity and changes in skin integrity. The reporting of data for this measure would affect the payment determination for FY 2018 and subsequent years. For the IRF setting, the measure assesses the percentage of patients with stage 2 through stage 4 pressure ulcers that are new or worsened since admission. Details regarding the specifications for this measure are available on the NQF web site at http://www.qualityforum.org/QPS/0678.

CMS proposes to adopt six additional quality measures beginning with the FY 2018 payment determination. These new proposed quality measures are:

1. (NQF #0674) An application of Percent of Residents Experiencing One or More Falls with Major Injury (Long Stay)
2. (NQF #2631; under review) Percent of LTCH Patients with an Admission and Discharge Functional Assessment and a Care Plan That Addresses Function
3. (NQF #2633; under review) IRF Functional Outcome Measure: Change in Self-Care Score for Medical Rehabilitation Patients
4. (NQF #2634; under review) IRF Functional Outcome Measure: Change in Mobility Score for Medical Rehabilitation Patients
5. (NQF #2635; under review) IRF Functional Outcome Measure: Discharge Self-Care Score for Medical Rehabilitation Patients
6. (NQF #2636; under review) IRF Functional Outcome Measure: Discharge Mobility Score for Medical Rehabilitation Patients

Data collection for the first item (NQF #0674) for the IRF QRP would begin on October 1, 2016, and would affect payment determination for FY 2018 and subsequent years.

The regulations in the IMPACT Act require the specification of quality measures and resource use and other measures that are standardized and interoperable across PAC settings as well as the reporting of standardized patient assessment data and other necessary data specified by the Secretary. The Percent of Residents Experiencing One or More Falls with Major Injury (Long Stay) (NQF #0674) measure is NQF-endorsed for long-stay residents in nursing homes and has been successfully implemented in nursing facilities for long-stay residents. The NQF-endorsed measure has been in use as part of CMS's Nursing Home Quality Initiative since 2011. In addition, the measure is currently reported on CMS's Nursing Home Compare web site at http://www.medicare.gov/nursinghomecompare/search.html.

Further, the measure was adopted for use in the LTCH QRP in the FY 2014 IPPS/LTCH PPS final rule (78 FR 50874 through 50877). In the FY 2015 IPPS/LTCH PPS final rule (79 FR 50290), CMS revised the data collection period for this measure with data collection to begin starting April 1, 2016.

CMS reviewed the NQF's consensus endorsed measures and were unable to identify any NQF-endorsed cross-setting quality measures focused on falls with a major injury. The agency is unaware of any other cross-setting quality measures for falls with major injury that have been endorsed or adopted by another consensus organization. Therefore, the agency is proposing an application of the measure, the Percent of Residents Experiencing One or More Falls with Major Injury (Long Stay) (NQF #0674), under the Secretary's authority to select non-NQF-endorsed measures.

For more information on the Percent of Residents Experiencing One or More Falls with Major Injury (Long Stay), visit the NQF web site: http://www.qualityforum.org/QPS/0674. CMS proposes that data for this quality measure would be collected using the IRF-PAI with submission through the QIES ASAP system. More information on IRF reporting using the QIES ASAP system is located at the web site: http://www.cms.gov/Medicare/Quality-Initiatives-Patient-Assessment-Instruments/NursingHomeQualityInits/SNF-Quality-Reporting.html. Data collected through a revised IRF-PAI would be used to calculate this quality measure. Consistent with the IRF-PAI reporting requirements, the application of the Percent of Residents Experiencing One or More Falls with Major Injury (Long Stay) (NQF #0674), will apply to all Medicare patients discharged from IRFs. Data items in the revised IRF-PAI would include: J1800: Any Falls Since Admission, and J1900: Number of Falls Since Admission.

The calculation of the proposed application of the measure would be based on item J1900C: Number of Falls with Major Injury since Admission.

Data collection will begin October 1, 2016, for the IRF QRP for FY 2018 payment determination and subsequent years to fulfill the requirements in the IMPACT Act.

Application of Percent of Long-Term Care Hospital Patients With an Admission and Discharge Functional Assessment and a Care Plan That Addresses Function (NQF #2631; under review)

CMS proposes to adopt an application of the quality measure Percent of LTCH Patients with an Admission and Discharge Functional Assessment and a Care Plan that Addresses Function (NQF #2631; under review) in the IRF QRP as a cross-setting quality measure that addresses the domain of functional status, cognitive function, and changes in function and cognitive function. The reporting of data for this measure would affect the payment determination for FY 2018 and subsequent years. This quality measure reports the percent of patients with both an admission and a discharge functional assessment and a goal that addresses function.

The cross-setting function quality measure proposed for the FY 2018 payment determination and subsequent years is a process measure that is an application of the quality measure Percent of LTCH Patients with an Admission and Discharge Functional Assessment and a Care Plan that Addresses Function (NQF #2631; under review). This quality measure was developed by CMS. It reports the percentage of patients with both an admission and a discharge functional assessment and a treatment goal that addresses function. The treatment goal provides documentation that a care plan with a goal has been established for the patient.

This process measure requires the collection of admission and discharge functional status data using standardized clinical assessment items, or data elements, that assess specific functional activities, such as self-care, mobility activities. The self-care and mobility function activities are coded using a six-level rating scale that indicates the patient's level of independence with the activity; higher scores indicate more independence. For this quality measure, documentation of a goal for one of the function items reflects that the patient's care plan addresses function. The function goal is recorded at admission for at least one of the standardized self-care or mobility function items using the six-level rating scale.

When a patient has an incomplete stay (for example, for the purpose of being admitted to an acute care facility), collection of discharge functional status data might not be feasible. For patients with incomplete stays, admission functional status data and at least one treatment goal would be required; discharge functional status data would not be required to be reported. This quality measure was developed by CMS.

CMS is proposing to specify and adopt this functional assessment measure for use in the IRF QRP for the FY 2018 payment determination and subsequent years under the Secretary's authority to select non-NQF-endorsed measures. The proposed first data collection period is three months (October 1, 2016, to December 31, 2016), and the proposed subsequent data collection periods are 12 months in length and follow the calendar year (that is, January 1 to December 31).

Data for this proposed quality measure must be collected using the IRF-PAI, with submission through the QIES ASAP system. For more information on IRF QRP reporting through the QIES ASAP system, go to the CMS web site at: http://www.cms.gov/Medicare/Quality-Initiatives-Patient-Assessment-Instruments/NursingHomeQualityInits/NHQIMDS30Technical Information.html.

For purposes of assessment data collection, CMS proposes to add a new section to the IRF-PAI. The new proposed section will include new functional status items that will be used to calculate the application of the Percent of LTCH Patients with an Admission and Discharge Functional Assessment and a Care Plan that Addresses Function (NQF #2631; under review) if this quality measure is adopted.

Data collection will start on October 1, 2016, for the FY 2018 payment determination and subsequent years.

IRF Functional Outcome Measure: Change in Self-Care Score for Medical Rehabilitation Patients (NQF #2633; Under Review)

The third proposed quality measure for the FY 2018 payment determination and subsequent years is an outcome measure entitled IRF Functional Outcome Measure: Change in Self-Care Score for Medical Rehabilitation Patients (NQF

#2633; under review). This quality measure estimates the risk-adjusted mean change in self-care score between admission and discharge among IRF patients. A summary of the measure specifications can be accessed on the NQF web site: http://www.qualityforum.org/qps/2633.

IRFs are designed to provide intensive rehabilitation services to patients. Patients seeking care in IRFs are those whose illness, injury, or condition has resulted in a loss of function, and for whom rehabilitative care is expected to help regain that function. Examples of conditions treated in IRFs include stroke, spinal cord injury, hip fracture, brain injury, neurological disorders, and other diagnoses characterized by loss of function.

The functional assessment items included in this quality measure were originally developed and tested as part of the Post-Acute Care Payment Reform Demonstration version of the CARE Tool, most of which was designed to standardize assessment of patients' status across acute and post-acute providers, including IRFs, SNFs, HHAs, and LTCHs.

This measure is proposed for adoption for the IRF QRP for the FY 2018 payment determination and subsequent years. CMS is proposing that data for the proposed quality measure be collected using the IRF-PAI, with the submission through the QIES ASAP system. For more information on IRF QRP reporting through the QIES ASAP system, refer to the CMS web site. If this measure is adopted, the IRF-PAI will be revised to include new items that assess functional status and the risk factor items.

Data collection would start on October 1, 2016, for the FY 2018 payment determination and subsequent years.

The fourth quality measure proposed for the FY 2018 payment determination and subsequent years is an outcome quality measure entitled IRF Functional Outcome Measure: Change in Mobility Score for Medical Rehabilitation Patients (NQF #2634; under review). This quality measure estimates the risk-adjusted mean change in mobility score between admission and discharge among IRF patients.

This outcome measure requires the collection of admission and discharge functional status data by trained clinicians using standardized clinical assessment items, or data elements that assess specific functional mobility activities (for example, toilet transfer and walking). The mobility function items are coded using a six-level rating scale that indicates the patient's level of independence with the activity; higher scores indicate more independence. In addition, this measure requires the collection of risk factors data, such as patient functioning prior to the current reason for admission, history of falls, bladder continence, communication ability and cognitive function, at the time of admission.

The fifth quality measure proposed for the FY 2018 payment determination and subsequent years is an outcome quality measure entitled IRF Functional Outcome Measure: Discharge Self-Care Score for Medical Rehabilitation Patients (NQF #2635; under review). This quality measure estimates the percentage of IRF patients who meet or exceed an expected discharge self-care score.

This outcome measure requires the collection of admission and discharge functional status data by trained clinicians using standardized clinical assessment items, or data elements that assess specific functional mobility activities (that is, eating, oral hygiene, and dressing). The self-care function items are coded using a six-level rating scale that indicates the patient's level of independence with the activity; higher scores indicate more independence. In addition, this measure requires the collection of risk factors data, such as patient functioning prior to the current reason for admission, bladder continence, communication ability, and cognitive function, at the time of admission. The data collection required for this measure is the same data required for the measure IRF Functional Outcome Measure: Change in Self-Care Score for Medical Rehabilitation Patients (NQF #2635; under review).

Also proposed for adoption for the FY 2018 payment determination and subsequent years is the quality measure entitled IRF Functional Outcome Measure: Discharge Self-Care Score for Medical Rehabilitation Patients (NQF #2635; under review).

The proposed first data collection period is three months (October 1, 2016, to December 31, 2016), and the proposed subsequent data collection periods are 12 months in length and follow the calendar year (that is, January 1 to December 31).

Data for the proposed quality measure be collected using the IRF-PAI, with submission through the QIES ASAP system.

The sixth quality measure proposed is the IRF Functional Outcome Measure: Discharge Mobility Score for Medical Rehabilitation Patients (NQF #2636; Under Review). It is proposed for FY 2016 implementation and the FY 2018 payment determination and subsequent years. This quality measure estimates the percentage of IRF patients who meet or exceed an expected discharge mobility score. It requires the collection of admission and discharge functional status data by trained clinicians using standardized clinical assessment items, or data elements that assess specific functional mobility activities (that is, bed mobility and walking). The mobility function items are coded using a six-level rating scale that indicates the patient's level of independence with the activity; higher scores indicate more independence. In addition, this measure requires the collection of risk factors data, such as patient functioning prior to the current reason for admission, history of falls, bladder continence, communication ability, and cognitive function, at the time of admission. Note that the data collection required for this measure is the same data required for the measure IRF Functional Outcome Measure: Mobility in Self-Care Score for Medical Rehabilitation Patients (NQF #2634; under review).

The proposed first data collection period is three months (October 1, 2016, to December 31, 2016), and the proposed subsequent data collection periods are 12 months in length and follow the calendar year (that is, January 1 to December 31). Data for this quality measure be collected using the IRF-PAI, with submission through the QIES ASAP system

Inpatient Rehabilitation Facility Requirements

Title 42 Code of Federal Regulations (CFR) 412.23(b)(2) specifies the requirements for IRFs. Beginning on or after July 1, 2007, the facility must service an inpatient population of whom at least 75 percent require intensive rehabilitative services for one or more of the following conditions:

- Stroke
- Spinal cord injury
- Congenital deformity
- Amputation
- Major multiple trauma
- Femur fracture (hip fracture)
- Brain injury
- Neurological disorders, including multiple sclerosis, motor neuron diseases, polyneuropathy, muscular dystrophy, and Parkinson's disease
- Burns
- Active polyarticular rheumatoid arthritis, psoriatic arthritis, and seronegative arthropathies, which result in significant functional impairment of ambulation and other activities of daily living that have not improved after an appropriate, aggressive, and sustained course of outpatient therapy services
- Systemic vasculidities with joint inflammation, which result in significant functional impairment of ambulation and other activities of daily living that have not improved after an appropriate, aggressive, and sustained course of outpatient therapy services
- Severe or advanced osteoarthritis involving two or more major weight bearing joints (elbow, shoulder, hip, knee, but not counting a joint with a prosthesis) with joint deformity and substantial loss of range of motion, and atrophy of muscles surrounding the joint
- Knee or hip joint replacement, or both, during an acute hospitalization immediately preceding the inpatient rehabilitation stay

The *Federal Register* final rule for IRF PPS, released on August 6, 2013, contains several revisions that provide clarity and ensure that the regulations reflect current medical practices. Among the revised rules are the following:

- IRFs must provide rehabilitation nursing, physical therapy, occupational therapy, speech-language pathology, social services, psychological services, and prosthetic and orthotic services using qualified personnel, and the services must be ordered by a rehabilitation physician.

- Comprehensive preadmission screening must be conducted for each patient to evaluate the appropriateness of IRF-level of care. The screening must be conducted within the 48 hours immediately preceding the IRF admission to give the most accurate picture of the patient upon admission to the IRF. The rehabilitation physician must review and document his or her concurrence with the findings and results of the preadmission screening.

- A post-admission evaluation is required to document the status of the patient after admission to the IRF, to compare it to that noted in the preadmission screening documentation, and to begin development of the patient's overall plan of care. This evaluation must be performed within 24 hours of admission.

- An overall plan of care is required to establish the responsibility of the rehabilitation physician in the care planning process. The plan must be individualized to the unique needs of the patient to ensure that each patient's individual goals can be met. The plan must be developed and

present in the patient's medical record within 72 hours of the patient's admission.

- Requirements also involve an interdisciplinary team, the members of which are defined, along with requirements for the minimum content to be covered at team meetings and the required frequency of meetings (at least once per week per patient). The members will work cooperatively to define a set of coordinated goals for each patient.

- Requirements necessitate that the IRF patient must be able and willing to actively participate in an intensive rehabilitation program that is provided through a coordinated interdisciplinary team approach. The patient should also be expected to make measurable improvement that will be of practical value in terms of improving the patient's functional capacity or adaptation to impairments.

- Services related to the following areas are to be provided for a minimum of three hours per day:
  - rehabilitation nursing
  - physical therapy (PT), occupational therapy (OT), speech-language therapy (ST), etc.
  - psychosocial/social work interventions
  - orthotic and prosthetic services

- The "close medical supervision" requirement may generally be met by having a rehabilitation physician (or other licensed treating physician with specialized training and experience in inpatient rehabilitation) conduct face-to-face visits with the patient a minimum of at least three days per week throughout the patient's stay.

In an IRF, a patient's condition must require the 24-hour availability of a physician with special training or experience in the field of rehabilitation. The patient's medical record should reflect frequent, direct, and medically necessary physician involvement in the patient's care, e.g., at least every two to three days during the patient's stay. This degree of physician involvement is generally greater than that provided to a skilled nursing facility patient and is indicative of a need for services available only in a hospital setting. While in an IRF, a patient must require and receive at least three hours of physical and/or occupational therapy each day, according to the patient's condition and needs. In some cases a combination of therapy and other services (e.g., prosthetic-orthotic services) may be provided in lieu of the three-hour requirement.

Patient Screening and Assessment

A preadmission screening is typically performed prior to admission to an IRF. The screening provides a preliminary overview of the patient's condition and previous medical history to determine whether the patient would benefit from an intensive rehabilitation stay. At the time of a Medicare Part A IRF admission, a physician's order must be present, outlining the care required. The Centers for Medicare and Medicaid Services (CMS) has provided a patient assessment instrument (PAI) to assess the appropriateness of the IRF stay upon admission and at discharge for Medicare patients. The PAI consists of nine sections, each designed to collect different categories of patient information. The categories include identification and demographic information, medical information, information related to quality of care, and basic patient safety. IRFs must be computerized and electronically report the IRF-PAI data, which must be electronically entered into the IRF-PAI software product.

In general, the admission assessment must be based on observations performed on the first three days of the IRF stay and be completed by the fourth day of stay. The PAI reference date should be day three of the IRF stay. The discharge assessment must have an assessment reference date that is the actual day that the patient is discharged from the IRF (or the day the patient expires). This assessment is based upon observations made in the three calendar days prior to and including the assessment reference date on the discharge assessment. The discharge assessment must be completed by the fifth calendar day that follows the discharge assessment reference date, with the discharge assessment reference date being counted as the first day of the five calendar day period.

Medicare will cover the inpatient assessment as a part of the IRF stay only if it was reasonable and necessary to perform the assessment in the hospital. It is performed based on information in the patient's medical record but is more than a paperwork review. It should be an onsite professional review of the patient's condition by the necessary disciplines. Inpatient assessments conducted by a rehabilitation team usually require from three to 10 calendar days, during which time the patient typically receives therapies rather than simple screening assessments. An inpatient assessment may be covered even if the assessment subsequently determines that a patient is not suitable for an IRF program, if the patient's condition on admission was such that an extensive inpatient

Appendix K: Inpatient Rehabilitation Facility Prospective Payment System (PPS) Overview *(vertical side text)*

assessment was considered reasonable and necessary for a final determination to be made on a patient's actual rehabilitation potential.

Case-Mix Groups

The clinical characteristics of the Medicare patient are used to group the case into a case-mix group (CMG). CMGs are based on rehabilitation impairment categories (RICs), functional measurements, age, and comorbidities. The RICs are codes that indicate the primary cause of the rehabilitation hospitalization and are clinically homogenous. Cases that are similar in clinical characteristics and resource use most often group into the same RIC. Examples of RICs include:

01 Stroke

02 Traumatic brain injury (TBI)

08 Replacement of lower extremity (LE) joint

The first two digits of the CMG indicate the RIC, and the CMGs are further subdivided using functional measures of motor and cognitive scores, or age. The following table is an example of a RIC and its corresponding associated impairment group codes (IGCs).

Rehabilitation Impairment Category	Associated Impairment Group Codes
01 Stroke	01.1 Left body involvement (right brain)
	01.2 Right body involvement (left brain)
	01.3 Bilateral involvement
	01.4 No paresis
	01.9 Other stroke

A RIC may be divided into many separate CMGs, depending upon the differentiating clinical factors. For example, a patient with a stroke may be classified into one of the following CMGs:

CMG	CMG Description
0101	Stroke with motor score > 51.05
0102	Stroke with motor score from 44.45-51.05 & cognitive score >18.5
0103	Stroke with motor score from 44.45-51.05 & cognitive score <18.5
0104	Stroke with motor score from 38.85-44.45
0105	Stroke with motor score from 34.25-38.85
0106	Stroke with motor score from 30.05-34.25
0107	Stroke with motor score from 26.15-30.05
0108	Stroke with motor score < 26.15 & patient is 84.5 years old or older
0109	Stroke with motor score from 22.35-26.15 & patient is younger than 84.5 years old

Comorbidities

A comorbidity is a secondary condition that is typically complex and affects the cost of providing services to a beneficiary. Analysis indicated that the effect of specific comorbidities varied significantly among different principal diagnosis conditions. When it was found that the comorbidities substantially increased the average cost of a CMG and were clinically relevant, CMG relative weights were adjusted accordingly. Conditions that were deemed to be irrelevant to the inpatient rehabilitation population were excluded, as were those that were determined to be preventable by good medical care (e.g., urinary tract infections). Conditions that were considered to be inherent to a specific RIC were excluded as comorbidities for that RIC. Conditions with demonstrably higher costs were included.

In specific CMGs, comorbidities were found to substantially increase the average cost; these comorbidities were arranged in three tiers based on whether the costs are considered high, medium, or low. To compute payments for the comorbidity tiers, a regression analysis was performed to determine whether the comorbidity tiers affect costs per case by RIC. If a case has more than one comorbidity, the CMG payment rate will be based on the comorbidity that results in the highest payment.

The IRF-PAI software grouper generates a five-digit CMG number. The first digit is an alpha character that indicates the comorbidity tier, and the last four digits represent the specific CMG number. There are currently 21 RICs and 100 CMGs. Reimbursement may also be affected by adjustments for such factors as interrupted stays, transfers, short stays, and patient expiration. In addition, IRF providers are also subject to adjustments for wage index, percentage of low-income patients, rural location, and outlier payments.

Proposed Wage Adjustment

The IRF PPS wage index must be updated on the basis of information available to the Secretary on the wages and wage-related costs to furnish rehabilitation services. Any adjustment or updates for a fiscal year must be made in a budget-neutral manner. For FY 2016, CMS proposes to maintain the policies and methodologies described in the FY 2012 IRF PPS final rule related to the labor market area definitions and the wage index methodology for areas with wage data.

CMS proposes to use the Core-Based Statistical Areas (CBSA) labor market area definitions and the FY 2015 pre-reclassification and pre-floor hospital wage index data. The FY 2015 pre-reclassification and pre-floor hospital wage index is based on data submitted for hospital cost reporting periods beginning on or after October 1, 2010, and before October 1, 2011 (FY 2011 cost report data).

The labor market designations made by the OMB include some geographic areas where there are no hospitals and, thus, no hospital wage index data on which to base the calculation of the IRF PPS wage index. CMS will continue to use the same methodology as in the FY 2008 IRF PPS final rule to address those geographic areas where there are no hospitals and, thus, no hospital wage index data on which to base the calculation for the FY 2016 IRF PPS wage index.

The wage index used for the IRF PPS is calculated using the pre-reclassification and pre-floor acute care hospital wage index data and is assigned to the IRF on the basis of the labor market area in which the IRF is geographically located. IRF labor market areas are delineated based on the CBSA established by the Office of Management and Budget (OMB). The current CBSA labor market definitions used in FY 2015 are based on OMB standards published on December 27, 2000.

CMS is proposing to include the 2010 Census-based CBSA changes in the IRF PPS wage index for FY 2016. On February 28, 2013, the OMB issued OMB Bulletin No. 13–01, which established revised delineations for metropolitan statistical areas, micropolitan statistical areas, and combined statistical areas, and provided guidance on the use of the delineations of these statistical areas.

While the revisions OMB published on February 28, 2013, are not as sweeping as the changes made when adopted for the CBSA geographic designations in the FY 2006 IRF PPS final rule, the February 28, 2013, OMB bulletin does contain a number of significant changes. For example, there are new CBSAs, urban counties that become rural, rural counties that become urban, and existing CBSAs that are being split apart. The bulletin was not issued until February 28, 2013, with supporting data not available until later, and because the changes made by the bulletin and their ramifications needed to be extensively reviewed and verified, these changes were not incorporated into the hospital wage index until FY 2015 and are proposed for implementation in the IRF PPS beginning in FY 2016.

CMS is proposing a one-year transition with a blended wage index for all providers and a three-year phase-out of the rural adjustment for a subset of providers in FY 2016 to help providers adapt to the new OMB delineations.

The OMB defines a "micropolitan statistical area" as a CBSA associated with at least one urban cluster that has a population of at least 10,000 but less than 50,000. After extensive impact analysis, consistent with the treatment of these areas under the IPPS, CMS determined the best course of action would be to treat micropolitan areas as "rural" and include them in the calculation of each state's IRF PPS rural wage index. This means the IRF PPS statewide rural wage index is determined using IPPS hospital data from hospitals located in non-MSA areas, and the statewide rural wage index is assigned to IRFs located in those areas. Micropolitan areas tend to encompass smaller population centers and contain fewer hospitals than MSAs. CMS determined that if micropolitan areas were to be treated as separate labor market areas, the IRF PPS wage index would have included significantly more single-provider labor market areas, which would generally increase the potential for dramatic shifts in year-to-year wage index values as a single hospital (or group of hospitals) could have a disproportionate effect on the wage index of an area. For these reasons, CMS adopted a policy to include micropolitan areas in the state's rural wage area for purposes of the IRF PPS wage index and have continued this policy through the present.

The 2010 decennial census data contain a number of urban counties that have switched status and have joined or became micropolitan areas, and some counties that once were part of a micropolitan area have become urban. Overall, there are fewer micropolitan areas (541) under the new OMB delineations based on the 2010 Census than existed under the latest data from the prior data. CMS believes that the best course of action would be to continue the policy established in the FY 2006 IRF PPS final rule and include micropolitan areas in each state's rural wage index. These areas continue to be defined as having relatively small urban cores (populations of 10,000 to 49,999).

CMS's analysis based on the new OMB delineations shows that a total of 37 counties (and county equivalents) that are currently considered part of an urban CBSA would be considered located in a rural area for IRF PPS payment beginning in FY 2016. CMS proposes that these hospitals now be considered rural when their respective state's rural wage index value is calculated. This rural wage index value would be used under the IRF PPS.

CMS analysis of the new OMB delineations (based upon the 2010 decennial Census data) shows that, based on the new OMB delineations, a total of 105 counties (and county equivalents) that are currently located in rural areas would be located in urban areas. CMS proposes that these hospitals now be considered urban.

In addition to rural counties becoming urban and urban counties becoming rural, several urban counties would shift from one urban CBSA to another urban CBSA under the proposal to adopt the new OMB delineations. In other cases, applying the new OMB delineations would involve a change only in CBSA name or number, while the CBSA continues to encompass the same constituent counties. For example, CBSA 29140 (Lafayette, Ind.), would experience a change to both its number and its name, and would become CBSA 29200 (Lafayette-West Lafayette, Ind.), while all of its three constituent counties would remain the same. CMS considers some of these changes to be inconsequential changes to the IRF PPS wage index. However, in other cases, new OMB delineations would cause counties to shift between existing and new CBSAs, changing the constituent makeup of the CBSAs. Some CBSAs have counties that would split off to become part of, or to form, entirely new labor market areas. Finally, in some cases, a CBSA would lose counties to another existing CBSA.

The movement of these CBSAs may have both negative and positive impacts upon their specific wage index values. CMS proposes to implement a transition wage index to adjust for these possible impacts.

CMS's analysis indicates that a majority of IRFs expect either no change in the wage index or an increase in the wage index based on the new CBSA delineations. However, the agency found that 188 facilities will experience a decline in their wage index, with 29 facilities experiencing a decline of 5 percent or more based on the CBSA changes. CMS is proposing a similar transition methodology to that used in FY 2006. For the FY 2016 IRF PPS, CMS is proposing to implement a budget-neutral one-year transition policy. All IRF providers would receive a one-year blended wage index using 50 percent of their FY 2016 wage index based on the proposed new OMB delineations and 50 percent of their FY 2016 wage index based on the OMB delineations used in FY 2015. This one-year blended wage index would be applied in FY 2016 for all geographic areas to assist providers in adapting to these proposed changes. This transition policy would be for a one-year period, October 1, 2016, through September 30, 2017.

CMS's analysis for the FY 2016 proposed rule indicates that 22 IRFs will experience a change in either rural or urban designations. Of these, 19 facilities designated as rural in FY 2015 would be designated as urban in FY 2016. While 16 of these rural IRFs that would be designated as urban under the new CBSA delineations will experience an increase in their wage index, these IRFs will lose the 14.9 percent rural adjustment. In many cases, this loss exceeds the urban CBSA-based increase in the wage index. CMS feels that a phase-out of the rural adjustment for these facilities specifically is appropriate as these IRFs would experience a steeper and more abrupt reduction in their payments compared with other IRFs. Therefore, in addition to the one-year transition policy noted, CMS is proposing a budget-neutral three-year phase-out of the rural adjustment for existing FY 2015 rural IRFs that will become urban in FY 2016 and that experience a loss in payments due to changes from the new CBSA delineations. The loss of the FY 2015 rural adjustment of 14.9 percent will be phased out over FYs 2016, 2017, and 2018. This policy will allow rural IRFs that would be classified as urban in FY 2016 to receive two-thirds of the 2015 rural adjustment for FY 2016, as well as the blended wage index. For FY 2017, these IRFs will receive the full FY 2017 wage index and one-third of the FY 2015 rural adjustment. For FY 2018, these IRFs will receive the full FY 2018 wage index without a rural adjustment.

There is no transition policy for urban facilities that become rural in FY 2016 because these IRFs will receive the full rural adjustment of 14.9 percent beginning October 1, 2015.

Proposed Budget Neutrality, Market Basket Adjustments and Conversion Factor

Adjustments or updates to the IRF wage index made under section must be made in a budget-neutral manner. The proposed 2016 budget-neutral wage adjustment factor is 1.0027.

CMS began by applying the proposed adjusted market basket increase factor for FY 2016 that was adjusted in accordance with the Affordable Care Act, to the standard payment conversion factor for FY 2015 ($15,198).

To calculate the proposed standard payment conversion factor for FY 2016, the proposed 1.9 percent adjusted market basket increase for FY 2016 was applied to the standard payment conversion factor for FY 2015 of $15,198, yielding a standard payment amount of $15,487. Next the proposed budget neutrality factor for the FY 2016 wage index and labor-related share are applied, which results in a proposed standard payment amount of $15,529. The labor related portion is proposed to be 0.696.

The proposed budget neutrality factors for the revised CMG relative weights of 1.0000 are applied next, which results in the proposed standard payment conversion factor of $15,529 for FY 2016. After the application of the proposed CMG relative weights, the results are the proposed unadjusted IRF prospective payment rates for FY 2016.

Adjusting the proposed wage-adjusted federal payment by the facility-level adjustments involves several steps. First, the wage-adjusted federal prospective payment is multiplied by the appropriate rural and LIP adjustments (if applicable). Second, to determine the appropriate amount of additional payment for the teaching status adjustment (if applicable), the teaching status adjustment is multiplied by the wage-adjusted and rural-adjusted amount (if applicable). Finally, add the additional teaching status payments (if applicable) to the wage, rural, and LIP adjusted federal prospective payment rates.

Beginning with the FY 2006 IRF PPS final rule, the market basket index used to update IRF payments was a market basket reflecting the operating and capital cost structures for freestanding IRFs, freestanding inpatient psychiatric facilities (IPFs), and long-term care hospitals (LTCHs) (hereafter referred to as the rehabilitation, psychiatric, and long-term care [RPL] market basket).

Outliers

The Secretary has the authority to make payments in addition to the basic IRF prospective payments for cases incurring extraordinarily high costs. A case qualifies for an outlier payment if the estimated cost of the case exceeds the adjusted outlier threshold. The adjusted outlier threshold is calculated by adding the IRF PPS payment for the case (the CMG payment adjusted by all of the relevant facility-level adjustments) and the adjusted threshold amount (also adjusted by all of the relevant facility-level adjustments).

The estimated cost of a case is then calculated by multiplying the IRF's overall CCR by the Medicare allowable covered charge. If the estimated cost of the case is higher than the adjusted outlier threshold, CMS will make an outlier payment for the case equal to 80 percent of the difference between the estimated cost of the case and the outlier threshold.

The IRF outlier threshold amount has been updated annually to maintain estimated outlier payments at 3 percent of total estimated payments. To update the IRF outlier threshold amount for FY 2016, CMS proposes to use FY 2014 claims data and the same methodology that was used to set and update the outlier threshold amounts. The agency estimates that IRF outlier payments as a percentage of total estimated payments are approximately 3.2 percent in FY 2015. CMS proposes to update the outlier threshold amount to $9,698 to maintain estimated outlier payments at approximately 3 percent of total estimated aggregate IRF payments for FY 2016.

Cost-to-Charge Ratio (CCR) Changes

As has been past practice, CMS will apply a ceiling to IRF's CCRs. Using past methodology, CMS proposes to update the national urban and rural CCRs for IRFs, as well as the national CCR ceiling for FY 2016.

National urban and rural CCRs are applied in the following situations:

- New IRFs that have not yet submitted their first Medicare cost report
- IRFs whose overall CCR is in excess of the national CCR ceiling for FY 2016
- Other IRFs for which accurate data to calculate an overall CCR are not available

For FY 2016, CMS proposes to estimate a national average CCR of 0.569 for rural IRFs, which is the average of the CCRs for all rural IRFs using their most recently submitted cost report data. Similarly, a national average CCR of 0.437 is estimated for urban IRFs.

As has been past methodology, the national CCR ceiling is proposed at 3 standard deviations above the mean CCR. Using this method, the proposed national CCR ceiling would be 1.36 for FY 2016. This means that, if an individual IRF's CCR exceeds this proposed ceiling of 1.36 for FY 2016, CMS would replace the IRF's CCR with the appropriate proposed national average CCR (either rural or urban, depending on the geographic location of the IRF).

Multifactor Productivity

The Affordable Care Act provided a productivity adjustment for fiscal year 2012 and each subsequent fiscal year. The statute defines the productivity adjustment as equal to the 10-year moving average of changes in annual economywide private nonfarm business MFP (as projected by the Secretary for the 10-year

Appendix K: Inpatient Rehabilitation Facility Prospective Payment System (PPS) Overview

period ending with the applicable fiscal year, year, cost reporting period, or other annual period) (the "MFP adjustment"). MFP is derived by subtracting the contribution of labor and capital input growth from output growth.

For the FY 2016 rule-making cycle, the MFP adjustment is calculated using a revised series developed to proxy the aggregate capital inputs. CMS is using IGI IHS Global Insight's most recent forecast of the BLS capital input series in the MFP calculations beginning with the FY 2016 rule-making cycle. A complete description of the MFP projection methodology is available on CMS web site at: http://www.cms.gov/Research-Statistics-Data-and-Systems/ Statistics-Trends-and-Reports/MedicareProgramRatesStats/MarketBasketResear ch.html.

Using first quarter 2015 forecast, the MFP adjustment for FY 2016 (the 10-year moving average of MFP for the period ending FY 2016) is projected to be 0.6 percent. This leads CMS to propose basing the FY 2016 market basket update, which is used to determine the applicable percentage increase for the IRF payments, on the most recent estimate of the proposed 2012-based IRF market basket. Currently this is estimated to be 2.7 percent based on IGI's first quarter 2015 forecast. This would then be reduced by the current estimate of the MFP adjustment for FY 2016 by a 0.6 percentage point (the 10-year moving average of MFP for the period ending FY 2016 based on IGI's first quarter 2015 forecast). Following application of the MFP, the applicable percentage increases by 0.2 percentage point, as required by sections of the Affordable Care Act. Together the current estimate of the FY 2016 IRF update is 1.9 percent (2.7 percent market basket update, less a 0.6 percentage point MFP adjustment, less a 0.2 percentage point legislative adjustment).

If more recent data becomes available subsequently (for example, a more recent estimate of the market basket and MFP adjustment), the FY 2016 market basket update and MFP adjustment will be recalculated in the final rule.

The Affordable Care Act requires an additional 0.2 percentage point adjustment to the IRF increase factor for FY 2016. The application of these adjustments to the market basket update may result in an update that is less than 0.0 for a fiscal year and in payment rates for a fiscal year being less than such payment rates for the preceding fiscal year. Beginning in FY 2014, there is a 2 percentage point reduction of the applicable market basket increase factor for IRFs that fail to comply with the quality data submission requirements. Application of the 2 percentage point reduction may result in an update that is less than 0.0 for a fiscal year and in payment rates for a fiscal year being less than such payment rates for the preceding fiscal year. Reporting-based reductions to the market basket increase factor will not be cumulative; they will apply only for the fiscal year involved.

Appendix L: Rehabilitation Impairment Categories (RIC)

A case is assigned to a rehabilitation impairment category (RIC) based upon the primary reason for inpatient rehabilitation. The intent of this resource was to provide the RIC and the primary reason for inpatient rehabilitation (e.g., the ICD-10-CM diagnosis code(s)) for that RIC. Unfortunately the ICD-10-CM code information was not available at the time of publication.

CMS reports: "We are reviewing Section 6: ICD-9-CM Codes Related to Specific Impairment Groups and plan to have an updated table in the IRF-PAI training manual prior to when ICD-10-CM becomes the required medical data code set (October 1, 2015)."

Refer to the IRF Patient Assessment Instrument Training Manual found at the following link, for finalization and future updates on ICD-10-CM codes:

http://www.cms.gov/Medicare/Medicare-Fee-for-Service-Payment/InpatientRehabFacPPS/IRFPAI.html or go to Optum 360's customer support page at https://www.optumcoding.com/ProductUpdates, where we will post an updated table once the codes have been finalized.

Rehabilitation Impairment Categories (RIC)	Primary Reason for Inpatient Rehabilitation – Diagnosis Codes
01 Stroke Case with etiology of cerebral ischemia due to vascular thrombosis, embolism or hemorrhage	ICD-10-CM code information was not available at time of publication
02 Brain dysfunction - Non-traumatic brain dysfunction Cases with etiology of neoplasm including metastases, encephalitis, inflammation, anoxia, metabolic toxicity, or degenerative processes	ICD-10-CM code information was not available at time of publication
02 Brain dysfunction - Traumatic brain dysfunction Cases with motor and/or cognitive disorders secondary to brain trauma	ICD-10-CM code information was not available at time of publication
03 Neurologic conditions (except Guillain-Barré syndrome) Cases with neurologic or neuromuscular dysfunctions of various etiologies	ICD-10-CM code information was not available at time of publication
03 Neurologic conditions - Guillain-Barré syndrome	ICD-10-CM code information was not available at time of publication
04 Spinal cord dysfunction – Non-traumatic spinal cord dysfunction Cases with quadriplegia/paresis and paraplegia/paresis of non-traumatic (i.e., medical or postoperative) origin	ICD-10-CM code information was not available at time of publication
04 Spinal cord dysfunction – Traumatic spinal cord dysfunction Cases with quadriplegia/paresis and paraplegia/paresis secondary to trauma	ICD-10-CM code information was not available at time of publication
05 Amputation of limb Cases in which the major deficit is partial or complete absence of a limb	ICD-10-CM code information was not available at time of publication
06 Arthritis Cases in which the major disorder is arthritis of all etiologies	ICD-10-CM code information was not available at time of publication
07 Pain syndromes Cases in which the major disorder is pain of various etiologies, unaccompanied by a neurologic deficit	ICD-10-CM code information was not available at time of publication
08 Orthopaedic disorders Cases in which the major disorder is post-fracture of bone or post-arthroplasty (joint replacement)	ICD-10-CM code information was not available at time of publication
09 Cardiac Cases in which the major disorder is poor activity tolerance secondary to cardiac insufficiency or general deconditioning due to a cardiac disorder	ICD-10-CM code information was not available at time of publication
10 Pulmonary disorders Cases in which the major disorder is poor activity tolerance secondary to pulmonary insufficiency	ICD-10-CM code information was not available at time of publication
11 Burns Cases in which the major disorder is thermal injury to major areas of the skin and/or underlying tissue	ICD-10-CM code information was not available at time of publication
12 Congenital deformities Cases in which the major disorder is an anomaly or deformity of the nervous or musculoskeletal system that has been present since birth	ICD-10-CM code information was not available at time of publication
13 Other disabling impairments To be used only for cases that cannot be classified into any of the other Impairment Groups	ICD-10-CM code information was not available at time of publication

Appendix L: Rehabilitation Impairment Categories (RIC)

Rehabilitation Impairment Categories (RIC)	Primary Reason for Inpatient Rehabilitation – Diagnosis Codes
14 Major multiple trauma Cases with more complex management due to involvement of multiple systems or sites	ICD-10-CM code information was not available at time of publication
15 Developmental disability Cases in which the major disorder is impaired cognitive and/or motor function resulting in developmental delay	ICD-10-CM code information was not available at time of publication
16 Debility Cases with generalized deconditioning not attributable to any of the other Impairment Groups	ICD-10-CM code information was not available at time of publication
17 Medically complex conditions – Infections Cases admitted primarily for medical management of infections	ICD-10-CM code information was not available at time of publication
17 Medically complex conditions – Neoplasms Cases that require continuing care after surgery, chemotherapy, radiation, and immunotherapy or hormone therapy as a result of a neoplasm; care may include management of complications from the illness or the treatment	ICD-10-CM code information was not available at time of publication
17 Medically complex conditions – Nutrition Cases that require care and monitoring related to fluids and nutrition; care may include management of complications from endocrine, metabolic or neoplastic disorders	ICD-10-CM code information was not available at time of publication
17 Medically complex conditions – Circulatory disorders Cases that have complications of the circulatory system (heart, blood vessels) or need continuing management after surgery or treatment for circulatory conditions; may include acute myocardial infarction and cerebrovascular disease (stroke) if the time since onset of the circulatory disorder is greater than 2 months	ICD-10-CM code information was not available at time of publication
17 Medically complex conditions – Respiratory disorders, ventilator dependent Cases that are dependent on a ventilator upon admission, regardless of whether a weaning program is planned or is in effect	ICD-10-CM code information was not available at time of publication
17 Medically complex conditions – Respiratory disorders, non-ventilator dependent Cases that are not dependent on a ventilator	ICD-10-CM code information was not available at time of publication
17 Medically complex conditions – Terminal care Includes, but is not limited to, cases at the end stages of cancer, Alzheimer's disease, renal failure, congestive heart failure, stroke, acquired immunodeficiency syndrome (AIDS), Parkinsonism and emphysema; care typically focuses on comfort measures and pain relief as desired by the person	ICD-10-CM code information was not available at time of publication

[Source Document: *IRF-PAI Training Manual Section 6 ICD-9-CM Codes Related to Specific Impairment Groups* Effective 10/01/2014]

Appendix M: RIC Comorbid Conditions

The following lists the comorbid conditions that may qualify a case for payment adjustment when reported as a secondary diagnosis during admission. The rehabilitation impairment category (RIC) exclusions are identified as well as the comorbidity payment tier for each condition.

Note: A three-, four-, or five-character code followed by a dash indicates that all codes in that category/subcategory are included.

Note: For those T codes to which a 7th character is needed to complete the code, only the initial encounter (7th character A) is considered a CC.

Code	Title	Tier	RIC Excl
A02.1	Salmonella sepsis	3	
A04.7	Enterocolitis d/t C. diff	2	
A04.8	Oth spec bact intestinal infect	2	
A15.0	TB of lung	3	15
A15.4	TB of intrathoracic ln	3	15
A15.5	TB of larynx/trachea/bronchus	3	15
A15.6	TB pleurisy	3	15
A15.8	Oth respir TB	3	15
A15.9	Respir TB unsp	3	15
A17.0	TB meningitis	3	03, 05
A17.1	Meningeal tuberculoma	3	03, 05
A17.81	Tuberculoma brain/spinal cord	3	03, 05
A17.82	TB meningoencephalitis	3	03
A17.83	TB neuritis	3	03
A17.89	Other TB of nervous system	3	03, 05
A17.9	TB of nervous system, unsp	3	03, 05
A18.01	TB of spine	3	03, 09
A18.02	TB arthritis of oth joints	3	09
A18.03	TB of oth bones	3	09, 10, 11
A18.09	Oth musculoskeletal TB	3	09
A18.1-	TB of GU system	3	
A18.2	TB peripheral lymphadenopathy	3	
A18.3-	TB of intestines/peritoneum/mesenteric glands	3	
A18.4	TB of skin/subcu tissue	3	
A18.5-	TB of eye	3	
A18.6	TB of ear	3	
A18.7	TB of adrenal glands	3	
A18.8-	TB of oth spec organs	3	
A19.-	Miliary TB	3	
A22.1	Pulmonary anthrax	3	15
A22.7	Anthrax sepsis	3	
A26.-	Erysipeloid	3	
A28.0	Pasteurellosis	3	
A28.2	Extraintestinal yersiniosis	3	
A28.8	Oth spec zoo bact dis, nec	3	
A28.9	Zoo bact dis, unsp	3	
A32.-	Listeriosis	3	
A35	Oth tetanus	3	06

Code	Title	Tier	RIC Excl
A37.01	Whoop cough d/t Bordetella pertussis w pneu	3	
A37.11	Whoop cough d/t Bordetella parapertussis w pneu	3	
A37.81	Whoop cough d/t oth Bordetella species w pneu	3	15
A37.91	Whoop cough, unsp species w pneu	3	15
A39.0	Meningococcal meningitis	3	03, 05
A39.1	Waterhouse-Friderichsen syndrome	3	05
A39.2	Acute meningococcemia	3	03, 05
A39.3	Chronic meningococcemia	3	03, 05
A39.4	Meningococcemia, unsp	3	03, 05
A39.50	Meningococcal carditis, unsp	3	14
A39.51	Meningococcal endocarditis	3	14
A39.52	Meningococcal myocarditis	3	14
A40.-	Strep sepsis	3	
A41.-	Other sepsis	3	
A42.7	Actinomycotic sepsis	3	
A48.1	Legionnaires' disease	3	15
A50.41	Late congenital syphilitic meningitis	3	03, 05
A52.03	Syphilitic endocarditis	3	14
A52.06	Other syphilitic heart involvement	3	14
A52.13	Late syphilitic meningitis	3	03, 05
A52.19	Other symptomatic neurosyphilis	3	01, 03
A54.82	Gonococcal brain abscess	3	
A54.84	Gonococcal pneumonia	3	
A54.86	Gonococcal sepsis	3	
A54.89	Other gonococcal infections	3	
A54.9	Gonococcal infection, unsp	3	
A86	Unsp viral encephalitis	3	03
A87.0	Enteroviral meningitis	3	03, 05
A87.2	Lymphocytic choriomeningitis	3	03, 05
A87.8	Other viral meningitis	3	03, 05
A87.9	Viral meningitis, unsp	3	03, 05
A88.0	Enteroviral exanthematous fever	3	03, 05
A89	Unsp viral infection of cns	3	03
B00.3	Herpesviral meningitis	3	03, 05
B00.4	Herpesviral encephalitis	3	03
B00.7	Disseminated herpesviral disease	3	03
B00.82	Herpes simplex myelitis	3	

Code	Title	Tier	RIC Excl
B00.89	Oth herpesviral infection	3	
B01.11	Varicella encephalitis/encephalomyelitis	3	03
B01.2	Varicella pneumonia	3	15
B02.1	Zoster meningitis	3	03, 05
B02.23	Postherpetic polyneuropathy	3	06
B05.0	Measles complicated by encephalitis	3	03
B05.2	Measles complicated by pneumonia	3	15
B10.0-	Oth human herpesvirus encephalitis	3	03
B16.0	Ac hep B w delta w hep coma	3	03
B16.2	Ac hep B wo delta w hep coma	3	03
B17.0	Ac delta-(super) infection of hep B carrier	3	03
B17.11	Ac hep C w hep coma	3	03
B17.2	Ac hep E	3	03
B17.8	Oth spec ac viral hep	3	03
B18.0	Chr viral hep B w delta	3	03
B18.1	Chr viral hep B wo delta	3	03
B18.2	Chr viral hep C	3	03
B19.0	Unsp viral hep w hep coma	3	03
B19.11	Unsp viral hep B w hep coma	3	03
B19.21	Unsp viral hep C w hep coma	3	03
B20	HIV	3	
B25.0	Cytomegaloviral pneumonitis	3	15
B26.1	Mumps meningitis	3	03, 05
B26.2	Mumps encephalitis	3	03
B26.3	Mumps pancreatitis	3	
B33.3	Retrovirus infections, nec	3	
B37.1	Pulmonary candidiasis	3	15
B37.5	Candidal meningitis	3	03, 05
B37.6	Candidal endocarditis	3	14
B37.7	Candidal sepsis	3	
B37.81	Candidal esophagitis	3	
B38.4	Coccidioidomycosis meningitis	3	03, 05
B39.0	Ac pulmonary histoplasm capsulati	3	15
B39.1	Chr pulmonary histoplasm capsulati	3	15
B39.2	Pulm histoplasm capsulati, unsp	3	15
B39.3	Disseminated histoplasm capsulati	3	15
B39.4	Histoplasm capsulati, unsp	3	15
B39.5	Histoplasm duboisii	3	
B39.9	Histoplasm, unsp	3	15
B44.0	Invasive pulm aspergillosis	3	15
B45.1	Cerebral cryptococcosis	3	03, 05
B58.2	Toxoplasma meningoencephalitis	3	03, 05
B58.3	Pulmonary toxoplasmosis	3	15
B58.81	Toxoplasma myocarditis	3	14
B59	Pneumocystosis	3	15

Code	Title	Tier	RIC Excl
B77.81	Ascariasis pneumonia	3	15
B94.1	Sequelae of viral encephalitis	3	03
B96.5	Pseudomonas as the cause of dis class elwh	2	
B97.30	Unsp retrovirus as the cause of dis class elwh	3	
B97.31	Lentivirus as the cause of dis class elwh	3	
B97.32	Oncovirus as the cause of dis class elwh	3	
B97.33	HTLV-I as the cause of dis class elwh	3	06
B97.34	HTLV-II as the cause of dis class elwh	3	06
B97.35	HIV 2 as the cause of dis class elwh	3	
B97.39	Oth retrovirus as cause of dis class elwh	3	
C91.00	Ac lymphoblastic leuk no remis	3	
C91.02	Ac lymphoblastic leuk, in relapse	3	
C92.00	Ac myeloblastic leuk, no remis	3	
C92.02	Ac myeloblastic leuk, in relapse	3	
C92.40	Ac promyelocytic leuk, no remis	3	
C92.42	Ac promyelocytic leuk, in relapse	3	
C92.50	Ac myelomonocytic leuk, no remis	3	
C92.52	Ac myelomonocytic leuk, in relapse	3	
C92.60	Ac myeloid leuk w 11q23-abnormality no remis	3	
C92.62	Ac myeloid leuk w 11q23-abnormality in relapse	3	
C92.A0	Ac myeloid leuk w multilineage dysplasia, no remis	3	
C92.A2	Ac myeloid leuk w multilineage dysplasia, in relapse	3	
C93.00	Ac monoblastic/monocytic leuk, no remis	3	
C93.02	Ac monoblastic/monocytic leuk, in relapse	3	
C94.00	Ac erythroid leuk, no remis	3	
C94.02	Ac erythroid leuk, in relapse	3	
C95.00	Ac leuk of unsp cell type no remis	3	
C95.02	Ac leuk of unsp cell type, in relapse	3	
D57.0-	Hb-SS w crisis	3	
D57.1	Sickle-cell wo crisis	3	
D57.20	Sickle-cell/Hb-C wo crisis	3	
D57.21-	Sickle-cell/Hb-C w crisis	3	
D57.411	Sickle-cell thal w ac chest synd	3	
D57.80	Oth sickle-cell d/o wo crisis	3	
D57.81-	Oth sickle-cell d/o w crisis	3	
D60.-	Acq pure red cell aplasia	3	
D61.-	Oth aplastic anemia/oth bone marrow fail syndr	3	
D64.81	Anemia d/t antineo chemo	3	
D65	DIC	3	
D66	Hereditary factor VIII deficiency	3	
D67	Hereditary factor IX deficiency	3	

Code	Title	Tier	RIC Excl
E08.2-	DM d/t underlying condition w kidney complications	3	
E08.3-	DM d/t underlying condition w ophthalmic complications	3	
E08.40	DM d/t underlying condition w diabetic neuro, unsp	3	06
E08.41	DM d/t underlying condition w diabetic mononeuro	3	
E08.42	DM d/t underlying condition w diabetic polyneuro	3	06
E08.43	DM d/t underlying condition w diabetic autonomic (poly)neuro	3	
E08.44	DM d/t underlying condition w diabetic amyotrophy	3	
E08.49	DM d/t underlying condition w oth diabetic neuro complication	3	
E08.5-	DM d/t underlying condition w circulatory complications	3	
E08.61-	DM d/t underlying condition w diabetic arthropathy	3	
E08.62-	DM d/t underlying condition w skin complications	3	
E08.63-	DM d/t underlying condition w oral complications	3	
E08.649	DM d/t underlying condition w hypoglycemia wo coma	3	
E08.65	DM d/t underlying condition w hyperglycemia	3	
E08.69	DM d/t underlying condition w oth spec complication	3	
E09.2-	Drug/chem induced DM w kidney complications	3	
E09.3-	Drug/chem induced DM w ophthalmic complications	3	
E09.40	Drug/chem induced DM w neuro compl w diabetic neuro, unsp	3	06
E09.41	Drug/chem induced DM w neuro compl w diabetic mononeuro	3	
E09.42	Drug/chem induced DM w neuro compl w diabetic polyneuro	3	06
E09.43	Drug/chem induced DM w neuro compl w diabetic auto neuro	3	
E09.44	Drug/chem induced DM w neuro compl w diabetic amyotrophy	3	
E09.49	Drug/chem induced DM w neuro compl w oth diab neuro compl	3	
E09.5-	Drug/chem induced DM w circulatory complications	3	
E09.61-	Drug/chem induced DM w diabetic arthropathy	3	
E09.62-	Drug/chem induced DM w skin complications	3	
E09.63-	Drug/chem induced DM w oral complications	3	
E09.649	Drug/chem induced DM w hypoglycemia wo coma	3	

Code	Title	Tier	RIC Excl
E09.65	Drug/chem induced DM w hyperglycemia	3	
E09.69	Drug/chem induced DM w oth spec complication	3	
E10.2-	T1 DM w kidney complications	3	
E10.3-	T1 DM w ophthalmic complications	3	
E10.4-	T1 DM w neuro complications	3	06
E10.5-	T1 DM w circulatory complications	3	
E10.610	T1 DM w diabetic neuropathic arthropathy	3	06
E10.618	T1 DM w oth diabetic arthropathy	3	
E10.62-	T1 DM w skin complications	3	
E10.63-	T1 DM w oral complications	3	
E10.649	T1 DM w hypoglycemia wo coma	3	
E10.65	T1 DM w hyperglycemia	3	
E10.69	T1 DM w oth spec complication	3	
E10.8	T1 DM w unsp complications	3	
E10.9	T1 DM wo complications	3	
E11.2-	T2 DM w kidney complications	3	
E11.3-	T2 DM w ophthalmic complications	3	
E11.4-	T2 DM w neuro complications	3	06
E11.5-	T2 DM w circulatory complications	3	
E11.610	T2 DM w diabetic neuro arthropathy	3	06
E11.618	T2 DM w oth diabetic arthropathy	3	
E11.62-	T2 DM w skin complications	3	
E11.63-	T2 DM w oral complications	3	
E11.649	T2 DM w hypoglycemia wo coma	3	
E11.65	T2 DM w hyperglycemia	3	
E11.69	T2 DM w oth spec complication	3	
E13.2-	Oth spec DM w kidney complications	3	
E13.3-	Oth spec DM w ophthalmic complications	3	
E13.4-	Oth spec DM w neuro complications	3	06
E13.5-	Oth spec DM w circulatory complications	3	
E13.610	Oth spec DM w diabetic neuro arthropathy	3	06
E13.618	Oth spec DM w oth diabetic arthropathy	3	
E13.62-	Oth spec DM w skin complications	3	
E13.63-	Oth spec DM w oral complications	3	
E13.649	Oth spec DM w hypoglycemia wo coma	3	
E13.65	Oth spec DM w hyperglycemia	3	
E13.69	Oth spec DM w oth spec complication	3	
E66.01	Morbid (severe) obesity	3	
E84.0	Cystic fibrosis w pulm manifestations	3	15
E84.11	Meconium ileus in cystic fibrosis	3	15
E84.19	Cystic fibrosis w oth intestinal manifestations	3	15
E84.8	Cystic fibrosis w oth manifestations	3	15
E84.9	Cystic fibrosis, unsp	3	15
G00.-	Bact menigitis, nec	3	03, 05

Code	Title	Tier	RIC Excl	Code	Title	Tier	RIC Excl
G01	Meningitis in bact dis class elwh	3	03, 05	I46.-	Cardiac arrest	3	14
G02	Meningitis in oth infect/parasitic dis class elwh	3	03, 05	I49.01	Ventricular fibrillation	3	14
G03.0	Nonpyogenic meningitis	3	03, 05	I50.1	Left ventricular failure	3	14
G03.1	Chronic meningitis	3	03, 05	I50.2-	Systolic heart failure	3	14
G03.2	Benign recurrent meningitis	3	03, 05	I50.3-	Diastolic heart failure	3	14
G03.9	Meningitis, unsp	3	03, 05	I50.4-	Combined systolic/diastolic heart failure	3	14
G04.00	Ac disseminated encephalitis/encephalomyelitis, unsp	3	03	I60.-	Nontraumatic subarachnoid hemor	3	01, 02, 03
G04.01	Postinfect ac disseminated encephalitis/encephalomyelitis	3	03	I61.-	Nontraumatic intracerebral hemor	3	01, 02, 03
G04.2	Bact meningoencephalitis/meningomyelitis, nec	3	03, 05	I62.0-	Nontraumatic subdural hemor	3	01, 02, 03
				I62.1	Nontraumatic extradural hemor	3	01, 02, 03
G04.30	Ac necrotizing hemorrhagic encephalo, unsp	3	03	I63.-	Cerebral infarction	3	01
G04.31	Postinfect ac necrotizing hemorrhagic encephalo	3	03	I67.89	Oth cerebrovascular dis	3	01
G04.39	Oth ac necrotizing hemorrhagic encephalo	3	03	I69.091	Dysphagia following nontraum subarachnoid hemor	2	01
G04.8-	Oth encephalitis/myelitis/encephalomyelitis	3	03	I69.191	Dysphagia following nontraum intracerebral hemor	2	01
G04.9-	Encephalitis/myelitis/encephalomyelitis, unsp	3	03	I69.291	Dysphagia following oth nontraum intracranial hemor	2	01
G05.4	Myelitis in dis class elwh	3	03	I69.391	Dysphagia following cerebral infarction	2	01
G06.-	Intracranial/intraspinal abscess/granuloma	3	03	I69.891	Dysphagia following oth cerebrovascular dis	2	01
G07	Intracranial/intraspinal abscess/granuloma in dis class elwh	3	03	I69.991	Dysphagia following unsp cerebrovascular dis	2	01
G37.3	Ac transverse myelitis in demyelinating dis of cns	3	03	I70.23-	Athero of native arteries right leg w ulceration	3	10, 11
G37.4	Subac necrotizing myelitis of cns	3	03	I70.24-	Athero of native arteries left leg w ulceration	3	10, 11
G40.301	Gen idio epilepsy/epileptic synd, not intract, w status epil	3	02, 03	I70.25	Athero of native arteries oth extremities w ulceration	3	10, 11
G40.31-	Gen idio epilepsy/epileptic synd, intract	3	02, 03	I70.26-	Athero of native arteries extremities w gangrene	3	10, 11
G40.41-	Oth gen epilepsy/epileptic synd, intract	3	02, 03	I70.92	Chr total occlusion of artery of the extremities	3	10, 11
G81.-	Hemiplegia and hemiparesis	3	01	I71.0-	Dissection of aorta	3	05
G93.1	Anoxic brain damage, nec	3	02, 03	I71.1	Thoracic aortic aneurysm, rupt	3	05
H05.01-	Cellulitis of orbit	3		I71.3	Abdominal aortic aneurysm, rupt	3	05
H05.02-	Osteomyelitis of orbit	3		I71.5	Thoracoabdominal aortic aneurysm, rupt	3	05
H05.03-	Periostitis of orbit	3		I71.8	Aortic aneurysm of unsp site, rupt	3	
I09.0	Rheumatic myocarditis	3	14	I76	Septic arterial embolism	3	
I12.0	Htn ckd w stage 5 ckd or esrd	3		I81	Portal vein thrombosis	3	
I13.0	Htn heart/ckd w hf and stage 1 - 4 ckd, or unsp ckd	3	14	I82.0	Budd-Chiari syndrome	3	
I13.2	Htn heart/ckd w hf and stage 5 ckd, or esrd	3	14	I82.1	Thrombophlebitis migrans	3	
I26.-	Pulm embolism	3	15	I82.22-	Embolism/thrombosis inferior vena cava	3	
I27.82	Chr pulm embolism	3	15	I82.3	Embolism/thrombosis renal vein	3	
I33.-	Ac and subac infective endocarditis	3	14	I96	Gangrene, nec	3	10, 11
I39	Endocarditis/heart valve d/o in dis class elwh	3	14	J04.11	Ac tracheitis w obstruction	3	15
I40.-	Ac myocarditis	3	14	J05.0	Ac obstructive laryngitis	3	15
I41	Myocarditis in dis class elwh	3	14	J05.11	Ac epiglottitis w obstruction	3	15
				J09.X-	Influ d/t identified novel influ A virus	3	15

Code	Title	Tier	RIC Excl
J10.00	Influ d/t oth identified influ virus w unsp pneu	3	15
J10.08	Influ d/t oth identified influ virus w oth spec pneu	3	15
J10.1	Influ d/t oth identified influ virus w oth resp manif	3	15
J11.0-	Influ d/t unidentified influ virus w pneu	3	15
J12.0	Adenoviral pneu	3	15
J12.1	Resp syncytial virus pneu	3	15
J12.2	Parainfluenza virus pneu	3	15
J12.3	Human metapneumovirus pneu	3	15
J12.89	Other viral pneumonia	3	15
J12.9	Viral pneumonia, unsp	3	15
J13	Pneu d/t Streptococcus pneumoniae	3	15
J14	Pneu d/t H. influenzae	3	15
J15.-	Bact pneumonis, nec	3	15
J16.-	Pneu d/t oth infect org, nec	3	15
J17	Pneumonia in dis class elsw	3	15
J18.-	Pneumonia, unsp organism	3	15
J21.-	Acute bronchiolitis	3	15
J38.0-	Dix of vocal cords/larynx, nec	3	15
J38.4	Edema of larynx	1	15
J68.0	Bronchitis/pneumonitis d/t chem/gas/fume/vapor	3	15
J68.1	Pulm edema d/t chem/gas/fume/vapor	3	15
J69.-	Pneumonitis d/t inhalation of food/vomit	3	15
J81.1	Chronic pulmonary edema	3	15
J82	Pulmonary eosinophilia, nec	3	15
J84.10	Pulmonary fibrosis, unsp	3	15
J84.112	Idiop pulmonary fibrosis	3	15
J84.113	Idiop non-specific interstitial pneumonitis	3	15
J84.114	Acute interstitial pneumonitis	3	15
J84.115	Resp bronchiolitis interstitial lung dis	3	15
J84.17	Oth interstitial pulm dis w fibrosis in dis class elwh	3	15
J84.89	Oth spec interstitial pulmonary dis	3	15
J85.-	Abscess of lung/mediastinum	3	15
J86.-	Pyothorax	3	15
J90	Pleural effusion, nec	3	15
J94.2	Hemothorax	3	15
J95.1	Ac pulm insuff following thoracic surg	3	15
J95.2	Ac pulm insuff following nonthoracic surg	3	15
J95.3	Chr pulm insuff following surg	3	15
J95.82-	Postproc resp failure	3	15
J96.0-	Acute resp failure	3	15
J96.2-	Ac and chr resp failure	3	15
J96.9-	Resp failure, unsp	3	15

Code	Title	Tier	RIC Excl
J98.5	Diseases of mediastinum, nec	3	15
K12.2	Cellulitis/abscess of mouth	3	
K22.3	Perforation of esophagus	3	
K22.8	Oth spec dis of esophagus	3	15
K25.0	Ac gastric ulcer w hemor	3	
K25.1	Ac gastric ulcer w perf	3	
K25.2	Ac gastric ulcer w both hemor/perf	3	
K25.4	Chr/unsp gastric ulcer w hemor	3	
K25.5	Chr/unsp gastric ulcer w perf	3	
K25.6	Chr/unsp gastric ulcer w both hemor/perf	3	
K26.0	Ac duodenal ulcer w hemor	3	
K26.1	Ac duodenal ulcer w perf	3	
K26.2	Ac duodenal ulcer w hemor/perf	3	
K26.4	Chr/unsp duodenal ulcer w hemor	3	
K26.5	Chr/unsp duodenal ulcer w perf	3	
K26.6	Chr/unsp duodenal ulcer w hemor/perf	3	
K27.0	Ac peptic ulcer, site unsp, w hemor	3	
K27.1	Ac peptic ulcer, site unsp, w perf	3	
K27.2	Ac peptic ulcer, site unsp, w hemor/perf	3	
K27.4	Chr/unsp peptic ulcer, site unsp w hemor	3	
K27.5	Chr/unsp peptic ulcer, site unsp w perf	3	
K27.6	Chr/unsp peptic ulcer, site unsp w hemor/perf	3	
K28.0	Ac gastrojejunal ulcer w hemor	3	
K28.1	Ac gastrojejunal ulcer w perf	3	
K28.2	Ac gastrojejunal ulcer w hemor/perf	3	
K28.4	Chr/unsp gastrojejunal ulcer w hemor	3	
K28.5	Chr/unsp gastrojejunal ulcer w perf	3	
K28.6	Chr/unsp gastrojejunal ulcer w hemor/perf	3	
K29.01	Acute gastritis w bleeding	3	
K29.21	Alcoholic gastritis w bleeding	3	
K29.31	Chr superficial gastritis w bleed	3	
K29.41	Chr atrophic gastritis w bleed	3	
K29.51	Unsp chr gastritis w bleed	3	
K29.61	Oth gastritis w bleed	3	
K29.71	Gastritis, unsp, w bleed	3	
K29.81	Duodenitis w bleed	3	
K29.91	Gastroduodenitis, unsp, w bleed	3	
K31.6	Fistula of stomach/duodenum	3	
K31.811	Angiodysplasia of stomach/duod w bleed	3	
K31.82	Dieulafoy lesion of stomach/duod	3	
K35.2	Ac appendicitis w gen peritonitis	3	
K52.81	Eosinophilic gastritis or gastroenteritis	3	
K55.0	Ac vascular d/o of intestine	3	
K55.21	Angiodysplasia of colon w hemor	3	

Code	Title	Tier	RIC Excl
K57.01	Diverticulitis sm intest w perf/abscess w bleed	3	
K57.11	Diverticulosis sm intest wo perf/abscess w bleed	3	
K57.13	Diverticulitis sm intest wo perf/abscess w bleed	3	
K57.21	Diverticulitis lg intest w perf/abscess w bleed	3	
K57.31	Diverticulosis lg intest wo perf/abscess w bleed	3	
K57.33	Diverticulitis lg intest wo perf/abscess w bleed	3	
K57.41	Diverticulitis sm/lg intest w perf/abscess w bleed	3	
K57.51	Diverticulosis sm/lg intest wo perf/abscess w bleed	3	
K57.53	Diverticulitis sm/lg intest wo perf/abscess w bleed	3	
K57.81	Diverticulitis intest, part unsp, w perf/abscess w bleed	3	
K57.91	Diverticulosis intest, part unsp, wo perf/abscess w bleed	3	
K57.93	Diverticulitis intest, part unsp, wo perf/abscess w bleed	3	
K63.1	Perforation of intestine (nontraumatic)	3	
K65.-	Peritonitis	3	
K67	D/o of peritoneum in infect dis class elwh	3	
K68.11	Postproc retroperitoneal abscess	3	
K68.19	Oth retroperitoneal abscess	3	
K68.9	Oth d/o of retroperitoneum	3	
K72.0-	Hepatic failure, nec	3	
K75.0	Abscess of liver	3	
K76.2	Central hemor necrosis of liver	3	
K76.3	Infarction of liver	3	
K76.7	Hepatorenal syndrome	3	
K82.2	Perforation of gallbladder	3	
K83.2	Perforation of bile duct	3	
K86.2	Cyst of pancreas	3	
K86.3	Pseudocyst of pancreas	3	
K91.2	Postsurgl malabsorption, nec	2	
K94.0-	Colostomy complication, unsp	3	
K94.1-	Enterostomy complication, unsp	3	
L02.01	Cutaneous abscess face	3	
L02.11	Cutaneous abscess neck	3	
L02.21-	Cutaneous abscess abdominal wall	3	
L02.31	Cutaneous abscess buttock	3	
L02.411	Cutaneous abscess right axilla	3	
L02.412	Cutaneous abscess left axilla	3	
L02.413	Cutaneous abscess right upper limb	3	
L02.414	Cutaneous abscess left upper limb	3	

Code	Title	Tier	RIC Excl
L02.415	Cutaneous abscess right lower limb	3	10
L02.416	Cutaneous abscess left lower limb	3	10
L02.419	Cutaneous abscess limb, unsp	3	10
L02.51-	Cutaneous abscess hand	3	
L02.61-	Cutaneous abscess foot	3	10
L02.811	Cutaneous abscess head, exc face	3	
L02.818	Cutaneous abscess of oth sites	3	
L03.111	Cellulitis of right axilla	3	
L03.112	Cellulitis of left axilla	3	
L03.113	Cellulitis of right upper limb	3	
L03.114	Cellulitis of left upper limb	3	
L03.115	Cellulitis of right lower limb	3	10
L03.116	Cellulitis of left lower limb	3	10
L03.119	Cellulitis of unsp part of limb	3	10
L03.121	Ac lymphangitis right axilla	3	
L03.122	Ac lymphangitis left axilla	3	
L03.123	Ac lymphangitis right upper limb	3	
L03.124	Ac lymphangitis left upper limb	3	
L03.125	Ac lymphangitis right lower limb	3	10
L03.126	Ac lymphangitis left lower limb	3	10
L03.129	Ac lymphangitis unsp part of limb	3	10
L03.2-	Cellulitis/ac lymphangitis face/neck	3	
L03.31-	Cellulitis trunk	3	
L03.32-	Ac lymphangitis trunk	3	
L03.811	Cellulitis of head, exc face	3	
L03.818	Cellulitis of oth sites	3	
L03.891	Ac lymphangitis of head, exc face	3	
L03.898	Ac lymphangitis of oth sites	3	
M31.2	Lethal midline granuloma	3	
N00.-	Acute nephritic syndrome	3	
N01.-	Rapid progressive nephritic synd	3	
N05.9	Unsp nephritic synd w unsp morphologic changes	3	
N08	Glomerular d/o in dis class elwh	3	
N15.1	Renal/perinephric abscess	3	
N17.-	Acute kidney failure	3	
N32.89	Oth spec d/o of bladder	3	
O71.0-	Rupture of uterus before onset labor	3	
O71.1	Rupture of uterus during labor	3	
O75.1	Shock during or following labor/delivery	3	03
O75.3	Other infection during labor	3	01
O88.01-	Obstetric air embolism in preg	3	01
O88.02	Air embolism in childbirth	3	01
O88.03	Air embolism in the puerperium	3	01
O88.11-	Amniotic fluid emoblism in preg	3	01

Code	Title	Tier	RIC Excl
O88.12	Amniotic fluid embolism in childbirth	3	01
O88.13	Amniotic fluid embolism in puerperium	3	01
O88.21-	Thromboembolism in pregnancy	3	15
O88.22	Thromboembolism in childbirth	3	15
O88.23	Thromboembolism in the puerperium	3	15
O88.31-	Pyemic/septic embolism in preg	3	03
O88.32	Pyemic/septic embolism in childbirth	3	03
O88.33	Pyemic/septic embolism in puerperium	3	03
O88.81-	Oth embolism in pregnancy	3	15
O88.82	Oth embolism in childbirth	3	15
O88.83	Oth embolism in puerperium	3	15
O90.4	Postpartum acute kidney failure	3	
O99.419	Dis of circ system complicating preg, unsp tri	3	01, 03
P07.01	Extremely low birth weight nb, less than 500 grams	3	
P07.02	Extremely low birth weight nb, 500-749 grams	3	
P07.03	Extremely low birth weight nb, 750-999 grams	3	
R09.2	Respiratory arrest	3	15
R13.-	Aphagia/dysphagia	2	01
R29.0	Tetany	3	06
R50.82	Postprocedural fever	3	
R50.84	Febrile nonhemolytic transfusion reaction	3	
R57.0	Cardiogenic shock	3	14
R57.1	Hypovolemic shock	3	
R57.8	Other shock	3	
R65.-	Symp/signs ass w systemic inflam/infect	3	
R91.8	Oth nonspecific abnormal finding of lung field	3	15
T79.0XX	Air embolism (traumatic)	3	02, 03
T79.1XX	Fat embolism (traumatic)	3	02, 03
T79.5XX	Traumatic anuria	3	
T80.0XX	Air embol following infusion/transfusion/thera inj	3	03
T80.21-	Infection due to central venous cath	3	
T81.1-	Postprocedural shock	3	
T81.3-	Disruption of wound, nec	3	
T81.4XX	Infection following a procedure	3	
T81.83X	Persistent postprocedural fistula	3	
T82.0-	Mech complication heart valve prosth	3	14
T82.6XX	Infect/inflam react d/t cardiac valve prosthesis	3	14
T82.7XX	Infect/inflam react d/t oth cardiac/vasc dev/implant/gft	3	
T84.5-	Infect/inflam react d/t unsp internal jt prosth	3	08

Code	Title	Tier	RIC Excl
T84.6-	Infect/inflam react d/t internal fix dev unsp site	3	09
T84.7XX	Infect/inflam react d/t oth int ortho prosth dev/implant/gft	3	09
T85.7-	Infect/inflam react d/t oth int prosth dev/implant/gft	3	09
T86.842	Corneal transplant infection	3	09
T87.4-	Infection amputation stump	3	09, 10, 11
Z43.0	Encounter for attention to trach	1	
Z93.0	Tracheostomy status	1	
Z99.2	Dependence on renal dialysis	1	

Appendix M: RIC Comorbid Conditions

Code	Choice	Title	Tier	RIC Excl
B39.4	A	Histoplasm capsulati, unsp	3	03, 05
G02	B	Meningitis in oth infect/parasitic dis class elwh		
B39.4	A	Histoplasm capsulati, unsp	3	
H32	B	Chorioretinal d/o in dis class elwh		
B39.4	A	Histoplasm capsulati, unsp	3	14
I32	B	Pericarditis in dis class elwh		
B39.4	A	Histoplasm capsulati, unsp	3	14
I39	B	Endocarditis/heart valve d/o in dis class elwh		
B39.5	A	Histoplasm duboisii	3	03, 05
G02	B	Meningitis in oth infect/parasitic dis class elwh		
B39.5	A	Histoplasm duboisii	3	
H32	B	Chorioretinal d/o in dis class elwh		
B39.5	A	Histoplasmduboisii	3	14
I32	B	Pericarditis in dis class elwh		
B39.5	A	Histoplasm duboisii	3	14
I39	B	Endocarditis/heart valve d/o in dis class elwh		
B39.5	A	Histoplasm duboisii	3	15
J17	B	Pneumonia in dis class elwh		
B39.9	A	Histoplasmosis, unspecified	3	03, 05
G02	B	Meningitis in oth infect/parasitic dis class elwh		
B39.9	A	Histoplasm, unsp	3	
H32	B	Chorioretinal d/o in dis class elwh		
B39.9	A	Histoplasm, unsp	3	14
I32	B	Pericarditis in dis class elwh		
B39.9	A	Histoplasm, unsp	3	14
I39	B	Endocarditis/heart valve d/o in dis class elwh		
B39.9	A	Histoplasm, unsp	3	15
J17	B	Pneumonia in dis class elwh		
E08.21	A	DM d/t underlying cond w dm nephro	3	
E09.21	A	Drug/chem induced DM w diabetic nephro		
E08.65	B	DM d/t underlying condition w hyperglycemia		
E08.40	A	DM d/t underlying condition w diabetic neuro, unsp	3	
E09.40	A	Drug/chem induced DM w neuro complications w diabetic neuro, unsp		
E08.65	B	DM d/t underlying condition w hyperglycemia		

Code	Choice	Title	Tier	RIC Excl
E08.51	A	DM d/t underlying condition w diabetic peripheral angiopathy wo gangrene	3	
E09.51	A	Drug/chem induced DM w diabetic peripheral angiopathy wo gangrene		
E08.65	B	DM d/t underlying condition w hyperglycemia		
E08.69	A	DM d/t underlying condition w oth spec complication	3	
E09.69	A	Drug/chem induced DM w oth spec complication		
E08.65	B	DM d/t underlying condition w hyperglycemia		
E08.8	A	DM d/t underlying condition w unsp complications	3	
E09.8	A	Drug/chem induced DM w unsp complications		
E08.65	B	DM d/t underlying condition w hyperglycemia		
E11.21	A	T2 DM w diabetic nephro	3	
E11.65	B	T2 DM w hyperglycemia		
E10.21	A	T1 DM w diabetic nephro	3	
E10.65	B	T1 DM w hyperglycemia		
E11.311	A	T2 DM w unsp diabetic retinopathy w macular edema	3	
E11.319	A	T2 DM w unsp diabetic retinopathy wo macular edema		
E11.36	A	T2 DM w diabetic cataract		
E11.39	A	T2 DM w oth diabetic ophthalmic complication		
E11.65	B	T2 DM w hyperglycemia		
E10.311	A	T1 DM w unsp diabetic retinopathy w macular edema	3	
E10.319	A	T1 DM w unsp diabetic retinopathy wo macular edema		
E10.36	A	T1 DM w diabetic cataract		
E10.39	A	T1 DM w oth diabetic ophthalmic complication		
E10.65	B	T1 DM w hyperglycemia		
E11.40	A	T2 DM w diabetic neuro, unsp	3	06
E11.65	B	T2 DM w hyperglycemia		
E10.40	A	T1 DM w diabetic neuro, unsp	3	06
E10.65	B	T1 DM w hyperglycemia		
E11.51	A	T2 DM w diabetic peripheral angiopathy wo gangrene	3	
E11.65	B	T2 DM w hyperglycemia		
E10.51	A	T1 DM w diabetic peripheral angiopathy wo gangrene	3	
E10.65	B	T1 DM w hyperglycemia		
E11.69	A	T2 DM w oth spec complication	3	
E11.65	B	T2 DM w hyperglycemia		

Code	Choice	Title	Tier	RIC Excl	Code	Choice	Title	Tier	RIC Excl
E10.69	A	T1 DM w oth spec complication	3		K56.60	B	Unsp intestinal obst		
E10.65	B	T1 DM w hyperglycemia			K26.4	A	Chr/unsp duod ulcer w hemor	3	
E11.8	A	T2 DM w unsp complications	3		K56.60	B	Unsp intestinal obst		
E11.65	B	T2 DM w hyperglycemia			K26.5	A	Chr/unsp duod ulcer w perf	3	
K25.0	A	Ac gastric ulcer w hemor	3		K56.60	B	Unsp intestinal obst		
K56.60	B	Unsp intestinal obst			K26.6	A	Chr/unsp duod ulcer w both hemor/perf	3	
K25.1	A	Ac gastric ulcer w perf	3						
K56.60	B	Unsp intestinal obst			K56.60	B	Unsp intestinal obst		
K25.2	A	Ac gastric ulcer w both hemor/perf	3		T80.0XX	A	Air embol following infusion/transfusion/therap inj	3	15
K56.60	B	Unsp intestinal obst			T81.718	A	Complication of oth artery following a procedure, nec		
K25.4	A	Chr/unsp gastric ulcer w hemor	3						
K56.60	B	Unsp intestinal obst			T81.72X	A	Complication of vein following a procedure, nec		
K25.5	A	Chr/unsp gastric ulcer w perf	3						
K56.60	B	Unsp intestinal obst			T82.817	A	Embolism of cardiac prosthetic dev/implant/gft		
K25.6	A	Chr/unsp gastric ulcer w both hemor/perf	3						
K56.60	B	Unsp intestinal obst			T82.818	A	Embolism of vascular prosthetic dev/implant/gft		
K26.0	A	Ac duod ulcer w hemor	3		I26.90	B	Septic pulm embolism wo acute cor pulmonale		
K56.60	B	Unsp intestinal obst							
K26.1	A	Ac duod ulcer w perf	3		I26.99	B	Other pulm embolism wo acute cor pulmonale		
K56.60	B	Unsp intestinal obst							
K26.2	A	Ac duod ulcer w both hemor/perf	3						

Illustrations

Peripheral Nervous System

Brain

Cranial Nerves

Eye

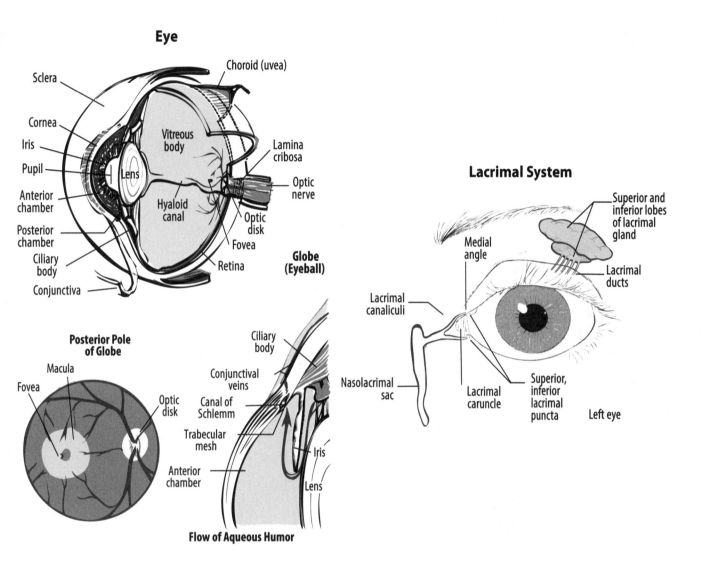

Sclera
Cornea
Iris
Pupil
Anterior chamber
Posterior chamber
Ciliary body
Conjunctiva

Choroid (uvea)
Vitreous body
Lamina cribosa
Lens
Hyaloid canal
Optic nerve
Optic disk
Fovea
Retina

Globe (Eyeball)

Posterior Pole of Globe

Macula
Fovea
Optic disk

Ciliary body
Conjunctival veins
Canal of Schlemm
Trabecular mesh
Anterior chamber
Iris
Lens

Flow of Aqueous Humor

Lacrimal System

Medial angle
Lacrimal canaliculi
Nasolacrimal sac

Superior and inferior lobes of lacrimal gland
Lacrimal ducts
Superior, inferior lacrimal puncta
Lacrimal caruncle

Left eye

Ear and Mastoid

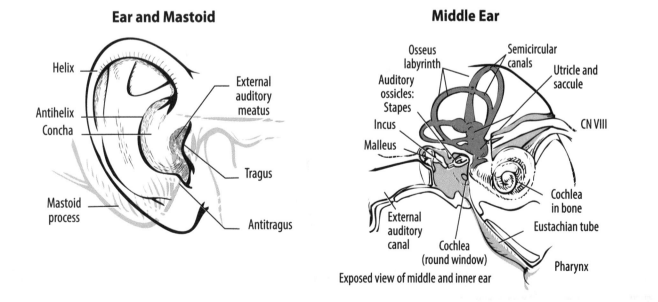

Helix
Antihelix
Concha
Mastoid process

External auditory meatus
Tragus
Antitragus

Middle Ear

Osseus labyrinth
Auditory ossicles:
Stapes
Incus
Malleus

Semicircular canals
Utricle and saccule
CN VIII
Cochlea in bone
Eustachian tube
Pharynx

External auditory canal
Cochlea (round window)

Exposed view of middle and inner ear

Arteries

Veins

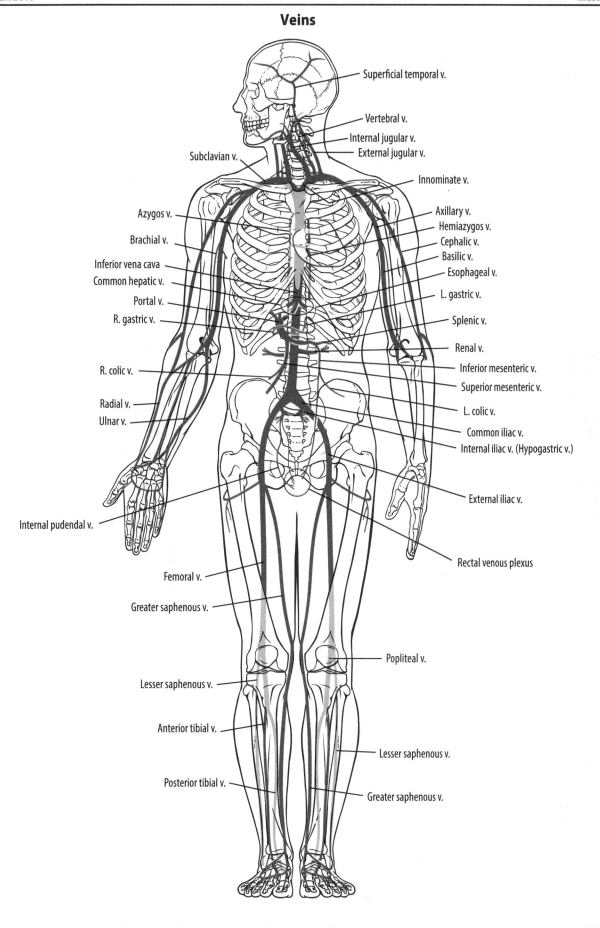

Superficial temporal v.

Vertebral v.

Internal jugular v.

External jugular v.

Subclavian v.

Innominate v.

Azygos v.

Axillary v.

Hemiazygos v.

Brachial v.

Cephalic v.

Basilic v.

Inferior vena cava

Esophageal v.

Common hepatic v.

L. gastric v.

Portal v.

R. gastric v.

Splenic v.

Renal v.

R. colic v.

Inferior mesenteric v.

Superior mesenteric v.

Radial v.

L. colic v.

Ulnar v.

Common iliac v.

Internal iliac v. (Hypogastric v.)

External iliac v.

Internal pudendal v.

Rectal venous plexus

Femoral v.

Greater saphenous v.

Popliteal v.

Lesser saphenous v.

Anterior tibial v.

Lesser saphenous v.

Posterior tibial v.

Greater saphenous v.

Anatomy of Heart

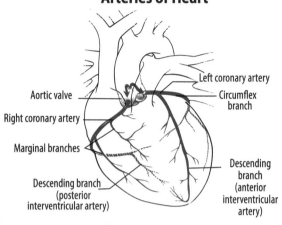

Arteries of Heart

Cerebrovascular Arteries

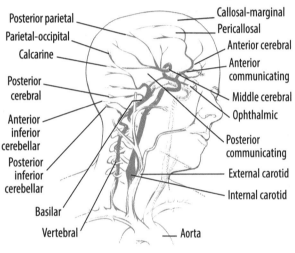

Veins of Head and Neck

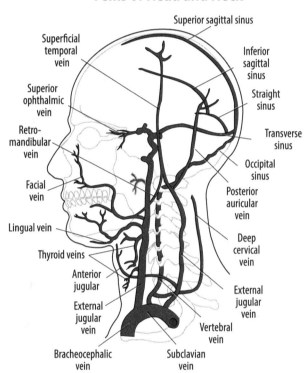

Lymphatic System of Head and Neck

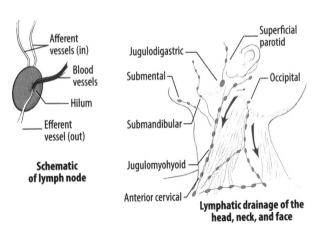

Schematic of lymph node

Lymphatic drainage of the head, neck, and face

Lymph Nodes

Respiratory System

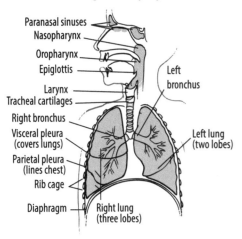

Paranasal sinuses
Nasopharynx
Oropharynx
Epiglottis
Larynx
Tracheal cartilages
Right bronchus
Visceral pleura (covers lungs)
Parietal pleura (lines chest)
Rib cage
Diaphragm
Left bronchus
Left lung (two lobes)
Right lung (three lobes)

Paranasal Sinuses

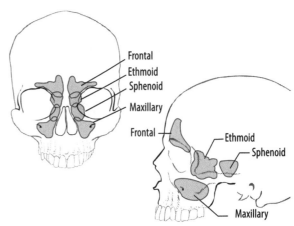

Frontal
Ethmoid
Sphenoid
Maxillary
Frontal
Ethmoid
Sphenoid
Maxillary

Oral Cavity

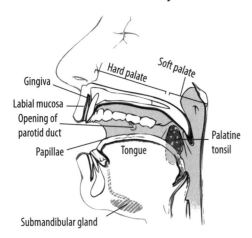

Gingiva
Labial mucosa
Opening of parotid duct
Papillae
Hard palate
Soft palate
Tongue
Palatine tonsil
Submandibular gland

Pancreas

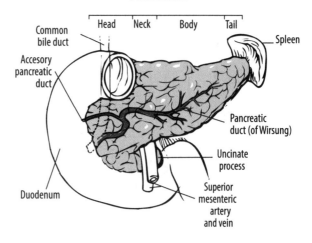

Head   Neck   Body   Tail
Common bile duct
Accesory pancreatic duct
Duodenum
Spleen
Pancreatic duct (of Wirsung)
Uncinate process
Superior mesenteric artery and vein

Gallbladder and Bile Ducts

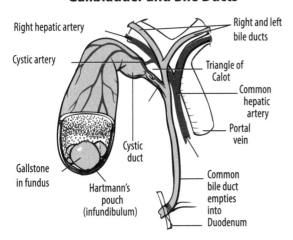

Right hepatic artery
Cystic artery
Gallstone in fundus
Hartmann's pouch (infundibulum)
Cystic duct
Right and left bile ducts
Triangle of Calot
Common hepatic artery
Portal vein
Common bile duct empties into Duodenum

Liver

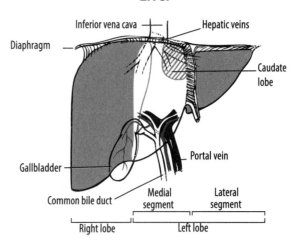

Inferior vena cava
Diaphragm
Gallbladder
Common bile duct
Hepatic veins
Caudate lobe
Portal vein
Medial segment
Lateral segment
Right lobe
Left lobe

Gastrointestinal System

Ethmoid sinus

Frontal sinus

Sphenoid sinus

Maxillary sinus

Upper esophagus

Esophageal region:

Cervical portion

Thoracic portion

Lower esophagus

Fundus

Esophagogastric junction

Abdominal portion

Stomach

Diaphragm

Pylorus

Left colic (splenic) flexure

Transverse colon

Right colic (hepatic) flexure

Duodenum

Large intestine

Ascending colon

Descending colon

Jejunum

Ileocecal junction

Cecum

Appendix

Small intestine

Ileum

Rectum

Sigmoid colon

Anus

Anal sphincter

Endocrine System

Kidney

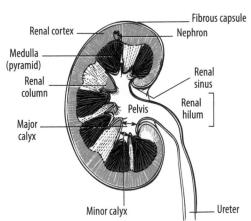

Dorsal View of Parathyroid Gland

Urinary System

Male Pelvic Organs

Female Genitourinary System

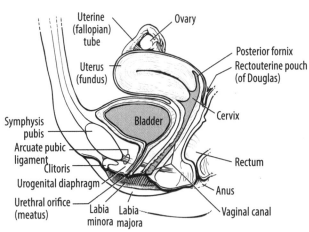

Joints

Shoulder (Anterior View)

Shoulder (Posterior View)

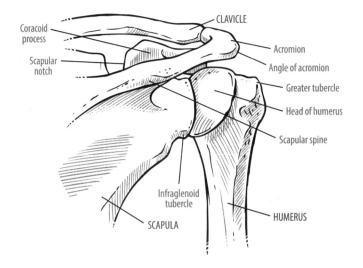

Joints
Elbow (Anterior View)

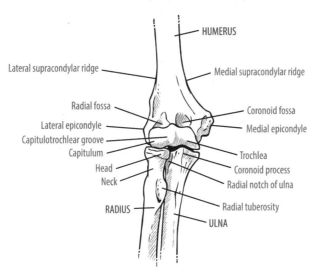

- HUMERUS
- Lateral supracondylar ridge
- Medial supracondylar ridge
- Radial fossa
- Coronoid fossa
- Lateral epicondyle
- Medial epicondyle
- Capitulotrochlear groove
- Capitulum
- Trochlea
- Head
- Coronoid process
- Neck
- Radial notch of ulna
- RADIUS
- Radial tuberosity
- ULNA

Elbow (Posterior View)

- HUMERUS
- Medial supracondylar ridge
- Lateral border
- Lateral supracondylar ridge
- Medial epicondyle
- Olecranon fossa
- Olecranon
- Lateral epicondyle
- Groove for Ulnar nerve
- Head of radius (articular circumference)
- Neck
- ULNA
- RADIUS

Hand

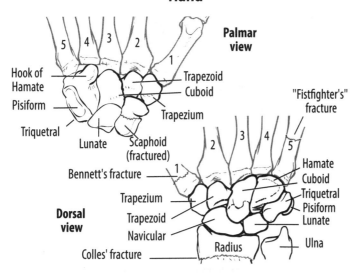

Palmar view

- Hook of Hamate
- Pisiform
- Triquetral
- Lunate
- Scaphoid (fractured)
- Trapezoid
- Cuboid
- Trapezium

Dorsal view

- Bennett's fracture
- Trapezium
- Trapezoid
- Navicular
- Colles' fracture
- "Fistfighter's" fracture
- Hamate
- Cuboid
- Triquetral
- Pisiform
- Lunate
- Radius
- Ulna

Joints

Hip (Anterior View)

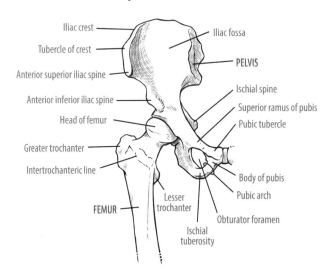

Iliac crest
Tubercle of crest
Anterior superior iliac spine
Anterior inferior iliac spine
Head of femur
Greater trochanter
Intertrochanteric line
FEMUR
Lesser trochanter
Ischial tuberosity
Iliac fossa
PELVIS
Ischial spine
Superior ramus of pubis
Pubic tubercle
Body of pubis
Pubic arch
Obturator foramen

Hip (Posterior View)

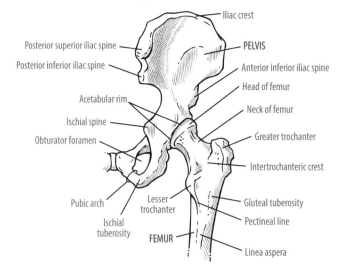

Iliac crest
Posterior superior iliac spine
Posterior inferior iliac spine
Acetabular rim
Ischial spine
Obturator foramen
Pubic arch
Ischial tuberosity
Lesser trochanter
FEMUR
PELVIS
Anterior inferior iliac spine
Head of femur
Neck of femur
Greater trochanter
Intertrochanteric crest
Gluteal tuberosity
Pectineal line
Linea aspera

Joints

Knee (Anterior View)

Knee (Posterior View)

Right Foot

Bones/Joints

Muscles

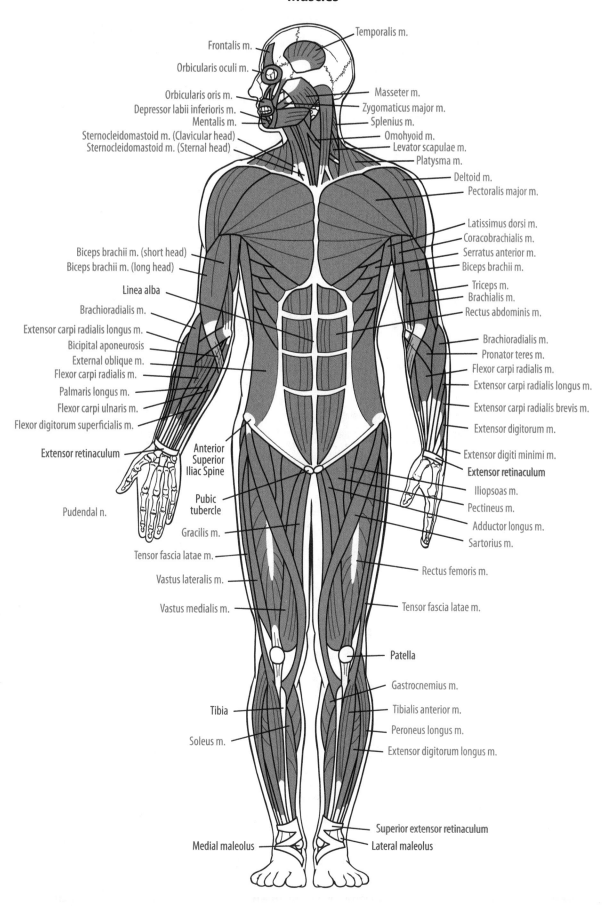